M000192338

GERIATRIC DOSAGE HANDBOOK

Including Clinical Recommendations and Monitoring Guidelines

Senior Editors:
Todd P. Semla, MS, PharmD, BCPS, FCCP, AGSF
Judith L. Beizer, PharmD, CGP, FASCP
Martin D. Higbee, PharmD

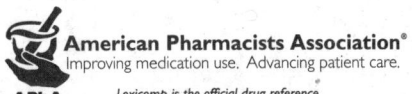

American Pharmacists Association®
Improving medication use. Advancing patient care.

APhA *Lexicomp is the official drug reference
for the American Pharmacists Association*

18th Edition

Lexicomp®

GERIATRIC DOSAGE HANDBOOK

Including Clinical Recommendations and Monitoring Guidelines

Todd P. Semla, MS, PharmD, BCPS, FCCP, AGSF
Senior Editor
Clinical Pharmacy Specialist
Department of Veterans Affairs
Pharmacy Benefits Management Services
Associate Professor, Clinical
Departments of Medicine and Psychiatry and Behavioral Health
Feinberg School of Medicine
Northwestern University
Chicago, Illinois

Judith L. Beizer, PharmD, CGP, FASCP
Senior Editor
Clinical Professor
Department of Clinical Pharmacy Practice
St John's University College of Pharmacy and Health Sciences
Jamaica, New York

Martin D. Higbee, PharmD
Senior Editor
Adjunct Professor
Department of Pharmacy Practice and Science
The University of Arizona
Tucson, Arizona

Lexicomp®

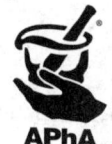

APhA

NOTICE

This data is intended to serve the user as a handy reference and not as a complete drug information resource. It does not include information on every therapeutic agent available. The publication covers 999 commonly used drugs and is specifically designed to present important aspects of drug data in a more concise format than is typically found in medical literature or product material supplied by manufacturers.

The nature of drug information is that it is constantly evolving because of ongoing research and clinical experience and is often subject to interpretation. While great care has been taken to ensure the accuracy of the information and recommendations presented, the reader is advised that the authors, editors, reviewers, contributors, and publishers cannot be responsible for the continued currency of the information or for any errors, omissions, or the application of this information, or for any consequences arising therefrom. Therefore, the author(s) and/or publisher shall have no liability to any person or entity with regard to claims, loss, or damage caused, or alleged to be caused, directly or indirectly, by the use of information contained herein. Because of the dynamic nature of drug information, readers are advised that decisions regarding drug therapy must be based on the independent judgment of the clinician, changing information about a drug (eg, as reflected in the literature and manufacturer's most current product information), and changing medical practices. Therefore, this data is designed to be used in conjunction with other necessary information and is not designed to be solely relied upon by any user. The user of this data hereby and forever releases the authors and publishers of this data from any and all liability of any kind that might arise out of the use of this data. The editors are not responsible for any inaccuracy of quotation or for any false or misleading implication that may arise due to the text or formulas as used or due to the quotation of revisions no longer official.

Certain of the authors, editors, and contributors have written this book in their private capacities. No official support or endorsement by any federal or state agency or pharmaceutical company is intended or inferred.

The publishers have made every effort to trace any third party copyright holders, if any, for borrowed material. If they have inadvertently overlooked any, they will be pleased to make the necessary arrangements at the first opportunity.

If you have any suggestions or questions regarding any information presented in this data, please contact our drug information pharmacists at (330) 650-6506. Book revisions are available at our website at http://www.lexi.com/home/revisions/.

This manual was produced using Lexi-Comp's Information Management System™ (LIMS) — A complete publishing service of Lexi-Comp, Inc.

Lexicomp®

1100 Terex Road • Hudson, Ohio • 44236
(330) 650-6506

ISBN 978-1-59195-316-6

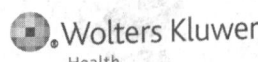

®.Wolters Kluwer
Health

TABLE OF CONTENTS

EDITORIAL ADVISORY PANEL

Laura Cummings, PharmD, BCPS
Pharmacotherapy Specialist
Lexi-Comp, Inc

William J. Dana, PharmD, FASHP
Pharmacy Quality Assurance
Harris County Hospital District

Beth Deen, PharmD, BDNSP
Senior Pediatric Clinical Pharmacy Specialist
Cook Children's Medical Center

Julie A. Dopheide, PharmD, BCPP
Associate Professor of Clinical Pharmacy, Psychiatry and the Behavioral Sciences
Schools of Pharmacy and Medicine
University of Southern California

Teri Dunsworth, PharmD, FCCP, BCPS
Pharmacotherapy Specialist
Lexi-Comp, Inc

Eve Echt, MD
Medical Staff
Department of Radiology
Akron General Medical Center

Michael S. Edwards, PharmD, MBA, BCOP
Chief, Oncology Pharmacy
and *Director, Oncology Pharmacy Residency Program*
Walter Reed Army Medical Center

Vicki L. Ellingrod, PharmD, BCPP
Head, Clinical Pharmacogenomics Laboratory
and *Associate Professor*
Department of Psychiatry
Colleges of Pharmacy and Medicine
University of Michigan

Kelley K. Engle, BSPharm
Medical Science Pharmacist
Lexi-Comp, Inc

Christopher Ensor, PharmD, BCPS (AQ-CV)
Clinical Specialist
Cardiothoracic Transplantation and Mechanical Circulatory Support
The Johns Hopkins Hospital

Erin Fabian, PharmD, RPh
Pharmacotherapy Specialist
Lexi-Comp, Inc

Elizabeth A. Farrington, PharmD, FCCP, FCCM, FPPAG, BCPS
Pharmacist III - Pediatrics
New Hanover Regional Medical Center

Margaret A. Fitzgerald, MS, APRN, BC, NP-C, FAANP
President
Fitzgerald Health Education Associates, Inc.
Family Nurse Practitioner
Greater Lawrence Family Health Center

Lawrence A. Frazee, PharmD, BCPS
Pharmacotherapy Specialist in Internal Medicine
Akron General Medical Center

Matthew A. Fuller, PharmD, BCPS, BCPP, FASHP
Clinical Pharmacy Specialist, Psychiatry
Cleveland Department of Veterans Affairs Medical Center
Associate Clinical Professor of Psychiatry and *Clinical Instructor of Psychology*
Case Western Reserve University
Adjunct Associate Professor of Clinical Pharmacy
University of Toledo

Jason C. Gallagher, PharmD, BCPS
Clinical Pharmacy Specialist, Infectious Diseases
and *Clinical Associate Professor*
Temple University Hospital

Jennifer L. Gardner, PharmD
Neonatal Clinical Pharmacy Specialist
Texas Children's Hospital

Meredith D. Girard, MD, FACP
Medical Staff
Department of Internal Medicine
Summa Health Systems
Assistant Professor Internal Medicine
Northeast Ohio Medical University (NEOMED)

Morton P. Goldman, RPh, PharmD, BCPS, FCCP
Senior Editor
Lexi-Comp, Inc

Julie A. Golembiewski, PharmD
Clinical Associate Professor and *Clinical Pharmacist, Anesthesia/Pain*
Colleges of Pharmacy and Medicine
University of Illinois

Jeffrey P. Gonzales, PharmD, BCPS
Critical Care Clinical Pharmacy Specialist
University of Maryland Medical Center

Roland Grad, MDCM, MSc, CCFP, FCFP
Associate Professor
Department of Family Medicine
McGill University

Tim T.Y. Lau, PharmD, ACPR, FCSHP
Pharmacotherapeutic Specialist in Infectious Diseases
Pharmaceutical Sciences
Vancouver General Hospital

Mandy C. Leonard, PharmD, BCPS
Assistant Professor
Cleveland Clinic Lerner College of Medicine of Case Western University
Assistant Director, Drug Information Services
The Cleveland Clinic Foundation

John J. Lewin III, PharmD, BCPS
Clinical Specialist, Neurosciences Critical Care
The Johns Hopkins Hospital

Jeffrey D. Lewis, PharmD, MACM
Associate Dean and Associate Professor of Pharmacy Practice
Cedarville University School of Pharmacy

John Lindsley, PharmD, BCPS
Cardiology Clinical Pharmacy Specialist
The Johns Hopkins Hospital

Nicholas A. Link, PharmD, BCOP
Clinical Specialist, Oncology
Hillcrest Hospital

Jennifer Fisher Lowe, PharmD, BCOP
Pharmacotherapy Contributor
Lexi-Comp, Inc

Sherry Luedtke, PharmD
Associate Professor
Department of Pharmacy Practice
Texas Tech University HSC School of Pharmacy

Melissa Makii, PharmD, BCPS
Clinical Pharmacy Specialist
Pediatric Oncology
Rainbow Babies & Children's Hospital

Vincent F. Mauro, BS, PharmD, FCCP
Professor of Clinical Pharmacy
and *Adjunct Professor of Medicine*
Colleges of Pharmacy and Medicine
The University of Toledo

Barrie McCombs, MD, FCFP
Medical Information Service Coordinator
The Alberta Rural Physician Action Plan

Christopher McPherson, PharmD
Clinical Pharmacist
Neonatal Intensive Care Unit
St. Louis Children's Hospital

Timothy F. Meiller, DDS, PhD
Professor
Oncology and Diagnostic Sciences
Baltimore College of Dental Surgery
Professor of Oncology
Marlene and Stewart Greenebaum Cancer Center
University of Maryland Medical System

Geralyn M. Meny, MD
Medical Director
American Red Cross, Penn-Jersey Region

Charla E. Miller, RPh, PharmD
Neonatal Clinical Pharmacy Specialist
Wolfson Children's Hospital

Julie Miller, PharmD
Pharmacy Clinical Specialist, Cardiology
Columbus Children's Hospital

Katherine Mills, PharmD
Pharmacotherapy Contributor
Lexi-Comp, Inc

Leah Millstein, MD
Assistant Professor
Division of General Internal Medicine
University of Maryland School of Medicine

Stephanie S. Minich, PharmD, BCOP
Pharmacotherapy Specialist
Lexi-Comp, Inc

Kim Moeller, RN, MSN, OCN, ACNS-BC
Advanced Practice Nurse
Summit Oncology Associates

Kevin M. Mulieri, BS, PharmD
Pediatric Hematology/Oncology Clinical Specialist
Penn State Milton S. Hershey Medical Center
Instructor of Pharmacology
Penn State College of Medicine

Elizabeth A. Neuner, PharmD, BCPS
Infectious Diseases Clinical Specialist
The Cleveland Clinic Foundation

Tom Palma, MS, RPh
Medical Science Pharmacist
Lexi-Comp, Inc

Susie H. Park, PharmD, BCPP
Assistant Professor of Clinical Pharmacy
University of Southern California

Nicole Passerrello, PharmD, BCPS
Pharmacotherapy Specialist
Lexi-Comp, Inc

Alpa Patel, PharmD
Antimicrobial Clinical Pharmacist
University of Louisville Hospital

5

John N. van den Anker, MD, PhD, FCP, FAAP
Vice Chair of Pediatrics for Experimental Therapeutics
and Chief and Professor of Evan and Cindy Jones Pediatric Clinical Pharmacology
Children's National Medical Center
Professor of Pediatrics, Pharmacology & Physiology
George Washington University School of Medicine and Health Sciences

Heather L. VandenBussche, PharmD
Professor of Pharmacy, Pediatrics
Pharmacy Practice
Ferris State University College of Pharmacy

Amy Van Orman, PharmD, BCPS
Pharmacotherapy Specialist
Lexi-Comp, Inc

Kristin Watson, PharmD, BCPS
Assistant Professor, Cardiology
and Clinical Pharmacist, Cardiology Service
Heart Failure Clinic
University of Maryland Medical Center

David M. Weinstein, PhD, RPh
Manager
Metabolism, Interactions, and Genomics Group
Lexi-Comp, Inc

Anne Marie Whelan, PharmD
Associate Professor
College of Pharmacy
Dalhousie University

Sherri J. Willard Argyres, MA, PharmD
Medical Science Pharmacist
Lexi-Comp, Inc

John C. Williamson, PharmD, BCPS
Pharmacy Clinical Coordinator, Infectious Diseases
Wake Forest Baptist Health

Nathan Wirick, PharmD
Infectious Disease and Antibiotic Management Clinical Specialist
Hillcrest Hospital

Richard L. Wynn, BSPharm, PhD
Professor of Pharmacology
Baltimore College of Dental Surgery
University of Maryland

Sallie Young, PharmD, BCPS, AQ Cardiology
Clinical Pharmacy Specialist, Cardiology
Penn State Milton S. Hershey Medical Center

Jennifer Zimmer-Young, PharmD, CCRP
Educator, Clinical Pharmacist
ThedaCare

ABOUT THE EDITORS

Todd P. Semla, MS, PharmD, BCPS, FCCP, AGSF

Dr Semla received his Bachelor of Science in Pharmacy, his Master of Science in Clinical Pharmacy, and his Doctor of Pharmacy degrees from the University of Iowa. After earning his doctorate, Dr Semla was awarded the American Society of Health-System Pharmacists Fellowship in Geriatric Pharmacotherapy which he completed at the University of Iowa.

Dr Semla has more than 30 years experience in geriatric pharmacotherapy in a variety of clinical settings including ambulatory care, acute care and rehabilitation, and the nursing home. He is a Clinical Pharmacy Specialist in the Department of Veterans Affairs Pharmacy Benefits Management Service and an Associate Professor of Medicine and Clinical Psychiatry at the Feinberg School of Medicine, Northwestern University.

Dr Semla is the Editor for the section "Drugs and Pharmacology," for the *Journal of the American Geriatrics Society* and Chair of the Panel on Alzheimer's Disease for *The Annals of Pharmacotherapy*. He is an active member of several professional organizations, including the American College of Clinical Pharmacy (ACCP). He is a past President and Chair of the Board of Directors of the American Geriatrics Society.

Judith L. Beizer, PharmD, CGP, FASCP

Dr Beizer received her Bachelor of Science in Pharmacy from the St Louis College of Pharmacy and then earned a Doctor of Pharmacy degree from the University of Tennessee. After pursuing a residency in clinical pharmacy at the Hospital of the University of Pennsylvania, she completed a fellowship in geriatric pharmacy at Montefiore Medical Center, Bronx, NY. During her fellowship, Dr Beizer was involved in a National Institute on Aging (NIA) grant concerning medication use and pharmacist intervention in community-dwelling elderly.

Dr Beizer is a Clinical Professor in the Department of Clinical Pharmacy Practice at St John's University College of Pharmacy and Health Sciences. As part of her teaching responsibilities, she serves as the Clinical Pharmacist at the Center for Extended Care and Rehabilitation, a long-term care facility in Manhasset, NY. At this facility, Dr Beizer has expanded clinical pharmacy services and precepts pharmacy students. Dr Beizer speaks regularly on the topic of medication use in the elderly and has published articles and abstracts on various issues in geriatric pharmacotherapy.

Dr Beizer is a member of a number of professional organizations, including the American Society of Health-System Pharmacists (ASHP), American Society of Consultant Pharmacists (ASCP), American College of Clinical Pharmacy (ACCP), American Pharmacists Association (APhA), and the American Geriatrics Society (AGS). She is a past president of ASCP. She previously served on the Board of Commissioners for the Commission for Certification in Geriatric Pharmacy. She is a past chairperson of the ASHP Special Interest Group on Geriatric Pharmacy Practice. Dr Beizer is on the Editorial Advisory Board of *The Consultant Pharmacist*.

Martin D. Higbee, PharmD

Dr Higbee received his Bachelor of Science in Pharmacy from The University of Utah in 1973. After a year of pharmacy practice and clinical pharmacy experience at The University of Utah, he entered the Doctor of Pharmacy degree program at The University of Texas at San Antonio. After graduation in 1977, he joined the University of Utah College of Pharmacy faculty. He became involved in development of the Salt Lake Veteran Administration Medical Center's Geriatric Treatment and Evaluation Unit, and after the establishment of this unit, Dr Higbee created an ASHP accredited post-doctoral Geriatric Residency through the Veteran's Administration Medical Center and The University of Utah College of Pharmacy. Dr Higbee was also on the editorial staff for the Eli Lily - AACP Geriatric Curriculum for Pharmacists project which created a geriatric textbook and curriculum for educators.

Dr Higbee joined the faculty at The University of Arizona in 1987. As part of his teaching responsibilities, he was a Clinical Pharmacist Consultant for the Hospital-Based Primary Care Team (division of Geriatric Care Center) at the Veterans Administration Medical Center in Tucson, Arizona, where he is preceptor for doctor of pharmacy students. Currently, he serves as an adjunct professor for the university. Dr Higbee has joined a nursing home consulting group, Donohue and Associates, a long-term care and assisted living consulting group based in Arizona. In addition, Dr Higbee frequently is called upon as an expert witness in legal proceedings.

Dr Higbee regularly speaks locally and nationally on geriatric drug therapy topics and has published articles, chapters, and abstracts on various geriatric research and pharmacotherapy topics. He is a member of numerous professional organizations. He is a past chairman of the ASHP Special Interest Group on Geriatric Pharmacy Practice and past member of the AACP Task Force on Aging.

DESCRIPTION OF SECTIONS AND FIELDS IN THIS HANDBOOK

The *Geriatric Dosage Handbook* is organized into four sections: Introductory information, drug information section, appendix, and pharmacologic category index.

Alphabetical Listing of Drugs

The drug information section of the handbook, wherein all drug monographs are arranged alphabetically by generic name, details information pertinent to geriatric use for each drug. U.S. brand names and index terms are cross-referenced between monographs and marked with diamonds ♦ for easy visibility.

Individual monographs contain most or all of the following fields of information:

Generic Name	U.S. adopted name
Pronunciation	Phonetic pronunciation guide
Related Information	Cross-reference to other pertinent information found elsewhere in this handbook
Medication Safety Issues	In an effort to promote the safe use of medications, this field is intended to highlight possible sources of medication errors such as look-alike/sound-alike drugs or highly concentrated formulations which require vigilance on the part of healthcare professionals. In addition, medications which have been associated with severe consequences in the event of a medication error are also identified in this field.
Brand Names: U.S.	Trade names (manufacturer-specific) found in the United States. The symbol [DSC] appears after trade names that have been recently discontinued.
Brand Names: Canada	Trade name(s) found in Canada
Index Terms	Includes names or accepted abbreviations of the generic drug; may include common brand names no longer available; this field is used to create cross-references to monographs
Generic Availability (U.S.)	Indicates availability of generic products in the United States
Pharmacologic Category	Unique systematic classification of medications
Use	Information pertaining to appropriate FDA-approved indications of the drug.
Unlabeled Use	Information pertaining to non-FDA-approved indications of the drug.
Prescribing and Access Restrictions	Provides information on any special requirements regarding the prescribing, obtaining or dispensing of drugs, including access restrictions pertaining to drugs with REMS elements and those drugs whose access restrictions are not REMS-related.
Medication Guide Available	Identifies drugs that have an FDA-approved Medication Guide.
Contraindications	Information pertaining to the inappropriate use of the drug as dictated by approved labeling; however, contraindications that pertain to certain special populations (eg, pediatric patients, pregnant women, or women of childbearing potential) which do not affect the geriatric population have been removed to maintain the scope and purpose of the Geriatric Dosage Handbook. Consult product labeling through the manufacturer or the FDA website for all contraindications.

Warnings/Precautions

Precautionary considerations, hazardous conditions related to use of the drug, and disease states or patient populations in which the drug should be cautiously used. Boxed warnings, when present, are clearly identified and are adapted from the FDA approved labeling; however, certain boxed warnings that pertain to certain special populations (eg, pediatric patients, pregnant women, or women of childbearing potential) which do not affect the geriatric population have been removed to maintain the scope and purpose of the Geriatric Dosage Handbook. Consult the product labeling for all boxed warnings and/or the exact language of the black box warning through the manufacturer or the FDA website.

Adverse Reactions

Side effects are grouped by percentage of incidence (if known) and/or body system; <1% effects are not listed, please consult manufacturer's product labeling regarding rare serious or life threatening events; **percentages are reflective of the adult population in general, not specific for older adults**

Drug Interactions

Metabolism/Transport Effects

If a drug has demonstrated involvement with cytochrome P450 enzymes, or other metabolism or transport proteins, this field will identify the drug as an inhibitor, inducer, or substrate of the specific enzyme(s) (eg, CYP1A2 or UGT1A1). CYP450 isoenzymes are identified as substrates (minor or major), inhibitors (weak, moderate, or strong), and inducers (weak or strong).

Avoid Concomitant Use

Designates drug combinations which should not be used concomitantly, due to an unacceptable risk:benefit assessment. Frequently, the concurrent use of the agents is explicitly prohibited or contraindicated by the product labeling.

Increased Effect/Toxicity

Drug combinations that result in an increased or toxic therapeutic effect between the drug listed in the monograph and other drugs or drug classes.

Decreased Effect

Drug combinations that result in a decreased therapeutic effect between the drug listed in the monograph and other drugs or drug classes.

Ethanol/Nutrition/Herb Interactions

Presents a description of the interaction between the drug listed in the monograph and ethanol, food, or herb/nutraceuticals.

Stability

Information regarding storage of product or steps for reconstitution. Provides the time and conditions for which a solution or mixture will maintain full potency. For example, some solutions may require refrigeration after reconstitution while stored at room temperature prior to preparation. Also includes compatibility information. **Note:** Professional judgment of the individual pharmacist in application of this information is imperative. While drug products may exhibit stability over longer durations of time, it may not be appropriate to utilize the drug product due to concerns in sterility.

Mechanism of Action

How drugs work in the body to elicit a response

Pharmacodynamics/Kinetics

The magnitude of a drug's effect depends on the drug concentration at the site of action. The pharmacodynamics are expressed in terms of onset of action and duration of action. Pharmacokinetics are expressed in terms of absorption, distribution (including appearance in breast milk and crossing of the placenta), protein binding, metabolism, bioavailability, half-life, time to peak serum concentration, and elimination.

Dosage

The amount of drug to be typically given or taken during therapy; may include the following:

Geriatric

Suggested amount of drug to be given to geriatric patients; for the purpose of this publication, the terms *elderly*, *geriatric*, or *older adult* include patients ≥65 years of age unless otherwise specified; may include adjustments from adult dosing; lack of this information in the monograph may imply that the drug is not used in the elderly patient or that no specific adjustments could be identified

Geriatric & Adult

This combined field is only used to indicate that no specific adjustments for elderly patients were identified. However, other issues should be considered (ie, renal or hepatic impairment). Also refer to Special Geriatric Considerations for additional information related to the elderly.

Adult	The recommended amount of drug to be given to adult patients
Renal Impairment	Suggested dosage adjustments or comments based on compromised renal function; may include dosing instructions for patients on dialysis
Hepatic Impairment	Suggested dosage adjustments or comments based on compromised liver function
Administration	Information regarding the recommended final concentrations, rates of administration for parenteral drugs, or other guidelines when giving the medication
Monitoring Parameters	Laboratory tests and patient physical parameters that should be monitored for safety and efficacy of drug therapy
Reference Range	Therapeutic and toxic serum concentrations listed including peak and trough levels
Test Interactions	Listing of assay interference when relevant
Pharmacotherapy Pearls	Information about sodium content and/or pertinent information about specific brands
Special Geriatric Considerations	Pertinent information specific to older adults
Product Availability	Provides availability information on products that have been approved by the FDA, but not yet available for use. Estimates for when a product may be available are included, when this information is known. May also provide any unique or critical drug availability issues.
Controlled Substance	Contains controlled substance schedule information as assigned by the United States Drug Enforcement Administration (DEA) or Canadian Controlled Substance Act (CDSA). CDSA information is only provided for drugs available in Canada and not available in the U.S.
Dosage Forms	Information with regard to form, strength, and availability of the drug in the United States. **Note:** Additional formulation information (eg, excipients, preservatives) is included when available. Please consult product labeling for further information.
Dosage Forms: Canada	Information with regard to form, strength, and availability of products that are uniquely available in Canada, but currently not available in the United States.
Extemporaneously Prepared	Directions for preparing liquid formulations from solid drug products. May include stability information and references.

Appendix

The appendix offers a compilation of tables, guidelines, and conversion information which can often be helpful when considering patient care.

Pharmacologic Category Index

This index provides a useful listing of drugs by their pharmacologic classification.

PREVENTING PRESCRIBING ERRORS

Prescribing errors account for the majority of reported medication errors and have prompted healthcare professionals to focus on the development of steps to make the prescribing process safer. Prescription legibility has been attributed to a portion of these errors and legislation has been enacted in several states to address prescription legibility. However, eliminating handwritten prescriptions and ordering medications through the use of technology [eg, computerized prescriber order entry (CPOE)] has been the primary recommendation. Whether a prescription is electronic, typed, or hand-printed, additional safe practices should be considered for implementation to maximize the safety of the prescribing process. Listed below are suggestions for safer prescribing:

- Ensure correct patient by using at least 2 patient identifiers on the prescription (eg, full name, birth date, or address). Review prescription with the patient or patient's caregiver.

- If geriatric patient, document patient's birth date or age.

- Prevent drug name confusion:

  - Use TALLman lettering (eg, buPROPion, busPIRone, predniSONE, predniso-LONE). For more information see http://www.fda.gov/Drugs/DrugSafety/MedicationErrors/ucm164587.htm.

  - Avoid abbreviated drug names (eg, MSO₄, MgSO₄, MS, HCT, 6MP, MTX), as they may be misinterpreted and cause error.

  - Avoid investigational names for drugs with FDA approval (eg, FK-506, CBDCA).

  - Avoid chemical names such as 6-mercaptopurine or 6-thioguanine, as sixfold overdoses have been given when these were not recognized as chemical names. The proper names of these drugs are mercaptopurine or thioguanine.

  - Use care when prescribing drugs that look or sound similar (eg, look- alike, sound-alike drugs). Common examples include: Celebrex® vs Celexa®, hydroxyzine vs hydralazine, Zyprexa® vs Zyrtec®.

- Avoid dangerous, error-prone abbreviations (eg, regardless of letter-case: U, IU, QD, QOD, μg, cc, @). Do not use apothecary system or symbols. Additionally, text messaging abbreviations (eg, "2Day") should never be used.

  - For more information see http://www.ismp.org/Tools/errorproneabbreviations.pdf

- Always use a leading zero for numbers less than 1 (0.5 mg is correct and .5 mg is **incorrect**) and never use a trailing zero for whole numbers (2 mg is correct and 2.0 mg is **incorrect**).

- Always use a space between a number and its units as it is easier to read. There should be no periods after the abbreviations mg or mL (10 mg is correct and 10mg is **incorrect**).

- For doses that are greater than 1,000 dosing units, use properly placed commas to prevent 10-fold errors (100,000 units is correct and 100000 units is **incorrect**).

- Do not prescribe drug dosage by the type of container in which the drug is available (eg, do not prescribe "1 amp", "2 vials", etc).

- Do not write vague or ambiguous orders which have the potential for misinterpretation by other healthcare providers. Examples of vague orders to avoid: "Resume pre-op medications," "give drug per protocol," or "continue home medications."

- Review each prescription with patient (or patient's caregiver) including the medication name, indication, and directions for use.

- Take extra precautions when prescribing *high alert drugs* (drugs that can cause significant patient harm when prescribed in error). Common examples of these drugs include: Anticoagulants, chemotherapy, insulins, opiates, and sedatives.

  - For more information see http://www.ismp.org/Tools/highalertmedications.pdf

To Err Is Human: Building a Safer Health System, Kohn LT, Corrigan JM, and Donaldson MS, eds, Washington, D.C.: National Academy Press, 2000.

A Complete Outpatient Prescription[1]

A complete outpatient prescription can prevent the prescriber, the pharmacist, and/or the patient from making a mistake and can eliminate the need for further clarification. The complete outpatient prescription should contain:

- Patient's full name
- Medication indication
- Allergies
- Prescriber name and telephone or pager number
- For geriatric patients: Their birth date or age
- Drug name, dosage form and strength
- Number or amount to be dispensed
- Complete instructions for the patient or caregiver, including the purpose of the medication, directions for use (including dose), dosing frequency, route of administration, duration of therapy, and number of refills.
- Dose should be expressed in convenient units of measure.
- When there are recognized contraindications for a prescribed drug, the prescriber should indicate knowledge of this fact to the pharmacist (ie, when prescribing a potassium salt for a patient receiving an ACE inhibitor, the prescriber should write "K serum leveling being monitored").

Upon dispensing of the final product, the pharmacist should ensure that the patient or caregiver can effectively demonstrate the appropriate administration technique. An appropriate measuring device should be provided or recommended. Household teaspoons and tablespoons should not be used to measure liquid medications due to their variability and inaccuracies in measurement; oral medication syringes are recommended.

For additional information see http://www.ppag.org/attachments/files/111/Guidelines_Peds.pdf
[1]Levine SR, Cohen MR, Blanchard NR, et al, "Guidelines for Preventing Medication Errors in Pediatrics," *J Pediatr Pharmacol Ther*, 2001, 6:426-42.

FDA NAME DIFFERENTIATION PROJECT: THE USE OF TALL-MAN LETTERS

Confusion between similar drug names is an important cause of medication errors. For years, The Institute For Safe Medication Practices (ISMP), has urged generic manufacturers to use a combination of large and small letters as well as bolding (ie, chlorpro**MAZINE** and chlorpro**PA-MIDE**) to help distinguish drugs with look-alike names, especially when they share similar strengths. Recently the FDA's Division of Generic Drugs began to issue recommendation letters to manufacturers suggesting this novel way to label their products to help reduce this drug name confusion. Although this project has had marginal success, the method has successfully eliminated problems with products such as diphenhydr**AMINE** and dimenhy**DRINATE**. Hospitals should also follow suit by making similar changes in their own labels, preprinted order forms, computer screens and printouts, and drug storage location labels.

Lexi-Comp, Inc. Medical Publishing will use "Tall-Man" letters for the drugs suggested by the FDA or recommended by ISMP.

The following is a list of generic and brand name product names and recommended revisions.

Drug Product	Recommended Revision
acetazolamide	aceta**ZOLAMIDE**
alprazolam	**ALPRAZ**olam
amiloride	a**MIL**oride
amlodipine	am**LODIP**ine
aripiprazole	**ARIP**iprazole
atomoxetine	ato**MOX**etine
atorvastatin	atorva**STAT**in
Avinza	**AVIN**za
azacitidine	aza**CITID**ine
azathioprine	aza**THIO**prine
bupropion	bu**PROP**ion
buspirone	bus**PIR**one
carbamazepine	car**BAM**azepine
carboplatin	**CARBO**platin
cefazolin	ce**FAZ**olin
cefotetan	cefo**TE**tan
cefoxitin	cef**OX**itin
ceftazidime	cef**TAZ**idime
ceftriaxone	cef**TRIAX**one
Celebrex	Cele**BREX**
Celexa	Cele**XA**
chlordiazepoxide	chlordiaze**POXIDE**
chlorpromazine	chlorpro**MAZINE**
chlorpropamide	chlorpro**PAMIDE**
cisplatin	**CIS**platin
clomiphene	clomi**PHENE**
clomipramine	clomi**PRAMINE**
clonazepam	clonaze**PAM**
clonidine	clo**NID**ine
clozapine	clo**ZAP**ine
cycloserine	cyclo**SERINE**
cyclosporine	cyclo**SPORINE**

FDA NAME DIFFERENTIATION PROJECT: THE USE OF TALL-MAN LETTERS

Drug Product	Recommended Revision
dactinomycin	**DACTIN**omycin
daptomycin	**DAPTO**mycin
daunorubicin	**DAUNO**rubicin
dimenhydrinate	dimenhy**DRINATE**
diphenhydramine	diphenhydr**AMINE**
dobutamine	**DOBUT**amine
docetaxel	**DOCE**taxel
dopamine	**DOP**amine
doxorubicin	**DOXO**rubicin
duloxetine	**DUL**oxetine
ephedrine	e**PHED**rine
epinephrine	**EPINEPH**rine
epirubicin	**EPI**rubicin
eribulin	eri**BUL**in
fentanyl	fenta**NYL**
flavoxate	flavox**ATE**
fluoxetine	**FLU**oxetine
fluphenazine	flu**PHENAZ**ine
fluvoxamine	fluvoxa**MINE**
glipizide	glipi**ZIDE**
glyburide	gly**BURIDE**
guaifenesin	guai**FEN**esin
guanfacine	guan**FACINE**
Humalog	Huma**LOG**
Humulin	Humu**LIN**
hydralazine	hydr**ALAZINE**
hydrocodone	**HYDRO**codone
hydromorphone	**HYDRO**morphone
hydroxyzine	hydr**OXY**zine
idarubicin	**IDA**rubicin
infliximab	in**FLIX**imab
Invanz	**INV**anz
isotretinoin	**ISO**tretinoin
Klonopin	Klono**PIN**
Lamictal	La**MIC**tal
Lamisil	Lam**ISIL**
lamivudine	lami**VUD**ine
lamotrigine	lamo**TRI**gine
levetiracetam	Lev**ETIRA**cetam
levocarnitine	lev**OCARN**itine
lorazepam	**LOR**azepam
medroxyprogesterone	medroxy**PROGESTER**one
metformin	met**FORMIN**
methylprednisolone	methyl**PREDNIS**olone
methyltestosterone	methyl**TESTOSTER**one
metronidazole	metro**NIDAZOLE**
mitomycin	mito**MY**cin
mitoxantrone	Mito**XAN**trone
Nexavar	Nex**AVAR**
Nexium	Nex**IUM**

Drug Product	Recommended Revision
nicardipine	niCARdipine
nifedipine	NIFEdipine
nimodipine	niMODipine
Novolin	NovoLIN
Novolog	NovoLOG
olanzapine	OLANZapine
oxcarbazepine	OXcarbazepine
oxycodone	oxyCODONE
Oxycontin	OxyCONTIN
paclitaxel	PACLitaxel
paroxetine	PARoxetine
pemetrexed	PEMEtrexed
penicillamine	penicillAMINE
pentobarbital	PENTobarbital
phenobarbital	PHENobarbital
pralatrexate	PRALAtrexate
prednisolone	prednisoLONE
prednisone	predniSONE
Prilosec	PriLOSEC
Prozac	PROzac
quetiapine	QUEtiapine
quinidine	quiNIDine
quinine	quiNINE
rabeprazole	RABEprazole
Risperdal	RisperDAL
risperidone	risperiDONE
rituximab	riTUXimab
romidepsin	romiDEPsin
romiplostim	romiPLOStim
ropinirole	rOPINIRole
Sandimmune	sandIMMUNE
Sandostatin	SandoSTATIN
Seroquel	SEROquel
Sinequan	SINEquan
sitagliptin	sitaGLIPtin
Solu-Cortef	Solu-CORTEF
Solu-Medrol	Solu-MEDROL
sorafenib	SORAfenib
sufentanil	SUFentanil
sulfadiazine	sulfADIAZINE
sulfasalazine	sulfaSALAzine
sumatriptan	SUMAtriptan
sunitinib	SUNItinib
Tegretol	TEGretol
tiagabine	tiaGABine
tizanidine	tiZANidine
tolazamide	TOLAZamide
tolbutamide	TOLBUTamide
tramadol	traMADol
trazodone	traZODone

FDA NAME DIFFERENTIATION PROJECT: THE USE OF TALL-MAN LETTERS

Drug Product	Recommended Revision
Trental	**TREN**tal
valacyclovir	val**ACY**clovir
valganciclovir	val**GAN**ciclovir
vinblastine	vin**BLAS**tine
vincristine	vin**CRIS**tine
zolmitriptan	**ZOLM**itriptan
Zyprexa	Zy**PREXA**
Zyrtec	Zyr**TEC**

"FDA and ISMP Lists of Look-Alike Drug Names with Recommended Tall Man Letter." Available at http://www.ismp. org/tools/tallmanletters.pdf. Last accessed January 6, 2011.

"Name Differentiation Project." Available at http://www.fda.gov/Drugs/DrugSafety/MedicationErrors/ucm164587.htm. Last accessed January 6, 2011.

U.S. Pharmacopeia, "USP Quality Review: Use Caution-Avoid Confusion," March 2001, No. 76. Available at http://www.usp.org

ALPHABETICAL LISTING OF DRUGS

♦ **A200® Lice [OTC]** *see* Permethrin *on page 1512*

Abatacept (ab a TA sept)

Medication Safety Issues
Sound-alike/look-alike issues:
  Orencia® may be confused with Oracea®
Brand Names: U.S. Orencia®
Brand Names: Canada Orencia®
Index Terms BMS-188667; CTLA-4Ig
Generic Availability (U.S.) No
Pharmacologic Category Antirheumatic, Disease Modifying; Selective T-Cell Costimulation Blocker
Use
Treatment of moderately- to severely-active adult rheumatoid arthritis (RA); may be used as monotherapy or in combination with other DMARDs
Treatment of moderately- to severely-active juvenile idiopathic arthritis (JIA); may be used as monotherapy or in combination with methotrexate
Note: Abatacept should **not** be used in combination with anakinra or TNF-blocking agents
Contraindications There are no contraindications listed within the manufacturer's U.S. labeling.

Canadian labeling: Hypersensitivity to abatacept or any component of the formulation; patients with, or at risk of sepsis syndrome (eg, immunocompromised, HIV positive)
Warnings/Precautions Serious and potentially fatal infections (including tuberculosis and sepsis) have been reported, particularly in patients receiving concomitant immunosuppressive therapy. RA patients receiving a concomitant TNF antagonist experienced an even higher rate of serious infection. Caution should be exercised when considering the use of abatacept in any patient with a history of recurrent infections, with conditions that predispose them to infections, or with chronic, latent, or localized infections. Patients who develop a new infection while undergoing treatment should be monitored closely. If a patient develops a serious infection, abatacept should be discontinued. Screen patients for latent tuberculosis infection prior to initiating abatacept; safety in tuberculosis-positive patients has not been established. Treat patients testing positive according to standard therapy prior to initiating abatacept. Adult patients receiving abatacept in combination with TNF-blocking agents had higher rates of infections (including serious infections) than patients on TNF-blocking agents alone. The manufacturer does not recommend concurrent use with anakinra or TNF-blocking agents. Monitor for signs and symptoms of infection when transitioning from TNF-blocking agents to abatacept. Due to the effect of T-cell inhibition on host defenses, abatacept may affect immune responses against infections and malignancies; impact on the development and course of malignancies is not fully defined.

Use caution with chronic obstructive pulmonary disease (COPD), higher incidences of adverse effects (COPD exacerbation, cough, rhonchi, dyspnea) have been observed; monitor closely. Rare cases of hypersensitivity, anaphylaxis, or anaphylactoid reactions have been reported; medications for the treatment of hypersensitivity reactions should be available for immediate use. Patients should be screened for viral hepatitis prior to use; antirheumatic therapy may cause reactivation of hepatitis B. Patients should be brought up to date with all immunizations before initiating therapy. Live vaccines should not be given concurrently or within 3 months of discontinuation of therapy; there is no data available concerning secondary transmission of live vaccines in patients receiving therapy. Powder for injection may contain maltose, which may result in falsely-elevated serum glucose readings on the day of infusion. Higher incidences of infection and malignancy were observed in the elderly; use with caution.
Adverse Reactions (Reflective of adult population; not specific for elderly) Note: Percentages not always reported; COPD patients experienced a higher frequency of COPD-related adverse reactions (COPD exacerbation, cough, dyspnea, pneumonia, rhonchi)

>10%:
  Central nervous system: Headache (≤18%)
  Gastrointestinal: Nausea
  Respiratory: Nasopharyngitis (12%), upper respiratory tract infection
  Miscellaneous: Infection (54%), antibody formation (2% to 41%)
1% to 10%:
  Cardiovascular: Hypertension (7%)
  Central nervous system: Dizziness (9%), fever
  Dermatologic: Rash (4%)
  Gastrointestinal: Dyspepsia (6%), abdominal pain, diarrhea
  Genitourinary: Urinary tract infection (6%)

Local: Injection site reaction (3%)

Neuromuscular & skeletal: Back pain (7%), limb pain (3%)

Respiratory: Cough (8%), bronchitis, pneumonia, rhinitis, sinusitis

Miscellaneous: Infusion-related reactions (≤9%), herpes simplex, immunogenicity (1% to 2%), influenza

Drug Interactions

Metabolism/Transport Effects None known.

Avoid Concomitant Use

Avoid concomitant use of Abatacept with any of the following: Anti-TNF Agents; BCG; Belimumab; Natalizumab; Pimecrolimus; Tacrolimus (Topical); Vaccines (Live)

Increased Effect/Toxicity

Abatacept may increase the levels/effects of: Belimumab; Leflunomide; Natalizumab; Vaccines (Live)

The levels/effects of Abatacept may be increased by: Anti-TNF Agents; Denosumab; Pimecrolimus; Roflumilast; Tacrolimus (Topical); Trastuzumab

Decreased Effect

Abatacept may decrease the levels/effects of: BCG; Coccidioidin Skin Test; Sipuleucel-T; Vaccines (Inactivated); Vaccines (Live)

The levels/effects of Abatacept may be decreased by: Echinacea

Ethanol/Nutrition/Herb Interactions Herb/Nutraceutical: Avoid echinacea (has immunostimulant properties; consider therapy modifications).

Stability

Prefilled syringe: Store at 2°C to 8°C (36°F to 46°F); do not freeze. Protect from light.

Powder for injection: Prior to reconstitution, store at 2°C to 8°C (36°F to 46°F); do not freeze. Protect from light. Reconstitute each vial with 10 mL SWFI using the provided silicone-free disposable syringe (discard solutions accidentally reconstituted with siliconized syringe as they may develop translucent particles). Inject SWFI down the side of the vial to avoid foaming. The reconstituted solution contains 25 mg/mL abatacept. Further dilute (using a silicone-free syringe) in 100 mL NS to a final concentration of ≤10 mg/mL. Prior to adding abatacept to the 100 mL bag, the manufacturer recommends withdrawing a volume of NS equal to the abatacept volume required, resulting in a final volume of 100 mL. Mix gently; do not shake.

After dilution, may be stored for up to 24 hours at room temperature or refrigerated at 2°C to 8°C (36°F to 46°F). Must be used within 24 hours of reconstitution.

Mechanism of Action Selective costimulation modulator; inhibits T-cell (T-lymphocyte) activation by binding to CD80 and CD86 on antigen presenting cells (APC), thus blocking the required CD28 interaction between APCs and T cells. Activated T lymphocytes are found in the synovium of rheumatoid arthritis patients.

Pharmacodynamics/Kinetics

Bioavailability: SubQ: 78.6% (relative to I.V. administration)

Distribution: V_{ss}: 0.02-0.13 L/kg

Half-life elimination: 8-25 days

Dosage

Geriatric Refer to adult dosing. Due to potential for higher rates of infections and malignancies, use caution.

Adult Rheumatoid arthritis (RA): I.V.: Dosing is according to body weight:

<60 kg: 500 mg

60-100 kg: 750 mg

>100 kg: 1000 mg

I.V. regimen: Following the initial I.V. infusion, repeat I.V. dose (using the same weight-based dosing) at 2 weeks and 4 weeks after the initial infusion, and every 4 weeks thereafter.

SubQ regimen: Following the initial I.V. infusion (using the weight-based dosing), administer 125 mg subcutaneously within 24 hours of the infusion, followed by 125 mg subcutaneously once weekly thereafter. **Note:** Patients unable to receive I.V. infusions may omit the initial I.V. loading dose and initiate once weekly SubQ therapy directly.

Transitioning from I.V. therapy to SubQ therapy: Administer the first SubQ dose instead of the next scheduled I.V. dose.

Administration

I.V.: Infuse over 30 minutes. Administer through a 0.2-1.2 micron low protein-binding filter

SubQ: Allow prefilled syringe to warm to room temperature (for 30-60 minutes) prior to administration. Inject into the front of the thigh (preferred), abdomen (except for 2-inch area around the navel), or the outer area of the upper arms (if administered by a caregiver). Rotate injection sites (≥1 inch apart); do not administer into tender, bruised, red, or hard skin.

Monitoring Parameters Signs and symptoms of infection, signs and symptoms of hypersensitivity reaction; hepatitis and TB screening prior to therapy initiation

Test Interactions Contains maltose; may result in falsely elevated blood glucose levels with dehydrogenase pyrroloquinolinequinone or glucose-dye-oxidoreductase testing methods on the day of infusion. Glucose monitoring methods which utilize glucose dehydrogenase nicotine adenine dinucleotide (GDH-NAD), glucose oxidase, or glucose hexokinase are recommended.

Special Geriatric Considerations The number of elderly (≥65 years of age) were insufficient to draw significant clinical conclusions. The studies to date have not demonstrated any differences in safety and efficacy between young adults and elderly. However, the frequency of infections and malignancy was higher in those >65 years of age than those <65 years. Since elderly experience a higher incidence of infections and malignancies, use abatacept with caution in this population.

Dosage Forms Excipient information presented when available (limited, particularly for generics); consult specific product labeling.

Injection, powder for reconstitution [preservative free]:
  Orencia®: 250 mg [contains maltose]
Injection, solution [preservative free]:
  Orencia®: 125 mg/mL (1 mL) [contains sucrose 170 mg/mL]

Abiraterone Acetate (a bir A ter one AS e tate)

Brand Names: U.S. Zytiga™
Brand Names: Canada Zytiga™
Index Terms Abiraterone; CB7630
Generic Availability (U.S.) No
Pharmacologic Category Antiandrogen; Antineoplastic Agent, Antiandrogen
Use Treatment of metastatic, castration-resistant prostate cancer (in combination with prednisone) in patients previously treated with docetaxel
Contraindications Canadian labeling: Additional contraindication (not in U.S. labeling): Hypersensitivity to abiraterone acetate or any component of the formulation or container
Warnings/Precautions Hazardous agent; use appropriate precautions for handling and disposal. Significant increases in liver enzymes have been reported; may require dosage reduction or discontinuation. ALT, AST, and bilirubin should be monitored prior to treatment, every 2 weeks for 3 months and monthly thereafter; patients with hepatic impairment, elevations in liver function tests, or experiencing hepatotoxicity require more frequent monitoring (see Dosage: Hepatic Impairment and Monitoring Parameters). Evaluate liver function promptly with signs or symptoms of hepatotoxicity. The safety of retreatment after significant elevations (ALT or AST >20 times the upper limit of normal [ULN] or total bilirubin >10 times ULN) has not been evaluated. Avoid use in patients with pre-existing severe hepatic impairment; dosage reduction is recommended in patients with baseline moderate impairment. Canadian labeling (not in U.S. labeling) also recommends avoiding use in patients with pre-existing moderate hepatic impairment.

Concurrent infection, stress, or interruption of daily corticosteroids is associated with reports of adrenocortical insufficiency. Monitor closely for signs and symptoms of adrenocorticoid insufficiency, which could be masked by adverse events associated with mineralocorticoid excess. Diagnostic testing for insufficiency may be clinically indicated. Increased corticosteroid doses may be required before, during, and after stress. May cause increased mineralocorticoid levels, which may result in hypertension, hypokalemia and fluid retention. Concomitant administration with corticosteroids reduces the incidence and severity of these adverse events. Due to potential for hypertension, hypokalemia, or fluid retention, use with caution in patients with cardiovascular disease (particularly heart failure, recent MI, or ventricular arrhythmia); patients with left ventricular ejection fraction (LVEF) <50% or NYHA class III or IV heart failure were excluded from clinical trials. Monitor at least monthly for hypertension, hypokalemia, and fluid retention.

Must be administered on an empty stomach (administer at least 1 hour before and 2 hours after any food). Avoid (or use caution) with concomitant CYP3A4 strong inhibitors and inducers. Avoid concurrent administration with CYP2D6 substrates with a narrow therapeutic index (eg, thioridazine); if concurrent administration cannot be avoided, consider a dose reduction of the CYP2D6 substrate.

Adverse Reactions (Reflective of adult population; not specific for elderly) Note: Adverse reactions reported for use in combination with prednisone.

>10%:

Cardiovascular: Edema (27%)

Endocrine & metabolic: Triglycerides increased (63%), hypokalemia (28%; grades 3/4: 5%), hypophosphatemia (24%; grades 3/4: 7%), hot flush (19%)

Gastrointestinal: Diarrhea (18%)

Genitourinary: Urinary tract infection (12%)

Hepatic: AST increased (31%; grades 3/4: 2%), ALT increased (11%; grades 3/4: 1%)

Neuromuscular & skeletal: Joint swelling/discomfort (30%), muscle discomfort (26%)

Respiratory: Cough (11%)

1% to 10%:

Cardiovascular: Hypertension (9%; grades 3/4: 1%), arrhythmia (7%), chest pain/discomfort (4%), heart failure (2%)

Gastrointestinal: Dyspepsia (6%)

Genitourinary: Polyuria (7%), nocturia (6%)

Hepatic: Bilirubin increased (7%; grades 3/4: <1%)

Respiratory: Upper respiratory infection (5%)

Drug Interactions

Metabolism/Transport Effects Substrate of CYP3A4 (major); **Note:** Assignment of Major/Minor substrate status based on clinically relevant drug interaction potential; **Inhibits** CYP1A2 (strong), CYP2C19 (moderate), CYP2C9 (moderate), CYP2D6 (strong), CYP3A4 (moderate), P-glycoprotein

Avoid Concomitant Use

Avoid concomitant use of Abiraterone Acetate with any of the following: Clopidogrel; Conivaptan; Pimozide; Silodosin; Tamoxifen; Thioridazine; Tolvaptan; Topotecan

Increased Effect/Toxicity

Abiraterone Acetate may increase the levels/effects of: ARIPiprazole; AtoMOXetine; Avanafil; Bendamustine; Budesonide (Systemic, Oral Inhalation); Carvedilol; Citalopram; Colchicine; CYP1A2 Substrates; CYP2C19 Substrates; CYP2C9 Substrates; CYP2D6 Substrates; CYP3A4 Substrates; Dabigatran Etexilate; Eplerenone; Everolimus; FentaNYL; Fesoterodine; Halofantrine; Iloperidone; Ivacaftor; Lurasidone; Nebivolol; P-glycoprotein/ABCB1 Substrates; Pimecrolimus; Pimozide; Propafenone; Prucalopride; Ranolazine; Rivaroxaban; Salmeterol; Saxagliptin; Silodosin; Tetrabenazine; Thioridazine; Tolvaptan; Topotecan; Vilazodone; Zuclopenthixol

The levels/effects of Abiraterone Acetate may be increased by: Conivaptan; CYP3A4 Inhibitors (Moderate); CYP3A4 Inhibitors (Strong); Dasatinib; Ivacaftor; Mifepristone

Decreased Effect

Abiraterone Acetate may decrease the levels/effects of: Clopidogrel; Codeine; Ifosfamide; Iloperidone; Tamoxifen; TraMADol

The levels/effects of Abiraterone Acetate may be decreased by: CYP3A4 Inducers (Strong); Deferasirox; Herbs (CYP3A4 Inducers); Tocilizumab

Ethanol/Nutrition/Herb Interactions Food: Taking with food will increase systemic exposure. Management: Do not administer with food. Must be taken on an empty stomach, at least 1 hour before and 2 hours after food.

Stability Store at 20°C to 25°C (68°F to 77°F); excursions permitted to 15°C to 30°C (59°F to 86°F).

Mechanism of Action Selectively and irreversibly inhibits CYP17 (17 alpha-hydroxylase/C17,20-lyase), an enzyme required for androgen biosynthesis which is expressed in testicular, adrenal, and prostatic tumor tissues. Inhibits the formation of the testosterone precursors dehydroepiandrosterone (DHEA) and androstenedione.

Pharmacodynamics/Kinetics

Distribution: V_{dss}: 19,669 ± 13,358 L

Protein binding: >99%; to albumin and alpha$_1$-acid glycoprotein

Metabolism: Abiraterone acetate is hydrolyzed to the active metabolite abiraterone; further metabolized to inactive metabolites abiraterone sulphate and N-oxide abiraterone sulphate via CYP3A4 and SULT2A1

Bioavailability: Systemic exposure is increased by food

Half-life elimination: 12 ± 5 hours

Time to peak: 2 hours

Excretion: Feces (~88%); urine (~5%)

Dosage

Geriatric & Adult Prostate cancer, metastatic, castration-resistant: Oral: 1000 mg once daily (in combination with prednisone 5 mg twice daily)

Renal Impairment No adjustment required.

◀ **Hepatic Impairment**
Hepatic impairment *prior to* treatment initiation:
Mild (Child-Pugh class A): No adjustment required
Moderate (Child-Pugh class B): 250 mg once daily (**Note:** Canadian labeling does not recommend use). Permanently discontinue treatment if ALT and/or AST >5 times the upper limit of normal (ULN) or total bilirubin >3 times ULN.
Severe (Child-Pugh class C): Avoid use
Hepatotoxicity *during* treatment:
U.S. labeling:
ALT and/or AST >5 times ULN or total bilirubin >3 times ULN: Withhold treatment until liver function tests return to baseline or ALT and AST ≤2.5 times ULN and total bilirubin ≤1.5 times ULN, then reinitiate at 750 mg once daily.
Recurrent hepatotoxicity on 750 mg/day: Withhold treatment until liver function tests return to baseline or ALT and AST ≤2.5 times ULN and total bilirubin ≤1.5 times ULN, then reinitiate at 500 mg once daily.
Recurrent hepatotoxicity on 500 mg/day: Discontinue treatment
Canadian labeling:
ALT and/or AST >5 times ULN or total bilirubin >3 times ULN:
Withhold treatment until liver function tests return to baseline, then reinitiate at 500 mg once daily
Recurrent hepatotoxicity on 500 mg/day: Discontinue treatment
ALT >20 times ULN (any time during treatment): Discontinue permanently.
Administration Administer orally on an empty stomach, at least 1 hour before and 2 hours after food. Swallow tablets whole with water.
Monitoring Parameters ALT, AST, and bilirubin prior to treatment, every 2 weeks for 3 months and monthly thereafter; if baseline moderate hepatic impairment (Child-Pugh class B), monitor ALT, AST, and bilirubin prior to treatment, weekly for the first month, every 2 weeks for 2 months then monthly thereafter. If hepatotoxicity develops during treatment (and only after therapy is interrupted and liver function tests have returned to safe levels), monitor ALT, AST, and bilirubin every 2 weeks for 3 months and monthly thereafter. Monitoring of testosterone levels is not necessary.

Monitor for signs and symptoms of adrenocorticoid insufficiency; monthly for hypertension, hypokalemia, and fluid retention.
Special Geriatric Considerations According to the manufacturer, 71% of men in clinical trials were ≥65 years; 28% were ≥75 years. No difference in efficacy or safety was noted between younger and older men.
Dosage Forms Excipient information presented when available (limited, particularly for generics); consult specific product labeling.
Tablet, oral:
Zytiga™: 250 mg

♦ **ABLC** *see* Amphotericin B (Lipid Complex) *on page 124*

AbobotulinumtoxinA (aye bo BOT yoo lin num TOKS in aye)

Medication Safety Issues
Other safety concerns:
Botulinum products are not interchangeable; potency differences may exist between the products.
Brand Names: U.S. Dysport™
Index Terms Botulinum Toxin Type A
Generic Availability (U.S.) No
Pharmacologic Category Neuromuscular Blocker Agent, Toxin
Use Treatment of cervical dystonia in both toxin-naive and previously treated patients; temporary improvement in the appearance of moderate-severe glabellar lines associated with procerus and corrugator muscle activity
Medication Guide Available Yes
Dosage
Geriatric
Cervical dystonia: Refer to adult dosing. No specific adjustment recommended.
Glabellar lines: Not recommended in patients ≥65 years of age.
Adult
Cervical dystonia: I.M.: Initial: 500 units divided among affected muscles in toxin-naïve or toxin-experienced patients. May re-treat at intervals of ≥12 weeks
Dosage adjustments: Adjust dosage in 250-unit increments; do not administer at intervals <12 weeks; dosage range used in studies: 250-1000 units

Glabellar lines: Adults <65 years: I.M.: Inject 10 units (0.05 mL or 0.08 mL) into each of 5 sites (2 injections in each corrugator muscle and 1 injection in the procerus muscle) for a total dose of 50 units; do not administer at intervals <3 months; efficacy has been demonstrated up to 4 repeated administrations

Renal Impairment No adjustment necessary.

Hepatic Impairment No adjustment necessary.

Special Geriatric Considerations No specific dosage adjustment recommended.

Dosage Forms Excipient information presented when available (limited, particularly for generics); consult specific product labeling.

Injection, powder for reconstitution:

Dysport™: 500 units [contains albumin (human), lactose 2.5 mg]

◆ **Abstral®** see FentaNYL on page 761
◆ **ABT-335** see Fenofibric Acid on page 755
◆ **AC 2993** see Exenatide on page 734

Acamprosate (a kam PROE sate)

Brand Names: U.S. Campral®
Brand Names: Canada Campral®
Index Terms Acamprosate Calcium; Calcium Acetylhomotaurinate
Generic Availability (U.S.) No
Pharmacologic Category GABA Agonist/Glutamate Antagonist
Use Maintenance of alcohol abstinence
Contraindications Hypersensitivity to acamprosate or any component of the formulation; severe renal impairment (Cl_{cr} <30 mL/minute)

Warnings/Precautions Should be used as part of a comprehensive program to treat alcohol dependence. Treatment should be initiated as soon as possible following the period of alcohol withdrawal, when the patient has achieved abstinence. Acamprosate does not eliminate or diminish the symptoms of alcohol withdrawal. Use caution in moderate renal impairment (Cl_{cr} 30-50 mL/minute). Contraindicated in patients with severe renal impairment (Cl_{cr} 30 mL/minute). Suicidal ideation, attempted and completed suicides have occurred in acamprosate-treated patients; monitor for depression and/or suicidal thinking. May cause CNS depression, which may impair physical or mental abilities; patients must be cautioned about performing tasks which require mental alertness (eg, operating machinery or driving). Use caution in the elderly due to age-related decrease in renal function. Traces of sulfites may be present in the formulation.

Adverse Reactions (Reflective of adult population; not specific for elderly) Note: Many adverse effects associated with treatment may be related to alcohol abstinence; reported frequency range may overlap with placebo.

>10%: Gastrointestinal: Diarrhea (10% to 17%)

1% to 10%:

Cardiovascular: Chest pain, edema (peripheral), hypertension, palpitation, syncope, vasodilatation

Central nervous system: Insomnia (6% to 9%), anxiety (5% to 8%), depression (4% to 8%), dizziness (3% to 4%), pain (2% to 4%), paresthesia (2% to 3%), abnormal thinking, amnesia, chills, headache, somnolence, tremor

Dermatologic: Pruritus (3% to 4%), rash

Endocrine & metabolic: Libido decreased

Gastrointestinal: Anorexia (2% to 5%), nausea (3% to 4%), flatulence (1% to 4%), xerostomia (1% to 3%), abdominal pain, appetite increased, constipation, dyspepsia, taste perversion, vomiting, weight gain

Genitourinary: Impotence

Neuromuscular & skeletal: Weakness (5% to 7%), arthralgia, back pain, myalgia

Ocular: Abnormal vision

Respiratory: Bronchitis, cough increased, dyspnea, pharyngitis, rhinitis

Miscellaneous: Diaphoresis (2% to 3%), flu-like syndrome, infection, suicide attempt

Drug Interactions

Metabolism/Transport Effects None known.

Avoid Concomitant Use There are no known interactions where it is recommended to avoid concomitant use.

Increased Effect/Toxicity There are no known significant interactions involving an increase in effect.

Decreased Effect There are no known significant interactions involving a decrease in effect. ▶

Ethanol/Nutrition/Herb Interactions

Ethanol: Abstinence is required during treatment. Ethanol does not affect the pharmacokinetics of acamprosate; however, the continued use of ethanol will decrease desired efficacy of acamprosate.

Food: Food decreases absorption of acamprosate (not clinically significant).

Stability Store at 25°C (77°F); excursions permitted to 15°C to 30°C (59°F to 86°F).

Mechanism of Action Mechanism not fully defined. Structurally similar to gamma-amino butyric acid (GABA), acamprosate appears to increase the activity of the GABA-ergic system, and decreases activity of glutamate within the CNS, including a decrease in activity at N-methyl D-aspartate (NMDA) receptors; may also affect CNS calcium channels. Restores balance to GABA and glutamate activities which appear to be disrupted in alcohol dependence. During therapeutic use, reduces alcohol intake, but does not cause a disulfiram-like reaction following alcohol ingestion. Insignificant CNS activity, outside its effect on alcohol dependence, was observed including no anxiolytic, anticonvulsant, or antidepressant activity.

Pharmacodynamics/Kinetics

Distribution: V_d: 1 L/kg
Protein binding: Negligible
Metabolism: Not metabolized
Bioavailability: 11%
Half-life elimination: 20-33 hours
Excretion: Urine (as unchanged drug)

Dosage

Geriatric & Adult Alcohol abstinence: Oral: 666 mg 3 times/day (a lower dose may be effective in some patients). **Note:** Treatment should be initiated as soon as possible following the period of alcohol withdrawal, when the patient has achieved abstinence and should be maintained if patient relapses.

Renal Impairment

Cl_{cr} 30-50 mL/minute: 333 mg 3 times/day
Cl_{cr} <30 mL/minute: Contraindicated in severe renal impairment.

Hepatic Impairment

Mild-to-moderate impairment: No dosage adjustments are recommended.
Severe impairment: There are no dosage adjustments provided in manufacturer's labeling.

Administration May be administered without regard to meals (administered with meals during clinical trials to possibly increase compliance). Tablet should be swallowed whole; do not crush or chew.

Special Geriatric Considerations Initial studies did not include sufficient geriatric patients to be able to derive sufficient data to compare elderly to younger adults. Only 41 out of 4234 patients in clinical trials were ≥65 years of age with none ≥75 years. However, since this medication is cleared renally exclusively, caution should be used since many elderly have Cl_{cr} 30-50 mL/minute where dosage reduction is required (see Dosage).

Dosage Forms Excipient information presented when available (limited, particularly for generics); consult specific product labeling.

Tablet, delayed release, enteric coated, oral, as calcium:
Campral®: 333 mg [contains calcium 33 mg/tablet, sulfites]

◆ **Acamprosate Calcium** see Acamprosate on page 25

Acarbose (AY car bose)

Related Information

Diabetes Mellitus Management, Adults on page 2193

Medication Safety Issues

Sound-alike/look-alike issues:

Precose® may be confused with PreCare®

High alert medication:

The Institute for Safe Medication Practices (ISMP) includes this medication among its list of drug classes which have a heightened risk of causing significant patient harm when used in error.

International issues:

Precose® [U.S., Malaysia] may be confused with Precosa brand name for *Saccharomyces boulardii* [Finland, Sweden]

Brand Names: U.S. Precose®

Brand Names: Canada Glucobay™

Generic Availability (U.S.) Yes

Pharmacologic Category Antidiabetic Agent, Alpha-Glucosidase Inhibitor

Use Adjunct to diet and exercise to lower blood glucose in patients with type 2 diabetes mellitus (noninsulin dependent, NIDDM)

Contraindications Hypersensitivity to acarbose or any component of the formulation; patients with diabetic ketoacidosis or cirrhosis; patients with inflammatory bowel disease, colonic ulceration, partial intestinal obstruction, or in patients predisposed to intestinal obstruction; patients who have chronic intestinal diseases associated with marked disorders of digestion or absorption, and in patients who have conditions that may deteriorate as a result of increased gas formation in the intestine

Warnings/Precautions Acarbose given in combination with a sulfonylurea or insulin will cause a further lowering of blood glucose and may increase the hypoglycemic potential of the sulfonylurea or insulin. Treatment-emergent elevations of serum transaminases (AST and/or ALT) occurred in up to 14% of acarbose-treated patients in long-term studies. These serum transaminase elevations appear to be dose related and were asymptomatic, reversible, more common in females, and, in general, were not associated with other evidence of liver dysfunction. Fulminant hepatitis has been reported rarely. It may be necessary to discontinue acarbose and administer insulin if the patient is exposed to stress (ie, fever, trauma, infection, surgery). Use not recommended in patients with significant impairment (S_{cr} >2 mg/dL); use with caution in other patients with renal impairment.

Adverse Reactions (Reflective of adult population; not specific for elderly) >10%:
Gastrointestinal: Diarrhea (31%) and abdominal pain (19%) tend to return to pretreatment levels over time; frequency and intensity of flatulence (74%) tend to abate with time
Hepatic: Transaminases increased (≤4%)

Drug Interactions

Metabolism/Transport Effects None known.

Avoid Concomitant Use There are no known interactions where it is recommended to avoid concomitant use.

Increased Effect/Toxicity
Acarbose may increase the levels/effects of: Hypoglycemic Agents

The levels/effects of Acarbose may be increased by: Herbs (Hypoglycemic Properties); MAO Inhibitors; Neomycin; Pegvisomant; Salicylates; Selective Serotonin Reuptake Inhibitors

Decreased Effect
Acarbose may decrease the levels/effects of: Digoxin

The levels/effects of Acarbose may be decreased by: Corticosteroids (Orally Inhaled); Corticosteroids (Systemic); Loop Diuretics; Luteinizing Hormone-Releasing Hormone Analogs; Somatropin; Thiazide Diuretics

Ethanol/Nutrition/Herb Interactions Ethanol: Limit ethanol.

Stability Store at <25°C (77°F). Protect from moisture.

Mechanism of Action Competitive inhibitor of pancreatic α-amylase and intestinal brush border α-glucosidases, resulting in delayed hydrolysis of ingested complex carbohydrates and disaccharides and absorption of glucose; dose-dependent reduction in postprandial serum insulin and glucose peaks; inhibits the metabolism of sucrose to glucose and fructose

Pharmacodynamics/Kinetics
Absorption: <2% as active drug; ~35% as metabolites
Metabolism: Exclusively via GI tract, principally by intestinal bacteria and digestive enzymes; 13 metabolites identified (major metabolites are sulfate, methyl, and glucuronide conjugates)
Bioavailability: Low systemic bioavailability of parent compound; acts locally in GI tract
Half-life elimination: ~2 hours
Time to peak: Active drug: ~1 hour
Excretion: Urine (~34% as inactive metabolites, <2% parent drug and active metabolite); feces (~51% as unabsorbed drug)

Dosage
Geriatric & Adult Type 2 diabetes: Oral:
Initial: 25 mg 3 times/day with the first bite of each main meal; to reduce GI effects, some patients may benefit from initiating at 25 mg once daily with gradual titration to 25 mg 3 times/day as tolerated
Maintenance dose: Should be adjusted at 4- to 8-week intervals based on 1-hour postprandial glucose levels and tolerance until maintenance dose is reached; maintenance dose: 50-100 mg 3 times/day. Dosage must be individualized on the basis of effectiveness and tolerance while not exceeding the maximum recommended dose.
Maximum:
≤60 kg: 50 mg 3 times/day
>60 kg: 100 mg 3 times/day
Patients receiving sulfonylureas or insulin: Acarbose given in combination with a sulfonylurea or insulin will cause a further lowering of blood glucose and may increase the hypoglycemic potential of the sulfonylurea or insulin. If hypoglycemia occurs, appropriate adjustments in the dosage of these agents should be made.

◀ **Renal Impairment**
Cl$_{cr}$ <25 mL/minute: Peak plasma concentrations were 5 times higher and AUCs were 6 times larger than in volunteers with normal renal function.
Significant renal dysfunction (S$_{cr}$ >2 mg/dL): Use is not recommended.

Administration Should be administered with the first bite of each main meal.

Monitoring Parameters Postprandial glucose, glycosylated hemoglobin levels, serum transaminase levels should be checked every 3 months during the first year of treatment and periodically thereafter, renal function (serum creatinine); blood pressure

Reference Range
Recommendations for glycemic control in adults with diabetes:
Hb A$_{1c}$: <7%
Preprandial capillary plasma glucose: 70-130 mg/dL
Peak postprandial capillary blood glucose: <180 mg/dL
Blood pressure: <130/80 mm Hg
Recommendations for glycemic control in older adults with diabetes:
Relatively healthy, cognitively intact, and with a ≥5-year life expectancy: See Adults
Frail, life expectancy <5 years or those for whom the risks of intensive glucose control outweigh the benefits:
Hb A$_{1c}$: <8% to 9%
Blood pressure: <140/80 mm Hg or <130/80 mm Hg if tolerated

Special Geriatric Considerations Intensive glucose control (Hb A$_{1c}$ <6.5%) has been linked to increased all-cause and cardiovascular mortality, hypoglycemia requiring assistance, and weight gain in adult type 2 diabetes. How "tightly" to control a geriatric patient's blood glucose needs to be individualized. Such a decision should be based on several factors, including the patient's functional and cognitive status, how well he/she recognizes hypoglycemic or hyperglycemic symptoms, and how to respond to them and other disease states. An Hb A$_{1c}$ <7.5% is an acceptable endpoint for a healthy older adult, while <8% is acceptable for frail elderly patients, those with a duration of illness >10 years, or those with comorbid conditions and requiring combination diabetes medications. For elderly patients with diabetes who are relatively healthy, attaining target goals for aspirin use, blood pressure, lipids, smoking cessation, and diet and exercise may be more important than normalized glycemic control.

Dosage Forms Excipient information presented when available (limited, particularly for generics); consult specific product labeling.
Tablet, oral: 25 mg, 50 mg, 100 mg
Precose®: 25 mg, 50 mg, 100 mg

◆ **Accolate®** see Zafirlukast on page 2041
◆ **AccuNeb®** see Albuterol on page 49
◆ **Accupril®** see Quinapril on page 1649
◆ **Accuretic®** see Quinapril and Hydrochlorothiazide on page 1652
◆ **ACE** see Captopril on page 282

Acebutolol (a se BYOO toe lole)

Related Information
Beta-Blockers on page 2108

Medication Safety Issues
Sound-alike/look-alike issues:
Sectral® may be confused with Seconal®, Septra®

Brand Names: U.S. Sectral®

Brand Names: Canada Apo-Acebutolol®; Ava-Acebutolol; Mylan-Acebutolol; Mylan-Acebutolol (Type S); Nu-Acebutolol; Rhotral; Sandoz-Acebutolol; Sectral®; Teva-Acebutolol

Index Terms Acebutolol Hydrochloride

Generic Availability (U.S.) Yes

Pharmacologic Category Antiarrhythmic Agent, Class II; Beta-Blocker With Intrinsic Sympathomimetic Activity

Use Treatment of hypertension; management of ventricular arrhythmias

Unlabeled Use Treatment of chronic stable angina (**Note:** Not recommended for patients with prior MI)

Contraindications Overt cardiac failure; cardiogenic shock; persistently-severe bradycardia or second- and third-degree heart block (except in patients with a functioning artificial pacemaker)

Warnings/Precautions Consider pre-existing conditions such as sick sinus syndrome before initiating. Beta-blocker therapy should not be withdrawn abruptly (particularly in patients with CAD), but gradually tapered to avoid acute tachycardia, hypertension, and/or ischemia. Chronic beta-blocker therapy should not be routinely withdrawn prior to major surgery. Use with caution in diabetic patients. Beta-blockers may impair glucose tolerance, potentiate hypoglycemia, and/or mask symptoms of hypoglycemia in a diabetic patient. Use with caution in bronchospastic lung disease, hepatic impairment, myasthenia gravis, psychiatric disease (may cause CNS depression), or renal dysfunction. May precipitate or aggravate symptoms of arterial insufficiency in patients with PVD and Raynaud's disease; use with caution and monitor for progression of arterial obstruction. Use reduced doses in the elderly since metabolism and elimination are reduced. Beta-blockers with intrinsic sympathomimetic activity (eg, acebutolol) are likely to worsen survival in HF and should be avoided. Adequate alpha$_1$-receptor blockade is required prior to use of any beta-blocker for patients with untreated pheochromocytoma. May mask signs of hyperthyroidism (eg, tachycardia); use caution if hyperthyroidism is suspected, abrupt withdrawal may precipitate thyroid storm. Alterations in thyroid function tests may be observed. May induce or exacerbate psoriasis. Use caution with history of severe anaphylaxis to allergens; patients taking beta-blockers may become more sensitive to repeated challenges. Treatment of anaphylaxis (eg, epinephrine) in patients taking beta-blockers may be ineffective or promote undesirable effects. Use with caution in patients on concurrent digoxin, verapamil, or diltiazem; bradycardia or heart block can occur. Use with caution in patients receiving inhaled anesthetic agents known to depress myocardial contractility.

Adverse Reactions (Reflective of adult population; not specific for elderly)
>10%: Central nervous system: Fatigue (11%)
1% to 10%:
  Cardiovascular: Chest pain (2%), edema (2%), bradycardia, hypotension, CHF
  Central nervous system: Headache (6%), dizziness (6%), insomnia (3%), depression (2%), abnormal dreams (2%), anxiety, hyper-/hypoesthesia
  Dermatologic: Rash (2%), pruritus
  Gastrointestinal: Constipation (4%), diarrhea (4%), dyspepsia (4%), nausea (4%), flatulence (3%), abdominal pain, vomiting
  Genitourinary: Micturition frequency (3%), dysuria, impotence, nocturia
  Neuromuscular & skeletal: Myalgia (2%), back pain, joint pain
  Ocular: Abnormal vision (2%), conjunctivitis, dry eyes, eye pain
  Respiratory: Dyspnea (4%), rhinitis (2%), cough (1%), pharyngitis, wheezing

Potential adverse effects (based on experience with other beta-blocking agents) include agranulocytosis, allergic reactions, alopecia (reversible), catatonia, claudication, depression (reversible), disorientation, emotional lability, erythematous rash, ischemic colitis, laryngospasm, mesenteric artery thrombosis, Peyronie's disease, purpura, respiratory distress, short-term memory loss, slightly clouded sensorium, thrombocytopenia

Drug Interactions
  Metabolism/Transport Effects Inhibits CYP2D6 (weak)
  Avoid Concomitant Use
    Avoid concomitant use of Acebutolol with any of the following: Floctafenine; Methacholine
  Increased Effect/Toxicity
    Acebutolol may increase the levels/effects of: Alpha-/Beta-Agonists (Direct-Acting); Alpha1-Blockers; Alpha2-Agonists; Amifostine; Antihypertensives; Antipsychotic Agents (Phenothiazines); ARIPiprazole; Bupivacaine; Cardiac Glycosides; Cholinergic Agonists; Fingolimod; Hypotensive Agents; Insulin; Lidocaine; Lidocaine (Systemic); Lidocaine (Topical); Mepivacaine; Methacholine; Midodrine; RiTUXimab; Sulfonylureas

    The levels/effects of Acebutolol may be increased by: Acetylcholinesterase Inhibitors; Aminoquinolines (Antimalarial); Amiodarone; Anilidopiperidine Opioids; Antipsychotic Agents (Phenothiazines); Calcium Channel Blockers (Dihydropyridine); Calcium Channel Blockers (Nondihydropyridine); Diazoxide; Dipyridamole; Disopyramide; Dronedarone; Floctafenine; Herbs (Hypotensive Properties); MAO Inhibitors; Pentoxifylline; Phosphodiesterase 5 Inhibitors; Propafenone; Prostacyclin Analogues; QuiNIDine; Reserpine
  Decreased Effect
    Acebutolol may decrease the levels/effects of: Beta2-Agonists; Theophylline Derivatives

    The levels/effects of Acebutolol may be decreased by: Barbiturates; Herbs (Hypertensive Properties); Methylphenidate; Nonsteroidal Anti-Inflammatory Agents; Rifamycin Derivatives; Yohimbine
Ethanol/Nutrition/Herb Interactions
  Food: Peak serum acebutolol levels may be slightly decreased if taken with food.
  Herb/Nutraceutical: Avoid dong quai if using for hypertension (has estrogenic activity). Avoid yohimbe, ginseng (may worsen hypertension).
Stability Store at controlled room temperature of 20°C to 25°C (68°F to 77°F). Protect from light and dispense in a light-resistant, tight container.

◀ **Mechanism of Action** Competitively blocks beta$_1$-adrenergic receptors with little or no effect on beta$_2$-receptors except at high doses; exhibits membrane stabilizing and intrinsic sympathomimetic activity

Pharmacodynamics/Kinetics

Onset of action: 1-2 hours

Duration: 12-24 hours

Absorption: Oral: 40%

Distribution: V$_d$: 1.2 L/kg

Protein binding: ~26%

Metabolism: Extensive first-pass effect to equipotent and cardioselective diacetolol metabolite

Bioavailability: Acebutolol: 40%

Half-life elimination: Parent drug: 3-4 hours; Metabolite: 8-13 hours

Time to peak: 2-4 hours

Excretion: Feces (50% to 60%); urine (30% to 40%); diacetolol eliminated primarily in the urine

Dosage

Geriatric Refer to adult dosing. Consider dose reduction due to age-related increase in bioavailability; do not exceed 800 mg/day. In the management of hypertension, consider lower initial dose (eg, 200-400 mg/day) and titrate to response (Aronow, 2011).

Adult

Angina, ventricular arrhythmia: Oral: 400 mg/day in 2 divided doses; maintenance: 600-1200 mg/day in divided doses; maximum: 1200 mg/day

Hypertension: Oral: 400-800 mg/day (larger doses may be divided); maximum: 1200 mg/day; usual dose range (JNC 7): 200-800 mg/day in 2 divided doses

Chronic stable angina (unlabeled use): Oral: Usual dose: 400-1200 mg/day in 2 divided doses (Gibbons, 2002); low doses (ie, 400 mg/day) may also be given as once daily (Pina, 1988)

Renal Impairment

Cl$_{cr}$ 25-49 mL/minute: Reduce dose by 50%.

Cl$_{cr}$ <25 mL/minute: Reduce dose by 75%.

Hepatic Impairment There are no dosage adjustments provided in manufacturer's labeling; use with caution.

Administration May be administered without regard to meals.

Monitoring Parameters Blood glucose (especially in patients with diabetes mellitus); blood pressure, orthostatic hypotension, heart rate, CNS effects, ECG

Special Geriatric Considerations Since bioavailability increased in elderly about twofold, geriatric patients may require lower maintenance doses, therefore, as serum and tissue concentrations increase beta$_1$ selectivity diminishes; due to alterations in the beta-adrenergic autonomic nervous system, beta-adrenergic blockade may result in less hemodynamic response than seen in younger adults. Studies indicate that despite decreased sensitivity to the chronotropic effects of beta-blockade with age, there appears to be an increased myocardial sensitivity to the negative inotropic effect during stress (ie, exercise). Controlled trials have shown the overall response rate for propranolol to be only 20% to 50% in elderly populations. Therefore, all beta-adrenergic blocking drugs may result in a decreased response as compared to younger adults. Adjust dose for renal function.

Dosage Forms Excipient information presented when available (limited, particularly for generics); consult specific product labeling.

Capsule, oral, as hydrochloride: 200 mg, 400 mg

Sectral®: 200 mg, 400 mg

◆ **Acebutolol Hydrochloride** see Acebutolol on page 28
◆ **Aceon®** see Perindopril Erbumine on page 1509
◆ **Acephen™ [OTC]** see Acetaminophen on page 31
◆ **Acerola [OTC]** see Ascorbic Acid on page 149

Acetaminophen (a seet a MIN oh fen)

Medication Safety Issues

Sound-alike/look-alike issues:

Acephen® may be confused with AcipHex®

FeverALL® may be confused with Fiberall®

Triaminic™ Children's Fever Reducer Pain Reliever may be confused with Triaminic® cough and cold products

Tylenol® may be confused with atenolol, timolol, Tylenol® PM, Tylox®

Other safety concerns:

Duplicate therapy issues: This product contains acetaminophen, which may be a component of combination products. Do not exceed the maximum recommended daily dose of acetaminophen.

Injection: Reports of 10-fold overdose errors using the parenteral product have occurred in the U.S. and Europe; calculation of doses in "mg" and subsequent administration of the dose in "mL" using the commercially available concentration of 10 mg/mL contributed to these errors. Expressing doses as mg **and** mL, as well as pharmacy preparation of doses, may decrease error potential (Dart, 2012; ISMP, 2012).

International issues:

Depon [Greece] may be confused with Depen brand name for penicillamine [U.S.]; Depin brand name for nifedipine [India]; Dipen brand name for diltiazem [Greece]

Duorol [Spain] may be confused with Diuril brand name for chlorothiazide [U.S., Canada]

Paralen [Czech Republic] may be confused with Aralen brand name for chloroquine [U.S., Mexico]

Brand Names: U.S. Acephen™ [OTC]; APAP 500 [OTC]; Aspirin Free Anacin® Extra Strength [OTC]; Cetafen® Extra [OTC]; Cetafen® [OTC]; Excedrin® Tension Headache [OTC]; Feverall® [OTC]; Infantaire [OTC]; Little Fevers™ [OTC]; Mapap® Arthritis Pain [OTC]; Mapap® Children's [OTC]; Mapap® Extra Strength [OTC]; Mapap® Infant's [OTC]; Mapap® Junior Rapid Tabs [OTC]; Mapap® [OTC]; Non-Aspirin Pain Reliever [OTC]; Nortemp Children's [OTC]; Ofirmev™; Pain & Fever Children's [OTC]; Pain Eze [OTC]; Q-Pap Children's [OTC]; Q-Pap Extra Strength [OTC]; Q-Pap Infant's [OTC]; Q-Pap [OTC]; RapiMed® Children's [OTC]; RapiMed® Junior [OTC]; Silapap Children's [OTC]; Silapap Infant's [OTC]; Triaminic™ Children's Fever Reducer Pain Reliever [OTC]; Tylenol® 8 Hour [OTC]; Tylenol® Arthritis Pain Extended Relief [OTC]; Tylenol® Children's Meltaways [OTC]; Tylenol® Children's [OTC]; Tylenol® Extra Strength [OTC]; Tylenol® Infant's Concentrated [OTC]; Tylenol® Jr. Meltaways [OTC]; Tylenol® [OTC]; Valorin Extra [OTC]; Valorin [OTC]

Brand Names: Canada Abenol®; Apo-Acetaminophen®; Atasol®; Novo-Gesic; Pediatrix; Tempra®; Tylenol®

Index Terms APAP (abbreviation is not recommended); N-Acetyl-P-Aminophenol; Paracetamol

Generic Availability (U.S.) Yes: Excludes extended release products; injectable formulation

Pharmacologic Category Analgesic, Miscellaneous

Use Treatment of mild-to-moderate pain and fever (analgesic/antipyretic)

I.V.: Additional indication: Management of moderate-to-severe pain when combined with opioid analgesia

Contraindications Hypersensitivity to acetaminophen or any component of the formulation; severe hepatic impairment or severe active liver disease (Ofirmev™)

Warnings/Precautions Limit dose to <4 g/day. May cause severe hepatotoxicity on acute overdose; in addition, chronic daily dosing in adults has resulted in liver damage in some patients. Use with caution in patients with alcoholic liver disease; consuming ≥3 alcoholic drinks/day may increase the risk of liver damage. Use caution in patients with hepatic impairment or active liver disease. Use of intravenous formulation is contraindicated in patients with severe hepatic impairment or severe active liver disease. Use caution in patients with known G6PD deficiency; rare reports of hemolysis have occurred. Use caution in patients with chronic malnutrition and hypovolemia (intravenous formulation). Use caution in patients with severe renal impairment; consider dosing adjustments. Hypersensitivity and anaphylactic reactions have been reported; discontinue immediately if symptoms of allergic or hypersensitivity reactions occur.

OTC labeling: When used for self-medication, patients should be instructed to contact healthcare provider if used for fever lasting >3 days or for pain lasting >10 days in adults.

Adverse Reactions (Reflective of adult population; not specific for elderly) Oral, Rectal: Frequency not defined:

Dermatologic: Rash

Endocrine & metabolic: May increase chloride, uric acid, glucose; may decrease sodium, bicarbonate, calcium

Hematologic: Anemia; blood dyscrasias (neutropenia, pancytopenia, leukopenia)

Hepatic: Bilirubin increased, alkaline phosphatase increased

Renal: Ammonia increased, nephrotoxicity with chronic overdose, analgesic nephropathy

Miscellaneous: Hypersensitivity reactions (rare)

I.V.:

>10%: Gastrointestinal: Nausea (adults 34%; children ≥5%), vomiting (adults 15%; children ≥5%)

1% to 10%:

Cardiovascular: Edema (peripheral), hypervolemia, hypo/hypertension, tachycardia

Central nervous system: Headache (adults 10%; children ≥1%), insomnia (adults 7%; children ≥1%), agitation (children ≥5%), anxiety, fatigue

Dermatologic: Pruritus (children ≥5%), rash

Endocrine & metabolic: Hypoalbuminemia, hypokalemia, hypomagnesemia, hypophosphatemia

Gastrointestinal: Constipation (children ≥5%), abdominal pain, diarrhea

Hematologic: Anemia

Hepatic: Transaminases increased

Local: Infusion site pain

Neuromuscular & skeletal: Muscle spasms, pain in extremity, trismus

Ocular: Periorbital edema

Renal: Oliguria (children ≥1%)

Respiratory: Atelectasis (children ≥5%), breath sounds abnormal, dyspnea, hypoxia, pleural effusion, pulmonary edema, stridor, wheezing

Drug Interactions

Metabolism/Transport Effects Substrate of CYP1A2 (minor), CYP2A6 (minor), CYP2C9 (minor), CYP2D6 (minor), CYP2E1 (minor), CYP3A4 (minor); **Note:** Assignment of Major/Minor substrate status based on clinically relevant drug interaction potential; **Inhibits** CYP3A4 (weak)

Avoid Concomitant Use

Avoid concomitant use of Acetaminophen with any of the following: Pimozide

Increased Effect/Toxicity

Acetaminophen may increase the levels/effects of: ARIPiprazole; Busulfan; Dasatinib; Imatinib; Pimozide; Prilocaine; SORAfenib; Vitamin K Antagonists

The levels/effects of Acetaminophen may be increased by: Dasatinib; Imatinib; Isoniazid; Metyrapone; Probenecid; SORAfenib

Decreased Effect

The levels/effects of Acetaminophen may be decreased by: Anticonvulsants (Hydantoin); Barbiturates; CarBAMazepine; Cholestyramine Resin; Peginterferon Alfa-2b; Tocilizumab

Ethanol/Nutrition/Herb Interactions

Ethanol: Excessive intake of ethanol may increase the risk of acetaminophen-induced hepatotoxicity. Avoid ethanol or limit to <3 drinks/day.

Food: Rate of absorption may be decreased when given with food.

Herb/Nutraceutical: St John's wort may decrease acetaminophen levels.

Stability

Injection: Store intact vials at room temperature of 20°C to 25°C (68°F to 77°F); do not refrigerate or freeze. Injectable solution may be administered directly from the vial without further dilution. For doses <1000 mg, withdraw the appropriate volume and transfer to a separate sterile container (eg, glass bottle, plastic I.V. container, syringe) for administration. Use within 6 hours of opening vial or transferring to another container. Discard any unused portion; single use vials only.

Oral formulations: Store at controlled room temperature.

Suppositories: Store at <27°C (80°F); do not freeze.

Mechanism of Action Although not fully elucidated, believed to inhibit the synthesis of prostaglandins in the central nervous system and work peripherally to block pain impulse generation; produces antipyresis from inhibition of hypothalamic heat-regulating center

Pharmacodynamics/Kinetics

Onset of action:

Oral: <1 hour

I.V.: Analgesia: 5-10 minutes; Antipyretic: Within 30 minutes

Peak effect: I.V.: Analgesic: 1 hour

Duration:
  I.V., Oral: Analgesia: 4-6 hours
  I.V.: Antipyretic: ≥6 hours
Absorption: Primarily absorbed in small intestine (rate of absorption dependent upon gastric emptying); minimal absorption from stomach; varies by dosage form
Distribution: ~1 L/kg at therapeutic doses
Protein binding: 10% to 25% at therapeutic concentrations; 8% to 43% at toxic concentrations
Metabolism: At normal therapeutic dosages, primarily hepatic metabolism to sulfate and glucuronide conjugates, while a small amount is metabolized by CYP2E1 to a highly reactive intermediate, N-acetyl-p-benzoquinone imine (NAPQI), which is conjugated rapidly with glutathione and inactivated to nontoxic cysteine and mercapturic acid conjugates. At toxic doses (as little as 4 g daily) glutathione conjugation becomes insufficient to meet the metabolic demand causing an increase in NAPQI concentrations, which may cause hepatic cell necrosis. Oral administration is subject to first pass metabolism.
Half-life elimination: Prolonged following toxic doses; ~2 hours (range: 2-3 hours); may be slightly prolonged in severe renal insufficiency (Cl_{cr}<30 mL/minute): 2-5.3 hours
Time to peak, serum: Oral: Immediate release: 10-60 minutes (may be delayed in acute overdoses); I.V.: 15 minutes
Excretion: Urine (<5% unchanged; 60% to 80% as glucuronide metabolites; 20% to 30% as sulphate metabolites; ~8% cysteine and mercapturic acid metabolites)

Dosage

Geriatric & Adult Note: No dose adjustment required if converting between different acetaminophen formulations. Limit acetaminophen dose from all sources (prescription and OTC) to <4 g daily.

Pain or fever:
  Oral: **Note:** OTC dosing recommendations may vary by product and/or manufacturer.
    Regular release: 325-650 mg every 4-6 hours or 1000 mg 3-4 times daily (maximum: 4 g daily)
    Extended release: 1300 mg every 8 hours (maximum: 3.9 g daily)
  Rectal: 325-650 mg every 4-6 hours or 1000 mg 3-4 times daily (maximum: 4 g daily)
  I.V.:
    <50 kg: 15 mg/kg every 6 hours or 12.5 mg/kg every 4 hours; maximum single dose: 750 mg/dose; maximum daily dose: 75 mg/kg/day (≤3.75 g daily)
    ≥50 kg: 650 mg every 4 hours or 1000 mg every 6 hours; maximum single dose: 1000 mg/dose; maximum daily dose: 4 g daily

Renal Impairment

Oral (Aronoff, 2007):
  Adults:
    Cl_{cr} 10-50 mL/minute: Administer every 6 hours.
    Cl_{cr} <10 mL/minute: Administer every 8 hours.
    Intermittent hemodialysis or peritoneal dialysis: No adjustment necessary.
    CRRT: Administer every 8 hours.
  I.V.: Cl_{cr} ≤30 mL/minute: Use with caution; consider decreasing daily dose and extending dosing interval.

Hepatic Impairment Use with caution. Limited, low-dose therapy is usually well tolerated in hepatic disease/cirrhosis. However, cases of hepatotoxicity at daily acetaminophen dosages <4 g/day have been reported. Avoid chronic use in hepatic impairment.

Administration

Suspension, oral: Shake well before pouring a dose.
Injection: For I.V. infusion only. May administer undiluted over 15 minutes.
  Doses <1000 mg (<50 kg): Withdraw appropriate dose from vial and place into separate empty, sterile container prior to administration.
  Doses of 1000 mg (≥50 kg): Insert vented I.V. set through vial stopper.

Monitoring Parameters Relief of pain or fever

Test Interactions Acetaminophen may cause false-positive urinary 5-hydroxyindoleacetic acid.

Pharmacotherapy Pearls In 2011, McNeil Consumer Healthcare announced it had voluntarily reduced the maximum doses and increased the dosing interval on the labeling of some of their acetaminophen OTC products in an attempt to protect consumers from inadvertent overdoses. For example, the maximum dose of Extra Strength Tylenol® OTC was lowered from 4 g/day to 3 g/day and the maximum dose of Regular Strength Tylenol® OTC was lowered from 3900 mg/day to 3250 mg/day. In addition, the dosing interval for Extra Strength Tylenol® OTC was increased from every 4-6 hours to every 6 hours. Healthcare professionals may still prescribe or recommend the 4 g/day maximum to patients (but are advised to use their own discretion and clinical judgment).

Special Geriatric Considerations No specific information for use in elderly.

Dosage Forms Excipient information presented when available (limited, particularly for generics); consult specific product labeling. [DSC] = Discontinued product
Caplet, oral: 500 mg
  Cetafen® Extra: 500 mg
  Mapap® Extra Strength: 500 mg
  Mapap® Extra Strength: 500 mg [scored]
  Pain Eze: 650 mg
  Tylenol®: 325 mg
  Tylenol® Extra Strength: 500 mg
Caplet, extended release, oral:
  Mapap® Arthritis Pain: 650 mg
  Tylenol® 8 Hour: 650 mg
  Tylenol® Arthritis Pain Extended Relief: 650 mg
Capsule, oral:
  Mapap® Extra Strength: 500 mg
Captab, oral: 500 mg
Elixir, oral:
  Mapap® Children's: 160 mg/5 mL (118 mL, 480 mL) [ethanol free; contains benzoic acid, propylene glycol, sodium benzoate; cherry flavor]
Gelcap, oral: 500 mg
  Mapap®: 500 mg
Gelcap, rapid release, oral: 500 mg
  Tylenol® Extra Strength: 500 mg
Geltab, oral: 500 mg
  Excedrin® Tension Headache: 500 mg [contains caffeine 65 mg/geltab]
Injection, solution [preservative free]:
  Ofirmev™: 10 mg/mL (100 mL)
Liquid, oral: 160 mg/5 mL (120 mL, 473 mL); 500 mg/5 mL (240 mL)
  APAP 500: 500 mg/5 mL (237 mL) [ethanol free, sugar free; cherry flavor]
  Q-Pap Children's: 160 mg/5 mL (118 mL, 473 mL) [ethanol free; contains propylene glycol, sodium 2 mg/5 mL, sodium benzoate; cherry flavor]
  Q-Pap Children's: 160 mg/5 mL (118 mL, 473 mL) [ethanol free; contains propylene glycol, sodium 2 mg/5 mL, sodium benzoate; grape flavor]
  Silapap Children's: 160 mg/5 mL (118 mL, 237 mL, 473 mL) [ethanol free, sugar free; contains propylene glycol, sodium benzoate; cherry flavor]
  Tylenol® Extra Strength: 500 mg/15 mL (240 mL) [ethanol free; contains propylene glycol, sodium benzoate; cherry flavor]
Solution, oral: 160 mg/5 mL (5 mL, 10 mL, 20 mL)
  Pain & Fever Children's: 160 mg/5 mL (118 mL, 473 mL) [ethanol free, sugar free; contains propylene glycol, sodium 1 mg/5 mL, sodium benzoate; cherry flavor]
Solution, oral [drops]: 80 mg/0.8 mL (15 mL)
  Infantaire: 80 mg/0.8 mL (15 mL, 30 mL)
  Little Fevers™: 80 mg/mL (30 mL) [dye free, ethanol free, gluten free; contains propylene glycol, sodium benzoate; berry flavor]
  Mapap®: 80 mg/0.8 mL (15 mL) [fruit flavor]
  Q-Pap Infant's: 80 mg/0.8 mL (15 mL) [ethanol free; contains propylene glycol; fruit flavor]
  Silapap Infant's: 80 mg/0.8 mL (15 mL, 30 mL) [ethanol free; contains propylene glycol, sodium benzoate; cherry flavor]
Suppository, rectal: 120 mg (12s); 325 mg (12s); 650 mg (12s)
  Acephen™: 120 mg (12s, 50s, 100s); 325 mg (6s, 12s, 50s, 100s); 650 mg (12s, 50s, 100s)
  Feverall®: 80 mg (6s, 50s); 120 mg (6s, 50s); 325 mg (6s, 50s); 650 mg (50s)
Suspension, oral: 160 mg/5 mL (5 mL, 10 mL [DSC], 10.15 mL, 20 mL [DSC], 20.3 mL)
  Mapap® Children's: 160 mg/5 mL (118 mL) [ethanol free; contains propylene glycol, sodium benzoate; cherry flavor]
  Nortemp Children's: 160 mg/5 mL (118 mL) [ethanol free; contains propylene glycol, sodium benzoate; cotton candy flavor]
  Pain & Fever Children's: 160 mg/5 mL (60 mL) [ethanol free; contains propylene glycol, sodium benzoate; cherry flavor]
  Q-Pap Children's: 160 mg/5 mL (118 mL) [ethanol free; contains sodium 2 mg/5 mL, sodium benzoate; bubblegum flavor]
  Q-Pap Children's: 160 mg/5 mL (118 mL) [ethanol free; contains sodium 2 mg/5 mL, sodium benzoate; cherry flavor]
  Q-Pap Children's: 160 mg/5 mL (118 mL) [ethanol free; contains sodium 2 mg/5 mL, sodium benzoate; grape flavor]
  Tylenol® Children's: 160 mg/5 mL (120 mL) [dye free, ethanol free; contains propylene glycol, sodium benzoate; cherry flavor]
  Tylenol® Children's: 160 mg/5 mL (120 mL) [ethanol free; contains propylene glycol, sodium 2 mg/5 mL, sodium benzoate; bubblegum flavor]

Tylenol® Children's: 160 mg/5 mL (60 mL, 120 mL) [ethanol free; contains propylene glycol, sodium 2 mg/5 mL, sodium benzoate; cherry flavor]

Tylenol® Children's: 160 mg/5 mL (120 mL) [ethanol free; contains propylene glycol, sodium 2 mg/5 mL, sodium benzoate; grape flavor]

Tylenol® Children's: 160 mg/5 mL (120 mL) [ethanol free; contains propylene glycol, sodium 2 mg/5 mL, sodium benzoate; strawberry flavor]

Suspension, oral [drops]: 80 mg/0.8 mL (0.8 mL, 2 mL)

Mapap® Infant's: 80 mg/0.8 mL (15 mL, 30 mL) [ethanol free; contains propylene glycol, sodium benzoate; cherry flavor]

Tylenol® Infant's Concentrated: 80 mg/0.8 mL (30 mL) [dye free; contains propylene glycol; cherry flavor]

Tylenol® Infant's Concentrated: 80 mg/0.8 mL (15 mL, 30 mL) [ethanol free; contains sodium benzoate; cherry flavor]

Tylenol® Infant's Concentrated: 80 mg/0.8 mL (15 mL, 30 mL) [ethanol free; contains sodium benzoate; grape flavor]

Syrup, oral:

Triaminic™ Children's Fever Reducer Pain Reliever: 160 mg/5 mL (118 mL) [contains benzoic acid, sodium 6 mg/5 mL; bubblegum flavor]

Triaminic™ Children's Fever Reducer Pain Reliever: 160 mg/5 mL (118 mL) [contains sodium 5 mg/5 mL, sodium benzoate; grape flavor]

Tablet, oral: 325 mg, 500 mg

Aspirin Free Anacin® Extra Strength: 500 mg

Cetafen®: 325 mg

Mapap®: 325 mg

Non-Aspirin Pain Reliever: 325 mg

Q-Pap: 325 mg [scored]

Q-Pap Extra Strength: 500 mg [scored]

Tylenol®: 325 mg

Tylenol® Extra Strength: 500 mg

Valorin: 325 mg [sugar free]

Valorin Extra: 500 mg [sugar free]

Tablet, chewable, oral: 80 mg

Mapap® Children's: 80 mg [fruit flavor]

Tablet, orally disintegrating, oral: 80 mg, 160 mg

Mapap® Children's: 80 mg [bubblegum flavor]

Mapap® Children's: 80 mg [grape flavor]

Mapap® Junior Rapid Tabs: 160 mg [bubblegum flavor]

RapiMed® Children's: 80 mg [gluten free, sugar free; bubblegum flavor]

RapiMed® Children's: 80 mg [gluten free, sugar free; wild grape flavor]

RapiMed® Junior: 160 mg [gluten free, sugar free; bubblegum flavor]

RapiMed® Junior: 160 mg [gluten free, sugar free; wild grape flavor]

Tylenol® Children's Meltaways: 80 mg [scored; bubblegum flavor]

Tylenol® Children's Meltaways: 80 mg [scored; grape flavor]

Tylenol® Jr. Meltaways: 160 mg [bubblegum flavor]

Tylenol® Jr. Meltaways: 160 mg [grape flavor]

Acetaminophen and Codeine (a seet a MIN oh fen & KOE deen)

Related Information
Acetaminophen *on page 31*
Codeine *on page 433*

Medication Safety Issues
Sound-alike/look-alike issues:
Tylenol® may be confused with atenolol, timolol, Tylox®

High alert medication:
The Institute for Safe Medication Practices (ISMP) includes this medication among its list of drug classes which have a heightened risk of causing significant patient harm when used in error.

Other safety concerns:
Duplicate therapy issues: This product contains acetaminophen, which may be a component of other combination products. Do not exceed the maximum recommended daily dose of acetaminophen.

T3 is an error-prone abbreviation (mistaken as liothyronine)

International issues:
Codex: Brand name for acetaminophen/codeine [Brazil], but also the brand name for *saccharomyces boulardii* [Italy]

ACETAMINOPHEN AND CODEINE

Codex [Brazil] may be confused with Cedax brand name for ceftibuten [U.S. and multiple international markets]

Brand Names: U.S. Capital® and Codeine; Tylenol® with Codeine No. 3; Tylenol® with Codeine No. 4

Brand Names: Canada ratio-Emtec; ratio-Lenoltec; Triatec-30; Triatec-8; Triatec-8 Strong; Tylenol Elixir with Codeine; Tylenol No. 1; Tylenol No. 1 Forte; Tylenol No. 2 with Codeine; Tylenol No. 3 with Codeine; Tylenol No. 4 with Codeine

Index Terms Codeine and Acetaminophen; Tylenol #2; Tylenol #3; Tylenol Codeine

Generic Availability (U.S.) Yes

Pharmacologic Category Analgesic Combination (Opioid)

Use Relief of mild-to-moderate pain

Dosage

Geriatric Doses should be titrated to appropriate analgesic effect.
One Tylenol® No. 3 tablet every 4 hours; do **not** exceed 4 g/day acetaminophen.

Adult Doses should be adjusted according to severity of pain and response of the patient. Adult doses ≥60 mg codeine fail to give commensurate relief of pain but merely prolong analgesia and are associated with an appreciably increased incidence of side effects.

Cough (Antitussive): Oral: Based on codeine (15-30 mg/dose) every 4-6 hours (maximum: 360 mg/24 hours based on codeine component)

Pain (Analgesic): Oral: Based on codeine (30-60 mg/dose) every 4-6 hours (maximum: 4000 mg/24 hours based on acetaminophen component)
1-2 tablets every 4 hours to a maximum of 12 tablets/24 hours

Renal Impairment See individual agents.

Hepatic Impairment Use with caution. Limited, low-dose therapy is usually well tolerated in hepatic disease/cirrhosis; however, cases of hepatotoxicity at daily acetaminophen dosages <4 g/day have been reported. Avoid chronic use in hepatic impairment.

Special Geriatric Considerations See individual agents.

Controlled Substance C-III; C-V

Dosage Forms Excipient information presented when available (limited, particularly for generics); consult specific product labeling.
Solution, oral [C-V]: Acetaminophen 120 mg and codeine phosphate 12 mg per 5 mL (5 mL, 10 mL, 12.5 mL, 15 mL, 120 mL, 480 mL) [contains alcohol 7%]
Suspension, oral [C-V] (Capital® and Codeine): Acetaminophen 120 mg and codeine phosphate 12 mg per 5 mL (480 mL) [alcohol free; contains propylene glycol, sodium benzoate; fruit punch flavor]
Tablet, oral [C-III]: Acetaminophen 300 mg and codeine phosphate 15 mg; acetaminophen 300 mg and codeine phosphate 30 mg; acetaminophen 300 mg and codeine phosphate 60 mg
Tylenol® with Codeine No. 3: Acetaminophen 300 mg and codeine phosphate 30 mg [contains sodium metabisulfite]
Tylenol® with Codeine No. 4: Acetaminophen 300 mg and codeine phosphate 60 mg [contains sodium metabisulfite]

Dosage Forms: Canada Excipient information presented when available (limited, particularly for generics); consult specific product labeling. **Note:** In countries outside of the U.S., some formulations of Tylenol® with Codeine include caffeine.
Caplet:
ratio-Lenoltec No. 1, Tylenol No. 1: Acetaminophen 300 mg, codeine phosphate 8 mg, and caffeine 15 mg
Tylenol No. 1 Forte: Acetaminophen 500 mg, codeine phosphate 8 mg, and caffeine 15 mg
Solution, oral:
Tylenol Elixir with Codeine: Acetaminophen 160 mg and codeine phosphate 8 mg per 5 mL (500 mL) [contains alcohol 7%, sucrose 31%; cherry flavor]
Tablet:
ratio-Emtec, Triatec-30: Acetaminophen 300 mg and codeine phosphate 30 mg
ratio-Lenoltec No. 1: Acetaminophen 300 mg, codeine phosphate 8 mg, and caffeine 15 mg
ratio-Lenoltec No. 2, Tylenol No. 2 with Codeine: Acetaminophen 300 mg, codeine phosphate 15 mg, and caffeine 15 mg
ratio-Lenoltec No. 3, Tylenol No. 3 with Codeine: Acetaminophen 300 mg, codeine phosphate 30 mg, and caffeine 15 mg
ratio-Lenoltec No. 4, Tylenol No. 4 with Codeine: Acetaminophen 300 mg and codeine phosphate 60 mg
Triatec-8: Acetaminophen 325 mg, codeine phosphate 8 mg, and caffeine 30 mg
Triatec-8 Strong: Acetaminophen 500 mg, codeine phosphate 8 mg, and caffeine 30 mg

♦ **Acetaminophen and Hydrocodone** see Hydrocodone and Acetaminophen on page 937
♦ **Acetaminophen and Oxycodone** see Oxycodone and Acetaminophen on page 1449

Acetaminophen and Phenylephrine (a seet a MIN oh fen & fen il EF rin)

Related Information
Acetaminophen *on page 31*

Medication Safety Issues
Other safety concerns:
Duplicate therapy issues: This product contains acetaminophen, which may be a component of combination products. Do not exceed the maximum recommended daily dose of acetaminophen.

Brand Names: U.S. Cetafen Cold® [OTC]; Contac® Cold + Flu Maximum Strength Non-Drowsy [OTC]; Excedrin® Sinus Headache [OTC]; Mapap® Sinus PE [OTC]; Robitussin® Peak Cold Nasal Relief [OTC]; Sinus Pain & Pressure [OTC]; Sudafed PE® Pressure + Pain [OTC]; Tylenol® Sinus Congestion & Pain Daytime [OTC]; Vicks® DayQuil® Sinex® Daytime Sinus [OTC]

Index Terms Phenylephrine Hydrochloride and Acetaminophen

Generic Availability (U.S.) Yes: Caplet, tablet

Pharmacologic Category Analgesic, Miscellaneous; Decongestant

Use Temporary relief of sinus/nasal congestion and pressure, headache, and minor aches and pains

Dosage
Geriatric & Adult Sinus pain/pressure: Oral: General dosing guidelines, refer to specific product labeling: Acetaminophen 325 mg and phenylephrine 5 mg/caplet: Take 2 caplets every 4 hours as needed; maximum: 12 caplets/24 hours

Special Geriatric Considerations Elderly are more predisposed to the adverse effects of sympathomimetics since they frequently have cardiovascular disease and diabetes mellitus as well as multiple drug therapies. Since oral and topical phenylephrine can be obtained OTC, elderly patients should be counseled about their proper use and in what disease states they should be avoided.

Dosage Forms Excipient information presented when available (limited, particularly for generics); consult specific product labeling.
Caplet, oral:
Contac® Cold + Flu Maximum Strength Non Drowsy: Acetaminophen 500 mg and phenylephrine hydrochloride 5 mg
Excedrin® Sinus Headache: Acetaminophen 325 mg and phenylephrine hydrochloride 5 mg
Mapap® Sinus PE, Sudafed PE® Pressure + Pain: Acetaminophen 325 mg and phenylephrine hydrochloride 5 mg
Tylenol® Sinus Congestion & Pain Daytime: Acetaminophen 325 mg and phenylephrine hydrochloride 5 mg [Cool Burst® flavor]
Capsule, liquid filled, oral:
Vicks® DayQuil® Sinex® Daytime Sinus: Acetaminophen 325 mg and phenylephrine hydrochloride 5 mg
Gelcap, rapid release, oral:
Tylenol® Sinus Congestion & Pain Daytime: Acetaminophen 325 mg and phenylephrine hydrochloride 5 mg
Tablet, oral:
Cetafen Cold®: Acetaminophen 500 mg and phenylephrine hydrochloride 5 mg
Robitussin® Peak Cold Nasal Relief: Acetaminophen 325 mg and phenylephrine hydrochloride 5 mg
Sinus Pain & Pressure: Acetaminophen 500 mg and phenylephrine hydrochloride 5 mg

AcetaZOLAMIDE (a set a ZOLE a mide)

Related Information
Glaucoma Drug Therapy *on page 2115*

Medication Safety Issues
International issues:
Diamox [Canada and multiple international markets] may be confused with Diabinese brand name for chlorpropamide [Multiple international markets]; Dobutrex brand name for dobutamine [Multiple international markets]; Trimox brand name for amoxicillin [Brazil]; Zimox brand name for amoxicillin [Italy] and carbidopa/levodopa [Greece]

Brand Names: U.S. Diamox® Sequels®

Brand Names: Canada Acetazolam; Diamox®

Generic Availability (U.S.) Yes

Pharmacologic Category Anticonvulsant, Miscellaneous; Carbonic Anhydrase Inhibitor; Diuretic, Carbonic Anhydrase Inhibitor; Ophthalmic Agent, Antiglaucoma

Use Treatment of glaucoma (chronic simple open-angle, secondary glaucoma, preoperatively in acute angle-closure); drug-induced edema or edema due to congestive heart failure (adjunctive therapy; I.V. and immediate release dosage forms); centrencephalic epilepsies (I.V. and immediate release dosage forms); prevention or amelioration of symptoms associated with acute mountain sickness (immediate and extended release dosage forms)

Unlabeled Use Metabolic alkalosis; respiratory stimulant in stable hypercapnic COPD

Contraindications Hypersensitivity to acetazolamide, sulfonamides, or any component of the formulation; hepatic disease or insufficiency; decreased sodium and/or potassium levels; adrenocortical insufficiency; cirrhosis; hyperchloremic acidosis, severe renal disease or dysfunction; long-term use in noncongestive angle-closure glaucoma

Warnings/Precautions Use with caution in patients with hepatic dysfunction; in cirrhosis, avoid electrolyte and acid/base imbalances that might lead to hepatic encephalopathy. Use with caution in patients with respiratory acidosis and diabetes mellitus (may change glucose control). Use with caution or avoid in patients taking high-dose aspirin concurrently; may lead to severe adverse effects including tachypnea, anorexia, lethargy, coma, and death. Use with caution in the elderly; may be more sensitive to side effects. Impairment of mental alertness and/or physical coordination may occur. Chemical similarities are present among sulfonamides, sulfonylureas, carbonic anhydrase inhibitors, thiazides, and loop diuretics (except ethacrynic acid). Use in patients with sulfonamide allergy is specifically contraindicated in product labeling, however, a risk of cross-reaction exists in patients with allergy to any of these compounds; avoid use when previous reaction has been severe. Discontinue if signs of hypersensitivity are noted. Increasing the dose does not increase diuresis and may increase the incidence of drowsiness and/or paresthesia; often results in a reduction of diuresis.

I.M. administration is painful because of the alkaline pH of the drug; use by this route is not recommended.

Adverse Reactions (Reflective of adult population; not specific for elderly) Frequency not defined.

Cardiovascular: Flushing

Central nervous system: Ataxia, confusion, convulsions, depression, dizziness, drowsiness, excitement, fatigue, fever, headache, malaise

Dermatologic: Allergic skin reactions, photosensitivity, Stevens-Johnson syndrome, toxic epidermal necrolysis, urticaria

Endocrine & metabolic: Electrolyte imbalance, hyperglycemia, hypoglycemia, hypokalemia, hyponatremia, metabolic acidosis

Gastrointestinal: Appetite decreased, diarrhea, melena, nausea, taste alteration, vomiting

Genitourinary: Crystalluria, glycosuria, hematuria, polyuria, renal failure

Hematologic: Agranulocytosis, aplastic anemia, leukopenia, thrombocytopenia, thrombocytopenic purpura

Hepatic: Cholestatic jaundice, fulminant hepatic necrosis, hepatic insufficiency, liver function tests abnormal

Local: Pain at injection site

Neuromuscular & skeletal: Flaccid paralysis, paresthesia

Ocular: Myopia

Otic: Hearing disturbance, tinnitus

Miscellaneous: Anaphylaxis

Drug Interactions

Metabolism/Transport Effects Inhibits CYP3A4 (weak)

Avoid Concomitant Use

Avoid concomitant use of AcetaZOLAMIDE with any of the following: Azelastine; Azelastine (Nasal); Carbonic Anhydrase Inhibitors; Methadone; Mirtazapine; Paraldehyde; Pimozide

Increased Effect/Toxicity

AcetaZOLAMIDE may increase the levels/effects of: Alcohol (Ethyl); Alpha-/Beta-Agonists; Amifostine; Amphetamines; Anticonvulsants (Barbiturate); Anticonvulsants (Hydantoin); Antihypertensives; ARIPiprazole; Azelastine; Azelastine (Nasal); Buprenorphine; CarBAMazepine; Carbonic Anhydrase Inhibitors; CNS Depressants; CycloSPORINE; CycloSPORINE (Systemic); Flecainide; Hypotensive Agents; Memantine; MetFORMIN; Methadone; Methotrimeprazine; Metyrosine; Mirtazapine; Paraldehyde; Pimozide; Primidone; QuiNIDine; RiTUXimab; Selective Serotonin Reuptake Inhibitors; Sodium Bicarbonate; Sodium Phosphates; Zolpidem

The levels/effects of AcetaZOLAMIDE may be increased by: Alfuzosin; Diazoxide; Droperidol; Herbs (Hypotensive Properties); HydrOXYzine; MAO Inhibitors; Methotrimeprazine; Pentoxifylline; Phosphodiesterase 5 Inhibitors; Prostacyclin Analogues; Salicylates

Decreased Effect

AcetaZOLAMIDE may decrease the levels/effects of: Lithium; Methenamine; Primidone; Trientine

The levels/effects of AcetaZOLAMIDE may be decreased by: Herbs (Hypertensive Properties); Ketorolac; Ketorolac (Nasal); Ketorolac (Systemic); Mefloquine; Methylphenidate; Yohimbine

Stability

Capsules, tablets: Store at controlled room temperature.

Injection: Store vial for injection (prior to reconstitution) at controlled room temperature. Reconstitute with at least 5 mL sterile water to provide a solution containing not more than 100 mg/mL. Reconstituted solution may be refrigerated (2°C to 8°C) for 1 week, however, use within 12 hours is recommended. Further dilute in D_5W or NS for I.V. infusion. Stability of IVPB solutions in D_5W or NS is 5 days at room temperature (25°C) and 44 days under refrigeration (5°C).

Mechanism of Action Reversible inhibition of the enzyme carbonic anhydrase resulting in reduction of hydrogen ion secretion at renal tubule and an increased renal excretion of sodium, potassium, bicarbonate, and water. Decreases production of aqueous humor and inhibits carbonic anhydrase in central nervous system to retard abnormal and excessive discharge from CNS neurons.

Pharmacodynamics/Kinetics

Onset of action: Capsule (extended release), tablet (immediate release): 2 hours; I.V.: 5-10 minutes

Peak effect: Capsule (extended release): 8-18 hours; I.V.: 15 minutes; Tablet: 2-4 hours

Duration: Inhibition of aqueous humor secretion: Capsule (extended release): 18-24 hours; I.V.: 4-5 hours; Tablet: 8-12 hours

Distribution: Erythrocytes, kidneys; blood-brain barrier

Time to peak, plasma: Capsule (extended release): 3-6 hours; Tablet: 1-4 hours

Excretion: Urine (70% to 100% as unchanged drug)

Dosage

Geriatric Refer to adult dosing. Oral: Initial doses should begin at the low end of the dosage range.

Adult Note: I.M. administration is not recommended because of pain secondary to the alkaline pH.

Altitude illness: Oral: Manufacturer's labeling: 500-1000 mg/day in divided doses every 8-12 hours (immediate release tablets) or divided every 12-24 hours (extended release capsules). These doses are associated with more frequent and/or increased side effects. Alternative dosing has been recommended:

Prevention: 125 mg twice daily; beginning either the day before (preferred) or on the day of ascent; may be discontinued after staying at the same elevation for 2-3 days or if descent initiated (Basnyat, 2006; Luks, 2010). **Note:** In situations of rapid ascent (such as rescue or military operations), 1000 mg/day is recommended by the manufacturer. The Wilderness Medical Society recommends consideration of using dexamethasone in addition to acetazolamide in these situations (Luks, 2010).

Treatment: 250 mg twice daily. **Note:** With high altitude cerebral edema, dexamethasone is the primary treatment; however, acetazolamide may be used adjunctively with the same treatment dose (Luks, 2010).

Edema: Oral, I.V.: 250-375 mg once daily

Epilepsy: Oral: 8-30 mg/kg/day in divided doses. A lower dosing range of 4-16 mg/kg/day in 1-4 divided doses has also been recommended; maximum dose: 30 mg/kg/day or 1 g/day (Oles, 1989; Reiss, 1996). **Note:** Minimal additional benefit with doses >16 mg/kg/day. **Extended release capsule is not recommended for treatment of epilepsy.**

Glaucoma: Oral, I.V.:

Chronic simple (open-angle): 250 mg 1-4 times/day or 500 mg extended release capsule twice daily

Secondary or acute (closed-angle): Initial: 250-500 mg; maintenance: 125-250 mg every 4 hours (250 mg every 12 hours has been effective in short-term treatment of some patients)

Metabolic alkalosis (unlabeled use): I.V.: 500 mg as a single dose; reassess need based upon acid-base status (Marik, 1991; Mazur, 1999)

Respiratory stimulant in stable hypercapnic COPD (unlabeled use): Oral: 250 mg twice daily (Wagenaar, 2003)

Renal Impairment Note: Use is contraindicated in marked renal impairment; creatinine clearance cutoff not specified in manufacturer's labeling.

Cl_{cr} 10-50 mL/minute: Administer every 12 hours.

Cl_{cr} <10 mL/minute: Avoid use.

Hemodialysis: Moderately dialyzable (20% to 50%).

Peritoneal dialysis: Supplemental dose is not necessary (Schwenk, 1994).

Administration

Oral: May be administered with food. May cause an alteration in taste, especially carbonated beverages. Short-acting tablets may be crushed and suspended in cherry or chocolate syrup to disguise the bitter taste of the drug; do not use fruit juices. Alternatively, submerge tablet in 10 mL of hot water and add 10 mL honey or syrup.

I.M.: I.M. administration is painful because of the alkaline pH of the drug; use by this route is not recommended.

I.V.: No specific guidance given by manufacturer, but I.V. push at a rate of up to 500 mg over 3 minutes has been reported in a clinical trial (Mazur, 1999); a study to assess cerebrovascular reserve has used rapid I.V. push of up to 1 g over ≤1 minute (Piepgras, 1990)

Monitoring Parameters Intraocular pressure; serum electrolytes, periodic CBC with differential

Test Interactions May cause false-positive results for urinary protein with Albustix®, Labstix®, Albutest®, Bumintest®; interferes with HPLC theophylline assay and serum uric acid levels

Special Geriatric Considerations Oral carbonic anhydrase inhibitors are an alternative for patients who have difficulty administering ophthalmic drugs, who do not achieve sufficient lowering of intraocular pressure, or who cannot tolerate other agents. Malaise and complaints of tiredness and myalgia are signs of excessive dosing and acidosis in older adults. Orthostatic hypotension may occur; assess blood pressure. Note renal impairment recommendations; many elderly have Cl_{cr} <50 mL/minute.

Dosage Forms Excipient information presented when available (limited, particularly for generics); consult specific product labeling.

Capsule, extended release, oral: 500 mg

Capsule, sustained release, oral:
   Diamox® Sequels®: 500 mg

Injection, powder for reconstitution: 500 mg

Tablet, oral: 125 mg, 250 mg

♦ **Acetoxymethylprogesterone** see MedroxyPROGESTERone on page 1190
♦ **Acetylcysteine, Methylcobalamin, and Methylfolate** see Methylfolate, Methylcobalamin, and Acetylcysteine on page 1246
♦ **Acetylcysteine, Methylfolate, and Methylcobalamin** see Methylfolate, Methylcobalamin, and Acetylcysteine on page 1246
♦ **Acetylsalicylic Acid** see Aspirin on page 154
♦ **Achromycin** see Tetracycline on page 1872
♦ **Aciclovir** see Acyclovir (Systemic) on page 41
♦ **Aciclovir** see Acyclovir (Topical) on page 44
♦ **Acid Gone [OTC]** see Aluminum Hydroxide and Magnesium Carbonate on page 79
♦ **Acid Gone Extra Strength [OTC]** see Aluminum Hydroxide and Magnesium Carbonate on page 79
♦ **Acidulated Phosphate Fluoride** see Fluoride on page 806
♦ **AcipHex®** see RABEprazole on page 1659
♦ **Aclovate®** see Alclometasone on page 52
♦ **Act® [OTC]** see Fluoride on page 806
♦ **Actemra®** see Tocilizumab on page 1918
♦ **Actigall®** see Ursodiol on page 1986
♦ **Actiq®** see FentaNYL on page 761
♦ **Activase®** see Alteplase on page 73
♦ **Activated Dimethicone** see Simethicone on page 1776
♦ **Activated Ergosterol** see Ergocalciferol on page 657
♦ **Activated Methylpolysiloxane** see Simethicone on page 1776
♦ **Act® Kids [OTC]** see Fluoride on page 806
♦ **Actonel®** see Risedronate on page 1707
♦ **Actoplus Met®** see Pioglitazone and Metformin on page 1545
♦ **Actoplus Met® XR** see Pioglitazone and Metformin on page 1545
♦ **Actos®** see Pioglitazone on page 1542
♦ **Act® Restoring™ [OTC]** see Fluoride on page 806
♦ **Act® Total Care™ [OTC]** see Fluoride on page 806
♦ **Acular®** see Ketorolac (Ophthalmic) on page 1076
♦ **Acular LS®** see Ketorolac (Ophthalmic) on page 1076
♦ **Acuvail®** see Ketorolac (Ophthalmic) on page 1076
♦ **ACV** see Acyclovir (Systemic) on page 41
♦ **ACV** see Acyclovir (Topical) on page 44
♦ **Acycloguanosine** see Acyclovir (Systemic) on page 41
♦ **Acycloguanosine** see Acyclovir (Topical) on page 44

Acyclovir (Systemic) (ay SYE kloe veer)

Medication Safety Issues
Sound-alike/look-alike issues:
Acyclovir may be confused with ganciclovir, Retrovir®, valacyclovir
Zovirax® may be confused with Doribax®, Valtrex®, Zithromax®, Zostrix®, Zyloprim®, Zyvox®

Brand Names: U.S. Zovirax®
Brand Names: Canada Apo-Acyclovir®; Mylan-Acyclovir; Nu-Acyclovir; ratio-Acyclovir; Teva-Acyclovir; Zovirax®
Index Terms Aciclovir; ACV; Acycloguanosine
Generic Availability (U.S.) Yes
Pharmacologic Category Antiviral Agent
Use Treatment of genital herpes simplex virus (HSV) and HSV encephalitis
Unlabeled Use Prevention of HSV reactivation in HIV-positive patients; prevention of HSV reactivation in hematopoietic stem cell transplant (HSCT); prevention of HSV reactivation during periods of neutropenia in patients with cancer; prevention of varicella zoster virus (VZV) reactivation in allogenic HSCT; prevention of CMV reactivation in low-risk allogeneic HSCT; treatment of disseminated HSV or VZV in immunocompromised patients with cancer; empiric treatment of suspected encephalitis in immunocompromised patients with cancer; treatment of initial and prophylaxis of recurrent mucosal and cutaneous herpes simplex (HSV-1 and HSV-2) infections in immunocompromised patients
Contraindications Hypersensitivity to acyclovir, valacyclovir, or any component of the formulation
Warnings/Precautions Use with caution in immunocompromised patients; thrombocytopenic purpura/hemolytic uremic syndrome (TTP/HUS) has been reported. Use caution in the elderly, pre-existing renal disease (may require dosage modification), or in those receiving other nephrotoxic drugs. Renal failure (sometimes fatal) has been reported. Maintain adequate hydration during oral or intravenous therapy. Use I.V. preparation with caution in patients with underlying neurologic abnormalities, serious hepatic or electrolyte abnormalities, or substantial hypoxia.

Varicella-zoster: Treatment should begin within 24 hours of appearance of rash.
Adverse Reactions (Reflective of adult population; not specific for elderly)
Oral:
>10%: Central nervous system: Malaise (≤12%)
1% to 10%:
Central nervous system: Headache (≤2%)
Gastrointestinal: Nausea (2% to 5%), vomiting (≤3%), diarrhea (2% to 3%)
Parenteral:
1% to 10%:
Dermatologic: Hives (2%), itching (2%), rash (2%)
Gastrointestinal: Nausea/vomiting (7%)
Hepatic: Liver function tests increased (1% to 2%)
Local: Inflammation at injection site or phlebitis (9%)
Renal: BUN increased (5% to 10%), creatinine increased (5% to 10%), acute renal failure
Drug Interactions
Metabolism/Transport Effects None known.
Avoid Concomitant Use
Avoid concomitant use of Acyclovir (Systemic) with any of the following: Zoster Vaccine
Increased Effect/Toxicity
Acyclovir (Systemic) may increase the levels/effects of: Mycophenolate; Tenofovir; Zidovudine

The levels/effects of Acyclovir (Systemic) may be increased by: Mycophenolate
Decreased Effect
Acyclovir (Systemic) may decrease the levels/effects of: Zoster Vaccine
Ethanol/Nutrition/Herb Interactions Food: Does not affect absorption of oral acyclovir.
Stability
Capsule, tablet: Store at controlled room temperature of 15°C to 25°C (59°F to 77°F); protect from moisture.
Injection: Store powder at controlled room temperature of 15°C to 25°C (59°F to 77°F). Reconstitute acyclovir 500 mg powder with SWFI 10 mL; do not use bacteriostatic water containing benzyl alcohol or parabens. For intravenous infusion, dilute in D₅W, D₅NS, D₅¼NS, D₅½NS, LR, or NS to a final concentration ≤7 mg/mL. Concentrations >10 mg/mL increase the risk of phlebitis. Reconstituted solutions remain stable for 12 hours at room

. temperature. Do not refrigerate reconstituted solutions or solutions diluted for infusion as they may precipitate. Once diluted for infusion, use within 24 hours.

Mechanism of Action Acyclovir is converted to acyclovir monophosphate by virus-specific thymidine kinase then further converted to acyclovir triphosphate by other cellular enzymes. Acyclovir triphosphate inhibits DNA synthesis and viral replication by competing with deoxyguanosine triphosphate for viral DNA polymerase and being incorporated into viral DNA.

Pharmacodynamics/Kinetics

Absorption: Oral: 15% to 30%

Distribution: V_d: 0.8 L/kg (63.6 L): Widely (eg, brain, kidney, lungs, liver, spleen, muscle, uterus, vagina, CSF)

Protein binding: 9% to 33%

Metabolism: Converted by viral enzymes to acyclovir monophosphate, and further converted to diphosphate then triphosphate (active form) by cellular enzymes

Bioavailability: Oral: 10% to 20% with normal renal function (bioavailability decreases with increased dose)

Half-life elimination: Terminal: Adults: 3 hours

Time to peak, serum: Oral: Within 1.5-2 hours

Excretion: Urine (62% to 90% as unchanged drug and metabolite)

Dosage

Geriatric & Adult Note: Obese patients should be dosed using ideal body weight

Genital herpes simplex virus (HSV) infection:

I.V.: Immunocompetent: Initial episode, severe: 5 mg/kg/dose every 8 hours for 5-7 days **or** 5-10 mg/kg/dose every 8 hours for 2-7 days, follow with oral therapy to complete at least 10 days of therapy (CDC, 2010)

Oral:

Initial episode: 200 mg every 4 hours while awake (5 times/day) for 10 days **or** 400 mg 3 times/day for 7-10 days (CDC, 2010)

Recurrence: 200 mg every 4 hours while awake (5 times/day) for 5 days (per manufacturer's labeling; begin at earliest signs of disease)

Alternatively, the following regimens are also recommended by the CDC: 400 mg 3 times/day for 5 days; 800 mg twice daily for 5 days; 800 mg 3 times/day for 2 days (CDC, 2010)

Chronic suppression: 400 mg twice daily or 200 mg 3-5 times/day, for up to 12 months followed by re-evaluation (per manufacturer's labeling)

Herpes zoster (shingles):

Oral: Immunocompetent: 800 mg every 4 hours (5 times/day) for 7-10 days

I.V.: Immunocompromised: 10 mg/kg/dose or 500 mg/m^2/dose every 8 hours for 7 days

HSV encephalitis: I.V.: 10 mg/kg/dose every 8 hours for 10 days (per manufacturer's labeling); 10-15 mg/kg/dose every 8 hours for 14-21 days also reported

Mucocutaneous HSV:

I.V.: Immunocompromised: Treatment: 5 mg/kg/dose every 8 hours for 7 days (Leflore, 2000); dosing for up to 14 days also reported

Oral (unlabeled use): Immunocompromised: 400 mg 5 times/day for 7 days (Leflore, 2000)

Orolabial HSV (unlabeled use): Oral (immunocompetent):

Treatment: 200-400 mg 5 times/day for 5 days (Cernik, 2008; Leflore, 2000; Spruance, 1990) for episodic/recurrent treatment; for initial treatment, limited data are available, 200 mg 5 times/day or 400 mg 3 times/day for 7-10 days has been recommended by some clinicians.

Chronic suppression: 400 mg 2 times/day (has been clinically evaluated for up to 1 year) (Cernik, 2008; Rooney, 1993)

Varicella-zoster (chickenpox): Begin treatment within the first 24 hours of rash onset:

Oral: >40 kg (immunocompetent): 800 mg/dose 4 times/day for 5 days

I.V.:

Manufacturer's labeling (immunocompromised): 10 mg/kg/dose every 8 hours for 7 days

CDC HIV guidelines (immunocompromised): 10-15 mg/kg/dose every 8 hours for 7-10 days

Prevention of HSV reactivation in HIV-positive patients (unlabeled use): Oral: 400-800 mg 2-3 times/day (CDC, 2010)

Prevention of HSV reactivation in HSCT (unlabeled use): CDC recommendation: **Note:** Start at the beginning of conditioning therapy and continue until engraftment or until mucositis resolves (~30 days)

Oral: 200 mg 3 times/day

I.V.: 250 mg/m^2/dose every 12 hours

Prevention of VZV reactivation in allogeneic HSCT (unlabeled use): NCCN guidelines:

Oral: 800 mg twice a day

Prevention of CMV reactivation in low-risk allogeneic HSCT (unlabeled use): *NCCN guidelines:* **Note:** Requires close monitoring (due to weak activity); not for use in patients at high risk for CMV disease: Oral: 800 mg 4 times/day

Treatment of disseminated HSV or VZV or empiric treatment of suspected encephalitis in immunocompromised patients with cancer: (unlabeled use): *NCCN guidelines:* I.V.: 10-12 mg/kg/dose every 8 hours

Treatment of episodic HSV infection in HIV-positive patient (unlabeled use): Oral: 400 mg 3 times/day for 5-10 days (CDC, 2010)

Renal Impairment

Oral:

Cl_{cr} 10-25 mL/minute/1.73 m^2: Normal dosing regimen 800 mg every 4 hours: Administer 800 mg every 8 hours

Cl_{cr} <10 mL/minute/1.73 m^2:

Normal dosing regimen 200 mg every 4 hours or 400 mg every 12 hours: Administer 200 mg every 12 hours

Normal dosing regimen 800 mg every 4 hours: Administer 800 mg every 12 hours

I.V.:

Cl_{cr} 25-50 mL/minute/1.73 m^2: Administer recommended dose every 12 hours

Cl_{cr} 10-25 mL/minute/1.73 m^2: Administer recommended dose every 24 hours

Cl_{cr} <10 mL/minute/1.73 m^2: Administer 50% of recommended dose every 24 hours

Intermittent hemodialysis (IHD) (administer after hemodialysis on dialysis days): Dialyzable (60% reduction following a 6-hour session): I.V.: 2.5-5 mg/kg every 24 hours (Heintz, 2009). **Note:** Dosing dependent on the assumption of 3 times/week, complete IHD sessions.

Peritoneal dialysis (PD): Administer 50% of normal dose once daily; no supplemental dose needed

Continuous renal replacement therapy (CRRT) (Heintz, 2009; Trotman, 2005): Drug clearance is highly dependent on the method of renal replacement, filter type, and flow rate. Appropriate dosing requires close monitoring of pharmacologic response, signs of adverse reactions due to drug accumulation, as well as drug concentrations in relation to target trough (if appropriate). The following are general recommendations only (based on dialysate flow/ultrafiltration rates of 1-2 L/hour and minimal residual renal function) and should not supersede clinical judgment:

CVVH: I.V.: 5-10 mg/kg every 24 hours

CVVHD/CVVHDF: I.V.: 5-10 mg/kg every 12-24 hours

Note: The higher end of dosage range (eg, 10 mg/kg every 12 hours for CVVHDF) is recommended for viral meningoencephalitis and varicella-zoster virus infections.

Administration

Oral: May be administered with or without food.

I.V.: Avoid rapid infusion; infuse over 1 hour to prevent renal damage; maintain adequate hydration of patient; check for phlebitis and rotate infusion sites. Avoid I.M. or SubQ administration.

Monitoring Parameters Urinalysis, BUN, serum creatinine, liver enzymes, CBC

Special Geriatric Considerations For herpes zoster, acyclovir should be started within 72 hours of the appearance of the rash to be effective. Dose adjustment may be necessary depending on creatinine clearance.

Dosage Forms Excipient information presented when available (limited, particularly for generics); consult specific product labeling.

Capsule, oral: 200 mg

Zovirax®: 200 mg

Injection, powder for reconstitution, as sodium [strength expressed as base]: 500 mg, 1000 mg

Injection, solution, as sodium [strength expressed as base, preservative free]: 50 mg/mL (10 mL, 20 mL)

Suspension, oral: 200 mg/5 mL (473 mL)

Zovirax®: 200 mg/5 mL (473 mL) [banana flavor]

Tablet, oral: 400 mg, 800 mg

Zovirax®: 400 mg

Zovirax®: 800 mg [scored]

Acyclovir (Topical) (ay SYE kloe veer)

Medication Safety Issues
Sound-alike/look-alike issues:
Acyclovir may be confused with ganciclovir, Retrovir®, valacyclovir
Zovirax® may be confused with Doribax®, Valtrex®, Zithromax®, Zostrix®, Zyloprim®, Zyvox®
International issues:
Opthavir [Mexico] may be confused with Optivar brand name for azelastine [U.S.]
Brand Names: U.S. Zovirax®
Brand Names: Canada Zovirax®
Index Terms Aciclovir; ACV; Acycloguanosine
Generic Availability (U.S.) No
Pharmacologic Category Antiviral Agent, Topical
Use Treatment of herpes labialis (cold sores), mucocutaneous HSV in immunocompromised patients
Dosage
Geriatric & Adult
Genital HSV: Topical: Immunocompromised: Ointment: Initial episode: 1/2" ribbon of ointment for a 4" square surface area every 3 hours (6 times/day) for 7 days
Herpes labialis (cold sores): Topical: Apply 5 times/day for 4 days
Mucocutaneous HSV: Topical: Ointment: Non-life-threatening, immunocompromised: 1/2" ribbon of ointment for a 4" square surface area every 3 hours (6 times/day) for 7 days
Special Geriatric Considerations No specific information concerning elderly patients.
Dosage Forms Excipient information presented when available (limited, particularly for generics); consult specific product labeling.
Cream, topical:
Zovirax®: 5% (2 g, 5 g)
Ointment, topical:
Zovirax®: 5% (15 g, 30 g)

◆ **Adacel®** see Diphtheria and Tetanus Toxoids, and Acellular Pertussis Vaccine on page 567
◆ **Adalat® CC** see NIFEdipine on page 1375

Adalimumab (a da LIM yoo mab)

Medication Safety Issues
Sound-alike/look-alike issues:
Humira® may be confused with Humulin®, Humalog®
Humira® Pen may be confused with HumaPen® Memoir®
Brand Names: U.S. Humira®; Humira® Pen
Brand Names: Canada Humira®
Index Terms Antitumor Necrosis Factor Alpha (Human); D2E7; Human Antitumor Necrosis Factor Alpha
Generic Availability (U.S.) No
Pharmacologic Category Antirheumatic, Disease Modifying; Gastrointestinal Agent, Miscellaneous; Monoclonal Antibody; Tumor Necrosis Factor (TNF) Blocking Agent
Use
Treatment of active rheumatoid arthritis (moderate-to-severe) and active psoriatic arthritis; may be used alone or in combination with disease-modifying antirheumatic drugs (DMARDs); treatment of ankylosing spondylitis
Treatment of moderately- to severely-active Crohn's disease in patients with inadequate response to conventional treatment, or patients who have lost response to or are intolerant of infliximab
Treatment of moderate-to-severe plaque psoriasis
Medication Guide Available Yes
Contraindications There are no contraindications listed within the FDA-approved labeling.

Canadian labeling: Additional contraindications (not in U.S. labeling): Hypersensitivity to adalimumab or any component of the formulation; severe infection (eg, sepsis, tuberculosis, opportunistic infection)
Warnings/Precautions [U.S. Boxed Warnings]: Patients should be evaluated for latent tuberculosis infection with a tuberculin skin test prior to therapy. Treatment of latent tuberculosis should be initiated before adalimumab is used. Tuberculosis (disseminated or extrapulmonary) has been reactivated while on adalimumab. Most cases have

been reported within the first 8 months of treatment. Doses higher than recommended are associated with an increased risk for tuberculosis reactivation. **Patients with initial negative tuberculin skin tests should receive continued monitoring for tuberculosis throughout treatment; active tuberculosis has developed in this population during treatment.** Rare reactivation of hepatitis B virus (HBV) has occurred in chronic virus carriers; use with caution; evaluate prior to initiation and during treatment.

[U.S. Boxed Warning]: Patients receiving adalimumab are at increased risk for serious infections which may result in hospitalization and/or fatality; infections usually developed in patients receiving concomitant immunosuppressive agents (eg, methotrexate or corticosteroids) and may present as disseminated (rather than local) disease. Active tuberculosis (or reactivation of latent tuberculosis), invasive fungal (including aspergillosis, blastomycosis, candidiasis, coccidioidomycosis, histoplasmosis, and pneumocystosis) and bacterial, viral or other opportunistic infections (including legionellosis and listeriosis) have been reported in patients receiving TNF-blocking agents, including adalimumab. Monitor closely for signs/symptoms of infection. Discontinue for serious infection or sepsis. Consider risks versus benefits prior to use in patients with a history of chronic or recurrent infection. Consider empiric antifungal therapy in patients who are at risk for invasive fungal infection and develop severe systemic illness. Caution should be exercised when considering use in the elderly or in patients with conditions that predispose them to infections (eg, diabetes) or residence/travel from areas of endemic mycoses (blastomycosis, coccidioidomycosis, histoplasmosis), or with latent or localized infections. Do not initiate adalimumab therapy with clinically important active infection. Patients who develop a new infection while undergoing treatment should be monitored closely. **[U.S. Boxed Warning]: Lymphoma and other malignancies have been reported in children and adolescent patients receiving other TNF-blocking agents.** Half the cases are lymphomas (Hodgkin's and non-Hodgkin's) and the other cases are varied, but include malignancies not typically observed in this population. Most patients were receiving concomitant immunosuppressants. **[U.S. Boxed Warning]: Hepatosplenic T-cell lymphoma (HSTCL), a rare T-cell lymphoma, has also been reported primarily in patients with Crohn's disease or ulcerative colitis treated with adalimumab and who received concomitant azathioprine or mercaptopurine; reports occurred predominantly in adolescent and young adult males.** Rare cases of lymphoma have also been reported in association with adalimumab. A higher incidence of nonmelanoma skin cancers was noted in adalimumab treated patients, when compared to the control group. Impact on the development and course of malignancies is not fully defined. May exacerbate pre-existing or recent-onset central or peripheral nervous system demyelinating disorders. Consider discontinuing use in patients who develop peripheral or central nervous system demyelinating disorders during treatment.

May exacerbate pre-existing or recent-onset demyelinating CNS disorders. Worsening and new-onset heart failure (HF) has been reported; use caution in patients with decreased left ventricular function. Use caution in patients with HF. Patients should be brought up to date with all immunizations before initiating therapy. No data are available concerning the effects of adalimumab on vaccination. Live vaccines should not be given concurrently. No data are available concerning secondary transmission of live vaccines in patients receiving adalimumab. Rare cases of pancytopenia (including aplastic anemia) have been reported with TNF-blocking agents; with significant hematologic abnormalities, consider discontinuing therapy. Positive antinuclear antibody titers have been detected in patients (with negative baselines) treated with adalimumab. Rare cases of autoimmune disorder, including lupus-like syndrome, have been reported; monitor and discontinue adalimumab if symptoms develop. May cause hypersensitivity reactions, including anaphylaxis; monitor. Infection and malignancy has been reported at a higher incidence in elderly patients compared to younger adults; use caution in elderly patients. The packaging (needle cover of prefilled syringe) may contain latex. Product may contain polysorbate 80.

Adverse Reactions (Reflective of adult population; not specific for elderly)
>10%:
Central nervous system: Headache (12%)
Dermatologic: Rash (6% to 12%)
Local: Injection site reaction (12% to 20%; includes erythema, itching, hemorrhage, pain, swelling)
Neuromuscular & skeletal: CPK increased (15%)
Respiratory: Upper respiratory tract infection (17%), sinusitis (11%)
Miscellaneous: Serious infection (adults 1.4-6.7 events/100 person years, children 2 events/100 person years [Burmester, 2012]), antibodies to adalimumab (3% to 26%; significance unknown), positive ANA (12%)

45

5% to 10%:
  Cardiovascular: Hypertension (5%)
  Endocrine & metabolic: Hyperlipidemia (7%), hypercholesterolemia (6%)
  Gastrointestinal: Nausea (9%), abdominal pain (7%)
  Genitourinary: Urinary tract infection (8%)
  Hepatic: Alkaline phosphatase increased (5%)
  Local: Injection site reaction (8%; other than erythema, itching, hemorrhage, pain, swelling)
  Neuromuscular & skeletal: Back pain (6%)
  Renal: Hematuria (5%)
  Miscellaneous: Accidental injury (10%), flu-like syndrome (7%), hypersensitivity reactions (children 6%; adults <1%)
1% to 5%:
  Cardiovascular: Arrhythmia, atrial fibrillation, chest pain, CHF, coronary artery disorder, deep vein thrombosis, heart arrest, MI, palpitation, pericardial effusion, pericarditis, peripheral edema, syncope, tachycardia, vascular disorder
  Central nervous system: Confusion, fever, hypertensive encephalopathy, multiple sclerosis, subdural hematoma
  Dermatologic: Alopecia, cellulitis, erysipelas
  Endocrine & metabolic: Dehydration, menstrual disorder, parathyroid disorder
  Gastrointestinal: Diverticulitis, esophagitis, gastroenteritis, gastrointestinal hemorrhage, vomiting
  Genitourinary: Cystitis, pelvic pain
  Hematologic: Agranulocytosis, granulocytopenia, leukopenia, pancytopenia, paraproteinemia, polycythemia
  Hepatic: Cholecystitis, cholelithiasis, hepatic necrosis
  Neuromuscular & skeletal: Arthralgia, arthritis, bone fracture, bone necrosis, joint disorder, muscle cramps, myasthenia, pain in extremity, paresthesia, pyogenic arthritis, synovitis, tendon disorder, tremor
  Ocular: Cataract
  Renal: Kidney calculus, pyelonephritis
  Respiratory: Asthma, bronchospasm, dyspnea, lung function decreased, pleural effusion, pneumonia
  Miscellaneous: Adenoma, allergic reactions (1%), carcinoma (including breast, gastrointestinal, skin, urogenital), healing abnormality, herpes zoster, ketosis, lupus erythematosus syndrome, lymphoma, melanoma, postsurgical infection, sepsis, tuberculosis (reactivation of latent infection; miliary, lymphatic, peritoneal and pulmonary)

Drug Interactions
  Metabolism/Transport Effects None known.
  Avoid Concomitant Use
    Avoid concomitant use of Adalimumab with any of the following: Abatacept; Anakinra; BCG; Belimumab; Canakinumab; Certolizumab Pegol; Natalizumab; Pimecrolimus; Rilonacept; Tacrolimus (Topical); Vaccines (Live)
  Increased Effect/Toxicity
    Adalimumab may increase the levels/effects of: Abatacept; Anakinra; Belimumab; Canakinumab; Certolizumab Pegol; Leflunomide; Natalizumab; Rilonacept; Vaccines (Live)

    The levels/effects of Adalimumab may be increased by: Abciximab; Denosumab; Pimecrolimus; Roflumilast; Tacrolimus (Topical); Trastuzumab
  Decreased Effect
    Adalimumab may decrease the levels/effects of: BCG; Coccidioidin Skin Test; Sipuleucel-T; Vaccines (Inactivated); Vaccines (Live)

    The levels/effects of Adalimumab may be decreased by: Echinacea
  Ethanol/Nutrition/Herb Interactions Herb/nutraceutical: Echinacea may decrease the therapeutic effects of adalimumab; avoid concurrent use.
  Stability Store under refrigeration at 2°C to 8°C (36°F to 46°F); do not freeze. Protect from light.
  Mechanism of Action Adalimumab is a recombinant monoclonal antibody that binds to human tumor necrosis factor alpha (TNF-alpha), thereby interfering with binding to TNFα receptor sites and subsequent cytokine-driven inflammatory processes. Elevated TNF levels in the synovial fluid are involved in the pathologic pain and joint destruction in immune-mediated arthritis. Adalimumab decreases signs and symptoms of psoriatic arthritis, rheumatoid arthritis, and ankylosing spondylitis. It inhibits progression of structural damage of rheumatoid and psoriatic arthritis. Reduces signs and symptoms and maintains clinical remission in Crohn's disease; reduces epidermal thickness and inflammatory cell infiltration in plaque psoriasis.

Pharmacodynamics/Kinetics

Distribution: V_d: 4.7-6 L; Synovial fluid concentrations: 31% to 96% of serum

Bioavailability: Absolute: 64%

Half-life elimination: Terminal: ~2 weeks (range: 10-20 days)

Time to peak, serum: SubQ: 131 ± 56 hours

Excretion: Clearance increased in the presence of anti-adalimumab antibodies; decreased in patients ≥40 years of age

Dosage

Geriatric & Adult

Rheumatoid arthritis: SubQ: 40 mg every other week; may be administered with other DMARDs; patients not taking methotrexate may increase dose to 40 mg every week

Ankylosing spondylitis, psoriatic arthritis: SubQ: 40 mg every other week

Crohn's disease: SubQ: Initial: 160 mg (given as 4 injections on day 1 or as 2 injections/day over 2 consecutive days), then 80 mg 2 weeks later (day 15); Maintenance: 40 mg every other week beginning day 29. **Note:** Some patients may require 40 mg every week as maintenance therapy (Lichtenstein, 2009).

Plaque psoriasis: SubQ: Initial: 80 mg as a single dose; maintenance: 40 mg every other week beginning 1 week after initial dose

Administration For SubQ injection; rotate injection sites. Do not use if solution is discolored. Do not administer to skin which is red, tender, bruised, or hard. Needle cap of the prefilled syringe may contain latex.

Monitoring Parameters Monitor improvement of symptoms and physical function assessments. Latent TB screening prior to initiating and during therapy; signs/symptoms of infection (prior to, during, and following therapy); CBC with differential; signs/symptoms/worsening of heart failure; HBV screening prior to initiating (all patients); HBV carriers (during and for several months following therapy); signs and symptoms of hypersensitivity reaction; symptoms of lupus-like syndrome; signs/symptoms of malignancy (eg, splenomegaly, hepatomegaly, abdominal pain, persistent fever, night sweats, weight loss)

Special Geriatric Considerations In studies, the elderly have an increased incidence of infection and malignancy compared to younger adults <65 years of age. Given the higher incidence of infections and malignancies in the elderly population, caution and close monitoring are recommended when using adalimumab in this population. Additionally, elderly patients with a history of HF may be at risk for HF exacerbation.

Dosage Forms Excipient information presented when available (limited, particularly for generics); consult specific product labeling.

Injection, solution [preservative free]:

Humira®: 40 mg/0.8 mL (0.8 mL) [contains natural rubber/natural latex in packaging, polysorbate 80; prefilled syringe]

Humira® Pen: 40 mg/0.8 mL (0.8 mL) [contains natural rubber/natural latex in packaging, polysorbate 80]

Injection, solution [pediatric, preservative free]:

Humira®: 20 mg/0.4 mL (0.4 mL) [contains natural rubber/natural latex in packaging, polysorbate 80; prefilled syringe]

Aflibercept (Ophthalmic) (a FLIB er sept)

Medication Safety Issues
  Sound-alike/look-alike issues:
    Aflibercept may be confused with Ziv-aflibercept
Brand Names: U.S. Eylea™
Index Terms AVE 0005; AVE 005; AVE-0005; VEGF Trap; VEGF Trap-Eye
Pharmacologic Category Ophthalmic Agent; Vascular Endothelial Growth Factor (VEGF) Inhibitor
Use Treatment of neovascular (wet) age-related macular degeneration (AMD)
Contraindications Hypersensitivity to aflibercept or any component of the formulation; current ocular or periocular infection; active intraocular inflammation
Warnings/Precautions Administer injection using proper aseptic technique. Intravitreal injections may be associated with endophthalmitis, retinal detachment, increased intraocular pressure, infections, or thromboembolic events (eg, nonfatal stroke/MI, vascular death); postprocedure monitoring for these adverse effects should be completed.
Adverse Reactions (Reflective of adult population; not specific for elderly)
  >10%: Ocular: Conjunctival hemorrhage (25%)
  1% to 10%:
    Local: Injection site pain (3%), injection site hemorrhage (1%)
    Ocular: Eye pain (9%), cataract (7%), vitreous detachment (6%), vitreous floaters (6%), intraocular pressure increased (5%), conjunctival hyperemia (4%), corneal erosion (4%), foreign body sensation (3%), lacrimation increased (3%), retinal pigment epithelium detachment (3%), blurred vision (2%), retinal pigment epithelium tear (2%), eyelid edema (1%), corneal edema (1%)
    Miscellaneous: Aflibercept antibodies (1% to 3%)
Drug Interactions
  Metabolism/Transport Effects None known.
  Avoid Concomitant Use There are no known interactions where it is recommended to avoid concomitant use.
  Increased Effect/Toxicity There are no known significant interactions involving an increase in effect.
  Decreased Effect There are no known significant interactions involving a decrease in effect.
Stability Store at 2°C to 8°C (36°F to 46°F); do not freeze. Store in original container prior to use; protect from light.
Mechanism of Action Aflibercept is a recombinant fusion protein that acts as a decoy receptor for vascular endothelial growth factor-A (VEGF-A) and placental growth factor (PIGF). Decoy receptor binding prevents VEGF-A and PIGF from binding and activating endothelial cell receptors, thereby suppressing neovascularization and slowing vision loss.
Pharmacodynamics/Kinetics
  Absorption: Low levels are detected in the serum following intravitreal injection
  Half-life elimination: Plasma: 5-6 days
Dosage
  Geriatric & Adult Age-related macular degeneration (AMD): Intravitreal injection: 2 mg (0.05 mL) every 4 weeks for 3 months then every 8 weeks thereafter
  Renal Impairment No dosage adjustment necessary.
  Hepatic Impairment No dosage adjustment provided in manufacturer's labeling (has not been studied); however, no adjustment expected due to minimal systemic absorption.
Administration For ophthalmic intravitreal injection only. Remove contents from vial using a 5 micron, 19-gauge 1½ inch filter needle (supplied) attached to a 1 mL syringe (supplied). Discard filter needle and replace with a sterile 30 gauge ½ inch needle (supplied) for intravitreal injection procedure (do not use filter needle for intravitreal injection). Depress plunger to expel excess air and medication (plunger tip should align with the 0.05 mL marking on syringe). Adequate anesthesia and a broad-spectrum antimicrobial agent should be administered prior to the procedure.
Monitoring Parameters Intraocular pressure immediately following injection; signs of infection/inflammation (for first week following injection); retinal perfusion; endophthalmitis; visual acuity
Special Geriatric Considerations Age-related macular degeneration primarily affects older adults. The mean age in the two Phase 3 approval trials was 78 and 74 years, respectively; range 49-99 years. Eighty-nine percent were ≥65 years and 63% were ≥75 years. No difference in outcomes were noted based on patient age.

Dosage Forms Excipient information presented when available (limited, particularly for generics); consult specific product labeling.

Injection, solution, intravitreal [preservative free]:

Eylea™: 40 mg/mL (0.05 mL) [derived from or manufactured using Chinese hamster ovary cells]

Albuterol (al BYOO ter ole)

Related Information

Inhalant Agents on page 2117

Medication Safety Issues

Sound-alike/look-alike issues:

Albuterol may be confused with Albutein®, atenolol

Proventil® may be confused with Bentyl®, PriLOSEC®, Prinivil®

Salbutamol may be confused with salmeterol

Ventolin® may be confused with phentolamine, Benylin®, Vantin

Brand Names: U.S. AccuNeb®; ProAir® HFA; Proventil® HFA; Ventolin® HFA; VoSpire ER®

Brand Names: Canada Airomir; Apo-Salvent®; Apo-Salvent® AEM; Apo-Salvent® CFC Free; Apo-Salvent® Sterules; Dom-Salbutamol; Mylan-Salbutamol Respirator Solution; Mylan-Salbutamol Sterinebs P.F.; Novo-Salbutamol HFA; Nu-Salbutamol; PHL-Salbutamol; PMS-Salbutamol; ratio-Ipra-Sal; ratio-Salbutamol; Sandoz-Salbutamol; Teva-Salbutamol; Ventolin®; Ventolin® Diskus; Ventolin® HFA; Ventolin® I.V. Infusion; Ventolin® Nebules P.F.

Index Terms Albuterol Sulfate; Salbutamol; Salbutamol Sulphate

Generic Availability (U.S.) Yes

Pharmacologic Category Beta$_2$ Agonist

Use Treatment or prevention of bronchospasm in patients with reversible obstructive airway disease; prevention of exercise-induced bronchospasm

Contraindications Hypersensitivity to albuterol, adrenergic amines, or any component of the formulation

Injection formulation (not available in U.S.): Patients with tachyarrhythmias

Warnings/Precautions Optimize anti-inflammatory treatment before initiating maintenance treatment with albuterol. Do not use as a component of chronic therapy without an anti-inflammatory agent. Only the mildest forms of asthma (Step 1 and/or exercise-induced) would not require concurrent use based upon asthma guidelines. Patient must be instructed to seek medical attention in cases where acute symptoms are not relieved or a previous level of response is diminished. The need to increase frequency of use may indicate deterioration of asthma, and treatment must not be delayed.

◀ Use caution in patients with cardiovascular disease (arrhythmia or hypertension or HF), convulsive disorders, diabetes, glaucoma, hyperthyroidism, or hypokalemia. Beta-agonists may cause elevation in blood pressure, heart rate, and result in CNS stimulation/excitation. Beta$_2$-agonists may increase risk of arrhythmia, increase serum glucose, or decrease serum potassium.

Immediate hypersensitivity reactions (urticaria, angioedema, rash, bronchospasm) have been reported. Do not exceed recommended dose; serious adverse events, including fatalities, have been associated with excessive use of inhaled sympathomimetics. Rarely, paradoxical bronchospasm may occur with use of inhaled bronchodilating agents; this should be distinguished from inadequate response. All patients should utilize a spacer device or valved holding chamber when using a metered-dose inhaler.

Adverse Reactions (Reflective of adult population; not specific for elderly) Incidence of adverse effects is dependent upon age of patient, dose, and route of administration.

Cardiovascular: Angina, atrial fibrillation, arrhythmias, chest discomfort, chest pain, extrasystoles, flushing, hyper-/hypotension, palpitation, supraventricular tachycardia, tachycardia

Central nervous system: CNS stimulation, dizziness, drowsiness, headache, insomnia, irritability, lightheadedness, migraine, nervousness, nightmares, restlessness, seizure

Dermatologic: Angioedema, rash, urticaria

Endocrine & metabolic: Hyperglycemia, hypokalemia, lactic acidosis

Gastrointestinal: Diarrhea, dry mouth, dyspepsia, gastroenteritis, nausea, unusual taste, vomiting

Genitourinary: Micturition difficulty

Local: Injection: Pain, stinging

Neuromuscular & skeletal: Muscle cramps, musculoskeletal pain, tremor, weakness

Otic: Otitis media, vertigo

Respiratory: Asthma exacerbation, bronchospasm, cough, epistaxis, laryngitis, oropharyngeal drying/irritation, oropharyngeal edema, pharyngitis, rhinitis, upper respiratory inflammation, viral respiratory infection

Miscellaneous: Allergic reaction, anaphylaxis, diaphoresis, lymphadenopathy

Drug Interactions

Metabolism/Transport Effects None known.

Avoid Concomitant Use

Avoid concomitant use of Albuterol with any of the following: Beta-Blockers (Nonselective); Iobenguane I 123

Increased Effect/Toxicity

Albuterol may increase the levels/effects of: Loop Diuretics; Sympathomimetics; Thiazide Diuretics

The levels/effects of Albuterol may be increased by: AtoMOXetine; Cannabinoids; MAO Inhibitors; Tricyclic Antidepressants

Decreased Effect

Albuterol may decrease the levels/effects of: Iobenguane I 123

The levels/effects of Albuterol may be decreased by: Alpha-/Beta-Blockers; Beta-Blockers (Beta1 Selective); Beta-Blockers (Nonselective); Betahistine

Ethanol/Nutrition/Herb Interactions

Food: Avoid or limit caffeine (may cause CNS stimulation).

Herb/Nutraceutical: Avoid ephedra, yohimbe (may cause CNS stimulation). Avoid St John's wort (may decrease the levels/effects of albuterol).

Stability

HFA aerosols: Store at 15°C to 25°C (59°F to 77°F).

Ventolin® HFA: Discard when counter reads 000 or 12 months after removal from protective pouch, whichever comes first. Store with mouthpiece down.

Infusion solution (Canadian labeling; product not available in U.S.): Ventolin® I.V.: Store at 15°C to 30°C (59°F to 86°F). Protect from light. After dilution, discard unused portion after 24 hours.

Inhalation solution: Solution for nebulization (0.5%): Store at 2°C to 25°C (36°F to 77°F). To prepare a 2.5 mg dose, dilute 0.5 mL of solution to a total of 3 mL with normal saline; also compatible with cromolyn or ipratropium nebulizer solutions.

AccuNeb®: Store at 2°C to 25°C (36°F to 77°F). Do not use if solution changes color or becomes cloudy. Use within 1 week of opening foil pouch.

Syrup: Store at 20°C to 25°C (68°F to 77°F).

Tablet: Store at 20°C to 25°C (68°F to 77°F).

Tablet, extended release: Store at 20°C to 25°C (68°F to 77°F)

Mechanism of Action Relaxes bronchial smooth muscle by action on beta$_2$-receptors with little effect on heart rate

Pharmacodynamics/Kinetics
Onset of action: Peak effect:
  Nebulization/oral inhalation: 0.5-2 hours
    CFC-propelled albuterol: 10 minutes
      Ventolin® HFA: 25 minutes
    Oral: 2-3 hours
Duration: Nebulization/oral inhalation: 3-4 hours; Oral: 4-6 hours
Metabolism: Hepatic to an inactive sulfate
Half-life elimination: Inhalation: 3.8 hours; Oral: 3.7-5 hours
Excretion: Urine (30% as unchanged drug)

Dosage
Geriatric
Inhalation: Refer to adult dosing.
Bronchospasm (treatment): Oral: 2 mg 3-4 times/day; maximum: 8 mg 4 times/day

Adult
Bronchospasm:
Metered-dose inhaler: 2 puffs every 4-6 hours as needed (NIH Guidelines, 2007):
Solution for nebulization: 2.5 mg 3-4 times daily as needed; Quick relief: 1.25-5 mg every 4 to 8 hours as needed (NIH Guidelines, 2007)
Oral: 2-4 mg/dose 3-4 times/day; maximum dose not to exceed 32 mg/day (divided doses)
  Extended release: 8 mg every 12 hours; maximum dose not to exceed 32 mg/day (divided doses). A 4 mg dose every 12 hours may be sufficient in some patients, such as adults of low body weight.
I.V. continuous infusion (Canadian labeling; product not available in U.S.): Severe bronchospasm and status asthmaticus: Initial: 5 mcg/minute; may increase up to 10-20 mcg/minute at 15- to 30-minute intervals if needed

Exacerbation of asthma (acute, severe) (NIH Guidelines, 2007):
Metered-dose inhaler: 4-8 puffs every 20 minutes for up to 4 hours, then every 1-4 hours as needed
Solution for nebulization: 2.5-5 mg every 20 minutes for 3 doses, then 2.5-10 mg every 1-4 hours as needed, **or** 10-15 mg/hour by continuous nebulization

Exercise-induced bronchospasm (prevention): *Metered-dose inhaler:* 2 puffs 5-30 minutes prior to exercise

Renal Impairment Use with caution in patients with renal impairment. No dosage adjustment required (including patients on hemodialysis, peritoneal dialysis, or CRRT; Aronoff, 2007).

Administration
Metered-dose inhaler: Shake well before use; prime prior to first use, and whenever inhaler has not been used for >2 weeks or when it has been dropped, by releasing 3-4 test sprays into the air (away from face). HFA inhalers should be cleaned with warm water at least once per week; allow to air dry completely prior to use. A spacer device or valved holding chamber is recommended for use with metered-dose inhalers.

Solution for nebulization: Concentrated solution should be diluted prior to use. Blow-by administration is not recommended, use a mask device if patient unable to hold mouthpiece in mouth for administration.

Infusion solution (Canadian labeling; product not available in U.S.): Do not inject undiluted. Reduce concentration by at least 50% before infusing. Administer as a continuous infusion via infusion pump.

Oral: Do not crush or chew extended release tablets.

Monitoring Parameters FEV_1, peak flow, and/or other pulmonary function tests; blood pressure, heart rate; CNS stimulation; serum glucose, serum potassium; asthma symptoms; arterial or capillary blood gases (if patients condition warrants)

Test Interactions Increased renin (S), increased aldosterone (S)

Pharmacotherapy Pearls The 2007 National Heart, Lung, and Blood Institute Guidelines for the Diagnosis and Management of Asthma do not recommend the use of oral systemic albuterol as a quick-relief medication and do not recommend regularly scheduled daily, chronic use of inhaled beta-agonists for long-term control of asthma.

Special Geriatric Considerations Because of its minimal effect on $beta_1$-receptors and its relatively long duration of action, albuterol is a rational choice in elderly when a beta-agonist is indicated. Elderly patients may find it beneficial to utilize a spacer device when using a metered dose inhaler. Oral use should be avoided due to adverse effects.

◀ **Dosage Forms** Excipient information presented when available (limited, particularly for generics); consult specific product labeling.
Aerosol, for oral inhalation:
  ProAir® HFA: 90 mcg/inhalation (8.5 g) [chlorofluorocarbon free; 200 metered actuations]
  Proventil® HFA: 90 mcg/inhalation (6.7 g) [chlorofluorocarbon free; 200 metered actuations]
  Ventolin® HFA: 90 mcg/inhalation (18 g) [chlorofluorocarbon free; 200 metered actuations]
  Ventolin® HFA: 90 mcg/inhalation (8 g) [chlorofluorocarbon free; 60 metered actuations]
Solution, for nebulization: 0.083% [2.5 mg/3 mL] (25s, 30s, 60s); 0.5% [100 mg/20 mL] (1s)
Solution, for nebulization [preservative free]: 0.021% [0.63 mg/3 mL] (25s); 0.042% [1.25 mg/3 mL] (25s, 30s); 0.083% [2.5 mg/3 mL] (25s, 30s, 60s); 0.5% [2.5 mg/0.5 mL] (30s)
  AccuNeb®: 0.021% [0.63 mg/3 mL] (25s); 0.042% [1.25 mg/3 mL] (25s)
Syrup, oral: 2 mg/5 mL (473 mL)
Tablet, oral: 2 mg, 4 mg
Tablet, extended release, oral: 4 mg, 8 mg
  VoSpire ER®: 4 mg, 8 mg
Dosage Forms: Canada Excipient information presented when available (limited, particularly for generics); consult specific product labeling.
Injection, solution, as sulphate:
  Ventolin® I.V.: 1 mg/1mL (5 mL)

◆ **Albuterol and Ipratropium** *see* Ipratropium and Albuterol *on page 1037*
◆ **Albuterol Sulfate** *see* Albuterol *on page 49*

Alcaftadine (al KAF ta deen)

Brand Names: U.S. Lastacaft™
Generic Availability (U.S.) No
Pharmacologic Category Histamine H_1 Antagonist; Histamine H_1 Antagonist, Second Generation; Mast Cell Stabilizer
Use Prevention of itching associated with allergic conjunctivitis
Dosage
  Geriatric & Adult Allergic conjunctivitis: Ophthalmic: Instill 1 drop into each eye once daily.
Special Geriatric Considerations Evaluate the patient's or caregiver's ability to safely administer the correct dose of ophthalmic medication.
Dosage Forms Excipient information presented when available (limited, particularly for generics); consult specific product labeling.
Solution, ophthalmic [drops]:
  Lastacaft™: 0.25% (3 mL) [contains benzalkonium chloride]

◆ **Alcalak [OTC]** *see* Calcium Carbonate *on page 262*

Alclometasone (al kloe MET a sone)

Related Information
  Topical Corticosteroids *on page 2113*
Medication Safety Issues
  Sound-alike/look-alike issues:
    Aclovate® may be confused with Accolate®
  International issues:
    Cloderm: Brand name for alclometasone [Indonesia], but also brand name for clobetasol [China, India, Malaysia, Singapore, Thailand]; clocortolone [U.S., Canada]; clotrimazole [Germany]
Brand Names: U.S. Aclovate®
Index Terms Alclometasone Dipropionate
Generic Availability (U.S.) Yes
Pharmacologic Category Corticosteroid, Topical
Use Treatment of inflammation of corticosteroid-responsive dermatosis (low to medium potency topical corticosteroid)
Dosage
  Geriatric & Adult Steroid-responsive dermatoses: Topical: Apply a thin film to the affected area 2-3 times/day. **Note:** Therapy should be discontinued when control is achieved; if no improvement is seen within 2 weeks, reassessment of diagnosis may be necessary.
Special Geriatric Considerations Due to age-related changes in skin, limit use of topical corticosteroids.

Dosage Forms Excipient information presented when available (limited, particularly for generics); consult specific product labeling.
Cream, topical, as dipropionate: 0.05% (15 g, 45 g, 60 g)
Aclovate®: 0.05% (15 g, 60 g)
Ointment, topical, as dipropionate: 0.05% (15 g, 45 g, 60 g)
Aclovate®: 0.05% (15 g, 60 g)

◆ **Alclometasone Dipropionate** see Alclometasone on page 52
◆ **Aldactazide®** see Hydrochlorothiazide and Spironolactone on page 936
◆ **Aldactone®** see Spironolactone on page 1805
◆ **Aldomet** see Methyldopa on page 1243
◆ **Aldroxicon I [OTC]** see Aluminum Hydroxide, Magnesium Hydroxide, and Simethicone on page 82
◆ **Aldroxicon II [OTC]** see Aluminum Hydroxide, Magnesium Hydroxide, and Simethicone on page 82

Alendronate (a LEN droe nate)

Related Information
Osteoporosis Management on page 2136
Medication Safety Issues
Sound-alike/look-alike issues:
Alendronate may be confused with risedronate
Fosamax® may be confused with Flomax®, Fosamax Plus D®, fosinopril, Zithromax®
International issues:
Fosamax [U.S., Canada, and multiple international markets] may be confused with Fisamox brand name for amoxicillin [Australia]
Brand Names: U.S. Fosamax®
Brand Names: Canada Alendronate-FC; Apo-Alendronate®; CO Alendronate; Dom-Alendronate; Fosamax®; JAMP-Alendronate; Mylan-Alendronate; PHL-Alendronate; PMS-Alendronate; PMS-Alendronate-FC; Q-Alendronate; ratio-Alendronate; Riva-Alendronate; Sandoz-Alendronate; Teva-Alendronate
Index Terms Alendronate Sodium; Alendronic Acid Monosodium Salt Trihydrate; Binosto™; MK-217
Generic Availability (U.S.) Yes
Pharmacologic Category Bisphosphonate Derivative
Use Treatment and prevention of osteoporosis in postmenopausal females; treatment of osteoporosis in males; Paget's disease of the bone in patients who are symptomatic, at risk for future complications, or with alkaline phosphatase ≥2 times the upper limit of normal; treatment of glucocorticoid-induced osteoporosis in males and females with low bone mineral density who are receiving a daily dosage ≥7.5 mg of prednisone (or equivalent)
Medication Guide Available Yes
Contraindications Hypersensitivity to alendronate, other bisphosphonates, or any component of the formulation; hypocalcemia; abnormalities of the esophagus which delay esophageal emptying such as stricture or achalasia; inability to stand or sit upright for at least 30 minutes
Warnings/Precautions Use caution in patients with renal impairment (not recommended for use in patients with Cl_{cr} <35 mL/minute); hypocalcemia must be corrected before therapy initiation; ensure adequate calcium and vitamin D intake. May cause irritation to upper gastrointestinal mucosa. Esophagitis, dysphagia, esophageal ulcers, esophageal erosions, and esophageal stricture (rare) have been reported; risk increases in patients unable to comply with dosing instructions. Use with caution in patients with dysphagia, esophageal disease, gastritis, duodenitis, or ulcers (may worsen underlying condition). Discontinue use if new or worsening symptoms develop.

Osteonecrosis of the jaw (ONJ) has been reported in patients receiving bisphosphonates. Risk factors include invasive dental procedures (eg, tooth extraction, dental implants, boney surgery); a diagnosis of cancer, with concomitant chemotherapy or corticosteroids; poor oral hygiene, ill-fitting dentures; and comorbid disorders (anemia, coagulopathy, infection, pre-existing dental disease). Most reported cases occurred after I.V. bisphosphonate therapy; however, cases have been reported following oral therapy. A dental exam and preventative dentistry should be performed prior to placing patients with risk factors on chronic bisphosphonate therapy. The manufacturer's labeling states that discontinuing bisphosphonates in patients requiring invasive dental procedures may reduce the risk of ONJ. However, other experts suggest that there is no evidence that discontinuing therapy reduces the risk of developing ONJ (Assael, 2009). The benefit/risk must be assessed by the treating physician and/or dentist/surgeon prior to any invasive dental procedure. Patients developing ONJ while on bisphosphonates should receive care by an oral surgeon.

Atypical femur fractures have been reported in patients receiving bisphosphonates for treatment/prevention of osteoporosis. The fractures include subtrochanteric femur (bone just below the hip joint) and diaphyseal femur (long segment of the thigh bone). Some patients experience prodromal pain weeks or months before the fracture occurs. It is unclear if bisphosphonate therapy is the cause for these fractures, although the majority have been reported in patients taking bisphosphonates. Patients receiving long-term (>3-5 years) therapy may be at an increased risk. Discontinue bisphosphonate therapy in patients who develop a femoral shaft fracture.

Severe (and occasionally debilitating) bone, joint, and/or muscle pain have been reported during bisphosphonate treatment. The onset of pain ranged from a single day to several months. Consider discontinuing therapy in patients who experience severe symptoms; symptoms usually resolve upon discontinuation. Some patients experienced recurrence when rechallenged with same drug or another bisphosphonate; avoid use in patients with a history of these symptoms in association with bisphosphonate therapy.

Adverse Reactions (Reflective of adult population; not specific for elderly) Note: Incidence of adverse effects (mostly GI) increases significantly in patients treated for Paget's disease at 40 mg/day.

>10%: Endocrine & metabolic: Hypocalcemia (transient, mild, 18%); hypophosphatemia (transient, mild, 10%)

1% to 10%:
Central nervous system: Headache (up to 3%)
Gastrointestinal: Abdominal pain (1% to 7%), acid reflux (1% to 4%), dyspepsia (1% to 4%), nausea (1% to 4%), flatulence (up to 4%), diarrhea (1% to 3%), gastroesophageal reflux disease (1% to 3%), constipation (up to 3%), esophageal ulcer (up to 2%), abdominal distension (up to 1%), gastritis (up to 1%), vomiting (up to 1%), dysphagia (up to 1%), gastric ulcer (1%), melena (1%)
Neuromuscular & skeletal: Musculoskeletal pain (up to 6%), muscle cramps (up to 1%)

Drug Interactions
Metabolism/Transport Effects None known.
Avoid Concomitant Use There are no known interactions where it is recommended to avoid concomitant use.
Increased Effect/Toxicity
Alendronate may increase the levels/effects of: Deferasirox; Phosphate Supplements; SUNItinib

The levels/effects of Alendronate may be increased by: Aminoglycosides; Aspirin; Non-steroidal Anti-Inflammatory Agents
Decreased Effect
The levels/effects of Alendronate may be decreased by: Antacids; Calcium Salts; Iron Salts; Magnesium Salts; Proton Pump Inhibitors
Ethanol/Nutrition/Herb Interactions
Ethanol: May increase risk of osteoporosis and gastric irritation. Management: Avoid ethanol.
Food: All food and beverages interfere with absorption. Coadministration with caffeine may reduce alendronate efficacy. Coadministration with dairy products may decrease alendronate absorption. Beverages (especially orange juice and coffee) and food may reduce the absorption of alendronate as much as 60%. Management: Alendronate must be taken with 6-8 oz of plain water first thing in the morning and ≥30 minutes before the first food, beverage, or other medication of the day. Do not take with mineral water or with other beverages.
Stability Store at room temperature of 15°C to 30°C (59°F to 86°F). Keep in well-closed container.
Mechanism of Action A bisphosphonate which inhibits bone resorption via actions on osteoclasts or on osteoclast precursors; decreases the rate of bone resorption, leading to an indirect increase in bone mineral density. In Paget's disease, characterized by disordered resorption and formation of bone, inhibition of resorption leads to an indirect decrease in bone formation; but the newly-formed bone has a more normal architecture.
Pharmacodynamics/Kinetics
Distribution: 28 L (exclusive of bone)
Protein binding: ~78%
Metabolism: None
Bioavailability: Fasting: 0.6%; reduced up to 60% with food or drink
Half-life elimination: Exceeds 10 years
Excretion: Urine; feces (as unabsorbed drug)

Dosage

Geriatric & Adult Note: Patients should receive supplemental calcium and vitamin D if dietary intake is inadequate.

Osteoporosis in postmenopausal females: Oral:
Prophylaxis: 5 mg once daily **or** 35 mg once weekly
Treatment: 10 mg once daily **or** 70 mg once weekly

Osteoporosis in males: Oral: 10 mg once daily **or** 70 mg once weekly

Osteoporosis secondary to glucocorticoids in males and females: Oral: Treatment: 5 mg once daily; a dose of 10 mg once daily should be used in postmenopausal females who are not receiving estrogen

Paget's disease of bone in males and females: Oral: 40 mg once daily for 6 months
Retreatment: Relapses during the 12 months following therapy occurred in 9% of patients who responded to treatment. Specific retreatment data are not available. Following a 6-month post-treatment evaluation period, treatment with alendronate may be considered in patients who have relapsed based on increases in serum alkaline phosphatase, which should be measured periodically. Retreatment may also be considered in those who failed to normalize their serum alkaline phosphatase.

Renal Impairment
Cl_{cr} ≥35 mL/minute: No dosage adjustment necessary.
Cl_{cr} <35 mL/minute: Use not recommended.

Hepatic Impairment No dosage adjustment necessary.

Administration Alendronate must be taken with 6-8 oz of plain water first thing in the morning and ≥30 minutes before the first food, beverage, or other medication of the day. Do not take with mineral water or with other beverages. Patients should be instructed to stay upright (not to lie down) for at least 30 minutes **and** until after first food of the day (to reduce esophageal irritation).

Monitoring Parameters

Osteoporosis: Bone mineral density as measured by central dual-energy x-ray absorptiometry (DXA) of the hip or spine (prior to initiation of therapy and at least every 2 years; after 6-12 months of combined glucocorticoid and alendronate treatment); annual measurements of height and weight, assessment of chronic back pain; serum calcium and 25(OH)D; may consider monitoring biochemical markers of bone turnover

Paget's disease: Alkaline phosphatase; pain; serum calcium and 25(OH)D

Reference Range Calcium (total): Adults: 9.0-11.0 mg/dL (2.05-2.54 mmol/L), may slightly decrease with aging; phosphorus: 2.5-4.5 mg/dL (0.81-1.45 mmol/L)

Test Interactions Bisphosphonates may interfere with diagnostic imaging agents such as technetium-99m-diphosphonate in bone scans.

Special Geriatric Considerations The elderly are frequently treated long-term for osteoporosis. Elderly patients should be advised to report any lower extremity, jaw (osteonecrosis), or muscle pain that cannot be explained or lasts longer than 2 weeks. Additionally, elderly often receive concomitant diuretic therapy and therefore their electrolyte status (eg, calcium, phosphate) should be periodically evaluated.

Due to the reports of atypical femur fractures and osteonecrosis of the jaw, recommendations for duration of bisphosphonate use in osteoporosis have been modified. Based on available data, consider discontinuing bisphosphonates after 5 years of use in low-risk patients, since the risk of nonvertebral fracture is the same as those patients taking bisphosphonates for 10 years. Those patients with high risk (fracture history) may be continued for a longer period, taking into consideration the risks vs benefits associated with continued therapy.

Product Availability Binosto™: FDA approved March 2012; availability anticipated September 2012. Consult prescribing information for additional information.

Dosage Forms Excipient information presented when available (limited, particularly for generics); consult specific product labeling.
Tablet, oral: 5 mg, 10 mg, 35 mg, 40 mg, 70 mg
Fosamax®: 70 mg

Alendronate and Cholecalciferol (a LEN droe nate & kole e kal SI fer ole)

Related Information
Alendronate *on page 53*
Cholecalciferol *on page 365*
Osteoporosis Management *on page 2136*

Medication Safety Issues
Sound-alike/look-alike issues:
Fosamax Plus D® may be confused with Fosamax®

Brand Names: U.S. Fosamax Plus D®

Brand Names: Canada Fosavance

ALENDRONATE AND CHOLECALCIFEROL

Index Terms Alendronate Sodium and Cholecalciferol; Cholecalciferol and Alendronate; Vitamin D_3 and Alendronate

Generic Availability (U.S.) No

Pharmacologic Category Bisphosphonate Derivative; Vitamin D Analog

Use Treatment of osteoporosis in postmenopausal females; increase bone mass in males with osteoporosis

Medication Guide Available Yes

Dosage

Geriatric & Adult Osteoporosis: Oral: One tablet (alendronate 70 mg/cholecalciferol 2800 units **or** alendronate 70 mg/cholecalciferol 5600 units) once weekly. Appropriate dose in most osteoporotic women or men: Alendronate 70 mg/cholecalciferol 5600 units once weekly. Supplemental calcium and vitamin D may be necessary if dietary intake is inadequate.

Renal Impairment

Cl_{cr} 35-60 mL/minute: No adjustment needed.

Cl_{cr} <35 mL/minute: Not recommended.

Hepatic Impairment Alendronate: None necessary. Cholecalciferol: May not be adequately absorbed in patients who have malabsorption due to inadequate bile production.

Special Geriatric Considerations The elderly are frequently treated long-term for osteoporosis. Elderly patients should be advised to report any lower extremity, jaw (osteonecrosis), or muscle pain that cannot be explained or lasts longer than 2 weeks. Additionally, elderly often receive concomitant diuretic therapy and therefore their electrolyte status (eg, calcium, phosphate) should be periodically evaluated.

Due to the reports of atypical femur fractures and osteonecrosis of the jaw, recommendations for duration of bisphosphonate use in osteoporosis have been modified. Based on available data, consider discontinuing bisphosphonates after 5 years of use in low-risk patients, since the risk of nonvertebral fracture is the same as those patients taking bisphosphonates for 10 years. Those patients with high risk (fracture history) may be continued for a longer period, taking into consideration the risks vs benefits associated with continued therapy.

Dosage Forms Excipient information presented when available (limited, particularly for generics); consult specific product labeling.

Tablet:

Fosamax Plus D® 70/2800: Alendronate 70 mg and cholecalciferol 2800 units

Fosamax Plus D® 70/5600: Alendronate 70 mg and cholecalciferol 5600 units

◆ **Alendronate Sodium** *see* Alendronate *on page 53*
◆ **Alendronate Sodium and Cholecalciferol** *see* Alendronate and Cholecalciferol *on page 55*
◆ **Alendronic Acid Monosodium Salt Trihydrate** *see* Alendronate *on page 53*
◆ **Aler-Cap [OTC]** *see* DiphenhydrAMINE (Systemic) *on page 556*
◆ **Aler-Dryl [OTC]** *see* DiphenhydrAMINE (Systemic) *on page 556*
◆ **Aler-Tab [OTC]** *see* DiphenhydrAMINE (Systemic) *on page 556*
◆ **Aleve® [OTC]** *see* Naproxen *on page 1338*

Alfuzosin (al FYOO zoe sin)

Related Information

Pharmacotherapy of Urinary Incontinence *on page 2141*

Brand Names: U.S. Uroxatral®

Brand Names: Canada Apo-Alfuzosin®; Sandoz-Alfuzosin; Teva-Alfuzosin PR; Xatral

Index Terms Alfuzosin Hydrochloride

Generic Availability (U.S.) Yes

Pharmacologic Category Alpha$_1$ Blocker

Use Treatment of the functional symptoms of benign prostatic hyperplasia (BPH)

Unlabeled Use Facilitation of expulsion of ureteral stones

Contraindications Hypersensitivity to alfuzosin or any component of the formulation; moderate or severe hepatic insufficiency (Child-Pugh class B and C); concurrent use with potent CYP3A4 inhibitors (eg, itraconazole, ketoconazole, ritonavir) or other alpha$_1$-blocking agents

Warnings/Precautions Not intended for use as an antihypertensive drug. May cause significant orthostatic hypotension and syncope, especially with first dose; anticipate a similar effect if therapy is interrupted for a few days, if dosage is rapidly increased, or used with antihypertensives (particularly vasodilators), PDE-5 inhibitors, nitrates or other medications which may result in hypotension. Discontinue if symptoms of angina occur or worsen. Alfuzosin has been shown to prolong the QT interval alone (minimal) and with other drugs with comparable effects on the QT interval (additive); use with caution in patients with known QT prolongation (congenital or acquired). Patients should be cautioned about performing hazardous tasks when starting new therapy or adjusting dosage upward. Discontinue if symptoms of angina occur or worsen. Rule out prostatic carcinoma before beginning therapy. Use caution with severe renal or mild hepatic impairment; contraindicated in moderate-to-severe hepatic impairment. Intraoperative floppy iris syndrome has been observed in cataract surgery patients who were on or were previously treated with alpha$_1$-blockers. Causality has not been established and there appears to be no benefit in discontinuing alpha-blocker therapy prior to surgery. May cause priapism. Contraindicated in patients taking strong CYP3A4 inhibitors or other alpha$_1$-blockers.

Adverse Reactions (Reflective of adult population; not specific for elderly) 1% to 10%:

Central nervous system: Dizziness (6%), fatigue (3%), headache (3%), pain (1% to 2%)

Gastrointestinal: Abdominal pain (1% to 2%), constipation (1% to 2%), dyspepsia (1% to 2%), nausea (1% to 2%)

Genitourinary: Impotence (1% to 2%)

Respiratory: Upper respiratory tract infection (3%), bronchitis (1% to 2%), pharyngitis (1% to 2%), sinusitis (1% to 2%)

Drug Interactions

Metabolism/Transport Effects Substrate of CYP3A4 (major); **Note:** Assignment of Major/Minor substrate status based on clinically relevant drug interaction potential

Avoid Concomitant Use

Avoid concomitant use of Alfuzosin with any of the following: Alpha1-Blockers; CYP3A4 Inhibitors (Strong); Highest Risk QTc-Prolonging Agents; Mifepristone; Protease Inhibitors; Telaprevir

Increased Effect/Toxicity

Alfuzosin may increase the levels/effects of: Alpha1-Blockers; Antihypertensives; Calcium Channel Blockers; Highest Risk QTc-Prolonging Agents; Moderate Risk QTc-Prolonging Agents; Nitroglycerin

The levels/effects of Alfuzosin may be increased by: Beta-Blockers; CYP3A4 Inhibitors (Moderate); CYP3A4 Inhibitors (Strong); Ivacaftor; MAO Inhibitors; Mifepristone; Phosphodiesterase 5 Inhibitors; Protease Inhibitors; QTc-Prolonging Agents (Indeterminate Risk and Risk Modifying); Telaprevir

Decreased Effect

The levels/effects of Alfuzosin may be decreased by: CYP3A4 Inducers (Strong); Deferasirox; Herbs (CYP3A4 Inducers); Tocilizumab

Ethanol/Nutrition/Herb Interactions

Food: Food increases the extent of absorption. Management: Administer immediately following a meal at the same time each day.

Herb/Nutraceutical: St John's wort may decrease alfuzosin levels. Management: Avoid St John's wort.

Stability Store at room temperature of 25°C (77°F); excursions permitted to 15°C to 30°C (59°F to 86°F). Protect from light and moisture.

Mechanism of Action An antagonist of alpha$_1$-adrenoreceptors in the lower urinary tract. Smooth muscle tone is mediated by the sympathetic nervous stimulation of alpha$_1$-adrenoreceptors, which are abundant in the prostate, prostatic capsule, prostatic urethra, and bladder neck. Blockade of these adrenoreceptors can cause smooth muscles in the bladder neck and prostate to relax, resulting in an improvement in urine flow rate and a reduction in BPH symptoms.

Pharmacodynamics/Kinetics

Absorption: Decreased 50% under fasting conditions

Distribution: V_d: 3.2 L/kg

Protein binding: 82% to 90%

Metabolism: Hepatic, primarily via CYP3A4; metabolism includes oxidation, O-demethylation, and N-dealkylation; forms metabolites (inactive)

Bioavailability: 49% following a meal

Half-life elimination: 10 hours

Time to peak, plasma: 8 hours following a meal

Excretion: Feces (69%); urine (24%; 11% as unchanged drug)

Dosage

Geriatric & Adult

Benign prostatic hyperplasia (BPH): Oral: 10 mg once daily

Ureteral stones, expulsion (unlabeled use): Oral: 10 mg once daily, discontinue after successful expulsion (average time to expulsion 1-2 weeks) (Agrawal, 2009; Ahmed, 2010; Gurbuz, 2011). **Note:** Patients with stones >10 mm were excluded from studies.

Renal Impairment Bioavailability and maximum serum concentrations are increased by ~50% with mild (Cl_{cr} 60-80 mL/minute), moderate (Cl_{cr} 30-59 mL/minute), or severe (Cl_{cr} <30 mL/minute) renal impairment.

◀ **Note:** Safety data is limited in patients with severe renal impairment (Cl$_{cr}$ <30 mL/minute). Use with caution.

Hepatic Impairment
Mild hepatic impairment: Use has not been studied; use caution.
Moderate or severe hepatic impairment (Child-Pugh class B or C): Clearance is decreased $1/3$ to $1/4$ and serum concentration is increased three- to fourfold; use is contraindicated.

Administration Tablet should be swallowed whole; do not crush or chew. Administer once daily (immediately following a meal); should be taken at the same time each day.

Monitoring Parameters Urine flow, blood pressure, PSA

Special Geriatric Considerations Alfuzosin is a functionally uroselective alpha-blocker, therefore, having minimal effects on the cardiovascular system. Alfuzosin appears to be well tolerated in elderly. In one study, orthostatic changes were minimal and not influenced by age.

Dosage Forms Excipient information presented when available (limited, particularly for generics); consult specific product labeling.
Tablet, extended release, oral, as hydrochloride: 10 mg
 Uroxatral®: 10 mg

◆ **Alfuzosin Hydrochloride** see Alfuzosin on page 56
◆ **Aliclen™** see Salicylic Acid on page 1743

Aliskiren (a lis KYE ren)

Related Information
 Angiotensin Agents on page 2093
Medication Safety Issues
 Sound-alike/look-alike issues:
 Tekturna® may be confused with Valturna®
Brand Names: U.S. Tekturna®
Brand Names: Canada Rasilez®
Index Terms Aliskiren Hemifumarate; SPP100
Generic Availability (U.S.) No
Pharmacologic Category Renin Inhibitor
Use Treatment of hypertension, alone or in combination with other antihypertensive agents
Unlabeled Use Treatment of persistent proteinuria in patients with type 2 diabetes mellitus, hypertension, and nephropathy despite administration of optimized recommended renoprotective therapy (eg, angiotensin II receptor blocker)
Contraindications
U.S. labeling: Concomitant use with an ACE inhibitor or ARB in patients with diabetes mellitus

Canada labeling: Additional contraindications (not in U.S. labeling): Hypersensitivity to aliskiren or any component of the formulation; history of angioedema with aliskiren, ACE inhibitors, or ARBs; hereditary or idiopathic angioedema; concomitant use with ACE inhibitors or ARBs in patients with GFR <60 mL/minute/1.73m^2

Warnings/Precautions Since the effect of aliskiren on bradykinin levels is unknown, the risk of kinin-mediated etiologies of angioedema occurring is also unknown. Use with caution in any patient with a history of angioedema (of any etiology) as angioedema, some cases necessitating hospitalization and intubation, has been observed (rarely) with aliskiren use. Discontinue immediately following any signs and symptoms of angioedema; do not readminister. Prolonged frequent monitoring may be required especially if tongue, glottis, or larynx are involved as they are associated with airway obstruction. Patients with a history of airway surgery may have a higher risk of airway obstruction. Early, aggressive, and appropriate management is critical. Hyperkalemia may occur (rarely) during monotherapy; risk may increase in patients with predisposing factors (eg, renal dysfunction, diabetes mellitus or concomitant use with ACE inhibitors, potassium-sparing diuretics, potassium supplements, and/or potassium-containing salts). Symptomatic hypotension may occur (rarely) during the initiation of therapy, particularly in patients with an activated renin-angiotensin system (ie, volume or salt-depleted patients). Use with caution or avoid in patients with deteriorating renal function or low renal blood flow (eg, renal artery stenosis, severe heart failure); may increase risk of developing acute renal failure and hyperkalemia. Concomitant use with an ACE inhibitor or ARB may increase risk of developing acute renal failure and should be avoided in patient with GFR <60 mL/minute. Use (monotherapy or combined with ACE inhibitors or ARBs) in patients with type 2 diabetes mellitus has demonstrated an increased incidence of renal impairment, hypotension, and hyperkalemia; use is contraindicated in patients with diabetes mellitus who are taking an ACE inhibitor or ARB. Avoid concurrent use with strong inhibitors of P-glycoprotein (eg, cyclosporine, itraconazole).

Adverse Reactions (Reflective of adult population; not specific for elderly) 1% to 10%:

Dermatologic: Rash (1%)

Endocrine & metabolic: Hyperkalemia (monotherapy ≤1%; may be increased with concurrent ACE inhibitor or ARB)

Gastrointestinal: Diarrhea (2%)

Hematologic: Creatine kinase increased (>300%: 1%)

Renal: BUN increased (≤7%), serum creatinine increased (≤7%)

Respiratory: Cough (1%)

Drug Interactions

Metabolism/Transport Effects Substrate of CYP3A4 (minor), P-glycoprotein; **Note:** Assignment of Major/Minor substrate status based on clinically relevant drug interaction potential

Avoid Concomitant Use

Avoid concomitant use of Aliskiren with any of the following: CycloSPORINE; Cyclo-SPORINE (Systemic); Itraconazole

Increased Effect/Toxicity

Aliskiren may increase the levels/effects of: ACE Inhibitors; Amifostine; Angiotensin II Receptor Blockers; Antihypertensives; Hypotensive Agents; RiTUXimab

The levels/effects of Aliskiren may be increased by: Alfuzosin; AtorvaSTATin; CycloSPOR-INE; CycloSPORINE (Systemic); Diazoxide; Herbs (Hypotensive Properties); Itraconazole; Ketoconazole; Ketoconazole (Systemic); MAO Inhibitors; Nonsteroidal Anti-Inflammatory Agents; Pentoxifylline; P-glycoprotein/ABCB1 Inhibitors; Phosphodiesterase 5 Inhibitors; Prostacyclin Analogues; Verapamil

Decreased Effect

Aliskiren may decrease the levels/effects of: Furosemide

The levels/effects of Aliskiren may be decreased by: Grapefruit Juice; Herbs (Hypertensive Properties); Methylphenidate; Nonsteroidal Anti-Inflammatory Agents; P-glycoprotein/ABCB1 Inducers; Tocilizumab; Yohimbine

Ethanol/Nutrition/Herb Interactions

Food: High-fat meals decrease absorption. Grapefruit juice may decrease the serum concentration of aliskiren. Management: Administer at the same time each day; may take with or without a meal, but consistent administration with regards to meals is recommended. Avoid concomitant use of aliskiren and grapefruit juice.

Herb/Nutraceutical: Some herbal medications may worsen hypertension (eg, licorice); others may increase the antihypertensive effect of aliskiren (eg, shepherd's purse). Management: Avoid bayberry, blue cohosh, cayenne, ephedra, ginger, ginseng (American), kola, licorice, and yohimbe. Avoid black cohosh, California poppy, coleus, golden seal, hawthorn, mistletoe, periwinkle, quinine, and shepherd's purse.

Stability Store at 25°C (77°F); excursions permitted to 15°C to 30°C (59°F to 86°F). Protect from moisture.

Mechanism of Action Aliskiren is a direct renin inhibitor, resulting in blockade of the conversion of angiotensinogen to angiotensin I. Angiotensin I suppression decreases the formation of angiotensin II (Ang II), a potent blood pressure-elevating peptide (via direct vasoconstriction, aldosterone release, and sodium retention). Ang II also functions within the Renin-Angiotensin-Aldosterone System (RAAS) as a negative inhibitory feedback mediator within the renal parenchyma to suppress the further release of renin. Thus, reductions in Ang II levels suppress this feedback loop, leading to further increased plasma renin concentrations (PRC) and subsequent activity (PRA). This disinhibition effect can be potentially problematic for ACE inhibitor and ARB therapy, as increased PRA could partially overcome the pharmacologic inhibition of the RAAS. As aliskiren is a direct inhibitor of renin activity, blunting of PRA despite the increased PRC (from loss of the negative feedback) may be clinically advantageous. The effect of aliskiren on bradykinin levels is unknown.

Pharmacodynamics/Kinetics

Onset of action: Maximum antihypertensive effect: Within 2 weeks

Absorption: Poor; absorption decreased by high-fat meal. Aliskiren is a substrate of P-glycoprotein; concurrent use of P-glycoprotein inhibitors may increase absorption.

Metabolism: Extent of metabolism unknown; *in vitro* studies indicate metabolism via CYP3A4

Bioavailability: ~3%

Half-life elimination: ~24 hours (range: 16-32 hours)

Time to peak, plasma: 1-3 hours

Excretion: Urine (~25% of absorbed dose excreted unchanged in urine); feces (unchanged via biliary excretion)

Dosage

Geriatric Refer to adult dosing. No initial dosage adjustment required.

Adult Hypertension: Initial: 150 mg once daily; may increase to 300 mg once daily (maximum: 300 mg/day). **Note:** Prior to initiation, correct hypovolemia and/or closely monitor volume status in patients on concurrent diuretics during treatment initiation.

Renal Impairment

Cl_{cr} ≥30 mL/minute: Initial: No dosage adjustment necessary

Cl_{cr} <30 mL/minute: No dosage adjustment provided in manufacturer's labeling; safety and efficacy has not been established; risk of hyperkalemia and progressive renal dysfunction may occur; use with caution.

ESRD (requiring hemodialysis): Based on a single dose pharmacokinetic study compared to patients with normal renal function, the manufacturer recommends no dosage adjustment necessary; however with chronic therapy, risk of hyperkalemia is increased; use with extreme caution.

Hepatic Impairment Initial: No dosage adjustment necessary.

Administration Administer at the same time daily; may take with or without a meal, but consistent administration with regards to meals is recommended.

Monitoring Parameters Blood pressure; serum potassium, BUN, serum creatinine

Special Geriatric Considerations The pharmacokinetic studies in elderly (≥65 years of age) demonstrated an increased AUC; however, adjustments in starting dose are not necessary. Blood pressure response and adverse effects were similar to younger adults in studies where 19% of patients were >65 years of age.

Dosage Forms Excipient information presented when available (limited, particularly for generics); consult specific product labeling.

Tablet, oral:

Tekturna®: 150 mg, 300 mg

Aliskiren, Amlodipine, and Hydrochlorothiazide

(a lis KYE ren, am LOE di peen, & hye droe klor oh THYE a zide)

Related Information

Aliskiren *on page 58*

AmLODIPine *on page 104*

Hydrochlorothiazide *on page 933*

Medication Safety Issues

Sound-alike/look-alike issues:

Amturnide™ may be confused with AMILoride

Brand Names: U.S. Amturnide™

Index Terms Aliskiren, Hydrochlorothiazide, and Amlodipine; Amlodipine Besylate, Aliskiren Hemifumarate, and Hydrochlorothiazide; Amlodipine, Aliskiren, and Hydrochlorothiazide; Amlodipine, Hydrochlorothiazide, and Aliskiren; Hydrochlorothiazide, Aliskiren, and Amlodipine; Hydrochlorothiazide, Amlodipine, and Aliskiren

Generic Availability (U.S.) No

Pharmacologic Category Antianginal Agent; Calcium Channel Blocker; Calcium Channel Blocker, Dihydropyridine; Diuretic, Thiazide; Renin Inhibitor

Use Treatment of hypertension (not for initial therapy)

Dosage

Geriatric Hypertension: Oral:

Patients ≥65 and <75 years: Refer to adult dosing.

Patients ≥75 years: Initial: Amlodipine 2.5 mg (strength not available in combination product)

Adult Note: Not for initial therapy. Dose is individualized; combination product may be substituted for individual components in patients currently maintained on all three agents separately, used to switch a patient on any dual combination of the components who is experiencing dose-limiting adverse reactions from an individual component (to a lower dose of that component), or used as add-on therapy in patients not adequately controlled with any two of the following: Aliskiren, dihydropyridine calcium channel blockers, and thiazide diuretics.

Hypertension: Oral: *Add-on/switch therapy/replacement therapy:* Aliskiren 150-300 mg and amlodipine 5-10 mg and hydrochlorothiazide 12.5-25 mg once daily; dose may be titrated after 2 weeks of therapy. Maximum recommended daily dose: Aliskiren 300 mg; amlodipine 10 mg; hydrochlorothiazide 25 mg

Renal Impairment

Cl_{cr} ≥30 mL/minute: Initial: No dosage adjustment necessary.

Cl_{cr} <30 mL/minute: No dosage adjustment provided in manufacturer's labeling; safety and efficacy has not been established; risk of aliskiren-induced hyperkalemia and progressive renal dysfunction may occur; use with caution. Use is contraindicated in patients who are anuric.

ESRD (requiring hemodialysis): Based on an aliskiren single dose pharmacokinetic study compared to patients with normal renal function, the manufacturer recommends no dosage adjustment necessary; however with chronic therapy, risk of hyperkalemia is increased; use with extreme caution. Use is contraindicated in patients who are anuric.

Hepatic Impairment

Mild-to-moderate impairment: No dosage adjustment necessary.

Severe impairment: Initial: Amlodipine 2.5 mg daily (strength not available in combination product).

Special Geriatric Considerations No overall differences in safety or efficacy were observed in older adults compared to younger adults receiving aliskiren, amlodipine, and hydrochlorothiazide (Amturnide™) during short-term clinical trials involving 19% of patients ≥65 years of age. Also see individual agents.

Dosage Forms Excipient information presented when available (limited, particularly for generics); consult specific product labeling.

Tablet, oral:

Amturnide™: Aliskiren 150 mg, amlodipine 5 mg, and hydrochlorothiazide 12.5 mg

Amturnide™: Aliskiren 300 mg, amlodipine 5 mg, and hydrochlorothiazide 12.5 mg

Amturnide™: Aliskiren 300 mg, amlodipine 5 mg, and hydrochlorothiazide 25 mg

Amturnide™: Aliskiren 300 mg, amlodipine 10 mg, and hydrochlorothiazide 12.5 mg

Amturnide™: Aliskiren 300 mg, amlodipine 10 mg, and hydrochlorothiazide 25 mg

Aliskiren and Amlodipine (a lis KYE ren & am LOE di peen)

Related Information

Aliskiren *on page 58*

AmLODIPine *on page 104*

Brand Names: U.S. Tekamlo™

Index Terms Aliskiren Hemifumarate and Amlodipine Besylate; Amlodipine and Aliskiren

Generic Availability (U.S.) No

Pharmacologic Category Antianginal Agent; Calcium Channel Blocker; Calcium Channel Blocker, Dihydropyridine; Renin Inhibitor

Use Treatment of hypertension, alone or in combination with other antihypertensive agents, including use as initial therapy in patients likely to need multiple antihypertensives for adequate control

Dosage

Geriatric Refer to adult dosing. No initial dosage adjustment required.

Adult

Hypertension: Oral: Dosage must be individualized. Combination product may be used as initial therapy or substituted for individual components in patients currently maintained on both agents separately or in patients not adequately controlled with monotherapy (using one of the agents or an agent within same antihypertensive class).

Initial therapy: Aliskiren 150 mg and amlodipine 5 mg once daily; dose may be titrated at 2- to 4-week intervals; maximum recommended daily doses: Aliskiren 300 mg; amlodipine 10 mg

Add-on therapy: Initiate by adding the lowest available dose of the alternative component (aliskiren 150 mg or amlodipine 5 mg); dose may be titrated at 2- to 4-week intervals; maximum recommended daily doses: Aliskiren 300 mg; amlodipine 10 mg

Replacement therapy: Substitute for the individually titrated components

Note: Prior to initiation, correct hypovolemia and/or closely monitor volume status in patients on concurrent diuretics during treatment initiation.

Renal Impairment

Cl_{cr} ≥30 mL/minute: Initial: No dosage adjustment necessary.

Cl_{cr} <30 mL/minute: No dosage adjustment provided in manufacturer's labeling; safety and efficacy has not been established; risk of hyperkalemia and progressive renal dysfunction may occur; use with caution.

ESRD (requiring hemodialysis): Based on an aliskiren single dose pharmacokinetic study compared to patients with normal renal function, the manufacturer recommends no dosage adjustment necessary; however with chronic therapy, risk of aliskiren-induced hyperkalemia is increased; use with extreme caution.

Hepatic Impairment

Mild-to-moderate impairment: Initial: No dosage adjustment necessary; titrate slowly.

Severe impairment: Use with caution; amlodipine elimination prolonged; lower initial dose should be considered (possibly requiring use of the individual agents).

◀ **Special Geriatric Considerations** No overall differences in safety or efficacy were observed in older adults compared to younger adults receiving aliskiren and amlodipine (Tekamlo™) during short-term clinical trials involving 17% of patients ≥65 years of age. Also see individual agents.

Dosage Forms Excipient information presented when available (limited, particularly for generics); consult specific product labeling.
Tablet, oral:
Tekamlo™ 150/5: Aliskiren 150 mg and amlodipine 5 mg
Tekamlo™ 150/10: Aliskiren 150 mg and amlodipine 10 mg
Tekamlo™ 300/5: Aliskiren 300 mg and amlodipine 5 mg
Tekamlo™ 300/10: Aliskiren 300 mg and amlodipine 10 mg

Aliskiren and Valsartan (a lis KYE ren & val SAR tan)

Related Information
Aliskiren *on page 58*
Valsartan *on page 1996*
Medication Safety Issues
Sound-alike/look-alike issues:
Valturna® may be confused with Tekturna®, valsartan
Brand Names: U.S. Valturna® [DSC]
Index Terms Aliskiren Hemifumarate and Valsartan; Valsartan and Aliskiren
Generic Availability (U.S.) No
Pharmacologic Category Angiotensin II Receptor Blocker; Renin Inhibitor
Use Treatment of hypertension, including use as initial therapy in patients likely to need multiple antihypertensives for adequate control
Dosage
Geriatric & Adult Hypertension: Oral: Dose is individualized; combination product may be used as initial therapy or substituted for individual components in patients currently maintained on both agents separately or in patients not adequately controlled with monotherapy (using one of the agents or an agent within same antihypertensive class). Titrate at 2- to 4-week intervals as necessary.
Initial therapy: Aliskiren 150 mg and valsartan 160 mg once daily; titrate to effect (maximum daily aliskiren dose: 300 mg; maximum daily valsartan dose: 320 mg)
Patients not controlled with single-agent therapy: Aliskiren 150 mg and valsartan 160 mg once daily; titrate to effect (maximum daily aliskiren dose: 300 mg; maximum daily valsartan dose: 320 mg)
Renal Impairment
Cl_{cr} ≥60 mL/minute: No dosage adjustment necessary.
Cl_{cr} <60 mL/minute: Avoid use.
Hepatic Impairment Initial:
Mild-to-moderate impairment: Initial: No dosage adjustment necessary.
Severe impairment: Use with caution; clinical experience is limited.
Special Geriatric Considerations See individual agents. Combination products are not recommended as first-line treatment. Use only if doses of individual agents correspond to the combination available.
Dosage Forms Excipient information presented when available (limited, particularly for generics); consult specific product labeling.
Tablet:
Valturna®:
150/160: Aliskiren 150 mg and valsartan 160 mg [DSC]
300/320: Aliskiren 300 mg and valsartan 320 mg [DSC]

Allopurinol (al oh PURE i nole)

Medication Safety Issues
Sound-alike/look-alike issues:
Allopurinol may be confused with Apresoline
Zyloprim® may be confused with ZORprin®, Zovirax®
Brand Names: U.S. Aloprim®; Zyloprim®
Brand Names: Canada Alloprin®; Novo-Purol; Zyloprim®
Index Terms Allopurinol Sodium
Generic Availability (U.S.) Yes
Pharmacologic Category Antigout Agent; Xanthine Oxidase Inhibitor
Use
Oral: Management of primary or secondary gout (acute attack, tophi, joint destruction, uric acid lithiasis, and/or nephropathy); management of hyperuricemia associated with cancer treatment for leukemia, lymphoma, or solid tumor malignancies; management of recurrent calcium oxalate calculi (with uric acid excretion >800 mg/day in men and >750 mg/day in women)

I.V.: Management of hyperuricemia associated with cancer treatment for leukemia, lymphoma, or solid tumor malignancies
Contraindications Hypersensitivity to allopurinol or any component of the formulation
Warnings/Precautions Do not use to treat asymptomatic hyperuricemia. Has been associated with a number of hypersensitivity reactions, including severe reactions (vasculitis and Stevens-Johnson syndrome); discontinue at first sign of rash. Reversible hepatotoxicity has been reported; use with caution in patients with pre-existing hepatic impairment. Bone marrow suppression has been reported; use caution with other drugs causing myelosuppression. Caution in renal impairment, dosage adjustments needed. Use with caution in patients taking diuretics concurrently. Risk of skin rash may be increased in patients receiving amoxicillin or ampicillin. The risk of hypersensitivity may be increased in patients receiving thiazides, and possibly ACE inhibitors. Use caution with mercaptopurine or azathioprine; dosage adjustment necessary. Full effect on serum uric acid levels in chronic gout may take several weeks to become evident; gradual titration is recommended.
Adverse Reactions (Reflective of adult population; not specific for elderly)
Dermatologic: Rash
Endocrine & metabolic: Gout (acute)
Gastrointestinal: Diarrhea, nausea
Hepatic: Alkaline phosphatase increased, liver enzymes increased
Drug Interactions
Metabolism/Transport Effects None known.
Avoid Concomitant Use
Avoid concomitant use of Allopurinol with any of the following: Didanosine
Increased Effect/Toxicity
Allopurinol may increase the levels/effects of: Amoxicillin; Ampicillin; Anticonvulsants (Hydantoin); AzaTHIOprine; CarBAMazepine; ChlorproPAMIDE; Cyclophosphamide; Didanosine; Mercaptopurine; Theophylline Derivatives; Vitamin K Antagonists

The levels/effects of Allopurinol may be increased by: ACE Inhibitors; Loop Diuretics; Thiazide Diuretics
Decreased Effect
The levels/effects of Allopurinol may be decreased by: Antacids
Ethanol/Nutrition/Herb Interactions
Ethanol: May decrease effectiveness.
Iron supplements: Hepatic iron uptake may be increased.
Vitamin C: Large amounts of vitamin C may acidify urine and increase kidney stone formation.
Stability
Powder for injection: Store at controlled room temperature of 20°C to 25°C (68°F to 77°F). Reconstitute powder for injection with SWFI. Further dilution with NS or D_5W (50-100 mL) to ≤6 mg/mL is recommended. Following preparation, intravenous solutions should be stored

at 20°C to 25°C (68°F to 77°F). Do not refrigerate reconstituted and/or diluted product. Must be administered within 10 hours of solution preparation.

Tablet: Store at controlled room temperature of 20°C to 25°C (68°F to 77°F). Protect from moisture and light.

Mechanism of Action Allopurinol inhibits xanthine oxidase, the enzyme responsible for the conversion of hypoxanthine to xanthine to uric acid. Allopurinol is metabolized to oxypurinol which is an inhibitor of xanthine oxidase; allopurinol acts on purine catabolism, reducing the production of uric acid without disrupting the biosynthesis of vital purines.

Pharmacodynamics/Kinetics

Onset of action: Peak effect: 1-2 weeks

Absorption: Oral: ~80%; Rectal: Poor and erratic

Distribution: V_d: ~1.6 L/kg; V_{ss}: 0.84-0.87 L/kg; enters breast milk

Protein binding: <1%

Metabolism: ~75% to active metabolites, chiefly oxypurinol

Bioavailability: 49% to 53%

Half-life elimination:

Normal renal function: Parent drug: 1-3 hours; Oxypurinol: 18-30 hours

End-stage renal disease: Prolonged

Time to peak, plasma: Oral: 30-120 minutes

Excretion: Urine (76% as oxypurinol, 12% as unchanged drug)

Allopurinol and oxypurinol are dialyzable

Dosage

Geriatric & Adult Note: Oral doses >300 mg should be given in divided doses.

Gout (chronic): Oral:

Manufacturer's labeling: Mild: 200-300 mg/day; Severe: 400-600 mg/day; to reduce the possibility of acute gouty attacks, initiate dose at 100 mg/day and increase weekly to recommended dosage, also consider using low-dose colchicine or an NSAID to reduce the risk of a gouty attack. Maximum daily dose: 800 mg/day.

Alternative recommendations (unlabeled dosing): Initial: 100 mg/day, increasing the dose gradually every 4 weeks, while monitoring plasma uric acid levels to achieve a goal of <6 mg/dL; dosages of 600 mg/day and rarely, 900 mg/day may be required (McGill, 2010) **or** Initial: 100 mg/day, increasing the dose by 100 mg/day at 2-4 weeks intervals as required to achieve desired uric acid level of ≤6 mg/dL (EULAR gout guidelines; Zhang, 2006).

Management of hyperuricemia associated with chemotherapy:

Oral:

Manufacturer's labeling: 600-800 mg/day in 2-3 divided doses

Alternative recommendations (unlabeled dosing; intermediate-risk for tumor lysis syndrome): Intermediate-risk for tumor lysis syndrome: 10 mg/kg/day (maximum dose/day: 800 mg) in 3 divided doses **or** 50-100 mg/m² every 8 hours (maximum dose: 300 mg/m²/day), begin 1-2 days before initiation of induction chemotherapy; may continue for 3-7 days after chemotherapy (Coiffier, 2008)

I.V.:

Manufacturer's labeling: 200-400 mg/m²/day (maximum: 600 mg/day) beginning 1-2 days before chemotherapy

Alternative recommendations (unlabeled dosing; intermediate-risk for tumor lysis syndrome): 200-400 mg/m²/day (maximum dose/day: 600 mg) in 1-3 divided doses beginning 1-2 days before the start of induction chemotherapy; may continue for 3-7 days after chemotherapy (Coiffier, 2008)

Note: Intravenous daily dose can be given as a single infusion or in equally divided doses at 6-, 8-, or 12-hour intervals. A fluid intake sufficient to yield a daily urinary output of at least 2 L in adults is desirable.

Recurrent calcium oxalate stones: Oral: 200-300 mg/day in single or divided doses

Renal Impairment

Manufacturer's labeling: Oral, I.V.: Lower doses are required in renal impairment due to potential for accumulation of allopurinol and metabolites.

Cl_{cr} 10-20 mL/minute: 200 mg/day

Cl_{cr} 3-10 mL/minute: ≤100 mg/day

Cl_{cr} <3 mL/minute: 100 mg/dose at extended intervals

Alternative recommendations (unlabeled dosing):

Management of hyperuricemia associated with chemotherapy: Dosage reduction of 50% is recommended in renal impairment (Coiffier, 2008)

Gout: Oral:

Initiate therapy with 50-100 mg daily, and gradually increase to a maintenance dose to achieve a serum uric acid level of ≤6 mg/dL (with close monitoring of serum uric acid levels and for hypersensitivity) (Dalbeth, 2007).

Hemodialysis: Initial: 100 mg alternate days given postdialysis, increase cautiously to 300 mg based on response. If dialysis is on a daily basis, an additional 50% of the dose may be required postdialysis (Dalbeth, 2007)

Administration

Oral: Do not initiate or discontinue allopurinol during an acute gout attack. Should administer oral forms after meals with plenty of fluid.

I.V.: The rate of infusion depends on the volume of the infusion; infuse maximum single daily doses (600 mg/day) over ≥30 minutes. Whenever possible, therapy should be initiated at 24-48 hours before the start of chemotherapy known to cause tumor lysis (including adrenocorticosteroids). I.V. daily dose can be administered as a single infusion or in equally divided doses at 6-, 8-, or 12-hour interval.

Monitoring Parameters CBC, serum uric acid levels, I & O, hepatic and renal function, especially at start of therapy; signs and symptoms of hypersensitivity

Reference Range Adults:

Males: 3.4-7 mg/dL or slightly more

Females: 2.4-6 mg/dL or slightly more

Target: ≤6 mg/dL

Values >7 mg/dL are sometimes arbitrarily regarded as hyperuricemia, but there is no sharp line between normals on the one hand, and the serum uric acid of those with clinical gout. Normal ranges cannot be adjusted for purine ingestion, but high purine diet increases uric acid. Uric acid may be increased with body size, exercise, and stress.

Special Geriatric Considerations Adjust dose based on renal function.

Dosage Forms Excipient information presented when available (limited, particularly for generics); consult specific product labeling.

Injection, powder for reconstitution, as sodium: 500 mg (base)

Aloprim®: 500 mg (base)

Tablet, oral: 100 mg, 300 mg

Zyloprim®: 100 mg, 300 mg [scored]

◆ **Allopurinol Sodium** see Allopurinol on page 63

◆ **Almacone® [OTC]** see Aluminum Hydroxide, Magnesium Hydroxide, and Simethicone on page 82

◆ **Almacone Double Strength® [OTC]** see Aluminum Hydroxide, Magnesium Hydroxide, and Simethicone on page 82

◆ **Almora® [OTC]** see Magnesium Salts (Various Salts) on page 1182

Almotriptan (al moh TRIP tan)

Medication Safety Issues

Sound-alike/look-alike issues:

Axert® may be confused with Antivert®

Brand Names: U.S. Axert®

Brand Names: Canada Axert®

Index Terms Almotriptan Malate

Generic Availability (U.S.) No

Pharmacologic Category Antimigraine Agent; Serotonin 5-HT$_{1B, 1D}$ Receptor Agonist

Use Acute treatment of migraine with or without aura in adults (with a history of migraine)

Contraindications Hypersensitivity to almotriptan or any component of the formulation; hemiplegic or basilar migraine; known or suspected ischemic heart disease (eg, angina pectoris, MI, documented silent ischemia, coronary artery vasospasm, Prinzmetal's variant angina); cerebrovascular syndromes (eg, stroke, transient ischemic attacks); peripheral vascular disease (eg, ischemic bowel disease); uncontrolled hypertension; use within 24 hours of another 5-HT$_1$ agonist; use within 24 hours of ergotamine derivatives and/or ergotamine-containing medications (eg, dihydroergotamine, ergotamine)

Warnings/Precautions Almotriptan is only indicated for the treatment of acute migraine headache; not indicated for migraine prophylaxis, or the treatment of cluster headaches, hemiplegic migraine, or basilar migraine. If a patient does not respond to the first dose, the diagnosis of acute migraine should be reconsidered.

Almotriptan should not be given to patients with documented ischemic or vasospastic CAD. Patients with risk factors for CAD (eg, hypertension, hypercholesterolemia, smoker, obesity, diabetes, strong family history of CAD, menopause, male >40 years of age) should undergo adequate cardiac evaluation prior to administration; if the cardiac evaluation is "satisfactory," the first dose of almotriptan should be given in the healthcare provider's office (consider ECG monitoring). All patients should undergo periodic evaluation of cardiovascular status during treatment. Cardiac events (coronary artery vasospasm, transient ischemia, myocardial infarction, ventricular tachycardia/fibrillation, cardiac arrest, and death), cerebral/subarachnoid hemorrhage, stroke, peripheral vascular ischemia, and colonic ischemia have been reported with 5-HT$_1$ agonist administration. Patients who experience sensations of chest pain/pressure/tightness or symptoms suggestive of angina following dosing should be evaluated for coronary artery disease or Prinzmetal's angina before receiving additional doses; if dosing is resumed and similar symptoms recur, monitor with ECG. Significant elevation in blood pressure, including hypertensive crisis, has also been reported on rare occasions following 5-HT$_1$ agonist administration in patients with and without a history of hypertension.

Transient and permanent blindness and partial vision loss have been reported (rare) with 5-HT$_1$ agonist administration. Almotriptan contains a sulfonyl group which is structurally different from a sulfonamide. Cross-reactivity in patients with sulfonamide allergy has not been evaluated; however, the manufacturer recommends that caution be exercised in this patient population. Use with caution in liver or renal dysfunction. Symptoms of agitation, confusion, hallucinations, hyper-reflexia, myoclonus, shivering, and tachycardia (serotonin syndrome) may occur with concomitant proserotonergic drugs (ie, SSRIs/SNRIs or triptans) or agents which reduce almotriptan's metabolism. Concurrent use of serotonin precursors (eg, tryptophan) is not recommended. If concomitant administration with SSRIs is warranted, monitor closely, especially at initiation and with dose increases. Efficacy has not been demonstrated in improvement of migraine-associated symptoms (eg, phonophobia, nausea, photophobia) in patients aged 12-17 years (Linder, 2008).

Adverse Reactions (Reflective of adult population; not specific for elderly) 1% to 10%:
Central nervous system: Somnolence (≤5%), dizziness (≤4%), headache (≤2%)
Gastrointestinal: Nausea (1% to 3%), vomiting (≤2%), xerostomia (1%)
Neuromuscular & skeletal: Paresthesia (≤1%)

Drug Interactions

Metabolism/Transport Effects Substrate of CYP2D6 (minor), CYP3A4 (minor); **Note:** Assignment of Major/Minor substrate status based on clinically relevant drug interaction potential

Avoid Concomitant Use
Avoid concomitant use of Almotriptan with any of the following: Ergot Derivatives; MAO Inhibitors

Increased Effect/Toxicity
Almotriptan may increase the levels/effects of: Ergot Derivatives; Metoclopramide; Serotonin Modulators

The levels/effects of Almotriptan may be increased by: Antipsychotics; CYP3A4 Inhibitors (Strong); Ergot Derivatives; MAO Inhibitors

Decreased Effect
The levels/effects of Almotriptan may be decreased by: Peginterferon Alfa-2b; Tocilizumab

Stability Store at 25°C (77°F); excursions permitted to 15°C to 30°C (59°F to 86°F).

Mechanism of Action Selective agonist for serotonin (5-HT$_{1B}$ and 5-HT$_{1D}$ receptors) in cranial arteries; causes vasoconstriction and reduces sterile inflammation associated with antidromic neuronal transmission correlating with relief of migraine

Pharmacodynamics/Kinetics Geriatrics: Pharmacokinetic disposition is similar to that in young adults.
Absorption: Well absorbed
Distribution: V_d: 180-200 L
Protein binding: ~35%
Metabolism: MAO type A oxidative deamination (~27% of dose)
Bioavailability: 12.5 mg dose - 80%; 25 mg dose - 70%
Half-life: 3-4 hours
Time to peak: 1-3 hours
Elimination: Urine (40% as unchanged drug); feces (13% unchanged and metabolized)

Dosage

Geriatric & Adult Migraine: Oral: Initial: 6.25-12.5 mg in a single dose; if the headache returns, repeat the dose after 2 hours; no more than 2 doses (maximum daily dose: 25 mg) **Note:** The safety of treating more than 4 migraines/month has not been established.

Dosage adjustment with concomitant use of an enzyme inhibitor:
Patients receiving a potent CYP3A4 inhibitor: Initial: 6.25 mg in a single dose; maximum daily dose: 12.5 mg
Patients with renal impairment and concomitant use of a potent CYP3A4 inhibitor: Avoid use
Patients with hepatic impairment and concomitant use of a potent CYP3A4 inhibitor: Avoid use

Renal Impairment Severe renal impairment (Cl$_{cr}$ ≤30 mL/minute): Initial: 6.25 mg in a single dose; maximum daily dose: 12.5 mg

Hepatic Impairment Initial: 6.25 mg in a single dose; maximum daily dose: 12.5 mg
Administration Administer without regard to meals.
Special Geriatric Considerations Use cautiously in elderly, particularly since many have cardiovascular disease, which would put them at risk for cardiovascular adverse effects. Safety and efficacy in elderly patients >65 years of age have not been established.
Dosage Forms Excipient information presented when available (limited, particularly for generics); consult specific product labeling.
Tablet, oral, as maleate:
  Axert®: 6.25 mg, 12.5 mg

- ◆ **Almotriptan Malate** see Almotriptan on page 65
- ◆ **Alocril®** see Nedocromil on page 1350
- ◆ **Alodox™** see Doxycycline on page 606
- ◆ **Aloe Vesta® Antifungal [OTC]** see Miconazole (Topical) on page 1276
- ◆ **Alomide®** see Lodoxamide on page 1152
- ◆ **Alophen® [OTC]** see Bisacodyl on page 214
- ◆ **Aloprim®** see Allopurinol on page 63
- ◆ **Alora®** see Estradiol (Systemic) on page 681

Alpha-Galactosidase (AL fa ga lak TOE si days)

Medication Safety Issues
  Sound-alike/look-alike issues:
    beano® may be confused with B&O (belladonna and opium)
Brand Names: U.S. beano® Meltaways [OTC]; beano® [OTC]
Index Terms Aspergillus niger
Generic Availability (U.S.) No
Pharmacologic Category Enzyme
Use Prevention of flatulence and bloating attributed to a variety of grains, cereals, nuts, and vegetables
Dosage
  Geriatric & Adult Flatulence and bloating: Oral: Adjust dose according to the number of problem foods per meal:
    Tablet, chewable (beano®): Usual dose: 2-3 tablets/meal
    Tablet, orally disintegrating (beano® Meltaways): One tablet per meal
Dosage Forms Excipient information presented when available (limited, particularly for generics); consult specific product labeling.
Tablet, chewable, oral:
  beano®: 150 Galactosidase units [scored]
Tablet, orally disintegrating, oral:
  beano® Meltaways: 300 Galactosidase units [strawberry flavor]

- ◆ **Alphagan® P** see Brimonidine on page 220
- ◆ **1α-Hydroxyergocalciferol** see Doxercalciferol on page 604
- ◆ **Alph-E [OTC]** see Vitamin E on page 2027
- ◆ **Alph-E-Mixed [OTC]** see Vitamin E on page 2027

ALPRAZolam (al PRAY zoe lam)

Related Information
  Anxiolytic, Sedative/Hypnotic, and Miscellaneous Benzodiazepines on page 2106
  Beers Criteria – Potentially Inappropriate Medications for Geriatrics on page 2183
Medication Safety Issues
  Sound-alike/look-alike issues:
    ALPRAZolam may be confused with alprostadil, LORazepam, triazolam
    Xanax® may be confused with Fanapt®, Lanoxin®, Tenex®, Tylox®, Xopenex®, Zantac®, ZyrTEC®
  BEERS Criteria medication:
    This drug may be potentially inappropriate for use in geriatric patients (Quality of evidence - high; Strength of recommendation - strong).
Brand Names: U.S. Alprazolam Intensol™; Niravam™; Xanax XR®; Xanax®
Brand Names: Canada Apo-Alpraz®; Apo-Alpraz® TS; Mylan-Alprazolam; NTP-Alprazolam; Nu-Alpraz; Teva-Alprazolam; Xanax TS™; Xanax®
Generic Availability (U.S.) Yes: Excludes oral solution
Pharmacologic Category Benzodiazepine
Use Treatment of anxiety disorder (GAD); short-term relief of symptoms of anxiety; panic disorder, with or without agoraphobia; anxiety associated with depression

Contraindications Hypersensitivity to alprazolam or any component of the formulation (cross-sensitivity with other benzodiazepines may exist); narrow-angle glaucoma; concurrent use with ketoconazole or itraconazole

Warnings/Precautions Rebound or withdrawal symptoms, including seizures, may occur following abrupt discontinuation or large decreases in dose (more common in patients receiving >4 mg/day or prolonged treatment); the risk of seizures appears to be greatest 24-72 hours following discontinuation of therapy. Breakthrough anxiety may occur at the end of dosing interval. Use with caution in patients receiving concurrent CYP3A4 inhibitors, moderate or strong CYP3A4 inducers, and major CYP3A4 substrates; consider alternative agents that avoid or lessen the potential for CYP-mediated interactions. Use with caution in renal impairment or predisposition to urate nephropathy; has weak uricosuric properties. In older adults, benzodiazepines increase the risk of impaired cognition, delirium, falls, fractures, and motor vehicle accidents. Due to increased sensitivity in this age group, avoid use for treatment of insomnia, agitation, or delirium (Beers Criteria). Use with caution in or debilitated patients, patients with hepatic disease (including alcoholics) or respiratory disease, or obese patients.

Causes CNS depression (dose related) which may impair physical and mental capabilities. Patients must be cautioned about performing tasks that require mental alertness (eg, operating machinery or driving). Effects with other sedative drugs or ethanol may be potentiated. Benzodiazepines have been associated with falls and traumatic injury and should be used with extreme caution in patients who are at risk of these events.

Use caution in patients with depression, particularly if suicidal risk may be present. Episodes of mania or hypomania have occurred in depressed patients treated with alprazolam. May cause physical or psychological dependence. Acute withdrawal may be precipitated in patients after administration of flumazenil.

Benzodiazepines have been associated with anterograde amnesia. Paradoxical reactions have been reported with benzodiazepines, particularly in adolescent/pediatric or psychiatric patients. Does not have analgesic, antidepressant, or antipsychotic properties.

Adverse Reactions (Reflective of adult population; not specific for elderly)
>10%:
Central nervous system: Abnormal coordination, cognitive disorder, depression, drowsiness, fatigue, irritability, lightheadedness, memory impairment, sedation, somnolence
Endocrine & metabolic: Libido decreased
Gastrointestinal: Appetite increased/decreased, constipation, weight gain/loss, xerostomia
Genitourinary: Micturition difficulty
Neuromuscular & skeletal: Dysarthria
Respiratory: Nasal congestion
1% to 10%:
Cardiovascular: Chest pain, hypotension, palpitation, sinus tachycardia
Central nervous system: Agitation, akathisia, ataxia, attention disturbance, confusion, depersonalization, derealization, disorientation, disinhibition, dizziness, dream abnormalities, fear, hallucination, headache, hypersomnia, hypoesthesia, insomnia, lethargy, malaise, mental impairment, nervousness, nightmares, restlessness, seizure, syncope, talkativeness, vertigo
Dermatologic: Dermatitis, rash
Endocrine & metabolic: Dysmenorrhea, libido increased, menstrual disorders, sexual dysfunction
Gastrointestinal: Abdominal pain, anorexia, diarrhea, dyspepsia, nausea, salivation increased, vomiting
Genitourinary: Incontinence
Hepatic: Bilirubin increased, jaundice, liver enzymes increased
Neuromuscular & skeletal: Arthralgia, back pain, dyskinesia, dystonia, muscle cramps, muscle twitching, myalgia, paresthesia, tremor, weakness
Ocular: Blurred vision
Respiratory: Allergic rhinitis, dyspnea, hyperventilation, upper respiratory infection
Miscellaneous: Diaphoresis

Drug Interactions
Metabolism/Transport Effects Substrate of CYP3A4 (major); **Note:** Assignment of Major/ Minor substrate status based on clinically relevant drug interaction potential
Avoid Concomitant Use
Avoid concomitant use of ALPRAZolam with any of the following: Azelastine; Azelastine (Nasal); Conivaptan; Indinavir; Methadone; Mirtazapine; OLANZapine; Paraldehyde
Increased Effect/Toxicity
ALPRAZolam may increase the levels/effects of: Alcohol (Ethyl); Azelastine; Azelastine (Nasal); Buprenorphine; CloZAPine; CNS Depressants; Methadone; Methotrimeprazine; Metyrosine; Mirtazapine; Paraldehyde; Selective Serotonin Reuptake Inhibitors; Zolpidem

The levels/effects of ALPRAZolam may be increased by: Antifungal Agents (Azole Derivatives, Systemic); Aprepitant; Boceprevir; Calcium Channel Blockers (Nondihydropyridine); Cimetidine; Conivaptan; Contraceptives (Estrogens); Contraceptives (Progestins); CYP3A4 Inhibitors (Moderate); CYP3A4 Inhibitors (Strong); Dasatinib; Droperidol; Fosaprepitant; Grapefruit Juice; HydrOXYzine; Indinavir; Isoniazid; Ivacaftor; Macrolide Antibiotics; Methotrimeprazine; Mifepristone; OLANZapine; Protease Inhibitors; Proton Pump Inhibitors; Selective Serotonin Reuptake Inhibitors; Telaprevir

Decreased Effect

The levels/effects of ALPRAZolam may be decreased by: CarBAMazepine; CYP3A4 Inducers (Strong); Deferasirox; Rifamycin Derivatives; St Johns Wort; Theophylline Derivatives; Tocilizumab; Yohimbine

Ethanol/Nutrition/Herb Interactions

Cigarette: Smoking may decrease alprazolam concentrations up to 50%.

Ethanol: Ethanol may increase CNS depression. Management: Avoid ethanol.

Food: Alprazolam serum concentration is unlikely to be increased by grapefruit juice because of alprazolam's high oral bioavailability. The C_{max} of the extended release formulation is increased by 25% when a high-fat meal is given 2 hours before dosing. T_{max} is decreased 33% when food is given immediately prior to dose and increased by 33% when food is given ≥1 hour after dose.

Herb/Nutraceutical: St John's wort may decrease alprazolam levels. Valerian, kava kava, and gotu kola may increase CNS depression. Management: Avoid St John's wort. Avoid valerian, kava kava, and gotu kola.

Stability

Immediate release tablets: Store at 20°C to 25°C (68°F to 77°F).

Extended release tablets: Store at 25°C (77°F); excursions permitted to 15°C to 30°C (59°F to 86°F).

Orally-disintegrating tablet: Store at room temperature of 20°C to 25°C (68°F to 77°F). Protect from moisture. Seal bottle tightly and discard any cotton packaged inside bottle.

Mechanism of Action Binds to stereospecific benzodiazepine receptors on the postsynaptic GABA neuron at several sites within the central nervous system, including the limbic system, reticular formation. Enhancement of the inhibitory effect of GABA on neuronal excitability results by increased neuronal membrane permeability to chloride ions. This shift in chloride ions results in hyperpolarization (a less excitable state) and stabilization.

Pharmacodynamics/Kinetics

Onset of action: Immediate release and extended release formulations: 1 hour

Duration: Immediate release: 5.1 ± 1.7 hours; Extended release: 11.3 ± 4.2 hours

Absorption: Extended release: Slower relative to immediate release formulation resulting in a concentration that is maintained 5-11 hours after dosing

Distribution: V_d: 0.9-1.2 L/kg

Protein binding: 80%; primarily to albumin

Metabolism: Hepatic via CYP3A4; forms two active metabolites (4-hydroxyalprazolam and α-hydroxyalprazolam)

Bioavailability: 90%

Half-life elimination:

Adults: 11.2 hours (Immediate release range: 6.3-26.9 hours; Extended release range: 10.7-15.8 hours); Orally-disintegrating tablet range: 7.9-19.2 hours)

Elderly: 16.3 hours (range: 9-26.9 hours)

Alcoholic liver disease: 19.7 hours (range: 5.8-65.3 hours)

Obesity: 21.8 hours (range: 9.9-40.4 hours)

Race: Asians: Increased by ~25% (as compared to Caucasians)

Time to peak, serum:

Immediate release: 1-2 hours

Extended release: ~9 hours (Glue, 2006); decreased by 1 hour when administered at bedtime (as compared to morning administration); decreased by 33% when administered with a high-fat meal; increased by 33% when administered ≥1 hour after a high-fat meal

Orally-disintegrating tablet: 1.5-2 hours; occurs ~15 minutes earlier when administered with water; decreased by 2 hours when administered with a high-fat meal

Excretion: Urine (as unchanged drug and metabolites)

Dosage

Geriatric Note: Elderly patients may be more sensitive to the effects of alprazolam including ataxia and oversedation. The elderly may also have impaired renal function leading to decreased clearance. Titrate gradually, if needed and tolerated.

Immediate release: Initial 0.25 mg 2-3 times/day

Extended release: Initial: 0.5 mg once daily

Adult Note: Treatment >4 months should be re-evaluated to determine the patient's continued need for the drug

◀

Anxiety: Oral: *Immediate release:* Initial: 0.25-0.5 mg 3 times/day; titrate dose upward every 3-4 days; usual maximum: 4 mg/day. Patients requiring doses >4 mg/day should be increased cautiously. Periodic reassessment and consideration of dosage reduction is recommended.

Panic disorder: Oral:

Immediate release: Initial: 0.5 mg 3 times/day; dose may be increased every 3-4 days in increments ≤1 mg/day. Mean effective dosage: 5-6 mg/day; some patients may require much as 10 mg/day

Extended release: 0.5-1 mg once daily; may increase dose every 3-4 days in increments ≤1 mg/day (range: 3-6 mg/day)

Switching from immediate release to extended release: Patients may be switched to extended release tablets by taking the total daily dose of the immediate release tablets and giving it once daily using the extended release preparation.

Preoperative anxiety (unlabeled use): Oral: 0.5 mg 60-90 minutes before procedure (De Witte, 2002)

Dose reduction: Abrupt discontinuation should be avoided. Daily dose may be decreased by 0.5 mg every 3 days; however, some patients may require a slower reduction. If withdrawal symptoms occur, resume previous dose and discontinue on a less rapid schedule.

Renal Impairment No dosage adjustment provided in manufacturer's labeling; however, use caution.

Hepatic Impairment Advanced liver disease:

Immediate release: 0.25 mg 2-3 times/day; titrate gradually if needed and tolerated.

Extended release: 0.5 mg once daily; titrate gradually if needed and tolerate

Administration

Immediate release preparations: Can be administered sublingually if oral administration is not possible; absorption and onset of effect are comparable to oral administration (Scavone,1987; Scavone, 1992)

Extended release tablet: Should be taken once daily in the morning; do not crush, break, or chew.

Orally-disintegrating tablets: Using dry hands, place tablet on top of tongue and allow to disintegrate. If using one-half of tablet, immediately discard remaining half (may not remain stable). Administration with water is not necessary.

Monitoring Parameters Respiratory and cardiovascular status

Pharmacotherapy Pearls Not intended for management of anxieties and minor distresses associated with everyday life. Treatment longer than 4 months should be re-evaluated to determine the patient's need for the drug. Patients who become physically dependent on alprazolam tend to have a difficult time discontinuing it; withdrawal symptoms may be severe. To minimize withdrawal symptoms, taper dosage slowly; do not discontinue abruptly. Abrupt discontinuation after sustained use (generally >10 days) may cause withdrawal symptoms.

Special Geriatric Considerations This medication is considered to be potentially inappropriate in this patient population (Beers Criteria: Quality of evidence - high; Strength of recommendation - strong).

Controlled Substance C-IV

Dosage Forms Excipient information presented when available (limited, particularly for generics); consult specific product labeling.

Solution, oral [concentrate]:

Alprazolam Intensol™: 1 mg/mL (30 mL) [dye free, ethanol free, sugar free; contains propylene glycol]

Tablet, oral: 0.25 mg, 0.5 mg, 1 mg, 2 mg

Xanax®: 0.25 mg, 0.5 mg, 1 mg, 2 mg [scored]

Tablet, extended release, oral: 0.5 mg, 1 mg, 2 mg, 3 mg

Xanax XR®: 0.5 mg, 1 mg, 2 mg, 3 mg

Tablet, orally disintegrating, oral: 0.25 mg, 0.5 mg, 1 mg, 2 mg

Niravam™: 0.25 mg, 0.5 mg, 1 mg, 2 mg [scored; orange flavor]

◆ **Alprazolam Intensol™** *see* ALPRAZolam *on page* 67

Alprostadil (al PROS ta dill)

Medication Safety Issues

Sound-alike/look-alike issues:

Alprostadil may be confused with alPRAZolam

Brand Names: U.S. Caverject Impulse®; Caverject®; Edex®; Muse®

Brand Names: Canada Caverject®; Muse® Pellet

Index Terms PGE_1; Prostaglandin E_1

Generic Availability (U.S.) Yes: Solution for injection

Pharmacologic Category Prostaglandin; Vasodilator

Use

Caverject®: Treatment of erectile dysfunction of vasculogenic, psychogenic, or neurogenic etiology; adjunct in the diagnosis of erectile dysfunction

Edex®, Muse®: Treatment of erectile dysfunction of vasculogenic, psychogenic, or neurogenic etiology

Contraindications Hypersensitivity to alprostadil or any component of the formulation; conditions predisposing patients to priapism (sickle cell anemia, multiple myeloma, leukemia); patients with anatomical deformation of the penis, penile implants; use in men for whom sexual activity is inadvisable or contraindicated

Warnings/Precautions When used in erectile dysfunction, priapism may occur; treat prolonged priapism (erection persisting for >4 hours) immediately to avoid penile tissue damage and permanent loss of potency; discontinue therapy if signs of penile fibrosis develop (penile angulation, cavernosal fibrosis, or Peyronie's disease). When used in erectile dysfunction (Muse®), syncope occurring within 1 hour of administration has been reported. The potential for drug-drug interactions may occur when Muse® is prescribed concomitantly with antihypertensives.

Adverse Reactions (Reflective of adult population; not specific for elderly)

Intraurethral:

>10%: Genitourinary: Penile pain, urethral burning

2% to 10%:

Central nervous system: Headache, dizziness, pain

Genitourinary: Vaginal itching (female partner), testicular pain, urethral bleeding (minor)

Intracavernosal injection:

>10%: Genitourinary: Penile pain

1% to 10%:

Cardiovascular: Hypertension

Central nervous system: Headache, dizziness

Genitourinary: Prolonged erection (>4 hours, 4%), penile fibrosis, penis disorder, penile rash, penile edema

Local: Injection site hematoma and/or bruising

Drug Interactions

Metabolism/Transport Effects None known.

Avoid Concomitant Use

Avoid concomitant use of Alprostadil with any of the following: Phosphodiesterase 5 Inhibitors

Increased Effect/Toxicity

The levels/effects of Alprostadil may be increased by: Phosphodiesterase 5 Inhibitors

Decreased Effect There are no known significant interactions involving a decrease in effect.

Ethanol/Nutrition/Herb Interactions Ethanol: Avoid concurrent use (vasodilating effect).

Stability

Caverject® Impulse™: Store at controlled room temperature of 15°C to 30°C (59°F to 86°F). Provided as a dual-chamber syringe with diluent in one chamber. To mix, hold syringe with needle pointing upward and turn plunger clockwise; turn upside down several times to mix. Device can be set to deliver specified dose, each device can be set at various increments. Following reconstitution, use within 24 hours and discard any unused solution.

Caverject® powder: The 5 mcg, 10 mcg, and 20 mcg vials should be stored at or below 25°C (77°F). The 40 mcg vial should be stored at 2°C to 8°C until dispensed. After dispensing, stable for up to 3 months at or below 25°C. Use only the supplied diluent for reconstitution (ie, bacteriostatic/sterile water with benzyl alcohol 0.945%). Following reconstitution, all strengths should be stored at or below 25°C (77°F); do not refrigerate or freeze; use within 24 hours.

Caverject® solution: Prior to dispensing, store frozen at -20°C to -10°C (-4°F to -14°F); once dispensed, may be stored frozen for up to 3 months, or under refrigeration at 2°C to 8°C (36°F to 46°F) for up to 7 days. Do not refreeze. Once removed from foil wrap, solution may be allowed to warm to room temperature prior to use. If not used immediately, solution should be discarded. Shake well prior to use.

Edex®: Store at controlled room temperature of 15°C to 30°C (59°F to 86°F); following reconstitution with NS, use immediately and discard any unused solution.

Muse®: Refrigerate at 2°C to 8°C (36°F to 46°F); may be stored at room temperature for up to 14 days.

Mechanism of Action Causes vasodilation by means of direct effect on vascular and ductus arteriosus smooth muscle; relaxes trabecular smooth muscle by dilation of cavernosal arteries when injected along the penile shaft, allowing blood flow to and entrapment in the lacunar spaces of the penis (ie, corporeal veno-occlusive mechanism)

Pharmacodynamics/Kinetics
Onset of action: Rapid
Duration: <1 hour
Distribution: Insignificant following penile injection
Protein binding, plasma: 81% to albumin
Metabolism: ~75% by oxidation in one pass via lungs
Half-life elimination: 5-10 minutes
Excretion: Urine (90% as metabolites) within 24 hours

Dosage
Geriatric Elderly patients may have a greater frequency of renal dysfunction; lowest effective dose should be used. In clinical studies with Edex®, higher minimally effective doses and a higher rate of lack of effect were noted.

Adult
Erectile dysfunction:
Intracavernous (Caverject®, Edex®): Individualize dose by careful titration; doses >40 mcg (Edex®) or >60 mcg (Caverject®) are not recommended: Initial dose must be titrated in physician's office. Patient must stay in the physician's office until complete detumescence occurs; if there is no response, then the next higher dose may be given within 1 hour; if there is still no response, a 1-day interval before giving the next dose is recommended; increasing the dose or concentration in the treatment of impotence results in increasing pain and discomfort.

Vasculogenic, psychogenic, or mixed etiology: Initiate dosage titration at 2.5 mcg, increasing by 2.5 mcg to a dose of 5 mcg and then in increments of 5-10 mcg depending on the erectile response until the dose produces an erection suitable for intercourse, not lasting >1 hour; if there is absolutely no response to initial 2.5 mcg dose, the second dose may be increased to 7.5 mcg, followed by increments of 5-10 mcg

Neurogenic etiology (eg, spinal cord injury): Initiate dosage titration at 1.25 mcg, increasing to a dose of 2.5 mcg and then 5 mcg; increase further in increments 5 mcg until the dose is reached that produces an erection suitable for intercourse, not lasting >1 hour

Maintenance: Once appropriate dose has been determined, patient may self-administer injections at a frequency of no more than 3 times/week with at least 24 hours between doses

Intraurethral (Muse® Pellet):
Initial: 125-250 mcg

Maintenance: Administer as needed to achieve an erection; duration of action is about 30-60 minutes; use only two systems per 24-hour period

Administration Erectile dysfunction: Use a ¹/₂", 27- to 30-gauge needle; inject into the dorsolateral aspect of the proximal third of the penis, avoiding visible veins; alternate side of the penis for injections

Monitoring Parameters Arterial pressure, respiratory rate, heart rate, temperature, degree of penile pain, length of erection, signs of infection

Special Geriatric Considerations Elderly may have concomitant diseases which would contraindicate the use of alprostadil. Other forms of attaining penile tumescence are recommended.

Dosage Forms Excipient information presented when available (limited, particularly for generics); consult specific product labeling. [DSC] = Discontinued product

Injection, powder for reconstitution:
Caverject®: 20 mcg, 40 mcg [contains lactose; diluent contains benzyl alcohol]
Caverject Impulse®: 10 mcg, 20 mcg [prefilled injection system; contains lactose; diluent contains benzyl alcohol]
Edex®: 10 mcg, 20 mcg, 40 mcg [contains lactose; packaged in kits containing diluent, syringe, and alcohol swab]
Pellet, urethral:
Muse®: 125 mcg (6s) [DSC], 250 mcg (6s), 500 mcg (6s), 1000 mcg (6s)

Alteplase (AL te plase)

Medication Safety Issues

Sound-alike/look-alike issues:

Activase® may be confused with Cathflo® Activase®, TNKase®

Alteplase may be confused with Altace®

"tPA" abbreviation should not be used when writing orders for this medication; has been misread as TNKase (tenecteplase)

High alert medication:

The Institute for Safe Medication Practices (ISMP) includes this medication (I.V.) among its list of drugs which have a heightened risk of causing significant patient harm when used in error.

Brand Names: U.S. Activase®; Cathflo® Activase®

Brand Names: Canada Activase® rt-PA; Cathflo® Activase®

Index Terms Alteplase, Recombinant; Alteplase, Tissue Plasminogen Activator, Recombinant; tPA

Generic Availability (U.S.) No

Pharmacologic Category Thrombolytic Agent

Use Management of ST-elevation myocardial infarction (STEMI) for the lysis of thrombi in coronary arteries; management of acute ischemic stroke (AIS); management of acute pulmonary embolism (PE)

Recommended criteria for treatment:

STEMI: Chest pain ≥20 minutes duration, onset of chest pain within 12 hours of treatment (or within prior 12-24 hours in patients with continuing ischemic symptoms), and ST-segment elevation >0.1 mV in at least two contiguous precordial leads or two adjacent limb leads on ECG or new or presumably new left bundle branch block (LBBB)

AIS: Onset of stroke symptoms within 3 hours of treatment

Acute pulmonary embolism: Age ≤75 years: Documented massive PE (defined as acute PE with sustained hypotension [SBP <90 mm Hg for ≤15 minutes or requiring inotropic support], persistent profound bradycardia [HR <40 bpm with signs or symptoms of shock], or pulselessness); alteplase may be considered for submassive PE with clinical evidence of adverse prognosis (eg, new hemodynamic instability, worsening respiratory insufficiency, severe RV dysfunction, or major myocardial necrosis) and low risk of bleeding complications. **Note:** Not recommended for patients with low-risk PE (eg, normotensive, no RV dysfunction, normal biomarkers) or submassive acute PE with minor RV dysfunction, minor myocardial necrosis, and no clinical worsening (Jaff, 2011).

Cathflo® Activase®: Restoration of central venous catheter function

Unlabeled Use Acute ischemic stroke presenting 3-4.5 hours after symptom onset; acute peripheral arterial occlusion; infected parapneumonic effusion (with [adult] or without [pediatric] dornase alfa); prosthetic valve thrombosis

Contraindications Hypersensitivity to alteplase or any component of the formulation

Treatment of STEMI or PE: Active internal bleeding; history of CVA; ischemic stroke within 3 months (Antman, 2004; Jaff, 2011); recent intracranial or intraspinal surgery or trauma; intracranial neoplasm; prior intracranial hemorrhage (Antman, 2004; Jaff, 2011); arteriovenous malformation or aneurysm; known bleeding diathesis; severe uncontrolled hypertension (listed as a relative contraindication in STEMI [Antman, 2004] and PE [Jaff, 2011] guidelines); suspected aortic dissection (Antman, 2004; Jaff, 2011); significant closed head or facial trauma (Antman, 2004; Jaff, 2011) within 3 months with radiographic evidence of bony fracture or brain injury (Jaff, 2011)

Treatment of acute ischemic stroke: Evidence of intracranial hemorrhage or suspicion of subarachnoid hemorrhage on pretreatment evaluation; intracranial or intraspinal surgery within 3 months; stroke or serious head injury within 3 months; history of intracranial hemorrhage; uncontrolled hypertension at time of treatment (eg, >185 mm Hg systolic or >110 mm Hg diastolic); seizure at the onset of stroke; active internal bleeding; intracranial neoplasm; arteriovenous malformation or aneurysm; multilobar cerebral infarction (hypodensity >1/3 cerebral hemisphere; Adams, 2007); clinical presentation suggesting post-MI pericarditis; known bleeding diathesis including but not limited to current use of oral anticoagulants producing an INR >1.7, an INR >1.7, administration of heparin within 48 hours preceding the onset of stroke with an elevated aPTT at presentation, platelet count <100,000/mm³.

Additional exclusion criteria within clinical trials:

Presentation <3 hours after initial symptoms (NINDS, 1995): Time of symptom onset unknown, rapidly improving or minor symptoms, major surgery within 2 weeks, GI or urinary tract hemorrhage within 3 weeks, aggressive treatment required to lower blood pressure, glucose level <50 or >400 mg/dL, and arterial puncture at a noncompressible site or lumbar puncture within 1 week.

Presentation 3-4.5 hours after initial symptoms (del Zoppo, 2009; ECASS-III; Hacke, 2008): Age >80 years, time of symptom onset unknown, rapidly improving or minor symptoms, current use of oral anticoagulants regardless of INR, glucose level <50 or >400 mg/dL, aggressive intravenous treatment required to lower blood pressure, major surgery or severe trauma within 3 months, baseline National Institutes of Health Stroke Scale (NIHSS) score >25, and history of both stroke and diabetes.

Warnings/Precautions The total dose should not exceed 90 mg for acute ischemic stroke or 100 mg for acute myocardial infarction or pulmonary embolism. Doses ≥150 mg associated with significantly increased risk of intracranial hemorrhage compared to doses ≤100 mg. Concurrent heparin anticoagulation may contribute to bleeding. In the treatment of acute ischemic stroke, concurrent use of anticoagulants was not permitted during the initial 24 hours of the <3 hour window trial (NINDS, 1995). Initiation of SubQ heparin (≤10,000 units) or equivalent doses of low molecular weight heparin for prevention of DVT during the first 24 hours of the 3-4.5 hour window trial was permitted and did not increase the incidence of intracerebral hemorrhage (Hacke, 2008). For acute PE, withhold heparin during the 2-hour infusion period. Monitor all potential bleeding sites. Intramuscular injections and nonessential handling of the patient should be avoided. Venipunctures should be performed carefully and only when necessary. If arterial puncture is necessary, use an upper extremity vessel that can be manually compressed. If serious bleeding occurs, the infusion of alteplase and heparin should be stopped. Avoid aspirin for 24 hours following administration of alteplase; administration within 24 hours increases the risk of hemorrhagic transformation.

For the following conditions, the risk of bleeding is higher with use of thrombolytics and should be weighed against the benefits of therapy: Recent major surgery (eg, CABG, organ biopsy, previous puncture of noncompressible vessels), prolonged CPR with evidence of thoracic trauma, lumbar puncture within 1 week, cerebrovascular disease, recent gastrointestinal or genitourinary bleeding, recent trauma, hypertension (systolic BP >175 mm Hg and/or diastolic BP >110 mm Hg), high likelihood of left heart thrombus (eg, mitral stenosis with atrial fibrillation), acute pericarditis, subacute bacterial endocarditis, hemostatic defects including ones caused by severe renal or hepatic dysfunction, significant hepatic dysfunction, diabetic hemorrhagic retinopathy or other hemorrhagic ophthalmic conditions, septic thrombophlebitis or occluded AV cannula at seriously infected site, advanced age (eg, >75 years), any other condition in which bleeding constitutes a significant hazard or would be particularly difficult to manage because of location. When treating acute MI or pulmonary embolism, use with caution in patients receiving oral anticoagulants. In the treatment of acute ischemic stroke within 3 hours of stroke symptom onset, the current use of oral anticoagulants producing an INR >1.7 is contraindicated.

Coronary thrombolysis may result in reperfusion arrhythmias. Patients who present **within 3 hours** of stroke symptom onset should be treated with alteplase unless contraindications exist. A longer time window (**3-4.5 hours** after symptom onset) has now been formally evaluated and shown to be safe and efficacious for select individuals (del Zoppo, 2009; Hacke, 2008). Treatment of patients with minor neurological deficit or with rapidly improving symptoms is not recommended. Follow standard management for STEMI while infusing alteplase.

Cathflo® Activase®: When used to restore catheter function, use Cathflo® cautiously in those patients with known or suspected catheter infections. Evaluate catheter for other causes of dysfunction before use. Avoid excessive pressure when instilling into catheter.

Adverse Reactions (Reflective of adult population; not specific for elderly) As with all drugs which may affect hemostasis, bleeding is the major adverse effect associated with alteplase. Hemorrhage may occur at virtually any site. Risk is dependent on multiple variables, including the dosage administered, concurrent use of multiple agents which alter hemostasis, and patient predisposition. Rapid lysis of coronary artery thrombi by thrombolytic agents may be associated with reperfusion-related atrial and/or ventricular arrhythmia. **Note:** Lowest rate of bleeding complications expected with dose used to restore catheter function.

1% to 10%:
Cardiovascular: Hypotension
Central nervous system: Fever
Dermatologic: Bruising (1%)
Gastrointestinal: GI hemorrhage (5%), nausea, vomiting
Genitourinary: GU hemorrhage (4%)
Hematologic: Bleeding (0.5% major, 7% minor: GUSTO trial)
Local: Bleeding at catheter puncture site (15.3%, accelerated administration)
Additional cardiovascular events associated **with use in STEMI:** AV block, cardiogenic shock, heart failure, cardiac arrest, recurrent ischemia/infarction, myocardial rupture,

electromechanical dissociation, pericardial effusion, pericarditis, mitral regurgitation, cardiac tamponade, thromboembolism, pulmonary edema, asystole, ventricular tachycardia, bradycardia, ruptured intracranial AV malformation, seizure, hemorrhagic bursitis, cholesterol crystal embolization

Additional events associated **with use in pulmonary embolism:** Pulmonary re-embolization, pulmonary edema, pleural effusion, thromboembolism

Additional events associated **with use in stroke:** Cerebral edema, cerebral herniation, seizure, new ischemic stroke

Drug Interactions

Metabolism/Transport Effects None known.

Avoid Concomitant Use There are no known interactions where it is recommended to avoid concomitant use.

Increased Effect/Toxicity

Alteplase may increase the levels/effects of: Anticoagulants; Dabigatran Etexilate; Drotrecogin Alfa (Activated)

The levels/effects of Alteplase may be increased by: Antiplatelet Agents; Herbs (Anticoagulant/Antiplatelet Properties); Nonsteroidal Anti-Inflammatory Agents; Salicylates

Decreased Effect

The levels/effects of Alteplase may be decreased by: Aprotinin; Nitroglycerin

Ethanol/Nutrition/Herb Interactions Herb/Nutraceutical: Avoid cat's claw, dong quai, evening primrose, feverfew, red clover, horse chestnut, garlic, green tea, ginseng, ginkgo (all have additional antiplatelet activity).

Stability

Activase®: The lyophilized product may be stored at room temperature (not to exceed 30°C/ 86°F), or under refrigeration. Once reconstituted, it should be used within 8 hours. Reconstitution:

50 mg vial: Use accompanying diluent; mix by gentle swirling or slow inversion; do not shake. Vacuum is present in 50 mg vial. Final concentration: 1 mg/mL.

100 mg vial: Use transfer set with accompanying diluent (100 mL vial of sterile water for injection). No vacuum is present in 100 mg vial. Final concentration: 1 mg/mL.

Cathflo® Activase®: Store lyophilized product under refrigeration.

To reconstitute, add 2.2 mL SWFI to vial; do not shake. Final concentration: 1 mg/mL. Once reconstituted, store at 2°C to 30°C (36°F to 86°F) and use within 8 hours. Do not mix other medications into infusion solution.

Mechanism of Action Initiates local fibrinolysis by binding to fibrin in a thrombus (clot) and converts entrapped plasminogen to plasmin

Pharmacodynamics/Kinetics

Duration: >50% present in plasma cleared ~5 minutes after infusion terminated, ~80% cleared within 10 minutes

Excretion: Clearance: Rapidly from circulating plasma (550-650 mL/minute), primarily hepatic; >50% present in plasma is cleared within 5 minutes after the infusion is terminated, ~80% cleared within 10 minutes

Dosage

Geriatric & Adult

ST-elevation myocardial infarction (STEMI): I.V. (Activase®): **Note:** Manufacturer's labeling recommends 3-hour infusion regimen; however, accelerated regimen preferred by the ACC/AHA (Antman, 2004).

Accelerated regimen (weight-based):

Patients >67 kg: Total dose: 100 mg over 1.5 hours; administered as a 15 mg I.V. bolus over 1-2 minutes followed by infusions of 50 mg over 30 minutes, then 35 mg over 1 hour. Maximum total dose: 100 mg

Patients ≤67 kg: Infuse 15 mg I.V. bolus over 1-2 minutes followed by infusions of 0.75 mg/kg (not to exceed 50 mg) over 30 minutes then 0.5 mg/kg (not to exceed 35 mg) over 1 hour. Maximum total dose: 100 mg

Note: All patients should receive 162-325 mg of chewable nonenteric coated aspirin as soon as possible and then daily. Administer concurrently with heparin 60 units/kg bolus (maximum: 4000 units) followed by continuous infusion of 12 units/kg/hour (maximum: 1000 units/hour) and adjust to aPTT target of 50-70 seconds (or 1.5-2 times the upper limit of control).

Acute massive or submassive pulmonary embolism (PE): I.V. (Activase®): 100 mg over 2 hours; may be administered as a 10 mg bolus followed by 90 mg over 2 hours as was done in patients with submassive PE (Konstantinides, 2002). **Note:** Not recommended for submassive PE with minor RV dysfunction, minor myocardial necrosis, and no clinical worsening or low-risk PE (ie, normotensive, no RV dysfunction, normal biomarkers) (Jaff, 2011).

ALTEPLASE

Acute ischemic stroke: I.V. (Activase®): Within 3 hours of the onset of symptom onset (labeled use) **or** within 3-4.5 hours of symptom onset (unlabeled use; del Zoppo, 2009; Hacke, 2008): **Note:** Initiation of anticoagulants (eg, heparin) or antiplatelet agents (eg, aspirin) within 24 hours after starting alteplase is not recommended; however, initiation of aspirin between 24-48 hours after stroke onset is recommended (Adams, 2007). Initiation of SubQ heparin (≤10,000 units) or equivalent doses of low molecular weight heparin for prevention of DVT during the first 24 hours of the 3-4.5 hour window trial did not increase incidence of intracerebral hemorrhage (Hacke, 2008).

Recommended total dose: 0.9 mg/kg (maximum total dose: 90 mg)

Patients ≤100 kg: Load with 0.09 mg/kg (10% of 0.9 mg/kg dose) as an I.V. bolus over 1 minute, followed by 0.81 mg/kg (90% of 0.9 mg/kg dose) as a continuous infusion over 60 minutes.

Patients >100 kg: Load with 9 mg (10% of 90 mg) as an I.V. bolus over 1 minute, followed by 81 mg (90% of 90 mg) as a continuous infusion over 60 minutes.

Central venous catheter clearance: Intracatheter (Cathflo® Activase® 1 mg/mL):

Patients <30 kg: 110% of the internal lumen volume of the catheter, not to exceed 2 mg/2 mL; retain in catheter for 0.5-2 hours; may instill a second dose if catheter remains occluded

Patients ≥30 kg: 2 mg (2 mL); retain in catheter for 0.5-2 hours; may instill a second dose if catheter remains occluded

Acute peripheral arterial occlusion (unlabeled use): Intra-arterial:

Weight-based regimen: 0.001-0.02 mg/kg/hour (maximum dose: 2 mg/hour) (Semba, 2000)

or

Fixed-dose regimen: 0.12-2 mg/hour (Semba, 2000)

Note: The ACC/AHA guidelines state that thrombolysis is an effective and beneficial therapy for those with acute limb ischemia (Rutherford categories I and IIa) of <14 days duration (Hirsch, 2006). The optimal dosage and concentration has not been established; a number of intra-arterial delivery techniques are employed with continuous infusion being the most common (Ouriel, 2004). The Advisory Panel to the Society for Cardiovascular and Interventional Radiology on Thrombolytic Therapy recommends dosing of ≤2 mg/hour and concomitant administration of subtherapeutic heparin (aPTT 1.25-1.5 times baseline) (Semba, 2000). Duration of alteplase infusion dependent upon size and location of the thrombus; typically between 6-48 hours (Disini, 2008).

Complicated parapneumonic effusion (unlabeled use): Intrapleural: 10 mg in 30 mL NS administered twice daily with a 1 hour dwell time for a total of 3 days; each dose followed in >2 hours by intrapleural dornase alfa (Rahman, 2011). Some clinicians suggest consideration of fibrinolytic use when patients have failed at least 24 hours of chest tube drainage and are poor surgical candidates (Hamblin, 2010).

Prosthetic valve thrombosis, right-sided (any size thrombus) or left-sided (thrombus area <0.8 cm², or left-sided (thrombus area ≥0.8 cm²) when contraindications to surgery exist (unlabeled use) (Alpert, 2003; Guyatt, 2012; Roudaut, 2003): I.V.:

High-dose regimen: Load with 10 mg, followed by 90 mg over 90-180 minutes (without heparin during infusion)

Low-dose regimen (preferred for very small adults): Load with 20 mg, followed by 10 mg/hour for 3 hours (without heparin during infusion)

Note: After successful administration of alteplase, heparin infusion should be introduced until warfarin achieves therapeutic INR (aortic: 3.0-4.0; mitral: 3.5-4.5) (Bonow, 2008). The 2012 ACCP guidelines for antithrombotic therapy make no recommendation regarding INR range after prosthetic valve thrombosis.

Administration

Activase®: ST-elevation MI: Accelerated infusion: Bolus dose may be prepared by one of three methods:

1) Removal of 15 mL reconstituted (1 mg/mL) solution from vial

2) Removal of 15 mL from a port on the infusion line after priming

3) Programming an infusion pump to deliver a 15 mL bolus at the initiation of infusion

Activase®: Acute ischemic stroke: Bolus dose (10% of total dose) may be prepared by one of three methods:

1) Removal of the appropriate volume from reconstituted solution (1 mg/mL)

2) Removal of the appropriate volume from a port on the infusion line after priming

3) Programming an infusion pump to deliver the appropriate volume at the initiation of infusion

Note: Remaining dose for STEMI, AIS, or total dose for acute pulmonary embolism may be administered as follows: Any quantity of drug not to be administered to the patient must be removed from vial(s) prior to administration of remaining dose.

50 mg vial: Either PVC bag or glass vial and infusion set

100 mg vial: Insert spike end of the infusion set through the same puncture site created by transfer device and infuse from vial

If further dilution is desired, may be diluted in equal volume of 0.9% sodium chloride or D$_5$W to yield a final concentration of 0.5 mg/mL.

Cathflo® Activase®: Intracatheter: Instill dose into occluded catheter. Do not force solution into catheter. After a 30-minute dwell time, assess catheter function by attempting to aspirate blood. If catheter is functional, aspirate 4-5 mL of blood in patients ≥10 kg or 3 mL in patients <10 kg to remove Cathflo® Activase® and residual clots. Gently irrigate the catheter with NS. If catheter remains nonfunctional, let Cathflo® Activase® dwell for another 90 minutes (total dwell time: 120 minutes) and reassess function. If catheter function is not restored, a second dose may be instilled.

Monitoring Parameters

Acute ischemic stroke (AIS): Baseline: Neurologic examination, head CT (without contrast), blood pressure, CBC, aPTT, PT/INR, glucose. During and after initiation: In addition to monitoring for bleeding complications, the 2007 AHA/ASA guidelines for the early management of AIS recommends the following:

Perform neurological assessments every 15 minutes during infusion and every 30 minutes thereafter for the next 6 hours, then hourly until 24 hours after treatment.

If severe headache, acute hypertension, nausea, or vomiting occurs, discontinue the infusion and obtain emergency CT scan.

Measure BP every 15 minutes for the first 2 hours then every 30 minutes for the next 6 hours, then hourly until 24 hours after initiation of alteplase. Increase frequency if a systolic BP is ≥180 mm Hg or if a diastolic BP is ≥105 mm Hg; administer antihypertensive medications to maintain BP at or below these levels.

Obtain a follow-up CT scan at 24 hours before starting anticoagulants or antiplatelet agents.

Central venous catheter clearance: Assess catheter function by attempting to aspirate blood.

ST-elevation MI: Baseline: Blood pressure, serum cardiac biomarkers, CBC, PT/INR, aPTT. During and after initiation: Assess for evidence of cardiac reperfusion through resolution of chest pain, resolution of baseline ECG changes, preserved left ventricular function, cardiac enzyme washout phenomenon, and/or the appearance of reperfusion arrhythmias; assess for bleeding potential through clinical evidence of GI bleeding, hematuria, gingival bleeding, fibrinogen levels, fibrinogen degradation products, PT and aPTT.

Reference Range Not routinely measured; literature supports therapeutic levels of 0.52-1.8 mcg/mL

Fibrinogen: 200-400 mg/dL

Activated partial thromboplastin time (aPTT): 22.5-38.7 seconds

Prothrombin time (PT): 10.9-12.2 seconds

Test Interactions Altered results of coagulation and fibrinolytic activity tests

Special Geriatric Considerations No specific changes in use in elderly patients are necessary.

Dosage Forms Excipient information presented when available (limited, particularly for generics); consult specific product labeling.

Injection, powder for reconstitution [recombinant]:

Activase®: 50 mg, 100 mg [contains polysorbate 80; derived from or manufactured using Chinese hamster ovary cells; supplied with diluent]

Cathflo® Activase®: 2 mg [contains polysorbate 80; derived from or manufactured using Chinese hamster ovary cells]

♦ Alteplase, Recombinant see Alteplase on page 73
♦ Alteplase, Tissue Plasminogen Activator, Recombinant see Alteplase on page 73
♦ ALternaGel® [OTC] see Aluminum Hydroxide on page 77
♦ Altoprev® see Lovastatin on page 1164

Aluminum Hydroxide (a LOO mi num hye DROKS ide)

Brand Names: U.S. ALternaGel® [OTC]; Dermagran® [OTC]

Brand Names: Canada Amphojel®; Basaljel®

Generic Availability (U.S.) Yes: Suspension

Pharmacologic Category Antacid; Antidote; Protectant, Topical

Use Treatment of hyperacidity; hyperphosphatemia; temporary protection of minor cuts, scrapes, and burns

Contraindications Hypersensitivity to aluminum salts or any component of the formulation

Warnings/Precautions Oral: Hypophosphatemia may occur with prolonged administration or large doses; aluminum intoxication and osteomalacia may occur in patients with uremia. Use with caution in patients with HF, renal failure, edema, cirrhosis, and low sodium diets, and patients who have recently suffered gastrointestinal hemorrhage; uremic patients not receiving dialysis may develop osteomalacia and osteoporosis due to phosphate depletion.

Elderly may be predisposed to constipation and fecal impaction. Careful evaluation of possible drug interactions must be done. When used as an antacid in ulcer treatment, consider buffer capacity (mEq/mL) to calculate dose.

Topical: Not for application over deep wounds, puncture wounds, infected areas, or lacerations. When used for self medication (OTC use), consult with healthcare provider if needed for >7 days.

Adverse Reactions (Reflective of adult population; not specific for elderly) Frequency not defined.

Gastrointestinal: Constipation, discoloration of feces (white speckles), fecal impaction, nausea, stomach cramps, vomiting

Endocrine & metabolic: Hypomagnesemia, hypophosphatemia

Drug Interactions

Metabolism/Transport Effects None known.

Avoid Concomitant Use

Avoid concomitant use of Aluminum Hydroxide with any of the following: Deferasirox; QuiNINE; Vitamin D Analogs

Increased Effect/Toxicity

Aluminum Hydroxide may increase the levels/effects of: Amphetamines; Calcium Polystyrene Sulfonate; Dexmethylphenidate; Methylphenidate; Sodium Polystyrene Sulfonate

The levels/effects of Aluminum Hydroxide may be increased by: Ascorbic Acid; Calcium Polystyrene Sulfonate; Citric Acid Derivatives; Sodium Polystyrene Sulfonate; Vitamin D Analogs

Decreased Effect

Aluminum Hydroxide may decrease the levels/effects of: ACE Inhibitors; Allopurinol; Anticonvulsants (Hydantoin); Antipsychotic Agents (Phenothiazines); Atazanavir; Bisacodyl; Bisphosphonate Derivatives; Cefditoren; Cefpodoxime; Cefuroxime; Chenodiol; Chloroquine; Corticosteroids (Oral); Dabigatran Etexilate; Dasatinib; Deferasirox; Deferiprone; Delavirdine; Eltrombopag; Erlotinib; Ethambutol; Fexofenadine; Gabapentin; HMG-CoA Reductase Inhibitors; Iron Salts; Isoniazid; Itraconazole; Ketoconazole; Ketoconazole (Systemic); Levothyroxine; Mesalamine; Methenamine; Mycophenolate; Nilotinib; PenicillAMINE; Phosphate Supplements; Protease Inhibitors; QuiNINE; Quinolone Antibiotics; Rilpivirine; Tetracycline Derivatives; Trientine; Ursodiol; Vismodegib

Ethanol/Nutrition/Herb Interactions Food: Aluminum hydroxide may cause constipation with inadequate hydration. Management: Maintain proper hydration unless instructed otherwise by physician. Take preferably 1-3 hours after meals (when used as an antacid). When used to decrease phosphorus, take within 20 minutes of a meal.

Mechanism of Action Neutralizes hydrochloride in stomach to form Al $(Cl)_3$ salt + H_2O

Dosage

Geriatric & Adult

Hyperphosphatemia: Oral: Initial: 300-600 mg 3 times/day with meals

Hyperacidity: Oral: 600-1200 mg between meals and at bedtime

Skin protectant: Topical: Apply to affected area as needed; reapply at least every 12 hours

Renal Impairment Aluminum may accumulate in renal impairment.

Administration

Oral: Dose should be followed with water.

Topical: Apply as needed to affected area; reapply at least every 12 hours

Monitoring Parameters Monitor phosphorus levels periodically when patient is on chronic therapy.

Test Interactions Decreased phosphorus, inorganic (S)

Pharmacotherapy Pearls When used primarily as a phosphate binder, dose should be followed with water; when used for peptic ulcer treatment, deliver 144 mEq neutralizing capacity 1 and 3 hours after meals as needed to control symptoms; often alternated with aluminum and magnesium combinations to decrease diarrhea

Special Geriatric Considerations Elderly, due to disease and/or drug therapy, may be predisposed to constipation and fecal impaction. Careful evaluation of possible drug interactions must be done. When used as an antacid in ulcer treatment, consider buffer capacity (mEq/mL) to calculate dose. Consider renal insufficiency (<30 mL/minute) as predisposition to aluminum toxicity.

Dosage Forms Excipient information presented when available (limited, particularly for generics); consult specific product labeling. [DSC] = Discontinued product

Ointment, topical:

Dermagran®: 0.275% (113 g)

Suspension, oral: 320 mg/5 mL (30 mL, 355 mL [DSC], 360 mL, 473 mL, 480 mL); 600 mg/5 mL (355 mL [DSC])

ALternaGel®: 600 mg/5 mL (360 mL) [sugar free]

Aluminum Hydroxide and Magnesium Carbonate
(a LOO mi num hye DROKS ide & mag NEE zhum KAR bun nate)

Related Information
Aluminum Hydroxide *on page 77*

Medication Safety Issues
International issues:
Remegel [Netherlands] may be confused with Renagel brand name for sevelamer [U.S., Canada, and multiple international markets]
Remegel: Brand name for aluminum hydroxide and magnesium carbonate [Netherlands], but also the brand name for calcium carbonate [Great Britain, Hungary, and Ireland]

Brand Names: U.S. Acid Gone Extra Strength [OTC]; Acid Gone [OTC]; Gaviscon® Extra Strength [OTC]; Gaviscon® Liquid [OTC]

Index Terms Magnesium Carbonate and Aluminum Hydroxide

Generic Availability (U.S.) Yes

Pharmacologic Category Antacid

Use Temporary relief of symptoms associated with gastric acidity

Adverse Reactions (Reflective of adult population; not specific for elderly) 1% to 10%:
Endocrine & metabolic: Hypermagnesemia, aluminum intoxication (prolonged use and concomitant renal failure), hypophosphatemia
Gastrointestinal: Constipation, diarrhea
Neuromuscular & skeletal: Osteomalacia

Drug Interactions
Metabolism/Transport Effects None known.

Avoid Concomitant Use
Avoid concomitant use of Aluminum Hydroxide and Magnesium Carbonate with any of the following: Deferasirox; QuiNINE; Vitamin D Analogs

Increased Effect/Toxicity
Aluminum Hydroxide and Magnesium Carbonate may increase the levels/effects of: Alpha-/Beta-Agonists; Amphetamines; Calcium Polystyrene Sulfonate; Dexmethylphenidate; Methylphenidate; Misoprostol; QuiNIDine; Sodium Polystyrene Sulfonate

The levels/effects of Aluminum Hydroxide and Magnesium Carbonate may be increased by: Ascorbic Acid; Calcium Polystyrene Sulfonate; Citric Acid Derivatives; Sodium Polystyrene Sulfonate; Vitamin D Analogs

Decreased Effect
Aluminum Hydroxide and Magnesium Carbonate may decrease the levels/effects of: ACE Inhibitors; Allopurinol; Anticonvulsants (Hydantoin); Antipsychotic Agents (Phenothiazines); Atazanavir; Bisacodyl; Bisphosphonate Derivatives; Cefditoren; Cefpodoxime; Cefuroxime; Chenodiol; Chloroquine; Corticosteroids (Oral); Dabigatran Etexilate; Dasatinib; Deferasirox; Deferiprone; Delavirdine; Eltrombopag; Erlotinib; Ethambutol; Fexofenadine; Gabapentin; HMG-CoA Reductase Inhibitors; Iron Salts; Isoniazid; Itraconazole; Ketoconazole; Ketoconazole (Systemic); Levothyroxine; Mesalamine; Methenamine; Mycophenolate; Nilotinib; PenicillAMINE; Phosphate Supplements; Protease Inhibitors; QuiNINE; Quinolone Antibiotics; Rilpivirine; Tetracycline Derivatives; Trientine; Ursodiol; Vismodegib

Dosage
Geriatric & Adult Dyspepsia, gastric acidity: Oral:
Liquid:
Gaviscon® Regular Strength: 15-30 mL 4 times/day after meals and at bedtime
Gaviscon® Extra Strength: 15-30 mL 4 times/day after meals
Tablet (Gaviscon® Extra Strength): Chew 2-4 tablets 4 times/day

Renal Impairment Aluminum and/or magnesium may accumulate in renal impairment.

Administration Administer 1-3 hours after meals with water, milk or juice.

Special Geriatric Considerations Elderly, due to disease or drug therapy, may be predisposed to diarrhea or constipation. Diarrhea may result in electrolyte imbalance. Decreased renal function (Cl_{cr} <30 mL/minute) may result in toxicity of aluminum or magnesium. Drug interactions must be considered. If possible, administer antacid 1-2 hours apart from other drugs. When treating ulcers, consider buffer capacity (mEq/mL) to calculate dose of antacid.

Dosage Forms Excipient information presented when available (limited, particularly for generics); consult specific product labeling.
Liquid:
Acid Gone: Aluminum hydroxide 31.7 mg and magnesium carbonate 119.3 mg per 5 mL (360 mL)

ALUMINUM HYDROXIDE AND MAGNESIUM CARBONATE

Gaviscon®: Aluminum hydroxide 31.7 mg and magnesium carbonate 119.3 mg per 5 mL (355 mL) [contains sodium 0.57 mEq/5 mL and benzyl alcohol; cool mint flavor]
Gaviscon® Extra Strength: Aluminum hydroxide 84.6 mg and magnesium carbonate 79.1 mg per 5 mL (355 mL) [contains sodium 0.9 mEq/5 mL and benzyl alcohol; cool mint flavor]

Tablet, chewable:
Acid Gone Extra Strength: Aluminum hydroxide 160 mg and magnesium carbonate 105 mg
Gaviscon® Extra Strength: Aluminum hydroxide 160 mg and magnesium carbonate 105 mg [contains sodium 19 mg/tablet (1.3 mEq/tablet); cherry and original flavors]

Aluminum Hydroxide and Magnesium Hydroxide
(a LOO mi num hye DROKS ide & mag NEE zhum hye DROK side)

Related Information
Aluminum Hydroxide *on page 77*
Magnesium Hydroxide *on page 1177*
Brand Names: U.S. Alamag [OTC]; Mag-Al Ultimate [OTC]; Mag-Al [OTC]
Brand Names: Canada Diovol®; Diovol® Ex; Gelusil® Extra Strength; Mylanta™
Index Terms Magnesium Hydroxide and Aluminum Hydroxide
Generic Availability (U.S.) No
Pharmacologic Category Antacid
Use Antacid for symptoms related to hyperacidity associated with heartburn, hiatal hernia, upset stomach, peptic ulcer, peptic esophagitis, or gastritis
Warnings/Precautions Prolonged antacid therapy may result in hypophosphatemia; aluminum in antacid may form insoluble complexes with phosphate leading to decreased phosphate absorption in the GI tract. Rarely, severe hypophosphatemia can lead to anorexia, muscle weakness, malaise, and osteomalacia. Use with caution in patients with renal impairment; avoid use in severe renal impairment; hypermagnesemia or aluminum intoxication may occur in severe renal impairment, particularly with prolonged use. Aluminum intoxication may lead to osteomalacia or dialysis encephalopathy. Use with caution in the elderly; the population group may be predisposed to diarrhea or constipation. Some products may contain phenylalanine.

Self-medication (OTC use): Patients with renal disease or on a magnesium-restricted diet should consult a healthcare provider prior to use. Unless directed by a physician, do not use for >2 weeks or exceed the recommended daily dose.
Adverse Reactions (Reflective of adult population; not specific for elderly) Frequency not defined.
Gastrointestinal: Constipation, chalky taste, cramping, fecal discoloration (white speckles), fecal impaction, nausea, vomiting
Endocrine & metabolic: Hypophosphatemia (rare), hypermagnesemia (rare)
Drug Interactions
Metabolism/Transport Effects None known.
Avoid Concomitant Use
Avoid concomitant use of Aluminum Hydroxide and Magnesium Hydroxide with any of the following: Calcium Polystyrene Sulfonate; Deferasirox; QuiNINE; Sodium Polystyrene Sulfonate; Vitamin D Analogs
Increased Effect/Toxicity
Aluminum Hydroxide and Magnesium Hydroxide may increase the levels/effects of: Alpha-/Beta-Agonists; Amphetamines; Calcium Channel Blockers; Calcium Polystyrene Sulfonate; Dexmethylphenidate; Methylphenidate; Misoprostol; Neuromuscular-Blocking Agents; QuiNIDine; Sodium Polystyrene Sulfonate

The levels/effects of Aluminum Hydroxide and Magnesium Hydroxide may be increased by: Alfacalcidol; Ascorbic Acid; Calcitriol; Calcium Channel Blockers; Calcium Polystyrene Sulfonate; Citric Acid Derivatives; Sodium Polystyrene Sulfonate; Vitamin D Analogs
Decreased Effect
Aluminum Hydroxide and Magnesium Hydroxide may decrease the levels/effects of: ACE Inhibitors; Allopurinol; Anticonvulsants (Hydantoin); Antipsychotic Agents (Phenothiazines); Atazanavir; Bisacodyl; Bisphosphonate Derivatives; Cefditoren; Cefpodoxime; Cefuroxime; Chenodiol; Chloroquine; Corticosteroids (Oral); Dabigatran Etexilate; Dasatinib; Deferasirox; Deferiprone; Delavirdine; Eltrombopag; Erlotinib; Ethambutol; Fexofenadine; Gabapentin; HMG-CoA Reductase Inhibitors; Iron Salts; Isoniazid; Itraconazole; Ketoconazole; Ketoconazole (Systemic); Levothyroxine; Mesalamine; Methenamine; Mycophenolate; Nilotinib; PenicillAMINE; Phosphate Supplements; Protease Inhibitors; QuiNINE; Quinolone Antibiotics; Rilpivirine; Tetracycline Derivatives; Trientine; Ursodiol; Vismodegib

The levels/effects of Aluminum Hydroxide and Magnesium Hydroxide may be decreased by: Trientine

Dosage

Geriatric & Adult Hyperacidity: Oral: OTC labeling:

Liquid (aluminum hydroxide 200 mg and magnesium hydroxide 200 mg per 5 mL): 10-20 mL 4 times/day (maximum:80 mL/day)

Suspension (aluminum hydroxide 500 mg and magnesium hydroxide 500 mg per 5 mL): 10-20 mL 4 times/day, between meals and at bedtime (maximum: 45 mL/day)

Tablet (aluminum hydroxide 300 mg and magnesium hydroxide 150 mg): 1-2 tablets after meals or at bedtime, or as needed (maximum: 16 tablets/day)

Renal Impairment Aluminum and/or magnesium may accumulate in severe renal impairment.

Administration

Liquid, suspension: Shake well before use; administer 1-3 hours after meals when stomach acidity is highest

Tablet: Chew tablet thoroughly before swallowing or allow tablets to dissolve slowly in mouth. Follow with a full glass of water.

Pharmacotherapy Pearls Sodium content varies with product; check for each product if important for patient

Special Geriatric Considerations Elderly, due to disease or drug therapy, may be predisposed to diarrhea or constipation. Diarrhea may result in electrolyte imbalance. Decreased renal function (Cl_{cr} <30 mL/minute) may result in toxicity of aluminum or magnesium. Drug interactions must be considered. If possible, administer antacid 1-2 hours apart from other drugs. When treating ulcers, consider buffer capacity (mEq/mL) to calculate dose of antacid.

Dosage Forms Excipient information presented when available (limited, particularly for generics); consult specific product labeling. [DSC] = Discontinued product

Liquid, oral:

Mag-Al: Aluminum hydroxide 200 mg and magnesium hydroxide 200 mg per 5 mL (30 mL) [dye free, ethanol free, sugar free; contains propylene glycol, sodium 4 mg/5 mL; peppermint flavor]

Suspension, oral:

Mag-Al Ultimate: Aluminum hydroxide 500 mg and magnesium hydroxide 500 mg per 5 mL (20 mL) [contains propylene glycol, sodium 4 mg/5 mL; peppermint flavor]

Tablet, chewable:

Alamag: Aluminum hydroxide 300 mg and magnesium hydroxide 150 mg [contains phenylalanine 2.63 mg; wild cherry flavor]

Aluminum Hydroxide and Magnesium Trisilicate
(a LOO mi num hye DROKS ide & mag NEE zhum trye SIL i kate)

Related Information

Aluminum Hydroxide *on page 77*

Brand Names: U.S. Gaviscon® Tablet [OTC]

Index Terms Magnesium Trisilicate and Aluminum Hydroxide

Generic Availability (U.S.) Yes

Pharmacologic Category Antacid

Use Temporary relief of hyperacidity

Drug Interactions

Metabolism/Transport Effects None known.

Avoid Concomitant Use

Avoid concomitant use of Aluminum Hydroxide and Magnesium Trisilicate with any of the following: Deferasirox; Nitrofurantoin; QuiNINE; Vitamin D Analogs

Increased Effect/Toxicity

Aluminum Hydroxide and Magnesium Trisilicate may increase the levels/effects of: Alpha-/ Beta-Agonists; Amphetamines; Calcium Polystyrene Sulfonate; Dexmethylphenidate; Methylphenidate; Misoprostol; QuiNIDine; Sodium Polystyrene Sulfonate

The levels/effects of Aluminum Hydroxide and Magnesium Trisilicate may be increased by: Ascorbic Acid; Calcium Polystyrene Sulfonate; Citric Acid Derivatives; Sodium Polystyrene Sulfonate; Vitamin D Analogs

Decreased Effect

Aluminum Hydroxide and Magnesium Trisilicate may decrease the levels/effects of: ACE Inhibitors; Allopurinol; Anticonvulsants (Hydantoin); Antipsychotic Agents (Phenothiazines); Atazanavir; Bisacodyl; Bisphosphonate Derivatives; Cefditoren; Cefpodoxime; Cefuroxime; Chenodiol; Chloroquine; Corticosteroids (Oral); Dabigatran Etexilate; Dasatinib; Deferasirox; Deferiprone; Delavirdine; Eltrombopag; Erlotinib; Ethambutol; Fexofenadine; Gabapentin;

◄ .HMG-CoA Reductase Inhibitors; Iron Salts; Isoniazid; Itraconazole; Ketoconazole; Ketoconazole (Systemic); Levothyroxine; Mesalamine; Methenamine; Mycophenolate; Nilotinib; Nitrofurantoin; PenicillAMINE; Phosphate Supplements; Protease Inhibitors; QuiNINE; Quinolone Antibiotics; Rilpivirine; Tetracycline Derivatives; Trientine; Ursodiol; Vismodegib

Dosage

Geriatric & Adult Dyspepsia, gastric acidity: Oral: Chew 2-4 tablets 4 times/day or as directed by healthcare provider

Renal Impairment Aluminum and/or magnesium may accumulate in renal impairment.

Administration Tablets should be chewed and not swallowed whole.

Special Geriatric Considerations Elderly, due to disease or drug therapy, may be predisposed to diarrhea or constipation. Diarrhea may result in electrolyte imbalance. Decreased renal function (Cl_{cr} <30 mL/minute) may result in toxicity of aluminum or magnesium. Drug interactions must be considered. If possible, administer antacid 1-2 hours apart from other drugs. When treating ulcers, consider buffer capacity (mEq/mL) to calculate dose of antacid.

Dosage Forms Excipient information presented when available (limited, particularly for generics); consult specific product labeling. [DSC] = Discontinued product

Tablet, chewable: Aluminum hydroxide 80 mg and magnesium trisilicate 20 mg

Gaviscon®: Aluminum hydroxide 80 mg and magnesium trisilicate 20 mg [contains sodium 0.8 mEq/tablet; butterscotch flavor]

Aluminum Hydroxide, Magnesium Hydroxide, and Simethicone
(a LOO ni num hye DROKS ide, mag NEE zhum hye DROKS ide, & sye METH i kone)

Related Information

Aluminum Hydroxide on page 77

Magnesium Hydroxide on page 1177

Simethicone on page 1776

Medication Safety Issues

Sound-alike/look-alike issues:

Maalox® may be confused with Maox®, Monodox®

Mylanta® may be confused with Mynatal®

Other safety concerns:

Liquid Maalox® products contain a different formulation than Maalox® Total Relief® which contains bismuth subsalicylate.

Brand Names: U.S. Alamag Plus [OTC]; Aldroxicon I [OTC]; Aldroxicon II [OTC]; Almacone Double Strength® [OTC]; Almacone® [OTC]; Gelusil® [OTC]; Maalox® Advanced Maximum Strength [OTC]; Maalox® Advanced Regular Strength [OTC]; Mi-Acid Maximum Strength [OTC] [DSC]; Mi-Acid [OTC]; Mintox Plus [OTC]; Mylanta® Classic Maximum Strength Liquid [OTC]; Mylanta® Classic Regular Strength Liquid [OTC]; Rulox [OTC]

Brand Names: Canada Diovol Plus®; Gelusil®; Mylanta® Double Strength; Mylanta® Extra Strength; Mylanta® Regular Strength

Index Terms Magnesium Hydroxide, Aluminum Hydroxide, and Simethicone; Simethicone, Aluminum Hydroxide, and Magnesium Hydroxide

Generic Availability (U.S.) Yes

Pharmacologic Category Antacid; Antiflatulent

Use Temporary relief of hyperacidity associated with gas; may also be used for indications associated with other antacids

Adverse Reactions (Reflective of adult population; not specific for elderly)

>10%: Gastrointestinal: Chalky taste, stomach cramps, constipation, bowel motility decreased, fecal impaction, hemorrhoids

1% to 10%: Gastrointestinal: Nausea, vomiting, discoloration of feces (white speckles)

Drug Interactions

Metabolism/Transport Effects None known.

Avoid Concomitant Use

Avoid concomitant use of Aluminum Hydroxide, Magnesium Hydroxide, and Simethicone with any of the following: Calcium Polystyrene Sulfonate; Deferasirox; QuiNINE; Sodium Polystyrene Sulfonate; Vitamin D Analogs

Increased Effect/Toxicity

Aluminum Hydroxide, Magnesium Hydroxide, and Simethicone may increase the levels/effects of: Alpha-/Beta-Agonists; Amphetamines; Calcium Channel Blockers; Calcium Polystyrene Sulfonate; Dexmethylphenidate; Methylphenidate; Misoprostol; Neuromuscular-Blocking Agents; QuiNIDine; Sodium Polystyrene Sulfonate

The levels/effects of Aluminum Hydroxide, Magnesium Hydroxide, and Simethicone may be increased by: Alfacalcidol; Ascorbic Acid; Calcitriol; Calcium Channel Blockers; Calcium Polystyrene Sulfonate; Citric Acid Derivatives; Sodium Polystyrene Sulfonate; Vitamin D Analogs

Decreased Effect

Aluminum Hydroxide, Magnesium Hydroxide, and Simethicone may decrease the levels/ effects of: ACE Inhibitors; Allopurinol; Anticonvulsants (Hydantoin); Antipsychotic Agents (Phenothiazines); Atazanavir; Bisacodyl; Bisphosphonate Derivatives; Cefditoren; Cefpodoxime; Cefuroxime; Chenodiol; Chloroquine; Corticosteroids (Oral); Dabigatran Etexilate; Dasatinib; Deferasirox; Deferiprone; Delavirdine; Eltrombopag; Erlotinib; Ethambutol; Fexofenadine; Gabapentin; HMG-CoA Reductase Inhibitors; Iron Salts; Isoniazid; Itraconazole; Ketoconazole; Ketoconazole (Systemic); Levothyroxine; Mesalamine; Methenamine; Mycophenolate; Nilotinib; PenicillAMINE; Phosphate Supplements; Protease Inhibitors; QuiNINE; Quinolone Antibiotics; Rilpivirine; Tetracycline Derivatives; Trientine; Ursodiol; Vismodegib

The levels/effects of Aluminum Hydroxide, Magnesium Hydroxide, and Simethicone may be decreased by: Trientine

Dosage

Geriatric & Adult Dyspepsia, abdominal bloating: Oral: 10-20 mL or 2-4 tablets 4-6 times/ day between meals and at bedtime; may be used every hour for severe symptoms

Renal Impairment Aluminum and/or magnesium may accumulate in renal impairment.

Administration Administer 1-2 hours apart from oral drugs; administer 1-3 hours after meals.

Dosage Forms Excipient information presented when available (limited, particularly for generics); consult specific product labeling. [DSC] = Discontinued product

Liquid, oral: Aluminum hydroxide 200 mg, magnesium hydroxide 200 mg, and simethicone 20 mg per 5 mL (360 mL); aluminum hydroxide 400 mg, magnesium hydroxide 400 mg, and simethicone 40 mg per 5 mL (360 mL)

Aldroxicon I: Aluminum hydroxide 200 mg, magnesium hydroxide 200 mg, and simethicone 20 mg per 5 mL (30 mL)

Aldroxicon II: Aluminum hydroxide 400 mg, magnesium hydroxide 400 mg, and simethicone 40 mg per 5 mL (30 mL)

Almacone®: Aluminum hydroxide 200 mg, magnesium hydroxide 200 mg, and simethicone 20 mg per 5 mL (360 mL)

Almacone Double Strength®: Aluminum hydroxide 400 mg, magnesium hydroxide 400 mg, and simethicone 40 mg per 5 mL (360 mL)

Maalox® Advanced Maximum Strength: Aluminum hydroxide 400 mg, magnesium hydroxide 400 mg, and simethicone 40 mg per 5 mL (355 mL, 769 mL) [contains magnesium 167 mg/5 mL; cherry flavor]

Maalox® Advanced Maximum Strength: Aluminum hydroxide 400 mg, magnesium hydroxide 400 mg, and simethicone 40 mg per 5 mL (355 mL, 769 mL) [contains magnesium 167 mg/5 mL; lemon flavor]

Maalox® Advanced Maximum Strength: Aluminum hydroxide 400 mg, magnesium hydroxide 400 mg, and simethicone 40 mg per 5 mL (355 mL) [contains magnesium 167 mg/5 mL; mint flavor]

Maalox® Advanced Maximum Strength: Aluminum hydroxide 400 mg, magnesium hydroxide 400 mg, and simethicone 40 mg per 5 mL (355 mL) [contains magnesium 167 mg/5 mL; vanilla crème flavor]

Maalox® Advanced Regular Strength: Aluminum hydroxide 200 mg, magnesium hydroxide 200 mg, and simethicone 20 mg per 5 mL (360 mL, 780 mL) [contains magnesium 75 mg/5 mL, potassium 5 mg/5 mL, propylene glycol; mint flavor]

Mi-Acid: Aluminum hydroxide 200 mg, magnesium hydroxide 200 mg, and simethicone 20 mg per 5 mL (360 mL)

Mi-Acid Maximum Strength: Aluminum hydroxide 400 mg, magnesium hydroxide 400 mg, and simethicone 40 mg per 5 mL (360 mL)

Mylanta® Classic Maximum Strength: Aluminum hydroxide 400 mg, magnesium hydroxide 400 mg, and simethicone 40 mg per 5 mL (360 mL, 720 mL) [original, cherry, orange creme, and mint flavors]

Mylanta® Classic Regular Strength: Aluminum hydroxide 200 mg, magnesium hydroxide 200 mg, and simethicone 20 mg per 5 mL (360 mL) [original and mint flavors]

Suspension, oral: Aluminum hydroxide 225 mg, magnesium hydroxide 200 mg, and simethicone 25 mg per 5 mL (360 mL)

Rulox: Aluminum hydroxide 200 mg, magnesium hydroxide 200 mg, and simethicone 25 mg per 5 mL (355 mL) [contains magnesium 85 mg/5 mL; mint flavor]

Tablet, chewable: Aluminum hydroxide 200 mg, magnesium hydroxide 200 mg, and simethicone 25 mg

Alamag Plus: Aluminum hydroxide 200 mg, magnesium hydroxide 200 mg, and simethicone 25 mg [contains magnesium 83 mg/tablet, phenylalanine 2.6 mg/tablet; cherry flavor]

Almacone®: Aluminum hydroxide 200 mg, magnesium hydroxide 200 mg, and simethicone 20 mg [dye free; contains magnesium 82 mg/tablet; peppermint flavor]

Gelusil®: Aluminum hydroxide 200 mg, magnesium hydroxide 200 mg, and simethicone 25 mg [peppermint flavor]

Mintox Plus: Aluminum hydroxide 200 mg, magnesium hydroxide 200 mg, and simethicone 25 mg [lemon crème flavor]

◆ **Aluminum Sucrose Sulfate, Basic** *see* Sucralfate *on page 1810*

Aluminum Sulfate and Calcium Acetate
(a LOO mi num SUL fate & KAL see um AS e tate)

Related Information
Calcium Acetate *on page 259*
Brand Names: U.S. Domeboro® [OTC]; Gordon Boro-Packs [OTC]; Pedi-Boro® [OTC]
Index Terms Calcium Acetate and Aluminum Sulfate
Generic Availability (U.S.) Yes
Pharmacologic Category Topical Skin Product
Use Astringent wet dressing for relief of inflammatory conditions of the skin; reduce weeping that may occur in dermatitis
Dosage
Geriatric & Adult Dermal inflammation, dermatitis: Topical: Soak affected area in the solution 2-4 times/day for 15-30 minutes or apply wet dressing soaked in the solution for more extended periods; rewet dressing with solution 2-4 times/day every 15-30 minutes
Special Geriatric Considerations No special considerations necessary
Dosage Forms Excipient information presented when available (limited, particularly for generics); consult specific product labeling.
Powder, for solution, topical: Aluminum sulfate 1191 mg and calcium acetate 839 mg per packet (12s)
Domeboro®: Aluminum sulfate tetradecahydrate 1347 mg and calcium acetate monohydrate 952 mg per packet (12s, 100s)
Gordon Boro-Packs: Aluminum sulfate 49% and calcium acetate 51% per packet (100s)
Pedi-Boro®: Aluminum sulfate tetradecahydrate 1191 mg and calcium acetate monohydrate 839 mg per packet (12s, 100s)

◆ **Alupent** *see* Metaproterenol *on page 1220*
◆ **Alvesco®** *see* Ciclesonide (Oral Inhalation) *on page 370*

Amantadine (a MAN ta deen)

Related Information
Antiparkinsonian Agents *on page 2101*
Medication Safety Issues
Sound-alike/look-alike issues:
Amantadine may be confused with ranitidine, rimantadine
Symmetrel may be confused with Synthroid®
Brand Names: Canada Dom-Amantadine; Mylan-Amantadine; PHL-Amantadine; PMS-Amantadine
Index Terms Adamantanamine Hydrochloride; Amantadine Hydrochloride; Symmetrel
Generic Availability (U.S.) Yes
Pharmacologic Category Anti-Parkinson's Agent, Dopamine Agonist; Antiviral Agent; Antiviral Agent, Adamantane
Use Prophylaxis and treatment of influenza A viral infection (per manufacturer's labeling; also refer to current ACIP guidelines for recommendations during current flu season); treatment of parkinsonism; treatment of drug-induced extrapyramidal symptoms
Contraindications Hypersensitivity to amantadine or any component of the formulation
Warnings/Precautions May cause CNS depression, which may impair physical or mental abilities; patients must be cautioned about performing tasks which require mental alertness (eg, operating machinery or driving). There have been reports of suicidal ideation/attempt in patients with and without a history of psychiatric illness. Use with caution in patients with liver disease, a history of recurrent and eczematoid dermatitis, uncontrolled psychosis or severe psychoneurosis, seizures and in those receiving CNS stimulant drugs; reduce dose in renal disease; when treating Parkinson's disease, do not discontinue abruptly. In many patients, the therapeutic benefits of amantadine are limited to a few months. Abrupt discontinuation may cause agitation, anxiety, delirium, delusions, depression, hallucinations, paranoia, parkinsonian crisis, slurred speech, or stupor. Upon discontinuation of amantadine therapy, gradually taper dose. Elderly patients may be more susceptible to the CNS effects (using 2 divided daily

doses may minimize this effect); may require dosage reductions based on renal function. Use with caution in patients with HF, peripheral edema, or orthostatic hypotension; dosage reduction may be required. Avoid in untreated angle closure glaucoma.

Dopamine agonists have been associated with compulsive behaviors and/or loss of impulse control, which has manifested as pathological gambling, libido increases (hypersexuality), and/or binge eating. Causality has not been established, and controversy exists as to whether this phenomenon is related to the underlying disease, prior behaviors/addictions, and/or drug therapy. Dose reduction or discontinuation of therapy has been reported to reverse these behaviors in some, but not all cases. Risk for melanoma development is increased in Parkinson's disease patients; drug causation or factors contributing to risk have not been established. Patients should be monitored closely and periodic skin examinations should be performed.

Due to increased resistance, the ACIP has recommended that rimantadine and amantadine no longer be used for the treatment or prophylaxis of influenza A in the United States until susceptibility has been re-established; consult current guidelines.

Adverse Reactions (Reflective of adult population; not specific for elderly) 1% to 10%:
Cardiovascular: Orthostatic hypotension, peripheral edema
Central nervous system: Agitation, anxiety, ataxia, confusion, delirium, depression, dizziness, dream abnormality, fatigue, hallucinations, headache, insomnia, irritability, lightheadedness, nervousness, somnolence
Dermatologic: Livedo reticularis
Gastrointestinal: Anorexia, constipation, diarrhea, nausea, xerostomia
Respiratory: Dry nose

Drug Interactions

Metabolism/Transport Effects None known.

Avoid Concomitant Use There are no known interactions where it is recommended to avoid concomitant use.

Increased Effect/Toxicity
Amantadine may increase the levels/effects of: Glycopyrrolate; Highest Risk QTc-Prolonging Agents; Moderate Risk QTc-Prolonging Agents; Trimethoprim

The levels/effects of Amantadine may be increased by: MAO Inhibitors; Methylphenidate; Mifepristone; Trimethoprim

Decreased Effect
Amantadine may decrease the levels/effects of: Antipsychotics (Typical); Influenza Virus Vaccine (Live/Attenuated)

The levels/effects of Amantadine may be decreased by: Antipsychotics (Atypical); Antipsychotics (Typical); Metoclopramide

Ethanol/Nutrition/Herb Interactions Ethanol: Avoid ethanol (may increase CNS adverse effects).

Stability Store at 25°C (77°F); excursions permitted to 15°C to 30°C (59°F to 86°F).

Mechanism of Action As an antiviral, blocks the uncoating of influenza A virus preventing penetration of virus into host; antiparkinsonian activity may be due to its blocking the reuptake of dopamine into presynaptic neurons or by increasing dopamine release from presynaptic fibers

Pharmacodynamics/Kinetics
Onset of action: Antidyskinetic: Within 48 hours
Absorption: Well absorbed
Distribution: V_d: Normal: 1.5-6.1 L/kg; Renal failure: 5.1 ± 0.2 L/kg; in saliva, tear film, and nasal secretions; in animals, tissue (especially lung) concentrations higher than serum concentrations; crosses blood-brain barrier
Protein binding: Normal renal function: ~67%; Hemodialysis: ~59%
Metabolism: Not appreciable; small amounts of an acetyl metabolite identified
Bioavailability: 86% to 90%
Half-life elimination: Normal renal function: 16 ± 6 hours (9-31 hours); Healthy, older (≥60 years) males: 29 hours (range: 20-41 hours); End-stage renal disease: 7-10 days
Time to peak, plasma: 2-4 hours
Excretion: Urine (80% to 90% unchanged) by glomerular filtration and tubular secretion

Dosage
Geriatric Patients ≥65 years: Adjust dose based on renal function; some patients tolerate the drug better when it is given in 2 divided daily doses (to avoid adverse neurologic reactions).
Influenza A treatment/prophylaxis: 100 mg once daily

◄ **Adult**
Influenza A treatment/prophylaxis: Note: Due to issues of resistance, amantadine is no longer recommended for the treatment or prophylaxis of influenza A. Please refer to the current ACIP recommendations. The following is based on the manufacturer's labeling:
Influenza A treatment: Oral: 200 mg once daily **or** 100 mg twice daily (may be preferred to reduce CNS effects); **Note:** Initiate within 24-48 hours after onset of symptoms; continue for 24-48 hours after symptom resolution (duration of therapy is generally 3-5 days).
Influenza A prophylaxis: Oral: 200 mg once daily **or** 100 mg twice daily (may be preferred to reduce CNS effects). **Note:** Continue prophylaxis throughout the peak influenza activity in the community or throughout the entire influenza season in patients who cannot be vaccinated. Development of immunity following vaccination takes ~2 weeks; amantadine therapy should be considered for high-risk patients from the time of vaccination until immunity has developed.
Drug-induced extrapyramidal symptoms: Oral: 100 mg twice daily; may increase to 300 mg/day in divided doses, if needed
Parkinson's disease: Oral: Usual dose: 100 mg twice daily as monotherapy; may increase to 400 mg/day in divided doses, if needed, with close monitoring. **Note:** Patients with a serious concomitant illness or those receiving high doses of other anti-parkinson drugs should be started at 100 mg/day; may increase to 100 mg twice daily, if needed, after one to several weeks.
Renal Impairment
Cl_{cr} 30-50 mL/minute: Administer 200 mg on day 1, then 100 mg/day
Cl_{cr} 15-29 mL/minute: Administer 200 mg on day 1, then 100 mg on alternate days
Cl_{cr} <15 mL/minute: Administer 200 mg every 7 days
Hemodialysis: Administer 200 mg every 7 days
Peritoneal dialysis: No supplemental dose is needed
Continuous arteriovenous or venous-venous hemofiltration: No supplemental dose is needed
Monitoring Parameters Renal function, Parkinson's symptoms, mental status, influenza symptoms, blood pressure
Test Interactions May interfere with urine detection of amphetamines/methamphetamines (false-positive).
Special Geriatric Considerations Amantadine is no longer recommended for the treatment or chemoprophylaxis of influenza A infection. Elderly patients may be more susceptible to the CNS effects of amantadine. Adjust dose based on renal function. Liquid forms may be used to administer doses <100 mg.
Dosage Forms Excipient information presented when available (limited, particularly for generics); consult specific product labeling.
Capsule, oral, as hydrochloride: 100 mg
Capsule, softgel, oral, as hydrochloride: 100 mg
Solution, oral, as hydrochloride: 50 mg/5 mL (473 mL)
Syrup, oral, as hydrochloride: 50 mg/5 mL (10 mL, 473 mL, 480 mL)
Tablet, oral, as hydrochloride: 100 mg

◆ **Amantadine Hydrochloride** *see* Amantadine *on page 84*
◆ **Amaryl®** *see* Glimepiride *on page 877*
◆ **Ambien®** *see* Zolpidem *on page 2064*
◆ **Ambien CR®** *see* Zolpidem *on page 2064*

Amcinonide (am SIN oh nide)

Related Information
Topical Corticosteroids *on page 2113*
Brand Names: Canada Amcort®; Cyclocort®; ratio-Amcinonide; Taro-Amcinonide
Generic Availability (U.S.) Yes
Pharmacologic Category Corticosteroid, Topical
Use Relief of the inflammatory and pruritic manifestations of corticosteroid-responsive dermatoses (high potency corticosteroid)
Dosage
Geriatric & Adult Steroid-responsive dermatoses: Topical: Apply in a thin film 2-3 times/day. Therapy should be discontinued when control is achieved; if no improvement is seen, reassessment of diagnosis may be necessary.
Special Geriatric Considerations Due to age-related changes in skin, limit use of topical corticosteroids.
Dosage Forms Excipient information presented when available (limited, particularly for generics); consult specific product labeling. [DSC] = Discontinued product
Cream, topical: 0.1% (15 g, 30 g, 60 g)

Lotion, topical: 0.1% (60 mL)
Ointment, topical: 0.1% (30 g [DSC], 60 g)

◆ **Amerge®** see Naratriptan on page 1344
◆ **A-Methapred** see MethylPREDNISolone on page 1252
◆ **A-Methapred®** see MethylPREDNISolone on page 1252
◆ **Amethopterin** see Methotrexate on page 1236
◆ **AMG 073** see Cinacalcet on page 379
◆ **AMG-162** see Denosumab on page 502

Amikacin (am i KAY sin)

Related Information
Antimicrobial Drugs of Choice on page 2163
Medication Safety Issues
Sound-alike/look-alike issues:
Amikacin may be confused with Amicar®, anakinra
Amikin® may be confused with Amicar®, Kineret®
Brand Names: Canada Amikacin Sulfate Injection, USP; Amikin®
Index Terms Amikacin Sulfate
Generic Availability (U.S.) Yes
Pharmacologic Category Antibiotic, Aminoglycoside
Use Treatment of serious infections (bone infections, respiratory tract infections, endocarditis, and septicemia) due to organisms resistant to gentamicin and tobramycin, including *Pseudomonas, Proteus, Serratia,* and other gram-negative bacilli; documented infection of mycobacterial organisms susceptible to amikacin
Unlabeled Use Bacterial endophthalmitis
Contraindications Hypersensitivity to amikacin sulfate or any component of the formulation; cross-sensitivity may exist with other aminoglycosides
Warnings/Precautions [U.S. Boxed Warning]: Amikacin may cause neurotoxicity, nephrotoxicity, and/or neuromuscular blockade and respiratory paralysis; usual risk factors include pre-existing renal impairment, concomitant neuro-/nephrotoxic medications, advanced age and dehydration. Dose and/or frequency of administration must be monitored and modified in patients with renal impairment. Drug should be discontinued if signs of ototoxicity, nephrotoxicity, or hypersensitivity occur. Ototoxicity is proportional to the amount of drug given and the duration of treatment. Tinnitus or vertigo may be indications of vestibular injury and impending bilateral irreversible damage. Renal damage is usually reversible. Use with caution in patients with neuromuscular disorders, hearing loss and hypocalcemia. Prolonged use may result in fungal or bacterial superinfection, including *C. difficile*-associated diarrhea (CDAD) and pseudomembranous colitis; CDAD has been observed >2 months postantibiotic treatment. Solution contains sodium metabisulfate; use caution in patients with sulfite allergy.
Adverse Reactions (Reflective of adult population; not specific for elderly) 1% to 10%:
Central nervous system: Neurotoxicity
Otic: Ototoxicity (auditory), ototoxicity (vestibular)
Renal: Nephrotoxicity
Drug Interactions
Metabolism/Transport Effects None known.
Avoid Concomitant Use
Avoid concomitant use of Amikacin with any of the following: BCG; Gallium Nitrate
Increased Effect/Toxicity
Amikacin may increase the levels/effects of: AbobotulinumtoxinA; Bisphosphonate Derivatives; CARBOplatin; Colistimethate; CycloSPORINE; CycloSPORINE (Systemic); Gallium Nitrate; Neuromuscular-Blocking Agents; OnabotulinumtoxinA; RimabotulinumtoxinB

The levels/effects of Amikacin may be increased by: Amphotericin B; Capreomycin; Cephalosporins (2nd Generation); Cephalosporins (3rd Generation); Cephalosporins (4th Generation); CISplatin; Loop Diuretics; Nonsteroidal Anti-Inflammatory Agents; Vancomycin
Decreased Effect
Amikacin may decrease the levels/effects of: BCG; Typhoid Vaccine

The levels/effects of Amikacin may be decreased by: Penicillins
Stability Store at controlled room temperature. Following admixture at concentrations of 0.25-5 mg/mL, amikacin is stable for 24 hours at room temperature and 2 days at refrigeration when mixed in D_5W, NS, and LR.
Mechanism of Action Inhibits protein synthesis in susceptible bacteria by binding to 30S ribosomal subunits

Pharmacodynamics/Kinetics

Absorption: I.M.: Aminoglycosides may be delayed in the bedridden patient

Half-life:

Adults: 2-3 hours

Anuria: 28-86 hours

Half-life and clearance are dependent on renal function primarily distributed into extracellular fluid (highly hydrophilic); penetrates the blood-brain barrier when meninges are inflamed

Time to peak serum concentration:

I.M.: Within 45-120 minutes

I.V.: Within 30 minutes

Elimination: 94% to 98% excreted unchanged in urine via glomerular filtration within 24 hours

Clearance (renal) may be reduced and half-life prolonged in geriatric patients

The pharmacokinetics of the aminoglycosides are heterogeneous in older adults; it is best to assume that clearance is reduced and half-life prolonged in older adults, while volume of distribution is usually unchanged. The establishment of each patient's pharmacokinetic parameters is important for proper dosing in order to achieve optimal therapeutic benefit and minimize the risk of toxicity.

Dosage

Geriatric & Adult Individualization is critical because of the low therapeutic index

Note: Use of ideal body weight (IBW) for determining the mg/kg/dose appears to be more accurate than dosing on the basis of total body weight (TBW)

In morbid obesity, dosage requirement may best be estimated using a dosing weight of IBW + 0.4 (TBW - IBW)

Initial and periodic peak and trough plasma drug levels should be determined, particularly in critically-ill patients with serious infections or in disease states known to significantly alter aminoglycoside pharmacokinetics (eg, cystic fibrosis, burns, or major surgery). Manufacturer recommends a maximum daily dose of 15 mg/kg/day (or 1.5 g/day in heavier patients). Higher doses may be warranted based on therapeutic drug monitoring or susceptibility information.

Usual dosage range:

I.M., I.V.: 5-7.5 mg/kg/dose every 8 hours; **Note:** Some clinicians suggest a daily dose of 15-20 mg/kg for all patients with normal renal function. This dose is at least as efficacious with similar, if not less, toxicity than conventional dosing.

Intrathecal/intraventricular (unlabeled route): Meningitis (susceptible gram-negative organisms): 5-50 mg/day

Indication-specific dosing:

Endophthalmitis, bacterial (unlabeled use): Intravitreal: 0.4 mg/0.1 mL NS in combination with vancomycin

Hospital-acquired pneumonia (HAP): I.V.: 20 mg/kg/day with antipseudomonal beta-lactam or carbapenem (American Thoracic Society/ATS guidelines)

Meningitis (susceptible gram-negative organisms):

I.V.: 5 mg/kg every 8 hours (administered with another bacteriocidal drug)

Intrathecal/intraventricular (unlabeled route): Usual dose: 30 mg/day (IDSA, 2004); Range: 5-50 mg/day (with concurrent systemic antimicrobial therapy) (Gilbert, 1986; Guardado, 2008; IDSA, 2004; Kasiakou, 2005)

Mycobacterium fortuitum, M. chelonae, or M. abscessus: I.V.: 10-15 mg/kg daily for at least 2 weeks with high dose cefoxitin

Renal Impairment Some patients may require larger or more frequent doses if serum levels document the need (ie, cystic fibrosis or febrile granulocytopenic patients).

Cl_{cr} ≥60 mL/minute: Administer every 8 hours

Cl_{cr} 40-60 mL/minute: Administer every 12 hours

Cl_{cr} 20-40 mL/minute: Administer every 24 hours

Cl_{cr} <20 mL/minute: Loading dose, then monitor levels

Intermittent hemodialysis (IHD) (administer after hemodialysis on dialysis days): Dialyzable (20%; variable; dependent on filter, duration, and type of HD): 5-7.5 mg/kg every 48-72 hours. Follow levels. Redose when pre-HD concentration <10 mg/L; redose when post-HD concentration <6-8 mg/L (Heintz, 2009). **Note:** Dosing dependent on the assumption of 3 times/week, complete IHD sessions.

Peritoneal dialysis (PD): Dose as Cl_{cr} <20 mL/minute: Follow levels.

Continuous renal replacement therapy (CRRT) (Heintz, 2009; Trotman, 2005): Drug clearance is highly dependent on the method of renal replacement, filter type, and flow rate. Appropriate dosing requires close monitoring of pharmacologic response, signs of adverse reactions due to drug accumulation, as well as drug concentrations in relation to target trough (if appropriate). The following are general recommendations only (based on dialysate flow/ultrafiltration rates of 1-2 L/hour and minimal residual renal function) and should not supersede clinical judgment:

CVVH/CVVHD/CVVHDF: Loading dose of 10 mg/kg followed by maintenance dose of 7.5 mg/kg every 24-48 hours

Note: For severe gram-negative rod infections, target peak concentration of 15-30 mg/L; redose when concentration <10 mg/L (Heintz, 2009).

Administration Administer I.M. injection in large muscle mass

Monitoring Parameters Urinalysis, BUN, serum creatinine, appropriately timed peak and trough concentrations, vital signs, temperature, weight, I & O, hearing parameters

Some penicillin derivatives may accelerate the degradation of aminoglycosides *in vitro*. This may be clinically-significant for certain penicillin (ticarcillin, piperacillin, carbenicillin) and aminoglycoside (gentamicin, tobramycin) combination therapy in patients with significant renal impairment. Close monitoring of aminoglycoside levels is warranted.

Reference Range

Sample size: 0.5-2 mL blood (red top tube) or 0.1-1 mL serum (separated)

Therapeutic levels:

Peak:

Life-threatening infections: 25-40 mcg/mL

Serious infections: 20-25 mcg/mL

Urinary tract infections: 15-20 mcg/mL

Trough: <8 mcg/mL

The American Thoracic Society (ATS) recommends trough levels of <4-5 mcg/mL for patients with hospital-acquired pneumonia.

Toxic concentration: Peak: >40 mcg/mL; Trough: >10 mcg/mL

Timing of serum samples: Draw peak 30 minutes after completion of 30-minute infusion or at 1 hour following initiation of infusion or I.M. injection; draw trough within 30 minutes prior to next dose

Test Interactions Some penicillin derivatives may accelerate the degradation of aminoglycosides *in vitro*, leading to a potential underestimation of aminoglycoside serum concentration.

Pharmacotherapy Pearls Drug should be discontinued if signs of ototoxicity, nephrotoxicity, or hypersensitivity occurs; hearing should be tested before, during, and after treatment, when indicated; sodium content of 1 g: 29.9 mg (1.3 mEq). Aminoglycoside serum concentrations measured from blood taken from silastic central catheters can sometimes give falsely high readings.

Special Geriatric Considerations The aminoglycosides are important therapeutic interventions for infections due to susceptible organisms and as empiric therapy in seriously ill patients. Their use is not without risk of toxicity whose risks can be minimized if initial dosing is adjusted for estimated renal function and appropriate monitoring performed. High dose, once daily aminoglycosides have been advocated as an alternative to traditional dosing regimens. Once daily or extended interval dosing is as effective and may be safer than traditional dosing.

Dosage Forms Excipient information presented when available (limited, particularly for generics); consult specific product labeling.

Injection, solution, as sulfate: 250 mg/mL (2 mL, 4 mL)

♦ **Amikacin Sulfate** *see* Amikacin *on page 87*

AMILoride (a MIL oh ride)

Medication Safety Issues

Sound-alike/look-alike issues:

AMILoride may be confused with amiodarone, amLODIPine, inamrinone

Brand Names: Canada Apo-Amiloride®; Midamor

Index Terms Amiloride Hydrochloride

Generic Availability (U.S.) Yes

Pharmacologic Category Diuretic, Potassium-Sparing

Use Counteracts potassium loss induced by other diuretics in the treatment of hypertension or edematous conditions including CHF, hepatic cirrhosis, and hypoaldosteronism; usually used in conjunction with more potent diuretics such as thiazides or loop diuretics

Unlabeled Use Investigational: Cystic fibrosis; reduction of lithium-induced polyuria

Contraindications Hypersensitivity to amiloride or any component of the formulation; presence of elevated serum potassium levels (>5.5 mEq/L); if patient is receiving other potassium-conserving agents (eg, spironolactone, triamterene) or potassium supplementation (medicine, potassium-containing salt substitutes, potassium-rich diet); anuria; acute or chronic renal insufficiency; evidence of diabetic nephropathy. Patients with evidence of renal impairment or diabetes mellitus should not receive this medicine without close, frequent monitoring of serum electrolytes and renal function.

Warnings/Precautions [U.S. Boxed Warning]: Hyperkalemia can occur; patients at risk include those with renal impairment, diabetes, the elderly, and the severely ill. Serum potassium levels must be monitored at frequent intervals especially when dosages are changed or with any illness that may cause renal dysfunction. Excess amounts can lead to profound diuresis with fluid and electrolyte loss; close medical supervision and dose evaluation are required. Watch for and correct electrolyte disturbances; adjust dose to avoid dehydration. In cirrhosis, avoid electrolyte and acid/base imbalances that might lead to hepatic encephalopathy. Use with extreme caution in patients with diabetes mellitus; monitor closely. Discontinue amiloride 3 days prior to glucose tolerance testing. Use with caution in patients who are at risk for metabolic or respiratory acidosis (eg, cardiopulmonary disease, uncontrolled diabetes).

Adverse Reactions (Reflective of adult population; not specific for elderly) 1% to 10%:

Central nervous system: Headache, fatigue, dizziness

Endocrine & metabolic: Hyperkalemia (up to 10%; risk reduced in patients receiving kaliuretic diuretics), hyperchloremic metabolic acidosis, dehydration, hyponatremia, gynecomastia

Gastrointestinal: Nausea, diarrhea, vomiting, abdominal pain, gas pain, appetite changes, constipation

Genitourinary: Impotence

Neuromuscular & skeletal: Muscle cramps, weakness

Respiratory: Cough, dyspnea

Drug Interactions

Metabolism/Transport Effects None known.

Avoid Concomitant Use

Avoid concomitant use of AMILoride with any of the following: CycloSPORINE; Cyclo-SPORINE (Systemic); Tacrolimus; Tacrolimus (Systemic)

Increased Effect/Toxicity

AMILoride may increase the levels/effects of: ACE Inhibitors; Amifostine; Ammonium Chloride; Antihypertensives; Cardiac Glycosides; CycloSPORINE; CycloSPORINE (Systemic); Dofetilide; Hypotensive Agents; RiTUXimab; Sodium Phosphates; Tacrolimus; Tacrolimus (Systemic)

The levels/effects of AMILoride may be increased by: Alfuzosin; Angiotensin II Receptor Blockers; Diazoxide; Drospirenone; Eplerenone; Herbs (Hypotensive Properties); MAO Inhibitors; Nonsteroidal Anti-Inflammatory Agents; Pentoxifylline; Phosphodiesterase 5 Inhibitors; Potassium Salts; Prostacyclin Analogues; Tolvaptan

Decreased Effect

AMILoride may decrease the levels/effects of: Cardiac Glycosides; QuiNIDine

The levels/effects of AMILoride may be decreased by: Herbs (Hypertensive Properties); Methylphenidate; Nonsteroidal Anti-Inflammatory Agents; Yohimbine

Ethanol/Nutrition/Herb Interactions Food: Hyperkalemia may result if amiloride is taken with potassium-containing foods.

Mechanism of Action Blocks epithelial sodium channels in the late distal convoluted tubule (DCT), and collecting duct which inhibits sodium reabsorption from the lumen. This effectively reduces intracellular sodium, decreasing the function of Na+/K+ATPase, leading to potassium retention and decreased calcium, magnesium, and hydrogen excretion. As sodium uptake capacity in the DCT/collecting duct is limited, the natriuretic, diuretic, and antihypertensive effects are generally considered weak.

Pharmacodynamics/Kinetics

Onset of action: 2 hours

Duration: 24 hours

Absorption: ~15% to 25%

Distribution: V_d: 350-380 L

Protein binding: 23%

Metabolism: No active metabolites

Half-life elimination: Normal renal function: 6-9 hours; End-stage renal disease: 8-144 hours

Time to peak, serum: 6-10 hours

Excretion: Urine and feces (equal amounts as unchanged drug)

Dosage
  Geriatric Oral: Initial: 5 mg once daily or every other day
  Adult Hypertension, edema (to limit potassium loss): Oral: Initial: 5-10 mg/day (up to 20 mg)
    Hypertension (JNC 7): 5-10 mg/day in 1-2 divided doses
  Renal Impairment Oral:
    Cl_{cr} 10-50 mL/minute: Administer 50% of normal dose.
    Cl_{cr} <10 mL/minute: Avoid use.
Administration Administer with food or meals to avoid GI upset.
Monitoring Parameters I & O, daily weights, blood pressure, serum electrolytes, renal function
Test Interactions May falsely elevate serum digoxin levels done by radioimmunoassay
Pharmacotherapy Pearls Medication should be discontinued if potassium level exceeds 6.5 mEq/L. Combined with hydrochlorothiazide as Moduretic®. Amiloride is considered an alternative to triamterene or spironolactone.
Special Geriatric Considerations Use lower initial dose, and adjust dose for renal impairment. Potassium excretion may be decreased in the elderly, increasing the risk of hyperkalemia, which may occur with potassium-sparing diuretics such as amiloride.
Dosage Forms Excipient information presented when available (limited, particularly for generics); consult specific product labeling.
  Tablet, oral, as hydrochloride: 5 mg

Amiloride and Hydrochlorothiazide
(a MIL oh ride & hye droe klor oh THYE a zide)

Related Information
  AMILoride *on page 89*
  Hydrochlorothiazide *on page 933*
Brand Names: Canada Ami-Hydro; Apo-Amilzide®; Gen-Amilazide; Moduret; Novamilor; Nu-Amilzide
Index Terms Hydrochlorothiazide and Amiloride
Generic Availability (U.S.) Yes
Pharmacologic Category Diuretic, Combination
Use Potassium-sparing diuretic; antihypertensive
Dosage
  Geriatric Oral: Initial: 1/2 to 1 tablet/day
  Adult Hypertension, edema: Oral: Initial: 1 tablet/day; may be increased to 2 tablets/day if needed; usually given in a single dose
  Renal Impairment See individual agents.
Special Geriatric Considerations See individual agents. Hydrochlorothiazide is not effective in patients with a Cl_{cr} <30 mL/minute; therefore, it may not be a useful agent in many elderly patients. Potassium excretion may be decreased in the elderly, increasing the risk of hyperkalemia with potassium-sparing diuretics such as amiloride.
Dosage Forms Excipient information presented when available (limited, particularly for generics); consult specific product labeling.
  Tablet, 5/50: Amiloride hydrochloride 5 mg and hydrochlorothiazide 50 mg

◆ **Amiloride Hydrochloride** *see* AMILoride *on page 89*
◆ **2-Amino-6-Trifluoromethoxy-benzothiazole** *see* Riluzole *on page 1703*
◆ **Aminobenzylpenicillin** *see* Ampicillin *on page 127*

Aminolevulinic Acid (a MEE noh lev yoo lin ik AS id)

Medication Safety Issues
  Sound-alike/look-alike issues:
    Aminolevulinic acid may be confused with methyl aminolevulinate
Brand Names: U.S. Levulan® Kerastick®
Brand Names: Canada Levulan® Kerastick®
Index Terms 5-ALA; 5-Aminolevulinic Acid; ALA; Amino Levulinic Acid; Aminolevulinic Acid Hydrochloride
Generic Availability (U.S.) No
Pharmacologic Category Photosensitizing Agent, Topical; Topical Skin Product
Use Treatment of minimally to moderately thick actinic keratoses (grade 1 or 2) of the face or scalp; to be used in conjunction with blue light illumination
Unlabeled Use Photodynamic treatment of low-risk superficial basal cell skin cancer and low-risk squamous cell skin cancer *in situ* (Bowen's disease)

Dosage
Geriatric & Adult Actinic keratoses: Topical: Apply to actinic keratoses (**not** perilesional skin) followed 14-18 hours later by blue light illumination. Application/treatment may be repeated at a treatment site (once) after 8 weeks.
Special Geriatric Considerations Complaints by elderly with skin lesions increase with age. Common skin lesions are actinic keratoses, squamous cell carcinoma, and basal cell carcinoma. Although other agents for treatment are commonly used for these diseases, this agent is an alternative agent.
Dosage Forms Excipient information presented when available (limited, particularly for generics); consult specific product labeling.
Powder for solution, topical, as hydrochloride:
  Levulan® Kerastick®: 20% (6s) [contains ethanol 48% (in diluent); supplied with diluent]

◆ **Amino Levulinic Acid** *see* Aminolevulinic Acid *on page 91*
◆ **5-Aminolevulinic Acid** *see* Aminolevulinic Acid *on page 91*
◆ **Aminolevulinic Acid Hydrochloride** *see* Aminolevulinic Acid *on page 91*

Aminophylline (am in OFF i lin)

Medication Safety Issues
Sound-alike/look-alike issues:
  Aminophylline may be confused with amitriptyline, ampicillin
Brand Names: Canada Aminophylline Injection; JAA-Aminophylline
Index Terms Theophylline Ethylenediamine
Generic Availability (U.S.) Yes: Excludes tablet
Pharmacologic Category Phosphodiesterase Enzyme Inhibitor, Nonselective
Use Treatment of symptoms and reversible airway obstruction due to asthma or other chronic lung diseases (eg, emphysema, chronic bronchitis)

Note: The National Heart, Lung, and Blood Institute Guidelines (2007) do not recommend aminophylline I.V. for the treatment of asthma exacerbations.
Unlabeled Use Reversal of adenosine-, dipyridamole-, or regadenoson-induced adverse reactions (eg, angina, hypotension) during nuclear cardiac stress testing
Contraindications Hypersensitivity to theophylline, ethylenediamine, or any component of the formulation

Canadian labeling: Additional contraindications (not in U.S. labeling): Coronary artery disease where cardiac stimulation might prove harmful; patients with peptic ulcer disease
Warnings/Precautions If a patient develops signs and symptoms of theophylline toxicity, a serum level should be measured and subsequent doses held. Theophylline clearance may be decreased in patients with acute pulmonary edema, congestive heart failure, cor pulmonale, fever, hepatic disease, acute hepatitis, cirrhosis, hypothyroidism, sepsis with multiorgan failure, and shock; clearance may also be decreased in the elderly >60 years of age and patients following cessation of smoking. Due to potential saturation of theophylline clearance at serum levels within (or in some patients less than) the therapeutic range, dosage adjustment should be made in small increments (maximum: 25% dose increase). Due to wide interpatient variability, theophylline serum level measurements must be used to optimize therapy and prevent serious toxicity. Use caution with peptic ulcer (use is contraindicated in the Canadian labeling), hyperthyroidism, seizure disorder, hypertension, or tachyarrhythmias.
Adverse Reactions (Reflective of adult population; not specific for elderly) Frequency not defined. Adverse events observed at therapeutic serum levels:
Cardiovascular: Flutter, tachycardia
Central nervous system: Behavior alterations (children), headache, insomnia, irritability, restlessness, seizures
Dermatologic: Allergic skin reactions, exfoliative dermatitis
Gastrointestinal: Diarrhea, nausea, vomiting
Neuromuscular & skeletal: Tremor
Renal: Diuresis (transient)
Drug Interactions
Metabolism/Transport Effects Substrate of CYP1A2 (major); **Note:** Assignment of Major/Minor substrate status based on clinically relevant drug interaction potential
Avoid Concomitant Use
  Avoid concomitant use of Aminophylline with any of the following: Iobenguane I 123
Increased Effect/Toxicity
  Aminophylline may increase the levels/effects of: Formoterol; Indacaterol; Pancuronium; Sympathomimetics

The levels/effects of Aminophylline may be increased by: Abiraterone Acetate; Allopurinol; Antithyroid Agents; AtoMOXetine; Cannabinoids; Cimetidine; Contraceptives (Estrogens); CYP1A2 Inhibitors (Moderate); CYP1A2 Inhibitors (Strong); Deferasirox; Disulfiram; Febuxostat; FluvoxaMINE; Interferons; Isoniazid; Linezolid; Macrolide Antibiotics; Methotrexate; Mexiletine; Pentoxifylline; Propafenone; QuiNINE; Quinolone Antibiotics; Thiabendazole; Ticlopidine; Zafirlukast

Decreased Effect

Aminophylline may decrease the levels/effects of: Adenosine; Benzodiazepines; CarBAMazepine; Fosphenytoin; Iobenguane I 123; Lithium; Pancuronium; Phenytoin; Regadenoson; Zafirlukast

The levels/effects of Aminophylline may be decreased by: Aminoglutethimide; Barbiturates; Beta-Blockers (Beta1 Selective); Beta-Blockers (Nonselective); CarBAMazepine; CYP1A2 Inducers (Strong); Cyproterone; Fosphenytoin; Isoproterenol; Phenytoin; Protease Inhibitors; Thyroid Products

Ethanol/Nutrition/Herb Interactions Food: Food does not appreciably affect absorption. Avoid extremes of dietary protein and carbohydrate intake. Changes in diet may affect the elimination of theophylline; charcoal-broiled foods may increase elimination, reducing half-life by 50%. Ethanol may decrease theophylline clearance.

Stability

Solution: Vials should be stored at room temperature of 20°C to 25°C (68°F to 77°F). Protect from light. Do not use solutions if discolored or if crystals are present.

Tablet: Store at room temperature of 20°C to 25°C (68°F to 77°F). Protect from light and moisture.

Mechanism of Action Causes bronchodilatation, diuresis, CNS and cardiac stimulation, and gastric acid secretion by blocking phosphodiesterase which increases tissue concentrations of cyclic adenine monophosphate (cAMP) which in turn promote catecholamine stimulation of lipolysis, glycogenolysis, and gluconeogenesis and induce release of epinephrine from adrenal medulla cells

Pharmacodynamics/Kinetics

Theophylline:

Absorption: Oral: Immediate release tablet: Rapid and complete

Distribution: 0.45 L/kg based on ideal body weight

Protein binding: 40%, primarily to albumin

Metabolism: Adults: Hepatic; involves CYP1A2, 2E1, and 3A4; forms active metabolites (caffeine and 3-methylxanthine)

Half-life elimination: Highly variable and dependent upon age, liver function, cardiac function, lung disease, and smoking history

Adults 16-60 years with asthma, nonsmoking, otherwise healthy: 8.7 hours (range: 6.1-12.8 hours)

Time to peak, serum:

Oral: Immediate release tablet: 1-2 hours; Sustained release tablet (Canadian labeling; not available in U.S.): 4-5 hours

I.V.: Within 30 minutes

Excretion: Adults: Urine (10% as unchanged drug)

Dosage

Geriatric Adults >60 years: Refer to adult dosing. Do not exceed a dose of aminophylline 507 mg/day (equivalent to theophylline 400 mg/day)

Adult Note: Doses should be individualized based on peak serum concentrations and should be based on ideal body weight. Theophylline dose is 80% of aminophylline dose.

Acute symptoms: Loading dose: Oral, I.V.:

Patients **not currently receiving** aminophylline or theophylline: Aminophylline 5.7 mg/kg (equivalent to theophylline 4.6 mg/kg) administered I.V. or theophylline 5 mg/kg administered orally.

Patients **currently receiving** aminophylline or theophylline: A loading dose is not recommended without first obtaining a serum theophylline concentration in patients who have received aminophylline or theophylline within the past 24 hours. The loading dose should be calculated as follows:

Dose = (desired serum theophylline concentration - measured serum theophylline concentration) (V_d)

Acute symptoms: Maintenance dose: I.V.: **Note:** To achieve a target theophylline concentration of 10 mcg/mL unless otherwise noted. Lower initial doses may be required in patients with reduced theophylline clearance. Dosage should be adjusted according to serum level measurements during the first 12- to 24-hour period.

Adults 16-60 years (otherwise healthy, nonsmokers): 0.51 mg/kg/hour (equivalent to theophylline 0.4 mg/kg/hour); maximum: 900 mg/day unless serum levels indicate need for larger dose

Adults >60 years: 0.38 mg/kg/hour (equivalent to theophylline 0.3 mg/kg/hour); maximum: 400 mg/day unless serum levels indicate need for larger dose

Dosage adjustment for cardiac decompensation, cor pulmonale, hepatic dysfunction, sepsis with multiorgan failure, shock: 0.25 mg/kg hour (equivalent to theophylline 0.2 mg/kg/hour); maximum: 400 mg/day unless serum levels indicate need for larger dose

Dosage adjustment after serum theophylline measurement:

Within normal limits: Asthma: 5-15 mcg/mL: Maintain dosage if tolerated. Recheck serum theophylline concentration at 24-hour intervals (for acute I.V. dosing) or at 6- to 12-month intervals (for oral dosing). Finer adjustments in dosage may be needed for some patients. If levels ≥15 mcg/mL, consider 10% dose reduction to improve safety margin.

Too high:

20-24.9 mcg/mL: Decrease dose by ~25%. Recheck serum theophylline concentrations (see "**Note**").

25-30 mcg/mL: Skip next dose (oral) or stop infusion for 24 hours and decrease subsequent doses by ~25%. Recheck serum theophylline concentrations (see "**Note**").

>30 mcg/mL: Stop dosing and treat overdose; if resumed, decrease subsequent doses by 50%. Recheck serum theophylline concentrations (see "**Note**").

Too low: <9.9 mcg/mL: If tolerated, but symptoms remain, increase dose by ~25%. Recheck serum theophylline concentrations (see "**Note**").

Note: Recheck serum theophylline levels after 3 days when using oral dosing, or after 24 hours when dosing intravenously. Patients maintained with oral therapy may be reassessed at 6- to 12-month intervals.

Chronic conditions: Oral:

Immediate release tablets: **Note:** Increase dose only if tolerated. Consider lowering dose or using a slower titration if caffeine-like adverse events occur. Smaller doses given more frequently may be used in patients with a more rapid metabolism to prevent breakthrough symptoms which could occur due to low trough concentration prior to the next dose.

Adults 16-60 years **without** risk factors for impaired theophylline clearance:

Aminophylline 380 mg/day (equivalent to theophylline 300 mg/day) in divided doses every 6-8 hours for 3 days;

Then increase to 507 mg/day (equivalent to theophylline 400 mg/day) in divided doses every 6-8 hours for 3 days

Maintenance dose: 760 mg/day (equivalent to theophylline 600 mg/day) in divided doses every 6-8 hours

Dose adjustment in patients **with** risk factors for impaired theophylline clearance and patients in whom monitoring serum theophylline levels is not feasible: Do not exceed a dose of aminophylline 507 mg/day (equivalent to theophylline 400 mg/day)

Sustained release tablets: Canadian labeling: Initial: 1 tablet (225-350 mg) every 12 hours (equivalent to theophylline 182.25-283.5 mg every 12 hours); may increase dose by 1/2 tablet per dose at 3- to 4-day intervals; maximum dose: 1125 mg/day (equivalent to theophylline 900 mg/day); do not exceed maximum dose without monitoring theophylline concentrations.

Reversal of adenosine-, dipyridamole-, or regadenoson-induced adverse reactions (eg, angina, hypotension) during nuclear cardiac stress testing (unlabeled use): I.V.: 50-250 mg administered over 30-60 seconds, repeat as necessary. **Note:** Since adenosine-induced side effects are short lived after discontinuation of the infusion, aminophylline administration is only very rarely required.

Administration

I.M.: Not recommended

I.V.: Loading doses should be administered I.V. over 30 minutes. Infusion rate should not exceed 21 mg/hour (equivalent to theophylline 17 mg/hour) in patients with cor pulmonale, cardiac decompensation, liver dysfunction, patients >60 years of age, or patients taking medications which reduce theophylline clearance.

For reversal of adenosine-, dipyridamole-, or regadenoson-induced adverse events during nuclear cardiac stress testing, administer I.V. undiluted over 30-60 seconds, repeat as necessary. Since adenosine-induced side effects are short lived after discontinuation of the infusion, aminophylline administration is only very rarely required.

Tablet: If dose is missed, administer the next dose at the scheduled time (do not make up missed dose).

Monitoring Parameters Monitor heart rate; CNS effects (insomnia, irritability); respiratory rate (COPD patients often have resting controlled respiratory rates in low 20s); arterial or capillary blood gases (if applicable)

Theophylline levels: Serum theophylline levels should be monitored prior to making dose increases; in the presence of signs or symptoms of toxicity; or when a new illness, worsening of a present illness, or medication changes occur that may change theophylline clearance

I.V. loading dose: Measure serum concentrations 30 minutes after the end of an I.V. loading dose

I.V. infusion: Measure serum concentrations one half-life after starting a continuous infusion, then every 12-24 hours

Reference Range
Therapeutic levels: Asthma: 5-15 mcg/mL (peak level)
Toxic concentration: >20 mcg/mL

Test Interactions Plasma glucose, uric acid, free fatty acids, total cholesterol, HDL, HDL/LDL ratio, and urinary free cortisol excretion may be increased by theophylline. Theophylline may decrease triiodothyronine.

Pharmacotherapy Pearls 100 mg aminophylline = 79 mg theophylline
Older adults, the acutely ill, and patients with severe respiratory problems, pulmonary edema, or liver dysfunction are at greater risk of toxicity because of reduced drug clearance.

Special Geriatric Considerations Although there is a great intersubject variability for half-lives of methylxanthines (2-10 hours), elderly, as a group, have slower hepatic clearance. Therefore, use lower initial doses and monitor closely for response and adverse reactions. Additionally, elderly patients are at greater risk for toxicity due to concomitant disease (eg, congestive heart failure, arrhythmias), and drug use (eg, cimetidine, ciprofloxacin, etc).

Dosage Forms Excipient information presented when available (limited, particularly for generics); consult specific product labeling. [DSC] = Discontinued product
Injection, solution, as dihydrate: 25 mg/mL (10 mL, 20 mL)
Injection, solution, as dihydrate [preservative free]: 25 mg/mL (10 mL, 20 mL)
Tablet, oral, as dihydrate: 100 mg [DSC], 200 mg [DSC]

Dosage Forms: Canada Excipient information presented when available (limited, particularly for generics); consult specific product labeling.
Injection, solution [preservative free]: 25 mg/mL (10 mL); 50 mg/mL (10 mL)
Tablet, oral: 100 mg

◆ **4-aminopyridine** *see* Dalfampridine *on page* 474
◆ **Aminosalicylate Sodium** *see* Aminosalicylic Acid *on page* 95

Aminosalicylic Acid (a mee noe sal i SIL ik AS id)

Related Information
Antimicrobial Drugs of Choice *on page* 2163

Brand Names: U.S. Paser®

Index Terms 4-Aminosalicylic Acid; Aminosalicylate Sodium; Para-Aminosalicylate Sodium; PAS; Sodium PAS

Generic Availability (U.S.) No

Pharmacologic Category Antitubercular Agent

Use Adjunctive treatment of tuberculosis used in combination with other antitubercular agents

Unlabeled Use Treatment of Crohn's disease

Dosage

Geriatric & Adult Tuberculosis: Oral: 8-12 g/day in 2-3 divided doses (**Note:** Studies have shown administration of 4 g twice daily is adequate to achieve the target serum concentration) (*MMWR*, 2003)

Renal Impairment No dosage adjustment provided in manufacturer's labeling; however, the following adjustments have been used by some clinicians:
Aronoff, 2007:
Cl_{cr} >50 mL/minute: No dosage adjustment necessary
Cl_{cr} 10-50 mL/minute: Administer 50% to 75% of dose
Cl_{cr} <10 mL/minute: Administer 50% of dose
Administer after hemodialysis: Administer 50% of dose
Continuous arteriovenous hemofiltration: Dose for Cl_{cr} <10 mL/minute
MMWR, 2003:
Cl_{cr} ≥30 mL/minute: No dosage adjustment necessary
Cl_{cr} <30 mL/minute: 4 g twice daily

Hepatic Impairment Use with caution

Special Geriatric Considerations The elderly may require a lower recommended dose due to age-related changes in renal function.

Dosage Forms Excipient information presented when available (limited, particularly for generics); consult specific product labeling.
Granules, delayed release, oral:
Paser®: 4 g/packet (30s) [sugar free]

◆ **4-Aminosalicylic Acid** *see* Aminosalicylic Acid *on page* 95
◆ **5-Aminosalicylic Acid** *see* Mesalamine *on page* 1217

♦ **Aminoxin® [OTC]** *see* Pyridoxine *on page 1640*

Amiodarone (a MEE oh da rone)

Related Information
  Beers Criteria − Potentially Inappropriate Medications for Geriatrics *on page 2183*
Medication Safety Issues
  Sound-alike/look-alike issues:
    Amiodarone may be confused with aMILoride, inamrinone
    Cordarone® may be confused with Cardura®, Cordran®
  High alert medication:
    The Institute for Safe Medication Practices (ISMP) includes this medication among its list of drugs which have a heightened risk of causing significant patient harm when used in error.
  BEERS Criteria medication:
    This drug may be potentially inappropriate for use in geriatric patients (Quality of evidence - high; Strength of recommendation - strong).
Brand Names: U.S. Cordarone®; Nexterone®; Pacerone®
Brand Names: Canada Amiodarone Hydrochloride Injection; Apo-Amiodarone®; Ava-Amiodarone; Cordarone®; Dom-Amiodarone; Mylan-Amiodarone; PHL-Amiodarone; PMS-Amiodarone; PRO-Amiodarone; ratio-Amiodarone; Riva-Amiodarone; Sandoz-Amiodarone; Teva-Amiodarone
Index Terms Amiodarone Hydrochloride
Generic Availability (U.S.) Yes
Pharmacologic Category Antiarrhythmic Agent, Class III
Use Management of life-threatening recurrent ventricular fibrillation (VF) or hemodynamically-unstable ventricular tachycardia (VT) refractory to other antiarrhythmic agents or in patients intolerant of other agents used for these conditions
Unlabeled Use
  Atrial fibrillation (AF): Pharmacologic conversion of AF to and maintenance of normal sinus rhythm; treatment of AF in patients with heart failure [no accessory pathway] who require heart rate control (ACC/AHA/ESC Practice Guidelines) or in patients with hypertrophic cardiomyopathy (ACCF/AHA Practice Guidelines); prevention of postoperative AF associated with cardiothoracic surgery
  Paroxysmal supraventricular tachycardia (SVT) (not initial drug of choice)
  Ventricular tachyarrhythmias (ACLS/PALS guidelines): Cardiac arrest with persistent VT or VF if defibrillation, CPR, and vasopressor administration have failed; control of hemodynamically-stable monomorphic VT, polymorphic VT with a normal baseline QT interval, or wide-complex tachycardia of uncertain origin; control of rapid ventricular rate due to accessory pathway conduction in pre-excited atrial arrhythmias (ACLS guidelines) or stable narrow-complex tachycardia (ACLS guidelines)
    Adjunct to ICD therapy to suppress symptomatic ventricular tachyarrhythmias in otherwise optimally-treated patients with heart failure (ACC/AHA/ESC Practice Guidelines)
Medication Guide Available Yes
Contraindications Hypersensitivity to amiodarone, iodine, or any component of the formulation; severe sinus-node dysfunction; second- and third-degree heart block (except in patients with a functioning artificial pacemaker); bradycardia causing syncope (except in patients with a functioning artificial pacemaker); cardiogenic shock
Warnings/Precautions **[U.S. Boxed Warning]: Only indicated for patients with life-threatening arrhythmias because of risk of toxicity. Alternative therapies should be tried first before using amiodarone. Patients should be hospitalized when amiodarone is initiated.** Currently, the 2005 ACLS guidelines recommend I.V. amiodarone as the preferred antiarrhythmic for the treatment of pulseless VT/VF, both life-threatening arrhythmias. In patients with non-life-threatening arrhythmias (eg, atrial fibrillation), amiodarone should be used only if the use of other antiarrhythmics has proven ineffective or are contraindicated.

[U.S. Boxed Warning]: Lung damage (abnormal diffusion capacity) may occur without symptoms. Monitor for pulmonary toxicity. Evaluate new respiratory symptoms; pre-existing pulmonary disease does not increase risk of developing pulmonary toxicity, but if pulmonary toxicity develops then the prognosis is worse. The lowest effective dose should be used as appropriate for the acuity/severity of the arrhythmia being treated. **[U.S. Boxed Warning]: Liver toxicity is common, but usually mild with evidence of increased liver enzymes. Severe liver toxicity can occur and has been fatal in a few cases.**

[U.S. Boxed Warning]: Amiodarone can exacerbate arrhythmias, by making them more difficult to tolerate or reverse; other types of arrhythmias have occurred, including significant heart block, sinus bradycardia new ventricular fibrillation, incessant ventricular tachycardia, increased resistance to cardioversion, and polymorphic ventricular tachycardia associated with QT_c prolongation (torsade de pointes [TdP]). Risk may be increased with concomitant use of other antiarrhythmic agents or drugs that prolong the QT_c interval. Proarrhythmic effects may be prolonged.

Monitor pacing or defibrillation thresholds in patients with implantable cardiac devices (eg, pacemakers, defibrillators). Use very cautiously and with close monitoring in patients with thyroid or liver disease. May cause hyper- or hypothyroidism. Hyperthyroidism may result in thyrotoxicosis and may aggravate or cause breakthrough arrhythmias. If any new signs of arrhythmia appear, hyperthyroidism should be considered. Thyroid function should be monitored prior to treatment and periodically thereafter.

May cause optic neuropathy and/or optic neuritis, usually resulting in visual impairment. Corneal microdeposits occur in a majority of patients, and may cause visual disturbances in some patients (blurred vision, halos); these are not generally considered a reason to discontinue treatment. Corneal refractive laser surgery is generally contraindicated in amiodarone users. Avoid excessive exposure to sunlight; may cause photosensitivity.

Amiodarone is a potent inhibitor of CYP enzymes and transport proteins (including p-glycoprotein), which may lead to increased serum concentrations/toxicity of a number of medications. Particular caution must be used when a drug with QT_c-prolonging potential relies on metabolism via these enzymes, since the effect of elevated concentrations may be additive with the effect of amiodarone. Carefully assess risk:benefit of coadministration of other drugs which may prolong QT_c interval. Patients may still be at risk for amiodarone–related drug interactions after the drug has been discontinued. The pharmacokinetics are complex (due to prolonged duration of action and half-life) and difficult to predict. Correct electrolyte disturbances, especially hypokalemia or hypomagnesemia, prior to use and throughout therapy. Use caution when initiating amiodarone in patients on warfarin. Cases of increased INR with or without bleeding have occurred in patients treated with warfarin; monitor INR closely after initiating amiodarone in these patients.

In the treatment of atrial fibrillation in older adults, avoid antiarrhythmics as first-line treatment. In older adults, data suggests rate control may provide more benefits than risks compared to rhythm control for most patients (Beers Criteria).

May cause hypotension and bradycardia (infusion-rate related). Hypotension with rapid administration has been attributed to the emulsifier polysorbate 80. Commercially-prepared premixed solutions do not contain polysorbate 80 and may have a lower incidence of hypotension. Caution in surgical patients; may enhance hemodynamic effect of anesthetics; associated with increased risk of adult respiratory distress syndrome (ARDS) postoperatively. Vials for injection contain benzyl alcohol. Commercially-prepared premixed solutions do not contain benzyl alcohol. Commercially-prepared premixed infusion contains the excipient cyclodextrin (sulfobutyl ether beta-cyclodextrin), which may accumulate in patients with renal insufficiency.

Adverse Reactions (Reflective of adult population; not specific for elderly) In a recent meta-analysis, adult patients taking lower doses of amiodarone (152-330 mg daily for at least 12 months) were more likely to develop thyroid, neurologic, skin, ocular, and bradycardic abnormalities than those taking placebo (Vorperian, 1997). Pulmonary toxicity was similar in both the low-dose amiodarone group and in the placebo group, but there was a trend towards increased toxicity in the amiodarone group. Gastrointestinal and hepatic events were seen to a similar extent in both the low-dose amiodarone group and placebo group. As the frequency of adverse events varies considerably across studies as a function of route and dose, a consolidation of adverse event rates is provided by Goldschlager, 2000.

>10%:
  Cardiovascular: Hypotension (I.V. 16%, refractory in rare cases)
  Central nervous system (3% to 40%): Abnormal gait/ataxia, dizziness, fatigue, headache, malaise, impaired memory, involuntary movement, insomnia, poor coordination, peripheral neuropathy, sleep disturbances, tremor
  Dermatologic: Photosensitivity (10% to 75%)
  Endocrine & Metabolic: Hypothyroidism (1% to 22%)
  Gastrointestinal: Nausea, vomiting, anorexia, and constipation (10% to 33%)
  Hepatic: AST or ALT level >2x normal (15% to 50%)
  Ocular: Corneal microdeposits (>90%; causes visual disturbance in <10%)
1% to 10%:
  Cardiovascular: CHF (3%), bradycardia (3% to 5%), AV block (5%), conduction abnormalities, SA node dysfunction (1% to 3%), cardiac arrhythmia, flushing, edema. Additional effects associated with I.V. administration include asystole, atrial fibrillation, cardiac arrest, electromechanical dissociation, pulseless electrical activity (PEA), ventricular tachycardia, and cardiogenic shock.

Dermatologic: Slate blue skin discoloration (<10%)

Endocrine & metabolic: Hyperthyroidism (3% to 10%; more common in iodine-deficient regions of the world), libido decreased

Gastrointestinal: Abdominal pain, abnormal salivation, abnormal taste (oral), diarrhea, nausea (I.V.)

Hematologic: Coagulation abnormalities

Hepatic: Hepatitis and cirrhosis (<3%)

Local: Phlebitis (I.V., with concentrations >3 mg/mL)

Ocular: Visual disturbances (2% to 9%), halo vision (<5% occurring especially at night), optic neuritis (1%)

Respiratory: Pulmonary toxicity has been estimated to occur at a frequency between 2% and 7% of patients (some reports indicate a frequency as high as 17%). Toxicity may present as hypersensitivity pneumonitis; pulmonary fibrosis (cough, fever, malaise); pulmonary inflammation; interstitial pneumonitis; or alveolar pneumonitis. ARDS has been reported in up to 2% of patients receiving amiodarone, and postoperatively in patients receiving oral amiodarone.

Miscellaneous: Abnormal smell (oral)

Drug Interactions

Metabolism/Transport Effects Substrate of CYP1A2 (minor), CYP2C19 (minor), CYP2C8 (major), CYP2D6 (minor), CYP3A4 (major), P-glycoprotein; **Note:** Assignment of Major/Minor substrate status based on clinically relevant drug interaction potential; **Inhibits** CYP1A2 (weak), CYP2A6 (moderate), CYP2B6 (weak), CYP2C9 (moderate), CYP2D6 (moderate), CYP3A4 (moderate), P-glycoprotein

Avoid Concomitant Use

Avoid concomitant use of Amiodarone with any of the following: Agalsidase Alfa; Agalsidase Beta; Conivaptan; Fingolimod; Grapefruit Juice; Highest Risk QTc-Prolonging Agents; Mifepristone; Moderate Risk QTc-Prolonging Agents; Propafenone; Protease Inhibitors; Silodosin; Tolvaptan; Topotecan

Increased Effect/Toxicity

Amiodarone may increase the levels/effects of: Antiarrhythmic Agents (Class Ia); ARIPiprazole; Avanafil; Beta-Blockers; Budesonide (Systemic, Oral Inhalation); Cardiac Glycosides; Colchicine; CycloSPORINE; CycloSPORINE (Systemic); CYP2A6 Substrates; CYP2C9 Substrates; CYP2D6 Substrates; CYP3A4 Substrates; Dabigatran Etexilate; Eplerenone; Everolimus; FentaNYL; Fesoterodine; Flecainide; Fosphenytoin; Highest Risk QTc-Prolonging Agents; HMG-CoA Reductase Inhibitors; Ivacaftor; Lidocaine; Lidocaine (Systemic); Lidocaine (Topical); Loratadine; Lurasidone; P-glycoprotein/ABCB1 Substrates; Phenytoin; Pimecrolimus; Porfimer; Propafenone; Prucalopride; Rivaroxaban; Salmeterol; Saxagliptin; Silodosin; Tolvaptan; Topotecan; Vilazodone; Vitamin K Antagonists

The levels/effects of Amiodarone may be increased by: Azithromycin; Azithromycin (Systemic); Boceprevir; Calcium Channel Blockers (Nondihydropyridine); Cimetidine; Conivaptan; CYP2C8 Inhibitors (Moderate); CYP2C8 Inhibitors (Strong); CYP3A4 Inhibitors (Moderate); CYP3A4 Inhibitors (Strong); Deferasirox; EriBULin; Fingolimod; Grapefruit Juice; Ivacaftor; Lidocaine (Topical); Mifepristone; Moderate Risk QTc-Prolonging Agents; P-glycoprotein/ABCB1 Inhibitors; Propafenone; Protease Inhibitors; QTc-Prolonging Agents (Indeterminate Risk and Risk Modifying); Telaprevir

Decreased Effect

Amiodarone may decrease the levels/effects of: Agalsidase Alfa; Agalsidase Beta; Clopidogrel; Codeine; Ifosfamide; Sodium Iodide I131; TraMADol

The levels/effects of Amiodarone may be decreased by: Bile Acid Sequestrants; CYP2C8 Inducers (Strong); CYP3A4 Inducers (Strong); Deferasirox; Etravirine; Fosphenytoin; Grapefruit Juice; Herbs (CYP3A4 Inducers); Orlistat; Peginterferon Alfa-2b; P-glycoprotein/ABCB1 Inducers; Phenytoin; Rifamycin Derivatives; Tocilizumab

Ethanol/Nutrition/Herb Interactions

Food: Increases the rate and extent of absorption of amiodarone. Grapefruit juice increases bioavailability of oral amiodarone by 50% and decreases the conversion of amiodarone to N-DEA (active metabolite); altered effects are possible. Management: Take consistently with regard to meals; grapefruit juice should be avoided during therapy.

Herb/Nutraceutical: St John's wort may decrease amiodarone levels or enhance photosensitization. Ephedra may worsen arrythmia. Management: Avoid St John's wort, ephedra and dong quai.

Stability Store undiluted vials and premixed solutions at 20°C to 25°C (68°F to 77°F). Protect from light.

Vials for injection: When admixed in D_5W to a final concentration of 1-6 mg/mL, the solution is stable at room temperature for 24 hours in polyolefin or glass, or for 2 hours in PVC. Infusions >2 hours must be administered in a non-PVC container (eg, glass or polyolefin). Do not use evacuated glass containers; buffer may cause precipitation.

Mechanism of Action Class III antiarrhythmic agent which inhibits adrenergic stimulation (alpha- and beta-blocking properties), affects sodium, potassium, and calcium channels, prolongs the action potential and refractory period in myocardial tissue; decreases AV conduction and sinus node function

Pharmacodynamics/Kinetics

Absorption: Slow and variable

Onset of action: Oral: 2 days to 3 weeks; I.V.: May be more rapid
  Peak effect: 1 week to 5 months

Duration after discontinuing therapy: 7-50 days

Distribution: V_d: 66 L/kg (range: 18-148 L/kg)

Protein binding: 96%

Metabolism: Hepatic via CYP2C8 and 3A4 to active N-desethylamiodarone metabolite; possible enterohepatic recirculation

Bioavailability: Oral: 35% to 65%

Half-life elimination: Terminal: 40-55 days (range: 26-107 days)

Time to peak, serum: 3-7 hours

Excretion: Feces; urine (<1% as unchanged drug)

Dosage

Geriatric Refer to adult dosing. No specific guidelines available. Dose selection should be cautious, at low end of dosage range, and titration should be slower to evaluate response. Although not supported by clinical evidence, a maintenance dose of 100 mg/day is commonly used especially for the elderly or patients with low body mass (Fuster, 2006; Zimetbaum, 2007).

Adult Note: Lower loading and maintenance doses are preferable in women and all patients with low body weight.

Atrial fibrillation pharmacologic cardioversion (ACC/AHA/ESC Practice Guidelines) (unlabeled use):

Oral: *Inpatient:* 1.2-1.8 g/day in divided doses until 10 g total, then 200-400 mg/day maintenance. *Outpatient:* 600-800 mg/day in divided doses until 10 g total, then 200-400 mg/day maintenance; although not supported by clinical evidence, a maintenance dose of 100 mg/day is commonly used especially for the elderly or patients with low body mass (Fuster, 2006; Zimetbaum, 2007). **Note:** Other regimens have been described and may be used clinically:
  400 mg 3 times/day for 5-7 days, then 400 mg/day for 1 month, then 200 mg/day
  or
  10 mg/kg/day for 14 days, followed by 300 mg/day for 4 weeks, followed by maintenance dosage of 200 mg/day (Roy, 2000)

I.V.: 5-7 mg/kg over 30-60 minutes, then 1.2-1.8 g/day continuous infusion or in divided oral doses until 10 g total. Maintenance: See oral dosing.

Atrial fibrillation prophylaxis following open heart surgery (unlabeled use): Note: A variety of regimens have been used in clinical trials, including oral and intravenous regimens:

Oral: Starting in postop recovery, 400 mg twice daily for up to 7 days. Alternative regimen of amiodarone: 600 mg/day for 7 days prior to surgery, followed by 200 mg/day until hospital discharge, has also been shown to decrease the risk of postoperative atrial fibrillation.

I.V.: Starting at postop recovery, 1000 mg infused over 24 hours for 2 days has been shown to reduce the risk of postoperative atrial fibrillation.

Recurrent atrial fibrillation (unlabeled use): No standard regimen defined; examples of regimens include: Oral: Initial: 10 mg/kg/day for 14 days; followed by 300 mg/day for 4 weeks, followed by maintenance dosage of 200 mg/day (Roy, 2000). Other regimens have been described and are used clinically (ie, 400 mg 3 times/day for 5-7 days, then 400 mg/day for 1 month, then 200 mg/day).

Ventricular arrhythmias: Oral: 800-1600 mg/day in 1-2 doses for 1-3 weeks, then when adequate arrhythmia control is achieved, decrease to 600-800 mg/day in 1-2 doses for 1 month; maintenance: 400 mg/day; lower doses are recommended for supraventricular arrhythmias.

Pulseless VT or VF (ACLS, 2010): I.V. push, I.O.: Initial: 300 mg rapid bolus; if pulseless VT or VF continues after subsequent defibrillation attempt or recurs, administer supplemental dose of 150 mg. **Note:** In this setting, administering **undiluted** is preferred (Dager, 2006; Skrifvars, 2004). *The Handbook of Emergency Cardiovascular Care* (Hazinski, 2010) and the 2010 ACLS guidelines, do not make any specific recommendations regarding dilution of amiodarone in this setting. Experience limited with I.O. administration of amiodarone (ACLS, 2010).

Upon return of spontaneous circulation, follow with an infusion of 1 mg/minute for 6 hours, then 0.5 mg/minute for 18 hours (mean daily doses >2.1 g/day have been associated with hypotension).

Stable VT or SVT (unlabeled use): First 24 hours: 1050 mg according to following regimen
Step 1: 150 mg (100 mL) over first 10 minutes (mix 3 mL in 100 mL D_5W)
Step 2: 360 mg (200 mL) over next 6 hours (mix 18 mL in 500 mL D_5W): 1 mg/minute
Step 3: 540 mg (300 mL) over next 18 hours: 0.5 mg/minute
Note: After the first 24 hours: 0.5 mg/minute utilizing concentration of 1-6 mg/mL
Breakthrough stable VT or SVT: 150 mg supplemental doses in 100 mL D_5W or NS over 10 minutes (mean daily doses >2.1 g/day have been associated with hypotension)

I.V. to oral therapy conversion: Use the following as a guide:
<1-week I.V. infusion: 800-1600 mg/day
1- to 3-week I.V. infusion: 600-800 mg/day
>3-week I.V. infusion: 400 mg
Note: Conversion from I.V. to oral therapy has not been formally evaluated. Some experts recommend a 1-2 day overlap when converting from I.V. to oral therapy especially when treating ventricular arrhythmias.

Recommendations for conversion to intravenous amiodarone after oral administration: During long-term amiodarone therapy (ie, ≥4 months), the mean plasma-elimination half-life of the active metabolite of amiodarone is 61 days. Replacement therapy may not be necessary in such patients if oral therapy is discontinued for a period <2 weeks, since any changes in serum amiodarone concentrations during this period may **not** be clinically significant.

Renal Impairment No dosage adjustment necessary.
Hemodialysis: Not dialyzable (0% to 5%); supplemental dose is not necessary
Peritoneal dialysis: Not dialyzable (0% to 5%); supplemental dose is not necessary
Hepatic Impairment Dosage adjustment is probably necessary in substantial hepatic impairment. No specific guidelines available. If hepatic enzymes exceed 3 times normal or double in a patient with an elevated baseline, consider decreasing the dose or discontinuing amiodarone.

Administration
Oral: Administer consistently with regard to meals. Take in divided doses with meals if GI upset occurs or if taking large daily dose. If GI intolerance occurs with single-dose therapy, use twice daily dosing.
I.V.: For infusions >1 hour, use concentrations ≤2 mg/mL unless a central venous catheter is used; commercially-prepared premixed solutions in concentrations of 1.5 mg/mL and 1.8 mg/mL are available. Use only volumetric infusion pump; use of drop counting may lead to underdosage. Administer through an I.V. line located as centrally as possible. For continuous infusions, an in-line filter has been recommended during administration to reduce the incidence of phlebitis. During pulseless VT/VF, administering **undiluted** is preferred (Dager, 2006; Skrifvars, 2004). *The Handbook of Emergency Cardiovascular Care* (Hazinski, 2010) and the 2010 ACLS guidelines do not make any specific recommendations regarding dilution of amiodarone in this setting.
Adjust administration rate to urgency (give more slowly when perfusing arrhythmia present). Slow the infusion rate if hypotension or bradycardia develops. Infusions >2 hours must be administered in a non-PVC container (eg, glass or polyolefin). PVC tubing is recommended for administration regardless of infusion duration. **Note:** I.V. administration at lower flow rates (potentially associated with use in pediatrics) and higher concentrations than recommended may result in leaching of plasticizers (DEHP) from intravenous tubing. DEHP may adversely affect male reproductive tract development. Alternative means of dosing and administration (1 mg/kg aliquots) may need to be considered.
Monitoring Parameters Blood pressure, heart rate (ECG) and rhythm throughout therapy; assess patient for signs of lethargy, edema of the hands or feet, weight loss, and pulmonary toxicity (baseline pulmonary function tests and chest X-ray; continue monitoring chest X-ray annually during therapy); liver function tests (semiannually); monitor serum electrolytes, especially potassium and magnesium. Assess thyroid function tests before initiation of treatment and then periodically thereafter (some experts suggest every 3-6 months). If signs or symptoms of thyroid disease or arrhythmia breakthrough/exacerbation occur then immediate re-evaluation is necessary. Amiodarone partially inhibits the peripheral conversion of thyroxine (T_4) to triiodothyronine (T_3); serum T_4 and reverse triiodothyronine (rT_3) concentrations may be increased and serum T_3 may be decreased; most patients remain clinically euthyroid, however, clinical hypothyroidism or hyperthyroidism may occur.

Perform regular ophthalmic exams.

Patients with implantable cardiac devices: Monitor pacing or defibrillation thresholds with initiation of amiodarone and during treatment.
Reference Range Therapeutic: 0.5-2.5 mg/L (SI: 1-4 micromole/L) (parent); desethyl metabolite is active and is present in equal concentration to parent drug

Special Geriatric Considerations Information describing the clinical use and pharmacokinetics in the elderly is lacking; however, the elderly may be predisposed to toxicity. Half-life may be prolonged due to decreased clearance; monitor closely. It is recommended to start dosing at the lower end of the dosing range. Elderly patients may be predisposed to toxicity due to reduced renal, hepatic, or cardiac function. It is recommended to monitor thyroid function (TSH) quarterly for those elderly taking amiodarone for extended periods.

This medication is considered to be potentially inappropriate in this patient population (Beers Criteria: Quality of evidence - high; Strength of recommendation - strong).

Dosage Forms Excipient information presented when available (limited, particularly for generics); consult specific product labeling.

Infusion, premixed iso-osmotic dextrose solution, as hydrochloride:

Nexterone®: 150 mg (100 mL); 360 mg (200 mL) [contains cyclodextrin]

Injection, solution, as hydrochloride: 50 mg/mL (3 mL, 9 mL, 18 mL)

Tablet, oral, as hydrochloride: 200 mg, 400 mg

Cordarone®: 200 mg [scored]

Pacerone®: 100 mg

Pacerone®: 200 mg, 400 mg [scored]

◆ **Amiodarone Hydrochloride** *see* Amiodarone *on page 96*

◆ **Amitiza®** *see* Lubiprostone *on page 1170*

Amitriptyline (a mee TRIP ti leen)

Related Information

Antidepressant Agents *on page 2097*

Beers Criteria – Potentially Inappropriate Medications for Geriatrics *on page 2183*

Medication Safety Issues

Sound-alike/look-alike issues:

Amitriptyline may be confused with aminophylline, imipramine, nortriptyline

Elavil® may be confused with Aldoril®, Eldepryl®, enalapril, Equanil®, Plavix®

BEERS Criteria medication:

This drug may be potentially inappropriate for use in geriatric patients (Quality of evidence - high [moderate for SIADH]; Strength of recommendation - strong).

Brand Names: Canada Bio-Amitriptyline; Dom-Amitriptyline; Elavil; Levate®; Novo-Triptyn; PMS-Amitriptyline

Index Terms Amitriptyline Hydrochloride; Elavil

Generic Availability (U.S.) Yes

Pharmacologic Category Antidepressant, Tricyclic (Tertiary Amine)

Use Relief of symptoms of depression

Unlabeled Use Analgesic for certain chronic and neuropathic pain (including diabetic neuropathy); prophylaxis against migraine headaches; post-traumatic stress disorder (PTSD)

Medication Guide Available Yes

Contraindications Hypersensitivity to amitriptyline or any component of the formulation (cross-sensitivity with other tricyclics may occur); use of MAO inhibitors within past 14 days; acute recovery phase following myocardial infarction; concurrent use of cisapride

Warnings/Precautions [U.S. Boxed Warning]: Antidepressants increase the risk of suicidal thinking and behavior in children, adolescents, and young adults (18-24 years of age) with major depressive disorder (MDD) and other psychiatric disorders; consider risk prior to prescribing. Short-term studies did not show an increased risk in patients >24 years of age and showed a decreased risk in patients ≥65 years. Closely monitor for clinical worsening, suicidality, or unusual changes in behavior; the patient's family or caregiver should be instructed to closely observe the patient and communicate condition with healthcare provider. Such observation would generally include at least weekly face-to-face contact with patients or their family members or caregivers during the first 4 weeks of treatment, then every other week visits for the next 4 weeks, then at 12 weeks, and as clinically indicated beyond 12 weeks. Additional contact by telephone may be appropriate between face-to-face visits. Adults treated with antidepressants should be observed similarly for clinical worsening and suicidality, especially during the initial few months of a course of drug therapy, or at times of dose changes, either increases or decreases. A medication guide should be dispensed with each prescription.

The possibility of a suicide attempt is inherent in major depression and may persist until remission occurs. Monitor for worsening of depression or suicidality, especially during initiation of therapy (generally first 1-2 months) or with dose increases or decreases. Worsening depression and severe abrupt suicidality that are not part of the presenting symptoms may require discontinuation or modification of drug therapy. The patient's family or caregiver should be alerted to monitor patients for the emergence of suicidality and associated behaviors (such as agitation, irritability, hostility, impulsivity, and hypomania) and notify healthcare provider.

May worsen psychosis in some patients or precipitate a shift to mania or hypomania in patients with bipolar disorder. Patients presenting with depressive symptoms should be screened for bipolar disorder. Monotherapy in patients with bipolar disorder should be avoided. **Amitriptyline is not FDA approved for bipolar depression.**

The degree of sedation, anticholinergic effects, orthostasis, and conduction abnormalities are high relative to other antidepressants. Amitriptyline often causes drowsiness/sedation, resulting in impaired performance of tasks requiring alertness (eg, operating machinery or driving). Sedative effects may be additive with other CNS depressants and/or ethanol. Use with caution in patients with a history of cardiovascular disease (including previous MI, stroke, tachycardia, or conduction abnormalities). Use with caution in patients with urinary retention, benign prostatic hyperplasia, narrow-angle glaucoma, xerostomia, visual problems, constipation, or a history of bowel obstruction.

TCAs may rarely cause bone marrow suppression; monitor for any signs of infection and obtain CBC if symptoms (eg, fever, sore throat) evident. May alter glucose control - use with caution in patients with diabetes. Consider discontinuing, when possible, prior to elective surgery. Therapy should not be abruptly discontinued in patients receiving high doses for prolonged periods. May lower seizure threshold - use caution in patients with a previous seizure disorder or condition predisposing to seizures such as brain damage, alcoholism, or concurrent therapy with other drugs which lower the seizure threshold. Hyperpyrexia has been observed with TCAs in combination with anticholinergics and/or neuroleptics, particularly during hot weather. May increase the risks associated with electroconvulsive therapy. Use with caution in hyperthyroid patients or those receiving thyroid supplementation. Use with caution in patients with hepatic or renal dysfunction. Avoid use in the elderly due to its potent anticholinergic and sedative properties, and potential to cause orthostatic hypotension. In addition, may cause or exacerbate syndrome of inappropriate antidiuretic hormone secretion or hyponatremia; monitor sodium closely with initiation or dosage adjustments in older adults (Beers Criteria).

Adverse Reactions (Reflective of adult population; not specific for elderly) Anticholinergic effects may be pronounced; moderate to marked sedation can occur (tolerance to these effects usually occurs).

Frequency not defined.

Cardiovascular: Orthostatic hypotension, tachycardia, ECG changes (nonspecific), AV conduction changes, cardiomyopathy (rare), MI, stroke, heart block, arrhythmia, syncope, hypertension, palpitation

Central nervous system: Restlessness, dizziness, insomnia, sedation, fatigue, anxiety, cognitive function (impaired), seizure, extrapyramidal symptoms, coma, hallucinations, confusion, disorientation, coordination impaired, ataxia, headache, nightmares, hyperpyrexia

Dermatologic: Allergic rash, urticaria, photosensitivity, alopecia

Endocrine & metabolic: Syndrome of inappropriate ADH secretion

Gastrointestinal: Weight gain, xerostomia, constipation, paralytic ileus, nausea, vomiting, anorexia, stomatitis, peculiar taste, diarrhea, black tongue

Genitourinary: Urinary retention

Hematologic: Bone marrow depression, purpura, eosinophilia

Neuromuscular & skeletal: Numbness, paresthesia, peripheral neuropathy, tremor, weakness

Ocular: Blurred vision, mydriasis, ocular pressure increased

Otic: Tinnitus

Miscellaneous: Diaphoresis, withdrawal reactions (nausea, headache, malaise)

Drug Interactions

Metabolism/Transport Effects Substrate of CYP1A2 (minor), CYP2B6 (minor), CYP2C19 (minor), CYP2C9 (minor), CYP2D6 (major), CYP3A4 (minor); **Note:** Assignment of Major/Minor substrate status based on clinically relevant drug interaction potential; **Inhibits** CYP1A2 (weak), CYP2C19 (weak), CYP2C9 (weak), CYP2D6 (weak), CYP2E1 (weak)

Avoid Concomitant Use

Avoid concomitant use of Amitriptyline with any of the following: Cisapride; Iobenguane I 123; MAO Inhibitors; Methylene Blue

Increased Effect/Toxicity

Amitriptyline may increase the levels/effects of: Alpha-/Beta-Agonists (Direct-Acting); Alpha1-Agonists; Amphetamines; Anticholinergics; Aspirin; Beta2-Agonists; Cisapride; Desmopressin; Highest Risk QTc-Prolonging Agents; Methylene Blue; Metoclopramide; Moderate Risk QTc-Prolonging Agents; NSAID (COX-2 Inhibitor); NSAID (Nonselective); QuiNIDine; Serotonin Modulators; Sodium Phosphates; Sulfonylureas; TraMADol; Vitamin K Antagonists; Yohimbine

The levels/effects of Amitriptyline may be increased by: Abiraterone Acetate; Altretamine; Antipsychotics; BuPROPion; Cimetidine; Cinacalcet; CYP2D6 Inhibitors (Moderate); CYP2D6 Inhibitors (Strong); Dexmethylphenidate; Divalproex; DULoxetine; Linezolid; Lithium; MAO Inhibitors; Methylphenidate; Metoclopramide; Metyrosine; Mifepristone; Pramlintide; Protease Inhibitors; QuiNIDine; Selective Serotonin Reuptake Inhibitors; Terbinafine; Terbinafine (Systemic); Valproic Acid

Decreased Effect

Amitriptyline may decrease the levels/effects of: Acetylcholinesterase Inhibitors (Central); Alpha2-Agonists; Iobenguane I 123

The levels/effects of Amitriptyline may be decreased by: Acetylcholinesterase Inhibitors (Central); Barbiturates; CarBAMazepine; Peginterferon Alfa-2b; St Johns Wort; Tocilizumab

Ethanol/Nutrition/Herb Interactions

Ethanol: May increase CNS depression; monitor for increased effects with coadministration. Caution patients about effects.

Food: Grapefruit juice may inhibit the metabolism of some TCAs and clinical toxicity may result.

Herb/Nutraceutical: St John's wort may decrease amitriptyline levels. Avoid valerian, St John's wort, kava kava, gotu kola (may increase CNS depression).

Mechanism of Action Increases the synaptic concentration of serotonin and/or norepinephrine in the central nervous system by inhibition of their reuptake by the presynaptic neuronal membrane

Pharmacodynamics/Kinetics

Onset of action: Migraine prophylaxis: 6 weeks, higher dosage may be required in heavy smokers because of increased metabolism; Depression: 4-6 weeks, reduce dosage to lowest effective level

Metabolism: Hepatic to nortriptyline (active), hydroxy and conjugated derivatives; may be impaired in the elderly

Half-life elimination: Adults: 9-27 hours (average: 15 hours)

Time to peak, serum: ~4 hours

Excretion: Urine (18% as unchanged drug); feces (small amounts)

Dosage

Geriatric Depression: Oral: Initial: 10-25 mg at bedtime; dose should be increased in 10-25 mg increments every week if tolerated; dose range: 25-150 mg/day. See Renal/Hepatic Impairment.

Adult

Depression: Oral: 50-150 mg/day single dose at bedtime or in divided doses; dose may be gradually increased up to 300 mg/day.

Chronic pain management (unlabeled use): Oral: Initial: 25 mg at bedtime; may increase as tolerated to 100 mg/day.

Diabetic neuropathy (unlabeled use): Oral: 25-100 mg/day (Bril, 2011)

Migraine prophylaxis (unlabeled use): Oral: Initial: 10-25 mg at bedtime; usual dose: 150 mg; reported dosing ranges: 10-400 mg/day

Post-traumatic stress disorder (PTSD) (unlabeled use): Oral: 75-200 mg/day

Renal Impairment Nondialyzable

Hepatic Impairment Use with caution and monitor plasma levels and patient response.

Monitoring Parameters Monitor blood pressure and pulse rate prior to and during initial therapy; evaluate mental status, suicide ideation (especially at the beginning of therapy or when doses are increased or decreased); ECG in older adults and patients with cardiac disease

Reference Range Therapeutic: Amitriptyline and nortriptyline 100-250 ng/mL (SI: 360-900 nmol/L); nortriptyline 50-150 ng/mL (SI: 190-570 nmol/L); Toxic: >0.5 mcg/mL; plasma levels do not always correlate with clinical effectiveness

Test Interactions May cause false-positive reaction to EMIT immunoassay for imipramine

Special Geriatric Considerations Not a drug of choice for the elderly. The most anticholinergic and sedating of the antidepressants; pronounced effects on the cardiovascular system (hypotension).

A systematic review and meta-analysis of antidepressant placebo-controlled trials in persons with depression and dementia found evidence "suggestive" of efficacy but not of sufficient strength to "confirm" efficacy. Antidepressant trials in this patient population are small and underpowered. Older patients with depression being treated with an antidepressant should be closely monitored for response and adverse effects. Treatment should be switched or augmented when response is inadequate with a therapeutic dose. Antidepressants that are not tolerated should be discontinued and an alternative agent should be started.

◄ This medication is considered to be potentially inappropriate in this patient population (Beers Criteria: Quality of evidence - high [moderate for SIADH]; Strength of recommendation - strong).

Dosage Forms Excipient information presented when available (limited, particularly for generics); consult specific product labeling.

Tablet, oral, as hydrochloride: 10 mg, 25 mg, 50 mg, 75 mg, 100 mg, 150 mg

◆ **Amitriptyline Hydrochloride** see Amitriptyline on page 101

AmLODIPine (am LOE di peen)

Related Information

Calcium Channel Blockers – Comparative Pharmacokinetics on page 2111

Medication Safety Issues

Sound-alike/look-alike issues:

AmLODIPine may be confused with aMILoride

Norvasc® may be confused with Navane®, Norvir®, Vascor®

International issues:

Norvasc [U.S., Canada, and multiple international markets] may be confused with Vascor brand name for imidapril [Philippines] and simvastatin [Malaysia, Singapore, and Thailand]

Brand Names: U.S. Norvasc®

Brand Names: Canada Accel-Amlodipine; Amlodipine-Odan; Apo-Amlodipine®; CO Amlodipine; Dom-Amlodipine; GD-Amlodipine; JAMP-Amlodipine; Manda-Amlodipine; Mint-Amlodipine; Mylan-Amlodipine; Norvasc®; PHL-Amlodipine; PMS-Amlodipine; Q-Amlodipine; RAN™-Amlodipine; ratio-Amlodipine; Riva-Amlodipine; Sandoz Amlodipine; Septa-Amlodipine; Teva-Amlodipine; ZYM-Amlodipine

Index Terms Amlodipine Besylate

Generic Availability (U.S.) Yes

Pharmacologic Category Antianginal Agent; Calcium Channel Blocker; Calcium Channel Blocker, Dihydropyridine

Use Treatment of hypertension; treatment of symptomatic chronic stable angina, vasospastic (Prinzmetal's) angina (confirmed or suspected); prevention of hospitalization due to angina with documented CAD (limited to patients without heart failure or ejection fraction <40%)

Contraindications Hypersensitivity to amlodipine or any component of the formulation

Warnings/Precautions Increased angina and/or MI has occurred with initiation or dosage titration of calcium channel blockers. Symptomatic hypotension with or without syncope can rarely occur; blood pressure must be lowered at a rate appropriate for the patient's clinical condition. Use caution in severe aortic stenosis and/or hypertrophic cardiomyopathy with outflow tract obstruction. Use caution in patients with hepatic impairment; may require lower starting dose; titrate slowly with severe hepatic impairment. The most common side effect is peripheral edema; occurs within 2-3 weeks of starting therapy. Reflex tachycardia may occur with use. Peak antihypertensive effect is delayed; dosage titration should occur after 7-14 days on a given dose. Initiate at a lower dose in the elderly.

Adverse Reactions (Reflective of adult population; not specific for elderly)

>10%: Cardiovascular: Peripheral edema (2% to 15% dose related); HF patients: 27% [Packer, 1996])

1% to 10%:

Cardiovascular: Flushing (1% to 5% dose related), palpitation (1% to 5% dose related)

Central nervous system: Dizziness (1% to 3% dose related), fatigue (5%), somnolence (1% to 2%)

Dermatologic: Rash (1% to 2%), pruritus (1% to 2%)

Endocrine & metabolic: Male sexual dysfunction (1% to 2%)

Gastrointestinal: Nausea (3%), abdominal pain (1% to 2%), dyspepsia (1% to 2%)

Neuromuscular & skeletal: Muscle cramps (1% to 2%), weakness (1% to 2%)

Respiratory: Dyspnea (1% to 2%), pulmonary edema (HF patients: 27% [Packer, 1996])

Drug Interactions

Metabolism/Transport Effects Substrate of CYP3A4 (major); **Note:** Assignment of Major/Minor substrate status based on clinically relevant drug interaction potential; **Inhibits** CYP1A2 (moderate), CYP2A6 (weak), CYP2B6 (weak), CYP2C8 (weak), CYP2C9 (weak), CYP2D6 (weak), CYP3A4 (weak)

Avoid Concomitant Use

Avoid concomitant use of AmLODIPine with any of the following: Conivaptan; Pimozide

Increased Effect/Toxicity

AmLODIPine may increase the levels/effects of: Amifostine; Antihypertensives; ARIPiprazole; Beta-Blockers; Calcium Channel Blockers (Nondihydropyridine); CYP1A2 Substrates; Fosphenytoin; Hypotensive Agents; Magnesium Salts; Neuromuscular-Blocking Agents

(Nondepolarizing); Nitroprusside; Phenytoin; Pimozide; QuiNIDine; RiTUXimab; Simvastatin; Tacrolimus; Tacrolimus (Systemic)

The levels/effects of AmLODIPine may be increased by: Alpha1-Blockers; Antifungal Agents (Azole Derivatives, Systemic); Calcium Channel Blockers (Nondihydropyridine); Conivaptan; CycloSPORINE; CycloSPORINE (Systemic); CYP3A4 Inhibitors (Moderate); CYP3A4 Inhibitors (Strong); Dasatinib; Diazoxide; Fluconazole; Grapefruit Juice; Herbs (Hypotensive Properties); Ivacaftor; Macrolide Antibiotics; Magnesium Salts; MAO Inhibitors; Mifepristone; Pentoxifylline; Phosphodiesterase 5 Inhibitors; Prostacyclin Analogues; Protease Inhibitors; QuiNIDine

Decreased Effect
AmLODIPine may decrease the levels/effects of: Clopidogrel; QuiNIDine

The levels/effects of AmLODIPine may be decreased by: Barbiturates; Calcium Salts; CarBAMazepine; CYP3A4 Inducers (Strong); Deferasirox; Herbs (CYP3A4 Inducers); Herbs (Hypertensive Properties); Methylphenidate; Nafcillin; Rifamycin Derivatives; Tocilizumab; Yohimbine

Ethanol/Nutrition/Herb Interactions
Food: Grapefruit juice may modestly increase amlodipine levels.
Herb/Nutraceutical: St John's wort may decrease amlodipine levels. Avoid herbs with *hypertensive* properties (bayberry, blue cohosh, cayenne, ephedra, ginger, ginseng [American], kola, licorice). Avoid herbs with *hypotensive* properties (black cohosh, California poppy, coleus, garlic, goldenseal, hawthorn, mistletoe, periwinkle, quinine, shepherd's purse).

Stability Store at room temperature of 15°C to 30°C (59°F to 86°F).

Mechanism of Action Inhibits calcium ion from entering the "slow channels" or select voltage-sensitive areas of vascular smooth muscle and myocardium during depolarization, producing a relaxation of coronary vascular smooth muscle and coronary vasodilation; increases myocardial oxygen delivery in patients with vasospastic angina. Amlodipine directly acts on vascular smooth muscle to produce peripheral arterial vasodilation reducing peripheral vascular resistance and blood pressure.

Pharmacodynamics/Kinetics
Duration of antihypertensive effect: 24 hours
Absorption: Oral: Well absorbed
Distribution: V_d: 21 L/kg
Protein binding: 93% to 98%
Metabolism: Hepatic (>90%) to inactive metabolites
Bioavailability: 64% to 90%
Half-life elimination: Terminal: 30-50 hours; increased with hepatic dysfunction
Time to peak, plasma: 6-12 hours
Excretion: Urine (10% of total dose as unchanged drug, 60% of total dose as metabolites)

Dosage
Geriatric Dosing should start at the lower end of dosing range and titrated to response due to possible increased incidence of hepatic, renal, or cardiac impairment. Elderly patients also show decreased clearance of amlodipine.
Hypertension: Oral: 2.5 mg once daily
Angina: Oral: 5 mg once daily

Adult
Hypertension: Oral: Initial dose: 5 mg once daily; maximum dose: 10 mg once daily. In general, titrate in 2.5 mg increments over 7-14 days. Usual dosage range (JNC 7): 2.5-10 mg once daily.
Angina: Oral: Usual dose: 5-10 mg; most patients require 10 mg for adequate effect.
Renal Impairment Dialysis: Hemodialysis and peritoneal dialysis do not enhance elimination. Supplemental dose is not necessary.

Hepatic Impairment
Hypertension: Administer 2.5 mg once daily
Angina: Administer 5 mg once daily

Administration May be administered without regard to meals.

Monitoring Parameters Heart rate, blood pressure, peripheral edema

Special Geriatric Considerations Elderly may experience a greater hypotensive response. Constipation may be more of a problem in elderly. Calcium channel blockers are no more effective in elderly than other therapies, however, they do not cause significant CNS effects which is an advantage over some antihypertensive agents.

Dosage Forms Excipient information presented when available (limited, particularly for generics); consult specific product labeling.
Tablet, oral: 2.5 mg, 5 mg, 10 mg
Norvasc®: 2.5 mg, 5 mg, 10 mg

◆ **Amlodipine, Aliskiren, and Hydrochlorothiazide** *see* Aliskiren, Amlodipine, and Hydrochlorothiazide *on page 60*

◆ **Amlodipine and Aliskiren** *see* Aliskiren and Amlodipine *on page 61*

Amlodipine and Benazepril (am LOE di peen & ben AY ze pril)

Related Information
AmLODIPine *on page 104*
Benazepril *on page 197*
Brand Names: U.S. Lotrel®
Index Terms Benazepril Hydrochloride and Amlodipine Besylate
Generic Availability (U.S.) Yes
Pharmacologic Category Angiotensin-Converting Enzyme (ACE) Inhibitor; Antianginal Agent; Calcium Channel Blocker; Calcium Channel Blocker, Dihydropyridine
Use Treatment of hypertension
Dosage
  Geriatric Initial dose: 2.5 mg (based on amlodipine component). Refer to adult dosing.
  Adult Note: Dose is individualized; combination product may be substituted for individual components in patients currently maintained on both agents separately or in patients not adequately controlled with monotherapy (using one of the agents or an agent within same antihypertensive class).
    Hypertension: Oral: 2.5-10 mg (amlodipine) and 10-40 mg (benazepril) once daily; maximum: Amlodipine: 10 mg/day; benazepril: 80 mg/day
  Renal Impairment Cl_{cr} ≤30 mL/minute: Use of combination product is not recommended.
  Hepatic Impairment Initial dose: 2.5 mg based on amlodipine component.
Special Geriatric Considerations See individual agents. Combination products are not recommended as first-line treatment. Use only if doses of individual agents correspond to the combination available.
Dosage Forms Excipient information presented when available (limited, particularly for generics); consult specific product labeling.
  Capsule, oral:
    2.5/10: Amlodipine 2.5 mg and benazepril hydrochloride 10 mg
    5/10: Amlodipine 5 mg and benazepril hydrochloride 10 mg
    5/20: Amlodipine 5 mg and benazepril hydrochloride 20 mg
    5/40: Amlodipine 5 mg and benazepril hydrochloride 40 mg
    10/20: Amlodipine 10 mg and benazepril hydrochloride 20 mg
    10/40: Amlodipine 10 mg and benazepril hydrochloride 40 mg
      Lotrel® 2.5/10: Amlodipine 2.5 mg and benazepril hydrochloride 10 mg
      Lotrel® 5/10: Amlodipine 5 mg and benazepril hydrochloride 10 mg
      Lotrel® 5/20: Amlodipine 5 mg and benazepril hydrochloride 20 mg
      Lotrel® 5/40: Amlodipine 5 mg and benazepril hydrochloride 40 mg
      Lotrel® 10/20: Amlodipine 10 mg and benazepril hydrochloride 20 mg
      Lotrel® 10/40: Amlodipine 10 mg and benazepril hydrochloride 40 mg

Amlodipine and Olmesartan (am LOE di peen & olme SAR tan)

Related Information
AmLODIPine *on page 104*
Olmesartan *on page 1411*
Brand Names: U.S. Azor™
Index Terms Amlodipine Besylate and Olmesartan Medoxomil; Olmesartan and Amlodipine
Generic Availability (U.S.) No
Pharmacologic Category Angiotensin II Receptor Blocker; Antianginal Agent; Calcium Channel Blocker; Calcium Channel Blocker, Dihydropyridine
Use Treatment of hypertension, including initial treatment in patients who will require multiple antihypertensives for adequate control
Dosage
  Geriatric Initial therapy is not recommended in patients ≥75 years of age.
  Adult Dose is individualized; combination product may be substituted for individual components in patients currently maintained on both agents separately or in patients not adequately controlled with monotherapy (using one of the agents or an agent within the same antihypertensive class). May also be used as initial therapy in patients who are likely to need >1 antihypertensive to control blood pressure.

Hypertension: Oral:

Initial therapy (antihypertensive naive): Amlodipine 5 mg/olmesartan 20 mg once daily; dose may be increased after 1-2 weeks of therapy. Maximum recommended dose: Amlodipine 10 mg/day; olmesartan 40 mg/day.

Add-on/replacement therapy: Amlodipine 5-10 mg and olmesartan 20-40 mg once daily depending upon previous doses, current control, and goals of therapy; dose may be titrated after 2 weeks of therapy. Maximum recommended dose: Amlodipine 10 mg/day; olmesartan 40 mg/day.

Renal Impairment No specific guidelines for dosage adjustment.

Hepatic Impairment Initial therapy is not recommended.

Special Geriatric Considerations See individual agents. Combination products are not recommended as first-line treatment. Use only if doses of individual agents correspond to the combination available.

Dosage Forms Excipient information presented when available (limited, particularly for generics); consult specific product labeling.

Tablet:

Azor™ 5/20: Amlodipine 5 mg and olmesartan medoxomil 20 mg

Azor™ 5/40: Amlodipine 5 mg and olmesartan medoxomil 40 mg

Azor™ 10/20: Amlodipine 10 mg and olmesartan medoxomil 20 mg

Azor™ 10/40: Amlodipine 10 mg and olmesartan medoxomil 40 mg

♦ **Amlodipine and Telmisartan** *see* Telmisartan and Amlodipine *on page 1848*

Amlodipine and Valsartan (am LOE di peen & val SAR tan)

Related Information

AmLODIPine *on page 104*

Valsartan *on page 1996*

Brand Names: U.S. Exforge®

Index Terms Amlodipine Besylate and Valsartan; Valsartan and Amlodipine

Generic Availability (U.S.) No

Pharmacologic Category Angiotensin II Receptor Blocker; Antianginal Agent; Calcium Channel Blocker; Calcium Channel Blocker, Dihydropyridine

Use Treatment of hypertension

Dosage

Geriatric Refer to adult dosing. Initiate amlodipine at 2.5 mg/day; due to decreased clearance.

Adult Note: Dose is individualized; combination product may be used as initial therapy or substituted for individual components in patients currently maintained on both agents separately or in patients not adequately controlled with monotherapy (using one of the agents or an agent within same antihypertensive class).

Hypertension: Oral:

Initial therapy: Amlodipine 5 mg and valsartan 160 mg once daily, dose may be titrated after 1-2 weeks of therapy. Maximum recommended doses: Amlodipine 10 mg/day; valsartan 320 mg/day

Add-on/replacement therapy: Amlodipine 5-10 mg and valsartan 160-320 mg once daily; dose may be titrated after 3-4 weeks of therapy. Maximum recommended doses: Amlodipine 10 mg/day; valsartan 320 mg/day

Renal Impairment

Cl_{cr} >10 mL/minute: No dosage adjustment necessary.

Cl_{cr} ≤10 mL/minute: Use caution; titrate slowly.

Hepatic Impairment Mild-to-moderate hepatic impairment: No initial dosage adjustment required, titrate slowly. Amlodipine and valsartan exposure increased in presence of hepatic impairment.

Amlodipine: Use caution in severe hepatic impairment; lower initial doses may be required.

Valsartan: Mild-to-moderate hepatic impairment: No dosage adjustment required; however, patients with mild-to-moderate chronic disease have twice the exposure as healthy volunteers.

Special Geriatric Considerations See individual agents. Combination products are not recommended as first-line treatment. Use only if doses of individual agents correspond to the combination available.

Dosage Forms Excipient information presented when available (limited, particularly for generics); consult specific product labeling.
Tablet:
Exforge®:
5/160: Amlodipine 5 mg and valsartan 160 mg
5/320 mg: Amlodipine 5 mg and valsartan 320 mg
10/160: Amlodipine 10 mg and valsartan 160 mg
10/320: Amlodipine 10 mg and valsartan 320 mg

◆ **Amlodipine Besylate** *see* AmLODIPine *on page* 104
◆ **Amlodipine Besylate, Aliskiren Hemifumarate, and Hydrochlorothiazide** *see* Aliskiren, Amlodipine, and Hydrochlorothiazide *on page* 60
◆ **Amlodipine Besylate and Olmesartan Medoxomil** *see* Amlodipine and Olmesartan *on page* 106
◆ **Amlodipine Besylate and Telmisartan** *see* Telmisartan and Amlodipine *on page* 1848
◆ **Amlodipine Besylate and Valsartan** *see* Amlodipine and Valsartan *on page* 107
◆ **Amlodipine Besylate, Olmesartan Medoxomil, and Hydrochlorothiazide** *see* Olmesartan, Amlodipine, and Hydrochlorothiazide *on page* 1412
◆ **Amlodipine Besylate, Valsartan, and Hydrochlorothiazide** *see* Amlodipine, Valsartan, and Hydrochlorothiazide *on page* 108
◆ **Amlodipine, Hydrochlorothiazide, and Aliskiren** *see* Aliskiren, Amlodipine, and Hydrochlorothiazide *on page* 60
◆ **Amlodipine, Hydrochlorothiazide, and Olmesartan** *see* Olmesartan, Amlodipine, and Hydrochlorothiazide *on page* 1412
◆ **Amlodipine, Hydrochlorothiazide, and Valsartan** *see* Amlodipine, Valsartan, and Hydrochlorothiazide *on page* 108

Amlodipine, Valsartan, and Hydrochlorothiazide
(am LOE di peen, val SAR tan, & hye droe klor oh THYE a zide)

Related Information
AmLODIPine *on page* 104
Hydrochlorothiazide *on page* 933
Valsartan *on page* 1996
Brand Names: U.S. Exforge HCT®
Index Terms Amlodipine Besylate, Valsartan, and Hydrochlorothiazide; Amlodipine, Hydrochlorothiazide, and Valsartan; Hydrochlorothiazide, Amlodipine, and Valsartan; Valsartan, Hydrochlorothiazide, and Amlodipine
Generic Availability (U.S.) No
Pharmacologic Category Angiotensin II Receptor Blocker; Antianginal Agent; Calcium Channel Blocker; Calcium Channel Blocker, Dihydropyridine; Diuretic, Thiazide
Use Treatment of hypertension (not for initial therapy)
Dosage
Geriatric & Adult Note: Not for initial therapy. Dose is individualized; combination product may be substituted for individual components in patients currently maintained on all three agents separately or in patients not adequately controlled with any two of the following antihypertensive classes: Calcium channel blockers, angiotensin II receptor blockers, and diuretics.

Hypertension: Oral: Add-on/switch/replacement therapy: Amlodipine 5-10 mg and valsartan 160-320 mg and hydrochlorothiazide 12.5-25 mg once daily; dose may be titrated after 2 weeks of therapy. Maximum recommended daily dose: Amlodipine 10 mg/valsartan 320 mg/hydrochlorothiazide 25 mg

Renal Impairment
Cl_{cr} >30 mL/minute: No adjustment needed.
Cl_{cr} ≤30 mL/minute: Use of combination not recommended; contraindicated in patients with anuria.
Hepatic Impairment Use of combination is not recommended in severe hepatic impairment. Use with caution in mild-to-moderate hepatic impairment; monitor for worsening of hepatic or renal function and adverse reactions.
Special Geriatric Considerations See individual agents. Combination products are not recommended as first-line treatment. Use only if doses of individual agents correspond to the combination available.

Dosage Forms Excipient information presented when available (limited, particularly for generics); consult specific product labeling.
Tablet, oral:
  Exforge HCT®:
    Amlodipine 5 mg, valsartan 160 mg, and hydrochlorothiazide 12.5 mg
    Amlodipine 5 mg, valsartan 160 mg, and hydrochlorothiazide 25 mg
    Amlodipine 10 mg, valsartan 160 mg, and hydrochlorothiazide 12.5 mg
    Amlodipine 10 mg, valsartan 160 mg, and hydrochlorothiazide 25 mg
    Amlodipine 10 mg, valsartan 320 mg, and hydrochlorothiazide 25 mg

Ammonium Chloride (a MOE nee um KLOR ide)

Generic Availability (U.S.) Yes
Pharmacologic Category Electrolyte Supplement, Parenteral
Use Treatment of hypochloremic states or metabolic alkalosis
Contraindications Severe hepatic or renal dysfunction
Warnings/Precautions Monitor closely for signs and symptoms of ammonia toxicity, including diaphoresis, altered breathing, bradycardia, arrhythmias, retching, twitching, and coma. Use caution in patients with primary respiratory acidosis or pulmonary insufficiency.
Adverse Reactions (Reflective of adult population; not specific for elderly) Frequency not defined.
Central nervous system: Coma, drowsiness, EEG abnormalities, headache, mental confusion, seizure
Dermatologic: Rash
Endocrine & metabolic: Calcium-deficient tetany, hyperchloremia, hypokalemia, metabolic acidosis, potassium may be decreased, sodium may be decreased
Gastrointestinal: Abdominal pain, gastric irritation, nausea, vomiting
Hepatic: Ammonia may be increased
Local: Pain at site of injection
Neuromuscular & skeletal: Twitching
Respiratory: Hyperventilation
Drug Interactions
Metabolism/Transport Effects None known.
Avoid Concomitant Use There are no known interactions where it is recommended to avoid concomitant use.
Increased Effect/Toxicity
Ammonium Chloride may increase the levels/effects of: Salicylates

The levels/effects of Ammonium Chloride may be increased by: Potassium-Sparing Diuretics
Decreased Effect
Ammonium Chloride may decrease the levels/effects of: Amphetamines; Analgesics (Opioid)
Stability Prior to use, vials should be stored at controlled room temperature of 15°C to 30°C (59°F to 86°F). Solution may crystallize if exposed to low temperatures. If crystals are observed, warm vial to room temperature in a water bath prior to use. Dilute prior to use; final concentration should not exceed 1% to 2% ammonium chloride. Suggested dilution: Mix contents of 1-2 vials (100-200 mEq) in 500-1000 mL NS.
Mechanism of Action Increases acidity by increasing free hydrogen ion concentration
Pharmacodynamics/Kinetics
Metabolism: Hepatic; forms urea and hydrochloric acid
Excretion: Urine
Dosage
Geriatric & Adult Metabolic alkalosis: The following equations represent different methods of correction utilizing either the serum HCO_3^-, the serum chloride, or the base excess

Dosing of mEq NH_4 Cl via the chloride-deficit method (hypochloremia):
Dose of mEq NH_4Cl = [0.2 L/kg x body weight (kg)] x [103 - observed serum chloride]; administer 50% of dose over 12 hours, then re-evaluate
Note: 0.2 L/kg is the estimated chloride volume of distribution and 103 is the average normal serum chloride concentration (mEq/L)
Dosing of mEq NH_4 Cl via the bicarbonate-excess method (refractory hypochloremic metabolic alkalosis):
Dose of NH_4Cl = [0.5 L/kg x body weight (kg)] x (observed serum HCO_3^- - 24); administer 50% of dose over 12 hours, then re-evaluate

Note: 0.5 L/kg is the estimated bicarbonate volume of distribution and 24 is the average normal serum bicarbonate concentration (mEq/L)

These equations will yield different requirements of ammonium chloride

Administration Administer by slow intravenous infusion to avoid local irritation and adverse effects. Rate of infusion should not exceed 5 mL/minute in an adult.

Monitoring Parameters Serum bicarbonate; signs and symptoms of ammonia toxicity

Pharmacotherapy Pearls Do not exceed a 1% to 2% concentration of ammonium chloride or an administration rate of more than 5 mL/minute; administer over approximately 3 hours for I.V. infusion

Special Geriatric Considerations No specific data available for elderly; monitor closely with hepatic disease for signs of toxicity.

Dosage Forms Excipient information presented when available (limited, particularly for generics); consult specific product labeling.

Injection, solution: Ammonium 5 mEq/mL and chloride 5 mEq/mL (20 mL) [equivalent to ammonium chloride 267.5 mg/mL]

◆ **Amoclan** see Amoxicillin and Clavulanate on page 115

Amoxapine (a MOKS a peen)

Related Information

Antidepressant Agents on page 2097

Beers Criteria – Potentially Inappropriate Medications for Geriatrics on page 2183

Medication Safety Issues

Sound-alike/look-alike issues:

Amoxapine may be confused with amoxicillin, Amoxil

Asendin may be confused with aspirin

BEERS Criteria medication:

This drug may be potentially inappropriate for use in geriatric patients (Quality of evidence - moderate; Strength of recommendation - strong).

Index Terms Asendin [DSC]

Generic Availability (U.S.) Yes

Pharmacologic Category Antidepressant, Tricyclic (Secondary Amine)

Use Treatment of depression (including endogenous, neurotic, psychotic, and reactive depression); treatment of depression accompanied by anxiety or agitation

Medication Guide Available Yes

Contraindications Hypersensitivity to amoxapine or any component of the formulation; use with or within 14 days of MAO inhibitors; acute recovery phase following myocardial infarction

Warnings/Precautions [U.S. Boxed Warning]: Antidepressants increase the risk of suicidal thinking and behavior in children, adolescents, and young adults (18-24 years of age) with major depressive disorder (MDD) and other psychiatric disorders; consider risk prior to prescribing. Short-term studies did not show an increased risk in patients >24 years of age and showed a decreased risk in patients ≥65 years. Closely monitor for clinical worsening, suicidality, or unusual changes in behavior; the patient's family or caregiver should be instructed to closely observe the patient and communicate condition with healthcare provider. A medication guide should be dispensed with each prescription.

The possibility of a suicide attempt is inherent in major depression and may persist until remission occurs. Monitor for worsening of depression or suicidality, especially during initiation of therapy (generally first 1-2 months) or with dose increases or decreases. Use caution in high-risk patients. Worsening depression and severe abrupt suicidality that are not part of the presenting symptoms may require discontinuation or modification of drug therapy. The patient's family or caregiver should be alerted to monitor patients for the emergence of suicidality and associated behaviors (such as agitation, irritability, hostility, impulsivity, and hypomania) and notify the healthcare provider.

May worsen psychosis in some patients or precipitate a shift to mania or hypomania in patients with bipolar disorder. Patients presenting with depressive symptoms should be screened for bipolar disorder. Monotherapy in patients with bipolar disorder should be avoided. **Amoxapine is not FDA approved for bipolar depression.** May cause extrapyramidal symptoms, including pseudoparkinsonism, acute dystonic reactions, akathisia, and tardive dyskinesia (risk of these reactions is low). The risk for tardive dyskinesia (may be irreversible) increases with long-term treatment and higher cumulative doses. Therapy should be discontinued in any patient if signs/symptoms of tardive dyskinesia appear. May be associated with neuroleptic malignant syndrome.

The degree of sedation, anticholinergic effects, orthostasis, and conduction abnormalities are moderate relative to other antidepressants. May cause drowsiness/sedation, resulting in impaired performance of tasks requiring alertness (eg, operating machinery or driving). Sedative effects may be additive with other CNS depressants and/or ethanol. Use with caution in patients with a history of cardiovascular disease (including previous MI, stroke, tachycardia, or conduction abnormalities). Use with caution in patients with urinary retention, benign prostatic hyperplasia, narrow-angle glaucoma, xerostomia, visual problems, constipation, or a history of bowel obstruction.

Consider discontinuing, when possible, prior to elective surgery. Therapy should not be abruptly discontinued in patients receiving high doses for prolonged periods. May lower seizure threshold - use caution in patients with a previous seizure disorder or condition predisposing to seizures such as brain damage, alcoholism, or concurrent therapy with other drugs which lower the seizure threshold. May increase the risks associated with electroconvulsive therapy. Use with caution in hyperthyroid patients or those receiving thyroid supplementation.

Use caution in elderly patients; may cause or exacerbate syndrome of inappropriate antidiuretic hormone secretion or hyponatremia; monitor sodium closely with initiation or dosage adjustments in older adults. May be inappropriate in older adults depending on comorbidities (eg, dementia, delirium) due to its potent anticholinergic effects (Beers Criteria). May also have increased risk of adverse events, including tardive dyskinesia (particularly older women) and sedation.

Adverse Reactions (Reflective of adult population; not specific for elderly)
>10%:
  Central nervous system: Drowsiness (14%)
  Gastrointestinal: Xerostomia (14%), constipation (12%)
1% to 10%:
  Cardiovascular: Palpitations
  Central nervous system: Anxiety, ataxia, confusion, dizziness, EEG abnormalities, excitement, fatigue, headache, insomnia, nervousness, nightmares, restlessness
  Dermatologic: Edema, skin rash
  Endocrine: Prolactin levels increased
  Gastrointestinal: Appetite increased, nausea
  Neuromuscular & skeletal: Tremor, weakness
  Ocular: Blurred vision (7%)
  Miscellaneous: Diaphoresis

Drug Interactions
  Metabolism/Transport Effects Substrate of CYP2D6 (major); **Note:** Assignment of Major/Minor substrate status based on clinically relevant drug interaction potential
  Avoid Concomitant Use
    Avoid concomitant use of Amoxapine with any of the following: Iobenguane I 123; MAO Inhibitors; Methylene Blue
  Increased Effect/Toxicity
    Amoxapine may increase the levels/effects of: Alpha-/Beta-Agonists (Direct-Acting); Alpha1-Agonists; Amphetamines; Anticholinergics; Beta2-Agonists; Desmopressin; Highest Risk QTc-Prolonging Agents; Methylene Blue; Metoclopramide; Moderate Risk QTc-Prolonging Agents; QuiNIDine; Serotonin Modulators; Sodium Phosphates; Sulfonylureas; TraMADol; Vitamin K Antagonists; Yohimbine

    The levels/effects of Amoxapine may be increased by: Abiraterone Acetate; Altretamine; Antipsychotics; Cimetidine; Cinacalcet; CYP2D6 Inhibitors (Moderate); CYP2D6 Inhibitors (Strong); Dexmethylphenidate; Divalproex; DULoxetine; Linezolid; Lithium; MAO Inhibitors; Methylphenidate; Metoclopramide; Metyrosine; Mifepristone; Pramlintide; Protease Inhibitors; QuiNIDine; Selective Serotonin Reuptake Inhibitors; Terbinafine; Terbinafine (Systemic); Valproic Acid
  Decreased Effect
    Amoxapine may decrease the levels/effects of: Acetylcholinesterase Inhibitors (Central); Alpha2-Agonists; Iobenguane I 123

    The levels/effects of Amoxapine may be decreased by: Acetylcholinesterase Inhibitors (Central); Barbiturates; CarBAMazepine; Peginterferon Alfa-2b; St Johns Wort
Ethanol/Nutrition/Herb Interactions
  Ethanol: May increase CNS depression; monitor for increased effects with coadministration. Caution patients about effects.
  Food: Grapefruit juice may inhibit the metabolism of some TCAs and clinical toxicity may result.
  Herb/Nutraceutical: Avoid valerian, St John's wort, SAMe, kava kava.
Stability Store at 20°C to 25°C (68°F to 77°F).

Mechanism of Action Reduces the reuptake of serotonin and norepinephrine. The metabolite, 7-OH-amoxapine has significant dopamine receptor blocking activity similar to haloperidol.

Pharmacodynamics/Kinetics

Onset of antidepressant effect: Usually occurs after 1-2 weeks, but may require 4-6 weeks

Absorption: Rapid and well absorbed

Distribution: V_d: 0.9-1.2 L/kg

Protein binding: ~90%

Metabolism: Extensively metabolized; hepatic hydroxylation produces two active metabolites, 7-hydroxyamoxapine (7-OH-amoxapine) and 8-hydroxyamoxapine (8-OH-amoxapine); metabolites undergo conjugation to form glucuronides

Half-life elimination: 8 hours; 7-hydroxyamoxapine metabolite: 4-6 hours; 8-hydroxyamoxapine metabolite: 30 hours

Time to peak, serum: ~90 minutes

Excretion: Urine (as unchanged drug and metabolites)

Dosage

Geriatric Depression: Oral: Use caution or avoid in the elderly. Initial: 25 mg 2-3 times/day; dose may be increased to 50 mg 2-3 times/day by the end of the first week, if tolerated; usual effective dose: 100-150 mg/day; if dose is ineffective, may further increase cautiously to 300 mg/day; once an effective dose is reached, doses ≤300 mg may be given once daily at bedtime. Maintenance: Once symptoms are controlled, gradually decrease to the lowest dose that will maintain remission.

Adult Depression: Oral:

Outpatients: Initial: 50 mg 2-3 times/day; dose may be increased to 100 mg 2-3 times/day by the end of the first week, if tolerated. Usual effective dose: 200-300 mg/day; if 300 mg daily has been reached and maintained for at least 2 weeks and no response is observed, may further increase to 400 mg/day. Once an effective dose is reached, doses ≤300 mg may be given once daily at bedtime and doses >300 mg/day should be divided.

Inpatients: Hospitalized patients refractory to antidepressant therapy (and no history of seizures) may be cautiously titrated to 600 mg/day in divided doses.

Maintenance: Outpatients and Inpatients: Once symptoms are controlled, gradually decrease to lowest dose that will maintain remission.

Monitoring Parameters Monitor blood pressure and pulse rate prior to and during initial therapy evaluate mental status, suicide ideation (especially at the beginning of therapy or when doses are increased or decreased); ECG in older adults and patients with cardiac disease

Test Interactions Increased glucose, liver function tests; decreased WBC

Pharmacotherapy Pearls Extrapyramidal reactions and tardive dyskinesia may occur.

Special Geriatric Considerations Amoxapine is not the drug of choice in the elderly. Significant anticholinergic and orthostatic effects can occur and there is a risk for tardive dyskinesia and neuroleptic malignant syndrome.

A systematic review and meta-analysis of antidepressant placebo-controlled trials in persons with depression and dementia found evidence "suggestive" of efficacy but not of sufficient strength to "confirm" efficacy. Antidepressant trials in this patient population are small and underpowered. Older patients with depression being treated with an antidepressant should be closely monitored for response and adverse effects. Treatment should be switched or augmented when response is inadequate with a therapeutic dose. Antidepressants that are not tolerated should be discontinued and an alternative agent should be started.

This medication is considered to be potentially inappropriate for use in geriatric patients (Beers Criteria: Quality of evidence - moderate; Strength of recommendation - strong).

Dosage Forms Excipient information presented when available (limited, particularly for generics); consult specific product labeling.

Tablet, oral: 25 mg, 50 mg, 100 mg, 150 mg

Amoxicillin (a moks i SIL in)

Related Information

Medication Safety Issues

Sound-alike/look-alike issues:

Amoxicillin may be confused with amoxapine, Augmentin®

Amoxil may be confused with amoxapine

International issues:

Fisamox [Australia] may be confused with Fosamax brand name for alendronate [U.S., Canada, and multiple international markets] and Vigamox brand name for moxifloxacin [U.S., Canada, and multiple international markets]

Limoxin [Mexico] may be confused with Lanoxin brand name for digoxin [U.S., Canada, and multiple international markets]; Lincocin brand name for lincomycin [U.S., Canada, and multiple international markets]

Zimox: Brand name for amoxicillin [Italy], but also the brand name for carbidopa/levodopa [Greece]

Zimox [Italy] may be confused with Diamox which is the brand name for acetazolamide [Canada and multiple international markets]

Brand Names: U.S. Moxatag™

Brand Names: Canada Apo-Amoxi®; Mylan-Amoxicillin; Novamoxin®; NTP-Amoxicillin; Nu-Amoxi; PHL-Amoxicillin; PMS-Amoxicillin; Pro-Amox-250; Pro-Amox-500

Index Terms p-Hydroxyampicillin; Amoxicillin Trihydrate; Amoxil; Amoxycillin

Generic Availability (U.S.) Yes: Excludes extended-release formulation

Pharmacologic Category Antibiotic, Penicillin

Use Treatment of otitis media, sinusitis, and infections caused by susceptible organisms involving the upper and lower respiratory tract, skin, and urinary tract; prophylaxis of infective endocarditis in patients undergoing surgical or dental procedures; as part of a multidrug regimen for *H. pylori* eradication; periodontitis

Unlabeled Use Postexposure prophylaxis for anthrax exposure with documented susceptible organisms

Contraindications Hypersensitivity to amoxicillin, penicillin, other beta-lactams, or any component of the formulation

Warnings/Precautions In patients with renal impairment, doses and/or frequency of administration should be modified in response to the degree of renal impairment; in addition, use of certain dosage forms (eg, extended release 775 mg tablet and immediate release 875 mg tablet) should be avoided in patients with Cl_{cr} <30 mL/minute or patients requiring hemodialysis. A high percentage of patients with infectious mononucleosis have developed rash during therapy with amoxicillin; ampicillin-class antibiotics not recommended in these patients. Serious and occasionally severe or fatal hypersensitivity (anaphylactoid) reactions have been reported in patients on penicillin therapy, especially with a history of beta-lactam hypersensitivity, history of sensitivity to multiple allergens, or previous IgE-mediated reactions (eg, anaphylaxis, angioedema, urticaria). Use with caution in asthmatic patients. Prolonged use may result in fungal or bacterial superinfection, including *C. difficile*-associated diarrhea (CDAD) and pseudomembranous colitis; CDAD has been observed >2 months postantibiotic treatment. Chewable tablets contain phenylalanine.

Adverse Reactions (Reflective of adult population; not specific for elderly) Frequency not defined.

Central nervous system: Agitation, anxiety, behavioral changes, confusion, dizziness, headache, hyperactivity (reversible), insomnia, seizure

Dermatologic: Acute exanthematous pustulosis, erythematous maculopapular rash, erythema multiforme, exfoliative dermatitis, hypersensitivity vasculitis, mucocutaneous candidiasis, Stevens-Johnson syndrome, toxic epidermal necrolysis, urticaria

Gastrointestinal: Black hairy tongue, diarrhea, hemorrhagic colitis, nausea, pseudomembranous colitis, tooth discoloration (brown, yellow, or gray; rare), vomiting

Hematologic: Agranulocytosis, anemia, eosinophilia, hemolytic anemia, leukopenia, thrombocytopenia, thrombocytopenia purpura

Hepatic: Acute cytolytic hepatitis, ALT increased, AST increased, cholestatic jaundice, hepatic cholestasis

Renal: Crystalluria

Miscellaneous: Anaphylaxis, serum sickness-like reaction

Drug Interactions

Metabolism/Transport Effects None known.

Avoid Concomitant Use

Avoid concomitant use of Amoxicillin with any of the following: BCG

Increased Effect/Toxicity

Amoxicillin may increase the levels/effects of: Methotrexate; Vitamin K Antagonists

The levels/effects of Amoxicillin may be increased by: Allopurinol; Probenecid

Decreased Effect

Amoxicillin may decrease the levels/effects of: BCG; Mycophenolate; Typhoid Vaccine

The levels/effects of Amoxicillin may be decreased by: Fusidic Acid; Tetracycline Derivatives

Stability

Amoxil®: Oral suspension remains stable for 14 days at room temperature or if refrigerated (refrigeration preferred). Unit-dose antibiotic oral syringes are stable at room temperature for at least 72 hours (Tu, 1988).

Moxatag™: Store at 25°C (77°F); excursions permitted to 15°C to 30°C (59°F to 86°F).

Mechanism of Action Inhibits bacterial cell wall synthesis by binding to one or more of the penicillin-binding proteins (PBPs) which in turn inhibits the final transpeptidation step of peptidoglycan synthesis in bacterial cell walls, thus inhibiting cell wall biosynthesis. Bacteria eventually lyse due to ongoing activity of cell wall autolytic enzymes (autolysins and murein hydrolases) while cell wall assembly is arrested.

Pharmacodynamics/Kinetics

Absorption: Oral: Rapid and nearly complete; food does not interfere

Extended-release tablet: Rate of absorption is slower compared to immediate-release formulations; food decreases the rate but not extent of absorption

Distribution: Widely to most body fluids and bone; poor penetration into cells, eyes, and across normal meninges

Pleural fluids, lungs, and peritoneal fluid; high urine concentrations are attained; also into synovial fluid, liver, prostate, muscle, and gallbladder; penetrates into middle ear effusions, maxillary sinus secretions, tonsils, sputum, and bronchial secretions

CSF:blood level ratio: Normal meninges: <1%; Inflamed meninges: 8% to 90%

Protein binding: 17% to 20%

Metabolism: Partially hepatic

Half-life elimination:

Adults: Normal renal function: 0.7-1.4 hours

Cl_{cr} <10 mL/minute: 7-21 hours

Time to peak: Capsule: 2 hours; Extended-release tablet: 3.1 hours; Suspension: 1 hour

Excretion: Urine (60% as unchanged drug)

Note: Extended-release tablets: In healthy volunteers, serum drug concentrations were below 0.25 mcg/mL and undetectable at 16 hours following dosing.

Dosage

Geriatric & Adult

Usual dosage range: Oral: 250-500 mg every 8 hours or 500-875 mg twice daily **or** extended-release tablet 775 mg once daily

Ear, nose, throat, genitourinary tract, or skin/skin structure infections:

Mild-to-moderate: Oral: 500 mg every 12 hours **or** 250 mg every 8 hours

Severe: Oral: 875 mg every 12 hours **or** 500 mg every 8 hours

Tonsillitis and/or pharyngitis: Oral: Extended release tablet: 775 mg once daily

***Helicobacter pylori* eradication:** Oral: 1000 mg twice daily; requires combination therapy with at least one other antibiotic and an acid-suppressing agent (proton pump inhibitor or H_2 blocker)

Lower respiratory tract infections: Oral: 875 mg every 12 hours **or** 500 mg every 8 hours

Lyme disease: Oral: 500 mg every 6-8 hours (depending on size of patient) for 21-30 days

Postexposure inhalational anthrax prophylaxis (ACIP recommendations): Oral: 500 mg every 8 hours. **Note:** Use **only** if isolates of the specific *B. anthracis* are sensitive to amoxicillin (MIC ≤0.125 mcg/mL). Duration of antibiotic postexposure prophylaxis (PEP) is ≥60 days in a previously unvaccinated exposed person. Antimicrobial therapy should continue for 14 days after the third dose of PEP vaccine. Those who are partially or fully vaccinated should receive at least a 30-day course of antimicrobial PEP and continue with licensed vaccination regimen. Unvaccinated workers, even those wearing personal protective equipment with adequate respiratory protection, should receive antimicrobial PEP. Antimicrobial PEP is not required for fully vaccinated people (five-dose I.M. vaccination series with a yearly booster) who enter an anthrax area clothed in personal protective equipment. If respiratory protection is disrupted, a 30-day course of antimicrobial therapy is recommended (ACIP, 2010).

Prophylaxis against infective endocarditis: Oral: 2 g 30-60 minutes before procedure. **Note:** American Heart Association (AHA) guidelines now recommend prophylaxis only in patients undergoing invasive procedures and in whom underlying cardiac conditions may predispose to a higher risk of adverse outcomes should infection occur. As of April 2007, routine prophylaxis for GI/GU procedures is no longer recommended by the AHA.

Prophylaxis in total joint replacement patients undergoing dental procedures which produce bacteremia: 2 g 1 hour prior to procedure

Renal Impairment

Use of certain dosage forms (eg, extended-release 775 mg tablet and immediate-release 875 mg tablet) should be avoided in patients with Cl$_{cr}$ <30 mL/minute or patients requiring hemodialysis

Cl$_{cr}$ 10-30 mL/minute: 250-500 mg every 12 hours

Cl$_{cr}$ <10 mL/minute: 250-500 mg every 24 hours

Moderately dialyzable (20% to 50%) by hemodialysis or peritoneal dialysis; approximately 50 mg of amoxicillin per liter of filtrate is removed by continuous arteriovenous or venovenous hemofiltration. Dose as per Cl$_{cr}$ <10 mL/minute guidelines.

Administration Administer around-the-clock to promote less variation in peak and trough serum levels. The appropriate amount of suspension may be mixed with formula, milk, fruit juice, water, ginger ale, or cold drinks; administer dose immediately after mixing.

Moxatag™ extended release tablet: Administer within 1 hour of finishing a meal.

Some penicillins (eg, carbenicillin, ticarcillin, and piperacillin) have been shown to inactivate aminoglycosides *in vitro*. This has been observed to a greater extent with tobramycin and gentamicin, while amikacin has shown greater stability against inactivation. Concurrent use of these agents may pose a risk of reduced antibacterial efficacy *in vivo*, particularly in the setting of profound renal impairment. However, definitive clinical evidence is lacking. If combination penicillin/aminoglycoside therapy is desired in a patient with renal dysfunction, separation of doses (if feasible), and routine monitoring of aminoglycoside levels, CBC, and clinical response should be considered.

Monitoring Parameters With prolonged therapy, monitor renal, hepatic, and hematologic function periodically; assess patient at beginning and throughout therapy for infection; monitor for signs of anaphylaxis during first dose

Test Interactions May interfere with urinary glucose tests using cupric sulfate (Benedict's solution, Clinitest®)

Some penicillin derivatives may accelerate the degradation of aminoglycosides *in vitro*, leading to a potential underestimation of aminoglycoside serum concentration.

Special Geriatric Considerations Resistance to amoxicillin has been a problem in patients on frequent antibiotics or in nursing homes. Alternative antibiotics may be necessary in these populations. Adjust dose based on renal function.

Dosage Forms Excipient information presented when available (limited, particularly for generics); consult specific product labeling.

Capsule, oral: 250 mg, 500 mg

Powder for suspension, oral: 125 mg/5 mL (80 mL, 100 mL, 150 mL); 200 mg/5 mL (50 mL, 75 mL, 100 mL); 250 mg/5 mL (80 mL, 100 mL, 150 mL); 400 mg/5 mL (50 mL, 75 mL, 100 mL)

Tablet, oral: 500 mg, 875 mg

Tablet, chewable, oral: 125 mg, 200 mg, 250 mg, 400 mg

Tablet, extended release, oral:

Moxatag™: 775 mg

Amoxicillin and Clavulanate (a moks i SIL in & klav yoo LAN ate)

Related Information

Amoxicillin *on page 112*

Antimicrobial Drugs of Choice *on page 2163*

Community-Acquired Pneumonia in Adults *on page 2171*

Medication Safety Issues

Sound-alike/look-alike issues:

Augmentin® may be confused with amoxicillin, Azulfidine®

Brand Names: U.S. Amoclan; Augmentin XR®; Augmentin®

Brand Names: Canada Amoxi-Clav; Apo-Amoxi-Clav®; Clavulin®; Novo-Clavamoxin; ratio-Aclavulanate

Index Terms Amoxicillin and Clavulanate Potassium; Amoxicillin and Clavulanic Acid; Clavulanic Acid and Amoxicillin

Generic Availability (U.S.) Yes

Pharmacologic Category Antibiotic, Penicillin

Use Treatment of otitis media, sinusitis, and infections caused by susceptible organisms involving the lower respiratory tract, skin and skin structure, and urinary tract; spectrum same as amoxicillin with additional coverage of beta-lactamase producing *B. catarrhalis*, *H. influenzae*, *N. gonorrhoeae*, and *S. aureus* (not MRSA). The expanded coverage of this combination makes it a useful alternative when amoxicillin resistance is present and patients cannot tolerate alternative treatments.

Contraindications Hypersensitivity to amoxicillin, clavulanic acid, penicillin, or any component of the formulation; history of cholestatic jaundice or hepatic dysfunction with amoxicillin/clavulanate potassium therapy; Augmentin XR™: severe renal impairment (Cl_{cr} <30 mL/minute) and hemodialysis patients

Warnings/Precautions Hypersensitivity reactions, including anaphylaxis (some fatal), have been reported. Prolonged use may result in fungal or bacterial superinfection, including *C. difficile*-associated diarrhea (CDAD) and pseudomembranous colitis; CDAD has been observed >2 months postantibiotic treatment. In patients with renal impairment, doses and/or frequency of administration should be modified in response to the degree of renal impairment. High percentage of patients with infectious mononucleosis have developed rash during therapy; ampicillin-class antibiotics not recommended in these patients. Incidence of diarrhea is higher than with amoxicillin alone. Due to differing content of clavulanic acid, not all formulations are interchangeable. Low incidence of cross-allergy with cephalosporins exists. Some products contain phenylalanine.

Adverse Reactions (Reflective of adult population; not specific for elderly)
>10%: Gastrointestinal: Diarrhea (3% to 34%; incidence varies upon dose and regimen used)
1% to 10%:
  Dermatologic: Diaper rash, skin rash, urticaria
  Gastrointestinal: Abdominal discomfort, loose stools, nausea, vomiting
  Genitourinary: Vaginitis, vaginal mycosis
  Miscellaneous: Moniliasis
Additional adverse reactions seen with **ampicillin-class antibiotics:** Agitation, agranulocytosis, alkaline phosphatase increased, anemia, angioedema, anxiety, behavioral changes, bilirubin increased, black "hairy" tongue, confusion, convulsions, crystalluria, dizziness, enterocolitis, eosinophilia, erythema multiforme, exanthematous pustulosis, exfoliative dermatitis, gastritis, glossitis, hematuria, hemolytic anemia, hemorrhagic colitis, indigestion, insomnia, hyperactivity, interstitial nephritis, leukopenia, mucocutaneous candidiasis, pruritus, pseudomembranous colitis, serum sickness-like reaction, Stevens-Johnson syndrome, stomatitis, transaminases increased, thrombocytopenia, thrombocytopenic purpura, tooth discoloration, toxic epidermal necrolysis

Drug Interactions
  Metabolism/Transport Effects None known.
  Avoid Concomitant Use
    Avoid concomitant use of Amoxicillin and Clavulanate with any of the following: BCG
  Increased Effect/Toxicity
    Amoxicillin and Clavulanate may increase the levels/effects of: Methotrexate; Vitamin K Antagonists

    The levels/effects of Amoxicillin and Clavulanate may be increased by: Allopurinol; Probenecid
  Decreased Effect
    Amoxicillin and Clavulanate may decrease the levels/effects of: BCG; Mycophenolate; Typhoid Vaccine

    The levels/effects of Amoxicillin and Clavulanate may be decreased by: Fusidic Acid; Tetracycline Derivatives

Stability
  Powder for oral suspension: Store dry powder at room temperature of 25°C (77°F). Reconstitute powder for oral suspension with appropriate amount of water as specified on the bottle. Shake vigorously until suspended. Reconstituted oral suspension should be kept in refrigerator. Discard unused suspension after 10 days. Unit-dose antibiotic oral syringes are stable under refrigeration for 24 hours (Tu, 1988).
  Tablet: Store at room temperature of 25°C (77°F).

Mechanism of Action Clavulanic acid binds and inhibits beta-lactamases that inactivate amoxicillin resulting in amoxicillin having an expanded spectrum of activity. Amoxicillin inhibits bacterial cell wall synthesis by binding to one or more of the penicillin-binding proteins (PBPs) which in turn inhibits the final transpeptidation step of peptidoglycan synthesis in bacterial cell walls, thus inhibiting cell wall biosynthesis. Bacteria eventually lyse due to ongoing activity of cell wall autolytic enzymes (autolysins and murein hydrolases) while cell wall assembly is arrested.

Pharmacodynamics/Kinetics Amoxicillin pharmacokinetics are not affected by clavulanic acid.
  Amoxicillin: See Amoxicillin monograph.

Clavulanic acid:
  Protein binding: ~25%
  Metabolism: Hepatic
  Half-life elimination: 1 hour
  Time to peak: 1 hour
  Excretion: Urine (30% to 40% as unchanged drug)
Dosage
  Geriatric & Adult Note: Dose is based on the amoxicillin component; see "Augmentin®
  Product-Specific Considerations" table.
  Susceptible infections: Adults: Oral: 250-500 mg every 8 hours or 875 mg every 12 hours

Augmentin® Product-Specific Considerations

Strength	Form	Consideration
125 mg	S	q8h dosing
	S	For adults having difficulty swallowing tablets, 125 mg/5 mL suspension may be substituted for 500 mg tablet.
200 mg	CT, S	q12h dosing
	CT	Contains phenylalanine
	S	For adults having difficulty swallowing tablets, 200 mg/5 mL suspension may be substituted for 875 mg tablet.
250 mg	S, T	q8h dosing
	T	Not for use in patients <40 kg
	S	For adults having difficulty swallowing tablets, 250 mg/5 mL suspension may be substituted for 500 mg tablet.
400 mg	CT, S	q12h dosing
	CT	Contains phenylalanine
	S	For adults having difficulty swallowing tablets, 400 mg/5 mL suspension may be substituted for 875 mg tablet.
500 mg	T	q8h or q12h dosing
600 mg	S	q12h dosing
		Not for use in adults ≥40 kg
		600 mg/5 mL suspension is not equivalent to or interchangeable with 200 mg/5 mL or 400 mg/5 mL due to differences in clavulanic acid.
875 mg	T	q12h dosing; not for use in Cl_{cr} <30 mL/minute
1000 mg	XR	q12h dosing
		Not interchangeable with two 500 mg tablets
		Not for use if Cl_{cr} <30 mL/minute or hemodialysis

Legend: CT = chewable tablet, S = suspension, T = tablet, XR = extended release.

  Acute bacterial sinusitis: Oral: Extended release tablet: Two 1000 mg tablets every 12
  hours for 10 days
  Bite wounds (animal/human): Oral: 875 mg every 12 hours **or** 500 mg every 8 hours
  Chronic obstructive pulmonary disease: Oral: 875 mg every 12 hours **or** 500 mg every 8
  hours
  Diabetic foot: Oral: Extended release tablet: Two 1000 mg tablets every 12 hours for
  7-14 days
  Diverticulitis, perirectal abscess: Oral: Extended release tablet: Two 1000 mg tablets
  every 12 hours for 7-10 days
  Erysipelas: Oral: 875 mg every 12 hours **or** 500 mg every 8 hours
  Febrile neutropenia: Oral: 875 mg every 12 hours
  Pneumonia:
    Aspiration: Oral: 875 mg every 12 hours
    Community-acquired: Oral: Extended release tablet: Two 1000 mg tablets every 12 hours
    for 7-10 days
  Pyelonephritis (acute, uncomplicated): Oral: 875 mg every 12 hours **or** 500 mg every 8
  hours
  Skin abscess: Oral: 875 mg every 12 hours

AMOXICILLIN AND CLAVULANATE

Renal Impairment
Cl$_{cr}$ <30 mL/minute: Do not use 875 mg tablet or extended release tablets.
Cl$_{cr}$ 10-30 mL/minute: 250-500 mg every 12 hours
Cl$_{cr}$ <10 mL/minute: 250-500 every 24 hours
Hemodialysis: Moderately dialyzable (20% to 50%)
  250-500 mg every 24 hours; administer dose during and after dialysis. Do not use extended release tablets.
Peritoneal dialysis: Moderately dialyzable (20% to 50%)
  Amoxicillin: Administer 250 mg every 12 hours
  Clavulanic acid: Dose for Cl$_{cr}$ <10 mL/minute
Continuous arteriovenous or venovenous hemofiltration effects:
  Amoxicillin: ~50 mg of amoxicillin/L of filtrate is removed
  Clavulanic acid: Dose for Cl$_{cr}$ <10 mL/minute

Administration Administer around-the-clock to promote less variation in peak and trough serum levels. Administer with food to increase absorption and decrease stomach upset; shake suspension well before use. Extended release tablets should be administered with food.

Some penicillins (eg, carbenicillin, ticarcillin, and piperacillin) have been shown to inactivate aminoglycosides *in vitro*. This has been observed to a greater extent with tobramycin and gentamicin, while amikacin has shown greater stability against inactivation. Concurrent use of these agents may pose a risk of reduced antibacterial efficacy *in vivo*, particularly in the setting of profound renal impairment. However, definitive clinical evidence is lacking. If combination penicillin/aminoglycoside therapy is desired in a patient with renal dysfunction, separation of doses (if feasible), and routine monitoring of aminoglycoside levels, CBC, and clinical response should be considered.

Monitoring Parameters Assess patient at beginning and throughout therapy for infection; with prolonged therapy, monitor renal, hepatic, and hematologic function periodically; monitor for signs of anaphylaxis during first dose

Test Interactions May interfere with urinary glucose tests using cupric sulfate (Benedict's solution, Clinitest®, Fehling's solution).
Some penicillin derivatives may accelerate the degradation of aminoglycosides *in vitro*, leading to a potential underestimation of aminoglycoside serum concentration.

Pharmacotherapy Pearls Two 250 mg tablets are not equivalent to a 500 mg tablet (both tablet sizes contain equivalent clavulanate). Two 500 mg tablets are not equivalent to a single 1000 mg extended release tablet.

Special Geriatric Considerations Expanded coverage of this combination makes it a useful alternative when amoxicillin resistance is present and patients cannot tolerate alternative treatments; consider renal function. Considered one of the drugs of choice in the outpatient treatment of community-acquired pneumonia in elderly.

Dosage Forms Excipient information presented when available (limited, particularly for generics); consult specific product labeling. [DSC] = Discontinued product
Powder for suspension, oral: 200: Amoxicillin 200 mg and clavulanate potassium 28.5 mg per 5 mL (50 mL, 75 mL, 100 mL); 250: Amoxicillin 250 mg and clavulanate potassium 62.5 mg per 5 mL (75 mL, 100 mL, 150 mL); 400: Amoxicillin 400 mg and clavulanate potassium 57 mg per 5 mL (50 mL, 75 mL, 100 mL); 600: Amoxicillin 600 mg and clavulanate potassium 42.9 mg per 5 mL (75 mL, 125 mL, 200 mL)
Amoclan:
  200: Amoxicillin 200 mg and clavulanate potassium 28.5 mg per 5 mL (50 mL, 75 mL, 100 mL) [contains phenylalanine 7 mg/5 mL and potassium 0.14 mEq/5 mL; fruit flavor]
  400: Amoxicillin 400 mg and clavulanate potassium 57 mg per 5 mL (50 mL, 75 mL, 100 mL) [contains phenylalanine 7 mg/5 mL and potassium 0.29 mEq/5 mL; fruit flavor]
  600: Amoxicillin 600 mg and clavulanate potassium 42.9 mg per 5 mL (75 mL, 125 mL 200 mL) [contains phenylalanine 7 mg/5 mL, potassium 0.248 mEq/5 mL; orange flavor]
Augmentin®:
  125: Amoxicillin 125 mg and clavulanate potassium 31.25 mg per 5 mL (75 mL, 100 mL, 150 mL) [contains potassium 0.16 mEq/5 mL; banana flavor]
  200: Amoxicillin 200 mg and clavulanate potassium 28.5 mg per 5 mL (50 mL, 75 mL, 100 mL) [contains phenylalanine 7 mg/5 mL and potassium 0.14 mEq/5 mL; orange flavor] [DSC]
  250: Amoxicillin 250 mg and clavulanate potassium 62.5 mg per 5 mL (75 mL, 100 mL, 150 mL) [contains potassium 0.32 mEq/5 mL; orange flavor]
  400: Amoxicillin 400 mg and clavulanate potassium 57 mg per 5 mL (50 mL, 75 mL, 100 mL) [contains phenylalanine 7 mg/5 mL and potassium 0.29 mEq/5 mL; orange flavor] [DSC]
Tablet, oral: 250: Amoxicillin 250 mg and clavulanate potassium 125 mg; 500: Amoxicillin 500 mg and clavulanate potassium 125 mg; 875: Amoxicillin 875 mg and clavulanate potassium 125 mg

Augmentin®:

250: Amoxicillin 250 mg and clavulanate potassium 125 mg [contains potassium 0.63 mEq/tablet] [DSC]

500: Amoxicillin 500 mg and clavulanate potassium 125 mg [contains potassium 0.63 mEq/tablet]

875: Amoxicillin 875 mg and clavulanate potassium 125 mg [contains potassium 0.63 mEq/tablet]

Tablet, chewable, oral: 200: Amoxicillin 200 mg and clavulanate potassium 28.5 mg [contains phenylalanine]; 400: Amoxicillin 400 mg and clavulanate potassium 57 mg [contains phenylalanine]

Tablet, extended release, oral: Amoxicillin 1000 mg and clavulanate acid 62.5 mg

Augmentin XR®: 1000: Amoxicillin 1000 mg and clavulanate acid 62.5 mg [contains potassium 12.6 mg (0.32 mEq) and sodium 29.3 mg (1.27 mEq) per tablet; packaged in either a 7-day or 10-day package]

◆ **Amoxicillin and Clavulanate Potassium** *see* Amoxicillin and Clavulanate *on page 115*

◆ **Amoxicillin and Clavulanic Acid** *see* Amoxicillin and Clavulanate *on page 115*

◆ **Amoxicillin Trihydrate** *see* Amoxicillin *on page 112*

◆ **Amoxil** *see* Amoxicillin *on page 112*

◆ **Amoxycillin** *see* Amoxicillin *on page 112*

◆ **Amphadase™** *see* Hyaluronidase *on page 931*

◆ **Amphotec®** *see* Amphotericin B Cholesteryl Sulfate Complex *on page 119*

Amphotericin B Cholesteryl Sulfate Complex

(am foe TER i sin bee kole LES te ril SUL fate KOM plecks)

Medication Safety Issues

High alert medication:

The Institute for Safe Medication Practices (ISMP) includes this medication among its list of drugs which have a heightened risk of causing significant patient harm when used in error.

Other safety concerns:

Lipid-based amphotericin formulations (Amphotec®) may be confused with conventional formulations (Amphocin®, Fungizone®)

Large overdoses have occurred when conventional formulations were dispensed inadvertently for lipid-based products. Single daily doses of conventional amphotericin formulation never exceed 1.5 mg/kg.

Brand Names: U.S. Amphotec®

Brand Names: Canada Amphotec®

Index Terms ABCD; Amphotericin B Colloidal Dispersion

Generic Availability (U.S.) No

Pharmacologic Category Antifungal Agent, Parenteral

Use Treatment of invasive aspergillosis in patients who have failed amphotericin B deoxycholate treatment, or who have renal impairment or experience unacceptable toxicity which precludes treatment with amphotericin B deoxycholate in effective doses.

Unlabeled Use Effective in patients with serious *Candida* species infections

Contraindications Hypersensitivity to amphotericin B or any component of the formulation (unless the benefits outweigh the possible risk to the patient)

Warnings/Precautions Anaphylaxis has been reported with amphotericin B-containing drugs. If severe respiratory distress occurs, the infusion should be immediately discontinued; the patient should not receive further infusions. During the initial dosing, the drug should be administered under close clinical observation. Acute infusion reactions, sometimes severe, may occur 1-3 hours after starting infusion. These reactions are usually more common with the first few doses and generally diminish with subsequent doses. Pretreatment with antihistamines/corticosteroids and/or decreasing the rate of infusion can be used to manage reactions. Avoid rapid infusion.

Adverse Reactions (Reflective of adult population; not specific for elderly)

>10%:

Cardiovascular: Hypotension, tachycardia

Central nervous system: Chills, fever

Endocrine & metabolic: Hypokalemia

Gastrointestinal: Vomiting

Hepatic: Hyperbilirubinemia

Renal: Creatinine increased

5% to 10%:

Cardiovascular: Chest pain, facial edema, hypertension

Central nervous system: Abnormal thinking, headache, insomnia, somnolence, tremor

Dermatologic: Pruritus, rash, sweating

◀ Endocrine & metabolic: Hyperglycemia, hypocalcemia, hypomagnesemia, hypophosphatemia

Gastrointestinal: Abdominal enlargement, abdominal pain, diarrhea, dry mouth, hematemesis, jaundice, nausea, stomatitis

Hematologic: Anemia, hemorrhage, thrombocytopenia

Hepatic: Alkaline phosphatase increased, liver function test abnormal

Neuromuscular & skeletal: Back pain, rigor

Respiratory: Cough increased, dyspnea, epistaxis, hypoxia, rhinitis

Note: Amphotericin B colloidal dispersion has an improved therapeutic index compared to conventional amphotericin B, and has been used safely in patients with amphotericin B-related nephrotoxicity; however, continued decline of renal function has occurred in some patients.

Drug Interactions

Metabolism/Transport Effects None known.

Avoid Concomitant Use

Avoid concomitant use of Amphotericin B Cholesteryl Sulfate Complex with any of the following: Gallium Nitrate

Increased Effect/Toxicity

Amphotericin B Cholesteryl Sulfate Complex may increase the levels/effects of: Aminoglycosides; Colistimethate; CycloSPORINE; CycloSPORINE (Systemic); Flucytosine; Gallium Nitrate

The levels/effects of Amphotericin B Cholesteryl Sulfate Complex may be increased by: Corticosteroids (Orally Inhaled); Corticosteroids (Systemic)

Decreased Effect

Amphotericin B Cholesteryl Sulfate Complex may decrease the levels/effects of: Saccharomyces boulardii

The levels/effects of Amphotericin B Cholesteryl Sulfate Complex may be decreased by: Antifungal Agents (Azole Derivatives, Systemic)

Stability Store intact vials at 15°C to 30°C (59°F to 86°F). Reconstitute 50 mg and 100 mg vials with 10 mL and 20 mL of SWI, respectively. The reconstituted vials contain 5 mg/mL of amphotericin B. Shake the vial gently by hand until all solid particles have dissolved. After reconstitution, the solution should be refrigerated at 2°C to 8°C (36°F to 46°F) and used within 24 hours. Further dilute amphotericin B colloidal dispersion with D_5W. Concentrations of 0.1-2 mg/mL in D_5W are stable for 24 hours at 2°C to 8°C (36°F to 46°F).

Mechanism of Action Binds to ergosterol altering cell membrane permeability in susceptible fungi and causing leakage of cell components with subsequent cell death. Proposed mechanism suggests that amphotericin causes an oxidation-dependent stimulation of macrophages (Lyman, 1992).

Pharmacodynamics/Kinetics

Distribution: V_d: Total volume increases with higher doses, reflects increasing uptake by tissues (with 4 mg/kg/day = 4 L/kg); predominantly distributed in the liver; concentrations in kidneys and other tissues are lower than observed with conventional amphotericin B

Half-life elimination: ~28 hours; prolonged with higher doses

Dosage

Geriatric & Adult Aspergillosis (invasive), treatment: *Usual dosage range:* 3-4 mg/kg/day. **Note:** 6 mg/kg/day has been used for treatment of life-threatening invasive aspergillosis in immunocompromised patients (Bowden, 2002).

Premedication: For patients who experience chills, fever, hypotension, nausea, or other nonanaphylactic infusion-related immediate reactions, premedicate with the following drugs 30-60 minutes prior to drug administration: A nonsteroidal with or without diphenhydramine **or** acetaminophen with diphenhydramine **or** hydrocortisone 50-100 mg with or without a nonsteroidal and diphenhydramine (Paterson, 2008).

Test dose: For patients receiving their first dose in a new treatment course, a small amount (10 mL of the final preparation, containing between 1.6-8.3 mg) infused over 15-30 minutes is recommended. The patient should then be observed for an additional 30 minutes.

Administration Initially infuse at 1 mg/kg/hour. Rate of infusion may be increased with subsequent doses as patient tolerance allows (minimum infusion time: 2 hours). For a patient who experiences chills, fever, hypotension, nausea, or other nonanaphylactic infusion-related reactions, premedicate with the following drugs 30-60 minutes prior to drug administration: A nonsteroidal with or without diphenhydramine **or** acetaminophen with diphenhydramine **or** hydrocortisone 50-100 mg with or without a nonsteroidal and diphenhydramine (Paterson, 2008). If the patient experiences rigors during the infusion, meperidine may be administered. If severe respiratory distress occurs, the infusion should be immediately discontinued.

Monitoring Parameters Liver function tests, electrolytes, BUN, serum creatinine, CBC, prothrombin time; temperature, I/O; signs of hypokalemia (muscle weakness, cramping, drowsiness, ECG changes)

Pharmacotherapy Pearls Controlled trials which compare the original formulation of amphotericin B to the newer liposomal formulations (ie, Amphotec®) are lacking. Thus, comparative data discussing differences among the formulations should be interpreted cautiously. Although the risk of nephrotoxicity and infusion-related adverse effects may be less with Amphotec®, the efficacy profiles of Amphotec® and the original amphotericin formulation are comparable. Consequently, Amphotec® should be restricted to those patients who cannot tolerate or fail a standard amphotericin B formulation.

Special Geriatric Considerations The pharmacokinetics and dosing of amphotericin have not been studied in the elderly. Caution should be exercised and renal function and desired effect monitored closely.

Dosage Forms Excipient information presented when available (limited, particularly for generics); consult specific product labeling.
Injection, powder for reconstitution:
Amphotec®: 50 mg [contains edetate disodium, lactose 950 mg]
Amphotec®: 100 mg [contains edetate disodium, lactose 1900 mg]

◆ **Amphotericin B Colloidal Dispersion** *see* Amphotericin B Cholesteryl Sulfate Complex *on page 119*

Amphotericin B (Conventional) (am foe TER i sin bee con VEN sha nal)

Medication Safety Issues
High alert medication:
The Institute for Safe Medication Practices (ISMP) includes this medication (intrathecal administration) among its list of drugs which have a heightened risk of causing significant patient harm when used in error.
Other safety concerns:
Conventional amphotericin formulations (Amphocin®, Fungizone®) may be confused with lipid-based formulations (AmBisome®, Abelcet®, Amphotec®).
Large overdoses have occurred when conventional formulations were dispensed inadvertently for lipid-based products. Single daily doses of conventional amphotericin formulation never exceed 1.5 mg/kg.

Brand Names: Canada Fungizone®

Index Terms Amphotericin B Deoxycholate; Amphotericin B Desoxycholate; Conventional Amphotericin B

Generic Availability (U.S.) Yes

Pharmacologic Category Antifungal Agent, Parenteral

Use Treatment of severe systemic and central nervous system infections caused by susceptible fungi such as *Candida* species, *Histoplasma capsulatum*, *Cryptococcus neoformans*, *Aspergillus* species, *Blastomyces dermatitidis*, *Torulopsis glabrata*, and *Coccidioides immitis*; fungal peritonitis; irrigant for bladder fungal infections; used in fungal infection in patients with bone marrow transplantation, amebic meningoencephalitis, ocular aspergillosis (intraocular injection), candidal cystitis (bladder irrigation), chemoprophylaxis (low-dose I.V.), immunocompromised patients at risk of aspergillosis (intranasal/nebulized), refractory meningitis (intrathecal), coccidioidal arthritis (intra-articular/I.M.).

Low-dose amphotericin B has been administered after bone marrow transplantation to reduce the risk of invasive fungal disease.

Contraindications Hypersensitivity to amphotericin or any component of the formulation

Warnings/Precautions Anaphylaxis has been reported with amphotericin B-containing drugs. During the initial dosing, the drug should be administered under close clinical observation. May cause nephrotoxicity; usual risk factors include underlying renal disease, concomitant nephrotoxic medications and daily and/or cumulative dose of amphotericin. Avoid use with other nephrotoxic drugs; drug-induced renal toxicity usually improves with interrupting therapy, decreasing dosage, or increasing dosing interval. However permanent impairment may occur, especially in patients receiving large cumulative dose (eg, >5 g) and in those also receiving other nephrotoxic drugs. Hydration and sodium repletion prior to administration may reduce the risk of developing nephrotoxicity. Frequent monitoring of renal function is recommended. Acute reactions (eg, fever, shaking chills, hypotension, anorexia, nausea, vomiting, headache, tachypnea) are most common 1-3 hours after starting the infusion and diminish with continued therapy. Avoid rapid infusion to prevent hypotension, hypokalemia, arrhythmias, and shock. If therapy is stopped for >7 days, restart at the lowest dose recommended and increase gradually. Leukoencephalopathy has been reported following administration of amphotericin. Total body irradiation has been reported to be a possible predisposition.

AMPHOTERICIN B (CONVENTIONAL)

[U.S. Boxed Warning]: Should be used primarily for treatment of progressive, potentially life-threatening fungal infections, not noninvasive forms of infection. **[U.S. Boxed warning]:** Verify the product name and dosage if dose exceeds 1.5 mg/kg.

Adverse Reactions (Reflective of adult population; not specific for elderly)

>10%:
  Central nervous system: Fever, chills, headache, malaise, generalized pain
  Endocrine & metabolic: Hypokalemia, hypomagnesemia
  Gastrointestinal: Anorexia
  Hematologic: Anemia
  Renal: Nephrotoxicity
1% to 10%:
  Cardiovascular: Hypotension, hypertension, flushing
  Central nervous system: Delirium, arachnoiditis, pain along lumbar nerves
  Gastrointestinal: Nausea, vomiting
  Genitourinary: Urinary retention
  Hematologic: Leukocytosis
  Local: Thrombophlebitis
  Neuromuscular & skeletal: Paresthesia (especially with I.T. therapy)
  Renal: Renal tubular acidosis, renal failure

Drug Interactions
  Metabolism/Transport Effects None known.
  Avoid Concomitant Use
    Avoid concomitant use of Amphotericin B (Conventional) with any of the following: Gallium Nitrate
  Increased Effect/Toxicity
    Amphotericin B (Conventional) may increase the levels/effects of: Aminoglycosides; Colistimethate; CycloSPORINE; CycloSPORINE (Systemic); Flucytosine; Gallium Nitrate

    The levels/effects of Amphotericin B (Conventional) may be increased by: Corticosteroids (Orally Inhaled); Corticosteroids (Systemic)
  Decreased Effect
    Amphotericin B (Conventional) may decrease the levels/effects of: Saccharomyces boulardii

    The levels/effects of Amphotericin B (Conventional) may be decreased by: Antifungal Agents (Azole Derivatives, Systemic)

Stability Store intact vials under refrigeration. Protect from light. Add 10 mL of SWFI (without a bacteriostatic agent) to each vial of amphotericin B. Further dilute with 250-500 mL D_5W; final concentration should not exceed 0.1 mg/mL (peripheral infusion) or 0.25 mg/mL (central infusion).

Reconstituted vials are stable, protected from light, for 24 hours at room temperature and 1 week when refrigerated. Parenteral admixtures are stable, protected from light, for 24 hours at room temperature and 2 days under refrigeration. Short-term exposure (<24 hours) to light during I.V. infusion does **not** appreciably affect potency.

Mechanism of Action Binds to ergosterol altering cell membrane permeability in susceptible fungi and causing leakage of cell components with subsequent cell death. Proposed mechanism suggests that amphotericin causes an oxidation-dependent stimulation of macrophages (Lyman, 1992).

Pharmacodynamics/Kinetics
  Distribution: Minimal amounts enter the aqueous humor, bile, CSF (inflamed or noninflamed meninges), pericardial fluid, pleural fluid, and synovial fluid
  Protein binding, plasma: 90%
  Half-life elimination: Biphasic: Initial: 15-48 hours; Terminal: 15 days
  Time to peak: Within 1 hour following a 4- to 6-hour dose
  Excretion: Urine (2% to 5% as biologically active form); ~40% eliminated over a 7-day period and may be detected in urine for at least 7 weeks after discontinued use

Dosage
  Geriatric & Adult Note: Premedication: For patients who experience infusion-related immediate reactions, premedicate with the following drugs 30-60 minutes prior to drug administration: NSAID ± diphenhydramine **or** acetaminophen with diphenhydramine **or** hydrocortisone. If the patient experiences rigors during the infusion, meperidine may be administered.
  Test dose: I.V.: 1 mg infused over 20-30 minutes. Many clinicians believe a test dose is unnecessary.
  Susceptible fungal infections: I.V.: Adults: 0.3-1.5 mg/kg/day; 1-1.5 mg/kg over 4-6 hours every other day may be given once therapy is established; aspergillosis, rhinocerebral mucormycosis, often require 1-1.5 mg/kg/day; do not exceed 1.5 mg/kg/day
  Aspergillosis, disseminated: I.V.: 0.6-0.7 mg/kg/day for 3-6 months

Bone marrow transplantation (prophylaxis): I.V.: Low-dose amphotericin B 0.1-0.25 mg/kg/day has been administered after bone marrow transplantation to reduce the risk of invasive fungal disease.

Candidemia (neutropenic or non-neutropenic): I.V.: 0.5-1 mg/kg/day until 14 days after first negative blood culture and resolution of signs and symptoms (Pappas, 2009)

Candidiasis, chronic, disseminated: I.V.: 0.5-0.7 mg/kg/day for 3-6 months and reso- lution of radiologic lesions (Pappas, 2009)

Dematiaceous fungi: I.V.: 0.7 mg/kg/day in combination with an azole

Endocarditis: I.V.: 0.6-1 mg/kg/day (with or without flucytosine) for 6 weeks after valve replacement; **Note:** If isolates susceptible and/or clearance demonstrated, guidelines recommend step-down to fluconazole; also for long-term suppression therapy if valve replacement is not possible (Pappas, 2009)

Endophthalmitis, fungal:
Intravitreal (unlabeled use): 10 mcg in 0.1 mL (in conjunction with systemic therapy)
I.V.: 0.7-1 mg/kg/day (with or without flucytosine) for at least 4-6 weeks (Pappas, 2009)

Esophageal candidiasis: I.V.: 0.3-0.7 mg/kg/day for 14-21 days after clinical improve- ment (Pappas, 2009)

Histoplasmosis: Chronic, severe pulmonary or disseminated: I.V.: 0.5-1 mg/kg/day for 7 days, then 0.8 mg/kg every other day (or 3 times/week) until total dose of 10-15 mg/kg; may continue itraconazole as suppressive therapy (lifelong for immunocompromised patients)

Meningitis:
Candidal: I.V.: 0.7-1 mg/kg/day (with or without flucytosine) for at least 4 weeks; **Note:** Liposomal amphotericin favored by IDSA guidelines based on decreased risk of nephrotoxicity and potentially better CNS penetration (Pappas, 2009)
Cryptococcal or Coccidioides: I.T.: Initial: 0.01-0.05 mg as single daily dose; may increase daily in increments of 0.025-0.1 mg as tolerated (maximum: 1.5 mg/day; most patients will tolerate a maximum dose of ~0.5 mg/treatment). Once titration to a maximum tolerated dose is achieved, that dose is administered daily. Once CSF improvement noted, may decrease frequency on a weekly basis (eg, 5 times/week, then 3 times/week, then 2 times/week, then once weekly, then once every other week, then once every 2 weeks, etc) until administration occurs once every 6 weeks. Typically, concurrent oral azole therapy is maintained (Stevens, 2001). **Note:** IDSA notes that the use of I.T. amphotericin for cryptococcal meningitis is generally discouraged and rarely necessary (Perfect, 2010).
Histoplasma: I.V.: 0.5-1 mg/kg/day for 7 days, then 0.8 mg/kg every other day (or 3 times/ week) for 3 months total duration; follow with fluconazole suppressive therapy for up to 12 months

Meningoencephalitis, cryptococcal (Perfect, 2010): I.V.:
HIV positive: Induction: 0.7-1 mg/kg/day (plus flucytosine 100 mg/kg/day) for 2 weeks, then change to oral fluconazole for at least 8 weeks; alternatively, amphotericin (0.7-1 mg/kg/day) may be continued uninterrupted for 4-6 weeks; maintenance: ampho- tericin 1 mg/kg/week for ≥1 year may be considered, but inferior to use of azoles
HIV negative: Induction: 0.7-1 mg/kg/day (plus flucytosine 100 mg/kg/day) for 2 weeks (low-risk patients), ≥4 weeks (non-low-risk, but without neurologic complication, immu- nosuppression, underlying disease, and negative CSF culture at 2 weeks), >6 weeks (neurologic complication or patients intolerant of flucytosine) Follow with azole con- solidation/maintenance treatment.

Oropharyngeal candidiasis: I.V.: 0.3 mg/kg/day for 7-14 days (Pappas, 2009)

Osteoarticular candidiasis: I.V.: 0.5-1 mg/kg/day for several weeks, followed by fluco- nazole for 6-12 months (osteomyelitis) or 6 weeks (septic arthritis) (Pappas, 2009)

Penicillium marneffei: I.V.: 0.6 mg/kg/day for 2 weeks

Pneumonia: Cryptococcal (mild-to-moderate): I.V.:
HIV positive: 0.5-1 mg/kg/day
HIV negative: 0.5-0.7 mg/kg/day (plus flucytosine) for 2 weeks

Sporotrichosis: Pulmonary, meningeal, osteoarticular or disseminated: I.V.: Total dose of 1-2 g, then change to oral itraconazole or fluconazole for suppressive therapy

Urinary tract candidiasis (Pappas, 2009):
Fungus balls: I.V.: 0.5-0.7 mg/kg/day with or without flucytosine 25 mg/kg 4 times daily
Pyelonephritis: I.V.: 0.5-0.7 mg/kg/day with or without flucytosine 25 mg/kg 4 times daily for 2 weeks
Symptomatic cystitis: I.V.: 0.3-0.6 mg/kg/day for 1-7 days
Bladder irrigation: Irrigate with 50 mcg/mL solution instilled periodically or continuously for 5-10 days or until cultures are clear for fluconazole-resistant *Candida*

Renal Impairment

If renal dysfunction is due to the drug, the daily total can be decreased by 50% or the dose can be given every other day. I.V. therapy may take several months.

Renal replacement therapy: Poorly dialyzed; no supplemental dose or dosage adjustment necessary, including patients on intermittent hemodialysis or CRRT.

Peritoneal dialysis (PD): Administration in dialysate: 1-2 mg/L of peritoneal dialysis fluid either with or without low-dose I.V. amphotericin B (a total dose of 2-10 mg/kg given over 7-14 days). Precipitate may form in ionic dialysate solutions.

Administration May be infused over 4-6 hours. For a patient who experiences chills, fever, hypotension, nausea, or other nonanaphylactic infusion-related reactions, premedicate with the following drugs 30-60 minutes prior to drug administration: A nonsteroidal (eg, ibuprofen, choline magnesium trisalicylate) ± diphenhydramine **or** acetaminophen with diphenhydramine **or** hydrocortisone. If the patient experiences rigors during the infusion, meperidine may be administered. Bolus infusion of normal saline immediately preceding, or immediately preceding and following amphotericin B may reduce drug-induced nephrotoxicity. Risk of nephrotoxicity increases with amphotericin B doses >1 mg/kg/day. Infusion of admixtures more concentrated than 0.25 mg/mL should be limited to patients absolutely requiring volume contraction.

Monitoring Parameters Renal function (monitor frequently during therapy), electrolytes (especially potassium and magnesium), liver function tests, temperature, PT/PTT, CBC; monitor input and output; monitor for signs of hypokalemia (muscle weakness, cramping, drowsiness, ECG changes, etc)

Reference Range Therapeutic: 1-2 mcg/mL (SI: 1-2.2 micromole/L)

Test Interactions Increased BUN (S), serum creatinine, alkaline phosphate, bilirubin; decreased magnesium, potassium (S)

Pharmacotherapy Pearls Premedication with diphenhydramine and acetaminophen may reduce the severity of acute infusion-related reactions. Meperidine reduces the duration of amphotericin B-induced rigors and chilling. Hydrocortisone may be used in patients with severe or refractory infusion-related reactions. Bolus infusion of normal saline immediately preceding, or immediately preceding and following amphotericin B may reduce drug-induced nephrotoxicity. Risk of nephrotoxicity increases with amphotericin B doses >1 mg/kg/day. Infusion of admixtures more concentrated than 0.25 mg/mL should be limited to patients absolutely requiring volume restriction. Amphotericin B does not have a bacteriostatic constituent, subsequently admixture expiration is determined by sterility more than chemical stability.

Special Geriatric Considerations The pharmacokinetics and dosing of amphotericin have not been studied in elderly. Caution should be exercised and renal function and desired effect monitored closely.

Dosage Forms Excipient information presented when available (limited, particularly for generics); consult specific product labeling.

Injection, powder for reconstitution, as desoxycholate: 50 mg

◆ **Amphotericin B Deoxycholate** see Amphotericin B (Conventional) on page 121
◆ **Amphotericin B Desoxycholate** see Amphotericin B (Conventional) on page 121

Amphotericin B (Lipid Complex) (am foe TER i sin bee LIP id KOM pleks)

Medication Safety Issues
High alert medication:
The Institute for Safe Medication Practices (ISMP) includes this medication among its list of drugs which have a heightened risk of causing significant patient harm when used in error.

Other safety concerns:
Lipid-based amphotericin formulations (Abelcet®) may be confused with conventional formulations (Fungizone®) or with other lipid-based amphotericin formulations (amphotericin B liposomal [AmBisome®]; amphotericin B cholesteryl sulfate complex [Amphotec®]) Large overdoses have occurred when conventional formulations were dispensed inadvertently for lipid-based products. Single daily doses of conventional amphotericin formulation never exceed 1.5 mg/kg.

Brand Names: U.S. Abelcet®
Brand Names: Canada Abelcet®
Index Terms ABLC
Generic Availability (U.S.) No
Pharmacologic Category Antifungal Agent, Parenteral
Use Treatment of invasive fungal infection in patients who are refractory to or intolerant of conventional amphotericin B (amphotericin B deoxycholate) therapy
Contraindications Hypersensitivity to amphotericin or any component of the formulation
Warnings/Precautions Anaphylaxis has been reported with amphotericin B-containing drugs. If severe respiratory distress occurs, the infusion should be immediately discontinued. During the initial dosing, the drug should be administered under close clinical observation. Acute reactions (including fever and chills) may occur 1-2 hours after starting an intravenous

infusion. These reactions are usually more common with the first few doses and generally diminish with subsequent doses. Infusion has been rarely associated with hypotension, bronchospasm, arrhythmias, and shock. Acute pulmonary toxicity has been reported in patients receiving leukocyte transfusions and amphotericin B; amphotericin B lipid complex and concurrent leukocyte transfusions are not recommended. Concurrent use with antineoplastic agents may enhance the potential for renal toxicity, bronchospasm or hypotension; use with caution. Concurrent use of amphotericin B with other nephrotoxic drugs may enhance the potential for drug-induced renal toxicity.

Adverse Reactions (Reflective of adult population; not specific for elderly) Nephrotoxicity and infusion-related hyperpyrexia, rigor, and chilling are reduced relative to amphotericin deoxycholate.

>10%:
Central nervous system: Chills (18%), fever (14%)
Renal: Serum creatinine increased (11%)
Miscellaneous: Multiple organ failure (11%)

1% to 10%:
Cardiovascular: Hypotension (8%), cardiac arrest (6%), hypertension (5%), chest pain (3%)
Central nervous system: Headache (6%), pain (5%)
Dermatologic: Rash (4%)
Endocrine & metabolic: Hypokalemia (5%), bilirubinemia (4%)
Gastrointestinal: Nausea (9%), vomiting (8%), diarrhea (6%), gastrointestinal hemorrhage (4%), abdominal pain (4%)
Hematologic: Thrombocytopenia (5%), anemia (4%), leukopenia (4%)
Renal: Renal failure (5%)
Respiratory: Respiratory failure (8%), dyspnea (6%), respiratory disorder (4%)
Miscellaneous: Sepsis (7%), infection (5%)

Drug Interactions

Metabolism/Transport Effects None known.

Avoid Concomitant Use

Avoid concomitant use of Amphotericin B (Lipid Complex) with any of the following: Gallium Nitrate

Increased Effect/Toxicity

Amphotericin B (Lipid Complex) may increase the levels/effects of: Aminoglycosides; Colistimethate; CycloSPORINE; CycloSPORINE (Systemic); Flucytosine; Gallium Nitrate

The levels/effects of Amphotericin B (Lipid Complex) may be increased by: Corticosteroids (Orally Inhaled); Corticosteroids (Systemic)

Decreased Effect

Amphotericin B (Lipid Complex) may decrease the levels/effects of: Saccharomyces boulardii

The levels/effects of Amphotericin B (Lipid Complex) may be decreased by: Antifungal Agents (Azole Derivatives, Systemic)

Stability Intact vials should be stored at 2°C to 8°C (35°F to 46°F); do not freeze. Protect intact vials from exposure to light. Solutions for infusion are stable for 48 hours under refrigeration and for an additional 6 hours at room temperature. To prepare the infusion, shake the vial gently until there is no evidence of any yellow sediment at the bottom. Withdraw the appropriate dose from the vial using an 18-gauge needle. Remove the 18-gauge needle and attach the provided 5-micron filter needle to filter, and dilute the dose with D_5W to a final concentration of 1 mg/mL. Each filter needle may be used to filter up to four 100 mg vials. A final concentration of 2 mg/mL may be used for pediatric patients and patients with cardiovascular disease.

Do not dilute with saline solutions or mix with other drugs or electrolytes - compatibility has not been established

Mechanism of Action Binds to ergosterol altering cell membrane permeability in susceptible fungi and causing leakage of cell components with subsequent cell death. Proposed mechanism suggests that amphotericin causes an oxidation-dependent stimulation of macrophages.

Pharmacodynamics/Kinetics Note: Exhibits nonlinear kinetics; volume of distribution and clearance from blood increases with increasing dose.

Distribution: V_d: Increases with higher doses (likely reflects increased uptake by tissues); 131 L/kg with 5 mg/kg/day

Half-life elimination: 173 hours following multiple doses

Excretion: 0.9% of dose excreted in urine over 24 hours; effects of hepatic and renal impairment on drug disposition are unknown

Dialysis: Amphotericin B (lipid complex) is not hemodialyzable

AMPHOTERICIN B (LIPID COMPLEX)

◀ **Dosage**

Geriatric & Adult Note: Premedication: For patients who experience infusion-related immediate reactions, premedicate with the following drugs 30-60 minutes prior to drug administration: A nonsteroidal anti-inflammatory agent ± diphenhydramine **or** acetaminophen with diphenhydramine **or** hydrocortisone. If the patient experiences rigors during the infusion, meperidine may be administered.

Usual dose: I.V.: 5 mg/kg once daily

Manufacturer's labeling: Invasive fungal infections (when patients are intolerant or refractory to conventional amphotericin B): I.V.: 5 mg/kg/day

Indication-specific dosing:

Aspergillosis, invasive (HIV positive or HIV negative patients) (alternative to preferred therapy): I.V.: 5 mg/kg/day; duration of treatment in HIV-negative patients depends on site of infection, extent of disease and level of immunosuppression; in HIV-positive patients, treat until CD4 count >200 cells/mm^3 and evidence of clinical response (CDC [adults], 2009; Walsh, 2008)

Blastomycosis, moderately-severe-to-severe (unlabeled dose): I.V.: 3-5 mg/kg/day for 1-2 weeks or until improvement, followed by oral itraconazole (Chapman, 2008)

Candidiasis (unlabeled dose): I.V.:

Chronic disseminated candidiasis, pericarditis or myocarditis due to Candida, suppurative thrombophlebitis: 3-5 mg/kg/day. **Note:** In chronic disseminated candidiasis, transition to fluconazole after several weeks in stable patients is preferred (Pappas, 2009)

CNS candidiasis: 3-5 mg/kg/day (with or without flucytosine) for several weeks, followed by fluconazole (Pappas, 2009)

Endocarditis due to Candida, infected pacemaker, ICD, or VAD: 3-5 mg/kg/day (with or without flucytosine); continue to treat for 4-6 weeks after device removal unless device cannot be removed then chronic suppression with fluconazole is recommended (Pappas, 2009)

Coccidioidomycosis (unlabeled dose): I.V.:

Progressive, disseminated: (alternative to preferred therapy): 2-5 mg/kg/day (Galgiani, 2005)

HIV-positive patients with severe, nonmeningeal infection: 4-6 mg/kg/day until clinical improvement, then switch to fluconazole or itraconazole (CDC, 2009)

Cryptococcosis: I.V.:

Cryptococcal meningoencephalitis in HIV-positive patients (as an alternative to conventional amphotericin B in patients with renal concerns): Induction therapy: 4-6 mg/kg/day (unlabeled dose; CDC [adult], 2009) or 5 mg/kg/day (Perfect, 2010) with flucytosine for at least 2 weeks, followed by oral fluconazole. **Note:** If flucytosine is not given due to intolerance, duration of amphotericin B lipid complex therapy should be 4-6 weeks (Perfect, 2010).

Cryptococcal meningoencephalitis in HIV-negative patients and nontransplant patients (as an alternative to conventional amphotericin B): Induction therapy: 5 mg/kg/day (with flucytosine if possible) for ≥4 weeks followed by oral fluconazole. **Note:** If flucytosine is not given or treatment is interrupted, consider prolonging induction therapy for an additional 2 weeks (Perfect, 2010).

Cryptococcal meningoencephalitis in transplant recipients: Induction therapy: 5 mg/kg/day (with flucytosine) for at least 2 weeks, followed by oral fluconazole **Note:** If flucytosine is not given, duration of amphotericin B lipid complex therapy should be 4-6 weeks (Perfect, 2010).

Nonmeningeal cryptococcosis: Induction therapy: 5 mg/kg/day (with flucytosine if possible) for ≥4 weeks may be used for severe pulmonary cryptococcosis or for cryptococcemia with evidence of high fungal burden, followed by oral fluconazole. **Note:** If flucytosine is not given or treatment is interrupted, consider prolonging induction therapy for an additional 2 weeks (Perfect, 2010).

Histoplasmosis: I.V.:

Acute pulmonary (moderately-severe-to-severe): 5 mg/kg/day for 1-2 weeks, followed by oral itraconazole (Wheat, 2007)

Progressive disseminated (alternative to preferred therapy): 5 mg/kg/day for 1-2 weeks, followed by oral itraconazole (Wheat, 2007)

Sporotrichosis (unlabeled dose): I.V.:

Meningeal: 5 mg/kg/day for 4-6 weeks, followed by oral itraconazole (Kauffman, 2007)

Pulmonary, osteoarticular, and disseminated: 3-5 mg/kg/day, followed by oral itraconazole after a favorable response is seen with amphotericin initial therapy (Kauffman, 2007)

Renal Impairment

Manufacturer's recommendations: No dosage adjustment provided in manufacturer's labeling (has not been studied).

Alternate recommendations (Aronoff, 2007):

Intermittent hemodialysis: No supplemental dosage necessary.

Peritoneal dialysis: No supplemental dosage necessary.

Continuous renal replacement therapy (CRRT): No supplemental dosage necessar.

Hepatic Impairment No dosage adjustment provided in manufacturer's labeling (has not been studied).

Administration For patients who experience nonanaphylactic infusion-related reactions, premedicate 30-60 minutes prior to drug administration with a nonsteroidal anti-inflammatory agent ± diphenhydramine **or** acetaminophen with diphenhydramine **or** hydrocortisone. If the patient experiences rigors during the infusion, meperidine may be administered.

Administer at an infusion rate of 2.5 mg/kg/hour (eg, over 2 hours for 5 mg/kg). Invert infusion container several times prior to administration and every 2 hours during infusion if it exceeds 2 hours. **Do not use an in-line filter during administration.** Flush line with dextrose; normal saline may cause precipitate.

Monitoring Parameters Renal function (monitor frequently during therapy), electrolytes (especially potassium and magnesium), liver function tests, temperature, PT/PTT, CBC; monitor input and output; monitor for signs of hypokalemia (muscle weakness, cramping, drowsiness, ECG changes, etc)

Pharmacotherapy Pearls As a modification of dimyristoyl phosphatidylcholine:dimyristoyl phosphatidylglycerol 7:3 (DMPC:DMPG) liposome, amphotericin B lipid-complex has a higher drug to lipid ratio and the concentration of amphotericin B is 33 M. ABLC is a ribbon-like structure, not a liposome.

Controlled trials which compare the original formulation of amphotericin B to the newer liposomal formulations (ie, Abelcet®) are lacking. Thus, comparative data discussing differences among the formulations should be interpreted cautiously. Although the risk of nephrotoxicity and infusion-related adverse effects may be less with Abelcet®, the efficacy profiles of Abelcet® and the original amphotericin formulation are comparable. Consequently, Abelcet® should be restricted to those patients who cannot tolerate or fail a standard amphotericin B formulation.

Special Geriatric Considerations The pharmacokinetics and dosing of amphotericin have not been studied in elderly. It appears that use is similar to young adults; caution should be exercised and renal function and desired effect monitored closely.

Dosage Forms Excipient information presented when available (limited, particularly for generics); consult specific product labeling.

Injection, suspension [preservative free]:

Abelcet®: 5 mg/mL (20 mL)

Ampicillin (am pi SIL in)

Related Information

Antibiotic Treatment of Adults With Infective Endocarditis *on page 2157*
Antimicrobial Drugs of Choice *on page 2163*
Prevention of Infective Endocarditis *on page 2175*

Medication Safety Issues

Sound-alike/look-alike issues:

Ampicillin may be confused with aminophylline

Brand Names: Canada Ampicillin for Injection; Apo-Ampi®; Novo-Ampicillin; Nu-Ampi

Index Terms Aminobenzylpenicillin; Ampicillin Sodium; Ampicillin Trihydrate

Generic Availability (U.S.) Yes

Pharmacologic Category Antibiotic, Penicillin

Use Treatment of susceptible bacterial infections (nonbeta-lactamase-producing organisms); treatment or prophylaxis of infective endocarditis; susceptible bacterial infections caused by streptococci, pneumococci, nonpenicillinase-producing staphylococci, *Listeria*, meningococci; some strains of *H. influenzae*, *Salmonella*, *Shigella*, *E. coli*, *Enterobacter*, and *Klebsiella*

Contraindications Hypersensitivity to ampicillin, any component of the formulation, or other penicillins

Warnings/Precautions Dosage adjustment may be necessary in patients with renal impairment. Serious and occasionally severe or fatal hypersensitivity (anaphylactoid) reactions have been reported in patients on penicillin therapy, especially with a history of beta-lactam hypersensitivity, history of sensitivity to multiple allergens, or previous IgE-mediated reactions (eg, anaphylaxis, angioedema, urticaria). Use with caution in asthmatic patients. High percentage of patients with infectious mononucleosis have developed rash during therapy with ampicillin; ampicillin-class antibiotics not recommended in these patients. Appearance of a rash should be carefully evaluated to differentiate a nonallergic ampicillin rash from a hypersensitivity reaction. Prolonged use may result in fungal or bacterial superinfection, including *C. difficile*-associated diarrhea (CDAD) and pseudomembranous colitis; CDAD has been observed >2 months postantibiotic treatment.

Adverse Reactions (Reflective of adult population; not specific for elderly) Frequency not defined.

Central nervous system: Fever, penicillin encephalopathy, seizure

Dermatologic: Erythema multiforme, exfoliative dermatitis, rash, urticaria

Note: Appearance of a rash should be carefully evaluated to differentiate (if possible) nonallergic ampicillin rash from hypersensitivity reaction. Incidence is higher in patients with viral infection, *Salmonella* infection, lymphocytic leukemia, or patients that have hyperuricemia.

Gastrointestinal: Black hairy tongue, diarrhea, enterocolitis, glossitis, nausea, oral candidiasis, pseudomembranous colitis, sore mouth or tongue, stomatitis, vomiting

Hematologic: Agranulocytosis, anemia, hemolytic anemia, eosinophilia, leukopenia, thrombocytopenia purpura

Hepatic: AST increased

Renal: Interstitial nephritis (rare)

Respiratory: Laryngeal stridor

Miscellaneous: Anaphylaxis, serum sickness-like reaction

Drug Interactions

Metabolism/Transport Effects None known.

Avoid Concomitant Use

Avoid concomitant use of Ampicillin with any of the following: BCG

Increased Effect/Toxicity

Ampicillin may increase the levels/effects of: Methotrexate; Vitamin K Antagonists

The levels/effects of Ampicillin may be increased by: Allopurinol; Probenecid

Decreased Effect

Ampicillin may decrease the levels/effects of: Atenolol; BCG; Mycophenolate; Typhoid Vaccine

The levels/effects of Ampicillin may be decreased by: Chloroquine; Fusidic Acid; Lanthanum; Tetracycline Derivatives

Ethanol/Nutrition/Herb Interactions Food: Food decreases ampicillin absorption rate; may decrease ampicillin serum concentration. Management: Take at equal intervals around-the-clock, preferably on an empty stomach (1 hour before or 2 hours after meals). Maintain adequate hydration, unless instructed to restrict fluid intake.

Stability

Oral: Oral suspension is stable for 7 days at room temperature or for 14 days under refrigeration.

I.V.:

I.V. minimum volume: Concentration should not exceed 30 mg/mL due to concentration-dependent stability restrictions. Solutions for I.M. or direct I.V. should be used within 1 hour. Solutions for I.V. infusion will be inactivated by dextrose at room temperature. If dextrose-containing solutions are to be used, the resultant solution will only be stable for 2 hours versus 8 hours in the 0.9% sodium chloride injection. D_5W has limited stability.

Stability of parenteral admixture in NS at room temperature (25°C) is 8 hours.

Stability of parenteral admixture in NS at refrigeration temperature (4°C) is 2 days.

Standard diluent: 500 mg/50 mL NS; 1 g/50 mL NS; 2 g/100 mL NS

Mechanism of Action Inhibits bacterial cell wall synthesis by binding to one or more of the penicillin-binding proteins (PBPs) which in turn inhibits the final transpeptidation step of peptidoglycan synthesis in bacterial cell walls, thus inhibiting cell wall biosynthesis. Bacteria eventually lyse due to ongoing activity of cell wall autolytic enzymes (autolysins and murein hydrolases) while cell wall assembly is arrested.

Pharmacodynamics/Kinetics

Absorption: Oral: 50%

Distribution: Bile, blister, and tissue fluids; penetration into CSF occurs with inflamed meninges only, good only with inflammation (exceeds usual MICs)

Normal meninges: Nil; Inflamed meninges: 5% to 10%

Protein binding: 15% to 25%

Half-life elimination:

Adults: 1-1.8 hours

Anuria/end-stage renal disease: 7-20 hours

Time to peak: Oral: Within 1-2 hours

Excretion: Urine (~90% as unchanged drug) within 24 hours

Dosage
Geriatric & Adult
Usual dosage range:
Oral: 250-500 mg every 6 hours

I.M., I.V.: 1-2 g every 4-6 hours or 50-250 mg/kg/day in divided doses (maximum: 12 g/day)

Cholangitis (acute): I.V.: 2 g every 4 hours with gentamicin

Diverticulitis: I.M., I.V.: 2 g every 6 hours with metronidazole

Endocarditis:

Infective: I.V.: 12 g/day via continuous infusion or divided every 4 hours

Prophylaxis: Dental, oral, or respiratory tract procedures: I.M., I.V.: 2 g within 30-60 minutes prior to procedure in patients not allergic to penicillin and unable to take oral amoxicillin. Intramuscular injections should be avoided in patients who are receiving anticoagulant therapy. In these circumstances, orally administered regimens should be given whenever possible. Intravenously administered antibiotics should be used for patients who are unable to tolerate or absorb oral medications. **Note:** American Heart Association (AHA) guidelines now recommend prophylaxis only in patients undergoing invasive procedures and in whom underlying cardiac conditions may predispose to a higher risk of adverse outcomes should infection occur.

Prophylaxis in total joint replacement patient: I.M., I.V.: 2 g 1 hour prior to the procedure

Genitourinary and gastrointestinal tract procedures: I.M., I.V.:

High-risk patients: 2 g within 30 minutes prior to procedure, followed by ampicillin 1 g (or amoxicillin 1 g orally) 6 hours later; must be used in combination with gentamicin. **Note:** As of April 2007, routine prophylaxis for GI/GU procedures is no longer recommended by the AHA.

Moderate-risk patients: 2 g within 30 minutes prior to procedure

Group B strep prophylaxis (intrapartum): I.V.: 2 g initial dose, then 1 g every 4 hours until delivery

***Listeria* infections:** I.V.: 2 g every 4 hours (consider addition of aminoglycoside)

Mild-to-moderate infections: Oral: 250-500 mg every 6 hours

Sepsis/meningitis: I.M., I.V.: 150-250 mg/kg/day divided every 3-4 hours (range: 6-12 g/day)

Urinary tract infections (*Enterococcus* suspected): I.V.: 1-2 g every 6 hours with gentamicin

Renal Impairment
Cl_{cr} >50 mL/minute: Administer every 6 hours

Cl_{cr} 10-50 mL/minute: Administer every 6-12 hours

Cl_{cr} <10 mL/minute: Administer every 12-24 hours

Intermittent hemodialysis (IHD) (administer after hemodialysis on dialysis days): Dialyzable (20% to 50%): I.V.: 1-2 g every 12-24 hours (Heintz, 2009). **Note:** Dosing dependent on the assumption of 3 times/week, complete IHD sessions.

Peritoneal dialysis (PD): 250 mg every 12 hours

Continuous renal replacement therapy (CRRT) (Heintz, 2009): Drug clearance is highly dependent on the method of renal replacement, filter type, and flow rate. Appropriate dosing requires close monitoring of pharmacologic response, signs of adverse reactions due to drug accumulation, as well as drug concentrations in relation to target trough (if appropriate). The following are general recommendations only (based on dialysate flow/ultrafiltration rates of 1-2 L/hour and minimal residual renal function) and should not supersede clinical judgment:

CVVH: Loading dose of 2 g followed by 1-2 g every 8-12 hours

CVVHD: Loading dose of 2 g followed by 1-2 g every 8 hours

CVVHDF: Loading dose of 2 g followed by 1-2 g every 6-8 hours

Administration Administer around-the-clock to promote less variation in peak and trough serum levels.

Oral: Administer on an empty stomach (ie, 1 hour prior to, or 2 hours after meals) to increase total absorption.

I.V.: Administer over 3-5 minutes (125-500 mg) or over 10-15 minutes (1-2 g). More rapid infusion may cause seizures. Ampicillin and gentamicin should not be mixed in the same I.V. tubing.

Some penicillins (eg, carbenicillin, ticarcillin, and piperacillin) have been shown to inactivate aminoglycosides *in vitro*. This has been observed to a greater extent with tobramycin and gentamicin, while amikacin has shown greater stability against inactivation. Concurrent use of these agents may pose a risk of reduced antibacterial efficacy *in vivo*, particularly in the setting of profound renal impairment. However, definitive clinical evidence is lacking. If combination penicillin/aminoglycoside therapy is desired in a patient with renal dysfunction, separation of doses (if feasible), and routine monitoring of aminoglycoside levels, CBC, and clinical response should be considered.

◀ **Monitoring Parameters** With prolonged therapy, monitor renal, hepatic, and hematologic function periodically; observe signs and symptoms of anaphylaxis during first dose

Test Interactions May interfere with urinary glucose tests using cupric sulfate (Benedict's solution, Clinitest®)

Some penicillin derivatives may accelerate the degradation of aminoglycosides *in vitro*, leading to a potential underestimation of aminoglycoside serum concentration.

Special Geriatric Considerations Resistance to ampicillin has been a problem in patients on frequent antibiotics or in nursing homes. Alternative antibiotics may be necessary in these populations. Adjust dose for renal function.

Dosage Forms Excipient information presented when available (limited, particularly for generics); consult specific product labeling.

Capsule, oral: 250 mg, 500 mg

Injection, powder for reconstitution, as sodium [strength expressed as base]: 125 mg, 250 mg, 500 mg, 1 g, 2 g, 10 g

Powder for suspension, oral: 125 mg/5 mL (100 mL, 200 mL); 250 mg/5 mL (100 mL, 200 mL)

Ampicillin and Sulbactam (am pi SIL in & SUL bak tam)

Related Information
Ampicillin *on page 127*
Antibiotic Treatment of Adults With Infective Endocarditis *on page 2157*
Antimicrobial Drugs of Choice *on page 2163*
Community-Acquired Pneumonia in Adults *on page 2171*

Brand Names: U.S. Unasyn®

Brand Names: Canada Unasyn®

Index Terms Sulbactam and Ampicillin

Generic Availability (U.S.) Yes

Pharmacologic Category Antibiotic, Penicillin

Use Treatment of susceptible bacterial infections involved with skin and skin structure, intra-abdominal infections, gynecological infections; spectrum is that of ampicillin plus organisms producing beta-lactamases such as *S. aureus*, *H. influenzae*, *E. coli*, *Klebsiella*, *Acinetobacter*, *Enterobacter*, and anaerobes

Unlabeled Use Acute bacterial rhinosinusitis (ABRS)

Contraindications Hypersensitivity to ampicillin, sulbactam, penicillins, or any component of the formulations

Warnings/Precautions Dosage adjustment may be necessary in patients with renal impairment. Serious and occasionally severe or fatal hypersensitivity (anaphylactoid) reactions have been reported in patients on penicillin therapy, especially with a history of beta-lactam hypersensitivity, history of sensitivity to multiple allergens, or previous IgE-mediated reactions (eg, anaphylaxis, angioedema, urticaria). Use with caution in asthmatic patients. High percentage of patients with infectious mononucleosis have developed rash during therapy with ampicillin; ampicillin-class antibiotics not recommended in these patients. Appearance of a rash should be carefully evaluated to differentiate a nonallergic ampicillin rash from a hypersensitivity reaction. Prolonged use may result in fungal or bacterial superinfection, including *C. difficile*-associated diarrhea (CDAD) and pseudomembranous colitis; CDAD has been observed >2 months postantibiotic treatment.

Adverse Reactions (Reflective of adult population; not specific for elderly) Also see Ampicillin.

>10%: Local: Pain at injection site (I.M.)

1% to 10%:
Dermatologic: Rash
Gastrointestinal: Diarrhea
Local: Pain at injection site (I.V.), thrombophlebitis
Miscellaneous: Allergic reaction (may include serum sickness, urticaria, bronchospasm, hypotension, etc)

Drug Interactions
Metabolism/Transport Effects None known.

Avoid Concomitant Use
Avoid concomitant use of Ampicillin and Sulbactam with any of the following: BCG

Increased Effect/Toxicity
Ampicillin and Sulbactam may increase the levels/effects of: Methotrexate; Vitamin K Antagonists

The levels/effects of Ampicillin and Sulbactam may be increased by: Allopurinol; Probenecid

Decreased Effect

Ampicillin and Sulbactam may decrease the levels/effects of: Atenolol; BCG; Mycophenolate; Typhoid Vaccine

The levels/effects of Ampicillin and Sulbactam may be decreased by: Chloroquine; Fusidic Acid; Lanthanum; Tetracycline Derivatives

Stability Prior to reconstitution, store at ≤30°C (86°F).

I.M. and direct I.V. administration: Use within 1 hour after preparation. Reconstitute with sterile water for injection or 0.5% or 2% lidocaine hydrochloride injection (I.M.). Sodium chloride 0.9% (NS) is the diluent of choice for I.V. piggyback use. Solutions made in NS are stable up to 72 hours when refrigerated whereas dextrose solutions (same concentration) are stable for only 4 hours.

Mechanism of Action The addition of sulbactam, a beta-lactamase inhibitor, to ampicillin extends the spectrum of ampicillin to include some beta-lactamase-producing organisms; inhibits bacterial cell wall synthesis by binding to one or more of the penicillin-binding proteins (PBPs) which in turn inhibits the final transpeptidation step of peptidoglycan synthesis in bacterial cell walls, thus inhibiting cell wall biosynthesis. Bacteria eventually lyse due to ongoing activity of cell wall autolytic enzymes (autolysins and murein hydrolases) while cell wall assembly is arrested.

Pharmacodynamics/Kinetics

Ampicillin: See Ampicillin.

Sulbactam:

Distribution: Bile, blister, and tissue fluids

Protein binding: 38%

Half-life elimination: Normal renal function: 1-1.3 hours

Excretion: Urine (~75% to 85% as unchanged drug) within 8 hours

Dosage

Geriatric & Adult Doses expressed as ampicillin/sulbactam combination.

Susceptible infections: I.M., I.V.: 1.5-3 g every 6 hours (maximum: Unasyn® 12 g)

Acute bacterial rhinosinusitis, severe infection requiring hospitalization (unlabeled use): I.V.: 1.5-3 g every 6 hours for 5-7 days (Chow, 2012)

Amnionitis, cholangitis, diverticulitis, endometritis, endophthalmitis, epididymitis/ orchitis, liver abscess, osteomyelitis (diabetic foot), peritonitis: I.V.: 3 g every 6 hours; **Note:** Due to high rates of *E. coli* resistance, not recommended for the treatment of community-acquired intra-abdominal infections (Solomkin, 2010)

Endocarditis: I.V.: 3 g every 6 hours with gentamicin or vancomycin for 4-6 weeks

Orbital cellulitis: I.V.: 1.5 g every 6 hours

Parapharyngeal space infections: I.V.: 3 g every 6 hours

***Pasteurella multocida* (human, canine/feline bites):** I.V.: 1.5-3 g every 6 hours

Pelvic inflammatory disease: I.V.: 3 g every 6 hours with doxycycline

Peritonitis associated with CAPD: Intraperitoneal:

Anuric, intermittent: 3 g every 12 hours (Li, 2010)

Anuric, continuous: Loading dose: 1.5 g per liter of dialysate; maintenance dose: 150 mg per liter of dialysate (Li, 2010)

Pneumonia:

Aspiration, community-acquired: I.V.: 1.5-3 g every 6 hours

Hospital-acquired: I.V.: 3 g every 6 hours

Urinary tract infections, pyelonephritis: I.V.: 3 g every 6 hours for 14 days

Renal Impairment Note: Estimation of renal function for the purpose of drug dosing should be done using the Cockcroft-Gault formula.

Cl_{cr} 15-29 mL/minute/1.73 m^2: 1.5-3 g every 12 hours

Cl_{cr} 5-14 mL/minute/1.73 m^2: 1.5-3 g every 24 hours

Intermittent hemodialysis (IHD) (administer after hemodialysis on dialysis days): 1.5-3 g every 12-24 hours (Heintz, 2009). **Note:** Dosing dependent on the assumption of 3 times/week, complete IHD sessions.

Peritoneal dialysis (PD): 3 g every 24 hours

Continuous renal replacement therapy (CRRT): Drug clearance is highly dependent on the method of renal replacement, filter type, and flow rate. Appropriate dosing requires close monitoring of pharmacologic response, signs of adverse reactions due to drug accumulation, as well as drug levels in relation to target trough (if appropriate). The following are general recommendations only (based on dialysate flow/ultrafiltration rates of 1-2 L/hour and minimal residual renal function) and should not supersede clinical judgment (Heintz, 2009; Trotman, 2005):

CVVH: Initial: 3 g; maintenance: 1.5-3 g every 8-12 hours

CVVHD: Initial: 3 g; maintenance: 1.5-3 g every 8 hours

CVVHDF: Initial: 3 g; maintenance: 1.5-3 g every 6-8 hours

Administration Administer around-the-clock to promote less variation in peak and trough serum levels. Administer by slow injection over 10-15 minutes or I.V. over 15-30 minutes. Ampicillin and gentamicin should not be mixed in the same I.V. tubing.

Some penicillins (eg, carbenicillin, ticarcillin, and piperacillin) have been shown to inactivate aminoglycosides *in vitro*. This has been observed to a greater extent with tobramycin and gentamicin, while amikacin has shown greater stability against inactivation. Concurrent use of these agents may pose a risk of reduced antibacterial efficacy *in vivo*, particularly in the setting of profound renal impairment. However, definitive clinical evidence is lacking. If combination penicillin/aminoglycoside therapy is desired in a patient with renal dysfunction, separation of doses (if feasible), and routine monitoring of aminoglycoside levels, CBC, and clinical response should be considered.

Monitoring Parameters With prolonged therapy, monitor hematologic, renal, and hepatic function; monitor for signs of anaphylaxis during first dose

Test Interactions May interfere with urinary glucose tests using cupric sulfate (Benedict's solution, Clinitest®).

Some penicillin derivatives may accelerate the degradation of aminoglycosides *in vitro*, leading to a potential underestimation of aminoglycoside serum concentration.

Special Geriatric Considerations Adjust dose for renal function.

Dosage Forms Excipient information presented when available (limited, particularly for generics); consult specific product labeling.

Injection, powder for reconstitution: 1.5 g: Ampicillin 1 g and sulbactam 0.5 g; 3 g: Ampicillin 2 g and sulbactam 1 g; 15 g: Ampicillin 10 g and sulbactam 5 g

Unasyn®:

1.5 g: Ampicillin 1 g and sulbactam 0.5 g [contains sodium 115 mg (5 mEq)/1.5 g)]

3 g: Ampicillin 2 g and sulbactam 1 g [contains sodium 115 mg (5 mEq)/1.5 g)]

15 g: Ampicillin 10 g and sulbactam 5 g [bulk package; contains sodium 115 mg (5 mEq)/1.5 g)]

◆ **Ampicillin Sodium** *see* Ampicillin *on page 127*

◆ **Ampicillin Trihydrate** *see* Ampicillin *on page 127*

◆ **Ampyra™** *see* Dalfampridine *on page 474*

◆ **Amrix®** *see* Cyclobenzaprine *on page 454*

◆ **Amturnide™** *see* Aliskiren, Amlodipine, and Hydrochlorothiazide *on page 60*

◆ **Amylase, Lipase, and Protease** *see* Pancrelipase *on page 1466*

◆ **Anafranil®** *see* ClomiPRAMINE *on page 408*

Anakinra (an a KIN ra)

Medication Safety Issues

Sound-alike/look-alike issues:

Anakinra may be confused with amikacin, Ampyra™

Kineret® may be confused with Amikin®

Brand Names: U.S. Kineret®

Brand Names: Canada Kineret®

Index Terms IL-1Ra; Interleukin-1 Receptor Antagonist

Generic Availability (U.S.) No

Pharmacologic Category Antirheumatic, Disease Modifying; Interleukin-1 Receptor Antagonist

Use Treatment of moderately- to severely-active rheumatoid arthritis in adult patients who have failed one or more disease-modifying antirheumatic drugs (DMARDs); may be used alone or in combination with DMARDs (other than tumor necrosis factor-blocking agents)

Contraindications Hypersensitivity to *E. coli*-derived proteins, anakinra, or any component of the formulation

Warnings/Precautions Anakinra may affect defenses against infections and malignancies. Safety and efficacy in patients with immunosuppression or chronic infections have not been evaluated. Discontinue administration if patient develops a serious infection. Do not start drug administration in patients with an active infection. Patients with asthma may be at an increased risk of serious infections. Use is not recommended in combination with tumor necrosis factor antagonists. Impact on the development and course of malignancies is not fully defined. As compared to the general population, an increased risk of lymphoma has been noted in clinical trials; however, rheumatoid arthritis has been previously associated with an increased rate of lymphoma.

Use caution in patients with a history of significant hematologic abnormalities; has been associated with uncommon, but significant decreases in hematologic parameters (particularly neutrophil counts). Patients must be advised to seek medical attention if they develop signs and symptoms suggestive of blood dyscrasias. Discontinue if significant hematologic abnormalities are confirmed.

Use is not recommended in combination with tumor necrosis factor antagonists. Patients should be brought up to date with all immunizations before initiating therapy. Live vaccines should not be given concurrently. Patients with a significant exposure to varicella virus should temporarily discontinue anakinra. Hypersensitivity reactions may occur; discontinue use if severe hypersensitivity occurs. Impact on the development and course of malignancies is not fully defined. Use caution in patients with renal impairment; consider extended dosing intervals for severe renal dysfunction (Cl_{cr} <30 mL/minute). Use with caution in patients with asthma; may have increased risk of serious infection. Use caution in the elderly due to the potential for higher risk of infections. The packaging (needle cover) contains latex.

Adverse Reactions (Reflective of adult population; not specific for elderly)
>10%:
  Central nervous system: Headache (12%)
  Local: Injection site reaction (majority mild, typically lasting 14-28 days, characterized by erythema, ecchymosis, inflammation, and pain; up to 71%)
  Miscellaneous: Infection (39% versus 37% in placebo; serious infection 2% to 3%)
1% to 10%:
  Gastrointestinal: Nausea (8%), diarrhea (7%)
  Hematologic: Neutropenia (8%; grades 3/4: 0.4%)

Drug Interactions
Metabolism/Transport Effects None known.
Avoid Concomitant Use
  Avoid concomitant use of Anakinra with any of the following: Anti-TNF Agents; BCG; Canakinumab; Natalizumab; Pimecrolimus; Tacrolimus (Topical); Vaccines (Live)
Increased Effect/Toxicity
  Anakinra may increase the levels/effects of: Canakinumab; Leflunomide; Natalizumab; Vaccines (Live)

  The levels/effects of Anakinra may be increased by: Anti-TNF Agents; Denosumab; Pimecrolimus; Roflumilast; Tacrolimus (Topical); Trastuzumab
Decreased Effect
  Anakinra may decrease the levels/effects of: BCG; Coccidioidin Skin Test; Sipuleucel-T; Vaccines (Inactivated); Vaccines (Live)

  The levels/effects of Anakinra may be decreased by: Echinacea
Stability Store in refrigerator at 2°C to 8°C (36°F to 46°F); do not freeze. Do not shake. Protect from light.
Mechanism of Action Antagonist of the interleukin-1 (IL-1) receptor. Endogenous IL-1 is induced by inflammatory stimuli and mediates a variety of immunological responses, including degradation of cartilage (loss of proteoglycans) and stimulation of bone resorption.
Pharmacodynamics/Kinetics
Bioavailability: SubQ: 95%
Half-life elimination: Terminal: 4-6 hours; Severe renal impairment (Cl_{cr} <30 mL/minute): ~7 hours; ESRD: 9.7 hours (Yang, 2003)
Time to peak: SubQ: 3-7 hours
Dosage
Geriatric & Adult Rheumatoid arthritis: SubQ: 100 mg once daily (administer at approximately the same time each day)
Renal Impairment Cl_{cr} <30 mL/minute and/or end-stage renal disease: 100 mg every other day
Hepatic Impairment There are no dosage adjustments recommended in manufacturer's labeling.
Administration Rotate injection sites (thigh, abdomen, upper arm, buttocks); injection should be given at least 1 inch away from previous injection site. Allow solution to warm to room temperature prior to use (60-90 minutes). Do not shake. Provided in single-use, preservative free syringes with 27-gauge needles; discard any unused portion.
Monitoring Parameters CBC with differential (baseline, then monthly for 3 months, then every 3 months for a period up to 1 year); serum creatinine
Pharmacotherapy Pearls Anakinra is produced by recombinant DNA/*E. coli* technology.
Special Geriatric Considerations Clinical trials with older adults (65% to 75%) demonstrated no clinical differences between elderly patients and younger adults in safety and efficacy. Since elderly may be more liable to infections in general, use with caution. Also, since

many elderly patients may have Cl$_{cr}$ <30 mL/minute, close monitoring should be followed with calculation of creatinine clearance prior to initiating therapy with anakinra.

Dosage Forms Excipient information presented when available (limited, particularly for generics); consult specific product labeling.

Injection, solution [preservative free]:

Kineret®: 100 mg/0.67 mL (0.67 mL) [contains edetate disodium, natural rubber/natural latex in packaging, polysorbate 80]

◆ **Anaprox®** see Naproxen on page 1338
◆ **Anaprox® DS** see Naproxen on page 1338
◆ **Anaspaz®** see Hyoscyamine on page 960

Anastrozole (an AS troe zole)

Medication Safety Issues
Sound-alike/look-alike issues:
Anastrozole may be confused with anagrelide, letrozole
Arimidex® may be confused with Aromasin®

Brand Names: U.S. Arimidex®
Brand Names: Canada Arimidex®
Index Terms ICI-D1033; ZD1033
Generic Availability (U.S.) Yes
Pharmacologic Category Antineoplastic Agent, Aromatase Inhibitor
Use First-line treatment of locally-advanced or metastatic breast cancer (hormone receptor-positive or unknown) in postmenopausal women; treatment of advanced breast cancer in postmenopausal women with disease progression following tamoxifen therapy; adjuvant treatment of early hormone receptor-positive breast cancer in postmenopausal women
Unlabeled Use Treatment of recurrent or metastatic endometrial or uterine cancers, treatment of recurrent ovarian cancer
Contraindications Hypersensitivity to anastrozole or any component of the formulation
Warnings/Precautions Hazardous agent - use appropriate precautions for handling and disposal. Anastrozole offers no clinical benefit in premenopausal women with breast cancer. Patients with pre-existing ischemic cardiac disease have an increased risk for ischemic cardiovascular events.

Due to decreased circulating estrogen levels, anastrozole is associated with a reduction in bone mineral density (BMD); decreases (from baseline) in total hip and lumbar spine BMD have been reported. Patients with pre-existing osteopenia are at higher risk for developing osteoporosis (Eastell, 2008). When initiating anastrozole treatment, follow available guidelines for bone mineral density management in postmenopausal women with similar fracture risk; concurrent use of bisphosphonates may be useful in patients at risk for fractures.

Elevated total cholesterol levels (contributed to by LDL cholesterol increases) have been reported in patients receiving anastrozole; use with caution in patients with hyperlipidemias; cholesterol levels should be monitored/managed in accordance with current guidelines for patients with LDL elevations. Plasma concentrations in patients with stable hepatic cirrhosis were within the range of concentrations seen in normal subjects across all clinical trials; use has not been studied in patients with severe hepatic impairment.

Adverse Reactions (Reflective of adult population; not specific for elderly)
>10%:
Cardiovascular: Vasodilatation (25% to 36%), ischemic cardiovascular disease (4%; 17% in patients with pre-existing ischemic heart disease), hypertension (2% to 13%), angina (2%; 12% in patients with pre-existing ischemic heart disease)
Central nervous system: Mood disturbance (19%), fatigue (19%), pain (11% to 17%), headache (9% to 13%), depression (5% to 13%)
Dermatologic: Rash (6% to 11%)
Endocrine & metabolic: Hot flashes (12% to 36%)
Gastrointestinal: Nausea (11% to 19%), vomiting (8% to 13%)
Neuromuscular & skeletal: Weakness (16% to 19%), arthritis (17%), arthralgia (2% to 15%), back pain (10% to 12%), bone pain (6% to 11%), osteoporosis (11%)
Respiratory: Pharyngitis (6% to 14%), cough increased (8% to 11%)
1% to 10%:
Cardiovascular: Peripheral edema (5% to 10%), chest pain (5% to 7%), edema (7%), venous thromboembolic events (2% to 4%), ischemic cerebrovascular events (2%), MI (1%)
Central nervous system: Insomnia (2% to 10%), dizziness (6% to 8%), anxiety (2% to 6%), fever (2% to 5%), malaise (2% to 5%), confusion (2% to 5%), nervousness (2% to 5%), somnolence (2% to 5%), lethargy (1%)
Dermatologic: Alopecia (2% to 5%), pruritus (2% to 5%)

Endocrine & metabolic: Hypercholesterolemia (9%), breast pain (2% to 8%)

Gastrointestinal: Diarrhea (8% to 9%), constipation (7% to 9%), abdominal pain (7% to 9%), weight gain (2% to 9%), anorexia (5% to 7%), xerostomia (6%), dyspepsia (7%), weight loss (2% to 5%)

Genitourinary: Urinary tract infection (2% to 8%), vulvovaginitis (6%), pelvic pain (5%), vaginal bleeding (1% to 5%), vaginitis (4%), vaginal discharge (4%), vaginal hemorrhage (2% to 4%), leukorrhea (2% to 3%), vaginal dryness (2% to 5%)

Hematologic: Anemia (2% to 5%), leukopenia (2% to 5%)

Hepatic: Liver function tests increased (1% to 10%), alkaline phosphatase increased (1% to 10%), gamma GT increased (≤5%)

Local: Thrombophlebitis (2% to 5%)

Neuromuscular & skeletal: Fracture (1% to 10%), arthrosis (7%), paresthesia (5% to 7%), joint disorder (6%), myalgia (2% to 6%), neck pain (2% to 5%), carpal tunnel syndrome (3%), hypertonia (3%)

Ocular: Cataracts (6%)

Respiratory: Dyspnea (8% to 10%), sinusitis (2% to 6%), bronchitis (2% to 5%), rhinitis (2% to 5%)

Miscellaneous: Lymphedema (10%), infection (2% to 9%), flu-like syndrome (2% to 7%), diaphoresis (2% to 5%), cyst (5%), neoplasm (5%), tumor flare (3%)

Drug Interactions

Metabolism/Transport Effects Inhibits CYP1A2 (weak), CYP2C8 (weak), CYP2C9 (weak), CYP3A4 (weak)

Avoid Concomitant Use

Avoid concomitant use of Anastrozole with any of the following: Estrogen Derivatives; Pimozide

Increased Effect/Toxicity

Anastrozole may increase the levels/effects of: ARIPiprazole; Pimozide

Decreased Effect

The levels/effects of Anastrozole may be decreased by: Estrogen Derivatives; Tamoxifen

Stability Store at 20°C to 25°C (68°F to 77°F).

Mechanism of Action Potent and selective nonsteroidal aromatase inhibitor. By inhibiting aromatase, the conversion of androstenedione to estrone, and testosterone to estradiol, is prevented, thereby decreasing tumor mass or delaying progression in patients with tumors responsive to hormones. Anastrozole causes an 85% decrease in estrone sulfate levels.

Pharmacodynamics/Kinetics

Onset of estradiol reduction: 70% reduction after 24 hours; 80% after 2 weeks therapy

Duration of estradiol reduction: 6 days

Absorption: Well absorbed; extent of absorption not affected by food

Protein binding, plasma: 40%

Metabolism: Extensively hepatic (~85%) via N-dealkylation, hydroxylation, and glucuronidation; primary metabolite (triazole) inactive

Half-life elimination: ~50 hours

Time to peak, plasma: ~2 hours without food; 5 hours with food

Excretion: Feces; urine (urinary excretion accounts for ~10% of total elimination, mostly as metabolites)

Dosage

Geriatric & Adult Females: Postmenopausal:

Breast cancer, advanced: Oral: 1 mg once daily; continue until tumor progression

Breast cancer, early (adjuvant treatment): Oral: 1 mg once daily; optimal duration unknown, duration in clinical trial is 5 years

Renal Impairment Dosage adjustment is not necessary.

Hepatic Impairment

Mild-to-moderate impairment or stable hepatic cirrhosis: Dosage adjustment is not required.

Severe hepatic impairment: Has not been studied in this population.

Administration May be administered with or without food.

Monitoring Parameters Bone mineral density; total cholesterol and LDL

Pharmacotherapy Pearls Oncology Comment: The American Society of Clinical Oncology (ASCO) guidelines for adjuvant endocrine therapy in postmenopausal women with HR-positive breast cancer (Burstein, 2010) recommend considering aromatase inhibitor (AI) therapy at some point in the treatment course (primary, sequentially, or extended). Optimal duration at this time is not known; however, treatment with an AI should not exceed 5 years in primary and extended therapies, and 2-3 years if followed by tamoxifen in sequential therapy (total of 5 years). If initial therapy with AI has been discontinued before the 5 years, consideration should be taken to receive tamoxifen for a total of 5 years. The optimal time to switch to an AI is also not known, so options switching after 2-3 years of tamoxifen (sequential) or after 5 years of tamoxifen (extended). If patient becomes intolerant or has poor adherence, consideration should be made to switch to another AI or initiate tamoxifen.

Special Geriatric Considerations No age-related changes in pharmacokinetics were noted in clinical trials.

Dosage Forms Excipient information presented when available (limited, particularly for generics); consult specific product labeling.

Tablet, oral: 1 mg

Arimidex®: 1 mg

◆ **Ancef** see CeFAZolin on page 309
◆ **Ancobon®** see Flucytosine on page 799
◆ **Androderm®** see Testosterone on page 1861
◆ **AndroGel®** see Testosterone on page 1861
◆ **Android®** see MethylTESTOSTERone on page 1256
◆ **AneCream™ [OTC]** see Lidocaine (Topical) on page 1128
◆ **Anestafoam™ [OTC]** see Lidocaine (Topical) on page 1128
◆ **Aneurine Hydrochloride** see Thiamine on page 1878
◆ **Angeliq®** see Drospirenone and Estradiol on page 616
◆ **Ansamycin** see Rifabutin on page 1696
◆ **Antara®** see Fenofibrate on page 752
◆ **Anti-Diarrheal [OTC]** see Loperamide on page 1153
◆ **Antidiuretic Hormone** see Vasopressin on page 2008
◆ **Anti-Fungal™ [OTC]** see Clotrimazole (Topical) on page 426
◆ **Anti-Hist [OTC]** see DiphenhydrAMINE (Systemic) on page 556
◆ **Antitumor Necrosis Factor Alpha (Human)** see Adalimumab on page 44
◆ **Antivert®** see Meclizine on page 1186
◆ **Anucort-HC™** see Hydrocortisone (Topical) on page 943
◆ **Anu-Med [OTC]** see Phenylephrine (Topical) on page 1527
◆ **Anu-med HC** see Hydrocortisone (Topical) on page 943
◆ **Anusol-HC®** see Hydrocortisone (Topical) on page 943
◆ **Anzemet®** see Dolasetron on page 589
◆ **4-AP** see Dalfampridine on page 474
◆ **APAP 500 [OTC]** see Acetaminophen on page 31
◆ **APAP (abbreviation is not recommended)** see Acetaminophen on page 31
◆ **APC8015** see Sipuleucel-T on page 1780
◆ **Apidra®** see Insulin Glulisine on page 1014
◆ **Apidra® SoloStar®** see Insulin Glulisine on page 1014
◆ **Aplenzin™** see BuPROPion on page 241
◆ **Aplisol®** see Tuberculin Tests on page 1980
◆ **Aplonidine** see Apraclonidine on page 138
◆ **APO-066** see Deferiprone on page 497
◆ **Apokyn®** see Apomorphine on page 136

Apomorphine (a poe MOR feen)

Related Information

Antiparkinsonian Agents on page 2101

Brand Names: U.S. Apokyn®

Index Terms Apomorphine Hydrochloride; Apomorphine Hydrochloride Hemihydrate

Generic Availability (U.S.) No

Pharmacologic Category Anti-Parkinson's Agent, Dopamine Agonist

Use Treatment of hypomobility, "off" episodes with Parkinson's disease

Unlabeled Use Treatment of erectile dysfunction

Prescribing and Access Restrictions Apokyn® is only available through a select group of specialty pharmacies and cannot be obtained through a retail pharmacy. Apokyn® may be obtained from the following specialty pharmacies: Accredo Nova Factor or PharmaCare. To obtain the medication, contact the APOKYN Call Center at 1-877-7APOKYN (1-877-727-6596).

Contraindications Hypersensitivity to apomorphine or any component of the formulation; **concomitant use with 5HT₃ antagonists**; intravenous administration

Warnings/Precautions May cause orthostatic hypotension, especially during dosage escalation; use extreme caution, especially in patients on antihypertensives and/or vasodilators. If patient develops clinically-significant orthostatic hypotension with test dose then apomorphine should not be used. Ergot-derived dopamine agonists have also been associated with fibrotic complications (eg, retroperitoneal fibrosis, pleural thickening, and pulmonary infiltrates). **Pretreatment with antiemetic is necessary.** Monitor patients for drowsiness. May cause hallucinations/psychosis. Use caution in patients with risk factors for torsade de pointes. Use caution in cardiovascular and cerebrovascular disease. Use caution in patients with hepatic or renal dysfunction. Use with caution in patients with pre-existing dyskinesias; may be exacerbated.

Dopamine agonists have been associated with compulsive behaviors and/or loss of impulse control, which has manifested as pathological gambling, libido increases (hypersexuality), and/or binge eating. Causality has not been established, and controversy exists as to whether this phenomenon is related to the underlying disease, prior behaviors/addictions and/or drug therapy. Dose reduction or discontinuation of therapy has been reported to reverse these behaviors in some, but not all cases. Dopaminergic agents have been associated with a syndrome resembling neuroleptic malignant syndrome on abrupt withdrawal or significant dosage reduction after long-term use. Retinal degeneration has been observed in animal studies when using dopamine agonists for prolonged periods. Rare cases of abuse have been reported. Risk for melanoma development is increased in Parkinson's disease patients; drug causation or factors contributing to risk have not been established. Patients should be monitored closely and periodic skin examinations should be performed. Contains metabisulfite. Do not give intravenously; thrombus formation or pulmonary embolism may occur.

Adverse Reactions (Reflective of adult population; not specific for elderly)
>10%:
  Cardiovascular: Chest pain/pressure or angina (15%)
  Central nervous system: Drowsiness or somnolence (35%), dizziness or orthostatic hypotension (20%)
  Gastrointestinal: Nausea and/or vomiting (30%)
  Neuromuscular & skeletal: Falls (30%), dyskinesias (24% to 35%)
  Respiratory: Yawning (40%), rhinorrhea (20%)
1% to 10%:
  Cardiovascular: Edema (10%), vasodilation (3%), hypotension (2%), syncope (2%), CHF
  Central nervous system: Hallucinations or confusion (10%), anxiety, depression, fatigue, headache, insomnia, pain
  Dermatologic: Bruising
  Endocrine & metabolic: Dehydration
  Gastrointestinal: Constipation, diarrhea
  Local: Injection site reactions
  Neuromuscular & skeletal: Arthralgias, weakness
  Miscellaneous: Diaphoresis increased

Drug Interactions
Metabolism/Transport Effects Substrate of COMT, CYP1A2 (minor), CYP2C19 (minor), CYP3A4 (minor); **Note:** Assignment of Major/Minor substrate status based on clinically relevant drug interaction potential; **Inhibits** CYP1A2 (weak), CYP2C19 (weak), CYP3A4 (weak)

Avoid Concomitant Use
Avoid concomitant use of Apomorphine with any of the following: Antiemetics (5HT3 Antagonists)

Increased Effect/Toxicity
Apomorphine may increase the levels/effects of: Highest Risk QTc-Prolonging Agents; Moderate Risk QTc-Prolonging Agents

The levels/effects of Apomorphine may be increased by: Antiemetics (5HT3 Antagonists); COMT Inhibitors; MAO Inhibitors; Methylphenidate; Mifepristone

Decreased Effect
Apomorphine may decrease the levels/effects of: Antipsychotics (Typical)

The levels/effects of Apomorphine may be decreased by: Antipsychotics (Atypical); Antipsychotics (Typical); Metoclopramide; Tocilizumab

Ethanol/Nutrition/Herb Interactions Ethanol: Caution with ethanol consumption; may increase risk of hypotension.

Stability Store at 15°C to 30°C (59°F to 86°F).

Mechanism of Action Stimulates postsynaptic D2-type receptors within the caudate putamen in the brain.

Pharmacodynamics/Kinetics
Onset of action: SubQ: Rapid
Distribution: V_d: Mean: 218 L
Metabolism: Not established; potential routes of metabolism include sulfation, N-demethylation, glucuronidation, and oxidation; catechol-O methyltransferase and nonenzymatic oxidation. CYP isoenzymes do not appear to play a significant role.
Half-life elimination: Terminal: 40 minutes
Time to peak, plasma: Improved motor scores: 20 minutes
Excretion: Urine 93% (as metabolites); feces 16%

Dosage
Geriatric & Adult Begin antiemetic therapy 3 days prior to initiation and continue for 2 months before reassessing need.

Parkinson's disease, "off" episode: SubQ: Initial test dose 2 mg, **medical supervision required; see "Note".** Subsequent dosing is based on both tolerance and response to initial test dose.

If patient tolerates test dose and responds: Starting dose: 2 mg as needed; may increase dose in 1 mg increments every few days; maximum dose: 6 mg

If patient tolerates but does not respond to 2 mg test dose: Second test dose: 4 mg

If patient tolerates and responds to 4 mg test dose: Starting dose: 3 mg, as needed for "off" episodes; may increase dose in 1 mg increments every few days; maximum dose 6 mg

If patient does not tolerate 4 mg test dose: Third test dose: 3 mg

If patient tolerates 3 mg test dose: Starting dose: 2 mg as needed for "off" episodes; may increase dose in 1 mg increments to a maximum of 3 mg

If therapy is interrupted for >1 week, restart at 2 mg and gradually titrate dose.

Note: Medical supervision is required for all test doses with standing and supine blood pressure monitoring predose and 20-, 40-, and 60 minutes postdose. If subsequent test doses are required, wait >2 hours before another test dose is given; next test dose should be timed with another "off" episode. If a single dose is ineffective for a particular "off" episode, then a second dose should not be given. The average dosing frequency was 3 times/day in the development program with limited experience in dosing >5 times/day and with total daily doses >20 mg. Apomorphine is intended to treat the "off" episodes associated with levodopa therapy of Parkinson's disease and has not been studied in levodopa-naive Parkinson's patients.

Renal Impairment
Mild-to-moderate impairment: Reduce test dose and starting dose: 1 mg
Severe impairment: Has not been studied

Hepatic Impairment
Mild-to-moderate impairment: Use caution
Severe impairment: Has not been studied

Administration SubQ: Initiate antiemetic 3 days before test dose of apomorphine and continue for 2 months (if patient to be treated) before reassessment. Administer in abdomen, upper arm, or upper leg; change site with each injection. 3 mL cartridges are used with a manual, reusable, multidose injector pen. Injector pen can deliver doses up to 1 mL in 0.02 mL increments. Do not give intravenously; thrombus formation or pulmonary embolism may occur.

Monitoring Parameters Each test dose: Supine and standing blood pressure predose and 20, 40, and 60 minutes postdose; drowsiness

Special Geriatric Considerations No specific information for use in elderly.

Dosage Forms Excipient information presented when available (limited, particularly for generics); consult specific product labeling.

Injection, solution, as hydrochloride:
Apokyn®: 10 mg/mL (3 mL) [contains benzyl alcohol, sodium metabisulfite]

◆ **Apomorphine Hydrochloride** see Apomorphine on page 136
◆ **Apomorphine Hydrochloride Hemihydrate** see Apomorphine on page 136
◆ **APPG** see Penicillin G Procaine on page 1502

Apraclonidine (a pra KLOE ni deen)

Related Information
Glaucoma Drug Therapy on page 2115

Medication Safety Issues
Sound-alike/look-alike issues:
Iopidine® may be confused with indapamide, iodine, Lodine®

Brand Names: U.S. Iopidine®

Brand Names: Canada Iopidine®

Index Terms Aplonidine; Apraclonidine Hydrochloride; p-Aminoclonidine

Generic Availability (U.S.) Yes

Pharmacologic Category Alpha$_2$ Agonist, Ophthalmic

Use Prevention and treatment of postsurgical intraocular pressure (IOP) elevation; short-term, adjunctive therapy in patients who require additional reduction of IOP

Dosage
Geriatric & Adult Postsurgical intraocular pressure elevation (prevention/treatment): Ophthalmic:
0.5%: Instill 1-2 drops in the affected eye(s) 3 times/day
1%: Instill 1 drop in operative eye 1 hour prior to anterior segment laser surgery, second drop in eye immediately upon completion of procedure

Renal Impairment Although the topical use of apraclonidine has not been studied in renal failure patients, structurally-related clonidine undergoes a significant increase in half-life in patients with severe renal impairment. Close monitoring of cardiovascular parameters in patients with impaired renal function is advised.

Hepatic Impairment Close monitoring of cardiovascular parameters in patients with impaired liver function is advised because the systemic dosage form of clonidine is partially metabolized in the liver.

Special Geriatric Considerations Evaluate the patient's or caregiver's ability to safely administer the correct dose of ophthalmic medication.

Dosage Forms Excipient information presented when available (limited, particularly for generics); consult specific product labeling.

Solution, ophthalmic [drops]: 0.5% (5 mL, 10 mL)

Iopidine®: 0.5% (5 mL, 10 mL); 1% (0.1 mL) [contains benzalkonium chloride]

◆ **Apraclonidine Hydrochloride** *see* Apraclonidine *on page 138*

Aprepitant (ap RE pi tant)

Medication Safety Issues

Sound-alike/look-alike issues:

Aprepitant may be confused with fosaprepitant

Emend® (aprepitant) oral capsule formulation may be confused with Emend® for injection (fosaprepitant)

Brand Names: U.S. Emend®

Brand Names: Canada Emend®

Index Terms L 754030; MK 869

Generic Availability (U.S.) No

Pharmacologic Category Antiemetic; Substance P/Neurokinin 1 Receptor Antagonist

Use Prevention of acute and delayed nausea and vomiting associated with moderately- and highly-emetogenic chemotherapy (in combination with other antiemetics); prevention of post-operative nausea and vomiting (PONV)

Contraindications Hypersensitivity to aprepitant or any component of the formulation; concurrent use with cisapride or pimozide

Warnings/Precautions Use caution with agents primarily metabolized via CYP3A4; aprepitant is a 3A4 inhibitor. Effect on orally administered 3A4 substrates is greater than those administered intravenously. Chronic continuous use is not recommended; however, a single 40 mg aprepitant oral dose is not likely to alter plasma concentrations of CYP3A4 substrates. Use caution with severe hepatic impairment; has not been studied in patients with severe hepatic impairment (Child-Pugh class C). Not studied for treatment of existing nausea and vomiting. Chronic continuous administration is not recommended.

Adverse Reactions (Reflective of adult population; not specific for elderly) Note: Adverse reactions reported as part of a combination chemotherapy regimen or with general anesthesia.

>10%:

Central nervous system: Fatigue (≤18%)

Gastrointestinal: Nausea (6% to 13%), constipation (9% to 10%)

Neuromuscular & skeletal: Weakness (≤18%)

Miscellaneous: Hiccups (11%)

1% to 10%:

Cardiovascular: Hypotension (≤6%), bradycardia (≤4%)

Central nervous system: Dizziness (≤7%)

Endocrine & metabolic: Dehydration (≤6%)

Gastrointestinal: Diarrhea (≤10%), dyspepsia (≤6%), abdominal pain (≤5%), epigastric discomfort (4%), gastritis (4%), stomatitis (3%)

Hepatic: ALT increased (≤6%), AST increased (3%)

Renal: Proteinuria (7%), BUN increased (5%)

Drug Interactions

Metabolism/Transport Effects Substrate of CYP1A2 (minor), CYP2C19 (minor), CYP3A4 (major); **Note:** Assignment of Major/Minor substrate status based on clinically relevant drug interaction potential; **Inhibits** CYP2C19 (weak), CYP2C9 (weak), CYP3A4 (moderate); **Induces** CYP2C9 (strong), CYP3A4 (weak/moderate)

Avoid Concomitant Use

Avoid concomitant use of Aprepitant with any of the following: Axitinib; Cisapride; Con-ivaptan; Pimozide; Tolvaptan

Increased Effect/Toxicity

Aprepitant may increase the levels/effects of: ARIPiprazole; Avanafil; Benzodiazepines (metabolized by oxidation); Budesonide (Systemic, Oral Inhalation); Cisapride; Colchicine; Corticosteroids (Systemic); CYP3A4 Substrates; Diltiazem; Eplerenone; Everolimus; FentaNYL; Halofantrine; Ivacaftor; Lurasidone; Pimecrolimus; Pimozide; Propafenone; Ranolazine; Salmeterol; Saxagliptin; Tolvaptan; Vilazodone; Zuclopenthixol

The levels/effects of Aprepitant may be increased by: Antifungal Agents (Azole Derivatives, Systemic); Conivaptan; CYP3A4 Inhibitors (Moderate); CYP3A4 Inhibitors (Strong); Dasatinib; Diltiazem; Ivacaftor; Mifepristone

Decreased Effect

Aprepitant may decrease the levels/effects of: ARIPiprazole; Axitinib; Contraceptives (Estrogens); Contraceptives (Progestins); CYP2C9 Substrates; Diclofenac; Ifosfamide; PARoxetine; Saxagliptin; TOLBUTamide; Warfarin

The levels/effects of Aprepitant may be decreased by: CYP3A4 Inducers (Strong); Deferasirox; Herbs (CYP3A4 Inducers); PARoxetine; Rifamycin Derivatives; Tocilizumab

Ethanol/Nutrition/Herb Interactions

Food: Aprepitant serum concentration may be increased when taken with grapefruit juice; avoid concurrent use.

Herb/Nutraceutical: Avoid St John's wort (may decrease aprepitant levels).

Stability Store at room temperature of 20°C to 25°C (68°F to 77°F).

Mechanism of Action Prevents acute and delayed vomiting by inhibiting the substance P/ neurokinin 1 (NK_1) receptor; augments the antiemetic activity of 5-HT_3 receptor antagonists and corticosteroids to inhibit acute and delayed phases of chemotherapy-induced emesis.

Pharmacodynamics/Kinetics

Distribution: V_d: ~70 L; crosses the blood-brain barrier

Protein binding: >95%

Metabolism: Extensively hepatic via CYP3A4 (major); CYP1A2 and CYP2C19 (minor); forms 7 metabolites (weakly active)

Bioavailability: ~60% to 65%

Half-life elimination: Terminal: ~9-13 hours

Time to peak, plasma: ~3-4 hours

Dosage

Geriatric & Adult

Prevention of chemotherapy-induced nausea/vomiting: Oral: 125 mg 1 hour prior to chemotherapy on day 1, followed by 80 mg once daily on days 2 and 3 (in combination with a corticosteroid and 5-HT_3 antagonist antiemetic)

Prevention of PONV: Oral: 40 mg within 3 hours prior to induction

Renal Impairment No dose adjustment necessary in patients with renal disease or end-stage renal disease maintained on hemodialysis.

Hepatic Impairment

Mild-to-moderate impairment (Child-Pugh class A or B): No adjustment necessary.

Severe impairment (Child-Pugh class C): Use caution; no data available.

Administration Administer with or without food.

Chemotherapy induced nausea/vomiting: First dose should be given 1 hour prior to antineoplastic therapy; subsequent doses should be given in the morning.

PONV: Administer within 3 hours prior to induction

Pharmacotherapy Pearls Oncology Comment: Aprepitant is recommended in the American Society of Clinical Oncology (ASCO) oncology antiemetic guidelines for use in combination with a serotonin receptor antagonist and dexamethasone for chemotherapy with high emetic risk and for chemotherapy regimens of moderate emetic risk which contain an anthracycline and cyclophosphamide (Kris, 2006). The National Comprehensive Cancer Network (NCCN) Clinical Practice Guidelines in Oncology for Antiemesis (version 2.2009) recommend the same use of aprepitant as is in the ASCO recommendation. In addition to the moderately emetogenic chemotherapy listed above, the NCCN guidelines suggest that aprepitant may also be used for select moderately emetogenic regimens containing carboplatin, cisplatin, doxorubicin, epirubicin, ifosfamide, irinotecan and methotrexate. Either fosaprepitant 115 mg or aprepitant (125 mg orally) are administered on day 1; for day 2 and 3, patients should receive aprepitant 80 mg orally.

Special Geriatric Considerations In two studies by the manufacturer, with a total of 544 patients, 31% were >65 years of age, while 5% were >75 years. No differences in safety and efficacy were noted between elderly subjects and younger adults. No dosing adjustment is necessary.

Dosage Forms Excipient information presented when available (limited, particularly for generics); consult specific product labeling.

Capsule, oral:

Emend®: 40 mg, 80 mg, 125 mg

Combination package, oral [each package contains]:

Emend®: Capsule: 80 mg (2s) and Capsule: 125 mg (1s)

- ◆ **Aprepitant Injection** see Fosaprepitant on page 844
- ◆ **Apresoline [DSC]** see HydrALAZINE on page 931
- ◆ **Apriso™** see Mesalamine on page 1217
- ◆ **Aprodine [OTC]** see Triprolidine and Pseudoephedrine on page 1975
- ◆ **Aqua Gem-E™ [OTC]** see Vitamin E on page 2027
- ◆ **Aquanil HC® [OTC]** see Hydrocortisone (Topical) on page 943
- ◆ **Aquasol E® [OTC]** see Vitamin E on page 2027
- ◆ **Aqueous Procaine Penicillin G** see Penicillin G Procaine on page 1502
- ◆ **Aquoral™** see Saliva Substitute on page 1748
- ◆ **Aranesp®** see Darbepoetin Alfa on page 488
- ◆ **Aranesp® SingleJect®** see Darbepoetin Alfa on page 488
- ◆ **Arava®** see Leflunomide on page 1098
- ◆ **Arcapta™ Neohaler™** see Indacaterol on page 989
- ◆ **Aredia®** see Pamidronate on page 1462

Arformoterol (ar for MOE ter ol)

Related Information

Inhalant Agents on page 2117

Brand Names: U.S. Brovana®

Index Terms (R,R)-Formoterol L-Tartrate; Arformoterol Tartrate

Generic Availability (U.S.) No

Pharmacologic Category Beta$_2$-Adrenergic Agonist; Beta$_2$-Adrenergic Agonist, Long-Acting

Use Long-term maintenance treatment of bronchoconstriction in chronic obstructive pulmonary disease (COPD), including chronic bronchitis and emphysema

Medication Guide Available Yes

Contraindications Hypersensitivity to arformoterol, racemic formoterol, or any component of the formulation

Additional contraindication for all long-acting beta$_2$-agonists: Use in patients with asthma (without concomitant use of a long-term asthma control medication)

Warnings/Precautions [U.S. Boxed Warning]: Long-acting beta$_2$-agonists (LABAs) increase the risk of asthma-related deaths. Monotherapy with an LABA is contraindicated in the treatment of asthma. In a large, randomized, placebo-controlled U.S. clinical trial (SMART, 2006), salmeterol was associated with an increase in asthma-related deaths (when added to usual asthma therapy); risk is considered a class effect among all LABAs. LABAs should not be used for acute bronchospasm. **Safety and efficacy of arformoterol in patients with asthma have not been established.** Do not exceed recommended dose; serious adverse events, including fatalities, have been associated with excessive use of inhaled sympathomimetics.

Use with caution in patients with cardiovascular disease (eg, arrhythmia, hypertension, HF); beta-agonists may cause elevation in blood pressure, heart rate and result in CNS stimulation/ excitation. Beta$_2$-agonists may also increase risk of arrhythmias and prolong QT$_c$ interval. Do **not** use for acute episodes of COPD. Do not initiate in patients with significantly worsening or acutely deteriorating COPD. Data are not available to determine if LABA use increases the risk of death in patients with COPD. Use with caution in patients with diabetes mellitus; beta$_2$-agonists may increase serum glucose. Use caution in hepatic impairment; systemic clearance prolonged in hepatic dysfunction. Use with caution in hyperthyroidism; may stimulate thyroid activity. Use with caution in patients with hypokalemia; beta$_2$-agonists may decrease serum potassium. Use with caution in patients with seizure disorders; beta$_2$-agonists may result in CNS stimulation/excitation.

Tolerance/tachyphylaxis to the bronchodilator effect, measured by FEV$_1$, has been observed in studies. Patients using inhaled, short-acting beta$_2$-agonists (eg, albuterol) should be instructed to discontinue routine use of these medications prior to beginning treatment; short-acting agents should be reserved for symptomatic relief of acute symptoms. Patients must be instructed to seek medical attention in cases where acute symptoms are not relieved or a previous level of response is diminished. The need to increase frequency of use may indicate deterioration of COPD, and treatment must not be delayed.

Adverse Reactions (Reflective of adult population; not specific for elderly) 2% to 10%:

Cardiovascular: Chest pain (7%), peripheral edema (3%)

Central nervous system: Pain (8%)

Dermatologic: Rash (4%)

Gastrointestinal: Diarrhea (6%)

Neuromuscular & skeletal: Back pain (6%), leg cramps (4%)

Respiratory: Dyspnea (4%), sinusitis (5%), congestive conditions (2%)

Miscellaneous: Flu-like syndrome (3%)

Drug Interactions

Metabolism/Transport Effects None known.

Avoid Concomitant Use

Avoid concomitant use of Arformoterol with any of the following: Beta-Blockers (Non-selective); Iobenguane I 123

Increased Effect/Toxicity

Arformoterol may increase the levels/effects of: Loop Diuretics; Sympathomimetics; Thiazide Diuretics

The levels/effects of Arformoterol may be increased by: AtoMOXetine; Cannabinoids; MAO Inhibitors; Tricyclic Antidepressants

Decreased Effect

Arformoterol may decrease the levels/effects of: Iobenguane I 123

The levels/effects of Arformoterol may be decreased by: Alpha-/Beta-Blockers; Beta-Blockers (Beta1 Selective); Beta-Blockers (Nonselective); Betahistine

Stability Prior to dispensing, store in protective foil pouch under refrigeration at 2°C to 8°C (36°F to 46°F). Protect from light and excessive heat. After dispensing, unopened foil pouches may be stored at room temperature at 20°C to 25°C (68°F to 77°F) for up to 6 weeks. Only remove vial from foil pouch immediately before use.

Mechanism of Action Arformoterol, the (R,R)-enantiomer of the racemic formoterol, is a long-acting beta$_2$-agonist that relaxes bronchial smooth muscle by selective action on beta$_2$-receptors with little effect on cardiovascular system.

Pharmacodynamics/Kinetics

Onset of action: 7-20 minutes

Peak effect: 1-3 hours

Absorption: A portion of inhaled dose is absorbed into systemic circulation

Protein binding: 52% to 65%

Metabolism: Hepatic via direct glucuronidation and secondarily via O-demethylation; CYP2D6 and CYP2C19 (to a lesser extent) involved in O-demethylation

Half-life elimination: 26 hours

Time to peak: 0.5-3 hours

Dosage

Geriatric & Adult COPD: Nebulization: 15 mcg twice daily; maximum: 30 mcg/day

Renal Impairment No adjustment required.

Hepatic Impairment No dosage adjustment required, but use caution; systemic drug exposure prolonged (1.3- to 2.4-fold).

Administration Nebulization: Remove each vial from individually sealed foil pouch immediately before use. Use with standard jet nebulizer connected to an air compressor, administer with mouthpiece or face mask. Administer vial undiluted and do not mix with other medications in nebulizer.

Monitoring Parameters FEV$_1$, peak flow, and/or other pulmonary function tests; blood pressure, heart rate; CNS stimulation; serum glucose, serum potassium. Monitor for increased use of short-acting beta$_2$-agonist inhalers; may be marker of a deteriorating COPD condition.

Special Geriatric Considerations In clinical trials, no significant difference was seen in the AUC and C$_{max}$ between younger and older subjects. In addition, no significant difference in clinical response was noted.

Dosage Forms Excipient information presented when available (limited, particularly for generics); consult specific product labeling.

Solution, for nebulization:

Brovana®: 15 mcg/2 mL (30s, 60s)

◆ **Arformoterol Tartrate** *see* Arformoterol *on page* 141
◆ **8-Arginine Vasopressin** *see* Vasopressin *on page* 2008
◆ **Aricept®** *see* Donepezil *on page* 591
◆ **Aricept® ODT** *see* Donepezil *on page* 591
◆ **Arimidex®** *see* Anastrozole *on page* 134

ARIPiprazole (ay ri PIP ray zole)

Related Information
Antipsychotic Agents *on page 2103*
Atypical Antipsychotics *on page 2107*
Beers Criteria − Potentially Inappropriate Medications for Geriatrics *on page 2183*
Medication Safety Issues
Sound-alike/look-alike issues:
Abilify® may be confused with Ambien®
ARIPiprazole may be confused with proton pump inhibitors (dexlansoprazole, esomeprazole, lansoprazole, omeprazole, pantoprazole, RABEprazole)
BEERS Criteria medication:
This drug may be potentially inappropriate for use in geriatric patients (Quality of evidence - moderate; Strength of recommendation - strong).
Brand Names: U.S. Abilify Discmelt®; Abilify®
Brand Names: Canada Abilify®
Index Terms BMS 337039; OPC-14597
Generic Availability (U.S.) No
Pharmacologic Category Antipsychotic Agent, Atypical
Use
Oral: Acute and maintenance treatment of schizophrenia; acute (manic and mixed episodes) and maintenance treatment of bipolar I disorder as monotherapy or as an adjunct to lithium or valproic acid; adjunctive treatment of major depressive disorder; treatment of irritability associated with autistic disorder
Injection: Agitation associated with schizophrenia or bipolar I disorder
Unlabeled Use Depression with psychotic features; psychosis/agitation related to Alzheimer's dementia
Medication Guide Available Yes
Contraindications Hypersensitivity to aripiprazole or any component of the formulation
Warnings/Precautions [U.S. Boxed Warning]: Elderly patients with dementia-related psychosis treated with antipsychotics are at an increased risk of death compared to placebo. Most deaths appeared to be either cardiovascular (eg, heart failure, sudden death) or infectious (eg, pneumonia) in nature. In addition, an increased incidence of cerebrovascular effects (eg, transient ischemic attack, cerebrovascular accidents) has been reported in studies of placebo-controlled trials of aripiprazole in elderly patients with dementia-related psychosis. Aripiprazole is not approved for the treatment of dementia-related psychosis.

The possibility of a suicide attempt is inherent in major depression and may persist until remission occurs. Patients treated with antidepressants should be observed for clinical worsening and suicidality, especially during the initial few months of a course of drug therapy, or at times of dose changes, either increases or decreases. Prescriptions should be written for the smallest quantity consistent with good patient care. The patient's family or caregiver should be alerted to monitor patients for the emergence of suicidality and associated behaviors; patients should be instructed to notify their healthcare provider if any of these symptoms or worsening depression or psychosis occur.

Leukopenia, neutropenia, and agranulocytosis (sometimes fatal) have been reported in clinical trials and postmarketing reports with antipsychotic use; presence of risk factors (eg, pre-existing low WBC or history of drug-induced leuko-/neutropenia) should prompt periodic blood count assessment. Discontinue therapy at first signs of blood dyscrasias or if absolute neutrophil count <1000/mm^3.

A medication guide concerning the use of antidepressants should be dispensed with each prescription.

May cause extrapyramidal symptoms (EPS), including pseudoparkinsonism, acute dystonic reactions, akathisia, and tardive dyskinesia (risk of these reactions is very low relative to typical/conventional antipsychotics, frequencies reported are similar to placebo). Risk of dystonia (and probably other EPS) may be greater with increased doses, use of conventional antipsychotics, and males. May be associated with neuroleptic malignant syndrome (NMS).

May be sedating, use with caution in disorders where CNS depression is a feature. May cause orthostatic hypotension (although reported rates are similar to placebo); use caution in patients at risk of this effect or those who would not tolerate transient hypotensive episodes (cerebrovascular disease, cardiovascular disease, or other medications which may predispose).

Use caution in patients with Parkinson's disease; predisposition to seizures; and severe cardiac disease. May alter cardiac conduction; life-threatening arrhythmias have occurred with therapeutic doses of antipsychotics. Esophageal dysmotility and aspiration have been associated with antipsychotic use; use caution in patients at risk of pneumonia (eg, Alzheimer's disease). May alter temperature regulation. Significant weight gain has been observed with antipsychotic therapy; incidence varies with product. Monitor waist circumference and BMI.

Atypical antipsychotics have been associated with development of hyperglycemia; in some cases, may be extreme and associated with ketoacidosis, hyperosmolar coma, or death. Reports of hyperglycemia with aripiprazole therapy have been few and specific risk associated with this agent is not known. Use caution in patients with diabetes or other disorders of glucose regulation; monitor for worsening of glucose control.

Use in elderly patients with dementia is associated with an increased risk of mortality and cerebrovascular accidents; avoid antipsychotic use for behavioral problems associated with dementia unless alternative nonpharmacologic therapies have failed and patient may harm self or others. In addition, use may cause or exacerbate syndrome of inappropriate antidiuretic hormone secretion or hyponatremia; monitor sodium closely with initiation or dosage adjustments in older adults (Beers Criteria).

Tablets contain lactose; avoid use in patients with galactose intolerance or glucose-galactose malabsorption.

Abilify Discmelt®: Use caution in phenylketonuria; contains phenylalanine.

Adverse Reactions (Reflective of adult population; not specific for elderly) Unless otherwise noted, frequency of adverse reactions is shown as reported for adult patients receiving oral administration. Spectrum and incidence of adverse effects similar in children; exceptions noted when incidence much higher in children.

>10%:
  Central nervous system: Headache (27%; injection 12%), agitation (19%), insomnia (18%), anxiety (17%), EPS (dose related; 5% to 16%; children 6% to 26%), akathisia (dose related; 8% to 13%; injection 2%), sedation (dose related; 5% to 11%; children 8% to 24%; injection 3% to 9%)
  Gastrointestinal: Weight gain (2% to 30%; highest frequency in patients with baseline BMI <23 and prolonged use), nausea (15%; injection 9%), constipation (11%), vomiting (11%; children 9% to 14%; injection 3%), dyspepsia (9%)
1% to 10%:
  Cardiovascular: Orthostatic hypotension (1% to 4%; injection 1% to 3%), tachycardia (injection 2%), chest pain, hypertension, peripheral edema
  Central nervous system: Dizziness (10%; injection 8%), pyrexia (children 5% to 9%), restlessness (5% to 6%), fatigue (dose related; 6%; children 8% to 17%; injection 2%), lethargy (children 2% to 5%), lightheadedness (4%), pain (3%), dystonia (children 1%), hypersomnia (1%), irritability (children 1%), coordination impaired, suicidal ideation
  Dermatologic: Rash (children 2%), hyperhidrosis
  Endocrine & metabolic: Dysmenorrhea (children 2%)
  Gastrointestinal: Salivation increased (dose related; children 4% to 9%), appetite decreased (children 4% to 7%), appetite increased (children 7%), xerostomia (5%), toothache (4%), abdominal discomfort (3%), diarrhea (children 5%), weight loss
  Local: Injection site reaction (injection)
  Neuromuscular & skeletal: Tremor (dose related; 5% to 6%; children 6% to 10%), extremity pain (4%), stiffness (4%), myalgia (2%), spasm (2%), arthralgia (children 1%), dyskinesia (children 1%), CPK increased, weakness
  Ocular: Blurred vision (3%; children 3% to 8%)
  Respiratory: Nasopharyngitis (children 6%), pharyngolaryngeal pain (3%), cough (3%), rhinorrhea (children 2%), aspiration pneumonia, dyspnea, nasal congestion
  Miscellaneous: Thirst (children 1%)

Drug Interactions
  Metabolism/Transport Effects Substrate of CYP2D6 (major), CYP3A4 (major); **Note:** Assignment of Major/Minor substrate status based on clinically relevant drug interaction potential
  Avoid Concomitant Use
    Avoid concomitant use of ARIPiprazole with any of the following: Azelastine; Azelastine (Nasal); Methadone; Metoclopramide; Paraldehyde
  Increased Effect/Toxicity
    ARIPiprazole may increase the levels/effects of: Alcohol (Ethyl); Azelastine; Azelastine (Nasal); Buprenorphine; CNS Depressants; DULoxetine; FLUoxetine; Methadone; Methotrimeprazine; Methylphenidate; Paraldehyde; PARoxetine; Serotonin Modulators; Zolpidem

The levels/effects of ARIPiprazole may be increased by: Abiraterone Acetate; Acetylcholinesterase Inhibitors (Central); CYP2D6 Inhibitors (Moderate); CYP2D6 Inhibitors (Strong); CYP2D6 Inhibitors (Weak); CYP3A4 Inhibitors (Moderate); CYP3A4 Inhibitors (Strong); CYP3A4 Inhibitors (Weak); Dasatinib; Droperidol; DULoxetine; FLUoxetine; HydrOXYzine; Ivacaftor; Lithium formulations; Methotrimeprazine; Methylphenidate; Metoclopramide; Metyrosine; Mifepristone; PARoxetine; Tetrabenazine

Decreased Effect

ARIPiprazole may decrease the levels/effects of: Amphetamines; Anti-Parkinson's Agents (Dopamine Agonist); Quinagolide

The levels/effects of ARIPiprazole may be decreased by: CYP3A4 Inducers; Deferasirox; Lithium formulations; Peginterferon Alfa-2b; Tocilizumab

Ethanol/Nutrition/Herb Interactions

Ethanol: May increase CNS depression; monitor for increased effects with coadministration. Caution patients about effects.

Food: Ingestion with a high-fat meal delays time to peak plasma level.

Herb/Nutraceutical: St John's wort may decrease aripiprazole levels. Avoid kava kava, gotu kola, valerian, St John's wort (may increase CNS depression).

Stability

Injection solution: Store at controlled room temperature of 25°C (77°F); excursions permitted to 15°C to 30°C (59°F to 86°F). Protect from light.

Oral solution: Store at controlled room temperature of 25°C (77°F); excursions permitted to 15°C to 30°C (59°F to 86°F). Use within 6 months after opening.

Tablet: Store at controlled room temperature of 25°C (77°F); excursions permitted to 15°C to 30°C (59°F to 86°F).

Mechanism of Action Aripiprazole is a quinolinone antipsychotic which exhibits high affinity for D_2, D_3, 5-HT$_{1A}$, and 5-HT$_{2A}$ receptors; moderate affinity for D_4, 5-HT$_{2C}$, 5-HT$_7$, alpha$_1$ adrenergic, and H_1 receptors. It also possesses moderate affinity for the serotonin reuptake transporter; has no affinity for muscarinic (cholinergic) receptors. Aripiprazole functions as a partial agonist at the D_2 and 5-HT$_{1A}$ receptors, and as an antagonist at the 5-HT$_{2A}$ receptor.

Pharmacodynamics/Kinetics

Onset of action: Initial: 1-3 weeks

Absorption: Well absorbed

Distribution: V_d: 4.9 L/kg

Protein binding: ≥99%, primarily to albumin

Metabolism: Hepatic, via CYP2D6, CYP3A4 (dehydro-aripiprazole metabolite has affinity for D_2 receptors similar to the parent drug and represents 40% of the parent drug exposure in plasma)

Bioavailability: I.M.: 100%; Tablet: 87%

Half-life elimination: Aripiprazole: 75 hours; dehydro-aripiprazole: 94 hours

CYP2D6 poor metabolizers: Aripiprazole: 146 hours

Time to peak, plasma: I.M.: 1-3 hours; Tablet: 3-5 hours

With high-fat meal: Aripiprazole: Delayed by 3 hours; dehydro-aripiprazole: Delayed by 12 hours

Excretion: Feces (55%, ~18% of the total dose as unchanged drug); urine (25%, <1% of the total dose as unchanged drug)

Dosage

Geriatric & Adult Note: Oral solution may be substituted for the oral tablet on a mg-per-mg basis, up to 25 mg. Patients receiving 30 mg tablets should be given 25 mg oral solution. Orally disintegrating tablets (Abilify Discmelt®) are bioequivalent to the immediate release tablets (Abilify®).

Acute agitation (schizophrenia/bipolar mania): I.M.: 9.75 mg as a single dose (range: 5.25-15 mg); repeated doses may be given at ≥2-hour intervals to a maximum of 30 mg/day. **Note:** If ongoing therapy with aripiprazole is necessary, transition to oral therapy as soon as possible.

Bipolar I disorder (acute manic or mixed episodes): Oral:

Stabilization:

Monotherapy: Initial: 15 mg once daily. May increase to 30 mg once daily if clinically indicated; safety of doses >30 mg/day has not been evaluated

Adjunct to lithium or valproic acid: Initial: 10-15 mg once daily. May increase to 30 mg once daily if clinically indicated; safety of doses >30 mg/day has not been evaluated

Maintenance: Continue stabilization dose for up to 6 weeks; efficacy of continued treatment >6 weeks has not been established.

Depression (adjunctive with antidepressants): Oral: Initial: 2-5 mg/day (range: 2-15 mg/day); dose adjustments of up to 5 mg/day may be made in intervals of ≥1 week. **Note:** Dosing based on patients already receiving antidepressant therapy.

Schizophrenia: Oral: 10-15 mg once daily; may be increased to a maximum of 30 mg once daily (efficacy at dosages above 10-15 mg has not been shown to be increased). Dosage titration should not be more frequent than every 2 weeks.

Dosage adjustment with concurrent CYP450 inducer or inhibitor therapy: Oral:
CYP3A4 inducers (eg, carbamazepine): Aripiprazole dose should be doubled; dose should be subsequently reduced if concurrent inducer agent discontinued.

Strong CYP3A4 inhibitors (eg, ketoconazole): Aripiprazole dose should be reduced to 50% of the usual dose, and proportionally increased upon discontinuation of the inhibitor agent.

Strong CYP2D6 inhibitors (eg, fluoxetine, paroxetine): Aripiprazole dose should be reduced to 50% of the usual dose, and proportionally increased upon discontinuation of the inhibitor agent. **Note:** Dose reduction does not apply to patients with major depressive disorder; follow usual dosing recommendations.

CYP3A4 and CYP2D6 inhibitors: Aripiprazole dose should be reduced to 25% of the usual dose. In patients receiving inhibitors of differing (eg, moderate 3A4/strong 2D6) or same (eg, moderate 3A4/moderate 2D6) potencies (excluding concurrent strong inhibitors), further dosage adjustments can be made to achieve the desired clinical response. In patients receiving strong CYP3A4 and 2D6 inhibitors, aripiprazole dose is proportionally increased upon discontinuation of one or both inhibitor agents.

Dosage adjustment based on CYP2D6 metabolizer status: Oral: Aripiprazole dose should be reduced to 50% of the usual dose in CYP2D6 poor metabolizers and to 25% of the usual dose in poor metabolizers receiving a concurrent strong CYP3A4 inhibitor; subsequently adjust dose for favorable clinical response.

Renal Impairment No dosage adjustment necessary.

Hepatic Impairment No dosage adjustment necessary.

Administration

Injection: For I.M. use only; do not administer SubQ or I.V.; inject slowly into deep muscle mass

Oral: May be administered with or without food. Tablet and oral solution may be interchanged on a mg-per-mg basis, up to 25 mg. Doses using 30 mg tablets should be exchanged for 25 mg oral solution. Orally-disintegrating tablets (Abilify Discmelt®) are bioequivalent to the immediate release tablets (Abilify®).

Orally-disintegrating tablet: Remove from foil blister by peeling back (do not push tablet through the foil). Place tablet in mouth immediately upon removal. Tablet dissolves rapidly in saliva and may be swallowed without liquid. If needed, can be taken with liquid. Do not split tablet.

Monitoring Parameters Vital signs; fasting lipid profile and fasting blood glucose/Hb A_{1c} (prior to treatment, at 3 months, then annually); CBC frequently during first few months of therapy in patients with pre-existing low WBC or a history of drug-induced leukopenia/ neutropenia; BMI, personal/family history of diabetes, waist circumference, blood pressure, mental status, abnormal involuntary movement scale (AIMS), extrapyramidal symptoms (EPS). Weight should be assessed prior to treatment, at 4 weeks, 8 weeks, 12 weeks, and then at quarterly intervals. Consider titrating to a different antipsychotic agent for a weight gain ≥5% of the initial weight.

Special Geriatric Considerations Elderly patients have an increased risk of adverse response to side effects or adverse reactions to antipsychotics. Aripiprazole has been studied in elderly patients with psychosis associated with Alzheimer's disease. The package insert does not provide the outcomes of this study other than somnolence was more frequent with aripiprazole (8%) than placebo (1%). Clinical data have shown an increased incidence of serious cerebrovascular events in the elderly, some fatal. In light of significant risks and adverse effects in the elderly population (compared with limited data demonstrating efficacy in the treatment of dementia-related psychosis, aggression, and agitation), an extensive risk: benefit analysis should be performed prior to use. Aripiprazole's delayed onset of action and long half-life may limit its role in treating older persons with psychosis. Not approved for the treatment of patients with dementia-related psychosis.

This medication is considered to be potentially inappropriate for use in geriatric patients (Beers Criteria: Quality of evidence - moderate; Strength of recommendation - strong).

Dosage Forms Excipient information presented when available (limited, particularly for generics); consult specific product labeling.

Injection, solution:
Abilify®: 7.5 mg/mL (1.3 mL)

Solution, oral:
Abilify®: 1 mg/mL (150 mL) [contains fructose 200 mg/mL, propylene glycol, sucrose 400 mg/mL; orange cream flavor]

Tablet, oral:
Abilify®: 2 mg, 5 mg, 10 mg, 15 mg, 20 mg, 30 mg

Tablet, orally disintegrating, oral:
  Abilify Discmelt®: 10 mg [contains phenylalanine 1.12 mg/tablet; creme de vanilla flavor]
  Abilify Discmelt®: 15 mg [contains phenylalanine 1.68 mg/tablet; creme de vanilla flavor]

◆ **Aristospan®** *see* Triamcinolone (Systemic) *on page 1957*
◆ **Arixtra®** *see* Fondaparinux *on page 837*

Armodafinil (ar moe DAF i nil)

Brand Names: U.S. Nuvigil®
Index Terms R-modafinil
Generic Availability (U.S.) No
Pharmacologic Category Stimulant
Use Improve wakefulness in patients with excessive daytime sleepiness associated with narcolepsy and shift work sleep disorder (SWSD); adjunctive therapy for obstructive sleep apnea/hypopnea syndrome (OSAHS)
Medication Guide Available Yes
Contraindications Hypersensitivity to armodafinil, modafinil, or any component of the formulation
Warnings/Precautions For use following complete evaluation of sleepiness and in conjunction with other standard treatments (eg, CPAP). The degree of sleepiness should be reassessed frequently; some patients may not return to a normal level of wakefulness. Use is not recommended with a history of angina, cardiac ischemia, recent history of myocardial infarction, left ventricular hypertrophy, or patients with mitral valve prolapse who have developed mitral valve prolapse syndrome with previous CNS stimulant use. Blood pressure monitoring may be required in patients on armodafinil. New or additional antihypertensive therapy may be needed.

Serious and life-threatening rashes including Stevens-Johnson syndrome, toxic epidermal necrolysis, and drug rash with eosinophilia and systemic symptoms have been reported with modafinil, the racemate of armodafinil. In clinical trials of modafinil, these rashes were more likely to occur in children; however, in the postmarketing period, serious reactions have occurred in both adults and children. Most cases have been reported within the first 5 weeks of initiating therapy; however, rare cases have occurred after prolonged therapy.

Caution should be exercised when modafinil is given to patients with a history of psychosis; may impair the ability to engage in potentially hazardous activities. Stimulants may unmask tics in individuals with coexisting Tourette's syndrome. Use caution with renal or hepatic impairment (dosage adjustment in hepatic dysfunction is recommended). Use reduced doses in elderly patients.

Adverse Reactions (Reflective of adult population; not specific for elderly)
>10%: Central nervous system: Headache (14% to 23%; dose-related)
1% to 10%:
  Cardiovascular: Palpitation (2%), increased heart rate (1%)
  Central nervous system: Dizziness (5%), insomnia (4% to 6%; dose related), anxiety (4%), depression (1% to 3%; dose related), fatigue (2%), agitation (1%), attention disturbance (1%), depressed mood (1%), migraine (1%), nervousness (1%), pain (1%), pyrexia (1%), tremor (1%)
  Dermatologic: Rash (1% to 4%; dose related), contact dermatitis (1%), hyperhidrosis (1%)
  Gastrointestinal: Nausea (6% to 9%; dose related), xerostomia (2% to 7%; dose related), diarrhea (4%), abdominal pain (2%), dyspepsia (2%), anorexia (1%), appetite decreased (1%), constipation (1%), loose stools (1%), vomiting (1%)
  Genitourinary: Polyuria (1%)
  Hepatic: GGT increased (1%)
  Neuromuscular & skeletal: Paresthesia (1%)
  Respiratory: Dyspnea (1%)
  Miscellaneous: Flu-like syndrome (1%), thirst (1%)
Drug Interactions
  Metabolism/Transport Effects Substrate of CYP3A4 (major); **Note:** Assignment of Major/Minor substrate status based on clinically relevant drug interaction potential; **Inhibits** CYP2C19 (moderate); **Induces** CYP3A4 (weak/moderate)
  Avoid Concomitant Use
    Avoid concomitant use of Armodafinil with any of the following: Axitinib; Clopidogrel; Conivaptan; Iobenguane I 123
  Increased Effect/Toxicity
    Armodafinil may increase the levels/effects of: Citalopram; CYP2C19 Substrates; Sympathomimetics

The levels/effects of Armodafinil may be increased by: AtoMOXetine; Cannabinoids; Conivaptan; CYP3A4 Inhibitors (Moderate); CYP3A4 Inhibitors (Strong); Dasatinib; Ivacaftor; Linezolid; Mifepristone

Decreased Effect

Armodafinil may decrease the levels/effects of: ARIPiprazole; Axitinib; Clopidogrel; Contraceptives (Estrogens); CycloSPORINE; CycloSPORINE (Systemic); Iobenguane I 123; Saxagliptin

The levels/effects of Armodafinil may be decreased by: CYP3A4 Inducers (Strong); Deferasirox; Herbs (CYP3A4 Inducers); Tocilizumab

Ethanol/Nutrition/Herb Interactions

Ethanol: Avoid or limit ethanol.

Food: Delays absorption, but minimal effects on bioavailability. Food may affect the onset and time course of armodafinil.

Stability Store at 20°C to 25°C (68°F to 77°F).

Mechanism of Action The exact mechanism of action of armodafinil is unknown. It is the R-enantiomer of modafinil. Armodafinil binds to the dopamine transporter and inhibits dopamine reuptake, which may result in increased extracellular dopamine levels in the brain. However, it does not appear to be a dopamine receptor agonist and also does not appear to bind to or inhibit the most common receptors or enzymes that are relevant for sleep/wake regulation.

Pharmacodynamics/Kinetics

Absorption: Readily absorbed

Distribution: V_d: 42 L

Protein binding: ~60% (based on modafinil; primarily albumin)

Metabolism: Hepatic, multiple pathways, including CYP3A4/5; metabolites include R-modafinil acid and modafinil sulfone

Clearance: 33 mL/minute, mainly via hepatic metabolism

Half-life elimination: 15 hours; Steady state: ~7 days

Time to peak, plasma: 2 hours (fasted)

Excretion: Urine (80% predominantly as metabolites; <10% as unchanged drug)

Dosage

Geriatric Refer to adult dosing. Consider lower initial dosage. Concentrations were almost doubled in clinical trials (based on modafinil).

Adult

Narcolepsy: Oral: 150-250 mg once daily in the morning

Obstructive sleep apnea/hypopnea syndrome (OSAHS): Oral: 150-250 mg once daily in the morning; 250 mg was not shown to have any increased benefit over 150 mg

Shift work sleep disorder (SWSD): Oral: 150 mg given once daily ~1 hour prior to work shift

Renal Impairment Inadequate data to determine safety and efficacy in severe renal impairment.

Hepatic Impairment Severe hepatic impairment (Child-Pugh class B or C): Based on modafinil, dose should be reduced by half.

Administration May be administered without regard to food.

Monitoring Parameters Signs of hypersensitivity, rash, psychiatric symptoms, levels of sleepiness, blood pressure, and drug abuse

Special Geriatric Considerations There are no specific pharmacokinetic data for armodafinil, but the clearance of modafinil may be reduced in the elderly. Safety and effectiveness in persons >65 years of age have not been established.

Controlled Substance C-IV

Dosage Forms Excipient information presented when available (limited, particularly for generics); consult specific product labeling.

Tablet, oral:

Nuvigil®: 50 mg, 150 mg, 250 mg

◆ **Armour® Thyroid** *see* Thyroid, Desiccated *on page 1885*
◆ **Aromasin®** *see* Exemestane *on page 732*
◆ **Artane** *see* Trihexyphenidyl *on page 1968*
◆ **Arthropan®** *see* Salicylates (Various Salts) *on page 1742*
◆ **Arthrotec®** *see* Diclofenac and Misoprostol *on page 537*
◆ **Artificial Saliva** *see* Saliva Substitute *on page 1748*

Artificial Tears (ar ti FISH il tears)

Medication Safety Issues

Sound-alike/look-alike issues:

Isopto® Tears may be confused with Isoptin®

Brand Names: U.S. Advanced Eye Relief™ Dry Eye Environmental [OTC]; Advanced Eye Relief™ Dry Eye Rejuvenation [OTC]; Bion® Tears [OTC]; HypoTears [OTC]; Murine Tears® [OTC]; Soothe® Hydration [OTC]; Soothe® [OTC]; Systane® Ultra [OTC]; Systane® [OTC]; Tears Again® [OTC]; Tears Naturale® Forte [OTC]; Tears Naturale® Free [OTC]; Tears Naturale® II [OTC]; Viva-Drops® [OTC]

Brand Names: Canada Teardrops®

Index Terms Hydroxyethylcellulose; Polyvinyl Alcohol

Generic Availability (U.S.) Yes

Pharmacologic Category Ophthalmic Agent, Miscellaneous

Use Ophthalmic lubricant; for temporary relief of burning and eye irritation due to dry eyes

Dosage

Geriatric & Adult Ocular dryness/irritation: Ophthalmic: 1-2 drops into eye(s) as needed to relieve symptoms

Special Geriatric Considerations Evaluate the patient's or caregiver's ability to safely administer the correct dose of ophthalmic medication.

Dosage Forms Excipient information presented when available (limited, particularly for generics); consult specific product labeling.

Solution, ophthalmic:

Advanced Eye Relief™ Dry Eye Environmental: Glycerin 1% (15 mL) [contains benzalkonium chloride]

Advanced Eye Relief™ Dry Eye Rejuvenation: Glycerin 0.3% and propylene glycol 1.0% (30 mL) [contains benzalkonium chloride]

HypoTears: Polyvinyl alcohol 1% and polyethylene glycol 400 1% (30 mL) [contains benzalkonium chloride]

Murine Tears®: Polyvinyl alcohol 0.5% and povidone 0.6% (15 mL) [contains benzalkonium chloride]

Soothe® Hydration: Povidone 1.25% (15 mL)

Systane® Ultra: Polyethylene glycol 400 0.4% and propylene glycol 0.3% (5 mL, 10 mL)

Systane®: Polyethylene glycol 400 0.4% and propylene glycol 0.3% (5 mL, 15 mL, 30 mL)

Tears Again®: Polyvinyl alcohol 1.4% (30 mL)

Tears Naturale® II: Dextran 70 0.1% and hydroxypropyl methylcellulose 2910 0.3% (30 mL)

Tears Naturale® Forte: Dextran 70 1%, glycerin 0.2%, and hydroxypropyl methylcellulose 2910 0.3% (30 mL)

Solution, ophthalmic [preservative free]:

Bion® Tears: Dextran 70 0.1% and hydroxypropyl methylcellulose 2910 0.3% per 0.4 mL (28s)

Soothe®: Glycerin 0.6% and propylene glycol 0.6% per 0.6 mL (28s)

Systane® Ultra: Polyethylene glycol 400 0.4% and propylene glycol 0.3% per 0.4 mL (24s)

Tears Naturale® Free: Dextran 70 0.1% and hydroxypropyl methylcellulose 2910 0.3% per 0.5 mL (36s, 60s)

Viva-Drops®: Polysorbate 80 1% (0.5 mL, 10 mL)

◆ **ASA** see Aspirin on page 154
◆ **5-ASA** see Mesalamine on page 1217
◆ **Asacol®** see Mesalamine on page 1217
◆ **Asacol® HD** see Mesalamine on page 1217
◆ **Asco-Caps-500 [OTC]** see Ascorbic Acid on page 149
◆ **Asco-Caps-1000 [OTC]** see Ascorbic Acid on page 149
◆ **Ascocid® [OTC]** see Ascorbic Acid on page 149
◆ **Ascocid®-500 [OTC]** see Ascorbic Acid on page 149
◆ **Ascor L 500® [DSC]** see Ascorbic Acid on page 149
◆ **Ascor L NC® [DSC]** see Ascorbic Acid on page 149

Ascorbic Acid (a SKOR bik AS id)

Medication Safety Issues

International issues:

Rubex [Ireland] may be confused with Brivex brand name for brivudine [Switzerland]

Rubex: Brand name for ascorbic acid [Ireland], but also the brand name for doxorubicin [Brazil]

Brand Names: U.S. Acerola [OTC]; Asco-Caps-1000 [OTC]; Asco-Caps-500 [OTC]; Asco-Tabs-1000 [OTC]; Ascocid® [OTC]; Ascocid®-500 [OTC]; Ascor L 500® [DSC]; Ascor L NC® [DSC]; C-Gel [OTC]; C-Gram [OTC]; C-Time [OTC]; Cemill 1000 [OTC]; Cemill 500 [OTC]; Chew-C [OTC]; Dull-C® [OTC]; Mild-C® [OTC]; One Gram C [OTC]; Time-C® [OTC]; Vicks® Vitamin C [OTC]; Vita-C® [OTC]

Brand Names: Canada Proflavanol C™; Revitalose C-1000®

Index Terms Vitamin C

Generic Availability (U.S.) Yes

Pharmacologic Category Vitamin, Water Soluble

Use Prevention and treatment of scurvy; acidify the urine

Unlabeled Use Investigational: In large doses to decrease the severity of "colds"; dietary supplementation; a 20-year study was recently completed involving 730 individuals which indicates a possible decreased risk of death by stroke when ascorbic acid at doses ≥45 mg/day was administered

Warnings/Precautions Patients with diabetes and patients prone to recurrent renal calculi (eg, dialysis patients) should not take excessive doses for extended periods of time. Some parenteral products contain aluminum; use caution in patients with impaired renal function.

Adverse Reactions (Reflective of adult population; not specific for elderly) 1% to 10%: Renal: Hyperoxaluria with large doses

Drug Interactions

Metabolism/Transport Effects None known.

Avoid Concomitant Use There are no known interactions where it is recommended to avoid concomitant use.

Increased Effect/Toxicity

Ascorbic Acid may increase the levels/effects of: Aluminum Hydroxide; Deferoxamine; Estrogen Derivatives

Decreased Effect

Ascorbic Acid may decrease the levels/effects of: Amphetamines; Bortezomib; Cyclo-SPORINE; CycloSPORINE (Systemic)

The levels/effects of Ascorbic Acid may be decreased by: Copper

Stability Injectable form should be stored under refrigeration (2°C to 8°C). Protect oral dosage forms from light. Rapidly oxidized when in solution in air and alkaline media.

Mechanism of Action Not fully understood; necessary for collagen formation and tissue repair; involved in some oxidation-reduction reactions as well as other metabolic pathways, such as synthesis of carnitine, steroids, and catecholamines and conversion of folic acid to folinic acid

Pharmacodynamics/Kinetics

Absorption: Oral: Readily absorbed; an active process thought to be dose dependent

Distribution: Large

Metabolism: Hepatic via oxidation and sulfation

Excretion: Urine (with high blood levels)

Dosage

Geriatric & Adult

Recommended daily allowance (RDA): Upper limit of intake should not exceed 2000 mg/day

Male: 90 mg

Female: 75 mg;

Adult smoker: Add an additional 35 mg/day

Scurvy: Oral, I.M., I.V., SubQ: 100-250 mg 1-2 times/day for at least 2 weeks

Urinary acidification: Oral, I.V.: 4-12 g/day in 3-4 divided doses

Prevention and treatment of colds: Oral: 1-3 g/day

Dietary supplement: Oral: 50-200 mg/day

Administration Avoid rapid I.V. injection

Monitoring Parameters Monitor pH of urine when using as an acidifying agent

Test Interactions False-positive urinary glucose with cupric sulfate reagent, false-negative urinary glucose with glucose oxidase method; false-negative stool occult blood 48-72 hours after ascorbic acid ingestion

Pharmacotherapy Pearls Sodium content of 1 g of sodium ascorbate: ~5 mEq

Special Geriatric Considerations Minimum RDA for elderly is not established. Vitamin C is provided mainly in citrus fruits and tomatoes. The elderly, however, avoid citrus fruits due to cost and difficulty preparing (peeling). Daily replacement through a single multiple vitamin is recommended. Use of natural vitamin C or rose hips offers no advantages. Acidity may produce GI complaints.

Dosage Forms Excipient information presented when available (limited, particularly for generics); consult specific product labeling. [DSC] = Discontinued product

Caplet, oral: 1000 mg

Caplet, timed release, oral: 500 mg, 1000 mg

Capsule, oral:

Mild-C®: 500 mg

Capsule, softgel, oral:

C-Gel: 1000 mg

Capsule, sustained release, oral:

C-Time: 500 mg

Capsule, timed release, oral: 500 mg
  Asco-Caps-500: 500 mg
  Asco-Caps-1000: 1000 mg [sugar free]
  Time-C®: 500 mg
Crystals for solution, oral: (170 g, 1000 g)
  Mild-C®: (170 g, 1000 g)
  Vita-C®: (113 g, 454 g) [dye free, gluten free, sugar free]
Injection, solution: 500 mg/mL (50 mL)
  Ascor L 500®: 500 mg/mL (50 mL [DSC]) [contains edetate disodium]
Injection, solution [preservative free]: 500 mg/mL (50 mL)
  Ascor L NC®: 500 mg/mL (50 mL [DSC]) [contains edetate disodium]
Liquid, oral: 500 mg/5 mL (118 mL, 473 mL)
Lozenge, oral:
  Vicks® Vitamin C: 25 mg (20s) [contains sodium 5 mg/lozenge; orange flavor]
Powder for solution, oral:
  Ascocid®: (227 g, 454 g)
  Dull-C®: (113 g, 454 g) [dye free, gluten free, sugar free]
Tablet, oral: 100 mg, 250 mg, 500 mg, 1000 mg
  Asco-Tabs-1000: 1000 mg [sugar free]
  Ascocid®-500: 500 mg [sugar free]
  C-Gram: 1000 mg [dye free, gluten free, sugar free]
  One Gram C: 1000 mg
Tablet, chewable, oral: 250 mg, 500 mg
  Acerola: 500 mg [cherry flavor]
  Mild-C®: 250 mg [orange-tangerine flavor]
Tablet, chewable, oral [buffered]:
  Chew-C: 500 mg [orange flavor]
Tablet, timed release, oral: 500 mg, 1000 mg
  Cemill 500: 500 mg
  Cemill 1000: 1000 mg
  Mild-C®: 1000 mg

◆ **Asco-Tabs-1000 [OTC]** *see* Ascorbic Acid *on page 149*
◆ **Ascriptin® Maximum Strength [OTC]** *see* Aspirin *on page 154*
◆ **Ascriptin® Regular Strength [OTC]** *see* Aspirin *on page 154*

Asenapine (a SEN a peen)

Related Information
  Antipsychotic Agents *on page 2103*
  Atypical Antipsychotics *on page 2107*
  Beers Criteria – Potentially Inappropriate Medications for Geriatrics *on page 2183*
Medication Safety Issues
  BEERS Criteria medication:
    This drug may be potentially inappropriate for use in geriatric patients (Quality of evidence - moderate; Strength of recommendation - strong).
Brand Names: U.S. Saphris®
Brand Names: Canada Saphris®
Pharmacologic Category Antimanic Agent; Antipsychotic Agent, Atypical
Use Acute and maintenance treatment of schizophrenia; treatment of acute mania or mixed episodes associated with bipolar I disorder (as monotherapy or in combination with lithium or valproate)
Contraindications Hypersensitivity to asenapine or any component of the formulation
Warnings/Precautions **[U.S. Boxed Warning]: Elderly patients with dementia-related psychosis treated with atypical antipsychotics are at an increased risk of death compared to placebo.** Most deaths appeared to be either cardiovascular (eg, heart failure, sudden death) or infectious (eg, pneumonia) in nature. In addition, an increased incidence of cerebrovascular effects (eg, transient ischemic attack, cerebrovascular accidents) has been reported in studies of placebo-controlled trials of antipsychotics in elderly patients with dementia-related psychosis. Asenapine is not approved for the treatment of dementia-related psychosis.

Use in elderly patients with dementia is associated with an increased risk of mortality and cerebrovascular accidents; avoid antipsychotic use for behavioral problems associated with dementia unless alternative nonpharmacologic therapies have failed and patient may harm self or others. In addition, use may cause or exacerbate syndrome of inappropriate antidiuretic hormone secretion or hyponatremia; monitor sodium closely with initiation or dosage adjustments in older adults (Beers Criteria). Pharmacokinetic studies showed a decrease in clearance in older adults (65-85 years of age) with psychosis compared to younger adults; increased risk of adverse effects and orthostasis may occur.

Leukopenia, neutropenia, and agranulocytosis (sometimes fatal) have been reported in clinical trials and postmarketing reports with antipsychotic use; presence of risk factors (eg, pre-existing low WBC or history of drug-induced leuko/neutropenia) should prompt periodic blood count assessment. Discontinue therapy at first signs of blood dyscrasias or if absolute neutrophil count <1000/mm³.

May be sedating; use with caution in disorders where CNS depression is a feature. Use with caution in Parkinson's disease. Use with caution in patients at risk of seizures, including those with a history of seizures, head trauma, brain damage, alcoholism, or concurrent therapy with medications which may lower seizure threshold. Use is not recommended in severe hepatic impairment; increased drug concentrations may occur. Esophageal dysmotility and aspiration have been associated with antipsychotic use; use with caution in patients at risk of aspiration pneumonia (ie, Alzheimer's disease). Elevates prolactin levels; use with caution in breast cancer or other prolactin-dependent tumors. May alter temperature regulation.

Use with caution in patients with cardiovascular diseases (eg, heart failure, history of myocardial infarction or ischemia, cerebrovascular disease, conduction abnormalities). May cause orthostatic hypotension; use with caution in patients at risk of this effect (eg, concurrent medication use which may predispose to hypotension/bradycardia or presence of hypovolemia) or in those who would not tolerate transient hypotensive episodes. May result in QT_c prolongation. Risk may be increased by conditions or concomitant medications which cause bradycardia, hypokalemia, and/or hypomagnesemia. Avoid use in combination with QT_c-prolonging drugs and in patients with congenital long QT syndrome or patients with history of cardiac arrhythmia.

May cause extrapyramidal symptoms (EPS), including pseudoparkinsonism, acute dystonic reactions, akathisia, and tardive dyskinesia. Risk of dystonia (and probably other EPS) may be greater with increased doses, use of conventional antipsychotics, males, and younger patients. Risk of neuroleptic malignant syndrome (NMS) may be increased in patients with Parkinson's disease or Lewy body dementia. May cause hyperglycemia; in some cases may be extreme and associated with ketoacidosis, hyperosmolar coma, or death. Use with caution in patients with diabetes or other disorders of glucose regulation; monitor for worsening of glucose control. Dyslipidemia has been reported with atypical antipsychotics; risk profile may differ between agents. In clinical trials, the incidence of hypertriglyceridemia observed with asenapine was greater than that observed with placebo, while total cholesterol elevations were similar. Significant weight gain has been observed with antipsychotic therapy; incidence varies with product. Monitor waist circumference and BMI. May cause anaphylaxis or hypersensitivity reactions.

The possibility of a suicide attempt is inherent in psychotic illness or bipolar disorder; use caution in high-risk patients during initiation of therapy. Prescriptions should be written for the smallest quantity consistent with good patient care.

Adverse Reactions (Reflective of adult population; not specific for elderly) Actual frequency may be dependent upon dose and/or indication.
>10%:
  Central nervous system: Somnolence (13% to 24%), insomnia (6% to 16%), extrapyramidal symptoms (6% to 12%), headache (12%), akathisia (4% to 11%; dose related), dizziness (3% to 11%)
  Endocrine & metabolic: Hypertriglyceridemia (13% to 15%)
1% to 10%:
  Cardiovascular: Peripheral edema (3%), hypertension (2% to 3%)
  Central nervous system: Hypoesthesia (4% to 7%), fatigue (3% to 4%), anxiety (4%), depression (2%), irritability (1% to 2%)
  Endocrine & metabolic: Cholesterol increased (8% to 9%), glucose increased (5% to 7%), hyperprolactinemia (2% to 3%)
  Gastrointestinal: Constipation (4% to 7%), vomiting (4% to 7%), weight gain (2% to 5%), dyspepsia (3% to 4%), appetite increased (≤4%), salivation increased (≤4%), abnormal taste (3%), toothache (3%), abdominal discomfort (≤3%), xerostomia (1% to 3%)
  Hematologic: Creatine kinase increased (6%)
  Hepatic: Transaminases increased (<1% to 3%)
  Neuromuscular & skeletal: Arthralgia (3%), extremity pain (2%)

Drug Interactions
  Metabolism/Transport Effects Substrate of CYP1A2 (major), CYP2D6 (minor), CYP3A4 (minor); **Note:** Assignment of Major/Minor substrate status based on clinically relevant drug interaction potential; **Inhibits** CYP2D6 (weak)

Avoid Concomitant Use
Avoid concomitant use of Asenapine with any of the following: Azelastine; Azelastine (Nasal); Highest Risk QTc-Prolonging Agents; Metoclopramide; Mifepristone; Moderate Risk QTc-Prolonging Agents; Paraldehyde

Increased Effect/Toxicity
Asenapine may increase the levels/effects of: Alcohol (Ethyl); ARIPiprazole; Azelastine; Azelastine (Nasal); Buprenorphine; CNS Depressants; Highest Risk QTc-Prolonging Agents; Methylphenidate; Paraldehyde; PARoxetine; Serotonin Modulators; Zolpidem

The levels/effects of Asenapine may be increased by: Abiraterone Acetate; Acetylcholinesterase Inhibitors (Central); CYP1A2 Inhibitors (Moderate); CYP1A2 Inhibitors (Strong); Deferasirox; FluvoxaMINE; HydrOXYzine; Lithium formulations; MAO Inhibitors; Methylphenidate; Metoclopramide; Metyrosine; Mifepristone; Moderate Risk QTc-Prolonging Agents; QTc-Prolonging Agents (Indeterminate Risk and Risk Modifying); Tetrabenazine

Decreased Effect
Asenapine may decrease the levels/effects of: Amphetamines; Anti-Parkinson's Agents (Dopamine Agonist); Quinagolide

The levels/effects of Asenapine may be decreased by: CYP1A2 Inducers (Strong); Cyproterone; Lithium formulations; Peginterferon Alfa-2b; Tocilizumab

Ethanol/Nutrition/Herb Interactions Ethanol: May increase CNS depression; monitor for increased effects with coadministration. Caution patients about effects.

Stability Store at 15°C to 30°C (59°F to 86°F).

Mechanism of Action Asenapine is a dibenzo-oxepino pyrrole atypical antipsychotic with mixed serotonin-dopamine antagonist activity. It exhibits high affinity for $5-HT_{1A}$, $5-HT_{1B}$, $5-HT_{2A}$, $5-HT_{2B}$, $5-HT_{2C}$, $5-HT_{5-7}$, D_{1-4}, H_1 and, alpha$_1$- and alpha$_2$-adrenergic receptors; moderate affinity for H_2 receptors. Asenapine has no significant affinity for muscarinic receptors. The binding affinity to the D_2 receptor is 19 times lower than the $5-HT_{2A}$ affinity (Weber, 2009). The addition of serotonin antagonism to dopamine antagonism (classic neuroleptic mechanism) is thought to improve negative symptoms of psychoses and reduce the incidence of extrapyramidal side effects as compared to typical antipsychotics.

Pharmacodynamics/Kinetics
Absorption: Rapid

Distribution: V_d: ~20-25 L/kg

Protein binding: 95% (including albumin and α_1-acid glycoprotein)

Metabolism: Hepatic via CYP1A2 oxidation and UGT1A4 glucuronidation

Bioavailability: Sublingual: 35%; decreased if swallowed (<2%); decreased if administered with food or liquid

Half-life elimination: Terminal: ~24 hours

Time to peak, plasma: 0.5-1.5 hours

Excretion: Urine (~50%); feces (~40%)

Dosage
Geriatric & Adult Note: Safety of doses >20 mg/day has not been evaluated:

Schizophrenia: Sublingual:

Acute treatment: Initial: 5 mg twice daily. Daily doses >20 mg/day in clinical trials did not appear to offer any additional benefits and increased risk of adverse effects.

Maintenance treatment: Initial: 5 mg twice daily; may increase to 10 mg twice daily after 1 week based on tolerability

Bipolar disorder: Sublingual:

Monotherapy: Initial: 10 mg twice daily; decrease to 5 mg twice daily if dose not tolerated

Combination therapy (with lithium or valproate): 5 mg twice daily; may increase to 10 mg twice daily based on tolerability

Renal Impairment No dosage adjustment is necessary.

Hepatic Impairment

Mild-to-moderate hepatic impairment (Child-Pugh class A or B): No dosage adjustment is necessary

Severe hepatic impairment (Child-Pugh class C): Use is not recommended

Administration Sublingual tablets should be placed under the tongue and allowed to disintegrate. Do not crush, chew, or swallow. Avoid eating or drinking for at least 10 minutes after administration.

Monitoring Parameters
Vital signs; fasting lipid profile and fasting blood glucose/Hgb A_{1c} (baseline and periodically); CBC frequently during first few months of therapy in patients with pre-existing low WBC or a history of drug-induced leukopenia/neutropenia; BMI, personal/family history of obesity, waist circumference; blood pressure; mental status, abnormal involuntary movement scale (AIMS), extrapyramidal symptoms; orthostatic blood pressure changes for 3-5 days after starting or increasing dose. Weight should be assessed prior to treatment and regularly throughout therapy. Consider titrating to a different antipsychotic agent for a weight gain ≥5% of the initial weight.

ASENAPINE

Special Geriatric Considerations Studies to date have not had sufficient numbers of patients to determine if elderly respond differently than younger adults. Given the high percentages of CNS adverse effects, patients should be monitored closely for somnolence, insomnia, EPS, akathisia, and dizziness. Elderly (with dementia-related psychosis) were determined, in initial studies with antipsychotics, to have an increased risk of death (1.6-1.7 times that seen in placebo groups). Asenapine is not approved for the treatment of dementia-related psychosis.

This medication is considered to be potentially inappropriate in this patient population (Beers Criteria: Quality of evidence - moderate; Strength of recommendation - strong).

Dosage Forms Excipient information presented when available (limited, particularly for generics); consult specific product labeling.
Tablet, sublingual:
Saphris®: 5 mg [unflavored]
Saphris®: 5 mg [black cherry flavor]
Saphris®: 10 mg [unflavored]
Saphris®: 10 mg [black cherry flavor]

◆ **Asendin [DSC]** see Amoxapine on page 110
◆ **Asmanex® Twisthaler®** see Mometasone (Oral Inhalation) on page 1304
◆ **Aspart Insulin** see Insulin Aspart on page 1005
◆ **Aspercin [OTC]** see Aspirin on page 154
◆ **Aspergillus niger** see Alpha-Galactosidase on page 67
◆ **Aspergum® [OTC]** see Aspirin on page 154

Aspirin (AS pir in)

Related Information
Antithrombotic Therapy in Adult Patients With Prosthetic Heart Valves on page 2182
Beers Criteria – Potentially Inappropriate Medications for Geriatrics on page 2183
Perioperative/Periprocedural Management of Anticoagulant and Antiplatelet Therapy on page 2209

Medication Safety Issues
Sound-alike/look-alike issues:
Aspirin may be confused with Afrin®
Ascriptin® may be confused with Aricept®
Ecotrin® may be confused with Edecrin®, Epogen®
Halfprin® may be confused with Haltran®
ZORprin® may be confused with Zyloprim®
International issues:
Cartia [multiple international markets] may be confused with Cartia XT brand name for diltiazem [U.S.]
BEERS Criteria medication:
This drug may be potentially inappropriate for use in geriatric patients (Quality of evidence - moderate; Strength of recommendation - strong).

Brand Names: U.S. Ascriptin® Maximum Strength [OTC]; Ascriptin® Regular Strength [OTC]; Aspercin [OTC]; Aspergum® [OTC]; Aspir-low [OTC]; Aspirtab [OTC]; Bayer® Aspirin Extra Strength [OTC]; Bayer® Aspirin Regimen Adult Low Strength [OTC]; Bayer® Aspirin Regimen Children's [OTC]; Bayer® Aspirin Regimen Regular Strength [OTC]; Bayer® Genuine Aspirin [OTC]; Bayer® Plus Extra Strength [OTC]; Bayer® Women's Low Dose Aspirin [OTC]; Buffasal [OTC]; Bufferin® Extra Strength [OTC]; Bufferin® [OTC]; Buffinol [OTC]; Ecotrin® Arthritis Strength [OTC]; Ecotrin® Low Strength [OTC]; Ecotrin® [OTC]; Halfprin® [OTC]; St Joseph® Adult Aspirin [OTC]; Tri-Buffered Aspirin [OTC]

Brand Names: Canada Asaphen; Asaphen E.C.; Entrophen®; Novasen; Praxis ASA EC 81 Mg Daily Dose

Index Terms Acetylsalicylic Acid; ASA; Baby Aspirin

Generic Availability (U.S.) Yes: Excludes gum

Pharmacologic Category Antiplatelet Agent; Salicylate

Use Treatment of mild-to-moderate pain, inflammation, and fever; prevention and treatment of acute coronary syndromes (ST-elevation MI, non-ST-elevation MI, unstable angina), acute ischemic stroke, and transient ischemic episodes; management of rheumatoid arthritis, rheumatic fever, osteoarthritis; adjunctive therapy in revascularization procedures (coronary artery bypass graft [CABG], percutaneous transluminal coronary angioplasty [PTCA], carotid endarterectomy), stent implantation

Unlabeled Use Low doses have been used in the prevention of pre-eclampsia, complications associated with autoimmune disorders such as lupus or antiphospholipid syndrome; colorectal cancer; Kawasaki disease; alternative therapy for prevention of thromboembolism associated with atrial fibrillation in patients not candidates for warfarin; pericarditis associated with MI; thromboprophylaxis for aortic valve repair, Blalock-Taussig shunt placement, carotid artery stenosis, coronary artery disease, Fontan surgery, peripheral arterial occlusive disease, peripheral artery percutaneous transluminal angioplasty, peripheral artery bypass graft surgery, prosthetic valves, ventricular assist device (VAD) placement

Contraindications Hypersensitivity to salicylates, other NSAIDs, or any component of the formulation; asthma; rhinitis; nasal polyps; inherited or acquired bleeding disorders (including factor VII and factor IX deficiency)

Warnings/Precautions Use with caution in patients with platelet and bleeding disorders, renal dysfunction, dehydration, erosive gastritis, or peptic ulcer disease. Heavy ethanol use (>3 drinks/day) can increase bleeding risks. Avoid use in severe renal failure or in severe hepatic failure. Low-dose aspirin for cardioprotective effects is associated with a two- to fourfold increase in UGI events (eg, symptomatic or complicated ulcers); risks of these events increase with increasing aspirin dose; during the chronic phase of aspirin dosing, doses >81 mg are not recommended unless indicated (Bhatt, 2008).

Discontinue use if tinnitus or impaired hearing occurs. Caution in mild-to-moderate renal failure (only at high dosages). Patients with sensitivity to tartrazine dyes, nasal polyps, and asthma may have an increased risk of salicylate sensitivity. In the treatment of acute ischemic stroke, avoid aspirin for 24 hours following administration of alteplase; administration within 24 hours increases the risk of hemorrhagic transformation. Concurrent use of aspirin and clopidogrel is not recommended for secondary prevention of ischemic stroke or TIA in patients unable to take oral anticoagulants due to hemorrhagic risk (Furie, 2011). Surgical patients should avoid ASA if possible, for 1-2 weeks prior to surgery, to reduce the risk of excessive bleeding (except in patients with cardiac stents that have not completed their full course of dual antiplatelet therapy [aspirin, clopidogrel]; patient-specific situations need to be discussed with cardiologist; AHA/ACC/SCAI/ACS/ADA Science Advisory provides recommendations). When used concomitantly with ≤325 mg of aspirin, NSAIDs (including selective COX-2 inhibitors) substantially increase the risk of gastrointestinal complications (eg, ulcer); concomitant gastroprotective therapy (eg, proton pump inhibitors) is recommended (Bhatt, 2008).

Elderly: Avoid chronic use of doses >325 mg/day (unless alternative agents ineffective and patient can receive concomitant gastroprotective agent); nonselective oral NSAID use is associated with an increased risk of GI bleeding and peptic ulcer disease in older adults in high risk category (eg, >75 years or age or receiving concomitant oral/parenteral corticosteroids, anticoagulants, or antiplatelet agents) (Beers Criteria).

When used for self-medication (OTC labeling): Changes in behavior (along with nausea and vomiting) may be an early sign of Reye's syndrome; patients should be instructed to contact their healthcare provider if these occur.

Adverse Reactions (Reflective of adult population; not specific for elderly) As with all drugs which may affect hemostasis, bleeding is associated with aspirin. Hemorrhage may occur at virtually any site. Risk is dependent on multiple variables including dosage, concurrent use of multiple agents which alter hemostasis, and patient susceptibility. Many adverse effects of aspirin are dose related, and are rare at low dosages. Other serious reactions are idiosyncratic, related to allergy or individual sensitivity. Accurate estimation of frequencies is not possible. The reactions listed below have been reported for aspirin (frequency not defined).

Cardiovascular: Hypotension, tachycardia, dysrhythmias, edema

Central nervous system: Fatigue, insomnia, nervousness, agitation, confusion, dizziness, headache, lethargy, cerebral edema, hyperthermia, coma

Dermatologic: Rash, angioedema, urticaria

Endocrine & metabolic: Acidosis, hyperkalemia, dehydration, hypoglycemia (children), hyperglycemia, hypernatremia (buffered forms)

Gastrointestinal: Nausea, vomiting, dyspepsia, epigastric discomfort, heartburn, stomach pain, gastrointestinal ulceration (6% to 31%), gastric erosions, gastric erythema, duodenal ulcers

Hematologic: Anemia, disseminated intravascular coagulation (DIC), prothrombin times prolonged, coagulopathy, thrombocytopenia, hemolytic anemia, bleeding, iron deficiency anemia

Hepatic: Hepatotoxicity, transaminases increased, hepatitis (reversible)

Neuromuscular & skeletal: Rhabdomyolysis, weakness, acetabular bone destruction (OA)

Otic: Hearing loss, tinnitus

Renal: Interstitial nephritis, papillary necrosis, proteinuria, renal impairment, renal failure (including cases caused by rhabdomyolysis), BUN increased, serum creatinine increased

Respiratory: Asthma, bronchospasm, dyspnea, laryngeal edema, hyperpnea, tachypnea, respiratory alkalosis, noncardiogenic pulmonary edema

Miscellaneous: Anaphylaxis, prolonged pregnancy and labor, stillbirths, low birth weight, peripartum bleeding, Reye's syndrome

Drug Interactions

Metabolism/Transport Effects Substrate of CYP2C9 (minor); **Note:** Assignment of Major/Minor substrate status based on clinically relevant drug interaction potential

Avoid Concomitant Use

Avoid concomitant use of Aspirin with any of the following: Floctafenine; Influenza Virus Vaccine (Live/Attenuated); Ketorolac; Ketorolac (Nasal); Ketorolac (Systemic)

Increased Effect/Toxicity

Aspirin may increase the levels/effects of: Alendronate; Anticoagulants; Carbonic Anhydrase Inhibitors; Collagenase (Systemic); Corticosteroids (Systemic); Dabigatran Etexilate; Divalproex; Dasatinib; Drotrecogin Alfa (Activated); Heparin; Hypoglycemic Agents; Ibritumomab; Methotrexate; PRALAtrexate; Rivaroxaban; Salicylates; Thrombolytic Agents; Ticagrelor; Tositumomab and Iodine I 131 Tositumomab; Valproic Acid; Varicella Virus-Containing Vaccines; Vitamin K Antagonists

The levels/effects of Aspirin may be increased by: Ammonium Chloride; Antidepressants (Tricyclic, Tertiary Amine); Antiplatelet Agents; Calcium Channel Blockers (Nondihydropyridine); Dasatinib; Floctafenine; Ginkgo Biloba; Glucosamine; Herbs (Anticoagulant/Antiplatelet Properties); Influenza Virus Vaccine (Live/Attenuated); Ketorolac; Ketorolac (Nasal); Ketorolac (Systemic); Loop Diuretics; Nonsteroidal Anti-Inflammatory Agents; NSAID (Nonselective); Omega-3-Acid Ethyl Esters; Pentosan Polysulfate Sodium; Pentoxifylline; Potassium Acid Phosphate; Prostacyclin Analogues; Selective Serotonin Reuptake Inhibitors; Serotonin/Norepinephrine Reuptake Inhibitors; Tipranavir; Treprostinil; Vitamin E

Decreased Effect

Aspirin may decrease the levels/effects of: ACE Inhibitors; Hyaluronidase; Loop Diuretics; NSAID (Nonselective); Probenecid; Ticagrelor; Tiludronate

The levels/effects of Aspirin may be decreased by: Corticosteroids (Systemic); Nonsteroidal Anti-Inflammatory Agents; NSAID (Nonselective)

Ethanol/Nutrition/Herb Interactions

Ethanol: Avoid ethanol (may enhance gastric mucosal damage).

Food: Food may decrease the rate but not the extent of oral absorption.

Folic acid: Hyperexcretion of folate; folic acid deficiency may result, leading to macrocytic anemia.

Iron: With chronic aspirin use and at doses of 3-4 g/day, iron-deficiency anemia may result.

Sodium: Hypernatremia resulting from buffered aspirin solutions or sodium salicylate containing high sodium content. Avoid or use with caution in CHF or any condition where hypernatremia would be detrimental.

Benedictine liqueur, prunes, raisins, tea, and gherkins: Potential salicylate accumulation.

Fresh fruits containing vitamin C: Displace drug from binding sites, resulting in increased urinary excretion of aspirin.

Herb/Nutraceutical: Avoid cat's claw, dong quai, evening primrose, feverfew, garlic, ginger, ginkgo, red clover, horse chestnut, green tea, ginseng (all have additional antiplatelet activity). Limit curry powder, paprika, licorice; may cause salicylate accumulation. These foods contain 6 mg salicylate/100 g. An ordinary American diet contains 10-200 mg/day of salicylate.

Stability Keep suppositories in refrigerator; do not freeze. Hydrolysis of aspirin occurs upon exposure to water or moist air, resulting in salicylate and acetate, which possess a vinegar-like odor. Do not use if a strong odor is present.

Mechanism of Action Irreversibly inhibits cyclooxygenase-1 and 2 (COX-1 and 2) enzymes, via acetylation, which results in decreased formation of prostaglandin precursors; irreversibly inhibits formation of prostaglandin derivative, thromboxane A_2, via acetylation of platelet cyclooxygenase, thus inhibiting platelet aggregation; has antipyretic, analgesic, and anti-inflammatory properties

Pharmacodynamics/Kinetics

Duration: 4-6 hours

Absorption: Rapid

Distribution: V_d: 10 L; readily into most body fluids and tissues

Metabolism: Hydrolyzed to salicylate (active) by esterases in GI mucosa, red blood cells, synovial fluid, and blood; metabolism of salicylate occurs primarily by hepatic conjugation; metabolic pathways are saturable

Bioavailability: 50% to 75% reaches systemic circulation

Half-life elimination: Parent drug: 15-20 minutes; Salicylates (dose dependent): 3 hours at lower doses (300-600 mg), 5-6 hours (after 1 g), 10 hours with higher doses

Time to peak, serum: ~1-2 hours

Excretion: Urine (75% as salicyluric acid, 10% as salicylic acid)

Dosage

Geriatric & Adult Note: For most cardiovascular uses, typical maintenance dosing of aspirin is 81 mg once daily.

Acute coronary syndrome (ST-segment elevation myocardial infarction [STEMI], unstable angina (UA)/non-ST-segment elevation myocardial infarction [NSTEMI]):
Oral: Initial: 162-325 mg given on presentation (patient should chew nonenteric-coated aspirin especially if not taking before presentation); for patients unable to take oral, may use rectal suppository (300 mg). Maintenance (secondary prevention): 75-162 mg once daily indefinitely (Anderson, 2007; Antman, 2004). **Note:** When aspirin is used with ticagrelor, the recommended maintenance dose of aspirin is 81 mg/day (Jneid, 2012).

UA/NSTEMI: Concomitant antiplatelet therapy (Jneid, 2012):

If invasive strategy chosen: Aspirin is recommended in combination with either clopidogrel, ticagrelor, (or prasugrel if at the time of PCI) or an I.V. GP IIb/IIIa inhibitor (if given before PCI, eptifibatide and tirofiban are preferred agents).

If noninvasive strategy chosen: Aspirin is recommended in combination with clopidogrel or ticagrelor.

Analgesic and antipyretic:
Oral: 325-650 mg every 4-6 hours up to 4 g/day
Rectal: 300-600 mg every 4-6 hours up to 4 g/day

Anti-inflammatory: Oral: Initial: 2.4-3.6 g/day in divided doses; usual maintenance: 3.6-5.4 g/day; monitor serum concentrations

Aortic valve repair (unlabeled use): Oral: 50-100 mg once daily (Guyatt, 2012)

Atrial fibrillation (in patients not candidates for oral anticoagulation or at low risk of ischemic stroke) (unlabeled use): Oral: 75-325 mg once daily (Furie, 2011; Fuster, 2006). **Note:** Combination therapy with clopidogrel has been suggested over aspirin alone for those patients who are unsuitable for or choose not to take oral anticoagulant for reasons other than concerns for bleeding (Guyatt, 2012).

As an alternative to adjusted-dose warfarin in patients with atrial fibrillation and mitral stenosis: 75-325 mg once daily with (preferred) or without clopidogrel (Guyatt, 2012)

CABG: Oral: 100-325 mg once daily initiated either preoperatively or within 6 hours postoperatively; continue indefinitely (Hillis, 2011)

Carotid artery stenosis (unlabeled use): Oral: 75-100 mg once daily. **Note:** When symptomatic (including recent carotid endarterectomy), the use of clopidogrel or aspirin/extended-release dipyridamole has been suggested over aspirin alone (Guyatt, 2012).

Coronary artery disease (CAD), established: Oral: 75-100 mg once daily (Guyatt, 2012)

PCI: Oral: Preprocedure: 81-325 mg (325 mg [nonenteric coated] in aspirin-naive patients) starting at least 2 hours (preferably 24 hours) before procedure. Postprocedure: 81 mg once daily continued indefinitely (in combination with a $P2Y_{12}$ inhibitor [eg, clopidogrel, prasugrel, ticagrelor] up to 12 months) (Levine, 2011)

Alternatively, in patients who have undergone elective PCI with either bare metal or drug-eluting stent placement: The American College of Chest Physicians recommends the use of 75-325 mg once daily (in combination with clopidogrel) for 1 month (BMS) or 3-6 months (dependent upon DES type) followed by 75-100 mg once daily (in combination with clopidogrel) for up to12 months. For patients who underwent PCI but did not have stent placement, 75-325 mg once daily (in combination with clopidogrel) for 1 month is recommended. In either case, single antiplatelet therapy (either aspirin or clopidogrel) is recommended indefinitely (Guyatt, 2012).

Pericarditis associated with myocardial infarction (unlabeled use): Oral: 162-325 mg once daily; doses as high as 650 mg every 4-6 hours may be required; enteric-coated recommended (Antman, 2004)

Peripheral arterial disease (unlabeled use): Oral: 75-100 mg once daily (Guyatt, 2012) **or** 75-325 mg once daily; may use in conjunction with clopidogrel in those who are not at an increased risk of bleeding but are of high cardiovascular risk. **Note:** These recommendations also pertain to those with intermittent claudication or critical limb ischemia, prior lower extremity revascularization, or prior amputation for lower extremity ischemia (Rooke, 2011).

Peripheral artery percutaneous transluminal angioplasty (with or without stenting) or peripheral artery bypass graft surgery, postprocedure (unlabeled use): Oral: 75-100 mg once daily (Guyatt, 2012). **Note:** For below-knee bypass graft surgery with prosthetic grafts, combine with clopidogrel (Guyatt, 2012).

Pre-eclampsia prevention (women at risk) (unlabeled use): Oral: 75-100 mg once daily starting in the second trimester (Guyatt, 2012)

Primary prevention: Oral:

American College of Cardiology/American Heart Association: Prevention of myocardial infarction: 75-162 mg once daily. **Note:** Patients are most likely to benefit if their 10-year coronary heart disease risk is ≥6% (Antman, 2004).

American College of Chest Physicians: Prevention of myocardial infarction and stroke: Select individuals ≥50 years of age (without symptomatic cardiovascular disease): 75-100 mg once daily (Guyatt, 2012; Grade 2B, weak recommendation)

Prosthetic heart valve: Oral:

Bioprosthetic aortic valve (patient in normal sinus rhythm) (unlabeled use): 50-100 mg once daily. **Note:** If mitral bioprosthetic valve, oral anticoagulation with warfarin (instead of aspirin) is recommended for the first 3 months postoperatively, followed by aspirin alone (Guyatt, 2012).

Mechanical aortic or mitral valve (unlabeled use):
Low risk of bleeding: 50-100 mg once daily (in combination with warfarin) (Guyatt, 2012)
History of thromboembolism while receiving oral anticoagulants: 75-100 mg once daily (in combination with warfarin) (Furie, 2011)

Transcatheter aortic bioprosthetic valve (unlabeled use): 50-100 mg once daily (in combination with clopidogrel) (Guyatt, 2012)

Stroke/TIA: Oral:

Acute ischemic stroke/TIA: Initial: 160-325 mg within 48 hours of stroke/TIA onset, followed by 75-100 mg once daily (Adams, 2007; Guyatt, 2012)

Cardioembolic, secondary prevention (oral anticoagulation unsuitable): 75-100 mg once daily (in combination with clopidogrel) (Guyatt, 2012)

Cryptogenic with patent foramen ovale (PFO) or atrial septal aneurysm: 50-100 mg once daily (Guyatt, 2012)

Noncardioembolic, secondary prevention: 75-325 mg once daily (Smith, 2011) **or** 75-100 mg once daily (Guyatt, 2012). **Note:** Combination aspirin/extended release dipyridamole or clopidogrel is preferred over aspirin alone (Guyatt, 2012).

Women at high risk, primary prevention: 81 mg once daily **or** 100 mg every other day (Goldstein, 2010)

Renal Impairment
Cl_{cr} <10 mL/minute: Avoid use.
Dialyzable (50% to 100%)

Hepatic Impairment Avoid use in severe liver disease.

Administration Do not crush enteric coated tablet. Administer with food or a full glass of water to minimize GI distress. For acute myocardial infarction, have patient chew tablet.

Reference Range Timing of serum samples: Peak levels usually occur 2 hours after ingestion. Salicylate serum concentrations correlate with the pharmacological actions and adverse effects observed. The serum salicylate concentration (mcg/mL) and the corresponding clinical correlations are as follows: See table.

Serum Salicylate: Clinical Correlations

Serum Salicylate Concentration (mcg/mL)	Desired Effects	Adverse Effects / Intoxication
~100	Antiplatelet Antipyresis Analgesia	GI intolerance and bleeding, hypersensitivity, hemostatic defects
150-300	Anti-inflammatory	Mild salicylism
250-400	Treatment of rheumatic fever	Nausea/vomiting, hyperventilation, salicylism, flushing, sweating, thirst, headache, diarrhea, and tachycardia
>400-500		Respiratory alkalosis, hemorrhage, excitement, confusion, asterixis, pulmonary edema, convulsions, tetany, metabolic acidosis, fever, coma, cardiovascular collapse, renal and respiratory failure

Test Interactions False-negative results for glucose oxidase urinary glucose tests (Clinistix®); false-positives using the cupric sulfate method (Clinitest®); also, interferes with Gerhardt test, VMA determination; 5-HIAA, xylose tolerance test and T_3 and T_4

Special Geriatric Considerations Elderly are a high-risk population for adverse effects from nonsteroidal anti-inflammatory agents. As much as 60% of elderly with GI complications to NSAIDs can develop peptic ulceration and/or hemorrhage asymptomatically. The concomitant use of H_2 blockers and sucralfate is not effective as prophylaxis with the exception of NSAID-induced duodenal ulcers which may be prevented by the use of ranitidine. Misoprostol and proton pump inhibitors are the only prophylactic agents proven to help prevent the development of NSAID-induced ulcers. Also, concomitant disease and drug use contribute to the risk for GI adverse effects. Use lowest effective dose for shortest period possible. Consider renal function decline with age. Use of NSAIDs can compromise existing renal function especially when Cl_{cr} is ≤30 mL/minute. Tinnitus may be a difficult and unreliable indication of toxicity due to age-related hearing loss or eighth cranial nerve damage. CNS adverse effects such as confusion, agitation, and hallucination are generally seen in overdose or high dose situations, but elderly may demonstrate these adverse effects at lower doses than younger adults.

This medication is considered to be potentially inappropriate in this patient population (Beers Criteria: Quality of evidence - moderate; Strength of recommendation - strong).

Dosage Forms Excipient information presented when available (limited, particularly for generics); consult specific product labeling.

Caplet, oral: 500 mg
  Bayer® Aspirin Extra Strength: 500 mg
  Bayer® Genuine Aspirin: 325 mg
  Bayer® Women's Low Dose Aspirin: 81 mg [contains elemental calcium 300 mg]
Caplet, oral [buffered]:
  Ascriptin® Maximum Strength: 500 mg [contains aluminum hydroxide, calcium carbonate, magnesium hydroxide]
  Bayer® Plus Extra Strength: 500 mg [contains calcium carbonate]
Caplet, enteric coated, oral:
  Bayer® Aspirin Regimen Regular Strength: 325 mg
Gum, chewing, oral:
  Aspergum®: 227 mg (12s) [cherry flavor]
  Aspergum®: 227 mg (12s) [orange flavor]
Suppository, rectal: 300 mg (12s); 600 mg (12s)
Tablet, oral: 325 mg
  Aspercin: 325 mg
  Aspirtab: 325 mg
  Bayer® Genuine Aspirin: 325 mg
Tablet, oral [buffered]: 325 mg
  Ascriptin® Regular Strength: 325 mg [contains aluminum hydroxide, calcium carbonate, magnesium hydroxide]
  Buffasal: 325 mg [contains magnesium oxide]
  Bufferin®: 325 mg [contains calcium carbonate, magnesium carbonate, magnesium oxide]
  Bufferin® Extra Strength: 500 mg [contains calcium carbonate, magnesium carbonate, magnesium oxide]
  Buffinol: 324 mg [sugar free; contains magnesium oxide]
  Tri-Buffered Aspirin: 325 mg [contains calcium carbonate, magnesium carbonate, magnesium oxide]
Tablet, chewable, oral: 81 mg
  Bayer® Aspirin Regimen Children's: 81 mg [cherry flavor]
  Bayer® Aspirin Regimen Children's: 81 mg [orange flavor]
  St Joseph® Adult Aspirin: 81 mg
Tablet, enteric coated, oral: 81 mg, 325 mg, 650 mg
  Aspir-low: 81 mg
  Bayer® Aspirin Regimen Adult Low Strength: 81 mg
  Ecotrin®: 325 mg
  Ecotrin® Arthritis Strength: 500 mg
  Ecotrin® Low Strength: 81 mg
  Halfprin®: 81 mg, 162 mg
  St Joseph® Adult Aspirin: 81 mg

Aspirin and Dipyridamole (AS pir in & dye peer ID a mole)

Related Information
  Aspirin *on page 154*
  Dipyridamole *on page 572*
Medication Safety Issues
  Sound-alike/look-alike issues:
    Aggrenox® may be confused with Aggrastat®
Brand Names: U.S. Aggrenox®
Brand Names: Canada Aggrenox®
Index Terms Aspirin and Extended-Release Dipyridamole; Dipyridamole and Aspirin
Generic Availability (U.S.) No
Pharmacologic Category Antiplatelet Agent
Use Reduction in the risk of stroke in patients who have had transient ischemia of the brain or ischemic stroke due to thrombosis
Unlabeled Use Hemodialysis graft patency; symptomatic carotid artery stenosis (including recent carotid endarterectomy)

Contraindications Hypersensitivity to dipyridamole, aspirin, or any component of the formulation; allergy to NSAIDs; patients with the syndrome of asthma, rhinitis, and nasal polyps

Canadian labeling: Additional contraindications (not in U.S. labeling): Patients with hereditary fructose and/or galactose intolerance

Warnings/Precautions Patients who consume ≥3 alcoholic drinks per day may be at risk of bleeding. Use cautiously in patients with inherited or acquired bleeding disorders, renal impairment, hypotension, unstable angina, recent MI or hepatic dysfunction. Avoid use in patients with a history of active peptic ulcer disease, severe hepatic failure, or severe renal impairment (Cl_{cr} <10 mL/minute). Monitor for signs and symptoms of GI ulcers and bleeding. Discontinue use if dizziness, tinnitus, or impaired hearing occurs. Discontinue use 24 hours prior to pharmacologic (I.V. dipyridamole) stress testing. Discontinue 1-2 weeks before elective surgical procedures to reduce the risk of bleeding. Use caution in the elderly who are at high risk for adverse events. Dose of aspirin in this combination may not be adequate to prevent for cardiac indications (eg, MI prophylaxis). Formulation may contain lactose and/or sucrose. Use in patients with fructose and/or galactose intolerance is contraindicated in the Canadian labeling.

Adverse Reactions (Reflective of adult population; not specific for elderly)
>10%:
Central nervous system: Headache (39%; tolerance usually develops)
Gastrointestinal: Abdominal pain (18%), dyspepsia (18%), nausea (16%), diarrhea (13%)
1% to 10%:
Cardiovascular: Cardiac failure (2%), syncope (1%)
Central nervous system: Fatigue (6%), pain (6%), amnesia (2%), malaise (2%), seizure (2%), confusion (1%), somnolence (1%)
Dermatologic: Purpura (1%)
Gastrointestinal: Vomiting (8%), GI bleeding (4%), melena (2%), rectal bleeding (2%), hemorrhoids (1%), GI hemorrhage (1%), anorexia (1%)
Hematologic: Hemorrhage (3%), anemia (2%)
Neuromuscular & skeletal: Arthralgia (6%), back pain (5%), weakness (2%), arthritis (2%), arthrosis (1%), myalgia (1%)
Respiratory: Cough (2%), epistaxis (2%), upper respiratory tract infection (1%)

Drug Interactions

Metabolism/Transport Effects Refer to individual components.

Avoid Concomitant Use
Avoid concomitant use of Aspirin and Dipyridamole with any of the following: Floctafenine; Influenza Virus Vaccine (Live/Attenuated); Ketorolac; Ketorolac (Nasal); Ketorolac (Systemic); Silodosin

Increased Effect/Toxicity
Aspirin and Dipyridamole may increase the levels/effects of: Adenosine; Alendronate; Anticoagulants; Beta-Blockers; Carbonic Anhydrase Inhibitors; Colchicine; Collagenase (Systemic); Corticosteroids (Systemic); Dabigatran Etexilate; Divalproex; Drotrecogin Alfa (Activated); Everolimus; Heparin; Hypoglycemic Agents; Hypotensive Agents; Ibritumomab; Methotrexate; P-glycoprotein/ABCB1 Substrates; PRALAtrexate; Prucalopride; Regadenoson; Rivaroxaban; Salicylates; Silodosin; Thrombolytic Agents; Ticagrelor; Topotecan; Tositumomab and Iodine I 131 Tositumomab; Valproic Acid; Varicella Virus-Containing Vaccines; Vitamin K Antagonists

The levels/effects of Aspirin and Dipyridamole may be increased by: Ammonium Chloride; Antidepressants (Tricyclic, Tertiary Amine); Antiplatelet Agents; Calcium Channel Blockers (Nondihydropyridine); Dasatinib; Floctafenine; Ginkgo Biloba; Glucosamine; Herbs (Anticoagulant/Antiplatelet Properties); Influenza Virus Vaccine (Live/Attenuated); Ketorolac; Ketorolac (Nasal); Ketorolac (Systemic); Loop Diuretics; Nonsteroidal Anti-Inflammatory Agents; NSAID (Nonselective); Omega-3-Acid Ethyl Esters; Pentosan Polysulfate Sodium; Pentoxifylline; Potassium Acid Phosphate; Prostacyclin Analogues; Selective Serotonin Reuptake Inhibitors; Serotonin/Norepinephrine Reuptake Inhibitors; Tipranavir; Treprostinil; Vitamin E

Decreased Effect
Aspirin and Dipyridamole may decrease the levels/effects of: ACE Inhibitors; Acetylcholinesterase Inhibitors; Hyaluronidase; Loop Diuretics; NSAID (Nonselective); Probenecid; Ticagrelor; Tiludronate

The levels/effects of Aspirin and Dipyridamole may be decreased by: Corticosteroids (Systemic); Nonsteroidal Anti-Inflammatory Agents; NSAID (Nonselective)

Ethanol/Nutrition/Herb Interactions Ethanol: Avoid ethanol (due to GI irritation).

Stability Store at 25°C (77°F); excursions permitted to 15°C to 30°C (59°F to 86°F). Protect from excessive moisture.

Mechanism of Action The antithrombotic action results from additive antiplatelet effects. Dipyridamole inhibits the uptake of adenosine into platelets, endothelial cells, and erythrocytes. Aspirin inhibits platelet aggregation by irreversible inhibition of platelet cyclooxygenase and thus inhibits the generation of thromboxane A_2.

Pharmacodynamics/Kinetics See individual agents.

Dosage

Geriatric & Adult

Stroke prevention: Oral: One capsule (dipyridamole 200 mg, aspirin 25 mg) twice daily

Alternative regimen for patients with intolerable headache: Oral: One capsule at bedtime and low-dose aspirin in the morning. Return to usual dose (1 capsule twice daily) as soon as tolerance to headache develops (usually within a week).

Carotid artery stenosis, symptomatic (including recent carotid endarterectomy) (unlabeled use): Oral: One capsule (dipyridamole 200 mg, aspirin 25 mg) twice daily (Guyatt, 2012)

Hemodialysis graft patency (unlabeled use): Oral: One capsule (dipyridamole 200 mg, aspirin 25 mg) twice daily

Renal Impairment Avoid use in patients with severe renal dysfunction (Cl_{cr} <10 mL/minute).

Hepatic Impairment Avoid use in patients with severe hepatic impairment.

Administration Capsule should be swallowed whole; do not crush or chew. May be administered with or without food.

Monitoring Parameters Hemoglobin, hematocrit, signs or symptoms of bleeding, signs or symptoms of stroke or transient ischemic attack

Test Interactions See individual agents.

Special Geriatric Considerations Plasma concentrations were 40% higher, but specific dosage adjustments have not been recommended. Some evidence suggests that the doses of dipyridamole commonly used are ineffective for prevention of platelet aggregation, however, the addition of aspirin will add substantial efficacy. The dose of aspirin is effective for platelet inhibition, but low enough to offer a low adverse drug reaction rate.

Dosage Forms Excipient information presented when available (limited, particularly for generics); consult specific product labeling.

Capsule, variable release:

Aggrenox®: Aspirin 25 mg [immediate release] and dipyridamole 200 mg [extended release] [contains lactose, sucrose]

Atenolol (a TEN oh lole)

Related Information

Beta-Blockers on page 2108

Medication Safety Issues

Sound-alike/look-alike issues:

Atenolol may be confused with albuterol, Altenol®, timolol, Tylenol®

Tenormin® may be confused with Imuran®, Norpramin®, thiamine, Trovan®

Brand Names: U.S. Tenormin®

Brand Names: Canada Apo-Atenol®; Ava-Atenolol; CO Atenolol; Dom-Atenolol; JAMP-Atenolol; Mint-Atenolol; Mylan-Atenolol; Nu-Atenol; PMS-Atenolol; RAN™-Atenolol; ratio-Atenolol; Riva-Atenolol; Sandoz-Atenolol; Septa-Atenolol; Tenormin®; Teva-Atenolol

Generic Availability (U.S.) Yes

Pharmacologic Category Antianginal Agent; Beta-Blocker, Beta-1 Selective

Use Treatment of hypertension, alone or in combination with other agents; management of angina pectoris; secondary prevention postmyocardial infarction

Unlabeled Use Acute ethanol withdrawal (in combination with a benzodiazepine), supraventricular and ventricular arrhythmias, and migraine headache prophylaxis

ATENOLOL

Contraindications Hypersensitivity to atenolol or any component of the formulation; sinus bradycardia; sinus node dysfunction; heart block greater than first-degree (except in patients with a functioning artificial pacemaker); cardiogenic shock; uncompensated cardiac failure; pulmonary edema

Warnings/Precautions Consider pre-existing conditions such as sick sinus syndrome before initiating. Administer cautiously in compensated heart failure and monitor for a worsening of the condition (efficacy of atenolol in heart failure has not been established). **[U.S. Boxed Warning]: Beta-blocker therapy should not be withdrawn abruptly (particularly in patients with CAD), but gradually tapered to avoid acute tachycardia, hypertension, and/or ischemia.** Chronic beta-blocker therapy should not be routinely withdrawn prior to major surgery. Beta-blockers should be avoided in patients with bronchospastic disease (asthma). Atenolol, with B_1 selectivity, has been used cautiously in bronchospastic disease with close monitoring. May precipitate or aggravate symptoms of arterial insufficiency in patients with PVD and Raynaud's disease; use with caution and monitor for progression of arterial obstruction. Use cautiously in patients with diabetes - may mask hypoglycemic symptoms. May mask signs of hyperthyroidism (eg, tachycardia); use caution if hyperthyroidism is suspected, abrupt withdrawal may precipitate thyroid storm. Alterations in thyroid function tests may be observed. Use cautiously in the renally impaired (dosage adjustment required). Caution in myasthenia gravis or psychiatric disease (may cause CNS depression). Bradycardia may be observed more frequently in elderly patients (>65 years of age); dosage reductions may be necessary. Adequate alpha-blockade is required prior to use of any beta-blocker for patients with untreated pheochromocytoma. May induce or exacerbate psoriasis. Use caution with history of severe anaphylaxis to allergens; patients taking beta-blockers may become more sensitive to repeated challenges. Treatment of anaphylaxis (eg, epinephrine) in patients taking beta-blockers may be ineffective or promote undesirable effects. Use with caution in patients on concurrent digoxin, verapamil, or diltiazem; bradycardia or heart block can occur. Use with caution in patients receiving inhaled anesthetic agents known to depress myocardial contractility.

Adverse Reactions (Reflective of adult population; not specific for elderly) 1% to 10%:

Cardiovascular: Persistent bradycardia, hypotension, chest pain, edema, heart failure, second- or third-degree AV block, Raynaud's phenomenon

Central nervous system: Dizziness, fatigue, insomnia, lethargy, confusion, mental impairment, depression, headache, nightmares

Gastrointestinal: Constipation, diarrhea, nausea

Genitourinary: Impotence

Miscellaneous: Cold extremities

Drug Interactions

Metabolism/Transport Effects None known.

Avoid Concomitant Use

Avoid concomitant use of Atenolol with any of the following: Floctafenine; Methacholine

Increased Effect/Toxicity

Atenolol may increase the levels/effects of: Alpha-/Beta-Agonists (Direct-Acting); Alpha1-Blockers; Alpha2-Agonists; Amifostine; Antihypertensives; Bupivacaine; Cardiac Glycosides; Cholinergic Agonists; Fingolimod; Hypotensive Agents; Insulin; Lidocaine; Lidocaine (Systemic); Lidocaine (Topical); Mepivacaine; Methacholine; Midodrine; RiTUXimab; Sulfonylureas

The levels/effects of Atenolol may be increased by: Acetylcholinesterase Inhibitors; Amiodarone; Anilidopiperidine Opioids; Calcium Channel Blockers (Dihydropyridine); Calcium Channel Blockers (Nondihydropyridine); Diazoxide; Dipyridamole; Disopyramide; Dronedarone; Floctafenine; Glycopyrrolate; Herbs (Hypotensive Properties); MAO Inhibitors; Pentoxifylline; Phosphodiesterase 5 Inhibitors; Prostacyclin Analogues; Reserpine

Decreased Effect

Atenolol may decrease the levels/effects of: Beta2-Agonists; Theophylline Derivatives

The levels/effects of Atenolol may be decreased by: Ampicillin; Herbs (Hypertensive Properties); Methylphenidate; Nonsteroidal Anti-Inflammatory Agents; Yohimbine

Ethanol/Nutrition/Herb Interactions

Food: Atenolol serum concentrations may be decreased if taken with food.

Herb/Nutraceutical: Dong quai has estrogenic activity. Ephedra, yohimbe, and ginseng may worsen hypertension. Garlic may have increased antihypertensive effect. Management: Avoid dong quai, ephedra, yohimbe, ginseng, and garlic.

Stability Protect from light.

Mechanism of Action Competitively blocks response to beta-adrenergic stimulation, selectively blocks beta$_1$-receptors with little or no effect on beta$_2$-receptors except at high doses

Pharmacodynamics/Kinetics
Onset of action: Peak effect: Oral: 2-4 hours
Duration: Normal renal function: 12-24 hours
Absorption: Oral: Rapid, incomplete (~50%)
Distribution: Low lipophilicity; does not cross blood-brain barrier
Protein binding: 6% to 16%
Metabolism: Limited hepatic
Half-life elimination: Beta: Normal renal function: 6-7 hours, prolonged with renal impairment;
  End-stage renal disease: 15-35 hours
Time to peak, plasma: Oral: 2-4 hours
Excretion: Feces (50%); urine (40% as unchanged drug)

Dosage
Geriatric Refer to adult dosing. In the management of hypertension, consider lower initial doses and titrate to response (Aronow, 2011).

Adult

Hypertension: Oral: 25-50 mg once daily, may increase to 100 mg/day. Doses >100 mg are unlikely to produce any further benefit.

Angina pectoris: Oral: 50 mg once daily; may increase to 100 mg/day. Some patients may require 200 mg/day.

Postmyocardial infarction: Oral: 100 mg/day or 50 mg twice daily for 6-9 days postmyocardial infarction

Thyrotoxicosis (unlabeled use): Oral: 25-100 mg once or twice daily (Bahn, 2011)

Renal Impairment
Cl_{cr} 15-35 mL/minute: Administer 50 mg/day maximum.
Cl_{cr} <15 mL/minute: Administer 50 mg every other day maximum.
Hemodialysis effects: Moderately dialyzable (20% to 50%) via hemodialysis. Administer dose postdialysis or administer 25-50 mg supplemental dose. Elimination is not enhanced with peritoneal dialysis. Supplemental dose is not necessary.

Administration When administered acutely for cardiac treatment, monitor ECG and blood pressure. May be administered without regard to meals.

Monitoring Parameters Acute cardiac treatment: Monitor ECG and blood pressure

Test Interactions Increased glucose; decreased HDL

Special Geriatric Considerations Due to alterations in the beta-adrenergic autonomic nervous system, beta-adrenergic blockade may result in less hemodynamic response than seen in younger adults. Studies indicate that despite decreased sensitivity to the chronotropic effects of beta-blockade with age, there appears to be an increased myocardial sensitivity to the negative inotropic effect during stress (ie, exercise). Controlled trials have shown the overall response rate for propranolol to be only 20% to 50% in the elderly. Therefore, all beta-adrenergic blocking drugs may result in a decreased response as compared to younger adults. Since many elderly have Cl_{cr} <35 mL/minute, creatinine clearance should be estimated or measured such that appropriate dose adjustment can be made.

Dosage Forms Excipient information presented when available (limited, particularly for generics); consult specific product labeling.
Tablet, oral: 25 mg, 50 mg, 100 mg
  Tenormin®: 25 mg
  Tenormin®: 50 mg [scored]
  Tenormin®: 100 mg

◆ **Ativan®** *see* LORazepam *on page 1157*
◆ **Atlizumab** *see* Tocilizumab *on page 1918*

AtorvaSTATin (a TORE va sta tin)

Related Information
Hyperlipidemia Management *on page 2130*

Medication Safety Issues
Sound-alike/look-alike issues:
AtorvaSTATin may be confused with atoMOXetine, lovastatin, nystatin, pitavastatin, pravastatin, rosuvastatin, simvastatin

Lipitor® may be confused with labetalol, Levatol®, lisinopril, Loniten®, Lopid®, Mevacor®, Zocor®, ZyrTEC®

Brand Names: U.S. Lipitor®

Brand Names: Canada Apo-Atorvastatin®; Ava-Atorvastatin; CO Atorvastatin; Dom-Atorvastatin; GD-Atorvastatin; Lipitor®; Mylan-Atorvastatin; Novo-Atorvastatin; PMS-Atorvastatin; RAN™-Atorvastatin; ratio-Atorvastatin; Sandoz-Atorvastatin

Index Terms Atorvastatin Calcium

Generic Availability (U.S.) Yes

Pharmacologic Category Antilipemic Agent, HMG-CoA Reductase Inhibitor

Use Treatment of dyslipidemias or primary prevention of cardiovascular disease (atherosclerotic) as detailed below:

Primary prevention of cardiovascular disease (high-risk for CVD): To reduce the risk of MI or stroke in patients without evidence of heart disease who have multiple CVD risk factors or type 2 diabetes. Treatment reduces the risk for angina or revascularization procedures in patients with multiple risk factors.

Secondary prevention of cardiovascular disease: To reduce the risk of nonfatal MI, nonfatal stroke, revascularization procedures, hospitalization for heart failure, and angina in patients with evidence of coronary heart disease.

Treatment of dyslipidemias: To reduce elevations in total cholesterol (C), LDL-C, apolipoprotein B, and triglycerides in patients with elevations of one or more components, and/or to increase low HDL-C as present in Fredrickson type IIa, IIb, III, and IV hyperlipidemias, heterozygous familial and nonfamilial hypercholesterolemia, and homozygous familial hypercholesterolemia

Unlabeled Use Secondary prevention in patients who have experienced a noncardioembolic stroke/TIA or following an ACS event regardless of baseline LDL-C using intensive lipid-lowering therapy

Contraindications Hypersensitivity to atorvastatin or any component of the formulation; active liver disease; unexplained persistent elevations of serum transaminases

Note: Telaprevir Canadian product monograph contraindicates use with atorvastatin.

Warnings/Precautions Secondary causes of hyperlipidemia should be ruled out prior to therapy. Atorvastatin has not been studied when the primary lipid abnormality is chylomicron elevation (Fredrickson types I and V). Liver function tests must be obtained prior to initiating therapy, repeat if clinically indicated thereafter. May cause hepatic dysfunction. Use with caution in patients who consume large amounts of ethanol or have a history of liver disease; use is contraindicated in patients with active liver disease or unexplained persistent elevations of serum transaminases. Monitoring is recommended. Patients with a history of hemorrhagic stroke may be at increased risk for another hemorrhagic stroke with use.

Rhabdomyolysis with acute renal failure has occurred. Risk is dose related and is increased with concurrent use of lipid-lowering agents which may cause rhabdomyolysis (fibric acid derivatives or niacin at doses ≥1 g/day) or during concurrent use with potent CYP3A4 inhibitors (including amiodarone, clarithromycin, erythromycin, itraconazole, ketoconazole, nefazodone, grapefruit juice in large quantities, verapamil, or protease inhibitors such as indinavir, nelfinavir, or ritonavir). Ensure patient is on the lowest effective atorvastatin dose. If concurrent use of clarithromycin or combination protease inhibitors (eg, lopinavir/ritonavir or ritonavir/saquinavir) is warranted consider dose adjustment of atorvastatin. Do not use with cyclosporine, gemfibrozil, tipranavir plus ritonavir, or telaprevir. Monitor closely if used with other drugs associated with myopathy. Weigh the risk versus benefit when combining any of these drugs with atorvastatin. Discontinue in any patient in which CPK levels are markedly elevated (>10 times ULN) or if myopathy is suspected/diagnosed. The manufacturer recommends temporary discontinuation for elective major surgery, acute medical or surgical conditions, or in any patient experiencing an acute or serious condition predisposing to renal failure (eg, sepsis, hypotension, trauma, uncontrolled seizures). However, based upon current evidence, HMG-CoA reductase inhibitor therapy should be continued in the perioperative period unless risk outweighs cardioprotective benefit. Use with caution in patients with advanced age, these patients are predisposed to myopathy. Safety and efficacy have not been established in patients <10 years of age or in premenarcheal girls.

Adverse Reactions (Reflective of adult population; not specific for elderly)

>10%:
  Gastrointestinal: Diarrhea (5% to 14%)
  Neuromuscular & skeletal: Arthralgia (4% to 12%)
  Respiratory: Nasopharyngitis (4% to 13%)

2% to 10%:
  Central nervous system: Insomnia (1% to 5%)
  Gastrointestinal: Nausea (4% to 7%), dyspepsia (3% to 6%)
  Genitourinary: Urinary tract infection (4% to 8%)
  Hepatic: Transaminases increased (2% to 3% with 80 mg/day dosing)
  Neuromuscular & skeletal: Limb pain (3% to 9%), myalgia (3% to 8%), muscle spasms (2% to 5%), musculoskeletal pain (2% to 5%)
  Respiratory: Pharyngolaryngeal pain (1% to 4%)

Additional class-related events or case reports (not necessarily reported with atorvastatin therapy): Cataracts, cirrhosis, dermatomyositis, eosinophilia, erectile dysfunction, extraocular muscle movement impaired, fulminant hepatic necrosis, gynecomastia, hemolytic anemia, interstitial lung disease, ophthalmoplegia, peripheral nerve palsy, polymyalgia

ATORVASTATIN

rheumatica, positive ANA, renal failure (secondary to rhabdomyolysis), systemic lupus erythematosus-like syndrome, thyroid dysfunction, tremor, vasculitis, vertigo

Drug Interactions

Metabolism/Transport Effects Substrate of CYP3A4 (major), P-glycoprotein, SLCO1B1; **Note:** Assignment of Major/Minor substrate status based on clinically relevant drug interaction potential; **Inhibits** CYP3A4 (weak), P-glycoprotein

Avoid Concomitant Use

Avoid concomitant use of AtorvaSTATin with any of the following: Conivaptan; Cyclo-SPORINE; CycloSPORINE (Systemic); Gemfibrozil; Pimozide; Red Yeast Rice; Silodosin; Telaprevir; Topotecan

Increased Effect/Toxicity

AtorvaSTATin may increase the levels/effects of: Aliskiren; ARIPiprazole; DAPTOmycin; Digoxin; Diltiazem; Everolimus; Ketoconazole; Ketoconazole (Systemic); Midazolam; Pazopanib; P-glycoprotein/ABCB1 Substrates; Pimozide; Prucalopride; Rivaroxaban; Silodosin; Topotecan; Trabectedin; Verapamil

The levels/effects of AtorvaSTATin may be increased by: Amiodarone; Boceprevir; Colchicine; Conivaptan; CycloSPORINE; CycloSPORINE (Systemic); CYP3A4 Inhibitors (Moderate); CYP3A4 Inhibitors (Strong); Cyproterone; Danazol; Dasatinib; Diltiazem; Dronedarone; Eltrombopag; Fenofibrate; Fenofibric Acid; Fluconazole; Fusidic Acid; Gemfibrozil; Grapefruit Juice; Itraconazole; Ivacaftor; Ketoconazole; Ketoconazole (Systemic); Macrolide Antibiotics; Mifepristone; Niacin; Niacinamide; P-glycoprotein/ABCB1 Inhibitors; Posaconazole; Protease Inhibitors; QuiNINE; Red Yeast Rice; Sildenafil; Telaprevir; Verapamil; Voriconazole

Decreased Effect

AtorvaSTATin may decrease the levels/effects of: Dabigatran Etexilate; Lanthanum

The levels/effects of AtorvaSTATin may be decreased by: Antacids; Bexarotene; Bexarotene (Systemic); Bosentan; CYP3A4 Inducers (Strong); Deferasirox; Efavirenz; Etravirine; Fosphenytoin; P-glycoprotein/ABCB1 Inducers; Phenytoin; Rifamycin Derivatives; St Johns Wort; Tocilizumab

Ethanol/Nutrition/Herb Interactions

Ethanol: Ethanol may enhance the potential of adverse hepatic effects. Management: Avoid excessive ethanol consumption.

Food: Atorvastatin serum concentrations may be increased by grapefruit juice. Management: Avoid concurrent intake of large quantities of grapefruit juice (>1 quart/day). Red yeast rice contains an estimated 2.4 mg lovastatin per 600 mg rice.

Herb/Nutraceutical: St John's wort may decrease atorvastatin levels.

Stability Store at controlled room temperature of 20°C to 25°C (68°F to 77°F).

Mechanism of Action Inhibitor of 3-hydroxy-3-methylglutaryl coenzyme A (HMG-CoA) reductase, the rate-limiting enzyme in cholesterol synthesis (reduces the production of mevalonic acid from HMG-CoA); this then results in a compensatory increase in the expression of LDL receptors on hepatocyte membranes and a stimulation of LDL catabolism

Pharmacodynamics/Kinetics

Onset of action: Initial changes: 3-5 days; Maximal reduction in plasma cholesterol and triglycerides: 2 weeks

Absorption: Rapid

Distribution: V_d: ~381 L

Protein binding: ≥98%

Metabolism: Hepatic; forms active ortho- and parahydroxylated derivates and an inactive beta-oxidation product

Bioavailability: ~14% (parent drug); ~30% (parent drug and equipotent metabolites)

Half-life elimination: Parent drug: 14 hours; Equipotent metabolites: 20-30 hours

Time to peak, serum: 1-2 hours

Excretion: Bile; urine (<2% as unchanged drug)

Dosage

Geriatric & Adult

Primary prevention: **Note:** Doses should be individualized according to the baseline LDL-cholesterol concentrations, the recommended goal of therapy, and patient response; adjustments should be made at intervals of 2-4 weeks

Hypercholesterolemia (heterozygous familial and nonfamilial) and mixed hyperlipidemia (Fredrickson types IIa and IIb): Oral: Initial: 10-20 mg once daily; patients requiring >45% reduction in LDL-C may be started at 40 mg once daily; range: 10-80 mg once daily

Homozygous familial hypercholesterolemia: Oral: 10-80 mg once daily

Secondary prevention:

Clinically-evident coronary heart disease: Oral: Initial: 80 mg once daily; adjust based on patient tolerability and recommended goal LDL-C (LaRosa, 2005)

Intensive lipid-lowering after an ACS event regardless of baseline LDL (unlabeled use): Oral: Initial: 80 mg once daily; adjust based on patient tolerability and recommended goal LDL-C (Cannon, 2004; Pederson, 2005; Schwartz, 2001). **Note:** Currently, the ACC/AHA guidelines for UA/NSTEMI do not specify which statin to use (Anderson, 2007).

Noncardioembolic stroke/TIA (unlabeled use): Oral: Initial: 80 mg once daily; adjust based on patient tolerability and recommended goal LDL-C (Adams, 2008; Amarenco, 2006)

Dosage adjustment for atorvastatin with concomitant medications:
Clarithromycin, itraconazole, fosamprenavir, ritonavir (plus darunavir, fosamprenavir, lopinavir, or saquinavir): Lowest effective atorvastatin dose (not to exceed 20 mg/day) should be used.

Nelfinavir: Lowest effective atorvastatin dose (not to exceed 40 mg/day) should be used.

Renal Impairment No adjustment is necessary.

Hepatic Impairment Contraindicated in active liver disease or in patients with unexplained persistent elevations of serum transaminases.

Administration May be administered with food if desired; may take without regard to time of day.

Monitoring Parameters Baseline CPK (recheck CPK in any patient with symptoms suggestive of myopathy; discontinue therapy if markedly elevated); baseline liver function tests (LFTs) and repeat when clinically indicated thereafter. Patients with elevated transaminase levels should have a second (confirmatory) test and frequent monitoring until values normalize; discontinue if increase in ALT/AST is persistently >3 times ULN (NCEP, 2002).

Lipid panel (total cholesterol, HDL, LDL, triglycerides):
ATP III recommendations (NCEP, 2002): Baseline; 6-8 weeks after initiation of drug therapy; if dose increased, then at 6-8 weeks until final dose determined. Once treatment goal achieved, follow-up intervals may be reduced to every 4-6 months. Lipid panel should be assessed at least annually, and preferably at each clinic visit.

Manufacturer recommendation: Upon initiation or titration, lipid panel should be analyzed within 2-4 weeks.

Special Geriatric Considerations Effective and well tolerated in the elderly. The definition of and, therefore, when to treat hyperlipidemia in the elderly is a controversial issue. The National Cholesterol Education Program recommends that all adults maintain a plasma cholesterol <160 mg/dL. For elderly patients with one additional risk factor, goal LDL would be <130 mg/dL. It is the authors' belief that pharmacologic treatment be reserved for those who are unable to obtain a desirable plasma cholesterol concentration by diet alone and for whom the benefits of treatment are believed to outweigh the potential adverse effects, drug interactions, and cost of treatment. Age ≥65 years is a risk factor for myopathy.

Dosage Forms Excipient information presented when available (limited, particularly for generics); consult specific product labeling.
Tablet, oral: 10 mg, 20 mg, 40 mg, 80 mg
Lipitor®: 10 mg, 20 mg, 40 mg, 80 mg

◆ **Atorvastatin Calcium** *see* AtorvaSTATin *on page* 163
◆ **AtroPen®** *see* Atropine *on page* 166

Atropine (A troe peen)

Related Information
Beers Criteria − Potentially Inappropriate Medications for Geriatrics *on page* 2183
Medication Safety Issues
BEERS Criteria medication:
This drug may be potentially inappropriate for use in geriatric patients (Quality of evidence - varies based on comorbidity; Strength of recommendation - varies based on comorbidity)
Brand Names: U.S. AtroPen®; Atropine Care™; Isopto® Atropine
Brand Names: Canada Dioptic's Atropine Solution; Isopto® Atropine
Index Terms Atropine Sulfate
Generic Availability (U.S.) Yes
Pharmacologic Category Anticholinergic Agent; Anticholinergic Agent, Ophthalmic; Antidote; Antispasmodic Agent, Gastrointestinal; Ophthalmic Agent, Mydriatic
Use
Injection: Preoperative medication to inhibit salivation and secretions; treatment of symptomatic sinus bradycardia, AV block (nodal level); antidote for anticholinesterase poisoning (carbamate insecticides, nerve agents, organophosphate insecticides); adjuvant use with anticholinesterases (eg, edrophonium, neostigmine) to decrease their side effects during reversal of neuromuscular blockade

Note: Use is no longer recommended in the management of asystole or pulseless electrical activity (PEA) (ACLS, 2010).

Ophthalmic: Produce mydriasis and cycloplegia for examination of the retina and optic disc and accurate measurement of refractive errors; produce papillary dilation in inflammatory conditions (eg, uveitis)

Prescribing and Access Restrictions The AtroPen® formulation is available for use primarily by the Department of Defense.

Contraindications Hypersensitivity to atropine or any component of the formulation; narrow-angle glaucoma; adhesions between the iris and lens (ophthalmic product); pyloric stenosis; prostatic hypertrophy

Note: No contraindications exist in the treatment of life-threatening organophosphate or carbamate insecticide or nerve agent poisoning.

Warnings/Precautions Heat prostration may occur in the presence of high environmental temperatures. Psychosis may occur in sensitive individuals or following use of excessive doses. Avoid use if possible in patients with obstructive uropathy or in other conditions resulting in urinary retention; use is contraindicated in patients with prostatic hypertrophy. Avoid use in patients with paralytic ileus, intestinal atony of the elderly or debilitated patient, severe ulcerative colitis, and toxic megacolon complicating ulcerative colitis. Use with caution in patients with autonomic neuropathy, hyperthyroidism, renal or hepatic impairment, myocardial ischemia, HF, tachyarrhythmias (including sinus tachycardia), hypertension, and hiatal hernia associated with reflux esophagitis. Treatment-related blood pressure increases and tachycardia may lead to ischemia, precipitate an MI, or increase arrhythmogenic potential. In heart transplant recipients, atropine will likely be ineffective in treatment of bradycardia due to lack of vagal innervation of the transplanted heart; cholinergic reinnervation may occur over time (years), so atropine may be used cautiously; however, some may experience paradoxical slowing of the heart rate and high-degree AV block upon administration (ACLS, 2010; Bernheim, 2004).

Avoid relying on atropine for effective treatment of type II second-degree or third-degree AV block (with or without a new wide QRS complex). Asystole or bradycardic pulseless electrical activity (PEA): Although no evidence exists for significant detrimental effects, routine use is unlikely to have a therapeutic benefit and is no longer recommended (ACLS, 2010).

AtroPen®: There are no absolute contraindications for the use of atropine in severe organophosphate or carbamate insecticide or nerve agent poisonings; however in mild poisonings, use caution in those patients where the use of atropine would be otherwise contraindicated. Formulation for use by trained personnel only. Clinical symptoms consistent with highly-suspected organophosphate or carbamate insecticides or nerve agent poisoning should be treated with antidote immediately; administration should not be delayed for confirmatory laboratory tests. Signs of atropinization include flushing, mydriasis, tachycardia, and dryness of the mouth or nose. Monitor effects closely when administering subsequent injections as necessary. The presence of these effects is not indicative of the success of therapy; inappropriate use of mydriasis as an indicator of successful treatment has resulted in atropine toxicity. Reversal of bronchial secretions is the preferred indicator of success. Adjunct treatment with a cholinesterase reactivator (eg, pralidoxime) may be required in patients with toxicity secondary to organophosphorus insecticides or nerve agents. Treatment should always include proper evacuation and decontamination procedures; medical personnel should protect themselves from inadvertent contamination. Antidote administration is intended only for initial management; definitive and more extensive medical care is required following administration. Individuals should not rely solely on antidote for treatment, as other supportive measures (eg, artificial respiration) may still be required. Atropine reverses the muscarinic but not the nicotinic effects associated with anticholinesterase toxicity.

May be inappropriate in older adults depending on comorbidities (eg, dementia, delirium) due to its potent anticholinergic effects (Beers Criteria).

Adverse Reactions (Reflective of adult population; not specific for elderly) Severity and frequency of adverse reactions are dose related and vary greatly; listed reactions are limited to significant and/or life-threatening.

Cardiovascular: Arrhythmia, flushing, hypotension, palpitation, tachycardia

Central nervous system: Ataxia, coma, delirium, disorientation, dizziness, drowsiness, excitement, fever, hallucinations, headache, insomnia, nervousness

Dermatologic: Anhidrosis, urticaria, rash, scarlatiniform rash

Gastrointestinal: Bloating, constipation, delayed gastric emptying, loss of taste, nausea, paralytic ileus, vomiting, xerostomia, dry throat, nasal dryness

Genitourinary: Urinary hesitancy, urinary retention

Neuromuscular & skeletal: Weakness

Ocular: Angle-closure glaucoma, blurred vision, cycloplegia, dry eyes, mydriasis, ocular tension increased

Respiratory: Dyspnea, laryngospasm, pulmonary edema

Miscellaneous: Anaphylaxis

◀ **Drug Interactions**

Metabolism/Transport Effects None known.

Avoid Concomitant Use There are no known interactions where it is recommended to avoid concomitant use.

Increased Effect/Toxicity

Atropine may increase the levels/effects of: AbobotulinumtoxinA; Anticholinergics; Cannabinoids; OnabotulinumtoxinA; Potassium Chloride; RimabotulinumtoxinB

The levels/effects of Atropine may be increased by: Pramlintide

Decreased Effect

Atropine may decrease the levels/effects of: Acetylcholinesterase Inhibitors (Central); Secretin

The levels/effects of Atropine may be decreased by: Acetylcholinesterase Inhibitors (Central)

Stability Store injection at controlled room temperature of 15°C to 30°C (59°F to 86°F); avoid freezing. In addition, AtroPen® should be protected from light.

Preparation of bulk atropine solution for mass chemical terrorism: Add atropine sulfate powder to 100 mL NS in polyvinyl chloride bags to yield a final concentration of 1 mg/mL. Stable for 72 hours at 4°C to 8°C (39°F to 46°F); 20°C to 25°C (68°F to 77°F); 32°C to 36°C (90°F to 97°F) (Dix, 2003).

Mechanism of Action Blocks the action of acetylcholine at parasympathetic sites in smooth muscle, secretory glands, and the CNS; increases cardiac output, dries secretions. Atropine reverses the muscarinic effects of cholinergic poisoning due to agents with acetylcholinesterase inhibitor activity by acting as a competitive antagonist of acetylcholine at muscarinic receptors. The primary goal in cholinergic poisonings is reversal of bronchorrhea and bronchoconstriction. Atropine has no effect on the nicotinic receptors responsible for muscle weakness, fasciculations, and paralysis.

Pharmacodynamics/Kinetics

Onset of action: I.M., I.V.: Rapid

Absorption: I.M.: Rapid and well absorbed

Distribution: Widely throughout the body; crosses blood-brain barrier

Metabolism: Hepatic via enzymatic hydrolysis

Half-life elimination: 2-3 hours; Elderly 65-75 years of age: 10 hours

Time to peak: I.M.: 3 minutes

Excretion: Urine (30% to 50% as unchanged drug and metabolites)

Dosage

Geriatric Refer to adult dosing.

Nerve agent toxicity management: See **Note**. I.M.: Elderly and frail patients:

Prehospital ("in the field"): Mild-to-moderate symptoms: 1 mg; severe symptoms: 2-4 mg

Hospital/emergency department: Mild-to-moderate symptoms: 1 mg; severe symptoms: 2 mg

Note: Pralidoxime is a component of the management of nerve agent toxicity.

Prehospital ("in the field") management: Repeat atropine I.M. (2 mg) at 5-10 minute intervals until secretions have diminished and breathing is comfortable or airway resistance has returned to near normal.

Hospital management: Repeat atropine I.M. (2 mg) at 5-10 minute intervals until secretions have diminished and breathing is comfortable or airway resistance has returned to near normal.

Adult Doses <0.5 mg have been associated with paradoxical bradycardia.

Inhibit salivation and secretions (preanesthesia): *I.M., I.V., SubQ:* 0.4-0.6 mg 30-60 minutes preop and repeat every 4-6 hours as needed.

Bradycardia (Note: Atropine may be ineffective in heart transplant recipients): *I.V.:* 0.5 mg every 3-5 minutes, not to exceed a total of 3 mg or 0.04 mg/kg (ACLS, 2010)

Neuromuscular blockade reversal: *I.V.:* 25-30 mcg/kg 30-60 seconds before neostigmine or 7-10 mcg/kg 30-60 seconds before edrophonium

Organophosphate or carbamate insecticide or nerve agent poisoning: Note: The dose of atropine required varies considerably with the severity of poisoning. The total amount of atropine used for carbamate poisoning is usually less than with organophosphate insecticide or nerve agent poisoning. Severely poisoned patients may exhibit significant tolerance to atropine; ≥2 times the suggested doses may be needed. Titrate to pulmonary status (decreased bronchial secretions); consider administration of atropine via continuous I.V. infusion in patients requiring large doses of atropine. Once patient is stable for a period of time, the dose/dosing frequency may be decreased. If atropinization occurs after 1-2 mg of atropine then re-evaluate working diagnosis (Reigart, 1999).

I.V., I.M. (unlabeled dose): Initial: 1-6 mg (ATSDR, 2011; Roberts, 2007); repeat every 3-5 minutes as needed, doubling the dose if previous dose did not induce atropinization (Eddleston, 2004b; Roberts, 2007). Maintain atropinization by administering repeat doses as needed for ≥2-12 hours based on recurrence of symptoms (Reigart, 1999).

I.V. Infusion (unlabeled dose): Following atropinization, administer 10% to 20% of the total loading dose required to induce atropinization as a continuous I.V. infusion per hour; adjust as needed to maintain adequate atropinization without atropine toxicity (Eddleston, 2004b; Roberts, 2007)

I.M. (AtroPen®):

Mild symptoms (≥2 mild symptoms): Administer 2 mg as soon as an exposure is known or strongly suspected. If severe symptoms develop after the first dose, 2 additional doses should be repeated in rapid succession 10 minutes after the first dose; do not administer more than 3 doses. If profound anticholinergic effects occur in the absence of excessive bronchial secretions, further doses of atropine should be withheld.

Severe symptoms (≥1 severe symptoms): Immediately administer **three** 2 mg doses in rapid succession.

Symptoms of insecticide or nerve agent poisoning, as provided by manufacturer in the AtroPen® product labeling, to guide therapy:

Mild symptoms: Blurred vision, bradycardia, breathing difficulties, chest tightness, coughing, drooling, miosis, muscular twitching, nausea, runny nose, salivation increased, stomach cramps, tachycardia, teary eyes, tremor, vomiting, or wheezing

Severe symptoms: Breathing difficulties (severe), confused/strange behavior, defecation (involuntary), muscular twitching/generalized weakness (severe), respiratory secretions (severe), seizure, unconsciousness, urination (involuntary)

Mydriasis, cycloplegia (preprocedure): Ophthalmic (1% solution): Instill 1-2 drops 1 hour before the procedure.

Uveitis: *Ophthalmic:*

1% solution: Instill 1-2 drops up to 4 times/day.

Ointment: Apply a small amount in the conjunctival sac up to 3 times/day. Compress the lacrimal sac by digital pressure for 1-3 minutes after instillation.

Administration

I.M.: AtroPen®: Administer to the outer thigh. Firmly grasp the autoinjector with the green tip (0.5 mg, 1 mg, and 2 mg autoinjector) or black tip (0.25 mg autoinjector) pointed down; remove the yellow safety release (0.5 mg, 1 mg, and 2 mg autoinjector) or gray safety release (0.25 mg autoinjector). Jab the green tip at a 90° angle against the outer thigh; may be administered through clothing as long as pockets at the injection site are empty. In thin patients or patients <6.8 kg (15 lb), bunch up the thigh prior to injection. Hold the autoinjector in place for 10 seconds following the injection; remove the autoinjector and massage the injection site. After administration, the needle will be visible; if the needle is not visible, repeat the above steps. After use, bend the needle against a hard surface (needle does not retract) to avoid accidental injury.

I.V.: Administer undiluted by rapid I.V. injection; slow injection may result in paradoxical bradycardia. In bradycardia, atropine administration should not delay treatment with external pacing.

Endotracheal: Dilute in NS or sterile water. Absorption may be greater with sterile water. Stop compressions (if using for cardiac arrest), spray the drug quickly down the tube. Follow immediately with several quick insufflations and continue chest compressions.

Monitoring Parameters Heart rate, blood pressure, pulse, mental status; intravenous administration requires a cardiac monitor

Organophosphate or carbamate insecticide or nerve agent poisoning: Heart rate, blood pressure, respiratory status, oxygenation secretions. Maintain atropinization with repeated dosing as indicated by clinical status. Crackles in lung bases, or continuation of cholinergic signs, may be signs of inadequate dosing. Pulmonary improvement may not parallel other signs of atropinization. Monitor for signs and symptoms of atropine toxicity (eg, fever, muscle fasciculations, delirium); if toxicity occurs, discontinue atropine and monitor closely.

Special Geriatric Considerations Anticholinergic agents are generally not well tolerated in the elderly and their use should be avoided when possible.

This medication is considered to be potentially inappropriate in this patient population (Beers Criteria: Quality of evidence - varies based on comorbidity; Strength of recommendation - varies based on comorbidity).

Dosage Forms Excipient information presented when available (limited, particularly for generics); consult specific product labeling. [DSC] = Discontinued product

Injection, solution, as sulfate: 0.05 mg/mL (5 mL); 0.1 mg/mL (5 mL, 10 mL); 0.4 mg/mL (20 mL)

AtroPen®: 0.25 mg/0.3 mL (0.3 mL); 0.5 mg/0.7 mL (0.7 mL); 1 mg/0.7 mL (0.7 mL); 2 mg/0.7 mL (0.7 mL)

Injection, solution, as sulfate [preservative free]: 0.4 mg/0.5 mL (0.5 mL [DSC]); 0.4 mg/mL (1 mL); 1 mg/mL (1 mL)
Ointment, ophthalmic, as sulfate: 1% (3.5 g)
Solution, ophthalmic, as sulfate [drops]: 1% (2 mL, 5 mL, 15 mL)
  Atropine Care™: 1% (2 mL, 5 mL, 15 mL) [contains benzalkonium chloride]
  Isopto® Atropine: 1% (5 mL, 15 mL) [contains benzalkonium chloride]

◆ **Atropine and Diphenoxylate** see Diphenoxylate and Atropine on page 560
◆ **Atropine Care™** see Atropine on page 166
◆ **Atropine, Hyoscyamine, Phenobarbital, and Scopolamine** see Hyoscyamine, Atropine, Scopolamine, and Phenobarbital on page 963
◆ **Atropine Sulfate** see Atropine on page 166
◆ **Atrovent®** see Ipratropium (Nasal) on page 1036
◆ **Atrovent® HFA** see Ipratropium (Oral Inhalation) on page 1035
◆ **Augmentin®** see Amoxicillin and Clavulanate on page 115
◆ **Augmentin XR®** see Amoxicillin and Clavulanate on page 115

Auranofin (au RANE oh fin)

Medication Safety Issues
Sound-alike/look-alike issues:
Ridaura® may be confused with Cardura®
Brand Names: U.S. Ridaura®
Brand Names: Canada Ridaura®
Generic Availability (U.S.) No
Pharmacologic Category Gold Compound
Use Management of active stage classic or definite rheumatoid arthritis in patients who do not respond to or tolerate other agents
Contraindications History of severe toxicity to gold compounds including anaphylaxis, bone marrow aplasia, severe hematologic disorders, exfoliative dermatitis, necrotizing enterocolitis, or pulmonary fibrosis.
Warnings/Precautions [U.S. Boxed Warning]: May cause significant toxicity involving dermatologic, gastrointestinal, hematologic, pulmonary, renal and hepatic systems; patient education is required. Dermatitis and lesions of the mucous membranes are common and may be serious; pruritus may precede the early development of a skin reaction. Signs of toxicity include hematologic depression (depressed hemoglobin, leukocytes, granulocytes, or platelets); stomatitis, persistent diarrhea, enterocolitis, cholestatic jaundice; proteinuria (nephritic syndrome), and interstitial pulmonary fibrosis. Avoid use in patients with prior inflammatory bowel disease.

Concurrent use of gold products with ACE inhibitors may increase the risk of nitritoid reactions. Laboratory monitoring should be completed prior to each new prescription. Frequent monitoring of patients for signs and symptoms of toxicity will prevent serious adverse reactions.
Adverse Reactions (Reflective of adult population; not specific for elderly)
>10%:
  Dermatologic: Rash (24%), pruritus (17%)
  Gastrointestinal: Diarrhea/loose stools (47%), abdominal pain (14%), stomatitis (13%)
1% to 10%:
  Dermatologic: Alopecia (1% to 3%), urticaria (1% to 3%)
  Gastrointestinal: Nausea (10%), vomiting (10%), anorexia (3% to 9%), dyspepsia (3% to 9%), flatulence (3% to 9%), constipation (1% to 3%), dysgeusia (1% to 3%), glossitis (1% to 3%)
  Hematologic: Anemia (1% to 3%), eosinophilia (1% to 3%), leukopenia (1% to 3%), thrombocytopenia (1% to 3%)
  Hepatic: Transaminases increased (1% to 3%)
  Ocular: Conjunctivitis (3% to 9%)
  Renal: Proteinuria (3% to 9%), hematuria (1% to 3%)
Drug Interactions
Metabolism/Transport Effects None known.
Avoid Concomitant Use There are no known interactions where it is recommended to avoid concomitant use.
Increased Effect/Toxicity There are no known significant interactions involving an increase in effect.
Decreased Effect There are no known significant interactions involving a decrease in effect.
Stability Store at 15°C to 30°C (59°F to 86°F). Protect from light.

Mechanism of Action The exact mechanism of action of gold is unknown; gold is taken up by macrophages which results in inhibition of phagocytosis and lysosomal membrane stabilization; other actions observed are decreased serum rheumatoid factor and alterations in immunoglobulins. Additionally, complement activation is decreased, prostaglandin synthesis is inhibited, and lysosomal enzyme activity is decreased.

Pharmacodynamics/Kinetics

Onset of action: Delayed; therapeutic response may require as long as 3-4 months

Duration: Prolonged

Absorption: Oral: ~25% gold in dose is absorbed

Protein binding: 60%

Half-life elimination (single or multiple dose dependent): 21-31 days

Time to peak, serum: ~2 hours

Excretion: Urine (~60% of absorbed gold); remainder in feces

Dosage

Geriatric & Adult Rheumatoid arthritis: Oral: Initial: 6 mg/day in 1-2 divided doses; after 6 months may be increased to 9 mg/day in 3 divided doses; discontinue therapy if no response after 3 months at 9 mg/day

Note: Signs of clinical improvement may not be evident until after 3 months of therapy.

Renal Impairment There are no dosage adjustments provided in the manufacturer's labeling. The following guidelines have been used by some clinicians (Aronoff, 2007):

Cl_{cr} 50-80 mL/minute: Administer 50% of dose.

Cl_{cr} <50 mL/minute: Avoid use.

Monitoring Parameters Patients should have baseline CBC with differential, platelet count, renal function tests, liver function tests, and urinalysis; CBC with differential, platelet count and urinalysis should also be monitored monthly during therapy. Skin and oral mucosa should be inspected for skin rash, bruising or oral ulceration/stomatitis. Specific questioning for symptoms such as pruritus, rash, stomatitis or metallic taste should be included. Dosing should be withheld in patients with significant gastrointestinal, renal, dermatologic, or hematologic effects (platelet count falls to <100,000/mm^3, WBC <4000, granulocytes <1500/mm^3

Reference Range Gold: Normal: 0-0.1 mcg/mL (SI: 0-0.0064 micromole/L); Therapeutic: 1-3 mcg/mL (SI: 0.06-0.18 micromole/L); Urine: <0.1 mcg/24 hours

Test Interactions May enhance the response to a tuberculin skin test

Special Geriatric Considerations Tolerance to gold decreases with advanced age; use cautiously only after traditional therapy and other disease modifying antirheumatic drugs (DMARDs) have been attempted.

Dosage Forms Excipient information presented when available (limited, particularly for generics); consult specific product labeling.

Capsule, oral:

Ridaura®: 3 mg [gold 29%]

◆ **Auraphene B® [OTC]** *see* Carbamide Peroxide *on page 291*
◆ **Auro® [OTC]** *see* Carbamide Peroxide *on page 291*
◆ **Auvi-Q™** *see* EPINEPHrine (Systemic, Oral Inhalation) *on page 645*
◆ **Avalide®** *see* Irbesartan and Hydrochlorothiazide *on page 1039*

Avanafil (a VAN a fil)

Medication Safety Issues

Sound-alike/look-alike issues:

Avanafil may be confused with sildenafil, tadalafil, vardenafil

Index Terms Stendra™

Generic Availability (U.S.) No

Pharmacologic Category Phosphodiesterase-5 Enzyme Inhibitor

Use Treatment of erectile dysfunction (ED)

Contraindications Hypersensitivity to avanafil or any component of the formulation; concurrent (regular or intermittent) use of organic nitrates in any form (eg, nitroglycerin, isosorbide dinitrate)

Warnings/Precautions There is a degree of cardiac risk associated with sexual activity; therefore, physicians may wish to consider the patient's cardiovascular status prior to initiating any treatment for erectile dysfunction. Use caution in patients with anatomical deformation of the penis (angulation, cavernosal fibrosis, or Peyronie's disease) and in patients who have conditions which may predispose them to priapism (sickle cell anemia, multiple myeloma, leukemia). Instruct patients to seek immediate medical attention if erection persists >4 hours.

Use is not recommended in patients with hypotension (<90/50 mm Hg); uncontrolled hypertension (>170/100 mm Hg); unstable angina or angina during intercourse; life-threatening arrhythmias, stroke, or MI within the last 6 months; cardiac failure or coronary artery disease causing unstable angina. Safety and efficacy have not been studied in these patients. Use caution in patients with left ventricular outflow obstruction (eg, aortic stenosis). Use caution with alpha-blockers; dosage adjustment is needed. Avoid or limit concurrent substantial alcohol consumption as this may increase the risk of symptomatic hypotension.

Rare cases of nonarteritic ischemic optic neuropathy (NAION) have been reported; risk may be increased with history of vision loss. Other risk factors for NAION include heart disease, diabetes, hypertension, smoking, age >50 years, or history of certain eye problems. Sudden decrease or loss of hearing has been reported rarely; hearing changes may be accompanied by tinnitus and dizziness.

Safety and efficacy have not been studied in patients with the following conditions, therefore, use in these patients is not recommended at this time: Severe hepatic impairment (Child-Pugh class C); severe renal impairment; end-stage renal disease requiring dialysis; retinitis pigmentosa or other degenerative retinal disorders. The safety and efficacy of avanafil with other treatments for erectile dysfunction have not been studied and are not recommended as combination therapy. Concomitant use with all forms of nitrates is contraindicated. If nitrate administration is medically necessary, at least 12 hours should elapse from time of last dose of avanafil to time of nitrate administration; administer only under close medical supervision with appropriate hemodynamic monitoring. Avoid use in patients taking strong CYP3A4 inhibitors (see Drug Interactions); dosage reduction recommended in patients taking moderate CYP3A4 inhibitors. Potential underlying causes of erectile dysfunction should be evaluated prior to treatment.

Adverse Reactions (Reflective of adult population; not specific for elderly)
>10%: Central nervous system: Headache (5% to 12%)
2% to 10%:
Cardiovascular: Flushing (3% to 10%), ECG abnormal (1% to 3%)
Central nervous system: Dizziness (1% to 2%)
Neuromuscular & skeletal: Back pain (1% to 3%)
Respiratory: Nasopharyngitis (1% to 5%), nasal congestion (1% to 3%), upper respiratory infection (1% to 3%)

Drug Interactions
Metabolism/Transport Effects Substrate of CYP3A4 (major); **Note:** Assignment of Major/Minor substrate status based on clinically relevant drug interaction potential

Avoid Concomitant Use
Avoid concomitant use of Avanafil with any of the following: Alprostadil; Amyl Nitrite; CYP3A4 Inhibitors (Strong); Itraconazole; Ketoconazole (Systemic); Phosphodiesterase 5 Inhibitors; Posaconazole; Vasodilators (Organic Nitrates); Voriconazole

Increased Effect/Toxicity
Avanafil may increase the levels/effects of: Alpha1-Blockers; Alprostadil; Amyl Nitrite; Antihypertensives; Bosentan; Phosphodiesterase 5 Inhibitors; Vasodilators (Organic Nitrates)

The levels/effects of Avanafil may be increased by: Alcohol (Ethyl); CYP3A4 Inhibitors (Moderate); CYP3A4 Inhibitors (Strong); Dasatinib; Fluconazole; Itraconazole; Ivacaftor; Ketoconazole (Systemic); Mifepristone; Posaconazole; Sapropterin; Voriconazole

Decreased Effect
The levels/effects of Avanafil may be decreased by: Bosentan; CYP3A4 Inducers (Strong); Deferasirox; Etravirine; Herbs (CYP3A4 Inducers); Tocilizumab

Ethanol/Nutrition/Herb Interactions Ethanol: Substantial consumption of ethanol may increase the risk of hypotension and orthostasis. Lower ethanol consumption has not been associated with significant changes in blood pressure or increase in orthostatic symptoms. Management: Avoid or limit ethanol consumption.
Food: Avoid grapefruit juice.

Stability Store at 20°C to 25°C (68°F to 77°F); excursions permitted to 30°C (86°F). Protect from light.

Mechanism of Action Does not directly cause penile erections, but affects the response to sexual stimulation. The physiologic mechanism of erection of the penis involves release of nitric oxide (NO) in the corpus cavernosum during sexual stimulation. NO then activates the enzyme guanylate cyclase, which results in increased levels of cyclic guanosine monophosphate (cGMP), producing smooth muscle relaxation and inflow of blood to the corpus cavernosum. Avanafil enhances the effect of NO by inhibiting phosphodiesterase type 5 (PDE-5), which is responsible for degradation of cGMP in the corpus cavernosum; when sexual stimulation causes local release of NO, inhibition of PDE-5 by avanafil causes increased levels of cGMP in the corpus cavernosum, resulting in smooth muscle relaxation and inflow of blood to the corpus cavernosum; at recommended doses, it has no effect in the absence of sexual stimulation.

Pharmacodynamics/Kinetics

Absorption: Rapid

Protein binding: ~99%

Metabolism: Hepatic via CYP3A4 (major), CYP2C (minor); forms metabolites (active and inactive)

Half-life elimination: Terminal: ~5 hours

Time to peak, plasma: 30-45 minutes (fasting); 1.12-1.25 hours (high-fat meal)

Excretion: Feces (~62%); urine (~21%)

Dosage

Geriatric Elderly ≥65 years: Refer to adult dosing.

Adult Erectile dysfunction: Oral: Initial: 100 mg 30 minutes prior to sexual activity; to be given as one single dose and not given more than once daily; dosing range: 50-200 mg once daily

Dosing adjustment with concomitant medications:

Alpha-blocker (dose should be stable at time of avanafil initiation): Initial avanafil dose: 50 mg every 24 hours

Moderate CYP34A inhibitors (including aprepitant, diltiazem, erythromycin, fluconazole, fosamprenavir, verapamil): Maximum avanafil dose: 50 mg every 24 hours

Renal Impairment

Cl_{cr} ≥30 mL/minute: No dosage adjustment necessary.

Cl_{cr} <30 mL/minute: Has not been studied; use is not recommended by the manufacturer.

ESRD requiring hemodialysis: Has not been studied; use is not recommended by the manufacturer.

Hepatic Impairment

Mild-to-moderate hepatic impairment (Child-Pugh class A or B): No adjustment required.

Severe hepatic impairment (Child-Pugh class C): Has not been studied; use is not recommended by the manufacturer.

Administration May be administered with or without food, 30 minutes prior to sexual activity.

Monitoring Parameters Monitor for response, adverse reactions, blood pressure, and heart rate.

Product Availability Stendra™: FDA approved April 2012; availability currently undetermined.

AzaTHIOprine (ay za THYE oh preen)

Medication Safety Issues

Sound-alike/look-alike issues:

AzaTHIOprine may be confused with azaCITIDine, azidothymidine, azithromycin, Azulfidine®

Imuran® may be confused with Elmiron®, Enduron, Imdur®, Inderal®, Tenormin®

Other safety concerns:

Azathioprine is metabolized to mercaptopurine; concurrent use of these commercially-available products has resulted in profound myelosuppression.

Brand Names: U.S. Azasan®; Imuran®

Brand Names: Canada Apo-Azathioprine®; Imuran®; Mylan-Azathioprine; Teva-Azathioprine

Index Terms Azathioprine Sodium

Generic Availability (U.S.) Yes

Pharmacologic Category Immunosuppressant Agent

Use Adjunctive therapy in prevention of rejection of kidney transplants; management of active rheumatoid arthritis (RA)

Unlabeled Use Adjunct in prevention of rejection of solid organ (nonrenal) transplants; remission maintenance or reduction of steroid use in Crohn's disease (CD) and in ulcerative colitis (UC); dermatomyositis/polymyositis; erythema multiforme; pemphigus vulgaris, lupus nephritis, chronic refractory immune (idiopathic) thrombocytopenic purpura, relapsed/remitting multiple sclerosis

Contraindications Hypersensitivity to azathioprine or any component of the formulation; patients with rheumatoid arthritis and a history of treatment with alkylating agents (eg, cyclophosphamide, chlorambucil, melphalan) may have a prohibitive risk of neoplasia with azathioprine treatment

Warnings/Precautions [U.S. Boxed Warning]: Immunosuppressive agents, including azathioprine, are associated with the development of lymphoma and other malignancies, especially of the skin. Hepatosplenic T-Cell Lymphoma (HSTCL), a rare white blood cell cancer that is usually fatal, has predominantly occurred in adolescents and young adults treated for Crohn's disease or ulcerative colitis and receiving TNF blockers (eg, adalimumab, certolizumab pegol, etanercept, golimumab), azathioprine, and/or mercaptopurine. Most cases have occurred in patients treated with a combination of immunosuppressant agents, although there have been reports of HSTCL in patients receiving azathioprine or mercaptopurine monotherapy. Renal transplant patients are also at increased risk for malignancy (eg, skin cancer, lymphoma); limit sun and ultraviolet light exposure and use appropriate sun protection. Dose-related hematologic toxicities (leukopenia, thrombocytopenia, and anemias, including macrocytic anemia, or pancytopenia) may occur; delayed toxicities may also occur. May be more severe with renal transplants undergoing rejection; dosage modification for hematologic toxicity may be necessary. Chronic immunosuppression increases the risk of serious infections; may require dosage reduction. Use with caution in patients with liver disease or renal impairment; monitor hematologic function closely. Azathioprine is metabolized to mercaptopurine; concomitant use may result in profound myelosuppression and should be avoided. Patients with genetic deficiency of thiopurine methyltransferase (TPMT) or concurrent therapy with drugs which may inhibit TPMT may be sensitive to myelosuppressive effects. Patients with intermediate TPMT activity may be at risk for increased myelosuppression; those with low or absent TPMT activity are at risk for developing severe myelotoxicity. TPMT genotyping or phenotyping may assist in identifying patients at risk for developing toxicity. Consider TPMT testing in patients with abnormally low CBC unresponsive to dose reduction. TPMT testing does not substitute for CBC monitoring. Xanthine oxidase inhibitors may increase risk for hematologic toxicity; reduce azathioprine dose when used concurrently with allopurinol; patients with low or absent TPMT activity may require further dose reductions or discontinuation.

Hepatotoxicity (transaminase, bilirubin, and alkaline phosphatase elevations) may occur, usually in renal transplant patients and generally within 6 months of transplant; normally reversible with discontinuation; monitor liver function periodically. Rarely, hepatic sinusoidal obstruction syndrome (SOS; formerly called veno-occlusive disease) has been reported; discontinue if hepatic SOS is suspected. Severe nausea, vomiting, diarrhea, rash, fever, malaise, myalgia, hypotension, and liver enzyme abnormalities may occur within the first several weeks of treatment and are generally reversible upon discontinuation. **[U.S. Boxed Warning]: Should be prescribed by physicians familiar with the risks, including hematologic toxicities and mutagenic potential.** Immune response to vaccines may be diminished. Hazardous agent - use appropriate precautions for handling and disposal.

Adverse Reactions (Reflective of adult population; not specific for elderly) Frequency not always defined; dependent upon dose, duration, indication, and concomitant therapy.

Central nervous system: Fever, malaise

Gastrointestinal: Nausea/vomiting (RA 12%), diarrhea

Hematologic: Leukopenia (renal transplant >50%; RA 28%), thrombocytopenia

Hepatic: Alkaline phosphatase increased, bilirubin increased, hepatotoxicity, transaminases increased

Neuromuscular & skeletal: Myalgia

Miscellaneous: Infection (renal transplant 20%; RA <1%; includes bacterial, fungal, protozoal, viral), neoplasia (renal transplant 3% [other than lymphoma], 0.5% [lymphoma])

Drug Interactions

Metabolism/Transport Effects None known.

Avoid Concomitant Use

Avoid concomitant use of AzaTHIOprine with any of the following: BCG; Febuxostat; Mercaptopurine; Natalizumab; Pimecrolimus; Tacrolimus (Topical)

Increased Effect/Toxicity

AzaTHIOprine may increase the levels/effects of: Leflunomide; Mercaptopurine; Natalizumab; Vaccines (Live)

The levels/effects of AzaTHIOprine may be increased by: 5-ASA Derivatives; ACE Inhibitors; Allopurinol; Denosumab; Febuxostat; Pimecrolimus; Ribavirin; Roflumilast; Sulfamethoxazole; Tacrolimus (Topical); Trastuzumab; Trimethoprim

Decreased Effect

AzaTHIOprine may decrease the levels/effects of: BCG; Coccidioidin Skin Test; Sipuleucel-T; Vaccines (Inactivated); Vitamin K Antagonists

The levels/effects of AzaTHIOprine may be decreased by: Echinacea

Ethanol/Nutrition/Herb Interactions Herb/Nutraceutical: Avoid cat's claw, echinacea (have immunostimulant properties).

Stability

Tablet: Store at room temperature of 15°C to 25°C (59°F to 77°F). Protect from light and moisture.

Powder for injection: Store intact vials at room temperature of 15°C to 25°C (59°F to 77°F). Protect from light. Reconstitute each vial with 10 mL sterile water for injection; may further dilute for infusion (in D_5W, 1/2NS, or NS). Reconstituted solution should be used within 24 hours; solutions diluted in D_5W, 1/2NS, or NS for infusion are stable at room temperature or refrigerated for up to 16 days (Johnson, 1981); however, the manufacturer recommends use within 24 hours of reconstitution. Use appropriate precautions for handling and disposal.

Mechanism of Action Azathioprine is an imidazolyl derivative of mercaptopurine; antagonizes purine metabolism and may inhibit synthesis of DNA, RNA, and proteins; may also interfere with cellular metabolism and inhibit mitosis. The 6-thioguanine nucleotides appear to mediate the majority of azathioprine's immunosuppressive and toxic effects.

Pharmacodynamics/Kinetics

Absorption: Oral: Well absorbed

Protein binding: ~30%

Metabolism: Hepatic, to 6-mercaptopurine (6-MP), possibly by glutathione S-transferase (GST). Further metabolism of 6-MP (in the liver and GI tract), via three major pathways: Hypoxanthine guanine phosphoribosyltransferase (to 6-thioguanine-nucleotides, or 6-TGN), xanthine oxidase (to 6-thiouric acid), and thiopurine methyltransferase (TPMT), which forms 6-methylmercaptopurine (6-MMP).

Half-life elimination: Parent drug: 12 minutes; mercaptopurine: 0.7-3 hours; End-stage renal disease: Slightly prolonged

Time to peak, plasma: 1-2 hours (including metabolites)

Excretion: Urine (primarily as metabolites)

Dosage

Geriatric & Adult Note: Patients with intermediate TPMT activity may be at risk for increased myelosuppression; those with low or absent TPMT activity receiving conventional azathioprine doses are at risk for developing severe, life-threatening myelotoxicity. Dosage reductions are recommended for patients with reduced TPMT activity.

I.V. dose is equivalent to oral dose (dosing should be transitioned from I.V. to oral as soon as tolerated):

Renal transplantation (treatment usually started the day of transplant, however, has been initiated [rarely] 1-3 days prior to transplant): Oral, I.V.: Initial: 3-5 mg/kg/day usually given as a single daily dose, then 1-3 mg/kg/day maintenance

Rheumatoid arthritis: Oral:

Initial: 1 mg/kg/day (50-100 mg) given once daily or divided twice daily for 6-8 weeks; may increase by 0.5 mg/kg every 4 weeks until response or up to 2.5 mg/kg/day; an adequate trial should be a minimum of 12 weeks

Maintenance dose: Reduce dose by 0.5 mg/kg (~25 mg daily) every 4 weeks until lowest effective dose is reached; optimum duration of therapy not specified; may be discontinued abruptly

Crohn's disease, remission maintenance or reduction of steroid use (unlabeled use): Oral: 2-3 mg/kg/day (Lichtenstein, 2009)

Dermatomyositis/polymyositis, adjunctive management (unlabeled use): Oral: 50 mg/day in conjunction with prednisone; increase by 50 mg/week to total dose of 2-3 mg/kg/day (Briemberg, 2003); **Note:** Onset of beneficial effects may take 3-6 months; however, may be preferred over methotrexate in patients with pulmonary or hepatic toxicity.

Immune (idiopathic) thrombocytopenic purpura, chronic refractory (unlabeled use): Oral: Maintenance: 100-200 mg/day (Boruchov, 2007)

Lupus nephritis (unlabeled use): Oral: Initial: 2 mg/kg/day; may reduce to 1.5 mg/kg/day after 1 month (if proteinuria <1 g/day and serum creatinine stable) (Moroni, 2006) **or** target dose: 2 mg/kg/day (Houssiau, 2010)

Ulcerative colitis, remission maintenance or reduction of steroid use (unlabeled use): Oral: 1.5-2.5 mg/kg/day (Kornbluth, 2010)

Dosage adjustment for concomitant use with allopurinol: Reduce azathioprine dose to one-third or one-fourth the usual dose when used concurrently with allopurinol. Patients with low or absent TPMT activity may require further dose reductions or discontinuation.

Renal Impairment Although dosage reductions are recommended, specific guidelines are not available in the FDA-approved labeling; the following guidelines have been used by some clinicians (Aronoff, 2007):

Cl_{cr} >50 mL/minute: No adjustment recommended.

Cl_{cr} 10-50 mL/minute: Administer 75% of normal dose.

Cl_{cr} <10 mL/minute: Administer 50% of normal dose.

Hemodialysis (dialyzable; ~45% removed in 8 hours): Supplement: 0.25 mg/kg

CAPD: Unknown

CRRT: Administer 75% of normal dose

Administration

I.V.: Azathioprine can be administered IVP over 5 minutes at a concentration not to exceed 10 mg/mL **or** azathioprine can be further diluted with normal saline, $^1/_2$NS, or D_5W and administered by intermittent infusion usually over 30-60 minutes or by an extended infusion up to 8 hours.

Oral: Administering tablets after meals or in divided doses may decrease adverse GI events.

Monitoring Parameters CBC with differential and platelets (weekly during first month, twice monthly for months 2 and 3, then monthly; monitor more frequently with dosage modifications), total bilirubin, liver function tests, creatinine clearance, TPMT genotyping or phenotyping (consider TPMT testing in patients with abnormally low CBC unresponsive to dose reduction); monitor for symptoms of infection

For use as immunomodulatory therapy in CD or UC, monitor CBC with differential weekly for 1 month, then biweekly for 1 month, followed by monitoring every 1-2 months throughout the course of therapy; monitor more frequently if symptomatic. LFTs should be assessed every 3 months. Monitor for signs/symptoms of malignancy (eg, splenomegaly, hepatomegaly, abdominal pain, persistent fever, night sweats, weight loss).

Test Interactions TPMT phenotyping results will not be accurate following recent blood transfusions.

Special Geriatric Considerations Toxicity to immunosuppressives is increased in elderly. Start with lowest recommended adult doses. Signs of infection, such as fever and WBC rise, may not occur. Lethargy and confusion may be more prominent signs of infection. In the elderly, adjust dose to creatinine clearance.

Dosage Forms Excipient information presented when available (limited, particularly for generics); consult specific product labeling.

Injection, powder for reconstitution: 100 mg

Tablet, oral: 50 mg

Azasan®: 75 mg, 100 mg [scored]

Imuran®: 50 mg [scored]

◆ **Azathioprine Sodium** see AzaTHIOprine on page 174

◆ **AZD6140** see Ticagrelor on page 1888

Azelastine (Nasal) (a ZEL as teen)

Medication Safety Issues
Sound-alike/look-alike issues:
Astelin® may be confused with Astepro®
Brand Names: U.S. Astelin®; Astepro®
Brand Names: Canada Astelin®
Index Terms Azelastine Hydrochloride
Generic Availability (U.S.) Yes
Pharmacologic Category Histamine H_1 Antagonist; Histamine H_1 Antagonist, Second Generation
Use Treatment of the symptoms of seasonal allergic rhinitis such as rhinorrhea, sneezing, and nasal pruritus; treatment of the symptoms of vasomotor rhinitis
Dosage
Geriatric & Adult
Seasonal allergic rhinitis (Astelin®, Astepro®): Intranasal: 1-2 sprays each nostril twice daily.
Vasomotor rhinitis (Astelin®): Intranasal: 2 sprays each nostril twice daily.
Special Geriatric Considerations Evaluate the patient's or caregiver's ability to safely administer the correct dose of nasal medication. Only a small number of older subjects were included in premarketing trials. In those patients, side effects were no different than in younger patients.
Dosage Forms Excipient information presented when available (limited, particularly for generics); consult specific product labeling.
Solution, intranasal, as hydrochloride [spray]: 0.1% [137 mcg/spray] (30 mL)
Astelin®: 0.1% [137 mcg/spray] (30 mL) [contains benzalkonium chloride; 200 metered sprays]
Astepro®: 0.15% [205.5 mcg/spray] (30 mL) [contains benzalkonium chloride; 200 metered sprays]

Azelastine (Ophthalmic) (a ZEL as teen)

Medication Safety Issues
Sound-alike/look-alike issues:
Optivar® may be confused with Optiray®, Optive™
International issues:
Optivar [U.S.] may be confused with Opthavir brand name for acyclovir [Mexico]
Brand Names: U.S. Optivar®
Index Terms Azelastine Hydrochloride
Generic Availability (U.S.) Yes
Pharmacologic Category Histamine H_1 Antagonist; Histamine H_1 Antagonist, Second Generation
Use Treatment of itching of the eye associated with seasonal allergic conjunctivitis
Dosage
Geriatric & Adult Seasonal allergic conjunctivitis: Ophthalmic: Instill 1 drop into affected eye(s) twice daily.
Special Geriatric Considerations Evaluate the patient's or caregiver's ability to safely administer the correct dose of ophthalmic medication.
Dosage Forms Excipient information presented when available (limited, particularly for generics); consult specific product labeling.
Solution, ophthalmic, as hydrochloride [drops]: 0.05% (6 mL)
Optivar®: 0.05% (6 mL) [contains benzalkonium chloride]

◆ **Azelastine Hydrochloride** see Azelastine (Nasal) on page 177
◆ **Azelastine Hydrochloride** see Azelastine (Ophthalmic) on page 177
◆ **Azilect®** see Rasagiline on page 1680

Azilsartan (ay zil SAR tan)

Related Information
Angiotensin Agents on page 2093
Brand Names: U.S. edarbi™
Index Terms Azilsartan Medoxomil; AZL-M
Generic Availability (U.S.) No
Pharmacologic Category Angiotensin II Receptor Blocker

◀ **Use** Treatment of hypertension; may be used alone or in combination with other antihypertensives

Contraindications There are no contraindications listed in manufacturer's labeling.

Warnings/Precautions Angiotensin II receptor blockers may cause hyperkalemia; avoid potassium supplementation unless specifically required by healthcare provider. Avoid use or use a smaller dose in patients who are volume depleted; correct depletion first. May be associated with deterioration of renal function and/or increases in serum creatinine, particularly in patients with low renal blood flow (eg, renal artery stenosis, heart failure, volume depletion) whose glomerular filtration rate (GFR) is dependent on efferent arteriolar vasoconstriction by angiotensin II. Use with caution in unstented unilateral/bilateral renal artery stenosis. When unstented bilateral renal artery stenosis is present, use is generally avoided due to the elevated risk of deterioration in renal function unless possible benefits outweigh risks. Use with caution in pre-existing renal insufficiency; significant aortic/mitral stenosis. Concurrent use with ACE inhibitors may increase the risk of clinically-significant adverse events (eg, renal dysfunction, hyperkalemia).

Adverse Reactions (Reflective of adult population; not specific for elderly)
Cardiovascular: Hypotension, orthostatic hypotension
Central nervous system: Dizziness, fatigue
Gastrointestinal: Diarrhea (2%), nausea
Hematologic: Hemoglobin decreased, hematocrit decreased, leukopenia (rare), RBC decreased, thrombocytopenia (rare)
Neuromuscular & skeletal: Muscle spasm, weakness
Renal: Serum creatinine increased
Respiratory: Cough

Drug Interactions

Metabolism/Transport Effects Substrate of CYP2C9 (minor); **Note:** Assignment of Major/Minor substrate status based on clinically relevant drug interaction potential

Avoid Concomitant Use There are no known interactions where it is recommended to avoid concomitant use.

Increased Effect/Toxicity
Azilsartan may increase the levels/effects of: ACE Inhibitors; Amifostine; Antihypertensives; Hypotensive Agents; Lithium; Nonsteroidal Anti-Inflammatory Agents; Potassium-Sparing Diuretics; RiTUXimab; Sodium Phosphates

The levels/effects of Azilsartan may be increased by: Alfuzosin; Aliskiren; Diazoxide; Eplerenone; Herbs (Hypotensive Properties); MAO Inhibitors; Pentoxifylline; Phosphodiesterase 5 Inhibitors; Potassium Salts; Prostacyclin Analogues; Tolvaptan; Trimethoprim

Decreased Effect
The levels/effects of Azilsartan may be decreased by: Herbs (Hypertensive Properties); Methylphenidate; Nonsteroidal Anti-Inflammatory Agents; Rifamycin Derivatives; Yohimbine

Ethanol/Nutrition/Herb Interactions Herb/Nutraceutical: Avoid ephedra, yohimbe, ginseng (may worsen hypertension). Avoid garlic (may have increased antihypertensive effect).

Stability Store at 25°C (77°F); excursions permitted to 15°C to 30°C (59°F to 86°F). Protect from moisture and light. Dispense and store in original container.

Mechanism of Action Angiotensin II (which is formed by enzymatic conversion from angiotensin I) is the primary pressor agent of the renin-angiotensin system. Effects of angiotensin II include vasoconstriction, stimulation of aldosterone synthesis/release, cardiac stimulation, and renal sodium reabsorption. Azilsartan inhibits angiotensin II's vasoconstrictor and aldosterone-secreting effects by selectively blocking the binding of angiotensin II to the AT_1 receptor in vascular smooth muscle and adrenal gland tissues (azilsartan has a stronger affinity for the AT_1 receptor than the AT_2 receptor). The action is independent of the angiotensin II synthesis pathways. Azilsartan does not inhibit ACE (kininase II), therefore it does not affect the response to bradykinin (the clinical relevance of this is unknown) and does not bind to or inhibit other receptors or ion channels of importance in cardiovascular regulation.

Pharmacodynamics/Kinetics
Distribution: V_d: ~16 L
Protein binding: >99%; primarily to serum albumin
Metabolism: Gut: prodrug hydrolyzed to active metabolite; Hepatic: primarily via CYP2C9 to inactive metabolites
Bioavailability: ~60%
Half-life elimination: ~11 hours
Time to peak, serum: 1.5-3 hours
Excretion: Feces (~55%); urine (~42%, 15% as unchanged drug)
Clearance: 2.3 mL/minute

Dosage

Geriatric & Adult Hypertension: Oral: 80 mg once daily; consider initial dose of 40 mg once daily in patients with volume depletion (eg, patients receiving high-dose diuretics)

Renal Impairment No starting dosage adjustment is necessary; however, carefully monitor the patient.

Hepatic Impairment No starting dosage adjustment is necessary in patients with mild-to-moderate impairment; however, carefully monitor the patient. Not studied in patients with severe impairment.

Administration Administer without regard to food.

Monitoring Parameters Electrolytes, serum creatinine, BUN; blood pressure

Special Geriatric Considerations No dosage adjustment based on age is necessary with azilsartan. In clinical studies with this drug, 26% of the patients were elderly (≥65 years of age), with 5% of these being ≥75 years. Significant increases in serum creatinine was seen more often in those ≥75 years. No other differences in safety and efficacy were noted between elderly and younger adults. Recommend monitoring serum creatinine when employing this agent in the geriatric population.

Dosage Forms Excipient information presented when available (limited, particularly for generics); consult specific product labeling.

Tablet, oral, as medoxomil:
edarbi™: 40 mg, 80 mg

Azilsartan and Chlorthalidone (ay zil SAR tan & klor THAL i done)

Brand Names: U.S. edarbyclor™

Index Terms Azilsartan Medoxomil and Chlorthalidone; Chlorthalidone and Azilsartan

Generic Availability (U.S.) No

Pharmacologic Category Angiotensin II Receptor Blocker; Diuretic, Thiazide

Use Treatment of hypertension

Dosage

Geriatric & Adult Dose is individualized; combination product may be substituted for individual components in patients currently maintained on both agents separately or in patients not adequately controlled with monotherapy (using one of the agents or an agent within the same antihypertensive class). May also be used as initial therapy in patients who are likely to need >1 antihypertensive to control blood pressure.

Hypertension: Oral: *Initial therapy:* Azilsartan 40 mg/chlorthalidone 12.5 mg once daily; dose may be increased after 2-4 weeks of therapy to azilsartan 40 mg/chlorthalidone 25 mg once daily. Maximum recommended dose: Azilsartan 40 mg/day; chlorthalidone 25 mg/day

Renal Impairment

Mild-to-moderate renal impairment (eGFR 30-90 mL/minute/1.73 m^2): No dosage adjustment necessary.

Severe renal impairment (eGFR <30 mL/minute/1.73 m^2): Safety and effectiveness not established.

Hepatic Impairment

Mild-to-moderate hepatic impairment: No initial dosage adjustment necessary; monitor patient carefully.

Severe hepatic impairment: Safety and effectiveness not established; use with caution in patients with severe hepatic impairment.

Special Geriatric Considerations No dosage adjustment based on age is necessary with azilsartan and chlorthalidone. In clinical studies with this drug, 24% of the patients were elderly (≥65 years of age), with 5.7% of these being ≥75 years. No overall differences in safety and efficacy were noted between elderly and younger adults. Recommend monitoring renal function when employing this agent in the geriatric population.

Studies have found chlorthalidone to be effective in the treatment of isolated systolic hypertension in the elderly. The use of chlorthalidone as a step one medication reduced the incidence of stroke in the SHEP trial.

Dosage Forms Excipient information presented when available (limited, particularly for generics); consult specific product labeling.

Tablet, oral:
edarbyclor™: 40/12.5: Azilsartan medoxomil 40 mg and chlorthalidone 12.5 mg
edarbyclor™: 40/25: Azilsartan medoxomil 40 mg and chlorthalidone 25 mg

◆ **Azilsartan Medoxomil** *see* Azilsartan *on page 177*
◆ **Azilsartan Medoxomil and Chlorthalidone** *see* Azilsartan and Chlorthalidone *on page 179*

Azithromycin (Systemic) (az ith roe MYE sin)

Related Information
Antimicrobial Drugs of Choice *on page 2163*
Community-Acquired Pneumonia in Adults *on page 2171*
Prevention of Infective Endocarditis *on page 2175*

Medication Safety Issues
Sound-alike/look-alike issues:
Azithromycin may be confused with azathioprine, erythromycin
Zithromax® may be confused with Fosamax®, Zinacef®, Zovirax®

Brand Names: U.S. Zithromax®; Zithromax® TRI-PAK™; Zithromax® Z-PAK®; Zmax®

Brand Names: Canada Apo-Azithromycin®; Ava-Azithromycin; Azithromycin for Injection; CO Azithromycin; Dom-Azithromycin; GD-Azithromycin; Mylan-Azithromycin; Novo-Azithromycin; PHL-Azithromycin; PMS-Azithromycin; PRO-Azithromycin; ratio-Azithromycin; Riva-Azithromycin; Sandoz-Azithromycin; Zithromax®; Zmax SR™

Index Terms Azithromycin Dihydrate; Azithromycin Monohydrate; Z-Pak; Zithromax TRI-PAK™; Zithromax Z-PAK®

Generic Availability (U.S.) Yes: Excludes extended release microspheres

Pharmacologic Category Antibiotic, Macrolide

Use Oral, I.V.: Treatment of acute otitis media due to *H. influenzae, M. catarrhalis,* or *S. pneumoniae*; pharyngitis/tonsillitis due to *S. pyogenes*; treatment of mild-to-moderate upper and lower respiratory tract infections, infections of the skin and skin structure, community-acquired pneumonia, pelvic inflammatory disease (PID), sexually-transmitted diseases (urethritis/cervicitis), and genital ulcer disease (chancroid) due to susceptible strains of *Chlamydophila pneumoniae, C. trachomatis, M. catarrhalis, H. influenzae, S. aureus, S. pneumoniae, Mycoplasma genitalium, Mycoplasma pneumoniae,* and *C. psittaci*; acute bacterial exacerbations of chronic obstructive pulmonary disease (COPD) due to *H. influenzae, M. catarrhalis,* or *S. pneumoniae*; acute bacterial sinusitis; prevention, alone or in combination with rifabutin, of MAC in patients with advanced HIV infection; treatment, in combination with ethambutol, of disseminated MAC in patients with advanced HIV infection

Unlabeled Use Prophylaxis of infective endocarditis in patients who are allergic to penicillin and undergoing surgical or dental procedures; pertussis

Contraindications Hypersensitivity to azithromycin, other macrolide (eg, azalide or ketolide) antibiotics, or any component of the formulation; history of cholestatic jaundice/hepatic dysfunction associated with prior azithromycin use

Note: The manufacturer does not list concurrent use of pimozide as a contraindication; however, azithromycin is listed as a contraindication in the manufacturer's labeling for pimozide.

Warnings/Precautions Use with caution in patients with pre-existing liver disease; hepatocellular and/or cholestatic hepatitis, with or without jaundice, hepatic necrosis, failure and death have occurred. Discontinue immediately if symptoms of hepatitis occur (malaise, nausea, vomiting, abdominal colic, fever). Allergic reactions have been reported (rare); reappearance of allergic reaction may occur shortly after discontinuation without further azithromycin exposure. May mask or delay symptoms of incubating gonorrhea or syphilis, so appropriate culture and susceptibility tests should be performed prior to initiating azithromycin. Prolonged use may result in fungal or bacterial superinfection, including *C. difficile*-associated diarrhea (CDAD); CDAD has been observed >2 months postantibiotic treatment. Use caution with renal dysfunction. Prolongation of the QT_c interval has been reported with macrolide antibiotics; use caution in patients at risk of prolonged cardiac repolarization. Use with caution in patients with myasthenia gravis.

Oral suspensions (immediate release and extended release) are not interchangeable.

Adverse Reactions (Reflective of adult population; not specific for elderly)
>10%: Gastrointestinal: Diarrhea (4% to 9%; high single-dose regimens 12% to 14%), nausea (≤7%; high single-dose regimens 18%)
2% to 10%:
Dermatologic: Pruritus, rash
Gastrointestinal: Abdominal pain, anorexia, cramping, vomiting (especially with high single-dose regimens)
Genitourinary: Vaginitis
Local: (with I.V. administration): Injection site pain, inflammation

Drug Interactions
Metabolism/Transport Effects Substrate of CYP3A4 (minor); **Note:** Assignment of Major/Minor substrate status based on clinically relevant drug interaction potential; **Inhibits** CYP1A2 (weak)

Avoid Concomitant Use

Avoid concomitant use of Azithromycin (Systemic) with any of the following: BCG; Pimozide; QuiNINE; Terfenadine

Increased Effect/Toxicity

Azithromycin (Systemic) may increase the levels/effects of: Amiodarone; Cardiac Glycosides; CycloSPORINE; CycloSPORINE (Systemic); Highest Risk QTc-Prolonging Agents; Ivermectin; Ivermectin (Systemic); Moderate Risk QTc-Prolonging Agents; Pimozide; QuiNINE; Rivaroxaban; Tacrolimus; Tacrolimus (Systemic); Tacrolimus (Topical); Terfenadine; Vitamin K Antagonists

The levels/effects of Azithromycin (Systemic) may be increased by: Mifepristone; Nelfinavir

Decreased Effect

Azithromycin (Systemic) may decrease the levels/effects of: BCG; Typhoid Vaccine

The levels/effects of Azithromycin (Systemic) may be decreased by: Tocilizumab

Ethanol/Nutrition/Herb Interactions Food: Rate and extent of GI absorption may be altered depending upon the formulation. Azithromycin suspension, not tablet form, has significantly increased absorption (46%) with food.

Stability

Injection (Zithromax®): Store intact vials of injection at room temperature. Reconstitute the 500 mg vial with 4.8 mL of sterile water for injection and shake until all of the drug is dissolved. Each mL contains 100 mg azithromycin. Reconstituted solution is stable for 24 hours when stored below 30°C (86°F). Use of a standard syringe is recommended due to the vacuum in the vial (which may draw additional solution through an automated syringe).

The initial solution should be further diluted to a concentration of 1 mg/mL (500 mL) to 2 mg/mL (250 mL) in 0.9% sodium chloride, 5% dextrose in water, or lactated Ringer's. The diluted solution is stable for 24 hours at or below room temperature (30°C or 86°F) and for 7 days if stored under refrigeration (5°C or 41°F).

Suspension, immediate release (Zithromax®): Store dry powder below 30°C (86°F). Following reconstitution, store at 5°C to 30°C (41°F to 86°F).

Suspension, extended release (Zmax®): Store dry powder ≤30°C (86°F). Following reconstitution, store at 25°C (77°F); excursions permitted to 15°C to 30°C (59°F to 86°F); do not refrigerate or freeze. Should be consumed within 12 hours following reconstitution.

Tablet (Zithromax®): Store between 15°C to 30°C (59°F to 86°F).

Mechanism of Action Inhibits RNA-dependent protein synthesis at the chain elongation step; binds to the 50S ribosomal subunit resulting in blockage of transpeptidation

Pharmacodynamics/Kinetics

Absorption: Oral: Rapid

Distribution: Extensive tissue; distributes well into skin, lungs, sputum, tonsils, and cervix; penetration into CSF is poor; I.V.: 33.3 L/kg; Oral: 31.1 L/kg

Protein binding (concentration dependent): Oral, I.V.: 7% to 51%

Metabolism: Hepatic

Bioavailability: Oral: 38%, decreased by 17% with extended release suspension; variable effect with food (increased with immediate or delayed release oral suspension, unchanged with tablet)

Half-life elimination: Oral, I.V.: Terminal: Immediate release: 68-72 hours; Extended release: 59 hours

Time to peak, serum: Oral: Immediate release: 2-3 hours; Extended release: 5 hours

Excretion: Oral, I.V.: Biliary (major route); urine (6%)

Dosage

Geriatric & Adult Note: Extended release suspension (Zmax®) is not interchangeable with immediate release formulations. Use should be limited to approved indications. All doses are expressed as immediate release azithromycin unless otherwise specified.

Bacterial sinusitis: Oral: 500 mg/day for a total of 3 days
  Extended release suspension (Zmax®): 2 g as a single dose

Cat scratch disease (unlabeled use): Oral: >45.5 kg: 500 mg as a single dose, then 250 mg once daily for 4 days

Chancroid due to H. ducreyi: Oral: 1 g as a single dose (CDC, 2010)

C. trachomatis urethritis/cervicitis: Oral: 1 g as a single dose

Community-acquired pneumonia:
  Oral: 500 mg on day 1 followed by 250 mg once daily on days 2-5
  Extended release suspension (Zmax®): 2 g as a single dose
  I.V.: 500 mg as a single dose for at least 2 days, follow I.V. therapy by the oral route with a single daily dose of 500 mg to complete a 7- to 10-day course of therapy.

Disseminated *M. avium* complex disease in patients with advanced HIV infection: Oral:
Treatment: 600 mg/day in combination with ethambutol
Primary prophylaxis: 1200 mg once weekly (preferred), with or without rifabutin **or**
alternatively, 600 mg twice weekly (CDC, 2009)
Secondary prophylaxis: 500-600 mg/day in combination with ethambutol (CDC, 2009)

Gonococcal infection, uncomplicated (cervix, pharynx, rectum, urethra): Oral: 1 g as a
single dose (in combination with a cephalosporin) (CDC, 2010)
Note: Monotherapy with azithromycin (1 g and 2 g) have been associated with resistance
and/or treatment failure; use in combination with a cephalosporin (CDC, 2010). However,
a single 2 g azithromycin dose is still an FDA-approved dose for gonococcal urethritis
and cervicitis and also may be appropriate for treatment of a gonococcal infection in
pregnant women who cannot tolerate a cephalosporin (CDC, 2010).

Granuloma inguinale (donovanosis): Oral: 1 g once a week for at least 3 weeks (and until
lesions have healed) (CDC, 2010)

Mild-to-moderate respiratory tract, skin, and soft tissue infections: Oral: 500 mg in a
single loading dose on day 1 followed by 250 mg/day as a single dose on days 2-5
Alternative regimen: Bacterial exacerbation of COPD: 500 mg/day for a total of 3 days

***M. genitalium* infections** (confirmed cases in males or females or clinically significant
persistent urethritis in males): Oral: 1 g as a single dose or 500 mg on day 1, followed by
250 mg/day on days 2-5 (Manhart, 2011):
Note: Follow up patients on either regimen in 3-4 weeks for test of cure; consider
moxifloxacin for treatment failures (Manhart, 2011)

Pelvic inflammatory disease (PID): I.V.: 500 mg as a single dose for 1-2 days, follow I.V.
therapy by the oral route with a single daily dose of 250 mg to complete a 7-day course of
therapy.

Pertussis (CDC, 2005): Oral: 500 mg on day 1 followed by 250 mg/day on days 2-5
(maximum: 500 mg/day)

Prophylaxis against infective endocarditis (unlabeled use): Oral: 500 mg 30-60 minutes
prior to the procedure. **Note:** American Heart Association (AHA) guidelines now recommend prophylaxis only in patients undergoing invasive procedures and in whom underlying
cardiac conditions may predispose to a higher risk of adverse outcomes should infection
occur. As of April 2007, routine prophylaxis for GI/GU procedures is no longer recommended by the AHA.

Prophylaxis against sexually-transmitted diseases following sexual assault: Oral: 1 g
as a single dose (in combination with a cephalosporin and metronidazole) (CDC, 2010)

Renal Impairment Use caution in patients with GFR <10 mL/minute.
Poorly dialyzed; no supplemental dose or dosage adjustment necessary, including patients
on intermittent hemodialysis, peritoneal dialysis, or continuous renal replacement therapy
(eg, CVVHD).

Hepatic Impairment Use with caution due to potential for hepatotoxicity (rare). Specific
guidelines for dosing in hepatic impairment have not been established.

Administration
I.V.: Infusate concentration and rate of infusion for azithromycin for injection should be either
1 mg/mL over 3 hours or 2 mg/mL over 1 hour. Other medications should not be infused
simultaneously through the same I.V. line.
Oral: Immediate release suspension and tablet may be taken without regard to food; extended
release suspension should be taken on an empty stomach (at least 1 hour before or 2 hours
following a meal), within 12 hours of reconstitution.

Monitoring Parameters Liver function tests, CBC with differential

Pharmacotherapy Pearls Zithromax® tablets and immediate release suspension may be
interchanged (eg, two Zithromax® 250 mg tablets may be substituted for one Zithromax®
500 mg tablet or the tablets may be substituted with the immediate release suspension);
however, the extended release suspension (Zmax®) is not bioequivalent with Zithromax® and
therefore should not be interchanged.

Azithromycin is not recommended for treatment of early syphilis; the 23S rRNA mutation,
which has been associated with macrolide resistance, has been documented in multiple
geographic areas and in the MSM population. If a penicillin allergic patient cannot take
doxycycline (preferred alternative to penicillin), azithromycin (single 2 g dose orally) may be
considered but close clinical follow-up is needed (Ghanem, 2011).

Special Geriatric Considerations Dosage adjustment does not appear to be necessary in
the elderly. Considered to be one of the drugs of choice in the outpatient treatment of
community-acquired pneumonia in elderly.

Dosage Forms Excipient information presented when available (limited, particularly for
generics); consult specific product labeling. [DSC] = Discontinued product
Injection, powder for reconstitution, as dihydrate [strength expressed as base]: 500 mg [DSC]
Zithromax®: 500 mg [contains sodium 114 mg (4.96 mEq)/vial]
Injection, powder for reconstitution, as monohydrate [strength expressed as base]: 500 mg

Microspheres for suspension, extended release, oral, as dihydrate [strength expressed as base]:
Zmax®: 2 g/bottle (60 mL) [contains sodium 148 mg/bottle, sucrose 19 g/bottle; cherry-banana flavor; product contains azithromycin 27 mg/mL after constitution]
Powder for suspension, oral, as dihydrate [strength expressed as base]: 100 mg/5 mL (15 mL); 200 mg/5 mL (15 mL, 22.5 mL, 30 mL); 1 g/packet (3s)
Zithromax®: 100 mg/5 mL (15 mL) [contains sodium 3.7 mg/5 mL; cherry-crème de vanilla-banana flavor]
Zithromax®: 200 mg/5 mL (15 mL, 22.5 mL, 30 mL) [contains sodium 7.4 mg/5 mL; cherry-crème de vanilla-banana flavor]
Zithromax®: 1 g/packet (3s, 10s) [contains sodium 37 mg/packet; banana-cherry flavor]
Powder for suspension, oral, as monohydrate [strength expressed as base]: 100 mg/5 mL (15 mL); 200 mg/5 mL (15 mL, 22.5 mL, 30 mL)
Tablet, oral, as anhydrous: 250 mg, 500 mg, 600 mg
Tablet, oral, as dihydrate [strength expressed as base]: 250 mg, 500 mg, 600 mg
Zithromax®: 250 mg [contains sodium 0.9 mg/tablet]
Zithromax®: 500 mg [contains sodium 1.8 mg/tablet]
Zithromax®: 600 mg [contains sodium 2.1 mg/tablet]
Zithromax® TRI-PAK™: 500 mg [contains sodium 1.8 mg/tablet]
Zithromax® Z-PAK®: 250 mg [contains sodium 0.9 mg/tablet]
Tablet, oral, as monohydrate [strength expressed as base]: 250 mg, 500 mg, 600 mg

Azithromycin (Ophthalmic) (az ith roe MYE sin)

Medication Safety Issues
Sound-alike/look-alike issues:
Azithromycin may be confused with azathioprine, erythromycin
Brand Names: U.S. AzaSite®
Generic Availability (U.S.) No
Pharmacologic Category Antibiotic, Macrolide; Antibiotic, Ophthalmic
Use Treatment of bacterial conjunctivitis caused by susceptible microorganisms
Dosage
Geriatric & Adult Bacterial conjunctivitis: Ophthalmic: Instill 1 drop into affected eye(s) twice daily (8-12 hours apart) for 2 days, then 1 drop into affected eye(s) once daily for 5 days
Special Geriatric Considerations Evaluate the patient's or caregiver's ability to safely administer the correct dose of ophthalmic medication.
Dosage Forms Excipient information presented when available (limited, particularly for generics); consult specific product labeling.
Solution, ophthalmic [drops]:
AzaSite®: 1% (2.5 mL) [contains benzalkonium chloride]

♦ **Azithromycin Dihydrate** see Azithromycin (Systemic) on page 180
♦ **Azithromycin Monohydrate** see Azithromycin (Systemic) on page 180
♦ **AZL-M** see Azilsartan on page 177
♦ **Azo-Gesic™ [OTC]** see Phenazopyridine on page 1516
♦ **Azopt®** see Brinzolamide on page 221
♦ **Azor™** see Amlodipine and Olmesartan on page 106
♦ **AZO Standard® [OTC] [DSC]** see Phenazopyridine on page 1516
♦ **AZO Standard® Maximum Strength [OTC] [DSC]** see Phenazopyridine on page 1516
♦ **AZO Urinary Pain Relief™ [OTC]** see Phenazopyridine on page 1516
♦ **AZO Urinary Pain Relief™ Maximum Strength [OTC]** see Phenazopyridine on page 1516
♦ **Azthreonam** see Aztreonam on page 183

Aztreonam (AZ tree oh nam)

Related Information
Antimicrobial Drugs of Choice on page 2163
Community-Acquired Pneumonia in Adults on page 2171
Medication Safety Issues
Sound-alike/look-alike issues:
Aztreonam may be confused with azidothymidine
Brand Names: U.S. Azactam®; Cayston®
Brand Names: Canada Cayston®
Index Terms Azthreonam
Generic Availability (U.S.) Yes: Injection (powder for reconstitution)

Pharmacologic Category Antibiotic, Miscellaneous

Use

Injection: Treatment of patients with urinary tract infections, lower respiratory tract infections, septicemia, skin/skin structure infections, intra-abdominal infections, and gynecological infections caused by susceptible gram-negative bacilli

Inhalation: Improve respiratory symptoms in cystic fibrosis (CF) patients with *Pseudomonas aeruginosa*

Prescribing and Access Restrictions Cayston® (aztreonam inhalation solution) is only available through a select group of specialty pharmacies and cannot be obtained through a retail pharmacy. Because Cayston® may only be used with the Altera® Nebulizer System, it can only be obtained from the following specialty pharmacies: Cystic Fibrosis Services, Inc; IV Solutions; Foundation Care; and Pharmaceutical Specialties, Inc. This network of specialty pharmacies ensures proper access to both the drug and device. To obtain the medication and proper nebulizer, contact the Cayston Access Program at 1-877-7CAYSTON (1-877-722-9786) or at www.cayston.com.

Contraindications Hypersensitivity to aztreonam or any component of the formulation

Warnings/Precautions Rare cross-allergenicity to penicillins and cephalosporins has been reported. Use caution in renal impairment; dosing adjustment required for the injectable formulation. Prolonged use may result in fungal or bacterial superinfection, including *C. difficile*-associated diarrhea (CDAD) and pseudomembranous colitis; CDAD has been observed >2 months postantibiotic treatment. Patients colonized with *Burkholderia cepacia* have not been studied. Safety and efficacy has not been established in patients with FEV$_1$ <25% or >75% predicted. To reduce the development of resistant bacteria and maintain efficacy reserve use for CF patients with known *Pseudomonas aeruginosa*. Bronchospasm may occur occur following nebulization; administer a bronchodilator prior to treatment.

Adverse Reactions (Reflective of adult population; not specific for elderly)

Inhalation:

>10%:

Central nervous system: Fever (13%; more common in children)

Respiratory: Cough (54%), nasal congestion (16%), pharyngeal pain (12%), wheezing (16%)

1% to 10%:

Cardiovascular: Chest discomfort (8%)

Dermatologic: Rash (2%)

Gastrointestinal: Abdominal pain (7%), vomiting (6%)

Respiratory: Bronchospasm (3%)

Injection:

>10%:

Hematologic: Neutropenia (children 3% to 11%)

Hepatic: ALT/AST increased (children 4% to 6%; >3 times ULN: 15% to 20%, high dose)

Local: Pain at injection site (children 12%, adults 2%)

1% to 10%:

Central nervous system: Fever (≤1%)

Dermatologic: Rash (children 4%, adults 1%)

Gastrointestinal: Diarrhea (1%), nausea (1%), vomiting (1%)

Hematologic: Eosinophilia (children 6%, adults <1%), thrombocytosis (children 4%, adults <1%), neutropenia (adults <1%)

Local: Injection site reactions (1% to 3%) (erythema, induration; more common in children), phlebitis/thrombophlebitis (2%)

Renal: Serum creatinine increased (children 6%)

Drug Interactions

Metabolism/Transport Effects None known.

Avoid Concomitant Use

Avoid concomitant use of Aztreonam with any of the following: BCG

Increased Effect/Toxicity There are no known significant interactions involving an increase in effect.

Decreased Effect

Aztreonam may decrease the levels/effects of: BCG; Typhoid Vaccine

Stability

Inhalation: Prior to reconstitution, store at 2°C to 8°C (36°F to 46°F). Once removed from refrigeration, aztreonam and the diluent may be stored at room temperature (up to 25°C/77°F) for ≤28 days. Protect from light. Reconstitute immediately prior to use. Squeeze diluent into opened glass vial. Replace rubber stopper and gently swirl vial until contents have completely dissolved. Use immediately after reconstitution.

Injection: Prior to reconstitution, store at room temperature; avoid excessive heat. Reconstituted solutions are colorless to light yellow straw and may turn pink upon standing without affecting potency. Use reconstituted solutions and I.V. solutions (in NS and D_5W) within 48 hours if kept at room temperature (25°C) or 7 days under refrigeration (4°C).

I.M.: Reconstitute with at least 3 mL SWFI, sterile bacteriostatic water for injection, NS, or bacteriostatic sodium chloride.

I.V.:

Bolus injection: Reconstitute with 6-10 mL SWFI.

Infusion: Reconstitute to a final concentration ≤2%; the final concentration should not exceed 20 mg/mL. Solution for infusion may be frozen at less than -2°C (less than -4°F) for up to 3 months. Thawed solution should be used within 24 hours if thawed at room temperature or within 72 hours if thawed under refrigeration. **Do not refreeze.**

Mechanism of Action Inhibits bacterial cell wall synthesis by binding to one or more of the penicillin-binding proteins (PBPs) which in turn inhibits the final transpeptidation step of peptidoglycan synthesis in bacterial cell walls, thus inhibiting cell wall biosynthesis. Bacteria eventually lyse due to ongoing activity of cell wall autolytic enzymes (autolysins and murein hydrolases) while cell wall assembly is arrested. Monobactam structure makes cross-allergenicity with beta-lactams unlikely.

Pharmacodynamics/Kinetics

Absorption: I.M.: Well absorbed

Distribution: V_d (adults): 0.2 L/kg

Protein binding: 56%

Half-life: 1.3-2.2 hours (half-life prolonged in renal failure)

Time to peak serum concentration: Within 60 minutes following a dose

Elimination: 60% to 70% excreted unchanged in urine and partially excreted in feces

In healthy older adults with normal renal function (mean Cl_{cr}: 99 mL/minute), there were no significant changes in pharmacokinetic parameters. However, in older adults with impaired renal function (mean Cl_{cr}: 24 mL/minute) serum concentrations were inversely related to Cl_{cr}

Dosage

Geriatric & Adult

Urinary tract infection: I.M., I.V.: 500 mg to 1 g every 8-12 hours

Moderately severe systemic infections:

I.M.: 1 g every 8-12 hours

I.V.: 1-2 g every 8-12 hours

Severe systemic or life-threatening infections (especially caused by _Pseudomonas aeruginosa_): I.V.: 2 g every 6-8 hours; maximum: 8 g/day

Meningitis (gram-negative): I.V.: 2 g every 6-8 hours

Pseudomonas aeruginosa **infection in cystic fibrosis:** Inhalation (nebulizer): 75 mg 3 times daily (at least 4 hours apart) for 28 days. Do not repeat for 28 days after completion.

Renal Impairment

Oral inhalation: Dosage adjustment not required for mild, moderate or severe renal impairment.

I.M., I.V.: Adults: Following initial dose, maintenance doses should be given as follows:

Cl_{cr} 10-30 mL/minute: 50% of usual dose at the usual interval

Cl_{cr} <10 mL/minute: 25% of usual dosage at the usual interval

Intermittent hemodialysis (IHD): Dialyzable (20% to 50%): Loading dose of 500 mg, 1 g, or 2 g, followed by 25% of initial dose at usual interval; for serious/life-threatening infections, administer one-eighth ($^1/_8$) of initial dose after each hemodialysis session (given in addition to the maintenance doses). Alternatively, may administer 500 mg every 12 hours (Heintz, 2009). **Note:** Dosing dependent on the assumption of 3 times/week, complete IHD sessions.

Peritoneal dialysis (PD): Administer as for Cl_{cr} <10 mL/minute

Continuous renal replacement therapy (CRRT) (Heintz, 2009; Trotman, 2005): Drug clearance is highly dependent on the method of renal replacement, filter type, and flow rate. Appropriate dosing requires close monitoring of pharmacologic response, signs of adverse reactions due to drug accumulation, as well as drug concentrations in relation to target trough (if appropriate). The following are general recommendations only (based on dialysate flow/ultrafiltration rates of 1-2 L/hour and minimal residual renal function) and should not supersede clinical judgment:

CVVH: Loading dose of 2 g followed by 1-2 g every 12 hours

CVVHD/CVVHDF: Loading dose of 2 g followed by either 1 g every 8 hours **or** 2 g every 12 hours (Heintz, 2009)

Administration

Inhalation: Administer using only an Altera® nebulizer system; **administer alone; do not mix with other nebulizer medications.** Administer a bronchodilator before administration of aztreonam (short-acting: 15 minutes to 4 hours before; long-acting: 30 minutes to 12 hours before). For patients on multiple inhaled therapies, administer bronchodilator first, then mucolytic, and lastly, aztreonam.

To administer Cayston®, pour reconstituted solution into the handset of the nebulizer system, turn unit on. Place the mouthpiece in the patient's mouth and encourage to breath normally through the mouth. Administration time is usually 2-3 minutes. Administer doses ≥4 hours apart.

Injection: Doses >1 g should be administered I.V.

I.M.: Administer by deep injection into large muscle mass, such as upper outer quadrant of gluteus maximus or the lateral part of the thigh

I.V.: Administer by slow I.V. push over 3-5 minutes or by intermittent infusion over 20-60 minutes.

Monitoring Parameters

Injection: Periodic liver function test; monitor for signs of anaphylaxis during first dose

Inhalation: Consider measuring FEV_1 prior to initiation of therapy

Test Interactions May interfere with urine glucose tests containing cupric sulfate (Benedict's solution, Clinitest®); positive Coombs' test

Pharmacotherapy Pearls Normally used with other antibiotics in life-threatening situations; member of new class of antibiotics called monobactams, with excellent gram-negative bacteria effectiveness, without ototoxicity or nephrotoxicity

Special Geriatric Considerations Injection: Adjust dose relative to renal function.

Dosage Forms Excipient information presented when available (limited, particularly for generics); consult specific product labeling.

Infusion, premixed iso-osmotic solution:
  Azactam®: 1 g (50 mL); 2 g (50 mL)
Injection, powder for reconstitution: 1 g, 2 g
  Azactam®: 1 g, 2 g
Powder for reconstitution, for oral inhalation [preservative free]:
  Cayston®: 75 mg [supplied with diluent]

◆ **Azulfidine®** see SulfaSALAzine on page 1817
◆ **Azulfidine EN-tabs®** see SulfaSALAzine on page 1817
◆ **B6** see Pyridoxine on page 1640
◆ **Baby Aspirin** see Aspirin on page 154
◆ **Bacid® [OTC]** see Lactobacillus on page 1084

Baclofen (BAK loe fen)

Medication Safety Issues

Sound-alike/look-alike issues:

Baclofen may be confused with Bactroban®

Lioresal® may be confused with lisinopril, Lotensin®

High alert medication:

The Institute for Safe Medication Practices (ISMP) includes this medication (intrathecal administration) among its list of drugs which have a heightened risk of causing significant patient harm when used in error.

Brand Names: U.S. Gablofen®; Lioresal®

Brand Names: Canada Apo-Baclofen®; Ava-Baclofen; Dom-Baclofen; Lioresal®; Lioresal® D.S.; Lioresal® Intrathecal; Med-Baclofen; Mylan-Baclofen; Novo-Baclofen; Nu-Baclo; PHL-Baclofen; PMS-Baclofen; ratio-Baclofen; Riva-Baclofen

Generic Availability (U.S.) Yes: Tablets

Pharmacologic Category Skeletal Muscle Relaxant

Use Treatment of reversible spasticity associated with multiple sclerosis or spinal cord lesions

Orphan drug: Intrathecal: Treatment of intractable spasticity caused by spinal cord injury, multiple sclerosis, and other spinal disease (spinal ischemia or tumor, transverse myelitis, cervical spondylosis, degenerative myelopathy)

Unlabeled Use Treatment of intractable hiccups, intractable pain relief, bladder spasticity, trigeminal neuralgia, cerebral palsy, Huntington's chorea

Contraindications Hypersensitivity to baclofen or any component of the formulation

Warnings/Precautions Use with caution in patients with seizure disorder or impaired renal function. **[U.S. Boxed Warning]: Avoid abrupt withdrawal of the drug; abrupt withdrawal of intrathecal baclofen has resulted in severe sequelae (hyperpyrexia, obtundation, rebound/exaggerated spasticity, muscle rigidity, and rhabdomyolysis), leading to organ failure and some fatalities.** Risk may be higher in patients with injuries at T-6 or above, history of baclofen withdrawal, or limited ability to communicate. May cause CNS depression, which may impair physical or mental abilities; patients must be cautioned about performing tasks which require mental alertness (eg, operating machinery or driving). Elderly are more sensitive to the effects of baclofen and are more likely to experience adverse CNS effects at higher doses.

Cases (most from pharmacy compounded preparations) of intrathecal mass formation at the implanted catheter tip have been reported; may lead to loss of clinical response, pain or new/ worsening neurological effects. Neurosurgical evaluation and/or an appropriate imaging study should be considered if a mass is suspected.

Adverse Reactions (Reflective of adult population; not specific for elderly)
>10%:
　Central nervous system: Drowsiness, vertigo, psychiatric disturbances, insomnia, slurred speech, ataxia, hypotonia
　Neuromuscular & skeletal: Weakness
1% to 10%:
　Cardiovascular: Hypotension
　Central nervous system: Fatigue, confusion, headache
　Dermatologic: Rash
　Gastrointestinal: Nausea, constipation
　Genitourinary: Polyuria

Drug Interactions
　Metabolism/Transport Effects None known.
　Avoid Concomitant Use
　　Avoid concomitant use of Baclofen with any of the following: Azelastine; Azelastine (Nasal); Methadone; Mirtazapine; Paraldehyde
　Increased Effect/Toxicity
　　Baclofen may increase the levels/effects of: Alcohol (Ethyl); Azelastine; Azelastine (Nasal); Buprenorphine; CNS Depressants; Methadone; Methotrimeprazine; Metyrosine; Mirtazapine; Paraldehyde; Selective Serotonin Reuptake Inhibitors; Zolpidem

　　The levels/effects of Baclofen may be increased by: Droperidol; HydrOXYzine; Methotrimeprazine
　Decreased Effect There are no known significant interactions involving a decrease in effect.

Ethanol/Nutrition/Herb Interactions
　Ethanol: May increase CNS depression; monitor for increased effects with coadministration. Caution patients about effects.
　Herb/Nutraceutical: Avoid valerian, St John's wort, kava kava, gotu kola.

Mechanism of Action Inhibits the transmission of both monosynaptic and polysynaptic reflexes at the spinal cord level, possibly by hyperpolarization of primary afferent fiber terminals, with resultant relief of muscle spasticity

Pharmacodynamics/Kinetics
　Onset of action: 3-4 days
　　Peak effect: 5-10 days
　Absorption (dose dependent): Oral: Rapid
　Protein binding: 30%
　Metabolism: Hepatic (15% of dose)
　Half-life elimination: 3.5 hours
　Time to peak, serum: Oral: Within 2-3 hours
　Excretion: Urine and feces (85% as unchanged drug)

Dosage
　Geriatric Oral (the lowest effective dose is recommended): Initial: 5 mg 2-3 times/day, increasing gradually as needed; if benefits are not seen withdraw the drug slowly.
　Adult
　　Spasticity:
　　　Oral: 5 mg 3 times/day, may increase 5 mg/dose every 3 days to a maximum of 80 mg/day
　　　Intrathecal:
　　　　Test dose: 50-100 mcg, doses >50 mcg should be given in 25 mcg increments, separated by 24 hours. A screening dose of 25 mcg may be considered in very small patients. Patients not responding to screening dose of 100 mcg should not be considered for chronic infusion/implanted pump.
　　　　Maintenance: After positive response to test dose, a maintenance intrathecal infusion can be administered via an implanted intrathecal pump. Initial dose via pump: Infusion at a 24-hourly rate dosed at twice the test dose. Avoid abrupt discontinuation.
　　Hiccups (unlabeled use): Oral: 10-20 mg 2-3 times/day

Renal Impairment May be necessary to reduce dosage; no specific guidelines have been established
　Hemodialysis: Poor water solubility allows for accumulation during chronic hemodialysis. Low-dose therapy is recommended. There have been several case reports of accumulation of baclofen resulting in toxicity symptoms (organic brain syndrome, myoclonia, deceleration and steep potentials in EEG) in patients with renal failure who have received normal doses of baclofen.

Administration Intrathecal: For screening dosages, dilute with preservative-free sodium chloride to a final concentration of 50 mcg/mL for bolus injection into the subarachnoid space. For maintenance infusions, concentrations of 500-2000 mcg/mL may be used.

Test Interactions Increased alkaline phosphatase, AST, glucose, ammonia (B); decreased bilirubin (S)

Special Geriatric Considerations The elderly are more sensitive to the effects of baclofen and are more likely to experience adverse CNS effects at higher doses.

Dosage Forms Excipient information presented when available (limited, particularly for generics); consult specific product labeling.
Injection, solution, intrathecal [preservative free]:
  Gablofen®: 500 mcg/mL (20 mL); 1000 mcg/mL (20 mL); 2000 mcg/mL (20 mL)
  Lioresal®: 500 mcg/mL (20 mL); 2000 mcg/mL (5 mL, 20 mL)
Injection, solution, intrathecal [for screening, preservative free]:
  Gablofen®: 50 mcg/mL (1 mL)
  Lioresal®: 50 mcg/mL (1 mL)
Tablet, oral: 10 mg, 20 mg

Becaplermin (be KAP ler min)

Medication Safety Issues
Sound-alike/look-alike issues:
  Regranex® may be confused with Granulex®, Repronex®
Brand Names: U.S. Regranex®
Index Terms Recombinant Human Platelet-Derived Growth Factor B; rPDGF-BB
Generic Availability (U.S.) No
Pharmacologic Category Growth Factor, Platelet-Derived; Topical Skin Product
Use Adjunctive treatment of diabetic neuropathic ulcers occurring on the lower limbs and feet that extend into subcutaneous tissue (or beyond) and have adequate blood supply
Contraindications Hypersensitivity to becaplermin or any component of the formulation; known neoplasm(s) at the site(s) of application
Warnings/Precautions For external use only; do not use in wounds that close by primary intention. Use with caution in ulcer wounds related to arterial or venous insufficiency and when there are thermal, electrical, or radiation burns at wound site. **[U.S. Boxed Warning]: In a retrospective study, an increase in mortality secondary to malignancy has been observed in patients treated with ≥3 tubes of becaplermin.** Malignancies of varying types have been reported; all were remote from the becaplermin treatment site; use with caution in patients with known malignancy. Effects on exposed joints, tendons, ligaments, and bone have not been established.
Adverse Reactions (Reflective of adult population; not specific for elderly) 1% to 10%: Dermatologic: Erythematous rash (2%)

Drug Interactions

Metabolism/Transport Effects None known.

Avoid Concomitant Use There are no known interactions where it is recommended to avoid concomitant use.

Increased Effect/Toxicity There are no known significant interactions involving an increase in effect.

Decreased Effect There are no known significant interactions involving a decrease in effect.

Stability Refrigerate at 2°C to 8°C (36°F to 46°F); do not freeze. The following stability information has also been reported: May be stored at room temperature for up to 6 days (Cohen, 2007).

Mechanism of Action Recombinant B-isoform homodimer of human platelet-derived growth factor (rPDGF-BB) which enhances formation of new granulation tissue, induces fibroblast proliferation and differentiation to promote wound healing; also promotes angiogenesis.

Pharmacodynamics/Kinetics

Onset of action: Complete healing: 15% of patients within 8 weeks, 25% at 10 weeks

Absorption: Minimal

Distribution: Binds to PDGF beta-receptors in normal skin and granulation tissue

Dosage

Geriatric & Adult Diabetic ulcers (lower extremity): Topical: Apply appropriate amount of gel once daily with a cotton swab or similar tool, as a coating over the ulcer. The amount of becaplermin to be applied will vary depending on the size of the ulcer area.

Note: If the ulcer does not decrease in size by ~30% after 10 weeks of treatment or complete healing has not occurred in 20 weeks, continued treatment with becaplermin gel should be reassessed.

Estimation of gel requirement: To calculate the length of gel applied to the ulcer, measure the greatest length of the ulcer by the greatest width of the ulcer. Tube size and unit of measure will determine the formula used in the calculation. Recalculate amount of gel needed every 1-2 weeks, depending on the rate of change in ulcer area.

Centimeters:

15 g tube: [ulcer length (cm) x width (cm)] divided by 4 = length of gel (cm)

2 g tube: [ulcer length (cm) x width (cm)] divided by 2 = length of gel (cm)

Inches:

15 g tube: [length (in) x width (in)] x 0.6 = length of gel (in)

2 g tube: [length (in) x width (in)] x 1.3 = length of gel (in)

Administration For external use only. Squeeze appropriate amount of gel onto clean measuring surface (eg, wax paper), spread onto entire ulcer area in a thin, continuous layer ~1/16 inch thick. Cover with saline moistened dressing; leave dressing in place ~12 hours. After 12 hours, remove dressing, rinse with saline or water to remove residual becaplermin gel and cover with saline moistened dressing (without becaplermin gel) for remainder of the day. Continue use once daily until ulcer is completely healed.

Monitoring Parameters Ulcer volume (pressure ulcers); wound area; evidence of closure; drainage (diabetic ulcers); signs/symptoms of toxicity (erythema, local infections)

Special Geriatric Considerations No specific information for use in elderly.

Dosage Forms Excipient information presented when available (limited, particularly for generics); consult specific product labeling. [DSC] = Discontinued product

Gel, topical:

Regranex®: 0.01% (2 g [DSC], 15 g)

Beclomethasone (Oral Inhalation) (be kloe METH a sone)

Related Information

Asthma *on page 2125*

Inhalant Agents *on page 2117*

Brand Names: U.S. QVAR®

Brand Names: Canada QVAR®

Index Terms Vanceril

Generic Availability (U.S.) No

Pharmacologic Category Corticosteroid, Inhalant (Oral)

Use Oral inhalation: Maintenance and prophylactic treatment of asthma; includes those who require corticosteroids and those who may benefit from a dose reduction/elimination of systemically-administered corticosteroids. Not for relief of acute bronchospasm.

BECLOMETHASONE (ORAL INHALATION)

◄ **Contraindications** Hypersensitivity to beclomethasone or any component of the formulation; status asthmaticus, or other acute asthma episodes requiring intensive measures

Canadian labeling: Additional contraindications (not in U.S. labeling): Moderate-to-severe bronchiectasis requiring intensive measures; untreated fungal, bacterial, or tubercular infections of the respiratory tract

Warnings/Precautions May cause hypercorticism or suppression of hypothalamic-pituitary-adrenal (HPA) axis, particularly in patients receiving high doses for prolonged periods. HPA axis suppression may lead to adrenal crisis. Withdrawal and discontinuation of a corticosteroid should be done slowly and carefully. Particular care is required when patients are transferred from systemic corticosteroids to inhaled products due to possible adrenal insufficiency or withdrawal from steroids, including an increase in allergic symptoms. Patients receiving >20 mg per day of prednisone (or equivalent) may be most susceptible. Fatalities have occurred due to adrenal insufficiency in asthmatic patients during and after transfer from systemic corticosteroids to aerosol steroids; aerosol steroids do **not** provide the systemic steroid needed to treat patients having trauma, surgery, or infections.

Bronchospasm may occur with wheezing after inhalation; if this occurs, stop steroid and treat with a fast-acting bronchodilator. Supplemental steroids (oral or parenteral) may be needed during stress or severe asthma attacks. Not to be used in status asthmaticus or for the relief of acute bronchospasm. Corticosteroid use may cause psychiatric disturbances, including depression, euphoria, insomnia, mood swings, and personality changes. Pre-existing psychiatric conditions may be exacerbated by corticosteroid use. Prolonged use of corticosteroids may also increase the incidence of secondary infection, mask acute infection (including fungal infections), prolong or exacerbate viral infections, or limit response to vaccines. Avoid use in patients with ocular herpes or untreated viral, fungal, parasitic or bacterial systemic infections (Canadian labeling contraindicates use with untreated respiratory infections). Exposure to chickenpox should be avoided. Close observation is required in patients with latent tuberculosis and/or TB reactivity; restrict use in active TB (only in conjunction with antituberculosis treatment). Prolonged treatment with corticosteroids has been associated with the development of Kaposi's sarcoma (case reports); if noted, discontinuation of therapy should be considered.

Use with caution in patients with thyroid disease, hepatic impairment, renal impairment, cardiovascular disease, diabetes, glaucoma, cataracts, myasthenia gravis, patients at risk for osteoporosis, patients at risk for seizures, or GI diseases (diverticulitis, peptic ulcer, ulcerative colitis) due to perforation risk. Use caution following acute MI (corticosteroids have been associated with myocardial rupture). Because of the risk of adverse effects, systemic corticosteroids should be used cautiously in the elderly in the smallest possible effective dose for the shortest duration.

There have been reports of systemic corticosteroid withdrawal symptoms (eg, joint/muscle pain, lassitude, depression) when withdrawing oral inhalation therapy.

Adverse Reactions (Reflective of adult population; not specific for elderly)
>10%: Central nervous system: Headache (12%)
1% to 10%:
  Central nervous system: Dysphonia (1% to 3%), pain (2%)
  Endocrine & metabolic: Dysmenorrhea (1% to 3%)
  Gastrointestinal: Nausea (1%)
  Neuromuscular & skeletal: Back pain (1%)
  Respiratory: Upper respiratory tract infection (9%), pharyngitis (8%), rhinitis (6%), sinusitis (3%), cough (1% to 3%)

Drug Interactions
  Metabolism/Transport Effects None known.
  Avoid Concomitant Use
    Avoid concomitant use of Beclomethasone (Oral Inhalation) with any of the following: Aldesleukin; BCG; Natalizumab; Pimecrolimus; Tacrolimus (Topical)
  Increased Effect/Toxicity
    Beclomethasone (Oral Inhalation) may increase the levels/effects of: Amphotericin B; Deferasirox; Leflunomide; Loop Diuretics; Natalizumab; Thiazide Diuretics

    The levels/effects of Beclomethasone (Oral Inhalation) may be increased by: Denosumab; Pimecrolimus; Tacrolimus (Topical); Telaprevir; Trastuzumab
  Decreased Effect
    Beclomethasone (Oral Inhalation) may decrease the levels/effects of: Aldesleukin; Antidiabetic Agents; BCG; Coccidioidin Skin Test; Corticorelin; Hyaluronidase; Sipuleucel-T; Telaprevir; Vaccines (Inactivated)

    The levels/effects of Beclomethasone (Oral Inhalation) may be decreased by: Echinacea

Stability Do not store near heat or open flame. Do not puncture canisters. Store at 25°C (77°F); excursions permitted between 15°C to 30°C (59°F to 86°F). Rest QVAR® on concave end of canister with actuator on top.

Mechanism of Action Controls the rate of protein synthesis; depresses the migration of polymorphonuclear leukocytes, fibroblasts; reverses capillary permeability and lysosomal stabilization at the cellular level to prevent or control inflammation

Pharmacodynamics/Kinetics

Onset of action: Therapeutic effect: 1-4 weeks

Absorption: Readily; quickly hydrolyzed by pulmonary esterases to active metabolite (beclomethasone-17-monoproprionate [17-BMP]) during absorption

Protein binding: 17-BMP: 94% to 96%

Metabolism: Pro-drug; undergoes rapid conversion to 17-BMP during absorption; followed by additional metabolism via CYP3A4 to other, less active metabolites (beclomethasone-21-monopropionate [21-BMP] and beclomethasone [BOH])

Half-life elimination: 17-BMP: 3 hours

Time to peak, plasma: Oral inhalation: BDP: 0.5 hours; 17-BMP: 0.7 hours

Excretion: Mainly in feces; urine (<10%)

Dosage

Geriatric & Adult

Asthma: Inhalation, oral (doses should be titrated to the lowest effective dose once asthma is controlled):

U.S. labeling:

Patients previously on bronchodilators only: Initial dose 40-80 mcg twice daily; maximum dose: 320 mcg twice day

Patients previously on inhaled corticosteroids: Initial dose 40-160 mcg twice daily; maximum dose: 320 mcg twice daily

NIH Asthma Guidelines (NIH, 2007):

"Low" dose: 80-240 mcg/day

"Medium" dose: >240-480 mcg/day

"High" dose: >480 mcg/day

Canadian labeling:

Mild asthma: 50-100 mcg twice daily; maximum dose: 100 mcg twice daily

Moderate asthma: 100-250 mcg twice daily; maximum dose: 250 mcg twice daily

Severe asthma: 300-400 mcg twice daily; maximum dose: 400 mcg twice daily

Conversion from oral systemic corticosteroid to orally inhaled corticosteroid: Initiation of oral inhalation therapy should begin in patients whose asthma is reasonably stabilized on oral corticosteroids (OCS). A gradual dose reduction of OCS should begin ~7 days after starting inhaled therapy. U.S. labeling recommends reducing prednisone dose no more rapidly than ≤2.5 mg/day (or equivalent of other OCS) every 1-2 weeks. The Canadian labeling recommends decreasing the daily dose of prednisone by 1 mg (or equivalent of other OCS) every 7 days or more in closely monitored patients. If adrenal insufficiency occurs, temporarily increase the OCS dose and follow with a more gradual withdrawal. **Note:** When transitioning from systemic to inhaled corticosteroids, supplemental systemic corticosteroid therapy may be necessary during periods of stress or during severe asthma attacks.

Administration Canister does not need shaken prior to use. Prime canister by spraying twice into the air prior to initial use or if not in use for >10 days. Avoid spraying in face or eyes. Exhale fully prior to bringing inhaler to mouth. Place inhaler in mouth, close lips around mouthpiece, and inhale slowly and deeply. Remove inhaler and hold breath for approximately 5-10 seconds. Rinse mouth and throat after use to prevent *Candida* infection. Do not wash or put inhaler in water; mouth piece may be cleaned with a dry tissue or cloth. Discard after the "discard by" date or after labeled number of doses has been used, even if container is not completely empty. Patients using a spacer should inhale immediately due to decreased amount of medication that is delivered with a delayed inspiration.

Monitoring Parameters Signs/symptoms of HPA axis suppression/adrenal insufficiency; signs/symptoms of oral candidiasis; ocular effects (eg, cataracts, increased intraocular pressure, glaucoma)

Pharmacotherapy Pearls Not used in status asthmaticus; shake thoroughly before using; oral inhalation and nasal inhalation dosage forms are **not** to be used interchangeably

Special Geriatric Considerations Elderly patients may have difficulty with oral metered dose inhalers and may benefit from the use of a spacer or chamber device.

Dosage Forms Excipient information presented when available (limited, particularly for generics); consult specific product labeling. [DSC] = Discontinued product

Aerosol, for oral inhalation, as dipropionate:

QVAR®: 40 mcg/inhalation (7.3 g [DSC]) [chlorofluorocarbon free; contains ethanol; 100 metered actuations]

QVAR®: 40 mcg/inhalation (8.7 g) [chlorofluorocarbon free; contains ethanol; 120 metered actuations]

QVAR®: 80 mcg/inhalation (7.3 g [DSC]) [chlorofluorocarbon free; contains ethanol; 100 metered actuations]

QVAR®: 80 mcg/inhalation (8.7 g) [chlorofluorocarbon free; contains ethanol; 120 metered actuations]

Dosage Forms: Canada Excipient information presented when available (limited, particularly for generics); consult specific product labeling.

Aerosol, for oral inhalation, as dipropionate:

QVAR™: 50 mcg/inhalation (6.5 g) [chlorofluorocarbon free; contains ethanol; 100 metered actuations]

QVAR™: 50 mcg/inhalation (12.4 g) [chlorofluorocarbon free; contains ethanol; 200 metered actuations]

QVAR™: 100 mcg/inhalation (6.5 g) [chlorofluorocarbon free; contains ethanol; 100 metered actuations]

QVAR™: 100 mcg/inhalation (12.4 g) [chlorofluorocarbon free; contains ethanol; 200 metered actuations]

Beclomethasone (Nasal) (be kloe METH a sone)

Brand Names: U.S. Beconase AQ®; Qnasl™

Brand Names: Canada Apo-Beclomethasone®; Mylan-Beclo AQ; Nu-Beclomethasone; Rivanase AQ

Index Terms Beclomethasone Dipropionate

Generic Availability (U.S.) No

Pharmacologic Category Corticosteroid, Nasal

Use

Beconase AQ®: Symptomatic treatment of seasonal or perennial allergic rhinitis; nonallergic (vasomotor) rhinitis; prevent recurrence of nasal polyps following surgery

Qnasl™: Symptomatic treatment of seasonal or perennial allergic rhinitis

Unlabeled Use Adjunct to antibiotics in empiric treatment of acute bacterial rhinosinusitis (ABRS) (Chow, 2012)

Dosage

Geriatric & Adult

Allergic rhinitis: Inhalation, nasal:

Beconase® AQ: 1-2 inhalations each nostril twice daily (total dose: 168-336 mcg/day)

Qnasl™: Two inhalations each nostril once daily (total dose: 320 mcg/day)

Nasal polyps (postsurgical prophylaxis), vasomotor rhinitis (Beconase AQ®): Inhalation, nasal: 1-2 inhalations each nostril twice daily (total dose: 168-336 mcg/day)

Special Geriatric Considerations Evaluate the patient's or caregiver's ability to safely administer the correct dose of nasal medication.

Dosage Forms Excipient information presented when available (limited, particularly for generics); consult specific product labeling.

Aerosol, spray, intranasal, as dipropionate:

Qnasl™: 80 mcg/inhalation (8.7 g) [contains dehydrated ethanol; 120 metered actuations]

Suspension, intranasal, as dipropionate [spray]:

Beconase AQ®: 42 mcg/inhalation (25 g) [contains benzalkonium chloride, ethanol 0.25%; 180 metered actuations]

◆ **Beclomethasone Dipropionate** see Beclomethasone (Nasal) on page 192

◆ **Beconase AQ®** see Beclomethasone (Nasal) on page 192

Belatacept (bel AT a sept)

Brand Names: U.S. Nulojix®

Index Terms BMS-224818; LEA29Y

Generic Availability (U.S.) No

Pharmacologic Category Selective T-Cell Costimulation Blocker

Use Prophylaxis of organ rejection concomitantly with basiliximab, mycophenolate, and corticosteroids in Epstein-Barr virus (EBV) seropositive kidney transplant recipients

Prescribing and Access Restrictions The ENLiST registry has been created to further determine the safety of belatacept, particularly the incidence of post-transplant lymphoproliferative disorder (PTLD) and progressive multifocal leukoencephalopathy (PML), in EBV-seropositive kidney transplant patients. Transplant centers are encouraged to participate (1-800-321-1335).

Medication Guide Available Yes

Contraindications Transplant patients who are Epstein-Barr virus (EBV) seronegative or with unknown EBV status

Warnings/Precautions [U.S. Boxed Warning]: Risk of post-transplant lymphoprolifer-ative disorder (PTLD) is increased, primarily involving the CNS, in patients receiving belatacept compared to patients receiving cyclosporine-based regimens. Degree of immuno-suppression is a risk factor for PTLD developing; do not exceed recommended dosing. Patients who are Epstein-Barr virus seronegative (EBV) are at an even higher risk; use is contraindicated in patients without evidence of immunity to EBV. Therapy is only appropriate in patients who are EBV seropositive via evidence of acquired immunity, such as presence of IgG antibodies to viral capsid antigen [VCA] and EBV nuclear antigen [EBNA]. Cytomegalo-virus (CMV) infection also increases the risk for PTLD; CMV prophylaxis is recommended for a minimum of 3 months following transplantation. Although CMV disease is a risk for PTLD and CMV seronegative patients are at an increased risk for CMV disease, the clinical role, if any, of determining CMV serology to determine risk of PTLD development has not been determined.

[U.S. Boxed Warning]: Risk for infection is increased. Immunosuppressive therapy may lead to opportunistic infections, sepsis, and/or fatal infections. Tuberculosis (TB) is increased; test patients for latent TB prior to initiation, and treat latent TB infection prior to use. Patients receiving immunosuppressive therapy are at an increased risk of activation of latent viral infections, including John Cunningham virus (JCV) and BK virus infection. Activation of JCV may result in progressive multifocal leukoencephalopathy (PML), a rare and potentially fatal condition affecting the CNS. Symptoms of PML include apathy, ataxia, cognitive deficiencies, confusion, and hemiparesis. Polyoma virus-associated nephropathy (PVAN), primarily from activation of BK virus, may also occur and lead to the deterioration of renal function and/or renal graft loss. Risk factors for the development of PML and PVAN include immunosup-pression and treatment with immunosuppressant therapy. The onset of PML or PVAN may warrant a reduction in immunosuppressive therapy; however, in transplant recipients, the risk of reduced immunosuppression and graft rejection should be considered.

[U.S. Boxed Warning]: Risk for malignancy is increased. Malignancy, including skin malignancy and post-transplant lymphoproliferative disease, is associated with the use of immunosuppressants, including belatacept; higher than recommended doses or more fre-quent dosing is not recommended; patients should be advised to limit their exposure to sunlight/UV light.

[U.S. Boxed Warning]: Therapy is not recommended in liver transplant patients due to increased risk of graft loss and death. [U.S. Boxed Warning]: Should be administered under the supervision of a physician experienced in immunosuppressive therapy. Patients should not be immunized with attenuated or live viral vaccines during or shortly after treatment; safety of immunization following therapy has not been studied.

Adverse Reactions (Reflective of adult population; not specific for elderly) Inci-dences reported occurred during clinical trials using belatacept compared to a cyclosporine control regimen. All patients also received basiliximab induction, mycophenolate mofetil, and corticosteroids, and were followed up to 3 years.

>10%:
 Cardiovascular: Peripheral edema (34%), hypertension (32%), hypotension (18%)
 Central nervous system: Fever (28%), headache (21%), insomnia (15%)
 Endocrine & metabolic: Hypokalemia (21%), hyperkalemia (20%), hypophosphatemia (19%), dyslipidemia (19%), hyperglycemia (16%), hypocalcemia (13%), hypercholester-olemia (11%)
 Gastrointestinal: Diarrhea (39%), constipation (33%), nausea (24%), vomiting (22%), abdominal pain (19%)
 Genitourinary: Urinary tract infection (37%), dysuria (11%)
 Hematologic: Anemia (45%), leukopenia (20%)
 Neuromuscular & skeletal: Arthralgia (17%), back pain (13%)
 Renal: Proteinuria (16%; up to 33% 2+ proteinuria at 1 month post-transplant), renal graft dysfunction (25%), hematuria (16%), serum creatinine increased (15%)
 Respiratory: Cough (24%), upper respiratory infection (15%), nasopharyngitis (13%), dyspnea (12%)
 Miscellaneous: Infection (72% to 82%; serious infection: 24% to 36%), herpes (7% to 14%), CMV (11% to 13%), influenza (11%)
1% to 10%:
 Cardiovascular: Arteriovenous fistula thrombosis (<10%), atrial fibrillation (<10%)
 Central nervous system: Anxiety (10%), dizziness (9%)
 Dermatologic: Alopecia (<10%), hyperhidrosis (<10%), acne (8%)
 Endocrine & metabolic: New-onset diabetes (5% to 8%), hypomagnesemia (7%), hyper-uricemia (5%)
 Gastrointestinal: Stomatitis (<10%), upper abdominal pain (9%)

Genitourinary: Urinary incontinence (<10%)

Hematologic: Hematoma (<10%), neutropenia (<10%)

Neuromuscular & skeletal: Musculoskeletal pain (<10%), tremor (8%)

Renal: Chronic allograft nephropathy (<10%), hydronephrosis (<10%), renal impairment (<10%), renal artery stenosis (<10%), renal tubular necrosis (9%)

Respiratory: Bronchitis (10%)

Miscellaneous: Guillain-Barré syndrome (<10%), lymphocele (<10%), infusion reactions (5%), malignancy (4%), polyoma virus (3% to 4%), antibelatacept antibody development (2%), nonmelanoma skin cancer (2%), tuberculosis (1% to 2%), BK virus-associated nephropathy (1%)

Drug Interactions

Metabolism/Transport Effects None known.

Avoid Concomitant Use

Avoid concomitant use of Belatacept with any of the following: BCG; Belimumab; Natalizumab; Pimecrolimus; Tacrolimus (Topical); Vaccines (Live)

Increased Effect/Toxicity

Belatacept may increase the levels/effects of: Belimumab; Leflunomide; Mycophenolate; Natalizumab; Vaccines (Live)

The levels/effects of Belatacept may be increased by: Denosumab; Pimecrolimus; Roflumilast; Tacrolimus (Topical); Trastuzumab

Decreased Effect

Belatacept may decrease the levels/effects of: BCG; Coccidioidin Skin Test; Sipuleucel-T; Vaccines (Inactivated); Vaccines (Live)

The levels/effects of Belatacept may be decreased by: Echinacea

Stability Prior to use, store refrigerated at 2°C to 8°C (36°F to 46°F). Protect from light. After dilution, the infusion solution (reconstituted solution must be further diluted immediately) may be stored refrigerated for up to 24 hours, with a maximum of 4 hours of the 24 hours at room temperature, 20°C to 25°C (68°F to 77°F), and room light. Infusion must be completed within 24 hours of reconstitution.

Reconstitute each vial with 10.5 mL of diluent (SWFI, NS, or D_5W) using the provided silicone-free disposable syringe, and an 18- to 21-gauge needle. Reconstituted using **only** the silicone-free syringe provided (discard if powder is inadvertently mixed using a siliconized syringe, translucent particles may develop). Inject the diluent down the side of the vial to avoid foaming. Rotate the vial and invert with gentle swirling until completely dissolved; do **not** shake vial. The reconstituted solution should be clear to slightly opalescent and colorless to pale yellow. Immediately transfer the reconstituted solution using the same silicone-free syringe to an infusion bag or bottle with NS or D_5W (if NS or D_5W were used to reconstitute, the same fluid should be used to further dilute). The final concentration should range from 2 mg/mL and 10 mg/mL (typical infusion volume is 100 mL). Prior to adding belatacept to the infusion solution, the manufacturer recommends withdrawing a volume equal to the amount of belatacept to be added. Mix gently; do not shake.

Mechanism of Action Fusion protein which acts as a selective T-cell (lymphocyte) costimulation blocker by binding to CD80 and CD86 receptors on antigen presenting cells (APC), blocking the required CD28 mediated interaction between APCs and T cells needed to activate T lymphocytes. T-cell stimulation results in cytokine production and proliferation, mediators in immunologic rejection associated with kidney transplantation.

Pharmacodynamics/Kinetics

Distribution: V_{ss}: 0.11 L/kg (transplant patients)

Half-life elimination: ~10 days (healthy patients and kidney transplant patients)

Dosage

Adult Note: Dosing is based on actual body weight at the time of transplantation; do not modify weight-based dosing during course of therapy unless the change in body weight is >10%. The prescribed dose must be evenly divisible by 12.5 mg to allow accurate preparation of the reconstituted solution using the provided required disposable syringe for preparation. For example, the calculated dose for a 64 kg patient: 64 kg x 10 mg per kg = 640 mg. The nearest doses to 640 mg that are evenly divisible by 12.5 mg would be 637.5 mg or 650 mg; the closest dose to the calculated dose is 637.5 mg, therefore, 637.5 should be the actual prescribed dose for the patient.

Kidney transplant, prophylaxis of organ rejection: I.V.:

Initial phase: 10 mg/kg/dose on Day 1 (day of transplant, prior to implantation) and on day 5 (~96 hours after Day 1 dose), followed by 10 mg/kg/dose given at the end of Week 2, Week 4, Week 8, and Week 12 following transplantation

Maintenance phase: 5 mg/kg/dose every 4 weeks (plus or minus 3 days) beginning at Week 16 following transplantation

Renal Impairment There are no dosage adjustments provided in manufacturer's labeling. Pharmacokinetic studies in kidney transplant patients indicated that renal function did not affect the clearance of belatacept.

Hepatic Impairment There are no dosage adjustments provided in manufacturer's labeling. Pharmacokinetic studies in kidney transplant patients indicated that hepatic function did not affect the clearance of belatacept.

Administration Administer as an I.V. infusion over 30 minutes using an infusion set with a 0.2-1.2 micron low protein-binding filter. Prior to administration, inspect visually and do not use if solution is discolored or contains particulate matter.

Monitoring Parameters New-onset or worsening neurological, cognitive, or behavioral signs/ symptoms; signs/symptoms of infection; TB screening prior to therapy initiation; EBV sero-positive verification prior to therapy initiation

Pharmacotherapy Pearls If additional silicone-free disposable syringes are needed, contact Bristol-Myers Squibb at 1-888-NULOJIX.

Special Geriatric Considerations Insufficient studies including elderly patients to offer geriatric-specific comments.

Dosage Forms Excipient information presented when available (limited, particularly for generics); consult specific product labeling.
Injection, powder for reconstitution:
Nulojix®: 250 mg [contains sucrose 500 mg/vial]

Belimumab (be LIM yoo mab)

Brand Names: U.S. Benlysta®
Brand Names: Canada Benlysta®
Pharmacologic Category Monoclonal Antibody
Use Treatment of autoantibody-positive (antinuclear antibody [ANA] and/or antidouble-stranded DNA [anti-ds-DNA]) active systemic lupus erythematosus (SLE) in addition to standard therapy
Medication Guide Available Yes
Contraindications Hypersensitivity (anaphylaxis) to belimumab or any component of the formulation
Warnings/Precautions Hazardous agent - use appropriate precautions for handling and disposal. Deaths due to infection, cardiovascular disease, and suicide were higher in belimumab patients compared to placebo during clinical trials. Serious and potentially fatal infections may occur during treatment. Use with caution in patients with chronic infections; treatment should not be undertaken if receiving therapy for chronic infection. Consider interrupting belimumab in patients who develop new infections and initiate appropriate anti-infective treatment; monitor closely.

Serious hypersensitivity reactions including anaphylaxis (with fatalities) and infusion-related reactions (eg, bradycardia, hypotension, myalgia, headache, rash, and urticaria) have been associated with use; onset may be delayed. Monitor for an appropriate time following administration. Discontinue for severe reactions (anaphylaxis, angioedema); infusion may be slowed or temporarily interrupted for other infusion-related reactions. Risk for hypersensitivity reactions may be increased with history of multiple drug allergies or significant hypersensitivity. Immunosuppressants may increase risk of malignancy. May cause psychiatric adverse effects, including anxiety, insomnia, or new/worsening depression. Combined use with other immune modifying biologic therapy (including those targeting B-cells) or with intravenous cyclophosphamide is not recommended. Live vaccines should not be given within 30 days before or concurrently with belimumab. Black/African-American patients may have a lower response rate. Has not been studied in patients with severe active lupus nephritis or severe active CNS lupus; use not recommended.

Adverse Reactions (Reflective of adult population; not specific for elderly)
>10%:
Gastrointestinal: Nausea (15%), diarrhea (12%)
Miscellaneous: Infusion-related reaction (17%), hypersensitivity (13%)
≥3% to 10%:
Central nervous system: Fever (10%), insomnia (6% to 7%), migraine (5%), depression (5% to 6%), anxiety (4%), headache (≥3%)
Dermatologic: Skin reactions (≥3%)
Gastrointestinal: Viral gastroenteritis (3%)
Genitourinary: Urinary tract infection (site not specified >5%), cystitis (4%)
Hematologic: Leukopenia (4%)
Neuromuscular & skeletal: Pain in extremity (6%)
Respiratory: Bronchitis (9%), nasopharyngitis (9%), pharyngitis (5%), sinusitis (>5%), upper respiratory infection (>5%)
Miscellaneous: Influenza (>5%)

Drug Interactions
Metabolism/Transport Effects None known.
Avoid Concomitant Use
Avoid concomitant use of Belimumab with any of the following: Abatacept; Alefacept; BCG; Belatacept; Cyclophosphamide; Denileukin Diftitox; Etanercept; Monoclonal Antibodies; Natalizumab; Pimecrolimus; Tacrolimus (Topical); Vaccines (Live)
Increased Effect/Toxicity
Belimumab may increase the levels/effects of: Cyclophosphamide; Leflunomide; Natalizumab; Vaccines (Live)

The levels/effects of Belimumab may be increased by: Abatacept; Abciximab; Alefacept; Belatacept; Denileukin Diftitox; Denosumab; Etanercept; Monoclonal Antibodies; Pimecrolimus; Roflumilast; Tacrolimus (Topical); Trastuzumab
Decreased Effect
Belimumab may decrease the levels/effects of: BCG; Coccidioidin Skin Test; Sipuleucel-T; Vaccines (Inactivated); Vaccines (Live)

The levels/effects of Belimumab may be decreased by: Echinacea
Stability Prior to reconstitution, store unused vials between 2°C to 8°C (36°F to 46°F); do not freeze. Protect from light. To reconstitute, allow vial to reach room temperature. Reconstitute 120 mg vial with 1.5 mL of SWFI. Reconstitute 400 mg vial with 4.8 mL of SWFI. To minimize foaming, direct SWFI toward the side of the vial. Gently swirl for 60 seconds every 5 minutes until powder has dissolved (usual reconstitution time is 10-15 minutes, but may take up to 30 minutes); do not shake. If utilizing a mechanical reconstitution device, do not exceed 500 rpm or 30 minutes. Further dilute reconstituted solution in 250 mL of 0.9% sodium chloride by first removing and discarding the volume equivalent to the volume of the reconstituted solution to be added to prepare the appropriate dose; add the appropriate volume of the reconstituted solution to the infusion container and gently invert to mix solution. Protect from light. Prior to further dilution, the reconstituted solution must be stored under refrigeration. The diluted solution may be stored refrigerated or at room temperature. Infusion must be completed within 8 hours of reconstitution.
Mechanism of Action Belimumab is an IgG1-lambda monoclonal antibody that prevents the survival of B lymphocytes by blocking the binding of soluble human B lymphocyte stimulator protein (BLyS) to receptors on B lymphocytes. This reduces the activity of B-cell mediated immunity and the autoimmune response.
Pharmacodynamics/Kinetics
Onset of action: B cells: 8 weeks; Clinical improvement (SLE Responder Index and flare reduction): 16 weeks (Navarra, 2011)
Distribution: V_d: 5.29 L
Half-life elimination: 19.4 days
Dosage
Geriatric & Adult Systemic lupus erythematosus (SLE): I.V.: Initial: 10 mg/kg every 2 weeks for 3 doses; Maintenance: 10 mg/kg every 4 weeks
Renal Impairment No dosage adjustment is necessary for Cl_{cr} ≥15 mL/minute; has not been studied in Cl_{cr}<15 mL/minute
Hepatic Impairment No dosage adjustment provided in manufacturer's labeling (has not been studied).
Administration Administer intravenously over 1 hour through a dedicated I.V. line. Do **NOT** administer as an I.V. push or bolus. Discontinue infusion for severe hypersensitivity reaction (eg, anaphylaxis, angioedema). The infusion may be slowed or temporarily interrupted for minor reactions. Consider premedicating with an antihistamine and antipyretic for prophylaxis against hypersensitivity or infusion reactions.
Monitoring Parameters Monitor for hypersensitivity or infusion reactions; infections; worsening of depression, mood changes, or suicidal thoughts
Special Geriatric Considerations Clinical studies did not include sufficient numbers of elderly subjects to note differences in efficacy or toxicity; therefore, use with caution in the elderly.
Dosage Forms Excipient information presented when available (limited, particularly for generics); consult specific product labeling.
Injection, powder for reconstitution:
Benlysta®: 120 mg, 400 mg [contains polysorbate 80, sucrose 80 mg/mL]

◆ **Belladonna Alkaloids With Phenobarbital** *see* Hyoscyamine, Atropine, Scopolamine, and Phenobarbital *on page 963*
◆ **Benadryl® Allergy [OTC]** *see* DiphenhydrAMINE (Systemic) *on page 556*
◆ **Benadryl® Allergy Quick Dissolve [OTC]** *see* DiphenhydrAMINE (Systemic) *on page 556*
◆ **Benadryl® Children's Allergy [OTC]** *see* DiphenhydrAMINE (Systemic) *on page 556*

- **Benadryl® Children's Allergy FastMelt® [OTC]** *see* DiphenhydrAMINE (Systemic) *on page 556*
- **Benadryl® Children's Allergy Perfect Measure™ [OTC]** *see* DiphenhydrAMINE (Systemic) *on page 556*
- **Benadryl® Children's Dye Free Allergy [OTC]** *see* DiphenhydrAMINE (Systemic) *on page 556*
- **Benadryl® Dye-Free Allergy [OTC]** *see* DiphenhydrAMINE (Systemic) *on page 556*
- **Benadryl® Extra Strength Itch Stopping [OTC]** *see* DiphenhydrAMINE (Topical) *on page 559*
- **Benadryl® Itch Relief Extra Strength [OTC]** *see* DiphenhydrAMINE (Topical) *on page 559*
- **Benadryl® Itch Stopping [OTC]** *see* DiphenhydrAMINE (Topical) *on page 559*
- **Benadryl® Itch Stopping Extra Strength [OTC]** *see* DiphenhydrAMINE (Topical) *on page 559*

Benazepril (ben AY ze pril)

Related Information
Angiotensin Agents *on page 2093*
Medication Safety Issues
Sound-alike/look-alike issues:
Benazepril may be confused with Benadryl®
Lotensin® may be confused with Lioresal®, lovastatin
Brand Names: U.S. Lotensin®
Brand Names: Canada Lotensin®
Index Terms Benazepril Hydrochloride
Generic Availability (U.S.) Yes
Pharmacologic Category Angiotensin-Converting Enzyme (ACE) Inhibitor
Use Treatment of hypertension, either alone or in combination with other antihypertensive agents
Unlabeled Use Treatment of left ventricular dysfunction after myocardial infarction
Contraindications Hypersensitivity to benazepril or any component of the formulation; patients with a history of angioedema (with or without prior ACE inhibitor therapy)
Warnings/Precautions Anaphylactic reactions may occur rarely with ACE inhibitors. At any time during treatment (especially following first dose) angioedema may occur rarely with ACE inhibitors. It may involve the head and neck (potentially compromising airway) or the intestine (presenting with abdominal pain). African-Americans and patients with idiopathic or hereditary angioedema may be at an increased risk. Prolonged frequent monitoring may be required especially if tongue, glottis, or larynx are involved as they are associated with airway obstruction. Patients with a history of airway surgery may have a higher risk of airway obstruction. Aggressive early and appropriate management is critical. Contraindicated in patients with history of angioedema with or without prior ACE inhibitor therapy. Hypersensitivity reactions may be seen during hemodialysis (eg, CVVHD) with high-flux dialysis membranes (eg, AN69), and rarely, during low density lipoprotein apheresis with dextran sulfate cellulose. Rare cases of anaphylactoid reactions have been reported in patients undergoing sensitization treatment with hymenoptera (bee, wasp) venom while receiving ACE inhibitors.

Symptomatic hypotension with or without syncope can occur with ACE inhibitors (usually with the first several doses); effects are most often observed in volume depleted patients; close monitoring of patient is required especially with initial dosing and dosing increases; blood pressure must be lowered at a rate appropriate for the patient's clinical condition. Initiation of therapy in patients with ischemic heart disease or cerebrovascular disease warrants close observation due to the potential consequences posed by falling blood pressure (eg, MI, stroke). Use with caution in hypertrophic cardiomyopathy with outflow tract obstruction, severe aortic stenosis, or before, during, or immediately after major surgery.

Hyperkalemia may occur with ACE inhibitors; risk factors include renal dysfunction, diabetes mellitus, concomitant use of potassium-sparing diuretics, potassium supplements and/or potassium containing salts. Use cautiously, if at all, with these agents and monitor potassium closely. Cough may occur with ACE inhibitors. Other causes of cough should be considered (eg, pulmonary congestion in patients with heart failure) and excluded prior to discontinuation. Use with caution in patients with diabetes receiving insulin or oral antidiabetic agents; may be at increased risk for episodes of hypoglycemia.

◀ May be associated with deterioration of renal function and/or increases in serum creatinine, particularly in patients with low renal blood flow (eg, renal artery stenosis, heart failure) whose glomerular filtration rate (GFR) is dependent on efferent arteriolar vasoconstriction by angiotensin II; deterioration may result in oliguria, acute renal failure, and progressive azotemia. Small increases in serum creatinine may occur following initiation; consider discontinuation only in patients with progressive and/or significant deterioration in renal function. Use with caution in patients with unstented unilateral/bilateral renal artery stenosis. When unstented bilateral renal artery stenosis is present, use is generally avoided due to the elevated risk of deterioration in renal function unless possible benefits outweigh risks. Concurrent use of angiotensin receptor blockers may increase the risk of clinically-significant adverse events (eg, renal dysfunction, hyperkalemia).

Rare toxicities associated with ACE inhibitors include cholestatic jaundice (which may progress to fulminant hepatic necrosis), agranulocytosis, neutropenia, or leukopenia with myeloid hypoplasia. Patients with collagen vascular diseases (especially with concomitant renal impairment) or renal impairment alone may be at increased risk for hematologic toxicity; periodically monitor CBC with differential in these patients.

Adverse Reactions (Reflective of adult population; not specific for elderly)

1% to 10%:

Cardiovascular: Postural dizziness (2%)

Central nervous system: Headache (6%), dizziness (4%), somnolence (2%)

Renal: Serum creatinine increased (2%), worsening of renal function may occur in patients with bilateral renal artery stenosis or hypovolemia

Respiratory: Cough (1% to 10%)

Eosinophilic pneumonitis, anaphylaxis, renal insufficiency, and renal failure have been reported with other ACE inhibitors. In addition, a syndrome including fever, myalgia, arthralgia, interstitial nephritis, vasculitis, rash, eosinophilia, and elevated ESR has been reported to be associated with ACE inhibitors.

Drug Interactions

Metabolism/Transport Effects None known.

Avoid Concomitant Use There are no known interactions where it is recommended to avoid concomitant use.

Increased Effect/Toxicity

Benazepril may increase the levels/effects of: Allopurinol; Amifostine; Antihypertensives; AzaTHIOprine; CycloSPORINE; CycloSPORINE (Systemic); Ferric Gluconate; Gold Sodium Thiomalate; Hypotensive Agents; Iron Dextran Complex; Lithium; Nonsteroidal Anti-Inflammatory Agents; RiTUXimab; Sodium Phosphates

The levels/effects of Benazepril may be increased by: Alfuzosin; Aliskiren; Angiotensin II Receptor Blockers; Diazoxide; DPP-IV Inhibitors; Eplerenone; Everolimus; Herbs (Hypotensive Properties); Hydrochlorothiazide; Loop Diuretics; MAO Inhibitors; Pentoxifylline; Phosphodiesterase 5 Inhibitors; Potassium Salts; Potassium-Sparing Diuretics; Prostacyclin Analogues; Sirolimus; Temsirolimus; Thiazide Diuretics; TiZANidine; Tolvaptan; Trimethoprim

Decreased Effect

Benazepril may decrease the levels/effects of: Hydrochlorothiazide

The levels/effects of Benazepril may be decreased by: Antacids; Aprotinin; Herbs (Hypertensive Properties); Icatibant; Lanthanum; Methylphenidate; Nonsteroidal Anti-Inflammatory Agents; Salicylates; Yohimbine

Ethanol/Nutrition/Herb Interactions

Food: Potassium supplements and/or potassium-containing salts may cause or worsen hyperkalemia. Management: Consult prescriber before consuming a potassium-rich diet, potassium supplements, or salt substitutes.

Herb/Nutraceutical: Some herbal medications may worsen hypertension (eg, licorice); others may increase the antihypertensive effect of benazepril (eg, shepherd's purse). Management: Avoid bayberry, blue cohosh, cayenne, ephedra, ginger, ginseng (American), kola, licorice, and yohimbe. Avoid black cohosh, California poppy, coleus, golden seal, hawthorn, mistletoe, periwinkle, quinine, and shepherd's purse.

Stability Store at ≤30°C (86°F). Protect from moisture.

Mechanism of Action Competitive inhibition of angiotensin I being converted to angiotensin II, a potent vasoconstrictor, through the angiotensin I-converting enzyme (ACE) activity, with resultant lower levels of angiotensin II which causes an increase in plasma renin activity and a reduction in aldosterone secretion

Pharmacodynamics/Kinetics

Reduction in plasma angiotensin-converting enzyme (ACE) activity:

Onset of action: Peak effect: 1-2 hours after 2-20 mg dose

Duration: >90% inhibition for 24 hours after 5-20 mg dose

Reduction in blood pressure:
  Peak effect: Single dose: 2-4 hours; Continuous therapy: 2 weeks
Absorption: Rapid (37%); food does not alter significantly; metabolite (benazeprilat) itself unsuitable for oral administration due to poor absorption
Distribution: V_d: ~8.7 L
Protein binding:
  Benazepril: ~97%
  Benazeprilat: ~95%
Metabolism: Rapidly and extensively hepatic to its active metabolite, benazeprilat, via enzymatic hydrolysis; extensive first-pass effect
Half-life elimination: Benazeprilat: Effective: 10-11 hours; Terminal: Adults: 22 hours
Time to peak: Parent drug: 0.5-1 hour
Excretion:
  Urine (trace amounts as benazepril; 20% as benazeprilat; 12% as other metabolites)
  Clearance: Nonrenal clearance (ie, biliary, metabolic) appears to contribute to the elimination of benazeprilat (11% to 12%), particularly patients with severe renal impairment; hepatic clearance is the main elimination route of unchanged benazepril
  Dialysis: ~6% of metabolite removed within 4 hours of dialysis following 10 mg of benazepril administered 2 hours prior to procedure; parent compound not found in dialysate

Dosage

Geriatric Oral: Initial: 5-10 mg/day in single or divided doses; usual range: 20-40 mg/day; adjust for renal function. Also see "Note" in adult dosing.

Adult Hypertension: Oral: Initial: 10 mg/day in patients not receiving a diuretic; 20-80 mg/day as a single dose or 2 divided doses; the need for twice-daily dosing should be assessed by monitoring peak (2-6 hours after dosing) and trough responses.

Note: Patients taking diuretics should have them discontinued 2-3 days prior to starting benazepril. If they cannot be discontinued, then initial dose should be 5 mg; restart after blood pressure is stabilized if needed.

Renal Impairment

Cl_{cr} <30 mL/minute: Administer 5 mg/day initially; maximum daily dose: 40 mg.

Hemodialysis: Moderately dialyzable (20% to 50%); administer dose postdialysis or administer 25% to 35% supplemental dose.

Peritoneal dialysis: Supplemental dose is not necessary.

Monitoring Parameters Blood pressure; serum creatinine and potassium; if patient has collagen vascular disease and/or renal impairment, periodically monitor CBC with differential

Special Geriatric Considerations Due to frequent decreases in glomerular filtration (also Cl_{cr}) with aging, elderly patients may have exaggerated responses to ACE inhibitors; differences in clinical response due to hepatic changes are not observed. ACE inhibitors may be preferred agents in elderly patients with congestive heart failure and diabetes mellitus. Diabetic proteinuria is reduced and insulin sensitivity is enhanced. In general, the side effect profile is favorable in elderly and causes little or no CNS confusion; use lowest dose recommendations initially. Many elderly may be volume depleted due to diuretic use and/or blunted thirst reflex resulting in inadequate fluid intake.

Benazepril and benazeprilat are substantially excreted by the kidney. Because elderly are more likely to have decreased renal function, care should be taken in dose selection, and it may be useful to monitor renal function.

Dosage Forms Excipient information presented when available (limited, particularly for generics); consult specific product labeling. [DSC] = Discontinued product

Tablet, oral, as hydrochloride: 5 mg, 10 mg, 20 mg, 40 mg
  Lotensin®: 5 mg [DSC], 10 mg, 20 mg, 40 mg

Extemporaneously Prepared To prepare a 2 mg/mL suspension, mix 15 benazepril 20 mg tablets in a bottle with Ora-Plus® 75 mL. Shake for 2 minutes, allow suspension to stand for ≥1 hour, then shake again for at least 1 additional minute. Add Ora-Sweet® 75 mL to suspension and shake to disperse. Will make 150 mL of a 2 mg/mL suspension. Store under refrigeration at 2°C to 8°C (36°F to 46°F) for up to 30 days. Shake prior to each use.

Benazepril and Hydrochlorothiazide
(ben AY ze pril & hye droe klor oh THYE a zide)

Related Information
Benazepril *on page 197*
Hydrochlorothiazide *on page 933*
Brand Names: U.S. Lotensin HCT®
Index Terms Benazepril Hydrochloride and Hydrochlorothiazide; Hydrochlorothiazide and Benazepril
Generic Availability (U.S.) Yes

Pharmacologic Category Angiotensin-Converting Enzyme (ACE) Inhibitor; Diuretic, Thiazide

Use Treatment of hypertension

Dosage

  Geriatric Dose is individualized.

  Adult Note: Not for initial therapy; dose should be individualized.

    Hypertension: Oral: Range: Benazepril: 5-20 mg; Hydrochlorothiazide: 6.25-25 mg/day

      Add-on therapy:

        Patients not adequately controlled on benazepril monotherapy: Initiate benazepril 10-20 mg/hydrochlorothiazide 12.5 mg; titrate to effect at 2- to 3-week intervals

        Patients controlled on hydrochlorothiazide 25 mg/day but experience significant potassium loss with this regimen: Initiate benazepril 5 mg/hydrochlorothiazide 6.25 mg

      Replacement therapy: Substitute for the individually titrated components

  Renal Impairment $Cl_{cr} \leq 30$ mL/minute: Not recommended; loop diuretics are preferred.

Special Geriatric Considerations See individual agents. Combination products are not recommended as first-line treatment. Use only if doses of individual agents correspond to the combination available.

Dosage Forms Excipient information presented when available (limited, particularly for generics); consult specific product labeling.

  Tablet: 5/6.25: Benazepril hydrochloride 5 mg and hydrochlorothiazide 6.25 mg; 10/12.5: Benazepril hydrochloride 10 mg and hydrochlorothiazide 12.5 mg; 20/12.5: Benazepril hydrochloride 20 mg and hydrochlorothiazide 12.5 mg; 20/25: Benazepril hydrochloride 20 mg and hydrochlorothiazide 25 mg

  Lotensin HCT® 10/12.5: Benazepril hydrochloride 10 mg and hydrochlorothiazide 12.5 mg

  Lotensin HCT® 20/12.5: Benazepril hydrochloride 20 mg and hydrochlorothiazide 12.5 mg

  Lotensin HCT® 20/25: Benazepril hydrochloride 20 mg and hydrochlorothiazide 25 mg

♦ **Benazepril Hydrochloride** see Benazepril on page 197
♦ **Benazepril Hydrochloride and Amlodipine Besylate** see Amlodipine and Benazepril on page 106
♦ **Benazepril Hydrochloride and Hydrochlorothiazide** see Benazepril and Hydrochlorothiazide on page 199
♦ **Benefiber® [OTC]** see Wheat Dextrin on page 2039
♦ **Benefiber® Plus Calcium [OTC]** see Wheat Dextrin on page 2039
♦ **Benemid [DSC]** see Probenecid on page 1604
♦ **Benicar®** see Olmesartan on page 1411
♦ **Benicar HCT®** see Olmesartan and Hydrochlorothiazide on page 1413
♦ **Benlysta®** see Belimumab on page 195
♦ **Bentyl®** see Dicyclomine on page 539
♦ **Benzathine Benzylpenicillin** see Penicillin G Benzathine on page 1497
♦ **Benzathine Penicillin G** see Penicillin G Benzathine on page 1497
♦ **Benzene Hexachloride** see Lindane on page 1135
♦ **Benzhexol Hydrochloride** see Trihexyphenidyl on page 1968

Benzonatate (ben ZOE na tate)

Brand Names: U.S. Tessalon®; Zonatuss™

Index Terms Tessalon Perles

Generic Availability (U.S.) Yes: Capsule (softgel)

Pharmacologic Category Antitussive

Use Symptomatic relief of nonproductive cough

Contraindications Hypersensitivity to benzonatate, related compounds (such as tetracaine), or any component of the formulation

Warnings/Precautions Severe reactions, including bronchospasm, cardiovascular collapse and laryngospasm have been reported. May be related to localized anesthetic effects due to sucking or chewing the capsule. Isolated cases of abnormal behavior including mental confusion and visual hallucinations have been reported; may be related to prior sensitivity to related agents (eg, tetracaine, procaine) or interaction with concurrent medications. Signs and symptoms of overdose (restlessness, tremors, convulsion, coma, cardiac arrest) may occur within 15-20 minutes after ingestion. Death has been reported within 1 hour.

Adverse Reactions (Reflective of adult population; not specific for elderly) Frequency not defined.

  Central nervous system: Confusion, dizziness, hallucinations, headache, sedation

  Dermatologic: Pruritus, skin eruptions

  Gastrointestinal: Constipation, GI upset, nausea

  Neuromuscular & skeletal: Chest numbness

  Ocular: Burning sensation in eyes

Respiratory: Nasal congestion

Miscellaneous: Chill sensation, hypersensitivity reactions (bronchospasm, laryngospasm, cardiovascular collapse)

Drug Interactions

Metabolism/Transport Effects None known.

Avoid Concomitant Use There are no known interactions where it is recommended to avoid concomitant use.

Increased Effect/Toxicity There are no known significant interactions involving an increase in effect.

Decreased Effect There are no known significant interactions involving a decrease in effect.

Stability Store at room temperature of 25°C (77°F); excursions permitted to 15°C to 30°C (59°F to 86°F).

Mechanism of Action Tetracaine congener with antitussive properties; suppresses cough by topical anesthetic action on the respiratory stretch receptors

Pharmacodynamics/Kinetics

Onset of action: Therapeutic: 15-20 minutes

Duration: 3-8 hours

Dosage

Geriatric & Adult Cough: Oral: 100-200 mg 3 times/day as needed; maximum dose: 600 mg/day

Administration Swallow capsule whole (do not break. chew, dissolve, cut, or crush).

Monitoring Parameters Monitor patient's chest sounds and respiratory pattern

Special Geriatric Considerations No specific geriatric information is available about benzonatate. Avoid use in patients with impaired gag reflex or who cannot swallow the capsule whole.

Dosage Forms Excipient information presented when available (limited, particularly for generics); consult specific product labeling.

Capsule, oral:

Zonatuss™: 150 mg

Capsule, softgel, oral: 100 mg, 200 mg

Tessalon®: 100 mg, 200 mg

Benztropine (BENZ troe peen)

Related Information

Antiparkinsonian Agents *on page 2101*

Beers Criteria – Potentially Inappropriate Medications for Geriatrics *on page 2183*

Medication Safety Issues

Sound-alike/look-alike issues:

Benztropine may be confused with bromocriptine

BEERS Criteria medication:

This drug may be potentially inappropriate for use in geriatric patients (Parkinson's disease: Quality of evidence - moderate; Strength of recommendation - strong).

Brand Names: U.S. Cogentin®

Brand Names: Canada Apo-Benztropine®; Benztropine Omega; PMS-Benztropine

Index Terms Benztropine Mesylate

Generic Availability (U.S.) Yes

Pharmacologic Category Anti-Parkinson's Agent, Anticholinergic; Anticholinergic Agent

Use Adjunctive treatment of Parkinson's disease; treatment of drug-induced extrapyramidal symptoms (except tardive dyskinesia)

Contraindications Hypersensitivity to benztropine or any component of the formulation; pyloric or duodenal obstruction, stenosing peptic ulcers; bladder neck obstructions; achalasia; myasthenia gravis

Warnings/Precautions Use with caution in hot weather or during exercise. May cause anhydrosis and hyperthermia, which may be severe. The risk is increased in hot environments, particularly in the elderly, alcoholics, patients with CNS disease, and those with prolonged outdoor exposure.

Avoid use of oral benztropine in older adults for prevention of extrapyramidal symptoms with antipsychotics and alternative agents preferred in the treatment of Parkinson's disease. May be inappropriate in older adults depending on comorbidities (eg, dementia, delirium) due to its potent anticholinergic effects (Beers Criteria).

Use with caution in patients with tachycardia, cardiac arrhythmias, hypertension, hypotension, glaucoma, prostatic hyperplasia (especially in the elderly), any tendency toward urinary retention, liver or kidney disorders, and obstructive disease of the GI or GU tract. When given in large doses or to susceptible patients, may cause weakness and inability to move particular muscle groups.

May be associated with confusion or hallucinations (generally at higher dosages). Intensification of symptoms or toxic psychosis may occur in patients with mental disorders. May cause CNS depression, which may impair physical or mental abilities; patients must be cautioned about performing tasks which require mental alertness (eg, operating machinery or driving). Benztropine does not relieve symptoms of tardive dyskinesia.

Adverse Reactions (Reflective of adult population; not specific for elderly) Frequency not defined.

Cardiovascular: Tachycardia

Central nervous system: Confusion, disorientation, memory impairment, toxic psychosis, visual hallucinations

Dermatologic: Rash

Endocrine & metabolic: Heat stroke, hyperthermia

Gastrointestinal: Constipation, dry throat, ileus, nasal dryness, nausea, vomiting, xerostomia

Genitourinary: Urinary retention, dysuria

Ocular: Blurred vision, mydriasis

Miscellaneous: Fever

Drug Interactions

Metabolism/Transport Effects Substrate of CYP2D6 (minor); **Note:** Assignment of Major/Minor substrate status based on clinically relevant drug interaction potential

Avoid Concomitant Use There are no known interactions where it is recommended to avoid concomitant use.

Increased Effect/Toxicity

Benztropine may increase the levels/effects of: AbobotulinumtoxinA; Anticholinergics; Cannabinoids; OnabotulinumtoxinA; Potassium Chloride; RimabotulinumtoxinB

The levels/effects of Benztropine may be increased by: Pramlintide

Decreased Effect

Benztropine may decrease the levels/effects of: Acetylcholinesterase Inhibitors (Central); Ioflupane I 123; Secretin

The levels/effects of Benztropine may be decreased by: Acetylcholinesterase Inhibitors (Central); Peginterferon Alfa-2b

Ethanol/Nutrition/Herb Interactions Ethanol: Avoid ethanol (may increase CNS depression).

Mechanism of Action Possesses both anticholinergic and antihistaminic effects. *In vitro* anticholinergic activity approximates that of atropine; *in vivo* it is only about half as active as atropine. Animal data suggest its antihistaminic activity and duration of action approach that of pyrilamine maleate. May also inhibit the reuptake and storage of dopamine, thereby prolonging the action of dopamine.

Pharmacodynamics/Kinetics

Onset of action: Oral: Within 1 hour; Parenteral: Within 15 minutes

Duration: 6-48 hours

Metabolism: Hepatic (N-oxidation, N-dealkylation, and ring hydroxylation)

Bioavailability: 29%

Dosage

Geriatric Refer to adult dosing. Use caution or avoid; anticholinergics generally not tolerated in older adults.

Adult

Acute dystonia: I.M., I.V.: 1-2 mg

Drug-induced extrapyramidal symptom: Oral, I.M., I.V.: 1-4 mg 1-2 times/day or 1-2 mg 2-3 times/day for reactions developing soon after initiation of antipsychotic medication; usually provides relief within 1-2 days, but may continue for up to 1-2 weeks; withdraw after 1-2 weeks to reassess continued need for therapy

Parkinsonism, idiopathic or postencephalitic: Oral, I.M., I.V.: Usual dose: 1-2 mg/day; range: 0.5-6 mg/day in a single dose at bedtime or divided in 2-4 doses; titrate dose in 0.5 mg increments at 5- to 6-day intervals up to a maximum of 6 mg.

Administration

Oral: May be given with or without food.

Injectable: May administer I.M or I.V. if oral route is unacceptable. Manufacturer's labeling states there is no difference in onset of effect after I.V. or I.M. injection and therefore there is usually no need to use the I.V. route. No specific instructions on administering benztropine I.V. are provided in the labeling. The I.V. route has been reported in the literature (slow I.V. push when reported), although specific instructions are lacking (Duncan, 2001; Lydon, 1998; Sachdev, 1993; Schramm, 2002).

Monitoring Parameters Symptoms of EPS or Parkinson's, pulse, anticholinergic effects

Special Geriatric Considerations Anticholinergic agents are generally not well tolerated in the elderly (often results in bowel, bladder, and CNS adverse effects) and their use should be avoided when possible. In the elderly, anticholinergic agents should not be used as prophylaxis against extrapyramidal symptoms.

This medication is considered to be potentially inappropriate in this patient population (Beers Criteria: Parkinson's disease: Quality of evidence - moderate; Strength of recommendation - strong).

Dosage Forms Excipient information presented when available (limited, particularly for generics); consult specific product labeling.

Injection, solution, as mesylate: 1 mg/mL

Cogentin®: 1 mg/mL

Tablet, oral, as mesylate: 0.5 mg, 1 mg, 2 mg

♦ **Benztropine Mesylate** see Benztropine on page 201
♦ **Benzylpenicillin Benzathine** see Penicillin G Benzathine on page 1497
♦ **Benzylpenicillin Potassium** see Penicillin G (Parenteral/Aqueous) on page 1500
♦ **Benzylpenicillin Sodium** see Penicillin G (Parenteral/Aqueous) on page 1500

Bepotastine (be poe TAS teen)

Brand Names: U.S. Bepreve®
Index Terms Bepotastine Besilate
Generic Availability (U.S.) No
Pharmacologic Category Histamine H_1 Antagonist; Histamine H_1 Antagonist, Second Generation; Mast Cell Stabilizer
Use Treatment of itching associated with allergic conjunctivitis
Dosage
Geriatric & Adult Allergic conjunctivitis: Ophthalmic: Instill 1 drop into the affected eye(s) twice daily
Special Geriatric Considerations Evaluate the patient's or caregiver's ability to safely administer the correct dose of ophthalmic medication.
Dosage Forms Excipient information presented when available (limited, particularly for generics); consult specific product labeling.

Solution, ophthalmic, as besilate [drops]:

Bepreve®: 1.5% (5 mL, 10 mL) [contains benzalkonium chloride]

♦ **Bepotastine Besilate** see Bepotastine on page 203
♦ **Bepreve®** see Bepotastine on page 203

Besifloxacin (be si FLOX a sin)

Brand Names: U.S. Besivance™
Index Terms Besifloxacin Hydrochloride; BOL-303224-A; SS734
Generic Availability (U.S.) No
Pharmacologic Category Antibiotic, Ophthalmic; Antibiotic, Quinolone
Use Treatment of bacterial conjunctivitis
Dosage
Geriatric & Adult Bacterial conjunctivitis: Ophthalmic: Instill 1 drop into affected eye(s) 3 times/day (4-12 hours apart) for 7 days
Special Geriatric Considerations Evaluate the patient's or caregiver's ability to safely administer the correct dose of ophthalmic medication.
Dosage Forms Excipient information presented when available (limited, particularly for generics); consult specific product labeling.

Suspension, ophthalmic [drops]:

Besivance™: 0.6% (5 mL) [contains benzalkonium chloride]

♦ **Besifloxacin Hydrochloride** see Besifloxacin on page 203
♦ **Besivance™** see Besifloxacin on page 203
♦ **β,β-Dimethylcysteine** see PenicillAMINE on page 1493
♦ **Betagan®** see Levobunolol on page 1112
♦ **Beta-HC® [OTC]** see Hydrocortisone (Topical) on page 943

Betamethasone (bay ta METH a sone)

Related Information
Corticosteroids Systemic Equivalencies *on page 2112*
Topical Corticosteroids *on page 2113*

Medication Safety Issues
Sound-alike/look-alike issues:
Luxiq® may be confused with Lasix®
International issues:
Beta-Val [U.S.] may be confused with Betanol brand name for metipranolol [Monaco]

Brand Names: U.S. Celestone®; Celestone® Soluspan®; Diprolene®; Diprolene® AF; Luxiq®

Brand Names: Canada Betaderm; Betaject™; Betnesol®; Betnovate®; Celestone® Soluspan®; Diprolene®; Diprolene® Glycol; Diprosone®; Ectosone; Prevex® B; ratio-Ectosone; Ratio-Topilene; ratio-Topilene; Ratio-Topisone; ratio-Topisone; Rivasone; Rolene; Rosone; Taro-Sone; Valisone® Scalp Lotion

Index Terms Betamethasone Dipropionate; Betamethasone Dipropionate, Augmented; Betamethasone Sodium Phosphate; Betamethasone Valerate; Flubenisolone

Generic Availability (U.S.) Yes: Excludes foam, solution

Pharmacologic Category Corticosteroid, Systemic; Corticosteroid, Topical

Use Inflammatory dermatoses such as seborrheic or atopic dermatitis, neurodermatitis, anogenital pruritus, psoriasis, inflammatory phase of xerosis

Unlabeled Use Accelerate fetal lung maturation in patients with preterm labor

Contraindications Hypersensitivity to betamethasone, other corticosteroids, or any component of the formulation; systemic fungal infections; I.M. administration contraindicated in idiopathic thrombocytopenia purpura

Warnings/Precautions Very high potency topical products are not for treatment of rosacea, perioral dermatitis; not for use on face, groin, or axillae; not for use in a diapered area. Avoid concurrent use of other corticosteroids.

May cause hypercorticism or suppression of hypothalamic-pituitary-adrenal (HPA) axis, particularly in patients receiving high doses for prolonged periods. HPA axis suppression may lead to adrenal crisis. Withdrawal and discontinuation of a corticosteroid should be done slowly and carefully. Particular care is required when patients are transferred from systemic corticosteroids to inhaled products due to possible adrenal insufficiency or withdrawal from steroids, including an increase in allergic symptoms. Patients receiving >20 mg per day of prednisone (or equivalent) may be most susceptible. Fatalities have occurred due to adrenal insufficiency in asthmatic patients during and after transfer from systemic corticosteroids to aerosol steroids; aerosol steroids do not provide the systemic steroid needed to treat patients having trauma, surgery, or infections. In stressful situations, HPA axis-suppressed patients should receive adequate supplementation with natural glucocorticoids (hydrocortisone or cortisone) rather than betamethasone (due to lack of mineralocorticoid activity).

Acute myopathy has been reported with high dose corticosteroids, usually in patients with neuromuscular transmission disorders; may involve ocular and/or respiratory muscles; monitor creatine kinase; recovery may be delayed. Corticosteroid use may cause psychiatric disturbances, including depression, euphoria, insomnia, mood swings, and personality changes. Pre-existing psychiatric conditions may be exacerbated by corticosteroid use. Prolonged use of corticosteroids may also increase the incidence of secondary infection, mask acute infection (including fungal infections), prolong or exacerbate viral infections, or limit response to vaccines. Exposure to chickenpox should be avoided; corticosteroids should not be used to treat ocular herpes simplex. Corticosteroids should not be used for cerebral malaria or viral hepatitis. Close observation is required in patients with latent tuberculosis and/or TB reactivity; restrict use in active TB (only in conjunction with antituberculosis treatment). Prolonged treatment with corticosteroids has been associated with the development of Kaposi's sarcoma (case reports); if noted, discontinuation of therapy should be considered. High-dose corticosteroids should not be used to manage acute head injury.

Use with caution in patients with thyroid disease, hepatic impairment, renal impairment, cardiovascular disease, diabetes, glaucoma, cataracts, myasthenia gravis, patients at risk for osteoporosis, patients at risk for seizures, or GI diseases (diverticulitis, peptic ulcer, ulcerative colitis) due to perforation risk. Use caution following acute MI (corticosteroids have been associated with myocardial rupture). Because of the risk of adverse effects, systemic corticosteroids should be used cautiously in the elderly in the smallest possible effective dose for the shortest duration. Do not use occlusive dressings on weeping or exudative lesions and general caution with occlusive dressings should be observed; adverse effects may be

BETAMETHASONE

increased. Discontinue if skin irritation or contact dermatitis should occur; do not use in patients with decreased skin circulation. Withdraw therapy with gradual tapering of dose.

Adverse Reactions (Reflective of adult population; not specific for elderly)

Systemic:

Cardiovascular: Congestive heart failure, edema, hyper-/hypotension

Central nervous system: Dizziness, headache, insomnia, intracranial pressure increased, lightheadedness, nervousness, pseudotumor cerebri, seizure, vertigo

Dermatologic: Ecchymoses, facial erythema, fragile skin, hirsutism, hyper-/hypopigmentation, perioral dermatitis (oral), petechiae, striae, wound healing impaired

Endocrine & metabolic: Amenorrhea, Cushing's syndrome, diabetes mellitus, growth suppression, hyperglycemia, hypokalemia, menstrual irregularities, pituitary-adrenal axis suppression, protein catabolism, sodium retention, water retention

Local: Injection site reactions (intra-articular use), sterile abscess

Neuromuscular & skeletal: Arthralgia, muscle atrophy, fractures, muscle weakness, myopathy, osteoporosis, necrosis (femoral and humeral heads)

Ocular: Cataracts, glaucoma, intraocular pressure increased

Miscellaneous: Anaphylactoid reaction, diaphoresis, hypersensitivity, secondary infection

Topical:

Dermatologic: Acneiform eruptions, allergic dermatitis, burning, dry skin, erythema, folliculitis, hypertrichosis, irritation, miliaria, pruritus, skin atrophy, striae, vesiculation

Endocrine and metabolic effects have occasionally been reported with topical use.

Drug Interactions

Metabolism/Transport Effects None known.

Avoid Concomitant Use

Avoid concomitant use of Betamethasone with any of the following: Aldesleukin; BCG; Mifepristone; Natalizumab; Pimecrolimus; Tacrolimus (Topical)

Increased Effect/Toxicity

Betamethasone may increase the levels/effects of: Acetylcholinesterase Inhibitors; Amphotericin B; Deferasirox; Leflunomide; Loop Diuretics; Natalizumab; NSAID (COX-2 Inhibitor); NSAID (Nonselective); Thiazide Diuretics; Vaccines (Live); Warfarin

The levels/effects of Betamethasone may be increased by: Antifungal Agents (Azole Derivatives, Systemic); Aprepitant; Calcium Channel Blockers (Nondihydropyridine); Denosumab; Estrogen Derivatives; Fluconazole; Fosaprepitant; Indacaterol; Macrolide Antibiotics; Mifepristone; Neuromuscular-Blocking Agents (Nondepolarizing); Pimecrolimus; Quinolone Antibiotics; Roflumilast; Salicylates; Tacrolimus (Topical); Telaprevir; Trastuzumab

Decreased Effect

Betamethasone may decrease the levels/effects of: Aldesleukin; Antidiabetic Agents; BCG; Calcitriol; Coccidioidin Skin Test; Corticorelin; Hyaluronidase; Isoniazid; Salicylates; Sipuleucel-T; Telaprevir; Vaccines (Inactivated)

The levels/effects of Betamethasone may be decreased by: Aminoglutethimide; Antacids; Barbiturates; Bile Acid Sequestrants; Echinacea; Mifepristone; Mitotane; Primidone; Rifamycin Derivatives

Ethanol/Nutrition/Herb Interactions

Ethanol: Avoid ethanol (may enhance gastric mucosal irritation).

Food: Betamethasone interferes with calcium absorption.

Herb/Nutraceutical: Avoid cat's claw, echinacea (have immunostimulant properties).

Mechanism of Action Controls the rate of protein synthesis; depresses the migration of polymorphonuclear leukocytes, fibroblasts; reverses capillary permeability and lysosomal stabilization at the cellular level to prevent or control inflammation

Pharmacodynamics/Kinetics

Protein binding: 64%

Metabolism: Hepatic

Half-life elimination: 6.5 hours

Time to peak, serum: I.V.: 10-36 minutes

Excretion: Urine (<5% as unchanged drug)

Dosage

Geriatric Refer to adult dosing. Use the lowest effective dose.

Adult Base dosage on severity of disease and patient response

Inflammatory conditions:

Oral: 2.4-4.8 mg/day in 2-4 doses; range: 0.6-7.2 mg/day

I.M.: Betamethasone sodium phosphate and betamethasone acetate: 0.6-9 mg/day (generally, 1/3 to 1/2 of oral dose) divided every 12-24 hours

Psoriasis (scalp): Topical (foam): Apply to the scalp twice daily, once in the morning and once at night.

Rheumatoid arthritis/osteoarthritis:
Intrabursal, intra-articular, intradermal: 0.25-2 mL
Intralesional:
Very large joints: 1-2 mL
Large joints: 1 mL
Medium joints: 0.5-1 mL
Small joints: 0.25-0.5 mL
Steroid-responsive dermatoses: Therapy should be discontinued when control is achieved; if no improvement is seen, reassessment of diagnosis may be necessary.
Gel, augmented formulation: Apply once or twice daily; rub in gently. **Note:** Do not exceed 2 weeks of treatment or 50 g/week.
Lotion: Apply a few drops twice daily
Augmented formulation: Apply a few drops once or twice daily; rub in gently. **Note:** Do not exceed 2 weeks of treatment or 50 mL/week.
Cream/ointment: Apply once or twice daily
Augmented formulation: Apply once or twice daily. **Note:** Do not exceed 2 weeks of treatment or 45 g/week.
Hepatic Impairment Adjustments may be necessary in patients with liver failure because betamethasone is extensively metabolized in the liver

Administration
Oral: Not for alternate day therapy; once daily doses should be given in the morning.
I.M.: Do **not** give injectable sodium phosphate/acetate suspension I.V.
Topical: Apply topical sparingly to areas. Not for use on broken skin or in areas of infection. Do not apply to wet skin unless directed; do not cover with occlusive dressing. Do not apply very high potency agents to face, groin, axillae, or perianal area.
Foam: Invert can and dispense a small amount onto a saucer or other cool surface. Do not dispense directly into hands. Pick up small amounts of foam and gently massage into affected areas until foam disappears. Repeat until entire affected scalp area is treated.

Monitoring Parameters Blood pressure, blood glucose, electrolytes

Test Interactions May suppress the wheal and flare reactions to skin test antigens

Pharmacotherapy Pearls
Very High Potency: Augmented betamethasone dipropionate ointment, lotion
High Potency: Augmented betamethasone dipropionate cream, betamethasone dipropionate cream and ointment
Intermediate Potency: Betamethasone dipropionate lotion, betamethasone valerate cream

Special Geriatric Considerations Because of the risk of adverse effects, systemic corticosteroids should be used cautiously in the elderly, in the smallest possible dose, and for the shortest possible time.

Dosage Forms Excipient information presented when available (limited, particularly for generics); consult specific product labeling.
Aerosol, foam, topical, as valerate:
Luxiq®: 0.12% (50 g, 100 g) [contains ethanol 60.4%]
Cream, topical, as dipropionate [strength expressed as base]: 0.05% (15 g, 45 g, 50 g)
Cream, topical, as dipropionate [strength expressed as base, augmented]: 0.05% (15 g, 50 g)
Diprolene® AF: 0.05% (15 g, 50 g)
Cream, topical, as valerate [strength expressed as base]: 0.1% (15 g, 45 g)
Gel, topical, as dipropionate [strength expressed as base, augmented]: 0.05% (15 g, 50 g)
Injection, suspension: Betamethasone sodium phosphate 3 mg and betamethasone acetate 3 mg per 1 mL (5 mL)
Celestone® Soluspan®: Betamethasone sodium phosphate 3 mg and betamethasone acetate 3 mg per 1 mL (5 mL) [contains benzalkonium chloride, edetate disodium; total of 6 mg/mL]
Lotion, topical, as dipropionate [strength expressed as base]: 0.05% (60 mL)
Lotion, topical, as dipropionate [strength expressed as base, augmented]: 0.05% (30 mL, 60 mL)
Diprolene®: 0.05% (30 mL, 60 mL) [contains isopropyl alcohol 30%]
Lotion, topical, as valerate [strength expressed as base]: 0.1% (60 mL)
Ointment, topical, as dipropionate [strength expressed as base]: 0.05% (15 g, 45 g)
Ointment, topical, as dipropionate [strength expressed as base, augmented]: 0.05% (15 g, 45 g, 50 g)
Diprolene®: 0.05% (15 g, 50 g)
Ointment, topical, as valerate [strength expressed as base]: 0.1% (15 g, 45 g)
Solution, oral, as base:
Celestone®: 0.6 mg/5 mL (118 mL) [contains ethanol <1%, propylene glycol, sodium benzoate]

◆ **Betamethasone Dipropionate** see Betamethasone on page 204
◆ **Betamethasone Dipropionate, Augmented** see Betamethasone on page 204

- **Betamethasone Sodium Phosphate** *see* Betamethasone *on page* 204
- **Betamethasone Valerate** *see* Betamethasone *on page* 204
- **Betapace®** *see* Sotalol *on page* 1800
- **Betapace AF®** *see* Sotalol *on page* 1800
- **Beta Sal® [OTC]** *see* Salicylic Acid *on page* 1743
- **Betaseron®** *see* Interferon Beta-1b *on page* 1032

Betaxolol (Systemic) (be TAKS oh lol)

Related Information
Beta-Blockers *on page* 2108

Medication Safety Issues
Sound-alike/look-alike issues:
Betaxolol may be confused with bethanechol, labetalol

Brand Names: U.S. Kerlone®

Index Terms Betaxolol Hydrochloride

Generic Availability (U.S.) Yes

Pharmacologic Category Beta-Blocker, Beta-1 Selective

Use Management of hypertension

Unlabeled Use Treatment of coronary artery disease

Contraindications Hypersensitivity to betaxolol or any component of the formulation; sinus bradycardia; heart block greater than first-degree (except in patients with a functioning artificial pacemaker); cardiogenic shock; uncompensated cardiac failure

Warnings/Precautions Consider pre-existing conditions (such as sick sinus syndrome) before initiating. Administer cautiously in compensated heart failure and monitor for a worsening of the condition. Beta-blocker therapy should not be withdrawn abruptly (particularly in patients with CAD), but gradually tapered to avoid acute tachycardia, hypertension, and/or ischemia. Chronic beta-blocker therapy should not be routinely withdrawn prior to major surgery. Use caution with concurrent use of digoxin, verapamil, or diltiazem; bradycardia or heart block can occur. Use with caution in patients receiving inhaled anesthetic agents known to depress myocardial contractility. Bradycardia may be observed more frequently in elderly patients (>65 years of age); dosage reductions may be necessary.

May precipitate or aggravate symptoms of arterial insufficiency in patients with peripheral vascular disease (PVD) and Raynaud's disease; use with caution; monitor for progression of arterial obstruction. In general, beta-blockers should be avoided in patients with bronchospastic disease. Betaxolol, with beta$_1$ selectivity, may be used cautiously in bronchospastic disease with the lowest possible dose (eg, 5-10 mg/day), availability of a bronchodilator, and close monitoring; if dosage increase is indicated, administer in divided doses. Use cautiously in patients with diabetes because it may potentiate and/or mask prominent hypoglycemic symptoms. May mask signs of hyperthyroidism (eg, tachycardia); use caution if hyperthyroidism is suspected, abrupt withdrawal may precipitate thyroid storm. May induce or exacerbate psoriasis. Use with caution in patients with cerebrovascular insufficiency; hypotension and decreased heart rate may reduce cerebral blood flow. Dosage adjustment required in severe renal impairment and in patients on dialysis. Use with caution in patients with myasthenia gravis (may potentiate myasthenia-related muscle weakness, including diplopia and ptosis) or psychiatric disease (may cause CNS depression). Adequate alpha-blockade is required prior to use of any beta-blocker for patients with untreated pheochromocytoma. Use caution with history of severe anaphylaxis to allergens; patients taking beta-blockers may become more sensitive to repeated challenges. Treatment of anaphylaxis (eg, epinephrine) in patients taking beta-blockers may be ineffective or promote undesirable effects.

Adverse Reactions (Reflective of adult population; not specific for elderly) 2% to 10%:
Cardiovascular: Bradycardia (6% to 8%; symptomatic bradycardia: <1% to 2%; dose-dependent), chest pain (2% to 7%), palpitation (2%), edema (≤2%; similar to placebo)
Central nervous system: Fatigue (3% to 10%), insomnia (1% to 5%), lethargy (3%)
Gastrointestinal: Nausea (2% to 6%), dyspepsia (4% to 5%), diarrhea (2%)
Neuromuscular & skeletal: Arthralgia (3% to 5%), paresthesia (2%)
Respiratory: Dyspnea (2%), pharyngitis (2%)
Miscellaneous: Antinuclear antibody positive (5%), cold extremities (2%)

Drug Interactions
Metabolism/Transport Effects Substrate of CYP1A2 (major), CYP2D6 (minor); **Note:** Assignment of Major/Minor substrate status based on clinically relevant drug interaction potential; **Inhibits** CYP2D6 (weak)

Avoid Concomitant Use
Avoid concomitant use of Betaxolol (Systemic) with any of the following: Floctafenine; Methacholine

Increased Effect/Toxicity

Betaxolol (Systemic) may increase the levels/effects of: Alpha-/Beta-Agonists (Direct-Acting); Alpha1-Blockers; Alpha2-Agonists; Amifostine; Antihypertensives; Antipsychotic Agents (Phenothiazines); ARIPiprazole; Bupivacaine; Cardiac Glycosides; Cholinergic Agonists; Fingolimod; Hypotensive Agents; Insulin; Lidocaine; Lidocaine (Systemic); Lidocaine (Topical); Mepivacaine; Methacholine; Midodrine; RiTUXimab; Sulfonylureas

The levels/effects of Betaxolol (Systemic) may be increased by: Abiraterone Acetate; Acetylcholinesterase Inhibitors; Aminoquinolines (Antimalarial); Amiodarone; Anilidopiperidine Opioids; Antipsychotic Agents (Phenothiazines); Calcium Channel Blockers (Dihydropyridine); Calcium Channel Blockers (Nondihydropyridine); CYP1A2 Inhibitors (Moderate); CYP1A2 Inhibitors (Strong); Deferasirox; Diazoxide; Dipyridamole; Disopyramide; Dronedarone; Floctafenine; Herbs (Hypotensive Properties); MAO Inhibitors; Pentoxifylline; Phosphodiesterase 5 Inhibitors; Propafenone; Prostacyclin Analogues; QuiNIDine; Reserpine

Decreased Effect

Betaxolol (Systemic) may decrease the levels/effects of: Beta2-Agonists; Theophylline Derivatives

The levels/effects of Betaxolol (Systemic) may be decreased by: Barbiturates; CYP1A2 Inducers (Strong); Cyproterone; Herbs (Hypertensive Properties); Methylphenidate; Nonsteroidal Anti-Inflammatory Agents; Peginterferon Alfa-2b; Rifamycin Derivatives; Yohimbine

Ethanol/Nutrition/Herb Interactions Herb/Nutraceutical: Avoid bayberry; blue cohosh, cayenne, ephedra, ginger, ginseng (American), gotu kola, and licorice (may worsen hypertension). Avoid black cohosh, California poppy, coleus, golden seal, hawthorn, mistletoe, periwinkle, quinine, shepherd's purse (may have increased antihypertensive effects).

Stability Avoid freezing. Store tablets at room temperature of 15°C to 25°C (59°F to 77°F).

Mechanism of Action Competitively blocks beta$_1$-receptors, with little or no effect on beta$_2$-receptors

Pharmacodynamics/Kinetics

Onset of action: 1-1.5 hours

Absorption: ~100%

Metabolism: Hepatic to multiple metabolites

Protein binding: ~50%

Bioavailability: 89%

Half-life elimination: 14-22 hours; prolonged in hepatic disease and/or chronic renal failure

Time to peak: 1.5-6 hours

Excretion: Urine (>80%, as unchanged drug [15%] and inactive metabolites)

Dosage

Geriatric Hypertension: Oral: Refer to adult dosing. Initial: 5 mg/day.

Adult Hypertension (labeled use), coronary artery disease (unlabeled use): Oral: 5-10 mg/day; may increase dose to 20 mg/day after 7-14 days if desired response is not achieved

Renal Impairment

Severe impairment: Initial dose: 5 mg/day; may increase every 2 weeks up to a maximum of 20 mg/day.

Hemodialysis: Initial dose: 5 mg/day; may increase every 2 weeks up to a maximum of 20 mg/day. Supplemental dose not required.

Administration Absorption is not affected by food.

Monitoring Parameters Blood pressure, pulse; baseline renal function

Test Interactions Oral betaxolol may interfere with glaucoma screening tests.

Special Geriatric Considerations Due to alterations in the beta-adrenergic autonomic nervous system, beta-adrenergic blockade may result in less hemodynamic response than seen in younger adults. Studies indicate that despite decreased sensitivity to the chronotropic effects of beta-blockade with age, there appears to be an increased myocardial sensitivity to the negative inotropic effect during stress (ie, exercise). Controlled trials have shown the overall response rate for propranolol to be only 20% to 50% in elderly populations. Therefore, all beta-adrenergic blocking drugs may result in a decreased response as compared to younger adults.

Dosage Forms Excipient information presented when available (limited, particularly for generics); consult specific product labeling.

Tablet, oral, as hydrochloride: 10 mg, 20 mg

Kerlone®: 10 mg [scored]

Kerlone®: 20 mg

Betaxolol (Ophthalmic) (be TAKS oh lol)

Related Information
Glaucoma Drug Therapy *on page 2115*
Medication Safety Issues
Sound-alike/look-alike issues:
  Betoptic® S may be confused with Betagan®, Timoptic®
Brand Names: U.S. Betoptic S®
Brand Names: Canada Betoptic® S; Sandoz-Betaxolol
Index Terms Betaxolol Hydrochloride
Generic Availability (U.S.) Yes: Solution
Pharmacologic Category Ophthalmic Agent, Antiglaucoma
Use Treatment of chronic open-angle glaucoma or ocular hypertension
Dosage
  Geriatric & Adult
    Glaucoma: Ophthalmic:
      Solution: Instill 1-2 drops into affected eye(s) twice daily.
      Suspension (Betoptic® S): Instill 1 drop into affected eye(s) twice daily.
Special Geriatric Considerations Evaluate the patient's or caregiver's ability to safely administer the correct dose of ophthalmic medication.
Dosage Forms Excipient information presented when available (limited, particularly for generics); consult specific product labeling.
  Solution, ophthalmic [drops]: 0.5% (5 mL, 10 mL, 15 mL) [contains benzalkonium chloride]
  Suspension, ophthalmic [drops]:
    Betoptic S®: 0.25% (10 mL, 15 mL) [contains benzalkonium chloride]

◆ **Betaxolol Hydrochloride** *see* Betaxolol (Ophthalmic) *on page 209*
◆ **Betaxolol Hydrochloride** *see* Betaxolol (Systemic) *on page 207*

Bethanechol (be THAN e kole)

Medication Safety Issues
Sound-alike/look-alike issues:
  Bethanechol may be confused with betaxolol
Brand Names: U.S. Urecholine®
Brand Names: Canada Duvoid®; PHL-Bethanechol; PMS-Bethanechol
Index Terms Bethanechol Chloride
Generic Availability (U.S.) Yes
Pharmacologic Category Cholinergic Agonist
Use Treatment of acute postoperative and postpartum nonobstructive (functional) urinary retention; treatment of neurogenic atony of the urinary bladder with retention
Unlabeled Use Gastroesophageal reflux
Contraindications Hypersensitivity to bethanechol or any component of the formulation; mechanical obstruction of the GI or GU tract or when the strength or integrity of the GI or bladder wall is in question; hyperthyroidism, peptic ulcer disease, epilepsy, asthma, bradycardia, vasomotor instability, coronary artery disease, hypotension, or parkinsonism
Warnings/Precautions Potential for reflux infection if the sphincter fails to relax as bethanechol contracts the bladder.
Adverse Reactions (Reflective of adult population; not specific for elderly) Frequency not defined.
  Cardiovascular: Hypotension, tachycardia, flushed skin
  Central nervous system: Headache, malaise, seizure
  Gastrointestinal: Abdominal cramps, belching, borborygmi, colicky pain, diarrhea, nausea, vomiting, salivation
  Genitourinary: Urinary urgency
  Ocular: Lacrimation, miosis
  Respiratory: Asthmatic attacks, bronchial constriction
  Miscellaneous: Diaphoresis
Drug Interactions
  Metabolism/Transport Effects None known.
  Avoid Concomitant Use There are no known interactions where it is recommended to avoid concomitant use.
  Increased Effect/Toxicity
    The levels/effects of Bethanechol may be increased by: Acetylcholinesterase Inhibitors; Beta-Blockers
  Decreased Effect There are no known significant interactions involving a decrease in effect.

Stability Store at room temperature of 15°C to 30°C (59°F to 86°F).

Mechanism of Action Due to stimulation of the parasympathetic nervous system, betha-nechol increases bladder muscle tone causing contractions which initiate urination. Betha-nechol also stimulates gastric motility, increases gastric tone and may restore peristalsis.

Pharmacodynamics/Kinetics
Onset of action: 30-90 minutes
Duration: Up to 6 hours
Absorption: Variable

Dosage
Geriatric Refer to adult dosing. Use the lowest effective dose.
Adult
Urinary retention, neurogenic bladder: Oral: Initial: 10-50 mg 3-4 times/day (some patients may require dosages of 50-100 mg 4 times/day). To determine effective dose, may initiate at a dose of 5-10 mg, with additional doses of 5-10 mg hourly until an effective cumulative dose is reached. Cholinergic effects at higher oral dosages may be cumulative.
Gastroesophageal reflux (unlabeled): Oral: 25 mg 4 times/day

Administration Should be administered 1 hour before meals or 2 hours after meals.

Monitoring Parameters Urinary output, blood pressure, pulse

Test Interactions Increased lipase, amylase (S), bilirubin, aminotransferase [ALT/AST] (S)

Special Geriatric Considerations Urinary incontinence in elderly patients should be investigated. Bethanechol may be used for overflow incontinence (ie, dribbling) caused by an atonic or hypotonic bladder, but clinical efficacy is variable.

Dosage Forms Excipient information presented when available (limited, particularly for generics); consult specific product labeling.
Tablet, oral, as chloride: 5 mg, 10 mg, 25 mg, 50 mg
Urecholine®: 5 mg, 10 mg, 25 mg, 50 mg [scored]

Dosage Forms: Canada Excipient information presented when available (limited, particularly for generics); consult specific product labeling.
Tablet, as chloride:
Duvoid®: 10 mg, 25 mg, 50 mg

- ◆ **Bethanechol Chloride** see Bethanechol on page 209
- ◆ **Betimol®** see Timolol (Ophthalmic) on page 1902
- ◆ **Betoptic S®** see Betaxolol (Ophthalmic) on page 209
- ◆ **BI-1356** see Linagliptin on page 1130
- ◆ **Biaxin®** see Clarithromycin on page 392
- ◆ **Biaxin® XL** see Clarithromycin on page 392

Bicalutamide (bye ka LOO ta mide)

Medication Safety Issues
Sound-alike/look-alike issues:
Casodex® may be confused with Kapidex [DSC]
International issues:
Casodex [U.S., Canada, and multiple international markets] may be confused with Capadex brand name for propoxyphene/acetaminophen [Australia, New Zealand]

Brand Names: U.S. Casodex®

Brand Names: Canada Apo-Bicalutamide®; Ava-Bicalutamide; Casodex®; CO Bicaluta-mide; Dom-Bicalutamide; JAMP-Bicalutamide; Mylan-Bicalutamide; Novo-Bicalutamide; PHL-Bicalutamide; PMS-Bicalutamide; PRO-Bicalutamide; ratio-Bicalutamide; Sandoz-Bica-lutamide

Index Terms CDX; ICI-176334

Generic Availability (U.S.) Yes

Pharmacologic Category Antineoplastic Agent, Antiandrogen

Use Treatment of metastatic prostate cancer (in combination with an LHRH agonist)

Unlabeled Use Monotherapy for locally-advanced prostate cancer

Contraindications Hypersensitivity to bicalutamide or any component of the formulation; use in women

Warnings/Precautions Hazardous agent - use appropriate precautions for handling and disposal. Rare cases of death or hospitalization due to hepatitis have been reported postmarketing. Use with caution in moderate-to-severe hepatic dysfunction. Hepatotoxicity generally occurs within the first 3-4 months of use; patients should be monitored for signs and symptoms of liver dysfunction. Bicalutamide should be discontinued if patients have jaundice or ALT is >2 times the upper limit of normal. Androgen-deprivation therapy may increase the risk for cardiovascular disease (Levine, 2010). May cause gynecomastia, breast pain, or lead to spermatogenesis inhibition. When used in combination with LHRH agonists, a loss of glycemic control and decrease in glucose tolerance has been reported in patients with diabetes; monitor. May cause gynecomastia or breast pain (at higher, unlabeled doses), or lead to spermatogenesis inhibition.

Adverse Reactions (Reflective of adult population; not specific for elderly) Adverse reaction percentages reported as part of combination regimen with an LHRH analogue unless otherwise noted.

>10%:
Cardiovascular: Peripheral edema (13%)
Central nervous system: Pain (35%)
Endocrine & metabolic: Hot flashes (53%), breast pain (6%; monotherapy [150 mg]: 39% to 85%), gynecomastia (9%; monotherapy [150 mg]: 38% to 73%)
Gastrointestinal: Constipation (22%), nausea (15%), diarrhea (12%), abdominal pain (11%)
Genitourinary: Pelvic pain (21%), hematuria (12%), nocturia (12%)
Hematologic: Anemia (11%)
Neuromuscular & skeletal: Back pain (25%), weakness (22%)
Respiratory: Dyspnea (13%)
Miscellaneous: Infection (18%)

≥2% to 10%:
Cardiovascular: Chest pain (8%), hypertension (8%), angina pectoris (2% to <5%), cardiac arrest (2% to <5%), CHF (2% to <5%), edema (2% to <5%), MI (2% to <5%), coronary artery disorder (2% to <5%), syncope (2% to <5%)
Central nervous system: Dizziness (10%), headache (7%), insomnia (7%), anxiety (5%), depression (4%), chills (2% to <5%), confusion (2% to <5%), fever (2% to <5%), nervousness (2% to <5%), somnolence (2% to <5%)
Dermatologic: Rash (9%), alopecia (2% to <5%), dry skin (2% to <5%), pruritus (2% to <5%), skin carcinoma (2% to <5%)
Endocrine & metabolic: Hyperglycemia (6%), dehydration (2% to <5%), gout (2% to <5%), hypercholesterolemia (2% to <5%), libido decreased (2% to <5%)
Gastrointestinal: Dyspepsia (7%), weight loss (7%), anorexia (6%), flatulence (6%), vomiting (6%), weight gain (5%), dysphagia (2% to <5%), gastrointestinal carcinoma (2% to <5%), melena (2% to <5%), periodontal abscess (2% to <5%), rectal hemorrhage (2% to <5%), xerostomia (2% to <5%)
Genitourinary: Urinary tract infection (9%), impotence (7%), polyuria (6%), urinary retention (5%), urinary impairment (5%), urinary incontinence (4%), dysuria (2% to <5%), urinary urgency (2% to <5%)
Hepatic: LFTs increased (7%), alkaline phosphatase increased (5%)
Neuromuscular & skeletal: Bone pain (9%), paresthesia (8%), myasthenia (7%), arthritis (5%), pathological fracture (4%), hypertonia (2% to <5%), leg cramps (2% to <5%), myalgia (2% to <5%), neck pain (2% to <5%), neuropathy (2% to <5%)
Ocular: Cataract (2% to <5%)
Renal: BUN increased (2% to <5%), creatinine increased (2% to <5%), hydronephrosis (2% to <5%)
Respiratory: Cough (8%), pharyngitis (8%), bronchitis (6%), pneumonia (4%), rhinitis (4%), asthma (2% to <5%), epistaxis (2% to <5%), sinusitis (2% to <5%)
Miscellaneous: Flu-like syndrome (7%), diaphoresis (6%), cyst (2% to <5%), hernia (2% to <5%), herpes zoster (2% to <5%), sepsis (2% to <5%)

Drug Interactions
Metabolism/Transport Effects Inhibits CYP3A4 (moderate)
Avoid Concomitant Use
Avoid concomitant use of Bicalutamide with any of the following: Pimozide; Tolvaptan
Increased Effect/Toxicity
Bicalutamide may increase the levels/effects of: ARIPiprazole; Avanafil; Budesonide (Systemic, Oral Inhalation); Colchicine; CYP3A4 Substrates; Eplerenone; Everolimus; FentaNYL; Halofantrine; Ivacaftor; Lurasidone; Pimecrolimus; Pimozide; Propafenone; Ranolazine; Salmeterol; Saxagliptin; Tolvaptan; Vilazodone; Vitamin K Antagonists; Zuclopenthixol
Decreased Effect
Bicalutamide may decrease the levels/effects of: Ifosfamide
Stability Store at room temperature of 20°C to 25°C (68°F to 77°F).
Mechanism of Action Androgen receptor inhibitor; pure nonsteroidal antiandrogen that binds to androgen receptors; specifically a competitive inhibitor for the binding of dihydrotestosterone and testosterone; prevents testosterone stimulation of cell growth in prostate cancer

◀ **Pharmacodynamics/Kinetics**
  Absorption: Rapid and complete; unaffected by food
  Protein binding: 96%
  Metabolism: Extensively hepatic; glucuronidation and oxidation of the R (active) enantiomer to inactive metabolites; the S enantiomer is inactive
  Half-life elimination: Active enantiomer: ~6 days, ~10 days in severe liver disease
  Time to peak, plasma: Active enantiomer: ~31 hours
  Excretion: Urine (36%, as inactive metabolites); feces (42%, as unchanged drug and inactive metabolites)

Dosage
  Geriatric & Adult
    Prostate cancer, metastatic: Oral: 50 mg once daily (in combination with an LHRH analogue)
    Prostate cancer, locally-advanced (unlabeled use): Oral: 150 mg once daily (as monotherapy) (McLeod, 2006)
  Renal Impairment No adjustment required
  Hepatic Impairment No adjustment required for mild, moderate, or severe hepatic impairment; use caution with moderate-to-severe impairment. Discontinue if ALT >2 times ULN or patient develops jaundice.

Administration Dose should be taken at the same time each day with or without food. Treatment for metastatic cancer should be started concomitantly with an LHRH analogue.

Monitoring Parameters Periodically monitor CBC, ECG, echocardiograms, serum testosterone, luteinizing hormone, and prostate specific antigen (PSA). Liver function tests should be obtained at baseline and repeated regularly during the first 4 months of treatment, and periodically thereafter; monitor for signs and symptoms of liver dysfunction (discontinue if jaundice is noted or ALT is >2 times the upper limit of normal). Monitor blood glucose in patients with diabetes. If initiating bicalutamide in patients who are on warfarin, closely monitor prothrombin time.

Pharmacotherapy Pearls Oncology Comment: According to the 2007 update of the American Society of Clinical Oncology (ASCO) guidelines for initial hormonal management of androgen-sensitive advanced prostate cancer, the standard of care is initial treatment with a luteinizing hormone-releasing hormone (LHRH) agonist, however, bicalutamide should be considered in combination with an LHRH agonist for combined androgen blockade (CAB) treatment. Although the incidence of adverse effects is increased, the addition of a non-steroidal antiandrogen (NSAA) such a s bicalutamide, increases overall survival (OS) (Loblaw, 2007).

The National Comprehensive Cancer Network (NCCN) Guidelines for Prostate Cancer (v.2.2009) also recommend an LHRH agonist as medical castration, which may be given alone or in combination with an NSAA. Certain patients (with evidence of metastases) receiving LHRH agonists are at risk for tumor flare, a condition in which an initial transient increase in testosterone levels induced by an LHRH agonist, results in worsening symptoms. These patients, according to the NCCN guidelines, should receive an antiandrogen with the LHRH agonist for at least 7 days, which may begin with or just prior to the LHRH agonist. The NCCN guidelines also address monotherapy with bicalutamide (150 mg orally daily) and while, to date, no OS advantage has been demonstrated in early, localized, or locally advanced prostate cancer, an improvement in progression-free survival has been demonstrated in locally advanced prostate cancer.

Special Geriatric Considerations Renal impairment has no clinically-significant changes in elimination of the parent compound or active metabolite; therefore, no dosage adjustment is needed in the elderly. In dosage studies, no difference was found between young adults and elderly with regard to steady-state serum concentrations for bicalutamide and its active R-enantiomer metabolite.

Dosage Forms Excipient information presented when available (limited, particularly for generics); consult specific product labeling.
  Tablet, oral: 50 mg
    Casodex®: 50 mg

◆ **Bicillin® L-A** see Penicillin G Benzathine on page 1497
◆ **Bicillin® C-R** see Penicillin G Benzathine and Penicillin G Procaine on page 1498
◆ **Bicillin® C-R 900/300** see Penicillin G Benzathine and Penicillin G Procaine on page 1498
◆ **Bicitra** see Sodium Citrate and Citric Acid on page 1790
◆ **Bidex®-400 [OTC]** see GuaiFENesin on page 904
◆ **BiDil®** see Isosorbide Dinitrate and Hydralazine on page 1052

Bimatoprost (bi MAT oh prost)

Related Information
Glaucoma Drug Therapy *on page 2115*
Brand Names: U.S. Latisse®; Lumigan®
Brand Names: Canada Latisse®; Lumigan®; Lumigan® RC
Generic Availability (U.S.) No
Pharmacologic Category Ophthalmic Agent, Antiglaucoma; Prostaglandin, Ophthalmic
Use Reduction of intraocular pressure (IOP) in patients with open-angle glaucoma or ocular hypertension; hypotrichosis treatment of the eyelashes
Contraindications
Latisse®: Hypersensitivity to bimatoprost or any component of the formulation
Lumigan®: There are no contraindications listed in the manufacturer's prescribing information.
Warnings/Precautions May cause permanent changes in eye color (increases the amount of brown pigment in the iris), the eyelid skin, and eyelashes. In addition, may increase the length and/or number of eyelashes (may vary between eyes). Use caution in patients with intraocular inflammation, aphakic patients, pseudophakic patients with a torn posterior lens capsule, or patients with risk factors for macular edema. Contains benzalkonium chloride (may be adsorbed by contact lenses). Safety and efficacy have not been determined for use in patients with angle-closure, inflammatory, or neovascular glaucoma.

Latisse®: Additional warnings: Patients receiving medications to reduce intraocular pressure should consult their healthcare provider prior to using; may interfere with desired reduction of intraocular pressure. Unintentional hair growth may occur on skin that has repeated contact with solution; apply to upper eyelid only, blot away excess.
Adverse Reactions (Reflective of adult population; not specific for elderly) Adverse reactions and percentages are for Lumigan® unless noted:
>10%: Ocular: Conjunctival hyperemia (25% to 45%; Latisse®: <4%), growth of eyelashes, ocular pruritus (>10%; Latisse®: <4%)
1% to 10%:
Central nervous system: Headache (1% to 5%)
Dermatologic: Skin hyperpigmentation (Latisse®: <4%), abnormal hair growth
Hepatic: Liver function tests abnormal (1% to 5%)
Neuromuscular & skeletal: Weakness (1% to 5%)
Ocular: Dry eyes (1% to 10%; Latisse®: <4%), erythema (eyelid/periorbital region; 1% to 10%; Latisse®: <4%), irritation (1% to 10%; Latisse®: <4%), allergic conjunctivitis, asthenopia, blepharitis, burning, cataract, conjunctival edema, conjunctival hemorrhage, discharge, eyelash darkening, foreign body sensation, iris pigmentation increased (may be delayed), pain, photophobia, pigmentation of periocular skin, superficial punctate keratitis, tearing, visual disturbance
Miscellaneous: Infections (10% [primarily colds and upper respiratory tract infections])
Drug Interactions
Metabolism/Transport Effects None known.
Avoid Concomitant Use There are no known interactions where it is recommended to avoid concomitant use.
Increased Effect/Toxicity
The levels/effects of Bimatoprost may be increased by: Latanoprost
Decreased Effect There are no known significant interactions involving a decrease in effect.
Stability Store between 2°C to 25°C (36°F to 77°F).
Mechanism of Action As a synthetic analog of prostaglandin with ocular hypotensive activity, bimatoprost decreases intraocular pressure by increasing the outflow of aqueous humor. Bimatoprost may increase the percent and duration of hairs in the growth phase, resulting in eyelash growth.
Pharmacodynamics/Kinetics
Onset of action: Reduction of IOP: ~4 hours
Peak effect: Maximum reduction of IOP: ~8-12 hours
Distribution: V_d: 0.67 L/kg
Protein binding: ~88%
Metabolism: Undergoes oxidation, N-deethylation, and glucuronidation after reaching systemic circulation; forms metabolites
Half-life elimination: I.V.: ~45 minutes
Time to peak: ≤10 minutes
Excretion: Urine (≤67%); feces (25%)

Dosage
Geriatric & Adult
Open-angle glaucoma or ocular hypertension: Ophthalmic: Instill 1 drop into affected eye(s) once daily in the evening; do not exceed once-daily dosing (may decrease IOP-lowering effect). If used with other topical ophthalmic agents, separate administration by at least 5 minutes.

Hypotrichosis of the eyelashes: Ophthalmic, topical: Place one drop on applicator and apply evenly along the skin of the upper eyelid at base of eyelashes once daily at bedtime; repeat procedure for second eye (use a clean applicator).

Administration
Latisse®: Remove make-up and contact lenses prior to application; ensure face is clean. Apply with the sterile applicator provided only; do not use other brushes or applicators. Use a tissue or cloth to blot any excess solution on the outside of the upper eyelid margin; do not apply to lower eyelash line. Do not reuse applicators; use new applicator for second eye. Applying more than once nightly will not increase eyelash growth; eyelash growth is expected to return to baseline when therapy is discontinued. May reinsert contacts 15 minutes after application.

Lumigan®: May be used with other eye drops to lower intraocular pressure. If using more than one ophthalmic product, wait at least 5 minutes in between application of each medication. Remove contact lenses prior to administration and wait 15 minutes before reinserting.

Pharmacotherapy Pearls The IOP-lowering effect was shown to be 7-8 mm Hg in clinical studies.

Special Geriatric Considerations Evaluate the patient's or caregiver's ability to safely administer the correct dose of ophthalmic medication.

Dosage Forms Excipient information presented when available (limited, particularly for generics); consult specific product labeling.

Solution, ophthalmic [drops]:
Latisse®: 0.03% (3 mL) [contains benzalkonium chloride]
Lumigan®: 0.01% (2.5 mL, 5 mL, 7.5 mL); 0.03% (2.5 mL, 5 mL, 7.5 mL) [contains benzalkonium chloride]

♦ **Binosto™** see Alendronate on page 53
♦ **Bio-D-Mulsion® [OTC]** see Cholecalciferol on page 365
♦ **Bio-D-Mulsion Forte® [OTC]** see Cholecalciferol on page 365
♦ **Bion® Tears [OTC]** see Artificial Tears on page 148
♦ **Biotene® Moisturizing Mouth Spray [OTC]** see Saliva Substitute on page 1748
♦ **Biotene® Oral Balance® [OTC]** see Saliva Substitute on page 1748
♦ **Bird Flu Vaccine** see Influenza Virus Vaccine (H5N1) on page 996
♦ **Bisac-Evac™ [OTC]** see Bisacodyl on page 214

Bisacodyl (bis a KOE dil)

Related Information
Laxatives, Classification and Properties on page 2121
Treatment Options for Constipation on page 2142
Medication Safety Issues
Sound-alike/look-alike issues:
Doxidan® may be confused with doxepin
Dulcolax® (bisacodyl) may be confused with Dulcolax® (docusate)
Brand Names: U.S. Alophen® [OTC]; Bisac-Evac™ [OTC]; Biscolax™ [OTC]; Correctol® Tablets [OTC]; Dacodyl™ [OTC]; Doxidan® [OTC]; Dulcolax® [OTC]; ex-lax® Ultra [OTC]; Femilax™ [OTC]; Fleet® Bisacodyl [OTC]; Fleet® Stimulant Laxative [OTC]; Veracolate® [OTC]
Brand Names: Canada Apo-Bisacodyl® [OTC]; Bisacodyl-Odan [OTC]; Bisacolax [OTC]; Carter's Little Pills® [OTC]; Codulax [OTC]; Dulcolax® [OTC]; PMS-Bisacodyl [OTC]; ratio-Bisacodyl [OTC]; Silver Bullet Suppository [OTC]; Soflax [OTC]; The Magic Bullet [OTC]; Woman's Laxative [OTC]
Generic Availability (U.S.) Yes: Excludes enema
Pharmacologic Category Laxative, Stimulant
Use Treatment of constipation; colonic evacuation prior to procedures or examination
Contraindications Hypersensitivity to bisacodyl or any component of the formulation; abdominal pain or obstruction, nausea, or vomiting
Drug Interactions
Metabolism/Transport Effects None known.
Avoid Concomitant Use There are no known interactions where it is recommended to avoid concomitant use.

Increased Effect/Toxicity There are no known significant interactions involving an increase in effect.

Decreased Effect

The levels/effects of Bisacodyl may be decreased by: Antacids

Ethanol/Nutrition/Herb Interactions Food: Milk or dairy products may disrupt enteric coating, increasing stomach irritation.

Mechanism of Action Stimulates peristalsis by directly irritating the smooth muscle of the intestine, possibly the colonic intramural plexus; alters water and electrolyte secretion producing net intestinal fluid accumulation and laxation

Pharmacodynamics/Kinetics

Onset of action: Oral: 6-10 hours; Rectal: 0.25-1 hour

V_d: BHPM: 289 L (after multiple doses) (Friedrich, 2011)

Half-life: BHPM: ~8 hours (Friedrich, 2011)

Metabolism: Bisacodyl is metabolized to an active metabolite (BHPM) in the colon; BHPM is then converted in the liver to a glucuronide salt (Friedrich, 2011)

Absorption: Oral, rectal: Systemic, <5% (Wald, 2003)

Excretion: BHPM: Urine, bile (Friedrich, 2011)

Dosage

Geriatric & Adult

Relief of constipation:

Oral: 5-15 mg as single dose (up to 30 mg when complete evacuation of bowel is required)

Rectal: Suppository: 10 mg as single dose

Administration Administer tablet with a glass of water on an empty stomach for rapid effect. To protect the enteric coating, tablet should not be administered within 1 hour of milk, any dairy products, or taking an antacid.

Special Geriatric Considerations The chronic use of stimulant cathartics is inappropriate and should be avoided; although constipation is a common complaint from elderly, such complaints require evaluation; elderly are often predisposed to constipation due to disease, drugs, immobility, and a decreased fluid intake, partially because they have a blunted "thirst reflex" with aging; short-term use of stimulants is best; if prophylaxis is desired, this can be accomplished with bulk agents (psyllium), stool softeners, and hyperosmotic agents (sorbitol 70%); stool softeners are unnecessary if stools are well hydrated, soft, or "mushy".

Dosage Forms Excipient information presented when available (limited, particularly for generics); consult specific product labeling.

Solution, rectal [enema]:

Fleet® Bisacodyl: 10 mg/30 mL (37 mL)

Suppository, rectal: 10 mg (12s, 50s, 100s)

Bisac-Evac™: 10 mg (8s, 12s, 50s, 100s, 500s, 1000s)

Biscolax™: 10 mg (12s, 100s)

Dulcolax®: 10 mg (4s, 8s, 16s, 28s, 50s)

Tablet, oral: 5 mg, 10 mg

Tablet, delayed release, oral: 5 mg

Doxidan®: 5 mg

Fleet® Stimulant Laxative: 5 mg

Tablet, enteric coated, oral: 5 mg

Alophen®: 5 mg

Bisac-Evac™: 5 mg

Correctol® Tablets: 5 mg

Dacodyl™: 5 mg

Dulcolax®: 5 mg

ex-lax® Ultra: 5 mg [contains sodium 0.1 mg/tablet]

Femilax™: 5 mg

Veracolate®: 5 mg

◆ **Bisacodyl and Polyethylene Glycol-Electrolyte Solution** *see* Polyethylene Glycol-Electrolyte Solution and Bisacodyl *on page 1565*

◆ **Biscolax™ [OTC]** *see* Bisacodyl *on page 214*

◆ **Bismatrol** *see* Bismuth *on page 216*

◆ **Bismatrol [OTC]** *see* Bismuth *on page 216*

◆ **Bismatrol Maximum Strength [OTC]** *see* Bismuth *on page 216*

Bismuth (BIZ muth)

Related Information
Antimicrobial Drugs of Choice *on page 2163*
H. pylori Treatment in Adult Patients *on page 2116*

Medication Safety Issues
Sound-alike/look-alike issues:
Kaopectate® may be confused with Kayexalate®
Other safety concerns:
Maalox® Total Relief® is a different formulation than other Maalox® liquid antacid products which contain aluminum hydroxide, magnesium hydroxide, and simethicone.
Canadian formulation of Kaopectate® does not contain bismuth; the active ingredient in the Canadian formulation is attapulgite.

Brand Names: U.S. Bismatrol Maximum Strength [OTC]; Bismatrol [OTC]; Diotame [OTC]; Kao-Tin [OTC]; Kaopectate® Extra Strength [OTC]; Kaopectate® [OTC]; Peptic Relief [OTC]; Pepto Relief [OTC]; Pepto-Bismol® Maximum Strength [OTC]; Pepto-Bismol® [OTC]

Index Terms Bismatrol; Bismuth Subsalicylate; Pink Bismuth

Generic Availability (U.S.) Yes

Pharmacologic Category Antidiarrheal

Use Subsalicylate formulation: Symptomatic treatment of mild, nonspecific diarrhea; control of traveler's diarrhea (enterotoxigenic *Escherichia coli*); as part of a multidrug regimen for *H. pylori* eradication to reduce the risk of duodenal ulcer recurrence

Contraindications Hypersensitivity to bismuth or any component of the formulation

Subsalicylate formulation: Do not use subsalicylate in patients with influenza or chickenpox because of risk of Reye's syndrome; hypersensitivity to salicylates or any component of the formulation; history of severe GI bleeding; history of coagulopathy

Warnings/Precautions Bismuth subsalicylate should be used with caution if patient is taking aspirin. Bismuth products may be neurotoxic with very large doses.

When used for self-medication (OTC labeling): Changes in behavior (along with nausea and vomiting) may be an early sign of Reye's syndrome; patients should be instructed to contact their healthcare provider if these occur. Patients should be instructed to contact healthcare provider for diarrhea lasting >2 days, hearing loss, or ringing in the ears.

Adverse Reactions (Reflective of adult population; not specific for elderly) Frequency not defined; subsalicylate formulation:
Central nervous system: Anxiety, confusion, headache, mental depression, slurred speech
Gastrointestinal: Discoloration of the tongue (darkening), grayish black stools, impaction may occur in infants and debilitated patients
Neuromuscular & skeletal: Muscle spasms, weakness
Otic: Hearing loss, tinnitus

Drug Interactions
Metabolism/Transport Effects None known.
Avoid Concomitant Use There are no known interactions where it is recommended to avoid concomitant use.
Increased Effect/Toxicity There are no known significant interactions involving an increase in effect.
Decreased Effect
Bismuth may decrease the levels/effects of: Tetracycline Derivatives

Mechanism of Action Bismuth subsalicylate exhibits both antisecretory and antimicrobial action. This agent may provide some anti-inflammatory action as well. The salicylate moiety provides antisecretory effect and the bismuth exhibits antimicrobial directly against bacterial and viral gastrointestinal pathogens.

Pharmacodynamics/Kinetics
Absorption: Bismuth: <1%; Subsalicylate: >90%
Metabolism: Bismuth subsalicylate is converted to salicylic acid and insoluble bismuth salts in the GI tract.
Half-life elimination: Terminal: Bismuth: Highly variable
Excretion: Bismuth: Urine and feces; Salicylate: Urine

Dosage
Geriatric & Adult
Treatment of nonspecific diarrhea, control/relieve traveler's diarrhea: Subsalicylate: Oral: 524 mg every 30 minutes to 1 hour as needed up to 8 doses/24 hours
Helicobacter pylori **eradication:** Oral: Subsalicylate: 524 mg 4 times/day with meals and at bedtime; requires combination therapy

Renal Impairment Bismuth has been associated with nephrotoxicity in overdose (Leussnik, 2002); although there are no specific recommendations by the manufacturer, consider using with caution in patients with renal impairment.

Administration Liquids must be shaken prior to use. Chewable tablets should be chewed thoroughly. Nonchewable caplets should be swallowed whole with a full glass of water.

Monitoring Parameters Signs/symptoms of nausea, diarrhea, tinnitus, CNS toxic effects, GI bleeding

Test Interactions Increased uric acid, increased AST; bismuth absorbs x-rays and may interfere with diagnostic procedures of GI tract

Pharmacotherapy Pearls Pepto-Bismol® contains bismuth 58% and salicylate 42%; do not exceed 4.2 g/day dosage; bismuth is radiopaque; 2 tablets yield 204 mg salicylate; 30 mL of suspension yields 258 mg

Special Geriatric Considerations Tinnitus and CNS side effects (confusion, dizziness, high tone deafness, delirium, psychosis) may be difficult to assess in some elderly patients. Limit use of this agent in elderly.

Dosage Forms Excipient information presented when available (limited, particularly for generics); consult specific product labeling.

Caplet, oral, as subsalicylate:
  Pepto-Bismol®: 262 mg [sugar free; contains sodium 2 mg/caplet]
Liquid, oral, as subsalicylate: 262 mg/15 mL (120 mL, 240 mL, 360 mL, 480 mL); 525 mg/15 mL (240 mL, 360 mL)
  Bismatrol: 262 mg/15 mL (240 mL)
  Bismatrol Maximum Strength: 525 mg/15 mL (240 mL)
  Diotame: 262 mg/15 mL (30 mL) [sugar free]
  Kao-Tin: 262 mg/15 mL (240 mL, 473 mL) [contains sodium benzoate]
  Kaopectate®: 262 mg/15 mL (236 mL) [contains potassium 5 mg/15 mL, sodium 5 mg/15 mL; peppermint flavor]
  Kaopectate®: 262 mg/15 mL (177 mL) [contains sodium 4 mg/15 mL; cherry flavor]
  Kaopectate®: 262 mg/15 mL (236 mL, 354 mL) [contains sodium 4 mg/15 mL; vanilla flavor]
  Kaopectate® Extra Strength: 525 mg/15 mL (236 mL) [contains potassium 5 mg/15 mL, sodium 5 mg/15 mL; peppermint flavor]
  Peptic Relief: 262 mg/15 mL (237 mL) [sugar free; mint flavor]
  Pepto-Bismol®: 262 mg/15 mL (240 mL, 360 mL, 480 mL) [sugar free; contains benzoic acid, sodium 6 mg/15 mL; cherry flavor]
  Pepto-Bismol®: 262 mg/15 mL (120 mL, 240 mL, 360 mL, 480 mL) [sugar free; contains benzoic acid, sodium 6 mg/15 mL; wintergreen flavor]
  Pepto-Bismol® Maximum Strength: 525 mg/15 mL (120 mL, 240 mL, 360 mL) [sugar free; contains benzoic acid, sodium 6 mg/15 mL; wintergreen flavor]
Suspension, oral, as subsalicylate: 262 mg/15 mL (30 mL)
Tablet, chewable, oral, as subsalicylate: 262 mg
  Bismatrol: 262 mg
  Diotame: 262 mg [sugar free]
  Peptic Relief: 262 mg
  Pepto Relief: 262 mg
  Pepto-Bismol®: 262 mg [sugar free; contains sodium <1 mg/tablet; cherry flavor]
  Pepto-Bismol®: 262 mg [sugar free; contains sodium <1 mg/tablet; wintergreen flavor]

◆ **Bismuth Subsalicylate** *see* Bismuth *on page 216*

Bisoprolol (bis OH proe lol)

Related Information
  Beta-Blockers *on page 2108*
  Heart Failure (Systolic) *on page 2203*
Medication Safety Issues
  Sound-alike/look-alike issues:
    Zebeta® may be confused with DiaBeta®, Zetia®
Brand Names: U.S. Zebeta®
Brand Names: Canada Apo-Bisoprolol®; Ava-Bisoprolol; Mylan-Bisoprolol; Novo-Bisoprolol; PHL-Bisoprolol; PMS-Bisoprolol; PRO-Bisoprolol; Sandoz-Bisoprolol
Index Terms Bisoprolol Fumarate
Generic Availability (U.S.) Yes
Pharmacologic Category Beta-Blocker, Beta-1 Selective
Use Treatment of hypertension, alone or in combination with other agents
Unlabeled Use Chronic stable angina, supraventricular arrhythmias, PVCs, heart failure (HF)
Contraindications Cardiogenic shock; overt cardiac failure; marked sinus bradycardia or heart block greater than first-degree (except in patients with a functioning artificial pacemaker)

Warnings/Precautions Consider pre-existing conditions such as sick sinus syndrome before initiating. Use caution in patients with heart failure; use gradual and careful titration; monitor for symptoms of congestive heart failure. Use with caution in patients with myasthenia gravis, psychiatric disease (may cause CNS depression), bronchospastic disease, undergoing anesthesia; and in those with impaired hepatic function. Bradycardia may be observed more frequently in elderly patients (>65 years of age); dosage reductions may be necessary. Beta-blocker therapy should not be withdrawn abruptly (particularly in patients with CAD), but gradually tapered to avoid acute tachycardia, hypertension, and/or ischemia. Chronic beta-blocker therapy should not be routinely withdrawn prior to major surgery. Can precipitate or aggravate symptoms of arterial insufficiency in patients with PVD and Raynaud's disease; use with caution and monitor for progression of arterial obstruction. Use caution with concurrent use of digoxin, verapamil, or diltiazem; bradycardia or heart block may occur. Use with caution in patients receiving inhaled anesthetic agents known to depress myocardial contractility. Bisoprolol, with beta$_1$-selectivity, may be used cautiously in bronchospastic disease with close monitoring. Use cautiously in patients with diabetes because it can mask prominent hypoglycemic symptoms. May mask signs of hyperthyroidism (eg, tachycardia); use caution if hyperthyroidism is suspected, abrupt withdrawal may precipitate thyroid storm. Dosage adjustment is required in patients with significant hepatic or renal dysfunction. Adequate alpha-blockade is required prior to use of any beta-blocker for patients with untreated pheochromocytoma. May induce or exacerbate psoriasis. Use caution with history of severe anaphylaxis to allergens; patients taking beta-blockers may become more sensitive to repeated challenges. Treatment of anaphylaxis (eg, epinephrine) in patients taking beta-blockers may be ineffective or promote undesirable effects.

Adverse Reactions (Reflective of adult population; not specific for elderly) 1% to 10%:

Cardiovascular: Chest pain (1% to 2%)

Central nervous system: Fatigue (dose related; 6% to 8%), insomnia (2% to 3%), hypoesthesia (1% to 2%)

Gastrointestinal: Diarrhea (dose related; 3% to 4%), nausea (2%), vomiting (1% to 2%)

Neuromuscular & skeletal: Arthralgia, weakness (dose related; ≤2%)

Respiratory: Upper respiratory infection (5%), rhinitis (3% to 4%), sinusitis (dose related; 2%), dyspnea (1% to 2%)

Drug Interactions

Metabolism/Transport Effects Substrate of CYP2D6 (minor), CYP3A4 (major); **Note:** Assignment of Major/Minor substrate status based on clinically relevant drug interaction potential

Avoid Concomitant Use

Avoid concomitant use of Bisoprolol with any of the following: Conivaptan; Floctafenine; Methacholine

Increased Effect/Toxicity

Bisoprolol may increase the levels/effects of: Alpha-/Beta-Agonists (Direct-Acting); Alpha1-Blockers; Alpha2-Agonists; Amifostine; Antihypertensives; Antipsychotic Agents (Phenothiazines); Bupivacaine; Cardiac Glycosides; Cholinergic Agonists; Fingolimod; Hypotensive Agents; Insulin; Lidocaine; Lidocaine (Systemic); Lidocaine (Topical); Mepivacaine; Methacholine; Midodrine; RiTUXimab; Sulfonylureas

The levels/effects of Bisoprolol may be increased by: Acetylcholinesterase Inhibitors; Aminoquinolines (Antimalarial); Amiodarone; Anilidopiperidine Opioids; Antipsychotic Agents (Phenothiazines); Calcium Channel Blockers (Dihydropyridine); Calcium Channel Blockers (Nondihydropyridine); Conivaptan; CYP3A4 Inhibitors (Moderate); CYP3A4 Inhibitors (Strong); Dasatinib; Diazoxide; Dipyridamole; Disopyramide; Dronedarone; Floctafenine; Herbs (Hypotensive Properties); Ivacaftor; MAO Inhibitors; Mifepristone; Pentoxifylline; Phosphodiesterase 5 Inhibitors; Propafenone; Prostacyclin Analogues; QuiNIDine; Reserpine

Decreased Effect

Bisoprolol may decrease the levels/effects of: Beta2-Agonists; Theophylline Derivatives

The levels/effects of Bisoprolol may be decreased by: Barbiturates; CYP3A4 Inducers (Strong); Deferasirox; Herbs (CYP3A4 Inducers); Herbs (Hypertensive Properties); Methylphenidate; Nonsteroidal Anti-Inflammatory Agents; Peginterferon Alfa-2b; Rifamycin Derivatives; Tocilizumab; Yohimbine

Ethanol/Nutrition/Herb Interactions Herb/Nutraceutical: Avoid dong quai if using for hypertension (has estrogenic activity). Avoid ephedra, yohimbe, ginseng (may worsen hypertension). Avoid garlic (may have increased antihypertensive effect).

Stability Store at controlled room temperature 20°C to 25°C (68°F to 77°F). Protect from moisture.

Mechanism of Action Selective inhibitor of beta$_1$-adrenergic receptors; competitively blocks beta$_1$-receptors, with little or no effect on beta$_2$-receptors at doses ≤20 mg

Pharmacodynamics/Kinetics

Onset of action: 1-2 hours

Absorption: Rapid and almost complete

Distribution: Widely; highest concentrations in heart, liver, lungs, and saliva; crosses blood-brain barrier

Protein binding: ~30%

Metabolism: Extensively hepatic; significant first-pass effect (~20%)

Bioavailability: ~80%

Half-life elimination: Normal renal function: 9-12 hours; Cl_{cr} <40 mL/minute: 27-36 hours; Hepatic cirrhosis: 8-22 hours

Time to peak: 2-4 hours

Excretion: Urine (50% as unchanged drug, remainder as inactive metabolites); feces (<2%)

Dosage

Geriatric & Adult

Hypertension: Oral: Initial: 2.5-5 mg once daily; may be increased to 10 mg and then up to 20 mg once daily, if necessary; usual dose range (JNC 7): 2.5-10 mg once daily

Heart failure (unlabeled use): Oral: Initial: 1.25 mg once daily; maximum recommended dose: 10 mg once daily. **Note:** Increase dose gradually and monitor for signs and symptoms of CHF (Hunt, 2009; Lindenfeld, 2010)

Renal Impairment

Cl_{cr} <40 mL/minute: Oral: Initial: 2.5 mg/day; increase cautiously

Not dialyzable

Administration
May be administered without regard to meals.

Monitoring Parameters
Blood pressure, heart rate, ECG; serum glucose regularly (in patients with diabetes)

Special Geriatric Considerations
Due to alterations in the beta-adrenergic autonomic nervous system, beta-adrenergic blockade may result in less hemodynamic response than seen in younger adults. Studies indicate that despite decreased sensitivity to the chronotropic effects of beta-blockade with age, there appears to be an increased myocardial sensitivity to the negative inotropic effect during stress (ie, exercise). Controlled trials have shown the overall response rate for propranolol to be only 20% to 50% in elderly populations. Therefore, all beta-adrenergic blocking drugs may result in a decreased response as compared to younger adults.

Dosage Forms
Excipient information presented when available (limited, particularly for generics); consult specific product labeling.

Tablet, oral, as fumarate: 5 mg, 10 mg

Zebeta®: 5 mg [scored]

Zebeta®: 10 mg

BRIMONIDINE

Brimonidine (bri MOE ni deen)

Related Information
Glaucoma Drug Therapy *on page 2115*
Medication Safety Issues
Sound-alike/look-alike issues:
Brimonidine may be confused with bromocriptine
Brand Names: U.S. Alphagan® P
Brand Names: Canada Alphagan®; Apo-Brimonidine P®; Apo-Brimonidine®; PMS-Brimonidine Tartrate; ratio-Brimonidine; Sandoz-Brimonidine
Index Terms Brimonidine Tartrate
Generic Availability (U.S.) Yes
Pharmacologic Category Alpha$_2$ Agonist, Ophthalmic; Ophthalmic Agent, Antiglaucoma
Use Lowering of intraocular pressure (IOP) in patients with open-angle glaucoma or ocular hypertension
Contraindications Hypersensitivity to brimonidine tartrate or any component of the formulation; during or within 14 days of MAO inhibitor therapy
Warnings/Precautions Exercise caution in treating patients with severe cardiovascular disease. Use with caution in patients with depression, cerebral or coronary insufficiency, Raynaud's phenomenon, orthostatic hypotension, or thromboangiitis obliterans. Use with caution in patients with hepatic or renal impairment. Systemic absorption has been reported. May cause CNS depression, which may impair physical or mental abilities; patients must be cautioned about performing tasks which require mental alertness (eg, operating machinery or driving).

Some formulations may contain benzalkonium chloride which may be absorbed by soft contact lenses; remove contacts prior to administration and wait 15 minutes before reinserting. The IOP-lowering efficacy observed with brimonidine tartrate during the first of month of therapy may not always reflect the long-term level of IOP reduction. Routinely monitor IOP.

Adverse Reactions (Reflective of adult population; not specific for elderly) Actual frequency of adverse reactions may be formulation dependent; percentages reported with Alphagan® P:

>10%:
Central nervous system: Somnolence (adults 1% to 4%; children 25% to 83%)
Ocular: Allergic conjunctivitis, conjunctival hyperemia, eye pruritus
1% to 10% (unless otherwise noted 1% to 4%):
Cardiovascular: Hypertension (5% to 9%), hypotension
Central nervous system: Alertness decreased (children), dizziness, fatigue, headache, insomnia
Dermatologic: Rash
Endocrine & metabolic: Hypercholesterolemia
Gastrointestinal: Xerostomia (5% to 9%), dyspepsia
Neuromuscular & skeletal: Weakness
Ocular: Burning sensation (5% to 9%), conjunctival folliculosis (5% to 9%), ocular allergic reaction (5% to 9%), visual disturbance (5% to 9%), blepharitis, blepharoconjunctivitis, blurred vision, cataract, conjunctival edema, conjunctival hemorrhage, conjunctivitis, dry eye, epiphora, eye discharge, eyelid disorder, eyelid edema, eyelid erythema, follicular conjunctivitis, foreign body sensation, irritation, keratitis, pain, photophobia, stinging, superficial punctate keratopathy, visual acuity worsened, visual field defect, vitreous detachment, vitreous floaters, watery eyes
Respiratory: Bronchitis, cough, dyspnea, pharyngitis, rhinitis, sinus infection, sinusitis
Miscellaneous: Allergic reaction, flu-like syndrome, infection
Drug Interactions
Metabolism/Transport Effects None known.
Avoid Concomitant Use
Avoid concomitant use of Brimonidine with any of the following: Azelastine; Azelastine (Nasal); MAO Inhibitors; Methadone; Mirtazapine; Paraldehyde
Increased Effect/Toxicity
Brimonidine may increase the levels/effects of: Alcohol (Ethyl); Azelastine; Azelastine (Nasal); Buprenorphine; CNS Depressants; Hypotensive Agents; Methadone; Methotrimeprazine; Metyrosine; Mirtazapine; Paraldehyde; Selective Serotonin Reuptake Inhibitors; Zolpidem

The levels/effects of Brimonidine may be increased by: Droperidol; HydrOXYzine; MAO Inhibitors; Methotrimeprazine
Decreased Effect There are no known significant interactions involving a decrease in effect.

Ethanol/Nutrition/Herb Interactions Herb/Nutraceutical: Avoid herbs with **hypertensive** properties (bayberry, blue cohosh, cayenne, ephedra, ginger, ginseng, gotu kola, licorice); may diminish antihypertensive effect. Avoid herbs with **hypotensive** properties (black cohosh, California poppy, coleus, golden seal, hawthorn, mistletoe, periwinkle, quinine, shepherd's purse); may enhance hypotensive effect.

Stability Store between 15°C to 25°C (59°F to 77°F).

Mechanism of Action Selective agonism for alpha$_2$-receptors; causes reduction of aqueous humor formation and increased uveoscleral outflow

Pharmacodynamics/Kinetics
Onset of action: Peak effect: 2 hours
Metabolism: Hepatic
Half-life elimination: ~2 hours
Time to peak, plasma: 0.5-2.5 hours
Excretion: Urine (74%)

Dosage
Geriatric & Adult Glaucoma, ocular hypertension: Ophthalmic: Instill 1 drop in affected eye(s) 3 times/day (approximately every 8 hours)

Administration Remove contact lenses prior to administration; wait 15 minutes before reinserting if using products containing benzalkonium chloride. Separate administration of other ophthalmic agents by 5 minutes.

Monitoring Parameters Closely monitor patients who develop fatigue or drowsiness; IOP

Pharmacotherapy Pearls The use of Purite® as a preservative in Alphagan® P has lead to a reduced incidence of certain adverse effects associated with products using benzalkonium chloride as a preservative. The 0.1% and 0.15% solutions are comparable to the 0.2% solution in lowering intraocular pressure.

Special Geriatric Considerations Evaluate the patient's or caregiver's ability to safely administer the correct dose of ophthalmic medication.

Dosage Forms Excipient information presented when available (limited, particularly for generics); consult specific product labeling.
Solution, ophthalmic, as tartrate [drops]: 0.15% (5 mL, 10 mL, 15 mL); 0.2% (5 mL, 10 mL, 15 mL)
Alphagan® P: 0.1% (5 mL, 10 mL, 15 mL); 0.15% (5 mL, 10 mL, 15 mL) [contains Purite®]

♦ **Brimonidine Tartrate** see Brimonidine on page 220

Brinzolamide (brin ZOH la mide)

Related Information
Glaucoma Drug Therapy on page 2115
Brand Names: U.S. Azopt®
Brand Names: Canada Azopt®
Generic Availability (U.S.) No
Pharmacologic Category Carbonic Anhydrase Inhibitor; Ophthalmic Agent, Antiglaucoma
Use Treatment of elevated intraocular pressure in patients with ocular hypertension or open-angle glaucoma
Contraindications Hypersensitivity to brinzolamide or any component of the formulation
Warnings/Precautions Brinzolamide is a sulfonamide; although administered ocularly, systemic absorption may occur and could result in hypersensitivity; discontinue use if signs of hypersensitivity or a serious reaction occur. Use with caution in patients with low endothelial cell counts; may be at increased risk of corneal edema. Use has not been studied in acute angle-closure glaucoma. Use not recommended in patients with severe renal impairment (has not been studied; parent and metabolite may accumulate). Product contains benzalkonium chloride which may be absorbed by soft contact lenses; remove lens prior to administration and wait 15 minutes before reinserting. Concurrent use with oral carbonic anhydrase inhibitors may result in additive systemic effects and is not recommended.
Adverse Reactions (Reflective of adult population; not specific for elderly) 1% to 10%:
Cardiovascular: Hyperemia (1% to 5%)
Central nervous system: Headache (1% to 5%)
Dermatologic: Dermatitis (1% to 5%)
Gastrointestinal: Taste disturbances (5% to 10%)
Ocular: Ocular: Blurred vision (5% to 10%), blepharitis (1% to 5%), dry eye (1% to 5%), eye discharge (1% to 5%), eye discomfort (1% to 5%), eye pain (1% to 5%), foreign body sensation (1% to 5%), itching of eye (1% to 5%), keratitis (1% to 5%)
Respiratory: Rhinitis (1% to 5%)

Drug Interactions
Metabolism/Transport Effects Substrate of CYP3A4 (minor); **Note:** Assignment of Major/Minor substrate status based on clinically relevant drug interaction potential
Avoid Concomitant Use
Avoid concomitant use of Brinzolamide with any of the following: Carbonic Anhydrase Inhibitors
Increased Effect/Toxicity
Brinzolamide may increase the levels/effects of: Carbonic Anhydrase Inhibitors

The levels/effects of Brinzolamide may be increased by: CYP3A4 Inhibitors (Strong)
Decreased Effect
The levels/effects of Brinzolamide may be decreased by: Tocilizumab
Stability Store at 4°C to 30°C (39°F to 86°F). Shake well before use.
Mechanism of Action Brinzolamide inhibits carbonic anhydrase, leading to decreased aqueous humor secretion. This results in a reduction of intraocular pressure.
Pharmacodynamics/Kinetics
Absorption: Topical: Into systemic circulation
Distribution: Accumulates extensively in red blood cells, binding to carbonic anhydrase (brinzolamide and metabolite)
Protein binding: ~60%
Metabolism: To N-desethyl brinzolamide
Excretion: Urine (as unchanged drug and metabolites)
Dosage
Geriatric & Adult Ocular hypertension or open-angle glaucoma: Ophthalmic: Instill 1 drop in affected eye(s) 3 times/day
Renal Impairment Severe renal impairment (Cl_{cr} <30 mL/minute): Use is not recommended (has not been studied; brinzolamide and metabolite are excreted predominantly by the kidney).
Administration Remove contact lenses prior to administration; wait 15 minutes before reinserting. If more than one topical ophthalmic drug is being used, administer drugs at least 10 minutes apart. Shake well before use.
Monitoring Parameters Intraocular pressure
Special Geriatric Considerations Evaluate the patient's or caregiver's ability to safely administer the correct dose of ophthalmic medication.
Dosage Forms Excipient information presented when available (limited, particularly for generics); consult specific product labeling.
Suspension, ophthalmic [drops]:
Azopt®: 1% (10 mL, 15 mL) [contains benzalkonium chloride]

◆ **Brioschi® [OTC]** *see* Sodium Bicarbonate *on page* 1785
◆ **BRL 43694** *see* Granisetron *on page* 900
◆ **Bromax [DSC]** *see* Brompheniramine *on page* 226
◆ **Bromday™** *see* Bromfenac *on page* 222

Bromfenac (BROME fen ak)

Brand Names: U.S. Bromday™
Index Terms Bromfenac Sodium
Generic Availability (U.S.) Yes
Pharmacologic Category Nonsteroidal Anti-inflammatory Drug (NSAID), Ophthalmic
Use Treatment of postoperative inflammation and reduction in ocular pain following cataract removal
Contraindications There are no contraindications listed in the manufacturer's prescribing information.
Warnings/Precautions Use with caution in patients with previous sensitivity to acetylsalicylic acid and phenylacetic acid derivatives, including patients who experience bronchospasm, asthma, rhinitis, or urticaria following NSAID or aspirin therapy. May slow/delay healing or prolong bleeding time following surgery. Use caution in patients with a predisposition to bleeding (bleeding tendencies or medications which interfere with coagulation).

May cause keratitis; continued use of bromfenac in a patient with keratitis may cause severe corneal adverse reactions, potentially resulting in loss of vision. Immediately discontinue use in patients with evidence of corneal epithelial damage.

Use caution in patients with complicated ocular surgeries, corneal denervation, corneal epithelial defects, diabetes mellitus, ocular surface disease, rheumatoid arthritis, or repeat ocular surgeries (within a short timeframe); may be at risk of corneal adverse events, potentially resulting in loss of vision. Patients using ophthalmic drops should not wear contact lenses during administration. Use for more than 1 day prior to surgery or for 14 days beyond surgery may increase risk and severity of corneal adverse events.

Contains sulfites, which may cause allergic reactions.

Adverse Reactions (Reflective of adult population; not specific for elderly) 2% to 7%:

Central nervous system: Headache

Ocular: Abnormal sensation, conjunctival hyperemia, iritis, irritation (burning/stinging), pain, pruritus, redness

Drug Interactions

Metabolism/Transport Effects None known.

Avoid Concomitant Use There are no known interactions where it is recommended to avoid concomitant use.

Increased Effect/Toxicity There are no known significant interactions involving an increase in effect.

Decreased Effect

Bromfenac may decrease the levels/effects of: Latanoprost

Stability Store at 15°C to 25°C (59°F to 77°F).

Mechanism of Action Inhibits prostaglandin synthesis by decreasing the activity of the enzyme, cyclooxygenase, which results in decreased formation of prostaglandin precursors.

Pharmacodynamics/Kinetics

Absorption: Theoretically, systemic absorption may occur following ophthalmic use (not characterized); anticipated levels are below the limits of assay detection

Metabolism: Hepatic

Half-life elimination: 0.5-4 hours (following oral administration)

Dosage

Geriatric & Adult Pain, inflammation associated with cataract surgery: Ophthalmic: Instill 1 drop into affected eye(s) once daily beginning 1 day prior to surgery and continuing on the day of surgery and for 2 weeks postoperatively

Administration Remove contact lenses prior to administration and wait 15 minutes before reinserting. May be used with other eye drops. If using more than 1 ophthalmic product, wait at least 5 minutes between application of each medication.

Special Geriatric Considerations No differences in safety and efficacy noted between elderly and younger adults. No dosage adjustment necessary. Elderly may be taking other medications that will increase bleeding.

Dosage Forms Excipient information presented when available (limited, particularly for generics); consult specific product labeling.

Solution, ophthalmic [drops]: 0.09% (2.5 mL, 5 mL)

Bromday™: 0.09% (1.7 mL) [contains benzalkonium chloride, sodium sulfite]

◆ **Bromfenac Sodium** *see* Bromfenac *on page 222*

Bromocriptine (broe moe KRIP teen)

Related Information

Antiparkinsonian Agents *on page 2101*

Diabetes Mellitus Management, Adults *on page 2193*

Medication Safety Issues

Sound-alike/look-alike issues:

Bromocriptine may be confused with benztropine, brimonidine

Cycloset® may be confused with Glyset®

Parlodel® may be confused with pindolol, Provera®

Brand Names: U.S. Cycloset®; Parlodel®; Parlodel® SnapTabs®

Brand Names: Canada Dom-Bromocriptine; PMS-Bromocriptine

Index Terms Bromocriptine Mesylate; Cycloset®

Generic Availability (U.S.) Yes: Excludes Cycloset®

Pharmacologic Category Anti-Parkinson's Agent, Dopamine Agonist; Antidiabetic Agent, Dopamine Agonist; Ergot Derivative

Use Treatment of hyperprolactinemia associated with amenorrhea with or without galactorrhea, infertility, or hypogonadism; treatment of prolactin-secreting adenomas; treatment of acromegaly; treatment of Parkinson's disease

Cycloset®: Management of type 2 diabetes mellitus (noninsulin dependent, NIDDM) as an adjunct to diet and exercise

Unlabeled Use Treatment of neuroleptic malignant syndrome

◄ **Contraindications** Hypersensitivity to bromocriptine, ergot alkaloids, or any component of the formulation; ergot alkaloids are contraindicated with potent inhibitors of CYP3A4 (includes protease inhibitors, azole antifungals, and some macrolide antibiotics); uncontrolled hypertension; severe ischemic heart disease or peripheral vascular disorders

Warnings/Precautions Complete evaluation of pituitary function should be completed prior to initiation of treatment of any hyperprolactinemia-associated dysfunction. Use caution in patients with a history of peptic ulcer disease, dementia, or cardiovascular disease (myocardial infarction, arrhythmia). Use with extreme caution or avoid in patients with psychosis. Symptomatic hypotension may occur in a significant number of patients. In addition, hypertension, seizures, MI, and stroke have been rarely associated with bromocriptine therapy. Severe headache or visual changes may precede events. The onset of reactions may be immediate or delayed (often may occur in the second week of therapy). Sudden sleep onset and somnolence have been reported with use, primarily in patients with Parkinson's disease. Patients must be cautioned about performing tasks which require mental alertness.

Use with caution in patients taking strong CYP3A4 inhibitors and/or major CYP3A4 substrates (includes protease inhibitors, azole antifungals, and some macrolide antibiotics); consider alternative agents that avoid or lessen the potential for CYP-mediated interactions. Concurrent antihypertensives or drugs which may alter blood pressure should be used with caution. Concurrent use with levodopa has been associated with an increased risk of hallucinations. Consider dosage reduction and/or discontinuation in patients with hallucinations. Hallucinations may require weeks to months before resolution.

Dopamine agonists have been associated with compulsive behaviors and/or loss of impulse control, which has manifested as pathological gambling, libido increases (hypersexuality), and/or binge eating. Causality has not been established, and controversy exists as to whether this phenomenon is related to the underlying disease, prior behaviors/addictions and/or drug therapy. Dose reduction or discontinuation of therapy has been reported to reverse these behaviors in some, but not all cases. Risk for melanoma development is increased in Parkinson's disease patients; drug causation or factors contributing to risk have not been established. Patients should be monitored closely and periodic skin examinations should be performed.

In the treatment of acromegaly, discontinuation is recommended if tumor expansion occurs during therapy. Digital vasospasm (cold sensitive) may occur in some patients with acromegaly; may require dosage reduction. Use of bromocriptine in patients with uncontrolled hypertension is not recommended.

Monitoring and careful evaluation of visual changes during the treatment of hyperprolactinemia is recommended to differentiate between tumor shrinkage and traction on the optic chiasm; rapidly progressing visual field loss requires neurosurgical consultation. Discontinuation of bromocriptine in patients with macroadenomas has been associated with rapid regrowth of tumor and increased prolactin serum levels. Pleural and retroperitoneal fibrosis have been reported with prolonged daily use. Cardiac valvular fibrosis has also been associated with ergot alkaloids.

In the management of type 2 diabetes mellitus, Cycloset® ('quick-release' tablet) should not be interchanged with any other bromocriptine product due to formulation differences and resulting pharmacokinetics. Therapy is not appropriate in patients with diabetic ketoacidosis (DKA) or type 1 diabetes mellitus due to lack of efficacy in these patient populations. There is limited efficacy of use in combination with thiazolidinediones or in combination with insulin. Combination therapy with other hypoglycemic agents may increase risk for hypoglycemic events; dose reduction of concomitant hypoglycemics may be warranted.

Safety and efficacy have not been established in patients with hepatic or renal dysfunction.

Adverse Reactions (Reflective of adult population; not specific for elderly) Note: Frequency of adverse effects may vary by dose and/or indication.

>10%:
  Central nervous system: Dizziness, fatigue, headache
  Gastrointestinal: Constipation, nausea
  Neuromuscular & skeletal: Weakness
  Respiratory: Rhinitis
1% to 10%:
  Cardiovascular: Hypotension (including postural/orthostatic), Raynaud's syndrome exacerbation, syncope
  Central nervous system: Drowsiness, lightheadedness, somnolence
  Endocrine & metabolic: Hypoglycemia (4%; in combination with sulfonylureas or other antidiabetic agents: 7% to 9%)
  Gastrointestinal: Abdominal cramps, anorexia, diarrhea, dyspepsia, GI bleeding, vomiting, xerostomia

Neuromuscular & skeletal: Digital vasospasm
Ocular: Amblyopia
Respiratory: Nasal congestion, sinusitis
Miscellaneous: Infection, flu-like syndrome

Drug Interactions

Metabolism/Transport Effects Substrate of CYP3A4 (major); **Note:** Assignment of Major/Minor substrate status based on clinically relevant drug interaction potential; **Inhibits** CYP1A2 (weak), CYP3A4 (weak)

Avoid Concomitant Use

Avoid concomitant use of Bromocriptine with any of the following: Alpha-/Beta-Agonists; Alpha1-Agonists; Conivaptan; Nitroglycerin; Protease Inhibitors; Serotonin 5-HT1D Receptor Agonists

Increased Effect/Toxicity

Bromocriptine may increase the levels/effects of: Alcohol (Ethyl); Alpha-/Beta-Agonists; Alpha1-Agonists; CycloSPORINE; CycloSPORINE (Systemic); Metoclopramide; Serotonin 5-HT1D Receptor Agonists; Serotonin Modulators

The levels/effects of Bromocriptine may be increased by: Alcohol (Ethyl); Alpha-/Beta-Agonists; Antipsychotics; Conivaptan; CYP3A4 Inhibitors (Moderate); CYP3A4 Inhibitors (Strong); Dasatinib; Ivacaftor; Macrolide Antibiotics; MAO Inhibitors; Methylphenidate; Mifepristone; Nitroglycerin; Protease Inhibitors; Serotonin 5-HT1D Receptor Agonists

Decreased Effect

Bromocriptine may decrease the levels/effects of: Antipsychotics (Typical); Nitroglycerin

The levels/effects of Bromocriptine may be decreased by: Antipsychotics (Atypical); Antipsychotics (Typical); Metoclopramide; Tocilizumab

Ethanol/Nutrition/Herb Interactions

Ethanol: Avoid ethanol (may increase GI side effects or ethanol intolerance).
Herb/Nutraceutical: St John's wort may decrease bromocriptine levels.

Stability Store at or below 25°C (77°F).

Mechanism of Action Semisynthetic ergot alkaloid derivative and a dopamine receptor agonist which activates postsynaptic dopamine receptors in the tuberoinfundibular (inhibiting pituitary prolactin secretion) and nigrostriatal pathways (enhancing coordinated motor control).

In the treatment of type 2 diabetes mellitus, the mechanism of action is unknown; however, bromocriptine is believed to affect circadian rhythms which are mediated, in part, by dopaminergic activity, and are believed to play a role in obesity and insulin resistance. It is postulated that bromocriptine (when administered during the morning and released into the systemic circulation in a rapid, 'pulse-like' dose) may reset hypothalamic circadian activities which have been altered by obesity, thereby resulting in the reversal of insulin resistance and decreases in glucose production, without increasing serum insulin concentrations.

Pharmacodynamics/Kinetics

Onset of action: Parlodel®: Prolactin decreasing effect: 1-2 hours
Distribution: V_d: ~61L
Protein binding: 90% to 96% (primarily albumin)
Metabolism: Primarily hepatic via CYP3A; extensive first-pass biotransformation (Cycloset®: ~93%)
Bioavailability: Parlodel®: 28%; Cycloset®: 65% to 95%
Half-life elimination: Cycloset®: ~6 hours; Parlodel®: Biphasic: Terminal: 15 hours (range: 8-20 hours)
Time to peak, serum: Parlodel®: 1-3 hours; Cycloset®: 53 minutes
Excretion: Feces; urine (2% to 6% as unchanged drug and metabolites)

Dosage

Geriatric & Adult

Acromegaly: Oral: Initial: 1.25-2.5 mg daily increasing by 1.25-2.5 mg daily as necessary every 3-7 days; usual dose: 20-30 mg/day (maximum: 100 mg/day)

Hyperprolactinemia: Oral: Initial: 1.25-2.5 mg/day; may be increased by 2.5 mg/day as tolerated every 2-7 days until optimal response (range: 2.5-15 mg/day)

Parkinsonism: Oral: 1.25 mg twice daily, increased by 2.5 mg/day in 2- to 4-week intervals as needed (maximum: 100 mg/day)

Type 2 diabetes (Cycloset®): Oral: Initial: 0.8 mg once daily; may increase at weekly intervals in 0.8 mg increments as tolerated; usual dose: 1.6-4.8 mg/day (maximum: 4.8 mg/day)

Neuroleptic malignant syndrome (unlabeled use): Oral: 2.5 mg (orally or via gastric tube) every 8-12 hours, increased to a maximum of 45 mg/day, if needed; continue therapy until NMS is controlled, then taper slowly (Gortney, 2009; Strawn, 2007)

Hepatic Impairment No guidelines are available; however, adjustment may be necessary due to extensive hepatic metabolism.

◀ **Administration** Administer with food to decrease GI distress.
Cycloset®: Administer within 2 hours of waking in the morning.

Monitoring Parameters Monitor blood pressure closely as well as hepatic, hematopoietic, and cardiovascular function

Reference Range Recommendations for glycemic control in adults with diabetes:
Hb A$_{1c}$: <7%
Preprandial capillary plasma glucose: 70-130 mg/dL
Peak postprandial capillary blood glucose: <180 mg/dL

Pharmacotherapy Pearls Usually used with levodopa or levodopa/carbidopa to treat Parkinson's disease. When adding bromocriptine, the dose of levodopa/carbidopa can usually be decreased.

Special Geriatric Considerations No special considerations are recommended since drug is dosed to response; however, elderly patients may have concomitant diseases or drug therapy which may complicate therapy. Because more dopamine-specific agonists have fewer side effects, bromocriptine is rarely the drug of choice in Parkinson's disease.

Dosage Forms Excipient information presented when available (limited, particularly for generics); consult specific product labeling.
Capsule, oral: 5 mg
Parlodel®: 5 mg
Tablet, oral: 2.5 mg
Cycloset®: 0.8 mg
Parlodel® SnapTabs®: 2.5 mg [scored]

◆ **Bromocriptine Mesylate** *see* Bromocriptine *on page 223*

Brompheniramine (brome fen IR a meen)

Related Information
Beers Criteria – Potentially Inappropriate Medications for Geriatrics *on page 2183*

Medication Safety Issues
BEERS Criteria medication:
This drug may be potentially inappropriate for use in geriatric patients (Quality of evidence - moderate; Strength of recommendation - strong).

Brand Names: U.S. Bromax [DSC]; J-Tan PD [OTC]; LoHist-12 [DSC]

Index Terms Brompheniramine Maleate; Brompheniramine Tannate

Generic Availability (U.S.) Yes

Pharmacologic Category Alkylamine Derivative; Histamine H$_1$ Antagonist; Histamine H$_1$ Antagonist, First Generation

Use Symptomatic relief of perennial and seasonal allergic rhinitis, vasomotor rhinitis, and other respiratory allergies

Contraindications Hypersensitivity to brompheniramine or any component of the formulation; use with or within 14 days of MAO inhibitor therapy; narrow-angle glaucoma; urinary retention; peptic ulcer disease; during acute asthmatic attacks

Warnings/Precautions Causes sedation; caution must be used in performing tasks which require alertness (eg, operating machinery or driving). Sedative effects of CNS depressants or ethanol are potentiated. Use with caution in patients with hyperthyroidism, increased intraocular pressure, prostatic hyperplasia, history of asthma, and cardiovascular disease (including hypertension and ischemic heart disease). In the elderly, avoid use of this potent anticholinergic agent due to increased risk of confusion, dry mouth, constipation, and other anticholinergic effects; clearance decreases in patients of advanced age (Beers Criteria). Some products may contain tartrazine.

Adverse Reactions (Reflective of adult population; not specific for elderly) Frequency not defined.
Cardiovascular: Angina, blood pressure increased, chest tightness, circulatory collapse, extrasystoles, hypotension, palpitation, tachycardia
Central nervous system: Anxiety, chills, confusion, coordination impaired, dizziness, drowsiness, euphoria, excitation, fatigue, headache, hysteria, insomnia, irritability, nervousness, neuritis, restlessness, sedation, seizure, stimulation, tension, vertigo
Dermatologic: Photosensitivity, rash, urticaria
Endocrine & metabolic: Early menses
Gastrointestinal: Abdominal cramps, anorexia, constipation, diarrhea, dry throat, epigastric distress, heartburn, nausea, vomiting, xerostomia
Genitourinary: Dysuria, polyuria, urinary retention
Hematologic: Agranulocytosis, hemolytic anemia, hypoplastic anemia, thrombocytopenia
Neuromuscular & skeletal: Paresthesia, tremor, weakness
Ocular: Blurred vision, diplopia, mydriasis
Otic: Labyrinthitis (acute), tinnitus

Respiratory: Dry nose, nasal congestion, thickening of bronchial secretions, wheezing

Miscellaneous: Anaphylactic shock, diaphoresis

Drug Interactions

Metabolism/Transport Effects None known.

Avoid Concomitant Use

Avoid concomitant use of Brompheniramine with any of the following: Azelastine; Azelastine (Nasal); Methadone; Mirtazapine; Paraldehyde

Increased Effect/Toxicity

Brompheniramine may increase the levels/effects of: Alcohol (Ethyl); Anticholinergics; Azelastine; Azelastine (Nasal); Buprenorphine; CNS Depressants; Methadone; Methotrimeprazine; Metyrosine; Mirtazapine; Paraldehyde; Selective Serotonin Reuptake Inhibitors; Zolpidem

The levels/effects of Brompheniramine may be increased by: Droperidol; HydrOXYzine; Methotrimeprazine; Pramlintide

Decreased Effect

Brompheniramine may decrease the levels/effects of: Acetylcholinesterase Inhibitors (Central); Benzylpenicilloyl Polylysine; Betahistine; Hyaluronidase

The levels/effects of Brompheniramine may be decreased by: Acetylcholinesterase Inhibitors (Central); Amphetamines

Ethanol/Nutrition/Herb Interactions Ethanol: May increase CNS depression; monitor for increased effects with coadministration. Caution patients about effect.

Stability Store between 15°C to 30°C (59°F to 86°F). Protect from light.

Mechanism of Action Competes with histamine for H_1-receptor sites on effector cells

Pharmacodynamics/Kinetics

Distribution: V_d: Adults: ~12 L/kg (Simons, 1982)

Protein binding: 39% to 49% (Martínez-Gómez, 2007)

Metabolism: Hepatic (Simons, 2004)

Half-life, elimination: Adults: ~25 hours (Simons, 1982)

Time to peak, serum: Adults: 2-4 hours (Simons, 1982)

Excretion: Urine (Bruce, 1968)

Dosage

Adult Allergic rhinitis, allergic symptoms, vasomotor rhinitis: Oral:

Bromax: One tablet twice daily

LoHist-12: 1-2 tablets every 12 hours (maximum: 4 tablets/day)

Administration Extended release tablets are to be swallowed whole; do not crush or chew.

Test Interactions May interfere with urine detection of amphetamine/methamphetamine (false-positive). May interfere with skin tests using allergen extracts.

Special Geriatric Considerations Anticholinergic action may cause significant confusional symptoms, constipation, or problems voiding urine. If an antihistamine is indicated, a second generation nonsedating antihistamine would be a more appropriate choice.

This medication is considered to be potentially inappropriate in this patient population (Beers Criteria: Quality of evidence - moderate; Strength of recommendation - strong).

Dosage Forms Excipient information presented when available (limited, particularly for generics); consult specific product labeling. [DSC] = Discontinued product

Liquid, oral, as maleate [drops]:

J-Tan PD: 1 mg/mL (30 mL) [dye free, ethanol free, sugar free; contains propylene glycol; strawberry-banana flavor]

Tablet, extended release, oral, as maleate:

Bromax: 11 mg [DSC] [dye free]

LoHist-12: 6 mg [DSC] [scored; dye free]

♦ **Brompheniramine Maleate** *see* Brompheniramine *on page 226*

♦ **Brompheniramine Tannate** *see* Brompheniramine *on page 226*

♦ **Brovana®** *see* Arformoterol *on page 141*

♦ **BTX-A** *see* OnabotulinumtoxinA *on page 1423*

♦ **B-type Natriuretic Peptide (Human)** *see* Nesiritide *on page 1361*

♦ **Budeprion XL®** *see* BuPROPion *on page 241*

♦ **Budeprion SR®** *see* BuPROPion *on page 241*

Budesonide (Systemic, Oral Inhalation) (byoo DES oh nide)

Related Information

Asthma *on page 2125*

Inhalant Agents *on page 2117*

Brand Names: U.S. Entocort® EC; Pulmicort Flexhaler®; Pulmicort Respules®

BUDESONIDE (SYSTEMIC, ORAL INHALATION)

Brand Names: Canada Entocort®; Pulmicort® Turbuhaler®

Generic Availability (U.S.) Yes: Capsule; suspension for nebulization

Pharmacologic Category Corticosteroid, Inhalant (Oral); Corticosteroid, Systemic

Use

Nebulization: Maintenance and prophylactic treatment of asthma

Oral capsule: Treatment of active Crohn's disease (mild-to-moderate) involving the ileum and/ or ascending colon; maintenance of remission (for up to 3 months) of Crohn's disease (mild-to-moderate) involving the ileum and/or ascending colon

Oral inhalation: Maintenance and prophylactic treatment of asthma; includes patients who require oral corticosteroids and those who may benefit from systemic dose reduction/ elimination

Contraindications Hypersensitivity to budesonide or any component of the formulation; primary treatment of status asthmaticus, acute episodes of asthma; not for relief of acute bronchospasm

Canadian labeling: Additional contraindications (not in U.S. labeling): Moderate-to-severe bronchiectasis, pulmonary tuberculosis (active or quiescent), untreated respiratory infection (bacterial, fungal, or viral)

Warnings/Precautions May cause hypercorticism or suppression of hypothalamic-pituitary-adrenal (HPA) axis, particularly in patients receiving high doses for prolonged periods. HPA axis suppression may lead to adrenal crisis. Withdrawal and discontinuation of a corticosteroid should be done slowly and carefully. Particular care is required when patients are transferred from systemic corticosteroids to inhaled products due to possible adrenal insufficiency or withdrawal from steroids, including an increase in allergic symptoms. Patients receiving >20 mg per day of prednisone (or equivalent) may be most susceptible. Fatalities have occurred due to adrenal insufficiency in asthmatic patients during and after transfer from systemic corticosteroids to aerosol steroids; aerosol steroids do not provide the systemic steroid needed to treat patients having trauma, surgery, or infections. Do not use this product to transfer patients directly from oral corticosteroid therapy.

Bronchospasm may occur with wheezing after inhalation; if this occurs stop steroid and treat with a fast-acting bronchodilator (eg, albuterol). Supplemental steroids (oral or parenteral) may be needed during stress or severe asthma attacks. Not to be used in status asthmaticus or for the relief of acute bronchospasm. Acute myopathy has been reported with high-dose corticosteroids, usually in patients with neuromuscular transmission disorders; may involve ocular and/or respiratory muscles; monitor creatine kinase; recovery may be delayed. Corticosteroid use may cause psychiatric disturbances, including depression, euphoria, insomnia, mood swings, and personality changes. Pre-existing psychiatric conditions may be exacerbated by corticosteroid use. Prolonged use of corticosteroids may also increase the incidence of secondary infection, mask acute infection (including fungal infections), prolong or exacerbate viral infections, or limit response to vaccines. Exposure to chickenpox should be avoided; corticosteroids should not be used to treat ocular herpes simplex. Corticosteroids should not be used for cerebral malaria or viral hepatitis. Close observation is required in patients with latent tuberculosis and/or TB reactivity; restrict use in active TB (only in conjunction with antituberculosis treatment). *Candida albicans* infections may occur in the mouth and pharynx; rinsing (and spitting) with water after inhaler use may decrease risk. Prolonged treatment with corticosteroids has been associated with the development of Kaposi's sarcoma (case reports); if noted, discontinuation of therapy should be considered.

Use with caution in patients with thyroid disease, hepatic impairment, renal impairment, cardiovascular disease, diabetes, glaucoma, cataracts, myasthenia gravis, patients at risk for osteoporosis, patients at risk for seizures, or GI diseases (diverticulitis, peptic ulcer, ulcerative colitis) due to perforation risk. Use caution following acute MI (corticosteroids have been associated with myocardial rupture). Because of the risk of adverse effects, systemic corticosteroids should be used cautiously in the elderly in the smallest possible effective dose for the shortest duration.

Pulmicort Flexhaler™ contains lactose; very rare anaphylactic reactions have been reported in patients with severe milk protein allergy.

Adverse Reactions (Reflective of adult population; not specific for elderly) Reaction severity varies by dose and duration; not all adverse reactions have been reported with each dosage form.

>10%:

Central nervous system: Headache (≤21%)

Gastrointestinal: Nausea (≤11%)

Respiratory: Respiratory infection, rhinitis

Miscellaneous: Symptoms of HPA axis suppression and/or hypercorticism may occur in >10% of patients following administration of dosage forms which result in higher systemic exposure (ie, oral capsule), but may be less frequent than rates observed with comparator drugs (prednisolone). These symptoms may be rare (<1%) following administration via methods which result in lower exposures (topical).

1% to 10%:

Cardiovascular: Chest pain, edema, flushing, hypertension, palpitation, syncope, tachycardia

Central nervous system: Amnesia, dizziness, dysphonia, emotional lability, fatigue, fever, insomnia, malaise, migraine, nervousness, pain, sleep disorder, somnolence, vertigo

Dermatologic: Acne, alopecia, bruising, contact dermatitis, eczema, hirsutism, pruritus, pustular rash, rash, striae

Endocrine & metabolic: Adrenal insufficiency, hypokalemia, menstrual disorder

Gastrointestinal: Abdominal pain, anorexia, diarrhea, dyspepsia, flatulence, gastroenteritis (including viral), glossitis, intestinal obstruction, oral candidiasis, taste perversion, tongue edema, vomiting, weight gain, xerostomia

Genitourinary: Dysuria, hematuria, nocturia, pyuria

Hematologic: Cervical lymphadenopathy, leukocytosis, purpura

Hepatic: Alkaline phosphatase increased

Neuromuscular & skeletal: Arthralgia, back pain, fracture, hyperkinesis, hypertonia, myalgia, neck pain, paresthesia, weakness

Ocular: Conjunctivitis, eye infection

Otic: Earache, ear infection, external ear infection

Respiratory: Bronchitis, bronchospasm, cough, epistaxis, hoarseness, nasal congestion, nasal irritation, pharyngitis, sinusitis, stridor, throat irritation

Miscellaneous: Abscess, allergic reaction, C-reactive protein increased, erythrocyte sedimentation rate increased, fat distribution (moon face, buffalo hump); flu-like syndrome, herpes simplex, infection, moniliasis, viral infection, voice alteration

Drug Interactions

Metabolism/Transport Effects Substrate of CYP3A4 (major); **Note:** Assignment of Major/Minor substrate status based on clinically relevant drug interaction potential

Avoid Concomitant Use

Avoid concomitant use of Budesonide (Systemic, Oral Inhalation) with any of the following: Aldesleukin; BCG; Grapefruit Juice; Natalizumab; Pimecrolimus; Tacrolimus (Topical)

Increased Effect/Toxicity

Budesonide (Systemic, Oral Inhalation) may increase the levels/effects of: Amphotericin B; Deferasirox; Leflunomide; Loop Diuretics; Natalizumab; Thiazide Diuretics

The levels/effects of Budesonide (Systemic, Oral Inhalation) may be increased by: CYP3A4 Inhibitors (Moderate); CYP3A4 Inhibitors (Strong); Dasatinib; Denosumab; Grapefruit Juice; Ivacaftor; Mifepristone; Pimecrolimus; Tacrolimus (Topical); Telaprevir; Trastuzumab

Decreased Effect

Budesonide (Systemic, Oral Inhalation) may decrease the levels/effects of: Aldesleukin; Antidiabetic Agents; BCG; Coccidioidin Skin Test; Corticorelin; Hyaluronidase; Sipuleucel-T; Telaprevir; Vaccines (Inactivated)

The levels/effects of Budesonide (Systemic, Oral Inhalation) may be decreased by: Antacids; Bile Acid Sequestrants; Echinacea; Tocilizumab

Ethanol/Nutrition/Herb Interactions

Food: Grapefruit juice may double systemic exposure of orally administered budesonide. Administration of capsules with a high-fat meal delays peak concentration, but does not alter the extent of absorption. Management: Avoid grapefruit juice when using oral capsules.

Herb/Nutraceutical: Echinacea may diminish the therapeutic effect of budesonide. Management: Avoid echinacea.

Stability

Suspension for nebulization: Store upright at 20°C to 25°C (68°F to 77°F). Protect from light. Do not refrigerate or freeze. Once aluminum package is opened, solution should be used within 2 weeks. Continue to protect from light.

Oral inhaler (Pulmicort Flexhaler™): Store at controlled room temperature of 20°C to 25°C (68°F to 77°F). Protect from moisture.

Mechanism of Action Controls the rate of protein synthesis; depresses the migration of polymorphonuclear leukocytes, fibroblasts; reverses capillary permeability and lysosomal stabilization at the cellular level to prevent or control inflammation. Has potent glucocorticoid activity and weak mineralocorticoid activity.

Pharmacodynamics/Kinetics

Onset of action: Pulmicort Respules®: 2-8 days; Inhalation: 24 hours

Peak effect: Pulmicort Respules®: 4-6 weeks; Inhalation: 1-2 weeks

Distribution: 2.2-3.9 L/kg

Protein binding: 85% to 90%

Metabolism: Hepatic via CYP3A4 to two metabolites: 16 alpha-hydroxyprednisolone and 6 beta-hydroxybudesonide; minor activity

Bioavailability: Limited by high first-pass effect; Capsule: 9% to 21%; Pulmicort Respules®: 6%; Inhalation: 6% to 13%

Half-life elimination: 2-3.6 hours

Time to peak: Capsule: 0.5-10 hours (variable in Crohn's disease); Pulmicort Respules®: 10-30 minutes; Inhalation: 1-2 hours

Excretion: Urine (60%) and feces as metabolites

Dosage

Geriatric & Adult

Asthma: Oral inhalation: Titrate to lowest effective dose once patient is stable.

U.S. labeling: Pulmicort Flexhaler™: Initial: 360 mcg twice daily (selected patients may be initiated at 180 mcg twice daily); maximum: 720 mcg twice daily; **Note:** May increase dose after 1-2 weeks of therapy in patients who are not adequately controlled:

NIH Asthma Guidelines (NIH, 2007) (administer in divided doses twice daily):

"Low" dose: 180-600 mcg/day

"Medium" dose: >600-1200 mcg/day

"High" dose: >1200 mcg/day

Canadian labeling: Pulmicort® Turbuhaler®:

Initial (or during periods of severe asthma or when switching from oral corticosteroid therapy): 400-2400 mcg daily in 2-4 divided doses

Maintenance: 200-400 mcg twice daily (higher doses may be needed for some patients). Patients taking 400 mcg/day may take as a single daily dose.

Conversion from oral systemic corticosteroid to orally inhaled corticosteroid: Initiation of oral inhalation therapy should begin in patients whose asthma is reasonably stabilized on oral corticosteroids (OCS). A gradual dose reduction of OCS should begin ~7-10 days after starting inhaled therapy. U.S. labeling recommends reducing prednisone dose by 2.5 mg/day (or equivalent of other OCS) on a weekly basis (patients using oral inhaler) or by ≤25% every 1-2 weeks (patients using respules). Canadian labeling recommends reducing prednisone dose by 2.5 mg/day (or equivalent of other OCS) every 4 days in closely monitored patients or every 10 days if not closely monitored. If adrenal insufficiency occurs, temporarily increase the OCS dose and follow with a more gradual withdrawal. **Note:** When transitioning from systemic to inhaled corticosteroids, supplemental systemic corticosteroid therapy may be necessary during periods of stress or during severe asthma attacks.

Crohn's disease (active): Oral: 9 mg once daily in the morning for up to 8 weeks; recurring episodes may be treated with a repeat 8-week course of treatment. **Note:** Patients receiving CYP3A4 inhibitors should be monitored closely for signs and symptoms of hypercorticism; dosage reduction may be required. If switching from oral prednisolone, prednisolone dosage should be tapered while budesonide (Entocort™ EC) treatment is initiated.

Maintenance of remission: Following treatment of active disease (control of symptoms with CDAI <150), treatment may be continued at a dosage of 6 mg once daily for up to 3 months. If symptom control is maintained for 3 months, tapering of the dosage to complete cessation is recommended. Continued dosing beyond 3 months has not been demonstrated to result in substantial benefit.

Renal Impairment Inhalation, Nebulization, Oral: No dosage adjustment provided in manufacturer's labeling; has not been studied.

Hepatic Impairment Inhalation, Nebulization, Oral: No specific dosage adjustment provided in manufacturer's labeling; has not been studied. Manufacturer's labeling for oral budesonide suggests a dosage reduction may be necessary with moderate to severe impairment. Budesonide undergoes hepatic metabolism; monitor closely for signs and symptoms of hypercorticism.

Administration

Oral capsule: Capsule should be swallowed whole; do not crush or chew.

Powder for inhalation:

Pulmicort Flexhaler™: Hold inhaler in upright position (mouthpiece up) to load dose. Do not shake prior to use. Unit should be primed prior to first use only. It will not need primed again, even if not used for a long time. Place mouthpiece between lips and inhale forcefully and deeply. Do not exhale through inhaler; do not use a spacer. Dose indicator does not move with every dose, usually only after 5 doses. Discard when dose indicator reads "0". Rinse mouth with water after each use to reduce incidence of candidiasis.

Pulmicort® Turbuhaler® [CAN, not available in the U.S.]: Hold inhaler in upright position (mouthpiece up) to load dose. Do not shake inhaler after dose is loaded. Unit should be primed prior to first use. Place mouthpiece between lips and inhale forcefully and deeply; mouthpiece should face up. Do not exhale through inhaler; do not use a spacer. When a red mark appears in the dose indicator window, 20 doses are left. When the red mark reaches the bottom of the window, the inhaler should be discarded. Rinse mouth with water after use to reduce incidence of candidiasis.

Suspension for nebulization: Shake well before using. Use Pulmicort Respules® with jet nebulizer connected to an air compressor; administer with mouthpiece or facemask. Do not use ultrasonic nebulizer. Do not mix with other medications in nebulizer. Rinse mouth following treatments to decrease risk of oral candidiasis (wash face if using face mask).

Monitoring Parameters Monitor blood pressure, serum glucose, weight with high-dose or long-term oral use

Asthma: FEV_1, peak flow, and/or other pulmonary function tests

Pharmacotherapy Pearls No geriatric-specific information.

Special Geriatric Considerations Ensure that patients can correctly use inhaler.

Dosage Forms Excipient information presented when available (limited, particularly for generics); consult specific product labeling.

Capsule, enteric coated, oral: 3 mg
  Entocort® EC: 3 mg
Powder, for oral inhalation:
  Pulmicort Flexhaler®: 90 mcg/inhalation (165 mg) [contains lactose; delivers ~80 mcg/inhalation; 60 actuations]
  Pulmicort Flexhaler®: 180 mcg/inhalation (225 mg) [contains lactose; delivers ~160 mcg/inhalation; 120 actuations]
Suspension, for nebulization: 0.25 mg/2 mL (30s); 0.5 mg/2 mL (30s)
  Pulmicort Respules®: 0.25 mg/2 mL (30s); 0.5 mg/2 mL (30s); 1 mg/2 mL (30s)

Dosage Forms: Canada Excipient information presented when available (limited, particularly for generics); consult specific product labeling.

Powder for oral inhalation:
  Pulmicort® Turbuhaler®: 100 mcg/inhalation [delivers 200 metered actuations]; 200 mcg/inhalation [delivers 200 metered actuations]; 400 mcg/inhalation [delivers 200 metered actuations]

Budesonide (Nasal) (byoo DES oh nide)

Brand Names: U.S. Rhinocort Aqua®:
Brand Names: Canada Mylan-Budesonide AQ; Rhinocort® Aqua®; Rhinocort® Turbuhaler®
Generic Availability (U.S.) No
Pharmacologic Category Corticosteroid, Nasal
Use Management of symptoms of seasonal or perennial rhinitis

Canadian labeling: Additional use (not in U.S. labeling): Prevention and treatment of nasal polyps

Unlabeled Use Adjunct to antibiotics in empiric treatment of acute bacterial rhinosinusitis (ABRS) (Chow, 2012)

Dosage

Geriatric & Adult

Nasal polyps: *Nasal inhalation:*
  Canadian labeling:
    Rhinocort® Aqua®: 256 mcg/day administered as a single 64 mcg spray in each nostril twice daily; maximum dose: 256 mcg/day
    Rhinocort® Turbuhaler®: 100 mcg into each nostril twice daily; maximum: 400 mcg/day

Rhinitis: *Nasal inhalation:*
  U.S. labeling (Rhinocort® Aqua®): 64 mcg/day as a single 32 mcg spray in each nostril. Some patients who do not achieve adequate control may benefit from increased dosage. A reduced dosage may be effective after initial control is achieved
  Maximum dose: 256 mcg/day)
  Canadian labeling:
    Rhinocort® Aqua®: Initial: 256 mcg/day administered as two 64 mcg sprays in each nostril once daily or a single 64 mcg spray in each nostril twice daily; Maintenance: Individualize, lowest effective dose (maximum dose: 256 mcg/day)
    Rhinocort® Turbuhaler®: Initial: 200 mcg into each nostril once daily; Maintenance: Individualize, lowest effective dose (maximum: 400 mcg/day)

Hepatic Impairment Monitor closely for signs and symptoms of hypercorticism; dosage reduction may be required.

Special Geriatric Considerations Evaluate the patient's or caregiver's ability to safely administer the correct dose of nasal medication.

Dosage Forms Excipient information presented when available (limited, particularly for generics); consult specific product labeling.

Suspension, intranasal [spray]:
  Rhinocort Aqua®: 32 mcg/inhalation (8.6 g) [120 metered actuations]

◀ **Dosage Forms: Canada** Excipient information presented when available (limited, particularly for generics); consult specific product labeling.

Powder for nasal inhalation:
  Rhinocort® Turbuhaler®: 100 mcg/inhalation [delivers 200 metered actuations]
Suspension, intranasal [spray]:
  Rhinocort® Aqua®: 64 mcg/inhalation [120 metered actuations]

◆ **Budesonide and Eformoterol** *see* Budesonide and Formoterol *on page* 232

Budesonide and Formoterol (byoo DES oh nide & for MOH te rol)

Brand Names: U.S. Symbicort®
Brand Names: Canada Symbicort®
Index Terms Budesonide and Eformoterol; Eformoterol and Budesonide; Formoterol and Budesonide; Formoterol Fumarate Dihydrate and Budesonide
Pharmacologic Category Beta$_2$ Agonist; Beta$_2$-Adrenergic Agonist, Long-Acting; Corticosteroid, Inhalant (Oral)
Use Treatment of asthma in patients ≥12 years of age where combination therapy is indicated; maintenance treatment of airflow obstruction associated with chronic obstructive pulmonary disease (COPD; including chronic bronchitis and emphysema)
Medication Guide Available Yes
Contraindications Hypersensitivity to budesonide, formoterol, or any component of the formulation; need for acute bronchodilation in COPD or asthma (including status asthmaticus)

Canadian labeling: Additional contraindications (not in U.S. labeling): Hypersensitivity to inhaled lactose
Warnings/Precautions [U.S. Boxed Warning]: Long-acting beta$_2$-agonists (LABAs), such as formoterol, increase the risk of asthma-related deaths; budesonide and formoterol should only be used in patients not adequately controlled on a long-term asthma control medication (ie, inhaled corticosteroid) or whose disease severity requires initiation of two maintenance therapies. In a large, randomized, placebo-controlled U.S. clinical trial (SMART, 2006), salmeterol was associated with an increase in asthma-related deaths (when added to usual asthma therapy); risk is considered a class effect among all LABAs. Data are not available to determine if the addition of an inhaled corticosteroid lessens this increased risk of death associated with LABA use. Assess patients at regular intervals once asthma control is maintained on combination therapy to determine if step-down therapy is appropriate (without loss of asthma control), and the patient can be maintained on an inhaled corticosteroid only. LABAs are not appropriate in patients whose asthma is adequately controlled on low- or medium-dose inhaled corticosteroids.

Do **not** use for acute bronchospasm or acute symptomatic COPD. Short-acting beta$_2$-agonist (eg, albuterol) should be used for acute symptoms and symptoms occurring between treatments. Do **not** initiate in patients with significantly worsening or acutely deteriorating asthma or COPD. Increased use and/or ineffectiveness of short-acting beta$_2$-agonists may indicate rapidly deteriorating disease and should prompt re-evaluation of the patient's condition. Patients must be instructed to seek medical attention in cases where acute symptoms are not relieved by short-acting beta-agonist (not formoterol) or a previous level of response is diminished. Medical evaluation must not be delayed. Patients using inhaled, short acting beta$_2$-agonists should be instructed to discontinue routine use of these medications prior to beginning treatment with Symbicort®; short acting agents should be reserved for symptomatic relief of acute symptoms. Data are not available to determine if LABA use increases the risk of death in patients with COPD.

Immediate hypersensitivity reactions (urticaria, angioedema, rash, bronchospasm) have been reported. Do not exceed recommended dose; serious adverse events, including fatalities, have been associated with excessive use of inhaled sympathomimetics. Rarely, paradoxical bronchospasm may occur with use of inhaled bronchodilating agents; this should be distinguished from inadequate response. Pneumonia and other lower respiratory tract infections have been reported in patients with COPD following the use of inhaled corticosteroids; monitor COPD patients closely since pneumonia symptoms may overlap symptoms of exacerbations.

Use caution in patients with cardiovascular disease (arrhythmia or hypertension or HF), seizure disorders, diabetes, hepatic impairment, ocular disease, osteoporosis, thyroid disease, or hypokalemia. Beta agonists may cause elevation in blood pressure, heart rate, and result in CNS stimulation/excitation. Beta$_2$-agonists may increase risk of arrhythmia, increase serum glucose, or decrease serum potassium. Long-term use may affect bone mineral density in adults. Infections with *Candida albicans* in the mouth and throat (thrush) have been reported with use. Use with caution in patients taking strong CYP3A4 inhibitors (see Drug

Interactions); consider alternative agents that avoid or lessen the potential for CYP-mediated interactions.

Budesonide may cause hypercorticism and/or suppression of hypothalamic-pituitary-adrenal (HPA) axis, particularly in younger children or in patients receiving high doses for prolonged periods. Caution is required when patients are transferred from systemic corticosteroids to products with lower systemic bioavailability (ie, inhalation). May lead to possible adrenal insufficiency or withdrawal symptoms, including an increase in allergic symptoms. Patients receiving prolonged therapy ≥20 mg per day of prednisone (or equivalent) may be most susceptible. Aerosol steroids do **not** provide the systemic steroid needed to treat patients having trauma, surgery, or infections.

Prolonged use of corticosteroids may also increase the incidence of secondary infection, mask acute infection (including fungal infections), prolong or exacerbate viral infections, or limit response to vaccines. Exposure to chickenpox should be avoided; corticosteroids should not be used to treat ocular herpes simplex. Corticosteroids should not be used for cerebral malaria. Close observation is required in patients with latent tuberculosis and/or TB reactivity restrict use in active TB (only in conjunction with antituberculosis treatment).

Some products available in Canada contain lactose; very rare anaphylactic reactions have been reported in patients with severe milk protein allergy. Withdraw systemic therapy with gradual tapering of dose. There have been reports of systemic corticosteroid withdrawal symptoms (eg, joint/muscle pain, lassitude, depression) when withdrawing oral inhalation therapy.

Adverse Reactions (Reflective of adult population; not specific for elderly) Note: Percentage of adverse events may be dose related; causation not established. Also see individual agents.
>10%:
  Central nervous system: Headache (7% to 11%)
  Respiratory: Nasopharyngitis (7% to 11%), upper respiratory tract infections (4% to 11%)
1% to 10%:
  Central nervous system: Dizziness (<3%)
  Gastrointestinal: Stomach discomfort (1% to 7%), oral candidiasis (1% to 6%), vomiting (1% to 3%)
  Neuromuscular & skeletal: Back pain (2% to 3%)
  Respiratory: Pharyngolaryngeal pain (6% to 9%), lower respiratory tract infection (3% to 8%), sinusitis (4% to 6%), bronchitis (5%), nasal congestion (3%)
  Miscellaneous: Influenza (2% to 3%)

Drug Interactions
  Metabolism/Transport Effects Refer to individual components.
  Avoid Concomitant Use
  Avoid concomitant use of Budesonide and Formoterol with any of the following: Aldesleukin; BCG; Beta-Blockers (Nonselective); Grapefruit Juice; Iobenguane I 123; Natalizumab; Pimecrolimus; Tacrolimus (Topical)
  Increased Effect/Toxicity
  Budesonide and Formoterol may increase the levels/effects of: Amphotericin B; Deferasirox; Leflunomide; Loop Diuretics; Natalizumab; Sympathomimetics; Thiazide Diuretics

  The levels/effects of Budesonide and Formoterol may be increased by: AtoMOXetine; Caffeine; Cannabinoids; CYP3A4 Inhibitors (Moderate); CYP3A4 Inhibitors (Strong); Dasatinib; Denosumab; Grapefruit Juice; Ivacaftor; MAO Inhibitors; Mifepristone; Pimecrolimus; Tacrolimus (Topical); Telaprevir; Theophylline Derivatives; Trastuzumab; Tricyclic Antidepressants
  Decreased Effect
  Budesonide and Formoterol may decrease the levels/effects of: Aldesleukin; Antidiabetic Agents; BCG; Coccidioidin Skin Test; Corticorelin; Hyaluronidase; Iobenguane I 123; Sipuleucel-T; Telaprevir; Vaccines (Inactivated)

  The levels/effects of Budesonide and Formoterol may be decreased by: Alpha-/Beta-Blockers; Antacids; Beta-Blockers (Beta1 Selective); Beta-Blockers (Nonselective); Betahistine; Bile Acid Sequestrants; Echinacea; Tocilizumab

Stability
  Symbicort® 80/4.5, Symbicort® 160/4.5: Store at room temperature of 20°C to 25°C (68°F to 77°F) with mouthpiece down. Do not puncture, incinerate, or store near heat or open flame. Discard inhaler after the labeled number of inhalations have been used or within 3 months after removal from foil pouch.
  Symbicort® Turbuhaler®: Store at room temperature of 15°C to 30°C. Protect from heat and moisture.

BUDESONIDE AND FORMOTEROL

◀ **Mechanism of Action** Formoterol relaxes bronchial smooth muscle by selective action on beta$_2$-receptors with little effect on heart rate. Formoterol has a long-acting effect. Budesonide is a corticosteroid which controls the rate of protein synthesis, depresses the migration of polymorphonuclear leukocytes/fibroblasts, and reverses capillary permeability and lysosomal stabilization at the cellular level to prevent or control inflammation.

Pharmacodynamics/Kinetics See individual agents.

Onset of action: Asthma: 15 minutes; maximum benefit: may take ≥2 weeks

Dosage

Geriatric & Adult

Asthma: Oral inhalation:

U.S. labeling: Symbicort® 80/4.5, Symbicort® 160/4.5: Two inhalations twice daily (maximum: 4 inhalations/day). Recommended starting dose combination is determined according to asthma severity. In patients not adequately controlled on the lower combination dose following 1-2 weeks of therapy, consider the higher dose combination.

Canadian labeling:

Symbicort® 100 Turbuhaler® [CAN; not available in U.S.], Symbicort® 200 Turbuhaler® [CAN; not available in U.S.]:

Initial: 1-2 inhalations twice daily until symptom control, then titrate to lowest effective dosage to maintain control

Maintenance: 1-2 inhalations once or twice daily (maximum: 8 inhalations/day as temporary treatment in periods of worsening asthma)

Symbicort® Maintenance and Reliever Therapy (Symbicort® SMART): **Note:** Not approved in the U.S.:

Maintenance: Symbicort® 100 Turbuhaler® [CAN] **or** Symbicort® 200 Turbuhaler® [CAN]: 1-2 inhalations twice daily **or** 2 inhalations once daily

Reliever therapy: Symbicort® 100 Turbuhaler [CAN] **or** Symbicort® 200 Turbuhaler® [CAN]: 1 additional inhalation as needed, may repeat if no relief for up to 6 inhalations total (maximum: 8 inhalations/day)

COPD: Oral inhalation:

U.S. labeling: Symbicort® 160/4.5: Two inhalations twice daily (maximum: 4 inhalations/day)

Canadian labeling: Symbicort® 200 Turbuhaler® [CAN; not available in U.S.]: Two inhalations twice daily (maximum: 4 inhalations/day)

Hepatic Impairment Use of this combination has not been studied in patients with hepatic impairment; however, the manufacturer recommends close monitoring of patients with hepatic disease.

Administration

Symbicort® 80/4.5, Symbicort® 160/4.5: Prior to first use, inhaler must be primed by releasing 2 test sprays into the air; shake well for 5 seconds before each spray. Inhaler must be reprimed if not used for >7 days or if it has been dropped. Shake well for 5 seconds before each use. Discard inhaler after the labeled number of inhalations have been used or within 3 months after removal from foil pouch (do not use the "float test" to determine amount remaining in canister).

Symbicort® Turbuhaler® [CAN; not available in U.S.]:

To "load" inhaler: Turn grip on inhaler as far as it will move in one direction, then turn in opposite direction as far as it will go (inhaler is "loaded" with a dose, indicated by a "click"). Prior to first use, this procedure should be done twice, it does not need to be repeated with subsequent uses even when not used regularly.

Delivery of dose: Instruct patient to place mouthpiece gently between teeth, closing lips around inhaler. Instruct patient to inhale deeply and hold breath held for 5-10 seconds. The amount of drug delivered is small, and the individual will not sense the medication as it is inhaled. Remove mouthpiece prior to exhalation. Patient should not breathe out through the mouthpiece. After use of the inhaler, patient should rinse mouth/oropharynx with water and spit out rinse solution.

Monitoring Parameters FEV$_1$, peak flow meter and/or other pulmonary function tests; monitor for increased use if short-acting beta$_2$-adrenergic agonists (may be a sign of asthma or COPD deterioration)

Dosage Forms Excipient information presented when available (limited, particularly for generics); consult specific product labeling.

Aerosol for oral inhalation:

Symbicort® 80/4.5: Budesonide 80 mcg and formoterol fumarate dihydrate 4.5 mcg per actuation (6.9 g) [60 metered inhalations]; budesonide 80 mcg and formoterol fumarate dihydrate 4.5 mcg per actuation (10.2 g) [120 metered inhalations]

Symbicort® 160/4.5: Budesonide 160 mcg and formoterol fumarate dihydrate 4.5 mcg per actuation (6 g) [60 metered inhalations]; budesonide 160 mcg and formoterol fumarate dihydrate 4.5 mcg per actuation (10.2 g) [120 metered inhalations]

Dosage Forms: Canada Excipient information presented when available (limited, particularly for generics); consult specific product labeling.

Powder for oral inhalation:

Symbicort® 100 Turbuhaler®: Budesonide 100 mcg and formoterol dihydrate 6 mcg per inhalation (available in 60 or 120 metered doses) [delivers ~80 mcg budesonide and 4.5 mcg formoterol per inhalation; contains lactose]

Symbicort® 200 Turbuhaler®: Budesonide 200 mcg and formoterol dihydrate 6 mcg per inhalation (available in 60 or 120 metered doses) [delivers ~160 mcg budesonide and 4.5 mcg formoterol per inhalation; contains lactose]

◆ **Buffasal [OTC]** see Aspirin on page 154
◆ **Bufferin® [OTC]** see Aspirin on page 154
◆ **Bufferin® Extra Strength [OTC]** see Aspirin on page 154
◆ **Buffinol [OTC]** see Aspirin on page 154
◆ **Bulk-K [OTC]** see Psyllium on page 1635

Bumetanide (byoo MET a nide)

Medication Safety Issues

Sound-alike/look-alike issues:

Bumetanide may be confused with Buminate®

Bumex® may be confused with Brevibloc®, Buprenex®

International issues:

Bumex [U.S.] may be confused with Permax brand name for pergolide [multiple international markets]

Brand Names: Canada Burinex®

Index Terms Bumex

Generic Availability (U.S.) Yes

Pharmacologic Category Diuretic, Loop

Use Management of edema secondary to heart failure or hepatic or renal disease (including nephrotic syndrome)

Unlabeled Use Treatment of hypertension

Contraindications Hypersensitivity to bumetanide or any component of the formulation; anuria; patients with hepatic coma or in states of severe electrolyte depletion until the condition improves or is corrected

Warnings/Precautions [U.S. Boxed Warning]: Excessive amounts can lead to profound diuresis with fluid and electrolyte loss; close medical supervision and dose evaluation are required. Potassium supplementation and/or use of potassium-sparing diuretics may be necessary to prevent hypokalemia. In cirrhosis, initiate bumetanide therapy with conservative dosing and close monitoring of electrolytes; avoid sudden changes in fluid and electrolyte balance and acid/base status which may lead to hepatic encephalopathy. Coadministration of antihypertensives may increase the risk of hypotension.

Monitor fluid status and renal function in an attempt to prevent oliguria, azotemia, and reversible increases in BUN and creatinine; close medical supervision of aggressive diuresis required. Bumetanide-induced ototoxicity (usually transient) may occur with rapid I.V. administration, renal impairment, excessive doses, and concurrent use of other ototoxins (eg, aminoglycosides). Asymptomatic hyperuricemia has been reported with use.

Chemical similarities are present among sulfonamides, sulfonylureas, carbonic anhydrase inhibitors, thiazides, and loop diuretics (except ethacrynic acid); the manufacturer's labeling states that bumetanide may be used in patients allergic to furosemide. Use in patients with sulfonylurea allergy is not specifically contraindicated in product labeling; however, a risk of cross-reaction exists in patients with allergy to any of these compounds; avoid use when previous reaction has been severe. Discontinue if signs of hypersensitivity are noted.

Adverse Reactions (Reflective of adult population; not specific for elderly)

>10%:

Endocrine & metabolic: Hyperuricemia (18%), hypochloremia (15%), hypokalemia (15%)

Renal: Azotemia (11%)

1% to 10%:

Central nervous system: Dizziness (1%)

Endocrine & metabolic: Hyponatremia (9%), hyperglycemia (7%), phosphorus altered (5%), CO_2 content altered (4%), bicarbonate altered (3%), calcium altered (2%)

Neuromuscular & skeletal: Muscle cramps (1%)

Renal: Serum creatinine increased (7%)

Miscellaneous: LDH altered (1%)

Drug Interactions

Metabolism/Transport Effects None known.

Avoid Concomitant Use There are no known interactions where it is recommended to avoid concomitant use.

Increased Effect/Toxicity

Bumetanide may increase the levels/effects of: ACE Inhibitors; Allopurinol; Amifostine; Aminoglycosides; Antihypertensives; Cardiac Glycosides; CISplatin; Dofetilide; Hypotensive Agents; Lithium; Methotrexate; Neuromuscular-Blocking Agents; RisperiDONE; RiTUXimab; Salicylates; Sodium Phosphates

The levels/effects of Bumetanide may be increased by: Alfuzosin; Beta2-Agonists; Corticosteroids (Orally Inhaled); Corticosteroids (Systemic); CycloSPORINE (Systemic); Diazoxide; Herbs (Hypotensive Properties); Licorice; MAO Inhibitors; Methotrexate; Pentoxifylline; Phosphodiesterase 5 Inhibitors; Probenecid; Prostacyclin Analogues

Decreased Effect

Bumetanide may decrease the levels/effects of: Hypoglycemic Agents; Lithium; Neuromuscular-Blocking Agents

The levels/effects of Bumetanide may be decreased by: Bile Acid Sequestrants; Fosphenytoin; Herbs (Hypertensive Properties); Methotrexate; Methylphenidate; Nonsteroidal Anti-Inflammatory Agents; Phenytoin; Probenecid; Salicylates; Yohimbine

Ethanol/Nutrition/Herb Interactions

Food: Bumetanide serum levels may be decreased if taken with food. It has been recommended that bumetanide be administered without food (Bard, 2004).

Herb/Nutraceutical: Avoid ephedra, yohimbe, ginseng (may worsen hypertension). Avoid dong quai if using for hypertension (has estrogenic activity). Avoid garlic (may have increased antihypertensive effect).

Stability

I.V.: Store vials at 15°C to 30°C (59°F to 86°F). Infusion solutions should be used within 24 hours after preparation. Light sensitive; discoloration may occur when exposed to light.

Tablet: Store at 15°C to 30°C (59°F to 86°F).

Mechanism of Action Inhibits reabsorption of sodium and chloride in the ascending loop of Henle and proximal renal tubule, interfering with the chloride-binding cotransport system, thus causing increased excretion of water, sodium, chloride, magnesium, phosphate, and calcium; it does not appear to act on the distal tubule

Pharmacodynamics/Kinetics

Onset of action: Oral, I.M.: 0.5-1 hour; I.V.: 2-3 minutes

Peak effect: Oral: 1-2 hours; I.V.: 15-30 minutes

Duration: 4-6 hours

Distribution: V_d: Adults: 9-25 L

Protein binding: 94% to 96%

Metabolism: Partially hepatic

Bioavailability: 59% to 89% (median: 80%)

Half-life elimination: Adults: 1-1.5 hours

Excretion: Urine (81% of total dose; 45% of which is unchanged drug); feces (2% of total dose)

Dosage

Geriatric & Adult

Edema:

Oral: 0.5-2 mg/dose 1-2 times/day; if diuretic response to initial dose is not adequate, may repeat in 4-5 hours for up to 2 doses (maximum dose: 10 mg/day)

I.M., I.V.: 0.5-1 mg/dose; if diuretic response to initial dose is not adequate, may repeat in 2-3 hours for up to 2 doses (maximum dose: 10 mg/day)

Continuous I.V. infusion (unlabeled dose): Initial: 1 mg I.V. load then 0.5-2 mg/hour (Hunt, 2009)

Hypertension (unlabeled use): *Oral:* 0.5 mg daily (maximum dose: 5 mg/day); usual dosage range (JNC 7): 0.5-2 mg/day in 2 divided doses (Chobanian, 2003)

Administration

I.V.: Administer slowly, over 1-2 minutes.

Oral: An alternate-day schedule or a 3-4 daily dosing regimen with rest periods of 1-2 days in between may be the most tolerable and effective regimen for the continued control of edema.

Monitoring Parameters Blood pressure; serum electrolytes, renal function; fluid status (weight and I & O), blood pressure

Pharmacotherapy Pearls Can be used in furosemide-allergic patients; 1 mg = 40 mg furosemide. Administer I.V. slowly, over 1-2 minutes.

Special Geriatric Considerations Loop diuretics are potent diuretics; excess amounts can lead to profound diuresis with fluid and electrolyte loss; close medical supervision and dose evaluation is required, particularly in the elderly. Severe loss of sodium and/or increases in BUN can cause confusion; for any change in mental status in patients on bumetanide, monitor electrolytes and renal function.

Dosage Forms Excipient information presented when available (limited, particularly for generics); consult specific product labeling.
Injection, solution: 0.25 mg/mL (2 mL, 4 mL, 10 mL)
Tablet, oral: 0.5 mg, 1 mg, 2 mg

♦ **Bumex** see Bumetanide on page 235
♦ **Buprenex®** see Buprenorphine on page 237

Buprenorphine (byoo pre NOR feen)

Related Information
Opioid Analgesics on page 2122
Medication Safety Issues
Sound-alike/look-alike issues:
Buprenex® may be confused with Brevibloc®, Bumex®
High alert medication:
The Institute for Safe Medication Practices (ISMP) includes this medication among its list of drug classes which have a heightened risk of causing significant patient harm when used in error.
Brand Names: U.S. Buprenex®; Butrans®; Subutex® [DSC]
Brand Names: Canada Buprenex®; Subutex®
Index Terms Buprenorphine Hydrochloride
Generic Availability (U.S.) Yes: Excludes patch
Pharmacologic Category Analgesic, Opioid; Analgesic, Opioid Partial Agonist
Use
Injection: Management of moderate-to-severe pain
Sublingual tablet: Treatment of opioid dependence
Transdermal patch: Management of moderate-to-severe chronic pain in patients requiring an around-the-clock opioid analgesic for an extended period of time
Unlabeled Use Injection: Management of opioid withdrawal in heroin-dependent hospitalized patients
Prescribing and Access Restrictions Prescribing of tablets for opioid dependence is limited to physicians who have met the qualification criteria and have received a DEA number specific to prescribing this product. Tablets will be available through pharmacies and wholesalers which normally provide controlled substances.
Medication Guide Available Yes
Contraindications Hypersensitivity to buprenorphine or any component of the formulation

Transdermal patch: Additional contraindications: Significant respiratory depression; severe asthma; known or suspected paralytic ileus; management of mild, acute, or intermittent pain; management of pain requiring short-term opioid analgesia; management of postoperative pain
Warnings/Precautions An opioid-containing analgesic regimen should be tailored to each patient's needs and based upon the type of pain being treated (acute versus chronic), the route of administration, degree of tolerance for opioids (naive versus chronic user), age, weight, and medical condition. The optimal analgesic dose varies widely among patients. Doses should be titrated to pain relief/prevention.

May cause CNS depression, which may impair physical or mental abilities. Effects with other sedative drugs or ethanol may be potentiated. Elderly may be more sensitive to CNS depressant and constipating effects. May cause respiratory depression - use caution in patients with respiratory disease or pre-existing respiratory depression. Hypersensitivity reactions, including bronchospasm, angioneurotic edema, and anaphylactic shock, have also been reported. Potential for drug dependency exists, abrupt cessation may precipitate withdrawal. Use caution in elderly, debilitated, depression or suicidal tendencies. Tolerance, psychological and physical dependence may occur with prolonged use. Partial antagonist activity may precipitate acute narcotic withdrawal in opioid-dependent individuals.

Hepatitis has been reported with buprenorphine use; hepatic events ranged from transient, asymptomatic transaminase elevations to hepatic failure; in many cases, patients had preexisting hepatic dysfunction. Monitor liver function tests in patients at increased risk for hepatotoxicity (eg, history of alcohol abuse, pre-existing hepatic dysfunction, I.V. drug abusers) prior to and during therapy. Use with caution in patients with hepatic impairment; dosage adjustments are recommended in hepatic impairment.

Use with caution in patients with pulmonary or renal function impairment. Also use caution in patients with head injury or increased ICP, biliary tract dysfunction, patients with history of hyperthyroidism, morbid obesity, adrenal insufficiency, prostatic hyperplasia, urinary stricture, CNS depression, toxic psychosis, pancreatitis, alcoholism, delirium tremens, or kyphoscoliosis. May cause hypotension; use with caution in patients with hypovolemia, cardiovascular disease (including acute MI), or drugs which may exaggerate hypotensive effects (including phenothiazines or general anesthetics). May obscure diagnosis or clinical course of patients with acute abdominal conditions. Opioid therapy may lower seizure threshold; use caution in patients with a history of seizure disorders.

Transdermal patch: **[U.S. Boxed Warning]: Do not exceed one 20 mcg/hour transdermal patch due to the risk of QT$_c$-interval prolongation.** Avoid using in patients with history of long QT syndrome or in patients with predisposing factors increasing the risk of QT abnormalities (eg, concurrent medications such as antiarrhythmics, hypokalemia, unstable heart failure, unstable atrial fibrillation). **[U.S. Boxed Warning]: Healthcare provider should be alert to problems of abuse, misuse, and diversion.**

Sublingual tablets, which are used for induction treatment of opioid dependence, should not be started until effects of withdrawal are evident.

Adverse Reactions (Reflective of adult population; not specific for elderly)
Injection:
>10%: Central nervous system: Sedation
1% to 10%:
Cardiovascular: Hypotension
Central nervous system: Respiratory depression, dizziness, headache
Gastrointestinal: Vomiting, nausea
Ocular: Miosis
Otic: Vertigo
Miscellaneous: Diaphoresis

Tablet:
>10%:
Central nervous system: Headache (30%), pain (24%), insomnia (21% to 25%), anxiety (12%), depression (11%)
Gastrointestinal: Nausea (10% to 14%), abdominal pain (12%), constipation (8% to 11%)
Neuromuscular & skeletal: Back pain (14%), weakness (14%)
Respiratory: Rhinitis (11%)
Miscellaneous: Withdrawal syndrome (19%; placebo 37%), infection (12% to 20%), diaphoresis (12% to 13%)
1% to 10%:
Central nervous system: Chills (6%), nervousness (6%), somnolence (5%), dizziness (4%), fever (3%)
Gastrointestinal: Vomiting (5% to 8%), diarrhea (5%), dyspepsia (3%)
Ocular: Lacrimation (5%)
Respiratory: Cough (4%), pharyngitis (4%)
Miscellaneous: Flu-like syndrome (6%)

Transdermal patch:
>10%:
Central nervous system: Headache (16%), dizziness (16%), somnolence (14%),
Gastrointestinal: Nausea (23%), constipation (14%), vomiting (11%)
Local: Application site pruritus (15%)
1% to 10%:
Cardiovascular: Peripheral edema (7%), chest pain, hypertension
Central nervous system: Fatigue (5%), insomnia (3%), hypoesthesia (2%), anxiety, depression, fever, migraine
Dermatologic: Pruritus (4%), rash (2%)
Gastrointestinal: Xerostomia (7%), diarrhea (3%), abdominal discomfort (2%), anorexia (2%), upper abdominal pain
Genitourinary: Urinary tract infection (3%)
Local: Application site erythema (7%); application site rash (6%), application site irritation
Neuromuscular & skeletal: Pain in extremity (3%), back pain (3%), joint swelling (3%), paresthesia (2%), tremor (2%), muscles spasms, musculoskeletal pain, myalgia, neck pain, weakness
Respiratory: Dyspnea (3%), bronchitis, cough, nasopharyngitis, pharyngolaryngeal pain, sinusitis, upper respiratory tract infection
Miscellaneous: Hyperhidrosis (4%), fall (4%), flu-like syndrome

Drug Interactions

Metabolism/Transport Effects Substrate of CYP3A4 (major); **Note:** Assignment of Major/ Minor substrate status based on clinically relevant drug interaction potential; **Inhibits** CYP1A2 (weak), CYP2A6 (weak), CYP2C19 (weak), CYP2D6 (weak)

Avoid Concomitant Use

Avoid concomitant use of Buprenorphine with any of the following: Atazanavir; Azelastine; Azelastine (Nasal); Conivaptan; MAO Inhibitors; Mirtazapine; Paraldehyde

Increased Effect/Toxicity

Buprenorphine may increase the levels/effects of: Alvimopan; ARIPiprazole; Azelastine; Azelastine (Nasal); Desmopressin; MAO Inhibitors; Metyrosine; Mirtazapine; Paraldehyde; Selective Serotonin Reuptake Inhibitors; Thiazide Diuretics; Zolpidem

The levels/effects of Buprenorphine may be increased by: Alcohol (Ethyl); Amphetamines; Antipsychotic Agents (Phenothiazines); Atazanavir; Boceprevir; CNS Depressants; Conivaptan; CYP3A4 Inhibitors (Moderate); CYP3A4 Inhibitors (Strong); Dasatinib; Droperidol; HydrOXYzine; Ivacaftor; Mifepristone; Succinylcholine

Decreased Effect

Buprenorphine may decrease the levels/effects of: Analgesics (Opioid); Atazanavir; Pegvisomant

The levels/effects of Buprenorphine may be decreased by: Ammonium Chloride; Boceprevir; CYP3A4 Inducers (Strong); Deferasirox; Efavirenz; Etravirine; Herbs (CYP3A4 Inducers); Mixed Agonist / Antagonist Opioids; Tocilizumab

Ethanol/Nutrition/Herb Interactions

Ethanol: May increase CNS depression; monitor for increased effects with coadministration. Caution patients about effect.

Herb/Nutraceutical: Avoid valerian, St John's wort, kava kava, gotu kola (may increase CNS depression).

Stability

Injection: Protect from excessive heat >40°C (>104°F). Protect from light.

Patch, tablet: Store at room temperature of 25°C (77°F).

Mechanism of Action Buprenorphine exerts its analgesic effect via high affinity binding to μ opiate receptors in the CNS; displays partial mu agonist and weak kappa antagonist activity

Pharmacodynamics/Kinetics

Onset of action: Analgesic: I.M: Within 15 minutes

Peak effect: I.M.: ~1 hour; Transdermal patch: Steady state achieved by day 3

Duration: I.M.: ≥6 hours

Absorption: I.M., SubQ: 30% to 40%

Distribution: V_d: 97-187 L/kg

Protein binding: High (~96%, primarily to alpha- and beta globulin)

Metabolism: Primarily hepatic via N-dealkylation by CYP3A4 to norbuprenorphine (active metabolite), and to a lesser extent via glucuronidation by UGT1A1 and 2B7 to buprenorphine-3-O-glucuronide; the major metabolite, norbuprenorphine, also undergoes glucuronidation via UGT1A3; extensive first-pass effect

Bioavailability (relative to I.V. administration): I.M.: 70%; Sublingual tablet: 29%; Transdermal patch: ~15%

Half-life elimination: I.V.: 2.2-3 hours; Apparent terminal half-life: Sublingual tablet: ~37 hours; Transdermal patch: ~26 hours. **Note:** Extended elimination half-life for sublingual administration may be due to depot effect (Kuhlman, 1996).

Time to peak, plasma: Sublingual: 30 minutes to 1 hour (Kuhlman, 1996)

Excretion: Feces (~70%); urine (27% to 30%)

Dosage

Geriatric

Acute pain (moderate-to-severe): I.M., slow I.V.: 0.15 mg every 6 hours; elderly patients are more likely to suffer from confusion and drowsiness compared to younger patients. **Long-term use is not recommended.**

Chronic pain (moderate-to-severe): Transdermal patch: No specific dosage adjustments required; use caution due to potential for increased risk of adverse events.

Adult

Acute pain (moderate-to-severe): Note: Long-term use is not recommended. The following recommendations are guidelines and do not represent the maximum doses that may be required in all patients. Doses should be titrated to pain relief/prevention. In high-risk patients (eg, elderly, debilitated, presence of respiratory disease) and/or concurrent CNS depressant use, reduce dose by one-half. Buprenorphine has an analgesic ceiling.

I.M.: Initial: Opiate-naive: 0.3 mg every 6-8 hours as needed; initial dose (up to 0.3 mg) may be repeated once in 30-60 minutes after the initial dose if needed; usual dosage range: 0.15-0.6 mg every 4-8 hours as needed

◀

Slow I.V.: Initial: Opiate-naive: 0.3 mg every 6-8 hours as needed; initial dose (up to 0.3 mg) may be repeated once in 30-60 minutes after the initial dose if needed

Chronic pain (moderate-to-severe): Transdermal patch:

Opioid-naive patients: Initial: 5 mcg/hour applied once every 7 days

Opioid-experienced patients (conversion from other opioids to buprenorphine): Taper the current around-the-clock opioid for up to 7 days to ≤30 mg/day of oral morphine or equivalent before initiating therapy. Short-acting analgesics as needed may be continued until analgesia with transdermal buprenorphine is attained. There is a potential for buprenorphine to precipitate withdrawal in patients already receiving opioids.

Patients who were receiving daily dose of <30 mg of oral morphine equivalents: Initial: 5 mcg/hour applied once every 7 days

Patients who were receiving daily dose of 30-80 mg of oral morphine equivalents: Initial: 10 mcg/hour applied once every 7 days

Dose titration (opioid-naive or opioid-experienced patients): May increase dose, based on patient's supplemental short-acting analgesic requirements, with a minimum titration interval of 72 hours (maximum dose: 20 mcg/hour applied once every 7 days; risk for QT_c prolongation increases with doses ≥20 mcg/hour patch).

Discontinuation of therapy: Taper dose gradually to prevent withdrawal; consider initiating immediate-release opioids, if needed.

Opiate withdrawal in heroin-dependent hospitalized patients (unlabeled use): I.V. infusion: 0.3-0.9 mg (diluted in 50-100 mL of NS) over 20-30 minutes every 6-12 hours (Welsh, 2002)

Opioid dependence: Sublingual tablet: **Note:** The combination product, buprenorphine and naloxone, is preferred therapy over buprenorphine monotherapy for induction treatment (and stabilization/maintenance treatment) for short-acting opioid dependence (U.S. Department of Health and Human Services, 2005).

Manufacturer's labeling:

Induction: Day 1: 8 mg; Day 2 and subsequent induction days: 16 mg; usual induction dosage range: 12-16 mg/day (induction usually accomplished over 3-4 days). Treatment should begin at least 4 hours after last use of heroin or other short-acting opioids, preferably when first signs of withdrawal appear. Titrating dose to clinical effectiveness should be done as rapidly as possible to prevent undue withdrawal symptoms and patient drop-out during the induction period. There is little controlled experience with induction in patients on methadone or other long-acting opioids; consult expert physician experienced with this procedure.

Maintenance: Target dose: 16 mg/day; in some patients 12 mg/day may be effective; patients should be switched to the buprenorphine/naloxone combination product for maintenance and unsupervised therapy

Hepatic Impairment

Injection, sublingual tablet: Use caution due to extensive hepatic metabolism; dosage adjustments recommended although no specific recommendations are provided by the manufacturer.

Transdermal patch:

Mild-to-moderate impairment: Initial: 5 mcg/hour applied once every 7 days.

Severe impairment: Not studied; consider alternative therapy with more flexibility for dosing adjustments.

Administration

I.M.: Administer via deep I.M. injection

I.V.: Administer slowly, over at least 2 minutes. Administration over 20-30 minutes preferred when managing opioid withdrawal in heroin-dependent hospitalized patients (Welsh, 2002).

Oral: Sublingual tablet: Tablet should be placed under the tongue until dissolved; should not be swallowed. If two or more tablets are needed per dose, all may be placed under the tongue at once, or two at a time. To ensure consistent bioavailability, subsequent doses should always be taken the same way.

Transdermal patch: Apply to patch to intact, nonirritated skin only. Apply to a hairless or nearly hairless skin site. If hairless site is not available, do not shave skin; hair at application site should be clipped. Prior to application, if the site must be cleaned, clean with clear water and allow to dry completely; do not use soaps, alcohol, lotions or abrasives due to potential for increased skin absorption. Do not use any patch that has been damaged, cut or manipulated in any way. Remove patch from protective pouch immediately before application. Remove the protective backing, and apply the sticky side of the patch to one of eight possible application sites (upper outer arm, upper chest, upper back or the side of the chest [on either side of the body]). Firmly press patch in place and hold for ~15 seconds. Change patch every 7 days. Rotate patch application sites; wait ≥21 days before reapplying another patch to the same skin site. Avoid exposing application site to external heat sources (eg, heating pad, electric blanket, heat lamp, hot tub). If there is difficulty with patch adhesion, the edges of the system may be taped in place with first-aid tape. If the patch falls off during the 7-day dosing interval, dispose of the patch and apply a new patch to a different skin site.

Monitoring Parameters Pain relief, respiratory and mental status, CNS depression, blood pressure; LFTs (prior to initiation and during therapy); symptoms of withdrawal; application site reactions (transdermal patch)

Special Geriatric Considerations One postmarketing study found that elderly patients were more likely to suffer from confusion and drowsiness after buprenorphine as compared to younger patients. Use transdermal system with caution in the elderly. Respiratory depression occurs more frequently in the elderly. In clinical trials, the incidence of adverse events was higher in older subjects.

Controlled Substance C-III

Dosage Forms Excipient information presented when available (limited, particularly for generics); consult specific product labeling. [DSC] = Discontinued product
Injection, solution: 0.3 mg/mL (1 mL)
  Buprenex®: 0.3 mg/mL (1 mL)
Injection, solution [preservative free]: 0.3 mg/mL (1 mL)
Patch, transdermal:
  Butrans®: 5 mcg/hr (4s) [total buprenorphine 5 mg]
  Butrans®: 10 mcg/hr (4s) [total buprenorphine 10 mg]
  Butrans®: 20 mcg/hr (4s) [total buprenorphine 20 mg]
Tablet, sublingual: 2 mg, 8 mg
  Subutex®: 2 mg [DSC], 8 mg [DSC]

♦ **Buprenorphine Hydrochloride** see Buprenorphine on page 237
♦ **Buproban®** see BuPROPion on page 241

BuPROPion (byoo PROE pee on)

Related Information
Antidepressant Agents on page 2097
Medication Safety Issues
Sound-alike/look-alike issues:
Aplenzin™ may be confused with Albenza®, Relenza®
BuPROPion may be confused with busPIRone
Wellbutrin XL® may be confused with Wellbutrin SR®
Zyban® may be confused with Diovan®

Brand Names: U.S. Aplenzin™; Budeprion SR®; Budeprion XL®; Buproban®; Wellbutrin SR®; Wellbutrin XL®; Wellbutrin®; Zyban®

Brand Names: Canada Ava-Bupropion SR; Bupropion SR®; Novo-Bupropion SR; PMS-Bupropion SR; ratio-Bupropion SR; Sandoz-Bupropion SR; Wellbutrin® SR; Wellbutrin® XL; Zyban®

Index Terms Bupropion Hydrobromide; Bupropion Hydrochloride

Generic Availability (U.S.) Yes: Excludes bupropion hydrobromide tablet, sustained release hydrochloride tablet

Pharmacologic Category Antidepressant, Dopamine-Reuptake Inhibitor; Smoking Cessation Aid

Use Treatment of major depressive disorder, including seasonal affective disorder (SAD); adjunct in smoking cessation

Unlabeled Use Attention-deficit/hyperactivity disorder (ADHD); depression associated with bipolar disorder

Medication Guide Available Yes

Contraindications Hypersensitivity to bupropion or any component of the formulation; seizure disorder; history of anorexia/bulimia; use of MAO inhibitors within 14 days; patients undergoing abrupt discontinuation of ethanol or sedatives (including benzodiazepines); patients receiving other dosage forms of bupropion

Warnings/Precautions [U.S. Boxed Warning]: Use in treating psychiatric disorders; consider risk prior to prescribing. Short-term studies did not show an increased risk in patients >24 years of age and showed a decreased risk in patients ≥65 years. All patients must be closely monitored for clinical worsening, suicidality, or unusual changes in behavior, especially during the initiation of therapy (generally first 1-2 months) or following an increase or decrease in dosage. The patient's family or caregiver should be instructed to closely observe the patient and communicate condition with healthcare provider. A medication guide should be dispensed with each prescription.

[U.S. Boxed Warning]: Use in smoking cessation: Serious neuropsychiatric events, including depression, suicidal thoughts, and suicide, have been reported with use; some cases may have been complicated by symptoms of nicotine withdrawal following smoking cessation. Smoking cessation (with or without treatment) is associated with nicotine withdrawal symptoms and the exacerbation of underlying psychiatric illness; however, some of the behavioral disturbances were reported in treated patients who continued to smoke. These neuropsychiatric symptoms (eg, mood disturbances, psychosis, hostility) have occurred in patients with and without pre-existing psychiatric disease; many cases resolved following therapy discontinuation although in some cases, symptoms persisted. Monitor all patients for behavioral changes and psychiatric symptoms (eg, agitation, depression, suicidal behavior, suicidal ideation); inform patients to discontinue treatment and contact their healthcare provider immediately if they experience any behavioral and/or mood changes.

The possibility of a suicide attempt is inherent in major depression and may persist until remission occurs. Use caution in high-risk patients. Worsening depression and severe abrupt suicidality that are not part of the presenting symptoms may require discontinuation or modification of drug therapy. The patient's family or caregiver should be alerted to monitor patients for the emergence of suicidality and associated behaviors (such as agitation, irritability, hostility, impulsivity, and hypomania) and notify the healthcare provider.

May worsen psychosis in some patients or precipitate a shift to mania or hypomania in patients with bipolar disorder. Patients presenting with depressive symptoms should be screened for bipolar disorder. Monotherapy in patients with bipolar disorder should be avoided. **Bupropion is not FDA approved for bipolar depression.**

The risk of seizures is dose-dependent and increased in patients with a history of seizures, anorexia/bulimia, head trauma, CNS tumor, severe hepatic cirrhosis, abrupt discontinuation of sedative-hypnotics or ethanol, medications which lower seizure threshold (antipsychotics, antidepressants, theophyllines, systemic steroids), stimulants, or hypoglycemic agents. Risk of seizures may also be increased by chewing, crushing, or dividing long-acting products. Risk may be reduced by limiting the daily dose to bupropion hydrochloride ≤450 mg or bupropion hydrobromide 522 mg. Gradually increase dose incrementally to reduce risk. Discontinue and do not restart in patients experiencing a seizure.

May cause CNS stimulation (restlessness, anxiety, insomnia) or anorexia. May increase the risks associated with electroconvulsive therapy. Consider discontinuing, when possible, prior to elective surgery. May cause weight loss; use caution in patients where weight loss is not desirable. The incidence of sexual dysfunction with bupropion is generally lower than with SSRIs.

Use caution in patients with cardiovascular disease, history of hypertension, or coronary artery disease; treatment-emergent hypertension (including some severe cases) has been reported, both with bupropion alone and in combination with nicotine transdermal systems. Use with caution in patients with hepatic or renal dysfunction and in elderly patients; reduced dose and/or frequency may be recommended. Elderly patients may be at greater risk of accumulation during chronic dosing. May cause motor or cognitive impairment in some patients; use with caution if tasks requiring alertness such as operating machinery or driving are undertaken. Arthralgia, myalgia, and fever with rash and other symptoms suggestive of delayed hypersensitivity resembling serum sickness have been reported.

Extended release tablet: Insoluble tablet shell may remain intact and be visible in the stool.
Adverse Reactions (Reflective of adult population; not specific for elderly) Frequencies, when reported, reflect highest incidence reported with sustained release product.

>10%:
  Cardiovascular: Tachycardia (11%)
  Central nervous system: Headache (25% to 34%), insomnia (11% to 20%), dizziness (6% to 11%)
  Gastrointestinal: Xerostomia (17% to 26%), weight loss (14% to 23%), nausea (1% to 18%)
  Respiratory: Pharyngitis (3% to 13%)
1% to 10%:
  Cardiovascular: Palpitation (2% to 6%), arrhythmias (5%), chest pain (3% to 4%), hypertension (2% to 4%; may be severe), flushing (1% to 4%), hypotension (3%)
  Central nervous system: Agitation (2% to 9%), confusion (8%), anxiety (5% to 7%), hostility (6%), nervousness (3% to 5%), sleep disturbance (4%), sensory disturbance (4%), migraine (1% to 4%), abnormal dreams (3%), irritability (2% to 3%), somnolence (2% to 3%), pain (2% to 3%), memory decreased (≤3%), fever (1% to 2%), CNS stimulation (1% to 2%), depression
  Dermatologic: Rash (1% to 5%), pruritus (2% to 4%), urticaria (1% to 2%)
  Endocrine & metabolic: Menstrual complaints (2% to 5%), hot flashes (1% to 3%), libido decreased (3%)
  Gastrointestinal: Constipation (5% to 10%), abdominal pain (2% to 9%), diarrhea (5% to 7%), flatulence (6%), anorexia (3% to 5%), appetite increased (4%), taste perversion (2% to 4%), vomiting (2% to 4%), dyspepsia (3%), dysphagia (≤2%)
  Genitourinary: Polyuria (2% to 5%), urinary urgency (≤2%), vaginal hemorrhage (≤2%), UTI (≤1%)

Neuromuscular & skeletal: Tremor (3% to 6%), myalgia (2% to 6%), weakness (2% to 4%), arthralgia (1% to 4%), arthritis (2%), akathisia (≤2%), paresthesia (1% to 2%), twitching (1% to 2%), neck pain

Ocular: Blurred vision (2% to 3%), amblyopia (2%)

Otic: Tinnitus (3% to 6%), auditory disturbance (5%)

Respiratory: Upper respiratory infection (9%), cough increased (1% to 4%), sinusitis (1% to 5%)

Miscellaneous: Infection (8% to 9%), diaphoresis (5% to 6%), allergic reaction (including anaphylaxis, pruritus, urticaria)

Drug Interactions

Metabolism/Transport Effects Substrate of CYP1A2 (minor), CYP2A6 (minor), CYP2B6 (major), CYP2C9 (minor), CYP2D6 (minor), CYP2E1 (minor), CYP3A4 (minor); **Note:** Assignment of Major/Minor substrate status based on clinically relevant drug interaction potential; **Inhibits** CYP2D6 (strong)

Avoid Concomitant Use

Avoid concomitant use of BuPROPion with any of the following: MAO Inhibitors; Methylene Blue; Pimozide; Tamoxifen; Thioridazine

Increased Effect/Toxicity

BuPROPion may increase the levels/effects of: Alcohol (Ethyl); ARIPiprazole; AtoMOXetine; CYP2D6 Substrates; Fesoterodine; Iloperidone; Methylene Blue; Nebivolol; Pimozide; Propafenone; Tetrabenazine; Thioridazine; Tricyclic Antidepressants

The levels/effects of BuPROPion may be increased by: Alcohol (Ethyl); CYP2B6 Inhibitors (Moderate); CYP2B6 Inhibitors (Strong); MAO Inhibitors; Mifepristone; Quazepam

Decreased Effect

BuPROPion may decrease the levels/effects of: Codeine; Iloperidone; Ioflupane I 123; Tamoxifen; TraMADol

The levels/effects of BuPROPion may be decreased by: CYP2B6 Inducers (Strong); Efavirenz; Lopinavir; Peginterferon Alfa-2b; Ritonavir; Tocilizumab

Ethanol/Nutrition/Herb Interactions

Ethanol: May increase CNS depression; monitor for increased effects with coadministration. Caution patients about effects.

Herb/Nutraceutical: Avoid valerian, St John's wort, SAMe, gotu kola, kava kava (may increase CNS depression).

Stability Store at controlled room temperature of 20°C to 25°C (68°F to 77°F). Aplenzin™, Wellbutrin XL®: Store at 15°C to 30°C (59°F to 86°F).

Mechanism of Action Aminoketone antidepressant structurally different from all other marketed antidepressants; like other antidepressants the mechanism of bupropion's activity is not fully understood. Bupropion is a relatively weak inhibitor of the neuronal uptake of norepinephrine and dopamine, and does not inhibit monoamine oxidase or the reuptake of serotonin. Metabolite inhibits the reuptake of norepinephrine. The primary mechanism of action is thought to be dopaminergic and/or noradrenergic.

Pharmacodynamics/Kinetics

Absorption: Rapid

Distribution: V_d: ~20-47 L/kg (Laizure, 1985)

Protein binding: 84%

Metabolism: Extensively hepatic via CYP2B6 to hydroxybupropion; non-CYP-mediated metabolism to erythrohydrobupropion and threohydrobupropion. Metabolite activity ranges from 20% to 50% potency of bupropion.

Half-life:

Distribution: 3-4 hours

Elimination: 21 ± 9 hours; Metabolites: Hydroxybupropion: 20 ± 5 hours; Erythrohydrobupropion: 33 ± 10 hours; Threohydrobupropion: 37 ± 13 hours

Extended release (Aplenzin™): 21 ± 7 hours; Metabolites: Hydroxybupropion: 24 ± 5 hours; Erythrohydrobupropion: 31 ± 8 hours; Threohydrobupropion: 51 ± 9 hours

Time to peak, serum:

Bupropion: Immediate release: Within 2 hours; Sustained release: Within 3 hours; Extended release: ~5 hours

Metabolite: Hydroxybupropion: Immediate release: ~3 hours; Extended release, sustained release: ~6-7 hours

Excretion: Urine (87%, primarily as metabolites); feces (10%, primarily as metabolites)

Dosage

Geriatric

Depression: Oral (hydrochloride salt): Initial: 37.5 mg of immediate release tablets twice daily or 100 mg/day of sustained release tablets; increase by 37.5-100 mg every 3-4 days as tolerated. There is evidence that the elderly respond at 150 mg/day in divided doses, but some may require a higher dose. **Note:** Patients with Alzheimer's dementia-related ▶

depression may require a lower starting dosage of 37.5 mg once or twice daily (100 mg/day sustained release), increased as needed up to 300 mg/day in divided doses (300 mg/day for sustained release)

Smoking cessation: Refer to adult dosing.

Adult

Depression: Oral:

Immediate release hydrochloride salt: 100 mg 3 times/day; begin at 100 mg twice daily; may increase to a maximum dose of 450 mg/day

Sustained release hydrochloride salt: Initial: 150 mg/day in the morning; may increase to 150 mg twice daily by day 4 if tolerated; target dose: 300 mg/day given as 150 mg twice daily; maximum dose: 400 mg/day given as 200 mg twice daily

Extended release:

Hydrochloride salt: Initial: 150 mg/day in the morning; may increase as early as day 4 of dosing to 300 mg/day; maximum dose: 450 mg/day

Hydrobromide salt (Aplenzin™): Target dose: 348 mg/day in the morning. Patients not previously on bupropion: Initial: 174 mg/day in the morning; may increase as early as day 4 of dosing to 348 mg/day; maximum dose: 522 mg/day. **Note:** 174 mg strength not currently available; 348 mg tablet cannot be split.

Switching from hydrochloride salt formulation (eg, Wellbutrin® immediate release, SR®, XL®) to hydrobromide salt formulation (Aplenzin™): **Note:** Patients being treated twice daily with bupropion hydrochloride would be switched to the equivalent once daily dose of bupropion hydrobromide.

Bupropion hydrochloride 150 mg is equivalent to bupropion hydrobromide 174 mg
Bupropion hydrochloride 300 mg is equivalent to bupropion hydrobromide 348 mg
Bupropion hydrochloride 450 mg is equivalent to bupropion hydrobromide 522 mg

SAD (Wellbutrin XL®): Oral: Initial: 150 mg/day in the morning; if tolerated, may increase after 1 week to 300 mg/day

Note: Prophylactic treatment should be reserved for those patients with frequent depressive episodes and/or significant impairment. Initiate treatment in the Autumn prior to symptom onset, and discontinue in early Spring with dose tapering to 150 mg/day for 2 weeks

Smoking cessation (Zyban®): Oral: Initiate with 150 mg once daily for 3 days; increase to 150 mg twice daily; treatment should continue for 7-12 weeks.

Note: Therapy should begin at least 1 week before target quit date. Target quit dates are generally in the second week of treatment. If patient successfully quits smoking after 7-12 weeks, may consider ongoing maintenance therapy based on individual patient risk: benefit. Efficacy of maintenance therapy (300 mg/day) has been demonstrated for up to 6 months. Conversely, if significant progress has not been made by the seventh week of therapy, success is unlikely and treatment discontinuation should be considered.

Dosing conversion between hydrochloride salt (eg, Wellbutrin®) immediate, sustained, and extended release products: Convert using same total daily dose (up to the maximum recommended dose for a given dosage form), but adjust frequency as indicated for sustained (twice daily) or extended (once daily) release products.

Renal Impairment Use with caution and consider a reduction in dosing frequency; limited pharmacokinetic information suggests elimination of bupropion and/or the active metabolites may be reduced.

Moderate-to-severe renal impairment: Bupropion exposure was approximately twofold higher compared to normal subjects following a 150 mg single dose administration.

End-stage renal failure: Per the manufacturer, the elimination of hydroxybupropion and threohydrobupropion are reduced in patients with end-stage renal failure.

Hepatic Impairment

Mild-to-moderate hepatic impairment: Use with caution and/or reduced dose/frequency

Severe hepatic cirrhosis: Use with extreme caution; maximum dose:

Aplenzin™: 174 mg every other day
Wellbutrin®: 75 mg/day;
Wellbutrin SR®: 100 mg/day or 150 mg every other day
Wellbutrin XL®: 150 mg every other day
Zyban®: 150 mg every other day

Note: The mean AUC increased by ~1.5-fold for hydroxybupropion and ~2.5-fold for erythro/threohydrobupropion; median T_{max} was observed 19 hours later for hydroxybupropion, 31 hours later for erythro/threohydrobupropion; mean half-life for hydroxybupropion increased fivefold, and increased twofold for erythro/threohydrobupropion in patients with severe hepatic cirrhosis compared to healthy volunteers.

Administration May be taken without regard to meals. Zyban® and extended release tablets (hydrochloride and hydrobromide salt formulations) should be swallowed whole; do not crush, chew, or divide. The insoluble shell of the extended-release tablet may remain intact during GI transit and is eliminated in the feces.

Monitoring Parameters Body weight; mental status for depression, suicidal ideation (especially at the beginning of therapy or when doses are increased or decreased), anxiety, social functioning, mania, panic attacks

Reference Range Therapeutic levels (trough, 12 hours after last dose): 50-100 ng/mL

Test Interactions
May interfere with urine detection of amphetamine/methamphetamine (false-positive). Decreased prolactin levels.

Pharmacotherapy Pearls Risk of seizures: When using bupropion hydrochloride immediate release tablets, seizure risk is increased at total daily dosage >450 mg, individual dosages >150 mg, or by sudden, large increments in dose. Data for the immediate-release formulation of bupropion revealed a seizure incidence of 0.4% in patients treated at doses in the 300-450 mg/day range. The estimated seizure incidence increases almost 10-fold between 450 mg and 600 mg per day. Data for the sustained release dosage form revealed a seizure incidence of 0.1% in patients treated at a dosage range of 100-300 mg/day, and increases to ~0.4% at the maximum recommended dose of 400 mg/day.

Special Geriatric Considerations Studies have found bupropion effective as an antidepressant for older persons with major depressive disorder and as effective as paroxetine and imipramine. Its side effect profile (minimal anticholinergic and blood pressure effects) is favorable and makes it an alternative to other first-line antidepressants. A single- and multiple-dose pharmacokinetic study suggested that accumulation of bupropion and its metabolites may occur in the elderly.

A systematic review and meta-analysis of antidepressant placebo-controlled trials in persons with depression and dementia found evidence "suggestive" of efficacy but not of sufficient strength to "confirm" efficacy. Antidepressant trials in this patient population are small and underpowered. Older patients with depression being treated with an antidepressant should be closely monitored for response and adverse effects. Treatment should be switched or augmented when response is inadequate with a therapeutic dose. Antidepressants that are not tolerated should be discontinued and an alternative agent should be started.

Dosage Forms Excipient information presented when available (limited, particularly for generics); consult specific product labeling. [DSC] = Discontinued product
Tablet, oral, as hydrochloride: 75 mg [generic for Wellbutrin®], 100 mg [generic for Wellbutrin®]
  Wellbutrin®: 75 mg, 100 mg
Tablet, extended release, oral, as hydrobromide:
  Aplenzin™: 174 mg, 348 mg, 522 mg
Tablet, extended release, oral, as hydrochloride: 100 mg [generic for Wellbutrin SR®], 150 mg [generic for Wellbutrin SR®], 150 mg [generic for Wellbutrin XL®], 150 mg [generic for Zyban®], 200 mg [generic for Wellbutrin SR®], 300 mg [generic for Wellbutrin XL®]
  Budeprion SR®: 100 mg [contains tartrazine; generic for Wellbutrin SR®]
  Budeprion SR®: 150 mg [generic for Wellbutrin SR®]
  Budeprion XL®: 150 mg [DSC] [generic for Wellbutrin XL®]
  Budeprion XL®: 300 mg [contains tartrazine; generic for Wellbutrin XL®]
  Buproban®: 150 mg [generic for Zyban®]
  Wellbutrin XL®: 150 mg, 300 mg
Tablet, sustained release, oral, as hydrochloride:
  Wellbutrin SR®: 100 mg, 150 mg, 200 mg
  Zyban®: 150 mg

◆ **Bupropion Hydrobromide** see BuPROPion on page 241
◆ **Bupropion Hydrochloride** see BuPROPion on page 241
◆ **Burn Jel® [OTC]** see Lidocaine (Topical) on page 1128
◆ **Burn Jel Plus [OTC]** see Lidocaine (Topical) on page 1128
◆ **BuSpar** see BusPIRone on page 245

BusPIRone (byoo SPYE rone)

Medication Safety Issues
  Sound-alike/look-alike issues:
    BusPIRone may be confused with buPROPion

Brand Names: Canada Apo-Buspirone®; BuSpar®; Bustab®; Dom-Buspirone; Novo-Buspirone; Nu-Buspirone; PMS-Buspirone; Riva-Buspirone

Index Terms BuSpar; Buspirone Hydrochloride

Generic Availability (U.S.) Yes

Pharmacologic Category Antianxiety Agent, Miscellaneous

Use Management of generalized anxiety disorder (GAD)

BUSPIRONE

◀ **Unlabeled Use** Management of aggression in mental retardation and secondary mental disorders, major depression; potential augmenting agent for antidepressants

Contraindications Hypersensitivity to buspirone or any component of the formulation

Warnings/Precautions Use in severe hepatic or renal impairment is not recommended; does not prevent or treat withdrawal from benzodiazepines. Low potential for cognitive or motor impairment. Use with MAO inhibitors may result in hypertensive reactions. Restlessness syndrome has been reported in small number of patients; monitor for signs of any dopamine-related movement disorders. Buspirone does not exhibit cross-tolerance with benzodiazepines or other sedative/hypnotic agents. If substituting buspirone for any of these agents, gradually withdraw the drug(s) prior to initiating buspirone.

Adverse Reactions (Reflective of adult population; not specific for elderly)
>10%: Central nervous system: Dizziness (12%)
1% to 10%:
   Cardiovascular: Chest pain (≥1%)
   Central nervous system: Drowsiness (10%), headache (6%), nervousness (5%), light-headedness (3%), anger/hostility (2%), confusion (2%), excitement (2%), dream disturbance (≥1%)
   Dermatologic: Rash (1%)
   Gastrointestinal: Nausea (8%), diarrhea (2%)
   Neuromuscular & skeletal: Numbness (2%), weakness (2%), musculoskeletal pain (1%), paresthesia (1%), incoordination (1%), tremor (1%)
   Ocular: Blurred vision (2%)
   Otic: Tinnitus (≥1%)
   Respiratory: Nasal congestion (≥1%), sore throat (≥1%)
   Miscellaneous: Diaphoresis (1%)

Drug Interactions

Metabolism/Transport Effects Substrate of CYP2D6 (minor), CYP3A4 (major); **Note:** Assignment of Major/Minor substrate status based on clinically relevant drug interaction potential

Avoid Concomitant Use
   Avoid concomitant use of BusPIRone with any of the following: Azelastine; Azelastine (Nasal); Conivaptan; MAO Inhibitors; Methadone; Methylene Blue; Paraldehyde

Increased Effect/Toxicity
   BusPIRone may increase the levels/effects of: Alcohol (Ethyl); Antidepressants (Serotonin Reuptake Inhibitor/Antagonist); Azelastine; Azelastine (Nasal); Buprenorphine; CNS Depressants; MAO Inhibitors; Methadone; Methylene Blue; Metoclopramide; Metyrosine; Paraldehyde; Selective Serotonin Reuptake Inhibitors; Serotonin Modulators; Zolpidem

   The levels/effects of BusPIRone may be increased by: Antifungal Agents (Azole Derivatives, Systemic); Antipsychotics; Calcium Channel Blockers (Nondihydropyridine); Conivaptan; CYP3A4 Inhibitors (Moderate); CYP3A4 Inhibitors (Strong); Dasatinib; Grapefruit Juice; HydrOXYzine; Ivacaftor; Macrolide Antibiotics; Mifepristone; Selective Serotonin Reuptake Inhibitors

Decreased Effect
   BusPIRone may decrease the levels/effects of: Ioflupane I 123

   The levels/effects of BusPIRone may be decreased by: CYP3A4 Inducers (Strong); Deferasirox; Peginterferon Alfa-2b; Rifamycin Derivatives; Tocilizumab; Yohimbine

Ethanol/Nutrition/Herb Interactions
   Ethanol: Ethanol may increase CNS depression. Management: Monitor for increased effects with coadministration. Caution patients about effects.
   Food: Food may decrease the absorption of buspirone, but it may also decrease the first-pass metabolism, thereby increasing the bioavailability of buspirone. Grapefruit juice may cause increased buspirone concentrations. Management: Avoid intake of large quantities of grapefruit juice.
   Herb/Nutraceutical: St John's wort may decrease buspirone levels or increase CNS depression. Kava kava, valerian, and gotu kola may increase CNS depression; yohimbe may diminish the therapeutic effect of buspirone. Management: Avoid St John's wort, kava kava, valerian, gotu kola, and yohimbe.

Stability Store at USP controlled room temperature of 25°C (77°F). Protect from light.

Mechanism of Action The mechanism of action of buspirone is unknown. Buspirone has a high affinity for serotonin 5-HT$_{1A}$ and 5-HT$_2$ receptors, without affecting benzodiazepine-GABA receptors. Buspirone has moderate affinity for dopamine D$_2$ receptors.

Pharmacodynamics/Kinetics
   Absorption: Rapid
   Distribution: V$_d$: 5.3 L/kg
   Protein binding: 86% to 95%
   Metabolism: Hepatic oxidation, primarily via CYP3A4; extensive first-pass effect

Bioavailability: ~4%

Half-life elimination: 2-3 hours

Time to peak, serum: 40-90 minutes

Excretion: Urine: 29% to 63% (<0.1% dose excreted unchanged); feces: 18% to 38%

Dosage

Geriatric Oral: Initial: 5 mg twice daily, increase by 5 mg/day every 2-3 days as needed up to 20-30 mg/day; maximum daily dose: 60 mg/day

Adult Anxiety disorders (GAD): Oral: 15 mg/day (7.5 mg twice daily); may increase in increments of 5 mg/day every 2-3 days to a maximum of 60 mg/day. Target dose for most people is 20-30 mg/day (10-15 mg twice daily).

Renal Impairment Patients with impaired renal function demonstrated increased plasma levels and a prolonged half-life of buspirone. Use in patients with severe renal impairment not recommended.

Hepatic Impairment Patients with impaired hepatic function demonstrated increased plasma levels and a prolonged half-life of buspirone. Use in patients with severe hepatic impairment not recommended.

Monitoring Parameters Mental status, symptoms of anxiety

Pharmacotherapy Pearls Has shown little potential for abuse; not effective when used prn; maximal effect may not be achieved until 3-4 weeks after adequate dose is achieved. Some response may be seen in 1-2 weeks after initiation of therapy. Buspirone, in the treatment of agitation, has been shown to be effective in older adults at an average daily dose of 30-35 mg; slow titration, as described in Dosage, is necessary to avoid side effects and achieve maximum tolerable doses for individual patients.

Special Geriatric Considerations Because buspirone is less sedating than other anxiolytics, it may be a useful agent in geriatric patients when an anxiolytic is indicated.

Dosage Forms Excipient information presented when available (limited, particularly for generics); consult specific product labeling.

Tablet, oral, as hydrochloride: 5 mg, 7.5 mg, 10 mg, 15 mg, 30 mg

♦ **Buspirone Hydrochloride** see BusPIRone on page 245
♦ **Bussulfam** see Busulfan on page 247

Busulfan (byoo SUL fan)

Medication Safety Issues

Sound-alike/look-alike issues:

Myleran® may be confused with Alkeran®, Leukeran®, melphalan, Mylicon®

High alert medication:

This medication is in a class the Institute for Safe Medication Practices (ISMP) includes among its list of drug classes which have a heightened risk of causing significant patient harm when used in error.

Brand Names: U.S. Busulfex®; Myleran®

Brand Names: Canada Busulfex®; Myleran®

Index Terms Bussulfam; Busulfanum; Busulphan

Generic Availability (U.S.) No

Pharmacologic Category Antineoplastic Agent, Alkylating Agent

Use Palliative treatment of chronic myelogenous leukemia (CML) (oral); conditioning regimen prior to allogeneic hematopoietic progenitor cell transplantation (I.V.) for CML

Unlabeled Use Conditioning regimen prior to hematopoietic stem cell transplant (HSCT) (oral); treatment of polycythemia vera and essential thrombocytosis

Contraindications Hypersensitivity to busulfan or any component of the formulation; oral busulfan is contraindicated in patients without a definitive diagnosis of CML

Warnings/Precautions Hazardous agent - use appropriate precautions for handling and disposal. **[U.S. Boxed Warning]: Severe bone marrow suppression is common; reduce dose or discontinue oral busulfan for unusual suppression; may require bone marrow biopsy.** May result in severe neutropenia, thrombocytopenia, anemia, bone marrow failure, and/or pancytopenia; pancytopenia may be prolonged (1 month up to 2 years) and may be reversible. Use with caution in patients with compromised bone marrow reserve (due to prior treatment or radiation therapy). Monitor closely for signs of infection (due to neutropenia) or bleeding (due to thrombocytopenia) Seizures have been reported with use; use caution in patients predisposed to seizures, history of seizures or head trauma; when using as a conditioning regimen for transplant, initiate prophylactic anticonvulsant therapy (eg, phenytoin) prior to treatment. Phenytoin increases busulfan clearance by ≥15%; busulfan kinetics and dosing recommendations for high-dose HSCT conditioning were studied with concomitant phenytoin. If alternate anticonvulsants are used, busulfan clearance may be decreased and dosing should be monitored accordingly.

Bronchopulmonary dysplasia with pulmonary fibrosis ("busulfan lung") is associated with busulfan; onset is delayed with symptoms occurring at an average of 4 years (range: 4 months to 10 years) after treatment; may be fatal. Symptoms generally include a slow onset of cough, dyspnea, and fever (low-grade), although acute symptomatic onset may also occur. Diminished diffusion capacity and decreased pulmonary compliance have been noted with pulmonary function testing. Differential diagnosis should rule out opportunistic pulmonary infection or leukemic pulmonary infiltrates; may require lung biopsy. Discontinue busulfan if toxicity develops. Pulmonary toxicity may be additive if administered with other cytotoxic agents also associated with pulmonary toxicity. Busulfan has been causally related to the development of secondary malignancies (tumors and acute leukemias); chromosomal alterations may also occur.

High busulfan area under the concentration versus time curve (AUC) values (>1500 micromolar•minute) are associated with increased risk of hepatic sinusoidal obstruction syndrome (SOS; formerly called veno-occlusive disease [VOD]) due to conditioning for allogenic HSCT; patients with a history of radiation therapy, prior chemotherapy (≥3 cycles), or prior stem cell transplantation are at increased risk; monitor liver function tests periodically. Oral busulfan doses above 16 mg/kg (based on IBW) and concurrent use with alkylating agents may also increase the risk for hepatic SOS. The solvent in I.V. busulfan, DMA, may impair fertility. DMA may also be associated with hepatotoxicity, hallucinations, somnolence, lethargy, and confusion. **[U.S. Boxed Warning]: Should be administered under the supervision of an experienced cancer chemotherapy physician; for the I.V. formulation, should be experienced in management of HSCT and management of patients with severe pancytopenia; according to the manufacturer, oral busulfan should not be used until CML diagnosis has been established.** Cellular dysplasia in many organs has been observed (in addition to lung dysplasia); giant hyperchromatic nuclei have been noted in adrenal glands, liver, lymph nodes, pancreas, thyroid, and bone marrow. May obscure routine diagnostic cytologic exams (eg, cervical smear).

Adverse Reactions (Reflective of adult population; not specific for elderly)

I.V.:
>10%:

Cardiovascular: Tachycardia (44%), hypertension (36%; grades 3/4: 7%), edema (28% to 79%), thrombosis (33%), chest pain (26%), vasodilation (25%), hypotension (11%; grades 3/4: 3%)

Central nervous system: Insomnia (84%), fever (80%), anxiety (72% to 75%), headache (69%), chills (46%), pain (44%), dizziness (30%), depression (23%), confusion (11%)

Dermatologic: Rash (57%), pruritus (28%), alopecia (17%)

Endocrine & metabolic: Hypomagnesemia (77%), hyperglycemia (66% to 67%; grades 3/4: 15%), hypokalemia (64%), hypocalcemia (49%), hypophosphatemia (17%)

Gastrointestinal: Vomiting (43% to 100%), nausea (83% to 98%), mucositis/stomatitis (79% to 97%; grades 3/4: 26%), anorexia (85%), diarrhea (84%; grades 3/4: 5%), abdominal pain (72%), dyspepsia (44%), constipation (38%), xerostomia (26%), rectal disorder (25%), abdominal fullness (23%)

Hematologic: Myelosuppression (≤100%), neutropenia (100%; onset: 4 days; median recovery: 13 days [with G-CSF support]), thrombocytopenia (98%; median onset: 5-6 days), lymphopenia (children: 79%), anemia (69%)

Hepatic: Hyperbilirubinemia (49%; grades 3/4: 30%), ALT increased (31%; grades 3/4: 7%), hepatic sinusoidal obstruction syndrome (SOS; veno-occlusive disease) (adults: 8% to 12%; children: 21%), alkaline phosphatase increased (15%), jaundice (12%)

Local: Injection site inflammation (25%), injection site pain (15%)

Neuromuscular & skeletal: Weakness (51%), back pain (23%), myalgia (16%), arthralgia (13%)

Renal: Creatinine increased (21%), oliguria (15%)

Respiratory: Rhinitis (44%), lung disorder (34%), cough (28%), epistaxis (25%), dyspnea (25%), pneumonia (children: 21%), hiccup (18%), pharyngitis (18%)

Miscellaneous: Infection (51%; includes severe bacterial, viral [CMV], and fungal infections), allergic reaction (26%)

1% to 10%:

Cardiovascular: Arrhythmia (5%), cardiomegaly (5%), atrial fibrillation (2%), ECG abnormal (2%), heart block (2%), heart failure (grade 3/4: 2%), pericardial effusion (2%), tamponade (children with thalassemia: 2%), ventricular extrasystoles (2%), hypervolemia

Central nervous system: Lethargy (7%), hallucination (5%), agitation (2%), delirium (2%), encephalopathy (2%), seizure (2%), somnolence (2%), cerebral hemorrhage (1%)

Dermatologic: Vesicular rash (10%), vesiculobullous rash (10%), skin discoloration (8%), maculopapular rash (8%), acne (7%), exfoliative dermatitis (5%), erythema nodosum (2%)

Endocrine & metabolic: Hyponatremia (2%)

Gastrointestinal: Ileus (8%), weight gain (8%), esophagitis (grade 3: 2%), hematemesis (2%), pancreatitis (2%)

Hematologic: Prothrombin time increased (2%)
Hepatic: Hepatomegaly (6%)
Renal: Hematuria (8%), dysuria (7%), hemorrhagic cystitis (grade 3/4: 7%), BUN increased (3%; grades 3/4: 2%)
Respiratory: Asthma (8%), alveolar hemorrhage (5%), hyperventilation (5%), hemoptysis (3%), pleural effusion (3%), sinusitis (3%), atelectasis (2%), hypoxia (2%)

Oral: Frequency not defined:
Dermatologic: Hyperpigmentation of skin (5% to 10%), rash
Endocrine & metabolic: Amenorrhea, ovarian suppression
Gastrointestinal: Xerostomia
Hematologic: Myelosuppression (anemia, leukopenia, thrombocytopenia)

Drug Interactions

Metabolism/Transport Effects Substrate of CYP3A4 (major); **Note:** Assignment of Major/Minor substrate status based on clinically relevant drug interaction potential

Avoid Concomitant Use

Avoid concomitant use of Busulfan with any of the following: BCG; CloZAPine; Conivaptan; Natalizumab; Pimecrolimus; Tacrolimus (Topical); Vaccines (Live)

Increased Effect/Toxicity

Busulfan may increase the levels/effects of: CloZAPine; Ifosfamide; Leflunomide; Natalizumab; Vaccines (Live); Vitamin K Antagonists

The levels/effects of Busulfan may be increased by: Acetaminophen; Antifungal Agents (Azole Derivatives, Systemic); Conivaptan; CYP3A4 Inhibitors (Moderate); CYP3A4 Inhibitors (Strong); Dasatinib; Denosumab; Ivacaftor; MetroNIDAZOLE; MetroNIDAZOLE (Systemic); Mifepristone; Pimecrolimus; Roflumilast; Tacrolimus (Topical); Trastuzumab

Decreased Effect

Busulfan may decrease the levels/effects of: BCG; Coccidioidin Skin Test; Sipuleucel-T; Vaccines (Inactivated); Vaccines (Live); Vitamin K Antagonists

The levels/effects of Busulfan may be decreased by: CYP3A4 Inducers (Strong); Deferasirox; Echinacea; Fosphenytoin; Herbs (CYP3A4 Inducers); Phenytoin; Tocilizumab

Ethanol/Nutrition/Herb Interactions

Ethanol: Avoid ethanol due to GI irritation.
Food: No clear or firm data on the effect of food on busulfan bioavailability.
Herb/Nutraceutical: Avoid St John's wort (may decrease busulfan levels).

Stability

Injection: Store intact vials under refrigeration at 2°C to 8°C (36°F to 46°F). Dilute in 0.9% sodium chloride (NS) injection or dextrose 5% in water (D_5W). The dilution volume should be ten times the volume of busulfan injection, ensuring that the final concentration of busulfan is 0.5 mg/mL. Always add busulfan to the diluent, and not the diluent to the busulfan. Mix with several inversions. Solutions diluted in NS or D_5W for infusion are stable for up to 8 hours at room temperature (25°C [77°F]); the infusion must also be completed within that 8-hour timeframe. Dilution of busulfan injection in NS is stable for up to 12 hours at refrigeration (2°C to 8°C); the infusion must be completed within that 12-hour timeframe. Do not use polycarbonate syringes or filters for preparation or administration.
Tablet: Store at 25°C (77°F); excursions permitted to 15°C to 30°C (59°F to 86°F).

Mechanism of Action Busulfan is an alkylating agent which reacts with the N-7 position of guanosine and interferes with DNA replication and transcription of RNA. Busulfan has a more marked effect on myeloid cells than on lymphoid cells and is also very toxic to hematopoietic stem cells. Busulfan exhibits little immunosuppressive activity. Interferes with the normal function of DNA by alkylation and cross-linking the strands of DNA.

Pharmacodynamics/Kinetics

Absorption: Rapid and complete
Distribution: V_d: ~1 L/kg; distributes into CSF with levels equal to plasma
Protein binding: 32% to plasma proteins and 47% to red blood cells
Metabolism: Extensively hepatic (may increase with multiple doses); glutathione conjugation followed by oxidation
Bioavailability: Oral: Adults: 80% ± 20%
Half-life elimination: 2-3 hours
Time to peak, serum: Oral: ~1 hour; I.V.: Within 5 minutes
Excretion: Urine (25% to 60% predominantly as metabolites; <2% as unchanged drug)

Dosage

Geriatric Oral (refer to individual protocols): Start with lowest recommended doses for adults.
Adult Note: Premedicate with prophylactic anticonvulsant therapy (eg, phenytoin) prior to high-dose busulfan treatment. Prophylactic antiemetics may be necessary for high-dose (HSCT) regimens.

Chronic myelogenous leukemia (CML), palliation (manufacturer's labeling): *Oral:*
Remission induction: 60 mcg/kg/day or 1.8 mg/m²/day; usual range: 4-8 mg/day; titrate dose (or withhold) to maintain leukocyte counts ≥15,000/mm³ (doses >4 mg/day should be reserved for patients with the most compelling symptoms)
Maintenance: When leukocyte count ≥50,000/mm³: Resume induction dose **or** (if remission <3 months) 1-3 mg/day (to control hematologic status and prevent relapse)

Hematopoietic stem cell (HSCT) conditioning regimen:
I.V.:
0.8 mg/kg every 6 hours for 4 days (a total of 16 doses); **Note:** Use ideal body weight or actual body weight, (whichever is lower) for dosing. For obese or severely-obese patients, use of an adjusted body weight [IBW + 0.25 x (actual – IBW)] is recommended.
Reduced intensity conditioning regimen (unlabeled dosing): 0.8 mg/kg/day for 4 days starting 5 days prior to transplant (in combinations with fludarabine) (Ho, 2009)
Oral (unlabeled use): 1 mg/kg/dose every 6 hours for 16 doses (in combination with cyclophosphamide) (Socié, 2001) **or** 1 mg/kg/dose every 6 hours for 16 doses beginning 9 days prior to transplant (in combination with cyclophosphamide) (Cassileth, 1993) **or** 0.44 mg/kg/dose every 6 hours for 16 doses (in combination with cyclophosphamide) (Anderson, 1996) **or** 1 mg/kg/dose every 6 hours for 16 doses beginning 6 days prior to transplant (in combination with melphalan) (Fermand, 2005)

Polycythemia vera and essential thrombocythemia (unlabeled uses): Oral: 2-4 mg/day (Fabris, 2009; Tefferi, 2011)

Renal Impairment
I.V.: No dosage adjustment provided in the manufacturer's labeling (has not been studied).
Oral: No dosage adjustment provided in the manufacturer's labeling (elimination appears to be independent of renal function); however, some clinicians suggest adjustment is not necessary (Aronoff, 2007).

Hepatic Impairment
I.V.: No dosage adjustment provided in the manufacturer's labeling (has not been studied).
Oral: No dosage adjustment provided in the manufacturer's labeling.

Administration Intravenous busulfan should be infused over 2 hours via central line. Flush line before and after each infusion with 5 mL D₅W or NS. Do not use polycarbonate syringes or filters for preparation or administration

HSCT only: To facilitate ingestion of high oral doses, may insert multiple tablets into gelatin capsules.

Monitoring Parameters CBC with differential and platelet count (weekly for palliative treatment; daily until engraftment for HSCT); liver function tests (evaluate transaminases, alkaline phosphatase, and bilirubin daily for at least 28 days post transplant). If conducting therapeutic drug monitoring for AUC calculations in HSCT, monitor blood samples at appropriate collections times (record collection times).

Special Geriatric Considerations Toxicity is increased in the elderly. Start with lowest recommended adult doses. Signs of infection, such as fever and rise in WBCs, may not occur. Lethargy and confusion may be more prominent signs of infection. Patients should report any development of persistent cough, dyspnea, and fever.

Dosage Forms Excipient information presented when available (limited, particularly for generics); consult specific product labeling.
Injection, solution:
Busulfex®: 6 mg/mL (10 mL) [contains N,N-dimethylacetamide (DMA), polyethylene glycol 400]
Tablet, oral:
Myleran®: 2 mg [scored]

◆ **Busulfanum** *see* Busulfan *on page 247*
◆ **Busulfex®** *see* Busulfan *on page 247*
◆ **Busulphan** *see* Busulfan *on page 247*

Butorphanol (byoo TOR fa nole)

Related Information
Opioid Analgesics *on page 2122*

Medication Safety Issues
Sound-alike/look-alike issues:
Stadol may be confused with Haldol®, sotalol

High alert medication:
The Institute for Safe Medication Practices (ISMP) includes this medication among its list of drug classes which have a heightened risk of causing significant patient harm when used in error.

Brand Names: Canada Apo-Butorphanol®; PMS-Butorphanol

Index Terms Butorphanol Tartrate; Stadol

Generic Availability (U.S.) Yes

Pharmacologic Category Analgesic, Opioid; Analgesic, Opioid Partial Agonist

Use

Parenteral: Management of moderate-to-severe pain; preoperative medication; supplement to balanced anesthesia; management of pain during labor

Nasal spray: Management of moderate-to-severe pain, including migraine headache pain

Contraindications Hypersensitivity to butorphanol or any component of the formulation; avoid use in opiate-dependent patients who have not been detoxified, may precipitate opiate withdrawal

Warnings/Precautions An opioid-containing analgesic regimen should be tailored to each patient's needs and based upon the type of pain being treated (acute versus chronic), the route of administration, degree of tolerance for opioids (naive versus chronic user), age, weight, and medical condition. The optimal analgesic dose varies widely among patients. Doses should be titrated to pain relief/prevention. May cause CNS depression; use with caution in patients with head trauma, morbid obesity, thyroid dysfunction, hepatic/renal dysfunction, adrenal insufficiency, prostatic hyperplasia and/or urinary stricture, may elevate CSF pressure, may increase cardiac workload; tolerance of drug dependence may result from extended use. Use with caution in patients with biliary tract dysfunction; acute pancreatitis may cause constriction of sphincter of Oddi.

Partial antagonist activity may precipitate acute narcotic withdrawal in opioid-dependent individuals. Use with caution in patients with pre-existing respiratory compromise (hypoxia and/or hypercapnia), COPD or other obstructive pulmonary disease; critical respiratory depression may occur, even at therapeutic dosages. May cause hypotension; use with caution in patients with hypovolemia, cardiovascular disease (including acute MI), or drugs which may exaggerate hypotensive effects (including phenothiazines or general anesthetics). May obscure diagnosis or clinical course of patients with acute abdominal conditions.

Concurrent use of sumatriptan nasal spray and butorphanol nasal spray may increase risk of transient high blood pressure. Healthcare provider should be alert to problems of abuse, misuse, and diversion. Use with caution in the elderly and debilitated patients; may be more sensitive to adverse effects.

Adverse Reactions (Reflective of adult population; not specific for elderly)

>10%:

Central nervous system: Somnolence (43%), dizziness (19%), insomnia (nasal spray 11%)

Gastrointestinal: Nausea/vomiting (13%)

Respiratory: Nasal congestion (nasal spray 13%)

1% to 10%:

Cardiovascular: Palpitation, vasodilation

Central nervous system: Anxiety, confusion, headache, lethargy, lightheadedness

Dermatologic: Pruritus

Gastrointestinal: Anorexia, constipation, stomach pain, unpleasant aftertaste, xerostomia

Neuromuscular & skeletal: Tremor, paresthesia, weakness

Ocular: Blurred vision

Otic: Ear pain, tinnitus

Respiratory: Bronchitis, cough, dyspnea, epistaxis, nasal irritation, pharyngitis, rhinitis, sinus congestion, sinusitis, upper respiratory infection

Miscellaneous: Diaphoresis increased

Drug Interactions

Metabolism/Transport Effects None known.

Avoid Concomitant Use

Avoid concomitant use of Butorphanol with any of the following: Azelastine; Azelastine (Nasal); Mirtazapine; Paraldehyde

Increased Effect/Toxicity

Butorphanol may increase the levels/effects of: Alcohol (Ethyl); Alvimopan; Azelastine; Azelastine (Nasal); CNS Depressants; Desmopressin; Metyrosine; Mirtazapine; Paraldehyde; Selective Serotonin Reuptake Inhibitors; Thiazide Diuretics; Zolpidem

The levels/effects of Butorphanol may be increased by: Amphetamines; Antipsychotic Agents (Phenothiazines); Droperidol; HydrOXYzine; Succinylcholine

Decreased Effect

Butorphanol may decrease the levels/effects of: Analgesics (Opioid); Pegvisomant

The levels/effects of Butorphanol may be decreased by: Ammonium Chloride; Mixed Agonist/Antagonist Opioids

Ethanol/Nutrition/Herb Interactions

Ethanol: May increase CNS depression; monitor for increased effects with coadministration. Caution patients about effects.

Herb/Nutraceutical: Avoid valerian, St John's wort, kava kava, gotu kola (may increase CNS depression).

Stability Store at room temperature; protect from freezing.

Mechanism of Action Agonist of kappa opiate receptors and partial agonist of mu opiate receptors in the CNS, causing inhibition of ascending pain pathways, altering the perception of and response to pain; produces analgesia, respiratory depression, and sedation similar to opioids

Pharmacodynamics/Kinetics

Onset of action: I.M.: 5-10 minutes; I.V.: <10 minutes; Nasal: Within 15 minutes

Peak effect: I.M.: 0.5-1 hour; I.V.: 4-5 minutes

Duration: I.M., I.V.: 3-4 hours; Nasal: 4-5 hours

Absorption: Rapid and well absorbed

Protein binding: 80%

Metabolism: Hepatic

Bioavailability: Nasal: 60% to 70%

Half-life elimination:

Geriatrics: 5.5 hours

Adults: 2.5-4 hours

Excretion: Primarily urine

Dosage

Geriatric

I.M., I.V.: Initial dosage should generally be ¹/₂ of the recommended dose; repeated dosing must be based on initial response rather than fixed intervals, but generally should be at least 6 hours apart

Nasal spray: Initial dose should not exceed 1 mg; a second dose may be given after 90-120 minutes

Adult Note: These are guidelines and do not represent the maximum doses that may be required in all patients. Doses should be titrated to pain relief/prevention. Butorphanol has an analgesic ceiling.

Acute pain (moderate-to-severe):

I.M.: Initial: 2 mg, may repeat every 3-4 hours as needed; usual range: 1-4 mg every 3-4 hours as needed

I.V.: Initial: 1 mg, may repeat every 3-4 hours as needed; usual range: 0.5-2 mg every 3-4 hours as needed

Intranasal (spray) (includes use for migraine headache pain): Initial: 1 spray (~1 mg per spray) in 1 nostril; if adequate pain relief is not achieved within 60-90 minutes, an additional 1 spray in 1 nostril may be given; may repeat initial dose sequence in 3-4 hours after the last dose as needed

Alternatively, an initial dose of 2 mg (1 spray in each nostril) may be used in patients who will be able to remain recumbent (in the event drowsiness or dizziness occurs); additional 2 mg doses should not be given for 3-4 hours

Note: In some clinical trials, an initial dose of 2 mg (as 2 doses 1 hour apart or 2 mg initially - 1 spray in each nostril) has been used, followed by 1 mg in 1 hour; side effects were greater at these dosages

Migraine: *Nasal spray:* Refer to "moderate-to-severe pain" indication

Preoperative medication: *I.M.:* 2 mg 60-90 minutes before surgery

Supplement to balanced anesthesia: *I.V.:* 2 mg shortly before induction and/or an incremental dose of 0.5-1 mg (up to 0.06 mg/kg), depending on previously administered sedative, analgesic, and hypnotic medications

Renal Impairment

I.M., I.V.: Initial dosage should generally be ¹/₂ of the recommended dose; repeated dosing must be based on initial response rather than fixed intervals, but generally should be at least 6 hours apart

Nasal spray: Initial dose should not exceed 1 mg; a second dose may be given after 90-120 minutes

Hepatic Impairment

I.M., I.V.: Initial dosage should generally be ¹/₂ of the recommended dose; repeated dosing must be based on initial response rather than fixed intervals, but generally should be at least 6 hours apart

Nasal spray: Initial dose should not exceed 1 mg; a second dose may be given after 90-120 minutes

Administration Intranasal: Consider avoiding simultaneous intranasal migraine sprays; may want to separate by at least 30 minutes

Monitoring Parameters Pain relief, respiratory and mental status, blood pressure

Reference Range 0.7-1.5 ng/mL

Special Geriatric Considerations Adjust dose for renal function in the elderly.

Controlled Substance C-IV

Dosage Forms Excipient information presented when available (limited, particularly for generics); consult specific product labeling.

Injection, solution, as tartrate: 1 mg/mL (1 mL); 2 mg/mL (1 mL, 2 mL, 10 mL)

Injection, solution, as tartrate [preservative free]: 1 mg/mL (1 mL); 2 mg/mL (1 mL, 2 mL)

Solution, intranasal, as tartrate [spray]: 10 mg/mL (2.5 mL)

Calcipotriene (kal si POE try een)

Brand Names: U.S. Calcitrene™; Dovonex®; Sorilux™

Brand Names: Canada Dovonex®

Generic Availability (U.S.) Yes: Excludes cream, foam

Pharmacologic Category Topical Skin Product; Vitamin D Analog

Use Treatment of plaque psoriasis (cream, foam, ointment); chronic, moderate-to-severe psoriasis of the scalp (solution)

Contraindications Hypersensitivity to calcipotriene or any component of the formulation; patients with demonstrated hypercalcemia or evidence of vitamin D toxicity; use on the face (cream, ointment); patients with acute psoriatic eruptions (scalp solution)

Warnings/Precautions Discontinue use if irritation occurs. May cause transient increases in serum calcium (reversible); if hypercalcemia occurs, discontinue treatment until levels return to normal. For external use only; not for ophthalmic, oral, or intravaginal use. Avoid or limit excessive exposure to natural or artificial sunlight, or phototherapy. Use with caution in elderly patients; severity of skin related adverse reactions may be increased compared to younger adults. Foam product is flammable; keep away from fire, flame, or smoking during and immediately following application.

Adverse Reactions (Reflective of adult population; not specific for elderly) Frequency may vary with site of application.

>10%: Dermatologic: Burning, itching, rash, skin irritation, stinging, tingling

1% to 10%: Dermatologic: Dermatitis, dry skin, erythema, peeling, pruritus, worsening of psoriasis

Drug Interactions

Metabolism/Transport Effects None known.

Avoid Concomitant Use

Avoid concomitant use of Calcipotriene with any of the following: Aluminum Hydroxide; Sucralfate; Vitamin D Analogs

Increased Effect/Toxicity

Calcipotriene may increase the levels/effects of: Aluminum Hydroxide; Cardiac Glycosides; Sucralfate; Vitamin D Analogs

The levels/effects of Calcipotriene may be increased by: Calcium Salts; Danazol; Thiazide Diuretics

Decreased Effect

The levels/effects of Calcipotriene may be decreased by: Orlistat

CALCIPOTRIENE

Stability
Cream, ointment, solution: Store at controlled room temperature of 15°C to 25°C (59°F to 77°F); do not freeze. Solution should be kept away from open flame; avoid sunlight.
Foam: Store at 25°C (77°F); excursions permitted to 15°C to 30°C (59°F to 86°F). Contents are flammable; keep away from heat and flame.

Mechanism of Action Synthetic vitamin D_3 analog which regulates skin cell production and proliferation

Pharmacodynamics/Kinetics
Onset of action: Improvement begins after 2 weeks; marked improvement seen after 8 weeks
Absorption: When applied to psoriasis plaques: Cream, foam: Undetermined; Ointment: ~6%; Solution: <1%
Metabolism: Converted in the skin to inactive metabolites

Dosage
Geriatric & Adult Psoriasis: Topical:
Cream, foam: Apply a thin film to the affected skin twice daily
Ointment: Apply a thin film to the affected skin once or twice daily
Solution: Apply to the affected scalp twice daily

Administration For external use only.
Cream, foam, ointment: Apply to affected skin; rub in gently and completely. Wash hands thoroughly before and after use.
Solution: Prior to using scalp solution, comb hair to remove debris; apply only to lesions. Rub in gently and completely. Avoid solution spreading or dripping onto forehead. Avoid contact with eyes. Wash hands thoroughly before and after use.

Monitoring Parameters Serum calcium

Special Geriatric Considerations Use caution in older adults, severity of skin-related adverse reactions may be increased compared to younger adults.

Dosage Forms Excipient information presented when available (limited, particularly for generics); consult specific product labeling.
Aerosol, foam, topical:
Sorilux™: 0.005% (60 g, 120 g) [ethanol free]
Cream, topical: 0.005% (60 g, 120 g)
Dovonex®: 0.005% (60 g, 120 g)
Ointment, topical:
Calcitrene™: 0.005% (60 g)
Solution, topical: 0.005% (60 mL)
Dovonex®: 0.005% (60 mL) [contains isopropyl alcohol 51% v/v]

Calcitonin (kal si TOE nin)

Related Information
Osteoporosis Management *on page 2136*

Medication Safety Issues
Sound-alike/look-alike issues:
Calcitonin may be confused with calcitriol
Miacalcin® may be confused with Micatin®

Administration issues:
Calcitonin nasal spray is administered as a single spray into **one** nostril daily, using alternate nostrils each day.

Brand Names: U.S. Fortical®; Miacalcin®

Brand Names: Canada Apo-Calcitonin®; Calcimar®; Caltine®; Miacalcin® NS; PRO-Calcitonin; Sandoz-Calcitonin

Index Terms Calcitonin (Salmon)

Generic Availability (U.S.) Yes: Intranasal solution

Pharmacologic Category Antidote; Hormone

Use Treatment of Paget's disease of bone (osteitis deformans); adjunctive therapy for hypercalcemia; treatment of osteoporosis in women >5 years postmenopause

Contraindications Hypersensitivity to calcitonin salmon or any component of the formulation

Warnings/Precautions A skin test should be performed prior to initiating therapy of calcitonin salmon in patients with suspected sensitivity; have epinephrine immediately available for a possible hypersensitivity reaction. A detailed skin testing protocol is available from the manufacturers. Temporarily withdraw use of nasal spray if ulceration of nasal mucosa occurs. Discontinue for ulcerations >1.5 mm or those that penetrate below the mucosa. Patients >65 years of age may experience a higher incidence of nasal adverse events with calcitonin nasal spray.

Adverse Reactions (Reflective of adult population; not specific for elderly) Unless otherwise noted, frequencies reported are with nasal spray.

>10%: Respiratory: Rhinitis (≤12%, including ulcerative)

1% to 10%:

Cardiovascular: Flushing (nasal spray: <1%; injection: 2% to 5%), angina (1% to 3%), hypertension (1% to 3%)

Central nervous system: Depression (1% to 3%), dizziness (1% to 3%), fatigue (1% to 3%)

Dermatologic: Erythematous rash (1% to 3%)

Gastrointestinal: Nausea (injection: 10%; nasal spray: 2%), abdominal pain (1% to 3%), constipation (1% to 3%), diarrhea (1% to 3%), dyspepsia (1% to 3%)

Genitourinary: Cystitis (1% to 3%)

Local: Injection site reactions (injection: 10%)

Neuromuscular & skeletal: Back pain (5%), arthrosis (1% to 3%), myalgia (1% to 3%), paresthesia (1% to 3%)

Ocular: Conjunctivitis (1% to 3%), lacrimation abnormality (1% to 3%)

Respiratory: Nasal ulcerations (3%), bronchospasm (1% to 3%), sinusitis (1% to 3%), upper respiratory tract infection (1% to 3%)

Miscellaneous: Flu-like syndrome (1% to 3%), infection (1% to 3%), lymphadenopathy (1% to 3%)

Drug Interactions

Metabolism/Transport Effects None known.

Avoid Concomitant Use There are no known interactions where it is recommended to avoid concomitant use.

Increased Effect/Toxicity There are no known significant interactions involving an increase in effect.

Decreased Effect

Calcitonin may decrease the levels/effects of: Lithium

Ethanol/Nutrition/Herb Interactions Ethanol: Avoid ethanol (may increase risk of osteoporosis).

Stability

Injection: Store under refrigeration at 2°C to 8°C (36°F to 46°F); protect from freezing. NS has been recommended for the dilution to prepare a skin test in patients with suspected sensitivity. The following stability information has also been reported: May be stored at room temperature for up to 14 days (Cohen, 2007).

Nasal: Store unopened bottle under refrigeration at 2°C to 8°C (36°F to 46°F); do not freeze.

Fortical®: After opening, store for up to 30 days at 20°C to 25°C (68°F to 77°F); excursions permitted to 15°C to 30°C (59°F to 86°F). Store in upright position.

Miacalcin®: After opening, store for up to 35 days at room temperature of 15°C to 30°C (59°F to 86°F). Store in upright position.

Mechanism of Action Peptide sequence similar to human calcitonin; functionally antagonizes the effects of parathyroid hormone. Directly inhibits osteoclastic bone resorption; promotes the renal excretion of calcium, phosphate, sodium, magnesium, and potassium by decreasing tubular reabsorption; increases the jejunal secretion of water, sodium, potassium, and chloride

Pharmacodynamics/Kinetics

Onset of action:

Hypercalcemia: I.M., SubQ: ~2 hours

Paget's disease: Within a few months; may take up to 1 year for neurologic symptom improvement

Duration: Hypercalcemia: I.M., SubQ: 6-8 hours

Distribution: V_d: 0.15-0.3 L/kg

Metabolism: Metabolized in kidneys, blood and peripheral tissue

Bioavailability: I.M.: 66%; SubQ: 71%; Nasal: ~3% to 5% (relative to I.M.)

Half-life elimination (terminal): I.M. 58 minutes; SubQ 59-64 minutes; Nasal: ~18 minutes

Time to peak, plasma: SubQ ~23 minutes; Nasal: ~13 minutes

Excretion: Urine (as inactive metabolites)

Dosage

Geriatric & Adult

Paget's disease *(Miacalcin®)*: I.M., SubQ: Initial: 100 units/day; maintenance: 50 units/day or 50-100 units every 1-3 days

Hypercalcemia *(Miacalcin®)*: Initial: I.M., SubQ: 4 units/kg every 12 hours; may increase up to 8 units/kg every 12 hours; if the response remains unsatisfactory, a further increase up to a maximum of 8 units/kg every 6 hours may be considered

Postmenopausal osteoporosis:

Miacalcin®: I.M., SubQ: 100 units/every other day

Fortical®, Miacalcin®: Intranasal: 200 units (1 spray) in one nostril daily

CALCITONIN

Administration

Injection solution: May be administered I.M. or SubQ. I.M route is preferred if the injection volume is >2 mL. SubQ route is preferred for outpatient self-administration unless the injection volume is >2 mL.

Nasal spray: Before first use, allow bottle to reach room temperature, then prime pump by releasing at least 5 sprays until full spray is produced. To administer, place nozzle into nostril with head in upright position. Alternate nostrils daily. Do not prime pump before each daily use. Discard after 30 doses.

Monitoring Parameters Serum electrolytes and calcium; alkaline phosphatase and 24-hour urine collection for hydroxyproline excretion (Paget's disease), urinalysis (urine sediment); bone mineral density

Nasal formulation: Visualization of nasal mucosa, turbinate, septum, and mucosal blood vessels (at baseline and with nasal complaints)

Special Geriatric Considerations Studies have shown calcitonin's effects on bone density and fracture rates are positive, but less than other treatments. Calcium and vitamin D supplements should also be given. Calcitonin may also be effective in steroid-induced osteoporosis and other states associated with high bone turnover. Nasal spray may provide faster onset of analgesic effects than I.M.

Dosage Forms Excipient information presented when available (limited, particularly for generics); consult specific product labeling.

Injection, solution [calcitonin-salmon]:
 Miacalcin®: 200 units/mL (2 mL)
Solution, intranasal [calcitonin-salmon/rDNA origin/spray]:
 Fortical®: 200 units/actuation (3.7 mL) [contains benzyl alcohol; delivers 30 doses]
Solution, intranasal [calcitonin-salmon/spray]: 200 units/actuation (3.7 mL)
 Miacalcin®: 200 units/actuation (3.7 mL) [contains benzalkonium chloride; delivers 30 doses]

◆ **Calcitonin (Salmon)** see Calcitonin on page 254
◆ **Calcitrate [OTC]** see Calcium Citrate on page 268
◆ **Cal-Citrate™ 225 [OTC]** see Calcium Citrate on page 268
◆ **Calcitrene™** see Calcipotriene on page 253

Calcitriol (kal si TRYE ole)

Medication Safety Issues

Sound-alike/look-alike issues:
 Calcitriol may be confused with alfacalcidol, Calciferol™, calcitonin, calcium carbonate, captopril, colestipol, paricalcitol, ropinirole

Administration issues:
 Dosage is expressed in mcg (micrograms), **not** mg (milligrams); rare cases of acute overdose have been reported

Brand Names: U.S. Calcijex®; Rocaltrol®; Vectical®
Brand Names: Canada Calcijex®; Rocaltrol®
Index Terms 1,25 Dihydroxycholecalciferol
Generic Availability (U.S.) Yes: Excludes ointment
Pharmacologic Category Vitamin D Analog

Use
Oral, injection: Management of hypocalcemia in patients on chronic renal dialysis; management of secondary hyperparathyroidism in patients with chronic kidney disease (CKD); management of hypocalcemia in hypoparathyroidism and pseudohypoparathyroidism
Topical: Management of mild-to-moderate plaque psoriasis

Unlabeled Use Decrease severity of psoriatic lesions in psoriatic vulgaris; vitamin D-dependent rickets

Contraindications Hypersensitivity to calcitriol or any component of the formulation; hypercalcemia, vitamin D toxicity
Topical: There are no contraindications listed in the manufacturer's labeling.

Warnings/Precautions
Oral, injection: Adequate dietary (supplemental) calcium is necessary for clinical response to vitamin D. Excessive vitamin D may cause severe hypercalcemia, hypercalciuria, and hyperphosphatemia; calcium-phosphate product (serum calcium times phosphorus) must not exceed 70 mg^2/dL^2. Other forms of vitamin D should be withheld during therapy. Immobilization may increase risk of hypercalcemia and/or hypercalciuria. Maintain adequate hydration. Use caution in patients with malabsorption syndromes (efficacy may be limited and/or response may be unpredictable). Use of calcitriol for the treatment of secondary hyperparathyroidism associated with CKD is not recommended in patients with rapidly worsening kidney function or in noncompliant patients. Increased serum phosphate levels in patients with

256

renal failure may lead to calcification; the use of an aluminum-containing phosphate binder is recommended along with a low phosphate diet in these patients. Use with caution in patients taking cardiac glycosides; digitalis toxicity is potentiated by hypocalcemia. Products may contain coconut (capsule) or palm seed oil (oral solution). Some products may contain tartrazine.

Topical: May cause hypercalcemia; if alterations in calcium occur, discontinue treatment until levels return to normal. For external use only; not for ophthalmic, oral, or intravaginal use. Do not apply to facial skin, eyes, or lips. Absorption may be increased with occlusive dressings. Avoid or limit excessive exposure to natural or artificial sunlight, or phototherapy. The safety and effectiveness has not been evaluated in patients with erythrodermic, exfoliative, or pustular psoriasis.

Adverse Reactions (Reflective of adult population; not specific for elderly)

Oral, I.V.: Frequency not defined.

Cardiovascular: Cardiac arrhythmia, hypertension

Central nervous system: Apathy, headache, hypothermia, psychosis, sensory disturbances, somnolence

Dermatologic: Erythema multiforme, pruritus

Endocrine & metabolic: Dehydration, growth suppression, hypercalcemia, hypercholesterolemia, hypermagnesemia, hyperphosphatemia, libido decreased, polydipsia

Gastrointestinal: Abdominal pain, anorexia, constipation, metallic taste, nausea, pancreatitis, stomach ache, vomiting, weight loss, xerostomia

Genitourinary: Nocturia, urinary tract infection

Hepatic: ALT increased, AST increased

Local: Injection site pain (mild)

Neuromuscular & skeletal: Bone pain, myalgia, dystrophy, soft tissue calcification, weakness

Ocular: Conjunctivitis, photophobia

Renal: Albuminuria, BUN increased, creatinine increased, hypercalciuria, nephrocalcinosis, polyuria

Respiratory: Rhinorrhea

Miscellaneous: Allergic reaction

Topical:

>10%: Endocrine: Hypercalcemia (≤24%)

1% to 10%:

Dermatologic: Skin discomfort (3%), pruritus (1% to 3%)

Genitourinary: Urine abnormality (4%)

Renal: Hypercalciuria (3%)

Drug Interactions

Metabolism/Transport Effects Substrate of CYP3A4 (major); **Note:** Assignment of Major/Minor substrate status based on clinically relevant drug interaction potential; **Induces** CYP3A4 (weak/moderate)

Avoid Concomitant Use

Avoid concomitant use of Calcitriol with any of the following: Aluminum Hydroxide; Axitinib; Conivaptan; Sucralfate; Vitamin D Analogs

Increased Effect/Toxicity

Calcitriol may increase the levels/effects of: Aluminum Hydroxide; Cardiac Glycosides; Magnesium Salts; Sucralfate; Vitamin D Analogs

The levels/effects of Calcitriol may be increased by: Calcium Salts; Conivaptan; CYP3A4 Inhibitors (Moderate); CYP3A4 Inhibitors (Strong); Danazol; Dasatinib; Ivacaftor; Mifepristone; Thiazide Diuretics

Decreased Effect

Calcitriol may decrease the levels/effects of: ARIPiprazole; Axitinib; Saxagliptin

The levels/effects of Calcitriol may be decreased by: Bile Acid Sequestrants; Corticosteroids (Systemic); CYP3A4 Inducers (Strong); Deferasirox; Herbs (CYP3A4 Inducers); Mineral Oil; Orlistat; Sevelamer; Tocilizumab

Stability

Injection: Store at room temperature of 15°C to 30°C (59°F to 86°F). Protect from light.

Oral capsule, solution: Store at room temperature of 20°C to 25°C (68°F to 77°F). Protect from light.

Topical: Store at room temperature of 25°C (77°F); excursions permitted to 15°C to 30°C (59°F to 86°F); do not refrigerate; do not freeze.

Mechanism of Action
Calcitriol is a potent active metabolite of vitamin D. Vitamin D promotes absorption of calcium in the intestines and retention at the kidneys thereby increasing calcium levels in the serum; decreases excessive serum phosphatase levels, parathyroid hormone levels, and decreases bone resorption; increases renal tubule phosphate resorption

The mechanism by which calcitriol is beneficial in the treatment of psoriasis has not been established.

Pharmacodynamics/Kinetics

Onset of action: Oral: ~2-6 hours

Duration: Oral, I.V.: 3-5 days

Absorption: Oral: Rapid

Protein binding: 99.9%

Metabolism: Primarily to 1,24,25-trihydroxycholecalciferol and 1,24,25-trihydroxy ergocalciferol

Half-life elimination: Normal adults: 5-8 hours; Hemodialysis: 16-22 hours

Time to peak, serum: Oral: 3-6 hours; Hemodialysis: 8-12 hours

Excretion: Primarily feces; urine

Dosage

Geriatric Refer to adult dosing. No dosage recommendations, but start at the lower end of the dosage range.

Adult

Hypocalcemia in patients on chronic renal dialysis (manufacturer's labeling):

Oral: 0.25 mcg/day or every other day (may require 0.5-1 mcg/day); increases should be made at 4- to 8-week intervals

I.V.: Initial: 1-2 mcg 3 times/week (0.02 mcg/kg) approximately every other day. Adjust dose at 2-4 week intervals; dosing range: 0.5-4 mcg 3 times/week

Hypocalcemia in hypoparathyroidism/pseudohypoparathyroidism (manufacturer's labeling): Oral (evaluate dosage at 2- to 4-week intervals): Initial: 0.25 mcg/day, range: 0.5-2 mcg once daily

Secondary hyperparathyroidism associated with moderate-to-severe CKD in patients not on dialysis (manufacturer's labeling): Oral: 0.25 mcg/day; may increase to 0.5 mcg/day

K/DOQI guidelines for vitamin D therapy in CKD:

CKD stage 3: Oral: 0.25 mcg/day. Treatment should only be started with serum 25(OH) D >30 ng/mL, serum iPTH >70 pg/mL, serum calcium <9.5 mg/dL and serum phosphorus <4.6 mg/dL

CKD stage 4: Oral: 0.25 mcg/day. Treatment should only be started with serum 25(OH) D >30 ng/mL, serum iPTH >110 pg/mL, serum calcium <9.5 mg/dL and serum phosphorus <4.6 mg/dL

CKD stage 5:

Peritoneal dialysis: Oral: Initial: 0.5-1 mcg 2-3 times/week or 0.25 mcg/day

Hemodialysis: **Note:** The following initial doses are based on plasma PTH and serum calcium levels for patients with serum phosphorus <5.5 mg/dL and Ca-P product <55. Adjust dose based on serum phosphate, calcium, and PTH levels. Intermittent I.V. administration may be more effective than daily oral dosing.

Plasma PTH 300-600 pg/mL and serum Ca <9.5 mg/dL: Oral, I.V.: 0.5-1.5 mcg

Plasma PTH 600-1000 pg/mL and serum Ca <9.5 mg/dL:

Oral: 1-4 mcg

I.V.: 1-3 mcg

Plasma PTH >1000 pg/mL and serum Ca <10 mg/dL:

Oral: 3-7 mcg

I.V.: 3-5 mcg

Psoriasis: Topical: Apply twice daily to affected areas (maximum: 200 g/week)

Vitamin D-dependent rickets (unlabeled use): Oral: 1 mcg once daily

Administration

I.V.: May be administered as a bolus dose I.V. through the catheter at the end of hemodialysis.

Oral: May be administered without regard to food. Administer with meals to reduce GI problems.

Topical: Apply externally; not for ophthalmic, oral, or intravaginal use. Do not apply to eyes, lips, or facial skins. Rub in gently so that no medication remains visible. Limit application to only the areas of skin affected by psoriasis.

Monitoring Parameters

Serum calcium and phosphorus: Frequency of measurement may be dependent upon the presence and magnitude of abnormalities, the rate of progression of CKD, and the use of treatments for CKD-mineral and bone disorders (KDIGO, 2009):

CKD stage 3: Every 6-12 months

CKD stage 4: Every 3-6 months

CKD stage 5 and 5D: Every 1-3 months

Periodic 24-hour urinary calcium and phosphorus; magnesium; alkaline phosphatase every 12 months or more frequently in the presence of elevated PTH; creatinine, BUN, albumin; intact parathyroid hormone (iPTH) every 3-12 months depending on CKD severity

Reference Range

Corrected total serum calcium (K/DOQI, 2003): CKD stages 3 and 4: 8.4-10.2 mg/dL (2.1-2.6 mmol/L); CKD stage 5: 8.4-9.5 mg/dL (2.1-2.37 mmol/L); KDIGO guidelines recommend maintaining normal ranges for all stages of CKD (3-5D) (KDIGO, 2009)

Phosphorus (K/DOQI, 2003):

CKD stages 3 and 4: 2.7-4.6 mg/dL (0.87-1.48 mmol/L) (adults)

CKD stage 5 (including those treated with dialysis): 3.5-5.5 mg/dL (1.13-1.78 mmol/L) (adults)

KDIGO guidelines recommend maintaining normal ranges for CKD stages 3-5 and lowering elevated phosphorus levels toward the normal range for CKD stage 5D (KDIGO, 2009)

Serum calcium-phosphorus product (K/DOQI, 2003): CKD stage 3-5: <55 mg^2/dL^2 (adults)

PTH: Whole molecule, immunochemiluminometric assay (ICMA): 1.0-5.2 pmol/L; whole molecule, radioimmunoassay (RIA): 10.0-65.0 pg/mL; whole molecule, immunoradiometric, double antibody (IRMA): 1.0-6.0 pmol/L

Target ranges by stage of chronic kidney disease (KDIGO, 2009): CKD stage 3-5: Optimal iPTH is unknown; maintain normal range (assay-dependent); CKD stage 5D: Maintain iPTH within 2-9 times the upper limit of normal for the assay used

Special Geriatric Considerations Vitamin D, folate, and B$_{12}$ (cyanocobalamin) have decreased absorption with age (clinical significance unknown); studies in ill geriatrics demonstrated that low serum concentrations of vitamin D result in greater bone loss. Calorie requirements decrease with age and therefore, nutrient density must be increased to ensure adequate nutrient intake, including vitamins and minerals. The use of a daily supplement with a multiple vitamin with minerals is recommended because elderly consume less vitamin D, absorption may be decreased, and many have decreased sun exposure. This is a recommendation of particular need to those with high risk for osteoporosis.

Vitamin D supplementation has been shown to increase muscle function and strength, as well as improve balance. Patients at risk for falls should have vitamin D serum concentrations measured and be evaluated for supplementation.

Dosage Forms Excipient information presented when available (limited, particularly for generics); consult specific product labeling.

Capsule, softgel, oral: 0.25 mcg, 0.5 mcg

Rocaltrol®: 0.25 mcg, 0.5 mcg [contains coconut oil]

Injection, solution: 1 mcg/mL (1 mL)

Calcijex®: 1 mcg/mL (1 mL) [contains aluminum]

Ointment, topical:

Vectical®: 3 mcg/g (100 g)

Solution, oral: 1 mcg/mL (15 mL)

Rocaltrol®: 1 mcg/mL (15 mL) [contains palm oil]

Calcium Acetate (KAL see um AS e tate)

Related Information

Osteoporosis Management *on page 2136*

Medication Safety Issues

Sound-alike/look-alike issues:

PhosLo® may be confused with Phos-Flur®, ProSom

Brand Names: U.S. Eliphos™; PhosLo®; Phoslyra™

Brand Names: Canada PhosLo®

Generic Availability (U.S.) Yes: Gelcap

Pharmacologic Category Antidote; Calcium Salt; Phosphate Binder

Use Control of hyperphosphatemia in end-stage renal failure; does not promote aluminum absorption

Contraindications Hypersensitivity to any component of the formulation; hypercalcemia, renal calculi

Warnings/Precautions Constipation, bloating, and gas are common with calcium supplements. Hypercalcemia and hypercalciuria are most likely to occur in hypoparathyroid patients receiving high doses of vitamin D. Use with caution in patients who may be at risk of cardiac arrhythmias. Use with caution in digitalized patients; hypercalcemia may precipitate cardiac arrhythmias. Calcium administration interferes with absorption of some minerals and drugs; use with caution. Oral solution may contain maltitol (a sugar substitute) which may cause a laxative effect.

Adverse Reactions (Reflective of adult population; not specific for elderly)

$>10\%$:

Endocrine & metabolic: Hypercalcemia

Gastrointestinal: Diarrhea (oral solution)

1% to 10%: Gastrointestinal: Nausea, vomiting

Drug Interactions

Metabolism/Transport Effects None known.

Avoid Concomitant Use

Avoid concomitant use of Calcium Acetate with any of the following: Calcium Salts

Increased Effect/Toxicity

Calcium Acetate may increase the levels/effects of: CefTRIAXone; Vitamin D Analogs

The levels/effects of Calcium Acetate may be increased by: Calcium Salts; Thiazide Diuretics

Decreased Effect

Calcium Acetate may decrease the levels/effects of: Bisphosphonate Derivatives; Calcium Channel Blockers; Deferiprone; DOBUTamine; Eltrombopag; Estramustine; Phosphate Supplements; Quinolone Antibiotics; Tetracycline Derivatives; Thyroid Products; Trientine

The levels/effects of Calcium Acetate may be decreased by: Trientine

Ethanol/Nutrition/Herb Interactions

Ethanol: Ethanol may decrease calcium absorption.

Food: Caffeine may decrease calcium absorption and increase calcium excretion. Foods that contain maltitol may have an additive laxative effect with the oral solution formulation (contains maltitol).

Mechanism of Action Combines with dietary phosphate to form insoluble calcium phosphate which is excreted in feces

Pharmacodynamics/Kinetics

Absorption: Requires vitamin D; minimal unless chronic, high doses are given; calcium is absorbed in soluble, ionized form; solubility of calcium is increased in an acid environment

Excretion: Primarily feces (as unabsorbed calcium); urine (20%)

Dosage

Geriatric Control of hyperphosphatemia (ESRD, on dialysis): Refer to adult dosing.

Adult Control of hyperphosphatemia (ESRD, on dialysis): Oral: Initial: 1334 mg with each meal, can be increased gradually (ie, every 2-3 weeks) to bring the serum phosphate value <6 mg/dL as long as hypercalcemia does not develop (usual dose: 2001-2668 mg calcium acetate with each meal); do not give additional calcium supplements

Administration Administer with meals.

Monitoring Parameters Serum calcium (twice weekly during initial dose adjustments), serum phosphorus; serum calcium-phosphorus product; intact parathyroid hormone (iPTH)

Reference Range

Corrected total serum calcium (K/DOQI, 2003): CKD stages 3 and 4: 8.4-10.2 mg/dL (2.1-2.6 mmol/L); CKD stage 5: 8.4-9.5 mg/dL (2.1-2.37 mmol/L); KDIGO guidelines recommend maintaining normal ranges for all stages of CKD (3-5D) (KDIGO, 2009)

Phosphorus (K/DOQI, 2003):

CKD stages 3 and 4: 2.7-4.6 mg/dL (0.87-1.48 mmol/L) (adults)

CKD stage 5 (including those treated with dialysis): 3.5-5.5 mg/dL (1.13-1.78 mmol/L) (adults)

KDIGO guidelines recommend maintaining normal ranges for CKD stages 3-5 and lowering elevated phosphorus levels toward the normal range for CKD stage 5D (KDIGO, 2009)

Serum calcium-phosphorus product (K/DOQI, 2003): CKD stage 3-5: <55 mg^2/dL^2 (adults)

PTH: Whole molecule, immunochemiluminometric assay (ICMA): 1.0-5.2 pmol/L; whole molecule, radioimmunoassay (RIA): 10.0-65.0 pg/mL; whole molecule, immunoradiometric, double antibody (IRMA): 1.0-6.0 pmol/L

Target ranges by stage of chronic kidney disease (KDIGO, 2009): CKD stage 3-5: Optimal iPTH is unknown; maintain normal range (assay-dependent); CKD stage 5D: Maintain iPTH within 2-9 times the upper limit of normal for the assay used

Pharmacotherapy Pearls Calcium acetate binds to phosphorus in the GI tract better than other calcium salts due to its lower solubility and subsequent reduced absorption and increased formation of calcium phosphate.

12.7 mEq calcium/g; 250 mg/g elemental calcium (25% elemental calcium)

Special Geriatric Considerations Constipation and gas can be significant in the elderly, but are usually mild.

Dosage Forms Excipient information presented when available (limited, particularly for generics); consult specific product labeling.

Gelcap, oral: 667 mg [equivalent to elemental calcium 169 mg (8.45 mEq)]

PhosLo®: 667 mg [equivalent to elemental calcium 169 mg (8.45 mEq)]

Solution, oral:

Phoslyra™: 667 mg/5 mL (473 mL) [contains maltitol (1 g/5 mL), propylene glycol; black cherry-menthol flavor; equivalent to elemental calcium 169 mg (8.45 mEq)/5 mL]

Tablet, oral:

Eliphos™: 667 mg [equivalent to elemental calcium 169 mg (8.45 mEq)]

♦ **Calcium Acetate and Aluminum Sulfate** *see* Aluminum Sulfate and Calcium Acetate on page 84
♦ **Calcium Acetylhomotaurinate** *see* Acamprosate on page 25

Calcium and Vitamin D (KAL see um & VYE ta min dee)

Medication Safety Issues
Sound-alike/look-alike issues:
Os-Cal® may be confused with Asacol®
Brand Names: U.S. Cal-CYUM [OTC]; Caltrate® 600+D [OTC]; Caltrate® 600+Soy™ [OTC]; Caltrate® ColonHealth™ [OTC]; Chew-Cal [OTC]; Citracal® Maximum [OTC]; Citracal® Petites [OTC]; Citracal® Regular [OTC]; Liqua-Cal [OTC]; Os-Cal® 500+D [OTC]; Oysco 500+D [OTC]; Oysco D [OTC]; Oyst-Cal-D 500 [OTC]
Index Terms Calcium Citrate and Vitamin D; Vitamin D and Calcium Carbonate
Generic Availability (U.S.) Yes
Pharmacologic Category Calcium Salt; Electrolyte Supplement, Oral; Vitamin, Fat Soluble
Use Dietary supplement, antacid
Contraindications Hypersensitivity to any component of the formulation; hypophosphatemia, hypercalcemia, evidence of vitamin D toxicity; history of kidney stones
Warnings/Precautions Constipation, bloating, and gas are common with calcium supplements. Use with caution patients with respiratory failure, renal impairment or respiratory acidosis. Use with caution in patients with renal failure to avoid hypercalcemia; frequent monitoring of serum calcium and phosphorus is necessary. Use caution when administering calcium supplements to patients with a history of kidney stones. Hypercalcemia and hypercalciuria are most likely to occur in hypoparathyroid patients receiving high doses of vitamin D. Calcium absorption is impaired in achlorhydria; common in elderly, use an alternate salt (eg, citrate) and administer with food. Calcium administration interferes with absorption of some minerals and drugs; use with caution. Taking calcium (≤500 mg) with food improves absorption.

Some products may contain soy, tartrazine, or phenylalanine, or may be derived from shellfish.

Adverse Reactions (Reflective of adult population; not specific for elderly) Frequency not defined; also see individual agents
Central nervous system: Headache
Endocrine & metabolic: Hypercalcemia, hypercalciuria
Gastrointestinal: Gastrointestinal discomfort
Drug Interactions
Metabolism/Transport Effects None known.
Avoid Concomitant Use
Avoid concomitant use of Calcium Carbonate and Vitamin D with any of the following: Calcium Acetate
Increased Effect/Toxicity
Calcium Carbonate and Vitamin D may increase the levels/effects of: Alpha-/Beta-Agonists; Amphetamines; Calcium Acetate; Calcium Polystyrene Sulfonate; Dexmethylphenidate; Methylphenidate; QuiNIDine; Sodium Polystyrene Sulfonate; Vitamin D Analogs

The levels/effects of Calcium Carbonate and Vitamin D may be increased by: Thiazide Diuretics
Decreased Effect
Calcium Carbonate and Vitamin D may decrease the levels/effects of: ACE Inhibitors; Allopurinol; Anticonvulsants (Hydantoin); Antipsychotic Agents (Phenothiazines); Atazanavir; Bisacodyl; Bisphosphonate Derivatives; Calcium Channel Blockers; Cefditoren; Cefpodoxime; Cefuroxime; Chloroquine; Corticosteroids (Oral); Dabigatran Etexilate; Dasatinib; Deferiprone; Delavirdine; DOBUTamine; Eltrombopag; Erlotinib; Estramustine; Gabapentin; HMG-CoA Reductase Inhibitors; Iron Salts; Isoniazid; Itraconazole; Ketoconazole; Ketoconazole (Systemic); Mesalamine; Methenamine; Mycophenolate; Nilotinib; PenicillAMINE; Phosphate Supplements; Protease Inhibitors; Quinolone Antibiotics; Rilpivirine; Tetracycline Derivatives; Thyroid Products; Trientine; Vismodegib

The levels/effects of Calcium Carbonate and Vitamin D may be decreased by: Trientine
Ethanol/Nutrition/Herb Interactions
Ethanol: Avoid ethanol (may increase risk of osteoporosis).
Food: Food may increase calcium absorption. Calcium may decrease iron absorption. Bran, foods high in oxalates, or whole grain cereals may decrease calcium absorption.

Dosage
  Geriatric & Adult Calcium supplement, hyperphosphatemia: Oral: Refer to individual monographs for dietary reference intake.
  Renal Impairment Use caution in severe renal impairment.
  Administration Administer, preferably with food, 2 hours before or after other medications.
  Monitoring Parameters Monitor serum calcium (particularly if used in patients with severe renal impairment)
  Special Geriatric Considerations Constipation and gas with calcium supplements can be significant in the elderly but are usually mild.

  Vitamin D supplementation has been shown to increase muscle function and strength, as well as improve balance. Patients at risk for falls should have vitamin D serum concentrations measured and be evaluated for supplementation.
  Dosage Forms Excipient information presented when available (limited, particularly for generics); consult specific product labeling.
  Caplet, oral:
    Citracal® Maximum: Calcium 315 mg and vitamin D 250 units [gluten free]
  Capsule, softgel, oral: Calcium 500 mg and vitamin D 500 units; calcium 600 mg and vitamin D 100 units; calcium 600 mg and vitamin D 200 units
    Liqua-Cal: Calcium 600 mg and vitamin D 200 units [contains beeswax, lecithin, and soybean oil]
  Tablet, oral: Calcium 250 mg and vitamin D 125 units; calcium 500 mg and vitamin D 125 units; calcium 500 mg and vitamin D 200 units; calcium 600 mg and vitamin D 125 units; calcium 600 mg and vitamin D 200 units
    Caltrate® 600+D: Calcium 600 mg and vitamin D 200 units [contains soybean oil]
    Caltrate® 600+Soy™: Calcium 600 mg and vitamin D 200 units [contains soy isoflavones 25 mg]
    Caltrate® ColonHealth™: Calcium 600 mg and vitamin D 200 units [contains soybean oil]
    Citracal® Petites: Calcium 200 mg and vitamin D 250 units [gluten free]
    Citracal® Regular: Calcium 250 mg and vitamin D 200 units [gluten free]
    Oysco D: Calcium 250 mg and vitamin D 125 units
    Oysco 500+D: Calcium 500 mg and vitamin D 200 units [contains tartrazine]
    Oyst-Cal-D 500: Calcium 500 mg and vitamin D 200 units [sodium free, sugar free; contains tartrazine]
  Tablet, chewable: Calcium 500 mg and vitamin D 100 units; Calcium 600 mg and vitamin D 400 units
    Os-Cal® 500+D: Calcium 500 mg and vitamin D 400 units [sugar free; contains phenylalanine; light lemon flavor]
  Wafer, chewable:
    Cal-CYUM: Calcium 519 mg and vitamin D 150 units (50s) [dye free; vanilla flavor]
    Chew-Cal: Calcium 333 mg and vitamin D 40 units (100s, 250s)

Calcium Carbonate (KAL see um KAR bun ate)

Related Information
  Calculations *on page 2087*
  Osteoporosis Management *on page 2136*
Medication Safety Issues
  Sound-alike/look-alike issues:
    Calcium carbonate may be confused with calcitriol
    Florical® may be confused with Fiorinal®
    Mylanta® may be confused with Mynatal®
    Nephro-Calci® may be confused with Nephrocaps®
  International issues:
    Remegel [Hungary, Great Britain, and Ireland] may be confused with Renagel brand name for sevelamer [U.S., Canada, and multiple international markets]
    Remegel: Brand name for calcium carbonate [Hungary, Great Britain, and Ireland], but also the brand name for aluminum hydroxide and magnesium carbonate [Netherlands]
  Brand Names: U.S. Alcalak [OTC]; Alka-Mints® [OTC]; Cal-Gest [OTC]; Cal-Mint [OTC]; Calci-Chew® [OTC]; Calci-Mix® [OTC]; Caltrate® 600 [OTC]; Children's Pepto [OTC]; Chooz® [OTC]; Florical® [OTC]; Maalox® Children's [OTC]; Maalox® Regular Strength [OTC]; Nephro-Calci® [OTC]; Nutralox® [OTC]; Oysco 500 [OTC]; Oystercal™ 500 [OTC]; Rolaids® Extra Strength [OTC]; Super Calcium 600 [OTC]; Titralac™ [OTC]; Tums® E-X [OTC]; Tums® Extra Strength Sugar Free [OTC]; Tums® Quickpak [OTC]; Tums® Smoothies™ [OTC]; Tums® Ultra [OTC]; Tums® [OTC]

Brand Names: Canada Apo-Cal®; Calcite-500; Caltrate®; Caltrate® Select; Os-Cal®; Tums Extra Strength; Tums Smoothies; Tums® Chews Extra Strength; Tums® Regular Strength; Tums® Ultra Strength

Index Terms Oscal

Generic Availability (U.S.) Yes

Pharmacologic Category Antacid; Antidote; Calcium Salt; Electrolyte Supplement, Oral

Use As an antacid; treatment and prevention of calcium deficiency or hyperphosphatemia (eg, osteoporosis, osteomalacia, mild/moderate renal insufficiency, hypoparathyroidism, postmenopausal osteoporosis, rickets); has been used to bind phosphate

Contraindications Hypercalcemia, renal calculi, hypophosphatemia; patients with suspected digoxin toxicity

Warnings/Precautions Constipation, bloating, and gas are common with calcium supplements. Calcium absorption is impaired in achlorhydria; administration is followed by increased gastric acid secretion within 2 hours of administration especially with high doses. Common in the elderly, use an alternate salt (eg, citrate) and administer with food. Hypercalcemia and hypercalciuria are most likely to occur in hypoparathyroid patients receiving high doses of vitamin D. Use caution when administering calcium supplements to patients with a history of kidney stones. Calcium administration interferes with absorption of some minerals and drugs; use with caution. It is recommended to concomitantly administer vitamin D for optimal calcium absorption. Taking calcium (≤500 mg) with food improves absorption.

Adverse Reactions (Reflective of adult population; not specific for elderly) Well tolerated

1% to 10%:

  Central nervous system: Headache

  Endocrine & metabolic: Hypophosphatemia, hypercalcemia

  Gastrointestinal: Constipation, laxative effect, acid rebound, nausea, vomiting, anorexia, abdominal pain, xerostomia, flatulence

  Miscellaneous: Milk-alkali syndrome with very high, chronic dosing and/or renal failure (headache, nausea, irritability, weakness, alkalosis, hypercalcemia, renal impairment)

Drug Interactions

  Metabolism/Transport Effects None known.

  Avoid Concomitant Use

   Avoid concomitant use of Calcium Carbonate with any of the following: Calcium Acetate

  Increased Effect/Toxicity

   Calcium Carbonate may increase the levels/effects of: Alpha-/Beta-Agonists; Amphetamines; Calcium Acetate; Calcium Polystyrene Sulfonate; Dexmethylphenidate; Methylphenidate; QuiNIDine; Sodium Polystyrene Sulfonate; Vitamin D Analogs

   The levels/effects of Calcium Carbonate may be increased by: Thiazide Diuretics

  Decreased Effect

   Calcium Carbonate may decrease the levels/effects of: ACE Inhibitors; Allopurinol; Anticonvulsants (Hydantoin); Antipsychotic Agents (Phenothiazines); Atazanavir; Bisacodyl; Bisphosphonate Derivatives; Calcium Channel Blockers; Cefditoren; Cefpodoxime; Cefuroxime; Chloroquine; Corticosteroids (Oral); Dabigatran Etexilate; Dasatinib; Deferiprone; Delavirdine; DOBUTamine; Eltrombopag; Erlotinib; Estramustine; Gabapentin; HMG-CoA Reductase Inhibitors; Iron Salts; Isoniazid; Itraconazole; Ketoconazole; Ketoconazole (Systemic); Mesalamine; Methenamine; Mycophenolate; Nilotinib; PenicillAMINE; Phosphate Supplements; Protease Inhibitors; Quinolone Antibiotics; Rilpivirine; Tetracycline Derivatives; Thyroid Products; Trientine; Vismodegib

   The levels/effects of Calcium Carbonate may be decreased by: Trientine

Ethanol/Nutrition/Herb Interactions

  Ethanol: Avoid ethanol (may increase risk of osteoporosis).

  Food: Food may increase calcium absorption. Calcium may decrease iron absorption. Bran, foods high in oxalates, or whole grain cereals may decrease calcium absorption.

Mechanism of Action As dietary supplement, used to prevent or treat negative calcium balance; in osteoporosis, it helps to prevent or decrease the rate of bone loss. The calcium in calcium salts moderates nerve and muscle performance and allows normal cardiac function. Also used to treat hyperphosphatemia in patients with advanced renal insufficiency by combining with dietary phosphate to form insoluble calcium phosphate, which is excreted in feces. Calcium salts as antacids neutralize gastric acidity resulting in increased gastric and duodenal bulb pH; they additionally inhibit proteolytic activity of peptic if the pH is increased >4 and increase lower esophageal sphincter tone.

Pharmacodynamics/Kinetics

  Absorption: Requires vitamin D; minimal unless chronic, high doses are given; calcium is absorbed in soluble, ionized form; solubility of calcium is increased in an acid environment

  Excretion: Primarily feces (as unabsorbed calcium); urine (20%)

Dosage
Geriatric
Dietary Reference Intake for Calcium:
Females: Refer to adult dosing.
Males ≤70 years: Refer to adult dosing.
Males >70 years: 1200 mg/day
All other indications: Refer to adult dosing.
Adult Dosage is in terms of **elemental** calcium:
Dietary Reference Intake for Calcium: Oral: Adults, Females/Males: RDA:
19-50 years: 1000 mg/day
≥51 years, females: 1200 mg/day
51-70 years, males: 1000 mg/day
Hypocalcemia (dose depends on clinical condition and serum calcium level): Oral:
Dose expressed in mg of **elemental calcium:** 1-2 g or more/day in 3-4 divided doses
Dietary supplementation: Oral: 500 mg to 2 g divided 2-4 times/day
Antacid: Oral: Dosage based on acid-neutralizing capacity of specific product; generally, 1-2 tablets or 5-10 mL every 2 hours; maximum: 7000 mg calcium carbonate per 24 hours; specific product labeling should be consulted
Osteoporosis: Oral: Adults >51 years: 1200 mg/day
Renal Impairment Cl_{cr} <25 mL/minute: Dosage adjustments may be necessary depending on the serum calcium levels.

Reference Range
Serum calcium: 8.5-10.5 mg/dL. Monitor plasma calcium levels if using calcium salts as electrolyte supplements for deficiency.
Due to a poor correlation between the serum ionized calcium (free) and total serum calcium, particularly in states of low albumin or acid/base imbalances, direct measurement of ionized calcium is recommended
In low albumin states, the corrected **total** serum calcium may be estimated by:
Corrected total calcium = total serum calcium + 0.8 (4.0 - measured serum albumin)

Test Interactions Increased calcium (S); decreased magnesium

Pharmacotherapy Pearls 20 mEq calcium/g; 400 mg elemental calcium/g calcium carbonate (40% elemental calcium)

Dosage Forms Excipient information presented when available (limited, particularly for generics); consult specific product labeling. [DSC] = Discontinued product
Capsule, oral:
Calci-Mix®: 1250 mg [equivalent to elemental calcium 500 mg]
Florical®: 364 mg [equivalent to elemental calcium 145 mg; contains fluoride]
Gum, chewing, oral:
Chooz®: 500 mg (12s) [sugar free; contains phenylalanine 1.4 mg/tablet; mint flavor; equivalent to elemental calcium 200 mg]
Powder, oral: (480 g)
Tums® Quickpak: 1000 mg/packet (24s) [contains sodium <5 mg/packet; berry fusion flavor; equivalent to elemental calcium 400 mg]
Suspension, oral: 1250 mg/5 mL (5 mL, 500 mL, 16 oz) [equivalent to elemental calcium 500 mg/5 mL]
Tablet, oral: 648 mg [equivalent to elemental calcium 260 mg], 650 mg [equivalent to elemental calcium 260 mg], 1250 mg [equivalent to elemental calcium 500 mg], 1500 mg [equivalent to elemental calcium 600 mg]
Caltrate® 600: 1500 mg [scored; equivalent to elemental calcium 600 mg]
Florical®: 364 mg [equivalent to elemental calcium 145 mg; contains fluoride]
Nephro-Calci®: 1500 mg [equivalent to elemental calcium 600 mg]
Oysco 500: 1250 mg [equivalent to elemental calcium 500 mg]
Oystercal™ 500: 1250 mg [equivalent to elemental calcium 500 mg]
Super Calcium 600: 1500 mg [gluten free, sugar free; equivalent to elemental calcium 600 mg]
Super Calcium 600: 1500 mg [sugar free; equivalent to elemental calcium 600 mg]
Tablet, chewable, oral: 420 mg [equivalent to elemental calcium 168 mg], 500 mg [equivalent to elemental calcium 200 mg], 500 mg, 600 mg [DSC] [equivalent to elemental calcium 222 mg], 650 mg [equivalent to elemental calcium 260 mg], 750 mg [equivalent to elemental calcium 300 mg], 1250 mg [equivalent to elemental calcium 500 mg]
Alcalak: 420 mg [aluminum free; mint flavor; equivalent to elemental calcium 168 mg]
Alka-Mints®: 850 mg [spearmint flavor; equivalent to elemental calcium 340 mg]
Cal-Gest: 500 mg [equivalent to elemental calcium 200 mg]
Cal-Mint: 650 mg [aluminum free, dye free, gluten free, sugar free; mint flavor; equivalent to elemental calcium 260 mg]
Calci-Chew®: 1250 mg [cherry flavor; equivalent to elemental calcium 500 mg]
Children's Pepto: 400 mg [bubblegum flavor; equivalent to elemental calcium 161 mg]

Children's Pepto: 400 mg [watermelon flavor; equivalent to elemental calcium 161 mg]
Maalox® Children's: 400 mg [contains phenylalanine 0.3 mg/tablet; wildberry flavor; equivalent to elemental calcium 160 mg]
Maalox® Regular Strength: 600 mg [contains phenylalanine 0.5 mg/tablet; wildberry flavor; equivalent to elemental calcium 240 mg]
Nutralox®: 420 mg [sugar free; mint flavor; equivalent to elemental calcium 168 mg]
Titralac™: 420 mg [sugar free; contains sodium 1.1 mg/tablet; spearmint flavor; equivalent to elemental calcium 168 mg]
Tums®: 500 mg [contains tartrazine; assorted fruit flavor; equivalent to elemental calcium 200 mg]
Tums®: 500 mg [contains tartrazine; peppermint flavor; equivalent to elemental calcium 200 mg]
Tums® E-X: 750 mg [tropical fruit flavor; equivalent to elemental calcium 300 mg]
Tums® E-X: 750 mg [wintergreen flavor; equivalent to elemental calcium 300 mg]
Tums® E-X: 750 mg [contains tartrazine; assorted berries flavor; equivalent to elemental calcium 300 mg]
Tums® E-X: 750 mg [contains tartrazine; assorted fruit flavor; equivalent to elemental calcium 300 mg]
Tums® E-X: 750 mg [contains tartrazine; cool relief mint flavor; equivalent to elemental calcium 300 mg]
Tums® E-X: 750 mg [contains tartrazine; fresh blend flavor; equivalent to elemental calcium 300 mg]
Tums® E-X: 750 mg [contains tartrazine; tropical fruit flavor; equivalent to elemental calcium 300 mg]
Tums® Extra Strength Sugar Free: 750 mg [sugar free; contains phenylalanine <1 mg/tablet; orange cream flavor; equivalent to elemental calcium 300 mg]
Tums® Smoothies™: 750 mg [contains tartrazine; assorted fruit flavor; equivalent to elemental calcium 300 mg]
Tums® Smoothies™: 750 mg [contains tartrazine; peppermint flavor; equivalent to elemental calcium 300 mg]
Tums® Smoothies™: 750 mg [contains tartrazine; tropical assorted fruits flavor; equivalent to elemental calcium 300 mg]
Tums® Ultra: 1000 mg [contains tartrazine; assorted berries flavor; equivalent to elemental calcium 400 mg]
Tums® Ultra: 1000 mg [contains tartrazine; assorted fruit flavor; equivalent to elemental calcium 400 mg]
Tums® Ultra: 1000 mg [contains tartrazine; peppermint flavor; equivalent to elemental calcium 400 mg]
Tums® Ultra: 1000 mg [contains tartrazine; spearmint flavor; equivalent to elemental calcium 400 mg]
Tums® Ultra: 1000 mg [contains tartrazine; tropical assorted fruits flavor; equivalent to elemental calcium 400 mg]
Tablet, softchew, oral:
Rolaids® Extra Strength: 1177 mg [contains coconut oil, soya lecithin; vanilla crème flavor; equivalent to elemental calcium 471 mg]
Rolaids® Extra Strength: 1177 mg [contains coconut oil, soya lecithin; wild cherry flavor; equivalent to elemental calcium 471 mg]

♦ **Calcium Carbonate, Magnesium Hydroxide, and Famotidine** *see* Famotidine, Calcium Carbonate, and Magnesium Hydroxide *on page 746*

Calcium Chloride (KAL see um KLOR ide)

Related Information
Calculations *on page 2087*
Medication Safety Issues
Sound-alike/look-alike issues:
Calcium chloride may be confused with calcium gluconate
Administration issues:
Calcium chloride may be confused with calcium gluconate.
Confusion with the different intravenous salt forms of calcium has occurred. There is a threefold difference in the primary cation concentration between calcium chloride (in which 1 g = 14 mEq [270 mg] of elemental Ca++) and calcium gluconate (in which 1 g = 4.65 mEq [90 mg] of elemental Ca++).
Prescribers should specify which salt form is desired. Dosages should be expressed either as mEq, mg, or grams of the salt form.
Generic Availability (U.S.) Yes
Pharmacologic Category Calcium Salt; Electrolyte Supplement, Parenteral

CALCIUM CHLORIDE

Use Treatment of hypocalcemia and conditions secondary to hypocalcemia (eg, tetany, seizures, arrhythmias); emergent treatment of severe hypermagnesemia

Unlabeled Use Calcium channel blocker overdose; beta-blocker overdose (refractory to glucagon and high-dose vasopressors); severe hyperkalemia (K+ >6.5 mEq/L with toxic ECG changes) [ACLS guidelines]; malignant arrhythmias (including cardiac arrest) associated with hypermagnesemia [ACLS guidelines]

Contraindications Known or suspected digoxin toxicity; not recommended as routine treatment in cardiac arrest (includes asystole, ventricular fibrillation, pulseless ventricular tachycardia, or pulseless electrical activity)

Warnings/Precautions For I.V. use only; do not inject SubQ or I.M.; avoid rapid I.V. administration (<100 mg/minute) unless being given emergently. Avoid extravasation. Use with caution in patients with hyperphosphatemia, respiratory acidosis, renal impairment, or respiratory failure; acidifying effect of calcium chloride may potentiate acidosis. Use with caution in patients with chronic renal failure to avoid hypercalcemia; frequent monitoring of serum calcium and phosphorus is necessary. Use with caution in hypokalemic or digitalized patients since acute rises in serum calcium levels may precipitate cardiac arrhythmias. Solutions may contain aluminum; toxic levels may occur following prolonged administration in patients with renal impairment. Avoid metabolic acidosis (ie, administer only 2-3 days then change to another calcium salt).

Adverse Reactions (Reflective of adult population; not specific for elderly) Frequency not defined. I.V.:

Cardiovascular (following rapid I.V. injection): Arrhythmia, bradycardia, cardiac arrest, hypotension, syncope, vasodilation

Central nervous system: Sense of oppression (with rapid I.V. injection)

Endocrine & metabolic: Hypercalcemia

Gastrointestinal: Irritation, chalky taste

Hepatic: Serum amylase increased

Local (following extravasation): Tissue necrosis

Neuromuscular & skeletal: Tingling sensation (with rapid I.V. injection)

Renal: Renal calculi

Miscellaneous: Hot flashes (with rapid I.V. injection)

Postmarketing and/or case reports: Calcinosis cutis

Drug Interactions

Metabolism/Transport Effects None known.

Avoid Concomitant Use

Avoid concomitant use of Calcium Chloride with any of the following: Calcium Acetate

Increased Effect/Toxicity

Calcium Chloride may increase the levels/effects of: Calcium Acetate; CefTRIAXone; Vitamin D Analogs

The levels/effects of Calcium Chloride may be increased by: Thiazide Diuretics

Decreased Effect

Calcium Chloride may decrease the levels/effects of: Bisphosphonate Derivatives; Calcium Channel Blockers; Deferiprone; DOBUTamine; Eltrombopag; Phosphate Supplements; Tetracycline Derivatives; Thyroid Products; Trientine

The levels/effects of Calcium Chloride may be decreased by: Trientine

Stability Do not refrigerate solutions; I.V. infusion solutions are stable for 24 hours at room temperature.

Although calcium chloride is not routinely used in the preparation of parenteral nutrition, it is important to note that phosphate salts may precipitate when mixed with calcium salts. Solubility is improved in amino acid parenteral nutrition solutions. Check with a pharmacist to determine compatibility.

Mechanism of Action Moderates nerve and muscle performance via action potential excitation threshold regulation

Pharmacodynamics/Kinetics

Protein binding: ~40%, primarily to albumin (Wills, 1971)

Excretion: Primarily feces (80% as insoluble calcium salts); urine (20%)

Dosage

Geriatric & Adult Note: One gram of calcium chloride salt is equal to 270 mg of elemental calcium.

Dosages are expressed in terms of the <u>calcium chloride salt</u> based on a solution concentration of 100 mg/mL (10%) containing 1.4 mEq (27 mg)/mL elemental calcium.

Hypocalcemia: I.V.:

Acute, symptomatic: Manufacturer's recommendations: 200-1000 mg every 1-3 days

Severe, symptomatic (eg, seizure, tetany): 1000 mg over 10 minutes; repeat every 60 minutes until symptoms resolve (French, 2012)

Note: In general, I.V. calcium gluconate is preferred over I.V. calcium chloride in non-emergency settings due to the potential for extravasation with calcium chloride.

Cardiac arrest or cardiotoxicity in the presence of hyperkalemia, hypocalcemia, or hypermagnesemia: I.V.: 500-1000 mg over 2-5 minutes; may repeat as necessary (Vanden Hoek, 2010)

Note: Routine use in cardiac arrest is not recommended due to the lack of improved survival (Neumar, 2010).

Beta-blocker overdose, refractory to glucagon and high-dose vasopressors (unlabeled use): Note: Optimal dose has not been established (DeWitt, 2004): I.V.: 20 mg/kg over 5-10 minutes followed by an infusion of 20 mg/kg/hour titrated to adequate hemodynamic response (Vanden Hoek, 2010)

Calcium channel blocker overdose (unlabeled use): Note: Optimal dose has not been established (DeWitt, 2004).

I.V.: Initial: 1000-2000 mg over 5 minutes; may repeat every 10-20 minutes with 3-4 additional doses **or** 1000 mg every 2-3 minutes until clinical effect is achieved (DeWitt, 2004); if favorable response obtained, consider I.V. infusion

I.V. infusion: 20-40 mg/kg/hour (DeWitt, 2004; Salhanick, 2003)

Renal Impairment No initial dosage adjustment necessary; however, accumulation may occur with renal impairment and subsequent doses may require adjustment based on serum calcium concentrations.

Hepatic Impairment No initial dosage adjustment necessary; subsequent doses should be guided by serum calcium concentrations.

Administration For I.V. administration only; avoid extravasation. Avoid rapid administration (do not exceed 100 mg/minute except in emergency situations). For intermittent I.V. infusion, dilute to a maximum concentration of 20 mg/mL and infuse over 1 hour or no greater than 45-90 mg/kg/hour (0.6-1.2 mEq/kg/hour); administration via a central or deep vein is preferred; do not use scalp, small hand or foot veins for I.V. administration since severe necrosis and sloughing may occur. Monitor ECG if calcium is infused faster than 2.5 mEq/minute; **stop the infusion if the patient complains of pain or discomfort.** Warm solution to body temperature prior to administration. **Do not infuse calcium chloride in the same I.V. line as phosphate-containing solutions.** Not for I.M. or SubQ administration (severe necrosis and sloughing may occur).

Monitoring Parameters Monitor infusion site, ECG when appropriate; serum calcium and ionized calcium (normal: 8.5-10.2 mg/dL [total]; 4.5-5.0 mg/dL [ionized]), albumin, serum phosphate; magnesium (to facilitate calcium repletion)

Calcium channel blocker overdose, beta-blocker overdose: Hemodynamic response, serum ionized calcium concentration

Reference Range

Serum total calcium: 8.4-10.2 mg/dL (2.1-2.55 mmol/L). **Note:** Due to a poor correlation between the serum ionized calcium (free) and total serum calcium, particularly in states of low albumin or acid/base imbalances, direct measurement of ionized calcium is recommended.

In low albumin states, the corrected **total** serum calcium may be estimated by the following equation (assuming a normal albumin of 4 g/dL [40 g/L]).

Corrected total calcium (mg/dL) = measured total calcium (mg/mL) + 0.8 [4 - measured serum albumin(g/dL)]

or

Corrected total calcium (mmol/L) = measured total calcium (mmol/L) + 0.02 [40-measured serum albumin (g/L)]

Pharmacotherapy Pearls 14 mEq calcium/g (10 mL); 270 mg elemental calcium/g calcium chloride (27% elemental calcium)

Special Geriatric Considerations When using in the elderly, check albumin status and make appropriate decisions concerning reference serum concentrations. Elderly, especially the ill, often have low albumin due to malnutrition.

Dosage Forms Excipient information presented when available (limited, particularly for generics); consult specific product labeling.

Injection, solution: 10% (10 mL) [equivalent to elemental calcium 27 mg (1.4 mEq)/mL]

Injection, solution [preservative free]: 10% (10 mL) [equivalent to elemental calcium 27 mg (1.4 mEq)/mL]

Calcium Citrate (KAL see um SIT rate)

Related Information
Osteoporosis Management *on page 2136*

Medication Safety Issues
Sound-alike/look-alike issues:
Citracal® may be confused with Citrucel®

Brand Names: U.S. Cal-C-Caps [OTC]; Cal-Cee [OTC]; Cal-Citrate™ 225 [OTC]; Calcitrate [OTC]

Brand Names: Canada Osteocit®

Generic Availability (U.S.) Yes

Pharmacologic Category Calcium Salt

Use Dietary supplement

Contraindications Hypersensitivity to any component of the formulation

Warnings/Precautions Constipation, bloating, and gas are common with calcium supplements. Use with caution in patients with renal failure to avoid hypercalcemia; frequent monitoring of serum calcium and phosphorus is necessary. Use caution when administering calcium supplements to patients with a history of kidney stones. Hypercalcemia and hypercalciuria are most likely to occur in hypoparathyroid patients receiving high doses of vitamin D. Calcium absorption is impaired in achlorhydria; common in elderly. Citrate may be preferred because better absorbed. Calcium administration interferes with absorption of some minerals and drugs; use with caution. It is recommended to concomitantly administer vitamin D for optimal calcium absorption. Taking calcium (≤500 mg) with food improves absorption.

Adverse Reactions (Reflective of adult population; not specific for elderly) Frequency not defined.
Mild hypercalcemia (calcium: >10.5 mg/dL) may be asymptomatic or manifest itself as constipation, anorexia, nausea, and vomiting
More severe hypercalcemia (calcium: >12 mg/dL) is associated with confusion, delirium, stupor, and coma
Central nervous system: Headache
Endocrine & metabolic: Hypophosphatemia, hypercalcemia
Gastrointestinal: Nausea, anorexia, vomiting, abdominal pain, constipation
Miscellaneous: Thirst

Drug Interactions
Metabolism/Transport Effects None known.
Avoid Concomitant Use
Avoid concomitant use of Calcium Citrate with any of the following: Calcium Acetate
Increased Effect/Toxicity
Calcium Citrate may increase the levels/effects of: Aluminum Hydroxide; Calcium Acetate; Vitamin D Analogs

The levels/effects of Calcium Citrate may be increased by: Thiazide Diuretics
Decreased Effect
Calcium Citrate may decrease the levels/effects of: Bisphosphonate Derivatives; Calcium Channel Blockers; Deferiprone; DOBUTamine; Eltrombopag; Estramustine; Phosphate Supplements; Quinolone Antibiotics; Tetracycline Derivatives; Thyroid Products; Trientine

The levels/effects of Calcium Citrate may be decreased by: Trientine

Ethanol/Nutrition/Herb Interactions Ethanol: Avoid ethanol (may increase risk of osteoporosis).

Mechanism of Action Moderates nerve and muscle performance via action potential excitation threshold regulation

Pharmacodynamics/Kinetics Absorption: Requires vitamin D

Dosage
Geriatric Dietary Reference Intake for Calcium: RDA:
Females: Refer to adult dosing.
Males ≤70 years: Refer to adult dosing.
Males >70 years: 1200 mg/day
Adult Oral: Dosage is in terms of **elemental** calcium
Dietary Reference Intake for Calcium: Adults, Females/Males: RDA:
19-50 years: 1000 mg/day
≥51 years, females: 1200 mg/day
51-70 years, males: 1000 mg/day

Reference Range

Serum calcium: 8.5-10.5 mg/dL. Monitor plasma calcium levels if using calcium salts as electrolyte supplements for deficiency.

Due to a poor correlation between the serum ionized calcium (free) and total serum calcium, particularly in states of low albumin or acid/base imbalances, direct measurement of ionized calcium is recommended

In low albumin states, the corrected **total** serum calcium may be estimated by:

Corrected total calcium = total serum calcium + 0.8 (4.0 - measured serum albumin)

Dosage Forms Excipient information presented when available (limited, particularly for generics); consult specific product labeling. [DSC] = Discontinued product

Capsule, oral:

Cal-C-Caps: Elemental calcium 180 mg

Cal-Citrate™ 225: Elemental calcium 225 mg

Granules, oral: (480 g)

Tablet, oral: Elemental calcium 200 mg [DSC], Elemental calcium 250 mg

Cal-Cee: Elemental calcium 250 mg

Calcitrate: Elemental calcium 200 mg

◆ **Calcium Citrate and Vitamin D** see Calcium and Vitamin D on page 261

Calcium Glubionate (KAL see um gloo BYE oh nate)

Related Information

Osteoporosis Management on page 2136

Medication Safety Issues

Sound-alike/look-alike issues:

Calcium glubionate may be confused with calcium gluconate

Brand Names: U.S. Calcionate [OTC]

Generic Availability (U.S.) Yes

Pharmacologic Category Calcium Salt

Use Dietary supplement

Contraindications Hypersensitivity to any component of the formulation

Warnings/Precautions Constipation, bloating, and gas are common with calcium supplements. Calcium absorption is impaired in achlorhydria; administration is followed by increased gastric acid secretion within 2 hours of administration especially with high doses. Common in the elderly, use an alternate salt (eg, citrate) and administer with food. Hypercalcemia and hypercalciuria are most likely to occur in hypoparathyroid patients receiving high doses of vitamin D. Use caution when administering calcium supplements to patients with a history of kidney stones. Calcium administration interferes with absorption of some minerals and drugs; use with caution. It is recommended to concomitantly administer vitamin D for optimal calcium absorption. Taking calcium (≤500 mg) with food improves absorption.

Adverse Reactions (Reflective of adult population; not specific for elderly) Frequency not defined; symptoms reported with hypercalcemia:

Gastrointestinal: Abdominal pain, anorexia, constipation, nausea, thirst, vomiting, xerostomia

Genitourinary: Polyuria

Drug Interactions

Metabolism/Transport Effects None known.

Avoid Concomitant Use

Avoid concomitant use of Calcium Glubionate with any of the following: Calcium Acetate

Increased Effect/Toxicity

Calcium Glubionate may increase the levels/effects of: Calcium Acetate; Vitamin D Analogs

The levels/effects of Calcium Glubionate may be increased by: Thiazide Diuretics

Decreased Effect

Calcium Glubionate may decrease the levels/effects of: Bisphosphonate Derivatives; Calcium Channel Blockers; Deferiprone; DOBUTamine; Eltrombopag; Estramustine; Phosphate Supplements; Quinolone Antibiotics; Tetracycline Derivatives; Thyroid Products; Trientine

The levels/effects of Calcium Glubionate may be decreased by: Trientine

Ethanol/Nutrition/Herb Interactions

Ethanol: Avoid ethanol (may increase risk of osteoporosis).

Food: Food may increase calcium absorption. Calcium may decrease iron absorption. Bran, foods high in oxalates, or whole grain cereals may decrease calcium absorption.

Mechanism of Action As dietary supplement, used to prevent or treat negative calcium balance. The calcium in calcium salts moderates nerve and muscle performance and allows normal cardiac function.

◄ **Pharmacodynamics/Kinetics**
Absorption: Requires vitamin D; calcium is absorbed in soluble, ionized form; solubility of calcium is increased in an acid environment
Excretion: Primarily feces (as unabsorbed calcium); urine

Dosage

Geriatric

Dietary Reference Intake for Calcium: RDA: Oral:
Females: Refer to adult dosing.
Males ≤70 years: Refer to adult dosing.
Males >70 years: 1200 mg/day
Dietary supplement: Refer to adult dosing.

Adult Dosage is in terms of **elemental** calcium

Dietary Reference Intake for Calcium: Oral: Adults, Females/Males: RDA:
19-50 years: 1000 mg/day
≥51 years, females: 1200 mg/day
51-70 years, males: 1000 mg/day
Dietary supplement: Oral: 15 mL 3 times/day

Administration Take with a full glass of water or juice, 1-3 hours after meals and other medications, and 1-2 hours before any approved iron supplements.

Reference Range
Serum calcium: 8.5-10.5 mg/dL. Monitor plasma calcium levels if using calcium salts as electrolyte supplements for deficiency.
Due to a poor correlation between the serum ionized calcium (free) and total serum calcium, particularly in states of low albumin or acid/base imbalances, direct measurement of ionized calcium is recommended
In low albumin states, the corrected **total** serum calcium may be estimated by:
Corrected total calcium = total serum calcium + 0.8 (4.0 - measured serum albumin)

Test Interactions Decreased magnesium

Dosage Forms Excipient information presented when available (limited, particularly for generics); consult specific product labeling.
Syrup, oral:
Calcionate: 1.8 g/5 mL (473 mL) [contains benzoic acid; caramel-orange flavor; equivalent to elemental calcium 115 mg/5 mL]

Calcium Gluconate (KAL see um GLOO koe nate)

Related Information
Calculations *on page* 2087
Osteoporosis Management *on page* 2136

Medication Safety Issues
Sound-alike/look-alike issues:
Calcium gluconate may be confused with calcium glubionate, cupric sulfate
Administration issues:
Calcium gluconate may be confused with calcium chloride.
Confusion with the different intravenous salt forms of calcium has occurred. There is a threefold difference in the primary cation concentration between calcium gluconate (in which 1 g = 4.65 mEq [90 mg] of elemental Ca++) and calcium chloride (in which 1 g = 14 mEq [270 mg] of elemental Ca++).
Prescribers should specify which salt form is desired. Dosages should be expressed either as mEq, mg, or grams of the salt form.

Brand Names: U.S. Cal-G [OTC] [DSC]; Cal-GLU™ [OTC]

Generic Availability (U.S.) Yes

Pharmacologic Category Calcium Salt; Electrolyte Supplement, Oral; Electrolyte Supplement, Parenteral

Use
I.V.: Treatment of hypocalcemia and conditions secondary to hypocalcemia (eg, tetany, seizures, arrhythmias); treatment of cardiac disturbances secondary to hyperkalemia; adjunctive treatment of rickets, osteomalacia, and magnesium sulfate overdose; decrease capillary permeability in allergic conditions, nonthrombocytopenic purpura, and exudative dermatoses (eg, dermatitis herpetiformis, pruritus secondary to certain drugs)
Oral: Dietary calcium supplementation

Unlabeled Use Calcium channel blocker overdose; treatment of hydrofluoric acid exposure

Contraindications Ventricular fibrillation; hypercalcemia

Warnings/Precautions Injection solution is for I.V. use only; do not inject SubQ or I.M. Avoid too rapid I.V. administration and avoid extravasation. Use with caution in digitalized patients, severe hyperphosphatemia, respiratory failure, or acidosis. May produce cardiac arrest.

Hypercalcemia may occur in patients with renal failure; frequent determination of serum calcium is necessary. Use caution with renal disease. Use caution when administering calcium supplements to patients with a history of kidney stones. Solutions may contain aluminum; toxic levels may occur following prolonged administration in patients with renal dysfunction. Oral: Constipation, bloating, and gas are common with oral calcium supplements (especially carbonate salt). Taking calcium (≤500 mg) with food improves absorption. Calcium administration interferes with absorption of some minerals and drugs; use with caution. It is recommended to concomitantly administer vitamin D for optimal calcium absorption.

Adverse Reactions (Reflective of adult population; not specific for elderly) Frequency not defined.

I.V.:

Cardiovascular (with rapid I.V. injection): Arrhythmia, bradycardia, cardiac arrest, hypotension, syncope, vasodilation

Central nervous system: Sense of oppression (with rapid I.V. injection)

Endocrine & metabolic: Hypercalcemia

Gastrointestinal: Chalky taste

Neuromuscular & skeletal: Tingling sensation (with rapid I.V. injection)

Miscellaneous: Heat waves (with rapid I.V. injection)

Postmarketing and/or case reports: Calcinosis cutis

Oral: Gastrointestinal: Constipation

Drug Interactions

Metabolism/Transport Effects None known.

Avoid Concomitant Use

Avoid concomitant use of Calcium Gluconate with any of the following: Calcium Acetate

Increased Effect/Toxicity

Calcium Gluconate may increase the levels/effects of: Calcium Acetate; CefTRIAXone; Vitamin D Analogs

The levels/effects of Calcium Gluconate may be increased by: Thiazide Diuretics

Decreased Effect

Calcium Gluconate may decrease the levels/effects of: Bisphosphonate Derivatives; Calcium Channel Blockers; Deferiprone; DOBUTamine; Eltrombopag; Estramustine; Phosphate Supplements; Quinolone Antibiotics; Tetracycline Derivatives; Thyroid Products; Trientine

The levels/effects of Calcium Gluconate may be decreased by: Trientine

Stability

I.V.: Store at 20°C to 25°C (68°F to 77°F); excursions permitted to 15°C to 30°C (59°F to 86°F). If crystallization has occurred, place vial in a warm water bath for 15-30 minutes and occasionally shake to dissolve; cool to body temperature before use.

Usual concentrations: 1 g/100 mL D_5W or NS; 2 g/100 mL D_5W or NS.

Maximum concentration in parenteral nutrition solutions is variable depending upon concentration and solubility (consult detailed reference).

Mechanism of Action Moderates nerve and muscle performance via action potential threshold regulation.

In hydrogen fluoride exposures, calcium gluconate provides a source of calcium ions to complex free fluoride ions and prevent or reduce toxicity; administration also helps to correct fluoride-induced hypocalcemia.

Pharmacodynamics/Kinetics

Absorption: Oral: Requires vitamin D; calcium is absorbed in soluble, ionized form; solubility of calcium is increased in an acid environment

Protein binding: ~40%, primarily to albumin (Wills, 1971)

Excretion: Primarily feces (as unabsorbed calcium salts); urine (20%)

Dosage

Geriatric Note: One gram of calcium gluconate salt is equal to 93 mg of elemental calcium.

Dosages are expressed in terms of the calcium gluconate salt (unless otherwise specified as elemental calcium). Dosages expressed in terms of the calcium gluconate salt are based on a solution concentration of 100 mg/mL (10%) containing 0.465 mEq (9.3 mg)/mL elemental calcium, except where noted.

Dietary Reference Intake for Calcium: Oral: **Note:** Expressed in terms of elemental calcium: RDA

Females: Refer to adult dosing.

Males ≤70 years: Refer to adult dosing.

Males >70 years: 1200 mg **elemental calcium** daily

All other indications: Refer to adult dosing.

CALCIUM GLUCONATE

Adult

Dietary Reference Intake for Calcium:

Adults, Female/Male: RDA:

19-50 years: 1000 mg/day

≥51 years, females: 1200 mg/day

51-70 years, males: 1000 mg/day

Dosage note: Calcium chloride has 3 times more elemental calcium than calcium gluconate. Calcium chloride is 27% elemental calcium; calcium gluconate is 9% elemental calcium. One gram of calcium chloride is equal to 270 mg of elemental calcium; 1 gram of calcium gluconate is equal to 90 mg of elemental calcium. The following dosages are expressed in terms of the calcium gluconate salt based on a solution concentration of 100 mg/mL (10%) containing 0.465 mEq (9.3 mg)/mL elemental calcium:

Hypocalcemia:

I.V.: 2-15 g/24 hours as a continuous infusion or in divided doses

Oral: 500 mg to 2 g 2-4 times/day

Hypocalcemia secondary to citrated blood infusion: I.V.: 500 mg to 1 g per 500 mL of citrated blood (infused into another vein). Single doses up to 2 g have also been recommended.

Note: Routine administration of calcium, in the absence of signs/symptoms of hypocalcemia, is generally not recommended. A number of recommendations have been published seeking to address potential hypocalcemia during massive transfusion of citrated blood; however, many practitioners recommend replacement only as guided by clinical evidence of hypocalcemia and/or serial monitoring of ionized calcium.

Hypocalcemic tetany: I.V.: 1-3 g/dose may be administered until therapeutic response occurs

Magnesium intoxication or cardiac arrest in the presence of hyperkalemia or hypocalcemia: I.V.: 500-800 mg/dose (maximum: 3 g/dose)

Maintenance electrolyte requirements for TPN: I.V.: Daily requirements: 1.7-3.4 g/1000 kcal/24 hours

Calcium channel blocker overdose (unlabeled use): I.V. infusion: 10% solution: 0.6-1.2 mL/kg/hour or I.V. 0.2-0.5 ml/kg every 15-20 minutes for 4 doses (maximum: 2-3 g/dose). In life-threatening situations, 1 g has been given every 1-10 minutes until clinical effect is achieved (case reports of resistant hypotension reported use of 12-18 g total).

Renal Impairment No initial dosage adjustment necessary; however, accumulation may occur with renal impairment and subsequent doses may require adjustment based on serum calcium concentrations.

Hepatic Impairment No initial dosage adjustment necessary; subsequent doses should be guided by serum calcium concentrations. In patients in the anhepatic stage of liver transplantation, equal rapid increases in ionized concentrations occur suggesting that calcium gluconate does not require hepatic metabolism for release of ionized calcium (Martin, 1990).

Administration

I.V.: Administer slowly (~1.5 mL calcium gluconate 10% per minute; not to exceed 200 mg/minute except in emergency situations) through a small needle into a large vein in order to avoid too rapid increases in the serum calcium and extravasation. Not for I.M. administration; not for routine SubQ administration (exception: treatment of hydrofluoric acid burns [unlabeled route/use]).

Treatment of hydrofluoric acid burns (unlabeled use):

SubQ infiltration (unlabeled route): Using a 27- or 30-gauge needle, approach the wound from the distal point of injury and infiltrate directly into the affected dermis and subcutaneous tissue. The infiltration should be carried 0.5 cm away from the margin of the injured tissue into the surrounding uninjured areas (Dibbell, 1970). Avoid excessive administration as it can cause compartment syndrome and further exacerbate tissue damage. Following subungual exposure, administer to the affected area via the lateral or volar route through the fat pad (under digital nerve block); administration may also require removal of the nailbed, splitting the distal nail from the nailbed, or trimming the nail to the nailbed to reach the affected area (Kirkpatrick, 1995; Roberts, 1989).

Intra-arterial (unlabeled route): Requires radiology to place an arterial catheter in an artery supplying blood to the area of exposure; infuse over four hours (Vance, 1986). **This intervention should be used only by those accustomed to this technique. Care should be taken to avoid the extravasation.** A poison information center or clinical toxicologist should be consulted prior to implementation.

Inhalation: Mix 1 **mL** of 10% calcium gluconate solution with 4 mL NS to make a 2.5% solution and administer via nebulization.

Reference Range

Serum total calcium: 8.4-10.2 mg/dL (2.1-2.55 mmol/L). **Note:** Due to a poor correlation between the serum ionized calcium (free) and total serum calcium, particularly in states of low albumin or acid/base imbalances, direct measurement of ionized calcium is recommended.

In low albumin states, the corrected **total** serum calcium may be estimated by the following equation (assuming a normal albumin of 4 g/dL [40 g/L]).

Corrected total calcium (mg/dL) = measured total calcium (mg/mL) + 0.8 [4 - measured serum albumin(g/dL)]

or

Corrected total calcium (mmol/L) = measured total calcium (mmol/L) + 0.02 [40-measured serum albumin (g/L)]

Test Interactions I.V. administration may produce falsely decreased serum and urine magnesium concentrations

Special Geriatric Considerations Constipation and gas can be significant in elderly, but are usually mild.

Dosage Forms Excipient information presented when available (limited, particularly for generics); consult specific product labeling. [DSC] = Discontinued product

Capsule, oral:

Cal-G: 700 mg [DSC] [gluten free; equivalent to elemental calcium 65 mg]

Cal-GLU™: 515 mg [dye free, sugar free; equivalent to elemental calcium 50 mg]

Injection, solution [preservative free]: 10% (10 mL, 50 mL, 100 mL) [equivalent to elemental calcium 9.3 mg (0.465 mEq)/mL]

Powder, oral: (480 g)

Tablet, oral: 500 mg [equivalent to elemental calcium 45 mg], 648 mg [equivalent to elemental calcium 60 mg]

Calcium Lactate (KAL see um LAK tate)

Related Information

Calculations *on page 2087*

Osteoporosis Management *on page 2136*

Generic Availability (U.S.) Yes

Pharmacologic Category Calcium Salt

Use Treatment and prevention of calcium depletion

Warnings/Precautions Constipation, bloating, and gas are common with calcium supplements. Use with caution in patients with renal failure to avoid hypercalcemia; frequent monitoring of serum calcium and phosphorus is necessary. Use caution when administering calcium supplements to patients with a history of kidney stones. Hypercalcemia and hypercalciuria are most likely to occur in hypoparathyroid patients receiving high doses of vitamin D. Calcium absorption is impaired in achlorhydria; common in elderly, use an alternate salt (eg, citrate) and administer with food. Calcium administration interferes with absorption of some minerals and drugs; use with caution. It is recommended to concomitantly administer vitamin D for optimal calcium absorption. Taking calcium (≤500 mg) with food improves absorption.

Drug Interactions

Metabolism/Transport Effects None known.

Avoid Concomitant Use

Avoid concomitant use of Calcium Lactate with any of the following: Calcium Acetate

Increased Effect/Toxicity

Calcium Lactate may increase the levels/effects of: Calcium Acetate; Vitamin D Analogs

The levels/effects of Calcium Lactate may be increased by: Thiazide Diuretics

Decreased Effect

Calcium Lactate may decrease the levels/effects of: Bisphosphonate Derivatives; Calcium Channel Blockers; Deferiprone; DOBUTamine; Eltrombopag; Estramustine; Phosphate Supplements; Quinolone Antibiotics; Tetracycline Derivatives; Thyroid Products; Trientine

The levels/effects of Calcium Lactate may be decreased by: Trientine

Ethanol/Nutrition/Herb Interactions Ethanol: Avoid ethanol (may increase risk of osteoporosis).

Mechanism of Action As dietary supplement, used to prevent or treat negative calcium balance; in osteoporosis, it helps to prevent or decrease the rate of bone loss. The calcium in calcium salts moderates nerve and muscle performance and allows normal cardiac function.

Pharmacodynamics/Kinetics Absorption: Requires vitamin D

Dosage
 Geriatric Dosage in terms of elemental calcium:
  Dietary Reference Intake for Calcium: RDA:
   Females: Refer to adult dosing.
   Males ≤70 years: Refer to adult dosing.
   Males >70 years: 1200 mg/day
 Adult Dosage in terms of elemental calcium:
  Dietary Reference Intake for Calcium: Oral: Adults, Females/Males: RDA:
   19-50 years: 1000 mg/day
   ≥51 years, females: 1200 mg/day
   51-70 years, males: 1000 mg/day

Reference Range
 Serum calcium: 8.5-10.5 mg/dL. Monitor plasma calcium levels if using calcium salts as electrolyte supplements for deficiency.
 Due to a poor correlation between the serum ionized calcium (free) and total serum calcium, particularly in states of low albumin or acid/base imbalances, direct measurement of ionized calcium is recommended
 In low albumin states, the corrected **total** serum calcium may be estimated by:
  Corrected total calcium = total serum calcium + 0.8 (4.0 - measured serum albumin)

Dosage Forms Excipient information presented when available (limited, particularly for generics); consult specific product labeling. [DSC] = Discontinued product
 Tablet, oral: 648 mg [equivalent to elemental calcium 84.5 mg], 650 mg [DSC] [equivalent to elemental calcium 84.5 mg]

Calcium Phosphate (Tribasic) (KAL see um FOS fate tri BAY sik)

Brand Names: U.S. Posture® [OTC]
Index Terms Tricalcium Phosphate
Generic Availability (U.S.) No
Pharmacologic Category Calcium Salt
Use Dietary supplement
Warnings/Precautions Constipation, bloating, and gas are common with calcium supplements. Calcium absorption is impaired in achlorhydria; common in elderly, use an alternate salt (eg, citrate) and administer with food. Hypercalcemia and hypercalciuria are most likely to occur in hypoparathyroid patients receiving high doses of vitamin D. Use caution when administering calcium supplements to patients with a history of kidney stones. Use with caution in patients with renal failure to avoid hypercalcemia; frequent monitoring of serum calcium and phosphorus is necessary. Calcium administration interferes with absorption of some minerals and drugs; use with caution. It is recommended to concomitantly administer vitamin D for optimal calcium absorption. Taking calcium (≤500 mg) with food improves absorption.
Drug Interactions
 Metabolism/Transport Effects None known.
 Avoid Concomitant Use
  Avoid concomitant use of Calcium Phosphate (Tribasic) with any of the following: Calcium Acetate
 Increased Effect/Toxicity
  Calcium Phosphate (Tribasic) may increase the levels/effects of: Calcium Acetate; Vitamin D Analogs

  The levels/effects of Calcium Phosphate (Tribasic) may be increased by: Bisphosphonate Derivatives; Thiazide Diuretics
 Decreased Effect
  Calcium Phosphate (Tribasic) may decrease the levels/effects of: Bisphosphonate Derivatives; Calcium Channel Blockers; Deferiprone; DOBUTamine; Eltrombopag; Estramustine; Phosphate Supplements; Quinolone Antibiotics; Tetracycline Derivatives; Thyroid Products; Trientine

  The levels/effects of Calcium Phosphate (Tribasic) may be decreased by: Antacids; Calcium Salts; Iron Salts; Magnesium Salts; Sucralfate; Trientine
Ethanol/Nutrition/Herb Interactions Ethanol: Avoid ethanol (may increase risk of osteoporosis).
Mechanism of Action As dietary supplement, used to prevent or treat negative calcium balance; in osteoporosis, it helps to prevent or decrease the rate of bone loss. The calcium in calcium salts moderates nerve and muscle performance and allows normal cardiac function.

Dosage

Geriatric

Dietary Reference Intake for Calcium: RDA: Oral:
Females: Refer to adult dosing.
Males ≤70 years: Refer to adult dosing.
Males >70 years: 1200 mg/day
Dietary supplement: Refer to adult dosing.

Adult

Dietary Reference Intake for Calcium: Oral: Adults, Females/Males: RDA:
19-50 years: 1000 mg/day
≥51 years, females: 1200 mg/day
51-70 years, males: 1000 mg/day
Dietary supplement: Oral: 2 tablets daily

Reference Range

Serum calcium: 8.5-10.5 mg/dL. Monitor plasma calcium levels if using calcium salts as electrolyte supplements for deficiency.

Due to a poor correlation between the serum ionized calcium (free) and total serum calcium, particularly in states of low albumin or acid/base imbalances, direct measurement of ionized calcium is recommended

In low albumin states, the corrected **total** serum calcium may be estimated by:
Corrected total calcium = total serum calcium + 0.8 (4.0 - measured serum albumin)

Dosage Forms Excipient information presented when available (limited, particularly for generics); consult specific product labeling.
Caplet:
Posture®: Calcium 600 mg and phosphorus 280 mg [as tricalcium phosphate]

♦ **Cal-CYUM [OTC]** see Calcium and Vitamin D on page 261
♦ **Caldecort® [OTC]** see Hydrocortisone (Topical) on page 943
♦ **Caldolor™** see Ibuprofen on page 966
♦ **Cal-G [OTC] [DSC]** see Calcium Gluconate on page 270
♦ **Cal-Gest [OTC]** see Calcium Carbonate on page 262
♦ **Cal-GLU™ [OTC]** see Calcium Gluconate on page 270
♦ **Cal-Mint [OTC]** see Calcium Carbonate on page 262
♦ **Caltrate® 600 [OTC]** see Calcium Carbonate on page 262
♦ **Caltrate® 600+D [OTC]** see Calcium and Vitamin D on page 261
♦ **Caltrate® 600+Soy™ [OTC]** see Calcium and Vitamin D on page 261
♦ **Caltrate® ColonHealth™ [OTC]** see Calcium and Vitamin D on page 261
♦ **Cambia™** see Diclofenac (Systemic) on page 531
♦ **Campral®** see Acamprosate on page 25
♦ **Canasa®** see Mesalamine on page 1217
♦ **Cancidas®** see Caspofungin on page 304

Candesartan (kan de SAR tan)

Related Information

Angiotensin Agents on page 2093
Heart Failure (Systolic) on page 2203

Medication Safety Issues

Sound-alike/look-alike issues:
Atacand® may be confused with antacid

Brand Names: U.S. Atacand®

Brand Names: Canada Apo-Candesartan; Atacand®; CO Candesartan; JAMP-Candesartan; Mylan-Candesartan; Sandoz-Candesartan; Teva-Candesartan

Index Terms Candesartan Cilexetil

Generic Availability (U.S.) No

Pharmacologic Category Angiotensin II Receptor Blocker; Antihypertensive

Use Alone or in combination with other antihypertensive agents in treating hypertension; treatment of heart failure (NYHA class II-IV)

Contraindications Hypersensitivity to candesartan or any component of the formulation

Warnings/Precautions May cause hyperkalemia; avoid potassium supplementation unless specifically required by healthcare provider. Avoid use or use a smaller dose in patients who are volume depleted; correct depletion first. May be associated with deterioration of renal function and/or increases in serum creatinine, particularly in patients with low renal blood flow (eg, renal artery stenosis, heart failure) whose glomerular filtration rate (GFR) is dependent on efferent arteriolar vasoconstriction by angiotensin II. Use with caution in unstented unilateral/bilateral renal artery stenosis, pre-existing renal insufficiency, or significant aortic/mitral stenosis. Use with caution in patients with moderate hepatic impairment. Contraindicated with severe hepatic impairment and/or cholestasis. Use caution when initiating in heart failure; may need to adjust dose, and/or concurrent diuretic therapy, because of candesartan-induced hypotension. Hypotension may occur during major surgery and anesthesia; use cautiously before, during, and immediately after such interventions. Although concurrent therapy with an ACE inhibitor may be rational in select patients, concurrent use of ACE inhibitors may increase the risk of clinically-significant adverse events (eg, renal dysfunction, hyperkalemia).

Adverse Reactions (Reflective of adult population; not specific for elderly)
Cardiovascular: Angina, hypotension (heart failure 19%), MI, palpitation, tachycardia
Central nervous system: Anxiety, depression, dizziness, drowsiness, fever, headache, light-headedness, somnolence, vertigo
Dermatologic: Angioedema, rash
Endocrine & metabolic: Hyperglycemia, hyperkalemia (heart failure <1% to 6%), hyper-triglyceridemia, hyperuricemia
Gastrointestinal: Dyspepsia, gastroenteritis
Neuromuscular & skeletal: Back pain, CPK increased, myalgia, paresthesia, weakness
Renal: Serum creatinine increased (up to 13% in patients with heart failure with drug discontinuation required in 6%), hematuria
Respiratory: Dyspnea, epistaxis, pharyngitis, rhinitis, upper respiratory tract infection
Miscellaneous: Diaphoresis increased

Drug Interactions
Metabolism/Transport Effects Substrate of CYP2C9 (minor); **Note:** Assignment of Major/Minor substrate status based on clinically relevant drug interaction potential; **Inhibits** CYP2C8 (weak), CYP2C9 (weak)
Avoid Concomitant Use There are no known interactions where it is recommended to avoid concomitant use.
Increased Effect/Toxicity
Candesartan may increase the levels/effects of: ACE Inhibitors; Amifostine; Antihypertensives; Hypotensive Agents; Lithium; Nonsteroidal Anti-Inflammatory Agents; Potassium-Sparing Diuretics; RiTUXimab; Sodium Phosphates

The levels/effects of Candesartan may be increased by: Alfuzosin; Aliskiren; Diazoxide; Eplerenone; Herbs (Hypotensive Properties); MAO Inhibitors; Pentoxifylline; Phosphodiesterase 5 Inhibitors; Potassium Salts; Prostacyclin Analogues; Tolvaptan; Trimethoprim
Decreased Effect
The levels/effects of Candesartan may be decreased by: Herbs (Hypertensive Properties); Methylphenidate; Nonsteroidal Anti-Inflammatory Agents; Yohimbine

Ethanol/Nutrition/Herb Interactions
Food: Potassium supplements and/or potassium-containing salts may cause or worsen hyperkalemia. Management: Consult prescriber before consuming a potassium-rich diet, potassium supplements, or salt substitutes.
Herb/Nutraceutical: Dong quai has estrogenic activity. Ephedra, yohimbe, and ginseng may worsen hypertension. Garlic may increase antihypertensive effect of candesartan. Management: Avoid dong quai if using for hypertension. Avoid ephedra, yohimbe, ginseng, and garlic.

Stability Store at 25°C (77°F); excursions permitted to 15°C to 30°C (59°F to 86°F).
Mechanism of Action Candesartan is an angiotensin receptor antagonist. Angiotensin II acts as a vasoconstrictor. In addition to causing direct vasoconstriction, angiotensin II also stimulates the release of aldosterone. Once aldosterone is released, sodium as well as water are reabsorbed. The end result is an elevation in blood pressure. Candesartan binds to the AT1 angiotensin II receptor. This binding prevents angiotensin II from binding to the receptor thereby blocking the vasoconstriction and the aldosterone secreting effects of angiotensin II.

Pharmacodynamics/Kinetics
Onset of action: 2-3 hours
 Peak effect: 6-8 hours
Duration: >24 hours
Distribution: V_d: 0.13 L/kg
Protein binding: >99%
Metabolism: Parent compound bioactivated during absorption via ester hydrolysis within intestinal wall to candesartan
Bioavailability: 15%
Half-life elimination (dose dependent): 5-9 hours
Time to peak: 3-4 hours
Excretion: Urine (26%)

Dosage

Geriatric Refer to adult dosing. No initial dosage adjustment is necessary for elderly patients (although higher concentrations (C_{max}) and AUC were observed in these populations), for patients with mildly impaired renal function, or for patients with mildly impaired hepatic function.

Adult

Hypertension: Oral: Dosage must be individualized. Initial: 16 mg once daily; titrate to response (within 2 weeks, antihypertensive effect usually observed); usual range: 8-32 mg/day in 1-2 divided doses; maximum daily dose: 32 mg/day.

Heart failure: Oral: Initial: 4 mg once daily; double the dose at 2-week intervals, as tolerated; target dose: 32 mg once daily

Note: In selected cases, concurrent therapy with an ACE inhibitor may provide additional benefit.

Renal Impairment Adults: No initial dosage adjustment necessary; however, in patients with severe renal impairment (Cl_{cr} <30 mL/minute/1.73m^2) AUC and C_{max} were approximately doubled after repeated dosing.

Hepatic Impairment

Mild impairment: No initial dosage adjustment necessary.

Moderate impairment: Consider initiation at lower dosages (AUC increased by 145%).

Severe impairment: No dosage adjustment provided in manufacturer's labeling (has not been studied).

Administration Administer without regard to meals.

Monitoring Parameters Supine blood pressure, electrolytes, serum creatinine, BUN, urinalysis, symptomatic hypotension, and tachycardia; in heart failure, serum potassium during dose escalation and periodically thereafter

Pharmacotherapy Pearls May have an advantage over losartan due to minimal metabolism requirements and consequent use in mild-to-moderate hepatic impairment

Special Geriatric Considerations High concentrations occur in the elderly compared to younger subjects. AUC may be doubled in patients with renal impairment. No initial dose adjustment necessary since repeated dose did not demonstrate accumulation of drug or metabolites in elderly.

Dosage Forms Excipient information presented when available (limited, particularly for generics); consult specific product labeling.

Tablet, oral, as cilexetil:

Atacand®: 4 mg, 8 mg, 16 mg, 32 mg [scored]

Candesartan and Hydrochlorothiazide
(kan de SAR tan & hye droe klor oh THYE a zide)

Related Information

Candesartan *on page 275*

Hydrochlorothiazide *on page 933*

Brand Names: U.S. Atacand HCT®

Brand Names: Canada Atacand® Plus

Index Terms Candesartan Cilexetil and Hydrochlorothiazide; Hydrochlorothiazide and Candesartan

Generic Availability (U.S.) No

Pharmacologic Category Angiotensin II Receptor Blocker; Diuretic, Thiazide

Use Treatment of hypertension; combination product should not be used for initial therapy

Dosage

Geriatric & Adult Hypertension, replacement therapy: Oral: Combination product can be substituted for individual agents; maximum therapeutic effect would be expected within 4 weeks

Usual dosage range:

Candesartan: 16-32 mg/day, given once daily or twice daily in divided doses

Hydrochlorothiazide: 12.5-25 mg once daily

Renal Impairment Serum levels of candesartan are increased and the half-life of hydrochlorothiazide is prolonged in patients with renal impairment. Contraindicated with severe renal impairment (Cl_{cr} <30 mL/minute).

Hepatic Impairment Use with caution with moderate hepatic impairment. Contraindicated with severe hepatic impairment and/or cholestasis.

Special Geriatric Considerations See individual agents. Combination products are not recommended as first-line treatment. Use only if doses of individual agents correspond to the combination available.

◀ **Dosage Forms** Excipient information presented when available (limited, particularly for generics); consult specific product labeling.

Tablet:

Atacand HCT®:

16/12.5: Candesartan cilexetil 16 mg and hydrochlorothiazide 12.5 mg

32/12.5: Candesartan cilexetil 32 mg and hydrochlorothiazide 12.5 mg

32/25: Candesartan cilexetil 32 mg and hydrochlorothiazide 25 mg

- ◆ **Candesartan Cilexetil** *see* Candesartan *on page 275*
- ◆ **Candesartan Cilexetil and Hydrochlorothiazide** *see* Candesartan and Hydrochlorothiazide *on page 277*
- ◆ **Cankaid® [OTC]** *see* Carbamide Peroxide *on page 291*
- ◆ **Capastat® Sulfate** *see* Capreomycin *on page 278*
- ◆ **Capex®** *see* Fluocinolone (Topical) *on page 803*
- ◆ **Caphosol®** *see* Saliva Substitute *on page 1748*
- ◆ **Capital® and Codeine** *see* Acetaminophen and Codeine *on page 35*

Capreomycin (kap ree oh MYE sin)

Related Information

Antimicrobial Drugs of Choice *on page 2163*

Medication Safety Issues

Sound-alike/look-alike issues:

Capastat® may be confused with Cepastat®

Brand Names: U.S. Capastat® Sulfate

Index Terms Capreomycin Sulfate

Generic Availability (U.S.) No

Pharmacologic Category Antibiotic, Miscellaneous; Antitubercular Agent

Use Treatment of tuberculosis in conjunction with at least one other antituberculosis agent

Contraindications Hypersensitivity to capreomycin or any component of the formulation

Warnings/Precautions [U.S. Boxed Warnings]: Use in patients with renal insufficiency or pre-existing auditory impairment must be undertaken with great caution, and the risk of additional eighth nerve impairment or renal injury should be weighed against the benefits to be derived from therapy. Since other parenteral antituberculous agents (eg, streptomycin) also have similar and sometimes irreversible toxic effects, particularly on eighth cranial nerve and renal function, simultaneous administration of these agents with capreomycin is not recommended. Use with nonantituberculous drugs (ie, aminoglycoside antibiotics) having ototoxic or nephrotoxic potential should be undertaken only with great caution. Use caution with renal dysfunction and in the elderly; dosage reductions are recommended for known or suspected renal impairment. Electrolyte imbalances (hypocalcemia, hypokalemia, and hypomagnesemia) have been reported with use. Prolonged use may result in fungal or bacterial superinfection, including *C. difficile*-associated diarrhea (CDAD) and pseudomembranous colitis; CDAD has been observed >2 months postantibiotic treatment.

Adverse Reactions (Reflective of adult population; not specific for elderly)

>10%:

Otic: Ototoxicity (subclinical hearing loss: 11%; clinical loss: 3%)

Renal: Nephrotoxicity (36%, increased BUN)

1% to 10%: Hematologic: Eosinophilia (dose related, mild)

Drug Interactions

Metabolism/Transport Effects None known.

Avoid Concomitant Use

Avoid concomitant use of Capreomycin with any of the following: BCG

Increased Effect/Toxicity

Capreomycin may increase the levels/effects of: Aminoglycosides; Colistimethate; Neuromuscular-Blocking Agents; Polymyxin B

Decreased Effect

Capreomycin may decrease the levels/effects of: BCG

Stability Powder for injection should be stored at room temperature of 15°C to 30°C (59°F to 86°F). Dissolve powder with 2 mL of NS or SWFI; allow 2-3 minutes for dissolution.
For I.V. administration: Further dilute in NS 100 mL.
For I.M. administration:
  1 g dose: Administer contents of reconstituted vial
  <1 g dose: See table:

Capreomycin Dilution for Doses <1 g (I.M. Administration)

Diluent Volume (mL)	Capreomycin Solution Volume (mL)	Final Concentration (approximate)
2.15	2.85	370 mg/mL
2.63	3.33	315 mg/mL
3.3	4	260 mg/mL
4.3	5	210 mg/mL

Following reconstitution, may store under refrigeration for up to 24 hours.

Mechanism of Action Capreomycin is a cyclic polypeptide antimicrobial. It is administered as a mixture of capreomycin IA and capreomycin IB. The mechanism of action of capreomycin is not well understood. Mycobacterial species that have become resistant to other agents are usually still sensitive to the action of capreomycin. However, significant cross-resistance with viomycin, kanamycin, and neomycin occurs.

Pharmacodynamics/Kinetics
Half-life elimination: Normal renal function: 4-6 hours; Cl_{cr} 100-110 mL/minute: 5-6 hours; Cl_{cr} 50-80 mL/minute: 7-10 hours; Cl_{cr} 20-40 mL/minute: 12-20 hours; Cl_{cr} 10 mL/minute: 29 hours; Cl_{cr} 0 mL/minute: 55 hours
Time to peak, serum: I.M.: 1-2 hours
Excretion: Urine (52% within 12 hours)

Dosage
  Geriatric Refer to adult dosing. Use with caution due to the increased potential for pre-existing renal dysfunction or impaired hearing. The manufacturer recommends initiating at lower end of dosing range. Adults >59 years of age: 10 mg/kg (maximum: 750 mg/dose) for 5-7 days per week for 2-4 months, followed by 10 mg/kg (maximum: 750 mg/dose) 2-3 times/week (*MMWR*, 2003).
  Adult Tuberculosis: I.M., I.V.: 1 g/day (maximum: 20 mg/kg/day) for 60-120 days, followed by 1 g 2-3 times/week **or** 15 mg/kg/day (maximum: 1 g/dose) for 2-4 months, followed by 15 mg/kg (maximum: 1 g/dose) 2-3 times/week (*MMWR*, 2003)
  Renal Impairment Adults:
   The FDA-approved labeling contains the following renal dosing adjustment guidelines (maximum: 1 g/dose):
   Cl_{cr} 110 mL/minute: Administer 13.9 mg/kg every 24 hours
   Cl_{cr} 100 mL/minute: Administer 12.7 mg/kg every 24 hours
   Cl_{cr} 80 mL/minute: Administer 10.4 mg/kg every 24 hours
   Cl_{cr} 60 mL/minute: Administer 8.2 mg/kg every 24 hours
   Cl_{cr} 50 mL/minute: Administer 7 mg/kg every 24 hours **or** 14 mg/kg every 48 hours
   Cl_{cr} 40 mL/minute: Administer 5.9 mg/kg every 24 hours **or** 11.7 mg/kg every 48 hours
   Cl_{cr} 30 mL/minute: Administer 4.7 mg/kg every 24 hours **or** 9.5 mg/kg every 48 hours **or** 14.2 mg/kg every 72 hours
   Cl_{cr} 20 mL/minute: Administer 3.6 mg/kg every 24 hours **or** 7.2 mg/kg every 48 hours **or** 10.7 mg/kg every 72 hours
   Cl_{cr} 10 mL/minute: Administer 2.4 mg/kg every 24 hours **or** 4.9 mg/kg every 48 hours **or** 7.3 mg/kg every 72 hours
   Cl_{cr} 0 mL/minute: Administer 1.3 mg/kg every 24 hours **or** 2.6 mg/kg every 48 hours **or** 3.9 mg/kg every 72 hours

   The following (unlabeled) guidelines may also be used:
   MMWR, 2003:
    Cl_{cr} ≥30 mL/minute: No adjustment required
    Cl_{cr} <30 mL/minute and hemodialysis: 12-15 mg/kg (maximum: 1 g/dose) 2-3 days per week (**NOT** daily)
   Aronoff, 2007:
    Cl_{cr} ≥10 mL/minute: 1 g every 24 hours
    Cl_{cr} <10 mL/minute: 1 g every 48 hours
   Hemodialysis: Administer dose after hemodialysis only
   Continuous renal replacement therapy (CRRT): 5 mg/kg every 24 hours

Administration Administer by deep I.M. injection into large muscle mass

◀ **Monitoring Parameters** Audiometric measurements and vestibular function at baseline and during therapy; renal function at baseline and weekly during therapy; frequent assessment of serum electrolytes (including calcium, magnesium, and potassium), liver function tests

Reference Range Recommended concentration for susceptibility testing: 10 mcg/mL

Special Geriatric Considerations Has not been studied in the elderly. I.M. administration may limit use due to painful injection or lack of sites in patients with decreased muscle mass. Use with caution in patients with pre-existing hearing impairment due to potential ototoxicity.

Dosage Forms Excipient information presented when available (limited, particularly for generics); consult specific product labeling.

Injection, powder for reconstitution, as sulfate:
   Capastat® Sulfate: 1 g

◆ **Capreomycin Sulfate** see Capreomycin on page 278

Capsaicin (kap SAY sin)

Medication Safety Issues
   Sound-alike/look-alike issues:
      Zostrix® may be confused with Zestril®, Zovirax®

Brand Names: U.S. Capzasin-HP® [OTC]; Capzasin-P® [OTC]; DiabetAid® Pain and Tingling Relief [OTC]; Qutenza™; Salonpas® Gel-Patch Hot [OTC]; Salonpas® Hot [OTC]; Trixaicin HP [OTC]; Trixaicin [OTC]; Zostrix® Diabetic Foot Pain [OTC]; Zostrix® [OTC]; Zostrix®-HP [OTC]

Brand Names: Canada Zostrix®; Zostrix® H.P.

Index Terms NGX-4010

Generic Availability (U.S.) Yes: Cream

Pharmacologic Category Analgesic, Topical; Topical Skin Product; Transient Receptor Potential Vanilloid 1 (TRPV1) Agonist

Use
   Topical patch (Qutenza™): Management of postherpetic neuralgia (PHN)
   OTC labeling: Temporary treatment of minor pain associated with muscles and joints due to backache, strains, sprains, bruises, cramps, or arthritis; temporary relief of pain associated with diabetic neuropathy

Unlabeled Use Diabetic neuropathy; treatment of pain associated with psoriasis and intractable pruritus. Potential use as topical agent in burning mouth syndrome and oral mucositis.

Contraindications There are no contraindications listed in the manufacturer's labeling.

Warnings/Precautions
   Topical high-concentration capsaicin patch (Qutenza™): Do not apply to face, scalp, or allow contact with eyes or mucous membranes. If an unintended area of skin is inadvertently exposed, the cleansing gel should be used. Post-application pain should be treated with local cooling methods and/or analgesics (opioids may be necessary). Avoid rapid removal of patches to decrease risk of aerosolization of capsaicin; inhalation of airborne capsaicin may result in coughing or sneezing; if shortness of breath occurs, medical care is required; remove patches gently and slowly to decrease risk of aerosolization. Use with caution in patients with uncontrolled hypertension, or a history of cardiovascular or cerebrovascular events; transient increases in blood pressure due to treatment-related pain have occurred during and after application of patch.

   Topical OTC products: Apply externally; avoid contact with eyes or mucous membranes. Should not be applied to broken or irritated skin. Treated area should not be exposed to heat or direct sunlight. Affected area should not be bandaged. Transient burning may occur and generally disappears after several days; discontinue use if severe burning develops. Stop use and consult a healthcare provider if redness or irritation develops, symptoms get worse, or symptoms resolve and then recur.

Adverse Reactions (Reflective of adult population; not specific for elderly) Topical patch (Qutenza™, capsaicin 8%):
   >10%: Local: Erythema (63%), pain (42%)
   1% to 10%:
      Cardiovascular: Hypertension (2%; transient)
      Dermatologic: Pruritus (2%)
      Gastrointestinal: Nausea (5%), vomiting (3%)
      Local: Pruritus (6%), papules (6%), edema (4%), dryness (2%), swelling (2%)
      Respiratory: Nasopharyngitis (4%), sinusitis (3%), bronchitis (2%)

Drug Interactions
   Metabolism/Transport Effects Substrate of CYP2E1 (minor); **Note:** Assignment of Major/Minor substrate status based on clinically relevant drug interaction potential

Avoid Concomitant Use There are no known interactions where it is recommended to avoid concomitant use.

Increased Effect/Toxicity There are no known significant interactions involving an increase in effect.

Decreased Effect There are no known significant interactions involving a decrease in effect.

Stability Qutenza™: Store at room temperature between 20°C to 25°C (68°F to 77°F).

Mechanism of Action Capsaicin, a transient receptor potential vanilloid 1 receptor (TRPV1) agonist, activates TRPV1 ligand-gated cation channels on nociceptive nerve fibers, resulting in depolarization, initiation of action potential, and pain signal transmission to the spinal cord; capsaicin exposure results in subsequent desensitization of the sensory axons and inhibition of pain transmission initiation. In arthritis, capsaicin induces release of substance P, the principal chemomediator of pain impulses from the periphery to the CNS, from peripheral sensory neurons; after repeated application, capsaicin depletes the neuron of substance P and prevents reaccumulation. The functional link between substance P and the capsaicin receptor, TRPV1, is not well understood.

Pharmacodynamics/Kinetics

Absorption: Topical patch (capsaicin 8%): Systemic absorption is transient and low (<5 ng/mL) in approximately one-third of patients when measured following 60-minute application. In patients with quantifiable levels, most fell below the limit of quantitation at 3-6 hours post application.

Half-life elimination: Topical patch (capsaicin 8%): 1.64 hours (Babbar, 2009)

Dosage

Geriatric & Adult

Pain relief: OTC labeling:

Patch (Salonpas®-Hot): Apply patch to affected area up to 3-4 times/day for 7 days. Patch may remain in place for up to 8 hours.

Topical products (cream, gel, liquid, lotion): Apply to affected area 3-4 times/day; efficacy may be decreased if used less than 3 times/day; best results seen after 2-4 weeks of continuous use

Postherpetic neuralgia: Patch (Qutenza™ [capsaicin 8%]): Apply patch to most painful area for 60 minutes. Up to 4 patches may be applied in a single application. Treatment may be repeated ≥3 months as needed for return of pain (do not apply more frequently than every 3 months). Area should be pretreated with a topical anesthetic prior to patch application.

Diabetic neuropathy (unlabeled use): Cream (0.075%): Apply 4 times/day (Bril, 2011)

Administration

Topical products (cream, gel, liquid, lotion): Wear gloves to apply; wash hands with soap and water after applying to avoid spreading to eyes or other sensitive areas of the body.

Topical patch (Salonpas®-Hot): Apply patch externally to clean and dry affected area. Backing film should be removed prior to application. Do not use within 1 hour prior to a bath or immediately after bathing. Do not use with a heating pad.

Topical patch (Qutenza™[capsaicin 8%]): Patch should only be applied by a physician or by a healthcare professional under the close supervision of a physician. The treatment area must be identified and marked by a physician. The patch can be cut to match size/shape of treatment area. If necessary, excessive hair present on and surrounding the treatment area, may be clipped (not shaved) to promote adherence. Prior to application, the treatment area should be cleansed with mild soap and water and dried thoroughly. The treatment area should be anesthetized with a topical anesthetic prior to patch application. Anesthetic should be removed with a dry wipe, and area should be cleansed again with soap/water, and dried. Patch may then be applied to dry, intact skin within 2 hours of opening the patch; apply patch using nitrile gloves (latex gloves should **not** be used). During application, slowly peel back the release liner under the patch. Patch should remain in place for 60 minutes. Remove patches gently and slowly. Following patch removal, apply cleansing gel to the treatment area and leave in place for at least 1 minute. All treatment materials should be disposed of according to biomedical waste procedures.

Special Geriatric Considerations Capsaicin products are available over-the-counter. Counsel patients about the appropriate use of these products. The American College of Rheumatology recommends capsaicin for the symptomatic treatment of osteoarthritis of the knee.

Dosage Forms Excipient information presented when available (limited, particularly for generics); consult specific product labeling. [DSC] = Discontinued product

Cream, topical: 0.025% (60 g); 0.075% (60 g [DSC])

Capzasin-HP®: 0.1% (42.5 g) [contains benzyl alcohol]

Capzasin-P®: 0.035% (42.5 g) [contains benzyl alcohol]

Trixaicin: 0.025% (60 g) [contains benzyl alcohol]

Trixaicin HP: 0.075% (60 g) [contains benzyl alcohol]

Zostrix®: 0.025% (60 g) [contains benzyl alcohol]

◀

Zostrix® Diabetic Foot Pain: 0.075% (60 g) [contains benzyl alcohol]
Zostrix®-HP: 0.075% (60 g) [contains benzyl alcohol]
Gel, topical:
Capzasin-P®: 0.025% (42.5 g) [contains menthol]
Liquid, topical:
Capzasin-P®: 0.15% (29.5 mL)
Lotion, topical:
DiabetAid® Pain and Tingling Relief: 0.025% (120 mL)
Patch, topical:
Qutenza™: 8% (1s, 2s) [contains metal; supplied with cleansing gel]
Salonpas® Gel-Patch Hot: 0.025% (3s, 6s) [contains menthol]
Salonpas® Hot: 0.025% (1s) [contains natural rubber/natural latex in packaging]

Captopril (KAP toe pril)

Related Information
Angiotensin Agents *on page 2093*
Heart Failure (Systolic) *on page 2203*
Medication Safety Issues
Sound-alike/look-alike issues:
Captopril may be confused with calcitriol, Capitrol®, carvedilol
International issues:
Acepril [Great Britain] may be confused with Accupril which is a brand name for quinapril in the U.S.
Acepril: Brand name for captopril [Great Britain], but also the brand name for enalapril [Hungary, Switzerland]; lisinopril [Malaysia]
Brand Names: Canada Apo-Capto®; Capoten®; Dom-Captopril; Mylan-Captopril; Nu-Capto; PMS-Captopril; Teva-Captopril
Index Terms ACE
Generic Availability (U.S.) Yes
Pharmacologic Category Angiotensin-Converting Enzyme (ACE) Inhibitor
Use Management of hypertension; treatment of heart failure, left ventricular dysfunction after myocardial infarction, diabetic nephropathy
Unlabeled Use To delay the progression of nephropathy and reduce risks of cardiovascular events in hypertensive patients with type 1 or 2 diabetes mellitus; treatment of hypertensive crisis, rheumatoid arthritis; diagnosis of anatomic renal artery stenosis, hypertension secondary to scleroderma renal crisis; diagnosis of aldosteronism, idiopathic edema, Bartter's syndrome, postmyocardial infarction for prevention of ventricular failure; increase circulation in Raynaud's phenomenon, hypertension secondary to Takayasu's disease
Contraindications Hypersensitivity to captopril, any other ACE inhibitor, or any component of the formulation; angioedema related to previous treatment with an ACE inhibitor
Warnings/Precautions Anaphylactic reactions may occur rarely with ACE inhibitors. At any time during treatment (especially following first dose) angioedema may occur rarely with ACE inhibitors; may involve the head and neck (potentially compromising airway) or the intestine (presenting with abdominal pain). African-Americans and patients with idiopathic or hereditary angioedema may be at an increased risk. Prolonged frequent monitoring may be required especially if tongue, glottis, or larynx are involved as they are associated with airway obstruction. Patients with a history of airway surgery may have a higher risk of airway obstruction. Aggressive early and appropriate management is critical. Use in patients with previous angioedema associated with ACE inhibitor therapy is contraindicated. Severe anaphylactoid reactions may be seen during hemodialysis (eg, CVVHD) with high-flux dialysis membranes (eg, AN69), and rarely, during low density lipoprotein apheresis with dextran sulfate cellulose. Rare cases of anaphylactoid reactions have been reported in patients undergoing sensitization treatment with hymenoptera (bee, wasp) venom while receiving ACE inhibitors.

Symptomatic hypotension with or without syncope can occur with ACE inhibitors (usually with the first several doses); effects are most often observed in volume depleted patients; close monitoring of patient is required especially with initial dosing and dosing increases; blood pressure must be lowered at a rate appropriate for the patient's clinical condition. Initiation of therapy in patients with ischemic heart disease or cerebrovascular disease warrants close observation due to the potential consequences posed by falling blood pressure (eg, MI, stroke). Use with caution in hypertrophic cardiomyopathy with outflow tract obstruction, severe aortic stenosis, or before, during, or immediately after major surgery.

Hyperkalemia may occur with ACE inhibitors; risk factors include renal dysfunction, diabetes mellitus, concomitant use of potassium-sparing diuretics, potassium supplements and/or potassium containing salts. Use cautiously, if at all, with these agents and monitor potassium closely. Cough may occur with ACE inhibitors. Other causes of cough should be considered (eg, pulmonary congestion in patients with heart failure) and excluded prior to discontinuation.

May be associated with deterioration of renal function and/or increases in serum creatinine, particularly in patients with low renal blood flow (eg, renal artery stenosis, heart failure) whose glomerular filtration rate (GFR) is dependent on efferent arteriolar vasoconstriction by angiotensin II; deterioration may result in oliguria, acute renal failure, and progressive azotemia. Small increases in serum creatinine may occur following initiation; consider discontinuation only in patients with progressive and/or significant deterioration in renal function. Use with caution in patients with unstented unilateral/bilateral renal artery stenosis. When unstented bilateral renal artery stenosis is present, use is generally avoided due to the elevated risk of deterioration in renal function unless possible benefits outweigh risks. Concurrent use of angiotensin receptor blockers may increase the risk of clinically-significant adverse events (eg, renal dysfunction, hyperkalemia).

Rare toxicities associated with ACE inhibitors include cholestatic jaundice (which may progress to fulminant hepatic necrosis), agranulocytosis, neutropenia, or leukopenia with myeloid hypoplasia. Patients with collagen vascular diseases (especially with concomitant renal impairment) or renal impairment alone may be at increased risk for hematologic toxicity; closely monitor CBC with differential for the first 3 months of therapy and periodically thereafter in these patients.

Adverse Reactions (Reflective of adult population; not specific for elderly)
Frequency not defined:
Cardiovascular: Angioedema, cardiac arrest, cerebrovascular insufficiency, rhythm disturbances, orthostatic hypotension, syncope, flushing, pallor, angina, MI, Raynaud's syndrome, CHF
Central nervous system: Ataxia, confusion, depression, nervousness, somnolence
Dermatologic: Bullous pemphigus, erythema multiforme, Stevens-Johnson syndrome, exfoliative dermatitis
Endocrine & metabolic: Alkaline phosphatase increased, bilirubin increased, gynecomastia
Gastrointestinal: Pancreatitis, glossitis, dyspepsia
Genitourinary: Urinary frequency, impotence
Hematologic: Anemia, thrombocytopenia, pancytopenia, agranulocytosis, anemia
Hepatic: Jaundice, hepatitis, hepatic necrosis (rare), cholestasis, hyponatremia (symptomatic), transaminases increased
Neuromuscular & skeletal: Asthenia, myalgia, myasthenia
Ocular: Blurred vision
Renal: Renal insufficiency, renal failure, nephrotic syndrome, polyuria, oliguria
Respiratory: Bronchospasm, eosinophilic pneumonitis, rhinitis
Miscellaneous: Anaphylactoid reactions
1% to 10%:
Cardiovascular: Hypotension (1% to 3%), tachycardia (1%), chest pain (1%), palpitation (1%)
Dermatologic: Rash (maculopapular or urticarial) (4% to 7%), pruritus (2%); in patients with rash, a positive ANA and/or eosinophilia has been noted in 7% to 10%
Endocrine & metabolic: Hyperkalemia (1% to 11%)
Hematologic: Neutropenia may occur in up to 4% of patients with renal insufficiency or collagen-vascular disease
Renal: Proteinuria (1%), serum creatinine increased, worsening of renal function (may occur in patients with bilateral renal artery stenosis or hypovolemia)
Respiratory: Cough (<1% to 2%)
Miscellaneous: Hypersensitivity reactions (rash, pruritus, fever, arthralgia, and eosinophilia) have occurred in 4% to 7% of patients (depending on dose and renal function); dysgeusia - loss of taste or diminished perception (2% to 4%)
Drug Interactions
Metabolism/Transport Effects Substrate of CYP2D6 (major); **Note:** Assignment of Major/Minor substrate status based on clinically relevant drug interaction potential
Avoid Concomitant Use There are no known interactions where it is recommended to avoid concomitant use.
Increased Effect/Toxicity
Captopril may increase the levels/effects of: Allopurinol; Amifostine; Antihypertensives; AzaTHIOprine; CycloSPORINE; CycloSPORINE (Systemic); Ferric Gluconate; Gold Sodium Thiomalate; Hypotensive Agents; Iron Dextran Complex; Lithium; Nonsteroidal Anti-Inflammatory Agents; RiTUXimab; Sodium Phosphates

The levels/effects of Captopril may be increased by: Abiraterone Acetate; Alfuzosin; Aliskiren; Angiotensin II Receptor Blockers; CYP2D6 Inhibitors (Moderate); CYP2D6 Inhibitors (Strong); Darunavir; Diazoxide; DPP-IV Inhibitors; Eplerenone; Everolimus; Herbs (Hypotensive Properties); Loop Diuretics; MAO Inhibitors; Pentoxifylline; Phosphodiesterase 5 Inhibitors; Potassium Salts; Potassium-Sparing Diuretics; Prostacyclin Analogues; Sirolimus; Temsirolimus; Thiazide Diuretics; TiZANidine; Tolvaptan; Trimethoprim

Decreased Effect

The levels/effects of Captopril may be decreased by: Antacids; Aprotinin; Herbs (Hypertensive Properties); Icatibant; Lanthanum; Methylphenidate; Nonsteroidal Anti-Inflammatory Agents; Peginterferon Alfa-2b; Salicylates; Yohimbine

Ethanol/Nutrition/Herb Interactions

Food: Captopril serum concentrations may be decreased if taken with food. Long-term use of captopril may lead to a zinc deficiency which can result in altered taste perception. Potassium supplements and/or potassium-containing salts may cause or worsen hyperkalemia. Management: Take on an empty stomach 1 hour before or 2 hours after meals. Consult prescriber before consuming a potassium-rich diet, potassium supplements, or salt substitutes.

Herb/Nutraceutical: Some herbal medications may worsen hypertension (eg, licorice); others may increase the antihypertensive effect of captopril (eg, shepherd's purse). Management: Avoid bayberry, blue cohosh, cayenne, ephedra, ginger, ginseng (American), kola, yohimbe, and licorice. Avoid black cohosh, california poppy, coleus, golden seal, hawthorn, mistletoe, periwinkle, quinine, and shepherd's purse.

Mechanism of Action Competitive inhibitor of angiotensin-converting enzyme (ACE); prevents conversion of angiotensin I to angiotensin II, a potent vasoconstrictor; results in lower levels of angiotensin II which causes an increase in plasma renin activity and a reduction in aldosterone secretion

Pharmacodynamics/Kinetics

Onset of action: Peak effect: Blood pressure reduction: 1-1.5 hours after dose

Duration: Dose related, may require several weeks of therapy before full hypotensive effect

Absorption: 60% to 75%; reduced 30% to 40% by food

Protein binding: 25% to 30%

Metabolism: 50%

Half-life elimination (renal and cardiac function dependent):

Adults, healthy volunteers: 1.9 hours; Heart failure: 2.06 hours; Anuria: 20-40 hours

Time to peak: 1 hour

Excretion: Urine (>95%) within 24 hours (40% to 50% as unchanged drug)

Dosage

Geriatric Refer to adult dosing. In the management of hypertension, consider lower initial doses and titrate to response (Aronow, 2011).

Adult Note: Titrate dose according to patient's response; use lowest effective dose.

Acute hypertension (urgency/emergency): Oral: 12.5-25 mg, may repeat as needed (may be given sublingually, but no therapeutic advantage demonstrated)

Heart failure: Oral:

Initial dose: 6.25-12.5 mg 3 times/day in conjunction with cardiac glycoside and diuretic therapy; initial dose depends upon patient's fluid/electrolyte status

Target dose: 50 mg 3 times/day

Hypertension: Oral: Initial dose: 25 mg 2-3 times/day (a lower initial dose of 12.5 mg 3 times/day may also be considered [VA Cooperative Study Group, 1984]); may increase by 12.5-25 mg/dose at 1- to 2-week intervals up to 50 mg 3 times/day; add thiazide diuretic, unless severe renal impairment coexists then consider loop diuretic, before further dosage increases or consider other treatment options; maximum dose: 150 mg 3 times/day

Usual dose range (JNC 7): 25-100 mg/day in 2 divided doses

LV dysfunction following MI: Oral: Initial: 6.25 mg; if tolerated, follow with 12.5 mg 3 times/day; then increase to 25 mg 3 times/day during next several days and then gradually increase over next several weeks to target dose of 50 mg 3 times/day (some dose schedules are more aggressive to achieve an increased goal dose within the first few days of initiation.)

Diabetic nephropathy: Oral: Initial: 25 mg 3 times/day. May be taken with other antihypertensive therapy if required to further lower blood pressure.

Renal Impairment

Manufacturers recommendations: Reduce initial daily dose and titrate slowly (1- to 2-week intervals) with smaller increments. Slowly back titrate to determine the minimum effective dose once the desired therapeutic effect has been reached.

Alternative recommendations (Aronoff 2007): Adults:
Cl$_{cr}$ 10-50 mL/minute: Administer at 75% of normal dose every 12-18 hours.
Cl$_{cr}$ <10 mL/minute: Administer at 50% of normal dose every 24 hours.
Intermittent hemodialysis (IHD): Administer after hemodialysis on dialysis days
Peritoneal dialysis: Dose for Cl$_{cr}$ 10-50 mL/minute; supplemental dose is not necessary

Administration Unstable in aqueous solutions; to prepare solution for oral administration, mix prior to administration and use within 10 minutes.

Monitoring Parameters BUN, electrolytes, serum creatinine; blood pressure. In patients with renal impairment and/or collagen vascular disease, closely monitor CBC with differential for the first 3 months of therapy and periodically thereafter.

Test Interactions Positive Coombs' [direct]; may cause false-positive results in urine acetone determinations using sodium nitroprusside reagent

Special Geriatric Considerations Due to frequent decreases in glomerular filtration (also Cl$_{cr}$) with aging, elderly patients may have exaggerated responses to ACE inhibitors; differences in clinical response due to hepatic changes are not observed. ACE inhibitors may be preferred agents in elderly patients with congestive heart failure and diabetes mellitus. Diabetic proteinuria is reduced and insulin sensitivity is enhanced. In general, the side effect profile is favorable in the elderly and causes little or no CNS confusion; use lowest dose recommendations initially. Many elderly may be volume depleted due to diuretic use and/or blunted thirst reflex resulting in inadequate fluid intake.

Dosage Forms Excipient information presented when available (limited, particularly for generics); consult specific product labeling.
Tablet, oral: 12.5 mg, 25 mg, 50 mg, 100 mg

Captopril and Hydrochlorothiazide (KAP toe pril & hye droe klor oh THYE a zide)

Related Information
Captopril *on page 282*
Hydrochlorothiazide *on page 933*
Index Terms Hydrochlorothiazide and Captopril
Generic Availability (U.S.) Yes
Pharmacologic Category Angiotensin-Converting Enzyme (ACE) Inhibitor; Diuretic, Thiazide
Use Management of hypertension
Dosage
Geriatric Refer to dosing in individual monographs.
Adult Hypertension, CHF: May be substituted for previously titrated dosages of the individual components; alternatively, may initiate as follows: Oral:
Initial: Single tablet (captopril 25 mg/hydrochlorothiazide 15 mg) taken once daily; daily dose of captopril should not exceed 150 mg; daily dose of hydrochlorothiazide should not exceed 50 mg
Renal Impairment May respond to smaller or less frequent doses.
Special Geriatric Considerations See individual agents. Combination products are not recommended as first-line treatment. Use only if doses of individual agents correspond to the combination available.

Divided doses of diuretics may increase the incidence of nocturia in the elderly.

Dosage Forms Excipient information presented when available (limited, particularly for generics); consult specific product labeling.
Tablet: 25/15: Captopril 25 mg and hydrochlorothiazide 15 mg; 25/25: Captopril 25 mg and hydrochlorothiazide 25 mg; 50/15: Captopril 50 mg and hydrochlorothiazide 15 mg; 50/25: Captopril 50 mg and hydrochlorothiazide 25 mg

♦ **Capzasin-HP® [OTC]** *see* Capsaicin *on page 280*
♦ **Capzasin-P® [OTC]** *see* Capsaicin *on page 280*
♦ **Carafate®** *see* Sucralfate *on page 1810*

Carbachol (KAR ba kole)

Related Information
Glaucoma Drug Therapy *on page 2115*
Medication Safety Issues
Sound-alike/look-alike issues:
Isopto® Carbachol may be confused with Isopto® Carpine
Brand Names: U.S. Isopto® Carbachol; Miostat®
Brand Names: Canada Isopto® Carbachol; Miostat®

◄ **Index Terms** Carbacholine; Carbamylcholine Chloride

Generic Availability (U.S.) No

Pharmacologic Category Cholinergic Agonist; Ophthalmic Agent, Antiglaucoma; Ophthalmic Agent, Miotic

Use Lowers intraocular pressure in the treatment of glaucoma; cause miosis during surgery

Contraindications Hypersensitivity to carbachol or any component of the formulation; acute iritis, acute inflammatory disease of the anterior chamber

Warnings/Precautions Use with caution in patients undergoing general anesthesia and in presence of corneal abrasion. Use caution with acute cardiac failure, asthma, peptic ulcer, hyperthyroidism, gastrointestinal spasm, urinary tract obstruction, and Parkinson's disease.

Adverse Reactions (Reflective of adult population; not specific for elderly) Frequency not defined.

Cardiovascular: Arrhythmia, flushing, hypotension, syncope

Central nervous system: Headache

Gastrointestinal: Abdominal cramps, diarrhea, epigastric distress, salivation, vomiting

Genitourinary: Urinary bladder tightness

Ocular: Bullous keratopathy, burning (transient), ciliary spasm, conjunctival injection, corneal clouding, irritation, postoperative iritis (following cataract extraction), retinal detachment, stinging (transient)

Respiratory: Asthma

Miscellaneous: Diaphoresis

Drug Interactions

Metabolism/Transport Effects None known.

Avoid Concomitant Use There are no known interactions where it is recommended to avoid concomitant use.

Increased Effect/Toxicity

The levels/effects of Carbachol may be increased by: Acetylcholinesterase Inhibitors; Beta-Blockers

Decreased Effect There are no known significant interactions involving a decrease in effect.

Stability

Intraocular: Store at room temperature of 15°C to 30°C (59°F to 86°F).

Topical: Store at 8°C to 27°C (46°F to 80°F).

Mechanism of Action Synthetic direct-acting cholinergic agent that causes miosis by stimulating muscarinic receptors in the eye

Pharmacodynamics/Kinetics

Ophthalmic instillation:

Onset of action: Miosis: 10-20 minutes

Duration: Reduction in intraocular pressure: 4-8 hours

Intraocular administration:

Onset of action: Miosis: 2-5 minutes

Duration: 24 hours

Dosage

Geriatric & Adult

Glaucoma: Ophthalmic: Instill 1-2 drops up to 3 times/day

Ophthalmic surgery (miosis): Intraocular: 0.5 mL instilled into anterior chamber before or after securing sutures

Administration Finger pressure should be applied on the lacrimal sac for 1-2 minutes following topical instillation; remove excess around the eye with a tissue

Special Geriatric Considerations Evaluate the patient's or caregiver's ability to safely administer the correct dose of ophthalmic medication.

Dosage Forms Excipient information presented when available (limited, particularly for generics); consult specific product labeling.

Solution, intraocular:

Miostat®: 0.01% (1.5 mL)

Solution, ophthalmic:

Isopto® Carbachol: 1.5% (15 mL); 3% (15 mL) [contains benzalkonium chloride]

◆ **Carbacholine** see Carbachol on page 285

CarBAMazepine (kar ba MAZ e peen)

Related Information

Beers Criteria – Potentially Inappropriate Medications for Geriatrics on page 2183

CARBAMAZEPINE

Medication Safety Issues
Sound-alike/look-alike issues:
CarBAMazepine may be confused with OXcarbazepine
Epitol® may be confused with Epinal®
TEGretol®, TEGretol®-XR may be confused with Mebaral®, Toprol-XL®, Toradol®, TRENtal®

BEERS Criteria medication:
This drug may be potentially inappropriate for use in geriatric patients (Quality of evidence - moderate; Strength of recommendation - strong).

Brand Names: U.S. Carbatrol®; Epitol®; Equetro®; TEGretol®; TEGretol®-XR
Brand Names: Canada Apo-Carbamazepine®; Dom-Carbamazepine; Mapezine®; Mylan-Carbamazepine CR; Nu-Carbamazepine; PMS-Carbamazepine; Sandoz-Carbamazepine; Taro-Carbamazepine Chewable; Tegretol®; Teva-Carbamazepine
Index Terms CBZ; SPD417
Generic Availability (U.S.) Yes
Pharmacologic Category Anticonvulsant, Miscellaneous
Use
Carbatrol®, Tegretol®, Tegretol®-XR: Partial seizures with complex symptomatology (psychomotor, temporal lobe), generalized tonic-clonic seizures (grand mal), mixed seizure patterns, trigeminal neuralgia
Equetro®: Acute manic and mixed episodes associated with bipolar 1 disorder
Unlabeled Use Treatment of restless leg syndrome and post-traumatic stress disorders
Medication Guide Available Yes
Contraindications Hypersensitivity to carbamazepine, tricyclic antidepressants, or any component of the formulation; bone marrow depression; with or within 14 days of MAO inhibitor use; concurrent use of nefazodone

Warnings/Precautions Hazardous agent - use appropriate precautions for handling and disposal. **[U.S. Boxed Warning]: Potentially fatal blood cell abnormalities have been reported.** Patients with a previous history of adverse hematologic reaction to any drug may be at increased risk.

Antiepileptics are associated with an increased risk of suicidal behavior/thoughts with use (regardless of indication); patients should be monitored for signs/symptoms of depression, suicidal tendencies, and other unusual behavior changes during therapy and instructed to inform their healthcare provider immediately if symptoms occur.

Administer carbamazepine with caution to patients with history of cardiac damage, ECG abnormalities (or at risk for ECG abnormalities), hepatic or renal disease. When used to treat bipolar disorder, the smallest effective dose is suggested to reduce the risk for overdose/suicide; high-risk patients should be monitored for suicidal ideations. Prescription should be written for the smallest quantity consistent with good patient care. May activate latent psychosis and/or cause confusion or agitation; elderly patients may be at an increased risk for psychiatric effects. Potentially serious, sometimes fatal multiorgan hypersensitivity reactions have been reported with some antiepileptic drugs; monitor for signs and symptoms of possible disparate manifestations associated with lymphatic, hepatic, renal, and/or hematologic organ systems; gradual discontinuation and conversion to alternate therapy may be required.

Carbamazepine is not effective in absence, myoclonic, or akinetic seizures; exacerbation of certain seizure types have been seen after initiation of carbamazepine therapy in children with mixed seizure disorders. Abrupt discontinuation is not recommended in patients being treated for seizures. Dizziness or drowsiness may occur; caution should be used when performing tasks which require alertness until the effects are known. Effects with other sedative drugs or ethanol may be potentiated. Carbamazepine has a high potential for drug interactions; use caution in patients taking strong CYP3A4 inducers or inhibitors or medications significantly metabolized via CYP1A2, 2B6, 2C9, 2C19, and 3A4. Coadministration of carbamazepine and nefazodone may lead to insufficient plasma levels of nefazodone; combination is contraindicated. Carbamazepine has mild anticholinergic activity; use with caution in patients with increased intraocular pressure, or sensitivity to anticholinergic effects. Severe dermatologic reactions, including toxic epidermal necrolysis and Stevens-Johnson syndrome, although rarely reported, have resulted in fatalities. **[U.S. Boxed Warning]: Use caution and screen for the genetic susceptibility genotype (*HLA-B*1502* allele) in Asian patients. Patients with a positive result should not be started on carbamazepine.** Discontinue if there are any signs of hypersensitivity. Use caution in elderly patients; may cause or exacerbate syndrome of inappropriate antidiuretic hormone secretion or hyponatremia; monitor sodium closely with initiation or dosage adjustments in older adults (Beers Criteria).

Administration of the suspension will yield higher peak and lower trough serum levels than an equal dose of the tablet form; consider a lower starting dose given more frequently (same total daily dose) when using the suspension.

Adverse Reactions (Reflective of adult population; not specific for elderly) Frequency not defined, unless otherwise specified.

Cardiovascular: Arrhythmias, AV block, bradycardia, chest pain (bipolar use), CHF, edema, hyper-/hypotension, lymphadenopathy, syncope, thromboembolism, thrombophlebitis

Central nervous system: Amnesia (bipolar use), anxiety (bipolar use), aseptic meningitis (case report), ataxia (bipolar use 15%), confusion, depression (bipolar use), dizziness (bipolar use 44%), fatigue, headache (bipolar use 22%), sedation, slurred speech, somnolence (bipolar use 32%)

Dermatologic: Alopecia, alterations in skin pigmentation, erythema multiforme, exfoliative dermatitis, photosensitivity reaction, pruritus (bipolar use 8%), purpura, rash, Stevens-Johnson syndrome, toxic epidermal necrolysis, urticaria

Endocrine & metabolic: Chills, fever, hyponatremia, syndrome of inappropriate ADH secretion (SIADH)

Gastrointestinal: Abdominal pain, anorexia, constipation, diarrhea, dyspepsia (bipolar use), gastric distress, nausea (bipolar use 29%), pancreatitis, vomiting (bipolar use 18%), xerostomia (bipolar use)

Genitourinary: Azotemia, impotence, renal failure, urinary frequency, urinary retention

Hematologic: Acute intermittent porphyria, agranulocytosis, aplastic anemia, bone marrow suppression, eosinophilia, leukocytosis, leukopenia, pancytopenia, thrombocytopenia

Hepatic: Abnormal liver function tests, hepatic failure, hepatitis, jaundice

Neuromuscular & skeletal: Back pain, pain (bipolar use 12%), peripheral neuritis, weakness

Ocular: Blurred vision, conjunctivitis, lens opacities, nystagmus

Otic: Hyperacusis, tinnitus

Miscellaneous: Diaphoresis, hypersensitivity (including multiorgan reactions, may include disorders mimicking lymphoma, eosinophilia, hepatosplenomegaly, vasculitis); infection (bipolar use 12%)

Drug Interactions

Metabolism/Transport Effects Substrate of CYP2C8 (minor), CYP3A4 (major); **Note:** Assignment of Major/Minor substrate status based on clinically relevant drug interaction potential; **Induces** CYP1A2 (strong), CYP2B6 (strong), CYP2C19 (strong), CYP2C8 (strong), CYP2C9 (strong), CYP3A4 (strong), P-glycoprotein

Avoid Concomitant Use

Avoid concomitant use of CarBAMazepine with any of the following: Axitinib; Azelastine; Azelastine (Nasal); Boceprevir; Bortezomib; CloZAPine; Conivaptan; Crizotinib; Dabigatran Etexilate; Dronedarone; Etravirine; Everolimus; Lapatinib; Lurasidone; MAO Inhibitors; Mifepristone; Mirtazapine; Nefazodone; Nilotinib; Paraldehyde; Pazopanib; Praziquantel; Ranolazine; Rilpivirine; Rivaroxaban; Roflumilast; RomiDEPsin; SORAfenib; Telaprevir; Ticagrelor; Tolvaptan; Toremifene; TraMADol; Vandetanib; Voriconazole

Increased Effect/Toxicity

CarBAMazepine may increase the levels/effects of: Adenosine; Alcohol (Ethyl); Azelastine; Azelastine (Nasal); Buprenorphine; ClomiPRAMINE; CloZAPine; CNS Depressants; Desmopressin; Fosphenytoin; Ifosfamide; Lithium; MAO Inhibitors; Methotrimeprazine; Metyrosine; Mirtazapine; Paraldehyde; Phenytoin

The levels/effects of CarBAMazepine may be increased by: Allopurinol; Antifungal Agents (Azole Derivatives, Systemic); Calcium Channel Blockers (Nondihydropyridine); Carbonic Anhydrase Inhibitors; Cimetidine; Conivaptan; CYP3A4 Inhibitors (Moderate); CYP3A4 Inhibitors (Strong); Danazol; Darunavir; Dasatinib; Droperidol; Fluconazole; Grapefruit Juice; HydrOXYzine; Isoniazid; Ivacaftor; LamoTRIgine; Macrolide Antibiotics; Methotrimeprazine; Mifepristone; Nefazodone; Protease Inhibitors; QuiNINE; Selective Serotonin Reuptake Inhibitors; Telaprevir; Thiazide Diuretics; TraMADol; Zolpidem

Decreased Effect

CarBAMazepine may decrease the levels/effects of: Acetaminophen; Apixaban; ARIPiprazole; Axitinib; Bendamustine; Benzodiazepines (metabolized by oxidation); Boceprevir; Bortezomib; Brentuximab Vedotin; Calcium Channel Blockers (Dihydropyridine); Calcium Channel Blockers (Nondihydropyridine); Caspofungin; CloZAPine; Contraceptives (Estrogens); Contraceptives (Progestins); Crizotinib; CycloSPORINE; CycloSPORINE (Systemic); CYP1A2 Substrates; CYP2B6 Substrates; CYP2C19 Substrates; CYP2C8 Substrates; CYP2C9 Substrates; CYP3A4 Substrates; Dabigatran Etexilate; Dasatinib; Diclofenac; Divalproex; Doxycycline; Dronedarone; Etravirine; Everolimus; Exemestane; Felbamate; Flunarizine; Fosphenytoin; Gefitinib; GuanFACINE; Haloperidol; Imatinib; Irinotecan; Ixabepilone; Lacosamide; LamoTRIgine; Lapatinib; Linagliptin; Lopinavir; Lurasidone; Maraviroc; Mebendazole; Methadone; MethylPREDNISolone; Mifepristone; Nefazodone; Nilotinib; Paliperidone; Pazopanib; P-glycoprotein/ABCB1 Substrates; Phenytoin; Praziquantel; Protease Inhibitors; QuiNINE; Ranolazine; Rilpivirine; RisperiDONE; Rivaroxaban; Roflumilast;

RomiDEPsin; Rufinamide; Saxagliptin; Selective Serotonin Reuptake Inhibitors; SORAfenib; SUNItinib; Tadalafil; Telaprevir; Temsirolimus; Theophylline Derivatives; Thyroid Products; Ticagrelor; Tolvaptan; Topiramate; Toremifene; TraMADol; Treprostinil; Tricyclic Antidepressants; Ulipristal; Valproic Acid; Vandetanib; Vecuronium; Vemurafenib; Vitamin K Antagonists; Voriconazole; Ziprasidone; Zolpidem; Zuclopenthixol

The levels/effects of CarBAMazepine may be decreased by: CYP3A4 Inducers (Strong); Deferasirox; Divalproex; Felbamate; Fosphenytoin; Herbs (CYP3A4 Inducers); Ketorolac; Ketorolac (Nasal); Ketorolac (Systemic); Mefloquine; Methylfolate; Phenytoin; Rufinamide; Theophylline Derivatives; Tocilizumab; TraMADol; Valproic Acid

Ethanol/Nutrition/Herb Interactions

Ethanol: Ethanol may increase CNS depression. Management: Avoid concurrent use of ethanol.

Food: Carbamazepine serum levels may be increased if taken with food and/or grapefruit juice. Management Avoid concurrent ingestion of grapefruit juice. Maintain adequate hydration, unless instructed to restrict fluid intake.

Herb/Nutraceutical: Evening primrose may decrease seizure threshold. Valerian, St John's wort, kava kava, and gotu kola may increase CNS depression. Management: Avoid evening primrose. Avoid valerian, St John's wort, kava kava, and gotu kola.

Mechanism of Action In addition to anticonvulsant effects, carbamazepine has anticholinergic, antineuralgic, antidiuretic, muscle relaxant, antimanic, antidepressive, and antiarrhythmic properties; may depress activity in the nucleus ventralis of the thalamus or decrease synaptic transmission or decrease summation of temporal stimulation leading to neural discharge by limiting influx of sodium ions across cell membrane or other unknown mechanisms; stimulates the release of ADH and potentiates its action in promoting reabsorption of water; chemically related to tricyclic antidepressants

Pharmacodynamics/Kinetics

Absorption: Slow

Distribution: V_d: Adults: 0.59-2 L/kg

Protein binding: Carbamazepine: 75% to 90%; Epoxide metabolite: 50%

Metabolism: Hepatic via CYP3A4 to active epoxide metabolite; induces hepatic enzymes to increase metabolism

Bioavailability: 85%

Half-life elimination: **Note:** Half-life is variable because of autoinduction which is usually complete 3-5 weeks after initiation of a fixed carbamazepine regimen.

Carbamazepine: Initial: 25-65 hours; Extended release: 35-40 hours; Multiple doses: Adults: 12-17 hours

Epoxide metabolite: Initial: 25-43 hours

Time to peak, serum: Unpredictable:

Immediate release: Suspension: 1.5 hour; tablet: 4-5 hours

Extended release: Carbatrol®, Equetro®: 12-26 hours (single dose), 4-8 hours (multiple doses); Tegretol®-XR: 3-12 hours

Excretion: Urine 72% (1% to 3% as unchanged drug); feces (28%)

Dosage

Geriatric & Adult Dosage must be adjusted according to patient's response and serum concentrations. Administer tablets (chewable or conventional) in 2-3 divided doses daily and suspension in 4 divided doses daily. Oral:

Epilepsy: Initial: 400 mg/day in 2 divided doses (tablets or extended release tablets) or 4 divided doses (oral suspension); increase by up to 200 mg/day at weekly intervals using a twice daily regimen of extended release tablets or capsules, or a 3-4 times/day regimen of other formulations until optimal response and therapeutic levels are achieved; usual dose: 800-1200 mg/day

Maximum recommended dose: 1600 mg/day; however, some patients have required up to 1.6-2.4 g/day

Trigeminal or glossopharyngeal neuralgia: Initial: 200 mg/day in 2 divided doses (tablets, extended release tablets, or extended release capsules) or 4 divided doses (oral suspension) with food, gradually increasing in increments of 200 mg/day as needed.

Maintenance: Usual: 400-800 mg daily in 2 divided doses (tablets, extended release tablets, or extended release capsules) or 4 divided doses (oral suspension); maximum dose: 1200 mg/day

Bipolar disorder: Initial: 400 mg/day in 2 divided doses (tablets, extended release tablets, or extended release capsules) or 4 divided doses (oral suspension), may adjust by 200 mg/day increments; maximum dose: 1600 mg/day.

Note: Equetro® is the only formulation specifically approved by the FDA for the management of bipolar disorder.

◀ **Renal Impairment** Dosage adjustments are not required or recommended in the manufacturer's labeling; however, the following guidelines have been used by some clinicians (Aronoff, 2007):

Adults:

GFR <10 mL/minute: Administer 75% of dose.

Hemodialysis, peritoneal dialysis: Administer 75% of dose.

Continuous renal replacement therapy (CRRT): Adults: No dosage adjustment recommended.

Hepatic Impairment Use with caution in hepatic impairment; metabolized primarily in the liver.

Administration

Suspension: Must be given on a 3-4 times/day schedule versus tablets which can be given 2-4 times/day. Since a given dose of suspension will produce higher peak and lower trough levels than the same dose given as the tablet form, patients given the suspension should be started on lower doses given more frequently (same total daily dose) and increased slowly to avoid unwanted side effects. When carbamazepine suspension has been combined with chlorpromazine or thioridazine solutions, a precipitate forms which may result in loss of effect. Therefore, it is recommended that the carbamazepine suspension dosage form not be administered at the same time with other liquid medicinal agents or diluents. Should be administered with meals.

Extended release capsule (Carbatrol®, Equetro®): Consists of three different types of beads: Immediate release, extended-release, and enteric release. The bead types are combined in a ratio to allow twice daily dosing. May be opened and contents sprinkled over food such as a teaspoon of applesauce; may be administered with or without food; do not crush or chew.

Extended release tablet: Should be inspected for damage. Damaged extended release tablets (without release portal) should not be administered. Should be administered with meals; swallow whole, do not crush or chew.

Monitoring Parameters CBC with platelet count, reticulocytes, serum iron, lipid panel, liver function tests, urinalysis, BUN, serum carbamazepine levels, thyroid function tests, serum sodium; ophthalmic exams (pupillary reflexes); observe patient for excessive sedation, especially when instituting or increasing therapy; signs of rash; *HLA-B*1502* genotype screening prior to therapy initiation in patients of Asian descent; suicidality (eg, suicidal thoughts, depression, behavioral changes)

Reference Range

Timing of serum samples: Absorption is slow, peak levels occur 6-8 hours after ingestion of the first dose; the half-life ranges from 8-60 hours, therefore, steady-state is achieved in 2-5 days

Therapeutic levels: 4-12 mcg/mL (SI: 17-51 micromole/L)

Toxic concentration: >15 mcg/mL; patients who require higher levels of 8-12 mcg/mL (SI: 34-51 micromole/L) should be watched closely. Side effects including CNS effects occur commonly at higher dosage levels. If other anticonvulsants are given therapeutic range is 4-8 mcg/mL.

Test Interactions May cause false-positive serum TCA screen

Special Geriatric Considerations Elderly may have increased risk of SIADH-like syndrome. Elderly are more susceptible to carbamazepine-induced confusion and agitation, AV block, and bradycardia.

This medication is considered to be potentially inappropriate in this patient population (Beers Criteria: Quality of evidence - moderate; Strength of recommendation - strong).

Dosage Forms Excipient information presented when available (limited, particularly for generics); consult specific product labeling.

Capsule, extended release, oral: 100 mg, 200 mg, 300 mg

Carbatrol®: 100 mg, 200 mg, 300 mg

Equetro®: 100 mg, 200 mg, 300 mg

Suspension, oral: 100 mg/5 mL (5 mL, 10 mL, 450 mL)

TEGretol®: 100 mg/5 mL (450 mL) [contains propylene glycol; citrus-vanilla flavor]

Tablet, oral: 200 mg

Epitol®: 200 mg [scored]

TEGretol®: 200 mg [scored]

Tablet, chewable, oral: 100 mg

TEGretol®: 100 mg [scored]

Tablet, extended release, oral: 200 mg, 400 mg

TEGretol®-XR: 100 mg, 200 mg, 400 mg

Carbamide Peroxide (KAR ba mide per OKS ide)

Brand Names: U.S. Auraphene B® [OTC]; Auro® [OTC]; Cankaid® [OTC]; Debrox® [OTC]; E-R-O® [OTC]; Gly-Oxide® [OTC]; Murine® Ear Wax Removal Kit [OTC]; Murine® Ear [OTC]; Otix® [OTC]; Wax Away [OTC]

Index Terms Urea Peroxide

Generic Availability (U.S.) Yes

Pharmacologic Category Anti-inflammatory, Locally Applied; Otic Agent, Cerumenolytic

Use Relief of minor inflammation of gums, oral mucosal surfaces, and lips including canker sores and dental irritation; emulsify and disperse ear wax

Dosage

Geriatric & Adult

Minor inflammation of gums, oral mucosal surfaces, and lips: Topical: Oral solution (should not be used for >7 days): Apply several drops undiluted on affected area 4 times/ day after meals and at bedtime; expectorate after 2-3 minutes **or** place 10 drops onto tongue, mix with saliva, swish for several minutes, expectorate

Ear wax removal: Otic: Tilt head sideways and instill 5-10 drops twice daily up to 4 days, tip of applicator should not enter ear canal; keep drops in ear for several minutes by keeping head tilted and placing cotton in ear

Special Geriatric Considerations Avoid contact with hearing aids.

Dosage Forms Excipient information presented when available (limited, particularly for generics); consult specific product labeling.

Liquid, oral: 10% (60 mL)
 Cankaid®: 10% (15 mL)
 Gly-Oxide®: 10% (15 mL, 60 mL)
Solution, otic [drops]: 6.5% (15 mL)
 Auraphene B®: 6.5% (15 mL)
 Auro®: 6.5% (22.2 mL)
 Debrox®: 6.5% (15 mL, 30 mL)
 E-R-O®: 6.5% (15 mL) [ethanol free]
 Murine® Ear: 6.5% (15 mL) [contains ethanol 6.3%]
 Murine® Ear Wax Removal Kit: 6.5% (15 mL) [contains ethanol 6.3%]
 Otix®: 6.5% (15 mL)
 Wax Away: 6.5% (15 mL)

♦ **Carbamylcholine Chloride** see Carbachol on page 285
♦ **Carbatrol®** see CarBAMazepine on page 286

Carbidopa (kar bi DOE pa)

Medication Safety Issues

International issues:
 Lodosyn [U.S.] may be confused with Lidosen brand name for lidocaine [Italy]

Brand Names: U.S. Lodosyn®

Generic Availability (U.S.) No

Pharmacologic Category Anti-Parkinson's Agent, Decarboxylase Inhibitor

Use Given with carbidopa-levodopa in the treatment of parkinsonism to enable a lower dosage of levodopa to be used and a more rapid response to be obtained and to decrease side effects; use with carbidopa-levodopa in patients requiring additional carbidopa; has no effect without levodopa

Contraindications Hypersensitivity to carbidopa or any component of the formulation; use of nonselective MAO inhibitor therapy with or within prior 14 days (however, may be administered concomitantly with the manufacturer's recommended dose of an MAO inhibitor with selectivity for MAO type B); narrow-angle glaucoma; history of melanoma or undiagnosed skin lesions

Warnings/Precautions Use with caution in patients with history of cardiovascular disease (including myocardial infarction and arrhythmias), psychosis, pulmonary diseases (such as asthma), endocrine disease, peptic ulcer disease, as well as in severe renal and hepatic dysfunction. Observe patients closely for development of depression with concomitant suicidal tendencies. Use with extreme caution in patients with psychotic disorders; observe patients closely for development of depression with concomitant suicidal tendencies.

Dopamine agonists have been associated with compulsive behaviors and/or loss of impulse control, which has manifested as pathological gambling, libido increases (hypersexuality), and/or binge eating. Causality has not been established, and controversy exists as to whether this phenomenon is related to the underlying disease, prior behaviors/addictions and/or drug therapy. Dose reduction or discontinuation of therapy has been reported to reverse these behaviors in some, but not all cases. Risk for melanoma development is increased in Parkinson's disease patients; drug causation or factors contributing to risk have not been established. Patients should be monitored closely and periodic skin examinations should be performed. Use with caution in patients with wide-angle glaucoma; monitor IOP carefully. Dopaminergic agents have been associated with a syndrome resembling neuroleptic malignant syndrome on abrupt withdrawal or significant dosage reduction after long-term use. Protein in the diet should be distributed throughout the day to avoid fluctuations in levodopa absorption. Carbidopa has no antiparkinsonian activity when administered alone.

Adverse Reactions (Reflective of adult population; not specific for elderly) Adverse reactions are associated with concomitant administration with levodopa.

Cardiovascular: Arrhythmia, chest pain, edema, flushing, hypotension, hypertension, MI, orthostatic hypotension, palpitation, phlebitis, syncope

Central nervous system: Agitation, anxiety, ataxia, confusion, delusions, dementia, depression (with or without suicidal tendencies), disorientation, dizziness, dreams abnormal, EPS, euphoria, faintness, falling, fatigue, gait abnormalities, headache, hallucinations, impulse control symptoms, insomnia, malaise, memory impairment, mental acuity decreased, nervousness, neuroleptic malignant syndrome, nightmares, on-off phenomena, paranoid ideation, pathological gambling, psychosis, seizure (causal relationship not established), somnolence

Dermatologic: Alopecia, malignant melanoma, rash

Endocrine & metabolic: Hot flashes, hyperglycemia, hypokalemia, libido increased (including hypersexuality), uric acid increased

Gastrointestinal: Abdominal pain, abdominal distress, anorexia, bruxism, constipation, diarrhea, discoloration of saliva, duodenal ulcer, dyspepsia, dysphagia, flatulence, GI bleeding, heartburn, nausea, sialorrhea, taste alterations, tongue burning sensation, weight gain/loss, vomiting, xerostomia

Genitourinary: Discoloration of urine, glycosuria, urinary frequency, priapism, proteinuria, urinary incontinence, urinary retention, urinary tract infection

Hematologic: Agranulocytosis, anemia, Coombs' test abnormal, hematocrit decreased, hemoglobin decreased, hemolytic anemia, leukopenia, thrombocytopenia

Hepatic: Alkaline phosphatase abnormal, ALT abnormal, AST abnormal, bilirubin abnormal, LDH abnormal

Neuromuscular & skeletal: Back pain, dyskinesias (including choreiform, dystonic and other involuntary movements), leg pain, muscle cramps, muscle twitching, numbness, paresthesia, peripheral neuropathy, shoulder pain, tremor increased, trismus, weakness

Ocular: Blepharospasm, blurred vision, diplopia, Horner's syndrome reactivation, mydriasis, oculogyric crises (may be associated with acute dystonic reactions)

Renal: BUN increased, serum creatinine increased

Respiratory: Cough, dyspnea, hoarseness, pharyngeal pain, upper respiratory infection

Miscellaneous: Discoloration of sweat, diaphoresis increased, hiccups, hypersensitivity reactions (including angioedema, pruritus, urticaria, bullous lesions [including pemphigus-like reactions], Henoch-Schönlein purpura)

Drug Interactions

Metabolism/Transport Effects None known.

Avoid Concomitant Use There are no known interactions where it is recommended to avoid concomitant use.

Increased Effect/Toxicity There are no known significant interactions involving an increase in effect.

Decreased Effect There are no known significant interactions involving a decrease in effect.

Stability Store at room temperature of 25°C (77°F); excursions permitted to 15°C to 30°C (59°F to 86°F).

Mechanism of Action Carbidopa is a peripheral decarboxylase inhibitor with little or no pharmacological activity when given alone in usual doses. It inhibits the peripheral decarboxylation of levodopa to dopamine; and as it does not cross the blood-brain barrier, unlike levodopa, effective brain concentrations of dopamine are produced with lower doses of levodopa. At the same time, reduced peripheral formation of dopamine reduces peripheral side-effects, notably nausea and vomiting, and cardiac arrhythmias, although the dyskinesias and adverse mental effects associated with levodopa therapy tend to develop earlier.

Pharmacodynamics/Kinetics Distribution: Does not cross the blood-brain barrier

Dosage

Geriatric & Adult Parkinson's disease: Oral: Note: Optimal daily dosage determined by careful titration; generally if carbidopa is ≥70 mg/day, a 1:10 proportion of carbidopa:levodopa provides the most patient response.

Carbidopa augmentation in patients receiving carbidopa-levodopa:
Patients receiving Sinemet® 10/100: 25 mg carbidopa daily with first daily dose of Sinemet® 10/100; if necessary, 12.5-25 carbidopa mg may be given with each subsequent dose of Sinemet® 10/100; maximum: 200 mg carbidopa/day (including carbidopa from Sinemet®)
Patients receiving Sinemet® 25/250 or Sinemet® 25/100: 25 mg carbidopa with any dose of Sinemet® 25/250 or Sinemet® 25/100 throughout the day; maximum: 200 mg carbidopa/day (including carbidopa from Sinemet®)
Individual titration of carbidopa and levodopa: Initial: 25 mg carbidopa 3-4 times/day; administer at the same time as levodopa, initial dose of levodopa should be 20% to 25% of the previous levodopa dose in carbidopa-naive patients; first dose of carbidopa should be taken ≥12 hours after the last dose of levodopa in carbidopa-naive patients; increase or decrease dose by 1/2 or 1 tablet/day

Administration Administer with meals to decrease GI upset.

Monitoring Parameters Signs and symptoms of Parkinson's disease; CBC, liver function tests, renal function; blood pressure, mental status; signs and symptoms of neuroleptic malignant syndrome if abrupt discontinuation required (as with surgery); periodic intraocular pressure (in patients with wide-angle glaucoma)

Test Interactions False-positive reaction for urinary glucose with Clinitest®; false-negative reaction using Clinistix®; false-positive urine ketones with Acetest®, Ketostix®, Labstix®

Special Geriatric Considerations No specific information for use in elderly.

Dosage Forms Excipient information presented when available (limited, particularly for generics); consult specific product labeling.
Tablet, oral:
Lodosyn®: 25 mg [scored]

Carbidopa and Levodopa (kar bi DOE pa & lee voe DOE pa)

Related Information
Antiparkinsonian Agents *on page 2101*
Carbidopa *on page 291*

Medication Safety Issues
Sound-alike/look-alike issues:
Sinemet® may be confused with Serevent®
International issues:
Zimox: Brand name for carbidopa and levodopa [Greece], but also the brand name for amoxicillin [Italy]
Zimox [Greece] may be confused with Diamox which is a brand name for acetazolamide [Canada and multiple international markets]

Brand Names: U.S. Parcopa®; Sinemet®; Sinemet® CR

Brand Names: Canada Apo-Levocarb®; Apo-Levocarb® CR; Dom-Levo-Carbidopa; Duodopa™; Levocarb CR; Nu-Levocarb; PRO-Levocarb; Sinemet®; Sinemet® CR; Teva-Levocarbidopa

Index Terms Levodopa and Carbidopa

Generic Availability (U.S.) Yes

Pharmacologic Category Anti-Parkinson's Agent, Decarboxylase Inhibitor; Anti-Parkinson's Agent, Dopamine Precursor

Use Idiopathic Parkinson's disease; postencephalitic parkinsonism; symptomatic parkinsonism

Duodopa™ intestinal gel: Canadian labeling (not available in U.S.): Treatment of advanced levodopa-responsive Parkinson's disease in which severe motor symptoms are not controlled by other Parkinson's agents

Unlabeled Use Restless leg syndrome

Prescribing and Access Restrictions Duodopa™ intestinal gel (Canadian labeling; product not available in U.S.): In Canada, the Duodopa™ Education Program is a risk mitigation program established to provide safe and effective use of Duodopa™ in advanced Parkinson's patients. The program involves:
- Education of prescribing neurologists and other healthcare providers on suitable candidates for treatment, surgical procedures (PEG tube placement), and follow-up care including infusion device education.
- Distribution of educational materials to patients and caregivers describing Duodopa™ intestinal gel and its proper use, PEG tube placement, and complications associated with the mode of administration and/or PEG tube placement.

Contraindications Hypersensitivity to levodopa, carbidopa, or any component of the formulation; narrow-angle glaucoma; use of MAO inhibitors within prior 14 days (however, may be administered concomitantly with the manufacturer's recommended dose of an MAO inhibitor with selectivity for MAO type B); history of melanoma or undiagnosed skin lesions

Canadian labeling: Additional contraindications: Clinical or laboratory evidence of uncompensated cardiovascular, cerebrovascular, endocrine, renal, hepatic, hematologic or pulmonary disease; when administration of a sympathomimetic amine (eg, epinephrine, norepinephrine or isoproterenol) is contraindicated; intestinal gel therapy in patients with any condition preventing the required placement of a PEG tube for administration.

Warnings/Precautions Use with caution in patients with history of cardiovascular disease (including myocardial infarction and arrhythmias), pulmonary diseases (such as asthma), psychosis, wide-angle glaucoma, peptic ulcer disease, seizure disorder or prone to seizures, and in severe renal and hepatic dysfunction. Use with caution when interpreting plasma/urine catecholamine levels; falsely diagnosed pheochromocytoma has been rarely reported. Severe cases or rhabdomyolysis have been reported. Sudden discontinuation of levodopa may cause a worsening of Parkinson's disease. Elderly may be more sensitive to CNS effects of levodopa. May cause or exacerbate dyskinesias. Patients have reported falling asleep while engaging in activities of daily living; this has been reported to occur without significant warning signs. May cause orthostatic hypotension; Parkinson's disease patients appear to have an impaired capacity to respond to a postural challenge; use with caution in patients at risk of hypotension (such as those receiving antihypertensive drugs) or where transient hypotensive episodes would be poorly tolerated (cardiovascular disease or cerebrovascular disease). Observe patients closely for development of depression with concomitant suicidal tendencies.

Dopamine agonists have been associated with compulsive behaviors and/or loss of impulse control, which has manifested as pathological gambling, libido increases (hypersexuality), and/or binge eating. Causality has not been established, and controversy exists as to whether this phenomenon is related to the underlying disease, prior behaviors/addictions and/or drug therapy. Dose reduction or discontinuation of therapy has been reported to reverse these behaviors in some, but not all cases. Risk for melanoma development is increased in Parkinson's disease patients; drug causation or factors contributing to risk have not been established. Patients should be monitored closely and periodic skin examinations should be performed. Dopaminergic agents have been associated with a syndrome resembling neuroleptic malignant syndrome on abrupt withdrawal or significant dosage reduction after long-term use. Protein in the diet should be distributed throughout the day to avoid fluctuations in levodopa absorption.

Intestinal gel (available in Canada, not available in U.S.): Product should be prescribed only by neurologists experienced in the treatment of Parkinson's disease and who have completed the Duodopa™ Education Program. Response to levodopa/carbidopa intestinal gel therapy should be assessed with a test period (~3 days) of administration via a temporary nasoduodenal tube prior to placement of a percutaneous endoscopic gastrostomy (PEG) tube for permanent access and administration. Sudden deterioration in therapy response with recurring motor symptoms may indicate PEG tube complications (eg, displacement) or obstruction of the infusion device. Tube or infusion device complications may require initiation of oral levodopa/carbidopa therapy until complications are resolved. Discontinue therapy 2-3 hours prior to surgical procedures requiring general anesthesia, if possible. May resume therapy postoperatively when oral fluid intake is permitted.

Adverse Reactions (Reflective of adult population; not specific for elderly) Frequency not defined.

Cardiovascular: Arrhythmia, chest pain, edema, flushing, hypotension, hypertension, MI, orthostatic hypotension, palpitation, phlebitis, syncope

Central nervous system: Agitation, anxiety, ataxia, confusion, delusions, dementia, depression (with or without suicidal tendencies), disorientation, dizziness, dreams abnormal, EPS, euphoria, faintness, falling, fatigue, gait abnormalities, headache, hallucinations, impulse control symptoms, insomnia, malaise, memory impairment, mental acuity decreased, nervousness, neuroleptic malignant syndrome, nightmares, on-off phenomena, paranoid ideation, pathological gambling, psychosis, seizure (causal relationship not established), somnolence

Dermatologic: Alopecia, malignant melanoma, rash

Endocrine & metabolic: Hot flashes, hyperglycemia, hypokalemia, libido increased (including hypersexuality), uric acid increased

Gastrointestinal: Abdominal pain, abdominal distress, anorexia, bruxism, constipation, diarrhea, discoloration of saliva, duodenal ulcer, dyspepsia, dysphagia, flatulence, GI bleeding, heartburn, nausea, sialorrhea, taste alterations, tongue burning sensation, weight gain/loss, vomiting, xerostomia

Genitourinary: Discoloration of urine, glycosuria, urinary frequency, priapism, proteinuria, urinary incontinence, urinary retention, urinary tract infection

Hematologic: Agranulocytosis, anemia, Coombs' test abnormal, hematocrit decreased, hemoglobin decreased, hemolytic anemia, leukopenia

Hepatic: Alkaline phosphatase abnormal, ALT abnormal, AST abnormal, bilirubin abnormal, LDH abnormal

Neuromuscular & skeletal: Back pain, dyskinesias (including choreiform, dystonic and other involuntary movements), leg pain, muscle cramps, muscle twitching, numbness, paresthesia, peripheral neuropathy, shoulder pain, tremor increased, trismus, weakness

Ocular: Blepharospasm, blurred vision, diplopia, Horner's syndrome reactivation, mydriasis, oculogyric crises (may be associated with acute dystonic reactions)

Renal: Difficult urination

Respiratory: Cough, dyspnea, hoarseness, pharyngeal pain, upper respiratory infection

Miscellaneous: Discoloration of sweat, diaphoresis increased, hiccups, hypersensitivity reactions (angioedema, pruritus, urticaria, bullous lesions [including pemphigus-like reactions], Henoch-Schönlein purpura)

Drug Interactions

Metabolism/Transport Effects None known.

Avoid Concomitant Use There are no known interactions where it is recommended to avoid concomitant use.

Increased Effect/Toxicity

Carbidopa and Levodopa may increase the levels/effects of: MAO Inhibitors

The levels/effects of Carbidopa and Levodopa may be increased by: MAO Inhibitors; Methylphenidate; Sapropterin

Decreased Effect

Carbidopa and Levodopa may decrease the levels/effects of: Antipsychotics (Typical)

The levels/effects of Carbidopa and Levodopa may be decreased by: Antipsychotics (Atypical); Antipsychotics (Typical); Fosphenytoin; Glycopyrrolate; Iron Salts; Methionine; Metoclopramide; Phenytoin; Pyridoxine

Ethanol/Nutrition/Herb Interactions

Ethanol: Avoid ethanol (due to CNS depression).

Food: Avoid high protein diets due to potential for impaired levodopa absorption; levodopa competes with certain amino acids for transport across the gut wall or across the blood-brain barrier.

Herb/Nutraceutical: Avoid kava kava (may decrease effects). Pyridoxine (vitamin B_6) in doses >10-25 mg (for levodopa alone) may decrease efficacy. Iron supplements or iron-containing multivitamins may reduce absorption of levodopa.

Stability

Tablet: Store at 20°C to 25°C (68°F to 77°F); excursions permitted between 15°C to 30°C (59°F to 86°F). Protect from light and moisture.

Intestinal gel (Canadian labeling; not available in U.S.): Store in refrigerator at 2°C to 8°C (36°F to 46°F). Keep in outer carton to protect from light. Cassettes are for single use only and should be discarded daily following infusion (up to 16 hours).

Mechanism of Action Parkinson's symptoms are due to a lack of striatal dopamine; levodopa circulates in the plasma to the blood-brain-barrier (BBB), where it crosses, to be converted by striatal enzymes to dopamine; carbidopa inhibits the peripheral plasma breakdown of levodopa by inhibiting its decarboxylation, and thereby increases available levodopa at the BBB

Pharmacodynamics/Kinetics

Carbidopa:
Absorption: Oral: 40% to 70%
Protein binding: 36%
Half-life: 1-2 hours
Elimination: Excreted unchanged

Levodopa:
Absorption: May be decreased if given with a high protein meal
Half-life: 1.2-2.3 hours
Elimination: Primarily in urine (80%) as dopamine, norepinephrine, and homovanillic acid

Dosage

Geriatric & Adult

Parkinson's disease:

Oral:

Immediate release tablet, orally-disintegrating tablet:

Initial: Carbidopa 25 mg/levodopa 100 mg 3 times/day

Dosage adjustment: Alternate tablet strengths may be substituted according to individual carbidopa/levodopa requirements. Increase by 1 tablet every 1-2 days as necessary, except when using the carbidopa 25 mg/levodopa 250 mg tablets where increases should be made using 1/2-1 tablet every 1-2 days. Use of more than 1 dosage strength or dosing 4 times/day may be required (maximum: 8 tablets of any strength/day or 200 mg of carbidopa and 2000 mg of levodopa)

Controlled release tablet:

Patients not currently receiving levodopa: Initial: Carbidopa 50 mg/levodopa 200 mg 2 times/day, at intervals not <6 hours

Patients converting from immediate release formulation to controlled release: Initial: Dosage should be substituted at an amount that provides ~10% more of levodopa/day; total calculated dosage is administered in divided doses 2-3 times/day (or ≥3 times/day for patients maintained on levodopa ≥700 mg). Intervals between doses should be 4-8 hours while awake; when divided doses are not equal, smaller doses should be given toward the end of the day. Depending on clinical response, dosage may need to be increased to provide up to 30% more levodopa/day.

Dosage adjustment: May adjust every 3 days; intervals should be between 4-8 hours during the waking day (maximum dose: 8 tablets/day)

Intestinal infusion via PEG tube: Intestinal gel (Canadian labeling; not available in U.S.):

Note: Conversion to/from oral levodopa tablet formulations and the intestinal gel formulation can be done on a 1:1 ratio. Total daily dose (expressed in terms of levodopa) consists of a morning bolus dose, a continuous maintenance dose, and additional bolus doses when necessary. Nighttime dosing may be necessary in certain rare situations (eg, nocturnal akinesia). Dosage adjustments should be carried out over a period of a few weeks.

Morning bolus dose (based on previous morning levodopa intake and volume to fill intestinal tubing): Usual: Levodopa 100-200 mg (5-10 mL); Maximum: Levodopa 300 mg (15 mL)

Continuous maintenance dose: Adjustable in increments of 2 mg/hour (0.1 mL/hour) and based on previous daily intake of levodopa: Usual: Levodopa 40-120 mg/hour (2-6 mL/hour) infused up to 16 hours; Range: Levodopa 20-200 mg/hour (1-10 mL/hour)

Additional bolus doses: Usual: Levodopa: 10-40 mg (0.5-2 mL), if needed for daytime hypokinesia; in patients requiring >5 additional boluses/day, the maintenance dose should be increased

Restless leg syndrome (RLS) (unlabeled use; Silber, 2004): Oral:

Immediate release tablet: Carbidopa 25 mg/levodopa 100 mg (0.5-1 tablet) given in the evening, at bedtime, or upon waking during the night with RLS symptoms

Controlled release tablet: Carbidopa 25 mg/levodopa 100 mg (1 tablet) before bedtime for RLS symptoms that awaken patient during the night

Renal Impairment Use with caution; manufacturer's labeling makes no specific dosing recommendations.

Hepatic Impairment Use with caution; manufacturer's labeling makes no specific dosing recommendations.

Administration

Oral tablet formulations: Space doses evenly over the waking hours. Give with meals to decrease GI upset. Controlled release product should not be chewed or crushed. Orally-disintegrating tablets do not require water; the tablet should disintegrate on the tongue's surface before swallowing.

Intestinal gel (Canadian labeling; not available in U.S.): Gel is administered directly to the duodenum via a portable infusion pump (CADD-legacy Duodopa™ pump). Administer through a temporary nasoduodenal tube for at least 3 days to evaluate patient response and for dose optimization. Long-term administration requires placement of PEG tube for intestinal infusion. Continuous maintenance dose is infused throughout the day for up to 16 hours.

Monitoring Parameters Periodic hepatic function tests, BUN, creatinine, and CBC; periodic skin examinations; blood pressure, standing and sitting/supine; symptoms of parkinsonism, dyskinesias, mental status

Test Interactions False-positive reaction for urinary glucose with Clinitest®; false-negative reaction using Clinistix®; false-positive urine ketones with Acetest®, Ketostix®, Labstix®

Pharmacotherapy Pearls To block the peripheral conversion of levodopa to dopamine, ≥70 mg/day of carbidopa is needed. "On-off" (a clinical syndrome characterized by sudden periods of drug activity/inactivity), can be managed by giving smaller, more frequent doses of Sinemet® or adding a dopamine agonist or selegiline; when adding a new agent, doses of Sinemet® can usually be decreased. Protein in the diet should be distributed throughout the day to avoid fluctuations in levodopa absorption. Levodopa is the drug of choice when rigidity is the predominant presenting symptom.

Conversion from levodopa to carbidopa/levodopa: **Note:** Levodopa must be discontinued at least 12 hours prior to initiation of levodopa/carbidopa:

Initial dose: Levodopa portion of carbidopa/levodopa should be at least 25% of previous levodopa therapy.

Levodopa <1500 mg/day: Sinemet® or Parcopa™ (levodopa 25 mg/carbidopa 100 mg) 3-4 times/day

Levodopa ≥1500 mg/day: Sinemet® or Parcopa™ (levodopa 25 mg/carbidopa 250 mg) 3-4 times/day

Conversion from immediate release carbidopa/levodopa (Sinemet® or Parcopa™) to Sinemet® CR (50/200):

Sinemet® or Parcopa™ [total daily dose of levodopa]/Sinemet® CR:

Sinemet® or Parcopa™ (levodopa 300-400 mg/day): Sinemet® CR (50/200) 1 tablet twice daily

Sinemet® or Parcopa™ (levodopa 500-600 mg/day): Sinemet® CR (50/200) 1 1/2 tablets twice daily or 1 tablet 3 times/day

Sinemet® or Parcopa™ (levodopa 700-800 mg/day): Sinemet® CR (50/200) 4 tablets in 3 or more divided doses

Sinemet® or Parcopa™ (levodopa 900-1000 mg/day): Sinemet® CR (50/200) 5 tablets in 3 or more divided doses

Intervals between doses of Sinemet® CR should be 4-8 hours while awake; when divided doses are not equal, smaller doses should be given toward the end of the day

Special Geriatric Considerations The elderly may be more sensitive to the CNS effects of levodopa.

Dosage Forms Excipient information presented when available (limited, particularly for generics); consult specific product labeling.

Tablet: 10/100: Carbidopa 10 mg and levodopa 100 mg; 25/100: Carbidopa 25 mg and levodopa 100 mg; 25/250: Carbidopa 25 mg and levodopa 250 mg

Sinemet®:

10/100: Carbidopa 10 mg and levodopa 100 mg

25/100: Carbidopa 25 mg and levodopa 100 mg

25/250: Carbidopa 25 mg and levodopa 250 mg

Tablet, extended release: 25/100: Carbidopa 25 mg and levodopa 100 mg; 50/200: Carbidopa 50 mg and levodopa 200 mg

Tablet, orally disintegrating: 10/100: Carbidopa 10 mg and levodopa 100 mg; 25/100: Carbidopa 25 mg and levodopa 100 mg; 25/250: Carbidopa 25 mg and levodopa 250 mg

Parcopa®:

10/100: Carbidopa 10 mg and levodopa 100 mg [contains phenylalanine 3.4 mg/tablet; mint flavor]

25/100: Carbidopa 25 mg and levodopa 100 mg [contains phenylalanine 3.4 mg/tablet; mint flavor]

25/250: Carbidopa 25 mg and levodopa 250 mg [contains phenylalanine 8.4 mg/tablet; mint flavor]

Tablet, sustained release: 25/100: Carbidopa 25 mg and levodopa 100 mg; 50/200: Carbidopa 50 mg and levodopa 200 mg

Sinemet® CR:

25/100: Carbidopa 25 mg and levodopa 100 mg

50/200: Carbidopa 50 mg and levodopa 200 mg

Dosage Forms: Canada Excipient information presented when available (limited, particularly for generics); consult specific product labeling.

Intestinal gel:

Duodopa™: Carbidopa 5 mg and levodopa 20 mg/1 mL (100 mL)

◆ **Carbidopa, Entacapone, and Levodopa** see Levodopa, Carbidopa, and Entacapone on page 1115

◆ **Carbidopa, Levodopa, and Entacapone** see Levodopa, Carbidopa, and Entacapone on page 1115

◆ **Carboxypeptidase-G2** see Glucarpidase on page 885

◆ **Cardene® I.V.** see NiCARdipine on page 1368

◆ **Cardene® SR** see NiCARdipine on page 1368

◆ **Cardizem®** see Diltiazem on page 550

◆ **Cardizem® CD** see Diltiazem on page 550

◆ **Cardizem® LA** see Diltiazem on page 550

◆ **Cardura®** see Doxazosin on page 598

◆ **Cardura® XL** see Doxazosin on page 598

◆ **Carimune® NF** see Immune Globulin on page 982

◆ **Carisoprodate** see Carisoprodol on page 298

Carisoprodol (kar eye soe PROE dole)

Related Information
Beers Criteria − Potentially Inappropriate Medications for Geriatrics *on page 2183*

Medication Safety Issues
BEERS Criteria medication:
This drug may be potentially inappropriate for use in geriatric patients (Quality of evidence - moderate; Strength of recommendation - strong).

Brand Names: U.S. Soma®
Index Terms Carisoprodate; Isobamate
Generic Availability (U.S.) Yes
Pharmacologic Category Skeletal Muscle Relaxant
Use Short-term (2-3 weeks) treatment of acute musculoskeletal pain
Contraindications Hypersensitivity to carisoprodol, meprobamate, or any component of the formulation; acute intermittent porphyria
Warnings/Precautions Can cause CNS depression, which may impair physical or mental abilities. Patients must be cautioned about performing tasks which require mental alertness (eg, operating machinery or driving); postmarketing reports of motor vehicle accidents have been associated with use. Effects with other CNS-depressant drugs or ethanol may be potentiated. Use with caution in patients with hepatic/renal dysfunction. Tolerance or drug dependence may result from extended use. Limit use to 2-3 weeks; use caution in patients who may be prone to addiction. May precipitate withdrawal after abrupt cessation of prolonged use.

Idiosyncratic reactions and/or severe allergic reactions may occur. Idiosyncratic reactions occur following the initial dose and may include severe weakness, transient quadriplegia, euphoria, or vision loss (temporary). Has been associated (rarely) with seizures in patients with and without seizure history. Carisoprodol should be used with caution in patients who are poor CYP2C19 metabolizers; poor metabolizers have been shown to have a fourfold increase in exposure to carisoprodol and a 50% reduced exposure to the metabolite meprobamate compared to normal metabolizers. Muscle relaxants are poorly tolerated by the elderly due to potent anticholinergic effects, sedation, and risk of fracture. Efficacy is questionable at dosages tolerated by elderly patients; avoid use (Beers Criteria).

Adverse Reactions (Reflective of adult population; not specific for elderly)
>10%: Central nervous system: Drowsiness (13% to 17%)
1% to 10%: Central nervous system: Dizziness (7% to 8%), headache (3% to 5%)

Drug Interactions
Metabolism/Transport Effects Substrate of CYP2C19 (major); **Note:** Assignment of Major/Minor substrate status based on clinically relevant drug interaction potential
Avoid Concomitant Use
Avoid concomitant use of Carisoprodol with any of the following: Azelastine; Azelastine (Nasal); Methadone; Mirtazapine; Paraldehyde
Increased Effect/Toxicity
Carisoprodol may increase the levels/effects of: Alcohol (Ethyl); Azelastine; Azelastine (Nasal); Buprenorphine; CNS Depressants; Methadone; Methotrimeprazine; Metyrosine; Mirtazapine; Paraldehyde; Selective Serotonin Reuptake Inhibitors; Zolpidem

The levels/effects of Carisoprodol may be increased by: CYP2C19 Inhibitors (Moderate); CYP2C19 Inhibitors (Strong); Droperidol; HydrOXYzine; Methotrimeprazine
Decreased Effect
The levels/effects of Carisoprodol may be decreased by: CYP2C19 Inducers (Strong)
Ethanol/Nutrition/Herb Interactions Ethanol: May increase CNS depression; monitor for increased effects with coadministration. Caution patients about effects.
Stability Store at controlled room temperature of 20°C to 25°C (68°F to 77°F).
Mechanism of Action Precise mechanism is not yet clear, but many effects have been ascribed to its central depressant actions. In animals, carisoprodol blocks interneuronal activity and depresses polysynaptic neuron transmission in the spinal cord and reticular formation of the brain. It is also metabolized to meprobamate, which has anxiolytic and sedative effects.
Pharmacodynamics/Kinetics
Onset of action: ~30 minutes
Duration: 4-6 hours
Metabolism: Hepatic, via CYP2C19 to active metabolite (meprobamate)
Half-life elimination: ~2 hours; Meprobamate: 10 hours
Time to peak, plasma: 1.5-2 hours
Excretion: Urine, as metabolite

Dosage
Geriatric Not recommended for use in the elderly.
Adult Note: Carisoprodol should only be used for short periods (2-3 weeks) due to lack of evidence of effectiveness with prolonged use.
Acute musculoskeletal pain: Oral: 250-350 mg 3 times/day and at bedtime
Renal Impairment Use in renal impairment has not been studied; use with caution.
Dialysis: Removed by hemo- and peritoneal dialysis
Hepatic Impairment Use in hepatic impairment has not been studied; use with caution.
Administration Administer with or without food.
Monitoring Parameters CNS effects (eg, mental status, excessive drowsiness); relief of pain and/or muscle spasm; signs of drug abuse in addiction-prone individuals
Special Geriatric Considerations Avoid or use with caution in the elderly; not considered a drug of choice because of the risk of orthostatic hypotension and CNS depression.

This medication is considered to be potentially inappropriate in this patient population (Beers Criteria: Quality of evidence - moderate; Strength of recommendation - strong).
Controlled Substance C-IV
Dosage Forms Excipient information presented when available (limited, particularly for generics); consult specific product labeling.
Tablet, oral: 350 mg
Soma®: 250 mg, 350 mg

♦ **Carrington® Antifungal [OTC]** see Miconazole (Topical) on page 1276

Carteolol (Ophthalmic) (KAR tee oh lole)

Related Information
Glaucoma Drug Therapy on page 2115
Medication Safety Issues
Sound-alike/look-alike issues:
Carteolol may be confused with carvedilol
Index Terms Carteolol Hydrochloride
Generic Availability (U.S.) Yes
Pharmacologic Category Ophthalmic Agent, Antiglaucoma
Use Treatment of chronic open-angle glaucoma and intraocular hypertension
Contraindications Hypersensitivity to carteolol or any component of the formulation; sinus bradycardia; heart block greater than first-degree (except in patients with a functioning artificial pacemaker); cardiogenic shock; bronchial asthma, bronchospasm, or COPD; uncompensated cardiac failure; pulmonary edema
Warnings/Precautions Consider pre-existing conditions such as sick sinus syndrome before initiating. Use caution in patients with PVD (can aggravate arterial insufficiency) or myasthenia gravis. In general, patients with bronchospastic disease should not receive beta-blockers; if used at all, should be used cautiously with close monitoring. Use cautiously in diabetics because it can mask prominent hypoglycemic symptoms. Systemic absorption and adverse effects may occur with ophthalmic product, including bradycardia and/or hypotension. Should not be used alone in angle-closure glaucoma (has no effect on pupillary constriction). Adequate alpha-blockade is required prior to use of any beta-blocker for patients with untreated pheochromocytoma.
Adverse Reactions (Reflective of adult population; not specific for elderly)
>10%: Ocular: Conjunctival hyperemia
1% to 10%: Ocular: Anisocoria, corneal punctate keratitis, corneal sensitivity decreased, corneal staining, eye pain, vision disturbances
Drug Interactions
Metabolism/Transport Effects Substrate of CYP2D6 (minor); **Note:** Assignment of Major/Minor substrate status based on clinically relevant drug interaction potential
Avoid Concomitant Use
Avoid concomitant use of Carteolol (Ophthalmic) with any of the following: Beta2-Agonists; Floctafenine; Methacholine
Increased Effect/Toxicity
Carteolol (Ophthalmic) may increase the levels/effects of: Alpha-/Beta-Agonists (Direct-Acting); Alpha1-Blockers; Alpha2-Agonists; Amifostine; Antihypertensives; Antipsychotic Agents (Phenothiazines); Bupivacaine; Cardiac Glycosides; Cholinergic Agonists; Fingolimod; Hypotensive Agents; Insulin; Lidocaine; Lidocaine (Systemic); Lidocaine (Topical); Mepivacaine; Methacholine; Midodrine; RiTUXimab; Sulfonylureas

The levels/effects of Carteolol (Ophthalmic) may be increased by: Acetylcholinesterase Inhibitors; Amiodarone; Anilidopiperidine Opioids; Antipsychotic Agents (Phenothiazines); Calcium Channel Blockers (Dihydropyridine); Calcium Channel Blockers (Nondihydropyridine); Diazoxide; Dipyridamole; Disopyramide; Dronedarone; Floctafenine; Herbs (Hypotensive Properties); MAO Inhibitors; Pentoxifylline; Phosphodiesterase 5 Inhibitors; Prostacyclin Analogues; Reserpine

Decreased Effect

Carteolol (Ophthalmic) may decrease the levels/effects of: Beta2-Agonists; Theophylline Derivatives

The levels/effects of Carteolol (Ophthalmic) may be decreased by: Barbiturates; Herbs (Hypertensive Properties); Methylphenidate; Nonsteroidal Anti-Inflammatory Agents; Yohimbine

Mechanism of Action Blocks both beta$_1$- and beta$_2$-receptors and has mild intrinsic sympathomimetic activity; reduces intraocular pressure by decreasing aqueous humor production

Dosage

Geriatric & Adult Glaucoma or intraocular hypertension: Ophthalmic: Instill 1 drop in affected eye(s) twice daily

Administration Intended for twice daily dosing. Keep eye open and do not blink for 30 seconds after instillation. Wear sunglasses to avoid photophobic discomfort. Apply gentle pressure to lacrimal sac during and immediately following instillation (1 minute).

Monitoring Parameters Intraocular pressure

Pharmacotherapy Pearls When treating glaucoma/intraocular hypertension, if the desired IOP is not achieved, consider adding concomitant therapy with pilocarpine, dipivefrin, etc.

Special Geriatric Considerations Evaluate the patient's ability to self-administer the ophthalmic product.

Dosage Forms Excipient information presented when available (limited, particularly for generics); consult specific product labeling.
Solution, ophthalmic, as hydrochloride [drops]: 1% (5 mL, 10 mL, 15 mL) [contains benzalkonium chloride]

◆ **Carteolol Hydrochloride** see Carteolol (Ophthalmic) on page 299
◆ **Cartia XT®** see Diltiazem on page 550

Carvedilol (KAR ve dil ole)

Related Information
Beta-Blockers on page 2108
Heart Failure (Systolic) on page 2203

Medication Safety Issues

Sound-alike/look-alike issues:
Carvedilol may be confused with atenolol, captopril, carbidopa, carteolol
Coreg® may be confused with Corgard®, Cortef®, Cozaar®

Brand Names: U.S. Coreg CR®; Coreg®

Brand Names: Canada Apo-Carvedilol®; Ava-Carvedilol; Dom-Carvedilol; JAMP-Carvedilol; Mylan-Carvedilol; Novo-Carvedilol; PMS-Carvedilol; RAN™-Carvedilol; ratio-Carvedilol; ZYM-Carvedilol

Generic Availability (U.S.) Yes: Tablet

Pharmacologic Category Beta-Blocker With Alpha-Blocking Activity

Use Mild-to-severe heart failure of ischemic or cardiomyopathic origin (usually in addition to standard therapy); left ventricular dysfunction following myocardial infarction (MI) (clinically stable with LVEF ≤40%); management of hypertension

Unlabeled Use Angina pectoris

Contraindications Serious hypersensitivity to carvedilol or any component of the formulation; decompensated cardiac failure requiring intravenous inotropic therapy; bronchial asthma or related bronchospastic conditions; second- or third-degree AV block, sick sinus syndrome, and severe bradycardia (except in patients with a functioning artificial pacemaker); cardiogenic shock; severe hepatic impairment

Warnings/Precautions Consider pre-existing conditions such as sick sinus syndrome before initiating. Heart failure patients may experience a worsening of renal function (rare); risk factors include ischemic heart disease, diffuse vascular disease, underlying renal dysfunction, and systolic BP <100 mm Hg. Initiate cautiously and monitor for possible deterioration in patient status (eg, symptoms of HF). Worsening heart failure or fluid retention may occur during upward titration; dose reduction or temporary discontinuation may be necessary. Adjustment of other medications (ACE inhibitors and/or diuretics) may also be required.

Bradycardia may be observed more frequently in elderly patients (>65 years of age); dosage reductions may be necessary.

Symptomatic hypotension with or without syncope may occur with carvedilol (usually within the first 30 days of therapy); close monitoring of patient is required especially with initial dosing and dosing increases; blood pressure must be lowered at a rate appropriate for the patient's clinical condition. Initiation with a low dose, gradual up-titration, and administration with food may help to decrease the occurrence of hypotension or syncope. Patients should be advised to avoid driving or other hazardous tasks during initiation of therapy due to the risk of syncope. Beta-blocker therapy should not be withdrawn abruptly (particularly in patients with CAD), but gradually tapered to avoid acute tachycardia, hypertension, and/or ischemia. Chronic beta-blocker therapy should not be routinely withdrawn prior to major surgery.

In general, patients with bronchospastic disease should not receive beta-blockers; if used at all, should be used cautiously with close monitoring. May precipitate or aggravate symptoms of arterial insufficiency in patients with PVD and Raynaud's disease; use with caution and monitor for progression of arterial obstruction. Use caution with concurrent use of digoxin, verapamil or diltiazem; bradycardia or heart block can occur. Use with caution in patients receiving inhaled anesthetic agents known to depress myocardial contractility. Use cautiously in patients with diabetes because it can mask prominent hypoglycemic symptoms. In patients with heart failure and diabetes, use of carvedilol may worsen hyperglycemia; may require adjustment of antidiabetic agents. May mask signs of hyperthyroidism (eg, tachycardia); if hyperthyroidism is suspected, carefully manage and monitor; abrupt withdrawal may exacerbate symptoms of hyperthyroidism or precipitate thyroid storm. May induce or exacerbate psoriasis. Use with caution in patients with myasthenia gravis or psychiatric disease (may cause CNS depression). Use with caution in patients with mild-to-moderate hepatic impairment; use is contraindicated in patients with severe impairment. Manufacturer recommends discontinuation of therapy if liver injury occurs (confirmed by laboratory testing). Adequate alpha-blockade is required prior to use of any beta-blocker for patients with untreated pheochromocytoma. Use caution with history of severe anaphylaxis to allergens; patients taking beta-blockers may become more sensitive to repeated challenges. Treatment of anaphylaxis (eg, epinephrine) in patients taking beta-blockers may be ineffective or promote undesirable effects.

Intraoperative floppy iris syndrome has been observed in cataract surgery patients who were on or were previously treated with alpha$_1$-blockers; causality has not been established and there appears to be no benefit in discontinuing alpha-blocker therapy prior to surgery. Instruct patients to inform ophthalmologist of carvedilol use when considering eye surgery.

Adverse Reactions (Reflective of adult population; not specific for elderly) Note: Frequency ranges include data from hypertension and heart failure trials. Higher rates of adverse reactions have generally been noted in patients with heart failure. However, the frequency of adverse effects associated with placebo is also increased in this population.

>10%:
  Cardiovascular: Hypotension (9% to 20%)
  Central nervous system: Dizziness (2% to 32%), fatigue (4% to 24%)
  Endocrine & metabolic: Hyperglycemia (5% to 12%)
  Gastrointestinal: Diarrhea (1% to 12%), weight gain (10% to 12%)
  Neuromuscular & skeletal: Weakness (7% to 11%)
1% to 10%:
  Cardiovascular: Bradycardia (2% to 10%), syncope (3% to 8%), peripheral edema (1% to 7%), generalized edema (5% to 6%), angina (1% to 6%), dependent edema (≤4%), AV block, cerebrovascular accident, hypertension, hyper-/hypovolemia, orthostatic hypotension, palpitation
  Central nervous system: Headache (5% to 8%), depression, fever, hypoesthesia, hypotonia, insomnia, malaise, somnolence, vertigo
  Endocrine & metabolic: Hypercholesterolemia (1% to 4%), hypertriglyceridemia (1%), diabetes mellitus, gout, hyperkalemia, hyperuricemia, hypoglycemia, hyponatremia
  Gastrointestinal: Nausea (2% to 9%), vomiting (1% to 6%), abdominal pain, melena, periodontitis, weight loss
  Genitourinary: Impotence
  Hematologic: Anemia, prothrombin decreased, purpura, thrombocytopenia
  Hepatic: Alkaline phosphatase increased (1% to 3%), GGT increased, transaminases increased
  Neuromuscular & skeletal: Back pain (2% to 7%), arthralgia (1% to 6%), arthritis, muscle cramps, paresthesia
  Ocular: Blurred vision (1% to 5%)
  Renal: BUN increased (≤6%), nonprotein nitrogen increased (6%), albuminuria, creatinine increased, glycosuria, hematuria, renal insufficiency

◀ Respiratory: Cough (5% to 8%), nasopharyngitis (4%), rales (4%), dyspnea (>3%), pulmonary edema (>3%), rhinitis (2%), nasal congestion (1%), sinus congestion (1%)

Miscellaneous: Injury (3% to 6%), allergy, flu-like syndrome, sudden death

Drug Interactions

Metabolism/Transport Effects Substrate of CYP1A2 (minor), CYP2C9 (minor), CYP2D6 (major), CYP2E1 (minor), CYP3A4 (minor), P-glycoprotein; **Note:** Assignment of Major/Minor substrate status based on clinically relevant drug interaction potential; **Inhibits** P-glycoprotein

Avoid Concomitant Use

Avoid concomitant use of Carvedilol with any of the following: Beta2-Agonists; Floctafenine; Methacholine; Topotecan

Increased Effect/Toxicity

Carvedilol may increase the levels/effects of: Alpha-/Beta-Agonists (Direct-Acting); Alpha1-Blockers; Alpha2-Agonists; Amifostine; Antihypertensives; Antipsychotic Agents (Phenothiazines); Bupivacaine; Cardiac Glycosides; Cholinergic Agonists; Colchicine; CycloSPORINE; CycloSPORINE (Systemic); Dabigatran Etexilate; Digoxin; Everolimus; Fingolimod; Hypotensive Agents; Insulin; Lidocaine; Lidocaine (Systemic); Lidocaine (Topical); Mepivacaine; Methacholine; Midodrine; P-glycoprotein/ABCB1 Substrates; Prucalopride; RiTUXimab; Rivaroxaban; Sulfonylureas; Topotecan

The levels/effects of Carvedilol may be increased by: Abiraterone Acetate; Acetylcholinesterase Inhibitors; Aminoquinolines (Antimalarial); Amiodarone; Anilidopiperidine Opioids; Antipsychotic Agents (Phenothiazines); Calcium Channel Blockers (Dihydropyridine); Calcium Channel Blockers (Nondihydropyridine); Cimetidine; CYP2C9 Inhibitors (Moderate); CYP2C9 Inhibitors (Strong); CYP2D6 Inhibitors (Moderate); CYP2D6 Inhibitors (Strong); Darunavir; Diazoxide; Digoxin; Dipyridamole; Disopyramide; Dronedarone; Floctafenine; Herbs (Hypotensive Properties); MAO Inhibitors; Pentoxifylline; P-glycoprotein/ABCB1 Inhibitors; Phosphodiesterase 5 Inhibitors; Propafenone; Prostacyclin Analogues; QuiNIDine; Reserpine; Selective Serotonin Reuptake Inhibitors

Decreased Effect

Carvedilol may decrease the levels/effects of: Beta2-Agonists; Theophylline Derivatives

The levels/effects of Carvedilol may be decreased by: Barbiturates; Herbs (Hypertensive Properties); Methylphenidate; Nonsteroidal Anti-Inflammatory Agents; Peginterferon Alfa-2b; P-glycoprotein/ABCB1 Inducers; Rifamycin Derivatives; Tocilizumab; Yohimbine

Ethanol/Nutrition/Herb Interactions

Food: Food decreases rate but not extent of absorption. Administration with food minimizes risks of orthostatic hypotension.

Herb/Nutraceutical: Avoid herbs with hypertensive properties (bayberry, blue cohosh, cayenne, ephedra, ginger, ginseng [American], kola, licorice); may diminish the antihypertensive effect of carvedilol. Avoid herbs with hypotensive properties (black cohosh, California poppy, coleus, golden seal, hawthorn, mistletoe, periwinkle, quinine, shepherd's purse); may enhance the hypotensive effect of carvedilol.

Stability

Coreg® Store at <30°C (<86°F). Protect from moisture.

Coreg CR®: Store at 25°C (77°F); excursions permitted to 15°C to 30°C (59°F to 86°F).

Mechanism of Action As a racemic mixture, carvedilol has nonselective beta-adrenoreceptor and alpha-adrenergic blocking activity. No intrinsic sympathomimetic activity has been documented. Associated effects in hypertensive patients include reduction of cardiac output, exercise- or beta-agonist-induced tachycardia, reduction of reflex orthostatic tachycardia, vasodilation, decreased peripheral vascular resistance (especially in standing position), decreased renal vascular resistance, reduced plasma renin activity, and increased levels of atrial natriuretic peptide. In CHF, associated effects include decreased pulmonary capillary wedge pressure, decreased pulmonary artery pressure, decreased heart rate, decreased systemic vascular resistance, increased stroke volume index, and decreased right arterial pressure (RAP).

Pharmacodynamics/Kinetics

Onset of action: 1-2 hours
  Peak antihypertensive effect: ~1-2 hours

Absorption: Rapid and extensive

Distribution: V_d: 115 L

Protein binding: >98%, primarily to albumin

Metabolism: Extensively hepatic, via CYP2C9, 2D6, 3A4, and 2C19 (2% excreted unchanged); three active metabolites (4-hydroxyphenyl metabolite is 13 times more potent than parent drug for beta-blockade); first-pass effect; plasma concentrations in the elderly and those with cirrhotic liver disease are 50% and 4-7 times higher, respectively

Bioavailability: Immediate release: 25% to 35% (due to significant first-pass metabolism); Extended release: 85% of immediate release

Half-life elimination: 7-10 hours
Time to peak, plasma: Extended release: 5 hours
Excretion: Primarily feces

Dosage

Geriatric Refer to adult dosing. In the management of hypertension, consider lower initial doses and titrate to response (Aronow, 2011).

Adult Reduce dosage if heart rate drops to <55 beats/minute.

Hypertension: Oral:

Immediate release: 6.25 mg twice daily; if tolerated, dose should be maintained for 1-2 weeks, then increased to 12.5 mg twice daily. If necessary, dosage may be increased to a maximum of 25 mg twice daily after 1-2 weeks.

Extended release: Initial: 20 mg once daily, if tolerated, dose should be maintained for 1-2 weeks then increased to 40 mg once daily if necessary; maximum dose: 80 mg once daily

Heart failure: Oral:

Immediate release: 3.125 mg twice daily for 2 weeks; if this dose is tolerated, may increase to 6.25 mg twice daily. Double the dose every 2 weeks to the highest dose tolerated by patient. (Prior to initiating therapy, other heart failure medications should be stabilized and fluid retention minimized.)

Maximum recommended dose:
Mild-to-moderate heart failure:
<85 kg: 25 mg twice daily
>85 kg: 50 mg twice daily
Severe heart failure: 25 mg twice daily

Extended release: Initial: 10 mg once daily for 2 weeks; if the dose is tolerated, increase dose to 20 mg, 40 mg, and 80 mg over successive intervals of at least 2 weeks. Maintain on lower dose if higher dose is not tolerated.

Left ventricular dysfunction following MI: Oral: **Note:** Should be initiated only after patient is hemodynamically stable and fluid retention has been minimized.

Immediate release: Initial 3.125-6.25 mg twice daily; increase dosage incrementally (ie, from 6.25-12.5 mg twice daily) at intervals of 3-10 days, based on tolerance, to a target dose of 25 mg twice daily.

Extended release: Initial: Extended release: Initial: 10-20 mg once daily; increase dosage incrementally at intervals of 3-10 days, based on tolerance, to a target dose of 80 mg once daily.

Angina pectoris (unlabeled use): Oral: *Immediate release:* 25-50 mg twice daily

Conversion from immediate release to extended release (Coreg CR®):
Current dose immediate release tablets 3.125 mg twice daily: Convert to extended release capsules 10 mg once daily
Current dose immediate release tablets 6.25 mg twice daily: Convert to extended release capsules 20 mg once daily
Current dose immediate release tablets 12.5 mg twice daily: Convert to extended release capsules 40 mg once daily
Current dose immediate release tablets 25 mg twice daily: Convert to extended release capsules 80 mg once daily

Renal Impairment None necessary

Hepatic Impairment Use is contraindicated in severe liver dysfunction.

Administration Administer with food to minimize the risk of orthostatic hypotension. Extended release capsules should not be crushed or chewed. Capsules may be opened and sprinkled on applesauce for immediate use.

Monitoring Parameters Heart rate, blood pressure (base need for dosage increase on trough blood pressure measurements and for tolerance on standing systolic pressure 1 hour after dosing); renal studies, BUN, liver function; in patient with increase risk for developing renal dysfunction, monitor during dosage titration.

Pharmacotherapy Pearls Fluid retention during therapy should be treated with an increase in diuretic dosage.

Special Geriatric Considerations Due to alterations in the beta-adrenergic autonomic nervous system, beta-adrenergic blockade may result in less hemodynamic response than seen in younger adults. In U.S. trials conducted by the manufacturer, hypertension patients who were elderly (>65%) had a higher incidence of dizziness (8.8% vs 6%) than seen in younger patients. No other differences noted between young and old in these trials.

Dosage Forms Excipient information presented when available (limited, particularly for generics); consult specific product labeling.
Capsule, extended release, oral, as phosphate:
Coreg CR®: 10 mg, 20 mg, 40 mg, 80 mg
Tablet, oral: 3.125 mg, 6.25 mg, 12.5 mg, 25 mg
Coreg®: 3.125 mg, 6.25 mg, 12.5 mg, 25 mg

◆ **Casodex®** *see* Bicalutamide *on page 210*

Caspofungin (kas poe FUN jin)

Brand Names: U.S. Cancidas®
Brand Names: Canada Cancidas®
Index Terms Caspofungin Acetate
Generic Availability (U.S.) No
Pharmacologic Category Antifungal Agent, Parenteral; Echinocandin

Use Treatment of invasive *Aspergillus* infections in patients who are refractory or intolerant of other therapy; treatment of candidemia and other *Candida* infections (intra-abdominal abscesses, esophageal, peritonitis, pleural space); empirical treatment for presumed fungal infections in febrile neutropenic patient

Contraindications Hypersensitivity to caspofungin or any component of the formulation

Warnings/Precautions Concurrent use of cyclosporine should be limited to patients for whom benefit outweighs risk, due to a high frequency of hepatic transaminase elevations observed during concurrent use. Use caution in hepatic impairment; increased transaminases and rare cases of liver impairment have been reported in pediatric and adult patients. Dosage reduction required in adults with moderate hepatic impairment; safety and efficacy have not been established in adults with severe hepatic impairment.

Adverse Reactions (Reflective of adult population; not specific for elderly)

>10%:
  Cardiovascular: Hypotension (3% to 20%), peripheral edema (6% to 11%), tachycardia (4% to 11%)
  Central nervous system: Fever (6% to 30%), chills (9% to 23%), headache (5% to 15%)
  Dermatologic: Rash (4% to 23%)
  Endocrine & metabolic: Hypokalemia (5% to 23%)
  Gastrointestinal: Diarrhea (6% to 27%), vomiting (6% to 17%), nausea (4% to 15%)
  Hematologic: Hemoglobin decreased (18% to 21%), hematocrit decreased (13% to 18%), WBC decreased (12%), anemia (2% to 11%)
  Hepatic: Serum alkaline phosphatase increased (9% to 22%), transaminases increased (2% to 18%), bilirubin increased (5% to 13%)
  Local: Phlebitis/thrombophlebitis (18%)
  Renal: Serum creatinine increased (3% to 11%)
  Respiratory: Respiratory failure (2% to 20%), cough (6% to 11%), pneumonia (4% to 11%)
  Miscellaneous: Infusion reactions (20% to 35%), septic shock (11% to 14%)

5% to 10%:
  Cardiovascular: Hypertension (5% to 6%; children 9% to 10%)
  Dermatologic: Erythema (4% to 9%), pruritus (6% to 7%)
  Endocrine & metabolic: Hypomagnesemia (7%), hyperglycemia (6%)
  Gastrointestinal: Mucosal inflammation (4% to 10%), abdominal pain (4% to 9%)
  Hepatic: Albumin decreased (7%)
  Local: Infection (1% to 9%, central line)
  Renal: Hematuria (10%), blood urea nitrogen increased (4% to 9%)
  Respiratory: Dyspnea (9%), pleural effusion (9%), respiratory distress (≤8%), rales (7%)
  Miscellaneous: Sepsis (5% to 7%)

Drug Interactions

Metabolism/Transport Effects None known.

Avoid Concomitant Use There are no known interactions where it is recommended to avoid concomitant use.

Increased Effect/Toxicity
  The levels/effects of Caspofungin may be increased by: CycloSPORINE; CycloSPORINE (Systemic)

Decreased Effect
  Caspofungin may decrease the levels/effects of: Saccharomyces boulardii; Tacrolimus; Tacrolimus (Systemic)

  The levels/effects of Caspofungin may be decreased by: Inducers of Drug Clearance; Rifampin

Stability Store vials at 2°C to 8°C (36°F to 46°F). Reconstituted solution may be stored at ≤25°C (≤77°F) for 1 hour prior to preparation of infusion solution. Infusion solutions may be stored at ≤25°C (≤77°F) and should be used within 24 hours; up to 48 hours if stored at 2°C to 8°C (36°F to 46°F).

Bring refrigerated vial to room temperature. Reconstitute vials using 0.9% sodium chloride for injection, SWFI, or bacteriostatic water for injection. Mix gently until clear solution is formed;

do not use if cloudy or contains particles. Solution should be further diluted with 0.9%, 0.45%, or 0.225% sodium chloride or LR (do not exceed final concentration of 0.5 mg/mL).

Mechanism of Action Inhibits synthesis of β(1,3)-D-glucan, an essential component of the cell wall of susceptible fungi. Highest activity in regions of active cell growth. Mammalian cells do not require β(1,3)-D-glucan, limiting potential toxicity.

Pharmacodynamics/Kinetics

Protein binding: ~97% to albumin

Metabolism: Slowly, via hydrolysis and *N*-acetylation as well as by spontaneous degradation, with subsequent metabolism to component amino acids. Overall metabolism is extensive.

Half-life elimination: Beta (distribution): 9-11 hours; Terminal: 40-50 hours

Excretion: Urine (41%; primarily as metabolites, ~1% of total dose as unchanged drug); feces (35%; primarily as metabolites)

Dosage

Geriatric & Adult Note: Duration of caspofungin treatment should be determined by patient status and clinical response. Empiric therapy should be given until neutropenia resolves. In patients with positive cultures, treatment should continue until 14 days after last positive culture. In neutropenic patients, treatment should be given at least 7 days after both signs and symptoms of infection **and** neutropenia resolve.

Aspergillosis, invasive: I.V.: Initial dose: 70 mg on day 1; subsequent dosing: 50 mg/day. If clinical response inadequate, may increase up to 70 mg/day if tolerated, but increased efficacy not demonstrated. **Note:** Duration of therapy should be a minimum of 6-12 weeks or throughout period of immunosuppression.

Candidiasis: I.V.: Initial dose: 70 mg on day 1; subsequent dosing: 50 mg/day; higher doses (150 mg once daily infused over ~2 hours) compared to the standard adult dosing regimen (50 mg once daily) have not demonstrated additional benefit or toxicity in patients with invasive candidiasis (Betts, 2009).

Esophageal: 50 mg/day; **Note:** The majority of patients studied for this indication also had oropharyngeal involvement.

Empiric therapy: I.V.: Initial dose: 70 mg on day 1; subsequent dosing: 50 mg/day; if clinical response inadequate, may increase up to 70 mg/day if tolerated, but increased efficacy not demonstrated

Dosage adjustment with concomitant use of an enzyme inducer:

Patients receiving rifampin: 70 mg caspofungin daily

Patients receiving carbamazepine, dexamethasone, efavirenz, nevirapine, or phenytoin (and possibly other enzyme inducers) may require an increased daily dose of caspofungin (70 mg/day).

Renal Impairment No dosage adjustment required in renal impairment.

Poorly dialyzed; no supplemental dose or dosage adjustment necessary, including patients on intermittent hemodialysis, peritoneal dialysis, or continuous renal replacement therapy (eg, CVVHD).

Hepatic Impairment Adults:

Mild hepatic insufficiency (Child-Pugh score 5-6): No adjustment necessary.

Moderate hepatic insufficiency (Child-Pugh score 7-9): 70 mg on day 1 (where recommended), followed by 35 mg once daily.

Severe hepatic insufficiency (Child-Pugh score >9): No information available.

Administration Infuse slowly, over 1 hour (manufacturer); recent study, using doses of 50-150 mg, infused over ~2 hours (Betts, 2009); monitor during infusion. Isolated cases of possible histamine-related reactions have occurred during clinical trials (rash, flushing, pruritus, facial edema).

Monitoring Parameters Liver function

Special Geriatric Considerations The number of patients >65 years of age in clinical studies was not sufficient to establish whether a difference in response may be anticipated.

Dosage Forms Excipient information presented when available (limited, particularly for generics); consult specific product labeling.

Injection, powder for reconstitution, as acetate:

Cancidas®: 50 mg [contains sucrose 39 mg]

Cancidas®: 70 mg [contains sucrose 54 mg]

♦ **Caspofungin Acetate** see Caspofungin on page 304

Castor Oil (KAS tor oyl)

Related Information

Laxatives, Classification and Properties on page 2121

Index Terms Oleum Ricini

Generic Availability (U.S.) Yes: Oil

Pharmacologic Category Laxative, Miscellaneous

Use Preparation for rectal or bowel examination or surgery; rarely used to relieve constipation; also applied to skin as emollient and protectant

Dosage

Geriatric & Adult Bowel evacuation, constipation: Oil: Oral: 15-60 mL as a single dose

Special Geriatric Considerations Not a drug of first choice for constipation in the elderly.

Elderly are often predisposed to constipation due to disease, immobility, drugs, low residue diets, and a decreased fluid intake usually due to a decreased "thirst reflex" with age. Avoid stimulant cathartic use on a chronic basis if possible. Use osmotic, lubricant, stool softeners, and bulk agents as prophylaxis. Patients should be instructed for proper dietary fiber and fluid intake as well as regular exercise. Monitor closely for fluid/electrolyte imbalance, CNS signs of fluid/electrolyte loss, and hypotension. Strong and chronic purging may cause severe fluid and electrolyte loss which may affect mental function (CNS).

Dosage Forms Excipient information presented when available (limited, particularly for generics); consult specific product labeling.

Oil, oral: 100% (60 mL, 120 mL, 180 mL, 480 mL, 3840 mL)

Cefaclor (SEF a klor)

Related Information

Antimicrobial Drugs of Choice on page 2163

Medication Safety Issues

Sound-alike/look-alike issues:

Cefaclor may be confused with cephalexin

Brand Names: Canada Apo-Cefaclor®; Ceclor®; Novo-Cefaclor; Nu-Cefaclor; PMS-Cefaclor

Generic Availability (U.S.) Yes

Pharmacologic Category Antibiotic, Cephalosporin (Second Generation)

Use Treatment of susceptible bacterial infections including otitis media, lower respiratory tract infections, acute exacerbations of chronic bronchitis, pharyngitis and tonsillitis, urinary tract infections, skin and skin structure infections

Contraindications Hypersensitivity to cefaclor, any component of the formulation, or other cephalosporins

Warnings/Precautions Modify dosage in patients with severe renal impairment. Prolonged use may result in fungal or bacterial superinfection, including C. difficile-associated diarrhea (CDAD) and pseudomembranous colitis; CDAD has been observed >2 months postantibiotic treatment. Use with caution in patients with a history of penicillin allergy, especially IgE-mediated reactions (eg, anaphylaxis, urticaria). Beta-lactamase-negative, ampicillin-resistant (BLNAR) strains of H. influenzae should be considered resistant to cefaclor. Some products may contain phenylalanine.

Adverse Reactions (Reflective of adult population; not specific for elderly)
1% to 10%:
  Dermatologic: Rash (maculopapular, erythematous, or morbilliform) (1% to 2%)
  Gastrointestinal: Diarrhea (3%)
  Genitourinary: Vaginitis (2%)
  Hematologic: Eosinophilia (2%)
  Hepatic: Transaminases increased (3%)
  Miscellaneous: Moniliasis (2%)
Reactions reported with other cephalosporins: Fever, abdominal pain, superinfection, renal dysfunction, toxic nephropathy, hemorrhage, cholestasis

Drug Interactions
  Metabolism/Transport Effects None known.
  Avoid Concomitant Use
    Avoid concomitant use of Cefaclor with any of the following: BCG
  Increased Effect/Toxicity
    Cefaclor may increase the levels/effects of: Aminoglycosides

    The levels/effects of Cefaclor may be increased by: Probenecid
  Decreased Effect
    Cefaclor may decrease the levels/effects of: BCG; Typhoid Vaccine

Ethanol/Nutrition/Herb Interactions Food: Cefaclor serum levels may be decreased slightly if taken with food. The bioavailability of cefaclor extended release tablets is decreased 23% and the maximum concentration is decreased 67% when taken on an empty stomach.

Stability Store at controlled room temperature. Refrigerate suspension after reconstitution. Discard after 14 days. Do not freeze.

Mechanism of Action Inhibits bacterial cell wall synthesis by binding to one or more of the penicillin-binding proteins (PBPs) which in turn inhibits the final transpeptidation step of peptidoglycan synthesis in bacterial cell walls, thus inhibiting cell wall biosynthesis. Bacteria eventually lyse due to ongoing activity of cell wall autolytic enzymes (autolysins and murein hydrolases) while cell wall assembly is arrested.

Pharmacodynamics/Kinetics
  Absorption: Well absorbed, acid stable
  Distribution: Widely throughout the body and reaches therapeutic concentration in most tissues and body fluids, including synovial, pericardial, pleural, peritoneal fluids; bile, sputum, and urine; bone, myocardium, gallbladder, skin and soft tissue
  Protein binding: 25%
  Metabolism: Partially hepatic
  Half-life elimination: 0.5-1 hour; prolonged with renal impairment
  Time to peak: Capsule: 60 minutes; Suspension: 45 minutes
  Excretion: Urine (80% as unchanged drug)

Dosage
  Geriatric & Adult Treatment of infections: Oral: Dosing range: 250-500 mg every 8 hours
  Renal Impairment
    Cl_{cr} 10-50 mL/minute: Administer 50% to 100% of dose
    Cl_{cr} <10 mL/minute: Administer 50% of dose
    Hemodialysis: Moderately dialyzable (20% to 50%)

Administration Administer around-the-clock to promote less variation in peak and trough serum levels.
  Oral suspension: Shake well before using.

Monitoring Parameters Assess patient at beginning and throughout therapy for infection; monitor for signs of anaphylaxis during first dose

Test Interactions Positive direct Coombs', false-positive urinary glucose test using cupric sulfate (Benedict's solution, Clinitest®, Fehling's solution), false-positive serum or urine creatinine with Jaffé reaction

Special Geriatric Considerations Has not been studied in the elderly. Adjust dose for renal function in elderly. Considered to be one of the drugs of choice in the outpatient treatment of community-acquired pneumonia in elderly.

Dosage Forms Excipient information presented when available (limited, particularly for generics); consult specific product labeling.
  Capsule, oral: 250 mg, 500 mg
  Powder for suspension, oral: 125 mg/5 mL (75 mL, 150 mL); 250 mg/5 mL (75 mL, 150 mL); 375 mg/5 mL (50 mL, 100 mL)
  Tablet, extended release, oral: 500 mg

Cefadroxil (sef a DROKS il)

Brand Names: Canada Apo-Cefadroxil®; PRO-Cefadroxil; Teva-Cefadroxil

Index Terms Cefadroxil Monohydrate; Duricef
Generic Availability (U.S.) Yes
Pharmacologic Category Antibiotic, Cephalosporin (First Generation)
Use Treatment of susceptible bacterial infections, including those caused by group A beta-hemolytic *Streptococcus*
Contraindications Hypersensitivity to cefadroxil, any component of the formulation, or other cephalosporins
Warnings/Precautions Modify dosage in patients with severe renal impairment. Use with caution in patients with a history of penicillin allergy, especially IgE-mediated reactions (eg, anaphylaxis, angioedema, urticaria). Prolonged use may result in fungal or bacterial super-infection, including *C. difficile*-associated diarrhea (CDAD) and pseudomembranous colitis; CDAD has been observed >2 months postantibiotic treatment.
Adverse Reactions (Reflective of adult population; not specific for elderly)
1% to 10%: Gastrointestinal: Diarrhea
Reactions reported with other cephalosporins: Toxic epidermal necrolysis, abdominal pain, superinfection, renal dysfunction, toxic nephropathy, aplastic anemia, hemolytic anemia, hemorrhage, prothrombin time prolonged, BUN increased, creatinine increased, eosinophilia, pancytopenia, seizure
Drug Interactions
Metabolism/Transport Effects None known.
Avoid Concomitant Use
Avoid concomitant use of Cefadroxil with any of the following: BCG
Increased Effect/Toxicity
The levels/effects of Cefadroxil may be increased by: Probenecid
Decreased Effect
Cefadroxil may decrease the levels/effects of: BCG; Typhoid Vaccine
Ethanol/Nutrition/Herb Interactions Food: Concomitant administration with food or cow's milk does **not** significantly affect absorption.
Stability Refrigerate suspension after reconstitution; discard after 14 days.
Mechanism of Action Inhibits bacterial cell wall synthesis by binding to one or more of the penicillin-binding proteins (PBPs) which in turn inhibits the final transpeptidation step of peptidoglycan synthesis in bacterial cell walls, thus inhibiting cell wall biosynthesis. Bacteria eventually lyse due to ongoing activity of cell wall autolytic enzymes (autolysins and murein hydrolases) while cell wall assembly is arrested.
Pharmacodynamics/Kinetics
Absorption: Rapid and well absorbed
Distribution: Widely throughout the body and reaches therapeutic concentrations in most tissues and body fluids, including synovial, pericardial, pleural, and peritoneal fluids; bile, sputum, and urine; bone, myocardium, gallbladder, skin, and soft tissue
Protein binding: 20%
Half-life elimination: 1-2 hours; Renal failure: 20-24 hours
Time to peak, serum: 70-90 minutes
Excretion: Urine (>90% as unchanged drug)
Dosage
Geriatric & Adult
Susceptible infections: Oral: 1-2 g/day in 2 divided doses
Orofacial infections: Oral: 250-500 mg every 8 hours
Renal Impairment
Cl_{cr} 10-25 mL/minute: Administer every 24 hours.
Cl_{cr} <10 mL/minute: Administer every 36 hours.
Administration Administer around-the-clock to promote less variation in peak and trough serum levels.
Monitoring Parameters Observe for signs and symptoms of anaphylaxis during first dose.
Test Interactions Positive direct Coombs', false-positive urinary glucose test using cupric sulfate (Benedict's solution, Clinitest®, Fehling's solution), false-positive serum or urine creatinine with Jaffé reaction
Special Geriatric Considerations Adjust dose for renal function.
Dosage Forms Excipient information presented when available (limited, particularly for generics); consult specific product labeling. [DSC] = Discontinued product
Capsule, oral, as hemihydrate [strength expressed as base]: 500 mg [DSC]
Capsule, oral, as monohydrate [strength expressed as base]: 500 mg
Powder for suspension, oral, as monohydrate [strength expressed as base]: 250 mg/5 mL (50 mL, 100 mL); 500 mg/5 mL (75 mL, 100 mL)
Tablet, oral, as hemihydrate [strength expressed as base]: 1 g
Tablet, oral, as monohydrate [strength expressed as base]: 1 g

◆ **Cefadroxil Monohydrate** *see* Cefadroxil *on page 307*

CeFAZolin (sef A zoe lin)

Related Information
Antibiotic Treatment of Adults With Infective Endocarditis *on page 2157*
Prevention of Infective Endocarditis *on page 2175*
Medication Safety Issues
Sound-alike/look-alike issues:
CeFAZolin may be confused with cefoTEtan, cefOXitin, cefprozil, cefTAZidime, cefTRIAXone, cephalexin
Index Terms Ancef; Cefazolin Sodium
Generic Availability (U.S.) Yes
Pharmacologic Category Antibiotic, Cephalosporin (First Generation)
Use Treatment of respiratory tract, skin, genital, urinary tract, biliary tract, bone and joint infections, and septicemia due to susceptible gram-positive cocci (except *Enterococcus*); some gram-negative bacilli including *E. coli*, *Proteus*, and *Klebsiella* may be susceptible; surgical prophylaxis
Unlabeled Use Prophylaxis against infective endocarditis
Contraindications Hypersensitivity to cefazolin sodium, any component of the formulation, or other cephalosporins
Warnings/Precautions Modify dosage in patients with severe renal impairment. Use with caution in patients with a history of penicillin allergy, especially IgE-mediated reactions (eg, anaphylaxis, angioedema, urticaria). Prolonged use may result in fungal or bacterial superinfection, including *C. difficile*-associated diarrhea (CDAD) and pseudomembranous colitis; CDAD has been observed >2 months postantibiotic treatment. May be associated with increased INR, especially in nutritionally-deficient patients, prolonged treatment, hepatic or renal disease. Use with caution in patients with a history of seizure disorder; high levels, particularly in the presence of renal impairment, may increase risk of seizures.
Adverse Reactions (Reflective of adult population; not specific for elderly) Frequency not defined.
Central nervous system: Fever, seizure
Dermatologic: Rash, pruritus, Stevens-Johnson syndrome
Gastrointestinal: Diarrhea, nausea, vomiting, abdominal cramps, anorexia, pseudomembranous colitis, oral candidiasis
Genitourinary: Vaginitis
Hepatic: Transaminases increased, hepatitis
Hematologic: Eosinophilia, neutropenia, leukopenia, thrombocytopenia, thrombocytosis
Local: Pain at injection site, phlebitis
Renal: BUN increased, serum creatinine increased, renal failure
Miscellaneous: Anaphylaxis
Reactions reported with other cephalosporins: Toxic epidermal necrolysis, abdominal pain, cholestasis, superinfection, toxic nephropathy, aplastic anemia, hemolytic anemia, hemorrhage, prothrombin time prolonged, pancytopenia
Drug Interactions
Metabolism/Transport Effects None known.
Avoid Concomitant Use
Avoid concomitant use of CeFAZolin with any of the following: BCG
Increased Effect/Toxicity
CeFAZolin may increase the levels/effects of: Fosphenytoin; Phenytoin; Vitamin K Antagonists

The levels/effects of CeFAZolin may be increased by: Probenecid
Decreased Effect
CeFAZolin may decrease the levels/effects of: BCG; Typhoid Vaccine
Stability Store intact vials at room temperature and protect from temperatures exceeding 40°C. Dilute large vial with 2.5 mL SWFI; 10 g vial may be diluted with 45 mL to yield 1 g/5 mL or 96 mL to yield 1 g/10 mL. May be injected or further dilution for I.V. administration in 50-100 mL compatible solution. Standard diluent is 1 g/50 mL D_5W or 2 g/50 mL D_5W.

Reconstituted solutions of cefazolin are light yellow to yellow. Protection from light is recommended for the powder and for the reconstituted solutions. Reconstituted solutions are stable for 24 hours at room temperature and for 10 days under refrigeration. Stability of parenteral admixture at room temperature (25°C) is 48 hours. Stability of parenteral admixture at refrigeration temperature (4°C) is 14 days.

DUPLEX™: Store at 20°C to 25°C (68°F to 77°F); excursions permitted to 15°C to 30°C (59°F to 86°F) prior to activation. Following activation, stable for 24 hours at room temperature and for 7 days under refrigeration.

Mechanism of Action Inhibits bacterial cell wall synthesis by binding to one or more of the penicillin-binding proteins (PBPs) which in turn inhibits the final transpeptidation step of peptidoglycan synthesis in bacterial cell walls, thus inhibiting cell wall biosynthesis. Bacteria eventually lyse due to ongoing activity of cell wall autolytic enzymes (autolysins and murein hydrolases) while cell wall assembly is arrested.

Pharmacodynamics/Kinetics

Distribution: Widely into most body tissues and fluids including gallbladder, liver, kidneys, bone, sputum, bile, pleural, and synovial; CSF penetration is poor

Protein binding: 74% to 86%

Metabolism: Minimally hepatic

Half-life elimination: 90-150 minutes; prolonged with renal impairment

Time to peak, serum: I.M.: 0.5-2 hours

Excretion: Urine (80% to 100% as unchanged drug)

Dosage

Geriatric & Adult

Usual dosage range: I.M., I.V.: 1-1.5 g every 8 hours, depending on severity of infection; maximum: 12 g/day

Cholecystitis, mild-to-moderate: I.V.: 1-2 g every 8 hours for 4-7 days (provided source controlled)

Endocarditis due to MSSA (without prosthesis) (unlabeled use): I.V.: 2 g every 8 hours; **Note:** Recommended for penicillin-allergic (nonanaphylactoid) patients (Baddour, 2005)

Intra-abdominal infection, complicated, community-acquired, mild-to-moderate (in combination with metronidazole): I.V.: 1-2 g every 8 hours for 4-7 days (provided source controlled)

Moderate-to-severe infections: 500 mg to 1 g every 6-8 hours

Mild infection with gram-positive cocci: 250-500 mg every 8 hours

Perioperative prophylaxis: 1-2 g within 60 minutes prior to surgery (may repeat in 2-5 hours intraoperatively); followed by 500 mg to 1 g every 6-8 hours for 24 hours post-operatively

Cardiothoracic surgery: 1 g (see **"Note"**) within 60 minutes prior to incision, followed by 1 g at sternotomy and 1 g after cardiopulmonary bypass; may continue 1 g every 6 hours for 24-48 hours postoperatively (Eagle, 2004)

  Note: For patients weighing >60 kg, the Society of Thoracic Surgeons recommends a preoperative dose of 2 g administered within 60 minutes of skin incision. If the surgical incision remains open in the operating room, follow with 1 g every 3-4 hours unless cardiopulmonary bypass is to be discontinued within 4 hours then delay administration (Engelman, 2007).

Cholecystectomy: 1-2 g every 8 hours, discontinue within 24 hours unless infection outside gallbladder suspected

Total joint replacement: 1 g 1 hour prior to the procedure

Pneumococcal pneumonia: 500 mg every 12 hours

Severe infection: 1-1.5 g every 6 hours

Prophylaxis against infective endocarditis (unlabeled use): 1 g 30-60 minutes before procedure. **Note:** Intramuscular injections should be avoided in patients who are receiving anticoagulant therapy. In these circumstances, orally administered regimens should be given whenever possible. Intravenously administered antibiotics should be used for patients who are unable to tolerate or absorb oral medications.

  Note: American Heart Association (AHA) guidelines now recommend prophylaxis only in patients undergoing invasive procedures and in whom underlying cardiac conditions may predispose to a higher risk of adverse outcomes should infection occur. As of April 2007, routine prophylaxis for GI/GU procedures is no longer recommended by the AHA.

UTI (uncomplicated): 1 g every 12 hours

Renal Impairment

Cl_{cr} 35-54 mL/minute: Administer full dose in intervals of ≥8 hours

Cl_{cr} 11-34 mL/minute: Administer 50% of usual dose every 12 hours

Cl_{cr} ≤10 mL/minute: Administer 50% of usual dose every 18-24 hours

Intermittent hemodialysis (IHD) (administer after hemodialysis on dialysis days): Dialyzable (20% to 50%): 0.5-1 g every 24 hours **or** use 1-2 g every 48-72 hours (Heintz, 2009); **Note:** Dosing dependent on the assumption of 3 times/week, complete IHD sessions. Alternatively, may administer 15-20 mg/kg (maximum dose: 2 g) after dialysis without regularly scheduled dosing (Ahern, 2003; Sowinski, 2001).

Peritoneal dialysis (PD): 0.5 g every 12 hours

Continuous renal replacement therapy (CRRT) (Heintz, 2009; Trotman, 2005): Drug clearance is highly dependent on the method of renal replacement, filter type, and flow rate. Appropriate dosing requires close monitoring of pharmacologic response, signs of adverse reactions due to drug accumulation, as well as drug concentrations in relation to target trough (if appropriate). The following are general recommendations only (based on dialysate flow/ultrafiltration rates of 1-2 L/hour and minimal residual renal function) and should not supersede clinical judgment:

CVVH: Loading dose of 2 g followed by 1-2 g every 12 hours

CVVHD/CVVHDF: Loading dose of 2 g followed by either 1 g every 8 hours **or** 2 g every 12 hours. **Note:** Dosage of 1 g every 8 hours results in similar steady-state concentrations as 2 g every 12 hours and is more cost effective (Heintz, 2009).

Administration

I.M.: Inject deep I.M. into large muscle mass.

I.V.: Inject direct I.V. over 5 minutes. Infuse intermittent infusion over 30-60 minutes.

Some penicillins (eg, carbenicillin, ticarcillin and piperacillin) have been shown to inactivate aminoglycosides *in vitro*. This has been observed to a greater extent with tobramycin and gentamicin, while amikacin has shown greater stability against inactivation. Concurrent use of these agents may pose a risk of reduced antibacterial efficacy *in vivo*, particularly in the setting of profound renal impairment. However, definitive clinical evidence is lacking. If combination penicillin/aminoglycoside therapy is desired in a patient with renal dysfunction, separation of doses (if feasible), and routine monitoring of aminoglycoside levels, CBC, and clinical response should be considered.

Monitoring Parameters Renal function periodically when used in combination with other nephrotoxic drugs, hepatic function tests, CBC; monitor for signs of anaphylaxis during first dose

Test Interactions Positive direct Coombs', false-positive urinary glucose test using cupric sulfate (Benedict's solution, Clinitest®, Fehling's solution), false-positive serum or urine creatinine with Jaffé reaction.

Some penicillin derivatives may accelerate the degradation of aminoglycosides *in vitro*, leading to a potential underestimation of aminoglycoside serum concentration.

Special Geriatric Considerations Adjust dose for renal function.

Dosage Forms Excipient information presented when available (limited, particularly for generics); consult specific product labeling.

Infusion, premixed iso-osmotic dextrose solution: 1 g (50 mL) [products contain sodium ~48 mg (2mEq)/g]

Injection, powder for reconstitution: 500 mg, 1 g, 2 g, 10 g, 20 g, 100 g, 300 g [products contain sodium ~48 mg (2mEq)/g]

◆ **Cefazolin Sodium** *see* CeFAZolin *on page 309*

Cefdinir (SEF di ner)

Brand Names: U.S. Omnicef® [DSC]

Index Terms CFDN

Generic Availability (U.S.) Yes

Pharmacologic Category Antibiotic, Cephalosporin (Third Generation)

Use Treatment of community-acquired pneumonia, acute exacerbations of chronic bronchitis, acute bacterial otitis media, acute maxillary sinusitis, pharyngitis/tonsillitis, and uncomplicated skin and skin structure infections.

Contraindications Hypersensitivity to cefdinir, any component of the formulation, other cephalosporins, or related antibiotics

Warnings/Precautions Administer cautiously to penicillin-sensitive patients, especially IgE-mediated reactions (eg, anaphylaxis, urticaria). Prolonged use may result in fungal or bacterial superinfection, including *C. difficile*-associated diarrhea (CDAD) and pseudomembranous colitis; CDAD has been observed >2 months postantibiotic treatment. Use caution with renal dysfunction (Cl$_{cr}$ <30 mL/minute); dose adjustment may be required.

Adverse Reactions (Reflective of adult population; not specific for elderly)

>10%: Gastrointestinal: Diarrhea (8% to 15%)

1% to 10%:

Central nervous system: Headache (2%)

Dermatologic: Rash (≤3%)

Endocrine & metabolic: Bicarbonate decreased (≤1%), hyperglycemia (≤1%), hyperphosphatemia (≤1%)

Gastrointestinal: Nausea (≤3%), abdominal pain (≤1%), vomiting (≤1%)

Genitourinary: Vaginal moniliasis (≤4%), urine leukocytes increased (≤2%), urine pH increased (≤1%), urine specific gravity increased (≤1%), vaginitis (≤1%)

Hematologic: Lymphocytes increased (≤2%), eosinophils increased (1%), lymphocytes decreased (1%), platelets increased (≤1%), PMN changes (≤1%), WBC decreased/increased (≤1%)

Hepatic: Alkaline phosphatase increased (≤1%), ALT increased (≤1%)

Renal: Proteinuria (1% to 2%), microhematuria (≤1%), glycosuria (≤1%)

Miscellaneous: GGT increased (≤1%), lactate dehydrogenase increased (≤1%)

Additional reactions reported with other cephalosporins: Agranulocytosis, angioedema, aplastic anemia, asterixis, encephalopathy, hemorrhage, interstitial nephritis, neuromuscular excitability, PT prolonged, seizure, superinfection, and toxic nephropathy

Drug Interactions

Metabolism/Transport Effects None known.

Avoid Concomitant Use

Avoid concomitant use of Cefdinir with any of the following: BCG

Increased Effect/Toxicity

Cefdinir may increase the levels/effects of: Aminoglycosides

The levels/effects of Cefdinir may be increased by: Probenecid

Decreased Effect

Cefdinir may decrease the levels/effects of: BCG; Typhoid Vaccine

The levels/effects of Cefdinir may be decreased by: Iron Salts

Stability Capsules and unmixed powder should be stored at 25°C (77°F); excursions permitted to 15°C to 30°C (59°F to 86°F). Oral suspension should be mixed with 38 mL water for the 60 mL bottle and 63 mL of water for the 100 mL bottle. After mixing, the suspension can be stored at room temperature of 25°C (77°F) for 10 days.

Mechanism of Action Inhibits bacterial cell wall synthesis by binding to one or more of the penicillin-binding proteins (PBPs) which in turn inhibits the final transpeptidation step of peptidoglycan synthesis in bacterial cell walls, thus inhibiting cell wall biosynthesis. Bacteria eventually lyse due to ongoing activity of cell wall autolytic enzymes (autolysins and murein hydrolases) while cell wall assembly is arrested.

Pharmacodynamics/Kinetics

Distribution: V_d: Adults: 0.06-0.64 L/kg

Protein binding: 60% to 70%

Metabolism: Minimally hepatic

Bioavailability: Capsule: 16% to 21%; suspension 25%

Half-life elimination: 100 minutes

Excretion: Primarily urine

Dosage

Geriatric & Adult

Acute exacerbations of chronic bronchitis, pharyngitis/tonsillitis: Oral: 300 mg twice daily for 5-10 days **or** 600 mg once daily for 10 days

Acute maxillary sinusitis: Oral: 300 mg twice daily **or** 600 mg once daily for 10 days

Community-acquired pneumonia, uncomplicated skin and skin structure infections: Oral: 300 mg twice daily for 10 days

Renal Impairment Adults: 300 mg once daily

Hepatic Impairment No adjustment necessary.

Administration Twice daily doses should be given every 12 hours. May be administered with or without food. Manufacturer recommends administering at least 2 hours before or after antacids or iron supplements. Shake suspension well before use.

Monitoring Parameters Observe for signs and symptoms of anaphylaxis during first dose.

Test Interactions False-positive reaction for urinary ketones may occur with nitroprusside-but not nitroferricyanide-based tests. False-positive urine glucose results may occur when using Clinitest®, Benedict's solution, or Fehling's solution; glucose-oxidase-based reaction systems (eg, Clinistix®, Tes-Tape®) are recommended. May cause positive direct Coombs' test.

Special Geriatric Considerations Cefdinir has not been studied exclusively in the elderly. Patients ≥65 years of age have been included in clinical. No information is available on their response or tolerance.

Dosage Forms Excipient information presented when available (limited, particularly for generics); consult specific product labeling. [DSC] = Discontinued product

Capsule, oral: 300 mg

Omnicef®: 300 mg [DSC]

Powder for suspension, oral: 125 mg/5 mL (60 mL, 100 mL); 250 mg/5 mL (60 mL, 100 mL)

Omnicef®: 125 mg/5 mL (60 mL [DSC], 100 mL [DSC]); 250 mg/5 mL (60 mL [DSC], 100 mL [DSC]) [contains sodium benzoate, sucrose 2.86 g/5 mL; strawberry flavor]

Cefditoren (sef de TOR en)

Medication Safety Issues

International issues:

Spectracef [U.S., Great Britain, Mexico, Portugal, Spain] may be confused with Spectrocef brand name for cefotaxime [Italy]

Brand Names: U.S. Spectracef®

Index Terms Cefditoren Pivoxil

Generic Availability (U.S.) Yes

Pharmacologic Category Antibiotic, Cephalosporin (Third Generation)

Use Treatment of acute bacterial exacerbation of chronic bronchitis or community-acquired pneumonia (due to susceptible organisms including *Haemophilus influenzae, Haemophilus parainfluenzae, Streptococcus pneumoniae*-penicillin susceptible only, *Moraxella catarrhalis*); pharyngitis or tonsillitis (*Streptococcus pyogenes*); and uncomplicated skin and skin-structure infections (*Staphylococcus aureus* - not MRSA, *Streptococcus pyogenes*)

Contraindications Hypersensitivity to cefditoren, any component of the formulation, other cephalosporins, or milk protein; carnitine deficiency

Warnings/Precautions Use with caution in patients with a history of penicillin allergy, especially IgE-mediated reactions (eg, anaphylaxis, urticaria). Prolonged use may result in fungal or bacterial superinfection, including *C. difficile*-associated diarrhea (CDAD) and pseudomembranous colitis; CDAD has been observed >2 months postantibiotic treatment. Caution in individuals with seizure disorders; high levels, particularly in the presence of renal impairment, may increase risk of seizures. Use caution in patients with renal or hepatic impairment; modify dosage in patients with severe renal impairment. Cefditoren causes renal excretion of carnitine; do not use in patients with carnitine deficiency; not for long-term therapy due to the possible development of carnitine deficiency over time. May prolong prothrombin time; use with caution in patients with a history of bleeding disorder. Cefditoren tablets contain sodium caseinate, which may cause hypersensitivity reactions in patients with milk protein hypersensitivity; this does not affect patients with lactose intolerance.

Adverse Reactions (Reflective of adult population; not specific for elderly)

>10%: Gastrointestinal: Diarrhea (11% to 15%)

1% to 10%:

Central nervous system: Headache (2% to 3%)

Endocrine & metabolic: Glucose increased (1% to 2%)

Gastrointestinal: Nausea (4% to 6%), abdominal pain (2%), dyspepsia (1% to 2%), vomiting (1%)

Genitourinary: Vaginal moniliasis (3% to 6%)

Hematologic: Hematocrit decreased (2%)

Renal: Hematuria (3%), urinary white blood cells increased (2%)

Reactions reported with other cephalosporins: Anaphylaxis, aplastic anemia, cholestasis, hemorrhage, hemolytic anemia, renal dysfunction, reversible hyperactivity, serum sickness-like reaction, toxic nephropathy

Drug Interactions

Metabolism/Transport Effects None known.

Avoid Concomitant Use There are no known interactions where it is recommended to avoid concomitant use.

Increased Effect/Toxicity

The levels/effects of Cefditoren may be increased by: Probenecid

Decreased Effect

The levels/effects of Cefditoren may be decreased by: Antacids; H2-Antagonists; Proton Pump Inhibitors

Ethanol/Nutrition/Herb Interactions Food: Moderate- to high-fat meals increase bioavailability and maximum plasma concentration. Management: Take with meals. Maintain adequate hydration, unless instructed to restrict fluid intake.

Stability Store at controlled room temperature of 15°C to 30°C (59°F to 86°F). Protect from light and moisture.

Mechanism of Action Inhibits bacterial cell wall synthesis by binding to one or more of the penicillin-binding proteins (PBPs) which in turn inhibits the final transpeptidation step of peptidoglycan synthesis in bacterial cell walls, thus inhibiting cell wall biosynthesis. Bacteria eventually lyse due to ongoing activity of cell wall autolytic enzymes (autolysins and murein hydrolases) while cell wall assembly is arrested.

Pharmacodynamics/Kinetics

Distribution: 9.3 ± 1.6 L

Protein binding: 88% (*in vitro*), primarily to albumin

Metabolism: Cefditoren pivoxil is hydrolyzed to cefditoren (active) and pivalate

Bioavailability: ~14% to 16%, increased by moderate- to high-fat meal

Half-life elimination: 1.6 ± 0.4 hours
Time to peak: 1.5-3 hours
Excretion: Urine (as cefditoren and pivaloylcarnitine)

Dosage

Geriatric & Adult

Acute bacterial exacerbation of chronic bronchitis: Oral: 400 mg twice daily for 10 days
Community-acquired pneumonia: Oral: 400 mg twice daily for 14 days
Dental infections (unlabeled use): Oral: 400 mg twice daily for 10 days
Pharyngitis, tonsillitis, uncomplicated skin and skin structure infections: Oral: 200 mg twice daily for 10 days

Renal Impairment

Cl_{cr} 30-49 mL/minute/1.73 m^2: Maximum dose: 200 mg twice daily
Cl_{cr} <30 mL/minute/1.73 m^2: Maximum dose: 200 mg once daily
End-stage renal disease: Appropriate dosing not established

Hepatic Impairment

Mild-to-moderate impairment: Adjustment not required
Severe impairment (Child-Pugh class C): Specific guidelines not available

Administration Should be administered with meals.

Monitoring Parameters Assess patient at beginning and throughout therapy for infection; monitor for signs of anaphylaxis during first dose.

Test Interactions May induce a positive direct Coomb's test. May cause a false-negative ferricyanide test. Glucose oxidase or hexokinase methods recommended for blood/plasma glucose determinations. False-positive urine glucose test when using copper reduction based assays (eg, Clinitest®).

Special Geriatric Considerations Adjust dose for renal function.

Dosage Forms Excipient information presented when available (limited, particularly for generics); consult specific product labeling.
Tablet, oral: 200 mg, 400 mg
  Spectracef®: 200 mg, 400 mg [contains sodium caseinate]

◆ **Cefditoren Pivoxil** *see* Cefditoren *on page* 313

Cefepime (SEF e pim)

Related Information

Antimicrobial Drugs of Choice *on page* 2163
Community-Acquired Pneumonia in Adults *on page* 2171

Medication Safety Issues

Sound-alike/look-alike issues:
Cefepime may be confused with cefixime, cefTAZidime

Brand Names: U.S. Maxipime® [DSC]
Brand Names: Canada Maxipime®
Index Terms Cefepime Hydrochloride
Generic Availability (U.S.) Yes
Pharmacologic Category Antibiotic, Cephalosporin (Fourth Generation)

Use Treatment of uncomplicated and complicated urinary tract infections, including pyelonephritis caused by typical urinary tract pathogens; monotherapy for febrile neutropenia; uncomplicated skin and skin structure infections caused by *Streptococcus pyogenes*; moderate-to-severe pneumonia caused by pneumococcus, *Pseudomonas aeruginosa*, and other gram-negative organisms; complicated intra-abdominal infections (in combination with metronidazole). Also active against methicillin-susceptible staphylococci, *Enterobacter* sp, and many other gram-negative bacilli.

Unlabeled Use Brain abscess (postneurosurgical prevention); malignant otitis externa; septic lateral/cavernous sinus thrombosis

Contraindications Hypersensitivity to cefepime, other cephalosporins, penicillins, other beta-lactam antibiotics, or any component of the formulation

Warnings/Precautions Modify dosage in patients with renal impairment (Cl_{cr} ≤60 mL/minute); may increase risk of encephalopathy, myoclonus, and seizures. Use with caution in patients with a history of penicillin or cephalosporin allergy, especially IgE-mediated reactions (eg, anaphylaxis, urticaria). Prolonged use may result in fungal or bacterial superinfection, including *C. difficile*-associated diarrhea (CDAD) and pseudomembranous colitis; CDAD has been observed >2 months postantibiotic treatment. Use with caution in patients with a history of gastrointestinal disease, especially colitis. May be associated with increased INR, especially in nutritionally-deficient patients, prolonged treatment, hepatic or renal disease. Use with caution in patients with a history of seizure disorder; high levels, particularly in the presence of renal impairment, may increase risk of seizures.

Adverse Reactions (Reflective of adult population; not specific for elderly)

>10%: Hematologic: Positive Coombs' test without hemolysis (16%)

1% to 10%:

Central nervous system: Fever (1%), headache (1%)

Dermatologic: Rash (1% to 4%), pruritus (1%)

Endocrine & metabolic: Hypophosphatemia (3%)

Gastrointestinal: Diarrhea (≤3%), nausea (≤2%), vomiting (≤1%)

Hematologic: Eosinophils (2%)

Hepatic: ALT increased (3%), AST increased (2%), PTT abnormal (2%), PT abnormal (1%)

Local: Inflammation, phlebitis, and pain (1%)

Reactions reported with other cephalosporins: Aplastic anemia, erythema multiforme, hemolytic anemia, hemorrhage, pancytopenia, PT prolonged, renal dysfunction, Stevens-Johnson syndrome, superinfection, toxic epidermal necrolysis, toxic nephropathy, vaginitis

Drug Interactions

Metabolism/Transport Effects None known.

Avoid Concomitant Use

Avoid concomitant use of Cefepime with any of the following: BCG

Increased Effect/Toxicity

Cefepime may increase the levels/effects of: Aminoglycosides

The levels/effects of Cefepime may be increased by: Probenecid

Decreased Effect

Cefepime may decrease the levels/effects of: BCG; Typhoid Vaccine

Stability

Vials: Store at 20°C to 25°C (68°F to 77°F). Protect from light. After reconstitution, stable in normal saline, D_5W, and a variety of other solutions for 24 hours at room temperature and 7 days refrigerated.

Premixed solution: Store frozen at -20°C (-4°F). Thawed solution is stable for 24 hours at room temperature or 7 days under refrigeration; do not refreeze.

Mechanism of Action

Inhibits bacterial cell wall synthesis by binding to one or more of the penicillin-binding proteins (PBPs) which in turn inhibits the final transpeptidation step of peptidoglycan synthesis in bacterial cell walls, thus inhibiting cell wall biosynthesis. Bacteria eventually lyse due to ongoing activity of cell wall autolytic enzymes (autolysins and murein hydrolases) while cell wall assembly is arrested.

Pharmacodynamics/Kinetics

Note: A longer half-life (mean: 3 hours) and reduced renal and total clearances have been reported in older adults compared to younger subjects

Absorption: I.M.: Rapid and complete

Distribution: V_d: Adults: 16-20 L; penetrates into inflammatory fluid at concentrations ~80% of serum levels and into bronchial mucosa at levels ~60% of those reached in the plasma; crosses blood-brain barrier

Protein binding, plasma: ~20%

Metabolism: Minimally hepatic

Half-life elimination: 2 hours

Time to peak: I.M.: 1-2 hours; I.V.: 0.5 hours

Excretion: Urine (85% as unchanged drug)

Dosage

Geriatric & Adult

Brain abscess, postneurosurgical prevention (unlabeled use): I.V.: 2 g every 8 hours with vancomycin

Febrile neutropenia, monotherapy: I.V: 2 g every 8 hours for 7 days or until the neutropenia resolves

Intra-abdominal infections, complicated, severe (in combination with metronidazole): I.V.: 2 g every 12 hours for 7-10 days. **Note:** 2010 IDSA guidelines recommend 2 g every 8-12 hours for 4-7 days (provided source controlled). Not recommended for hospital-acquired intra-abdominal infections (IAI) associated with multidrug-resistant gram negative organisms or in mild-to-moderate community-acquired IAIs due to risk of toxicity and the development of resistant organisms (Solomkin, 2010).

Otitis externa, malignant (unlabeled use): I.V.: 2 g every 12 hours

Pneumonia: I.V.:

Nosocomial (HAP/VAP): 1-2 g every 8-12 hours; **Note:** Duration of therapy may vary considerably (7-21 days); usually longer courses are required if *Pseudomonas*. In absence of *Pseudomonas*, and if appropriate empiric treatment used and patient responsive, it may be clinically appropriate to reduce duration of therapy to 7-10 days (American Thoracic Society Guidelines, 2005).

Community-acquired (including pseudomonal): 1-2 g every 12 hours for 10 days

Septic lateral/cavernous sinus thrombosis (unlabeled use): I.V.: 2 g every 8-12 hours; with metronidazole for lateral

Skin and skin structure, uncomplicated: I.V.: 2 g every 12 hours for 10 days

Urinary tract infections, complicated and uncomplicated:

Mild-to-moderate: I.M., I.V.: 0.5-1 g every 12 hours for 7-10 days

Severe: I.V.: 2 g every 12 hours for 10 days

Renal Impairment

Cefepime Hydrochloride

Creatinine Clearance (mL/minute)	Recommended Maintenance Schedule			
>60 (normal recommended dosing schedule)	500 mg every 12 hours	1 g every 12 hours	2 g every 12 hours	2 g every 8 hours
30-60	500 mg every 24 hours	1 g every 24 hours	2 g every 24 hours	2 g every 12 hours
11-29	500 mg every 24 hours	500 mg every 24 hours	1 g every 24 hours	2 g every 24 hours
<11	250 mg every 24 hours	250 mg every 24 hours	500 mg every 24 hours	1 g every 24 hours

Intermittent hemodialysis (IHD) (administer after hemodialysis on dialysis days): I.V.: Initial: 1 g (single dose) on day 1. Maintenance: 0.5-1 g every 24 hours **or** 1-2 g every 48-72 hours (Heintz, 2009). **Note:** Dosing dependent on the assumption of 3 times/week, complete IHD sessions.

Peritoneal dialysis (PD): Removed to a lesser extent than hemodialysis; administer normal recommended dose every 48 hours

Continuous renal replacement therapy (CRRT) (Heintz, 2009; Trotman, 2005): Drug clearance is highly dependent on the method of renal replacement, filter type, and flow rate. Appropriate dosing requires close monitoring of pharmacologic response, signs of adverse reactions due to drug accumulation, as well as drug concentrations in relation to target trough (if appropriate). The following are general recommendations only (based on dialysate flow/ultrafiltration rates of 1-2 L/hour and minimal residual renal function) and should not supersede clinical judgment:

CVVH: Loading dose of 2 g followed by 1-2 g every 12 hours

CVVHD/CVVHDF: Loading dose of 2 g followed by either 1 g every 8 hours **or** 2 g every 12 hours. **Note:** Dosage of 1 g every 8 hours results in similar steady-state concentrations as 2 g every 12 hours and is more cost effective (Heintz, 2009).

Note: Consider higher dosage of 4 g/day if treating *Pseudomonas* or life-threatening infections in order to maximize time above MIC (Trotman, 2005). Dosage of 2 g every 8 hours may be needed for gram-negative rods with MIC ≥4 mg/L (Heintz, 2009).

Administration May be administered either I.M. or I.V.

Inject deep I.M. into large muscle mass. Inject direct I.V. over 5 minutes. Infuse intermittent infusion over 30 minutes.

Monitoring Parameters Obtain specimen for culture and susceptibility prior to the first dose. Monitor for signs of anaphylaxis during first dose.

Test Interactions Positive direct Coombs', false-positive urinary glucose test using cupric sulfate (Benedict's solution, Clinitest®, Fehling's solution), false-positive serum or urine creatinine with Jaffé reaction, false-positive urinary proteins and steroids

Special Geriatric Considerations Adjust dose for renal function.

Dosage Forms Excipient information presented when available (limited, particularly for generics); consult specific product labeling. [DSC] = Discontinued product

Infusion, premixed iso-osmotic dextrose solution, as hydrochloride: 1 g (50 mL); 2 g (100 mL)

Injection, powder for reconstitution, as hydrochloride: 500 mg, 1 g, 2 g

Maxipime®: 500 mg [DSC], 1 g [DSC], 2 g [DSC]

◆ **Cefepime Hydrochloride** *see* Cefepime *on page 314*

Cefixime (sef IKS eem)

Related Information

Antimicrobial Drugs of Choice *on page 2163*

Medication Safety Issues

Sound-alike/look-alike issues:

Cefixime may be confused with cefepime

Suprax® may be confused with Sporanox®

International issues:
Cefiton: Brand name for cefixime [Portugal] may be confused with Ceftim brand name for ceftazidime [Portugal]; Ceftime brand name for ceftazidime [Thailand]; Ceftin brand name for cefuroxime [U.S., Canada]

Brand Names: U.S. Suprax®

Brand Names: Canada Suprax®

Index Terms Cefixime Trihydrate

Generic Availability (U.S.) No

Pharmacologic Category Antibiotic, Cephalosporin (Third Generation)

Use Treatment of urinary tract infections, otitis media, respiratory infections due to susceptible organisms including *S. pneumoniae* and *S. pyogenes, H. influenzae,* and many Enterobacteriaceae; uncomplicated cervical/urethral gonorrhea due to *N. gonorrhoeae*

Contraindications Hypersensitivity to cefixime, any component of the formulation, or other cephalosporins

Warnings/Precautions Prolonged use may result in fungal or bacterial superinfection, including *C. difficile*-associated diarrhea (CDAD) and pseudomembranous colitis; CDAD has been observed >2 months postantibiotic treatment. Modify dosage in patients with renal impairment. Use with caution in patients with a history of penicillin allergy, especially IgE-mediated reactions (eg, anaphylaxis, urticaria).

Adverse Reactions (Reflective of adult population; not specific for elderly)
>10%: Gastrointestinal: Diarrhea (16%)
2% to 10%: Gastrointestinal: Abdominal pain, nausea, dyspepsia, flatulence, loose stools
Reactions reported with other cephalosporins: Interstitial nephritis, aplastic anemia, hemolytic anemia, hemorrhage, pancytopenia, agranulocytosis, colitis, superinfection

Drug Interactions

Metabolism/Transport Effects None known.

Avoid Concomitant Use
Avoid concomitant use of Cefixime with any of the following: BCG

Increased Effect/Toxicity
Cefixime may increase the levels/effects of: Aminoglycosides

The levels/effects of Cefixime may be increased by: Probenecid

Decreased Effect
Cefixime may decrease the levels/effects of: BCG; Typhoid Vaccine

Ethanol/Nutrition/Herb Interactions Food: Delays cefixime absorption.

Stability After reconstitution, suspension may be stored for 14 days at room temperature or under refrigeration.

Mechanism of Action Inhibits bacterial cell wall synthesis by binding to one or more of the penicillin-binding proteins (PBPs); which in turn inhibits the final transpeptidation step of peptidoglycan synthesis in bacterial cell walls, thus inhibiting cell wall biosynthesis. Bacteria eventually lyse due to ongoing activity of cell wall autolytic enzymes (autolysins and murein hydrolases) while cell wall assembly is arrested.

Pharmacodynamics/Kinetics
Absorption: 40% to 50%
Distribution: Widely throughout the body and reaches therapeutic concentration in most tissues and body fluids, including synovial, pericardial, pleural, peritoneal; bile, sputum, and urine; bone, myocardium, gallbladder, and skin and soft tissue
Protein binding: 65%
Half-life elimination: Normal renal function: 3-4 hours; Renal failure: Up to 11.5 hours
Time to peak, serum: 2-6 hours; delayed with food
Excretion: Urine (50% of absorbed dose as active drug); feces (10%)

Dosage

Geriatric & Adult
Susceptible infections: Oral: 400 mg/day divided every 12-24 hours
Gonococcal infections: Oral:
Uncomplicated cervical/urethral gonorrhea due to *N. gonorrhoeae:* 400 mg as a single dose
Note: Due to increased antimicrobial resistance, the Public Health Agency of Canada recommends 800 mg/day as a single dose (unlabeled dose) for treatment of uncomplicated gonococcal infections.
Disseminated (after appropriate I.V. or I.M. antibiotics and improvement noted) (unlabeled use): 800 mg/day in 2 divided doses to complete a total of 7 days of therapy (CDC, 2010)
S. pyogenes infections: Oral: 400 mg/day divided every 12-24 hours for 10 days
Typhoid fever (unlabeled use): Oral: 20-30 mg/kg/day in 2 divided doses for 7-14 days after I.V. therapy

◀

Renal Impairment
Cl$_{cr}$ 21-60 mL/minute: Administer 75% of the standard dose.
Cl$_{cr}$ <20 mL/minute: Administer 50% of the standard dose.
10% removed by hemodialysis

Administration May be administered with or without food; administer with food to decrease GI distress. Shake oral suspension well before use.

Monitoring Parameters With prolonged therapy, monitor renal and hepatic function periodically. Observe for signs and symptoms of anaphylaxis during first dose.

Test Interactions Positive direct Coombs', false-positive urinary glucose test using cupric sulfate (Benedict's solution, Clinitest®, Fehling's solution), false-positive serum or urine creatinine with Jaffé reaction; false-positive urine ketones using tests with nitroprusside

Special Geriatric Considerations Adjust dose for renal function.

Dosage Forms Excipient information presented when available (limited, particularly for generics); consult specific product labeling. [DSC] = Discontinued product

Powder for suspension, oral, as trihydrate:
   Suprax®: 100 mg/5 mL (50 mL, 100 mL [DSC]); 200 mg/5 mL (50 mL, 75 mL) [contains sodium benzoate; strawberry flavor]

Tablet, oral, as trihydrate:
   Suprax®: 400 mg [scored]

◆ **Cefixime Trihydrate** *see* Cefixime *on page* 316
◆ **Cefotan** *see* CefoTEtan *on page* 320

Cefotaxime (sef oh TAKS eem)

Related Information
Antibiotic Treatment of Adults With Infective Endocarditis *on page* 2157
Antimicrobial Drugs of Choice *on page* 2163
Community-Acquired Pneumonia in Adults *on page* 2171

Medication Safety Issues
Sound-alike/look-alike issues:
  Cefotaxime may be confused with cefOXitin, cefuroxime
International issues:
  Spectrocef [Italy] may be confused with Spectracef brand name for cefditoren [U.S., Great Britain, Mexico, Portugal, Spain]

Brand Names: U.S. Claforan®

Brand Names: Canada Cefotaxime Sodium For Injection; Claforan®

Index Terms Cefotaxime Sodium

Generic Availability (U.S.) Yes: Powder

Pharmacologic Category Antibiotic, Cephalosporin (Third Generation)

Use Treatment of susceptible organisms in lower respiratory tract, skin and skin structure, bone and joint, urinary tract, intra-abdominal, gynecologic as well as bacteremia/septicemia, and documented or suspected central nervous system infections (eg, meningitis). Active against most gram-negative bacilli (not *Pseudomonas* spp) and gram-positive cocci (not enterococcus). Active against many penicillin-resistant pneumococci.

Unlabeled Use Acute bacterial rhinosinusitis (ABRS)

Contraindications Hypersensitivity to cefotaxime, any component of the formulation, or other cephalosporins

Warnings/Precautions Modify dosage in patients with severe renal impairment. Prolonged use may result in superinfection. A potentially life-threatening arrhythmia has been reported in patients who received a rapid (<1 minute) bolus injection via central venous catheter. Granulocytopenia and more rarely agranulocytosis may develop during prolonged treatment (>10 days). Minimize tissue inflammation by changing infusion sites when needed. Use with caution in patients with a history of penicillin allergy, especially IgE-mediated reactions (eg, anaphylaxis, urticaria). Prolonged use may result in fungal or bacterial superinfection, including *C. difficile*-associated diarrhea (CDAD) and pseudomembranous colitis; CDAD has been observed >2 months postantibiotic treatment.

Adverse Reactions (Reflective of adult population; not specific for elderly)
1% to 10%:
  Dermatologic: Pruritus, rash
  Gastrointestinal: Colitis, diarrhea, nausea, vomiting
  Local: Pain at injection site
Reactions reported with other cephalosporins: Aplastic anemia, hemorrhage, pancytopenia, renal dysfunction, seizure, superinfection, toxic nephropathy.

Drug Interactions
Metabolism/Transport Effects None known.

Avoid Concomitant Use
Avoid concomitant use of Cefotaxime with any of the following: BCG

Increased Effect/Toxicity
Cefotaxime may increase the levels/effects of: Aminoglycosides

The levels/effects of Cefotaxime may be increased by: Probenecid

Decreased Effect
Cefotaxime may decrease the levels/effects of: BCG; Typhoid Vaccine

Stability Reconstituted solution is stable for 12-24 hours at room temperature and 7-10 days when refrigerated and for 13 weeks when frozen. For I.V. infusion in NS or D_5W, solution is stable for 24 hours at room temperature, 5 days when refrigerated, or 13 weeks when frozen in Viaflex® plastic containers. Thawed solutions previously of frozen premixed bags are stable for 24 hours at room temperature or 10 days when refrigerated.

Mechanism of Action Inhibits bacterial cell wall synthesis by binding to one or more of the penicillin-binding proteins (PBPs) which in turn inhibits the final transpeptidation step of peptidoglycan synthesis in bacterial cell walls, thus inhibiting cell wall biosynthesis. Bacteria eventually lyse due to ongoing activity of cell wall autolytic enzymes (autolysins and murein hydrolases) while cell wall assembly is arrested.

Pharmacodynamics/Kinetics
Distribution: Widely to body tissues and fluids including aqueous humor, ascitic and prostatic fluids, bone; penetrates CSF best when meninges are inflamed

Metabolism: Partially hepatic to active metabolite, desacetylcefotaxime

Half-life elimination:

Cefotaxime: Adults: 1-1.5 hours; prolonged with renal and/or hepatic impairment

Desacetylcefotaxime: 1.5-1.9 hours; prolonged with renal impairment

Time to peak, serum: I.M.: Within 30 minutes

Excretion: Urine (~60% as unchanged drug and metabolites)

Dosage
Geriatric & Adult
Usual dosage range: I.M., I.V.: 1-2 g every 4-12 hours

Uncomplicated infections: I.M., I.V.: 1 g every 12 hours

Moderate-to-severe infections: I.M., I.V.: 1-2 g every 8 hours

Life-threatening infections: I.V.: 2 g every 4 hours

Acute bacterial rhinosinusitis, severe infection requiring hospitalization: I.V.: 2 g every 4-6 hours for 5-7 days (Chow, 2012)

Arthritis (septic): I.V.: 1 g every 8 hours

Brain abscess, meningitis: I.V.: 2 g every 4-6 hours in combination with other antimicrobial therapy as warranted (Kowlessar, 2006; Tunkel, 2004)

Caesarean section: I.M., I.V.: 1 g as soon as the umbilical cord is clamped, then 1 g at 6- and 12-hour intervals

Complicated community-acquired intra-abdominal infection of mild-to-moderate severity, including hepatic abscess (in combination with metronidazole): I.V.: 1-2 g every 6-8 hours for 4-7 days (provided source controlled). **Note:** For severe infections consider other antimicrobial agents (Bradley, 1987; Kim, 2010; Solomkin, 2010).

Gonorrhea (CDC, 2010) (as an alternative to ceftriaxone):

Uncomplicated: I.M.: 0.5 g as a single dose; may also administer 1 g as a single dose for rectal gonorrhea in males (per the manufacturer)

Disseminated: I.V.: 1 g every 8 hours; may switch to cefixime (after improvement noted) to complete a total of 7 days of therapy

Lyme disease (as an alternative to ceftriaxone):

Cardiac manifestations: I.V.: 2 g every 8 hours for 14-21 days (Wormser, 2006)

CNS manifestations: I.V.: 2 g every 8 hours for 10-28 days (Halperin, 2007; Wormser, 2006)

Peritonitis (spontaneous): I.V.: 2 g every 8 hours, unless life-threatening then 2 g every 4 hours (Gilbert, 2011; Runyon, 2009)

Sepsis: I.V.: 2 g every 6-8 hours

Skin and soft tissue:

Bite wounds (animal): I.V.: 2 g every 6 hours

Mixed, necrotizing: I.V.: 2 g every 6 hours, with metronidazole or clindamycin (Stevens, 2005)

Renal Impairment
Manufacturer's labeling: **Note:** Renal function may be estimated using Cockcroft-Gault formula for dosage adjustment purposes.

Cl_{cr} <20 mL/minute/1.73 m^2: Dose should be decreased by 50%.

Alternate recommendations:

Adults: The following dosage adjustments have been used by some clinicians (Aronoff, 2007; Heintz, 2009; Trotman, 2005):

GFR >50 mL/minute: Administer every 6 hours (Aronoff, 2007)

GFR 10-50 mL/minute: Administer every 6-12 hours (Aronoff, 2007)

GFR <10 mL/minute: Administer every 24 hours **or** decrease the dose by 50% (and administer at usual intervals) (Aronoff, 2007)

Intermittent hemodialysis (IHD): Administer 1-2 g every 24 hours (on dialysis days, administer after hemodialysis). **Note:** Dosing dependent on the assumption of 3 times/week, complete IHD sessions (Heintz, 2009).

Peritoneal dialysis (PD): 1 g every 24 hours (Aronoff, 2007)

Continuous renal replacement therapy (CRRT) (Heintz, 2009; Trotman, 2005): Drug clearance is highly dependent on the method of renal replacement, filter type, and flow rate. Appropriate dosing requires close monitoring of pharmacologic response, signs of adverse reactions due to drug accumulation, as well as drug concentrations in relation to target trough (if appropriate). The following are general recommendations only (based on dialysate flow/ultrafiltration rates of 1-2 L/hour and minimal residual renal function) and should not supersede clinical judgment:

CVVH: 1-2 g every 8-12 hours

CVVHD: 1-2 g every 8 hours

CVVHDF: 1-2 g every 6-8 hours

Hepatic Impairment Dosage reduction generally not necessary unless concurrent severe renal impairment. Consider dose reduction to 0.5 g every 12 hours in patients with Cl_{cr} <5 mL/minute (Wise, 1985).

Administration Can be administered IVP over at least 3-5 minutes or I.V. intermittent infusion over 15-30 minutes.

Monitoring Parameters Observe for signs and symptoms of anaphylaxis during first dose; CBC with differential (especially with long courses); renal function

Test Interactions Positive direct Coombs', false-positive urinary glucose test using cupric sulfate (Benedict's solution, Clinitest®, Fehling's solution), false-positive serum or urine creatinine with Jaffé reaction

Special Geriatric Considerations Adjust dose for renal function.

Dosage Forms Excipient information presented when available (limited, particularly for generics); consult specific product labeling.

Infusion, premixed iso-osmotic solution:

Claforan®: 1 g (50 mL); 2 g (50 mL) [contains sodium ~50.5 mg (2.2 mEq) per cefotaxime 1 g]

Injection, powder for reconstitution: 500 mg, 1 g, 2 g, 10 g

Claforan®: 500 mg, 1 g, 2 g, 10 g [contains sodium ~50.5 mg (2.2 mEq) per cefotaxime 1 g]

♦ **Cefotaxime Sodium** see Cefotaxime on page 318

CefoTEtan (SEF oh tee tan)

Related Information
Antimicrobial Drugs of Choice on page 2163

Medication Safety Issues
Sound-alike/look-alike issues:
CefoTEtan may be confused with ceFAZolin, cefOXitin, cefTAZidime, Ceftin®, cefTRIAXone

Index Terms Cefotan; Cefotetan Disodium

Generic Availability (U.S.) Yes

Pharmacologic Category Antibiotic, Cephalosporin (Second Generation)

Use Surgical prophylaxis; intra-abdominal infections and other mixed infections; respiratory tract, skin and skin structure, bone and joint, urinary tract and gynecologic as well as septicemia; active against gram-negative enteric bacilli including E. coli, Klebsiella, and Proteus; less active against staphylococci and streptococci than first generation cephalosporins, but active against anaerobes including Bacteroides fragilis

Contraindications Hypersensitivity to cefotetan, any component of the formulation, or other cephalosporins; previous cephalosporin-associated hemolytic anemia

Warnings/Precautions Modify dosage in patients with severe renal impairment. Although cefotetan contains the methyltetrazolethiol side chain, bleeding has not been a significant problem. Use with caution in patients with a history of penicillin allergy, especially IgE-mediated reactions (eg, anaphylaxis, urticaria). Cefotetan has been associated with a higher risk of hemolytic anemia relative to other cephalosporins (approximately threefold); monitor carefully during use and consider cephalosporin-associated immune anemia in patients who have received cefotetan within 2-3 weeks (either as treatment or prophylaxis). Prolonged use may result in fungal or bacterial superinfection, including C. difficile-associated diarrhea (CDAD) and pseudomembranous colitis; CDAD has been observed >2 months postantibiotic treatment. May be associated with increased INR, especially in nutritionally-deficient patients, prolonged treatment, hepatic or renal disease.

Adverse Reactions (Reflective of adult population; not specific for elderly)

1% to 10%:
Gastrointestinal: Diarrhea (1%)
Hepatic: Transaminases increased (1%)
Miscellaneous: Hypersensitivity reactions (1%)

Reactions reported with other cephalosporins: Seizure, Stevens-Johnson syndrome, toxic epidermal necrolysis, renal dysfunction, toxic nephropathy, cholestasis, aplastic anemia, hemolytic anemia, hemorrhage, pancytopenia, agranulocytosis, colitis, superinfection

Drug Interactions

Metabolism/Transport Effects None known.

Avoid Concomitant Use
Avoid concomitant use of CefoTEtan with any of the following: BCG

Increased Effect/Toxicity
CefoTEtan may increase the levels/effects of: Alcohol (Ethyl); Aminoglycosides; Vitamin K Antagonists

The levels/effects of CefoTEtan may be increased by: Probenecid

Decreased Effect
CefoTEtan may decrease the levels/effects of: BCG; Typhoid Vaccine

Ethanol/Nutrition/Herb Interactions Ethanol: Avoid ethanol (may cause a disulfiram-like reaction).

Stability Reconstituted solution is stable for 24 hours at room temperature and 96 hours when refrigerated. For I.V. infusion in NS or D_5W solution and after freezing, thawed solution is stable for 24 hours at room temperature or 96 hours when refrigerated. Frozen solution is stable for 12 weeks.

Mechanism of Action Inhibits bacterial cell wall synthesis by binding to one or more of the penicillin-binding proteins (PBPs) which in turn inhibits the final transpeptidation step of peptidoglycan synthesis in bacterial cell walls, thus inhibiting cell wall biosynthesis. Bacteria eventually lyse due to ongoing activity of cell wall autolytic enzymes (autolysins and murein hydrolases) while cell wall assembly is arrested.

Pharmacodynamics/Kinetics

Distribution: Widely to body tissues and fluids including bile, sputum, prostatic, peritoneal; low concentrations enter CSF
Protein binding: 76% to 90%
Half-life elimination: 3-5 hours
Time to peak, serum: I.M.: 1.5-3 hours
Excretion: Primarily urine (as unchanged drug); feces (20%)

Dosage

Geriatric & Adult

Susceptible infections: I.M., I.V.: 1-6 g/day in divided doses every 12 hours; usual dose: 1-2 g every 12 hours for 5-10 days; 1-2 g may be given every 24 hours for urinary tract infection; **Note:** Due to high rates of B. fragilis group resistance, not recommended for the treatment of community-acquired intra-abdominal infections (Solomkin, 2010)

Orbital cellulitis, odontogenic infections: I.V.: 2 g every 12 hours

Pelvic inflammatory disease: I.V.: 2 g every 12 hours; used in combination with doxycycline

Preoperative prophylaxis: I.M., I.V.: 1-2 g 30-60 minutes prior to surgery; when used for cesarean section, dose should be given as soon as umbilical cord is clamped

Urinary tract infection: I.M., I.V.: 1-2 g may be given every 24 hours

Renal Impairment I.M., I.V.:
Cl_{cr} 10-30 mL/minute: Administer every 24 hours
Cl_{cr} <10 mL/minute: Administer every 48 hours
Hemodialysis: Dialyzable (5% to 20%); administer 1/4 the usual dose every 24 hours on days between dialysis; administer 1/2 the usual dose on the day of dialysis.
Continuous arteriovenous or venovenous hemodiafiltration effects: Administer 750 mg every 12 hours

Administration I.M. doses should be given in a large muscle mass (ie, gluteus maximus)

Monitoring Parameters Observe for signs and symptoms of anaphylaxis during first dose; monitor for signs and symptoms of hemolytic anemia, including hematologic parameters where appropriate.

Test Interactions Positive direct Coombs', false-positive urinary glucose test using cupric sulfate (Benedict's solution, Clinitest®, Fehling's solution), false-positive serum or urine creatinine with Jaffé reaction

Pharmacotherapy Pearls Sodium content of 1 g: 3.5 mEq

Special Geriatric Considerations Cefotetan has not been studied in the elderly. Adjust dose for renal function.

◀ **Dosage Forms** Excipient information presented when available (limited, particularly for generics); consult specific product labeling.

Injection, powder for reconstitution: 1 g, 2 g, 10 g [products contain sodium 80 mg (3.5 mEq)/g]

◆ **Cefotetan Disodium** see CefoTEtan on page 320

CefOXitin (se FOKS i tin)

Related Information
Antimicrobial Drugs of Choice on page 2163

Medication Safety Issues
Sound-alike/look-alike issues:
CefOXitin may be confused with ceFAZolin, cefotaxime, cefoTEtan, cefTAZidime, cefTRIAX-one, Cytoxan
Mefoxin® may be confused with Lanoxin®

Brand Names: U.S. Mefoxin®

Brand Names: Canada Cefoxitin For Injection

Index Terms Cefoxitin Sodium

Generic Availability (U.S.) Yes: Excludes infusion

Pharmacologic Category Antibiotic, Cephalosporin (Second Generation)

Use Less active against staphylococci and streptococci than first generation cephalosporins, but active against anaerobes including *Bacteroides fragilis*; active against gram-negative enteric bacilli including *E. coli*, *Klebsiella*, and *Proteus*; used predominantly for respiratory tract, skin, bone and joint, urinary tract and gynecologic as well as septicemia; surgical prophylaxis; intra-abdominal infections and other mixed infections; indicated for bacterial *Eikenella corrodens* infections

Contraindications Hypersensitivity to cefoxitin, any component of the formulation, or other cephalosporins

Warnings/Precautions Modify dosage in patients with severe renal impairment. Prolonged use may result in superinfection. Use with caution in patients with a history of penicillin allergy, especially IgE-mediated reactions (eg, anaphylaxis, urticaria). Prolonged use may result in fungal or bacterial superinfection, including *C. difficile*-associated diarrhea (CDAD) and pseudomembranous colitis; CDAD has been observed >2 months postantibiotic treatment.

Adverse Reactions (Reflective of adult population; not specific for elderly)
1% to 10%: Gastrointestinal: Diarrhea
Reactions reported with other cephalosporins: Agranulocytosis, aplastic anemia, cholestasis, colitis, erythema multiforme, hemolytic anemia, hemorrhage, pancytopenia, renal dysfunction, serum-sickness reactions, seizure, Stevens-Johnson syndrome, superinfection, toxic nephropathy, vaginitis

Drug Interactions
Metabolism/Transport Effects None known.
Avoid Concomitant Use
Avoid concomitant use of CefOXitin with any of the following: BCG
Increased Effect/Toxicity
CefOXitin may increase the levels/effects of: Aminoglycosides; Vitamin K Antagonists

The levels/effects of CefOXitin may be increased by: Probenecid
Decreased Effect
CefOXitin may decrease the levels/effects of: BCG; Typhoid Vaccine

Stability Reconstitute vials with SWFI, bacteriostatic water for injection, NS, or D_5W. For I.V. infusion, solutions may be further diluted in NS, $D_5\frac{1}{4}NS$, $D_5\frac{1}{2}NS$, D_5NS, D_5W, $D_{10}W$, LR, D_5LR, mannitol 10%, or sodium bicarbonate 5%. Reconstituted solution is stable for 6 hours at room temperature or 7 days when refrigerated; I.V. infusion in NS or D_5W solution is stable for 18 hours at room temperature or 48 hours when refrigerated. Premixed frozen solution, when thawed, is stable for 24 hours at room temperature or 21 days when refrigerated.

Mechanism of Action Inhibits bacterial cell wall synthesis by binding to one or more of the penicillin-binding proteins (PBPs) which in turn inhibits the final transpeptidation step of peptidoglycan synthesis in bacterial cell walls, thus inhibiting cell wall biosynthesis. Bacteria eventually lyse due to ongoing activity of cell wall autolytic enzymes (autolysins and murein hydrolases) while cell wall assembly is arrested.

Pharmacodynamics/Kinetics
Distribution: Widely to body tissues and fluids including pleural, synovial, ascitic, bile; poorly penetrates into CSF even with inflammation of the meninges
Protein binding: 65% to 79%
Half-life elimination: 45-60 minutes; significantly prolonged with renal impairment
Time to peak, serum: I.M.: 20-30 minutes

Excretion: Urine (85% as unchanged drug)

Compared to younger patients (<55 years), older patients (66-94 years) have been reported to have a reduced total body clearance, prolonged half-life, increased volume of distribution, and reduced protein binding.

Dosage

Geriatric & Adult

Susceptible infections: I.M., I.V.: 1-2 g every 6-8 hours (I.M. injection is painful); up to 12 g/day

Amnionitis and endomyometritis: I.M., I.V.: 2 g every 6-8 hours

Aspiration pneumonia, empyema, orbital cellulitis, parapharyngeal space, and human bites: I.M., I.V.: 2 g every 8 hours

Intra-abdominal infection, complicated, community acquired, mild-to-moderate: I.V.: 2 g every 6 hours for 4-7 days (provided source controlled)

Liver abscess: I.V.: 1 g every 4 hours

Mycobacterium species, not MTB or MAI: I.V.: 12 g/day with amikacin

Pelvic inflammatory disease:

Inpatients: I.V.: 2 g every 6 hours **plus** doxycycline 100 mg I.V. or 100 mg orally every 12 hours until improved, followed by doxycycline 100 mg orally twice daily to complete 14 days

Outpatients: I.M.: 2 g **plus** probenecid 1 g orally as a single dose, followed by doxycycline 100 mg orally twice daily for 14 days

Perioperative prophylaxis: I.M., I.V.: 1-2 g 30-60 minutes prior to surgery (may repeat in 2-5 hours intraoperatively) followed by 1-2 g every 6-8 hours for no more than 24 hours after surgery depending on the procedure

Renal Impairment I.M., I.V.:

Cl_{cr} 30-50 mL/minute: Administer 1-2 g every 8-12 hours

Cl_{cr} 10-29 mL/minute: Administer 1-2 g every 12-24 hours

Cl_{cr} 5-9 mL/minute: Administer 0.5-1 g every 12-24 hours

Cl_{cr} <5 mL/minute: Administer 0.5-1 g every 24-48 hours

Hemodialysis: Moderately dialyzable (20% to 50%); administer a loading dose of 1-2 g after each hemodialysis; maintenance dose as noted above based on Cl_{cr}

Continuous arteriovenous or venovenous hemodiafiltration effects: Dose as for Cl_{cr} 10-50 mL/minute

Administration

I.M.: Inject deep I.M. into large muscle mass.

I.V.: Can be administered IVP over 3-5 minutes at a maximum concentration of 100 mg/mL or I.V. intermittent infusion over 10-60 minutes at a final concentration for I.V. administration not to exceed 40 mg/mL

Monitoring Parameters Monitor renal function periodically when used in combination with other nephrotoxic drugs; observe for signs and symptoms of anaphylaxis during first dose

Test Interactions Positive direct Coombs', false-positive urinary glucose test using cupric sulfate (Benedict's solution, Clinitest®, Fehling's solution), false-positive serum or urine creatinine with Jaffé reaction

Pharmacotherapy Pearls Sodium content of 1 g: 53 mg (2.3 mEq)

Special Geriatric Considerations Adjust dose for renal function.

Dosage Forms Excipient information presented when available (limited, particularly for generics); consult specific product labeling.

Infusion, premixed iso-osmotic dextrose solution:

Mefoxin®: 1 g (50 mL); 2 g (50 mL) [contains sodium 53.8 mg (2.3 mEq)/g]

Injection, powder for reconstitution: 1 g, 2 g, 10 g

♦ **Cefoxitin Sodium** *see* CefOXitin *on page 322*

Cefpodoxime (sef pode OKS eem)

Related Information

Antimicrobial Drugs of Choice *on page 2163*

Community-Acquired Pneumonia in Adults *on page 2171*

Medication Safety Issues

Sound-alike/look-alike issues:

Vantin may be confused with Ventolin®

Index Terms Cefpodoxime Proxetil; Vantin

Generic Availability (U.S.) Yes

Pharmacologic Category Antibiotic, Cephalosporin (Third Generation)

Use Treatment of susceptible acute, community-acquired pneumonia caused by *S. pneumoniae* or nonbeta-lactamase producing *H. influenzae*; acute uncomplicated gonorrhea caused by *N. gonorrhoeae*; uncomplicated skin and skin structure infections caused by *S. aureus* or

CEFPODOXIME

S. pyogenes; acute otitis media caused by *S. pneumoniae, H. influenzae,* or *M. catarrhalis*; pharyngitis or tonsillitis; and uncomplicated urinary tract infections caused by *E. coli, Klebsiella,* and *Proteus*

Contraindications Hypersensitivity to cefpodoxime, any component of the formulation, or other cephalosporins

Warnings/Precautions Modify dosage in patients with severe renal impairment. Prolonged use may result in fungal or bacterial superinfection, including *C. difficile*-associated diarrhea (CDAD) and pseudomembranous colitis; CDAD has been observed >2 months postantibiotic treatment. Use with caution in patients with a history of penicillin allergy, especially IgE-mediated reactions (eg, anaphylaxis, urticaria).

Adverse Reactions (Reflective of adult population; not specific for elderly)
>10%:
  Dermatologic: Diaper rash (12%)
  Gastrointestinal: Diarrhea in infants and toddlers (15%)
1% to 10%:
  Central nervous system: Headache (1%)
  Dermatologic: Rash (1%)
  Gastrointestinal: Diarrhea (7%), nausea (4%), abdominal pain (2%), vomiting (1% to 2%)
  Genitourinary: Vaginal infection (3%)
Reactions reported with other cephalosporins: Seizure, Stevens-Johnson syndrome, toxic epidermal necrolysis, erythema multiforme, urticaria, serum-sickness reactions, renal dysfunction, interstitial nephritis toxic nephropathy, cholestasis, aplastic anemia, hemolytic anemia, hemorrhage, pancytopenia, agranulocytosis, colitis, vaginitis, superinfection

Drug Interactions
  Metabolism/Transport Effects None known.
  Avoid Concomitant Use
    Avoid concomitant use of Cefpodoxime with any of the following: BCG
  Increased Effect/Toxicity
    Cefpodoxime may increase the levels/effects of: Aminoglycosides

    The levels/effects of Cefpodoxime may be increased by: Probenecid
  Decreased Effect
    Cefpodoxime may decrease the levels/effects of: BCG; Typhoid Vaccine

    The levels/effects of Cefpodoxime may be decreased by: Antacids; H2-Antagonists

Ethanol/Nutrition/Herb Interactions Food: Food and/or low gastric pH delays absorption and may increase serum levels. Management: Take with or without food at regular intervals on an around-the-clock schedule to promote less variation in peak and trough serum levels.

Stability Shake well before using. After mixing, keep suspension in refrigerator. Discard unused portion after 14 days.

Mechanism of Action Inhibits bacterial cell wall synthesis by binding to one or more of the penicillin-binding proteins (PBPs) which in turn inhibits the final transpeptidation step of peptidoglycan synthesis in bacterial cell walls, thus inhibiting cell wall biosynthesis. Bacteria eventually lyse due to ongoing activity of cell wall autolytic enzymes (autolysins and murein hydrolases) while cell wall assembly is arrested.

Pharmacodynamics/Kinetics
  Absorption: Rapid and well absorbed (50%), acid stable; enhanced in the presence of food or low gastric pH
  Distribution: Good tissue penetration, including lung and tonsils; penetrates into pleural fluid
  Protein binding: 18% to 23%
  Metabolism: De-esterified in GI tract to active metabolite, cefpodoxime
  Half-life elimination: 2.2 hours; prolonged with renal impairment
  Time to peak: Within 1 hour
  Excretion: Urine (80% as unchanged drug) in 24 hours

Dosage
  Geriatric & Adult
    Acute community-acquired pneumonia and bacterial exacerbations of chronic bronchitis: Oral: 200 mg every 12 hours for 14 days and 10 days, respectively
    Acute maxillary sinusitis: Oral: 200 mg every 12 hours for 10 days
    Pharyngitis/tonsillitis: Oral: 100 mg every 12 hours for 5-10 days
    Skin and skin structure: Oral: 400 mg every 12 hours for 7-14 days
    Uncomplicated gonorrhea (male and female) and rectal gonococcal infections (female): Oral: 200 mg as a single dose
    Uncomplicated urinary tract infection: Oral: 100 mg every 12 hours for 7 days
  Renal Impairment
    Cl_cr <30 mL/minute: Administer every 24 hours.
    Hemodialysis: Dose 3 times/week following dialysis.
  Hepatic Impairment Dose adjustment is not necessary in patients with cirrhosis.

Administration Administer around-the-clock to promote less variation in peak and trough serum levels.

Monitoring Parameters Observe for signs and symptoms of anaphylaxis during first dose

Test Interactions Positive direct Coombs', false-positive urinary glucose test using cupric sulfate (Benedict's solution, Clinitest®, Fehling's solution), false-positive serum or urine creatinine with Jaffé reaction

Pharmacotherapy Pearls Dose adjustment is not necessary in patients with cirrhosis

Special Geriatric Considerations Considered one of the drugs of choice for outpatient treatment of community-acquired pneumonia in the elderly. Adjust dosage with renal function.

Dosage Forms Excipient information presented when available (limited, particularly for generics); consult specific product labeling.

Granules for suspension, oral: 50 mg/5 mL (50 mL, 100 mL); 100 mg/5 mL (50 mL, 100 mL)

Tablet, oral: 100 mg, 200 mg

◆ **Cefpodoxime Proxetil** *see Cefpodoxime on page 323*

Cefprozil (sef PROE zil)

Medication Safety Issues

Sound-alike/look-alike issues:

Cefprozil may be confused with ceFAZolin, cefuroxime

Cefzil may be confused with Ceftin®

Brand Names: Canada Apo-Cefprozil®; Auro-Cefprozil; Ava-Cefprozil; Cefzil®; RAN™-Cefprozil; Sandoz-Cefprozil

Index Terms Cefzil

Generic Availability (U.S.) Yes

Pharmacologic Category Antibiotic, Cephalosporin (Second Generation)

Use Treatment of otitis media and infections involving the respiratory tract and skin and skin structure; active against methicillin-sensitive staphylococci, many streptococci, and various gram-negative bacilli including *E. coli*, some *Klebsiella*, *P. mirabilis*, *H. influenzae*, and *Moraxella*.

Contraindications Hypersensitivity to cefprozil, any component of the formulation, or other cephalosporins

Warnings/Precautions Modify dosage in patients with severe renal impairment. Use with caution in patients with a history of penicillin allergy, especially IgE-mediated reactions (eg, anaphylaxis, urticaria). Prolonged use may result in fungal or bacterial superinfection, including *C. difficile*-associated diarrhea (CDAD) and pseudomembranous colitis; CDAD has been observed >2 months postantibiotic treatment. Some products may contain phenyl-alanine.

Adverse Reactions (Reflective of adult population; not specific for elderly)

1% to 10%:

Central nervous system: Dizziness (1%)

Dermatologic: Diaper rash (2%)

Gastrointestinal: Diarrhea (3%), nausea (4%), vomiting (1%), abdominal pain (1%)

Genitourinary: Vaginitis, genital pruritus (2%)

Hepatic: Transaminases increased (2%)

Miscellaneous: Superinfection

Reactions reported with other cephalosporins: Seizure, toxic epidermal necrolysis, renal dysfunction, interstitial nephritis, toxic nephropathy, aplastic anemia, hemolytic anemia, hemorrhage, pancytopenia, agranulocytosis, colitis, vaginitis, superinfection

Drug Interactions

Metabolism/Transport Effects None known.

Avoid Concomitant Use

Avoid concomitant use of Cefprozil with any of the following: BCG

Increased Effect/Toxicity

Cefprozil may increase the levels/effects of: Aminoglycosides

The levels/effects of Cefprozil may be increased by: Probenecid

Decreased Effect

Cefprozil may decrease the levels/effects of: BCG; Typhoid Vaccine

Ethanol/Nutrition/Herb Interactions Food: Food delays cefprozil absorption.

Mechanism of Action Inhibits bacterial cell wall synthesis by binding to one or more of the penicillin-binding proteins (PBPs) which in turn inhibits the final transpeptidation step of peptidoglycan synthesis in bacterial cell walls, thus inhibiting cell wall biosynthesis. Bacteria eventually lyse due to ongoing activity of cell wall autolytic enzymes (autolysins and murein hydrolases) while cell wall assembly is arrested.

Pharmacodynamics/Kinetics A mixture of *cis-* (90%) and *trans-* (10%) isomers; well absorbed from the GI tract (90%); food does not delay or reduce absorption; distribution is to most body tissues including the aqueous humor, bone, soft tissues, and the CSF. Elimination is primarily renal with 60% to 70% of the drug excreted in the urine in 24 hours; hepatic dysfunction does not appear to significantly alter elimination. Significantly greater peak concentrations and area under the curve is found in patients with Cl_{cr} <30 mL/minute; also, the half-life is prolonged 1.7 vs 5.9 hours and renal clearance reduced 198 mL/minute vs 18.8 mL/minute compared to patients with normal renal function.

Dosage

Geriatric & Adult

Pharyngitis/tonsillitis: Oral: 500 mg every 24 hours for 10 days

Secondary bacterial infection of acute bronchitis or acute bacterial exacerbation of chronic bronchitis: Oral: 500 mg every 12 hours for 10 days

Uncomplicated skin and skin structure infections: Oral: 250 mg every 12 hours, or 500 mg every 12-24 hours for 10 days

Renal Impairment

Cl_{cr} <30 mL/minute: Reduce dose by 50%.

Hemodialysis effects: 55% is removed by hemodialysis.

Administration Administer around-the-clock to promote less variation in peak and trough serum levels. Chilling the reconstituted oral suspension improves flavor (do not freeze).

Monitoring Parameters Assess patient at beginning and throughout therapy for infection; monitor for signs of anaphylaxis during first dose

Test Interactions Positive direct Coombs', false-positive urinary glucose test using cupric sulfate (Benedict's solution, Clinitest®, Fehling's solution), false-positive serum or urine creatinine with Jaffé reaction

Special Geriatric Considerations Has not been studied exclusively in the elderly. Adjust dose for renal function.

Dosage Forms Excipient information presented when available (limited, particularly for generics); consult specific product labeling.

Powder for suspension, oral: 125 mg/5 mL (50 mL, 75 mL, 100 mL); 250 mg/5 mL (50 mL, 75 mL, 100 mL)

Tablet, oral: 250 mg, 500 mg

Ceftaroline Fosamil (sef TAR oh leen FOS a mil)

Brand Names: U.S. Teflaro™
Index Terms PPI-0903; PPI-0903M; T-91825; TAK-599
Generic Availability (U.S.) No
Pharmacologic Category Antibiotic, Cephalosporin (Fifth Generation)
Use Treatment of acute bacterial skin and skin structure infections (ABSSSI) caused by susceptible isolates of *Staphylococcus aureus* (including methicillin-susceptible and -resistant isolates), *Streptococcus pyogenes*, *Streptococcus agalactiae*, *Escherichia coli*, *Klebsiella pneumoniae,* and *Klebsiella oxytoca,* and community-acquired pneumonia (CAP) caused by *Streptococcus pneumoniae* (including cases with concurrent bacteremia), *Staphylococcus aureus* (methicillin-susceptible isolates only), *Haemophilus influenzae, Klebsiella pneumoniae, Klebsiella oxytoca,* and *Escherichia coli*
Contraindications Hypersensitivity to ceftaroline, other cephalosporins, or any component of the formulation
Warnings/Precautions Use with caution in patients with a history of penicillin allergy, especially IgE-mediated reactions (eg, anaphylaxis, angioedema, urticaria). Prolonged use may result in fungal or bacterial superinfection, including *C. difficile*-associated diarrhea (CDAD) and pseudomembranous colitis; CDAD has been observed >2 months postantibiotic treatment. Use with caution in patients with renal impairment (Cl_{cr} ≤50 mL/minute); dosage adjustments recommended.
Adverse Reactions (Reflective of adult population; not specific for elderly)
>10%: Hematologic: Positive Coombs' test without hemolysis (~11%)
2% to 10%:
Central nervous system: Headache (3% to 5%), insomnia (3% to 4%)
Dermatologic: Pruritus (3% to 4%), rash (3%)
Endocrine & metabolic: Hypokalemia (2%)
Gastrointestinal: Diarrhea (5%), nausea (4%), constipation (2%), vomiting (2%)
Hepatic: Transaminases increased (2%)
Local: Phlebitis (2%)

Drug Interactions

Metabolism/Transport Effects None known.

Avoid Concomitant Use

Avoid concomitant use of Ceftaroline Fosamil with any of the following: BCG

Increased Effect/Toxicity

The levels/effects of Ceftaroline Fosamil may be increased by: Probenecid

Decreased Effect

Ceftaroline Fosamil may decrease the levels/effects of: BCG; Typhoid Vaccine

Stability Store unused vials at 2°C to 8°C (36°F to 46°F); unused vials may be stored at room temperature, up to 25°C (77°F), for ≤7 days. Reconstitute 400 mg or 600 mg vial with 20 mL SWFI; mix gently; reconstituted solution should be further diluted for I.V. administration in 50-250 mL of a compatible solution (eg, D_5W, NS); use within 6 hours at room temperature or within 24 hours if refrigerated; color of infusion solutions ranges from clear and light to dark yellow depending on concentration and storage conditions.

Mechanism of Action Inhibits bacterial cell wall synthesis by binding to penicillin-binding proteins (PBPs) 1 through 3. This action blocks the final transpeptidation step of peptidoglycan synthesis in bacterial cell walls and inhibits cell wall biosynthesis. Bacteria eventually lyse due to ongoing activity of cell wall autolytic enzymes (autolysis and murein hydrolases) while cell wall assembly is arrested. Ceftaroline has a strong affinity for PBP2a, a modified PBP in MRSA, and PBP2x in *S. pneumoniae*, contributing to its spectrum of activity against these bacteria.

Pharmacodynamics/Kinetics

Distribution: V_d: 18.3-21.6 L

Protein binding: ~20%

Metabolism: Ceftaroline fosamil (inactive prodrug) undergoes rapid conversion to bioactive ceftaroline in plasma by phosphatase enzyme; ceftaroline is hydrolyzed to form inactive ceftaroline M-1 metabolite

Half-life elimination: Normal renal function: 2.4 hours; Moderate renal impairment (Cl_{cr} 30-50 ml/minute): 4.5 hours

Time to peak: 1 hour

Excretion: Urine (~88%); feces (~6%)

Dosage

Geriatric & Adult

Usual dosage range: I.V.: 600 mg every 12 hours

Indication-specific dosage: I.V.:

Pneumonia, community-acquired: 600 mg every 12 hours for 5-7 days

Skin and skin structure, complicated: 600 mg every 12 hours for 5-14 days

Renal Impairment

Cl_{cr} 31-50 mL/minute: Administer 400 mg every 12 hours

Cl_{cr} 15-30 mL/minute: Administer 300 mg every 12 hours

Cl_{cr} <15mL/minute and ESRD patients receiving hemodialysis: Administer 200 mg every 12 hours; should be given after hemodialysis, if applicable

Administration Administer by slow I.V. infusion over 60 minutes.

Monitoring Parameters Obtain specimen for culture and susceptibility prior to the first dose. Monitor for signs of anaphylaxis during first dose. Monitor renal function.

Pharmacotherapy Pearls Considered to be ineffective against *Pseudomonas aeruginosa*, *Enterococcus* species (including vancomycin-susceptible and -resistant isolates), extended-spectrum beta-lactamase (ESBL) producing or AmpC overexpressing Enterobacteriaceae.

Special Geriatric Considerations Patients 65 years and older accounted for 30.5% of the participants (n=397) in the clinical trials leading to FDA's approval of ceftaroline. Similar cure rates for ABSSI and CABP were reported for those 65 years and older compared to younger adults. Adverse drug events were reported in 52.4% of older participants compared to 42.8% in patients less than 65 years of age. A 33% increase in ceftaroline's AUC was found in healthy older adults (65 and older) compared to younger adults. The increase in AUC was attributed to age-related decrease in kidney function. Adjust dose for renal function.

Dosage Forms Excipient information presented when available (limited, particularly for generics); consult specific product labeling.

Injection, powder for reconstitution:

Teflaro™: 600 mg

CefTAZidime (SEF tay zi deem)

Related Information
Antimicrobial Drugs of Choice *on page 2163*

Medication Safety Issues
Sound-alike/look-alike issues:
CefTAZidime may be confused with ceFAZolin, cefepime, cefoTEtan, cefOXitin, cefTRIAX-one
Ceptaz® may be confused with Septra®
Tazicef® may be confused with Tazidime®

International issues:
Ceftim [Portugal] and Ceftime [Thailand] brand names for ceftazidime may be confused with Ceftin brand name for cefuroxime [U.S., Canada]; Cefiton brand name for cefixime [Portugal]

Brand Names: U.S. Fortaz®; Tazicef®

Brand Names: Canada Ceftazidime For Injection; Fortaz®

Generic Availability (U.S.) Yes: Injection

Pharmacologic Category Antibiotic, Cephalosporin (Third Generation)

Use Treatment of documented susceptible *Pseudomonas aeruginosa* infection and infections due to other susceptible aerobic gram-negative organisms; empiric therapy of a febrile, granulocytopenic patient

Unlabeled Use Bacterial endophthalmitis

Contraindications Hypersensitivity to ceftazidime, any component of the formulation, or other cephalosporins

Warnings/Precautions Modify dosage in patients with severe renal impairment. Use with caution in patients with a history of penicillin allergy, especially IgE-mediated reactions (eg, anaphylaxis, urticaria). Prolonged use may result in fungal or bacterial superinfection, including *C. difficile*-associated diarrhea (CDAD) and pseudomembranous colitis; CDAD has been observed >2 months postantibiotic treatment. May be associated with increased INR, especially in nutritionally-deficient patients, prolonged treatment, hepatic or renal disease. Use with caution in patients with a history of seizure disorder; high levels, particularly in the presence of renal impairment, may increase risk of seizures.

Adverse Reactions (Reflective of adult population; not specific for elderly)
1% to 10%:
Gastrointestinal: Diarrhea (1%)
Local: Pain at injection site (1%)
Miscellaneous: Hypersensitivity reactions (2%)
Reactions reported with other cephalosporins: Seizure, urticaria, serum-sickness reactions, renal dysfunction, interstitial nephritis, toxic nephropathy, BUN increased, creatinine increased, cholestasis, aplastic anemia, hemolytic anemia, pancytopenia, agranulocytosis, colitis, prolonged PT, hemorrhage, superinfection

Drug Interactions
Metabolism/Transport Effects None known.

Avoid Concomitant Use
Avoid concomitant use of CefTAZidime with any of the following: BCG

Increased Effect/Toxicity
CefTAZidime may increase the levels/effects of: Aminoglycosides

The levels/effects of CefTAZidime may be increased by: Probenecid

Decreased Effect
CefTAZidime may decrease the levels/effects of: BCG; Typhoid Vaccine

Stability
Fortaz®: Store dry vials at 15°C to 30°C (59°F to 86°F). Protect from light. Reconstituted solution and solution further diluted for I.V. infusion are stable for 12 hours at room temperature, for 3 days when refrigerated, or for 12 weeks when frozen at -20°C (-4°F). After freezing, thawed solution in SWFI for I.M. administration is stable for 3 hours at room temperature or for 3 days when refrigerated; thawed solution in NS in a Viaflex® small volume container for I.V. administration is stable for 12 hours at room temperature or for 3 days when refrigerated; and thawed solution in SWFI in the original container is stable for 8 hours at room temperature or for 3 days when refrigerated.
Premixed frozen solution: Store frozen at -20°C (-4°F). Thawed solution is stable for 8 hours at room temperature or for 3 days under refrigeration; do not refreeze.

Fortaz®, Tazicef®: ADD-Vantage® vials: Diluted in 50 or 100 mL of D$_5$W, NS, or 0.45% sodium chloride in an ADD-Vantage® flexible diluent container only, may be stored for up to 12 hours at room temperature or for 3 days under refrigeration. Freezing solutions in the ADD-Vantage® system is not recommended. Joined vials that have not been activated may be used within 14 days.

Tazicef® vials: Store dry vials at 20°C to 25°C (68°F to 77°F). Protect from light. Reconstituted vials and solution further diluted for I.V. infusion are stable for 24 hours at room temperature, for 7 days when refrigerated, or for 12 weeks when frozen at -20°C (-4°F). When thawed, solution is stable for 8 hours at room temperature and 4 days when refrigerated.

Reconstitution:

I.M.: Using SWFI, bacteriostatic water, lidocaine 0.5%, or lidocaine 1%, reconstitute the 500 mg vials with 1.5 mL or the 1 g vials with 3 mL; final concentration of ~280 mg/mL

I.V.: Using SWFI, reconstitute as follows (**Note:** After reconstitution, may dilute further with a compatible solution to administer via I.V. infusion):

Fortaz®:

~100 mg/mL solution:

500 mg vial: 5.3 mL SWFI (withdraw 5 mL from the reconstituted vial to obtain a 500 mg dose)

1 g vial: 10 mL SWFI (withdraw 10 mL from the reconstituted vial to obtain a 1 g dose)

6 g vial: 56 mL SWFI (withdraw 10 mL from the reconstituted vial to obtain a 1 g dose)

~170 mg/mL solution: 2 g vial: 10 mL SWFI (withdraw 11.5 mL from the reconstituted vial to obtain a 2 g dose)

~200 mg/mL solution: 6 g vial: 26 mL SWFI (withdraw 5 mL from the reconstituted vial to obtain a 1 g dose)

Tazicef®:

~95 mg/mL solution: 1 g vial: 10 mL SWFI (withdraw 10.6 mL from the reconstituted vial to obtain a 1 g dose)

~180 mg/mL solution: 2 g vial: 10 mL SWFI (withdraw 11.2 mL from the reconstituted vial to obtain a 2 g dose)

Fortaz®, Tazicef®: ADD-Vantage® vials: Dilute in 50 or 100 mL of D$_5$W, NS, or 0.45% sodium chloride in an ADD-Vantage® flexible diluent container only.

Mechanism of Action Inhibits bacterial cell wall synthesis by binding to one or more of the penicillin-binding proteins (PBPs) which in turn inhibits the final transpeptidation step of peptidoglycan synthesis in bacterial cell walls, thus inhibiting cell wall biosynthesis. Bacteria eventually lyse due to ongoing activity of cell wall autolytic enzymes (autolysins and murein hydrolases) while cell wall assembly is arrested.

Pharmacodynamics/Kinetics

Distribution: Widely throughout the body including bone, bile, skin, CSF (diffuses into CSF with higher concentrations when the meninges are inflamed) endometrium, heart, pleural and lymphatic fluids

Protein binding: 17%, <10% protein binding in older adults; in older adults half-life increased, volume of distribution decreased, and AUC increased

Half-life: 1-2 hours (prolonged with renal impairment)

Time to peak serum concentration: I.M.: Within 60 minutes

Elimination: By glomerular filtration with 80% to 90% of the dose excreted as unchanged drug within 24 hours

Dosage

Geriatric I.M., I.V.: Dosage should be based on renal function with a dosing interval not more frequent then every 12 hours.

Adult

Bacterial arthritis (gram negative bacilli): I.V.: 1-2 g every 8 hours

Bone and joint infections: I.V.: 2 g every 12 hours

Cystic fibrosis, lung infection caused by *Pseudomonas* **spp:** I.V.: 30-50 mg/kg/dose every 8 hours (maximum: 6 g/day)

Endophthalmitis, bacterial (unlabeled use): Intravitreal: 2.25 mg/0.1 mL NS in combination with vancomycin

Intra-abdominal infection, severe (in combination with metronidazole): I.V.: 2 g every 8 hours for 4-7 days (provided source controlled). Not recommended for hospital-acquired intra-abdominal infections (IAI) associated with multidrug-resistant gram negative organisms or in mild-to-moderate community-acquired IAIs due to risk of toxicity and the development of resistant organisms (Solomkin, 2010).

Melioidosis: I.V.: 40 mg/kg/dose every 8 hours for 10 days, followed by oral therapy with doxycycline or TMP/SMX

Otitis externa: I.V.: 2 g every 8 hours

Peritonitis (CAPD):
Anuric, intermittent: 1000-1500 mg/day
Anuric, continuous (per liter exchange): Loading dose: 250 mg; maintenance dose: 125 mg

Pneumonia: I.V.:
Uncomplicated: 500 mg to 1 g every 8 hours
Complicated or severe: 2 g every 8 hours

Skin and soft tissue infections: I.V., I.M.: 500 mg to 1 g every 8 hours

Severe infections, including meningitis, complicated pneumonia, endophthalmitis, CNS infection, osteomyelitis, gynecological, skin and soft tissue: I.V.: 2 g every 8 hours

Urinary tract infections: I.V., I.M.:
Uncomplicated: 250 mg every 12 hours
Complicated: 500 mg every 8-12 hours

Renal Impairment

Cl_{cr} 30-50 mL/minute: Administer every 12 hours

Cl_{cr} 10-30 mL/minute: Administer every 24 hours

Cl_{cr} <10 mL/minute: Administer every 48-72 hours

Intermittent hemodialysis (IHD) (administer after hemodialysis on dialysis days): Dialyzable (50% to 100%): 0.5-1 g every 24 hours **or** 1-2 g every 48-72 hours (Heintz, 2009). **Note:** Dosing dependent on the assumption of 3 times/week, complete IHD sessions.

Peritoneal dialysis (PD): Loading dose of 1 g, followed by 500 mg every 24 hours

Continuous renal replacement therapy (CRRT) (Heintz, 2009; Trotman, 2005): Drug clearance is highly dependent on the method of renal replacement, filter type, and flow rate. Appropriate dosing requires close monitoring of pharmacologic response, signs of adverse reactions due to drug accumulation, as well as drug concentrations in relation to target trough (if appropriate). The following are general recommendations only (based on dialysate flow/ultrafiltration rates of 1-2 L/hour and minimal residual renal function) and should not supersede clinical judgment:

CVVH: Loading dose of 2 g followed by 1-2 g every 12 hours

CVVHD/CVVHDF: Loading dose of 2 g followed by either 1 g every 8 hours **or** 2 g every 12 hours. **Note:** Dosage of 1 g every 8 hours results in similar steady-state concentrations as 2 g every 12 hours and is more cost effective. Dosage of 2 g every 8 hours may be needed for gram-negative rods with MIC ≥4 mg/L (Heintz, 2009).

Note: For patients receiving CVVHDF, some recommend giving a loading dose of 2 g followed by 3 g over 24 hours as a continuous I.V. infusion to maintain concentrations ≥4 times the MIC for susceptible pathogens (Heintz, 2009).

Administration Any carbon dioxide bubbles that may be present in the withdrawn solution should be expelled prior to injection. Ceftazidime can be administered IVP over 3-5 minutes, or I.V. retrograde or I.V. intermittent infusion over 15-30 minutes; final concentration for I.V. administration should not exceed 100 mg/mL; can be reconstituted for I.M. administration with 0.5% or 1% lidocaine if volume tolerated.

Monitoring Parameters Observe for signs and symptoms of anaphylaxis during first dose

Test Interactions Positive direct Coombs', false-positive urinary glucose test using cupric sulfate (Benedict's solution, Clinitest®, Fehling's solution), false-positive serum or urine creatinine with Jaffé reaction

Pharmacotherapy Pearls Sodium content of 1 g: 54 mg (2.3 mEq). For most older adults; weak third generation cephalosporin strongest against anaerobes and gram-positive bacteria; *Pseudomonas* sp.

Special Geriatric Considerations Changes in renal function associated with aging and corresponding alterations in pharmacokinetics result in every 12-hour dosing being an adequate dosing interval. Adjust dose based on renal function.

Dosage Forms Excipient information presented when available (limited, particularly for generics); consult specific product labeling. [DSC] = Discontinued product

Infusion, premixed iso-osmotic solution, as sodium [strength expressed as base]:
Fortaz®: 1 g (50 mL); 2 g (50 mL) [contains sodium ~54 mg (2.3 mEq)/g]

Injection, powder for reconstitution: 500 mg [DSC], 1 g, 2 g, 6 g
Fortaz®: 500 mg, 1 g, 2 g, 6 g [contains sodium ~54 mg (2.3 mEq)/g]
Tazicef®: 1 g, 2 g, 6 g [contains sodium ~54 mg (2.3 mEq)/g]

Ceftibuten (sef TYE byoo ten)

Medication Safety Issues
Sound-alike/look-alike issues:
Cedax® may be confused with Cidex®
International issues:
Cedax [U.S. and multiple international markets] may be confused with Codex brand name for acetaminophen/codeine [Brazil] and *Saccharomyces boulardii* [Italy]

Brand Names: U.S. Cedax®
Generic Availability (U.S.) No
Pharmacologic Category Antibiotic, Cephalosporin (Third Generation)
Use Treatment of acute exacerbations of chronic bronchitis, acute bacterial otitis media, and pharyngitis/tonsillitis
Contraindications Hypersensitivity to ceftibuten, any component of the formulation, or other cephalosporins
Warnings/Precautions Modify dosage in patients with moderate-to-severe renal impairment. Prolonged use may result in fungal or bacterial superinfection, including *C. difficile*-associated diarrhea (CDAD) and pseudomembranous colitis; CDAD has been observed >2 months postantibiotic treatment. Use with caution in patients with a history of colitis and other gastrointestinal diseases. Use with caution in patients with a history of penicillin allergy, especially IgE-mediated reactions (eg, anaphylaxis, urticaria). Oral suspension formulation contains sucrose.

Adverse Reactions (Reflective of adult population; not specific for elderly)
1% to 10%:
Central nervous system: Headache (≤3%), dizziness (≤1%)
Gastrointestinal: Nausea (≤4%), diarrhea (3% to 4%), dyspepsia (≤2%), loose stools (≤2%), abdominal pain (1% to 2%), vomiting (1% to 2%)
Hematologic: Eosinophils increased (3%), hemoglobin decreased (1% to 2%), platelets increased (≤1%)
Hepatic: ALT increased (≤1%), bilirubin increased (≤1%)
Renal: BUN increased (2% to 4%)
Additional reactions reported with other cephalosporins: Allergic reaction, agranulocytosis, angioedema, aplastic anemia, anaphylaxis, asterixis, cholestasis, drug fever, encephalopathy, erythema multiforme, hemolytic anemia, hemorrhage, interstitial nephritis, neuromuscular excitability, neutropenia, pancytopenia, prolonged PT, renal dysfunction, seizure, superinfection, toxic nephropathy

Drug Interactions
Metabolism/Transport Effects None known.
Avoid Concomitant Use
Avoid concomitant use of Ceftibuten with any of the following: BCG
Increased Effect/Toxicity
Ceftibuten may increase the levels/effects of: Aminoglycosides

The levels/effects of Ceftibuten may be increased by: Probenecid
Decreased Effect
Ceftibuten may decrease the levels/effects of: BCG; Typhoid Vaccine
Stability Store capsules and powder for suspension at 2°C to 25°C (36°F to 77°F). Reconstituted suspension is stable for 14 days when refrigerated at 2°C to 8°C (36°F to 46°F).
Mechanism of Action Inhibits bacterial cell wall synthesis by binding to one or more of the penicillin-binding proteins (PBPs) which in turn inhibits the final transpeptidation step of peptidoglycan synthesis in bacterial cell walls, thus inhibiting cell wall biosynthesis. Bacteria eventually lyse due to ongoing activity of cell wall autolytic enzymes (autolysins and murein hydrolases) while cell wall assembly is arrested.

Pharmacodynamics/Kinetics
Absorption: Rapid; food decreases peak concentrations, delays T_{max}, and lowers AUC
Distribution: V_d: Adults: 0.21 L/kg
Protein binding: 65%
Half-life elimination: 2 hours; Cl_{cr} 30-49 mL/minute: 7 hours; Cl_{cr} 5-29 mL/minute: 13 hours; Cl_{cr} <5 mL/minute: 22 hours
Time to peak: 2-3 hours
Excretion: Urine (~56%); feces (39%)

Dosage
  Geriatric & Adult Susceptible infections: Oral: 400 mg once daily for 10 days
  Renal Impairment
    Cl_{cr} ≥50 mL//minute: No adjustment needed
    Cl_{cr} 30-49 mL//minute: Administer 4.5 mg/kg or 200 mg every 24 hours.
    Cl_{cr} 5-29 mL/minute: Administer 2.25 mg/kg or 100 mg every 24 hours.
    Hemodialysis: Administer 400 mg or 9 mg/kg (maximum: 400 mg) after each hemodialysis session.

Administration
  Capsule: Administer without regard to food.
  Suspension: Administer 2 hours before or 1 hour after meals. Shake well before use.

Monitoring Parameters Observe for signs and symptoms of anaphylaxis during first dose; with prolonged therapy, monitor renal, hepatic, and hematologic function periodically

Test Interactions Positive direct Coombs', false-positive urinary glucose test using cupric sulfate (Benedict's solution, Clinitest®, Fehling's solution), false-positive serum or urine creatinine with Jaffé reaction

Special Geriatric Considerations Has not been studied specifically in the elderly. Adjust dose for renal function.

Dosage Forms Excipient information presented when available (limited, particularly for generics); consult specific product labeling.
  Capsule, oral:
    Cedax®: 400 mg
  Powder for suspension, oral:
    Cedax®: 90 mg/5 mL (60 mL, 90 mL, 120 mL); 180 mg/5 mL (60 mL) [contains sodium benzoate, sucrose ~1 g/5 mL; cherry flavor]

◆ **Ceftin®** *see* Cefuroxime *on page 336*

CefTRIAXone (sef trye AKS one)

Related Information
  Antibiotic Treatment of Adults With Infective Endocarditis *on page 2157*
  Antimicrobial Drugs of Choice *on page 2163*
  Community-Acquired Pneumonia in Adults *on page 2171*
  Prevention of Infective Endocarditis *on page 2175*
Medication Safety Issues
  Sound-alike/look-alike issues:
    CefTRIAXone may be confused with CeFAZolin, cefoTEtan, cefOXitin, cefTAZidime, Cetraxal®
    Rocephin® may be confused with Roferon®
Brand Names: U.S. Rocephin®
Brand Names: Canada Ceftriaxone for Injection; Ceftriaxone Sodium for Injection BP; Rocephin®
Index Terms Ceftriaxone Sodium
Generic Availability (U.S.) Yes
Pharmacologic Category Antibiotic, Cephalosporin (Third Generation)
Use Treatment of lower respiratory tract infections, acute bacterial otitis media, skin and skin structure infections, bone and joint infections, intra-abdominal and urinary tract infections, pelvic inflammatory disease (PID), uncomplicated gonorrhea, bacterial septicemia, and meningitis; used in surgical prophylaxis
Unlabeled Use Treatment of chancroid, epididymitis, complicated gonococcal infections; sexually-transmitted diseases (STD); periorbital or buccal cellulitis; salmonellosis or shigellosis; atypical community-acquired pneumonia; acute bacterial rhinosinusitis (ABRS); epiglottitis, Lyme disease; used in chemoprophylaxis for high-risk contacts (close exposure to patients with invasive meningococcal disease); sexual assault; typhoid fever, Whipple's disease
Contraindications Hypersensitivity to ceftriaxone sodium, any component of the formulation, or other cephalosporins
Warnings/Precautions Use with caution in patients with a history of penicillin allergy, especially IgE-mediated reactions (eg, anaphylaxis, urticaria). Abnormal gallbladder sonograms have been reported, possibly due to cetriaxone-calcium precipitates; discontinue in patients who develop signs and symptoms of gallbladder disease. Secondary to biliary obstruction, pancreatitis has been reported rarely. Use with caution in patients with a history of GI disease, especially colitis. Severe cases (including some fatalities) of immune-related

hemolytic anemia have been reported in patients receiving cephalosporins, including ceftriaxone. Prolonged use may result in fungal or bacterial superinfection, including *C. difficile*-associated diarrhea (CDAD) and pseudomembranous colitis; CDAD has been observed >2 months postantibiotic treatment.

May be associated with increased INR (rarely), especially in nutritionally-deficient patients, prolonged treatment, hepatic or renal disease. No adjustment is generally necessary in patients with renal impairment; use with caution in patients with concurrent hepatic dysfunction and significant renal disease, dosage should not exceed 2 g/day. Ceftriaxone may complex with calcium causing precipitation. Ceftriaxone should not be diluted or administered simultaneously with any calcium-containing solution via a Y-site in any patient. However, ceftriaxone and calcium-containing solution may be administered sequentially of one another for use in patients **other than neonates** if infusion lines are thoroughly flushed, with a compatible fluid, between infusions

Adverse Reactions (Reflective of adult population; not specific for elderly)

>10%: Local: Induration (I.M. 5% to 17%), warmth (I.M.), tightness (I.M.)

1% to 10%:

Dermatologic: Rash (2%)

Gastrointestinal: Diarrhea (3%)

Hematologic: Eosinophilia (6%), thrombocytosis (5%), leukopenia (2%)

Hepatic: Transaminases increased (3%)

Local: Tenderness at injection site (I.V. 1%), pain

Renal: BUN increased (1%)

Reactions reported with other cephalosporins: Angioedema, allergic reaction, aplastic anemia, asterixis, cholestasis, encephalopathy, hemorrhage, hepatic dysfunction, hyperactivity (reversible), hypertonia, interstitial nephritis, LDH increased, neuromuscular excitability, pancytopenia, paresthesia, renal dysfunction, superinfection, toxic nephropathy

Drug Interactions

Metabolism/Transport Effects None known.

Avoid Concomitant Use

Avoid concomitant use of CefTRIAXone with any of the following: BCG

Increased Effect/Toxicity

CefTRIAXone may increase the levels/effects of: Aminoglycosides; Vitamin K Antagonists

The levels/effects of CefTRIAXone may be increased by: Calcium Salts (Intravenous); Probenecid; Ringer's Injection (Lactated)

Decreased Effect

CefTRIAXone may decrease the levels/effects of: BCG; Typhoid Vaccine

Stability

Powder for injection: Prior to reconstitution, store at room temperature ≤25°C (≤77°F). Protect from light.

Premixed solution (manufacturer premixed): Store at -20°C. Once thawed, solutions are stable for 3 days at room temperature of 25°C (77°F) or for 21 days refrigerated at 5°C (41°F). Do not refreeze.

Stability of reconstituted solutions:

10-40 mg/mL: Reconstituted in D_5W, $D_{10}W$, NS, or SWFI: Stable for 2 days at room temperature of 25°C (77°F) or for 10 days when refrigerated at 4°C (39°F). Stable for 26 weeks when frozen at -20°C when reconstituted with D_5W or NS. Once thawed (at room temperature), solutions are stable for 2 days at room temperature of 25°C (77°F) or for 10 days when refrigerated at 4°C (39°F); does not apply to manufacturer's premixed bags. Do not refreeze.

100 mg/mL:

Reconstituted in D_5W, SWFI, or NS: Stable for 2 days at room temperature of 25°C (77°F) or for 10 days when refrigerated at 4°C (39°F).

Reconstituted in lidocaine 1% solution or bacteriostatic water: Stable for 24 hours at room temperature of 25°C (77°F) or for 10 days when refrigerated at 4°C (39°F).

250-350 mg/mL: Reconstituted in D_5W, NS, lidocaine 1% solution, bacteriostatic water, or SWFI: Stable for 24 hours at room temperature of 25°C (77°F) or for 3 days when refrigerated at 4°C (39°F).

Reconstitution:

I.M. injection: Vials should be reconstituted with appropriate volume of diluent (including D_5W, NS, SWFI, bacteriostatic water, or 1% lidocaine) to make a final concentration of 250 mg/mL or 350 mg/mL.

Volume to add to create a **250 mg/mL** solution:
250 mg vial: 0.9 mL
500 mg vial: 1.8 mL
1 g vial: 3.6 mL
2 g vial: 7.2 mL
Volume to add to create a **350 mg/mL** solution:
500 mg vial: 1.0 mL
1 g vial: 2.1 mL
2 g vial: 4.2 mL
I.V. infusion: Infusion is prepared in two stages: Initial reconstitution of powder, followed by dilution to final infusion solution.
Vials: Reconstitute powder with appropriate I.V. diluent (including SWFI, D_5W, $D_{10}W$, NS) to create an initial solution of ~100 mg/mL. Recommended volume to add:
250 mg vial: 2.4 mL
500 mg vial: 4.8 mL
1 g vial: 9.6 mL
2 g vial: 19.2 mL
Note: After reconstitution of powder, further dilution into a volume of compatible solution (eg, 50-100 mL of D_5W or NS) is recommended.
Piggyback bottle: Reconstitute powder with appropriate I.V. diluent (D_5W or NS) to create a resulting solution of ~100 mg/mL. Recommended initial volume to add:
1 g bottle:10 mL
2 g bottle: 20 mL
Note: After reconstitution, to prepare the final infusion solution, further dilution to 50 mL or 100 mL volumes with the appropriate I.V. diluent (including D_5W or NS) is recommended.

Mechanism of Action Inhibits bacterial cell wall synthesis by binding to one or more of the penicillin-binding proteins (PBPs) which in turn inhibits the final transpeptidation step of peptidoglycan synthesis in bacterial cell walls, thus inhibiting cell wall biosynthesis. Bacteria eventually lyse due to ongoing activity of cell wall autolytic enzymes (autolysins and murein hydrolases) while cell wall assembly is arrested.

Pharmacodynamics/Kinetics
Absorption: I.M.: Well absorbed
Distribution: V_d: 6-14 L; widely throughout the body including gallbladder, lungs, bone, bile, CSF (higher concentrations achieved when meninges are inflamed)
Protein binding: 85% to 95%
Half-life elimination: Normal renal and hepatic function: 5-9 hours; Renal impairment (mild-to-severe): 12-16 hours
Time to peak, serum: I.M.: 2-3 hours
Excretion: Urine (33% to 67% as unchanged drug); feces (as inactive drug)

Dosage
Geriatric & Adult
Dosage range: Usual dose: 1-2 g every 12-24 hours, depending on the type and severity of infection
Acute bacterial rhinosinusitis, severe infection requiring hospitalization (unlabeled use): I.V.: 1-2 g every 12-24 hours for 5-7 days (Chow, 2012)
Arthritis, septic (unlabeled use): I.V.: 1-2 g once daily
Brain abscess (unlabeled use): I.V.: 2 g every 12 hours with metronidazole
Cavernous sinus thrombosis (unlabeled use): I.V.: 2 g once daily with vancomycin or linezolid
Chancroid (unlabeled use): I.M.: 250 mg as single dose (CDC, 2010)
Chemoprophylaxis for high-risk contacts (close exposure to patients with invasive meningococcal disease) (unlabeled use): I.M.: 250 mg in a single dose
Cholecystitis, mild-to-moderate: 1-2 g every 12-24 hours for 4-7 days (provided source controlled)
Gonococcal infections (CDC, 2010):
Conjunctivitis, complicated (unlabeled use): I.M., I.V.: 1 g in a single dose
Disseminated (unlabeled use): I.M., I.V.: 1 g once daily for 24-48 hours may switch to cefixime (after improvement noted) to complete a total of 7 days of therapy
Endocarditis (unlabeled use): I.M., I.V.: 1-2 g every 24 hours for at least 28 days
Epididymitis, acute (unlabeled use): I.M.: 250 mg in a single dose with doxycycline
Meningitis: I.M., I.V.: 1-2 g every 12 hours for 10-14 days
Proctitis (unlabeled use): I.M.: 250 mg in a single dose with doxycycline
Prostatitis (unlabeled use): I.M.: 125-250 mg in a single dose with doxycycline
Uncomplicated cervicitis, pharyngitis, urethritis (unlabeled use): I.M.: 250 mg in a single dose with doxycycline or azithromycin

Infective endocarditis: I.M., I.V.:

Native valve: 2 g once daily for 2-4 weeks; **Note:** If using 2-week regimen, concurrent gentamicin is recommended

Prosthetic valve: I.M., I.V.: 2 g once daily for 6 weeks (with or without 2 weeks of gentamicin [dependent on penicillin MIC]); **Note:** For HACEK organisms, duration of therapy is 4 weeks

Enterococcus faecalis (resistant to penicillin, aminoglycoside, and vancomycin), native or prosthetic valve: 2 g twice daily for ≥8 weeks administered concurrently with ampicillin

Prophylaxis: I.M., I.V.: 1 g 30-60 minutes before procedure. Intramuscular injections should be avoided in patients who are receiving anticoagulant therapy. In these circumstances, orally administered regimens should be given whenever possible. Intravenously administered antibiotics should be used for patients who are unable to tolerate or absorb oral medications.

Note: American Heart Association (AHA) guidelines now recommend prophylaxis only in patients undergoing invasive procedures and in whom underlying cardiac conditions may predispose to a higher risk of adverse outcomes should infection occur. As of April 2007, routine prophylaxis for GI/GU procedures is no longer recommended by the AHA.

Intra-abdominal infection, complicated, community-acquired, mild-to-moderate (in combination with metronidazole): 1-2 g every 12-24 hours for 4-7 days (provided source controlled)

Lyme disease (unlabeled use): I.V.: 2 g once daily for 14-28 days

Mastoiditis (hospitalized; unlabeled use): I.V.: 2 g once daily; >60 years old: 1 g once daily

Meningitis: I.V.: 2 g every 12 hours for 7-14 days (longer courses may be necessary for selected organisms)

Orbital cellulitis (unlabeled use) and endophthalmitis: I.V.: 2 g once daily

Pelvic inflammatory disease: I.M.: 250 mg in a single dose plus doxycycline (with or without metronidazole) (CDC, 2010)

Pneumonia, community-acquired: I.V.: 1 g once daily, usually in combination with a macrolide; consider 2 g/day for patients at risk for more severe infection and/or resistant organisms (ICU status, age >65 years, disseminated infection)

Prophylaxis against sexually-transmitted diseases following sexual assault: I.M.: 250 mg as a single dose (in combination with azithromycin and metronidazole) (CDC, 2010)

Pyelonephritis (acute, uncomplicated): Females: I.V.: 1-2 g once daily (Stamm, 1993). Many physicians administer a single parenteral dose before initiating oral therapy (Warren, 1999).

Septic/toxic shock/necrotizing fasciitis (unlabeled use): I.V.: 2 g once daily; with clindamycin for toxic shock

Surgical prophylaxis: I.V.: 1 g 30 minutes to 2 hours before surgery

Cholecystectomy: 1-2 g every 12-24 hours, discontinue within 24 hours unless infection outside gallbladder suspected

Syphilis (unlabeled use): I.M., I.V.: 1 g once daily for 10-14 days; **Note:** Alternative treatment for early syphilis, optimal dose, and duration have not been defined (CDC, 2010)

Typhoid fever (unlabeled use): I.V.: 2 g once daily for 14 days

Whipple's disease (unlabeled use): Initial: 2 g once daily for 10-14 days, then oral therapy for ~1 year.

Renal Impairment No dosage adjustment is generally necessary in renal impairment; **Note:** Concurrent renal and hepatic dysfunction: Maximum dose: ≤2 g/day

Poorly dialyzed; no supplemental dose or dosage adjustment necessary, including patients on intermittent hemodialysis, peritoneal dialysis, or continuous renal replacement therapy (eg, CVVHD).

Hepatic Impairment No adjustment necessary unless there is concurrent renal dysfunction (see Dosage: Renal Impairment).

Administration Do not admix with aminoglycosides in same bottle/bag. Do not reconstitute, admix, or coadminister with calcium-containing solutions. Infuse intermittent infusion over 30 minutes.

I.M.: Inject deep I.M. into large muscle mass; a concentration of 250 mg/mL or 350 mg/mL is recommended for all vial sizes except the 250 mg size (250 mg/mL is suggested); can be diluted with 1:1 water and 1% lidocaine for I.M. administration.

I.V.: Infuse intermittent infusion over 30 minutes.

Monitoring Parameters Observe for signs and symptoms of anaphylaxis

Test Interactions Positive direct Coombs', false-positive urinary glucose test using cupric sulfate (Benedict's solution, Clinitest®, Fehling's solution), false-positive serum or urine creatinine with Jaffé reaction

Special Geriatric Considerations No adjustment for changes in renal function necessary.

◀ **Dosage Forms** Excipient information presented when available (limited, particularly for generics); consult specific product labeling.

Infusion, premixed in D$_5$W: 1 g (50 mL); 2 g (50 mL)

Injection, powder for reconstitution: 250 mg, 500 mg, 1 g, 2 g, 10 g

Rocephin®: 500 mg, 1 g [contains sodium ~83 mg (3.6 mEq) per ceftriaxone 1 g]

◆ **Ceftriaxone Sodium** *see* CefTRIAXone *on page* 332

Cefuroxime (se fyoor OKS eem)

Related Information
Antimicrobial Drugs of Choice *on page* 2163
Community-Acquired Pneumonia in Adults *on page* 2171

Medication Safety Issues

Sound-alike/look-alike issues:
Cefuroxime may be confused with cefotaxime, cefprozil, deferoxamine
Ceftin® may be confused with Cefzil®, Cipro®
Zinacef® may be confused with Zithromax®

International issues:
Ceftin [U.S., Canada] may be confused with Cefiton brand name for cefixime [Portugal]; Ceftim brand name for ceftazidime [Portugal]; Ceftime brand name for ceftazidime [Thailand]

Brand Names: U.S. Ceftin®; Zinacef®

Brand Names: Canada Apo-Cefuroxime®; Auro-Cefuroxime; Ceftin®; Cefuroxime For Injection; PRO-Cefuroxime; ratio-Cefuroxime

Index Terms Cefuroxime Axetil; Cefuroxime Sodium

Generic Availability (U.S.) Yes

Pharmacologic Category Antibiotic, Cephalosporin (Second Generation)

Use Treatment of infections caused by staphylococci, group B streptococci, *H. influenzae* (type A and B), *E. coli*, *Enterobacter*, *Salmonella*, and *Klebsiella*; treatment of susceptible infections of the upper and lower respiratory tract, otitis media, urinary tract, uncomplicated skin and soft tissue, bone and joint, sepsis, uncomplicated gonorrhea, and early Lyme disease; surgical prophylaxis

Contraindications Hypersensitivity to cefuroxime, any component of the formulation, or other cephalosporins

Warnings/Precautions Modify dosage in patients with severe renal impairment. Use with caution in patients with a history of penicillin allergy, especially IgE-mediated reactions (eg, anaphylaxis, urticaria). Prolonged use may result in fungal or bacterial superinfection, including *C. difficile*-associated diarrhea (CDAD) and pseudomembranous colitis; CDAD has been observed >2 months postantibiotic treatment. May be associated with increased INR, especially in nutritionally-deficient patients, prolonged treatment, hepatic or renal disease. Tablets and oral suspension are not bioequivalent (do not substitute on a mg-per-mg basis). Some products may contain phenylalanine.

Adverse Reactions (Reflective of adult population; not specific for elderly)
>10%: Gastrointestinal: Diarrhea (4% to 11%, duration-dependent)
1% to 10%:
Dermatologic: Diaper rash (3%)
Endocrine & metabolic: Alkaline phosphatase increased (2%), lactate dehydrogenase increased (1%)
Gastrointestinal: Nausea/vomiting (3% to 7%)
Genitourinary: Vaginitis (≤5%)
Hematologic: Eosinophilia (7%), hemoglobin and hematocrit decreased (10%)
Hepatic: Transaminases increased (2% to 4%)
Local: Thrombophlebitis (2%)
Reactions reported with other cephalosporins: Agranulocytosis, aplastic anemia, asterixis, encephalopathy, hemorrhage, neuromuscular excitability, serum-sickness reactions, superinfection, toxic nephropathy

Drug Interactions

Metabolism/Transport Effects None known.

Avoid Concomitant Use
Avoid concomitant use of Cefuroxime with any of the following: BCG

Increased Effect/Toxicity
Cefuroxime may increase the levels/effects of: Aminoglycosides

The levels/effects of Cefuroxime may be increased by: Probenecid

Decreased Effect
Cefuroxime may decrease the levels/effects of: BCG; Typhoid Vaccine

The levels/effects of Cefuroxime may be decreased by: Antacids; H2-Antagonists

Ethanol/Nutrition/Herb Interactions Food: Bioavailability is increased with food; cefuroxime serum levels may be increased if taken with food or dairy products.

Stability
Injection: Reconstituted solution is stable for 24 hours at room temperature and 48 hours when refrigerated. I.V. infusion in NS or D_5W solution is stable for 24 hours at room temperature, 7 days when refrigerated, or 26 weeks when frozen. After freezing, thawed solution is stable for 24 hours at room temperature or 21 days when refrigerated.

Oral suspension: Prior to reconstitution, store at 2°C to 30°C (36°F to 86°F). Reconstituted suspension is stable for 10 days at 2°C to 8°C (36°F to 46°F).

Tablet: Store at 15°C to 30°C (59°F to 86°F).

Mechanism of Action Inhibits bacterial cell wall synthesis by binding to one or more of the penicillin-binding proteins (PBPs) which in turn inhibits the final transpeptidation step of peptidoglycan synthesis in bacterial cell walls, thus inhibiting cell wall biosynthesis. Bacteria eventually lyse due to ongoing activity of cell wall autolytic enzymes (autolysins and murein hydrolases) while cell wall assembly is arrested.

Pharmacodynamics/Kinetics
Absorption: Oral (cefuroxime axetil): Increases with food

Distribution: Widely to body tissues and fluids; crosses blood-brain barrier; therapeutic concentrations achieved in CSF even when meninges are not inflamed

Protein binding: 33% to 50%

Bioavailability: Tablet: Fasting: 37%; Following food: 52%

Half-life elimination: 1-2 hours; prolonged with renal impairment

Time to peak, serum: I.M.: ~15-60 minutes; I.V.: 2-3 minutes; Oral: 2-3 hours

Excretion: Urine (66% to 100% as unchanged drug)

Dosage
Geriatric & Adult Note: Cefuroxime axetil film-coated tablets and oral suspension are not bioequivalent and are not substitutable on a mg/mg basis. All oral doses listed are for tablet formulation:

Bronchitis, acute (and exacerbations of chronic bronchitis):
Oral: 250-500 mg every 12 hours for 10 days
I.V.: 500-750 mg every 8 hours (complete therapy with oral dosing)

Cellulitis, orbital: I.V.: 1.5 g every 8 hours

Cholecystitis, mild-to-moderate: I.V.: 1.5 g every 8 hours for 4-7 days (provided source controlled)

Gonorrhea:
Disseminated: I.M., I.V.: 750 mg every 8 hours
Uncomplicated:
Oral: 1 g as a single dose
I.M.: 1.5 g as single dose (administer in two different sites with probenecid)

Intra-abdominal infection, complicated, community-acquired, mild-to-moderate (in combination with metronidazole): I.V.: 1.5 g every 8 hours for 4-7 days (provided source controlled)

Lyme disease (early): Oral: 500 mg twice daily for 20 days

Pharyngitis/tonsillitis and sinusitis: Oral: 250 mg twice daily for 10 days

Skin/skin structure infection, uncomplicated:
Oral: 250-500 mg every 12 hours for 10 days
I.M., I.V.: 750 mg every 8 hours

Pneumonia, uncomplicated: I.M., I.V.: 750 mg every 8 hours

Severe or complicated infections: I.M., I.V.: 1.5 g every 8 hours (up to 1.5 g every 6 hours in life-threatening infections)

Surgical prophylaxis: I.V.: 1.5 g 30 minutes to 1 hour prior to procedure (if procedure is prolonged can give 750 mg every 8 hours I.M.)
Cholecystectomy: I.V.: 1.5 g every 8 hours, discontinue within 24 hours unless infection outside gallbladder suspected
Open heart: I.V.: 1.5 g every 12 hours to a total of 6 g

Urinary tract infection, uncomplicated:
Oral: 125-250 mg twice daily for 7-10 days
I.V., I.M.: 750 mg every 8 hours

Renal Impairment
Cl_{cr} 10-20 mL/minute: Administer every 12 hours.

Cl_{cr} <10 mL/minute: Administer every 24 hours.

Hemodialysis: Dialyzable (25%)

Peritoneal dialysis: Dose every 24 hours

Continuous renal replacement therapy (CRRT): 1 g every 12 hours

Note: Cefuroxime axetil film-coated tablets and oral suspension are not bioequivalent and are not substitutable on a mg/mg basis.

Administration Tablets can be crushed and given with soft foods to mask the bitter taste; I.M. doses should be given deep into a large muscle (ie, gluteus maximus)

Monitoring Parameters Observe for signs and symptoms of anaphylaxis during first dose; with prolonged therapy, monitor renal, hepatic, and hematologic function periodically; monitor prothrombin time in patients at risk of prolongation during cephalosporin therapy (nutritionally-deficient, prolonged treatment, renal or hepatic disease)

Test Interactions Positive direct Coombs', false-positive urinary glucose test using cupric sulfate (Benedict's solution, Clinitest®, Fehling's solution); false-negative may occur with ferricyanide test. Glucose oxidase or hexokinase-based methods should be used.

Pharmacotherapy Pearls Sodium content of 1 g: 54.2 mg (2.4 mEq)

Special Geriatric Considerations Adjust dose for renal function. Considered one of the drugs of choice for outpatient treatment of community-acquired pneumonia in the elderly.

Dosage Forms Excipient information presented when available (limited, particularly for generics); consult specific product labeling.

Infusion, premixed iso-osmotic solution, as sodium [strength expressed as base]:
Zinacef®: 750 mg (50 mL); 1.5 g (50 mL) [contains sodium 4.8 mEq (111 mg) per 750 mg]

Injection, powder for reconstitution, as sodium [strength expressed as base]: 750 mg, 1.5 g, 7.5 g, 75 g
Zinacef®: 750 mg, 1.5 g, 7.5 g [contains sodium ~1.8 mEq (41 mg) per 750 mg]

Powder for suspension, oral, as axetil [strength expressed as base]: 125 mg/5 mL (100 mL); 250 mg/5 mL (50 mL, 100 mL)
Ceftin®: 125 mg/5 mL (100 mL) [contains phenylalanine 11.8 mg/5 mL; tutti frutti flavor]
Ceftin®: 250 mg/5 mL (50 mL, 100 mL) [contains phenylalanine 25.2 mg/5 mL; tutti frutti flavor]

Tablet, oral, as axetil [strength expressed as base]: 250 mg, 500 mg
Ceftin®: 250 mg, 500 mg

♦ **Cefuroxime Axetil** see Cefuroxime on page 336
♦ **Cefuroxime Sodium** see Cefuroxime on page 336
♦ **Cefzil** see Cefprozil on page 325
♦ **CeleBREX®** see Celecoxib on page 338

Celecoxib (se le KOKS ib)

Medication Safety Issues
Sound-alike/look-alike issues:
CeleBREX® may be confused with CeleXA®, Cerebyx®, Cervarix®, Clarinex®

Brand Names: U.S. CeleBREX®
Brand Names: Canada Celebrex®
Generic Availability (U.S.) No
Pharmacologic Category Nonsteroidal Anti-inflammatory Drug (NSAID), COX-2 Selective
Use Relief of the signs and symptoms of osteoarthritis, ankylosing spondylitis, and rheumatoid arthritis; management of acute pain
Medication Guide Available Yes
Contraindications Hypersensitivity to celecoxib, sulfonamides, aspirin, other NSAIDs, or any component of the formulation; perioperative pain in the setting of coronary artery bypass graft (CABG) surgery

Canadian labeling: Additional contraindications (not in U.S. labeling): Severe, uncontrolled heart failure; active gastrointestinal ulcer (gastric, duodenal, peptic) or bleeding; inflammatory bowel disease; cerebrovascular bleeding; severe liver impairment or active hepatic disease; severe renal impairment (Cl$_{cr}$ <30 mL/minute) or deteriorating renal disease; known hyperkalemia

Warnings/Precautions [U.S. Boxed Warning]: NSAIDs are associated with an increased risk of serious (and potentially fatal) adverse cardiovascular thrombotic events, including MI and stroke. Risk may be increased with duration of use or pre-existing cardiovascular risk factors or disease. Carefully evaluate individual cardiovascular risk profiles prior to prescribing. New-onset or exacerbation of hypertension may occur (NSAIDS may impair response to thiazide or loop diuretics); may contribute to cardiovascular events; monitor blood pressure; use with caution in patients with hypertension. May cause sodium and fluid retention; use with caution in patients with edema, cerebrovascular disease, or ischemic heart disease. Avoid use in heart failure.

[U.S. Boxed Warning]: Celecoxib is contraindicated for treatment of perioperative pain in the setting of coronary artery bypass graft (CABG) surgery. Risk of MI and stroke may be increased with use following CABG surgery.

[U.S. Boxed Warning]: NSAIDs may increase risk of serious gastrointestinal ulceration, bleeding, and perforation (may be fatal). These events may occur at any time during therapy and without warning. Use caution with a history of GI disease (bleeding or ulcers), concurrent therapy with aspirin, anticoagulants and/or corticosteroids, smoking, use of alcohol, the elderly or debilitated patients. When used concomitantly with ≤325 mg of aspirin, a substantial increase in the risk of gastrointestinal complications (eg, ulcer) occurs; concomitant gastroprotective therapy (eg, proton pump inhibitors) is recommended (Bhatt, 2008).

Use the lowest effective dose for the shortest duration of time, consistent with individual patient goals, to reduce risk of cardiovascular or GI adverse events. Alternate therapies should be considered for patients at high risk.

NSAIDs may cause serious skin adverse events including exfoliative dermatitis, Stevens-Johnson syndrome (SJS), and toxic epidermal necrolysis (TEN); may occur without warning and in patients without prior known sulfa allergy. Anaphylactoid reactions may occur, even without prior exposure; patients with "aspirin triad" (bronchial asthma, aspirin intolerance, rhinitis) may be at increased risk. Do not use in patients who experience bronchospasm, asthma, rhinitis, or urticaria with NSAID or aspirin therapy. Use with caution in other forms of asthma.

Use with caution in patients with decreased hepatic (dosage adjustments are recommended for moderate hepatic impairment; not recommended for patients with severe hepatic impairment) or renal function. Transaminase elevations have been reported with use; closely monitor patients with any abnormal LFT. Severe hepatic reactions (eg, fulminant hepatitis, liver failure) have occurred with NSAID use, rarely; discontinue if signs or symptoms of liver disease develop, if systemic manifestations occur, or with persistent or worsening abnormal hepatic function tests. NSAID use may compromise existing renal function; dose-dependent decreases in prostaglandin synthesis may result from NSAID use, causing a reduction in renal blood flow which may cause renal decompensation (usually reversible). Patients with impaired renal function, dehydration, heart failure, liver dysfunction, those taking diuretics, ACE inhibitors, angiotensin II receptor blockers, and the elderly are at greater risk for renal toxicity. Rehydrate patient before starting therapy; monitor renal function closely. Not recommended for use in patients with advanced renal disease or severe renal insufficiency; discontinue use with persistent or worsening abnormal renal function tests. Long-term NSAID use may result in renal papillary necrosis. Should not be considered a treatment or replacement of corticosteroid-dependent diseases.

Anaphylactoid reactions may occur, even with no prior exposure to celecoxib. Use with caution in patients with known or suspected deficiency of cytochrome P450 isoenzyme 2C9; poor metabolizers may have higher plasma levels due to reduced metabolism; consider reduced initial doses.

Anemia may occur with use; monitor hemoglobin or hematocrit in patients on long-term treatment. Celecoxib does not affect PT, PTT or platelet counts; does not inhibit platelet aggregation at approved doses.

Adverse Reactions (Reflective of adult population; not specific for elderly)

≥2%
  Cardiovascular: Peripheral edema
  Central nervous system: Dizziness, fever, headache, insomnia
  Dermatologic: Rash
  Gastrointestinal: Abdominal pain, diarrhea, dyspepsia, flatulence, nausea, vomiting
  Neuromuscular & skeletal: Arthralgia, back pain
  Respiratory: Cough, nasopharyngitis, pharyngitis, rhinitis, sinusitis, upper respiratory tract infection

0.1% to 1.9%:
  Cardiovascular: Angina, aortic valve incompetence, chest pain, coronary artery disorder, edema, facial edema, hypertension (aggravated), MI, palpitation, sinus bradycardia, tachycardia, ventricular hypertrophy
  Central nervous system: Anxiety, depression, fatigue, hypoesthesia, migraine, nervousness, pain, somnolence, vertigo
  Dermatologic: Alopecia, bruising, cellulitis, dermatitis, dry skin, photosensitivity, pruritus, rash (erythematous), rash (maculopapular), urticaria
  Endocrine & metabolic: Hot flashes, hypercholesterolemia, hyperglycemia, hypokalemia, ovarian cyst, testosterone decreased
  Gastrointestinal: Anorexia, appetite increased, constipation, diverticulitis, dysphagia, eructation, esophagitis, gastritis, gastroenteritis, gastroesophageal reflux, gastrointestinal ulcer, hemorrhoids, hiatal hernia, melena, stomatitis, tenesmus, weight gain, xerostomia
  Genitourinary: Cystitis, dysuria, urinary frequency
  Hematologic: Anemia, thrombocythemia
  Hepatic: Alkaline phosphatase increased, transaminases increased

Neuromuscular & skeletal: Arthrosis, CPK increased, hypertonia, leg cramps, myalgia, paresthesia, synovitis, tendonitis

Ocular: Conjunctival hemorrhage, vitreous floaters

Otic: Deafness, labyrinthitis, tinnitus

Renal: Albuminuria, BUN increased, creatinine increased, hematuria, nonprotein nitrogen increased, renal calculi

Respiratory: Bronchitis, bronchospasm, dyspnea, epistaxis, laryngitis, pneumonia

Miscellaneous: Allergic reactions, allergy aggravated, cyst, diaphoresis, flu-like syndrome

Drug Interactions

Metabolism/Transport Effects Substrate of CYP2C9 (major), CYP3A4 (minor); **Note:** Assignment of Major/Minor substrate status based on clinically relevant drug interaction potential; **Inhibits** CYP2C8 (moderate), CYP2D6 (moderate)

Avoid Concomitant Use

Avoid concomitant use of Celecoxib with any of the following: Floctafenine; Ketorolac; Ketorolac (Nasal); Ketorolac (Systemic); Thioridazine

Increased Effect/Toxicity

Celecoxib may increase the levels/effects of: Aliskiren; Aminoglycosides; Anticoagulants; Antiplatelet Agents; ARIPiprazole; Bisphosphonate Derivatives; CycloSPORINE; CycloSPORINE (Systemic); CYP2C8 Substrates; CYP2D6 Substrates; Deferasirox; Desmopressin; Digoxin; Eplerenone; Fesoterodine; Haloperidol; Lithium; Methotrexate; Nebivolol; Nonsteroidal Anti-Inflammatory Agents; Porfimer; Potassium-Sparing Diuretics; PRALAtrexate; Prilocaine; Quinolone Antibiotics; Thioridazine; Thrombolytic Agents; Vancomycin; Vitamin K Antagonists

The levels/effects of Celecoxib may be increased by: ACE Inhibitors; Angiotensin II Receptor Blockers; Antidepressants (Tricyclic, Tertiary Amine); Corticosteroids (Systemic); CycloSPORINE; CycloSPORINE (Systemic); CYP2C9 Inhibitors (Moderate); CYP2C9 Inhibitors (Strong); Floctafenine; Herbs (Anticoagulant/Antiplatelet Properties); Ketorolac; Ketorolac (Nasal); Ketorolac (Systemic); Mifepristone; Probenecid; Propafenone; Selective Serotonin Reuptake Inhibitors; Sodium Phosphates; Treprostinil

Decreased Effect

Celecoxib may decrease the levels/effects of: ACE Inhibitors; Aliskiren; Angiotensin II Receptor Blockers; Antiplatelet Agents; Beta-Blockers; Codeine; Eplerenone; HydrALA-ZINE; Loop Diuretics; Potassium-Sparing Diuretics; Selective Serotonin Reuptake Inhibitors; Tamoxifen; Thiazide Diuretics; TraMADol

The levels/effects of Celecoxib may be decreased by: Bile Acid Sequestrants; CYP2C9 Inducers (Strong); Peginterferon Alfa-2b; Tocilizumab

Ethanol/Nutrition/Herb Interactions

Ethanol: Avoid ethanol (increased GI irritation).

Food: Peak concentrations are delayed and AUC is increased by 10% to 20% when taken with a high-fat meal.

Herb/Nutraceutical: Avoid concomitant use with herbs possessing anticoagulation/antiplatelet properties, including alfalfa, anise, bilberry, bladderwrack, bromelain, cat's claw, celery, chamomile, coleus, cordyceps, dong quai, evening primrose, fenugreek, feverfew, garlic, ginger, ginkgo biloba, ginseng (American, Panax, Siberian), grapeseed, green tea, guggul, horse chestnuts, horseradish, licorice, prickly ash, red clover, reishi, SAMe (S-adenosylmethionine), sweet clover, turmeric, white willow.

Stability Store at 25°C (77°F); excursions permitted to 15°C to 30°C (59°F to 86°F).

Mechanism of Action Inhibits prostaglandin synthesis by decreasing the activity of the enzyme, cyclooxygenase-2 (COX-2), which results in decreased formation of prostaglandin precursors; has antipyretic, analgesic, and anti-inflammatory properties. Celecoxib does not inhibit cyclooxygenase-1 (COX-1) at therapeutic concentrations.

Pharmacodynamics/Kinetics

Distribution: V_d (apparent): ~400 L

Protein binding: ~97% primarily to albumin

Metabolism: Hepatic via CYP2C9; forms inactive metabolites

Bioavailability: Absolute: Unknown

Half-life elimination: ~11 hours (fasted)

Time to peak: ~3 hours

Excretion: Feces (~57% as metabolites, <3% as unchanged drug); urine (27% as metabolites, <3% as unchanged drug)

Dosage

Geriatric Refer to adult dosing. No specific adjustment based on age is recommended. However, the AUC in elderly patients may be increased by 50% as compared to younger subjects. Initiate at the lowest recommended dose in patients weighing <50 kg.

Adult Note: Use the lowest effective dose for the shortest duration of time, consistent with individual patient treatment goals.

Osteoarthritis: Oral: 200 mg/day as a single dose or in divided doses twice daily
Ankylosing spondylitis: Oral: 200 mg/day as a single dose or in divided doses twice daily; if no effect after 6 weeks, may increase to 400 mg/day. If no response following 6 weeks of treatment with 400 mg/day, consider discontinuation and alternative treatment.
Canadian labeling; Recommended maximum dose: 200 mg/day
Rheumatoid arthritis: Oral: 100-200 mg twice daily
Acute pain: Oral: Initial dose: 400 mg, followed by an additional 200 mg if needed on day 1; maintenance dose: 200 mg twice daily as needed
Canadian labeling; Recommended maximum dose for treatment of acute pain: 400 mg/day up to 7 days
Dosing adjustment in poor CYP2C9 metabolizers (eg, CYP2C9*3/*3): Consider reducing initial dose by 50%
Canadian labeling: Recommended maximum dose: 100 mg/day.
Renal Impairment
Advanced renal disease: Use is not recommended; however, if celecoxib treatment cannot be avoided, monitor renal function closely.
Severe renal insufficiency: Use is not recommended.
Canadian labeling: Cl_{cr} <30 mL/minute: Use is contraindicated.
Abnormal renal function tests (persistent or worsening): Discontinue use.
Hepatic Impairment
Moderate hepatic impairment (Child-Pugh class B): Reduce dose by 50%.
Severe hepatic impairment (Child-Pugh class C): Use is not recommended.
Canadian labeling: Use is contraindicated.
Abnormal liver function tests (persistent or worsening): Discontinue use.
Administration May be administered without regard to meals. Capsules may be swallowed whole or the entire contents emptied onto a teaspoon of cool or room temperature applesauce. The contents of the capsules sprinkled onto applesauce may be stored under refrigeration for up to 6 hours.
Monitoring Parameters CBC; blood chemistry profile; occult blood loss and periodic liver function tests; monitor renal function (urine output, serum BUN and creatinine; monitor response (pain, range of motion, grip strength, mobility, ADL function), inflammation; blood pressure (baseline and during treatment); observe for weight gain, edema; observe for bleeding, bruising; evaluate gastrointestinal effects (abdominal pain, bleeding, dyspepsia)
Special Geriatric Considerations The elderly are at increased risk for adverse effects from NSAIDs. As many as 60% of elderly can develop peptic ulceration and/or hemorrhage asymptomatically; however, elderly patients may demonstrate these adverse effects at lower doses than younger adults. The elderly are also at increased risk of renal toxicity. Although celecoxib is associated with a decreased incidence of GI side effects, use the lowest recommended dose in patients weighing <50 kg.
Dosage Forms Excipient information presented when available (limited, particularly for generics); consult specific product labeling.
Capsule, oral:
CeleBREX®: 50 mg, 100 mg, 200 mg, 400 mg

◆ **Celestone®** *see* Betamethasone *on page 204*
◆ **Celestone® Soluspan®** *see* Betamethasone *on page 204*
◆ **CeleXA®** *see* Citalopram *on page 387*
◆ **Celontin®** *see* Methsuximide *on page 1242*
◆ **Cemill 500 [OTC]** *see* Ascorbic Acid *on page 149*
◆ **Cemill 1000 [OTC]** *see* Ascorbic Acid *on page 149*
◆ **Cenestin®** *see* Estrogens (Conjugated A/Synthetic) *on page 696*
◆ **Centany®** *see* Mupirocin *on page 1324*
◆ **Centany® AT** *see* Mupirocin *on page 1324*

Cephalexin (sef a LEKS in)

Related Information
Prevention of Infective Endocarditis *on page 2175*
Medication Safety Issues
Sound-alike/look-alike issues:
Cephalexin may be confused with cefaclor, ceFAZolin, ciprofloxacin
Keflex® may be confused with Keppra®, Valtrex®
Brand Names: U.S. Keflex®
Brand Names: Canada Apo-Cephalex®; Dom-Cephalexin; Keflex®; Novo-Lexin; Nu-Cephalex; PMS-Cephalexin
Index Terms Cephalexin Monohydrate
Generic Availability (U.S.) Yes

CEPHALEXIN

Pharmacologic Category Antibiotic, Cephalosporin (First Generation)

Use Treatment of susceptible bacterial infections including respiratory tract infections, otitis media, skin and skin structure infections, bone infections, and genitourinary tract infections, including acute prostatitis; alternative therapy for acute infective endocarditis prophylaxis

Contraindications Hypersensitivity to cephalexin, any component of the formulation, or other cephalosporins

Warnings/Precautions Modify dosage in patients with severe renal impairment. Use with caution in patients with a history of penicillin allergy, especially IgE-mediated reactions (eg, anaphylaxis, urticaria). Prolonged use may result in fungal or bacterial superinfection, including *C. difficile*-associated diarrhea (CDAD) and pseudomembranous colitis; CDAD has been observed >2 months postantibiotic treatment. May be associated with increased INR, especially in nutritionally-deficient patients, prolonged treatment, hepatic or renal disease.

Adverse Reactions (Reflective of adult population; not specific for elderly) Frequency not defined.

Central nervous system: Agitation, confusion, dizziness, fatigue, hallucinations, headache

Dermatologic: Angioedema, erythema multiforme (rare), rash, Stevens-Johnson syndrome (rare), toxic epidermal necrolysis (rare), urticaria

Gastrointestinal: Abdominal pain, diarrhea, dyspepsia, gastritis, nausea (rare), pseudomembranous colitis, vomiting (rare)

Genitourinary: Genital pruritus, genital moniliasis, vaginitis, vaginal discharge

Hematologic: Eosinophilia, hemolytic anemia, neutropenia, thrombocytopenia

Hepatic: ALT increased, AST increased, cholestatic jaundice (rare), transient hepatitis (rare)

Neuromuscular & skeletal: Arthralgia, arthritis, joint disorder

Renal: Interstitial nephritis (rare)

Miscellaneous: Allergic reactions, anaphylaxis

Drug Interactions

Metabolism/Transport Effects None known.

Avoid Concomitant Use

Avoid concomitant use of Cephalexin with any of the following: BCG

Increased Effect/Toxicity

Cephalexin may increase the levels/effects of: MetFORMIN

The levels/effects of Cephalexin may be increased by: Probenecid

Decreased Effect

Cephalexin may decrease the levels/effects of: BCG; Typhoid Vaccine

The levels/effects of Cephalexin may be decreased by: Zinc Salts

Ethanol/Nutrition/Herb Interactions Food: Peak antibiotic serum concentration is lowered and delayed, but total drug absorbed is not affected. Cephalexin serum levels may be decreased if taken with food.

Stability

Capsule: Store at 15°C to 30°C (59°F to 86°F).

Powder for oral suspension: Refrigerate suspension after reconstitution; discard after 14 days.

Mechanism of Action Inhibits bacterial cell wall synthesis by binding to one or more of the penicillin-binding proteins (PBPs) which in turn inhibits the final transpeptidation step of peptidoglycan synthesis in bacterial cell walls, thus inhibiting cell wall biosynthesis. Bacteria eventually lyse due to ongoing activity of cell wall autolytic enzymes (autolysins and murein hydrolases) while cell wall assembly is arrested.

Pharmacodynamics/Kinetics

Absorption: Rapid (90%)

Distribution: Widely into most body tissues and fluids, including gallbladder, liver, kidneys, bone, sputum, bile, and pleural and synovial fluids; CSF penetration is poor

Protein binding: 6% to 15%

Half-life elimination: Adults: 0.5-1.2 hours; prolonged with renal impairment

Time to peak, serum: ~1 hour

Excretion: Urine (80% to 100% as unchanged drug) within 8 hours

Dosage

Geriatric & Adult

Dosing range: Oral: 250-1000 mg every 6 hours (maximum: 4 g/day)

Indication-specific dosing:

Cellulitis and mastitis: Oral 500 mg every 6 hours

Furunculosis/skin abscess: Oral: 250 mg 4 times/day

Prophylaxis against infective endocarditis (dental, oral, or respiratory tract procedures): Oral: 2 g 30-60 minutes prior to procedure. **Note:** American Heart Association (AHA) guidelines now recommend prophylaxis only in patients undergoing invasive procedures and in whom underlying cardiac conditions may predispose to a higher risk of adverse outcomes should infection occur.

Prophylaxis in total joint replacement patients undergoing dental procedures which produce bacteremia: Oral: 2 g 1 hour prior to procedure

Streptococcal pharyngitis, skin and skin structure infections: Oral: 500 mg every 12 hours

Uncomplicated cystitis: Oral: 500 mg every 12 hours for 7-14 days

Renal Impairment Adults:

Cl_{cr} 10-50 mL/minute: 500 mg every 8-12 hours

Cl_{cr} <10: 250-500 mg every 12-24 hours

Hemodialysis: 250 mg every 12-24 hours; moderately dialyzable (20% to 50%); give dose after dialysis session

Administration Take without regard to food. If GI distress, take with food. Give around-the-clock to promote less variation in peak and trough serum levels.

Monitoring Parameters With prolonged therapy monitor renal, hepatic, and hematologic function periodically; monitor for signs of anaphylaxis during first dose

Test Interactions Positive direct Coombs', false-positive urinary glucose test using cupric sulfate (Benedict's solution, Clinitest®, Fehling's solution), false-positive serum or urine creatinine with Jaffé reaction, false-positive urinary proteins and steroids

Special Geriatric Considerations Adjust dose for renal function.

Dosage Forms Excipient information presented when available (limited, particularly for generics); consult specific product labeling.

Capsule, oral: 250 mg, 500 mg

Keflex®: 250 mg, 500 mg, 750 mg

Powder for suspension, oral: 125 mg/5 mL (100 mL, 200 mL); 250 mg/5 mL (100 mL, 200 mL)

Tablet, oral: 250 mg, 500 mg

◆ **Cephalexin Monohydrate** see Cephalexin on page 341

◆ **Cerebyx®** see Fosphenytoin on page 849

◆ **Cerefolin® NAC** see Methylfolate, Methylcobalamin, and Acetylcysteine on page 1246

Certolizumab Pegol (cer to LIZ u mab PEG ol)

Brand Names: U.S. Cimzia®

Brand Names: Canada Cimzia®

Index Terms CDP870

Generic Availability (U.S.) No

Pharmacologic Category Antirheumatic, Disease Modifying; Gastrointestinal Agent, Miscellaneous; Tumor Necrosis Factor (TNF) Blocking Agent

Use Treatment of moderately- to severely-active Crohn's disease in patients who have inadequate response to conventional therapy; moderately- to severely-active rheumatoid arthritis (as monotherapy or in combination with nonbiological disease-modifying antirheumatic drugs [DMARDS])

Medication Guide Available Yes

Contraindications There are no contraindications listed within the manufacturer's labeling.

Warnings/Precautions [U.S. Boxed Warning]: Patients receiving certolizumab are at increased risk for serious infections which may result in hospitalization and/or fatality; infections usually developed in patients receiving concomitant immunosuppressive agents (eg, methotrexate or corticosteroids) and may present as disseminated (rather than local) disease. Active tuberculosis (or reactivation of latent tuberculosis), invasive fungal (including aspergillosis, blastomycosis, candidiasis, coccidioidomycosis, histoplasmosis, and pneumocystosis) and bacterial, viral or other opportunistic infections (including legionellosis and listeriosis) have been reported in patients receiving TNF-blocking agents, including certolizumab. Monitor closely for signs/symptoms of infection. Discontinue for serious infection or sepsis. Consider risks versus benefits prior to use in patients with a history of chronic or recurrent infection. Consider empiric antifungal therapy in patients who are at risk for invasive fungal infection and develop severe systemic illness. Caution should be exercised when considering use in the elderly or in patients with conditions that predispose them to infections (eg, diabetes) or residence/travel from areas of endemic mycoses (blastomycosis, coccidioidomycosis, histoplasmosis), or with latent or localized infections. Do not initiate certolizumab therapy with clinically important active infection. Patients who develop a new infection while undergoing treatment should be monitored closely. **[U.S. Boxed Warning]: Lymphoma and other malignancies have been reported in children and adolescent patients receiving other TNF-blocking agents.** Use of TNF blockers may affect defenses against malignancies; impact on the development and course of malignancies is not fully defined. Lymphoma has been noted in clinical trials. Chronic immunosuppressant therapy use may be a predisposing factor for malignancy development; rheumatoid arthritis alone has been previously associated with an increased rate of lymphoma. Hepatosplenic T-cell lymphoma (HSTCL), a rare T-cell lymphoma, has also been associated with TNF-blocking agents, primarily reported in adolescent and young adult males with Crohn's disease or ulcerative colitis.

Tuberculosis has been reported with certolizumab treatment. **[U.S. Boxed Warnings]: Patients should be evaluated for tuberculosis risk factors and for latent tuberculosis infection (with a tuberculin skin test) prior to therapy. Treatment of latent tuberculosis should be initiated before use. Patients with initial negative tuberculin skin tests should receive continued monitoring for tuberculosis throughout treatment;** active tuberculosis has developed in this population during treatment. Use with caution in patients who have resided in regions where tuberculosis is endemic. If appropriate, antituberculosis therapy should be considered (prior to certolizumab treatment) in patients with several or with highly significant risk factors for tuberculosis development.

Rare reactivation of hepatitis B virus (HBV) has occurred in chronic virus carriers; use with caution; evaluate prior to initiation and during treatment.

Hypersensitivity reactions, including angioedema, dyspnea, rash, serum sickness and urticaria have been reported (rarely) with treatment; discontinue and do not resume therapy if hypersensitivity occurs. Use with caution in patients who have experienced hypersensitivity with other TNF blockers. Use with caution in heart failure patients; worsening heart failure and new onset heart failure have been reported with TNF blockers, including certolizumab pegol; monitor closely. Rare cases of pancytopenia and other significant cytopenias, including aplastic anemia and have been reported with TNF-blocking agents. Leukopenia and thrombocytopenia have occurred with certolizumab; use with caution in patients with underlying hematologic disorders; consider discontinuing therapy with significant hematologic abnormalities. Autoantibody formation may develop; rarely resulting in autoimmune disorder, including lupus-like syndrome; monitor and discontinue if symptoms develop. A small number of patients (8%) develop antibodies to certolizumab during therapy. Antibody-positive patients may have an increased incidence of adverse events (including injection site pain/erythema, abdominal pain and erythema nodosum). Use with caution in patients with pre-existing or recent-onset CNS demyelinating disorders; rare cases of optic neuritis, seizure, peripheral neuropathy, and demyelinating disease (new onset or exacerbation) have been reported.

The manufacturer does not recommend concurrent use with anakinra or other tumor necrosis factor (TNF) blocking agents due to the risk of serious infections. Do not use in combination with biologic DMARDS. Patients should be up to date with all immunizations before initiating therapy; live vaccines should not be given concurrently. There is no data available concerning the effects of therapy on vaccination or secondary transmission of live vaccines in patients receiving therapy. Use has not been studied in patients with renal impairment; however, the pharmacokinetics of the pegylated (polyethylene glycol) component may be dependent on renal function. Use with caution in the elderly, may be at higher risk for infections.

Adverse Reactions (Reflective of adult population; not specific for elderly)

>10%:
  Central nervous system: Headache (5% to 18%)
  Gastrointestinal: Nausea (≤11%)
  Respiratory: Upper respiratory infection (6% to 20%), nasopharyngitis (4% to 13%)
  Miscellaneous: Infection (14% to 38%; serious: 3%)

1% to 10%:
  Cardiovascular: Hypertension (≤5%)
  Central nervous system: Dizziness (≤6%), fever (≤5%), fatigue (≤3%)
  Dermatologic: Rash (9%)
  Gastrointestinal: Abdominal pain (≤6%), vomiting (5%)
  Genitourinary: Urinary tract infection (≤8%)
  Local: Injection site reactions (includes bleeding, burning, erythema, inflammation, pain, rash: ≤7%; incidence higher with placebo)
  Neuromuscular & skeletal: Arthralgia (6% to 7%), back pain (≤4%)
  Respiratory: Cough (≤6%), bronchitis (≤3%), pharyngitis (≤3%)
  Miscellaneous: Antibody formation (7% to 8%), positive ANA (≤4%)

Drug Interactions

Metabolism/Transport Effects None known.

Avoid Concomitant Use
  Avoid concomitant use of Certolizumab Pegol with any of the following: Abatacept; Anakinra; Anti-TNF Agents; BCG; Canakinumab; Natalizumab; Pimecrolimus; Rilonacept; RiTUXimab; Tacrolimus (Topical); Vaccines (Live)

Increased Effect/Toxicity
  Certolizumab Pegol may increase the levels/effects of: Abatacept; Anakinra; Canakinumab; Leflunomide; Natalizumab; Rilonacept; Vaccines (Live)

The levels/effects of Certolizumab Pegol may be increased by: Anti-TNF Agents; Denosumab; Pimecrolimus; RiTUXimab; Roflumilast; Tacrolimus (Topical); Trastuzumab

Decreased Effect

Certolizumab Pegol may decrease the levels/effects of: BCG; Coccidioidin Skin Test; Sipuleucel-T; Vaccines (Inactivated); Vaccines (Live)

The levels/effects of Certolizumab Pegol may be decreased by: Echinacea; Pegloticase

Ethanol/Nutrition/Herb Interactions Herb/Nutraceutical: Echinacea may decrease the therapeutic effects of certolizumab; avoid concurrent use.

Stability Prior to reconstitution, store refrigerated at 2°C to 8°C (36°F to 46°F); do not freeze. Bring to room temperature prior to administration.

Prefilled syringe: Protect from light.

Vials: Allow to reach room temperature prior to reconstitution. Using aseptic technique, reconstitute each vial with 1 mL sterile water for injection (provided) to a concentration of ~200 mg/mL; the manufacturer recommends using a 20-gauge needle (provided). Gently swirl to facilitate wetting of powder; do not shake. Allow vials to set undisturbed (may take up to 30 minutes) until fully reconstituted. Reconstituted solutions should not contain visible particles or gels in the solution. Reconstituted vials may be retained at room temperature for ≤2 hours or refrigerated (do not freeze) for ≤24 hours prior to administration.

Mechanism of Action Certolizumab pegol is a pegylated humanized antibody Fab' fragment of tumor necrosis factor alpha (TNF-alpha) monoclonal antibody. Certolizumab pegol binds to and selectively neutralizes human TNF-alpha activity. (Elevated levels of TNF-alpha have a role in the inflammatory process associated with Crohn's disease and in joint destruction associated with rheumatoid arthritis.) Since it is not a complete antibody (lacks Fc region), it does not induce complement activation, antibody-dependent cell-mediated cytotoxicity, or apoptosis. Pegylation of certolizumab allows for delayed elimination and therefore an extended half-life.

Pharmacodynamics/Kinetics

Distribution: V_{ss}: 6-8 L

Bioavailability: SubQ: ~80% (range: 76% to 88%)

Half-life elimination: ~14 days

Time to peak, plasma: 54-171 hours

Dosage

Geriatric & Adult Note: Each 400 mg dose should be administered as 2 injections of 200 mg each.

Crohn's disease: SubQ: Initial: 400 mg, repeat dose 2 and 4 weeks after initial dose; Maintenance: 400 mg every 4 weeks

Rheumatoid arthritis: SubQ: Initial: 400 mg, repeat dose 2 and 4 weeks after initial dose; Maintenance: 200 mg every other week. May consider maintenance dose of 400 mg every 4 weeks.

Renal Impairment Moderate-to-severe renal impairment: The pharmacokinetics of the pegylated (polyethylene glycol) component may be dependent on renal function; however, data is insufficient to provide a dosing recommendation.

Administration SubQ: Bring to room temperature prior to administration. Total dose requires 2 vials **or** 2 prefilled syringes. After reconstitution (of vials), draw each vial into separate syringes (using 20-gauge needles).

Administer each syringe subcutaneously (using provided 23-gauge needle) to separate sites on abdomen or thigh. Rotate injections sites; do not administer to areas where skin is tender, bruised, red, or hard.

Monitoring Parameters Monitor improvement of symptoms and physical function assessments. Latent TB screening prior to initiating and during therapy; signs/symptoms of infection (prior to, during, and following therapy); CBC with differential; signs/symptoms/worsening of heart failure; HBV screening prior to initiating (all patients), HBV carriers (during and for several months following therapy); signs and symptoms of hypersensitivity reaction; symptoms of lupus-like syndrome; signs/symptoms of malignancy (eg, splenomegaly, hepatomegaly, abdominal pain, persistent fever, night sweats, weight loss).

Test Interactions Tests for latent tuberculosis may be falsely negative while on certolizumab pegol treatment. Falsely elevated aPTT assays have been reported with PTT-Lupus Anticoagulant (LA) and Standard Target Activated Partial Thromboplastin time (STA-PTT) tests from Diagnostica Stago, and with HemosiL APTT-SP liquid and HemosiL lyophilized silica tests from Instrumentation Laboratories.

Special Geriatric Considerations Studies to date have insufficient data to make conclusions for use in elderly. Anecdotal reports in clinical settings do not demonstrate any clinical difference between elderly and younger adults. Since elderly have a higher incidence of infection, use with caution and close monitoring.

Dosage Forms Excipient information presented when available (limited, particularly for generics); consult specific product labeling.
Injection, powder for reconstitution [preservative free]:
  Cimzia®: 200 mg [contains sucrose 100 mg]
Injection, solution [preservative free]:
  Cimzia®: 200 mg/mL (1 mL)

- ◆ **C.E.S.** *see* Estrogens (Conjugated/Equine, Systemic) *on page* 703
- ◆ **C.E.S.** *see* Estrogens (Conjugated/Equine, Topical) *on page* 707
- ◆ **Cetafen® [OTC]** *see* Acetaminophen *on page* 31
- ◆ **Cetafen Cold® [OTC]** *see* Acetaminophen and Phenylephrine *on page* 37
- ◆ **Cetafen® Extra [OTC]** *see* Acetaminophen *on page* 31

Cetirizine (se TI ra zeen)

Medication Safety Issues
Sound-alike/look-alike issues:
ZyrTEC® may be confused with Lipitor®, Serax, Xanax®, Zantac®, Zerit®, Zocor®, ZyPREXA®, ZyrTEC-D®
ZyrTEC® (cetirizine) may be confused with ZyrTEC® Itchy Eye (ketotifen)
Brand Names: U.S. All Day Allergy [OTC]; ZyrTEC® Allergy [OTC]; ZyrTEC® Children's Allergy [OTC]; ZyrTEC® Children's Hives Relief [OTC]
Brand Names: Canada Aller-Relief [OTC]; Apo-Cetirizine® [OTC]; Extra Strength Allergy Relief [OTC]; PMS-Cetirizine; Reactine [OTC]; Reactine™
Index Terms Cetirizine Hydrochloride; P-071; UCB-P071
Generic Availability (U.S.) Yes: Excludes liquid gel capsule
Pharmacologic Category Histamine H_1 Antagonist; Histamine H_1 Antagonist, Second Generation; Piperazine Derivative
Use Perennial and seasonal allergic rhinitis and other allergic symptoms including urticaria; chronic idiopathic urticaria
Contraindications Hypersensitivity to cetirizine, hydroxyzine, or any component of the formulation
Warnings/Precautions Cetirizine should be used cautiously in patients with hepatic or renal dysfunction; dosage adjustment recommended. Use with caution in the elderly; may be more sensitive to adverse effects. May cause drowsiness; use caution performing tasks which require alertness (eg, operating machinery or driving). Effects may be potentiated when used with other sedative drugs or ethanol.
Adverse Reactions (Reflective of adult population; not specific for elderly)
>10%: Central nervous system: Headache (children 11% to 14%, placebo 12%), somnolence (adults 14%, children 2% to 4%)
2% to 10%:
  Central nervous system: Insomnia (children 9%, adults <2%), fatigue (adults 6%), malaise (4%), dizziness (adults 2%)
  Gastrointestinal: Abdominal pain (children 4% to 6%), dry mouth (adults 5%), diarrhea (children 2% to 3%), nausea (children 2% to 3%, placebo 2%), vomiting (children 2% to 3%)
  Respiratory: Epistaxis (children 2% to 4%, placebo 3%), pharyngitis (children 3% to 6%, placebo 3%), bronchospasm (children 2% to 3%, placebo 2%)
Drug Interactions
  Metabolism/Transport Effects Substrate of CYP3A4 (minor), P-glycoprotein; **Note:** Assignment of Major/Minor substrate status based on clinically relevant drug interaction potential
  Avoid Concomitant Use
  Avoid concomitant use of Cetirizine with any of the following: Azelastine; Azelastine (Nasal); Methadone; Mirtazapine; Paraldehyde
  Increased Effect/Toxicity
  Cetirizine may increase the levels/effects of: Alcohol (Ethyl); Anticholinergics; Azelastine; Azelastine (Nasal); Buprenorphine; CNS Depressants; Methadone; Methotrimeprazine; Metyrosine; Mirtazapine; Paraldehyde; Selective Serotonin Reuptake Inhibitors; Zolpidem

  The levels/effects of Cetirizine may be increased by: Droperidol; HydrOXYzine; Methotrimeprazine; P-glycoprotein/ABCB1 Inhibitors; Pramlintide
  Decreased Effect
  Cetirizine may decrease the levels/effects of: Acetylcholinesterase Inhibitors (Central); Benzylpenicilloyl Polylysine; Betahistine; Hyaluronidase

  The levels/effects of Cetirizine may be decreased by: Acetylcholinesterase Inhibitors (Central); Amphetamines; P-glycoprotein/ABCB1 Inducers; Tocilizumab

Ethanol/Nutrition/Herb Interactions Ethanol: May increase CNS depression; monitor for increased effects with coadministration. Caution patients about effects.

Stability Store at room temperature.
Syrup: Store at room temperature of 15°C to 30°C (59°F to 86°F), or under refrigeration at 2°C to 8°C (36°F to 46°F).

Mechanism of Action Competes with histamine for H_1-receptor sites on effector cells in the gastrointestinal tract, blood vessels, and respiratory tract

Pharmacodynamics/Kinetics
Distribution: Minimal penetration into central nervous system
Protein binding: 93%
Metabolism: **Not** extensively metabolized by the liver
Half-life: 7.4-9 hours; in mild-moderate renal failure the half-life is increased to 19-21 hours
Time to peak: 0.5-1 hour; food may delay time to peak and decrease C_{max}
Elimination: 60% of dose is excreted unchanged in urine within 24 hours
Note: In older adults, there was a 50% increase in half-life and a 40% decrease in clearance, most likely due to change in renal function; not removed by hemodialysis

Dosage
Geriatric Oral: Initial: 5 mg once daily; may increase to 10 mg/day
Note: Manufacturer recommends 5 mg/day in patients ≥77 years of age.
Adult Perennial or seasonal allergic rhinitis, chronic urticaria: Oral: 5-10 mg once daily, depending upon symptom severity
Renal Impairment Adults:
Cl_{cr} 11-31 mL/minute or hemodialysis: Administer 5 mg once daily
Cl_{cr} <11 mL/minute, not on dialysis: Cetirizine use not recommended.
Hepatic Impairment Adults: Administer 5 mg once daily

Administration May be administered with or without food.

Monitoring Parameters Relief of symptoms, sedation and anticholinergic effects

Test Interactions May cause false-positive serum TCA screen. May suppress the wheal and flare reactions to skin test antigens.

Special Geriatric Considerations Adjust dose for renal function. Because of its OTC status, counsel patients on appropriate use.

Dosage Forms Excipient information presented when available (limited, particularly for generics); consult specific product labeling.
Capsule, liquid gel, oral, as hydrochloride:
ZyrTEC® Allergy: 10 mg
Solution, oral, as hydrochloride: 5 mg/5 mL (5 mL)
Syrup, oral, as hydrochloride: 5 mg/5 mL (5 mL, 118 mL, 120 mL, 473 mL, 480 mL)
ZyrTEC® Children's Allergy: 5 mg/5 mL (118 mL) [contains propylene glycol; grape flavor]
ZyrTEC® Children's Allergy: 5 mg/5 mL (118 mL) [dye free, sugar free; contains propylene glycol, sodium benzoate; bubblegum flavor]
ZyrTEC® Children's Hives Relief: 5 mg/5 mL (118 mL) [contains propylene glycol; grape flavor]
Tablet, oral, as hydrochloride: 5 mg, 10 mg
All Day Allergy: 10 mg
ZyrTEC® Allergy: 10 mg
Tablet, chewable, oral, as hydrochloride: 5 mg, 10 mg
All Day Allergy: 5 mg, 10 mg [fruit flavor]
ZyrTEC® Children's Allergy: 5 mg, 10 mg [grape flavor]

◆ **Cetirizine Hydrochloride** *see* Cetirizine *on page 346*
◆ **Cetraxal®** *see* Ciprofloxacin (Otic) *on page 386*

Cevimeline (se vi ME leen)

Medication Safety Issues
Sound-alike/look-alike issues:
Cevimeline may be confused with Savella®
Evoxac® may be confused with Eurax®

Brand Names: U.S. Evoxac®
Brand Names: Canada Evoxac®
Index Terms Cevimeline Hydrochloride
Generic Availability (U.S.) No
Pharmacologic Category Cholinergic Agonist
Use Treatment of symptoms of dry mouth in patients with Sjögren's syndrome

Contraindications Hypersensitivity to cevimeline or any component of the formulation; uncontrolled asthma; narrow-angle glaucoma; acute iritis; other conditions where miosis is undesirable

Warnings/Precautions May alter cardiac conduction and/or heart rate; use caution in patients with significant cardiovascular disease, including angina, myocardial infarction, or conduction disturbances. Cevimeline has the potential to increase bronchial smooth muscle tone, airway resistance, and bronchial secretions; use with caution in patients with controlled asthma, COPD, or chronic bronchitis. May cause decreased visual acuity (particularly at night and in patients with central lens changes) and impaired depth perception. Patients should be cautioned about driving at night or performing hazardous activities in reduced lighting. May cause a variety of parasympathomimetic effects, which may be particularly dangerous in elderly patients; excessive sweating may lead to dehydration in some patients.

Use with caution in patients with a history of biliary stones or nephrolithiasis; cevimeline may induce smooth muscle spasms, precipitating cholangitis, cholecystitis, biliary obstruction, renal colic, or ureteral reflux in susceptible patients. Patients with a known or suspected deficiency of CYP2D6 may be at higher risk of adverse effects.

Adverse Reactions (Reflective of adult population; not specific for elderly)

>10%:

Gastrointestinal: Nausea (14%)
Respiratory: Sinusitis (12%), rhinitis (11%), upper respiratory infection (11%)
Miscellaneous: Diaphoresis increased (19%)

1% to 10%:

Cardiovascular: Chest pain, edema, palpitation, peripheral edema
Central nervous system: Fatigue (3%), insomnia (2%), depression, fever, hypoesthesia, migraine, vertigo
Dermatologic: Erythematous rash, pruritus, skin disorder
Endocrine & metabolic: Hot flashes (2%)
Gastrointestinal: Abdominal pain (8%), vomiting (5%), excessive salivation (2%), amylase increased, anorexia, constipation, eructation, flatulence, gastroesophageal reflux, salivary gland pain, sialoadenitis, toothache, ulcerative stomatitis, xerostomia
Genitourinary: Urinary tract infection (6%), cystitis, vaginitis
Hematologic: Anemia
Local: Abscess
Neuromuscular & skeletal: Back pain (5%), arthralgia (4%), skeletal pain (3%), weakness (1%), hypertonia, hyporeflexia, leg cramps, myalgia, tremor
Ocular: Abnormal vision, eye abnormality, eye infection, eye pain, xerophthalmia
Otic: Earache, otitis media
Respiratory: Coughing (6%), bronchitis (4%), epistaxis, pneumonia
Miscellaneous: Allergy, flu-like syndrome, fungal infection, hiccups, infection, moniliasis

Drug Interactions

Metabolism/Transport Effects Substrate of CYP2D6 (minor), CYP3A4 (minor); **Note:** Assignment of Major/Minor substrate status based on clinically relevant drug interaction potential

Avoid Concomitant Use There are no known interactions where it is recommended to avoid concomitant use.

Increased Effect/Toxicity
The levels/effects of Cevimeline may be increased by: Acetylcholinesterase Inhibitors; Beta-Blockers

Decreased Effect
The levels/effects of Cevimeline may be decreased by: Peginterferon Alfa-2b; Tocilizumab

Stability Store at 25°C (77°F); excursions permitted to 15°C to 30°C (59°F to 86°F).

Mechanism of Action Binds to muscarinic (cholinergic) receptors, causing an increase in secretion of exocrine glands (including salivary glands)

Pharmacodynamics/Kinetics

Absorption: Rapid
Distribution: V_d: 6 L/kg
Protein binding: <20%
Metabolism: Hepatic via CYP2D6 and CYP3A4
Half-life elimination: 4-6 hours
Time to peak: 1.5-2 hours
Excretion: Urine (as metabolites and unchanged drug)

Dosage

Geriatric Refer to adult dosing. No specific dosage adjustment is recommended; however, use caution when initiating due to potential for increased sensitivity.

Adult Xerostomia (in Sjögren's syndrome): Oral: 30 mg 3 times/day

Renal Impairment No dosage adjustment provided in the manufacturer's labeling.

Hepatic Impairment No dosage adjustment provided in the manufacturer's labeling.

Administration Administer with or without food.

Special Geriatric Considerations No specific studies in the elderly are available. However, elderly often have cardiovascular, pulmonary, and gastrointestinal diseases which may restrict or contraindicate the use of this agent. The use of saliva substitutes should be considered initially. Although the clinical studies included elderly patients (>65 years of age), the number of elderly was insufficient to determine any significant differences between young adults and elderly.

Dosage Forms Excipient information presented when available (limited, particularly for generics); consult specific product labeling.

Capsule, oral, as hydrochloride:

Evoxac®: 30 mg

- ◆ **Cevimeline Hydrochloride** see Cevimeline on page 347
- ◆ **CFDN** see Cefdinir on page 311
- ◆ **CG5503** see Tapentadol on page 1836
- ◆ **C-Gel [OTC]** see Ascorbic Acid on page 149
- ◆ **CGP 33101** see Rufinamide on page 1739
- ◆ **CGP-39393** see Desirudin on page 508
- ◆ **CGP-42446** see Zoledronic Acid on page 2057
- ◆ **C-Gram [OTC]** see Ascorbic Acid on page 149
- ◆ **CGS-20267** see Letrozole on page 1101
- ◆ **Chantix®** see Varenicline on page 2006
- ◆ **Cheracol® D [OTC]** see Guaifenesin and Dextromethorphan on page 906
- ◆ **Cheracol® Plus [OTC]** see Guaifenesin and Dextromethorphan on page 906
- ◆ **Cheratussin** see GuaiFENesin on page 904
- ◆ **Chew-C [OTC]** see Ascorbic Acid on page 149
- ◆ **Chew-Cal [OTC]** see Calcium and Vitamin D on page 261
- ◆ **Children's Nasal Decongestant [OTC]** see Pseudoephedrine on page 1633
- ◆ **Children's Pepto [OTC]** see Calcium Carbonate on page 262
- ◆ **Chloral** see Chloral Hydrate on page 349

Chloral Hydrate (KLOR al HYE drate)

Related Information

Beers Criteria – Potentially Inappropriate Medications for Geriatrics on page 2183

Medication Safety Issues

High alert medication:

The Institute for Safe Medication Practices (ISMP) includes this medication among its list of drugs which have a heightened risk of causing significant patient harm when used in error.

BEERS Criteria medication:

This drug may be potentially inappropriate for use in geriatric patients (Quality of evidence - low; Strength of recommendation - strong).

Brand Names: U.S. Somnote®

Brand Names: Canada PMS-Chloral Hydrate

Index Terms Chloral; Hydrated Chloral; Trichloroacetaldehyde Monohydrate

Generic Availability (U.S.) No

Pharmacologic Category Hypnotic, Miscellaneous

Use Short-term sedative and hypnotic (<2 weeks); sedative/hypnotic for diagnostic procedures; sedative prior to EEG evaluations

Dosage

Geriatric Hypnotic: Initial: Oral: 250 mg at bedtime; adjust for renal impairment.

Adult

Sedation, anxiety: Oral: 250 mg 3 times/day

Hypnotic: Oral: 500-1000 mg at bedtime or 30 minutes prior to procedure, not to exceed 2 g/24 hours

Discontinuation: Withdraw gradually over 2 weeks if patient has been maintained on high doses for prolonged period of time. Do not stop drug abruptly; sudden withdrawal may result in delirium.

Renal Impairment

Cl_{cr} <50 mL/minute: Avoid use.

Hemodialysis effects: Supplemental dose is not necessary; dialyzable (50% to 100%).

Hepatic Impairment Avoid use in patients with severe hepatic impairment.

Special Geriatric Considerations Chloral hydrate is not a hypnotic agent of choice in the elderly. Guidelines from the Centers for Medicare and Medicaid Services (CMS) discourage the use of chloral hydrate in residents of long-term care facilities.

CHLORAL HYDRATE

◄ This medication is considered to be potentially inappropriate in this patient population (Beers Criteria: Quality of evidence - low; Strength of recommendation - strong).

Controlled Substance C-IV

Dosage Forms Excipient information presented when available (limited, particularly for generics); consult specific product labeling. [DSC] = Discontinued product

Capsule, oral:

Somnote®: 500 mg

Syrup, oral: 500 mg/5 mL (5 mL [DSC], 473 mL [DSC])

Chlorambucil (klor AM byoo sil)

Medication Safety Issues

Sound-alike/look-alike issues:

Chlorambucil may be confused with Chloromycetin®

Leukeran® may be confused with Alkeran®, leucovorin, Leukine®, Myleran®

High alert medication:

This medication is in a class the Institute for Safe Medication Practices (ISMP) includes among its list of drug classes which have a heightened risk of causing significant patient harm when used in error.

Brand Names: U.S. Leukeran®

Brand Names: Canada Leukeran®

Index Terms CB-1348; Chlorambucilum; Chloraminophene; Chlorbutinum; WR-139013

Generic Availability (U.S.) No

Pharmacologic Category Antineoplastic Agent, Alkylating Agent

Use Management of chronic lymphocytic leukemia (CLL), Hodgkin lymphoma, non-Hodgkin's lymphomas (NHL)

Canadian labeling: Additional uses (not in U.S. labeling): Management of Waldenström's macroglobulinemia

Unlabeled Use Nephrotic syndrome, Waldenström's macroglobulinemia

Contraindications Hypersensitivity to chlorambucil or any component of the formulation; hypersensitivity to other alkylating agents (may have cross-hypersensitivity); prior (demonstrated) resistance to chlorambucil

Canadian labeling: Additional contraindications (not in U.S. labeling): Use within 4 weeks of a full course of radiation or chemotherapy

Warnings/Precautions Hazardous agent - use appropriate precautions for handling and disposal. Seizures have been observed; use with caution in patients with seizure disorder or head trauma; history of nephrotic syndrome and high pulse doses are at higher risk of seizures. **[U.S. Boxed Warning]: May cause severe bone marrow suppression;** neutropenia may be severe. Reduce initial dosage if patient has received myelosuppressive or radiation therapy within the previous 4 weeks, or has a depressed baseline leukocyte or platelet count. Irreversible bone marrow damage may occur with total doses approaching 6.5 mg/kg. Progressive lymphopenia may develop (recovery is generally rapid after discontinuation). Avoid administration of live vaccines to immunocompromised patients. Rare instances of severe skin reactions (eg, erythema multiforme, Stevens-Johnson syndrome, toxic epidermal necrolysis) have been reported; discontinue promptly if skin reaction occurs.

Chlorambucil is primarily metabolized in the liver. Dosage reductions should be considered in patients with hepatic impairment. **[U.S. Boxed Warning]: Affects human fertility; carcinogenic in humans and probably mutagenic and teratogenic as well;** chromosomal damage has been documented. Reversible and irreversible sterility (when administered to prepubertal and pubertal males), azoospermia (in adult males) and amenorrhea (in females) have been observed. **[U.S. Boxed Warning]: Carcinogenic;** acute myelocytic leukemia and secondary malignancies may be associated with chronic therapy. Duration of treatment and higher cumulative doses are associated with a higher risk for development of leukemia.

Adverse Reactions (Reflective of adult population; not specific for elderly) Frequency not always defined.

Central nervous system: Agitation (rare), ataxia (rare), confusion (rare), drug fever, fever, focal/generalized seizure (rare), hallucinations (rare)

Dermatologic: Angioneurotic edema, erythema multiforme (rare), rash, skin hypersensitivity, Stevens-Johnson syndrome (rare), toxic epidermal necrolysis (rare), urticaria

Endocrine & metabolic: Amenorrhea, infertility, SIADH (rare)

Gastrointestinal: Diarrhea (infrequent), nausea (infrequent), oral ulceration (infrequent), vomiting (infrequent)

Genitourinary: Azoospermia, cystitis (sterile)

Hematologic: Neutropenia (onset: 3 weeks; recovery: 10 days after last dose), bone marrow failure (irreversible), bone marrow suppression, anemia, leukemia (secondary), leukopenia, lymphopenia, pancytopenia, thrombocytopenia

Hepatic: Hepatotoxicity, jaundice

Neuromuscular & skeletal: Flaccid paresis (rare), muscular twitching (rare), myoclonia (rare), peripheral neuropathy, tremor (rare)

Respiratory: Interstitial pneumonia, pulmonary fibrosis

Miscellaneous: Allergic reactions, malignancies (secondary)

Drug Interactions

Metabolism/Transport Effects None known.

Avoid Concomitant Use

Avoid concomitant use of Chlorambucil with any of the following: BCG; CloZAPine; Natalizumab; Pimecrolimus; Tacrolimus (Topical); Vaccines (Live)

Increased Effect/Toxicity

Chlorambucil may increase the levels/effects of: CloZAPine; Leflunomide; Natalizumab; Vaccines (Live)

The levels/effects of Chlorambucil may be increased by: Denosumab; Pimecrolimus; Roflumilast; Tacrolimus (Topical); Trastuzumab

Decreased Effect

Chlorambucil may decrease the levels/effects of: BCG; Coccidioidin Skin Test; Sipuleucel-T; Vaccines (Inactivated); Vaccines (Live)

The levels/effects of Chlorambucil may be decreased by: Echinacea

Ethanol/Nutrition/Herb Interactions Food: Absorption is decreased when administered with food.

Stability Store in refrigerator at 2°C to 8°C (36°F to 46°F).

Mechanism of Action Alkylating agent; interferes with DNA replication and RNA transcription by alkylation and cross-linking the strands of DNA

Pharmacodynamics/Kinetics

Absorption: Rapid and complete (>70%); reduced with food

Distribution: V_d: ~0.3 L/kg

Protein binding: ~99%; primarily to albumin

Metabolism: Hepatic (extensively); primarily to active metabolite, phenylacetic acid mustard

Half-life elimination: ~1.5 hours; Phenylacetic acid mustard: ~1.8 hours

Time to peak, plasma: Within 1 hour; Phenylacetic acid mustard: 1.2-2.6 hours

Excretion: Urine (~20% to 60%, primarily as inactive metabolites, <1% as unchanged drug or phenylacetic acid mustard)

Dosage

Geriatric Refer to adult dosing. Begin at the lower end of dosing range(s)

Adult Note: With bone marrow lymphocytic infiltration involvement (in CLL, Hodgkin lymphoma, or NHL), the maximum dose is 0.1 mg/kg/day. While short treatment courses are preferred, if maintenance therapy is required, the maximum dose is 0.1 mg/kg/day.

Chronic lymphocytic leukemia (CLL): Oral:

U.S. labeling: 0.1 mg/kg/day for 3-6 weeks **or** 0.4 mg/kg pulsed doses administered intermittently, biweekly, or monthly (increased by 0.1 mg/kg/dose until response/toxicity observed)

Canadian labeling: Initial: 0.15 mg/kg/day until WBC is 10,000/mm³; interrupt treatment for 4 weeks, then may resume at 0.1 mg/kg/day until response (generally ~2 years)/toxicity observed

Unlabeled dosing: 30 mg/m² day 1 every 2 weeks (in combination with prednisone) (Raphael, 1991) **or** 0.4 mg/kg day 1 every 2 weeks; if tolerated may increase by 0.1 mg/kg with each treatment course to a maximum dose of 0.8 mg/kg and maximum of 24 cycles (Eichhorst, 2009) **or** 40 mg/m² day 1 every 4 weeks until disease progression or complete remission or response plateau for up to a maximum of 12 cycles (Rai, 2000)

Hodgkin lymphoma: Oral:

U.S. labeling: 0.2 mg/kg/day for 3-6 weeks

Canadian labeling: 0.2 mg/kg/day for 4-8 weeks

Non-Hodgkin lymphomas (NHL): Oral

U.S. labeling: 0.1 mg/kg/day for 3-6 weeks

Canadian labeling: Initial: 0.1-0.2 mg/kg/day for 4-8 weeks; for maintenance treatment, reduce dose or administer intermittently

Waldenström's macroglobulinemia (U.S. unlabeled use): Oral: 0.1 mg/kg/day (continuously) for at least 6 months **or** 0.3 mg/kg/day for 7 days every 6 weeks for at least 6 months (Kyle, 2000)

Renal Impairment No dosage adjustment provided in manufacturer's labeling; however, renal elimination of unchanged chlorambucil and active metabolite (phenylacetic acid mustard) is minimal and renal impairment is not likely to affect elimination. The following adjustments have been recommended: Adults:

Aronoff, 2007:

Cl_{cr} >50 mL/minute: No adjustment necessary.

Cl_{cr} 10-50 mL/minute: Administer 75% of dose.

Cl_{cr} <10 mL/minute: Administer 50% of dose.

Peritoneal dialysis (PD): Administer 50% of dose.

Kintzel, 1995: Based on the pharmacokinetics, dosage adjustment is not indicated

Hepatic Impairment Chlorambucil undergoes extensive hepatic metabolism. Although dosage reduction should be considered in patients with hepatic impairment, no dosage adjustment is provided in the manufacturer's labeling (data is insufficient).

Administration Usually administered as a single dose; preferably on an empty stomach.

Monitoring Parameters Liver function tests, CBC with differential (weekly, with WBC monitored twice weekly during the first 3-6 weeks of treatment)

Special Geriatric Considerations Toxicity to immunosuppressives is increased in the elderly. Start with lowest recommended adult doses. Signs of infection, such as fever and rise in WBCs, may not occur. Lethargy and confusion may be more prominent signs of infection.

Dosage Forms Excipient information presented when available (limited, particularly for generics); consult specific product labeling.

Tablet, oral:

Leukeran®: 2 mg

♦ **Chlorambucilum** see Chlorambucil on page 350

♦ **Chloraminophene** see Chlorambucil on page 350

Chloramphenicol (klor am FEN i kole)

Related Information

Antimicrobial Drugs of Choice on page 2163

Medication Safety Issues

Sound-alike/look-alike issues:

Chloromycetin® may be confused with chlorambucil, Chlor-Trimeton®

Brand Names: Canada Chloromycetin®; Chloromycetin® Succinate; Diochloram®; Pentam-ycetin®

Generic Availability (U.S.) Yes

Pharmacologic Category Antibiotic, Miscellaneous

Use Treatment of serious infections due to organisms resistant to other less toxic antibiotics or when its penetrability into the site of infection is clinically superior to other antibiotics to which the organism is sensitive; useful in infections caused by *Bacteroides*, *H. influenzae*, *Neisseria meningitidis*, *Salmonella*, and *Rickettsia*; active against many vancomycin-resistant enterococci

Contraindications Hypersensitivity to chloramphenicol or any component of the formulation; treatment of trivial or viral infections; bacterial prophylaxis

Warnings/Precautions Hazardous agent - use appropriate precautions for handling and disposal. Gray syndrome characterized by circulatory collapse, cyanosis, acidosis, abdominal distention, myocardial depression, coma, and death has occurred. Use with caution in patients with impaired renal or hepatic function. Reduce dose with impaired liver function. Use with care in patients with glucose 6-phosphate dehydrogenase deficiency. **[U.S. Boxed Warning]: Serious and fatal blood dyscrasias (aplastic anemia, hypoplastic anemia, thrombocy-topenia, and granulocytopenia) have occurred after both short-term and prolonged therapy. Monitor CBC frequently in all patients;** discontinue if evidence of myelosuppres-sion. Irreversible bone marrow suppression may occur weeks or months after therapy. Avoid repeated courses of treatment. Should not be used for minor infections or when less potentially toxic agents are effective. Prolonged use may result in fungal or bacterial super-infection, including *C. difficile*-associated diarrhea (CDAD) and pseudomembranous colitis; CDAD has been observed >2 months postantibiotic treatment.

Adverse Reactions (Reflective of adult population; not specific for elderly) Fre-quency not defined.

Central nervous system: Confusion, delirium, depression, fever, headache

Dermatologic: Angioedema, rash, urticaria

Gastrointestinal: Diarrhea, enterocolitis, glossitis, nausea, stomatitis, vomiting

Hematologic: Aplastic anemia, bone marrow suppression, granulocytopenia, hypoplastic anemia, pancytopenia, thrombocytopenia

Ocular: Optic neuritis

Miscellaneous: Anaphylaxis, hypersensitivity reactions, Gray syndrome

Drug Interactions

Metabolism/Transport Effects Inhibits CYP2C19 (strong), CYP2C9 (weak), CYP3A4 (strong)

Avoid Concomitant Use

Avoid concomitant use of Chloramphenicol with any of the following: Alfuzosin; Avanafil; Axitinib; BCG; Clopidogrel; CloZAPine; Conivaptan; Crizotinib; Dronedarone; Eplerenone; Everolimus; Fluticasone (Oral Inhalation); Halofantrine; Lapatinib; Lovastatin; Lurasidone; Nilotinib; Nisoldipine; Pimozide; Ranolazine; Red Yeast Rice; Rivaroxaban; RomiDEPsin; Salmeterol; Silodosin; Simvastatin; Tamsulosin; Ticagrelor; Tolvaptan; Toremifene

Increased Effect/Toxicity

Chloramphenicol may increase the levels/effects of: Alfuzosin; Almotriptan; Alosetron; Anticonvulsants (Hydantoin); ARIPiprazole; Avanafil; Axitinib; Barbiturates; Bortezomib; Brentuximab Vedotin; Brinzolamide; Budesonide (Nasal); Budesonide (Systemic, Oral Inhalation); Ciclesonide; Citalopram; CloZAPine; Colchicine; Conivaptan; Corticosteroids (Orally Inhaled); Crizotinib; CycloSPORINE; CycloSPORINE (Systemic); CYP2C19 Substrates; CYP3A4 Substrates; Dienogest; Dronedarone; Dutasteride; Eplerenone; Everolimus; FentaNYL; Fesoterodine; Fluticasone (Nasal); Fluticasone (Oral Inhalation); GuanFACINE; Halofantrine; Iloperidone; Ivacaftor; Ixabepilone; Lapatinib; Lovastatin; Lumefantrine; Lurasidone; Maraviroc; MethylPREDNISolone; Mifepristone; Nilotinib; Nisoldipine; Paricalcitol; Pazopanib; Pimecrolimus; Pimozide; Propafenone; Ranolazine; Red Yeast Rice; Rivaroxaban; RomiDEPsin; Ruxolitinib; Salmeterol; Saxagliptin; Sildenafil; Silodosin; Simvastatin; SORAfenib; Sulfonylureas; Tacrolimus; Tacrolimus (Systemic); Tadalafil; Tamsulosin; Ticagrelor; Tolterodine; Tolvaptan; Toremifene; Vardenafil; Vemurafenib; Vilazodone; Vitamin K Antagonists; Voriconazole; Zuclopenthixol

Decreased Effect

Chloramphenicol may decrease the levels/effects of: BCG; Clopidogrel; Cyanocobalamin; Ifosfamide; Prasugrel; Ticagrelor; Typhoid Vaccine

The levels/effects of Chloramphenicol may be decreased by: Anticonvulsants (Hydantoin); Barbiturates; Rifampin

Ethanol/Nutrition/Herb Interactions Food: May decrease intestinal absorption of vitamin B_{12} may have increased dietary need for riboflavin, pyridoxine, and vitamin B_{12}.

Stability Store at room temperature prior to reconstitution. Reconstituted solutions remain stable for 30 days. Use only clear solutions. Frozen solutions remain stable for 6 months.

Mechanism of Action Reversibly binds to 50S ribosomal subunits of susceptible organisms preventing amino acids from being transferred to growing peptide chains thus inhibiting protein synthesis

Pharmacodynamics/Kinetics

Distribution: To most tissues and body fluids
  Chloramphenicol: V_d: 0.5-1 L/kg
  Chloramphenicol succinate: V_d: 0.2-3.1 L/kg; decreased with hepatic or renal dysfunction
Protein binding: Chloramphenicol: ~60%; decreased with hepatic or renal dysfunction
Metabolism:
  Chloramphenicol: Hepatic to metabolites (inactive)
  Chloramphenicol succinate: Hydrolyzed in the liver, kidney and lungs to chloramphenicol (active)
Bioavailability:
  Chloramphenicol: Oral: ~80%
  Chloramphenicol succinate: I.V.: ~70%; highly variable, dependant upon rate and extent of metabolism to chloramphenicol
Half-life elimination:
  Normal renal function:
    Chloramphenicol: Adults: ~4 hours
    Chloramphenicol succinate: Adults: ~3 hours
  End-stage renal disease: Chloramphenicol: 3-7 hours
  Hepatic disease: Prolonged
Excretion: Urine (~30% as unchanged chloramphenicol succinate in adults; 5% to 15% as chloramphenicol)

Dosage

Geriatric & Adult Systemic infections: I.V.: 50-100 mg/kg/day in divided doses every 6 hours; maximum daily dose: 4 g/day.

Renal Impairment Use with caution; monitor serum concentrations.

Hepatic Impairment Use with caution; monitor serum concentrations.

Administration Do not administer I.M.; can be administered IVP over at least 1 minute at a concentration of 100 mg/mL, or I.V. intermittent infusion over 15-30 minutes at a final concentration for administration of ≤20 mg/mL

◀ **Monitoring Parameters** CBC with differential (baseline and every 2 days during therapy), periodic liver and renal function tests, serum drug concentration

Reference Range
Therapeutic levels:
Meningitis:
Peak: 15-25 mcg/mL; toxic concentration: >40 mcg/mL
Trough: 5-15 mcg/mL
Other infections:
Peak: 10-20 mcg/mL
Trough: 5-10 mcg/mL
Timing of serum samples: Draw levels 0.5-1.5 hours after completion of I.V. dose

Test Interactions May cause false-positive results in urine glucose tests when using cupric sulfate (Benedict's solution, Clinitest®).

Pharmacotherapy Pearls Sodium content of 1 g (injection): 51.8 mg (2.25 mEq)

Special Geriatric Considerations Chloramphenicol has not been studied in the elderly. Dose adjustment for renal function. Chloramphenicol should be reserved for serious infections.

Dosage Forms Excipient information presented when available (limited, particularly for generics); consult specific product labeling.
Injection, powder for reconstitution: 1 g [contains sodium [~52 mg (2.25 mEq)/g]]

◆ **Chlorbutinum** see Chlorambucil on page 350

ChlordiazePOXIDE (klor dye az e POKS ide)

Related Information
Anxiolytic, Sedative/Hypnotic, and Miscellaneous Benzodiazepines on page 2106
Beers Criteria − Potentially Inappropriate Medications for Geriatrics on page 2183

Medication Safety Issues
Sound-alike/look-alike issues:
ChlordiazePOXIDE may be confused with chlorproMAZINE
Librium may be confused with Librax®
BEERS Criteria medication:
This drug may be potentially inappropriate for use in geriatric patients (Quality of evidence - high; Strength of recommendation - strong).

Index Terms Librium; Methaminodiazepoxide Hydrochloride
Generic Availability (U.S.) Yes
Pharmacologic Category Benzodiazepine
Use Management of anxiety disorder or for the short-term relief of symptoms of anxiety; withdrawal symptoms of acute alcoholism; preoperative apprehension and anxiety
Contraindications Hypersensitivity to chlordiazepoxide or any component of the formulation (cross-sensitivity with other benzodiazepines may also exist)
Warnings/Precautions Active metabolites with extended half-lives may lead to delayed accumulation and adverse effects. Use with caution in elderly or debilitated patients, patients with hepatic disease (including alcoholics) or renal impairment, patients with respiratory disease or impaired gag reflex, patients with porphyria.

Causes CNS depression (dose related) resulting in sedation, dizziness, confusion, or ataxia which may impair physical and mental capabilities. Patients must be cautioned about performing tasks which require mental alertness (eg, operating machinery or driving). Use with caution in patients receiving other CNS depressants or psychoactive agents (lithium, phenothiazines). Effects with other sedative drugs or ethanol may be potentiated. Benzodiazepines have been associated with falls and traumatic injury and should be used with extreme caution in patients who are at risk of these events. In older adults, benzodiazepines increase the risk of impaired cognition, delirium, falls, fractures, and motor vehicle accidents. Due to increased sensitivity in this age group and slower metabolism of long-acting agents (such as chlordiazepoxide), avoid use for treatment of insomnia, agitation, or delirium (Beers Criteria).

Use caution in patients with depression, particularly if suicidal risk may be present. Use with caution in patients with a history of drug dependence. Benzodiazepines have been associated with dependence and acute withdrawal symptoms on discontinuation or reduction in dose. Acute withdrawal, including seizures, may be precipitated in patients after administration of flumazenil to patients receiving long-term benzodiazepine therapy.

Benzodiazepines have been associated with anterograde amnesia. Paradoxical reactions, including hyperactive or aggressive behavior have been reported with benzodiazepines, particularly in adolescent/pediatric or psychiatric patients. Does not have analgesic, anti-depressant, or antipsychotic properties.

Adverse Reactions (Reflective of adult population; not specific for elderly)

>10%:

Central nervous system: Drowsiness, fatigue, ataxia, lightheadedness, memory impairment, dysarthria, irritability

Dermatologic: Rash

Endocrine & metabolic: Libido decreased, menstrual disorders

Gastrointestinal: Xerostomia, salivation decreased, appetite increased or decreased, weight gain/loss

Genitourinary: Micturition difficulties

1% to 10%:

Cardiovascular: Hypotension

Central nervous system: Confusion, dizziness, disinhibition, akathisia

Dermatologic: Dermatitis

Endocrine & metabolic: Libido increased

Gastrointestinal: Salivation increased

Genitourinary: Sexual dysfunction, incontinence

Neuromuscular & skeletal: Rigidity, tremor, muscle cramps

Otic: Tinnitus

Respiratory: Nasal congestion

Drug Interactions

Metabolism/Transport Effects Substrate of CYP3A4 (major); **Note:** Assignment of Major/Minor substrate status based on clinically relevant drug interaction potential

Avoid Concomitant Use

Avoid concomitant use of ChlordiazePOXIDE with any of the following: Azelastine; Azelastine (Nasal); Conivaptan; Methadone; Mirtazapine; OLANZapine; Paraldehyde

Increased Effect/Toxicity

ChlordiazePOXIDE may increase the levels/effects of: Alcohol (Ethyl); Azelastine; Azelastine (Nasal); Buprenorphine; CloZAPine; CNS Depressants; Fosphenytoin; Methadone; Methotrimeprazine; Metyrosine; Mirtazapine; Paraldehyde; Phenytoin; Selective Serotonin Reuptake Inhibitors; Zolpidem

The levels/effects of ChlordiazePOXIDE may be increased by: Antifungal Agents (Azole Derivatives, Systemic); Aprepitant; Calcium Channel Blockers (Nondihydropyridine); Cimetidine; Conivaptan; Contraceptives (Estrogens); Contraceptives (Progestins); CYP3A4 Inhibitors (Moderate); CYP3A4 Inhibitors (Strong); Dasatinib; Disulfiram; Droperidol; Fosaprepitant; Grapefruit Juice; HydrOXYzine; Isoniazid; Ivacaftor; Macrolide Antibiotics; MAO Inhibitors; Methotrimeprazine; Mifepristone; OLANZapine; Proton Pump Inhibitors; Selective Serotonin Reuptake Inhibitors

Decreased Effect

The levels/effects of ChlordiazePOXIDE may be decreased by: CarBAMazepine; CYP3A4 Inducers (Strong); Deferasirox; Rifamycin Derivatives; St Johns Wort; Theophylline Derivatives; Tocilizumab; Yohimbine

Ethanol/Nutrition/Herb Interactions

Ethanol: May increase CNS depression; monitor for increased effects with coadministration. Caution patients about effects.

Food: Serum concentrations/effects may be increased with grapefruit juice, but unlikely because of high oral bioavailability of chlordiazepoxide.

Herb/Nutraceutical: Avoid valerian, St John's wort, kava kava, gotu kola (may increase CNS depression).

Stability Store at controlled room temperature. Protect from light and moisture.

Mechanism of Action Binds to stereospecific benzodiazepine receptors on the postsynaptic GABA neuron at several sites within the central nervous system, including the limbic system, reticular formation. Enhancement of the inhibitory effect of GABA on neuronal excitability results by increased neuronal membrane permeability to chloride ions. This shift in chloride ions results in hyperpolarization (a less excitable state) and stabilization.

Pharmacodynamics/Kinetics

Distribution: V_d: 3.3 L/kg

Protein binding: 90% to 98%

Metabolism: Extensively hepatic to desmethyldiazepam (active and long-acting)

Half-life elimination: 6.6-25 hours; End-stage renal disease: 5-30 hours; Cirrhosis: 30-63 hours

Time to peak, serum: Within 2 hours

Excretion: Urine (minimal as unchanged drug)

Dosage
Geriatric Oral: 5 mg 2-4 times/day. Avoid use if possible due to long-acting metabolite.
Adult
Anxiety; Oral:
Mild-moderate anxiety: Usual daily dose: 5-10 mg 3-4 times/day
Severe anxiety: Usual daily dose: 20-25 mg 3-4 times/day
Preoperative anxiety: Oral: 5-10 mg 3-4 times/day on the days preceding surgery
Ethanol withdrawal symptoms: Oral: 50-100 mg to start; dose may be repeated in 2-4 hours as necessary to a maximum of 300 mg/24 hours. **Note:** Frequency of repeat doses is often based on institution-specific protocols.
Renal Impairment Dosage adjustments are not provided in the manufacturer's labeling; however, the following guidelines have been used by some clinicians (Aronoff, 2007): Adults: Cl$_{cr}$ <10 mL/minute: Administer 50% of dose.
Peritoneal dialysis: Administer 50% of the dose.
Hepatic Impairment There are no specific hepatic dosage adjustments provided in the manufacturer's labeling. Use with caution or avoid use in hepatic impairment; hepatic metabolism occurs.
Administration Administer orally in divided doses.
Monitoring Parameters Respiratory and cardiovascular status, mental status, check for orthostasis
Reference Range Therapeutic: 0.1-3 mcg/mL (SI: 0-10 micromole/L); Toxic: >23 mcg/mL (SI: >77 micromole/L)
Pharmacotherapy Pearls The parenteral formulation of chlordiazepoxide is no longer commercially available in the U.S. or Canada.
Special Geriatric Considerations Due to its long-acting metabolite, chlordiazepoxide is not considered a drug of choice in the elderly. Long-acting benzodiazepines have been associated with falls in the elderly. Guidelines from the Centers for Medicare and Medicaid Services (CMS) discourage the use of this agent in residents of long-term care facilities.

This medication is considered to be potentially inappropriate in this patient population (Beers Criteria: Quality of evidence - high; Strength of recommendation - strong).
Controlled Substance C-IV
Dosage Forms Excipient information presented when available (limited, particularly for generics); consult specific product labeling.
Capsule, oral, as hydrochloride: 5 mg, 10 mg, 25 mg

♦ **Chlordiazepoxide and Clidinium** *see* Clidinium and Chlordiazepoxide *on page 398*
♦ **Chlor Hist [OTC]** *see* Chlorpheniramine *on page 357*
♦ **Chlormeprazine** *see* Prochlorperazine *on page 1609*

Chlorothiazide (klor oh THYE a zide)

Medication Safety Issues
International issues:
Diuril [U.S., Canada] may be confused with Duorol brand name for acetaminophen [Spain]
Brand Names: U.S. Diuril®; Sodium Diuril®
Brand Names: Canada Diuril®
Generic Availability (U.S.) Yes: Excludes oral suspension
Pharmacologic Category Diuretic, Thiazide
Use Management of mild-to-moderate hypertension; adjunctive treatment of edema
Dosage
Geriatric Oral: 500 mg once daily **or** 1 g 3 times/week
Adult Note: The manufacturer states that I.V. and oral dosing are equivalent. Some clinicians may use lower I.V. doses; however, because of chlorothiazide's poor oral absorption.

Hypertension: Oral: 500-2000 mg/day divided in 1-2 doses (manufacturer's labeling); doses of 125-500 mg/day have also been recommended (JNC 7)
Edema: Oral, I.V.: 500-1000 mg once or twice daily; intermittent treatment (eg, therapy on alternative days) may be appropriate for some patients
ACC/AHA 2009 Heart Failure guidelines:
Oral: 250-500 mg once or twice daily (maximum daily dose: 1000 mg)
I.V.: 500-1000 mg once or twice daily plus a loop diuretic
Renal Impairment Cl$_{cr}$ <10 mL/minute: Avoid use. Ineffective with Cl$_{cr}$ <30 mL/minute unless in combination with a loop diuretic (Aronoff, 2007)
Note: ACC/AHA 2009 Heart Failure Guidelines suggest that thiazides lose their efficacy when Cl$_{cr}$ <40 mL/minute

Special Geriatric Considerations Chlorothiazide is minimally effective in patients with a Cl_{cr} <30 mL/minute. This may limit the usefulness of chlorothiazide in the elderly.

Dosage Forms Excipient information presented when available (limited, particularly for generics); consult specific product labeling.

Injection, powder for reconstitution, as sodium [strength expressed as base]: 500 mg
  Sodium Diuril®: 0.5 g
Suspension, oral:
  Diuril®: 250 mg/5 mL (237 mL) [contains benzoic acid, ethanol 0.5%]
Tablet, oral: 250 mg, 500 mg

◆ **Chlorphen [OTC]** *see* Chlorpheniramine *on page 357*
◆ **Chlorphen-12™ [OTC]** *see* Chlorpheniramine *on page 357*

Chlorpheniramine (klor fen IR a meen)

Related Information
  Beers Criteria – Potentially Inappropriate Medications for Geriatrics *on page 2183*
Medication Safety Issues
  Sound-alike/look-alike issues:
    Chlor-Trimeton® may be confused with Chloromycetin®
  BEERS Criteria medication:
    This drug may be potentially inappropriate for use in geriatric patients (Quality of evidence - moderate; Strength of recommendation - strong).

Brand Names: U.S. Aller-chlor® [OTC]; Allergy Relief [OTC]; Chlor Hist [OTC]; Chlor-Trimeton® Allergy [OTC]; Chlorphen [OTC]; Chlorphen-12™ [OTC]; ED Chlorped Jr [OTC]; Ed ChlorPed [OTC]; Ed-Chlortan [OTC]

Brand Names: Canada Chlor-Tripolon®; Novo-Pheniram

Index Terms Chlorpheniramine Maleate; CTM

Generic Availability (U.S.) Yes

Pharmacologic Category Alkylamine Derivative; Histamine H_1 Antagonist; Histamine H_1 Antagonist, First Generation

Use Perennial and seasonal allergic rhinitis and other allergic symptoms including urticaria

Contraindications Hypersensitivity to chlorpheniramine maleate or any component of the formulation; narrow-angle glaucoma; bladder neck obstruction; symptomatic prostate hypertrophy; during acute asthmatic attacks; stenosing peptic ulcer; pyloroduodenal obstruction.

Warnings/Precautions Causes sedation, caution must be used in performing tasks which require alertness (eg, operating machinery or driving). Sedative effects of CNS depressants or ethanol are potentiated. Use with caution in patients with urinary tract obstruction, symptomatic prostatic hyperplasia, thyroid dysfunction, increased intraocular pressure, and cardiovascular disease (including hypertension and ischemic heart disease). In the elderly, avoid use of this potent anticholinergic agent due to increased risk of confusion, dry mouth, constipation, and other anticholinergic effects; clearance decreases in patients of advanced age (Beers Criteria).

Adverse Reactions (Reflective of adult population; not specific for elderly)
>10%:
  Central nervous system: Slight to moderate drowsiness
  Respiratory: Thickening of bronchial secretions
1% to 10%:
  Central nervous system: Headache, excitability, fatigue, nervousness, dizziness
  Gastrointestinal: Nausea, xerostomia, diarrhea, abdominal pain, appetite increase, weight gain
  Genitourinary: Urinary retention
  Neuromuscular & skeletal: Arthralgia, weakness
  Ocular: Diplopia
  Renal: Polyuria
  Respiratory: Pharyngitis

Drug Interactions
  Metabolism/Transport Effects Substrate of CYP2D6 (minor), CYP3A4 (major); **Note:** Assignment of Major/Minor substrate status based on clinically relevant drug interaction potential; **Inhibits** CYP2D6 (weak)
  Avoid Concomitant Use
    Avoid concomitant use of Chlorpheniramine with any of the following: Azelastine; Azelastine (Nasal); Conivaptan; Methadone; Mirtazapine; Paraldehyde

Increased Effect/Toxicity

Chlorpheniramine may increase the levels/effects of: Alcohol (Ethyl); Anticholinergics; ARIPiprazole; Azelastine; Azelastine (Nasal); Buprenorphine; CNS Depressants; Methadone; Methotrimeprazine; Metyrosine; Mirtazapine; Paraldehyde; Selective Serotonin Reuptake Inhibitors; Zolpidem

The levels/effects of Chlorpheniramine may be increased by: Conivaptan; CYP3A4 Inhibitors (Moderate); CYP3A4 Inhibitors (Strong); Dasatinib; Droperidol; HydrOXYzine; Ivacaftor; Methotrimeprazine; Mifepristone; Pramlintide

Decreased Effect

Chlorpheniramine may decrease the levels/effects of: Acetylcholinesterase Inhibitors (Central); Benzylpenicilloyl Polylysine; Betahistine; Hyaluronidase

The levels/effects of Chlorpheniramine may be decreased by: Acetylcholinesterase Inhibitors (Central); Amphetamines; Peginterferon Alfa-2b; Tocilizumab

Ethanol/Nutrition/Herb Interactions Ethanol: May increase CNS depression; monitor for increased effects with coadministration. Caution patients about effects.

Stability Protect from light.

Mechanism of Action Competes with histamine for H_1-receptor sites on effector cells in the gastrointestinal tract, blood vessels, and respiratory tract

Pharmacodynamics/Kinetics

Distribution: V_d: Adults: 6-12 L/kg (Paton, 1985)

Protein bindng: 33% (range: 29% to 37%) (Martínez-Gómez, 2007)

Metabolism: Hepatic via CYP450 enzymes (including CYP2D6 and other unidentified enzymes) to active and inactive metabolites; significant first-pass effect (Sharma, 2003)

Half-life elimination: Serum: Adults: 14-24 hours (Paton, 1985)

Time to peak: 2-3 hours (Sharma, 2003)

Excretion: Urine (Sharma, 2003)

Dosage

Adult Allergic symptoms, allergic rhinitis: Oral: **Chlorpheniramine maleate:**

Immediate release: 4 mg every 4-6 hours; do not exceed 24 mg/24 hours

Extended release: 12 mg every 12 hours; do not exceed 24 mg/24 hours

Administration May be administered with food or water. Timed release oral forms are to be swallowed whole, not crushed or chewed.

Test Interactions May suppress the wheal and flare reactions to skin test antigens.

Pharmacotherapy Pearls Not effective for nasal stuffiness.

Special Geriatric Considerations Anticholinergic action may cause significant confusional symptoms, constipation, or problems voiding urine. If an antihistamine is indicated, a second generation nonsedating antihistamine would be a more appropriate choice.

This medication is considered to be potentially inappropriate in this patient population (Beers Criteria: Quality of evidence - moderate; Strength of recommendation - strong).

Dosage Forms Excipient information presented when available (limited, particularly for generics); consult specific product labeling.

Liquid, oral, as maleate [drops]:

Ed ChlorPed: 2 mg/mL (60 mL) [contains propylene glycol, sodium benzoate; cotton candy flavor]

Syrup, oral, as maleate:

Aller-chlor®: 2 mg/5 mL (118 mL) [contains ethanol 5%, menthol, propylene glycol; cherry flavor]

ED Chlorped Jr: 2 mg/5 mL (473 mL) [ethanol free, sugar free; contains propylene glycol; cherry flavor]

Tablet, oral, as maleate: 4 mg

Aller-chlor®: 4 mg [scored]

Allergy Relief: 4 mg

Chlor Hist: 4 mg

Chlor-Trimeton® Allergy: 4 mg

Chlorphen: 4 mg

Ed-Chlortan: 4 mg [scored]

Tablet, extended release, oral, as maleate:

Chlorphen-12™: 12 mg [contains calcium 28 mg/tablet]

◆ **Chlorpheniramine Maleate** *see* Chlorpheniramine *on page 357*

ChlorproMAZINE (klor PROE ma zeen)

Related Information

Antipsychotic Agents *on page 2103*

Beers Criteria – Potentially Inappropriate Medications for Geriatrics *on page 2183*

Medication Safety Issues

Sound-alike/look-alike issues:

ChlorproMAZINE may be confused with chlordiazePOXIDE, chlorproPAMIDE, clomiPR-AMINE, prochlorperazine, promethazine

Thorazine may be confused with thiamine, thioridazine

BEERS Criteria medication:

This drug may be potentially inappropriate for use in geriatric patients (Quality of evidence - moderate; Strength of recommendation - strong).

Brand Names: Canada Chlorpromazine Hydrochloride Inj; Teva-Chlorpromazine

Index Terms Chlorpromazine Hydrochloride; CPZ; Thorazine

Generic Availability (U.S.) Yes

Pharmacologic Category Antimanic Agent; Antipsychotic Agent, Typical, Phenothiazine

Use Management of psychotic disorders (control of mania, treatment of schizophrenia); control of nausea and vomiting; relief of restlessness and apprehension before surgery; acute intermittent porphyria; adjunct in the treatment of tetanus; intractable hiccups

Unlabeled Use Behavioral symptoms associated with dementia (elderly); psychosis/agitation related to Alzheimer's dementia

Contraindications Hypersensitivity to chlorpromazine or any component of the formulation (cross-reactivity between phenothiazines may occur); severe CNS depression; coma

Warnings/Precautions [U.S. Boxed Warning]: Elderly patients with dementia-related psychosis treated with antipsychotics are at an increased risk of death compared to placebo. Most deaths appeared to be either cardiovascular (eg, heart failure, sudden death) or infectious (eg, pneumonia) in nature. Chlorpromazine is not approved for the treatment of dementia-related psychosis. Highly sedating, use with caution in disorders where CNS depression is a feature and in patients with Parkinson's disease. Use with caution in patients with hemodynamic instability, predisposition to seizures, subcortical brain damage, severe cardiac, hepatic, or renal disease. Use caution in respiratory disease (eg, severe asthma, emphysema) due to potential for CNS effects.

Leukopenia, neutropenia, and agranulocytosis (sometimes fatal) have been reported in clinical trials and postmarketing reports with antipsychotic use; presence of risk factors (eg, pre-existing low WBC or history of drug-induced leuko/neutropenia) should prompt periodic blood count assessment. Discontinue therapy at first signs of blood dyscrasias or if absolute neutrophil count <1000/mm^3.

Esophageal dysmotility and aspiration have been associated with antipsychotic use; use with caution in patients at risk of aspiration pneumonia (ie, Alzheimer's disease). Use associated with increased prolactin levels; clinical significance of hyperprolactinemia in patients with breast cancer or other prolactin-dependent tumors is unknown. May alter temperature regulation or mask toxicity of other drugs due to antiemetic effects. May alter cardiac conduction; life-threatening arrhythmias have occurred with therapeutic doses of neuroleptics. May cause QT prolongation and subsequent torsade de pointes; avoid use in patients with diagnosed or suspected congenital long QT syndrome. Avoid concurrent use with other drugs known to prolong QT$_c$ interval.

Use with caution in patients at risk of hypotension (orthostasis is common) or those who would tolerate transient hypotensive episodes (cerebrovascular disease, cardiovascular disease, or other medications which may predispose). Significant hypotension may occur, particularly with parenteral administration. Injection contains sulfites.

Use with caution in patients with decreased gastrointestinal motility, urinary retention, BPH, xerostomia, or visual problems (ie, narrow-angle glaucoma), and myasthenia gravis. Relative to other neuroleptics, chlorpromazine has a moderate potency of cholinergic blockade. May cause pigmentary retinopathy, and lenticular and corneal deposits, particularly with prolonged therapy.

May cause extrapyramidal symptoms (EPS), including pseudoparkinsonism, acute dystonic reactions, akathisia, and tardive dyskinesia. Risk of dystonia (and possibly other EPS) may be greater with increased doses, use of conventional antipsychotics, males, and younger patients. May cause neuroleptic malignant syndrome (NMS).

Use in elderly patients with dementia is associated with an increased risk of mortality and cerebrovascular accidents; avoid antipsychotic use for behavioral problems associated with dementia unless alternative nonpharmacologic therapies have failed and patient may harm self or others. In addition, may cause or exacerbate syndrome of inappropriate antidiuretic hormone secretion or hyponatremia; monitor sodium closely with initiation or dosage adjustments in older adults. May be inappropriate in older adults depending on comorbidities (eg, delirium) due to its potent anticholinergic effects (Beers Criteria). Increased risk for developing tardive dyskinesia, particularly in elderly women.

Adverse Reactions (Reflective of adult population; not specific for elderly) Frequency not defined.

Cardiovascular: Orthostatic hypotension, tachycardia, dizziness, nonspecific QT changes

Central nervous system: Drowsiness, dystonias, akathisia, pseudoparkinsonism, tardive dyskinesia, neuroleptic malignant syndrome, seizure

Dermatologic: Photosensitivity, dermatitis, skin pigmentation (slate gray)

Endocrine & metabolic: Lactation, breast engorgement, false-positive pregnancy test, amenorrhea, gynecomastia, hyper- or hypoglycemia

Gastrointestinal: Xerostomia, constipation, nausea

Genitourinary: Urinary retention, ejaculatory disorder, impotence

Hematologic: Agranulocytosis, eosinophilia, leukopenia, hemolytic anemia, aplastic anemia, thrombocytopenic purpura

Hepatic: Jaundice

Ocular: Blurred vision, corneal and lenticular changes, epithelial keratopathy, pigmentary retinopathy

Drug Interactions

Metabolism/Transport Effects Substrate of CYP1A2 (minor), CYP2D6 (major), CYP3A4 (minor); **Note:** Assignment of Major/Minor substrate status based on clinically relevant drug interaction potential; **Inhibits** CYP2D6 (moderate), CYP2E1 (weak)

Avoid Concomitant Use

Avoid concomitant use of ChlorproMAZINE with any of the following: Azelastine; Azelastine (Nasal); Highest Risk QTc-Prolonging Agents; Metoclopramide; Mifepristone; Paraldehyde

Increased Effect/Toxicity

ChlorproMAZINE may increase the levels/effects of: Alcohol (Ethyl); Analgesics (Opioid); Anticholinergics; Antidepressants (Serotonin Reuptake Inhibitor/Antagonist); ARIPiprazole; Azelastine; Azelastine (Nasal); Beta-Blockers; CNS Depressants; CYP2D6 Substrates; Desmopressin; Divalproex; Fesoterodine; Haloperidol; Highest Risk QTc-Prolonging Agents; Methylphenidate; Moderate Risk QTc-Prolonging Agents; Paraldehyde; Porfimer; Serotonin Modulators; Valproic Acid; Zolpidem

The levels/effects of ChlorproMAZINE may be increased by: Abiraterone Acetate; Acetylcholinesterase Inhibitors (Central); Antidepressants (Serotonin Reuptake Inhibitor/Antagonist); Antimalarial Agents; Beta-Blockers; CYP2D6 Inhibitors (Moderate); CYP2D6 Inhibitors (Strong); Darunavir; Haloperidol; HydrOXYzine; Lithium formulations; Methylphenidate; Metoclopramide; Metyrosine; Mifepristone; Pramlintide; QTc-Prolonging Agents (Indeterminate Risk and Risk Modifying); Tetrabenazine

Decreased Effect

ChlorproMAZINE may decrease the levels/effects of: Amphetamines; Anti-Parkinson's Agents (Dopamine Agonist); Quinagolide

The levels/effects of ChlorproMAZINE may be decreased by: Antacids; Anti-Parkinson's Agents (Dopamine Agonist); Lithium formulations; Peginterferon Alfa-2b; Tocilizumab

Ethanol/Nutrition/Herb Interactions

Ethanol: May increase CNS depression; monitor for increased effects with coadministration. Caution patients about effects.

Herb/Nutraceutical: Avoid St John's wort (may decrease chlorpromazine levels, increase photosensitization, or enhance sedative effect). Avoid dong quai (may enhance photosensitization). Avoid kava kava, gotu kola, valerian (may increase CNS depression).

Stability Injection: Protect from light. A slightly yellowed solution does not indicate potency loss, but a markedly discolored solution should be discarded. Diluted injection (1 mg/mL) with NS and stored in 5 mL vials remains stable for 30 days.

Mechanism of Action Chlorpromazine is an aliphatic phenothiazine antipsychotic which blocks postsynaptic mesolimbic dopaminergic receptors in the brain; exhibits a strong alpha-adrenergic blocking effect and depresses the release of hypothalamic and hypophyseal hormones; believed to depress the reticular activating system, thus affecting basal metabolism, body temperature, wakefulness, vasomotor tone, and emesis

Pharmacodynamics/Kinetics

Onset of action: I.M.: 15 minutes; Oral: 30-60 minutes

Absorption: Rapid

Distribution: V_d: 20 L/kg

Protein binding: 92% to 97%

Metabolism: Extensively hepatic to active and inactive metabolites

Bioavailability: 20%

Half-life, biphasic: Initial: 2 hours; Terminal: 30 hours

Excretion: Urine (<1% as unchanged drug) within 24 hours

Dosage

Geriatric

Behavioral symptoms associated with dementia (unlabeled use): Initial: 10-25 mg 1-2 times/day; increase at 4- to 7-day intervals by 10-25 mg/day. Increase dose intervals (eg, twice daily, 3 times/day) as necessary to control behavior response or side effects; maximum daily dose: 800 mg; gradual increases (titration) may prevent some side effects or decrease their severity.

Other indications: Refer to adult dosing.

Adult

Schizophrenia/psychoses:

Oral: Range: 30-800 mg/day in 1-4 divided doses, initiate at lower doses and titrate as needed; usual dose: 200-600 mg/day; some patients may require 1-2 g/day

I.M., I.V.: Initial: 25 mg, may repeat (25-50 mg) in 1-4 hours, gradually increase to a maximum of 400 mg/dose every 4-6 hours until patient is controlled; usual dose: 300-800 mg/day

Intractable hiccups:

Oral, I.M.: 25-50 mg 3-4 times/day

I.V. (refractory to oral or I.M. treatment): 25-50 mg via slow I.V. infusion

Nausea and vomiting:

Oral: 10-25 mg every 4-6 hours

I.M., I.V.: 25-50 mg every 4-6 hours

Renal Impairment Not dialyzable (0% to 5%)

Hepatic Impairment Avoid use in severe hepatic dysfunction.

Administration Do not administer SubQ (tissue damage and irritation may occur); for direct I.V. injection: Dilute with normal saline to a maximum concentration of 1 mg/mL, administer slow I.V. at a rate not to exceed 1 mg/minute in adults. For treatment of intractable hiccups the manufacturer recommends diluting 25-50 mg of chlorpromazine in 500-1000 ml of normal saline. To reduce the risk of hypotension, patients receiving I.V. chlorpromazine must remain lying down during and for 30 minutes after the injection. **Note:** Avoid skin contact with solution; may cause contact dermatitis.

Monitoring Parameters Vital signs (especially with parenteral use); lipid profile, fasting blood glucose/Hgb A_{1c}; BMI; mental status; abnormal involuntary movement scale (AIMS); extrapyramidal symptoms (EPS); CBC in patients with risk factors for leukopenia/neutropenia

Reference Range

Therapeutic: 50-300 ng/mL (SI: 157-942 nmol/L)

Toxic: >750 ng/mL (SI: >2355 nmol/L); serum concentrations poorly correlate with expected response

Test Interactions False-positives for phenylketonuria, amylase, uroporphyrins, urobilinogen. May interfere with urine detection of amphetamine/methamphetamine and methadone (false-positives).

Special Geriatric Considerations Many elderly patients receive antipsychotic medications for inappropriate nonpsychotic behavior. Before initiating antipsychotic medication, the clinician should investigate any possible reversible cause; any stress or stress from any disease can cause acute "confusion" or worsening of baseline nonpsychotic behavior. Most commonly acute changes in behavior are due to increases in drug dose or addition of new drug to regimen; fluid electrolyte loss; infections; and changes in environment.

Any changes in disease status in any organ system can result in behavior changes.

In the treatment of agitated, demented, elderly patients, authors of meta-analysis of controlled trials of the response to the traditional antipsychotics (phenothiazines, butyrophenones) in controlling agitation have concluded that the use of neuroleptics results in a response rate of 18%. Clearly neuroleptic therapy for behavior control should be limited with frequent attempts to withdraw the agent given for behavior control.

This medication is considered to be potentially inappropriate in this patient population (Beers Criteria: Quality of evidence - moderate; Strength of recommendation - strong).

Dosage Forms Excipient information presented when available (limited, particularly for generics); consult specific product labeling.

Injection, solution, as hydrochloride: 25 mg/mL (1 mL, 2 mL)

Tablet, oral, as hydrochloride: 10 mg, 25 mg, 50 mg, 100 mg, 200 mg

◆ **Chlorpromazine Hydrochloride** *see* ChlorproMAZINE *on page 359*

ChlorproPAMIDE (klor PROE pa mide)

Related Information

Beers Criteria – Potentially Inappropriate Medications for Geriatrics *on page 2183*

Diabetes Mellitus Management, Adults *on page 2193*

Medication Safety Issues

Sound-alike/look-alike issues:

ChlorproPAMIDE may be confused with chlorproMAZINE

Diabinese may be confused with DiaBeta®, Diamox®

High alert medication:

The Institute for Safe Medication Practices (ISMP) includes this medication among its list of drugs which have a heightened risk of causing significant patient harm when used in error.

BEERS Criteria medication:

This drug may be potentially inappropriate for use in geriatric patients (Quality of evidence - high; Strength of recommendation - strong).

Brand Names: Canada Apo-Chlorpropamide®

Generic Availability (U.S.) Yes

Pharmacologic Category Antidiabetic Agent, Sulfonylurea

Use Management of blood sugar in type 2 diabetes mellitus (noninsulin dependent, NIDDM)

Unlabeled Use Neurogenic diabetes insipidus

Contraindications Hypersensitivity to chlorpropamide, sulfonylureas, sulfonamides, or any component of the formulation; type 1 diabetes mellitus (insulin dependent, IDDM); diabetic ketoacidosis

Warnings/Precautions All sulfonylurea drugs are capable of producing severe hypoglycemia. Hypoglycemia is more likely to occur when caloric intake is deficient, after severe or prolonged exercise, when ethanol is ingested, or when more than one glucose-lowering drug is used. It is also more likely in elderly patients, malnourished patients and in patients with impaired renal or hepatic function; use with caution. Avoid use in the elderly due to prolonged half-life/hypoglycemia and risk of causing SIADH (Beers Criteria).

Loss of efficacy may be observed following prolonged use as a result of the progression of type 2 diabetes mellitus which results in continued beta cell destruction. In patients who were previously responding to sulfonylurea therapy, consider additional factors which may be contributing to decreased efficacy (eg, inappropriate dose, nonadherence to diet and exercise regimen). If no contributing factors can be identified, consider discontinuing use of the sulfonylurea due to secondary failure of treatment. Additional antidiabetic therapy (eg, insulin) will be required. It may be necessary to discontinue therapy and administer insulin if the patient is exposed to stress (fever, trauma, infection, surgery).

Chemical similarities are present among sulfonamides, sulfonylureas, carbonic anhydrase inhibitors, thiazides, and loop diuretics (except ethacrynic acid). Use in patients with sulfonylurea or sulfonamide allergy is specifically contraindicated in product labeling, however, a risk of cross-reaction exists in patients with allergy to any of these compounds; avoid use when previous reaction has been severe. Patients with G6PD deficiency may be at an increased risk of sulfonylurea-induced hemolytic anemia; however, cases have also been described in patients without G6PD deficiency during postmarketing surveillance. Use with caution and consider a nonsulfonylurea alternative in patients with G6PD deficiency.

Product labeling states oral hypoglycemic drugs may be associated with an increased cardiovascular mortality as compared to treatment with diet alone or diet plus insulin. Data to support this association are limited, and several studies, including a large prospective trial (UKPDS) have not supported an association.

Adverse Reactions (Reflective of adult population; not specific for elderly) Frequency not defined.

Central nervous system: Dizziness, headache

Dermatologic: Erythema multiforme, exfoliative dermatitis, maculopapular eruptions, photosensitivity, pruritus, urticaria

Endocrine & metabolic: Disulfiram-like reactions, hypoglycemia, SIADH

Gastrointestinal: Anorexia, diarrhea, hunger, nausea, proctocolitis, vomiting

Hematologic: Agranulocytosis, aplastic anemia, eosinophilia, hemolytic anemia, leukopenia, pancytopenia, porphyria cutanea tarda, thrombocytopenia

Hepatic: Cholestatic jaundice, hepatic porphyria, hepatitis, liver failure

Drug Interactions

Metabolism/Transport Effects Substrate of CYP2C9 (major); **Note:** Assignment of Major/Minor substrate status based on clinically relevant drug interaction potential

Avoid Concomitant Use There are no known interactions where it is recommended to avoid concomitant use.

Increased Effect/Toxicity

ChlorproPAMIDE may increase the levels/effects of: Alcohol (Ethyl); Hypoglycemic Agents; Porfimer; Vitamin K Antagonists

The levels/effects of ChlorproPAMIDE may be increased by: Allopurinol; Beta-Blockers; Chloramphenicol; Cimetidine; Cyclic Antidepressants; CYP2C9 Inhibitors (Moderate); CYP2C9 Inhibitors (Strong); Fibric Acid Derivatives; Fluconazole; GLP-1 Agonists; Herbs (Hypoglycemic Properties); MAO Inhibitors; Mifepristone; Pegvisomant; Probenecid; Quinolone Antibiotics; Ranitidine; Salicylates; Selective Serotonin Reuptake Inhibitors; Sulfonamide Derivatives; Vitamin K Antagonists; Voriconazole

Decreased Effect

The levels/effects of ChlorproPAMIDE may be decreased by: Corticosteroids (Orally Inhaled); Corticosteroids (Systemic); CYP2C9 Inducers (Strong); Loop Diuretics; Luteinizing Hormone-Releasing Hormone Analogs; Peginterferon Alfa-2b; Quinolone Antibiotics; Rifampin; Somatropin; Thiazide Diuretics

Ethanol/Nutrition/Herb Interactions

Ethanol: Avoid ethanol (possible disulfiram-like reaction).

Herb/Nutraceutical: Herbs with hypoglycemic properties may enhance the hypoglycemic effect of chlorpropamide. This includes alfalfa, aloe, bilberry, bitter melon, burdock, celery, damiana, fenugreek, garcinia, garlic, ginger, ginseng (American), gymnema, marshmallow, stinging nettle

Mechanism of Action

Stimulates insulin release from the pancreatic beta cells; reduces glucose output from the liver; insulin sensitivity is increased at peripheral target sites

Pharmacodynamics/Kinetics

Onset of action: 1 hour
  Peak effect: 3-6 hours
Duration: 24 hours
Absorption: Rapid
Distribution: V_d: 0.13-0.23 L/kg
Protein binding: 90%
Metabolism: Extensively hepatic (~80%), primarily via CYP2C9; forms metabolites
Half-life elimination: ~36 hours; prolonged in elderly or with renal impairment
  End-stage renal disease: 50-200 hours
Time to peak, serum: 2-4 hours
Excretion: Urine

Dosage

Geriatric Reduce initial dose to 100-125 mg/day in older patients; subsequent dosages may be increased or decreased by 50-125 mg/day at 3- to 5-day intervals (slower upward titration may be appropriate in older patients)

Adult Type 2 diabetes: Oral: The dosage of chlorpropamide is variable and should be individualized based upon the patient's response

Initial dose: 250 mg/day in mild-to-moderate diabetes in middle-aged, stable diabetic; 100-125 mg/day in older patients
Titration: Subsequent dosages may be increased or decreased by 50-125 mg/day at 3- to 5-day intervals
Maintenance dose: 100-250 mg/day; severe patients with diabetes may require 500 mg/day; avoid doses >750 mg/day

Renal Impairment
Cl_{cr} <50 mL/minute: Avoid use.
Hemodialysis: Removed with hemoperfusion.
Peritoneal dialysis: Supplemental dose is not necessary.

Hepatic Impairment Dosage reduction is recommended. Conservative initial and maintenance doses are recommended in patients with liver impairment because chlorpropamide undergoes extensive hepatic metabolism.

Administration May be administered with food to reduce GI upset. Patients that are NPO or require decreased caloric intake may need doses held to avoid hypoglycemia.

Monitoring Parameters Blood glucose, Hgb A_{1c}; monitor for signs and symptoms of hypoglycemia (fatigue, sweating, numbness of extremities)

Reference Range Recommendations for glycemic control in adults with diabetes:
Hb A_{1c}: <7%
Preprandial capillary plasma glucose: 70-130 mg/dL
Peak postprandial capillary blood glucose: <180 mg/dL
Blood pressure: <130/80 mm Hg

Special Geriatric Considerations Because of chlorpropamide's long half-life, duration of action, drug interactions, and the increased risk for hypoglycemia, it is not considered a hypoglycemic agent of choice in the elderly. Intensive glucose control (Hb A_{1c} <6.5%) has been linked to increased all-cause and cardiovascular mortality, hypoglycemia requiring assistance, and weight gain in adult type 2 diabetes. How "tightly" to control a geriatric patient's blood glucose needs to be individualized. Such a decision should be based on several factors, including the patient's functional and cognitive status, how well he/she recognizes hypoglycemic or hyperglycemic symptoms, and how to respond to them and other disease states. An Hb A_{1c} <7.5% is an acceptable endpoint for a healthy older adult, while <8% is acceptable for frail elderly patients, those with a duration of illness >10 years, or those with comorbid conditions and requiring combination diabetes medications. For elderly patients with diabetes who are relatively healthy, attaining target goals for aspirin use, blood pressure, lipids, smoking cessation, and diet and exercise may be more important than normalized glycemic control.

This medication is considered to be potentially inappropriate in this patient population (Beers Criteria: Quality of evidence - high; Strength of recommendation - strong).

Dosage Forms Excipient information presented when available (limited, particularly for generics); consult specific product labeling.
Tablet, oral: 100 mg, 250 mg

Chlorthalidone (klor THAL i done)

Brand Names: U.S. Thalitone®
Brand Names: Canada Apo-Chlorthalidone®
Index Terms Hygroton
Generic Availability (U.S.) Yes
Pharmacologic Category Diuretic, Thiazide
Use Management of mild-to-moderate hypertension when used alone or in combination with other agents; treatment of edema associated with heart failure or nephrotic syndrome. Recent studies have found chlorthalidone effective in the treatment of isolated systolic hypertension in the elderly.
Dosage
Geriatric Oral: Initial: 12.5-25 mg/day or every other day; there is little advantage to using doses >25 mg/day.
Adult
Hypertension: Oral: 25-100 mg/day or 100 mg 3 times/week; usual dosage range (JNC 7): 12.5-25 mg/day
Edema: Initial: 50-100 mg/day or 100 mg on alternate days; maximum dose: 200 mg/day
Heart failure-associated edema: 12.5-25 mg once daily; maximum daily dose: 100 mg (ACC/AHA 2009 Heart Failure Guidelines)
Renal Impairment Cl_{cr} <10 mL/minute: Avoid use. Ineffective with low GFR (Aronoff, 2002)
Note: ACC/AHA 2009 Heart Failure Guidelines suggest that thiazides lose their efficacy when Cl_{cr} <40 mL/minute
Special Geriatric Considerations Studies have found chlorthalidone effective in the treatment of isolated systolic hypertension in the elderly. The use of chlorthalidone as a step 1 medication reduced the incidence of stroke in the SHEP trial.
Dosage Forms Excipient information presented when available (limited, particularly for generics); consult specific product labeling. [DSC] = Discontinued product
Tablet, oral: 25 mg, 50 mg, 100 mg [DSC]
Thalitone®: 15 mg

◆ **Chlorthalidone and Azilsartan** see Azilsartan and Chlorthalidone on page 179
◆ **Chlor-Trimeton® Allergy [OTC]** see Chlorpheniramine on page 357

Chlorzoxazone (klor ZOKS a zone)

Related Information
Beers Criteria – Potentially Inappropriate Medications for Geriatrics on page 2183
Medication Safety Issues
BEERS Criteria medication:
This drug may be potentially inappropriate for use in geriatric patients (Quality of evidence - moderate; Strength of recommendation - strong).
Brand Names: U.S. Lorzone™; Parafon Forte® DSC
Brand Names: Canada Parafon Forte®; Strifon Forte®
Generic Availability (U.S.) Yes
Pharmacologic Category Skeletal Muscle Relaxant
Use Symptomatic treatment of muscle spasm and pain associated with acute musculoskeletal conditions

Contraindications Hypersensitivity to chlorzoxazone or any component of the formulation; impaired liver function

Warnings/Precautions Muscle relaxants are poorly tolerated by the elderly due to potent anticholinergic effects, sedation, and risk of fracture. Efficacy is questionable at dosages tolerated by elderly patients; avoid use (Beers Criteria).

Adverse Reactions (Reflective of adult population; not specific for elderly) Frequency not defined.

Central nervous system: Dizziness, drowsiness lightheadedness, paradoxical stimulation, malaise

Dermatologic: Rash, petechiae, ecchymoses (rare), angioneurotic edema

Gastrointestinal: Nausea, vomiting, stomach cramps

Genitourinary: Urine discoloration

Hepatic: Liver dysfunction

Miscellaneous: Anaphylaxis (very rare)

Drug Interactions

Metabolism/Transport Effects Substrate of CYP1A2 (minor), CYP2A6 (minor), CYP2D6 (minor), CYP2E1 (minor), CYP3A4 (minor); **Note:** Assignment of Major/Minor substrate status based on clinically relevant drug interaction potential; **Inhibits** CYP2E1 (weak), CYP3A4 (weak)

Avoid Concomitant Use

Avoid concomitant use of Chlorzoxazone with any of the following: Azelastine; Azelastine (Nasal); Methadone; Mirtazapine; Paraldehyde; Pimozide

Increased Effect/Toxicity

Chlorzoxazone may increase the levels/effects of: Alcohol (Ethyl); ARIPiprazole; Azelastine; Azelastine (Nasal); Buprenorphine; CNS Depressants; Methadone; Methotrimeprazine; Metyrosine; Mirtazapine; Paraldehyde; Pimozide; Selective Serotonin Reuptake Inhibitors; Zolpidem

The levels/effects of Chlorzoxazone may be increased by: Disulfiram; Droperidol; HydrOXYzine; Isoniazid; Methotrimeprazine

Decreased Effect

The levels/effects of Chlorzoxazone may be decreased by: Peginterferon Alfa-2b; Tocilizumab

Ethanol/Nutrition/Herb Interactions Ethanol: May increase CNS depression; monitor for increased effects with coadministration. Caution patients about effects.

Mechanism of Action Acts on the spinal cord and subcortical levels by depressing polysynaptic reflexes

Pharmacodynamics/Kinetics

Onset of action: ~1 hour

Duration: 6-12 hours

Absorption: Readily absorbed

Metabolism: Extensively hepatic via glucuronidation

Excretion: Urine (as conjugates)

Dosage

Geriatric Oral: Initial: 250 mg 2-4 times/day; increase as necessary to 750 mg 3-4 times/day.

Adult Muscle spasm: Oral: 250-500 mg 3-4 times/day up to 750 mg 3-4 times/day

Monitoring Parameters Periodic liver functions tests

Special Geriatric Considerations Start dosing low and increase as necessary. Because it can cause unpredictable, fatal hepatic toxicity, the use of chlorzoxazone should be avoided.

This medication is considered to be potentially inappropriate in this patient population (Beers Criteria: Quality of evidence - moderate; Strength of recommendation - strong).

Dosage Forms Excipient information presented when available (limited, particularly for generics); consult specific product labeling.

Caplet, oral:

Parafon Forte® DSC: 500 mg [scored]

Tablet, oral: 500 mg

Lorzone™: 375 mg

Lorzone™: 750 mg [scored]

Cholecalciferol (kole e kal SI fer ole)

Medication Safety Issues

Sound-alike/look-alike issues:

Cholecalciferol may be confused with alfacalcidol, ergocalciferol

Brand Names: U.S. Bio-D-Mulsion Forte® [OTC]; Bio-D-Mulsion® [OTC]; D-3 [OTC]; D3-50™ [OTC]; D3-5™ [OTC]; DDrops® Baby [OTC]; DDrops® Kids [OTC]; DDrops® [OTC]; Delta® D3 [OTC]; Enfamil® D-Vi-Sol™ [OTC]; Maximum D3® [OTC]; Vitamin D3 [OTC]

Brand Names: Canada D-Vi-Sol®

Index Terms D3

Generic Availability (U.S.) Yes

Pharmacologic Category Vitamin D Analog

Use Dietary supplement, treatment of vitamin D deficiency, or prophylaxis of deficiency

Unlabeled Use Osteoporosis prevention

Contraindications Hypercalcemia; hypersensitivity to cholecalciferol or any component of the formulation; malabsorption syndrome; evidence of vitamin D toxicity

Adverse Reactions (Reflective of adult population; not specific for elderly) Frequency not defined: Endocrine & metabolic: Hypervitaminosis D (signs and symptoms include hypercalcemia, resulting in headache, nausea, vomiting, lethargy, confusion, sluggishness, abdominal pain, bone pain, polyuria, polydipsia, weakness, cardiac arrhythmias [eg, QT shortening, sinus tachycardia], soft tissue calcification, calciuria, and nephrocalcinosis)

Drug Interactions

Metabolism/Transport Effects Inhibits CYP2C19 (weak), CYP2C9 (weak), CYP2D6 (weak)

Avoid Concomitant Use

Avoid concomitant use of Cholecalciferol with any of the following: Aluminum Hydroxide; Sucralfate; Vitamin D Analogs

Increased Effect/Toxicity

Cholecalciferol may increase the levels/effects of: Aluminum Hydroxide; ARIPiprazole; Cardiac Glycosides; Sucralfate; Vitamin D Analogs

The levels/effects of Cholecalciferol may be increased by: Calcium Salts; Danazol; Thiazide Diuretics

Decreased Effect

The levels/effects of Cholecalciferol may be decreased by: Bile Acid Sequestrants; Mineral Oil; Orlistat

Ethanol/Nutrition/Herb Interactions

Food: Olestra may impair the absorption of vitamin D.

Pharmacodynamics/Kinetics

Distribution: Primarily hepatic

Protein binding: Extensively to vitamin D-binding protein

Metabolism: Primary liver and kidney hydroxylation; glucuronidation (minimal)

Half-life elimination: 14 hours

Time to peak, plasma: 11 hours

Excretion: As metabolites, urine (2.4%) and feces (4.9%)

Dosage

Geriatric

Dietary Reference Intake for Vitamin D: Oral:

≤70 years: Refer to adult dosing.

>70 years: RDA: 800 units/day

Osteoporosis prevention (unlabeled use) Refer to adult dosing.

Vitamin D deficiency treatment (unlabeled dose): Refer to adult dosing.

Adult

Dietary Reference Intake for Vitamin D: Oral:

Adults: 19-70 years: RDA: 600 int. units/day

Osteoporosis prevention (unlabeled): Adults ≥50 years: Oral: 800-1000 int. units/day (NOF guidelines, 2010)

Vitamin D deficiency treatment (unlabeled dose): Oral: 1000 int. units/day (Holick, 2007)

Reference Range

Serum calcium times phosphorus should not exceed 70 mg^2/dL^2 to avoid ectopic calcification

Vitamin D deficiency: There is no clear consensus on a reference range for total serum 25 (OH)D concentrations or the validity of this level as it relates clinically to bone health. In addition, there is significant variability in the reporting of serum 25 (OH)D levels as a result of different assay types in use. However, the following ranges have been suggested: Adults (NAS, 2011):

<30 nmol/L (12 ng/mL): At risk for deficiency

30-50 nmol/L (12-20 ng/mL): Potentially at risk for inadequacy

≥50 nmol/L (20 ng/mL): Sufficient levels in practically all persons

>125 nmol/L (50 ng/mL): Concern for risk of toxicity

Special Geriatric Considerations Vitamin D, folate, and B$_{12}$ (cyanocobalamin) have decreased absorption with age (clinical significance unknown); studies in ill geriatrics demonstrated that low serum concentrations of vitamin D result in greater bone loss. Calorie requirements decrease with age and therefore, nutrient density must be increased to ensure adequate nutrient intake, including vitamins and minerals. The use of a daily supplement with a multiple vitamin with minerals is recommended because elderly consume less vitamin D, absorption may be decreased, and many have decreased sun exposure. This is a recommendation of particular need to those with high risk for osteoporosis.

Vitamin D supplementation has been shown to increase muscle function and strength, as well as improve balance. Patients at risk for falls should have vitamin D serum concentrations measured and be evaluated for supplementation.

Dosage Forms Excipient information presented when available (limited, particularly for generics); consult specific product labeling.

Capsule, oral: 5000 units
  D-3: 1000 units
  D3-50™: 50,000 units
  D3-5™: 5000 units
  Maximum D3®: 10,000 units [contains soybean lecithin]
Capsule, softgel, oral:
  D-3: 2000 units
Solution, oral [drops]:
  Bio-D-Mulsion Forte®: 2000 units/drop (30 mL) [contains sesame oil]
  Bio-D-Mulsion®: 400 units/drop (30 mL) [contains sesame oil]
  DDrops®: 1000 units/drop (10 mL); 2000 units/drop (10 mL)
  DDrops® Baby: 400 units/drop (10 mL)
  DDrops® Kids: 400 units/drop (10 mL)
  Enfamil® D-Vi-Sol™: 400 units/mL (50 mL) [gluten free, sugar free; citrus flavor]
Tablet, oral: 400 units, 1000 units
  Delta® D3: 400 units [sugar free]
  Vitamin D3: 1000 units [sugar free]

◆ **Cholecalciferol and Alendronate** see Alendronate and Cholecalciferol on page 55

Cholestyramine Resin (koe LES teer a meen REZ in)

Related Information
Hyperlipidemia Management on page 2130

Brand Names: U.S. Prevalite®; Questran®; Questran® Light

Brand Names: Canada Novo-Cholamine; Novo-Cholamine Light; Olestyr; PMS-Cholestyramine; Questran®; Questran® Light Sugar Free; ZYM-Cholestyramine-Light; ZYM-Cholestyramine-Regular

Generic Availability (U.S.) Yes

Pharmacologic Category Antilipemic Agent, Bile Acid Sequestrant

Use Adjunct in the management of primary hypercholesterolemia; pruritus associated with elevated levels of bile acids; regression of arteriolosclerosis

Unlabeled Use Diarrhea associated with excess fecal bile acids (Westergaard, 2007); may be used to enhance elimination of digoxin when non-life-threatening toxicity occurs (Henderson, 1988)

Contraindications Hypersensitivity to bile acid sequestering resins or any component of the formulation; complete biliary obstruction

Warnings/Precautions Use caution in patients with renal impairment. Not to be taken simultaneously with many other medicines (decreased absorption). Treat any diseases contributing to hypercholesterolemia first. Use with caution in patients susceptible to fat-soluble vitamin deficiencies. Absorption of fat soluble vitamins A, D, E, and K and folic acid may be decreased; patients should take vitamins ≥4 hours before cholestyramine. Chronic use may be associated with bleeding problems (especially in high doses); may be prevented with use of oral vitamin K therapy. May produce or exacerbate constipation problems; fecal impaction may occur; initiate therapy at a reduced dose in patients with a history of constipation. Hemorrhoids may be worsened. Some products may contain phenylalanine.

Adverse Reactions (Reflective of adult population; not specific for elderly) Frequency not defined.

Cardiovascular: Edema, syncope

Central nervous system: Anxiety, dizziness, drowsiness, eructation, fatigue, headache, vertigo

Dermatologic: Bruising, rash, skin irritation, urticaria

Endocrine & metabolic: Hyperchloremic acidosis (children), libido increased

Gastrointestinal: Abdominal pain, anorexia, biliary colic, black stools, constipation, dental bleeding, dental caries, dental erosion, diarrhea, diverticulitis, duodenal ulcer bleeding, dysphagia, eructation, flatulence, gallbladder calcification, GI hemorrhage, intestinal obstruction (rare), hemorrhoidal bleeding, nausea, pancreatitis, perianal irritation, rectal bleeding, rectal pain, steatorrhea, taste disturbance, tongue irritation, tooth discoloration, ulcer, vomiting, weight gain/loss

Hepatic: Hypothrombinemia, liver function abnormalities, prothrombin time increased

Hematologic: Anemia, bleeding

Neuromuscular & skeletal: Arthritis, backache, joint/muscle/nerve pain, osteoporosis, paresthesia

Ocular: Night blindness (rare), uveitis

Otic: Tinnitus

Renal: Diuresis, dysuria, hematuria

Respiratory: Asthma, dyspnea, wheezing

Miscellaneous: Hiccups, swollen glands

Drug Interactions

Metabolism/Transport Effects None known.

Avoid Concomitant Use

Avoid concomitant use of Cholestyramine Resin with any of the following: Mycophenolate

Increased Effect/Toxicity There are no known significant interactions involving an increase in effect.

Decreased Effect

Cholestyramine Resin may decrease the levels/effects of: Acetaminophen; Amiodarone; Antidiabetic Agents (Thiazolidinedione); Cardiac Glycosides; Chenodiol; Contraceptives (Estrogens); Contraceptives (Progestins); Corticosteroids (Oral); Deferasirox; Ezetimibe; Fibric Acid Derivatives; Fluvastatin; Leflunomide; Loop Diuretics; Methotrexate; Methylfolate; Mycophenolate; Niacin; Nonsteroidal Anti-Inflammatory Agents; PHENobarbital; Pravastatin; Propranolol; Raloxifene; Tetracycline Derivatives; Thiazide Diuretics; Thyroid Products; Ursodiol; Vancomycin; Vitamin D Analogs; Vitamin K Antagonists

Ethanol/Nutrition/Herb Interactions

Food: Cholestyramine (especially high doses or long-term therapy) may decrease the absorption of folic acid, calcium, and iron.

Herb/Nutraceutical: Cholestyramine (especially high doses or long-term therapy) may decrease the absorption of fat-soluble vitamins (vitamins A, D, E, and K).

Stability Store at 20°C to 25°C (68°F to 77°F); excursions permitted to 15°C to 30°C (59°F to 86°F).

Mechanism of Action Forms a nonabsorbable complex with bile acids in the intestine, releasing chloride ions in the process; inhibits enterohepatic reuptake of intestinal bile salts and thereby increases the fecal loss of bile salt-bound low density lipoprotein cholesterol

Pharmacodynamics/Kinetics

Onset of action: Peak effect: 21 days

Absorption: None

Excretion: Feces (as insoluble complex with bile acids)

Dosage

Geriatric & Adult Dosages are expressed in terms of anhydrous resin:

Dyslipidemia: Oral: Initial: 4 g 1-2 times/day; increase gradually over ≥1-month intervals; maintenance: 8-16 g/day divided in 2 doses; maximum: 24 g/day

Renal Impairment No dosage adjustment provided in manufacturer's labeling; however, use with caution in renal impairment; may cause hyperchloremic acidosis.

Hepatic Impairment No dosage adjustment necessary; not absorbed from the gastrointestinal tract.

Administration Mix powder with 60-180 mL water or other noncarbonated liquid prior to administration and mix well; may also be taken with highly fluid soups, applesauce or crushed pineapple; not to be taken in dry form. Suspension should not be sipped or held in mouth for prolonged periods (may cause tooth discoloration or enamel decay). Administration at mealtime is recommended. Twice-daily dosing is recommended, but may be administered in 1-6 doses/day.

Monitoring Parameters Serum cholesterol and triglyceride levels before initiating treatment and periodically throughout treatment (in accordance with NCEP guidelines)

Test Interactions Increased prothrombin time

Special Geriatric Considerations The definition of and, therefore, when to treat hyperlipidemia in the elderly is a controversial issue. The National Cholesterol Education Program recommends that all adults maintain a plasma cholesterol <160 mg/dL. Elderly with one additional risk factor, goal LDL would be <130 mg/dL. It is the authors' belief that pharmacologic treatment be reserved for those who are unable to obtain a desirable plasma cholesterol concentration by diet alone and for whom the benefits of treatment are believed to outweigh the potential adverse effects, drug interactions, and cost of treatment.

Dosage Forms Excipient information presented when available (limited, particularly for generics); consult specific product labeling.

Powder for suspension, oral: Cholestyramine resin 4 g/5 g of powder (210 g); Cholestyramine resin 4 g/5.7 g of powder (239.4 g); Cholestyramine resin 4 g/9 g of powder (378 g);

Cholestyramine resin 4 g/5 g packet (60s); Cholestyramine resin 4 g/5.7 g packet (60s); Cholestyramine resin 4 g/9 g packet (60s)

Prevalite®: Cholestyramine resin 4 g/5.5 g of powder (231 g); Cholestyramine resin 4 g/ 5.5 g packet (42s, 60s) [contains phenylalanine 14.1 mg/5.5 g; orange flavor]

Questran®: Cholestyramine resin 4 g/9 g of powder (378 g); Cholestyramine resin 4 g/9 g packet (60s) [orange flavor]

Questran® Light: Cholestyramine resin 4 g/5 g of powder (210 g); Cholestyramine resin 4 g/ 5 g packet (60s) [contains phenylalanine 14 mg/5 g; orange flavor]

◆ **Choline Fenofibrate** *see* Fenofibric Acid *on page 755*

Choline Magnesium Trisalicylate (KOE leen mag NEE zhum trye sa LIS i late)

Index Terms Tricosal; Trilisate

Generic Availability (U.S.) Yes

Pharmacologic Category Salicylate

Use Management of osteoarthritis, rheumatoid arthritis, and other arthritis; acute painful shoulder

Contraindications Hypersensitivity to salicylates, other nonacetylated salicylates, other NSAIDs, or any component of the formulation; bleeding disorders

Warnings/Precautions Salicylate salts may not inhibit platelet aggregation and, therefore, should not be substituted for aspirin in the prophylaxis of thrombosis. Use with caution in patients with impaired hepatic or renal function, dehydration, erosive gastritis, asthma, or peptic ulcer.

Elderly are a high-risk population for adverse effects from NSAIDs. As many as 60% of elderly can develop peptic ulceration and/or hemorrhage asymptomatically. Use lowest effective dose for shortest period possible. Tinnitus or impaired hearing may indicate toxicity. Tinnitus may be a difficult and unreliable indication of toxicity due to age-related hearing loss or eighth cranial nerve damage. CNS adverse effects may be observed in the elderly at lower doses than younger adults.

Adverse Reactions (Reflective of adult population; not specific for elderly)
<20%:
Gastrointestinal: Nausea, vomiting, diarrhea, heartburn, dyspepsia, epigastric pain, constipation
Otic: Tinnitus
<2%:
Central nervous system: Headache, lightheadedness, dizziness, drowsiness, lethargy
Otic: Hearing impairment

Drug Interactions

Metabolism/Transport Effects None known.

Avoid Concomitant Use
Avoid concomitant use of Choline Magnesium Trisalicylate with any of the following: Influenza Virus Vaccine (Live/Attenuated)

Increased Effect/Toxicity
Choline Magnesium Trisalicylate may increase the levels/effects of: Anticoagulants; Carbonic Anhydrase Inhibitors; Corticosteroids (Systemic); Divalproex; Drotrecogin Alfa (Activated); Hypoglycemic Agents; Methotrexate; PRALAtrexate; Salicylates; Thrombolytic Agents; Valproic Acid; Varicella Virus-Containing Vaccines; Vitamin K Antagonists

The levels/effects of Choline Magnesium Trisalicylate may be increased by: Ammonium Chloride; Antiplatelet Agents; Calcium Channel Blockers (Nondihydropyridine); Ginkgo Biloba; Herbs (Anticoagulant/Antiplatelet Properties); Influenza Virus Vaccine (Live/Attenuated); Loop Diuretics; Potassium Acid Phosphate; Treprostinil

Decreased Effect
Choline Magnesium Trisalicylate may decrease the levels/effects of: ACE Inhibitors; Hyaluronidase; Loop Diuretics; Probenecid

The levels/effects of Choline Magnesium Trisalicylate may be decreased by: Corticosteroids (Systemic)

Ethanol/Nutrition/Herb Interactions
Ethanol: Avoid ethanol (may enhance gastric mucosal irritation).
Food: May decrease the rate but not the extent of oral absorption.
Herb/Nutraceutical: Avoid cat's claw, dong quai, evening primrose, feverfew, garlic, ginger, ginkgo, red clover, horse chestnut, green tea, ginseng (all have additional antiplatelet activity). Limit curry powder, paprika, licorice, Benedictine liqueur, prunes, raisins, tea, and gherkins; may cause salicylate accumulation. These foods contain 6 mg salicylate/100 g.

Stability Store at controlled room temperature of 15°C to 30°C (59°F to 86°F).

Mechanism of Action Weakly inhibits cyclooxygenase enzymes, which results in decreased formation of prostaglandin precursors; antipyretic, analgesic, and anti-inflammatory properties.

Other proposed mechanisms not fully elucidated (and possibly contributing to the anti-inflammatory effect to varying degrees) include inhibiting chemotaxis, altering lymphocyte activity, inhibiting neutrophil aggregation/activation, and decreasing proinflammatory cytokine levels.

Pharmacodynamics/Kinetics
Absorption: From the stomach and small intestine
Distribution: Readily into most body fluids and tissues
Half-life: Dose-dependent ranging from 2-3 hours at low doses to 30 hours at high doses
Time to peak plasma concentrations: Within ~2 hours

Dosage
Geriatric Usual dose: 750 mg 3 times/day.
Adult Arthritis, pain: Oral (based on total salicylate content): 500 mg to 1.5 g 2-3 times/day **or** 3 g at bedtime; usual maintenance dose: 1-4.5 g/day
Renal Impairment Avoid use in severe renal impairment.

Administration Liquid may be mixed with fruit juice just before drinking. Do not administer with antacids. Take with a full glass of water and remain in an upright position for 15-30 minutes after administration.

Monitoring Parameters Serum concentrations, renal function; hearing changes or tinnitus; monitor for response (ie, pain, inflammation, range of motion, grip strength); observe for abnormal bleeding, bruising, weight gain

Reference Range Salicylate blood levels for anti-inflammatory effect: 150-300 mcg/mL; analgesia and antipyretic effect: 30-50 mcg/mL

Test Interactions False-negative results for glucose oxidase urinary glucose tests (Clinistix®); false-positives using the cupric sulfate method (Clinitest®); also, interferes with Gerhardt test (urinary ketone analysis), VMA determination; 5-HIAA, xylose tolerance test, and T_3 and T_4; increased PBI

Pharmacotherapy Pearls Salicylate salts do not inhibit platelet aggregation and, therefore, should not be substituted for aspirin in the prophylaxis of thrombosis; use caution in patients with renal failure or reduced renal function (ie, older adults - magnesium accumulation)

Special Geriatric Considerations Elderly are a high-risk population for adverse effects from nonsteroidal anti-inflammatory agents. As much as 60% of elderly can develop peptic ulceration and/or hemorrhage asymptomatically. The concomitant use of H_2 blockers and sucralfate is not effective as prophylaxis with the exception of NSAID-induced duodenal ulcers which may be prevented by the use of ranitidine. Misoprostol and proton pump inhibitors are the only agents proven to help prevent the development of NSAID-induced ulcers. Also, concomitant disease and drug use contribute to the risk for GI adverse effects. Avoid use of multiple drugs (OTCs) which contain salicylates (eg, bismuth subsalicylate with other salicylates). Use lowest effective dose for shortest period possible. Consider renal function decline with age. Use of NSAIDs can compromise existing renal function especially when Cl_{cr} is ≤30 mL/minute. There is the consideration that the use of choline magnesium salicylate may cause less gastrointestinal and renal adverse effects than ASA or other NSAIDs in the elderly. Tinnitus may be a difficult and unreliable indication of toxicity due to age-related hearing loss or eighth cranial nerve damage. CNS adverse effects such as confusion, agitation, and hallucination are generally seen in overdose or high dose situations, but elderly may demonstrate these adverse effects at lower doses than younger adults.

Dosage Forms Excipient information presented when available (limited, particularly for generics); consult specific product labeling.
Liquid, oral: 500 mg/5 mL (240 mL) [choline salicylate 293 mg and magnesium salicylate 362 mg per 5 mL]

◆ **Choline Salicylate** *see* Salicylates (Various Salts) *on page* 1742
◆ **Chooz® [OTC]** *see* Calcium Carbonate *on page* 262
◆ **CI-1008** *see* Pregabalin *on page* 1598
◆ **Cialis®** *see* Tadalafil *on page* 1826

Ciclesonide (Oral Inhalation) (sye KLES oh nide)

Brand Names: U.S. Alvesco®
Brand Names: Canada Alvesco®
Generic Availability (U.S.) No
Pharmacologic Category Corticosteroid, Inhalant (Oral)
Use Prophylactic management of bronchial asthma

Contraindications Hypersensitivity to ciclesonide or any component of the formulation; primary treatment of acute asthma or status asthmaticus

Canadian labeling: Additional contraindications (not in U.S. labeling): Untreated fungal, bacterial, or tuberculosis infections of the respiratory tract; moderate-to-severe bronchiectasis

Warnings/Precautions May cause hypercorticism or suppression of hypothalamic-pituitary-adrenal (HPA) axis, particularly in patients receiving high doses for prolonged periods. HPA axis suppression may lead to adrenal crisis. Withdrawal and discontinuation of a corticosteroid should be done slowly and carefully. Particular care is required when patients are transferred from systemic corticosteroids to inhaled products due to possible adrenal insufficiency or withdrawal from steroids, including an increase in allergic symptoms. Patients receiving >20 mg per day of prednisone (or equivalent) may be most susceptible. Fatalities have occurred due to adrenal insufficiency in asthmatic patients during and after transfer from systemic corticosteroids to aerosol steroids; aerosol steroids do **not** provide the systemic steroid needed to treat patients having trauma, surgery, or infections.

Bronchospasm may occur with wheezing after inhalation; if this occurs stop steroid and treat with a fast-acting bronchodilator. Supplemental steroids (oral or parenteral) may be needed during stress or severe asthma attacks. Not to be used in status asthmaticus or for the relief of acute bronchospasm. Oropharyngeal thrush due to candida albicans infection may occur with use. Prolonged use of corticosteroids may also increase the incidence of secondary infection, mask acute infection (including fungal infections), prolong or exacerbate viral infections, or limit response to vaccines. Corticosteroids should not be used to treat ocular herpes simplex. Close observation is required in patients with latent tuberculosis and/or TB reactivity; restrict use in active TB (only in conjunction with antituberculosis treatment). Use in patients with TB is contraindicated in the Canadian labeling. Prolonged treatment with corticosteroids has been associated with the development of Kaposi's sarcoma (case reports); if noted, discontinuation of therapy should be considered.

Use with caution in patients with cardiovascular disease, diabetes, severe hepatic impairment, thyroid disease, psychiatric disturbances, myasthenia gravis, glaucoma, cataracts, patients at risk for osteoporosis, and patients at risk for seizures. Use in renally-impaired patients has not been studied; however, ≤20% of drug is eliminated renally. Use with caution in elderly patients.

To minimize the systemic effects of orally inhaled corticosteroids, each patient should be titrated to the lowest effective dose.

Adverse Reactions (Reflective of adult population; not specific for elderly)
>10%:
Central nervous system: Headache (≤11%)
Respiratory: Nasopharyngitis (≤11%)
1% to 10%:
Cardiovascular: Facial edema (≥3%)
Central nervous system: Dizziness (≥3%), fatigue (≥3%), dysphonia (1%)
Dermatologic: Urticaria (≥3%)
Gastrointestinal: Gastroenteritis (≥3%), oral candidiasis (≥3%)
Neuromuscular & skeletal: Arthralgia (≥3%), musculoskeletal chest pain (≥3%), back pain (≥3%), extremity pain (≥3%)
Ocular: Conjunctivitis (≥3%)
Otic: Ear pain (2%)
Respiratory: Upper respiratory infection (≤9%), nasal congestion (≤6%), pharyngolaryngeal pain (≤5%), hoarseness (≥3%), pneumonia (≥3%), sinusitis (≥3%), paradoxical bronchospasm (2%)
Miscellaneous: Influenza (≥3%)
Drug Interactions
Metabolism/Transport Effects Substrate of CYP3A4 (major); **Note:** Assignment of Major/Minor substrate status based on clinically relevant drug interaction potential
Avoid Concomitant Use
Avoid concomitant use of Ciclesonide (Oral Inhalation) with any of the following: Aldesleukin
Increased Effect/Toxicity
Ciclesonide (Oral Inhalation) may increase the levels/effects of: Deferasirox

The levels/effects of Ciclesonide (Oral Inhalation) may be increased by: CYP3A4 Inhibitors (Moderate); Dasatinib; Ivacaftor; Mifepristone; Telaprevir
Decreased Effect
Ciclesonide (Oral Inhalation) may decrease the levels/effects of: Aldesleukin; Corticorelin; Hyaluronidase; Telaprevir

The levels/effects of Ciclesonide (Oral Inhalation) may be decreased by: Tocilizumab
Stability Store at 15°C to 30°C (59°F to 86°F); do not freeze.

◀ **Mechanism of Action** Ciclesonide is a nonhalogenated, glucocorticoid prodrug that is hydrolyzed to the pharmacologically active metabolite des-ciclesonide following administration. Des-ciclesonide has a high affinity for the glucocorticoid receptor and exhibits anti-inflammatory activity. The mechanism of action for corticosteroids is believed to be a combination of three important properties – anti-inflammatory activity, immunosuppressive properties, and antiproliferative actions.

Pharmacodynamics/Kinetics

Absorption: 52% (lung deposition)

Protein binding: ≥99%

Metabolism: Ciclesonide hydrolyzed to its active metabolite, des-ciclesonide via esterases in nasal mucosa and lungs; des-ciclesonide undergoes further hepatic metabolism primarily via CYP3A4 and to a lesser extent via CYP2D6

Bioavailability: 63% (active metabolite)

Half-life elimination: ~6-7 hours (active metabolite)

Time to peak: ~1 hour (active metabolite)

Excretion: Feces (66%); urine (≤20% as active metabolite)

Dosage

Geriatric & Adult Asthma: Oral inhalation (Alvesco®): **Note:** Titrate to the lowest effective dose once asthma stability is achieved:

U.S. labeling:

Prior therapy with bronchodilators alone: Initial: 80 mcg twice daily (maximum dose: 320 mcg/day)

Prior therapy with inhaled corticosteroids: Initial: 80 mcg twice daily (maximum dose: 640 mcg/day)

Prior therapy with oral corticosteroids: Initial: 320 mcg twice daily (maximum dose: 640 mcg/day)

Canadian labeling: Initial: 400 mcg once daily; maintenance: 100-800 mcg/day (1-2 puffs once daily; more severe asthma may require 400 mcg twice daily). **Note:** Canadian Thoracic Society 2010 Asthma Management guidelines recommendation: Doses >200 mcg/day may provide minimal additional benefit while increasing risks for adverse events; add-on therapy should be considered prior to dose increases >200 mcg/day (Lougheed, 2010).

Global Strategy for Asthma Management and Prevention, 2011:

"Low" dose: 80-160 mcg/day

"Medium" dose: >160-320 mcg/day

"High" dose: >320 mcg/day

Conversion from oral to orally-inhaled steroid: Initiation of oral inhalation therapy should begin in patients who have previously been stabilized on oral corticosteroids (OCS). A gradual dose reduction of OCS should begin ~7-10 days after starting inhaled therapy. U.S. labeling recommends reducing prednisone dose no more rapidly than ≤2.5 mg/day on a weekly basis. The Canadian labeling recommends decreasing the daily dose of prednisone by 1 mg (or equivalent of other OCS) every 7 days in closely monitored patients, and every 10 days in patients whom close monitoring is not possible. In the presence of withdrawal symptoms, resume previous OCS dose for 1 week before attempting further dose reductions.

Renal Impairment There are no dosage adjustments provided in the manufacturer's labeling (has not been studied); however, dose adjustments may not be necessary as ≤20% of drug is eliminated renally.

Hepatic Impairment Dosage adjustments are not necessary.

Administration Remove mouthpiece cover, place inhaler in mouth, close lips around mouthpiece, and inhale slowly and deeply. Press down on top of inhaler after slow inhalation has begun. Remove inhaler while holding breath for approximately 10 seconds. Breathe out slowly and replace mouthpiece on inhaler. Rinse mouth with water (and spit out) after inhalation. Do not wash or place inhaler in water. Clean mouthpiece using a dry cloth or tissue once weekly. Discard after the "discard by" date or after labeled number of doses has been used, even if container is not completely empty.

Shaking is not necessary since drug is formulated as a solution aerosol. Prime inhaler prior to initial use or if not in use for ≥7-10 days by releasing 3 puffs into the air.

Monitoring Parameters Signs/symptoms of HPA axis suppression/adrenal insufficiency; ocular effects (eg, cataracts, increased intraocular pressure, glaucoma)

Pharmacotherapy Pearls The incidence of oral candidiasis, as well as other localized oropharyngeal effects, observed with ciclesonide use has been reported to be approximately one-half of that seen with other commonly inhaled corticosteroids such as budesonide and fluticasone. Small particle size, minimal activation, and deposition in the oropharynx may explain this decreased incidence.

Special Geriatric Considerations Ensure proper use of inhaler.

Dosage Forms Excipient information presented when available (limited, particularly for generics); consult specific product labeling.
Aerosol, for oral inhalation:
Alvesco®: 80 mcg/inhalation (6.1 g); 160 mcg/inhalation (6.1 g) [contains ethanol; 60 metered actuations]
Dosage Forms: Canada Excipient information presented when available (limited, particularly for generics); consult specific product labeling.
Aerosol for oral inhalation:
Alvesco®: 100 mcg/inhalation [30-, 60-, and 120 metered actuations]; 200 mcg/inhalation [30-, 60-, and 120 metered actuations]

Ciclesonide (Nasal) (sye KLES oh nide)

Brand Names: U.S. Omnaris®; Zetonna™
Brand Names: Canada Omnaris®
Generic Availability (U.S.) No
Pharmacologic Category Corticosteroid, Nasal
Use Management of seasonal and perennial allergic rhinitis
Unlabeled Use Adjunct to antibiotics in empiric treatment of acute bacterial rhinosinusitis (ABRS) (Chow, 2012)
Dosage
Geriatric & Adult Perennial allergic rhinitis, seasonal allergic rhinitis:
Omnaris®: 2 sprays (50 mcg/spray) per nostril once daily; maximum: 200 mcg/day
Zetonna™: 1 spray (37 mcg/spray) per nostril once daily; maximum: 74 mcg/day
Special Geriatric Considerations Evaluate the patient's or caregiver's ability to safely administer the correct dose of nasal medication.

No specific information is available for the elderly patient.
Dosage Forms Excipient information presented when available (limited, particularly for generics); consult specific product labeling.
Aerosol, intranasal:
Zetonna™: 37 mcg/inhalation (6.1 g) [contains ethanol; 60 metered actuations]
Suspension, intranasal [spray]:
Omnaris®: 50 mcg/inhalation (12.5 g) [120 metered actuations]

◆ Ciclodan™ *see* Ciclopirox *on page 373*
◆ Ciclodan™ Kit *see* Ciclopirox *on page 373*

Ciclopirox (sye kloe PEER oks)

Brand Names: U.S. Ciclodan™; Ciclodan™ Kit; Loprox®; Pedipirox™ -4 Kit; Penlac®
Brand Names: Canada Apo-Ciclopirox®; Loprox®; Penlac®; Stieprox®; Taro-Ciclopirox
Index Terms Ciclopirox Olamine
Generic Availability (U.S.) Yes
Pharmacologic Category Antifungal Agent, Topical
Use
Cream/suspension: Treatment of tinea pedis (athlete's foot), tinea cruris (jock itch), tinea corporis (ringworm), cutaneous candidiasis, and tinea versicolor (pityriasis)
Gel: Treatment of tinea pedis (athlete's foot), tinea corporis (ringworm); seborrheic dermatitis of the scalp
Lacquer (solution): Topical treatment of mild-to-moderate onychomycosis of the fingernails and toenails due to *Trichophyton rubrum* (not involving the lunula) and the immediately-adjacent skin
Shampoo: Treatment of seborrheic dermatitis of the scalp
Contraindications Hypersensitivity to ciclopirox or any component of the formulation; avoid occlusive wrappings or dressings
Warnings/Precautions For external use only; avoid contact with eyes. Nail lacquer is for topical use only and has not been studied in conjunction with systemic therapy or in patients with type 1 diabetes mellitus (insulin dependent, IDDM). Use has not been evaluated in immunosuppressed or immunocompromised patients. Discontinue treatment if signs and/or symptoms of hypersensitivity are noted.
Adverse Reactions (Reflective of adult population; not specific for elderly)
Central nervous system: Headache
Dermatologic: Alopecia, dry skin, erythema, facial edema, hair discoloration (rare; shampoo formulation in light-haired individuals), nail disorder (shape or color change with lacquer), pruritus, rash
Local: Burning sensation (gel: 34%; ≤1% with other forms), irritation, redness, or pain

CICLOPIROX

Drug Interactions
  Metabolism/Transport Effects None known.
  Avoid Concomitant Use There are no known interactions where it is recommended to avoid concomitant use.
  Increased Effect/Toxicity There are no known significant interactions involving an increase in effect.
  Decreased Effect There are no known significant interactions involving a decrease in effect.

Stability
  Cream, suspension: Store between 5°C to 25°C (41°F to 77°F).
  Lacquer (solution): Store at room temperature of 15°C to 30°C (59°F to 86°F); protect from light. Flammable; keep away from heat and flame.
  Gel, shampoo: Store at room temperature of 15°C to 30°C (59°F to 86°F).

Mechanism of Action Inhibiting transport of essential elements in the fungal cell disrupting the synthesis of DNA, RNA, and protein

Pharmacodynamics/Kinetics
  Absorption: Cream, suspension: <2% through intact skin; increased with gel; <5% with lacquer
  Distribution: Scalp application: To epidermis, corium (dermis), including hair, hair follicles, and sebaceous glands
  Protein binding: 94% to 98%
  Half-life elimination: Biologic: 1.7 hours (suspension); elimination: 5.5 hours (gel)
  Excretion: Urine (gel: 3% to 10%); feces (small amounts)

Dosage
  Geriatric & Adult
    Tinea pedis, tinea corporis: Topical:
      Cream and suspension: Apply twice daily, gently massage into affected areas; if no improvement after 4 weeks of treatment, re-evaluate the diagnosis.
      Gel: Apply twice daily, gently massage into affected areas and surrounding skin; if no improvement after 4 weeks of treatment, re-evaluate diagnosis
    Tinea cruris, cutaneous candidiasis, and tinea versicolor: Topical: *Cream and suspension:* Apply twice daily, gently massage into affected areas; if no improvement after 4 weeks of treatment, re-evaluate the diagnosis.
    Onychomycosis of the fingernails and toenails: Topical: *Lacquer (solution):* Apply to adjacent skin and affected nails daily (as a part of a comprehensive management program for onychomycosis). Remove with alcohol every 7 days.
    Seborrheic dermatitis of the scalp: Topical:
      Gel: Apply twice daily, gently massage into affected areas and surrounding skin; if no improvement after 4 weeks of treatment, re-evaluate diagnosis.
      Shampoo: Apply ~5 mL to wet hair; lather, and leave in place ~3 minutes; rinse. May use up to 10 mL for longer hair. Repeat twice weekly for 4 weeks; allow a minimum of 3 days between applications.

  Administration Topical:
    Cream, suspension: Gently massage into affected areas.
    Gel: Gently massage into affected areas and adjacent skin.
    Lacquer (solution): Apply evenly over nail and surrounding skin at bedtime (or allow 8 hours before washing); apply daily over previous coat for 7 days; after 7 days, may remove with alcohol and continue cycle.
    Shampoo: Apply to wet hair; lather and leave in place for ~3 minutes; rinse.

Special Geriatric Considerations
  Instruct patient or caregiver on appropriate use of topical ciclopirox products.

Dosage Forms Excipient information presented when available (limited, particularly for generics); consult specific product labeling.
  Cream, topical, as olamine: 0.77% (15 g, 30 g, 90 g)
  Gel, topical: 0.77% (30 g, 45 g, 100 g)
    Loprox®: 0.77% (30 g, 45 g, 100 g) [contains isopropyl alcohol]
  Shampoo, topical: 1% (120 mL)
    Loprox®: 1% (120 mL)
  Solution, topical [nail lacquer]: 8% (6.6 mL)
    Ciclodan™: 8% (6.6 mL) [contains isopropyl alcohol]
    Ciclodan™ Kit: 8% (6.6 mL) [contains isopropyl alcohol; packaged with Toetal Fresh™]
    Pedipirox™ -4 Kit: 8% (1s) [contains isopropyl alcohol; kit contains one Pedipirox™ 6.6 mL, one Pedipirox ™3.3 mL, 15 nail lacquer removal pads, nail file, and pedi-sorb™ foot powder]
    Penlac®: 8% (6.6 mL) [contains isopropyl alcohol]
  Suspension, topical, as olamine: 0.77% (30 mL, 60 mL)

◆ **Ciclopirox Olamine** *see* Ciclopirox *on page* 373

◆ **Cidecin** *see* DAPTOmycin *on page 485*

Cilostazol (sil OH sta zol)

Medication Safety Issues
Sound-alike/look-alike issues:
Pletal® may be confused with Plendil®

Brand Names: U.S. Pletal®

Index Terms OPC-13013

Generic Availability (U.S.) Yes

Pharmacologic Category Antiplatelet Agent; Phosphodiesterase-3 Enzyme Inhibitor

Use Symptomatic management of peripheral vascular disease, primarily intermittent claudication

Unlabeled Use Investigational: Treatment of acute coronary syndromes and for graft patency improvement in percutaneous coronary interventions with or without stenting

Contraindications Hypersensitivity to cilostazol or any component of the formulation; heart failure (HF) of any severity; hemostatic disorders or active bleeding

Warnings/Precautions [U.S. Boxed Warning]: The use of this drug is contraindicated in patients with heart failure. Use with caution in severe underlying heart disease. Use with caution in patients receiving other platelet aggregation inhibitors or in patients with thrombocytopenia. Discontinue therapy if thrombocytopenia or leukopenia occur; progression to agranulocytosis (reversible) has been reported when cilostazol was not immediately stopped. When cilostazol and clopidogrel are used concurrently, manufacturer recommends checking bleeding times. Withhold for at least 4-6 half-lives prior to elective surgical procedures. Use with caution in patients receiving CYP3A4 inhibitors (eg, ketoconazole or erythromycin) or CYP2C19 inhibitors (eg, omeprazole). If concurrent use is warranted, consider dosage adjustment of cilostazol. Use caution in moderate-to-severe hepatic impairment. Use cautiously in severe renal impairment (Cl_{cr} <25 mL/minute).

Adverse Reactions (Reflective of adult population; not specific for elderly)
>10%:
Central nervous system: Headache (27% to 34%)
Gastrointestinal: Abnormal stools (12% to 15%), diarrhea (12% to 19%)
Respiratory: Rhinitis (7% to 12%)
Miscellaneous: Infection (10% to 14%)

2% to 10%:
Cardiovascular: Peripheral edema (7% to 9%), palpitation (5% to 10%), tachycardia (4%)
Central nervous system: Dizziness (9% to 10%), vertigo (up to 3%)
Gastrointestinal: Dyspepsia (6%), nausea (6% to 7%), abdominal pain (4% to 5%), flatulence (2% to 3%)
Neuromuscular & skeletal: Back pain (6% to 7%), myalgia (2% to 3%)
Respiratory: Pharyngitis (7% to 10%), cough (3% to 4%)

Drug Interactions
Metabolism/Transport Effects Substrate of CYP1A2 (minor), CYP2C19 (major), CYP2D6 (minor), CYP3A4 (major); **Note:** Assignment of Major/Minor substrate status based on clinically relevant drug interaction potential

Avoid Concomitant Use
Avoid concomitant use of Cilostazol with any of the following: Conivaptan

Increased Effect/Toxicity
Cilostazol may increase the levels/effects of: Anticoagulants; Antiplatelet Agents; Collagenase (Systemic); Dabigatran Etexilate; Drotrecogin Alfa (Activated); Ibritumomab; Rivaroxaban; Salicylates; Thrombolytic Agents; Tositumomab and Iodine I 131 Tositumomab

The levels/effects of Cilostazol may be increased by: Antifungal Agents (Azole Derivatives, Systemic); Conivaptan; CYP2C19 Inhibitors (Moderate); CYP2C19 Inhibitors (Strong); CYP3A4 Inhibitors (Moderate); CYP3A4 Inhibitors (Strong); Dasatinib; Esomeprazole; Glucosamine; Herbs (Anticoagulant/Antiplatelet Properties); Ivacaftor; Macrolide Antibiotics; Mifepristone; Nonsteroidal Anti-Inflammatory Agents; Omega-3-Acid Ethyl Esters; Omeprazole; Pentosan Polysulfate Sodium; Pentoxifylline; Prostacyclin Analogues; Tipranavir; Vitamin E

Decreased Effect
The levels/effects of Cilostazol may be decreased by: CYP3A4 Inducers (Strong); Deferasirox; Herbs (CYP3A4 Inducers); Nonsteroidal Anti-Inflammatory Agents; Peginterferon Alfa-2b; Tocilizumab

Ethanol/Nutrition/Herb Interactions

Food: Taking cilostazol with a high-fat meal may increase peak concentration by 90%. Grapefruit juice may increase serum levels of cilostazol and enhance toxic effects. Management: Administer cilostazol on an empty stomach 30 minutes before or 2 hours after meals. Avoid concurrent ingestion of grapefruit juice.

Herb/Nutraceutical: St John's wort may decrease the levels/effects of cilostazol. Other herbs/nutraceuticals have additional antiplatelet activity. Management: Avoid alfalfa, anise, bilberry, bladderwrack, bromelain, cat's claw, chamomile, coleus, cordyceps, dong quai, evening primrose oil, fenugreek, feverfew, garlic, ginger, ginkgo biloba, ginseng (American), ginseng (Panax), ginseng (Siberian), grapeseed, green tea, guggul, horse chestnut seed, horseradish, licorice, prickly ash, red clover, reishi, SAMe (S-adenosylmethionine), St John's wort, sweet clover, turmeric, and white willow.

Stability Store at 25°C (77°F); excursions permitted to 15°C to 30°C (59°F to 86°F).

Mechanism of Action Cilostazol and its metabolites are inhibitors of phosphodiesterase III. As a result, cyclic AMP is increased leading to reversible inhibition of platelet aggregation, vasodilation, and inhibition of vascular smooth muscle cell proliferation.

Pharmacodynamics/Kinetics

Onset of action: 2-4 weeks; may require up to 12 weeks

Protein binding: Cilostazol 95% to 98%; active metabolites 66% to 97%

Metabolism: Hepatic via CYP3A4 (primarily), 1A2, 2C19, and 2D6; at least one metabolite has significant activity

Half-life elimination: 11-13 hours

Excretion: Urine (74%) and feces (20%) as metabolites

Dosage

Geriatric & Adult

Intermittent claudication: Oral: 100 mg twice daily (when refractory to exercise therapy and smoking cessation, use in combination with either aspirin or clopidogrel) (Guyatt, 2012)

PCI (following elective stent placement) (unlabeled use): Oral: 100 mg twice daily in combination with aspirin or clopidogrel. Note: Only recommended in patients with an allergy or intolerance to either aspirin or clopidogrel (Guyatt, 2012).

Secondary prevention of noncardioembolic stroke or TIA (unlabeled use): Oral: 100 mg twice daily. Note: Clopidogrel or aspirin/extended release dipyridamole recommended over the use of cilostazol (Guyatt, 2012).

Dosage adjustment for cilostazol with concomitant medications:

CYP2C19 inhibitors (eg, omeprazole): Dosage of cilostazol should be reduced to 50 mg twice daily

CYP3A4 inhibitors (eg, ketoconazole, itraconazole, erythromycin, diltiazem): Dosage of cilostazol should be reduced to 50 mg twice daily

Administration Administer cilostazol 30 minutes before or 2 hours after meals.

Monitoring Parameters Monitor response (increased walking distance, increased mobility)

Special Geriatric Considerations Elderly must be evaluated for cardiac status. Since CHF is common, this disease cannot be overlooked.

Dosage Forms Excipient information presented when available (limited, particularly for generics); consult specific product labeling.

Tablet, oral: 50 mg, 100 mg

Pletal®: 50 mg, 100 mg

◆ **Ciloxan®** see Ciprofloxacin (Ophthalmic) on page 385

Cimetidine (sye MET i deen)

Medication Safety Issues

Sound-alike/look-alike issues:

Cimetidine may be confused with simethicone

Brand Names: U.S. Tagamet HB 200® [OTC]

Brand Names: Canada Apo-Cimetidine®; Dom-Cimetidine; Mylan-Cimetidine; Novo-Cimetidine; Nu-Cimet; PMS-Cimetidine

Generic Availability (U.S.) Yes

Pharmacologic Category Histamine H_2 Antagonist

Use Short-term treatment of active duodenal ulcers and benign gastric ulcers; maintenance therapy of duodenal ulcer; treatment of gastric hypersecretory states; treatment of gastroesophageal reflux disease (GERD)

OTC labeling: Prevention or relief of heartburn, acid indigestion, or sour stomach

Unlabeled Use Part of a multidrug regimen for H. pylori eradication to reduce the risk of duodenal ulcer recurrence

Contraindications Hypersensitivity to cimetidine, any component of the formulation, or other H_2 antagonists

Warnings/Precautions Reversible confusional states, usually clearing within 3-4 days after discontinuation, have been linked to use. Increased age (>50 years) and renal or hepatic impairment are thought to be associated. Use caution in the elderly due to risk of confusion and other CNS effects. Dosage should be adjusted in renal/hepatic impairment or in patients receiving drugs metabolized through the P450 system.

Over the counter (OTC) cimetidine should not be taken by individuals experiencing painful swallowing, vomiting with blood, or bloody or black stools; medical attention should be sought. A physician should be consulted prior to use when pain in the stomach, shoulder, arms or neck is present; if heartburn has occurred for >3 months; or if unexplained weight loss, or nausea and vomiting occur. Frequent wheezing, shortness of breath, lightheadedness, or sweating, especially with chest pain or heartburn, should also be reported. Consultation of a healthcare provider should occur by patients if also taking theophylline, phenytoin, or warfarin; if heartburn or stomach pain continues or worsens; or if use is required for >14 days. Symptoms of GI distress may be associated with a variety of conditions; symptomatic response to H_2 antagonists does not rule out the potential for significant pathology (eg, malignancy).

Adverse Reactions (Reflective of adult population; not specific for elderly)
1% to 10%:
Central nervous system: Headache (2% to 4%), dizziness (1%), somnolence (1%), agitation
Endocrine & metabolic: Gynecomastia (<1% to 4%)
Gastrointestinal: Diarrhea (1%)
Frequency not defined:
Cardiovascular: AV block, bradycardia, hypotension, tachycardia, vasculitis
Central nervous system: Confusion, fever
Dermatologic: Alopecia, erythema multiforme, exfoliative dermatitis, Stevens-Johnson syndrome, toxic epidermal necrolysis, rash
Endocrine & metabolic: Edema of the breasts, sexual ability decreased
Gastrointestinal: Nausea, pancreatitis, vomiting
Hematologic: Agranulocytosis, aplastic anemia, hemolytic anemia (immune-based), neutropenia, pancytopenia, thrombocytopenia
Hepatic: ALT increased, AST increased, hepatic fibrosis (case report)
Neuromuscular & skeletal: Arthralgia, myalgia, polymyositis
Renal: Creatinine increased, interstitial nephritis
Miscellaneous: Anaphylaxis, pneumonia (causal relationship not established)

Drug Interactions

Metabolism/Transport Effects Substrate of P-glycoprotein; **Inhibits** CYP1A2 (moderate), CYP2C19 (moderate), CYP2C9 (weak), CYP2D6 (moderate), CYP2E1 (weak), CYP3A4 (moderate)

Avoid Concomitant Use
Avoid concomitant use of Cimetidine with any of the following: Clopidogrel; Delavirdine; Dofetilide; EPIrubicin; Pimozide; Thioridazine; Tolvaptan

Increased Effect/Toxicity
Cimetidine may increase the levels/effects of: Alfentanil; Amiodarone; Anticonvulsants (Hydantoin); ARIPiprazole; Benzodiazepines (metabolized by oxidation); Bromazepam; Budesonide (Systemic, Oral Inhalation); Calcium Channel Blockers; CarBAMazepine; Carmustine; Carvedilol; Cisapride; CloZAPine; Colchicine; CYP1A2 Substrates; CYP2C19 Substrates; CYP2D6 Substrates; CYP3A4 Substrates; Dalfampridine; Dexmethylphenidate; Dofetilide; EPIrubicin; Eplerenone; Escitalopram; Everolimus; Fesoterodine; Halofantrine; Ivacaftor; Lurasidone; Mebendazole; MetFORMIN; Methylphenidate; Moclobemide; Nebivolol; Nicotine; Pentoxifylline; Pimecrolimus; Pimozide; Pramipexole; Praziquantel; Procainamide; Propafenone; QuiNIDine; QuiNINE; Ranolazine; Roflumilast; Salmeterol; Saquinavir; Saxagliptin; Selective Serotonin Reuptake Inhibitors; Sulfonylureas; Theophylline Derivatives; Thioridazine; Tolvaptan; Tricyclic Antidepressants; Varenicline; Vitamin K Antagonists; Zaleplon; ZOLMitriptan; Zuclopenthixol

The levels/effects of Cimetidine may be increased by: P-glycoprotein/ABCB1 Inhibitors

Decreased Effect
Cimetidine may decrease the levels/effects of: Atazanavir; Cefditoren; Cefpodoxime; Cefuroxime; Clopidogrel; Dasatinib; Delavirdine; Erlotinib; Fosamprenavir; Gefitinib; Ifosfamide; Indinavir; Iron Salts; Itraconazole; Ketoconazole; Ketoconazole (Systemic); Mesalamine; Nelfinavir; Nilotinib; Posaconazole; Rilpivirine; Tamoxifen; Vismodegib

The levels/effects of Cimetidine may be decreased by: P-glycoprotein/ABCB1 Inducers

CIMETIDINE

Ethanol/Nutrition/Herb Interactions
Ethanol: Avoid ethanol (may enhance gastric mucosal irritation).
Food: Cimetidine may increase serum caffeine levels if taken with caffeine. Cimetidine peak serum levels may be decreased if taken with food.
Herb/Nutraceutical: St John's wort may decrease cimetidine levels.

Stability Tablet: Store between 15°C and 30°C (59°F to 86°F). Protect from light.

Mechanism of Action Competitive inhibition of histamine at H_2 receptors of the gastric parietal cells resulting in reduced gastric acid secretion, gastric volume and hydrogen ion concentration reduced

Pharmacodynamics/Kinetics
Onset of action: 1 hour
Duration: 80% reduction in gastric acid secretion for 4-5 hours after 300 mg dose
Absorption: Rapid
Distribution: 1.3 L/kg
Protein binding: 20%
Metabolism: Partially hepatic, forms metabolites
Bioavailability: 60% to 70%
Half-life elimination: Adults: 2 hours
Time to peak, serum: Oral: 1-2 hours
Excretion: Primarily urine (48% as unchanged drug); feces (some)

Dosage
Geriatric & Adult
Short-term treatment of active ulcers: Oral: 300 mg 4 times/day or 800 mg at bedtime or 400 mg twice daily for up to 8 weeks
  Note: Higher doses of 1600 mg at bedtime for 4 weeks may be beneficial for a subpopulation of patients with larger duodenal ulcers (>1 cm defined endoscopically) who are also heavy smokers (≥1 pack/day).
Duodenal ulcer prophylaxis: 400 mg at bedtime
Gastric hypersecretory conditions: 300-600 mg every 6 hours; dosage not to exceed 2.4 g/day
Gastroesophageal reflux disease: 400 mg 4 times/day or 800 mg twice daily for 12 weeks
Peptic ulcer disease eradication of *Helicobacter pylori* (unlabeled use): 400 mg twice daily; requires combination therapy with antibiotics
Heartburn, acid indigestion, sour stomach (OTC labeling): 200 mg up to twice daily; may take 30 minutes prior to eating foods or beverages expected to cause heartburn or indigestion

Renal Impairment
Cl_{cr} 10-50 mL/minute: Administer 50% of normal dose
Cl_{cr} <10 mL/minute: Administer 25% of normal dose
Slightly dialyzable (5% to 20%); administer after dialysis

Hepatic Impairment Usual dose is safe in mild liver disease but use with caution and in reduced dosage in severe liver disease. Increased risk of CNS toxicity in cirrhosis suggested by enhanced penetration of CNS.

Administration Administer with meals so that the drug's peak effect occurs at the proper time (peak inhibition of gastric acid secretion occurs at 1 and 3 hours after dosing in fasting subjects and approximately 2 hours in nonfasting subjects; this correlates well with the time food is no longer in the stomach offering a buffering effect)

Monitoring Parameters CBC, gastric pH, occult blood with GI bleeding; monitor renal function to correct dose.

Special Geriatric Considerations Patients diagnosed with PUD should be evaluated for *Helicobacter pylori*. H_2 blockers are the preferred drugs for treating PUD in elderly due to cost and ease of administration. These agents are no less or more effective than any other therapy. The preferred agents, due to favorable pharmacokinetic, side effect and drug interaction profiles are ranitidine, famotidine, and nizatidine. Due to the potential for confusion and drug interactions, cimetidine has been identified by a panel of experts as a drug to avoid in the elderly. Consider evaluating creatinine clearance before initiating H_2-blocker therapy.

Dosage Forms Excipient information presented when available (limited, particularly for generics); consult specific product labeling. [DSC] = Discontinued product
Solution, oral, as hydrochloride [strength expressed as base]: 300 mg/5 mL (237 mL, 473 mL [DSC])
Tablet, oral: 200 mg, 300 mg, 400 mg, 800 mg
  Tagamet HB 200®: 200 mg

◆ **Cimzia®** *see* Certolizumab Pegol *on page 343*

Cinacalcet (sin a KAL cet)

Brand Names: U.S. Sensipar®
Brand Names: Canada Sensipar®
Index Terms AMG 073; Cinacalcet Hydrochloride
Generic Availability (U.S.) No
Pharmacologic Category Calcimimetic

Use Treatment of secondary hyperparathyroidism in patients with chronic kidney disease (CKD) on dialysis; treatment of hypercalcemia in patients with parathyroid carcinoma; treatment of severe hypercalcemia in patients with primary hyperparathyroidism who are unable to undergo parathyroidectomy

Contraindications Hypocalcemia (serum calcium lower than the lower limit of normal range)

Canadian labeling: Additional contraindications (not in U.S. labeling): Hypersensitivity to any component of the formulation

Warnings/Precautions Use is contraindicated in hypocalcemia. Monitor serum calcium and for symptoms of hypocalcemia (eg, cramps, myalgia, paresthesia, seizure, tetany); may require treatment interruption, dose reduction, or initiation (or dose increases) of calcium-based phosphate binder or vitamin D to raise serum calcium depending on calcium levels or symptoms of hypocalcemia. Use with caution in patients with a seizure disorder (seizure threshold is lowered by significant serum calcium reductions); monitor calcium levels closely. Adynamic bone disease may develop if intact parathyroid hormone (iPTH) levels are suppressed (<100 pg/mL).

Use caution in patients with moderate-to-severe hepatic impairment (Child-Pugh classes B and C); monitor serum calcium, serum phosphorus and iPTH closely. In the U.S., the long-term safety and efficacy of cinacalcet has not been evaluated in chronic kidney disease (CKD) patients with hyperparathyroidism not requiring dialysis. Not indicated for CKD patients not receiving dialysis. Although possibly related to lower baseline calcium levels, clinical studies have shown an increased incidence of hypocalcemia (<8.4 mg/dL) in patients not requiring dialysis. Monitor serum calcium and iPTH concentrations closely in patients on concurrent CYP2D6 inhibitors; dosage adjustment may be required. Cinacalcet is a strong inhibitor of CYP2D6; if on concurrent therapy with a CYP2D6 substrate, dosage adjustment of the CYP2D6 substrate may be necessary. May cause a decrease in testosterone levels (free and total); although below normal testosterone levels may occur in patients with end-stage renal disease, the clinical significance has not been determined. Use with caution in patients with cardiovascular disease; idiosyncratic hypotension, worsening of heart failure, and/or arrhythmia have been reported in patients with impaired cardiovascular function; may correlate with decreased serum calcium.

Adverse Reactions (Reflective of adult population; not specific for elderly)
>10%:
  Central nervous system: Fatigue (12% to 21%), headache (≤21%), depression (10% to 18%)
  Endocrine & metabolic: Hypocalcemia (≤66%), dehydration (≤24%), hypercalcemia (12% to 21%)
  Gastrointestinal: Nausea (31% to 66%), vomiting (27% to 52%), diarrhea (≤21%), anorexia (6% to 21%), constipation (10% to 18%)
  Hematologic: Anemia (6% to 17%)
  Neuromuscular & skeletal: Parasthesia (14% to 29%), fracture (12% to 21%), weakness (7% to 17%), arthralgia (6% to 17%), myalgia (≤15%), limb pain (10% to 12%)
  Respiratory: Upper respiratory infection (10% to 12%)
1% to 10%:
  Cardiovascular: Hypertension (≤7%)
  Central nervous system: Dizziness (≤10%), seizure (1%)
  Endocrine & metabolic: Testosterone decreased
  Neuromuscular & skeletal: Chest pain (noncardiac; ≤6%)
Drug Interactions
Metabolism/Transport Effects Substrate of CYP1A2 (minor), CYP2D6 (minor), CYP3A4 (major); **Note:** Assignment of Major/Minor substrate status based on clinically relevant drug interaction potential; **Inhibits** CYP2D6 (strong)
Avoid Concomitant Use
Avoid concomitant use of Cinacalcet with any of the following: Conivaptan; Pimozide; Tamoxifen; Thioridazine

Increased Effect/Toxicity
Cinacalcet may increase the levels/effects of: ARIPiprazole; AtoMOXetine; CYP2D6 Substrates; Fesoterodine; Iloperidone; Nebivolol; Pimozide; Propafenone; Tetrabenazine; Thioridazine; Tricyclic Antidepressants

The levels/effects of Cinacalcet may be increased by: Antifungal Agents (Azole Derivatives, Systemic); Conivaptan; CYP3A4 Inhibitors (Moderate); CYP3A4 Inhibitors (Strong); Dasatinib; Ivacaftor; Mifepristone

Decreased Effect
Cinacalcet may decrease the levels/effects of: Codeine; Iloperidone; Tacrolimus; Tacrolimus (Systemic); Tamoxifen; TraMADol

The levels/effects of Cinacalcet may be decreased by: Peginterferon Alfa-2b; Tocilizumab

Ethanol/Nutrition/Herb Interactions Food: Food increases bioavailability. Management: Administer with food or shortly after a meal.

Stability Store at 25°C (77°F); excursions permitted to 15°C to 30°C (59°F to 86°F).

Mechanism of Action Increases the sensitivity of the calcium-sensing receptor on the parathyroid gland thereby, concomitantly lowering parathyroid hormone (PTH), serum calcium, and serum phosphorus levels, preventing progressive bone disease and adverse events associated with mineral metabolism disorders.

Pharmacodynamics/Kinetics
Distribution: V_d: ~1000 L
Protein binding: ~93% to 97%
Metabolism: Hepatic (extensive) via CYP3A4, 2D6, 1A2; forms inactive metabolites
Half-life elimination: Terminal: 30-40 hours; moderate hepatic impairment: 65 hours; severe hepatic impairment: 84 hours
Time to peak, plasma: ~2-6 hours
Excretion: Urine ~80% (as metabolites); feces ~15%

Dosage
Geriatric Refer to adult dosing. No adjustment required.

Adult Note: Do not titrate dose more frequently than every 2-4 weeks. Dosage adjustment may be required in patients on concurrent CYP3A4 inhibitors.

Secondary hyperparathyroidism: Oral: Initial: 30 mg once daily (maximum daily dose: 180 mg); increase dose incrementally (60 mg, 90 mg, 120 mg, 180 mg once daily) as necessary to maintain intact parathyroid hormone (iPTH) level between 150-300 pg/mL.

Parathyroid carcinoma, primary hyperparathyroidism: Oral: Initial: 30 mg twice daily (maximum daily dose: 360 mg daily as 90 mg 4 times/day); increase dose incrementally (60 mg twice daily, 90 mg twice daily, 90 mg 3-4 times/day) as necessary to normalize serum calcium levels.

Renal Impairment No adjustment required.

Hepatic Impairment Patients with moderate-to-severe dysfunction (Child-Pugh class B or C) have an increased exposure to cinacalcet and increased half-life. Dosage adjustments may be necessary based on serum calcium, serum phosphorus and/or iPTH.

Administration Administer with food or shortly after a meal. Do not break or divide tablet; should be taken whole.

Monitoring Parameters
Secondary hyperparathyroidism: Serum calcium and phosphorus levels prior to initiation and within a week of initiation or dosage adjustment; iPTH should be measured 1-4 weeks after initiation or dosage adjustment. After the maintenance dose is established, monthly calcium and phosphorus levels and iPTH every 1-3 months are required. Wait at least 12 hours after dose before drawing iPTH levels.

Parathyroid carcinoma and primary hyperparathyroidism: Serum calcium levels prior to initiation and within a week of initiation or dosage adjustment; once maintenance dose is established, obtain serum calcium every 2 months.

Reference Range
CKD K/DOQI guidelines definition of stages; chronic disease is kidney damage or GFR <60 mL/minute/1.73 m^2 for ≥3 months:
Stage 2: GFR 60-89 mL/minute/1.73 m^2 (kidney damage with mild decrease GFR)
Stage 3: GFR 30-59 mL/minute/1.73 m^2 (moderate decrease GFR)
Stage 4: GFR 15-29 mL/minute/1.73 m^2 (severe decrease GFR)
Stage 5: GFR <15 mL/minute/1.73 m^2 or dialysis (kidney failure)
Target range for iPTH: Adults:
Stage 3 CKD: 35-70 pg/mL
Stage 4 CKD: 70-110 pg/mL
Stage 5 CKD: 150-300 pg/mL
Serum phosphorus: Adults:
Stage 3 and 4 CKD: ≥2.7 to <4.6 mg/dL
Stage 5 CKD: 3.5-5.5 mg/dL
Serum calcium-phosphorus product: Adults: Stage 3-5 CKD: <55 mg^2/dL^2

Dosage Forms Excipient information presented when available (limited, particularly for generics); consult specific product labeling.
Tablet, oral:
Sensipar®: 30 mg, 60 mg, 90 mg

♦ **Cinacalcet Hydrochloride** see Cinacalcet on page 379
♦ **Cipro®** see Ciprofloxacin (Systemic) on page 381
♦ **Ciprodex®** see Ciprofloxacin and Dexamethasone on page 386

Ciprofloxacin (Systemic) (sip roe FLOKS a sin)

Related Information
Antibiotic Treatment of Adults With Infective Endocarditis on page 2157
Antimicrobial Drugs of Choice on page 2163
Community-Acquired Pneumonia in Adults on page 2171
Medication Safety Issues
Sound-alike/look-alike issues:
Ciprofloxacin may be confused with cephalexin
Cipro® may be confused with Ceftin®
Brand Names: U.S. Cipro®; Cipro® I.V.; Cipro® XR
Brand Names: Canada Apo-Ciproflox®; Auro-Ciprofloxacin; Ciprofloxacin Injection; Cipro-floxacin Intravenous Infusion; Cipro®; Cipro® XL; CO Ciprofloxacin; Dom-Ciprofloxacin; JAMP-Ciprofloxacin; Mint-Ciprofloxacin; Mylan-Ciprofloxacin; Novo-Ciprofloxacin; PHL-Cipro-floxacin; PMS-Ciprofloxacin; PRO-Ciprofloxacin; RAN™-Ciprofloxacin; ratio-Ciprofloxacin; Riva-Ciprofloxacin; Sandoz-Ciprofloxacin; Taro-Ciprofloxacin
Index Terms Ciprofloxacin Hydrochloride
Generic Availability (U.S.) Yes: Excludes suspension
Pharmacologic Category Antibiotic, Quinolone
Use
Adults: To reduce incidence or progression of disease following exposure to aerolized *Bacillus anthracis*. Treatment of the following infections when caused by susceptible bacteria: Urinary tract infections; acute uncomplicated cystitis in females; chronic bacterial prostatitis; lower respiratory tract infections (including acute exacerbations of chronic bronchitis); acute sinusitis; skin and skin structure infections; bone and joint infections; complicated intra-abdominal infections (in combination with metronidazole); infectious diarrhea; typhoid fever due to *Salmonella typhi* (eradication of chronic typhoid carrier state has not been proven); uncomplicated cervical and urethra gonorrhea (due to *N. gonorrhoeae*); nosocomial pneumonia; empirical therapy for febrile neutropenic patients (in combination with piperacillin)
Note: As of April 2007, the CDC no longer recommends the use of fluoroquinolones for the treatment of gonococcal disease.
Unlabeled Use Cutaneous/gastrointestinal/oropharyngeal anthrax; disseminated gonococcal infection; chancroid; prophylaxis to *Neisseria meningitidis* following close contact with an infected person; empirical therapy (oral) for febrile neutropenia in low-risk cancer patients; HACEK group endocarditis; periodontitis
Medication Guide Available Yes
Contraindications Hypersensitivity to ciprofloxacin, any component of the formulation, or other quinolones; concurrent administration of tizanidine
Warnings/Precautions [U.S. Boxed Warning]: There have been reports of tendon inflammation and/or rupture with quinolone antibiotics; risk may be increased with concurrent corticosteroids, organ transplant recipients, and in patients >60 years of age. Rupture of the Achilles tendon sometimes requiring surgical repair has been reported most frequently; but other tendon sites (eg, rotator cuff, biceps) have also been reported. Strenuous physical activity, rheumatoid arthritis, and renal impairment may be an independent risk factor for tendonitis. Discontinue at first sign of tendon inflammation or pain. May occur even after discontinuation of therapy. Use with caution in patients with rheumatoid arthritis; may increase risk of tendon rupture. CNS effects may occur (tremor, restlessness, confusion, and very rarely hallucinations, increased intracranial pressure [including pseudotumor cerebri] or seizures). Use with caution in patients with known or suspected CNS disorder. Potential for seizures, although very rare, may be increased with concomitant NSAID therapy. Use with caution in individuals at risk of seizures. Fluoroquinolones may prolong QT$_c$ interval; avoid use in patients with a history of QT$_c$ prolongation, uncorrected hypokalemia, hypomagnesemia, or concurrent administration of other medications known to prolong the QT interval (including Class Ia and Class III antiarrhythmics, cisapride, erythromycin, antipsychotics, and tricyclic antidepressants). Prolonged use may result in fungal or bacterial superinfection, including *C. difficile*-associated diarrhea (CDAD) and pseudomembranous colitis; CDAD has been observed >2 months postantibiotic treatment. Rarely crystalluria has occurred; urine alkalinity

may increase the risk. Ensure adequate hydration during therapy. Rare cases of peripheral neuropathy may occur.

Fluoroquinolones have been associated with the development of serious, and sometimes fatal, hypoglycemia, most often in elderly diabetics but also in patients without diabetes. This occurred most frequently with gatifloxacin (no longer available systemically), but may occur at a lower frequency with other quinolones.

Severe hypersensitivity reactions, including anaphylaxis, have occurred with quinolone therapy. Reactions may present as typical allergic symptoms after a single dose, or may manifest as severe idiosyncratic dermatologic, vascular, pulmonary, renal, hepatic, and/or hematologic events, usually after multiple doses. Prompt discontinuation of drug should occur if skin rash or other symptoms arise. **[U.S. Boxed Warning]: Quinolones may exacerbate myasthenia gravis; avoid use (rare, potentially life-threatening weakness of respiratory muscles may occur).** Use caution in renal impairment. Avoid excessive sunlight and take precautions to limit exposure (eg, loose fitting clothing, sunscreen); may cause moderate-to-severe phototoxicity reactions. Discontinue use if photosensitivity occurs. Since ciprofloxacin is ineffective in the treatment of syphilis and may mask symptoms, all patients should be tested for syphilis at the time of gonorrheal diagnosis and 3 months later. Hemolytic reactions may (rarely) occur with quinolone use in patients with latent or actual G6PD deficiency.

Ciprofloxacin is a potent inhibitor of CYP1A2. Coadministration of drugs which depend on this pathway may lead to substantial increases in serum concentrations and adverse effects.

Adverse Reactions (Reflective of adult population; not specific for elderly) 1% to 10%:

Central nervous system: Neurologic events (children 2%, includes dizziness, insomnia, nervousness, somnolence); fever (children 2%); headache (I.V. administration); restlessness (I.V. administration)

Dermatologic: Rash (children 2%, adults 1%)

Gastrointestinal: Nausea (3%); diarrhea (children 5%, adults 2%); vomiting (children 5%, adults 1%); abdominal pain (children 3%, adults <1%); dyspepsia (children 3%)

Hepatic: ALT increased, AST increased (adults 1%)

Local: Injection site reactions (I.V. administration)

Respiratory: Rhinitis (children 3%)

Drug Interactions

Metabolism/Transport Effects Substrate of P-glycoprotein; **Inhibits** CYP1A2 (strong), CYP3A4 (weak)

Avoid Concomitant Use

Avoid concomitant use of Ciprofloxacin (Systemic) with any of the following: BCG; TiZANidine

Increased Effect/Toxicity

Ciprofloxacin (Systemic) may increase the levels/effects of: ARIPiprazole; Bendamustine; Caffeine; Corticosteroids (Systemic); CYP1A2 Substrates; Erlotinib; Highest Risk QTc-Prolonging Agents; Methotrexate; Moderate Risk QTc-Prolonging Agents; Pentoxifylline; Porfimer; Roflumilast; ROPINIRole; Ropivacaine; Sulfonylureas; Theophylline Derivatives; TiZANidine; Varenicline; Vitamin K Antagonists

The levels/effects of Ciprofloxacin (Systemic) may be increased by: Insulin; Mifepristone; Nonsteroidal Anti-Inflammatory Agents; P-glycoprotein/ABCB1 Inhibitors; Probenecid

Decreased Effect

Ciprofloxacin (Systemic) may decrease the levels/effects of: BCG; Fosphenytoin; Mycophenolate; Phenytoin; Sulfonylureas; Typhoid Vaccine

The levels/effects of Ciprofloxacin (Systemic) may be decreased by: Antacids; Calcium Salts; Didanosine; Iron Salts; Lanthanum; Magnesium Salts; P-glycoprotein/ABCB1 Inducers; Quinapril; Sevelamer; Sucralfate; Zinc Salts

Ethanol/Nutrition/Herb Interactions

Food: Food decreases rate, but not extent, of absorption. Ciprofloxacin serum levels may be decreased if taken with divalent or trivalent cations. Ciprofloxacin may increase serum caffeine levels if taken concurrently. Rarely, crystalluria may occur. Enteral feedings may decrease plasma concentrations of ciprofloxacin probably by >30% inhibition of absorption. Management: May administer with food to minimize GI upset. Avoid or take ciprofloxacin 2 hours before or 6 hours after antacids, dairy products, or calcium-fortified juices alone or in a meal containing >800 mg calcium, oral multivitamins, or mineral supplements containing divalent and/or trivalent cations. Restrict caffeine intake if excessive cardiac or CNS stimulation occurs. Ensure adequate hydration during therapy. Ciprofloxacin should not be administered with enteral feedings. The feeding would need to be discontinued for 1-2 hours prior to and after ciprofloxacin administration. Nasogastric administration produces a greater loss of ciprofloxacin bioavailability than does nasoduodenal administration.

Herb/Nutraceutical: Dong quai and St John's wort may also cause photosensitization. Management: Avoid dong quai and St John's wort.

Stability

Injection:

Premixed infusion: Store between 5°C to 25°C (41°F to 77°F); avoid freezing. Protect from light.

Vial: Store between 5°C to 30°C (41°F to 86°F); avoid freezing. Protect from light. May be diluted with NS, D_5W, SWFI, $D_{10}W$, $D_5^1/_4NS$, $D_5^1/_2NS$, LR. Diluted solutions of 0.5-2 mg/mL are stable for up to 14 days refrigerated or at room temperature.

Microcapsules for oral suspension: Prior to reconstitution, store below 25°C (77°F); protect from freezing. Following reconstitution, store below 30°C (86°F) for up to 14 days; protect from freezing.

Tablet:

Immediate release: Store below 30°C (86°F).

Extended release: Store at room temperature of 15°C to 30°C (59°F to 86°F).

Mechanism of Action

Inhibits DNA-gyrase in susceptible organisms; inhibits relaxation of supercoiled DNA and promotes breakage of double-stranded DNA

Pharmacodynamics/Kinetics

Absorption: Oral: Immediate release tablet: Rapid (~50% to 85%)

Distribution: V_d: 2.1-2.7 L/kg; tissue concentrations often exceed serum concentrations especially in kidneys, gallbladder, liver, lungs, gynecological tissue, and prostatic tissue; CSF concentrations: 10% of serum concentrations (noninflamed meninges), 14% to 37% (inflamed meninges)

Protein binding: 20% to 40%

Metabolism: Partially hepatic; forms 4 metabolites (limited activity)

Half-life elimination: Adults: Normal renal function: 3-5 hours

Time to peak: Oral:

Immediate release tablet: 0.5-2 hours

Extended release tablet: Cipro® XR: 1-2.5 hours

Excretion: Urine (30% to 50% as unchanged drug); feces (15% to 43%)

Dosage

Geriatric Refer to adult dosing. Adjust dose carefully based on renal function.

Adult Note: Extended release tablets and immediate release formulations are not interchangeable. Unless otherwise specified, oral dosing reflects the use of immediate release formulations.

Anthrax:

Inhalational (postexposure prophylaxis):

Oral: 500 mg every 12 hours for 60 days

I.V.: 400 mg every 12 hours for 60 days

Cutaneous (treatment, CDC guidelines): Oral: Immediate release formulation: 500 mg every 12 hours for 60 days. **Note:** In the presence of systemic involvement, extensive edema, lesions on head/neck, refer to I.V. dosing for treatment of inhalational/gastrointestinal/oropharyngeal anthrax.

Inhalational/gastrointestinal/oropharyngeal (treatment, CDC guidelines): I.V.: 400 mg every 12 hours. **Note:** Initial treatment should include two or more agents predicted to be effective (per CDC recommendations). Continue combined therapy for 60 days.

Bone/joint infections:

Oral: 500-750 mg twice daily for 4-6 weeks

I.V.:

Mild/moderate: 400 mg every 12 hours for 4-6 weeks

Severe/complicated: 400 mg every 8 hours for 4-6 weeks

Chancroid (unlabeled use): Oral: 500 mg twice daily for 3 days (CDC, 2010)

Endocarditis due to HACEK organisms (AHA guidelines, unlabeled use): Note: Not first-line option; use only if intolerant of beta-lactam therapy:

Oral: 500 mg every 12 hours for 4 weeks

I.V.: 400 mg every 12 hours for 4 weeks

Epididymitis, chlamydial (unlabeled use): Oral: 500 mg single dose (Canadian STI Guidelines, 2008)

Febrile neutropenia: I.V.: 400 mg every 8 hours for 7-14 days (combination therapy generally recommended)

Gonococcal infections:

Urethral/cervical gonococcal infections: Oral: 250-500 mg as a single dose (CDC recommends concomitant doxycycline or azithromycin due to possible coinfection with *Chlamydia*); **Note:** As of April 2007, the CDC no longer recommends the use of fluoroquinolones for the treatment of uncomplicated gonococcal disease.

Disseminated gonococcal infection (CDC guidelines): Oral: 500 mg twice daily to complete 7 days of therapy (initial treatment with ceftriaxone 1 g I.M./I.V. daily for 24-48 hours after improvement begins); **Note:** As of April 2007, the CDC no longer recommends the use of fluoroquinolones for the treatment of more serious gonococcal disease, unless no other options exist and susceptibility can be confirmed via culture.

Granuloma inguinale (donovanosis) (unlabeled use): Oral: 750 mg twice daily for at least 3 weeks (and until lesions have healed) (CDC, 2010)

Infectious diarrhea: Oral:

Salmonella: 500 mg twice daily for 5-7 days

Shigella: 500 mg twice daily for 3 days

Traveler's diarrhea: Mild: 750 mg for one dose; Severe: 500 mg twice daily for 3 days

Vibrio cholerae: 1 g for one dose

Intra-abdominal, complicated, community-acquired (in combination with metronidazole): Note: Avoid using in settings where *E. coli* susceptibility to fluoroquinolones is <90%:

Oral: 500 mg every 12 hours for 7-14 days

I.V.: 400 mg every 12 hours for 7-14 days; **Note:** 2010 IDSA guidelines recommend treatment duration of 4-7 days (provided source controlled)

Lower respiratory tract, skin/skin structure infections:

Oral: 500-750 mg twice daily for 7-14 days

I.V.:

Mild/moderate: 400 mg every 12 hours for 7-14 days

Severe/complicated: 400 mg every 8 hours for 7-14 days

Meningococcal meningitis prophylaxis (unlabeled use): Oral: 500 mg as a single dose (CDC, 2005)

Nosocomial pneumonia: I.V.: 400 mg every 8 hours for 10-14 days

Periodontitis (unlabeled use): Oral: 500 mg every 12 hours for 8-10 days

Prostatitis (chronic, bacterial): Oral: 500 mg every 12 hours for 28 days

Sinusitis (acute): Oral: 500 mg every 12 hours for 10 days

Typhoid fever: Oral: 500 mg every 12 hours for 10 days

Urinary tract infection:

Acute uncomplicated, cystitis:

Oral:

Immediate release formulation: 250 mg every 12 hours for 3 days

Extended release formulation (Cipro® XR): 500 mg every 24 hours for 3 days

I.V.: 200 mg every 12 hours for 7-14 days

Complicated (including pyelonephritis):

Oral:

Immediate release formulation: 500 mg every 12 hours for 7-14 days

Extended release formulation (Cipro® XR): 1000 mg every 24 hours for 7-14 days

I.V.: 400 mg every 12 hours for 7-14 days

Renal Impairment Adults:

Manufacturer's recommendations:

Oral, immediate release:

Cl_{cr} >50 mL/minute: No dosage adjustment necessary.

Cl_{cr} 30-50 mL/minute: 250-500 mg every 12 hours

Cl_{cr} 5-29 mL/minute: 250-500 mg every 18 hours

Hemodialysis/peritoneal dialysis (PD) (administer after dialysis on dialysis days): 250-500 mg every 24 hours

Oral, extended release:

Cl_{cr} ≥30 mL/minute: No dosage adjustment necessary.

Cl_{cr} <30 mL/minute: 500 mg every 24 hours

Hemodialysis/peritoneal dialysis (PD) (administer after dialysis on dialysis days): 500 mg every 24 hours

I.V.:

Cl_{cr} ≥30 mL/minute: No dosage adjustment necessary.

Cl_{cr} 5-29 mL/minute: 200-400 mg every 18-24 hours

Alternate recommendations: Oral (immediate release), I.V.:

Cl_{cr} >50 mL/minute: No dosage adjustment necessary (Aronoff, 2007).

Cl_{cr} 10-50 mL/minute: Administer 50% to 75% of usual dose every 12 hours (Aronoff, 2007).

Cl_{cr} <10 mL/minute: Administer 50% of usual dose every 12 hours (Aronoff, 2007).

Intermittent hemodialysis (IHD) (administer after hemodialysis on dialysis days): Minimally dialyzable (<10%): Oral: 250-500 mg every 24 hours **or** I.V.: 200-400 mg every 24 hours (Heintz, 2009). **Note:** Dosing dependent on the assumption of 3 times/week, complete IHD sessions.

Continuous renal replacement therapy (CRRT) (Heintz, 2009; Trotman, 2005): Drug clearance is highly dependent on the method of renal replacement, filter type, and flow rate. Appropriate dosing requires close monitoring of pharmacologic response, signs of adverse reactions due to drug accumulation, as well as drug concentrations in relation to target trough (if appropriate). The following are general recommendations only (based on dialysate flow/ultrafiltration rates of 1-2 L/hour and minimal residual renal function) and should not supersede clinical judgment:

CVVH/CVVHD/CVVHDF: I.V.: 200-400 mg every 12-24 hours

Administration

Oral: May administer with food to minimize GI upset; avoid antacid use; maintain proper hydration and urine output. Administer immediate release ciprofloxacin and Cipro® XR at least 2 hours before or 6 hours after antacids or other products containing calcium, iron, or zinc (including dairy products or calcium-fortified juices). Separate oral administration from drugs which may impair absorption (see Drug Interactions).

Oral suspension: Should not be administered through feeding tubes (suspension is oil-based and adheres to the feeding tube). Patients should avoid chewing on the microcapsules.

Nasogastric/orogastric tube: Crush immediate-release tablet and mix with water. Flush feeding tube before and after administration. Hold tube feedings at least 1 hour before and 2 hours after administration.

Tablet, extended release: Do not crush, split, or chew. May be administered with meals containing dairy products (calcium content <800 mg), but not with dairy products alone.

Parenteral: Administer by slow I.V. infusion over 60 minutes to reduce the risk of venous irritation (burning, pain, erythema, and swelling); final concentration for administration should not exceed 2 mg/mL.

Monitoring Parameters CBC, renal and hepatic function during prolonged therapy

Reference Range Therapeutic: 2.6-3 mcg/mL; Toxic: >5 mcg/mL

Test Interactions Some quinolones may produce a false-positive urine screening result for opiates using commercially-available immunoassay kits. This has been demonstrated most consistently for levofloxacin and ofloxacin, but other quinolones have shown cross-reactivity in certain assay kits. Confirmation of positive opiate screens by more specific methods should be considered.

Pharmacotherapy Pearls No geriatric-specific information.

Special Geriatric Considerations Ciprofloxacin should not be used as first-line therapy unless the culture and sensitivity findings show resistance to usual therapy. The interactions with caffeine and theophylline can result in serious toxicity in the elderly. Adjust dose for renal function. The risk of torsade de pointes and tendon inflammation and/or rupture associated with the concomitant use of corticosteroids and quinolones is increased in the elderly population. See Warnings/Precautions regarding tendon rupture in patients >60 years of age.

Dosage Forms Excipient information presented when available (limited, particularly for generics); consult specific product labeling. [DSC] = Discontinued product

Infusion, premixed in D₅W: 200 mg (100 mL); 400 mg (200 mL)

Cipro® I.V.: 200 mg (100 mL [DSC]); 400 mg (200 mL)

Infusion, premixed in D₅W [preservative free]: 200 mg (100 mL); 400 mg (200 mL)

Injection, solution: 10 mg/mL (20 mL, 40 mL)

Injection, solution [preservative free]: 10 mg/mL (20 mL, 40 mL [DSC])

Microcapsules for suspension, oral:

Cipro®: 250 mg/5 mL (100 mL); 500 mg/5 mL (100 mL) [strawberry flavor]

Tablet, oral, as hydrochloride [strength expressed as base]: 100 mg, 250 mg, 500 mg, 750 mg

Cipro®: 250 mg, 500 mg

Tablet, extended release, oral, as base and hydrochloride [strength expressed as base]: 500 mg, 1000 mg

Cipro® XR: 500 mg, 1000 mg

Ciprofloxacin (Ophthalmic) (sip roe FLOKS a sin)

Medication Safety Issues

Sound-alike/look-alike issues:

Ciprofloxacin may be confused with cephalexin

Ciloxan® may be confused with Cytoxan

Brand Names: U.S. Ciloxan®

Brand Names: Canada Ciloxan®

Index Terms Ciprofloxacin Hydrochloride

Generic Availability (U.S.) Yes: Excludes ointment

Pharmacologic Category Antibiotic, Ophthalmic; Antibiotic, Quinolone

Use Treatment of superficial ocular infections (corneal ulcers, conjunctivitis) due to susceptible strains

Dosage

Geriatric & Adult

Bacterial conjunctivitis:

Ophthalmic solution: Instill 1-2 drops in eye(s) every 2 hours while awake for 2 days and 1-2 drops every 4 hours while awake for the next 5 days

Ophthalmic ointment: Apply a 1/2" ribbon into the conjunctival sac 3 times/day for the first 2 days, followed by a 1/2" ribbon applied twice daily for the next 5 days

Corneal ulcer: *Ophthalmic solution:* Instill 2 drops into affected eye every 15 minutes for the first 6 hours, then 2 drops into the affected eye every 30 minutes for the remainder of the first day. On day 2, instill 2 drops into the affected eye hourly. On days 3-14, instill 2 drops into affected eye every 4 hours. Treatment may continue after day 14 if re-epithelialization has not occurred.

Special Geriatric Considerations Evaluate the patient's or caregiver's ability to safely administer the correct dose of ophthalmic medication.

Dosage Forms Excipient information presented when available (limited, particularly for generics); consult specific product labeling.

Ointment, ophthalmic, as hydrochloride:

Ciloxan®: 3.33 mg/g (3.5 g) [equivalent to ciprofloxacin base 0.3%]

Solution, ophthalmic, as hydrochloride [drops]: 3.5 mg/mL (2.5 mL, 5 mL, 10 mL) [equivalent to ciprofloxacin base 0.3%]

Ciloxan®: 3.5 mg/mL (5 mL) [contains benzalkonium chloride; equivalent to ciprofloxacin base 0.3%]

Ciprofloxacin (Otic) (sip roe FLOKS a sin)

Medication Safety Issues

Sound-alike/look-alike issues:

Cetraxal® may be confused with cefTRIAXone

Ciprofloxacin may be confused with cephalexin

Brand Names: U.S. Cetraxal®

Index Terms Ciprofloxacin Hydrochloride

Generic Availability (U.S.) No

Pharmacologic Category Antibiotic, Otic; Antibiotic, Quinolone

Use Treatment of acute otitis externa due to susceptible strains of *Pseudomonas aeruginosa* or *Staphylococcus aureus*

Dosage

Geriatric & Adult Acute otitis externa: Otic solution: Instill 0.25 mL (contents of 1 single-dose container) into affected ear twice daily for 7 days

Special Geriatric Considerations Evaluate the patient's or caregiver's ability to safetly administer the correct dose of otic medication.

Dosage Forms Excipient information presented when available (limited, particularly for generics); consult specific product labeling.

Solution, otic, as hydrochloride [preservative free]:

Cetraxal®: 0.5 mg/0.25 mL (14s) [equivalent to ciprofloxacin base 0.2%]

Ciprofloxacin and Dexamethasone (sip roe FLOKS a sin & deks a METH a sone)

Related Information

Ciprofloxacin (Otic) *on page 386*

Brand Names: U.S. Ciprodex®

Brand Names: Canada Ciprodex®

Index Terms Ciprofloxacin Hydrochloride and Dexamethasone; Dexamethasone and Ciprofloxacin

Generic Availability (U.S.) No

Pharmacologic Category Antibiotic, Otic; Antibiotic/Corticosteroid, Otic; Corticosteroid, Otic

Use Treatment of acute otitis externa

Dosage

Geriatric & Adult Acute otitis externa: Otic: Instill 4 drops into affected ear(s) twice daily for 7 days

Special Geriatric Considerations Evaluate the patient's or caregiver's ability to safely administer the correct dose of otic medication.

Dosage Forms Excipient information presented when available (limited, particularly for generics); consult specific product labeling.

Suspension, otic:

Ciprodex®: Ciprofloxacin 0.3% and dexamethasone 0.1% (7.5 mL) [contains benzalkonium chloride]

Ciprofloxacin and Hydrocortisone (sip roe FLOKS a sin & hye droe KOR ti sone)

Related Information

Ciprofloxacin (Otic) *on page 386*

Brand Names: U.S. Cipro® HC

Brand Names: Canada Cipro® HC

Index Terms Ciprofloxacin Hydrochloride and Hydrocortisone; Hydrocortisone and Ciprofloxacin

Generic Availability (U.S.) No

Pharmacologic Category Antibiotic/Corticosteroid, Otic

Use Treatment of acute otitis externa, sometimes known as "swimmer's ear"

Dosage

Geriatric & Adult Otitis externa: Otic: The recommended dosage for all patients is three drops of the suspension in the affected ear twice daily for 7 days; twice-daily dosing schedule is more convenient for patients than that of existing treatments with hydrocortisone, which are typically administered three or four times a day

Special Geriatric Considerations Evaluate the patient's or caregiver's ability to safely administer the correct dose of otic medication.

Dosage Forms Excipient information presented when available (limited, particularly for generics); consult specific product labeling.

Suspension, otic:

Cipro® HC: Ciprofloxacin hydrochloride 0.2% and hydrocortisone 1% (10 mL) [contains benzyl alcohol]

♦ **Ciprofloxacin Hydrochloride** *see* Ciprofloxacin (Ophthalmic) *on page 385*
♦ **Ciprofloxacin Hydrochloride** *see* Ciprofloxacin (Otic) *on page 386*
♦ **Ciprofloxacin Hydrochloride** *see* Ciprofloxacin (Systemic) *on page 381*
♦ **Ciprofloxacin Hydrochloride and Dexamethasone** *see* Ciprofloxacin and Dexamethasone *on page 386*
♦ **Ciprofloxacin Hydrochloride and Hydrocortisone** *see* Ciprofloxacin and Hydrocortisone *on page 387*
♦ **Cipro® HC** *see* Ciprofloxacin and Hydrocortisone *on page 387*
♦ **Cipro® I.V.** *see* Ciprofloxacin (Systemic) *on page 381*
♦ **Cipro® XR** *see* Ciprofloxacin (Systemic) *on page 381*

Citalopram (sye TAL oh pram)

Related Information

Antidepressant Agents *on page 2097*

Medication Safety Issues

Sound-alike/look-alike issues:

CeleXA® may be confused with CeleBREX®, Cerebyx®, Ranexa™, ZyPREXA®

BEERS Criteria medication:

This drug may be potentially inappropriate for use in geriatric patients (Quality of evidence - moderate; Strength of recommendation - strong).

Brand Names: U.S. CeleXA®

Brand Names: Canada Apo-Citalopram®; Auro-Citalopram; Ava-Citalopram; Celexa®; Citalopram-Odan; CO Citalopram; CTP 30; Dom-Citalopram; JAMP-Citalopram; Manda-Citalopram; Mint-Citalopram; Mylan-Citalopram; PHL-Citalopram; PMS-Citalopram; Q-Citalopram; RAN™-Citalo; ratio-Citalopram; Riva-Citalopram; Sandoz-Citalopram; Septa-Citalopram; Teva-Citalopram

Index Terms Citalopram Hydrobromide; Nitalapram

Generic Availability (U.S.) Yes

Pharmacologic Category Antidepressant, Selective Serotonin Reuptake Inhibitor

Use Treatment of depression

Unlabeled Use Obsessive-compulsive disorder (OCD)

Medication Guide Available Yes

Contraindications Hypersensitivity to citalopram or any component of the formulation; concomitant use with MAO inhibitors or within 2 weeks of discontinuing MAO inhibitors; concomitant use with pimozide

Warnings/Precautions Short-term studies did not show an increased risk in patients >24 years of age and showed a decreased risk in patients ≥65 years. Closely monitor patients for clinical worsening, suicidality, or unusual changes in behavior, particularly during the initial 1-2 months of therapy or during periods of dosage adjustments (increases or decreases); the patient's family or caregiver should be instructed to closely observe the patient and communicate condition with healthcare provider. A medication guide concerning the use of antidepressants should be dispensed with each prescription.

The possibility of a suicide attempt is inherent in major depression and may persist until remission occurs. Use caution in high-risk patients. Worsening depression and severe abrupt suicidality that are not part of the presenting symptoms may require discontinuation or modification of drug therapy. The patient's family or caregiver should be alerted to monitor patients for the emergence of suicidality and associated behaviors (such as agitation, irritability, hostility, impulsivity, and hypomania) and call healthcare provider.

May worsen psychosis in some patients or precipitate a shift to mania or hypomania in patients with bipolar disorder. Patients presenting with depressive symptoms should be screened for bipolar disorder. Monotherapy in patients with bipolar disorder should be avoided. **Citalopram is not FDA approved for the treatment of bipolar depression.**

Serotonin syndrome and neuroleptic malignant syndrome (NMS)-like reactions have occurred with serotonin/norepinephrine reuptake inhibitors (SNRIs) and selective serotonin reuptake inhibitors (SSRIs) when used alone, and particularly when used in combination with serotonergic agents (eg, triptans) or antidopaminergic agents (eg, antipsychotics). Concurrent use with MAO inhibitors is contraindicated. May increase the risks associated with electroconvulsive therapy. Has a low potential to impair cognitive or motor performance; caution operating hazardous machinery or driving.

Citalopram causes dose-dependent QT_c prolongation; torsade de pointes, ventricular tachycardia, and sudden death have been reported. Use is not recommended in patients with congenital long QT syndrome, bradycardia, recent MI, uncompensated heart failure, hypokalemia, and/or hypomagnesemia, or patients receiving concomitant medications that prolong the QT interval; if use is essential and cannot be avoided in these patients, ECG monitoring is recommended. Discontinue therapy in any patient with persistent QT_c measurements >500 msec. Serum electrolytes, particularly potassium and magnesium, should be monitored prior to initiation and periodically during therapy in any patient at increased risk for significant electrolyte disturbances; hypokalemia and/or hypomagnesemia should be corrected prior to use. Due to the QT prolongation risk, doses >40 mg/day are not recommended. Additionally, the maximum daily dose should not exceed 20 mg/day in certain populations (eg, CYP2C19 poor metabolizers, patients with hepatic impairment, elderly patients). Concomitant use of citalopram with moderate-to-strong inhibitors of CYP2C19 (eg, omeprazole, cimetidine) may decrease citalopram clearance; lower maximum daily doses of citalopram may be advised.

Use with caution in patients with a previous seizure disorder or condition predisposing to seizures such as brain damage or alcoholism. Use caution with concomitant use of aspirin, NSAIDs, warfarin, or other drugs that affect coagulation; the risk of bleeding may be potentiated. May cause or exacerbate sexual dysfunction. Upon discontinuation of citalopram therapy, gradually taper dose. If intolerable symptoms occur following a decrease in dosage or upon discontinuation of therapy, then resuming the previous dose with a more gradual taper should be considered. May cause hyponatremia/SIADH (elderly at increased risk); volume depletion and diuretics may increase risk. Monitor sodium closely with initiation or dosage adjustments in older adults (Beers Criteria).

Adverse Reactions (Reflective of adult population; not specific for elderly)
>10%:
Central nervous system: Somnolence (18%; dose related), insomnia (15%; dose related)
Gastrointestinal: Nausea (21%), xerostomia (20%)
Miscellaneous: Diaphoresis (11%; dose related)
1% to 10%:
Cardiovascular: QT prolongation (2%), hypotension (≥1%), orthostatic hypotension (≥1%), tachycardia (≥1%), bradycardia (1%)
Central nervous system: Fatigue (5%; dose related), anxiety (4%), agitation (3%), fever (2%), yawning (2%; dose related), amnesia (≥1%), apathy (≥1%), concentration impaired (≥1%), confusion (≥1%), depression (≥1%), migraine (≥1%), suicide attempt (≥1%)
Dermatologic: Rash (≥1%), pruritus (≥1%)
Endocrine & metabolic: Libido decreased (1% to 4%), dysmenorrhea (3%), amenorrhea (≥1%)
Gastrointestinal: Diarrhea (8%), dyspepsia (5%), anorexia (4%), vomiting (4%), abdominal pain (3%), appetite increased (≥1%), flatulence (≥1%), salivation increased (≥1%), taste perversion (≥1%), weight gain/loss (≥1%)

Genitourinary: Ejaculation disorder (6%), impotence (3%; dose related), polyuria (≥1%)

Neuromuscular & skeletal: Tremor (8%), arthralgia (2%), myalgia (2%), paresthesia (≥1%)

Ocular: Abnormal accommodation (≥1%)

Respiratory: Rhinitis (5%), upper respiratory tract infection (5%), sinusitis (3%), cough (≥1%)

Drug Interactions

Metabolism/Transport Effects Substrate of CYP2C19 (major), CYP2D6 (minor), CYP3A4 (major); **Note:** Assignment of Major/Minor substrate status based on clinically relevant drug interaction potential; **Inhibits** CYP1A2 (weak), CYP2B6 (weak), CYP2C19 (weak), CYP2D6 (weak)

Avoid Concomitant Use

Avoid concomitant use of Citalopram with any of the following: Conivaptan; Highest Risk QTc-Prolonging Agents; Iobenguane I 123; MAO Inhibitors; Methylene Blue; Mifepristone; Moderate Risk QTc-Prolonging Agents; Pimozide; Tryptophan

Increased Effect/Toxicity

Citalopram may increase the levels/effects of: Alpha-/Beta-Blockers; Anticoagulants; Antidepressants (Serotonin Reuptake Inhibitor/Antagonist); Antiplatelet Agents; Aspirin; BusPIRone; CarBAMazepine; CloZAPine; Collagenase (Systemic); Dabigatran Etexilate; Desmopressin; Dextromethorphan; Drotrecogin Alfa (Activated); Highest Risk QTc-Prolonging Agents; Hypoglycemic Agents; Ibritumomab; Lithium; Methadone; Methylene Blue; Metoclopramide; Mexiletine; NSAID (COX-2 Inhibitor); NSAID (Nonselective); Pimozide; RisperiDONE; Rivaroxaban; Salicylates; Serotonin Modulators; Thrombolytic Agents; Tositumomab and Iodine I 131 Tositumomab); TraMADol; Tricyclic Antidepressants; Vitamin K Antagonists

The levels/effects of Citalopram may be increased by: Alcohol (Ethyl); Analgesics (Opioid); Antipsychotics; BusPIRone; Cimetidine; CNS Depressants; Conivaptan; CYP2C19 Inhibitors (Moderate); CYP2C19 Inhibitors (Strong); CYP3A4 Inhibitors (Moderate); CYP3A4 Inhibitors (Strong); Fluconazole; Glucosamine; Herbs (Anticoagulant/Antiplatelet Properties); Ivacaftor; Linezolid; Macrolide Antibiotics; MAO Inhibitors; Metoclopramide; Metyrosine; Mifepristone; Moderate Risk QTc-Prolonging Agents; Omega-3-Acid Ethyl Esters; Pentosan Polysulfate Sodium; Pentoxifylline; Prostacyclin Analogues; QTc-Prolonging Agents (Indeterminate Risk and Risk Modifying); Tipranavir; TraMADol; Tryptophan; Vitamin E

Decreased Effect

Citalopram may decrease the levels/effects of: Iobenguane I 123; Ioflupane I 123

The levels/effects of Citalopram may be decreased by: CarBAMazepine; CYP2C19 Inducers (Strong); CYP3A4 Inducers (Strong); Cyproheptadine; Deferasirox; NSAID (COX-2 Inhibitor); NSAID (Nonselective); Peginterferon Alfa-2b; Tocilizumab

Ethanol/Nutrition/Herb Interactions

Ethanol: May increase CNS depression; monitor for increased effects with coadministration. Caution patients about effects.

Herb/Nutraceutical: Avoid valerian, St John's wort, SAMe, kava kava, and gotu kola (may increase CNS depression).

Stability Store at 25°C (77°F); excursions permitted to 15°C to 30°C (59°F to 86°F). Protect from moisture.

Mechanism of Action A racemic bicyclic phthalane derivative, citalopram selectively inhibits serotonin reuptake in the presynaptic neurons and has minimal effects on norepinephrine or dopamine. Uptake inhibition of serotonin is primarily due to the S-enantiomer of citalopram. Displays little to no affinity for serotonin, dopamine, adrenergic, histamine, GABA, or muscarinic receptor subtypes.

Pharmacodynamics/Kinetics

Onset of action: Depression: The onset of action is 1-4 weeks; however, individual response varies greatly and full response may not be seen until 8-12 weeks after initiation of treatment.

Distribution: V_d: 12 L/kg

Protein binding, plasma: ~80%

Metabolism: Extensively hepatic, via CYP3A4 and 2C19 (major pathways), and 2D6 (minor pathway); metabolized to demethylcitalopram (DCT), didemethylcitalopram (DDCT), citalopram-N-oxide, and a deaminated propionic acid derivative, which are at least eight times less potent than citalopram

Bioavailability: 80%; tablets and oral solution are bioequivalent

Half-life elimination: 24-48 hours (average: 35 hours); doubled with hepatic impairment and increased by 30% (following multiple doses) to 50% (following single dose) in elderly patients (≥60 years)

Time to peak, serum: 1-6 hours, average within 4 hours

Excretion: Urine (Citalopram 10% and DCT 5%)

Note: Clearance was decreased, while half-life was significantly increased in patients with hepatic impairment. Mild-to-moderate renal impairment may reduce clearance (17%) and prolong half-life of citalopram. No pharmacokinetic information is available concerning patients with severe renal impairment. AUC and half-life were significantly increased in elderly patients (≥60 years), and in poor CYP2C19 metabolizers, steady state C_{max} and AUC was increased by 68% and 107%, respectively.

Dosage

Geriatric Depression: Elderly ≥60 years: Oral: Initial: 20 mg once daily; maximum dose in adults ≥60 years: 20 mg daily due to increased exposure and the risk of QT prolongation. Refer to adult dosing.

Adult Depression: Adults <60 years: Oral: Initial: 20 mg once daily; increase the dose by 20 mg at an interval of ≥1 week to a maximum dose of 40 mg daily. **Note:** Doses >40 mg daily are not recommended due to the risk of QT prolongation; additional efficacy with doses >40 mg daily has not been demonstrated in clinical trials.

Poor metabolizers of CYP2C19 or concurrent use of moderate-to-strong CYP2C19 inhibitors (eg, cimetidine, omeprazole): Maximum dose: 20 mg daily

Renal Impairment

Mild-to-moderate impairment: No dosage adjustment necessary.

Severe impairment: Cl_{cr} <20 mL/minute: No dosage adjustment provided in manufacturer's labeling (has not been studied); use caution.

Hepatic Impairment Initial: 20 mg once daily; maximum recommended dose: 20 mg daily due to decreased clearance and the risk of QT prolongation

Administration May be administered without regard to food.

Monitoring Parameters ECG (patients at increased risk for QT-prolonging effects due to certain conditions); electrolytes (potassium and magnesium concentrations [prior to initiation and periodically during therapy in patients at increased risk for electrolyte abnormalities]); signs/symptoms of arrhythmias (eg, dizziness, palpitations, syncope); liver function tests and CBC with continued therapy; monitor patient periodically for symptom resolution; mental status for depression, suicidal ideation (especially at the beginning of therapy or when doses are increased or decreased), anxiety, social functioning, mania, panic attacks; akathisia

Special Geriatric Considerations AUC was increased by 23% to 30% and half-life increased by 30% to 50% in older adults ≥60 years of age compared to younger adults. Due to the risk of QT prolongation associated with higher doses of citalopram, a lower maximum daily dose of 20 mg/day in recommended in all older adults.

A seven- to eightfold variation in citalopram S(+) (active) and R(-) enantiomer concentrations have been reported in the elderly. The racemic citalopram concentration-to-dose ratio was 1.8 times greater in elderly patients compared to younger patients. The elderly are also more prone to SSRI/SNRI-induced hyponatremia.

In patients with hepatic impairment, clearance was decreased, while half-life was significantly increased. Mild-to-moderate renal impairment may reduce clearance of citalopram (17% reduction noted in trials). No pharmacokinetic information is available concerning patients with severe renal impairment. Pharmacokinetics was also significantly altered in poor CYP2C19 metabolizers.

A systematic review and meta-analysis of antidepressant placebo-controlled trials in persons with depression and dementia found evidence "suggestive" of efficacy but not of sufficient strength to "confirm" efficacy. Antidepressant trials in this patient population are small and underpowered. Older patients with depression being treated with an antidepressant should be closely monitored for response and adverse effects. Treatment should be switched or augmented when response is inadequate with a therapeutic dose. Antidepressants that are not tolerated should be discontinued and an alternative agent should be started.

This medication is considered to be potentially inappropriate in this patient population (Beers Criteria: Quality of evidence - moderate; Strength of recommendation - strong).

Dosage Forms Excipient information presented when available (limited, particularly for generics); consult specific product labeling.

Solution, oral: 10 mg/5 mL (240 mL)

Tablet, oral: 10 mg, 20 mg, 40 mg

CeleXA®: 10 mg

CeleXA®: 20 mg, 40 mg [scored]

Citric Acid, Sodium Citrate, and Potassium Citrate
(SIT rik AS id, SOW dee um SIT rate, & poe TASS ee um SIT rate)

Medication Safety Issues
Sound-alike/look-alike issues:
Polycitra may be confused with Bicitra
Brand Names: U.S. Cytra-3; Tricitrates

Index Terms Polycitra; Potassium Citrate, Citric Acid, and Sodium Citrate; Sodium Citrate, Citric Acid, and Potassium Citrate

Generic Availability (U.S.) Yes

Pharmacologic Category Alkalinizing Agent

Use Conditions where long-term maintenance of an alkaline urine is desirable as in control and dissolution of uric acid and cystine calculi of the urinary tract

Contraindications Severe renal impairment with oliguria or azotemia; untreated Addison's disease; severe myocardial damage.

Warnings/Precautions Use with caution in patients with heart failure, peripheral or pulmonary edema, and renal impairment; contains sodium. Conversion to bicarbonate may be impaired in patients who are severely ill, in shock, or with hepatic failure. Use with caution in digitalized patients or those who are receiving concomitant medications that increase potassium.

Adverse Reactions (Reflective of adult population; not specific for elderly) Frequency not defined.
Cardiovascular: Cardiac abnormalities
Endocrine & metabolic: Metabolic alkalosis, calcium levels, hyperkalemia, hypernatremia
Gastrointestinal: Diarrhea
Neuromuscular & skeletal: Tetany

Drug Interactions
Metabolism/Transport Effects None known.

Avoid Concomitant Use There are no known interactions where it is recommended to avoid concomitant use.

Increased Effect/Toxicity
Citric Acid, Sodium Citrate, and Potassium Citrate may increase the levels/effects of: ACE Inhibitors; Aluminum Hydroxide; Angiotensin II Receptor Blockers; Potassium-Sparing Diuretics

The levels/effects of Citric Acid, Sodium Citrate, and Potassium Citrate may be increased by: Eplerenone

Decreased Effect There are no known significant interactions involving a decrease in effect.

Stability Store at controlled room temperature of 20°C to 25°C (68°F to 77°F); do not freeze. Protect from excessive heat.

Dosage
Geriatric & Adult Alkalinizing agent/bicarbonate precursor/potassium supplement: Oral: 15-30 mL diluted in water after meals and at bedtime

Administration Administer after meals. Dilute with water prior to administration. Chilling solution prior to dosing helps to enhance palatability. May follow dose with additional water.

Monitoring Parameters Blood gas (pH and bicarbonate); serum bicarbonate

Reference Range Note: Reference ranges may vary depending on the laboratory
Urinary pH: 4.6-8.0

Special Geriatric Considerations
Use with caution in the elderly because of sodium and potassium content.

Dosage Forms Excipient information presented when available (limited, particularly for generics); consult specific product labeling. [DSC] = Discontinued product
Solution, oral:
Cytra-3: Citric acid 334 mg, sodium citrate 500 mg, and potassium citrate 550 mg per 5 mL (480 mL [DSC]) [equivalent to potassium 1 mEq, sodium 1 mEq, and bicarbonate 2 mEq per 1 mL; alcohol free, sugar free; contains sodium benzoate and propylene glycol; raspberry flavor]
Tricitrates: Citric acid 334 mg, sodium citrate 500 mg, and potassium citrate 550 mg per 5 mL (480 mL) [equivalent to potassium 1 mEq, sodium 1 mEq, and bicarbonate 2 mEq per 1 mL; alcohol free; contains sodium benzoate; raspberry flavor]
Tricitrates: Citric acid 334 mg, sodium citrate 500 mg, and potassium citrate 550 mg per 5 mL (15 mL [DSC]; 30 mL [DSC]; 480 mL [DSC]) [equivalent to potassium 1 mEq, sodium 1 mEq, and bicarbonate 2 mEq per 1 mL; alcohol free, sugar free; contains sodiuim benzoate and propylene glycol; raspberry flavor]

◆ **Citroma® [OTC]** *see* Magnesium Citrate *on page* 1175
◆ **CL-118,532** *see* Triptorelin *on page* 1976

◆ **CI-719** *see* Gemfibrozil *on page* 869
◆ **Claforan®** *see* Cefotaxime *on page* 318
◆ **Clarinex®** *see* Desloratadine *on page* 510

Clarithromycin (kla RITH roe mye sin)

Related Information

Antimicrobial Drugs of Choice *on page* 2163
Community-Acquired Pneumonia in Adults *on page* 2171
H. pylori Treatment in Adult Patients *on page* 2116
Prevention of Infective Endocarditis *on page* 2175

Medication Safety Issues

Sound-alike/look-alike issues:
Clarithromycin may be confused with Claritin®, clindamycin, erythromycin

Brand Names: U.S. Biaxin®; Biaxin® XL

Brand Names: Canada Apo-Clarithromycin®; Ava-Clarithromycin; Biaxin®; Biaxin® XL; Dom-Clarithromycin; Mylan-Clarithromycin; PMS-Clarithromycin; RAN™-Clarithromycin; ratio-Clarithromycin; Riva-Clarithromycin; Sandoz-Clarithromycin

Generic Availability (U.S.) Yes

Pharmacologic Category Antibiotic, Macrolide

Use

Adults:

Pharyngitis/tonsillitis due to susceptible *S. pyogenes*

Acute maxillary sinusitis due to susceptible *H. influenzae, M. catarrhalis,* or *S. pneumoniae*

Acute exacerbation of chronic bronchitis due to susceptible *H. influenzae, H. parainfluenzae, M. catarrhalis,* or *S. pneumoniae*

Community-acquired pneumonia due to susceptible *H. influenzae, H. parainfluenzae, Mycoplasma pneumoniae, S. pneumoniae,* or *Chlamydia pneumoniae* (TWAR), *Moraxella catarrhalis*

Uncomplicated skin/skin structure infections due to susceptible *S. aureus, S. pyogenes*

Disseminated mycobacterial infections due to *M. avium* or *M. intracellulare*

Prevention of disseminated mycobacterial infections due to *M. avium* complex (MAC) disease (eg, patients with advanced HIV infection)

Duodenal ulcer disease due to *H. pylori* in regimens with other drugs including amoxicillin and lansoprazole or omeprazole, ranitidine bismuth citrate, bismuth subsalicylate, tetracycline, and/or an H_2 antagonist

Unlabeled Use Pertussis (CDC guidelines); alternate antibiotic for prophylaxis of infective endocarditis in patients who are allergic to penicillin and undergoing surgical or dental procedures (ACC/AHA guidelines)

Contraindications Hypersensitivity to clarithromycin, erythromycin, or any macrolide antibiotic; use with ergot derivatives, pimozide, cisapride, astemizole, terfenadine, colchicine (if patient has concomitant renal or hepatic impairment); history of cholestatic jaundice or hepatic dysfunction with prior clarithromycin use

Warnings/Precautions Dosage adjustment required with severe renal impairment; decreased dosage or prolonged dosing interval may be appropriate. May cause hepatotoxicity (elevated liver function tests, hepatitis, jaundice, hepatic failure); use caution with pre-existing hepatic disease or hepatotoxic medications. Use with caution in patients with myasthenia gravis. Colchicine toxicity (including fatalities) has been reported with concomitant use; concomitant use is contraindicated in patients with renal or hepatic impairment. Prolonged use may result in fungal or bacterial superinfection, including *C. difficile*-associated diarrhea (CDAD) and pseudomembranous colitis; CDAD has been observed >2 months postantibiotic treatment. Macrolides (including clarithromycin) have been associated with rare QT prolongation and ventricular arrhythmias, including torsade de pointes. Use caution in patients with coronary artery disease. Avoid use of extended release tablets (Biaxin® XL) in patients with known stricture/narrowing of the GI tract.

Adverse Reactions (Reflective of adult population; not specific for elderly) 1% to 10%:

Central nervous system: Headache (adults and children 2%)

Dermatologic: Rash (children 3%)

Gastrointestinal: Abnormal taste (adults 3% to 7%), diarrhea (adults 3% to 6%; children 6%), vomiting (children 6%), nausea (adults 3%), abdominal pain (adults 2%; children 3%), dyspepsia (adults 2%)

Hepatic: Prothrombin time increased (adults 1%)

Renal: BUN increased (4%)

Drug Interactions

Metabolism/Transport Effects Substrate of CYP3A4 (major); **Note:** Assignment of Major/ Minor substrate status based on clinically relevant drug interaction potential; **Inhibits** CYP1A2 (weak), CYP3A4 (strong), P-glycoprotein

Avoid Concomitant Use

Avoid concomitant use of Clarithromycin with any of the following: Alfuzosin; Avanafil; Axitinib; BCG; Cisapride; Conivaptan; Crizotinib; Dihydroergotamine; Disopyramide; Dronedarone; Eplerenone; Ergotamine; Everolimus; Fluticasone (Oral Inhalation); Halofantrine; Highest Risk QTc-Prolonging Agents; Lapatinib; Lovastatin; Lurasidone; Mifepristone; Nilotinib; Nisoldipine; Pimozide; QuiNINE; Ranolazine; Red Yeast Rice; Rivaroxaban; RomiDEPsin; Salmeterol; Silodosin; Simvastatin; Tamsulosin; Terfenadine; Ticagrelor; Tolvaptan; Topotecan; Toremifene

Increased Effect/Toxicity

Clarithromycin may increase the levels/effects of: Alfentanil; Alfuzosin; Almotriptan; Alosetron; Antifungal Agents (Azole Derivatives, Systemic); Antineoplastic Agents (Vinca Alkaloids); ARIPiprazole; Avanafil; Axitinib; Benzodiazepines (metabolized by oxidation); Boceprevir; Bortezomib; Brentuximab Vedotin; Brinzolamide; Budesonide (Nasal); Budesonide (Systemic, Oral Inhalation); BusPIRone; Calcium Channel Blockers; CarBAMazepine; Cardiac Glycosides; Ciclesonide; Cilostazol; Cisapride; CloZAPine; Colchicine; Conivaptan; Corticosteroids (Orally Inhaled); Corticosteroids (Systemic); Crizotinib; CycloSPORINE; CycloSPORINE (Systemic); CYP3A4 Inducers (Strong); CYP3A4 Substrates; Dabigatran Etexilate; Dienogest; Dihydroergotamine; Disopyramide; Dronedarone; Dutasteride; Eletriptan; Eplerenone; Ergot Derivatives; Ergotamine; Everolimus; FentaNYL; Fesoterodine; Fluticasone (Nasal); Fluticasone (Oral Inhalation); GlipiZIDE; GlyBURIDE; GuanFACINE; Halofantrine; Highest Risk QTc-Prolonging Agents; HMG-CoA Reductase Inhibitors; Iloperidone; Ivacaftor; Ixabepilone; Lapatinib; Lovastatin; Lumefantrine; Lurasidone; Maraviroc; MethylPREDNISolone; Mifepristone; Moderate Risk QTc-Prolonging Agents; Nilotinib; Nisoldipine; Paricalcitol; Pazopanib; P-glycoprotein/ABCB1 Substrates; Pimecrolimus; Pimozide; Propafenone; Protease Inhibitors; Prucalopride; QuiNIDine; QuiNINE; Ranolazine; Red Yeast Rice; Repaglinide; Rifamycin Derivatives; Rivaroxaban; RomiDEPsin; Ruxolitinib; Salmeterol; Saxagliptin; Selective Serotonin Reuptake Inhibitors; Sildenafil; Silodosin; Simvastatin; Sirolimus; SORAfenib; Tacrolimus; Tacrolimus (Systemic); Tacrolimus (Topical); Tadalafil; Tamsulosin; Telaprevir; Temsirolimus; Terfenadine; Theophylline Derivatives; Ticagrelor; Tolterodine; Tolvaptan; Topotecan; Toremifene; Vardenafil; Vemurafenib; Vilazodone; Vitamin K Antagonists; Zidovudine; Zopiclone; Zuclopenthixol

The levels/effects of Clarithromycin may be increased by: Antifungal Agents (Azole Derivatives, Systemic); Boceprevir; CYP3A4 Inducers (Strong); CYP3A4 Inhibitors (Moderate); CYP3A4 Inhibitors (Strong); Mifepristone; Protease Inhibitors; QTc-Prolonging Agents (Indeterminate Risk and Risk Modifying); Telaprevir

Decreased Effect

Clarithromycin may decrease the levels/effects of: BCG; Clopidogrel; Ifosfamide; Prasugrel; Ticagrelor; Typhoid Vaccine; Zidovudine

The levels/effects of Clarithromycin may be decreased by: CYP3A4 Inducers (Strong); Deferasirox; Etravirine; Herbs (CYP3A4 Inducers); Protease Inhibitors; Tocilizumab

Ethanol/Nutrition/Herb Interactions

Food: Immediate release: Food delays rate, but not extent of absorption; Extended release: Food increases clarithromycin AUC by ~30% relative to fasting conditions.

Herb/Nutraceutical: St John's wort may decrease clarithromycin levels.

Stability

Immediate release 250 mg tablets and granules for oral suspension: Store at controlled room temperature of 15°C to 30°C (59°F to 86°F). Reconstituted oral suspension should not be refrigerated because it might gel; microencapsulated particles of clarithromycin in suspension are stable for 14 days when stored at room temperature. Protect tablets from light.

Immediate release 500 mg tablets and Biaxin® XL: Store at controlled room temperature of 20°C to 25°C (68°F to 77°F); excursions permitted to 15°C to 30°C (59°F to 86°F).

Mechanism of Action Exerts its antibacterial action by binding to 50S ribosomal subunit resulting in inhibition of protein synthesis. The 14-OH metabolite of clarithromycin is twice as active as the parent compound against certain organisms.

Pharmacodynamics/Kinetics

Absorption: Immediate release: Rapid; food delays rate, but not extent of absorption

Distribution: Widely into most body tissues except CNS

Protein binding: 42% to 50%

Metabolism: Partially hepatic via CYP3A4; converted to 14-OH clarithromycin (active metabolite)

Bioavailability: ~50%

◀ Half-life elimination: Immediate release: Clarithromycin: 3-7 hours; 14-OH-clarithromycin: 5-9 hours

Time to peak: Immediate release: 2-3 hours

Excretion: Primarily urine (20% to 40% as unchanged drug; additional 10% to 15% as metabolite)

Clearance: Approximates normal GFR

Dosage

Geriatric & Adult

Usual dosage range: Oral: 250-500 mg every 12 hours **or** 1000 mg (two 500 mg extended release tablets) once daily for 7-14 days

Acute exacerbation of chronic bronchitis: Oral:

M. catarrhalis and *S. pneumoniae*: 250 mg every 12 hours for 7-14 days **or** 1000 mg (two 500 mg extended release tablets) once daily for 7 days

H. influenzae: 500 mg every 12 hours for 7-14 days **or** 1000 mg (two 500 mg extended release tablets) once daily for 7 days

H. parainfluenzae: 500 mg every 12 hours for 7 days **or** 1000 mg (two 500 mg extended release tablets) once daily for 7 days

Acute maxillary sinusitis: Oral: 500 mg every 12 hours **or** 1000 mg (two 500 mg extended release tablets) once daily for 14 days

Mycobacterial infection (prevention and treatment): Oral: 500 mg twice daily (use with other antimycobacterial drugs, eg, ethambutol or rifampin)

Peptic ulcer disease: Eradication of *Helicobacter pylori*: Dual or triple combination regimens with bismuth subsalicylate, amoxicillin, an H_2-receptor antagonist, or proton-pump inhibitor: 500 mg every 8-12 hours for 10-14 days

Pertussis (unlabeled use; CDC, 2005): Oral: 500 mg twice daily for 7 days

Pharyngitis, tonsillitis: Oral: 250 mg every 12 hours for 10 days

Pneumonia: Oral:

C. pneumoniae, M. pneumoniae, and *S. pneumoniae*: 250 mg every 12 hours for 7-14 days **or** 1000 mg (two 500 mg extended release tablets) once daily for 7 days

H. influenzae: 250 mg every 12 hours for 7 days **or** 1000 mg (two 500 mg extended release tablets) once daily for 7 days

H. parainfluenzae and *M. catarrhalis*: 1000 mg (two 500 mg extended release tablets) once daily for 7 days

Prophylaxis against infective endocarditis (unlabeled use): Oral: 500 mg 30-60 minutes prior to procedure. **Note:** American Heart Association (AHA) guidelines now recommend prophylaxis only in patients undergoing invasive procedures and in whom underlying cardiac conditions may predispose to a higher risk of adverse outcomes should infection occur. As of April 2007, routine prophylaxis for GI/GU procedures is no longer recommended by the AHA.

Skin and skin structure infection, uncomplicated: Oral: 250 mg every 12 hours for 7-14 days

Renal Impairment

Cl_{cr} <30 mL/minute: Decrease clarithromycin dose by 50%

Hemodialysis: Administer after HD session is completed (Aronoff, 2007).

In combination with atazanavir or ritonavir:

Cl_{cr} 30-60 mL/minute: Decrease clarithromycin dose by 50%.

Cl_{cr} <30 mL/minute: Decrease clarithromycin dose by 75%.

Hepatic Impairment No dosing adjustment is needed as long as renal function is normal.

Administration Clarithromycin immediate release tablets and oral suspension may be administered with or without meals. Give every 12 hours rather than twice daily to avoid peak and trough variation. Shake suspension well before each use.

Extended release tablets: Should be given with food. Do not crush or chew extended release tablet.

Monitoring Parameters CBC with differential, BUN, creatinine; perform culture and sensitivity studies prior to initiating drug therapy

Special Geriatric Considerations Considered one of the drugs of choice in the outpatient treatment of community-acquired pneumonia in elderly. After doses of 500 mg every 12 hours for 5 days, 12 healthy elderly subjects had significantly increased C_{max} and C_{min}, elimination half-lives of clarithromycin and 14-OH clarithromycin compared to 12 healthy young subjects. These changes were attributed to a significant decrease in renal clearance; at a dose of 1000 mg twice daily, 100% of 13 elderly subjects experienced an adverse event compared to only 10% taking 500 mg twice daily.

Dosage Forms Excipient information presented when available (limited, particularly for generics); consult specific product labeling.

Granules for suspension, oral: 125 mg/5 mL (50 mL, 100 mL); 250 mg/5 mL (50 mL, 100 mL)
  Biaxin®: 125 mg/5 mL (50 mL, 100 mL); 250 mg/5 mL (50 mL, 100 mL) [fruit-punch flavor]
Tablet, oral: 250 mg, 500 mg
  Biaxin®: 250 mg, 500 mg
Tablet, extended release, oral: 500 mg
  Biaxin® XL: 500 mg

◆ **Claritin® 24 Hour Allergy [OTC]** *see* Loratadine *on page 1155*
◆ **Claritin® Children's Allergy [OTC]** *see* Loratadine *on page 1155*
◆ **Claritin™ Eye [OTC]** *see* Ketotifen (Ophthalmic) *on page 1076*
◆ **Claritin® Liqui-Gels® 24 Hour Allergy [OTC]** *see* Loratadine *on page 1155*
◆ **Claritin® RediTabs® 24 Hour Allergy [OTC]** *see* Loratadine *on page 1155*
◆ **Clavulanic Acid and Amoxicillin** *see* Amoxicillin and Clavulanate *on page 115*
◆ **Clean & Clear® Advantage® Acne Cleanser [OTC]** *see* Salicylic Acid *on page 1743*
◆ **Clean & Clear® Advantage® Acne Spot Treatment [OTC]** *see* Salicylic Acid *on page 1743*
◆ **Clean & Clear® Advantage® Invisible Acne Patch [OTC]** *see* Salicylic Acid *on page 1743*
◆ **Clean & Clear® Advantage® Oil-Free Acne [OTC]** *see* Salicylic Acid *on page 1743*
◆ **Clean & Clear® Blackhead Clearing Daily Cleansing [OTC]** *see* Salicylic Acid *on page 1743*
◆ **Clean & Clear® Blackhead Clearing Scrub [OTC]** *see* Salicylic Acid *on page 1743*
◆ **Clean & Clear® Deep Cleaning [OTC]** *see* Salicylic Acid *on page 1743*
◆ **Clean & Clear® Dual Action Moisturizer [OTC]** *see* Salicylic Acid *on page 1743*
◆ **Clean & Clear® Invisible Blemish Treatment [OTC]** *see* Salicylic Acid *on page 1743*
◆ **Clear eyes® for Dry Eyes Plus ACR Relief [OTC]** *see* Naphazoline (Ophthalmic) *on page 1337*
◆ **Clear eyes® for Dry Eyes plus Redness Relief [OTC]** *see* Naphazoline (Ophthalmic) *on page 1337*
◆ **Clear eyes® Redness Relief [OTC]** *see* Naphazoline (Ophthalmic) *on page 1337*
◆ **Clear eyes® Seasonal Relief [OTC]** *see* Naphazoline (Ophthalmic) *on page 1337*

Clemastine (KLEM as teen)

Related Information
  Beers Criteria – Potentially Inappropriate Medications for Geriatrics *on page 2183*
Medication Safety Issues
  BEERS Criteria medication:
    This drug may be potentially inappropriate for use in geriatric patients (Quality of evidence - moderate; Strength of recommendation - strong).
Brand Names: U.S. Tavist® Allergy [OTC]
Index Terms Clemastine Fumarate
Generic Availability (U.S.) Yes
Pharmacologic Category Ethanolamine Derivative; Histamine H_1 Antagonist; Histamine H_1 Antagonist, First Generation
Use Perennial and seasonal allergic rhinitis and other allergic symptoms including urticaria
Contraindications Hypersensitivity to clemastine or any component of the formulation; narrow-angle glaucoma
Warnings/Precautions Use caution with bladder neck obstruction, symptomatic prostate hypertrophy, asthmatic attacks, stenosing peptic ulcer, increased intraocular pressure, hyperthyroidism, cardiovascular disease, hypertension, and in the elderly. May cause drowsiness; use caution in performing tasks which require alertness. Effects may be potentiated when used with other sedative drugs or ethanol. In the eldery, avoid use of this potent anticholinergic agent due to increased risk of confusion, dry mouth, constipation, and other anticholinergic effects; clearance decreases in patients of advanced age (Beers Criteria).
Adverse Reactions (Reflective of adult population; not specific for elderly) Frequency not defined.
  Cardiovascular: Palpitation, hypotension, tachycardia
  Central nervous system: Dyscoordination, sedation, somnolence slight to moderate, sleepiness, confusion, restlessness, nervousness, insomnia, irritability, fatigue, headache, dizziness increased
  Dermatologic: Rash, photosensitivity
  Gastrointestinal: Diarrhea, nausea, xerostomia, epigastric distress, vomiting, constipation
  Genitourinary: Urinary frequency, difficult urination, urinary retention
  Hematologic: Hemolytic anemia, thrombocytopenia, agranulocytosis
  Ocular: Blurred vision
  Otic: Tinnitus

◄ Respiratory: Thickening of bronchial secretions
Miscellaneous: Anaphylaxis

Drug Interactions

Metabolism/Transport Effects Inhibits CYP2D6 (weak), CYP3A4 (weak)

Avoid Concomitant Use

Avoid concomitant use of Clemastine with any of the following: Azelastine; Azelastine (Nasal); Methadone; Mirtazapine; Paraldehyde; Pimozide

Increased Effect/Toxicity

Clemastine may increase the levels/effects of: Alcohol (Ethyl); Anticholinergics; ARIPiprazole; Azelastine; Azelastine (Nasal); Buprenorphine; CNS Depressants; Methadone; Methotrimeprazine; Metyrosine; Mirtazapine; Paraldehyde; Pimozide; Selective Serotonin Reuptake Inhibitors; Zolpidem

The levels/effects of Clemastine may be increased by: Droperidol; HydrOXYzine; Methotrimeprazine; Pramlintide

Decreased Effect

Clemastine may decrease the levels/effects of: Acetylcholinesterase Inhibitors (Central); Benzylpenicilloyl Polylysine; Betahistine; Hyaluronidase

The levels/effects of Clemastine may be decreased by: Acetylcholinesterase Inhibitors (Central); Amphetamines

Ethanol/Nutrition/Herb Interactions Ethanol: May increase CNS depression; monitor for increased effects with coadministration. Caution patients about effects.

Mechanism of Action Competes with histamine for H_1-receptor sites on effector cells in the gastrointestinal tract, blood vessels, and respiratory tract

Pharmacodynamics/Kinetics

Onset of action: Peak effect: Therapeutic: 5-7 hours
Duration: 8-12 hours; may persist for 24 hours
Absorption: Well absorbed
Distribution: V_d: ~800 L (range: 500-1000 L) (Sharma, 2003)
Metabolism: Hepatic; metabolized via unidentified enzymes by O-dealkylation followed by alcohol dehydration, aliphatic oxidation, aromatic oxidation, and direct oxidation; significant first-pass effect (Sharma, 2003)
Bioavailability: ~40% (Sharma, 2003)
Half-life elimination: ~21 hours (range: 10-33 hours) (Sharma, 2003)
Time to peak: 2-4 hours
Excretion: Urine (~42% as metabolites) (Sharma, 2003)

Dosage

Geriatric Lower doses should be considered in patients >60 years of age.

Adult

Rhinitis or allergic symptoms (including urticaria): Oral:
1.34 mg clemastine fumarate (1 mg base) twice daily to 2.68 mg (2 mg base) 3 times/day; do not exceed 8.04 mg/day (6 mg base)
OTC labeling: 1.34 mg clemastine fumarate (1 mg base) twice daily; do not exceed 2 mg base/24 hours

Monitoring Parameters Look for a reduction of rhinitis, urticaria, eczema, pruritus, or other allergic symptoms

Special Geriatric Considerations Elderly patients may be more susceptible to adverse effects.

This medication is considered to be potentially inappropriate in this patient population (Beers Criteria: Quality of evidence - moderate; Strength of recommendation - strong).

Dosage Forms Excipient information presented when available (limited, particularly for generics); consult specific product labeling.
Syrup, oral, as fumarate: 0.67 mg/5 mL (120 mL) [equivalent to clemastine base 0.5 mg/5 mL; prescription formulation]
Tablet, oral, as fumarate: 1.34 mg [equivalent to clemastine base 1 mg; OTC], 2.68 mg [equivalent to clemastine base 2 mg; prescription formulation]
Tavist® Allergy: 1.34 mg [scored; equivalent to clemastine base 1 mg]

◆ **Clemastine Fumarate** *see* Clemastine *on page 395*
◆ **Cleocin®** *see* Clindamycin (Topical) *on page 402*
◆ **Cleocin HCl®** *see* Clindamycin (Systemic) *on page 399*
◆ **Cleocin Pediatric®** *see* Clindamycin (Systemic) *on page 399*
◆ **Cleocin Phosphate®** *see* Clindamycin (Systemic) *on page 399*
◆ **Cleocin T®** *see* Clindamycin (Topical) *on page 402*
◆ **Cleocin® Vaginal Ovule** *see* Clindamycin (Topical) *on page 402*

Clevidipine (klev ID i peen)

Related Information
Calcium Channel Blockers – Comparative Pharmacokinetics *on page 2111*

Medication Safety Issues
Sound-alike/look-alike issues:
Clevidipine may be confused with cladribine, clofarabine, clomiPRAMINE
Cleviprex® may be confused with Claravis™

Brand Names: U.S. Cleviprex®

Index Terms Clevidipine Butyrate

Generic Availability (U.S.) No

Pharmacologic Category Calcium Channel Blocker; Calcium Channel Blocker, Dihydropyridine

Use Management of hypertension

Contraindications Hypersensitivity to clevidipine or any component of the formulation (soybeans, soy products, eggs, egg products); hypertriglyceridemia or complications of hypertriglyceridemia (eg, acute pancreatitis); lipoid nephrosis; severe aortic stenosis

Warnings/Precautions Symptomatic hypotension with or without syncope and reflex tachycardia may rarely occur. Blood pressure must be lowered at a rate appropriate for the patient's clinical condition; dosage reductions may be necessary. Treatment of clevidipine-induced tachycardia with beta-blockers is **not** recommended. After prolonged use, discontinuation may cause rebound hypertension; monitor closely for ≥8 hours after discontinuation. Use with caution in patients with heart failure (may worsen symptoms). Clevidipine is formulated within a 20% fat emulsion (0.2 g/mL); hypertriglyceridemia is an expected side effect with high-dose or extended treatment periods; median infusion duration in clinical trials was approximately 6.5 hours (Aronson, 2008). Patients who develop hypertriglyceridemia (eg, >500 mg/dL) are at risk of developing pancreatitis. A reduction in the quantity of concurrently administered lipids may be necessary. Use is contraindicated in patients with hypertriglyceridemia or complications associated with hypertriglyceridemia (eg, acute pancreatitis) and lipoid nephrosis. Withdrawal from concomitant beta-blocker therapy should be done gradually. Initiate therapy at the low end of the dosage range in the elderly, with careful upward titration if needed. Use within 12 hours of puncturing vial; maintain aseptic technique while handling.

Adverse Reactions (Reflective of adult population; not specific for elderly)
>10%:
Cardiovascular: Atrial fibrillation (21%)
Central nervous system: Fever (19%), insomnia (12%)
Gastrointestinal: Nausea (5% to 21%)
1% to 10%:
Central nervous system: Headache (6%)
Gastrointestinal: Vomiting (3%)
Hematologic: Postprocedural hemorrhage (3%)
Renal: Acute renal failure (9%)
Respiratory: Pneumonia (3%), respiratory failure (3%)

Drug Interactions
Metabolism/Transport Effects None known.

Avoid Concomitant Use There are no known interactions where it is recommended to avoid concomitant use.

Increased Effect/Toxicity
Clevidipine may increase the levels/effects of: Amifostine; Antihypertensives; Beta-Blockers; Calcium Channel Blockers (Nondihydropyridine); Hypotensive Agents; Magnesium Salts; Neuromuscular-Blocking Agents (Nondepolarizing); Nitroprusside; QuiNIDine; RiTUXimab

The levels/effects of Clevidipine may be increased by: Alpha1-Blockers; Calcium Channel Blockers (Nondihydropyridine); Diazoxide; Herbs (Hypotensive Properties); Magnesium Salts; MAO Inhibitors; Pentoxifylline; Phosphodiesterase 5 Inhibitors; Prostacyclin Analogues; QuiNIDine

Decreased Effect
Clevidipine may decrease the levels/effects of: QuiNIDine

The levels/effects of Clevidipine may be decreased by: Calcium Salts; Herbs (Hypertensive Properties); Methylphenidate; Yohimbine

Ethanol/Nutrition/Herb Interactions Herb/Nutraceutical: Avoid bayberry, blue cohosh, cayenne, ephedra, ginger, ginseng (American), kola, licorice (may worsen hypertension). Avoid black cohosh, California poppy, coleus, golden seal, hawthorn, mistletoe, periwinkle, quinine, shepherd's purse (may have increased antihypertensive effect).

Stability Store in refrigerator at 2°C to 8°C (36°F to 46°F). Unopened vials are stable for 2 months at room temperature. Vials are stable for 12 hours once opened. Protect from light during storage. Do not freeze.

Mechanism of Action Dihydropyridine calcium channel blocker with potent arterial vaso-dilating activity. Inhibits calcium ion influx through the L-type calcium channels during depolarization in arterial smooth muscle, producing a decrease in mean arterial pressure (MAP) by reducing systemic vascular resistance.

Pharmacodynamics/Kinetics
Onset of action: 2-4 minutes after start of infusion
Duration: I.V.: 5-15 minutes
Distribution: V_{dss}: 0.17 L/kg
Protein binding: >99.5%
Metabolism: Rapid hydrolysis primarily by esterases in blood and extravascular tissues to an inactive carboxylic acid metabolite and formaldehyde
Half-life elimination: Biphasic: Initial: 1 minute (predominant); Terminal: 15 minutes
Excretion: Urine (63% to 74% as metabolites); feces (7% to 22% as metabolites)

Dosage
Geriatric Refer to adult dosing. Initiate at the low end of the dosage range.
Adult Management of hypertension: I.V.: Initial: 1-2 mg/hour
Titration: Initial: dose may be doubled at 90-second intervals toward blood pressure goal. As blood pressure approaches goal, dose may be increased by less than double every 5-10 minutes. **Note:** For every 1-2 mg/hour increase in dose, an approximate reduction of 2-4 mm Hg in systolic blood pressure may occur.
Usual maintenance: 4-6 mg/hour; maximum: 21 mg/hour (1000 mL within a 24-hour period due to lipid load restriction). There is limited short-term experience with doses up to 32 mg/hour. Data is limited beyond 72 hours.

Renal Impairment No adjustment required with initial infusion rate.
Hepatic Impairment No adjustment required with initial infusion rate.

Administration I.V.: Maintain aseptic technique. Do not use if contamination is suspected. Do not dilute. Invert vial gently several times to ensure uniformity of emulsion prior to administration. Administer as a slow continuous infusion via central or peripheral line, using infusion device allowing for calibrated infusion rates. Use within 12 hours of puncturing vial; discard any tubing and unused portion, including that currently being infused.

Monitoring Parameters Blood pressure, heart rate; patients who receive prolonged infusions of clevidipine and are not transitioned to other antihypertensive therapy should be monitored for at least 8 hours after discontinuation

Special Geriatric Considerations No overall differences in safety or efficacy noted in the initial studies in elderly. Doses should be started at low end of dosage range and titrated slowly since elderly may experience a greater hypotensive response, reflecting their greater frequency of renal and cardiac disease with decreased function and concomitant drug therapy.

Dosage Forms Excipient information presented when available (limited, particularly for generics); consult specific product labeling. [DSC] = Discontinued product
Injection, emulsion:
Cleviprex®: 0.5 mg/mL (50 mL, 100 mL) [contains edetate disodium, egg yolk phospholipid, soybean oil]
Cleviprex®: 0.5 mg/mL (50 mL [DSC], 100 mL [DSC]) [contains egg yolk phospholipid, soybean oil]

◆ **Clevidipine Butyrate** see Clevidipine on page 397
◆ **Cleviprex®** see Clevidipine on page 397

Clidinium and Chlordiazepoxide (kli DI nee um & klor dye az e POKS ide)

Related Information
Beers Criteria – Potentially Inappropriate Medications for Geriatrics on page 2183
ChlordiazePOXIDE on page 354
Medication Safety Issues
Sound-alike/look-alike issues:
Librax® may be confused with Librium
BEERS Criteria medication:
This drug may be inappropriate for use in geriatric patients (Quality of evidence: moderate [clidinium]/high [chlordiazepoxide]; Strength of recommendation - strong).
Brand Names: U.S. Librax®
Brand Names: Canada Apo-Chlorax®; Librax®
Index Terms Chlordiazepoxide and Clidinium
Generic Availability (U.S.) Yes

Pharmacologic Category Antispasmodic Agent, Gastrointestinal; Benzodiazepine
Use Adjunct treatment of peptic ulcer; treatment of irritable bowel syndrome
Dosage
  Geriatric & Adult Adjunct treatment of peptic ulcer; treatment of IBS: Oral: 1-2 capsules 3-4 times/day, before meals or food and at bedtime. **Caution:** Do not abruptly discontinue after prolonged use; taper dose gradually.
  Special Geriatric Considerations The use of anticholinergic agents may cause problems with bladder emptying, constipation, or confusion. The addition of chlordiazepoxide may enhance confusion potential. Avoid use in the elderly; if it must be used, monitor closely.

  This medication is considered to be potentially inappropriate in this patient population (Beers Criteria: Quality of evidence: moderate [clidinium]/high [chlordiazepoxide]; Strength of recommendation - strong)
  Dosage Forms Excipient information presented when available (limited, particularly for generics); consult specific product labeling.
    Capsule: Clidinium bromide 2.5 mg and chlordiazepoxide hydrochloride 5 mg
      Librax®: Clidinium bromide 2.5 mg and chlordiazepoxide hydrochloride 5 mg

♦ **Climara®** see Estradiol (Systemic) *on page 681*
♦ **Clindagel®** see Clindamycin (Topical) *on page 402*
♦ **ClindaMax®** see Clindamycin (Topical) *on page 402*

Clindamycin (Systemic) (klin da MYE sin)

Related Information
  Antimicrobial Drugs of Choice *on page 2163*
  Community-Acquired Pneumonia in Adults *on page 2171*
  Prevention of Infective Endocarditis *on page 2175*
Medication Safety Issues
  Sound-alike/look-alike issues:
    Cleocin® may be confused with bleomycin, Clinoril®, Cubicin®, Lincocin®
    Clindamycin may be confused with clarithromycin, Claritin®, vancomycin
Brand Names: U.S. Cleocin HCl®; Cleocin Pediatric®; Cleocin Phosphate®
Brand Names: Canada Apo-Clindamycin®; Ava-Clindamycin; Clindamycin Injection, USP; Clindamycine; Dalacin™ C; Mylan-Clindamycin; PMS-Clindamycin; Riva-Clindamycin; Teva-Clindamycin
Index Terms Clindamycin Hydrochloride; Clindamycin Palmitate
Generic Availability (U.S.) Yes
Pharmacologic Category Antibiotic, Lincosamide
Use Treatment of susceptible bacterial infections, mainly those caused by anaerobes, streptococci, pneumococci, and staphylococci; pelvic inflammatory disease (I.V.)
Unlabeled Use May be useful in PCP; alternate treatment for toxoplasmosis; bacterial vaginosis (oral); alternate treatment for MRSA infections; alternate antibiotic for prophylaxis of infective endocarditis in patients who are allergic to penicillin and undergoing surgical or dental procedures (ACC/AHA guidelines); treatment of severe or uncomplicated malaria; treatment of babesiosis
Contraindications Hypersensitivity to clindamycin, lincomycin, or any component of the formulation
Warnings/Precautions Dosage adjustment may be necessary in patients with severe hepatic dysfunction. **[U.S. Boxed Warning]: Can cause severe and possibly fatal colitis.** Prolonged use may result in fungal or bacterial superinfection, including *C. difficile*-associated diarrhea (CDAD) and pseudomembranous colitis; CDAD has been observed >2 months postantibiotic treatment. Use with caution in patients with a history of gastrointestinal disease. Discontinue drug if significant diarrhea, abdominal cramps, or passage of blood and mucus occurs. Some dosage forms contain benzyl alcohol or tartrazine. Use caution in atopic patients. Not appropriate for use in the treatment of meningitis due to inadequate penetration into the CSF.
Adverse Reactions (Reflective of adult population; not specific for elderly) Frequency not defined.
  Cardiovascular: Cardiac arrest (rare; I.V. administration), hypotension (rare; I.V. administration)
  Dermatologic: Erythema multiforme (rare), exfoliative dermatitis (rare), pruritus, rash, Stevens-Johnson syndrome (rare), urticaria
  Gastrointestinal: Abdominal pain, diarrhea, esophagitis, nausea, pseudomembranous colitis, vomiting
  Genitourinary: Vaginitis

399

Hematologic: Agranulocytosis, eosinophilia (transient), neutropenia (transient), thrombocytopenia

Hepatic: Jaundice, liver function test abnormalities

Local: Induration/pain/sterile abscess (I.M.), thrombophlebitis (I.V.)

Neuromuscular & skeletal: Polyarthritis (rare)

Renal: Renal dysfunction (rare)

Miscellaneous: Anaphylactoid reactions (rare)

Drug Interactions

Metabolism/Transport Effects None known.

Avoid Concomitant Use

Avoid concomitant use of Clindamycin (Systemic) with any of the following: BCG; Erythromycin; Erythromycin (Systemic)

Increased Effect/Toxicity

Clindamycin (Systemic) may increase the levels/effects of: Neuromuscular-Blocking Agents

Decreased Effect

Clindamycin (Systemic) may decrease the levels/effects of: BCG; Erythromycin (Systemic); Typhoid Vaccine

The levels/effects of Clindamycin (Systemic) may be decreased by: Erythromycin; Kaolin

Ethanol/Nutrition/Herb Interactions

Food: Peak concentrations may be delayed with food.

Herb/Nutraceutical: St John's wort may decrease clindamycin levels.

Stability

Capsule: Store at room temperature of 20°C to 25°C (68°F to 77°F).

I.V.: Infusion solution in NS or D_5W solution is stable for 16 days at room temperature, 32 days refrigerated, or 8 weeks frozen. Prior to use, store vials and premixed bags at controlled room temperature 20°C to 25°C (68°F to 77°F). After initial use, discard any unused portion of vial after 24 hours.

Oral solution: Do not refrigerate reconstituted oral solution (it will thicken); following reconstitution, oral solution is stable for 2 weeks at room temperature of 20°C to 25°C (68°F to 77°F).

Mechanism of Action Reversibly binds to 50S ribosomal subunits preventing peptide bond formation thus inhibiting bacterial protein synthesis; bacteriostatic or bactericidal depending on drug concentration, infection site, and organism

Pharmacodynamics/Kinetics

Absorption: Oral, hydrochloride: Rapid (90%)

Distribution: High concentrations in bone and urine; no significant levels in CSF, even with inflamed meninges

V_d: ~2 L/kg

Metabolism: Hepatic; forms metabolites (variable activity); Clindamycin phosphate is converted to clindamycin HCl (active)

Half-life elimination: Adults: ~2-3 hours; Elderly 4 hours (range 3.4-5.1 hours)

Time to peak, serum: Oral: Within 60 minutes; I.M.: 1-3 hours

Excretion: Urine (10%) and feces (~4%) as active drug and metabolites

Dosage

Geriatric & Adult

Usual dose:

Oral: 150-450 mg/dose every 6-8 hours; maximum dose: 1.8 g/day

I.M., I.V.: 1.2-2.7 g/day in 2-4 divided doses; maximum dose: 4.8 g/day

Amnionitis: *I.V.:* 450-900 mg every 8 hours

Anthrax (unlabeled use): *I.V.:* 900 mg every 8 hours with ciprofloxacin or doxycycline

Babesiosis (unlabeled use):

Oral: 600 mg 3 times/day for 7-10 days with quinine (*Medical Letter*, 2007)

I.V.: 1.2 g twice daily for 7-10 days with quinine (*Medical Letter*, 2007)

Bacterial vaginosis (unlabeled use): *Oral:* 300 mg twice daily for 7 days (CDC, 2010)

Bite wounds (canine): *Oral:* 300 mg 4 times/day with a fluoroquinolone

Cellulitis due to MRSA (unlabeled use): Oral: 300-450 mg 3 times/day for 5-10 days (Liu, 2011)

Complicated skin/soft tissue infection due to MRSA (unlabeled use): I.V., Oral: 600 mg 3 times/day for 7-14 days (Liu, 2011)

Gangrenous pyomyositis: *I.V.:* 900 mg every 8 hours with penicillin G

Group B streptococcus (neonatal prophylaxis): *I.V.:* 900 mg every 8 hours until delivery

Malaria, severe (unlabeled use): I.V.: Load: 10 mg/kg followed by 15 mg/kg/day divided every 8 hours *plus* I.V. quinidine gluconate; switch to oral therapy (clindamycin *plus* quinine) when able for total clindamycin treatment duration of 7 days (**Note:** Quinine duration is region specific, consult CDC for current recommendations) (CDC, 2009)

Malaria, uncomplicated treatment (unlabeled use): Oral: 20 mg/kg/day divided every 8 hours for 7 days *plus* quinine (CDC, 2009)

Orofacial/parapharyngeal space infections:
Oral: 150-450 mg every 6 hours for at least 7 days; maximum dose: 1.8 g/day
I.V.: 600-900 mg every 8 hours

Osteomyelitis due to MRSA (unlabeled use): *I.V., Oral:* 600 mg 3 times/day for a minimum of 8 weeks (some experts combine with rifampin) (Liu, 2011)

Pelvic inflammatory disease: *I.V.:* 900 mg every 8 hours with gentamicin (conventional or single daily dosing); 24 hours after clinical improvement may convert to oral doxycycline 100 mg twice daily **or** clindamycin 450 mg 4 times/day to complete 14 days of total therapy. Avoid doxycycline if tubo-ovarian abscess is present (CDC, 2010).

Pneumocystis jirovecii **pneumonia (unlabeled use):**
I.V.: 600-900 mg every 6-8 hours with primaquine for 21 days (CDC, 2009)
Oral: 300-450 mg every 6-8 hours with primaquine for 21 days (CDC, 2009)

Pneumonia due to MRSA (unlabeled use): *I.V., Oral:* 600 mg 3 times/day for 7-21 days (Liu, 2011)

Prophylaxis against infective endocarditis (unlabeled use):
Oral: 600 mg 30-60 minutes before procedure with no follow-up dose needed (Wilson, 2007)
I.M., I.V.: 600 mg 30-60 minutes before procedure. Intramuscular injections should be avoided in patients who are receiving anticoagulant therapy. In these circumstances, orally administered regimens should be given whenever possible. Intravenously administered antibiotics should be used for patients who are unable to tolerate or absorb oral medications (Wilson, 2007).
Note: American Heart Association (AHA) guidelines now recommend prophylaxis only in patients undergoing invasive procedures and in whom underlying cardiac conditions may predispose to a higher risk of adverse outcomes should infection occur. As of April 2007, routine prophylaxis for GI/GU procedures is no longer recommended by the AHA.

Prophylaxis in total joint replacement patients undergoing dental procedures which produce bacteremia (unlabeled use):
Oral: 600 mg 1 hour prior to procedure (ADA, 2003)
I.V.: 600 mg 1 hour prior to procedure (for patients unable to take oral medication) (ADA, 2003)

Septic arthritis due to MRSA (unlabeled use): *I.V., Oral:* 600 mg 3 times/day for 3-4 weeks (Liu, 2011)

Toxic shock syndrome: *I.V.:* 900 mg every 8 hours with penicillin G or ceftriaxone

Toxoplasmosis (HIV-exposed/positive; secondary prevention [unlabeled use]): *Oral:* 600 mg every 8 hours (with pyrimethamine and leucovorin calcium) (CDC, 2009)

Renal Impairment No dosage adjustment required in renal impairment.
Poorly dialyzed; no supplemental dose or dosage adjustment necessary, including patients on intermittent hemodialysis, peritoneal dialysis, or continuous renal replacement therapy (eg, CVVHD).

Hepatic Impairment Systemic use: No adjustment required. Use caution with severe hepatic impairment.

Administration
I.M.: Deep I.M. sites, rotate sites; do not exceed 600 mg in a single injection.
I.V.: **Never administer as bolus**; administer by I.V. intermittent infusion over at least 10-60 minutes, at a rate **not** to exceed 30 mg/minute (do not exceed 1200 mg/hour); final concentration for administration should not exceed 18 mg/mL.
Oral: Administer with a full glass of water to minimize esophageal ulceration; give around-the-clock to promote less variation in peak and trough serum levels.

Monitoring Parameters Observe for changes in bowel frequency. Monitor for colitis and resolution of symptoms. During prolonged therapy monitor CBC, liver and renal function tests periodically.

Pharmacotherapy Pearls *In vitro* susceptibility rates to clindamycin are higher in community acquired versus hospital acquired MRSA, although this may vary by geographic region. The D-zone test is recommended for detection of inducible resistance to clindamycin in erythromycin-resistant but clindamycin-susceptible isolates (Liu, 2011).

Special Geriatric Considerations Clindamycin has not been studied in the elderly; however, since it is eliminated principally by nonrenal mechanisms, major alteration in its pharmacokinetics are not expected. Elderly patients are often at a higher risk for developing serious colitis and require close monitoring.

Dosage Forms Excipient information presented when available (limited, particularly for generics); consult specific product labeling.
Capsule, oral, as hydrochloride [strength expressed as base]: 75 mg, 150 mg, 300 mg
Cleocin HCl®: 75 mg, 150 mg [contains tartrazine]
Cleocin HCl®: 300 mg

Granules for solution, oral, as palmitate hydrochloride [strength expressed as base]: 75 mg/5 mL (100 mL)
 Cleocin Pediatric®: 75 mg/5 mL (100 mL) [cherry flavor]
Infusion, premixed in D₅W, as phosphate [strength expressed as base]:
 Cleocin Phosphate®: 300 mg (50 mL); 600 mg (50 mL); 900 mg (50 mL) [contains edetate disodium]
Injection, solution, as phosphate [strength expressed as base]: 150 mg/mL (2 mL, 4 mL, 6 mL, 60 mL)
 Cleocin Phosphate®: 150 mg/mL (2 mL, 4 mL, 6 mL, 60 mL) [contains benzyl alcohol, edetate disodium]

Clindamycin (Topical) (klin da MYE sin)

Related Information
Antimicrobial Drugs of Choice *on page 2163*
Medication Safety Issues
Sound-alike/look-alike issues:
 Cleocin® may be confused with bleomycin, Clinoril®, Cubicin®, Lincocin®
 Clindamycin may be confused with clarithromycin, Claritin®, vancomycin
Brand Names: U.S. Cleocin T®; Cleocin®; Cleocin® Vaginal Ovule; Clindagel®; Clinda-Max®; ClindaReach® [DSC]; Clindesse®; Evoclin®
Brand Names: Canada Clinda-T; Clindasol™; Clindets; Dalacin® C; Dalacin® T; Dalacin® Vaginal; Taro-Clindamycin
Index Terms Clindamycin Phosphate
Generic Availability (U.S.) Yes: Excludes vaginal suppositories
Pharmacologic Category Antibiotic, Lincosamide; Topical Skin Product, Acne
Use Treatment of bacterial vaginosis (vaginal cream, vaginal suppository); topically in treatment of severe acne
Dosage
Geriatric & Adult
Acne: *Topical:*
 Gel (Cleocin T®, ClindaMax®), pledget, lotion, solution: Apply a thin film twice daily
 Gel (Clindagel®), foam (Evoclin®): Apply once daily
Bacterial vaginosis: *Intravaginal:*
 Suppositories: Insert one ovule (100 mg clindamycin) daily into vagina at bedtime for 3 days
 Cream:
  Cleocin®: One full applicator inserted intravaginally once daily before bedtime for 3 or 7 consecutive days
  Clindesse®: One full applicator inserted intravaginally as a single dose at anytime during the day in nonpregnant patients
Special Geriatric Considerations This formulation has not been studied in a sufficient number of elderly patients to draw conclusions.
Dosage Forms Excipient information presented when available (limited, particularly for generics); consult specific product labeling. [DSC] = Discontinued product
Aerosol, foam, topical, as phosphate [strength expressed as base]: 1% (50 g, 100 g)
 Evoclin®: 1% (50 g, 100 g) [contains ethanol 58%]
Cream, vaginal, as phosphate [strength expressed as base]: 2% (40 g)
 Cleocin®: 2% (40 g) [contains benzyl alcohol, mineral oil]
 Clindesse®: 2% (5 g) [contains mineral oil]
Gel, topical, as phosphate [strength expressed as base]: 1% (30 g, 60 g)
 Cleocin T®: 1% (30 g, 60 g)
 Clindagel®: 1% (40 mL, 75 mL)
 ClindaMax®: 1% (30 g, 60 g)
Lotion, topical, as phosphate [strength expressed as base]: 1% (60 mL)
 Cleocin T®: 1% (60 mL)
 ClindaMax®: 1% (60 mL)
Pledget, topical, as phosphate [strength expressed as base]: 1% (60s, 69s [DSC])
 Cleocin T®: 1% (60s) [contains isopropyl alcohol 50%]
 ClindaReach®: 1% (120s [DSC]) [contains isopropyl alcohol 50%]
Solution, topical, as phosphate [strength expressed as base]: 1% (30 mL, 60 mL)
 Cleocin T®: 1% (30 mL, 60 mL) [contains isopropyl alcohol 50%]
Suppository, vaginal, as phosphate [strength expressed as base]:
 Cleocin® Vaginal Ovule: 100 mg (3s) [contains oleaginous base]

Clindamycin and Tretinoin (klin da MYE sin & TRET i noyn)

Brand Names: U.S. Veltin™; Ziana®
Index Terms Clindamycin Phosphate and Tretinoin; Tretinoin and Clindamycin; Veltin™
Generic Availability (U.S.) No
Pharmacologic Category Acne Products; Retinoic Acid Derivative; Topical Skin Product; Topical Skin Product, Acne
Use Treatment of acne vulgaris
Dosage
  Adult Acne: Topical: Apply once daily
Special Geriatric Considerations This formulation has not been studied in a sufficient number of elderly patients to draw conclusions.
Dosage Forms Excipient information presented when available (limited, particularly for generics); consult specific product labeling.
  Gel, topical:
    Veltin™: Clindamycin phosphate 1.2% and tretinoin 0.025% (30 g, 60 g)
    Ziana®: Clindamycin phosphate 1.2% and tretinoin 0.025% (30 g, 60 g)

- **Clindamycin Hydrochloride** see Clindamycin (Systemic) on page 399
- **Clindamycin Palmitate** see Clindamycin (Systemic) on page 399
- **Clindamycin Phosphate** see Clindamycin (Topical) on page 402
- **Clindamycin Phosphate and Tretinoin** see Clindamycin and Tretinoin on page 403
- **ClindaReach® [DSC]** see Clindamycin (Topical) on page 402
- **Clindesse®** see Clindamycin (Topical) on page 402
- **Clinoril®** see Sulindac on page 1819
- **Clinpro™ 5000** see Fluoride on page 806

Clobazam (KLOE ba zam)

Medication Safety Issues
  Sound-alike/look-alike issues:
    Clobazam may be confused with clonazePAM
Brand Names: U.S. Onfi™
Brand Names: Canada Apo-Clobazam®; Clobazam-10; Dom-Clobazam; Frisium®; Novo-Clobazam; PMS-Clobazam
Pharmacologic Category Benzodiazepine
Use Adjunctive treatment of seizures associated with Lennox-Gastaut syndrome

Canadian labeling: Adjunctive treatment of epilepsy
Unlabeled Use Catamenial epilepsy; epilepsy (monotherapy)
Medication Guide Available Yes
Contraindications There are no contraindications in the manufacturer's labeling.

Canadian labeling (not in U.S. labeling): Hypersensitivity to clobazam or any component of the formulation (cross sensitivity with other benzodiazepines may exist); myasthenia gravis; narrow-angle glaucoma; severe hepatic or respiratory disease; sleep apnea; history of substance abuse

Warnings/Precautions Rebound or withdrawal symptoms may occur following abrupt discontinuation or large decreases in dose (more common with prolonged treatment). Cautiously taper dose if drug discontinuation is required. Use with caution in elderly or debilitated patients, patients with mild-to-moderate hepatic impairment or with pre-existing muscle weakness or ataxia (may cause muscle weakness).

Causes CNS depression (dose related) resulting in sedation, dizziness, confusion, or ataxia which may impair physical and mental capabilities. Patients must be cautioned about performing tasks which require mental alertness (eg, operating machinery or driving). Use with caution in patients receiving other CNS depressants or psychoactive agents. Effects with other sedative drugs or ethanol may be potentiated. Use with caution in patients with an impaired gag reflex or respiratory disease.

Tolerance, psychological and physical dependence may occur with prolonged use. Where possible, avoid use in patients with drug abuse, alcoholism, or psychiatric disease (eg, depression, psychosis). May increase risk of suicidal thoughts/behavior.

Acute withdrawal, including seizures, may be precipitated in patients after administration of flumazenil to patients receiving long-term benzodiazepine therapy.

403

◀ Benzodiazepines have been associated with anterograde amnesia. Paradoxical reactions, including hyperactive or aggressive behavior, have been reported with benzodiazepines, particularly in psychiatric patients. Does not have analgesic, antidepressant, or antipsychotic properties.

Adverse Reactions (Reflective of adult population; not specific for elderly)
>10%:
Central nervous system: Somnolence (22%), fever (13%), lethargy (10%)
Respiratory: Upper respiratory tract infection (12%)
1% to 10%:
Central nervous system: Aggressiveness (8%), irritability (7%), ataxia (5%), fatigue (5%), insomnia (5%), sedation (5%), psychomotor hyperactivity (4%)
Gastrointestinal: Salivation increased (9%), vomiting (7%), constipation (5%), appetite increased (3%), dysphagia (2%)
Genitourinary: Urinary tract infection (4%)
Neuromuscular & skeletal: Dysarthria (3%)
Respiratory: Cough (5%), pneumonia (4%), bronchitis (2%)

Drug Interactions
Metabolism/Transport Effects Substrate of CYP2B6 (minor), CYP2C19 (major), CYP3A4 (minor), P-glycoprotein; **Note:** Assignment of Major/Minor substrate status based on clinically relevant drug interaction potential; **Inhibits** CYP2C9 (weak), CYP2D6 (moderate), UGT1A4, UGT1A6, UGT2B4; **Induces** CYP3A4 (weak/moderate)

Avoid Concomitant Use
Avoid concomitant use of Clobazam with any of the following: Axitinib; Azelastine; Azelastine (Nasal); Methadone; Mirtazapine; OLANZapine; Paraldehyde; Thioridazine

Increased Effect/Toxicity
Clobazam may increase the levels/effects of: ARIPiprazole; Azelastine; Azelastine (Nasal); Buprenorphine; CloZAPine; CNS Depressants; CYP2D6 Substrates; Deferiprone; Fesoterodine; Fosphenytoin; Methadone; Methotrimeprazine; Metyrosine; Mirtazapine; Nebivolol; Paraldehyde; Phenytoin; Selective Serotonin Reuptake Inhibitors; Thioridazine; Zolpidem

The levels/effects of Clobazam may be increased by: Alcohol (Ethyl); Antifungal Agents (Azole Derivatives, Systemic); Aprepitant; Calcium Channel Blockers (Nondihydropyridine); Cimetidine; Contraceptives (Estrogens); Contraceptives (Progestins); CYP2C19 Inhibitors (Moderate); CYP2C19 Inhibitors (Strong); Droperidol; Fosaprepitant; Grapefruit Juice; HydrOXYzine; Isoniazid; Macrolide Antibiotics; Methotrimeprazine; OLANZapine; Propafenone; Proton Pump Inhibitors; Selective Serotonin Reuptake Inhibitors

Decreased Effect
Clobazam may decrease the levels/effects of: ARIPiprazole; Axitinib; Codeine; Contraceptives (Estrogens); Contraceptives (Progestins); Saxagliptin; Tamoxifen; TraMADol

The levels/effects of Clobazam may be decreased by: CarBAMazepine; CYP2C19 Inducers (Strong); Rifamycin Derivatives; St Johns Wort; Theophylline Derivatives; Tocilizumab; Yohimbine

Ethanol/Nutrition/Herb Interactions
Ethanol: Concomitant administration may increase bioavailability of clobazam by 50%. Ethanol may also increase CNS depression; monitor for increased effects with coadministration. Caution patients about effects.
Food: Serum concentrations may be increased by grapefruit juice.
Herb/Nutraceutical: St John's wort may decrease benzodiazepine levels. Avoid valerian, St John's wort, kava kava, gotu kola (may increase CNS depression).

Stability Store at 20°C to 25°C (68°F to 77°F).

Mechanism of Action Clobazam is a 1,5 benzodiazepine which binds to stereospecific benzodiazepine receptors on the postsynaptic GABA neuron at several sites within the central nervous system, including the limbic system, reticular formation. Enhancement of the inhibitory effect of GABA on neuronal excitability results by increased neuronal membrane permeability to chloride ions. This shift in chloride ions results in hyperpolarization (a less excitable state) and stabilization.

Pharmacodynamics/Kinetics
Absorption: Rapid; ~87%
Protein binding: 80% to 90%
Metabolism: Hepatic via CYP3A4 and to a lesser extent via CYP2C19 and 2B6 (N-demethylation to active metabolite [N-desmethyl] with ~20% activity of clobazam). CYP2C19 primarily mediates subsequent hydroxylation of the N-desmethyl metabolite.
Half-life elimination: 36-42 hours; N-desmethyl (active): 71-82 hours
Time to peak: 30 minutes to 4 hours
Excretion: Urine (~94%), as metabolites

Dosage

Geriatric Lennox-Gastaut (adjunctive): Oral:

≤30 kg: Initial: 5 mg once daily for ≥2 weeks, then increase to 5 mg twice daily; after ≥1 week may increase to 10 mg twice daily based on patient tolerability and response

>30 kg: Initial: 5 mg once daily for ≥1 week, then increase to 5 mg twice daily for ≥1 week, then increase to 10 mg twice daily; after ≥1 week may increase to 20 mg twice daily based on patient tolerability and response

Adult

Lennox-Gastaut (adjunctive): U.S. labeling: Oral: **Note:** Dose should be titrated according to patient tolerability and response.

≤30 kg: Initial: 5 mg once daily for ≥1 week, then increase to 5 mg twice daily for ≥1 week, then increase to 10 mg twice daily thereafter

>30 kg: Initial: 5 mg twice daily for ≥1 week, then increase to 10 mg twice daily for ≥1 week, then increase to 20 mg twice daily thereafter

CYP2C19 poor metabolizers:

≤30 kg: Initial: 5 mg once daily for ≥2 weeks, then increase to 5 mg twice daily; after ≥1 week may increase to 10 mg twice daily

>30 kg: Initial: 5 mg once daily for ≥1 week, then increase to 5 mg twice daily for ≥1 week, then increase to 10 mg twice daily; after ≥1 week may increase to 20 mg twice daily

Epilepsy (adjunctive): Canadian labeling (not in U.S. labeling): Oral: Initial: 5-15 mg/day; dosage may be gradually adjusted (based on tolerance and seizure control) to a maximum of 80 mg/day. **Note:** Daily doses of up to 30 mg may be taken as a single dose at bedtime; higher doses should be divided.

Catamenial epilepsy (unlabeled use): Oral: 20-30 mg daily for 10 days during the perimenstrual period (Feely, 1984)

Renal Impairment

U.S. labeling:

Cl_{cr} ≥30 mL/minute: No dosage adjustment necessary.

Cl_{cr} <30 mL/minute: No dosage adjustment provided in manufacturer's labeling (has not been studied); use with caution.

Canadian labeling: No dosage adjustment provided in manufacturer's labeling; however, a reduced dosage is recommended.

Hepatic Impairment

U.S. labeling:

Mild-to-moderate impairment:

≤30 kg: Initial: 5 mg once daily for ≥2 weeks, then increase to 5 mg twice daily; after ≥1 week may increase to 10 mg twice daily based on patient tolerability and response

>30 kg: Initial: 5 mg once daily for ≥1 week, then increase to 5 mg twice daily for ≥1 week, then increase to 10 mg twice daily; after ≥1 week may increase to 20 mg twice daily based on patient tolerability and response

Severe impairment: No dosage adjustment provided in manufacturer's labeling (has not been studied). Use with caution; undergoes extensive hepatic metabolism.

Canadian labeling:

Mild-to-moderate impairment: No dosage adjustment provided in manufacturer's labeling; however, a reduced dosage is recommended.

Severe impairment: Use is contraindicated.

Administration May be administered with or without food. Tablets can be crushed and mixed in applesauce.

Monitoring Parameters Respiratory and mental status/suicidality (eg, suicidal thoughts, depression, behavioral changes). The Canadian labeling recommends periodic CBC, liver function, renal function and thyroid function tests.

Special Geriatric Considerations Plasma concentrations of clobazam are generally higher in the elderly. Titrate the dose slowly, starting with 5 mg/day, regardless of weight. Titrate to 10-20 mg/day, depending on weight, in divided doses. If tolerated, the dose may be increased to a maximum of 40 mg/day (depending on weight). Since clobazam is a benzodiazepine with a relatively long half-life and active metabolite, elderly patients should be monitored for CNS depression.

Controlled Substance C-IV

Dosage Forms Excipient information presented when available (limited, particularly for generics); consult specific product labeling.

Tablet, oral:

Onfi™: 5 mg, 10 mg, 20 mg

Dosage Forms: Canada Excipient information presented when available (limited, particularly for generics); consult specific product labeling.

Tablet:

Alti-Clobazam, Apo-Clobazam®, Clobazam-10, Dom-Clobazam, Frisium®, Novo-Clobazam, PMS-Clobazam, ratio-Clobazam: 10 mg

Clobetasol (kloe BAY ta sol)

Related Information
Topical Corticosteroids *on page 2113*

Medication Safety Issues
International issues:
Clobex [U.S., Canada, and multiple international markets] may be confused with Codex brand name for *Saccharomyces boulardii* [Italy]
Cloderm: Brand name for clobetasol [China, India, Malaysia, Singapore, Thailand], but also brand name for alclometasone [Indonesia]; clocortolone [U.S., Canada]; clotrimazole [Germany]

Brand Names: U.S. Clobex®; Cormax®; Olux-E™; Olux®; Temovate E®; Temovate®

Brand Names: Canada Clobex®; Dermovate®; Mylan-Clobetasol Cream; Mylan-Clobetasol Ointment; Mylan-Clobetasol Scalp Application; Novo-Clobetasol; PMS-Clobetasol; ratio-Clobetasol; Taro-Clobetasol

Index Terms Clobetasol Propionate

Generic Availability (U.S.) Yes: Excludes spray

Pharmacologic Category Corticosteroid, Topical

Use Short-term relief of inflammation of moderate-to-severe corticosteroid-responsive dermatoses (very high potency topical corticosteroid)

Contraindications Hypersensitivity to clobetasol or any component of the formulation; viral, fungal, or tubercular skin lesions

Warnings/Precautions Systemic absorption of topical corticosteroids may cause hypothalamic-pituitary-adrenal (HPA) axis suppression (reversible). HPA axis suppression may lead to adrenal crisis. Risk is increased when used over large surface areas, for prolonged periods, or with occlusive dressings. Allergic contact dermatitis can occur, it is usually diagnosed by failure to heal rather than clinical exacerbation. Prolonged treatment with corticosteroids has been associated with the development of Kaposi's sarcoma (case reports); if noted, discontinuation of therapy should be considered. Adverse systemic effects including hyperglycemia, glycosuria, fluid and electrolyte changes, and HPA suppression may occur when used on large surface areas, for prolonged periods, or with an occlusive dressing. Do not use on the face, axillae, or groin.

Adverse Reactions (Reflective of adult population; not specific for elderly) Frequency not defined; may depend upon formulation used, length of application, surface area covered, and the use of occlusive dressings.

Central nervous system: Intracranial hypertension (systemic effect reported in children treated with topical corticosteroids)
Endocrine & metabolic: Adrenal suppression, Cushing's syndrome, hyperglycemia
Local: Application site: Burning, cracking/fissuring of the skin, dryness, erythema, folliculitis, irritation, numbness, pruritus, skin atrophy, stinging, telangiectasia
Renal: Glycosuria
Effects reported with other high-potency topical steroids: Acneiform eruptions, allergic contact dermatitis, hypertrichosis, hypopigmentation, maceration of the skin, miliaria, perioral dermatitis, secondary infection

Drug Interactions
Metabolism/Transport Effects None known.
Avoid Concomitant Use
Avoid concomitant use of Clobetasol with any of the following: Aldesleukin
Increased Effect/Toxicity
Clobetasol may increase the levels/effects of: Deferasirox

The levels/effects of Clobetasol may be increased by: Telaprevir
Decreased Effect
Clobetasol may decrease the levels/effects of: Aldesleukin; Corticorelin; Hyaluronidase; Telaprevir

Stability
Cream, emollient cream, ointment: Store at room temperature, between 15°C to 30°C (59°F to 86°F); do not refrigerate.
Foam: Store at room temperature; do not expose to temperatures >49°C (120°F). Avoid fire, flame, or smoking during and immediately following application.
Gel: Store between 2°C to 30°C (36°F to 86°F).
Lotion, shampoo, spray: Store at room temperature of 20°C to 25°C (68°F to 77°F). Spray is flammable; do not use near open flame.
Solution: Store between 4°C to 25°C (39°F to 77°F). Do not use near an open flame.

Mechanism of Action Stimulates the synthesis of enzymes needed to decrease inflammation, suppress mitotic activity, and cause vasoconstriction

Pharmacodynamics/Kinetics
Absorption: Percutaneous absorption is variable and dependent upon many factors including vehicle used, integrity of epidermis, dose, and use of occlusive dressings
Metabolism: Hepatic
Excretion: Urine and feces

Dosage
Geriatric & Adult Note: Discontinue when control achieved; if improvement not seen within 2 weeks, reassessment of diagnosis may be necessary.

Oral mucosal inflammation (unlabeled use): Topical: Cream: Apply twice daily for up to 2 weeks (maximum dose: 50 g/week); discontinue application when control is achieved; if no improvement is seen, reassessment of diagnosis may be necessary

Steroid-responsive dermatoses: Topical:
Cream, emollient cream, gel, lotion, ointment: Apply twice daily for up to 2 weeks (maximum dose: 50 g/week)
Foam (Olux-E™): Apply to affected area twice daily for up to 2 weeks (maximum dose: 50 g/week); do not apply to face or intertriginous areas

Steroid-responsive dermatoses of the scalp: Topical: Foam (Olux®), solution: Apply to affected scalp twice daily for up to 2 weeks (maximum dose: 50 g or 50 mL/week)

Mild-to-moderate plaque-type psoriasis of nonscalp areas: Topical: Foam (Olux®): Apply to affected area twice daily for up to 2 weeks (maximum dose: 50 g/week); do not apply to face or intertriginous areas

Moderate-to-severe plaque-type psoriasis: Topical:
Emollient cream, lotion: Apply twice daily for up to 2 weeks, has been used for up to 4 weeks when application is <10% of body surface area; use with caution (maximum dose: 50 g/week)
Spray: Apply by spraying directly onto affected area twice daily; should be gently rubbed into skin. Should be used for not longer than 4 weeks; treatment beyond 2 weeks should be limited to localized lesions which have not improved sufficiently. Total dose should not exceed 50 g/week or 59 mL/week.

Scalp psoriasis: Topical: Shampoo: Apply thin film to dry scalp once daily; leave in place for 15 minutes, then add water, lather; rinse thoroughly

Administration
Cream, gel, lotion, ointment, solution: Apply the smallest amount that will cover affected area. Do not apply to face or intertriginous areas. Total dose should not exceed 50 g/week (or 50 mL/week of lotion or solution).

Foam: Turn can upside down and spray a small amount (golf ball size) of foam into the cap or another cool surface. If fingers are warm, rinse with cool water and dry prior to handling (foam will melt on contact with warm skin). Massage foam into affected area. If the can is warm or the foam is runny, run can under cold water.

Monitoring Parameters Adrenal suppression with extensive/prolonged use (ACTH stimulation test, morning plasma cortisol test, urinary free cortisol test)

Pharmacotherapy Pearls Considered a super high potency steroid; avoid use on face

Special Geriatric Considerations Due to age-related changes in skin, limit use of topical corticosteroids.

Dosage Forms Excipient information presented when available (limited, particularly for generics); consult specific product labeling. [DSC] = Discontinued product
Aerosol, foam, topical, as propionate: 0.05% (50 g, 100 g)
  Olux-E™: 0.05% (50 g, 100 g) [chlorofluorocarbon free, ethanol free]
  Olux®: 0.05% (50 g, 100 g) [chlorofluorocarbon free; contains ethanol 60%; for scalp application]
Cream, topical, as propionate: 0.05% (15 g, 30 g, 45 g, 60 g)
  Temovate®: 0.05% (30 g, 60 g)
Cream, topical, as propionate [emollient-based]: 0.05% (15 g, 30 g, 60 g)
  Temovate E®: 0.05% (60 g)
Gel, topical, as propionate: 0.05% (15 g, 30 g, 60 g)
  Temovate®: 0.05% (60 g)
Lotion, topical, as propionate: 0.05% (59 mL, 118 mL)
  Clobex®: 0.05% (30 mL, 59 mL, 118 mL)
Ointment, topical, as propionate: 0.05% (15 g, 30 g, 45 g, 60 g)
  Cormax®: 0.05% (15 g [DSC], 45 g [DSC])
  Temovate®: 0.05% (15 g, 30 g)
Shampoo, topical, as propionate: 0.05% (118 mL)
  Clobex®: 0.05% (118 mL) [contains ethanol]
Solution, topical, as propionate [for scalp application]: 0.05% (25 mL, 50 mL)
  Cormax®: 0.05% (25 mL [DSC], 50 mL) [contains isopropyl alcohol 40%]
  Temovate®: 0.05% (50 mL) [contains isopropyl alcohol 39.3%]
Solution, topical, as propionate [spray]:
  Clobex®: 0.05% (59 mL, 125 mL) [contains ethanol]

♦ **Clobetasol Propionate** *see* Clobetasol *on page 406*
♦ **Clobex®** *see* Clobetasol *on page 406*

ClomiPRAMINE (kloe MI pra meen)

Related Information
Antidepressant Agents *on page 2097*
Beers Criteria – Potentially Inappropriate Medications for Geriatrics *on page 2183*

Medication Safety Issues
Sound-alike/look-alike issues:
ClomiPRAMINE may be confused with chlorproMAZINE, clevidipine, clomiPHENE, desipramine, Norpramin®
Anafranil® may be confused with alfentanil, enalapril, nafarelin

BEERS Criteria medication:
This drug may be potentially inappropriate for use in geriatric patients (Quality of evidence - high [moderate for SIADH]; Strength of recommendation - strong).

Brand Names: U.S. Anafranil®

Brand Names: Canada Anafranil®; Apo-Clomipramine®; CO Clomipramine; Dom-Clomipramine; Novo-Clomipramine

Index Terms Clomipramine Hydrochloride

Generic Availability (U.S.) Yes

Pharmacologic Category Antidepressant, Tricyclic (Tertiary Amine)

Use Treatment of obsessive-compulsive disorder (OCD)

Unlabeled Use Depression, panic attacks, chronic pain

Medication Guide Available Yes

Contraindications Hypersensitivity to clomipramine, other tricyclic agents, or any component of the formulation; use of MAO inhibitors within 14 days; use in a patient during the acute recovery phase of MI

Warnings/Precautions [U.S. Boxed Warning]: Antidepressants increase the risk of suicidal thinking and behavior in children, adolescents, and young adults (18-24 years of age) with major depressive disorder (MDD) and other psychiatric disorders; consider risk prior to prescribing. Short-term studies did not show an increased risk in patients >24 years of age and showed a decreased risk in patients ≥65 years. Closely monitor for clinical worsening, suicidality, or unusual changes in behavior; the patient's family or caregiver should be instructed to closely observe the patient and communicate condition with healthcare provider. A medication guide should be dispensed with each prescription.

The possibility of a suicide attempt is inherent in major depression and may persist until remission occurs. Monitor for worsening of depression or suicidality, especially during initiation of therapy (generally first 1-2 months) or with dose increases or decreases. Use caution in high-risk patients. Worsening depression and severe abrupt suicidality that are not part of the presenting symptoms may require discontinuation or modification of drug therapy. The patient's family or caregiver should be alerted to monitor patients for the emergence of suicidality and associated behaviors (such as agitation, irritability, hostility, impulsivity, and hypomania) and notify the healthcare provider.

May worsen psychosis in some patients or precipitate a shift to mania or hypomania in patients with bipolar disorder. Patients presenting with depressive symptoms should be screened for bipolar disorder. Monotherapy in patients with bipolar disorder should be avoided. **Clomipramine is not FDA approved for bipolar depression.**

TCAs may rarely cause bone marrow suppression; monitor for any signs of infection and obtain CBC if symptoms (eg, fever, sore throat) evident. May cause seizures (relationship to dose and/or duration of therapy) - do not exceed maximum doses. Use caution in patients with a previous seizure disorder or condition predisposing to seizures such as brain damage, alcoholism, or concurrent therapy with other drugs which lower the seizure threshold. May increase the risks associated with electroconvulsive therapy. Has been associated with a high incidence of sexual dysfunction. Weight gain may occur. Hyperpyrexia has been observed with TCAs in combination with anticholinergics and/or neuroleptics, particularly during hot weather.

The degree of sedation, anticholinergic effects, and conduction abnormalities are high relative to other antidepressants. Clomipramine often causes drowsiness/sedation, resulting in impaired performance of tasks requiring alertness (eg, operating machinery or driving). Sedative effects may be additive with other CNS depressants and/or ethanol. The risk of orthostasis is moderate to high relative to other antidepressants. Use with caution in patients with a history of cardiovascular disease (including previous MI, stroke, tachycardia, or conduction abnormalities). Use with caution in patients with urinary retention, benign prostatic hyperplasia, narrow-angle glaucoma, xerostomia, visual problems, constipation, or a history of bowel obstruction.

Consider discontinuing, when possible, prior to elective surgery. Therapy should not be abruptly discontinued in patients receiving high doses for prolonged periods. Use with caution in hyperthyroid patients or those receiving thyroid supplementation. Use with caution in patients with hepatic or renal dysfunction. Avoid use in the elderly due to its potent anticholinergic and sedative properties, and potential to cause orthostatic hypotension. In addition, may also cause or exacerbate syndrome of inappropriate antidiuretic hormone secretion or hyponatremia; monitor sodium closely with initiation or dosage adjustments in older adults (Beers Criteria).

Adverse Reactions (Reflective of adult population; not specific for elderly) Data shown for children reflects both children and adolescents studied in clinical trials.
>10%:
  Central nervous system: Dizziness (54%), somnolence (54%), drowsiness, headache (52%; children 28%), fatigue (39%), insomnia (25%; children 11%), malaise, nervousness (18%; children 4%)
  Endocrine & metabolic: Libido changes (21%), hot flushes (5%)
  Gastrointestinal: Xerostomia (84%, children 63%) constipation (47%; children 22%), nausea (33%; children 9%), dyspepsia (22%; children 13%), weight gain (18%; children 2%), diarrhea (13%; children 7%), anorexia (12%; children 22%), abdominal pain (11%), appetite increased (11%)
  Genitourinary: Ejaculation failure (42%), impotence (20%), micturition disorder (14%; children 4%)
  Neuromuscular & skeletal: Tremor (54%), myoclonus (13%; children 2%), myalgia (13%)
  Ocular: Abnormal vision (18%; children 7%)
  Respiratory: Pharyngitis (14%), rhinitis (12%)
  Miscellaneous: Diaphoresis increased (29%; children 9%)
1% to 10%:
  Cardiovascular: Flushing (8%), orthostatic hypotension (6%), palpitation (4%), tachycardia (4%; children 2%), chest pain (4%), edema (2%)
  Central nervous system: Anxiety (9%), memory impairment (9%), twitching (7%), depression (5%), concentration impaired (5%), fever (4%), hypertonia (4%), abnormal dreaming (3%), agitation (3%), confusion (3%), migraine (3%), pain (3%), psychosomatic disorder (3%), speech disorder (3%), yawning (3%), aggressiveness (children 2%), chills (2%), depersonalization (2%), emotional lability (2%), irritability (2%), panic reaction (1%)
  Dermatologic: Rash (8%), pruritus (6%), purpura (3%), dermatitis (2%), acne (2%), dry skin (2%), urticaria (1%)
  Endocrine & metabolic: Amenorrhea (1%), breast enlargement (2%), breast pain (1%), hot flashes (5%), lactation (nonpuerperal) (1%)
  Gastrointestinal: Taste disturbance (8%), vomiting (7%), flatulence (6%), dental caries and teeth grinding (5%), dysphagia (2%), esophagitis (1%)
  Genitourinary: UTI (2% to 6%), micturition frequency (5%), dysuria (2%), leucorrhea (2%), vaginitis (2%), urinary retention (2%)
  Neuromuscular & skeletal: Paresthesia (9%), back pain (6%), arthralgia (3%), paresis (children 2%), weakness (1%)
  Ocular: Lacrimation abnormal (3%), mydriasis (2%), conjunctivitis (1%)
  Otic: Tinnitus (6%)
  Respiratory: Sinusitis (6%), coughing (6%), bronchospasm (2%; children 7%), epistaxis (2%)
Drug Interactions
  Metabolism/Transport Effects Substrate of CYP1A2 (major), CYP2C19 (major), CYP2D6 (major), CYP3A4 (minor); **Note:** Assignment of Major/Minor substrate status based on clinically relevant drug interaction potential; **Inhibits** CYP2D6 (moderate)
  Avoid Concomitant Use
    Avoid concomitant use of ClomiPRAMINE with any of the following: Iobenguane I 123; MAO Inhibitors; Methylene Blue
  Increased Effect/Toxicity
    ClomiPRAMINE may increase the levels/effects of: Alpha-/Beta-Agonists (Direct-Acting); Alpha1-Agonists; Amphetamines; Anticholinergics; Aspirin; Beta2-Agonists; CYP2D6 Substrates; Desmopressin; Fesoterodine; Highest Risk QTc-Prolonging Agents; Methylene Blue; Metoclopramide; Milnacipran; Moderate Risk QTc-Prolonging Agents; Nebivolol; NSAID (COX-2 Inhibitor); NSAID (Nonselective); QuiNIDine; Serotonin Modulators; Sodium Phosphates; Sulfonylureas; TraMADol; Vitamin K Antagonists; Yohimbine

    The levels/effects of ClomiPRAMINE may be increased by: Abiraterone Acetate; Altretamine; Antipsychotics; BuPROPion; CarBAMazepine; Cimetidine; Cinacalcet; CYP1A2

Inhibitors (Moderate); CYP1A2 Inhibitors (Strong); CYP2C19 Inhibitors (Moderate); CYP2C19 Inhibitors (Strong); CYP2D6 Inhibitors (Moderate); CYP2D6 Inhibitors (Strong); Deferasirox; Dexmethylphenidate; Divalproex; DULoxetine; Grapefruit Juice; Linezolid; Lithium; MAO Inhibitors; Methylphenidate; Metoclopramide; Metyrosine; Mifepristone; Pramlintide; Protease Inhibitors; QuiNIDine; Selective Serotonin Reuptake Inhibitors; Terbinafine; Terbinafine (Systemic); Valproic Acid

Decreased Effect

ClomiPRAMINE may decrease the levels/effects of: Acetylcholinesterase Inhibitors (Central); Alpha2-Agonists; Codeine; Iobenguane I 123

The levels/effects of ClomiPRAMINE may be decreased by: Acetylcholinesterase Inhibitors (Central); Barbiturates; CYP1A2 Inducers (Strong); CYP2C19 Inducers (Strong); Cyproterone; Peginterferon Alfa-2b; St Johns Wort; Tocilizumab

Ethanol/Nutrition/Herb Interactions

Ethanol: Ethanol may increase CNS depression. Management: Avoid ethanol.

Food: Serum concentrations/toxicity may be increased by grapefruit juice. Management: Avoid grapefruit juice.

Herb/Nutraceutical: St John's wort may increase the metabolism of clomipramine. Clomipramine may increase the serum concentration of yohimbe. Avoid valerian, St John's wort, SAMe, kava kava, and yohimbe.

Mechanism of Action Clomipramine appears to affect serotonin uptake while its active metabolite, desmethylclomipramine, affects norepinephrine uptake

Pharmacodynamics/Kinetics

Absorption: Rapid

Protein binding: 97%, primarily to albumin

Metabolism: Hepatic to desmethylclomipramine (DMI; active); extensive first-pass effect

Half-life elimination: Clomipramine: mean 32 hours (19-37 hours); DMI: mean 69 hours (range 54-77 hours)

Time to peak, plasma: 2-6 hours

Excretion: Urine and feces

Dosage

Geriatric & Adult Treatment of OCD: Oral: Initial: 25 mg/day; may gradually increase as tolerated over the first 2 weeks to 100 mg/day in divided doses; Maintenance: May further increase to recommended maximum of 250 mg/day; may give as a single daily dose at bedtime once tolerated

Administration During titration, may divide doses and administer with meals to decrease gastrointestinal side effects. After titration, may administer total daily dose at bedtime to decrease daytime sedation.

Monitoring Parameters Pulse rate and blood pressure prior to and during therapy; ECG/cardiac status in older adults and patients with cardiac disease; suicidal ideation (especially at the beginning of therapy, after initiation, or when doses are increased or decreased)

Test Interactions Increased glucose; may interfere with urine detection of methadone (false-positive)

Special Geriatric Considerations Clomipramine's anticholinergic and hypotensive effects limit its use versus other preferred antidepressants. Elderly patients were found to have higher dose-normalized plasma concentrations as a result of decreased demethylation (decreased 50%) and hydroxylation (25%).

A systematic review and meta-analysis of antidepressant placebo-controlled trials in persons with depression and dementia found evidence "suggestive" of efficacy but not of sufficient strength to "confirm" efficacy. Antidepressant trials in this patient population are small and underpowered. Older patients with depression being treated with an antidepressant should be closely monitored for response and adverse effects. Treatment should be switched or augmented when response is inadequate with a therapeutic dose. Antidepressants that are not tolerated should be discontinued and an alternative agent should be started.

This medication is considered to be potentially inappropriate in this patient population (Beers Criteria: Quality of evidence - high [moderate for SIADH]; Strength of recommendation - strong).

Dosage Forms Excipient information presented when available (limited, particularly for generics); consult specific product labeling.

Capsule, oral, as hydrochloride: 25 mg, 50 mg, 75 mg

Anafranil®: 25 mg, 50 mg, 75 mg

◆ **Clomipramine Hydrochloride** *see* ClomiPRAMINE *on page 408*

ClonazePAM (kloe NA ze pam)

Related Information
Anxiolytic, Sedative/Hypnotic, and Miscellaneous Benzodiazepines *on page 2106*
Beers Criteria – Potentially Inappropriate Medications for Geriatrics *on page 2183*

Medication Safety Issues
Sound-alike/look-alike issues:
ClonazePAM may be confused with clobazam, cloNIDine, clorazepate, cloZAPine, LORazepam

KlonoPIN® may be confused with cloNIDine, clorazepate, cloZAPine, LORazepam

BEERS Criteria medication:
This drug may be potentially inappropriate for use in geriatric patients (Quality of evidence - high; Strength of recommendation - strong).

Brand Names: U.S. KlonoPIN®

Brand Names: Canada Apo-Clonazepam®; Clonapam; CO Clonazepam; Dom-Clonazepam; Mylan-Clonazepam; Novo-Clonazepam; Nu-Clonazepam; PHL-Clonazepam; PMS-Clonazepam; PRO-Clonazepam; ratio-Clonazepam; Riva-Clonazepam; Rivotril®; Sandoz-Clonazepam; ZYM-Clonazepam

Generic Availability (U.S.) Yes

Pharmacologic Category Benzodiazepine

Use Alone or as an adjunct in the treatment of petit mal variant (Lennox-Gastaut), akinetic, and myoclonic seizures; petit mal (absence) seizures unresponsive to succimides; panic disorder with or without agoraphobia

Unlabeled Use Restless legs syndrome; neuralgia; multifocal tic disorder; parkinsonian dysarthria; bipolar disorder; adjunct therapy for schizophrenia; burning mouth syndrome

Medication Guide Available Yes

Contraindications Hypersensitivity to clonazepam or any component of the formulation (cross-sensitivity with other benzodiazepines may exist); significant liver disease; narrow-angle glaucoma

Warnings/Precautions Hazardous agent - use appropriate precautions for handling and disposal. Antiepileptics are associated with an increased risk of suicidal behavior/thoughts with use (regardless of indication); patients should be monitored for signs/symptoms of depression, suicidal tendencies, and other unusual behavior changes during therapy and instructed to inform their healthcare provider immediately if symptoms occur.

Use with caution in elderly or debilitated patients, patients with hepatic disease (including alcoholics), or renal impairment. Use with caution in patients with respiratory disease or impaired gag reflex or ability to protect the airway from secretions (salivation may be increased). Worsening of seizures may occur when added to patients with multiple seizure types. Concurrent use with valproic acid may result in absence status. Monitoring of CBC and liver function tests has been recommended during prolonged therapy.

Causes CNS depression (dose related) resulting in sedation, dizziness, confusion, or ataxia which may impair physical and mental capabilities. Patients must be cautioned about performing tasks which require mental alertness (eg, operating machinery or driving). Use with caution in patients receiving other CNS depressants or psychoactive agents. Effects with other sedative drugs or ethanol may be potentiated. Benzodiazepines have been associated with falls and traumatic injury and should be used with extreme caution in patients who are at risk of these events.

Use caution in patients with depression, particularly if suicidal risk may be present. Use with caution in patients with a history of drug dependence. Benzodiazepines have been associated with dependence and acute withdrawal symptoms, including seizures, on discontinuation or reduction in dose. Acute withdrawal, including seizures, may be precipitated in patients after administration of flumazenil to patients receiving long-term benzodiazepine therapy.

Benzodiazepines have been associated with anterograde amnesia. Paradoxical reactions, including hyperactive or aggressive behavior, have been reported with benzodiazepines, particularly in adolescent/pediatric or psychiatric patients. Does not have analgesic, anti-depressant, or antipsychotic properties.

In older adults, benzodiazepines increase the risk of impaired cognition, delirium, falls, fractures, and motor vehicle accidents. Due to increased sensitivity in this age group and slower metabolism of long-acting agents (such as clonazepam), avoid use for treatment of insomnia, agitation, or delirium (Beers Criteria).

Adverse Reactions (Reflective of adult population; not specific for elderly) Reactions reported in patients with seizure and/or panic disorder. Frequency not always defined.
Cardiovascular: Edema (ankle or facial), palpitation

CLONAZEPAM

Central nervous system: Amnesia, ataxia (seizure disorder ~30%; panic disorder 5%), behavior problems (seizure disorder ~25%), coma, confusion, depression, dizziness, drowsiness (seizure disorder ~50%), emotional lability, fatigue, fever, hallucinations, headache, hypotonia, hysteria, insomnia, intellectual ability reduced, memory disturbance, nervousness; paradoxical reactions (including aggressive behavior, agitation, anxiety, excitability, hostility, irritability, nervousness, nightmares, sleep disturbance, vivid dreams); psychosis, slurred speech, somnolence (panic disorder 37%), suicidal attempt, suicide ideation, vertigo

Dermatologic: Hair loss, hirsutism, skin rash

Endocrine & metabolic: Dysmenorrhea, libido increased/decreased

Gastrointestinal: Abdominal pain, anorexia, appetite increased/decreased, coated tongue, constipation, dehydration, diarrhea, gastritis, gum soreness, nausea, weight changes (loss/gain), xerostomia

Genitourinary: Colpitis, dysuria, ejaculation delayed, enuresis, impotence, micturition frequency, nocturia, urinary retention, urinary tract infection

Hematologic: Anemia, eosinophilia, leukopenia, thrombocytopenia

Hepatic: Alkaline phosphatase increased (transient), hepatomegaly, serum transaminases increased (transient)

Neuromuscular & skeletal: Choreiform movements, coordination abnormal, dysarthria, muscle pain, muscle weakness, myalgia, tremor

Ocular: Blurred vision, eye movements abnormal, diplopia, nystagmus

Respiratory: Chest congestion, cough, bronchitis, hypersecretions, pharyngitis, respiratory depression, respiratory tract infection, rhinitis, rhinorrhea, shortness of breath, sinusitis

Miscellaneous: Allergic reaction, aphonia, dysdiadochokinesis, encopresis, "glassy-eyed" appearance, hemiparesis, lymphadenopathy

Drug Interactions

Metabolism/Transport Effects Substrate of CYP3A4 (major); **Note:** Assignment of Major/Minor substrate status based on clinically relevant drug interaction potential

Avoid Concomitant Use

Avoid concomitant use of ClonazePAM with any of the following: Azelastine; Azelastine (Nasal); Conivaptan; Methadone; Mirtazapine; OLANZapine; Paraldehyde

Increased Effect/Toxicity

ClonazePAM may increase the levels/effects of: Alcohol (Ethyl); Azelastine; Azelastine (Nasal); Buprenorphine; CloZAPine; CNS Depressants; Fosphenytoin; Methadone; Methotrimeprazine; Metyrosine; Mirtazapine; Paraldehyde; Phenytoin; Selective Serotonin Reuptake Inhibitors; Zolpidem

The levels/effects of ClonazePAM may be increased by: Antifungal Agents (Azole Derivatives, Systemic); Aprepitant; Calcium Channel Blockers (Nondihydropyridine); Cimetidine; Conivaptan; Contraceptives (Estrogens); Contraceptives (Progestins); CYP3A4 Inhibitors (Moderate); CYP3A4 Inhibitors (Strong); Dasatinib; Droperidol; Fosaprepitant; Grapefruit Juice; HydrOXYzine; Isoniazid; Ivacaftor; Macrolide Antibiotics; Methotrimeprazine; Mifepristone; OLANZapine; Proton Pump Inhibitors; Selective Serotonin Reuptake Inhibitors

Decreased Effect

The levels/effects of ClonazePAM may be decreased by: CarBAMazepine; CYP3A4 Inducers (Strong); Deferasirox; Rifamycin Derivatives; St Johns Wort; Theophylline Derivatives; Tocilizumab; Yohimbine

Ethanol/Nutrition/Herb Interactions

Ethanol: May increase CNS depression; monitor for increased effects with coadministration. Caution patients about effects.

Food: Clonazepam serum concentration is unlikely to be increased by grapefruit juice because of clonazepam's high oral bioavailability.

Herb/Nutraceutical: St John's wort may decrease clonazepam levels. Avoid valerian, St John's wort, kava kava, gotu kola (may increase CNS depression).

Mechanism of Action The exact mechanism is unknown, but believed to be related to its ability to enhance the activity of GABA; suppresses the spike-and-wave discharge in absence seizures by depressing nerve transmission in the motor cortex

Pharmacodynamics/Kinetics

Onset of action: 20-60 minutes

Duration: Adults: ≤12 hours

Absorption: Well absorbed

Distribution: Adults: V_d: 1.5-4.4 L/kg

Protein binding: 85%

Metabolism: Extensively hepatic via glucuronide and sulfate conjugation

Half-life elimination: Adults: 19-50 hours

Time to peak, serum: 1-3 hours; Steady-state: 5-7 days

Excretion: Urine (<2% as unchanged drug); metabolites excreted as glucuronide or sulfate conjugates

Dosage

Geriatric Refer to adult dosing. Initiate with low doses and observe closely.

Adult

Burning mouth syndrome (unlabeled use): Oral: 0.25-3 mg/day in 2 divided doses, in morning and evening.

Seizure disorders: Oral:

Initial daily dose not to exceed 1.5 mg given in 3 divided doses; may increase by 0.5-1 mg every third day until seizures are controlled or adverse effects seen (maximum: 20 mg/day)

Usual maintenance dose: 0.05-0.2 mg/kg; do not exceed 20 mg/day

Panic disorder: Oral: 0.25 mg twice daily; increase in increments of 0.125-0.25 mg twice daily every 3 days; target dose: 1 mg/day (maximum: 4 mg/day)

Discontinuation of treatment: To discontinue, treatment should be withdrawn gradually. Decrease dose by 0.125 mg twice daily every 3 days until medication is completely withdrawn.

Renal Impairment Hemodialysis: Supplemental dose is not necessary.

Administration Orally-disintegrating tablet: Open pouch and peel back foil on the blister; do not push tablet through foil. Use dry hands to remove tablet and place in mouth. May be swallowed with or without water. Use immediately after removing from package.

Monitoring Parameters CBC, liver function tests; observe patient for excess sedation, respiratory depression; suicidality (eg, suicidal thoughts, depression, behavioral changes)

Reference Range Relationship between serum concentration and seizure control is not well established

Timing of serum samples: Peak serum levels occur 1-3 hours after oral ingestion; the half-life is 20-40 hours; therefore, steady-state occurs in 5-7 days

Therapeutic levels: 20-80 ng/mL; Toxic concentration: >80 ng/mL

Pharmacotherapy Pearls Ethosuximide or valproic acid may be preferred for treatment of absence (petit mal) seizures. Clonazepam-induced behavioral disturbances may be more frequent in mentally handicapped patients. Abrupt discontinuation after sustained use (generally >10 days) may cause withdrawal symptoms. Flumazenil, a competitive benzodiazepine antagonist at the CNS receptor site, reverses benzodiazepine-induced CNS depression.

Special Geriatric Considerations Hepatic clearance may be decreased allowing accumulation of active drug. Also, metabolites of clonazepam are renally excreted and may accumulate in the elderly as renal function declines with age. Observe for signs of CNS and pulmonary toxicity.

This medication is considered to be potentially inappropriate in this patient population (Beers Criteria: Quality of evidence - high; Strength of recommendation - strong).

Controlled Substance C-IV

Dosage Forms Excipient information presented when available (limited, particularly for generics); consult specific product labeling.

Tablet, oral: 0.5 mg, 1 mg, 2 mg

KlonoPIN®: 0.5 mg [scored]

KlonoPIN®: 1 mg, 2 mg

Tablet, orally disintegrating, oral: 0.125 mg, 0.25 mg, 0.5 mg, 1 mg, 2 mg

CloNIDine (KLON i deen)

Related Information

Beers Criteria – Potentially Inappropriate Medications for Geriatrics *on page 2183*

Medication Safety Issues

Sound-alike/look-alike issues:

CloNIDine may be confused with Clomid®, clomiPHENE, clonazePAM, cloZAPine, KlonoPIN®, quiNIDine

Catapres® may be confused with Cataflam®, Combipres

High alert medication:
The Institute for Safe Medication Practices (ISMP) includes this medication (epidural administration) among its list of drug classes which have a heightened risk of causing significant patient harm when used in error.

BEERS Criteria medication:
This drug may be potentially inappropriate for use in geriatric patients (Quality of evidence - low; Strength of recommendation - strong).

Administration issues:
Use caution when interpreting dosing information.

Other safety concerns:
Transdermal patch may contain conducting metal (eg, aluminum); remove patch prior to MRI. Errors have occurred when the inactive, optional adhesive cover has been applied instead of the active clonidine-containing patch.

Brand Names: U.S. Catapres-TTS®-1; Catapres-TTS®-2; Catapres-TTS®-3; Catapres®; Duraclon®; Kapvay®; Nexiclon™ XR

Brand Names: Canada Apo-Clonidine®; Catapres®; Dixarit®; Dom-Clonidine; Novo-Clonidine; Nu-Clonidine

Index Terms Clonidine Hydrochloride

Generic Availability (U.S.) Yes: Excludes extended release tablets, oral suspension

Pharmacologic Category Alpha$_2$-Adrenergic Agonist

Use
Oral:
Immediate release: Management of hypertension (monotherapy or as adjunctive therapy)
Extended release:
Kapvay™: Treatment of attention-deficit/hyperactivity disorder (ADHD) (monotherapy or as adjunctive therapy)
Nexiclon™ XR: Management of hypertension (monotherapy or as adjunctive therapy)
Epidural (Duraclon®): For continuous epidural administration as adjunctive therapy with opioids for treatment of severe cancer pain in patients tolerant to or unresponsive to opioids alone; epidural clonidine is generally more effective for neuropathic pain and less effective (or possibly ineffective) for somatic or visceral pain
Transdermal patch: Management of hypertension (monotherapy or as adjunctive therapy)

Unlabeled Use Heroin or nicotine withdrawal; severe pain; dysmenorrhea; vasomotor symptoms associated with menopause; ethanol dependence; prophylaxis of migraines; glaucoma; diabetes-associated diarrhea; impulse control disorder, clozapine-induced sialorrhea; aid in the diagnosis of growth hormone deficiency; aggression associated with conduct disorder

Contraindications Hypersensitivity to clonidine hydrochloride or any component of the formulation

Epidural administration: Injection site infection; concurrent anticoagulant therapy; bleeding diathesis; administration above the C4 dermatome

Warnings/Precautions May cause CNS depression, which may impair physical or mental abilities; patients must be cautioned about performing tasks which require mental alertness (eg, operating machinery or driving). Sedating effects may be potentiated when used with other CNS-depressant drugs or ethanol. Use with caution in patients with severe coronary insufficiency; conduction disturbances; recent MI, CVA, or chronic renal insufficiency. May cause dose dependent reductions in heart rate; use with caution in patients with preexisting bradycardia or those predisposed to developing bradycardia. Caution in sinus node dysfunction. Use with caution in patients concurrently receiving agents known to reduce SA node function and/or AV nodal conduction (eg, digoxin, diltiazem, metoprolol, verapamil). May cause significant xerostomia. Clonidine may cause eye dryness in patients who wear contact lenses.

[U.S. Boxed Warning]: Must dilute concentrated epidural injectable (500 mcg/mL) solution prior to use. Epidural clonidine is not recommended for perioperative, obstetrical, or postpartum pain due to risk of hemodynamic instability. Clonidine injection should be administered via a continuous epidural infusion device. Monitor closely for catheter-related infection such as meningitis or epidural abscess. Epidural clonidine is not recommended for use in patients with severe cardiovascular disease or hemodynamic instability; may lead to cardiovascular instability (hypotension, bradycardia). Symptomatic hypotension may occur with use; in all patients, use epidural clonidine with caution due to the potential for severe hypotension especially in women and those of low body weight. Most hypotensive episodes occur within the first 4 days of initiation; however, episodes may occur throughout the duration of therapy.

Gradual withdrawal is needed (taper oral immediate release or epidural dose gradually over 2-4 days to avoid rebound hypertension) if drug needs to be stopped. Patients should be instructed about abrupt discontinuation (causes rapid increase in BP and symptoms of sympathetic overactivity). In patients on both a beta-blocker and clonidine where withdrawal of clonidine is necessary, withdraw the beta-blocker first and several days before clonidine withdrawal, then slowly decrease clonidine. Discontinue oral immediate release formulations within 4 hours of surgery then restart as soon as possible afterwards. Discontinue oral extended release formulations up to 28 hours prior to surgery, then restart the following day.

Oral formulations of clonidine (immediate release versus extended release) are not interchangeable on a mg:mg basis due to different pharmacokinetic profiles. This includes commercially available oral suspension (Nexiclon™ XR) which is an extended release preparation and should not be used interchangeably with any extemporaneously prepared clonidine oral suspension.

Transdermal patch may contain conducting metal (eg, aluminum); remove patch prior to MRI. Due to the potential for altered electrical conductivity, remove transdermal patch before cardioversion or defibrillation. Localized contact sensitization to the transdermal system has been reported; in these patients, allergic reactions (eg, generalized rash, urticaria, angioedema) have also occurred following subsequent substitution of oral therapy.

In the elderly, avoid use as first-line antihypertensive due to high risk of CNS adverse effects; may also cause orthostatic hypotension and bradycardia (Beers Criteria).

Adverse Reactions (Reflective of adult population; not specific for elderly) Frequency not always defined.

Oral, Transdermal: Incidence of adverse events may be less with transdermal compared to oral due to the lower peak/trough ratio.

Cardiovascular: Bradycardia (≤4%), palpitation (1%), tachycardia (1%), arrhythmia, atrioventricular block, chest pain, CHF, ECG abnormalities, flushing, orthostatic hypotension, pallor, Raynaud's phenomenon, syncope

Central nervous system: Drowsiness (12% to 38%), headache (1% to 29%), fatigue (4% to 16%), dizziness (2% to 16%), sedation (3% to 10%), insomnia (≤6%), lethargy (3%), nervousness (1% to 3%), mental depression (1%), aggression, agitation, anxiety, behavioral changes, CVA, delirium, delusional perception, fever, hallucinations (visual and auditory), irritability, malaise, nightmares, restlessness, vivid dreams

Dermatologic: Transient localized skin reactions characterized by pruritus and erythema (transdermal 15% to 50%), contact dermatitis (transdermal 8% to 34%), vesiculation (transdermal 7%), allergic contact sensitization (transdermal 5%), hyperpigmentation (transdermal 5%), burning (transdermal 3%), edema (3%), excoriation (transdermal 3%), blanching (transdermal 1%), generalized macular rash (1%), papules (transdermal 1%), throbbing (transdermal 1%), alopecia, angioedema, hives, localized hypopigmentation (transdermal), rash, urticaria

Endocrine & metabolic: Sexual dysfunction (3%), gynecomastia (1%), creatine phosphokinase increased (transient; oral), hyperglycemia (transient; oral), libido decreased

Gastrointestinal: Xerostomia (≤40%), constipation (2% to 10%), anorexia (1%), taste perversion (1%), weight gain (<1%), abdominal pain (oral), diarrhea, nausea, parotid gland pain (oral), parotitis (oral), pseudo-obstruction (oral), throat pain, vomiting

Genitourinary: Erectile dysfunction (2% to 3%), nocturia (1%), dysuria, enuresis, urinary retention

Hematologic: Thrombocytopenia (oral)

Hepatic: Liver function test (mild transient abnormalities; ≤1%), hepatitis

Neuromuscular & skeletal: Weakness (10%), arthralgia (1%), myalgia (1%), leg cramps (<1%), numbness (localized, transdermal), pain in extremities, paresthesia, tremor

Ocular: Accommodation disorder, blurred vision, burning eyes, dry eyes, lacrimation decreased, lacrimation increased

Otic: Ear pain, otitis media

Renal: Pollakiuria

Respiratory: Asthma, epistaxis, nasal congestion, nasal dryness, nasopharyngitis, respiratory tract infection, rhinorrhea

Miscellaneous: Withdrawal syndrome (1%), flu-like syndrome, thirst

Epidural: Note: The following adverse events occurred more often than placebo in cancer patients with intractable pain being treated with concurrent epidural morphine.

>10%:

Cardiovascular: Hypotension (45%), orthostatic hypotension (32%)

Central nervous system: Confusion (13%), dizziness (13%)

Gastrointestinal: Xerostomia (13%)

◄ 1% to 10%:
Cardiovascular: Chest pain (5%)
Central nervous system: Hallucinations (5%)
Gastrointestinal: Nausea/vomiting (8%)
Otic: Tinnitus (5%)
Miscellaneous: Diaphoresis (5%)

Drug Interactions

Metabolism/Transport Effects None known.

Avoid Concomitant Use

Avoid concomitant use of CloNIDine with any of the following: Iobenguane I 123

Increased Effect/Toxicity

CloNIDine may increase the levels/effects of: Amifostine; Antihypertensives; Hypotensive Agents; RiTUXimab

The levels/effects of CloNIDine may be increased by: Alfuzosin; Beta-Blockers; Diazoxide; Herbs (Hypotensive Properties); MAO Inhibitors; Methylphenidate; Pentoxifylline; Phosphodiesterase 5 Inhibitors; Prostacyclin Analogues

Decreased Effect

CloNIDine may decrease the levels/effects of: Iobenguane I 123

The levels/effects of CloNIDine may be decreased by: Antidepressants (Alpha2-Antagonist); Herbs (Hypertensive Properties); Serotonin/Norepinephrine Reuptake Inhibitors; Tricyclic Antidepressants; Yohimbine

Ethanol/Nutrition/Herb Interactions

Ethanol: Avoid ethanol (may increase CNS depression). *In vitro* studies have shown high concentrations of alcohol may increase the rate of release of Nexiclon™ XR.

Herb/Nutraceutical: Avoid dong quai if using for hypertension (has estrogenic activity). Avoid ephedra, yohimbe, ginseng (may worsen hypertension). Avoid valerian, St John's wort, kava kava, gotu kola (may increase CNS depression).

Stability

Epidural formulation: Store at 25°C (77°F); excursions permitted to 15°C to 30°C (59°F to 86°F). **Preservative free;** discard unused portion. Prior to administration, the 500 mcg/mL concentration must be diluted in 0.9% sodium chloride for injection (preservative-free) to a final concentration of 100 mcg/mL.

Oral suspension, tablets: Store at 25°C (77°F); excursions permitted to 15°C to 30°C (59°F to 86°F). Protect from light.

Transdermal patches: Store below 30°C (86°F).

Mechanism of Action Stimulates alpha$_2$-adrenoceptors in the brain stem, thus activating an inhibitory neuron, resulting in reduced sympathetic outflow from the CNS, producing a decrease in peripheral resistance, renal vascular resistance, heart rate, and blood pressure; epidural clonidine may produce pain relief at spinal presynaptic and postjunctional alpha$_2$-adrenoceptors by preventing pain signal transmission; pain relief occurs only for the body regions innervated by the spinal segments where analgesic concentrations of clonidine exist. For the treatment of ADHD, the mechanism of action is unknown; it has been proposed that postsynaptic alpha$_2$-agonist stimulation regulates subcortical activity in the prefrontal cortex, the area of the brain responsible for emotions, attentions, and behaviors and causes reduced hyperactivity, impulsiveness, and distractibility.

Pharmacodynamics/Kinetics

Onset of action: Oral: 0.5-1 hour; Transdermal: Initial application: 2-3 days

Duration: 6-10 hours

Absorption: Oral: Extended release tablets (Kapvay™) are not bioequivalent with immediate release formulations; peak plasma concentrations are 50% lower compared to immediate release formulations

Distribution: V_d: Adults: 2.1 L/kg; highly lipid soluble; distributes readily into extravascular sites

Note: Epidurally administered clonidine readily distributes into plasma via the epidural veins and attains clinically significant systemic concentrations.

Protein binding: 20% to 40%

Metabolism: Extensively hepatic to inactive metabolites; undergoes enterohepatic recirculation

Bioavailability: Oral: Immediate release: 75% to 85%; Extended release (Kapvay™): 89% (relative to immediate release formulation)

Half-life elimination: Adults: Normal renal function: 12-16 hours; Renal impairment: Up to 41 hours

Epidural administration: CSF half-life elimination: 0.8-1.8 hours

Time to peak: Oral: Immediate release: 3-5 hours; Extended release: 7-8 hours

Excretion: Urine (40% to 60%as unchanged drug)

Dosage

Geriatric Hypertension: Oral:

Immediate release: Initial: 0.1 mg once daily at bedtime, increase gradually as needed.

Extended release (Nexiclon™ XR): No specific recommendations are provided by the manufacturer although a lower initial dose is recommended.

Adult Note: Dosing is expressed as the salt (clonidine hydrochloride) unless otherwise noted. Formulations of clonidine (immediate release versus extended release) are not interchangeable on a mg:mg basis due to different pharmacokinetic profiles. This includes commercially available oral suspension (Nexiclon™ XR) which is an extended release preparation and should not be used interchangeably with any extemporaneously prepared clonidine oral suspension.

Hypertension:

Oral:

Immediate release: Initial dose: 0.1 mg twice daily (maximum recommended dose: 2.4 mg/day); usual dose range (JNC 7): 0.1-0.8 mg/day in 2 divided doses

Extended release (Nexiclon™ XR): Initial: 0.17 mg clonidine base once daily at bedtime; may increase increments of 0.09 mg/day every 7 days; maintenance: usual dose range: 0.17-0.52 mg clonidine base once daily; maximum: 0.52 mg/day clonidine base

Conversion between immediate release clonidine hydrochloride and extended release (Nexiclon™ XR) clonidine base:

Current dose immediate release tablets 0.05 mg twice daily: Convert to extended release tablet of 0.09 mg clonidine base once daily

Current dose immediate release tablets 0.1 mg twice daily: Convert to extended release tablet of 0.17 mg clonidine base once daily

Current dose immediate release tablets 0.2 mg twice daily: Convert to extended release tablet of 0.34 mg clonidine base once daily

Current dose immediate release tablets 0.3 mg twice daily: convert to extended release tablets of 0.52 mg clonidine base once daily

Transdermal: Initial: 0.1 mg/24 hour patch applied once every 7 days and increase by 0.1 mg at 1- to 2-week intervals (dosages >0.6 mg/24 hours do not improve efficacy); usual dose range (JNC 7): 0.1-0.3 mg/24 hour patch applied applied once every 7 days

Acute hypertension (urgency) (unlabeled use): Oral: Initial 0.1-0.2 mg; may be followed by additional doses of 0.1 mg every hour, if necessary, to a maximum total dose of 0.7 mg (Atkin, 1992; Jaker, 1989)

Unlabeled route of administration: Sublingual: Initial: 0.1-0.2 mg; followed by 0.05-0.1 mg every hour until blood pressure controlled or a cumulative dose of 0.7 mg is reached (Cunningham, 1994; Matuschka, 1999)

Nicotine withdrawal symptoms (unlabeled use; Fiore, 2008):

Oral: Initial: 0.1 mg twice daily; titreate by 0.1 mg/day every 7 days if needed; dosage range used in clinical trials: 0.15-0.75 mg/day; duration of therapy ranged from 3-10 weeks in clinical trials

Transdermal: Initial; 0.1 mg/24 hour patch applied once every 7 days and increase by 0.1 mg at 1-week intervals if necessary; dosage range used in clinical trials: 0.1-0.2 mg/24 hour patch applied once every 7 days; duration of therapy ranged from 3-10 weeks in clinical trials

Pain management: Epidural infusion: Reserved for cancer patients with severe intractable pain, unresponsive to other opioid analgesics: Starting dose: 30 mcg/hour; titrate as required for relief of pain or presence of side effects; experience with doses >40 mcg/hour is limited; should be considered an adjunct to opioid therapy

Conversion from oral to transdermal: **Note:** If transitioning from oral to transdermal therapy, overlap oral regimen for 1-2 days; transdermal route takes 2-3 days to achieve therapeutic effects. An example transition is below:

Day 1: Place Catapres-TTS® 1; administer 100% of oral dose.

Day 2: Administer 50% of oral dose.

Day 3: Administer 25% of oral dose.

Day 4: Patch remains, no further oral supplement necessary.

Conversion from transdermal to oral: After transdermal patch removal, therapeutic clonidine levels persist for ~8 hours and then slowly decrease over several days. Consider starting oral clonidine no sooner than 8 hours after patch removal.

Renal Impairment Bradycardia, sedation, and hypotension may be more likely to occur in patients with renal failure; may consider using doses at the lower end of the dosing range and monitor closely.

Not dialyzable (0% to 5%) via hemodialysis; supplemental dose is not necessary; unclear how much is removed via peritoneal dialysis. Oral antihypertensive drugs given preferentially at night may reduce the nocturnal surge of blood pressure and minimize the intradialytic hypotension that may occur when taken the morning before a dialysis session (K/DOQI, 2005).

Oral: Extended release (Nexiclon™ XR):
 Moderate-to-severe impairment (not on dialysis): No dosage adjustment recommended; titrate slowly
 End-stage kidney disease (on maintenance dialysis): Initial: 0.09 mg clonidine base/day; titrate slowly

Administration
 Epidural: Specialized techniques are required for continuous epidural administration; administration via this route should only be performed by qualified individuals familiar with the techniques of epidural administration and patient management problems associated with this route. Familiarization of the epidural infusion device is essential. Do not discontinue clonidine abruptly; if needed, gradually reduce dose over 2-4 days to avoid withdrawal symptoms.
 Oral: May be taken with or without food. Do not discontinue clonidine abruptly. If needed, gradually reduce dose over 2-4 days to avoid rebound hypertension.
  Extended release products:
   Kapvay™: Swallow whole; do not crush, split, or chew.
   Nexiclon™ XR: Tablets may be split. Shake suspension well before use.
 Transdermal patch: Patches should be applied weekly at a consistent time to a clean, hairless area of the upper outer arm or chest. Rotate patch sites weekly. Redness under patch may be reduced if a topical corticosteroid spray is applied to the area before placement of the patch.

Monitoring Parameters Blood pressure, standing and sitting/supine, mental status, heart rate

When used for the treatment of ADHD, thoroughly evaluate for cardiovascular risk. Monitor heart rate, blood pressure (when started and weaned), and consider obtaining ECG prior to initiation (Vetter, 2008).

Clonidine tolerance test: In addition to growth hormone concentrations, monitor blood pressure and blood glucose (Huang, 2001).

Epidural: Carefully monitor infusion pump; inspect catheter tubing for obstruction or dislodgement to reduce risk of inadvertent abrupt withdrawal of infusion. Monitor closely for catheter-related infection (eg, meningitis or epidural abscess).

Test Interactions Positive Coombs' test

Pharmacotherapy Pearls Each 0.1 mg of clonidine hydrochloride (salt form) is equivalent to 0.087 mg of the free base.
 Transdermal clonidine should only be used in patients unable to take oral medication. The transdermal product is much more expensive than oral clonidine and produces no better therapeutic effects.
 When used for ADHD treatment, clonidine is recommended to be used as part of a comprehensive treatment program (eg, psychological, educational, and social) for attention-deficit disorder.

Special Geriatric Considerations Because of its potential CNS adverse effects, clonidine may not be considered a drug of choice in the elderly. If the decision is to use clonidine, adjust dose based on response and adverse reactions. In patients on the transdermal system, monitor for appropriate placement of the patch.

This medication is considered to be potentially inappropriate in this patient population (Beers Criteria: Quality of evidence - low; Strength of recommendation - strong).

Dosage Forms Excipient information presented when available (limited, particularly for generics); consult specific product labeling.
 Injection, solution, as hydrochloride [epidural, preservative free]: 100 mcg/mL (10 mL); 500 mcg/mL (10 mL)
  Duraclon®: 100 mcg/mL (10 mL); 500 mcg/mL (10 mL)
 Patch, transdermal: 0.1 mg/24 hours (4s); 0.2 mg/24 hours (4s); 0.3 mg/24 hours (4s)
  Catapres-TTS®-1: 0.1 mg/24 hours (4s) [contains metal]
  Catapres-TTS®-2: 0.2 mg/24 hours (4s) [contains metal]
  Catapres-TTS®-3: 0.3 mg/24 hours (4s) [contains metal]
 Suspension, extended release, oral, as base:
  Nexiclon™ XR: 0.09 mg/mL (118 mL)
 Tablet, oral, as hydrochloride: 0.1 mg, 0.2 mg, 0.3 mg
  Catapres®: 0.1 mg, 0.2 mg, 0.3 mg [scored]

Tablet, extended release, oral, as base:
Nexiclon™ XR: 0.17 mg [scored]
Tablet, extended release, oral, as hydrochloride:
Kapvay®: 0.1 mg, 0.2 mg
Tablet, extended release, oral, as hydrochloride [dose-pack]:
Kapvay®: 0.1 mg AM dose, 0.2 mg PM dose

♦ **Clonidine Hydrochloride** *see* CloNIDine *on page* 413

Clopidogrel (kloh PID oh grel)

Related Information
Antithrombotic Therapy in Adult Patients With Prosthetic Heart Valves *on page* 2182
Perioperative/Periprocedural Management of Anticoagulant and Antiplatelet Therapy *on page* 2209

Medication Safety Issues
Sound-alike/look-alike issues:
Plavix® may be confused with Elavil®, Paxil®, Pradax™ (Canada), Pradaxa®

Brand Names: U.S. Plavix®

Brand Names: Canada Apo-Clopidogrel®; CO Clopidogrel; Mylan-Clopidogrel; Plavix®; PMS-Clopidogrel; Sandoz-Clopidogrel; Teva-Clopidogrel

Index Terms Clopidogrel Bisulfate

Generic Availability (U.S.) Yes

Pharmacologic Category Antiplatelet Agent; Antiplatelet Agent, Thienopyridine

Use Reduces rate of atherothrombotic events (myocardial infarction, stroke, vascular deaths) in patients with recent MI or stroke, or established peripheral arterial disease; reduces rate of atherothrombotic events in patients with unstable angina (UA) or non-ST-segment elevation (NSTEMI) managed medically or with percutaneous coronary intervention (PCI) (with or without stent) or CABG; reduces rate of death and atherothrombotic events in patients with ST-segment elevation MI (STEMI) managed medically

Canadian labeling: Additional use (not in U.S. labeling): Prevention of atherothrombotic and thromboembolic events, including stroke, in patients with atrial fibrillation with at least 1 risk factor for vascular events who are not suitable for treatment with an anticoagulant and are at a low risk for bleeding.

Unlabeled Use In patients with allergy or major gastrointestinal intolerance to aspirin, initial treatment of acute coronary syndromes (ACS) or prevention of coronary artery bypass graft closure (saphenous vein); stable coronary artery disease (in combination with aspirin); in patients having undergone peripheral artery percutaneous transluminal angioplasty; symptomatic carotid artery stenosis (including recent carotid endarterectomy)

Medication Guide Available Yes

Contraindications Hypersensitivity to clopidogrel or any component of the formulation; active pathological bleeding such as peptic ulcer or intracranial hemorrhage

Canadian labeling: Additional contraindications (not in U.S. labeling): Significant liver impairment or cholestatic jaundice

Warnings/Precautions [U.S. Boxed Warning]: Patients with one or more copies of the variant *CYP2C19*2* and/or *CYP2C19*3* alleles (and potentially other reduced-function variants) may have reduced conversion of clopidogrel to its active thiol metabolite. Lower active metabolite exposure may result in reduced platelet inhibition and, thus, a higher rate of cardiovascular events following MI or stent thrombosis following PCI. Although evidence is insufficient to recommend routine genetic testing, tests are available to determine CYP2C19 genotype and may be used to determine therapeutic strategy; alternative treatment or treatment strategies may be considered if patient is identified as a CYP2C19 poor metabolizer. Genetic testing may be considered prior to initiating clopidogrel in patients at moderate or high risk for poor outcomes (eg, PCI in patients with extensive and/or very complex disease). The optimal dose for CYP2C19 poor metabolizers has yet to be determined. After initiation of clopidogrel, functional testing (eg, VerifyNow® P2Y12 assay) may also be done to determine clopidogrel responsiveness (Holmes, 2010).

Use with caution in patients who may be at risk of increased bleeding, including patients with PUD, trauma, or surgery. In patients with coronary stents, premature interruption of therapy may result in stent thrombosis with subsequent fatal and nonfatal MI. Duration of therapy, in general, is determined by the type of stent placed (bare metal or drug eluting) and whether an ACS event was ongoing at the time of placement. Consider discontinuing 5 days before elective surgery (except in patients with cardiac stents that have not completed their full course of dual antiplatelet therapy; patient-specific situations need to be discussed with cardiologist; AHA/ACC/SCAI/ACS/ADA Science Advisory provides recommendations). ▶

◄ Discontinue at least 5 days before elective CABG; when urgent CABG is necessary, the ACCF/AHA CABG guidelines recommend discontinuation for at least 24 hours prior to surgery (Hillis, 2011).

Because of structural similarities, cross-reactivity is possible among the thienopyridines (clopidogrel, prasugrel, and ticlopidine); use with caution or avoid in patients with previous thienopyridine hypersensitivity. Use of clopidogrel is contraindicated in patients with hypersensitivity to clopidogrel, although desensitization may be considered for mild-to-moderate hypersensitivity.

Use caution in concurrent treatment with anticoagulants (eg, heparin, warfarin) or other antiplatelet drugs; bleeding risk is increased. Concurrent use with drugs known to inhibit CYP2C19 (eg, proton pump inhibitors) may reduce levels of active metabolite and subsequently reduce clinical efficacy and increase the risk of cardiovascular events; if possible, avoid concurrent use of moderate-to-strong CYP2C19 inhibitors. In patients requiring antacid therapy, consider use of an acid-reducing agent lacking (eg, ranitidine) with less CYP2C19 inhibition. According to the manufacturer, avoid concurrent use of omeprazole or esomeprazole; if a PPI is necessary, the use of pantoprazole, a weak CYP2C19 inhibitor, is recommended since it has been shown to have less of an effect on the pharmacologic activity of clopidogrel; lansoprazole exhibits the most potent CYP2C19 inhibition (Li, 2004). Others have recommended the continued use of PPIs, regardless of the degree of inhibition, in patients with multiple risk factors for GI bleeding who are also receiving clopidogrel since no evidence has established clinically meaningful differences in outcome; however, a clinically-significant interaction cannot be excluded in those who are poor metabolizers of clopidogrel. Staggering PPIs with clopidogrel is not recommended until further evidence is available (Abraham, 2010). Concurrent use of aspirin and clopidogrel is not recommended for secondary prevention of ischemic stroke or TIA in patients unable to take oral anticoagulants due to hemorrhagic risk (Furie, 2011).

Use with caution in patients with severe liver or renal disease (experience is limited). Cases of TTP (usually occurring within the first 2 weeks of therapy), resulting in some fatalities, have been reported; urgent plasmapheresis is required. Use in patients with severe hepatic impairment or cholestatic jaundice is contraindicated in the Canadian labeling. Cases of TTP (usually occurring within the first 2 weeks of therapy), resulting in some fatalities, have been reported; urgent plasmapheresis is required. In patients with recent lacunar stroke (within 180 days), the use of clopidogrel in addition to aspirin did not significantly reduce the incidence of the primary outcome of stroke recurrence (any ischemic stroke or intracranial hemorrhage) compared to aspirin alone; the use of clopidogrel in addition to aspirin did however increase the risk of major hemorrhage and the rate of all-cause mortality (SPS3 Investigators, 2012).

Assess bleeding risk carefully prior to initiating therapy in patients with atrial fibrillation (Canadian labeling; not an approved use in U.S. labeling); in clinical trials, a significant increase in major bleeding events (including intracranial hemorrhage and fatal bleeding events) were observed in patients receiving clopidogrel plus aspirin versus aspirin alone. Vitamin K antagonist (VKA) therapy (in suitable patients) has demonstrated a greater benefit in stroke reduction than aspirin (with or without clopidogrel).

Adverse Reactions (Reflective of adult population; not specific for elderly) As with all drugs which may affect hemostasis, bleeding is associated with clopidogrel. Hemorrhage may occur at virtually any site. Risk is dependent on multiple variables, including the concurrent use of multiple agents which alter hemostasis and patient susceptibility.

3% to 10%:
Dermatologic: Rash (4%), pruritus (3%)
Hematologic: Bleeding (major 4%; minor 5%), purpura/bruising (5%), epistaxis (3%)
1% to 3%:
Gastrointestinal: GI hemorrhage (2%)
Hematologic: Hematoma

Drug Interactions
Metabolism/Transport Effects Substrate of CYP2C19 (major), CYP3A4 (minor); **Note:** Assignment of Major/Minor substrate status based on clinically relevant drug interaction potential; **Inhibits** CYP2B6 (moderate), CYP2C9 (weak)
Avoid Concomitant Use
Avoid concomitant use of Clopidogrel with any of the following: CYP2C19 Inhibitors (Moderate); CYP2C19 Inhibitors (Strong); Omeprazole
Increased Effect/Toxicity
Clopidogrel may increase the levels/effects of: Anticoagulants; Antiplatelet Agents; Collagenase (Systemic); CYP2B6 Substrates; Dabigatran Etexilate; Drotrecogin Alfa (Activated); Ibritumomab; Rivaroxaban; Salicylates; Thrombolytic Agents; Tositumomab and Iodine I 131 Tositumomab; Warfarin

The levels/effects of Clopidogrel may be increased by: Dasatinib; Glucosamine; Herbs (Anticoagulant/Antiplatelet Properties); Nonsteroidal Anti-Inflammatory Agents; Omega-3-Acid Ethyl Esters; Pentosan Polysulfate Sodium; Pentoxifylline; Prostacyclin Analogues; Rifamycin Derivatives; Tipranavir; Vitamin E

Decreased Effect

The levels/effects of Clopidogrel may be decreased by: Amiodarone; Calcium Channel Blockers; CYP2C19 Inhibitors (Moderate); CYP2C19 Inhibitors (Strong); Dexlansoprazole; Esomeprazole; Lansoprazole; Macrolide Antibiotics; Nonsteroidal Anti-Inflammatory Agents; Omeprazole; Pantoprazole; RABEprazole; Tocilizumab

Ethanol/Nutrition/Herb Interactions Herb/Nutraceutical: Avoid alfalfa, anise, bilberry, bladderwrack, bromelain, cat's claw, chamomile, coleus, cordyceps, dong quai, evening primrose oil, fenugreek, feverfew, garlic, ginger, ginkgo biloba, ginseng (American), ginseng (Panax), ginseng (Siberian), grape seed, green tea, guggul, horse chestnut seed, horse-radish, licorice, prickly ash, red clover, reishi, SAMe (S-adenosylmethionine), sweet clover, turmeric, white willow (all have additional antiplatelet activity).

Stability Store at 25°C (77°F); excursions permitted to 15°C to 30°C (59°F to 86°F).

Mechanism of Action Clopidogrel requires *in vivo* biotransformation to an active thiol metabolite. The active metabolite irreversibly blocks the $P2Y_{12}$ component of ADP receptors on the platelet surface, which prevents activation of the GPIIb/IIIa receptor complex, thereby reducing platelet aggregation. Platelets blocked by clopidogrel are affected for the remainder of their lifespan (~7-10 days).

Pharmacodynamics/Kinetics

Onset of action: Inhibition of platelet aggregation (IPA): Dose-dependent:

300-600 mg loading dose: Detected within 2 hours

50-100 mg/day: Detected by the second day of treatment

Peak effect: Time to maximal IPA: Dose-dependent: **Note:** Degree of IPA based on adenosine diphosphate (ADP) concentration used during light aggregometry:

300-600 mg loading dose:

ADP 5 micromole/L: 20% to 30% IPA at 6 hours post administration (Montelescot, 2006)

ADP 20 micromole/L: 30% to 37% IPA at 6 hours post administration (Montelescot, 2006)

50-100 mg/day: ADP 5 micromole/L: 50% to 60% IPA at 5-7 days (Herbert, 1993)

Absorption: Well absorbed

Protein binding: Parent drug: 98%; Inactive metabolite: 94%

Metabolism: Extensively hepatic via esterase-mediated hydrolysis to a carboxylic acid derivative (inactive) and via CYP450-mediated (CYP2C19 primarily) oxidation to a thiol metabolite (active)

Half-life elimination: Parent drug: ~6 hours; Active metabolite: ~30 minutes

Time to peak, serum: ~0.75 hours

Excretion: Urine (50%); feces (46%)

Dosage

Geriatric & Adult

Recent MI, recent stroke, or established peripheral arterial disease (PAD): Oral: 75 mg once daily. **Note:** The ACCF/AHA guidelines for PAD recommend clopidogrel as an alternative to aspirin (Class Ib recommendation) or in conjunction with aspirin for those who are not at an increased risk of bleeding but are of high cardiovascular risk (Class IIb recommendation). These recommendations also pertain to those with intermittent claudication or critical limb ischemia, prior lower extremity revascularization, or prior amputation for lower extremity ischemia (Rooke, 2011).

Coronary artery disease (CAD), established: Oral: 75 mg once daily. **Note:** Established CAD defined as patients 1-year post ACS, with prior revascularization, coronary stenosis >50% by angiogram, and/or evidence for cardiac ischemia on diagnostic testing (includes patients after the first year post-ACS and/or with prior CABG surgery) (Guyatt, 2012).

Secondary prevention of cardioembolic stroke (patient not candidate for oral anti-coagulation): Oral: 75 mg once daily (in combination with aspirin) (Guyatt, 2012)

Acute coronary syndrome (ACS): Oral:

Unstable angina, non-ST-segment elevation myocardial infarction (UA/NSTEMI): Initial: 300 mg loading dose, followed by 75 mg once daily for up to 12 months (in combination with aspirin indefinitely) (Jneid, 2012). The American College of Chest Physicians recommends combination aspirin dose of 75-100 mg (Guyatt, 2012).

ST-segment elevation myocardial infarction (STEMI): 75 mg once daily (in combination with aspirin 162-325 mg initially followed by 81-162 mg/day or 75-100 mg/day [Guyatt, 2012]). **Note:** CLARITY-TIMI 28 used a 300 mg loading dose (with thrombolysis) demonstrating an improvement in the patency rate of the infarct related artery and reduction in ischemic complications. The duration of therapy was <28 days (usually until hospital discharge) unless nonprimary percutaneous coronary intervention (PCI) was performed (Sabatine, 2005).

Percutaneous coronary intervention (PCI) for acute coronary syndrome (eg, UA/NSTEMI or STEMI): Loading dose: 600 mg given as early as possible before or at the time of PCI, followed by 75 mg once daily (in combination with aspirin 81 mg/day). **Note:** If fibrinolytic administered within the previous 24 hours, administer 300 mg loading dose instead (Levine, 2011). The use of ticagrelor (instead of clopidogrel) in combination with aspirin has been suggested (Guyatt, 2012).

Higher versus standard maintenance dosing: May consider a maintenance dose of 150 mg once daily for 6 days, then 75 mg once daily thereafter in patients not at high risk for bleeding (CURRENT-OASIS 7 Investigators, 2010; Jneid, 2012); however, in another study, in patients with high on-treatment platelet reactivity, the use of 150 mg once daily for 6 months did not demonstrate a difference in 6-month incidence of death from cardiovascular causes, nonfatal MI, or stent thrombosis compared to standard dose therapy (Price, 2011).

Duration of clopidogrel (in combination with aspirin) after stent placement for ACS and non-ACS indications: **Premature interruption of therapy may result in stent thrombosis with subsequent fatal and nonfatal MI.** At least 12 months of clopidogrel is recommended for those with ACS receiving either stent type (bare metal [BMS] or drug eluting stent [DES]) or those receiving a DES for a non-ACS indication (ie, elective PCI). Those receiving a BMS for a non-ACS indication should be given at least 1 month and ideally up to 12 months; if patient is at increased risk of bleeding, give for a minimum of 2 weeks. A duration >12 months, regardless of indication, may be considered in patients with DES placement (Jneid, 2012; Levine, 2011).

CYP2C19 poor metabolizers (ie, *CYP2C19*2* or *3* carriers): Although routine genetic testing is not recommended in patients treated with clopidogrel undergoing PCI, testing may be considered to identify poor metabolizers who would be at risk for poor outcomes while receiving clopidogrel; if identified, these patients may be considered for an alternative P2Y$_{12}$ inhibitor (Levine, 2011). An appropriate regimen for this patient population has not been established in clinical outcome trials. Although the manufacturer suggests a 600 mg loading dose, followed by 150 mg once daily, it does not appear that this dosing strategy improves outcomes for this patient population (Price, 2011).

Atrial fibrillation (in patients not candidates for warfarin and at a low risk of bleeding) (Canadian labeling; ACTIVE Investigators, 2009; unlabeled use in U.S.): Oral: 75 mg once daily (in combination with aspirin 75-100 mg once daily). **Note:** Combination may also be used as an alternative for patients with atrial fibrillation and mitral stenosis (Guyatt, 2012).

Carotid artery stenosis, symptomatic (including recent carotid endarterectomy) (unlabeled use): Oral: 75 mg once daily (Guyatt, 2012)

Peripheral artery percutaneous transluminal angioplasty (with or without stenting) or peripheral artery bypass graft surgery, postprocedure (unlabeled use): Oral: 75 mg once daily. **Note:** For below-knee bypass graft surgery with prosthetic grafts, combine with aspirin 75-100 mg/day (Guyatt, 2012).

Prevention of coronary artery bypass graft closure (saphenous vein) and postoperative adverse cardiovascular events (unlabeled use): Oral: Aspirin-allergic patients: 75 mg once daily (Hillis, 2011)

Renal Impairment No adjustment is necessary.

Hepatic Impairment Use with caution; experience is limited. **Note:** Inhibition of ADP-induced platelet aggregation and mean bleeding time prolongation were similar in patients with severe hepatic impairment compared to healthy subjects after repeated doses of 75 mg once daily for 10 days.

Administration May be administered without regard to meals.

Monitoring Parameters Signs of bleeding; hemoglobin and hematocrit periodically. May consider platelet function testing to determine platelet inhibitory response or genotyping for CYP2C19 loss of function variant if results of testing may alter management (Jneid, 2012).

Special Geriatric Considerations Plasma concentrations of the main metabolite of clopidogrel were significantly higher in the elderly (≥75 years). This was not associated with changes in bleeding time or platelet aggregation. No dosage adjustment is recommended.

Dosage Forms Excipient information presented when available (limited, particularly for generics); consult specific product labeling.

Tablet, oral: 75 mg, 300 mg

Plavix®: 75 mg, 300 mg

◆ **Clopidogrel Bisulfate** *see* Clopidogrel *on page 419*

Clorazepate (klor AZ e pate)

Related Information
Anxiolytic, Sedative/Hypnotic, and Miscellaneous Benzodiazepines *on page 2106*

Medication Safety Issues
Sound-alike/look-alike issues:
Clorazepate may be confused with clofibrate, clonazepam, KlonoPIN®

BEERS Criteria medication:
This drug may be potentially inappropriate for use in geriatric patients (Quality of evidence - high; Strength of recommendation - strong).

Brand Names: U.S. Tranxene® T-Tab®

Brand Names: Canada Apo-Clorazepate®; Novo-Clopate

Index Terms Clorazepate Dipotassium; Tranxene T-Tab

Generic Availability (U.S.) Yes

Pharmacologic Category Benzodiazepine

Use Treatment of generalized anxiety disorder; management of ethanol withdrawal; adjunct anticonvulsant in management of partial seizures

Medication Guide Available Yes

Contraindications Hypersensitivity to clorazepate or any component of the formulation (cross-sensitivity with other benzodiazepines may exist); narrow-angle glaucoma

Warnings/Precautions Antiepileptics are associated with an increased risk of suicidal behavior/thoughts with use (regardless of indication); patients should be monitored for signs/symptoms of depression, suicidal tendencies, and other unusual behavior changes during therapy and instructed to inform their healthcare provider immediately if symptoms occur.

Not recommended for use in patients with depressive or psychotic disorders. Use with caution in elderly or debilitated patients, patients with hepatic disease (including alcoholics), or renal impairment. Active metabolites with extended half-lives may lead to delayed accumulation and adverse effects. Use with caution in patients with respiratory disease or impaired gag reflex. Avoid use in patients with sleep apnea.

Causes CNS depression (dose related) resulting in sedation, dizziness, confusion, or ataxia which may impair physical and mental capabilities. Patients must be cautioned about performing tasks which require mental alertness (eg, operating machinery or driving). Use with caution in patients receiving other CNS depressants or psychoactive agents. Effects with other sedative drugs or ethanol may be potentiated. Benzodiazepines have been associated with falls and traumatic injury and should be used with extreme caution in patients who are at risk of these events. In older adults, benzodiazepines increase the risk of impaired cognition, delirium, falls, fractures, and motor vehicle accidents. Due to increased sensitivity in this age group and slower metabolism of long-acting agents (such as clorazepate), avoid use for treatment of insomnia, agitation, or delirium (Beers Criteria).

Use caution in patients with depression, particularly if suicidal risk may be present. Use with caution in patients with a history of drug dependence. Benzodiazepines have been associated with dependence and acute withdrawal symptoms on discontinuation or reduction in dose. Acute withdrawal, including seizures, may be precipitated in patients after administration of flumazenil to patients receiving long-term benzodiazepine therapy.

Benzodiazepines have been associated with anterograde amnesia. Paradoxical reactions, including hyperactive or aggressive behavior, have been reported with benzodiazepines, particularly in adolescent/pediatric or psychiatric patients. Does not have analgesic, antidepressant, or antipsychotic properties.

Adverse Reactions (Reflective of adult population; not specific for elderly) Frequency not defined.

Cardiovascular: Hypotension

Central nervous system: Drowsiness, fatigue, ataxia, lightheadedness, memory impairment, insomnia, anxiety, headache, depression, slurred speech, confusion, nervousness, dizziness, irritability

Dermatologic: Rash

Endocrine & metabolic: Libido decreased

Gastrointestinal: Xerostomia, constipation, diarrhea, nausea, salivation decreased, vomiting, appetite increased or decreased

Hepatic: Jaundice, transaminase increased

Neuromuscular & skeletal: Dysarthria, tremor

Ocular: Blurred vision, diplopia

◀ **Drug Interactions**

Metabolism/Transport Effects Substrate of CYP3A4 (major); **Note:** Assignment of Major/Minor substrate status based on clinically relevant drug interaction potential

Avoid Concomitant Use

Avoid concomitant use of Clorazepate with any of the following: Azelastine; Azelastine (Nasal); Conivaptan; Methadone; Mirtazapine; OLANZapine; Paraldehyde

Increased Effect/Toxicity

Clorazepate may increase the levels/effects of: Alcohol (Ethyl); Azelastine; Azelastine (Nasal); Buprenorphine; CloZAPine; CNS Depressants; Fosphenytoin; Methadone; Methotrimeprazine; Metyrosine; Mirtazapine; Paraldehyde; Phenytoin; Selective Serotonin Reuptake Inhibitors; Zolpidem

The levels/effects of Clorazepate may be increased by: Antifungal Agents (Azole Derivatives, Systemic); Aprepitant; Calcium Channel Blockers (Nondihydropyridine); Cimetidine; Conivaptan; Contraceptives (Estrogens); Contraceptives (Progestins); CYP3A4 Inhibitors (Moderate); CYP3A4 Inhibitors (Strong); Dasatinib; Droperidol; Fosamprenavir; Fosaprepitant; Grapefruit Juice; HydrOXYzine; Isoniazid; Ivacaftor; Macrolide Antibiotics; MAO Inhibitors; Methotrimeprazine; Mifepristone; OLANZapine; Proton Pump Inhibitors; Ritonavir; Saquinavir; Selective Serotonin Reuptake Inhibitors

Decreased Effect

The levels/effects of Clorazepate may be decreased by: CarBAMazepine; CYP3A4 Inducers (Strong); Deferasirox; Rifamycin Derivatives; St Johns Wort; Theophylline Derivatives; Tocilizumab; Yohimbine

Ethanol/Nutrition/Herb Interactions

Ethanol: May increase CNS depression; monitor for increased effects with coadministration. Caution patients about effects.

Food: Serum concentrations/toxicity may be increased by grapefruit juice.

Herb/Nutraceutical: Avoid valerian, St John's wort, kava kava, gotu kola (may increase CNS depression).

Stability Store at controlled room temperature at 20°C to 25°C (68°F to 77°F). Protect from moisture; keep bottle tightly closed; dispense in tightly closed, light-resistant container.

Mechanism of Action Binds to stereospecific benzodiazepine receptors on the postsynaptic GABA neuron at several sites within the central nervous system, including the limbic system, reticular formation. Enhancement of the inhibitory effect of GABA on neuronal excitability results by increased neuronal membrane permeability to chloride ions. This shift in chloride ions results in hyperpolarization (a less excitable state) and stabilization.

Pharmacodynamics/Kinetics

Onset of action: 1-2 hours

Duration: Variable, 8-24 hours

Distribution: Appears in urine

Protein binding: Nordiazepam 97% to 98%

Metabolism: Rapidly decarboxylated to nordiazepam (active) in acidic stomach prior to absorption; hepatically to oxazepam (active)

Half-life elimination: Adults: Nordiazepam: 40-50 hours; Oxazepam: 6-8 hours

Time to peak, serum: ~1 hour

Excretion: Primarily urine

Dosage

Geriatric Oral: Anxiety: 7.5 mg 1-2 times/day; use is not recommended in the elderly.

Adult

Anxiety: Oral: 7.5-15 mg 2-4 times/day

Ethanol withdrawal: Oral: Initial: 30 mg, then 15 mg 2-4 times/day on first day; maximum daily dose: 90 mg; gradually decrease dose over subsequent days.

Seizures (anticonvulsant): Oral: Initial: Up to 7.5 mg/dose 2-3 times/day; increase dose by 7.5 mg at weekly intervals; not to exceed 90 mg/day

Monitoring Parameters Respiratory and cardiovascular status, excess CNS depression; suicidality (eg, suicidal thoughts, depression, behavioral changes)

Reference Range Therapeutic: 0.12-1 mcg/mL (SI: 0.36-3.01 micromole/L)

Test Interactions Decreased hematocrit; abnormal liver and renal function tests

Pharmacotherapy Pearls Abrupt discontinuation after sustained use (generally >10 days) may cause withdrawal symptoms.

Special Geriatric Considerations Due to its long-acting metabolite, clorazepate is not considered a drug of choice in the elderly. Long-acting benzodiazepines have been associated with falls in the elderly. Guidelines from the Centers for Medicare and Medicaid Services (CMS) discourage the use of this agent in residents of long-term care facilities.

This medication is considered to be potentially inappropriate in this patient population (Beers Criteria: Quality of evidence - high; Strength of recommendation - strong).

Controlled Substance C-IV

Dosage Forms Excipient information presented when available (limited, particularly for generics); consult specific product labeling.
Tablet, oral, as dipotassium: 3.75 mg, 7.5 mg, 15 mg
Tranxene® T-Tab®: 3.75 mg, 7.5 mg, 15 mg [scored]

♦ **Clorazepate Dipotassium** *see* Clorazepate *on page 423*

Clotrimazole (Oral) (kloe TRIM a zole)

Medication Safety Issues
Sound-alike/look-alike issues:
Clotrimazole may be confused with co-trimoxazole
Mycelex may be confused with Myoflex®
International issues:
Cloderm: Brand name for clotrimazole [Germany], but also brand name for alclomethasone [Indonesia]; clobetasol [China, India, Malaysia, Singapore, Thailand]; clocortolone [U.S., Canada]

Canesten [multiple international markets] may be confused with Canesten Bifonazol Comp brand name for bifonazole/urea [Austria]; Canesten Extra brand name for bifonazole [China, Germany]; Canesten Extra Nagelset brand name for bifonazole/urea [Denmark]; Canesten Fluconazol brand name for fluconazole [New Zealand]; Canesten Oasis brand name for sodium citrate [Great Britain]; Canesten Once Daily brand name for bifonazole [Australia]; Canesten Oral brand name for fluconazole [United Kingdom]; Cenestin brand name for estrogens (conjugated A/synthetic) [U.S., Canada]

Mycelex: Brand name for clotrimazole [U.S.] may be confused with Mucolex brand name for bromhexine [Malaysia]; carbocisteine [Thailand]
Index Terms Mycelex
Generic Availability (U.S.) Yes
Pharmacologic Category Antifungal Agent, Oral Nonabsorbed
Use Treatment of susceptible fungal infections, including oropharyngeal candidiasis; limited data suggest that clotrimazole troches may be effective for prophylaxis against oropharyngeal candidiasis in neutropenic patients
Contraindications Hypersensitivity to clotrimazole or any component of the formulation
Warnings/Precautions Clotrimazole should not be used for treatment of systemic fungal infection.

Adverse Reactions (Reflective of adult population; not specific for elderly)
>10%: Hepatic: Abnormal liver function tests
Frequency not defined:
Dermatologic: Pruritus
Gastrointestinal: Nausea, vomiting

Drug Interactions
Metabolism/Transport Effects Inhibits CYP1A2 (weak), CYP2A6 (weak), CYP2B6 (weak), CYP2C19 (weak), CYP2C8 (weak), CYP2C9 (weak), CYP2D6 (weak), CYP2E1 (weak), CYP3A4 (moderate)
Avoid Concomitant Use
Avoid concomitant use of Clotrimazole (Oral) with any of the following: Pimozide; Tolvaptan
Increased Effect/Toxicity
Clotrimazole (Oral) may increase the levels/effects of: ARIPiprazole; Avanafil; Budesonide (Systemic, Oral Inhalation); Colchicine; CYP3A4 Substrates; Eplerenone; Everolimus; FentaNYL; Halofantrine; Ivacaftor; Lurasidone; Pimecrolimus; Pimozide; Propafenone; Ranolazine; Salmeterol; Saxagliptin; Tacrolimus; Tacrolimus (Systemic); Tolvaptan; Vilazodone; Zuclopenthixol
Decreased Effect
Clotrimazole (Oral) may decrease the levels/effects of: Ifosfamide; Saccharomyces boulardii
Mechanism of Action Binds to phospholipids in the fungal cell membrane altering cell wall permeability resulting in loss of essential intracellular elements

Pharmacodynamics/Kinetics
Distribution: Oral (troche): Inhibitory concentrations remain in the saliva for up to 3 hours after dissolution of the troche
Excretion: Feces (as metabolites)

Dosage
Geriatric & Adult Oropharyngeal candidiasis: Oral:
Prophylaxis: 10 mg troche dissolved 3 times/day for the duration of chemotherapy or until steroids are reduced to maintenance levels
Treatment: 10 mg troche dissolved slowly 5 times/day for 14 consecutive days
Administration Oral: Allow troche to dissolve slowly over 15-30 minutes.

◀ **Monitoring Parameters** Periodic liver function tests during oral therapy with clotrimazole troche

Special Geriatric Considerations Localized fungal infections frequently follow broad-spectrum antimicrobial therapy. Specifically, oral and vaginal infections due to *Candida*.

Dosage Forms Excipient information presented when available (limited, particularly for generics); consult specific product labeling.

Troche, oral: 10 mg

Clotrimazole (Topical) (kloe TRIM a zole)

Medication Safety Issues

Sound-alike/look-alike issues:
Clotrimazole may be confused with co-trimoxazole

Lotrimin® may be confused with Lotrisone®

International issues:
Cloderm: Brand name for clotrimazole [Germany], but also brand name for alclomethasone [Indonesia]; clobetasol [China, India, Malaysia, Singapore, Thailand]; clocortolone [U.S., Canada]

Canesten: Brand name for clotrimazole [multiple international markets] may be confused with Canesten Bifonazol Comp brand name for bifonazole/urea [Austria]; Canesten Extra brand name for bifonazole [China, Germany]; Canesten Extra Nagelset brand name for bifonazole/urea [Denmark]; Canesten Fluconazole brand name for fluconazole [New Zealand]; Canesten Oasis brand name for sodium citrate [Great Britain]; Canesten Once Daily brand name for bifonazole [Australia]; Canesten Oral brand name for fluconazole [United Kingdom]; Cenestin® brand name for estrogens (conjugated A/synthetic) [U.S., Canada]

Brand Names: U.S. Anti-Fungal™ [OTC]; Cruex® [OTC]; Gyne-Lotrimin 3 [OTC]; Gyne-Lotrimin® 7 [OTC]; Lotrimin® AF Athlete's Foot [OTC]; Lotrimin® AF for Her [OTC]; Lotrimin® AF Jock Itch [OTC]

Brand Names: Canada Canesten® Topical; Canesten® Vaginal; Clotrimaderm; Trivagizole-3®

Generic Availability (U.S.) Yes

Pharmacologic Category Antifungal Agent, Topical; Antifungal Agent, Vaginal

Use Treatment of susceptible fungal infections, including dermatophytoses, superficial mycoses, and cutaneous candidiasis, as well as vulvovaginal candidiasis

Dosage

Geriatric & Adult

Dermatophytosis, cutaneous candidiasis: Topical (cream, solution): Apply twice daily; if no improvement occurs after 4 weeks of therapy, re-evaluate diagnosis.

Vulvovaginal candidiasis: Intravaginal:

Cream (1%): Insert 1 applicatorful of 1% vaginal cream daily (preferably at bedtime) for 7 consecutive days.

Cream (2%): Insert 1 applicatorful of 2% vaginal cream daily (preferably at bedtime) for 3 consecutive days.

Dermatologic infection (superficial): Topical (cream, solution): Apply to affected area twice daily (morning and evening) for 7 consecutive days.

Special Geriatric Considerations Localized fungal infections frequently follow broad-spectrum antimicrobial therapy. Specifically, oral and vaginal infections due to *Candida*.

Dosage Forms Excipient information presented when available (limited, particularly for generics); consult specific product labeling.

Cream, topical: 1% (15 g, 30 g, 45 g)

Anti-Fungal™: 1% (113 g)

Cruex®: 1% (15 g) [contains benzyl alcohol]

Lotrimin® AF Athlete's Foot: 1% (12 g) [contains benzyl alcohol]

Lotrimin® AF for Her: 1% (24 g) [contains benzyl alcohol]

Lotrimin® AF Jock Itch: 1% (12 g) [contains benzyl alcohol]

Cream, vaginal: 1% (45 g); 2% (21 g)

Gyne-Lotrimin® 7: 1% (45 g) [contains benzyl alcohol]

Gyne-Lotrimin® 3: 2% (21 g) [contains benzyl alcohol]

Solution, topical: 1% (10 mL, 30 mL)

Cloxacillin (kloks a SIL in)

Brand Names: Canada Apo-Cloxi®; Novo-Cloxin; Nu-Cloxi

Index Terms Cloxacillin Sodium

Pharmacologic Category Antibiotic, Penicillin

Use Treatment of bacterial infections including endocarditis, pneumonia, bone and joint infections, skin and soft-tissue infections, and sepsis that are caused by susceptible strains of penicillinase-producing staphylococci. **Note:** Exhibits good activity against *Staphylococcus aureus*; has activity against many streptococci, but is less active than penicillin and is generally not used in clinical practice to treat streptococcal infections.

Contraindications Hypersensitivity to cloxacillin, other penicillins, cephalosporins, or any component of the formulation

Warnings/Precautions Serious and occasionally severe or fatal hypersensitivity (anaphylactoid) reactions have been reported in patients on penicillin therapy, especially with a history of beta-lactam hypersensitivity, history of sensitivity to multiple allergens, or previous IgE-mediated reactions (eg, anaphylaxis, angioedema, urticaria). Use with caution in renal impairment as the rate of elimination is decreased. Use with caution in asthmatic patients. Prolonged use may result in fungal or bacterial superinfection, including *C. difficile*-associated diarrhea (CDAD) and pseudomembranous colitis; CDAD has been observed >2 months postantibiotic treatment. Use with caution in patients with a history of seizure disorders, particularly in the presence of renal impairment as increased serum levels may increase risk for seizures. Penicillin transport across the blood-brain barrier may be enhanced by inflamed meninges or during cardiopulmonary bypass increasing the risk of myoclonia, seizures, or reduced consciousness especially in patients with renal failure. Penicillin use has been associated with hematologic disorders (eg, agranulocytosis, neutropenia, thrombocytopenia) believed to be a hypersensitivity phenomena. Reactions are most often reversible upon discontinuing therapy.

Adverse Reactions (Reflective of adult population; not specific for elderly) Frequency not defined.

Cardiovascular: Hypotension

Central nervous system: Confusion, fever, lethargy, seizure (high doses and/or renal failure)

Dermatologic: Pruritus, rash, urticaria

Gastrointestinal: Abdominal pain, black or hairy tongue, diarrhea, flatulence, nausea, oral candidiasis, pseudomembranous colitis, stomatitis, vomiting

Hematologic: Agranulocytosis, bone marrow depression, eosinophilia, granulocytopenia, hemolytic anemia, leukopenia, neutropenia, thrombocytopenia

Hepatic: Alkaline phosphatase increased, ALT increased, AST increased, hepatotoxicity

Local: Thrombophlebitis

Neuromuscular & skeletal: Arthralgia, myalgia, myoclonus

Renal: Hematuria, interstitial nephritis, proteinuria, renal insufficiency, renal tubular damage

Respiratory: Bronchospasm, laryngeal edema, laryngospasm, sneezing, wheezing

Miscellaneous: Anaphylaxis, angioedema, allergic reaction, serum sickness-like reaction

Drug Interactions

Metabolism/Transport Effects None known.

Avoid Concomitant Use

Avoid concomitant use of Cloxacillin with any of the following: BCG

Increased Effect/Toxicity

Cloxacillin may increase the levels/effects of: Methotrexate; Vitamin K Antagonists

The levels/effects of Cloxacillin may be increased by: Probenecid

Decreased Effect

Cloxacillin may decrease the levels/effects of: BCG; Mycophenolate; Typhoid Vaccine

The levels/effects of Cloxacillin may be decreased by: Fusidic Acid; Tetracycline Derivatives

Ethanol/Nutrition/Herb Interactions Food: Food decreases cloxacillin absorption; serum levels are reduced by ~50%. Management: Administer with water on an empty stomach 1 hour before or 2 hours after meals.

Stability

Capsule: Store at room temperature not exceeding 25°C (77°F).

Powder for injection: Store at controlled room temperature not exceeding 25°C (77°F). Upon reconstitution the resulting solution is stable for up to 24 hours at controlled room temperature and 48 hours under refrigeration.

I.M. injection: Vials should be reconstituted with appropriate volume of SWFI to make a final concentration of 125 mg/mL or 250 mg/mL

I.V. injection: Vials should be reconstituted with appropriate volume of SWFI to make a final concentration of 50 mg/mL or 100 mg/mL

I.V. infusion: Infusion is prepared in 2 stages: Initial reconstitution of powder, followed by dilution to final infusion solution.

Note: After reconstitution of powder with appropriate volume of sterile water for injection, the manufacturer suggests further dilution to concentrations of 1-2 mg/mL in a compatible solution (eg, D_5W, NS); solutions are stable for up to 12 hours at controlled room temperature.

◄ Powder for oral solution: Prior to mixing, store powder at room temperature not exceeding 25°C (77°F). Refrigerate oral solution after reconstitution; discard after 14 days.

Mechanism of Action Inhibits bacterial cell wall synthesis by binding to one or more of the penicillin-binding proteins (PBPs) which in turn inhibit the final transpeptidation step of peptidoglycan synthesis in bacterial cell walls, thus inhibiting cell wall biosynthesis. Bacteria eventually lyse due to ongoing activity of cell wall autolytic enzymes (autolysins and murein hydrolases) while cell wall assembly is arrested.

Pharmacodynamics/Kinetics

Absorption: Oral: ~50%; reduced by food

Distribution: Widely to most body fluids and bone; penetration into cells, into eye, and across normal meninges is poor; inflammation increases amount that crosses blood-brain barrier

Protein binding: ~94% (primarily albumin)

Metabolism: Extensively hepatic to active and inactive metabolites

Half-life elimination: 0.5-1.5 hours; prolonged with renal impairment

Time to peak, serum: ~1 hour

Excretion: Urine and feces

Dosage

Geriatric & Adult Note: Dose and duration of therapy can vary depending on infecting organism, severity of infection, and clinical response of patient. Treat severe staphylococcal infections for at least 14 days; endocarditis and osteomyelitis require an extended duration of therapy for 4-6 weeks. The intravenous route should be used for severe infections.

Susceptible infections:

Oral: 250-500 mg every 6 hours (manufacturer recommended maximum adult dose: 6 g/day)

I.M., I.V.: 250-500 mg every 6 hours (manufacturer recommended maximum adult dose: 6 g/day)

Dosing recommendations of World Health Organization unless otherwise noted:

Arthritis (septic), methicillin-sensitive *Staphylococcus aureus* (MSSA) (unlabeled dosing): I.M., I.V.: 2 g every 6 hours for 2-3 weeks; **Note:** Oral therapy of 1 g every 6 hours may be used to complete therapy if parenteral therapy is discontinued prior to 2-3 week duration

Endocarditis (MSSA) (unlabeled dosing): I.V.:

Native valve: 2 g every 4 hours for 6 weeks; may give with gentamicin for initial 5 days (Choudri, 2000)

Prosthetic valve: 2 g every 4 hours for 6 weeks; give with gentamicin for 2 weeks and rifampin for 6 weeks (Choudri, 2000)

Uncomplicated endocarditis in I.V. drug users: 2 g every 4 hours for 4 weeks and gentamicin for initial 5 days **or** 2 g every 4 hours and gentamicin both given for 2 weeks total (Choudri, 2000)

Osteomyelitis (MSSA) (unlabeled dosing): I.M., I.V.: 2 g every 6 hours for 4-6 weeks (preferred) **or** for a minimum of 14 days, **followed by** 1 g every 6 hours orally to complete 4-6 weeks of therapy

Pneumonia (MSSA) (unlabeled dosing): I.M., I.V.: 1-2 g every 6 hours for 10-14 days

Renal Impairment No dosage adjustment necessary.

Administration

Oral: Administer with water 1 hour before or 2 hours after meals

I.M.: Administer slowly over 2-4 minutes

I.V.:

I.V. push: Administer slowly over 2-4 minutes

I.V. infusion: Administer over 30-40 minutes

Monitoring Parameters Observe for signs and symptoms of anaphylaxis during first dose; CBC with differential (prior to initiating therapy and weekly thereafter), periodic BUN, creatinine, hepatic function

Test Interactions May interfere with urinary glucose tests using cupric sulfate (Benedict's solution, Clinitest®); may inactivate aminoglycosides *in vitro*; false-positive urine and serum proteins; false-positive in uric acid, urinary steroids

Special Geriatric Considerations Dosage adjustment for renal function is not necessary.

Product Availability Not available in U.S.

Dosage Forms: Canada Excipient information presented when available (limited, particularly for generics); consult specific product labeling.

Capsule, oral, as sodium: 250 mg, 500 mg

Injection, powder for reconstitution: 250 mg, 500 mg, 1000 mg, 2000 mg

Powder for suspension, oral, as sodium: 125 mg/5 mL (60 mL, 100 mL, 200 mL)

◆ **Cloxacillin Sodium** *see* Cloxacillin *on page 426*

CloZAPine (KLOE za peen)

Related Information
Antipsychotic Agents *on page 2103*
Atypical Antipsychotics *on page 2107*
Beers Criteria – Potentially Inappropriate Medications for Geriatrics *on page 2183*

Medication Safety Issues
Sound-alike/look-alike issues:
CloZAPine may be confused with clonazePAM, cloNIDine, KlonoPIN®
Clozaril® may be confused with Clinoril®, Colazal®

BEERS Criteria medication:
This drug may be potentially inappropriate for use in geriatric patients (Quality of evidence - moderate; Strength of recommendation - strong).

Brand Names: U.S. Clozaril®; FazaClo®

Brand Names: Canada Apo-Clozapine®; Clozaril®; Gen-Clozapine

Generic Availability (U.S.) Yes

Pharmacologic Category Antipsychotic Agent, Atypical

Use Treatment-refractory schizophrenia; to reduce risk of recurrent suicidal behavior in schizophrenia or schizoaffective disorder

Unlabeled Use Schizoaffective disorder, bipolar disorder, severe obsessive-compulsive disorder; psychosis/agitation related to Alzheimer's dementia

Prescribing and Access Restrictions
U.S.: Clozaril® is deemed to have an approved REMS program. As a requirement of the REMS program, access to this medication is restricted. Patient-specific registration is required to dispense clozapine. Monitoring systems for individual clozapine manufacturers are independent. If a patient is switched from one brand/manufacturer of clozapine to another, the patient must be entered into a new registry (must be completed by the prescriber and delivered to the dispensing pharmacy). Healthcare providers, including pharmacists dispensing clozapine, should verify the patient's hematological status and qualification to receive clozapine with all existing registries. The manufacturer of Clozaril® requests that healthcare providers submit all WBC/ANC values following discontinuation of therapy to the Clozaril National Registry for all nonrechallengable patients until WBC is $\geq 3500/\text{mm}^3$ and ANC is $\geq 2000/\text{mm}^3$.

Canada: Currently, there are multiple manufacturers that distribute clozapine and each manufacturer has its own registry and distribution system. Patients must be registered in a database that includes their location, prescribing physician, testing laboratory, and dispensing pharmacist before using clozapine. Information specific to each monitoring program is available from the individual manufacturers.

Contraindications Hypersensitivity to clozapine or any component of the formulation; history of agranulocytosis or severe granulocytopenia with clozapine; uncontrolled epilepsy, severe central nervous system depression or comatose state; paralytic ileus; myeloproliferative disorders or use with other agents which have a well-known risk of agranulocytosis or bone marrow suppression

Canadian labeling: Additional contraindications (not in U.S. labeling): Active hepatic disease associated with nausea, anorexia, or jaundice; progressive hepatic disease or hepatic failure; severe renal impairment; severe cardiac disease (eg, myocarditis); patients unable to undergo blood testing

Warnings/Precautions [U.S. Boxed Warning]: Elderly patients with dementia-related psychosis treated with antipsychotics are at an increased risk of death compared to placebo. Most deaths appeared to be either cardiovascular (eg, heart failure, sudden death) or infectious (eg, pneumonia) in nature. Clozapine is not approved for the treatment of dementia-related psychosis.

[U.S. Boxed Warning]: Significant risk of potentially life-threatening agranulocytosis. Due to the significant risk of agranulocytosis, treatment should be reserved for patients who fail at least two trials of other primary medications for the treatment of schizophrenia (of adequate dose and duration) or for those at risk of reexperiencing suicidal behavior. Therapy should not be initiated in patients with WBC <3500 cells/mm³ or ANC <2000 cells/mm³, a history of myeloproliferative disorder, or clozapine-induced agranulocytosis or granulocytopenia. WBC testing should occur periodically on an on-going basis (see prescribing information for monitoring details) to ensure that acceptable WBC/ANC counts are maintained. Initial episodes of moderate leukopenia or granulopoietic suppression confer up to a 12-fold increased risk for subsequent episodes of agranulocytosis. WBCs must be monitored weekly for at least 4 weeks after therapy discontinuation or until WBC is $\geq 3500/\text{mm}^3$ and ANC is $\geq 2000/\text{mm}^3$. Use with caution in patients receiving other marrow suppressive agents. Eosinophilia has been reported to occur with clozapine. Interrupt therapy for eosinophil count >4000/mm^3. May resume therapy when eosinophil count <3000/mm^3. (Note: The Canadian labeling recommends discontinuing therapy for eosinophil count >3000/mm^3; may resume therapy when eosinophil count <1000/mm^3).The restricted distribution system ensures appropriate WBC and ANC monitoring.

Cognitive and/or motor impairment (sedation) is common with clozapine, resulting in impaired performance of tasks requiring alertness (eg, operating machinery or driving); use caution in patients receiving general anesthesia. **[U.S. Boxed Warning]: Seizures have been associated with clozapine use in a dose-dependent manner;** use with caution in patients at risk of seizures, including those with a history of seizures, head trauma, brain damage, alcoholism, or concurrent therapy with medications which may lower seizure threshold. Benign transient temperature elevation (>100.4°F) may occur; peaking within the first 3 weeks of treatment. Rule out infection, agranulocytosis, and neuroleptic malignant syndrome (NMS) in patients presenting with fever. However, clozapine may also be associated with severe febrile reactions, including neuroleptic malignant syndrome (NMS). Clozapine's potential for extrapyramidal symptoms (including tardive dyskinesia) appears to be extremely low. Risk of dystonia (and probably other EPS) may be greater with increased doses, use of conventional antipsychotics, males, and younger patients.

Deep vein thrombosis, myocarditis, pericarditis, pericardial effusion, cardiomyopathy, and HF have also been associated with clozapine. **[U.S. Boxed Warning]: Fatalities due to myocarditis have been reported; highest risk in the first month of therapy, however, later cases also reported.** Myocarditis or cardiomyopathy should be considered in patients who present with signs/symptoms of heart failure (dyspnea, fatigue, orthopnea, paroxysmal nocturnal dyspnea, peripheral edema), chest pain, palpitations, new electrocardiographic abnormalities (arrhythmias, ST-T wave abnormalities), or unexplained fever. Patients with tachycardia during the first month of therapy should be closely monitored for other signs of myocarditis. Discontinue clozapine if myocarditis is suspected; do not rechallenge in patients with clozapine-related myocarditis. The reported rate of myocarditis in clozapine-treated patients appears to be 17-322 times greater than in the general population. Clozapine should be discontinued in patients with confirmed cardiomyopathy unless benefit clearly outweighs risk. Rare cases of thromboembolism, including pulmonary embolism and stroke resulting in fatalities, have been associated with clozapine. Clozapine is associated with QT prolongation and ventricular arrhythmias including torsade de pointes; cardiac arrest and sudden death may occur. Use caution in patients with a history of QT syndrome, conditions which may increase the risk of QT prolongation (cardiovascular disease, recent MI, uncompensated heart failure, clinically significant arrhythmias, family history of QT syndrome) or concomitant use of medications known to prolong the QT interval. Hypokalemia and/or hypomagnesemia may increase the risk; correct electrolyte abnormalities prior to initiating therapy. Discontinue clozapine if QT$_c$ interval >500 msec.

An increased incidence of cerebrovascular effects (eg, transient ischemic attack, stroke), including fatalities, has been reported in placebo-controlled trials of atypical antipsychotics in elderly patients with dementia-related psychosis.

Clozapine is metabolized by CYP1A2, 2D6, and 3A4; use caution with medications which inhibit CYP activity. Use with other medications which may prolong the QT$_c$ interval (eg, some antipsychotic medications, some antibiotics, class 1a or III antiarrhythmics).

May cause anticholinergic effects; use with caution in patients with urinary retention, benign prostatic hyperplasia, narrow-angle glaucoma, xerostomia, visual problems, constipation, or history of bowel obstruction. May cause hyperglycemia; in some cases may be extreme and associated with ketoacidosis, hyperosmolar coma, or death. Use with caution in patients with diabetes or other disorders of glucose regulation; monitor for worsening of glucose control. Antipsychotic use has been associated with esophageal dysmotility and aspiration; use with caution in patients at risk of pneumonia (eg, Alzheimer's disease). Use with caution in patients with hepatic disease or impairment; monitor hepatic function regularly. Hepatitis has been reported as a consequence of therapy. Discontinuation of therapy may be necessary with significant elevations in liver function tests; may reinitiate with close monitoring and if values return to normal. Use with caution in patients with renal disease.

Use caution with cardiovascular or pulmonary disease; gradually increase dose. **[U.S. Boxed Warning]: May cause orthostatic hypotension (with or without syncope);** generally occurs more frequently with initial titration and in association with rapid dose increases; use with caution in patients at risk of hypotension or in patients where transient hypotensive episodes would be poorly tolerated (cardiovascular disease or cerebrovascular disease). Concurrent use with benzodiazepines may increase the risk of severe cardiopulmonary reactions. May cause tachycardia (including sustained); sustained tachycardia is not limited to a reflex response to orthostatic hypotension, and is present in all positions.

The possibility of a suicide attempt is inherent in psychotic illness or bipolar disorder; use caution in high-risk patients during initiation of therapy. Prescriptions should be written for the smallest quantity consistent with good patient care.

Use in elderly patients with dementia is associated with an increased risk of mortality and cerebrovascular accidents; avoid antipsychotic use for behavioral problems associated with dementia unless alternative nonpharmacologic therapies have failed and patient may harm self or others. In addition, use may cause or exacerbate syndrome of inappropriate antidiuretic hormone secretion or hyponatremia; monitor sodium closely with initiation or dosage adjustments in older adults. May also be inappropriate in older adults depending on comorbidities (eg, dementia, delirium) due to its potent anticholinergic effects (Beers Criteria). The elderly are more susceptible to adverse effects (including agranulocytosis, cardiovascular, anticholinergic, and tardive dyskinesia).

Medication should not be stopped abruptly; taper off over 1-2 weeks. If conditions warrant abrupt discontinuation (leukopenia, myocarditis, cardiomyopathy), monitor patient for psychosis and cholinergic rebound (headache, nausea, vomiting, diarrhea). Significant weight gain has been observed with antipsychotic therapy; incidence varies with product. Monitor waist circumference and BMI. Clozapine levels may be lower in patients who smoke. Smoking cessation may cause toxicity in a patient stabilized on clozapine. Monitor change in smoking. FazaClo® oral disintegrating tablets contain phenylalanine.

Adverse Reactions (Reflective of adult population; not specific for elderly)

>10%:
  Cardiovascular: Tachycardia (25%)
  Central nervous system: Drowsiness (39% to 46%), dizziness (19% to 27%), insomnia (2% to 20%)
  Gastrointestinal: Sialorrhea (31% to 48%), weight gain (4% to 31%), constipation (14% to 25%), nausea/vomiting (3% to 17%), abdominal discomfort/heartburn (4% to 14%)

1% to 10%:
  Cardiovascular: Hypotension (9%), syncope (6%), hypertension (4%), angina (1%), ECG changes (1%)
  Central nervous system: Headache (7%), agitation (4%), akinesia (4%), nightmares (4%), restlessness (4%), akathisia (3%), confusion (3%), seizure (3%), fatigue (2%), anxiety (1%), ataxia (1%), depression (1%), lethargy (1%), myoclonic jerks (1%), slurred speech (1%)
  Dermatologic: Rash (2%)
  Gastrointestinal: Xerostomia (6%), diarrhea (2%), anorexia (1%), throat discomfort (1%)
  Genitourinary: Urinary abnormalities (eg, abnormal ejaculation, retention, urgency, incontinence; 1% to 2%)
  Hematologic: Leukopenia (3%), agranulocytosis (1%), eosinophilia (1%)
  Hepatic: Liver function tests abnormal (1%)
  Neuromuscular & skeletal: Tremor (6%), hypokinesia (4%), rigidity (3%), hyperkinesia (1%), weakness (1%), pain (1%), spasm (1%)
  Ocular: Visual disturbances (5%)
  Respiratory: Dyspnea (1%), nasal congestion (1%)
  Miscellaneous: Diaphoresis (6%), tongue numbness (1%)

Drug Interactions

Metabolism/Transport Effects Substrate of CYP1A2 (major), CYP2A6 (minor), CYP2C19 (minor), CYP2C9 (minor), CYP2D6 (minor), CYP3A4 (minor); **Note:** Assignment of Major/Minor substrate status based on clinically relevant drug interaction potential; **Inhibits** CYP1A2 (weak), CYP2C19 (weak), CYP2C9 (weak), CYP2D6 (moderate), CYP2E1 (weak), CYP3A4 (weak)

Avoid Concomitant Use

Avoid concomitant use of CloZAPine with any of the following: Azelastine; Azelastine (Nasal); Highest Risk QTc-Prolonging Agents; Metoclopramide; Mifepristone; Myelosuppressive Agents; Paraldehyde

Increased Effect/Toxicity

CloZAPine may increase the levels/effects of: Alcohol (Ethyl); Anticholinergics; ARIPiprazole; Azelastine; Azelastine (Nasal); Buprenorphine; CNS Depressants; CYP2D6 Substrates; Fesoterodine; Highest Risk QTc-Prolonging Agents; Methylphenidate; Moderate Risk QTc-Prolonging Agents; Nebivolol; Paraldehyde; Serotonin Modulators; Zolpidem

The levels/effects of CloZAPine may be increased by: Abiraterone Acetate; Acetylcholinesterase Inhibitors (Central); Benzodiazepines; Cimetidine; CYP1A2 Inhibitors (Moderate); CYP1A2 Inhibitors (Strong); Deferasirox; HydrOXYzine; Lithium formulations; Macrolide Antibiotics; MAO Inhibitors; Methylphenidate; Metoclopramide; Metyrosine; Mifepristone; Myelosuppressive Agents; Nefazodone; Omeprazole; Pramlintide; QTc-Prolonging Agents (Indeterminate Risk and Risk Modifying); Selective Serotonin Reuptake Inhibitors; Tetrabenazine

◀ **Decreased Effect**

CloZAPine may decrease the levels/effects of: Amphetamines; Anti-Parkinson's Agents (Dopamine Agonist); Codeine; Quinagolide

The levels/effects of CloZAPine may be decreased by: CarBAMazepine; CYP1A2 Inducers (Strong); Cyproterone; Fosphenytoin; Lithium formulations; Omeprazole; Phenytoin; Tocilizumab

Ethanol/Nutrition/Herb Interactions

Ethanol: May increase CNS depression; monitor for increased effects with coadministration. Caution patients about effects.

Herb/Nutraceutical: St John's wort may decrease clozapine levels. Avoid kava kava, gotu kola, valerian, St John's wort (may increase CNS depression).

Stability Store at ≤30°C (86°F).

FazaClo®: Store at 25°C (77°F); excursions permitted to 15°C to 30°C (59°F to 86°F). Protect from moisture; do not remove from package until ready to use.

Mechanism of Action Clozapine (dibenzodiazepine antipsychotic) exhibits weak antagonism of D_1, D_2, D_3, and D_5 dopamine receptor subtypes, but shows high affinity for D_4; in addition, it blocks the serotonin ($5HT_2$), alpha-adrenergic, histamine H_1, and cholinergic receptors

Pharmacodynamics/Kinetics

Protein binding: 97% to serum proteins

Metabolism: Extensively hepatic; forms metabolites with limited or no activity

Bioavailability: 50% to 60% (not affected by food)

Half-life elimination: Steady state: 12 hours (range: 4-66 hours)

Time to peak: 2.5 hours (range: 1-6 hours)

Excretion: Urine (~50%) and feces (30%) with trace amounts of unchanged drug

Dosage

Geriatric

Schizophrenia: Oral: Experience in the elderly is limited; initial dose should be 12.5-25 mg/day; increase as tolerated by 25 mg/day to desired response. Elderly may require slower titration and daily increases may not be tolerated.

Psychosis/agitation related to Alzheimer's dementia (unlabeled use): Oral: Initial: 12.5 mg/day; if necessary, gradually increase as tolerated not to exceed 75-100 mg/day (Rabins, 2007)

Adult

Schizophrenia: Initial: 12.5 mg once or twice daily; increased, as tolerated, in increments of 25-50 mg/day to a target dose of 300-450 mg/day after 2 weeks; may further titrate in increments not exceeding 100 mg and no more frequently than once or twice weekly. May require doses as high as 600-900 mg/day (maximum dose: 900 mg/day). **Note:** In some efficacy studies, total daily dosage was administered in 3 divided doses.

Suicidal behavior in schizophrenia or schizoaffective disorder: Initial: 12.5 mg once or twice daily; increased, as tolerated, in increments of 25-50 mg/day to a target dose of 300-450 mg/day after 2 weeks; mean dose is ~300 mg/day (range: 12.5-900 mg); treatment duration 2 years then reassess need. **Note:** If no longer a suicide risk, may resume prior antipsychotic therapy after gradually tapering off clozapine over 1-2 weeks.

Termination of therapy: If dosing is interrupted for ≥48 hours, therapy must be reinitiated at 12.5-25 mg/day; may be increased more rapidly than with initial titration, unless cardio-pulmonary arrest occurred during initial titration.

In the event of planned termination of clozapine, gradual reduction in dose over a 1- to 2-week period is recommended. If conditions warrant abrupt discontinuation (leukopenia), monitor patient for psychosis and cholinergic rebound (headache, nausea, vomiting, diarrhea).

Administration May be taken without regard to food. Total daily dose may be divided into uneven doses with larger dose administered at bedtime.

Canadian labeling: Maintenance dosing ≤200 mg/day may be administered as single dose in the evening.

Orally-disintegrating tablet: Should be removed from foil blister by peeling apart (do not push tablet through the foil). Remove immediately prior to use. Place tablet in mouth and allow to dissolve; swallow with saliva. If dosing requires splitting tablet, throw unused portion away.

Monitoring Parameters Note: The Canadian labeling recommends initiating treatment in an inpatient setting or an outpatient setting with medical supervision and monitoring of vital signs for at least 6-8 hours after the first few doses.

Mental status, ECG, WBC (see below), vital signs, fasting lipid profile and fasting blood glucose/Hgb A_{1c} (prior to treatment, at 3 months, then annually; liver function tests; BMI; personal/family history of obesity; waist circumference (weight should be assessed prior to treatment, at 4 weeks, 8 weeks, 12 weeks, and then at quarterly intervals. Consider titrating to a different antipsychotic agent for a weight gain ≥5% of the initial weight); blood pressure; abnormal involuntary movement scale (AIMS).

WBC and ANC should be obtained at baseline and at least weekly for the first 6 months (26 weeks) of continuous treatment. If counts remain acceptable (WBC ≥3500/mm^3, ANC ≥2000/mm^3) during this time period, then they may be monitored every other week for the next 6 months (26 weeks). If WBC/ANC continue to remain within these acceptable limits after the second 6 months (26 weeks) of therapy, monitoring can be decreased to every 4 weeks. If clozapine is discontinued, a weekly WBC should be conducted for an additional 4 weeks or until WBC is ≥3500/mm^3 and ANC is ≥2000/mm^3. If clozapine therapy is interrupted due to moderate leukopenia, weekly WBC/ANC monitoring is required for 12 months in patients restarted on clozapine treatment. (Note: When therapy is interrupted for >3 days, the Canadian labeling recommends weekly hematologic testing for an additional 6 weeks). If therapy is interrupted for reasons other than leukopenia/granulocytopenia, the 6-month time period for initiation of biweekly WBCs may need to be reset. This determination depends upon the treatment duration, the length of the break in therapy, and whether or not an abnormal blood event occurred.

Consult manufacturer prescribing information for determination of appropriate WBC/ANC monitoring interval.

Special Geriatric Considerations Not recommended for use in nonpsychotic patients (eg, dimentia-related psychotic symptoms). Studies in subjects >65 years of age have not been done. Orthostatic hypotension and sustained tachycardia have been noted in up to 25% of patients taking clozapine; therefore, elderly with cardiovascular disease may be at risk. The anticholinergic effects of clozapine may be prominent in elderly (eg, constipation, confusion, urinary retention).

This medication is considered to be potentially inappropriate in this patient population (Beers Criteria: Quality of evidence - moderate; Strength of recommendation - strong).

Dosage Forms Excipient information presented when available (limited, particularly for generics); consult specific product labeling.

Tablet, oral: 25 mg, 50 mg, 100 mg, 200 mg
  Clozaril®: 25 mg, 100 mg [scored]
Tablet, orally disintegrating, oral: 12.5 mg, 25 mg, 100 mg
  FazaClo®: 12.5 mg [contains phenylalanine 0.87 mg/tablet; mint flavor]
  FazaClo®: 25 mg [contains phenylalanine 1.74 mg/tablet; mint flavor]
  FazaClo®: 100 mg [contains phenylalanine 6.96 mg/tablet; mint flavor]
  FazaClo®: 150 mg [contains phenylalanine 10.44 mg/tablet; mint flavor]
  FazaClo®: 200 mg [contains phenylalanine 13.92 mg/tablet; mint flavor]

◆ **Clozaril®** see CloZAPine on page 429
◆ **CNTO-148** see Golimumab on page 895
◆ **CNTO 1275** see Ustekinumab on page 1987
◆ **Codar® GF** see Guaifenesin and Codeine on page 906

Codeine (KOE deen)

Medication Safety Issues
Sound-alike/look-alike issues:
Codeine may be confused with Cardene®, Cordran®, iodine, Lodine
High alert medication:
The Institute for Safe Medication Practices (ISMP) includes this medication among its list of drug classes which have a heightened risk of causing significant patient harm when used in error.

Brand Names: Canada Codeine Contin®; PMS-Codeine; ratio-Codeine
Index Terms Codeine Phosphate; Codeine Sulfate; Methylmorphine
Generic Availability (U.S.) Yes
Pharmacologic Category Analgesic, Opioid; Antitussive
Use Management of mild-to-moderately-severe pain
Unlabeled Use Short-term relief of cough in select patients
Medication Guide Available Yes
Contraindications Hypersensitivity to codeine or any component of the formulation; respiratory depression in the absence of resuscitative equipment; acute or severe bronchial asthma or hypercarbia; presence or suspicion of paralytic ileus

Canadian labeling: Additional contraindications (not in U.S. labeling): Hypersensitivity to other opioid analgesics; cor pulmonale; acute alcoholism; delirium tremens; severe CNS depression; convulsive disorders; increased cerebrospinal or intracranial pressure; head injury; suspected surgical abdomen; use with or within 14 days of MAO inhibitors.

Warnings/Precautions May cause dose-related respiratory depression. The risk is increased in elderly patients, debilitated patients, and patients with conditions associated with hypoxia, hypercapnia, or upper airway obstruction. Use with caution in patients with pre-existing respiratory compromise (hypoxia and/or hypercapnia), COPD or other obstructive pulmonary disease, and kyphoscoliosis or other skeletal disorder which may alter respiratory function; critical respiratory depression may occur, even at therapeutic dosages.

Use may cause or aggravate constipation; chronic use may result in obstructive bowel disease, particularly in those with underlying intestinal motility disorders. Avoid use in patients with gastrointestinal obstruction, particularly paralytic ileus. May cause hypotension; use with caution in patients with hypovolemia, cardiovascular disease (including acute MI), or drugs which may exaggerate hypotensive effects (including phenothiazines or general anesthetics). May cause CNS depression, which may impair physical or mental abilities; patients must be cautioned about performing tasks which require mental alertness (eg, operating machinery or driving).

Use with extreme caution in patients with head injury, intracranial lesions, or elevated intracranial pressure; exaggerated elevation of ICP may occur. Use with caution in patients with hypersensitivity reactions to other phenanthrene-derivative opioid agonists (hydrocodone, hydromorphone, levorphanol, oxycodone, oxymorphone), adrenal insufficiency (including Addison's disease), biliary tract dysfunction, CNS depression or coma, thyroid dysfunction, morbid obesity, prostatic hyperplasia and/or urinary stricture, or severe hepatic or renal impairment. Use may obscure diagnosis or clinical course of patients with acute abdominal conditions. May induce or aggravate seizures; use with caution in patients with seizure disorders.

Use with caution in patients with a history of drug abuse or acute alcoholism; potential for drug dependency exists. Tolerance, psychological and physical dependence may occur with prolonged use. Effects may be potentiated when used with other sedative drugs or ethanol. Concurrent use of agonist/antagonist analgesics may precipitate withdrawal symptoms and/or reduced analgesic efficacy in patients following prolonged therapy with mu opioid agonists. Abrupt discontinuation following prolonged use may also lead to withdrawal symptoms.

Use caution in patients with two or more copies of the variant CYP2D6*2 allele; may have extensive conversion to morphine and thus increased opioid-mediated effects.

Some preparations contain sulfites which may cause allergic reactions. Healthcare provider should be alert to the potential for abuse, misuse, and diversion.

Adverse Reactions (Reflective of adult population; not specific for elderly) Frequency not defined.

Cardiovascular: Bradycardia, cardiac arrest, circulatory depression, flushing, hyper-/hypotension, palpitation, shock, syncope, tachycardia

Central nervous system: Abnormal dreams, agitation, anxiety, apprehension, chills, coordination impaired, depression, disorientation, dizziness, drowsiness, dysphoria, euphoria, faintness, fatigue, hallucinations, headache, insomnia, intracranial pressure increased, lightheadedness, nervousness, sedation, shakiness, somnolence, vertigo

Dermatologic: Pruritus, rash, urticaria

Gastrointestinal: Abdominal cramps/pain, anorexia, biliary tract spasm, constipation, diarrhea, nausea, pancreatitis, taste disturbance, vomiting, xerostomia

Genitourinary: Urinary hesitancy/retention

Neuromuscular & skeletal: Paresthesia, rigidity, tremor, weakness

Ocular: Blurred vision, diplopia, miosis, nystagmus, visual disturbances

Respiratory: Bronchospasm, dyspnea, laryngospasm, respiratory arrest, respiratory depression

Miscellaneous: Allergic reaction, diaphoresis

Drug Interactions

Metabolism/Transport Effects Substrate of CYP2D6 (major); **Note:** Assignment of Major/Minor substrate status based on clinically relevant drug interaction potential

Avoid Concomitant Use

Avoid concomitant use of Codeine with any of the following: Azelastine; Azelastine (Nasal); Methadone; Mirtazapine; Paraldehyde

Increased Effect/Toxicity

Codeine may increase the levels/effects of: Alcohol (Ethyl); Alvimopan; Azelastine; Azelastine (Nasal); CNS Depressants; Desmopressin; Methadone; Metyrosine; Mirtazapine; Paraldehyde; Selective Serotonin Reuptake Inhibitors; Thiazide Diuretics; Zolpidem

The levels/effects of Codeine may be increased by: Amphetamines; Antipsychotic Agents (Phenothiazines); Droperidol; HydrOXYzine; Somatostatin Analogs; Succinylcholine

Decreased Effect

Codeine may decrease the levels/effects of: Pegvisomant

The levels/effects of Codeine may be decreased by: Ammonium Chloride; CYP2D6 Inhibitors (Moderate); CYP2D6 Inhibitors (Strong); Mixed Agonist / Antagonist Opioids

Ethanol/Nutrition/Herb Interactions

Ethanol: May increase CNS depression; monitor for increased effects with coadministration. Caution patients about effects.

Herb/Nutraceutical: St John's wort may decrease codeine levels. Avoid valerian, St John's wort, kava kava, gotu kola (may increase CNS depression).

Stability

Oral solution, tablet: Store at controlled room temperature.

Mechanism of Action

Binds to opioid receptors in the CNS, causing inhibition of ascending pain pathways, altering the perception of and response to pain; causes cough suppression by direct central action in the medulla; produces generalized CNS depression

Pharmacodynamics/Kinetics

Onset of action: Oral: Immediate release: 0.5-1 hour

Peak effect: Oral: Immediate release: 1-1.5 hours

Duration: Immediate release: 4-6 hours

Distribution: ~3-6 L/kg

Protein binding: ~7% to 25%

Metabolism: Hepatic via UGT2B7 and UGT2B4 to codeine-6-glucuronide, via CYP2D6 to morphine (active), and via CYP3A4 to norcodeine. Morphine is further metabolized via glucuronidation to morphine-3-glucuronide and morphine-6-glucuronide (active).

Bioavailability: 53%

Half-life elimination: ~3 hours

Time to peak, plasma: Immediate release: 1 hour; Controlled release (Canadian availability; not available in the U.S.): 3.3 hours

Excretion: Urine (~90%, ~10% of the total dose as unchanged drug); feces

Dosage

Geriatric & Adult Note: These are guidelines and do not represent the maximum doses that may be required in all patients. Doses should be titrated to pain relief/prevention.

Pain management (analgesic): Oral:

Immediate release (tablet, oral solution): Initial: 15-60 mg every 4 hours as needed; maximum total daily dose: 360 mg/day; patients with prior opioid exposure may require higher initial doses. **Note:** The American Pain Society recommends an initial dose of 30-60 mg for adults with moderate pain (American Pain Society, 2008).

Controlled release: Codeine Contin® (Canadian availability; not available in U.S.): **Note:** Titrate at intervals of ≥48 hours until adequate analgesia has been achieved. Daily doses >600 mg/day should not be used; patients requiring higher doses should be switched to an opioid approved for use in severe pain. In patients who receive both Codeine Contin® and an immediate release or combination codeine product for breakthrough pain, the rescue dose of immediate release codeine product should be ≤12.5% of the total daily Codeine Contin® dose.

Opioid-naive patients: Initial: 50 mg every 12 hours

Conversion from immediate release codeine preparations: Immediate release codeine preparations contain ~75% codeine base. Therefore, patients who are switching from immediate release codeine preparations may be transferred to a ~25% lower total daily dose of Codeine Contin®, equally divided into 2 daily doses.

Conversion from a combination codeine product (eg, codeine with acetaminophen or aspirin): See table:

Number of 30 mg Codeine Combination Tablets Daily	Initial Dose of Codeine Contin®	Maintenance Dose of Codeine Contin®
≤6	50 mg every 12 h	100 mg every 12 h
7-9	100 mg every 12 h	150 mg every 12 h
10-12	150 mg every 12 h	200 mg every 12 h
>12	200 mg every 12 h	200-300 every 12 h (maximum: 300 mg every 12 h)

Conversion from another opioid analgesic: Using the patient's current opioid dose, calculate an equivalent daily dose of immediate release codeine. A ~25% lower dose of Codeine Contin® should then be initiated, equally divided into 2 daily doses.

Discontinuation of therapy: **Note:** Gradual dose reduction is recommended if clinically appropriate. Initially reduce the total daily dose by 50% and administer equally divided into 2 daily doses for 2 days followed by a 25% reduction every 2 days thereafter.

Treatment of cough (unlabeled use): Oral: Reported doses vary; range: 7.5-120 mg/day as a single dose or in divided doses (Bolser, 2006; Smith, 2010); **Note:** The American College of Chest Physicians does not recommend the routine use of codeine as an antitussive in patients with upper respiratory infections (Bolser, 2006).

Renal Impairment
Manufacturer's recommendations: Clearance may be reduced; active metabolites may accumulate. Initiate at lower doses or longer dosing intervals followed by careful titration.
Alternate recommendations: The following guidelines have been used by some clinicians (Aronoff, 2007):
Cl_{cr} 10-50 mL/minute: Administer 75% of dose
Cl_{cr} <10 mL/minute: Administer 50% of dose

Hepatic Impairment No dosage adjustment provided in manufacturer's labeling (has not been studied); however, initial lower doses or longer dosing intervals followed by careful titration are recommended.

Administration May administer without regard to meals. Take with food or milk to decrease adverse GI effects.
Controlled release tablets: Codeine Contin® (Canadian availability; not available in U.S.): Tablets should be swallowed whole; do not chew, dissolve, or crush. All strengths may be halved, **except** the 50 mg tablets; half tablets should also be swallowed intact.

Monitoring Parameters Pain relief, respiratory and mental status, blood pressure, heart rate

Reference Range Therapeutic: Not established

Test Interactions Some quinolones may produce a false-positive urine screening result for opioids using commercially-available immunoassay kits. This has been demonstrated most consistently for levofloxacin and ofloxacin, but other quinolones have shown cross-reactivity in certain assay kits. Confirmation of positive opioid screens by more specific methods should be considered.

Special Geriatric Considerations The elderly may be particularly susceptible to CNS depression and confusion as well as the constipating effects of narcotics.

Controlled Substance C-II

Dosage Forms Excipient information presented when available (limited, particularly for generics); consult specific product labeling. [DSC] = Discontinued product
Powder, for prescription compounding, as phosphate: USP: 100% (10 g, 25 g)
Solution, oral, as phosphate: 30 mg/5 mL (500 mL)
Solution, oral, as sulfate: 30 mg/5 mL (500 mL)
Tablet, oral, as phosphate: 30 mg [DSC], 60 mg [DSC]
Tablet, oral, as sulfate: 15 mg, 30 mg, 60 mg

Dosage Forms: Canada Excipient information presented when available (limited, particularly for generics); consult specific product labeling.
Tablet, controlled release:
Codeine Contin®: 50 mg, 100 mg, 150 mg, 200 mg

◆ **Codeine and Acetaminophen** *see* Acetaminophen and Codeine *on page* 35
◆ **Codeine and Guaifenesin** *see* Guaifenesin and Codeine *on page* 906
◆ **Codeine Phosphate** *see* Codeine *on page* 433
◆ **Codeine Sulfate** *see* Codeine *on page* 433
◆ **Cogentin®** *see* Benztropine *on page* 201
◆ **Colace® [OTC]** *see* Docusate *on page* 583
◆ **ColBenemid** *see* Colchicine and Probenecid *on page* 440

Colchicine (KOL chi seen)

Medication Safety Issues
Sound-alike/look-alike issues:
Colchicine may be confused with Cortrosyn®

Brand Names: U.S. Colcrys®

Brand Names: Canada Jamp-Colchicine

Generic Availability (U.S.) No

Pharmacologic Category Antigout Agent

Use Prevention and treatment of acute gout flares; treatment of familial Mediterranean fever (FMF)

Unlabeled Use Primary biliary cirrhosis; pericarditis

Medication Guide Available Yes

Contraindications Concomitant use of a P-glycoprotein (P-gp) or strong CYP3A4 inhibitor in presence of renal or hepatic impairment

Canadian labeling: Additional contraindications (not in U.S. labeling): Hypersensitivity to colchicine; serious gastrointestinal, hepatic, renal, and cardiac disease

Warnings/Precautions Hazardous agent - use appropriate precautions for handling and disposal. Myelosuppression (eg, thrombocytopenia, leukopenia, granulocytopenia, pancyto-penia) and aplastic anemia have been reported in patients receiving therapeutic doses. Neuromuscular toxicity (including rhabdomyolysis) has been reported in patients receiving therapeutic doses; patients with renal dysfunction and elderly patients are at increased risk. Concomitant use of cyclosporine, diltiazem, verapamil, fibrates, and statins may increase the risk of myopathy. Clearance is decreased in renal or hepatic impairment; monitor closely for adverse effects/toxicity. Dosage adjustments may be required depending on degree of impairment or indication, and may be affected by the use of concurrent medication (CYP3A4 or P-gp inhibitors). Concurrent use of P-gp or strong CYP3A4 inhibitors is contraindicated in renal impairment; fatal toxicity has been reported. Colchicine does not have analgesic activity and should not be used to treat pain from other causes. Colchicine requires dosage adjust-ment when used concurrently with protease inhibitor regimens. Colchicine does not have analgesic activity and should not be used to treat pain from other causes.

Adverse Reactions (Reflective of adult population; not specific for elderly)
>10%: Gastrointestinal: Gastrointestinal disorders including abdominal pain, cramping, nau-sea, vomiting (up to 26%), diarrhea (up to 23%)
1% to 10%: Respiratory: Pharyngolaryngeal pain (3%)

Drug Interactions

Metabolism/Transport Effects Substrate of CYP3A4 (major), P-glycoprotein; **Note:** Assignment of Major/Minor substrate status based on clinically relevant drug interaction potential; **Induces** CYP2C9 (weak/moderate), CYP2E1 (weak/moderate), CYP3A4 (weak/moderate)

Avoid Concomitant Use
Avoid concomitant use of Colchicine with any of the following: Axitinib

Increased Effect/Toxicity
Colchicine may increase the levels/effects of: HMG-CoA Reductase Inhibitors

The levels/effects of Colchicine may be increased by: CYP3A4 Inhibitors (Moderate); CYP3A4 Inhibitors (Strong); Dasatinib; Digoxin; Fibric Acid Derivatives; Fosamprenavir; Ivacaftor; Mifepristone; P-glycoprotein/ABCB1 Inhibitors; Telaprevir

Decreased Effect
Colchicine may decrease the levels/effects of: ARIPiprazole; Axitinib; Cyanocobalamin; Saxagliptin

The levels/effects of Colchicine may be decreased by: P-glycoprotein/ABCB1 Inducers; Tocilizumab

Ethanol/Nutrition/Herb Interactions
Ethanol: Management: Avoid ethanol.
Food: Grapefruit juice may increase colchicine serum concentrations. Management: Admin-ister orally with water and maintain adequate fluid intake. Dose adjustment may be required based on indication if ingesting grapefruit juice. Avoid grapefruit juice with hepatic or renal impairment.
Herb/Nutraceutical: Cyanocobalamin (vitamin B_{12}) absorption may be decreased by colchi-cine and result in macrocytic anemia or neurologic dysfunction. Management: Consider supplementing with vitamin B_{12}.

Stability Store at 20°C to 25°C (68°F to 77°F). Protect from light.

Mechanism of Action Disrupts cytoskeletal functions by inhibiting β-tubulin polymerization into microtubules, preventing activation, degranulation, and migration of neutrophils associ-ated with mediating some gout symptoms. In familial Mediterranean fever, may interfere with intracellular assembly of the inflammasome complex present in neutrophils and monocytes that mediate activation of interleukin-1β.

Pharmacodynamics/Kinetics
Onset of action: Oral: Pain relief: ~18-24 hours
Distribution: Concentrates in leukocytes, kidney, spleen, and liver; does not distribute in heart, skeletal muscle, and brain
V_d: 5-8 L/kg
Protein binding: ~39%
Metabolism: Hepatic via CYP3A4; 3 metabolites (2 primary, 1 minor)
Bioavailability: ~45%
Half-life elimination: 27-31 hours (multiple oral doses; young, healthy volunteers)
Time to peak, serum: Oral: 0.5-3 hours

Excretion: Urine (40% to 65% as unchanged drug); enterohepatic recirculation and biliary excretion also possible

Dosage

Geriatric Use caution; reduce prophylactic daily dose by 50% in individuals >70 years (Terkeltaub, 2009)

Adult

Familial Mediterranean fever (FMF): Oral: 1.2-2.4 mg/day in 1-2 divided doses. Titration: Increase or decrease dose in 0.3 mg/day increments based on efficacy or adverse effects; maximum: 2.4 mg/day

Gout: Oral:

U.S. labeling:

Flare treatment: Initial: 1.2 mg at the first sign of flare, followed in 1 hour with a single dose of 0.6 mg (maximum: 1.8 mg within 1 hour). Patients receiving prophylaxis therapy may receive treatment dosing; wait 12 hours before resuming prophylaxis dose. **Note:** Current FDA-approved dose for gout flare is substantially lower than what has been historically used clinically. Doses larger than the currently recommended dosage for gout flare have not been proven to be more effective.

Prophylaxis: 0.6 mg once or twice daily; maximum: 1.2 mg/day

Canadian labeling:

Flare treatment: Initial: 1-1.2 mg at the first sign of flare, followed by 0.5-0.6 mg dose every 2 hours until pain relief; maximum: 3 mg/24 hours

Prophylaxis: 0.5-0.6 mg 1-4 times/week (mild-moderate cases) or 0.5-0.6 mg once or twice daily (severe cases); maximum: 1.2 mg/24 hours

Pericarditis post-STEMI (unlabeled use): Oral: 0.6 mg twice daily (Antman, 2004)

Recurrent pericarditis due to previous autoimmune or idiopathic cause (unlabeled use): Note: Dosage strength not available in the U.S.: Oral: 0.5-1 mg every 12 hours for 1 day, followed by 0.25-0.5 mg every 12 hours for 6 months (in combination with high-dose aspirin or ibuprofen) (Imazio, 2011)

Patients <70 kg or unable to tolerate higher dosing regimen: 0.5 mg every 12 hours for 1 day followed by 0.5 mg once daily.

Primary biliary cirrhosis (unlabeled use): Oral: 0.6 mg twice daily (Kaplan, 2005); **Note:** Use reserved for patients refractory to ursodiol.

Dosage adjustment for concomitant therapy with CYP3A4 or P-glycoprotein (P-gp) inhibitors: *Dosage adjustment also required in patients receiving CYP3A4 or P-gp inhibitors up to 14 days prior to initiation of colchicine.* **Note:** Treatment of gout flare with colchicine is not recommended in patients receiving prophylactic colchicine and CYP3A4 inhibitors.

Coadministration of **strong** CYP3A4 inhibitor (eg, atazanavir, clarithromycin, darunavir, indinavir, itraconazole, ketoconazole, lopinavir/ritonavir, nefazodone, nelfinavir, ritonavir, saquinavir, telithromycin, tipranavir):

FMF: Maximum dose: 0.6 mg/day (0.3 mg twice daily)

Gout prophylaxis:

If original dose is 0.6 mg twice daily, adjust dose to 0.3 mg once daily

If original dose is 0.6 mg once daily, adjust dose to 0.3 mg every other day

Gout flare treatment: Initial: 0.6 mg, followed in 1 hour by a single dose of 0.3 mg; do not repeat for at least 3 days

Coadministration of **moderate** CYP3A4 inhibitor (eg, aprepitant, diltiazem, erythromycin, fluconazole, fosamprenavir, grapefruit juice, verapamil):

FMF: Maximum dose: 1.2 mg/day (0.6 mg twice daily)

Gout prophylaxis:

If original dose is 0.6 mg twice daily, adjust dose to 0.3 mg twice daily **or** 0.6 mg once daily

If original dose is 0.6 mg once daily, adjust dose to 0.3 mg once daily

Gout flare treatment: 1.2 mg as a single dose; do not repeat for at least 3 days

Coadministration of P-gp inhibitor (eg, cyclosporine, ranolazine):

FMF: Maximum dose: 0.6 mg/day (0.3 mg twice daily)

Gout prophylaxis:

If original dose is 0.6 mg twice daily, adjust dose to 0.3 mg once daily

If original dose is 0.6 mg once daily, adjust dose to 0.3 mg every other day

Gout flare treatment: Initial: 0.6 mg as a single dose; do not repeat for at least 3 days

Renal Impairment Concurrent use of colchicine and P-gp or strong CYP3A4 inhibitors is **contraindicated** in renal impairment. Fatal toxicity has been reported. Treatment of gout flares is not recommended in patients with renal impairment receiving prophylactic colchicine.

FMF:

Cl_{cr} 30-80 mL/minute: Monitor closely for adverse effects; dose reduction may be necessary.

Cl_{cr} <30 mL/minute: Initial dose: 0.3 mg/day; use caution if dose titrated; monitor for adverse effects.

Dialysis: 0.3 mg as a single dose; use caution if dose titrated; dosing can be increased with close monitoring; monitor for adverse effects. Not removed by dialysis.

Gout prophylaxis:

Cl_{cr} 30-80 mL/minute: Dosage adjustment not required; monitor closely for adverse effects.

Cl_{cr} <30 mL/minute: Initial dose: 0.3 mg/day; use caution if dose titrated; monitor for adverse effects.

Dialysis: 0.3 mg twice weekly; monitor closely for adverse effects.

Gout flare treatment:

Cl_{cr} 30-80 mL/minute: Dosage adjustment not required; monitor closely for adverse effects.

Cl_{cr} <30 mL/minute: Dosage reduction not required but may be considered; treatment course should not be repeated more frequently than every 14 days.

Dialysis: 0.6 mg as a single dose; treatment course should not be repeated more frequently than every 14 days. Not removed by dialysis.

Hemodialysis: Avoid chronic use of colchicine.

Hepatic Impairment Concurrent use of colchicine and P-glycoprotein or strong CYP3A4 inhibitors is **contraindicated** in hepatic impairment. Fatal toxicity has been reported. Treatment of gout flare with colchicine is not recommended in patients with hepatic impairment receiving prophylactic colchicine.

FMF:

Mild-to-moderate impairment: Use caution; monitor closely for adverse effects.

Severe impairment: Consider dosage reduction.

Gout prophylaxis:

Mild-to-moderate impairment: Dosage adjustment not required; monitor closely for adverse effects.

Severe impairment: Dosage adjustment should be considered.

Gout flare treatment:

Mild-to-moderate impairment: Dosage adjustment not required; monitor closely for adverse effects.

Severe impairment: Dosage reduction not required but may be considered; treatment course should not be repeated more frequently than every 14 days.

Administration Administer orally with water and maintain adequate fluid intake. May be administered without regard to meals.

Monitoring Parameters CBC, renal and hepatic function tests

Test Interactions May cause false-positive results in urine tests for erythrocytes or hemoglobin

Pharmacotherapy Pearls Oral colchicine had been available as an unapproved medication without FDA-approved prescribing information. In August 2009, the FDA approved prescribing information for a brand name colchicine product. The currently approved prescribing information recommends a lower than historically used dosage for the treatment of acute gout. This recommendation is based on data from the AGREE trial. In this trial, low-dose colchicine (1.8 mg total) had similar efficacy to high dose colchicine (4.8 mg total). Additionally, the low dosage regimen was associated with a lower incidence (26% vs 77%) of GI adverse events. Parenteral formulation of colchicine is no longer available in the U.S.; serious life-threatening complications (eg, neutropenia, acute renal failure, thrombocytopenia, heart failure) associated with intravenous colchicine have occurred prior to market withdrawal. The risks associated with oral colchicine are believed to be lower compared to intravenous use.

Special Geriatric Considerations Colchicine appears to be more toxic in older adults, particularly in the presence of renal, gastrointestinal, or cardiac disease. The most predictable oral side effects are gastrointestinal (eg, vomiting, abdominal pain, and nausea). If colchicine is stopped at this point, other more severe adverse effects may be avoided, such as bone marrow suppression, peripheral neuritis, etc.

Dosage Forms Excipient information presented when available (limited, particularly for generics); consult specific product labeling.

Tablet, oral: 0.6 mg

Colcrys®: 0.6 mg [scored]

Dosage Forms: Canada Excipient information presented when available (limited, particularly for generics); consult specific product labeling.

Tablet, oral: 1 mg [scored]

Colchicine and Probenecid (KOL chi seen & proe BEN e sid)

Related Information
Colchicine *on page 436*
Probenecid *on page 1604*
Index Terms ColBenemid; Probenecid and Colchicine
Generic Availability (U.S.) Yes
Pharmacologic Category Anti-inflammatory Agent; Antigout Agent; Uricosuric Agent
Use Treatment of chronic gouty arthritis when complicated by frequent, recurrent acute attacks of gout
Dosage
  Geriatric & Adult Gout: Oral: One tablet/day for 1 week, then 1 tablet twice daily thereafter
    Note: Current prescribing information states a maximum dose of 4 tablets per day; however this exceeds the usual maximum dose of colchicine for gout prophylaxis (1.2 mg per day).
  Renal Impairment See individual agents.
  Special Geriatric Considerations See individual agents.
  Dosage Forms Excipient information presented when available (limited, particularly for generics); consult specific product labeling.
    Tablet: Colchicine 0.5 mg and probenecid 0.5 g

◆ **Colcrys®** *see* Colchicine *on page 436*

Colesevelam (koh le SEV a lam)

Related Information
Diabetes Mellitus Management, Adults *on page 2193*
Hyperlipidemia Management *on page 2130*
Brand Names: U.S. Welchol®
Brand Names: Canada Welchol®
Generic Availability (U.S.) No
Pharmacologic Category Antilipemic Agent, Bile Acid Sequestrant
Use Management of elevated LDL in primary hypercholesterolemia (Fredrickson type IIa) when used alone or in combination with an HMG-CoA reductase inhibitor; improve glycemic control in type 2 diabetes mellitus (noninsulin dependent, NIDDM) in conjunction with diet, exercise, and insulin or oral antidiabetic agents
Contraindications History of bowel obstruction; serum triglyceride concentration >500 mg/dL; history of hypertriglyceridemia-induced pancreatitis
Warnings/Precautions Use with caution in treating patients with serum triglyceride concentrations >300 mg/dL and in patients using insulin or sulfonylureas (may cause increased concentrations) or in patients susceptible to fat-soluble vitamin deficiencies. Discontinue if triglyceride concentrations exceed 500 mg/dL or hypertriglyceridemia-induced pancreatitis occurs. Use in patients with gastroparesis, other severe GI motility disorders, or a history of major GI tract surgery is not recommended due to constipating effects of colesevelam. Patients with dysphagia or swallowing disorders should use the oral suspension form of colesevelam due to large tablet size and risk for esophageal obstruction.

Minimal effects are seen on HDL-C and triglyceride levels. Secondary causes of hypercholesterolemia should be excluded before initiation. Colesevelam has not been studied in Fredrickson Type I, III, IV, or V dyslipidemias. Colesevelam is not indicated for the management of type 1 diabetes, particularly in the acute management (eg, DKA). It is also not indicated in type 2 diabetes mellitus as monotherapy and must be used as an adjunct to diet, exercise, and glycemic control with insulin or oral antidiabetic agents. Combination with dipeptidyl peptidase 4 inhibitors or thiazolidinediones has not been studied extensively.

Use with caution in patients susceptible to fat-soluble vitamin deficiencies. Absorption of fat soluble vitamins A, D, E, and K may be decreased; patients should take vitamins ≥4 hours before colesevelam. Not to be taken simultaneously with many other medicines (decreased absorption). Some products may contain phenylalanine.
Adverse Reactions (Reflective of adult population; not specific for elderly) Actual frequency may be dependent upon indication. Unless otherwise noted, frequency of adverse effects is reported for adult patients.
>10%: Gastrointestinal: Constipation (9% to 11%)
1% to 10%:
  Cardiovascular: Hypertension (3%)
  Central nervous system:Headache (children 4% to 8%), fatigue (children 4%)

Endocrine & metabolic: Hypertriglyceridemia (4% to 5%), hypoglycemia (3%), CPK increased (children 2%)

Gastrointestinal: Dyspepsia (4% to 8%), nausea (3%), vomiting (children 2%)

Neuromuscular & skeletal: Weakness (4%), myalgia (2%)

Respiratory: Nasopharyngitis (children 5% to 6%), upper respiratory tract infection (children 5%), pharyngitis (3%), rhinitis (children 2%)

Miscellaneous: Flu-like syndrome (children 4%)

Drug Interactions

Metabolism/Transport Effects None known.

Avoid Concomitant Use There are no known interactions where it is recommended to avoid concomitant use.

Increased Effect/Toxicity There are no known significant interactions involving an increase in effect.

Decreased Effect

Colesevelam may decrease the levels/effects of: Amiodarone; Antidiabetic Agents (Thiazolidinedione); Chenodiol; Contraceptives (Estrogens); Contraceptives (Progestins); Corticosteroids (Oral); CycloSPORINE; CycloSPORINE (Systemic); Ethinyl Estradiol; Ezetimibe; Glimepiride; GlipiZIDE; GlyBURIDE; Leflunomide; Loop Diuretics; Methotrexate; Niacin; Nonsteroidal Anti-Inflammatory Agents; Norethindrone; Olmesartan; Phenytoin; Pravastatin; Propranolol; Raloxifene; Tetracycline Derivatives; Thiazide Diuretics; Thyroid Products; Ursodiol; Vancomycin; Vitamin D Analogs; Vitamin K Antagonists

Stability Store at 25°C (77°F); excursions permitted to 15°C to 30°C (59°F to 86°F). Protect from moisture.

Mechanism of Action Cholesterol is the major precursor of bile acid. Colesevelam binds with bile acids in the intestine to form an insoluble complex that is eliminated in feces. This increased excretion of bile acids results in an increased oxidation of cholesterol to bile acid and a lowering of the serum cholesterol.

Pharmacodynamics/Kinetics

Onset of action:

Lipid lowering: Therapeutic: ~2 weeks

Reduction of hemoglobin A_{1c} (Type II diabetes): 4-6 weeks initial onset; 12-18 weeks maximal effect

Absorption: None

Excretion: Urine (0.05%)

Dosage

Geriatric & Adult Dyslipidemia, type 2 diabetes (combination therapy with insulin or oral antidiabetic agents): Oral:

Once-daily dosing: 3.75 g (oral suspension or 6 tablets)

Twice-daily dosing: 1.875 g (3 tablets)

Renal Impairment No dosage adjustment necessary; not absorbed from the gastrointestinal tract.

Hepatic Impairment No dosage adjustment necessary; not absorbed from the gastro-intestinal tract.

Administration Educate the patient on dietary guidelines.

Tablets: Administer with meal(s) and a liquid. Due to tablet size, it is recommended that any patient who has trouble swallowing tablets should use the oral suspension form.

Granules for oral suspension: Administer with meal(s). Empty 1 packet into a glass; add 1/2-1 cup (4-8 ounces) of water, fruit juice, or a diet soft drink and mix well. Powder is not to be taken in dry form (to avoid GI distress).

Monitoring Parameters Serum cholesterol, LDL, and triglyceride levels should be obtained before initiating treatment and periodically thereafter (in accordance with NCEP guidelines)

Test Interactions Increased prothrombin time

Special Geriatric Considerations The definition of and, therefore, when to treat hyperlipidemia in elderly is a controversial issue. The National Cholesterol Education Program recommends that all adults maintain a plasma cholesterol <160 mg/dL. Elderly with one additional risk factor, goal LDL would be <130 mg/dL. It is the authors' belief that pharmacologic treatment be reserved for those who are unable to obtain a desirable plasma cholesterol concentration by diet alone and for whom the benefits of treatment are believed to outweigh the potential adverse effects, drug interactions, and cost of treatment.

Dosage Forms Excipient information presented when available (limited, particularly for generics); consult specific product labeling.

Granules for suspension, oral, as hydrochloride:

Welchol®: 3.75 g/packet (30s) [contains phenylalanine 48 mg/packet; citrus flavor]

Tablet, oral, as hydrochloride:

Welchol®: 625 mg

♦ **Colestid®** see Colestipol on page 442

◆ **Colestid® Flavored** see Colestipol on page 442

Colestipol (koe LES ti pole)

Related Information
Hyperlipidemia Management on page 2130
Medication Safety Issues
Sound-alike/look-alike issues:
Colestipol may be confused with calcitriol
Brand Names: U.S. Colestid®; Colestid® Flavored
Brand Names: Canada Colestid®
Index Terms Colestipol Hydrochloride
Generic Availability (U.S.) Yes
Pharmacologic Category Antilipemic Agent, Bile Acid Sequestrant
Use Adjunct in management of primary hypercholesterolemia
Unlabeled Use Diarrhea associated with excess fecal bile acids (Westergaard, 2007); relief of pruritus associated with elevated levels of bile acids (Datta, 1963; Scaldaferri, 2011)
Contraindications Hypersensitivity to bile acid sequestering resins or any component of the formulation
Warnings/Precautions Secondary causes of hyperlipidemia should be ruled out prior to therapy. Not to be taken simultaneously with many other medicines (decreased absorption). Use with caution in patients susceptible to fat-soluble vitamin deficiencies. Absorption of fat soluble vitamins A, D, E, and K and folic acid may be decreased; patients should take vitamins ≥4 hours before colestipol. Chronic use may be associated with bleeding problems; may be prevented with use of oral vitamin K therapy. May produce or exacerbate constipation; fecal impaction may occur, initiate therapy at a reduced dose in patients with a history of constipation. Hemorrhoids may be worsened. Some products may contain phenylalanine.
Adverse Reactions (Reflective of adult population; not specific for elderly) Frequency not defined.
Cardiovascular: Angina, chest pain, edema of hands or feet, tachycardia
Central nervous system: Dizziness, fatigue, headache (including migraine and sinus), light-headedness, insomnia
Dermatologic: Dermatitis, rash, urticaria
Gastrointestinal: Abdominal pain and cramping, anorexia, bloating, constipation, cholecystitis, cholelithiasis, diarrhea, dysphagia, esophageal obstruction, flatulence, indigestion, heart-burn, hemorrhoids (bleeding), nausea, peptic ulceration, vomiting
Hepatic: Alkaline phosphatase increased, ALT increased, AST increased
Neuromuscular & skeletal: Arthritis, backache, joint/muscle pain, weakness
Respiratory: Dyspnea
Drug Interactions
Metabolism/Transport Effects None known.
Avoid Concomitant Use There are no known interactions where it is recommended to avoid concomitant use.
Increased Effect/Toxicity There are no known significant interactions involving an increase in effect.
Decreased Effect
Colestipol may decrease the levels/effects of: Amiodarone; Antidiabetic Agents (Thiazolidinedione); Cardiac Glycosides; Chenodiol; Contraceptives (Estrogens); Contraceptives (Progestins); Corticosteroids (Oral); Diltiazem; Ezetimibe; Fibric Acid Derivatives; Leflunomide; Loop Diuretics; Methotrexate; Methylfolate; Niacin; Nonsteroidal Anti-Inflammatory Agents; Pravastatin; Propranolol; Raloxifene; Tetracycline Derivatives; Thiazide Diuretics; Thyroid Products; Ursodiol; Vancomycin; Vitamin D Analogs; Vitamin K Antagonists
Stability Store at 20°C to 25°C (68°F to 77°F).
Mechanism of Action Binds with bile acids to form an insoluble complex that is eliminated in feces; it thereby increases the fecal loss of bile acid-bound low density lipoprotein cholesterol
Pharmacodynamics/Kinetics
Absorption: None
Excretion: Feces
Dosage
Geriatric & Adult Dyslipidemia: Oral:
Granules: Initial: 5 g 1-2 times/day; maintenance: 5-30 g/day given once or in divided doses; increase by 5 g/day at 1- to 2-month intervals
Tablets: Initial: 2 g 1-2 times/day; maintenance: 2-16 g/day given once or in divided doses; increase by 2 g once or twice daily at 1- to 2-month intervals
Renal Impairment No dosage adjustment necessary; not absorbed from the gastrointestinal tract.

Hepatic Impairment No dosage adjustment necessary; not absorbed from the gastro-intestinal tract.

Administration Other drugs should be administered at least 1 hour before or 4 hours after colestipol.

Granules: Do not administer in dry form (to avoid GI distress). Dry granules should be added to at least 90 mL of liquid and stirred until completely mixed; may be mixed with any beverage or added to soups, cereal, or pulpy fruits. Rinse glass with a small amount of liquid to ensure all medication is taken.

Tablets: Administer tablets 1 at a time, swallowed whole, with plenty of liquid. Do not cut, crush, or chew tablets.

Monitoring Parameters Serum cholesterol, LDL, and triglyceride levels should be obtained before initiating treatment and periodically thereafter (in accordance with NCEP guidelines)

Test Interactions Increased prothrombin time

Special Geriatric Considerations The definition of and, therefore, when to treat hyper-lipidemia in the elderly is a controversial issue. The National Cholesterol Education Program recommends that all adults maintain a plasma cholesterol <160 mg/dL. Elderly with one additional risk factor, goal LDL would be <130 mg/dL. It is the authors' belief that pharmaco-logic treatment be reserved for those who are unable to obtain a desirable plasma cholesterol concentration by diet alone and for whom the benefits of treatment are believed to outweigh the potential adverse effects, drug interactions, and cost of treatment.

Dosage Forms Excipient information presented when available (limited, particularly for generics); consult specific product labeling.

Granules for suspension, oral, as hydrochloride: 5 g/scoop (500 g); 5 g/packet (30s, 90s)
Colestid®: 5 g/scoop (300 g, 500 g); 5 g/packet (30s, 90s) [unflavored]
Colestid® Flavored: 5 g/scoop (450 g) [contains phenylalanine 18.2 mg/scoop; orange flavor]
Colestid® Flavored: 5 g/packet (60s) [contains phenylalanine 18.2 mg/packet; orange flavor]

Tablet, oral, as hydrochloride: 1 g
Tablet, oral, as hydrochloride [micronized]: 1 g
Colestid®: 1 g

♦ **Colestipol Hydrochloride** see Colestipol on page 442
♦ **Colistin, Hydrocortisone, Neomycin, and Thonzonium** see Neomycin, Colistin, Hydro-cortisone, and Thonzonium on page 1355

Collagenase (Topical) (KOL la je nase)

Medication Safety Issues
Sound-alike/look-alike issues:
Topical collagenase formulation (Santyl®) may be confused with the injectable collagenase clostridium histolyticum (Xiaflex®)

Brand Names: U.S. Santyl®
Brand Names: Canada Santyl®
Generic Availability (U.S.) No
Pharmacologic Category Enzyme, Topical Debridement
Use Promotes debridement of necrotic tissue in dermal ulcers and severe burns
Contraindications Hypersensitivity to collagenase or any component of the formulation
Warnings/Precautions For external use only. Avoid contact with eyes. Monitor debilitated patients for systemic bacterial infections because debriding enzymes may increase the risk of bacteremia.

Adverse Reactions (Reflective of adult population; not specific for elderly) Frequency not defined.
Local: Irritation, pain and burning may occur at site of application

Drug Interactions
Metabolism/Transport Effects None known.
Avoid Concomitant Use There are no known interactions where it is recommended to avoid concomitant use.
Increased Effect/Toxicity There are no known significant interactions involving an increase in effect.
Decreased Effect There are no known significant interactions involving a decrease in effect.

Mechanism of Action Collagenase is an enzyme derived from the fermentation of Clostri-dium histolyticum and differs from other proteolytic enzymes in that its enzymatic action has a high specificity for native and denatured collagen. Collagenase will not attack collagen in healthy tissue or newly formed granulation tissue. In addition, it does not act on fat, fibrin, keratin, or muscle.

Dosage
  Geriatric & Adult Dermal ulcers, burns: Topical: Apply once daily (or more frequently if the dressing becomes soiled).
Administration For external use only. Clean target area of all interfering agents listed above. If infection is persistent, apply powdered antibiotic first. Do not introduce into major body cavities. Monitor debilitated patients for systemic bacterial infections.
Special Geriatric Considerations Preventive skin care should be instituted in all older patients at high risk for pressure ulcers. Collagenase is indicated in stage 3 and 4 pressure ulcers.
Dosage Forms Excipient information presented when available (limited, particularly for generics); consult specific product labeling.
  Ointment, topical:
    Santyl®: 250 units/g (30 g)

- **Colocort®** see Hydrocortisone (Topical) on page 943
- **Coly-Mycin® S** see Neomycin, Colistin, Hydrocortisone, and Thonzonium on page 1355
- **Combivent®** see Ipratropium and Albuterol on page 1037
- **Commit® [OTC]** see Nicotine on page 1372
- **Compazine** see Prochlorperazine on page 1609
- **Compound E** see Cortisone on page 446
- **Compound F** see Hydrocortisone (Systemic) on page 940
- **Compound F** see Hydrocortisone (Topical) on page 943
- **Compound W® [OTC]** see Salicylic Acid on page 1743
- **Compound W® One Step Invisible Strip [OTC]** see Salicylic Acid on page 1743
- **Compound W® One-Step Wart Remover [OTC]** see Salicylic Acid on page 1743
- **Compound W® One Step Wart Remover for Feet [OTC]** see Salicylic Acid on page 1743
- **Compound W® One-Step Wart Remover for Kids [OTC]** see Salicylic Acid on page 1743
- **Compoz® [OTC]** see DiphenhydrAMINE (Systemic) on page 556
- **Compro®** see Prochlorperazine on page 1609
- **Comtan®** see Entacapone on page 641
- **Concerta®** see Methylphenidate on page 1247

Conivaptan (koe NYE vap tan)

Brand Names: U.S. Vaprisol®
Index Terms Conivaptan Hydrochloride; YM087
Generic Availability (U.S.) No
Pharmacologic Category Vasopressin Antagonist
Use Treatment of euvolemic and hypervolemic hyponatremia in hospitalized patients
Contraindications Hypersensitivity to conivaptan, corn or corn products, or any component of the formulation; use in hypovolemic hyponatremia; concurrent use with strong CYP3A4 inhibitors (eg, ketoconazole, itraconazole, ritonavir, indinavir, and clarithromycin); anuria
Warnings/Precautions Monitor closely for rate of serum sodium increase and neurological status; overly rapid serum sodium correction (>12 mEq/L/24 hours) can lead to seizures, permanent neurological damage, coma, or death. Discontinue use if rate of serum sodium increase is undesirable; may reinitiate infusion (at reduced dose) if hyponatremia persists in the absence of neurological symptoms typically associated with rapid sodium rise. Of note, raising serum sodium concentrations with conivaptan has not demonstrated symptomatic benefit. Discontinue if hypovolemia or hypotension occurs. Safety and efficacy in patients with hypervolemic hyponatremia associated with heart failure have not been established. Use in small numbers of hypervolemic, hyponatremic heart failure patients led to increased adverse events. In other heart failure studies, conivaptan did not show significant improvements in outcomes over placebo. Coadministration with digoxin may increase digoxin concentrations; monitor digoxin concentrations. Use with caution in patients with hepatic impairment; dosage adjustment may be required. May cause injection-site reactions.
Adverse Reactions (Reflective of adult population; not specific for elderly)
  >10%:
    Cardiovascular: Orthostatic hypotension (6% to 14%)
    Central nervous system: Fever (5% to 11%)
    Endocrine & metabolic: Hypokalemia (10% to 22%)
    Local: Injection site reactions including pain, erythema, phlebitis, swelling (63% to 73%)
  1% to 10%:
    Cardiovascular: Hypertension (6% to 8%), hypotension (5% to 8%), peripheral edema (3% to 8%), phlebitis (5%), atrial fibrillation (2% to 5%), ECG abnormality (≤5%)
    Central nervous system: Headache (8% to 10%), insomnia (4% to 5%), confusion (≤5%), pain (2%)
    Dermatologic: Pruritus (1% to 5%), erythema (3%)

Endocrine & metabolic: Hyponatremia (6% to 8%), hypomagnesemia (2% to 5%), hyper-/hypoglycemia (3%)

Gastrointestinal: Constipation (6% to 8%), vomiting (5% to 7%), diarrhea (≤7%), nausea (3% to 5%), dry mouth (4%), dehydration (2%), oral candidiasis (2%)

Genitourinary: Urinary tract infection (4% to 5%)

Hematologic: Anemia (5% to 6%)

Renal: Polyuria (5% to 6%), hematuria (2%)

Respiratory: Pneumonia (2% to 5%), pharyngolaryngeal pain (1% to 5%)

Miscellaneous: Thirst (3% to 6%)

Drug Interactions

Metabolism/Transport Effects Substrate of CYP3A4 (major); **Note:** Assignment of Major/Minor substrate status based on clinically relevant drug interaction potential; **Inhibits** CYP3A4 (strong)

Avoid Concomitant Use

Avoid concomitant use of Conivaptan with any of the following: Alfuzosin; Antifungal Agents (Azole Derivatives, Systemic); Avanafil; Axitinib; Crizotinib; CYP3A4 Inhibitors (Strong); CYP3A4 Substrates; Dronedarone; Eplerenone; Everolimus; Fluticasone (Oral Inhalation); Halofantrine; Lapatinib; Lovastatin; Lurasidone; Nilotinib; Nisoldipine; Pimozide; Ranolazine; Red Yeast Rice; Rivaroxaban; RomiDEPsin; Salmeterol; Silodosin; Simvastatin; Tamsulosin; Ticagrelor; Tolvaptan; Toremifene

Increased Effect/Toxicity

Conivaptan may increase the levels/effects of: Alfuzosin; Almotriptan; Alosetron; ARIPiprazole; Avanafil; Axitinib; Bortezomib; Brentuximab Vedotin; Brinzolamide; Budesonide (Nasal); Budesonide (Systemic, Oral Inhalation); Ciclesonide; Colchicine; Corticosteroids (Orally Inhaled); Crizotinib; CYP3A4 Substrates; Dienogest; Digoxin; Dronedarone; Dutasteride; Eplerenone; Everolimus; FentaNYL; Fesoterodine; Fluticasone (Nasal); Fluticasone (Oral Inhalation); GuanFACINE; Halofantrine; Iloperidone; Ivacaftor; Ixabepilone; Lapatinib; Lovastatin; Lumefantrine; Lurasidone; Maraviroc; MethylPREDNISolone; Mifepristone; Nilotinib; Nisoldipine; Paricalcitol; Pazopanib; Pimecrolimus; Pimozide; Propafenone; Ranolazine; Red Yeast Rice; Rivaroxaban; RomiDEPsin; Ruxolitinib; Salmeterol; Saxagliptin; Sildenafil; Silodosin; Simvastatin; SORAfenib; Tadalafil; Tamsulosin; Ticagrelor; Tolterodine; Tolvaptan; Toremifene; Vardenafil; Vemurafenib; Vilazodone; Zuclopenthixol

The levels/effects of Conivaptan may be increased by: Antifungal Agents (Azole Derivatives, Systemic); CYP3A4 Inhibitors (Moderate); CYP3A4 Inhibitors (Strong); Dasatinib

Decreased Effect

Conivaptan may decrease the levels/effects of: Ifosfamide; Prasugrel; Ticagrelor

The levels/effects of Conivaptan may be decreased by: CYP3A4 Inducers (Strong); Deferasirox; Herbs (CYP3A4 Inducers); Tocilizumab

Ethanol/Nutrition/Herb Interactions Herb/Nutraceutical: St John's wort may decrease the levels/effects of conivaptan.

Stability Store at 25°C (77°F); brief excursions permitted up to 40°C (104°F). Protect from light and freezing. Do not remove protective overwrap until ready for use.

Mechanism of Action Conivaptan is an arginine vasopressin (AVP) receptor antagonist with affinity for AVP receptor subtypes V_{1A} and V_2. The antidiuretic action of AVP is mediated through activation of the V_2 receptor, which functions to regulate water and electrolyte balance at the level of the collecting ducts in the kidney. Serum levels of AVP are commonly elevated in euvolemic or hypervolemic hyponatremia, which results in the dilution of serum sodium and the relative hyponatremic state. Antagonism of the V_2 receptor by conivaptan promotes the excretion of free water (without loss of serum electrolytes) resulting in net fluid loss, increased urine output, decreased urine osmolality, and subsequent restoration of normal serum sodium concentrations.

Pharmacodynamics/Kinetics

Protein binding: 99%

Metabolism: Hepatic via CYP3A4 to four minimally-active metabolites

Half-life elimination: ~5-8 hours

Excretion: Feces (83%); urine (12%, primarily as metabolites)

Dosage

Geriatric & Adult Euvolemic or hypervolemic hyponatremia: I.V.: 20 mg infused over 30 minutes as a loading dose, followed by a continuous infusion of 20 mg over 24 hours (0.83 mg/hour) for 2-4 days; may increase to a maximum dose of 40 mg over 24 hours (1.7 mg/hour) if serum sodium not rising sufficiently; total duration of therapy not to exceed 4 days. **Note:** If patient requires 40 mg/24 hours, may administer two consecutive 20 mg/100 mL premixed solutions over 24 hours (ie, 20 mg over 12 hours followed by 20 mg over 12 hours).

Renal Impairment
Cl$_{cr}$ ≥30mL/minute: No dosage adjustment necessary.
Cl$_{cr}$ <30 mL/minute: Use not recommended; clinical response reduced; contraindicated in anuria (no benefit expected).

Hepatic Impairment
Mild impairment: No dosage adjustment necessary.
Moderate impairment: 10 mg infused over 30 minutes as a loading dose, followed by a continuous infusion of 10 mg over 24 hours (0.42 mg/hour) for 2-4 days; may increase to a maximum dose of 20 mg over 24 hours (0.83 mg/hour) if serum sodium not rising sufficiently; total duration of therapy not to exceed 4 days.
Severe impairment: Use not recommended (not studied).

Administration For intravenous use only; infuse into large veins and change infusion site every 24 hours to minimize vascular irritation. Do not administer with any other product in the same intravenous line or container.

Monitoring Parameters Rate of serum sodium increase, blood pressure, volume status, urine output

Special Geriatric Considerations Adverse events in elderly patients were generally similar to those seen in younger patients. In clinical studies, 52% of patients were >65 years of age and 34% were >75 years of age.

Dosage Forms Excipient information presented when available (limited, particularly for generics); consult specific product labeling.
Infusion, premixed in D$_5$W, as hydrochloride:
Vaprisol®: 20 mg (100 mL)

◆ **Conivaptan Hydrochloride** *see* Conivaptan *on page 444*
◆ **Conjugated Estrogen** *see* Estrogens (Conjugated/Equine, Systemic) *on page 703*
◆ **Conjugated Estrogen** *see* Estrogens (Conjugated/Equine, Topical) *on page 707*
◆ **Constulose** *see* Lactulose *on page 1086*
◆ **Contac® Cold + Flu Maximum Strength Non-Drowsy [OTC]** *see* Acetaminophen and Phenylephrine *on page 37*
◆ **Contac® Cold + Flu Maximum Strength Non-Drowsy [OTC]** *see* Pseudoephedrine *on page 1633*
◆ **ControlRx™** *see* Fluoride *on page 806*
◆ **ControlRx™ Multi** *see* Fluoride *on page 806*
◆ **Conventional Amphotericin B** *see* Amphotericin B (Conventional) *on page 121*
◆ **ConZip™** *see* TraMADol *on page 1942*
◆ **Copegus®** *see* Ribavirin *on page 1691*
◆ **Cordarone®** *see* Amiodarone *on page 96*
◆ **Coreg®** *see* Carvedilol *on page 300*
◆ **Coreg CR®** *see* Carvedilol *on page 300*
◆ **Corgard®** *see* Nadolol *on page 1328*
◆ **Coricidin HBP® Chest Congestion and Cough [OTC]** *see* Guaifenesin and Dextromethorphan *on page 906*
◆ **Cormax®** *see* Clobetasol *on page 406*
◆ **Correctol® [OTC]** *see* Docusate *on page 583*
◆ **Correctol® Tablets [OTC]** *see* Bisacodyl *on page 214*
◆ **Cortaid® Advanced [OTC]** *see* Hydrocortisone (Topical) *on page 943*
◆ **Cortaid® Intensive Therapy [OTC]** *see* Hydrocortisone (Topical) *on page 943*
◆ **Cortaid® Maximum Strength [OTC]** *see* Hydrocortisone (Topical) *on page 943*
◆ **Cortef®** *see* Hydrocortisone (Systemic) *on page 940*
◆ **Cortenema®** *see* Hydrocortisone (Topical) *on page 943*
◆ **CortiCool® [OTC]** *see* Hydrocortisone (Topical) *on page 943*
◆ **Cortifoam®** *see* Hydrocortisone (Topical) *on page 943*
◆ **Cortisol** *see* Hydrocortisone (Systemic) *on page 940*
◆ **Cortisol** *see* Hydrocortisone (Topical) *on page 943*

Cortisone (KOR ti sone)

Related Information
Corticosteroids Systemic Equivalencies *on page 2112*

Medication Safety Issues
Sound-alike/look-alike issues:
Cortisone may be confused with Cardizem®, Cortizone®

Index Terms Compound E; Cortisone Acetate
Generic Availability (U.S.) Yes
Pharmacologic Category Corticosteroid, Systemic
Use Management of adrenocortical insufficiency

Contraindications Hypersensitivity to cortisone acetate or any component of the formulation; serious infections, except septic shock or tuberculous meningitis; administration of live virus vaccines

Warnings/Precautions Use with caution in patients with thyroid disease, hepatic impairment, renal impairment, cardiovascular disease, diabetes, glaucoma, cataracts, myasthenia gravis, patients at risk for osteoporosis, patients at risk for seizures, or GI diseases (diverticulitis, peptic ulcer, ulcerative colitis) due to perforation risk. Use caution following acute MI (corticosteroids have been associated with myocardial rupture). Because of the risk of adverse effects, systemic corticosteroids should be used cautiously in the elderly in the smallest possible effective dose for the shortest duration. May affect growth velocity. Withdraw therapy with gradual tapering of dose.

May cause hypercorticism or suppression of hypothalamic-pituitary-adrenal (HPA) axis, particularly in patients receiving high doses for prolonged periods. HPA axis suppression may lead to adrenal crisis. Withdrawal and discontinuation of a corticosteroid should be done slowly and carefully. Particular care is required when patients are transferred from systemic corticosteroids to inhaled products due to possible adrenal insufficiency or withdrawal from steroids, including an increase in allergic symptoms. Patients receiving >20 mg per day of prednisone (or equivalent) may be most susceptible. Fatalities have occurred due to adrenal insufficiency in asthmatic patients during and after transfer from systemic corticosteroids to aerosol steroids; aerosol steroids do not provide the systemic steroid needed to treat patients having trauma, surgery, or infections.

Acute myopathy has been reported with high dose corticosteroids, usually in patients with neuromuscular transmission disorders; may involve ocular and/or respiratory muscles; monitor creatine kinase; recovery may be delayed. Corticosteroid use may cause psychiatric disturbances, including depression, euphoria, insomnia, mood swings, and personality changes. Pre-existing psychiatric conditions may be exacerbated by corticosteroid use. Prolonged use of corticosteroids may also increase the incidence of secondary infection, mask acute infection (including fungal infections), prolong or exacerbate viral infections, or limit response to vaccines. Exposure to chickenpox should be avoided; corticosteroids should not be used to treat ocular herpes simplex. Corticosteroids should not be used for cerebral malaria or viral hepatitis. Close observation is required in patients with latent tuberculosis and/or TB reactivity; restrict use in active TB (only in conjunction with antituberculosis treatment). Prolonged treatment with corticosteroids has been associated with the development of Kaposi's sarcoma (case reports); if noted, discontinuation of therapy should be considered.

Adverse Reactions (Reflective of adult population; not specific for elderly)
>10%:
Central nervous system: Insomnia, nervousness
Gastrointestinal: Increased appetite, indigestion
1% to 10%:
Dermatologic: Hirsutism
Endocrine & metabolic: Diabetes mellitus
Neuromuscular & skeletal: Arthralgia
Ocular: Cataracts, glaucoma
Respiratory: Epistaxis

Drug Interactions

Metabolism/Transport Effects None known.

Avoid Concomitant Use
Avoid concomitant use of Cortisone with any of the following: Aldesleukin; BCG; Mifepristone; Natalizumab; Pimecrolimus; Tacrolimus (Topical)

Increased Effect/Toxicity
Cortisone may increase the levels/effects of: Acetylcholinesterase Inhibitors; Amphotericin B; Deferasirox; Leflunomide; Loop Diuretics; Natalizumab; NSAID (COX-2 Inhibitor); NSAID (Nonselective); Thiazide Diuretics; Vaccines (Live); Warfarin

The levels/effects of Cortisone may be increased by: Antifungal Agents (Azole Derivatives, Systemic); Aprepitant; Calcium Channel Blockers (Nondihydropyridine); Denosumab; Estrogen Derivatives; Fluconazole; Fosaprepitant; Indacaterol; Macrolide Antibiotics; Mifepristone; Neuromuscular-Blocking Agents (Nondepolarizing); Pimecrolimus; Quinolone Antibiotics; Roflumilast; Salicylates; Tacrolimus (Topical); Telaprevir; Trastuzumab

Decreased Effect
Cortisone may decrease the levels/effects of: Aldesleukin; Antidiabetic Agents; BCG; Calcitriol; Coccidioidin Skin Test; Corticorelin; Hyaluronidase; Isoniazid; Salicylates; Sipuleucel-T; Telaprevir; Vaccines (Inactivated)

The levels/effects of Cortisone may be decreased by: Aminoglutethimide; Antacids; Barbiturates; Bile Acid Sequestrants; Echinacea; Mifepristone; Mitotane; Primidone; Rifamycin Derivatives; Somatropin; Tesamorelin

CORTISONE

Ethanol/Nutrition/Herb Interactions Food: Limit caffeine intake.
Mechanism of Action Decreases inflammation by suppression of migration of polymorpho-nuclear leukocytes and reversal of increased capillary permeability
Pharmacodynamics/Kinetics
Onset of action: Peak effect: Oral: ~2 hours; I.M.: 20-48 hours
Duration: 30-36 hours
Absorption: Slow
Distribution: Muscles, liver, skin, intestines, and kidneys
Metabolism: Hepatic to inactive metabolites
Half-life elimination: 0.5-2 hours; End-stage renal disease: 3.5 hours
Excretion: Urine and feces
Dosage
Geriatric & Adult If possible, administer glucocorticoids before 9 AM to minimize adreno-cortical suppression; dosing depends upon the condition being treated and the response of the patient. **Note:** Supplemental doses may be warranted during times of stress in the course of withdrawing therapy.

Anti-inflammatory or immunosuppressive: Oral: 25-300 mg/day in divided doses every 12-24 hours
Physiologic replacement: Oral: 25-35 mg/day
Renal Impairment
Hemodialysis: Supplemental dose is not necessary.
Peritoneal dialysis: Supplemental dose is not necessary.
Administration Insoluble in water.
Monitoring Parameters Blood pressure, blood glucose, electrolytes, symptoms of fluid retention
Test Interactions May suppress the wheal and flare reactions to skin test antigens
Pharmacotherapy Pearls Approximately 80% the potency of cortisol; the maximum activity of the adrenal cortex is between 2 AM and 8 AM and it is minimal between 4 PM and midnight; if possible, administer glucocorticoids before 9 AM to minimize adrenocortical suppression; prolonged therapy (>5 days) of pharmacologic doses of corticosteroids may lead to hypo-thalamic-pituitary-adrenal suppression, the degree of adrenal suppression varies with the degree and duration of glucocorticoid therapy; this must be taken into consideration when taking patients off steroids; supplemental doses may be warranted during times of stress in the course of withdrawal therapy
Special Geriatric Considerations Because of the risk of adverse effects, systemic cortico-steroids should be used cautiously in the elderly, in the smallest possible dose, and for the shortest possible time.
Dosage Forms Excipient information presented when available (limited, particularly for generics); consult specific product labeling.
Tablet, oral, as acetate: 25 mg

- Cortisone Acetate see Cortisone on page 446
- Cortisporin®-TC see Neomycin, Colistin, Hydrocortisone, and Thonzonium on page 1355
- Cortizone-10® Hydratensive Healing [OTC] see Hydrocortisone (Topical) on page 943
- Cortizone-10® Hydratensive Soothing [OTC] see Hydrocortisone (Topical) on page 943
- Cortizone-10® Intensive Healing Eczema [OTC] see Hydrocortisone (Topical) on page 943
- Cortizone-10® Maximum Strength [OTC] see Hydrocortisone (Topical) on page 943
- Cortizone-10® Maximum Strength Cooling Relief [OTC] see Hydrocortisone (Topical) on page 943
- Cortizone-10® Maximum Strength Easy Relief [OTC] see Hydrocortisone (Topical) on page 943
- Cortizone-10® Maximum Strength Intensive Healing Formula [OTC] see Hydrocortisone (Topical) on page 943
- Cortizone-10® Plus Maximum Strength [OTC] see Hydrocortisone (Topical) on page 943
- Cosopt® see Dorzolamide and Timolol on page 598
- Cosopt® PF see Dorzolamide and Timolol on page 598
- Co-Trimoxazole see Sulfamethoxazole and Trimethoprim on page 1813
- Coumadin® see Warfarin on page 2033
- Covera-HS® [DSC] see Verapamil on page 2014
- Cozaar® see Losartan on page 1160
- CPDG2 see Glucarpidase on page 885
- CPG2 see Glucarpidase on page 885
- CPM see Cyclophosphamide on page 456
- CPZ see ChlorproMAZINE on page 359
- Creomulsion® Adult Formula [OTC] see Dextromethorphan on page 525
- Creomulsion® for Children [OTC] see Dextromethorphan on page 525

448

Cromolyn (Systemic, Oral Inhalation) (KROE moe lin)

Brand Names: U.S. Gastrocrom®
Brand Names: Canada Nalcrom®; Nu-Cromolyn; PMS-Sodium Cromoglycate
Index Terms Cromoglycic Acid; Cromolyn Sodium; Disodium Cromoglycate; DSCG
Generic Availability (U.S.) Yes
Pharmacologic Category Mast Cell Stabilizer
Use
Inhalation: May be used as an adjunct in the prophylaxis of allergic disorders, including asthma; prevention of exercise-induced bronchospasm
Oral: Systemic mastocytosis
Unlabeled Use Oral: Food allergy, treatment of inflammatory bowel disease
Contraindications Hypersensitivity to cromolyn or any component of the formulation; acute asthma attacks
Warnings/Precautions Severe anaphylactic reactions may occur rarely; cromolyn is a prophylactic drug with no benefit for acute situations; caution should be used when withdrawing the drug or tapering the dose as symptoms may reoccur; use with caution in patients with a history of cardiac arrhythmias. Dosage of oral product should be decreased with hepatic or renal dysfunction.
Adverse Reactions (Reflective of adult population; not specific for elderly) Frequency not defined.
Cardiovascular: Angioedema, chest pain, edema, flushing, palpitation, premature ventricular contractions, tachycardia
Central nervous system: Anxiety, behavior changes, convulsions, depression, dizziness, fatigue, hallucinations, headache, irritability, insomnia, lethargy, migraine, nervousness, hypoesthesia, postprandial lightheadedness, psychosis
Dermatologic: Erythema, photosensitivity, pruritus, purpura, rash, urticaria
Gastrointestinal: Abdominal pain, constipation, diarrhea, dyspepsia, dysphagia, esophagospasm, flatulence, glossitis, nausea, stomatitis, vomiting
Genitourinary: Dysuria, urinary frequency
Hematologic: Neutropenia, pancytopenia, polycythemia
Hepatic: Liver function test abnormal
Local: Burning
Neuromuscular & skeletal: Arthralgia, leg stiffness, leg weakness, myalgia, paresthesia
Otic: Tinnitus
Respiratory: Dyspnea, pharyngitis
Miscellaneous: Lupus erythematosus
Drug Interactions
Metabolism/Transport Effects None known.
Avoid Concomitant Use There are no known interactions where it is recommended to avoid concomitant use.
Increased Effect/Toxicity There are no known significant interactions involving an increase in effect.
Decreased Effect There are no known significant interactions involving a decrease in effect.
Stability Store at room temperature of 15°C to 30°C (59°F to 86°F). Protect from light. Do not use oral solution if solution becomes discolored or forms a precipitate.
Mechanism of Action Prevents the mast cell release of histamine, leukotrienes, and slow-reacting substance of anaphylaxis by inhibiting degranulation after contact with antigens
Pharmacodynamics/Kinetics
Onset: Response to treatment: Oral: May occur within 2-6 weeks
Absorption:
Inhalation: ~8% reaches lungs upon inhalation; well absorbed
Oral: <1% of dose absorbed
Half-life elimination: 80-90 minutes
Time to peak, serum: Inhalation: ~15 minutes
Excretion: Urine and feces (equal amounts as unchanged drug); exhaled gases (small amounts)

Dosage

Geriatric & Adult

Asthma: For chronic control of asthma, taper frequency to the lowest effective dose (ie, 4 times/day to 3 times/day to twice daily). **Note:** Not effective for immediate relief of symptoms in acute asthmatic attacks; must be used at regular intervals for 2-4 weeks to be effective.

Nebulization solution: Initial: 20 mg 4 times/day; usual dose: 20 mg 3-4 times/day

Prophylaxis of bronchospasm (allergen- or exercise-induced):

Note: Administer 10-15 minutes prior to exercise or allergen exposure but no longer than 1 hour before:

Nebulization solution: Single dose of 20 mg

Mastocytosis: Oral: 200 mg 4 times/day; given ¹/₂ hour prior to meals and at bedtime. If control of symptoms is not seen within 2-3 weeks, dose may be increased to a maximum 40 mg/kg/day

Food allergy (unlabeled use), inflammatory bowel disease (unlabeled use): Oral: Initial dose: 200 mg 4 times/day; may double the dose if effect is not satisfactory within 2-3 weeks; up to 400 mg 4 times/day

Renal Impairment Specific guidelines not available; consider lower dose of oral product.

Hepatic Impairment Specific guidelines not available; consider lower dose of oral product.

Administration Oral solution: Open ampul and squeeze contents into glass of water; stir well; administer at least 30 minutes before meals and at bedtime

Monitoring Parameters Periodic pulmonary function tests

Special Geriatric Considerations Evaluate the patient's or caregiver's ability to safely administer the correct dose of medication.

Dosage Forms Excipient information presented when available (limited, particularly for generics); consult specific product labeling.

Solution, for nebulization, as sodium: 20 mg/2 mL (60s, 120s)

Solution, oral, as sodium [concentrate, preservative free]: 100 mg/5 mL (96s)

Gastrocrom®: 100 mg/5 mL (96s)

Cromolyn (Nasal) (KROE moe lin)

Medication Safety Issues

Sound-alike/look-alike issues:

NasalCrom® may be confused with Nasacort®, Nasalide®

Brand Names: U.S. NasalCrom® [OTC]

Brand Names: Canada Apo-Cromolyn Nasal Spray® [OTC]; Rhinaris-CS Anti-Allergic Nasal Mist

Index Terms Cromoglycic Acid; Cromolyn Sodium; Disodium Cromoglycate; DSCG

Generic Availability (U.S.) Yes

Pharmacologic Category Mast Cell Stabilizer

Use Prevention and treatment of seasonal and perennial allergic rhinitis

Dosage

Geriatric & Adult Allergic rhinitis (treatment and prophylaxis): Intranasal: Instill 1 spray in each nostril 3-4 times/day; may be increased to 6 times/day (symptomatic relief may require 2-4 weeks)

Special Geriatric Considerations Evaluate the patient's or caregiver's ability to safely administer the correct dose of nasal medication.

Dosage Forms Excipient information presented when available (limited, particularly for generics); consult specific product labeling.

Solution, intranasal, as sodium [spray]: 40 mg/mL (26 mL)

NasalCrom®: 40 mg/mL (13 mL) [contains benzalkonium chloride; 5.2 mg/inhalation]

Cromolyn (Ophthalmic) (KROE moe lin)

Brand Names: Canada Opticrom®

Index Terms Crolom; Cromoglycic Acid; Cromolyn Sodium; Disodium Cromoglycate; DSCG

Generic Availability (U.S.) Yes

Pharmacologic Category Mast Cell Stabilizer

Use Treatment of vernal keratoconjunctivitis, vernal conjunctivitis, and vernal keratitis

Dosage

Geriatric & Adult Conjunctivitis and keratitis: Ophthalmic: 1-2 drops in each eye 4-6 times/day

Special Geriatric Considerations Evaluate the patient's or caregiver's ability to safely administer the correct dose of ophthalmic medication.

Dosage Forms Excipient information presented when available (limited, particularly for generics); consult specific product labeling.
Solution, ophthalmic, as sodium [drops]: 4% (10 mL)

◆ **Cromolyn Sodium** see Cromolyn (Nasal) on page 450
◆ **Cromolyn Sodium** see Cromolyn (Ophthalmic) on page 450
◆ **Cromolyn Sodium** see Cromolyn (Systemic, Oral Inhalation) on page 449

Crotamiton (kroe TAM i tonn)

Medication Safety Issues
Sound-alike/look-alike issues:
Eurax® may be confused with Efudex®, Eulexin, Evoxac®, Serax, Urex
International issues:
Eurax [U.S., Canada, and multiple international markets] may be confused with Urex brand name for furosemide [Australia, China,Turkey] and methenamine [U.S., Canada]
Brand Names: U.S. Eurax®
Brand Names: Canada Eurax Cream
Generic Availability (U.S.) No
Pharmacologic Category Scabicidal Agent
Use Treatment of scabies (*Sarcoptes scabiei*) and symptomatic treatment of pruritus
Contraindications Hypersensitivity to crotamiton or any component of the formulation; patients who manifest a primary irritation response to topical medications
Warnings/Precautions Avoid contact with face, eyes, mucous membranes, and urethral meatus. Do not apply to acutely inflamed or raw skin. For external use only.
Adverse Reactions (Reflective of adult population; not specific for elderly) Frequency not defined. Topical:
Dermatologic: Contact dermatitis, pruritus, rash
Local: Local irritation
Miscellaneous: Allergic sensitivity reactions, warm sensation
Drug Interactions
Metabolism/Transport Effects None known.
Avoid Concomitant Use There are no known interactions where it is recommended to avoid concomitant use.
Increased Effect/Toxicity There are no known significant interactions involving an increase in effect.
Decreased Effect There are no known significant interactions involving a decrease in effect.
Stability Store at room temperature.
Mechanism of Action Crotamiton has scabicidal activity against *Sarcoptes scabiei*; mechanism of action unknown
Dosage
Geriatric & Adult
Scabies: Topical: Wash thoroughly and scrub away loose scales, then towel dry; apply a thin layer and massage drug onto skin of the entire body from the neck to the toes (with special attention to skin folds, creases, and interdigital spaces). Repeat application in 24 hours. Take a cleansing bath 48 hours after the final application. Treatment may be repeated after 7-10 days if live mites are still present.
Pruritus: Topical: Massage into affected areas until medication is completely absorbed; repeat as necessary
Administration Lotion: Shake well before using; avoid contact with face, eyes, mucous membranes, and urethral meatus
Special Geriatric Considerations If cure is not achieved after 2 doses, use alternative therapy.
Dosage Forms Excipient information presented when available (limited, particularly for generics); consult specific product labeling.
Cream, topical:
Eurax®: 10% (60 g)
Lotion, topical:
Eurax®: 10% (60 mL, 480 mL)

◆ **Cruex® [OTC]** see Clotrimazole (Topical) on page 426
◆ **Crystalline Penicillin** see Penicillin G (Parenteral/Aqueous) on page 1500
◆ **CS-747** see Prasugrel on page 1584
◆ **CsA** see CycloSPORINE (Ophthalmic) on page 467
◆ **CsA** see CycloSPORINE (Systemic) on page 460

- ◆ **C-Time [OTC]** *see* Ascorbic Acid *on page* 149
- ◆ **CTLA-4lg** *see* Abatacept *on page* 20
- ◆ **CTM** *see* Chlorpheniramine *on page* 357
- ◆ **CTX** *see* Cyclophosphamide *on page* 456
- ◆ **Cubicin®** *see* DAPTOmycin *on page* 485
- ◆ **Culturelle® [OTC]** *see* Lactobacillus *on page* 1084
- ◆ **Cuprimine®** *see* PenicillAMINE *on page* 1493
- ◆ **Curad® Mediplast® [OTC]** *see* Salicylic Acid *on page* 1743
- ◆ **Cutivate®** *see* Fluticasone (Topical) *on page* 827
- ◆ **Cuvposa™** *see* Glycopyrrolate *on page* 892
- ◆ **CVT-3146** *see* Regadenoson *on page* 1683
- ◆ **CyA** *see* CycloSPORINE (Ophthalmic) *on page* 467
- ◆ **CyA** *see* CycloSPORINE (Systemic) *on page* 460

Cyanocobalamin (sye an oh koe BAL a min)

Brand Names: U.S. Ener-B® [OTC]; Nascobal®; Twelve Resin-K [OTC]

Index Terms Vitamin B_{12}

Generic Availability (U.S.) Yes: Excludes nasal spray

Pharmacologic Category Vitamin, Water Soluble

Use Treatment of pernicious anemia; vitamin B_{12} deficiency due to dietary deficiencies or malabsorption diseases, inadequate secretion of intrinsic factor, and inadequate utilization of B_{12} (eg, during neoplastic treatment); increased B_{12} requirements due to thyrotoxicosis, hemorrhage, malignancy, liver or kidney disease

CaloMist™: Maintenance of vitamin B_{12} concentrations after initial correction in patients with B_{12} deficiency without CNS involvement

Contraindications Hypersensitivity to cyanocobalamin, cobalt, or any component of the formulation

Warnings/Precautions I.M./SubQ routes are used to treat pernicious anemia; oral and intranasal administration are not indicated until hematologic remission and no signs of nervous system involvement. Treatment of severe vitamin B_{12} megaloblastic anemia may result in thrombocytosis and severe hypokalemia, sometimes fatal, due to intracellular potassium shift upon anemia resolution. Vitamin B_{12} deficiency masks signs of polycythemia vera; use caution in other conditions where folic acid or vitamin B_{12} administration alone might mask true diagnosis, despite hematologic response. Vitamin B_{12} deficiency for >3 months results in irreversible degenerative CNS lesions; neurologic manifestations will not be prevented with folic acid unless vitamin B_{12} is also given. Spinal cord degeneration might also occur when folic acid used as a substitute for vitamin B_{12} in anemia prevention. Use caution in Leber's disease patients; B_{12} treatment may result in rapid optic atrophy. Some parenteral products contain aluminum; use caution in patients with impaired renal function. Some products contain benzyl alcohol. Avoid intravenous route; anaphylactic shock has occurred. Intradermal test dose of vitamin B_{12} is recommended for any patient suspected of cyanocobalamin sensitivity prior to intranasal or injectable administration. Efficacy of intranasal products in patients with nasal pathology or with other concomitant intranasal therapy has not been determined.

Adverse Reactions (Reflective of adult population; not specific for elderly) Frequency not defined.

Cardiovascular: CHF, peripheral vascular disorder, peripheral vascular thrombosis

Central nervous system: Anxiety, dizziness, headache, hypoesthesia, incoordination, pain, nervousness

Dermatologic: Itching, urticaria, exanthema (transient)

Gastrointestinal: Diarrhea, dyspepsia, glossitis, nausea, sore throat, vomiting

Hematologic: Polycythemia vera

Neuromuscular & skeletal: Abnormal gait, arthritis, back pain, myalgia, paresthesia, weakness

Respiratory: Dyspnea, pulmonary edema, rhinitis

Miscellaneous: Anaphylaxis (parenteral) and infection

Drug Interactions

Metabolism/Transport Effects None known.

Avoid Concomitant Use There are no known interactions where it is recommended to avoid concomitant use.

Increased Effect/Toxicity There are no known significant interactions involving an increase in effect.

Decreased Effect

The levels/effects of Cyanocobalamin may be decreased by: Chloramphenicol; Colchicine

Ethanol/Nutrition/Herb Interactions Ethanol: Heavy consumption >2 weeks may impair vitamin B_{12} absorption.

Stability

Injection: Clear pink to red solutions are stable at room temperature. Protect from light.

Intranasal spray: Store at 15°C to 30°C (59°F to 86°F); do not freeze. Protect from light.

Mechanism of Action Coenzyme for various metabolic functions, including fat and carbohydrate metabolism and protein synthesis, used in cell replication and hematopoiesis

Pharmacodynamics/Kinetics

Absorption: Oral: Variable from the terminal ileum; requires the presence of calcium and gastric "intrinsic factor" to transfer the compound across the intestinal mucosa

Distribution: Principally stored in the liver and bone marrow, also stored in the kidneys and adrenals

Protein binding: Transcobalamins

Metabolism: Converted in tissues to active coenzymes, methylcobalamin and deoxyadenosylcobalamin; undergoes some enterohepatic recycling

Bioavailability: Intranasal solution: Nascobal®: 6.1% (relative to I.M.)

Dosage

Geriatric & Adult

Recommended intake: 2.4 mcg/day

Vitamin B$_{12}$ deficiency:

Intranasal:

Nascobal®: 500 mcg in one nostril once weekly

CaloMist™: Maintenance therapy (following correction of vitamin B$_{12}$ deficiency): 25 mcg in each nostril daily (50 mcg/day). If inadequate response, 25 mcg in each nostril twice daily (100 mcg/day).

Oral: 250 mcg/day

I.M., deep SubQ: Initial: 30 mcg/day for 5-10 days; maintenance: 100-200 mcg/month

Pernicious anemia: I.M., deep SubQ (administer concomitantly with folic acid if needed, 1 mg/day for 1 month): 100 mcg/day for 6-7 days; if improvement, administer same dose on alternate days for 7 doses, then every 3-4 days for 2-3 weeks; once hematologic values have returned to normal, maintenance dosage: 100 mcg/month. **Note:** Alternative dosing of 1000 mcg/day for 5 days (followed by 500-1000 mcg/month) has been used.

Hematologic remission (without evidence of nervous system involvement):

Intranasal (Nascobal®): 500 mcg in one nostril once weekly

Oral: 1000-2000 mcg/day

I.M., SubQ: 100-1000 mcg/month

Schilling test: I.M.: 1000 mcg

Administration

I.M./SubQ: I.M. or deep SubQ are preferred routes of administration

Intranasal: Nasal spray:

Nascobal®: Prior to initial dose, activate (prime) spray nozzle by pumping unit quickly and firmly until first appearance of spray, then prime twice more. The unit must be reprimed once immediately before each subsequent use. Administer 1 hour before or after ingestion of hot foods/liquids.

CaloMist™: Prime unit by spraying 7 times. If ≥5 days since use, reprime with 2 sprays. Separate from other intranasal medications by several hours.

I.V.: Not recommended due to rapid elimination

Oral: Not recommended due to variable absorption; however, oral therapy of 1000-2000 mcg/day has been effective for anemia if I.M./SubQ routes refused or not tolerated.

Monitoring Parameters Vitamin B$_{12}$, hematocrit, reticulocyte count, folate and iron levels should be obtained prior to treatment; vitamin B$_{12}$ and peripheral blood counts should be monitored 1 month after beginning treatment, then every 3-6 months thereafter.

Megaloblastic anemia: In addition to normal hematological parameters, serum potassium and platelet counts should be monitored during therapy

Reference Range Normal range of serum B$_{12}$ is 150-750 pg/mL; this represents 0.1% of total body content. Metabolic requirements are 2-5 mcg/day; years of deficiency required before hematologic and neurologic signs and symptoms are seen. Occasional patients with significant neuropsychiatric abnormalities may have no hematologic abnormalities and normal serum cobalamin levels, 200 pg/mL (SI: >150 pmol/L), or more commonly between 100-200 pg/mL (SI: 75-150 pmol/L).

Test Interactions Methotrexate, pyrimethamine, and most antibiotics invalidate folic acid and vitamin B$_{12}$ diagnostic blood assays

Special Geriatric Considerations There exists evidence that people, particularly elderly whose serum cobalamin concentrations are <500 pg/mL, should receive replacement parenteral therapy or oral replacement (1000 mcg daily). This recommendation is based upon neuropsychiatric disorders and cardiovascular disorders associated with lower serum cobalamin concentrations.

Dosage Forms Excipient information presented when available (limited, particularly for generics); consult specific product labeling.
Injection, solution: 1000 mcg/mL (1 mL, 10 mL, 30 mL)
Lozenge, oral: 50 mcg (100s); 100 mcg (100s); 250 mcg (100s, 250s); 500 mcg (100s, 250s)
Lozenge, sublingual: 500 mcg (100s)
Solution, intranasal [spray]:
Nascobal®: 500 mcg/spray (2.3 mL) [contains benzalkonium chloride; delivers 8 doses]
Tablet, for buccal application/oral/sublingual:
Twelve Resin-K: 1000 mcg [gluten free]
Tablet, oral: 50 mcg, 100 mcg, 250 mcg, 500 mcg, 1000 mcg
Ener-B®: 100 mcg, 500 mcg, 1000 mcg
Tablet, sublingual: 1000 mcg, 2500 mcg, 5000 mcg
Tablet, timed release, oral: 1000 mcg
Ener-B®: 1500 mcg

◆ **Cyanokit®** see Hydroxocobalamin on page 951
◆ **Cyclivert® [OTC]** see Cyclizine on page 454

Cyclizine (SYE kli zeen)

Brand Names: U.S. Bonine® for Kids [OTC] [DSC]; Cyclivert® [OTC]; Marezine® [OTC]
Index Terms Cyclizine Hydrochloride; Cyclizine Lactate
Generic Availability (U.S.) No
Pharmacologic Category Histamine H_1 Antagonist; Histamine H_1 Antagonist, First Generation; Piperazine Derivative
Use Prevention and treatment of nausea, vomiting, and vertigo associated with motion sickness
Dosage
Geriatric & Adult Motion sickness (prophylaxis and treatment): Oral: 50 mg taken 30 minutes before departure; may repeat in 4-6 hours if needed, up to 200 mg/day
Special Geriatric Considerations Due to anticholinergic action, use lowest dose in divided doses to avoid side effects and their inconvenience; limit use if possible; may cause confusion or aggravate symptoms of confusion in those with dementia; constipation and difficulty voiding urine may occur
Dosage Forms Excipient information presented when available (limited, particularly for generics); consult specific product labeling. [DSC] = Discontinued product
Tablet, oral, as hydrochloride:
Cyclivert®: 25 mg [scored]
Marezine®: 50 mg
Tablet, chewable, oral, as hydrochloride:
Bonine® for Kids: 25 mg [DSC] [scored; berry blast flavor]

◆ **Cyclizine Hydrochloride** see Cyclizine on page 454
◆ **Cyclizine Lactate** see Cyclizine on page 454

Cyclobenzaprine (sye kloe BEN za preen)

Related Information
Beers Criteria – Potentially Inappropriate Medications for Geriatrics on page 2183
Medication Safety Issues
Sound-alike/look-alike issues:
Cyclobenzaprine may be confused with cycloSERINE, cyproheptadine
Flexeril® may be confused with Floxin®
BEERS Criteria medication:
This drug may be potentially inappropriate for use in geriatric patients (Quality of evidence - moderate; Strength of recommendation - strong).
International issues:
Flexin: Brand name for cyclobenzaprine [Chile], but also the brand name for diclofenac [Argentina] and orphenadrine [Israel]
Flexin [Chile] may be confused with Floxin brand name for flunarizine [Thailand], norfloxacin [South Africa], ofloxacin [U.S., Canada], and perfloxacin [Philippines]; Fluoxine brand name for fluoxetine [Thailand]
Brand Names: U.S. Amrix®; Fexmid®; Flexeril®
Brand Names: Canada Apo-Cyclobenzaprine®; Auro-Cyclobenzaprine; Ava-Cyclobenzaprine; Dom-Cyclobenzaprine; JAMP-Cyclobenzaprine; Mylan-Cyclobenzaprine; Novo-Cyclobenzaprine; Nu-Cyclobenzaprine; PHL-Cyclobenzaprine; PMS-Cyclobenzaprine; Q-Cyclobenzaprine; ratio-Cyclobenzaprine; Riva-Cycloprine; ZYM-Cyclobenzaprine

Index Terms Cyclobenzaprine Hydrochloride

Generic Availability (U.S.) Yes

Pharmacologic Category Skeletal Muscle Relaxant

Use Treatment of muscle spasm associated with acute, painful musculoskeletal conditions

Unlabeled Use Treatment of muscle spasm associated with acute temporomandibular joint pain (TMJ)

Contraindications Hypersensitivity to cyclobenzaprine or any component of the formulation; during or within 14 days of MAO inhibitors; hyperthyroidism; congestive heart failure; arrhythmias; heart block or conduction disturbances; acute recovery phase of MI

Warnings/Precautions May cause CNS depression, which may impair physical or mental abilities; patients must be cautioned about performing tasks which require mental alertness (eg, operating machinery or driving). Cyclobenzaprine shares the toxic potentials of the tricyclic antidepressants (including arrhythmias, tachycardia, and conduction time prolongation) and the usual precautions of tricyclic antidepressant therapy should be observed; use with caution in patients with urinary hesitancy or retention, angle-closure glaucoma or increased intraocular pressure, hepatic impairment, or in the elderly. Muscle relaxants are poorly tolerated by the elderly due to potent anticholinergic effects, sedation, and risk of fracture. Efficacy is questionable at dosages tolerated by elderly patients; avoid use (Beers Criteria). Extended release capsules not recommended for use in mild-to-severe hepatic impairment or in the elderly. Do not use concomitantly or within 14 days after MAO inhibitors; combination may cause hypertensive crisis, severe convulsions. Effects may be potentiated when used with other CNS depressants or ethanol.

Adverse Reactions (Reflective of adult population; not specific for elderly)

>10%:

Central nervous system: Drowsiness (29% to 39%), dizziness (1% to 11%)

Gastrointestinal: Xerostomia (21% to 32%)

1% to 10%:

Central nervous system: Fatigue (1% to 6%), headache (1% to 5%), confusion (1% to 3%), irritability (1% to 3%), mental acuity decreased (1% to 3%), nervousness (1% to 3%), somnolence (1% to 2%)

Gastrointestinal: Dyspepsia (≤4%), abdominal pain (1% to 3%), constipation (1% to 3%), diarrhea (1% to 3%), gastric regurgitation (1% to 3%), nausea (1% to 3%), unpleasant taste (1% to 3%)

Neuromuscular & skeletal: Weakness (1% to 3%)

Ocular: Blurred vision (1% to 3%)

Respiratory: Pharyngitis (1% to 3%), upper respiratory infection (1% to 3%)

Drug Interactions

Metabolism/Transport Effects Substrate of CYP1A2 (major), CYP2D6 (minor), CYP3A4 (minor); **Note:** Assignment of Major/Minor substrate status based on clinically relevant drug interaction potential

Avoid Concomitant Use

Avoid concomitant use of Cyclobenzaprine with any of the following: Azelastine; Azelastine (Nasal); MAO Inhibitors; Methadone; Paraldehyde

Increased Effect/Toxicity

Cyclobenzaprine may increase the levels/effects of: Alcohol (Ethyl); Anticholinergics; Azelastine; Azelastine (Nasal); Buprenorphine; CNS Depressants; MAO Inhibitors; Methadone; Metoclopramide; Metyrosine; Paraldehyde; Serotonin Modulators; Zolpidem

The levels/effects of Cyclobenzaprine may be increased by: Abiraterone Acetate; Antipsychotics; CYP1A2 Inhibitors (Moderate); CYP1A2 Inhibitors (Strong); Deferasirox; HydrOXYzine; Pramlintide

Decreased Effect

Cyclobenzaprine may decrease the levels/effects of: Acetylcholinesterase Inhibitors (Central)

The levels/effects of Cyclobenzaprine may be decreased by: Acetylcholinesterase Inhibitors (Central); Peginterferon Alfa-2b; Tocilizumab

Ethanol/Nutrition/Herb Interactions

Ethanol: May increase CNS depression; monitor for increased effects with coadministration. Caution patients about effects.

Food: Food increases bioavailability (peak plasma concentrations increased by 35% and area under the curve by 20%) of the extended release capsule.

Herb/Nutraceutical: Avoid valerian, kava kava, gotu kola (may increase CNS depression).

Stability

Amrix®, Flexeril®: Store at 25°C (77°F); excursions permitted to 15°C to 30°C (59°F to 86°F). Fexmid®: Store at 20°C to 25°C (68°F to 77°F).

Mechanism of Action Centrally-acting skeletal muscle relaxant pharmacologically related to tricyclic antidepressants; reduces tonic somatic motor activity influencing both alpha and gamma motor neurons

Pharmacodynamics/Kinetics

Metabolism: Hepatic via CYP3A4, 1A2, and 2D6; may undergo enterohepatic recirculation

Bioavailability: 33% to 55%

Half-life elimination: Range: 8-37 hours; Immediate release tablet: 18 hours; Extended release capsule: 32-33 hours

Time to peak, serum: Extended release capsule: 7-8 hours

Excretion: Urine (as inactive metabolites); feces (as unchanged drug)

Dosage

Geriatric

Capsule, extended release: Use not recommended

Tablet, immediate release: Initial: 5 mg; titrate dose slowly and consider less frequent dosing

Adult Muscle spasm: Oral: **Note:** Do not use longer than 2-3 weeks

Capsule, extended release: Usual: 15 mg once daily; some patients may require up to 30 mg once daily

Tablet, immediate release: Initial: 5 mg 3 times/day; may increase up to 10 mg 3 times/day if needed

Hepatic Impairment

Capsule, extended release: Mild-to-severe impairment: Use not recommended.

Tablet, immediate release:

Mild impairment: Initial: 5 mg; use with caution; titrate slowly and consider less frequent dosing

Moderate-to-severe impairment: Use not recommended

Administration Oral: Extended release capsules: Administer at the same time each day. Do not crush or chew.

Test Interactions May cause false-positive serum TCA screen.

Special Geriatric Considerations High doses in the elderly caused drowsiness and dizziness; therefore, use the lowest dose possible. Because cyclobenzaprine causes anti-cholinergic effects, it may not be the skeletal muscle relaxant of choice in the elderly.

This medication is considered to be potentially inappropriate in this patient population (Beers Criteria: Quality of evidence - moderate; Strength of recommendation - strong).

Dosage Forms Excipient information presented when available (limited, particularly for generics); consult specific product labeling.

Capsule, extended release, oral, as hydrochloride: 15 mg, 30 mg

Amrix®: 15 mg, 30 mg

Tablet, oral, as hydrochloride: 5 mg, 7.5 mg, 10 mg

Fexmid®: 7.5 mg

Flexeril®: 5 mg, 10 mg

◆ **Cyclobenzaprine Hydrochloride** see Cyclobenzaprine on page 454

Cyclophosphamide (sye kloe FOS fa mide)

Medication Safety Issues

Sound-alike/look-alike issues:

Cyclophosphamide may be confused with cycloSPORINE, ifosfamide

Cytoxan may be confused with cefOXitin, Ciloxan®, cytarabine, CytoGam®, Cytosar®, Cytosar-U, Cytotec®

High alert medication:

This medication is in a class the Institute for Safe Medication Practices (ISMP) includes among its list of drugs which have a heightened risk of causing significant patient harm when used in error.

Brand Names: Canada Procytox®

Index Terms CPM; CTX; CYT; Cytoxan; Neosar

Generic Availability (U.S.) Yes

Pharmacologic Category Antineoplastic Agent, Alkylating Agent

Use Treatment of Hodgkin's lymphoma, non-Hodgkin's lymphoma (including Burkitt's lymphoma), chronic lymphocytic leukemia (CLL), chronic myelocytic leukemia (CML), acute myelocytic leukemia (AML), acute lymphocytic leukemia (ALL), mycosis fungoides, multiple myeloma, neuroblastoma, retinoblastoma; breast cancer; ovarian adenocarcinoma

Unlabeled Use

Oncology-related uses: Ewing's sarcoma, rhabdomyosarcoma, Wilms tumor, ovarian germ cell tumors, small cell lung cancer, testicular cancer, pheochromocytoma, bone marrow transplantation conditioning regimen

Nononcology uses: Severe rheumatoid disorders, Wegener's granulomatosis, myasthenia gravis, multiple sclerosis, systemic lupus erythematosus, lupus nephritis, autoimmune hemolytic anemia, idiopathic thrombocytic purpura (ITP), and antibody-induced pure red cell aplasia; juvenile idiopathic arthritis (JIA)

Contraindications Hypersensitivity to cyclophosphamide or any component of the formulation

Warnings/Precautions Hazardous agent - use appropriate precautions for handling and disposal. Dosage adjustment may be needed for renal or hepatic failure. Hemorrhagic cystitis may occur; increased hydration and frequent voiding is recommended. Immunosuppression may occur; monitor for infections. May cause cardiotoxicity (HF, usually with higher doses); may potentiate the cardiotoxicity of anthracyclines. May impair fertility; interferes with oogenesis and spermatogenesis. Secondary malignancies (usually delayed) have been reported

Adverse Reactions (Reflective of adult population; not specific for elderly)
>10%:
Dermatologic: Alopecia (40% to 60%) but hair will usually regrow although it may be a different color and/or texture. Hair loss usually begins 3-6 weeks after the start of therapy.
Endocrine & metabolic: Fertility: May cause sterility; interferes with oogenesis and spermatogenesis; may be irreversible in some patients; gonadal suppression (amenorrhea)
Gastrointestinal: Nausea and vomiting (usually beginning 6-10 hours after administration; severe with high-dose therapy); anorexia, diarrhea, mucositis, and stomatitis are also seen
Genitourinary: Severe, potentially fatal, acute hemorrhagic cystitis or urinary fibrosis (7% to 40%)
Hematologic: Anemia, leukopenia (dose-related; recovery: 7-10 days after cessation), thrombocytopenia
1% to 10%:
Cardiovascular: Facial flushing
Central nervous system: Headache
Dermatologic: Skin rash
Respiratory: Nasal congestion occurs when I.V. doses are administered too rapidly; patients experience runny eyes, rhinorrhea, sinus congestion, and sneezing during or immediately after the infusion.

Drug Interactions
Metabolism/Transport Effects Substrate of CYP2A6 (minor), CYP2B6 (major), CYP2C19 (minor), CYP2C9 (minor), CYP3A4 (minor). **Note:** Assignment of Major/Minor substrate status based on clinically relevant drug interaction potential; **Inhibits** CYP3A4 (weak); **Induces** CYP2B6 (weak/moderate), CYP2C9 (weak/moderate)

Avoid Concomitant Use
Avoid concomitant use of Cyclophosphamide with any of the following: BCG; Belimumab; CloZAPine; Etanercept; Natalizumab; Pimecrolimus; Pimozide; Tacrolimus (Topical); Vaccines (Live)

Increased Effect/Toxicity
Cyclophosphamide may increase the levels/effects of: ARIPiprazole; CloZAPine; Leflunomide; Natalizumab; Pimozide; Succinylcholine; Vaccines (Live); Vitamin K Antagonists

The levels/effects of Cyclophosphamide may be increased by: Allopurinol; Belimumab; CYP2B6 Inhibitors (Moderate); CYP2B6 Inhibitors (Strong); Denosumab; Etanercept; Pentostatin; Pimecrolimus; Quazepam; Roflumilast; Tacrolimus (Topical); Trastuzumab

Decreased Effect
Cyclophosphamide may decrease the levels/effects of: BCG; Cardiac Glycosides; Coccidioidin Skin Test; Sipuleucel-T; Vaccines (Inactivated); Vaccines (Live); Vitamin K Antagonists

The levels/effects of Cyclophosphamide may be decreased by: CYP2B6 Inducers (Strong); Echinacea; Tocilizumab

Ethanol/Nutrition/Herb Interactions Herb/Nutraceutical: Avoid black cohosh, dong quai in estrogen-dependent tumors.

Stability Store intact vials of powder at room temperature of 15°C to 30°C (59°F to 86°F). Reconstitute vials with sterile water, normal saline, or 5% dextrose to a concentration of 20 mg/mL. Reconstituted solutions are stable for 24 hours at room temperature and 6 days under refrigeration at 2°C to 8°C (36°F to 46°F). Further dilutions in D_5W or NS are stable for 24 hours at room temperature and 6 days at refrigeration.

Mechanism of Action Cyclophosphamide is an alkylating agent that prevents cell division by cross-linking DNA strands and decreasing DNA synthesis. It is a cell cycle phase nonspecific agent. Cyclophosphamide also possesses potent immunosuppressive activity. Cyclophosphamide is a prodrug that must be metabolized to active metabolites in the liver.

Pharmacodynamics/Kinetics

Absorption: Oral: Well absorbed

Distribution: V_d: 0.48-0.71 L/kg; crosses into CSF (not in high enough concentrations to treat meningeal leukemia)

Protein binding: 10% to 60%

Metabolism: Hepatic to active metabolites acrolein, 4-aldophosphamide, 4-hydroperoxycyclophosphamide, and nor-nitrogen mustard; A large fraction of cyclophosphamide is eliminated by hepatic metabolism.

Half-life elimination: 3-12 hours

Time to peak, serum: Oral: ~1 hour

Elimination: Urine (<30% as unchanged drug, 85% to 90% as metabolites)

Dosage

Geriatric Details concerns dosing in combination regimens should also be consulted: Initial and maintenance for induction: 1-2 mg/kg/day; adjust for renal clearance.

Adult Details concerns dosing in combination regimens should also be consulted.

Single I.V. doses: 400-1800 mg/m^2 (30-50 mg/kg) per treatment course (1-5 days) which can be repeated at 2-4 week intervals

Continuous I.V. daily doses: 60-120 mg/m^2 (1-2.5 mg/kg) per day

Malignancy: Oral: Usual range (in the manufacturer's labeling): 1-5 mg/kg/day (initial and maintenance dosing)

Breast cancer (unlabeled dosing; combination chemotherapy): Oral:

CEF: 75 mg/m^2/day days 1-14 every 28 days (Levine, 1998)

CMF: 100 mg/m^2/day days 1-14 every 28 days (Bonadonna, 1995; Levine, 1998)

Nephrotic syndrome (refractory; unlabeled use): Oral: 2.5-3 mg/kg/day every day for 60-90 days (when refractory or intolerant to corticosteroid treatment)

JIA/vasculitis (unlabeled use): I.V.: 10 mg/kg every 2 weeks

SLE (unlabeled use): I.V.: 500 mg/m^2 every month; may increase up to a maximum dose of 1 g/m^2 every month (Austin, 1986)

Autologous BMT (unlabeled use): IVPB: 50 mg/kg/dose x 4 days **or** 60 mg/kg/dose for 2 days; total dose is usually divided over 2-4 days

High-dose BMT (unlabeled use):

I.V.:

60 mg/kg/day for 2 days (total dose: 120 mg/kg)

50 mg/kg/day for 4 days (total dose: 200 mg/kg)

1.8 g/m^2/day for 4 days (total dose: 7.2 g/m^2)

Continuous I.V.:

1.5 g/m^2/24 hours for 96 hours (total dose: 6 g/m^2)

1875 mg/m^2/24 hours for 72 hours (total dose: 5625 mg/m^2)

Note: Duration of infusion is 1-24 hours; generally combined with other high-dose chemotherapeutic drugs, lymphocyte immune globulin, or total body irradiation (TBI).

Renal Impairment The FDA-approved labeling states there is insufficient evidence to recommend dosage adjustment and therefore, does not contain renal dosing adjustment guidelines. The following guidelines have been used by some clinicians (Aronoff, 2007):

Cl_{cr} <10 mL/minute: Administer 75% of normal dose

Hemodialysis effects: Moderately dialyzable (20% to 50%)

Administer 50% of dose posthemodialysis

Continuous ambulatory peritoneal dialysis (CAPD): Administer 75% of normal dose

Continuous renal replacement therapy (CRRT): Administer 100% of normal dose

Hepatic Impairment The pharmacokinetics of cyclophosphamide are not significantly altered in the presence of hepatic insufficiency. The FDA-approved labeling does not contain hepatic dosing adjustment guidelines. The following guidelines have been used by some clinicians (Floyd, 2006):

Serum bilirubin 3.1-5 mg/dL or transaminases >3 times ULN: Administer 75% of dose

Serum bilirubin >5 mg/mL: Avoid use

Administration May be administered I.P., intrapleurally, IVPB, or continuous I.V. infusion; may also be administered slow IVP in doses ≤1 g.

I.V. infusions may be administered over 1-24 hours

Doses >500 mg to approximately 2 g may be administered over 20-30 minutes

To minimize bladder toxicity, increase normal fluid intake during and for 1-2 days after cyclophosphamide dose. Most adult patients will require a fluid intake of at least 2 L/day. High-dose regimens should be accompanied by vigorous hydration with or without mesna therapy.

Oral: Tablets are not scored and should not be cut or crushed. To minimize the risk of bladder irritation, do not administer tablets at bedtime.

Monitoring Parameters CBC with differential and platelet count, BUN, UA, serum electrolytes, serum creatinine

Pharmacotherapy Pearls In patients with CYP2B6 G516T variant allele, cyclophosphamide metabolism is markedly increased; metabolism is not influenced by CYP2C9 and CYP2C19 isotypes.

Special Geriatric Considerations Toxicity to immunosuppressives is increased in the elderly. Start with lowest recommended adult doses. Signs of infection, such as fever and WBC rise, may not occur. Lethargy and confusion may be more prominent signs of infection; adjust dose for renal function.

Dosage Forms Excipient information presented when available (limited, particularly for generics); consult specific product labeling.
Injection, powder for reconstitution: 500 mg, 1 g, 2 g
Tablet, oral: 25 mg, 50 mg

Extemporaneously Prepared A 2 mg/mL oral elixir was stable for 14 days when refrigerated when made as follows: Reconstitute a 200 mg vial with aromatic elixir, withdraw the solution, and add sufficient aromatic elixir to make a final volume of 100 mL (store in amber glass container).

Brook D, Davis RE, and Bequette RJ, "Chemical Stability of Cyclophosphamide in Aromatic Elixir U.S.P.," *Am J Health Syst Pharm*, 1973, 30:618-20.

CycloSERINE (sye kloe SER een)

Related Information
Antimicrobial Drugs of Choice *on page 2163*
Medication Safety Issues
Sound-alike/look-alike issues:
CycloSERINE may be confused with cyclobenzaprine, cycloSPORINE
Brand Names: U.S. Seromycin®
Generic Availability (U.S.) No
Pharmacologic Category Antibiotic, Miscellaneous; Antitubercular Agent
Use Adjunctive treatment in pulmonary or extrapulmonary tuberculosis
Unlabeled Use Treatment of Gaucher's disease
Contraindications Hypersensitivity to cycloserine or any component of the formulation; epilepsy; depression, severe anxiety, or psychosis; severe renal insufficiency; excessive concurrent use of alcohol
Warnings/Precautions Has been associated with CNS toxicity, including seizures, psychosis, depression, and confusion; decrease dosage or discontinue use if occurs. Use with caution in patients with epilepsy, depression, severe anxiety, psychosis, severe renal insufficiency, chronic alcoholism and patients with potential folate deficiency (malnourished, chronic anticonvulsant therapy, or elderly). Prolonged use may result in fungal or bacterial superinfection, including *C. difficile*-associated diarrhea (CDAD) and pseudomembranous colitis; CDAD has been observed >2 months postantibiotic treatment.
Adverse Reactions (Reflective of adult population; not specific for elderly) Frequency not defined.
Cardiovascular: Cardiac arrhythmia, heart failure
Central nervous system: Coma, confusion, dizziness, drowsiness, headache, paresis, psychosis, restlessness, seizures, vertigo
Dermatologic: Rash
Endocrine & metabolic: Vitamin B_{12} deficiency
Hematologic: Folate deficiency
Hepatic: Liver enzymes increased
Neuromuscular & skeletal: Dysarthria, hyperreflexia, paresthesia, tremor
Miscellaneous: Allergic manifestations
Drug Interactions
Metabolism/Transport Effects None known.
Avoid Concomitant Use
Avoid concomitant use of CycloSERINE with any of the following: Alcohol (Ethyl); BCG
Increased Effect/Toxicity
The levels/effects of CycloSERINE may be increased by: Alcohol (Ethyl); Ethionamide; Isoniazid
Decreased Effect
CycloSERINE may decrease the levels/effects of: BCG; Typhoid Vaccine
Ethanol/Nutrition/Herb Interactions
Ethanol: Avoid ethanol (may increase CNS depression).
Food: May increase vitamin B_{12} and folic acid dietary requirements.
Mechanism of Action Inhibits bacterial cell wall synthesis by competing with amino acid (D-alanine) for incorporation into the bacterial cell wall; bacteriostatic or bactericidal

Pharmacodynamics/Kinetics

Absorption: ~70% to 90%

Distribution: Widely to most body fluids and tissues including CSF, bile, sputum, lymph tissue, lungs, and ascitic, pleural, and synovial fluids

Metabolism: Hepatic

Half-life elimination: Normal renal function: 10 hours

Time to peak, serum: 4-8 hours

Excretion: Urine (60% to 70% as unchanged drug) within 72 hours; feces (small amounts); remainder metabolized

Dosage

Geriatric & Adult Note: In adults, some neurotoxic effects may be treated or prevented by concomitant administration of 200-300 mg of pyridoxine daily.

Tuberculosis: Oral: Initial: 250 mg every 12 hours for 14 days, then administer 500-1000 mg/day in 2 divided doses for 18-24 months (maximum daily dose: 1000 mg) **or** 10-15 mg/kg/day (1000 mg/day in 2 divided doses), usually 500-750 mg/day in 2 divided doses (*MMWR*, 2003). (**Note:** Experienced clinicians indicate most patients are unable to tolerate this dose. Serum concentrations targeted at 20-35 mcg/mL are often useful in determining the optimal dose.)

Renal Impairment No dosage adjustment provided in manufacturer's labeling; however, the following adjustments have been used by some clinicians:

Aronoff, 2007:

Cl_{cr} >50 mL/minute: No dosage adjustment necessary

Cl_{cr} 10-50 mL/minute: Administer every 24 hours

Cl_{cr} <10 mL/minute: Administer every 36-48 hours

MMWR, 2003:

Cl_{cr} <30 mL/minute and hemodialysis: 250 mg once daily, or 500 mg three times per week. (**Note:** Avoid in patients with Cl_{cr} <50 mL/minute unless the patient is receiving hemodialysis. The efficacy of 250 mg daily doses has not been established and careful monitoring is necessary for evidence of neurotoxicity. Monitor serum concentrations to minimize toxicity.)

Monitoring Parameters Periodic renal, hepatic, hematological tests, and plasma cycloserine concentrations

Reference Range

Therapeutic levels: Tuberculosis: 20-35 mcg/mL

Toxicity is greatly increased at levels >30 mcg/mL

Special Geriatric Considerations Adjust dose for renal function.

Dosage Forms Excipient information presented when available (limited, particularly for generics); consult specific product labeling.

Capsule, oral:

Seromycin®: 250 mg

- ◆ **Closet®** see Bromocriptine *on page 223*
- ◆ **Cyclosporin A** see CycloSPORINE (Ophthalmic) *on page 467*
- ◆ **Cyclosporin A** see CycloSPORINE (Systemic) *on page 460*

CycloSPORINE (Systemic) (SYE kloe spor een)

Medication Safety Issues

Sound-alike/look-alike issues:

CycloSPORINE may be confused with cyclophosphamide, Cyklokapron®, cycloSERINE

CycloSPORINE modified (Neoral®, Gengraf®) may be confused with cycloSPORINE non-modified (SandIMMUNE®)

Gengraf® may be confused with Prograf®

Neoral® may be confused with Neurontin®, Nizoral®

SandIMMUNE® may be confused with SandoSTATIN®

Brand Names: U.S. Gengraf®; Neoral®; SandIMMUNE®

Brand Names: Canada Apo-Cyclosporine®; Neoral®; Rhoxal-cyclosporine; Sandimmune® I.V.; Sandoz-Cyclosporine

Index Terms CsA; CyA; Cyclosporin A

Generic Availability (U.S.) Yes

Pharmacologic Category Calcineurin Inhibitor; Immunosuppressant Agent

Use Prophylaxis of organ rejection in kidney, liver, and heart transplants, has been used with azathioprine and/or corticosteroids; severe, active rheumatoid arthritis (RA) not responsive to methotrexate alone; severe, recalcitrant plaque psoriasis in nonimmunocompromised adults unresponsive to or unable to tolerate other systemic therapy

Unlabeled Use Allogenic stem cell transplants for prevention and treatment of graft-versus-host disease; also used in some cases of severe autoimmune disease (eg, SLE) that are resistant to corticosteroids and other therapy; focal segmental glomerulosclerosis; severe ulcerative colitis

Contraindications Hypersensitivity to cyclosporine or any component of the formulation. I.V. cyclosporine is contraindicated in hypersensitivity to polyoxyethylated castor oil (Cremophor® EL).

Rheumatoid arthritis and psoriasis: Abnormal renal function, uncontrolled hypertension, malignancies. Concomitant treatment with PUVA or UVB therapy, methotrexate, other immunosuppressive agents, coal tar, or radiation therapy are also contraindications for use in patients with psoriasis.

Warnings/Precautions Hazardous agent - use appropriate precautions for handling and disposal. **[U.S. Boxed Warning]: Renal impairment, including structural kidney damage has occurred (when used at high doses); monitor renal function closely.** Elevations in serum creatinine and BUN generally respond to dosage reductions. Use caution with other potentially nephrotoxic drugs (eg, acyclovir, aminoglycoside antibiotics, amphotericin B, ciprofloxacin). **[U.S. Boxed Warning]: Increased risk of lymphomas and other malignancies, particularly those of the skin;** risk is related to intensity/duration of therapy and the use of >1 immunosuppressive agent; all patients should avoid excessive sun/UV light exposure. **[U.S. Boxed Warning]: Increased risk of infection; fatal infections have been reported.** Latent viral infections may be activated (including BK virus which is associated with nephropathy) and result in serious adverse effects. **[U.S. Boxed Warning]: May cause hypertension.** Use caution when changing dosage forms. **[U.S. Boxed Warning]: Cyclosporine (modified) has increased bioavailability as compared to cyclosporine (non-modified) and cannot be used interchangeably without close monitoring.** Monitor cyclosporine concentrations closely following the addition, modification, or deletion of other medications; live, attenuated vaccines may be less effective; use should be avoided. Increased hepatic enzymes and bilirubin have occurred (when used at high doses); improvement usually seen with dosage reduction.

Transplant patients: To be used initially with corticosteroids. May cause significant hyperkalemia and hyperuricemia, seizures (particularly if used with high dose corticosteroids), and encephalopathy. Other neurotoxic events (eg, optic disc edema including papilledema and visual impairment) have been reported rarely. Make dose adjustments based on cyclosporine blood concentrations. **[U.S. Boxed Warning]: Adjustment of dose should only be made under the direct supervision of an experienced physician.** Anaphylaxis has been reported with I.V. use; reserve for patients who cannot take oral form. **[U.S. Boxed Warning]: Risk of skin cancer may be increased in transplant patients.** Due to the increased risk for nephrotoxicity in renal transplantation, avoid using standard doses of cyclosporine in combination with everolimus; reduced cyclosporine doses are recommended; monitor cyclosporine concentrations closely. Cyclosporine and everolimus combination therapy may increase the risk for proteinuria. Cyclosporine combined with either everolimus or sirolimus may increase the risk for thrombotic microangiopathy/thrombotic thrombocytopenic purpura/hemolytic uremic syndrome (TMA/TTP/HUS).

Psoriasis: Patients should avoid excessive sun exposure. **[U.S. Boxed Warning]: Risk of skin cancer may be increased with a history of PUVA and possibly methotrexate or other immunosuppressants, UVB, coal tar, or radiation.**

Rheumatoid arthritis: If receiving other immunosuppressive agents, radiation or UV therapy, concurrent use of cyclosporine is not recommended.

Products may contain corn oil, ethanol, or propylene glycol; injection also contains Cremophor® EL (polyoxyethylated castor oil), which has been associated with rare anaphylactic reactions.

Adverse Reactions (Reflective of adult population; not specific for elderly) Adverse reactions reported with systemic use, including rheumatoid arthritis, psoriasis, and transplantation (kidney, liver, and heart). Percentages noted include the highest frequency regardless of indication/dosage. Frequencies may vary for specific conditions or formulation.

>10%:
  Cardiovascular: Hypertension (8% to 53%), edema (5% to 14%)
  Central nervous system: Headache (2% to 25%)
  Dermatologic: Hirsutism (21% to 45%), hypertrichosis (5% to 19%)
  Endocrine & metabolic: Triglycerides increased (15%), female reproductive disorder (9% to 11%)
  Gastrointestinal: Nausea (23%), diarrhea (3% to 13%), gum hyperplasia (2% to 16%), abdominal discomfort (<1% to 15%), dyspepsia (2% to 12%)
  Neuromuscular & skeletal: Tremor (7% to 55%), paresthesia (1% to 11%), leg cramps/muscle contractions (2% to 12%)

Renal: Renal dysfunction/nephropathy (10% to 38%), creatinine increased (16% to ≥50%)
Respiratory: Upper respiratory infection (1% to 14%)
Miscellaneous: Infection (3% to 25%)

Kidney, liver, and heart transplant only (≤2% unless otherwise noted):
Cardiovascular: Flushes (<1% to 4%), MI
Central nervous system: Convulsions (1% to 5%), anxiety, confusion, fever, lethargy
Dermatologic: Acne (1% to 6%), brittle fingernails, hair breaking, pruritus
Endocrine & metabolic: Gynecomastia (<1% to 4%), hyperglycemia
Gastrointestinal: Nausea (2% to 10%), vomiting (2% to 10%), diarrhea (3% to 8%), abdominal discomfort (<1% to 7%), cramps (0% to 4%), anorexia, constipation, gastritis, mouth sores, pancreatitis, swallowing difficulty, upper GI bleed, weight loss
Hematologic: Leukopenia (<1% to 6%), anemia, thrombocytopenia
Hepatic: Hepatotoxicity (<1% to 7%)
Neuromuscular & skeletal: Paresthesia (1% to 3%), joint pain, muscle pain, tingling, weakness
Ocular: Conjunctivitis, visual disturbance
Otic: Hearing loss, tinnitus
Renal: Hematuria
Respiratory: Sinusitis (<1% to 7%)
Miscellaneous: Lymphoma (<1% to 6%), allergic reactions, hiccups, night sweats

Rheumatoid arthritis only (1% to <3% unless otherwise noted):
Cardiovascular: Hypertension (8%), edema (5%), chest pain (4%), arrhythmia (2%), abnormal heart sounds, cardiac failure, MI, peripheral ischemia
Central nervous system: Dizziness (8%), pain (6%), insomnia (4%), depression (3%), migraine (2%), anxiety, hypoesthesia, emotional lability, impaired concentration, malaise, nervousness, paranoia, somnolence, vertigo
Dermatologic: Purpura (3%), abnormal pigmentation, angioedema, cellulitis, dermatitis, dry skin, eczema, folliculitis, nail disorder, pruritus, skin disorder, urticaria
Endocrine & metabolic: Menstrual disorder (3%), breast fibroadenosis, breast pain, diabetes mellitus, goiter, hot flashes, hyperkalemia, hyperuricemia, hypoglycemia, libido increased/decreased
Gastrointestinal: Vomiting (9%), flatulence (5%), gingivitis (4%), gum hyperplasia (2%), constipation, dry mouth, dysphagia, enanthema, eructation, esophagitis, gastric ulcer, gastritis, gastroenteritis, gingival bleeding, glossitis, peptic ulcer, salivary gland enlargement, taste perversion, tongue disorder, gum hyperplasia, weight loss/gain
Genitourinary: Leukorrhea (1%), abnormal urine, micturition urgency, nocturia, polyuria, pyelonephritis, urinary incontinence, uterine hemorrhage
Hematologic: Anemia, leukopenia
Hepatic: Bilirubinemia
Neuromuscular & skeletal: Paresthesia (8%), tremor (8%), leg cramps/muscle contractions (2%), arthralgia, bone fracture, joint dislocation, myalgia, neuropathy, stiffness, synovial cyst, tendon disorder, weakness
Ocular: Abnormal vision, cataract, conjunctivitis, eye pain
Otic: Tinnitus, deafness, vestibular disorder
Renal: BUN increased, hematuria, renal abscess
Respiratory: Cough (5%), dyspnea (5%), sinusitis (4%), abnormal chest sounds, bronchospasm, epistaxis
Miscellaneous: Infection (9%), abscess, allergy, bacterial infection, carcinoma, fungal infection, herpes simplex, herpes zoster, lymphadenopathy, moniliasis, diaphoresis increased, tonsillitis, viral infection

Psoriasis only (1% to <3% unless otherwise noted):
Cardiovascular: Chest pain, flushes
Central nervous system: Psychiatric events (4% to 5%), pain (3% to 4%), dizziness, fever, insomnia, nervousness, vertigo
Dermatologic: Hypertrichosis (5% to 7%), acne, dry skin, folliculitis, keratosis, pruritus, rash, skin malignancies
Endocrine & metabolic: Hot flashes
Gastrointestinal: Nausea (5% to 6%), diarrhea (5% to 6%), gum hyperplasia (4% to 6%), abdominal discomfort (3% to 6%), dyspepsia (2% to 3%), abdominal distention, appetite increased, constipation, gingival bleeding
Genitourinary: Micturition increased
Hematologic: Bleeding disorder, clotting disorder, platelet disorder, red blood cell disorder
Hepatic: Hyperbilirubinemia
Neuromuscular & skeletal: Paresthesia (5% to 7%), arthralgia (1% to 6%)
Ocular: Abnormal vision
Respiratory: Bronchospasm (5%), cough (5%), dyspnea (5%), rhinitis (5%), respiratory infection
Miscellaneous: Flu-like syndrome (8% to 10%)

Drug Interactions

Metabolism/Transport Effects Substrate of CYP3A4 (major), P-glycoprotein; **Note:** Assignment of Major/Minor substrate status based on clinically relevant drug interaction potential; **Inhibits** CYP2C9 (weak), CYP3A4 (moderate), P-glycoprotein

Avoid Concomitant Use

Avoid concomitant use of CycloSPORINE (Systemic) with any of the following: Aliskiren; AtorvaSTATin; BCG; Bosentan; Conivaptan; Crizotinib; Dronedarone; Eplerenone; Lovastatin; Mifepristone; Natalizumab; Pimecrolimus; Pimozide; Pitavastatin; Potassium-Sparing Diuretics; Silodosin; Simvastatin; Sitaxentan; Tacrolimus; Tacrolimus (Systemic); Tacrolimus (Topical); Tolvaptan; Topotecan; Vaccines (Live)

Increased Effect/Toxicity

CycloSPORINE (Systemic) may increase the levels/effects of: Aliskiren; Ambrisentan; ARIPiprazole; AtorvaSTATin; Avanafil; Boceprevir; Bosentan; Budesonide (Systemic, Oral Inhalation); Calcium Channel Blockers (Dihydropyridine); Calcium Channel Blockers (Nondihydropyridine); Cardiac Glycosides; Caspofungin; Colchicine; CYP3A4 Substrates; Dabigatran Etexilate; Dexamethasone; Dexamethasone (Systemic); DOXOrubicin; Dronedarone; Etoposide; Etoposide Phosphate; Everolimus; Ezetimibe; FentaNYL; Fibric Acid Derivatives; Fluvastatin; Halofantrine; Imipenem; Ivacaftor; Leflunomide; Loop Diuretics; Lovastatin; Lurasidone; Methotrexate; MethylPREDNISolone; Minoxidil; Minoxidil (Systemic); Minoxidil (Topical); Natalizumab; Nonsteroidal Anti-Inflammatory Agents; P-glycoprotein/ABCB1 Substrates; Pimozide; Pitavastatin; Pravastatin; PrednisoLONE; PrednisoLONE (Systemic); PredniSONE; Propafenone; Protease Inhibitors; Prucalopride; Ranolazine; Repaglinide; Rivaroxaban; Rosuvastatin; Salmeterol; Saxagliptin; Silodosin; Simvastatin; Sirolimus; Sitaxentan; Tacrolimus; Tacrolimus (Systemic); Tacrolimus (Topical); Tolvaptan; Topotecan; Vaccines (Live); Vilazodone; Zuclopenthixol

The levels/effects of CycloSPORINE (Systemic) may be increased by: ACE Inhibitors; AcetaZOLAMIDE; Aminoglycosides; Amiodarone; Amphotericin B; Androgens; Antifungal Agents (Azole Derivatives, Systemic); Boceprevir; Bromocriptine; Calcium Channel Blockers (Nondihydropyridine); Carvedilol; Chloramphenicol; Conivaptan; Crizotinib; CYP3A4 Inhibitors (Moderate); CYP3A4 Inhibitors (Strong); Dasatinib; Denosumab; Dexamethasone; Dexamethasone (Systemic); Eplerenone; Ezetimibe; Fluconazole; GlyBURIDE; Grapefruit Juice; Imatinib; Imipenem; Ivacaftor; Macrolide Antibiotics; Melphalan; Methotrexate; MethylPREDNISolone; Metoclopramide; MetroNIDAZOLE; MetroNIDAZOLE (Systemic); Mifepristone; Nonsteroidal Anti-Inflammatory Agents; Norfloxacin; Omeprazole; P-glycoprotein/ABCB1 Inhibitors; Pimecrolimus; Potassium-Sparing Diuretics; Pravastatin; PrednisoLONE; PrednisoLONE (Systemic); PredniSONE; Protease Inhibitors; Pyrazinamide; Quinupristin; Roflumilast; Sirolimus; Sulfonamide Derivatives; Tacrolimus; Tacrolimus (Systemic); Tacrolimus (Topical); Telaprevir; Temsirolimus; Trastuzumab

Decreased Effect

CycloSPORINE (Systemic) may decrease the levels/effects of: BCG; Coccidioidin Skin Test; GlyBURIDE; Ifosfamide; Mycophenolate; Sipuleucel-T; Vaccines (Inactivated); Vaccines (Live)

The levels/effects of CycloSPORINE (Systemic) may be decreased by: Armodafinil; Ascorbic Acid; Barbiturates; Bosentan; CarBAMazepine; Colesevelam; CYP3A4 Inducers (Strong); Deferasirox; Dexamethasone; Dexamethasone (Systemic); Echinacea; Efavirenz; Fibric Acid Derivatives; Fosphenytoin; Griseofulvin; Imipenem; MethylPREDNISolone; Modafinil; Nafcillin; Orlistat; P-glycoprotein/ABCB1 Inducers; Phenytoin; PrednisoLONE; PrednisoLONE (Systemic); PredniSONE; Rifamycin Derivatives; Somatostatin Analogs; St Johns Wort; Sulfinpyrazone [Off Market]; Sulfonamide Derivatives; Terbinafine; Tocilizumab; Vitamin E

Ethanol/Nutrition/Herb Interactions

Food: Grapefruit juice increases cyclosporine serum concentrations. Management: Avoid grapefruit juice.

Herb/Nutraceutical: St John's wort may increase the metabolism of and decrease plasma levels of cyclosporine; organ rejection and graft loss have been reported. Cat's claw and echinacea have immunostimulant properties. Management: Avoid St John's wort, cat's claw, and echinacea.

Stability

Capsule: Store at controlled room temperature.

Injection: Store at controlled room temperature; do not refrigerate. Ampuls and vials should be protected from light. Stability of injection of parenteral admixture at room temperature (25°C) is 6 hours in PVC; 12-24 hours in Excel®, PAB® containers, or glass. To minimize leaching of DEHP, non-PVC containers and sets should be used for preparation and administration. Sandimmune® injection: Injection should be further diluted (1 mL [50 mg] of concentrate in 20-100 mL of D_5W or NS) for administration by intravenous infusion.

◀ Oral solution: Store at controlled room temperature; do not refrigerate. Use within 2 months after opening; should be mixed in glass containers.

Neoral® oral solution: Orange juice, apple juice; avoid changing diluents frequently; mix thoroughly and drink at once.

Sandimmune® oral solution: Milk, chocolate milk, orange juice; avoid changing diluents frequently; mix thoroughly and drink at once.

Mechanism of Action Inhibition of production and release of interleukin II and inhibits interleukin II-induced activation of resting T-lymphocytes.

Pharmacodynamics/Kinetics

Absorption: Oral:

Cyclosporine (non-modified): Erratic and incomplete; dependent on presence of food, bile acids, and GI motility

Cyclosporine (modified): Erratic and incomplete; increased absorption, up to 30% when compared to cyclosporine (non-modified); less dependent on food, bile acids, or GI motility when compared to cyclosporine (non-modified)

Distribution: Widely in tissues and body fluids including the liver, pancreas, and lungs

V_{dss}: 4-6 L/kg in renal, liver, and marrow transplant recipients (slightly lower values in cardiac transplant patients)

Protein binding: 90% to 98% to lipoproteins

Metabolism: Extensively hepatic via CYP3A4; forms at least 25 metabolites; extensive first-pass effect following oral administration

Bioavailability: Oral:

Cyclosporine (non-modified): Dependent on patient population and transplant type (<10% in adult liver transplant patients and as high as 89% in renal transplant patients); bioavailability of Sandimmune® capsules and oral solution are equivalent; bioavailability of oral solution is ~30% of the I.V. solution

Cyclosporine (modified): Bioavailability of Neoral® capsules and oral solution are equivalent: Adults: 23% greater than with cyclosporine (non-modified) in renal transplant patients; 50% greater in liver transplant patients

Half-life elimination: Oral: May be prolonged in patients with hepatic impairment

Cyclosporine (non-modified): Biphasic: Alpha: 1.4 hours; Terminal: 19 hours (range: 10-27 hours)

Cyclosporine (modified): Biphasic: Terminal: 8.4 hours (range: 5-18 hours)

Time to peak, serum: Oral:

Cyclosporine (non-modified): 2-6 hours; some patients have a second peak at 5-6 hours

Cyclosporine (modified): Renal transplant: 1.5-2 hours

Excretion: Primarily feces; urine (6%, 0.1% as unchanged drug and metabolites)

Dosage

Geriatric Refer to adult dosing. **Sandimmune® and Neoral®/Gengraf® are not bioequivalent and cannot be used interchangeably.**

Adult Neoral®/Gengraf® and Sandimmune® are not bioequivalent and cannot be used interchangeably.

Newly-transplanted patients: Adjunct therapy with corticosteroids is recommended. Initial dose should be given 4-12 hours prior to transplant or may be given postoperatively; adjust initial dose to achieve desired plasma concentration.

Oral: Dose is dependent upon type of transplant and formulation:

Cyclosporine (modified):

Renal: 9 ± 3 mg/kg/day, divided twice daily

Liver: 8 ± 4 mg/kg/day, divided twice daily

Heart: 7 ± 3 mg/kg/day, divided twice daily

Cyclosporine (non-modified): Initial doses of 10-14 mg/kg/day have been used for renal transplants (the manufacturer's labeling includes dosing from initial clinical trials of 15 mg/kg/day [range: 14-18 mg/kg/day]; however, this higher dosing level is rarely used any longer). Continue initial dose daily for 1-2 weeks; taper by 5% per week to a maintenance dose of 5-10 mg/kg/day; some renal transplant patients may be dosed as low as 3 mg/kg/day

Note: When using the non-modified formulation, cyclosporine levels may increase in liver transplant patients when the T-tube is closed; dose may need decreased

I.V.: Cyclosporine (non-modified): Manufacturer's labeling: Initial dose: 5-6 mg/kg/day or one-third of the oral dose as a single dose, infused over 2-6 hours; use should be limited to patients unable to take capsules or oral solution; patients should be switched to an oral dosage form as soon as possible

Note: Many transplant centers administer cyclosporine as "divided dose" infusions (in 2-3 doses/day) or as a continuous (24-hour) infusion; dosages range from 3-7.5 mg/kg/day. Specific institutional protocols should be consulted.

Note: Conversion to cyclosporine (modified) from cyclosporine (non-modified): Start with daily dose previously used and adjust to obtain preconversion cyclosporine trough concentration. Plasma concentrations should be monitored every 4-7 days and dose adjusted as necessary, until desired trough level is obtained. When transferring patients with previously poor absorption of cyclosporine (non-modified), monitor trough levels at least twice weekly (especially if initial dose exceeds 10 mg/kg/day); high plasma levels are likely to occur.

Rheumatoid arthritis: Oral: Cyclosporine (modified): Initial dose: 2.5 mg/kg/day, divided twice daily; salicylates, NSAIDs, and oral glucocorticoids may be continued (refer to Drug Interactions); dose may be increased by 0.5-0.75 mg/kg/day if insufficient response is seen after 8 weeks of treatment; additional dosage increases may be made again at 12 weeks (maximum dose: 4 mg/kg/day). Discontinue if no benefit is seen by 16 weeks of therapy.
Note: Increase the frequency of blood pressure monitoring after each alteration in dosage of cyclosporine. Cyclosporine dosage should be decreased by 25% to 50% in patients with no history of hypertension who develop sustained hypertension during therapy and, if hypertension persists, treatment with cyclosporine should be discontinued.

Psoriasis: Oral: Cyclosporine (modified): Initial dose: 2.5 mg/kg/day, divided twice daily; dose may be increased by 0.5 mg/kg/day if insufficient response is seen after 4 weeks of treatment; additional dosage increases may be made every 2 weeks if needed (maximum dose: 4 mg/kg/day). Discontinue if no benefit is seen by 6 weeks of therapy. Once patients are adequately controlled, the dose should be decreased to the lowest effective dose. Doses <2.5 mg/kg/day may be effective. Treatment longer than 1 year is not recommended.
Note: Increase the frequency of blood pressure monitoring after each alteration in dosage of cyclosporine. Cyclosporine dosage should be decreased by 25% to 50% in patients with no history of hypertension who develop sustained hypertension during therapy and, if hypertension persists, treatment with cyclosporine should be discontinued.

Focal segmental glomerulosclerosis (unlabeled use): Oral: Initial: 3.5-5 mg/kg/day divided every 12 hours (in combination with oral prednisone) (Braun, 2008; Cattran, 1999)

Lupus nephritis (unlabeled use): Oral: Initial: 4 mg/kg/day for 1 month (reduce dose if trough concentrations >200 ng/mL); reduce dose by 0.5 mg/kg every 2 weeks to a maintenance dose of 2.5-3 mg/kg/day (Moroni, 2006)

Severe ulcerative colitis (steroid-refractory) (unlabeled use):
I.V.: Cyclosporine (non-modified): 2-4 mg/kg/day, infused continuously over 24 hours. (Lichtiger, 1994; Van Assche, 2003). **Note:** Some studies suggest no therapeutic difference between low-dose (2 mg/kg) and high-dose (4 mg/kg) cyclosporine regimens (Van Assche, 2003).
Oral: Cyclosporine (modified): 2.3-3 mg/kg every 12 hours (De Saussure, 2005; Weber, 2006)
Note: Patients responsive to I.V. therapy should be switched to oral therapy when possible.

Renal Impairment For severe psoriasis:
Serum creatinine levels ≥25% above pretreatment levels: Take another sample within 2 weeks; if the level remains ≥25% above pretreatment levels, decrease dosage of cyclosporine (modified) by 25% to 50%. If two dosage adjustments do not reverse the increase in serum creatinine levels, treatment should be discontinued.
Serum creatinine levels ≥50% above pretreatment levels: Decrease cyclosporine dosage by 25% to 50%. If two dosage adjustments do not reverse the increase in serum creatinine levels, treatment should be discontinued.
Hemodialysis: Supplemental dose is not necessary.
Peritoneal dialysis: Supplemental dose is not necessary.

Hepatic Impairment Dosage adjustment is probably necessary; monitor levels closely

Administration
Oral solution: Do not administer liquid from plastic or styrofoam cup. May dilute Neoral® oral solution with orange juice or apple juice. May dilute Sandimmune® oral solution with milk, chocolate milk, or orange juice. Avoid changing diluents frequently. Mix thoroughly and drink at once. Use syringe provided to measure dose. Mix in a glass container and rinse container with more diluent to ensure total dose is taken. Do not rinse syringe before or after use (may cause dose variation).
Combination therapy with renal transplantation:
Everolimus: Administer cyclosporine at the same time as everolimus
Sirolimus: Administer cyclosporine 4 hours prior to sirolimus
I.V.: The manufacturer recommends that following dilution, intravenous admixture be administered over 2-6 hours. However, many transplant centers administer as divided doses (2-3 doses/day) or as a 24-hour continuous infusion. Discard solution after 24 hours. Anaphylaxis has been reported with I.V. use; reserve for patients who cannot take oral form. Patients should be under continuous observation for at least the first 30 minutes of the infusion, and should be monitored frequently thereafter. Maintain patent airway; other supportive measures and agents for treating anaphylaxis should be present when I.V. drug is given. To minimize leaching of DEHP, non-PVC sets should be used for administration.

◀ **Monitoring Parameters** Monitor blood pressure and serum creatinine after any cyclosporine dosage changes or addition, modification, or deletion of other medications. Monitor plasma concentrations periodically.

Transplant patients: Cyclosporine trough levels, serum electrolytes, renal function, hepatic function, blood pressure, lipid profile

Psoriasis therapy: Baseline blood pressure, serum creatinine (2 levels each), BUN, CBC, serum magnesium, potassium, uric acid, lipid profile. Biweekly monitoring of blood pressure, complete blood count, and levels of BUN, uric acid, potassium, lipids, and magnesium during the first 3 months of treatment for psoriasis. Monthly monitoring is recommended after this initial period. Also evaluate any atypical skin lesions prior to therapy. Increase the frequency of blood pressure monitoring after each alteration in dosage of cyclosporine. Cyclosporine dosage should be decreased by 25% to 50% in patients with no history of hypertension who develop sustained hypertension during therapy and, if hypertension persists, treatment with cyclosporine should be discontinued.

Rheumatoid arthritis: Baseline blood pressure, and serum creatinine (2 levels each); serum creatinine every 2 weeks for first 3 months, then monthly if patient is stable. Increase the frequency of blood pressure monitoring after each alteration in dosage of cyclosporine. Cyclosporine dosage should be decreased by 25% to 50% in patients with no history of hypertension who develop sustained hypertension during therapy and, if hypertension persists, treatment with cyclosporine should be discontinued.

Reference Range Reference ranges are method dependent and specimen dependent; use the same analytical method consistently

Method-dependent and specimen-dependent: Trough levels should be obtained:

Oral: 12-18 hours after dose (chronic usage)

I.V.: 12 hours after dose **or** immediately prior to next dose

Therapeutic range: Not absolutely defined, dependent on organ transplanted, time after transplant, organ function and CsA toxicity:

General range of 100-400 ng/mL

Toxic level: Not well defined, nephrotoxicity may occur at any level

Recommend cyclosporine therapeutic ranges when administered in combination with everolimus for renal transplant (Zortress® product labeling, 2010):

Month 1 post-transplant: 100-200 ng/mL

Months 2 and 3 post-transplant: 75-150 ng/mL

Months 4 and 5 post-transplant: 50-100 ng/mL

Months 6-12 post-transplant: 25-50 ng/mL

Test Interactions Specific whole blood assay for cyclosporine may be falsely elevated if sample is drawn from the same central venous line through which dose was administered (even if flush has been administered and/or dose was given hours before); cyclosporine metabolites cross-react with radioimmunoassay and fluorescence polarization immunoassay

Pharmacotherapy Pearls Cyclosporine (modified): Refers to the capsule dosage formulation of cyclosporine in an aqueous dispersion (previously referred to as "microemulsion"). Cyclosporine (modified) has increased bioavailability as compared to cyclosporine (non-modified) and cannot be used interchangeably without close monitoring.

Special Geriatric Considerations Cyclosporine has not been specifically studied in the elderly. Cyclosporine is being used in combination therapy for the treatment of severe rheumatoid arthritis.

Dosage Forms Excipient information presented when available (limited, particularly for generics); consult specific product labeling. [DSC] = Discontinued product

Capsule, oral [modified]:

Gengraf®: 25 mg, 100 mg [contains ethanol 12.8%]

Capsule, oral [non-modified]: 25 mg [DSC], 100 mg

Capsule, softgel, oral [modified]: 25 mg, 50 mg, 100 mg

Neoral®: 25 mg, 100 mg [contains corn oil, dehydrated ethanol 11.9%]

Capsule, softgel, oral [non-modified]:

SandIMMUNE®: 25 mg, 100 mg [contains corn oil, dehydrated ethanol 12.7%]

Injection, solution [non-modified]: 50 mg/mL (5 mL)

SandIMMUNE®: 50 mg/mL (5 mL) [contains ethanol 32.9%, polyoxyethylated castor oil]

Solution, oral [modified]: 100 mg/mL (50 mL)

Gengraf®: 100 mg/mL (50 mL) [contains propylene glycol]

Neoral®: 100 mg/mL (50 mL) [contains corn oil, dehydrated ethanol 11.9%, propylene glycol]

Solution, oral [non-modified]: 100 mg/mL (50 mL [DSC])

SandIMMUNE®: 100 mg/mL (50 mL) [contains ethanol 12.5%]

CycloSPORINE (Ophthalmic) (SYE kloe spor een)

Medication Safety Issues
Sound-alike/look-alike issues:
CycloSPORINE may be confused with cyclophosphamide, Cyklokapron®, cycloSERINE
Brand Names: U.S. Restasis®
Brand Names: Canada Restasis®
Index Terms CsA; CyA; Cyclosporin A
Generic Availability (U.S.) No
Pharmacologic Category Immunosuppressant Agent
Use Increase tear production when suppressed tear production is presumed to be due to keratoconjunctivitis sicca-associated ocular inflammation (in patients not already using topical anti-inflammatory drugs or punctal plugs)
Dosage
Geriatric & Adult Keratoconjunctivitis sicca: Ophthalmic (Restasis®): Instill 1 drop in each eye every 12 hours
Special Geriatric Considerations Evaluate the patient's or caregiver's ability to safely administer the correct dose of ophthalmic medication.
Dosage Forms Excipient information presented when available (limited, particularly for generics); consult specific product labeling.
Emulsion, ophthalmic [drops, preservative free]:
Restasis®: 0.05% (0.4 mL) [contains castor oil]

◆ Cymbalta® *see* DULoxetine *on page 620*

Cyproheptadine (si proe HEP ta deen)

Related Information
Beers Criteria − Potentially Inappropriate Medications for Geriatrics *on page 2183*
Medication Safety Issues
Sound-alike/look-alike issues:
Cyproheptadine may be confused with cyclobenzaprine
Periactin may be confused with Percodan®, Persantine®
BEERS Criteria medication:
This drug may be potentially inappropriate for use in geriatric patients (Quality of evidence - moderate; Strength of recommendation - strong).
International issues:
Periactin brand name for cyproheptadine [U.S., multiple international markets] may be confused with Perative brand name for an enteral nutrition preparation [multiple international markets] and brand name for ketoconazole [Argentina]
Brand Names: Canada Euro-Cyproheptadine; PMS-Cyproheptadine
Index Terms Cyproheptadine Hydrochloride; Periactin
Generic Availability (U.S.) Yes
Pharmacologic Category Histamine H$_1$ Antagonist; Histamine H$_1$ Antagonist, First Generation; Piperidine Derivative
Use Perennial and seasonal allergic rhinitis and other allergic symptoms including urticaria
Unlabeled Use Migraine headache prophylaxis, pruritus, spasticity associated with spinal cord damage
Contraindications Hypersensitivity to cyproheptadine or any component of the formulation; narrow-angle glaucoma; bladder neck obstruction; pyloroduodenal obstruction; symptomatic prostatic hyperplasia; stenosing peptic ulcer; concurrent use of MAO inhibitors; use in debilitated elderly patients
Warnings/Precautions May cause CNS depression, which may impair physical or mental abilities; patients must be cautioned about performing tasks which require mental alertness (eg, operating machinery or driving). Effects may be potentiated when used with other sedative drugs or ethanol. Use with caution in patients with cardiovascular disease; increased intraocular pressure; respiratory disease; or thyroid dysfunction. In the elderly, avoid use of this potent anticholinergic agent due to increased risk of confusion, dry mouth, constipation, and other anticholinergic effects; clearance decreases in patients of advanced age (Beers Criteria).
Adverse Reactions (Reflective of adult population; not specific for elderly) Frequency not defined.
Cardiovascular: Extrasystoles, hypotension, palpitation, tachycardia
Central nervous system: Confusion, coordination disturbed, dizziness, excitation, euphoria, faintness, hallucinations, headache, hysteria, insomnia, irritability, nervousness, neuritis, restlessness, sedation, seizure, sleepiness, tremor, vertigo

Dermatologic: Angioedema, photosensitivity, rash, urticaria

Gastrointestinal: Abdominal pain, anorexia, appetite increased, constipation, diarrhea, nausea, vomiting, xerostomia

Genitourinary: Difficult urination, urinary frequency, urinary retention

Hematologic: Agranulocytosis, hemolytic anemia, leukopenia, thrombocytopenia

Hepatic: Cholestasis, hepatic failure, hepatitis, jaundice

Neuromuscular & skeletal: Paresthesia

Ocular: Blurred vision, diplopia

Otic: Labyrinthitis (acute), tinnitus

Respiratory: Bronchial secretions (thickening), nasal congestion, pharyngitis

Miscellaneous: Allergic reactions, anaphylactic shock, chills, diaphoresis, fatigue

Drug Interactions

Metabolism/Transport Effects None known.

Avoid Concomitant Use

Avoid concomitant use of Cyproheptadine with any of the following: Azelastine; Azelastine (Nasal); Methadone; Mirtazapine; Paraldehyde

Increased Effect/Toxicity

Cyproheptadine may increase the levels/effects of: Alcohol (Ethyl); Anticholinergics; Azelastine; Azelastine (Nasal); Buprenorphine; CNS Depressants; Methadone; Methotrimeprazine; Metyrosine; Mirtazapine; Paraldehyde; Zolpidem

The levels/effects of Cyproheptadine may be increased by: Droperidol; HydrOXYzine; Methotrimeprazine; Pramlintide

Decreased Effect

Cyproheptadine may decrease the levels/effects of: Acetylcholinesterase Inhibitors (Central); Benzylpenicilloyl Polylysine; Betahistine; Hyaluronidase; Selective Serotonin Reuptake Inhibitors

The levels/effects of Cyproheptadine may be decreased by: Acetylcholinesterase Inhibitors (Central); Amphetamines

Ethanol/Nutrition/Herb Interactions Ethanol: May increase CNS depression; monitor for increased effects with coadministration. Caution patients about effects.

Mechanism of Action A potent antihistamine and serotonin antagonist, competes with histamine for H_1-receptor sites on effector cells in the gastrointestinal tract, blood vessels, and respiratory tract

Pharmacodynamics/Kinetics

Metabolism: Primarily by hepatic glucuronidation via UGT1A (Walker, 1996)

Half-life elimination: Metabolites: ~16 hours (Paton, 1985)

Time to peak, plasma: 6-9 hours (Paton, 1985)

Excretion: Urine (~40% primarily as metabolites); feces (2% to 20%)

Dosage

Geriatric Initiate therapy at the lower end of the dosage range.

Adult

Allergic conditions: Oral: 4-20 mg/day divided every 8 hours (not to exceed 0.5 mg/kg/day); some patients may require up to 32 mg/day for adequate control of symptoms

Spasticity associated with spinal cord damage (unlabeled use): Oral: Initial: 2-4 mg every 8 hours; maximum: 8 mg every 8 hours (Barbeau, 1982; Wainberg, 1990)

Test Interactions Diagnostic antigen skin test results may be suppressed; false positive serum TCA screen

Special Geriatric Considerations Elderly patients may not tolerate the anticholinergic effects of cyproheptadine.

This medication is considered to be potentially inappropriate in this patient population (Beers Criteria: Quality of evidence - moderate; Strength of recommendation - strong).

Dosage Forms Excipient information presented when available (limited, particularly for generics); consult specific product labeling.

Syrup, oral, as hydrochloride: 2 mg/5 mL (473 mL, 480 mL)

Tablet, oral, as hydrochloride: 4 mg

- ◆ **D3** *see* Cholecalciferol *on page 365*
- ◆ **D-3 [OTC]** *see* Cholecalciferol *on page 365*
- ◆ **D3-5™ [OTC]** *see* Cholecalciferol *on page 365*
- ◆ **D3-50™ [OTC]** *see* Cholecalciferol *on page 365*
- ◆ **D-3-Mercaptovaline** *see* PenicillAMINE *on page 1493*
- ◆ **D-23129** *see* Ezogabine *on page 740*

Dabigatran Etexilate (da BIG a tran ett EX ill ate)

Related Information
Beers Criteria – Potentially Inappropriate Medications for Geriatrics *on page 2183*
Medication Safety Issues
Sound-alike/look-alike issues:
Pradaxa® may be confused with Plavix®
Pradax™ (Canada) may be confused with Plavix®
High alert medication:
The Institute for Safe Medication Practices (ISMP) includes this medication among its list of drug classes which have a heightened risk of causing significant patient harm when used in error.
BEERS Criteria medication:
This drug may be potentially inappropriate for use in geriatric patients (Quality of evidence - moderate; Strength of recommendation - weak).
Brand Names: U.S. Pradaxa®
Brand Names: Canada Pradax™
Index Terms Dabigatran Etexilate Mesylate
Pharmacologic Category Anticoagulant, Thrombin Inhibitor
Use Prevention of stroke and systemic embolism in patients with nonvalvular atrial fibrillation
2011 ACCF/AHA/HRS atrial fibrillation guidelines: Not recommended for patients with coexisting prosthetic heart valve or hemodynamically significant valve disease, severe renal failure (Cl_{cr} <15 mL/minute), or advanced liver disease (impaired baseline clotting function)

Canadian labeling: Additional uses (not in U.S. labeling): Postoperative thromboprophylaxis in patients who have undergone total hip or knee replacement procedures
Medication Guide Available Yes
Contraindications Serious hypersensitivity (eg, anaphylaxis) to dabigatran or any component of the formulation; active pathological bleeding

Canadian labeling: Additional contraindications (not in U.S. labeling): Severe renal impairment (Cl_{cr} <30 mL/minute); bleeding diathesis or patients with spontaneous or pharmacological hemostatic impairment; lesions at risk of clinically significant bleeding (eg, hemorrhagic or ischemic cerebral infarction) within previous 6 months; concomitant therapy with oral ketoconazole
Warnings/Precautions The most common complication is bleeding, and sometimes fatal bleeding. Risk factors for bleeding include concurrent use of drugs that increase the risk of bleeding (eg, antiplatelet agents, heparin), renal impairment, impairment, and elderly patients (especially if low body weight). Monitor for signs and symptoms of bleeding; discontinue in patients with active pathological bleeding. **Important:** No specific antidote exists for dabigatran reversal. Therapy for severe hemorrhage may include transfusions of fresh frozen plasma, packed red blood cells, or surgical intervention when appropriate (Wann, 2011). The use of a PCC (Cofact ®, not available in the U.S.) has been shown to be **ineffective** for dabigatran reversal (Eerenberg, 2011); however, the manufacturer does suggest that activated PCC (eg, Feiba NF), recombinant factor VIIa, or concentrates of factors II, IX, or X may be considered, although their use has not been evaluated in clinical trials. Platelet concentrates should be considered when thrombocytopenia is present or long-acting antiplatelet drugs have been used. Use in patients with moderate hepatic impairment (Child-Pugh class B) demonstrated large inter-subject variability; however no consistent change in exposure or pharmacodynamics was seen. Use in patients with advanced liver disease (impaired baseline clotting function) is not recommended (Wann, 2011). Use in patients with a coexisting prosthetic heart valve or hemodynamically significant valve disease is not recommended (Wann, 2011).

Due to an increased risk of bleeding, avoid use with other direct thrombin inhibitors (eg, bivalirudin), unfractionated heparin or heparin derivatives, low molecular weight heparins (eg, enoxaparin), fondaparinux, thienopyridines (eg, clopidogrel, ticlopidine), GPIIb/IIIa antagonists (eg, eptifibatide), aspirin, coumarin derivatives, and sulfinpyrazone. NSAIDs should be used cautiously. Appropriate doses of unfractionated heparin may be used to maintain catheter patency. The concomitant use of P-gp inducers (eg, rifampin) may reduce dabigatran bioavailability and should be avoided. Concurrent use of certain P-gp inhibitors ((ie, verapamil, amiodarone, quinidine, and clarithromycin) does not require dosage adjustment if Cl_{cr} ≥30 mL/minute; however, this should not be extrapolated to other P-gp inhibitors. A dabigatran dose reduction should be considered with concurrent use of dronedarone or oral ketoconazole in patients with Cl_{cr} 30-50 mL/minute. Concurrent use of oral ketoconazole is contraindicated in the Canadian labeling. Use of any P-gp inhibitor should be avoided for Cl_{cr}<30 mL/minute.

Evaluate renal function prior to and during therapy, particularly if used in patients with any degree of pre-existing renal impairment or in any condition that may result in a decline in renal function (eg, hypovolemia, dehydration, concomitant use of medications with a potential to affect renal function); dabigatran concentrations may increase in any degree of renal impairment and increase the risk of bleeding. In moderate impairment, serum concentrations may increase 3 times higher than normal compared to concentrations in patients with normal renal function. However, U.S. labeling only requires dosage reduction in patients with severe renal impairment (Cl_{cr} 15-30 mL/minute) and recommends avoiding use in patients with Cl_{cr} <15 mL/minute due to insufficient evidence. Per the American College of Chest Physicians, dabigatran is considered contraindicated in patients with severe renal impairment (Cl_{cr} <30 mL/minute) (Guyatt, 2012). The Canadian labeling also contraindicates use in severe renal impairment (Cl_{cr} <30 mL/minute) and recommends indication-specific dose reductions in patients with moderate impairment (Cl_{cr} 30-50 mL/minute). Discontinue therapy in any patient who develops acute renal failure.

In the elderly, use with extreme caution or consider other treatment options. No dosage adjustment is recommended in the U.S. labeling based on age alone (unless renal impairment coexists); however, numerous case reports of hemorrhage, including hemorrhagic stroke, have been reported in elderly patients (median age: 80 years), with a quarter of these reports occurring in patients ≥84 years of age. Some reports have resulted in fatality, particularly in those with low body weight and mild-to-moderate renal impairment; the risk is expected to be higher in patients receiving interacting drugs (eg, amiodarone) (Legrand, 2011). The RE-LY trial, although not powered to assess safety in the elderly, employed 110 mg and 150 mg twice daily regiments. The 110 mg twice daily regimen was not approved for use in the United States. The Canadian labeling recommends a dose reduction for patients ≥80 years of age with atrial fibrillation and suggests that dose reductions be considered in patients >75 years of age receiving therapy for atrial fibrillation or postoperative thromboprophylaxis. In addition, due to the frequency of renal impairment in older adults, the Canadian labeling recommends monitoring renal function at a minimum of once per year in any patient >75 years of age; use of dabigatran is contraindicated in patients with Cl_{cr} <30 mL/minute. Per the Beers Criteria, there is a greater risk of bleeding in older adults aged ≥75 years (exceeds warfarin bleeding risk) and therapy should be used with caution in patients ≥75 years of age or in patients with Cl_{cr} <30 mL/minute (Beers Criteria).

If possible, discontinue dabigatran 1-2 days (Cl_{cr} ≥50 mL/minute) or 3-5 days (Cl_{cr} <50 mL/minute) before invasive or surgical procedures due to the risk of bleeding; consider longer times for patients undergoing major surgery, spinal puncture, or insertion of a spinal or epidural catheter or port. If surgery cannot be delayed, the risk of bleeding is elevated; weigh risk of bleeding with urgency of procedure. Bleeding risk can be assessed by the ecarin clotting time (ECT) if available; if ECT is not available, use of aPTT may provide an approximation of dabigatran's anticoagulant activity. When temporarily discontinuing anticoagulants, including dabigatran, for active bleeding, elective surgery, or invasive procedures, the risk of stroke may increase (dependent on amount of elapsed time); lapses in therapy should be minimized and reinitiation should begin as soon as possible.

Adverse Reactions (Reflective of adult population; not specific for elderly) Adverse reactions listed below are reflective of both the U.S. and Canadian product information. **Important:** No specific antidote exists for dabigatran reversal. Therapy for severe hemorrhage may include transfusions of fresh frozen plasma, packed red blood cells, or surgical intervention when appropriate (Wann, 2011). The use of a prothrombin complex concentrate (PCC) (Cofact®, not available in the U.S.) has been shown to be **ineffective** for dabigatran reversal (Eerenberg, 2011).

>10%:
 Gastrointestinal: Dyspepsia (11%; includes abdominal discomfort/pain, epigastric discomfort)
 Hematologic: Bleeding (8% to 33%; major: ≤6%)

1% to 10%:

Gastrointestinal: GI hemorrhage (≤6%), gastritis-like symptoms (eg, GERD, esophagitis, erosive gastritis, GI ulcer)

Hematologic: Anemia (1% to 4%), hematoma (1% to 2%), hemoglobin decreased (1% to 2%), hemorrhage (postprocedural or wound: 1% to 2%)

Hepatic: ALT increased (≥3 x ULN: 2% to 3%)

Renal: Hematuria (1%)

Miscellaneous: Wound secretion (5%), postprocedural discharge (1%)

Drug Interactions

Metabolism/Transport Effects Substrate of P-glycoprotein

Avoid Concomitant Use

Avoid concomitant use of Dabigatran Etexilate with any of the following: P-glycoprotein/ABCB1 Inducers; Rivaroxaban; Sulfinpyrazone [Off Market]

Increased Effect/Toxicity

Dabigatran Etexilate may increase the levels/effects of: Collagenase (Systemic); Deferasirox; Ibritumomab; Rivaroxaban; Tositumomab and Iodine I 131 Tositumomab

The levels/effects of Dabigatran Etexilate may be increased by: Amiodarone; Anticoagulants; Antiplatelet Agents; Dasatinib; Dronedarone; Herbs (Anticoagulant/Antiplatelet Properties); Ketoconazole; Ketoconazole (Systemic); Nonsteroidal Anti-Inflammatory Agents; Pentosan Polysulfate Sodium; P-glycoprotein/ABCB1 Inhibitors; Prostacyclin Analogues; QuiNIDine; Salicylates; Sulfinpyrazone [Off Market]; Thrombolytic Agents; Tipranavir; Verapamil

Decreased Effect

The levels/effects of Dabigatran Etexilate may be decreased by: Antacids; AtorvaSTATin; P-glycoprotein/ABCB1 Inducers; Proton Pump Inhibitors

Ethanol/Nutrition/Herb Interactions

Food: Food has no affect on the bioavailability of dabigatran, but delays the time to peak plasma concentrations by 2 hours.

Herb/Nutraceutical: St John's wort may decrease levels/effects of dabigatran (concomitant use is not recommended). Concomitant use of dabigatran with herbs possessing anticoagulant/antiplatelet properties may increase the risk for bleeding.

Stability

Blister: Store at 25°C (77°F); excursions permitted between 15°C to 30°C (59°F to 86°F). Protect from moisture.

Bottle: Store at 25°C (77°F); excursions permitted between 15°C to 30°C (59°F to 86°F). Dispense and store in original manufacturer's bottle to protect from moisture; discard 4 months after opening original container.

Mechanism of Action Prodrug lacking anticoagulant activity that is converted *in vivo* to the active dabigatran, a specific, reversible, direct thrombin inhibitor that inhibits both free and fibrin-bound thrombin. Inhibits coagulation by preventing thrombin-mediated effects, including cleavage of fibrinogen to fibrin monomers, activation of factors V, VIII, XI, and XIII, and inhibition of thrombin-induced platelet aggregation.

Pharmacodynamics/Kinetics

Absorption: Rapid; initially slow postoperatively

Distribution: V_d: 50-70 L

Protein binding: 35%

Metabolism: Hepatic; dabigatran etexilate is rapidly and completely hydrolyzed to dabigatran (active form) by plasma and hepatic esterases; dabigatran undergoes hepatic glucuronidation to active acylglucuronide isomers (similar activity to parent compound; accounts for <10% of total dabigatran in plasma)

Bioavailability: 3% to 7%

Half-life elimination: 12-17 hours; Elderly: 14-17 hours; Mild-to-moderate renal impairment: 15-18 hours; Severe renal impairment: 28 hours (Stangier, 2010)

Time to peak, plasma: Dabigatran: 1 hour; delayed 2 hours by food (no effect on bioavailability)

Excretion: Urine (80%)

Dosage

Geriatric

Nonvalvular atrial fibrillation (to prevent stroke and systemic embolism): Oral:

U.S. labeling:

Patients >65 years: Refer to adult dosing. No dosage adjustment required unless renal impairment exists; however, increased risk of bleeding has been observed, particularly in elderly patients with low body weight and/or concomitant renal impairment.

Patients ≥80 years: **Use with extreme caution or consider other treatment options;** no dosage adjustment provided in manufacturer's labeling; however, numerous cases of hemorrhage, including hemorrhagic stroke, have been reported postmarketing,

◀

particularly in this age group of octogenarians. Due to a lack of available dosing options available in the U.S., consider avoiding use of dabigatran in this population.

Canadian labeling:

Patients <80 years: 150 mg twice daily; **Note:** The manufacturer's labeling suggests that a dose reduction to 110 mg twice daily may be considered in patients >75 years with at least one other risk factor for bleeding (eg, moderate renal impairment [Cl_{cr} 30-50 mL/minute], concomitant treatment with strong P-gp inhibitors, or previous GI bleed); however, efficacy in stroke prevention may be lessened with this dose reduction.

Patients ≥80 years: 110 mg twice daily

Postoperative thromboprophylaxis (Canadian labeling): Oral: Patients >75 years: Use with caution; consider a dose of 150 mg daily

Adult

Nonvalvular atrial fibrillation (to prevent stroke and systemic embolism): Oral: 150 mg twice daily

Conversion from a parenteral anticoagulant: Initiate dabigatran ≤2 hours prior to the time of the next scheduled dose of the parenteral anticoagulant (eg, enoxaparin) or at the time of discontinuation for a continuously administered parenteral drug (eg, I.V. heparin); discontinue parenteral anticoagulant at the time of dabigatran initiation.

Conversion to a parenteral anticoagulant: Wait 12 hours (Cl_{cr} ≥30 mL/minute) or 24 hours (Cl_{cr} <30 mL/minute) after the last dose of dabigatran before initiating a parenteral anticoagulant.

Conversion from warfarin: Discontinue warfarin and initiate dabigatran when INR <2.0

Conversion to warfarin: Start time must be adjusted based on Cl_{cr}:

Cl_{cr} >50 mL/minute: Initiate warfarin 3 days before discontinuation of dabigatran

Cl_{cr} 31-50 mL/minute: Initiate warfarin 2 days before discontinuation of dabigatran

Cl_{cr} 15-30 mL/minute: Initiate warfarin 1 day before discontinuation of dabigatran

Cl_{cr} <15 mL/minute: No recommendations provided

Note: Since dabigatran contributes to INR elevation, warfarin's effect on the INR will be better reflected only after dabigatran has been stopped for ≥2 days

Secondary prevention of cardioembolic stroke or TIA: Oral: 150 mg twice daily initiated within 1-2 weeks after stroke onset or earlier in patients at low bleeding risk (Guyatt, 2012)

Postoperative thromboprophylaxis (Canadian labeling): Oral: **Note:** Therapy should not be initiated until hemostasis has been established.

Knee replacement: Initial: 110 mg given 1-4 hours after completion of surgery and establishment of hemostasis **OR** 220 mg as 1 dose in postoperative patients in whom therapy is not initiated on day of surgery regardless of reason; maintenance: 220 mg once daily (total duration of therapy: 10 days; ACCP recommendation [Guyatt, 2012]: Minimum of 10-14 days; extended duration of up to 35 days suggested)

Hip replacement: Initial: 110 mg given 1-4 hours after completion of surgery and establishment of hemostasis **OR** 220 mg as 1 dose in postoperative patients in whom therapy is not initiated on day of surgery regardless of reason; maintenance: 220 mg once daily (total duration of therapy: 28-35 days; ACCP recommendation [Guyatt, 2012]: Minimum of 10-14 days; extended duration of up to 35 days suggested)

Conversion information (Canadian labeling): When transitioning from parenteral anticoagulation therapy, initiate oral dabigatran therapy ≤2 hours prior to the time of next regularly scheduled dose of intermittent parenteral anticoagulant or at the time of discontinuation for continuously administered parenteral anticoagulation therapy. When transitioning from dabigatran to I.V. anticoagulation therapy, allow 24 hours after the last dabigatran dose before initiating I.V. anticoagulation therapy. When transitioning from warfarin, discontinue warfarin and initiate dabigatran when INR <2.0.

Dosing adjustment with concomitant medications:

U.S. labeling: Nonvalvular atrial fibrillation (to prevent stroke and systemic embolism):

Dronedarone with Cl_{cr} 30-50 mL/minute: Consider dabigatran dose reduction to 75 mg twice daily.

Ketoconazole (oral) with Cl_{cr} 30-50 mL/minute: Consider dabigatran dose reduction to 75 mg twice daily.

Any P-glycoprotein inhibitor (including dronedarone and oral ketoconazole) with Cl_{cr} 15-30 mL/minute: Avoid concurrent use.

Canadian labeling:

Nonvalvular atrial fibrillation (to prevent stroke and systemic embolism): *Verapamil:* No dosage adjustment recommended; however, for concomitant verapamil use, it is recommended that dabigatran be administered ≥2 hours before verapamil to minimize interaction potential (caution and monitoring is also recommended).

Postoperative thromboprophylaxis: *Amiodarone, quinidine, or verapamil:* Use caution and reduce dabigatran to 150 mg daily. In patients with Cl_{cr} 30-50 mL/minute and receiving verapamil, consider dabigatran dose reduction to 75 mg once daily.

Renal Impairment Note: Clinical trial evaluating safety and efficacy utilized the Cockcroft-Gault formula with the use of actual body weight (data on file; Boehringer Ingelheim Pharmaceuticals Inc, 2012).

Nonvalvular atrial fibrillation (to prevent stroke and systemic embolism):
U.S. labeling:

Cl_{cr} >30 mL/minute: No dosage adjustment provided in manufacturer's labeling (unless patient receiving certain concomitant medications); however, use with caution in mild-to-moderate renal impairment due to risk for increased dabigatran exposure (concentrations may be increased 3 times higher than normal concentrations in moderate impairment), particularly if patient is also of advanced age.

Cl_{cr} 30-50 mL/minute **and** patient receiving concomitant dronedarone or oral ketoconazole: Consider dose reduction to 75 mg twice daily.

Cl_{cr} 15-30 mL/minute: 75 mg twice daily; if concomitant administration with any P-gp inhibitor (including dronedarone or oral ketoconazole), avoid concurrent use. **Note:** Patients with Cl_{cr} <30 mL/minute were excluded from the RE-LY trial (Connolly, 2009). Per the American College of Chest Physicians, dabigatran is considered contraindicated in patients with severe renal impairment (Cl_{cr} <30 mL/minute) (Guyatt, 2012).

Cl_{cr} <15 mL/minute: Use not recommended (has not been studied). Per the American College of Chest Physicians, dabigatran is considered contraindicated in patients with severe renal impairment (Cl_{cr} <30 mL/minute) (Guyatt, 2012).

ESRD requiring hemodialysis: Use not recommended (has not been studied); **Note:** Hemodialysis removes ~60% over 2-3 hours.

Canadian labeling:

Cl_{cr} ≥30 mL/minute: No dosage adjustment recommended. **Note:** Patients with moderate renal impairment (Cl_{cr} 30-50 mL/minute) are at an increased risk for bleeding; routine assessment of renal status is recommended; use recommended unadjusted dosage of 150 mg twice daily with caution in these patients.

Severe renal impairment (Cl_{cr} <30 mL/minute): Use is contraindicated.

Postoperative thromboprophylaxis: Canadian labeling:
Moderate renal impairment (Cl_{cr} 30-50 mL/minute): Initial: 75 mg given 1-4 hours after completion of surgery and establishment of hemostasis; Maintenance: 150 mg/day
Severe renal impairment (Cl_{cr} <30 mL/minute): Use is contraindicated.

Hepatic Impairment Nonvalvular atrial fibrillation (to prevent stroke and systemic embolism): No dosage adjustment required.

Administration Do not break, chew, or open capsules, as this will lead to 75% increase in absorption and potentially serious adverse reactions. Administer with water. May be taken without regard to meals.

Monitoring Parameters Routine monitoring of coagulation tests not required. However, the measurement of activated partial thromboplastin time (aPTT) (values >2.5 x control may indicate overanticoagulation), ecarin clotting test (ECT) if available, or thrombin time (TT; most sensitive) may be useful to determine presence of dabigatran and level of coagulopathy; CBC with differential; renal function (prior to initiation and periodically as clinically indicated [ie, situations associated with a decline in renal function]); **Note:** Canadian labeling specifically recommends renal function be routinely assessed at least once per year in elderly patients (>75 years of age) or patients with moderate renal impairment (Cl_{cr} 30-50 mL/minute)

Reference Range
At therapeutic dabigatran doses, aPTT, ECT (ecarin clotting time), and TT (thrombin time) are prolonged. A median peak aPTT of ~2 x control and a median trough aPTT of 1.5 x control were observed in subjects taking dabigatran 150 mg twice daily in the RE-LY trail
A therapeutic range has not been established for aPTT or for other tests of anticoagulant activity

Special Geriatric Considerations In the RE-LY study, 82% of the patients enrolled were ≥65 years of age, with 40% ≥75 years of age. There was a trend towards increased risk of bleeding in elderly patients ≥75 years of age receiving 150 mg twice daily. Dabigatran is predominantly eliminated by the kidney; therefore, renal function should be closely monitored in elderly patients. No dosage adjustment based on age is recommended in the U.S. labeling (unless renal impairment coexists). However, case reports of serious bleeding including fatality has occurred in the elderly with low body weight and mild-moderate renal impairment. The risk is expected to be higher in patients receiving other interacting drugs (eg, amiodarone) (Legrand, 2011). Octogenarians may be at an even greater risk for serious bleeds, as indicated by a high number of postmarketing reports of hemorrhage, including hemorrhagic stroke, being reported in elderly patients with a median age of 80 years. A number of these reports occurred in patients ≥84 years of age. Impaired renal function may also play a significant role. Renal function should be assessed at least annually.

This medication is considered to be potentially inappropriate in this patient population (Beers Criteria: Quality of evidence - moderate; Strength of recommendation - weak).

Dosage Forms Excipient information presented when available (limited, particularly for generics); consult specific product labeling.

Capsule, oral:

Pradaxa®: 75 mg, 150 mg

Dosage Forms: Canada Excipient information presented when available (limited, particularly for generics); consult specific product labeling.

Capsule, oral:

Pradax™: 75 mg, 110 mg, 150 mg

♦ **Dabigatran Etexilate Mesylate** see Dabigatran Etexilate on page 469
♦ **Dacodyl™ [OTC]** see Bisacodyl on page 214

Dalfampridine (dal FAM pri deen)

Medication Safety Issues

Sound-alike/look-alike issues:

Ampyra™ may be confused with anakinra

Dalfampridine may be confused with delavirdine, desipramine

Dalfampridine (U.S.) and fampridine (Canada) are different generic names for the same chemical entity (4-aminopyridine)

Brand Names: U.S. Ampyra™

Brand Names: Canada Fampyra™

Index Terms 4-aminopyridine; 4-AP; EL-970; Fampridine; Fampridine-SR

Pharmacologic Category Potassium Channel Blocker

Use Treatment to improve walking in multiple sclerosis (MS) patients

Medication Guide Available Yes

Contraindications History of seizure; moderate or severe renal impairment (Cl_{cr} ≤50 mL/minute)

Canadian labeling: Additional contraindications (not in U.S. labeling): Hypersensitivity to fampridine or any component of the formulation or container; mild, moderate, severe renal impairment (Cl_{cr} ≤80 mL/minute); concomitant use with compounded 4-aminopyridine or other forms of fampridine; concomitant use with drugs that inhibit organic cation transporter 2 (OCT2), such as cimetidine or quinidine

Warnings/Precautions The chemical entity of 4-aminopyridine is referred to with a generic name of dalfampridine in the U.S. and with a generic name of fampridine in Canada. Administration is associated with a dose-dependent risk of seizure; assess risk of seizure prior to treatment initiation; use caution or avoid in patients who may have a lower seizure threshold due to predisposing factors. Seizures may occur within days to weeks after initiation of the recommended dose in patients with no history of seizures. Discontinue use and do not reinitiate therapy if seizure occurs during treatment. Use is contraindicated in patients with a history of seizures. Use in renal impairment is associated with an increased risk of seizure and other adverse events, primarily neurologic effects, due to increased serum concentrations; elimination is predominately via the kidneys as unchanged drug. U.S. labeling contraindicates use in moderate-to-severe renal impairment (Cl_{cr} ≤50 mL/minute). Canadian labeling contra-indicates use in mild, moderate, and severe renal impairment (Cl_{cr} ≤80 mL/minute). To avoid adverse reactions, sustained release products available in the U.S. (dalfampridine) or in Canada (fampridine) should not be administered with other 4-aminopyridine formulations (eg, compounded immediate release fampridine).

Adverse Reactions (Reflective of adult population; not specific for elderly)

>10%: Genitourinary: Urinary tract infection (12%)

1% to 10%:

Central nervous system: Insomnia (9%), dizziness (7%), headache (7%), multiple sclerosis relapse (4%), seizures (up to 4%; dose-dependent)

Gastrointestinal: Nausea (7%), constipation (3%), dyspepsia (2%)

Neuromuscular & skeletal: Weakness (7%), back pain (5%), balance disorder (5%), paresthesia (4%)

Respiratory: Nasopharyngitis (4%), pharyngolaryngeal pain (2%)

Drug Interactions

Metabolism/Transport Effects Substrate of CYP2E1 (minor); **Note:** Assignment of Major/Minor substrate status based on clinically relevant drug interaction potential; **Inhibits** CYP2E1 (weak)

Avoid Concomitant Use There are no known interactions where it is recommended to avoid concomitant use.

Increased Effect/Toxicity

Dalfampridine may increase the levels/effects of: MetFORMIN

The levels/effects of Dalfampridine may be increased by: Cimetidine; MetFORMIN; QuiNIDine

Decreased Effect There are no known significant interactions involving a decrease in effect.

Stability Store at 25°C (77°F); excursions permitted to 15°C to 30°C (59°F to 86°F).

Mechanism of Action Nonspecific potassium channel blocker which improves conduction in focally demyelinated axons by delaying repolarization and prolonging the duration of action potentials. Enhanced neuronal conduction is thought to strengthen skeletal muscle fiber twitch activity, thereby, improving peripheral motor neurologic function.

Pharmacodynamics/Kinetics

Absorption: Rapid and complete

Distribution: V_d: 2.6 L/kg

Protein binding: Negligible

Metabolism: Limited metabolism; *in vitro* data suggests hepatic metabolism to 3-hydroxy-4-aminopyridine occurs primarily via CYP2E1; further conjugated to 3-hydroxy-4-aminopyridine sulfate; metabolites are inactive

Bioavailability: 96% (relative to aqueous solution)

Half-life elimination: 5-7 hours; prolonged in severe renal impairment (~3 times longer)

Time to peak, plasma: 3-4 hours

Excretion: Urine (96%; 90% of total dose as unchanged drug); feces (0.5%)

Dosage

Geriatric & Adult Multiple sclerosis: Oral: 10 mg every 12 hours (maximum daily dose: 20 mg); no additional benefit seen with doses >20 mg/day

Renal Impairment Note: Creatinine clearance is estimated with Cockcroft-Gault formula.

U.S. labeling:

Mild renal impairment (Cl_{cr} 51-80 mL/minute): No specific adjustment recommended by the manufacturer; however, use with extreme caution as risk of seizure may be increased secondary to reduced clearance.

Moderate-to-severe renal impairment (Cl_{cr} ≤50 mL/minute): Use is contraindicated.

Canadian labeling:

Mild-to-severe impairment (Cl_{cr} ≤80 mL/minute): Use is contraindicated.

Hepatic Impairment No dosage adjustment required; drug undergoes minimal metabolism and is primarily excreted unchanged in the urine.

Administration May be administered with or without food. Do not chew, crush, dissolve, or divide tablet.

Monitoring Parameters Renal function (baseline and at least annually thereafter); EEG; walking ability

Special Geriatric Considerations U.S. labeling contraindicates use of dalfampridine in patients with a Cl_{cr} ≤50 mL/minute. Canadian labeling contraindicates use in patients with a Cl_{cr} ≤80 mL/minute. Because many older patients have impaired renal function, this medication should be used with extreme caution or avoided due to potential for increased adverse effects, particularly the risk of seizure.

Dosage Forms Excipient information presented when available (limited, particularly for generics); consult specific product labeling.

Tablet, extended release, oral:

Ampyra™: 10 mg

Dosage Forms: Canada Excipient information presented when available (limited, particularly for generics); consult specific product labeling.

Tablet, extended release, oral:

Fampyra™: 10 mg

◆ **Dalfopristin and Quinupristin** *see* Quinupristin and Dalfopristin *on page 1658*

◆ **d-Alpha Gems™ [OTC]** *see* Vitamin E *on page 2027*

◆ *d*-Alpha Tocopherol *see* Vitamin E *on page 2027*

Dalteparin (dal TE pa rin)

Related Information
Injectable Heparins/Heparinoids Comparison Table *on page 2119*

Medication Safety Issues
High alert medication:
The Institute for Safe Medication Practices (ISMP) includes this medication among its list of drugs which have a heightened risk of causing significant patient harm when used in error.

National Patient Safety Goals:
The Joint Commission (TJC) requires healthcare organizations that provide anticoagulant therapy to have a process in place to reduce the risk of anticoagulant-associated patient harm. Patients receiving anticoagulants should receive individualized care through a defined process that includes standardized ordering, dispensing, administration, monitoring and education. This does not apply to routine short-term use of anticoagulants for prevention of venous thromboembolism when the expectation is that the patient's laboratory values will remain within or close to normal values (NPSG.03.05.01).

Brand Names: U.S. Fragmin®

Brand Names: Canada Fragmin®

Index Terms Dalteparin Sodium

Generic Availability (U.S.) No

Pharmacologic Category Low Molecular Weight Heparin

Use Prevention of deep vein thrombosis (DVT) which may lead to pulmonary embolism, in patients requiring abdominal surgery who are at risk for thromboembolism complications (eg, patients >40 years of age, obesity, patients with malignancy, history of DVT or pulmonary embolism, and surgical procedures requiring general anesthesia and lasting >30 minutes); prevention of DVT in patients undergoing hip-replacement surgery; patients immobile during an acute illness; prevention of ischemic complications in patients with unstable angina or non-Q-wave myocardial infarction on concurrent aspirin therapy; in patients with cancer, extended treatment (6 months) of acute symptomatic venous thromboembolism (DVT and/or PE) to reduce the recurrence of venous thromboembolism

Canadian labeling: Additional use (unlabeled use in U.S.): Treatment of acute DVT; prevention of venous thromboembolism (VTE) in patients at risk of VTE undergoing general surgery; anticoagulant in extracorporeal circuit during hemodialysis and hemofiltration

Unlabeled Use Active treatment of deep vein thrombosis (noncancer patients)

Contraindications Hypersensitivity to dalteparin or any component of the formulation; history of heparin-induced thrombocytopenia (HIT) or HIT with thrombosis; hypersensitivity to heparin or pork products; patients with active major bleeding; patients with unstable angina, non-Q-wave MI, or acute venous thromboembolism undergoing epidural/neuraxial anesthesia

Canadian labeling: Additional contraindications (not in U.S. labeling): Septic endocarditis; major blood clotting disorders; acute gastroduodenal ulcer; cerebral hemorrhage; severe uncontrolled hypertension; diabetic or hemorrhagic retinopathy; other diseases that increase risk of hemorrhage; injuries to and operations on the CNS, eyes, and ears

Warnings/Precautions [U.S. Boxed Warning]: Spinal or epidural hematomas, including subsequent paralysis, may occur with recent or anticipated neuraxial anesthesia (epidural or spinal) or spinal puncture in patients anticoagulated with LMWH or heparinoids. Consider risk versus benefit prior to spinal procedures; risk is increased by the use of concomitant agents which may alter hemostasis, the use of indwelling epidural catheters for analgesia, a history of spinal deformity or spinal surgery, as well as traumatic or repeated epidural or spinal punctures. Use of dalteparin is contraindicated in patients undergoing epidural/neuraxial anesthesia. Patient should be observed closely for bleeding if enoxaparin is administered during or immediately following diagnostic lumbar puncture, epidural anesthesia, or spinal anesthesia.

Use with caution in patients with pre-existing thrombocytopenia, subacute bacterial endocarditis, peptic ulcer disease, pericarditis or pericardial effusion, liver or renal function impairment, recent lumbar puncture, vasculitis, concurrent use of aspirin (increased bleeding risk), previous hypersensitivity to heparin, heparin-associated thrombocytopenia. Monitor platelet count closely. Rare cases of thrombocytopenia (some with thrombosis) have occurred. Consider discontinuation of dalteparin in any patient developing significant thrombocytopenia related to initiation of dalteparin especially when associated with a positive *in vitro* test for antiplatelet antibodies. Use caution in patients with congenital or drug-induced thrombocytopenia or platelet defects. Cancer patients with thrombocytopenia may require dose adjustments for treatment of acute venous thromboembolism. In patients with a history of heparin-induced thrombocytopenia (HIT) or HIT with thrombosis, dalteparin is contraindicated.

Monitor patient closely for signs or symptoms of bleeding. Certain patients are at increased risk of bleeding. Risk factors include bacterial endocarditis; congenital or acquired bleeding disorders; active ulcerative or angiodysplastic GI diseases; severe uncontrolled hypertension; hemorrhagic stroke; or use shortly after brain, spinal, or ophthalmology surgery; in patients treated concomitantly with platelet inhibitors; recent GI bleeding; thrombocytopenia or platelet defects; severe liver disease; hypertensive or diabetic retinopathy; or in patients undergoing invasive procedures.

Use with caution in patients with severe renal impairment; accumulation may occur with repeated dosing increasing the risk for bleeding. Multidose vials contain benzyl alcohol. Heparin can cause hyperkalemia by affecting aldosterone. Similar reactions could occur with dalteparin. Monitor for hyperkalemia. Do **not** administer intramuscularly. Not to be used interchangeably (unit for unit) with heparin or any other low molecular weight heparins.

There is no consensus for adjusting/correcting the weight-based dosage of LMWH for patients who are morbidly obese (BMI ≥40 kg/m^2). The American College of Chest Physicians Practice Guidelines suggest consulting with a pharmacist regarding dosing in bariatric surgery patients and other obese patients who may require higher doses of LMWH (Gould, 2012).

Adverse Reactions (Reflective of adult population; not specific for elderly) Note: As with all anticoagulants, bleeding is the major adverse effect of dalteparin. Hemorrhage may occur at virtually any site. Risk is dependent on multiple variables.
>10%: Hematologic: Bleeding (3% to 14%), thrombocytopenia (including heparin-induced thrombocytopenia), <1%; cancer clinical trials: ~11%)
1% to 10%:
  Hematologic: Major bleeding (up to 6%), wound hematoma (up to 3%)
  Hepatic: AST >3 times upper limit of normal (5% to 9%), ALT >3 times upper limit of normal (4% to 10%)
  Local: Pain at injection site (up to 12%), injection site hematoma (up to 7%)

Drug Interactions
Metabolism/Transport Effects None known.
Avoid Concomitant Use
  Avoid concomitant use of Dalteparin with any of the following: Rivaroxaban
Increased Effect/Toxicity
  Dalteparin may increase the levels/effects of: Anticoagulants; Collagenase (Systemic); Dabigatran Etexilate; Deferasirox; Drotrecogin Alfa (Activated); Ibritumomab; Palifermin; Rivaroxaban; Tositumomab and Iodine I 131 Tositumomab

  The levels/effects of Dalteparin may be increased by: 5-ASA Derivatives; Antiplatelet Agents; Dasatinib; Herbs (Anticoagulant/Antiplatelet Properties); Nonsteroidal Anti-Inflammatory Agents; Pentosan Polysulfate Sodium; Pentoxifylline; Prostacyclin Analogues; Salicylates; Thrombolytic Agents; Tipranavir
Decreased Effect There are no known significant interactions involving a decrease in effect.
Ethanol/Nutrition/Herb Interactions Herb/Nutraceutical: Alfalfa, anise, bilberry, bladderwrack, bromelain, cat's claw, celery, chamomile, coleus, cordyceps, dong quai, evening primrose oil, fenugreek, feverfew, garlic, ginger, ginkgo biloba, ginseng (American), ginseng (panax), ginseng (Siberian), grapeseed, green tea, guggul, horse chestnut seed, horseradish, licorice, prickly ash, red clover, reishi, SAMe (s-adenosylmethionine), sweet clover, turmeric, white willow (all have additional antiplatelet/anticoagulant activity)
Stability Store at temperatures of 20°C to 25°C (68°F to 77°F). Multidose vials may be stored for up to 2 weeks at room temperature after entering.

Canadian labeling: If necessary, may dilute in isotonic sodium chloride or dextrose solutions to a concentration of 20 units/mL. Use within 24 hours of mixing.
Mechanism of Action Low molecular weight heparin analog with a molecular weight of 4000-6000 daltons; the commercial product contains 3% to 15% heparin with a molecular weight <3000 daltons, 65% to 78% with a molecular weight of 3000-8000 daltons and 14% to 26% with a molecular weight >8000 daltons; while dalteparin has been shown to inhibit both factor Xa and factor IIa (thrombin), the antithrombotic effect of dalteparin is characterized by a higher ratio of antifactor Xa to antifactor IIa activity (ratio = 4)
Pharmacodynamics/Kinetics
Onset of action: Anti-Xa activity: Within 1-2 hours
Duration: >12 hours
Distribution: V_d: 40-60 mL/kg
Protein binding: Low affinity for plasma proteins (Howard, 1997)
Bioavailability: SubQ: 81% to 93%
Half-life elimination (route dependent): Anti-Xa activity: 2-5 hours; prolonged in chronic renal insufficiency: 3.7-7.7 hours (following a single 5000 unit dose)
Time to peak, serum: Anti-Xa activity: ~4 hours
Excretion: Primarily renal (Howard, 1997)

◄ **Dosage**

Geriatric & Adult Note: Each 2500 units of anti-Xa activity is equal to 16 mg of dalteparin.

Anticoagulant for hemodialysis and hemofiltration: I.V.: Canadian labeling (not in U.S. labeling):

Chronic renal failure with no other bleeding risks:

Hemodialysis/filtration ≤4 hours: I.V. bolus: 5,000 units

Hemodialysis/filtration >4 hours: I.V. bolus: 30-40 units/kg, followed by an infusion of 10-15 units/kg/hour (typically produces plasma concentrations of 0.5-1 units anti-Xa/mL)

Acute renal failure and high bleeding risk: I.V. bolus: 5-10 units/kg, followed by an infusion of 4-5 units/kg/hour (typically produces plasma concentrations of 0.2-0.4 units anti-Xa/mL)

DVT prophylaxis: Note: In morbidly obese patients (BMI ≥40 kg/m^2), increasing the prophylactic dose by 30% may be appropriate (Nutescu, 2009):

Abdominal surgery:

Low-to-moderate DVT risk: SubQ: 2500 units 1-2 hours prior to surgery, then once daily for 5-10 days postoperatively

High DVT risk: SubQ: 5000 units the evening prior to surgery and then once daily for 5-10 days postoperatively. Alternatively in patients with malignancy: 2500 units 1-2 hours prior to surgery, 2500 units 12 hours later, then 5000 units once daily for 5-10 days postoperatively.

General surgery with risk factors for VTE: Canadian labeling (not in U.S. labeling):
2500 units 1-2 hours preoperatively followed by 2500-5000 int.units every morning (may administer 2500 units no sooner than 4 hours after surgery and 8 hours after previous dose provided hemostasis has been achieved) or if other risk factors are present (eg, malignancy, heart failure), then may administer 5000 units the evening prior to surgery followed by 5000 units every evening postoperatively; continue treatment until patient is mobilized (approximately ≥5-7 days)

Total hip replacement surgery: SubQ: **Note:** Three treatment options are currently available. Dose is given for 5-10 days, although up to 14 days of treatment have been tolerated in clinical trials. The American College of Chest Physicians (ACCP) recommends a minimum duration of at least 10-14 days; extended duration of up to 35 days is suggested (Guyatt, 2012).

Postoperative regimen:

Initial: 2500 units 4-8 hours after surgery (or later if hemostasis not achieved). The ACCP recommends initiation ≥12 hours after surgery if postoperative regimen chosen (Guyatt, 2012).

Maintenance: 5000 int. units once daily; allow at least 6 hours to elapse after initial postsurgical dose (adjust administration time accordingly)

Preoperative regimen (starting day of surgery):

Initial: 2500 int. units within 2 hours **before** surgery. The ACCP recommends initiation ≥12 hours before surgery if preoperative regimen chosen (Guyatt, 2012). At 4-8 hours **after** surgery (or later if hemostasis not achieved), administer 2500 int. units.

Maintenance: 5000 units once daily; allow at least 6 hours to elpase after initial postsurgical dose (adjust administration time accordingly)

Preoperative regimen (starting evening prior to surgery):

Initial: 5000 int. units 10-14 hours **before** surgery. The ACCP recommends initiation ≥12 hours before surgery if preoperative regimen chosen (Guyatt, 2012). At 4-8 hours **after** surgery (or later if hemostasis not achieved), administer 5000 int. units.

Maintenance: 5000 int. units once daily, allowing 24 hours between doses

Immobility during acute illness: 5000 units once daily

Unstable angina or non-Q-wave myocardial infarction: SubQ: 120 units/kg body weight (maximum dose: 10,000 units) every 12 hours for up to 5-8 days with concurrent aspirin therapy. Discontinue dalteparin once patient is clinically stable.

Obesity: Use actual body weight to calculate dose; dose capping at 10,000 units recommended (Nutescu, 2009)

Venous thromboembolism, extended treatment in cancer patients: SubQ:

Initial (month 1): 200 units/kg (maximum dose: 18,000 units) once daily for 30 days

Maintenance (months 2-6): ~150 units/kg (maximum dose: 18,000 units) once daily. If platelet count between 50,000-100,000/mm^3, reduce dose by 2,500 units until platelet count recovers to ≥100,000/mm^3. If platelet count <50,000/mm^3, discontinue dalteparin until platelet count recover to >50,000/mm^3.

Obesity: Use actual body weight to calculate dose; dose capping is not recommended (Nutescu, 2009). However, the manufacturer recommends a maximum dose of 18,000 units per day for the treatment of VTE in cancer patients.

DVT (with or without PE) treatment in noncancer patients (unlabeled use in U.S.): SubQ: 200 units/kg once daily (Feissinger, 1996; Jaff, 2011; Wells, 2005) **or** 100 units/kg twice daily (Jaff, 2011). Use of once daily administration is suggested (Guyatt, 2012).

Canadian labeling: SubQ: 200 units/kg once daily (maximum dose: 18,000 units/day) **or** alternatively, may adapt dose as follows (SubQ):
46-56 kg: 10,000 units once daily
57-68 kg: 12,500 units once daily
69-82 kg: 15,000 units once daily
≥83 kg: 18,000 units once daily
Note: If increased bleeding risk, may give 100 units/kg SubQ twice daily. Concomitant treatment with a vitamin-K antagonist is usually initiated immediately.

Obesity: Use actual body weight to calculate dose; dose capping is not recommended (Nutescu, 2009). One study demonstrated similar anti-Xa levels after 3 days of therapy in obese patients (>40% above IBW; range: 82-190 kg) compared to those ≤20% above IBW or between 20% to 40% above IBW (Wilson, 2001).

Renal Impairment Half-life is increased in patients with chronic renal failure, use with caution, accumulation can be expected; specific dosage adjustments have not been recommended. Accumulation was not observed in critically ill patients with severe renal insufficiency (Cl$_{cr}$ <30 mL/minute) receiving prophylactic doses (5000 units) for a median of 7 days (Douketis, 2008). In cancer patients, receiving treatment for venous thromboembolism, if Cl$_{cr}$ <30 mL/minute, manufacturer recommends monitoring anti-Xa levels to determine appropriate dose.

Hepatic Impairment No dosage adjustment provided in manufacturer's labeling; use with caution.

Administration

For deep SubQ injection; may be injected in a U-shape to the area surrounding the navel, the upper outer side of the thigh, or the upper outer quadrangle of the buttock. Use thumb and forefinger to lift a fold of skin when injecting dalteparin to the navel area or thigh. Insert needle at a 45- to 90-degree angle. The entire length of needle should be inserted. Do not expel air bubble from fixed-dose syringe prior to injection. Air bubble (and extra solution, if applicable) may be expelled from graduated syringes. In order to minimize bruising, do not rub injection site.

To convert from I.V. unfractionated heparin (UFH) infusion to SubQ dalteparin (Nutescu, 2007): Calculate specific dose for dalteparin based on indication, discontinue UFH and begin dalteparin within 1 hour

To convert from SubQ dalteparin to I.V. UFH infusion (Nutescu, 2007): Discontinue dalteparin; calculate specific dose for I.V. UFH infusion based on indication; omit heparin bolus/ loading dose

Converting from SubQ dalteparin dosed every 12 hours: Start I.V. UFH infusion 10-11 hours after last dose of dalteparin

Converting from SubQ dalteparin dosed every 24 hours: Start I.V. UFH infusion 22-23 hours after last dose of dalteparin

I.V. (Canadian labeling; not an approved route in U.S. labeling): Administer as bolus I.V. injection or as continuous infusion. Recommended concentration for infusion: 20 units/mL.

Monitoring Parameters Periodic CBC including platelet count; stool occult blood tests; monitoring of PT and PTT is not necessary. Once patient has received 3-4 doses, anti-Xa levels, drawn 4-6 hours after dalteparin administration, may be used to monitor effect in patients with severe renal dysfunction or if abnormal coagulation parameters or bleeding should occur. For patients >190 kg, if anti-Xa monitoring is available, adjusting dose based on anti-Xa levels is recommended; if anti-Xa monitoring is unavailable, reduce dose if bleeding occurs (Nutescu, 2009).

Reference Range Treatment of venous thromboembolism: Peak anti-Xa concentration target (measured 4 hours after administration): *Once-daily dosing:* 1.05 anti-Xa units/mL (Garcia, 2012); per the manufacturer, target anti-Xa range is 0.5-1.5 units/mL (measured 4-6 hours after administration and after patient received 3-4 doses)

Special Geriatric Considerations No specific recommendations are necessary for the elderly.

Dosage Forms Excipient information presented when available (limited, particularly for generics); consult specific product labeling.
Injection, solution:
Fragmin®: 25,000 anti-Xa units/mL (3.8 mL) [contains benzyl alcohol]
Injection, solution [preservative free]:
Fragmin®: 10,000 anti-Xa units/mL (1 mL); 2500 anti-Xa units/0.2 mL (0.2 mL); 5000 anti-Xa units/0.2 mL (0.2 mL); 7500 anti-Xa units/0.3 mL (0.3 mL); 12,500 anti-Xa units/0.5 mL (0.5 mL); 15,000 anti-Xa units/0.6 mL (0.6 mL); 18,000 anti-Xa units/0.72 mL (0.72 mL)

◆ **Dalteparin Sodium** see Dalteparin on page 476

Danaparoid (da NAP a roid)

Medication Safety Issues

Sound-alike/look-alike issues:

Orgaran® may be confused with argatroban

Brand Names: Canada Orgaran®

Index Terms Danaparoid Sodium

Pharmacologic Category Anticoagulant; Heparinoid

Use Prevention of postoperative deep vein thrombosis (DVT) following orthopedic or major abdominal and thoracic surgery; prevention of DVT in patients with confirmed diagnosis of non-hemorrhagic stroke; management of heparin-induced thrombocytopenia (HIT)

Contraindications Hypersensitivity to danaparoid, or any component of the formulation (including sulfites); history of thrombocytopenia while receiving danaparoid or when associated with a positive *in vitro* test for antiplatelet antibodies in the presence of danaparoid; hemorrhagic stroke (without systemic emboli); acute hemorrhagic stroke; patients with active major bleeding; severe hemorrhagic diathesis (hemophilia, idiopathic thrombocytopenic purpura); acute or subacute bacterial endocarditis; active gastric or duodenal ulcer; surgery of CNS, eyes, or ears; diabetic or hemorrhagic retinopathy; severe uncontrolled hypertension; other conditions or diseases that increase risk of hemorrhage; not for I.M. use

Warnings/Precautions Hemorrhagic stroke should be ruled out by CT scan prior to initiating therapy. Do not administer intramuscularly.

Spinal or epidural hematomas, including subsequent paralysis, may occur with recent or anticipated neuraxial anesthesia (epidural or spinal anesthesia) or spinal puncture in patients anticoagulated with LMWH or heparinoids. Consider risk versus benefit prior to spinal procedures; risk is increased by the use of concomitant agents which may alter hemostasis, the use of indwelling epidural catheters for analgesia, a history of spinal deformity or spinal surgery, as well as a history of traumatic or repeated epidural or spinal punctures. Spinal procedures should be avoided for 12 hours after the last danaparoid dose; allow at least 2 hours after procedure before resuming danaparoid therapy. Patient should be observed closely for bleeding and signs and symptoms of neurological impairment if therapy is administered during or immediately following diagnostic lumbar puncture, epidural anesthesia, or spinal anesthesia.

Use with caution in patients with history of peptic ulcer disease, hepatic impairment, and severe renal impairment. Monitor patient closely for signs or symptoms of bleeding. Certain patients are at increased risk of bleeding (eg, severe hepatic disease, patients undergoing knee surgery or other invasive procedures, concomitant therapy with platelet inhibitors, elderly). Discontinue use if bleeding occurs. Danaparoid is not effectively antagonized by protamine sulfate. No other antidote is available, so extreme caution is needed in monitoring dose given and resulting Xa inhibition effect.

Use caution in patients with or with a history of thrombocytopenia (heparin-induced, congenital) or platelet defects. The manufacturer's labeling recommends that patients with a history of heparin-induced thrombocytopenia be tested for cross-reactivity with danaparoid prior to initiating therapy; if test is positive, alternative therapy should be employed unless otherwise not available. If danaparoid is administered, therapy must be discontinued immediately with clinical signs of positive cross-reactivity (eg, increased reduction in platelet counts, thrombosis, skin necrosis). May resume therapy (if needed) only after laboratory confirmed negative test for danaparoid activated antiplatelet antibodies. Cutaneous allergy tests may help detect the presence of cross-reactivity between heparins and danaparoid (Grassegger, 2001).

Safety and efficacy have not been established for use as thromboprophylaxis in patients with prosthetic heart valves. Heparin can cause hyperkalemia by affecting aldosterone. A similar reaction could occur with danaparoid. Monitor for hyperkalemia. Not to be used interchangeably (unit for unit) with heparin or any other low molecular weight heparins.

This product contains sodium sulfite which may cause allergic-type reactions, including anaphylactic symptoms and life-threatening asthmatic episodes in susceptible people; this is seen more frequently in asthmatics.

Adverse Reactions (Reflective of adult population; not specific for elderly) As with all anticoagulants, bleeding is the major adverse effect of danaparoid. Hemorrhage may occur at virtually any site. Risk is dependent on multiple variables.

Frequency not always defined.

Cardiovascular: Arterial pressure decreased, atrial fibrillation, cerebral infarction, DVT, hypotension, peripheral edema

Central nervous system: Pain (5%), fever (2% to 5%), confusion, fatigue, insomnia, loss of consciousness, restlessness

Dermatologic: Rash (1%), bruising

Gastrointestinal: Nausea (3%), constipation (2%)

Genitourinary: Urinary retention (1%), urinary incontinence

Hematologic: Cerebral hemorrhage, hematoma, hemorrhage, spinal or epidural hematomas (may occur following neuraxial anesthesia or spinal puncture, resulting in paralysis), thrombocytopenia

Hepatic: Alkaline phosphatase increased, ALT increased (transient), AST increased (transient)

Local: Injection site hematoma (≤5%)

Neuromuscular & skeletal: Hemiparesis, involuntary muscle contractions, tremor

Renal: Hematuria

Respiratory: Apnea, asthma

Miscellaneous: Infection (2%), allergic reaction, sepsis

Drug Interactions

Metabolism/Transport Effects None known.

Avoid Concomitant Use

Avoid concomitant use of Danaparoid with any of the following: Rivaroxaban

Increased Effect/Toxicity

Danaparoid may increase the levels/effects of: Anticoagulants; Collagenase (Systemic); Dabigatran Etexilate; Deferasirox; Drotrecogin Alfa (Activated); Ibritumomab; Rivaroxaban; Tositumomab and Iodine I 131 Tositumomab

The levels/effects of Danaparoid may be increased by: Antiplatelet Agents; Dasatinib; Herbs (Anticoagulant/Antiplatelet Properties); Nonsteroidal Anti-Inflammatory Agents; Pentosan Polysulfate Sodium; Prostacyclin Analogues; Salicylates; Thrombolytic Agents; Tipranavir

Decreased Effect There are no known significant interactions involving a decrease in effect.

Ethanol/Nutrition/Herb Interactions Herb/Nutraceutical: Avoid cat's claw, dong quai, evening primrose, feverfew, garlic, ginger, ginkgo, red clover, horse chestnut, green tea, and ginseng (all have additional antiplatelet activity).

Stability Store at 2°C to 30°C (36°F to 86°F). Protect from light. Stable for up to 48 hours in the following I.V. solutions: D5NS, NS, Ringer's, LR, mannitol.

Mechanism of Action Inhibits factor Xa and IIa (anti-Xa effects >20 times anti-IIa effects). Prevents fibrin formation in the coagulation pathway via thrombin generation inhibition.

Pharmacodynamics/Kinetics

Onset of action: Peak effect: SubQ: Maximum antifactor Xa activities occur in 4-5 hours

Bioavailability: SubQ: ~100%

Half-life elimination: Anti-Xa activity: ~25 hours (renal impairment: 29-35 hours); Thrombin generation inhibition activity: ~7 hours

Excretion: Primarily urine

Dosage

Geriatric & Adult Note: Dosing recommendations per manufacturer's labeling unless otherwise noted. Dose expressed as anti-Xa units.

Prevention of DVT following orthopedic, major abdominal, or thoracic surgery: SubQ: 750 units twice daily for up to 14 days; it is recommended that patients begin prophylactic therapy preoperatively and receive their last preoperative dose 1-4 hours before surgery.

Prevention of DVT in stroke (nonhemorrhagic):

Initial: I.V.: Up to 1000 units as single dose

Maintenance: SubQ: 750 units every 12 hours for 7-14 days

Heparin-induced thrombocytopenia (HIT):

Prevention of DVT (with current or past HIT): **Note:** May administer I.V. bolus of 1250 units if clinically necessary (ie, current HIT) or may initiate maintenance regimen without a bolus as follows:

SubQ:

≤90 kg: Current HIT or past HIT: 750 units every 8-12 hours for 7-10 days

>90 kg: Current HIT: 1250 units every 8-12 hours for 7-10 days; Past HIT: 1250 units every 12 hours or 750 units every 8 hours for 7-10 days

Treatment of DVT/PE (see also Linkins, 2012):

Initial I.V. bolus: Thrombosis <5 days old: ≤55 kg: 1250-1500 units; 55-90 kg: 2250-2500 units; >90 kg: 3750 units; followed by a maintenance I.V. infusion or maintenance SubQ injections. **Note:** If thrombosis is ≥5 days old, administer an I.V. bolus dose of 1250 units followed by maintenance SubQ injections.

Maintenance: I.V. infusion (after I.V. bolus administered): Thrombosis <5 days old: 400 units/hour for 4 hours, then 300 units/hour for 4 hours, then 150-200 units/hour for 5-7 days; adjust rate according to target anti-Xa levels

or

Maintenance: SubQ injections (after I.V. bolus administered):

Thrombosis <5 days old: ≤55 kg: 1500 units every 12 hours; 55-90 kg: 2000 units every 12 hours; >90 kg: 1750 units every 8 hours for 4-7 days.

Thrombosis ≥5 days old: ≤90 kg: 750 units every 8-12 hours; >90 kg: 750 units every 8 hours or 1250 units every 8-12 hours

HIT/surgical thromboprophylaxis:

Nonvascular surgery: SubQ:

≤90 kg: 750 units 1-4 hours preoperatively and at ≥6 hours postop, followed by 750 units every 12 hours beginning day 1 post-op and continued for 7-10 days

>90 kg: 750 units 1-4 hours preoperatively and at ≥6 hours postop, followed by 750 units every 8 hours or 1250 units every 12 hours beginning day 1 post-op and continued for 7-10 days

Embolectomy:

55-90 kg: I.V.: 2250-2500 units as a bolus preoperatively, followed by SubQ: 1250 units every 12 hours beginning ≥6 hours postop. **Note:** After several days of I.V. therapy, may switch to SubQ: 750 units every 8-12 hours or oral anticoagulant therapy.

>90 kg: I.V.: 2250-2500 units as a bolus preoperatively, followed by 150-200 units/hour beginning ≥6 hours post-op for 5-7 days. **Note:** After several days of I.V. therapy, may switch to SubQ: 750 units every 8-12 hours or oral anticoagulant therapy.

HIT/cardiac procedures: Note: Other therapies may be preferred (eg, bivalirudin); long half-life and irreversibility of danaparoid make it a poor choice in these settings. Refer to product labeling for dosing recommendations.

Catheter patency: Mix 750 units with 50 mL normal saline. Flush catheter with 5-10 mL of resulting solution as needed.

Conversion to oral anticoagulant therapy (OAC): Establish adequate antithrombotic effect with danaparoid prior to initiation of oral anticoagulant (OAC) therapy. PT/INR should be therapeutic before discontinuing use of danaparoid. **Note:** Laboratory values taken within 5 hours of danaparoid administration may be unreliable.

Conversion of SubQ danaparoid to OAC (based on current danaparoid dose):

Danaparoid 750 units every 12 hours: Initiate OAC and maintain danaparoid therapy until PT/INR is therapeutic; may take up to 5 days.

Danaparoid 1250 units every 12 hours: Initiate OAC and decrease danaparoid to 750 units every 12 hours; maintain danaparoid therapy until PT/INR is therapeutic; may take up to 5 days.

Conversion of I.V. danaparoid to OAC: Initiate OAC with concurrent danaparoid I.V. infusion (maximum 300 units/hour); discontinue I.V. infusion once INR is therapeutic (maximum INR: 3.0). If bleeding risk is present, I.V. infusion should be reduced to 75 units/hour and OAC initiation withheld for 24 hours **or** danaparoid I.V. infusion may be switched to subcutaneous route at a dose of 1250 units every 12 hours and the recommended conversion of SubQ danaparoid to OAC regimen followed (ie, subsequent reduction to 750 units every 12 hours while OAC initiated).

Renal Impairment Note: Danaparoid half-life is significantly prolonged in renal impairment; anti-Xa levels should be closely monitored. Dosage reduction, especially with maintenance doses, may be required.

Mild or moderate impairment: There are no dosage adjustments provided in manufacturer's labeling.

Severe impairment (serum creatinine ≥220 micromol/L [≥2.5 mg/dL]): Following initial dose, dose reductions or temporary discontinuation of therapy may be necessary to prevent accumulation of plasma anti-Xa (indicated by consistent, steady state-plasma anti-Xa activity >0.5 anti-Xa units).

Hemodialysis: Adults: I.V.: 1500-3750 units before dialysis session. **Note:** Dose depends on frequency of dialysis regimen (eg, daily dialysis vs every-other-day or less frequently) and weight of patient with the lower dose recommended for patients <55 kg. Do not administer prior to dialysis if plasma antifactor Xa levels >400 units/L and not receiving daily dialysis; however, if fibrin threads are present in bubble chamber may administer 1500 units.

Hemofiltration: Adults: I.V.: 55-90 kg: 2500 units as a bolus, followed by 600 units/hour for 4 hours, then 400 units/hour for 4 hours, then 200-600 units/hour to maintain adequate anti-Xa levels. **Note:** If patient is <55 kg, reduce bolus dose to 2000 units, followed by 400 units/hour for 4 hours, then 150-400 units/hour to maintain adequate anti-Xa levels.

Hepatic Impairment There are no dosage adjustments provided in manufacturer's labeling.

Administration May administer intravenously as bolus or infusion, or by subcutaneous injection. When administered intravenously, do not mix with other drugs. For subcutaneous administration, rotate injection sites. Do **not** administer intramuscularly.

Dosage

Geriatric & Adult

Skin and/or skin structure infections (complicated): I.V.: 4 mg/kg once daily for 7-14 days

Bacteremia, right-sided native valve endocarditis caused by MSSA or MRSA: I.V.: 6 mg/kg once daily for 2-6 weeks (some experts recommend 8-10 mg/kg once daily for complicated bacteremia or infective endocarditis [Liu, 2011])

Osteomyelitis (unlabeled use): I.V.: 6 mg/kg once daily for a minimum of 8 weeks (some experts combine with rifampin) (Liu, 2011)

Septic arthritis (unlabeled use): I.V.: 6 mg/kg once daily for 3-4 weeks (Liu, 2011)

Renal Impairment

Cl_{cr} <30 mL/minute:

Skin and soft tissue infections: 4 mg/kg every 48 hours

Staphylococcal bacteremia: 6 mg/kg every 48 hours

Intermittent hemodialysis or peritoneal dialysis (PD): Dose as in Cl_{cr} <30 mL/minute (administer after hemodialysis on dialysis days) or (unlabeled dosing) may administer 6 mg/kg after hemodialysis 3 times weekly (Salama, 2010)

Note: High permeability intermittent hemodialysis removes ~50% during a 4-hour session (Salama, 2010).

Continuous renal replacement therapy (CRRT) (Heintz, 2009; Trotman, 2005): Drug clearance is highly dependent on the method of renal replacement, filter type, and flow rate. Appropriate dosing requires close monitoring of pharmacologic response, signs of adverse reactions due to drug accumulation, as well as drug concentrations in relation to target trough (if appropriate). The following are general recommendations only (based on dialysate flow/ultrafiltration rates of 1-2 L/hour and minimal residual renal function) and should not supersede clinical judgment:

Continuous veno-venous hemodialysis (CVVHD): 8 mg/kg every 48 hours (Vilay, 2010)

Note: For other forms of CRRT (eg, CVVH or CVVHDF), dosing as with Cl_{cr}<30 mL/minute may result in low C_{max}. May consider 4-6 mg/kg every 24 hours (or 8 mg/kg every 48 hours) depending on site or severity of infection or if not responding to standard dosing; therapeutic drug monitoring and/or more frequent serum CPK levels may be necessary (Heintz, 2009).

Slow extended daily dialysis (or extended dialysis): 6 mg/kg every 24 hours (Kielstein, 2010); **Note:** Dialysis should be initiated within 8 hours of administering daptomycin dose to avoid dose accumulation.

Hepatic Impairment No adjustment required for mild-to-moderate impairment (Child-Pugh class A or B). Not evaluated in severe hepatic impairment (Child-Pugh class C).

Administration May administer I.V. push over 2 minutes or infuse IVPB over 30 minutes. Do not use in conjunction with ReadyMED® elastomeric infusion pumps (Cardinal Health, Inc) due to an impurity (2-mercaptobenzothiazole) leaching from the pump system into the daptomycin solution.

Monitoring Parameters Monitor signs and symptoms of infection. CPK should be monitored at least weekly during therapy; more frequent monitoring if current or prior statin therapy, unexplained CPK increases, and/or renal impairment. Monitor for muscle pain or weakness, especially if noted in distal extremities. Canadian labeling recommends CPK monitoring every 48 hours with unexplained muscle pain, tenderness, weakness or cramps. Monitor for signs/symptoms of eosinophilic pneumonia.

Reference Range

Trough concentrations at steady-state:

4 mg/kg once daily: 5.9 ± 1.6 mcg/mL

6 mg/kg once daily: 6.7 ± 1.6 mcg/mL

Note: Trough concentrations are not predictive of efficacy/toxicity. Drug exhibits concentration-dependent bactericidal activity, so C_{max}:MIC ratios may be a more useful parameter.

Test Interactions Daptomycin may cause false prolongation of the PT and increase of INR with certain reagents. This appears to be a dose-dependent phenomenon. Therefore, it is recommended to obtain blood samples immediately prior to next daptomycin dose (eg, trough). If PT/INR elevated, clinicians should repeat PT/INR and evaluate for other causes of hypocoagulation.

Special Geriatric Considerations The manufacturer reports that in studies of complicated skin and skin structure infections, elderly patients had a lower clinical success rate and a higher incidence of adverse effects (no quantitative data provided in product labeling). Adjust dose in renal impairment.

Dosage Forms Excipient information presented when available (limited, particularly for generics); consult specific product labeling.

Injection, powder for reconstitution:

Cubicin®: 500 mg

Darbepoetin Alfa (dar be POE e tin AL fa)

Medication Safety Issues
Sound-alike/look-alike issues:
Aranesp® may be confused with Aralast, Aricept®
Darbepoetin alfa may be confused with dalteparin, epoetin alfa, epoetin beta
Brand Names: U.S. Aranesp®; Aranesp® SingleJect®
Brand Names: Canada Aranesp®
Index Terms Erythropoiesis-Stimulating Agent (ESA); Erythropoiesis-Stimulating Protein; NESP; Novel Erythropoiesis-Stimulating Protein
Generic Availability (U.S.) No
Pharmacologic Category Colony Stimulating Factor; Erythropoiesis-Stimulating Agent (ESA); Growth Factor; Recombinant Human Erythropoietin
Use Treatment of anemia due to concurrent myelosuppressive chemotherapy in patients with cancer (nonmyeloid malignancies) receiving chemotherapy (palliative intent) for a planned minimum of 2 additional months of chemotherapy; treatment of anemia due to chronic kidney disease (including patients on dialysis and not on dialysis)

Note: Darbepoetin is **not** indicated for use under the following conditions:
- Cancer patients receiving hormonal therapy, therapeutic biologic products, or radiation therapy unless also receiving concurrent myelosuppressive chemotherapy
- Cancer patients receiving myelosuppressive chemotherapy when the expected outcome is curative
- As a substitute for RBC transfusion in patients requiring immediate correction of anemia

Note: In clinical trials, darbepoetin has not demonstrated improved quality of life, fatigue, or well-being.

Unlabeled Use Treatment of symptomatic anemia in myelodysplastic syndrome (MDS)
Prescribing and Access Restrictions As a requirement of the REMS program, access to this medication is restricted. Healthcare providers and hospitals must be enrolled in the ESA APPRISE (Assisting Providers and Cancer Patients with Risk Information for the Safe use of ESAs) Oncology Program (866-284-8089; http://www.esa-apprise.com) to prescribe or dispense ESAs (ie, darbepoetin alfa, epoetin alfa) to patients with cancer.
Medication Guide Available Yes
Contraindications Hypersensitivity to darbepoetin or any component of the formulation; uncontrolled hypertension; pure red cell aplasia (due to darbepoetin or other erythropoietin protein drugs)
Warnings/Precautions [U.S. Boxed Warning]: Erythropoiesis-stimulating agents (ESAs) increased the risk of serious cardiovascular events, thromboembolic events, stroke, and/or tumor progression in clinical studies when administered to target hemoglobin levels >11 g/dL (and provide no additional benefit); a rapid rise in hemoglobin (>1 g/dL over 2 weeks) may also contribute to these risks. **[U.S. Boxed Warning]: A shortened overall survival and/or increased risk of tumor progression or recurrence has been reported in studies with breast, cervical, head and neck, lymphoid, and nonsmall cell lung cancer patients.** It is of note that in these studies, patients received ESAs to a target hemoglobin of ≥12 g/dL; although risk has not been excluded when dosed to achieve a target hemoglobin of <12 g/dL. **[U.S. Boxed Warnings]: To decrease these risks, and risk of cardio- and thrombovascular events, use ESAs in cancer patients only for the treatment of anemia related to concurrent myelosuppressive chemotherapy and use the lowest dose needed to avoid red blood cell transfusions. Discontinue ESA following completion of the chemotherapy course. ESAs are not indicated for patients receiving myelosuppressive therapy when the anticipated outcome is curative.** A dosage modification is appropriate if hemoglobin levels rise >1 g/dL per 2-week time period during treatment (Rizzo, 2010). Use of ESAs has been associated with an increased risk of venous thromboembolism (VTE) without a reduction in transfusions in patients >65 years of age with cancer (Hershman, 2009). Improved anemia symptoms, quality of life, fatigue, or well-being have not been demonstrated in controlled clinical trials. **[U.S. Boxed Warning]: Because of the risks of decreased survival and increased risk of tumor growth or progression, all healthcare providers and hospitals are required to enroll and comply with the ESA APPRISE (Assisting Providers and Cancer Patients with Risk Information for the Safe use of ESAs) Oncology Program prior to prescribing or dispensing ESAs to cancer patients.** Prescribers and patients will have to provide written documentation of discussed risks prior to each course.

[U.S. Boxed Warning]: An increased risk of death, serious cardiovascular events, and stroke was reported in patients with chronic kidney disease (CKD) administered ESAs to target hemoglobin levels ≥11 g/dL; use the lowest dose sufficient to reduce the need

for RBC transfusions. An optimal target hemoglobin level, dose or dosing strategy to reduce these risks has not been identified in clinical trials. Hemoglobin rising >1 g/dL in a 2-week period may contribute to the risk (dosage reduction recommended). CKD patients who exhibit an inadequate hemoglobin response to ESA therapy may be at a higher risk for cardiovascular events and mortality compared to other patients. ESA therapy may reduce dialysis efficacy (due to increase in red blood cells and decrease in plasma volume); adjustments in dialysis parameters may be needed. Patients treated with epoetin may require increased heparinization during dialysis to prevent clotting of the extracorporeal circuit. CKD patients not requiring dialysis may have a better response to darbepoetin and may require lower doses. An increased risk of DVT has been observed in patients treated with epoetin undergoing surgical orthopedic procedures. Darbepoetin is **not** approved for reduction in allogeneic red blood cell transfusions in patients scheduled for surgical procedures. The risk for seizures is increased with darbepoetin use in patients with CKD; use with caution in patients with a history of seizures. Monitor closely for neurologic symptoms during the first several months of therapy. Use with caution in patients with hypertension; hypertensive encephalopathy has been reported. Use is contraindicated in patients with uncontrolled hypertension. If hypertension is difficult to control, reduce or hold darbepoetin alfa. Due to the delayed onset of erythropoiesis, darbepoetin alfa is **not** recommended for acute correction of severe anemia or as a substitute for emergency transfusion. Consider discontinuing in patients who receive a renal transplant.

Prior to treatment, correct or exclude deficiencies of iron, vitamin B_{12}, and/or folate, as well as other factors which may impair erythropoiesis (inflammatory conditions, infections, bleeding). Prior to and during therapy, iron stores must be evaluated. Supplemental iron is recommended if serum ferritin <100 mcg/L or serum transferrin saturation <20%; most patients with CKD will require iron supplementation. Poor response should prompt evaluation of these potential factors, as well as possible malignant processes and hematologic disease (thalassemia, refractory anemia, myelodysplastic disorder), occult blood loss, hemolysis, osteitis fibrosa cystic, and/or bone marrow fibrosis. Severe anemia and pure red cell aplasia (PRCA) with associated neutralizing antibodies to erythropoietin has been reported, predominantly in patients with CKD receiving SubQ darbepoetin (the I.V. route is preferred for hemodialysis patients). Cases have also been reported in patients with hepatitis C who were receiving ESAs, interferon, and ribavirin. Patients with a sudden loss of response to darbepoetin (with severe anemia and a low reticulocyte count) should be evaluated for PRCA with associated neutralizing antibodies to erythropoietin; discontinue treatment (permanently) in patients with PRCA secondary to neutralizing antibodies to erythropoietin. Antibodies may cross-react; do not switch to another ESA in patients who develop antibody-mediated anemia.

Potentially serious allergic reactions have been reported (rarely). Discontinue immediately (and permanently) in patients who experience serious allergic/anaphylactic reactions. Some products may contain albumin and the packaging of some formulations may contain latex.

Adverse Reactions (Reflective of adult population; not specific for elderly)
>10%:
  Cardiovascular: Hypertension (31%), peripheral edema (17%), edema (6% to 13%)
  Gastrointestinal: Abdominal pain (10% to 13%)
  Respiratory: Dyspnea (17%), cough (12%)
1% to 10%:
  Cardiovascular: Angina, fluid overload, hypotension, MI, thromboembolic events
  Central nervous system: Cerebrovascular disorder
  Dermatologic: Rash/erythema
  Local: AV graft thrombosis, vascular access complications
  Respiratory: Pulmonary embolism
Drug Interactions
  Metabolism/Transport Effects None known.
  Avoid Concomitant Use There are no known interactions where it is recommended to avoid concomitant use.
  Increased Effect/Toxicity There are no known significant interactions involving an increase in effect.
  Decreased Effect There are no known significant interactions involving a decrease in effect.
Ethanol/Nutrition/Herb Interactions Ethanol: Should be avoided due to adverse effects on erythropoiesis.
Stability Store at 2°C to 8°C (36°F to 46°F); do not freeze. Do not shake. Protect from light. Store in original carton until use. The following stability information has also been reported: May be stored at room temperature for up to 7 days (Cohen, 2007). Do not dilute or administer with other solutions.

DARBEPOETIN ALFA

Mechanism of Action Induces erythropoiesis by stimulating the division and differentiation of committed erythroid progenitor cells; induces the release of reticulocytes from the bone marrow into the bloodstream, where they mature to erythrocytes. There is a dose response relationship with this effect. This results in an increase in reticulocyte counts followed by a rise in hematocrit and hemoglobin levels. When administered SubQ or I.V., darbepoetin's half-life is ~3 times that of epoetin alfa concentrations.

Pharmacodynamics/Kinetics

Onset of action: Increased hemoglobin levels not generally observed until 2-6 weeks after initiating treatment

Absorption: SubQ: Slow

Distribution: V_d: 0.06 L/kg

Bioavailability: CKD: SubQ: Adults: ~37% (range: 30% to 50%)

Half-life elimination:
CKD: Adults:
I.V.: 21 hours
SubQ: Nondialysis patients: 70 hours (range: 35-139 hours); Dialysis patients: 46 hours (range: 12-89 hours)
Cancer: Adults: SubQ: 74 hours (range: 24-144 hours)
Note: Darbepoetin half-life is approximately threefold longer than epoetin alfa following I.V. administration

Time to peak: SubQ:
CKD: Adults: 48 hours (range: 12-72 hours; independent of dialysis)
Cancer: Adults: 71-90 hours (range: 28-123 hours)

Dosage

Geriatric & Adult

Anemia associated with chronic kidney disease (CKD): Individualize dosing and use the lowest dose necessary to reduce the need for RBC transfusions.

Chronic kidney disease patients **ON** *dialysis* (I.V. route is preferred for hemodialysis patients; initiate treatment when hemoglobin is <10 g/dL; reduce dose or interrupt treatment if hemoglobin approaches or exceeds 11 g/dL): I.V., SubQ: Initial: 0.45 mcg/kg once weekly **or** 0.75 mcg/kg once every 2 weeks **or** epoetin alfa doses of <1500 to ≥90,000 units per week may be converted to doses ranging from 6.25-200 mcg darbepoetin alfa per week (see adult column in conversion table below).

Chronic kidney disease patients **NOT** *on dialysis* (consider initiating treatment when hemoglobin is <10 g/dL; use only if rate of hemoglobin decline would likely result in RBC transfusion and desire is to reduce risk of alloimmunization or other RBC transfusion-related risks; reduce dose or interrupt treatment if hemoglobin exceeds 10 g/dL): I.V., SubQ: Initial: 0.45 mcg/kg once every 4 weeks

Dosage adjustments for chronic kidney disease patients (either on dialysis or not on dialysis): Do not increase dose more frequently than every 4 weeks (dose decreases may occur more frequently).

If hemoglobin increases >1 g/dL in any 2-week period: Decrease dose by ≥25%

If hemoglobin does not increase by >1 g/dL after 4 weeks: Increase dose by 25%

Inadequate or lack of response: If adequate response is not achieved over 12 weeks, further increases are unlikely to be of benefit and may increase the risk for adverse events; use the minimum effective dose that will maintain a hemoglobin level sufficient to avoid red blood cell transfusions **and** evaluate patient for other causes of anemia; discontinue treatment if responsiveness does not improve

Anemia due to chemotherapy in cancer patients: Initiate treatment only if hemoglobin <10 g/dL and anticipated duration of myelosuppressive chemotherapy is ≥2 months. Titrate dosage to use the minimum effective dose that will maintain a hemoglobin level sufficient to avoid red blood cell transfusions. Discontinue darbepoetin following completion of chemotherapy.

SubQ: Initial: 2.25 mcg/kg once weekly **or** 500 mcg once every 3 weeks until completion of chemotherapy

Dosage adjustments:

Increase dose: If hemoglobin does not increase by 1 g/dL **and** remains below 10 g/dL after initial 6 weeks (for patients receiving weekly therapy only), increase dose to 4.5 mcg/kg once weekly (no dosage adjustment if using every 3 week dosing).

Reduce dose by 40% if hemoglobin increases >1g/dL in any 2-week period **or** hemoglobin reaches a level sufficient to avoid red blood cell transfusion.

Withhold dose if hemoglobin exceeds a level needed to avoid red blood cell transfusion. Resume treatment with a 40% dose reduction when hemoglobin approaches a level where transfusions may be required.

Discontinue: On completion of chemotherapy or if after 8 weeks of therapy there is no hemoglobin response or RBC transfusions still required

Symptomatic anemia associated with MDS (unlabeled use): SubQ: 150-300 mcg once weekly (NCCN MDS guidelines v.2.2011)

Conversion from epoetin alfa to darbepoetin alfa: See table.

Conversion From Epoetin Alfa to Darbepoetin Alfa (Initial Dose)

Previous Dosage of Epoetin Alfa (units/week)	Children Darbepoetin Alfa Dosage (mcg/week)	Adults Darbepoetin Alfa Dosage (mcg/week)
<1500	Not established	6.25
1500-2499	6.25	6.25
2500-4999	10	12.5
5000-10,999	20	25
11,000-17,999	40	40
18,000-33,999	60	60
34,000-89,999	100	100
≥90,000	200	200

Note: In patients receiving epoetin alfa 2-3 times per week, darbepoetin alfa is administered once weekly. In patients receiving epoetin alfa once weekly, darbepoetin alfa is administered once every 2 weeks. The darbepoetin dose to be administered every 2 weeks is derived by adding together 2 weekly epoetin alfa doses and then converting to the appropriate darbepoetin dose. Titrate dose to hemoglobin response thereafter.

Administration May be administered by SubQ or I.V. injection. The I.V. route is recommended in hemodialysis patients. Do not shake; vigorous shaking may denature darbepoetin alfa, rendering it biologically inactive. Do not dilute or administer in conjunction with other drug solutions. Discard any unused portion of the vial; do not pool unused portions.

Monitoring Parameters Hemoglobin (at least once per week until maintenance dose established and after dosage changes; monitor less frequently once hemoglobin is stabilized); CKD patients should be also be monitored at least monthly following hemoglobin stability); iron stores (transferrin saturation and ferritin) prior to and during therapy; serum chemistry (CKD patients); blood pressure; fluid balance (CKD patients); seizures (CKD patients following initiation for first few months, includes new-onset or change in seizure frequency or premonitory symptoms)

Cancer patients: Examinations recommended by the ASCO/ASH guidelines (Rizzo, 2010) prior to treatment include peripheral blood smear (in some situations a bone marrow exam may be necessary), assessment for iron, folate, or vitamin B_{12} deficiency, reticulocyte count, renal function status, and occult blood loss; during ESA treatment, assess baseline and periodic iron, total iron-binding capacity, and transferrin saturation or ferritin levels.

Pharmacotherapy Pearls Oncology Comment: The American Society of Clinical Oncology (ASCO) and American Society of Hematology (ASH) 2010 updates to the clinical practice guidelines for the use of erythropoiesis-stimulating agents (ESAs) in patients with cancer indicate that ESAs are appropriate when used according to the parameters identified within the Food and Drug Administration (FDA) approved labeling for epoetin and darbepoetin (Rizzo, 2010). ESAs are an option for chemotherapy associated anemia when the hemoglobin has fallen to <10 g/dL to decrease the need for RBC transfusions. ESAs should only be used in conjunction with concurrent chemotherapy. Although the FDA label now limits ESA use to the palliative setting, the ASCO/ASH guidelines suggest using clinical judgment in weighing risks versus benefits as formal outcomes studies of ESA use defined by intent of chemotherapy treatment have not been conducted.

The ASCO/ASH guidelines continue to recommend following the FDA approved dosing (and dosing adjustment) guidelines as alternate dosing and schedules have not demonstrated consistent differences in effectiveness with regard to hemoglobin response. In patients who do not have a response within 6-8 weeks (hemoglobin rise <1-2 g/dL or no reduction in transfusions) ESA therapy should be discontinued.

Prior to the initiation of ESAs, other sources of anemia (in addition to chemotherapy or underlying hematologic malignancy) should be investigated. Examinations recommended prior to treatment include peripheral blood smear (in some situations a bone marrow exam may be necessary), assessment for iron, folate, or vitamin B_{12} deficiency, reticulocyte count, renal function status, and occult blood loss. During ESA treatment, assess baseline and periodic iron, total iron-binding capacity, and transferrin saturation or ferritin levels. Iron supplementation may be necessary.

The guidelines note that patients with an increased risk of thromboembolism (generally includes previous history of thrombosis, surgery, and/or prolonged periods of immobilization) and patients receiving concomitant medications that may increase thromboembolic risk, should begin ESA therapy only after careful consideration. With the exception of low-risk myelodysplasia-associated anemia (which has evidence supporting the use of ESAs without concurrent chemotherapy), the guidelines do not support the use of ESAs in the absence of concurrent chemotherapy.

Special Geriatric Considerations Endogenous erythropoietin secretion has been reported to be decreased in elderly with normocytic or iron deficiency anemias or those with a serum hemoglobin concentration <12 g/dL; one study did not find such a relationship in the elderly with chronic anemia. A blunted erythropoietin response to anemia has been reported in patients with cancer, rheumatoid arthritis, and AIDS.

Dosage Forms Excipient information presented when available (limited, particularly for generics); consult specific product labeling.

Injection, solution [preservative free]:
Aranesp®: 25 mcg/mL (1 mL); 40 mcg/mL (1 mL); 60 mcg/mL (1 mL); 100 mcg/mL (1 mL); 150 mcg/0.75 mL (0.75 mL); 200 mcg/mL (1 mL); 300 mcg/mL (1 mL) [contains polysorbate 80]
Aranesp® SingleJect®: 25 mcg/0.42 mL (0.42 mL); 40 mcg/0.4 mL (0.4 mL); 60 mcg/0.3 mL (0.3 mL); 100 mcg/0.5 mL (0.5 mL); 150 mcg/0.3 mL (0.3 mL); 200 mcg/0.4 mL (0.4 mL); 300 mcg/0.6 mL (0.6 mL); 500 mcg/mL (1 mL) [contains natural rubber/natural latex in packaging, polysorbate 80]

Darifenacin (dar i FEN a sin)

Related Information
Beers Criteria – Potentially Inappropriate Medications for Geriatrics on page 2183
Pharmacotherapy of Urinary Incontinence on page 2141
Medication Safety Issues
BEERS Criteria medication:
This drug may be potentially inappropriate for use in geriatric patients (Quality of evidence - varies based on comorbidity; Strength of recommendation - varies based on comorbidity)
Brand Names: U.S. Enablex®
Brand Names: Canada Enablex®
Index Terms Darifenacin Hydrobromide; UK-88,525
Generic Availability (U.S.) No
Pharmacologic Category Anticholinergic Agent
Use Management of symptoms of bladder overactivity (urge incontinence, urgency, and frequency)
Contraindications Hypersensitivity to darifenacin or any component of the formulation; uncontrolled narrow-angle glaucoma; urinary retention, paralytic ileus, GI or GU obstruction
Warnings/Precautions May cause drowsiness and/or blurred vision, which may impair physical or mental abilities; patients must be cautioned about performing tasks which require mental alertness (eg, operating machinery or driving). May occur in the presence of increased environmental temperature; use caution in hot weather and/or exercise. Use with caution with hepatic impairment; dosage limitation is required in moderate hepatic impairment (Child-Pugh class B). Not recommended for use in severe hepatic impairment (Child-Pugh class C). Use with caution in patients with clinically-significant bladder outlet obstruction or prostatic hyperplasia (nonobstructive). Use caution in patients with decreased GI motility, constipation, hiatal hernia, reflux esophagitis, and ulcerative colitis. Use caution in patients with myasthenia gravis. In patients with controlled narrow-angle glaucoma, darifenacin should be used with extreme caution and only when the potential benefit outweighs risks of treatment. Use with caution in patients taking strong CYP3A4 inhibitors (see Drug Interactions); dosage limitation of darifenacin is required. This medication is associated with potent anticholinergic properties which may be inappropriate in older adults depending on comorbidities (eg, dementia, delirium) (Beers Criteria).
Adverse Reactions (Reflective of adult population; not specific for elderly)
>10%: Gastrointestinal: Xerostomia (19% to 35%), constipation (15% to 21%)
1% to 10%:
Cardiovascular: Hypertension (≥1%), peripheral edema (≥1%)
Central nervous system: Headache (7%), dizziness (<2%), pain (≥1%)
Dermatological: Dry skin (≥1%), pruritus (≥1%), rash (≥1%)
Gastrointestinal: Dyspepsia (3% to 8%), abdominal pain (2% to 4%), nausea (2% to 4%), vomiting (≥1%), weight gain (≥1%)

Genitourinary: Urinary tract infection (4% to 5%), vaginitis (≥1%), urinary retention (acute)
Neuromuscular & skeletal: Weakness (<3%), arthralgia (≥1%), back pain (≥1%)
Ocular: Dry eyes (2%), abnormal vision (≥1%)
Respiratory: Bronchitis (≥1%), pharyngitis (≥1%), rhinitis (≥1%), sinusitis (≥1%)
Miscellaneous: Flu-like syndrome (1% to 3%)

Drug Interactions

Metabolism/Transport Effects Substrate of CYP2D6 (minor), CYP3A4 (major); **Note:** Assignment of Major/Minor substrate status based on clinically relevant drug interaction potential; **Inhibits** CYP2D6 (moderate), CYP3A4 (weak)

Avoid Concomitant Use

Avoid concomitant use of Darifenacin with any of the following: Conivaptan; Pimozide; Thioridazine

Increased Effect/Toxicity

Darifenacin may increase the levels/effects of: AbobotulinumtoxinA; Anticholinergics; ARI-Piprazole; Cannabinoids; CYP2D6 Substrates; Fesoterodine; Nebivolol; Onabotulinumtoxin-inA; Pimozide; Potassium Chloride; RimabotulinumtoxinB; Thioridazine

The levels/effects of Darifenacin may be increased by: Conivaptan; CYP3A4 Inhibitors (Moderate); CYP3A4 Inhibitors (Strong); Dasatinib; Ivacaftor; Mifepristone; Pramlintide; Propafenone

Decreased Effect

Darifenacin may decrease the levels/effects of: Acetylcholinesterase Inhibitors (Central); Codeine; Secretin; Tamoxifen; TraMADol

The levels/effects of Darifenacin may be decreased by: Acetylcholinesterase Inhibitors (Central); CYP3A4 Inducers (Strong); Deferasirox; Herbs (CYP3A4 Inducers); Peginterferon Alfa-2b; Tocilizumab

Ethanol/Nutrition/Herb Interactions Herb/Nutraceutical: Darifenacin serum concentration may be decreased by St John's wort (avoid concurrent use.)

Stability Store at 25°C (77°F); excursions permitted to 15°C to 30°C (59°F to 86°F). Protect from light.

Mechanism of Action Selective antagonist of the M3 muscarinic (cholinergic) receptor subtype. Blockade of the receptor limits bladder contractions, reducing the symptoms of bladder irritability/overactivity (urge incontinence, urgency and frequency).

Pharmacodynamics/Kinetics

Distribution: V_{dss}: ~163 L
Protein binding: ~98% (primarily alpha$_1$-acid glycoprotein)
Metabolism: Hepatic, via CYP3A4 (major) and CYP2D6 (minor)
Bioavailability: 15% to 19%
Half-life elimination: ~13-19 hours
Time to peak, plasma: ~7 hours
Excretion: As metabolites (inactive); urine (60%), feces (40%)

Dosage

Geriatric & Adult

Symptoms of bladder overactivity: Oral: Initial: 7.5 mg once daily. If response is not adequate after a minimum of 2 weeks, dosage may be increased to 15 mg once daily.

Dosage adjustment with concomitant potent CYP3A4 inhibitors (eg, azole antifungals, erythromycin, isoniazid, protease inhibitors): Daily dosage should not exceed 7.5 mg/day

Renal Impairment No adjustment required.

Hepatic Impairment

Moderate impairment (Child-Pugh class B): Daily dosage should not exceed 7.5 mg/day
Severe impairment (Child-Pugh class C): Has not been evaluated; use is not recommended

Administration Tablet should be taken with liquid and swallowed whole; do not chew, crush, or split tablet. May be taken without regard to food.

Special Geriatric Considerations There is a trend for decreased clearance of darifenacin with age, though no change in dose is recommended. The selectivity of darifenacin for the M3 receptor on the bladder may offer an advantage (less CNS and cardiovascular effects) over other anticholinergic agents used in the treatment of overactive bladder.

This medication is considered to be potentially inappropriate in this patient population (Beers Criteria: Quality of evidence - varies based on comorbidity; Strength of recommendation - varies based on comorbidity)

Dosage Forms Excipient information presented when available (limited, particularly for generics); consult specific product labeling.
Tablet, extended release, oral:
Enablex®: 7.5 mg, 15 mg

◆ **Darifenacin Hydrobromide** *see* Darifenacin *on page 492*
◆ **1-Day™ [OTC]** *see* Tioconazole *on page 1906*

- ◆ **Daypro®** *see* Oxaprozin *on page 1435*
- ◆ **Daytrana®** *see* Methylphenidate *on page 1247*
- ◆ **DDAVP®** *see* Desmopressin *on page 511*
- ◆ **DDrops® [OTC]** *see* Cholecalciferol *on page 365*
- ◆ **DDrops® Baby [OTC]** *see* Cholecalciferol *on page 365*
- ◆ **DDrops® Kids [OTC]** *see* Cholecalciferol *on page 365*
- ◆ **1-Deamino-8-D-Arginine Vasopressin** *see* Desmopressin *on page 511*
- ◆ **Debrox® [OTC]** *see* Carbamide Peroxide *on page 291*
- ◆ **Decadron** *see* Dexamethasone (Systemic) *on page 517*
- ◆ **Decavac® [DSC]** *see* Diphtheria and Tetanus Toxoids *on page 562*
- ◆ **Declomycin** *see* Demeclocycline *on page 500*
- ◆ **Deep Sea [OTC]** *see* Sodium Chloride *on page 1787*

Deferasirox (de FER a sir ox)

Medication Safety Issues
Sound-alike/look-alike issues:
Deferasirox may be confused with deferiprone, deferoxamine
Brand Names: U.S. Exjade®
Brand Names: Canada Exjade®
Index Terms ICL670
Generic Availability (U.S.) No
Pharmacologic Category Chelating Agent
Use Treatment of chronic iron overload due to blood transfusions (transfusional hemosiderosis)
Prescribing and Access Restrictions Deferasirox (Exjade®) is only available through a restricted distribution program called EPASS™ Complete Care. Prescribers must enroll patients in this program in order to obtain the medication. For patient enrollment, contact 1-888-90-EPASS (1-888-903-7277).
Contraindications Hypersensitivity to deferasirox or any component of the formulation; platelet counts <50,000/mm^3; poor performance status and high-risk myelodysplastic syndromes or advanced malignancies; creatinine clearance <40 mL/minute or serum creatinine >2 x age-appropriate ULN

Canadian labeling: Additional contraindications (not in U.S. labeling): Cl$_{cr}$ <60 mL/minute
Warnings/Precautions [U.S. Boxed Warning]: Renal impairment and renal failure (some fatal) have been reported; observed more frequently in elderly patients, high-risk myelodysplastic syndromes (MDS), underlying renal dysfunction, and/or other comorbidities. Monitor serum creatinine and/or creatinine clearance at baseline and monthly thereafter; in patients with underlying renal dysfunction or at risk for renal dysfunction, monitor weekly during the first month. Dose reduction, interruption, or discontinuation should be considered for serum creatinine elevations; interrupt for progressive increases beyond the upper limit of normal; may reinitiate with dose reduction once serum creatinine returns to age-appropriate normal range. Monitor closely if creatinine clearance is between 40-<60 mL/minute. Acute renal failure (some have required dialysis) has been reported; generally occurs in patients with multiple comorbidities. May cause proteinuria; closely monitor. Renal tubulopathy has also been reported, primarily in pediatric patients with β-thalassemia and serum ferritin levels <1500 mcg/L.

[U.S. Boxed Warning]: Hepatic dysfunction or failure (including fatalities) have occurred; observed more frequently in elderly patients, high-risk myelodysplastic syndromes (MDS), underlying hepatic dysfunction, and/or other comorbidities. Monitor transaminases and bilirubin at baseline, every 2 weeks for 1 month, then monthly thereafter. Hepatitis and elevated transaminases have also been reported. Avoid use in severe hepatic impairment, reduce dose for moderate impairment, and monitor closely in mild or moderate impairment. **[U.S. Boxed Warning]: Gastrointestinal (GI) hemorrhage, including fatalities, has occurred with use; observed more frequently in elderly patients with high-risk myelodysplastic syndromes (MDS) and/or low platelet counts (<50,000/mm^3).** Other GI effects including irritation and ulceration have been reported. Use caution with concurrent medications that may increase risk of adverse GI effects (eg, NSAIDs, corticosteroids, anticoagulants, oral bisphosphonates). Monitor patients closely for signs/symptoms of GI ulceration/bleeding.

May cause skin rash (dose-related), including erythema multiforme; mild-to-moderate rashes may resolve without treatment interruption; for severe rash, interrupt and consider restarting at a lower dose with dose escalation and use of steroids. Hypersensitivity reactions, including severe reactions (anaphylaxis and angioedema) have been reported, onset is usually within the first month of treatment; discontinue if severe. Auditory (decreased hearing and high frequency hearing loss) or ocular disturbances (lens opacities, cataracts, intraocular pressure elevation, and retinal disorders) have been reported (rare); monitor and consider dose reduction or treatment interruption. Cytopenias (including agranulocytosis, neutropenia, and thrombocytopenia) have been reported, predominately in patients with preexisting hematologic disorders; monitor blood counts regularly; interrupt treatment for unexplained cytopenias (may reinitiate once cause of cytopenia has been excluded). Potent UGT inducers (eg, rifampin) or cholestyramine may decrease the efficacy of deferasirox; avoid concomitant use. If coadministration necessary, dosage modifications may be needed; monitor serum ferritin and clinical response. Not approved for use in combination with other iron chelation therapies; safety of combinations has not been established. Treatment should be initiated with evidence of chronic iron overload (eg, transfusion of ~100 mL/kg of packed RBCs [~20 units for a 40 kg individual] and serum ferritin consistently >1000 mcg/L). Prior to use, consider risk versus anticipated benefit with respect to individual patient's life expectancy and prognosis. Use with caution in the elderly due to the higher incidence of hepatic, renal and cardiac dysfunction in the elderly.

Adverse Reactions (Reflective of adult population; not specific for elderly)

>10%:
  Central nervous system: Fever (19%), headache (16%)
  Dermatologic: Rash (dose related; 8% to 11%)
  Gastrointestinal: Abdominal pain (dose related; 21% to 28%), diarrhea (dose related; 12% to 20%), nausea (dose related; 11% to 23%), vomiting (dose related; 10% to 21%)
  Renal: Serum creatinine increased (dose related; 7% to 38%), proteinuria (19%)
  Respiratory: Cough (14%), nasopharyngitis (13%), pharyngolaryngeal pain (11%)
  Miscellaneous: Influenza (11%)

1% to 10%:
  Central nervous system: Fatigue (6%)
  Dermatologic: Urticaria (4%)
  Hepatic: ALT increased (2% to 8%), transaminitis (4%)
  Neuromuscular & skeletal: Arthralgia (7%), back pain (6%)
  Otic: Ear infection (5%)
  Respiratory: Respiratory tract infection (10%), bronchitis (9%), pharyngitis (8%), acute tonsillitis (6%), rhinitis (6%)

Drug Interactions

Metabolism/Transport Effects Substrate of UGT1A1; **Inhibits** CYP1A2 (moderate), CYP2C8 (moderate); **Induces** CYP3A4 (weak/moderate)

Avoid Concomitant Use

Avoid concomitant use of Deferasirox with any of the following: Aluminum Hydroxide; Axitinib; Theophylline

Increased Effect/Toxicity

Deferasirox may increase the levels/effects of: CYP1A2 Substrates; CYP2C8 Substrates; Repaglinide; Theophylline

The levels/effects of Deferasirox may be increased by: Anticoagulants; Bisphosphonate Derivatives; Corticosteroids; Corticosteroids (Systemic); Nonsteroidal Anti-Inflammatory Agents

Decreased Effect

Deferasirox may decrease the levels/effects of: ARIPiprazole; Axitinib; CYP3A4 Substrates; Saxagliptin

The levels/effects of Deferasirox may be decreased by: Aluminum Hydroxide; Cholestyramine Resin; Fosphenytoin; PHENobarbital; Phenytoin; Rifampin; Ritonavir

Ethanol/Nutrition/Herb Interactions Food: Bioavailability is increased variably when taken with food. Management: Take on an empty stomach at the same time each day at least 30 minutes before food. Maintain adequate hydration, unless instructed to restrict fluid intake.

Stability Store at room temperature of 25°C (77°F); excursions permitted to 15°C and 30°C (59°F and 86°F). Protect from moisture.

Mechanism of Action Selectively binds iron, forming a complex which is excreted primarily through the feces.

Pharmacodynamics/Kinetics

Distribution: Adults: 14.4 ± 2.7L
Protein binding: ~99% to serum albumin
Metabolism: Hepatic via glucuronidation by UGT1A1(primarily) and UGT1A3; minor oxidation by CYP450; undergoes enterohepatic recirculation
Bioavailability: 70%
Half-life elimination: 8-16 hours
Time to peak, plasma: ~1.5-4 hours
Excretion: Feces (84%); urine (8%)

◀ **Dosage**

Geriatric & Adult Chronic iron overload due to blood transfusion: Oral: **Note:** Baseline serum ferritin and iron levels should be obtained prior to therapy; toxicity may be increased in patients with low iron burden or with only slightly elevated serum ferritin.

Initial: 20 mg/kg daily (calculate dose to nearest whole tablet); administer as a suspension (see **Administration**)

Maintenance: Adjust dose every 3-6 months based on serum ferritin trends; adjust by 5 or 10 mg/kg/day (calculate dose to nearest whole tablet); titrate to individual response and treatment goals. Usual range: 20-30 mg/kg/day; doses up to 40 mg/kg/day may be considered for serum ferritin levels persistently >2500 mcg/L (doses above 40 mg/kg/day are not recommended). **Note:** Consider interrupting therapy for serum ferritin <500 mcg/L and dose reduction or interruption for hearing loss or visual disturbances.

Dosage adjustment with concomitant cholestyramine or potent UGT inducers (eg, rifampin, phenytoin, phenobarbital, ritonavir): Avoid concomitant use; if coadministration necessary, consider increasing the initial dose of deferasirox dose to 30 mg/kg; monitor serum ferritin and clinical response. Doses above 40 mg/kg are not recommended.

Renal Impairment

Cl_{cr} ≥60 mL/minute: No initial adjustment necessary. Monitor renal function; increases in serum creatinine may require alteration or discontinuation of therapy.

Cl_{cr} ≥40 to <60 mL/minute: No initial adjustment necessary. Use caution; monitor renal function closely, particularly in patients at increased risk for further renal impairment (eg, concomitant nephrotoxic therapy, dehydration, severe infection); increases in serum creatinine may require alteration or discontinuation of therapy.

Cl_{cr} <40 mL/minute or serum creatinine >2 times age-appropriate ULN: Use is contra-indicated.

Increase in serum creatinine: Consider dose reduction, interruption, or discontinuation.

Progressive increase in serum creatinine above the age-appropriate ULN: Interrupt treatment; once serum creatinine recovers to within the normal range, reinitiate treatment at a reduced dose; gradually escalate the dose if the clinical benefit outweighs potential risk.

Adults: For increase in serum creatinine >33% above the average pretreatment level for 2 consecutive levels (and cannot be attributed to other causes), reduce daily dose by 10 mg/kg

Hepatic Impairment

Mild hepatic impairment (Child-Pugh class A): No adjustment necessary. Monitor closely for efficacy and for adverse reactions requiring dosage reduction.

Moderate hepatic impairment (Child-Pugh class B): Reduce dose by 50%; monitor closely for efficacy and for adverse reactions requiring dosage reduction.

Severe hepatic impairment (Child-Pugh class C): Avoid use.

Administration Oral: **Do not chew or swallow whole tablets.** Completely disperse tablets in water, orange juice, or apple juice (use 3.5 ounces for total doses <1 g; 7 ounces for doses ≥1 g); stir to form a fine suspension and drink entire contents. Rinse remaining residue with more fluid; drink. Administer at same time each day on an empty stomach, 30 minutes before food. Do not take simultaneously with aluminum-containing antacids.

Monitoring Parameters Serum ferritin (baseline, monthly thereafter), iron levels (baseline), CBC with differential, serum creatinine and/or creatinine clearance (2 baseline assessments then monthly thereafter; in patients who are at increased risk of complications [eg, pre-existing renal conditions, elderly, comorbid conditions, or receiving other potentially nephrotoxic medications]: weekly for the first month then monthly thereafter); urine protein (monthly); serum transaminases and bilirubin (baseline, every 2 weeks for the first month, then monthly); baseline and annual auditory and ophthalmic function (including slit lamp examinations and dilated fundoscopy); performance status (in patients with hematologic malignancies); signs and symptoms of GI ulcers or hemorrhage; number of RBC units received

Pharmacotherapy Pearls Deferasirox has a low affinity for binding with zinc and copper, may cause variable decreases in the serum concentration of these trace minerals.

Oncology Comment: The National Comprehensive Cancer Network (NCCN) guidelines for myelodysplastic syndromes (MDS) recommend considering iron chelation therapy in low- or intermediate-risk MDS patients to decrease iron overload due to multiple transfusions (v.2.2011). Treatment is generally recommended in MDS patients who have received >20-30 RBC transfusions and for those with serum ferritin levels >2500 mcg/L, with a goal to decrease ferritin levels to <1000 mcg/L.

Special Geriatric Considerations The majority of subjects ≥65 years of age studied have had myelodysplastic syndrome. In general, geriatric patients experienced a higher frequency of adverse events (compared to younger patients). Use caution in patients with mild-to-moderate liver dysfunction or low serum albumin. Monitor renal function. In general, this drug should be used with caution and close monitoring in elderly due to the greater incidence of decreased hepatic, renal, and cardiac function, as well as concomitant disease and drug therapy.

Dosage Forms Excipient information presented when available (limited, particularly for generics); consult specific product labeling.
Tablet for suspension, oral:
Exjade®: 125 mg, 250 mg, 500 mg

Deferiprone (de FER i prone)

Medication Safety Issues
Sound-alike/look-alike issues:
Deferiprone may be confused with deferoxamine, deferasirox
Brand Names: U.S. Ferriprox®
Index Terms APO-066; Ferriprox®
Pharmacologic Category Chelating Agent
Use Treatment of transfusional iron overload due to thalassemia syndromes with inadequate response to other chelation therapy
Medication Guide Available Yes
Contraindications Hypersensitivity to deferiprone or any component of the formulation
Warnings/Precautions [U.S. Boxed Warning]: May cause agranulocytosis, which may lead to serious infections (some fatal). Neutropenia may precede agranulocytosis; monitor absolute neutrophil count (ANC) prior to treatment initiation and weekly during therapy. If infection develops, interrupt treatment and monitor ANC more frequently. Patients should promptly report any symptoms which may indicate infection. Interrupt treatment if neutropenia (ANC <1500/mm^3) develops; withhold other medications which may also be associated with neutropenia; monitor CBC, corrected WBC, ANC, and platelets daily until ANC recovery. If ANC <500/mm^3, consider hospitalization (and other clinically appropriate management); do not resume or rechallenge unless the potential benefits outweigh potential risks. Neutropenia and agranulocytosis were generally reversible upon discontinuation. Avoid concurrent use with other agents associated with neutropenia (or agranulocytosis).

ALT elevations in have been observed; monitor ALT and consider treatment interruption for persistent elevations. Use with caution in patients at risk for QT prolongation (eg, bradycardia, cardiac hypertrophy, congestive HF, diuretic use, hypokalemia or hypomagnesemia). There has been a single case report of torsade de pointes in a patient with a history of QT prolongation. Patients should promptly report any symptoms suggestive of arrhythmias (eg, dizziness, light headedness, palpitations, seizure or syncope). Lower plasma zinc concentrations have been observed; monitor zinc levels and supplement if necessary.

Adverse Reactions (Reflective of adult population; not specific for elderly)
>10%:
Gastrointestinal: Nausea (13%)
Genitourinary: Chromaturia (15%)
1% to 10%:
Central nervous system: Headache (3%)
Gastrointestinal: Abdominal pain/discomfort (10%), vomiting (10%), appetite increased (4%), diarrhea (3%), dyspepsia (2%), weight gain (2%), appetite decreased (1%)
Hematologic: Neutropenia (6% to 7%), agranulocytosis (2%)
Hepatic: ALT increased (8%), AST increased (1%)
Neuromuscular and skeletal: Arthralgia (10%), back pain (2%), limb pain (2%), arthropathy (1%)
Drug Interactions
Metabolism/Transport Effects Substrate of UGT1A6, UGT1A9, UGT2B15, UGT2B7
Avoid Concomitant Use There are no known interactions where it is recommended to avoid concomitant use.
Increased Effect/Toxicity
The levels/effects of Deferiprone may be increased by: UGT1A6 Inhibitors
Decreased Effect
The levels/effects of Deferiprone may be decreased by: Antacids; Calcium Salts; Iron Salts; Magnesium Salts; Zinc Salts
Ethanol/Nutrition/Herb Interactions Herb/Nutraceutical: Deferiprone may bind with polyvalent cations (eg, aluminum, zinc). Allow at least 4 hours between other medications or supplements containing polyvalent cations.
Stability Store at 20°C to 25°C (68°F to 77°F); excursions permitted to 15°C to 30°C (59°F to 86°F).
Mechanism of Action Iron-chelating agent with affinity for ferric ion (iron III); binds to ferric ion and forms a 3:1 (deferiprone:iron) complex which is excreted in the urine. Has a lower affinity for other metals such as copper, aluminum, and zinc.

◀ **Pharmacodynamics/Kinetics**
Absorption: Rapid
Distribution: 1.6 L/kg (in thalassemia patients)
Protein binding: <10%
Metabolism: Primarily by UGT 1A6; major metabolite (3-O-glucuronide) lacks iron-binding capacity
Half life elimination: 1.9 hours
Time to peak: ~1-2 hours
Excretion: Urine (75% to 90%; as free deferiprone, the iron deferiprone complex, and glucuronide metabolite)

Dosage
Geriatric Refer to adult dosing. Begin at the low end of dosing range.
Adult Note: Round dose to the nearest 250 mg (or 1/2 tablet). If serum ferritin falls consistently below 500 mcg/L, consider temporary treatment interruption.
Transfusional iron overload: Oral: Initial: 25 mg/kg 3 times/day (75 mg/kg/day); individualize dose based on response and therapeutic goal; maximum dose: 33 mg/kg 3 times/day (99 mg/kg/day)
Renal Impairment No dosage adjustments are provided in the manufacturer's labeling (has not been studied).
Hepatic Impairment No dosage adjustments are provided in the manufacturer's labeling (has not been studied).
Administration Administer in the morning, at mid day and in the evening. Administration with food may decrease nausea.
Monitoring Parameters Serum ferritin (every 2-3 months); ANC (at baseline and weekly during treatment); if ANC <1500/mm^3, monitor CBC, WBC (corrected for nucleated RBCs), ANC, and platelets daily until ANC recovery; ALT (monthly); zinc levels; symptoms suggestive of QT prolongation; signs or symptoms of infection
Special Geriatric Considerations The elderly may be at risk for infection due to age-related declines in their immune system function or due to drug therapy which decreases their immune competence. Patients should report any symptoms of infections, including fever, sore throat, or cough.
Dosage Forms Excipient information presented when available (limited, particularly for generics); consult specific product labeling.
Tablet, oral:
Ferriprox®: 500 mg [scored]

Degarelix (deg a REL ix)

Medication Safety Issues
Sound-alike/look-alike issues:
Degarelix may be confused with cetrorelix, ganirelix
Brand Names: U.S. Firmagon®
Brand Names: Canada Firmagon®
Index Terms Degarelix Acetate; FE200486
Generic Availability (U.S.) No
Pharmacologic Category Antineoplastic Agent, Gonadotropin-Releasing Hormone Antagonist; Gonadotropin Releasing Hormone Antagonist
Use Treatment of advanced prostate cancer
Contraindications Hypersensitivity to degarelix or any component of the formulation
Warnings/Precautions Hazardous agent - use appropriate precautions for handling and disposal. Long-term androgen deprivation therapy may prolong the QT interval; use with caution in patients with a known history of QT prolongation or other risk factors for QT prolongation (eg, concomitant use of medications known to prolong QT interval, heart failure, and/or electrolyte abnormalities). Androgen-deprivation therapy may increase the risk for cardiovascular disease (Levine, 2010) and decreased bone mineral density. Androgen deprivation therapy may cause obesity and insulin resistance; the risk for diabetes is increased.

Degarelix exposure is decreased in patients with hepatic impairment, dosage adjustment is not recommended in patients with mild-to-moderate hepatic impairment, although testosterone levels should be monitored. Has not been studied in patients with severe hepatic impairment; use with caution. Data for use in patients with moderate-to-severe renal impairment (Cl_{cr} <50 mL/minute) is limited; use with caution.

Adverse Reactions (Reflective of adult population; not specific for elderly)

>10%:

Endocrine & metabolic: Hot flashes (26%)

Local: Injections site reactions (35%, grade 3: ≤2%; pain 28%, erythema 17%, swelling 6%, induration 4%, nodule 3%)

1% to 10%:

Cardiovascular: Hypertension (6%)

Central nervous system: Chills (5%), dizziness (1% to 5%), fever (1% to 5%), headache (1% to 5%), insomnia (1% to 5%), fatigue (3%)

Dermatologic: Hyperhydrosis

Endocrine & metabolic: Hypercholesterolemia (3%), gynecomastia, testicular atrophy

Gastrointestinal: Weight gain (9%), constipation (5%), nausea (1% to 5%), diarrhea

Genitourinary: Urinary tract infection (5%), erectile dysfunction

Hepatic: ALT increased (10%; grade 3: <1%), AST increased (5%; grade 3: <1%), GGT increased

Neuromuscular & skeletal: Back pain (6%), arthralgia (5%), weakness (1% to 5%)

Miscellaneous: Antidegarelix antibody formation (10%), night sweats (1% to 5%)

Drug Interactions

Metabolism/Transport Effects None known.

Avoid Concomitant Use

Avoid concomitant use of Degarelix with any of the following: Highest Risk QTc-Prolonging Agents; Mifepristone

Increased Effect/Toxicity

Degarelix may increase the levels/effects of: Highest Risk QTc-Prolonging Agents; Moderate Risk QTc-Prolonging Agents

The levels/effects of Degarelix may be increased by: Mifepristone; QTc-Prolonging Agents (Indeterminate Risk and Risk Modifying)

Decreased Effect There are no known significant interactions involving a decrease in effect.

Stability Store at 25°C (77°F); excursions permitted to 15°C to 30°C (59°F to 86°F). Use appropriate precautions (wear gloves for preparation and administration) for handling and disposal. Reconstitute with preservative free sterile water for injection (reconstitute each 120 mg vial with 3 mL; reconstitute the 80 mg vial with 4.2 mL). Swirl gently; do not shake (to prevent foaming). Dissolution may take up to 15 minutes. Keep vial upright at all times. Tilt vial slightly, keeping needle in lowest section of vial to withdraw for administration. Administer within 1 hour of reconstitution.

Mechanism of Action Gonadotropin-releasing hormone (GnRH) antagonist which reversibly binds to GnRH receptors in the anterior pituitary gland, blocking the receptor and decreasing secretion of luteinizing hormone (LH) and follicle stimulation hormone (FSH), resulting in rapid androgen deprivation by decreasing testosterone production, thereby decreasing testosterone levels. Testosterone levels do not exhibit an initial surge, or flare, as is typical with GnRH agonists.

Pharmacodynamics/Kinetics

Onset of action: Rapid; ~96% of patients had testosterone levels ≤50 ng/dL within 3 days (Klotz, 2008)

Distribution: V_d: >1000 L

Protein binding: ~90%

Metabolism: Hepatobiliary, via peptide hydrolysis

Bioavailability: Biphasic release: Rapid release initially, then slow release from depot formed after subcutaneous injection administration (Tornoe, 2007)

Half-life elimination: Loading dose: SubQ: ~53 days

Time to peak, plasma: Loading dose: SubQ: Within 2 days

Excretion: Feces (~70% to 80%, primarily as peptide fragments); urine (~20% to 30%)

Dosage

Geriatric & Adult Prostate cancer: SubQ:

Loading dose: 240 mg administered as two 120 mg (3 mL) injections

Maintenance dose: 80 mg every 28 days (beginning 28 days after initial loading dose)

Renal Impairment Cl_{cr} <50 mL/minute: Use with caution.

Hepatic Impairment

Mild-to-moderate hepatic impairment: No adjustment required; monitor serum testosterone levels.

Severe hepatic impairment: Has not been studied; use with caution.

Administration Not for I.V. use. Administer SubQ in the abdominal area by grasping skin and elevating SubQ tissue; insert the needle deeply at an angle not ≤45 degrees. Avoid pressure exposed areas (eg, waistband, belt, or near ribs); rotate injection site. Inject loading dose as two 3 mL injections (40 mg/mL); maintenance dose should be administered as a single 4 mL injection (20 mg/mL); begin maintenance dose 28 days after initial loading dose.

◀ **Monitoring Parameters** Prostate-specific antigen (PSA) periodically, serum testosterone levels (if PSA increases; in patients with hepatic impairment: monitor testosterone levels monthly until achieve castration levels, then consider monitoring every other month), liver function tests (at baseline), serum electrolytes (calcium, magnesium, potassium, sodium); bone mineral density

Screen for diabetes and cardiovascular risk prior to initiating treatment.

Test Interactions Suppression of pituitary-gonadal function may affect diagnostic tests of pituitary gonadotropic and gonadal functions.

Special Geriatric Considerations No dosage adjustments are necessary in elderly. Monitor serum lipids and for hypertension.

Dosage Forms Excipient information presented when available (limited, particularly for generics); consult specific product labeling.
Injection, powder for reconstitution, as acetate:
   Firmagon®: 80 mg, 120 mg

Demeclocycline (dem e kloe SYE kleen)

Index Terms Declomycin; Demeclocycline Hydrochloride; Demethylchlortetracycline
Generic Availability (U.S.) Yes
Pharmacologic Category Antibiotic, Tetracycline Derivative
Use Treatment of susceptible bacterial infections (eg, acne, urinary tract infections, respiratory infections) caused by both gram-negative and gram-positive organisms
   Note: Use of demeclocycline as an antibacterial agent is uncommon; alternative tetracycline agents (eg, doxycycline, minocycline, tetracycline) are generally preferred.
Unlabeled Use Treatment of chronic syndrome of inappropriate secretion of antidiuretic hormone (SIADH)
Contraindications Hypersensitivity to demeclocycline, tetracyclines, or any component of the formulation; concomitant use with methoxyflurane
Warnings/Precautions Photosensitivity reactions occur frequently with this drug; avoid prolonged exposure to sunlight and do not use tanning equipment. Use caution in patients with renal or hepatic impairment (eg, elderly); dosage modification required in patients with renal impairment. May act as an antianabolic agent and increase BUN. Pseudotumor cerebri has been reported with tetracycline use (usually resolves with discontinuation). Outdated drug can cause nephropathy. Prolonged use may result in fungal or bacterial superinfection, including *C. difficile*-associated diarrhea (CDAD) and pseudomembranous colitis; CDAD has been observed >2 months postantibiotic treatment.
Adverse Reactions (Reflective of adult population; not specific for elderly) Frequency not defined.
Cardiovascular: Pericarditis
Central nervous system: Bulging fontanels (infants), dizziness, headache, pseudotumor cerebri (adults)
Dermatologic: Angioedema, anogenital inflammatory lesions (with monilial overgrowth), erythema multiforme, erythematous rash, exfoliative dermatitis (rare), maculopapular rash, photosensitivity, pigmentation of skin, Stevens-Johnson syndrome (rare), urticaria
Endocrine & metabolic: Microscopic discoloration of thyroid gland (brown/black), nephrogenic diabetes insipidus, thyroid dysfunction (rare)
Gastrointestinal: Anorexia, diarrhea, dysphagia, enterocolitis, esophageal ulcerations, glossitis, nausea, pancreatitis, vomiting
Genitourinary: Balanitis
Hematologic: Eosinophilia, neutropenia, hemolytic anemia, thrombocytopenia
Hepatic: Hepatitis (rare), hepatotoxicity (rare), liver enzymes increased, liver failure (rare)
Neuromuscular & skeletal: Myasthenic syndrome, polyarthralgia, tooth discoloration (children <8 years, rarely in adults)
Ocular: Visual disturbances
Otic: Tinnitus

Renal: Acute renal failure, BUN increased

Respiratory: Pulmonary infiltrates

Miscellaneous: Anaphylaxis, anaphylactoid purpura, fixed drug eruptions (rare), lupus-like syndrome, superinfection, systemic lupus erythematosus exacerbation

Drug Interactions

Metabolism/Transport Effects None known.

Avoid Concomitant Use

Avoid concomitant use of Demeclocycline with any of the following: BCG; Retinoic Acid Derivatives

Increased Effect/Toxicity

Demeclocycline may increase the levels/effects of: Neuromuscular-Blocking Agents; Porfimer; Retinoic Acid Derivatives; Vitamin K Antagonists

Decreased Effect

Demeclocycline may decrease the levels/effects of: BCG; Desmopressin; Penicillins; Typhoid Vaccine

The levels/effects of Demeclocycline may be decreased by: Antacids; Bile Acid Sequestrants; Bismuth; Bismuth Subsalicylate; Calcium Salts; Iron Salts; Lanthanum; Magnesium Salts; Quinapril; Sucralfate; Zinc Salts

Ethanol/Nutrition/Herb Interactions

Food: Demeclocycline serum levels may be decreased if taken with food, milk, or dairy products. Management: Administer 1 hour before or 2 hours after food, milk, or dairy products.

Herb/Nutraceutical: Some herbal medications may cause photosensitization. Management: Avoid dong quai and St John's wort.

Stability Store at controlled room temperature at 20°C to 25°C (68°F to 77°F).

Mechanism of Action Inhibits protein synthesis by binding with the 30S and possibly the 50S ribosomal subunit(s) of susceptible bacteria; may also cause alterations in the cytoplasmic membrane; inhibits the action of ADH in patients with chronic SIADH

Pharmacodynamics/Kinetics

Onset of action: SIADH: 2-5 days

Absorption: 66%; extent of absorption is reduced by food and by certain antacids and dairy products containing aluminum, calcium, magnesium, or iron

Distribution: 1.7 L/kg

Protein binding: 40% to 90%

Metabolism: None

Half-life elimination: 10-16 hours

Time to peak, serum: ~4 hours

Excretion: Urine (44% as unchanged drug); feces (13% to 46% as unchanged drug)

Dosage

Geriatric & Adult

Susceptible infections: Manufacturer's labeling: Oral: 150 mg 4 times/day or 300 mg twice daily

SIADH (unlabeled use): Oral: 600-1200 mg/day (Goh, 2004; Gross, 2008)

Renal Impairment Use with caution; dosage adjustment and/or increase in time interval between doses recommended in manufacturer's labeling; no specific adjustment recommendations provided.

Hepatic Impairment Use with caution; dosage adjustment and/or increase in time interval between doses recommended in manufacturer's labeling; no specific adjustment recommendations provided.

Administration Administer 1 hour before or 2 hours after food or milk with plenty of fluid; avoid administration within 2-3 hours of antacids

Monitoring Parameters CBC, renal and hepatic function

Special Geriatric Considerations Has not been studied exclusively in the elderly.

Dosage Forms Excipient information presented when available (limited, particularly for generics); consult specific product labeling.

Tablet, oral, as hydrochloride: 150 mg, 300 mg

◆ **Demeclocycline Hydrochloride** see Demeclocycline on page 500
◆ **Demerol®** see Meperidine on page 1208
◆ **Demethylchlortetracycline** see Demeclocycline on page 500
◆ **Denorex® Extra Strength Protection [OTC]** see Salicylic Acid on page 1743
◆ **Denorex® Extra Strength Protection 2-in-1 [OTC]** see Salicylic Acid on page 1743

Denosumab (den OH sue mab)

Medication Safety Issues
Other safety concerns:
Duplicate therapy issues: Prolia® contains denosumab, which is the same ingredient contained in Xgeva®; patients receiving Xgeva® should not be treated with Prolia®

Brand Names: U.S. Prolia™; Xgeva®
Brand Names: Canada Prolia®; Xgeva®
Index Terms AMG-162
Generic Availability (U.S.) No
Pharmacologic Category Bone-Modifying Agent; Monoclonal Antibody
Use Treatment of osteoporosis in postmenopausal women at high risk for fracture; treatment of bone loss in men receiving androgen deprivation therapy (ADT) for nonmetastatic prostate cancer; treatment of bone loss in women receiving aromatase inhibitor (AI) therapy for breast cancer; prevention of skeletal-related events (eg, fracture, spinal cord compression, bone pain requiring surgery/radiation therapy) in patients with bone metastases from solid tumors
Unlabeled Use Treatment of bone destruction caused by rheumatoid arthritis
Medication Guide Available Yes
Contraindications
Prolia®: Hypersensitivity to denosumab or any component of the formulation; pre-existing hypocalcemia
Xgeva®: There are no contraindications listed in the manufacturer's labeling.
Warnings/Precautions Denosumab may cause or exacerbate hypocalcemia. Monitor calcium levels; correct pre-existing hypocalcemia prior to therapy. Use caution in patients with a history of hypoparathyroidism, thyroid surgery, parathyroid surgery, malabsorption syndromes, excision of small intestine, severe renal impairment/dialysis or other conditions which would predispose the patient to hypocalcemia; monitor calcium, phosphorus, and magnesium closely during therapy. Ensure adequate calcium and vitamin D intake; supplement with calcium and vitamin D; magnesium supplementation may also be necessary. Incidence of infections may be increased, including serious skin infections, abdominal, urinary, ear, or periodontal infections. Endocarditis has also been reported following use. Patients should be advised to contact healthcare provider if signs or symptoms of severe infection or cellulitis develop. Use with caution in patients with impaired immune systems or using concomitant immunosuppressive therapy; may be at increased risk for serious infections. Evaluate the need for continued treatment with serious infection. Osteonecrosis of the jaw (ONJ) has been reported in patients receiving denosumab. ONJ may manifest as jaw pain, osteomyelitis, osteitis, bone erosion, tooth/periodontal infection, toothache, gingival ulceration/erosion. Risk factors include invasive dental procedures (eg, tooth extraction, dental implants, dental surgery); a diagnosis of cancer, concomitant chemotherapy or corticosteroids, poor oral hygiene, ill-fitting dentures; and comorbid disorders (anemia, coagulopathy, infection, pre-existing dental disease). Patients should maintain good oral hygiene during treatment. A dental exam and preventative dentistry should be performed prior to therapy. The benefit/risk must be assessed by the treating physician and/or dentist/surgeon prior to any invasive dental procedure; avoid invasive procedures in patients with bone metastases receiving therapy for prevention of skeletal-related events. Patients developing ONJ while on denosumab therapy should receive care by a dentist or oral surgeon; extensive dental surgery to treat ONJ may exacerbate ONJ; evaluate individually and consider discontinuing if extensive dental surgery is necessary.

Postmenopausal osteoporosis: For use in women at high risk for fracture which is defined as a history of osteoporotic fracture or multiple risk factors for fracture. May also be used in women who failed or did not tolerate other therapies.

Bone metastases: Denosumab is not indicated for the prevention of skeletal-related events in patients with multiple myeloma. In trials of with multiple myeloma patients, denosumab was noninferior to zoledronic acid in delaying time to first skeletal-related event and mortality was increased in a subset of the denosumab-treated group.

Denosumab therapy results in significant suppression of bone turnover; the long term effects of treatment are not known but may contribute to adverse outcomes such as ONJ, atypical fractures, or delayed fracture healing; monitor. Use with caution in patients with renal impairment (Cl_{cr} <30 mL/minute) or patients on dialysis; risk of hypocalcemia is increased. Dose adjustment is not needed when administered at 60 mg every 6 months (Prolia®); once-monthly dosing has not been evaluated in patients with renal impairment (Xgeva®). Dermatitis, eczema, and rash (which are not necessarily specific to the injection site) have been reported; consider discontinuing if severe symptoms occur. Packaging may contain natural latex rubber. Do not administer Prolia® and Xgeva® to the same patient for different indications.

Adverse Reactions (Reflective of adult population; not specific for elderly) A postmarketing safety program for Prolia® is available to collect information on adverse events; more information is available at http://www.proliasafety.com. To report adverse events for either Prolia® or Xgeva®, prescribers may also call Amgen at 800-772-6436 or FDA at 800-332-1088.

Percentages noted with Prolia® (60 mg every 6 months) unless specified as Xgeva® (120 mg every 4 weeks):

>10%:

Central nervous system: Fatigue (Xgeva®: 45%), headache (Xgeva®: 13%)

Dermatologic: Dermatitis (11%), eczema (11%), rash (3% to 11%)

Endocrine & metabolic: Hypophosphatemia (Xgeva®: 32%; grade 3: 15%), hypocalcemia (2%; Xgeva®: 18%; grade 3: 3%)

Gastrointestinal: Nausea (Xgeva®: 31%), diarrhea (Xgeva®: 20%)

Neuromuscular & skeletal: Weakness (Xgeva®: 45%), arthralgia (14%), limb pain (10% to 12%), back pain (12%)

Respiratory: Dyspnea (Xgeva®: 21%), cough (Xgeva®: 15%)

1% to 10%:

Cardiovascular: Peripheral edema (5%), angina (3%)

Endocrine & metabolic: Hypercholesterolemia (7%)

Gastrointestinal: Flatulence (2%)

Neuromuscular & skeletal: Musculoskeletal pain (6%), sciatica (5%), bone pain (4%), myalgia (3%), osteonecrosis of the jaw (ONJ; ≤2%)

Ocular: Cataracts (≤5%)

Respiratory: Upper respiratory tract infection (5%)

Miscellaneous: New malignancies (5%), infections (nonfatal, serious; 4%)

Drug Interactions

Metabolism/Transport Effects None known.

Avoid Concomitant Use There are no known interactions where it is recommended to avoid concomitant use.

Increased Effect/Toxicity

Denosumab may increase the levels/effects of: Immunosuppressants

Decreased Effect There are no known significant interactions involving a decrease in effect.

Ethanol/Nutrition/Herb Interactions Ethanol: Avoid ethanol (may increase risk of osteoporosis).

Stability Prior to use, store in original carton under refrigeration, 2°C to 8°C (36°F to 46°F). Do not freeze. Prior to use, bring to room temperature of 25°C (77°F) in original container (usually takes 15-30 minutes); do not use any other methods for warming. Use within 14 days once at room temperature. Protect from direct heat and light; do not expose to temperatures >25°C (77°F). Avoid vigorous shaking.

Mechanism of Action Denosumab is a monoclonal antibody with affinity for nuclear factor-kappa ligand (RANKL). Osteoblasts secrete RANKL; RANKL activates osteoclast precursors and subsequent osteolysis which promotes release of bone-derived growth factors, such as insulin-like growth factor-1 (IGF1) and transforming growth factor-beta (TGF-beta), and increases serum calcium levels. Denosumab binds to RANKL, blocks the interaction between RANKL and RANK (a receptor located on osteoclast surfaces), and prevents osteoclast formation, leading to decreased bone resorption and increased bone mass in osteoporosis. In solid tumors with bony metastases, RANKL inhibition decreases osteoclastic activity leading to decreased skeletal related events and tumor-induced bone destruction.

Pharmacodynamics/Kinetics

Onset of action: Decreases markers of bone resorption by ~85% within 3 days; maximal reductions observed within 1 month

Duration: Markers of bone resorption return to baseline within 12 months of discontinuing therapy

Bioavailability: SubQ: 62%

Half-life elimination: ~25-28 days

Time to peak, serum: 10 days (range: 3-21 days)

Dosage

Geriatric & Adult

Prevention of skeletal-related events in bone metastases from solid tumors (Xgeva®): SubQ: 120 mg every 4 weeks

Treatment of androgen deprivation-induced bone loss in men with prostate cancer (Prolia®): SubQ: 60 mg as a single dose, once every 6 months (Smith, 2009)

Treatment of aromatase inhibitor-induced bone loss in women with breast cancer (Prolia®): SubQ: 60 mg as a single dose, once every 6 months (Ellis, 2008)

◀ **Treatment of osteoporosis in postmenopausal females (Prolia®):** SubQ: 60 mg as a single dose, once every 6 months

Renal Impairment Cl_{cr} <30 mL/minute (including dialysis-dependent): No adjustment necessary when administered every 6 months (Prolia®); once-monthly dosing has not been evaluated in patients with renal impairment (Xgeva®). Monitor patients with severe impairment (Cl_{cr} <30 mL/minute or on dialysis) due to increased risk of hypocalcemia.

Hepatic Impairment No dosage adjustment provided in manufacturer's labeling (has not been studied).

Administration SubQ: Prior to administration, bring to room temperature in original container (allow to stand ~15-30 minutes); do not warm by any other method. Solution may contain trace amounts of translucent to white protein particles; do not use if cloudy, discolored (normal solution should be clear and colorless to pale yellow), or contains excessive particles or foreign matter. Avoid vigorous shaking. Administer via SubQ injection in the upper arm, upper thigh, or abdomen.

Prolia®: If a dose is missed, administer as soon as possible, then continue dosing every 6 months from the date of the last injection.

Monitoring Parameters Recommend monitoring of serum creatinine, serum calcium, phosphorus and magnesium, signs and symptoms of hypocalcemia, especially in patients predisposed to hypocalcemia (severe renal impairment, thyroid/parathyroid surgery, malabsorption syndromes, hypoparathyroidism); infection, or dermatologic reactions; routine oral exam (prior to treatment); dental exam if risk factors for ONJ

Osteoporosis: Bone mineral density as measured by central dual-energy x-ray absorptiometry (DXA) of the hip or spine (prior to initiation of therapy and at least every 2 years; annual measurements of height and weight, assessment of chronic back pain; serum calcium and 25(OH)D; may consider monitoring biochemical markers of bone turnover (National Osteoporosis Foundation Guidelines, 2010)

Pharmacotherapy Pearls Oncology Comment: Metastatic breast cancer: The American Society of Clinical Oncology (ASCO) updated guidelines on the role of bone-modifying agents (BMAs) in the prevention and treatment of skeletal-related events for metastatic breast cancer patients (Van Poznak, 2011). The guidelines recommend initiating a BMA (denosumab, pamidronate, zoledronic acid) in patients with metastatic breast cancer to the bone. There is currently no literature indicating the superiority of one particular BMA. Optimal duration is not defined; however, the guidelines recommend continuing therapy until substantial decline in patient's performance status. In patients with normal creatinine clearance (Cl_{cr} >60 mL/minute), no dosage/interval/infusion rate changes for pamidronate or zoledronic acid are necessary. For patients with Cl_{cr} <30 mL/minute, pamidronate and zoledronic acid are not recommended. While no renal dose adjustments are recommended for denosumab, close monitoring is advised for risk of hypocalcemia in patients with Cl_{cr} <30 mL/minute or on dialysis. The ASCO guidelines are in alignment with package insert guidelines for dosing, renal dose adjustments, infusion times, prevention and management of osteonecrosis of the jaw, and monitoring of laboratory parameter recommendations. BMAs are not the first-line therapy for pain. BMAs are to be used as adjunctive therapy for cancer-related bone pain associated with bone metastasis, demonstrating a modest pain control benefit. BMAs should be used in conjunction with agents such as NSAIDs, opioid and nonopioid analgesics, corticosteroids, radiation/surgery, and interventional procedures.

Special Geriatric Considerations No specific information for use in elderly.

Dosage Forms Excipient information presented when available (limited, particularly for generics); consult specific product labeling.

Injection, solution [preservative free]:

Prolia™: 60 mg/mL (1 mL) [contains natural rubber/natural latex in packaging]

Xgeva®: 70 mg/mL (1.7 mL)

- **Deprenyl** *see* Selegiline *on page 1760*
- **DermaFungal [OTC]** *see* Miconazole (Topical) *on page 1276*
- **Dermagran® [OTC]** *see* Aluminum Hydroxide *on page 77*
- **Dermagran® AF [OTC]** *see* Miconazole (Topical) *on page 1276*
- **Dermamycin® [OTC]** *see* DiphenhydrAMINE (Topical) *on page 559*
- **Dermarest® Eczema Medicated [OTC]** *see* Hydrocortisone (Topical) *on page 943*
- **Dermarest® Psoriasis Medicated Moisturizer [OTC]** *see* Salicylic Acid *on page 1743*
- **Dermarest® Psoriasis Medicated Scalp Treatment [OTC]** *see* Salicylic Acid *on page 1743*
- **Dermarest® Psoriasis Medicated Shampoo/Conditioner [OTC]** *see* Salicylic Acid *on page 1743*
- **Dermarest® Psoriasis Medicated Skin Treatment [OTC]** *see* Salicylic Acid *on page 1743*
- **Dermarest® Psoriasis Overnight Treatment [OTC]** *see* Salicylic Acid *on page 1743*
- **Derma-Smoothe/FS®** *see* Fluocinolone (Topical) *on page 803*
- **Dermatop®** *see* Prednicarbate *on page 1591*
- **DermOtic®** *see* Fluocinolone (Otic) *on page 803*
- **Desiccated Thyroid** *see* Thyroid, Desiccated *on page 1885*

Desipramine (des IP ra meen)

Related Information
Antidepressant Agents *on page 2097*
Beers Criteria – Potentially Inappropriate Medications for Geriatrics *on page 2183*

Medication Safety Issues
Sound-alike/look-alike issues:
Desipramine may be confused with clomiPRAMINE, dalfampridine, diphenhydrAMINE, disopyramide, imipramine, nortriptyline
Norpramin® may be confused with clomiPRAMINE, imipramine, Normodyne®, Norpace®, nortriptyline, Tenormin®

BEERS Criteria medication:
This drug may be potentially inappropriate for use in geriatric patients (SIADH: Quality of evidence - moderate; Strength of recommendation - strong).

International issues:
Norpramin: Brand name for desipramine [U.S., Canada], but also the brand name for enalapril/hydrochlorothiazide [Portugal]; omeprazole [Spain]

Brand Names: U.S. Norpramin®

Brand Names: Canada Dom-Desipramine; Novo-Desipramine; Nu-Desipramine; PMS-Desipramine

Index Terms Desipramine Hydrochloride; Desmethylimipramine Hydrochloride

Generic Availability (U.S.) Yes

Pharmacologic Category Antidepressant, Tricyclic (Secondary Amine)

Use Treatment of depression

Unlabeled Use Analgesic adjunct in chronic pain; peripheral neuropathies (including diabetic neuropathy); attention-deficit/hyperactivity disorder (ADHD)

Medication Guide Available Yes

Contraindications Hypersensitivity to desipramine, drugs of similar chemical class, or any component of the formulation; use of MAO inhibitors with or within 14 days; use in a patient during the acute recovery phase of MI

Warnings/Precautions [U.S. Boxed Warning]: Antidepressants increase the risk of suicidal thinking and behavior in children, adolescents, and young adults (18-24 years of age) with major depressive disorder (MDD) and other psychiatric disorders; consider risk prior to prescribing. Short-term studies did not show an increased risk in patients >24 years of age and showed a decreased risk in patients ≥65 years. Closely monitor for clinical worsening, suicidality, or unusual changes in behavior; the patient's family or caregiver should be instructed to closely observe the patient and communicate condition with healthcare provider. A medication guide should be dispensed with each prescription.

The possibility of a suicide attempt is inherent in major depression and may persist until remission occurs. Monitor for worsening of depression or suicidality, especially during initiation of therapy (generally first 1-2 months) or with dose increases or decreases. Use caution in high-risk patients. Worsening depression and severe abrupt suicidality that are not part of the presenting symptoms may require discontinuation or modification of drug therapy. The patient's family or caregiver should be alerted to monitor patients for the emergence of suicidality and associated behaviors (such as agitation, irritability, hostility, impulsivity, and hypomania) and notify healthcare provider.

May worsen psychosis in some patients or precipitate a shift to mania or hypomania in patients with bipolar disorder. Patients presenting with depressive symptoms should be screened for bipolar disorder. Monotherapy in patients with bipolar disorder should be avoided. **Desipramine is not FDA approved for the treatment of bipolar depression.**

TCAs may rarely cause bone marrow suppression; monitor for any signs of infection and obtain CBC if symptoms (eg, fever, sore throat) evident. The degree of anticholinergic blockade produced by this agent is low relative to other cyclic antidepressants - however, extreme caution should be used in patients with urinary retention, benign prostatic hyperplasia, narrow-angle glaucoma, xerostomia, visual problems, constipation, or a history of bowel obstruction. The degree of sedation with desipramine are low relative to other antidepressants. However, desipramine may cause drowsiness/sedation, resulting in impaired performance of tasks requiring alertness (eg, operating machinery or driving). Sedative effects may be additive with other CNS depressants and/or ethanol. The risk of orthostasis is moderate relative to other antidepressants. Due to risk of conduction abnormalities, use with extreme caution in patients with a history of cardiovascular disease (including previous MI, stroke, tachycardia, or conduction abnormalities) or in patients with a family history of sudden death, dysrhythmias, or conduction abnormalities. Use with caution in patients with diabetes mellitus; may alter glucose regulation.

Consider discontinuing, when possible, prior to elective surgery. Therapy should not be abruptly discontinued. May lower seizure threshold - use extreme caution in patients with a previous seizure disorder or condition predisposing to seizures such as brain damage, alcoholism, or concurrent therapy with other drugs which lower the seizure threshold. In some patients, seizures may precede cardiac dysrhythmias and death. May increase the risks associated with electroconvulsive therapy. Use with extreme caution in hyperthyroid patients or those receiving thyroid supplementation. Use with caution in patients with glaucoma, hepatic or renal dysfunction.

Use caution in elderly patients; may cause or exacerbate syndrome of inappropriate antidiuretic hormone secretion or hyponatremia; monitor sodium closely with initiation or dosage adjustments in older adults. May be inappropriate in older adults depending on comorbidities (eg, dementia, delirium) due to its potent anticholinergic effects (Beers Criteria). May also increase risk of falling or confusional states.

Adverse Reactions (Reflective of adult population; not specific for elderly) Frequency not defined.

Cardiovascular: Arrhythmias, edema, flushing, heart block, hyper-/hypotension, MI, palpitation, stroke, tachycardia

Central nervous system: Agitation, anxiety, ataxia, confusion, delusions, disorientation, dizziness, drowsiness, EEG alterations, exacerbation of psychosis, extrapyramidal symptoms, fatigue, fever, hallucinations, headache, hypomania, incoordination, insomnia, neuroleptic malignant syndrome, nightmares, restlessness, seizure, suicidal thinking and behavior

Dermatologic: Alopecia, itching, petechiae, photosensitivity, skin rash, urticaria

Endocrine & metabolic: Breast enlargement, galactorrhea, gynecomastia, hyper-/hypoglycemia, impotence, libido changes, SIADH

Gastrointestinal: Abdominal cramps, anorexia, black tongue, constipation, diarrhea, epigastric distress, nausea, parotid edema, paralytic ileus, stomatitis, sublingual adenitis, unpleasant taste, vomiting, weight gain/loss, xerostomia

Genitourinary: Micturition delayed, nocturia, painful ejaculation, polyuria, testicular edema, urinary retention

Hematologic: Agranulocytosis, eosinophilia, purpura, thrombocytopenia

Hepatic: Alkaline phosphatase increased, cholestatic jaundice, hepatitis, liver enzymes increased

Neuromuscular & skeletal: Falling, numbness, paresthesia of extremities, peripheral neuropathy, tingling, tremor, weakness

Ocular: Blurred vision, disturbances of accommodation, intraocular pressure increased, mydriasis

Otic: Tinnitus

Miscellaneous: Allergic reaction, diaphoresis (excessive), withdrawal symptoms

Drug Interactions

Metabolism/Transport Effects Substrate of CYP1A2 (minor), CYP2D6 (major); **Note:** Assignment of Major/Minor substrate status based on clinically relevant drug interaction potential; **Inhibits** CYP2A6 (moderate), CYP2B6 (moderate), CYP2D6 (moderate), CYP2E1 (weak), CYP3A4 (moderate)

Avoid Concomitant Use

Avoid concomitant use of Desipramine with any of the following: Iobenguane I 123; MAO Inhibitors; Methylene Blue; Tolvaptan

Increased Effect/Toxicity

Desipramine may increase the levels/effects of: Alpha-/Beta-Agonists (Direct-Acting); Alpha1-Agonists; Amphetamines; Anticholinergics; Avanafil; Beta2-Agonists; Budesonide (Systemic, Oral Inhalation); Colchicine; CYP2B6 Substrates; CYP2D6 Substrates; CYP3A4 Substrates; Desmopressin; Eplerenone; Everolimus; FentaNYL; Fesoterodine; Highest Risk QTc-Prolonging Agents; Ivacaftor; Methylene Blue; Metoclopramide; Moderate Risk QTc-Prolonging Agents; Nebivolol; Pimecrolimus; QuiNIDine; Saxagliptin; Serotonin Modulators; Sodium Phosphates; Sulfonylureas; Tolvaptan; TraMADol; Vitamin K Antagonists; Yohimbine

The levels/effects of Desipramine may be increased by: Abiraterone Acetate; Altretamine; Antipsychotics; Boceprevir; BuPROPion; Cimetidine; Cinacalcet; CYP2D6 Inhibitors (Moderate); CYP2D6 Inhibitors (Strong); Dexmethylphenidate; Divalproex; DULoxetine; Linezolid; Lithium; MAO Inhibitors; Methylphenidate; Metoclopramide; Metyrosine; Mifepristone; Pramlintide; Protease Inhibitors; QuiNIDine; Selective Serotonin Reuptake Inhibitors; Telaprevir; Terbinafine; Terbinafine (Systemic); Valproic Acid

Decreased Effect

Desipramine may decrease the levels/effects of: Acetylcholinesterase Inhibitors (Central); Alpha2-Agonists; Codeine; Ifosfamide; Iobenguane I 123

The levels/effects of Desipramine may be decreased by: Acetylcholinesterase Inhibitors (Central); Barbiturates; CarBAMazepine; Peginterferon Alfa-2b; St Johns Wort

Ethanol/Nutrition/Herb Interactions

Ethanol: May increase CNS depression; monitor for increased effects with coadministration. Caution patients about effects.

Food: Grapefruit juice may inhibit the metabolism of some TCAs and clinical toxicity may result.

Herb/Nutraceutical: Avoid valerian, St John's wort, SAMe, kava kava (may increase risk of serotonin syndrome and/or excessive sedation).

Stability
Store at 20°C to 25°C (68°F to 77°F).

Mechanism of Action
Traditionally believed to increase the synaptic concentration of norepinephrine (and to a lesser extent, serotonin) in the central nervous system by inhibition of its reuptake by the presynaptic neuronal membrane. However, additional receptor effects have been found including desensitization of adenyl cyclase, down regulation of beta-adrenergic receptors, and down regulation of serotonin receptors.

Pharmacodynamics/Kinetics

Onset of action: Earliest therapeutic effects: 2-5 days; Maximum antidepressant effect: >2 weeks

Metabolism: Hepatic

Half-life elimination: Adults: 15-24 hours (Weiner, 1981)

Time to peak, plasma: ~6 hours (Weiner, 1981)

Excretion: Urine (~70%)

Dosage

Geriatric Depression: Oral: Initial dose: Start at the lower range and increase based on tolerance and response to 100 mg/day in divided or single dose; usual maintenance dose: 25-100 mg/day, but doses up to 150 mg/day may be necessary in severely depressed patients

Adult

Depression: Oral: Initial dose: Start at the lower range and increase based on tolerance and response; usual maintenance dose: 100-200 mg/day, but doses up to 300 mg/day may be necessary in severely depressed patients

Neuropathic pain (unlabeled use): Oral: Initial: 10-25 mg/day; increase dose every 3 days as necessary until the desired effect is obtained; usual effective dose: 50-150 mg/day (maximum dose: 150 mg/day)

Renal Impairment
Hemodialysis/peritoneal dialysis effects: Supplemental dose is not necessary.

Monitoring Parameters
Monitor blood pressure and pulse rate prior to and during initial therapy; evaluate mental status, suicide ideation (especially at the beginning of therapy or when doses are increased or decreased); monitor weight; ECG in older adults and those patients with cardiac disease

When used for the treatment of ADHD, thoroughly evaluate for cardiovascular risk. Monitor heart rate, blood pressure, and consider obtaining ECG prior to initiation (Vetter, 2008); ensure PR interval ≤200 ms, QRS duration ≤120 ms, and QT_c ≤460 ms.

Test Interactions
Increased glucose; decreased glucose has also been reported. May interfere with urine detection of amphetamines/methamphetamines (false-positive).

Special Geriatric Considerations Preferred tricyclic antidepressant because of its milder side effect profile; patients may experience excitation or stimulation; in such cases, administer as a single morning dose or divided dose.

A systematic review and meta-analysis of antidepressant placebo-controlled trials in persons with depression and dementia found evidence "suggestive" of efficacy but not of sufficient strength to "confirm" efficacy. Antidepressant trials in this patient population are small and underpowered. Older patients with depression being treated with an antidepressant should be closely monitored for response and adverse effects. Treatment should be switched or augmented when response is inadequate with a therapeutic dose. Antidepressants that are not tolerated should be discontinued and an alternative agent should be started.

This medication is considered to be potentially inappropriate in this patient population (Beers Criteria: SIADH: Quality of evidence - moderate; Strength of recommendation - strong).

Dosage Forms Excipient information presented when available (limited, particularly for generics); consult specific product labeling.

Tablet, oral, as hydrochloride: 10 mg, 25 mg, 50 mg, 75 mg, 100 mg, 150 mg

Norpramin®: 10 mg, 25 mg, 50 mg, 75 mg, 100 mg, 150 mg [contains soybean oil]

♦ **Desipramine Hydrochloride** see Desipramine on page 505

Desirudin (des i ROO din)

Medication Safety Issues

High alert medication:

The Institute for Safe Medication Practices (ISMP) includes this medication among its list of drugs which have a heightened risk of causing significant patient harm when used in error.

Brand Names: U.S. Iprivask®

Index Terms CGP-39393; Desulfato-Hirudin; Desulfatohirudin; Desulphatohirudin; r-Hirudin; Recombinant Desulfatohirudin; Recombinant Hirudin

Generic Availability (U.S.) No

Pharmacologic Category Anticoagulant, Thrombin Inhibitor

Use Prophylaxis of deep vein thrombosis (DVT) in patients undergoing surgery for hip replacement

Contraindications Hypersensitivity to natural or recombinant hirudins; active bleeding and/or irreversible coagulation disorders

Warnings/Precautions [U.S. Boxed Warning]: Patients with recent or anticipated neuraxial anesthesia (epidural or spinal anesthesia) are at risk of epidural or spinal hematoma and subsequent paralysis. Consider risk versus benefit prior to neuraxial anesthesia; risk is increased by concomitant agents which may alter hemostasis, as well as traumatic or repeated epidural or spinal puncture. Patient should be observed closely for bleeding and signs and symptoms of neurological impairment if therapy is administered during or immediately following diagnostic lumbar puncture, epidural anesthesia, or spinal anesthesia.

Allergic and hypersensitivity reactions, including anaphylaxis and fatal anaphylactoid reactions have been reported with other hirudin derivatives. Exercise caution when re-exposing patients (anaphylaxis has been reported). Monitor patient closely for signs or symptoms of bleeding. Certain patients are at increased risk of bleeding. Risk factors include bacterial endocarditis; congenital or acquired bleeding disorders; active ulcerative or angiodysplastic GI diseases; severe uncontrolled hypertension; history of hemorrhagic stroke; use shortly after brain, spinal, or ophthalmology surgery; patients treated concomitantly with platelet inhibitors; recent GI bleeding; thrombocytopenia or platelet defects; renal impairment; hepatic impairment; hypertensive or diabetic retinopathy; or in patients undergoing invasive procedures. Do not administer with other agents that increase the risk of hemorrhage unless coadministration cannot be avoided. Discontinue if bleeding occurs. Contraindicated with active bleeding and/or irreversible coagulation disorders.

Do **not** administer intramuscularly (I.M.). Do not use interchangeably (unit-for-unit) with other hirudins. Use with caution in patients with moderate-to-severe renal dysfunction (Cl_{cr} <60 mL/minute/1.73 m^2); dosage reduction is necessary; monitor aPTT and renal function daily.

Adverse Reactions (Reflective of adult population; not specific for elderly) As with all anticoagulants, bleeding is the major adverse effect. Hemorrhage may occur at any site. 2% to 10%:

Gastrointestinal: Nausea (2%)

Hematologic: Hematoma (6%), hemorrhage (major, <1% to 3%; may include cases of intracranial, retroperitoneal, intraocular, intraspinal, or prosthetic joint hemorrhage), anemia (3%)

Local: Injection site mass (4%), deep thrombophlebitis (2%)

Miscellaneous: Wound secretion (4%)

Drug Interactions

Metabolism/Transport Effects None known.

Avoid Concomitant Use

Avoid concomitant use of Desirudin with any of the following: Rivaroxaban

Increased Effect/Toxicity

Desirudin may increase the levels/effects of: Anticoagulants; Collagenase (Systemic); Dabigatran Etexilate; Deferasirox; Ibritumomab; Rivaroxaban; Tositumomab and Iodine I 131 Tositumomab

The levels/effects of Desirudin may be increased by: Antiplatelet Agents; Dasatinib; Herbs (Anticoagulant/Antiplatelet Properties); Nonsteroidal Anti-Inflammatory Agents; Pentosan Polysulfate Sodium; Prostacyclin Analogues; Salicylates; Thrombolytic Agents; Tipranavir

Decreased Effect There are no known significant interactions involving a decrease in effect.

Ethanol/Nutrition/Herb Interactions Herb/Nutraceutical: Avoid alfalfa, anise, bilberry, bladderwrack, bromelain, cat's claw, celery, coleus, cordyceps, dong quai, evening primrose oil, fenugreek, feverfew, garlic, ginger, ginkgo biloba, ginseng (American/Panax/Siberian), grapeseed, green tea, guggul, horse chestnut seed, horseradish, licorice, prickly ash, red clover, reishi, sweet clover, turmeric, white willow (all possess anticoagulant or antiplatelet activity and as such, may enhance the anticoagulant effects of desirudin).

Stability Store at 25°C (77°F); excursions permitted to 15°C to 30°C (59°F to 86°F). Protect from light. Following reconstitution, solution may be stored at room temperature for up to 24 hours. Discard unused solution after 24 hours.

Reconstitution: Attach enclosed vial adapter to vial containing desirudin. Remove syringe cap and attach provided syringe containing diluent to adapter on vial. Slowly push plunger down to transfer entire contents of syringe into vial. Do not remove syringe from vial adapter. Gently swirl solution; round tablet in vial will dissolve within 10 seconds. Resultant solution concentration is 31.5 mg/mL (15.75 mg/0.5 mL provides a 15 mg dose). Turn vial upside down; withdraw appropriate dose amount back into syringe. Remove syringe from vial. Attach enclosed Eclipse™ needle (or any needle appropriate for subcutaneous administration); pull pink lever down and uncap needle; ready for injection. After injection, flip up pink lever to cover needle until it snaps into place; dispose of syringe appropriately.

Mechanism of Action Desirudin is a direct, highly selective thrombin inhibitor. Reversibly binds to the active thrombin site of free and clot-associated thrombin. Inhibits fibrin formation, activation of coagulation factors V, VII, and XIII, and thrombin-induced platelet aggregation resulting in a dose-dependent prolongation of the activated partial thromboplastin time (aPTT).

Pharmacodynamics/Kinetics

Absorption: Subcutaneous: Complete

Distribution: V_{dss}: 0.25 L/kg

Half-life elimination: ~2 hours; Prolonged with renal impairment (Cl_{cr} <31 mL/minute/1.73m^2: Up to 12 hours)

Time to peak, plasma: 1-3 hours

Excretion: Urine (40% to 50% as unchanged drug)

Dosage

Geriatric & Adult DVT prophylaxis: SubQ: 15 mg every 12 hours; initial dose may be given up to 5-15 minutes prior to surgery (after induction of regional anesthesia, if used); has been administered for up to 12 days (average: 9-12 days) in clinical trials

Renal Impairment

Moderate renal impairment (Cl_{cr} ≥31-60 mL/minute/1.73 m^2): 5 mg every 12 hours

Severe renal impairment (Cl_{cr} <31 mL/minute/1.73 m^2): 1.7 mg every 12 hours

Administration Do **not** administer I.M.; for SubQ administration only. Administration should be alternated between the left and right anterolateral and left and right posterolateral thigh or abdominal wall. Insert needle into a skin fold held between the thumb and forefinger; the skin fold should be held throughout the injection. Do not rub injection site. Do not mix with other injections or infusions. Administer according to recommended regimen.

Monitoring Parameters Monitor aPTT, serum creatinine/creatinine clearance, CBC; stool occult blood tests. Serum creatinine and aPTT should be monitored daily in patients with moderate-to-severe renal insufficiency. Interrupt therapy if aPTT exceeds 2 times normal; resume at a reduced dose when aPTT is <2 times control.

Special Geriatric Considerations Serious adverse drug events are more common in persons ≥75 years of age. Dosage adjustment may be necessary based on kidney function.

Dosage Forms Excipient information presented when available (limited, particularly for generics); consult specific product labeling.

Injection, powder for reconstitution [preservative free]:

Iprivask®: 15 mg [supplied with prefilled diluent syringe]

Desloratadine (des lor AT a deen)

Medication Safety Issues
  Sound-alike/look-alike issues:
    Clarinex® may be confused with Celebrex®
Brand Names: U.S. Clarinex®
Brand Names: Canada Aerius®; Aerius® Kids; Desloratadine Allergy Control
Generic Availability (U.S.) Yes: Excludes syrup, orally disintegrating tablet
Pharmacologic Category Histamine H_1 Antagonist; Histamine H_1 Antagonist, Second Generation; Piperidine Derivative
Use Relief of nasal and non-nasal symptoms of seasonal allergic rhinitis (SAR) and perennial allergic rhinitis (PAR); treatment of chronic idiopathic urticaria (CIU)
Contraindications Hypersensitivity to desloratadine, loratadine, or any component of the formulation
Warnings/Precautions Dose should be adjusted in patients with liver or renal impairment. Use with caution in patients known to be slow metabolizers of desloratadine (incidence of side effects may be increased). Some products may contain phenylalanine.
Adverse Reactions (Reflective of adult population; not specific for elderly) Note: Frequency reported in children, unless otherwise noted.
  >10%:
    Central nervous system: Fever (12% to 17%), headache (adults 14%), irritability (12%)
    Gastrointestinal: Diarrhea (15% to 20%)
    Respiratory: Upper respiratory tract infection (11% to 21%), cough (11%)
  1% to 10%:
    Central nervous system: Somnolence (children 9%; adults 2%), insomnia (5%), fatigue (adults 2% to 5%), dizziness (adults 4%), emotional lability (3%)
    Dermatologic: Erythema (3%), maculopapular rash (3%)
    Endocrine & metabolic: Dysmenorrhea (adults 2%)
    Gastrointestinal: Vomiting (6%), anorexia (5%), nausea (children 3%; adults 5%), nausea (5%), appetite increased (3%), dyspepsia (adults 3%), xerostomia (adults 3%)
    Genitourinary: Urinary tract infection (4%)
    Neuromuscular & skeletal: Myalgia (adults 2% to 3%)
    Otic: Otitis media (children 6%)
    Respiratory: Bronchitis (6%), rhinorrhea (5%), pharyngitis (children 3% to 5%; adults 3% to 4%), epistaxis (3%)
    Miscellaneous: Varicella infection (4%), parasitic infection (3%)
Drug Interactions
  Metabolism/Transport Effects Substrate of P-glycoprotein
  Avoid Concomitant Use
    Avoid concomitant use of Desloratadine with any of the following: Azelastine; Azelastine (Nasal); Methadone; Mirtazapine; Paraldehyde
  Increased Effect/Toxicity
    Desloratadine may increase the levels/effects of: Alcohol (Ethyl); Anticholinergics; Azelastine; Azelastine (Nasal); Buprenorphine; CNS Depressants; Methadone; Methotrimeprazine; Metyrosine; Mirtazapine; Paraldehyde; Selective Serotonin Reuptake Inhibitors; Zolpidem

    The levels/effects of Desloratadine may be increased by: Droperidol; HydrOXYzine; Methotrimeprazine; P-glycoprotein/ABCB1 Inhibitors; Pramlintide
  Decreased Effect
    Desloratadine may decrease the levels/effects of: Acetylcholinesterase Inhibitors (Central); Benzylpenicilloyl Polylysine; Betahistine; Hyaluronidase

    The levels/effects of Desloratadine may be decreased by: Acetylcholinesterase Inhibitors (Central); Amphetamines; P-glycoprotein/ABCB1 Inducers
  Ethanol/Nutrition/Herb Interactions
    Ethanol: May increase CNS depression; monitor for increased effects with coadministration. Caution patients about effects.
    Food: Does not affect bioavailability.
Stability Syrup, tablet, orally-disintegrating tablet: Store at 25°C (77°F); excursions permitted between 15°C to 30°C (59°F to 85°F). Protect from moisture and excessive heat. Use orally-disintegrating tablet immediately after opening blister package. Syrup should be protected from light.
Mechanism of Action Desloratadine, a major active metabolite of loratadine, is a long-acting tricyclic antihistamine with selective peripheral histamine H_1 receptor antagonistic activity.

Pharmacodynamics/Kinetics

Onset of action: Within 1 hour

Duration: 24 hours

Protein binding: Desloratadine: 82% to 87%; 3-hydroxydesloratadine (active metabolite): 85% to 89%

Metabolism: Hepatic to active metabolite, 3-hydroxydesloratadine (specific enzymes not identified); subsequently undergoes glucuronidation. Decreased in slow metabolizers of desloratadine. Not expected to affect or be affected by medications metabolized by CYP with normal doses.

Half-life elimination: 27 hours

Time to peak: 3 hours

Excretion: Urine and feces (as metabolites)

Dosage

Geriatric & Adult Seasonal or perennial allergic rhinitis, chronic idiopathic urticaria: Oral: 5 mg once daily

Renal Impairment 5 mg every other day

Hepatic Impairment Adults: Mild-to-severe impairment: 5 mg every other day.

Administration May be taken with or without food. RediTabs® should be placed on the tongue; tablet will disintegrate immediately. May be taken with or without water.

Monitoring Parameters Relief of symptoms, mental status

Test Interactions May suppress the wheal and flare reactions to skin test antigens

Special Geriatric Considerations No specific dosing adjustment based on age. Adjust dose based on renal function.

Dosage Forms Excipient information presented when available (limited, particularly for generics); consult specific product labeling.

Syrup, oral:
Clarinex®: 0.5 mg/mL (480 mL) [contains propylene glycol, sodium benzoate; bubblegum flavor]

Tablet, oral: 5 mg
Clarinex®: 5 mg

Tablet, orally disintegrating, oral:
Clarinex®: 2.5 mg [contains phenylalanine 1.4 mg/tablet; tutti frutti flavor]
Clarinex®: 5 mg [contains phenylalanine 2.9 mg/tablet; tutti frutti flavor]

◆ **Desmethylimipramine Hydrochloride** see Desipramine on page 505

Desmopressin (des moe PRES in)

Brand Names: U.S. DDAVP®; Stimate®

Brand Names: Canada Apo-Desmopressin®; DDAVP®; DDAVP® Melt; Minirin®; Novo-Desmopressin; Octostim®; PMS-Desmopressin

Index Terms 1-Deamino-8-D-Arginine Vasopressin; Desmopressin Acetate

Generic Availability (U.S.) Yes

Pharmacologic Category Antihemophilic Agent; Hemostatic Agent; Vasopressin Analog, Synthetic

Use

Injection: Treatment of diabetes insipidus; maintenance of hemostasis and control of bleeding in hemophilia A with factor VIII coagulant activity levels >5% and mild-to-moderate classic von Willebrand's disease (type 1) with factor VIII coagulant activity levels >5%

Nasal solutions (DDAVP® Nasal Spray and DDAVP® Rhinal Tube): Treatment of central diabetes insipidus

Nasal spray (Stimate®): Maintenance of hemostasis and control of bleeding in hemophilia A with factor VIII coagulant activity levels >5% and mild-to-moderate classic von Willebrand's disease (type 1) with factor VIII coagulant activity levels >5%

Tablet: Treatment of central diabetes insipidus, temporary polyuria and polydipsia following pituitary surgery or head trauma, primary nocturnal enuresis

Unlabeled Use Uremic bleeding associated with acute or chronic renal failure; prevention of surgical bleeding in patients with uremia

Contraindications Hypersensitivity to desmopressin or any component of the formulation; hyponatremia or a history of hyponatremia; moderate-to-severe renal impairment (Cl_{cr}<50 mL/minute)

Canadian labeling: Additional contraindications (not in U.S. labeling): Type 2B or platelet-type (pseudo) von Willebrand's disease (injection, intranasal, oral, sublingual); known hyponatremia, habitual or psychogenic polydipsia, cardiac insufficiency or other conditions requiring diuretic therapy (intranasal, sublingual); nephrosis, severe hepatic dysfunction (sublingual); primary nocturnal enuresis (intranasal)

DESKMOPRESSIN

Warnings/Precautions Allergic reactions and anaphylaxis have been reported rarely with both the I.V. and intranasal formulations. Fluid intake should be adjusted downward in the elderly and very young patients to decrease the possibility of water intoxication and hyponatremia. Use may rarely lead to extreme decreases in plasma osmolality, resulting in seizures, coma, and death. Use caution with cystic fibrosis, heart failure, renal dysfunction, polydipsia (habitual or psychogenic [contraindicated in Canadian labeling]), or other conditions associated with fluid and electrolyte imbalance due to potential hyponatremia. Use caution with coronary artery insufficiency or hypertensive cardiovascular disease; may increase or decrease blood pressure leading to changes in heart rate. Consider switching from nasal to intravenous solution if changes in the nasal mucosa (scarring, edema) occur leading to unreliable absorption. Use caution in patients predisposed to thrombus formation; thrombotic events (acute cerebrovascular thrombosis, acute myocardial infarction) have occurred (rare).

Desmopressin (intranasal and I.V.), when used for hemostasis in hemophilia, is not for use in hemophilia B, type 2B von Willebrand disease, severe classic von Willebrand disease (type 1), or in patients with factor VIII antibodies. In general, desmopressin is also not recommended for use in patients with ≤5% factor VIII activity level, although it may be considered in selected patients with activity levels between 2% and 5%.

Consider switching from nasal to intravenous administration if changes in the nasal mucosa (scarring, edema) occur leading to unreliable absorption. Consider alternative rout of administration (I.V. or intranasal) with inadequate therapeutic response at maximum recommended oral doses. Therapy should be interrupted if patient experiences an acute illness (eg, fever, recurrent vomiting or diarrhea), vigorous exercise, or any condition associated with an increase in water consumption. Some patients may demonstrate a change in response after long-term therapy (>6 months) characterized as decreased response or a shorter duration of response.

Adverse Reactions (Reflective of adult population; not specific for elderly) Frequency may not be defined (may be dose or route related).
Cardiovascular: Blood pressure increased/decreased (I.V.), facial flushing
Central nervous system: Headache (2% to 5%), dizziness (intranasal; ≤3%), chills (intranasal; 2%)
Dermatologic: Rash
Endocrine & metabolic: Hyponatremia, water intoxication
Gastrointestinal: Abdominal pain (intranasal; 2%), gastrointestinal disorder (intranasal; ≤2%), nausea (intranasal; ≤2%), abdominal cramps, sore throat
Hepatic: Transient increases in liver transaminases (associated primarily with tablets)
Local: Injection: Burning pain, erythema, and swelling at the injection site
Neuromuscular & Skeletal: Weakness (intranasal; ≤2%)
Ocular: Conjunctivitis (intranasal; ≤2%), eye edema (intranasal; ≤2%), lacrimation disorder (intranasal; ≤2%)
Respiratory: Rhinitis (intranasal; 3% to 8%), epistaxis (intranasal; ≤3%), nostril pain (intranasal; ≤2%), cough, nasal congestion, upper respiratory infection

Drug Interactions
Metabolism/Transport Effects None known.
Avoid Concomitant Use There are no known interactions where it is recommended to avoid concomitant use.
Increased Effect/Toxicity
Desmopressin may increase the levels/effects of: Lithium

The levels/effects of Desmopressin may be increased by: Analgesics (Opioid); CarBAMazepine; ChlorproMAZINE; LamoTRIgine; Nonsteroidal Anti-Inflammatory Agents; Selective Serotonin Reuptake Inhibitors; Tricyclic Antidepressants
Decreased Effect
The levels/effects of Desmopressin may be decreased by: Demeclocycline; Lithium
Ethanol/Nutrition/Herb Interactions Ethanol: Avoid ethanol (may decrease antidiuretic effect).
Stability
DDAVP®:
Nasal spray: Store at controlled room temperature of 20°C to 25°C (68°F to 77°F). Keep nasal spray in upright position.
Rhinal Tube solution: Store refrigerated at 2°C to 8°C (36°F to 46°F). May store at controlled room temperature of 20°C to 25°C (68°F to 77°F) for up to 3 weeks.
Solution for injection: Store refrigerated at 2°C to 8°C (36°F to 46°F). Dilute solution for injection in 10-50 mL NS for I.V. infusion (50 mL for adults).
Tablet: Store at controlled room temperature of 20°C to 25°C (68°F to 77°F).

DESMOPRESSIN

DDAVP® Melt (CAN; not available in U.S.): Store at 15°C to 25°C (59°F to 77°F) in original container. Protect from moisture.

Stimate® nasal spray: Store at controlled room temperature of 20°C to 25°C (68°F to 77°F). Keep nasal spray in upright position. Discard 6 months after opening.

Mechanism of Action In a dose dependent manner, desmopressin increases cyclic adenosine monophosphate (cAMP) in renal tubular cells which increases water permeability resulting in decreased urine volume and increased urine osmolality; increases plasma levels of von Willebrand factor, factor VIII, and t-PA contributing to a shortened activated partial thromboplastin time (aPTT) and bleeding time.

Pharmacodynamics/Kinetics

Onset of action:

Intranasal: Antidiuretic: 15-30 minutes; Increased factor VIII and von Willebrand factor (vWF) activity (dose related): 30 minutes

Peak effect: Antidiuretic: 1 hour; Increased factor VIII and vWF activity: 1.5 hours

I.V. infusion: Increased factor VIII and vWF activity: 30 minutes (dose related)

Peak effect: 1.5-2 hours

Oral tablet: Antidiuretic: ~1 hour

Peak effect: 4-7 hours

Duration: Intranasal, I.V. infusion, Oral tablet: ~6-14 hours

Absorption: Sublingual: Rapid

Bioavailability: Intranasal: ~3.5%; Oral tablet: 5% compared to intranasal, 0.16% compared to I.V.

Half-life elimination: Intranasal: ~3.5 hours; I.V. infusion: 3 hours; Oral tablet: 2-3 hours

Renal impairment: ≤9 hours

Excretion: Urine

Dosage

Geriatric & Adult

Diabetes insipidus:

I.V., SubQ: U.S. labeling: 2-4 mcg/day (0.5-1 mL) in 2 divided doses or one-tenth ($^1/_{10}$) of the maintenance intranasal dose. Fluid restriction should be observed.

I.M., I.V., SubQ: Canadian labeling (not in U.S. labeling): 1-4 mcg (0.25-1 mL) once daily or one-tenth ($^1/_{10}$) of the maintenance intranasal dose. Fluid restriction should be observed.

Intranasal (100 mcg/mL nasal solution): 10-40 mcg/day (0.1-0.4 mL) divided 1-3 times/day; adjust morning and evening doses separately for an adequate diurnal rhythm of water turnover. **Note:** The nasal spray pump can only deliver doses of 10 mcg (0.1 mL) or multiples of 10 mcg (0.1 mL); if doses other than this are needed, the rhinal tube delivery system is preferred. Fluid restriction should be observed.

Oral:

U.S. labeling: Initial: 0.05 mg twice daily; total daily dose should be increased or decreased as needed to obtain adequate antidiuresis (range: 0.1-1.2 mg divided 2-3 times/day). Fluid restriction should be observed.

Canadian labeling (not in U.S. labeling): Initial: 0.1 mg 3 times/day; total daily dose should be increased or decreased as needed to obtain adequate antidiuresis (range: 0.3-1.2 mg divided 3 times/day). Fluid restriction should be observed.

Sublingual formulation: Canadian labeling (not in U.S. labeling): Initial: 60 mcg 3 times/day; total daily dose should be increased or decreased as needed to obtain adequate antidiuresis. Usual maintenance: 60-120 mcg 3 times/day (range: 120-720 mcg divided 2-3 times/day). Fluid restriction should be observed.

Nocturnal enuresis: *Oral:* 0.2 mg at bedtime; dose may be titrated up to 0.6 mg to achieve desired response.

Hemophilia A and mild-to-moderate von Willebrand disease (type 1):

I.V.: 0.3 mcg/kg by slow infusion; if used preoperatively, administer 30 minutes before procedure

Canadian labeling (not in U.S. labeling): Maximum I.V. dose: 20 mcg

Intranasal (using high concentration spray [1.5 mg/mL]): <50 kg: 150 mcg (1 spray); >50 kg: 300 mcg (1 spray each nostril); repeat use is determined by the patient's clinical condition and laboratory work. If using preoperatively, administer 2 hours before surgery.

Uremic bleeding associated with acute or chronic renal failure (unlabeled use) (Watson, 1984): I.V.: 0.4 mcg/kg over 10 minutes

Prevention of surgical bleeding in patients with uremia (unlabeled use) (Mannucci, 1983): I.V.: 0.3 mcg/kg over 30 minutes

Renal Impairment Cl$_{cr}$ <50 mL/minute: Use is contraindicated according to the manufacturer; however, has been used in acute and chronic renal failure patients experiencing uremic bleeding or for prevention of surgical bleeding (unlabeled uses) (Mannucci, 1983; Watson, 1984).

Administration
I.M., I.V. push, SubQ injection: Central diabetes insipidus: Withdraw dose from ampul into appropriate syringe size (eg, insulin syringe). Further dilution is not required. Administer as direct injection.
I.V. infusion:
    Hemophilia A, von Willebrand disease (type 1), and prevention of surgical bleeding in patients with uremia (unlabeled; Mannucci, 1983): Infuse over 15-30 minutes
    Acute uremic bleeding (unlabeled; Watson, 1984): May infuse over 10 minutes
Intranasal:
    DDAVP®: Nasal pump spray: Delivers 0.1 mL (10 mcg); for doses <10 mcg or for other doses which are not multiples, use rhinal tube. DDAVP® Nasal spray delivers fifty 10 mcg doses. For 10 mcg dose, administer in one nostril. Any solution remaining after 50 doses should be discarded. Pump must be primed prior to first use.
    DDAVP® Rhinal tube: Insert top of dropper into tube (arrow marked end) in downward position. Squeeze dropper until solution reaches desired calibration mark. Disconnect dropper. Grasp the tube ¾ inch from the end and insert tube into nostril until the fingertips reach the nostril. Place opposite end of tube into the mouth (holding breath). Tilt head back and blow with a strong, short puff into the nostril. Reseal dropper after use.

Monitoring Parameters Blood pressure and pulse should be monitored during I.V. infusion

Note: For all indications, fluid intake, urine volume, and signs and symptoms of hyponatremia should be closely monitored especially in high-risk patient subgroups (eg, young children, elderly, patients with heart failure).
Diabetes insipidus: Urine specific gravity, plasma and urine osmolality, serum electrolytes
Hemophilia A: Factor VIII coagulant activity, factor VIII ristocetin cofactor activity, and factor VIII antigen levels, aPTT
von Willebrand disease: Factor VIII coagulant activity, factor VIII ristocetin cofactor activity, and factor VIII von Willebrand antigen levels, bleeding time
Nocturnal enuresis: Serum electrolytes if used for >7 days

Pharmacotherapy Pearls 10 mcg of desmopressin acetate is equivalent to 40 units

Special Geriatric Considerations Elderly patients should be cautioned not to increase their fluid intake beyond that sufficient to satisfy their thirst in order to avoid water intoxication and hyponatremia. Under experimental conditions, the elderly have been shown to have a decreased responsiveness to vasopressin with respect to its effects on water homeostasis.

Dosage Forms Excipient information presented when available (limited, particularly for generics); consult specific product labeling.
Injection, solution, as acetate: 4 mcg/mL (1 mL, 10 mL)
    DDAVP®: 4 mcg/mL (1 mL)
    DDAVP®: 4 mcg/mL (10 mL) [contains chlorobutanol]
Solution, intranasal, as acetate: 0.1 mg/mL (2.5 mL)
    DDAVP®: 0.1 mg/mL (2.5 mL) [contains chlorobutanol; with rhinal tube]
Solution, intranasal, as acetate [spray]: 0.1 mg/mL (5 mL)
    DDAVP®: 0.1 mg/mL (5 mL) [contains benzalkonium chloride; delivers 10 mcg/spray]
    Stimate®: 1.5 mg/mL (2.5 mL) [contains benzalkonium chloride; delivers 150 mcg/spray]
Tablet, oral, as acetate: 0.1 mg, 0.2 mg
    DDAVP®: 0.1 mg, 0.2 mg [scored]

Dosage Forms: Canada Excipient information presented when available (limited, particularly for generics); consult specific product labeling.
Tablet, as acetate, sublingual:
    DDAVP® Melt: 60 mcg, 120 mcg, 240 mcg

- ◆ **Desmopressin Acetate** see Desmopressin on page 511
- ◆ **Desoxyphenobarbital** see Primidone on page 1601
- ◆ **Desulfato-Hirudin** see Desirudin on page 508
- ◆ **Desulphatohirudin** see Desirudin on page 508

Desvenlafaxine (des ven la FAX een)

Related Information
Antidepressant Agents on page 2097
Medication Safety Issues
    BEERS Criteria medication:
        This drug may be potentially inappropriate for use in geriatric patients (Quality of evidence - moderate; Strength of recommendation - strong).
Brand Names: U.S. Pristiq®
Brand Names: Canada Pristiq®
Index Terms O-desmethylvenlafaxine; ODV

Generic Availability (U.S.) No

Pharmacologic Category Antidepressant, Serotonin/Norepinephrine Reuptake Inhibitor

Use Treatment of major depressive disorder

Medication Guide Available Yes

Contraindications Hypersensitivity to desvenlafaxine, venlafaxine or any component of the formulation; use of MAO inhibitors within 14 days; should not initiate MAO inhibitor within 7 days of discontinuing desvenlafaxine

Warnings/Precautions [U.S. Boxed Warning]: Antidepressants increase the risk of suicidal thinking and behavior in children, adolescents, and young adults (18-24 years of age) with major depressive disorder (MDD) and other psychiatric disorders; consider risk prior to prescribing. Short-term studies did not show an increased risk in patients >24 years of age and showed a decreased risk in patients ≥65 years. Closely monitor for clinical worsening, suicidality, or unusual changes in behavior; the patient's family or caregiver should be instructed to closely observe the patient and communicate condition with healthcare provider. A medication guide should be dispensed with each prescription.

The possibility of a suicide attempt is inherent in major depression and may persist until remission occurs. Monitor for worsening of depression or suicidality, especially during initiation of therapy (generally first 1-2 months) or with dose increases or decreases. Use caution in high-risk patients. Worsening depression and severe abrupt suicidality that are not part of the presenting symptoms may require discontinuation or modification of drug therapy. The patient's family or caregiver should be alerted to monitor patients for the emergence of suicidality and associated behaviors (such as agitation, irritability, hostility, impulsivity, and hypomania) and call healthcare provider.

May worsen psychosis in some patients or precipitate a shift to mania or hypomania in patients with bipolar disorder. Patients presenting with depressive symptoms should be screened for bipolar disorder. Monotherapy in patients with bipolar disorder should be avoided. **Desvenlafaxine is not FDA approved for the treatment of bipolar depression.**

Serotonin syndrome and neuroleptic malignant syndrome (NMS)-like reactions have occurred with serotonin/norepinephrine reuptake inhibitors (SNRIs) and selective serotonin reuptake inhibitors (SSRIs) when used alone, and particularly when used in combination with serotonergic agents (eg, triptans) or antidopaminergic agents (eg, antipsychotics). Concurrent use with MAO inhibitors is contraindicated. Do not begin desvenlafaxine within 14 days of terminating MAO-I therapy; do not initiate MAO-I treatment within 7 days of discontinuing desvenlafaxine. May cause sustained increase in blood pressure or heart rate; dose related. Control pre-existing hypertension prior to initiation of desvenlafaxine. Use caution in patients with recent history of MI, unstable heart disease, or cerebrovascular disease; may cause increases in serum lipids (cholesterol, LDL, triglycerides). Use caution in patients with renal impairment; dose reduction required in severe renal impairment. Use caution in patients with hepatic impairment; clearance is decreased and average AUC is increased; dosage adjustment is recommended. May cause hyponatremia/SIADH (elderly at increased risk); volume depletion (diuretics may increase risk).

Interstitial lung disease and eosinophilic pneumonia have been rarely reported with venlafaxine (the parent drug of desvenlafaxine); may present as progressive dyspnea, cough, and/or chest pain. Prompt evaluation and possible discontinuation of therapy may be necessary. Use cautiously in patients with a history of seizures. The risks of cognitive or motor impairment are low. May cause or exacerbate sexual dysfunction. May impair platelet aggregation, resulting in bleeding.

Use caution in elderly patients; may cause or exacerbate syndrome of inappropriate antidiuretic hormone secretion or hyponatremia; monitor sodium closely with initiation or dosage adjustments in older adults (Beers Criteria).

Abrupt discontinuation or dosage reduction after extended (≥6 weeks) therapy may lead to agitation, dysphoria, nervousness, anxiety, and other symptoms; discontinuation symptoms may also occur when switching from another antidepressant. When discontinuing therapy or switching antidepressants, dosage should be tapered gradually over at least a 2-week period. If intolerable symptoms occur following a decrease in dosage or upon discontinuation of therapy, then resuming the previous dose with a more gradual taper should be considered. Use caution in patients with increased intraocular pressure or at risk of acute narrow-angle glaucoma.

Adverse Reactions (Reflective of adult population; not specific for elderly)
Reported for 50-100 mg/day.
>10%:
 Central nervous system: Dizziness (10% to 13%), insomnia (9% to 12%)
 Gastrointestinal: Nausea (22% to 26%), xerostomia (11% to 17%), diarrhea (9% to 11%)
 Miscellaneous: Diaphoresis (10% to 11%)

◀

1% to 10%:

Cardiovascular: Palpitation (≤3%), orthostatic hypotension (<2%; elderly 8%), syncope (<2%), hypertension (dose related; ≤1% of patients taking 50-100 mg daily had sustained diastolic BP ≥90 mm Hg)

Central nervous system: Somnolence (≤9%), fatigue (7%), anxiety (3% to 5%), abnormal dreams (2% to 3%), irritability (2%), vertigo (1% to 2%), feeling jittery (≤2%), depersonalization (<2%), extrapyramidal symptoms (<2%), hypomania (<2%), seizures (<2%), concentration decreased (≤1%)

Dermatologic: Rash (1%)

Endocrine & metabolic: Libido decreased (males 4% to 5%), cholesterol (increased by ≥50 mg/dL and ≥261 mg/dL: 3% to 4%), anorgasmia (females 1%; males ≤3%), hot flushes (1%), low density lipoprotein cholesterol (increased by ≥50 mg/dL and ≥190 mg/dL: ≤1%), sexual dysfunction (males ≤1%)

Gastrointestinal: Constipation (9%), anorexia (5% to 8%), vomiting (≤4%), weight loss (≤2%), weight gain (<2%)

Genitourinary: Urinary hesitancy (≤1%)

Hepatic: Liver function tests abnormal (<2%)

Neuromuscular & skeletal: Tremor (≤3%), paresthesia (2%), weakness (≤2%), stiffness (<2%)

Ocular: Blurred vision (3% to 4%), mydriasis (2%)

Otic: Tinnitus (≤2%)

Renal: Proteinuria (6% to 8%)

Respiratory: Epistaxis (<2%)

Miscellaneous: Ejaculation retarded (1% to 5%), erectile dysfunction (3% to 6%), bruxism (<2%), hypersensitivity reaction (<2%), yawning (1%), ejaculation failure (≤1%)

Class-wide adverse effects: Gastrointestinal hemorrhage, hallucinations, photosensitivity

Drug Interactions

Metabolism/Transport Effects Substrate of CYP3A4 (minor); **Note:** Assignment of Major/Minor substrate status based on clinically relevant drug interaction potential; **Inhibits** CYP2D6 (weak); **Induces** CYP3A4 (weak/moderate)

Avoid Concomitant Use

Avoid concomitant use of Desvenlafaxine with any of the following: Axitinib; Iobenguane I 123; MAO Inhibitors; Methylene Blue

Increased Effect/Toxicity

Desvenlafaxine may increase the levels/effects of: Alpha-/Beta-Agonists; Aspirin; Methylene Blue; Metoclopramide; NSAID (Nonselective); Serotonin Modulators; Vitamin K Antagonists

The levels/effects of Desvenlafaxine may be increased by: Alcohol (Ethyl); Antipsychotics; Linezolid; MAO Inhibitors

Decreased Effect

Desvenlafaxine may decrease the levels/effects of: Alpha2-Agonists; Axitinib; Iobenguane I 123; Ioflupane I 123; Saxagliptin

The levels/effects of Desvenlafaxine may be decreased by: Tocilizumab

Ethanol/Nutrition/Herb Interactions

Ethanol: May increase CNS depression; monitor for increased effects with coadministration. Caution patients about effects.

Herb/Nutraceutical: Avoid St John's wort (may increase risk of serotonin syndrome and/or excessive sedation).

Mechanism of Action Desvenlafaxine is a potent and selective serotonin and norepinephrine reuptake inhibitor.

Pharmacodynamics/Kinetics

Distribution: V_d: 3.4 L/kg

Protein binding: 30%

Metabolism: Hepatic via conjugation, and oxidation via CYP3A4 (minor pathway)

Bioavailability: ~80%

Half-life elimination: ~11 hours; prolonged in renal failure

Time to peak, serum: ~7.5 hours

Excretion: Urine (45% as unchanged drug; ~24% as metabolites)

Dosage

Geriatric & Adult Depression: Oral: 50 mg once daily; doses up to 400 mg once daily have been studied; however, the manufacturer states there is no evidence that doses >50 mg/day confer any additional benefit. A flat dose response curve for efficacy between 50-400 mg/day has been noted as well as an increase in adverse events.

Note: Gradually taper dose (by increasing dosing interval) if discontinuing.

Renal Impairment
Cl$_{cr}$ >50 mL/minute: No dosage adjustment required
Cl$_{cr}$ 30-50 mL/minute: 50 mg once daily (maximum)
Cl$_{cr}$ <30 mL/minute: 50 mg every other day (maximum)
Hemodialysis: 50 mg every other day (maximum). Supplemental doses not required after HD.

Hepatic Impairment 50 mg once daily; maximum dose: 100 mg/day

Administration May be taken with or without food. Swallow tablet whole; do not crush, chew, break, or dissolve. When discontinuing therapy, extend dosing interval to taper.

Monitoring Parameters Renal function for dosing purposes; blood pressure should be regularly monitored, especially in patients with a high baseline blood pressure; lipid panel (eg, total cholesterol, LDL, triglycerides); mental status for depression, suicide ideation (especially at the beginning of therapy or when doses are increased or decreased). Intraocular pressure should be monitored in those with baseline elevations or a history of glaucoma.

Test Interactions May interfere with urine detection of PCP and amphetamine (false-positive).

Special Geriatric Considerations No dose adjustment is necessary for age alone; adjust dose for renal function. According to desvenlafaxine's manufacturer, 5% of the 3292 patients in clinical trials were 65 years of age or older. No differences in safety or efficacy were reported between younger and older adults. The elderly are more prone to SSRI/SNRI-induced hyponatremia.

A systematic review and meta-analysis of antidepressant placebo-controlled trials in persons with depression and dementia found evidence "suggestive" of efficacy but not of sufficient strength to "confirm" efficacy. Antidepressant trials in this patient population are small and underpowered. Older patients with depression being treated with an antidepressant should be closely monitored for response and adverse effects. Treatment should be switched or augmented when response is inadequate with a therapeutic dose. Antidepressants that are not tolerated should be discontinued and an alternative agent should be started.

This medication is considered to be potentially inappropriate in this patient population (Beers Criteria: Quality of evidence - moderate; Strength of recommendation - strong).

Dosage Forms Excipient information presented when available (limited, particularly for generics); consult specific product labeling.
Tablet, extended release, oral:
Pristiq®: 50 mg, 100 mg

◆ **Desyrel** see TraZODone on page 1953
◆ **Detemir Insulin** see Insulin Detemir on page 1010
◆ **Detrol®** see Tolterodine on page 1931
◆ **Detrol® LA** see Tolterodine on page 1931
◆ **Detryptoreline** see Triptorelin on page 1976

Dexamethasone (Systemic) (deks a METH a sone)

Related Information
Corticosteroids Systemic Equivalencies on page 2112
Medication Safety Issues
Sound-alike/look-alike issues:
Dexamethasone may be confused with desoximetasone, dextroamphetamine
Decadron® may be confused with Percodan®

Brand Names: U.S. Baycadron™; Dexamethasone Intensol™; DexPak® 10 Day Taper-Pak®; DexPak® 13 Day TaperPak®; DexPak® 6 Day TaperPak®

Brand Names: Canada Apo-Dexamethasone®; Dexasone®; Dom-Dexamethasone; PHL-Dexamethasone; PMS-Dexamethasone; PRO-Dexamethasone; ratio-Dexamethasone

Index Terms Decadron; Dexamethasone Sodium Phosphate

Generic Availability (U.S.) Yes: Excludes concentrated oral solution

Pharmacologic Category Anti-inflammatory Agent; Antiemetic; Corticosteroid, Systemic

Use Primarily as an anti-inflammatory or immunosuppressant agent in the treatment of a variety of diseases including those of allergic, dermatologic, endocrine, hematologic, inflammatory, neoplastic, nervous system, renal, respiratory, rheumatic, and autoimmune origin; may be used in management of cerebral edema, chronic swelling, as a diagnostic agent, diagnosis of Cushing's syndrome, antiemetic

Unlabeled Use Dexamethasone suppression test as an indicator of depression and/or risk of suicide; prevention and treatment of acute mountain sickness and high altitude cerebral edema

Contraindications Hypersensitivity to dexamethasone or any component of the formulation; systemic fungal infections, cerebral malaria

◀ **Warnings/Precautions** Use with caution in patients with thyroid disease, hepatic impairment, renal impairment, cardiovascular disease, diabetes, glaucoma, cataracts, myasthenia gravis, patients at risk for osteoporosis, patients at risk for seizures, or GI diseases (diverticulitis, peptic ulcer, ulcerative colitis) due to perforation risk. Use caution following acute MI (corticosteroids have been associated with myocardial rupture). Because of the risk of adverse effects, systemic corticosteroids should be used cautiously in the elderly in the smallest possible effective dose for the shortest duration. Withdraw therapy with gradual tapering of dose.

May cause hypercorticism or suppression of hypothalamic-pituitary-adrenal (HPA) axis, particularly in patients receiving high doses for prolonged periods. HPA axis suppression may lead to adrenal crisis. Withdrawal and discontinuation of a corticosteroid should be done slowly and carefully. Particular care is required when patients are transferred from systemic corticosteroids to inhaled products due to possible adrenal insufficiency or withdrawal from steroids, including an increase in allergic symptoms. Patients receiving >20 mg per day of prednisone (or equivalent) may be most susceptible. Fatalities have occurred due to adrenal insufficiency in asthmatic patients during and after transfer from systemic corticosteroids to aerosol steroids; aerosol steroids do not provide the systemic steroid needed to treat patients having trauma, surgery, or infections. Dexamethasone does not provide adequate mineralocorticoid activity in adrenal insufficiency (may be employed as a single dose while cortisol assays are performed). The lowest possible dose should be used during treatment; discontinuation and/or dose reductions should be gradual.

Acute myopathy has been reported with high dose corticosteroids, usually in patients with neuromuscular transmission disorders; may involve ocular and/or respiratory muscles; monitor creatine kinase; recovery may be delayed. Corticosteroid use may cause psychiatric disturbances, including depression, euphoria, insomnia, mood swings, and personality changes. Pre-existing psychiatric conditions may be exacerbated by corticosteroid use. Prolonged use of corticosteroids may also increase the incidence of secondary infection, mask acute infection (including fungal infections), prolong or exacerbate viral infections, or limit response to vaccines. Exposure to chickenpox should be avoided; corticosteroids should not be used to treat ocular herpes simplex. Corticosteroids should not be used for cerebral malaria or viral hepatitis. Close observation is required in patients with latent tuberculosis and/or TB reactivity; restrict use in active TB (only in conjunction with antituberculosis treatment). Prolonged treatment with corticosteroids has been associated with the development of Kaposi's sarcoma (case reports); if noted, discontinuation of therapy should be considered. High-dose corticosteroids should not be used to manage acute head injury.

Adverse Reactions (Reflective of adult population; not specific for elderly) Frequency not defined.

Cardiovascular: Arrhythmia, bradycardia, cardiac arrest, cardiomyopathy, CHF, circulatory collapse, edema, hypertension, myocardial rupture (post-MI), syncope, thromboembolism, vasculitis

Central nervous system: Depression, emotional instability, euphoria, headache, intracranial pressure increased, insomnia, malaise, mood swings, neuritis, personality changes, pseudotumor cerebri (usually following discontinuation), psychic disorders, seizure, vertigo

Dermatologic: Acne, allergic dermatitis, alopecia, angioedema, bruising, dry skin, erythema, fragile skin, hirsutism, hyper-/hypopigmentation, hypertrichosis, perianal pruritus (following I.V. injection), petechiae, rash, skin atrophy, skin test reaction impaired, striae, urticaria, wound healing impaired

Endocrine & metabolic: Adrenal suppression, carbohydrate tolerance decreased, Cushing's syndrome, diabetes mellitus, glucose intolerance decreased, growth suppression (children), hyperglycemia, hypokalemic alkalosis, menstrual irregularities, negative nitrogen balance, pituitary-adrenal axis suppression, protein catabolism, sodium retention

Gastrointestinal: Abdominal distention, appetite increased, gastrointestinal hemorrhage, gastrointestinal perforation, nausea, pancreatitis, peptic ulcer, ulcerative esophagitis, weight gain

Genitourinary: Altered (increased or decreased) spermatogenesis

Hepatic: Hepatomegaly, transaminases increased

Local: Postinjection flare (intra-articular use), thrombophlebitis

Neuromuscular & skeletal: Arthropathy, aseptic necrosis (femoral and humoral heads), fractures, muscle mass loss, myopathy (particularly in conjunction with neuromuscular disease or neuromuscular-blocking agents), neuropathy, osteoporosis, parasthesia, tendon rupture, vertebral compression fractures, weakness

Ocular: Cataracts, exophthalmos, glaucoma, intraocular pressure increased

Renal: Glucosuria

Respiratory: Pulmonary edema

Miscellaneous: Abnormal fat deposition, anaphylactoid reaction, anaphylaxis, avascular necrosis, diaphoresis, hiccups, hypersensitivity, impaired wound healing, infections, Kaposi's sarcoma, moon face, secondary malignancy

Drug Interactions

Metabolism/Transport Effects Substrate of CYP3A4 (major), P-glycoprotein; **Note:** Assignment of Major/Minor substrate status based on clinically relevant drug interaction potential; **Inhibits** P-glycoprotein; **Induces** CYP2A6 (weak/moderate), CYP2B6 (weak/moderate), CYP2C9 (weak/moderate), CYP3A4 (strong), P-glycoprotein

Avoid Concomitant Use

Avoid concomitant use of Dexamethasone (Systemic) with any of the following: Aldesleukin; Axitinib; BCG; Conivaptan; Crizotinib; Dabigatran Etexilate; Dronedarone; Everolimus; Lapatinib; Lurasidone; Mifepristone; Natalizumab; Nilotinib; Nisoldipine; Pazopanib; Pimecrolimus; Praziquantel; Ranolazine; Rilpivirine; Rivaroxaban; RomiDEPsin; SORAfenib; Tacrolimus (Topical); Ticagrelor; Tolvaptan; Toremifene; Vandetanib

Increased Effect/Toxicity

Dexamethasone (Systemic) may increase the levels/effects of: Acetylcholinesterase Inhibitors; Amphotericin B; CycloSPORINE; CycloSPORINE (Systemic); Deferasirox; Ifosfamide; Leflunomide; Lenalidomide; Loop Diuretics; Natalizumab; NSAID (COX-2 Inhibitor); NSAID (Nonselective); Thalidomide; Thiazide Diuretics; Vaccines (Live); Warfarin

The levels/effects of Dexamethasone (Systemic) may be increased by: Antifungal Agents (Azole Derivatives, Systemic); Aprepitant; Asparaginase (E. coli); Asparaginase (Erwinia); Calcium Channel Blockers (Nondihydropyridine); Conivaptan; CycloSPORINE; CycloSPORINE (Systemic); CYP3A4 Inhibitors (Moderate); CYP3A4 Inhibitors (Strong); Dasatinib; Denosumab; Estrogen Derivatives; Fluconazole; Fosaprepitant; Indacaterol; Ivacaftor; Macrolide Antibiotics; Mifepristone; Neuromuscular-Blocking Agents (Nondepolarizing); P-glycoprotein/ABCB1 Inhibitors; Pimecrolimus; Quinolone Antibiotics; Roflumilast; Salicylates; Tacrolimus (Topical); Telaprevir; Trastuzumab

Decreased Effect

Dexamethasone (Systemic) may decrease the levels/effects of: Aldesleukin; Antidiabetic Agents; Apixaban; ARIPiprazole; Axitinib; BCG; Boceprevir; Brentuximab Vedotin; Calcitriol; Caspofungin; Coccidioidin Skin Test; Corticorelin; Crizotinib; CycloSPORINE; CycloSPORINE (Systemic); CYP3A4 Substrates; Dabigatran Etexilate; Dasatinib; Dronedarone; Everolimus; Exemestane; Gefitinib; GuanFACINE; Hyaluronidase; Imatinib; Isoniazid; Ixabepilone; Lapatinib; Lurasidone; Maraviroc; NIFEdipine; Nilotinib; Nisoldipine; Pazopanib; P-glycoprotein/ABCB1 Substrates; Praziquantel; Ranolazine; Rilpivirine; Rivaroxaban; RomiDEPsin; Salicylates; Sipuleucel-T; SORAfenib; SUNItinib; Tadalafil; Telaprevir; Ticagrelor; Tolvaptan; Toremifene; Ulipristal; Vaccines (Inactivated); Vandetanib; Vemurafenib; Zuclopenthixol

The levels/effects of Dexamethasone (Systemic) may be decreased by: Aminoglutethimide; Antacids; Barbiturates; Bile Acid Sequestrants; CYP3A4 Inducers (Strong); Echinacea; Herbs (CYP3A4 Inducers); Mifepristone; Mitotane; P-glycoprotein/ABCB1 Inducers; Primidone; Rifamycin Derivatives; Tocilizumab

Ethanol/Nutrition/Herb Interactions

Ethanol: Avoid ethanol (may enhance gastric mucosal irritation).

Food: Dexamethasone interferes with calcium absorption. Limit caffeine.

Herb/Nutraceutical: Avoid cat's claw, echinacea (have immunostimulant properties).

Stability Injection solution: Store at room temperature; protect from light and freezing.

Stability of injection of parenteral admixture at room temperature (25°C): 24 hours

Stability of injection of parenteral admixture at refrigeration temperature (4°C): 2 days; protect from light and freezing.

Injection should be diluted in 50-100 mL NS or D_5W.

Mechanism of Action Decreases inflammation by suppression of neutrophil migration, decreased production of inflammatory mediators, and reversal of increased capillary permeability; suppresses normal immune response. Dexamethasone's mechanism of antiemetic activity is unknown.

Pharmacodynamics/Kinetics

Onset of action: Acetate: Prompt

Duration of metabolic effect: 72 hours; acetate is a long-acting repository preparation

Metabolism: Hepatic

Half-life elimination: Normal renal function: 1.8-3.5 hours; Biological half-life: 36-54 hours

Time to peak, serum: Oral: 1-2 hours; I.M.: ~8 hours

Excretion: Urine and feces

DEXAMETHASONE (SYSTEMIC)

Dosage

Geriatric Refer to adult dosing. Use cautiously in the elderly in the smallest possible dose.

Adult

Anti-inflammatory:

Oral, I.M., I.V.: 0.75-9 mg/day in divided doses every 6-12 hours

Intra-articular, intralesional, or soft tissue: 0.4-6 mg/day

Extubation or airway edema: Oral, I.M., I.V.: 0.5-2 mg/kg/day in divided doses every 6 hours beginning 24 hours prior to extubation and continuing for 4-6 doses afterwards

Antiemetic:

Prophylaxis: Oral, I.V.: 10-20 mg 15-30 minutes before treatment on each treatment day

Continuous infusion regimen: Oral or I.V.: 10 mg every 12 hours on each treatment day

Mildly emetogenic therapy: Oral, I.M., I.V.: 4 mg every 4-6 hours

Delayed nausea/vomiting: Oral: 4-10 mg 1-2 times/day for 2-4 days **or**

8 mg every 12 hours for 2 days; then

4 mg every 12 hours for 2 days **or**

20 mg 1 hour before chemotherapy; then

10 mg 12 hours after chemotherapy; then

8 mg every 12 hours for 4 doses; then

4 mg every 12 hours for 4 doses

Multiple myeloma: Oral, I.V.: 40 mg/day, days 1 to 4, 9 to 12, and 17 to 20, repeated every 4 weeks (alone or as part of a regimen)

Cerebral edema: I.V. 10 mg stat, 4 mg I.M./I.V. (should be given as sodium phosphate) every 6 hours until response is maximized, then switch to oral regimen, then taper off if appropriate; dosage may be reduced after 2-4 days and gradually discontinued over 5-7 days

Dexamethasone suppression test (depression/suicide indicator) (unlabeled use): Oral: 1 mg at 11 PM, draw blood at 8 AM the following day for plasma cortisol determination

Cushing's syndrome, diagnostic: Oral: 1 mg at 11 PM, draw blood at 8 AM; greater accuracy for Cushing's syndrome may be achieved by the following:

Dexamethasone 0.5 mg by mouth every 6 hours for 48 hours (with 24-hour urine collection for 17-hydroxycorticosteroid excretion)

Differentiation of Cushing's syndrome due to ACTH excess from Cushing's due to other causes: Oral: Dexamethasone 2 mg every 6 hours for 48 hours (with 24-hour urine collection for 17-hydroxycorticosteroid excretion)

Multiple sclerosis (acute exacerbation): Oral: 30 mg/day for 1 week, followed by 4-12 mg/day for 1 month

Treatment of shock:

Addisonian crisis/shock (eg, adrenal insufficiency/responsive to steroid therapy): I.V.: 4-10 mg as a single dose, which may be repeated if necessary

Unresponsive shock (eg, unresponsive to steroid therapy): I.V.: 1-6 mg/kg as a single I.V. dose or up to 40 mg initially followed by repeat doses every 2-6 hours while shock persists

Physiological replacement: Oral, I.M., I.V. (should be given as sodium phosphate): 0.03-0.15 mg/kg/day **or** 0.6-0.75 mg/m^2/day in divided doses every 6-12 hours

Acute mountain sickness (AMS)/high altitude cerebral edema (HACE) (unlabeled use):

Prevention: Oral: 2 mg every 6 hours **or** 4 mg every 12 hours starting on the day of ascent; may be discontinued after staying at the same elevation for 2-3 days or if descent is initiated; do not exceed a 10 day duration (Luks, 2010). **Note:** In situations of rapid ascent to altitudes >3500 meters (such as rescue or military operations), 4 mg every 6 hours may be considered (Luks, 2010).

Treatment: Oral, I.M., I.V.:

AMS: 4 mg every 6 hours (Luks, 2010)

HACE: Initial: 8 mg as a single dose; Maintenance: 4 mg every 6 hours until symptoms resolve (Luks, 2010)

Renal Impairment Hemodialysis or peritoneal dialysis: Supplemental dose is not necessary.

Administration

Oral: Administer with meals to decrease GI upset. **Note:** Oral administration of dexamethasone for croup may be prepared using a parenteral dexamethasone formulation and mixing it with an oral flavored syrup. (Bjornson, 2004)

I.V.: Administer as a 5-10 minute bolus; rapid injection is associated with a high incidence of perineal discomfort.

Monitoring Parameters Hemoglobin, occult blood loss, serum potassium, glucose

Reference Range Dexamethasone suppression test, overnight: 8 AM cortisol <6 mcg/100 mL (dexamethasone 1 mg); plasma cortisol determination should be made on the day after giving dose

Test Interactions May suppress the wheal and flare reactions to skin test antigens

Pharmacotherapy Pearls Withdrawal/tapering of therapy: Corticosteroid tapering following short-term use is limited primarily by the need to control the underlying disease state; tapering may be accomplished over a period of days. Following longer-term use, tapering over weeks to months may be necessary to avoid signs and symptoms of adrenal insufficiency and to allow recovery of the HPA axis. Testing of HPA axis responsiveness may be of value in selected patients. Subtle deficits in HPA response may persist for months after discontinuation of therapy, and may require supplemental dosing during periods of acute illness or surgical stress.

Special Geriatric Considerations Because of the risk of adverse effects, systemic corticosteroids should be used cautiously in the elderly in the smallest possible dose, and for the shortest possible time.

Dosage Forms Excipient information presented when available (limited, particularly for generics); consult specific product labeling.

Elixir, oral: 0.5 mg/5 mL (237 mL)

Baycadron™: 0.5 mg/5 mL (237 mL) [contains benzoic acid, ethanol 5.1%, propylene glycol; raspberry flavor]

Injection, solution, as sodium phosphate: 4 mg/mL (1 mL, 5 mL, 30 mL); 10 mg/mL (1 mL, 10 mL)

Injection, solution, as sodium phosphate [preservative free]: 10 mg/mL (1 mL)

Solution, oral: 0.5 mg/5 mL (240 mL, 500 mL)

Solution, oral [concentrate]:

Dexamethasone Intensol™: 1 mg/mL (30 mL) [dye free, sugar free; contains benzoic acid, ethanol 30%, propylene glycol]

Tablet, oral: 0.5 mg, 0.75 mg, 1 mg, 1.5 mg, 2 mg, 4 mg, 6 mg

DexPak® 6 Day TaperPak®: 1.5 mg [scored; 21 tablets on taper dose card]
DexPak® 10 Day TaperPak®: 1.5 mg [scored; 35 tablets on taper dose card]
DexPak® 13 Day TaperPak®: 1.5 mg [scored; 51 tablets on taper dose card]

Dexamethasone (Ophthalmic) (deks a METH a sone)

Medication Safety Issues
Sound-alike/look-alike issues:
Dexamethasone may be confused with desoximetasone, dextroamphetamine
Maxidex® may be confused with Maxzide®

Brand Names: U.S. Maxidex®; Ozurdex®
Brand Names: Canada Diodex®; Maxidex®; Ozurdex®
Index Terms Dexamethasone Sodium Phosphate
Generic Availability (U.S.) Yes: Ophthalmic solution
Pharmacologic Category Anti-inflammatory Agent, Ophthalmic; Corticosteroid, Ophthalmic; Corticosteroid, Otic

Use Management of steroid-responsive inflammatory conditions such as allergic conjunctivitis, iritis, or cyclitis; symptomatic treatment of corneal injury from chemical, radiation, or thermal burns, or penetration of foreign bodies. The ophthalmic solution is also indicated for otic use to treat steroid-responsive inflammatory conditions of the external auditory meatus.

Ophthalmic intravitreal implant (Ozurdex®): Treatment of macular edema following branch retinal vein occlusion (BRVO) or central retinal vein occlusion (CRVO); treatment of non-infective uveitis

Dosage
Geriatric Refer to adult dosing. Solution/suspension: Use cautiously in the elderly in the smallest possible dose.

Adult

Anti-inflammatory:

Ophthalmic:

Solution: Instill 1-2 drops into conjunctival sac every hour during the day and every other hour during the night; gradually reduce dose to 1 drop every 4 hours, then to 3-4 times/day

Suspension: Instill 1-2 drops into conjunctival sac up to 4-6 times/day; may use hourly in severe disease; taper prior to discontinuation

Otic: Solution: Initial: Instill 3-4 drops into the aural canal 3-4 times a day; reduce dose gradually once a favorable response is obtained. Alternately, may pack the aural canal with a gauze wick saturated with the solution; remove from the ear after 12-24 hours. Repeat as necessary.

Macular edema (following BRVO or CRVO): Ocular implant (Ozurdex®): Intravitreal injection: 0.7 mg implant injected in affected eye

Noninfective uveitis: Ocular implant (Ozurdex®): Intravitreal injection: 0.7 mg implant injected in affected eye

◀ **Special Geriatric Considerations** Evaluate the patient's or caregiver's ability to safely administer the correct dose of ophthalmic medication.

Dosage Forms Excipient information presented when available (limited, particularly for generics); consult specific product labeling.

Implant, intravitreal:
Ozurdex®: 0.7 mg (1s)
Solution, ophthalmic, as phosphate [drops]: 0.1% (5 mL)
Suspension, ophthalmic [drops]:
Maxidex®: 0.1% (5 mL) [contains benzalkonium chloride]

◆ **Dexamethasone and Ciprofloxacin** see Ciprofloxacin and Dexamethasone on page 386
◆ **Dexamethasone and Tobramycin** see Tobramycin and Dexamethasone on page 1918
◆ **Dexamethasone Intensol™** see Dexamethasone (Systemic) on page 517
◆ **Dexamethasone, Neomycin, and Polymyxin B** see Neomycin, Polymyxin B, and Dexamethasone on page 1355
◆ **Dexamethasone Sodium Phosphate** see Dexamethasone (Ophthalmic) on page 521
◆ **Dexamethasone Sodium Phosphate** see Dexamethasone (Systemic) on page 517

Dexchlorpheniramine (deks klor fen EER a meen)

Related Information
Beers Criteria – Potentially Inappropriate Medications for Geriatrics on page 2183

Medication Safety Issues
BEERS Criteria medication:
This drug may be potentially inappropriate for use in geriatric patients (Quality of evidence - moderate; Strength of recommendation - strong).

Index Terms Dexchlorpheniramine Maleate

Generic Availability (U.S.) Yes

Pharmacologic Category Alkylamine Derivative; Histamine H_1 Antagonist; Histamine H_1 Antagonist, First Generation

Use Perennial and seasonal allergic rhinitis and other allergic symptoms including urticaria

Contraindications Hypersensitivity to dexchlorpheniramine or any component of the formulation; narrow-angle glaucoma

Warnings/Precautions Causes sedation, caution must be used in performing tasks which require alertness (eg, operating machinery or driving). Effects may be potentiated when used with other sedative drugs or ethanol. Use with caution in patients with angle-closure glaucoma, pyloroduodenal obstruction (including stenotic peptic ulcer), urinary tract obstruction (including bladder neck obstruction and symptomatic prostatic hyperplasia), hyperthyroidism, increased intraocular pressure, and cardiovascular disease (including hypertension and ischemic heart disease). In the elderly, avoid use of this potent anticholinergic agent due to increased risk of confusion, dry mouth, constipation, and other anticholinergic effects; clearance decreases in patients of advanced age (Beers Criteria).

Adverse Reactions (Reflective of adult population; not specific for elderly)
>10%:
Central nervous system: Slight to moderate drowsiness
Respiratory: Thickening of bronchial secretions
1% to 10%:
Central nervous system: Headache, fatigue, nervousness, dizziness
Gastrointestinal: Appetite increase, weight gain, nausea, diarrhea, abdominal pain, xerostomia
Neuromuscular & skeletal: Arthralgia
Respiratory: Pharyngitis

Drug Interactions
Metabolism/Transport Effects None known.

Avoid Concomitant Use
Avoid concomitant use of Dexchlorpheniramine with any of the following: Azelastine; Azelastine (Nasal); Methadone; Mirtazapine; Paraldehyde

Increased Effect/Toxicity
Dexchlorpheniramine may increase the levels/effects of: Alcohol (Ethyl); Anticholinergics; Azelastine; Azelastine (Nasal); Buprenorphine; CNS Depressants; Methadone; Methotrimeprazine; Metyrosine; Mirtazapine; Paraldehyde; Selective Serotonin Reuptake Inhibitors; Zolpidem

The levels/effects of Dexchlorpheniramine may be increased by: Droperidol; HydrOXYzine; Methotrimeprazine; Pramlintide

Decreased Effect

Dexchlorpheniramine may decrease the levels/effects of: Acetylcholinesterase Inhibitors (Central); Benzylpenicilloyl Polylysine; Betahistine; Hyaluronidase

The levels/effects of Dexchlorpheniramine may be decreased by: Acetylcholinesterase Inhibitors (Central); Amphetamines

Ethanol/Nutrition/Herb Interactions Ethanol: May increase CNS depression; monitor for increased effects with coadministration. Caution patients about effects.

Mechanism of Action Competes with histamine for H_1-receptor sites on effector cells in the gastrointestinal tract, blood vessels, and respiratory tract. Dexchlorpheniramine is the predominant active isomer of chlorpheniramine and is approximately twice as active as the racemic compound.

Pharmacodynamics/Kinetics

Metabolism: Hepatic (Simons, 2004)
Half-life elimination: 20-30 hours (Moreno, 2010)
Time to peak: ~3 hours (Moreno, 2010)
Excretion: Urine

Dosage

Geriatric & Adult Allergy symptoms: Oral: 2 mg every 4-6 hours or 4-6 mg timed release at bedtime or every 8-10 hours

Administration May be administered without regard to meals.

Special Geriatric Considerations Anticholinergic action may cause significant confusional symptoms, constipation, or problems voiding urine.

This medication is considered to be potentially inappropriate in this patient population (Beers Criteria: Quality of evidence - moderate; Strength of recommendation - strong).

Dosage Forms Excipient information presented when available (limited, particularly for generics); consult specific product labeling.
Syrup, oral, as maleate: 2 mg/5 mL (473 mL)

◆ **Dexchlorpheniramine Maleate** *see* Dexchlorpheniramine *on page 522*
◆ **Dexferrum®** *see* Iron Dextran Complex *on page 1039*
◆ **Dexilant™** *see* Dexlansoprazole *on page 523*

Dexlansoprazole (deks lan SOE pra zole)

Medication Safety Issues

Sound-alike/look-alike issues:
Dexlansoprazole may be confused with aripiprazole, lansoprazole
Kapidex [DSC] may be confused with Casodex®, Kadian®

International issues:
Kapidex [DSC] may be confused with Capadex which is a brand name for propoxyphene/acetaminophen combination product [Australia, New Zealand]

Brand Names: U.S. Dexilant™
Brand Names: Canada Dexilant™
Index Terms Kapidex; TAK-390MR
Generic Availability (U.S.) No
Pharmacologic Category Proton Pump Inhibitor; Substituted Benzimidazole

Use Short-term (4 weeks) treatment of heartburn associated with nonerosive GERD; short-term (up to 8 weeks) treatment of all grades of erosive esophagitis; to maintain healing of erosive esophagitis for up to 6 months

Contraindications Hypersensitivity to dexlansoprazole or any component of the formulation

Warnings/Precautions Use of proton pump inhibitors (PPIs) may increase the risk of gastrointestinal infections (eg, *Salmonella, Campylobacter*). Relief of symptoms does not preclude the presence of a gastric malignancy. Atrophic gastritis (by biopsy) has been noted with long-term omeprazole therapy; this may also occur with dexlansoprazole. No occurrences of enterochromaffin-like (ECL) cell carcinoids, dysplasia, or neoplasia, such as those seen in rodent studies, have been reported in humans. Patients with moderate hepatic impairment (Child-Pugh class B) may require dosage reductions; no studies have been conducted in patients with severe hepatic impairment.

PPIs may diminish the therapeutic effect of clopidogrel, thought to be due to reduced formation of the active metabolite of clopidogrel. The manufacturer of clopidogrel recommends either avoidance of omeprazole or use of a PPI with less potent CYP2C19 inhibition (eg, pantoprazole). Lansoprazole exhibits the most potent CYP2C19 inhibition; given the potency of CYP2C19 inhibitory activity, avoidance of dexlansoprazole would appear prudent. Others have recommended the continued use of PPIs, regardless of the degree of inhibition, in patients with a history of GI bleeding or multiple risk factors for GI bleeding who are also receiving clopidogrel since no evidence has established clinically meaningful differences in outcome; however, a clinically-significant interaction cannot be excluded in those who are poor metabolizers of clopidogrel (Abraham, 2010; Levine, 2011). Additionally, concomitant use of dexlansoprazole with some drugs may require cautious use, may not be recommended, or may require dosage adjustments.

Increased incidence of osteoporosis-related bone fractures of the hip, spine, or wrist may occur with PPI therapy. Patients on high-dose (multiple daily doses) or long-term therapy (≥1 year) should be monitored. Use the lowest effective dose for the shortest duration of time, use vitamin D and calcium supplementation, and follow appropriate guidelines to reduce risk of fractures in patients at risk.

Hypomagnesemia, reported rarely, usually with prolonged PPI use of >3 months (most cases >1 year of therapy); may be symptomatic or asymptomatic; severe cases may cause tetany, seizures, and cardiac arrhythmias. Consider obtaining serum magnesium concentrations prior to beginning long-term therapy, especially if taking concomitant digoxin, diuretics, or other drugs known to cause hypomagnesemia; and periodically thereafter. Hypomagnesemia may be corrected by magnesium supplementation, although discontinuation of dexlansoprazole may be necessary; magnesium levels typically return to normal within 1 week of stopping.

Adverse Reactions (Reflective of adult population; not specific for elderly) 2% to 10%:

Gastrointestinal: Diarrhea (5%), abdominal pain (4%), nausea (3%), flatulence (1% to 3%), vomiting (1% to 2%)

Respiratory: Upper respiratory tract infection (2% to 3%)

Drug Interactions

Metabolism/Transport Effects None known.

Avoid Concomitant Use

Avoid concomitant use of Dexlansoprazole with any of the following: Delavirdine; Erlotinib; Nelfinavir; Posaconazole; Rilpivirine

Increased Effect/Toxicity

Dexlansoprazole may increase the levels/effects of: Amphetamines; Benzodiazepines (metabolized by oxidation); Dexmethylphenidate; Methotrexate; Methylphenidate; Raltegravir; Saquinavir; Tacrolimus; Tacrolimus (Systemic); Voriconazole

The levels/effects of Dexlansoprazole may be increased by: Fluconazole; Ketoconazole; Ketoconazole (Systemic)

Decreased Effect

Dexlansoprazole may decrease the levels/effects of: Atazanavir; Bisphosphonate Derivatives; Cefditoren; Clopidogrel; Dabigatran Etexilate; Dasatinib; Delavirdine; Erlotinib; Gefitinib; Indinavir; Iron Salts; Itraconazole; Ketoconazole; Ketoconazole (Systemic); Mesalamine; Mycophenolate; Nelfinavir; Nilotinib; Posaconazole; Rilpivirine; Vismodegib

The levels/effects of Dexlansoprazole may be decreased by: Tipranavir

Ethanol/Nutrition/Herb Interactions Ethanol: Avoid ethanol (may cause gastric mucosal irritation).

Stability Store at 25°C (77°F); excursions permitted to 15°C to 30°C (59°F to 86°F).

Mechanism of Action Proton pump inhibitor; decreases acid secretion in gastric parietal cells through inhibition of (H+, K+)-ATPase enzyme system, blocking the final step in gastric acid production

Pharmacodynamics/Kinetics

Distribution: V_d: 40.3 L

Protein binding: ~96% to 99%

Metabolism: Hepatic via CYP2C19-mediated hydroxylation and CYP3A4-mediated oxidation; followed by reduction to sulfate, glucuronide, and glutathione conjugates (inactive)

Bioavailability: May be increased when administered with food

Half-life, elimination: ~1-2 hours

Time to peak, serum: **Note:** Two distinct peaks secondary to dual release formulation:

Peak 1: 1-2 hours

Peak 2: 4-5 hours

Excretion: Urine (~51% as metabolites); feces (~48% as metabolites)

Dosage

Geriatric & Adult

Erosive esophagitis: Oral: Short-term treatment: 60 mg once daily for up to 8 weeks; maintenance therapy: 30 mg once daily for up to 6 months

Symptomatic GERD: Oral: Short-term treatment: 30 mg once daily for 4 weeks

Renal Impairment No dosage adjustment is needed.

Hepatic Impairment

Mild hepatic impairment (Child-Pugh class A): No dosage adjustment is needed.

Moderate hepatic impairment (Child-Pugh class B): Consider a maximum dose of 30 mg/day.

Severe hepatic impairment (Child-Pugh class C): Use has not been studied in patients with severe hepatic impairment.

Administration May be administered without regard to meals; some patients may benefit from premeal administration if symptoms do not adequately respond to post-meal dosing. Capsules should be swallowed whole; alternatively, patients who are unable to swallow capsules may open the capsule, sprinkle the intact granules onto 1 tablespoon of applesauce, and swallow intact granules immediately.

Special Geriatric Considerations No dose adjustment is recommended based on age or renal function. An increased half-life (2.23 vs 1.5 hours) and greater AUC (34.5%) in elderly compared to younger subjects are not considered to be clinically significant.

An increased risk of fractures of the hip, spine, or wrist has been observed in epidemiologic studies with proton pump inhibitor (PPI) use, primarily in older adults ≥50 years of age. The greatest risk was seen in patients receiving high doses or on long-term therapy (≥1 year). Calcium and vitamin D supplementation and close monitoring are recommended to reduce the risk of fracture in high-risk patients. Additionally, long-term use of proton pump inhibitors has resulted in reports of hypomagnesemia and *Clostridium difficile* infections.

Dosage Forms Excipient information presented when available (limited, particularly for generics); consult specific product labeling.

Capsule, delayed release, oral:

Dexilant™: 30 mg, 60 mg

◆ **DexPak® 6 Day TaperPak®** *see* Dexamethasone (Systemic) *on page 517*
◆ **DexPak® 10 Day TaperPak®** *see* Dexamethasone (Systemic) *on page 517*
◆ **DexPak® 13 Day TaperPak®** *see* Dexamethasone (Systemic) *on page 517*
◆ **Dextrin** *see* Wheat Dextrin *on page 2039*

Dextromethorphan (deks troe meth OR fan)

Medication Safety Issues

Sound-alike/look-alike issues:

Benylin® may be confused with Benadryl®, Ventolin®

Delsym® may be confused with Delfen®, Desyrel

Brand Names: U.S. Creo-Terpin® [OTC]; Creomulsion® Adult Formula [OTC]; Creomulsion® for Children [OTC]; Delsym® [OTC]; Father John's® [OTC]; Hold® DM [OTC]; Nycoff [OTC]; PediaCare® Children's Long-Acting Cough [OTC]; Robafen Cough [OTC]; Robitussin® Children's Cough Long-Acting [OTC]; Robitussin® Cough Long Acting [OTC] [DSC]; Robitussin® CoughGels™ Long-Acting [OTC] [DSC]; Robitussin® Lingering Cold Long-Acting Cough [OTC]; Robitussin® Lingering Cold Long-Acting CoughGels® [OTC]; Scot-Tussin® Diabetes [OTC]; Silphen-DM [OTC]; Triaminic Thin Strips® Children's Long Acting Cough [OTC]; Triaminic® Children's Cough Long Acting [OTC]; Trocal® [OTC] [DSC]; Vicks® 44® Cough Relief [OTC]; Vicks® DayQuil® Cough [OTC]; Vicks® Nature Fusion™ Cough [OTC]

Generic Availability (U.S.) Yes: Excludes strip

Pharmacologic Category Antitussive; N-Methyl-D-Aspartate Receptor Antagonist

Use Symptomatic relief of coughs caused by the common cold or inhaled irritants

Unlabeled Use N-methyl-D-aspartate (NMDA) antagonist

Contraindications Concurrent administration with or within 2 weeks of discontinuing an MAO inhibitor

Warnings/Precautions Symptoms of agitation, confusion, hallucinations, hyper-reflexia, myoclonus, shivering, and tachycardia may occur with concomitant proserotonergic drugs (ie, SSRIs/SNRIs or triptans); especially with higher dextromethorphan doses.

Some products may contain sodium benzoate which may cause allergic reactions in susceptible individuals.

Healthcare providers should be alert to problems of abuse or misuse. Abuse can cause death, brain damage, seizure, loss of consciousness and irregular heartbeat. Use with caution in patients who are sedated, debilitated or confined to a supine position. Some products may contain tartrazine.

Self-medication (OTC use): When used for self medication (OTC) notify healthcare provider if symptoms do not improve within 7 days, or are accompanied by fever, rash or persistent headache. Do not use for persistent or chronic cough (as with smoking, asthma, chronic bronchitis, emphysema) or if cough is accompanied by excessive phlegm unless directed to do so by healthcare provider.

Drug Interactions

Metabolism/Transport Effects Substrate of CYP2B6 (minor), CYP2C19 (minor), CYP2C9 (minor), CYP2D6 (major), CYP2E1 (minor), CYP3A4 (minor); **Note:** Assignment of Major/Minor substrate status based on clinically relevant drug interaction potential; **Inhibits** CYP2D6 (weak)

Avoid Concomitant Use

Avoid concomitant use of Dextromethorphan with any of the following: MAO Inhibitors

Increased Effect/Toxicity

Dextromethorphan may increase the levels/effects of: Metoclopramide; Serotonin Modulators

The levels/effects of Dextromethorphan may be increased by: Abiraterone Acetate; Antipsychotics; CYP2D6 Inhibitors (Moderate); CYP2D6 Inhibitors (Strong); Darunavir; MAO Inhibitors; QuiNIDine; Selective Serotonin Reuptake Inhibitors

Decreased Effect

The levels/effects of Dextromethorphan may be decreased by: Peginterferon Alfa-2b; Tocilizumab

Mechanism of Action Decreases the sensitivity of cough receptors and interrupts cough impulse transmission by depressing the medullary cough center through sigma receptor stimulation; structurally related to codeine

Pharmacodynamics/Kinetics

Onset of action: Antitussive: 15-30 minutes

Duration: ≤6 hours

Metabolism: Hepatic via demethylation via CYP2D6 to dextrorphan (active); CYP3A4 and CYP3A5 form smaller amounts of 3-hydroxy and 3-methoxy derivatives

Half-life elimination: Dextromethorphan: Extensive metabolizers: 2-4 hours; poor metabolizers: 24 hours

Time to peak: 2-3 hours

Excretion: Primarily in urine as metabolites

Dosage

Geriatric & Adult Cough suppressant: Oral: 10-20 mg every 4 hours or 30 mg every 6-8 hours; extended release: 60 mg twice daily; maximum: 120 mg/day

Test Interactions False-positive phencyclidine (PCP), opiates, opioids and heroin urine drug screen

Special Geriatric Considerations No specific information for use in elderly.

Dosage Forms Excipient information presented when available (limited, particularly for generics); consult specific product labeling. [DSC] = Discontinued product

Capsule, liquid filled, oral, as hydrobromide:

Robafen Cough: 15 mg

Robitussin® CoughGels™ Long-Acting: 15 mg [DSC]

Robitussin® Lingering Cold Long-Acting CoughGels®: 15 mg [contains coconut oil]

Liquid, oral, as hydrobromide: 15 mg/5 mL (120 mL [DSC])

Creo-Terpin®: 10 mg/15 mL (120 mL) [contains ethanol 25%, tartrazine]

Scot-Tussin® Diabetes: 10 mg/5 mL (118 mL) [ethanol free, gluten free, sugar free; contains propylene glycol; cherry-strawberry flavor]

Vicks® 44® Cough Relief: 10 mg/5 mL (120 mL) [contains ethanol, propylene glycol, sodium 28 mg/15 mL, sodium benzoate]

Vicks® Nature Fusion™ Cough: 30 mg/30 mL (240 mL) [dye free, ethanol free, gluten free; contains sodium 36 mg/30 mL; honey flavor]

Lozenge, oral, as hydrobromide:

Hold® DM: 5 mg (10s) [cherry flavor]

Hold® DM: 5 mg (10s) [original flavor]

Trocal®: 7.5 mg (50s [DSC], 300s [DSC]) [cherry flavor]

Solution, oral, as hydrobromide:

PediaCare® Children's Long-Acting Cough: 7.5 mg/5 mL (118 mL) [ethanol free; contains sodium 15 mg/5 mL, sodium benzoate; grape flavor]

Vicks® DayQuil® Cough: 15 mg/15 mL (177 mL, 295 mL) [ethanol free; contains propylene glycol, sodium 15 mg/15 mL; citrus flavor]

Strip, orally disintegrating, oral, as hydrobromide:

Triaminic Thin Strips® Children's Long Acting Cough: 7.5 mg (14s, 16s) [contains ethanol; cherry flavor; equivalent to dextromethorphan 5.5 mg]

Suspension, extended release, oral:

Delsym®: Dextromethorphan polistirex [equivalent to dextromethorphan hydrobromide] 30 mg/5 mL (89 mL, 148 mL) [ethanol free; contains propylene glycol, sodium 7 mg/5 mL; grape flavor]

Delsym®: Dextromethorphan polistirex [equivalent to dextromethorphan hydrobromide] 30 mg/5 mL (89 mL, 148 mL) [ethanol free; contains propylene glycol, sodium 7 mg/5 mL; orange flavor]

Syrup, oral, as hydrobromide:

Creomulsion® Adult Formula: 20 mg/15 mL (120 mL) [ethanol free; contains sodium benzoate]

Creomulsion® for Children: 5 mg/5 mL (120 mL) [ethanol free; contains sodium benzoate; cherry flavor]

Father John's®: 10 mg/5 mL (118 mL, 236 mL) [ethanol free]

Robitussin® Children's Cough Long-Acting: 7.5 mg/5 mL (118 mL) [ethanol free; contains propylene glycol, sodium 5 mg/5 mL, sodium benzoate; fruit-punch flavor]

Robitussin® Cough Long Acting: 15 mg/5 mL (240 mL [DSC]) [contains ethanol, sodium benzoate]

Robitussin® Lingering Cold Long-Acting Cough: 15 mg/5 mL (118 mL) [contains ethanol 1.4%, menthol, sodium benzoate]

Silphen-DM: 10 mg/5 mL (120 mL) [strawberry flavor]

Triaminic® Children's Cough Long Acting: 7.5 mg/5 mL (118 mL) [contains benzoic acid, propylene glycol, sodium 7 mg/5 mL]

Tablet, oral, as hydrobromide:

Nycoff: 15 mg

- ◆ **Dextromethorphan and Guaifenesin** see Guaifenesin and Dextromethorphan on page 906
- ◆ **Dex-Tuss** see Guaifenesin and Codeine on page 906
- ◆ **DHE** see Dihydroergotamine on page 548
- ◆ **D.H.E. 45®** see Dihydroergotamine on page 548
- ◆ **DHPG Sodium** see Ganciclovir (Systemic) on page 865
- ◆ **DHS™ Sal [OTC]** see Salicylic Acid on page 1743
- ◆ **Diabeta** see GlyBURIDE on page 887
- ◆ **DiaBeta®** see GlyBURIDE on page 887
- ◆ **DiabetAid® Antifungal Foot Bath [OTC]** see Miconazole (Topical) on page 1276
- ◆ **DiabetAid® Pain and Tingling Relief [OTC]** see Capsaicin on page 280
- ◆ **Diabetic Siltussin DAS-Na [OTC]** see GuaiFENesin on page 904
- ◆ **Diabetic Siltussin-DM DAS-Na [OTC]** see Guaifenesin and Dextromethorphan on page 906
- ◆ **Diabetic Siltussin-DM DAS-Na Maximum Strength [OTC]** see Guaifenesin and Dextromethorphan on page 906
- ◆ **Diabetic Tussin® DM [OTC]** see Guaifenesin and Dextromethorphan on page 906
- ◆ **Diabetic Tussin® DM Maximum Strength [OTC]** see Guaifenesin and Dextromethorphan on page 906
- ◆ **Diabetic Tussin® EX [OTC]** see GuaiFENesin on page 904
- ◆ **Diamode [OTC]** see Loperamide on page 1153
- ◆ **Diamox® Sequels®** see AcetaZOLAMIDE on page 37
- ◆ **Diastat®** see Diazepam on page 527
- ◆ **Diastat® AcuDial™** see Diazepam on page 527

Diazepam (dye AZ e pam)

Related Information

Anxiolytic, Sedative/Hypnotic, and Miscellaneous Benzodiazepines on page 2106
Beers Criteria – Potentially Inappropriate Medications for Geriatrics on page 2183
Patient Information for Disposal of Unused Medications on page 2244

Medication Safety Issues

Sound-alike/look-alike issues:

Diazepam may be confused with diazoxide, diltiazem, Ditropan, LORazepam

Valium® may be confused with Valcyte®

BEERS Criteria medication:

This drug may be potentially inappropriate for use in geriatric patients (Quality of evidence - high; Strength of recommendation - strong).

Brand Names: U.S. Diastat®; Diastat® AcuDial™; Diazepam Intensol™; Valium®

Brand Names: Canada Apo-Diazepam®; Bio-Diazepam; Diastat®; Diazemuls®; Diazepam Auto Injector; Diazepam Injection USP; Novo-Dipam; PMS-Diazepam; Valium®

Generic Availability (U.S.) Yes

Pharmacologic Category Benzodiazepine

Use Management of anxiety disorders, ethanol withdrawal symptoms; skeletal muscle relaxant; treatment of convulsive disorders; preoperative or preprocedural sedation and amnesia

◀ Rectal gel: Management of selected, refractory epilepsy patients on stable regimens of antiepileptic drugs requiring intermittent use of diazepam to control episodes of increased seizure activity

Unlabeled Use Panic disorders; sedation for mechanically-ventilated patients in the intensive care unit

Contraindications Hypersensitivity to diazepam or any component of the formulation (cross-sensitivity with other benzodiazepines may exist); myasthenia gravis; severe respiratory insufficiency; severe hepatic insufficiency; sleep apnea syndrome; acute narrow-angle glaucoma

Warnings/Precautions Withdrawal has also been associated with an increase in the seizure frequency. Use with caution with drugs which may decrease diazepam metabolism. Use with caution in debilitated patients, obese patients, patients with hepatic disease (including alcoholics), or renal impairment. Active metabolites with extended half-lives may lead to delayed accumulation and adverse effects. Use with caution in patients with respiratory disease or impaired gag reflex.

Acute hypotension, muscle weakness, apnea, and cardiac arrest have occurred with parenteral administration. Acute effects may be more prevalent in patients receiving concurrent barbiturates, narcotics, or ethanol. Appropriate resuscitative equipment and qualified personnel should be available during administration and monitoring. Avoid use of the injection in patients with shock, coma, or acute ethanol intoxication. Intra-arterial injection or extravasation of the parenteral formulation should be avoided. Parenteral formulation contains propylene glycol, which has been associated with toxicity when administered in high dosages. Administration of rectal gel should only be performed by individuals trained to recognize characteristic seizure activity and monitor response.

Causes CNS depression (dose-related) resulting in sedation, dizziness, confusion, or ataxia which may impair physical and mental capabilities. Patients must be cautioned about performing tasks which require mental alertness (eg, operating machinery or driving). Use with caution in patients receiving other CNS depressants or psychoactive agents. Effects with other sedative drugs or ethanol may be potentiated. The dosage of narcotics should be reduced by approximately one-third when diazepam is added. Benzodiazepines have been associated with falls and traumatic injury and should be used with extreme caution in patients who are at risk of these events. Benzodiazepines with long half-lives may produce prolonged sedation and increase the risk of falls and fracture. In older adults, benzodiazepines increase the risk of impaired cognition, delirium, falls, fractures, and motor vehicle accidents. Due to increased sensitivity in this age group and slower metabolism of long-acting agents (such as diazepam), avoid use for treatment of insomnia, agitation, or delirium (Beers Criteria).

Use with caution in patients taking strong CYP3A4 inhibitors, moderate or strong CYP3A4 and CYP2C19 inducers and major CYP3A4 substrates.

Use caution in patients with depression or anxiety associated with depression, particularly if suicidal risk may be present. Use with caution in patients with a history of drug dependence. Benzodiazepines have been associated with dependence and acute withdrawal symptoms on discontinuation or reduction in dose. Acute withdrawal, including seizures, may be precipitated in patients after administration of flumazenil to patients receiving long-term benzodiazepine therapy.

Diazepam has been associated with anterograde amnesia. Psychiatric and paradoxical reactions, including hyperactive or aggressive behavior, have been reported with benzodiazepines, particularly in elderly patients. Does not have analgesic, antidepressant, or antipsychotic properties.

Adverse Reactions (Reflective of adult population; not specific for elderly) Frequency not defined. Adverse reactions may vary by route of administration.

Cardiovascular: Hypotension, vasodilatation

Central nervous system: Amnesia, ataxia, confusion, depression, drowsiness, fatigue, headache, slurred speech, paradoxical reactions (eg, aggressiveness, agitation, anxiety, delusions, hallucinations, inappropriate behavior, increased muscle spasms, insomnia, irritability, psychoses, rage, restlessness, sleep disturbances, stimulation), vertigo

Dermatologic: Rash

Endocrine & metabolic: Libido changes

Gastrointestinal: Constipation, diarrhea, nausea, salivation changes (dry mouth or hypersalivation)

Genitourinary: Incontinence, urinary retention

Hepatic: Jaundice

Local: Phlebitis, pain with injection

Neuromuscular & skeletal: Dysarthria, tremor, weakness

Ocular: Blurred vision, diplopia

Respiratory: Apnea, asthma, respiratory rate decreased

Drug Interactions

Metabolism/Transport Effects Substrate of CYP1A2 (minor), CYP2B6 (minor), CYP2C19 (major), CYP2C9 (minor), CYP3A4 (major); **Note:** Assignment of Major/Minor substrate status based on clinically relevant drug interaction potential; **Inhibits** CYP2C19 (weak), CYP3A4 (weak)

Avoid Concomitant Use

Avoid concomitant use of Diazepam with any of the following: Azelastine; Azelastine (Nasal); Conivaptan; Methadone; Mirtazapine; OLANZapine; Paraldehyde; Pimozide

Increased Effect/Toxicity

Diazepam may increase the levels/effects of: Alcohol (Ethyl); ARIPiprazole; Azelastine; Azelastine (Nasal); Buprenorphine; CloZAPine; CNS Depressants; Fosphenytoin; Methadone; Methotrimeprazine; Metyrosine; Mirtazapine; Paraldehyde; Phenytoin; Pimozide; Selective Serotonin Reuptake Inhibitors; Zolpidem

The levels/effects of Diazepam may be increased by: Antifungal Agents (Azole Derivatives, Systemic); Aprepitant; Calcium Channel Blockers (Nondihydropyridine); Cimetidine; Conivaptan; Contraceptives (Estrogens); Contraceptives (Progestins); CYP2C19 Inhibitors (Moderate); CYP2C19 Inhibitors (Strong); CYP3A4 Inhibitors (Moderate); CYP3A4 Inhibitors (Strong); Dasatinib; Disulfiram; Droperidol; Fosamprenavir; Fosaprepitant; Grapefruit Juice; HydrOXYzine; Isoniazid; Ivacaftor; Macrolide Antibiotics; Methotrimeprazine; Mifepristone; OLANZapine; Proton Pump Inhibitors; Ritonavir; Saquinavir; Selective Serotonin Reuptake Inhibitors

Decreased Effect

The levels/effects of Diazepam may be decreased by: CarBAMazepine; CYP2C19 Inducers (Strong); CYP3A4 Inducers (Strong); Deferasirox; Rifamycin Derivatives; St Johns Wort; Theophylline Derivatives; Tocilizumab; Yohimbine

Ethanol/Nutrition/Herb Interactions

Ethanol: Ethanol may increase CNS depression. Potential for drug dependency exists. Management: Avoid ethanol.

Food: Diazepam serum concentrations may be decreased if taken with food. Grapefruit juice may increase diazepam serum concentrations. Management: Avoid concurrent use of grapefruit juice. Maintain adequate hydration, unless instructed to restrict fluid intake.

Herb/Nutraceutical: St John's wort may decrease diazepam levels. Yohimbe may decrease the effectiveness of diazepam. Kava kava, valerian, and gotu kola may increase CNS depression. Avoid St John's wort, yohimbe, kava kava, valerian, and gotu kola.

Stability

Injection: Store at 20°C to 25°C (68°F to 77°F); excursions permitted to 15°C to 30°C (59°F to 86°F). Protect from light. Potency is retained for up to 3 months when kept at room temperature. Most stable at pH 4-8; hydrolysis occurs at pH <3. Per manufacturer, do not mix I.V. product with other medications.

Rectal gel: Store at 25°C (77°F); excursion permitted to 15°C to 30°C (59°F to 86°F).

Tablet: Store at 15°C to 30°C (59°F to 86°F).

Mechanism of Action Binds to stereospecific benzodiazepine receptors on the postsynaptic GABA neuron at several sites within the central nervous system, including the limbic system, reticular formation. Enhancement of the inhibitory effect of GABA on neuronal excitability results by increased neuronal membrane permeability to chloride ions. This shift in chloride ions results in hyperpolarization (a less excitable state) and stabilization.

Pharmacodynamics/Kinetics

Onset of action: I.V.: Almost immediate; Oral: Rapid

Duration: I.V.: 20-30 minutes; Oral: Variable (dose and frequency dependent)

Absorption: Oral: 85% to 100%, more reliable than I.M.

Protein binding: 98%

Metabolism: Hepatic

Half-life elimination: Parent drug: Adults: 20-50 hours; increased half-life in elderly and those with severe hepatic disorders; Active major metabolite (desmethyldiazepam): 50-100 hours

Time to peak: Oral: 15 minutes to 2 hours

Dosage

Geriatric Oral absorption is more reliable than I.M. Elderly and/or debilitated patients:

Oral: 2-2.5 mg 1-2 times/day initially; increase gradually as needed and tolerated.

Rectal gel: Due to the increased half-life in elderly and debilitated patients, consider reducing dose.

Adult Note: Oral absorption is more reliable than I.M.

Acute ethanol withdrawal: *Oral:* 10 mg 3-4 times during first 24 hours, then decrease to 5 mg 3-4 times/day as needed

Anticonvulsant (acute treatment): *Rectal gel:* 0.2 mg/kg. **Note:** Dosage should be rounded upward to the next available dose, 2.5, 5, 7.5, 10, 12.5, 15, 17.5, and 20 mg/ dose; dose may be repeated in 4-12 hours if needed; do not use for more than 5 episodes per month or more than one episode every 5 days.

Anxiety (symptoms/disorders): *Oral, I.M, I.V.:* 2-10 mg 2-4 times/day if needed

Muscle spasm: *I.V., I.M.:* Initial: 5-10 mg; then 5-10 mg in 3-4 hours, if necessary. Larger doses may be required if associated with tetanus.

Sedation in the ICU patient: *I.V.:* 0.03-0.1 mg/kg every 30 minutes to 6 hours (Jacobi, 2002)

Skeletal muscle relaxant (adjunct therapy): *Oral:* 2-10 mg 3-4 times/day

Status epilepticus:
I.V.: 5-10 mg every 5-10 minutes given over ≤5 mg/minute (maximum dose: 30 mg)
Rectal gel: Premonitory/Out-of-hospital treatment: 10 mg once; may repeat once if necessary (Kälviäinen, 2007)

Rapid tranquilization of agitated patient (administer every 30-60 minutes): *Oral:* 5-10 mg; average total dose for tranquilization: 20-60 mg

Renal Impairment No dose adjustment recommended; decrease dose if administered for prolonged periods.

I.V.: Risk of propylene glycol toxicity; monitor closely if using for prolonged periods or at high doses.

Hemodialysis: Not dialyzable (0% to 5%); supplemental dose is not necessary.

Hepatic Impairment Decrease maintenance dose by 50%; half-life significantly prolonged.

Administration Intensol™ should be diluted before use.

Continuous infusion is not recommended because of precipitation in I.V. fluids and absorption of drug into infusion bags and tubing.

Rectal gel: Prior to administration, confirm that prescribed dose is visible and correct, and that the green "ready" band is visible. Patient should be positioned on side (facing person responsible for monitoring), with top leg bent forward. Insert rectal tip (lubricated) into rectum and push in plunger gently over 3 seconds. Remove tip of rectal syringe after 3 additional seconds. Buttocks should be held together for 3 seconds after removal. Dispose of syringe appropriately.

Monitoring Parameters Respiratory, cardiovascular, and mental status; check for orthostasis

Reference Range Therapeutic: Diazepam: 0.2-1.5 mcg/mL (SI: 0.7-5.3 micromole/L); N-desmethyldiazepam (nordiazepam): 0.1-0.5 mcg/mL (SI: 0.35-1.8 micromole/L)

Test Interactions False-negative urinary glucose determinations when using Clinistix® or Diastix®

Pharmacotherapy Pearls Diazepam does not have any analgesic effects.

Diastat® AcuDial™: When dispensing, consult package information for directions on setting patient's dose; confirm green "ready" band is visible prior to dispensing product.

Special Geriatric Considerations Due to its long-acting metabolite, diazepam is not considered a drug of choice in the elderly. Long-acting benzodiazepines have been associated with falls in the elderly. Guidelines from the Centers for Medicare and Medicaid Services (CMS) strongly discourage the use of this agent in residents of long-term care facilities.

This medication is considered to be potentially inappropriate in this patient population (Beers Criteria: Quality of evidence - high; Strength of recommendation - strong).

Controlled Substance C-IV

Dosage Forms Excipient information presented when available (limited, particularly for generics); consult specific product labeling.

Gel, rectal [adult rectal tip (6 cm)]: 20 mg (4 mL) [delivers set doses of 12.5 mg, 15 mg, 17.5 mg, 20 mg]
Diastat® AcuDial™: 20 mg (4 mL) [contains benzoic acid, benzyl alcohol, ethanol 10%, propylene glycol, sodium benzoate; 5 mg/mL (delivers set doses of 12.5 mg, 15 mg, 17.5 mg, and 20 mg)]

Gel, rectal [pediatric rectal tip (4.4 cm)]: 5 mg/mL (0.5 mL)
Diastat®: 5 mg/mL (0.5 mL) [contains benzoic acid, benzyl alcohol, ethanol 10%, propylene glycol, sodium benzoate]

Gel, rectal [pediatric/adult rectal tip (4.4 cm)]: 10 mg (2 mL) [delivers set doses of 5 mg, 7.5 mg, 10 mg]
Diastat® AcuDial™: 10 mg (2 mL) [contains benzoic acid, benzyl alcohol, ethanol 10%, propylene glycol, sodium benzoate; 5 mg/mL (delivers set doses of 5 mg, 7.5 mg, and 10 mg)]

Injection, solution: 5 mg/mL (2 mL, 10 mL)

Solution, oral: 5 mg/5 mL (5 mL, 500 mL)

Solution, oral [concentrate]:
Diazepam Intensol™: 5 mg/mL (30 mL) [contains ethanol 19%, propylene glycol]

Tablet, oral: 2 mg, 5 mg, 10 mg
Valium®: 5 mg, 10 mg [scored]
Valium®: 2 mg [scored; dye free]

♦ **Diazepam Intensol™** *see* Diazepam *on page 527*
♦ **Dibenzyline®** *see* Phenoxybenzamine *on page 1523*

Diclofenac (Systemic) (dye KLOE fen ak)

Related Information
Beers Criteria – Potentially Inappropriate Medications for Geriatrics *on page 2183*

Medication Safety Issues
Sound-alike/look-alike issues:
Diclofenac may be confused with Diflucan®
Cataflam® may be confused with Catapres®
Voltaren may be confused with traMADol, Ultram®, Verelan®

BEERS Criteria medication:
This drug may be potentially inappropriate for use in geriatric patients (Quality of evidence - moderate; Strength of recommendation - strong).

International issues:
Diclofenac may be confused with Duphalac brand name for lactulose [multiple international markets]
Flexin: Brand name for diclofenac [Argentina], but also the brand name for cyclobenzaprine [Chile] and orphenadrine [Israel]
Flexin [Argentina] may be confused with Floxin brand name for flunarizine [Thailand], norfloxacin [South Africa], ofloxacin [U.S., Canada], and perfloxacin [Philippines]

Brand Names: U.S. Cambia™; Cataflam®; Voltaren®-XR; Zipsor®

Brand Names: Canada Apo-Diclo Rapide®; Apo-Diclo®; Apo-Diclo® SR®; Ava-Diclofenac; Ava-Diclofenac SR; Cambia®; Cataflam®; Diclofenac ECT; Diclofenac Sodium; Diclofenac Sodium SR; Diclofenac SR; Dom-Diclofenac; Dom-Diclofenac SR; NTP-Diclofenac; NTP-Diclofenac SR; Nu-Diclo; Nu-Diclo-SR; PMS-Diclofenac; PMS-Diclofenac SR; PMS-Diclofenac-K; PRO-Diclo-Rapide; Sandoz-Diclofenac; Sandoz-Diclofenac Rapide; Sandoz-Diclofenac SR; Teva-Diclofenac; Teva-Diclofenac K; Teva-Diclofenac SR; Voltaren Rapide®; Voltaren SR®; Voltaren®

Index Terms Diclofenac Potassium; Diclofenac Sodium; Voltaren

Generic Availability (U.S.) Yes: Excludes capsule, oral solution

Pharmacologic Category Nonsteroidal Anti-inflammatory Drug (NSAID); Nonsteroidal Anti-inflammatory Drug (NSAID), Oral

Use
Capsule: Relief of mild-to-moderate acute pain
Immediate-release tablet: Relief of mild-to-moderate pain; primary dysmenorrhea; acute and chronic treatment of rheumatoid arthritis, osteoarthritis
Delayed-release tablet: Acute and chronic treatment of rheumatoid arthritis, osteoarthritis, ankylosing spondylitis
Extended-release tablet: Chronic treatment of osteoarthritis, rheumatoid arthritis
Oral solution: Treatment of acute migraine with or without aura
Suppository (CAN; not available in U.S.): Symptomatic treatment of rheumatoid arthritis and osteoarthritis (including degenerative joint disease of hip)

Unlabeled Use Juvenile idiopathic arthritis (JIA)

Medication Guide Available Yes

Contraindications Hypersensitivity to diclofenac or any component of the formulation; hypersensitivity to bovine protein (capsule formulation only); patients who exhibit asthma, urticaria, or other allergic-type reactions after taking aspirin or other NSAIDs; perioperative pain in the setting of coronary artery bypass graft (CABG) surgery

Canadian labeling: Additional contraindications (not in U.S. labeling): Uncontrolled heart failure, active gastric/duodenal/peptic ulcer; active GI bleed or perforation; regional ulcer, gastritis, or ulcerative colitis; cerebrovascular bleeding or other bleeding disorders; inflammatory bowel disease; severe hepatic impairment; active hepatic disease; severe renal impairment (Cl_{cr} <30 mL/minute) or deteriorating renal disease; known hyperkalemia; use of diclofenac suppository if recent history of bleeding or inflammatory lesions of rectum/anus

Warnings/Precautions [U.S. Boxed Warning]: NSAIDs are associated with an increased risk of adverse cardiovascular thrombotic events, including MI and stroke. Risk may be increased with duration of use or pre-existing cardiovascular risk factors or disease. Carefully evaluate individual cardiovascular risk profiles prior to prescribing. May cause new-onset hypertension or worsening of existing hypertension. Monitor blood pressure closely. Use caution with fluid retention. Avoid use in heart failure. Concurrent administration of ibuprofen, and potentially other nonselective NSAIDs, may interfere with aspirin's cardioprotective effect.

[U.S. Boxed Warning]: Use is contraindicated for treatment of perioperative pain in the setting of coronary artery bypass graft (CABG) surgery. Risk of MI and stroke may be increased with use following CABG surgery.

NSAID use may compromise existing renal function; dose-dependent decreases in prostaglandin synthesis may result from NSAID use, reducing renal blood flow which may cause renal decompensation. NSAID use may increase the risk for hyperkalemia. Patients with impaired renal function, dehydration, heart failure, liver dysfunction, those taking diuretics and ACEI, and the elderly are at greater risk of renal toxicity and hyperkalemia. Rehydrate patient before starting therapy; monitor renal function closely. Not recommended for use in patients with advanced renal disease. Long-term NSAID use may result in renal papillary necrosis while persistent urinary symptoms (eg, dysuria, bladder pain), cystitis, or hematuria may occur anytime after initiating NSAID therapy. Discontinue therapy with symptom onset and evaluate for origin.

[U.S. Boxed Warning]: NSAIDs may increase risk of gastrointestinal irritation, inflammation, ulceration, bleeding, and perforation. These events may occur at any time during therapy and without warning. Use caution with a history of GI disease (bleeding or ulcers), concurrent therapy with aspirin, anticoagulants and/or corticosteroids, smoking, use of alcohol, the elderly or debilitated patients. When used concomitantly with ≤325 mg of aspirin, a substantial increase in the risk of gastrointestinal complications (eg, ulcer) occurs; concomitant gastroprotective therapy (eg, proton pump inhibitors) is recommended (Bhatt, 2008).

Use the lowest effective dose for the shortest duration of time, consistent with individual patient goals, to reduce risk of cardiovascular or GI adverse events. Alternate therapies should be considered for patients at high risk.

NSAIDs may cause photosensitivity or serious skin adverse events including exfoliative dermatitis, Stevens-Johnson syndrome (SJS), and toxic epidermal necrolysis (TEN); discontinue use at first sign of skin rash or hypersensitivity. Anaphylactoid reactions may occur, even without prior exposure; patients with "aspirin triad" (bronchial asthma, aspirin intolerance, rhinitis) may be at increased risk. Do not use in patients who experience bronchospasm, asthma, rhinitis, or urticaria with NSAID or aspirin therapy. Use caution in other forms of asthma. Platelet adhesion and aggregation may be decreased; may prolong bleeding time; patients with coagulation disorders or who are receiving anticoagulants should be monitored closely. Anemia may occur; patients on long-term NSAID therapy should be monitored for anemia. Rarely, NSAID use may cause severe blood dyscrasias (eg, agranulocytosis, aplastic anemia, thrombocytopenia).

Use with caution in patients with impaired hepatic function. Closely monitor patients with any abnormal LFT. Diclofenac can cause transaminase elevations; initiate monitoring 4-8 weeks into therapy. Rarely, severe hepatic reactions (eg, fulminant hepatitis, liver failure) have occurred; discontinue all formulations if signs or symptoms of liver disease develop, or if systemic manifestations occur. Use with caution in hepatic porphyria (may trigger attack).

NSAIDS may cause drowsiness, dizziness, blurred vision, and other neurologic effects which may impair physical or mental abilities; patients must be cautioned about performing tasks which require mental alertness (eg, operating machinery or driving). Discontinue use with blurred or diminished vision and perform ophthalmologic exam. Monitor vision with long-term therapy. May increase the risk of aseptic meningitis, especially in patients with systemic lupus erythematosus (SLE) and mixed connective tissue disorders. In the elderly, avoid chronic use (unless alternative agents ineffective and patient can receive concomitant gastroprotective agent); nonselective oral NSAID use is associated with an increased risk of GI bleeding and peptic ulcer disease in older adults in high risk category (eg, >75 years or age or receiving concomitant oral/parenteral corticosteroids, anticoagulants, or antiplatelet agents) (Beers Criteria).

Withhold for at least 4-6 half-lives prior to surgical or dental procedures.

Capsule: Contains gelatin; use is contraindicated in patients with history of hypersensitivity to bovine protein.

Oral solution: Only indicated for the acute treatment of migraine; not indicated for migraine prophylaxis or cluster headache. Not bioequivalent to other forms of diclofenac (even same dose); do not interchange products. Contains phenylalanine.

Adverse Reactions (Reflective of adult population; not specific for elderly)

Oral:

1% to 10%:

Cardiovascular: Edema

Central nervous system: Dizziness, headache

Dermatologic: Pruritus, rash

Endocrine & metabolic: Fluid retention

Gastrointestinal: Abdominal distension, abdominal pain, constipation, diarrhea, dyspepsia, flatulence, GI perforation, heartburn, nausea, peptic ulcer/GI bleed, vomiting

Hematologic: Anemia, bleeding time increased

Hepatic: Liver enzyme abnormalities (>3 x ULN; ≤4%)

Otic: Tinnitus

Renal: Renal function abnormal

Miscellaneous: Diaphoresis increased

Rectal suppository (CAN; not available in U.S.): Also refer to adverse reactions associated with oral formulations.

Drug Interactions

Metabolism/Transport Effects Substrate of CYP1A2 (minor), CYP2B6 (minor), CYP2C19 (minor), CYP2C8 (minor), CYP2C9 (minor), CYP2D6 (minor), CYP3A4 (minor); **Note:** Assignment of Major/Minor substrate status based on clinically relevant drug interaction potential; **Inhibits** CYP1A2 (weak), CYP2C9 (weak), CYP2E1 (weak), CYP3A4 (weak)

Avoid Concomitant Use

Avoid concomitant use of Diclofenac (Systemic) with any of the following: Floctafenine; Ketorolac; Ketorolac (Nasal); Ketorolac (Systemic); Pimozide

Increased Effect/Toxicity

Diclofenac (Systemic) may increase the levels/effects of: Aliskiren; Aminoglycosides; Anticoagulants; Antiplatelet Agents; ARIPiprazole; Bisphosphonate Derivatives; Collagenase (Systemic); CycloSPORINE; CycloSPORINE (Systemic); Dabigatran Etexilate; Deferasirox; Desmopressin; Digoxin; Drotrecogin Alfa (Activated); Eplerenone; Haloperidol; Ibritumomab; Lithium; Methotrexate; Nonsteroidal Anti-Inflammatory Agents; PEMEtrexed; Pimozide; Porfimer; Potassium-Sparing Diuretics; PRALAtrexate; Quinolone Antibiotics; Rivaroxaban; Salicylates; Thrombolytic Agents; Tositumomab and Iodine I 131 Tositumomab; Vancomycin; Vitamin K Antagonists

The levels/effects of Diclofenac (Systemic) may be increased by: ACE Inhibitors; Angiotensin II Receptor Blockers; Antidepressants (Tricyclic, Tertiary Amine); Corticosteroids (Systemic); CycloSPORINE; CycloSPORINE (Systemic); Dasatinib; Floctafenine; Glucosamine; Herbs (Anticoagulant/Antiplatelet Properties); Ketorolac; Ketorolac (Nasal); Ketorolac (Systemic); Nonsteroidal Anti-Inflammatory Agents; Omega-3-Acid Ethyl Esters; Pentosan Polysulfate Sodium; Pentoxifylline; Probenecid; Prostacyclin Analogues; Selective Serotonin Reuptake Inhibitors; Serotonin/Norepinephrine Reuptake Inhibitors; Sodium Phosphates; Tipranavir; Treprostinil; Vitamin E; Voriconazole

Decreased Effect

Diclofenac (Systemic) may decrease the levels/effects of: ACE Inhibitors; Aliskiren; Angiotensin II Receptor Blockers; Antiplatelet Agents; Beta-Blockers; Eplerenone; HydrALAZINE; Loop Diuretics; Potassium-Sparing Diuretics; Salicylates; Selective Serotonin Reuptake Inhibitors; Thiazide Diuretics

The levels/effects of Diclofenac (Systemic) may be decreased by: Bile Acid Sequestrants; Nonsteroidal Anti-Inflammatory Agents; Peginterferon Alfa-2b; Salicylates; Tocilizumab

Ethanol/Nutrition/Herb Interactions

Ethanol: Avoid ethanol (may enhance gastric mucosal irritation).

Herb/Nutraceutical: Avoid alfalfa, anise, bilberry, bladderwrack, bromelain, cat's claw, celery, chamomile, coleus, cordyceps, dong quai, evening primrose, fenugreek, feverfew, garlic, ginger, ginkgo biloba, grapeseed, green tea, ginseng (Siberian), guggul, horse chestnut, horseradish, licorice, prickly ash, red clover, reishi, SAMe (s-adenosylmethionine), sweet clover, turmeric, white willow (all have additional antiplatelet activity).

Stability

Capsule, oral solution: Store at 25°C (77°F); excursions permitted to 15°C to 30°C (59°F to 86°F). Protect from moisture.

Suppository (CAN; not available in U.S.): Store at 15°C to 30°C (59°F to 86°F); protect from heat.

Tablet: Store below 30°C (86°F). Protect from moisture; store in tight container.

Mechanism of Action Reversibly inhibits cyclooxygenase-1 and 2 (COX-1 and 2) enzymes, which results in decreased formation of prostaglandin precursors; has antipyretic, analgesic, and anti-inflammatory properties

Other proposed mechanisms not fully elucidated (and possibly contributing to the anti-inflammatory effect to varying degrees), include inhibiting chemotaxis, altering lymphocyte activity, inhibiting neutrophil aggregation/activation, and decreasing proinflammatory cytokine levels.

Pharmacodynamics/Kinetics

Onset of action:

Cataflam® (potassium salt) is more rapid than the sodium salt because it dissolves in the stomach instead of the duodenum

Suppository: More rapid onset, but slower rate of absorption when compared to enteric coated tablet

Distribution: ~1.4 L/kg

Protein binding: >99%, primarily to albumin

Metabolism: Hepatic; undergoes first-pass metabolism; forms several metabolites (1 with weak activity)

Bioavailability: 55%

Half-life elimination: ~2 hours

Time to peak, serum:

Cambia™: ~0.25 hours

Cataflam®: ~1 hour

Voltaren® XR ~5 hours

Zipsor™: ~0.5 hour

Suppository: ≤1 hour; **Note:** Suppository: C_{max}: Approximately two-thirds of that observed with enteric coated tablet (equivalent 50 mg dose)

Tablet, delayed release (diclofenac sodium): ~2 hours

Excretion: Urine (~65%); feces (~35%)

Dosage

Geriatric Refer to adult dosing. No specific dosing recommendations; elderly may demonstrate adverse effects at lower doses than younger adults, and >60% may develop asymptomatic peptic ulceration with or without hemorrhage; monitor renal function.

Adult

Analgesia: Oral:

Immediate release tablet: Starting dose: 50 mg 3 times/day (maximum dose: 150 mg/day); may administer 100 mg loading dose, followed by 50 mg every 8 hours (maximum dose day 1: 200 mg/day; maximum dose day 2 and thereafter: 150 mg/day)

Canadian labeling: Maximum loading dose day 1: 200 mg/day; maximum dose day 2 and up to 7 days: 150 mg/day (50 mg every 6-8 hours)

Immediate release capsule: 25 mg 4 times/day

Primary dysmenorrhea: Oral: Immediate release tablet: Starting dose: 50 mg 3 times/day (maximum dose: 150 mg/day); may administer 100 mg loading dose, followed by 50 mg every 8 hours

Canadian labeling: Maximum loading dose day 1: 200 mg/day; maximum dose day 2 and up to 7 days: 150 mg/day (50 mg every 6-8 hours)

Rheumatoid arthritis:

Oral: Immediate release tablet: 150-200 mg/day in 3-4 divided doses; Delayed release tablet: 150-200 mg/day in 2-4 divided doses; Extended release tablet: 100 mg/day (may increase dose to 200 mg/day in 2 divided doses)

Canadian labeling: 150 mg/day in 3 divided doses (75-150 mg/day of slow release tablet)

Rectal suppository (not available in U.S.): Canadian labeling: Insert 50 mg or 100 mg rectally as single dose to substitute for final (third) oral daily dose (maximum combined dose [rectal and oral]: 150 mg/day

Osteoarthritis:

Oral: Immediate release tablet: 150-200 mg/day in 3-4 divided doses; Delayed release tablet: 150-200 mg/day in 2-4 divided doses; Extended release tablet: 100 mg/day; may increase dose to 200 mg/day in 2 divided doses

Canadian labeling: 150 mg/day in 3 divided doses (75-150 mg/day of slow release tablet)

Rectal suppository (not available in U.S.): Canadian labeling: Insert 50 mg or 100 mg rectally as single dose to substitute for final (third) oral daily dose (maximum combined dose [rectal and oral]: 150 mg/day)

Ankylosing spondylitis: Oral: Delayed release tablet: 100-125 mg/day in 4-5 divided doses

Migraine: Oral: Oral solution: 50 mg (one packet) as a single dose at the time of migraine onset; safety and efficacy of a second dose have not been established.

Renal Impairment Not recommended in patients with advanced renal disease or significant renal impairment.

Hepatic Impairment May require dosage adjustment; use oral solution only if benefits outweigh risks.

Administration

Oral: Do not crush delayed or extended release tablets. Administer with food or milk to avoid gastric distress. Take with full glass of water to enhance absorption.

Oral solution: Empty contents of packet into 1-2 ounces (30-60 mL) of water (do not use other liquids), mix well and administer immediately; food may reduce effectiveness.

Rectal suppository: Remove entire plastic wrapping prior to inserting rectally.

Monitoring Parameters Monitor CBC, liver enzymes (periodically during chronic therapy starting 4-8 weeks after initiation), BUN/serum creatinine; monitor urine output; occult blood loss

Special Geriatric Considerations Elderly are a high-risk population for adverse effects from nonsteroidal anti-inflammatory agents. As much as 60% of the elderly can develop peptic ulceration and/or hemorrhage asymptomatically. The concomitant use of H_2 blockers and sucralfate is not effective as prophylaxis with the exception of NSAID-induced duodenal ulcers which may be prevented by the use of ranitidine. Misoprostol and proton pump inhibitors are the only agents proven to help prevent the development of NSAID-induced ulcers. Also, concomitant disease and drug use contribute to the risk for GI adverse effects. Use lowest effective dose for shortest period possible. Consider renal function decline with age. Use of NSAIDs can compromise existing renal function especially when Cl_{cr} is ≤30 mL/minute. CNS adverse effects such as confusion, agitation, and hallucination are generally seen in overdose or high dose situations, but elderly may demonstrate these adverse effects at lower doses than younger adults.

This medication is considered to be potentially inappropriate in this patient population (Beers Criteria: Quality of evidence - moderate; Strength of recommendation - strong).

Dosage Forms Excipient information presented when available (limited, particularly for generics); consult specific product labeling.

Capsule, liquid filled, oral, as potassium:
Zipsor®: 25 mg [contains gelatin]
Powder for solution, oral, as potassium:
Cambia™: 50 mg/packet (1s) [contains phenylalanine 25 mg/packet; anise-mint flavor]
Tablet, oral, as potassium: 50 mg
Cataflam®: 50 mg
Tablet, delayed release, enteric coated, oral, as sodium: 25 mg, 50 mg, 75 mg
Tablet, extended release, oral, as sodium: 100 mg
Voltaren®-XR: 100 mg

Dosage Forms: Canada Excipient information presented when available (limited, particularly for generics); consult specific product labeling.
Suppository:
Voltaren®: 50 mg, 100mg

Diclofenac (Ophthalmic) (dye KLOE fen ak)

Medication Safety Issues

Sound-alike/look-alike issues:
Diclofenac may be confused with Diflucan®

International Issues:
Diclofenac may be confused with Duphalac brand name for lactulose [multiple international markets]
Flexin: Brand name for diclofenac [Argentina], but also the brand name for cyclobenzaprine [Chile] and orphenadrine [Israel]
Flexin [Argentina] may be confused with Floxin brand name for flunarizine [Thailand], norfloxacin [South Africa], ofloxacin [U.S., Canada], and pefloxacin [Philippines]

Brand Names: U.S. Voltaren Ophthalmic®

Brand Names: Canada Voltaren Ophtha®

Index Terms Diclofenac Sodium

Generic Availability (U.S.) Yes

Pharmacologic Category Nonsteroidal Anti-inflammatory Drug (NSAID); Nonsteroidal Anti-inflammatory Drug (NSAID), Ophthalmic

Use Treatment of postoperative inflammation following cataract extraction; temporary relief of pain and photophobia in patients undergoing corneal refractive surgery

Dosage

Geriatric Refer to adult dosing. No specific dosing recommendations.

Adult

Cataract surgery: Ophthalmic: Instill 1 drop into affected eye 4 times/day beginning 24 hours after cataract surgery and continuing for 2 weeks

Corneal refractive surgery: Ophthalmic: Instill 1-2 drops into affected eye within the hour prior to surgery, within 15 minutes following surgery, and then continue for 4 times/day, up to 3 days

Special Geriatric Considerations Evaluate the patient's or caregiver's ability to safely administer the correct dose of ophthalmic medication.

Dosage Forms Excipient information presented when available (limited, particularly for generics); consult specific product labeling.

Solution, ophthalmic, as sodium [drops]: 0.1% (2.5 mL, 5 mL)

Voltaren Ophthalmic®: 0.1% (2.5 mL, 5 mL) [contains sorbic acid]

Diclofenac (Topical) (dye KLOE fen ak)

Medication Safety Issues
Sound-alike/look-alike issues:
Diclofenac may be confused with Diflucan®

Voltaren® may be confused with traMADol, Ultram®, Verelan®

Other safety concerns:
Transdermal patch (Flector®) contains conducting metal (eg, aluminum); remove patch prior to MRI.

International issues:
Diclofenac may be confused with Duphalac brand name for lactulose [multiple international markets]

Flexin: Brand name for diclofenac [Argentina], but also the brand name for cyclobenzaprine [Chile] and orphenadrine [Israel]

Flexin [Argentina] may be confused with Floxin brand name for flunarizine [Thailand], norfloxacin [South Africa], ofloxacin [U.S., Canada], and perfloxacin [Philippines]

Brand Names: U.S. Flector®; Pennsaid®; Solaraze®; Voltaren® Gel

Brand Names: Canada Pennsaid®; Voltaren® Emulgel™

Index Terms Diclofenac Diethylamine [CAN]; Diclofenac Epolamine; Diclofenac Sodium

Generic Availability (U.S.) No

Pharmacologic Category Nonsteroidal Anti-inflammatory Drug (NSAID); Nonsteroidal Anti-inflammatory Drug (NSAID), Topical

Use
Topical gel 1%: Relief of osteoarthritis pain in joints amenable to topical therapy (eg, ankle, elbow, foot, hand, knee, wrist)

Canadian labeling (not in U.S. labeling): Relief of pain associated with acute, localized joint/muscle injuries (eg, sports injuries, strains) in patients ≥16 years of age

Topical gel 3%: Actinic keratosis (AK) in conjunction with sun avoidance

Topical patch: Acute pain due to minor strains, sprains, and contusions

Topical solution: Relief of osteoarthritis pain of the knee

Medication Guide Available Yes

Dosage
Geriatric Refer to adult dosing. No specific dosing recommendations; elderly may demonstrate adverse effects at lower doses than younger adults, and >60% may develop asymptomatic peptic ulceration with or without hemorrhage; monitor renal function.

Adult
Osteoarthritis:
Topical gel (Voltaren®): **Note:** Maximum total body dose of 1% gel should not exceed 32 g per day

Lower extremities: Apply 4 g of 1% gel to affected area 4 times/day (maximum: 16 g per joint per day)

Upper extremities: Apply 2 g of 1% gel to affected area 4 times/day (maximum: 8 g per joint per day)

Topical solution: Knee:

U.S. labeling: Apply 40 drops 4 times/day to each affected knee

Canadian labeling: Apply 40 drops 4 times/day **or** 50 drops 3 times/day to each affected knee for up to 3 months

Actinic keratosis (AK): Topical (Solaraze® Gel): Apply 3% gel to lesion area twice daily for 60-90 days

Acute pain (strains, sprains, contusions): Topical:
Patch: Apply 1 patch twice daily to most painful area of skin

Gel (Voltaren® Emulgel™ [CAN; not available in U.S.]): Apply 2-4 g to the skin over affected area(s) 3 or 4 times/day for up to 7 days

Special Geriatric Considerations Instruct patient or caregiver on appropriate use of topical diclofenac products.

Dosage Forms Excipient information presented when available (limited, particularly for generics); consult specific product labeling.
Gel, topical, as sodium:
Solaraze®: 3% (100 g) [contains benzyl alcohol]
Voltaren® Gel: 1% (100 g) [contains isopropyl alcohol]
Patch, transdermal, as epolamine:
Flector®: 1.3% (30s) [contains metal; 180 mg]
Solution, topical, as sodium:
Pennsaid®: 1.5% (150 mL)
Dosage Forms: Canada Excipient information presented when available (limited, particularly for generics); consult specific product labeling.
Gel, topical, as diethylamine:
Voltaren® Emulgel™: 1.16% (20 g, 50 g, 100 g)
Solution, topical, as sodium:
Pennsaid®: 1.5% (15 ml, 30 mL, 60 mL, 120 mL)

Diclofenac and Misoprostol (dye KLOE fen ak & mye soe PROST ole)

Related Information
Diclofenac (Systemic) on page 531
Misoprostol on page 1297
Brand Names: U.S. Arthrotec®
Brand Names: Canada Arthrotec®
Index Terms Misoprostol and Diclofenac
Generic Availability (U.S.) No
Pharmacologic Category Nonsteroidal Anti-inflammatory Drug (NSAID), Oral; Prostaglandin
Use Treatment of osteoarthritis and rheumatoid arthritis in patients at high risk for NSAID-induced gastric and duodenal ulceration
Medication Guide Available Yes
Dosage
Geriatric & Adult
Osteoarthritis: Oral: Arthrotec® 50: 1 tablet 3 times/day
Rheumatoid arthritis: Oral: Arthrotec® 50: 1 tablet 3 or 4 times/day
Note: For both indications, may administer Arthrotec® 50 or Arthrotec® 75 one tablet twice daily if recommended dose is not tolerated; however, these options are less effective in preventing GI ulceration. May adjust dose using individual agents in combination with Arthrotec®. The maximum daily dose of misoprostal is 800 mcg and the maximum single dose of misoprostal is 200 mcg. The maximum daily dose of diclofenac is 150 mg/day (osteoarthritis) or 225 mg/day (rheumatoid arthritis).
Renal Impairment Not recommended for use in patients with advanced renal disease. In renal insufficiency, diclofenac should be used with caution due to potential detrimental effects on renal function, and misoprostol dosage reduction may be required if adverse effects occur (misoprostol is renally eliminated).
Hepatic Impairment May require dosage adjustment.
Special Geriatric Considerations See individual agents.
Dosage Forms Excipient information presented when available (limited, particularly for generics); consult specific product labeling.
Tablet, oral:
Arthrotec® 50: Diclofenac sodium 50 mg and misoprostol 200 mcg
Arthrotec® 75: Diclofenac sodium 75 mg and misoprostol 200 mcg

♦ **Diclofenac Diethylamine [CAN]** see Diclofenac (Topical) on page 536
♦ **Diclofenac Epolamine** see Diclofenac (Topical) on page 536
♦ **Diclofenac Potassium** see Diclofenac (Systemic) on page 531
♦ **Diclofenac Sodium** see Diclofenac (Ophthalmic) on page 535
♦ **Diclofenac Sodium** see Diclofenac (Systemic) on page 531
♦ **Diclofenac Sodium** see Diclofenac (Topical) on page 536

Dicloxacillin (dye kloks a SIL in)

Index Terms Dicloxacillin Sodium
Generic Availability (U.S.) Yes
Pharmacologic Category Antibiotic, Penicillin
Use Treatment of systemic infections such as pneumonia, skin and soft tissue infections, and osteomyelitis caused by penicillinase-producing staphylococci

◄ **Contraindications** Hypersensitivity to dicloxacillin, penicillin, or any component of the formulation

Warnings/Precautions Monitor PT if patient concurrently on warfarin. Serious and occasionally severe or fatal hypersensitivity (anaphylactoid) reactions have been reported in patients on penicillin therapy, especially with a history of beta-lactam hypersensitivity, history of sensitivity to multiple allergens, or previous IgE-mediated reactions (eg, anaphylaxis, angioedema, urticaria). Use with caution in asthmatic patients. Prolonged use may result in fungal or bacterial superinfection, including *C. difficile*-associated diarrhea and pseudomembranous colitis.

Adverse Reactions (Reflective of adult population; not specific for elderly) 1% to 10%: Gastrointestinal: Nausea, diarrhea, abdominal pain

Drug Interactions

Metabolism/Transport Effects Induces CYP3A4 (weak/moderate)

Avoid Concomitant Use

Avoid concomitant use of Dicloxacillin with any of the following: Axitinib; BCG

Increased Effect/Toxicity

Dicloxacillin may increase the levels/effects of: Methotrexate; Vitamin K Antagonists

The levels/effects of Dicloxacillin may be increased by: Probenecid

Decreased Effect

Dicloxacillin may decrease the levels/effects of: ARIPiprazole; Axitinib; BCG; Mycophenolate; Saxagliptin; Typhoid Vaccine; Vitamin K Antagonists

The levels/effects of Dicloxacillin may be decreased by: Fusidic Acid; Tetracycline Derivatives

Ethanol/Nutrition/Herb Interactions Food: Food decreases drug absorption rate and serum concentration. Management: Administer around-the-clock on an empty stomach with a large glass of water 1 hour before or 2 hours after meals.

Mechanism of Action Inhibits bacterial cell wall synthesis by binding to one or more of the penicillin-binding proteins (PBPs) which in turn inhibits the final transpeptidation step of peptidoglycan synthesis in bacterial cell walls, thus inhibiting cell wall biosynthesis. Bacteria eventually lyse due to ongoing activity of cell wall autolytic enzymes (autolysins and murein hydrolases) while cell wall assembly is arrested.

Pharmacodynamics/Kinetics

Absorption: 35% to 76% from GI tract

Half-life: 0.6-0.8 hours, half-life is slightly prolonged in patients with renal impairment Protein binding: 96%

Time to peak serum concentration: Within 0.5-2 hours

Elimination: Partially by the liver and excreted in bile, 56% to 70% is eliminated in urine as unchanged drug

The percent unbound has been reported to be increased in older adults compared to young healthy volunteers (8.8% vs 7.3%), but this is not felt to be clinically significant

Dosage

Geriatric & Adult

Susceptible infections: Oral: 125-500 mg every 6 hours

Erysipelas, furunculosis, mastitis, otitis externa, septic bursitis, skin abscess: Oral: 500 mg every 6 hours

Impetigo: 250 mg every 6 hours

Prosthetic joint (long-term suppression therapy): Oral: 250 mg twice daily

Staphylococcus aureus, methicillin susceptible infection if no I.V. access: Oral: 500-1000 mg every 6-8 hours

Renal Impairment

Dosage adjustment is not necessary.

Not dialyzable (0% to 5%); supplemental dose is not necessary.

Peritoneal dialysis effects: Supplemental dose is not necessary.

Continuous arteriovenous or venovenous hemofiltration: Supplemental dose is not necessary.

Administration Administer 1 hour before or 2 hours after meals; administer around-the-clock rather than 4 times/day, 3 times/day, etc (ie, 12-6-12-6, not 9-1-5-9) to promote less variation in peak and trough serum concentrations

Monitoring Parameters Monitor prothrombin time if patient concurrently on warfarin; monitor for signs of anaphylaxis during first dose

Test Interactions False-positive urine and serum proteins; false-positive in uric acid, urinary steroids; may interfere with urinary glucose tests using cupric sulfate (Benedict's solution, Clinitest®); may inactivate aminoglycosides *in vitro*

Special Geriatric Considerations No dosage adjustment for renal function is necessary.

Dosage Forms Excipient information presented when available (limited, particularly for generics); consult specific product labeling.
Capsule, oral: 250 mg, 500 mg

◆ **Dicloxacillin Sodium** *see* Dicloxacillin *on page 537*

Dicyclomine (dye SYE kloe meen)

Related Information
Beers Criteria – Potentially Inappropriate Medications for Geriatrics *on page 2183*
Pharmacotherapy of Urinary Incontinence *on page 2141*
Medication Safety Issues
Sound-alike/look-alike issues:
Dicyclomine may be confused with diphenhydrAMINE, doxycycline, dyclonine
Bentyl® may be confused with Aventyl®, Benadryl®, Bontril®, Cantil®, Proventil®, TRENtal®
BEERS Criteria medication:
This drug may be potentially inappropriate for use in geriatric patients (Quality of evidence - moderate; Strength of recommendation - strong).
Brand Names: U.S. Bentyl®
Brand Names: Canada Bentylol®; Dicyclomine Hydrochloride Injection; Formulex®; Jamp-Dicyclomine; Protylol; Riva-Dicyclomine
Index Terms Dicyclomine Hydrochloride; Dicycloverine Hydrochloride
Generic Availability (U.S.) Yes: Excludes syrup
Pharmacologic Category Anticholinergic Agent
Use Treatment of functional bowel/irritable bowel syndrome
Unlabeled Use Urinary incontinence
Dosage
Geriatric 10-20 mg 4 times/day; increasing as necessary to 160 mg/day
Adult Gastrointestinal motility disorders/irritable bowel:
Oral: Initiate with 80 mg/day in 4 equally divided doses, then increase up to 160 mg/day
I.M. **(should not be used I.V.):** 80 mg/day in 4 divided doses (20 mg/dose)
Special Geriatric Considerations Long-term use of antispasmodics should be avoided in the elderly. The potential for a toxic reaction is greater than the potential benefit. In addition, the anticholinergic effects of dicyclomine are not well tolerated in the elderly.

This medication is considered to be potentially inappropriate in this patient population (Beers Criteria: Quality of evidence - moderate; Strength of recommendation - strong).
Dosage Forms Excipient information presented when available (limited, particularly for generics); consult specific product labeling.
Capsule, oral, as hydrochloride: 10 mg
Bentyl®: 10 mg
Injection, solution, as hydrochloride: 10 mg/mL (2 mL)
Bentyl®: 10 mg/mL (2 mL)
Syrup, oral, as hydrochloride: 10 mg/5 mL (473 mL)
Bentyl®: 10 mg/5 mL (480 mL) [contains propylene glycol]
Tablet, oral, as hydrochloride: 20 mg
Bentyl®: 20 mg

◆ **Dicyclomine Hydrochloride** *see* Dicyclomine *on page 539*
◆ **Dicycloverine Hydrochloride** *see* Dicyclomine *on page 539*
◆ **Didronel®** *see* Etidronate *on page 728*
◆ **Dificid™** *see* Fidaxomicin *on page 786*
◆ **Difimicin** *see* Fidaxomicin *on page 786*
◆ **Diflucan®** *see* Fluconazole *on page 795*

Diflunisal (dye FLOO ni sal)

Related Information
Beers Criteria – Potentially Inappropriate Medications for Geriatrics *on page 2183*
Medication Safety Issues
BEERS Criteria medication:
This drug may be potentially inappropriate for use in geriatric patients (Quality of evidence - moderate; Strength of recommendation - strong).
Brand Names: Canada Apo-Diflunisal®; Novo-Diflunisal; Nu-Diflunisal
Index Terms Dolobid
Generic Availability (U.S.) Yes

◀ **Pharmacologic Category** Nonsteroidal Anti-inflammatory Drug (NSAID), Oral

Use Management of inflammatory disorders usually including rheumatoid arthritis and osteo-arthritis; can be used as an analgesic for treatment of mild-to-moderate pain

Medication Guide Available Yes

Contraindications Hypersensitivity to diflunisal, aspirin, other NSAIDs, or any component of the formulation; perioperative pain in the setting of coronary artery bypass graft (CABG) surgery

Warnings/Precautions [U.S. Boxed Warning]: NSAIDs are associated with an increased risk of adverse cardiovascular thrombotic events, including MI and stroke. Risk may be increased with duration of use or pre-existing cardiovascular risk factors or disease. Carefully evaluate individual cardiovascular risk profiles prior to prescribing. May cause new-onset hypertension or worsening of existing hypertension. Use caution with fluid retention. Avoid use in heart failure. Concurrent administration of ibuprofen, and potentially other nonselective NSAIDs, may interfere with aspirin's cardioprotective effect. **[U.S. Boxed Warning]: Use is contraindicated for treatment of perioperative pain in the setting of coronary artery bypass graft (CABG) surgery.** Risk of MI and stroke may be increased with use following CABG surgery.

[U.S. Boxed Warning]: NSAIDs may increase risk of gastrointestinal irritation, inflammation, ulceration, bleeding, and perforation. Use caution with a history of GI disease (bleeding or ulcers), concurrent therapy with aspirin, anticoagulants and/or corticosteroids, smoking, use of alcohol, the elderly or debilitated patients. When used concomitantly with ≤325 mg of aspirin, a substantial increase in the risk of gastrointestinal complications (eg, ulcer) occurs; concomitant gastroprotective therapy (eg, proton pump inhibitors) is recommended (Bhatt, 2008).

In the elderly, avoid chronic use (unless alternative agents ineffective and patient can receive concomitant gastroprotective agent); nonselective oral NSAID use is associated with an increased risk of GI bleeding and peptic ulcer disease in older adults in high risk category (eg, >75 years or age or receiving concomitant oral/parenteral corticosteroids, anticoagulants, or antiplatelet agents) (Beers Criteria).

Platelet adhesion and aggregation may be decreased; may prolong bleeding time; patients with coagulation disorders or who are receiving anticoagulants should be monitored closely. Anemia may occur; patients on long-term NSAID therapy should be monitored for anemia. Rarely, NSAID use may cause severe blood dyscrasias (eg, agranulocytosis, aplastic anemia, thrombocytopenia).

NSAID use may compromise existing renal function; dose-dependent decreases in prostaglandin synthesis may result from NSAID use, reducing renal blood flow which may cause renal decompensation. NSAID use may increase the risk for hyperkalemia. Patients with impaired renal function, dehydration, heart failure, liver dysfunction, those taking diuretics, and ACE inhibitors, and the elderly are at greater risk of renal toxicity and hyperkalemia. Rehydrate patient before starting therapy; monitor renal function closely. Not recommended for use in patients with advanced renal disease. Long-term NSAID use may result in renal papillary necrosis. Use with caution in patients with decreased hepatic function.

NSAIDS may cause drowsiness, dizziness, blurred vision and other neurologic effects which may impair physical or mental abilities; patients must be cautioned about performing tasks which require mental alertness (eg, operating machinery or driving). Discontinue use with blurred or diminished vision and perform ophthalmologic exam. Monitor vision with long-term therapy.

Use the lowest effective dose for the shortest duration of time, consistent with individual patient goals, to reduce risk of cardiovascular or GI adverse events.

NSAIDs may cause serious skin adverse events including exfoliative dermatitis, Stevens-Johnson syndrome (SJS), and toxic epidermal necrolysis (TEN); discontinue use at first sign of skin rash or hypersensitivity. Do not use in patients who experience bronchospasm, asthma, rhinitis, or urticaria with NSAID or aspirin therapy. Use caution in other forms of asthma.

A hypersensitivity syndrome has been reported; monitor for constitutional symptoms and cutaneous findings; other organ dysfunction may be involved.

Diflunisal is a derivative of acetylsalicylic acid and therefore may be associated with Reye's syndrome. Withhold for at least 4-6 half-lives prior to surgical or dental procedures.

Adverse Reactions (Reflective of adult population; not specific for elderly) 1% to 10%:

Central nervous system: Headache (3% to 9%), dizziness (1% to 3%), insomnia (1% to 3%), somnolence (1% to 3%), fatigue (1% to 3%)

Dermatologic: Rash (3% to 9%)

Gastrointestinal: Nausea (3% to 9%), dyspepsia (3% to 9%), GI pain (3% to 9%), diarrhea (3% to 9%), constipation (1% to 3%), flatulence (1% to 3%), vomiting (1% to 3%), GI ulceration

Otic: Tinnitus (1% to 3%)

Drug Interactions

Metabolism/Transport Effects None known.

Avoid Concomitant Use

Avoid concomitant use of Diflunisal with any of the following: Floctafenine; Ketorolac; Ketorolac (Nasal); Ketorolac (Systemic)

Increased Effect/Toxicity

Diflunisal may increase the levels/effects of: Aliskiren; Aminoglycosides; Anticoagulants; Antiplatelet Agents; Bisphosphonate Derivatives; Collagenase (Systemic); CycloSPORINE; CycloSPORINE (Systemic); Dabigatran Etexilate; Deferasirox; Desmopressin; Digoxin; Drotrecogin Alfa (Activated); Eplerenone; Haloperidol; Ibritumomab; Lithium; Methotrexate; Nonsteroidal Anti-Inflammatory Agents; PEMEtrexed; Porfimer; Potassium-Sparing Diuretics; PRALAtrexate; Quinolone Antibiotics; Rivaroxaban; Salicylates; Thrombolytic Agents; Tositumomab and Iodine I 131 Tositumomab; Vancomycin; Vitamin K Antagonists

The levels/effects of Diflunisal may be increased by: ACE Inhibitors; Angiotensin II Receptor Blockers; Antidepressants (Tricyclic, Tertiary Amine); Corticosteroids (Systemic); CycloSPORINE; CycloSPORINE (Systemic); Dasatinib; Floctafenine; Glucosamine; Herbs (Anticoagulant/Antiplatelet Properties); Ketorolac; Ketorolac (Nasal); Ketorolac (Systemic); Nonsteroidal Anti-Inflammatory Agents; Omega-3-Acid Ethyl Esters; Pentosan Polysulfate Sodium; Pentoxifylline; Probenecid; Prostacyclin Analogues; Selective Serotonin Reuptake Inhibitors; Serotonin/Norepinephrine Reuptake Inhibitors; Sodium Phosphates; Tipranavir; Treprostinil; Vitamin E

Decreased Effect

Diflunisal may decrease the levels/effects of: ACE Inhibitors; Aliskiren; Angiotensin II Receptor Blockers; Antiplatelet Agents; Beta-Blockers; Eplerenone; HydrALAZINE; Loop Diuretics; Potassium-Sparing Diuretics; Salicylates; Selective Serotonin Reuptake Inhibitors; Thiazide Diuretics

The levels/effects of Diflunisal may be decreased by: Bile Acid Sequestrants; Nonsteroidal Anti-Inflammatory Agents; Salicylates

Ethanol/Nutrition/Herb Interactions

Ethanol: Avoid ethanol (may enhance gastric mucosal irritation).

Herb/Nutraceutical: Avoid alfalfa, anise, bilberry, bladderwrack, bromelain, cat's claw, celery, chamomile, coleus, cordyceps, dong quai, evening primrose, fenugreek, feverfew, garlic, ginger, ginkgo biloba, ginseng (American, Panax, Siberian), grapeseed, green tea, guggul, horse chestnut seed, horseradish, licorice, prickly ash, red clover, reishi, SAMe (S-adenosylmethionine), sweet clover, turmeric, white willow (all have additional antiplatelet activity).

Mechanism of Action Reversibly inhibits cyclooxygenase-1 and 2 (COX-1 and 2) enzymes, which results in decreased formation of prostaglandin precursors; has antipyretic, analgesic, and anti-inflammatory properties.

Other proposed mechanisms not fully elucidated (and possibly contributing to the anti-inflammatory effect to varying degrees) include inhibiting chemotaxis, altering lymphocyte activity, inhibiting neutrophil aggregation/activation, and decreasing proinflammatory cytokine levels.

Pharmacodynamics/Kinetics

Onset of action: Analgesic: ~1 hour; maximal effect: 2-3 hours

Duration: 8-12 hours

Absorption: Well absorbed

Protein binding: >99%

Distribution: 0.11 L/kg

Metabolism: Extensively hepatic; metabolic pathways are saturable

Half-life elimination: 8-12 hours; prolonged with renal impairment

Time to peak, serum: 2-3 hours

Excretion: Urine (~3% as unchanged drug, 90% as glucuronide conjugates) within 72-96 hours

Dosage

Geriatric & Adult

Mild-to-moderate pain: Oral: Initial: 500-1000 mg followed by 250-500 mg every 8-12 hours; maximum daily dose: 1.5 g

Arthritis: Oral: 500-1000 mg/day in 2 divided doses; maximum daily dose: 1.5 g

Renal Impairment

Use with caution; Cl$_{cr}$ <50 mL/minute: Administer 50% of normal dose (Aronoff, 1998)

Hemodialysis: No supplement required

CAPD: No supplement require

CAVH: Dose for GFR 10-50

Administration Tablet should be swallowed whole; do not crush or chew.

Test Interactions Falsely elevated increase in serum salicylate levels

Pharmacotherapy Pearls Diflunisal is a salicylic acid derivative which is chemically different than aspirin and is not metabolized to salicylic acid. It is not considered a salicylate. Diflunisal 500 mg is equal in analgesic efficacy to aspirin 650 mg, acetaminophen 650 mg, and acetaminophen 650 mg/propoxyphene napsylate 100 mg, but has a longer duration of effect (8-12 hours). Not recommended as an antipyretic. Not found to be clinically useful to treat fever; at doses ≥2 g/day, platelets are reversibly inhibited in function. Diflunisal is uricosuric at 500-750 mg/day; causes less GI and renal toxicity than aspirin and other NSAIDs; fecal blood loss is 1/2 that of aspirin at 2.6 g/day.

Special Geriatric Considerations The elderly are a high-risk population for adverse effects from nonsteroidal anti-inflammatory agents. As much as 60% of elderly can develop peptic ulceration and/or hemorrhage asymptomatically. The concomitant use of H$_2$ blockers and sucralfate is not effective as prophylaxis with the exception of NSAID-induced duodenal ulcers which may be prevented by the use of ranitidine. Misoprostol and proton pump inhibitors are the only agents proven to help prevent the development of NSAID-induced ulcers. Also, concomitant disease and drug use contribute to the risk for GI adverse effects. Use lowest effective dose for shortest period possible. Consider renal function decline with age. Use of NSAIDs can compromise existing renal function especially when Cl$_{cr}$ is ≤30 mL/minute. Tinnitus may be a difficult and unreliable indication of toxicity due to age-related hearing loss or eighth cranial nerve damage. CNS adverse effects such as confusion, agitation, and hallucination are generally seen in overdose or high dose situations, but elderly may demonstrate these adverse effects at lower doses than younger adults.

This medication is considered to be potentially inappropriate in this patient population (Beers Criteria: Quality of evidence - moderate; Strength of recommendation - strong).

Dosage Forms Excipient information presented when available (limited, particularly for generics); consult specific product labeling.

Tablet, oral: 500 mg

Difluprednate (dye floo PRED nate)

Medication Safety Issues

Sound-alike/look-alike issues:

Durezol® may be confused with Durasal™

Brand Names: U.S. Durezol®

Generic Availability (U.S.) No

Pharmacologic Category Corticosteroid, Ophthalmic

Use Treatment of inflammation and pain following ocular surgery; treatment of endogenous anterior uveitis

Contraindications Active viral (including herpes simplex keratitis, vaccinia, varicella) infections of the cornea or conjunctiva, fungal infection of ocular structures, or mycobacterial ocular infections

Warnings/Precautions For ophthalmic use only; not for intraocular administration. Steroids may mask infection or enhance existing ocular infection; prolonged use may result in secondary infections due to immunosuppression. Fungal infections should be considered with persistent corneal ulceration during therapy. Use caution in patients with a history of herpes simplex infection. Prolonged use has been associated with the development of corneal or scleral perforation and posterior subcapsular cataracts; may mask or enhance the establishment of acute purulent untreated infections of the eye; may delay healing after cataract surgery; intraocular pressure should be monitored if this product is used ≥10 days. Initial prescription and renewal of medication for >28 days should be made by healthcare provider only after examination with the aid of magnification such as slit lamp biomicroscopy or fluorescein staining (if appropriate). Contains sorbic acid which may be absorbed by contact lenses; contact lenses should be removed prior to use.

Adverse Reactions (Reflective of adult population; not specific for elderly)

Adverse reactions following ocular surgery:

5% to 15%: Ocular: Anterior chamber cells/flare, blepharitis, ciliary and conjunctival hyperemia, conjunctival/corneal edema, pain, photophobia, posterior capsule opacification

1% to 5%: Ocular: Inflammation, iritis, punctuate keratitis, visual acuity reduced

Adverse reactions associated with treatment of endogenous anterior uveitis:

5% to 10%:

Central nervous system: Headache

Ocular: Blurred vision, hyperemia (conjunctival and limbal), intraocular pressure increased, irritation, pain, punctate keratitis, uveitis

2% to 5%: Ocular: Anterior chamber flare, corneal edema, dry eye, iridocyclitis, photophobia, visual acuity decreased

Drug Interactions

Metabolism/Transport Effects None known.

Avoid Concomitant Use There are no known interactions where it is recommended to avoid concomitant use.

Increased Effect/Toxicity There are no known significant interactions involving an increase in effect.

Decreased Effect There are no known significant interactions involving a decrease in effect.

Stability Store at 15°C to 25°C (59°F to 77°F); do not freeze. Protect from light.

Mechanism of Action Corticosteroids inhibit the inflammatory response including edema, capillary dilation, leukocyte migration, and scar formation. Difluprednate penetrates cells readily to induce the production of lipocortins. These proteins modulate the activity of prostaglandins and leukotrienes.

Pharmacodynamics/Kinetics

Absorption: Systemic: Exposure to active metabolite is negligible with ocular administration

Metabolism: Undergoes deacetylation to an active metabolite (DFB)

Dosage

Geriatric & Adult

Endogenous anterior uveitis: Ophthalmic: Instill 1 drop into conjunctival sac of the affected eye(s) 4 times/day for 14 days then taper as clinically indicated

Inflammation associated with ocular surgery: Ophthalmic: Instill 1 drop in conjunctival sac of the affected eye(s) 4 times/day beginning 24 hours after surgery, continue for 2 weeks, then decrease to 2 times/day for 1 week, then taper based on response

Administration Wash hands prior to use and avoid touching tip of dropper. Remove contact lenses prior to use. Do not reinsert contact lenses within 10 minutes of difluprednate eye drops. The use of the same bottle for both eyes is not recommended in surgical patients.

Monitoring Parameters Intraocular pressure and periodic examination of lens (with prolonged use >28 days)

Special Geriatric Considerations Evaluate the patient's or caregiver's ability to safely administer the correct dose of ophthalmic medication.

Dosage Forms Excipient information presented when available (limited, particularly for generics); consult specific product labeling.

Emulsion, ophthalmic [drops]:

Durezol®: 0.05% (5 mL) [contains sorbic acid]

◆ **Digitalis** see Digoxin on page 543

Digoxin (di JOKS in)

Related Information

Beers Criteria – Potentially Inappropriate Medications for Geriatrics on page 2183
Heart Failure (Systolic) on page 2203

Medication Safety Issues

Sound-alike/look-alike issues:

Digoxin may be confused with Desoxyn®, doxepin

◄ Lanoxin® may be confused with Lasix®, levothyroxine, Levoxyl®, Levsinex®, Lomotil®, Mefoxin®, naloxone, Xanax®

High alert medication:
The Institute for Safe Medication Practices (ISMP) includes this medication among its list of drugs which have a heightened risk of causing significant patient harm when used in error.

BEERS Criteria medication:
This drug may be potentially inappropriate for use in geriatric patients (Quality of evidence - moderate; Strength of recommendation - strong).

International issues:
Lanoxin [U.S., Canada, and multiple international markets] may be confused with Limoxin brand name for ambroxol [Indonesia] and amoxicillin [Mexico]

Brand Names: U.S. Lanoxin®

Brand Names: Canada Apo-Digoxin®; Digoxin Injection CSD; Lanoxin®; Pediatric Digoxin CSD; PMS-Digoxin; Toloxin®

Index Terms Digitalis

Generic Availability (U.S.) Yes

Pharmacologic Category Antiarrhythmic Agent, Miscellaneous; Cardiac Glycoside

Use Treatment of mild-to-moderate (or stage C as recommended by the ACCF/AHA) heart failure (HF); atrial fibrillation (rate-control)
Note: In treatment of atrial fibrillation (AF), use is not considered first-line unless AF coexistent with heart failure or in sedentary patients (Fuster, 2006).

Unlabeled Use Fetal tachycardia with or without hydrops; to slow ventricular rate in supraventricular tachyarrhythmias such as supraventricular tachycardia (SVT) excluding atrioventricular reciprocating tachycardia (AVRT)

Contraindications Hypersensitivity to digoxin (rare) or other forms of digitalis, or any component of the formulation; ventricular fibrillation

Warnings/Precautions Watch for proarrhythmic effects (especially with digoxin toxicity). Withdrawal in clinically stable patients with HF may lead to recurrence of HF symptoms. During an episode of atrial fibrillation or flutter in patients with an accessory bypass tract (eg, Wolff-Parkinson-White syndrome), use has been associated with increased anterograde conduction down the accessory pathway leading to ventricular fibrillation; avoid use in such patients. Avoid use in patients with second- or third-degree heart block (except in patients with a functioning artificial pacemaker); incomplete AV block (eg, Stokes-Adams attack) may progress to complete block with digoxin administration. HF patients with preserved left ventricular function including patients with restrictive cardiomyopathy, constrictive pericarditis, and amyloid heart disease may be susceptible to digoxin toxicity; use unless used to control ventricular response with atrial fibrillation. Digoxin should not be used in patients with low EF, sinus rhythm, and no HF symptoms since the risk of harm may be greater than clinical benefit. Avoid use in patients with hypertrophic cardiomyopathy (HCM) and outflow tract obstruction unless used to control ventricular response with atrial fibrillation; outflow obstruction may worsen due to the positive inotropic effects of digoxin.

Use with caution in patients with hyperthyroidism, hypothyroidism, recent acute MI (within 6 months), sinus nodal disease (eg, sick sinus syndrome). Reduce dose with renal impairment and when amiodarone, propafenone, quinidine, or verapamil are added to a patient on digoxin; use with caution in patients taking strong inducers or inhibitors of P-glycoprotein (eg, cyclosporine). Avoid rapid I.V. administration of calcium in digitalized patients; may produce serious arrhythmias.

Atrial arrhythmias associated with hypermetabolic states are very difficult to treat; treat underlying condition first; if digoxin is used, ensure digoxin toxicity does not occur. Patients with beri beri heart disease may fail to adequately respond to digoxin therapy; treat underlying thiamine deficiency concomitantly. Correct electrolyte disturbances, especially hypokalemia or hypomagnesemia, prior to use and throughout therapy; toxicity may occur despite therapeutic digoxin concentrations. Hypercalcemia may increase the risk of digoxin toxicity; maintain normocalcemia. It is not necessary to routinely reduce or hold digoxin therapy prior to elective electrical cardioversion for atrial fibrillation; however, exclusion of digoxin toxicity (eg, clinical and ECG signs) is necessary prior to cardioversion. If signs of digoxin excess exist, withhold digoxin and delay cardioversion until toxicity subsides; usually >24 hours. Use with caution in the elderly; decreases in renal clearance may result in toxic effects; in general, avoid doses >0.125 mg/day; in heart failure, higher doses may increase the risk of potential toxicity and have not been shown to provide additional benefit (Beers Criteria).

Adverse Reactions (Reflective of adult population; not specific for elderly) Incidence not always reported.
Cardiovascular: Accelerated junctional rhythm, asystole, atrial tachycardia with or without block, AV dissociation, first-, second- (Wenckebach), or third-degree heart block, facial edema, PR prolongation, PVCs (especially bigeminy or trigeminy), ST segment depression, ventricular tachycardia or ventricular fibrillation

Central nervous system: Dizziness (6%), mental disturbances (5%), headache (4%), apathy, anxiety, confusion, delirium, depression, fever, hallucinations

Dermatologic: Rash (erythematous, maculopapular [most common], papular, scarlatiniform, vesicular or bullous), pruritus, urticaria, angioneurotic edema

Gastrointestinal: Nausea (4%), vomiting (2%), diarrhea (4%), abdominal pain, anorexia

Neuromuscular & skeletal: Weakness

Ocular: Visual disturbances (blurred or yellow vision)

Respiratory: Laryngeal edema

Drug Interactions

Metabolism/Transport Effects Substrate of CYP3A4 (minor), P-glycoprotein; **Note:** Assignment of Major/Minor substrate status based on clinically relevant drug interaction potential

Avoid Concomitant Use There are no known interactions where it is recommended to avoid concomitant use.

Increased Effect/Toxicity

Digoxin may increase the levels/effects of: Adenosine; Carvedilol; Colchicine; Dronedarone; Midodrine

The levels/effects of Digoxin may be increased by: Aminoquinolines (Antimalarial); Amiodarone; Antithyroid Agents; AtorvaSTATin; Beta-Blockers; Boceprevir; Calcium Channel Blockers (Nondihydropyridine); Calcium Polystyrene Sulfonate; Carvedilol; Conivaptan; CycloSPORINE; CycloSPORINE (Systemic); Dronedarone; Etravirine; Glycopyrrolate; Itraconazole; Lenalidomide; Loop Diuretics; Macrolide Antibiotics; Mifepristone; Milnacipran; Nefazodone; Neuromuscular-Blocking Agents; NIFEdipine; Nonsteroidal Anti-Inflammatory Agents; Paricalcitol; P-glycoprotein/ABCB1 Inhibitors; Posaconazole; Potassium-Sparing Diuretics; Propafenone; Protease Inhibitors; QuiNIDine; QuiNINE; Ranolazine; Reserpine; SitaGLIPtin; Sodium Polystyrene Sulfonate; Spironolactone; Telaprevir; Telmisartan; Ticagrelor; Tolvaptan; Vitamin D Analogs

Decreased Effect

Digoxin may decrease the levels/effects of: Antineoplastic Agents (Anthracycline, Systemic)

The levels/effects of Digoxin may be decreased by: 5-ASA Derivatives; Acarbose; Aminoglycosides; Antineoplastic Agents; Antineoplastic Agents (Anthracycline, Systemic); Bile Acid Sequestrants; Kaolin; PenicillAMINE; P-glycoprotein/ABCB1 Inducers; Potassium-Sparing Diuretics; St Johns Wort; Sucralfate; Tocilizumab

Ethanol/Nutrition/Herb Interactions

Food: Digoxin peak serum concentrations may be decreased if taken with food. Meals containing increased fiber (bran) or foods high in pectin may decrease oral absorption of digoxin.

Herb/Nutraceutical: Avoid ephedra (risk of cardiac stimulation). Avoid natural licorice (causes sodium and water retention and increases potassium loss).

Stability Store at 25°C (77°F); excursions permitted to 15°C to 30°C (59°F to 86°F). Protect elixir, injection, and tablets from light.

Mechanism of Action

Heart failure: Inhibition of the sodium/potassium ATPase pump in myocardial cells results in a transient increase of intracellular sodium, which in turn promotes calcium influx via the sodium-calcium exchange pump leading to increased contractility.

Supraventricular arrhythmias: Direct suppression of the AV node conduction to increase effective refractory period and decrease conduction velocity - positive inotropic effect, enhanced vagal tone, and decreased ventricular rate to fast atrial arrhythmias. Atrial fibrillation may decrease sensitivity and increase tolerance to higher serum digoxin concentrations.

Pharmacodynamics/Kinetics

Onset of action: Heart rate control: Oral: 1-2 hours; I.V.: 5-60 minutes

Peak effect: Heart rate control: Oral: 2-8 hours; I.V.: 1-6 hours; **Note:** In patients with atrial fibrillation, median time to ventricular rate control in one study was 6 hours (range: 3-15 hours) (Siu, 2009)

Duration: Adults: 3-4 days

Absorption: By passive nonsaturable diffusion in the upper small intestine; food may delay, but does not affect extent of absorption

Distribution:

Normal renal function: 6-7 L/kg

V_d: Extensive to peripheral tissues, with a distinct distribution phase which lasts 6-8 hours; concentrates in heart, liver, kidney, skeletal muscle, and intestines. Heart/serum concentration is 70:1. Pharmacologic effects are delayed and do not correlate well with serum concentrations during distribution phase.

Hyperthyroidism: Increased V_d

Hyperkalemia, hyponatremia: Decreased digoxin distribution to heart and muscle

Hypokalemia: Increased digoxin distribution to heart and muscles

Concomitant quinidine therapy: Decreased V_d

Chronic renal failure: 4-6 L/kg

Decreased sodium/potassium ATPase activity - decreased tissue binding

Adults: 7 L/kg, decreased with renal disease

Protein binding: ~25%; in uremic patients, digoxin is displaced from plasma protein binding sites

Metabolism: Via sequential sugar hydrolysis in the stomach or by reduction of lactone ring by intestinal bacteria (in ~10% of population, gut bacteria may metabolize up to 40% of digoxin dose); once absorbed, only ~16% is metabolized to 3-beta-digoxigenin, 3-keto-digoxigenin, and glucuronide and sulfate conjugates; metabolites may contribute to therapeutic and toxic effects of digoxin; metabolism is reduced with decompensated HF

Bioavailability: Oral (formulation dependent): Elixir: 70% to 85%; Tablet: 60% to 80%

Half-life elimination (age, renal and cardiac function dependent):

Adults: 36-48 hours

Adults, anephric: 3.5-5 days

Half-life elimination: Parent drug: 38 hours; Metabolites: Digoxigenin: 4 hours; Monodigitoxoside: 3-12 hours

Time to peak, serum: Oral: 1-3 hours

Excretion: Urine (50% to 70% as unchanged drug)

Dosage

Geriatric Dose is based on assessment of lean body mass and renal function. Elderly patients with low lean body mass may experience higher digoxin concentrations due to reduced volume of distribution (Cheng, 2010). Decrease dose in patients with decreased renal function (see Dosage: Renal Impairment).

Heart failure: If patient is >70 years of age, low doses (eg, 0.125 mg daily or every other day) should be used (Hunt, 2009).

Adult Note: When changing from oral (tablets or liquid) or I.M. to I.V. therapy, dosage should be reduced by 20% to 25%.

Atrial fibrillation (rate control) in patients with heart failure: Loading dose: I.V.: 0.25 mg every 2 hours, up to 1.5 mg within 24 hours; for nonacute situations, may administer 0.5 mg orally once daily for 2 days followed by oral maintenance dose. Maintenance dose: I.V., Oral: 0.125-0.375 mg once daily (Fuster, 2006)

Heart failure: Daily maintenance dose (**Note:** Loading dose not recommended): Oral: 0.125-0.25 mg once daily; higher daily doses (up to 0.5 mg/day) are rarely necessary. If patient is >70 years of age, has impaired renal function, or has a low lean body mass, low doses (eg, 0.125 mg daily or every other day) should be used (Hunt, 2009).

Supraventricular tachyarrhythmias (rate control):

Initial: Total digitalizing dose:

Oral: 0.75-1.5 mg

I.V., I.M.: 0.5-1 mg (**Note:** I.M. not preferred due to severe injection site pain.)

Give ¹/₂ (one-half) of the total digitalizing dose (TDD) as the initial dose, then give ¹/₄ (one-quarter) of the TDD in each of 2 subsequent doses at 6- to 8-hour intervals. Obtain ECG 6 hours after each dose to assess potential toxicity.

Daily maintenance dose:

Oral: 0.125-0.5 mg once daily

I.V., I.M.: 0.1-0.4 mg once daily (**Note:** I.M. not preferred due to severe injection site pain.)

Renal Impairment

Loading dose:

ESRD: If loading dose necessary, reduce dose by 50%

Acute renal failure: Based on expert opinion, if patient in acute renal failure requires ventricular rate control (eg, in atrial fibrillation), consider alternative therapy. If loading digoxin becomes necessary, patient volume of distribution may be increased and reduction in loading dose may not be necessary; however, maintenance dosing will require adjustment as long as renal failure persists.

Maintenance dose:

Cl_{cr} 10-50 mL/minute: Administer 25% to 75% of dose or every 36 hours.

Cl_{cr} <10 mL/minute: Administer 10% to 25% of dose or every 48 hours.

Not dialyzable

Administration

I.M.: I.V. route preferred. If I.M. injection necessary, administer by deep injection followed by massage at the injection site. Inject no more than 2 mL per injection site. May cause intense pain.

I.V.: May be administered undiluted or diluted fourfold in D_5W, NS, or SWFI for direct injection. Less than fourfold dilution may lead to drug precipitation. Inject slowly over ≥5 minutes.

Monitoring Parameters

Heart rate and rhythm should be monitored along with periodic ECGs to assess desired effects and signs of toxicity; baseline and periodic serum creatinine. Periodically monitor serum potassium, magnesium, and calcium especially if on medications where these electrolyte disturbances can occur (eg, diuretics), or if patient has a history of hypokalemia or hypomagnesemia. Observe patients for noncardiac signs of toxicity, confusion, and depression.

When to draw serum digoxin concentrations: Digoxin serum concentrations are monitored because digoxin possesses a narrow therapeutic serum range; the therapeutic endpoint is difficult to quantify and digoxin toxicity may be life-threatening. Digoxin serum concentrations should be drawn **at least 6-8 hours after last dose, regardless of route of administration (optimally 12-24 hours after a dose). Note:** Serum digoxin concentrations may decrease in response to exercise due to increased skeletal muscle uptake; a period of rest (eg, ~2 hours) after exercise may be necessary prior to drawing serum digoxin concentrations.

Initiation of therapy:

If a loading dose is given: Digoxin serum concentration may be drawn within 12-24 hours after the initial loading dose administration. Concentrations drawn this early may confirm the relationship of digoxin plasma concentrations and response but are of little value in determining maintenance doses.

If a loading dose is not given: Digoxin serum concentration should be obtained after 3-5 days of therapy.

Maintenance therapy:

Trough concentrations should be followed just prior to the next dose or at a minimum of 6-8 hours after last dose.

Digoxin serum concentrations should be obtained within 5-7 days (approximate time to steady-state) after any dosage changes. Continue to obtain digoxin serum concentrations 7-14 days after any change in maintenance dose. **Note:** In patients with end-stage renal disease, it may take 15-20 days to reach steady-state.

Patients who are receiving electrolyte-depleting medications such as diuretics, serum potassium, magnesium, and calcium should be monitored closely.

Digoxin serum concentrations should be obtained whenever any of the following conditions occur:

Questionable patient compliance or to evaluate clinical deterioration following an initial good response

Changing renal function

Suspected digoxin toxicity

Initiation or discontinuation of therapy with drugs (eg, amiodarone, quinidine, verapamil) which potentially interact with digoxin.

Any disease changes (eg, thyroid disease)

Reference Range

Digoxin therapeutic serum concentrations:

Heart failure: 0.5-0.8 ng/mL

Adults: <0.5 ng/mL; probably indicates underdigitalization unless there are special circumstances

Toxic: >2 ng/mL

Digoxin-like immunoreactive substance (DLIS) may cross-react with digoxin immunoassay. DLIS has been found in patients with renal and liver disease and heart failure.

Test Interactions Spironolactone may interfere with digoxin radioimmunoassay.

Special Geriatric Considerations Digitalis preparations (primarily digoxin) are frequently used to treat common cardiac diseases in the elderly (heart failure, atrial fibrillation). Elderly are at risk for toxicity due to age-related changes; volume of distribution is diminished significantly; half-life is increased as a result of decreased total body clearance. Additionally, elderly frequently have concomitant diseases which affect the pharmacokinetics in digitalis glycosides; hypo- and hyperthyroidism and renal function decline will affect clearance of digoxin. Exercise in elderly will reduce serum concentrations of digoxin due to increased skeletal muscle uptake. Therefore, a knowledge of the physical activity of elderly helps interpret serum assays. Must be observant for noncardiac signs of toxicity in elderly such as anorexia, vision changes (blurred), confusion, and depression. Changes in dose may be necessary with declining renal function with age; monitor closely.

This medication is considered to be potentially inappropriate in this patient population (Beers Criteria: Quality of evidence - moderate; Strength of recommendation - strong).

◀ **Dosage Forms** Excipient information presented when available (limited, particularly for generics); consult specific product labeling.

Injection, solution: 250 mcg/mL (2 mL)

  Lanoxin®: 250 mcg/mL (2 mL) [contains ethanol 10%, propylene glycol 40%]

Injection, solution [pediatric]:

  Lanoxin®: 100 mcg/mL (1 mL) [contains ethanol 10%, propylene glycol 40%]

Solution, oral: 50 mcg/mL (60 mL)

Tablet, oral: 125 mcg, 250 mcg

  Lanoxin®: 125 mcg, 250 mcg [scored]

Dosage Forms: Canada Excipient information presented when available (limited, particularly for generics); consult specific product labeling.

Tablet, oral:

  Apo-Digoxin®: 62.5 mcg, 125 mcg, 250 mcg

Dihydroergotamine (dye hye droe er GOT a meen)

Brand Names: U.S. D.H.E. 45®; Migranal®

Brand Names: Canada Migranal®

Index Terms DHE; Dihydroergotamine Mesylate

Generic Availability (U.S.) Yes: Injection

Pharmacologic Category Antimigraine Agent; Ergot Derivative

Use Treatment of migraine headache with or without aura; injection also indicated for treatment of cluster headaches

Unlabeled Use Adjunct for DVT prophylaxis for hip surgery, for orthostatic hypotension, xerostomia secondary to antidepressant use, and pelvic congestion with pain

Contraindications Hypersensitivity to dihydroergotamine or any component of the formulation; uncontrolled hypertension, ischemic heart disease, angina pectoris, history of MI, silent ischemia, or coronary artery vasospasm including Prinzmetal's angina; hemiplegic or basilar migraine; peripheral vascular disease; sepsis; severe hepatic or renal dysfunction; following vascular surgery; avoid use within 24 hours of sumatriptan, zolmitriptan, other serotonin agonists, or ergot-like agents; avoid during or within 2 weeks of discontinuing MAO inhibitors; concurrent use of peripheral and central vasoconstrictors; ergot alkaloids are contraindicated with potent inhibitors of CYP3A4 (includes protease inhibitors, azole antifungals, and some macrolide antibiotics)

Warnings/Precautions [U.S. Boxed Warning]: Ergot alkaloids are contraindicated with potent inhibitors of CYP3A4 (includes protease inhibitors, azole antifungals, and some macrolide antibiotics); concomitant use associated with an increased risk of vasospasm leading to cerebral ischemia and/or ischemia of the extremities. Do not give to patients with risk factors for CAD until a cardiovascular evaluation has been performed; if evaluation is satisfactory, the healthcare provider should administer the first dose and cardiovascular status should be periodically evaluated. May cause vasospastic reactions; persistent vasospasm may lead to gangrene or death in patients with compromised circulation. Discontinue if signs of vasoconstriction develop. Rare reports of increased blood pressure in patients without history of hypertension. Rare reports of adverse cardiac events (acute MI, life-threatening arrhythmias, death) have been reported following use of the injection. Cerebral hemorrhage, subarachnoid hemorrhage, and stroke have also occurred following use of the injection. Not for prolonged use. Pleural and peritoneal fibrosis have been reported with prolonged daily use. Cardiac valvular fibrosis has also been associated with ergot alkaloids. Use with caution in the elderly.

Migranal® Nasal Spray: Local irritation to nose and throat (usually transient and mild-moderate in severity) can occur; long-term consequences on nasal or respiratory mucosa have not been extensively evaluated.

Adverse Reactions (Reflective of adult population; not specific for elderly)

>10%: Nasal spray: Respiratory: Rhinitis (26%)

1% to 10%: Nasal spray:

  Central nervous system: Dizziness (4%), somnolence (3%)

  Endocrine & metabolic: Hot flashes (1%)

  Gastrointestinal: Nausea (10%), taste disturbance (8%), vomiting (4%), diarrhea (2%)

  Local: Application site reaction (6%)

  Neuromuscular & skeletal: Weakness (1%), stiffness (1%)

  Respiratory: Pharyngitis (3%)

Drug Interactions

  Metabolism/Transport Effects Substrate of CYP3A4 (major); **Note:** Assignment of Major/Minor substrate status based on clinically relevant drug interaction potential; **Inhibits** CYP3A4 (weak)

Avoid Concomitant Use

Avoid concomitant use of Dihydroergotamine with any of the following: Alpha-/Beta-Agonists; Alpha1-Agonists; Boceprevir; Clarithromycin; Conivaptan; Crizotinib; Efavirenz; Itraconazole; Ketoconazole; Ketoconazole (Systemic); Mifepristone; Nitroglycerin; Posaconazole; Protease Inhibitors; Serotonin 5-HT1D Receptor Agonists; Telaprevir; Voriconazole

Increased Effect/Toxicity

Dihydroergotamine may increase the levels/effects of: Alpha-/Beta-Agonists; Alpha1-Agonists; Metoclopramide; Serotonin 5-HT1D Receptor Agonists; Serotonin Modulators

The levels/effects of Dihydroergotamine may be increased by: Antipsychotics; Boceprevir; Clarithromycin; Conivaptan; Crizotinib; CYP3A4 Inhibitors (Moderate); CYP3A4 Inhibitors (Strong); Dasatinib; Efavirenz; Itraconazole; Ivacaftor; Ketoconazole; Ketoconazole (Systemic); Macrolide Antibiotics; Mifepristone; Nitroglycerin; Posaconazole; Protease Inhibitors; Serotonin 5-HT1D Receptor Agonists; Telaprevir; Voriconazole

Decreased Effect

Dihydroergotamine may decrease the levels/effects of: Nitroglycerin

The levels/effects of Dihydroergotamine may be decreased by: Tocilizumab

Stability

Injection: Store below 25°C (77°F); do not refrigerate or freeze; protect from heat. Protect from light.

Nasal spray: Prior to use, store below 25°C (77°F); do not refrigerate or freeze. Once spray applicator has been prepared, use within 8 hours; discard any unused solution.

Mechanism of Action Ergot alkaloid alpha-adrenergic blocker directly stimulates vascular smooth muscle to vasoconstrict peripheral and cerebral vessels; also has effects on serotonin receptors

Pharmacodynamics/Kinetics

Onset of action: I.M.: 15-30 minutes

Duration: I.M.: 3-4 hours

Distribution: V_d: ~800 L

Protein binding: 93%

Metabolism: Extensively hepatic

Half-life elimination: ~9-10 hours

Time to peak, serum: I.M.: 24 minutes; I.V.: 1-2 minutes; Intranasal: 30-60 minutes; SubQ 15-45 minutes

Excretion: Primarily feces; urine (6% to 7% as unchanged drug)

Dosage

Geriatric Refer to adult dosing. Patients >65 years of age were not included in controlled clinical studies.

Adult

Migraine, cluster headache:

I.M., SubQ: 1 mg at first sign of headache; repeat hourly to a maximum dose of 3 mg/day; maximum dose: 6 mg/week

I.V.: 1 mg at first sign of headache; repeat hourly up to a maximum dose of 2 mg/day; maximum dose: 6 mg/week

Intranasal: 1 spray (0.5 mg) of nasal spray should be administered into each nostril; if needed, repeat after 15 minutes, up to a total of 4 sprays (2 mg). **Note:** Do not exceed 6 sprays (3 mg) in a 24-hour period and no more than 8 sprays (4 mg) in a week.

Intractable migraine (status migrainosus; >72 hours): *I.V.:* Raskin protocol (unlabeled dosing): Initial test dose: 0.5 mg (following premedication with metoclopramide); subsequent dosing is titrated (range: 0.2-1 mg) every 8 hours for 2-3 days and administered with or without metoclopramide based on response and tolerance (Raskin, 1986; Raskin, 1990). **Note:** Some clinicians use modified versions of this protocol, with additional adjunctive medications and/or alternate antiemetic agents.

Renal Impairment Contraindicated in severe renal impairment

Hepatic Impairment Dosage reductions are probably necessary but specific guidelines are not available; contraindicated in severe hepatic dysfunction.

Administration

Intranasal: Prior to administration of nasal spray, the nasal spray applicator must be primed (pumped 4 times); in order to let the drug be absorbed through the skin in the nose, patients should not inhale deeply through the nose while spraying or immediately after spraying; for best results, treatment should be initiated at the first symptom or sign of an attack; however, nasal spray can be used at any stage of a migraine attack.

I.M., SubQ: May administer by intramuscular or subcutaneous injection.

I.V.: Administer slowly over 2-3 minutes (Raskin protocol)

Reference Range Minimum concentration for vasoconstriction is reportedly 0.06 ng/mL

Special Geriatric Considerations Monitor cardiac and peripheral effects closely in the elderly since they often have cardiovascular disease and peripheral vascular impairment (ie, diabetes mellitus, PVD) that will complicate therapy and monitoring for adverse effects.

Dosage Forms Excipient information presented when available (limited, particularly for generics); consult specific product labeling.

Injection, solution, as mesylate: 1 mg/mL (1 mL)

D.H.E. 45®: 1 mg/mL (1 mL) [contains ethanol 6.2%]

Solution, intranasal, as mesylate [spray]:

Migranal®: 4 mg/mL (1 mL) [contains caffeine 10 mg/mL; 0.5 mg/spray]

◆ **Dihydroergotamine Mesylate** *see* Dihydroergotamine *on page* 548
◆ **Dihydroergotoxine** *see* Ergoloid Mesylates *on page* 659
◆ **Dihydrogenated Ergot Alkaloids** *see* Ergoloid Mesylates *on page* 659
◆ **Dihydrohydroxycodeinone** *see* OxyCODONE *on page* 1446
◆ **Dihydromorphinone** *see* HYDROmorphone *on page* 945
◆ **1,25 Dihydroxycholecalciferol** *see* Calcitriol *on page* 256
◆ **Dihydroxypropyl Theophylline** *see* Dyphylline *on page* 625
◆ **Diiodohydroxyquin** *see* Iodoquinol *on page* 1034
◆ **Dilacor XR®** *see* Diltiazem *on page* 550
◆ **Dilantin®** *see* Phenytoin *on page* 1527
◆ **Dilantin-125®** *see* Phenytoin *on page* 1527
◆ **Dilatrate®-SR** *see* Isosorbide Dinitrate *on page* 1050
◆ **Dilaudid®** *see* HYDROmorphone *on page* 945
◆ **Dilaudid-HP®** *see* HYDROmorphone *on page* 945
◆ **Dilt-CD** *see* Diltiazem *on page* 550
◆ **Diltia XT®** *see* Diltiazem *on page* 550

Diltiazem (dil TYE a zem)

Related Information

Calcium Channel Blockers – Comparative Pharmacokinetics *on page* 2111

Medication Safety Issues

Sound-alike/look-alike issues:

Cardizem® may be confused with Cardene®, Cardene SR®, Cardizem CD®, Cardizem SR®, cortisone

Cartia XT® may be confused with Procardia XL®

Diltiazem may be confused with Calan®, diazepam, Dilantin®

Tiazac® may be confused with Tigan®, Tiazac® XC [CAN], Ziac®

High alert medication:

The Institute for Safe Medication Practices (ISMP) includes this medication (I.V. formulation) among its list of drug classes which have a heightened risk of causing significant patient harm when used in error.

Administration issues:

Significant differences exist between oral and I.V. dosing. Use caution when converting from one route of administration to another.

International issues:

Cardizem [U.S., Canada, and multiple international markets] may be confused with Cardem brand name for celiprolol [Spain]

Cartia XT [U.S.] may be confused with Cartia brand name for aspirin [multiple international markets]

Dilacor XR [U.S.] may be confused with Dilacor brand name for verapamil [Brazil]

Dipen [Greece] may be confused with Depen brand name for penicillamine [U.S.]; Depin brand name for nifedipine [India]; Depon brand name for acetaminophen [Greece]

Tiazac: Brand name for diltiazem [U.S, Canada], but also the brand name for pioglitazone [Chile]

Brand Names: U.S. Cardizem®; Cardizem® CD; Cardizem® LA; Cartia XT®; Dilacor XR®; Dilt-CD; Dilt-XR; Diltia XT®; Diltzac; Matzim™ LA; Taztia XT®; Tiazac®

Brand Names: Canada Apo-Diltiaz CD®; Apo-Diltiaz SR®; Apo-Diltiaz TZ®; Apo-Diltiaz®; Apo-Diltiaz® Injectable; Ava-Diltiazem; Cardizem® CD; CO Diltiazem CD; CO Diltiazem T; Diltiazem HCl ER®; Diltiazem Hydrochloride Injection; Diltiazem TZ; Diltiazem-CD; Nu-Diltiaz; Nu-Diltiaz-CD; PMS-Diltiazem CD; ratio-Diltiazem CD; Sandoz-Diltiazem CD; Sandoz-Diltiazem T; Teva-Diltiazem; Teva-Diltiazem CD; Teva-Diltiazem HCL ER Capsules; Tiazac®; Tiazac® XC

Index Terms Diltiazem Hydrochloride

Generic Availability (U.S.) Yes

Pharmacologic Category Antianginal Agent; Antiarrhythmic Agent, Class IV; Calcium Channel Blocker; Calcium Channel Blocker, Nondihydropyridine

Use
Oral: Essential hypertension; chronic stable angina or angina from coronary artery spasm

Injection: Control of rapid ventricular rate in patients with atrial fibrillation or atrial flutter; conversion of paroxysmal supraventricular tachycardia (PSVT)

Unlabeled Use ACLS guidelines: Injection: Stable narrow-complex tachycardia uncontrolled or unconverted by adenosine or vagal maneuvers or if SVT is recurrent

Contraindications
Oral: Hypersensitivity to diltiazem or any component of the formulation; sick sinus syndrome (except in patients with a functioning artificial pacemaker); second- or third-degree AV block (except in patients with a functioning artificial pacemaker); severe hypotension (systolic <90 mm Hg); acute MI and pulmonary congestion

Intravenous (I.V.): Hypersensitivity to diltiazem or any component of the formulation; sick sinus syndrome (except in patients with a functioning artificial pacemaker); second- or third-degree AV block (except in patients with a functioning artificial pacemaker); severe hypotension (systolic <90 mm Hg); cardiogenic shock; administration concomitantly or within a few hours of the administration of I.V. beta-blockers; atrial fibrillation or flutter associated with accessory bypass tract (eg, Wolff-Parkinson-White syndrome); ventricular tachycardia (with wide-complex tachycardia, must determine whether origin is supraventricular or ventricular)

Warnings/Precautions Can cause first-, second-, and third-degree AV block or sinus bradycardia and risk increases with agents known to slow cardiac conduction. The most common side effect is peripheral edema; occurs within 2-3 weeks of starting therapy. Symptomatic hypotension with or without syncope can rarely occur; blood pressure must be lowered at a rate appropriate for the patient's clinical condition. Use caution when using diltiazem together with a beta-blocker; may result in conduction disturbances, hypotension, and worsened LV function. Simultaneous administration of I.V. diltiazem and an I.V. beta-blocker or administration within a few hours of each other may result in asystole and is contraindicated. Use with other agents known to either reduce SA node function and/or AV nodal conduction (eg, digoxin) or reduce sympathetic outflow (eg, clonidine) may increase the risk of serious bradycardia. Use caution in left ventricular dysfunction (may exacerbate condition). Avoid use of diltiazem in patients with heart failure and reduced ejection fraction (Hunt, 2009). Use with caution with hypertrophic obstructive cardiomyopathy; routine use is currently not recommended due to insufficient evidence (Maron, 2003). Use with caution in hepatic or renal dysfunction. Transient dermatologic reactions have been observed with use; if reaction persists, discontinue. May (rarely) progress to erythema multiforme or exfoliative dermatitis.

Adverse Reactions (Reflective of adult population; not specific for elderly) Note: Frequencies represent ranges for various dosage forms. Patients with impaired ventricular function and/or conduction abnormalities may have higher incidence of adverse reactions.

>10%:
  Cardiovascular: Edema (2% to 15%)
  Central nervous system: Headache (5% to 12%)
2% to 10%:
  Cardiovascular: AV block (first degree 2% to 8%), edema (lower limb 2% to 8%), pain (6%), bradycardia (2% to 6%), hypotension (<2% to 4%), vasodilation (2% to 3%), extrasystoles (2%), flushing (1% to 2%), palpitation (1% to 2%)
  Central nervous system: Dizziness (3% to 10%), nervousness (2%)
  Dermatologic: Rash (1% to 4%)
  Endocrine & metabolic: Gout (1% to 2%)
  Gastrointestinal: Dyspepsia (1% to 6%), constipation (<2% to 4%), vomiting (2%), diarrhea (1% to 2%)
  Local: Injection site reactions: Burning, itching (4%)
  Neuromuscular & skeletal: Weakness (1% to 4%), myalgia (2%)
  Respiratory: Rhinitis (<2% to 10%), pharyngitis (2% to 6%), dyspnea (1% to 6%), bronchitis (1% to 4%), cough (≤3%), sinus congestion (1% to 2%)

Drug Interactions
Metabolism/Transport Effects Substrate of CYP2C9 (minor), CYP2D6 (minor), CYP3A4 (major), P-glycoprotein; **Note:** Assignment of Major/Minor substrate status based on clinically relevant drug interaction potential; **Inhibits** CYP2C9 (weak), CYP2D6 (weak), CYP3A4 (moderate)

Avoid Concomitant Use
Avoid concomitant use of Diltiazem with any of the following: Conivaptan; Dantrolene; Pimozide; Tolvaptan

DILTIAZEM

Increased Effect/Toxicity
Diltiazem may increase the levels/effects of: Alfentanil; Amifostine; Amiodarone; Antihypertensives; Aprepitant; ARIPiprazole; AtorvaSTATin; Avanafil; Benzodiazepines (metabolized by oxidation); Beta-Blockers; Budesonide (Systemic, Oral Inhalation); BusPIRone; Calcium Channel Blockers (Dihydropyridine); CarBAMazepine; Cardiac Glycosides; Colchicine; Corticosteroids (Systemic); CycloSPORINE; CycloSPORINE (Systemic); CYP3A4 Substrates; Dronedarone; Eletriptan; Eplerenone; Everolimus; Fingolimod; Fosaprepitant; Fosphenytoin; Halofantrine; Hypotensive Agents; Ivacaftor; Lithium; Lovastatin; Lurasidone; Magnesium Salts; Midodrine; Neuromuscular-Blocking Agents (Nondepolarizing); Nitroprusside; Phenytoin; Pimecrolimus; Pimozide; Propafenone; QuiNIDine; Ranolazine; Red Yeast Rice; RiTUXimab; Rivaroxaban; Salicylates; Salmeterol; Saxagliptin; Simvastatin; Tacrolimus; Tacrolimus (Systemic); Tacrolimus (Topical); Tolvaptan; Vilazodone; Zuclopenthixol

The levels/effects of Diltiazem may be increased by: Alpha1-Blockers; Anilidopiperidine Opioids; Antifungal Agents (Azole Derivatives, Systemic); Aprepitant; AtorvaSTATin; Calcium Channel Blockers (Dihydropyridine); Cimetidine; Conivaptan; CycloSPORINE; CycloSPORINE (Systemic); CYP3A4 Inhibitors (Moderate); CYP3A4 Inhibitors (Strong); Dantrolene; Dasatinib; Diazoxide; Dronedarone; Fluconazole; Fosaprepitant; Grapefruit Juice; Herbs (Hypotensive Properties); Ivacaftor; Lovastatin; Macrolide Antibiotics; Magnesium Salts; MAO Inhibitors; Mifepristone; Pentoxifylline; P-glycoprotein/ABCB1 Inhibitors; Phosphodiesterase 5 Inhibitors; Prostacyclin Analogues; Protease Inhibitors; Simvastatin

Decreased Effect
Diltiazem may decrease the levels/effects of: Clopidogrel; Ifosfamide

The levels/effects of Diltiazem may be decreased by: Barbiturates; Calcium Salts; CarBAMazepine; Colestipol; CYP3A4 Inducers (Strong); Deferasirox; Herbs (CYP3A4 Inducers); Herbs (Hypertensive Properties); Methylphenidate; Nafcillin; Peginterferon Alfa-2b; P-glycoprotein/ABCB1 Inducers; Rifamycin Derivatives; Tocilizumab; Yohimbine

Ethanol/Nutrition/Herb Interactions
Ethanol: Ethanol may increase risk of hypotension or vasodilation. Management: Avoid ethanol.

Food: Diltiazem serum levels may be elevated if taken with food. Serum concentrations were not altered by grapefruit juice in small clinical trials.

Herb/Nutraceutical: St John's wort may decrease diltiazem levels. Some herbal medications may worsen hypertension (eg, licorice); others may increase the antihypertensive effect of diltiazem (eg, shepherd's purse). Management: Avoid St John's wort, bayberry, blue cohosh, cayenne, ephedra, ginger, ginseng (American), kola, licorice, and yohimbe. Avoid black cohosh, California poppy, coleus, golden seal, hawthorn, mistletoe, periwinkle, quinine, and shepherd's purse.

Stability
Capsule, tablet: Store at room temperature. Protect from light.

Solution for injection: Store in refrigerator at 2°C to 8°C (36°F to 46°F); do not freeze. May be stored at room temperature for up to 1 month. Following dilution to ≤1 mg/mL with $D_5^1/_2NS$, D_5W, or NS, solution is stable for 24 hours at room temperature or under refrigeration.

Mechanism of Action
Nondihydropyridine calcium channel blocker which inhibits calcium ion from entering the "slow channels" or select voltage-sensitive areas of vascular smooth muscle and myocardium during depolarization, producing a relaxation of coronary vascular smooth muscle and coronary vasodilation; increases myocardial oxygen delivery in patients with vasospastic angina

Pharmacodynamics/Kinetics
Onset of action: Oral: Immediate release tablet: 30-60 minutes; I.V.: 3 minutes

Duration: I.V.: Bolus: 1-3 hours; Continuous infusion (after discontinuation): 0.5-10 hours

Absorption: Immediate release tablet: >90%; Extended release capsule: ~93%

Distribution: V_d: 3-13 L/kg

Protein binding: 70% to 80%

Metabolism: Hepatic (extensive first-pass effect); following single I.V. injection, plasma concentrations of N-monodesmethyldiltiazem and desacetyldiltiazem are typically undetectable; however, these metabolites accumulate to detectable concentrations following 24-hour constant rate infusion. N-monodesmethyldiltiazem appears to have 20% of the potency of diltiazem; desacetyldiltiazem is about 25% to 50% as potent as the parent compound.

Bioavailability: Oral: ~40% (undergoes extensive first-pass metabolism)

Half-life elimination: Immediate release tablet: 3-4.5 hours, may be prolonged with renal impairment; Extended release tablet: 6-9 hours; Extended release capsules: 5-10 hours; I.V.: single dose: ~3.4 hours; continuous infusion: 4-5 hours

Time to peak, serum: Immediate release tablet: 2-4 hours; Extended release tablet: 11-18 hours; Extended release capsule: 10-14 hours

Excretion: Urine (2% to 4% as unchanged drug; 6% to 7% as metabolites); feces

Dosage

Geriatric Refer to adult dosing. In the management of hypertension, consider lower initial doses (eg, 120 mg once daily using extended release capsule) and titrate to response (Aronow, 2011).

Adult

Angina: Oral:

Capsule, extended release:

Dilacor XR®, Dilt-XR, Diltia XT®: Initial: 120 mg once daily; titrate over 7-14 days; usual dose range: 120-320 mg/day; maximum: 480 mg/day

Cardizem® CD, Cartia XT®, Dilt-CD: Initial: 120-180 mg once daily; titrate over 7-14 days; usual dose range: 120-320 mg/day; maximum: 480 mg/day

Tiazac®, Taztia XT®: Initial: 120-180 mg once daily; titrate over 7-14 days; usual dose range: 120-320 mg/day; maximum: 540 mg/day

Tablet, extended release (Cardizem® LA, Matzim™ LA, Tiazac® XC [CAN; not available in U.S.]): 180 mg once daily; may increase at 7- to 14-day intervals; usual dose range: 120-320 mg/day; maximum: 360 mg/day

Tablet, immediate release (Cardizem®): Usual starting dose: 30 mg 4 times/day; titrate dose gradually at 1- to 2-day intervals; usual dose range: 120-320 mg/day

Hypertension: Oral:

Capsule, extended release (once-daily dosing):

Cardizem® CD, Cartia XT®, Dilt-CD: Initial: 180-240 mg once daily; dose adjustment may be made after 14 days; usual dose range (JNC 7): 180-420 mg/day; maximum: 480 mg/day

Dilacor® XR, Diltia XT®, Dilt-XR: Initial: 180-240 mg once daily; dose adjustment may be made after 14 days; usual dose range (JNC 7): 180-420 mg/day; maximum: 540 mg/day

Tiazac®, Taztia XT®: Initial: 120-240 mg once daily; dose adjustment may be made after 14 days; usual dose range (JNC 7): 180-420 mg/day; maximum: 540 mg/day

Capsule, extended release (twice-daily dosing): Initial: 60-120 mg twice daily; dose adjustment may be made after 14 days; usual range: 240-360 mg/day

Note: Diltiazem is available as a generic intended for either once- or twice-daily dosing, depending on the formulation; verify appropriate extended release capsule formulation is administered.

Tablet, extended release (Cardizem® LA, Matzim™ LA, Tiazac® XC [CAN; not available in U.S.]): Initial: 180-240 mg once daily; dose adjustment may be made after 14 days; usual dose range (JNC 7): 120-540 mg/day

Atrial fibrillation, atrial flutter, PSVT: I.V.:

Initial bolus dose: 0.25 mg/kg actual body weight over 2 minutes (average adult dose: 20 mg); ACLS guideline recommends 15-20 mg

Repeat bolus dose (may be administered after 15 minutes if the response is inadequate): 0.35 mg/kg actual body weight over 2 minutes (average adult dose: 25 mg); ACLS guideline recommends 20-25 mg

Continuous infusion (infusions >24 hours or infusion rates >15 mg/hour are not recommended): Initial infusion rate of 10 mg/hour; rate may be increased in 5 mg/hour increments up to 15 mg/hour as needed; some patients may respond to an initial rate of 5 mg/hour.

If diltiazem injection is administered by continuous infusion for >24 hours, the possibility of decreased diltiazem clearance, prolonged elimination half-life, and increased diltiazem and/or diltiazem metabolite plasma concentrations should be considered.

Conversion from I.V. diltiazem to oral diltiazem:

Oral dose (mg/day) is approximately equal to [rate (mg/hour) x 3 + 3] x 10.

3 mg/hour = 120 mg/day

5 mg/hour = 180 mg/day

7 mg/hour = 240 mg/day

11 mg/hour = 360 mg/day

Renal Impairment Use with caution; no dosing adjustments recommended.

Dialysis: Not removed by hemo- or peritoneal dialysis; supplemental dose is not necessary.

Hepatic Impairment Use with caution; no specific dosing recommendations available; extensively metabolized by the liver; half-life is increased in patients with cirrhosis.

Administration

Oral:

Immediate release tablet (Cardizem®): Administer before meals and at bedtime.

Long acting dosage forms: Do not open, chew, or crush; swallow whole.

Cardizem® CD, Cardizem® LA, Cartia XT®, Dilt-CD, Matzim™ LA: May be administered without regards to meals.

Dilacor XR®, Dilt-XR, Diltia XT®: Administer on an empty stomach.

Taztia XT™, Tiazac®: Capsules may be opened and sprinkled on a spoonful of apple-sauce. Applesauce should not be hot and should be swallowed without chewing, followed by drinking a glass of water.

Tiazac® XC [CAN; not available in U.S.]: Administer at bedtime

I.V.: Bolus doses given over 2 minutes with continuous ECG and blood pressure monitoring. Continuous infusion should be via infusion pump.

Monitoring Parameters Liver function tests, blood pressure, ECG, heart rate

Special Geriatric Considerations Elderly may experience a greater hypotensive response; constipation may be encountered more often in elderly. Calcium channel blockers are no more effective in elderly than other therapies; however, they do not cause significant CNS effects which is an advantage over other antihypertensive agents (eg, beta-blockers, clonidine).

Dosage Forms Excipient information presented when available (limited, particularly for generics); consult specific product labeling.

Capsule, extended release, oral, as hydrochloride [once-daily dosing]: 120 mg, 180 mg, 240 mg, 300 mg, 360 mg, 420 mg

Cardizem® CD: 120 mg, 180 mg, 240 mg, 300 mg, 360 mg
Cartia XT®: 120 mg, 180 mg, 240 mg, 300 mg
Dilacor XR®: 240 mg
Dilt-CD: 120 mg, 180 mg, 240 mg, 300 mg
Dilt-XR: 120 mg, 180 mg, 240 mg
Diltia XT®: 120 mg, 180 mg, 240 mg
Diltzac: 120 mg, 180 mg, 240 mg, 300 mg, 360 mg
Taztia XT®: 120 mg, 180 mg, 240 mg, 300 mg, 360 mg
Tiazac®: 120 mg, 180 mg, 240 mg, 300 mg, 360 mg, 420 mg

Capsule, extended release, oral, as hydrochloride [twice-daily dosing]: 60 mg, 90 mg, 120 mg
Injection, powder for reconstitution, as hydrochloride: 100 mg
Injection, solution, as hydrochloride: 5 mg/mL (5 mL, 10 mL, 25 mL)
Tablet, oral, as hydrochloride: 30 mg, 60 mg, 90 mg, 120 mg

Cardizem®: 30 mg
Cardizem®: 60 mg, 90 mg, 120 mg [scored]

Tablet, extended release, oral, as hydrochloride [once-daily dosing]:
Cardizem® LA: 120 mg, 180 mg, 240 mg, 300 mg, 360 mg, 420 mg
Matzim™ LA: 180 mg, 240 mg, 300 mg, 360 mg, 420 mg

Dosage Forms: Canada Excipient information presented when available (limited, particularly for generics); consult specific product labeling.

Tablet, extended release, as hydrochloride:
Tiazac® XC: 120 mg, 180 mg, 240 mg, 300 mg, 360 mg

◆ **Diltiazem Hydrochloride** see Diltiazem on page 550
◆ **Dilt-XR** see Diltiazem on page 550
◆ **Diltzac** see Diltiazem on page 550

DimenhyDRINATE (dye men HYE dri nate)

Related Information
Beers Criteria – Potentially Inappropriate Medications for Geriatrics on page 2183

Medication Safety Issues
Sound-alike/look-alike issues:
DimenhyDRINATE may be confused with diphenhydrAMINE
BEERS Criteria medication:
This drug may be potentially inappropriate for use in geriatric patients (Quality of evidence - varies based on comorbidity; Strength of recommendation - varies based on comorbidity)

Brand Names: U.S. Dramamine® for kids [OTC]; Dramamine® [OTC]; Driminate [OTC]; TripTone® [OTC]

Brand Names: Canada Apo-Dimenhydrinate® [OTC]; Children's Motion Sickness Liquid [OTC]; Dimenhydrinate Injection; Dinate® [OTC]; Gravol IM; Gravol® [OTC]; Jamp-Dimenhydrinate [OTC]; Nauseatol [OTC]; Novo-Dimenate [OTC]; PMS-Dimenhydrinate [OTC]; Sandoz-Dimenhydrinate [OTC]; Travel Tabs [OTC]

Generic Availability (U.S.) Yes: Excludes chewable tablet

Pharmacologic Category Ethanolamine Derivative; Histamine H_1 Antagonist; Histamine H_1 Antagonist, First Generation

Use Treatment and prevention of nausea, vertigo, and vomiting associated with motion sickness

Contraindications Hypersensitivity to dimenhydrinate or any component of the formulation

Warnings/Precautions Causes sedation, caution must be used in performing tasks which require alertness (eg, operating machinery or driving). May mask the symptoms of ototoxicity, use caution if used in conjuction with antibiotics that have the potential to cause ototoxicity.

Effects may be potentiated when used with other sedative drugs or ethanol. Use with caution in patients with angle-closure glaucoma, asthma, pyloroduodenal obstruction (including stenotic peptic ulcer), urinary tract obstruction (including bladder neck obstruction and symptomatic prostatic hyperplasia), hyperthyroidism, increased intraocular pressure, and cardiovascular disease (including hypertension and tachycardia). May be inappropriate for use in older adults depending on comorbidities (eg, dementia, delirium, etc) due to its potent anticholinergic effects (Beers Criteria). Use with caution in the elderly; may be more sensitive to adverse effects. Parenteral formulation should not be injected intra-arterially.

Adverse Reactions (Reflective of adult population; not specific for elderly) Frequency not defined.

Cardiovascular: Tachycardia

Central nervous system: Dizziness, drowsiness, excitation, headache, insomnia, lassitude, nervousness, restlessness

Dermatologic: Rash

Gastrointestinal: Anorexia, epigastric distress, nausea, xerostomia

Genitourinary: Dysuria

Ocular: Blurred vision

Respiratory: Thickening of bronchial secretions

Drug Interactions

Metabolism/Transport Effects None known.

Avoid Concomitant Use

Avoid concomitant use of DimenhyDRINATE with any of the following: Azelastine; Azelastine (Nasal); Methadone; Mirtazapine; Paraldehyde

Increased Effect/Toxicity

DimenhyDRINATE may increase the levels/effects of: Alcohol (Ethyl); Anticholinergics; Azelastine; Azelastine (Nasal); Buprenorphine; CNS Depressants; Methadone; Methotrimeprazine; Metyrosine; Mirtazapine; Paraldehyde; Selective Serotonin Reuptake Inhibitors; Zolpidem

The levels/effects of DimenhyDRINATE may be increased by: Droperidol; HydrOXYzine; Methotrimeprazine; Pramlintide

Decreased Effect

DimenhyDRINATE may decrease the levels/effects of: Acetylcholinesterase Inhibitors (Central); Benzylpenicilloyl Polylysine; Betahistine; Hyaluronidase

The levels/effects of DimenhyDRINATE may be decreased by: Acetylcholinesterase Inhibitors (Central); Amphetamines

Ethanol/Nutrition/Herb Interactions Ethanol: May increase CNS depression; monitor for increased effects with coadministration. Caution patients about effects.

Stability Injection: Store at 20°C to 25°C (68°F to 77°F). Protect from light.

Mechanism of Action Competes with histamine for H_1-receptor sites on effector cells in the gastrointestinal tract, blood vessels, and respiratory tract; blocks chemoreceptor trigger zone, diminishes vestibular stimulation, and depresses labyrinthine function through its central anticholinergic activity

Pharmacodynamics/Kinetics Note: Dimenhydrinate is a salt of two drugs: Diphenhydramine (53% to 55.5%) and 8-chlorotheophylline (44% to 47%). Refer to DiphenhydrAMINE (Systemic) monograph on page 556.

Dosage

Geriatric & Adult Motion sickness (prevention/treatment):

Oral: 50-100 mg every 4-6 hours, not to exceed 400 mg/day

I.M., I.V.: 50 mg every 4 hours; maximum: 100 mg every 4 hours

Administration

Oral: To prevent motion sickness, administer 30-60 minutes prior to exposure.

Solution for injection:

I.M.: Administer undiluted

I.V.: Must dilute each 50 mg in 10 mL NS; inject over 2 minutes

Special Geriatric Considerations

Monitor for anticholinergic side effects (confusion, constipation, etc); if possible, limit use to short-term therapy

This medication is considered to be potentially inappropriate in this patient population (Beers Criteria: Quality of evidence - varies based on comorbidity; Strength of recommendation - varies based on comorbidity).

Dosage Forms Excipient information presented when available (limited, particularly for generics); consult specific product labeling.

Injection, solution: 50 mg/mL (1 mL) [contains benzyl alcohol]

DIMENHYDRINATE

Tablet, oral: 50 mg
  Dramamine®: 50 mg [scored]
  Driminate: 50 mg [scored]
  TripTone®: 50 mg
Tablet, chewable, oral:
  Dramamine®: 50 mg [scored; contains phenylalanine 0.84 mg/tablet; orange flavor]
  Dramamine® for kids: 25 mg [scored; dye free; contains phenylalanine 0.84 mg/tablet; grape flavor]

◆ **Diocto [OTC]** *see Docusate on page 583*
◆ **Dioctyl Calcium Sulfosuccinate** *see Docusate on page 583*
◆ **Dioctyl Sodium Sulfosuccinate** *see Docusate on page 583*
◆ **Diotame [OTC]** *see Bismuth on page 216*
◆ **Diovan®** *see Valsartan on page 1996*
◆ **Diovan HCT®** *see Valsartan and Hydrochlorothiazide on page 1998*
◆ **Dipentum®** *see Olsalazine on page 1414*
◆ **Diphen [OTC]** *see DiphenhydrAMINE (Systemic) on page 556*
◆ **Diphenhist® [OTC]** *see DiphenhydrAMINE (Systemic) on page 556*

DiphenhydrAMINE (Systemic) (dye fen HYE dra meen)

Related Information
  Beers Criteria – Potentially Inappropriate Medications for Geriatrics *on page 2183*
Medication Safety Issues
  Sound-alike/look-alike issues:
    DiphenhydrAMINE may be confused with desipramine, dicyclomine, dimenhyDRINATE
    Benadryl® may be confused with benazepril, Bentyl®, Benylin®, Caladryl®
  BEERS Criteria medication:
    This drug may be potentially inappropriate for use in geriatric patients (Quality of evidence - moderate; Strength of recommendation - strong).
  International issues:
    Sominex brand name for diphenhydramine [U.S., Canada], but also the brand name for promethazine [Great Britain]; valerian [Chile]
Brand Names: U.S. Aler-Cap [OTC]; Aler-Dryl [OTC]; Aler-Tab [OTC]; AllerMax® [OTC]; Altaryl [OTC]; Anti-Hist [OTC]; Banophen™ [OTC]; Benadryl® Allergy Quick Dissolve [OTC]; Benadryl® Allergy [OTC]; Benadryl® Children's Allergy FastMelt® [OTC]; Benadryl® Children's Allergy Perfect Measure™ [OTC]; Benadryl® Children's Allergy [OTC]; Benadryl® Children's Dye Free Allergy [OTC]; Benadryl® Dye-Free Allergy [OTC]; Compoz® [OTC]; Diphen [OTC]; Diphenhist® [OTC]; Geri-Dryl; Histaprin [OTC]; Nytol® Quick Caps [OTC]; Nytol® Quick Gels [OTC]; PediaCare® Children's Allergy [OTC]; PediaCare® Children's NightTime Cough [OTC]; Q-dryl [OTC]; Quenalin [OTC]; Siladryl Allergy [OTC]; Silphen [OTC]; Simply Sleep® [OTC]; Sleep-ettes D [OTC]; Sleep-Tabs [OTC]; Sleepinal® [OTC]; Sominex® Maximum Strength [OTC]; Sominex® [OTC]; Theraflu® Thin Strips® Multi Symptom [OTC]; Triaminic Thin Strips® Children's Cough & Runny Nose [OTC]; Twilite® [OTC]; Unisom® SleepGels® Maximum Strength [OTC]; Unisom® SleepMelts™ [OTC]; Vicks® ZzzQuil™ [OTC]
Brand Names: Canada Allerdryl®; Allernix; Benadryl®; Nytol®; Nytol® Extra Strength; PMS-Diphenhydramine; Simply Sleep®; Sominex®
Index Terms Diphenhydramine Citrate; Diphenhydramine Hydrochloride; Diphenhydramine Tannate
Generic Availability (U.S.) Yes: Excludes orally-disintegrating tablet, strip
Pharmacologic Category Ethanolamine Derivative; Histamine H_1 Antagonist; Histamine H_1 Antagonist, First Generation
Use Symptomatic relief of allergic symptoms caused by histamine release including nasal allergies and allergic dermatosis; adjunct to epinephrine in the treatment of anaphylaxis; nighttime sleep aid; prevention or treatment of motion sickness; antitussive; management of Parkinsonian syndrome including drug-induced extrapyramidal symptoms
Contraindications Hypersensitivity to diphenhydramine or any component of the formulation; acute asthma; use as a local anesthetic (injection)
Warnings/Precautions Causes sedation, caution must be used in performing tasks which require alertness (eg, operating machinery or driving). Sedative effects of CNS depressants or ethanol are potentiated. Use with caution in patients with angle-closure glaucoma, pyloro-duodenal obstruction (including stenotic peptic ulcer), urinary tract obstruction (including bladder neck obstruction and symptomatic prostatic hyperplasia), asthma, hyperthyroidism, increased intraocular pressure, and cardiovascular disease (including hypertension and tachycardia). Some preparations contain soy protein; avoid use in patients with soy protein or peanut allergies. Some products may contain phenylalanine.

Oral products: In the elderly, avoid use of this potent anticholinergic agent due to increased risk of confusion, dry mouth, constipation, and other anticholinergic effects; clearance decreases in patients of advanced age; tolerance develops to hypnotic effects; when used for severe allergic reaction, use may be appropriate (Beers Criteria).

Self-medication (OTC use): Do not use with other products containing diphenhydramine, even ones used on the skin.

Adverse Reactions (Reflective of adult population; not specific for elderly) Frequency not defined.

Cardiovascular: Chest tightness, extrasystoles, hypotension, palpitation, tachycardia

Central nervous system: Chills, confusion, convulsion, disturbed coordination, dizziness, euphoria, excitation, fatigue, headache, insomnia, irritability, nervousness, paradoxical excitement, restlessness, sedation, sleepiness, vertigo

Endocrine & metabolic: Menstrual irregularities (early menses)

Gastrointestinal: Anorexia, constipation, diarrhea, dry mucous membranes, epigastric distress, nausea, throat tightness, vomiting, xerostomia

Genitourinary: Difficult urination, urinary frequency, urinary retention

Hematologic: Agranulocytosis, hemolytic anemia, thrombocytopenia

Neuromuscular & skeletal: Neuritis, paresthesia, tremor

Ocular: Blurred vision, diplopia

Otic: Labyrinthitis (acute), tinnitus

Respiratory: Nasal stuffiness, thickening of bronchial secretions, wheezing

Miscellaneous: Anaphylactic shock, diaphoresis

Drug Interactions

Metabolism/Transport Effects Inhibits CYP2D6 (moderate)

Avoid Concomitant Use

Avoid concomitant use of DiphenhydrAMINE (Systemic) with any of the following: Azelastine; Azelastine (Nasal); Methadone; Mirtazapine; Paraldehyde; Thioridazine

Increased Effect/Toxicity

DiphenhydrAMINE (Systemic) may increase the levels/effects of: Alcohol (Ethyl); Anticholinergics; ARIPiprazole; Azelastine; Azelastine (Nasal); Buprenorphine; CNS Depressants; CYP2D6 Substrates; Fesoterodine; Methadone; Methotrimeprazine; Metyrosine; Mirtazapine; Nebivolol; Paraldehyde; Selective Serotonin Reuptake Inhibitors; Thioridazine; Zolpidem

The levels/effects of DiphenhydrAMINE (Systemic) may be increased by: Droperidol; HydrOXYzine; Methotrimeprazine; Pramlintide; Propafenone

Decreased Effect

DiphenhydrAMINE (Systemic) may decrease the levels/effects of: Acetylcholinesterase Inhibitors (Central); Benzylpenicilloyl Polylysine; Betahistine; Codeine; Hyaluronidase; Tamoxifen; TraMADol

The levels/effects of DiphenhydrAMINE (Systemic) may be decreased by: Acetylcholinesterase Inhibitors (Central); Amphetamines

Ethanol/Nutrition/Herb Interactions

Ethanol: May increase CNS depression; monitor for increased effects with coadministration. Caution patients about effects.

Herb/Nutraceutical: Avoid valerian, St John's wort, kava kava, gotu kola (may increase CNS depression).

Stability Injection: Store at room temperature of 15°C to 30°C (59°F to 86°F); protect from freezing. Protect from light.

Mechanism of Action Competes with histamine for H_1-receptor sites on effector cells in the gastrointestinal tract, blood vessels, and respiratory tract; anticholinergic and sedative effects are also seen

Pharmacodynamics/Kinetics

Duration:

Histamine-induced wheal suppression: ≤10 hours (Simons, 1990)

Histamine-induced flare suppression: ≤12 hours (Simons, 1990)

Distribution: V_d: Adults: 17 L/kg (range: 13-20 L/kg); Elderly: 14 L/kg (range: 7-20 L/kg) (Blyden, 1986; Simons, 1990)

Protein binding: 98.5% (Vozeh, 1988)

Metabolism: Extensively hepatic n-demethylation via CYP2D6; minor demethylation via CYP1A2, 2C9 and 2C19; smaller degrees in pulmonary and renal systems; significant first-pass effect (Akutsu, 2007)

Bioavailability: 42% to 62% (Paton, 1985)

Half-life elimination: Adults: 9 hours (range: 7-12 hours); Elderly: 13.5 hours (range: 9-18 hours) (Blyden, 1986; Simons, 1990)

Time to peak, serum: ~2 hours (Blyden, 1986; Simons, 1990)

Excretion: Urine (as metabolites and unchanged drug) (Albert, 1975; Maurer, 1988)

Dosage

Geriatric Initial: 25 mg 2-3 times/day increasing as needed

Adult Note: Dosages are expressed as the hydrochloride salt.

Allergic reactions or motion sickness:
Oral: 25-50 mg every 6-8 hours
I.M., I.V.: 10-50 mg per dose; single doses up to 100 mg may be used if needed; not to exceed 400 mg/day

Antitussive: Oral: 25 mg every 4 hours; maximum: 150 mg/24 hours

Night-time sleep aid: Oral: 50 mg at bedtime

Dystonic reaction: I.M., I.V.: 50 mg in a single dose; may repeat in 20-30 minutes if necessary

Administration When used to prevent motion sickness, first dose should be given 30 minutes prior to exposure. Injection solution is for I.V. or I.M. administration only; local necrosis may result with SubQ or intradermal use. For I.V. administration, inject at a rate ≤25 mg/minute.

Monitoring Parameters Relief of symptoms, mental alertness

Test Interactions May interfere with urine detection of methadone and PCP (false-positives); may cause false-positive serum TCA screen; may suppress the wheal and flare reactions to skin test antigens

Pharmacotherapy Pearls Diphenhydramine citrate 19 mg is equivalent to diphenhydramine hydrochloride 12.5 mg

Special Geriatric Considerations Diphenhydramine has high sedative and anticholinergic properties, so it may not be considered the antihistamine of choice for prolonged use in the elderly. Its use as a sleep aid is discouraged due to its anticholinergic effects. Guidelines from the Centers for Medicare and Medicaid Services (CMS) discourage the use of diphenhydramine as a sedative or anxiolytic in long-term care facilities.

This medication is considered to be potentially inappropriate in this patient population (Beers Criteria: Quality of evidence - moderate; Strength of recommendation - strong).

Dosage Forms Excipient information presented when available (limited, particularly for generics); consult specific product labeling. [DSC] = Discontinued product

Caplet, oral, as hydrochloride:
Aler-Dryl: 50 mg
AllerMax®: 50 mg
Anti-Hist: 25 mg
Compoz®: 50 mg
Histaprin: 25 mg
Nytol® Quick Caps: 25 mg
Simply Sleep®: 25 mg [contains calcium 20 mg/caplet]
Sleep-ettes D: 50 mg
Sominex® Maximum Strength: 50 mg
Twilite®: 50 mg

Capsule, oral, as hydrochloride: 25 mg, 50 mg
Aler-Cap: 25 mg
Banophen™: 25 mg
Benadryl® Allergy: 25 mg [contains calcium 35 mg/capsule]
Diphen: 25 mg
Diphenhist®: 25 mg
Q-dryl: 25 mg
Sleepinal®: 50 mg

Capsule, liquid filled, oral, as hydrochloride:
Vicks® ZzzQuil™: 25 mg

Capsule, softgel, oral, as hydrochloride:
Benadryl® Dye-Free Allergy: 25 mg [dye free]
Compoz®: 50 mg
Nytol® Quick Gels: 50 mg
Unisom® SleepGels® Maximum Strength: 50 mg

Captab, oral, as hydrochloride:
Diphenhist®: 25 mg

Elixir, oral, as hydrochloride:
Altaryl: 12.5 mg/5 mL (120 mL [DSC], 480 mL, 3840 mL) [ethanol free; cherry flavor]
Banophen™: 12.5 mg/5 mL (120 mL)
Banophen™: 12.5 mg/5 mL (480 mL) [sugar free]

Injection, solution, as hydrochloride: 50 mg/mL (1 mL, 10 mL)

Injection, solution, as hydrochloride [preservative free]: 50 mg/mL (1 mL)

Liquid, oral, as hydrochloride:
AllerMax®: 12.5 mg/5 mL (120 mL)

Benadryl® Children's Allergy: 12.5 mg/5 mL (118 mL, 236 mL) [ethanol free; contains sodium 14 mg/5 mL, sodium benzoate; cherry flavor]

Benadryl® Children's Allergy Perfect Measure™: 12.5 mg/5 mL (5 mL) [ethanol free; contains sodium 14 mg/5 mL, sodium benzoate; cherry flavor]

Benadryl® Children's Dye Free Allergy: 12.5 mg/5 mL (118 mL) [dye free, ethanol free, sugar free; contains sodium 11 mg/5 mL, sodium benzoate; bubblegum flavor]

Siladryl Allergy: 12.5 mg/5 mL (118 mL, 237 mL, 473 mL) [ethanol free, sugar free; black-cherry flavor]

Vicks® ZzzQuil™: 50 mg/30 mL (177 mL, 354 mL) [contains ethanol, propylene glycol, sodium 23 mg/30 mL, sodium benzoate; berry flavor]

Solution, oral, as hydrochloride: 12.5 mg/5 mL (5 mL, 10 mL)

Diphenhist®: 12.5 mg/5 mL (120 mL, 480 mL) [ethanol free; contains sodium benzoate]

Q-dryl: 12.5 mg/5 mL (120 mL, 240 mL, 480 mL) [ethanol free; contains sodium 5 mg/5 mL, sodium benzoate; cherry flavor]

Strip, orally disintegrating, oral, as hydrochloride:

Benadryl® Allergy Quick Dissolve: 25 mg (10s) [contains sodium 4 mg/strip; vanilla-mint flavor]

Theraflu® Thin Strips® Multi Symptom: 25 mg (12s, 24s) [contains ethanol; cherry flavor]

Triaminic Thin Strips® Children's Cough & Runny Nose: 12.5 mg (14s) [contains ethanol; grape flavor]

Syrup, oral, as hydrochloride:

PediaCare® Children's Allergy: 12.5 mg/5 mL (118 mL) [contains sodium 14 mg/5 mL, sodium benzoate; cherry flavor]

PediaCare® Children's NightTime Cough: 12.5 mg/5 mL (118 mL) [ethanol free; contains sodium 15 mg/5 mL, sodium benzoate; cherry flavor]

Quenalin: 12.5 mg/5 mL (118 mL) [contains ethanol 5%, propylene glycol; strawberry flavor]

Silphen: 12.5 mg/5 mL (118 mL, 237 mL, 473 mL) [contains ethanol 5%; strawberry flavor]

Tablet, oral, as hydrochloride: 25 mg, 50 mg

Aler-Tab: 25 mg

Banophen™: 25 mg

Benadryl® Allergy: 25 mg

Geri-Dryl: 25 mg

Sleep-Tabs: 25 mg

Sominex®: 25 mg

Tablet, orally dissolving, oral, as hydrochloride:

Benadryl® Children's Allergy FastMelt®: 12.5 mg [cherry flavor]

Benadryl® Children's Allergy FastMelt®: 12.5 mg [grape flavor]

Unisom® SleepMelts™: 25 mg [cherry flavor]

DiphenhydrAMINE (Topical) (dye fen HYE dra meen)

Medication Safety Issues

Sound-alike/look-alike issues:

DiphenhydrAMINE may be confused with desipramine, dicyclomine, dimenhyDRINATE

Benadryl® may be confused with benazepril, Bentyl®, Benylin®, Caladryl®

Administration issues:

Institute for Safe Medication Practices (ISMP) has reported cases of patients mistakenly swallowing Benadryl® Itch Stopping [OTC] gel intended for topical application. Unclear labeling and similar packaging of the topical gel in containers resembling an oral liquid are factors believed to be contributing to the administration errors. The topical gel contains camphor which can be toxic if swallowed. ISMP has requested the manufacturer to make the necessary changes to prevent further confusion.

Brand Names: U.S. Banophen™ Anti-Itch [OTC]; Benadryl® Extra Strength Itch Stopping [OTC]; Benadryl® Itch Relief Extra Strength [OTC]; Benadryl® Itch Stopping Extra Strength [OTC]; Benadryl® Itch Stopping [OTC]; Dermamycin® [OTC]

Brand Names: Canada Benadryl® Cream; Benadryl® Itch Relief Stick; Benadryl® Spray

Index Terms Diphenhydramine Hydrochloride

Generic Availability (U.S.) Yes: Excludes gel, liquid stick, spray

Pharmacologic Category Ethanolamine Derivative; Histamine H_1 Antagonist; Histamine H_1 Antagonist, First Generation; Topical Skin Product

Use Topically for relief of pain and itching associated with insect bites, minor cuts and burns, or rashes due to poison ivy, poison oak, and poison sumac

Dosage

Adult Relief of pain and itching: Topical: Apply 1% or 2% to affected area up to 3-4 times/day

Special Geriatric Considerations Instruct patient or caregiver on appropriate use of topical diphenhydramine products.

DIPHENHYDRAMINE (TOPICAL)

Dosage Forms Excipient information presented when available (limited, particularly for generics); consult specific product labeling.
Cream, topical, as hydrochloride: 2% (30 g)
  Banophen™ Anti-Itch: 2% (28.4 g) [contains zinc acetate 0.1%]
  Benadryl® Itch Stopping: 1% (14.2 g, 28.3 g) [contains zinc acetate 0.1%]
  Benadryl® Itch Stopping Extra Strength: 2% (14.2 g) [contains zinc acetate 0.1%]
  Dermamycin®: 2% (28 g)
Gel, topical, as hydrochloride:
  Benadryl® Extra Strength Itch Stopping: 2% (120 mL)
Liquid, topical, as hydrochloride [spray]:
  Benadryl® Itch Stopping Extra Strength: 2% (59 mL) [contains ethanol; contains zinc acetate 0.1%]
  Dermamycin®: 2% (60 mL) [contains menthol]
Liquid, topical, as hydrochloride [stick]:
  Benadryl® Itch Relief Extra Strength: 2% (14 mL) [contains ethanol; contains zinc acetate 0.1%]

◆ **Diphenhydramine Citrate** see DiphenhydrAMINE (Systemic) on page 556
◆ **Diphenhydramine Hydrochloride** see DiphenhydrAMINE (Systemic) on page 556
◆ **Diphenhydramine Hydrochloride** see DiphenhydrAMINE (Topical) on page 559
◆ **Diphenhydramine Tannate** see DiphenhydrAMINE (Systemic) on page 556

Diphenoxylate and Atropine (dye fen OKS i late & A troe peen)

Related Information
Atropine on page 166
Medication Safety Issues
Sound-alike/look-alike issues:
  Lomotil® may be confused with LaMICtal®, LamISIL®, lamoTRIgine, Lanoxin®, Lasix®, loperamide
International issues:
  Lomotil [U.S., Canada, and multiple international markets] may be confused with Ludiomil brand name for maprotiline [multiple international markets]
  Lomotil: Brand name for diphenoxylate [U.S., Canada, and multiple international markets], but also the brand name for loperamide [Mexico, Philippines]
Brand Names: U.S. Lomotil®
Brand Names: Canada Lomotil®
Index Terms Atropine and Diphenoxylate
Generic Availability (U.S.) Yes
Pharmacologic Category Antidiarrheal
Use Treatment of diarrhea
Contraindications Hypersensitivity to diphenoxylate, atropine, or any component of the formulation; obstructive jaundice; diarrhea associated with pseudomembranous enterocolitis or enterotoxin-producing bacteria
Warnings/Precautions Use in conjunction with fluid and electrolyte therapy when appropriate. In case of severe dehydration or electrolyte imbalance, withhold diphenoxylate/atropine treatment until corrective therapy has been initiated. Inhibiting peristalsis may lead to fluid retention in the intestine aggravating dehydration and electrolyte imbalance. Reduction of intestinal motility may be deleterious in diarrhea resulting from *Shigella, Salmonella*, toxigenic strains of *E. coli*, and pseudomembranous enterocolitis associated with broad-spectrum antibiotics; use is not recommended.

Use caution with acute ulcerative colitis, hepatic or renal dysfunction. If there is no response with 48 hours, this medication is unlikely to be effective and should be discontinued; if chronic diarrhea is not improved symptomatically within 10 days at maximum dosage, control is unlikely with further use. Physical and psychological dependence have been reported with higher than recommended dosing.

Adverse Reactions (Reflective of adult population; not specific for elderly) Frequency not defined.
Cardiovascular: Tachycardia
Central nervous system: Confusion, depression, dizziness, drowsiness, euphoria, flushing, headache, hyperthermia, lethargy, malaise, restlessness, sedation
Dermatologic: Angioneurotic edema, dry skin, pruritus, urticaria
Gastrointestinal: Abdominal discomfort, anorexia, gum swelling, nausea, pancreatitis, paralytic ileus, toxic megacolon, vomiting, xerostomia
Genitourinary: Urinary retention
Neuromuscular & skeletal: Numbness
Miscellaneous: Anaphylaxis

Drug Interactions

Metabolism/Transport Effects None known.

Avoid Concomitant Use

Avoid concomitant use of Diphenoxylate and Atropine with any of the following: Azelastine; Azelastine (Nasal); Methadone; Mirtazapine; Paraldehyde

Increased Effect/Toxicity

Diphenoxylate and Atropine may increase the levels/effects of: AbobotulinumtoxinA; Alcohol (Ethyl); Anticholinergics; Azelastine; Azelastine (Nasal); Buprenorphine; Cannabinoids; CNS Depressants; Methadone; Methotrimeprazine; Metyrosine; Mirtazapine; Onabotulinumtoxin-inA; Paraldehyde; Potassium Chloride; RimabotulinumtoxinB; Selective Serotonin Reuptake Inhibitors; Zolpidem

The levels/effects of Diphenoxylate and Atropine may be increased by: Droperidol; HydrOXYzine; Methotrimeprazine; Pramlintide

Decreased Effect

Diphenoxylate and Atropine may decrease the levels/effects of: Acetylcholinesterase Inhibitors (Central); Secretin

The levels/effects of Diphenoxylate and Atropine may be decreased by: Acetylcholinesterase Inhibitors (Central)

Ethanol/Nutrition/Herb Interactions Ethanol: May increase CNS depression; monitor for increased effects with coadministration. Caution patients about effects.

Mechanism of Action Diphenoxylate inhibits excessive GI motility and GI propulsion; commercial preparations contain a subtherapeutic amount of atropine to discourage abuse

Pharmacodynamics/Kinetics

Atropine: See Atropine monograph.

Diphenoxylate:

Onset of action: Antidiarrheal: 45-60 minutes

Duration: Antidiarrheal: 3-4 hours

Absorption: Well absorbed

Metabolism: Extensively hepatic via ester hydrolysis to diphenoxylic acid (active)

Half-life elimination: Diphenoxylate: 2.5 hours; Diphenoxylic acid: 12-14 hours

Time to peak, serum: 2 hours

Excretion: Primarily feces (49% as unchanged drug and metabolites); urine (~14%, <1% as unchanged drug)

Dosage

Geriatric & Adult Diarrhea: Oral: Diphenoxylate 5 mg 4 times/day until control achieved (maximum: 20 mg/day), then reduce dose as needed; some patients may be controlled on doses of 5 mg/day

Administration If there is no response within 48 hours of continuous therapy, this medication is unlikely to be effective and should be discontinued; if chronic diarrhea is not improved symptomatically within 10 days at maximum dosage, control is unlikely with further use.

Monitoring Parameters Watch for signs of atropinism (dryness of skin and mucous membranes, tachycardia, thirst, flushing); monitor number and consistency of stools; observe for signs of toxicity, fluid and electrolyte loss, hypotension, and respiratory depression

Pharmacotherapy Pearls If there is no response within 48 hours, the drug is unlikely to be effective and should be discontinued. If chronic diarrhea is not improved symptomatically within 10 days at maximum dosage of 20 mg/day, control is unlikely with further use. Diarrhea should also be treated with dietary measures (ie, clear liquids), and avoid milk products and high sodium foods such as bouillon and soups.

Special Geriatric Considerations Elderly are particularly sensitive to fluid and electrolyte loss. This generally results in lethargy, weakness, and confusion. Repletion and maintenance of electrolytes and water are essential in the treatment of diarrhea. Drug therapy must be limited in order to avoid toxicity with this agent.

Controlled Substance C-V

Dosage Forms Excipient information presented when available (limited, particularly for generics); consult specific product labeling. [DSC] = Discontinued product

Solution, oral: Diphenoxylate hydrochloride 2.5 mg and atropine sulfate 0.025 mg per 5 mL (5 mL, 10 mL, 60 mL)

Lomotil®: Diphenoxylate hydrochloride 2.5 mg and atropine sulfate 0.025 mg per 5 mL (60 mL) [contains alcohol 15%; cherry flavor] [DSC]

Tablet, oral: Diphenoxylate hydrochloride 2.5 mg and atropine sulfate 0.025 mg

Lomotil®: Diphenoxylate hydrochloride 2.5 mg and atropine sulfate 0.025 mg

♦ **Diphenylhydantoin** *see* Phenytoin *on page* 1527

Diphtheria and Tetanus Toxoids (dif THEER ee a & TET a nus TOKS oyds)

Related Information
  Immunization Administration Recommendations *on page 2144*
  Immunization Recommendations *on page 2149*
  Tetanus Toxoid (Adsorbed) *on page 1869*
Medication Safety Issues
  Sound-alike/look-alike issues:
    Diphtheria and Tetanus Toxoids (Td) may be confused with tuberculin purified protein derivative (PPD)
    Pediatric diphtheria and tetanus (DT) may be confused with adult tetanus and diphtheria (Td)
Brand Names: U.S. Decavac® [DSC]; Tenivac™
Brand Names: Canada Td Adsorbed
Index Terms DT; Td; Tetanus and Diphtheria Toxoid
Generic Availability (U.S.) Yes
Pharmacologic Category Vaccine, Inactivated (Bacterial)
Use Tetanus and diphtheria toxoids adsorbed for adult use (Td) (Decavac®, Tenivac™): Adults: Active immunization against diphtheria and tetanus; tetanus prophylaxis in wound management

The Advisory Committee on Immunization Practices (ACIP) recommends routine vaccination for the following:
• Adults should receive a booster dose of Td every 10 years; may substitute a single Td booster dose with Tdap
• Adults and the elderly (≥65 years) who are wounded in bombings or similar mass casualty events who have penetrating injuries or nonintact skin exposure and who cannot confirm receipt of a tetanus booster within the previous 5 years, may also receive a single dose of Td; adults may also receive Td if Tdap is unavailable

Contraindications Hypersensitivity to diphtheria, tetanus toxoid, or any component of the formulation
Warnings/Precautions Do not confuse pediatric diphtheria and tetanus (DT) with adult tetanus and diphtheria (Td). Immediate treatment for anaphylactic/anaphylactoid reaction should be available during administration. Patients with a history of severe local reaction (Arthus-type) following a previous dose should not be given further routine or emergency doses of Td more frequently than every 10 years even if using for wound management with wounds that are not clean or minor; these patients generally have high serum antitoxin levels. Continue use with caution if Guillain-Barré syndrome occurs within 6 weeks of prior tetanus toxoid. Syncope has been reported with use of injectable vaccines and may be accompanied by transient visual disturbances, weakness, or tonic-clonic movements. Procedures should be in place to avoid injuries from falling and to restore cerebral perfusion if syncope occurs.

For I.M. administration; use caution with history of bleeding disorders or anticoagulant therapy. Defer administration during moderate or severe illness (with or without fever). Immune response may be decreased in immunocompromised patients; in general, household and close contacts of persons with altered immunocompetence may receive all age appropriate vaccines. Some products may contain natural latex/natural rubber or thimerosal. In order to maximize vaccination rates, the ACIP recommends simultaneous administration of all age-appropriate vaccines (live or inactivated) for which a person is eligible at a single clinic visit, unless contraindications exist. The use of combination vaccines is generally preferred over separate injections, taking into consideration provider assessment, patient preference, and adverse events. When using combination vaccines, the minimum age for administration is the oldest minimum age for any individual component; the minimum interval between dosing is the greatest minimum interval between any individual component.

Adverse Reactions (Reflective of adult population; not specific for elderly) All serious adverse reactions must be reported to the U.S. Department of Health and Human Services (DHHS) Vaccine Adverse Event Reporting System (VAERS) 1-800-822-7967 or online at https://vaers.hhs.gov/esub/index. In Canada, adverse reactions may be reported to local provincial/territorial health agencies or to the Vaccine Safety Section at Public Health Agency of Canada (1-866-844-0018).

Note: Percentages noted within 2 weeks following booster dose of Decavac® in persons ≥11 years of age:
>10%:
  Central nervous system: Headache (34% to 40%), tiredness (21% to 27%), chills (7% to 13%)
  Gastrointestinal: Nausea (8% to 12%), diarrhea (10% to 11%)
  Local: Injection site: Pain (63% to 71%), erythema (20% to 22%), swelling (17% to 18%)

Neuromuscular & skeletal: Body ache/muscle weakness (19% to 30%), sore/swollen joints (7% to 12%)

1% to 10%:

Central nervous system: Fever (1% to 3%)

Dermatologic: Rash (2%)

Endocrine & metabolic: Lymph node swelling (4% to 5%)

Gastrointestinal: Vomiting (2% to 3%)

Drug Interactions

Metabolism/Transport Effects None known.

Avoid Concomitant Use There are no known interactions where it is recommended to avoid concomitant use.

Increased Effect/Toxicity There are no known significant interactions involving an increase in effect.

Decreased Effect

The levels/effects of Diphtheria and Tetanus Toxoids may be decreased by: Belimumab; Fingolimod; Immunosuppressants

Stability Store at 2°C to 8°C (35°F to 46°F). Do not freeze; discard if product has been frozen.

Dosage

Geriatric & Adult

Primary immunization (Td): I.M.:

Decavac®: Patients previously not immunized should receive 2 primary doses of 0.5 mL each, given at an interval of 4 weeks; third (reinforcing) dose of 0.5 mL 6 months later

Tenivac™: Patients previously not immunized should receive 2 primary doses of 0.5 mL each, given at an interval of 8 weeks; third (reinforcing) dose of 0.5 mL 6-8 months later

Booster immunization (Td): I.M.: 0.5 mL every 10 years (for routine booster in patients who have completed primary immunization series). The ACIP prefers Tdap for use in some situations if no contraindications exist; refer to Diphtheria and Tetanus Toxoids, and Acellular Pertussis Vaccine monograph on page 567 for additional information.

Tetanus prophylaxis in wound management: I.M.: Tetanus prophylaxis in patients with wounds should consider if the wound is clean or contaminated, the immunization status of the patient, proper use of tetanus toxoid and/or tetanus immune globulin (TIG), wound cleaning, and (if required) surgical debridement and the proper use of antibiotics. Patients with an uncertain or incomplete tetanus immunization status should have additional follow up to ensure a series is completed. Patients with a history of Arthus reaction following a previous dose of a tetanus toxoid-containing vaccine should not receive a tetanus toxoid-containing vaccine until >10 years after the most recent dose even if they have a wound that is neither clean nor minor. See table.

Tetanus Prophylaxis in Wound Management

History of Tetanus Immunization Doses	Clean, Minor Wounds		All Other Wounds[1]	
	Tetanus Toxoid[2]	TIG	Tetanus Toxoid[2]	TIG
Uncertain or <3 doses	Yes	No	Yes	Yes
3 or more doses	No[3]	No	No[4]	No

[1]Such as, but not limited to, wounds contaminated with dirt, feces, soil, and saliva; puncture wounds; wounds from crushing, tears, burns, and frostbite.

[2]Tetanus toxoid in this chart refers to a tetanus toxoid-containing vaccine. For children <7 years of age, DTaP (DT, if pertussis vaccine contraindicated) is preferred to tetanus toxoid alone. For children ≥7 years and adults, Td preferred to tetanus toxoid alone; Tdap may be preferred if the patient has not previously been vaccinated with Tdap.

[3]Yes, if ≥10 years since last dose.

[4]Yes, if ≥5 years since last dose.

Adapted from CDC "Yellow Book" (Health Information for International Travel 2010), "Routine Vaccine-Preventable Diseases, Tetanus" (available at http://www.cdc.gov/yellowbook) and MMWR 2006, 55(RR-17).

Abbreviations: **DT** = Diphtheria and Tetanus Toxoids (formulation for age ≤6 years); **DTaP** = Diphtheria and Tetanus Toxoids, and Acellular Pertussis (formulation for age ≤6 years; Daptacel®, Infanrix®); **Td** = Diphtheria and Tetanus Toxoids (formulation for age ≥7 years; Decavac®,Tenivac™); **TT** = Tetanus toxoid (adsorbed [formulation for age ≥7 years]); **Tdap** = Diphtheria and Tetanus Toxoids, and Acellular Pertussis (Adacel® or Boostrix® [formulations for age ≥7 years]); **TIG** = Tetanus Immune Globulin

Administration For I.M. administration; prior to use, shake suspension well

Td: Administer in the deltoid muscle; do not inject in the gluteal area

DT: Administer in the anterolateral aspect of the thigh or the deltoid muscle; do not inject in the gluteal area

For patients at risk of hemorrhage following intramuscular injection, the ACIP recommends "it should be administered intramuscularly if, in the opinion of the physician familiar with the patient's bleeding risk, the vaccine can be administered by this route with reasonable safety. If the patient receives antihemophilia or other similar therapy, intramuscular vaccination can be scheduled shortly after such therapy is administered. A fine needle (23 gauge or smaller) can be used for the vaccination and firm pressure applied to the site (without rubbing) for at least 2 minutes. The patient should be instructed concerning the risk of hematoma from the injection." Patients on anticoagulant therapy should be considered to have the same bleeding risks and treated as those with clotting factor disorders (CDC, 60[2], 2011).

Simultaneous administration of vaccines helps ensure the patients will be fully vaccinated by the appropriate age. Simultaneous administration of vaccines is defined as administering >1 vaccine on the same day at different anatomic sites. The use of licensed combination vaccines is generally preferred over separate injections of the equivalent components. Separate vaccines should not be combined in the same syringe unless indicated by product specific labeling. Separate needles and syringes should be used for each injection. The ACIP prefers each dose of a specific vaccine in a series come from the same manufacturer when possible. Adolescents and adults should be vaccinated while seated or lying down. In general, preterm infants should be vaccinated at the same chronological age as full-term infants (CDC, 60[2], 2011).

Antipyretics have not been shown to prevent febrile seizures. Antipyretics may be used to treat fever or discomfort following vaccination (CDC, 2011). One study reported that routine prophylactic administration of acetaminophen to prevent fever prior to vaccination decreased the immune response of some vaccines; the clinical significance of this reduction in immune response has not been established (Prymula, 2009).

Monitoring Parameters Monitor for syncope for 15 minutes following administration. If seizure-like activity associated with syncope occurs, maintain patient in supine or Trendelenburg position to reestablish adequate cerebral perfusion.

Pharmacotherapy Pearls Pediatric dosage form should only be used in patients ≤6 years of age. U.S. federal law requires that the name of medication, date of administration, the vaccine manufacturer, lot number of vaccine, and the administering person's name, title, and address be entered into the patient's permanent medical record.

DT contains higher proportions of diphtheria toxoid than Td.

Special Geriatric Considerations Since protective tetanus and diphtheria antibodies decline with age (only 31% of persons >70 years of age in the U.S. are believed to be immune to tetanus) and older adults have a disproportionate burden of illness from tetanus, it is advisable to offer Td to the elderly concurrent with their influenza and other immunization programs if history of vaccination is unclear; boosters should be given at 10-year intervals (earlier for wounds). ACIP has issued recommendations for the use of Tdap in adults ≥65 years who previously have not received a dose of Tdap. For patients who have or anticipate having close contact with an infant <12 months of age, a single dose of Tdap is recommended; for other adults ≥65 years, a single dose of Tdap may be given to replace a single dose of Td.

Dosage Forms Excipient information presented when available (limited, particularly for generics); consult specific product labeling. [DSC] = Discontinued product

Injection, suspension [Td, adult; preservative free]: Diphtheria 2 Lf units and tetanus 2 Lf units per 0.5 mL (0.5 mL)

Decavac® [DSC]: Diphtheria 2 Lf units and tetanus 5 Lf units per 0.5 mL (0.5 mL) [contains aluminum, may contain natural rubber/natural latex in prefilled syringe, thimerosal (may have trace amounts)]

Tenivac™: Diphtheria 2 Lf units and tetanus 5 Lf units per 0.5 mL (0.5 mL) [contains aluminum, may contain natural rubber/natural latex in prefilled syringe]

Injection, suspension [DT, pediatric; preservative free]: Diphtheria 6.7 Lf units and tetanus 5 Lf units per 0.5 mL (0.5 mL) [DSC]; Diphtheria 25 Lf units and tetanus 5 Lf units per 0.5 mL (0.5 mL) [contains aluminum]

Diphtheria and Tetanus Toxoids, Acellular Pertussis, and Poliovirus Vaccine

(dif THEER ee a & TET a nus TOKS oyds, ay CEL yoo lar per TUS sis & POE lee oh VYE rus vak SEEN)

Related Information

Immunization Administration Recommendations *on page 2144*

Immunization Recommendations *on page 2149*

Medication Safety Issues

Sound-alike/look-alike issues:

Adacel® (trade name for Diphtheria and Tetanus Toxoids, and Acellular Pertussis Vaccine) should not be confused with Adacel®-Polio (trade name for Diphtheria and Tetanus Toxoids, Acellular Pertussis, and Poliovirus Vaccine in Canada)

Brand Names: U.S. Kinrix®

Brand Names: Canada Adacel®-Polio

Index Terms Diphtheria and Tetanus Toxoids and Acellular Pertussis Adsorbed, and Inactivated Poliovirus Vaccine Combined; Diphtheria, Tetanus Toxoids, Acellular Pertussis (DTaP); DTaP-IPV; Poliovirus, Inactivated (IPV)

Generic Availability (U.S.) No

Pharmacologic Category Vaccine, Inactivated (Bacterial); Vaccine, Inactivated (Viral)

Use Kinrix®: Active immunization against diphtheria, tetanus, pertussis, and poliomyelitis, used as the fifth dose in the DTaP series and the 4th dose in the IPV series

Adacel®-Polio (Canadian availability): Active booster immunization against diphtheria, tetanus, pertussis, and poliomyelitis; alternative to fifth dose of DTaP-IPV; May be used for wound management when a tetanus toxoid-containing vaccine is needed for wound management [refer to current National Advisory Committee on Immunization (NACI) guidelines]

Contraindications Hypersensitivity to diphtheria and tetanus toxoids, pertussis, poliovirus vaccine, or any component of the vaccine; encephalopathy occurring within 7 days of a previous pertussis vaccine not (not attributable to another identifiable cause); progressive neurologic disorders (including uncontrolled epilepsy or progressive encephalopathy)

Warnings/Precautions Immediate treatment for anaphylactic/anaphylactoid reaction should be available during vaccine use. Use caution if one or more has occurred within 48 hours of whole-cell DTP or a vaccine containing acellular pertussis: Fever 40.5°C (≥105°F) within 48 hours not due to an identifiable cause; collapse or shock-like state (hypotonic-hyporesponsive episode [HHE]) occurring within 48 hours; persistent, inconsolable crying that occurs within 48 hours and lasts ≥3 hours; seizures with or without fever that occur within 3 days. Use caution if Guillain-Barré syndrome occurred within 6 weeks of prior vaccination with tetanus toxoid. May consider deferring administration in patients with moderate or severe acute illness (with or without fever); may administer to patients with mild acute illness (with or without fever).

Use with caution in patients with history of seizure disorder, progressive neurologic disease, or conditions predisposing to seizures; ACIP and AAP guidelines recommend deferring immunization until health status can be assessed and condition stabilized. Antipyretics may be considered at the time of and for 24 hours following vaccination to patients at high risk for seizures to reduce the possibility of postvaccination fever. Use caution with bleeding disorders. Use with caution in severely immunocompromised patients (eg, patients receiving chemo/radiation therapy or other immunosuppressive therapy [including high-dose corticosteroids]); may have a reduced response to vaccination. Contains aluminum, neomycin, polymyxin B, and polysorbate 80; packaging may contain latex. In order to maximize vaccination rates, the ACIP recommends simultaneous administration of all age-appropriate vaccines (live or inactivated) for which a person is eligible at a single clinic visit, unless contraindications exist. The use of combination vaccines is generally preferred over separate injections, taking into consideration provider assessment, patient preference, and adverse events.

Adverse Reactions (Reflective of adult population; not specific for elderly) All serious adverse reactions must be reported to the U.S. Department of Health and Human Services (DHHS) Vaccine Adverse Event Reporting System (VAERS) 1-800-822-7967 or online at https://vaers.hhs.gov/esub/index. In Canada, adverse reactions may be reported to local provincial/territorial health agencies or to the Vaccine Safety Section at Public Health Agency of Canada (1-866-844-0018).

◀ Adverse events reported within 4 days of vaccination: >10%:

Central nervous system: Drowsiness (19%, grade 3: 1%), fever (≥99.5°F: 16%, >100.4: 7%, >104: <1%)

Gastrointestinal: Loss of appetite (16%; grade 3: 1%)

Local: Injection site: Pain (57%; grade 3: 2%), redness (37%; ≥50 mm: 18%, ≥110 mm: 3%), arm circumference increase (36%, >20 mm: 7%, >30 mm: 2%), swelling (26%; ≥50 mm: 10%, ≥110 mm: 1%)

Drug Interactions

Metabolism/Transport Effects None known.

Avoid Concomitant Use There are no known interactions where it is recommended to avoid concomitant use.

Increased Effect/Toxicity There are no known significant interactions involving an increase in effect.

Decreased Effect

The levels/effects of Diphtheria and Tetanus Toxoids, Acellular Pertussis, and Poliovirus Vaccine may be decreased by: Belimumab; Fingolimod; Immunosuppressants

Stability

Kinrix®: Store under refrigeration of 2°C to 8°C (36°F to 46°F); do not freeze. Discard if frozen.

Adacel®-Polio: Store under refrigeration of 2°C to 8°C (36°F to 46°F); stable for 72 hours at temperatures up to 25°C (77°F); do not freeze. Discard if frozen.

Mechanism of Action Promotes active immunity to diphtheria, tetanus, pertussis, and poliovirus (types 1, 2 and 3) by inducing production of specific antibodies and antitoxins.

Pharmacodynamics/Kinetics Onset of action: Immune response observed to all components ~1 month following vaccination

Dosage

Adult Booster immunization: Adacel®-Polio (Canadian availability): I.M.: 0.5 mL

Administration For I.M. use only, preferably in the deltoid; Adacel®-Polio (Canadian availability) label recommends avoiding administration into the buttocks. Do not administer intradermally, I.V., or SubQ. Shake well prior to use; do not use unless a homogeneous, turbid, white suspension forms. Discard if the suspension is discolored or if there are cracks in the vial or syringe. Administer in the deltoid muscle of the upper arm. Do not administer additional vaccines or immunoglobulins at the same site, or using the same syringe.

For patients at risk of hemorrhage following intramuscular injection, the ACIP recommends "it should be administered intramuscularly if, in the opinion of the physician familiar with the patient's bleeding risk, the vaccine can be administered by this route with reasonable safety. If the patient receives antihemophilia or other similar therapy, intramuscular vaccination can be scheduled shortly after such therapy is administered. A fine needle (23 gauge or smaller) can be used for the vaccination and firm pressure applied to the site (without rubbing) for at least 2 minutes. The patient should be instructed concerning the risk of hematoma from the injection." Patients on anticoagulant therapy should be considered to have the same bleeding risks and treated as those with clotting factor disorders (CDC, 2011).

Simultaneous administration of vaccines helps ensure the patients will be fully vaccinated by the appropriate age. Simultaneous administration of vaccines is defined as administering >1 vaccine on the same day at different anatomic sites. The use of licensed combination vaccines is generally preferred over separate injections of the equivalent components. Separate vaccines should not be combined in the same syringe unless indicated by product specific labeling. Separate needles and syringes should be used for each injection. The ACIP prefers each dose of a specific vaccine in a series come from the same manufacturer when possible. Adolescents and adults should be vaccinated while seated or lying down. In general, preterm infants should be vaccinated at the same chronological age as full-term infants (CDC, 2011).

Antipyretics have not been shown to prevent febrile seizures. Antipyretics may be used to treat fever or discomfort following vaccination (CDC, 2011). One study reported that routine prophylactic administration of acetaminophen to prevent fever prior to vaccination decreased the immune response of some vaccines; the clinical significance of this reduction in immune response has not been established (Prymula, 2009).

Monitoring Parameters Monitor for syncope for 15 minutes following administration. If seizure-like activity associated with syncope occurs, maintain patient in supine or Trendelenburg position to reestablish adequate cerebral perfusion.

Pharmacotherapy Pearls U.S. federal law requires that the name of medication, date of administration, name of the vaccine manufacturer, lot number of vaccine, and the administering person's name, title, and address be entered into the patient's permanent medical record.

Kinrix®: Contains the following three pertussis antigens: Inactivated pertussis toxin (PT), filamentous hemagglutinin (FHA), and pertactin. Contains the same diphtheria, tetanus toxoids, and pertussis antigens found in Infanrix® and Pediarix®. Contains the same polio-virus antigens found in Infanrix®.

Special Geriatric Considerations Since protective tetanus and diphtheria antibodies decline with age, only 28% of persons >70 years of age in the U.S. are believed to be immune to tetanus, and most of the tetanus-induced deaths occur in people >60 years of age, it is advisable to offer Td, especially to elderly, concurrent with their influenza and other immunization programs if history of vaccination is unclear; boosters should be given at 10-year intervals (earlier for wounds). For the elderly who cannot document a primary immunization series or at risk due to contact or travel, administer the initial series. Boosters may be necessary for travel since antibody titers may diminish with age.

Dosage Forms Excipient information presented when available (limited, particularly for generics); consult specific product labeling.

Injection, suspension [preservative free]:

Kinrix®: Diphtheria toxoid 25 Lf, tetanus toxoid 10 Lf, acellular pertussis antigens [inacti-vated pertussis toxin 25 mcg, filamentous hemagglutinin 25 mcg, pertactin 8 mcg], type 1 poliovirus 40 D-antigen units, type 2 poliovirus 8 D-antigen units, and type 3 poliovirus 32 D-antigen units per 0.5 mL (0.5 mL) [contains aluminum, neomycin sulfate, polymyxin B, polysorbate 80; may contain natural rubber/natural latex in prefilled syringe]

Dosage Forms: Canada Excipient information presented when available (limited, particularly for generics); consult specific product labeling.

Injection, suspension [preservative free]:

Adacel®-Polio: Diphtheria toxoid 2 Lf, tetanus toxoid 5 Lf, acellular pertussis antigens [inactivated pertussis toxoid 2.5 mcg, filamentous hemagglutinin 5 mcg, pertactin 3 mcg, types 2 and 3 fimbriae 5 mcg], type 1 poliovirus 40 D-antigen units, type 2 poliovirus 8 D-antigen units, and type 3 poliovirus 32 D-antigen units per 0.5 mL (0.5 mL) [contains aluminum, neomycin sulfate, polymyxin B, polysorbate 80]

◆ **Diphtheria and Tetanus Toxoids and Acellular Pertussis Adsorbed, and Inactivated Poliovirus Vaccine Combined** see Diphtheria and Tetanus Toxoids, Acellular Pertussis, and Poliovirus Vaccine on page 565

Diphtheria and Tetanus Toxoids, and Acellular Pertussis Vaccine
(dif THEER ee a & TET a nus TOKS oyds & ay CEL yoo lar per TUS sis vak SEEN)

Related Information
Immunization Administration Recommendations on page 2144
Immunization Recommendations on page 2149

Medication Safety Issues
Sound-alike/look-alike issues:
Adacel® (Tdap) may be confused with Daptacel® (DTaP)
Tdap (Adacel®, Boostrix®) may be confused with DTaP (Daptacel®, Infanrix®, Tripedia®)
Administration issues:
Carefully review product labeling to prevent inadvertent administration of Tdap when DTaP is indicated. Tdap contains lower amounts of diphtheria toxoid and some pertussis antigens than DTaP.
DTaP is not indicated for use in persons ≥7 years of age
Guidelines are available in case of inadvertent administration of these products; refer to ACIP recommendations, February 2006 available at http://www.cdc.gov/mmwr/preview/mmwrhtml/rr55e223a1.htm
Other safety concerns:
DTaP: Diphtheria and tetanus toxoids and acellular pertussis vaccine
DTP: Diphtheria and tetanus toxoids and pertussis vaccine (unspecified pertussis antigens)
DTwP: Diphtheria and tetanus toxoids and whole-cell pertussis vaccine (no longer available on U.S. market)
Tdap: Tetanus toxoid, reduced diphtheria toxoid, and acellular pertussis vaccine

Brand Names: U.S. Adacel®; Boostrix®; Daptacel®; Infanrix®
Brand Names: Canada Adacel®; Boostrix®
Index Terms DTaP; Tdap; Tetanus Toxoid, Reduced Diphtheria Toxoid, and Acellular Pertussis, Adsorbed; Tripedia
Generic Availability (U.S.) No
Pharmacologic Category Vaccine, Inactivated (Bacterial)
Use
Daptacel®, Infanrix®, Tripedia® (DTaP): Active immunization against diphtheria, tetanus, and pertussis from age 6 weeks through 6 years of age (prior to seventh birthday)
Adacel®, Boostrix® (Tdap): Active booster immunization against diphtheria, tetanus, and pertussis

DIPHTHERIA AND TETANUS TOXOIDS, AND ACELLULAR PERTUSSIS VACCINE

The Advisory Committee on Immunization Practices (ACIP) recommends routine vaccination for the following:

Adolescents ≥11 years and Adults (Tdap):
- Persons wounded in bombings or similar mass casualty events and who cannot confirm receipt of a tetanus booster within the previous 5 years and who have penetrating injuries or nonintact skin exposure should receive a single dose of Tdap (CDC, 57 [RR6] 2008)

Adults 19-64 years (Tdap): A single dose of Tdap should be given to replace a single dose of the 10-year Td booster in patients who have not previously received Tdap or for whom vaccine status is not known, and as soon as feasible to all:
- Close contacts of children <12 months of age; Tdap should ideally be administered at least 2 weeks prior to beginning close contact (CDC, 60[4], 2011; CDC, 55[RR17], 2006)
- Healthcare providers with direct patient contact (CDC, 60[4], 2011; CDC, 55[RR17], 2006)

Adults ≥65 years who have not previously received Tdap:
- All adults ≥65 years may receive a single dose of Tdap in place of a dose of Td (CDC, 60 [1], 2011)
- Adults ≥65 years who anticipate close contact with children <12 months of age should receive a single dose of Tdap in place a of a dose of Td (CDC, 60[1], 2011)

Note: Tdap is currently recommended for a single dose only (all age groups) (CDC, 60 [1], 2011)

Contraindications Hypersensitivity to diphtheria, tetanus toxoids, pertussis, or any component of the formulation; history of any of the following effects from previous administration of pertussis-containing vaccine - progressive neurologic disorder, uncontrolled epilepsy or progressive epilepsy (postpone until condition stabilized); encephalopathy occurring within 7 days of administration and not attributable to another cause

Warnings/Precautions Defer administration during moderate or severe illness (with or without fever). Carefully consider use in patients with history of any of the following effects from previous administration of any pertussis-containing vaccine: Fever ≥105°F (40.5°C) within 48 hours of unknown cause; seizures with or without fever occurring within 3 days; shock or collapse within 48 hours. Carefully consider use in patients with history of Guillain-Barré syndrome occurring within 6 weeks of a vaccine containing tetanus toxoid. Td or Tdap vaccines and emergency doses of Td vaccine should not be given more frequently than every 10 years in patients who have experienced a serious Arthus-type hypersensitivity reaction following a prior use of tetanus toxoid even if using for wound management with wounds that are not clean or minor; these patients generally have high serum antitoxin levels. Syncope has been reported with use of injectable vaccines and may be accompanied by transient visual disturbances, weakness, or tonic-clonic movements. Procedures should be in place to avoid injuries from falling and to restore cerebral perfusion if syncope occurs.

Use caution in patients with coagulation disorders (including thrombocytopenia) where intramuscular injections should not be used. Patients who are immunocompromised may have reduced response; may be used in patients with HIV infection. In general, household and close contacts of persons with altered immunocompetence may receive all age appropriate vaccines. Use caution in patients with history of seizure disorder, progressive neurologic disease, or conditions predisposing to seizures; ACIP and APP guidelines recommend deferring immunization until health status can be assessed and condition stabilized. Antipyretics may be considered at the time of and for 24 hours following vaccination to patients at high risk for seizures to reduce the possibility of postvaccination fever. Products may contain thimerosal or gelatin; packaging may contain natural latex rubber. Immediate treatment for anaphylactic/anaphylactoid reaction should be available during vaccine use. In order to maximize vaccination rates, the ACIP recommends simultaneous administration of all age-appropriate vaccines (live or inactivated) for which a person is eligible at a single clinic visit, unless contraindications exist. The use of combination vaccines is generally preferred over separate injections, taking into consideration provider assessment, patient preference, and adverse events. When using combination vaccines, the minimum age for administration is the oldest minimum age for any individual component; the minimum interval between dosing is the greatest minimum interval between any individual component.

Adverse Reactions (Reflective of adult population; not specific for elderly) All serious adverse reactions must be reported to the U.S. Department of Health and Human Services (DHHS) Vaccine Adverse Event Reporting System (VAERS) 1-800-822-7967 or online at https://vaers.hhs.gov/esub/index. In Canada, adverse reactions may be reported to local provincial/territorial health agencies or to the Vaccine Safety Section at Public Health Agency of Canada (1-866-844-0018).

Daptacel®, Infanrix® (incidence of erythema, swelling, and fever increases with successive doses):

Frequency not defined:

Central nervous system: Drowsiness, fever, fussiness, irritability, lethargy

Gastrointestinal: Appetite decreased, vomiting

Local: Pain, redness, swelling, tenderness

Miscellaneous: Prolonged or persistent crying, refusal to play

Adacel®, Boostrix®: Note: Ranges presented, actual percent varies by product and age group

>10%:

Central nervous system: Fatigue, tiredness (24% to 37%; grade 3/severe: 1% to 4%), headache (12% to 44%; grade 3/severe: 1% to 4%), chills (8% to 15%; severe: <1%)

Gastrointestinal: Gastrointestinal symptoms, includes abdominal pain, diarrhea, nausea and/or vomiting (3% to 26%; grade 3/severe: ≤3%)

Local: Injection site pain (22% to 78%; grade 3/severe: ≤5%), arm circumference increased (28%; >40 mm: 0.5%), redness (11% to 25%; ≥50 mm: 2% to 4%), swelling (8% to 21%; ≥50 mm: ≤3%)

Neuromuscular & skeletal: Body aches/muscle weakness (22% to 30%; severe: 1%), soreness/swollen joints (9% to 11%; severe: <1%)

1% to 10%:

Central nervous system: Fever ≥38°C (≥100.4°F: 1% to 5%)

Dermatologic: Rash (2% to 3%)

Miscellaneous: Lymph node swelling (7%; severe: <1%)

Drug Interactions

Metabolism/Transport Effects None known.

Avoid Concomitant Use There are no known interactions where it is recommended to avoid concomitant use.

Increased Effect/Toxicity There are no known significant interactions involving an increase in effect.

Decreased Effect

The levels/effects of Diphtheria and Tetanus Toxoids, and Acellular Pertussis Vaccine may be decreased by: Belimumab; Fingolimod; Immunosuppressants

Stability Refrigerate at 2°C to 8°C (35°F to 46°F); do not freeze; discard if frozen. The following stability information has also been reported for Infanrix®: May be stored at room temperature for up to 72 hours (Cohen, 2007).

Mechanism of Action Promotes active immunity to diphtheria, tetanus, and pertussis by inducing production of specific antibodies.

Dosage

Geriatric

Booster Immunization: I.M.: Adults ≥65 years:

ACIP recommendations: Refer to adult dosing. In adults ≥65 years Boostrix® should be used if feasible; however, ACIP has concluded that either Tdap vaccine (Boostrix® or Adacel®) may be used (CDC, 61[25], 2012).

Manufacturer's recommendations: Boostrix®: 0.5 mL as a single dose, administered 5 years after last dose of tetanus toxoid, diphtheria toxoid, and/or pertussis-containing vaccine.

Wound Management: I.M.: Refer to adult dosing.

Adult Note: Tdap can be administered regardless of the interval between the last tetanus or diphtheria toxoid containing vaccine. Tdap is currently recommended for a single dose only (CDC, 60[1], 2011; CDC, 61[25], 2012).

Booster immunization: ACIP recommendations: I.M.: Adults ≥19 years: 0.5 mL per dose. A single dose of Tdap should be given to replace a single dose of the 10 year Td booster in patients who have not previously received Tdap or for whom vaccine status is not known. A single dose of Tdap is recommended for health care personnel who have not previously received Tdap and who have direct patient contact (CDC, 55[17], 2006; CDC, 61[4], 2012). Tdap should be administered regardless of interval since last tetanus- or diphtheria-containing vaccine (CDC, 61[25], 2012).

Booster immunization: Manufacturer's recommendations: I.M.: Adults ≤64 years (Adacel®, Boostrix®): 0.5 mL as a single dose, administered 5 years after last dose of tetanus toxoid, diphtheria toxoid, and/or pertussis-containing vaccine

Wound management: I.M.: Adacel® or Boostrix® may be used as an alternative to Td vaccine when a tetanus toxoid-containing vaccine is needed for wound management, and in whom the pertussis component is also indicated. Tetanus prophylaxis in patients with wounds should consider if the wound is clean or contaminated, the immunization status of the patient, proper use of tetanus toxoid and/or tetanus immune globulin (TIG), wound cleaning, and (if required) surgical debridement and the proper use of antibiotics. Patients with an uncertain or incomplete tetanus immunization status should have additional follow up to ensure a series is completed. Patients with a history of Arthus reaction following a previous dose of a tetanus toxoid-containing vaccine should not receive a tetanus toxoid-containing vaccine until >10 years after the most recent dose even if they have a wound that is neither clean nor minor. See table on next page.

DIPHTHERIA AND TETANUS TOXOIDS, AND ACELLULAR PERTUSSIS VACCINE

Tetanus Prophylaxis in Wound Management

History of Tetanus Immunization Doses	Clean, Minor Wounds		All Other Wounds[1]	
	Tetanus Toxoid[2]	TIG	Tetanus Toxoid[2]	TIG
Uncertain or <3 doses	Yes	No	Yes	Yes
3 or more doses	No[3]	No	No[4]	No

[1]Such as, but not limited to, wounds contaminated with dirt, feces, soil, and saliva; puncture wounds; wounds from crushing, tears, burns, and frostbite.

[2]Tetanus toxoid in this chart refers to a tetanus toxoid-containing vaccine. For children <7 years of age, DTaP (DT, if pertussis vaccine contraindicated) is preferred to tetanus toxoid alone. For children ≥7 years and adults, Td preferred to tetanus toxoid alone; Tdap may be preferred if the patient has not previously been vaccinated with Tdap.

[3]Yes, if ≥10 years since last dose.

[4]Yes, if ≥5 years since last dose.

Adapted from CDC "Yellow Book" (*Health Information for International Travel 2010*), "Routine Vaccine-Preventable Diseases, Tetanus" (available at http://www.cdc.gov/yellowbook) and *MMWR* 2006, 55(RR-17).

Abbreviations: **DT** = Diphtheria and Tetanus Toxoids (formulation for age ≤6 years); **DTaP** = Diphtheria and Tetanus Toxoids, and Acellular Pertussis (formulation for age ≤6 years; Daptacel®, Infanrix®); **Td** = Diphtheria and Tetanus Toxoids (formulation for age ≥7 years; Decavac®,Tenivac™); **TT**= Tetanus toxoid (adsorbed [formulation for age ≥7 years]); **Tdap** = Diphtheria and Tetanus Toxoids, and Acellular Pertussis (Adacel® or Boostrix® [formulations for age ≥7 years]); **TIG** = Tetanus Immune Globulin

Administration Shake suspension well.

Adacel®, Boostrix®: Administer only I.M. in deltoid muscle of upper arm.

Daptacel®, Infanrix®: Administer only I.M. in anterolateral aspect of thigh or deltoid muscle of upper arm.

If feasible, the same brand of DTaP should be used for all doses in the series (CDC, 60 [2], 2011).

For patients at risk of hemorrhage following intramuscular injection, the ACIP recommends "it should be administered intramuscularly if, in the opinion of the physician familiar with the patient's bleeding risk, the vaccine can be administered by this route with reasonable safety. If the patient receives antihemophilia or other similar therapy, intramuscular vaccination can be scheduled shortly after such therapy is administered. A fine needle (23 gauge or smaller) can be used for the vaccination and firm pressure applied to the site (without rubbing) for at least 2 minutes. The patient should be instructed concerning the risk of hematoma from the injection." Patients on anticoagulant therapy should be considered to have the same bleeding risks and treated as those with clotting factor disorders (CDC, 60[2], 2011).

Simultaneous administration of vaccines helps ensure the patients will be fully vaccinated by the appropriate age. Simultaneous administration of vaccines is defined as administering >1 vaccine on the same day at different anatomic sites. The use of licensed combination vaccines is generally preferred over separate injections of the equivalent components. Separate vaccines should not be combined in the same syringe unless indicated by product specific labeling. Separate needles and syringes should be used for each injection. The ACIP prefers each dose of a specific vaccine in a series come from the same manufacturer when possible. Adolescents and adults should be vaccinated while seated or lying down. In general, preterm infants should be vaccinated at the same chronological age as full-term infants (CDC, 60[2], 2011).

Antipyretics have not been shown to prevent febrile seizures. Antipyretics may be used to treat fever or discomfort following vaccination (CDC, 2011). One study reported that routine prophylactic administration of acetaminophen to prevent fever prior to vaccination decreased the immune response of some vaccines; the clinical significance of this reduction in immune response has not been established (Prymula, 2009).

Monitoring Parameters Monitor for syncope for 15 minutes following administration. If seizure-like activity associated with syncope occurs, maintain patient in supine or Trendelenburg position to reestablish adequate cerebral perfusion.

Pharmacotherapy Pearls Adacel® is formulated with the same antigens found in Daptacel® but with reduced quantities of pertussis and tetanus. It is intended for use as a booster dose in children and adults, 11-64 years of age, and **not** for primary immunization.

Boostrix® is formulated with the same antigens found in Infanrix® but in reduced quantities. It is intended for use as a booster dose in children and adults, 10-64 years of age, and is **not** for primary immunization.

Federal law requires that the name of medication, date of administration, the vaccine manufacturer, lot number of vaccine, and the administering person's name, title and address be entered into the patient's permanent medical record.

Special Geriatric Considerations Protective tetanus and diphtheria antibodies decline with age (only 31% of persons >70 years of age in the U.S. are believed to be immune to tetanus). The true incidence and burden of pertussis in older adults is unknown, but is believed to be significantly higher than actually reported. ACIP has issued recommendations for the use of Tdap in adults ≥65 years and recommends a single dose of Tdap be administered in all patients who have not previously received a dose of Tdap or for whom vaccine status is not known. Following Tdap administration, routine boosters using Td should be given every 10 years. Of the 2 Tdap vaccines available in the U.S., Boostrix® and Adacel®, only Boostrix® is FDA approved for use in adults ≥65 years; however, ACIP recommends use of either Tdap vaccine if Boostrix® administration is not feasible. ACIP concluded that Adacel® would likely provide protection and administration of either Tdap vaccine is considered valid. Providers should not miss an opportunity to vaccinate with Tdap. Adverse events in adults ≥65 years using either Tdap vaccine are reportedly comparable to patients <65 years (CDC, 61[25], 2012).

Dosage Forms Excipient information presented when available (limited, particularly for generics); consult specific product labeling.

Injection, suspension [Tdap, booster formulation]:

Adacel®: Diphtheria 2 Lf units, tetanus 5 Lf units, and acellular pertussis antigens [detoxified pertussis toxin 2.5 mcg, filamentous hemagglutinin 5 mcg, pertactin 3 mcg, fimbriae (types 2 and 3) 5 mcg] per 0.5 mL (0.5 mL) [contains aluminum; may contain natural rubber/natural latex in prefilled syringe]

Boostrix®: Diphtheria 2.5 Lf units, tetanus 5 Lf units, and acellular pertussis antigens [inactivated pertussis toxin 8 mcg, filamentous hemagglutinin 8 mcg, pertactin 2.5 mcg] per 0.5 mL (0.5 mL) [contains aluminum and polysorbate 80; may contain natural rubber/natural latex in prefilled syringe]

Injection, suspension [DTaP, active immunization formulation]:

Daptacel®: Diphtheria 15 Lf units, tetanus 5 Lf units, and acellular pertussis antigens [detoxified pertussis toxin 10 mcg, filamentous hemagglutinin 5 mcg, pertactin 3 mcg, fimbriae (types 2 and 3) 5 mcg] per 0.5 mL (0.5 mL) [preservative free; contains aluminum]

Infanrix®: Diphtheria 25 Lf units, tetanus 10 Lf units, and acellular pertussis antigens [inactivated pertussis toxin 25 mcg, filamentous hemagglutinin 25 mcg, pertactin 8 mcg] per 0.5 mL (0.5 mL) [preservative free; contains aluminum and polysorbate 80]

Infanrix®: Diphtheria 25 Lf units, tetanus 10 Lf units, and acellular pertussis antigens [inactivated pertussis toxin 25 mcg, filamentous hemagglutinin 25 mcg, pertactin 8 mcg] per 0.5 mL (0.5 mL) [preservative free; contains aluminum and polysorbate 80; prefilled syringes contain natural rubber/natural latex] [DSC]

◆ **Diphtheria, Tetanus Toxoids, Acellular Pertussis (DTaP)** see Diphtheria and Tetanus Toxoids, Acellular Pertussis, and Poliovirus Vaccine on page 565
◆ **Dipivalyl Epinephrine** see Dipivefrin on page 571

Dipivefrin (dye PI ve frin)

Related Information
Glaucoma Drug Therapy on page 2115
Brand Names: Canada Ophtho-Dipivefrin™; PMS-Dipivefrin; Propine®
Index Terms Dipivalyl Epinephrine; Dipivefrin Hydrochloride; DPE
Generic Availability (U.S.) No
Pharmacologic Category Alpha/Beta Agonist; Ophthalmic Agent, Antiglaucoma; Ophthalmic Agent, Vasoconstrictor
Use Reduces elevated intraocular pressure in chronic open-angle glaucoma; also used to treat ocular hypertension, low tension, and secondary glaucomas
Contraindications Hypersensitivity to dipivefrin, any component of the formulation, or epinephrine; angle-closure glaucoma
Warnings/Precautions Use with caution in patients with hypertension or cardiac disorders and in aphakic patients. Contains sodium metabisulfite.
Adverse Reactions (Reflective of adult population; not specific for elderly) 1% to 10%:
Central nervous system: Headache
Local: Burning, stinging
Ocular: Blepharoconjunctivitis, blurred vision, bulbar conjunctival follicles, cystoid macular edema, ocular congestion, ocular pain, mydriasis, photophobia
Drug Interactions
Metabolism/Transport Effects None known.
Avoid Concomitant Use
Avoid concomitant use of Dipivefrin with any of the following: Ergot Derivatives; Iobenguane I 123

Increased Effect/Toxicity

Dipivefrin may increase the levels/effects of: Sympathomimetics

The levels/effects of Dipivefrin may be increased by: AtoMOXetine; Cannabinoids; Ergot Derivatives; Linezolid; Serotonin/Norepinephrine Reuptake Inhibitors

Decreased Effect

Dipivefrin may decrease the levels/effects of: Iobenguane I 123

The levels/effects of Dipivefrin may be decreased by: Spironolactone

Stability Avoid exposure to light and air. Discolored or darkened solutions indicate loss of potency.

Mechanism of Action Dipivefrin is a prodrug of epinephrine which is the active agent that stimulates alpha- and/or beta-adrenergic receptors increasing aqueous humor outflow

Pharmacodynamics/Kinetics

Ocular pressure effect:
Onset of action: ~30 minutes
Duration: ≥12 hours
Mydriasis:
Onset of action: ~30 minutes
Duration: Several hours
Absorption: Rapid into aqueous humor
Metabolism: Converted to epinephrine

Dosage

Geriatric & Adult Glaucoma: Ophthalmic: Instill 1 drop every 12 hours into the eyes

Monitoring Parameters Intraocular pressure; heart rate and blood pressure

Special Geriatric Considerations Use with caution in patients with heart disease. Evaluate the patient's or caregiver's ability to safely administer the correct dose of ophthalmic medication.

Dosage Forms Excipient information presented when available (limited, particularly for generics); consult specific product labeling. [DSC] = Discontinued product

Solution, ophthalmic, as hydrochloride [drops]:
Propine®: 0.1% (10 mL [DSC]) [contains benzalkonium chloride]

♦ **Dipivefrin Hydrochloride** *see* Dipivefrin *on page* 571
♦ **Diprolene®** *see* Betamethasone *on page* 204
♦ **Diprolene® AF** *see* Betamethasone *on page* 204
♦ **Dipropylacetic Acid** *see* Valproic Acid *on page* 1991

Dipyridamole (dye peer ID a mole)

Related Information
Beers Criteria – Potentially Inappropriate Medications for Geriatrics *on page* 2183

Medication Safety Issues

Sound-alike/look-alike issues:
Dipyridamole may be confused with disopyramide
Persantine® may be confused with Periactin

BEERS Criteria medication:
This drug may be potentially inappropriate for use in geriatric patients (Quality of evidence - moderate; Strength of recommendation - strong).

International issues:
Persantine [U.S., Canada, Belgium, Denmark, France] may be confused with Permitil brand name for sildenafil [Argentina]

Brand Names: U.S. Persantine®

Brand Names: Canada Apo-Dipyridamole FC®; Dipyridamole For Injection; Persantine®

Generic Availability (U.S.) Yes

Pharmacologic Category Antiplatelet Agent; Vasodilator

Use

Oral: Used with warfarin to decrease thrombosis in patients after artificial heart valve replacement

I.V.: Diagnostic agent in CAD

Unlabeled Use Stroke prevention (in combination with aspirin); **Note:** For this indication, the use of aspirin/extended release dipyridamole is recommended (Guyatt, 2012).

Contraindications Hypersensitivity to dipyridamole or any component of the formulation

Warnings/Precautions Use with caution in patients with hypotension, unstable angina, and/ or recent MI. Use with caution in hepatic impairment. Avoid use of oral dipyridamole in this age group due to risk of orthostatic hypotension and availability of more efficacious alternative agents (Beers Criteria). Use caution in patients on other antiplatelet agents or anticoagulation. Severe adverse reactions have occurred with I.V. administration (rarely); use the I.V. form with caution in patients with bronchospastic disease or unstable angina. Aminophylline should be available in case of urgency or emergency with I.V. use.

Adverse Reactions (Reflective of adult population; not specific for elderly)
Oral:
>10%: Dizziness (14%)
1% to 10%:
  Central nervous system: Headache (2%)
  Dermatologic: Rash (2%)
  Gastrointestinal: Abdominal distress (6%)
Frequency not defined: Diarrhea, vomiting, flushing, pruritus, angina pectoris, liver dysfunction
I.V.:
>10%:
  Cardiovascular: Exacerbation of angina pectoris (20%)
  Central nervous system: Dizziness (12%), headache (12%)
1% to 10%:
  Cardiovascular: Hypotension (5%), hypertension (2%), blood pressure lability (2%), ECG abnormalities (ST-T changes, extrasystoles; 5% to 8%), pain (3%), tachycardia (3%)
  Central nervous system: Flushing (3%), fatigue (1%)
  Gastrointestinal: Nausea (5%)
  Neuromuscular & skeletal: Paresthesia (1%)
  Respiratory: Dyspnea (3%)

Drug Interactions
Metabolism/Transport Effects Inhibits BCRP, P-glycoprotein
Avoid Concomitant Use
  Avoid concomitant use of Dipyridamole with any of the following: Silodosin
Increased Effect/Toxicity
  Dipyridamole may increase the levels/effects of: Adenosine; Anticoagulants; Antiplatelet Agents; Beta-Blockers; Colchicine; Collagenase (Systemic); Dabigatran Etexilate; Drotrecogin Alfa (Activated); Everolimus; Hypotensive Agents; Ibritumomab; P-glycoprotein/ABCB1 Substrates; Prucalopride; Regadenoson; Rivaroxaban; Salicylates; Silodosin; Thrombolytic Agents; Topotecan; Tositumomab and Iodine I 131 Tositumomab

  The levels/effects of Dipyridamole may be increased by: Dasatinib; Glucosamine; Herbs (Anticoagulant/Antiplatelet Properties); Nonsteroidal Anti-Inflammatory Agents; Omega-3-Acid Ethyl Esters; Pentosan Polysulfate Sodium; Pentoxifylline; Prostacyclin Analogues; Tipranavir; Vitamin E
Decreased Effect
  Dipyridamole may decrease the levels/effects of: Acetylcholinesterase Inhibitors

  The levels/effects of Dipyridamole may be decreased by: Nonsteroidal Anti-Inflammatory Agents
Ethanol/Nutrition/Herb Interactions
Food: Management: Administer with water 1 hour before meals.
Herb/Nutraceutical: Many herbal medications may have additional antiplatelet activity. Management: Avoid cat's claw, dong quai, evening primrose, feverfew, garlic, ginger, ginkgo, glucosamine, omega-3-acid ethyl esters (fish oil), red clover, horse chestnut, green tea, and ginseng.

Stability I.V.: Store between 15°C to 25°C (59°F to 77°F); do not freeze. Protect from light. Prior to administration, dilute to a ≥1:2 ratio in NS, 1/2NS, or D_5W. Total volume should be ~20-50 mL.

Mechanism of Action Inhibits the activity of adenosine deaminase and phosphodiesterase, which causes an accumulation of adenosine, adenine nucleotides, and cyclic AMP; these mediators then inhibit platelet aggregation and may cause vasodilation; may also stimulate release of prostacyclin or PGD_2; causes coronary vasodilation

Pharmacodynamics/Kinetics
Absorption: Readily, but variable
Distribution: Adults: V_d: 2-3 L/kg
Protein binding: 91% to 99%
Metabolism: Hepatic
Half-life elimination: Terminal: 10-12 hours
Time to peak, serum: 2-2.5 hours
Excretion: Feces (as glucuronide conjugates and unchanged drug)

◄ **Dosage**
Geriatric & Adult
Adjunctive therapy for prophylaxis of thromboembolism with cardiac valve replacement: Oral: 75-100 mg 4 times/day
Evaluation of coronary artery disease: I.V.: 0.14 mg/kg/minute for 4 minutes; maximum dose: 60 mg

Following dipyridamole infusion, inject thallium-201 within 5 minutes. **Note:** Aminophylline should be available for urgent/emergent use; dosing of 50-100 mg (range: 50-250 mg) I.V. push over 30-60 seconds.

Administration
I.V.: Infuse diluted solution over 4 minutes.
Tablet: Administer with water 1 hour before meals.

Monitoring Parameters Blood pressure, heart rate, ECG (stress test)

Test Interactions Concurrent caffeine or theophylline use may demonstrate a false-negative result with dipyridamole-thallium myocardial imaging.

Special Geriatric Considerations Since evidence suggests that clinically used doses are ineffective for prevention of platelet aggregation, consideration for low-dose aspirin (81-325 mg/day) alone may be necessary. This will decrease cost as well as inconvenience.

This medication is considered to be potentially inappropriate in this patient population (Beers Criteria: Quality of evidence - moderate; Strength of recommendation - strong).

Dosage Forms Excipient information presented when available (limited, particularly for generics); consult specific product labeling. [DSC] = Discontinued product
Injection, solution: 5 mg/mL (2 mL [DSC], 10 mL)
Tablet, oral: 25 mg, 50 mg, 75 mg
Persantine®: 25 mg, 50 mg, 75 mg

◆ **Dipyridamole and Aspirin** see Aspirin and Dipyridamole *on page* 159
◆ **Disalicylic Acid** see Salsalate *on page* 1751
◆ **Disodium Cromoglycate** see Cromolyn (Nasal) *on page* 450
◆ **Disodium Cromoglycate** see Cromolyn (Ophthalmic) *on page* 450
◆ **Disodium Cromoglycate** see Cromolyn (Systemic, Oral Inhalation) *on page* 449
◆ **d-Isoephedrine Hydrochloride** see Pseudoephedrine *on page* 1633

Disopyramide (dye soe PEER a mide)

Related Information
Beers Criteria – Potentially Inappropriate Medications for Geriatrics *on page* 2183
Medication Safety Issues
Sound-alike/look-alike issues:
Disopyramide may be confused with desipramine, dipyridamole
Norpace® may be confused with Norpramin®
BEERS Criteria medication:
This drug may be potentially inappropriate for use in geriatric patients (Quality of evidence - low; Strength of recommendation - strong).
Brand Names: U.S. Norpace®; Norpace® CR
Brand Names: Canada Norpace®; Rythmodan®; Rythmodan®-LA
Index Terms Disopyramide Phosphate
Generic Availability (U.S.) Yes
Pharmacologic Category Antiarrhythmic Agent, Class Ia
Use Life-threatening ventricular arrhythmias (eg, sustained ventricular tachycardia)
Unlabeled Use Alternative agent for the prevention of recurrent symptomatic focal atrial tachycardia (in combination with an AV nodal blocking agent), atrial fibrillation (especially vagally-induced), or atrial flutter (in combination with an AV nodal-blocking agent); obstructive hypertrophic cardiomyopathy (HCM) in combination with ventricular rate-controlling agents (eg, beta blockers or verapamil) to control symptoms of angina or dyspnea who are unresponsive to rate-controlling agents alone; atrial fibrillation in patients with HCM in combination with rate-controlling agents
Contraindications Hypersensitivity to disopyramide or any component of the formulation; cardiogenic shock; pre-existing second- or third-degree heart block (except in patients with a functioning artificial pacemaker); congenital QT syndrome; sick sinus syndrome
Warnings/Precautions Watch for proarrhythmic effects; may cause QT_c prolongation and subsequent torsade de pointes; avoid use in patients with diagnosed or suspected congenital long QT syndrome. Monitor and adjust dose to prevent QT_c prolongation. Avoid concurrent use with other medications that prolong QT interval or decrease myocardial contractility. Correct hypokalemia before initiating therapy; may worsen toxicity. **[U.S. Boxed Warning]: In the Cardiac Arrhythmia Suppression Trial (CAST), recent (>6 days but <2 years ago)**

myocardial infarction patients with asymptomatic, non-life-threatening ventricular arrhythmias did not benefit and may have been harmed by attempts to suppress the arrhythmia with flecainide or encainide. An increased mortality or nonfatal cardiac arrest rate (7.7%) was seen in the active treatment group compared with patients in the placebo group (3%). The applicability of the CAST results to other populations is unknown. Antiarrhythmic agents should be reserved for patients with life-threatening ventricular arrhythmias. Use with caution or avoid in patients with any degree of left ventricular dysfunction or history of heart failure (HF); may precipitate or exacerbate HF. Due to significant anticholinergic effects, do not use in patients with urinary retention, BPH, glaucoma, or myasthenia gravis. Reduce dosage in renal or hepatic impairment. Avoid use in the elderly due to a risk of developing heart failure (potent negative inotrope) and adverse effects associated with potent anticholinergic properties; alternative antiarrhythmic agents preferred (Beers Criteria). Controlled release form is not recommended for Cl_{cr} ≤40 mL/ minute. In patients with atrial fibrillation or flutter, block the AV node before initiating. Use caution in Wolff-Parkinson-White syndrome or bundle branch block. Monitor closely for hypotension during the initiation of therapy.

Adverse Reactions (Reflective of adult population; not specific for elderly) The most common adverse effects are related to cholinergic blockade. The most serious adverse effects of disopyramide are hypotension and CHF.

>10%:
  Gastrointestinal: Xerostomia (32%), constipation (11%)
  Genitourinary: Urinary hesitancy (14% to 23%)
1% to 10%:
  Cardiovascular: CHF, hypotension, cardiac conduction disturbance, edema, syncope, chest pain
  Central nervous system: Fatigue, headache, malaise, dizziness, nervousness
  Dermatologic: Rash, generalized dermatoses, pruritus
  Endocrine & metabolic: Cholesterol increased, hypokalemia, triglycerides increased
  Gastrointestinal: Dry throat, nausea, abdominal distension, flatulence, abdominal bloating, anorexia, diarrhea, vomiting, weight gain
  Genitourinary: Urinary retention, urinary frequency, urinary urgency, impotence (1% to 3%)
  Neuromuscular & skeletal: Muscle weakness, muscular pain
  Ocular: Blurred vision, dry eyes
  Respiratory: Dyspnea

Drug Interactions
Metabolism/Transport Effects Substrate of CYP3A4 (major); **Note:** Assignment of Major/ Minor substrate status based on clinically relevant drug interaction potential

Avoid Concomitant Use
Avoid concomitant use of Disopyramide with any of the following: Conivaptan; Fingolimod; Highest Risk QTc-Prolonging Agents; Macrolide Antibiotics; Mifepristone; Moderate Risk QTc-Prolonging Agents; Propafenone; Verapamil

Increased Effect/Toxicity
Disopyramide may increase the levels/effects of: AbobotulinumtoxinA; Anticholinergics; Beta-Blockers; Cannabinoids; Highest Risk QTc-Prolonging Agents; Lidocaine; Lidocaine (Systemic); OnabotulinumtoxinA; Potassium Chloride; RimabotulinumtoxinB

The levels/effects of Disopyramide may be increased by: Amiodarone; Conivaptan; CYP3A4 Inhibitors (Moderate); CYP3A4 Inhibitors (Strong); EriBULin; Fingolimod; Ivacaftor; Lurasidone; Macrolide Antibiotics; Mifepristone; Moderate Risk QTc-Prolonging Agents; Pramlintide; Propafenone; QTc-Prolonging Agents (Indeterminate Risk and Risk Modifying); Verapamil

Decreased Effect
Disopyramide may decrease the levels/effects of: Acetylcholinesterase Inhibitors (Central); Secretin

The levels/effects of Disopyramide may be decreased by: Acetylcholinesterase Inhibitors (Central); Barbiturates; CYP3A4 Inducers (Strong); Deferasirox; Etravirine; Fosphenytoin; Herbs (CYP3A4 Inducers); Phenytoin; Rifamycin Derivatives; Tocilizumab

Ethanol/Nutrition/Herb Interactions
  Ethanol: Ethanol may increase CNS depression. Management: Avoid ethanol.
  Food: Management: Administer at the same time around-the-clock on an empty stomach.
  Herb/Nutraceutical: St John's wort may decrease disopyramide levels. Ephedra may worsen arrhythmia. Management: Avoid St John's wort and ephedra.

Stability Extemporaneously prepared suspension is stable for 4 weeks refrigerated.
Mechanism of Action Class Ia antiarrhythmic: Decreases myocardial excitability and conduction velocity; reduces disparity in refractory between normal and infarcted myocardium; possesses anticholinergic, peripheral vasoconstrictive, and negative inotropic effects

Pharmacodynamics/Kinetics

Onset of action: 0.5-3.5 hours

Duration: Immediate release: 1.5-8.5 hours

Absorption: 60% to 83%

Distribution: V_d: 0.8-2 L/kg

Protein binding (concentration dependent): 20% to 60%

Metabolism: Hepatic; N-dealkylation to the active metabolite N-despropyldisopyramide (or mono-N-dealkylated [MND] metabolite) and other inactive metabolites

Half-life elimination: Adults: 4-10 hours; prolonged with hepatic or renal impairment

Time to peak, serum: Immediate release: Within 2 hours; Controlled release: 4-7 hours

Excretion: Urine (~50% as unchanged drug; ~20% as MND; 10% other metabolites); feces (10% to 15%)

Dosage

Geriatric Refer to adult dosing. Dose with caution, starting at the lower end of dosing range.

Adult

Ventricular arrhythmias: Oral: **Note:** Since newer agents with less toxicity are available, the use of disopyramide for this indication has fallen out of favor. Controlled release formulation not to be used when rapid achievement of disopyramide plasma concentrations is desired. A maximum dose up to 400 mg every 6 hours (immediate release) may be required for patients with severe refractory ventricular tachycardia.

<50 kg:

Immediate release: An initial loading dose of 200 mg may be administered if rapid onset is required. Maintenance dose: 100 mg every 6 hours

Controlled release: Maintenance dose: 200 mg every 12 hours

≥50 kg:

Immediate release: An initial loading dose of 300 mg may be administered if rapid onset is required. Maintenance dose: 150 mg every 6 hours. If rapid control is necessary and no response seen within 6 hours of loading dose, may increase maintenance dose to 200 mg every 6 hours.

Controlled release: Maintenance dose: 300 mg every 12 hours

Hypertrophic cardiomyopathy (obstructive physiology) with or without atrial fibrillation (unlabeled use): Oral: Initial: *Controlled release:* 200-250 mg twice daily. If symptoms do not improve, increase by 100 mg/day at 2-week intervals to a maximum daily dose of 600 mg (Gersh, 2011; Sherrid, 2005).

Renal Impairment

Manufacturer recommendations:

Immediate release:

Cl_{cr} >40 mL/minute: 100 mg every 6 hours

Cl_{cr} 30-40 mL/minute: 100 mg every 8 hours

Cl_{cr} 15-30 mL/minute: 100 mg every 12 hours

Cl_{cr} <15 mL/minute: 100 mg every 24 hours

Controlled release:

Cl_{cr} >40 mL/minute: 200 mg every 12 hours

Cl_{cr} ≤40 mL/minute: Not recommended for use

Alternative recommendations (Aronoff, 2007): *Immediate release:*

Cl_{cr} >50 mL/minute: 100-200 mg every 8 hours

Cl_{cr} 10-50 mL/minute: 100-200 mg every 12-24 hours

Cl_{cr} <10 mL/minute: 100-200 mg every 24-48 hours

Dialysis: Not dialyzable (0% to 5%) by hemo- or peritoneal methods; supplemental dose is not necessary.

Hepatic Impairment Manufacturer's recommendations:

Immediate release: 100 mg every 6 hours

Controlled release: 200 mg every 12 hours

Administration Do not break or chew controlled release capsules. Administer around-the-clock rather than 4 times/day (ie, 12-6-12-6, not 9-1-5-9) to promote less variation in peak and trough serum levels. Should be taken on an empty stomach.

Monitoring Parameters ECG, blood pressure, urinary retention, CNS anticholinergic effects (confusion, agitation, hallucinations, etc); disopyramide drug level (if available)

Reference Range

Therapeutic concentration:

Atrial arrhythmias: 2.8-3.2 mcg/mL

Ventricular arrhythmias 3.3-7.5 mcg/mL

Toxic concentration: >7 mcg/mL

Special Geriatric Considerations Due to changes in total clearance (decreased) in the elderly, monitor closely; the anticholinergic action may be intolerable and require discontinuation; monitor for CNS anticholinergic effects (confusion, agitation, hallucinations, etc). **Note:** Dose needs to be altered with Cl$_{cr}$ <40 mL/minute which may be found frequently in older adults.

Clinical studies of Norpace®/Norpace® CR did not include sufficient numbers of subjects ≥65 years of age to determine whether they respond differently from younger subjects. Other reported clinical experience has not identified differences in responses between elderly and younger patients. In general, dose selection for an elderly patient should be cautious, usually starting at the low end of the dosing range, reflecting the greater frequency of decreased hepatic, renal, or cardiac function, and of concomitant disease or other drug therapy.

Because of its anticholinergic activity, disopyramide phosphate should not be used in patients with glaucoma, urinary retention, or benign prostatic hyperplasia (medical conditions commonly associated with the elderly) unless adequate overriding measures are taken. In the event of increased anticholinergic side effects, plasma levels of disopyramide should be monitored and the dose of the drug adjusted accordingly. A reduction of the dose by one third, from the recommended 600 mg/day to 400 mg/day, would be reasonable, without changing the dosing interval. This drug is known to be substantially excreted by the kidney, and the risk of toxic reactions to this drug may be greater in patients with impaired renal function. Because elderly patients are more likely to have decreased renal function, care should be taken in dose selection, and it may be useful to monitor renal function.

This medication is considered to be potentially inappropriate in this patient population (Beers Criteria: Quality of evidence - low; Strength of recommendation - strong).

Dosage Forms Excipient information presented when available (limited, particularly for generics); consult specific product labeling.
Capsule, oral: 100 mg, 150 mg
  Norpace®: 100 mg, 150 mg
Capsule, controlled release, oral:
  Norpace® CR: 100 mg, 150 mg

◆ **Disopyramide Phosphate** *see* Disopyramide *on page 574*
◆ **Ditropan** *see* Oxybutynin *on page 1443*
◆ **Ditropan XL®** *see* Oxybutynin *on page 1443*
◆ **Diuril®** *see* Chlorothiazide *on page 356*

Divalproex (dye VAL proe ex)

Medication Safety Issues
  Sound-alike/look-alike issues:
    Depakote® may be confused with Depakene®, Depakote® ER, Senokot®
    Depakote® ER may be confused with divalproex enteric coated
Brand Names: U.S. Depakote®; Depakote® ER; Depakote® Sprinkle
Brand Names: Canada Apo-Divalproex®; Dom-Divalproex; Epival®; Mylan-Divalproex; Novo-Divalproex; Nu-Divalproex; PHL-Divalproex; PMS-Divalproex
Index Terms Divalproex Sodium; Valproate Semisodium; Valproic Acid Derivative
Generic Availability (U.S.) Yes
Pharmacologic Category Anticonvulsant, Miscellaneous; Antimanic Agent; Histone Deacetylase Inhibitor
Use Monotherapy and adjunctive therapy in the treatment of patients with complex partial seizures; monotherapy and adjunctive therapy of simple and complex absence seizures; adjunctive therapy in patients with multiple seizure types that include absence seizures
  Depakote®, Depakote® ER: Mania associated with bipolar disorder; migraine prophylaxis
Unlabeled Use Diabetic neuropathy
Contraindications Hypersensitivity to divalproex, derivatives, or any component of the formulation; hepatic disease or significant impairment; urea cycle disorders
Warnings/Precautions [U.S. Boxed Warning]: Hepatic failure resulting in fatalities has occurred in patients. Other risk factors include organic brain disease, mental retardation with severe seizure disorders, congenital metabolic disorders, and patients on multiple anticonvulsants. Hepatotoxicity has usually been reported within 6 months of therapy initiation. Monitor patients closely for appearance of malaise, weakness, facial edema, anorexia, jaundice, and vomiting; discontinue immediately with signs/symptom of significant or suspected impairment. Liver function tests should be performed at baseline and at regular intervals after initiation of therapy, especially within the first 6 months. Hepatic dysfunction may progress despite discontinuing treatment. Should only be used as monotherapy in patients at high risk for hepatotoxicity. Contraindicated with severe impairment.

[U.S. Boxed Warning]: Cases of life-threatening pancreatitis, occurring at the start of therapy or following years of use, have been reported. Some cases have been hemorrhagic with rapid progression of initial symptoms to death. Promptly evaluate symptoms of abdominal pain, nausea, vomiting, and/or anorexia; should generally be discontinued if pancreatitis is diagnosed.

May cause severe thrombocytopenia, inhibition of platelet aggregation, and bleeding. Tremors may indicate overdosage; use with caution in patients receiving other anticonvulsants. Hypersensitivity reactions affecting multiple organs have been reported in association with divalproex use; may include dermatologic and/or hematologic changes (eosinophilia, neutropenia, thrombocytopenia) or symptoms of organ dysfunction.

Hyperammonemia and/or encephalopathy, sometimes fatal, have been reported following the initiation of divalproex therapy and may be present with normal transaminase levels. Ammonia levels should be measured in patients who develop unexplained lethargy and vomiting, changes in mental status, or in patients who present with hypothermia (unintentional drop in core body temperature to <35°C/95°F). Discontinue therapy if ammonia levels are increased and evaluate for possible urea cycle disorder (UCD); contraindicated in patients with UCD. Evaluation of UCD should be considered for the following patients prior to the start of therapy: History of unexplained encephalopathy or coma; encephalopathy associated with protein load; unexplained mental retardation; history of elevated plasma ammonia or glutamine; history of cyclical vomiting and lethargy; episodic extreme irritability, ataxia; low BUN or protein avoidance; family history of UCD or unexplained infant deaths (particularly male); or signs or symptoms of UCD (hyperammonemia, encephalopathy, respiratory alkalosis). Hypothermia has been reported with divalproex therapy; may or may not be associated with hyperammonemia; may also occur with concomitant topiramate therapy.

In vitro studies have suggested divalproex stimulates the replication of HIV and CMV viruses under experimental conditions. The clinical consequence of this is unknown, but should be considered when monitoring affected patients.

Antiepileptics are associated with an increased risk of suicidal behavior/thoughts with use (regardless of indication); patients should be monitored for signs/symptoms of depression, suicidal tendencies, and other unusual behavior changes during therapy and instructed to inform their healthcare provider immediately if symptoms occur.

Anticonvulsants should not be discontinued abruptly because of the possibility of increasing seizure frequency; divalproex should be withdrawn gradually to minimize the potential of increased seizure frequency, unless safety concerns require a more rapid withdrawal. Concomitant use with carbapenem antibiotics may reduce valproic acid levels to subtherapeutic levels; monitor levels frequently and consider alternate therapy if levels drop significantly or lack of seizure control occurs. Concomitant use with clonazepam may induce absence status. Patients treated for bipolar disorder should be monitored closely for clinical worsening or suicidality; prescriptions should be written for the smallest quantity consistent with good patient care.

CNS depression may occur with divalproex use. Patients must be cautioned about performing tasks which require mental alertness (operating machinery or driving). Effects with other sedative drugs or ethanol may be potentiated. Use with caution in the elderly.

Adverse Reactions (Reflective of adult population; not specific for elderly)

>10%:
  Central nervous system: Headache (≤31%), somnolence (≤30%), dizziness (12% to 25%), insomnia (>1% to 15%), nervousness (>1% to 11%), pain (1% to 11%)
  Dermatologic: Alopecia (>1% to 24%)
  Gastrointestinal: Nausea (15% to 48%), vomiting (7% to 27%), diarrhea (7% to 23%), abdominal pain (7% to 23%), dyspepsia (7% to 23%), anorexia (>1% to 12%)
  Hematologic: Thrombocytopenia (1% to 24%; dose related)
  Neuromuscular & skeletal: Tremor (≤57%), weakness (6% to 27%)
  Ocular: Diplopia (>1% to 16%), amblyopia/blurred vision (≤12%)
  Miscellaneous: Infection (≤20%), flu-like syndrome (12%)
1% to 10%:
  Cardiovascular: Peripheral edema (>1% to 8%), chest pain (>1% to <5%), edema (>1% to <5%), facial edema (>1% to <5%), hypertension (>1% to <5%), hypotension (>1% to <5%), orthostatic hypotension (>1% to <5%), palpitation (>1% to <5%), tachycardia (>1% to <5%), vasodilation(>1% to <5%), arrhythmia
  Central nervous system: Ataxia (>1% to 8%), amnesia (>1% to 7%), emotional lability (>1% to 6%), fever (>1% to 6%), abnormal thinking (≤6%), depression (>1% to 5%), abnormal dreams (>1% to <5%), agitation (>1% to <5%), anxiety (>1% to <5%), catatonia (>1% to <5%), chills (>1% to <5%), confusion (>1% to <5%), coordination abnormal (>1% to <5%), hallucination (>1% to <5%), malaise (>1% to <5%), personality disorder (>1% to <5%),

speech disorder (>1% to <5%), tardive dyskinesia (>1% to <5%), vertigo (>1% to <5%), euphoria (1%), hypoesthesia (1%)

Dermatologic: Rash (>1% to 6%), bruising (>1% to 5%), discoid lupus erythematosus (>1% to <5%), dry skin (>1% to <5%), furunculosis (>1% to <5%), petechia (>1% to <5%), pruritus (>1% to <5), seborrhea (>1% to <5%)

Endocrine & metabolic: Amenorrhea (>1% to <5%), dysmenorrhea (>1% to <5%), metrorrhagia (>1% to <5%), hypoproteinemia

Gastrointestinal: Weight gain (4% to 9%), weight loss (6%), appetite increased (≤6%), constipation (>1% to 5%), xerostomia (>1% to 5%), eructation (>1% to <5%), fecal incontinence (>1% to <5%), flatulence (>1% to <5%), gastroenteritis (>1% to <5%), glossitis (>1% to <5%), hematemesis (>1% to <5%), pancreatitis (>1% to <5%), periodontal abscess (>1% to <5%), stomatitis (>1% to <5%), taste perversion (>1% to <5%), dysphagia, gum hemorrhage, mouth ulceration

Genitourinary: Cystitis (>1% to 5%), dysuria (>1% to 5%), urinary frequency (>1% to <5%), urinary incontinence (>1% to <5%), vaginal hemorrhage (>1% to 5%), vaginitis (>1% to <5%)

Hepatic: ALT increased (>1% to <5%), AST increased (>1% to <5%)

Local: Injection site pain (3%), injection site reaction (2%), injection site inflammation (1%)

Neuromuscular & skeletal: Back pain (≤8%), abnormal gait (>1% to <5%), arthralgia (>1% to <5%), arthrosis (>1% to <5%), dysarthria (>1% to <5%), hypertonia (>1% to <5%), hypokinesia (>1% to <5%), leg cramps (>1% to <5%), myalgia (>1% to <5%), myasthenia (>1% to <5%), neck pain (>1% to <5%), neck rigidity (>1% to <5%), paresthesia (>1% to <5%), reflex increased (>1% to <5%), twitching (>1% to <5%)

Ocular: Nystagmus (1% to 8%), dry eyes (>1% to 5%), eye pain (>1% to 5%), abnormal vision (>1% to <5%), conjunctivitis (>1% to <5%)

Otic: Tinnitus (1% to 7%), ear pain (>1% to 5%), deafness (>1% to <5%), otitis media (>1% to <5%)

Respiratory: Pharyngitis (2% to 8%), bronchitis (5%), rhinitis (>1% to 5%), dyspnea (1% to 5%), cough (>1% to <5%), epistaxis (>1% to <5%), pneumonia (>1% to <5%), sinusitis (>1% to <5%)

Miscellaneous: Diaphoresis (1%), hiccups

Drug Interactions

Metabolism/Transport Effects Substrate of CYP2A6 (minor), CYP2B6 (minor), CYP2C19 (minor), CYP2C9 (minor), CYP2E1 (minor); **Note:** Assignment of Major/Minor substrate status based on clinically relevant drug interaction potential; **Inhibits** CYP2C9 (weak); **Induces** CYP2A6 (weak/moderate)

Avoid Concomitant Use There are no known interactions where it is recommended to avoid concomitant use.

Increased Effect/Toxicity

Divalproex may increase the levels/effects of: Barbiturates; Ethosuximide; LamoTRIgine; LORazepam; Paliperidone; Primidone; RisperiDONE; Rufinamide; Temozolomide; Topiramate; Tricyclic Antidepressants; Vorinostat; Zidovudine

The levels/effects of Divalproex may be increased by: ChlorproMAZINE; Felbamate; GuanFACINE; Salicylates

Decreased Effect

Divalproex may decrease the levels/effects of: CarBAMazepine; Fosphenytoin; OXcarbazepine; Phenytoin

The levels/effects of Divalproex may be decreased by: Barbiturates; CarBAMazepine; Carbapenems; Ethosuximide; Fosphenytoin; Methylfolate; Phenytoin; Primidone; Protease Inhibitors; Rifampin

Ethanol/Nutrition/Herb Interactions

Ethanol: Avoid ethanol (may increase CNS depression).

Food: Food may delay but does not affect the extent of absorption. Valproic acid serum concentrations may be decreased if taken with food. Milk has no effect on absorption.

Herb/Nutraceutical: Avoid evening primrose (seizure threshold decreased).

Stability

Depakote® tablet: Store below 30°C (86°F).

Depakote® Sprinkles: Store below 25°C (77°F).

Depakote® ER: Store at controlled room temperature of 25°C (77°F).

Mechanism of Action Causes increased availability of gamma-aminobutyric acid (GABA), an inhibitory neurotransmitter, to brain neurons or may enhance the action of GABA or mimic its action at postsynaptic receptor sites

◀ **Pharmacodynamics/Kinetics**
Distribution: Total valproate: 11 L/1.73 m^2; Free valproate: 92 L/1.73 m^2
Protein binding (dose dependent): 80% to 90%; decreased in the elderly and with hepatic or renal dysfunction
Metabolism: Extensively hepatic via glucuronide conjugation and mitochondrial beta-oxidation. The relationship between dose and total valproate concentration is nonlinear; concentration does not increase proportionally with the dose, but increases to a lesser extent due to saturable plasma protein binding. The kinetics of unbound drug are linear.
Bioavailability: Depakote® ER: ~90% relative to I.V. dose and ~89% relative to delayed release formulation
Half-life elimination (increased with liver disease): Adults: 9-16 hours
Time to peak, serum: Depakote® tablet: ~4 hours; Depakote® ER: 4-17 hours
Excretion: Urine (30% to 50% as glucuronide conjugate, 3% as unchanged drug)

Dosage
Geriatric Initiate at lower doses; dose escalation should be managed more slowly (in persons of advanced age). Refer to adult dosing.

Adult Equivalent oral dosages of divalproex and valproic acid deliver the same quantities of valproate ion.

Seizures: Oral: Administer doses >250 mg/day in divided doses.
Simple and complex absence seizure: Initial: 15 mg/kg/day; increase by 5-10 mg/kg/day at weekly intervals until therapeutic levels are achieved; maximum: 60 mg/kg/day.
Complex partial seizure: Initial: 10-15 mg/kg/day; increase by 5-10 mg/kg/day at weekly intervals until therapeutic levels are achieved; maximum: 60 mg/kg/day.
Note: Regular release and delayed release formulations are usually given in 2-4 divided doses/day; extended release formulation (Depakote® ER) is usually given once daily. Conversion to Depakote® ER from a stable dose of Depakote® may require an increase in the total daily dose between 8% and 20% to maintain similar serum concentrations.

Mania: Oral:
Depakote® tablet: Initial: 750 mg/day in divided doses; dose should be adjusted as rapidly as possible to desired clinical effect; maximum recommended dosage: 60 mg/kg/day
Depakote® ER: Initial: 25 mg/kg/day given once daily; dose should be adjusted as rapidly as possible to desired clinical effect; maximum recommended dose: 60 mg/kg/day.

Migraine prophylaxis: Oral:
Depakote® tablet: 250 mg twice daily; adjust dose based on patient response, up to 1000 mg/day
Depakote® ER: 500 mg once daily for 7 days, then increase to 1000 mg once daily; adjust dose based on patient response; usual dosage range: 500-1000 mg/day

Diabetic neuropathy (unlabeled use): Oral: 500-1200 mg/day (Bril, 2011)

Renal Impairment A 27% reduction in clearance of unbound valproate is seen in patients with Cl$_{cr}$ <10 mL/minute. Hemodialysis reduces valproate concentrations by 20%, therefore, no dose adjustment is needed in patients with renal failure. Protein binding is reduced, monitoring only total valproate concentrations may be misleading.

Hepatic Impairment Dosage reduction is required. Clearance is decreased with liver impairment. Hepatic disease is also associated with decreased albumin concentrations and 2- to 2.6-fold increase in the unbound fraction. Free concentrations of valproate may be elevated while total concentrations appear normal. Use is contraindicated in severe impairment.

Administration
Depakote® ER: Swallow whole; do not crush or chew. Patients who need dose adjustments smaller than 500 mg/day for migraine prophylaxis should be changed to Depakote® delayed release tablets.
Depakote® Sprinkle capsules may be swallowed whole or open capsule and sprinkle on small amount (1 teaspoonful) of soft food and use immediately (do not store or chew).

Monitoring Parameters Liver enzymes (at baseline and during therapy), CBC with platelets (baseline and periodic intervals), PT/PTT (especially prior to surgery), serum ammonia (with symptoms of lethargy, mental status change), serum valproate levels (trough for therapeutic levels); suicidality (eg, suicidal thoughts, depression, behavioral changes)

Reference Range Note: In general, trough concentrations should be used to assess adequacy of therapy; peak concentrations may also be drawn if clinically necessary (eg, concentration-related toxicity). Within 2-4 days of initiation or dose adjustment, trough concentrations should be drawn just before the next dose (extended-release preparations) or before the morning dose (for immediate-release preparations). Patients with epilepsy should **not** delay taking their dose for >2-3 hours. Additional patient-specific factors must be taken into consideration when interpreting drug levels, including indication, age, clinical response, adherence, comorbidities, adverse effects, and concomitant medications (Patsalos, 2008; Reed, 2006).

Therapeutic:

Epilepsy: 50-100 mcg/mL (SI: 350-700 micromole/L); although seizure control may improve at levels >100 mcg/mL (SI: 700 micromole/L), toxicity may occur at levels of 100-150 mcg/mL (SI: 700-1040 micromole/L)

Mania: 50-125 mcg/mL (SI: 350-875 micromole/L)

Toxic: Some laboratories may report >200 mcg/mL (SI: >1390 micromole/L) as a toxic threshold, although clinical toxicity can occur at lower concentrations. Probability of thrombocytopenia increases with total valproate levels ≥110 mcg/mL in females or ≥135 mcg/mL in males.

Epilepsy: Although seizure control may improve at levels >100 mcg/mL (SI: 700 micromole/L), toxicity may occur at levels of 100-150 mcg/mL (SI: 700-1050 micromole/L)

Mania: Clinical response seen with trough levels between 50-125 mcg/mL (SI: 350-875 micromole/L); risk of toxicity increases at levels >125 mcg/mL (SI: 875 micromole/L)

Test Interactions False-positive result for urine ketones

Pharmacotherapy Pearls Divalproex sodium is a compound of sodium valproate and valproic acid; divalproex dissociates to valproate in the GI tract.

Extended release tablets have 10% to 20% less fluctuation in serum concentration than delayed release tablets. Extended release tablets are not bioequivalent to delayed release tablets.

Special Geriatric Considerations Although there is little data in elderly for the use of divalproex in the treatment of seizures, there are a number of studies which demonstrate its benefit in the treatment of agitation and dementia and other psychiatric disorders. It is important that the clinician understand that serum concentrations do not correlate with behavior response; likewise, it is imperative to monitor LFTs and CBC during the first 6 months of therapy. See Warnings/Precautions, Monitoring Parameters, and Pharmacotherapy Pearls.

Elimination is decreased in elderly. Studies of older adults with dementia show a high incidence of somnolence (which is usually transient); cognitive side effects generally minimal. In some patients, this was associated with weight loss. Starting doses should be lower and increased slowly, with careful monitoring of nutritional intake and dehydration. Safety and efficacy for use in patients >65 years of age have not been studied for migraine prophylaxis.

Dosage Forms Excipient information presented when available (limited, particularly for generics); consult specific product labeling.

Capsule, sprinkle, oral: 125 mg [strength expressed as valproic acid]

Depakote® Sprinkle: 125 mg [strength expressed as valproic acid]

Tablet, delayed release, oral: 125 mg [strength expressed as valproic acid], 250 mg [strength expressed as valproic acid], 500 mg [strength expressed as valproic acid]

Depakote®: 125 mg, 250 mg, 500 mg [strength expressed as valproic acid]

Tablet, extended release, oral: 250 mg [strength expressed as valproic acid], 500 mg [strength expressed as valproic acid]

Depakote® ER: 250 mg, 500 mg [strength expressed as valproic acid]

◆ **Divalproex Sodium** see Divalproex on page 577

◆ **Divigel®** see Estradiol (Systemic) on page 681

◆ **5071-1DL(6)** see Megestrol on page 1194

◆ **dl-Alpha Tocopherol** see Vitamin E on page 2027

DOBUTamine (doe BYOO ta meen)

Medication Safety Issues

Sound-alike/look-alike issues:

DOBUTamine may be confused with DOPamine

High alert medication:

The Institute for Safe Medication Practices (ISMP) includes this medication among its list of drugs which have a heightened risk of causing significant patient harm when used in error.

Brand Names: Canada Dobutamine Injection, USP; Dobutrex®

Index Terms Dobutamine Hydrochloride

Generic Availability (U.S.) Yes

Pharmacologic Category Adrenergic Agonist Agent

Use Short-term management of patients with cardiac decompensation

Unlabeled Use Positive inotropic agent for use in myocardial dysfunction related to sepsis; stress echocardiography

Contraindications Hypersensitivity to dobutamine or sulfites (some contain sodium meta-bisulfate), or any component of the formulation; idiopathic hypertrophic subaortic stenosis (IHSS)

Warnings/Precautions May increase heart rate. Patients with atrial fibrillation may experience an increase in ventricular response. An increase in blood pressure is more common, but occasionally a patient may become hypotensive. May exacerbate ventricular ectopy. If needed, correct hypovolemia first to optimize hemodynamics. Ineffective therapeutically in the presence of mechanical obstruction such as severe aortic stenosis. Use caution post-MI (can increase myocardial oxygen demand). Use cautiously in the elderly starting at lower end of the dosage range. Use with extreme caution in patients taking MAO inhibitors. Dobutamine in combination with stress echo may be used diagnostically. Product may contain sodium sulfite.

Adverse Reactions (Reflective of adult population; not specific for elderly) Incidence of adverse events is not always reported.

Cardiovascular: Increased heart rate, increased blood pressure, increased ventricular ectopic activity, hypotension, premature ventricular beats (5%, dose related), anginal pain (1% to 3%), nonspecific chest pain (1% to 3%), palpitation (1% to 3%)

Central nervous system: Fever (1% to 3%), headache (1% to 3%), paresthesia

Endocrine & metabolic: Slight decrease in serum potassium

Gastrointestinal: Nausea (1% to 3%)

Hematologic: Thrombocytopenia (isolated cases)

Local: Phlebitis, local inflammatory changes and pain from infiltration, cutaneous necrosis (isolated cases)

Neuromuscular & skeletal: Mild leg cramps

Respiratory: Dyspnea (1% to 3%)

Drug Interactions

Metabolism/Transport Effects Substrate of COMT

Avoid Concomitant Use

Avoid concomitant use of DOBUTamine with any of the following: Iobenguane I 123

Increased Effect/Toxicity

DOBUTamine may increase the levels/effects of: Sympathomimetics

The levels/effects of DOBUTamine may be increased by: AtoMOXetine; Cannabinoids; COMT Inhibitors; Linezolid

Decreased Effect

DOBUTamine may decrease the levels/effects of: Iobenguane I 123

The levels/effects of DOBUTamine may be decreased by: Calcium Salts

Stability Remix solution every 24 hours. Store reconstituted solution under refrigeration for 48 hours or 6 hours at room temperature. Pink discoloration of solution indicates slight oxidation but **no** significant loss of potency. Stability of parenteral admixture at room temperature (25°C): 48 hours; at refrigeration (4°C): 7 days.

Mechanism of Action Stimulates beta$_1$-adrenergic receptors, causing increased contractility and heart rate, with little effect on beta$_2$- or alpha-receptors

Pharmacodynamics/Kinetics

Onset of action: I.V.: 1-10 minutes

Peak effect: 10-20 minutes

Metabolism: In tissues and hepatically to inactive metabolites

Half-life elimination: 2 minutes

Excretion: Urine (as metabolites)

Dosage

Geriatric & Adult Cardiac decompensation: I.V. infusion: 2.5-20 mcg/kg/minute; maximum: 40 mcg/kg/minute, titrate to desired response; see table.

Infusion Rates of Various Dilutions of Dobutamine

Desired Delivery Rate (mcg/kg/min)	Infusion Rate (mL/kg/min)	
	500 mcg/mL	1000 mcg/mL
2.5	0.005	0.0025
5	0.01	0.005
7.5	0.015	0.0075
10	0.02	0.01
12.5	0.025	0.0125
15	0.03	0.015

Administration Use infusion device to control rate of flow; administer into large vein. Do not administer through same I.V. line as heparin, hydrocortisone sodium succinate, cefazolin, or penicillin.

Monitoring Parameters Blood pressure, ECG, heart rate, CVP, RAP, MAP; serum glucose, renal function; urine output; if pulmonary artery catheter is in place, monitor CI, PCWP, and SVR

Pharmacotherapy Pearls Dobutamine lowers central venous pressure and wedge pressure but has little effect on pulmonary vascular resistance.

Dobutamine therapy should be avoided in patients with stable heart failure due to an increase in mortality. In patients with intractable heart failure, dobutamine may be used as a short-term infusion to provide symptomatic benefit. It is not known whether short-term dobutamine therapy in end-stage heart failure has any outcome benefit.

Dobutamine infusion during echocardiography is used as a cardiovascular stress. Wall motion abnormalities developing with increasing doses of dobutamine may help to identify ischemic and/or hibernating myocardium.

Special Geriatric Considerations One study demonstrated beneficial hemodynamic effects in elderly patients; monitor closely.

Dosage Forms Excipient information presented when available (limited, particularly for generics); consult specific product labeling.

Infusion, premixed in D_5W, as hydrochloride: 1 mg/mL (250 mL); 2 mg/mL (250 mL); 4 mg/mL (250 mL)

Injection, solution, as hydrochloride: 12.5 mg/mL (20 mL, 40 mL)

◆ **Dobutamine Hydrochloride** *see DOBUTamine on page 581*
◆ **Doc-Q-Lace [OTC]** *see Docusate on page 583*
◆ **Doc-Q-Lax [OTC]** *see Docusate and Senna on page 585*

Docusate (DOK yoo sate)

Related Information

Laxatives, Classification and Properties *on page 2121*
Treatment Options for Constipation *on page 2142*

Medication Safety Issues

Sound-alike/look-alike issues:

Colace® may be confused with Calan®, Cozaar®

Dulcolax® (docusate) may be confused with Dulcolax® (bisacodyl)

International issues:

Docusate may be confused with Doxinate brand name for doxylamine and pyridoxine [India]

Brand Names: U.S. Colace® [OTC]; Correctol® [OTC]; Diocto [OTC]; Doc-Q-Lace [OTC]; Docu-Soft [OTC]; DocuSoft S™ [OTC]; Dok™ [OTC]; DSS® [OTC]; Dulcolax® Stool Softener [OTC]; Dulcolax® [OTC]; Enemeez® Plus [OTC]; Enemeez® [OTC]; Fleet® Pedia-Lax™ Liquid Stool Softener [OTC]; Fleet® Sof-Lax® [OTC]; Kao-Tin [OTC]; Kaopectate® Stool Softener [OTC]; Phillips'® Liquid-Gels® [OTC]; Phillips'® Stool Softener Laxative [OTC]; Silace [OTC]

Brand Names: Canada Apo-Docusate-Sodium®; Colace®; Colax-C®; Novo-Docusate Calcium; Novo-Docusate Sodium; PMS-Docusate Calcium; PMS-Docusate Sodium; Regulex®; Selax®; Soflax™

Index Terms Dioctyl Calcium Sulfosuccinate; Dioctyl Sodium Sulfosuccinate; Docusate Calcium; Docusate Potassium; Docusate Sodium; DOSS; DSS

Generic Availability (U.S.) Yes: Excludes enema

Pharmacologic Category Stool Softener

Use Stool softener in patients who should avoid straining during defecation and constipation associated with hard, dry stools; prophylaxis for straining (Valsalva) following myocardial infarction. A safe agent to be used in elderly; some evidence that doses <200 mg are ineffective; stool softeners are unnecessary if stool is well hydrated or "mushy" and soft; shown to be ineffective used long-term.

Unlabeled Use Ceruminolytic

Contraindications Hypersensitivity to docusate or any component of the formulation; concomitant use of mineral oil; intestinal obstruction, acute abdominal pain, nausea, or vomiting

Warnings/Precautions Prolonged, frequent, or excessive use may result in dependence or electrolyte imbalance

Adverse Reactions (Reflective of adult population; not specific for elderly) 1% to 10%:

Gastrointestinal: Intestinal obstruction, diarrhea, abdominal cramping

Miscellaneous: Throat irritation

Drug Interactions

Metabolism/Transport Effects None known.

Avoid Concomitant Use There are no known interactions where it is recommended to avoid concomitant use.

Increased Effect/Toxicity There are no known significant interactions involving an increase in effect.

Decreased Effect There are no known significant interactions involving a decrease in effect.

Mechanism of Action Reduces surface tension of the oil-water interface of the stool resulting in enhanced incorporation of water and fat allowing for stool softening

Pharmacodynamics/Kinetics

Onset of action: 12-72 hours

Excretion: Feces

Dosage

Geriatric & Adult Note: Docusate salts are interchangeable; the amount of sodium, calcium, or potassium per dosage unit is clinically insignificant.

Stool softener:

Oral: 50-500 mg/day in 1-4 divided doses

Rectal: Add 50-100 mg of docusate liquid to enema fluid (saline or water); give as retention or flushing enema

Administration Ensure adequate fluid intake. Docusate syrup should be administered with 6-8 ounces of milk or juice to mask the bitter taste.

Test Interactions Decreased potassium (S), decreased chloride (S)

Special Geriatric Considerations A safe agent to be used in the elderly. Some evidence that doses <200 mg are ineffective. Stool softeners are unnecessary if stool is well hydrated or "mushy" and soft; shown to be ineffective used long-term.

Dosage Forms Excipient information presented when available (limited, particularly for generics); consult specific product labeling. [DSC] = Discontinued product

Capsule, oral, as sodium:

Colace®: 50 mg [contains sodium 3 mg/capsule]

Colace®: 100 mg [contains sodium 5 mg/capsule]

Doc-Q-Lace: 100 mg

Capsule, liquid, oral, as sodium:

DocuSoft S™: 100 mg [contains sodium 5 mg/capsule]

Capsule, softgel, oral, as calcium: 240 mg

Kao-Tin: 240 mg

Kaopectate® Stool Softener: 240 mg

Capsule, softgel, oral, as sodium: 50 mg, 100 mg, 250 mg

Correctol®: 100 mg

Docu-Soft: 100 mg

Dok™: 100 mg, 250 mg

DSS®: 100 mg, 250 mg

Dulcolax®: 100 mg [contains sodium 5 mg/capsule]

Dulcolax® Stool Softener: 100 mg [contains sodium 5 mg/capsule]

Fleet® Sof-Lax®: 100 mg [contains sodium 5 mg/capsule]

Phillips'® Liquid-Gels®: 100 mg [contains sodium 5.2 mg/capsule]

Phillips'® Stool Softener Laxative: 100 mg [contains sodium 5.2 mg/capsule]

Liquid, oral, as sodium: 50 mg/5 mL (10 mL, 25 mL, 473 mL [DSC]); 150 mg/5 mL (480 mL)

Diocto: 50 mg/15 mL (473 mL) [contains sodium 15 mg/5 mL]

Diocto: 150 mg/15 mL (480 mL [DSC])

Diocto: 150 mg/15 mL (480 mL) [vanilla flavor]

Fleet® Pedia-Lax™ Liquid Stool Softener: 50 mg/15 mL (118 mL) [contains propylene glycol, sodium 13 mg/15 mL; fruit-punch flavor]

Silace: 150 mg/15 mL (473 mL) [lemon-vanilla flavor]

Solution, rectal, as sodium [enema]:

Enemeez®: 283 mg/5 mL (5 mL)

Enemeez® Plus: 283 mg/5 mL (5 mL) [contains benzocaine]

Syrup, oral, as sodium: 20 mg/5 mL (25 mL, 473 mL)

Colace®: 60 mg/15 mL (473 mL) [ethanol free, sugar free; contains propylene glycol, sodium 34 mg/15 mL]

Diocto: 60 mg/15 mL (480 mL) [mint flavor]

Diocto: 60 mg/15 mL (473 mL) [contains propylene glycol, sodium 14 mg/5 mL, sodium benzoate]

Doc-Q-Lace: 60 mg/15 mL (480 mL) [contains propylene glycol; peppermint flavor]

Silace: 60 mg/15 mL (480 mL) [peppermint flavor]

Tablet, oral, as sodium: 100 mg

Dok™: 100 mg [scored]

Docusate and Senna (DOK yoo sate & SEN na)

Related Information
Docusate *on page 583*
Laxatives, Classification and Properties *on page 2121*
Senna *on page 1764*
Treatment Options for Constipation *on page 2142*
Medication Safety Issues
Sound-alike/look-alike issues:
Senokot® may be confused with Depakote®
Brand Names: U.S. Doc-Q-Lax [OTC]; Dok™ Plus [OTC]; Geri-Stool [OTC]; Peri-Colace® [OTC]; Senexon-S [OTC]; Senna Plus [OTC]; SennaLax-S [OTC]; Senokot-S® [OTC]; SenoSol™-SS [OTC]
Index Terms Senna and Docusate; Senna-S
Generic Availability (U.S.) Yes
Pharmacologic Category Laxative, Stimulant; Stool Softener
Use Short-term treatment of constipation
Unlabeled Use Evacuation of the colon for bowel or rectal examinations; management/prevention of opiate-induced constipation
Contraindications Hypersensitivity to any component; intestinal obstruction; acute intestinal inflammation (eg, Crohn's disease); ulcerative colitis; appendicitis; abdominal pain of unknown origin; concurrent use of mineral oil
Warnings/Precautions Not recommended for over-the-counter (OTC) use in patients experiencing stomach pain, nausea, vomiting, or a sudden change in bowel movements which lasts >2 weeks. OTC labeling does not recommend for use longer than 1 week.
Adverse Reactions (Reflective of adult population; not specific for elderly) Frequency not defined.
Gastrointestinal: Nausea, vomiting, diarrhea, abdominal cramps
Genitourinary: Urine discoloration (red/brown)
Mechanism of Action Docusate is a stool softener; sennosides are laxatives
Dosage
Geriatric Constipation: OTC ranges: Oral: Consider half the initial dose in older, debilitated patients
Adult Constipation: OTC ranges: Oral: Initial: 2 tablets (17.2 mg sennosides plus 100 mg docusate) once daily (maximum: 4 tablets twice daily)
Administration Oral: Once-daily doses should be taken at bedtime.
Pharmacotherapy Pearls Individual product labeling should be consulted prior to dosing.
Special Geriatric Considerations The chronic use of stimulant cathartics is inappropriate and should be avoided. Although the elderly commonly complain of constipation, such complaints require evaluation; short-term use of stimulant cathartics is best. If prophylaxis is desired, then the use of bulk agents (eg, psyllium), stool softeners, and hyperosmotic agents (eg, sorbitol 70%) is preferred. Stool softeners are unnecessary if stools are well-hydrated (as in use of hyperosmotics), soft or "mushy". Patients should be instructed for proper dietary fiber and fluid intake, as well as regular exercise. Monitor closely for fluid/electrolyte imbalance, CNS signs of fluid/electrolyte loss, and hypotension.
Dosage Forms Excipient information presented when available (limited, particularly for generics); consult specific product labeling.
Tablet, oral: Docusate sodium 50 mg and sennosides 8.6 mg
Doc-Q-Lax: Docusate sodium 50 mg and sennosides 8.6 mg
Dok™ Plus: Docusate sodium 50 mg and sennosides 8.6 mg
Geri-Stool: Docusate sodium 50 mg and sennosides 8.6 mg
Peri-Colace®: Docusate sodium 50 mg and sennosides 8.6 mg
Senexon-S: Docusate sodium 50 mg and sennosides 8.6 mg
SennaLax-S: Docusate sodium 50 mg and sennosides 8.6 mg [contains sodium benzoate]
Senna Plus: Docusate sodium 50 mg and sennosides 8.6 mg
Senokot-S®: Docusate sodium 50 mg and sennosides 8.6 mg [sugar free; contains sodium 4 mg/tablet]
SenoSol™-SS: Docusate sodium 50 mg and sennosides 8.6 mg [contains sodium 3 mg/tablet]

◆ **Docusate Calcium** *see Docusate on page 583*
◆ **Docusate Potassium** *see Docusate on page 583*
◆ **Docusate Sodium** *see Docusate on page 583*
◆ **Docu-Soft [OTC]** *see Docusate on page 583*
◆ **DocuSoft S™ [OTC]** *see Docusate on page 583*

Dofetilide (doe FET il ide)

Related Information
  Beers Criteria – Potentially Inappropriate Medications for Geriatrics *on page* 2183
Medication Safety Issues
  Sound-alike/look-alike issues:
    Dofetilide may be confused with defibrotide
Brand Names: U.S. Tikosyn®
Brand Names: Canada Tikosyn®
Generic Availability (U.S.) No
Pharmacologic Category Antiarrhythmic Agent, Class III
Use Maintenance of normal sinus rhythm in patients with chronic atrial fibrillation/atrial flutter of longer than 1-week duration who have been converted to normal sinus rhythm; conversion of atrial fibrillation and atrial flutter to normal sinus rhythm
Unlabeled Use Alternative antiarrhythmic for the treatment of atrial fibrillation in patients with hypertrophic cardiomyopathy (HCM)
Prescribing and Access Restrictions As a requirement of the REMS program, access to this medication is restricted. Tikosyn® is only available to prescribers and hospitals that have confirmed their participation in a designated Tikosyn® Education Program. The program provides comprehensive education about the importance of in-hospital treatment initiation and individualized dosing.

T.I.P.S. is the Tikosyn® In Pharmacy System designated to allow retail pharmacies to stock and dispense Tikosyn® once they have been enrolled. A participating pharmacy must confirm receipt of the T.I.P.S. program materials and educate its pharmacy staff about the procedures required to fill an outpatient prescription for Tikosyn®. The T.I.P.S. enrollment form is available at www.tikosyn.com. Tikosyn® is only available from a special mail order pharmacy, and enrolled retail pharmacies. Pharmacists must verify that the hospital/prescriber is a confirmed participant before Tikosyn® is provided. For participant verification, the pharmacist may call 1-800-788-7353 or use the web site located at www.tikosynlist.com. Further details and directions on the program are provided at www.tikosyn.com.

Dofetilide therapy must be initiated/adjusted in a hospital setting with proper monitoring under the guidance of experienced personnel.
Medication Guide Available Yes
Contraindications Hypersensitivity to dofetilide or any component of the formulation; patients with congenital or acquired long QT syndromes, do not use if baseline QT interval or QT_c is >440 msec (500 msec in patients with ventricular conduction abnormalities); severe renal impairment (Cl_{cr} <20 mL/minute [Cockcroft-Gault method]); concurrent use with verapamil, cimetidine, hydrochlorothiazide (alone or in combinations), trimethoprim (alone or in combination with sulfamethoxazole), itraconazole (according to itraconazole prescribing information) ketoconazole, prochlorperazine, or megestrol
Warnings/Precautions [U.S. Boxed Warning]: Must be initiated (or reinitiated) in a setting with continuous monitoring and staff familiar with the recognition and treatment of life-threatening arrhythmias. Patients must be monitored with continuous ECG for a minimum of 3 days, or for a minimum of 12 hours after electrical or pharmacological cardioversion to normal sinus rhythm, whichever is greater. Patients should be readmitted for continuous monitoring if dosage is later increased.

Reserve for patients who are highly symptomatic with atrial fibrillation/atrial flutter; risk of torsade de pointes (TdP) significantly increases with doses >500 mcg twice daily; hold Class I or Class III antiarrhythmics for at least three half-lives prior to starting dofetilide; use in patients previously on amiodarone therapy only if serum amiodarone level is <0.3 mg/L or if amiodarone was discontinued ≥3 months ago; correct hypokalemia or hypomagnesemia before initiating dofetilide and maintain within normal limits during treatment. The risk of TdP may be higher in certain patient subgroups (eg, patients with heart failure). Most episodes of TdP occur within the first 3 days of therapy. Risk of hypokalemia and/or hypomagnesemia may be increased by potassium-depleting diuretics, increasing the risk of TdP. Concurrent use with other drugs known to prolong QT_c interval is not recommended.

In the treatment of atrial fibrillation in the elderly, avoid antiarrhythmics as first-line treatment. In older adults, data suggests rate control may provide more benefits than risks compared to rhythm control for most patients (Beers Criteria).

Patients with sick sinus syndrome or with second or third-degree heart block should not receive dofetilide unless a functional pacemaker is in place. Defibrillation threshold is reduced in patients with ventricular tachycardia or ventricular fibrillation undergoing implantation of a cardioverter-defibrillator device. Use with caution in renal impairment; **dose adjustment**

required for patients with Cl_{cr} ≤60 mL/minute. Use with caution in patients with severe hepatic impairment; not studied.

Adverse Reactions (Reflective of adult population; not specific for elderly)

Supraventricular arrhythmia patients:

>10%: Central nervous system: Headache (11%)

2% to 10%:

Central nervous system: Dizziness (8%), insomnia (4%)

Cardiovascular: Ventricular tachycardia (2.6% to 3.7%), chest pain (10%), torsade de pointes (3.3% in HF patients and 0.9% in patients with a recent MI; up to 10.5% in patients receiving doses in excess of those recommended). Torsade de pointes occurs most frequently within the first 3 days of therapy.

Dermatologic: Rash (3%)

Gastrointestinal: Nausea (5%), diarrhea (3%), abdominal pain (3%)

Neuromuscular & skeletal: Back pain (3%)

Respiratory: Respiratory tract infection (7%), dyspnea (6%)

Miscellaneous: Flu-like syndrome (4%)

<2%:

Central nervous system: CVA, facial paralysis, flaccid paralysis, migraine, paralysis

Cardiovascular: AV block (0.4% to 1.5%), bundle branch block (0.1% to 0.5%), heart block (0.1% to 0.5%), ventricular fibrillation (0% to 0.4%), bradycardia, cardiac arrest, edema, MI, sudden death, syncope

Dermatologic: Angioedema

Gastrointestinal: Liver damage

Neuromuscular & skeletal: Paresthesia

Respiratory: Cough

Drug Interactions

Metabolism/Transport Effects Substrate of CYP3A4 (minor); **Note:** Assignment of Major/Minor substrate status based on clinically relevant drug interaction potential

Avoid Concomitant Use

Avoid concomitant use of Dofetilide with any of the following: Antifungal Agents (Azole Derivatives, Systemic); Cimetidine; Fingolimod; Highest Risk QTc-Prolonging Agents; Megestrol; Mifepristone; Moderate Risk QTc-Prolonging Agents; Prochlorperazine; Propafenone; Saquinavir; Thiazide Diuretics; Trimethoprim; Verapamil

Increased Effect/Toxicity

Dofetilide may increase the levels/effects of: Highest Risk QTc-Prolonging Agents; Lidocaine (Topical)

The levels/effects of Dofetilide may be increased by: AMILoride; Antifungal Agents (Azole Derivatives, Systemic); Cimetidine; EriBULin; Fingolimod; Lidocaine (Topical); Loop Diuretics; Megestrol; MetFORMIN; Mifepristone; Moderate Risk QTc-Prolonging Agents; Prochlorperazine; Propafenone; QTc-Prolonging Agents (Indeterminate Risk and Risk Modifying); Saquinavir; Thiazide Diuretics; Triamterene; Trimethoprim; Verapamil

Decreased Effect

The levels/effects of Dofetilide may be decreased by: Tocilizumab

Ethanol/Nutrition/Herb Interactions Herb/Nutraceutical: St John's wort may decrease dofetilide levels. Avoid ephedra (may worsen arrhythmia).

Mechanism of Action Vaughan Williams Class III antiarrhythmic activity. Blockade of the cardiac ion channel carrying the rapid component of the delayed rectifier potassium current. Dofetilide has no effect on sodium channels, adrenergic alpha-receptors, or adrenergic beta-receptors. It increases the monophasic action potential duration due to delayed repolarization. The increase in the QT interval is a function of prolongation of both effective and functional refractory periods in the His-Purkinje system and the ventricles. Changes in cardiac conduction velocity and sinus node function have not been observed in patients with or without structural heart disease. PR and QRS width remain the same in patients with pre-existing heart block and or sick sinus syndrome.

Pharmacodynamics/Kinetics

Absorption: Well absorbed

Distribution: V_d: 3 L/kg

Protein binding: 60% to 70%

Metabolism: Hepatic via CYP3A4, but low affinity for it; metabolites formed by N-dealkylation and N-oxidation

Bioavailability: >90%

Half-life elimination: ~10 hours; prolonged with renal impairment

Time to peak, serum: Fasting: 2-3 hours

Excretion: Urine (80%; 80% as unchanged drug, 20% as inactive or minimally active metabolites); renal elimination consists of glomerular filtration and active tubular secretion via cationic transport system

◄ **Dosage**

Geriatric Refer to adult dosing. No specific dosage adjustments are recommended based on age; however, careful assessment of renal function is particularly important in this population.

Adult Note: QT or QT_c must be determined prior to first dose. If QT_c >440 msec (>500 msec in patients with ventricular conduction abnormalities), dofetilide is contraindicated.

Antiarrhythmic: Oral:

Initial: 500 mcg twice daily. Initial dosage must be adjusted in patients with estimated Cl_{cr} <60 mL/minute (see Dosage: Renal Impairment). Dofetilide may be initiated at lower doses than recommended based on physician discretion.

Modification of dosage in response to **initial** *dose:* QT_c interval should be measured 2-3 hours after the initial dose. If the QT_c is >15% of baseline, or if the QT_c is >500 msec (550 msec in patients with ventricular conduction abnormalities), dofetilide should be reduced. If the starting dose was 500 mcg twice daily, then reduce to 250 mcg twice daily. If the starting dose was 250 mcg twice daily, then reduce to 125 mcg twice daily. If the starting dose was 125 mcg twice daily, then reduce to 125 mcg once daily. If at any time after the second dose is given the QT_c is >500 msec (550 msec in patients with ventricular conduction abnormalities), dofetilide should be discontinued.

Renal Impairment Note: Using the Modification of Diet in Renal Disease (MDRD) equation and subsequent eGFR to determine dose may lead to overestimation of creatinine clearance and overdose of medication; use only the Cockcroft-Gault equation to estimate creatinine clearance (Denetclaw, 2011). Use actual body weight when using the Cockcroft-Gault equation to calculate creatinine clearance.

Cl_{cr} >60 mL/minute: Administer 500 mcg twice daily.

Cl_{cr} 40-60 mL/minute: Administer 250 mcg twice daily.

Cl_{cr} 20-39 mL/minute: Administer 125 mcg twice daily.

Cl_{cr} <20 mL/minute: Contraindicated.

Hepatic Impairment No dosage adjustments required in Child-Pugh class A and B; patients with severe hepatic impairment were not studied.

Monitoring Parameters ECG monitoring with attention to QT (if heart rate <60 beats per minute) or QT_c and occurrence of ventricular arrhythmias, baseline serum creatinine and changes in serum creatinine. Upon initiation (or reinitiation) continuous ECG monitoring recommended for a minimum of 3 days, or for at least 12 hours after electrical or pharmacological conversion to normal sinus rhythm, whichever is greater. Check serum potassium and magnesium levels at baseline and throughout therapy especially if on medications where these electrolyte disturbances can occur, or if patient has a history of hypokalemia or hypomagnesemia. QT or QT_c must be monitored at baseline prior to the first dose and 2-3 hours afterwards. If at baseline, QT_c >440 msec (>500 msec in patients with ventricular conduction abnormalities), dofetilide is contraindicated. If dofetilide initiated, QT_c interval must be determined 2-3 hours after each subsequent dose of dofetilide for in-hospital doses 2-5. Thereafter, QT or QT_c and creatinine clearance should be evaluated every 3 months. If at any time during therapy after the second dose the measured QT_c is >500 msec (550 msec in patients with ventricular conduction abnormalities), dofetilide should be discontinued.

Special Geriatric Considerations No specific dosage adjustments are recommended based on age; however, evaluation for use of this drug in the elderly is imperative. A complete review of medications, to assure there is no inadvertent use of contraindicated medications and those with potential drug interactions, can be re-evaluated for continued need. Laboratory values must be assessed prior to initiating medication; careful assessment of renal function is particularly important in the elderly population. Since the elderly often have creatinine clearances <60 mL/minute, the dose of dofetilide must be carefully adjusted to renal function. Calculating a creatinine clearance prior to dosing is recommended.

This medication is considered to be potentially inappropriate in this patient population (Beers Criteria: Quality of evidence - high; Strength of recommendation - strong).

Dosage Forms Excipient information presented when available (limited, particularly for generics); consult specific product labeling.

Capsule, oral:

Tikosyn®: 125 mcg, 250 mcg, 500 mcg

◆ **Dofus [OTC]** see *Lactobacillus on page 1084*

◆ **Dok™ [OTC]** see Docusate *on page 583*

◆ **Dok™ Plus [OTC]** see Docusate and Senna *on page 585*

Dolasetron (dol A se tron)

Medication Safety Issues
Sound-alike/look-alike issues:
Anzemet® may be confused with Aldomet, Antivert®, Avandamet®
Dolasetron may be confused with granisetron, ondansetron, palonosetron

Brand Names: U.S. Anzemet®

Brand Names: Canada Anzemet®

Index Terms Dolasetron Mesylate; MDL 73,147EF

Generic Availability (U.S.) No

Pharmacologic Category Antiemetic; Selective 5-HT$_3$ Receptor Antagonist

Use
U.S. labeling:
Injection: Prevention and treatment of postoperative nausea and vomiting
Oral: Prevention of nausea and vomiting associated with emetogenic cancer chemotherapy (initial and repeat courses); prevention of postoperative nausea and vomiting

Canadian labeling: Oral: Prevention of nausea and vomiting associated with emetogenic cancer chemotherapy (initial and repeat courses)

Contraindications
U.S. labeling:
Injection: Hypersensitivity to dolasetron or any component of the formulation; use for the prevention of chemotherapy induced nausea and vomiting
Tablet: Hypersensitivity to dolasetron or any component of the formulation

Canadian labeling: Injection, tablet: Hypersensitivity to dolasetron or any component of the formulation; use for the prevention or treatment of postoperative nausea and vomiting

Warnings/Precautions Dolasetron is associated with a number of dose-dependent increases in ECG intervals (eg, PR, QRS duration, QT/QT$_c$, JT), usually occurring 1-2 hours after I.V. administration and usually lasting 6-8 hours; however, may last ≥24 hours and rarely lead to heart block or arrhythmia. Clinically relevant QT-interval prolongation may occur resulting in torsade de pointes, when used in conjunction with other agents that prolong the QT interval (eg, Class I and III antiarrhythmics). Avoid use in patients at greater risk for QT prolongation (eg, patients with congenital long QT syndrome, medications known to prolong QT interval, electrolyte abnormalities, and cumulative high-dose anthracycline therapy) and/or ventricular arrhythmia. Correct potassium or magnesium abnormalities prior to initiating therapy. I.V. formulations of 5-HT$_3$ antagonists have more association with ECG interval changes, compared to oral formulations. Reduction in heart rate may also occur with the 5-HT$_3$ antagonists.

Use with caution in patients allergic to other 5-HT$_3$ receptor antagonists; cross-reactivity has been reported with other 5-HT$_3$ receptor antagonists. **For chemotherapy-associated nausea and vomiting, should be used on a scheduled basis, not on an "as needed" (PRN) basis,** since data support the use of this drug only in the prevention of nausea and vomiting (due to antineoplastic therapy) and not in the rescue of nausea and vomiting. Not intended for treatment of nausea and vomiting or for chronic continuous therapy.

Adverse Reactions (Reflective of adult population; not specific for elderly) Adverse events may vary according to indication
>10%:
Central nervous system: Headache (7% to 24%)
Gastrointestinal: Diarrhea (2% to 12%)
1% to 10%:
Cardiovascular: Bradycardia (4% to 5%), hypertension (≤3%), tachycardia (2% to 3%)
Central nervous system: Dizziness (1% to 6%), fatigue (3% to 6%), fever (4%), pain (≤2%), chills/shivering (1% to 2%)
Gastrointestinal: Dyspepsia (≤3%), abdominal pain (≤3%)
Hepatic: Abnormal hepatic function (4%)
Renal: Oliguria (3%)

Drug Interactions
Metabolism/Transport Effects Substrate of CYP2C9 (minor), CYP3A4 (minor); **Note:** Assignment of Major/Minor substrate status based on clinically relevant drug interaction potential; **Inhibits** CYP2D6 (weak)

Avoid Concomitant Use
Avoid concomitant use of Dolasetron with any of the following: Apomorphine; Highest Risk QTc-Prolonging Agents; Mifepristone

Increased Effect/Toxicity
Dolasetron may increase the levels/effects of: Apomorphine; ARIPiprazole; Highest Risk QTc-Prolonging Agents; Moderate Risk QTc-Prolonging Agents

The levels/effects of Dolasetron may be increased by: Mifepristone; QTc-Prolonging Agents (Indeterminate Risk and Risk Modifying)

Decreased Effect
Dolasetron may decrease the levels/effects of: Tapentadol; TraMADol

The levels/effects of Dolasetron may be decreased by: Tocilizumab

Ethanol/Nutrition/Herb Interactions Food: Food does not affect the bioavailability of oral doses.

Stability Store intact vials and tablets at room temperature of 20°C to 25°C (68°F to 77°F). Protect from light. Dilute in 50 mL of a compatible solution (ie, 0.9% NS, D_5W, $D_5^{1/2}NS$, D_5LR, LR, and 10% mannitol injection). Solutions diluted for infusion are stable under normal lighting conditions at room temperature for 24 hours or under refrigeration for 48 hours.

Mechanism of Action Selective serotonin receptor ($5\text{-}HT_3$) antagonist, blocking serotonin both peripherally (primary site of action) and centrally at the chemoreceptor trigger zone

Pharmacodynamics/Kinetics
Absorption: Oral: Rapid and complete

Distribution: Hydrodolasetron: 5.8 L/kg

Protein binding: Hydrodolasetron: 69% to 77% (50% bound to $alpha_1$-acid glycoprotein)

Metabolism: Hepatic; rapid reduction by carbonyl reductase to hydrodolasetron (active metabolite); further metabolized by CYP2D6, CYP3A, and flavin monooxygenase

Bioavailability: Oral: ~75% (not affected by food)

Half-life elimination: Dolasetron: ≤10 minutes; hydrodolasetron: 6-8 hours; Severe renal impairment: 11 hours; Severe hepatic impairment: 11 hours

Time to peak, plasma: Hydrodolasetron: I.V.: 0.6 hours; Oral: ~1 hour

Excretion: Urine ~67% (53% to 61% of the total dose as active metabolite hydrodolasetron); feces ~33%

Dosage
Geriatric & Adult Note: Use of dolasetron injection is contraindicated for the prevention of chemotherapy induced nausea and vomiting. In Canada, use of dolasetron is also contra-indicated in the prevention and treatment of postoperative nausea and vomiting in adults.

Prevention of chemotherapy-associated nausea and vomiting (including initial and repeat courses): Oral: 100 mg within 1 hour before chemotherapy

Postoperative nausea and vomiting: *U.S. labeling:*
Prevention:
Oral: 100 mg within 2 hours before surgery
I.V.: 12.5 mg ~15 minutes before cessation of anesthesia
Treatment: I.V.: 12.5 mg as soon as nausea or vomiting present

Renal Impairment No dosage adjustment necessary.

Hepatic Impairment No dosage adjustment necessary.

Administration
I.V. injection may be given either undiluted IVP over 30 seconds or diluted in 50 mL of compatible fluid and infused over 15 minutes. Flush line before and after dolasetron administration.

Oral: When unable to administer in tablet form, dolasetron injection may be diluted in apple or apple-grape juice and taken orally; this dilution is stable for 2 hours at room temperature.

Monitoring Parameters ECG (in patients with cardiovascular disease, elderly, renally impaired, those at risk of developing hypokalemia and/or hypomagnesemia); potassium, magnesium

Pharmacotherapy Pearls Efficacy of dolasetron, for chemotherapy treatment, is enhanced with concomitant administration of dexamethasone 20 mg (increases complete response by 10% to 20%). Oral administration of the intravenous solution is equivalent to tablets.

Special Geriatric Considerations In controlled trials, no difference in overall safety and efficacy were observed between elderly and younger adults. Pharmacokinetics are similar in younger adults and elderly. No dosage adjustment necessary.

Dosage Forms Excipient information presented when available (limited, particularly for generics); consult specific product labeling.
Injection, solution, as mesylate:
Anzemet®: 20 mg/mL (0.625 mL, 5 mL, 25 mL) [contains mannitol]
Tablet, oral, as mesylate:
Anzemet®: 50 mg, 100 mg

Extemporaneously Prepared Dolasetron injection may be diluted in apple or apple-grape juice and taken orally; this dilution is stable for 2 hours at room temperature.

◆ **Dolasetron Mesylate** *see* Dolasetron *on page 589*

♦ **Dolobid** *see* Diflunisal *on page 539*
♦ **Dolophine®** *see* Methadone *on page 1225*
♦ **Domeboro® [OTC]** *see* Aluminum Sulfate and Calcium Acetate *on page 84*

Donepezil (doh NEP e zil)

Medication Safety Issues
Sound-alike/look-alike issues:
Aricept® may be confused with AcipHex®, Ascriptin®, and Azilect®
Brand Names: U.S. Aricept®; Aricept® ODT
Brand Names: Canada Aricept®; Aricept® RDT
Index Terms E2020
Generic Availability (U.S.) Yes
Pharmacologic Category Acetylcholinesterase Inhibitor (Central)
Use Treatment of mild, moderate, or severe dementia of the Alzheimer's type
Unlabeled Use Attention-deficit/hyperactivity disorder (ADHD); behavioral syndromes in dementia; mild-to-moderate dementia associated with Parkinson's disease; Lewy body dementia
Contraindications Hypersensitivity to donepezil, piperidine derivatives, or any component of the formulation
Warnings/Precautions Cholinesterase inhibitors may have vagotonic effects which may cause bradycardia and/or heart block with or without a history of cardiac disease; syncopal episodes have been associated with donepezil. Alzheimer's treatment guidelines consider bradycardia to be a relative contraindication for use of centrally-active cholinesterase inhibitors. Use with caution with sick sinus syndrome or other supraventricular cardiac conduction abnormalities, COPD, or asthma. Use with caution in patients with a history of seizure disorder; cholinomimetics may potentially cause generalized seizures, although seizure activity may also result from Alzheimer's disease. Use with caution in patients at risk of ulcer disease (eg, previous history or NSAID use), or in patients with bladder outlet obstruction. May cause dose-related diarrhea, nausea, and/or vomiting, which usually resolves in 1-3 weeks. May cause anorexia and/or weight loss (dose-related). May exaggerate neuromuscular blockade effects of depolarizing neuromuscular-blocking agents (eg, succinylcholine).

Adverse Reactions (Reflective of adult population; not specific for elderly)
>10%:
Central nervous system: Insomnia (2% to 14%)
Gastrointestinal: Nausea (3% to 19%; dose related), diarrhea (5% to 15%; dose related)
Miscellaneous: Accident (7% to 13%), infection (11%)
1% to 10%:
Cardiovascular: Hypertension (3%), chest pain (2%), hemorrhage (2%), syncope (2%), hypotension, atrial fibrillation, bradycardia, ECG abnormal, edema, heart failure, hot flashes, peripheral edema, vasodilation
Central nervous system: Headache (3% to 10%), pain (3% to 9%), fatigue (1% to 8%), dizziness (2% to 8%), abnormal dreams (3%), hostility (3%), nervousness (1% to 3%), hallucinations (3%), depression (2% to 3%), confusion (2%), emotional lability (2%), personality disorder (2%), fever (2%), somnolence (2%), abnormal crying, aggression, agitation, anxiety, aphasia, delusions, irritability, restlessness, seizure, vertigo
Dermatologic: Bruising (4% to 5%), eczema (3%), pruritus, rash, skin ulcer, urticaria
Endocrine & metabolic: Dehydration (1% to 2%), hyperlipemia (2%), libido increased
Gastrointestinal: Anorexia (2% to 8%), vomiting (3% to 9%; dose related), weight loss (3% to 5%; dose related), abdominal pain, bloating, constipation, dyspepsia, epigastric pain, fecal incontinence, gastroenteritis, GI bleeding, toothache
Genitourinary: Urinary frequency (2%), urinary incontinence (1% to 3%), cystitis, hematuria, glycosuria, nocturia, UTI
Hematologic: Contusion (≤2%), anemia
Hepatic: Alkaline phosphatase increased
Neuromuscular & skeletal: Muscle cramps (3% to 8%), back pain (3%), CPK increased (3%), arthritis (1% to 2%), ataxia, bone fracture, gait abnormal, lactate dehydrogenase increased, paresthesia, tremor, weakness (1% to 2%)
Ocular: Blurred vision, cataract, eye irritation
Respiratory: Bronchitis, cough increased, dyspnea, pharyngitis, pneumonia, sore throat
Miscellaneous: Diaphoresis, fungal infection, flu symptoms, wandering
Drug Interactions
Metabolism/Transport Effects Substrate of CYP2D6 (minor), CYP3A4 (minor); **Note:** Assignment of Major/Minor substrate status based on clinically relevant drug interaction potential

Avoid Concomitant Use There are no known interactions where it is recommended to avoid concomitant use.

Increased Effect/Toxicity

Donepezil may increase the levels/effects of: Antipsychotics; Beta-Blockers; Cholinergic Agonists; Succinylcholine

The levels/effects of Donepezil may be increased by: Corticosteroids (Systemic)

Decreased Effect

Donepezil may decrease the levels/effects of: Anticholinergics; Neuromuscular-Blocking Agents (Nondepolarizing)

The levels/effects of Donepezil may be decreased by: Anticholinergics; Dipyridamole; Peginterferon Alfa-2b; Tocilizumab

Ethanol/Nutrition/Herb Interactions Herb/Nutraceutical: St John's wort may decrease donepezil levels. Ginkgo biloba may increase adverse effects/toxicity of acetylcholinesterase inhibitors.

Stability Store at 15°C to 30°C (59°F to 86°F).

Mechanism of Action Alzheimer's disease is characterized by cholinergic deficiency in the cortex and basal forebrain, which contributes to cognitive deficits. Donepezil reversibly and noncompetitively inhibits centrally-active acetylcholinesterase, the enzyme responsible for hydrolysis of acetylcholine. This appears to result in increased concentrations of acetylcholine available for synaptic transmission in the central nervous system.

Pharmacodynamics/Kinetics Geriatrics: No formal pharmacokinetic studies have been done in older adults; mean donepezil plasma concentrations were no different in older Alzheimer patients as compared to younger adults.

Absorption: Well absorbed

Distribution: V_{dss}: 12-16 L/kg

Protein binding: 96%, primarily to albumin (75%) and α_1-acid glycoprotein (21%)

Metabolism: Extensively to four major metabolites (two are active) via CYP2D6 and 3A4; undergoes glucuronidation

Bioavailability: 100%

Half-life elimination: 70 hours; time to steady-state: 15 days

Time to peak, plasma: Tablet, 10 mg: 3 hours; Tablet, 23 mg: ~8 hours; **Note:** Peak plasma concentrations almost twofold higher for the 23 mg tablet compared to the 10 mg tablet

Excretion: Urine 57% (17% as unchanged drug); feces 15%

Dosage

Geriatric Refer to adult dosing. **Note:** The Canadian labeling recommends a maximum dose of 5 mg once daily in elderly women of low body weight.

Adult Alzheimer's dementia: Oral:

Mild-to-moderate: Initial: 5 mg once daily; may increase to 10 mg once daily after 4-6 weeks; effective dosage range in clinical studies: 5-10 mg/day

Moderate-to-severe: Initial: 5 mg once daily; may increase to 10 mg once daily after 4-6 weeks; may increase further to 23 mg once daily after ≥3 months; effective dosage range in clinical studies: 10-23 mg/day

Administration Administer at bedtime without regard to food.

Aricept® 5 mg or 10 mg tablet: Swallow whole with water; do not split or crush per manufacturer's labeling. However, data available from the manufacturer showed that bioavailability was not affected by disintegration or dissolution when administered as a solution compared to a tablet during a bioequivalence study (data on file, Eisai Inc).

Aricept® 23 mg tablet: Swallow whole with water; do **NOT** crush or chew due to an increased rate of absorption. The 23 mg strength is provided in a unique film-coated formulation different from the 5 mg or 10 mg tablet strengths, which results in an altered pharmacokinetic profile.

Aricept® ODT: Allow tablet to dissolve completely on tongue and follow with water.

Monitoring Parameters Behavior, mood, bowel function, cognitive function, general function (eg, activities of daily living)

Special Geriatric Considerations The majority of patients enrolled in clinical studies to determine safety and efficacy were elderly (mean age: 73 years) since Alzheimer's disease primarily affects patients >55 years.

Dosage Forms Excipient information presented when available (limited, particularly for generics); consult specific product labeling.

Tablet, oral, as hydrochloride: 5 mg, 10 mg

Aricept®: 5 mg, 10 mg, 23 mg

Tablet, orally disintegrating, oral, as hydrochloride: 5 mg, 10 mg

Aricept® ODT: 5 mg, 10 mg

◆ **Donnatal®** see Hyoscyamine, Atropine, Scopolamine, and Phenobarbital *on page 963*

◆ **Donnatal Extentabs®** *see* Hyoscyamine, Atropine, Scopolamine, and Phenobarbital *on page 963*

DOPamine (DOE pa meen)

Related Information
Parkinson's Disease Management *on page 2140*

Medication Safety Issues
Sound-alike/look-alike issues:
DOPamine may be confused with DOBUTamine, Dopram®
High alert medication:
The Institute for Safe Medication Practices (ISMP) includes this medication among its list of drugs which have a heightened risk of causing significant patient harm when used in error.

Index Terms Dopamine Hydrochloride; Intropin

Generic Availability (U.S.) Yes

Pharmacologic Category Adrenergic Agonist Agent

Use Adjunct in the treatment of shock (eg, MI, open heart surgery, renal failure, cardiac decompensation) which persists after adequate fluid volume replacement

Unlabeled Use Symptomatic bradycardia or heart block unresponsive to atropine or pacing

Contraindications Hypersensitivity to sulfites (commercial preparation contains sodium bisulfite); pheochromocytoma; ventricular fibrillation

Warnings/Precautions Use with caution in patients with cardiovascular disease or cardiac arrhythmias or patients with occlusive vascular disease. Correct hypovolemia and electrolytes when used in hemodynamic support. May cause increases in HR and arrhythmia. Use with caution in post-MI patients. Use has been associated with a higher incidence of adverse events (eg, tachyarrhythmias) in patients with shock compared to norepinephrine. Higher 28-day mortality was also seen in patients with septic shock; the use of norepinephrine in patients with shock may be preferred. Use with extreme caution in patients taking MAO inhibitors. Avoid extravasation; infuse into a large vein if possible. Avoid infusion into leg veins. Watch I.V. site closely. **[U.S. Boxed Warning]: If extravasation occurs, infiltrate the area with diluted phentolamine (5-10 mg in 10-15 mL of saline) with a fine hypodermic needle. Phentolamine should be administered as soon as possible after extravasation is noted.** Product may contain sodium metabisulfite.

Adverse Reactions (Reflective of adult population; not specific for elderly) Frequency not defined.
Cardiovascular: Anginal pain, ectopic beats, hypotension, palpitation, tachycardia, vasoconstriction
Central nervous system: Headache
Gastrointestinal: Nausea and vomiting
Respiratory: Dyspnea

Drug Interactions
Metabolism/Transport Effects Substrate of COMT
Avoid Concomitant Use
Avoid concomitant use of DOPamine with any of the following: Hyaluronidase; Inhalational Anesthetics; Iobenguane I 123; Lurasidone
Increased Effect/Toxicity
DOPamine may increase the levels/effects of: Lurasidone; Sympathomimetics

The levels/effects of DOPamine may be increased by: AtoMOXetine; Cannabinoids; COMT Inhibitors; Hyaluronidase; Inhalational Anesthetics; Linezolid
Decreased Effect
DOPamine may decrease the levels/effects of: Iobenguane I 123

Stability Protect from light; solutions that are darker than slightly yellow should not be used.

Mechanism of Action Stimulates both adrenergic and dopaminergic receptors, lower doses are mainly dopaminergic stimulating and produce renal and mesenteric vasodilation, higher doses also are both dopaminergic and beta$_1$-adrenergic stimulating and produce cardiac stimulation and renal vasodilation; large doses stimulate alpha-adrenergic receptors

Pharmacodynamics/Kinetics
Onset of action: Adults: 5 minutes
Duration: Adults: <10 minutes
Metabolism: Renal, hepatic, plasma; 75% to inactive metabolites by monoamine oxidase and 25% to norepinephrine
Half-life elimination: 2 minutes
Excretion: Urine (as metabolites)

◀ **Dosage**

Geriatric & Adult

Hemodynamic support: I.V. infusion (administration requires the use of an infusion pump): 1-5 mcg/kg/minute up to 20 mcg/kg/minute; titrate to desired response (maximum: 50 mcg/kg/minute; however, doses >20 mcg/kg/minute may not have a beneficial effect on blood pressure and increase the risk of tachyarrhythmias); infusion may be increased by 1-4 mcg/kg/minute at 10- to 30-minute intervals until optimal response is obtained

Note: If dosages >20-30 mcg/kg/minute are needed, a more direct-acting vasopressor may be more beneficial (ie, epinephrine, norepinephrine).

Hemodynamic effects of dopamine are dose dependent (however, this is relative and there is overlap of clinical effects between dosing ranges):

Low-dose: 1-5 mcg/kg/minute, increased renal blood flow and urine output

Intermediate-dose: 5-15 mcg/kg/minute, increased renal blood flow, heart rate, cardiac contractility, and cardiac output

High-dose: >15 mcg/kg/minute, alpha-adrenergic effects begin to predominate, vasoconstriction, increased blood pressure

Administration Administer into large vein to prevent the possibility of extravasation (central line administration); monitor continuously for free flow; use infusion device to control rate of flow; administration into an umbilical arterial catheter is not recommended; when discontinuing the infusion, gradually decrease the dose of dopamine (sudden discontinuation may cause hypotension).

Extravasation management: Due to short half-life, withdrawal of drug is often only necessary treatment. Use phentolamine as antidote. Mix 5 mg of phentolamine with 9 mL of NS; inject a small amount of this dilution into extravasated area. Blanching should reverse immediately. Monitor site. If blanching should recur, additional injections of phentolamine may be needed.

Monitoring Parameters Blood pressure, ECG, heart rate, CVP, RAP, MAP; serum glucose, renal function; urine output; if pulmonary artery catheter is in place, monitor CI, PCWP, SVR, and PVR

Pharmacotherapy Pearls Dopamine is most frequently used for treatment of hypotension because of its peripheral vasoconstrictor action. In this regard, dopamine is often used together with dobutamine and minimizes hypotension secondary to dobutamine-induced vasodilation. Thus, pressure is maintained by increased cardiac output (from dobutamine) and vasoconstriction (by dopamine). It is critical neither dopamine nor dobutamine be used in patients in the absence of correcting any hypovolemia as a cause of hypotension.

Low-dose dopamine is often used in the intensive care setting for presumed beneficial effects on renal function. However, there is no clear evidence that low-dose dopamine confers any renal or other benefit. Indeed, dopamine may act on dopamine receptors in the carotid bodies causing chemoreflex suppression. In patients with heart failure, dopamine may inhibit breathing and cause pulmonary shunting. Both these mechanisms would act to decrease minute ventilation and oxygen saturation. This could potentially be deleterious in patients with respiratory compromise and patients being weaned from ventilators.

Special Geriatric Considerations Has not been specifically studied in the elderly; monitor closely, especially due to increase in cardiovascular disease with age.

Dosage Forms Excipient information presented when available (limited, particularly for generics); consult specific product labeling.

Infusion, premixed in D_5W, as hydrochloride: 0.8 mg/mL (250 mL, 500 mL); 1.6 mg/mL (250 mL, 500 mL); 3.2 mg/mL (250 mL)

Injection, solution, as hydrochloride: 40 mg/mL (5 mL, 10 mL); 80 mg/mL (5 mL); 160 mg/mL (5 mL)

◆ **Dopamine Hydrochloride** *see* DOPamine *on page* 593
◆ **Doral®** *see* Quazepam *on page* 1642
◆ **Doribax®** *see* Doripenem *on page* 594

Doripenem (dore i PEN em)

Medication Safety Issues

Sound-alike/look-alike issues:

Doripenem may be confused with ertapenem

Doribax® may be confused with Zovirax®

Brand Names: U.S. Doribax®

Brand Names: Canada Doribax®

Index Terms S-4661

Generic Availability (U.S.) No

Pharmacologic Category Antibiotic, Carbapenem

Use Treatment of complicated intra-abdominal infections and complicated urinary tract infections (including pyelonephritis) due to susceptible aerobic gram-positive, aerobic gram-negative (including *Pseudomonas aeruginosa*), and anaerobic bacteria

Canadian labeling: Additional use (not in U.S. labeling): Treatment of healthcare-associated pneumonia (including ventilator-associated pneumonia)

Unlabeled Use Treatment of intravascular catheter-related bloodstream infection due to extended-spectrum β-lactamase (ESBL)-producing *Escherichia coli* and *Klebsiella* spp

Contraindications Known serious hypersensitivity to doripenem or other carbapenems (eg, ertapenem, imipenem, meropenem); anaphylactic reactions to beta-lactam antibiotics

Warnings/Precautions Serious hypersensitivity reactions, including anaphylaxis, and skin reactions have been reported in patients receiving beta-lactams. Use may result in fungal or bacterial superinfection, including *C. difficile*-associated diarrhea (CDAD) and pseudomembranous colitis; CDAD has been observed >2 months postantibiotic treatment. Not indicated for the treatment of pneumonia including ventilator-associated pneumonia; decreased efficacy and increased mortality associated with use. Use with caution in patients with renal impairment; dosage adjustment required in patients with moderate-to-severe renal dysfunction. Carbapenems have been associated with CNS adverse effects, including confusional states and seizures (myoclonic); use caution with CNS disorders (eg, brain lesions and history of seizures) and adjust dose in renal impairment to avoid drug accumulation, which may increase seizure risk. May decrease divalproex sodium/valproic acid concentrations leading to breakthrough seizures; concomitant use not recommended. Administer via intravenous infusion only. Per manufacturer's labeling, investigational experience of doripenem via inhalation resulted in pneumonitis.

Adverse Reactions (Reflective of adult population; not specific for elderly)
>10%:
   Central nervous system: Headache (4% to 16%)
   Gastrointestinal: Nausea (4% to 12%), diarrhea (6% to 11%)
1% to 10%:
   Dermatologic: Rash (1% to 5%; includes allergic/bullous dermatitis, erythema, macular/papular eruptions, urticaria, and erythema multiforme), pruritus (≤3%)
   Gastrointestinal: Oral candidiasis (1%)
   Hematologic: Anemia (2% to 10%)
   Hepatic: Transaminases increased (1% to 2%)
   Local: Phlebitis (4% to 8%)
   Renal: Renal impairment/failure (≤1%)
   Miscellaneous: Vulvomycotic infection (1% to 2%)

Drug Interactions
Metabolism/Transport Effects None known.
Avoid Concomitant Use
   Avoid concomitant use of Doripenem with any of the following: BCG; Probenecid
Increased Effect/Toxicity
   The levels/effects of Doripenem may be increased by: Probenecid
Decreased Effect
   Doripenem may decrease the levels/effects of: BCG; Divalproex; Typhoid Vaccine; Valproic Acid

Stability Store dry powder vials at 15°C to 30°C (59°F to 86°F). Reconstitute 250 mg vial with 10 mL of SWFI or NS, and further dilute for infusion with 50 mL or 100 mL of NS or D_5W. Reconstitute 500 mg vial with 10 mL of SWFI or NS, and further dilute for infusion with 100 mL of NS or D_5W. Shake gently until clear. Reconstituted vial may be stored for up to 1 hour prior to preparation of infusion solution. Stability of solution when diluted in NS is 12 hours at room temperature or 72 hours under refrigeration; stability in D_5W is 4 hours at room temperature and 24 hours under refrigeration. To prepare a 250 mg dose using a 500 mg vial, reconstitute the 500 mg vial with 10 mL of SWFI or NS and further dilute with 100 mL of compatible solution as above, but remove and discard 55 mL from the infusion bag to leave the remaining solution containing the 250 mg dose.

Mechanism of Action Inhibits bacterial cell wall synthesis by binding to several of the penicillin-binding proteins (PBP-2, PBP-3, PBP-4), which in turn inhibits the final transpeptidation step of peptidoglycan synthesis in bacterial cell walls, thus inhibiting cell wall biosynthesis; bacteria eventually lyse due to ongoing activity of cell wall autolytic enzymes (autolysins and murein hydrolases) while cell wall assembly is arrested.

Pharmacodynamics/Kinetics Note: As with other time-dependent antibiotics, doripenem shows bacteriostatic effects at T>MIC <40% and bactericidal effects at T>MIC>40%. Of note, prolonged infusion time (over 4 hours) was more effective in increasing T>MIC over 40% to up to 81%. Pharmacokinetics are linear (AUC directly proportional to dose) at doses administered over 1 hour.

◀

Distribution: Penetrates well into body fluids and tissues, including peritoneal and retroperitoneal fluids, gallbladder, bile, and urine

V_d: 16.8 L

Protein binding: 8% to 9%

Metabolism: Non-CYP-mediated metabolism via hydrolysis by dehydropeptidase-I to doripenem-M1 (inactive metabolite)

Half-life elimination: ~1 hour

Excretion: Urine (70% as unchanged drug; 15% as doripenem-M1 metabolite); feces (<1%) Dialyzable with reduction in systemic levels by 48% to 62%.

Dosage

Geriatric & Adult

Note: A switch to appropriate oral antimicrobial therapy may be considered after 3 days of parenteral therapy and demonstrated clinical improvement.

Intra-abdominal infection, complicated, severe: I.V.: 500 mg every 8 hours for 5-14 days. **Note:** 2010 IDSA guidelines recommend treatment duration of 4-7 days (provided source controlled). Not recommended for mild-to-moderate, community-acquired intra-abdominal infections due to risk of toxicity and the development of resistant organisms (Solomkin, 2010).

Pneumonia (healthcare-associated [HAP], including ventilator-associated [VAP]): Canadian labeling (U.S. unlabeled use [Chastre, 2008; Rea-Neto, 2008]): I.V.: 500 mg every 8 hours for 7-14 days. **Note:** A VAP trial showed numerically lower cure rate (versus a comparator antibiotic) and increased mortality; doses were twofold higher than the Canadian approved dose (FDA communication, 2012).

Urinary tract infection (complicated) or pyelonephritis: I.V.: 500 mg every 8 hours for 10-14 days

Intravenous catheter-related bloodstream infection (unlabeled use): I.V.: 500 mg every 8 hours for 7-14 days (IDSA, 2009)

Renal Impairment

Cl_{cr} >50 mL/minute: No adjustment necessary.

Cl_{cr} 30-50 mL/minute: 250 mg every 8 hours

Cl_{cr} 11-29 mL/minute: 250 mg every 12 hours

Hemodialysis: Dialyzable (~52% of dose removed during 4-hour session in ESRD patients)

Intermittent HD: 250 mg every 24 hours; if treating infections caused by *Pseudomonas aeruginosa*, administer 500 mg every 12 hours on day 1, followed by 500 mg every 24 hours (Tanoue, 2011)

CVVHDF: 250 mg every 12 hours (Hidaka, 2010).

Administration Infuse intravenously over 1 hour. Use of 4-hour infusion has been shown to increase %T>MIC. **Note:** The Canadian labeling recommends a 4-hour infusion in late-onset ventilator-associated pneumonia (>5 days ventilation [not an approved indication in the U.S. labeling])

Monitoring Parameters Monitor for signs of anaphylaxis during first dose; periodic renal assessment; consider hematologic monitoring during prolonged therapy

Pharmacotherapy Pearls One mechanism of resistance to doripenem is production of the Ambler's class B metallo-beta-lactamase, a potent carbapenemase produced by *Stenotrophomonas maltophilia*.

Special Geriatric Considerations Careful attention to dose adjustment based on renal function, as well as monitoring renal function during treatment is recommended. According to the manufacturer, 28% of clinical trial patients were ≥65 years and 12% were ≥75 years, with no differences in overall age-related safety findings.

Dosage Forms Excipient information presented when available (limited, particularly for generics); consult specific product labeling.

Injection, powder for reconstitution:

Doribax®: 250 mg, 500 mg

◆ **Doryx®** *see* Doxycycline *on page 606*

Dorzolamide (dor ZOLE a mide)

Related Information

Glaucoma Drug Therapy *on page 2115*

Brand Names: U.S. Trusopt®

Brand Names: Canada Sandoz-Dorzolamide; Trusopt®

Index Terms Dorzolamide Hydrochloride

Generic Availability (U.S.) Yes

Pharmacologic Category Carbonic Anhydrase Inhibitor; Ophthalmic Agent, Antiglaucoma

Use Treatment of elevated intraocular pressure in patients with ocular hypertension or open-angle glaucoma

Contraindications Hypersensitivity to dorzolamide or any component of the formulation

Warnings/Precautions Although administered topically, systemic absorption occurs. Similar adverse reactions attributed to sulfonamides may occur with topical administration. Chemical similarities are present among sulfonamides, sulfonylureas, carbonic anhydrase inhibitors, thiazides, and loop diuretics (except ethacrynic acid). In patients with allergy to one of these compounds, a risk of cross-reaction exists; avoid use when previous reaction has been severe.

Not recommended for use in patients with severe renal impairment (Cl_{cr} <30 mL/minute). Use with caution in patients with hepatic impairment. Concurrent use with oral carbonic anhydrase inhibitors is not recommended. Local ocular adverse effects (conjunctivitis and lid reactions) were reported with chronic administration. Many resolved with discontinuation of drug therapy. If such reactions occur, discontinue dorzolamide. Choroidal detachment has been reported after filtration procedures. Patients with low endothelial cell counts may have increased risk for corneal edema; use caution.

Inadvertent contamination of multiple-dose ophthalmic solutions, has caused bacterial keratitis. Some products contain benzalkonium chloride which may be absorbed by soft contact lenses. Dorzolamide should not be administered while wearing soft contact lenses.

Adverse Reactions (Reflective of adult population; not specific for elderly)
>10%:
  Gastrointestinal: Bitter taste following administration (25%)
  Ocular: Burning, stinging or discomfort immediately following administration (33%); superficial punctate keratitis (10% to 15%); signs and symptoms of ocular allergic reaction (10%)
  1% to 5%: Ocular: Blurred vision, conjunctivitis, dryness, lid reactions, photophobia, redness, tearing

Drug Interactions

Metabolism/Transport Effects Substrate of CYP2C9 (minor), CYP3A4 (minor); **Note:** Assignment of Major/Minor substrate status based on clinically relevant drug interaction potential

Avoid Concomitant Use
  Avoid concomitant use of Dorzolamide with any of the following: Carbonic Anhydrase Inhibitors

Increased Effect/Toxicity
  Dorzolamide may increase the levels/effects of: Carbonic Anhydrase Inhibitors

Decreased Effect
  The levels/effects of Dorzolamide may be decreased by: Tocilizumab

Stability Store at room temperature 15°C to 30°C (59°F to 86°F). Protect from light.

Mechanism of Action Reversible inhibition of the enzyme carbonic anhydrase resulting in reduction of hydrogen ion secretion at renal tubule and an increased renal excretion of sodium, potassium, bicarbonate, and water to decrease production of aqueous humor; also inhibits carbonic anhydrase in central nervous system to retard abnormal and excessive discharge from CNS neurons

Pharmacodynamics/Kinetics
  Onset of action: Peak effect: 2 hours
  Duration: 8-12 hours
  Absorption: Topical: Reaches systemic circulation where it accumulates in RBCs during chronic dosing as a result of binding to CA-II
  Distribution: In RBCs during chronic administration
  Protein binding: 33%
  Metabolism: To N-desethyl metabolite (less potent than parent drug)
  Half-life elimination: Terminal RBC: 147 days; washes out of RBCs nonlinearly, resulting in a rapid decline of drug concentration initially, followed by a slower elimination phase with a half-life of about 4 months
  Excretion: Urine (as unchanged drug and metabolite, N-desethyl)

Dosage
  Geriatric & Adult Reduction of intraocular pressure: Ophthalmic: Instill 1 drop in the affected eye(s) 3 times/day

Administration If more than one topical ophthalmic drug is being used, administer the drugs at least 10 minutes apart. Remove contact lens prior to administration and wait 15 minutes before reinserting. Instruct patients to avoid allowing the tip of the dispensing container to contact the eye or surrounding structures. Ocular solutions can become contaminated by common bacteria known to cause ocular infections. Serious damage to the eye and subsequent loss of vision may occur from using contaminated solutions.

Monitoring Parameters Ophthalmic exams and IOP periodically

Special Geriatric Considerations Evaluate the patient's or caregiver's ability to safely administer the correct dose of ophthalmic medication.

Dosage Forms Excipient information presented when available (limited, particularly for generics); consult specific product labeling.
Solution, ophthalmic [drops]: 2% (10 mL)
Trusopt®: 2% (10 mL) [contains benzalkonium chloride]
Dosage Forms: Canada Excipient information presented when available (limited, particularly for generics); consult specific product labeling.
Solution, ophthalmic [drops; preservative free]:
Trusopt®: 2% (0.2 mL)

Dorzolamide and Timolol (dor ZOLE a mide & TYE moe lole)

Related Information
Dorzolamide on page 596
Timolol (Ophthalmic) on page 1902
Brand Names: U.S. Cosopt®; Cosopt® PF
Brand Names: Canada Apo-Dorzo-Timop; Cosopt®; Cosopt® Preservative Free; Sandoz-Dorzolamide/Timolol
Index Terms Cosopt® PF; Timolol and Dorzolamide
Generic Availability (U.S.) Yes: Excludes preservative free ophthalmic solution
Pharmacologic Category Beta-Adrenergic Blocker, Nonselective; Carbonic Anhydrase Inhibitor; Ophthalmic Agent, Antiglaucoma
Use Treatment of elevated intraocular pressure in patients with ocular hypertension or open-angle glaucoma
Dosage
Geriatric & Adult Reduction of intraocular pressure: Ophthalmic: Instill 1 drop in affected eye(s) twice daily
Special Geriatric Considerations See individual agents. Evaluate the patient's or caregiver's ability to safely administer the correct dose of ophthalmic medication.
Dosage Forms Excipient information presented when available (limited, particularly for generics); consult specific product labeling. [DSC] = Discontinued product
Solution, ophthalmic [drops]: Dorzolamide 2% and timolol 0.5% (10 mL)
Cosopt®: Dorzolamide 2% and timolol 0.5% (5 mL [DSC]; 10 mL) [contains benzalkonium chloride]
Solution, ophthalmic [drops, preservative free]:
Cosopt® PF: Dorzolamide 2% and timolol 0.5% (0.2 mL)

◆ **Dorzolamide Hydrochloride** see Dorzolamide on page 596
◆ **DOSS** see Docusate on page 583
◆ **Double Tussin DM [OTC]** see Guaifenesin and Dextromethorphan on page 906
◆ **Dovonex®** see Calcipotriene on page 253

Doxazosin (doks AY zoe sin)

Related Information
Beers Criteria – Potentially Inappropriate Medications for Geriatrics on page 2183
Pharmacotherapy of Urinary Incontinence on page 2141
Medication Safety Issues
Sound-alike/look-alike issues:
Doxazosin may be confused with doxapram, doxepin, DOXOrubicin
Cardura® may be confused with Cardene®, Cordarone®, Cordran®, Coumadin®, K-Dur®, Ridaura®
BEERS Criteria medication:
This drug may be potentially inappropriate for use in geriatric patients (Quality of evidence - moderate; Strength of recommendation - strong).
Brand Names: U.S. Cardura®; Cardura® XL
Brand Names: Canada Alti-Doxazosin; Apo-Doxazosin®; Cardura-1™; Cardura-2™; Cardura-4™; Gen-Doxazosin; Mylan-Doxazosin; Novo-Doxazosin
Index Terms Doxazosin Mesylate
Generic Availability (U.S.) Yes: Excludes extended release tablet
Pharmacologic Category Alpha$_1$ Blocker
Use
Immediate release formulation: Treatment of hypertension as monotherapy or in conjunction with diuretics, ACE inhibitors, beta-blockers, or calcium antagonists
Immediate release and extended release formulations: Treatment of urinary outflow obstruction and/or obstructive and irritative symptoms associated with benign prostatic hyperplasia (BPH)

Contraindications Hypersensitivity to quinazolines (prazosin, terazosin), doxazosin, or any component of the formulation

Warnings/Precautions Can cause significant orthostatic hypotension and syncope, especially with first dose; anticipate a similar effect if therapy is interrupted for a few days, if dosage is rapidly increased, or if another antihypertensive drug (particularly vasodilators) or a PDE-5 inhibitor is introduced. Discontinue if symptoms of angina occur or worsen. Patients should be cautioned about performing hazardous tasks when starting new therapy or adjusting dosage upward. Prostate cancer should be ruled out before starting for BPH. Use with caution in mild-to-moderate hepatic impairment; not recommended in severe dysfunction. Intraoperative floppy iris syndrome has been observed in cataract surgery patients who were on or were previously treated with alpha$_1$-blockers. Causality has not been established and there appears to be no benefit in discontinuing alpha-blocker therapy prior to surgery. In the elderly, avoid use as an antihypertensive due to high risk of orthostatic hypotension; alternative agents preferred due to a more favorable risk/benefit profile (Beers Criteria).

The extended release formulation consists of drug within a nondeformable matrix; following drug release/absorption, the matrix/shell is expelled in the stool. The use of nondeformable products in patients with known stricture/narrowing of the GI tract has been associated with symptoms of obstruction. Use caution in patients with increased GI retention (eg, chronic constipation) as doxazosin exposure may be increased. Extended release formulation is not indicated for use in women or for the treatment of hypertension.

Adverse Reactions (Reflective of adult population; not specific for elderly) Note: Type and frequency of adverse reactions reflect combined data from BPH and hypertension trials and immediate release and extended release products.

>10%: Central nervous system: Dizziness (5% to 19%), headache (5% to 14%)

1% to 10%:

Cardiovascular: Orthostatic hypotension (dose related; 0.3% up to 2%), edema (3% to 4%), hypotension (1% to 2%), palpitation (1% to 2%), chest pain (1% to 2%), arrhythmia (1%), syncope (2%), flushing (1%)

Central nervous system: Fatigue (8% to 12%), somnolence (1% to 5%), nervousness (2%), pain (2%), vertigo (2% to 4%), insomnia (1%), anxiety (1%), paresthesia (1%), movement disorder (1%), ataxia (1%), hypertonia (1%), depression (1%)

Dermatologic: Rash (1%), pruritus (1%)

Endocrine & metabolic: Sexual dysfunction (2%)

Gastrointestinal: Abdominal pain (2%), diarrhea (2%), dyspepsia (1% to 2%), nausea (1% to 3%), xerostomia (1% to 2%), constipation (1%), flatulence (1%)

Genitourinary: Urinary tract infection (1%), impotence (1%), polyuria (2%), incontinence (1%)

Neuromuscular & skeletal: Back pain (2% to 3%), weakness (1% to 7%), arthritis (1%), muscle weakness (1%), myalgia (≤1%), muscle cramps (1%)

Ocular: Abnormal vision (1% to 2%), conjunctivitis (1%)

Otic: Tinnitus (1%)

Respiratory: Respiratory tract infection (5%), rhinitis (3%), dyspnea (1% to 3%), respiratory disorder (1%), epistaxis (1%)

Miscellaneous: Diaphoresis increased (1%), flu-like syndrome (1%)

Drug Interactions

Metabolism/Transport Effects Substrate of CYP2C19 (minor), CYP2D6 (minor), CYP3A4 (major); **Note:** Assignment of Major/Minor substrate status based on clinically relevant drug interaction potential

Avoid Concomitant Use

Avoid concomitant use of Doxazosin with any of the following: Alpha1-Blockers; Conivaptan

Increased Effect/Toxicity

Doxazosin may increase the levels/effects of: Alpha1-Blockers; Amifostine; Antihypertensives; Calcium Channel Blockers; Hypotensive Agents; RiTUXimab

The levels/effects of Doxazosin may be increased by: Beta-Blockers; Conivaptan; CYP3A4 Inhibitors (Moderate); CYP3A4 Inhibitors (Strong); Dasatinib; Diazoxide; Herbs (Hypotensive Properties); Ivacaftor; MAO Inhibitors; Mifepristone; Pentoxifylline; Phosphodiesterase 5 Inhibitors; Prostacyclin Analogues

Decreased Effect

The levels/effects of Doxazosin may be decreased by: CYP3A4 Inducers (Strong); Deferasirox; Herbs (CYP3A4 Inducers); Herbs (Hypertensive Properties); Methylphenidate; Peginterferon Alfa-2b; Tocilizumab; Yohimbine

Ethanol/Nutrition/Herb Interactions Herb/Nutraceutical: Avoid dong quai if using for hypertension (has estrogenic activity). Avoid ephedra, yohimbe, ginseng (may worsen hypertension). Avoid saw palmetto when used for BPH (due to limited experience with this combination). Avoid garlic (may have increased antihypertensive effect).

Stability Store at 25°C (77°F); excursions permitted to 15°C to 30°C (59°F to 86°F).

◀ **Mechanism of Action**

Hypertension: Competitively inhibits postsynaptic alpha₁-adrenergic receptors which results in vasodilation of veins and arterioles and a decrease in total peripheral resistance and blood pressure; ~50% as potent on a weight by weight basis as prazosin.

BPH: Competitively inhibits postsynaptic alpha₁-adrenergic receptors in prostatic stromal and bladder neck tissues. This reduces the sympathetic tone-induced urethral stricture causing BPH symptoms.

Pharmacodynamics/Kinetics Not significantly affected by increased age

Duration: >24 hours

Protein binding: ~98%

Metabolism: Extensively hepatic to active metabolites; primarily via CYP3A4; secondary pathways involve CYP2D6 and 2C19

Bioavailability: Immediate release: ~65%; Extended release relative to immediate release: 54% to 59%

Half-life elimination: Immediate release: ~22 hours; Extended release: 15-19 hours

Time to peak, serum: Immediate release: 2-3 hours; Extended release: 8-9 hours

Excretion: Feces (63%, primarily as metabolites); urine (9%, primarily as metabolites)

Dosage

Geriatric Refer to adult dosing. In the management of hypertension, consider lower initial doses (eg, immediate release: 0.5 mg once daily) and titrate to response (Aronow, 2011)

Adult

BPH: Oral:

Immediate release: 1 mg once daily in morning or evening; may be increased to 2 mg once daily. Thereafter titrate upwards, if needed, over several weeks, balancing therapeutic benefit with doxazosin-induced postural hypotension. Goal: 4-8 mg/day; maximum dose: 8 mg/day

Reinitiation of therapy: If therapy is discontinued for several days, restart at 1 mg dose and titrate as before

Extended release: 4 mg once daily with breakfast; titrate based on response and tolerability every 3-4 weeks to maximum recommended dose of 8 mg/day

Reinitiation of therapy: If therapy is discontinued for several days, restart at 4 mg dose and titrate as before

Note: Conversion to extended release from immediate release: Omit final evening dose of immediate release prior to starting morning dosing with extended release product; initiate extended release product using 4 mg once daily

Hypertension: Oral: *Immediate release:* 1 mg once daily in morning or evening; may be increased to 2 mg once daily. Thereafter titrate upwards, if needed, over several weeks, balancing therapeutic benefit with doxazosin-induced postural hypotension. Maximum dose: 16 mg/day

Reinitiation of therapy: If therapy is discontinued for several days, restart at 1 mg dose and titrate as before

Hepatic Impairment Use with caution in mild-to-moderate hepatic dysfunction. Do not use with severe impairment.

Administration Cardura® XL: Tablets should be swallowed whole; do not crush, chew, or divide. Administer with morning meal.

Monitoring Parameters Blood pressure, standing and sitting/supine; syncope may occur usually within 90 minutes of the initial dose

Pharmacotherapy Pearls First-dose hypotension occurs less frequently with doxazosin as compared to prazosin; this may be due to its slower onset of action.

Special Geriatric Considerations Adverse reactions such as orthostatic hypotension, dry mouth, and urinary problems can be particularly bothersome in the elderly. In studies of the extended-release tablets, the incidence of hypotension was higher in the elderly compared to younger patients.

This medication is considered to be potentially inappropriate in this patient population (Beers Criteria: Quality of evidence - moderate; Strength of recommendation - strong).

Dosage Forms Excipient information presented when available (limited, particularly for generics); consult specific product labeling.

Tablet, oral: 1 mg, 2 mg, 4 mg, 8 mg

Cardura®: 1 mg, 2 mg, 4 mg, 8 mg [scored]

Tablet, extended release, oral:

Cardura® XL: 4 mg, 8 mg

◆ **Doxazosin Mesylate** *see* Doxazosin *on page 598*

Doxepin (Systemic) (DOKS e pin)

Related Information

Antidepressant Agents on page 2097

Beers Criteria – Potentially Inappropriate Medications for Geriatrics on page 2183

Medication Safety Issues

Sound-alike/look-alike issues:

Doxepin may be confused with digoxin, doxapram, doxazosin, Doxidan®, doxycycline

SINEquan® may be confused with saquinavir, SEROquel®, Singulair®, Zonegran®

BEERS Criteria medication:

This drug may be potentially inappropriate for use in geriatric patients (Quality of evidence - high [moderate for SIADH]; Strength of recommendation - strong).

International issues:

Doxal [Finland] may be confused with Doxil brand name for doxorubicin (liposomal) [U.S., Israel]

Doxal brand name for doxepin [Finland] but also brand name for pyridoxine/thiamine [Brazil]

Brand Names: U.S. Silenor®

Brand Names: Canada Apo-Doxepin®; Doxepine; Novo-Doxepin; Sinequan®

Index Terms Doxepin Hydrochloride

Generic Availability (U.S.) Yes: Excludes tablet

Pharmacologic Category Antidepressant, Tricyclic (Tertiary Amine)

Use Depression; treatment of insomnia (with difficulty of sleep maintenance)

Unlabeled Use Analgesic for certain chronic and neuropathic pain; anxiety

Medication Guide Available Yes

Contraindications Hypersensitivity to doxepin, drugs from similar chemical class, or any component of the formulation; narrow-angle glaucoma; urinary retention; use of MAO inhibitors within 14 days

Warnings/Precautions [U.S. Boxed Warning]: Antidepressants increase the risk of suicidal thinking and behavior in children, adolescents, and young adults (18-24 years of age) with major depressive disorder (MDD) and other psychiatric disorders; consider risk prior to prescribing. Short-term studies did not show an increased risk in patients >24 years of age and showed a decreased risk in patients ≥65 years. Closely monitor for clinical worsening, suicidality, or unusual changes in behavior; the patient's family or caregiver should be instructed to closely observe the patient and communicate condition with healthcare provider. A medication guide should be dispensed with each prescription.

The possibility of a suicide attempt is inherent in major depression and may persist until remission occurs. Monitor for worsening of depression or suicidality, especially during initiation of therapy (generally first 1-2 months) or with dose increases or decreases. Use caution in high-risk patients. Worsening depression and severe abrupt suicidality that are not part of the presenting symptoms may require discontinuation or modification of drug therapy. The patient's family or caregiver should be alerted to monitor patients for the emergence of suicidality and associated behaviors (such as agitation, irritability, hostility, impulsivity, and hypomania) and call healthcare provider.

Risk of suicidal behavior may be increased regardless of doxepin dose; antidepressant doses of doxepin are 10- to 100-fold higher than doses for insomnia.

May worsen psychosis in some patients or precipitate a shift to mania or hypomania in patients with bipolar disorder. Patients presenting with depressive symptoms should be screened for bipolar disorder. Monotherapy in patients with bipolar disorder should be avoided. **Doxepin is not FDA approved for the treatment of bipolar depression.**

Should only be used for insomnia after evaluation of potential causes of sleep disturbance. Failure of sleep disturbance to resolve after 7-10 days may indicate psychiatric or medical illness. An increased risk for hazardous sleep-related activities has been noted; discontinue use with any sleep-related episodes. The risks of sedative and anticholinergic effects are high relative to other antidepressant agents. Doxepin frequently causes sedation, which may result in impaired performance of tasks requiring alertness (eg, operating machinery or driving). Sedative effects may be additive with other CNS depressants and/or ethanol. Also use caution in patients with benign prostatic hyperplasia, xerostomia, visual problems, constipation, or history of bowel obstruction.

May cause orthostatic hypotension or conduction disturbances (risks are moderate relative to other antidepressants). Use with caution in patients with a history of cardiovascular disease (including previous MI, stroke, tachycardia, or conduction abnormalities). Use with caution in patients with respiratory compromise or sleep apnea; use is generally not recommended with severe sleep apnea. Consider discontinuation, when possible, prior to elective surgery.

Therapy should not be abruptly discontinued in patients receiving high doses for prolonged periods.

Use caution in patients with a previous seizure disorder or condition predisposing to seizures such as brain damage, alcoholism, or concurrent therapy with other drugs which lower the seizure threshold. Use with caution in hyperthyroid patients or those receiving thyroid supplementation. Use with caution in patients with hepatic or renal dysfunction.

In the elderly, avoid doses >6 mg/day in this age group due to its potent anticholinergic and sedative properties, and potential to cause orthostatic hypotension; safety of doses ≤6 mg/day is comparable to placebo. In addition, may also cause or exacerbate syndrome of inappropriate antidiuretic hormone secretion or hyponatremia; monitor sodium closely with initiation or dosage adjustments in older adults (Beers Criteria).

Adverse Reactions (Reflective of adult population; not specific for elderly) Actual frequency may be dependent on diagnosis.

Cardiovascular: Flushing, hypertension (<3%), hypotension, tachycardia

Central nervous system: Ataxia, chills, confusion, disorientation, dizziness, drowsiness, fatigue, hallucinations, headache, seizure, somnolence/sedation (6% to 9%)

Dermatologic: Alopecia, photosensitivity, pruritus, rash

Endocrine & metabolic: Blood sugar increased/decreased, breast enlargement, galactorrhea, gynecomastia, libido increased/decreased, SIADH

Gastrointestinal: Anorexia, aphthous stomatitis, constipation, diarrhea, gastroenteritis (≤2%), indigestion, nausea (2%), trouble with gums, unpleasant taste, vomiting, weight gain, xerostomia; lower esophageal sphincter tone decrease may cause GE reflux

Genitourinary: Testicular edema, urinary retention

Hematologic: Agranulocytosis, eosinophilia, leukopenia, purpura, thrombocytopenia, purpura

Hepatic: Jaundice

Neuromuscular & skeletal: Extrapyramidal symptoms, numbness, paresthesia, tardive dyskinesia, tremor, weakness

Ocular: Blurred vision

Otic: Tinnitus

Respiratory: Asthma exacerbation, nasopharyngitis/upper respiratory tract infection (≤4%)

Miscellaneous: Allergic reactions, diaphoresis (excessive)

Drug Interactions

Metabolism/Transport Effects Substrate of CYP1A2 (minor), CYP2C19 (minor), CYP2D6 (major), CYP3A4 (minor); **Note:** Assignment of Major/Minor substrate status based on clinically relevant drug interaction potential

Avoid Concomitant Use

Avoid concomitant use of Doxepin (Systemic) with any of the following: Iobenguane I 123; MAO Inhibitors; Methylene Blue

Increased Effect/Toxicity

Doxepin (Systemic) may increase the levels/effects of: Alpha-/Beta-Agonists (Direct-Acting); Alpha1-Agonists; Amphetamines; Anticholinergics; Aspirin; Beta2-Agonists; Desmopressin; Methylene Blue; Metoclopramide; NSAID (COX-2 Inhibitor); NSAID (Nonselective); QuiNIDine; Serotonin Modulators; Sodium Phosphates; Sulfonylureas; TraMADol; Vitamin K Antagonists; Yohimbine

The levels/effects of Doxepin (Systemic) may be increased by: Abiraterone Acetate; Altretamine; Antipsychotics; BuPROPion; Cimetidine; Cinacalcet; CYP2D6 Inhibitors (Moderate); CYP2D6 Inhibitors (Strong); Dexmethylphenidate; Divalproex; DULoxetine; Linezolid; Lithium; MAO Inhibitors; Methylphenidate; Metoclopramide; Metyrosine; Pramlintide; Protease Inhibitors; QuiNIDine; Selective Serotonin Reuptake Inhibitors; Terbinafine; Terbinafine (Systemic); Valproic Acid

Decreased Effect

Doxepin (Systemic) may decrease the levels/effects of: Acetylcholinesterase Inhibitors (Central); Alpha2-Agonists; Iobenguane I 123

The levels/effects of Doxepin (Systemic) may be decreased by: Acetylcholinesterase Inhibitors (Central); Barbiturates; CarBAMazepine; Peginterferon Alfa-2b; St Johns Wort; Tocilizumab

Ethanol/Nutrition/Herb Interactions

Ethanol: May increase CNS depression; monitor for increased effects with coadministration. Caution patients about effects.

Food: A high-fat meal increases the bioavailability of Silenor® and delays the peak plasma concentration by ~3 hours

Herb/Nutraceutical: Avoid valerian, St John's wort, SAMe, kava kava (may increase risk of serotonin syndrome and/or excessive sedation).

Stability Store at 20°C to 25°C (68°F to 77°F). Protect from light.

Mechanism of Action Increases the synaptic concentration of serotonin and norepinephrine in the central nervous system by inhibition of their reuptake by the presynaptic neuronal membrane; antagonizes the histamine (H_1) receptor for sleep maintenance

Pharmacodynamics/Kinetics
Onset of action: Peak effect: Antidepressant: Usually >2 weeks; Anxiolytic: may occur sooner
Protein binding: ~80%
Metabolism: Hepatic via CYP2C19 and 2D6; metabolites include N-desmethyldoxepin (active)
Half-life elimination: Adults: Doxepin: ~15 hours; N-desmethyldoxepin: 31 hours
Time to peak, serum: Hypnotic: 3.5 hours
Excretion: Urine (<3% as unchanged drug or N-desmethyldoxepin)

Dosage
Geriatric
Depression and/or anxiety: Oral: Initial: 10-25 mg at bedtime; increase by 10-25 mg every 3 days for inpatients and weekly for outpatients if tolerated. Rarely does the maximum dose required exceed 75 mg/day; a single bedtime dose is recommended.
Insomnia: Oral: 3 mg once daily 30 minutes prior to bedtime; increase to 6 mg once daily if clinically needed

Adult
Depression and/or anxiety: Oral: Initial: 25-150 mg/day at bedtime or in 2-3 divided doses; may gradually increase up to 300 mg/day; single dose should not exceed 150 mg; select patients may respond to 25-50 mg/day.
Insomnia (Silenor®): Oral: 3-6 mg once daily 30 minutes prior to bedtime; maximum dose: 6 mg/day

Hepatic Impairment Use a lower dose and adjust gradually.
Silenor®: Initial: 3 mg once daily

Administration Oral: Do not mix oral concentrate with carbonated beverages (physically incompatible).
Silenor®: Administer within 30 minutes prior to bedtime; do not take within 3 hours of food

Monitoring Parameters Monitor blood pressure and pulse rate prior to and during initial therapy; monitor mental status, suicidal ideation (especially at the beginning of therapy or when doses are increased or decreased); weight; ECG in older adults

Insomnia: Re-evaluate diagnosis if insomnia does not remit within 7-10 days of treatment.

Reference Range Proposed therapeutic concentration (doxepin plus desmethyldoxepin): 110-250 ng/mL. Toxic concentration (doxepin plus desmethyldoxepin): >500 ng/mL. Utility of serum level monitoring is controversial.

Test Interactions Increased glucose

Special Geriatric Considerations Strong potential for anticholinergic effects. Dosing should be approached cautiously, initiated at the low end of the dosage range. Clinical trials with 3 mg and 6 mg to treat insomnia included patients 65 and 75 years of age and older. Confusion and oversedation remain a caution. The pharmacokinetics of doxepin have not been studied in elderly patients.

This medication is considered to be potentially inappropriate in this patient population (Beers Criteria: Quality of evidence - high [moderate for SIADH]; Strength of recommendation - strong).

Dosage Forms Excipient information presented when available (limited, particularly for generics); consult specific product labeling.
Capsule, oral: 10 mg, 25 mg, 50 mg, 75 mg, 100 mg, 150 mg
Solution, oral [concentrate]: 10 mg/mL (118 mL, 120 mL)
Tablet, oral:
Silenor®: 3 mg, 6 mg

Doxepin (Topical) (DOKS e pin)

Medication Safety Issues
Sound-alike/look-alike issues:
Doxepin may be confused with digoxin, doxapram, doxazosin, Doxidan®, doxycycline
Zonalon® may be confused with Zone-A®
International issues:
Doxal [Finland] may be confused with Doxil brand name for doxorubicin (liposomal) [U.S., Israel]
Doxal brand name for doxepin [Finland] but also brand name for pyridoxine/thiamine [Brazil]
Brand Names: U.S. Prudoxin™; Zonalon®
Brand Names: Canada Zonalon®
Index Terms Doxepin Hydrochloride
Generic Availability (U.S.) No

DOXEPIN (TOPICAL)

Pharmacologic Category Topical Skin Product

Use Short-term (<8 days) management of moderate pruritus in adults with atopic dermatitis or lichen simplex chronicus

Unlabeled Use Cream: Treatment of burning mouth syndrome and neuropathic pain

Dosage

Geriatric

Pruritus: Topical: Refer to adult dosing.

Adult

Burning mouth syndrome (unlabeled use): Oral topical: Cream: Apply 3-4 times daily.

Pruritus: Topical: Apply a thin film 4 times/day with at least 3- to 4-hour interval between applications; not recommended for use >8 days. (Oral administration of doxepin 25-50 mg has also been used, but systemic adverse effects are increased.)

Special Geriatric Considerations Systemic absorption with plasma concentrations sufficient to result in anticholinergic effects, sedation, urinary retention, and delirium has been reported. Risk is likely related to the frequency of application and the surface area of application. Persons ≥65 years were not sufficiently represented in clinical trials.

Dosage Forms Excipient information presented when available (limited, particularly for generics); consult specific product labeling.

Cream, topical, as hydrochloride:

Prudoxin™: 5% (45 g) [contains benzyl alcohol]

Zonalon®: 5% (30 g, 45 g) [contains benzyl alcohol]

◆ **Doxepin Hydrochloride** *see* Doxepin (Systemic) *on page 601*

◆ **Doxepin Hydrochloride** *see* Doxepin (Topical) *on page 603*

Doxercalciferol (doks er kal si fe FEER ole)

Brand Names: U.S. Hectorol®

Brand Names: Canada Hectorol®

Index Terms 1α-Hydroxyergocalciferol

Generic Availability (U.S.) No

Pharmacologic Category Vitamin D Analog

Use Treatment of secondary hyperparathyroidism in patients with chronic kidney disease

Contraindications History of hypercalcemia or evidence of vitamin D toxicity

Warnings/Precautions Other forms of vitamin D should be discontinued when doxercalciferol is started. Excessive administration may lead to over suppression of PTH, hypercalcemia, hypercalciuria, hyperphosphatemia and adynamic bone disease. Acute hypercalcemia may increase risk of cardiac arrhythmias and seizures; use caution with cardiac glycosides as digitalis toxicity may be increased. Chronic hypercalcemia may lead to generalized vascular and other soft-tissue calcification. Phosphate and vitamin D (and its derivatives) should be withheld during therapy to avoid hypercalcemia. Hyperphosphatemia should be corrected before initiating therapy. Use with caution in patients with hepatic impairment. Injection is intended for I.V. use only.

Adverse Reactions (Reflective of adult population; not specific for elderly)

Note: As reported in dialysis patients.

>10%:

Cardiovascular: Edema (34%)

Central nervous system: Headache (28%), malaise (28%), dizziness (12%)

Gastrointestinal: Nausea/vomiting (21%)

Respiratory: Dyspnea (12%)

1% to 10%:

Cardiovascular: Bradycardia (7%)

Central nervous system: Sleep disorder (3%)

Dermatologic: Pruritus (8%)

Endocrine & metabolic: Hypercalcemia (I.V. ~1%), hyperphosphatemia (I.V. 2% to 4%)

Gastrointestinal: Anorexia (5%), dyspepsia (5%), weight gain (5%)

Neuromuscular & skeletal: Arthralgia (5%)

Miscellaneous: Abscess (3%)

Drug Interactions

Metabolism/Transport Effects None known.

Avoid Concomitant Use

Avoid concomitant use of Doxercalciferol with any of the following: Aluminum Hydroxide; Sucralfate; Vitamin D Analogs

Increased Effect/Toxicity

Doxercalciferol may increase the levels/effects of: Aluminum Hydroxide; Cardiac Glycosides; Sucralfate; Vitamin D Analogs

The levels/effects of Doxercalciferol may be increased by: Calcium Salts; Danazol; Thiazide Diuretics

Decreased Effect

The levels/effects of Doxercalciferol may be decreased by: Bile Acid Sequestrants; Mineral Oil; Orlistat

Stability Store at controlled room temperature of 15°C to 30°C (59°F to 86°F). Protect injection from light.

Mechanism of Action Doxercalciferol is metabolized to the active form of vitamin D. The active form of vitamin D controls the intestinal absorption of dietary calcium, the tubular reabsorption of calcium by the kidneys, and in conjunction with PTH, the mobilization of calcium from the skeleton.

Pharmacodynamics/Kinetics

Metabolism: Hepatic via CYP27 to active metabolites

Half-life elimination: Active metabolite: 32-37 hours; up to 96 hours

Dosage

Geriatric & Adult Secondary hyperparathyroidism:

Oral:

Dialysis patients: Dose should be titrated to lower iPTH to 150-300 pg/mL; dose is adjusted at 8-week intervals (maximum dose: 20 mcg 3 times/week)

Initial dose: iPTH >400 pg/mL: 10 mcg 3 times/week at dialysis

Dose titration:

iPTH level decreased by 50% and >300 pg/mL: Dose can be increased to 12.5 mcg 3 times/week for 8 more weeks; this titration process can continue at 8-week intervals; each increase should be by 2.5 mcg/dose

iPTH level 150-300 pg/mL: Maintain current dose

iPTH level <100 pg/mL: Suspend doxercalciferol for 1 week; resume at a reduced dose; decrease each dose (not weekly dose) by at least 2.5 mcg

Predialysis patients: Dose should be titrated to lower iPTH to 35-70 pg/mL with stage 3 disease or to 70-110 pg/mL with stage 4 disease: Dose may be adjusted at 2-week intervals (maximum dose: 3.5 mcg/day)

Initial dose: 1 mcg/day

Dose titration:

iPTH level >70 pg/mL with stage 3 disease or >110 pg/mL with stage 4 disease: Increase dose by 0.5 mcg every 2 weeks as necessary

iPTH level 35-70 pg/mL with stage 3 disease or 70-110 pg/mL with stage 4 disease: Maintain current dose

iPTH level is <35 pg/mL with stage 3 disease or <70 pg/mL with stage 4 disease: Suspend doxercalciferol for 1 week, then resume at a reduced dose (at least 0.5 mcg lower)

I.V.:

Dialysis patients: Dose should be titrated to lower iPTH to 150-300 pg/mL; dose is adjusted at 8-week intervals (maximum dose: 18 mcg/week)

Initial dose: iPTH level >400 pg/mL: 4 mcg 3 times/week after dialysis, administered as a bolus dose

Dose titration:

iPTH level decreased by <50% and >300 pg/mL: Dose can be increased by 1-2 mcg at 8-week intervals, as necessary

iPTH level decreased by >50% and >300 pg/mL: Maintain current dose

iPTH level 150-300 pg/mL: Maintain current dose

iPTH level <100 pg/mL: Suspend doxercalciferol for 1 week; resume at a reduced dose (at least 1 mcg lower)

Hypercalcemia, hyperphosphatemia, or serum calcium times phosphorus product >55 mg^2/dL^2: Decrease or suspend dose and/or adjust dose of phosphate binders; if dose is suspended, resume at a reduced dose (at least 1 mcg lower)

Renal Impairment No adjustment is required.

Hepatic Impairment Use with caution; no guidelines for dosage adjustment.

Monitoring Parameters

Serum calcium and phosphorus: Frequency of measurement may be dependent upon the presence and magnitude of abnormalities, the rate of progression of CKD, and the use of treatments for CKD-mineral and bone disorders (KDIGO, 2009):

CKD stage 3: Every 6-12 months

CKD stage 4: Every 3-6 months

CKD stage 5 and 5D: Every 1-3 months

◄ Periodic 24-hour urinary calcium and phosphorus; magnesium; alkaline phosphatase every 12 months or more frequently in the presence of elevated PTH; creatinine, BUN, albumin; intact parathyroid hormone (iPTH) every 3-12 months depending on CKD severity

Reference Range

Corrected total serum calcium (K/DOQI, 2003): CKD stages 3 and 4: 8.4-10.2 mg/dL (2.1-2.6 mmol/L); CKD stage 5: 8.4-9.5 mg/dL (2.1-2.37 mmol/L); KDIGO guidelines recommend maintaining normal ranges for all stages of CKD (3-5D) (KDIGO, 2009)

Phosphorus (K/DOQI, 2003): CKD stages 3 and 4: 2.7-4.6 mg/dL (0.87-1.48 mmol/L); CKD stage 5 (including those treated with dialysis): 3.5-5.5 mg/dL (1.13-1.78 mmol/L); KDIGO guidelines recommend maintaining normal ranges for CKD stages 3-5 and lowering elevated phosphorus levels toward the normal range for CKD stage 5D (KDIGO, 2009)

Serum calcium-phosphorus product (K/DOQI, 2003): CKD stage 3-5: <55 mg^2/dL^2

PTH: Whole molecule, immunochemiluminometric assay (ICMA): 1.0-5.2 pmol/L; whole molecule, radioimmunoassay (RIA): 10.0-65.0 pg/mL; whole molecule, immunoradiometric, double antibody (IRMA): 1.0-6.0 pmol/L

Target ranges by stage of chronic kidney disease (KDIGO, 2009): CKD stage 3-5: Optimal iPTH is unknown; maintain normal range (assay-dependent); CKD stage 5D: Maintain iPTH within 2-9 times the upper limit of normal for the assay used

Special Geriatric Considerations No special changes in dose are required. Caution should be used in the elderly using magnesium products (MOM, magnesium containing antacids, etc). These should be stopped if possible before initiating doxercalciferol.

Dosage Forms Excipient information presented when available (limited, particularly for generics); consult specific product labeling.

Capsule, softgel, oral:
Hectorol®: 0.5 mcg, 1 mcg, 2.5 mcg [contains coconut oil]

Injection, solution:
Hectorol®: 2 mcg/mL (1 mL, 2 mL) [contains edetate disodium, ethanol]

♦ **Doxidan® [OTC]** *see* Bisacodyl *on page* 214
♦ **Doxy 100™** *see* Doxycycline *on page* 606

Doxycycline (doks i SYE kleen)

Related Information
Antimicrobial Drugs of Choice *on page* 2163
Community-Acquired Pneumonia in Adults *on page* 2171

Medication Safety Issues
Sound-alike/look-alike issues:
Doxycycline may be confused with dicyclomine, doxepin, doxylamine
Doxy100™ may be confused with Doxil®
Monodox® may be confused with Maalox®
Oracea® may be confused with Orencia®
Vibramycin® may be confused with vancomycin, Vibativ™

Brand Names: U.S. Adoxa®; Alodox™; Doryx®; Doxy 100™; Monodox®; Ocudox™; Oracea®; Oraxyl™; Periostat®; Vibramycin®

Brand Names: Canada Apo-Doxy Tabs®; Apo-Doxy®; Dom-Doxycycline; Doxycin; Doxytab; Novo-Doxylin; Nu-Doxycycline; Periostat®; PHL-Doxycycline; PMS-Doxycycline; Vibra-Tabs®; Vibramycin®

Index Terms Doxycycline Calcium; Doxycycline Hyclate; Doxycycline Monohydrate

Generic Availability (U.S.) Yes: Excludes capsule (variable release), powder for suspension, syrup

Pharmacologic Category Antibiotic, Tetracycline Derivative

Use Principally in the treatment of infections caused by susceptible *Rickettsia*, *Chlamydia*, and *Mycoplasma*; alternative to mefloquine for malaria prophylaxis; treatment for syphilis, uncomplicated *Neisseria gonorrhoeae*, *Listeria*, *Actinomyces israelii*, and *Clostridium* infections in penicillin-allergic patients; used for community-acquired pneumonia and other common infections due to susceptible organisms; anthrax due to *Bacillus anthracis*, including inhalational anthrax (postexposure); treatment of infections caused by uncommon susceptible gram-negative and gram-positive organisms including *Borrelia recurrentis*, *Ureaplasma urealyticum*, *Haemophilus ducreyi*, *Yersinia pestis*, *Francisella tularensis*, *Vibrio cholerae*, *Campylobacter fetus*, *Brucella* spp, *Bartonella bacilliformis*, and *Klebsiella granulomatis*, Q fever, Lyme disease; treatment of inflammatory lesions associated with rosacea; intestinal amebiasis; severe acne

Unlabeled Use Sclerosing agent for pleural effusion (injection); vancomycin-resistant enterococci (VRE); alternate treatment for MRSA infections; treatment of periodontitis (refractory); treatment of acute bacterial rhinosinusitis (ABRS) (adults)

Contraindications Hypersensitivity to doxycycline, tetracycline or any component of the formulation

Warnings/Precautions Photosensitivity reaction may occur with this drug; avoid prolonged exposure to sunlight or tanning equipment. Antianabolic effects of tetracyclines can increase BUN (dose-related). Autoimmune syndromes have been reported. Hepatotoxicity rarely occurs; if symptomatic, conduct LFT and discontinue drug. Pseudotumor cerebri has been (rarely) reported with tetracycline use; usually resolves with discontinuation. Prolonged use may result in fungal or bacterial superinfection, including C. difficile-associated diarrhea (CDAD) and pseudomembranous colitis; CDAD has been observed >2 months postantibiotic treatment. May cause tissue hyperpigmentation, enamel hypoplasia, or permanent tooth discoloration; use of tetracyclines should be avoided during tooth development unless other drugs are not likely to be effective or are contraindicated. However, recommended in treatment of anthrax exposure and tickborne rickettsial diseases. In addition to affecting tooth development, tetracycline use has been associated with retardation of skeletal development and reduced bone growth.

Additional specific warnings: Oracea®: Should not be used for the treatment or prophylaxis of bacterial infections, since the lower dose of drug per capsule may be subefficacious and promote resistance. Syrup contains sodium metabisulfite. Effectiveness of products intended for use in periodontitis has not been established in patients with coexistent oral candidiasis; use with caution in patients with a history or predisposition to oral candidiasis.

Adverse Reactions (Reflective of adult population; not specific for elderly) Frequency not defined.

Cardiovascular: Intracranial hypertension, pericarditis

Dermatologic: Angioneurotic edema, erythema multiforme, exfoliative dermatitis (rare), photosensitivity, rash, skin hyperpigmentation, Stevens-Johnson syndrome, toxic epidermal necrolysis, urticaria

Endocrine & metabolic: Brown/black discoloration of thyroid gland (no dysfunction reported), hypoglycemia

Gastrointestinal: Anorexia, diarrhea, dysphagia, enterocolitis, esophagitis (rare), esophageal ulcerations (rare), glossitis, inflammatory lesions in anogenital region, nausea, oral (mucosal) pigmentation, pseudomembranous colitis, tooth discoloration (children), vomiting

Hematologic: Eosinophilia, hemolytic anemia, neutropenia, thrombocytopenia

Hepatic: Hepatotoxicity (rare)

Renal: BUN increased (dose related)

Miscellaneous: Anaphylactoid purpura, anaphylaxis, bulging fontanels (infants), serum sickness, SLE exacerbation

Note: Adverse effects in clinical trials occurring at a frequency more than 1% greater than placebo:

Periostat®: Diarrhea, dyspepsia, joint pain, menstrual cramp, nausea, dyspepsia, pain

Oracea®: Abdominal distention, abdominal pain, anxiety, AST increased, back pain, fungal infection, hyperglycemia, influenza, LDH increased, nasal congestion, nasopharyngitis, pain, sinus headache, sinusitis, xerostomia

Drug Interactions

Metabolism/Transport Effects Inhibits CYP3A4 (weak)

Avoid Concomitant Use

Avoid concomitant use of Doxycycline with any of the following: BCG; Pimozide; Retinoic Acid Derivatives

Increased Effect/Toxicity

Doxycycline may increase the levels/effects of: ARIPiprazole; Neuromuscular-Blocking Agents; Pimozide; Porfimer; Retinoic Acid Derivatives; Vitamin K Antagonists

Decreased Effect

Doxycycline may decrease the levels/effects of: BCG; Penicillins; Typhoid Vaccine

The levels/effects of Doxycycline may be decreased by: Antacids; Barbiturates; Bile Acid Sequestrants; Bismuth; Bismuth Subsalicylate; Calcium Salts; CarBAMazepine; Fosphenytoin; Iron Salts; Lanthanum; Magnesium Salts; Phenytoin; Quinapril; Sucralfate

Ethanol/Nutrition/Herb Interactions

Ethanol: Chronic ethanol ingestion may reduce the serum concentration of doxycycline.

Food: Doxycycline serum levels may be slightly decreased if taken with food or milk. Administration with iron or calcium may decrease doxycycline absorption. May decrease absorption of calcium, iron, magnesium, zinc, and amino acids.

Herb/Nutraceutical: St John's wort may decrease doxycycline levels. Avoid dong quai, St John's wort (may also cause photosensitization).

Stability

Capsule, tablet: Store at controlled room temperature of 25°C (77°F); excursions permitted to 15°C to 30°C (59°F to 86°F). Protect from light.

I.V. infusion: Following reconstitution with sterile water for injection, dilute to a final concentration of 0.1-1 mg/mL using a compatible solution. Solutions for I.V. infusion may be prepared using 0.9% sodium chloride, D5W, Ringer's injection, lactated Ringer's, D5LR. Protect from light. Stability varies based on solution.

Mechanism of Action Inhibits protein synthesis by binding with the 30S and possibly the 50S ribosomal subunit(s) of susceptible bacteria; may also cause alterations in the cytoplasmic membrane

Periostat® capsules (proposed mechanism): Has been shown to inhibit collagenase activity *in vitro*. Also has been noted to reduce elevated collagenase activity in the gingival crevicular fluid of patients with periodontal disease. Systemic levels do not reach inhibitory concentrations against bacteria.

Pharmacodynamics/Kinetics

Absorption: Oral: Almost complete

Distribution: Widely into body tissues and fluids including synovial, pleural, prostatic, seminal fluids, and bronchial secretions; saliva, aqueous humor, and CSF penetration is poor

Protein binding: 90%

Metabolism: Not hepatic; partially inactivated in GI tract by chelate formation

Bioavailability: Reduced at high pH; may be clinically significant in patients with gastrectomy, gastric bypass surgery or who are otherwise deemed achlorhydric

Half-life elimination: 12-15 hours (usually increases to 22-24 hours with multiple doses); End-stage renal disease: 18-25 hours; Oracea®: 21 hours

Time to peak, serum: 1.5-4 hours

Excretion: Feces (30%); urine (23%)

Dosage

Geriatric & Adult

Usual dosage range: Oral, I.V.: 100-200 mg/day in 1-2 divided doses

Acute bacterial rhinosinusitis (unlabeled use): Oral: 200 mg/day in 1-2 divided doses for 5-7 days (Chow, 2012)

Anthrax:

Inhalational (postexposure prophylaxis): Oral, I.V. (use oral route when possible): 100 mg every 12 hours for 60 days (ACIP, 2010)

Cutaneous (treatment): Oral: 100 mg every 12 hours for 60 days. **Note:** In the presence of systemic involvement, extensive edema, lesions on head/neck, refer to I.V. dosing for treatment of inhalational/gastrointestinal/oropharyngeal anthrax

Inhalational/gastrointestinal/oropharyngeal (treatment): I.V.: Initial: 100 mg every 12 hours; switch to oral therapy when clinically appropriate; some recommend initial loading dose of 200 mg, followed by 100 mg every 8-12 hours (Franz, 1997). **Note:** Initial treatment should include two or more agents predicted to be effective (CDC, 2001). Agents suggested for use in conjunction with doxycycline or ciprofloxacin include rifampin, vancomycin, imipenem, penicillin, ampicillin, chloramphenicol, clindamycin, and clarithromycin. May switch to oral antimicrobial therapy when clinically appropriate. Continue combined therapy for 60 days

Brucellosis: Oral: 100 mg twice daily for 6 weeks with rifampin or streptomycin

Cellulitis (purulent) due to community-acquired MRSA (unlabeled use): Oral: 100 mg twice daily for 5-10 days (Liu, 2011)

Chlamydial infections, uncomplicated: Oral: 100 mg twice daily for ≥7 days

Community-acquired pneumonia, bronchitis: Oral, I.V.: 100 mg twice daily (Ailani, 1999; Mandell, 2007)

Epididymitis: Oral: 100 mg twice daily for 10 days (in combination with ceftriaxone) (CDC, 2010)

Gonococcal infection, uncomplicated (cervix, pharynx, rectum, urethra): Oral: 100 mg twice daily for 7 days (in combination with a cephalosporin) (CDC, 2010)

Alternatively, the manufacturer recommends a single-visit dose in nonanorectal infections in men: 300 mg initially, repeat dose in 1 hour (total dose: 600 mg)

Granuloma inguinale (donovanosis): Oral: 100 mg twice daily for at least 3 weeks (and until lesions have healed) (CDC, 2010)

Lyme disease: Oral (Halperin, 2007; Wormser, 2006):

Prevention: Initiate within 72 hours of tick removal: 200 mg administered as a single dose

Treatment (early lyme disease without neurologic manifestations): 100 mg twice daily for 10-21 days

Treatment (meningitis or other early neurologic manifestations): 100-200 mg twice daily for 14 days (range: 10-28 days)

Lymphogranuloma venereum: Oral: 100 mg twice daily for 21 days (CDC, 2010)

Malaria chemoprophylaxis: Oral: 100 mg/day. Start 1-2 days prior to travel to endemic area; continue daily during travel and for 4 weeks after leaving endemic area

Malaria, severe, treatment (unlabeled use): Oral, I.V.: 100 mg every 12 hours for 7 days with quinidine gluconate. **Note:** Quinidine gluconate duration is region specific; consult CDC for current recommendations (CDC, 2011).

Malaria, uncomplicated, treatment (unlabeled use): Oral: 100 mg twice daily for 7 days with quinine sulfate. **Note:** Quinine sulfate duration is region specific; consult CDC for current recommendations (CDC, 2011).

Nongonococcal urethritis: Oral: 100 mg twice daily for 7 days (CDC, 2010)

Pelvic inflammatory disease:

Treatment, inpatient: Oral, I.V.: 100 mg twice daily (in combination with cefoxitin or cefotetan); may transition to oral doxycycline (add clindamycin or metronidazole if tubo-ovarian abscess present) to complete 14 days of treatment (CDC, 2010)

Treatment, outpatient: Oral: 100 mg twice daily for 14 days (with or without metronidazole); preceded by a single I.M. dose of cefoxitin (plus oral probenecid) or ceftriaxone (CDC, 2010)

Periodontitis: Oral (Periostat®): 20 mg twice daily as an adjunct following scaling and root planing

Periodontitis, refractory (unlabeled use): Oral: 100-200 mg daily (Jolkovsky, 2006)

Proctitis: Oral: 100 mg twice daily for 7 days (in combination with ceftriaxone) (CDC, 2010)

Q fever: Oral: 100 mg every 12 hours for 15-21days (CDC, 2009)

Rosacea (Oracea®): Oral: 40 mg once daily in the morning

Sclerosing agent for pleural effusion (unlabeled use): Intrapleural: 500 mg as a single dose in 100 mL NS (Porcel, 2006); may require a repeat dose (Kvale, 2007)

Syphilis:

Primary/secondary syphilis: Oral: 100 mg twice daily for 14 days (CDC, 2010)

Latent syphilis: Oral: 100 mg twice daily for 28 days (CDC, 2010)

Tickborne rickettsial disease: Oral, I.V.: 100 mg twice daily for 5-7 days; severe or complicated disease may require longer treatment; human granulocytotropic anaplasmosis (HGA) should be treated for 10-14 days.

Tularemia: I.V. (may transition to oral if clinically appropriate): Initial: 100 mg every 12 hours for 14-21 days (Dennis, 2001)

Vibrio cholerae: Oral: 300 mg as a single dose (WHO, 2004)

Yersinia pestis **(plague):** Oral, I.V.: 200 mg initially then 100 mg twice daily **or** 200 mg once daily for 10 days (Daya, 2005; Inglesby, 2000)

Renal Impairment No dosage adjustment necessary in renal impairment.

Poorly dialyzed; no supplemental dose or dosage adjustment necessary, including patients on intermittent hemodialysis, peritoneal dialysis, or continuous renal replacement therapy (eg, CVVHD).

Administration Oral administration is preferable unless patient has significant nausea and vomiting; I.V. and oral routes are bioequivalent.

Oral: May give with meals to decrease GI upset. Capsule and tablet: Administer with at least 8 ounces of water and have patient sit up for at least 30 minutes after taking to reduce the risk of esophageal irritation and ulceration.

Oracea®: Take on an empty stomach 1 hour before or 2 hours after meals.

Doryx®: May be administered by carefully breaking up the tablet and sprinkling tablet contents on a spoonful of cold applesauce. The delayed release pellets must not be crushed or damaged when breaking up tablet. Should be administered immediately after preparation and without chewing.

I.V.: Infuse I.V. doxycycline over 1-4 hours; avoid extravasation

Intrapleural (unlabeled route): Add to 100 mL NS and instill into chest tube (Porcel, 2006)

Monitoring Parameters Perform culture and sensitivity testing prior to initiating therapy. CBC, renal and liver function tests periodically with prolonged therapy.

Test Interactions Injectable tetracycline formulations (if they contain large amounts of ascorbic acid) may result in a false-negative urine glucose using glucose oxidase tests (eg, Clinistix®, Diastix, Tes-Tape®); false elevations of urinary catecholamines with fluorescence

Pharmacotherapy Pearls Oracea® capsules are not bioequivalent to other doxycycline products.

Special Geriatric Considerations Dose adjustment for renal function is not necessary.

Dosage Forms Excipient information presented when available (limited, particularly for generics); consult specific product labeling.

Capsule, oral [strength expressed as base]:

Oracea®: 40 mg [30 mg (immediate release) and 10 mg (delayed release)]

◀

Capsule, oral, as hyclate [strength expressed as base]: 50 mg, 100 mg
Ocudox™: 50 mg [kit includes Ocudox™ capsules (60s), Ocusoft® Lid Scrub™ Plus eyelid cleanser pads, and Tears Again® advanced spray]
Oraxyl™: 20 mg
Vibramycin®: 100 mg
Capsule, oral, as monohydrate [strength expressed as base]: 50 mg, 75 mg, 100 mg, 150 mg
Adoxa®: 150 mg
Monodox®: 50 mg, 75 mg, 100 mg
Injection, powder for reconstitution, as hyclate [strength expressed as base]: 100 mg
Doxy 100™: 100 mg
Powder for suspension, oral, as monohydrate [strength expressed as base]:
Vibramycin®: 25 mg/5 mL (60 mL) [raspberry flavor]
Syrup, oral, as calcium [strength expressed as base]:
Vibramycin®: 50 mg/5 mL (473 mL) [contains propylene glycol, sodium metabisulfite; raspberry-apple flavor]
Tablet, oral, as hyclate [strength expressed as base]: 20 mg, 100 mg
Alodox™: 20 mg [kit includes Alodox™ tablets (60s), Ocusoft® Lid Scrub™ pads, eyelid cleanser, and goggles]
Periostat®: 20 mg
Tablet, oral, as monohydrate [strength expressed as base]: 50 mg, 75 mg, 100 mg, 150 mg
Tablet, delayed release coated beads, oral, as hyclate [strength expressed as base]: 75 mg, 100 mg, 150 mg
Tablet, delayed release coated pellets, oral, as hyclate [strength expressed as base]:
Doryx®: 150 mg [scored; contains sodium 9 mg (0.392 mEq)/tablet]

◆ **Doxycycline Calcium** see Doxycycline on page 606
◆ **Doxycycline Hyclate** see Doxycycline on page 606
◆ **Doxycycline Monohydrate** see Doxycycline on page 606
◆ **DPA** see Valproic Acid on page 1991
◆ **DPE** see Dipivefrin on page 571
◆ **D-Penicillamine** see PenicillAMINE on page 1493
◆ **DPH** see Phenytoin on page 1527
◆ **Dramamine® [OTC]** see DimenhyDRINATE on page 554
◆ **Dramamine® for kids [OTC]** see DimenhyDRINATE on page 554
◆ **Dramamine® Less Drowsy Formula [OTC]** see Meclizine on page 1186
◆ **Driminate [OTC]** see DimenhyDRINATE on page 554
◆ **Drisdol®** see Ergocalciferol on page 657
◆ **Dristan® [OTC]** see Oxymetazoline (Nasal) on page 1452

Dronabinol (droe NAB i nol)

Medication Safety Issues
Sound-alike/look-alike issues:
Dronabinol may be confused with droperidol
Brand Names: Canada Marinol®
Index Terms Delta-9 THC; Delta-9-tetrahydro-cannabinol; Tetrahydrocannabinol; THC
Generic Availability (U.S.) Yes
Pharmacologic Category Antiemetic; Appetite Stimulant
Use Chemotherapy-associated nausea and vomiting refractory to other antiemetic(s); AIDS-related anorexia
Unlabeled Use Cancer-related anorexia
Contraindications Hypersensitivity to dronabinol, cannabinoids, sesame oil, or any component of the formulation, or marijuana; should be avoided in patients with a history of schizophrenia
Warnings/Precautions Use with caution in patients with hepatic disease or seizure disorders. Reduce dosage in patients with severe hepatic impairment. May cause additive CNS effects with sedatives, hypnotics or other psychoactive agents; patients must be cautioned about performing tasks which require mental alertness (eg, operating machinery or driving).

May have potential for abuse; drug is psychoactive substance in marijuana; use caution in patients with a history of substance abuse or potential. May cause withdrawal symptoms upon abrupt discontinuation. Use with caution in patients with mania, depression, or schizophrenia; careful psychiatric monitoring is recommended. Use caution in elderly; they are more sensitive to adverse effects.

Adverse Reactions (Reflective of adult population; not specific for elderly) Frequency not always specified.

>1%:

Cardiovascular: Palpitations, tachycardia, vasodilation/facial flushing

Central nervous system: Euphoria (8% to 24%, dose related), abnormal thinking (3% to 10%), dizziness (3% to 10%), paranoia (3% to 10%), somnolence (3% to 10%), amnesia, anxiety, ataxia, confusion, depersonalization, hallucination

Gastrointestinal: Abdominal pain (3% to 10%), nausea (3% to 10%), vomiting (3% to 10%)

Neuromuscular & skeletal: Weakness

Drug Interactions

Metabolism/Transport Effects None known.

Avoid Concomitant Use

Avoid concomitant use of Dronabinol with any of the following: Azelastine; Azelastine (Nasal); Mirtazapine; Paraldehyde

Increased Effect/Toxicity

Dronabinol may increase the levels/effects of: Alcohol (Ethyl); Azelastine; Azelastine (Nasal); CNS Depressants; Methotrimeprazine; Metyrosine; Mirtazapine; Paraldehyde; Selective Serotonin Reuptake Inhibitors; Sympathomimetics; Zolpidem

The levels/effects of Dronabinol may be increased by: Anticholinergic Agents; Cocaine; Droperidol; HydrOXYzine; MAO Inhibitors; Methotrimeprazine; Ritonavir

Decreased Effect There are no known significant interactions involving a decrease in effect.

Ethanol/Nutrition/Herb Interactions

Ethanol: May increase CNS depression; monitor for increased effects with coadministration. Caution patients about effects.

Food: Administration with high-lipid meals may increase absorption.

Herb/Nutraceutical: St John's wort may decrease dronabinol levels.

Stability Store under refrigeration (or in a cool environment) between 8°C and 15°C (46°F and 59°F); protect from freezing.

Mechanism of Action Unknown, may inhibit endorphins in the brain's emetic center, suppress prostaglandin synthesis, and/or inhibit medullary activity through an unspecified cortical action. Some pharmacologic effects appear to involve sympathomometic activity; tachyphylaxis to some effect (eg, tachycardia) may occur, but appetite-stimulating effects do not appear to wane over time. Antiemetic activity may be due to effect on cannabinoid receptors (CB1) within the central nervous system.

Pharmacodynamics/Kinetics

Onset of action: Within 1 hour

Peak effect: 2-4 hours

Duration: 24 hours (appetite stimulation)

Absorption: Oral: 90% to 95%; 10% to 20% of dose gets into systemic circulation

Distribution: V_d: 10 L/kg; dronabinol is highly lipophilic and distributes to adipose tissue

Protein binding: 97% to 99%

Metabolism: Hepatic to at least 50 metabolites, some of which are active; 11-hydroxy-delta-9-tetrahydrocannabinol (11-OH-THC) is the major metabolite; extensive first-pass effect

Half-life elimination: Dronabinol: 25-36 hours (terminal); Dronabinol metabolites: 44-59 hours

Time to peak, serum: 0.5-4 hours

Excretion: Feces (50% as unconjugated metabolites, 5% as unchanged drug); urine (10% to 15% as acid metabolites and conjugates)

Dosage

Geriatric & Adult

Antiemetic: Oral: 5 mg/m^2 1-3 hours before chemotherapy, then give 5 mg/m^2/dose every 2-4 hours after chemotherapy for a total of 4-6 doses/day; dose may be increased up to a maximum of 15 mg/m^2/dose if needed (dosage may be increased by 2.5 mg/m^2 increments).

Appetite stimulant (AIDS-related): Oral: Initial: 2.5 mg twice daily (before lunch and dinner); titrate up to a maximum of 20 mg/day.

Hepatic Impairment Usual dose should be reduced in patients with severe liver failure.

Monitoring Parameters CNS effects, heart rate, blood pressure, behavioral profile

Reference Range Antinauseant effects: 5-10 ng/mL

Test Interactions Decreased FSH, LH, and testosterone

Special Geriatric Considerations Elderly patients may be more sensitive to the CNS effects and postural hypotensive effects of dronabinol. Titrate the dose slowly and monitor for adverse effects.

Controlled Substance C-III

◀ **Dosage Forms** Excipient information presented when available (limited, particularly for generics); consult specific product labeling.
Capsule, soft gelatin, oral: 2.5 mg [contains sesame oil], 5 mg [contains sesame oil], 10 mg [contains sesame oil]

Dronedarone (droe NE da rone)

Related Information
Beers Criteria – Potentially Inappropriate Medications for Geriatrics *on page 2183*
Medication Safety Issues
BEERS Criteria medication:
This drug may be potentially inappropriate for use in geriatric patients (Quality of evidence - moderate/high; Strength of recommendation - strong).
Brand Names: U.S. Multaq®
Brand Names: Canada Multaq®
Index Terms Dronedarone Hydrochloride; SR33589
Generic Availability (U.S.) No
Pharmacologic Category Antiarrhythmic Agent, Class III
Use To reduce the risk of hospitalization for atrial fibrillation (AF) in patients in sinus rhythm with a history of paroxysmal or persistent AF
Unlabeled Use Alternative antiarrhythmic for the treatment of atrial fibrillation in patients with hypertrophic cardiomyopathy (HCM)
Medication Guide Available Yes
Contraindications Permanent atrial fibrillation (patients in whom sinus rhythm will not or cannot be restored); symptomatic heart failure (HF with recent decompensation requiring hospitalization or NYHA Class IV symptoms; second- or third-degree heart block or sick sinus syndrome (except in patients with a functioning artificial pacemaker); bradycardia <50 bpm; concomitant use of strong CYP3A4 inhibitors (eg, ketoconazole, itraconazole, voriconazole, cyclosporine, telithromycin, clarithromycin, nefazodone, or ritonavir); concomitant use of drugs or herbal products known to prolong the QT interval increasing the risk for torsade de pointes (eg, phenothiazine antipsychotics, tricyclic antidepressants, certain oral macrolide antibiotics, or class I and III antiarrhythmics); QT$_c$ (Bazett) interval ≥500 msec or PR interval >280 msec; liver toxicity related to previous amiodarone use; severe hepatic impairment

Canadian labeling: Additional contraindications (not in U.S. labeling): Hypersensitivity to dronedarone or any component of the formulation; permanent atrial fibrillation of any duration where sinus rhythm cannot be restored and further attempts to restore it are no longer considered; history of or current heart failure regardless of NYHA class; left ventricular systolic dysfunction; sinus node dysfunction; atrial conduction defects; complete or distal bundle branch block, unstable hemodynamic conditions; pulmonary toxicity related to prior amiodarone use

Warnings/Precautions [U.S. Boxed Warning]: The risk of death is doubled when used in patients with symptomatic heart failure with recent decompensation requiring hospitalization or NYHA Class IV symptoms; use is contraindicated in these patients. New-onset or worsening HF symptoms have been observed in postmarketing studies. If patient develops new or worsening HF symptoms (eg, weight gain, dependent edema, or increasing shortness of breath) requiring hospitalization while on therapy, discontinue dronedarone. Canadian labeling contraindicates use of dronedarone in patients with a history of or current heart failure, regardless of NYHA class.

[U.S. Boxed Warning]: Use in patients with permanent atrial fibrillation doubles the risk of death, stroke and hospitalization for heart failure. Use is contraindicated in patients with AF who will not or can not be converted to normal sinus rhythm. Monitor ECG at least every 3 months. Cardiovert patients who are in AF (if clinically indicated) or discontinue dronedarone. Initiate appropriate antithrombotic therapy prior to starting dronedarone.

In the treatment of atrial fibrillation in the elderly, avoid antiarrhythmics as first-line treatment. In older adults, data suggests rate control may provide more benefits than risks compared to rhythm control for most patients. Avoid use in patients with permanent atrial fibrillation or heart failure (Beers Criteria).

Dronedarone induces a moderate prolongation of the QT interval (average ~10 msec); much greater effects have been observed. Use in patients with QT$_c$ (Bazett) interval ≥500 msec is contraindicated; discontinue use of dronedarone if this occurs during therapy. Following initiation, dronedarone may produce a slight increase in serum creatinine (~0.1 mg/dL) due to inhibition of tubular secretion; glomerular filtration rate is not affected; effect is reversible upon discontinuation. Interstitial lung disease (including pulmonary fibrosis and pneumonitis) has been reported with use. Evaluate patients with onset of dyspnea or nonproductive cough for pulmonary toxicity. Canadian labeling recommends discontinuing therapy with confirmed pulmonary toxicity.

Severe liver injury, including acute liver failure leading to liver transplant, has been rarely reported. If liver injury is suspected, discontinue therapy and evaluate liver enzymes/bilirubin. Appropriate treatment should be started and therapy should not be reinitiated if liver injury is confirmed. Advise patients to report any signs or symptoms of hepatic injury (unusual fatigue, jaundice, nausea, vomiting, abdominal pain, and/or fever). Consider periodic monitoring of serum liver enzymes and bilirubin, especially during the first 6 months of therapy. Use with caution in patients with mild-to-moderate hepatic impairment; use is contraindicated in severe hepatic impairment.

Chronic administration of antiarrhythmic drugs may affect defibrillation or pacing thresholds; assess when initiating dronedarone and during therapy. Correct electrolyte disturbances, especially hypokalemia or hypomagnesemia, prior to use and throughout therapy. Dronedarone is a moderate inhibitor of CYP3A4 and CYP2D6 enzymes and has potential to inhibit p-glycoprotein, which may lead to increased serum concentrations/toxicity of a number of medications. Use caution when initiating dronedarone in patients on warfarin. Cases of increased INR with or without bleeding have occurred in patients treated with warfarin; monitor INR closely after initiating dronedarone in these patients. Initiate appropriate antithrombotic therapy prior to starting dronedarone.

Adverse Reactions (Reflective of adult population; not specific for elderly)

>10%:

Cardiovascular: QT_c (Bazett) prolongation (28% [placebo: 19%]; defined as >450 msec in males or >470 msec in females)

Renal: Serum creatinine increased ≥10% (51%; occurred 5 days after initiation)

1% to 10%:

Cardiovascular: Bradycardia (3%)

Dermatologic: Allergic dermatitis (≤5%), dermatitis (≤5%), eczema (≤5%), pruritus (≤5%), rash (≤5%; described as generalized, macular, maculopapular, erythematous)

Gastrointestinal: Diarrhea (9%), nausea (5%), abdominal pain (4%), dyspepsia (2%), vomiting (2%)

Neuromuscular & skeletal: Weakness (7%)

Drug Interactions

Metabolism/Transport Effects Substrate of CYP3A4 (major); **Note:** Assignment of Major/Minor substrate status based on clinically relevant drug interaction potential; **Inhibits** CYP2D6 (moderate), CYP3A4 (moderate), P-glycoprotein

Avoid Concomitant Use

Avoid concomitant use of Dronedarone with any of the following: CycloSPORINE; CycloSPORINE (Systemic); CYP3A4 Inducers (Strong); CYP3A4 Inhibitors (Strong); Fingolimod; Grapefruit Juice; Highest Risk QTc-Prolonging Agents; Mifepristone; Moderate Risk QTc-Prolonging Agents; Propafenone; Silodosin; St Johns Wort; Tolvaptan; Topotecan

Increased Effect/Toxicity

Dronedarone may increase the levels/effects of: ARIPiprazole; AtorvaSTATin; Avanafil; Beta-Blockers; Budesonide (Systemic, Oral Inhalation); Calcium Channel Blockers (Nondihydropyridine); Colchicine; CYP2D6 Substrates; CYP3A4 Substrates; Dabigatran Etexilate; Digoxin; DOCEtaxel; Eplerenone; Everolimus; FentaNYL; Fesoterodine; Highest Risk QTc-Prolonging Agents; Ivacaftor; Lidocaine (Topical); Lovastatin; Lurasidone; P-glycoprotein/ABCB1 Substrates; Pimecrolimus; Prucalopride; Red Yeast Rice; Rivaroxaban; Salmeterol; Saxagliptin; Silodosin; Simvastatin; Tolvaptan; Topotecan; Vilazodone; Vitamin K Antagonists

The levels/effects of Dronedarone may be increased by: Calcium Channel Blockers (Nondihydropyridine); CycloSPORINE; CycloSPORINE (Systemic); CYP3A4 Inhibitors (Moderate); CYP3A4 Inhibitors (Strong); Digoxin; EriBULin; Fingolimod; Grapefruit Juice; Ivacaftor; Lidocaine (Topical); Mifepristone; Moderate Risk QTc-Prolonging Agents; Propafenone; QTc-Prolonging Agents (Indeterminate Risk and Risk Modifying)

Decreased Effect

Dronedarone may decrease the levels/effects of: Codeine; Ifosfamide; TraMADol

The levels/effects of Dronedarone may be decreased by: CYP3A4 Inducers (Strong); Deferasirox; St Johns Wort; Tocilizumab

Ethanol/Nutrition/Herb Interactions

Food: Food increases the rate and extent of absorption of dronedarone; bioavailability is increased 11% with a high-fat meal. Grapefruit juice increases bioavailability of dronedarone threefold; altered effects are possible. Management: Take with food. Grapefruit/grapefruit juice should be avoided during therapy.

Herb/Nutraceutical: St John's wort may decrease dronedarone levels; ephedra may worsen arrhythmia. Management: Avoid St John's wort, ephedra, and dong quai.

DRONEDARONE

Stability Store at 25°C (77°F); excursions permitted to 15°C to 30°C (59°F to 86°F).

Mechanism of Action A noniodinated antiarrhythmic agent structurally related to amiodarone exhibiting properties of all 4 antiarrhythmic classes. Dronedarone inhibits sodium (I_{Na}) and potassium (I_{kr}, I_{Ks}, I_{k1}, and I_{k-ACh}) channels resulting in prolongation of the action potential and refractory period in myocardial tissue without reverse-use dependent effects; decreases AV conduction and sinus node function through inhibition of calcium (I_{Ca-L}) channels and beta$_1$-receptor blocking activity. Similar to amiodarone, dronedarone also inhibits alpha$_1$-receptor mediated increases in blood pressure.

Pharmacodynamics/Kinetics
Distribution: V_d: ~20 L/kg (based on a 70 kg patient)
Protein binding: >98%
Metabolism: Hepatic via CYP3A4 to active N-debutyl metabolite ($^1/_{10}$ to $^1/_3$ as potent as dronedarone) and other inactive metabolites
Bioavailability: Oral: Without food: 4%; With high-fat meal: 15%
Half-life elimination: 13-19 hours
Time to peak, plasma: 3-6 hours
Excretion: Feces (84% mainly as metabolites); urine (~6% mainly as metabolites)

Dosage
Geriatric & Adult Atrial fibrillation/atrial flutter: Oral: 400 mg twice daily
Renal Impairment No dosage adjustment necessary.
Hepatic Impairment
Mild-to-moderate impairment: No dosage adjustment necessary
Severe impairment: Contraindicated

Administration Administer with morning and evening meal.

Monitoring Parameters ECG (at least every 3 months), blood pressure, heart rate and rhythm throughout therapy; assess patient for signs of lethargy, edema of the hands or feet; monitor serum electrolytes, especially potassium and magnesium; serum liver enzymes and bilirubin (periodically, especially during the first 6 months of therapy)

Patients with implantable cardiac devices: Monitor pacing or defibrillation thresholds with initiation of dronedarone and during treatment.

Canadian labeling: Additional monitoring recommendations: ECG at least every 6 months during therapy; serum creatinine 1 week after initiating therapy followed by periodic renal function tests; periodic pulmonary function assessment

Special Geriatric Considerations Clinical studies, involving over 2000 patients 75 years of age and older, did not demonstrate any difference in safety and efficacy between younger adults and elderly. No dosage adjustments necessary for age.

This medication is considered to be potentially inappropriate in this patient population (Beers Criteria: Quality of evidence - moderate/high; Strength of recommendation - strong).

Dosage Forms Excipient information presented when available (limited, particularly for generics); consult specific product labeling.
Tablet, oral:
Multaq®: 400 mg

◆ **Dronedarone Hydrochloride** see Dronedarone on page 612

Droperidol (droe PER i dole)

Medication Safety Issues
Sound-alike/look-alike issues:
Droperidol may be confused with dronabinol
Brand Names: Canada Droperidol Injection, USP
Index Terms Dehydrobenzperidol
Generic Availability (U.S.) Yes
Pharmacologic Category Antiemetic; Antipsychotic Agent, Typical
Use Prevention and/or treatment of nausea and vomiting from surgical and diagnostic procedures
Contraindications Hypersensitivity to droperidol or any component of the formulation; known or suspected QT prolongation, including congenital long QT syndrome (prolonged QT_c is defined as >440 msec in males or >450 msec in females)
Warnings/Precautions May alter cardiac conduction. **[U.S. Boxed Warning]: Cases of QT prolongation and torsade de pointes, including some fatal cases, have been reported.** Use extreme caution in patients with bradycardia (<50 bpm), cardiac disease, concurrent MAO inhibitor therapy, Class I and Class III antiarrhythmics or other drugs known to prolong QT interval, and electrolyte disturbances (hypokalemia or hypomagnesemia), including concomitant drugs which may alter electrolytes (diuretics).

Use with caution in patients with seizures or severe liver disease. May be sedating, use with caution in disorders where CNS depression is a feature. Caution in patients with hemodynamic instability, predisposition to seizures, subcortical brain damage, pheochromocytoma or renal disease. Esophageal dysmotility and aspiration have been associated with antipsychotic use - use with caution in patients at risk of pneumonia (ie, Alzheimer's disease). Caution in breast cancer or other prolactin-dependent tumors (may elevate prolactin levels). May alter temperature regulation or mask toxicity of other drugs due to antiemetic effects. May cause orthostatic hypotension - use with caution in patients at risk of this effect or those who would tolerate transient hypotensive episodes (cerebrovascular disease, cardiovascular disease, or other medications which may predispose). Significant hypotension may occur.

May cause anticholinergic effects (confusion, agitation, constipation, xerostomia, blurred vision, urinary retention). Therefore, they should be used with caution in patients with decreased gastrointestinal motility, urinary retention, BPH, xerostomia, or visual problems. Conditions which also may be exacerbated by cholinergic blockade include narrow-angle glaucoma (screening is recommended) and worsening of myasthenia gravis. Relative to other neuroleptics, droperidol has a low potency of cholinergic blockade.

May cause extrapyramidal symptoms (EPS), including pseudoparkinsonism, acute dystonic reactions, akathisia, and tardive dyskinesia. Risk of dystonia (and possibly other EPS) may be greater with increased doses, use of conventional antipsychotics, males, and younger patients. May be associated with neuroleptic malignant syndrome (NMS). May mask toxicity of other drugs or conditions (eg, intestinal obstruction, Reye's syndrome, brain tumor) due to antiemetic effects. Use with caution in the elderly; reduce initial dose.

Adverse Reactions (Reflective of adult population; not specific for elderly) Frequency not defined.
Cardiovascular: Cardiac arrest, hypertension, hypotension (especially orthostatic), QT_c prolongation (dose dependent), tachycardia, torsade de pointes, ventricular tachycardia
Central nervous system: Anxiety, chills, depression (postoperative, transient), dizziness, drowsiness (postoperative) increased, dysphoria, extrapyramidal symptoms (akathisia, dystonia, oculogyric crisis), hallucinations (postoperative), hyperactivity, neuroleptic malignant syndrome (NMS) (rare), restlessness
Respiratory: Bronchospasm, laryngospasm
Miscellaneous: Anaphylaxis, shivering

Drug Interactions
Metabolism/Transport Effects None known.
Avoid Concomitant Use
Avoid concomitant use of Droperidol with any of the following: Azelastine; Azelastine (Nasal); Highest Risk QTc-Prolonging Agents; Metoclopramide; Mifepristone; Paraldehyde
Increased Effect/Toxicity
Droperidol may increase the levels/effects of: Alcohol (Ethyl); Anticholinergics; Azelastine; Azelastine (Nasal); Buprenorphine; CNS Depressants; Highest Risk QTc-Prolonging Agents; Methylphenidate; Metoclopramide; Moderate Risk QTc-Prolonging Agents; Paraldehyde; Serotonin Modulators; Zolpidem

The levels/effects of Droperidol may be increased by: Acetylcholinesterase Inhibitors (Central); HydrOXYzine; Lithium formulations; MAO Inhibitors; Methylphenidate; Metoclopramide; Metyrosine; Mifepristone; Pramlintide; QTc-Prolonging Agents (Indeterminate Risk and Risk Modifying); Tetrabenazine
Decreased Effect
Droperidol may decrease the levels/effects of: Amphetamines; Anti-Parkinson's Agents (Dopamine Agonist); Quinagolide

The levels/effects of Droperidol may be decreased by: Anti-Parkinson's Agents (Dopamine Agonist); Lithium formulations
Stability Store at 20°C to 25°C (68°F to 77°F); excursions permitted to 15°C to 30°C (59°F to 86°F). Protect from light. Solutions diluted in NS or D_5W are stable at room temperature for up to 7 days in PVC bags or glass bottles. Solutions diluted in LR are stable at room temperature for 24 hours in PVC bags and up to 7 days in glass bottles.
Mechanism of Action Droperidol is a butyrophenone antipsychotic; antiemetic effect is a result of blockade of dopamine stimulation of the chemoreceptor trigger zone. Other effects include alpha-adrenergic blockade, peripheral vascular dilation, and reduction of the pressor effect of epinephrine resulting in hypotension and decreased peripheral vascular resistance; may also reduce pulmonary artery pressure
Pharmacodynamics/Kinetics
Onset of action: 3-10 minutes
Peak effect: ~30 minutes
Duration: 2-4 hours, may extend to 12 hours
Absorption: I.M.: Rapid

Distribution: Crosses blood-brain barrier and placenta
    Adults: ~1.5 L/kg
Protein binding: 85% to 90%
Metabolism: Hepatic, to *p*-fluorophenylacetic acid, benzimidazolone, *p*-hydroxypiperidine
Half-life elimination: ~2.3 hours
Excretion: Urine (75%, <1% as unchanged drug); feces (22%, 11% as unchanged drug)

Dosage

Geriatric & Adult Note: Titrate carefully to desired effect

Prevention of PONV: I.M., I.V.:
    Manufacturer's labeling: Maximum initial dose: 2.5 mg; additional doses of 1.25 mg may be administered with caution to achieve desired effect
    Consensus guideline recommendations: 0.625-1.25 mg I.V. administered at the end of surgery (Gan, 2007)

Canadian labeling:
    Prevention and treatment of PONV: I.V.: 0.625-1.25 mg 30 minutes prior to anticipated end of surgery, and then every 6 hours as needed for breakthrough PONV

Renal Impairment
    U.S. labeling: Specific dosing recommendations are not provided; use with caution.
    Canadian labeling: I.V.: 0.625 mg; additional dosing should be administered with caution.

Hepatic Impairment
    U.S. labeling: Specific dosing recommendations are not provided; use with caution.
    Canadian labeling: I.V.: 0.625 mg; additional dosing should be administered with caution.

Administration Administer I.M. or I.V.; according to the manufacturer, I.V. push administration should be slow (generally regarded as 2-5 minutes); however, many clinicians administer I.V. doses rapidly (over 30-60 seconds) in an effort to reduce the incidence of EPS. The effect, if any, of rapid administration on QT prolongation is unclear. For I.V. infusion, dilute in 50-100 mL NS or D_5W; ECG monitoring for 2-3 hours after administration is recommended regardless of rate of infusion.

Monitoring Parameters To identify QT prolongation, a 12-lead ECG prior to use is recommended; continued ECG monitoring for 2-3 hours following administration is recommended. Vital signs; serum magnesium and potassium; mental status, abnormal involuntary movement scale (AIMS); observe for dystonias, extrapyramidal side effects, and temperature changes

Pharmacotherapy Pearls Has good antiemetic effect as well as sedative and antianxiety effects

Special Geriatric Considerations Many elderly patients receive antipsychotic medications for inappropriate nonpsychotic behavior although the use of droperidol is seldom used for this indication. Since elderly frequently have cardiac disease which may result in QT prolongation, evaluation should be made prior to considering use of this agent.

Dosage Forms Excipient information presented when available (limited, particularly for generics); consult specific product labeling.
Injection, solution: 2.5 mg/mL (2 mL)
Injection, solution [preservative free]: 2.5 mg/mL (2 mL)

Drospirenone and Estradiol (droh SPYE re none & es tra DYE ole)

Related Information
Beers Criteria – Potentially Inappropriate Medications for Geriatrics *on page 2183*

Medication Safety Issues
BEERS Criteria medication:
This drug may be potentially inappropriate for use in geriatric patients (Quality of evidence - high [oral and transdermal patch]; Strength of recommendation - strong [oral and transdermal patch]).

Brand Names: U.S. Angeliq®
Brand Names: Canada Angeliq®
Index Terms E2 and DRSP; Estradiol and Drospirenone
Generic Availability (U.S.) No
Pharmacologic Category Estrogen and Progestin Combination
Use Treatment of moderate-to-severe vasomotor symptoms associated with menopause; treatment of vulvar and vaginal atrophy associated with menopause
Contraindications Hypersensitivity to drospirenone, estradiol, or any component of the formulation; undiagnosed abnormal vaginal bleeding; history of or current thrombophlebitis or venous thromboembolic disorders (including DVT, PE); active or recent (within 1 year) arterial thromboembolic disease (eg, stroke, MI); carcinoma of the breast; estrogen-dependent tumor; hepatic or renal dysfunction or disease; adrenal insufficiency

Warnings/Precautions Drospirenone has antimineralocorticoid activity that may lead to hyperkalemia in patients with renal insufficiency, hepatic dysfunction, or adrenal insufficiency. Use caution with medications that may increase serum potassium.

Cardiovascular-related considerations: Estrogens with or without progestin should not be used to prevent coronary heart disease. Use caution with cardiovascular disease or dysfunction. May increase the risks of hypertension, myocardial infarction (MI), stroke, pulmonary emboli (PE), and deep vein thrombosis; incidence of these effects was shown to be significantly increased in postmenopausal women using conjugated equine estrogens (CEE) in combination with medroxyprogesterone acetate (MPA). Nonfatal MI, PE, and thrombophlebitis have also been reported in males taking high doses of CEE (eg, for prostate cancer). Estrogen compounds are generally associated with lipid effects such as increased HDL-cholesterol and decreased LDL-cholesterol. Triglycerides may also be increased; use with caution in patients with familial defects of lipoprotein metabolism. Whenever possible, estrogens should be discontinued at least 4 weeks prior to and for 2 weeks following elective surgery associated with an increased risk of thromboembolism or during periods of prolonged immobilization.

Neurological considerations: The risk of dementia may be increased in postmenopausal women; increased incidence was observed in women ≥65 years of age taking CEE alone or in combination with MPA.

Cancer-related considerations: Unopposed estrogens may increase the risk of endometrial carcinoma in postmenopausal women. Estrogens may exacerbate endometriosis. Malignant transformation of residual endometrial implants has been reported posthysterectomy with estrogen only therapy. Estrogens may increase the risk of breast cancer. An increased risk of invasive breast cancer was observed in postmenopausal women using CEE in combination with MPA; a smaller increase in risk was seen with estrogen therapy alone in observational studies. An increase in abnormal mammograms has also been reported with estrogen and progestin therapy. Estrogen use may lead to severe hypercalcemia in patients with breast cancer and bone metastases; discontinue estrogen if hypercalcemia occurs. Postmenopausal estrogen therapy and combined estrogen/progesterone therapy may increase the risk of ovarian cancer; however, the absolute risk to an individual woman is small. Although results from various studies are not consistent, risk does not appear to be significantly associated with the duration, route, or dose of therapy. In one study, the risk decreased after 2 years following discontinuation of therapy.

Estrogens may cause retinal vascular thrombosis; discontinue permanently if papilledema or retinal vascular lesions are observed on examination. Use with caution in patients with diseases which may be exacerbated by fluid retention, including asthma, epilepsy, migraine, diabetes, or renal dysfunction. Use with caution in patients with a history of severe hypocalcemia, SLE, hepatic hemangiomas, porphyria, endometriosis, and gallbladder disease. Use caution with history of cholestatic jaundice associated with past estrogen use.

Before prescribing estrogen therapy to postmenopausal women, the risks and benefits must be weighed for each patient. Women should be informed of these risks and benefits, as well as possible effects of progestin when added to estrogen therapy. Estrogens with or without progestin should be used for shortest duration possible consistent with treatment goals. Conduct periodic risk:benefit assessments. When used solely for the treatment of vulvar and vaginal atrophy, topical vaginal products should be considered. Not for use prior to menopause.

Adverse Reactions (Reflective of adult population; not specific for elderly)
>10%:
  Endocrine & metabolic: Breast pain (6% to 18%)
  Genitourinary: Genital tract bleeding (3% to 14%)
1% to 10%:
  Central nervous system: Emotional lability (1%), migraine (≤1%)
  Gastrointestinal: Abdominal/GI pain (4% to 7%)
  Genitourinary: Cervical polyp (≤1%)
Drug Interactions
  Metabolism/Transport Effects Refer to individual components.
  Avoid Concomitant Use
  Avoid concomitant use of Drospirenone and Estradiol with any of the following: Anastrozole; Axitinib; Boceprevir; CycloSPORINE; CycloSPORINE (Systemic); Griseofulvin; Pimozide; Tacrolimus; Tacrolimus (Systemic)
  Increased Effect/Toxicity
  Drospirenone and Estradiol may increase the levels/effects of: ACE Inhibitors; Amifostine; Ammonium Chloride; Antihypertensives; ARIPiprazole; Benzodiazepines (metabolized by oxidation); Cardiac Glycosides; Corticosteroids (Systemic); CycloSPORINE;

CycloSPORINE (Systemic); Hypotensive Agents; Pimozide; Potassium-Sparing Diuretics; RiTUXimab; ROPINIRole; Selegiline; Sodium Phosphates; Tacrolimus; Tacrolimus (Systemic); Tipranavir; Tranexamic Acid; Voriconazole

The levels/effects of Drospirenone and Estradiol may be increased by: Alfuzosin; Angiotensin II Receptor Blockers; Ascorbic Acid; Boceprevir; Diazoxide; Eplerenone; Herbs (Estrogenic Properties); Herbs (Hypotensive Properties); Herbs (Progestogenic Properties); MAO Inhibitors; Mifepristone; Nonsteroidal Anti-Inflammatory Agents; Pentoxifylline; P-glycoprotein/ABCB1 Inhibitors; Phosphodiesterase 5 Inhibitors; Potassium Salts; Prostacyclin Analogues; Tolvaptan; Voriconazole

Decreased Effect

Drospirenone and Estradiol may decrease the levels/effects of: Anastrozole; ARIPiprazole; Axitinib; Cardiac Glycosides; Chenodiol; Hyaluronidase; QuiNIDine; Saxagliptin; Somatropin; Thyroid Products; Ursodiol; Vitamin K Antagonists

The levels/effects of Drospirenone and Estradiol may be decreased by: Acitretin; Aminoglutethimide; Aprepitant; Artemether; Barbiturates; Bexarotene; Bexarotene (Systemic); Bile Acid Sequestrants; Bosentan; CarBAMazepine; Clobazam; CYP1A2 Inducers (Strong); CYP3A4 Inducers (Strong); Cyproterone; Deferasirox; Felbamate; Fosaprepitant; Fosphenytoin; Griseofulvin; Herbs (Hypertensive Properties); LamoTRIgine; Methylphenidate; Mifepristone; Mycophenolate; Nevirapine; Nonsteroidal Anti-Inflammatory Agents; OXcarbazepine; Peginterferon Alfa-2b; P-glycoprotein/ABCB1 Inducers; Phenytoin; Prucalopride; Retinoic Acid Derivatives; Rifamycin Derivatives; St Johns Wort; Telaprevir; Tipranavir; Tocilizumab; Topiramate; Yohimbine

Ethanol/Nutrition/Herb Interactions Ethanol: Avoid ethanol (routine use increases estrogen level and risk of breast cancer). Ethanol may also increase the risk of osteoporosis.

Stability Store at controlled room temperature of 15°C to 30°C (59°F to 86°F).

Mechanism of Action

Drospirenone is a synthetic progestin and spironolactone analog with antimineralocorticoid and antiandrogenic activity. Counteracts estrogen effects causing endometrial thinning.

Estrogens are responsible for the development and maintenance of the female reproductive system and secondary sexual characteristics. Estradiol is the principal intracellular human estrogen and is more potent than estrone and estriol at the receptor level; it is the primary estrogen secreted prior to menopause. Following menopause, estrone and estrone sulfate are more highly produced. Estrogens modulate the pituitary secretion of gonadotropins, luteinizing hormone, and follicle-stimulating hormone through a negative feedback system; estrogen replacement reduces elevated levels of these hormones in postmenopausal women.

Pharmacodynamics/Kinetics

Distribution: Drospirenone: 4.2 L/kg

Protein binding:

Drospirenone: 97%; does not bind to sex hormone binding globulin or corticosteroid binding globulin

Estradiol: 37% bound to sex hormone binding globulin; 61% bound to albumin

Metabolism: Hepatic

Drospirenone forms two metabolites (inactive)

Estradiol: Converted to estrone and estriol; also undergoes enterohepatic recirculation; estrone sulfite is the main metabolite in postmenopausal women

Bioavailability: Drospirenone: 76% to 85%

Half-life elimination: Drospirenone: ~36-42 hours

Time to peak, plasma: Drospirenone: 1 hour; Estradiol: ~2 hours (range: 0.3-10 hours)

Excretion: Drospirenone: Urine and feces; Estradiol: Urine

Dosage

Geriatric & Adult

Moderate-to-severe vasomotor symptoms associated with menopause: Oral: Drospirenone 0.25 mg/estradiol 0.5 mg or drospirenone 0.5 mg/estradiol 1 mg per tablet: One tablet daily.

Atrophic vaginitis in females with an intact uterus: Oral: Drospirenone 0.5 mg/estradiol 1 mg per tablet: One tablet daily.

Note: The lowest dose of estrogen/progestin that will control symptoms should be used; medication should be discontinued as soon as possible. Patients should be re-evaluated periodically to see if treatment is still necessary.

Renal Impairment Use is contraindicated.

Hepatic Impairment Use is contraindicated.

Administration Tablets should be swallowed whole and taken at the same time each day. Bleeding may occur if several doses are missed. Women who are not taking estrogen or who are changing from a continuous combination product may start therapy at any time. Women who are switching from sequential or cyclic hormone therapy should complete the current cycle before switching to this product.

Monitoring Parameters Yearly physical examination that includes blood pressure and Papanicolaou smear, breast exam, mammogram. Monitor for signs of endometrial cancer. Adequate diagnostic measures, including endometrial sampling, if indicated, should be performed to rule out malignancy in all cases of undiagnosed abnormal vaginal bleeding. Monitor for loss of vision, sudden onset of proptosis, diplopia, migraine; signs and symptoms of thromboembolic disorders; glycemic control in patients with diabetes; lipid profiles in patients being treated for hyperlipidemias; thyroid function in patients on thyroid hormone replacement therapy.

Menopausal symptoms: Assess need for therapy periodically

Test Interactions Reduced response to metyrapone test.

Special Geriatric Considerations Before prescribing estrogen therapy to postmenopausal women, the risks and benefits must be weighed for each patient. Women should be informed of these risks and benefits, as well as possible side effects and the return of menstrual bleeding (when cycled with a progestin), and be involved in the decision to prescribe. A higher incidence of stroke and invasive breast cancer was observed in women >75 years in a WHI substudy. Oral therapy may be more convenient for vaginal atrophy and urinary incontinence.

This medication is considered to be potentially inappropriate in this patient population (Beers Criteria: Quality of evidence - high [oral and transdermal patch]; Strength of recommendation - strong [oral and transdermal patch]).

Product Availability Angeliq® (drospirenone 0.25 mg and estradiol 0.5 mg) tablets: FDA approved March 2012; anticipated availability currently undetermined

Dosage Forms Excipient information presented when available (limited, particularly for generics); consult specific product labeling.
Tablet:
Angeliq®: Drospirenone 0.5 mg and estradiol 1 mg

- ◆ **Droxia®** *see* Hydroxyurea *on page 955*
- ◆ **Dr. Scholl's® Callus Removers [OTC]** *see* Salicylic Acid *on page 1743*
- ◆ **Dr. Scholl's® Clear Away® One Step Wart Remover [OTC]** *see* Salicylic Acid *on page 1743*
- ◆ **Dr. Scholl's® Clear Away® Plantar Wart Remover For Feet [OTC]** *see* Salicylic Acid *on page 1743*
- ◆ **Dr. Scholl's® Clear Away® Wart Remover [OTC]** *see* Salicylic Acid *on page 1743*
- ◆ **Dr. Scholl's® Clear Away® Wart Remover Fast-Acting [OTC]** *see* Salicylic Acid *on page 1743*
- ◆ **Dr. Scholl's® Clear Away® Wart Remover Invisible Strips [OTC]** *see* Salicylic Acid *on page 1743*
- ◆ **Dr. Scholl's® Corn/Callus Remover [OTC]** *see* Salicylic Acid *on page 1743*
- ◆ **Dr. Scholl's® Corn Removers [OTC]** *see* Salicylic Acid *on page 1743*
- ◆ **Dr. Scholl's® Extra-Thick Callus Removers [OTC]** *see* Salicylic Acid *on page 1743*
- ◆ **Dr. Scholl's® Extra Thick Corn Removers [OTC]** *see* Salicylic Acid *on page 1743*
- ◆ **Dr. Scholl's® For Her Corn Removers [OTC]** *see* Salicylic Acid *on page 1743*
- ◆ **Dr. Scholl's® OneStep Callus Removers [OTC]** *see* Salicylic Acid *on page 1743*
- ◆ **Dr. Scholl's® OneStep Corn Removers [OTC]** *see* Salicylic Acid *on page 1743*
- ◆ **Dr. Scholl's® Small Corn Removers [OTC]** *see* Salicylic Acid *on page 1743*
- ◆ **Dr. Scholl's® Ultra-Thin Corn Removers [OTC]** *see* Salicylic Acid *on page 1743*
- ◆ **DSCG** *see* Cromolyn (Nasal) *on page 450*
- ◆ **DSCG** *see* Cromolyn (Ophthalmic) *on page 450*
- ◆ **DSCG** *see* Cromolyn (Systemic, Oral Inhalation) *on page 449*
- ◆ **DSS** *see* Docusate *on page 583*
- ◆ **DSS® [OTC]** *see* Docusate *on page 583*
- ◆ **DT** *see* Diphtheria and Tetanus Toxoids *on page 562*
- ◆ **DTaP** *see* Diphtheria and Tetanus Toxoids, and Acellular Pertussis Vaccine *on page 567*
- ◆ **DTaP-IPV** *see* Diphtheria and Tetanus Toxoids, Acellular Pertussis, and Poliovirus Vaccine *on page 565*
- ◆ **D-Trp(6)-LHRH** *see* Triptorelin *on page 1976*
- ◆ **Duetact™** *see* Pioglitazone and Glimepiride *on page 1544*
- ◆ **Duexis®** *see* Ibuprofen and Famotidine *on page 971*
- ◆ **Dulcolax® [OTC]** *see* Bisacodyl *on page 214*
- ◆ **Dulcolax® [OTC]** *see* Docusate *on page 583*
- ◆ **Dulcolax Balance® [OTC]** *see* Polyethylene Glycol 3350 *on page 1564*
- ◆ **Dulcolax® Stool Softener [OTC]** *see* Docusate *on page 583*
- ◆ **Dulera®** *see* Mometasone and Formoterol *on page 1307*
- ◆ **Dull-C® [OTC]** *see* Ascorbic Acid *on page 149*

DULoxetine (doo LOX e teen)

Related Information
Antidepressant Agents *on page 2097*

Medication Safety Issues
Sound-alike/look-alike issues:
Cymbalta® may be confused with Symbyax®
DULoxetine may be confused with FLUoxetine
BEERS Criteria medication:
This drug may be potentially inappropriate for use in geriatric patients (Quality of evidence - moderate; Strength of recommendation - strong).

Brand Names: U.S. Cymbalta®
Brand Names: Canada Cymbalta®
Index Terms (+)-(S)-N-Methyl-γ-(1-naphthyloxy)-2-thiophenepropylamine Hydrochloride; Duloxetine Hydrochloride; LY248686
Generic Availability (U.S.) No
Pharmacologic Category Antidepressant, Serotonin/Norepinephrine Reuptake Inhibitor
Use Acute and maintenance treatment of major depressive disorder (MDD); treatment of generalized anxiety disorder (GAD); management of diabetic peripheral neuropathic pain (DPNP); management of fibromyalgia (FM); chronic musculoskeletal pain (eg, chronic low back pain, osteoarthritis)
Unlabeled Use Treatment of stress incontinence
Medication Guide Available Yes
Contraindications Concomitant use or within 2 weeks of MAO inhibitors; uncontrolled narrow-angle glaucoma
Note: MAO inhibitor therapy must be stopped for 14 days before duloxetine is initiated. Treatment with MAO inhibitors should not be initiated until 5 days after the discontinuation of duloxetine.

Canadian labeling: Additional contraindications (not in U.S. labeling): Hypersensitivity to duloxetine or any component of the formulation; hepatic impairment; severe renal impairment (eg, Cl$_{cr}$ <30 mL/minute) or end-stage renal disease (ESRD); concomitant use with thioridazine or with CYP1A2 inhibitors

Warnings/Precautions Short-term studies did not show an increased risk in patients >24 years of age and showed a decreased risk in patients ≥65 years. Closely monitor for clinical worsening, suicidality, or unusual changes in behavior; the patient's family or caregiver should be instructed to closely observe the patient and communicate condition with healthcare provider.

The possibility of a suicide attempt is inherent in major depression and may persist until remission occurs. Patients treated with antidepressants should be observed for clinical worsening and suicidality, especially during the initial (generally first 1-2 months) few months of a course of drug therapy, or at times of dose changes, either increases or decreases. Use caution in high-risk patients. Worsening depression and severe abrupt suicidality that are not part of the presenting symptoms may require discontinuation or modification of drug therapy. The patient's family or caregiver should be alerted to monitor patients for the emergence of suicidality and associated behaviors (such as agitation, irritability, hostility, impulsivity, and hypomania) and call healthcare provider.

May worsen psychosis in some patients or precipitate a shift to mania or hypomania in patients with bipolar disorder. Patients presenting with depressive symptoms should be screened for bipolar disorder. Monotherapy in patients with bipolar disorder should be avoided. **Duloxetine is not FDA approved for the treatment of bipolar depression.**

May cause orthostatic hypotension/syncope at therapeutic doses especially within the first week of therapy and after dose increases. Monitor blood pressure with initiation of therapy, dose increases (especially in patients receiving >60 mg/day), or with concomitant use of vasodilators, CYP2D6 inhibitors/substrates, or CYP1A2 inhibitors. Use caution in patients with hypertension. May increase blood pressure. Rare cases of hypertensive crisis have been reported in patients with pre-existing hypertension; evaluate blood pressure prior to initiating therapy and periodically thereafter; consider dose reduction or gradual discontinuation of therapy in individuals with sustained hypertension during therapy.

Modest increases in serum glucose and hemoglobin A$_{1c}$ (Hb A$_{1c}$) levels have been observed in some diabetic patients receiving duloxetine therapy for diabetic peripheral neuropathic pain (DPNP). Duloxetine may cause increased urinary resistance; advise patient to report symptoms of urinary hesitation/difficulty. Has a low potential to impair cognitive or motor performance. Use caution with a previous seizure disorder or condition predisposing to seizures such as brain damage or alcoholism. Avoid use in patients with substantial ethanol intake, evidence of chronic liver disease, or hepatic impairment (contraindicated in Canadian labeling). Rare cases of hepatic failure (including fatalities) have been reported with use. Hepatitis with abdominal pain, hepatomegaly, elevated transaminase levels >20 times the upper limit of normal (ULN) with and without jaundice have been observed. Discontinue therapy with the presentation of jaundice or other signs of hepatic dysfunction and do not reinitiate therapy unless another source or cause is identified. Use caution in patients with impaired gastric motility (eg, some diabetics) may affect stability of the capsule's enteric coating.

May cause hyponatremia/SIADH (elderly at increased risk); volume depletion (diuretics may increase risk). Use with caution in patients with controlled narrow angle glaucoma. May cause or exacerbate sexual dysfunction. Use caution with renal impairment (contraindicated in Canadian labeling for severe renal impairment or ESRD). Use caution with concomitant CNS depressants. May impair platelet aggregation; use caution with concomitant use of NSAIDs, ASA, or other drugs that affect coagulation; the risk of bleeding may be potentiated.

Serotonin syndrome and neuroleptic malignant syndrome (NMS)-like reactions have occurred with serotonin/norepinephrine reuptake inhibitors (SNRIs) and selective serotonin reuptake inhibitors (SSRIs) when used alone, and particularly when used in combination with serotonergic agents (eg, triptans) or antidopaminergic agents (eg, antipsychotics). Concurrent use with MAO inhibitors is contraindicated. Use caution during concurrent therapy with triptans and drugs which lower the seizure threshold; concurrent use of serotonin precursors (eg, tryptophan) is not recommended. To discontinue therapy with duloxetine, gradually taper dose. If intolerable symptoms occur following a decrease in dosage or upon discontinuation of therapy, then resuming the previous dose with a more gradual taper should be considered. May increase the risks associated with electroconvulsive therapy. Consider discontinuing, when possible, prior to elective surgery. Use caution in elderly patients; may cause or exacerbate syndrome of inappropriate antidiuretic hormone secretion or hyponatremia; monitor sodium closely with initiation or dosage adjustments in older adults (Beers Criteria). Formulation contains sucrose; patients with fructose intolerance, glucose-galactose malabsorption, or sucrase-isomaltase deficiency should avoid use.

Adverse Reactions (Reflective of adult population; not specific for elderly)
>10%:
  Central nervous system: Headache (13% to 14%), somnolence (10% to 12%; dose related), fatigue (10% to 11%)
  Gastrointestinal: Nausea (23% to 25%), xerostomia (11% to 15%; dose related)
1% to 10%:
  Cardiovascular: Palpitation (1% to 2%)
  Central nervous system: Dizziness (10%), insomnia (10%; dose related), agitation (3% to 5%), anxiety (3%), dreams abnormal (1% to 2%), yawning (1% to 2%), hypoesthesia (≥1%), lethargy (≥1%), vertigo (≥1%), chills (1%), sleep disorder (1%)
  Dermatologic: Hyperhidrosis (6% to 7%)
  Endocrine & metabolic: Libido decreased (2% to 4%), hot flushes (1% to 3%), orgasm abnormality (1% to 3%)
  Gastrointestinal: Constipation (10%; dose related), diarrhea (9% to 10%), appetite decreased (7% to 9%; dose related), abdominal pain (4% to 6%), vomiting (3% to 5%), dyspepsia (2%), weight loss (2%), flatulence (≥1%), taste abnormal (≥1%), weight gain (≥1%)
  Genitourinary: Erectile dysfunction (4% to 5%), ejaculation delayed (3%; dose related), ejaculatory dysfunction (2%)
  Hepatic: ALT >3x ULN (1%)
  Neuromuscular & skeletal: Muscle spasms (3%), tremor (2% to 3%; dose related), musculoskeletal pain (≥1%), paresthesia (≥1%), rigors (≥1%)
  Ocular: Blurred vision (1% to 3%)
  Respiratory: Nasopharyngitis (5%), cough (3%)
  Miscellaneous: Influenza (3%)
Drug Interactions
  Metabolism/Transport Effects Substrate of CYP1A2 (major), CYP2D6 (major); **Note:** Assignment of Major/Minor substrate status based on clinically relevant drug interaction potential; **Inhibits** CYP2D6 (moderate)
  Avoid Concomitant Use
    Avoid concomitant use of DULoxetine with any of the following: Iobenguane I 123; MAO Inhibitors; Methylene Blue
  Increased Effect/Toxicity
    DULoxetine may increase the levels/effects of: Alpha-/Beta-Agonists; ARIPiprazole; Aspirin; CYP2D6 Substrates; Fesoterodine; Methylene Blue; Metoclopramide; Nebivolol; NSAID (Nonselective); Serotonin Modulators; Tricyclic Antidepressants

DULOXETINE

The levels/effects of DULoxetine may be increased by: Abiraterone Acetate; Alcohol (Ethyl); Antipsychotics; ARIPiprazole; CYP1A2 Inhibitors (Moderate); CYP1A2 Inhibitors (Strong); CYP2D6 Inhibitors (Moderate); CYP2D6 Inhibitors (Strong); Darunavir; Deferasirox; FluvoxaMINE; Linezolid; MAO Inhibitors; PARoxetine; Propafenone

Decreased Effect

DULoxetine may decrease the levels/effects of: Alpha2-Agonists; Codeine; Iobenguane I 123; Ioflupane I 123; Tamoxifen

The levels/effects of DULoxetine may be decreased by: CYP1A2 Inducers (Strong); Cyproterone; Peginterferon Alfa-2b

Ethanol/Nutrition/Herb Interactions

Ethanol: Ethanol may increase hepatotoxic potential of duloxetine and increase CNS depression. Management: Avoid ethanol.

Herb/Nutraceutical: Some herbal medications may increase CNS depression. Management: Avoid valerian, St John's wort, SAMe, kava kava, and gotu kola.

Stability Store at 25°C (77°F); excursions permitted to 15°C to 30°C (59°F to 86°F)

Mechanism of Action Duloxetine is a potent inhibitor of neuronal serotonin and norepinephrine reuptake and a weak inhibitor of dopamine reuptake. Duloxetine has no significant activity for muscarinic cholinergic, H_1-histaminergic, or alpha$_2$-adrenergic receptors. Duloxetine does not possess MAO-inhibitory activity.

Pharmacodynamics/Kinetics

Absorption: Well absorbed, 2-hour delay in absorption after ingestion; food decreases extent of absorption ~10% (no effect on C_{max})

Distribution: 1640 L (range: 701-3800 L)

Protein binding: >90%; primarily to albumin and α_1-acid glycoprotein

Metabolism: Hepatic, via CYP1A2 and CYP2D6; forms multiple metabolites (inactive)

Half-life elimination: 12 hours (range: 8-17 hours)

Time to peak: 6 hours; 10 hours when ingested with food

Excretion: Urine (~70%; <1% of total dose as unchanged drug); feces (~20%)

Dosage

Geriatric

Major depressive disorder: Oral: Manufacturer does not recommend specific dosage adjustment. Conservatively, may initiate at a dose of 20 mg 1-2 times/day; increase to 40-60 mg/day as a single daily dose or in divided doses **or** initiate therapy at 30 mg/day for 1 week then increase to 60 mg/day as tolerated.

Other indications: Refer to adult dosing.

Adult

Major depressive disorder: Oral: Initial: 40-60 mg/day; dose may be divided (ie, 20 or 30 mg twice daily) or given as a single daily dose of 60 mg; maintenance: 60 mg once daily; for doses >60 mg/day, titrate dose in increments of 30 mg/day over 1 week as tolerated to a maximum dose: 120 mg/day. **Note:** Doses >60 mg/day have not been demonstrated to be more effective.

Diabetic neuropathy: Oral: 60 mg once daily; lower initial doses may be considered in patients where tolerability is a concern and/or renal impairment is present. **Note:** Doses up to 120 mg/day administered in clinical trials offered no additional benefit and were less well tolerated than dose of 60 mg/day.

Fibromyalgia: Oral: 30 mg once daily for 1 week, then increase to 60 mg once daily as tolerated. **Note:** Doses up to 120 mg/day administered in clinical trials offered no additional benefit and were less well tolerated than dose of 60 mg/day.

Generalized anxiety disorder: Oral: Initial: 30-60 mg/day as a single daily dose; patients initiated at 30 mg/day should be titrated to 60 mg/day after 1 week; maximum dose: 120 mg/day. **Note:** Doses >60 mg/day have not been demonstrated to be more effective than 60 mg/day.

Chronic musculoskeletal pain: Oral: 30 mg once daily for 1 week, then increase to 60 mg once daily as tolerated

Stress incontinence (unlabeled use): Oral: 40 mg twice daily (Dmochowski, 2003)

Note: Upon discontinuation of duloxetine therapy, gradually taper dose. If intolerable symptoms occur following a dose reduction, consider resuming the previously prescribed dose and/or decrease dose at a more gradual rate.

Renal Impairment Not recommended for use in Cl_{cr} <30 mL/minute or ESRD (contraindicated in Canadian labeling). In mild-moderate impairment, lower initial doses may be considered with titration guided by response and tolerability.

Hepatic Impairment Not recommended for use in hepatic impairment (contraindicated in Canadian labeling).

Administration Capsule should be swallowed whole; do not crush or chew. Although the manufacturer does not recommend opening the capsule to facilitate administration; the contents of capsule may be sprinkled on applesauce or in apple juice and swallowed (without chewing) immediately. Do not sprinkle contents on chocolate pudding (Wells, 2008). Administer without regard to meals.

Monitoring Parameters Blood pressure should be checked prior to initiating therapy and then regularly monitored, especially in patients with a high baseline blood pressure; mental status for depression, suicidal ideation (especially at the beginning of therapy or when doses are increased or decreased), anxiety, social functioning, mania, panic attacks; glucose levels and Hb A_{1c} levels in diabetic patients, creatinine, BUN, transaminases

For musculoskeletal pain: Pain relief

Special Geriatric Considerations In an 8-week study of elderly patients with a history of recurrent major depressive disorder, improvements in verbal learning and memory, and depression response and remission rates were significantly greater in subjects randomized to duloxetine 60 mg per day compared to placebo. Duloxetine was well tolerated by older patients in clinical trials who accounted for nearly one-third of subjects. Response rate did not differ between younger and older subjects. No dose adjustment is necessary for age alone; adjust dose for renal function. Higher doses are generally required for treatment of general anxiety disorder, neuropathic pain and stress urinary incontinence (unlabeled use). The elderly are more prone to SSRI/SNRI-induced hyponatremia.

A systematic review and meta-analysis of antidepressant placebo-controlled trials in persons with depression and dementia found evidence "suggestive" of efficacy but not of sufficient strength to "confirm" efficacy. Antidepressant trials in this patient population are small and underpowered. Older patients with depression being treated with an antidepressant should be closely monitored for response and adverse effects. Treatment should be switched or augmented when response is inadequate with a therapeutic dose. Antidepressants that are not tolerated should be discontinued and an alternative agent should be started.

This medication is considered to be potentially inappropriate in this patient population (Beers Criteria: Quality of evidence - moderate; Strength of recommendation - strong).

Dosage Forms Excipient information presented when available (limited, particularly for generics); consult specific product labeling.
Capsule, delayed release, enteric coated pellets, oral:
Cymbalta®: 20 mg, 30 mg, 60 mg

Dutasteride (doo TAS teer ide)

Brand Names: U.S. Avodart®
Brand Names: Canada Avodart®
Generic Availability (U.S.) No
Pharmacologic Category 5 Alpha-Reductase Inhibitor
Use Treatment of symptomatic benign prostatic hyperplasia (BPH) as monotherapy or combination therapy with tamsulosin
Unlabeled Use Treatment of male pattern baldness
Contraindications Hypersensitivity to dutasteride, other 5α-reductase inhibitors (eg, finasteride), or any component of the formulation; not indicated for use in women; pregnant women or women trying to conceive should not handle the product
Warnings/Precautions Hazardous agent - use appropriate precautions for handling and disposal. Pregnant women or women trying to conceive should not handle the product; active ingredient can be absorbed through the skin and may negatively impact fetal development. Urological diseases, including prostate cancer, and/or obstructive uropathy should be ruled out before initiating. Avoid donating blood during or for 6 months following treatment due to risk of administration to a pregnant female transfusion recipient. Use caution in hepatic impairment and with concurrent use of potent, chronic CYP3A4 inhibitors. Reduces PSA by ~50% within 3-6 months of use; if following serial PSAs, re-establish a new baseline ≥3 months after treatment initiation and monitor PSA periodically thereafter. If interpreting an isolated PSA value in a patient treated for ≥3 months, then double the PSA value for comparison to a normal PSA value in an untreated man. Failure to demonstrate a meaningful

PSA decrease (<50%) or a PSA increase while on this medication may be associated with an increased risk for prostate cancer (NCCN Prostate Cancer Early Detection Guidelines, v.1.2011). Patients on a 5-alpha-reductase inhibitor (5-ARI) with any increase in PSA levels, even if within normal limits, should be evaluated; may indicate presence of prostate cancer. When compared to placebo, 5-ARIs have been shown to reduce the overall incidence of prostate cancer, although an increase in the incidence of high-grade prostate cancers has been observed; 5-ARIs are not approved in the U.S. or Canada for the prevention of prostate cancer.

Adverse Reactions (Reflective of adult population; not specific for elderly)

1% to 10%: Endocrine & metabolic: Impotence (1% to 5%), libido decreased (≤3%), ejaculation disorders (≤1%), gynecomastia (including breast tenderness, breast enlargement; ≤1%)

Note: Frequency of adverse events (except gynecomastia) tends to decrease with continued use (>6 months).

Drug Interactions

Metabolism/Transport Effects Substrate of CYP3A4 (minor); **Note:** Assignment of Major/Minor substrate status based on clinically relevant drug interaction potential

Avoid Concomitant Use There are no known interactions where it is recommended to avoid concomitant use.

Increased Effect/Toxicity
The levels/effects of Dutasteride may be increased by: CYP3A4 Inhibitors (Strong)

Decreased Effect
The levels/effects of Dutasteride may be decreased by: Tocilizumab

Ethanol/Nutrition/Herb Interactions

Ethanol: No effect or interaction noted.

Food: Maximum serum concentrations reduced by 10% to 15% when taken with food; not clinically significant.

Herb/Nutraceutical: St John's wort may decrease dutasteride levels. Avoid saw palmetto (concurrent use has not been adequately studied).

Stability Store at controlled room temperature of 25°C (77°F); excursions permitted to 15°C to 30°C (59°F to 86°F).

Mechanism of Action Dutasteride is a 4-azo analog of testosterone and is a competitive, selective inhibitor of both reproductive tissues (type 2) and skin and hepatic (type 1) 5α-reductase. This results in inhibition of the conversion of testosterone to dihydrotestosterone and markedly suppresses serum dihydrotestosterone levels.

Pharmacodynamics/Kinetics

Absorption: Absorbed via skin when handling capsules

Distribution: V_d: 300-500 L, ~12% of serum concentrations partitioned into semen

Protein binding: 99% to albumin; ~97% to α_1-acid glycoprotein; >96% to semen protein

Metabolism: Hepatic via CYP3A4 isoenzyme; forms metabolites: 6-hydroxydutasteride has activity similar to parent compound, 4'-hydroxydutasteride and 1,2-dihydrodutasteride are much less potent than parent in vitro

Bioavailability: ~60% (range: 40% to 94%)

Half-life elimination: Terminal: ~5 weeks

Time to peak: 2-3 hours

Excretion: Feces (40% as metabolites, ~5% as unchanged drug); urine (<1% as unchanged drug); ~55% of dose unaccounted for

Dosage

Geriatric & Adult Males: **Benign prostatic hyperplasia (BPH):** Oral: 0.5 mg once daily alone or in combination with tamsulosin

Renal Impairment No adjustment is required.

Hepatic Impairment Use caution; no specific adjustments recommended.

Administration May be administered without regard to meals. Capsule should be swallowed whole; do not chew or open; contact with opened capsule can cause oropharyngeal irritation. Should not be touched or handled by women who are pregnant or are of childbearing age.

Monitoring Parameters Objective and subjective signs of relief of benign prostatic hyperplasia, including improvement in urinary flow, reduction in symptoms of urgency, and relief of difficulty in micturition; for serial PSA monitoring, establish a new baseline PSA level after 3 months of therapy and monitor PSA periodically thereafter.

Test Interactions PSA levels decrease in treated patients. After 3 months of therapy, PSA levels stabilize to a new baseline that is ~50% of pretreatment values. If following serial PSAs in a patient, re-establish a new baseline after ≥3 months of use. If interpreting an isolated PSA value in a patient treated for ≥3 months, then double the PSA value for comparison.

Special Geriatric Considerations No dosage adjustment necessary.

Dosage Forms Excipient information presented when available (limited, particularly for generics); consult specific product labeling.

Capsule, softgel, oral:

Avodart®: 0.5 mg

Dutasteride and Tamsulosin (doo TAS teer ide & tam SOO loe sin)

Related Information
Dutasteride *on page 623*
Tamsulosin *on page 1834*
Brand Names: U.S. Jalyn™
Index Terms Tamsulosin and Dutasteride; Tamsulosin Hydrochloride and Dutasteride
Generic Availability (U.S.) No
Pharmacologic Category 5 Alpha-Reductase Inhibitor; Alpha$_1$ Blocker
Use Treatment of symptomatic benign prostatic hyperplasia (BPH)
Dosage
Geriatric & Adult Males:
Benign prostatic hyperplasia (BPH): Oral: One capsule (0.5 mg dutasteride/0.4 mg tamsulosin) once daily ~30 minutes after the same meal each day
Renal Impairment
Cl_{cr} 10-30 mL/minute/1.73 m^2: No adjustment needed
Cl_{cr} <10 mL/minute/1.73 m^2: Not studied
Hepatic Impairment Use caution; no specific adjustments recommended
Special Geriatric Considerations See individual agents.
Dosage Forms Excipient information presented when available (limited, particularly for generics); consult specific product labeling.
Capsule, oral:
Jalyn™: Dutasteride 0.5 mg and tamsulosin hydrochloride 0.4 mg

♦ **Dutoprol™** *see* Metoprolol and Hydrochlorothiazide *on page 1267*
♦ **DW286** *see* Gemifloxacin *on page 871*
♦ **Dyazide®** *see* Hydrochlorothiazide and Triamterene *on page 936*
♦ **Dynacin®** *see* Minocycline *on page 1289*
♦ **DynaCirc CR®** *see* Isradipine *on page 1055*

Dyphylline (DYE fi lin)

Brand Names: U.S. Lufyllin®
Index Terms Dihydroxypropyl Theophylline
Generic Availability (U.S.) No
Pharmacologic Category Phosphodiesterase Enzyme Inhibitor, Nonselective
Use Bronchodilator in reversible airway obstruction due to asthma, chronic bronchitis, or emphysema
Dosage
Geriatric & Adult Bronchoconstriction (asthma, COPD): Oral: Up to 15 mg/kg 4 times daily, individualize dosage
Renal Impairment No dosage adjustment provided in manufacturer's labeling; primarily undergoes renal elimination and an increase in systemic exposure is likely. The following adjustments have been recommended (Aronoff, 2007):
Cl_{cr} >50 mL/minute: Administer 75% of normal dose
Cl_{cr} 10-50 mL/minute: Administer 50% of normal dose
Cl_{cr} <10 mL/minute: Administer 25% of normal dose
Special Geriatric Considerations No specific information for use in elderly.
Dosage Forms Excipient information presented when available (limited, particularly for generics); consult specific product labeling.
Tablet, oral:
Lufyllin®: 200 mg, 400 mg [scored]

♦ **Dyrenium®** *see* Triamterene *on page 1962*
♦ **Dysport™** *see* AbobotulinumtoxinA *on page 24*
♦ **E2 and DRSP** *see* Drospirenone and Estradiol *on page 616*
♦ **E2020** *see* Donepezil *on page 591*
♦ **E 2080** *see* Rufinamide *on page 1739*

Echothiophate Iodide (ek oh THYE oh fate EYE oh dide)

Related Information
Glaucoma Drug Therapy *on page 2115*
Brand Names: U.S. Phospholine Iodide®
Index Terms Ecostigmine Iodide
Generic Availability (U.S.) No
Pharmacologic Category Acetylcholinesterase Inhibitor; Ophthalmic Agent, Antiglaucoma; Ophthalmic Agent, Miotic
Use Used as miotic in treatment of chronic, open-angle glaucoma; may be useful in specific cases of angle-closure glaucoma (postiridectomy or where surgery refused/contraindicated); postcataract surgery-related glaucoma; accommodative esotropia
Contraindications Hypersensitivity to echothiophate or any component of the formulation; most cases of angle-closure glaucoma; active uveal inflammation
Warnings/Precautions If general anesthesia required, use succinylcholine with great caution due to potential for respiratory or cardiovascular collapse. Use caution in patients on concomitant anticholinesterase agents; warn patients of possible additive effects if chronically exposed to organophosphate/carbamate pesticides/insecticides. Baseline measurement of anterior chamber angle recommended; routine lens examinations (for opacities) should be conducted. Do not use for tonometric glaucoma, or with active or history of uveitis, or retinal detachment. Discontinue if cardiac irregularities or symptoms of excess cholinergic activity (eg, salivation, sweating, urinary incontinence). Not generally recommended for use in patients with any of the following: Vagotonia, asthma GI disturbances, PUD, bradycardia or hypotension, recent MI, epilepsy, parkinsonism. Use cautiously prior to ophthalmic surgery due to risk of blood in the anterior chamber. May depress plasma and erythrocyte cholinesterase levels after a few weeks of therapy. Tolerance may develop after prolonged use; a rest period restores response to the drug.
Adverse Reactions (Reflective of adult population; not specific for elderly) Frequency not defined.
Cardiovascular: Bradycardia, cardiac irregularities, flushing, hypotension
Gastrointestinal: Diarrhea, nausea, vomiting
Neurologic & skeletal: Muscle weakness
Ocular: Blurred vision, browache, burning eyes, ciliary redness, conjunctival redness/thickening, intraocular pressure increases (paradoxical), iris cysts, lacrimation, lid muscle twitching, miosis, myopia, latent iritis or uveitis activation, lens opacities, retinal detachment, stinging
Respiratory: Dyspnea
Miscellaneous: Diaphoresis, nasolacrimal canal obstruction
Drug Interactions
Metabolism/Transport Effects None known.
Avoid Concomitant Use There are no known interactions where it is recommended to avoid concomitant use.
Increased Effect/Toxicity
Echothiophate Iodide may increase the levels/effects of: Succinylcholine
Decreased Effect There are no known significant interactions involving a decrease in effect.
Stability Store undiluted vials at 2°C to 8°C (36°F to 46°F). Reconstituted solutions remain stable for 30 days at room temperature; do not refrigerate.
Mechanism of Action Long-acting inhibition of cholinesterase enhances activity of endogenous acetylcholine. Reduced degradation of acetylcholine leads to continuous stimulation of the ciliary muscle producing miosis; other effects include potentiation of accommodation and facilitation of aqueous humor outflow, with attendant reduction in intraocular pressure.
Pharmacodynamics/Kinetics
Onset of action: Miosis: 10-30 minutes; Intraocular pressure decrease: 4-8 hours
Peak effect: Intraocular pressure decrease: 24 hours
Duration: Miosis: 1-4 weeks
Dosage
Geriatric & Adult Open-angle or secondary glaucoma: Ophthalmic:
Initial: Instill 1 drop (0.03%) twice daily into eyes with 1 dose just prior to bedtime
Maintenance: Some patients have been treated with 1 dose daily or every other day
Conversion from other ophthalmic agents: If IOP control was unsatisfactory, patients may be expected to require higher doses of echothiophate (eg, ≥0.06%); however, patients should be initially started on the 0.03% strength for a short period to better tolerance.
Administration Proper administration technique is required for maximal benefit. The nasolacrimal duct(s) should be compressed for 1-2 minutes after instillation of the drops. Excess fluid around the eye should be blotted with tissue, and any contact of medication to the hands should be immediately washed off.
Monitoring Parameters Intraocular pressure

Pharmacotherapy Pearls Tolerance may develop after prolonged use; a rest period restores response to the drug.

Special Geriatric Considerations Evaluate the patient's or caregiver's ability to safely administer the correct dose of ophthalmic medication.

Dosage Forms Excipient information presented when available (limited, particularly for generics); consult specific product labeling.

Powder for reconstitution, ophthalmic:

Phospholine Iodide®: 6.25 mg (5 mL) [0.125%]

Edrophonium (ed roe FOE nee um)

Brand Names: U.S. Enlon®

Brand Names: Canada Enlon®; Tensilon®

Index Terms Edrophonium Chloride

Generic Availability (U.S.) No

Pharmacologic Category Acetylcholinesterase Inhibitor; Antidote; Diagnostic Agent

Use Diagnosis of myasthenia gravis; differentiation of cholinergic crises from myasthenia crises; reversal of nondepolarizing neuromuscular blockers

Contraindications Hypersensitivity to edrophonium, sulfites, or any component of the formulation; GI or GU obstruction

Warnings/Precautions Use with caution in patients with bronchial asthma and those receiving a cardiac glycoside; atropine sulfate should always be readily available as an antagonist. Overdosage can cause cholinergic crisis which may be fatal. I.V. atropine should be readily available for treatment of cholinergic reactions. Use with caution in patients with cardiac arrhythmias (eg, bradyarrhythmias). Use with caution in myasthenia gravis; may exacerbate muscular weakness. Products may contain sodium sulfite.

Adverse Reactions (Reflective of adult population; not specific for elderly) Frequency not defined.

Cardiovascular: Arrhythmias (especially bradycardia), AV block, carbon monoxide decreased, cardiac arrest, ECG changes (nonspecific), flushing, hypotension, nodal rhythm, syncope, tachycardia

Central nervous system: Convulsions, dizziness, drowsiness, dysarthria, dysphonia, headache, loss of consciousness

Dermatologic: Skin rash, thrombophlebitis (I.V.), urticaria

Gastrointestinal: Diarrhea, dysphagia, flatulence, hyperperistalsis, nausea, salivation, stomach cramps, vomiting

Genitourinary: Urinary urgency

Neuromuscular & skeletal: Arthralgias, fasciculations, muscle cramps, spasms, weakness

Ocular: Lacrimation, small pupils

Respiratory: Bronchiolar constriction, bronchospasm, dyspnea, bronchial secretions increased, laryngospasm, respiratory arrest, respiratory depression, respiratory muscle paralysis

Miscellaneous: Allergic reactions, anaphylaxis, diaphoresis increased

Drug Interactions

Metabolism/Transport Effects None known.

Avoid Concomitant Use There are no known interactions where it is recommended to avoid concomitant use.

Increased Effect/Toxicity

Edrophonium may increase the levels/effects of: Beta-Blockers; Cholinergic Agonists; Succinylcholine

The levels/effects of Edrophonium may be increased by: Corticosteroids (Systemic)

Decreased Effect
Edrophonium may decrease the levels/effects of: Neuromuscular-Blocking Agents (Non-depolarizing)

The levels/effects of Edrophonium may be decreased by: Dipyridamole

Mechanism of Action Inhibits destruction of acetylcholine by acetylcholinesterase. This facilitates transmission of impulses across myoneural junction and results in increased cholinergic responses such as miosis, increased tonus of intestinal and skeletal muscles, bronchial and ureteral constriction, bradycardia, and increased salivary and sweat gland secretions.

Pharmacodynamics/Kinetics
Onset of action: I.M.: 2-10 minutes; I.V.: 30-60 seconds
Duration: I.M.: 5-30 minutes; I.V.: 10 minutes
Distribution: V_d: Adults: 1.1 L/kg
Half-life elimination: Adults: 1.2-2.4 hours; Anephric patients: 2.4-4.4 hours
Excretion: Adults: Primarily urine (67%)

Dosage
Geriatric & Adult Usually administered I.V., however, if not possible, I.M. or SubQ may be used.

Diagnosis of Myasthenia gravis:
I.V.: 2 mg test dose administered over 15-30 seconds; 8 mg given 45 seconds later if no response is seen. Test dose may be repeated after 30 minutes.
I.M.: Initial: 10 mg; if no cholinergic reaction occurs, give 2 mg 30 minutes later to rule out false-negative reaction.

Titration of oral anticholinesterase therapy: 1-2 mg given 1 hour after oral dose of anticholinesterase; if strength improves, an increase in neostigmine or pyridostigmine dose is indicated.

Differentiation of cholinergic from myasthenic crisis: I.V.: 1 mg; may repeat after 1 minute. **Note:** Intubation and controlled ventilation may be required if patient has cholinergic crisis.

Reversal of nondepolarizing neuromuscular blocking agents (neostigmine with atropine usually preferred): I.V.: 10 mg over 30-45 seconds; may repeat every 5-10 minutes up to 40 mg.

Termination of paroxysmal atrial tachycardia: I.V. rapid injection: 5-10 mg

Renal Impairment Dose may need to be reduced in patients with chronic renal failure.
Administration Edrophonium is administered by direct I.V. injection; see Dosage
Monitoring Parameters Pre- and postinjection strength (cranial musculature is most useful); heart rate, respiratory rate, blood pressure
Test Interactions Increased aminotransferase [ALT/AST] (S), amylase (S)
Pharmacotherapy Pearls In the diagnosis of myasthenia gravis, all anticholinesterase medications should be discontinued for at least 8 hours before administering neostigmine; monitor for signs of cholinergic crisis
Special Geriatric Considerations Many elderly will have diseases which may influence the use of edrophonium. Also, many elderly will need doses reduced 50% due to creatinine clearances in the 10-50 mL/minute range (common in the aged). Side effects or concomitant disease may warrant use of pyridostigmine.
Dosage Forms Excipient information presented when available (limited, particularly for generics); consult specific product labeling.
Injection, solution, as chloride:
Enlon®: 10 mg/mL (15 mL) [contains natural rubber/natural latex in packaging, sodium sulfite]

◆ **Eldepryl®** *see* Selegiline *on page 1760*
◆ **Electrolyte Lavage Solution** *see* Polyethylene Glycol-Electrolyte Solution and Bisacodyl *on page 1565*
◆ **Elestat®** *see* Epinastine *on page 645*
◆ **Elestrin®** *see* Estradiol (Systemic) *on page 681*

Eletriptan (el e TRIP tan)

Brand Names: U.S. Relpax®
Brand Names: Canada Relpax®
Index Terms Eletriptan Hydrobromide
Generic Availability (U.S.) No
Pharmacologic Category Antimigraine Agent; Serotonin 5-HT$_{1B, 1D}$ Receptor Agonist
Use Acute treatment of migraine, with or without aura
Contraindications Hypersensitivity to eletriptan or any component of the formulation; ischemic heart disease (angina pectoris, history of myocardial infarction, or proven silent ischemia) or in patients with symptoms consistent with ischemic heart disease, coronary artery vasospasm, or Prinzmetal's angina; cerebrovascular syndromes (including strokes, transient ischemic attacks); peripheral vascular syndromes (including ischemic bowel disease); uncontrolled hypertension; use within 24 hours of ergotamine derivatives; use within 24 hours of another 5-HT$_1$ agonist; management of hemiplegic or basilar migraine; severe hepatic impairment

Warnings/Precautions Only indicated for treatment of acute migraine; not indicated for migraine prophylaxis, or for the treatment of cluster headache, hemiplegic or basilar migraine. If a patient does not respond to the first dose, the diagnosis of migraine should be reconsidered. Do not give to patients with risk factors for CAD until a cardiovascular evaluation has been performed; if evaluation is satisfactory, the healthcare provider should administer the first dose (consider ECG monitoring) and cardiovascular status should be periodically evaluated. Cardiac events (coronary artery vasospasm, transient ischemia, MI, ventricular tachycardia/fibrillation, cardiac arrest, and death), cerebral/subarachnoid hemorrhage, stroke, peripheral vascular ischemia, and colonic ischemia have been reported with 5-HT$_1$ agonist administration. Patients who experience sensations of chest pain/pressure/tightness or symptoms suggestive of angina following dosing should be evaluated for coronary artery disease or Prinzmetal's angina before receiving additional doses; if dosing is resumed and similar symptoms recur, monitor with ECG. Significant elevation in blood pressure, including hypertensive crisis, has also been reported on rare occasions in patients with and without a history of hypertension. Use with caution with mild-to-moderate hepatic impairment. Symptoms of agitation, confusion, hallucinations, hyper-reflexia, myoclonus, shivering, and tachycardia (serotonin syndrome) may occur with concomitant proserotonergic drugs (ie, SSRIs/SNRIs or triptans) or agents which reduce eletriptan's metabolism. Concurrent use of serotonin precursors (eg, tryptophan) is not recommended. If concomitant administration with SSRIs is warranted, monitor closely, especially at initiation and with dose increases. Use not recommended within 72 hours in patients taking strong CYP3A4 inhibitors.

Adverse Reactions (Reflective of adult population; not specific for elderly) 1% to 10%:
Cardiovascular: Chest pain/tightness (1% to 4%; placebo 1%), palpitation
Central nervous system: Dizziness (3% to 7%; placebo 3%), somnolence (3% to 7%; placebo 4%), headache (3% to 4%; placebo 3%), chills, pain, vertigo
Gastrointestinal: Nausea (4% to 8%; placebo 5%), xerostomia (2% to 4%, placebo 2%), dysphagia (1% to 2%), abdominal pain/discomfort (1% to 2%; placebo 1%), dyspepsia (1% to 2%; placebo 1%)
Neuromuscular & skeletal: Weakness (4% to 10%), paresthesia (3% to 4%), back pain, hypertonia, hypoesthesia
Respiratory: Pharyngitis
Miscellaneous: Diaphoresis

Drug Interactions
Metabolism/Transport Effects Substrate of CYP3A4 (major); **Note:** Assignment of Major/Minor substrate status based on clinically relevant drug interaction potential
Avoid Concomitant Use
Avoid concomitant use of Eletriptan with any of the following: Conivaptan; Ergot Derivatives
Increased Effect/Toxicity
Eletriptan may increase the levels/effects of: Ergot Derivatives; Metoclopramide; Serotonin Modulators

The levels/effects of Eletriptan may be increased by: Antifungal Agents (Azole Derivatives, Systemic); Antipsychotics; Calcium Channel Blockers (Nondihydropyridine); Conivaptan;

CYP3A4 Inhibitors (Moderate); CYP3A4 Inhibitors (Strong); Dasatinib; Ergot Derivatives; Fluconazole; Ivacaftor; Macrolide Antibiotics; Mifepristone

Decreased Effect
The levels/effects of Eletriptan may be decreased by: Tocilizumab

Ethanol/Nutrition/Herb Interactions Food: High-fat meal increases bioavailability.

Stability Store at 25°C (77°F); excursions permitted to 15°C to 30°C (59°F to 86°F).

Mechanism of Action Selective agonist for serotonin (5-HT$_{1B}$ and 5-HT$_{1D}$ receptors) in cranial arteries; causes vasoconstriction and reduces sterile inflammation associated with antidromic neuronal transmission correlating with relief of migraine

Pharmacodynamics/Kinetics
Absorption: Well absorbed
Distribution: V$_d$: 138 L
Protein binding: ~85%
Metabolism: Hepatic via CYP3A4; forms one metabolite (active)
Bioavailability: ~50%, increased with high-fat meal
Half-life elimination: ~4 hours (Elderly: 4.4-5.7 hours); Metabolite: ~13 hours
Time to peak, plasma: 1.5-2 hours

Dosage
Geriatric & Adult Acute migraine: Oral: Initial: 20-40 mg (maximum: 40 mg/dose); if the headache improves but returns, dose may be repeated after 2 hours have elapsed since first dose (maximum: 80 mg/day)

Note: If the first dose is ineffective, diagnosis needs to be re-evaluated. Safety of treating >3 headaches/month has not been established.

Renal Impairment No dosing adjustment needed; monitor for increased blood pressure.

Hepatic Impairment
Mild-to-moderate impairment: No adjustment necessary.
Severe impairment: Use is contraindicated.

Special Geriatric Considerations Since elderly often have cardiovascular disease, careful evaluation of the use of 5-HT agonists is needed to avoid complications with the use of these agents. Safety and efficacy in elderly >65 years of age have not been established, however, pharmacokinetic disposition is similar to that in younger adults. Use lowest recommended doses initially.

Dosage Forms Excipient information presented when available (limited, particularly for generics); consult specific product labeling.
Tablet, oral:
Relpax®: 20 mg, 40 mg

◆ **Eletriptan Hydrobromide** *see* Eletriptan *on page 629*
◆ **Eligard®** *see* Leuprolide *on page 1103*
◆ **Elimite** *see* Permethrin *on page 1512*
◆ **Eliphos™** *see* Calcium Acetate *on page 259*
◆ **Elixophyllin® Elixir** *see* Theophylline *on page 1875*
◆ **Elocon®** *see* Mometasone (Topical) *on page 1307*
◆ **Emadine®** *see* Emedastine *on page 630*
◆ **EMD 68843** *see* Vilazodone *on page 2024*

Emedastine (em e DAS teen)

Brand Names: U.S. Emadine®
Index Terms Emedastine Difumarate
Pharmacologic Category Histamine H$_1$ Antagonist; Histamine H$_1$ Antagonist, Second Generation

Use Treatment of allergic conjunctivitis

Dosage
Geriatric & Adult Allergic conjunctivitis: Ophthalmic: Instill 1 drop in affected eye up to 4 times/day

Special Geriatric Considerations Evaluate the patient's or caregiver's ability to safely administer the correct dose of ophthalmic medication.

Dosage Forms Excipient information presented when available (limited, particularly for generics); consult specific product labeling.
Solution, ophthalmic, as difumarate [drops]:
Emadine®: 0.05% (5 mL) [contains benzalkonium chloride]

◆ **Emedastine Difumarate** *see* Emedastine *on page 630*
◆ **Emend®** *see* Aprepitant *on page 139*
◆ **Emend® for Injection** *see* Fosaprepitant *on page 844*
◆ **Emsam®** *see* Selegiline *on page 1760*

◆ **ENA 713** *see* Rivastigmine *on page* 1719
◆ **Enablex®** *see* Darifenacin *on page* 492

Enalapril (e NAL a pril)

Related Information
Angiotensin Agents *on page* 2093
Heart Failure (Systolic) *on page* 2203

Medication Safety Issues
Sound-alike/look-alike issues:
Enalapril may be confused with Anafranil®, Elavil®, Eldepryl®, ramipril
Administration issues:
Significant differences exist between oral and I.V. dosing. Use caution when converting from one route of administration to another.
International issues:
Acepril [Hungary, Switzerland] may be confused with Accupril which is a brand name for quinapril [U.S., Canada, multiple international markets]
Acepril: Brand name for enalapril [Hungary, Switzerland], but also brand name for captopril [Great Britain]; lisinopril [Malaysia]

Brand Names: U.S. Vasotec®

Brand Names: Canada Apo-Enalapril®; CO Enalapril; Mylan-Enalapril; Novo-Enalapril; PMS-Enalapril; PRO-Enalapril; RAN™-Enalapril; ratio-Enalapril; Riva-Enalapril; Sandoz-Enalapril; Sig-Enalapril; Taro-Enalapril; Teva-Enalapril; Vasotec®

Index Terms Enalapril Maleate

Generic Availability (U.S.) Yes

Pharmacologic Category Angiotensin-Converting Enzyme (ACE) Inhibitor

Use Treatment of hypertension; treatment of symptomatic heart failure; treatment of asymptomatic left ventricular dysfunction

Unlabeled Use To delay the progression of nephropathy and reduce risks of cardiovascular events in hypertensive patients with type 1 or 2 diabetes mellitus; hypertensive crisis, diabetic nephropathy, hypertension secondary to scleroderma renal crisis, diagnosis of aldosteronism, idiopathic edema, Bartter's syndrome, postmyocardial infarction for prevention of ventricular failure

Contraindications Hypersensitivity to enalapril or enalaprilat; angioedema related to previous treatment with an ACE inhibitor; patients with idiopathic or hereditary angioedema

Warnings/Precautions Anaphylactic reactions may occur rarely with ACE inhibitors. At any time during treatment (especially following first dose) angioedema may occur rarely with ACE inhibitors; it may involve the head and neck (potentially compromising airway) or the intestine (presenting with abdominal pain). African-Americans may be at an increased risk. Prolonged frequent monitoring may be required especially if tongue, glottis, or larynx are involved as they are associated with airway obstruction. Patients with a history of airway surgery may have a higher risk of airway obstruction. Aggressive early and appropriate management is critical. Use in patients with idiopathic or hereditary angioedema or previous angioedema associated with ACE inhibitor therapy is contraindicated. Severe anaphylactoid reactions may be seen during hemodialysis (eg, CVVHD) with high-flux dialysis membranes (eg, AN69), and rarely, during low density lipoprotein apheresis with dextran sulfate cellulose. Rare cases of anaphylactoid reactions have been reported in patients undergoing sensitization treatment with hymenoptera (bee, wasp) venom while receiving ACE inhibitors.

Symptomatic hypotension with or without syncope can occur with ACE inhibitors (usually with the first several doses); effects are most often observed in volume depleted patients; correct volume depletion prior to initiation; close monitoring of patient is required especially with initial dosing and dosing increases; blood pressure must be lowered at a rate appropriate for the patient's clinical condition. Initiation of therapy in patients with ischemic heart disease or cerebrovascular disease warrants close observation due to the potential consequences posed by falling blood pressure (eg, MI, stroke). Use with caution in hypertrophic cardiomyopathy with outflow tract obstruction, severe aortic stenosis, or before, during, or immediately after major surgery.

Hyperkalemia may occur with ACE inhibitors; risk factors include renal dysfunction, diabetes mellitus, concomitant use of potassium-sparing diuretics, potassium supplements, and/or potassium-containing salts. Use cautiously, if at all, with these agents and monitor potassium closely. Cough may occur with ACE inhibitors. Other causes of cough should be considered (eg, pulmonary congestion in patients with heart failure) and excluded prior to discontinuation.

May be associated with deterioration of renal function and/or increases in serum creatinine, particularly in patients with low renal blood flow (eg, renal artery stenosis, heart failure) whose glomerular filtration rate (GFR) is dependent on efferent arteriolar vasoconstriction by angiotensin II; deterioration may result in oliguria, acute renal failure, and progressive azotemia. Small increases in serum creatinine may occur following initiation; consider discontinuation only in patients with progressive and/or significant deterioration in renal function. Use with caution in patients with unstented unilateral/bilateral renal artery stenosis. When unstented bilateral renal artery stenosis is present, use is generally avoided due to the elevated risk of deterioration in renal function unless possible benefits outweigh risks. Concurrent use of angiotensin receptor blockers may increase the risk of clinically-significant adverse events (eg, renal dysfunction, hyperkalemia).

Rare toxicities associated with ACE inhibitors include cholestatic jaundice (which may progress to fulminant hepatic necrosis), agranulocytosis, neutropenia or leukopenia with myeloid hypoplasia. Patients with collagen vascular diseases (especially with concomitant renal impairment) or renal impairment alone may be at increased risk for hematologic toxicity; periodically monitor CBC with differential in these patients.

Adverse Reactions (Reflective of adult population; not specific for elderly) Note: Frequency ranges include data from hypertension and heart failure trials. Higher rates of adverse reactions have generally been noted in patients with CHF. However, the frequency of adverse effects associated with placebo is also increased in this population.

1% to 10%:
Cardiovascular: Hypotension (1% to 7%), chest pain (2%), syncope (≤2%), orthostasis (2%), orthostatic hypotension (2%)
Central nervous system: Headache (2% to 5%), dizziness (4% to 8%), fatigue (2% to 3%)
Dermatologic: Rash (2%)
Gastrointestinal: Abnormal taste, abdominal pain, vomiting, nausea, diarrhea, anorexia, constipation
Neuromuscular & skeletal: Weakness
Renal: Serum creatinine increased (≤20%), worsening of renal function (in patients with bilateral renal artery stenosis or hypovolemia)
Respiratory (1% to 2%): Bronchitis, cough, dyspnea

Drug Interactions

Metabolism/Transport Effects None known.

Avoid Concomitant Use There are no known interactions where it is recommended to avoid concomitant use.

Increased Effect/Toxicity
Enalapril may increase the levels/effects of: Allopurinol; Amifostine; Antihypertensives; AzaTHIOprine; CycloSPORINE; CycloSPORINE (Systemic); Ferric Gluconate; Gold Sodium Thiomalate; Hypotensive Agents; Iron Dextran Complex; Lithium; Nonsteroidal Anti-Inflammatory Agents; RiTUXimab; Sodium Phosphates

The levels/effects of Enalapril may be increased by: Alfuzosin; Aliskiren; Angiotensin II Receptor Blockers; Diazoxide; DPP-IV Inhibitors; Eplerenone; Everolimus; Herbs (Hypotensive Properties); Loop Diuretics; MAO Inhibitors; Pentoxifylline; Phosphodiesterase 5 Inhibitors; Potassium Salts; Potassium-Sparing Diuretics; Prostacyclin Analogues; Sirolimus; Temsirolimus; Thiazide Diuretics; TiZANidine; Tolvaptan; Trimethoprim

Decreased Effect
The levels/effects of Enalapril may be decreased by: Antacids; Aprotinin; Herbs (Hypertensive Properties); Icatibant; Lanthanum; Methylphenidate; Nonsteroidal Anti-Inflammatory Agents; Salicylates; Yohimbine

Ethanol/Nutrition/Herb Interactions
Food: Potassium supplements and/or potassium-containing salts may cause or worsen hyperkalemia. Management: Consult prescriber before consuming a potassium-rich diet, potassium supplements, or salt substitutes.
Herb/Nutraceutical: Some herbal medications may worsen hypertension (eg, licorice); others may increase the antihypertensive effect of enalapril (eg, shepherd's purse). Management: Avoid bayberry, blue cohosh, cayenne, ephedra, ginger, ginseng (American), kola, licorice, and yohimbe. Avoid black cohosh, California poppy, coleus, golden seal, hawthorn, mistletoe, periwinkle, quinine, and shepherd's purse.

Mechanism of Action Competitive inhibitor of angiotensin-converting enzyme (ACE); prevents conversion of angiotensin I to angiotensin II, a potent vasoconstrictor; results in lower levels of angiotensin II which causes an increase in plasma renin activity and a reduction in aldosterone secretion

Pharmacodynamics/Kinetics

Onset of action: ~1 hour
Peak effect: 4-6 hours
Duration: 12-24 hours
Absorption: 55% to 75%
Protein binding: ~50% (Davies, 1984)
Metabolism: Prodrug, undergoes hepatic biotransformation to enalaprilat
Half-life elimination:
Enalapril: Adults: Healthy: 2 hours; Congestive heart failure: 3.4-5.8 hours
Enalaprilat: Adults: ~35 hours (Till, 1984; Ulm, 1982)
Time to peak, serum: Oral: Enalapril: 0.5-1.5 hours; Enalaprilat (active metabolite): 3-4.5 hours
Excretion: Urine (61%; 18% of which was enalapril, 43% was enalaprilat); feces (33%; 6% of which was enalapril, 27% was enalaprilat) (Ulm, 1982)

Dosage

Geriatric & Adult Use lower listed initial dose in patients with hyponatremia, hypovolemia, severe congestive heart failure, decreased renal function, or in those receiving diuretics.

Asymptomatic left ventricular dysfunction: Oral: 2.5 mg twice daily, titrated as tolerated to 20 mg/day

Heart failure: Oral: Initial: 2.5 mg once or twice daily (usual range: 5-40 mg/day in 2 divided doses); titrate slowly at 1- to 2-week intervals. Target dose: 10-20 mg twice daily (ACC/AHA 2009 Heart Failure Guidelines)

Hypertension: Oral: 2.5-5 mg/day then increase as required, usually at 1- to 2-week intervals; usual dose range (JNC 7): 2.5-40 mg/day in 1-2 divided doses. **Note:** Initiate with 2.5 mg if patient is taking a diuretic which cannot be discontinued. May add a diuretic if blood pressure cannot be controlled with enalapril alone.

Conversion from I.V. **enalaprilat** to oral **enalapril** therapy: If not concurrently receiving diuretics, initiate enalapril 5 mg once daily; if concurrently receiving diuretics and responding to enalaprilat 0.625 mg I.V. every 6 hours, initiate with enalapril 2.5 mg once daily; subsequent titration as needed.

Renal Impairment Manufacturer's recommendations:
Cl_{cr} >30 mL/minute: No dosage adjustment necessary
Cl_{cr} ≤30 mL/minute: Administer 2.5 mg day; titrated upward until blood pressure is controlled.
Heart failure patients with sodium <130 mEq/L or serum creatinine >1.6 mg/dL: Initiate dosage with 2.5 mg/day, increasing to twice daily as needed. Increase further in increments of 2.5 mg/dose at >4-day intervals to a maximum daily dose of 40 mg.
Intermittent hemodialysis (IHD): Moderately dialyzable (20% to 50%): Initial: 2.5 mg on dialysis days; adjust dose on nondialysis days depending on blood pressure response.
Conversion from I.V. **enalaprilat** to oral **enalapril** therapy:
Cl_{cr} >30 mL/minute: May initiate enalapril 5 mg once daily.
Cl_{cr} ≤30 mL/minute: May initiate enalapril 2.5 mg once daily.
Alternate recommendations (Aronoff, 2007):
Cl_{cr} >50 mL/minute: No dosage adjustment necessary
Cl_{cr} 10-50 mL/minute: Administer 75-100% of usual dose
Cl_{cr} <10 mL/minute: Administer 50% of usual dose
Peritoneal dialysis: Supplemental dose is not necessary, although some removal of drug occurs.

Hepatic Impairment Hydrolysis of enalapril to enalaprilat may be delayed and/or impaired in patients with severe hepatic impairment, but the pharmacodynamic effects of the drug do not appear to be significantly altered. No dosage adjustment is necessary.

Monitoring Parameters Blood pressure; serum creatinine and potassium; if patient has collagen vascular disease and/or renal impairment, periodically monitor CBC with differential

Test Interactions Positive Coombs' [direct]; may cause false-positive results in urine acetone determinations using sodium nitroprusside reagent

Special Geriatric Considerations Due to frequent decreases in glomerular filtration (also creatinine clearance) with aging, elderly patients may have exaggerated responses to ACE inhibitors; differences in clinical response due to hepatic changes are not observed. ACE inhibitors may be preferred agents in elderly patients with congestive heart failure and diabetes mellitus. Diabetic proteinuria is reduced and insulin sensitivity is enhanced. In general, the side effect profile is favorable in the elderly and causes little or no CNS confusion; use lowest dose recommendations initially; adjust dose for renal function in the elderly. Many elderly may be volume depleted due to diuretic use and/or blunted thirst reflex resulting in inadequate fluid intake.

◀ **Dosage Forms** Excipient information presented when available (limited, particularly for generics); consult specific product labeling.

Tablet, oral, as maleate: 2.5 mg, 5 mg, 10 mg, 20 mg

Vasotec®: 2.5 mg, 5 mg, 10 mg, 20 mg [scored]

Extemporaneously Prepared An enalapril oral suspension (1 mg/mL) has been made using 20 mg tablets and Bicitra®. Add 50 mL Bicitra® to a polyethylene terephthalate (PET) bottle containing ten 20 mg tablets and shake for at least 2 minutes. Let concentrate stand for 60 minutes. Following the 60-minute hold time, shake the concentration for an additional minute. Add 150 mL Bicitra® to the concentrate and shake the suspension to disperse the ingredients. The suspension should refrigerated at 2°C to 8°C (36°F to 46°F); it can be stored for up to 30 days. Shake suspension well before use.

Package labeling, Merck & Co, Inc, issued October 2000.

Enalapril and Hydrochlorothiazide (e NAL a pril & hye droe klor oh THYE a zide)

Related Information

Enalapril *on page 631*

Hydrochlorothiazide *on page 933*

Medication Safety Issues

International issues:

Norpramin: Brand name for enalapril/hydrochlorothiazide [Portugal], but also the brand name for desipramine [U.S., Canada]; omeprazole [Spain]

Brand Names: U.S. Vaseretic®

Brand Names: Canada Vaseretic®

Index Terms Enalapril Maleate and Hydrochlorothiazide; Hydrochlorothiazide and Enalapril

Generic Availability (U.S.) Yes

Pharmacologic Category Angiotensin-Converting Enzyme (ACE) Inhibitor; Diuretic, Thiazide

Use Treatment of hypertension

Dosage

Geriatric Refer to dosing in individual monographs; adjust for renal impairment.

Adult Hypertension: Oral: Enalapril 5-10 mg and hydrochlorothiazide 12.5-25 mg once daily (maximum: 40 mg/day [enalapril]; 50 mg/day [hydrochlorothiazide])

Renal Impairment

Cl_{cr} >30 mL/minute: Administer usual dose.

Severe renal failure: Avoid; loop diuretics are recommended.

Special Geriatric Considerations See individual agents. Combination products are not recommended as first-line treatment. Use only if doses of individual agents correspond to the combination available.

Dosage Forms Excipient information presented when available (limited, particularly for generics); consult specific product labeling.

Tablet:

5/12.5: Enalapril maleate 5 mg and hydrochlorothiazide 12.5 mg

10/25: Enalapril maleate 10 mg and hydrochlorothiazide 25 mg

Vaseretic®:

10/25: Enalapril maleate 10 mg and hydrochlorothiazide 25 mg

Enalaprilat (en AL a pril at)

Related Information

Angiotensin Agents *on page 2093*

Medication Safety Issues

Administration issues:

Significant differences exist between oral and I.V. dosing. Use caution when converting from one route of administration to another.

Brand Names: Canada Vasotec® I.V

Generic Availability (U.S.) Yes

Pharmacologic Category Angiotensin-Converting Enzyme (ACE) Inhibitor

Use Treatment of hypertension when oral therapy is not practical

Unlabeled Use Acute cardiogenic pulmonary edema

Contraindications Hypersensitivity to enalapril or enalaprilat; angioedema related to previous treatment with an ACE inhibitor; patients with idiopathic or hereditary angioedema

Warnings/Precautions Anaphylactic reactions may occur rarely with ACE inhibitors. At any time during treatment (especially following first dose) angioedema may occur rarely with ACE inhibitors; it may involve the head and neck (potentially compromising airway) or the intestine (presenting with abdominal pain). African-Americans may be at an increased risk. Prolonged frequent monitoring may be required especially if tongue, glottis, or larynx are involved as they are associated with airway obstruction. Patients with a history of airway surgery may have a higher risk of airway obstruction. Aggressive early and appropriate management is critical. Use in patients with idiopathic or hereditary angioedema or previous angioedema associated with ACE inhibitor therapy is contraindicated. Severe anaphylactoid reactions may be seen during hemodialysis (eg, CVVHD) with high-flux dialysis membranes (eg, AN69), and rarely, during low density lipoprotein apheresis with dextran sulfate cellulose. Rare cases of anaphylactoid reactions have been reported in patients undergoing sensitization treatment with hymenoptera (bee, wasp) venom while receiving ACE inhibitors.

Symptomatic hypotension with or without syncope can occur with ACE inhibitors (usually with the first several doses); effects are most often observed in volume-depleted patients; correct volume depletion prior to initiation; close monitoring of patient is required especially with initial dosing and dosing increases; blood pressure must be lowered at a rate appropriate for the patient's clinical condition. Initiation of therapy in patients with ischemic heart disease or cerebrovascular disease warrants close observation due to the potential consequences posed by falling blood pressure (eg, MI, stroke). Use with caution in hypertrophic cardiomyopathy with outflow tract obstruction, severe aortic stenosis, or before, during, or immediately after major surgery.

Hyperkalemia may occur with ACE inhibitors; risk factors include renal dysfunction, diabetes mellitus, concomitant use of potassium-sparing diuretics, potassium supplements, and/or potassium-containing salts. Use cautiously, if at all, with these agents and monitor potassium closely. Cough may occur with ACE inhibitors. Other causes of cough should be considered (eg, pulmonary congestion in patients with heart failure) and excluded prior to discontinuation.

May be associated with deterioration of renal function and/or increases in serum creatinine, particularly in patients with low renal blood flow (eg, renal artery stenosis, heart failure) whose glomerular filtration rate (GFR) is dependent on efferent arteriolar vasoconstriction by angiotensin II; deterioration may result in oliguria, acute renal failure, and progressive azotemia. Small increases in serum creatinine may occur following initiation; consider discontinuation only in patients with progressive and/or significant deterioration in renal function. Use with caution in patients with unstented unilateral/bilateral renal artery stenosis. When unstented bilateral renal artery stenosis is present, use is generally avoided due to the elevated risk of deterioration in renal function unless possible benefits outweigh risks. Concurrent use of angiotensin receptor blockers may increase the risk of clinically-significant adverse events (eg, renal dysfunction, hyperkalemia).

Rare toxicities associated with ACE inhibitors include cholestatic jaundice (which may progress to fulminant hepatic necrosis), agranulocytosis, neutropenia, or leukopenia with myeloid hypoplasia. Patients with collagen vascular diseases (especially with concomitant renal impairment) or renal impairment alone may be at increased risk for hematologic toxicity; periodically monitor CBC with differential in these patients.

Adverse Reactions (Reflective of adult population; not specific for elderly) Note: Since enalapril is converted to enalaprilat, adverse reactions associated with enalapril may also occur with enalaprilat (also refer to Enalapril monograph). Frequency ranges include data from hypertension and heart failure trials. Higher rates of adverse reactions have generally been noted in patients with CHF. However, the frequency of adverse effects associated with placebo is also increased in this population.

1% to 10%:
Cardiovascular: Hypotension (2% to 5%)
Central nervous system: Headache (3%)
Gastrointestinal: Nausea (1%)

Drug Interactions

Metabolism/Transport Effects None known.

Avoid Concomitant Use There are no known interactions where it is recommended to avoid concomitant use.

Increased Effect/Toxicity

Enalaprilat may increase the levels/effects of: Allopurinol; Amifostine; Antihypertensives; AzaTHIOprine; CycloSPORINE; CycloSPORINE (Systemic); Ferric Gluconate; Gold Sodium Thiomalate; Hypotensive Agents; Iron Dextran Complex; Lithium; Nonsteroidal Anti-Inflammatory Agents; RiTUXimab; Sodium Phosphates

The levels/effects of Enalaprilat may be increased by: Alfuzosin; Aliskiren; Angiotensin II Receptor Blockers; Diazoxide; DPP-IV Inhibitors; Eplerenone; Everolimus; Herbs (Hypotensive Properties); Loop Diuretics; MAO Inhibitors; Pentoxifylline; Phosphodiesterase 5 Inhibitors; Potassium Salts; Potassium-Sparing Diuretics; Prostacyclin Analogues; Sirolimus; Temsirolimus; Thiazide Diuretics; TiZANidine; Tolvaptan; Trimethoprim

ENALAPRILAT

Decreased Effect
The levels/effects of Enalaprilat may be decreased by: Aprotinin; Herbs (Hypertensive Properties); Icatibant; Methylphenidate; Nonsteroidal Anti-Inflammatory Agents; Salicylates; Yohimbine

Ethanol/Nutrition/Herb Interactions Herb/Nutraceutical: Avoid bayberry, blue cohosh, cayenne, ephedra, ginger, ginseng (American), kola, licorice (may worsen hypertension). Avoid black cohosh, California poppy, coleus, golden seal, hawthorn, mistletoe, periwinkle, quinine, shepherd's purse (may have increased antihypertensive effect).

Stability Enalaprilat is a clear, colorless solution which should be stored at <30°C (°F). I.V. is stable for 24 hours at room temperature in D_5W, NS, D_5NS, or D_5LR.

Mechanism of Action Competitive inhibitor of angiotensin-converting enzyme (ACE); prevents conversion of angiotensin I to angiotensin II, a potent vasoconstrictor; results in lower levels of angiotensin II which causes an increase in plasma renin activity and a reduction in aldosterone secretion

Pharmacodynamics/Kinetics
Onset of action: I.V.: ≤15 minutes
Peak effect: I.V.: 1-4 hours
Duration: I.V.: ~6 hours
Protein binding: ~50% (Davies, 1984)
Half-life elimination: Adults: ~35 hours (Till, 1984; Ulm, 1982)
Excretion: Urine (>90% as unchanged drug)

Dosage
Geriatric & Adult Use lower listed initial dose in patients with hyponatremia, hypovolemia, severe congestive heart failure, decreased renal function, or in those receiving diuretics.
Heart failure: Avoid I.V. administration in patients with unstable heart failure or those suffering acute myocardial infarction
Hypertension: I.V.: 1.25 mg/dose, given over 5 minutes every 6 hours; doses as high as 5 mg/dose every 6 hours have been tolerated for up to 36 hours. **Note:** If patients are concomitantly receiving diuretic therapy, begin with 0.625 mg I.V. over 5 minutes; if the effect is not adequate after 1 hour, repeat the dose and administer 1.25 mg at 6-hour intervals thereafter; if adequate, administer 0.625 mg I.V. every 6 hours.
Conversion from I.V. **enalaprilat** *to oral* **enalapril** *therapy:* If not concurrently receiving diuretics, initiate enalapril 5 mg once daily; if concurrently receiving diuretics and responding to enalaprilat 0.625 mg I.V. every 6 hours, initiate with enalapril 2.5 mg once daily; subsequent titration as needed.

Renal Impairment
Manufacturer's recommendations:
Cl_{cr} >30 mL/minute: No dosage adjustment necessary
Cl_{cr} ≤30 mL/minute: Initiate with 0.625 mg; if after 1 hour clinical response is unsatisfactory, may repeat. May then administer 1.25 mg every 6 hours.
Intermittent hemodialysis (IHD): Moderately dialyzable (20% to 50%): Initial: 0.625 mg I.V. over a period of 5-60 minutes (60-minute infusion duration preferred)
Conversion from I.V. **enalaprilat** to oral **enalapril** therapy:
Cl_{cr} >30 mL/minute: May initiate enalapril 5 mg once daily.
Cl_{cr} ≤30 mL/minute: May initiate enalapril 2.5 mg once daily.
Alternate recommendations (Aronoff, 2007):
Cl_{cr} >50 mL/minute: No dosage adjustment necessary
Cl_{cr} 10-50 mL/minute: Administer 75% to 100% of usual dose
Cl_{cr} <10 mL/minute: Administer 50% of usual dose
Peritoneal dialysis: Supplemental dose is not necessary, although some removal of drug occurs.

Hepatic Impairment No dosage adjustment necessary for patients with hepatic impairment; enalaprilat does not undergo hepatic metabolism.

Administration Administer direct IVP over at least 5 minutes or dilute in up to 50 mL of a compatible solution and infuse; discontinue diuretic, if possible, for 2-3 days before beginning enalaprilat therapy.

Monitoring Parameters Blood pressure; serum creatinine and potassium; if patient has collagen vascular disease and/or renal impairment, periodically monitor CBC with differential

Special Geriatric Considerations Due to frequent decreases in glomerular filtration (also creatinine clearance) with aging, elderly patients may have exaggerated responses to ACE inhibitors; differences in clinical response due to hepatic changes are not observed. ACE inhibitors may be preferred agents in elderly patients with congestive heart failure and diabetes mellitus. Diabetic proteinuria is reduced and insulin sensitivity is enhanced. In general, the side effect profile is favorable in the elderly and causes little or no CNS confusion; use lowest dose recommendations initially; adjust dose for renal function in the elderly. Many elderly may be volume depleted due to diuretic use and/or blunted thirst reflex resulting in inadequate fluid intake.

Dosage Forms Excipient information presented when available (limited, particularly for generics); consult specific product labeling.
Injection, solution: 1.25 mg/mL (1 mL, 2 mL)

◆ **Enalapril Maleate** *see* Enalapril *on page 631*
◆ **Enalapril Maleate and Hydrochlorothiazide** *see* Enalapril and Hydrochlorothiazide *on page 634*
◆ **Enbrel®** *see* Etanercept *on page 720*
◆ **Enbrel® SureClick®** *see* Etanercept *on page 720*
◆ **Endocet®** *see* Oxycodone and Acetaminophen *on page 1449*
◆ **Endodan®** *see* Oxycodone and Aspirin *on page 1452*
◆ **Endometrin®** *see* Progesterone *on page 1612*
◆ **Enemeez® [OTC]** *see* Docusate *on page 583*
◆ **Enemeez® Plus [OTC]** *see* Docusate *on page 583*
◆ **Ener-B® [OTC]** *see* Cyanocobalamin *on page 452*
◆ **Enfamil® D-Vi-Sol™ [OTC]** *see* Cholecalciferol *on page 365*
◆ **Engerix-B®** *see* Hepatitis B Vaccine (Recombinant) *on page 926*
◆ **Engerix-B® and Havrix®** *see* Hepatitis A and Hepatitis B Recombinant Vaccine *on page 919*
◆ **Enhanced-Potency Inactivated Poliovirus Vaccine** *see* Poliovirus Vaccine (Inactivated) *on page 1561*
◆ **Enjuvia™** *see* Estrogens (Conjugated B/Synthetic) *on page 700*
◆ **Enlon®** *see* Edrophonium *on page 627*

Enoxaparin (ee noks a PA rin)

Related Information
Injectable Heparins/Heparinoids Comparison Table *on page 2119*
Medication Safety Issues
Sound-alike/look-alike issues:
Lovenox® may be confused with Lasix®, Levaquin®, Lotronex®, Protonix®
High alert medication:
The Institute for Safe Medication Practices (ISMP) includes this medication among its list of drugs which have a heightened risk of causing significant patient harm when used in error.
National Patient Safety Goals:
The Joint Commission (TJC) requires healthcare organizations that provide anticoagulant therapy to have a process in place to reduce the risk of anticoagulant-associated patient harm. Patients receiving anticoagulants should receive individualized care through a defined process that includes standardized ordering, dispensing, administration, monitoring and education. This does not apply to routine short-term use of anticoagulants for prevention of venous thromboembolism when the expectation is that the patient's laboratory values will remain within or close to normal values (NPSG.03.05.01).
Brand Names: U.S. Lovenox®
Brand Names: Canada Enoxaparin Injection; Lovenox®; Lovenox® HP
Index Terms Enoxaparin Sodium
Generic Availability (U.S.) Yes
Pharmacologic Category Low Molecular Weight Heparin
Use
Acute coronary syndromes: Unstable angina (UA), non-ST-elevation (NSTEMI), and ST-elevation myocardial infarction (STEMI)
DVT prophylaxis: Following hip or knee replacement surgery, abdominal surgery, or in medical patients with severely-restricted mobility during acute illness who are at risk for thromboembolic complications
DVT treatment (acute): Inpatient treatment (patients with and without pulmonary embolism) and outpatient treatment (patients without pulmonary embolism)
Note: High-risk patients include those with one or more of the following risk factors: >40 years of age, obesity, general anesthesia lasting >30 minutes, malignancy, history of deep vein thrombosis or pulmonary embolism
Unlabeled Use Anticoagulant bridge therapy during temporary interruption of vitamin K antagonist therapy in patients at high risk for thromboembolism; DVT prophylaxis following moderate-risk general surgery, major gynecologic surgery and following higher-risk general surgery for cancer; anticoagulant used during percutaneous coronary intervention (PCI)
Contraindications Hypersensitivity to enoxaparin, heparin, or any component of the formulation; thrombocytopenia associated with a positive *in vitro* test for antiplatelet antibodies in the presence of enoxaparin; hypersensitivity to pork products; active major bleeding; not for I.M. use

Warnings/Precautions [U.S. Boxed Warning]: Spinal or epidural hematomas, including subsequent paralysis, may occur with recent or anticipated neuraxial anesthesia (epidural or spinal anesthesia) or spinal puncture in patients anticoagulated with LMWH or heparinoids. Consider risk versus benefit prior to spinal procedures; risk is increased by the use of concomitant agents which may alter hemostasis, the use of indwelling epidural catheters for analgesia, a history of spinal deformity or spinal surgery, as well as a history of traumatic or repeated epidural or spinal punctures. Patient should be observed closely for bleeding and signs and symptoms of neurological impairment if therapy is administered during or immediately following diagnostic lumbar puncture, epidural anesthesia, or spinal anesthesia.

Do not administer intramuscularly. Not recommended for thromboprophylaxis in patients with prosthetic heart valves. Not to be used interchangeably (unit for unit) with heparin or any other low molecular weight heparins. Use caution in patients with history of heparin-induced thrombocytopenia. Monitor patient closely for signs or symptoms of bleeding. Certain patients are at increased risk of bleeding. Risk factors include bacterial endocarditis; congenital or acquired bleeding disorders; active ulcerative or angiodysplastic GI diseases; severe uncontrolled hypertension; history of hemorrhagic stroke; use shortly after brain, spinal, or ophthalmic surgery; patients treated concomitantly with platelet inhibitors; recent GI bleeding; thrombocytopenia or platelet defects; severe liver disease; hypertensive or diabetic retinopathy; or in patients undergoing invasive procedures. Monitor platelet count closely. Rare cases of thrombocytopenia have occurred. Discontinue therapy and consider alternative treatment if platelets are <100,000/mm^3 and/or thrombosis develops. Rare cases of thrombocytopenia with thrombosis has occurred. Use caution in patients with congenital or drug-induced thrombocytopenia or platelet defects. Risk of bleeding may be increased in women <45 kg and in men <57 kg. Use caution in patients with renal failure; dosage adjustment needed if Cl$_{cr}$ <30 mL/minute. Use with caution in the elderly (delayed elimination may occur); dosage alteration/adjustment may be required (eg, omission of I.V. bolus in acute STEMI in patients ≥75 years of age). Monitor for hyperkalemia; can cause hyperkalemia possibly by suppressing aldosterone production. Multiple-dose vials contain benzyl alcohol.

There is no consensus for adjusting/correcting the weight-based dosage of LMWH for patients who are morbidly obese (BMI ≥40 kg/m^2). The American College of Chest Physicians Practice Guidelines suggest consulting with a pharmacist regarding dosing in bariatric surgery patients and other obese patients who may require higher doses of LMWH (Gould, 2012).

Adverse Reactions (Reflective of adult population; not specific for elderly) As with all anticoagulants, bleeding is the major adverse effect of enoxaparin. Hemorrhage may occur at virtually any site. Risk is dependent on multiple variables. At the recommended doses, single injections of enoxaparin do not significantly influence platelet aggregation or affect global clotting time (ie, PT or aPTT).

1% to 10%:
Central nervous system: Fever (5% to 8%), confusion, pain
Dermatologic: Erythema, bruising
Gastrointestinal: Nausea (3%), diarrhea
Hematologic: Hemorrhage (major, <1% to 4%; includes cases of intracranial, retroperitoneal, or intraocular hemorrhage; incidence varies with indication/population), thrombocytopenia (moderate 1%; severe 0.1% - see "**Note**"), anemia (<2%)
Hepatic: ALT increased, AST increased
Local: Injection site hematoma (9%), local reactions (irritation, pain, ecchymosis, erythema)
Renal: Hematuria (<2%)
Note: Thrombocytopenia with thrombosis: Cases of heparin-induced thrombocytopenia (some complicated by organ infarction, limb ischemia, or death) have been reported.

Drug Interactions
Metabolism/Transport Effects None known.
Avoid Concomitant Use
Avoid concomitant use of Enoxaparin with any of the following: Rivaroxaban
Increased Effect/Toxicity
Enoxaparin may increase the levels/effects of: Anticoagulants; Collagenase (Systemic); Dabigatran Etexilate; Deferasirox; Drotrecogin Alfa (Activated); Ibritumomab; Palifermin; Rivaroxaban; Tositumomab and Iodine I 131 Tositumomab

The levels/effects of Enoxaparin may be increased by: 5-ASA Derivatives; Antiplatelet Agents; Dasatinib; Herbs (Anticoagulant/Antiplatelet Properties); Nonsteroidal Anti-Inflammatory Agents; Pentosan Polysulfate Sodium; Pentoxifylline; Prostacyclin Analogues; Salicylates; Thrombolytic Agents; Tipranavir
Decreased Effect There are no known significant interactions involving a decrease in effect.

Ethanol/Nutrition/Herb Interactions Herb/Nutraceutical: Avoid cat's claw, dong quai, evening primrose, feverfew, garlic, ginger, ginkgo, red clover, horse chestnut, green tea, ginseng (all have additional antiplatelet activity).

Stability Store at 25°C (77°F); excursions permitted to 15°C to 30°C (59°F to 86°F); do not freeze.

Mechanism of Action Standard heparin consists of components with molecular weights ranging from 4000-30,000 daltons with a mean of 16,000 daltons. Heparin acts as an anticoagulant by enhancing the inhibition rate of clotting proteases by antithrombin III impairing normal hemostasis and inhibition of factor Xa. Low molecular weight heparins have a small effect on the activated partial thromboplastin time and strongly inhibit factor Xa. Enoxaparin is derived from porcine heparin that undergoes benzylation followed by alkaline depolymerization. The average molecular weight of enoxaparin is 4500 daltons which is distributed as (≤20%) 2000 daltons (≥68%) 2000-8000 daltons, and (≤15%) >8000 daltons. Enoxaparin has a higher ratio of antifactor Xa to antifactor IIa activity than unfractionated heparin.

Pharmacodynamics/Kinetics

Onset of action: Peak effect: SubQ: Antifactor Xa and antithrombin (antifactor IIa): 3-5 hours

Duration: 40 mg dose: Antifactor Xa activity: ~12 hours

Distribution: 4.3 L (based on antifactor Xa activity)

Protein binding: Does not bind to heparin binding proteins

Metabolism: Hepatic, to lower molecular weight fragments (little activity)

Half-life elimination, plasma: 2-4 times longer than standard heparin, independent of dose; based on anti-Xa activity: 4.5-7 hours

Excretion: Urine (40% of dose; 10% as active fragments)

Dosage

Geriatric SubQ: Refer to adult dosing. Increased incidence of bleeding with doses of 1.5 mg/kg/day or 1 mg/kg every 12 hours; injection-associated bleeding and serious adverse reactions are also increased in the elderly. Careful attention should be paid to elderly patients, particularly those <45 kg. **Note:** Dosage alteration/adjustment may be required.

Adult One mg of enoxaparin is equal to 100 units of anti-Xa activity (World Health Organization First International Low Molecular Weight Heparin Reference Standard).

DVT prophylaxis: Note: In morbidly obese patients (BMI ≥40 kg/m^2), increasing the prophylactic dose by 30% may be appropriate for some indications (Nutescu, 2009). For bariatric surgery, dose increases may be >30% based on clinical trial data. SubQ:

Hip replacement surgery:

Twice-daily dosing: 30 mg every 12 hours, with initial dose within 12-24 hours after surgery, and every 12 hours for at least 10 days or until risk of DVT has diminished or the patient is adequately anticoagulated on warfarin. The American College of Chest Physicians recommends initiation ≥12 hours preoperatively **or** ≥12 hours postoperatively; extended duration of up to 35 days suggested (Guyatt, 2012).

Once-daily dosing: 40 mg once daily, with initial dose within 9-15 hours before surgery, and daily for at least 10 days (or up to 35 days postoperatively) or until risk of DVT has diminished or the patient is adequately anticoagulated on warfarin. The American College of Chest Physicians recommends initiation ≥12 hours preoperatively **or** ≥12 hours postoperatively; extended duration of up to 35 days suggested (Guyatt, 2012).

Knee replacement surgery: 30 mg every 12 hours, with initial dose within 12-24 hours after surgery, and every 12 hours for at least 10 days or until risk of DVT has diminished or the patient is adequately anticoagulated on warfarin. The American College of Chest Physicians recommends initiation ≥12 hours preoperatively **or** ≥12 hours postoperatively; extended duration of up to 35 days suggested (Guyatt, 2012).

Abdominal surgery: 40 mg once daily, with initial dose given 2 hours prior to surgery; continue until risk of DVT has diminished (usually 7-10 days).

Bariatric surgery: Roux-en-Y gastric bypass: Appropriate dosing strategies have not been clearly defined (Borkgren-Okonek, 2008; Scholten, 2002):

BMI ≤50 kg/m^2: 40 mg every 12 hours

BMI >50 kg/m^2: 60 mg every 12 hours

Note: Bariatric surgery guidelines suggest initiation 30-120 minutes before surgery and postoperatively until patient is fully mobile (Mechanick, 2009). Alternatively, limiting administration to the postoperative period may reduce perioperative bleeding.

Medical patients with severely-restricted mobility during acute illness: 40 mg once daily; continue until risk of DVT has diminished (usually 6-11 days).

DVT treatment (acute): SubQ: **Note:** Start warfarin on the first or second treatment day and continue enoxaparin until INR is ≥2 for at least 24 hours (usually 5-7 days) (Guyatt, 2012).

Inpatient treatment (with or without pulmonary embolism): 1 mg/kg/dose every 12 hours or 1.5 mg/kg once daily.

Outpatient treatment (without pulmonary embolism): 1 mg/kg/dose every 12 hours.

Obesity: Use actual body weight to calculate dose; dose capping not recommended; use of twice daily dosing preferred (Nutescu, 2009)

Percutaneous coronary intervention (PCI), adjunctive therapy (unlabeled use): I.V.: In patients treated with multiple doses of enoxaparin undergoing PCI, if PCI occurs within 8 hours after the last SubQ enoxaparin dose, no additional dosing is needed. If PCI occurs 8-12 hours after the last SubQ enoxaparin dose or the patient received only 1 therapeutic SubQ dose (eg, 1 mg/kg), a single I.V. dose of 0.3 mg/kg should be administered. If PCI occurs >12 hours after the last SubQ dose, it is prudent to use an established anticoagulation regimen (eg, unfractionated heparin or bivalirudin) (Levine, 2011).

If patient has not received prior anticoagulant therapy: 0.5-0.75 mg/kg bolus dose (Levine, 2011)

ST-elevation MI (STEMI):

Patients <75 years of age: Initial: 30 mg I.V. single bolus plus 1 mg/kg (maximum 100 mg for the first 2 doses only) SubQ every 12 hours. The first SubQ dose should be administered with the I.V. bolus. Maintenance: After first 2 doses, administer 1 mg/kg SubQ every 12 hours.

Patients ≥75 years of age: Initial: SubQ: 0.75 mg/kg every 12 hours (**Note:** No I.V. bolus is administered in this population); a maximum dose of 75 mg is recommended for the first 2 doses. Maintenance: After first 2 doses, administer 0.75 mg/kg SubQ every 12 hours

Obesity: Use weight-based dosing; a maximum dose of 100 mg is recommended for the first 2 doses (Nutescu, 2009)

Additional notes on STEMI treatment: Therapy was continued for 8 days or until hospital discharge; optimal duration not defined. Unless contraindicated, all patients received aspirin (75-325 mg daily) in clinical trials. In patients with STEMI receiving thrombolytics, initiate enoxaparin dosing between 15 minutes before and 30 minutes after fibrinolytic therapy.

Unstable angina or non-ST-elevation MI (NSTEMI): 1 mg/kg every 12 hours in conjunction with oral aspirin therapy (100-325 mg once daily); continue until clinical stabilization (a minimum of at least 2 days)

Obesity: Use actual body weight to calculate dose; dose capping not recommended (Nutescu, 2009)

Renal Impairment

Cl$_{cr}$ ≥30 mL/minute: No specific adjustment recommended (per manufacturer); monitor closely for bleeding.

Cl$_{cr}$ <30 mL/minute:

DVT prophylaxis in abdominal surgery, hip replacement, knee replacement, or in medical patients during acute illness: SubQ: 30 mg once daily

DVT treatment (inpatient or outpatient treatment in conjunction with warfarin): SubQ: 1 mg/kg once daily

STEMI:

<75 years: Initial: I.V.: 30 mg as a single dose with the first dose of the SubQ maintenance regimen administered at the same time as the I.V. bolus; Maintenance: SubQ: 1 mg/kg every 24 hours

≥75 years of age: Omit I.V. bolus; Maintenance: SubQ: 1 mg/kg every 24 hours

Unstable angina, NSTEMI: SubQ: 1 mg/kg once daily

Dialysis: Enoxaparin has not been FDA approved for use in dialysis patients. It's elimination is primarily via the renal route. Serious bleeding complications have been reported with use in patients who are dialysis dependent or have severe renal failure. LMWH administration at fixed doses without monitoring has greater unpredictable anticoagulant effects in patients with chronic kidney disease. If used, dosages should be reduced and anti-Xa levels frequently monitored, as accumulation may occur with repeated doses. Many clinicians would not use enoxaparin in this population especially without timely anti-Xa levels.

Hemodialysis: Supplemental dose is not necessary.

Peritoneal dialysis: Significant drug removal is unlikely based on physiochemical characteristics.

Administration Do **not** administer I.M.; should be administered by deep SubQ injection to the left or right anterolateral and left or right posterolateral abdominal wall. A single dose may be administered I.V. as part of treatment for ST-elevation myocardial infarction (STEMI) to patients <75 years of age; no I.V. bolus is given to patients ≥75 years of age. To avoid loss of drug from the 30 mg and 40 mg syringes, do not expel the air bubble from the syringe prior to injection. In order to minimize bruising, do not rub injection site. An automatic injector (Lovenox EasyInjector™) is available with the 30 mg and 40 mg syringes to aid the patient with self-injections. **Note:** Enoxaparin is available in 100 mg/mL and 150 mg/mL concentrations.

To convert from I.V. unfractionated heparin (UFH) infusion to SubQ enoxaparin (Nutescu, 2007): Calculate specific dose for enoxaparin based on indication, discontinue UFH and begin enoxaparin within 1 hour.

To convert from SubQ enoxaparin to I.V. UFH infusion (Nutescu, 2007): Discontinue enoxaparin, calculate specific dose for I.V. UFH infusion based on indication, omit heparin bolus/loading dose:

Converting from SubQ enoxaparin dosed every 12 hours: Start I.V. UFH infusion 10-11 hours after last dose of enoxaparin

Converting from SubQ enoxaparin dosed every 24 hours: Start I.V. UFH infusion 22-23 hours after last dose of enoxaparin

Monitoring Parameters Platelets, occult blood, anti-Xa levels, serum creatinine; monitoring of PT and/or aPTT is not necessary. Routine monitoring of anti-Xa levels is not required, but has been utilized in patients with obesity and/or renal insufficiency. Monitoring anti-Xa levels is recommended when receiving enoxaparin for the prevention of thromboembolism with mechanical heart valves (Guyatt, 2012). For patients >190 kg, if anti-Xa monitoring is available, adjusting dose based on anti-Xa levels is recommended; if anti-Xa monitoring is unavailable, reduce dose if bleeding occurs (Nutescu, 2009).

Reference Range The following therapeutic ranges for anti-Xa levels have been suggested, but have not been validated in a controlled trial. Anti-Xa level measured 4 hours postdose. Treatment of venous thromboembolism: Anti-Xa concentration target (Garcia, 2012):

Once-daily dosing: >1 anti-Xa units/mL; the manufacturer recommends a range of 1-2 anti-Xa units/mL

Twice-daily dosing: 0.6-1 anti-Xa units/mL

Special Geriatric Considerations No specific dosage adjustment recommendations for most indications, however, total clearance is lower and elimination is delayed in patients with renal failure. Adjustment may be necessary if renal impairment is present. In the treatment of STEMI, a lower dosage (0.75 mg/kg every 12 hours) and omission of the I.V. bolus, are recommended in patients ≥75 years of age.

In clinical trials, the efficacy of enoxaparin injection in elderly (≥65 years) was similar to that seen in younger patients (<65 years). The incidence of bleeding complications was similar between elderly and younger patients when 30 mg every 12 hours or 40 mg once daily doses of enoxaparin injection was administered at doses of 1.5 mg/kg/day or 1 mg/kg every 12 hours. The risk of enoxaparin injection associated bleeding increased with age. Serious adverse events increased with age for patients receiving enoxaparin injections. Other clinical experience has not revealed additional differences in the safety of enoxaparin injection between elderly and younger patients. Careful attention to dosing intervals and concomitant medications (especially antiplatelet medications) is advised. Monitoring of elderly patients with low body weight (<45 kg) and those predisposed to decreased renal function should be considered.

Dosage Forms Excipient information presented when available (limited, particularly for generics); consult specific product labeling.

Injection, solution, as sodium: 100 mg/mL (3 mL)

Lovenox®: 100 mg/mL (3 mL) [contains benzyl alcohol; vial]

Injection, solution, as sodium [preservative free]: 30 mg/0.3 mL (0.3 mL); 40 mg/0.4 mL (0.4 mL); 60 mg/0.6 mL (0.6 mL); 80 mg/0.8 mL (0.8 mL); 100 mg/mL (1 mL); 120 mg/0.8 mL (0.8 mL); 150 mg/mL (1 mL)

Lovenox®: 30 mg/0.3 mL (0.3 mL); 40 mg/0.4 mL (0.4 mL); 60 mg/0.6 mL (0.6 mL); 80 mg/0.8 mL (0.8 mL); 100 mg/mL (1 mL); 120 mg/0.8 mL (0.8 mL); 150 mg/mL (1 mL) [prefilled syringe]

◆ **Enoxaparin Sodium** *see* Enoxaparin *on page 637*

Entacapone (en TA ka pone)

Related Information
Antiparkinsonian Agents *on page 2101*
Brand Names: U.S. Comtan®
Brand Names: Canada Comtan®; Sandoz-Entacapone; Teva-Entacapone
Generic Availability (U.S.) No
Pharmacologic Category Anti-Parkinson's Agent, COMT Inhibitor
Use Adjunct to levodopa/carbidopa therapy in patients with idiopathic Parkinson's disease who experience "wearing-off" symptoms at the end of a dosing interval
Contraindications Hypersensitivity to entacapone or any of component of the formulation
Warnings/Precautions May cause orthostatic hypotension and syncope; Parkinson's disease patients appear to have an impaired capacity to respond to a postural challenge; use with caution in patients at risk of hypotension (such as those receiving antihypertensive drugs) or where transient hypotensive episodes would be poorly tolerated (cardiovascular disease or

cerebrovascular disease). Parkinson's patients being treated with dopaminergic agonists ordinarily require careful monitoring for signs and symptoms of postural hypotension, especially during dose escalation, and should be informed of this risk. May cause hallucinations, which may improve with reduction in levodopa therapy. Use with caution in patients with pre-existing dyskinesias; exacerbation of pre-existing dyskinesia and severe rhabdomyolysis has been reported. Levodopa dosage reduction may be required, particularly in patients with levodopa dosages >600 mg daily or with moderate-to-severe dyskinesia prior to initiation. Entacapone, in conjunction with other drug therapy that alters brain biogenic amine concentrations (eg, MAO inhibitors, SSRIs), has been associated with a syndrome resembling neuroleptic malignant syndrome (hyperpyrexia and confusion - some fatal) on abrupt withdrawal or dosage reduction. Concomitant use of entacapone and nonselective MAO inhibitors should be avoided. Selegiline is a selective MAO type B inhibitor (when given orally at ≤10 mg/day) and can be taken with entacapone.

Dopaminergic agents have been associated with compulsive behaviors and/or loss of impulse control, which has manifested as pathological gambling, libido increases (hypersexuality), and/or binge eating. Causality has not been established, and controversy exists as to whether this phenomenon is related to the underlying disease, prior behaviors/addictions and/or drug therapy. Dose reduction or discontinuation of therapy has been reported to reverse these behaviors in some, but not all cases. Risk for melanoma development is increased in Parkinson's disease patients; drug causation or factors contributing to risk have not been established. Patients should be monitored closely and periodic skin examinations should be performed. Dopaminergic agents from the ergot class have also been associated with fibrotic complications, such as retroperitoneal fibrosis, pulmonary infiltrates or effusion and pleural thickening. It is unknown whether non-ergot, pro-dopaminergic agents like entacapone confer this risk. Use caution in patients with hepatic impairment or severe renal impairment. Do not withdraw therapy abruptly. Discoloration of urine, saliva, or sweat to dark colors (red, brown, black) may be observed during therapy. Use with caution in patients with lower gastrointestinal disease or an increased risk of dehydration; has been associated with delayed development of diarrhea (usual onset after 4-12 weeks). Diarrhea may be a sign of drug-induced colitis. Discontinue use with prolonged diarrhea.

Adverse Reactions (Reflective of adult population; not specific for elderly)

>10%:
  Gastrointestinal: Nausea (14%)
  Neuromuscular & skeletal: Dyskinesia (25%), placebo (15%)

1% to 10%:
  Cardiovascular: Orthostatic hypotension (4%), syncope (1%)
  Central nervous system: Dizziness (8%), fatigue (6%), hallucinations (4%), anxiety (2%), somnolence (2%), agitation (1%)
  Dermatologic: Purpura (2%)
  Gastrointestinal: Diarrhea (10%), abdominal pain (8%), constipation (6%), vomiting (4%), dry mouth (3%), dyspepsia (2%), flatulence (2%), gastritis (1%), taste perversion (1%)
  Genitourinary: Brown-orange urine discoloration (10%)
  Neuromuscular & skeletal: Hyperkinesia (10%), hypokinesia (9%), back pain (4%), weakness (2%)
  Respiratory: Dyspnea (3%)
  Miscellaneous: Diaphoresis increased (2%), bacterial infection (1%)

Drug Interactions

Metabolism/Transport Effects Inhibits COMT, CYP1A2 (weak), CYP2A6 (weak), CYP2C19 (weak), CYP2C9 (weak), CYP2D6 (weak), CYP2E1 (weak), CYP3A4 (weak)

Avoid Concomitant Use
  Avoid concomitant use of Entacapone with any of the following: Azelastine; Azelastine (Nasal); Methadone; Mirtazapine; Paraldehyde; Pimozide

Increased Effect/Toxicity
  Entacapone may increase the levels/effects of: Alcohol (Ethyl); ARIPiprazole; Azelastine; Azelastine (Nasal); Buprenorphine; CNS Depressants; COMT Substrates; MAO Inhibitors; Methadone; Methotrimeprazine; Metyrosine; Mirtazapine; Paraldehyde; Pimozide; Selective Serotonin Reuptake Inhibitors; Zolpidem

  The levels/effects of Entacapone may be increased by: Droperidol; HydrOXYzine; Methotrimeprazine

Decreased Effect There are no known significant interactions involving a decrease in effect.

Ethanol/Nutrition/Herb Interactions

Ethanol: May increase CNS depression; monitor for increased effects with coadministration. Caution patients about effects.

Food: Entacapone has been reported to chelate iron and decreasing serum iron levels were noted in clinical trials; however, clinically significant anemia has not been observed.

Mechanism of Action Entacapone is a reversible and selective inhibitor of catechol-O-methyltransferase (COMT). When entacapone is taken with levodopa, the pharmacokinetics are altered, resulting in more sustained levodopa serum levels compared to levodopa taken alone. The resulting levels of levodopa provide for increased concentrations available for absorption across the blood-brain barrier, thereby providing for increased CNS levels of dopamine, the active metabolite of levodopa.

Pharmacodynamics/Kinetics

Onset of action: Rapid

Peak effect: 1 hour

Absorption: Rapid

Distribution: I.V.: V_{dss}: 20 L

Protein binding: 98%, primarily to albumin

Metabolism: Isomerization to the *cis*-isomer, followed by direct glucuronidation of the parent and *cis*-isomer

Bioavailability: 35%

Half-life elimination: B phase: 0.4-0.7 hours; Y phase: 2.4 hours

Time to peak, serum: 1 hour

Excretion: Feces (90%); urine (10%)

Dosage

Geriatric & Adult Parkinson's disease: Oral: 200 mg with each dose of levodopa/carbidopa, up to a maximum of 8 times/day (maximum daily dose: 1600 mg/day). To optimize therapy, the dosage of levodopa may need reduced or the dosing interval may need extended. Patients taking levodopa ≥800 mg/day or who had moderate-to-severe dyskinesias prior to therapy required an average decrease of 25% in the daily levodopa dose.

Renal Impairment No adjustment is required; dialysis patients were not studied.

Hepatic Impairment Dosage adjustment in chronic therapy with standard treatment has not been studied.

Administration Always administer in association with levodopa/carbidopa; can be combined with both the immediate and sustained release formulations of levodopa/carbidopa. May be administered without regard to meals. Should not be abruptly withdrawn from patient's therapy due to significant worsening of symptoms.

Monitoring Parameters Signs and symptoms of Parkinson's disease; liver function tests, blood pressure, patient's mental status; serum iron (if signs of anemia)

Pharmacotherapy Pearls No increase in LFTs has been noted; therefore, does not require LFT monitoring. Because of this, entacapone may be preferred over the other COMT inhibitor, tolcapone, in patients with "wearing off". Entacapone has not been studied in patients with stable Parkinson's disease.

Special Geriatric Considerations No difference in adverse effects was noted in the elderly. Monitor levodopa dose.

Dosage Forms Excipient information presented when available (limited, particularly for generics); consult specific product labeling.

Tablet, oral:

Comtan®: 200 mg

◆ **Entacapone, Carbidopa, and Levodopa** *see* Levodopa, Carbidopa, and Entacapone *on page 1115*

◆ **Entertainer's Secret® [OTC]** *see* Saliva Substitute *on page 1748*

◆ **Entocort® EC** *see* Budesonide (Systemic, Oral Inhalation) *on page 227*

◆ **Entsol® [OTC]** *see* Sodium Chloride *on page 1787*

◆ **Enulose** *see* Lactulose *on page 1086*

EPHEDrine (Systemic) (e FED rin)

Medication Safety Issues

Sound-alike/look-alike issues:

EPHEDrine may be confused with Epifrin®, EPINEPHrine

Index Terms Ephedrine Sulfate

Generic Availability (U.S.) Yes

Pharmacologic Category Alpha/Beta Agonist

Use Treatment of nasal congestion, anesthesia-induced hypotension

Unlabeled Use Postoperative nausea and vomiting (PONV) refractory to traditional antiemetics; idiopathic orthostatic hypotension

Contraindications Hypersensitivity to ephedrine or any component of the formulation; angle-closure glaucoma; concurrent use of other sympathomimetic agents

Warnings/Precautions Blood volume depletion should be corrected before injectable ephedrine therapy is instituted; use caution in patients with unstable vasomotor symptoms, diabetes, hyperthyroidism, prostatic hyperplasia or a history of seizures; also use caution in the elderly and those patients with cardiovascular disorders such as coronary artery disease, arrhythmias, and hypertension. Ephedrine may cause hypertension. Long-term use may cause anxiety and symptoms of paranoid schizophrenia. Use with caution in the elderly, since it crosses the blood-brain barrier and may cause confusion. Use with extreme caution in patients taking MAO inhibitors.

Adverse Reactions (Reflective of adult population; not specific for elderly) Frequency not defined.

Cardiovascular: Arrhythmias, chest pain, elevation or depression of blood pressure, hypertension, palpitation, tachycardia, unusual pallor

Central nervous system: Agitation, anxiety, apprehension, CNS stimulating effects, dizziness, excitation, fear, headache hyperactivity, insomnia, irritability, nervousness, restlessness, tension

Gastrointestinal: Anorexia, GI upset, nausea, vomiting, xerostomia

Genitourinary: Painful urination

Neuromuscular & skeletal: Trembling, tremor (more common in the elderly), weakness

Respiratory: Dyspnea

Miscellaneous: Diaphoresis increased

Drug Interactions

Metabolism/Transport Effects None known.

Avoid Concomitant Use

Avoid concomitant use of EPHEDrine (Systemic) with any of the following: Ergot Derivatives; Hyaluronidase; Iobenguane I 123; MAO Inhibitors

Increased Effect/Toxicity

EPHEDrine (Systemic) may increase the levels/effects of: Bromocriptine; Sympathomimetics

The levels/effects of EPHEDrine (Systemic) may be increased by: Antacids; AtoMOXetine; Cannabinoids; Carbonic Anhydrase Inhibitors; Ergot Derivatives; Hyaluronidase; MAO Inhibitors; Serotonin/Norepinephrine Reuptake Inhibitors

Decreased Effect

EPHEDrine (Systemic) may decrease the levels/effects of: Benzylpenicilloyl Polylysine; FentaNYL; Iobenguane I 123

The levels/effects of EPHEDrine (Systemic) may be decreased by: Spironolactone

Ethanol/Nutrition/Herb Interactions Herb/Nutraceutical: Avoid ephedra, yohimbe (may cause CNS stimulation).

Stability Protect all dosage forms from light.

Injection: Store at room temperature. **Note:** Storage guidelines vary; check product labeling for exact temperature range.

Mechanism of Action Releases tissue stores of norepinephrine and thereby produces an alpha- and beta-adrenergic stimulation; longer-acting and less potent than epinephrine

Pharmacodynamics/Kinetics

Duration: Oral: 3-6 hours

Metabolism: Minimally hepatic; metabolites include p-hydroxyephedrine, p-hydroxynorephedrine, norephedrine

Half-life elimination: 2.5-3.6 hours

Excretion: Urine (60% to 77% as unchanged drug) within 24 hours

Dosage

Geriatric & Adult

Hypotension induced by anesthesia: I.V.: 5-25 mg/dose slow I.V. push repeated after 5-10 minutes as needed, then every 3-4 hours (maximum: 150 mg/24 hours)

Idiopathic orthostatic hypotension (unlabeled use): Oral: 25-50 mg 3 times/day; maximum: 150 mg/day. **Note:** Not considered first-line for this indication.

PONV refractory to traditional antiemetics (unlabeled use): I.M.: 0.5 mg/kg at the end of surgery (Gan, 2007; Hagemann, 2000)

Administration Injection solution: Dilute to 5 or 10 mg/mL. Administer as a slow I.V. push. Do not administer unless solution is clear.

Monitoring Parameters Injection solution: Monitor blood pressure, pulse

Test Interactions Can cause a false-positive amphetamine EMIT assay

Special Geriatric Considerations Avoid as a bronchodilator. Use caution since it crosses the blood-brain barrier and may cause confusion.

Dosage Forms Excipient information presented when available (limited, particularly for generics); consult specific product labeling.

Capsule, oral, as sulfate: 25 mg

Injection, solution, as sulfate [preservative free]: 50 mg/mL (1 mL)

Epinastine (ep i NAS teen)

Brand Names: U.S. Elestat®
Index Terms Epinastine Hydrochloride
Generic Availability (U.S.) Yes
Pharmacologic Category Histamine H$_1$ Antagonist; Histamine H$_1$ Antagonist, Second Generation
Use Treatment of allergic conjunctivitis
Dosage
  Geriatric & Adult Allergic conjunctivitis: Ophthalmic: Instill 1 drop into each eye twice daily. Continue throughout period of exposure, even in the absence of symptoms.
  Special Geriatric Considerations No difference in safety and efficacy was observed between elderly and younger patients.
  Dosage Forms Excipient information presented when available (limited, particularly for generics); consult specific product labeling.
  Solution, ophthalmic, as hydrochloride [drops]: 0.05% (5 mL)
    Elestat®: 0.05% (5 mL) [contains benzalkonium chloride]

♦ **Epinastine Hydrochloride** *see* Epinastine *on page* 645

EPINEPHrine (Systemic, Oral Inhalation) (ep i NEF rin)

Medication Safety Issues
  Sound-alike/look-alike issues:
    EPINEPHrine may be confused with ePHEDrine
    Epifrin® may be confused with ephedrine, EpiPen®
  High alert medication:
    The Institute for Safe Medication Practices (ISMP) includes this medication among its list of drugs which have a heightened risk of causing significant patient harm when used in error.
  Administration issues:
    Medication errors have occurred due to confusion with epinephrine products expressed as ratio strengths (eg, 1:1000 vs 1:10,000).
    Epinephrine 1:1000 = 1 mg/mL and is most commonly used I.M.
    Epinephrine 1:10,000 = 0.1 mg/mL and is used I.V.
    Medication errors have occurred when topical epinephrine 1 mg/mL (1:1000) has been inadvertently injected. Vials of injectable and topical epinephrine look very similar. Epinephrine should always be appropriately labeled with the intended administration.
  International issues:
    EpiPen [U.S., Canada, and multiple international markets] may be confused with Epigen brand name for glycyrrhizinic acid [Argentina, Mexico, Russia] and Epopen brand name for epoetin alfa [Spain]
Brand Names: U.S. Adrenalin®; Asthmanefrin™ [OTC]; EpiPen 2-Pak®; EpiPen Jr 2-Pak®; Primatene® Mist [OTC] [DSC]; S2® [OTC]; Twinject®
Brand Names: Canada Adrenalin®; Epi E-Z Pen®; EpiPen®; EpiPen® Jr; Twinject®
Index Terms Adrenaline; Auvi-Q™; Epinephrine Bitartrate; Epinephrine Hydrochloride; Racemic Epinephrine; Racepinephrine
Generic Availability (U.S.) Yes: Solution for injection
Pharmacologic Category Alpha/Beta Agonist
Use Treatment of bronchospasms, bronchial asthma, viral croup, anaphylactic reactions, cardiac arrest; added to local anesthetics to decrease systemic absorption of intraspinal and local anesthetics and increase duration of action; decrease superficial hemorrhage
Unlabeled Use ACLS guidelines: Ventricular fibrillation (VF) or pulseless ventricular tachycardia (VT) unresponsive to initial defibrillation shocks; pulseless electrical activity; asystole; hypotension/shock unresponsive to volume resuscitation; symptomatic bradycardia unresponsive to atropine or pacing; inotropic support
Contraindications There are no absolute contraindications to the use of injectable epinephrine (including EpiPen®, EpiPen® Jr, and Twinject®) in a life-threatening situation.

Oral inhalation: Concurrent use or within 2 weeks of MAO inhibitors

Injectable solution: Per the manufacturer, contraindicated in narrow-angle glaucoma; shock; during general anesthesia with halogenated hydrocarbons or cyclopropane (currently not available in U.S.); individuals with organic brain damage; with local anesthesia of the digits; during labor; heart failure; coronary insufficiency

Warnings/Precautions Use with caution in elderly patients, patients with diabetes mellitus, cardiovascular diseases (eg, coronary artery disease, hypertension), thyroid disease, cerebrovascular disease, Parkinson's disease, or patients taking tricyclic antidepressants. Some products contain sulfites as preservatives; the presence of sulfites in some products (eg, EpiPen® and Twinject®) should not deter administration during a serious allergic or other emergency situation even if the patient is sulfite-sensitive. Accidental injection into digits, hands, or feet may result in local reactions, including injection site pallor, coldness and hypoesthesia or injury, resulting in bruising, bleeding, discoloration, erythema or skeletal injury; patient should seek immediate medical attention if this occurs. Rapid I.V. administration may cause death from cerebrovascular hemorrhage or cardiac arrhythmias; however, rapid I.V. administration during pulseless arrest is necessary.

Oral inhalation: Use with caution in patients with prostate enlargement or urinary retention; may cause temporary worsening of symptoms.

Self medication (OTC use): Oral inhalation: Prior to self-medication, patients should contact healthcare provider. The product should only be used in persons with a diagnosis of asthma. If symptoms are not relieved in 20 minutes or become worse do not continue to use the product - seek immediate medical assistance. The product should not be used more frequently or at higher doses than recommended unless directed by a healthcare provider. This product should not be used in patients who have required hospitalization for asthma or if a patient is taking prescription medication for asthma. Do not use if you have taken a MAO inhibitor (certain drugs used for depression, Parkinson's disease, or other conditions) within 2 weeks.

Adverse Reactions (Reflective of adult population; not specific for elderly) Frequency not defined.

Cardiovascular: Angina, cardiac arrhythmia, chest pain, flushing, hypertension, pallor, palpitation, sudden death, tachycardia (parenteral), vasoconstriction, ventricular ectopy

Central nervous system: Anxiety (transient), apprehensiveness, cerebral hemorrhage, dizziness, headache, insomnia, lightheadedness, nervousness, restlessness

Gastrointestinal: Dry throat, loss of appetite, nausea, vomiting, xerostomia

Genitourinary: Acute urinary retention in patients with bladder outflow obstruction

Neuromuscular & skeletal: Tremor, weakness

Ocular: Allergic lid reaction, burning, eye pain, ocular irritation, precipitation of or exacerbation of narrow-angle glaucoma, transient stinging

Respiratory: Dyspnea, pulmonary edema

Miscellaneous: Diaphoresis

Drug Interactions

Metabolism/Transport Effects Substrate of COMT

Avoid Concomitant Use

Avoid concomitant use of EPINEPHrine (Systemic, Oral Inhalation) with any of the following: Ergot Derivatives; Hyaluronidase; Iobenguane I 123; Lurasidone

Increased Effect/Toxicity

EPINEPHrine (Systemic, Oral Inhalation) may increase the levels/effects of: Bromocriptine; Lurasidone; Sympathomimetics

The levels/effects of EPINEPHrine (Systemic, Oral Inhalation) may be increased by: Antacids; AtoMOXetine; Beta-Blockers; Cannabinoids; Carbonic Anhydrase Inhibitors; COMT Inhibitors; Ergot Derivatives; Hyaluronidase; Inhalational Anesthetics; MAO Inhibitors; Serotonin/Norepinephrine Reuptake Inhibitors; Tricyclic Antidepressants

Decreased Effect

EPINEPHrine (Systemic, Oral Inhalation) may decrease the levels/effects of: Benzylpenicilloyl Polylysine; Iobenguane I 123

The levels/effects of EPINEPHrine (Systemic, Oral Inhalation) may be decreased by: Promethazine; Spironolactone

Ethanol/Nutrition/Herb Interactions Herb/Nutraceutical: Avoid ephedra, yohimbe (may cause CNS stimulation).

Stability Epinephrine is sensitive to light and air; protection from light is recommended. Oxidation turns drug pink, then a brown color. **Solutions should not be used if they are discolored or contain a precipitate.**

Adrenalin®: Store between 15°C to 25°C (59°F to 77°F); do not freeze. Protect from light. The 1:1000 solution should be discarded 30 days after initial use.

EpiPen® and EpiPen® Jr: Store at 25°C (77°F); excursions permitted to 15°C to 30°C (59°F to 86°F); do not freeze or refrigerate. Protect from light by storing in carrier tube provided.

Twinject®: Store between 20°C to 25°C (68°F to 77°F); excursions permitted to 15°C to 30°C (59°F to 86°F); do not freeze or refrigerate. Protect from light.

Primatene® Mist: Store between 20°C to 25°C (68°F to 77°F).

S2®: Store between 2°C to 20°C (36°F to 68°F). Protect from light. Dilution not required when administered via hand-bulb nebulizer; dilute with NS 3-5 mL if using jet nebulizer

Stability of injection of parenteral admixture at room temperature (25°C) or refrigeration (4°C) is 24 hours.

Mechanism of Action Stimulates alpha-, beta$_1$-, and beta$_2$-adrenergic receptors resulting in relaxation of smooth muscle of the bronchial tree, cardiac stimulation (increasing myocardial oxygen consumption), and dilation of skeletal muscle vasculature; small doses can cause vasodilation via beta$_2$-vascular receptors; large doses may produce constriction of skeletal and vascular smooth muscle

Pharmacodynamics/Kinetics

Onset of action: Bronchodilation: SubQ: ~5-10 minutes; Inhalation: ~1 minute

Metabolism: Taken up into the adrenergic neuron and metabolized by monoamine oxidase and catechol-o-methyltransferase; circulating drug hepatically metabolized

Excretion: Urine (as inactive metabolites, metanephrine, and sulfate and hydroxy derivatives of mandelic acid, small amounts as unchanged drug)

Dosage

Geriatric & Adult

Asystole/pulseless arrest, pulseless VT/VF (ACLS, 2010):

I.V., I.O.: 1 mg every 3-5 minutes until return of spontaneous circulation; if this approach fails, higher doses of epinephrine (up to 0.2 mg/kg) have been used for treatment of specific problems (eg, beta-blocker or calcium channel blocker overdose)

Endotracheal: 2-2.5 mg every 3-5 minutes until I.V./I.O access established or return of spontaneous circulation; dilute in 5-10 mL NS or sterile water. **Note:** Absorption may be greater with sterile water (Naganobu, 2000). May cause false-negative reading with exhaled CO_2 detectors; use second method to confirm tube placement if CO_2 is not detected (Neumar, 2010).

Bradycardia (symptomatic; unresponsive to atropine or pacing): *I.V. infusion:* 2-10 mcg/minute **or** 0.1-0.5 mcg/kg/minute (7-35 mcg/minute in a 70 kg patient); titrate to desired effect (ACLS, 2010)

Bronchodilator:

SubQ: 0.3-0.5 mg (**1:1000** [1 mg/mL] solution) every 20 minutes for 3 doses

Nebulization: S2® (racepinephrine, OTC labeling):

Hand-bulb nebulizer: Add 0.5 mL (~10 drops) to nebulizer; 1-3 inhalations up to every 3 hours if needed

Jet nebulizer: Add 0.5 mL (~10 drops) to nebulizer and dilute with 3 mL of NS; administer over ~15 minutes every 3-4 hours as needed

Inhalation: Primatene® Mist (OTC labeling): One inhalation, wait at least 1 minute; if not relieved, may use once more. Do not use again for at least 3 hours.

Hypersensitivity reaction: Note: SubQ administration results in slower absorption and is less reliable. I.M. administration in the anterolateral aspect of the middle third of the thigh is preferred in the setting of anaphylaxis (ACLS guidelines, 2010; Kemp, 2008).

I.M., SubQ: 0.2-0.5 mg (**1:1000** [1 mg/mL] solution) every 5-15 minutes in the absence of clinical improvement (ACLS 2010; Kemp, 2008; Lieberman, 2010). If clinician deems appropriate, the 5-minute interval between injections may be shortened to allow for more frequent administration (Lieberman, 2010).

I.V.: 0.1 mg (**1:10,000** [0.1 mg/mL] solution) over 5 minutes; may infuse at 1-4 mcg/minute to prevent the need to repeat injections frequently **or** may initiate with an infusion at 5-15 mcg/minute (with crystalloid administration) (ACLS, 2010; Brown, 2004). In general, I.V. administration should only be done in patients who are profoundly hypotensive or are in cardiopulmonary arrest refractory to volume resuscitation and several epinephrine injections (Lieberman, 2010).

Self-administration following severe allergic reactions (eg, insect stings, food): **Note:** The World Health Organization (WHO) and Anaphylaxis Canada recommend the availability of one dose for every 10-20 minutes of travel time to a medical emergency facility. More than 2 doses should only be administered under direct medical supervision.

Twinject®: I.M., SubQ: 0.3 mg; if anaphylactic symptoms persist, dose may be repeated in 5-15 minutes using the same device after partial disassembly

EpiPen®: I.M., SubQ: 0.3 mg; if anaphylactic symptoms persist, dose may be repeated in 5-15 minutes using an additional EpiPen®

Hypotension/shock, severe and fluid resistant (unlabeled use): *I.V. infusion:* Initial: 0.1-0.5 mcg/kg/minute (7-35 mcg/minute in a 70 kg patient); titrate to desired response (ACLS, 2010)

Administration When administering as a continuous infusion, central line administration is preferred. I.V. infusions require an infusion pump. Epinephrine solutions for injection can be administered I.M., I.O., endotracheally, I.V., or SubQ. **Note:** EpiPen® and EpiPen® Jr Auto-Injectors contain a single, fixed-dose of epinephrine. Twinject® Auto-Injectors contain two doses; the first fixed-dose is available for auto-injection; the second dose is available for manual injection following partial disassembly of device.

Subcutaneous: SubQ administration results in slower absorption and is less reliable.

I.M.: I.M. administration into the buttocks should be avoided. I.M. administration in the anterolateral aspect of the middle third of the thigh is preferred in the setting of anaphylaxis (ACLS guidelines, 2010; Kemp, 2008). EpiPen®, EpiPen® Jr, and Twinject® Auto-Injectors should only be injected into the anterolateral aspect of the thigh, through clothing if necessary.

Endotracheal: Dilute in NS or sterile water. Absorption may be greater with sterile water (Naganobu, 2000). Stop compressions, spray drug quickly down tube. Follow immediately with several quick insufflations and continue chest compressions. May cause false-negative reading with exhaled CO_2 detectors; use second method to confirm tube placement if CO_2 is not detected (Neumar, 2010).

Oral inhalation: S2®: If using jet nebulizer: Administer over ~15 minutes; must be diluted. If using hand-held rubber bulb nebulizer, dilution is not required.

Extravasation management: Use phentolamine as antidote. Mix 5 mg phentolamine with 9 mL of NS. Inject a small amount of this dilution into extravasated area. Blanching should reverse immediately. Monitor site. If blanching should recur, additional injections of phentolamine may be needed.

Monitoring Parameters Pulmonary function, heart rate, blood pressure, site of infusion for blanching, extravasation; cardiac monitor and blood pressure monitor required during continuous infusion. If using to treat hypotension, assess intravascular volume and support as needed.

Pharmacotherapy Pearls Twinject® and EpiPen® are not interchangeable due to packaging considerations.

Special Geriatric Considerations The use of epinephrine in the treatment of acute exacerbations of asthma was studied in the elderly. A dose of 0.3 mg SubQ every 20 minutes for three doses was well tolerated in elderly patients with no history of angina or recent myocardial infarction. There was no significant difference in the incidence of ventricular arrhythmias in elderly versus younger adults.

Product Availability Auvi-Q™: FDA approved August 2012; anticipated availability currently unknown. Consult prescribing information for additional information.

Dosage Forms Excipient information presented when available (limited, particularly for generics); consult specific product labeling. [DSC] = Discontinued product

Aerosol, for oral inhalation:
  Primatene® Mist: 0.22 mg/inhalation (15 mL [DSC]) [contains chlorofluorocarbon, dehydrated ethanol 34%]

Injection, solution: 0.1 mg/mL (10 mL) [1:10,000 solution]; 1 mg/mL (1 mL) [1:1000 solution]
  EpiPen 2-Pak®: 0.3 mg/0.3 mL (2 mL) [contains sodium metabisulfite; 1:1000 solution; delivers 0.3 mg per injection]
  EpiPen Jr 2-Pak®: 0.15 mg/0.3 mL (2 mL) [contains sodium metabisulfite; 1:2000 solution; delivers 0.15 mg per injection]
  Twinject®: 0.15 mg/0.15 mL (1.1 mL) [contains chlorobutanol, sodium bisulfite; 1:1000 solution; delivers 0.15 mg per injection]
  Twinject®: 0.3 mg/0.3 mL (1.1 mL) [contains chlorobutanol, sodium bisulfite; 1:1000 solution; delivers 0.3 mg per injection]

Injection, solution, as hydrochloride: 1 mg/mL (30 mL) [1:1000 solution]
  Adrenalin®: 1 mg/mL (30 mL) [contains chlorobutanol, sodium bisulfite; 1:1000 solution]
  Adrenalin®: 1 mg/mL (1 mL) [contains sodium bisulfite; 1:1000 solution]

Injection, solution, as hydrochloride [preservative free]: 1 mg/mL (1 mL) [1:1000 solution]

Solution, for oral inhalation [preservative free]:
  Asthmanefrin™: Racepinephrine 2.25% (0.5 mL)
  S2®: Racepinephrine 2.25% (0.5 mL)

◆ **Epinephrine Bitartrate** see EPINEPHrine (Systemic, Oral Inhalation) on page 645
◆ **Epinephrine Hydrochloride** see EPINEPHrine (Systemic, Oral Inhalation) on page 645
◆ **EpiPen 2-Pak®** see EPINEPHrine (Systemic, Oral Inhalation) on page 645
◆ **EpiPen Jr 2-Pak®** see EPINEPHrine (Systemic, Oral Inhalation) on page 645
◆ **Epitol®** see CarBAMazepine on page 286

Eplerenone (e PLER en one)

Medication Safety Issues
Sound-alike/look-alike issues:
Inspra™ may be confused with Spiriva®

Brand Names: U.S. Inspra™

Generic Availability (U.S.) Yes

Pharmacologic Category Diuretic, Potassium-Sparing; Selective Aldosterone Blocker

Use Treatment of hypertension (may be used alone or in combination with other antihypertensive agents); treatment of heart failure (HF) following acute MI

Contraindications Serum potassium >5.5 mEq/L at initiation; Cl_{cr} ≤30 mL/minute; concomitant use of strong CYP3A4 inhibitors (see Drug Interactions for details)

The following additional contraindications apply to patients with hypertension: Type 2 diabetes mellitus (noninsulin dependent, NIDDM) with microalbuminuria; serum creatinine >2.0 mg/dL in males or >1.8 mg/dL in females; Cl_{cr} <50 mL/minute; concomitant use with potassium supplements or potassium-sparing diuretics

Warnings/Precautions Dosage adjustment needed for patients on moderate CYP3A4 inhibitors. Monitor closely for hyperkalemia; increases in serum potassium were dose related during clinical trials and rates of hyperkalemia also increased with declining renal function. Safety and efficacy have not been established in patients with severe hepatic impairment. Use with caution in HF patients post-MI with diabetes (especially if patient has proteinuria); risk of hyperkalemia is increased. Risk of hyperkalemia is increased with declining renal function. Use with caution in patients with mild renal impairment; contraindicated with moderate-severe impairment (HTN: Cl_{cr} <50 mL/minute; other indications: Cl_{cr} ≤30 mL/minute).

Adverse Reactions (Reflective of adult population; not specific for elderly)
>10%: Endocrine & metabolic: Hyperkalemia ([HF post-MI: K >5.5 mEq/L: 16%; K ≥6 mEq/L: 6%] [HTN: K >5.5 mEq/L at doses ≤100 mg: ≤1%; doses >100 mg: 9%]), hypertriglyceridemia (1% to 15%, dose related)

1% to 10%:
Central nervous system: Dizziness (3%), fatigue (2%)
Endocrine & metabolic: Hyponatremia (2%, dose related), breast pain (males <1% to 1%), gynecomastia (males <1% to 1%), hypercholesterolemia (<1% to 1%)
Gastrointestinal: Diarrhea (2%), abdominal pain (1%)
Genitourinary: Abnormal vaginal bleeding (<1% to 2%)
Renal: Creatinine increased (HF post-MI: 6%), albuminuria (1%)
Respiratory: Cough (2%)
Miscellaneous: Flu-like syndrome (2%)

Drug Interactions
Metabolism/Transport Effects Substrate of CYP3A4 (major); **Note:** Assignment of Major/Minor substrate status based on clinically relevant drug interaction potential

Avoid Concomitant Use
Avoid concomitant use of Eplerenone with any of the following: CycloSPORINE; CycloSPORINE (Systemic); CYP3A4 Inhibitors (Strong); Itraconazole; Ketoconazole; Ketoconazole (Systemic); Posaconazole; Tacrolimus; Tacrolimus (Systemic); Voriconazole

Increased Effect/Toxicity
Eplerenone may increase the levels/effects of: ACE Inhibitors; Amifostine; Angiotensin II Receptor Blockers; Antihypertensives; CycloSPORINE; CycloSPORINE (Systemic); Hypotensive Agents; Potassium Salts; Potassium-Sparing Diuretics; RiTUXimab; Tacrolimus; Tacrolimus (Systemic)

The levels/effects of Eplerenone may be increased by: Alfuzosin; Calcium Channel Blockers (Nondihydropyridine); CYP3A4 Inhibitors (Moderate); CYP3A4 Inhibitors (Strong); Dasatinib; Diazoxide; Fluconazole; Herbs (Hypotensive Properties); Itraconazole; Ivacaftor; Ketoconazole; Ketoconazole (Systemic); Macrolide Antibiotics; MAO Inhibitors; Mifepristone; Nitrofurantoin; Nonsteroidal Anti-Inflammatory Agents; Pentoxifylline; Phosphodiesterase 5 Inhibitors; Posaconazole; Prostacyclin Analogues; Protease Inhibitors; Trimethoprim; Voriconazole

Decreased Effect
The levels/effects of Eplerenone may be decreased by: CYP3A4 Inducers (Strong); Deferasirox; Herbs (CYP3A4 Inducers); Herbs (Hypertensive Properties); Methylphenidate; Nonsteroidal Anti-Inflammatory Agents; Tocilizumab; Yohimbine

Ethanol/Nutrition/Herb Interactions

Food: Grapefruit juice increases eplerenone AUC ~25%.

Herb/Nutraceutical: St John's wort may decrease levels of eplerenone. Avoid black cohosh, California poppy, coleus, golden seal, hawthorn, mistletoe, periwinkle, quinine, shepherd's purse (may have increased antihypertensive effect). Avoid bayberry, blue cohosh, cayenne, ephedra, ginger, ginseng (American), kola, licorice (may diminish the antihypertensive effect).

Stability Store at controlled room temperature of 25°C (77°F).

Mechanism of Action Aldosterone, a mineralocorticoid, increases blood pressure primarily by inducing sodium and water retention. Overexpression of aldosterone is thought to contribute to myocardial fibrosis (especially following myocardial infarction) and vascular fibrosis. Mineralocorticoid receptors are located in the kidney, heart, blood vessels, and brain. Eplerenone selectively blocks mineralocorticoid receptors reducing blood pressure in a dose-dependent manner and appears to prevent myocardial and vascular fibrosis.

Pharmacodynamics/Kinetics

Distribution: V_d: 43-90 L

Protein binding: ~50%; primarily to alpha$_1$-acid glycoproteins

Metabolism: Primarily hepatic via CYP3A4; metabolites inactive

Bioavailability: 69%

Half-life elimination: 4-6 hours

Time to peak, plasma: ~1.5 hours; may take up to 4 weeks for full antihypertensive effect

Excretion: Urine (~67%); feces (32%); <5% as unchanged drug in urine and feces

Dosage

Geriatric & Adult

Hypertension: Oral: Initial: 50 mg once daily; may increase to 50 mg twice daily if response is not adequate; may take up to 4 weeks for full therapeutic response. Doses >100 mg/day are associated with increased risk of hyperkalemia and no greater therapeutic effect.

Dose modification during concurrent use with moderate CYP3A4 inhibitors: Initial: 25 mg once daily

Heart failure (post-MI): Oral: Initial: 25 mg once daily; dosage goal: Titrate to 50 mg once daily within 4 weeks, as tolerated

Dosage adjustment per serum potassium concentrations for HF (post-MI):

<5.0 mEq/L:
Increase dose from 25 mg every other day to 25 mg daily **or**
Increase dose from 25 mg daily to 50 mg daily

5.0-5.4 mEq/L: No adjustment needed

5.5-5.9 mEq/L:
Decrease dose from 50 mg daily to 25 mg daily **or**
Decrease dose from 25 mg daily to 25 mg every other day **or**
Decrease dose from 25 mg every other day to withhold medication

≥6.0 mEq/L: Withhold medication until potassium <5.5 mEq/L, then restart at 25 mg every other day

Renal Impairment

Hypertension: Cl_{cr} <50 mL/minute or serum creatinine >2.0 mg/dL in males or >1.8 mg/dL in females: Use is contraindicated; risk of hyperkalemia increases with declining renal function

All other indications: Cl_{cr} ≤30 mL/minute: Use is contraindicated.

Hepatic Impairment No dosage adjustment needed for mild-to-moderate impairment. Safety and efficacy not established for severe impairment.

Administration May be administered with or without food.

Monitoring Parameters Blood pressure; serum potassium (levels monitored prior to therapy, within the first week, and at 1 month after start of treatment or dose adjustment, then periodically [monthly in clinical trials]); renal function

Special Geriatric Considerations Since this medication is contraindicated in the treatment of hypertension in patients with a Cl_{cr} <50 mL/minute, it may have limited use in the elderly. Due to physiologic changes, elderly may be at increased risk of hyperkalemia when using this medication.

Dosage Forms Excipient information presented when available (limited, particularly for generics); consult specific product labeling.

Tablet, oral: 25 mg, 50 mg

Inspra™: 25 mg, 50 mg

◆ **EPO** *see* Epoetin Alfa *on page 651*

Epoetin Alfa (e POE e tin AL fa)

Medication Safety Issues
Sound-alike/look-alike issues:
Epoetin alfa may be confused with darbepoetin alfa, epoetin beta
Epogen® may be confused with Neupogen®
International issues:
Epopen [Spain] may be confused with EpiPen brand name for epinephrine [U.S., Canada, and multiple international markets]

Brand Names: U.S. Epogen®; Procrit®

Brand Names: Canada Eprex®

Index Terms rHuEPO; rHuEPO-α; EPO; Erythropoiesis-Stimulating Agent (ESA); Erythropoietin

Generic Availability (U.S.) No

Pharmacologic Category Colony Stimulating Factor; Erythropoiesis-Stimulating Agent (ESA); Growth Factor; Recombinant Human Erythropoietin

Use Treatment of anemia due to concurrent myelosuppressive chemotherapy in patients with cancer (nonmyeloid malignancies) receiving chemotherapy (palliative intent) for a planned minimum of 2 additional months of chemotherapy; treatment of anemia due to chronic kidney disease (including patients on dialysis and not on dialysis) to decrease the need for RBC transfusion; treatment of anemia associated with HIV (zidovudine) therapy when endogenous erythropoietin levels ≤500 mUnits/mL; reduction of allogeneic RBC transfusion for elective, noncardiac, nonvascular surgery when perioperative hemoglobin is >10 to ≤13 g/dL and there is a high risk for blood loss

Note: Epoetin is **not** indicated for use under the following conditions:
- Cancer patients receiving hormonal therapy, therapeutic biologic products, or radiation therapy unless also receiving concurrent myelosuppressive chemotherapy
- Cancer patients receiving myelosuppressive chemotherapy when the expected outcome is curative
- Surgery patients who are willing to donate autologous blood
- Surgery patients undergoing cardiac or vascular surgery
- As a substitute for RBC transfusion in patients requiring immediate correction of anemia

Note: In clinical trials (and one meta-analysis), epoetin has not demonstrated improved quality of life, fatigue, or well-being.

Unlabeled Use Treatment of symptomatic anemia in myelodysplastic syndrome (MDS)

Prescribing and Access Restrictions As a requirement of the REMS program, access to this medication is restricted. Healthcare providers and hospitals must be enrolled in the ESA APPRISE (Assisting Providers and Cancer Patients with Risk Information for the Safe use of ESAs) Oncology Program (866-284-8089; http://www.esa-apprise.com) to prescribe or dispense ESAs (ie, epoetin alfa, darbepoetin alfa) to patients with cancer.

Medication Guide Available Yes

Contraindications Hypersensitivity to epoetin or any component of the formulation; uncontrolled hypertension; pure red cell aplasia (due to epoetin or other epoetin protein drugs)

Warnings/Precautions [U.S. Boxed Warning]: Erythropoiesis-stimulating agents (ESAs) increased the risk of serious cardiovascular events, thromboembolic events, stroke, mortality, and/or tumor progression in clinical studies when administered to target hemoglobin levels >11 g/dL (and provide no additional benefit); a rapid rise in hemoglobin (>1 g/dL over 2 weeks) may also contribute to these risks. **[U.S. Boxed Warning]: A shortened overall survival and/or increased risk of tumor progression or recurrence has been reported in studies with breast, cervical, head and neck, lymphoid, and nonsmall cell lung cancer patients.** It is of note that in these studies, patients received ESAs to a target hemoglobin of ≥12 g/dL; although risk has not been excluded when dosed to achieve a target hemoglobin of <12 g/dL. **[U.S. Boxed Warnings]: To decrease these risks, and risk of cardio- and thrombovascular events, use the lowest dose needed to avoid red blood cell transfusions. Use ESAs in cancer patients only for the treatment of anemia related to concurrent myelosuppressive chemotherapy; discontinue ESA following completion of the chemotherapy course. ESAs are not indicated for patients receiving myelosuppressive therapy when the anticipated outcome is curative.** A dosage modification is appropriate if hemoglobin levels rise >1 g/dL per 2-week time period during treatment (Rizzo, 2010). Use of ESAs has been associated with an increased risk of venous thromboembolism (VTE) without a reduction in transfusions in patients with cancer (Hershman, 2009). Improved anemia symptoms, quality of life, fatigue, or well-being have not been demonstrated in controlled clinical trials. **[U.S. Boxed Warning]: Because of the risks of decreased survival and increased risk of tumor growth or progression, all healthcare providers and hospitals are required to enroll and comply with the ESA APPRISE**

◄ **(Assisting Providers and Cancer Patients with Risk Information for the Safe use of ESAs) Oncology Program** prior to prescribing or dispensing ESAs to cancer patients. Prescribers and patients will have to provide written documentation of discussed risks prior to each epoetin course.

[U.S. Boxed Warning]: An increased risk of death, serious cardiovascular events, and stroke was reported in chronic kidney disease (CKD) patients administered ESAs to target hemoglobin levels ≥11 g/dL; use the lowest dose sufficient to reduce the need for RBC transfusions. An optimal target hemoglobin level, dose or dosing strategy to reduce these risks has not been identified in clinical trials. Hemoglobin rising >1 g/dL in a 2-week period may contribute to the risk (dosage reduction recommended). Chronic kidney disease patients who exhibit an inadequate hemoglobin response to ESA therapy may be at a higher risk for cardiovascular events and mortality compared to other patients. ESA therapy may reduce dialysis efficacy (due to increase in red blood cells and decrease in plasma volume); adjustments in dialysis parameters may be needed. Patients treated with epoetin may require increased heparinization during dialysis to prevent clotting of the extracorporeal circuit. **[U.S. Boxed Warning]: DVT prophylaxis is recommended in perisurgery patients due to the risk of DVT.** Increased mortality was also observed in patients undergoing coronary artery bypass surgery who received epoetin alfa; these deaths were associated with thrombotic events. Epoetin is **not** approved for reduction of red blood cell transfusion in patients undergoing cardiac or vascular surgery and is **not** indicated for surgical patients willing to donate autologous blood.

Use with caution in patients with hypertension (contraindicated in uncontrolled hypertension) or with a history of seizures; hypertensive encephalopathy and seizures have been reported. If hypertension is difficult to control, reduce or hold epoetin alfa. An excessive rate of rise of hemoglobin is associated with hypertension or exacerbation of hypertension; decrease the epoetin dose if the hemoglobin increase exceeds 1 g/dL in any 2-week period. Blood pressure should be controlled prior to start of therapy and monitored closely throughout treatment. The risk for seizures is increased with epoetin use in patients with CKD; monitor closely for neurologic symptoms during the first several months of therapy. Due to the delayed onset of erythropoiesis, epoetin alfa is **not** recommended for acute correction of severe anemia or as a substitute for emergency transfusion.

Prior to treatment, correct or exclude deficiencies of iron, vitamin B_{12}, and/or folate, as well as other factors which may impair erythropoiesis (inflammatory conditions, infections). Prior to and periodically during therapy, iron stores must be evaluated. Supplemental iron is recommended if serum ferritin <100 mcg/L or serum transferrin saturation <20%; most patients with chronic kidney disease will require iron supplementation. Poor response should prompt evaluation of these potential factors, as well as possible malignant processes and hematologic disease (thalassemia, refractory anemia, myelodysplastic disorder), occult blood loss, hemolysis, ostetis fibrosa cystic, and/or bone marrow fibrosis. Severe anemia and pure red cell aplasia (PRCA) with associated neutralizing antibodies to erythropoietin has been reported, predominantly in patients with CKD receiving SubQ epoetin (the I.V. route is preferred for hemodialysis patients). Cases have also been reported in patients with hepatitis C who were receiving ESAs, interferon, and ribavirin. Patients with a sudden loss of response to epoetin alfa (with severe anemia and a low reticulocyte count) should be evaluated for PRCA with associated neutralizing antibodies to erythropoietin; discontinue treatment (permanently) in patients with PRCA secondary to neutralizing antibodies to epoetin.

Potentially serious allergic reactions have been reported (rarely). Discontinue immediately (and permanently) in patients who experience serious allergic/anaphylactic reactions. Some products may contain albumin. Multidose vials contain benzyl alcohol.

Adverse Reactions (Reflective of adult population; not specific for elderly)
>10%:
Cardiovascular: Hypertension (3% to 28%)
Central nervous system: Fever (10% to 42%), headache (5% to 18%)
Dermatologic: Pruritus (12% to 21%), rash (2% to 19%)
Gastrointestinal: Nausea (35% to 56%), vomiting (12% to 28%)
Local: Injection site reaction (7% to 13%)
Neuromuscular & skeletal: Arthralgia (10% to 16%)
Respiratory: Cough (4% to 26%)
1% to 10%:
Cardiovascular: Deep vein thrombosis, edema, thrombosis
Central nervous system: Chills, depression, dizziness, insomnia
Dermatologic: Urticaria
Endocrine & metabolic: Hyperglycemia, hypokalemia
Gastrointestinal: Dysphagia, stomatitis, weight loss
Hematologic: Leukopenia

Local: Clotted vascular access

Neuromuscular & skeletal: Bone pain, muscle spasm, myalgia

Respiratory: Pulmonary embolism, respiratory congestion, upper respiratory infection

Drug Interactions

Metabolism/Transport Effects None known.

Avoid Concomitant Use There are no known interactions where it is recommended to avoid concomitant use.

Increased Effect/Toxicity There are no known significant interactions involving an increase in effect.

Decreased Effect There are no known significant interactions involving a decrease in effect.

Stability

Vials should be stored at 2°C to 8°C (36°F to 46°F); **do not freeze or shake**. Protect from light.

Single-dose 1 mL vial contains no preservative: Use one dose per vial. Do not re-enter vial; discard unused portions.

Single-dose vials (except 40,000 units/mL vial) are stable for 2 weeks at room temperature (Cohen, 2007). Single-dose 40,000 units/mL vial is stable for 1 week at room temperature.

Multidose 1 mL or 2 mL vial contains preservative. Store at 2°C to 8°C after initial entry and between doses. Discard 21 days after initial entry.

Multidose vials (with preservative) are stable for 1 week at room temperature (Cohen, 2007). Prefilled syringes containing the 20,000 units/mL formulation with preservative are stable for 6 weeks refrigerated (2°C to 8°C) (Naughton, 2003).

Dilutions of 1:10 and 1:20 (1 part epoetin:19 parts sodium chloride) are stable for 18 hours at room temperature (Ohls, 1996).

Prior to SubQ administration, preservative free solutions may be mixed with bacteriostatic NS containing benzyl alcohol 0.9% in a 1:1 ratio (Corbo, 1992). Dilutions of 1:10 in $D_{10}W$ with human albumin 0.05% or 0.1% are stable for 24 hours.

Mechanism of Action Induces erythropoiesis by stimulating the division and differentiation of committed erythroid progenitor cells; induces the release of reticulocytes from the bone marrow into the bloodstream, where they mature to erythrocytes. There is a dose response relationship with this effect. This results in an increase in reticulocyte counts followed by a rise in hematocrit and hemoglobin levels.

Pharmacodynamics/Kinetics

Onset of action: Several days

Peak effect: Hemoglobin level: 2-6 weeks

Distribution: V_d: 9 L; rapid in the plasma compartment; concentrated in liver, kidneys, and bone marrow

Metabolism: Some degradation does occur

Bioavailability: SubQ: ~21% to 31%; intraperitoneal epoetin: 3% (Macdougall, 1989)

Half-life elimination: Cancer: SubQ: 16-67 hours; Chronic kidney disease: I.V.: 4-13 hours

Time to peak, serum: Chronic kidney disease: SubQ: 5-24 hours

Excretion: Feces (majority); urine (small amounts, 10% unchanged in normal volunteers)

Dosage

Geriatric & Adult

Anemia associated with chronic kidney disease: Individualize dosing and use the lowest dose necessary to reduce the need for RBC transfusions.

Chronic kidney disease patients ON dialysis (I.V. route is preferred for hemodialysis patients; initiate treatment when hemoglobin is <10 g/dL; reduce dose or interrupt treatment if hemoglobin approaches or exceeds 11 g/dL): I.V., SubQ: Initial dose: 50-100 units/kg 3 times/week

Chronic kidney disease patients NOT on dialysis (consider initiating treatment when hemoglobin is <10 g/dL; use only if rate of hemoglobin decline would likely result in RBC transfusion and desire is to reduce risk of alloimmunization or other RBC transfusion-related risks; reduce dose or interrupt treatment if hemoglobin exceeds 10 g/dL): I.V., SubQ: Initial dose: 50-100 units/kg 3 times/week

Dosage adjustments for chronic kidney disease patients (either on dialysis or not on dialysis):

If hemoglobin does not increase by >1 g/dL after 4 weeks: Increase dose by 25%; do not increase the dose more frequently than once every 4 weeks

If hemoglobin increases >1 g/dL in any 2-week period: Reduce dose by ≥25%; dose reductions can occur more frequently than once every 4 weeks; avoid frequent dosage adjustments

Inadequate or lack of response over a 12-week escalation period: Further increases are unlikely to improve response and may increase risks; use the minimum effective dose that will maintain a Hgb level sufficient to avoid RBC transfusions and evaluate patient for other causes of anemia. Discontinue therapy if responsiveness does not improve.

EPOETIN ALFA

Anemia due to chemotherapy in cancer patients: Initiate treatment only if hemoglobin <10 g/dL and anticipated duration of myelosuppressive chemotherapy is ≥2 months. Titrate dosage to use the minimum effective dose that will maintain a hemoglobin level sufficient to avoid red blood cell transfusions. Discontinue erythropoietin following completion of chemotherapy. SubQ: Initial dose: 150 units/kg 3 times/week or 40,000 units once weekly until completion of chemotherapy

Dosage adjustments:

If hemoglobin does not increase by >1 g/dL **and** remains below 10 g/dL after initial 4 weeks: Increase to 300 units/kg 3 times/week or 60,000 units weekly; discontinue after 8 weeks of treatment if RBC transfusions are still required or there is no hemoglobin response

If hemoglobin exceeds a level needed to avoid red blood cell transfusion: Withhold dose; resume treatment with a 25% dose reduction when hemoglobin approaches a level where transfusions may be required.

If hemoglobin increases >1 g/dL in any 2-week period **or** hemoglobin reaches a level sufficient to avoid red blood cell transfusion: Reduce dose by 25%.

Anemia due to zidovudine in HIV-infected patients: Titrate dosage to use the minimum effective dose that will maintain a hemoglobin level sufficient to avoid red blood cell transfusions. Hemoglobin levels should not exceed 12 g/dL.

Serum erythropoietin levels ≤500 mUnits/mL and zidovudine doses ≤4200 mg/week): I.V., SubQ: Initial: 100 units/kg 3 times/week; if hemoglobin does not increase after 8 weeks, increase dose by ~50-100 units/kg at 4-8 week intervals until hemoglobin reaches a level sufficient to avoid RBC transfusion; maximum dose: 300 units/kg. Withhold dose if hemoglobin exceeds 12 g/dL, may resume treatment with a 25% dose reduction once hemoglobin <11 g/dL. Discontinue if hemoglobin increase is not achieved with 300 units/kg for 8 weeks.

Surgery patients (perioperative hemoglobin should be >10 g/dL and ≤13 g/dL; DVT prophylactic anticoagulation is recommended): SubQ: Initial dose:

300 units/kg/day beginning 10 days before surgery, on the day of surgery, and for 4 days after surgery **or**

600 units/kg once weekly for 4 doses, given 21-, 14-, and 7 days before surgery, and on the day of surgery

Symptomatic anemia associated with myelodysplastic syndrome (unlabeled use): SubQ: 40,000-60,000 units 1-3 times/week (NCCN MDS guidelines v.2.2011)

Administration

SubQ is the preferred route of administration **except** in patients with CKD on hemodialysis; 1:1 dilution with bacteriostatic NS (containing benzyl alcohol) acts as a local anesthetic to reduce pain at the injection site

Patients with CKD on hemodialysis: I.V. route preferred; it may be administered into the venous line at the end of the dialysis procedure

Monitoring Parameters Transferrin saturation and serum ferritin (prior to and during treatment); hemoglobin (weekly after initiation and following dose adjustments until stable and sufficient to minimize need for RBC transfusion, CKD patients should be also be monitored at least monthly following hemoglobin stability); blood pressure; seizures (CKD patients following initiation for first few months, includes new-onset or change in seizure frequency or premonitory symptoms)

Cancer patients: Examinations recommended by the ASCO/ASH guidelines (Rizzo, 2010) prior to treatment include: peripheral blood smear (in some situations a bone marrow exam may be necessary), assessment for iron, folate, or vitamin B_{12} deficiency, reticulocyte count, renal function status, and occult blood loss; during ESA treatment, assess baseline and periodic iron, total iron-binding capacity, and transferrin saturation or ferritin levels.

Reference Range Zidovudine-treated HIV patients: Available evidence indicates patients with endogenous serum erythropoietin levels >500 mU/mL are unlikely to respond

Pharmacotherapy Pearls Oncology Comment: The American Society of Clinical Oncology (ASCO) and American Society of Hematology (ASH) 2010 updates to the clinical practice guidelines for the use of erythropoiesis-stimulating agents (ESAs) in patients with cancer indicate that ESAs are most appropriate when used according to the parameters identified within the Food and Drug Administration (FDA) approved labeling for epoetin and darbepoetin (Rizzo, 2010). ESAs are an option for chemotherapy associated anemia when the hemoglobin has fallen to <10 g/dL to decrease the need for RBC transfusions. ESAs should only be used in conjunction with concurrent chemotherapy. Although the FDA label now limits ESA use to the palliative setting, the ASCO/ASH guidelines suggest using clinical judgment in weighing risks versus benefits as formal outcomes studies of ESA use defined by intent of chemotherapy treatment have not been conducted.

The ASCO/ASH guidelines continue to recommend following the FDA approved dosing (and dosing adjustment) guidelines as alternate dosing and schedules have not demonstrated consistent differences in effectiveness with regard to hemoglobin response. In patients who do not have a response within 6-8 weeks (hemoglobin rise <1-2 g/dL or no reduction in transfusions) ESA therapy should be discontinued.

Prior to the initiation of ESAs, other sources of anemia (in addition to chemotherapy or underlying hematologic malignancy) should be investigated. Examinations recommended prior to treatment include peripheral blood smear (in some situations a bone marrow exam may be necessary), assessment for iron, folate, or vitamin B_{12} deficiency, reticulocyte count, renal function status, and occult blood loss. During ESA treatment, assess baseline and periodic iron, total iron-binding capacity, and transferrin saturation or ferritin levels. Iron supplementation may be necessary

The guidelines note that patients with an increased risk of thromboembolism (generally includes previous history of thrombosis, surgery, and/or prolonged periods of immobilization) and patients receiving concomitant medications that may increase thromboembolic risk, should begin ESA therapy only after careful consideration. With the exception of low-risk myelodysplasia-associated anemia (which has evidence supporting the use of ESAs without concurrent chemotherapy), the guidelines do not support the use of ESAs in the absence of concurrent chemotherapy.

Special Geriatric Considerations Endogenous erythropoietin secretion has been reported to be decreased in elderly with normocytic or iron deficiency anemias or those with a serum hemoglobin concentration <12 g/dL; one study did not find such a relationship in the elderly with chronic anemia. A blunted erythropoietin response to anemia has been reported in patients with cancer, rheumatoid arthritis, and AIDS.

Dosage Forms Excipient information presented when available (limited, particularly for generics); consult specific product labeling.
Injection, solution:
Epogen®: 10,000 units/mL (2 mL); 20,000 units/mL (1 mL) [contains albumin (human), benzyl alcohol]
Procrit®: 10,000 units/mL (2 mL); 20,000 units/mL (1 mL) [contains albumin (human), benzyl alcohol]
Injection, solution [preservative free]:
Epogen®: 2000 units/mL (1 mL); 3000 units/mL (1 mL); 4000 units/mL (1 mL); 10,000 units/mL (1 mL) [contains albumin (human)]
Procrit®: 2000 units/mL (1 mL); 3000 units/mL (1 mL); 4000 units/mL (1 mL); 10,000 units/mL (1 mL); 40,000 units/mL (1 mL) [contains albumin (human)]

Dosage Forms: Canada Excipient information presented when available (limited, particularly for generics); consult specific product labeling.
Injection, solution [preservative free]:
Eprex®: 1000 units/0.5 mL (0.5 mL), 2000 units/0.5 mL (0.5 mL), 3000 units/0.3 mL (0.3 mL), 4000 units/0.4 mL (0.4 mL), 5000 units/0.5 mL (0.5 mL), 6000 units/0.6 mL (0.6 mL), 8000 units/0.8 mL (0.8 mL), 10,000 units/mL (1 mL), 20,000 units/0.5 mL (0.5 mL), 30,000 units/0.75 mL (0.75 mL), 40,000 units/mL (1 mL) [contains polysorbate 80; prefilled syringe, free of human serum albumin]

◆ Epogen® *see* Epoetin Alfa *on page 651*

Eprosartan (ep roe SAR tan)

Related Information
Angiotensin Agents *on page 2093*
Brand Names: U.S. Teveten®
Brand Names: Canada Teveten®
Generic Availability (U.S.) Yes
Pharmacologic Category Angiotensin II Receptor Blocker
Use Treatment of hypertension; may be used alone or in combination with other antihypertensives
Contraindications Hypersensitivity to eprosartan or any component of the formulation
Warnings/Precautions May cause hyperkalemia; avoid potassium supplementation unless specifically required by healthcare provider. Avoid use or use a smaller dose in patients who are volume depleted; correct depletion first. May be associated with deterioration of renal function and/or increases in serum creatinine, particularly in patients with low renal blood flow (eg, renal artery stenosis, heart failure) whose glomerular filtration rate (GFR) is dependent on efferent arteriolar vasoconstriction by angiotensin II. Use with caution in unstented unilateral/bilateral renal artery stenosis. When unstented bilateral renal artery stenosis is present, use is generally avoided due to the elevated risk of deterioration in renal function unless possible

benefits outweigh risks. Use with caution in pre-existing renal insufficiency; significant aortic/mitral stenosis. Concurrent use of ACE inhibitors may increase the risk of clinically-significant adverse events (eg, renal dysfunction, hyperkalemia).

Adverse Reactions (Reflective of adult population; not specific for elderly) 1% to 10%:

Central nervous system: Fatigue (2%), depression (1%)

Endocrine & metabolic: Hypertriglyceridemia (1%)

Gastrointestinal: Abdominal pain (2%)

Genitourinary: Urinary tract infection (1%)

Respiratory: Upper respiratory tract infection (8%), rhinitis (4%), pharyngitis (4%), cough (4%)

Miscellaneous: Viral infection (2%), injury (2%)

Drug Interactions

Metabolism/Transport Effects Inhibits CYP2C9 (weak)

Avoid Concomitant Use There are no known interactions where it is recommended to avoid concomitant use.

Increased Effect/Toxicity

Eprosartan may increase the levels/effects of: ACE Inhibitors; Amifostine; Antihypertensives; Hypotensive Agents; Lithium; Nonsteroidal Anti-Inflammatory Agents; Potassium-Sparing Diuretics; RiTUXimab; Sodium Phosphates

The levels/effects of Eprosartan may be increased by: Alfuzosin; Aliskiren; Diazoxide; Eplerenone; Herbs (Hypotensive Properties); MAO Inhibitors; Pentoxifylline; Phosphodiesterase 5 Inhibitors; Potassium Salts; Prostacyclin Analogues; Tolvaptan; Trimethoprim

Decreased Effect

The levels/effects of Eprosartan may be decreased by: Herbs (Hypertensive Properties); Methylphenidate; Nonsteroidal Anti-Inflammatory Agents; Yohimbine

Ethanol/Nutrition/Herb Interactions Herb/Nutraceutical: Dong quai has estrogenic activity. Some herbal medications may worsen hypertension (eg, ephedra); garlic may have additional antihypertensive effects. Management: Avoid dong quai if using for hypertension. Avoid ephedra, yohimbe, ginseng, and garlic.

Mechanism of Action Angiotensin II is formed from angiotensin I in a reaction catalyzed by angiotensin-converting enzyme (ACE, kininase II). Angiotensin II is the principal pressor agent of the renin-angiotensin system, with effects that include vasoconstriction, stimulation of synthesis and release of aldosterone, cardiac stimulation, and renal reabsorption of sodium. Eprosartan blocks the vasoconstrictor and aldosterone-secreting effects of angiotensin II by selectively blocking the binding of angiotensin II to the AT1 receptor in many tissues, such as vascular smooth muscle and the adrenal gland. Its action is therefore independent of the pathways for angiotensin II synthesis. Blockade of the renin-angiotensin system with ACE inhibitors, which inhibit the biosynthesis of angiotensin II from angiotensin I, is widely used in the treatment of hypertension. ACE inhibitors also inhibit the degradation of bradykinin, a reaction also catalyzed by ACE. Because eprosartan does not inhibit ACE (kininase II), it does not affect the response to bradykinin. Whether this difference has clinical relevance is not yet known. Eprosartan does not bind to or block other hormone receptors or ion channels known to be important in cardiovascular regulation.

Pharmacodynamics/Kinetics

Protein binding: 98%

Metabolism: Minimally hepatic

Bioavailability: 300 mg dose: 13%

Half-life elimination: Terminal: 5-9 hours

Time to peak, serum: Fasting: 1-2 hours

Excretion: Feces (90%); urine (7%, mostly as unchanged drug)

Clearance: 7.9 L/hour

Dosage

Geriatric & Adult Hypertension: Oral: Dosage must be individualized. Can administer once or twice daily with total daily doses of 400-800 mg. Usual starting dose is 600 mg once daily as monotherapy in patients who are euvolemic. Limited clinical experience with doses >800 mg.

Renal Impairment

Moderate-to-severe impairment: No initial starting dosage adjustment is necessary; however, carefully monitor the patient. Maximum dose: 600 mg daily.

Hemodialysis: Poorly removed (Cl_{HD} <1 L/hour)

Hepatic Impairment No starting dosage adjustment is necessary; however, carefully monitor the patient.

Monitoring Parameters Electrolytes, serum creatinine, BUN, urinalysis

Special Geriatric Considerations No specific dose adjustments are necessary in the elderly due to the drug's major route of elimination. However, since many elderly may be volume depleted due to their "blunted thirst reflex" and use of diuretics, care and monitoring of blood pressure and volume status are necessary upon initiation.

Dosage Forms Excipient information presented when available (limited, particularly for generics); consult specific product labeling.

Tablet, oral: 600 mg
  Teveten®: 400 mg, 600 mg

Eprosartan and Hydrochlorothiazide
(ep roe SAR tan & hye droe klor oh THYE a zide)

Related Information
  Eprosartan *on page 655*
  Hydrochlorothiazide *on page 933*
Brand Names: U.S. Teveten® HCT
Brand Names: Canada Teveten® HCT; Teveten® Plus
Index Terms Eprosartan Mesylate and Hydrochlorothiazide; Hydrochlorothiazide and Eprosartan
Generic Availability (U.S.) No
Pharmacologic Category Angiotensin II Receptor Blocker; Diuretic, Thiazide
Use Treatment of hypertension (not indicated for initial treatment)
Dosage

  Geriatric & Adult Hypertension: Oral: Dose is individualized (combination substituted for individual components)
    Usual recommended dose: Eprosartan 600 mg/hydrochlorothiazide 12.5 mg once daily (maximum dose: Eprosartan 600 mg/hydrochlorothiazide 25 mg once daily)

  Renal Impairment Moderate-to-severe impairment: Initial dose adjustments are not necessary per manufacturer; however carefully monitor patient. Do not exceed a maximum dose of eprosartan 600 mg daily. Hydrochlorothiazide is ineffective in patients with Cl_{cr} <30 mL/minute.

  Hepatic Impairment Initial dose adjustments not recommended by manufacturer; carefully monitor patient.

Special Geriatric Considerations See individual agents. Combination products are not recommended as first-line treatment. Use only if doses of individual agents correspond to the combination available.

Dosage Forms Excipient information presented when available (limited, particularly for generics); consult specific product labeling.
  Tablet:
    600 mg/12.5 mg: Eprosartan 600 mg and hydrochlorothiazide 12.5 mg
    600 mg/25 mg: Eprosartan 600 mg and hydrochlorothiazide 25 mg

◆ **Eprosartan Mesylate and Hydrochlorothiazide** *see* Eprosartan and Hydrochlorothiazide *on page 657*
◆ **Epsom Salt [OTC]** *see* Magnesium Salts (Various Salts) *on page 1182*
◆ **Equalactin® [OTC]** *see* Polycarbophil *on page 1563*
◆ **Equalizer Gas Relief [OTC]** *see* Simethicone *on page 1776*
◆ **Equanil** *see* Meprobamate *on page 1211*
◆ **Equetro®** *see* CarBAMazepine *on page 286*

Ergocalciferol (er goe kal SIF e role)

Medication Safety Issues
  Sound-alike/look-alike issues:
    Calciferol™ may be confused with calcitriol
    Drisdol® may be confused with Drysol™
    Ergocalciferol may be confused with alfacalcidol, cholecalciferol
Brand Names: U.S. Calciferol™ [OTC]; Drisdol®; Drisdol® [OTC]
Brand Names: Canada Drisdol®; Ostoforte®
Index Terms Activated Ergosterol; D2; Viosterol; Vitamin D2
Generic Availability (U.S.) Yes
Pharmacologic Category Vitamin D Analog
Use Treatment of refractory rickets, hypophosphatemia, hypoparathyroidism; dietary supplement
Unlabeled Use Prevention and treatment of vitamin D deficiency in patients with chronic kidney disease (CKD); osteoporosis prevention

Contraindications Hypersensitivity to ergocalciferol or any component of the formulation; hypercalcemia; malabsorption syndrome; hypervitaminosis D or abnormal sensitivity to the toxic effects of vitamin D

Warnings/Precautions Adequate calcium supplementation is required; calcium and phosphorous levels must be monitored during therapy. The range between therapeutic and toxic doses is narrow in vitamin D-resistant rickets. Adjust dose based on clinical response to avoid toxicity. Use caution with cardiovascular disease, renal impairment, or diseases that may impair vitamin D metabolism. Effects of vitamin D can last ≥2 months after therapy is discontinued. Products may contain tartrazine which may cause allergic reactions in certain individuals.

Adverse Reactions (Reflective of adult population; not specific for elderly) Frequency not defined: Endocrine & metabolic: Hypervitaminosis D (signs and symptoms include hypercalcemia, resulting in headache, nausea, vomiting, lethargy, confusion, sluggishness, abdominal pain, bone pain, polyuria, polydipsia, weakness, cardiac arrhythmias [eg, QT shortening, sinus tachycardia], soft tissue calcification, calciuria, and nephrocalcinosis)

Drug Interactions

Metabolism/Transport Effects None known.

Avoid Concomitant Use

Avoid concomitant use of Ergocalciferol with any of the following: Aluminum Hydroxide; Sucralfate; Vitamin D Analogs

Increased Effect/Toxicity

Ergocalciferol may increase the levels/effects of: Aluminum Hydroxide; Cardiac Glycosides; Sucralfate; Vitamin D Analogs

The levels/effects of Ergocalciferol may be increased by: Calcium Salts; Danazol; Thiazide Diuretics

Decreased Effect

The levels/effects of Ergocalciferol may be decreased by: Bile Acid Sequestrants; Mineral Oil; Orlistat

Stability Store at room temperature of 15°C to 30°C (59°F to 86°F). Protect from light.

Mechanism of Action Stimulates calcium and phosphate absorption from the small intestine, promotes secretion of calcium from bone to blood; promotes renal tubule phosphate resorption

Pharmacodynamics/Kinetics

Onset of action: Peak effect:~1 month following daily doses

Absorption: Readily; requires bile

Metabolism: Inactive until hydroxylated hepatically and renally to calcifediol and then to calcitriol (most active form)

Dosage

Geriatric Note: 1 mcg = 40 units

Dietary Reference Intake for Vitamin D: Oral:

≤70 years: Refer to adult dosing.

>70 years: RDA: 800 units/day

Adult Note: 1 mcg = 40 int. units

Dietary Reference Intake for Vitamin D: Oral:

Adults 19-70 years: RDA: 600 int. units/day

Osteoporosis prevention (unlabeled use): Adults ≥50 years: 800-1000 int. units/day (NOF guidelines, 2010)

Vitamin D deficiency treatment (unlabeled dose): Oral: 50,000 int. units once per week for 8 weeks, followed by 50,000 int. units every 2-4 weeks thereafter for maintenance of adequate levels (Holick, 2007) **or** 50,000 int. units twice per week for 5 weeks (Stechschulte, 2009)

Vitamin D deficiency/insufficiency in patients with CKD stages 3-4 (K/DOQI guidelines):

Note: Dose is based on 25-hydroxyvitamin D serum level (25[OH]D): Oral (treatment duration should be a total of 6 months):

Serum 25(OH)D <5 ng/mL:

50,000 int. units/week for 12 weeks, then 50,000 int. units/month

Serum 25(OH)D 5-15 ng/mL:

50,000 int. units/week for 4 weeks, then 50,000 int. units/month

Serum 25(OH)D 16-30 ng/mL:

50,000 int. units/month

Hypoparathyroidism: Oral: 625 mcg to 5 mg/day (25,000-200,000 int. units) and calcium supplements

Nutritional rickets and osteomalacia: Oral:

Adults with normal absorption: 25-125 mcg/day (1000-5000 int. units)

Adults with malabsorption: 250-7500 mcg (10,000-300,000 int. units)

Vitamin D-*dependent* rickets: Oral: 250 mcg to 1.5 mg/day (10,000-60,000 int. units)

Vitamin D-*resistant* rickets: Oral: 12,000-500,000 int. units/day
Familial hypophosphatemia: Oral: 10,000-60,000 int. units plus phosphate supplements
Monitoring Parameters Serum calcium, creatinine, BUN, and phosphorus every 1-2 weeks; x-ray bones monthly until stabilized; signs and symptoms of vitamin D intoxication

Vitamin D deficiency/insufficiency in patients with CKD stages 3-4: Measure serum 25(OH)D levels after 6 months in adults. Discontinue ergocalciferol (or any vitamin D supplements) if the corrected total serum calcium level is >10.2 mg/dL.

Reference Range
Serum calcium times phosphorus should not exceed 70 mg^2/dL^2 to avoid ectopic calcification
Vitamin D deficiency: There is no clear consensus on a reference range for total serum 25 (OH)D concentrations or the validity of this level as it relates clinically to bone health. In addition, there is significant variability in the reporting of serum 25 (OH)D levels as a result of different assay types in use. However, the following ranges have been suggested: Adults (NAS, 2011):
<30 nmol/L (12 ng/mL): At risk for deficiency
30-50 nmol/L (12-20 ng/mL): Potentially at risk for inadequacy
≥50 nmol/L (20 ng/mL): Sufficient levels in practically all persons
>125 nmol/L (50 ng/mL): Concern for risk of toxicity

Special Geriatric Considerations Vitamin D, folate, and B$_{12}$ (cyanocobalamin) have decreased absorption with age (clinical significance unknown); studies in ill geriatrics demonstrated that low serum concentrations of vitamin D result in greater bone loss. Calorie requirements decrease with age and therefore, nutrient density must be increased to ensure adequate nutrient intake, including vitamins and minerals. The use of a daily supplement with a multiple vitamin with minerals is recommended because elderly consume less vitamin D, absorption may be decreased, and many have decreased sun exposure. This is a recommendation of particular need to those with high risk for osteoporosis.

Vitamin D supplementation has been shown to increase muscle function and strength, as well as improve balance. Patients at risk for falls should have vitamin D serum concentrations measured and be evaluated for supplementation.

Dosage Forms Excipient information presented when available (limited, particularly for generics); consult specific product labeling.
Capsule, oral: 50,000 units [1.25 mg]
  Drisdol®: 50,000 units [contains soybean oil, tartrazine; 1.25 mg]
Capsule, softgel, oral: 50,000 units [1.25 mg]
Solution, oral [drops]: 8000 units/mL (60 mL)
  Calciferol™: 8000 units/mL (60 mL) [contains propylene glycol; 200 mcg/mL]
  Drisdol®: 8000 units/mL (60 mL) [contains propylene glycol; 200 mcg/mL, OTC]
Tablet, oral: 400 units

Ergoloid Mesylates (ER goe loid MES i lates)

Related Information
Beers Criteria – Potentially Inappropriate Medications for Geriatrics *on page* 2183
Medication Safety Issues
  BEERS Criteria medication:
    This drug may be potentially inappropriate for use in geriatric patients (Quality of evidence - high; Strength of recommendation - strong).
Brand Names: Canada Hydergine®
Index Terms Dihydroergotoxine; Dihydrogenated Ergot Alkaloids; Hydergine [DSC]
Generic Availability (U.S.) Yes
Pharmacologic Category Ergot Derivative
Use Treatment of cerebrovascular insufficiency in primary progressive dementia, Alzheimer's dementia, and senile onset
Contraindications Hypersensitivity to ergot or any component of the formulation; acute or chronic psychosis; ergot alkaloids are contraindicated with potent inhibitors of CYP3A4 (includes protease inhibitors, azole antifungals, and some macrolide antibiotics)
Warnings/Precautions Pleural and peritoneal fibrosis have been reported with prolonged daily use. Cardiac valvular fibrosis has also been associated with ergot alkaloids. Concomitant use with potent inhibitors of CYP3A4 (includes protease inhibitors, azole antifungals, and some macrolide antibiotics) and ergot alkaloids has been associated with acute ergot toxicity (ergotism); certain ergot alkaloids (eg, ergotamine and dihydroergotamine) are contraindicated by the manufacturer. Avoid use in the elderly due to lack of efficacy (Beers Criteria).

Adverse Reactions (Reflective of adult population; not specific for elderly) Adverse effects are minimal; most common include transient nausea, gastrointestinal disturbances and sublingual irritation with SL tablets; other common side effects include:

Cardiovascular: Bradycardia, orthostatic hypotension
Dermatologic: Flushing, skin rash
Ocular: Blurred vision
Respiratory: Nasal congestion

Drug Interactions

Metabolism/Transport Effects Substrate of CYP3A4 (major); **Note:** Assignment of Major/Minor substrate status based on clinically relevant drug interaction potential

Avoid Concomitant Use

Avoid concomitant use of Ergoloid Mesylates with any of the following: Boceprevir; Conivaptan; Efavirenz; Itraconazole; Ketoconazole; Ketoconazole (Systemic); Nitroglycerin; Posaconazole; Protease Inhibitors; Serotonin 5-HT1D Receptor Agonists; Telaprevir; Voriconazole

Increased Effect/Toxicity

Ergoloid Mesylates may increase the levels/effects of: Metoclopramide; Serotonin 5-HT1D Receptor Agonists; Serotonin Modulators

The levels/effects of Ergoloid Mesylates may be increased by: Antipsychotics; Boceprevir; Conivaptan; CYP3A4 Inhibitors (Moderate); CYP3A4 Inhibitors (Strong); Dasatinib; Efavirenz; Itraconazole; Ivacaftor; Ketoconazole; Ketoconazole (Systemic); Macrolide Antibiotics; Mifepristone; Nitroglycerin; Posaconazole; Protease Inhibitors; Serotonin 5-HT1D Receptor Agonists; Telaprevir; Voriconazole

Decreased Effect

Ergoloid Mesylates may decrease the levels/effects of: Nitroglycerin

The levels/effects of Ergoloid Mesylates may be decreased by: Tocilizumab

Mechanism of Action Ergoloid mesylates do not have the vasoconstrictor effects of the natural ergot alkaloids; exact mechanism in dementia is unknown; originally classed as peripheral and cerebral vasodilator, now considered a "metabolic enhancer"; there is no specific evidence which clearly establishes the mechanism by which ergoloid mesylate preparations produce mental effects, nor is there conclusive evidence that the drug particularly affects cerebral arteriosclerosis or cerebrovascular insufficiency

Pharmacodynamics/Kinetics

Absorption: Rapid yet incomplete
Half-life elimination, serum: 3.5 hours
Time to peak, serum: ~1 hour

Dosage

Geriatric & Adult Primary progressive dementia, Alzheimer's dementia: Oral: 1 mg 3 times/day up to 4.5-12 mg/day; up to 6 months of therapy may be necessary

Special Geriatric Considerations Ergoloid mesylates have no role in the treatment of dementia. Most clinicians regard it as no better than placebo and most patients do not experience significant benefits. Improvement in social function has been shown in some older studies, but no consistent improvement in memory or cognitive function was reported.

This medication is considered to be potentially inappropriate in this patient population (Beers Criteria: Quality of evidence - high; Strength of recommendation - strong).

Dosage Forms Excipient information presented when available (limited, particularly for generics); consult specific product labeling.

Tablet, oral: 1 mg

◆ **Ergomar®** *see* Ergotamine *on page 660*

Ergotamine (er GOT a meen)

Brand Names: U.S. Ergomar®
Index Terms Ergotamine Tartrate
Generic Availability (U.S.) No
Pharmacologic Category Antimigraine Agent; Ergot Derivative
Use Abort or prevent vascular headaches, such as migraine, migraine variants, or so-called "histaminic cephalalgia"
Contraindications Hypersensitivity to ergotamine or any component of the formulation; peripheral vascular disease; hepatic or renal disease; coronary artery disease; hypertension; sepsis; ergot alkaloids are contraindicated with strong inhibitors of CYP3A4 (includes protease inhibitors, azole antifungals, and some macrolide antibiotics)

Warnings/Precautions Ergot alkaloids have been associated with fibrotic valve thickening (eg, aortic, mitral, tricuspid); usually associated with long-term, chronic use; vasospasm or vasoconstriction can occur; ergot alkaloid use may result in ergotism (intense vasoconstriction) resulting in peripheral vascular ischemia and possible gangrene; rare cases of pleural and/or retroperitoneal fibrosis have been reported with prolonged daily use. Discontinuation after extended use may result in withdrawal symptoms (eg, rebound headache). Use with caution in the elderly.

[U.S. Boxed Warning]: Ergot alkaloids are contraindicated with potent inhibitors of CYP3A4 (includes protease inhibitors, azole antifungals, and some macrolide antibiotics); concomitant use associated with acute ergot toxicity (ergotism).

Adverse Reactions (Reflective of adult population; not specific for elderly) Frequency not defined.

Cardiovascular: Absence of pulse, bradycardia, cardiac valvular fibrosis, cyanosis, edema, ECG changes, gangrene, hypertension, ischemia, precordial distress and pain, tachycardia, vasospasm

Central nervous system: Vertigo

Dermatologic: Itching

Gastrointestinal: Nausea, vomiting

Genitourinary: Retroperitoneal fibrosis

Neuromuscular & skeletal: Muscle pain, numbness, paresthesia, weakness

Respiratory: Pleuropulmonary fibrosis

Miscellaneous: Cold extremities

Drug Interactions

Metabolism/Transport Effects Substrate of CYP3A4 (major); **Note:** Assignment of Major/Minor substrate status based on clinically relevant drug interaction potential; **Inhibits** CYP3A4 (weak)

Avoid Concomitant Use

Avoid concomitant use of Ergotamine with any of the following: Alpha-/Beta-Agonists; Alpha1-Agonists; Boceprevir; Clarithromycin; Conivaptan; Crizotinib; Efavirenz; Itraconazole; Ketoconazole; Ketoconazole (Systemic); Mifepristone; Nitroglycerin; Posaconazole; Protease Inhibitors; Serotonin 5-HT1D Receptor Agonists; Telaprevir; Voriconazole

Increased Effect/Toxicity

Ergotamine may increase the levels/effects of: Alpha-/Beta-Agonists; Alpha1-Agonists; Metoclopramide; Serotonin 5-HT1D Receptor Agonists; Serotonin Modulators

The levels/effects of Ergotamine may be increased by: Antipsychotics; Boceprevir; Clarithromycin; Conivaptan; Crizotinib; CYP3A4 Inhibitors (Moderate); CYP3A4 Inhibitors (Strong); Dasatinib; Efavirenz; Itraconazole; Ivacaftor; Ketoconazole; Ketoconazole (Systemic); Macrolide Antibiotics; Mifepristone; Nitroglycerin; Posaconazole; Protease Inhibitors; Serotonin 5-HT1D Receptor Agonists; Telaprevir; Voriconazole

Decreased Effect

Ergotamine may decrease the levels/effects of: Nitroglycerin

The levels/effects of Ergotamine may be decreased by: Tocilizumab

Ethanol/Nutrition/Herb Interactions Food: Caffeine may increase GI absorption of ergotamine. Grapefruit juice may cause increased blood levels of ergotamine, leading to increased toxicity. Management: Avoid caffeinated tea, cola, coffee, or other significant sources of caffeine.

Stability Store sublingual tablet at room temperature; protect from heat. Protect from light.

Mechanism of Action Has partial agonist and/or antagonist activity against tryptaminergic, dopaminergic and alpha-adrenergic receptors depending upon their site; is a highly active uterine stimulant; it causes constriction of peripheral and cranial blood vessels and produces depression of central vasomotor centers

Pharmacodynamics/Kinetics

Absorption: Oral: Erratic; enhanced by caffeine coadministration

Metabolism: Extensively hepatic

Half-life elimination: 2 hours

Time to peak, serum: 0.5-3 hours

Excretion: Feces (90% as metabolites)

Dosage

Geriatric Not recommended for use in the elderly.

Adult Migraine: Sublingual: One tablet under tongue at first sign, then 1 tablet every 30 minutes if needed; maximum dose: 3 tablets/24 hours, 5 tablets/week

Administration Do not crush sublingual drug product.

Monitoring Parameters Relief of symptoms, blood pressure, pulse, peripheral circulation

Special Geriatric Considerations Not recommended for use in the elderly. May be harmful due to reduction in cerebral blood flow. May precipitate angina, myocardial infarction, or aggravate intermittent claudication.

Dosage Forms Excipient information presented when available (limited, particularly for generics); consult specific product labeling.

Tablet, sublingual, as tartrate:
  Ergomar®: 2 mg [peppermint flavor]

Ergotamine and Caffeine (er GOT a meen & KAF een)

Related Information
  Ergotamine *on page 660*

Medication Safety Issues
  Sound-alike/look-alike issues:
  Cafergot® may be confused with Carafate®

Brand Names: U.S. Cafergot®; Migergot®

Brand Names: Canada Cafergor®

Index Terms Caffeine and Ergotamine; Ergotamine Tartrate and Caffeine

Generic Availability (U.S.) Yes: Tablet

Pharmacologic Category Antimigraine Agent; Ergot Derivative; Stimulant

Use Abort or prevent vascular headaches, such as migraine, migraine variants, or so-called "histaminic cephalalgia"

Dosage

Adult Migraine:

  Oral: Two tablets at onset of attack; then 1 tablet every 30 minutes as needed; maximum: 6 tablets per attack; do not exceed 10 tablets/week.

  Rectal: One suppository rectally at first sign of an attack; follow with second dose after 1 hour, if needed; maximum: 2 per attack; do not exceed 5/week.

Special Geriatric Considerations Not recommended for use in the elderly. May be harmful due to reduction in cerebral blood flow. May precipitate angina, myocardial infarction, or aggravate intermittent claudication.

Dosage Forms Excipient information presented when available (limited, particularly for generics); consult specific product labeling.

Suppository, rectal:
  Migergot®: Ergotamine tartrate 2 mg and caffeine 100 mg (12s)

Tablet, oral: Ergotamine tartrate 1 mg and caffeine 100 mg
  Cafergot®: Ergotamine tartrate 1 mg and caffeine 100 mg

♦ **Ergotamine Tartrate** *see* Ergotamine *on page 660*
♦ **Ergotamine Tartrate and Caffeine** *see* Ergotamine and Caffeine *on page 662*
♦ **E-R-O® [OTC]** *see* Carbamide Peroxide *on page 291*

Ertapenem (er ta PEN em)

Related Information
  Antimicrobial Drugs of Choice *on page 2163*
  Community-Acquired Pneumonia in Adults *on page 2171*

Medication Safety Issues
  Sound-alike/look-alike issues:
  Ertapenem may be confused with doripenem, imipenem, meropenem
  INVanz® may be confused with AVINza®, I.V. vancomycin

Brand Names: U.S. INVanz®

Brand Names: Canada Invanz®

Index Terms Ertapenem Sodium; L-749,345; MK0826

Generic Availability (U.S.) No

Pharmacologic Category Antibiotic, Carbapenem

Use Treatment of the following moderate-to-severe infections: Complicated intra-abdominal infections, complicated skin and skin structure infections (including diabetic foot infections without osteomyelitis, animal and human bites), complicated UTI (including pyelonephritis), acute pelvic infections (including postpartum endomyometritis, septic abortion, postsurgical gynecologic infections), and community-acquired pneumonia. Prophylaxis of surgical site infection following elective colorectal surgery. Antibacterial coverage includes aerobic gram-positive organisms, aerobic gram-negative organisms, and anaerobic organisms.

ERTAPENEM

Note: Methicillin-resistant *Staphylococcus aureus, Enterococcus* spp, penicillin-resistant strains of *Streptococcus pneumoniae, Acinetobacter,* and *Pseudomonas aeruginosa,* are **resistant** to ertapenem while most extended-spectrum β-lactamase (ESBL)-producing bacteria remain sensitive to ertapenem.

Unlabeled Use Treatment of intravenous catheter-related bloodstream infection

Contraindications Hypersensitivity to ertapenem, other carbapenems (eg, doripenem, imipenem, meropenem), or any component of the formulation; anaphylactic reactions to beta-lactam antibiotics. If using intramuscularly, known hypersensitivity to local anesthetics of the amide type (lidocaine is the diluent).

Warnings/Precautions Use caution with renal impairment. Dosage adjustment required in patients with moderate-to-severe renal dysfunction; elderly patients often require lower doses (based upon renal function). Use may result in fungal or bacterial superinfection, including *C. difficile*-associated diarrhea (CDAD) and pseudomembranous colitis; CDAD has been observed >2 months postantibiotic treatment. Carbapenems have been associated with CNS adverse effects, including confusional states and seizures (myoclonic); use caution with CNS disorders (eg, brain lesions and history of seizures) and adjust dose in renal impairment to avoid drug accumulation, which may increase seizure risk. Serious hypersensitivity reactions, including anaphylaxis, have been reported (some without a history of previous allergic reactions to beta-lactams). Doses for I.M. administration are mixed with lidocaine; consult Lidocaine (Systemic) information for associated Warnings/Precautions. May decrease divalproex sodium/valproic acid concentrations leading to breakthrough seizures; concomitant use not recommended.

Adverse Reactions (Reflective of adult population; not specific for elderly)
>10%: Gastrointestinal: Diarrhea (2% to 12%)
1% to 10%:
Cardiovascular: Edema (3%), chest pain (1% to 2%), hypertension (1% to 2%), hypotension (1% to 2%), tachycardia (1% to 2%)
Central nervous system: Headache (4% to 7%); altered mental status (eg, agitation, confusion, disorientation, mental acuity decreased, somnolence, stupor) (3% to 5%); fever (2% to 5%), insomnia (3%), dizziness (2%), hypothermia (infants, children, and adolescents <2%), fatigue (1%), anxiety (1%)
Dermatologic: Diaper rash (infants and children 5%), rash (2% to 3%), pruritus (1% to 2%), erythema (1% to 2%), genital rash (infants, children, and adolescents <2%), skin lesions (infants, children, and adolescents <2%)
Endocrine & metabolic: Hypokalemia (2%), hyperglycemia (1% to 2%), hyperkalemia (≤1%)
Gastrointestinal: Vomiting (2% to 10%), nausea (6% to 9%), abdominal pain (4% to 5%), constipation (2% to 4%), acid regurgitation (1% to 2%), appetite decreased (infants, children, and adolescents <2%), dyspepsia (1%), oral candidiasis (≤1%)
Genitourinary: Urine WBCs increased (2% to 3%), urine RBCs increased (1% to 3%), vaginitis (1% to 3%)
Hematologic: Thrombocytosis (4% to 7%), hematocrit/hemoglobin decreased (3% to 5%), eosinophils increased (1% to 2%), leukopenia (1% to 2%), neutrophils decreased (1% to 2%), thrombocytopenia (1%), prothrombin time increased (≤1%)
Hepatic: Hepatic enzyme increased (7% to 9%), alkaline phosphatase increase (4% to 7%), albumin decreased (1% to 2%), bilirubin (total) increased (1% to 2%)
Local: Infused vein complications (5% to 7%), phlebitis/thrombophlebitis (2%), extravasation (1% to 2%)
Neuromuscular & skeletal: Arthralgia (infants, children, and adolescents <2%), weakness (1%), leg pain (≤1%)
Otic: Otitis media (infants, children, and adolescents <2%)
Renal: Serum creatinine increased (1%)
Respiratory: Cough (1% to 4%), dyspnea (1% to 3%), nasopharyngitis (infants, children, and adolescents <2%), rhinitis (infants, children, and adolescents <2%), rhinorrhea (infants, children, and adolescents <2%), upper respiratory tract infection (infants, children, and adolescents <2%), wheezing (infants, children, and adolescents <2%), pharyngitis (1%), rales/rhonchi (1%), respiratory distress (≤1%)
Miscellaneous: Herpes simplex (infants, children, and adolescents <2%)

Drug Interactions
Metabolism/Transport Effects None known.
Avoid Concomitant Use
Avoid concomitant use of Ertapenem with any of the following: BCG
Increased Effect/Toxicity
The levels/effects of Ertapenem may be increased by: Probenecid
Decreased Effect
Ertapenem may decrease the levels/effects of: BCG; Divalproex; Typhoid Vaccine; Valproic Acid

Stability Before reconstitution store at ≤25°C (77°F).

I.M.: Reconstitute 1 g vial with 3.2 mL of 1% lidocaine HCl injection (without epinephrine). Shake well. Use within 1 hour after preparation.

I.V.: Reconstitute 1 g vial with 10 mL of sterile water for injection, 0.9% sodium chloride injection, or bacteriostatic water for injection. Shake well. For adults, transfer dose to 50 mL of 0.9% sodium chloride injection. Reconstituted I.V. solution may be stored at room temperature and must be used within 6 hours **or** refrigerated, stored for up to 24 hours and used within 4 hours after removal from refrigerator. Do not freeze.

Mechanism of Action Inhibits bacterial cell wall synthesis by binding to one or more of the penicillin-binding proteins, which in turn inhibits the final transpeptidation step of peptidoglycan synthesis in bacterial cell walls, thus inhibiting cell wall biosynthesis. Bacteria eventually lyse due to ongoing activity of cell wall autolytic enzymes (autolysins and murein hydrolases) while cell wall assembly is arrested.

Pharmacodynamics/Kinetics

Absorption: I.M.: Almost complete

Distribution: V_{dss}: Adults: ~0.12 L/kg

Protein binding (concentration dependent, primarily to albumin): 85% at 300 mcg/mL, 95% at <100 mcg/mL

Metabolism: Non-CYP-mediated hydrolysis to inactive metabolite

Bioavailability: I.M.: ~90%

Half-life elimination: Adults: ~4 hours

Time to peak: I.M.: ~2.3 hours

Excretion: Urine (~80% as unchanged drug and metabolite); feces (~10%)

Dosage

Geriatric & Adult Note: I.V. therapy may be administered for up to 14 days; I.M. for up to 7 days

Community-acquired pneumonia and complicated urinary tract infections (including pyelonephritis): I.M., I.V.: 1 g/day; duration of total antibiotic treatment: 10-14 days; duration includes possible switch to appropriate oral therapy once clinical improvement demonstrated. **Note:** The carbapenems, including ertapenem, are preferred agents for *Enterobacter* spp and *Burkholderia pseudomallei,* and are considered alternative agents for anaerobes in aspiration pneumonia (IDSA, 2007).

Intra-abdominal infection: I.M., I.V.: 1 g/day for 5-14 days; **Note:** 2010 IDSA guidelines recommend a treatment duration of 4-7 days (provided source controlled) for community-acquired, mild-to-moderate IAI

Pelvic infections (acute): I.M., I.V.: 1 g/day for 3-10 days

Prophylaxis of surgical site following colorectal surgery: I.V.: 1 g given 1 hour preoperatively

Skin and skin structure infections (excluding diabetic foot infections with osteomyelitis): I.M., I.V.: 1 g/day for 7-14 days. **Notes:** For diabetic foot infections, recommended treatment duration is up to 4 weeks depending on severity of infection and response to therapy (Lipsky, 2012); guidelines recommend ertapenem as a preferred agent for animal bites. (IDSA, 2005).

Intravenous catheter-related bloodstream infection (unlabeled use): I.V. 1 g/day (**Note:** Carbapenems, including ertapenem, are preferred agents for extended-spectrum β-lactamase (ESBL)-positive *Escherichia coli* and *Klebsiella, Enterobacter,* and *Serratia* [IDSA, 2009].)

Renal Impairment Adults:

Cl_{cr} >30 mL/minute/1.73 m^2: No adjustment required

Cl_{cr} ≤30 mL/minute/1.73 m^2 and ESRD: 500 mg/day

Hemodialysis: When the daily dose is given within 6 hours prior to hemodialysis, a supplementary dose of 150 mg is required following hemodialysis.

CAPD: I.V.: 500 mg/day (Cardone, 2011)

Hepatic Impairment Adjustments cannot be recommended (lack of experience and research in this patient population).

Administration

I.M.: Avoid injection into a blood vessel. Make sure patient does not have an allergy to lidocaine or another anesthetic of the amide type. Administer by deep I.M. injection into a large muscle mass (eg, gluteal muscle or lateral part of the thigh). Do not administer I.M. preparation or drug reconstituted for I.M. administration intravenously.

I.V.: Infuse over 30 minutes

Monitoring Parameters Periodic renal, hepatic, and hematopoietic assessment during prolonged therapy; neurological assessment

Special Geriatric Considerations According to the package insert, the total and unbound AUCs were increased 37% and 67%, respectively, in healthy men and women ≥65 years of age compared to younger adults. No dose adjustment is required for patients with normal age-adjusted renal function.

Dosage Forms Excipient information presented when available (limited, particularly for generics); consult specific product labeling.
Injection, powder for reconstitution:
INVanz®: 1 g [contains sodium ~137 mg (~6 mEq)/g]

◆ **Ertapenem Sodium** *see* Ertapenem *on page 662*
◆ **EryPed®** *see* Erythromycin (Systemic) *on page 665*
◆ **Ery-Tab®** *see* Erythromycin (Systemic) *on page 665*
◆ **Erythrocin®** *see* Erythromycin (Systemic) *on page 665*
◆ **Erythrocin® Lactobionate-I.V.** *see* Erythromycin (Systemic) *on page 665*

Erythromycin (Systemic) (er ith roe MYE sin)

Related Information
Antimicrobial Drugs of Choice *on page 2163*
Community-Acquired Pneumonia in Adults *on page 2171*
Medication Safety Issues
Sound-alike/look-alike issues:
Erythromycin may be confused with azithromycin, clarithromycin
Eryc® may be confused with Emcyt®, Ery-Tab®
Brand Names: U.S. E.E.S.®; Ery-Tab®; EryPed®; Erythro-RX; Erythrocin®; Erythrocin® Lactobionate-I.V.; PCE®
Brand Names: Canada Apo-Erythro Base®; Apo-Erythro E-C®; Apo-Erythro-ES®; Apo-Erythro-S®; EES®; Erybid™; Eryc®; Novo-Rythro Estolate; Novo-Rythro Ethylsuccinate; Nu-Erythromycin-S; PCE®
Index Terms Erythromycin Base; Erythromycin Ethylsuccinate; Erythromycin Lactobionate; Erythromycin Stearate
Generic Availability (U.S.) Yes: Capsule, tablet (as base, ethylsuccinate, and stearate)
Pharmacologic Category Antibiotic, Macrolide
Use Treatment of susceptible bacterial infections including *S. pyogenes*, some *S. pneumoniae*, some *S. aureus*, *M. pneumoniae*, *Legionella pneumophila*, diphtheria, pertussis, *Chlamydia*, erythrasma, *N. gonorrhoeae*, *E. histolytica*, syphilis and nongonococcal urethritis, and *Campylobacter* gastroenteritis; used in conjunction with neomycin for decontaminating the bowel
Unlabeled Use Treatment of gastroparesis, chancroid; preoperative gut sterilization
Contraindications Hypersensitivity to erythromycin, any macrolide antibiotics, or any component of the formulation
Concomitant use with pimozide, cisapride, ergotamine or dihydroergotamine, terfenadine, astemizole
Warnings/Precautions Use caution with hepatic impairment with or without jaundice has occurred, it may be accompanied by malaise, nausea, vomiting, abdominal colic, and fever; discontinue use if these occur. Use caution with other medication relying on CYP3A4 metabolism; high potential for drug interactions exists. Prolonged use may result in fungal or bacterial superinfection, including *C. difficile*-associated diarrhea (CDAD) and pseudomembranous colitis; CDAD has been observed >2 months postantibiotic treatment. Macrolides have been associated with rare QT_c prolongation and ventricular arrhythmias, including torsade de pointes. Use caution in elderly patients, as risk of adverse events may be increased. Use caution in myasthenia gravis patients; erythromycin may aggravate muscular weakness.
Adverse Reactions (Reflective of adult population; not specific for elderly) Frequency not defined. Incidence may vary with formulation.
Cardiovascular: QT_c prolongation, torsade de pointes, ventricular arrhythmia, ventricular tachycardia
Central nervous system: Seizure
Dermatologic: Erythema multiforme, pruritus, rash, Stevens-Johnson syndrome, toxic epidermal necrolysis
Gastrointestinal: Abdominal pain, anorexia, diarrhea, ile hypertrophic pyloric stenosis, nausea, oral candidiasis, pancreatitis, pseudomembranous colitis, vomiting
Hepatic: Cholestatic jaundice (most common with estolate), hepatitis, liver function tests abnormal
Local: Phlebitis at the injection site, thrombophlebitis
Neuromuscular & skeletal: Weakness
Otic: Hearing loss
Miscellaneous: Allergic reactions, anaphylaxis, hypersensitivity reactions, interstitial nephritis, urticaria

Drug Interactions

Metabolism/Transport Effects Substrate of CYP2B6 (minor), CYP3A4 (major), P-glycoprotein; **Note:** Assignment of Major/Minor substrate status based on clinically relevant drug interaction potential; **Inhibits** CYP3A4 (moderate), P-glycoprotein

Avoid Concomitant Use

Avoid concomitant use of Erythromycin (Systemic) with any of the following: BCG; Cisapride; Conivaptan; Disopyramide; Highest Risk QTc-Prolonging Agents; Lincosamide Antibiotics; Mifepristone; Pimozide; QuiNINE; Silodosin; Terfenadine; Tolvaptan; Topotecan

Increased Effect/Toxicity

Erythromycin (Systemic) may increase the levels/effects of: Alfentanil; Antifungal Agents (Azole Derivatives, Systemic); Antineoplastic Agents (Vinca Alkaloids); ARIPiprazole; Avanafil; Benzodiazepines (metabolized by oxidation); Budesonide (Systemic, Oral Inhalation); BusPIRone; Calcium Channel Blockers; CarBAMazepine; Cardiac Glycosides; Cilostazol; Cisapride; CloZAPine; Colchicine; Corticosteroids (Systemic); CycloSPORINE; CycloSPORINE (Systemic); CYP3A4 Substrates; Dabigatran Etexilate; Disopyramide; Eletriptan; Eplerenone; Ergot Derivatives; Everolimus; FentaNYL; Fexofenadine; Highest Risk QTc-Prolonging Agents; HMG-CoA Reductase Inhibitors; Ivacaftor; Lurasidone; Moderate Risk QTc-Prolonging Agents; P-glycoprotein/ABCB1 Substrates; Pimecrolimus; Pimozide; QuiNIDine; QuiNINE; Repaglinide; Rifamycin Derivatives; Rivaroxaban; Salmeterol; Saxagliptin; Selective Serotonin Reuptake Inhibitors; Silodosin; Sirolimus; Tacrolimus; Tacrolimus (Systemic); Tacrolimus (Topical); Temsirolimus; Terfenadine; Theophylline Derivatives; Tolvaptan; Topotecan; Vitamin K Antagonists; Zopiclone

The levels/effects of Erythromycin (Systemic) may be increased by: Antifungal Agents (Azole Derivatives, Systemic); Conivaptan; CYP3A4 Inhibitors (Moderate); CYP3A4 Inhibitors (Strong); Ivacaftor; Mifepristone; P-glycoprotein/ABCB1 Inhibitors; QTc-Prolonging Agents (Indeterminate Risk and Risk Modifying)

Decreased Effect

Erythromycin (Systemic) may decrease the levels/effects of: BCG; Clopidogrel; Ifosfamide; Typhoid Vaccine; Zafirlukast

The levels/effects of Erythromycin (Systemic) may be decreased by: CYP3A4 Inducers (Strong); Deferasirox; Etravirine; Herbs (CYP3A4 Inducers); Lincosamide Antibiotics; P-glycoprotein/ABCB1 Inducers; Tocilizumab

Ethanol/Nutrition/Herb Interactions

Ethanol: Ethanol may decrease absorption of erythromycin or enhance effects of ethanol. Management: Avoid ethanol.

Food: Erythromycin serum levels may be altered if taken with food (formulation-dependent). GI upset, including diarrhea, is common. Management: May be taken with food to decrease GI upset, otherwise take around-the-clock with a full glass of water. Do not give with milk or acidic beverages (eg, soda, juice).

Herb/Nutraceutical: St John's wort may decrease erythromycin levels. Management: Avoid St John's wort.

Stability

Injection:

Store unreconstituted vials at 15°C to 30°C (59°F to 86°F). Erythromycin lactobionate should be reconstituted with sterile water for injection without preservatives to avoid gel formation. The reconstituted solution is stable for 2 weeks when refrigerated or for 8 hours at room temperature.

Erythromycin I.V. infusion solution is stable at pH 6-8. Stability of lactobionate is pH dependent. I.V. form has the longest stability in 0.9% sodium chloride (NS) and should be prepared in this base solution whenever possible. Do not use D_5W as a diluent unless sodium bicarbonate is added to solution. If I.V. must be prepared in D_5W, 0.5 mL of the 8.4% sodium bicarbonate solution should be added per each 100 mL of D_5W.

Stability of parenteral admixture at room temperature (25°C) and at refrigeration temperature (4°C) is 24 hours.

Standard diluent: 500 mg/250 mL D_5W/NS; 750 mg/250 mL D_5W/NS; 1 g/250 mL D_5W/NS.

Oral suspension:

Granules: Prior to mixing, store at <30°C (86°F). After mixing, store under refrigeration and use within 10 days.

Powder: Prior to mixing, store at <30°C (86°F). After mixing, store at ≤25°C (77°F) and use within 35 days.

Tablet and capsule formulations: Store at <30°C (86°F).

Mechanism of Action Inhibits RNA-dependent protein synthesis at the chain elongation step; binds to the 50S ribosomal subunit resulting in blockage of transpeptidation

Pharmacodynamics/Kinetics

Absorption: Oral: Variable but better with salt forms than with base form; 18% to 45%; ethylsuccinate may be better absorbed with food

Distribution:

Relative diffusion from blood into CSF: Minimal even with inflammation

CSF:blood level ratio: Normal meninges: 2% to 13%; Inflamed meninges: 7% to 25%

Protein binding: Base: 73% to 81%

Metabolism: Demethylation primarily via hepatic CYP3A4

Half-life elimination: Peak: 1.5-2 hours; End-stage renal disease: 5-6 hours

Time to peak, serum: Base: 4 hours; Ethylsuccinate: 0.5-2.5 hours; delayed with food due to differences in absorption

Excretion: Primarily feces; urine (2% to 15% as unchanged drug)

Dosage

Geriatric & Adult Note: Due to differences in absorption, 400 mg erythromycin ethylsuccinate produces the same serum levels as 250 mg erythromycin base or stearate.

Usual dosage range:

Oral:

Base: 250-500 mg every 6-12 hours

Ethylsuccinate: 400-800 mg every 6-12 hours

I.V.: Lactobionate: 15-20 mg/kg/day divided every 6 hours or 500 mg to 1 g every 6 hours, or given as a continuous infusion over 24 hours (maximum: 4 g/24 hours)

Indication-specific dosing:

Bartonella sp infections (bacillary angiomatosis [BA], peliosis hepatis [PH]) (unlabeled use): Oral: 500 mg (base) 4 times/day for 3 months (BA) or 4 months (PH)

Chancroid (unlabeled use): Oral: 500 mg (base) 3 times/day for 7 days; **Note:** Not a preferred agent; isolates with intermediate resistance have been documented (CDC, 2010)

Gastrointestinal prokinetic (unlabeled use): I.V.: 200 mg initially followed by 250 mg (base) orally 3 times/day 30 minutes before meals. Lower dosages have been used in some trials.

Granuloma inguinale (donovanosis) (unlabeled use): Oral: 500 mg (base) 4 times/day for 21 days (CDC, 2010)

Legionnaires' disease: Oral: 1.6-4 g (ethylsuccinate)/day or 1-4 g (base)/day in divided doses for 21 days. **Note:** No longer preferred therapy and only used in nonhospitalized patients.

Lymphogranuloma venereum: Oral: 500 mg (base) 4 times/day for 21 days

Nongonococcal urethritis (including coinfection with *C. trachomatis*): Oral: 500 mg (base) 4 times/day for 7 days or 800 mg (ethylsuccinate) 4 times/day for 7 days. **Note:** May use 250 mg (base) or 400 mg (ethylsuccinate) 4 times/day for 14 days if gastrointestinal intolerance.

Pertussis: Oral: 500 mg (base) every 6 hours for 14 days

Preop bowel preparation: Oral: 1 g erythromycin base at 1, 2, and 11 PM on the day before surgery combined with mechanical cleansing of the large intestine and oral neomycin

Renal Impairment Slightly dialyzable (5% to 20%); supplemental dose is not necessary in hemo- or peritoneal dialysis or in continuous arteriovenous or venovenous hemofiltration.

Administration

Oral: Do not crush enteric coated drug product. GI upset, including diarrhea, is common. May be administered with food to decrease GI upset. Do not give with milk or acidic beverages.

I.V.: Infuse 1 g over 20-60 minutes. I.V. infusion may be very irritating to the vein. If phlebitis/pain occurs with used dilution, consider diluting further (eg, 1:5) if fluid status of the patient will tolerate, or consider administering in larger available vein. The addition of lidocaine or bicarbonate does not decrease the irritation of erythromycin infusions.

Test Interactions False-positive urinary catecholamines, 17-hydroxycorticosteroids and 17-ketosteroids

Special Geriatric Considerations Dose does not need to be adjusted unless there is severe renal or hepatic impairment. Elderly may be at an increased risk for torsade de pointes, ototoxicity (particularly when dose is ≥4 g/day in conjunction with renal or hepatic impairment).

Dosage Forms Excipient information presented when available (limited, particularly for generics); consult specific product labeling.

Capsule, delayed release, enteric coated pellets, oral, as base: 250 mg

Granules for suspension, oral, as ethylsuccinate:

E.E.S.®: Erythromycin activity 200 mg/5 mL (100 mL, 200 mL) [contains sodium 25.9 mg (1.1 mEq)/5 mL; cherry flavor]

Injection, powder for reconstitution, as lactobionate:

Erythrocin® Lactobionate-I.V.: Erythromycin activity 500 mg

Powder, for prescription compounding:
  Erythro-RX: USP: 100% (50 g)
Powder for suspension, oral, as ethylsuccinate:
  EryPed®: Erythromycin activity 200 mg/5 mL (100 mL) [contains sodium 117.5 mg (5.1 mEq)/5 mL; fruit flavor]
  EryPed®: Erythromycin activity 400 mg/5 mL (100 mL) [contains sodium 117.5 mg (5.1 mEq)/5 mL; banana flavor]
Tablet, oral, as base: 250 mg, 500 mg
Tablet, oral, as ethylsuccinate: Erythromycin activity 400 mg
  E.E.S.®: Erythromycin activity 400 mg [contains potassium 10 mg (0.3 mEq)/tablet, sodium 47 mg (2 mEq)/tablet]
Tablet, oral, as stearate:
  Erythrocin®: Erythromycin activity 250 mg [contains potassium 5 mg (0.1 mEq)/tablet, sodium 56.7 mg (2.5 mEq)/tablet]
  Erythrocin®: Erythromycin activity 500 mg [sodium free; contains potassium 7 mg (0.2 mEq)/tablet]
Tablet, delayed release, enteric coated, oral, as base:
  Ery-Tab®: 250 mg [contains sodium 8.3 mg (0.4 mEq)/tablet]
  Ery-Tab®: 333 mg [contains sodium 11.2 mg (0.5 mEq)/tablet]
  Ery-Tab®: 500 mg [contains sodium 16.7 mg (0.7 mEq)/tablet]
Tablet, polymer coated particles, oral, as base:
  PCE®: 333 mg [contains sodium 0.5 mg (0.02mEq)/tablet]
  PCE®: 500 mg [dye free, sodium free]

Erythromycin and Sulfisoxazole (er ith roe MYE sin & sul fi SOKS a zole)

Related Information
  Erythromycin (Systemic) on page 665
Medication Safety Issues
  Sound-alike/look-alike issues:
    Pediazole® may be confused with Pediapred®
Brand Names: U.S. E.S.P.®
Brand Names: Canada Pediazole®
Index Terms Sulfisoxazole and Erythromycin
Generic Availability (U.S.) Yes
Pharmacologic Category Antibiotic, Macrolide; Antibiotic, Macrolide Combination; Antibiotic, Sulfonamide Derivative
Use Treatment of susceptible bacterial infections of the upper and lower respiratory tract and many other infections in patients allergic to penicillin
Contraindications Hypersensitivity to erythromycin, sulfonamides, or any component of the formulation; hepatic dysfunction; porphyria; concurrent use with pimozide or cisapride
Warnings/Precautions Use with caution in patients with impaired renal or hepatic function, myasthenia gravis, G6PD deficiency (hemolysis may occur). Macrolides have been associated with rare QT_c prolongation and ventricular arrhythmias, including torsade de pointes; use with caution in patients at risk of prolonged cardiac repolarization. Chemical similarities are present among sulfonamides, sulfonylureas, carbonic anhydrase inhibitors, thiazides, and loop diuretics (except ethacrynic acid). In patients with allergy to one of these compounds, a risk of cross-reaction exists; avoid use when previous reaction has been severe. Prolonged use may result in fungal or bacterial superinfection, including C. difficile-associated diarrhea (CDAD) and pseudomembranous colitis; CDAD has been observed >2 months postantibiotic treatment.
Adverse Reactions (Reflective of adult population; not specific for elderly) Frequency not defined.
  Cardiovascular: Ventricular arrhythmia,
  Central nervous system: Headache, fever
  Dermatologic: Rash, Stevens-Johnson syndrome, toxic epidermal necrolysis
  Gastrointestinal: Abdominal pain, cramping, nausea, vomiting, oral candidiasis, hypertrophic pyloric stenosis, diarrhea, pseudomembranous colitis
  Hematologic: Agranulocytosis, aplastic anemia, eosinophilia
  Hepatic: Hepatic necrosis, cholestatic jaundice
  Local: Phlebitis at the injection site, thrombophlebitis
  Renal: Toxic nephrosis, crystalluria
  Miscellaneous: Hypersensitivity reactions
Drug Interactions
  Metabolism/Transport Effects Refer to individual components.

Avoid Concomitant Use

Avoid concomitant use of Erythromycin and Sulfisoxazole with any of the following: BCG; Cisapride; Conivaptan; Disopyramide; Highest Risk QTc-Prolonging Agents; Lincosamide Antibiotics; Lovastatin; Methenamine; Mifepristone; Pimozide; Potassium P-Aminobenzoate; Procaine; QuiNINE; Silodosin; Simvastatin; Terfenadine; Tolvaptan; Topotecan

Increased Effect/Toxicity

Erythromycin and Sulfisoxazole may increase the levels/effects of: Alfentanil; Antifungal Agents (Azole Derivatives, Systemic); Antineoplastic Agents (Vinca Alkaloids); ARIPiprazole; Avanafil; Benzodiazepines (metabolized by oxidation); Budesonide (Systemic, Oral Inhalation); BusPIRone; Calcium Channel Blockers; CarBAMazepine; Cardiac Glycosides; Carvedilol; Cilostazol; Cisapride; CloZAPine; Colchicine; Corticosteroids (Systemic); Cyclo-SPORINE; CycloSPORINE (Systemic); CYP2C9 Substrates; CYP3A4 Substrates; Dabigatran Etexilate; Diclofenac; Disopyramide; Eletriptan; Eplerenone; Ergot Derivatives; Everolimus; FentaNYL; Fexofenadine; Fosphenytoin; Highest Risk QTc-Prolonging Agents; HMG-CoA Reductase Inhibitors; Ivacaftor; Lovastatin; Lurasidone; Methotrexate; Moderate Risk QTc-Prolonging Agents; P-glycoprotein/ABCB1 Substrates; Phenytoin; Pimecrolimus; Pimozide; Porfimer; QuiNIDine; QuiNINE; Repaglinide; Rifamycin Derivatives; Rivaroxaban; Salmeterol; Saxagliptin; Selective Serotonin Reuptake Inhibitors; Sildenafil; Silodosin; Simvastatin; Sirolimus; Sulfonylureas; Tacrolimus; Tacrolimus (Systemic); Tacrolimus (Topical); Telaprevir; Temsirolimus; Terfenadine; Theophylline Derivatives; Tolvaptan; Topotecan; Vardenafil; Vitamin K Antagonists; Zopiclone

The levels/effects of Erythromycin and Sulfisoxazole may be increased by: Antifungal Agents (Azole Derivatives, Systemic); Conivaptan; CYP2C9 Inhibitors (Moderate); CYP2C9 Inhibitors (Strong); CYP3A4 Inhibitors (Moderate); CYP3A4 Inhibitors (Strong); Ivacaftor; Methenamine; Mifepristone; P-glycoprotein/ABCB1 Inhibitors; QTc-Prolonging Agents (Indeterminate Risk and Risk Modifying); Telaprevir

Decreased Effect

Erythromycin and Sulfisoxazole may decrease the levels/effects of: BCG; Clopidogrel; CycloSPORINE; CycloSPORINE (Systemic); Ifosfamide; Lincosamide Antibiotics; Typhoid Vaccine; Zafirlukast

The levels/effects of Erythromycin and Sulfisoxazole may be decreased by: CYP2C9 Inducers (Strong); CYP3A4 Inducers (Strong); Deferasirox; Etravirine; Herbs (CYP3A4 Inducers); Peginterferon Alfa-2b; P-glycoprotein/ABCB1 Inducers; Potassium P-Aminobenzoate; Procaine; Tocilizumab

Stability Reconstituted suspension is stable for 14 days when refrigerated.

Mechanism of Action Erythromycin inhibits bacterial protein synthesis; sulfisoxazole competitively inhibits bacterial synthesis of folic acid from para-aminobenzoic acid

Pharmacodynamics/Kinetics See individual agents.

Dosage

Geriatric Not recommended for use in the elderly.

Adult Susceptible infections: Oral (dosage recommendation is based on the product's erythromycin content): 400 mg erythromycin and 1200 mg sulfisoxazole every 6 hours

Renal Impairment Sulfisoxazole must be adjusted in renal impairment.

Cl_{cr} 10-50 mL/minute: Administer every 8-12 hours.

Cl_{cr} <10 mL/minute: Administer every 12-24 hours.

Monitoring Parameters CBC, periodic liver function test

Test Interactions False-positive urinary protein; false-positive urinary catecholamines, 17-hydroxycorticosteroids and 17-ketosteroids

Special Geriatric Considerations

Elderly may be at an increased risk for torsade de pointes, ototoxicity (particularly when dose of erythromycin is ≥4 g/day in conjunction with renal or hepatic impairment).

Dosage Forms Excipient information presented when available (limited, particularly for generics); consult specific product labeling.

Powder for oral suspension: Erythromycin ethylsuccinate 200 mg and sulfisoxazole acetyl 600 mg per 5 mL (100 mL, 150 mL, 200 mL)

E.S.P.®: Erythromycin ethylsuccinate 200 mg and sulfisoxazole acetyl 600 mg per 5 mL (100 mL, 150 mL, 200 mL) [cheri beri flavor]

◆ **Erythromycin Base** *see* Erythromycin (Systemic) *on page 665*

◆ **Erythromycin Ethylsuccinate** *see* Erythromycin (Systemic) *on page 665*

◆ **Erythromycin Lactobionate** *see* Erythromycin (Systemic) *on page 665*

◆ **Erythromycin Stearate** *see* Erythromycin (Systemic) *on page 665*

◆ **Erythropoiesis-Stimulating Agent (ESA)** *see* Darbepoetin Alfa *on page 488*

◆ **Erythropoiesis-Stimulating Agent (ESA)** *see* Epoetin Alfa *on page 651*

◆ **Erythropoiesis-Stimulating Agent (ESA)** *see* Peginesatide *on page 1483*

◆ **Erythropoiesis-Stimulating Protein** *see* Darbepoetin Alfa *on page 488*

◆ **Erythropoietin** *see* Epoetin Alfa *on page 651*
◆ **Erythro-RX** *see* Erythromycin (Systemic) *on page 665*

Escitalopram (es sye TAL oh pram)

Related Information
Antidepressant Agents *on page 2097*
Medication Safety Issues
Sound-alike/look-alike issues:
Lexapro® may be confused with Loxitane®
BEERS Criteria medication:
This drug may be potentially inappropriate for use in geriatric patients (Quality of evidence - moderate; Strength of recommendation - strong).
International issues:
Zavesca: Brand name for escitalopram [in multiple international markets; ISMP April 21, 2010], but also brand name for miglustat [Canada, U.S., and multiple international markets]
Brand Names: U.S. Lexapro®
Brand Names: Canada Cipralex®
Index Terms Escitalopram Oxalate; Lu-26-054; S-Citalopram
Generic Availability (U.S.) Yes
Pharmacologic Category Antidepressant, Selective Serotonin Reuptake Inhibitor
Use Treatment of major depressive disorder; generalized anxiety disorders (GAD)

Canadian labeling: Additional use (not in U.S. labeling): Treatment of obsessive-compulsive disorder (OCD)
Unlabeled Use Treatment of mild dementia-associated agitation in nonpsychotic patients; treatment of vasomotor symptoms associated with menopause
Medication Guide Available Yes
Contraindications Hypersensitivity to escitalopram, citalopram, or any component of the formulation; concomitant use with pimozide; concomitant use or within 2 weeks of MAO inhibitors

Canadian labeling: Additional contraindications (not in U.S. labeling): Known QT-interval prolongation or congenital long QT syndrome
Warnings/Precautions Short-term studies did not show an increased risk in patients >24 years of age and showed a decreased risk in patients ≥65 years. Closely monitor patients for clinical worsening, suicidality, or unusual changes in behavior, particularly during the initial 1-2 months of therapy or during periods of dosage adjustments (increases or decreases); the patient's family or caregiver should be instructed to closely observe the patient and communicate condition with healthcare provider. A medication guide concerning the use of antidepressants should be dispensed with each prescription.

The possibility of a suicide attempt is inherent in major depression and may persist until remission occurs. Use caution in high-risk patients. Worsening depression and severe abrupt suicidality that are not part of the presenting symptoms may require discontinuation or modification of drug therapy. The patient's family or caregiver should be alerted to monitor patients for the emergence of suicidality and associated behaviors (such as agitation, irritability, hostility, impulsivity, and hypomania) and call healthcare provider.

May worsen psychosis in some patients or precipitate a shift to mania or hypomania in patients with bipolar disorder. Patients presenting with depressive symptoms should be screened for bipolar disorder. Monotherapy in patients with bipolar disorder should be avoided. Escitalopram is not FDA approved for the treatment of bipolar depression. Escitalopram is not FDA approved for the treatment of bipolar depression.

Serotonin syndrome and neuroleptic malignant syndrome (NMS)-like reactions have occurred with serotonin/norepinephrine reuptake inhibitors (SNRIs) and selective serotonin reuptake inhibitors (SSRIs) when used alone, and particularly when used in combination with serotonergic agents (eg, triptans) or antidopaminergic agents (eg, antipsychotics). Concurrent use or within 2 weeks of an MAO inhibitor is contraindicated. May increase the risks associated with electroconvulsive therapy. Has a low potential to impair cognitive or motor performance; caution operating hazardous machinery or driving.

Use with caution in patients with a recent history of MI or unstable heart disease. Use has been associated with dose-dependent QT-interval prolongation with doses of 10 mg and 30 mg/day in healthy subjects (mean change from baseline: 4.3 msec and 10.7 msec, respectively); prolongation of QT interval and ventricular arrhythmia (including torsade de pointes) have been reported, particularly in females with pre-existing QT prolongation or other risk factors (eg, hypokalemia, other cardiac disease).

Use caution with a previous seizure disorder or condition predisposing to seizures such as brain damage, alcoholism, or concurrent therapy with other drugs which lower the seizure threshold. May cause hyponatremia/SIADH (elderly at increased risk); volume depletion (diuretics may increase risk) may occur. Use caution in patients with metabolic disease. May cause or exacerbate sexual dysfunction. Use caution in elderly patients; may cause or exacerbate syndrome of inappropriate antidiuretic hormone secretion or hyponatremia; monitor sodium closely with initiation or dosage adjustments in older adults (Beers Criteria). Bioavailability and half-life are increased by 50% in the elderly. Use caution with severe renal impairment or liver impairment; concomitant CNS depressants. Use with caution in patients who are hemodynamically unstable. Use caution with concomitant use of aspirin, NSAIDs, warfarin, or other drugs that affect coagulation; the risk of bleeding may be potentiated.

Upon discontinuation of escitalopram therapy, gradually taper dose. If intolerable symptoms occur following a decrease in dosage or upon discontinuation of therapy, then resuming the previous dose with a more gradual taper should be considered.

Adverse Reactions (Reflective of adult population; not specific for elderly)

>10%:

Central nervous system: Headache (24%), somnolence (4% to 13%), insomnia (7% to 12%)

Gastrointestinal: Diarrhea (6% to 14%), nausea (15% to 18%)

Genitourinary: Ejaculation disorder (9% to 14%)

1% to 10%:

Central nervous system: Fatigue (2% to 8%), dizziness (4% to 7%), abnormal dreaming (3%), lethargy (3%), yawning (2%)

Endocrine & metabolic: Libido decreased (3% to 7%), anorgasmia (2% to 6%), menstrual disorder (2%)

Gastrointestinal: Xerostomia (4% to 9%), constipation (3% to 6%), indigestion (2% to 6%), appetite decreased (3%), vomiting (3%), abdominal pain (2%), flatulence (2%), toothache (2%)

Genitourinary: Impotence (2% to 3%), urinary tract infection (children ≥2%)

Neuromuscular & skeletal: Neck/shoulder pain (3%), back pain (children ≥2%), paresthesia (2%)

Respiratory: Rhinitis (5%), sinusitis (3%), nasal congestion (children ≥2%)

Miscellaneous: Diaphoresis (3% to 8%), flu-like syndrome (5%)

Drug Interactions

Metabolism/Transport Effects Substrate of CYP2C19 (major), CYP3A4 (major); **Note:** Assignment of Major/Minor substrate status based on clinically relevant drug interaction potential; **Inhibits** CYP2D6 (weak)

Avoid Concomitant Use

Avoid concomitant use of Escitalopram with any of the following: Conivaptan; Highest Risk QTc-Prolonging Agents; Iobenguane I 123; MAO Inhibitors; Methylene Blue; Mifepristone; Moderate Risk QTc-Prolonging Agents; Pimozide; Tryptophan

Increased Effect/Toxicity

Escitalopram may increase the levels/effects of: Alpha-/Beta-Blockers; Anticoagulants; Antidepressants (Serotonin Reuptake Inhibitor/Antagonist); Antiplatelet Agents; Aspirin; BusPIRone; CarBAMazepine; CloZAPine; Collagenase (Systemic); Dabigatran Etexilate; Desmopressin; Dextromethorphan; Drotrecogin Alfa (Activated); Highest Risk QTc-Prolonging Agents; Hypoglycemic Agents; Ibritumomab; Lithium; Methadone; Methylene Blue; Metoclopramide; Mexiletine; NSAID (COX-2 Inhibitor); NSAID (Nonselective); Pimozide; RisperiDONE; Rivaroxaban; Salicylates; Serotonin Modulators; Thrombolytic Agents; Tositumomab and Iodine I 131 Tositumomab; TraMADol; Tricyclic Antidepressants; Vitamin K Antagonists

The levels/effects of Escitalopram may be increased by: Alcohol (Ethyl); Analgesics (Opioid); Antipsychotics; BusPIRone; Cimetidine; CNS Depressants; Conivaptan; CYP2C19 Inhibitors (Moderate); CYP2C19 Inhibitors (Strong); CYP3A4 Inhibitors (Moderate); CYP3A4 Inhibitors (Strong); Glucosamine; Herbs (Anticoagulant/Antiplatelet Properties); Ivacaftor; Linezolid; Macrolide Antibiotics; MAO Inhibitors; Metoclopramide; Metyrosine; Mifepristone; Moderate Risk QTc-Prolonging Agents; Omega-3-Acid Ethyl Esters; Omeprazole; Pentosan Polysulfate Sodium; Pentoxifylline; Prostacyclin Analogues; QTc-Prolonging Agents (Indeterminate Risk and Risk Modifying); Tipranavir; TraMADol; Tryptophan; Vitamin E

Decreased Effect

Escitalopram may decrease the levels/effects of: Iobenguane I 123; Ioflupane I 123

The levels/effects of Escitalopram may be decreased by: Boceprevir; CarBAMazepine; CYP2C19 Inducers (Strong); CYP3A4 Inducers (Strong); Cyproheptadine; Deferasirox; NSAID (COX-2 Inhibitor); NSAID (Nonselective); Telaprevir; Tocilizumab

Ethanol/Nutrition/Herb Interactions
Ethanol: May increase CNS depression; monitor for increased effects with coadministration. Caution patients about effects.
Herb/Nutraceutical: Avoid valerian, St John's wort, SAMe, kava kava, and gotu kola (may increase CNS depression).
Stability Store at 25°C (77°F); excursions permitted to 15°C to 30°C (59°F to 86°F).
Mechanism of Action Escitalopram is the S-enantiomer of the racemic derivative citalopram, which selectively inhibits the reuptake of serotonin with little to no effect on norepinephrine or dopamine reuptake. It has no or very low affinity for 5-HT$_{1-7}$, alpha- and beta-adrenergic, D$_{1-5}$, H$_{1-3}$, M$_{1-5}$, and benzodiazepine receptors. Escitalopram does not bind to or has low affinity for Na$^+$, K$^+$, Cl$^-$, and Ca^{++} ion channels.

Pharmacodynamics/Kinetics
Onset of action: Depression: The onset of action is within a week; however, individual response varies greatly and full response may not be seen until 8-12 weeks after initiation of treatment.
Distribution: V$_d$: ~20 L/kg (Søgaard, 2005)
Protein binding: ~56% to plasma proteins
Metabolism: Hepatic via CYP2C19 and 3A4 to S-desmethylcitalopram (S-DCT); S-DCT is metabolized to S-didesmethylcitalopram (S-DDCT) via CYP2D6; *in vitro* data suggest metabolites do not contribute significantly to the antidepressant effects of escitalopram
Half-life elimination: ~27-32 hours (increased ~50% in the elderly and doubled in patients with hepatic impairment)
Time to peak: Escitalopram: ~5 hours
Excretion: Urine (8% as unchanged drug; S-DCT 10%)

Dosage
Geriatric
Major depressive disorder, generalized anxiety disorder: *U.S. labeling:* Oral: 10 mg once daily
Major depressive disorder, generalized anxiety disorder (GAD), obsessive compulsive disorder (OCD): *Canadian labeling:* Oral: Initial: 5 mg once daily; dose may be increased as tolerated to a maximum of 10 mg once daily.
Adult
Major depressive disorder, generalized anxiety disorder: *U.S. labeling:* Oral: Initial: 10 mg once daily; dose may be increased to a maximum of 20 mg once daily after at least 1 week
Major depressive disorder, generalized anxiety disorder (GAD), obsessive compulsive disorder (OCD): *Canadian labeling:* Oral: Initial: 10 mg once daily (may consider 5 mg once daily where sensitivity is a concern); dose may be increased as tolerated to a maximum of 20 mg once daily. Patients with GAD or OCD who require extended therapy should be maintained at the lowest effective dose and assessed periodically to determine the need for continued therapy. **Note:** Initiate treatment in poor CYP2C19 metabolizers at a dose of 5 mg once daily; may increase dose to a maximum of 10 mg once daily.
Vasomotor symptoms associated with menopause (unlabeled use): Initial: 10 mg once daily, increase to 20 mg once daily after 4 weeks if symptoms not adequately controlled (Carpenter, 2012; Freeman, 2011).

Dosage adjustment with concomitant medications: *Canadian labeling:* Escitalopram dose should not exceed 10 mg once daily in patients taking omeprazole or cimetidine.
Renal Impairment
Mild-to-moderate impairment: No dosage adjustment is necessary
Severe impairment: Cl$_{cr}$ <20 mL/minute (U.S. labeling) or Cl$_{cr}$ <30 mL/minute (Canadian labeling): Use with caution.
Hepatic Impairment
U.S. labeling: 10 mg once daily
Canadian labeling:
Mild or moderate impairment (Child-Pugh class A or B): Initial: 5 mg once daily; dose may be increased as tolerated to 10 mg once daily (maximum dose)
Severe Impairment (Child-Pugh class C): No dosage adjustment provided in manufacturer's labeling; has not been studied. Use with caution.
Administration Administer once daily (morning or evening), with or without food.
Monitoring Parameters Mental status for depression, suicidal ideation (especially at the beginning of therapy or when doses are increased or decreased), anxiety, social functioning, mania, panic attacks; akathisia
Pharmacotherapy Pearls The tablet and oral solution dosage forms are bioequivalent. Clinically, escitalopram 20 mg is equipotent to citalopram 40 mg. Do not coadminister with citalopram.

Special Geriatric Considerations Bioavailability and half-life are increased by 50% in the elderly. Clinical trials comparing escitalopram to placebo found no difference in the change in depression scales scores from baseline or relief of symptoms with either treatment. Escitalopram has been shown to delay the time to relapse compared to placebo over 6 months. The elderly are more prone to SSRI/SNRI-induced hyponatremia.

A systematic review and meta-analysis of antidepressant placebo-controlled trials in persons with depression and dementia found evidence "suggestive" of efficacy but not of sufficient strength to "confirm" efficacy. Antidepressant trials in this patient population are small and underpowered. Older patients with depression being treated with an antidepressant should be closely monitored for response and adverse effects. Treatment should be switched or augmented when response is inadequate with a therapeutic dose. Antidepressants that are not tolerated should be discontinued and an alternative agent should be started.

This medication is considered to be potentially inappropriate in this patient population (Beers Criteria: Quality of evidence - moderate; Strength of recommendation - strong).

Dosage Forms Excipient information presented when available (limited, particularly for generics); consult specific product labeling.
Solution, oral: 1 mg/mL (240 mL)
Lexapro®: 1 mg/mL (240 mL) [contains propylene glycol; peppermint flavor]
Tablet, oral: 5 mg, 10 mg, 20 mg
Lexapro®: 5 mg
Lexapro®: 10 mg, 20 mg [scored]

Dosage Forms: Canada Excipient information presented when available (limited, particularly for generics); consult specific product labeling.
Tablet:
Cipralex®: 10 mg, 20 mg

◆ **Escitalopram Oxalate** see Escitalopram on page 670
◆ **Eserine Salicylate** see Physostigmine on page 1533
◆ **Eskalith** see Lithium on page 1150

Esmolol (ES moe lol)

Related Information
Beta-Blockers on page 2108
Medication Safety Issues
Sound-alike/look-alike issues:
Esmolol may be confused with Osmitrol®
Brevibloc® may be confused with Brevital®, Bumex®, Buprenex®
High alert medication:
The Institute for Safe Medication Practices (ISMP) includes this medication among its list of drugs which have a heightened risk of causing significant patient harm when used in error.
Brand Names: U.S. Brevibloc
Brand Names: Canada Brevibloc®; Brevibloc® Premixed
Index Terms Esmolol Hydrochloride
Generic Availability (U.S.) Yes: Excludes infusion
Pharmacologic Category Antiarrhythmic Agent, Class II; Beta-Blocker, Beta-1 Selective
Use Treatment of supraventricular tachycardia (SVT) and atrial fibrillation/flutter (control ventricular rate); treatment of intraoperative and postoperative tachycardia and/or hypertension; treatment of noncompensatory sinus tachycardia
Unlabeled Use Arrhythmia/rate control during acute coronary syndrome (eg, acute myocardial infarction, unstable angina), aortic dissection, intubation, thyroid storm, pheochromocytoma, electroconvulsive therapy
Contraindications Sinus bradycardia; heart block greater than first degree (except in patients with a functioning artificial pacemaker); cardiogenic shock; uncompensated cardiac failure
Warnings/Precautions Consider pre-existing conditions such as sick sinus syndrome before initiating. Hypotension is common; patients need close blood pressure monitoring. Administer cautiously in compensated heart failure and monitor for a worsening of the condition. Can precipitate or aggravate symptoms of arterial insufficiency in patients with PVD and Raynaud's disease. Use with caution and monitor for progression of arterial obstruction. Use caution with concurrent use of digoxin, verapamil or diltiazem; bradycardia or heart block can occur. Use with caution in patients receiving inhaled anesthetic agents known to depress myocardial contractility. Use beta-blockers cautiously in patients with bronchospastic disease; monitor pulmonary status closely. Use cautiously in patients with diabetes because it can mask prominent hypoglycemic symptoms. Bradycardia may be observed more frequently in elderly patients (>65 years of age); dosage reductions may be necessary. May mask signs of hyperthyroidism (eg, tachycardia); if hyperthyroidism is suspected, carefully manage and

monitor; abrupt withdrawal may exacerbate symptoms of hyperthyroidism or precipitate thyroid storm. Use with caution in patients with myasthenia gravis. Use caution in patients with renal dysfunction (active metabolite retained). Adequate alpha-blockade is required prior to use of any beta-blocker for patients with untreated pheochromocytoma. Use caution with history of severe anaphylaxis to allergens; patients taking beta-blockers may become more sensitive to repeated challenges. Treatment of anaphylaxis (eg, epinephrine) in patients taking beta-blockers may be ineffective or promote undesirable effects. Beta-blocker therapy should not be withdrawn abruptly (particularly in patients with CAD), but gradually tapered to avoid acute tachycardia, hypertension, and/or ischemia. Do not use in the treatment of hypertension associated with vasoconstriction related to hypothermia. Extravasation can lead to skin necrosis and sloughing.

Adverse Reactions (Reflective of adult population; not specific for elderly)

>10%:

Cardiovascular: Asymptomatic hypotension (dose related: 25% to 38%), symptomatic hypotension (dose related: 12%)

Miscellaneous: Diaphoresis (10%)

1% to 10%:

Cardiovascular: Peripheral ischemia (1%)

Central nervous system: Dizziness (3%), somnolence (3%), confusion (2%), headache (2%), agitation (2%), fatigue (1%)

Gastrointestinal: Nausea (7%), vomiting (1%)

Local: Pain on injection (8%), infusion site reaction

Drug Interactions

Metabolism/Transport Effects None known.

Avoid Concomitant Use

Avoid concomitant use of Esmolol with any of the following: Floctafenine; Methacholine

Increased Effect/Toxicity

Esmolol may increase the levels/effects of: Alpha-/Beta-Agonists (Direct-Acting); Alpha1-Blockers; Alpha2-Agonists; Amifostine; Antihypertensives; Antipsychotic Agents (Phenothiazines); Bupivacaine; Cardiac Glycosides; Cholinergic Agonists; Fingolimod; Hypotensive Agents; Insulin; Lidocaine; Lidocaine (Systemic); Lidocaine (Topical); Mepivacaine; Methacholine; Midodrine; RiTUXimab; Sulfonylureas

The levels/effects of Esmolol may be increased by: Acetylcholinesterase Inhibitors; Aminoquinolines (Antimalarial); Amiodarone; Anilidopiperidine Opioids; Antipsychotic Agents (Phenothiazines); Calcium Channel Blockers (Dihydropyridine); Calcium Channel Blockers (Nondihydropyridine); Diazoxide; Dipyridamole; Disopyramide; Dronedarone; Floctafenine; Herbs (Hypotensive Properties); MAO Inhibitors; Pentoxifylline; Phosphodiesterase 5 Inhibitors; Propafenone; Prostacyclin Analogues; QuiNIDine; Reserpine

Decreased Effect

Esmolol may decrease the levels/effects of: Beta2-Agonists; Theophylline Derivatives

The levels/effects of Esmolol may be decreased by: Barbiturates; Herbs (Hypertensive Properties); Methylphenidate; Nonsteroidal Anti-Inflammatory Agents; Rifamycin Derivatives; Yohimbine

Stability Clear, colorless to light yellow solution which should be stored at 25°C (77°F); excursions permitted to 15°C to 30°C (59°F to 86°F); do not freeze. Protect from excessive heat.

Stability of parenteral admixture at room temperature (25°C) is 24 hours.

Mechanism of Action Class II antiarrhythmic: Competitively blocks response to beta$_1$-adrenergic stimulation with little or no effect of beta$_2$-receptors except at high doses, no intrinsic sympathomimetic activity, no membrane stabilizing activity

Pharmacodynamics/Kinetics

Onset of action: Beta-blockade: I.V.: 2-10 minutes (quickest when loading doses are administered)

Duration of hemodynamic effects: 10-30 minutes; prolonged following higher cumulative doses, extended duration of use

Distribution: V_d: Esmolol: ~3.4 L/kg; Acid metabolite: ~0.4 L/kg

Protein binding: Esmolol: 55%; Acid metabolite: 10%

Metabolism: In blood by red blood cell esterases; forms acid metabolite (negligible activity; produces no clinically important effects) and methanol (does not achieve concentrations associated with methanol toxicity)

Half-life elimination: Adults: Esmolol: 9 minutes; Acid metabolite: 3.7 hours; elimination of metabolite decreases with end-stage renal disease

Excretion: Urine (~73% to 88% as acid metabolite, <2% unchanged drug)

Dosage

Geriatric & Adult

Intraoperative tachycardia and/or hypertension (immediate control): I.V.: Initial bolus: 80 mg (1 mg/kg) over 30 seconds, followed by a 150 mcg/kg/minute infusion, if necessary. Adjust infusion rate as needed to maintain desired heart rate and/or blood pressure, up to 300 mcg/kg/minute.

For control of postoperative hypertension, as many as one-third of patients may require higher doses (250-300 mcg/kg/minute) to control blood pressure; the safety of doses >300 mcg/kg/minute has not been studied.

Supraventricular tachycardia (SVT), gradual control of postoperative tachycardia/ hypertension: I.V.: Loading dose: 500 mcg/kg over 1 minute; follow with a 50 mcg/kg/ minute infusion for 4 minutes; response to this initial infusion rate may be a rough indication of the responsiveness of the ventricular rate.

Infusion may be continued at 50 mcg/kg/minute or, if the response is inadequate, titrated upward in 50 mcg/kg/minute increments (increased no more frequently than every 4 minutes) to a maximum of 200 mcg/kg/minute.

Note: To achieve more rapid response, following the initial loading dose and 50 mcg/kg/ minute infusion, rebolus with a second 500 mcg/kg loading dose over 1 minute, and increase the maintenance infusion to 100 mcg/kg/minute for 4 minutes. If necessary, a third (and final) 500 mcg/kg loading dose may be administered, prior to increasing to an infusion rate of 150 mcg/kg/minute. After 4 minutes of the 150 mcg/kg/minute infusion, the infusion rate may be increased to a maximum rate of 200 mcg/kg/minute (without a bolus dose).

Acute coronary syndromes (when relative contraindications to beta-blockade exist; unlabeled use): I.V.: 500 mcg/kg over 1 minute; follow with a 50 mcg/kg/minute infusion; if tolerated and response inadequate, may titrate upward in 50 mcg/kg/minute increments every 5-15 minutes to a maximum of 300 mcg/kg/minute (Mitchell, 2002); an additional bolus (500 mcg/kg over 1 minute) may be administered prior to each increase in infusion rate (Mooss, 1994)

Electroconvulsive therapy (unlabeled use): I.V.: 1 mg/kg administered 1 minute prior to induction of anesthesia (Weinger, 1991)

Intubation (unlabeled use): I.V.: 1-2 mg/kg given 1.5-3 minutes prior to intubation (Kindler, 1996)

Thyrotoxicosis or thyroid storm (unlabeled use): I.V.: 50-100 mcg/kg/minute (Bahn, 2011)

Guidelines for transfer to oral therapy (beta-blocker, calcium channel blocker):
Infusion should be reduced by 50% 30 minutes following the first dose of the alternative agent

Manufacturer suggests following the second dose of the alternative drug, patient's response should be monitored and if control is adequate for the first hour, esmolol may be discontinued.

Renal Impairment Not removed by hemo- or peritoneal dialysis. Supplemental dose is not necessary.

Administration Infusions must be administered with an infusion pump. Infusion into small veins or through a butterfly catheter should be avoided (can cause thrombophlebitis). Decrease or discontinue infusion if hypotension or congestive heart failure occur. Medication port of premixed bags should be used to withdraw only the initial bolus, if necessary (not to be used for withdrawal of additional bolus doses).

Monitoring Parameters Blood pressure, MAP, heart rate, continuous ECG, respiratory rate, I.V. site

Special Geriatric Considerations Due to alterations in the beta-adrenergic autonomic nervous system, beta-adrenergic blockade may result in less hemodynamic response than seen in younger adults. Studies indicate that despite decreased sensitivity to the chronotropic effects of beta-blockade with age, there appears to be an increased myocardial sensitivity to the negative inotropic effect during stress (ie, exercise). Controlled trials have shown the overall response rate for propranolol to be only 20% to 50% in elderly populations. Therefore, all beta-adrenergic blocking drugs may result in a decreased response as compared to younger adults.

Dosage Forms Excipient information presented when available (limited, particularly for generics); consult specific product labeling. [DSC] = Discontinued product

Infusion, premixed in NS, as hydrochloride [preservative free]:
Brevibloc: 2000 mg (100 mL) [20 mg/mL; double strength]
Brevibloc: 2500 mg (250 mL) [10 mg/mL]

Injection, solution, as hydrochloride [preservative free]: 10 mg/mL (10 mL)
Brevibloc: 10 mg/mL (10 mL)
Brevibloc: 20 mg/mL (5 mL [DSC]) [double strength]

◆ **Esmolol Hydrochloride** see Esmolol on page 673

Esomeprazole (es oh ME pray zol)

Related Information
H. pylori Treatment in Adult Patients on page 2116
Medication Safety Issues
Sound-alike/look-alike issues:
Esomeprazole may be confused with ARIPiprazole
NexIUM® may be confused with NexAVAR®
Brand Names: U.S. NexIUM®; NexIUM® I.V.
Brand Names: Canada Apo-Esomeprazole®; Nexium®
Index Terms Esomeprazole Magnesium; Esomeprazole Sodium
Generic Availability (U.S.) No
Pharmacologic Category Proton Pump Inhibitor; Substituted Benzimidazole
Use
Oral: Short-term (4-8 weeks) treatment of erosive esophagitis; maintaining symptom resolution and healing of erosive esophagitis; treatment of symptomatic gastroesophageal reflux disease (GERD); as part of a multidrug regimen for *Helicobacter pylori* eradication in patients with duodenal ulcer disease (active or history of within the past 5 years); prevention of gastric ulcers in patients at risk (age ≥60 years and/or history of gastric ulcer) associated with continuous NSAID therapy; long-term treatment of pathological hypersecretory conditions including Zollinger-Ellison syndrome
Canadian labeling: Additional use (not in U.S. labeling): Oral: Treatment of nonerosive reflux disease (NERD)

I.V.: Short-term (≤10 days) treatment of gastroesophageal reflux disease (GERD) when oral therapy is not possible or appropriate
Unlabeled Use I.V.: Prevention of recurrent peptic ulcer bleeding postendoscopy
Contraindications Hypersensitivity to esomeprazole, substituted benzimidazoles (eg, omeprazole, lansoprazole), or any component of the formulation
Warnings/Precautions Use of proton pump inhibitors (PPIs) may increase the risk of gastrointestinal infections (eg, *Salmonella, Campylobacter*). Relief of symptoms does not preclude the presence of a gastric malignancy. Atrophic gastritis (by biopsy) has been noted with long-term omeprazole therapy; this may also occur with esomeprazole. No reports of enterochromaffin-like (ECL) cell carcinoids, dysplasia, or neoplasia have occurred. Severe liver dysfunction may require dosage reductions. Safety and efficacy of I.V. therapy >10 days have not been established; transition from I.V. to oral therapy as soon possible. Bioavailability may be increased in Asian populations, the elderly, and patients with hepatic dysfunction. Decreased *H. pylori* eradication rates have been observed with short-term (≤7 days) combination therapy. The American College of Gastroenterology recommends 10-14 days of therapy (triple or quadruple) for eradication of *H. pylori* (Chey, 2007).

PPIs may diminish the therapeutic effect of clopidogrel, thought to be due to reduced formation of the active metabolite of clopidogrel. The manufacturer of clopidogrel recommends either avoidance of omeprazole or use of a PPI with less potent CYP2C19 inhibition (eg, pantoprazole); avoidance of esomeprazole would appear prudent. Others have recommended the continued use of PPIs, regardless of the degree of inhibition, in patients with a history of GI bleeding or multiple risk factors for GI bleeding who are also receiving clopidogrel since no evidence has established clinically meaningful differences in outcome; however, a clinically-significant interaction cannot be excluded in those who are poor metabolizers of clopidogrel (Abraham, 2010; Levine, 2011). Additionally, concomitant use of esomeprazole with other drugs may require cautious use, may not be recommended, or may require dosage adjustments.

Increased incidence of osteoporosis-related bone fractures of the hip, spine, or wrist may occur with PPI therapy. Patients on high-dose or long-term therapy should be monitored. Use the lowest effective dose for the shortest duration of time, use vitamin D and calcium supplementation, and follow appropriate guidelines to reduce risk of fractures in patients at risk.

Hypomagnesemia, reported rarely, usually with prolonged PPI use of >3 months (most cases >1 year of therapy); may be symptomatic or asymptomatic; severe cases may cause tetany, seizures, and cardiac arrhythmias. Consider obtaining serum magnesium concentrations prior to beginning long-term therapy, especially if taking concomitant digoxin, diuretics, or other drugs known to cause hypomagnesemia; and periodically thereafter. Hypomagnesemia may be corrected by magnesium supplementation, although discontinuation of esomeprazole may be necessary; magnesium levels typically return to normal within 1 week of stopping. Serum chromogranin A levels may be increased if assessed while patient on esomeprazole; may lead to diagnostic errors related to neuroendocrine tumors.

Adverse Reactions (Reflective of adult population; not specific for elderly) Unless otherwise specified, percentages represent adverse reactions identified in clinical trials evaluating the oral formulation.

>10%: Central nervous system: Headache (I.V. 11%; oral ≤8%)

1% to 10%:

Cardiovascular: Hypertension (≤3%), chest pain (>1%)

Central nervous system: Pain (4%), dizziness (oral >1%; I.V. 3%), anxiety (2%), insomnia (2%), pyrexia (2%), fatigue (>1%)

Dermatologic: Rash (>1%), pruritus (I.V. ≤1%)

Endocrine & metabolic: Hypercholesterolemia (2%)

Gastrointestinal: Flatulence (oral ≤5%; I.V. 10%), diarrhea (oral ≤7%; I.V. 4%), abdominal pain (oral ≤6%; I.V. 6%), nausea (oral 5%; I.V. 6%), dyspepsia (oral >1%; I.V. 6%), gastritis (≤6%), constipation (oral 2%; I.V. 3%), vomiting (≤3%), benign GI neoplasm (>1%), dyspepsia (>1%), duodenitis (>1%), epigastric pain (>1%), esophageal disorder (>1%), gastroenteritis (>1%), GI mucosal discoloration (>1%), serum gastrin increased (>1%), xerostomia (1%)

Genitourinary: Urinary tract infection (4%)

Hematologic: Anemia (>1%)

Hepatic: Transaminases increased (>1%)

Local: Injection site reaction (I.V. 2%)

Neuromuscular & skeletal: Arthralgia (3%), back pain (>1%), fracture (>1%), arthropathy (1%), myalgia (1%)

Respiratory: Respiratory infection (oral ≤9%; I.V. 1%), bronchitis (4%), sinusitis (oral ≤4%; I.V. 2%), coughing (>1%), rhinitis (>1%), dyspnea (1%)

Miscellaneous: Accident/injury (≤8%), viral infection (4%), allergy (2%), ear infection (2%), hernia (>1%), flu-like syndrome (1%)

Drug Interactions

Metabolism/Transport Effects Substrate of CYP2C19 (major), CYP3A4 (minor); **Note:** Assignment of Major/Minor substrate status based on clinically relevant drug interaction potential; **Inhibits** CYP2C19 (moderate)

Avoid Concomitant Use

Avoid concomitant use of Esomeprazole with any of the following: Delavirdine; Erlotinib; Nelfinavir; Posaconazole; Rifampin; Rilpivirine; St Johns Wort

Increased Effect/Toxicity

Esomeprazole may increase the levels/effects of: Amphetamines; Benzodiazepines (metabolized by oxidation); Cilostazol; Citalopram; CYP2C19 Substrates; Dexmethylphenidate; Methotrexate; Methylphenidate; Raltegravir; Saquinavir; Tacrolimus; Tacrolimus (Systemic); Vitamin K Antagonists; Voriconazole

The levels/effects of Esomeprazole may be increased by: Fluconazole; Ketoconazole; Ketoconazole (Systemic)

Decreased Effect

Esomeprazole may decrease the levels/effects of: Atazanavir; Bisphosphonate Derivatives; Cefditoren; Clopidogrel; Dabigatran Etexilate; Dasatinib; Delavirdine; Erlotinib; Gefitinib; Indinavir; Iron Salts; Itraconazole; Ketoconazole; Ketoconazole (Systemic); Mesalamine; Mycophenolate; Nelfinavir; Nilotinib; Posaconazole; Rilpivirine; Vismodegib

The levels/effects of Esomeprazole may be decreased by: CYP2C19 Inducers (Strong); Rifampin; St Johns Wort; Tipranavir; Tocilizumab

Ethanol/Nutrition/Herb Interactions

Food: Absorption is decreased by 43% to 53% when taken with food. Management: Take at least 1 hour before meals at the same time each day, best if before breakfast.

Herb/Nutraceutical: St John's wort may decrease the efficacy of esomeprazole. Management: Avoid St John's wort.

Stability

Capsule, granules: Store at 15°C to 30°C (59°F to 86°F). Keep container tightly closed.

Powder for injection: Store at 25°C (77°F); excursions permitted to 15°C to 30°C (59°F to 86°F). Protect from light.

For I.V. injection: Adults: Reconstitute powder with 5 mL NS.

For I.V. infusion: Adults: Initially reconstitute powder with 5 mL of NS, LR, or D_5W, then further dilute to a final volume of 50 mL.

Per the manufacturer, following reconstitution, solution for injection prepared in NS, and solution for infusion prepared in NS or LR should be used within 12 hours. Following reconstitution, solution for infusion prepared in D_5W should be used within 6 hours. Refrigeration is not required following reconstitution.

Additional stability data: Following reconstitution, solutions for infusion prepared in D_5W, NS, or LR in PVC bags are chemically and physically stable for 48 hours at room temperature (25°C) and for at least 120 hours under refrigeration (4°C) (Kupiec, 2008).

Mechanism of Action Proton pump inhibitor suppresses gastric acid secretion by inhibition of the H^+/K^+-ATPase in the gastric parietal cell. Esomeprazole is the S-isomer of omeprazole.

Pharmacodynamics/Kinetics

Distribution: V_{dss}: 16 L

Protein binding: 97%

Metabolism: Hepatic via CYP2C19 primarily and (to a lesser extent) via 3A4 to hydroxy, desmethyl, and sulfone metabolites (all inactive)

Bioavailability: Oral: 90% with repeat dosing

Half-life elimination: ~1-1.5 hours

Time to peak: Oral: 1.5-2 hours

Excretion: Urine (80%, primarily as inactive metabolites; <1% as active drug); feces (20%)

Dosage

Geriatric Refer to adult dosing. No dosage adjustment needed.

Adult

Erosive esophagitis (healing): Oral: Initial: 20-40 mg once daily for 4-8 weeks; if incomplete healing, may continue for an additional 4-8 weeks; maintenance: 20 mg once daily (controlled studies did not extend beyond 6 months)

Nonerosive reflux disease (NERD) (Canadian labeling): Initial: 20 mg once daily for 2-4 weeks; lack of symptom control after 4 weeks warrants further evaluation; maintenance (in patients with successful initial therapy): 20 mg once daily as needed

Symptomatic gastroesophageal reflux: Oral: 20 mg once daily for 4 weeks; may consider an additional 4 weeks of treatment if symptoms do not resolve

Treatment of GERD (short-term): I.V.: 20 mg or 40 mg once daily. **Note:** Indicated only in cases where oral therapy is inappropriate or not possible;safety/efficacy ≥10 days has not been established.

Prevention of recurrent peptic ulcer bleeding postendoscopy (unlabeled use; Sung, 2009): I.V. 80 mg over 30 minutes, followed by 8 mg/hour infusion for 72 hours, then 40 mg *orally* once daily for 27 additional days

Helicobacter pylori **eradication:** Oral:

Manufacturer's labeling: 40 mg once daily administered with amoxicillin 1000 mg *and* clarithromycin 500 mg twice daily for 10 days

American College of Gastroenterology guidelines (Chey, 2007):

Nonpenicillin allergy: 40 mg once daily administered with amoxicillin 1000 mg *and* clarithromycin 500 mg twice daily for 10-14 days

Penicillin allergy: 40 mg once daily administered with clarithromycin 500 mg *and* metronidazole 500 mg twice daily for 10-14 days **or** 40 mg once daily administered with bismuth subsalicylate 525 mg *and* metronidazole 250 mg *plus* tetracycline 500 mg 4 times/day for 10-14 days

Canadian labeling: 20 mg twice daily for 7 days; requires combination therapy

Prevention of NSAID-induced gastric ulcers: 20-40 mg once daily for up to 6 months

Treatment of NSAID-induced gastric ulcers (Canadian labeling): 20 mg once daily for 4-8 weeks.

Pathological hypersecretory conditions (Zollinger-Ellison syndrome): 40 mg twice daily; adjust regimen to individual patient needs; doses up to 240 mg/day have been administered

Renal Impairment No dosage adjustment necessary.

Hepatic Impairment

Mild-to-moderate hepatic impairment (Child-Pugh class A or B): No dosage adjustment needed.

Severe hepatic impairment (Child-Pugh class C): Dose should not exceed 20 mg/day.

Administration

Oral:

Capsule: Should be swallowed whole and taken at least 1 hour before eating (best if taken before breakfast). Capsule can be opened and contents mixed with 1 tablespoon of applesauce. Swallow immediately; mixture should not be chewed or warmed. For patients with difficulty swallowing, use of granules may be more appropriate.

Granules: Empty the 2.5 mg or 5 mg packet into a container with 5 mL of water or the 10 mg, 20 mg, or 40 mg packet into a container with 15 mL of water and stir; leave 2-3 minutes to thicken. Stir and drink within 30 minutes. If any medicine remains after drinking, add more water, stir and drink immediately.

Tablet (Canadian formulation, not available in U.S.): Swallow whole or may be dispersed in a half a glass of noncarbonated water. Stir until tablets disintegrate, leaving a liquid containing pellets. Drink contents within 30 minutes. Do not chew or crush pellets. After drinking, rinse glass with water and drink.

I.V.: Flush line prior to and after administration with NS, LR, or D_5W: Adults: May be administered by injection (≥3 minutes), intermittent infusion (10-30 minutes), or continuous infusion for up to 72 hours (Sung, 2009).

Nasogastric tube:

Capsule: Open capsule and place intact granules into a 60 mL catheter-tip syringe; mix with 50 mL of water. Replace plunger and shake vigorously for 15 seconds. Ensure that no granules remain in syringe tip. Do not administer if pellets dissolve or disintegrate. Use immediately after preparation. After administration, flush nasogastric tube with additional water.

Granules: Delayed release oral suspension granules can also be given by nasogastric or gastric tube. If using a 2.5 mg or 5 mg packet, first add 5 mL of water to a catheter-tipped syringe, then add granules from packet. If using a 10 mg, 20 mg, or 40 mg packet, first add 15 mL of water to a catheter-tipped syringe, then add granules from packet. Shake the syringe, leave 2-3 minutes to thicken. Shake the syringe and administer through naso-gastric or gastric tube (size 6 French or greater) within 30 minutes. Refill the syringe with equal amount (5 mL or 15 mL) of water, shake and flush nasogastric/gastric tube.

Tablet (Canadian formulation, not available in U.S.): Disperse tablets in 50 mL of non-carbonated water. Stir until tablets disintegrate leaving a liquid containing pellets. After administration, flush with additional 25-50 mL of water to clear the syringe and tube.

Monitoring Parameters Susceptibility testing recommended in patients who fail *H. pylori* eradication regimen. Monitor for rebleeding in patients with peptic ulcer bleed.

Test Interactions Esomeprazole may falsely elevate serum chromogranin A (CgA) levels. The increased CgA level may cause false-positive results in the diagnosis of a neuro-endocrine tumor. Temporarily stop esomeprazole if assessing CgA level; repeat level if initially elevated; use the same laboratory for all testing of CgA levels.

Special Geriatric Considerations Dose adjustment is not necessary.

An increased risk of fractures of the hip, spine, or wrist has been observed in epidemiologic studies with proton pump inhibitor (PPI) use, primarily in older adults ≥50 years of age. The greatest risk was seen in patients receiving high doses or on long-term therapy (≥1 year). Calcium and vitamin D supplementation and close monitoring are recommended to reduce the risk of fracture in high-risk patients. Additionally, long-term use of proton pump inhibitors has resulted in reports of hypomagnesemia and *Clostridium difficile* infections.

Dosage Forms Excipient information presented when available (limited, particularly for generics); consult specific product labeling.

Capsule, delayed release, oral, as magnesium [strength expressed as base]:
NexIUM®: 20 mg, 40 mg

Granules for suspension, delayed release, oral, as magnesium [strength expressed as base]:
NexIUM®: 10 mg/packet (30s); 20 mg/packet (30s); 40 mg/packet (30s)

Injection, powder for reconstitution, as sodium [strength expressed as base]:
NexIUM® I.V.: 20 mg, 40 mg [contains edetate disodium]

Dosage Forms: Canada Excipient information presented when available (limited, particularly for generics); consult specific product labeling.

Note: Strength expressed as base

Granules, for oral suspension, delayed release, as magnesium:
Nexium®: 10 mg/packet (28s)

Tablet, extended release, as magnesium:
Nexium®: 20 mg, 40 mg

♦ **Esomeprazole and Naproxen** *see* Naproxen and Esomeprazole *on page 1342*
♦ **Esomeprazole Magnesium** *see* Esomeprazole *on page 676*
♦ **Esomeprazole Sodium** *see* Esomeprazole *on page 676*
♦ **E.S.P.®** *see* Erythromycin and Sulfisoxazole *on page 668*

Estazolam (es TA zoe lam)

Related Information

Anxiolytic, Sedative/Hypnotic, and Miscellaneous Benzodiazepines *on page 2106*
Beers Criteria – Potentially Inappropriate Medications for Geriatrics *on page 2183*

Medication Safety Issues

Sound-alike/look-alike issues:

ProSom® may be confused with PhosLo®, Proscar®, PROzac®, Psorcon®

BEERS Criteria medication:

This drug may be potentially inappropriate for use in geriatric patients (Quality of evidence - high; Strength of recommendation - strong).

Index Terms ProSom

Generic Availability (U.S.) Yes

Pharmacologic Category Benzodiazepine

ESTAZOLAM

◄ **Use** Short-term management of insomnia

Contraindications Hypersensitivity to estazolam or any component of the formulation (cross-sensitivity with other benzodiazepines may exist)

Note: Manufacturer states concurrent therapy with itraconazole or ketoconazole is contraindicated.

Warnings/Precautions As a hypnotic, should be used only after evaluation of potential causes of sleep disturbance. Failure of sleep disturbance to resolve after 7-10 days may indicate psychiatric or medical illness. Use is not recommended in patients with depressive disorders or psychoses. Avoid use in patients with sleep apnea. Postmarketing studies have indicated that the use of hypnotic/sedative agents for sleep has been associated with hypersensitivity reactions including anaphylaxis as well as angioedema. An increased risk for hazardous sleep-related activities such as sleep-driving; cooking and eating food, and making phone calls while asleep have also been noted. Use with caution in patients receiving concurrent CYP3A4 inhibitors, particularly when these agents are added to therapy. Use with caution in elderly or debilitated patients, patients with hepatic disease (including alcoholics), renal impairment, respiratory disease, impaired gag reflex, or obese patients. Rebound or withdrawal symptoms may occur following abrupt discontinuation or large decreases in dose. Use caution when reducing dose or withdrawing therapy; decrease slowly and monitor for withdrawal symptoms.

Causes CNS depression (dose related) which may impair physical and mental capabilities. Use with caution in patients receiving other CNS depressants or psychoactive agents. Benzodiazepines have been associated with falls and traumatic injury and should be used with extreme caution in patients who are at risk of these events. In older adults, benzodiazepines increase the risk of impaired cognition, delirium, falls, fractures, and motor vehicle accidents. Due to increased sensitivity in this age group, avoid use for treatment of insomnia, agitation, or delirium (Beers Criteria). May cause physical or psychological dependence - use with caution in patients with a history of drug dependence.

Benzodiazepines have been associated with anterograde amnesia. Paradoxical reactions, including hyperactive or aggressive behavior, have been reported with benzodiazepines, particularly in psychiatric patients. Does not have analgesic, antidepressant, or antipsychotic properties.

Adverse Reactions (Reflective of adult population; not specific for elderly)

>10%:
  Central nervous system: Somnolence
  Neuromuscular & skeletal: Weakness

1% to 10%:
  Cardiovascular: Flushing, palpitation
  Central nervous system: Anxiety, confusion, dizziness, hypokinesia, abnormal coordination, hangover effect, agitation, amnesia, apathy, emotional lability, euphoria, hostility, seizure, sleep disorder, stupor, twitch
  Dermatologic: Dermatitis, pruritus, rash, urticaria
  Gastrointestinal: Xerostomia, constipation, appetite increased/decreased, flatulence, gastritis, perverse taste
  Genitourinary: Frequent urination, menstrual cramps, urinary hesitancy, urinary frequency, vaginal discharge/itching
  Neuromuscular & skeletal: Paresthesia
  Ocular: Photophobia, eye pain, eye swelling
  Respiratory: Cough, dyspnea, asthma, rhinitis, sinusitis
  Miscellaneous: Diaphoresis

Drug Interactions

Metabolism/Transport Effects Substrate of CYP3A4 (minor); **Note:** Assignment of Major/Minor substrate status based on clinically relevant drug interaction potential

Avoid Concomitant Use
  Avoid concomitant use of Estazolam with any of the following: Azelastine; Azelastine (Nasal); Methadone; Mirtazapine; OLANZapine; Paraldehyde

Increased Effect/Toxicity
  Estazolam may increase the levels/effects of: Alcohol (Ethyl); Azelastine; Azelastine (Nasal); Buprenorphine; CloZAPine; CNS Depressants; Fosphenytoin; Methadone; Methotrimeprazine; Metyrosine; Mirtazapine; Paraldehyde; Phenytoin; Selective Serotonin Reuptake Inhibitors; Zolpidem

  The levels/effects of Estazolam may be increased by: Antifungal Agents (Azole Derivatives, Systemic); Aprepitant; Calcium Channel Blockers (Nondihydropyridine); Cimetidine; Contraceptives (Estrogens); Contraceptives (Progestins); Droperidol; Fosaprepitant; Grapefruit Juice; HydrOXYzine; Isoniazid; Macrolide Antibiotics; Methotrimeprazine; OLANZapine; Proton Pump Inhibitors; Ritonavir; Selective Serotonin Reuptake Inhibitors

Decreased Effect

The levels/effects of Estazolam may be decreased by: CarBAMazepine; Rifamycin Derivatives; St Johns Wort; Theophylline Derivatives; Tocilizumab; Yohimbine

Ethanol/Nutrition/Herb Interactions

Ethanol: May increase CNS depression; monitor for increased effects with coadministration. Caution patients about effects.

Food: Serum levels and/or toxicity may be increased by grapefruit juice.

Mechanism of Action Binds to stereospecific benzodiazepine receptors on the postsynaptic GABA neuron at several sites within the central nervous system, including the limbic system, reticular formation. Enhancement of the inhibitory effect of GABA on neuronal excitability results by increased neuronal membrane permeability to chloride ions. This shift in chloride ions results in hyperpolarization (a less excitable state) and stabilization.

Pharmacodynamics/Kinetics

Onset of action: ~1 hour

Duration: Variable

Metabolism: Extensively hepatic

Half-life elimination: 10-24 hours (no significant changes in elderly)

Time to peak, serum: 0.5-1.6 hours

Excretion: Urine (<5% as unchanged drug)

Dosage

Geriatric Start at doses of 0.5 mg in small elderly patients.

Adult Insomnia: Oral: 1 mg at bedtime, some patients may require 2 mg; start at doses of 0.5 mg in debilitated patients.

Hepatic Impairment Adjustment may be necessary.

Monitoring Parameters Respiratory and cardiovascular status

Pharmacotherapy Pearls Abrupt discontinuation after sustained use (generally >10 days) may cause withdrawal symptoms.

Special Geriatric Considerations Because of its lack of active metabolites, estazolam could be considered for elderly patients when a benzodiazepine hypnotic is indicated.

This medication is considered to be potentially inappropriate in this patient population (Beers Criteria: Quality of evidence - high; Strength of recommendation - strong).

Controlled Substance C-IV

Dosage Forms Excipient information presented when available (limited, particularly for generics); consult specific product labeling.

Tablet, oral: 1 mg, 2 mg

◆ **Ester-E™ [OTC]** *see* Vitamin E *on page 2027*
◆ **Esterified Estrogens** *see* Estrogens (Esterified) *on page 714*
◆ **Estrace®** *see* Estradiol (Systemic) *on page 681*
◆ **Estrace®** *see* Estradiol (Topical) *on page 689*
◆ **Estradiol** *see* Estradiol (Systemic) *on page 681*
◆ **17β-estradiol** *see* Estradiol (Topical) *on page 689*

Estradiol (Systemic) (es tra DYE ole)

Related Information

Beers Criteria – Potentially Inappropriate Medications for Geriatrics *on page 2183*

Medication Safety Issues

Sound-alike/look-alike issues:

Alora® may be confused with Aldara®

Elestrin® may be confused with alosetron

BEERS Criteria medication:

This drug may be potentially inappropriate for use in geriatric patients (Quality of evidence - high [oral and transdermal patch]; Strength of recommendation - strong [oral and transdermal patch]).

Other safety issues:

Transdermal patch may contain conducting metal (eg, aluminum); remove patch prior to MRI.

International issues:

Vivelle: Brand name for estradiol [U.S. and multiple international markets, but also the brand name for ethinyl estradiol and norgestimate [Austria]

Brand Names: U.S. Alora®; Climara®; Delestrogen®; Depo®-Estradiol; Divigel®; Elestrin®; Estrace®; Estrasorb®; EstroGel®; Evamist®; Femring®; Femtrace®; Menostar®; Vivelle-Dot®

◄

Brand Names: Canada Climara®; Depo®-Estradiol; Estraderm®; Estradot®; EstroGel®; Menostar®; Oesclim®; Sandoz-Estradiol Derm 100; Sandoz-Estradiol Derm 50; Sandoz-Estradiol Derm 75

Index Terms Estradiol; Estradiol Acetate; Estradiol Transdermal; Estradiol Valerate

Generic Availability (U.S.) Yes: Oral tablet, patch, valerate oil for injection

Pharmacologic Category Estrogen Derivative

Use Treatment of moderate-to-severe vasomotor symptoms associated with menopause; treatment of moderate-to-severe vulvar and vaginal atrophy associated with menopause; hypoestrogenism (due to hypogonadism, castration, or primary ovarian failure); advanced prostatic cancer (palliation); metastatic breast cancer (palliation) in men and postmenopausal women; postmenopausal osteoporosis (prophylaxis)

Contraindications Angioedema or anaphylactic reaction to estradiol or any component of the formulation; undiagnosed abnormal vaginal bleeding; DVT or PE (current or history of); active or history of arterial thromboembolic disease (eg, stroke, MI); carcinoma of the breast (known, suspected or history of), except in appropriately selected patients being treated for metastatic disease; estrogen-dependent tumor; hepatic dysfunction or disease; known protein C, protein S, antithrombin deficiency or other known thrombophilic disorders

Warnings/Precautions [U.S. Boxed Warning]: The use of unopposed estrogen in women with an intact uterus is associated with an increased risk of endometrial cancer. The addition of a progestin to estrogen therapy may decrease the risk of endometrial hyperplasia, a precursor to endometrial cancer. The use of a progestin is not generally required when low doses of estrogen are used locally for vaginal atrophy (NAMS, 2012). **Adequate diagnostic measures, including endometrial sampling if indicated, should be performed to rule out malignancy in postmenopausal women with undiagnosed abnormal vaginal bleeding.** Estrogens may exacerbate endometriosis. Malignant transformation of residual endometrial implants has been reported posthysterectomy with unopposed estrogen therapy. Consider adding a progestin in women with residual endometriosis posthysterectomy. Postmenopausal estrogen therapy and combined estrogen/progesterone therapy may increase the risk of ovarian cancer; however, the absolute risk to an individual woman is small. Although results from various studies are not consistent, risk does not appear to be significantly associated with the duration, route, or dose of therapy. In one study, the risk decreased after 2 years following discontinuation of therapy (Mørch, 2009). Although the risk of ovarian cancer is rare, women who are at an increased risk (eg, family history) should be counseled about the association (NAMS, 2012). **[U.S. Boxed Warning]: Based on data from the Women's Health Initiative (WHI) studies, an increased risk of invasive breast cancer was observed in postmenopausal women using conjugated estrogens (CE) in combination with medroxyprogesterone acetate (MPA).** This risk may be associated with duration of use and declines once combined therapy is discontinued (Chlebowski, 2009). The risk of invasive breast cancer was decreased in postmenopausal women with a hysterectomy using CE only, regardless of weight. However, the risk was not significantly decreased in women at high risk for breast cancer (family history of breast cancer, personal history of benign breast disease) (Anderson, 2012). An increase in abnormal mammogram findings has also been reported with estrogen alone or in combination with progestin therapy. Estrogen use may lead to severe hypercalcemia in patients with breast cancer and bone metastases; discontinue estrogen if hypercalcemia occurs.

[U.S. Boxed Warning]: Estrogens with or without progestin should not be used to prevent coronary heart disease. Using data from the Women's Health Initiative (WHI) studies, an increased risk of deep vein thrombosis (DVT) and stroke has been reported with CE and an increased risk of DVT, stroke, pulmonary emboli (PE) and myocardial infarction (MI) has been reported with CE with MPA in postmenopausal women. Additional risk factors include diabetes mellitus, hypercholesterolemia, hypertension, SLE, obesity, tobacco use, and/or history of venous thromboembolism (VTE). Adverse cardiovascular events have also been reported in males taking estrogens for prostate cancer. Risk factors should be managed appropriately; discontinue use if adverse cardiovascular events occur or are suspected. Women with inherited thrombophilias (eg, protein C or S deficiency) may have increased risk of venous thromboembolism (DeSancho, 2010; van Vlijmen, 2011). Use is contraindicated in women with protein C, protein S, antithrombin deficiency or other known thrombophilic disorders.

[U.S. Boxed Warning]: Estrogens with or without progestin should not be used to prevent dementia. In the Women's Health Initiative Memory Study (WHIMS), an increased incidence of dementia was observed in women ≥65 years of age taking CE alone or in combination with MPA.

[U.S. Boxed Warning]: Estrogens with or without progestin should be used for the shortest duration possible at the lowest effective dose consistent with treatment goals. Before prescribing estrogen therapy to postmenopausal women, the risks and benefits must be weighed for each patient. Women should be informed of these risks and benefits, as well as possible effects of progestin when added to estrogen therapy. Patients should be reevaluated as clinically appropriate to determine if treatment is still necessary. Available data related to treatment risks are from Women's Health Initiative (WHI) studies, which evaluated oral CE 0.625 mg with or without MPA 2.5 mg relative to placebo in postmenopausal women. Other combinations and dosage forms of estrogens and progestins were not studied. **Outcomes reported from clinical trials using CE with or without MPA should be assumed to be similar for other doses and other dosage forms of estrogens and progestins until comparable data becomes available.**

Estrogen compounds are generally associated with lipid effects such as increased HDL-cholesterol and decreased LDL-cholesterol. Triglycerides may also be increased; use with caution in patients with familial defects of lipoprotein metabolism. Estrogens may increase thyroid-binding globulin (TBG) levels leading to increased circulating total thyroid hormone levels. Women on thyroid replacement therapy may require higher doses of thyroid hormone while receiving estrogens.

Estrogens may cause retinal vascular thrombosis; discontinue if migraine, loss of vision, proptosis, diplopia, or other visual disturbances occur; discontinue permanently if papilledema or retinal vascular lesions are observed on examination. Estrogens are poorly metabolized in patients with hepatic dysfunction. Use caution in patients with a history of cholestatic jaundice associated with prior estrogen use or pregnancy. Discontinue if jaundice develops or if acute or chronic hepatic disturbances occur. Use is contraindicated with hepatic disease. Use caution in patients with asthma, epilepsy, hepatic hemangiomas, migraine, porphyria, or SLE; may exacerbate disease. May have adverse effects on glucose tolerance; use caution in women with diabetes. Use with caution in patients with diseases which may be exacerbated by fluid retention, including cardiac or renal dysfunction. Use of postmenopausal estrogen may be associated with an increased risk of gallbladder disease requiring surgery. Use with caution in patients with severe hypocalcemia. In the elderly, avoid oral and transdermal patch estrogen products (with or without progestins) due to potential of increased risk of breast and endometrial cancers, and lack of proven cardioprotection and cognitive protection (Beers Criteria). Prior to puberty, estrogens may cause premature closure of the epiphyses, premature breast development in girls or gynecomastia in boys. Vaginal bleeding and vaginal cornification may also be induced in girls. Whenever possible, estrogens should be discontinued at least 4-6 weeks prior to elective surgery associated with an increased risk of thromboembolism or during periods of prolonged immobilization. May exacerbate angioedema symptoms in women with hereditary angioedema. The use of estrogens and/or progestins may change the results of some laboratory tests (eg, coagulation factors, lipids, glucose tolerance, binding proteins). The dose, route, and the specific estrogen/progestin influences these changes. In addition, personal risk factors (eg, cardiovascular disease, smoking, diabetes, age) also contribute to adverse events; use of specific products may be contraindicated in women with certain risk factors.

Estradiol may be transferred to another person following skin-to-skin contact with the application site. **[U.S. Boxed Warning]: Breast budding and breast masses in prepubertal females and gynecomastia and breast masses in prepubertal males have been reported following unintentional contact with application sites of women using topical estradiol (Evamist®). Patients should strictly adhere to instructions for use in order to prevent secondary exposure. In most cases, conditions resolved with removal of estradiol exposure.** If unexpected changes in sexual development occur in prepubertal children, the possibility of unintentional estradiol exposure should be evaluated by a healthcare provider. Discontinue if conditions for the safe use of the topical spray cannot be met.

Some products may contain chlorobutanol (a chloral derivative) as a preservative, which may be habit forming; some products may contain tartrazine.

Topical emulsion, gel, spray: Absorption of the topical emulsion (Estrasorb®) and topical gel (Elestrin®) is increased by application of sunscreen; do not apply sunscreen within close proximity of estradiol. When sunscreen is applied ~1 hour prior to the topical spray (Evamist®), no change in absorption was observed (estradiol absorption was decreased when sunscreen is applied 1 hour after Evamist®). Application of Divigel® or EstroGel® with sunscreen has not been evaluated.

Transdermal patch: May contain conducting metal (eg, aluminum); remove patch prior to MRI.

Vaginal ring: Use may not be appropriate in women with narrow vagina, vaginal stenosis, vaginal infections, cervical prolapse, rectoceles, cystoceles, or other conditions which may increase the risk of vaginal irritation, ulceration, or increase the risk of expulsion. Ring should be removed in case of ulceration, erosion, or adherence to vaginal wall; do not reinsert until healing is complete. Ensure proper vaginal placement of the ring to avoid inadvertent urinary bladder insertion.

◀ Osteoporosis: For use only in women at significant risk of osteoporosis and for who other nonestrogen medications are not considered appropriate.

Vulvar and vaginal atrophy: When used solely for the treatment of vulvar and vaginal atrophy, topical vaginal products should be considered. Use caution applying topical products to severely atrophic vaginal mucosa. Use of a progestin is normally not required when low-dose estrogen is applied locally and only for this purpose (NAMS, 2007).

Adverse Reactions (Reflective of adult population; not specific for elderly) Frequency not defined. Some adverse reactions observed with estrogen and/or progestin combination therapy.

Cardiovascular: Chest pain, DVT, edema, hypertension, MI, stroke, syncope, TIA, vasodilation, venous thromboembolism

Central nervous system: Anxiety, dementia, dizziness, epilepsy exacerbation, headache, insomnia, irritability, mental depression, migraine, mood disturbances, nervousness

Dermatologic: Angioedema, chloasma, dermatitis, erythema multiforme, erythema nodosum, hemorrhagic eruption, hirsutism, loss of scalp hair, melasma, rash, pruritus, urticaria

Endocrine & metabolic: Breast cancer, breast enlargement, breast pain, breast tenderness, carbohydrate intolerance, fibrocystic breast changes, fluid retention, galactorrhea, hot flashes, hypocalcemia, libido changes, nipple discharge, nipple pain

Gastrointestinal: Abdominal cramps, abdominal pain, bloating, cholecystitis, cholelithiasis, constipation, diarrhea, dyspepsia, flatulence, gallbladder disease, gastritis, nausea, pancreatitis, vomiting, weight gain/loss

Genitourinary: Alterations in frequency and flow of bleeding patterns, breakthrough bleeding, cervical ectropion changes, cervical secretion changes, cystitis, dysmenorrhea, endometrial cancer, endometrial hyperplasia, genital eruption, menorrhagia, metrorrhagia, ovarian cancer, ovarian cyst, Pap smear suspicious, spotting, uterine leiomyomata size increased, leukorrhea, uterine cancer, uterine enlargement, uterine pain, urinary incontinence, urogenital pruritus, vaginal candidiasis, vaginal discharge, vaginal moniliasis, vaginitis

Hematologic: Aggravation of porphyria

Hepatic: Cholestatic jaundice, hepatic hemangioma enlargement

Local: Thrombophlebitis

Gel, spray: Application site reaction

Transdermal patches: Erythema, irritation

Neuromuscular & skeletal: Arthralgia, back pain, chorea, leg cramps, myalgia, muscle cramps, skeletal pain, weakness

Ocular: Blindness, contact lens intolerance, corneal curvature steepening, retinal vascular thrombosis

Respiratory: Asthma exacerbation, pulmonary thromboembolism

Miscellaneous: Anaphylactoid/anaphylactic reactions, hypersensitivity reactions

Drug Interactions

Metabolism/Transport Effects Substrate of CYP1A2 (major), CYP2A6 (minor), CYP2B6 (minor), CYP2C19 (minor), CYP2C9 (minor), CYP2D6 (minor), CYP2E1 (minor), CYP3A4 (major), P-glycoprotein; **Note:** Assignment of Major/Minor substrate status based on clinically relevant drug interaction potential; **Inhibits** CYP1A2 (weak), CYP2C8 (weak); **Induces** CYP3A4 (weak/moderate)

Avoid Concomitant Use

Avoid concomitant use of Estradiol (Systemic) with any of the following: Anastrozole; Axitinib

Increased Effect/Toxicity

Estradiol (Systemic) may increase the levels/effects of: Corticosteroids (Systemic); ROPINIRole; Tipranavir

The levels/effects of Estradiol (Systemic) may be increased by: Ascorbic Acid; Herbs (Estrogenic Properties); P-glycoprotein/ABCB1 Inhibitors

Decreased Effect

Estradiol (Systemic) may decrease the levels/effects of: Anastrozole; ARIPiprazole; Axitinib; Chenodiol; Hyaluronidase; Saxagliptin; Somatropin; Thyroid Products; Ursodiol

The levels/effects of Estradiol (Systemic) may be decreased by: CYP1A2 Inducers (Strong); CYP3A4 Inducers (Strong); Cyproterone; Deferasirox; Herbs (CYP3A4 Inducers); Peginterferon Alfa-2b; P-glycoprotein/ABCB1 Inducers; Tipranavir; Tocilizumab

Ethanol/Nutrition/Herb Interactions

Ethanol: Avoid ethanol (routine use increases estrogen level and risk of breast cancer). Ethanol may also increase the risk of osteoporosis.

Food: Folic acid absorption may be decreased

Herb/Nutraceutical: St John's wort may decrease levels. Herbs with estrogenic properties may enhance the adverse/toxic effect of estrogen derivatives; examples include alfalfa, black cohosh, bloodroot, hops, kudzu, licorice, red clover, saw palmetto, soybean, thyme, wild yam, yucca.

Stability Store all products at controlled room temperature. In addition:
Climara®, Estraderm®, Menostar®: Do not store >30°C (>86°F); store in protective pouch.

Mechanism of Action Estrogens are responsible for the development and maintenance of the female reproductive system and secondary sexual characteristics. Estradiol is the principle intracellular human estrogen and is more potent than estrone and estriol at the receptor level; it is the primary estrogen secreted prior to menopause. Following menopause, estrone and estrone sulfate are more highly produced. Estrogens modulate the pituitary secretion of gonadotropins, luteinizing hormone, and follicle-stimulating hormone through a negative feedback system; estrogen replacement reduces elevated levels of these hormones in postmenopausal women.

Pharmacodynamics/Kinetics

Absorption: Well absorbed from the gastrointestinal tract, mucous membranes, and the skin. Average serum estradiol concentrations (C_{avg}) vary by product

Oral: Femtrace®: C_{avg}: 23.5-92.1 pg/mL

Injection: Estradiol valerate and estradiol cypionate are absorbed over several weeks following I.M. injection

Topical:
Alora®: C_{avg}: 41-98 pg/mL
Climara®: C_{avg}: 22-106 pg/mL
Divigel®: C_{avg}: 9.8-30.5 pg/mL
Elestrin®: C_{avg}: 15.4-39.2 pg/mL; Exposure increased by 55% with application of sunscreen 10 minutes prior to dose
Estraderm® 0.1 mg/day: C_{avg}: 73 pg/mL
Estrasorb®: Mean serum concentration on day 22 of therapy: ~35-65 pg/mL; Exposure increased by 35% with application of sunscreen 10 minutes prior to dose
Estrogel®: C_{avg} on day 14 of therapy: 28.3 pg/mL
Evamist®: C_{avg}: 19.6-30.9 pg/mL
Menostar®: C_{avg}: 13.7 pg/mL
Vivelle-Dot®: C_{avg}: 34-104 pg/mL

Vaginal: Femring®: Rapid during the first hour following application, then declines to a steady rate over 3 months; C_{avg}: 40.6-76 pg/mL

Distribution: Widely distributed; high concentrations in the sex hormone target organs

Protein binding: Bound to sex hormone-binding globulin and albumin

Metabolism: Hepatic; partial metabolism via CYP3A4 enzymes; estradiol is reversibly converted to estrone and estriol; oral estradiol also undergoes enterohepatic recirculation by conjugation in the liver, followed by excretion of sulfate and glucuronide conjugates into the bile, then hydrolysis in the intestine and estrogen reabsorption. Sulfate conjugates are the primary form found in postmenopausal women. With transdermal application, less estradiol is metabolized leading to higher circulating concentrations of estradiol and lower concentrations of estrone and conjugates.

Half-life elimination: Femtrace®: 21-26 hours

Time to peak, plasma: Oral: Femtrace®: 0.4-0.75 hours

Excretion: Primarily urine (as estradiol, estrone, estriol and their glucuronide and sulfate conjugates)

Dosage

Geriatric & Adult All dosage needs to be adjusted based upon the patient's response:

Vulvar and vaginal atrophy associated with menopause:
I.M.: Valerate (Delestrogen®): 10-20 mg every 4 weeks
Intravaginal: Vaginal ring (Femring®): 0.05 mg intravaginally; following insertion, ring should remain in place for 3 months; dose may be increased to 0.1 mg if needed
Oral (Estrace®): 1-2 mg/day; administration should be cyclic (3 weeks on, 1 week off)
Topical gel (EstroGel®): 1.25 g/day applied at the same time each day
Transdermal (Alora®, Climara®, Estraderm®, Vivelle-Dot®): Refer to product-specific dosing.

Breast cancer, metastatic (appropriately selected patients): Oral (Estrace®): Males and postmenopausal females: 10 mg 3 times/day **or** (unlabeled dosing) postmenopausal women: 2 mg 3 times/day (Ellis, 2009)

Hypoestrogenism (female) due to hypogonadism, castration, or primary ovarian failure:
Oral (Estrace®): 1-2 mg/day; titrate as necessary to control symptoms using minimal effective dose for maintenance therapy
I.M: Valerate (Delestrogen®): 10-20 mg every 4 weeks
Transdermal (Alora®, Climara®, Estraderm®, Vivelle-Dot®): Refer to product-specific dosing.

Hypoestrogenism (female) due to hypogonadism: I.M: Cypionate (Depo®-Estradiol): 1.5-2 mg monthly

Osteoporosis prevention (females):

Oral (Estrace®): Lowest effective dose has not been determined; doses of 0.5 mg/day in a cyclic regimen for 23 days of a 28-week cycle were used in clinical studies

Transdermal (Alora®, Climara®, Estraderm®, Menostar®, Vivelle-Dot®): Refer to product-specific dosing.

Prostate cancer, advanced (androgen-dependent):

I.M.: Valerate (Delestrogen®): 30 mg or more every 1-2 weeks

Oral (Estrace®): 1-2 mg 3 times/day

Vasomotor symptoms associated with menopause:

Oral:

Estrace®: 1-2 mg daily, adjusted as necessary to limit symptoms; administration should be cyclic (3 weeks on, 1 week off)

Femtrace®: Initial dose: 0.45 mg/day; dosage range 0.45-1.8 mg/day

I.M. Cypionate (Depo®-Estradiol): 1-5 mg every 3-4 weeks

I.M. Valerate (Delestrogen®): 10-20 mg every 4 weeks

Topical emulsion (Estrasorb®): 3.48 g applied once daily in the morning

Topical gel:

Divigel®: 0.25 g/day; adjust dose based on patient response. Dosing range: 0.25-1 g/day

Elestrin®: 0.87 g/day applied at the same time each day; adjust dose based on patient response. Dosing range: 0.87-1.7 g/day.

EstroGel®: 1.25 g/day applied at the same time each day

Topical spray (Evamist®): Initial: One spray (1.53 mg) per day. Adjust dose based on patient response. Dosing range: 1-3 sprays per day.

Transdermal (Alora®, Climara®, Estraderm®, Vivelle-Dot®): See product-specific dosing (below)

Vaginal ring (Femring®): Initial: 0.05 mg intravaginally; following insertion, ring should remain in place for 3 months; dose may be increased to 0.1 mg if needed

Transdermal product-specific dosing:

Note: Indicated dose may be used continuously in patients without an intact uterus. May be given continuously or cyclically (3 weeks on, 1 week off) in patients with an intact uterus **(exception - Menostar®, see specific dosing instructions).** When changing patients from oral to transdermal therapy, start transdermal patch 1 week after discontinuing oral hormone (may begin sooner if symptoms reappear within 1 week):

Transdermal once-weekly patch:

Vasomotor symptoms associated with menopause, vulvar and vaginal atrophy associated with menopause, female hypoestrogenism (due to hypogonadism, castration, or primary ovarian failure):

Climara®: Initial: Apply 0.025 mg/day patch once weekly. Adjust dose as necessary to control symptoms.

Prevention of osteoporosis in postmenopausal women:

Climara®: Apply patch once weekly; minimum effective dose 0.025 mg/day; adjust dosage based on response to therapy as indicated by biological markers and bone mineral density.

Menostar®: Apply patch once weekly (0.014 mg/day). In women with a uterus, also administer a progestin for 14 days every 6-12 months.

Transdermal twice-weekly patch:

Vasomotor symptoms associated with menopause, vulvar and vaginal atrophy associated with menopause, female hypoestrogenism (due to hypogonadism, castration, or primary ovarian failure): Titrate to lowest dose possible to control symptoms, adjusting initial dose after the first month of therapy:

Alora®, Estraderm®: Apply 0.05 mg patch twice weekly

Vivelle-Dot®: Apply 0.0375 mg patch twice weekly

Prevention of osteoporosis in postmenopausal women:

Alora®, Vivelle-Dot®: Apply 0.025 mg patch twice weekly; increase dose as necessary

Estraderm®: Apply 0.05 mg patch twice weekly; increase dose as necessary

Administration The use of a progestin should be considered when administering estrogens to postmenopausal women with an intact uterus.

Injection formulation: Intramuscular use only. Estradiol valerate should be injected into the upper outer quadrant of the gluteal muscle; administer with a dry needle (solution may become cloudy with wet needle).

Emulsion (Estrasorb®): Apply to clean, dry skin while in a sitting position. Contents of two pouches (total 3.48 g) are to be applied individually, once daily in the morning. Apply contents of first pouch to left thigh; massage into skin of left thigh and calf until thoroughly absorbed (~3 minutes). Apply excess from both hands to the buttocks. Apply contents of second pouch to the right thigh; massage into skin of right thigh and calf until thoroughly absorbed (~3 minutes). Apply excess from both hands to buttocks. Wash hands with soap and water. Allow skin to dry before covering legs with clothing. Do not apply to other areas of body. Do not apply to red or irritated skin.

Gel: Apply to clean, dry, unbroken skin at the same time each day. Allow to dry for 5 minutes prior to dressing. Gel is flammable; avoid fire or flame until dry. After application, wash hands with soap and water. Prior to the first use, pump must be primed. Do not apply gel to breast.

Divigel®: Apply entire contents of packet to right or left upper thigh each day (alternate sites). Do not apply to face, breasts, vaginal area or irritated skin. Apply over an area ~5x7 inches. Do not wash application site for 1 hour. Allow gel to dry before dressing

Elestrin®: Apply to upper arm and shoulder area using two fingers to spread gel. Apply after bath or shower; allow at least 2 hours between applying gel and going swimming. Wait at least 25 minutes before applying sunscreen to application area. Do not apply sunscreen to application area for ≥7 days (may increase absorption of gel).

EstroGel®: Apply gel to the arm, from the wrist to the shoulder. Spread gel as thinly as possible over one arm.

Spray: Evamist®: Prior to first use, prime pump by spraying 3 sprays with the cover on. To administer dose, hold container upright and vertical and rest the plastic cone flat against the skin while spraying. Spray to the inner surface of the forearm, starting near the elbow. If more than one spray is needed, apply to adjacent but not overlapping areas. Apply at the same time each day. Allow spray to dry for ~2 minutes; do not rub into skin; do not cover with clothing until dry. Do not wash application site for at least 60 minutes. Apply to clean, dry, unbroken skin. Do not apply to skin other than that of the forearm. Make sure that children do not come in contact with any skin area where the drug was applied. If contact with children is unavoidable, wear a garment with long sleeves that covers the site of application. If direct exposure should occur, wash the child in the area of exposure with soap and water as soon as possible. Solution contained in the spray is flammable; avoid fire, flame, or smoking until spray has dried. If needed, sunscreen should be applied ~1 hour prior to application of Evamist®.

Transdermal patch: Do not apply transdermal system to breasts, but place on trunk of body (preferably abdomen). Rotate application sites allowing a 1-week interval between applications at a particular site. Do not apply to oily, damaged or irritated skin; avoid waistline or other areas where tight clothing may rub the patch off. Apply patch immediately after removing from protective pouch. In general, if patch falls off, the same patch may be reapplied or a new system may be used for the remainder of the dosing interval (not recommended with all products). When replacing patch, reapply to a new site. Swimming, bathing or showering are not expected to affect use of the patch. Note the following exceptions:

Estraderm®: Do not apply to an area exposed to direct sunlight.

Climara®, Menostar®: Swimming, bathing, or wearing patch while in a sauna have not been studied; adhesion of patch may be decreased or delivery of estradiol may be affected. Remove patch slowly after use to avoid skin irritation. If any adhesive remains on the skin after removal, first allow skin to dry for 15 minutes, then gently rub area with an oil-based cream or lotion. If patch falls off, a new patch should be applied for the remainder of the dosing interval.

Vaginal ring: Exact positioning is not critical for efficacy; however, patient should not feel anything once inserted. In case of discomfort, ring should be pushed further into vagina. If ring is expelled prior to 90 days, it may be rinsed off and reinserted. Ensure proper vaginal placement of the ring to avoid inadvertent urinary bladder insertion. If vaginal infection develops, Femring® may remain in place during local treatment of a vaginal infection.

Monitoring Parameters Routine physical examination that includes blood pressure and Papanicolaou smear, breast exam, mammogram. Monitor for signs of endometrial cancer in female patients with uterus. Adequate diagnostic measures, including endometrial sampling, if indicated, should be performed to rule out malignancy in all cases of undiagnosed abnormal vaginal bleeding. Monitor for loss of vision, sudden onset of proptosis, diplopia, migraine; signs and symptoms of thromboembolic disorders; glycemic control in patients with diabetes; lipid profiles in patients being treated for hyperlipidemias; thyroid function in patients on thyroid hormone replacement therapy.

Menostar®: When used in a woman with a uterus, endometrial sampling is recommended at yearly intervals or when clinically indicated.

Menopausal symptoms, vulvar and vaginal atrophy: Assess need for therapy at 3- to 6-month intervals

Prevention of osteoporosis: Bone density measurement

Reference Range

Males: 10-50 pg/mL (SI: 37-184 pmol/L)

Females:

Premenopausal: 30-400 pg/mL (SI: 110-1468 pmol/L) (depending on phase of menstrual cycle)

Postmenopausal: 0-30 pg/mL (SI: 0-110 pmol/L)

Test Interactions Reduced response to metyrapone test.

Special Geriatric Considerations Before prescribing estrogen therapy to postmenopausal women, the risks and benefits must be weighed for each patient. Women should be informed of these risks and benefits, as well as possible side effects and the return of menstrual bleeding (when cycled with a progestin), and be involved in the decision to prescribe.

This medication is considered to be potentially inappropriate in this patient population (Beers Criteria: Quality of evidence - high [oral and transdermal patch]; Strength of recommendation - strong [oral and transdermal patch]).

Dosage Forms Excipient information presented when available (limited, particularly for generics); consult specific product labeling. [DSC] = Discontinued product

Emulsion, topical, as hemihydrate:
  Estrasorb®: 2.5 mg/g (56s) [contains ethanol, soybean oil; each pouch contains estradiol hemihydrate 4.35 mg; contents of two pouches delivers estradiol 0.05 mg/day]

Gel, topical:
  Divigel®: 0.1% (30s) [contains ethanol; delivers estradiol 0.25 mg/0.25 g packet]
  Divigel®: 0.1% (30s) [contains ethanol; delivers estradiol 0.5 mg/0.5 g packet]
  Divigel®: 0.1% (30s) [contains ethanol; delivers estradiol 1 mg/1 g packet]
  Elestrin®: 0.06% (35 g [DSC]) [contains ethanol; delivers estradiol 0.52 mg/0.87 g; 30 actuations]
  Elestrin®: 0.06% (70 g) [contains ethanol; delivers estradiol 0.52 mg/0.87 g; 60 actuations; packaged as 2x35 g]
  EstroGel®: 0.06% (50 g) [contains ethanol; delivers estradiol 0.75 mg/1.25 g; 32 actuations]

Injection, oil, as cypionate:
  Depo®-Estradiol: 5 mg/mL (5 mL) [contains chlorobutanol, cottonseed oil]

Injection, oil, as valerate: 10 mg/mL (5 mL); 20 mg/mL (5 mL); 40 mg/mL (5 mL)
  Delestrogen®: 10 mg/mL (5 mL) [contains chlorobutanol, sesame oil]
  Delestrogen®: 20 mg/mL (5 mL); 40 mg/mL (5 mL) [contains benzyl alcohol, benzyl benzoate, castor oil]

Patch, transdermal [once-weekly patch]: 0.025 mg/24 hours (4s); 0.0375 mg/24 hours (4s); 0.05 mg/24 hours (4s); 0.06 mg/24 hours (4s); 0.075 mg/24 hours (4s); 0.1 mg/24 hours (4s)
  Climara®: 0.025 mg/24 hours (4s) [6.5 cm^2, total estradiol 2 mg]
  Climara®: 0.0375 mg/24 hours (4s) [9.375 cm^2, total estradiol 2.85 mg]
  Climara®: 0.05 mg/24 hours (4s) [12.5 cm^2, total estradiol 3.8 mg]
  Climara®: 0.06 mg/24 hours (4s) [15 cm^2, total estradiol 4.55 mg]
  Climara®: 0.075 mg/24 hours (4s) [18.75 cm^2, total estradiol 5.7 mg]
  Climara®: 0.1 mg/24 hours (4s) [25 cm^2, total estradiol 7.6 mg]
  Menostar®: 0.014 mg/24 hours (4s) [3.25 cm^2, total estradiol 1 mg]

Patch, transdermal [twice-weekly patch]:
  Alora®: 0.025 mg/24 hours (8s) [9 cm^2, total estradiol 0.77 mg]
  Alora®: 0.05 mg/24 hours (8s) [18 cm^2, total estradiol 1.5 mg]
  Alora®: 0.075 mg/24 hours (8s) [27 cm^2, total estradiol 2.3 mg]
  Alora®: 0.1 mg/24 hours (8s) [36 cm^2, total estradiol 3.1 mg]
  Vivelle-Dot®: 0.025 mg/24 hours (24s) [2.5 cm^2, total estradiol 0.39 mg]
  Vivelle-Dot®: 0.0375 mg/24 hours (24s) [3.75 cm^2, total estradiol 0.585 mg]
  Vivelle-Dot®: 0.05 mg/24 hours (24s) [5 cm^2, total estradiol 0.78 mg]
  Vivelle-Dot®: 0.075 mg/24 hours (24s) [7.5 cm^2, total estradiol 1.17 mg]
  Vivelle-Dot®: 0.1 mg/24 hours (24s) [10 cm^2, total estradiol 1.56 mg]

Ring, vaginal, as acetate:
  Femring®: 0.05 mg/24 hours (1s) [total estradiol 12.4 mg; releases 0.05 mg/24 hours over 3 months]
  Femring®: 0.1 mg/24 hours (1s) [total estradiol 24.8 mg; releases 0.1 mg/24 hours over 3 months]

Solution, topical [spray]:
  Evamist®: 1.53 mg/spray (8.1 mL) [contains ethanol; delivers 75 sprays after priming]

Tablet, oral [micronized]: 0.5 mg, 1 mg, 2 mg
  Estrace®: 0.5 mg, 1 mg [scored]
  Estrace®: 2 mg [scored; contains tartrazine]

Tablet, oral, as acetate:
  Femtrace®: 0.45 mg [DSC], 0.9 mg

Estradiol (Topical) (es tra DYE ole)

Related Information

Beers Criteria – Potentially Inappropriate Medications for Geriatrics *on page 2183*

Medication Safety Issues

BEERS Criteria medication:

This drug may be potentially inappropriate for use in geriatric patients (Quality of evidence - moderate [topical]; Strength of recommendation - weak [topical]).

International issues:

Estring [U.S., Canada, and multiple international markets] may be confused with Estrena [Finland]

Brand Names: U.S. Estrace®; Estring®; Vagifem®

Brand Names: Canada Estrace®; Estring®; Vagifem®; Vagifem® 10

Index Terms 17β-estradiol

Generic Availability (U.S.) No

Pharmacologic Category Estrogen Derivative

Use Treatment of moderate-to-severe vulvar and vaginal atrophy associated with menopause

Contraindications Angioedema or anaphylactic reaction to estradiol or any component of the formulation; undiagnosed abnormal vaginal bleeding; DVT or PE (current or history of); active or history of arterial thromboembolic disease (eg, stroke, MI); carcinoma of the breast (known, suspected or history of); estrogen-dependent tumor; hepatic dysfunction or disease; known protein C, protein S, antithrombin deficiency, or other known thrombophilic disorders

Warnings/Precautions [U.S. Boxed Warning]: The use of unopposed estrogen in women with an intact uterus is associated with an increased risk of endometrial cancer. The addition of a progestin to estrogen therapy may decrease the risk of endometrial hyperplasia, a precursor to endometrial cancer. Adequate diagnostic measures, including endometrial sampling if indicated, should be performed to rule out malignancy in postmenopausal women with undiagnosed abnormal vaginal bleeding. Estrogens may exacerbate endometriosis. Malignant transformation of residual endometrial implants has been reported posthysterectomy with unopposed estrogen therapy. Consider adding a progestin in women with residual endometriosis posthysterectomy. Postmenopausal estrogen therapy and combined estrogen/progesterone therapy may increase the risk of ovarian cancer; however, the absolute risk to an individual woman is small. Although results from various studies are not consistent, risk does not appear to be significantly associated with the duration, route, or dose of therapy. In one study, the risk decreased after 2 years following discontinuation of therapy (Mørch, 2009). Although the risk of ovarian cancer is rare, women who are at an increased risk (eg, family history) should be counseled about the association (NAMS, 2012).

[U.S. Boxed Warning]: Based on data from the Women's Health Initiative (WHI) studies, an increased risk of invasive breast cancer was observed in postmenopausal women using conjugated estrogens (CE) in combination with medroxyprogesterone acetate (MPA). This risk may be associated with duration of use and declines once combined therapy is discontinued (Chlebowski, 2009). The risk of invasive breast cancer was decreased in postmenopausal women with a hysterectomy using CE only, regardless of weight. However, the risk was not significantly decreased in women at high risk for breast cancer (family history of breast cancer, personal history of benign breast disease) (Anderson, 2012). An increase in abnormal mammogram findings has also been reported with estrogen alone or in combination with progestin therapy. Estrogen use may also lead to severe hypercalcemia in patients with breast cancer and bone metastases; discontinue estrogen if hypercalcemia occurs. Use is contraindicated in patients with known or suspected breast cancer.

[U.S. Boxed Warning]: Estrogens with or without progestin should not be used to prevent cardiovascular disease. Using data from the Women's Health Initiative (WHI) studies, an increased risk of deep vein thrombosis (DVT) and stroke has been reported with CE and an increased risk of DVT, stroke, pulmonary emboli (PE) and myocardial infarction (MI) has been reported with CE with MPA in postmenopausal women. Additional risk factors include diabetes mellitus, hypercholesterolemia, hypertension, SLE, obesity, tobacco use, and/or history of venous thromboembolism (VTE). Risk factors should be managed appropriately; discontinue use if adverse cardiovascular events occur or are suspected. Women with inherited thrombophilias (eg, protein C or S deficiency) may have increased risk of venous thromboembolism (DeSancho, 2010; van Vlijmen, 2011). Use is contraindicated in women with protein C, protein S, antithrombin deficiency, or other known thrombophilic disorders.

◀ **[U.S. Boxed Warning]: Estrogens with or without progestin should not be used to prevent dementia. In the Women's Health Initiative Memory Study (WHIMS), an increased incidence of dementia was observed in women ≥65 years of age taking CE alone or in combination with MPA.**

[U.S. Boxed Warning]: Estrogens with or without progestin should be used for the shortest duration possible at the lowest effective dose consistent with treatment goals. Before prescribing estrogen therapy to postmenopausal women, the risks and benefits must be weighed for each patient. Women should be informed of these risks and benefits, as well as possible effects of progestin when added to estrogen therapy. Patients should be reevaluated as clinically appropriate to determine if treatment is still necessary. Available data related to treatment risks are from Women's Health Initiative (WHI) studies, which evaluated oral CE 0.625 mg with or without MPA 2.5 mg relative to placebo in postmenopausal women. Other combinations and dosage forms of estrogens and progestins were not studied. **Outcomes reported from clinical trials using CE with or without MPA should be assumed to be similar for other doses and other dosage forms of estrogens and progestins until comparable data becomes available.** Systemic absorption occurs following vaginal use; warnings, precautions, and adverse events observed with oral therapy should be considered.

Estrogen compounds are generally associated with lipid effects such as increased HDL-cholesterol and decreased LDL-cholesterol. Triglycerides may also be increased; discontinue if pancreatitis occurs. Estrogens may increase thyroid-binding globulin (TBG) levels leading to increased circulating total thyroid hormone levels. Women on thyroid replacement therapy may require higher doses of thyroid hormone while receiving estrogens.

In the elderly, low-dose intravaginal estrogen may be appropriate for use in the management of vaginal symptoms, lower urinary tract infections, and dyspareunia; in addition, evidence has shown that vaginal estrogens (particularly at estradiol doses of <25 mcg twice weekly) in the treatment of vaginal dryness is safe and effective in women with breast cancer (Beers Criteria).

Estrogens may cause retinal vascular thrombosis; discontinue if migraine, loss of vision, proptosis, diplopia, or other visual disturbances occur; discontinue permanently if papilledema or retinal vascular lesions are observed on examination. Estrogens are poorly metabolized in patients with hepatic dysfunction. Use caution with a history of cholestatic jaundice associated with prior estrogen use or pregnancy. Discontinue if jaundice develops or if acute or chronic hepatic disturbances occur. Use is contraindicated with hepatic disease. Exogenous estrogens may exacerbate angioedema symptoms in women with hereditary angioedema. Use caution in patients with asthma, epilepsy, hepatic hemangiomas, migraine, porphyria, or SLE; may exacerbate disease. May have adverse effects on glucose tolerance; use caution in women with diabetes. Use with caution in patients with diseases which may be exacerbated by fluid retention, including cardiac or renal dysfunction. Use of postmenopausal estrogen may be associated with an increased risk of gallbladder disease requiring surgery. Use caution in patients with hypoparathyroidism; estrogen-induced hypocalcemia may occur. Whenever possible, estrogens should be discontinued at least 4-6 weeks prior to elective surgery associated with an increased risk of thromboembolism or during periods of prolonged immobilization. The use of estrogens and/or progestins may change the results of some laboratory tests (eg, coagulation factors, lipids, glucose tolerance, binding proteins). The dose, route, and the specific estrogen/progestin influences these changes. In addition, personal risk factors (eg, cardiovascular disease, smoking, diabetes, age) also contribute to adverse events; use of specific products may be contraindicated in women with certain risk factors.

Vaginal ring: Use may not be appropriate in women with narrow vagina, vaginal stenosis, vaginal infections, cervical prolapse, rectoceles, cystoceles, or other conditions which may increase the risk of vaginal irritation, ulceration, or increase the risk of expulsion. Ring should be removed in case of ulceration, erosion, or adherence to vaginal wall; do not reinsert until healing is complete. Ensure proper vaginal placement of the ring to avoid inadvertent urinary bladder insertion.

Moderate-to-severe symptoms of vulvar and vaginal atrophy include vaginal dryness, dyspareunia, and atrophic vaginitis. Use caution applying topical products to severely atrophic vaginal mucosa. Local abrasion caused by the vaginal applicator has been reported in women with severely atrophic vaginal mucosa.

Adverse Reactions (Reflective of adult population; not specific for elderly)

>10%: Central nervous system: Headache (13%)

1% to 10%:

Cardiovascular: Chest pain, edema, hypertension, leg edema, MI, stroke, syncope, venous thrombosis

Central nervous system: Insomnia (4%), anxiety, migraine

Dermatologic: Angioedema, chloasma, dermatitis, erythema multiforme, erythema nodosum, hemorrhagic eruption, hirsutism, loss of scalp hair, melasma, pruritus, rash, skin hypertrophy, urticaria

Endocrine & metabolic: Hot flashes (2%), breast pain (1%), breast cancer, breast enlargement, breast tenderness, carbohydrate tolerance decreased, endometrial carcinoma, endometrial hyperplasia, fibrocystic breast changes, galactorrhea, hypocalcemia, libido changes, nipple discharge, ovarian cancer

Gastrointestinal: Abdominal pain (4%), diarrhea (5%), nausea (3%), dyspepsia, flatulence, gastritis, hemorrhoids, toothache, weight changes

Genitourinary: Leukorrhea (7%), cervical ectropion changes, cervical secretion changes, cystitis, dysmenorrhea, dysuria, genital eruption, urinary incontinence, uterine leiomyomata change, vaginal bleeding pattern change (including abnormal flow, breakthrough bleeding, spotting)

Vaginal: Trauma from applicator insertion may occur in women with severely atrophic mucosa; burning, discomfort, hemorrhage, moniliasis, pain, pruritus, vaginitis, vulvovaginal infection

Hematologic: Porphyria aggravated

Local: Thrombophlebitis

Neuromuscular & skeletal: Back pain (6% to 7%), arthritis (4%), arthralgias (3%), skeletal pain (2%), leg cramps

Ocular: Contact lens intolerance, retinal vascular thrombosis

Otic: Otitis media

Respiratory: Respiratory tract infection: (5%), sinusitis (4%), pharyngitis (1%), asthma exacerbation, bronchitis, pulmonary embolism

Miscellaneous: Anaphylactoid/anaphylactic reactions, flu-like syndrome (3%), hypersensitivity

Drug Interactions

Metabolism/Transport Effects Substrate of CYP1A2 (major), CYP2A6 (minor), CYP2B6 (minor), CYP2C19 (minor), CYP2C9 (minor), CYP2D6 (minor), CYP2E1 (minor), CYP3A4 (major), P-glycoprotein; **Note:** Assignment of Major/Minor substrate status based on clinically relevant drug interaction potential; **Inhibits** CYP1A2 (weak), CYP2C8 (weak); **Induces** CYP3A4 (weak/moderate)

Avoid Concomitant Use

Avoid concomitant use of Estradiol (Topical) with any of the following: Anastrozole; Axitinib

Increased Effect/Toxicity

Estradiol (Topical) may increase the levels/effects of: Corticosteroids (Systemic); ROPINIRole; Tipranavir

The levels/effects of Estradiol (Topical) may be increased by: Ascorbic Acid; Herbs (Estrogenic Properties); P-glycoprotein/ABCB1 Inhibitors

Decreased Effect

Estradiol (Topical) may decrease the levels/effects of: Anastrozole; ARIPiprazole; Axitinib; Chenodiol; Hyaluronidase; Saxagliptin; Somatropin; Thyroid Products; Ursodiol

The levels/effects of Estradiol (Topical) may be decreased by: CYP1A2 Inducers (Strong); CYP3A4 Inducers (Strong); Cyproterone; Deferasirox; Herbs (CYP3A4 Inducers); Peginterferon Alfa-2b; P-glycoprotein/ABCB1 Inducers; Tipranavir; Tocilizumab

Stability

Vaginal cream (Estrace®): Store at room temperature; protect from temperatures in excess of 40°C (104°F).

Vaginal ring (Estring®): Store at 15°C to 30°C (59°F to 86°F).

Vaginal tablet (Vagifem®): Store at 25°C (77°F); do not refrigerate.

Mechanism of Action In studies for vulvar and vaginal atrophy in postmenopausal women, local estrogens have been shown to reduce vaginal pH levels and mature the vaginal and urethral mucosa after 12 weeks of therapy, thereby improving vaginal dryness and mucosal atrophy.

Pharmacodynamics/Kinetics

Absorption: Average serum estradiol concentrations (C_{avg}) vary by product

Vaginal: Vaginal absorption is typically low; any contribution to circulating estradiol concentrations via systemic absorption does not exceed normal postmenopausal ranges (Ulrich, 2010; Weisberg, 2005).

Estring®: Average steady state serum concentrations decrease from 11.2 pg/mL at 48 hours to 8 pg/mL at 12 weeks

Vagifem®: C_{avg}: 10.9 pg/mL on day 1, 5.5 pg/mL on day 83

Distribution: Widely distributed; high concentrations in the sex hormone target organs

Protein binding: Bound to sex hormone-binding globulin and albumin

Metabolism: Hepatic; partial metabolism via CYP3A4 enzymes; estradiol is reversibly converted to estrone and estriol. Sulfate conjugates are the primary form found in postmenopausal women.

Excretion: Primarily urine (as estradiol, estrone, estriol and their glucuronide and sulfate conjugates)

Dosage
Geriatric & Adult All dosage needs to be adjusted based upon the patient's response:
Vulvar and vaginal atrophy associated with menopause: Intravaginal:

Vaginal cream (Estrace®): Insert 2-4 g/day intravaginally for 1-2 weeks, then gradually reduce to ¹/₂ the initial dose for 1-2 weeks, followed by a maintenance dose of 1 g 1-3 times/week

Vaginal ring (Estring®): 2 mg intravaginally; following insertion, ring should remain in place for 90 days

Vaginal tablet (Vagifem®): Initial: Insert 1 tablet (10 mcg) once daily for 2 weeks; Maintenance: Insert 1 tablet twice weekly

Administration
Vaginal ring: Exact positioning is not critical for efficacy; however, patient should not feel anything once inserted. In case of discomfort, ring should be pushed further into vagina. If ring is expelled prior to 90 days, it may be rinsed off and reinserted. Ensure proper vaginal placement of the ring to avoid inadvertent urinary bladder insertion. If vaginal infection develops, Estring® should be removed; reinsert only after infection has been appropriately treated.

Vaginal tablet: Insert tablet with supplied applicator at the same time each day. Once inserted, press plunger until fully depressed, then remove applicator and discard. If tablet comes out of applicator prior to insertion, do not replace; use a new tablet filled applicator instead.

Monitoring Parameters Routine physical examination that includes blood pressure and Papanicolaou smear, breast exam, mammogram. Monitor for signs of endometrial cancer in female patients with uterus. Adequate diagnostic measures, including endometrial sampling, if indicated, should be performed to rule out malignancy in all cases of undiagnosed abnormal vaginal bleeding. Monitor for loss of vision, sudden onset of proptosis, diplopia, migraine; signs and symptoms of thromboembolic disorders; glycemic control in patients with diabetes; lipid profiles in patients being treated for hyperlipidemias; thyroid function in patients on thyroid hormone replacement therapy. Assess need for therapy at 3- to 6-month intervals.

Test Interactions Reduced response to metyrapone test.

Special Geriatric Considerations Topical estrogen is beneficial in the management of urogenital atrophy and prevention of recurrent urinary tract infections in postmenopausal women. Topical estrogens are not void of the risks associated with oral and transdermal forms; thus, the risks and benefits must be weighed for each patient.

This medication is considered to be potentially inappropriate in this patient population (Beers Criteria: Quality of evidence - moderate [topical]; Strength of recommendation - weak [topical]).

Dosage Forms Excipient information presented when available (limited, particularly for generics); consult specific product labeling.

Cream, vaginal:
Estrace®: 0.1 mg/g (42.5 g)

Ring, vaginal, as base:
Estring®: 2 mg (1s) [total estradiol 2 mg; releases 7.5 mcg/day over 90 days]

Tablet, vaginal, as base:
Vagifem®: 10 mcg

◆ **Estradiol Acetate** see Estradiol (Systemic) on page 681
◆ **Estradiol and Drospirenone** see Drospirenone and Estradiol on page 616
◆ **Estradiol and NGM** see Estradiol and Norgestimate on page 692

Estradiol and Norgestimate (es tra DYE ole & nor JES ti mate)

Related Information

Medication Safety Issues
BEERS Criteria medication:
This drug may be potentially inappropriate for use in geriatric patients (Quality of evidence - high [oral and transdermal patch]; Strength of recommendation - strong [oral and transdermal patch]).

Brand Names: U.S. Prefest™

Index Terms Estradiol and NGM; Norgestimate and Estradiol; Ortho Prefest

Generic Availability (U.S.) No

Pharmacologic Category Estrogen and Progestin Combination

Use Women with an intact uterus: Treatment of moderate-to-severe vasomotor symptoms associated with menopause; treatment of atrophic vaginitis; prevention of osteoporosis

Contraindications Hypersensitivity to estradiol, norgestimate, or any component of the formulation; undiagnosed abnormal vaginal bleeding; history of or current thrombophlebitis or venous thromboembolic disorders (including DVT, PE); active or recent (within 1 year) arterial thromboembolic disease (eg, stroke, MI); carcinoma of the breast; estrogen-dependent tumor; hepatic dysfunction or disease

Warnings/Precautions

Cardiovascular-related considerations: **[U.S. Boxed Warning]: Estrogens with or without progestin should not be used to prevent cardiovascular disease.** Using data from the Women's Health Initiative (WHI) studies, an increased risk of deep vein thrombosis (DVT) and stroke has been reported with conjugated estrogens (CE) and an increased risk of DVT, stroke, pulmonary emboli (PE) and myocardial infarction (MI) has been reported with CE with medroxyprogesterone acetate (MPA) in postmenopausal women. Additional risk factors include diabetes mellitus, hypercholesterolemia, hypertension, SLE, obesity, tobacco use, and/or history of venous thromboembolism (VTE). Risk factors should be managed appropriately; discontinue use if adverse cardiovascular events occur or are suspected. Estrogen compounds are generally associated with lipid effects such as increased HDL-cholesterol and decreased LDL-cholesterol. Triglycerides may also be increased; use with caution in patients with familial defects of lipoprotein metabolism. Whenever possible, combination hormonal contraceptives should be discontinued at least 4-6 weeks prior to elective surgery associated with an increased risk of thromboembolism or during periods of prolonged immobilization. Women with inherited thrombophilias (eg, protein C or S deficiency) may have increased risk of venous thromboembolism (DeSancho, 2010; van Vlijmen, 2011).

Neurological considerations: **[U.S. Boxed Warning]: Estrogens with or without progestin should not be used to prevent dementia. In the Women's Health Initiative Memory Study (WHIMS), an increased incidence of dementia was observed in women ≥65 years of age taking CE alone or in combination with MPA.**

Cancer-related considerations: **[U.S. Boxed Warning]: Based on data from the Women's Health Initiative (WHI) studies, an increased risk of invasive breast cancer was observed in postmenopausal women using conjugated estrogens (CE) in combination with medroxyprogesterone acetate (MPA).** This risk may be associated with duration of use and declines once combined therapy is discontinued (Chlebowski, 2009). The risk of invasive breast cancer was decreased in postmenopausal women with a hysterectomy using CE only, regardless of weight. However, the risk was not significantly decreased in women at high risk for breast cancer (family history of breast cancer, personal history of benign breast disease) (Anderson, 2012). An increase in abnormal mammogram findings has also been reported with estrogen alone or in combination with progestin therapy. Estrogen use may also lead to severe hypercalcemia in patients with breast cancer and bone metastases; discontinue estrogen if hypercalcemia occurs. Use is contraindicated in patients with known or suspected breast cancer. The use of unopposed estrogen in women with an intact uterus is associated with an increased risk of endometrial cancer. The addition of a progestin to estrogen therapy may decrease the risk of endometrial hyperplasia, a precursor to endometrial cancer. Adequate diagnostic measures, including endometrial sampling if indicated, should be performed to rule out malignancy in postmenopausal women with undiagnosed abnormal vaginal bleeding. Estrogens may exacerbate endometriosis. Malignant transformation of residual endometrial implants has been reported posthysterectomy with unopposed estrogen therapy. Consider adding a progestin in women with residual endometriosis posthysterectomy. Postmenopausal estrogen therapy and combined estrogen/progesterone therapy may increase the risk of ovarian cancer; however, the absolute risk to an individual woman is small. Although results from various studies are not consistent, risk does not appear to be significantly associated with the duration, route, or dose of therapy. In one study, the risk decreased after 2 years following discontinuation of therapy (Mørch, 2009). Although the risk of ovarian cancer is rare, women who are at an increased risk (eg, family history) should be counseled about the association (NAMS, 2012).

Estrogens may cause retinal vascular thrombosis; discontinue if migraine, loss of vision, proptosis, diplopia, or other visual disturbances occur; discontinue permanently if papilledema or retinal vascular lesions are observed on examination. Use caution in patients with asthma, epilepsy, hepatic hemangiomas, hereditary angioedema, migraine, porphyria, or SLE; may exacerbate disease. May have adverse effects on glucose tolerance; use caution in women with diabetes. Use with caution in patients with diseases which may be exacerbated by fluid retention, including cardiac or renal dysfunction. Use of postmenopausal estrogen may be associated with an increased risk of gallbladder disease requiring surgery. Estrogens are poorly metabolized in patients with hepatic dysfunction. Use caution with a history of cholestatic jaundice associated with prior estrogen use or pregnancy. Discontinue if jaundice develops or if acute or chronic hepatic disturbances occur. Use is contraindicated with hepatic disease. Use with caution in patients with severe hypocalcemia. Estrogens may increase thyroid-binding globulin (TBG) levels leading to increased circulating total thyroid hormone levels. Women on thyroid replacement therapy may require higher doses of thyroid hormone while receiving estrogens. Not for use prior to menopause. The use of estrogens and/or progestins may change the results of some laboratory tests (eg, coagulation factors, lipids, glucose tolerance, binding proteins). The dose, route, and the specific estrogen/progestin influences these changes. In addition, personal risk factors (eg, cardiovascular disease, smoking, diabetes, age) also contribute to adverse events; use of specific products may be contraindicated in women with certain risk factors.

[U.S. Boxed Warning]: Estrogens with or without progestin should be used for the shortest duration possible at the lowest effective dose consistent with treatment goals. Before prescribing estrogen therapy to postmenopausal women, the risks and benefits must be weighed for each patient. Women should be informed of these risks and benefits, as well as possible effects of progestin when added to estrogen therapy. Patients should be reevaluated as clinically appropriate to determine if treatment is still necessary. Available data related to treatment risks are from Women's Health Initiative (WHI) studies, which evaluated oral CE 0.625 mg with or without MPA 2.5 mg relative to placebo in postmenopausal women. Other combinations and dosage forms of estrogens and progestins were not studied. **Outcomes reported from clinical trials using CE with or without MPA should be assumed to be similar for other doses and other dosage forms of estrogens and progestins until comparable data becomes available.**

Osteoporosis use: For use only in women at significant risk of osteoporosis and for who other nonestrogen medications are not considered appropriate.

Vulvar and vaginal atrophy use: When used solely for the treatment of vulvar and vaginal atrophy, topical vaginal products should be considered.

Elderly considerations: Avoid oral and transdermal patch estrogen products (with or without progestins) in this age group due to potential of increased risk of breast and endometrial cancers, and lack of proven cardioprotection and cognitive protection (Beers Criteria).

Adverse Reactions (Reflective of adult population; not specific for elderly)
>10%:
  Central nervous system: Headache (23%)
  Endocrine & metabolic: Breast pain (16%)
  Gastrointestinal: Abdominal pain (12%)
  Neuromuscular & skeletal: Back pain (12%)
  Respiratory: Upper respiratory tract infection (21%)
  Miscellaneous: Flu-like syndrome (11%)
1% to 10%:
  Central nervous system: Fatigue (6%), pain (6%), depression (5%), dizziness (5%)
  Endocrine & metabolic: Vaginal bleeding (9%), dysmenorrhea (8%), vaginitis (7%)
  Gastrointestinal: Nausea (6%), flatulence (5%)
  Neuromuscular & skeletal: Arthralgia (9%), myalgia (5%)
  Respiratory: Sinusitis (8%), pharyngitis (7%), cough (5%)
  Miscellaneous: Viral infection (6%)
Additional adverse effects associated with **estrogens and progestins**; frequency not defined:
  Cardiovascular: Edema, hypertension, MI, stroke, venous thrombosis
  Central nervous system: Anxiety, epilepsy exacerbation, insomnia, irritability, migraine, mood disturbances, nervousness, pyrexia, somnolence
  Dermatologic: Acne, chloasma, erythema multiforme, erythema nodosum, hemorrhagic eruptions, hirsutism, itching, melasma, pruritus, rash, scalp hair loss, urticaria
  Endocrine & metabolic: Amenorrhea, breast cancer, breast discharge, breast enlargement, Breast tenderness, carbohydrate tolerance decreased, endometrial cancer, endometrial hyperplasia, fibrocystic breast changes, galactorrhea, hypocalcemia, libido changes, ovarian cancer, triglycerides increased
  Gastrointestinal: Abdominal cramps, appetite changes, bloating, gallbladder disease, pancreatitis, vomiting, weight gain/loss
  Genitourinary: Abnormal withdrawal bleeding/flow, breakthrough bleeding, cervical secretion changes, cystitis syndrome, uterine leiomyomata size increased, vaginal candidiasis, vaginal bleeding/spotting
  Hematologic: Anemia, porphyria
  Hepatic: Cholestatic jaundice
  Local: Thrombophlebitis
  Neuromuscular & skeletal: Chorea
  Ocular: Contact lens intolerance, corneal curvature steepening, neuro-ocular lesions

Respiratory: Asthma exacerbation, pulmonary embolism
Miscellaneous: Anaphylaxis

Drug Interactions

Metabolism/Transport Effects Refer to individual components.

Avoid Concomitant Use

Avoid concomitant use of Estradiol and Norgestimate with any of the following: Anastrozole; Axitinib; Griseofulvin

Increased Effect/Toxicity

Estradiol and Norgestimate may increase the levels/effects of: Benzodiazepines (metabolized by oxidation); Corticosteroids (Systemic); ROPINIRole; Selegiline; Tipranavir; Tranexamic Acid; Voriconazole

The levels/effects of Estradiol and Norgestimate may be increased by: Ascorbic Acid; Boceprevir; Herbs (Estrogenic Properties); Herbs (Progestogenic Properties); Mifepristone; P-glycoprotein/ABCB1 Inhibitors; Voriconazole

Decreased Effect

Estradiol and Norgestimate may decrease the levels/effects of: Anastrozole; ARIPiprazole; Axitinib; Chenodiol; Hyaluronidase; Saxagliptin; Somatropin; Thyroid Products; Ursodiol; Vitamin K Antagonists

The levels/effects of Estradiol and Norgestimate may be decreased by: Acitretin; Aminoglutethimide; Aprepitant; Artemether; Barbiturates; Bexarotene; Bexarotene (Systemic); Bile Acid Sequestrants; Bosentan; CarBAMazepine; Clobazam; CYP1A2 Inducers (Strong); CYP3A4 Inducers (Strong); Cyproterone; Deferasirox; Efavirenz; Felbamate; Fosaprepitant; Fosphenytoin; Griseofulvin; LamoTRIgine; Mifepristone; Mycophenolate; Nevirapine; OXcarbazepine; Peginterferon Alfa-2b; P-glycoprotein/ABCB1 Inducers; Phenytoin; Prucalopride; Retinoic Acid Derivatives; Rifamycin Derivatives; St Johns Wort; Telaprevir; Tipranavir; Tocilizumab; Topiramate

Ethanol/Nutrition/Herb Interactions

Ethanol: Avoid ethanol (routine use increases estrogen level and risk of breast cancer). Ethanol may also increase the risk of osteoporosis.

Food: CNS effects of caffeine may be enhanced if combination estrogen/progestins are used concurrently with caffeine. Grapefruit juice increases ethinyl estradiol concentrations and would be expected to increase progesterone serum levels as well; clinical implications are unclear.

Herb/Nutraceutical: St John's wort may decrease the plasma levels of combination estrogen/progestin combinations by inducing hepatic enzymes. Avoid dong quai and black cohosh (have estrogen activity). Avoid saw palmetto, red clover, ginseng.

Stability Store at 25°C (77°F).

Mechanism of Action Estrogens are responsible for the development and maintenance of the female reproductive system and secondary sexual characteristics. Estradiol is the principle intracellular human estrogen and is more potent than estrone and estriol at the receptor level; it is the primary estrogen secreted prior to menopause. Following menopause, estrone and estrone sulfate are more highly produced. Estrogens modulate the pituitary secretion of gonadotropins, luteinizing hormone, and follicle-stimulating hormone through a negative feedback system; estrogen replacement reduces elevated levels of these hormones in postmenopausal women.

Progestins inhibit gonadotropin production which then prevents follicular maturation and ovulation. In women with adequate estrogen, progestins transform a proliferative endometrium into a secretory endometrium; when administered with estradiol, reduces the incidence of endometrial hyperplasia and risk of adenocarcinoma.

Pharmacodynamics/Kinetics

Estradiol: See Estradiol (Systemic) monograph.

Norgestimate:

Protein binding: 17-deacetylnorgestimate: 99%

Metabolism: Forms 17-deacetylnorgestimate (major active metabolite) and other metabolites; first-pass effect

Half-life elimination: 17-deacetylnorgestimate: 37 hours

Excretion: Norgestimate metabolites: Urine and feces

Dosage

Geriatric & Adult Females with an intact uterus:

Treatment of menopausal symptoms, atrophic vaginitis, prevention of osteoporosis: Oral: Treatment is cyclical and consists of the following: One tablet of estradiol 1 mg (pink tablet) once daily for 3 days, followed by 1 tablet of estradiol 1 mg and norgestimate 0.09 mg (white tablet) once daily for 3 days; repeat sequence continuously. Note: This dose may not be the lowest effective combination for these indications. In case of a missed tablet, restart therapy with next available tablet in sequence (taking only 1 tablet each day).

Administration In case of a missed tablet, restart therapy with next available tablet in sequence (taking only 1 tablet each day).

Monitoring Parameters Yearly physical examination that includes blood pressure and Papanicolaou smear, breast exam, mammogram. Monitor for signs of endometrial cancer. Adequate diagnostic measures, including endometrial sampling, if indicated. should be performed to rule out malignancy in all cases of undiagnosed abnormal vaginal bleeding. Monitor for loss of vision, sudden onset of proptosis, diplopia, migraine; signs and symptoms of thromboembolic disorders; glycemic control in patients with diabetes; lipid profiles in patients being treated for hyperlipidemias; thyroid function in patients on thyroid hormone replacement therapy.

Menopausal symptoms: Assess need for therapy at 3- to 6-month intervals

Prevention of osteoporosis: Bone density measurement

Test Interactions Reduced response to metyrapone test.

Special Geriatric Considerations See Estradiol (Systemic) monograph on page 681.

Dosage Forms Excipient information presented when available (limited, particularly for generics); consult specific product labeling.

Tablet, oral:

Prefest™: Estradiol 1 mg [15 peach tablets] and estradiol 1 mg and norgestimate 0.09 mg [15 white tablets]

- ◆ **Estradiol Transdermal** see Estradiol (Systemic) on page 681
- ◆ **Estradiol Valerate** see Estradiol (Systemic) on page 681
- ◆ **Estrasorb®** see Estradiol (Systemic) on page 681
- ◆ **Estring®** see Estradiol (Topical) on page 689
- ◆ **EstroGel®** see Estradiol (Systemic) on page 681
- ◆ **Estrogenic Substances, Conjugated** see Estrogens (Conjugated/Equine, Systemic) on page 703
- ◆ **Estrogenic Substances, Conjugated** see Estrogens (Conjugated/Equine, Topical) on page 707

Estrogens (Conjugated A/Synthetic)

(ES troe jenz, KON joo gate ed, aye, sin THET ik)

Related Information

Beers Criteria – Potentially Inappropriate Medications for Geriatrics on page 2183

Osteoporosis Management on page 2136

Medication Safety Issues

Sound-alike/look-alike issues:

Cenestin® may be confused with Senexon®

BEERS Criteria medication:

This drug may be potentially inappropriate for use in geriatric patients (Quality of evidence - high; Strength of recommendation - strong).

International issues:

Cenestin [U.S., Canada] may be confused with Canesten which is a brand name for clotrimazole [multiple international markets]

Brand Names: U.S. Cenestin®

Brand Names: Canada Cenestin

Generic Availability (U.S.) No

Pharmacologic Category Estrogen Derivative

Use Treatment of moderate-to-severe vasomotor symptoms of menopause; treatment of vulvar and vaginal atrophy

Contraindications Hypersensitivity to estrogens or any component of the formulation; undiagnosed abnormal vaginal bleeding; history of or current thrombophlebitis or venous thromboembolic disorders (including DVT, PE); active or recent (within 1 year) arterial thromboembolic disease (eg, stroke, MI); carcinoma of the breast; estrogen-dependent tumor; hepatic dysfunction or disease

Warnings/Precautions

Cardiovascular-related considerations: **[U.S. Boxed Warning]: Estrogens with or without progestin should not be used to prevent cardiovascular disease.** Using data from the Women's Health Initiative (WHI) studies, an increased risk of deep vein thrombosis (DVT) and stroke has been reported with conjugated estrogens [CE] and an increased risk of DVT, stroke, pulmonary emboli (PE) and myocardial infarction (MI) has been reported with CE with medroxyprogesterone acetate [MPA] in postmenopausal women. Additional risk factors include diabetes mellitus, hypercholesterolemia, hypertension, SLE, obesity, tobacco use, and/or history of venous thromboembolism (VTE). Adverse cardiovascular events have also been reported in males taking estrogens for prostate cancer. Risk factors should be managed appropriately; discontinue use if adverse cardiovascular events occur or are suspected.

Estrogen compounds are generally associated with lipid effects such as increased HDL-cholesterol and decreased LDL-cholesterol. Triglycerides may also be increased; use with caution in patients with familial defects of lipoprotein metabolism. Whenever possible, estrogens should be discontinued at least 4-6 weeks prior to elective surgery associated with an increased risk of thromboembolism or during periods of prolonged immobilization. Women with inherited thrombophilias (eg, protein C or S deficiency) may have increased risk of venous thromboembolism (DeSancho, 2010; van Vlijmen, 2011).

Neurological considerations: **[U.S. Boxed Warning]: Estrogens with or without progestin should not be used to prevent dementia. In the Women's Health Initiative Memory Study (WHIMS), an increased incidence of dementia was observed in women ≥65 years of age taking CE alone or in combination with MPA.**

Cancer-related considerations: **[U.S. Boxed Warning]: Based on data from the Women's Health Initiative (WHI) studies, an increased risk of invasive breast cancer was observed in postmenopausal women using conjugated estrogens (CE) in combination with medroxyprogesterone acetate (MPA).** This risk may be associated with duration of use and declines once combined therapy is discontinued (Chlebowski, 2009). The risk of invasive breast cancer was decreased in postmenopausal women with a hysterectomy using CE only, regardless of weight. However, the risk was not significantly decreased in women at high risk for breast cancer (family history of breast cancer, personal history of benign breast disease) (Anderson, 2012). An increase in abnormal mammogram findings has also been reported with estrogen alone or in combination with progestin therapy. Estrogen use may also lead to severe hypercalcemia in patients with breast cancer and bone metastases; discontinue estrogen if hypercalcemia occurs. Use is contraindicated in patients with known or suspected breast cancer. **[U.S. Boxed Warning]: The use of unopposed estrogen in women with an intact uterus is associated with an increased risk of endometrial cancer. The addition of a progestin to estrogen therapy may decrease the risk of endometrial hyperplasia, a precursor to endometrial cancer. Adequate diagnostic measures, including endometrial sampling if indicated, should be performed to rule out malignancy in postmenopausal women with undiagnosed abnormal vaginal bleeding.** Estrogens may exacerbate endometriosis. Malignant transformation of residual endometrial implants has been reported posthysterectomy with unopposed estrogen therapy. Consider adding a progestin in women with residual endometriosis posthysterectomy. Postmenopausal estrogen therapy and combined estrogen/progesterone therapy may increase the risk of ovarian cancer; however, the absolute risk to an individual woman is small. Although results from various studies are not consistent, risk does not appear to be significantly associated with the duration, route, or dose of therapy. In one study, the risk decreased after 2 years following discontinuation of therapy (Mørch, 2009). Although the risk of ovarian cancer is rare, women who are at an increased risk (eg, family history) should be counseled about the association (NAMS, 2012).

Estrogens may cause retinal vascular thrombosis; discontinue if migraine, loss of vision, proptosis, diplopia, or other visual disturbances occur; discontinue permanently if papilledema or retinal vascular lesions are observed on examination. Use caution in patients with asthma, epilepsy, hepatic hemangiomas, hereditary angioedema, migraine, porphyria, or SLE; may exacerbate disease. May have adverse effects on glucose tolerance; use caution in women with diabetes. Use with caution in patients with diseases which may be exacerbated by fluid retention, including cardiac or renal dysfunction. Use of postmenopausal estrogen may be associated with an increased risk of gallbladder disease requiring surgery. Estrogens are poorly metabolized in patients with hepatic dysfunction. Use caution with a history of cholestatic jaundice associated with prior estrogen use or pregnancy. Discontinue if jaundice develops or if acute or chronic hepatic disturbances occur. Use is contraindicated with hepatic disease. Use with caution in patients with severe hypocalcemia. Estrogens may increase thyroid-binding globulin (TBG) levels leading to increased circulating total thyroid hormone levels. Women on thyroid replacement therapy may require higher doses of thyroid hormone while receiving estrogens.

Avoid use of oral estrogen (with or without progestins) in the elderly due to potential of increased risk of breast and endometrial cancers, and lack of proven cardioprotection and cognitive protection (Beers Criteria). Whenever possible, estrogens should be discontinued at least 4-6 weeks prior to elective surgery associated with an increased risk of thromboembolism or during periods of prolonged immobilization. The use of estrogens and/or progestins may change the results of some laboratory tests (eg, coagulation factors, lipids, glucose tolerance, binding proteins). The dose, route, and the specific estrogen/progestin influences these changes. In addition, personal risk factors (eg, cardiovascular disease, smoking, diabetes, age) also contribute to adverse events; use of specific products may be contraindicated in women with certain risk factors.

ESTROGENS (CONJUGATED A/SYNTHETIC)

[U.S. Boxed Warning]: Estrogens with or without progestin should be used for the shortest duration possible at the lowest effective dose consistent with treatment goals. Before prescribing estrogen therapy to postmenopausal women, the risks and benefits must be weighed for each patient. Women should be informed of these risks and benefits, as well as possible effects of progestin when added to estrogen therapy. Patients should be reevaluated as clinically appropriate to determine if treatment is still necessary. Available data related to treatment risks are from Women's Health Initiative (WHI) studies, which evaluated oral CE 0.625 mg with or without MPA 2.5 mg relative to placebo in postmenopausal women. Other combinations and dosage forms of estrogens and progestins were not studied. **Outcomes reported from clinical trials using CE with or without MPA should be assumed to be similar for other doses and other dosage forms of estrogens and progestins until comparable data becomes available.**

Vulvar and vaginal atrophy use: When used solely for the treatment of vulvar and vaginal atrophy, topical vaginal products should be considered.

Adverse Reactions (Reflective of adult population; not specific for elderly)
>10%:
  Central nervous system: Headache (11% to 68%), dizziness (11%), pain (11%)
  Endocrine & metabolic: Breast pain (29%), endometrial thickening (19%), metrorrhagia (14%)
  Gastrointestinal: Abdominal pain (9% to 28%), nausea (9% to 18%)
  Neuromuscular & skeletal: Paresthesia (8% to 33%), back pain (14%)
  Respiratory: Upper respiratory tract infection (13%)
  Miscellaneous: Infection (2% to 14%)
1% to 10%:
  Central nervous system: Anxiety (6%), fever (1%)
  Gastrointestinal: Dyspepsia (10%), vomiting (7%), constipation (6%), diarrhea (6%), weight gain (6%)
  Genitourinary: Vaginitis (8%)
  Neuromuscular & skeletal: Leg cramps (10%), hypertonia (6%)
  Respiratory: Rhinitis (6% to 8%), cough (6%)

In addition, the following have been reported with estrogen and/or progestin therapy:
  Cardiovascular: Edema, hypertension, MI, stroke, venous thromboembolism
  Central nervous system: Epilepsy exacerbation, irritability, mental depression, migraine, mood disturbances, nervousness
  Dermatologic: Angioedema, chloasma, erythema multiforme, erythema nodosum, hemorrhagic eruption, hirsutism, melasma, pruritus, rash, scalp hair loss, urticaria
  Endocrine & metabolic: Breast cancer, breast enlargement, breast tenderness, glucose tolerance impaired, HDL-cholesterol increased, hyper-/hypocalcemia, LDL-cholesterol decreased, libido changes, serum triglycerides/phospholipids increased, thyroid-binding globulin increased, total thyroid hormone (T_4) increased
  Gastrointestinal: Abdominal cramps, bloating, cholecystitis, cholelithiasis, gallbladder disease, pancreatitis, weight gain/loss
  Genitourinary: Alterations in frequency and flow of menses, cervical secretion changes, endometrial cancer, endometrial hyperplasia, uterine leiomyomata size increased, vaginal candidiasis
  Hematologic: Aggravation of porphyria, antithrombin III and antifactor Xa decreased, fibrinogen levels increased, platelet aggregability and platelet count increased; prothrombin and factors VII, VIII, IX, X increased
  Hepatic: Cholestatic jaundice, hepatic hemangiomas enlarged
  Neuromuscular & skeletal: Arthralgias, chorea, leg cramps
  Local: Thrombophlebitis
  Ocular: Contact lens intolerance, retinal vascular thrombosis, corneal curvature steepening
  Respiratory: Asthma exacerbation, pulmonary thromboembolism
  Miscellaneous: Anaphylactoid/anaphylactic reactions, carbohydrate intolerance

Drug Interactions
Metabolism/Transport Effects Substrate of CYP1A2 (major), CYP2A6 (minor), CYP2B6 (minor), CYP2C19 (minor), CYP2C9 (minor), CYP2D6 (minor), CYP2E1 (minor), CYP3A4 (major); **Note:** Assignment of Major/Minor substrate status based on clinically relevant drug interaction potential; **Inhibits** CYP1A2 (weak); **Induces** CYP3A4 (weak/moderate)

Avoid Concomitant Use
  Avoid concomitant use of Estrogens (Conjugated A/Synthetic) with any of the following: Anastrozole; Axitinib

Increased Effect/Toxicity
  Estrogens (Conjugated A/Synthetic) may increase the levels/effects of: Corticosteroids (Systemic); ROPINIRole; Tipranavir

The levels/effects of Estrogens (Conjugated A/Synthetic) may be increased by: Ascorbic Acid; Herbs (Estrogenic Properties)

Decreased Effect

Estrogens (Conjugated A/Synthetic) may decrease the levels/effects of: Anastrozole; ARIPiprazole; Axitinib; Chenodiol; Hyaluronidase; Saxagliptin; Somatropin; Thyroid Products; Ursodiol

The levels/effects of Estrogens (Conjugated A/Synthetic) may be decreased by: CYP1A2 Inducers (Strong); CYP3A4 Inducers (Strong); Cyproterone; Deferasirox; Herbs (CYP3A4 Inducers); Peginterferon Alfa-2b; Tipranavir; Tocilizumab

Ethanol/Nutrition/Herb Interactions

Ethanol: Avoid ethanol (routine use increases estrogen plasma concentrations and risk of breast cancer).

Food: Grapefruit juice may increase estrogen plasma concentrations, leading to increased adverse effects.

Herb/Nutraceutical: St John's wort may decrease levels. Herbs with estrogenic properties may enhance the adverse/toxic effect of estrogen derivatives; examples include alfalfa, black cohosh, bloodroot, hops, kudzu, licorice, red clover, saw palmetto, soybean, thyme, wild yam, yucca.

Stability Store at room temperature of 25°C (77°F).

Mechanism of Action Conjugated A/synthetic estrogens contain a mixture of 9 synthetic estrogen substances, including sodium estrone sulfate, sodium equilin sulfate, sodium 17 alpha-dihydroequilin, sodium 17 alpha-estradiol and sodium 17 beta-dihydroequilin. Estrogens are responsible for the development and maintenance of the female reproductive system and secondary sexual characteristics. Estradiol is the principle intracellular human estrogen and is more potent than estrone and estriol at the receptor level; it is the primary estrogen secreted prior to menopause. Following menopause, estrone and estrone sulfate are more highly produced. Estrogens modulate the pituitary secretion of gonadotropins, luteinizing hormone, and follicle-stimulating hormone through a negative feedback system; estrogen replacement reduces elevated levels of these hormones in postmenopausal women.

Pharmacodynamics/Kinetics

Absorption: Well absorbed over a period of several hours

Protein-binding: Sex hormone-binding globulin (SHBG) and albumin

Metabolism: Hepatic via CYP3A4; estradiol is converted to estrone and estriol; also undergoes enterohepatic recirculation; estrone sulfate is the main metabolite in postmenopausal women

Excretion: Urine (primarily estriol, also as estradiol, estrone, and conjugates)

Dosage

Geriatric Refer to adult dosing. A higher incidence of stroke and invasive breast cancer were observed in women >75 years in a WHI substudy using conjugated equine estrogen.

Adult The lowest dose that will control symptoms should be used. Medication should be discontinued as soon as possible.

Menopause, moderate-to-severe vasomotor symptoms: Oral: 0.45 mg/day; may be titrated up to 1.25 mg/day; attempts to discontinue medication should be made at 3- to 6-month intervals

Vulvar and vaginal atrophy: Oral: 0.3 mg/day

Monitoring Parameters Yearly physical examination that includes blood pressure and Papanicolaou smear, breast exam, mammogram. Monitor for signs of endometrial cancer in female patients with uterus. Adequate diagnostic measures, including endometrial sampling, if indicated, should be performed to rule out malignancy in all cases of undiagnosed abnormal vaginal bleeding. Monitor for loss of vision, sudden onset of proptosis, diplopia, migraine; signs and symptoms of thromboembolic disorders; glycemic control in patients with diabetes; lipid profiles in patients being treated for hyperlipidemias; thyroid function in patients on thyroid hormone replacement therapy.

Menopausal symptoms: Assess need for therapy at 3- to 6-month intervals

Test Interactions Reduced response to metyrapone test observed with conjugated estrogens (equine).

Pharmacotherapy Pearls Not biologically equivalent to conjugated estrogens from equine source. Contains 9 unique estrogenic compounds (equine source contains at least 10 active estrogenic compounds).

Special Geriatric Considerations Before prescribing estrogen therapy to postmenopausal women, the risks and benefits must be weighed for each patient. Women should be informed of these risks and benefits, as well as possible side effects and the return of menstrual bleeding (when cycled with a progestin), and be involved in the decision to prescribe. A higher incidence of stroke and invasive breast cancer were observed in women >75 years in a WHI substudy using conjugated equine estrogen.

This medication is considered to be potentially inappropriate in this patient population (Beers Criteria: Quality of evidence - high; Strength of recommendation - strong).

Dosage Forms Excipient information presented when available (limited, particularly for generics); consult specific product labeling.

Tablet, oral:

Cenestin®: 0.3 mg, 0.45 mg, 0.625 mg, 0.9 mg, 1.25 mg

Estrogens (Conjugated B/Synthetic)

(ES troe jenz, KON joo gate ed, bee, sin THET ik)

Related Information

Beers Criteria − Potentially Inappropriate Medications for Geriatrics *on page 2183*

Medication Safety Issues

Sound-alike/look-alike issues:

Enjuvia™ may be confused with Januvia®

BEERS Criteria medication:

This drug may be potentially inappropriate for use in geriatric patients (Quality of evidence - high; Strength of recommendation - strong).

Brand Names: U.S. Enjuvia™

Generic Availability (U.S.) No

Pharmacologic Category Estrogen Derivative

Use Treatment of moderate-to-severe vasomotor symptoms of menopause; treatment of vulvar and vaginal atrophy associated with menopause; treatment of moderate-to-severe vaginal dryness and pain with intercourse associated with menopause

Contraindications Hypersensitivity to estrogens or any component of the formulation; undiagnosed abnormal vaginal bleeding; history of or current thrombophlebitis or venous thromboembolic disorders (including DVT, PE); active or recent (within 1 year) arterial thromboembolic disease (eg, stroke, MI); carcinoma of the breast; estrogen-dependent tumor; hepatic dysfunction or disease

Warnings/Precautions

Cardiovascular-related considerations: **[U.S. Boxed Warning]: Estrogens with or without progestin should not be used to prevent cardiovascular disease.** Using data from the Women's Health Initiative (WHI) studies, an increased risk of deep vein thrombosis (DVT) and stroke has been reported with CE and an increased risk of DVT, stroke, pulmonary emboli (PE), and myocardial infarction (MI) has been reported with CE with MPA in postmenopausal women. Additional risk factors include diabetes mellitus, hypercholesterolemia, hypertension, SLE, obesity, tobacco use, and/or history of venous thromboembolism (VTE). Risk factors should be managed appropriately; discontinue use if adverse cardiovascular events occur or are suspected. Estrogen compounds are generally associated with lipid effects such as increased HDL-cholesterol and decreased LDL-cholesterol. Triglycerides may also be increased; use with caution in patients with familial defects of lipoprotein metabolism. Whenever possible, estrogens should be discontinued at least 4-6 weeks prior to elective surgery associated with an increased risk of thromboembolism or during periods of prolonged immobilization. Women with inherited thrombophilias (eg, protein C or S deficiency) may have increased risk of venous thromboembolism (DeSancho, 2010; van Vlijmen, 2011).

Neurological considerations: [U.S. Boxed Warning]: Estrogens with or without progestin should not be used to prevent dementia. In the Women's Health Initiative Memory Study (WHIMS), an increased incidence of dementia was observed in women ≥65 years of age taking CE alone or in combination with MPA.

Cancer-related considerations: **[U.S. Boxed Warning]: Based on data from the Women's Health Initiative (WHI) studies, an increased risk of invasive breast cancer was observed in postmenopausal women using conjugated estrogens (CE) in combination with medroxyprogesterone acetate (MPA).** This risk may be associated with duration of use and declines once combined therapy is discontinued (Chlebowski, 2009). The risk of invasive breast cancer was decreased in postmenopausal women with a hysterectomy using CE only, regardless of weight. However, the risk was not significantly decreased in women at high risk for breast cancer (family history of breast cancer, personal history of benign breast disease) (Anderson, 2012). An increase in abnormal mammogram findings has also been reported with estrogen alone or in combination with progestin therapy. Estrogen use may also lead to severe hypercalcemia in patients with breast cancer and bone metastases; discontinue estrogen if hypercalcemia occurs. Use is contraindicated in patients with known or suspected breast cancer. **[U.S. Boxed Warning]: The use of unopposed estrogen in women with an intact uterus is associated with an increased risk of endometrial cancer. The addition of a progestin to estrogen therapy may decrease the risk of endometrial hyperplasia, a precursor to endometrial cancer. Adequate diagnostic measures, including endometrial sampling if indicated, should be performed to rule out malignancy in postmenopausal**

women with undiagnosed abnormal vaginal bleeding. Estrogens may exacerbate endometriosis. Malignant transformation of residual endometrial implants has been reported posthysterectomy with unopposed estrogen therapy. Consider adding a progestin in women with residual endometriosis posthysterectomy. Postmenopausal estrogen therapy and combined estrogen/progesterone therapy may increase the risk of ovarian cancer; however, the absolute risk to an individual woman is small. Although results from various studies are not consistent, risk does not appear to be significantly associated with the duration, route, or dose of therapy. In one study, the risk decreased after 2 years following discontinuation of therapy (Mørch, 2009). Although the risk of ovarian cancer is rare, women who are at an increased risk (eg, family history) should be counseled about the association (NAMS, 2012).

Estrogens may cause retinal vascular thrombosis; discontinue if migraine, loss of vision, proptosis, diplopia, or other visual disturbances occur; discontinue permanently if papilledema or retinal vascular lesions are observed on examination. Use caution in patients with asthma, epilepsy, hepatic hemangiomas, hereditary angioedema, migraine, porphyria, or SLE; may exacerbate disease. May have adverse effects on glucose tolerance; use caution in women with diabetes. Use with caution in patients with diseases which may be exacerbated by fluid retention, including cardiac or renal dysfunction. Use of postmenopausal estrogen may be associated with an increased risk of gallbladder disease requiring surgery. Estrogens are poorly metabolized in patients with hepatic dysfunction. Use caution with a history of cholestatic jaundice associated with prior estrogen use. Discontinue if jaundice develops or if acute or chronic hepatic disturbances occur. Use is contraindicated with hepatic disease. Use with caution in patients with severe hypocalcemia. Estrogens may increase thyroid-binding globulin (TBG) levels leading to increased circulating total thyroid hormone levels. Women on thyroid replacement therapy may require higher doses of thyroid hormone while receiving estrogens. Avoid use of oral estrogen (with or without progestins) in the elderly due to potential of increased risk of breast and endometrial cancers, and lack of proven cardioprotection and cognitive protection (Beers Criteria). Whenever possible, estrogens should be discontinued at least 4-6 weeks prior to elective surgery associated with an increased risk of thromboembolism or during periods of prolonged immobilization. The use of estrogens and/or progestins may change the results of some laboratory tests (eg, coagulation factors, lipids, glucose tolerance, binding proteins). The dose, route, and the specific estrogen/progestin influences these changes. In addition, personal risk factors (eg, cardiovascular disease, smoking, diabetes, age) also contribute to adverse events; use of specific products may be contraindicated in women with certain risk factors.

[U.S. Boxed Warning]: Estrogens with or without progestin should be used for the shortest duration possible at the lowest effective dose consistent with treatment goals. Before prescribing estrogen therapy to postmenopausal women, the risks and benefits must be weighed for each patient. Women should be informed of these risks and benefits, as well as possible effects of progestin when added to estrogen therapy. Patients should be reevaluated as clinically appropriate to determine if treatment is still necessary. Available data related to treatment risks are from Women's Health Initiative (WHI) studies, which evaluated oral CE 0.625 mg with or without MPA 2.5 mg relative to placebo in postmenopausal women. Other combinations and dosage forms of estrogens and progestins were not studied. **Outcomes reported from clinical trials using CE with or without MPA should be assumed to be similar for other doses and other dosage forms of estrogens and progestins until comparable data becomes available.** When used solely for the treatment of vaginal dryness and pain with intercourse, or vulvar and vaginal atrophy, topical vaginal products should be considered.

Adverse Reactions (Reflective of adult population; not specific for elderly)
>10%:
  Central nervous system: Headache (15% to 25%), pain (10% to 19%)
  Endocrine & metabolic: Breast pain (up to 14%)
  Gastrointestinal: Abdominal pain (4% to 15%), nausea (7% to 12%)
1% to 10%:
  Central nervous system: Dizziness (1% to 7%)
  Endocrine & metabolic: Dysmenorrhea (1% to 8%)
  Gastrointestinal: Flatulence (4% to 7%)
  Genitourinary: Vaginitis (2% to 7%)
  Neuromuscular & skeletal: Paresthesia (up to 6%)
  Respiratory: Bronchitis (up to 7%), rhinitis (4% to 7%), sinusitis (3% to 7%)
  Miscellaneous: Flu-like syndrome (4% to 7%)
In addition, the following have been reported with estrogen and/or progestin therapy:
  Cardiovascular: Edema, hypertension, MI, stroke, venous thromboembolism
  Central nervous system: Epilepsy exacerbation, irritability, mental depression, migraine, mood disturbances, nervousness

ESTROGENS (CONJUGATED B/SYNTHETIC)

◄

Dermatologic: Angioedema, chloasma, erythema multiforme, erythema nodosum, hemorrhagic eruption, hirsutism, loss of scalp hair, melasma, pruritus, rash, urticaria

Endocrine & metabolic: Breast cancer, breast enlargement, breast tenderness, HDL-cholesterol increased, hyper-/hypocalcemia, impaired glucose tolerance, LDL-cholesterol decreased, libido (changes in), serum triglycerides/phospholipids increased, thyroid-binding globulin increased, total thyroid hormone (T_4) increased

Gastrointestinal: Abdominal cramps, bloating, cholecystitis, cholelithiasis, gallbladder disease, pancreatitis, weight gain/loss

Genitourinary: Alterations in frequency and flow of menses, changes in cervical secretions, endometrial cancer, endometrial hyperplasia, increased size of uterine leiomyomata, vaginal candidiasis

Hematologic: Aggravation of porphyria; antithrombin III and antifactor Xa decreased; fibrinogen levels increased; platelet aggregability and platelet count increased; prothrombin and factors VII, VIII, IX, X increased

Hepatic: Cholestatic jaundice, hepatic hemangiomas enlarged

Local: Thrombophlebitis

Neuromuscular & skeletal: Arthralgias, chorea, leg cramps

Ocular: Contact lens intolerance, corneal curvature steepening, retinal vascular thrombosis

Respiratory: Asthma exacerbation, pulmonary thromboembolism

Miscellaneous: Anaphylactoid/anaphylactic reactions, carbohydrate intolerance

Drug Interactions

Metabolism/Transport Effects Substrate of CYP3A4 (major); **Note:** Assignment of Major/Minor substrate status based on clinically relevant drug interaction potential

Avoid Concomitant Use

Avoid concomitant use of Estrogens (Conjugated B/Synthetic) with any of the following: Anastrozole

Increased Effect/Toxicity

Estrogens (Conjugated B/Synthetic) may increase the levels/effects of: Corticosteroids (Systemic); ROPINIRole; Tipranavir

The levels/effects of Estrogens (Conjugated B/Synthetic) may be increased by: Ascorbic Acid; Herbs (Estrogenic Properties)

Decreased Effect

Estrogens (Conjugated B/Synthetic) may decrease the levels/effects of: Anastrozole; Chenodiol; Hyaluronidase; Somatropin; Thyroid Products; Ursodiol

The levels/effects of Estrogens (Conjugated B/Synthetic) may be decreased by: CYP3A4 Inducers (Strong); Deferasirox; Herbs (CYP3A4 Inducers); Tipranavir; Tocilizumab

Ethanol/Nutrition/Herb Interactions

Ethanol: Avoid ethanol (routine use increases estrogen plasma concentrations and risk of breast cancer).

Food: Grapefruit juice may increase estrogen plasma concentrations, leading to increased adverse effects.

Herb/Nutraceutical: St John's wort may decrease levels. Herbs with estrogenic properties may enhance the adverse/toxic effect of estrogen derivatives; examples include alfalfa, black cohosh, bloodroot, hops, kudzu, licorice, red clover, saw palmetto, soybean, thyme, wild yam, and yucca.

Stability Store at room temperature of 25°C (77°F).

Mechanism of Action Conjugated B/synthetic estrogens contain a mixture of 10 synthetic estrogen substances, including sodium estrone sulfate, sodium equilin sulfate, sodium 17-alpha-dihydroequilin, sodium 17-alpha-estradiol, and sodium 17-beta-dihydroequilin. Estrogens are responsible for the development and maintenance of the female reproductive system and secondary sexual characteristics. Estradiol is the principle intracellular human estrogen and is more potent than estrone and estriol at the receptor level; it is the primary estrogen secreted prior to menopause. Following menopause, estrone and estrone sulfate are more highly produced. Estrogens modulate the pituitary secretion of gonadotropins, luteinizing hormone, and follicle-stimulating hormone through a negative feedback system; estrogen replacement reduces elevated levels of these hormones in postmenopausal women.

Pharmacodynamics/Kinetics

Absorption: Well absorbed over a period of several hours

Protein-binding: Sex hormone-binding globulin (SHBG) and albumin

Metabolism: Hepatic via CYP3A4; estradiol is converted to estrone and estriol; also undergoes enterohepatic recirculation; estrone sulfate is the main metabolite in postmenopausal women

Half-life elimination: Conjugated estrone: 8-20 hours; conjugated equilin: 5-17 hours

Excretion: Urine (primarily estriol, also as estradiol, estrone, and conjugates)

Dosage

Geriatric Refer to adult dosing. A higher incidence of stroke and invasive breast cancer were observed in women >75 years in a WHI substudy using conjugated equine estrogen.

Adult The lowest dose that will control symptoms should be used. Medication should be discontinued as soon as possible.

Menopause, moderate-to-severe vasomotor symptoms: Oral: 0.3 mg/day; may be titrated up to 1.25 mg/day. Attempts to discontinue medication should be made at 3- to 6-month intervals.

Vaginal dryness/vulvar and vaginal atrophy associated with menopause: Oral: 0.3 mg/day. Attempts to discontinue medication should be made at 3- to 6-month intervals.

Monitoring Parameters Yearly physical examination that may include blood pressure and Papanicolaou smear, breast exam, mammogram. Monitor for signs of endometrial cancer in female patients with uterus. Adequate diagnostic measures, including endometrial sampling, if indicated, should be performed to rule out malignancy in all cases of undiagnosed abnormal vaginal bleeding. Monitor for loss of vision, sudden onset of proptosis, diplopia, migraine; signs and symptoms of thromboembolic disorders; glycemic control in patients with diabetes; lipid profiles in patients being treated for hyperlipidemias; thyroid function in patients on thyroid hormone replacement therapy.

Test Interactions Reduced response to metyrapone test observed with conjugated estrogens (equine).

Pharmacotherapy Pearls Not biologically equivalent to conjugated estrogens from equine source. Contains 10 unique estrogenic compounds (equine source contains at least 10 active estrogenic compounds).

Special Geriatric Considerations Enjuvia™ has not been studied in an elderly population. Before prescribing estrogen therapy to postmenopausal women, the risks and benefits must be weighed for each patient. Women should be informed of these risks and benefits, as well as possible side effects and the return of menstrual bleeding (when cycled with a progestin), and be involved in the decision to prescribe. A higher incidence of stroke and invasive breast cancer was observed in women >75 years of age in a WHI substudy.

This medication is considered to be potentially inappropriate in this patient population (Beers Criteria: Quality of evidence - high; Strength of recommendation - strong).

Dosage Forms Excipient information presented when available (limited, particularly for generics); consult specific product labeling.

Tablet, oral:

Enjuvia™: 0.3 mg, 0.45 mg, 0.625 mg, 0.9 mg, 1.25 mg

Estrogens (Conjugated/Equine, Systemic)
(ES troe jenz KON joo gate ed, EE kwine)

Related Information

Beers Criteria – Potentially Inappropriate Medications for Geriatrics *on page 2183*

Medication Safety Issues

Sound-alike/look-alike issues:

Premarin® may be confused with Primaxin®, Provera®, Remeron®

BEERS Criteria medication:

This drug may be potentially inappropriate for use in geriatric patients (Quality of evidence - high [oral]; Strength of recommendation - strong [oral]).

Brand Names: U.S. Premarin®

Brand Names: Canada C.E.S.®; Congest; PMS-Conjugated Estrogens C.S.D.; Premarin®

Index Terms C.E.S.; CE; CEE; Conjugated Estrogen; Estrogenic Substances, Conjugated

Generic Availability (U.S.) No

Pharmacologic Category Estrogen Derivative

Use Treatment of moderate-to-severe vasomotor symptoms associated with menopause; treatment of vulvar and vaginal atrophy due to menopause; hypoestrogenism (due to hypogonadism, castration, or primary ovarian failure); prostatic cancer (palliation); breast cancer (palliation); postmenopausal osteoporosis (prophylaxis); abnormal uterine bleeding

Unlabeled Use Uremic bleeding

Contraindications Angioedema or anaphylactic reaction to estrogens or any component of the formulation; undiagnosed abnormal vaginal bleeding; history of or current thrombophlebitis or venous thromboembolic disorders (including DVT, PE); active or history of arterial thromboembolic disease (eg, stroke, MI); carcinoma of the breast (except in appropriately selected patients being treated for metastatic disease); estrogen-dependent tumor; hepatic dysfunction or disease; known protein C, protein S, antithrombin deficiency or other known thrombophilic disorders

Canadian labeling: Additional contraindications (not in U.S. labeling): Endometrial hyperplasia; partial or complete vision loss due to ophthalmic vascular disease; migraine with aura

Warnings/Precautions

Anaphylaxis requiring emergency medical management has been reported within minutes to hours of taking conjugated estrogen (CE) tablets. Angioedema involving the face, feet, hands, larynx, and tongue has also been reported. Exogenous estrogens may exacerbate symptoms in women with hereditary angioedema.

[U.S. Boxed Warning]: **Based on data from the Women's Health Initiative (WHI) studies, an increased risk of invasive breast cancer was observed in postmenopausal women using conjugated estrogens (CE) in combination with medroxyprogesterone acetate (MPA).** This risk may be associated with duration of use and declines once combined therapy is discontinued (Chlebowski, 2009). The risk of invasive breast cancer was decreased in postmenopausal women with a hysterectomy using CE only, regardless of weight. However, the risk was not significantly decreased in women at high risk for breast cancer (family history of breast cancer, personal history of benign breast disease) (Anderson, 2012). An increase in abnormal mammogram findings has also been reported with estrogen alone or in combination with progestin therapy. Estrogen use may lead to severe hypercalcemia in patients with breast cancer and bone metastases; discontinue estrogen if hypercalcemia occurs. [U.S. Boxed Warning]: **The use of unopposed estrogen in women with an intact uterus is associated with an increased risk of endometrial cancer. The addition of a progestin to estrogen therapy may decrease the risk of endometrial hyperplasia, a precursor to endometrial cancer. Adequate diagnostic measures, including endometrial sampling if indicated, should be performed to rule out malignancy in postmenopausal women with undiagnosed abnormal vaginal bleeding.** Estrogens may exacerbate endometriosis. Malignant transformation of residual endometrial implants has been reported posthysterectomy with unopposed estrogen therapy. Consider adding a progestin in women with residual endometriosis posthysterectomy. Postmenopausal estrogen therapy and combined estrogen/progesterone therapy may increase the risk of ovarian cancer; however, the absolute risk to an individual woman is small. Although results from various studies are not consistent, risk does not appear to be significantly associated with the duration, route, or dose of therapy. In one study, the risk decreased after 2 years following discontinuation of therapy (Mørch, 2009). Although the risk of ovarian cancer is rare, women who are at an increased risk (eg, family history) should be counseled about the association (NAMS, 2012).

[U.S. Boxed Warning]: **Estrogens with or without progestin should not be used to prevent cardiovascular disease.** Using data from the Women's Health Initiative (WHI) studies, an increased risk of deep vein thrombosis (DVT) and stroke has been reported with CE and an increased risk of DVT, stroke, pulmonary emboli (PE) and myocardial infarction (MI) has been reported with CE with MPA in postmenopausal women. Additional risk factors include diabetes mellitus, hypercholesterolemia, hypertension, SLE, obesity, tobacco use, and/or history of venous thromboembolism (VTE). Adverse cardiovascular events have also been reported in males taking estrogens for prostate cancer. Risk factors should be managed appropriately; discontinue use if adverse cardiovascular events occur or are suspected. Women with inherited thrombophilias (eg, protein C or S deficiency) may have increased risk of venous thromboembolism (DeSancho, 2010; van Vlijmen, 2011). Use is contraindicated in women with protein C, protein S, antithrombin deficiency, or other known thrombophilic disorders.

[U.S. Boxed Warning]: **Estrogens with or without progestin should not be used to prevent dementia. In the Women's Health Initiative Memory Study (WHIMS), an increased incidence of dementia was observed in women ≥65 years of age taking CE alone or in combination with MPA.**

Estrogen compounds are generally associated with lipid effects such as increased HDL-cholesterol and decreased LDL-cholesterol. Triglycerides may also be increased; discontinue if pancreatitis occurs. Use with caution in patients with familial defects of lipoprotein metabolism. Estrogens may increase thyroid-binding globulin (TBG) levels leading to increased circulating total thyroid hormone levels. Women on thyroid replacement therapy may require higher doses of thyroid hormone while receiving estrogens. Use caution in patients with hypoparathyroidism; estrogen-induced hypocalcemia may occur. May have adverse effects on glucose tolerance; use caution in women with diabetes. Use caution in patients with asthma, epilepsy, hepatic hemangiomas, porphyria, or SLE; may exacerbate disease. Use with caution in patients with diseases which may be exacerbated by fluid retention, including cardiac or renal dysfunction. Use of postmenopausal estrogen may be associated with an increased risk of gallbladder disease requiring surgery. Use caution with migraine; may exacerbate disease. Canadian labeling contraindicates use in migraine with aura. Estrogens may cause retinal vascular thrombosis; discontinue if migraine, loss of vision, proptosis, diplopia, or other visual disturbances occur; discontinue permanently if papilledema or retinal vascular lesions are observed on examination.

Estrogens are poorly metabolized in patients with hepatic dysfunction. Use caution with a history of cholestatic jaundice associated with prior estrogen use or pregnancy. Discontinue if jaundice develops or if acute or chronic hepatic disturbances occur. Use is contraindicated with hepatic disease.

Whenever possible, estrogens should be discontinued at least 4-6 weeks prior to elective surgery associated with an increased risk of thromboembolism or during periods of prolonged immobilization. Avoid use of oral estrogen (with or without progestins) in the elderly due to potential of increased risk of breast and endometrial cancers, and lack of proven cardioprotection and cognitive protection (Beers Criteria). Prior to puberty, estrogens may cause premature closure of the epiphyses, premature breast development in girls or gynecomastia in boys. Vaginal bleeding and vaginal cornification may also be induced in girls. The use of estrogens and/or progestins may change the results of some laboratory tests (eg, coagulation factors, lipids, glucose tolerance, binding proteins). The dose, route, and the specific estrogen/progestin influences these changes. In addition, personal risk factors (eg, cardiovascular disease, smoking, diabetes, age) also contribute to adverse events; use of specific products may be contraindicated in women with certain risk factors.

[U.S. Boxed Warning]: Estrogens with or without progestin should be used for the shortest duration possible at the lowest effective dose consistent with treatment goals. Before prescribing estrogen therapy to postmenopausal women, the risks and benefits must be weighed for each patient. Women should be informed of these risks and benefits, as well as possible effects of progestin when added to estrogen therapy. Patients should be reevaluated as clinically appropriate to determine if treatment is still necessary. Available data related to treatment risks are from Women's Health Initiative (WHI) studies, which evaluated oral CE 0.625 mg with or without MPA 2.5 mg relative to placebo in postmenopausal women. Other combinations and dosage forms of estrogens and progestins were not studied. **Outcomes reported from clinical trials using CE with or without MPA should be assumed to be similar for other doses and other dosage forms of estrogens and progestins until comparable data becomes available.**

Vulvar and vaginal atrophy use: Moderate-to-severe symptoms of vulvar and vaginal atrophy include vaginal dryness, dyspareunia, and atrophic vaginitis. When used solely for the treatment of vulvar and vaginal atrophy, topical vaginal products should be considered (NAMS, 2007).

Osteoporosis use: For use only in women at significant risk of osteoporosis and for who other nonestrogen medications are not considered appropriate.

Adverse Reactions (Reflective of adult population; not specific for elderly)
Note: Percentages reported in postmenopausal women following oral use.

>10%:
Central nervous system: Headache (26% to 32%; placebo 28%), pain (17% to 20%; placebo 18%)
Endocrine & metabolic: Breast pain (7% to 12%; placebo 9%)
Gastrointestinal: Abdominal pain (15% to 17%), diarrhea (6% to 7%; placebo 6%)
Genitourinary: Vaginal hemorrhage (2% to 14%)
Neuromuscular & skeletal: Back pain (13% to 14%), arthralgia (7% to 14%; placebo 12%)
Respiratory: Pharyngitis (10% to 12%; placebo 11%), sinusitis: (6% to 11%; placebo 7%)

1% to 10%:
Central nervous system: Depression (5% to 8%), dizziness (4% to 6%), nervousness (2% to 5%)
Dermatologic: Pruritus (4% to 5%)
Gastrointestinal: Flatulence (6% to 7%)
Genitourinary: Vaginitis (5% to 7%), leukorrhea (4% to 7%), vaginal moniliasis (5% to 6%)
Neuromuscular & skeletal: Weakness (7% to 8%), leg cramps (3% to 7%)
Respiratory: Cough increased (4% to 7%)

Additional adverse reactions reported with injection; frequency not defined: Local: injection site: Edema, pain, phlebitis

Drug Interactions
Metabolism/Transport Effects Substrate of CYP1A2 (major), CYP2A6 (minor), CYP2B6 (minor), CYP2C19 (minor), CYP2C9 (minor), CYP2D6 (minor), CYP2E1 (minor), CYP3A4 (major); **Note:** Assignment of Major/Minor substrate status based on clinically relevant drug interaction potential; **Inhibits** CYP1A2 (weak); **Induces** CYP3A4 (weak/moderate)

Avoid Concomitant Use
Avoid concomitant use of Estrogens (Conjugated/Equine, Systemic) with any of the following: Anastrozole; Axitinib

Increased Effect/Toxicity
Estrogens (Conjugated/Equine, Systemic) may increase the levels/effects of: Corticosteroids (Systemic); ROPINIRole; Tipranavir

The levels/effects of Estrogens (Conjugated/Equine, Systemic) may be increased by: Ascorbic Acid; Herbs (Estrogenic Properties)

Decreased Effect
Estrogens (Conjugated/Equine, Systemic) may decrease the levels/effects of: Anastrozole; ARIPiprazole; Axitinib; Chenodiol; Hyaluronidase; Saxagliptin; Somatropin; Thyroid Products; Ursodiol

The levels/effects of Estrogens (Conjugated/Equine, Systemic) may be decreased by: CYP1A2 Inducers (Strong); CYP3A4 Inducers (Strong); Cyproterone; Deferasirox; Herbs (CYP3A4 Inducers); Peginterferon Alfa-2b; Tipranavir; Tocilizumab

Ethanol/Nutrition/Herb Interactions
Ethanol: Avoid ethanol (routine use increases estrogen plasma concentrations and risk of breast cancer). Ethanol may also increase the risk of osteoporosis.

Food: Folic acid absorption may be decreased.

Herb/Nutraceutical: St John's wort may decrease levels. Herbs with estrogenic properties may enhance the adverse/toxic effect of estrogen derivatives; examples include alfalfa, black cohosh, bloodroot, hops, kudzu, licorice, red clover, saw palmetto, soybean, thyme, wild yam, yucca.

Stability
Injection: Refrigerate at 2°C to 8°C (36°F to 46°F) prior to reconstitution. Reconstitute with sterile water for injection; slowly inject diluent against side wall of the vial. Agitate gently; do not shake violently. Use immediately following reconstitution.

Tablets: Store at room temperature 20°C to 25°C (68°F to 77°F).

Mechanism of Action
Conjugated estrogens contain a mixture of estrone sulfate, equilin sulfate, 17 alpha-dihydroequilin, 17 alpha-estradiol and 17 beta-dihydroequilin. Estrogens are responsible for the development and maintenance of the female reproductive system and secondary sexual characteristics. Estradiol is the principle intracellular human estrogen and is more potent than estrone and estriol at the receptor level; it is the primary estrogen secreted prior to menopause. Following menopause, estrone and estrone sulfate are more highly produced. Estrogens modulate the pituitary secretion of gonadotropins, luteinizing hormone, and follicle-stimulating hormone through a negative feedback system; estrogen replacement reduces elevated levels of these hormones in postmenopausal women.

Pharmacodynamics/Kinetics
Absorption: Well absorbed

Protein binding: Binds to sex-hormone-binding globulin and albumin

Metabolism: Hepatic via CYP3A4; estradiol is converted to estrone and estriol; also undergoes enterohepatic recirculation (avoided with vaginal administration); estrone sulfate is the main metabolite in postmenopausal women

Half-life elimination: Total estrone: 27 hours

Time to peak, plasma: Total estrone: 7 hours

Excretion: Urine (primarily estriol, also as estradiol, estrone, and conjugates

Dosage
Geriatric Refer to adult dosing. A higher incidence of stroke and breast cancer was observed in women >75 years in a WHI substudy.

Adult

Breast cancer palliation, metastatic disease in selected patients (males and females): Oral: 10 mg 3 times/day for at least 3 months

Uremic bleeding (unlabeled use): I.V.: 0.6 mg/kg/day for 5 days (Livio, 1986)

Androgen-dependent prostate cancer palliation (males): Oral: 1.25-2.5 mg 3 times/day

Prevention of postmenopausal osteoporosis: Oral:
U.S. labeling: Initial: 0.3 mg/day cyclically* or daily, depending on medical assessment of patient. Dose may be adjusted based on bone mineral density and clinical response. The lowest effective dose should be used.

Canadian labeling: 0.625 mg once daily

Menopause (moderate-to-severe vasomotor symptoms): Oral: Initial: 0.3 mg/day. May be given cyclically* or daily, depending on medical assessment of patient. Adjust dose based on patient's response. The lowest dose that will control symptoms should be used.

Vulvar and vaginal atrophy: Oral: Initial: 0.3 mg/day. The lowest dose that will control symptoms should be used. May be given cyclically* or daily, depending on medical assessment of patient. Adjust dose based on patient's response.

Female hypogonadism: Oral: 0.3-0.625 mg/day given cyclically*; dose may be titrated in 6- to 12-month intervals; progestin treatment should be added to maintain bone mineral density once skeletal maturity is achieved.

Female castration, primary ovarian failure: Oral: 1.25 mg/day given cyclically*; adjust according to severity of symptoms and patient response. For maintenance, adjust to the lowest effective dose.

Abnormal uterine bleeding: Acute/heavy bleeding:

Oral (unlabeled route): 10-20 mg/day in 4 divided doses has been used in place of I.M./I.V. doses (ACOG, 2000)

I.M., I.V.: 25 mg, may repeat in 6-12 hours if needed (manufacturer's labeling) **or** 25 mg I.V. repeated every 4 hours for 24 hours (ACOG, 2000). Patients who do not respond to 1-2 doses should be re-evaluated (ACOG, 2000).

Note: Treatment should be followed by a low-dose oral contraceptive; medroxyprogesterone acetate along with or following estrogen therapy can also be given

*Cyclic administration: Either 3 weeks on, 1 week off **or** 25 days on, 5 days off

Renal Impairment No dosage adjustment provided in manufacturer's labeling (has not been studied). Use with caution; may increase risk of fluid retention.

Hepatic Impairment Use is contraindicated with hepatic dysfunction or disease.

Administration

Injection: May also be administered intramuscularly; when administered I.V., drug should be administered slowly to avoid the occurrence of a flushing reaction

Oral tablet: Administer at bedtime to minimize adverse effects. May be administered without regard to meals.

Abnormal uterine bleeding: High-dose therapy (eg. 10-20 mg/day) may cause nausea; consider concomitant use of an antiemetic

Monitoring Parameters Routine physical examination that includes blood pressure and Papanicolaou smear, breast exam, mammogram. Monitor for signs of endometrial cancer in female patients with uterus. Adequate diagnostic measures, including endometrial sampling, if indicated, should be performed to rule out malignancy in all cases of undiagnosed abnormal vaginal bleeding. Monitor for loss of vision, sudden onset of proptosis, diplopia, migraine; signs and symptoms of thromboembolic disorders; glycemic control in patients with diabetes; lipid profiles in patients being treated for hyperlipidemias; thyroid function in patients on thyroid hormone replacement therapy.

Menopausal symptoms: Assess need for therapy at 3- to 6-month intervals

Prevention of osteoporosis: Bone density measurement

Uremic bleeding: Bleeding time

Reference Range Adults:

Males: 15-40 mcg/24 hours (SI: 52-139 micromole/day)

Females: Postmenopausal: <20 mcg/24 hours (SI: <69 micromole/day)

Test Interactions Reduced response to metyrapone test.

Special Geriatric Considerations Before prescribing estrogen therapy to postmenopausal women, the risks and benefits must be weighed for each patient. Women should be informed of these risks and benefits, as well as possible side effects and the return of menstrual bleeding (when cycled with a progestin), and be involved in the decision to prescribe. A higher incidence of stroke and invasive breast cancer was observed in women >75 years in a WHI substudy.

This medication is considered to be potentially inappropriate in this patient population (Beers Criteria: Quality of evidence - high [oral]; Strength of recommendation - strong [oral]).

Dosage Forms Excipient information presented when available (limited, particularly for generics); consult specific product labeling.

Injection, powder for reconstitution:

Premarin®: 25 mg [contains lactose 200 mg]

Tablet, oral:

Premarin®: 0.3 mg, 0.45 mg, 0.625 mg, 0.9 mg, 1.25 mg

Estrogens (Conjugated/Equine, Topical)

(ES troe jenz KON joo gate ed, EE kwine)

Related Information

Beers Criteria – Potentially Inappropriate Medications for Geriatrics on page 2183

Medication Safety Issues

Sound-alike/look-alike issues:

Premarin® may be confused with Primaxin®, Provera®, Remeron®

BEERS Criteria medication:

This drug may be potentially inappropriate for use in geriatric patients (Quality of evidence - moderate [topical]; Strength of recommendation - weak [topical]).

Brand Names: U.S. Premarin®

Brand Names: Canada Premarin®

Index Terms C.E.S.; CE; CEE; Conjugated Estrogen; Estrogenic Substances, Conjugated

Generic Availability (U.S.) No

Pharmacologic Category Estrogen Derivative

Use Treatment of atrophic vaginitis and kraurosis vulvae; moderate-to-severe dyspareunia (pain during intercourse) due to vaginal/vulvar atrophy of menopause

Contraindications Undiagnosed abnormal vaginal bleeding; history of or current thrombophlebitis or venous thromboembolic disorders (including DVT, PE); active or history of arterial thromboembolic disease (eg, stroke, MI); carcinoma of the breast; estrogen-dependent tumor; hepatic dysfunction or disease; known protein C, protein S, antithrombin deficiency or other known thrombophilic disorders

Canadian labeling: Additional contraindications (not in U.S. labeling): Hypersensitivity to estrogens or any component of the formulation; endometrial hyperplasia; partial or complete vision loss due to ophthalmic vascular disease

Warnings/Precautions [U.S. Boxed Warning]: Based on data from the Women's Health Initiative (WHI) studies, an increased risk of invasive breast cancer was observed in postmenopausal women using conjugated estrogens (CE) in combination with medroxyprogesterone acetate (MPA). This risk may be associated with duration of use and declines once combined therapy is discontinued (Chlebowski, 2009). The risk of invasive breast cancer was decreased in postmenopausal women with a hysterectomy using CE only, regardless of weight. However, the risk was not significantly decreased in women at high risk for breast cancer (family history of breast cancer, personal history of benign breast disease) (Anderson, 2012). An increase in abnormal mammogram findings has also been reported with estrogen alone or in combination with progestin therapy. Estrogen use may lead to severe hypercalcemia in patients with breast cancer and bone metastases; discontinue estrogen if hypercalcemia occurs. Use is contraindicated in patients with known or suspected breast cancer. **[U.S. Boxed Warning]: The use of unopposed estrogen in women with an intact uterus is associated with an increased risk of endometrial cancer. The addition of a progestin to estrogen therapy may decrease the risk of endometrial hyperplasia, a precursor to endometrial cancer. Adequate diagnostic measures, including endometrial sampling if indicated, should be performed to rule out malignancy in postmenopausal women with undiagnosed abnormal vaginal bleeding.** Estrogens may exacerbate endometriosis. Malignant transformation of residual endometrial implants has been reported posthysterectomy with unopposed estrogen therapy. Consider adding a progestin in women with residual endometriosis posthysterectomy. Postmenopausal estrogen therapy and combined estrogen/progesterone therapy may increase the risk of ovarian cancer; however, the absolute risk to an individual woman is small. Although results from various studies are not consistent, risk does not appear to be significantly associated with the duration, route, or dose of therapy. In one study, the risk decreased after 2 years following discontinuation of therapy (Mørch, 2009). Although the risk of ovarian cancer is rare, women who are at an increased risk (eg, family history) should be counseled about the association (NAMS, 2012).

[U.S. Boxed Warning]: Estrogens with or without progestin should not be used to prevent cardiovascular disease. Using data from the Women's Health Initiative (WHI) studies, an increased risk of deep vein thrombosis (DVT) and stroke has been reported with CE and an increased risk of DVT, stroke, pulmonary emboli (PE) and myocardial infarction (MI) has been reported with CE with MPA in postmenopausal women. Additional risk factors include diabetes mellitus, hypercholesterolemia, hypertension, SLE, obesity, tobacco use, and/or history of venous thromboembolism (VTE). Risk factors should be managed appropriately; discontinue use if adverse cardiovascular events occur or are suspected. Women with inherited thrombophilias (eg, protein C or S deficiency) may have increased risk of venous thromboembolism (DeSancho, 2010; van Vlijmen 2011). Use is contraindicated in women with protein C, protein S, antithrombin deficiency, or other known thrombophilic disorders.

[U.S. Boxed Warning]: Estrogens with or without progestin should not be used to prevent dementia. In the Women's Health Initiative Memory Study (WHIMS), an increased incidence of dementia was observed in women ≥65 years of age taking CE alone or in combination with MPA.

Estrogen compounds are generally associated with lipid effects such as increased HDL-cholesterol and decreased LDL-cholesterol. Triglycerides may also be increased; discontinue if pancreatitis occurs. Use with caution in patients with familial defects of lipoprotein metabolism. Estrogens may increase thyroid-binding globulin (TBG) levels leading to increased circulating total thyroid hormone levels. Women on thyroid replacement therapy may require higher doses of thyroid hormone while receiving estrogens. Use caution in patients with hypoparathyroidism; estrogen induced hypocalcemia may occur. May have adverse effects on glucose tolerance; use caution in women with diabetes. Use caution in patients with asthma, epilepsy, hepatic hemangiomas, migraine, porphyria or SLE; may exacerbate disease. Use with caution in patients with diseases which may be exacerbated by fluid retention, including cardiac or renal dysfunction. Use of postmenopausal estrogen may be associated with an increased risk of gallbladder disease requiring surgery. Estrogens may cause retinal vascular thrombosis; discontinue if migraine, loss of vision, proptosis, diplopia, or other visual disturbances occur; discontinue permanently if papilledema or retinal vascular lesions are observed on examination. Exogenous estrogens may exacerbate angioedema symptoms in women with hereditary angioedema. The use of estrogens and/or progestins may change the results of some laboratory tests (eg, coagulation factors, lipids, glucose tolerance, binding proteins). The dose, route, and the specific estrogen/progestin influences these changes. In addition, personal risk factors (eg, cardiovascular disease, smoking, diabetes, age) also contribute to adverse events; use of specific products may be contra-indicated in women with certain risk factors.

Estrogens are poorly metabolized in patients with hepatic dysfunction. Use caution with a history of cholestatic jaundice associated with prior estrogen use or pregnancy. Discontinue if jaundice develops or if acute or chronic hepatic disturbances occur. Use is contraindicated with hepatic disease.

In the elderly, low-dose intravaginal estrogen may be appropriate for use in the management of vaginal symptoms, lower urinary tract infections, and dyspareunia; in addition, evidence has shown that vaginal estrogens (particularly at estradiol doses of <25 mcg twice weekly) in the treatment of vaginal dryness is safe and effective in women with breast cancer. (Beers Criteria).

Vulvar and vaginal atrophy use: When used solely for the treatment of vulvar and vaginal atrophy, topical vaginal products should be considered. Use caution applying topical products to severely atrophic vaginal mucosa.

Whenever possible, estrogens should be discontinued at least 4-6 weeks prior to elective surgery associated with an increased risk of thromboembolism or during periods of prolonged immobilization.

[U.S. Boxed Warning]: Estrogens with or without progestin should be used for the shortest duration possible at the lowest effective dose consistent with treatment goals. Before prescribing estrogen therapy to postmenopausal women, the risks and benefits must be weighed for each patient. Women should be informed of these risks and benefits, as well as possible effects of progestin when added to estrogen therapy. Patients should be reevaluated as clinically appropriate to determine if treatment is still necessary. Available data related to treatment risks are from Women's Health Initiative (WHI) studies, which evaluated oral CE 0.625 mg with or without MPA 2.5 mg relative to placebo in postmenopausal women. Other combinations and dosage forms of estrogens and progestins were not studied. Outcomes reported from clinical trials using CE with or without MPA should be assumed to be similar for other doses and other dosage forms of estrogens and progestins until comparable data becomes available.

Moderate-to-severe symptoms of vulvar and vaginal atrophy include vaginal dryness, dyspareunia, and atrophic vaginitis. When used solely for the treatment of vulvar and vaginal atrophy, topical vaginal products should be considered. Use caution applying topical products to severely atrophic vaginal mucosa. Use of a progestin is normally not required when low-dose estrogen is applied locally and only for this purpose (NAMS, 2007).

Use of the vaginal cream may weaken latex found in condoms, diaphragms or cervical caps. Systemic absorption occurs following vaginal use; warnings, precautions, and adverse events observed with oral therapy should be considered.

Adverse Reactions (Reflective of adult population; not specific for elderly) Due to systemic absorption, other adverse effects associated with systemic therapy may also occur. Frequency of adverse events reported with daily use: 1% to 10%:

Cardiovascular: Vasodilatation (4%)
Central nervous system: Pain (7%)
Endocrine & metabolic: Breast pain (6%)
Gastrointestinal: Abdominal pain (8%)
Genitourinary: Vaginitis (6%)
Neuromuscular & skeletal: Back pain (5%), weakness (6%)

Drug Interactions

Metabolism/Transport Effects Substrate of CYP1A2 (major), CYP2A6 (minor), CYP2B6 (minor), CYP2C19 (minor), CYP2C9 (minor), CYP2D6 (minor), CYP2E1 (minor), CYP3A4 (major); **Note:** Assignment of Major/Minor substrate status based on clinically relevant drug interaction potential; **Inhibits** CYP1A2 (weak); **Induces** CYP3A4 (weak/moderate)

Avoid Concomitant Use

Avoid concomitant use of Estrogens (Conjugated/Equine, Topical) with any of the following: Anastrozole; Axitinib

Increased Effect/Toxicity

Estrogens (Conjugated/Equine, Topical) may increase the levels/effects of: Corticosteroids (Systemic); ROPINIRole; Tipranavir

The levels/effects of Estrogens (Conjugated/Equine, Topical) may be increased by: Ascorbic Acid; Herbs (Estrogenic Properties)

Decreased Effect

Estrogens (Conjugated/Equine, Topical) may decrease the levels/effects of: Anastrozole; ARIPiprazole; Axitinib; Chenodiol; Hyaluronidase; Saxagliptin; Somatropin; Thyroid Products; Ursodiol

The levels/effects of Estrogens (Conjugated/Equine, Topical) may be decreased by: CYP1A2 Inducers (Strong); CYP3A4 Inducers (Strong); Cyproterone; Deferasirox; Herbs (CYP3A4 Inducers); Peginterferon Alfa-2b; Tipranavir; Tocilizumab

Stability Vaginal cream: Store at room temperature of 20°C to 25°C (68°F to 77°F); excursions permitted to 15°C to 30°C (59°F to 86°F).

Mechanism of Action Conjugated estrogens contain a mixture of estrone sulfate, equilin sulfate, 17 alpha-dihydroequilin, 17 alpha-estradiol and 17 beta-dihydroequilin. Estrogens are responsible for the development and maintenance of the female reproductive system and secondary sexual characteristics. Estradiol is the principle intracellular human estrogen and is more potent than estrone and estriol at the receptor level; it is the primary estrogen secreted prior to menopause. Following menopause, estrone and estrone sulfate are more highly produced. Estrogens modulate the pituitary secretion of gonadotropins, luteinizing hormone, and follicle-stimulating hormone through a negative feedback system; estrogen replacement reduces elevated levels of these hormones in postmenopausal women.

Pharmacodynamics/Kinetics

Absorption: Systemic absorption occurs

Protein binding: Binds to sex-hormone-binding globulin and albumin

Metabolism: Hepatic via CYP3A4; estradiol is converted to estrone and estriol; also undergoes enterohepatic recirculation (avoided with vaginal administration); estrone sulfate is the main metabolite in postmenopausal women

Time to peak, plasma: Total estrone: 6 hours

Excretion: Urine (primarily estriol, also as estradiol, estrone, and conjugates

Dosage

Geriatric Refer to adult dosing. A higher incidence of stroke and breast cancer was observed in women >75 years in a WHI substudy.

Adult

Atrophic vaginitis, kraurosis vulvae: Adult females: Intravaginal: 0.5 g/day (range 0.5-2 g/day) administered cyclically (21 days on, 7 days off). Adjust dose based on patient response. **Note:** Canadian labeling recommends oral estrogen therapy (~1.25 mg/day for 10 days) prior to initiating topical estrogen in severe atrophic vaginitis.

Moderate-to-severe dyspareunia due to menopause: Adult females: Intravaginal: 0.5 g twice weekly (eg, Monday and Thursday) **or** once daily cyclically (21 days on, 7 days off)

Renal Impairment No dosage adjustment provided in manufacturer's labeling (has not been studied). Use with caution; may increase risk of fluid retention.

Hepatic Impairment Use is contraindicated with hepatic dysfunction or disease.

Administration Administer at bedtime to minimize adverse effects. Applicator calibrated in 0.5 g increments up to 2 g. To clean applicator, remove plunger from barrel. Wash with mild soap and warm water; do not boil or use hot water.

Monitoring Parameters Routine physical examination that includes blood pressure and Papanicolaou smear, breast exam, mammogram. Monitor for signs of endometrial cancer in female patients with uterus. Adequate diagnostic measures, including endometrial sampling, if indicated, should be performed to rule out malignancy in all cases of undiagnosed abnormal vaginal bleeding. Monitor for loss of vision, sudden onset of proptosis, diplopia, migraine; signs and symptoms of thromboembolic disorders; glycemic control in patients with diabetes; lipid profiles in patients being treated for hyperlipidemias; thyroid function in patients on thyroid hormone replacement therapy.

Test Interactions Reduced response to metyrapone test.

Special Geriatric Considerations Topical estrogen is beneficial in the management of urogenital atrophy and prevention of recurrent urinary tract infections in postmenopausal women. Topical estrogens are not void of the risks associated with oral and transdermal forms; thus, the risks and benefits must be weighed for each patient.

This medication is considered to be potentially inappropriate in this patient population (Beers Criteria: Quality of evidence - moderate [topical]; Strength of recommendation - weak [topical]).

Dosage Forms Excipient information presented when available (limited, particularly for generics); consult specific product labeling. [DSC] = Discontinued product
Cream, vaginal:
Premarin®: 0.625 mg/g (30 g, 42.5 g [DSC])

Estrogens (Conjugated/Equine) and Medroxyprogesterone
(ES troe jenz KON joo gate ed/EE kwine & me DROKS ee proe JES te rone)

Related Information
Beers Criteria – Potentially Inappropriate Medications for Geriatrics *on page* 2183
Estrogens (Conjugated/Equine, Systemic) *on page* 703
MedroxyPROGESTERone *on page* 1190

Medication Safety Issues
BEERS Criteria medication:
This drug may be potentially inappropriate for use in geriatric patients (Quality of evidence - high [oral]; Strength of recommendation - strong [oral]).

Brand Names: U.S. Premphase®; Prempro®
Brand Names: Canada Premphase®; Premplus®; Prempro®
Index Terms Medroxyprogesterone and Estrogens (Conjugated); MPA and Estrogens (Conjugated)
Generic Availability (U.S.) No
Pharmacologic Category Estrogen and Progestin Combination
Use Women with an intact uterus: Treatment of moderate-to-severe vasomotor symptoms associated with menopause; treatment of moderate-to-severe vulvar and vaginal atrophy due to menopause; postmenopausal osteoporosis (prophylaxis)
Contraindications Angioedema or anaphylactic reaction to estrogens or any component of the formulation; undiagnosed abnormal vaginal bleeding; DVT or PE (current or history of); active or history of arterial thromboembolic disease (eg, stroke, MI); carcinoma of the breast (known, suspected or history of); estrogen-dependent tumor; hepatic dysfunction or disease; known protein C, protein S, antithrombin deficiency or other known thrombophilic disorders

Warnings/Precautions

Cardiovascular-related considerations: **[U.S. Boxed Warning]: Estrogens with or without progestin should not be used to prevent cardiovascular disease.** Using data from the Women's Health Initiative (WHI) studies, an increased risk of deep vein thrombosis (DVT) and stroke has been reported with CE and an increased risk of DVT, stroke, pulmonary emboli (PE) and myocardial infarction (MI) has been reported with CE with MPA in postmenopausal women. Additional risk factors include diabetes mellitus, hypercholesterolemia, hypertension, SLE, obesity, tobacco use, and/or history of venous thromboembolism (VTE). Risk factors should be managed appropriately; discontinue use if adverse cardiovascular events occur or are suspected. Estrogen compounds are generally associated with lipid effects such as increased HDL-cholesterol and decreased LDL-cholesterol. Triglycerides may also be increased; use with caution in patients with familial defects of lipoprotein metabolism. Discontinue if pancreatitis occurs. Whenever possible, estrogens should be discontinued at least 4-6 weeks prior to elective surgery associated with an increased risk of thromboembolism or during periods of prolonged immobilization. Women with inherited thrombophilias (eg, protein C or S deficiency) may have increased risk of venous thromboembolism (DeSancho, 2010; van Vlijmen, 2011). Use is contraindicated in women with protein C, protein S, antithrombin deficiency, or other known thrombophilic disorders.

Neurological considerations: **[U.S. Boxed Warning]: The risk of dementia may be increased in postmenopausal women; increased incidence was observed in women ≥65 years of age taking CE alone or in combination with MPA.**

Cancer-related considerations: **[U.S. Boxed Warning]: Based on data from the Women's Health Initiative (WHI) studies, an increased risk of invasive breast cancer was observed in postmenopausal women using conjugated estrogens (CE) in combination with medroxyprogesterone acetate (MPA).** This risk may be associated with duration of use and declines once combined therapy is discontinued (Chlebowski, 2009). The risk of invasive breast cancer was decreased in postmenopausal women with a hysterectomy using CE only, regardless of weight. However, the risk was not significantly decreased in women at high risk for breast cancer (family history of breast cancer, personal history of benign breast disease) (Anderson, 2012). An increase in abnormal mammogram findings has also been reported with estrogen alone or in combination with progestin therapy. Estrogen use may also lead to severe hypercalcemia in patients with breast cancer and bone metastases; discontinue estrogen if hypercalcemia occurs. Use is contraindicated in patients with known or suspected breast cancer. [U.S. Boxed Warning]: The use of unopposed estrogen in women with an intact uterus is associated with an increased risk of endometrial cancer. The addition of a progestin to estrogen therapy may decrease the risk of endometrial hyperplasia, a precursor to endometrial cancer. Adequate diagnostic measures, including endometrial sampling if indicated, should be performed to rule out malignancy in postmenopausal women with undiagnosed abnormal vaginal bleeding. Estrogens may exacerbate endometriosis. Malignant transformation of residual endometrial implants has been reported posthysterectomy with unopposed estrogen therapy. Consider adding a progestin in women with residual endometriosis posthysterectomy. Postmenopausal estrogen therapy and combined estrogen/progesterone therapy may increase the risk of ovarian cancer; however, the absolute risk to an individual woman is small. Although results from various studies are not consistent, risk does not appear to be significantly associated with the duration, route, or dose of therapy. In one study, the risk decreased after 2 years following discontinuation of therapy (Mørch, 2009). Although the risk of ovarian cancer is rare, women who are at an increased risk (eg, family history) should be counseled about the association (NAMS, 2012).

Estrogens may cause retinal vascular thrombosis; discontinue if migraine, loss of vision, proptosis, diplopia, or other visual disturbances occur; discontinue permanently if papilledema or retinal vascular lesions are observed on examination. Use caution in patients with asthma, epilepsy, hepatic hemangiomas, migraine, porphyria, or SLE; may exacerbate disease. May have adverse effects on glucose tolerance; use caution in women with diabetes. Use with caution in patients with diseases which may be exacerbated by fluid retention, including cardiac or renal dysfunction. Use of postmenopausal estrogen may be associated with an increased risk of gallbladder disease requiring surgery. Estrogens are poorly metabolized in patients with hepatic dysfunction. Use caution with a history of cholestatic jaundice associated with prior estrogen use or pregnancy. Discontinue if jaundice develops or if acute or chronic hepatic disturbances occur. Use is contraindicated with hepatic disease. Use with caution in patients with severe hypocalcemia. Estrogens may increase thyroid-binding globulin (TBG) levels leading to increased circulating total thyroid hormone levels. Women on thyroid replacement therapy may require higher doses of thyroid hormone while receiving estrogens. Whenever possible, should be discontinued at least 4-6 weeks prior to elective surgery associated with an increased risk of thromboembolism or during periods of prolonged immobilization. The use of estrogens and/or progestins may change the results of some laboratory tests (eg, coagulation factors, lipids, glucose tolerance, binding proteins). The dose, route, and the specific estrogen/progestin influences these changes. In addition, personal risk factors (eg, cardiovascular disease, smoking, diabetes, age) also contribute to adverse events; use of specific products may be contraindicated in women with certain risk factors.

[U.S. Boxed Warning]: Estrogens with or without progestin should be used for the shortest duration possible at the lowest effective dose consistent with treatment goals. Before prescribing estrogen therapy to postmenopausal women, the risks and benefits must be weighed for each patient. Women should be informed of these risks and benefits, as well as possible effects of progestin when added to estrogen therapy. Patients should be reevaluated as clinically appropriate to determine if treatment is still necessary. Available data related to treatment risks are from Women's Health Initiative (WHI) studies, which evaluated oral CE 0.625 mg with or without MPA 2.5 mg relative to placebo in postmenopausal women. Other combinations and dosage forms of estrogens and progestins were not studied. Outcomes reported from clinical trials using CE with or without MPA should be assumed to be similar for other doses and other dosage forms of estrogens and progestins until comparable data becomes available.

Osteoporosis use: For use only in women at significant risk of osteoporosis and for who other nonestrogen medications are not considered appropriate.

When used solely for the treatment of vulvar and vaginal atrophy, topical vaginal products should be considered.

Adverse Reactions (Reflective of adult population; not specific for elderly)

>10%:
  Central nervous system: Headache (15% to 19%)
  Endocrine & metabolic: Breast pain (13% to 36%), dysmenorrhea (3% to 13%)
  Gastrointestinal: Abdominal pain (7% to 17%)
1% to 10%:
  Cardiovascular: Edema (≤4%), peripheral edema (2% to 3%), hypertension (2%), vasodilation (≤2%), chest pain (1%), palpitation (≤1%)
  Central nervous system: Depression (7% to 8%), pain (5%), emotional lability (3%), dizziness (2% to 3%), migraine (2% to 3%), nervousness (1% to 3%), anxiety (2%), insomnia (1% to 2%)

Dermatologic: Pruritus (2% to 6%), rash (2%), acne (≤2%), alopecia (≤2%), skin discoloration (1% to 2%), dry skin (≤1%)

Endocrine & metabolic: Leukorrhea (3% to 8%), breast enlargement (2% to 5%), breakthrough bleeding (1% to 4%), breast cancer (≤1%), breast engorgement (≤1%), glucose tolerance decreased (≤1%), menorrhagia (≤1%)

Gastrointestinal: Nausea (6% to 8%), flatulence (4% to 8%), diarrhea (≤6%), weight gain (3%), constipation (2%), appetite increased (≤2%), eructation (≤1%)

Genitourinary: Pelvic pain (2% to 5%), vaginal hemorrhage (≤5%), vaginitis (2% to 4%), monilial vaginitis (1% to 4%), uterine spasm (1% to 4%), cervical changes (1% to 3%), Pap smear suspicious (≤2%), incontinence (≤1%)

Neuromuscular & skeletal: Weakness (3% to 6%), back pain (2% to 7%), leg cramps (2% to 4%), hypertonia (1% to 2%)

Respiratory: Pharyngitis (>5%), sinusitis (>5%)

Miscellaneous: Moniliasis (≤2%), diaphoresis (≤1%), flu-like syndrome (≤1%), infection (≤1%)

Drug Interactions

Metabolism/Transport Effects Refer to individual components.

Avoid Concomitant Use

Avoid concomitant use of Estrogens (Conjugated/Equine) and Medroxyprogesterone with any of the following: Anastrozole; Axitinib; Griseofulvin

Increased Effect/Toxicity

Estrogens (Conjugated/Equine) and Medroxyprogesterone may increase the levels/effects of: Benzodiazepines (metabolized by oxidation); Corticosteroids (Systemic); ROPINIRole; Selegiline; Tipranavir; Tranexamic Acid; Voriconazole

The levels/effects of Estrogens (Conjugated/Equine) and Medroxyprogesterone may be increased by: Ascorbic Acid; Boceprevir; Herbs (Estrogenic Properties); Herbs (Progestogenic Properties); Mifepristone; Voriconazole

Decreased Effect

Estrogens (Conjugated/Equine) and Medroxyprogesterone may decrease the levels/effects of: Anastrozole; ARIPiprazole; Axitinib; Chenodiol; Hyaluronidase; Saxagliptin; Somatropin; Thyroid Products; Ursodiol; Vitamin K Antagonists

The levels/effects of Estrogens (Conjugated/Equine) and Medroxyprogesterone may be decreased by: Acitretin; Aminoglutethimide; Aprepitant; Artemether; Barbiturates; Bexarotene; Bexarotene (Systemic); Bile Acid Sequestrants; Bosentan; CarBAMazepine; Clobazam; CYP1A2 Inducers (Strong); CYP3A4 Inducers (Strong); Cyproterone; Deferasirox; Felbamate; Fosaprepitant; Fosphenytoin; Griseofulvin; LamoTRIgine; Mifepristone; Mycophenolate; Nevirapine; OXcarbazepine; Peginterferon Alfa-2b; Phenytoin; Prucalopride; Retinoic Acid Derivatives; Rifamycin Derivatives; St Johns Wort; Telaprevir; Tipranavir; Tocilizumab; Topiramate

Ethanol/Nutrition/Herb Interactions

Ethanol: Avoid ethanol (routine use increases estrogen plasma concentrations and risk of breast cancer). Ethanol may also increase the risk of osteoporosis.

Food: Folic acid absorption may be decreased.

Herb/Nutraceutical: St John's wort may decrease levels. Avoid black cohosh, dong quai (has estrogenic activity). Avoid red clover, saw palmetto, ginseng (due to potential hormonal effects).

Stability Store at room temperature 20°C to 25°C (68°F to 77°F).

Mechanism of Action

Conjugated estrogens contain a mixture of estrone sulfate, equilin sulfate, 17 alpha-dihydroequilin, 17 alpha-estradiol, and 17 beta-dihydroequilin. Estrogens are responsible for the development and maintenance of the female reproductive system and secondary sexual characteristics. Estradiol is the principle intracellular human estrogen and is more potent than estrone and estriol at the receptor level; it is the primary estrogen secreted prior to menopause. Following menopause, estrone and estrone sulfate are more highly produced. Estrogens modulate the pituitary secretion of gonadotropins, luteinizing hormone, and follicle-stimulating hormone through a negative feedback system; estrogen replacement reduces elevated levels of these hormones in postmenopausal women.

MPA inhibits gonadotropin production which then prevents follicular maturation and ovulation. In women with adequate estrogen, MPA transforms a proliferative endometrium into a secretory endometrium; when administered with conjugated estrogens, reduces the incidence of endometrial hyperplasia and risk of adenocarcinoma.

Pharmacodynamics/Kinetics See individual agents.

▶

◀ **Dosage**

Geriatric Refer to adult dosing. A higher incidence of stroke and breast cancer was observed in women >75 years in a WHI substudy.

Adult

Treatment of moderate-to-severe vasomotor symptoms associated with menopause; treatment of vulvar and vaginal atrophy due to menopause in women with a uterus; osteoporosis prophylaxis in females with an intact uterus (Note: The lowest dose that will control symptoms should be used; medication should be discontinued as soon as possible):

Premphase®: Oral: One maroon conjugated estrogen 0.625 mg tablet daily on days 1 through 14 and 1 light blue conjugated estrogen 0.625 mg/mPA 5 mg tablet daily on days 15 through 28

Prempro®: Oral: One conjugated estrogen/MPA tablet once daily; maximum dose: 1 conjugated estrogen 0.625 mg/mPA 5 mg tablet daily

Monitoring Parameters Routine physical examination that includes blood pressure and Papanicolaou smear, breast exam, mammogram. Monitor for signs of endometrial cancer. Adequate diagnostic measures, including endometrial sampling, if indicated, should be performed to rule out malignancy in all cases of undiagnosed abnormal vaginal bleeding. Monitor for loss of vision, sudden onset of proptosis, diplopia, migraine; signs and symptoms of thromboembolic disorders; glycemic control in patients with diabetes; lipid profiles in patients being treated for hyperlipidemias; thyroid function in patients on thyroid hormone replacement therapy.

Menopausal symptoms: Assess need for therapy at 3- to 6-month intervals

Prevention of osteoporosis: Bone density measurement

Test Interactions Reduced response to metyrapone test.

Special Geriatric Considerations Before prescribing estrogen therapy to postmenopausal women, the risks and benefits must be weighed for each patient. Women should be informed of these risks and benefits, as well as possible side effects and the return of menstrual bleeding (when cycled with a progestin), and be involved in the decision to prescribe. A higher incidence of stroke and invasive breast cancer was observed in women >75 years in a WHI substudy.

This medication is considered to be potentially inappropriate in this patient population (Beers Criteria: Quality of evidence - high [oral]; Strength of recommendation - strong [oral]).

Dosage Forms Excipient information presented when available (limited, particularly for generics); consult specific product labeling.

Tablet:

Premphase® [therapy pack contains 2 separate tablet formulations]: Conjugated estrogens 0.625 mg [14 maroon tablets] and conjugated estrogen 0.625 mg/medroxyprogesterone acetate 5 mg [14 light blue tablets] (28s)

Prempro®:

0.3/1.5: Conjugated estrogens 0.3 mg and medroxyprogesterone acetate 1.5 mg (28s)

0.45/1.5: Conjugated estrogens 0.45 mg and medroxyprogesterone acetate 1.5 mg (28s)

0.625/2.5: Conjugated estrogens 0.625 mg and medroxyprogesterone acetate 2.5 mg (28s)

0.625/5: Conjugated estrogens 0.625 mg and medroxyprogesterone acetate 5 mg (28s)

Estrogens (Esterified) (ES troe jenz, es TER i fied)

Related Information

Beers Criteria – Potentially Inappropriate Medications for Geriatrics *on page* 2183
Osteoporosis Management *on page* 2136

Medication Safety Issues

BEERS Criteria medication:

This drug may be potentially inappropriate for use in geriatric patients (Quality of evidence - high [oral]; Strength of recommendation - strong [oral]).

Brand Names: U.S. Menest®

Brand Names: Canada Estragyn; Estratab®; Menest®

Index Terms Esterified Estrogens

Generic Availability (U.S.) No

Pharmacologic Category Estrogen Derivative

Use Treatment of moderate-to-severe vasomotor symptoms associated with menopause; treatment of moderate-to-severe vulvar and vaginal atrophy associated with menopause; hypoestrogenism (due to hypogonadism, castration, or primary ovarian failure); advanced prostatic cancer (palliation), metastatic breast cancer (palliation) in men and postmenopausal women

Contraindications Hypersensitivity to estrogens or any component of the formulation; undiagnosed abnormal vaginal bleeding; DVT or PE (current or history of); active or recent (within 1 year) arterial thromboembolic disease (eg, stroke, MI); carcinoma of the breast (known, suspected or history of), except in appropriately selected patients being treated for metastatic disease; estrogen-dependent tumor; hepatic dysfunction or disease

Warnings/Precautions [U.S. Boxed Warning]: Based on data from the Women's Health Initiative (WHI) studies, an increased risk of invasive breast cancer was observed in postmenopausal women using conjugated estrogens (CE) in combination with medrox-yprogesterone acetate (MPA). This risk may be associated with duration of use and declines once combined therapy is discontinued (Chlebowski, 2009). The risk of invasive breast cancer was decreased in postmenopausal women with a hysterectomy using CE only, regardless of weight. However, the risk was not significantly decreased in women at high risk for breast cancer (family history of breast cancer, personal history of benign breast disease) (Anderson, 2012). An increase in abnormal mammogram findings has also been reported with estrogen alone or in combination with progestin therapy. Estrogen use may also lead to severe hypercalcemia in patients with breast cancer and bone metastases; discontinue estrogen if hypercalcemia occurs. **[U.S. Boxed Warning]: The use of unopposed estrogen in women with an intact uterus is associated with an increased risk of endometrial cancer. The addition of a progestin to estrogen therapy may decrease the risk of endometrial hyperplasia, a precursor to endometrial cancer. Adequate diagnostic measures, including endometrial sampling if indicated, should be performed to rule out malignancy in postmenopausal women with undiagnosed abnormal vaginal bleeding.** Estrogens may exacerbate endometriosis. Malignant transformation of residual endometrial implants has been reported posthysterectomy with unopposed estrogen therapy. Consider adding a progestin in women with residual endometriosis posthysterectomy. Postmenopausal estrogen therapy and combined estrogen/progesterone therapy may increase the risk of ovarian cancer; however, the absolute risk to an individual woman is small. Although results from various studies are not consistent, risk does not appear to be significantly associated with the duration, route, or dose of therapy. In one study, the risk decreased after 2 years following discontinuation of therapy (Mørch, 2009). Although the risk of ovarian cancer is rare, women who are at an increased risk (eg, family history) should be counseled about the association (NAMS, 2012).

[U.S. Boxed Warning]: Estrogens with or without progestin should not be used to prevent cardiovascular disease. Using data from the Women's Health Initiative (WHI) studies, an increased risk of deep vein thrombosis (DVT) and stroke has been reported with CE and an increased risk of DVT, stroke, pulmonary emboli (PE) and myocardial infarction (MI) has been reported with CE with MPA in postmenopausal women. Additional risk factors include diabetes mellitus, hypercholesterolemia, hypertension, SLE, obesity, tobacco use, and/or history of venous thromboembolism (VTE). Adverse cardiovascular events have also been reported in males taking estrogens for prostate cancer. Risk factors should be managed appropriately; discontinue use if adverse cardiovascular events occur or are suspected. Women with inherited thrombophilias (eg, protein C or S deficiency) may have increased risk of venous thromboembolism (DeSancho, 2010; van Vlijmen, 2011).

[U.S. Boxed Warning]: Estrogens with or without progestin should not be used to prevent dementia. In the Women's Health Initiative Memory Study (WHIMS), an increased incidence of dementia was observed in women ≥65 years of age taking CE alone or in combination with MPA.

[U.S. Boxed Warning]: Estrogens with or without progestin should be used for the shortest duration possible at the lowest effective dose consistent with treatment goals. Before prescribing estrogen therapy to postmenopausal women, the risks and benefits must be weighed for each patient. Women should be informed of these risks and benefits, as well as possible effects of progestin when added to estrogen therapy. Patients should be reevaluated as clinically appropriate to determine if treatment is still necessary. Available data related to treatment risks are from Women's Health Initiative (WHI) studies, which evaluated oral CE 0.625 mg with or without MPA 2.5 mg relative to placebo in postmenopausal women. Other combinations and dosage forms of estrogens and progestins were not studied. **Outcomes reported from clinical trials using CE with or without MPA should be assumed to be similar for other doses and other dosage forms of estrogens and progestins until comparable data becomes available.**

Estrogen compounds are generally associated with lipid effects such as increased HDL-cholesterol and decreased LDL-cholesterol. Triglycerides may also be increased; use with caution in patients with familial defects of lipoprotein metabolism. Estrogens may increase thyroid-binding globulin (TBG) levels leading to increased circulating total thyroid hormone levels. Women on thyroid replacement therapy may require higher doses of thyroid hormone while receiving estrogens.

Estrogens may cause retinal vascular thrombosis; discontinue if migraine, loss of vision, proptosis, diplopia or other visual disturbances occur; discontinue permanently if papilledema or retinal vascular lesions are observed on examination. Estrogens are poorly metabolized in patients with hepatic dysfunction. Use caution with a history of cholestatic jaundice associated with prior estrogen use or pregnancy. Discontinue if jaundice develops or if acute or chronic hepatic disturbances occur. Use is contraindicated with hepatic disease. Use caution in patients with asthma, epilepsy, hepatic hemangiomas, migraine, porphyria, or SLE; may exacerbate disease. May have adverse effects on glucose tolerance; use caution in women with diabetes. Use with caution in patients with diseases which may be exacerbated by fluid retention, including cardiac or renal dysfunction. Use of postmenopausal estrogen may be associated with an increased risk of gallbladder disease requiring surgery. Use with caution in patients with severe hypocalcemia. Avoid use of oral estrogen (with or without progestins) in the elderly due to potential of increased risk of breast and endometrial cancers, and lack of proven cardioprotection and cognitive protection (Beers Criteria). Prior to puberty, estrogens may cause premature closure of the epiphyses, premature breast development in girls or gynecomastia in boys. Vaginal bleeding and vaginal cornification may also be induced in girls. Whenever possible, estrogens should be discontinued at least 4-6 weeks prior to elective surgery associated with an increased risk of thromboembolism or during periods of prolonged immobilization. The use of estrogens and/or progestins may change the results of some laboratory tests (eg, coagulation factors, lipids, glucose tolerance, binding proteins). The dose, route, and the specific estrogen/progestin influences these changes. In addition, personal risk factors (eg, cardiovascular disease, smoking, diabetes, age) also contribute to adverse events; use of specific products may be contraindicated in women with certain risk factors.

Adverse Reactions (Reflective of adult population; not specific for elderly) Frequency not defined.

Cardiovascular: Edema, hypertension, MI, stroke, venous thromboembolism

Central nervous system: Dementia exacerbation, dizziness, epilepsy exacerbation, headache, irritability, mental depression, migraine, mood disturbances, nervousness

Dermatologic: Angioedema, chloasma, erythema multiforme, erythema nodosum, hemorrhagic eruption, hirsutism, pruritus, loss of scalp hair, melasma, rash, urticaria

Endocrine & metabolic: Breast cancer, breast enlargement, breast tenderness, carbohydrate intolerance, fibrocystic breast changes, galactorrhea, hypocalcemia, libido (changes in), nipple discharge, premenstrual like syndrome

Gastrointestinal: Abdominal cramps, bloating, gallbladder disease, nausea, pancreatitis, vomiting, weight gain/loss

Genitourinary: Alterations in frequency and flow of menstrual patterns, breakthrough bleeding, changes in cervical secretions, cervical ectropion changes, cystitis-like syndrome, dysmenorrhea, endometrial hyperplasia, endometrial cancer, increased size of uterine leiomyomata, ovarian cancer, vaginal candidiasis, vaginitis

Hematologic: Aggravation of porphyria

Hepatic: Cholestatic jaundice, hemangioma enlargement

Local: Thrombophlebitis

Neuromuscular & skeletal: Arthralgia, chorea, leg cramps

Ocular: Contact lens intolerance, corneal curvature steepening, retinal vascular thrombosis

Respiratory: Asthma exacerbation, pulmonary embolism

Miscellaneous: Anaphylactoid/anaphylactic reactions

Drug Interactions

Metabolism/Transport Effects Substrate of CYP1A2 (major), CYP2B6 (minor), CYP2C9 (minor), CYP2E1 (minor), CYP3A4 (major); **Note:** Assignment of Major/Minor substrate status based on clinically relevant drug interaction potential

Avoid Concomitant Use

Avoid concomitant use of Estrogens (Esterified) with any of the following: Anastrozole

Increased Effect/Toxicity

Estrogens (Esterified) may increase the levels/effects of: Corticosteroids (Systemic); ROPINIRole; Tipranavir

The levels/effects of Estrogens (Esterified) may be increased by: Ascorbic Acid; Herbs (Estrogenic Properties)

Decreased Effect

Estrogens (Esterified) may decrease the levels/effects of: Anastrozole; Chenodiol; Hyaluronidase; Somatropin; Thyroid Products; Ursodiol

The levels/effects of Estrogens (Esterified) may be decreased by: CYP1A2 Inducers (Strong); CYP3A4 Inducers (Strong); Cyproterone; Deferasirox; Herbs (CYP3A4 Inducers); Tipranavir; Tocilizumab

Ethanol/Nutrition/Herb Interactions

Ethanol: Avoid ethanol (routine use increases estrogen plasma concentrations and risk of breast cancer). Ethanol may also increase the risk of osteoporosis.

Food: Folic acid absorption may be decreased.

Herb/Nutraceutical: St John's wort may decrease levels. Herbs with estrogenic properties may enhance the adverse/toxic effect of estrogen derivatives; examples include alfalfa, black cohosh, bloodroot, hops, kudzu, licorice, red clover, saw palmetto, soybean, thyme, wild yam, yucca.

Mechanism of Action Esterified estrogens contain a mixture of estrogenic substances; the principle component is estrone. Preparations contain 75% to 85% sodium estrone sulfate and 6% to 15% sodium equilin sulfate such that the total is not <90%. Estrogens are responsible for the development and maintenance of the female reproductive system and secondary sexual characteristics. Estradiol is the principle intracellular human estrogen and is more potent than estrone and estriol at the receptor level; it is the primary estrogen secreted prior to menopause. In males and following menopause in females, estrone and estrone sulfate are more highly produced. Estrogens modulate the pituitary secretion of gonadotropins, luteinizing hormone, and follicle-stimulating hormone through a negative feedback system; estrogen replacement reduces elevated levels of these hormones.

Pharmacodynamics/Kinetics

Absorption: Readily

Distribution: Widely distributed; high concentrations in the sex hormone target organs

Protein binding: Bound to sex hormone-binding globulin and albumin

Metabolism: Hepatic; partial metabolism via CYP3A4 enzymes; estradiol is reversibly converted to estrone and estriol; oral estradiol also undergoes enterohepatic recirculation by conjugation in the liver, followed by excretion of sulfate and glucuronide conjugates into the bile, then hydrolysis in the intestine and estrogen reabsorption. Sulfate conjugates are the primary form found in postmenopausal women.

Excretion: Primarily urine (as estradiol, estrone, estriol, and their glucuronide and sulfate conjugates)

Dosage

Geriatric & Adult

Prostate cancer, advanced: Oral: 1.25-2.5 mg 3 times/day

Female hypoestrogenism due to hypogonadism: Oral: 2.5-7.5 mg/day in divided doses for 20 days followed by a 10-day rest period. Administer cyclically (3 weeks on and 1 week off). If bleeding does not occur by the end of the 10-day period, repeat the same dosing schedule; the number of courses dependent upon the responsiveness of the endometrium. If bleeding occurs before the end of the 10-day period, begin an estrogen-progestin cyclic regimen of 2.5-7.5 mg/day in divided doses for 20 days; during the last 5 days of estrogen therapy, give an oral progestin. If bleeding occurs before regimen is concluded, discontinue therapy and resume on the fifth day of bleeding.

Female hypoestrogenism due to castration and primary ovarian failure: Oral: 1.25 mg/day, cyclically. Adjust dosage upward or downward, according to the severity of symptoms and patient response. For maintenance, adjust dosage to lowest level that will provide effective control.

Vasomotor symptoms associated with menopause: Oral: 1.25 mg/day administered cyclically (3 weeks on and 1 week off). If patient has not menstruated within the last 2 months or more, cyclic administration is started arbitrary. If the patient is menstruating, cyclical administration is started on day 5 of the bleeding. For short-term use only and should be discontinued as soon as possible. Re-evaluate at 3- to 6-month intervals for tapering or discontinuation of therapy.

Vulvar and vaginal atrophy associated with menopause: Oral: 0.3 to ≥1.25 mg/day, depending on the tissue response of the individual patient. Administer cyclically. For short-term use only and should be discontinued as soon as possible. Re-evaluate at 3- to 6-month intervals for tapering or discontinuation of therapy.

Breast cancer, metastatic (appropriately selected patients): Males and postmenopausal females: Oral: 10 mg 3 times/day for at least 3 months

Administration Administer with food at same time each day.

Monitoring Parameters Routine physical examination that includes blood pressure and Papanicolaou smear, breast exam, mammogram. Monitor for signs of endometrial cancer in female patients with uterus. Adequate diagnostic measures, including endometrial sampling, if indicated, should be performed to rule out malignancy in all cases of undiagnosed abnormal vaginal bleeding. Monitor for loss of vision, sudden onset of proptosis, diplopia, migraine; signs and symptoms of thromboembolic disorders; glycemic control in patients with diabetes; lipid profiles in patients being treated for hyperlipidemias; thyroid function in patients on thyroid hormone replacement therapy.

Menopausal symptoms; vulvar and vaginal atrophy: Assess need for therapy at 3- to 6-month intervals

◀ **Test Interactions** Reduced response to metyrapone test.

Special Geriatric Considerations Before prescribing estrogen therapy to postmenopausal women, the risks and benefits must be weighed for each patient. Women should be informed of these risks and benefits, as well as possible side effects and the return of menstrual bleeding (when cycled with a progestin), and be involved in the decision to prescribe. A higher incidence of stroke and invasive breast cancer were observed in women >75 years in a WHI substudy using conjugated equine estrogen.

This medication is considered to be potentially inappropriate in this patient population (Beers Criteria: Quality of evidence - high [oral]; Strength of recommendation - strong [oral]).

Dosage Forms Excipient information presented when available (limited, particularly for generics); consult specific product labeling.

Tablet, oral:

Menest® 0.3 mg, 0.625 mg, 1.25 mg, 2.5 mg

Eszopiclone (es zoe PIK lone)

Related Information

Beers Criteria – Potentially Inappropriate Medications for Geriatrics *on page 2183*

Medication Safety Issues

Sound-alike/look-alike issues:

Lunesta® may be confused with Neulasta®

BEERS Criteria medication:

This drug may be potentially inappropriate for use in geriatric patients (Quality of evidence - moderate; Strength of recommendation - strong).

Brand Names: U.S. Lunesta®

Generic Availability (U.S.) No

Pharmacologic Category Hypnotic, Miscellaneous

Use Treatment of insomnia

Medication Guide Available Yes

Contraindications There are no contraindications listed within the manufacturer's labeling.

Warnings/Precautions Symptomatic treatment of insomnia should be initiated only after careful evaluation of potential causes of sleep disturbance. Tolerance did not develop over 6 months of use. Use with caution in patients with depression or a history of drug dependence. Abrupt discontinuance may lead to withdrawal symptoms. Use with caution in patients receiving other CNS depressants or psychoactive medications. Hypnotics/sedatives have been associated with abnormal thinking and behavior changes including decreased inhibition, aggression, bizarre behavior, agitation, hallucinations, and depersonalization. These changes may occur unpredictably and may indicate previously unrecognized psychiatric disorders; evaluate appropriately. Amnesia may occur. May impair physical and mental capabilities. Postmarketing studies have indicated that the use of hypnotic/sedative agents for sleep has been associated with hypersensitivity reactions including anaphylaxis as well as angioedema. An increased risk for hazardous sleep-related activities such as sleep-driving (as well as cooking and eating food and making phone calls while asleep) has also been noted. Use caution in patients with respiratory compromise, hepatic dysfunction, or those taking strong CYP3A4 inhibitors. Because of the rapid onset of action, administer immediately prior to bedtime or after the patient has gone to bed and is having difficulty falling asleep.

Use with caution in the elderly; dosage adjustment recommended. Avoid chronic use (>90 days) in older adults; adverse events, including delirium, falls, fractures, have been observed with nonbenzodiazepine hypnotic use in the elderly similar to events observed with benzodiazepines. Data suggests improvements in sleep duration and latency are minimal (Beers Criteria).

Adverse Reactions (Reflective of adult population; not specific for elderly)

>10%:

Central nervous system: Headache (15% to 21%)

Gastrointestinal: Unpleasant taste (8% to 34%)

1% to 10%:

Cardiovascular: Chest pain, peripheral edema

Central nervous system: Somnolence (8% to 10%), dizziness (5% to 7%), pain (4% to 5%), nervousness (up to 5%), depression (1% to 4%), confusion (up to 3%), hallucinations (1% to 3%), anxiety (1% to 3%), abnormal dreams (1% to 3%), migraine

Dermatologic: Rash (3% to 4%), pruritus (1% to 4%)

Endocrine & metabolic: Libido decreased (up to 3%), dysmenorrhea (up to 3%), gynecomastia (males up to 3%)

Gastrointestinal: Xerostomia (3% to 7%), dyspepsia (2% to 6%), nausea (4% to 5%), diarrhea (2% to 4%), vomiting (up to 3%)

Genitourinary: Urinary tract infection (up to 3%)

Neuromuscular & skeletal: Neuralgia (up to 3%)

Miscellaneous: Infection (5% to 10%), viral infection (3%), accidental injury (up to 3%)

Drug Interactions

Metabolism/Transport Effects Substrate of CYP2E1 (minor), CYP3A4 (major); **Note:** Assignment of Major/Minor substrate status based on clinically relevant drug interaction potential

Avoid Concomitant Use

Avoid concomitant use of Eszopiclone with any of the following: Azelastine; Azelastine (Nasal); Conivaptan; Methadone; Mirtazapine; Paraldehyde

Increased Effect/Toxicity

Eszopiclone may increase the levels/effects of: Alcohol (Ethyl); Azelastine; Azelastine (Nasal); Buprenorphine; CNS Depressants; Methadone; Methotrimeprazine; Metyrosine; Mirtazapine; Paraldehyde; Selective Serotonin Reuptake Inhibitors; Zolpidem

The levels/effects of Eszopiclone may be increased by: Antifungal Agents (Azole Derivatives, Systemic); Conivaptan; CYP3A4 Inhibitors (Moderate); CYP3A4 Inhibitors (Strong); Dasatinib; Droperidol; HydrOXYzine; Ivacaftor; Methotrimeprazine; Mifepristone

Decreased Effect

The levels/effects of Eszopiclone may be decreased by: CYP3A4 Inducers (Strong); Deferasirox; Flumazenil; Herbs (CYP3A4 Inducers); Tocilizumab

Ethanol/Nutrition/Herb Interactions

Ethanol: Ethanol may increase CNS depression. Management: Avoid ethanol.

Food: Onset of action may be reduced if taken with or immediately after a heavy meal. Management: Take immediately prior to bedtime, not with or immediately after a heavy or high-fat meal.

Herb/Nutraceutical: Some herbal medications may increase CNS depression. Management: Avoid valerian, St John's wort, kava kava, and gotu kola.

Stability Store at controlled room temperature of 25°C (77°F).

Mechanism of Action May interact with GABA-receptor complexes at binding domains located close to or allosterically coupled to benzodiazepine receptors.

Pharmacodynamics/Kinetics

Absorption: Rapid; high-fat/heavy meal may delay absorption

Protein binding: 52% to 59%

Metabolism: Hepatic via oxidation and demethylation (CYP2E1, 3A4); 2 primary metabolites; one with activity less than parent.

Half-life elimination: ~6 hours; Elderly (≥65 years): ~9 hours

Time to peak, plasma: ~1 hour

Excretion: Urine (up to 75%, primarily as metabolites; <10% as parent drug)

Dosage

Geriatric

Difficulty **falling** asleep: Initial: 1 mg before immediately bedtime; maximum dose: 2 mg.

Difficulty **staying** asleep: 2 mg immediately before bedtime.

Adult

Insomnia: Oral: Initial: 2 mg immediately before bedtime (maximum dose: 3 mg)

Concurrent use with strong CYP3A4 inhibitor: 1 mg immediately before bedtime; if needed, dose may be increased to 2 mg

Renal Impairment No adjustment required.

Hepatic Impairment

Mild-to-moderate: Use with caution; dosage adjustment unnecessary

Severe: Initial dose: 1 mg; maximum dose: 2 mg

Administration Because of the rapid onset of action, eszopiclone should be administered immediately prior to bedtime or after the patient has gone to bed and is having difficulty falling asleep. Do not take with, or immediately following, a high-fat meal; do not crush or break tablet.

Special Geriatric Considerations In subjects >65 years of age, the AUC was increased by 41%. The manufacturer reports that in studies, the pattern of adverse reactions in elderly subjects was not different from that seen in younger adults.

This medication is considered to be potentially inappropriate in this patient population (Beers Criteria: Quality of evidence - moderate; Strength of recommendation - strong).

Controlled Substance C-IV

Dosage Forms Excipient information presented when available (limited, particularly for generics); consult specific product labeling.

Tablet, oral:

Lunesta®: 1 mg, 2 mg, 3 mg

Etanercept (et a NER sept)

Medication Safety Issues
  Sound-alike/look-alike issues:
    Enbrel® may be confused with Levbid®
Brand Names: U.S. Enbrel®; Enbrel® SureClick®
Brand Names: Canada Enbrel®
Generic Availability (U.S.) No
Pharmacologic Category Antirheumatic, Disease Modifying; Tumor Necrosis Factor (TNF) Blocking Agent
Use Treatment of moderately- to severely-active rheumatoid arthritis (RA); moderately- to severely-active polyarticular juvenile idiopathic arthritis (JIA); psoriatic arthritis; active ankylosing spondylitis (AS); moderate-to-severe chronic plaque psoriasis
Medication Guide Available Yes
Contraindications Hypersensitivity to etanercept or any component of the formulation; patients with sepsis (mortality may be increased)
Warnings/Precautions [U.S. Boxed Warning]: Patients receiving etanercept are at increased risk for serious infections which may result in hospitalization and/or fatality; infections usually developed in patients receiving concomitant immunosuppressive agents (eg, methotrexate or corticosteroids) and may present as disseminated (rather than local) disease. Active tuberculosis (or reactivation of latent tuberculosis), invasive fungal (including aspergillosis, blastomycosis, candidiasis, coccidioidomycosis, histoplasmosis, and pneumocystosis) and bacterial, viral or other opportunistic infections (including legionellosis and listeriosis) have been reported in patients receiving TNF-blocking agents, including etanercept. Monitor closely for signs/symptoms of infection. Discontinue for serious infection or sepsis. Consider risks versus benefits prior to use in patients with a history of chronic or recurrent infection. Consider empiric antifungal therapy in patients who are at risk for invasive fungal infection and develop severe systemic illness. Caution should be exercised when considering use in the elderly or in patients with conditions that predispose them to infections (eg, diabetes) or residence/travel from areas of endemic mycoses (blastomycosis, coccidioidomycosis, histoplasmosis), or with latent or localized infections. Do not initiate etanercept therapy with clinically important active infection. Patients who develop a new infection while undergoing treatment should be monitored closely. **[U.S. Boxed Warning]: Tuberculosis (disseminated or extrapulmonary) has been reported in patients receiving etanercept; both reactivation of latent infection and new infections have been reported.** Patients should be evaluated for tuberculosis risk factors and for latent tuberculosis infection with a tuberculin skin test prior to starting therapy. Treatment of latent tuberculosis should be initiated before etanercept therapy; consider antituberculosis treatment if adequate course of treatment cannot be confirmed in patients with a history of latent or active tuberculosis or with risk factors despite negative skin test. Some patients who tested negative prior to therapy have developed active infection; monitor for signs and symptoms of tuberculosis in all patients. Rare reactivation of hepatitis B virus (HBV) has occurred in chronic virus carriers; use with caution; evaluate prior to initiation and during treatment. Patients should be brought up to date with all immunizations before initiating therapy. Live vaccines should not be given concurrently with etanercept. Patients with a significant exposure to varicella virus should temporarily discontinue etanercept. Treatment with varicella zoster immune globulin should be considered.

[U.S. Boxed Warning]: Lymphoma and other malignancies have been reported in children and adolescent patients receiving TNF-blocking agents, including etanercept. Half of the malignancies reported in children were lymphomas (Hodgkin's and non-Hodgkin's) while other cases varied and included malignancies not typically observed in this population. The impact of etanercept on the development and course of malignancy is not fully defined. Compared to the general population, an increased risk of lymphoma has been noted in clinical trials; however, rheumatoid arthritis alone has been previously associated with an increased rate of lymphoma. Lymphomas and other malignancies were also observed (at rates higher than expected for the general population) in adult patients receiving etanercept. Etanercept is not recommended for use in patients with Wegener's granulomatosis who are receiving immunosuppressive therapy. Hepatosplenic T-cell lymphoma (HSTCL), a rare T-cell lymphoma, has also been associated with TNF-blocking agents, primarily reported in adolescent and young adult males with Crohn's disease or ulcerative colitis. Treatment may result in the formation of autoimmune antibodies; cases of autoimmune disease have not been described. Non-neutralizing antibodies to etanercept may also be formed. Rarely, a reversible lupus-like syndrome has occurred.

Allergic reactions may occur; if an anaphylactic reaction or other serious allergic reaction occurs, administration should be discontinued immediately and appropriate therapy initiated.

Use with caution in patients with pre-existing or recent onset CNS demyelinating disorders; rare cases of new onset or exacerbation of CNS demyelinating disorders have occurred; may present with mental status changes and some may be associated with permanent disability. Optic neuritis, transverse myelitis, multiple sclerosis, and new onset or exacerbation of seizures have been reported. Use with caution in patients with heart failure or decreased left ventricular function; worsening and new-onset heart failure has been reported. Use caution in patients with a history of significant hematologic abnormalities; has been associated with pancytopenia and aplastic anemia (rare). Discontinue if significant hematologic abnormalities are confirmed. Use with caution in patients with moderate to severe alcoholic hepatitis. Compared to placebo, the mortality rate in patients treated with etanercept was similar at one month but significantly higher after 6 months

Due to a higher incidence of serious infections, concomitant use with anakinra is not recommended. Some dosage forms may contain dry natural rubber (latex).

Adverse Reactions (Reflective of adult population; not specific for elderly) Percentages reported for adults except where specified.

>10%:
  Central nervous system: Headache (17%; children 19%)
  Dermatologic: Rash (3% to 13%)
  Gastrointestinal: Abdominal pain (5%; children 19%), vomiting (3%; children 13%)
  Local: Injection site reaction (14% to 43%; bleeding, bruising, erythema, itching, pain or swelling)
  Respiratory: Respiratory tract infection (upper; 38% to 65%), rhinitis (12%)
  Miscellaneous: Infection (50% to 81%; children 62%), positive ANA (11%), positive anti-double-stranded DNA antibodies (15% by RIA, 3% by *Crithidia luciliae* assay)

≥3% to 10%:
  Central nervous system: Dizziness (7%)
  Dermatologic: Pruritus (2% to 5%)
  Gastrointestinal: Nausea (children 9%), dyspepsia (4%), diarrhea (3%)
  Neuromuscular & skeletal: Weakness (5%)
  Respiratory: Pharyngitis (7%), cough (6%), respiratory disorder (5%), sinusitis (3%)

Drug Interactions
  Metabolism/Transport Effects None known.
  Avoid Concomitant Use
    Avoid concomitant use of Etanercept with any of the following: Abatacept; Anakinra; BCG; Belimumab; Canakinumab; Certolizumab Pegol; Cyclophosphamide; Natalizumab; Pimecrolimus; Rilonacept; Tacrolimus (Topical); Vaccines (Live)
  Increased Effect/Toxicity
    Etanercept may increase the levels/effects of: Abatacept; Anakinra; Belimumab; Canakinumab; Certolizumab Pegol; Cyclophosphamide; Leflunomide; Natalizumab; Rilonacept; Vaccines (Live)

    The levels/effects of Etanercept may be increased by: Denosumab; Pimecrolimus; Roflumilast; Tacrolimus (Topical); Trastuzumab
  Decreased Effect
    Etanercept may decrease the levels/effects of: BCG; Coccidioidin Skin Test; Sipuleucel-T; Vaccines (Inactivated); Vaccines (Live)

    The levels/effects of Etanercept may be decreased by: Echinacea

Ethanol/Nutrition/Herb Interactions Herb/Nutraceutical: Echinacea may decrease the therapeutic effects of etanercept (avoid concurrent use).

Stability
  Prefilled syringes, autoinjectors: Store prefilled syringes and autoinjectors at 2°C to 8°C (36°F to 46°F); do not freeze. Protect from light; do not shake. The following stability information has also been reported: May be stored at room temperature for up to 4 days (Cohen, 2007).
  Powder for reconstitution: Must be refrigerated at 2°C to 8°C (36°F to 46°F); do not freeze. The following stability information has also been reported: May be stored at room temperature for up to 7 days (Cohen, 2007). Reconstitute lyophilized powder aseptically with 1 mL sterile bacteriostatic water for injection, USP (supplied); swirl gently, do not shake. Do not filter reconstituted solution during preparation or administration. Upon reconstitution of vial, administer immediately. If not administered immediately after reconstitution, vial may be stored at 2°C to 8°C (36°F to 46°F) for up to 14 days.

Mechanism of Action Etanercept is a recombinant DNA-derived protein composed of tumor necrosis factor receptor (TNFR) linked to the Fc portion of human IgG1. Etanercept binds tumor necrosis factor (TNF) and blocks its interaction with cell surface receptors. TNF plays an important role in the inflammatory processes and the resulting joint pathology of rheumatoid arthritis (RA), polyarticular-course juvenile idiopathic arthritis (JIA), ankylosing spondylitis (AS), and plaque psoriasis.

Pharmacodynamics/Kinetics
Onset of action: ~2-3 weeks; RA: 1-2 weeks
Half-life elimination: RA: SubQ: 72-132 hours
Time to peak: RA: SubQ: 35-103 hours

Dosage

Geriatric SubQ: Refer to adult dosing. Although greater sensitivity of some elderly patients cannot be ruled out, no overall differences in safety or effectiveness were observed.

Adult

Rheumatoid arthritis, psoriatic arthritis, ankylosing spondylitis: SubQ:
Once-weekly dosing: 50 mg once weekly
Twice-weekly dosing: 25 mg given twice weekly (individual doses should be separated by 72-96 hours)

Plaque psoriasis: SubQ:
Initial: 50 mg twice weekly, 72-96 hours apart; maintain initial dose for 3 months (starting doses of 25 or 50 mg once weekly have also been used successfully)
Maintenance dose: 50 mg once weekly

Renal Impairment No dosage adjustment provided in manufacturer's labeling (has not been studied).

Hepatic Impairment No dosage adjustment provided in manufacturer's labeling (has not been studied).

Administration Administer subcutaneously. Rotate injection sites. New injections should be given at least one inch from an old site and never into areas where the skin is tender, bruised, red, or hard. **Note:** If the physician determines that it is appropriate, patients may self-inject after proper training in injection technique.
Powder for reconstitution: Follow package instructions carefully for reconstitution. The maximum amount injected at any single site should not exceed 25 mg.
Solution for injection: May be allowed to reach room temperature prior to injection.

Monitoring Parameters Monitor improvement of symptoms and physical function assessments. Latent TB screening prior to initiating and during therapy; signs/symptoms of infection (prior to, during, and following therapy); CBC with differential; signs/symptoms/worsening of heart failure; HBV screening prior to initiating (all patients), HBV carriers (during and for several months following therapy); signs and symptoms of hypersensitivity reaction; symptoms of lupus-like syndrome; signs/symptoms of malignancy (eg, splenomegaly, hepatomegaly, abdominal pain, persistent fever, night sweats, weight loss).

Special Geriatric Considerations Clinical trials including those ≥65 years of age with rheumatoid arthritis have not demonstrated any differences in safety and efficacy between elderly and younger adults to date. Since elderly have a higher incidence of infections in general, caution should be used, with close monitoring and patient education.

Dosage Forms Excipient information presented when available (limited, particularly for generics); consult specific product labeling.
Injection, powder for reconstitution [preservative free]:
Enbrel®: 25 mg [contains benzyl alcohol (in diluent), sucrose 10 mg; derived from or manufactured using Chinese hamster ovary cells]
Injection, solution [preservative free]:
Enbrel®: 50 mg/mL (0.51 mL, 0.98 mL) [contains natural rubber/natural latex in packaging, sucrose 1%; derived from or manufactured using Chinese hamster ovary cells; prefilled syringe]
Enbrel® SureClick®: 50 mg/mL (0.98 mL) [contains natural rubber/natural latex in packaging, sucrose 1%; derived from or manufactured using Chinese hamster ovary cells; autoinjector]

♦ **Ethacrynate Sodium** see Ethacrynic Acid on page 722

Ethacrynic Acid (eth a KRIN ik AS id)

Medication Safety Issues
Sound-alike/look-alike issues:
Edecrin® may be confused with Eulexin, Ecotrin®
Brand Names: U.S. Edecrin®; Sodium Edecrin®
Brand Names: Canada Edecrin®; Sodium Edecrin®
Index Terms Ethacrynate Sodium
Generic Availability (U.S.) No
Pharmacologic Category Diuretic, Loop
Use Management of edema associated with congestive heart failure; hepatic cirrhosis or renal disease; short-term management of ascites due to malignancy, idiopathic edema, and lymphedema

Dosage

Geriatric Oral: Initial: 25-50 mg/day

Adult I.V. formulation should be diluted in D_5W or NS (1 mg/mL) and infused over several minutes.

Edema:

Oral: 50-200 mg/day in 1-2 divided doses; may increase in increments of 25-50 mg at intervals of several days to a maximum of 400 mg/24 hours.

I.V.: 0.5-1 mg/kg/dose (maximum: 100 mg/dose); repeat doses not routinely recommended; however, if indicated, repeat doses every 8-12 hours.

Renal Impairment

Cl_{cr} <10 mL/minute: Avoid use.

Not removed by hemo- or peritoneal dialysis; supplemental dose is not necessary.

Special Geriatric Considerations Ethacrynic acid is rarely used because of its increased incidence of ototoxicity as compared to the other loop diuretics.

Dosage Forms Excipient information presented when available (limited, particularly for generics); consult specific product labeling.

Injection, powder for reconstitution, as ethacrynate sodium:

Sodium Edecrin®: 50 mg

Tablet, oral:

Edecrin®: 25 mg [scored]

Ethambutol (e THAM byoo tole)

Related Information

Antimicrobial Drugs of Choice *on page 2163*

Medication Safety Issues

Sound-alike/look-alike issues:

Myambutol® may be confused with Nembutal®

Brand Names: U.S. Myambutol®

Brand Names: Canada Etibi®

Index Terms Ethambutol Hydrochloride

Generic Availability (U.S.) Yes

Pharmacologic Category Antitubercular Agent

Use Treatment of pulmonary tuberculosis in conjunction with other antituberculosis agents

Unlabeled Use Other mycobacterial diseases in conjunction with other antimycobacterial agents

Contraindications Hypersensitivity to ethambutol or any component of the formulation; optic neuritis (risk vs benefit decision); use in unconscious patients or any other patient who may be unable to discern and report visual changes

Warnings/Precautions May cause optic neuritis (unilateral or bilateral), resulting in decreased visual acuity or other vision changes. Discontinue promptly in patients with changes in vision, color blindness, or visual defects (effects normally reversible, but reversal may require up to a year). Irreversible blindness has been reported. Monitor visual acuity prior to and during therapy. Evaluation of visual acuity changes may be more difficult in patients with cataracts, optic neuritis, diabetic retinopathy, and inflammatory conditions of the eye; consideration should be given to whether or not visual changes are related to disease progression or effects of therapy. Dosage modification is required in patients with renal insufficiency; monitor renal function prior to and during treatment. Hepatic toxicity has been reported, possibly due to concurrent therapy; monitor liver function prior to and during treatment.

Adverse Reactions (Reflective of adult population; not specific for elderly) Frequency not defined.

Cardiovascular: Myocarditis, pericarditis

Central nervous system: Confusion, disorientation, dizziness, fever, hallucinations, headache, malaise

Dermatologic: Dermatitis, erythema multiforme, exfoliative dermatitis, pruritus, rash

Endocrine & metabolic: Acute gout or hyperuricemia

Gastrointestinal: Abdominal pain, anorexia, GI upset, nausea, vomiting

Hematologic: Eosinophilia, leukopenia, lymphadenopathy, neutropenia, thrombocytopenia

Hepatic: Hepatitis, hepatotoxicity (possibly related to concurrent therapy), LFTs abnormal

Neuromuscular & skeletal: Arthralgia, peripheral neuritis

Ocular: Optic neuritis; symptoms may include decreased acuity, scotoma, color blindness, or visual defects (usually reversible with discontinuation, irreversible blindness has been described)

Renal: Nephritis

Respiratory: Infiltrates (with or without eosinophilia), pneumonitis

Miscellaneous: Anaphylaxis, anaphylactoid reaction; hypersensitivity syndrome (cutaneous reactions, eosinophilia, and organ-specific inflammation)

Drug Interactions

Metabolism/Transport Effects None known.

Avoid Concomitant Use There are no known interactions where it is recommended to avoid concomitant use.

Increased Effect/Toxicity There are no known significant interactions involving an increase in effect.

Decreased Effect

The levels/effects of Ethambutol may be decreased by: Aluminum Hydroxide

Stability Store at controlled room temperature of 20°C to 25°C (68°F to 77°F).

Mechanism of Action Inhibits arabinosyl transferase resulting in impaired mycobacterial cell wall synthesis

Pharmacodynamics/Kinetics

Absorption: ~80%

Distribution: Widely throughout body; concentrated in kidneys, lungs, saliva, and red blood cells

Relative diffusion from blood into CSF: Adequate with or without inflammation (exceeds usual MICs)

CSF:blood level ratio: Normal meninges: 0%; Inflamed meninges: 25%

Protein binding: 20% to 30%

Metabolism: Hepatic (20%) to inactive metabolite

Half-life elimination: 2.5-3.6 hours; End-stage renal disease: 7-15 hours

Time to peak, serum: 2-4 hours

Excretion: Urine (~50% as unchanged drug, 8% to 15% as metabolites); feces (~20% as unchanged drug)

Dosage

Geriatric & Adult

Disseminated *Mycobacterium avium* (MAC) treatment in patients with advanced HIV infection (unlabeled use; ATS/IDSA guidelines, 2007): Oral: 15 mg/kg ethambutol in combination with clarithromycin or azithromycin with/without rifabutin

Tuberculosis, active: Oral: FDA-approved labeling: Adolescents ≥13 years and Adults: Initial: 15 mg/kg once daily (maximum dose: 1.5 g); Retreatment (previous antituberculosis therapy): 25 mg/kg once daily (maximum dose: 2.5 g) for 60 days or until bacteriologic smears and cultures become negative, followed by 15 mg/kg daily.

Suggested doses by lean body weight (CDC, 2003):

Daily therapy: 15-25 mg/kg (maximum dose: 1.6 g)
40-55 kg: 800 mg
56-75 kg: 1200 mg
76-90 kg: 1600 mg

Twice weekly directly observed therapy (DOT): 50 mg/kg (maximum dose: 4 g)
40-55 kg: 2000 mg
56-75 kg: 2800 mg
76-90 kg: 4000 mg

Three times/week DOT: 25-30 mg/kg (maximum dose: 2.4 g)
40-55 kg: 1200 mg
56-75 kg: 2000 mg
76-90 kg: 2400 mg

Note: Used as part of a multidrug regimen. Treatment regimens consist of an initial 2 month phase, followed by a continuation phase of 4 or 7 additional months; frequency of dosing may differ depending on phase of therapy.

Nontuberculous mycobacterium *(M. kansasii)* (unlabeled use; ATS/IDSA guidelines, 2007): Oral: 15 mg/kg/day ethambutol for duration to include 12 months of culture-negative sputum; typically used in combination with rifampin and isoniazid; **Note:** Previous recommendations stated to use 25 mg/kg/day for the initial 2 months of therapy; however, IDSA guidelines state this may be unnecessary given the success of rifampin-based regimens with ethambutol 15 mg/kg/day or omitted altogether.

Renal Impairment

MMWR, 2003: Cl$_{cr}$ <30 mL/minute and hemodialysis: 15-25 mg/kg/dose 3 times weekly

Aronoff, 2007

Cl$_{cr}$ 10-50 mL/minute: Administer every 24-36 hours

Cl$_{cr}$ <10 mL/minute: Administer every 48 hours

Hemodialysis: Slightly dialyzable (5% to 20%); Administer dose postdialysis

Peritoneal dialysis: Dose for Cl$_{cr}$ <10 mL/minute: Administer every 48 hours

Continuous arteriovenous or venovenous hemofiltration: Dose for Cl$_{cr}$ 10-50 mL/minute: Administer every 24-36 hours

Monitoring Parameters Baseline and periodic (monthly) visual testing (each eye individually, as well as both eyes tested together) in patients receiving >15 mg/kg/day; baseline and periodic renal, hepatic, and hematopoietic tests

Special Geriatric Considerations Since most elderly patients acquired their tuberculosis before current antituberculin regimens were available, ethambutol is only indicated when patients are from areas where drug resistant *M. tuberculosis* is endemic, in HIV-infected elderly patients, and when drug resistant *M. tuberculosis* is suspected (see Dosage: Renal Impairment).

Dosage Forms Excipient information presented when available (limited, particularly for generics); consult specific product labeling.
Tablet, oral, as hydrochloride: 100 mg, 400 mg
Myambutol®: 100 mg
Myambutol®: 400 mg [scored]

◆ **Ethambutol Hydrochloride** see Ethambutol on page 723

Ethionamide (e thye on AM ide)

Related Information
Antimicrobial Drugs of Choice on page 2163
Brand Names: U.S. Trecator®
Brand Names: Canada Trecator®
Generic Availability (U.S.) No
Pharmacologic Category Antitubercular Agent
Use Treatment of tuberculosis and other mycobacterial diseases, in conjunction with other antituberculosis agents, when first-line agents have failed or resistance has been demonstrated

Contraindications Hypersensitivity to ethionamide or any component of the formulation; severe hepatic impairment

Warnings/Precautions Use with caution in patients with diabetes mellitus or thyroid dysfunction; use with caution in patients receiving cycloserine or isoniazid. Cross-resistance to isoniazid has been reported if inhA mutation is present. May cause hepatotoxicity; monitor liver function tests monthly. Use not recommended in patients with porphyria; animal and *in vitro* studies have shown porphyria-inducing effects. Periodic eye exams are recommended. Drug-resistant tuberculosis develops rapidly if ethionamide is used alone; must administer with at least one other antituberculosis agent.

Adverse Reactions (Reflective of adult population; not specific for elderly) Frequency not defined.
Cardiovascular: Orthostatic hypotension
Central nervous system: Depression, dizziness, drowsiness, headache, psychiatric disturbances, restlessness, seizure
Dermatologic: Acne, alopecia, photosensitivity, purpura, rash
Endocrine & metabolic: Gynecomastia, hypoglycemia, hypothyroidism or goiter, menstrual irregularities, pellagra-like syndrome
Gastrointestinal: Abdominal pain, anorexia, diarrhea, excessive salivation, metallic taste, nausea, stomatitis, vomiting, weight loss
Genitourinary: Impotence
Hematologic: Leukopenia, thrombocytopenia
Hepatic: Bilirubin increased, hepatitis, jaundice, liver function tests increased
Neuromuscular & skeletal: Arthralgia, peripheral neuritis
Ocular: Blurred vision, diplopia, optic neuritis
Respiratory: Olfactory disturbances
Miscellaneous: Hypersensitivity reaction
Drug Interactions
Metabolism/Transport Effects None known.
Avoid Concomitant Use There are no known interactions where it is recommended to avoid concomitant use.
Increased Effect/Toxicity
Ethionamide may increase the levels/effects of: CycloSERINE; Isoniazid

The levels/effects of Ethionamide may be increased by: Alcohol (Ethyl)
Decreased Effect There are no known significant interactions involving a decrease in effect.
Ethanol/Nutrition/Herb Interactions
Ethanol: Avoid excessive ethanol ingestion; psychotic reaction may occur.
Stability Store at 20°C to 25°C (68°F to 77°F). Keep containers tightly closed.
Mechanism of Action Inhibits peptide synthesis; bacteriostatic

◀ **Pharmacodynamics/Kinetics**
Absorption: Rapid, complete
Distribution: Crosses placenta; V_d: 93.5 L
Protein binding: ~30%
Metabolism: Prodrug; extensively hepatic to active and inactive metabolites
Bioavailability: 80%
Half-life elimination: 2 hours
Time to peak, serum: 1 hour
Excretion: Urine (<1% as unchanged drug; as active and inactive metabolites)

Dosage
Geriatric & Adult Tuberculosis: Oral: 15-20 mg/kg/day; initiate dose at 250 mg/day for 1-2 days, then increase to 250 mg twice daily for 1-2 days, with gradual increases to highest tolerated dose; average adult dose: 750 mg/day (maximum: 1 g/day in 3-4 divided doses)
Renal Impairment Cl_{cr} <30 mL/minute: 250-500 mg/day

Administration Neurotoxic effects may be prevented or relieved by the coadministration of pyridoxine (see Pyridoxine monograph on page 1640 for dosing). May be taken with or without meals. Gastrointestinal adverse effects may be decreased by administration at meals or bedtime, decreased dose, or giving antiemetics.

Monitoring Parameters Initial and periodic serum ALT and AST; blood glucose; TSH every 6 months; initial and periodic ophthalmic exams

Pharmacotherapy Pearls Neurotoxic effects may be relieved by the administration of pyridoxine.

Special Geriatric Considerations Since many elderly have Cl_{cr} <50 mL/minute, adjust dose for renal function.

Dosage Forms Excipient information presented when available (limited, particularly for generics); consult specific product labeling.
Tablet, oral:
Trecator®: 250 mg

Ethosuximide (eth oh SUKS i mide)

Medication Safety Issues
Sound-alike/look-alike issues:
Ethosuximide may be confused with methsuximide
Zarontin® may be confused with Neurontin®, Xalatan®, Zantac®, Zaroxolyn®

Brand Names: U.S. Zarontin®
Brand Names: Canada Zarontin®
Generic Availability (U.S.) Yes: Excludes syrup
Pharmacologic Category Anticonvulsant, Succinimide
Use Management of absence (petit mal) seizures
Medication Guide Available Yes
Contraindications History of hypersensitivity to succinimides

Warnings/Precautions Antiepileptics are associated with an increased risk of suicidal behavior/thoughts with use (regardless of indication); patients should be monitored for signs/symptoms of depression, suicidal tendencies, and other unusual behavior changes during therapy and instructed to inform their healthcare provider immediately if symptoms occur. Severe reactions, including Stevens-Johnson syndrome, have been reported with an onset usually within 28 days, but may be observed later. Drug should be discontinued if there are any signs of rash. If SJS is suspected do not resume ethosuximide and consider alternative therapy.

Use with caution in patients with hepatic or renal disease; abrupt withdrawal of the drug may precipitate absence status; ethosuximide may increase tonic-clonic seizures when used alone in patients with mixed seizure disorders; ethosuximide must be used in combination with other anticonvulsants in patients with both absence and tonic-clonic seizures. Succinimides have been associated with severe blood dyscrasias and cases of systemic lupus erythematosus. Consider evaluation of blood counts in patients with signs/symptoms of infection. May cause CNS depression, which may impair physical or mental abilities; patients must be cautioned about performing tasks which require mental alertness (eg, operating machinery or driving). Effects with other sedative drugs or ethanol may be potentiated.

Adverse Reactions (Reflective of adult population; not specific for elderly) Frequency not defined.
Central nervous system: Aggressiveness, ataxia, concentration impaired, dizziness, drowsiness, euphoria, fatigue, headache, hyperactivity, irritability, lethargy, mental depression (with cases of overt suicidal intentions), night terrors, paranoid psychosis, sleep disturbance
Dermatologic: Hirsutism, pruritus, rash, Stevens-Johnson syndrome, urticaria
Endocrine & metabolic: Libido increased

Gastrointestinal: Dyspepsia (10%), abdominal cramps (3% to 9%), diarrhea (3% to 9%), flatulence (3% to 9%), nausea (3% to 9%), vomiting (1% to 3%), constipation (1% to 3%), melena (1% to 3%), gastritis (1% to 3%)
Genitourinary: Dysuria (1% to 3%)
Neuromuscular & skeletal: Weakness (3% to 9%)
Ocular: Blurred vision (1% to 3%)
Otic: Tinnitus (1% to 3%)
Renal: Polyuria (1% to 3%)

Drug Interactions
Metabolism/Transport Effects None known.
Avoid Concomitant Use
Avoid concomitant use of Etodolac with any of the following: Floctafenine; Ketorolac; Ketorolac (Nasal); Ketorolac (Systemic)

Increased Effect/Toxicity
Etodolac may increase the levels/effects of: Aliskiren; Aminoglycosides; Anticoagulants; Antiplatelet Agents; Bisphosphonate Derivatives; Collagenase (Systemic); CycloSPORINE; CycloSPORINE (Systemic); Dabigatran Etexilate; Deferasirox; Desmopressin; Digoxin; Drotrecogin Alfa (Activated); Eplerenone; Haloperidol; Ibritumomab; Lithium; Methotrexate; Nonsteroidal Anti-Inflammatory Agents; PEMEtrexed; Porfimer; Potassium-Sparing Diuretics; PRALAtrexate; Quinolone Antibiotics; Rivaroxaban; Salicylates; Thrombolytic Agents; Tositumomab and Iodine I 131 Tositumomab; Vancomycin; Vitamin K Antagonists

The levels/effects of Etodolac may be increased by: ACE Inhibitors; Angiotensin II Receptor Blockers; Antidepressants (Tricyclic, Tertiary Amine); Corticosteroids (Systemic); Cyclo-SPORINE; CycloSPORINE (Systemic); Dasatinib; Floctafenine; Glucosamine; Herbs (Anti-coagulant/Antiplatelet Properties); Ketorolac; Ketorolac (Nasal); Ketorolac (Systemic); Nonsteroidal Anti-Inflammatory Agents; Omega-3-Acid Ethyl Esters; Pentosan Polysulfate Sodium; Pentoxifylline; Probenecid; Prostacyclin Analogues; Selective Serotonin Reuptake Inhibitors; Serotonin/Norepinephrine Reuptake Inhibitors; Sodium Phosphates; Tipranavir; Treprostinil; Vitamin E

Decreased Effect
Etodolac may decrease the levels/effects of: ACE Inhibitors; Aliskiren; Angiotensin II Receptor Blockers; Antiplatelet Agents; Beta-Blockers; Eplerenone; HydrALAZINE; Loop Diuretics; Potassium-Sparing Diuretics; Salicylates; Selective Serotonin Reuptake Inhibitors; Thiazide Diuretics

The levels/effects of Etodolac may be decreased by: Bile Acid Sequestrants; Nonsteroidal Anti-Inflammatory Agents; Salicylates

Ethanol/Nutrition/Herb Interactions
Ethanol: Avoid ethanol (may enhance gastric mucosal irritation).
Food: Etodolac peak serum levels may be decreased if taken with food.
Herb/Nutraceutical: Avoid alfalfa, anise, bilberry, bladderwrack, bromelain, cat's claw, celery, chamomile, coleus, cordyceps, dong quai, evening primrose, fenugreek, feverfew, garlic, ginger, ginkgo biloba, ginseng (American, Panax, Siberian), grapeseed, green tea, guggul, horse chestnut seed, horseradish, licorice, prickly ash, red clover, reishi, SAMe (S-adeno-sylmethionine), sweet clover, turmeric, white willow (all have additional antiplatelet activity).

Stability Store at 20°C to 25°C (68°F to 77°F). Protect from moisture.

Mechanism of Action Reversibly inhibits cyclooxygenase-1 and 2 (COX-1 and 2) enzymes, which results in decreased formation of prostaglandin precursors; has antipyretic, analgesic, and anti-inflammatory properties

Other proposed mechanisms not fully elucidated (and possibly contributing to the anti-inflammatory effect to varying degrees), include inhibiting chemotaxis, altering lymphocyte activity, inhibiting neutrophil aggregation/activation, and decreasing proinflammatory cytokine levels.

Pharmacodynamics/Kinetics
Onset of action: Analgesic: 2-4 hours; Maximum anti-inflammatory effect: A few days
Absorption: ≥80%
Distribution: V_d:
Immediate release: Adults: 0.4 L/kg
Extended release: Adults: 0.57 L/kg
Protein binding: ≥99%, primarily albumin
Metabolism: Hepatic
Bioavailability: 100%
Half-life elimination: Terminal: Adults: 5-8 hours
Time to peak, serum:
Immediate release: Adults: 1-2 hours
Extended release: 5-7 hours, increased 1.4-3.8 hours with food
Excretion: Urine 73% (1% unchanged); feces 16%

Dosage

Geriatric & Adult Note: For chronic conditions, response is usually observed within 2 weeks.

Acute pain: Oral: Immediate release formulation: 200-400 mg every 6-8 hours, as needed, not to exceed total daily doses of 1000 mg

Rheumatoid arthritis, osteoarthritis: Oral:

Immediate release formulation: 400 mg 2 times/day **or** 300 mg 2-3 times/day **or** 500 mg 2 times/day (doses >1000 mg/day have not been evaluated)

Extended release formulation: 400-1000 mg once daily

Renal Impairment

Mild-to-moderate: No adjustment required

Severe: Use not recommended; use with caution

Hemodialysis: Not removed

Hepatic Impairment No adjustment required.

Administration May be administered with food to decrease GI upset.

Monitoring Parameters Monitor CBC and chemistry profile, liver enzymes; in patients with an increased risk for renal failure (CHF or decreased renal function, taking ACE inhibitors or diuretics, elderly), monitor urine output and BUN/serum creatinine

Test Interactions False-positive for urinary bilirubin and ketone

Special Geriatric Considerations The elderly are a high-risk population for adverse effects from nonsteroidal anti-inflammatory agents. As much as 60% of older adults who experience GI side effects can develop peptic ulceration and/or hemorrhage asymptomatically. The concomitant use of H_2 blockers and sucralfate is not effective as prophylaxis with the exception of NSAID-induced duodenal ulcers which may be prevented by the use of ranitidine. Misoprostol and proton pump inhibitors are the only agents proven to help prevent the development of NSAID-induced ulcers. Also, concomitant disease and drug use contribute to the risk for GI adverse effects. Use lowest effective dose for shortest period possible. Consider renal function decline with age. Use of NSAIDs can compromise existing renal function especially when Cl_{cr} is ≤30 mL/minute.

Tinnitus may be a difficult and unreliable indication of toxicity due to age-related hearing loss or eighth cranial nerve damage. CNS adverse effects such as confusion, agitation, and hallucination are generally seen in overdose or high dose situations, but older adults may demonstrate these adverse effects at lower doses than younger adults. In patients ≥65 years, no substantial differences in the pharmacokinetics or side-effects profile were seen compared with the general population. Studies with etodolac in elderly demonstrated no difference in safety or efficacy compared to younger adults. No dosing adjustment necessary in elderly.

This medication is considered to be potentially inappropriate in this patient population (Beers Criteria: Quality of evidence - moderate; Strength of recommendation - strong).

Dosage Forms Excipient information presented when available (limited, particularly for generics); consult specific product labeling.

Capsule, oral: 200 mg, 300 mg

Tablet, oral: 400 mg, 500 mg

Tablet, extended release, oral: 400 mg, 500 mg, 600 mg

Exemestane (ex e MES tane)

Medication Safety Issues

Sound-alike/look-alike issues:

Aromasin® may be confused with Arimidex®

Exemestane may be confused with estramustine.

Gastrointestinal: Abdominal pain, anorexia, cramps, diarrhea, epigastric pain, gastric upset, gum hypertrophy, nausea, tongue swelling, vomiting, weight loss

Genitourinary: Hematuria (microscopic), vaginal bleeding

Hematologic: Agranulocytosis, eosinophilia, leukopenia, pancytopenia

Ocular: Myopia

Miscellaneous: Allergic reaction, drug rash with eosinophilia and systemic symptoms (DRESS), hiccups, systemic lupus erythematosus

Drug Interactions

Metabolism/Transport Effects Substrate of CYP3A4 (major); **Note:** Assignment of Major/Minor substrate status based on clinically relevant drug interaction potential

Avoid Concomitant Use

Avoid concomitant use of Ethosuximide with any of the following: Azelastine; Azelastine (Nasal); Conivaptan; Methadone; Mirtazapine; Paraldehyde

Increased Effect/Toxicity

Ethosuximide may increase the levels/effects of: Alcohol (Ethyl); Azelastine; Azelastine (Nasal); Buprenorphine; CNS Depressants; Fosphenytoin; Methadone; Methotrimeprazine; Metyrosine; Mirtazapine; Paraldehyde; Phenytoin; Selective Serotonin Reuptake Inhibitors; Zolpidem

The levels/effects of Ethosuximide may be increased by: Conivaptan; CYP3A4 Inhibitors (Moderate); CYP3A4 Inhibitors (Strong); Dasatinib; Divalproex; Droperidol; HydrOXYzine; Ivacaftor; Methotrimeprazine; Mifepristone; Valproic Acid

Decreased Effect

Ethosuximide may decrease the levels/effects of: Divalproex; Valproic Acid

The levels/effects of Ethosuximide may be decreased by: Amphetamines; CYP3A4 Inducers (Strong); Deferasirox; Fosphenytoin; Herbs (CYP3A4 Inducers); Ketorolac; Ketorolac (Nasal); Ketorolac (Systemic); Mefloquine; Phenytoin; Tocilizumab

Ethanol/Nutrition/Herb Interactions

Ethanol: May increase CNS depression; monitor for increased effects with coadministration. Caution patients about effects.

Herb/Nutraceutical: St John's wort may decrease ethosuximide levels.

Stability

Capsules: Store at 25°C (77°F); excursions permitted to 15°C to 30°C (59°F to 86°F).

Solution: Store below 30°C (86°F); do not freeze. Protect from light.

Mechanism of Action Increases the seizure threshold and suppresses paroxysmal spike-and-wave pattern in absence seizures; depresses nerve transmission in the motor cortex

Pharmacodynamics/Kinetics

Distribution: Adults: V_d: 0.62-0.72 L/kg

Metabolism: Hepatic (~80% to 3 inactive metabolites)

Half-life elimination, serum: Adults: 50-60 hours

Time to peak, serum: Capsule: ~2-4 hours; Syrup: <2-4 hours

Excretion: Urine, slowly (50% as metabolites, 10% to 20% as unchanged drug); feces (small amounts)

Dosage

Geriatric & Adult Management of absence (petit mal) seizures: Oral: Initial: 500 mg/day; increase by 250 mg as needed every 4-7 days up to 1.5 g/day in divided doses

Renal Impairment No dosage adjustment provided in manufacturer's labeling; use with caution.

Hepatic Impairment No dosage adjustment provided in manufacturer's labeling; use with caution.

Monitoring Parameters Seizure frequency; trough serum concentrations, CBC, platelets, liver enzymes (periodic), urinalysis (periodic); signs of rash; suicidality (eg, suicidal thoughts, depression, behavioral changes)

Reference Range Therapeutic: 40-100 mcg/mL

Special Geriatric Considerations No specific studies with the use of this medication in the elderly. Consider renal function and proceed slowly with dosing increases; monitor closely.

Dosage Forms Excipient information presented when available (limited, particularly for generics); consult specific product labeling. [DSC] = Discontinued product

Capsule, softgel, oral: 250 mg

Zarontin®: 250 mg

Solution, oral: 250 mg/5 mL (473 mL)

Zarontin®: 250 mg/5 mL (480 mL) [contains sodium benzoate; raspberry flavor]

Syrup, oral: 250 mg/5 mL (473 mL [DSC])

◆ **Ethoxynaphthamido Penicillin Sodium** see Nafcillin on page 1330

◆ **Ethyl Esters of Omega-3 Fatty Acids** see Omega-3-Acid Ethyl Esters on page 1416

Etidronate (e ti DROE nate)

Medication Safety Issues
Sound-alike/look-alike issues:
Etidronate may be confused with etomidate

Brand Names: U.S. Didronel®

Brand Names: Canada Co-Etidronate; Mylan-Etidronate

Index Terms EHDP; Etidronate Disodium; Sodium Etidronate

Generic Availability (U.S.) Yes

Pharmacologic Category Bisphosphonate Derivative

Use Symptomatic treatment of Paget's disease; prevention and treatment of heterotopic ossification due to spinal cord injury or after total hip replacement

Contraindications Hypersensitivity to bisphosphonates or any component of the formulation; overt osteomalacia; patients with abnormalities of the esophagus which delay esophageal emptying, such as stricture or achalasia

Warnings/Precautions Ensure adequate calcium and vitamin D intake. Etidronate may retard mineralization of bone; treatment may need delayed or interrupted until callus is present. Use caution in patients with renal impairment. Use caution with enterocolitis; diarrhea has been reported at high doses and therapy may need to be withheld.

Osteonecrosis of the jaw (ONJ) has been reported in patients receiving bisphosphonates. Risk factors include invasive dental procedures (eg, tooth extraction, dental implants, boney surgery); a diagnosis of cancer, with concomitant chemotherapy or corticosteroids; poor oral hygiene; ill-fitting dentures; and comorbid disorders (anemia, coagulopathy, infection, pre-existing dental disease). Most reported cases occurred after I.V. bisphosphonate therapy; however, cases have been reported following oral therapy. A dental exam and preventative dentistry should be performed prior to placing patients with risk factors on chronic bisphosphonate therapy. The manufacturer's labeling states that discontinuing bisphosphonates in patients requiring invasive dental procedures may reduce the risk of ONJ. However, other experts suggest that there is no evidence that discontinuing therapy reduces the risk of developing ONJ (Assael, 2009). The benefit/risk must be assessed by the treating physician and/or dentist/surgeon prior to any invasive dental procedure. Patients developing ONJ while on bisphosphonates should receive care by an oral surgeon.

Infrequently, severe (and occasionally debilitating) bone, joint, and/or muscle pain have been reported during bisphosphonate treatment. The onset of pain ranged from a single day to several months. Consider discontinuing therapy in patients who experience severe symptoms; symptoms usually resolve upon discontinuation. Some patients experienced recurrence when rechallenged with same drug or another bisphosphonate; avoid use in patients with a history of these symptoms in association with bisphosphonate therapy. Do not exceed recommended dose or use continuously for >6 months in patients with Paget's disease; risk of osteomalacia or fractures may be increased. Long bones with predominantly lytic lesions may be prone to fracture, particularly in patients unresponsive to treatment.

Adverse Reactions (Reflective of adult population; not specific for elderly) Frequency not defined.

Gastrointestinal: Diarrhea, nausea

Neuromuscular & skeletal: Bone pain

Drug Interactions

Metabolism/Transport Effects None known.

Avoid Concomitant Use There are no known interactions where it is recommended to avoid concomitant use.

Increased Effect/Toxicity

Etidronate may increase the levels/effects of: Deferasirox; Phosphate Supplements; SUNItinib

The levels/effects of Etidronate may be increased by: Aminoglycosides; Nonsteroidal Anti-Inflammatory Agents

Decreased Effect

The levels/effects of Etidronate may be decreased by: Antacids; Calcium Salts; Iron Salts; Magnesium Salts; Proton Pump Inhibitors

Ethanol/Nutrition/Herb Interactions Food: Food and/or supplements decrease the absorption and bioavailability of the drug. Management: Administer tablet on an empty stomach with a full glass of plain water or fruit juice (6-8 oz) 2 hours before food. Avoid administering foods/supplements with calcium, iron, or magnesium within 2 hours of drug. Do not take with mineral water or other beverages.

Stability Store at controlled room temperature of 15°C to 30°C (59°F to 86°F).

Brand Names: U.S. Aromasin®
Brand Names: Canada Aromasin®
Generic Availability (U.S.) Yes
Pharmacologic Category Antineoplastic Agent, Aromatase Inactivator
Use Treatment of advanced breast cancer in postmenopausal women whose disease has progressed following tamoxifen therapy; adjuvant treatment of postmenopausal estrogen receptor-positive early breast cancer following 2-3 years of tamoxifen (for a total of 5 years of adjuvant therapy)
Unlabeled Use Risk reduction for invasive breast cancer in postmenopausal women; treatment of endometrial cancer; treatment of uterine sarcoma
Contraindications Hypersensitivity to exemestane or any component of the formulation
Warnings/Precautions Hazardous agent - use appropriate precautions for handling and disposal. Due to decreased circulating estrogen levels, exemestane is associated with a reduction in bone mineral density; decreases (from baseline) in lumbar spine and femoral neck density have been observed. Grade 3 or 4 lymphopenia has been observed with exemestane use, although most patients had preexisting lower grade lymphopenia. Increases in bilirubin, alkaline phosphatase and serum creatinine have been observed. Not to be given with estrogen-containing agents. Dose adjustment recommended with concomitant CYP3A4 inducers.

Adverse Reactions (Reflective of adult population; not specific for elderly)
>10%:
  Cardiovascular: Hypertension (5% to 15%)
  Central nervous system: Fatigue (8% to 22%), insomnia (11% to 14%), pain (13%), headache (7% to 13%), depression (6% to 13%)
  Dermatological: Hyperhidrosis (4% to 18%), alopecia (15%)
  Endocrine & metabolic: Hot flashes (13% to 33%)
  Gastrointestinal: Nausea (9% to 18%), abdominal pain (6% to 11%)
  Hepatic: Alkaline phosphatase increased (14% to 15%)
  Neuromuscular & skeletal: Arthralgia (15% to 29%)
1% to 10%:
  Cardiovascular: Edema (6% to 7%); cardiac ischemic events (2%: MI, angina, myocardial ischemia); chest pain
  Central nervous system: Dizziness (8% to 10%), anxiety (4% to 10%), fever (5%), confusion, hypoesthesia
  Dermatologic: Dermatitis (8%), itching, rash
  Endocrine & metabolic: Weight gain (8%)
  Gastrointestinal: Diarrhea (4% to 10%), vomiting (7%), anorexia (6%), constipation (5%), appetite increased (3%), dyspepsia
  Genitourinary: Urinary tract infection (2% to 5%)
  Hepatic: Bilirubin increased (5% to 7%)
  Neuromuscular & skeletal: Back pain (9%), limb pain (9%), myalgia (6%), osteoarthritis (6%), weakness (6%), osteoporosis (5%), pathological fracture (4%), paresthesia (3%), carpal tunnel syndrome (2%), cramps (2%)
  Ocular: Visual disturbances (5%)
  Renal: Creatinine increased (6%)
  Respiratory: Dyspnea (10%), cough (6%), bronchitis, pharyngitis, rhinitis, sinusitis, upper respiratory infection
  Miscellaneous: Flu-like syndrome (6%), lymphedema, infection

A dose-dependent decrease in sex hormone-binding globulin has been observed with daily doses of ≥2.5 mg. Serum luteinizing hormone and follicle-stimulating hormone levels have increased with this medicine.

Drug Interactions
  Metabolism/Transport Effects **Substrate** of CYP3A4 (major); **Note:** Assignment of Major/Minor substrate status based on clinically relevant drug interaction potential; **Induces** CYP3A4 (weak/moderate)
  Avoid Concomitant Use
    Avoid concomitant use of Exemestane with any of the following: Axitinib
  Increased Effect/Toxicity There are no known significant interactions involving an increase in effect.
  Decreased Effect
    Exemestane may decrease the levels/effects of: ARIPiprazole; Axitinib; Saxagliptin

    The levels/effects of Exemestane may be decreased by: CYP3A4 Inducers (Strong); Deferasirox; Herbs (CYP3A4 Inducers); Tocilizumab

Ethanol/Nutrition/Herb Interactions

Food: Plasma levels increased by 40% when exemestane was taken with a fatty meal.

Herb/Nutraceutical: St John's wort may decrease exemestane levels. Avoid black cohosh, dong quai in estrogen-dependent tumors.

Stability Store at 25°C (77°F); excursions permitted to 15°C to 30°C (59°F to 86°F).

Mechanism of Action Exemestane is an irreversible, steroidal aromatase inactivator. It is structurally related to androstenedione, and is converted to an intermediate that irreversibly blocks the active site of the aromatase enzyme, leading to inactivation ("suicide inhibition") and thus preventing conversion of androgens to estrogens in peripheral tissues. In post-menopausal breast cancers where growth is estrogen-dependent, this medicine will lower circulating estrogens.

Pharmacodynamics/Kinetics

Absorption: Rapid and moderate (~42%) following oral administration; absorption increases ~40% following high-fat meal

Distribution: Extensive into tissues

Protein binding: 90%, primarily to albumin and α_1-acid glycoprotein

Metabolism: Extensively hepatic; oxidation (CYP3A4) of methylene group, reduction of 17-keto group with formation of many secondary metabolites; metabolites are inactive

Half-life elimination: 24 hours

Time to peak: Women with breast cancer: 1.2 hours

Excretion: Urine (<1% as unchanged drug, 39% to 45% as metabolites); feces (36% to 48%)

Dosage

Geriatric & Adult Females: Postmenopausal:

Breast cancer, advanced: Oral: 25 mg once daily; continue until tumor progression

Breast cancer, early (adjuvant treatment): Oral: 25 mg once daily (following 2-3 years of tamoxifen therapy) for a total duration of 5 years of endocrine therapy (in the absence of recurrence or contralateral breast cancer)

Breast cancer, risk reduction (unlabeled use): Oral: 25 mg once daily for up to 5 years (Goss, 2011)

Dosage adjustment with CYP3A4 inducers: U.S. labeling: 50 mg once daily when used with potent inducers (eg, rifampin, phenytoin)

Renal Impairment No adjustment necessary (although the safety of chronic doses in patients with moderate-to-severe renal impairment has not been studied, dosage adjustment does not appear necessary).

Hepatic Impairment No adjustment necessary (although the safety of chronic doses in patients with moderate-to-severe hepatic impairment has not been studied, dosage adjustment does not appear necessary).

Administration Administer after a meal.

Pharmacotherapy Pearls Oncology Comment: The American Society of Clinical Oncology (ASCO) guidelines for adjuvant endocrine therapy in postmenopausal women with HR-positive breast cancer (Burstein, 2010) recommend considering aromatase inhibitor (AI) therapy at some point in the treatment course (primary, sequentially, or extended). Optimal duration at this time is not known; however, treatment with an AI should not exceed 5 years in primary and extended therapies, and 2-3 years if followed by tamoxifen in sequential therapy (total of 5 years). If initial therapy with AI has been discontinued before the 5 years, consideration should be taken to receive tamoxifen for a total of 5 years. The optimal time to switch to an AI is also not known, but data supports switching after 2-3 years of tamoxifen (sequential) or after 5 years of tamoxifen (extended). If patient becomes intolerant or has poor adherence, consideration should be made to switch to another AI or initiate tamoxifen.

Special Geriatric Considerations In pharmacokinetic trials, no significant changes were seen in women <68 years of age.

Dosage Forms Excipient information presented when available (limited, particularly for generics); consult specific product labeling.

Tablet, oral: 25 mg

Aromasin®: 25 mg

Exenatide (ex EN a tide)

Related Information

Diabetes Mellitus Management, Adults *on page* 2193

Brand Names: U.S. Bydureon™; Byetta®

Brand Names: Canada Byetta®

Index Terms AC 2993; AC002993; Exendin-4; LY2148568

Generic Availability (U.S.) No

Pharmacologic Category Antidiabetic Agent, Glucagon-Like Peptide-1 (GLP-1) Receptor Agonist

Use Treatment of type 2 diabetes mellitus (noninsulin dependent, NIDDM) to improve glycemic control

Canadian labeling: In conjunction with metformin and/or sulfonylurea for treatment of type 2 diabetes mellitus (noninsulin dependent, NIDDM) to improve glycemic control

Medication Guide Available Yes

Contraindications Hypersensitivity to exenatide or any component of the formulation

Bydureon™: Additional contraindications: History of or family history of medullary thyroid carcinoma (MTC); patients with multiple endocrine neoplasia syndrome type 2 (MEN2)

Byetta™: Canadian labeling: Additional contraindications (not in U.S. labeling): End-stage renal disease or severe renal impairment (Cl_{cr} <30 mL/minute) including dialysis patients; diabetic ketoacidosis, diabetic coma/precoma or type 1 diabetes mellitus

Warnings/Precautions Bydureon™: **[U.S. Boxed Warning] Dose- and duration- dependent thyroid C-cell tumors have developed in animal studies with exenatide extended release therapy; relevance in humans unknown.** Patients should be counseled on the risk and symptoms (eg, neck mass, dysphagia, dyspnea, persistent hoarseness) of thyroid tumors. Consultation with an endocrinologist is recommended in patients who develop elevated calcitonin concentrations or have thyroid nodules detected during imaging studies or physical exam. Use is contraindicated in patients with a personal or a family history of medullary thyroid cancer and in patients with multiple endocrine neoplasia syndrome type 2 (MEN2). All cases of MTC should be reported to the applicable state cancer registry.

Mechanism requires the presence of insulin, therefore use in type 1 diabetes (insulin dependent, IDDM) or diabetic ketoacidosis is not recommended (use is contraindicated in the Canadian labeling); it is not a substitute for insulin in insulin-requiring patients. Concurrent use with insulin therapy has not been evaluated and is not recommended. (Exception: Safety and efficacy of concurrent insulin glargine and immediate release exenatide has been demonstrated in a clinical trial.) May increase the risk of hypoglycemia in patients receiving concomitant insulin secretagogues (eg, sulfonylureas, meglitinides); dosage reduction of sulfonylureas may be required. Clinicians should note that the risk of hypoglycemia is not increased when exenatide is added to metformin monotherapy. Avoid concurrent use of extended release (weekly) and immediate release (daily) exenatide formulations. Bydureon™ is not recommended for first-line therapy in patients inadequately controlled on diet and exercise alone.

Exenatide is frequently associated with gastrointestinal adverse effects and is not recommended for use in patients with gastroparesis or severe gastrointestinal disease. Gastrointestinal effects may be dose-related and may decrease in frequency/severity with gradual titration and continued use. Due to its effects on gastric emptying, exenatide may reduce the rate and extent of absorption of orally-administered drugs; use with caution in patients receiving medications with a narrow therapeutic window or require rapid absorption from the GI tract. Administer medications 1 hour prior to the use of immediate release (daily) exenatide when optimal drug absorption and peak levels are important to the overall therapeutic effect (eg, antibiotics, oral contraceptives); effects of extended release (weekly) exenatide on drug absorption have not been evaluated; use caution. Cases of acute pancreatitis (including hemorrhagic and necrotizing with some fatalities) have been reported; monitor for unexplained severe abdominal pain and if pancreatitis suspected, discontinue use. Do not resume unless an alternative etiology of pancreatitis is confirmed. Consider alternative antidiabetic therapy in patients with a history of pancreatitis. Use may be associated with the development of anti-exenatide antibodies. Low titers are not associated with a loss of efficacy; however, high titers (observed in 6% to 12% of patients in clinical studies) may result in an attenuation of response. May be associated with weight loss (due to reduced intake) independent of the change in hemoglobin A_{1c}.

Not recommended in severe renal impairment (Cl_{cr} <30 mL/minute) or end-stage renal disease (ESRD) (use in these patients and in dialysis patients is contraindicated in the Canadian labeling). Patients with ESRD receiving dialysis may be more susceptible to GI effects (eg, nausea, vomiting) which may result in hypovolemia and further reductions in renal function. Use with caution in patients with renal transplantation or in patients with moderate renal impairment (Cl_{cr} 30-50 mL/minute). Cases of acute renal failure and chronic renal failure exacerbation, including severe cases requiring hemodialysis, have been reported, predominately in patients with nausea/vomiting/diarrhea or dehydration; renal dysfunction was usually reversible with appropriate corrective measures, including discontinuation of exenatide. Risk may be increased in patients receiving concomitant medications affecting renal function and/or hydration status.

Adverse Reactions (Reflective of adult population; not specific for elderly)

>10%:

Endocrine & metabolic: Hypoglycemia (monotherapy 2% to 5%; combination therapy with sulfonylurea 14% to 36%, with metformin ≤4%, with thiazolidinedione 11%)

Gastrointestinal: Nausea (monotherapy 8% to 11%; combination therapy 13% to 44%; dose-dependent), vomiting (monotherapy 4%; combination therapy 11% to 13%), diarrhea (monotherapy <2% to 11%; combination therapy 6% to 20%), constipation (monotherapy 9%; combination therapy 6% to 10%)

Local: Injection site nodule (Bydureon™ 6% to 77%), injection site reactions (2% to 18%; includes erythema, hematoma, pruritus)

Miscellaneous: Anti-exenatide antibodies (low titers 38% to 49%, high titers 6% to 12%)

1% to 10%:

Central nervous system: Nervousness (9%), dizziness (monotherapy <2%; combination therapy 9%), headache (5% to 9%), fatigue (3% to 6%)

Dermatologic: Hyperhidrosis (3%)

Gastrointestinal: Viral gastroenteritis (6% to 9%), dyspepsia (monotherapy 3% to 7%; combination therapy 5% to 7%), GERD (3% to 7%), appetite decreased (1% to 5%)

Neuromuscular & skeletal: Weakness (4%)

Drug Interactions

Metabolism/Transport Effects None known.

Avoid Concomitant Use There are no known interactions where it is recommended to avoid concomitant use.

Increased Effect/Toxicity

Exenatide may increase the levels/effects of: Sulfonylureas; Vitamin K Antagonists

The levels/effects of Exenatide may be increased by: Pegvisomant

Decreased Effect

The levels/effects of Exenatide may be decreased by: Corticosteroids (Orally Inhaled); Corticosteroids (Systemic); Luteinizing Hormone-Releasing Hormone Analogs; Somatropin; Thiazide Diuretics

Ethanol/Nutrition/Herb Interactions

Ethanol: Ethanol may cause hypoglycemia. Management: Consume ethanol with caution.

Food: Administer Byetta® within 60 minutes of meals, not after meals. May administer Bydureon™ without regard to meals or time of day.

Stability

Bydureon™: Store under refrigeration at 2°C to 8°C (36°F to 46°F); vials may be stored at ≤25°C (≤77°F) for up to 4 weeks. Do not freeze (discard if freezing occurs). Protect from light. Reconstitute vial using provided diluent; use immediately.

Byetta®: Prior to initial use, store under refrigeration at 2°C to 8°C (36°F to 46°F); after initial use, may store at ≤25°C (≤77°F). Do not freeze (discard if freezing occurs). Protect from light. Pen should be discarded 30 days after initial use.

Mechanism of Action Exenatide is an analog of the hormone incretin (glucagon-like peptide 1 or GLP-1) which increases glucose-dependent insulin secretion, decreases inappropriate glucagon secretion, increases B-cell growth/replication, slows gastric emptying, and decreases food intake. Exenatide administration results in decreases in hemoglobin A_{1c} by approximately 0.5% to 1% (immediate release) or 1.5% to 1.9% (extended release).

Pharmacodynamics/Kinetics

Distribution: V_d: 28.3 L

Metabolism: Minimal systemic metabolism; proteolytic degradation may occur following glomerular filtration

Half-life elimination:

Immediate release (daily) formulation: 2.4 hours

Extended release (weekly) formulation: ~2 weeks

Time to peak, plasma: SubQ:

Immediate release (daily) formulation: 2.1 hours

Extended release (weekly) formulation: Triphasic: Phase 1: 2-5 hours; Phase 2: ~2 weeks; Phase 3: ~7 weeks

Excretion: Urine (majority of dose)

Dosage

Geriatric & Adult Adjunctive therapy of type 2 diabetes: SubQ:

Immediate release: Initial: 5 mcg twice daily within 60 minutes prior to a meal; after 1 month, may be increased to 10 mcg twice daily (based on response)

Extended release: 2 mg once weekly

Note: May administer a missed dose as soon as noticed if the next regularly scheduled dose is due in ≥3 days; resume normal schedule thereafter. To establish a new day of the week administration schedule, wait ≥3 days after last dose given, then administer next dose on new desired day of the week.

Conversion from immediate release to extended release: Initiate weekly administration of exenatide extended release the day after discontinuing exenatide immediate release. **Note:** May experience increased blood glucose levels for ~2 weeks after conversion. Pretreatment with immediate release exenatide is not required when initiating extended release exenatide.

Renal Impairment

Cl_{cr} ≥50 mL/minute: No dosage adjustment necessary

Cl_{cr} 30-50 mL/minute: No dosage adjustment provided in manufacturer's labeling; use caution.

Cl_{cr} <30 mL/minute:

U.S. labeling: Use is not recommended.

Canadian labeling: Use is contraindicated.

Hepatic Impairment No dosage adjustment provided in manufacturer's labeling (has not been studied); however, hepatic dysfunction is not expected to affect exenatide pharmacokinetics.

Administration SubQ:

Immediate release: Use only if clear, colorless, and free of particulate matter. Administer via injection in the upper arm, thigh, or abdomen. Administer within 60 minutes prior to morning and evening meal (or prior to the 2 main meals of the day, approximately ≥6 hours apart). Set up each new pen before the first use by priming it. See pen user manual for further details. Dial the dose into the dose window before each administration.

Extended release: Administer via injection in the upper arm, thigh, or abdomen; rotate injection sites weekly. Administer immediately after reconstitution. May administer without regard to meals or time of day.

Monitoring Parameters Serum glucose, hemoglobin A_{1c}, and renal function

Reference Range Recommendations for glycemic control in adults with diabetes (ADA, 2012):

Hb A_{1c}: <7%

Preprandial capillary plasma glucose: 70-130 mg/dL

Peak postprandial capillary blood glucose: <180 mg/dL

Pharmacotherapy Pearls A dosing strategy which employs progressive dose escalation of exenatide (initiating at 0.02 mcg/kg 3 times daily and increasing in increments of 0.02 mcg/kg every 3 days) has been described, limiting the frequency and severity of gastrointestinal adverse effects. The complexity of this regimen may limit its clinical application.

In animal models, exenatide has been a useful adjunctive therapy when added to immunotherapy protocols, resulting in recovery of beta cell function and sustained remission.

Special Geriatric Considerations In five clinical trials with exenatide once weekly, 16.6% (132 subjects) were ≥65 years; only 20 subjects were ≥75 years. There was no difference between younger and older subjects in outcomes. Use in patients ≥75 years is limited.

Intensive glucose control ($_{1c}$ <6.5%) has been linked to increased all-cause and cardiovascular mortality, hypoglycemia requiring assistance, and weight gain in adult type 2 diabetes. How "tightly" to control a geriatric patient's blood glucose needs to be individualized. Such a decision should be based on several factors, including the patient's functional and cognitive status, how well he/she recognizes hypoglycemic or hyperglycemic symptoms, and how to respond to them and other disease states. An Hb A_{1c} <7.5% is an acceptable endpoint for a healthy older adult, while <8% is acceptable for frail elderly patients, those with a duration of illness >10 years, or with those with comorbid conditions and requiring combination diabetes medications. Patients who are unable to accurately draw up their dose will need assistance, such as prefilled syringes. Initial doses may require considerations for renal function in the elderly with dosing adjusted subsequently based on blood glucose monitoring. For elderly patients with diabetes who are relatively healthy, attaining target goals for aspirin use, blood pressure, lipids, smoking cessation, and diet and exercise may be more important than normalized glycemic control.

Dosage Forms Excipient information presented when available (limited, particularly for generics); consult specific product labeling.

Injection, microspheres for suspension, extended release:

Bydureon™: 2 mg [contains polylactide-co-glycolide, sucrose 0.8 mg/vial; supplied with diluent]

Injection, solution:

Byetta®: 250 mcg/mL (2.4 mL) [10 mcg/0.04 mL; 60 doses]

Byetta®: 250 mcg/mL (1.2 mL) [5 mcg/0.02 mL; 60 doses]

- ◆ **ex-lax® Maximum Strength [OTC]** *see Senna on page 1764*
- ◆ **ex-lax® Ultra [OTC]** *see Bisacodyl on page 214*
- ◆ **Extavia®** *see Interferon Beta-1b on page 1032*
- ◆ **Extended Release Epidural Morphine** *see Morphine (Liposomal) on page 1317*
- ◆ **Extina®** *see Ketoconazole (Topical) on page 1065*
- ◆ **Extra Strength Doan's® [OTC]** *see Salicylates (Various Salts) on page 1742*
- ◆ **EYE001** *see Pegaptanib on page 1480*
- ◆ **Eylea™** *see Aflibercept (Ophthalmic) on page 48*

Ezetimibe (ez ET i mibe)

Related Information
Hyperlipidemia Management *on page 2130*

Medication Safety Issues
Sound-alike/look-alike issues:
Ezetimibe may be confused with ezogabine
Zetia® may be confused with Zebeta®, Zestril®

Brand Names: U.S. Zetia®

Brand Names: Canada Ezetrol®

Generic Availability (U.S.) No

Pharmacologic Category Antilipemic Agent, 2-Azetidinone

Use Use in combination with dietary therapy for the treatment of primary hypercholesterolemia (as monotherapy or in combination with HMG-CoA reductase inhibitors); homozygous sitosterolemia; homozygous familial hypercholesterolemia (in combination with atorvastatin or simvastatin); mixed hyperlipidemia (in combination with fenofibrate)

Contraindications Hypersensitivity to ezetimibe or any component of the formulation; concomitant use with an HMG-CoA reductase inhibitor in patients with active hepatic disease, unexplained persistent elevations in serum transaminases

Warnings/Precautions Secondary causes of hyperlipidemia should be ruled out prior to therapy. Use caution with severe renal (Cl_{cr} <30 mL/minute); if using concurrent simvastatin in patients with moderate-to-severe renal impairment, the manufacturer of ezetimibe recommends that simvastatin doses exceeding 20 mg be used with caution and close monitoring for adverse events (eg, myopathy). Use caution with mild hepatic impairment (Child-Pugh class A); not recommended for use with moderate or severe hepatic impairment (Child-Pugh classes B and C). Concurrent use of ezetimibe and fibric acid derivatives may increase the risk of cholelithiasis.

Adverse Reactions (Reflective of adult population; not specific for elderly) 1% to 10%:
Central nervous system: Fatigue (2%)
Gastrointestinal: Diarrhea (4%)
Hepatic: Transaminases increased (with HMG-CoA reductase inhibitors) (≥3 x ULN, 1%)
Neuromuscular & skeletal: Arthralgia (3%), pain in extremity (3%)
Respiratory: Upper respiratory tract infection (4%), sinusitis (3%)
Miscellaneous: Influenza (2%)

Drug Interactions
Metabolism/Transport Effects Substrate of SLCO1B1
Avoid Concomitant Use There are no known interactions where it is recommended to avoid concomitant use.
Increased Effect/Toxicity
Ezetimibe may increase the levels/effects of: CycloSPORINE; CycloSPORINE (Systemic)

The levels/effects of Ezetimibe may be increased by: CycloSPORINE; CycloSPORINE (Systemic); Eltrombopag; Fibric Acid Derivatives
Decreased Effect
The levels/effects of Ezetimibe may be decreased by: Bile Acid Sequestrants

Ethanol/Nutrition/Herb Interactions Food: Ezetimibe did not cause meaningful reductions in fat-soluble vitamin concentrations during a 2-week clinical trial. Effects of long-term therapy have not been evaluated.

Stability Store at controlled room temperature of 25°C (77°F). Protect from moisture.

Mechanism of Action Inhibits absorption of cholesterol at the brush border of the small intestine via the sterol transporter, Niemann-Pick C1-Like1 (NPC1L1). This leads to a decreased delivery of cholesterol to the liver, reduction of hepatic cholesterol stores and an increased clearance of cholesterol from the blood; decreases total C, LDL-cholesterol (LDL-C), ApoB, and triglycerides (TG) while increasing HDL-cholesterol (HDL-C).

Pharmacodynamics/Kinetics

Protein binding: >90% to plasma proteins

Metabolism: Undergoes glucuronide conjugation in the small intestine and liver; forms metabolite (active); may undergo enterohepatic recycling

Bioavailability: Variable

Half-life elimination: 22 hours (ezetimibe and metabolite)

Time to peak, plasma: 4-12 hours

Excretion: Feces (78%, 69% as ezetimibe); urine (11%, 9% as metabolite)

Dosage

Geriatric & Adult Hyperlipidemias, sitosterolemia: Oral: 10 mg/day

Renal Impairment AUC increased with severe impairment (Cl_{cr} <30 mL/minute); no dosing adjustment necessary.

Hepatic Impairment AUC increased with hepatic impairment:

Mild impairment (Child-Pugh class A): No dosing adjustment necessary.

Moderate-to-severe impairment (Child-Pugh class B or C): Use of ezetimibe not recommended.

Administration May be administered without regard to meals. May be taken at the same time as HMG-CoA reductase inhibitors. Administer ≥2 hours before or ≥4 hours after bile acid sequestrants.

Monitoring Parameters Total cholesterol profile prior to therapy, and when clinically indicated and/or periodically thereafter. When used in combination with fenofibrate, monitor LFTs and signs and symptoms of cholelithiasis.

Pharmacotherapy Pearls When studied in combination with fenofibrate for mixed hyperlipidemia, the dose of fenofibrate was 160 mg daily.

Special Geriatric Considerations The definition of and, therefore, when to treat hyperlipidemia in the elderly is a controversial issue. The National Cholesterol Education Program recommends that all adults maintain a plasma cholesterol <160 mg/dL. For elderly patients with one additional risk factor, goal LDL would be <130 mg/dL. It is the authors' belief that pharmacologic treatment be reserved for those who are unable to obtain a desirable plasma cholesterol concentration by diet alone and for whom the benefits of treatment are believed to outweigh the potential adverse effects, drug interactions, and cost of treatment.

Dosage Forms Excipient information presented when available (limited, particularly for generics); consult specific product labeling.

Tablet, oral:

Zetia®: 10 mg

Ezetimibe and Simvastatin (ez ET i mibe & SIM va stat in)

Related Information

Ezetimibe *on page 738*

Hyperlipidemia Management *on page 2130*

Simvastatin *on page 1777*

Medication Safety Issues

Sound-alike/look-alike issues:

Vytorin® may be confused with Vyvanse®

Brand Names: U.S. Vytorin®

Index Terms Simvastatin and Ezetimibe

Generic Availability (U.S.) No

Pharmacologic Category Antilipemic Agent, 2-Azetidinone; Antilipemic Agent, HMG-CoA Reductase Inhibitor

Use Used in combination with dietary modification for the treatment of primary hypercholesterolemia and homozygous familial hypercholesterolemia

Dosage

Geriatric & Adult

Note: Dosing limitation: Simvastatin 80 mg is limited to patients that have been taking this dose for >12 consecutive months without evidence of myopathy and are not currently taking or beginning to take a simvastatin dose-limiting or contraindicated interacting medication. If patient is unable to achieve low-density lipoprotein-cholesterol (LDL-C) goal using the 40 mg dose of simvastatin, increasing to 80 mg dose is not recommended. Instead, switch patient to an alternative LDL-C-lowering treatment providing greater LDL-C reduction. After initiation or titration, monitor lipid response after ≥2 weeks and adjust dose as necessary.

Homozygous familial hypercholesterolemia: Oral: Ezetimibe 10 mg and simvastatin 40 mg once daily in the evening.

Hyperlipidemias: Oral: Initial: Ezetimibe 10 mg and simvastatin 10-20 mg once daily in the evening. Dosing range: Ezetimibe 10 mg and simvastatin 10-40 mg once daily.
Patients who require less aggressive reduction in LDL-C: Initial: Ezetimibe 10 mg and simvastatin 10 mg once daily in the evening
Patients who require >55% reduction in LDL-C: Initial: Ezetimibe 10 mg and simvastatin 40 mg once daily in the evening

Dosage adjustment with concomitant medications: Oral: **Note:** Patients currently tolerating and requiring a dose of simvastatin 80 mg who require initiation of an interacting drug with a dose cap for simvastatin should be switched to an alternative statin with less potential for drug-drug interaction.
Amiodarone, amlodipine, or ranolazine: Simvastatin dose should **not** exceed 20 mg once daily.
Diltiazem or verapamil: Simvastatin dose should **not** exceed 10 mg once daily.

Dosage adjustment in Chinese patients on niacin doses ≥1 g/day: Oral: Use caution with simvastatin doses exceeding 20 mg/day; because of an increased risk of myopathy, do not administer simvastatin 80 mg

Renal Impairment Manufacturer's recommendations:
Mild-to-moderate renal impairment: No dosage adjustment necessary; neither ezetimibe or simvastatin undergo significant renal excretion
Severe renal impairment: **Note:** Degree of renal impairment (ie, creatinine clearance) not defined: Initiate therapy only if patient has already tolerated ≥5 mg daily of simvastatin; monitor closely.

Hepatic Impairment Manufacturer's recommendations:
Mild impairment: No dosage adjustment necessary.
Moderate-to-severe impairment: Use not recommended.

Special Geriatric Considerations See individual agents. According to the manufacturer, 32% (3242/10,189) of the patients in the clinical trials were >65 years of age, including 8% who were ≥75 years. The safety observed in this group was similar to the younger patients, although age ≥65 is a risk factor for myopathy. Adding ezetimibe to a statin will decrease LDL-C; however, benefit in event outcomes has not been demonstrated. No dose adjustment is necessary for initiation of treatment in the elderly.

Dosage Forms Excipient information presented when available (limited, particularly for generics); consult specific product labeling.
Tablet:
Vytorin® 10/10: Ezetimibe 10 mg and simvastatin 10 mg
Vytorin® 10/20: Ezetimibe 10 mg and simvastatin 20 mg
Vytorin® 10/40: Ezetimibe 10 mg and simvastatin 40 mg
Vytorin® 10/80: Ezetimibe 10 mg and simvastatin 80 mg

◆ **EZG** *see* Ezogabine *on page 740*

Ezogabine (e ZOG a been)

Medication Safety Issues
Sound-alike/look-alike issues:
Ezogabine may be confused with ezetimibe.
Potiga™ may be confused with Portia®

Brand Names: U.S. Potiga™
Index Terms D-23129; EZG; Retigabine; RTG
Generic Availability (U.S.)
No
Pharmacologic Category Anticonvulsant, Neuronal Potassium Channel Opener
Use Adjuvant treatment of partial-onset seizures
Medication Guide Available Yes
Contraindications There are no contraindications listed in the manufacturer's labeling.
Warnings/Precautions Urinary retention, including retention requiring catheterization, has been reported, generally within the first 6 months of treatment. All patients should be monitored for urologic symptoms; close monitoring is recommended in patients with other risk factors for urinary retention (eg, benign prostatic hyperplasia), patients unable to communicate clinical symptoms, or patients who use concomitant medications that may affect voiding (eg, anticholinergics). Dose-related neuropsychiatric disorders, including confusion, psychotic symptoms, and hallucinations, have been reported, generally within the first 8 weeks of treatment; some patients required hospitalization. Symptoms resolved in most patients within 7 days of discontinuation of ezogabine. The risk appears to be greatest with rapid titration at greater than the recommended doses. Dose-related dizziness and somnolence (generally mild-to-moderate) have been reported; effects generally occur during dose titration and appear to diminish with continued use. Patients must be cautioned about

performing tasks which require mental alertness (eg, operating machinery or driving). QT prolongation has been observed; monitor EKG in patients with electrolyte abnormalities (eg, hypokalemia, hypomagnesemia), hypothyroidism, familial long QT syndrome, concomitant medications which may augment QT prolongation, or any underlying cardiac abnormality which may also potentiate risk (eg, congestive heart failure, ventricular hypertrophy). Pooled analysis of trials involving various antiepileptics (regardless of indication) showed an increased risk of suicidal thoughts/behavior (incidence rate: 0.43% treated patients compared to 0.24% of patients receiving placebo); risk observed as early as 1 week after initiation and continued through duration of trials (most trials ≤24 weeks). Monitor all patients for notable changes in behavior that might indicate suicidal thoughts or depression; notify healthcare provider immediately if symptoms occur.

Dosage adjustment recommended in hepatic impairment; ezogabine exposure increases in moderate-to-severe impairment. Dosage adjustment recommended in renal impairment; ezogabine undergoes significant renal elimination. Use caution in elderly due to potential for urinary retention, particularly in older men with symptomatic BPH. Systemic exposure is increased in the elderly; dosage adjustment is recommended in patients ≥65 years of age.

Anticonvulsants should not be discontinued abruptly because of the possibility of increasing seizure frequency; therapy should be withdrawn gradually over a period of ≥3 weeks to minimize the potential of increased seizure frequency, unless safety concerns require a more rapid withdrawal.

Adverse Reactions (Reflective of adult population; not specific for elderly)

>10%: Central nervous system: Dizziness (dose related; 23%), somnolence (dose related; 22%), fatigue (15%)

2% to 10%:

Central nervous system: Confusion (dose related; 9%), vertigo (8%), coordination impaired (dose related; 7%), attention disturbance (6%), memory impairment (dose related; 6%), aphasia (dose related; 4%), balance disorder (dose related; 4%), anxiety (3%), amnesia (2%), disorientation (2%)

Gastrointestinal: Nausea (7%), constipation (dose related; 3%), weight gain (dose related; 3%), dysphagia (2%)

Ocular: Diplopia (7%), blurred vision (dose related; 5%)

Neuromuscular & skeletal: Tremor (dose related; 8%), weakness (5%), abnormal gait (dose related; 4%), dysarthria (4%), paresthesia (3%)

Renal: Chromaturia (dose related; 2%), dysuria (dose related; 2%), hematuria (2%), urinary hesitation (2%)

Miscellaneous: Influenza infection (3%)

Stability Store at 25°C (77°F); excursions permitted to 15°C to 30°C (59°F to 86°F).

Mechanism of Action Ezogabine binds the KCNQ (Kv7.2-7.5) voltage-gated potassium channels, thereby stabilizing the channels in the open formation and enhancing the M-current. As a result, neuronal excitability is regulated and epileptiform activity is suppressed. In addition, ezogabine may also exert therapeutic effects through augmentation of GABA-mediated currents.

Pharmacodynamics/Kinetics

Absorption: Rapid

Distribution: V_{dss}: 2-3 L/kg

Protein binding: Ezogabine: 80%; N-acetyl active metabolite (NAMR): 45%

Metabolism: Glucuronidation via UGT1A4, UGT1A1, UGT1A3, and UGT1A9 and acetylation via NAT2 to an N-acetyl active metabolite (NAMR) and other inactive metabolites (eg, N-glucuronides, N-glucoside)

Bioavailability: Oral: ~60%

Half-life elimination: Ezogabine and NAMR: 7-11 hours; increased by ~30% in elderly patients

Time to peak, plasma: 0.5-2 hours; delayed by 0.75 hours when administered with high-fat food

Excretion: Urine (85%, 36% of total dose as unchanged drug, 18% of total dose as NAMR); feces (14%, 3% of total dose as unchanged drug)

Dosage

Geriatric Partial-onset seizures, adjunct: Oral: Initial: 50 mg 3 times/day; may increase at weekly intervals in increments of ≤150 mg/day to a maximum daily dose of 750 mg/day

Adult Partial-onset seizures, adjunct: Oral: Initial: 100 mg 3 times/day; may increase at weekly intervals in increments of ≤150 mg/day to a maintenance dose of 200-400 mg 3 times/day (maximum: 1200 mg/day). In clinical trials, no additional benefit and an increase in adverse effects was observed with doses >900 mg/day.

Renal Impairment
Cl$_{cr}$ ≥50 mL/minute: No dosage adjustments are recommended.
Cl$_{cr}$ <50 mL/minute: Initial: 50 mg 3 times/day; may increase at weekly intervals in increments of ≤150 mg/day to a maximum daily dose of 600 mg/day.
ESRD requiring hemodialysis: Initial: 50 mg 3 times/ day; may increase at weekly intervals in increments of ≤150 mg/day to a maximum daily dose of 600 mg/day.

Hepatic Impairment
Mild impairment (Child-Pugh ≤7): No dosage adjustments are recommended.
Moderate impairment (Child-Pugh 7-9): Initial: 50 mg 3 times/day; may increase at weekly intervals in increments of ≤150 mg/day to a maximum daily dose of 750 mg/day.
Severe impairment (Child-Pugh >9): Initial: 50 mg 3 times/day; may increase at weekly intervals in increment of ≤150 mg/day to a maximum daily dose of 600 mg/day.

Administration Oral: May be administered with or without food; swallow tablets whole. If therapy is discontinued, gradually reduce dose over ≥3 weeks unless safety concerns require abrupt withdrawal.

Monitoring Parameters Seizures; electrolytes, bilirubin, ALT, AST, serum creatinine, QT interval; urinary retention; observe patient for excessive sedation, confusion, psychotic symptoms, and hallucinations; suicidality (eg, suicidal thoughts, depression, behavioral changes); evaluate for signs/symptoms of ezogabine toxicity

Test Interactions Falsely elevated: Bilirubin, serum; Bilirubin, urine

Special Geriatric Considerations Pharmacokinetic studies (single dose) have demonstrated that the elderly have an AUC that is approximately 40% to 50% higher than in younger adults, and a half-life that is prolonged by approximately 30%. As a result, a dose reduction is recommended when initiating this agent. Additionally, the dose must be adjusted for renal function for Cl$_{cr}$ <50 mL/minute, of which many elderly will be below. It would be recommended to calculate a creatinine clearance before initiating this drug in elderly.

Controlled Substance C-V

Dosage Forms Excipient information presented when available (limited, particularly for generics); consult specific product labeling.
Tablet, oral:
Potiga™: 50 mg, 200 mg, 300 mg, 400 mg

◆ **F$_3$T** see Trifluridine on page 1968
◆ **Factive®** see Gemifloxacin on page 871

Famciclovir (fam SYE kloe veer)

Medication Safety Issues
Sound-alike/look-alike issues:
Famvir® may be confused with Femara®

Brand Names: U.S. Famvir®

Brand Names: Canada Apo-Famciclovir®; Ava-Famciclovir; CO Famciclovir; Famvir®; PMS-Famciclovir; Sandoz-Famciclovir

Generic Availability (U.S.) Yes

Pharmacologic Category Antiviral Agent

Use Treatment of acute herpes zoster (shingles) in immunocompetent patients; treatment and suppression of recurrent episodes of genital herpes in immunocompetent patients; treatment of herpes labialis (cold sores) in immunocompetent patients; treatment of recurrent orolabial/genital (mucocutaneous) herpes simplex in HIV-infected patients

Contraindications Hypersensitivity to famciclovir, penciclovir, or any component of the formulation

Warnings/Precautions Has not been established for use in immunocompromised patients (except HIV-infected patients with orolabial or genital herpes, patients with ophthalmic or disseminated zoster or with initial episode of genital herpes, and in Black and African American patients with recurrent episodes of genital herpes. Acute renal failure has been reported with use of inappropriate high doses in patients with underlying renal disease. Dosage adjustment is required in patients with renal insufficiency. Tablets contain lactose; do not use with galactose intolerance, severe lactase deficiency, or glucose-galactose malabsorption syndromes.

Adverse Reactions (Reflective of adult population; not specific for elderly) Note: Frequencies vary with dose and duration.

>10%:
Central nervous system: Headache (9% to 39%)
Gastrointestinal: Nausea (2% to 13%)

1% to 10%:
  Central nervous system: Fatigue (1% to 5%), migraine (1% to 3%)
  Dermatologic: Pruritus (≤4%), rash (≤3%)
  Endocrine & metabolic: Dysmenorrhea (≤8%)
  Gastrointestinal: Diarrhea (2% to 9%), abdominal pain (≤8%), vomiting (1% to 5%), flatulence (≤5%)
  Hematologic: Neutropenia (3%)
  Hepatic: Transaminases increased (2% to 3%), bilirubin increased (2%)
  Neuromuscular & skeletal: Paresthesia (≤3%)
Drug Interactions
  Metabolism/Transport Effects None known.
  Avoid Concomitant Use
    Avoid concomitant use of Famciclovir with any of the following: Zoster Vaccine
  Increased Effect/Toxicity There are no known significant interactions involving an increase in effect.
  Decreased Effect
    Famciclovir may decrease the levels/effects of: Zoster Vaccine
  Ethanol/Nutrition/Herb Interactions Food: Rate of absorption and/or conversion to penciclovir and peak concentration are reduced with food, but bioavailability is not affected.
Stability Store at 25°C (77°F); excursions permitted to 15°C to 30°C (59°F to 86°F).
Mechanism of Action Famciclovir undergoes rapid biotransformation to the active compound, penciclovir (prodrug), which is phosphorylated by viral thymidine kinase in HSV-1, HSV-2, and VZV-infected cells to a monophosphate form; this is then converted to penciclovir triphosphate and competes with deoxyguanosine triphosphate to inhibit HSV-2 polymerase, therefore, herpes viral DNA synthesis/replication is selectively inhibited.
Pharmacodynamics/Kinetics
  Absorption: Food decreases maximum peak penciclovir concentration and delays time to penciclovir peak; AUC remains the same
  Distribution: V_d: Penciclovir: 0.91-1.25 L/kg
  Protein binding: Penciclovir: <20%
  Metabolism: Famciclovir is rapidly deacetylated and oxidized to penciclovir (active prodrug); *in vitro* data demonstrate that metabolism does not occur via CYP isoenzymes
  Bioavailability: Penciclovir: 69% to 85%
  Half-life elimination: Penciclovir: 2-4 hours; Prolonged in renal impairment: Cl_{cr} 20-39 mL/minute: 5-8 hours, Cl_{cr} <20 mL/minute: 3-24 hours
  Time to peak: Penciclovir: ~1 hour
  Excretion: Urine (73% primarily as penciclovir); feces (27%)
Dosage
  Geriatric & Adult
    Immunocompetent patients:
      Acute herpes zoster: Oral: 500 mg every 8 hours for 7 days (**Note:** Initiate therapy as soon as possible after diagnosis and within 72 hours of rash onset)
      Genital herpes simplex virus (HSV) infection: Oral:
        Initial episode: 250 mg 3 times/day for 7-10 days (CDC, 2010)
        Recurrence: 1000 mg twice daily for 1 day (**Note:** Initiate therapy as soon as possible and within 6 hours of symptoms/lesions onset)
          Alternatively, the following regimens are also recommended: 125 mg twice daily for 5 days or 500 mg as a single dose, followed by 250 mg twice daily for 2 days (CDC, 2010). **Note:** Canadian labeling recommends 125 mg twice daily for 5 days.
        Suppressive therapy: 250 mg twice daily for up to 1 year; **Note:** Duration not established, but efficacy/safety have been demonstrated for 1 year (CDC, 2010)
      Recurrent herpes labialis (cold sores): Oral: 1500 mg as a single dose; initiate therapy at first sign or symptom such as tingling, burning, or itching (initiated within 1 hour in clinical studies)
    HIV patients (**Note:** Initiate therapy as soon as possible and within 48 hours of symptoms/lesions onset):
      Recurrent orolabial/genital (mucocutaneous) HSV infection: Oral: 500 mg twice daily for 7 days or 5-10 days (CDC, 2010).
      Prevention of HSV reactivation: Oral: 500 mg twice daily (CDC, 2010)
  Renal Impairment
    Dosing adjustment in renal impairment:
    Herpes zoster:
      Cl_{cr} ≥60 mL/minute: No dosage adjustment necessary
      Cl_{cr} 40-59 mL/minute: Administer 500 mg every 12 hours
      Cl_{cr} 20-39 mL/minute: Administer 500 mg every 24 hours
      Cl_{cr} <20 mL/minute: Administer 250 mg every 24 hours
      Hemodialysis: Administer 250 mg after each dialysis session.

Recurrent genital herpes: Treatment:
U.S. labeling (single-day regimen):
Cl_{cr} ≥60 mL/minute: No dosage adjustment necessary
Cl_{cr} 40-59 mL/minute: Administer 500 mg every 12 hours for 1 day
Cl_{cr} 20-39 mL/minute: Administer 500 mg as a single dose
Cl_{cr} <20 mL/minute: Administer 250 mg as a single dose
Hemodialysis: Administer 250 mg as a single dose after a dialysis session.
Canadian labeling:
Cl_{cr} >20 mL/minute/1.73 m^2: No dosage adjustment necessary
Cl_{cr} <20 mL/minute/1.73 m^2: Administer 125 mg every 24 hours
Hemodialysis: Administer 125 mg after each dialysis session.

Recurrent genital herpes: Suppression:
Cl_{cr} ≥40 mL/minute: No dosage adjustment necessary
Cl_{cr} 20-39 mL/minute: Administer 125 mg every 12 hours
Cl_{cr} <20 mL/minute: Administer 125 mg every 24 hours
Hemodialysis: Administer 125 mg after each dialysis session.

Recurrent herpes labialis: Treatment (single-dose regimen):
Cl_{cr} ≥60 mL/minute: No dosage adjustment necessary
Cl_{cr} 40-59 mL/minute: Administer 750 mg as a single dose
Cl_{cr} 20-39 mL/minute: Administer 500 mg as a single dose
Cl_{cr} <20 mL/minute: Administer 250 mg as a single dose
Hemodialysis: Administer 250 mg as a single dose after a dialysis session.

Recurrent orolabial/genital (mucocutaneous) herpes in HIV-infected patients:
Cl_{cr} ≥40 mL/minute: No dosage adjustment necessary
Cl_{cr} 20-39 mL/minute: Administer 500 mg every 24 hours
Cl_{cr} <20 mL/minute: Administer 250 mg every 24 hours
Hemodialysis: Administer 250 mg after each dialysis session.

Hepatic Impairment
Mild-to-moderate impairment: No dosage adjustment is necessary
Severe impairment: No dosage adjustment provided in manufacturer's labeling; has not been studied. However, a 44% decrease in the C_{max} of penciclovir (active metabolite) was noted in patients with mild-to-moderate impairment; impaired conversion of famciclovir to penciclovir may affect efficacy.

Administration May be administered without regard to meals.

Monitoring Parameters Periodic CBC during long-term therapy

Pharmacotherapy Pearls Most effective for herpes zoster if therapy is initiated within 48 hours of initial lesion. Resistance may occur by alteration of thymidine kinase, resulting in loss of or reduced penciclovir phosphorylation (cross-resistance occurs between acyclovir and famciclovir). When treatment for herpes labialis is initiated within 1 hour of symptom onset, healing time is reduced by ~2 days.

Special Geriatric Considerations For herpes zoster (shingles) infections, famciclovir should be started within 72 hours of the appearance of the rash to be effective. Famciclovir has been shown to accelerate healing, reduce the duration of viral shedding, and resolve posthepatic neuralgia faster than placebo. Adjust dose for estimated renal function.

Dosage Forms Excipient information presented when available (limited, particularly for generics); consult specific product labeling.
Tablet, oral: 125 mg, 250 mg, 500 mg
Famvir®: 125 mg [contains lactose 26.9 mg/tablet]
Famvir®: 250 mg [contains lactose 53.7 mg/tablet]
Famvir®: 500 mg [contains lactose 107.4 mg/tablet]

Famotidine (fa MOE ti deen)

Medication Safety Issues
Sound-alike/look-alike issues:
Famotidine may be confused with FLUoxetine, furosemide

Brand Names: U.S. Heartburn Relief Maximum Strength [OTC]; Heartburn Relief [OTC]; Pepcid®; Pepcid® AC Maximum Strength [OTC]; Pepcid® AC [OTC]

Brand Names: Canada Acid Control; Apo-Famotidine®; Apo-Famotidine® Injectable; Famotidine Omega; Mylan-Famotidine; Novo-Famotidine; Nu-Famotidine; Pepcid®; Pepcid® AC; Pepcid® I.V.; Ulcidine

Generic Availability (U.S.) Yes: Infusion, Injection, oral suspension, tablet

Pharmacologic Category Histamine H_2 Antagonist

Use Maintenance therapy and treatment of duodenal ulcer; treatment of gastroesophageal reflux disease (GERD), active benign gastric ulcer; pathological hypersecretory conditions
OTC labeling: Relief of heartburn, acid indigestion, and sour stomach

Unlabeled Use Part of a multidrug regimen for *H. pylori* eradication to reduce the risk of duodenal ulcer recurrence; stress ulcer prophylaxis in critically-ill patients; symptomatic relief in gastritis

Contraindications Hypersensitivity to famotidine, other H_2 antagonists, or any component of the formulation

Warnings/Precautions Modify dose in patients with moderate-to-severe renal impairment. Prolonged QT interval has been reported in patients with renal dysfunction. The FDA has received reports of torsade de pointes occurring with famotidine (Poluzzi, 2009). Relief of symptoms does not preclude the presence of a gastric malignancy. Reversible confusional states, usually clearing within 3-4 days after discontinuation, have been linked to use. Increased age (>50 years) and renal or hepatic impairment are thought to be associated. Multidose vials for injection contain benzyl alcohol.

OTC labeling: When used for self-medication, patients should be instructed not to use if they have difficulty swallowing, are vomiting blood, or have bloody or black stools. Not for use with other acid reducers.

Adverse Reactions (Reflective of adult population; not specific for elderly) 1% to 10%:

Central nervous system: Headache (5%), dizziness (1%)

Gastrointestinal: Diarrhea (2%), constipation (1%)

Drug Interactions

Metabolism/Transport Effects None known.

Avoid Concomitant Use

Avoid concomitant use of Famotidine with any of the following: Delavirdine

Increased Effect/Toxicity

Famotidine may increase the levels/effects of: Dexmethylphenidate; Highest Risk QTc-Prolonging Agents; Methylphenidate; Moderate Risk QTc-Prolonging Agents; Saquinavir; Varenicline

The levels/effects of Famotidine may be increased by: Mifepristone

Decreased Effect

Famotidine may decrease the levels/effects of: Atazanavir; Cefditoren; Cefpodoxime; Cefuroxime; Dasatinib; Delavirdine; Erlotinib; Fosamprenavir; Gefitinib; Indinavir; Iron Salts; Itraconazole; Ketoconazole; Ketoconazole (Systemic); Mesalamine; Nelfinavir; Nilotinib; Posaconazole; Rilpivirine; Vismodegib

Ethanol/Nutrition/Herb Interactions

Ethanol: Avoid ethanol (may cause gastric mucosal irritation).

Food: Famotidine bioavailability may be increased if taken with food.

Stability

Oral:

Powder for oral suspension: Prior to mixing, dry powder should be stored at controlled room temperature of 25°C (77°F). Reconstituted oral suspension is stable for 30 days at room temperature; do not freeze.

Tablet: Store at controlled room temperature. Protect from moisture.

I.V.:

Solution for injection: Prior to use, store at 2°C to 8°C (36°F to 46°F). If solution freezes, allow to solubilize at controlled room temperature. May be stored at room temperature for up to 3 months (data on file [Bedford Laboratories, 2011]).

I.V. push: Dilute famotidine with NS (or another compatible solution) to a total of 5-10 mL (some centers also administer undiluted). Following preparation, solutions for I.V. push should be used immediately, or may be stored in refrigerator and used within 48 hours.

Infusion: Dilute with D_5W 100 mL or another compatible solution. Following preparation, the manufacturer states may be stored for up to 48 hours under refrigeration; however, solutions for infusion have been found to be physically and chemically stable for 7 days at room temperature.

Solution for injection, premixed bags: Store at controlled room temperature of 25°C (77°F); avoid excessive heat.

Mechanism of Action Competitive inhibition of histamine at H_2 receptors of the gastric parietal cells, which inhibits gastric acid secretion

Pharmacodynamics/Kinetics

Onset of action: Antisecretory effect: Oral: Within 1 hour; I.V.: Within 30 minutes

Peak effect: Antisecretory effect: Oral: Within 1-3 hours (dose-dependent)

Duration: Antisecretory effect: I.V., Oral: 10-12 hours

Absorption: Oral: Incompletely absorbed

Distribution: V_d: ~1 L/kg

Protein binding: 15% to 20%

Metabolism: Minimal first-pass metabolism; forms one metabolite (S-oxide)

Bioavailability: Oral: 40% to 45%

◀ Half-life elimination: 2.5-3.5 hours; prolonged with renal impairment; Oliguria: >20 hours
Time to peak, serum: Oral: ~1-3 hours
Excretion: Urine (25% to 30% [oral], 65% to 70% [I.V.] as unchanged drug)

Dosage
Geriatric & Adult
Duodenal ulcer: Oral: Acute therapy: 40 mg/day at bedtime (or 20 mg twice daily) for 4-8 weeks; maintenance therapy: 20 mg/day at bedtime

Gastric ulcer: Oral: Acute therapy: 40 mg/day at bedtime

Hypersecretory conditions: Oral: Initial: 20 mg every 6 hours, may increase in increments up to 160 mg every 6 hours

GERD: Oral: 20 mg twice daily for 6 weeks

Esophagitis and accompanying symptoms due to GERD: Oral: 20 mg or 40 mg twice daily for up to 12 weeks

Peptic ulcer disease: Eradication of *Helicobacter pylori* (unlabeled use): Oral: 40 mg once daily; requires combination therapy with antibiotics

Patients unable to take oral medication: I.V.: 20 mg every 12 hours

Heartburn, indigestion, sour stomach: OTC labeling: Oral: 10-20 mg every 12 hours; dose may be taken 15-60 minutes before eating foods known to cause heartburn

Renal Impairment Cl_{cr} <50 mL/minute: Manufacturer recommendation: Administer 50% of dose **or** increase the dosing interval to every 36-48 hours (to limit potential CNS adverse effects).

Administration
I.V. push: Inject over at least 2 minutes
Solution for infusion: Administer over 15-30 minutes

Special Geriatric Considerations H_2 blockers are the preferred drugs for treating PUD in the elderly due to cost and ease of administration. They are no less or more effective than any other therapy. Famotidine is one of the preferred agents (due to side effects, drug interaction profile, and pharmacokinetics). Treatment for PUD in the elderly is recommended for 12 weeks since their lesions are typically larger; therefore, take longer to heal. Always adjust dose based upon creatinine clearance, since slight accumulation may result in CNS side effects, mainly confusion.

Dosage Forms Excipient information presented when available (limited, particularly for generics); consult specific product labeling.
Infusion, premixed in NS [preservative free]: 20 mg (50 mL)
Injection, solution: 10 mg/mL (4 mL, 20 mL, 50 mL)
Injection, solution [preservative free]: 10 mg/mL (2 mL)
Powder for suspension, oral: 40 mg/5 mL (50 mL)
Pepcid®: 40 mg/5 mL (50 mL) [contains sodium benzoate; cherry-banana-mint flavor]
Tablet, oral: 10 mg, 20 mg, 40 mg
Heartburn Relief: 10 mg
Heartburn Relief Maximum Strength: 20 mg
Pepcid®: 20 mg, 40 mg
Pepcid® AC: 10 mg
Pepcid® AC Maximum Strength: 20 mg
Tablet, chewable, oral:
Pepcid® AC Maximum Strength: 20 mg [berries 'n' cream flavor]
Pepcid® AC Maximum Strength: 20 mg [cool mint flavor]

◆ **Famotidine and Ibuprofen** see Ibuprofen and Famotidine on page 971

Famotidine, Calcium Carbonate, and Magnesium Hydroxide
(fa MOE ti deen, KAL see um KAR bun ate, & mag NEE zhum hye DROKS ide)

Related Information
Calcium Carbonate on page 262
Famotidine on page 744
Magnesium Hydroxide on page 1177
Brand Names: U.S. Pepcid® Complete® [OTC]; Tums® Dual Action [OTC]
Brand Names: Canada Pepcid® Complete® [OTC]
Index Terms Calcium Carbonate, Magnesium Hydroxide, and Famotidine; Magnesium Hydroxide, Famotidine, and Calcium Carbonate
Generic Availability (U.S.) No
Pharmacologic Category Antacid; Histamine H_2 Antagonist
Use Relief of heartburn due to acid indigestion

Dosage

Geriatric & Adult Relief of heartburn due to acid indigestion: Oral: Pepcid® Complete: 1 tablet as needed; no more than 2 tablets in 24 hours; do **not** swallow whole, chew tablet completely before swallowing; do not use for longer than 14 days

Special Geriatric Considerations Use with caution in the elderly with reduced renal function (Cl$_{cr}$ <30 mL/minute), since accumulation of magnesium and famotidine may occur and potentiate side effects

Dosage Forms Excipient information presented when available (limited, particularly for generics); consult specific product labeling.

Tablet, chewable, oral:

Pepcid® Complete®: Famotidine 10 mg, calcium carbonate 800 mg, and magnesium hydroxide 165 mg [contains calcium 320 mg/tablet, magnesium 70 mg/tablet; berry flavor]

Pepcid® Complete®: Famotidine 10 mg, calcium carbonate 800 mg, and magnesium hydroxide 165 mg [contains calcium 320 mg/tablet, magnesium 70 mg/tablet; mint flavor]

Pepcid® Complete®: Famotidine 10 mg, calcium carbonate 800 mg, and magnesium hydroxide 165 mg [contains calcium 320 mg/tablet, magnesium 70 mg/tablet, tartrazine; tropical fruit flavor]

Tums® Dual Action: Famotidine 10 mg, calcium carbonate 800 mg, and magnesium hydroxide 165 mg [contains calcium 320 mg/tablet, magnesium 65 mg/tablet, phenylalanine 2.2 mg/tablet; berry flavor]

Tums® Dual Action: Famotidine 10 mg, calcium carbonate 800 mg, and magnesium hydroxide 165 mg [contains calcium 320 mg/tablet, magnesium 65 mg/tablet, phenylalanine 2.2 mg/tablet; mint flavor]

Febuxostat (feb UX oh stat)

Brand Names: U.S. Uloric®
Brand Names: Canada Uloric®
Index Terms TEI-6720; TMX-67
Generic Availability (U.S.) No
Pharmacologic Category Antigout Agent; Xanthine Oxidase Inhibitor
Use Chronic management of hyperuricemia in patients with gout
Contraindications Concurrent use with azathioprine or mercaptopurine

Canadian labeling: Additional contraindications (not in U.S. labeling): Hypersensitivity to febuxostat or any component of the formulation; concomitant administration with theophylline

Warnings/Precautions Administer concurrently with an NSAID or colchicine (up to 6 months) to prevent gout flare upon initiation of therapy. Do not use to treat asymptomatic or secondary hyperuricemia. Significant hepatic transaminase elevations (>3 x ULN), MI, stroke and cardiovascular deaths have been reported in controlled trials (causal relationship not established). Monitor patients for signs/symptoms of MI and stroke. Liver function tests should be monitored 2 and 4 months after initiation of therapy and then periodically. Use with caution in patients with severe hepatic impairment (Child-Pugh class C); not studied. Use with caution in patients with severe renal impairment (Cl$_{cr}$ <30 mL/minute); insufficient data.

Adverse Reactions (Reflective of adult population; not specific for elderly) 1% to 10%:

Dermatologic: Rash (1% to 2%)
Hepatic: Liver function abnormalities (5% to 7%)
Neuromuscular & skeletal: Arthralgia (1%)

Drug Interactions

Metabolism/Transport Effects None known.

Avoid Concomitant Use

Avoid concomitant use of Febuxostat with any of the following: AzaTHIOprine; Didanosine; Mercaptopurine

Increased Effect/Toxicity

Febuxostat may increase the levels/effects of: AzaTHIOprine; Didanosine; Mercaptopurine; Theophylline Derivatives

Decreased Effect There are no known significant interactions involving a decrease in effect.

Stability Store at 25°C (77°F); excursions permitted to 15°C to 30°C (59°F to 86°F). Protect from light.

Mechanism of Action Selectively inhibits xanthine oxidase, the enzyme responsible for the conversion of hypoxanthine to xanthine to uric acid thereby decreasing uric acid. At therapeutic concentration does not inhibit other enzymes involved in purine and pyrimidine synthesis.

Pharmacodynamics/Kinetics

Absorption: ≥49%

Distribution: V_{ss}: ~50 L

Protein binding: ~99%, primarily to albumin

Metabolism: Extensive conjugation via uridine diphosphate glucuronosyltransferases (UGTs) 1A1, 1A3, 1A9, and 2B7 and oxidation via cytochrome P450 (CYP) 1A2, 2C8, and 2C9 as well as non-P450 enzymes. Oxidation leads to formation of active metabolites (67M-1, 67M-2, 67M-4)

Half-life elimination: ~5-8 hours

Time to peak, plasma: 1-1.5 hours

Excretion: Urine (~49% mostly as metabolites, 3% as unchanged drug); feces (~45% mostly as metabolites, 12% as unchanged drug)

Dosage

Geriatric & Adult Management of hyperuricemia in patients with gout: Note: It is recommended to take an NSAID or colchicine with initiation of therapy and may continue for up to 6 months to help prevent gout flares. If a gout flare occurs, febuxostat does not need to be discontinued.

Oral:

U.S. labeling: Initial: 40 mg once daily; may increase to 80 mg once daily in patients who do not achieve a serum uric acid level <6 mg/dL after 2 weeks

Canadian labeling: 80 mg once daily

Renal Impairment

Mild-to-moderate impairment (Cl_{cr} 30-89 mL/minute): No adjustment needed

Severe impairment (Cl_{cr} <30 mL/minute): Insufficient data; use caution (use not recommended in the Canadian labeling)

Dialysis: Not studied (use not recommended in the Canadian labeling)

Hepatic Impairment

Mild-to-moderate impairment (Child-Pugh class A or B): No adjustment needed

Severe impairment (Child-Pugh class C): Not studied; use caution (use not recommended in the Canadian labeling)

Administration Administer with or without meals or antacids.

Monitoring Parameters Liver function tests 2 and 4 months after initiation and then periodically, serum uric acid levels (as early as 2 weeks after initiation)

Reference Range Uric acid, serum:

Adults:

Male: 3.4-7 mg/dL or slightly more

Female: 2.4-6 mg/dL or slightly more

Target: <6 mg/dL

Values >7 mg/dL are sometimes arbitrarily regarded as hyperuricemia, but there is no sharp line between normals on the one hand, and the serum uric acid of those with clinical gout. Normal ranges cannot be adjusted for purine ingestion, but high purine diet increases uric acid. Uric acid may be increased with body size, exercise, and stress.

Special Geriatric Considerations In clinical trials, no clinically significant differences in safety or effectiveness were observed in elderly subjects. See Dosage: Renal Impairment.

Dosage Forms Excipient information presented when available (limited, particularly for generics); consult specific product labeling.

Tablet, oral:

Uloric®: 40 mg, 80 mg

Felbamate (FEL ba mate)

Brand Names: U.S. Felbatol®

Generic Availability (U.S.) Yes

Pharmacologic Category Anticonvulsant, Miscellaneous

Use Not as a first-line antiepileptic treatment; only in those patients who respond inadequately to alternative treatments and whose epilepsy is so severe that a substantial risk of aplastic anemia and/or liver failure is deemed acceptable in light of the benefits conferred by its use. Patient must be fully advised of risk and provide signed written informed consent. Felbamate can be used as either monotherapy or adjunctive therapy in the treatment of partial seizures (with and without generalization) and in adults with epilepsy.

Prescribing and Access Restrictions A patient "informed consent" form should be completed and signed by the patient and physician. Copies are available from MEDA Pharmaceuticals by calling 800-526-3840.

Medication Guide Available Yes

Contraindications Hypersensitivity to felbamate or any component of the formulation; known sensitivity to other carbamates; history of any blood dyscrasia or hepatic dysfunction

Warnings/Precautions [U.S. Boxed Warning]: Felbamate is associated with an increased risk of aplastic anemia. [U.S. Boxed Warning]: Felbamate has been associated with rare cases of hepatic failure (estimated >6 cases per 75,000 patients per year). Do not initiate treatment in patients with pre-existing hepatic dysfunction. Use caution in patients with renal impairment (dose adjustment recommended); half-life may be increased. Not indicated for use as a first-line antiepileptic treatment; only recommended in those patients who respond inadequately to alternative treatments and whose epilepsy is so severe that a substantial risk of aplastic anemia and/or liver failure is deemed acceptable in light of the benefits conferred by its use. Antiepileptics are associated with an increased risk of suicidal behavior/thoughts with use (regardless of indication); patients should be monitored for signs/symptoms of depression, suicidal tendencies, and other unusual behavior changes during therapy and instructed to inform their healthcare provider immediately if symptoms occur. Antiepileptic drugs should not be suddenly discontinued because of the possibility of increasing seizure frequency.

Adverse Reactions (Reflective of adult population; not specific for elderly)
>10%:
Central nervous system: Somnolence (children 48%; adults 19%), headache (children 7%; adults 7% to 37%), fever (children 23%; adults 3%), dizziness (18%), insomnia (9% to 18%), fatigue (7% to 17%), nervousness (children 16%; adults 7%)
Dermatologic: Purpura (children 13%)
Gastrointestinal: Anorexia (children 55%; adults 19%), vomiting (children 39%; adults 9% to 17%), nausea (children 7%; adults 34%), dyspepsia (9% to 12%), constipation (7% to 11%)
Respiratory: Upper respiratory infection (children 45%; adults 5% to 9%)
1% to 10%:
Cardiovascular: Chest pain (3%), facial edema (3%), palpitation (≥1%), tachycardia (≥1%)
Central nervous system: Abnormal thinking (children 7%; adults 4%), ataxia (children 7%; adults 4%), emotional lability (children 7%), anxiety (5%), depression (5%), stupor (3%), malaise (≥1%), agitation (≥1%), psychological disturbances (≥1%), aggressive reaction (≥1%), euphoria (≤1%), hallucination (≤1%), migraine (≤1%), suicide attempt (≤1%)
Dermatologic: Skin rash (children 10%; adults 3% to 4%), acne (3%), pruritus (≥1%), bullous eruption (≤1%), urticaria (≤1%)
Endocrine and metabolic: Hypophosphatemia (≤1% to 3%), intramenstrual bleeding (3%), hypokalemia (≤1%), hyponatremia (≤1%)
Gastrointestinal: Hiccup (children 10%), weight loss (children 7%; adults 3%), taste perversion (6%), abdominal pain (5%), diarrhea (5%), xerostomia (3%), weight gain (≥1%), appetite increased (≤1%), esophagitis (≤1%)
Genitourinary: Urinary tract infection (3%)
Hematologic: Leukopenia (children 7%; adults ≤1%), granulocytopenia (≤1%), leukocytosis (≤1%), lymphadenopathy (≤1%), thrombocytopenia (≤1%)
Hepatic: Liver function tests increased (1% to 5%), alkaline phosphatase increased (≤1%)
Neuromuscular & skeletal: Abnormal gait (children 10%; adults 5%), pain (children 7%), tremor (6%), paresthesia (4%), myalgia (3%), weakness (≥1%), dystonia (≤1%)
Ocular: Miosis (children 7%), diplopia (3% to 6%), abnormal vision (5%)
Otic: Otitis media (children 10%; adults 3%)
Respiratory: Pharyngitis (children 10%; adults 3%), cough (children 7%), rhinitis (7%), sinusitis (4%)
Miscellaneous: Flu-like syndrome (≥1%), LDH increased (≤1%)

Drug Interactions
Metabolism/Transport Effects Substrate of CYP2E1 (minor), CYP3A4 (major); **Note:** Assignment of Major/Minor substrate status based on clinically relevant drug interaction potential; **Inhibits** CYP2C19 (weak); **Induces** CYP3A4 (weak/moderate)
Avoid Concomitant Use
Avoid concomitant use of Felbamate with any of the following: Axitinib; Azelastine; Azelastine (Nasal); Conivaptan; Methadone; Mirtazapine; Paraldehyde
Increased Effect/Toxicity
Felbamate may increase the levels/effects of: Alcohol (Ethyl); Azelastine; Azelastine (Nasal); Barbiturates; Buprenorphine; CNS Depressants; Divalproex; Fosphenytoin;

Methadone; Methotrimeprazine; Metyrosine; Mirtazapine; Paraldehyde; PHENobarbital; Phenytoin; Primidone; Selective Serotonin Reuptake Inhibitors; Valproic Acid; Zolpidem

The levels/effects of Felbamate may be increased by: Conivaptan; CYP3A4 Inhibitors (Moderate); CYP3A4 Inhibitors (Strong); Dasatinib; Droperidol; HydrOXYzine; Ivacaftor; Methotrimeprazine; Mifepristone

Decreased Effect

Felbamate may decrease the levels/effects of: ARIPiprazole; Axitinib; CarBAMazepine; Contraceptives (Estrogens); Contraceptives (Progestins); Saxagliptin

The levels/effects of Felbamate may be decreased by: Barbiturates; CarBAMazepine; CYP3A4 Inducers (Strong); Deferasirox; Fosphenytoin; Herbs (CYP3A4 Inducers); Ketorolac; Ketorolac (Nasal); Ketorolac (Systemic); Mefloquine; PHENobarbital; Phenytoin; Primidone; Tocilizumab

Ethanol/Nutrition/Herb Interactions

Ethanol: May increase CNS depression; monitor for increased effects with coadministration. Caution patients about effects.

Food: Tablet: Food does not affect absorption.

Herb/Nutraceutical: Avoid evening primrose (seizure threshold decreased).

Stability Store in tightly closed container at controlled room temperature of 20°C to 25°C (68°F to 77°F).

Mechanism of Action Mechanism of action is unknown but has properties in common with other marketed anticonvulsants; has weak inhibitory effects on GABA-receptor binding, benzodiazepine receptor binding, and is devoid of activity at the MK-801 receptor binding site of the NMDA receptor-ionophore complex.

Pharmacodynamics/Kinetics Geriatrics: Reduced clearance and prolonged half-life have been reported in persons 66-78 years of age, compared to persons 18-45 years of age.

Absorption: Rapid and almost complete; food has no effect upon the tablet's absorption

Distribution: V_d: 0.7-0.8 L/kg

Protein binding: 22% to 25%, primarily to albumin

Half-life: 20-23 hours (average); prolonged in renal dysfunction

Time to peak, serum: 3-5 hours

Elimination: Urine (40% to 50% as unchanged drug, 40% as inactive metabolites)

Dosage

Geriatric & Adult

Anticonvulsant, monotherapy: Oral:

Initial: 1200 mg/day in divided doses 3 or 4 times/day; titrate previously untreated patients under close clinical supervision, increasing the dosage in 600 mg increments every 2 weeks to 2400 mg/day based on clinical response and thereafter to 3600 mg/day if clinically indicated

Conversion to monotherapy: Initiate at 1200 mg/day in divided doses 3 or 4 times/day, reduce the dosage of the concomitant anticonvulsant(s) by 33% at the initiation of felbamate therapy; at week 2, increase the felbamate dosage to 2400 mg/day while reducing the dosage of the other anticonvulsant(s) up to an additional 33% of their original dosage; at week 3, increase the felbamate dosage up to 3600 mg/day and continue to reduce the dosage of the other anticonvulsant(s) as clinically indicated

Anticonvulsant, adjunctive therapy: Oral: Initial: 1200 mg/day in divided doses 3 or 4 times/day; increase once per week by 1200 mg/day increments up to 3600 mg/day in divided doses 3 or 4 times/day.

Note: Dose of concomitant carbamazepine, phenobarbital, phenytoin, or valproic acid should be decreased by 20% when initiating felbamate therapy. Further dosage reductions may be necessary as dose of felbamate is increased.

Renal Impairment Use caution; reduce initial and maintenance doses by 50%.

Hepatic Impairment Use is contraindicated.

Administration May be administered with or without food. Shake suspension prior to use.

Monitoring Parameters Monitor serum levels of concomitant anticonvulsant therapy; obtain transaminases (AST, ALT) levels before initiation of therapy and periodically thereafter. Hematologic evaluations before therapy begins, frequently during therapy, and for a significant period after discontinuation. Monitor for suicidality (eg, suicidal thoughts, depression, behavioral changes).

Pharmacotherapy Pearls Monotherapy has not been associated with gingival hyperplasia, impaired concentration, weight gain, or abnormal thinking. Because felbamate is the only drug shown effective in Lennox-Gastaut syndrome, it is considered an orphan drug for this indication.

Special Geriatric Considerations Clinical studies have not included large numbers of patients >65 years of age. Due to decreased hepatic and renal function, dosing should start at the lower end of the dosage range.

Dosage Forms Excipient information presented when available (limited, particularly for generics); consult specific product labeling.
Suspension, oral: 600 mg/5 mL (240 mL, 473 mL)
  Felbatol®: 600 mg/5 mL (240 mL, 960 mL)
Tablet, oral: 400 mg, 600 mg
  Felbatol®: 400 mg, 600 mg [scored]

♦ **Felbatol®** see Felbamate *on page 748*
♦ **Feldene®** see Piroxicam *on page 1552*

Felodipine (fe LOE di peen)

Related Information
  Calcium Channel Blockers – Comparative Pharmacokinetics *on page 2111*
Medication Safety Issues
  Sound-alike/look-alike issues:
    Plendil® may be confused with Isordil®, pindolol, Pletal®, PriLOSEC®, Prinivil®
Brand Names: Canada Plendil®; Renedil®; Sandoz-Felodipine
Index Terms Plendil
Generic Availability (U.S.) Yes
Pharmacologic Category Calcium Channel Blocker; Calcium Channel Blocker, Dihydropyridine
Use Treatment of hypertension
Contraindications Hypersensitivity to felodipine, any component of the formulation, or other calcium channel blocker
Warnings/Precautions Increased angina and/or MI has occurred with initiation or dosage titration of dihydropyridine calcium channel blockers, reflex tachycardia may occur resulting in angina and/or MI in patients with obstructive coronary disease especially in the absence of concurrent beta-blockade. Use with extreme caution in patients with severe aortic stenosis. Use caution in patients with heart failure and/or hypertrophic cardiomyopathy with outflow tract obstruction. Elderly patients and patients with hepatic impairment should start off with a lower dose. Peripheral edema (dose dependent) is the most common side effect (occurs within 2-3 weeks of starting therapy). Symptomatic hypotension with or without syncope can rarely occur; blood pressure must be lowered at a rate appropriate for the patient's clinical condition. Dosage titration should occur after 14 days on a given dose.
Adverse Reactions (Reflective of adult population; not specific for elderly)
  >10%: Central nervous system: Headache (11% to 15%)
  2% to 10%: Cardiovascular: Peripheral edema (2% to 17%), tachycardia (0.4% to 2.5%), flushing (4% to 7%)
Drug Interactions
  Metabolism/Transport Effects Substrate of CYP3A4 (major); **Note:** Assignment of Major/Minor substrate status based on clinically relevant drug interaction potential; **Inhibits** CYP2C8 (moderate), CYP2C9 (weak), CYP2D6 (weak), CYP3A4 (weak)
  Avoid Concomitant Use
    Avoid concomitant use of Felodipine with any of the following: Conivaptan; Pimozide
  Increased Effect/Toxicity
    Felodipine may increase the levels/effects of: Amifostine; Antihypertensives; ARIPiprazole; Beta-Blockers; Calcium Channel Blockers (Nondihydropyridine); CYP2C8 Substrates; Fosphenytoin; Hypotensive Agents; Magnesium Salts; Neuromuscular-Blocking Agents (Nondepolarizing); Nitroprusside; Phenytoin; Pimozide; RiTUXimab; Tacrolimus; Tacrolimus (Systemic)

    The levels/effects of Felodipine may be increased by: Alpha1-Blockers; Antifungal Agents (Azole Derivatives, Systemic); Calcium Channel Blockers (Nondihydropyridine); Cimetidine; Conivaptan; CycloSPORINE; CycloSPORINE (Systemic); CYP3A4 Inhibitors (Moderate); CYP3A4 Inhibitors (Strong); Dasatinib; Diazoxide; Fluconazole; Grapefruit Juice; Herbs (Hypotensive Properties); Ivacaftor; Macrolide Antibiotics; Magnesium Salts; MAO Inhibitors; Mifepristone; Pentoxifylline; Phosphodiesterase 5 Inhibitors; Prostacyclin Analogues; Protease Inhibitors
  Decreased Effect
    Felodipine may decrease the levels/effects of: Clopidogrel

    The levels/effects of Felodipine may be decreased by: Barbiturates; Calcium Salts; CarBAMazepine; CYP3A4 Inducers (Strong); Deferasirox; Herbs (CYP3A4 Inducers); Herbs (Hypertensive Properties); Methylphenidate; Nafcillin; Rifamycin Derivatives; Tocilizumab; Yohimbine

Ethanol/Nutrition/Herb Interactions
Ethanol: Ethanol increases felodipine absorption. Management: Monitor for a greater hypotensive effect if ethanol is consumed.

Food: Compared to a fasted state, felodipine peak plasma concentrations are increased up to twofold when taken after a meal high in fat or carbohydrates. Grapefruit juice similarly increases felodipine C_{max} by twofold. Increased therapeutic and vasodilator side effects, including severe hypotension and myocardial ischemia, may occur. Management: May be taken with a small meal that is low in fat and carbohydrates; avoid grapefruit juice during therapy.

Herb/Nutraceutical: St John's wort may decrease felodipine levels. Dong quai has estrogenic activity. Some herbal medications may worsen hypertension (eg, ephedra); garlic may have additional antihypertensive effects. Management: Avoid dong quai if using for hypertension. Avoid ephedra, yohimbe, ginseng, and garlic.

Mechanism of Action Inhibits calcium ions from entering the "slow channels" or select voltage-sensitive areas of vascular smooth muscle and myocardium during depolarization, producing a relaxation of coronary vascular smooth muscle and coronary vasodilation; increases myocardial oxygen delivery in patients with vasospastic angina

Pharmacodynamics/Kinetics
Onset of action: Antihypertensive: 2-5 hours
Duration of antihypertensive effect: 24 hours
Absorption: 100%; Absolute: 20% due to first-pass effect
Protein binding: >99%
Metabolism: Hepatic; CYP3A4 substrate (major); extensive first-pass effect
Half-life elimination: Immediate release: 11-16 hours
Excretion: Urine (70% as metabolites); feces 10%

Dosage
Geriatric Refer to adult dosing. In the management of hypertension, consider lower initial doses (eg, 2.5 mg once daily) and titrate to response (Aronow, 2011).

Adult Hypertension: Oral: 2.5-10 mg once daily; increase by 5 mg at 2-week intervals, as needed, to a maximum of 20 mg/day; usual dose range (JNC 7): 2.5-20 mg once daily.

Hepatic Impairment Initial: 2.5 mg/day; monitor blood pressure

Administration Do not crush or chew extended release tablets; swallow whole.

Monitoring Parameters Heart rate, blood pressure

Pharmacotherapy Pearls Felodipine maintains renal and mesenteric blood flow during hemorrhagic shock in animals.

Special Geriatric Considerations Elderly may experience a greater hypotensive response. Constipation may be more of a problem in the elderly. Calcium channel blockers are no more effective in the elderly than other therapies; however, they do not cause significant CNS effects which is an advantage over some antihypertensive agents.

Dosage Forms Excipient information presented when available (limited, particularly for generics); consult specific product labeling.
Tablet, extended release, oral: 2.5 mg, 5 mg, 10 mg

♦ Femara® see Letrozole on page 1101
♦ Femilax™ [OTC] see Bisacodyl on page 214
♦ Femiron® [OTC] see Ferrous Fumarate on page 775
♦ Femring® see Estradiol (Systemic) on page 681
♦ Femtrace® see Estradiol (Systemic) on page 681
♦ Fenesin DM IR [OTC] see Guaifenesin and Dextromethorphan on page 906
♦ Fenesin IR [OTC] see GuaiFENesin on page 904

Fenofibrate (fen oh FYE brate)

Related Information
Hyperlipidemia Management on page 2130
Medication Safety Issues
Sound-alike/look-alike issues:
TriCor® may be confused with Fibricor®, Tracleer®

Brand Names: U.S. Antara®; Fenoglide®; Lipofen®; Lofibra®; TriCor®; Triglide®

Brand Names: Canada Apo-Feno-Micro®; Apo-Feno-Super®; Apo-Fenofibrate®; Dom-Fenofibrate Micro; Feno-Micro-200; Fenofibrate Micro; Fenofibrate-S; Fenomax; Lipidil EZ®; Lipidil Micro®; Lipidil Supra®; Mylan-Fenofibrate Micro; Novo-Fenofibrate; Novo-Fenofibrate Micronized; Novo-Fenofibrate-S; Nu-Fenofibrate; PHL-Fenofibrate Micro; PHL-Fenofibrate Supra; PMS-Fenofibrate Micro; PRO-Feno-Super; ratio-Fenofibrate MC; Riva-Fenofibrate Micro; Sandoz-Fenofibrate S

Index Terms Procetofene; Proctofene
Generic Availability (U.S.) Yes: Micronized capsule and tablet

Pharmacologic Category Antilipemic Agent, Fibric Acid

Use Adjunct to dietary therapy for the treatment of adults with elevations of serum triglyceride levels (types IV and V hyperlipidemia); adjunct to dietary therapy for the reduction of low density lipoprotein cholesterol (LDL-C), total cholesterol (total-C), triglycerides, and apolipo-protein B (apo B), and to increase high density lipoprotein cholesterol (HDL-C) in adult patients with primary hypercholesterolemia or mixed dyslipidemia (Fredrickson types IIa and IIb)

Contraindications Hypersensitivity to fenofibrate or any component of the formulation; hepatic dysfunction including primary biliary cirrhosis and unexplained persistent liver function abnormalities; severe renal dysfunction; pre-existing gallbladder disease

Canadian labeling: Additional contraindications (not in U.S. labeling): Known photoallergy or phototoxic reaction during treatment with fibrates or ketoprofen; allergy to soya lecithin or peanut or arachis oil

Warnings/Precautions Secondary causes of hyperlipidemia should be ruled out prior to therapy. Hepatic transaminases can become significantly elevated (dose-related); hepatocellular, chronic active, and cholestatic hepatitis have been reported. Regular monitoring of liver function tests is required. Use with caution in patients with mild-to-moderate renal impairment; dosage adjustment may be required. Contraindicated with severe renal impairment including those receiving dialysis. Increases in serum creatinine (>2 mg/dL) have been observed with use; monitor renal function in patients with renal impairment and consider monitoring patients with increased risk for developing renal impairment. May cause cholelithiasis. Use with caution in patient taking oral anticoagulants (eg, warfarin); adjustments in anticoagulation therapy may be required. Use caution with HMG-CoA reductase inhibitors (may lead to myopathy, rhabdomyolysis). No incremental benefit of combination therapy on cardiovascular morbidity and mortality over statin monotherapy has been established. In combination with HMG-CoA reductase inhibitors, fenofibrate is generally regarded as safer than gemfibrozil due to limited pharmacokinetic interaction with statins. Therapy should be withdrawn if an adequate response is not obtained after 2-3 months of therapy at the maximal daily dose. The occurrence of pancreatitis may represent a failure of efficacy in patients with severely elevated triglycerides. May cause mild-to-moderate decreases in hemoglobin, hematocrit, and WBC upon initiation of therapy which usually stabilizes with long-term therapy. Agranulocytosis and thrombocytopenia have rarely been reported. Periodic monitoring of blood counts is recommended during the first year of therapy.

Rare hypersensitivity reactions may occur. Use has been associated with pulmonary embolism (PE) and deep vein thrombosis (DVT). Use with caution in patients with risk factors for VTE. Dose adjustment may be required for elderly patients.

Adverse Reactions (Reflective of adult population; not specific for elderly)
>10%: Hepatic: Liver function tests increased (dose related; 3% to 13%)
1% to 10%:
   Central nervous system: Headache (3%)
   Gastrointestinal: Abdominal pain (5%), constipation (2%), nausea (2%)
   Neuromuscular & skeletal: Back pain (3%), CPK increased (3%)
   Respiratory: Respiratory disorder (6%), rhinitis (2%)

Drug Interactions

Metabolism/Transport Effects Substrate of CYP3A4 (minor); **Note:** Assignment of Major/Minor substrate status based on clinically relevant drug interaction potential; **Inhibits** CYP2A6 (weak), CYP2C8 (weak), CYP2C9 (weak)

Avoid Concomitant Use There are no known interactions where it is recommended to avoid concomitant use.

Increased Effect/Toxicity

Fenofibrate may increase the levels/effects of: Colchicine; Ezetimibe; HMG-CoA Reductase Inhibitors; Sulfonylureas; Vitamin K Antagonists; Warfarin

The levels/effects of Fenofibrate may be increased by: CycloSPORINE; CycloSPORINE (Systemic)

Decreased Effect

Fenofibrate may decrease the levels/effects of: Chenodiol; CycloSPORINE; CycloSPORINE (Systemic); Ursodiol

The levels/effects of Fenofibrate may be decreased by: Bile Acid Sequestrants; Tocilizumab

Stability Store at 15°C to 30°C (59°F to 86°F). Protect from light and moisture. Store tablets in moisture-protective container.

Mechanism of Action Fenofibric acid, an agonist for the nuclear transcription factor peroxisome proliferator-activated receptor-alpha (PPAR-alpha), downregulates apoprotein C-III (an inhibitor of lipoprotein lipase) and upregulates the synthesis of apolipoprotein A-I, fatty acid transport protein, and lipoprotein lipase resulting in an increase in VLDL catabolism, fatty acid oxidation, and elimination of triglyceride-rich particles; as a result of a decrease in

FENOFIBRATE

VLDL levels, total plasma triglycerides are reduced by 30% to 60%; modest increase in HDL occurs in some hypertriglyceridemic patients.

Pharmacodynamics/Kinetics

Absorption: Increased when taken with meals

Distribution: Widely to most tissues

Protein binding: >99%

Metabolism: Tissue and plasma via esterases to active form, fenofibric acid; undergoes inactivation by glucuronidation hepatically or renally

Half-life elimination: Fenofibric acid: Mean: 20 hours (range: 10-35 hours)

Time to peak: 3-8 hours

Excretion: Urine (60% as metabolites); feces (25%); hemodialysis has no effect on removal of fenofibric acid from plasma

Dosage

Geriatric Oral: Initial:

Antara® (micronized): 43 mg/day

Fenoglide®: Adjust dosage based on creatinine clearance

Lipidil EZ® [CAN; not available in U.S.]: 48 mg/day

Lipidil Micro® [CAN; not available in U.S.]: Adjust dosage based on creatinine clearance

Lipidil Supra® [CAN; not available in U.S.]: Adjust dosage based on creatinine clearance

Lipofen®: 50 mg/day

Lofibra® (micronized): 67 mg/day

Lofibra® (tablets): 54 mg/day

TriCor®: Adjust dosage based on creatinine clearance

Triglide®: 50 mg/day

Adult

Hypertriglyceridemia: Oral Initial:

Antara® (micronized): 43-130 mg/day; maximum dose: 130 mg/day

Fenoglide®: 40-120 mg/day; maximum dose: 120 mg/day

Lipidil EZ® [CAN; not available in U.S.]: 145 mg/day; maximum dose: 145 mg/day

Lipidil Micro® [CAN; not available in U.S.]: 200 mg/day; maximum dose: 200 mg/day

Lipidil Supra® [CAN; not available in U.S.]: 160 mg/day; maximum dose: 200 mg/day

Lipofen®: 50-150 mg/day; maximum dose: 150 mg/day

Lofibra® (micronized): 67-200 mg/day with meals; maximum dose: 200 mg/day

Lofibra® (tablets): 54-160 mg/day; maximum dose: 160 mg/day

TriCor®: 48-145 mg/day; maximum dose: 145 mg/day

Triglide®: 50-160 mg/day; maximum dose: 160 mg/day

Hypercholesterolemia or mixed hyperlipidemia: Oral:

Antara® (micronized): 130 mg/day

Fenoglide®: 120 mg/day

Lipidil EZ® [CAN; not available in U.S.]: 145 mg/day; maximum dose: 145 mg/day

Lipidil Micro® [CAN; not available in U.S.]: 200 mg/day; maximum dose: 200 mg/day

Lipidil Supra® [CAN; not available in U.S.]: 160 mg/day; maximum dose: 200 mg/day

Lipofen®: 150 mg/day

Lofibra® (micronized): 200 mg/day

Lofibra® (tablets): 160 mg/day

TriCor®: 145 mg/day

Triglide®: 160 mg/day

Renal Impairment Dosage adjustment in renal impairment: Monitor renal function and lipid panel before adjusting. **Note:** Use in severe renal impairment (including patients on dialysis) is contraindicated (see specific product labeling):

Antara® (micronized):

Cl_{cr} ≥50 mL/minute: No dosage adjustment necessary.

Cl_{cr} <50 mL/minute: Initiate at 43 mg/day (contraindicated in severe impairment)

Fenoglide®:

Cl_{cr} >80 mL/minute: No dosage adjustment necessary.

Cl_{cr} 31-80 mL/minute: Initiate at 40 mg/day

Cl_{cr} ≤30 mL/minute: Use is contraindicated.

Lipidil EZ® [CAN; not available in U.S.]: Cl_{cr} ≥20-50 mL/minute: Initiate at 48 mg/day

Lipidil Micro® [CAN; not available in U.S.]: Cl_{cr} ≥20-100 mL/minute: Initiate at 67 mg/day; **Note:** Lipidil Micro® 67 mg capsules are discontinued in Canada. Micronized formulation at this dosage strength is available through other manufacturers in Canada.

Lipidil Supra® [CAN; not available in U.S.]: Cl_{cr} ≥20-100 mL/minute: Initiate at 100 mg/day

Lipofen®:

Cl_{cr} >80 mL/minute: No dosage adjustment necessary.

Cl_{cr} 31-80 mL/minute: Initiate at 50 mg/day

Cl_{cr} ≤30 mL/minute: Use is contraindicated.

FENOFIBRIC ACID

Lofibra® (micronized):
Cl_{cr} ≥50 mL/minute: No dosage adjustment necessary.
Cl_{cr} <50 mL/minute: Initiate at 67 mg/day (contraindicated in severe impairment).
Lofibra® (tablets):
Cl_{cr} >80 mL/minute: No dosage adjustment necessary.
Cl_{cr} 31-80 mL/minute: Initiate at 54 mg/day
Cl_{cr} ≤30 mL/minute: Use is contraindicated.
TriCor®:
Cl_{cr} >80 mL/minute: No dosage adjustment necessary.
Cl_{cr} 31-80 mL/minute: Initiate at 48 mg/day
Cl_{cr} ≤30 mL/minute: Use is contraindicated.
Triglide®:
Cl_{cr} ≥50 mL/minute: No dosage adjustment necessary.
Cl_{cr} <50 mL/minute: Initiate at 50 mg/day (contraindicated in severe impairment).
Hepatic Impairment Use is contraindicated.
Administration 6-8 weeks of therapy is required to determine efficacy.
Fenoglide®, Lofibra® (capsules [micronized] and tablets), Lipofen®: Administer with meals.
Antara®, TriCor®: May be administered with or without food.
Triglide®: Do not consume chipped or broken tablets. May be administered with or without food.
Canadian products [not available in U.S.]:
Lipidil Micro®, Lipidil Supra®: Administer with meals.
Lipidil EZ®: May be administered with or without food.
Monitoring Parameters Periodic blood counts during first year of therapy. Total cholesterol, LDL-C, triglycerides, and HDL-C should be measured periodically; if only marginal changes are noted in 6-8 weeks, the drug should be discontinued. Monitor LFTs regularly and discontinue therapy if levels remain >3 times normal limits. Monitor renal function in patients with renal impairment or in those at increased risk for developing renal impairment.
Special Geriatric Considerations Adjust dose based on renal function and product.

The definition of and, therefore, when to treat hyperlipidemia in the elderly is a controversial issue. The National Cholesterol Education Program recommends that all adults maintain a plasma cholesterol <160 mg/dL. Older adults with one additional risk factor, goal LDL would be <130 mg/dL. It is the authors' belief that pharmacologic treatment be reserved for those who are unable to obtain a desirable plasma cholesterol concentration by diet alone and for whom the benefits of treatment are believed to outweigh the potential adverse effects, drug interactions, and cost of treatment.
Dosage Forms Excipient information presented when available (limited, particularly for generics); consult specific product labeling.
Capsule, oral:
Lipofen®: 50 mg, 150 mg
Capsule, oral [micronized]: 67 mg, 134 mg, 200 mg
Antara®: 43 mg, 130 mg
Lofibra®: 67 mg, 134 mg, 200 mg
Tablet, oral: 54 mg, 160 mg
Fenoglide®: 40 mg, 120 mg
Lofibra®: 54 mg, 160 mg
TriCor®: 48 mg, 145 mg [contains soybean lecithin]
Triglide®: 50 mg, 160 mg [contains egg lecithin]

Fenofibric Acid (fen oh FYE brik AS id)

Medication Safety Issues
Sound-alike/look-alike issues:
Fibricor® may be confused with Tricor®
TriLipix® may be confused with Trileptal®, TriLyte®
Brand Names: U.S. Fibricor®; TriLipix®
Index Terms ABT-335; Choline Fenofibrate
Generic Availability (U.S.) Yes
Pharmacologic Category Antilipemic Agent, Fibric Acid
Use Adjunct to dietary therapy for the treatment of severely elevated serum triglyceride levels; adjunct to dietary therapy for the reduction of low density lipoprotein cholesterol (LDL-C), total cholesterol (total-C), triglycerides, and apolipoprotein B (apo B) and to increase high density lipoprotein cholesterol (HDL-C) in patients with primary hypercholesterolemia or mixed dyslipidemia

TriLipix™ is also indicated as adjunct to dietary therapy concomitantly with a statin to reduce triglyceride levels and increase HDL-C levels in patients with mixed dyslipidemia and coronary heart disease (CHD) or at risk for CHD

Medication Guide Available Yes

Contraindications Hypersensitivity to fenofibric acid, choline fenofibrate, fenofibrate, or any component of the formulation; hepatic dysfunction including primary biliary cirrhosis and unexplained persistent liver function abnormalities; severe renal dysfunction (including patients on dialysis); pre-existing gallbladder disease

Warnings/Precautions Secondary causes of hyperlipidemia should be ruled out prior to therapy. Has been associated with rare myositis or rhabdomyolysis; patients should be monitored closely. Risk increased in the elderly, patients with diabetes mellitus, renal failure, or hypothyroidism. Patients should be instructed to report unexplained muscle pain, tenderness, weakness, or brown urine. Hepatic transaminases can become significantly elevated (dose-related); hepatocellular, chronic active, and cholestatic hepatitis have been reported. Regular monitoring of liver function tests is required. Use with caution in patients with mild-to-moderate renal impairment; dosage adjustment may be required. Contraindicated with severe renal impairment including those receiving dialysis. Increases in serum creatinine (>2 mg/dL) have been observed with use; monitor renal function in patients with renal impairment and consider monitoring patients with increased risk for developing renal impairment. May cause cholelithiasis discontinue if gallstones found upon gallbladder studies. Use caution with oral anticoagulants; adjustments in therapy may be required.

Use caution with HMG-CoA reductase inhibitors (may lead to myopathy, rhabdomyolysis). No incremental benefit of combination therapy on cardiovascular morbidity and mortality over statin monotherapy has been established. In combination with HMG-CoA reductase inhibitors, fenofibric acid derivatives are generally regarded as safer than gemfibrozil due to limited pharmacokinetic interaction. Therapy should be withdrawn if an adequate response is not obtained after 2-3 months of therapy at the maximal daily dose. The occurrence of pancreatitis may represent a failure of efficacy in patients with severely elevated triglycerides. May cause mild-to-moderate decreases in hemoglobin, hematocrit, and WBC upon initiation of therapy, which usually stabilizes with long-term therapy. Rare hypersensitivity reactions may occur. Use has been associated with pulmonary embolism (PE) and deep vein thrombosis (DVT). Use with caution in patients with risk factors for VTE. Dose adjustment is required for renal impairment and elderly patients.

Adverse Reactions (Reflective of adult population; not specific for elderly) Adverse reactions and frequency reported as observed during monotherapy and concurrent administration with a statin (HMG-CoA reductase inhibitor).

>10%: Central nervous system: Headache (12% to 13%)

1% to 10%:

Central nervous system: Dizziness (3% to 4%), pain (1% to 4%), fatigue (2% to 3%)

Gastrointestinal: Nausea (4% to 6%), dyspepsia (3% to 5%), diarrhea (3% to 4%), constipation (3%)

Hepatic: ALT increased (monotherapy: 1%; coadministered with statin: 3%)

Neuromuscular & skeletal: Back pain (4% to 6%), pain in extremities (3% to 5%), arthralgia (4%), myalgia (3% to 4%), muscle spasm (2% to 3%)

Respiratory: Nasopharyngitis (4% to 5%), upper respiratory infection (4% to 5%), sinusitis (3% to 4%)

Additional adverse reactions when fenofibric acid coadministered with a statin (frequency not defined): AST increased, bronchitis, cough, CPK increased, hepatic enzymes increased, hypertension, influenza, insomnia, musculoskeletal pain, pharyngolaryngeal pain, urinary tract infection

Drug Interactions

Metabolism/Transport Effects Inhibits CYP2A6 (weak), CYP2C8 (weak), CYP2C9 (moderate)

Avoid Concomitant Use There are no known interactions where it is recommended to avoid concomitant use.

Increased Effect/Toxicity

Fenofibric Acid may increase the levels/effects of: Carvedilol; Colchicine; CYP2C9 Substrates; Ezetimibe; HMG-CoA Reductase Inhibitors; Sulfonylureas; Vitamin K Antagonists; Warfarin

The levels/effects of Fenofibric Acid may be increased by: CycloSPORINE; CycloSPORINE (Systemic)

Decreased Effect

Fenofibric Acid may decrease the levels/effects of: Chenodiol; CycloSPORINE; CycloSPORINE (Systemic); Ursodiol

The levels/effects of Fenofibric Acid may be decreased by: Bile Acid Sequestrants

Stability Store at 25°C (77°F); excursions permitted to 15°C to 30°C (59°F to 86°F). Protect from light and moisture.

Mechanism of Action Fenofibric acid, an agonist for the nuclear transcription factor peroxisome proliferator-activated receptor-alpha (PPAR-alpha), downregulates apoprotein C-III (an inhibitor of lipoprotein lipase) and upregulates the synthesis of apolipoprotein A-I, fatty acid transport protein, and lipoprotein lipase resulting in an increase in VLDL catabolism, fatty acid oxidation, and elimination of triglyceride-rich particles; as a result of a decrease in VLDL levels, total plasma triglycerides are reduced by 30% to 60%; modest increased in HDL occurs in some hypertriglyceridemia patients.

Pharmacodynamics/Kinetics

Absorption: Well absorbed

Protein binding: ~99%

Metabolism: Fenofibric acid (active form) undergoes inactivation by glucuronidation. The choline salt dissociates in the GI tract to form fenofibric acid (free acid)

Bioavailability: TriLipix™: ~81%

Half-life elimination: ~20 hours

Time to peak, plasma: Fibricor®: ~2.5 hours; TriLipix™: 4-5 hours

Excretion: Urine (as fenofibric acid and fenofibric acid glucuronide)

Dosage

Geriatric Oral: Dosage based on renal function

Adult

Mixed dyslipidemia (coadministered with a statin): Oral: TriLipix™: 135 mg once daily (maximum: 135 mg/day)

Hypertriglyceridemia: Oral:

Fibricor®: Initial: 35-105 mg once daily; Maintenance: Individualize according to patient response (maximum: 105 mg/day)

TriLipix™: Initial: 45-135 mg once daily; Maintenance: Individualize according to patient response (maximum: 135 mg/day)

Primary hypercholesterolemia or mixed dyslipidemia: Oral:

Fibricor®: 105 mg once daily (maximum: 105 mg/day)

TriLipix™: 135 mg once daily (maximum: 135 mg/day)

Renal Impairment

Cl_{cr} >80 mL/minute: No dosage adjustment necessary.

Cl_{cr} 30-80 mL/minute: Initial: Fibricor®: 35 mg once daily or TriLipix™: 45 mg once daily; only increase once effects on lipids and renal function evaluated.

Cl_{cr} <30 mL/minute (with or without dialysis): Use is contraindicated.

Hepatic Impairment Use is contraindicated.

Administration May be administered with or without food.

Monitoring Parameters Periodic blood counts during first year of therapy; total cholesterol, LDL-C, triglycerides, and HDL-C should be measured periodically; monitor LFTs (including ALT) regularly and discontinue therapy if levels remain >3 times normal limits; serum creatinine (in patients with or at risk for renal impairment)

Special Geriatric Considerations Adjust dose based on renal function and product.

The definition of and, therefore, when to treat hyperlipidemia in the elderly is a controversial issue. The National Cholesterol Education Program recommends that all adults maintain a plasma cholesterol <160 mg/dL. Older adults with one additional risk factor, goal LDL would be <130 mg/dL. It is the authors' belief that pharmacologic treatment be reserved for those who are unable to obtain a desirable plasma cholesterol concentration by diet alone and for whom the benefits of treatment are believed to outweigh the potential adverse effects, drug interactions, and cost of treatment.

Dosage Forms Excipient information presented when available (limited, particularly for generics); consult specific product labeling.

Capsule, delayed release, oral:

TriLipix®: 45 mg, 135 mg

Tablet, oral: 35 mg, 105 mg

Fibricor®: 35 mg, 105 mg

◆ **Fenoglide®** see Fenofibrate on page 752

Fenoprofen (fen oh PROE fen)

Related Information
Beers Criteria – Potentially Inappropriate Medications for Geriatrics *on page 2183*

Medication Safety Issues
Sound-alike/look-alike issues:
Fenoprofen may be confused with flurbiprofen
BEERS Criteria medication:
This drug may be potentially inappropriate for use in geriatric patients (Quality of evidence - moderate; Strength of recommendation - strong).

Brand Names: U.S. Nalfon®
Brand Names: Canada Nalfon®
Index Terms Fenoprofen Calcium
Generic Availability (U.S.) Yes: Tablet
Pharmacologic Category Nonsteroidal Anti-inflammatory Drug (NSAID), Oral
Use Symptomatic treatment of acute and chronic rheumatoid arthritis and osteoarthritis; relief of mild-to-moderate pain
Unlabeled Use Migraine prophylaxis
Medication Guide Available Yes
Contraindications Hypersensitivity to fenoprofen, aspirin, or other NSAIDs, or any component of the formulation; perioperative pain in the setting of coronary artery bypass graft (CABG) surgery; significant renal dysfunction
Warnings/Precautions [U.S. Boxed Warning]: NSAIDs are associated with an increased risk of adverse cardiovascular thrombotic events, including MI and stroke. Risk may be increased with duration of use or pre-existing cardiovascular risk factors or disease. Carefully evaluate individual cardiovascular risk profiles prior to prescribing. May cause new-onset hypertension or worsening of existing hypertension. Use caution with fluid retention. Avoid use in heart failure. Concurrent administration of ibuprofen, and potentially other nonselective NSAIDs, may interfere with aspirin's cardioprotective effect. **[U.S. Boxed Warning]: Use is contraindicated for treatment of perioperative pain in the setting of coronary artery bypass graft (CABG) surgery.** Risk of MI and stroke may be increased with use following CABG surgery.

NSAID use may compromise existing renal function; dose-dependent decreases in prostaglandin synthesis may result from NSAID use, reducing renal blood flow which may cause renal decompensation. NSAID use may increase the risk for hyperkalemia. Patients with impaired renal function, dehydration, heart failure, liver dysfunction, those taking diuretics and ACE inhibitors, and the elderly are at greater risk of renal toxicity and hyperkalemia. Rehydrate patient before starting therapy; monitor renal function closely. Not recommended for use in patients with advanced renal disease. Long-term NSAID use may result in renal papillary necrosis.

[U.S. Boxed Warning]: NSAIDs may increase risk of gastrointestinal irritation, inflammation, ulceration, bleeding, and perforation. These events may occur at any time during therapy and without warning. Use caution with a history of GI disease (bleeding or ulcers), concurrent therapy with aspirin, anticoagulants and/or corticosteroids, smoking, use of alcohol, the elderly or debilitated patients. When used concomitantly with ≤325 mg of aspirin, a substantial increase in the risk of gastrointestinal complications (eg, ulcer) occurs; concomitant gastroprotective therapy (eg, proton pump inhibitors) is recommended (Bhatt, 2008).

Platelet adhesion and aggregation may be decreased; may prolong bleeding time; patients with coagulation disorders or who are receiving anticoagulants should be monitored closely. Anemia may occur; patients on long-term NSAID therapy should be monitored for anemia. Rarely, NSAID use has been associated with potentially severe blood dyscrasias (eg, agranulocytosis, thrombocytopenia, aplastic anemia).

Use the lowest effective dose for the shortest duration of time, consistent with individual patient goals, to reduce risk of cardiovascular or GI adverse events. Alternate therapies should be considered for patients at high risk.

NSAIDs may cause serious skin adverse events including exfoliative dermatitis, Stevens-Johnson syndrome (SJS), and toxic epidermal necrolysis (TEN); discontinue use at first sign of skin rash or hypersensitivity. Anaphylactoid reactions may occur, even without prior exposure; patients with "aspirin triad" (bronchial asthma, aspirin intolerance, rhinitis) may be at increased risk. Do not use in patients who experience bronchospasm, asthma, rhinitis, or urticaria with NSAID or aspirin therapy. Use caution in other forms of asthma.

Use with caution in patients with decreased hepatic function. Closely monitor patients with any abnormal LFT. Severe hepatic reactions (eg, fulminant hepatitis, liver failure) have occurred with NSAID use, rarely; discontinue if signs or symptoms of liver disease develop, or if systemic manifestations occur.

NSAIDS may cause drowsiness, dizziness, blurred vision and other neurologic effects which may impair physical or mental abilities; patients must be cautioned about performing tasks which require mental alertness (eg, operating machinery or driving). Discontinue use with blurred or diminished vision and perform ophthalmologic exam. Monitor vision with long-term therapy.

In the elderly, avoid chronic use (unless alternative agents ineffective and patient can receive concomitant gastroprotective agent); nonselective oral NSAID use is associated with an increased risk of GI bleeding and peptic ulcer disease in older adults in high risk category (eg, >75 years or age or receiving concomitant oral/parenteral corticosteroids, anticoagulants, or antiplatelet agents) (Beers Criteria).

Withhold for at least 4-6 half-lives prior to surgical or dental procedures.

Adverse Reactions (Reflective of adult population; not specific for elderly) 1% to 10%:

Cardiovascular: Peripheral edema (5%), palpitation (3%)

Central nervous system: Headache (9%), somnolence (9%), dizziness (7%), nervousness (6%), fatigue (2%), confusion (1%)

Dermatologic: Itching (4%), rash (4%)

Gastrointestinal: Dyspepsia (10%), nausea (8%), constipation (7%), vomiting (3%), abdominal pain (2%)

Neuromuscular & skeletal: Weakness (5%), tremor (2%)

Ocular: Blurred vision (2%)

Otic: Tinnitus (5%), hearing decreased (2%)

Respiratory: Dyspnea (3%), nasopharyngitis (1%)

Miscellaneous: Diaphoresis (5%)

Drug Interactions

Metabolism/Transport Effects None known.

Avoid Concomitant Use

Avoid concomitant use of Fenoprofen with any of the following: Floctafenine; Ketorolac; Ketorolac (Nasal); Ketorolac (Systemic)

Increased Effect/Toxicity

Fenoprofen may increase the levels/effects of: Aliskiren; Aminoglycosides; Anticoagulants; Antiplatelet Agents; Bisphosphonate Derivatives; Collagenase (Systemic); CycloSPORINE; CycloSPORINE (Systemic); Dabigatran Etexilate; Deferasirox; Desmopressin; Digoxin; Drotrecogin Alfa (Activated); Eplerenone; Haloperidol; Ibritumomab; Lithium; Methotrexate; Nonsteroidal Anti-Inflammatory Agents; PEMEtrexed; Porfimer; Potassium-Sparing Diuretics; PRALAtrexate; Quinolone Antibiotics; Rivaroxaban; Salicylates; Thrombolytic Agents; Tositumomab and Iodine I 131 Tositumomab; Vancomycin; Vitamin K Antagonists

The levels/effects of Fenoprofen may be increased by: ACE Inhibitors; Angiotensin II Receptor Blockers; Antidepressants (Tricyclic, Tertiary Amine); Corticosteroids (Systemic); CycloSPORINE; CycloSPORINE (Systemic); Dasatinib; Floctafenine; Glucosamine; Herbs (Anticoagulant/Antiplatelet Properties); Ketorolac; Ketorolac (Nasal); Ketorolac (Systemic); Nonsteroidal Anti-Inflammatory Agents; Omega-3-Acid Ethyl Esters; Pentosan Polysulfate Sodium; Pentoxifylline; Probenecid; Prostacyclin Analogues; Selective Serotonin Reuptake Inhibitors; Serotonin/Norepinephrine Reuptake Inhibitors; Sodium Phosphates; Tipranavir; Treprostinil; Vitamin E

Decreased Effect

Fenoprofen may decrease the levels/effects of: ACE Inhibitors; Aliskiren; Angiotensin II Receptor Blockers; Antiplatelet Agents; Beta-Blockers; Eplerenone; HydrALAZINE; Loop Diuretics; Potassium-Sparing Diuretics; Salicylates; Selective Serotonin Reuptake Inhibitors; Thiazide Diuretics

The levels/effects of Fenoprofen may be decreased by: Bile Acid Sequestrants; Nonsteroidal Anti-Inflammatory Agents; Salicylates

Ethanol/Nutrition/Herb Interactions

Ethanol: Avoid ethanol (may enhance gastric mucosal irritation).

Food: Fenoprofen peak serum levels may be decreased if taken with food; total amount absorbed is not affected.

Herb/Nutraceutical: Avoid alfalfa, anise, bilberry, bladderwrack, bromelain, cat's claw, celery, chamomile, coleus, cordyceps, dong quai, evening primrose, fenugreek, feverfew, garlic, ginger, ginkgo biloba, ginseng (American, Panax, Siberian), grapeseed, green tea, guggul, horse chestnut seed, horseradish, licorice, prickly ash, red clover, reishi, SAMe (S-adeno-sylmethionine), sweet clover, turmeric, white willow (all have additional antiplatelet activity).

Stability Store at controlled room temperature of 20°C to 25°C (67°F to 77°F).

◀ **Mechanism of Action** Reversibly inhibits cyclooxygenase-1 and 2 (COX-1 and 2) enzymes, which results in decreased formation of prostaglandin precursors; has antipyretic, analgesic, and anti-inflammatory properties

Other proposed mechanisms not fully elucidated (and possibly contributing to the anti-inflammatory effect to varying degrees), include inhibiting chemotaxis, altering lymphocyte activity, inhibiting neutrophil aggregation/activation, and decreasing proinflammatory cytokine levels.

Pharmacodynamics/Kinetics

Onset of action: A few days; full benefit: up to 2-3 weeks

Absorption: Rapid, 80%

Protein binding: 99%; to albumin

Metabolism: Extensively hepatic

Half-life elimination: 2.5-3 hours

Time to peak, serum: ~2 hours

Excretion: Urine (2% to 5% as unchanged drug); feces (small amounts)

Dosage

Geriatric & Adult

Rheumatoid arthritis, osteoarthritis: Oral: 300-600 mg 3-4 times/day; maximum dose: 3.2 g/day

Mild-to-moderate pain: Oral: 200 mg every 4-6 hours as needed; maximum dose: 3.2 g/day

Renal Impairment Not recommended in patients with advanced renal disease.

Administration Do not crush tablets. Swallow whole with a full glass of water. Take with food to minimize stomach upset.

Monitoring Parameters Monitor CBC, liver enzymes; monitor urine output and BUN/serum creatinine in patients receiving diuretics; monitor blood pressure in patients receiving antihypertensives; audiogram (in patients with baseline hearing impairment)

Reference Range Therapeutic: 20-65 mcg/mL (SI: 82-268 micromole/L)

Test Interactions Fenoprofen may interfere with Amerlex-M kit assay values; falsely elevated values of total and free triiodothyronine have been reported.

Special Geriatric Considerations Elderly are a high-risk population for adverse effects from NSAIDs. As much as 60% of elderly can develop peptic ulceration and/or hemorrhage asymptomatically. The concomitant use of H_2 blockers and sucralfate is not effective as prophylaxis with the exception of NSAID-induced duodenal ulcers which may be prevented by the use of ranitidine. Misoprostol and proton pump inhibitors are the only agents proven to help prevent the development of NSAID-induced ulcers. Also, concomitant disease and drug use contribute to the risk for GI adverse effects. Use lowest effective dose for shortest period possible. Consider renal function decline with age. Use of NSAIDs can compromise existing renal function especially when Cl_{cr} is ≤30 mL/minute. Tinnitus may be a difficult and unreliable indication of toxicity due to age-related hearing loss or eighth cranial nerve damage. CNS adverse effects such as confusion, agitation, and hallucination are generally seen in overdose or high-dose situations, but elderly may demonstrate these adverse effects at lower doses than younger adults.

This medication is considered to be potentially inappropriate in this patient population (Beers Criteria: Quality of evidence - moderate; Strength of recommendation - strong).

Dosage Forms Excipient information presented when available (limited, particularly for generics); consult specific product labeling.

Capsule, oral:

Nalfon®: 200 mg, 400 mg

Tablet, oral: 600 mg

◆ **Fenoprofen Calcium** see Fenoprofen on page 758

FentaNYL (FEN ta nil)

Related Information
Opioid Analgesics *on page 2122*
Patient Information for Disposal of Unused Medications *on page 2244*

Medication Safety Issues

Sound-alike/look-alike issues:
FentaNYL may be confused with alfentanil, SUFentanil

High alert medication:
The Institute for Safe Medication Practices (ISMP) includes this medication among its list of drug classes which have a heightened risk of causing significant patient harm when used in error.

Administration issues:
Fentanyl transdermal system patches: Leakage of fentanyl gel from the patch has been reported; patch may be less effective; do not use. Thoroughly wash any skin surfaces coming into direct contact with gel with water (do not use soap). May contain conducting metal (eg, aluminum); remove patch prior to MRI.

Other safety concerns:
Fentanyl transdermal system patches:
Dosing of transdermal fentanyl patches may be confusing. Transdermal fentanyl patches should always be prescribed in mcg/hour, not size. Patch dosage form of Duragesic®-12 actually delivers 12.5 mcg/hour of fentanyl. Use caution, as orders may be written as "Duragesic 12.5" which can be erroneously interpreted as a 125 mcg dose.

Patches should be stored and disposed of with care to avoid accidental exposure to children. The FDA has issued numerous safety advisories to warn users of the possible consequences (including death) of inappropriate storage or disposal of patches.

Abstral®, Actiq®, Fentora®, Onsolis®, and Subsys® are not interchangeable; do not substitute doses on a mcg-per-mcg basis.

Brand Names: U.S. Abstral®; Actiq®; Duragesic®; Fentora®; Lazanda®; Onsolis®; Subsys®

Brand Names: Canada Abstral™; Actiq®; Duragesic®; Duragesic® MAT; Fentanyl Citrate Injection, USP; Novo-Fentanyl; PMS-Fentanyl MTX; RAN™-Fentanyl Matrix Patch; RAN™-Fentanyl Transdermal System; ratio-Fentanyl

Index Terms Fentanyl Citrate; Fentanyl Hydrochloride; Fentanyl Patch; OTFC (Oral Transmucosal Fentanyl Citrate)

Generic Availability (U.S.) Yes: Injection, lozenge, patch

Pharmacologic Category Analgesic, Opioid; Anilidopiperidine Opioid; General Anesthetic

Use
Injection: Relief of pain, preoperative medication, adjunct to general or regional anesthesia
Transdermal patch (eg, Duragesic®): Management of persistent moderate-to-severe chronic pain in opioid-tolerant patients when around-the clock analgesia is needed for an extended period of time
Transmucosal lozenge (eg, Actiq®), buccal tablet (Fentora®), buccal film (Onsolis®), nasal spray (Lazanda®), sublingual tablet (Abstral®), sublingual spray (Subsys®): Management of breakthrough cancer pain in opioid-tolerant patients
Note: "Opioid-tolerant" patients are defined as patients who are taking at least:
Oral morphine 60 mg/day, **or**
Transdermal fentanyl 25 mcg/hour, **or**
Oral oxycodone 30 mg/day, **or**
Oral hydromorphone 8 mg/day, **or**
Oral oxymorphone 25 mg/day, **or**
Equianalgesic dose of another opioid for at least 1 week

Prescribing and Access Restrictions As a requirement of the REMS program, access is restricted.
Transmucosal immediate-release fentanyl products (eg, sublingual tablets and spray, oral lozenges, buccal tablets and soluble film, nasal spray) are only available through the Transmucosal Immediate-Release Fentanyl (TIRF) REMS ACCESS program. Enrollment in the program is required for outpatients, prescribers for outpatient use, pharmacies (inpatient and outpatient), and distributors. Enrollment is not required for inpatient administration (eg, hospitals, hospices, long-term care facilities), inpatients, and prescribers who prescribe to inpatients. Further information is available at 1-866-822-1483 or at www.TIRFREMSaccess.com

Note: Effective December, 2011, individual REMs programs for TIRF products were combined into a single access program (TIRF REMS Access). Prescribers and pharmacies that were enrolled in at least one individual REMS program for these products will automatically be transitioned to the single access program.

Medication Guide Available Yes

Contraindications Hypersensitivity to fentanyl or any component of the formulation

Additional contraindications for transdermal patches (eg, Duragesic®): Severe respiratory disease or depression including acute asthma (unless patient is mechanically ventilated); paralytic ileus; patients requiring short-term therapy, management of acute or intermittent pain, postoperative or mild pain, and in patients who are **not** opioid tolerant

Additional contraindications for transmucosal buccal tablets (Fentora®), buccal films (Onsolis™), lozenges (eg, Actiq®), sublingual tablets (Abstral®), sublingual spray (Subsys®), nasal spray (Lazanda®): Contraindicated in the management of acute or postoperative pain (including headache, migraine, or dental pain), and in patients who are **not** opioid tolerant. Abstral® and Onsolis™ also are contraindicated for acute pain management in the emergency room.

Canadian labeling: Additional contraindication (not in U.S. labeling): Sublingual tablets (Abstral™): Severe respiratory depression or severe obstructive lung disease

Warnings/Precautions An opioid-containing analgesic regimen should be tailored to each patient's needs and based upon the type of pain being treated (acute versus chronic), the route of administration, degree of tolerance for opioids (naive versus chronic user), age, weight, and medical condition. The optimal analgesic dose varies widely among patients. Doses should be titrated to pain relief/prevention. May cause CNS depression, which may impair physical or mental abilities; patients must be cautioned about performing tasks which require mental alertness (eg, operating machinery or driving). When using with other CNS depressants, reduce dose of one or both agents. Fentanyl shares the toxic potentials of opiate agonists, and precautions of opiate agonist therapy should be observed; use with caution in patients with bradycardia or bradyarrhythmias; rapid I.V. infusion may result in skeletal muscle and chest wall rigidity leading to respiratory distress and/or apnea, bronchoconstriction, laryngospasm; inject slowly over 3-5 minutes. **[U.S. Boxed Warning]: Healthcare provider should be alert to problems of abuse, misuse, and diversion.** Tolerance or drug dependence may result from extended use. The elderly may be particularly susceptible to the CNS depressant and constipating effects of narcotics. Use extreme caution in patients with COPD or other chronic respiratory conditions. Use caution with head injuries, morbid obesity, renal impairment, or hepatic dysfunction. **[U.S. Boxed Warning]: Use with strong or moderate CYP3A4 inhibitors may result in increased effects and potentially fatal respiratory depression.** Use is not recommended with MAO inhibitors or within 14 days of MAO inhibitor use; severe and unpredictable adverse effects may result. Concurrent use of agonist/antagonist analgesics may precipitate withdrawal symptoms and/or reduced analgesic efficacy in patients following prolonged therapy with mu opioid agonists. Abrupt discontinuation following prolonged use may also lead to withdrawal symptoms.

[U.S. Boxed Warning]: Buccal film (Onsolis™), nasal spray (Lazanda®), sublingual tablet (Abstral®): Indicated only for cancer patients who are opioid tolerant and are ≥18 years of age.

[U.S. Boxed Warning] Abstral®, Actiq®, Duragesic®, Fentora®, Lazanda®, Onsolis™, Subsys®: May cause potentially life-threatening hypoventilation, respiratory depression, and/or death; Abstral®, Actiq®, Duragesic®, Fentora®, Lazanda®, Onsolis™, or Subsys® should only be prescribed for opioid-tolerant patients. Risk of respiratory depression increased in elderly patients, debilitated patients, and patients with conditions associated with hypoxia or hypercapnia; usually occurs after administration of initial dose in nontolerant patients or when given with other drugs that depress respiratory function.

Nasal spray (Lazanda®): **[U.S. Boxed Warning]: Should be used only for the care of opioid-tolerant cancer patients with breakthrough pain who are already receiving opioid therapy for their underlying persistent cancer pain. Intended to be prescribed only by health care professionals who are knowledgeable in treating cancer pain.** Use is contraindicated in opioid nontolerant patients or in the management of acute or postoperative pain, including headache/migraine, dental pain, or use in the ER. **[U.S. Boxed Warning]: Available only through the Lazanda REMS program. Prescribers who prescribe to outpatients, pharmacies (inpatient and outpatient), outpatients, and distributors are required to enroll in the program. [U.S. Boxed Warning]: Due to differing pharmacokinetics of fentanyl in the nasal spray formulation, do not substitute Lazanda® on a mcg-per-mcg basis for any other fentanyl product.** Serious adverse events, including death, may occur when used inappropriately (improper dose or patient selection). All patients must begin therapy with a 100 mcg dose and titrate, if needed.

During therapy, patients must wait at least 2 hours before taking another dose of nasal spray. Allergic rhinitis is not expected to alter fentanyl absorption following nasal administration; however, use of nasal decongestants (eg, oxymetazoline) during episodes of rhinitis may result in lower peak concentrations and delayed T_{max}, therefore, titration of the nasal spray is not recommended during use of nasal decongestants.

[U.S. Boxed Warning]: Lozenge (eg, Actiq®), buccal tablet (Fentora®), buccal film (Onsolis™), sublingual tablet (Abstral®): Should be used only for the care of opioid-tolerant cancer patients with breakthrough pain and is intended for use by specialists who are knowledgeable in treating cancer pain. Not approved for use in management of acute or postoperative pain.

Transmucosal: Buccal film (eg, Onsolis™): [U.S. Boxed Warning]: Available only through the FOCUS Program, a restricted distribution program with prescriber, pharmacy, and patient required enrollment. [U.S. Boxed Warning]: Onsolis™ is contraindicated in the management of acute or postoperative pain, including headache/migraine. [U.S. Boxed Warning]: Due to higher bioavailability of fentanyl in the buccal film formulation, do not substitute Onsolis™ on a mcg-per-mcg basis for any other fentanyl product. Serious adverse events, including death, may occur when used inappropriately (improper dose or patient selection). All patients must begin therapy with a 200 mcg dose and titrate, if needed. During therapy, patients must wait at least 2 hours before taking another dose.

Transmucosal: Buccal tablet (Fentora®): [U.S. Boxed Warning]: Available only through the FENTORA REMS program. Prescribers who prescribe to outpatients, outpatients, pharmacies, and distributors are required to enroll in the program. [U.S. Boxed Warning]: Due to the higher bioavailability of fentanyl in Fentora®, when converting patients from oral transmucosal fentanyl citrate (OTFC, Actiq®) to Fentora®, do not substitute Fentora®): on a mcg-per-mcg basis for any other fentanyl product. [U.S. Boxed Warning]: Fentora® is contraindicated in the management of acute or post-operative pain, including headache/migraine. Serious adverse events, including death, have been reported when used inappropriately (improper dose or patient selection). [U.S. Boxed Warning]: Patients using Fentora® who experience breakthrough pain may only take one additional dose using the same strength and must wait four hours before taking another dose.

Transmucosal: Lozenge (Actiq®): [U.S. Boxed Warning]: Available only through the ACTIQ REMS program. Prescribers who prescribe to outpatients, outpatients, pharmacies, and distributors are required to enroll in the program. [U.S. Boxed Warning]: The substitution of Actiq® for any other fentanyl product may result in a fatal overdose. Do not convert patients on a mcg-per-mcg basis to Actiq® from other fentanyl products. Do not substitute Actiq® for any other fentanyl product. [U.S. Boxed Warning]: Patients using fentanyl lozenges who experience breakthrough pain may only take 1 additional dose using the same strength and must wait 4 hours before taking another dose.

Transmucosal: Sublingual spray (Subsys®): [U.S. Boxed Warning]: Available only through the TIRF REMS ACCESS Program, a restricted distribution program with outpatients, prescribers who prescribe to outpatients, pharmacy (outpatient), and distributor-required enrollment. [U.S. Boxed Warning]: Subsys® is contraindicated in the management of acute or postoperative pain, including headache/migraine. [U.S. Boxed Warning]: Due to differing pharmacokinetics of fentanyl in the sublingual spray formulation, do not substitute Subsys® on a mcg-per-mcg basis for any other fentanyl product. Serious adverse events, including death, may occur when used inappropriately (improper dose or patient selection). All patients must begin therapy with a 100 mcg dose and titrate, if needed. Cancer patients with oral mucositis experienced increased fentanyl exposure following sublingual spray administration; avoid use in patients with grade 2 or higher mucositis; use with caution in patients with grade 1 mucositis, and closely monitor for respiratory and CNS depression.

Transmucosal: Sublingual tablet (Abstral®): [U.S. Boxed Warning]: Available only through the ABSTRAL REMS program. Prescribers who prescribe to outpatients, outpatients, pharmacies, and distributors are required to enroll in the program. [U.S. Boxed Warning]: Abstral® is contraindicated in opioid nontolerant patients. [U.S. Boxed Warning]: Due to differing pharmacokinetics of fentanyl in the sublingual tablet formulation, do not substitute Abstral® on a mcg-per-mcg basis for any other fentanyl product. Serious adverse events, including death, may occur when used inappropriately (improper dose or patient selection). All patients must begin therapy with a 100 mcg dose. During therapy, patients must wait at least 2 hours before treating another episode of breakthrough pain.

◀ Transdermal patches (eg, Duragesic®): **[U.S. Boxed Warning]: Indicated for the management of persistent moderate-to-severe pain when around the clock pain control is
needed for an extended time period. Should only be used in patients who are already
receiving opioid therapy, are opioid tolerant, and who require a total daily dose
equivalent to 25 mcg/hour transdermal patch. Contraindicated in patients who are
not opioid tolerant, in the management of short-term analgesia, or in the management
of postoperative pain. Should be applied only to intact skin. Use of a patch that has
been cut, damaged, or altered in any way may result in overdosage.** Serum fentanyl
concentrations may increase approximately one-third for patients with a body temperature of
40°C secondary to a temperature-dependent increase in fentanyl release from the patch and
increased skin permeability. **[U.S. Boxed Warning]: Avoid exposure of application site and
surrounding area to direct external heat sources.** Patients who experience fever or
increase in core temperature should be monitored closely. Patients who experience adverse
reactions should be monitored for at least 24 hours after removal of the patch. Transdermal
patch may contain conducting metal (eg, aluminum); remove patch prior to MRI.

Adverse Reactions (Reflective of adult population; not specific for elderly)

>10%:

Cardiovascular: Bradycardia, edema

Central nervous system: CNS depression, confusion, dizziness, drowsiness, fatigue, headache, sedation

Endocrine & metabolic: Dehydration

Gastrointestinal: Constipation, nausea, vomiting, xerostomia

Local: Application-site reaction erythema

Neuromuscular & skeletal: Chest wall rigidity (high dose I.V.), muscle rigidity, weakness

Ocular: Miosis

Respiratory: Dyspnea, respiratory depression

Miscellaneous: Diaphoresis

1% to 10%:

Cardiovascular: Cardiac arrhythmia, cardiorespiratory arrest, chest pain, DVT, flushing,
hyper-/hypotension, orthostatic hypotension, pallor, palpitation, peripheral edema, sinus
tachycardia, syncope, tachycardia, vasodilation

Central nervous system: Abnormal dreams, abnormal thinking, agitation, amnesia, anxiety,
attention disturbance, chills, depression, disorientation, dysphoria, euphoria, fever, hallucinations, hypoesthesia, insomnia, irritability, lethargy, malaise, mental status change,
migraine, nervousness, paranoid reaction, restlessness, somnolence, stupor, vertigo

Dermatologic: Alopecia, bruising, cellulitis, decubitus ulcer, erythema, hyperhidrosis, papules, pruritus, rash

Endocrine & metabolic: Breast pain, dehydration, hot flashes, hyper-/hypocalcemia, hyper-/
hypoglycemia, hypoalbuminemia, hypokalemia, hypomagnesemia, hyponatremia

Gastrointestinal: Abdominal distension, abdominal pain, abnormal taste, anorexia, appetite
decreased, biliary tract spasm, diarrhea, dyspepsia, dysphagia (buccal tablet/film/sublin-
gual spray), flatulence, gastritis, gastroenteritis, gastroesophageal reflux, GI hemorrhage,
gingival pain (buccal tablet), gingivitis (lozenge), glossitis (lozenge), hematemesis, ileus,
intestinal obstruction (buccal film), periodontal abscess (lozenge/buccal tablet), proctalgia,
stomatitis (lozenge/buccal tablet/sublingual tablet/sublingual spray), tongue disorder (sublingual tablet), ulceration (gingival, lip, mouth; transmucosal use/nasal spray), weight loss

Genitourinary: Dysuria, erectile dysfunction, urinary incontinence, urinary retention, urinary
tract infection, vaginitis, vaginal hemorrhage

Hematologic: Anemia, leukopenia, neutropenia, thrombocytopenia

Hepatic: Alkaline phosphatase increased, ascites, AST increased, jaundice

Local: Application site pain, application site irritation

Neuromuscular & skeletal: Abnormal coordination, abnormal gait, arthralgia, back pain, limb
pain, myalgia, neuropathy, paresthesia, rigors, tremor

Ocular: Blurred vision, diplopia, dry eye, swelling, ptosis, strabismus

Renal: Renal failure

Respiratory: Apnea, asthma, bronchitis, cough, dyspnea (exertional), epistaxis, hemoptysis,
hypoventilation, hypoxia, laryngitis, nasal congestion (nasal spray), nasal discomfort (nasal
spray), nasopharyngitis, pharyngolaryngeal pain, pharyngitis, pneumonia, postnasal drip
(nasal spray), pulmonary embolism (nasal spray), rhinitis, rhinorrhea (nasal spray), sinusitis, upper respiratory infection, wheezing

Miscellaneous: Flu-like syndrome, hiccups, hypersensitivity, lymphadenopathy, night
sweats, parosmia, speech disorder, withdrawal syndrome

Drug Interactions

Metabolism/Transport Effects Substrate of CYP3A4 (major); **Note:** Assignment of Major/
Minor substrate status based on clinically relevant drug interaction potential; **Inhibits**
CYP3A4 (weak)

Avoid Concomitant Use

Avoid concomitant use of FentaNYL with any of the following: Azelastine; Azelastine (Nasal); Crizotinib; MAO Inhibitors; Methadone; Mifepristone; Mirtazapine; Paraldehyde; Pimozide

Increased Effect/Toxicity

FentaNYL may increase the levels/effects of: Alcohol (Ethyl); Alvimopan; ARIPiprazole; Azelastine; Azelastine (Nasal); Beta-Blockers; Calcium Channel Blockers (Nondihydropyridine); CNS Depressants; Desmopressin; MAO Inhibitors; Methadone; Metyrosine; Mirtazapine; Paraldehyde; Pimozide; Selective Serotonin Reuptake Inhibitors; Thiazide Diuretics; Zolpidem

The levels/effects of FentaNYL may be increased by: Amphetamines; Antipsychotic Agents (Phenothiazines); Crizotinib; CYP3A4 Inhibitors (Moderate); CYP3A4 Inhibitors (Strong); Dasatinib; Droperidol; HydrOXYzine; Ivacaftor; MAO Inhibitors; Mifepristone; Succinylcholine

Decreased Effect

FentaNYL may decrease the levels/effects of: Ioflupane I 123; Pegvisomant

The levels/effects of FentaNYL may be decreased by: Alpha-/Beta-Agonists (Indirect-Acting); Alpha1-Agonists; Ammonium Chloride; Mixed Agonist / Antagonist Opioids; Rifamycin Derivatives; Tocilizumab

Ethanol/Nutrition/Herb Interactions

Ethanol: Ethanol may increase CNS depression. Management: Monitor for increased effects with coadministration. Caution patients about effects.

Food: Fentanyl concentrations may be increased by grapefruit juice. Management: Avoid concurrent intake of large quantities (>1 quart/day) of grapefruit juice.

Herb/Nutraceutical: St John's wort may decrease fentanyl levels; gotu kola, valerian, and kava kava may increase CNS depression. Management: Avoid St John's wort, gotu kola, valerian, and kava kava.

Stability

Injection formulation: Store at controlled room temperature of 20°C to 25°C (68°F to 77°F). Protect from light.

Nasal spray: Do not store above 25°C (77°F); do not freeze. Protect from light. Bottle should be stored in the provided child-resistant container when not in use and kept out of the reach of children at all times.

Transdermal patch: Do not store above 25°C (77°F). Keep out of the reach of children.

Transmucosal (buccal film, buccal tablet, lozenge, sublingual spray, sublingual tablet): Store at controlled room temperature of 20°C to 25°C (68°F to 77°F). Protect from freezing and moisture. Keep out of the reach of children.

Mechanism of Action Binds with stereospecific receptors at many sites within the CNS, increases pain threshold, alters pain reception, inhibits ascending pain pathways

Pharmacodynamics/Kinetics

Onset of action: Analgesic: I.M.: 7-8 minutes; I.V.: Almost immediate; Transdermal (initial placement): 6 hours; Transmucosal: 5-15 minutes

Peak effect: Analgesic: Transdermal (initial placement): 12 hours; Transmucosal: 15-30 minutes

Duration: I.M.: 1-2 hours; I.V.: 0.5-1 hour; Transdermal (removal of patch/no replacement): 12 hours; Transmucosal: Related to blood level; respiratory depressant effect may last longer than analgesic effect

Absorption:

Transdermal: Initial application: Gradually absorbed for the first 12-24 hours, followed by a constant absorption for the remainder of the dosing interval. Absorption is decreased in cachectic patients (compared to normal size patients).

Transmucosal, buccal tablet and buccal film: Rapid, ~50% from the buccal mucosa; remaining 50% swallowed with saliva and slowly absorbed from GI tract.

Transmucosal, lozenge: Rapid, ~25% from the buccal mucosa; 75% swallowed with saliva and slowly absorbed from GI tract

Distribution: 4-6 L/kg; Highly lipophilic, redistributes into muscle and fat

Protein binding: 80% to 85%

Metabolism: Hepatic, primarily via CYP3A4

Bioavailability:

Buccal film: 71% (mucositis did not have a clinically significant effect on C_{max} and AUC; however, bioavailability is expected to decrease if film is inappropriately chewed and swallowed)

Buccal tablet: 65% (range: 45% to 85%)

Lozenge: 47% (range: 37% to 57%)

Sublingual spray: 76%

Sublingual tablet: 54%

◀

Half-life elimination:
  I.V.: 2-4 hours
  Transdermal patch: 17 hours (13-22 hours, half-life is influenced by extended absorption rate)
  Transmucosal products: 3-14 hours (dose dependent); Nasal spray: 15-25 hours (based on a multiple-dose pharmacokinetic study when doses are administered in the same nostril and separated by a 1-, 2-, or 4-hour time lapse)
Time to peak:
  Buccal film: 0.75-4 hours (median: 1 hour)
  Buccal tablet: 20-240 minutes (median: 47 minutes)
  Lozenge: 20-480 minutes (median: 20-40 minutes)
  Nasal spray: Median: 15-21 minutes
  Sublingual spray: 10-120 minutes (median: 90 minutes)
  Sublingual tablet: 15-240 minutes (median: 30-60 minutes)
  Transdermal patch: 24-72 hours, after several sequential 72-hour applications, steady state serum concentrations are reached
Excretion: Urine 75% (primarily as metabolites, <7% to 10% as unchanged drug); feces ~9%

Dosage

Geriatric Elderly have been found to be twice as sensitive as younger patients to the effects of fentanyl. A wide range of doses may be used. When choosing a dose, take into consideration the following patient factors: age, weight, physical status, underlying disease states, other drugs used, type of anesthesia used, and the surgical procedure to be performed.

Transmucosal lozenge (eg, Actiq®): In clinical trials, patients who were >65 years of age were titrated to a mean dose that was 200 mcg less than that of younger patients.

Adult Note: Ranges listed may not represent the maximum doses that may be required in all patients. Doses and dosage intervals should be titrated to pain relief/prevention. Monitor vital signs routinely. Single I.M. doses have duration of 1-2 hours, single I.V. doses last 0.5-1 hour.

Surgery:
  Premedication: I.M., slow I.V.: 50-100 mcg/dose 30-60 minutes prior to surgery
    Adjunct to regional anesthesia: Slow I.V.: 25-100 mcg/dose over 1-2 minutes. **Note:** An I.V. should be in place with regional anesthesia so the I.M. route is rarely used but still maintained as an option in the package labeling.
  Adjunct to general anesthesia: Slow I.V.:
    Low dose: 0.5-2 mcg/kg/dose depending on the indication.
    Moderate dose: Initial: 2-20 mcg/kg/dose; Maintenance (bolus or infusion): 1-2 mcg/kg/**hour**. Discontinuing fentanyl infusion 30-60 minutes prior to the end of surgery will usually allow adequate ventilation upon emergence from anesthesia. For "fast-tracking" and early extubation following major surgery, total fentanyl doses are limited to 10-15 mcg/kg.
    High dose: 20-50 mcg/kg/dose; **Note:** High-dose fentanyl as an adjunct to general anesthesia is rarely used, but is still described in the manufacturer's label.

Pain management: Adults:
  I.V. (unlabeled use): Bolus at start of infusion: 1-2 mcg/kg **or** 25-100 mcg/dose; continuous infusion rate: 1-2 mcg/kg/**hour or** 25-200 mcg/hour
  Severe (unlabeled use): I.M, I.V.: 50-100 mcg/dose every 1-2 hours as needed; patients with prior opiate exposure may tolerate higher initial doses
  Patient-controlled analgesia (PCA) (unlabeled use): I.V.:
    Usual concentration: 10 mcg/mL
    Demand dose: Usual: 20 mcg; range: 10-50 mcg
    Lockout interval: 5-8 minutes
    Usual basal rate: ≤50 mcg/hour
  Critically-ill patients (unlabeled dose): Slow I.V.: 25-100 mcg (based on ~70 kg patient) **or** 0.35-1.5 mcg/kg every 30-60 minutes as needed. **Note:** More frequent dosing may be needed (eg, mechanically-ventilated patients).
    Continuous infusion: 50-700 mcg/hour (based on ~70 kg patient) **or** 0.7-10 mcg/kg/**hour**
  Intrathecal (I.T.) (unlabeled use; American Pain Society, 2008): **Must be preservative-free.** Doses must be adjusted for age, injection site, and patient's medical condition and degree of opioid tolerance.
    Single dose: 5-25 mcg/dose; may provide adequate relief for up to 6 hours
    Continuous infusion: Not recommended in acute pain management due to risk of excessive accumulation. For chronic cancer pain, infusion of very small doses may be practical (American Pain Society, 2008).

Epidural (unlabeled use; American Pain Society, 2008): **Must be preservative-free.** Doses must be adjusted for age, injection site, and patient's medical condition and degree of opioid tolerance

Single dose: 25-100 mcg/dose; may provide adequate relief for up to 8 hours

Continuous infusion: 25-100 mcg/hour

Breakthrough cancer pain: Transmucosal: For patients who are tolerant to and currently receiving opioid therapy for persistent cancer pain; dosing should be individually titrated to provide adequate analgesia with minimal side effects. Dose titration should be done if patient requires more than 1 dose/breakthrough pain episode for several consecutive episodes. Patients experiencing >4 breakthrough pain episodes/day should have the dose of their long-term opioid re-evaluated.

Lozenge: Initial dose: 200 mcg; the second dose may be started 15 minutes after completion of the first dose if pain unrelieved. A maximum of 1 additional dose can be given per pain episode; must wait at least 4 hours before treating another episode. Consumption should be limited to ≤4 units/day. Additional requirements suggest need for improved baseline therapy.

Buccal film (Onsolis™): Initial dose: 200 mcg for all patients **Note:** Patients previously using another transmucosal product should be initiated at doses of 200 mcg; do **not** switch patients using any other fentanyl product on a mcg-per-mcg basis.

Dose titration: If titration required, increase dose in 200 mcg increments once per episode using multiples of the 200 mcg film; do not redose within a single episode of breakthrough pain and separate single doses by ≥2 hours. During titration, do not exceed 4 simultaneous applications of the 200 mcg films (800 mcg). If >800 mcg required, treat next episode with one 1200 mcg film (maximum dose: 1200 mcg). Once maintenance dose is determined, all other unused films should be disposed of and that strength (using a single film) should be used. During any pain episode, if adequate relief is not achieved after 30 minutes following buccal film application, a rescue medication (as determined by healthcare provider) may be used.

Maintenance: Determined dose applied as a single film once per episode and separated by ≥2 hours (dose range: 200-1200 mcg); limit to 4 applications/day. Consider increasing the around-the-clock opioid therapy in patients experiencing >4 breakthrough pain episodes/day.

Buccal tablet (Fentora®): Initial dose: 100 mcg; a second 100 mcg dose, if needed, may be started 30 minutes after the start of the first dose. **Note:** For patients previously using the transmucosal lozenge (Actiq®), the initial dose should be selected using the conversions listed below (maximum: 2 doses per breakthrough pain episode every 4 hours).

Dose titration, if required, should be done using multiples of the 100 mcg tablets. Patient can take two 100 mcg tablets (one on each side of mouth). If that dose is not successful, can use four 100 mcg tablets (two on each side of mouth). If titration requires >400 mcg/dose, then use 200 mcg tablets.

Conversion from lozenge to buccal tablet (Fentora®):

Lozenge dose 200-400 mcg, then buccal tablet 100 mcg

Lozenge dose 600-800 mcg, then buccal tablet 200 mcg

Lozenge dose 1200-1600 mcg, then buccal tablet 400 mcg

Note: Four 100 mcg buccal tablets deliver approximately 12% and 13% higher values of C_{max} and AUC, respectively, compared to one 400 mcg buccal tablet. To prevent confusion, patient should only have one strength available at a time. Using more than four buccal tablets at a time has not been studied.

Nasal spray (Lazanda®):

Initial dose: 100 mcg (one 100 mcg spray in one nostril) for all patients. **Note:** Patients previously using another fentanyl product should be initiated at a dose of 100 mcg; do not convert patients from other fentanyl products to Lazanda® on a mcg-per-mcg basis.

Dose titration: If pain is relieved within 30 minutes, that same dose should be used to treat subsequent episodes. If pain is unrelieved, may increase to a higher dose using the recommended titration steps. **Must wait at least 2 hours before treating another episode with nasal spray.** Dose titration steps: If no relief with 100 mcg dose, increase to 200 mcg dose per episode (one 100 mcg spray in each nostril); if no relief with 200 mcg dose, increase to 400 mcg per episode (one 400 mcg spray); if no relief with 400 mcg dose, increase to 800 mcg dose per episode (one 400 mcg spray in each nostril). **Note:** Single doses >800 mcg have not been evaluated. There are no data supporting the use of a combination of dose strengths.

Maintenance dose: Once maintenance dose for breakthrough pain episode has been determined, use that dose for subsequent episodes. For pain that is not relieved after 30 minutes of Lazanda® administration or if a separate breakthrough pain episode occurs within the 2 hour window before the next Lazanda® dose is permitted, a rescue medication may be used. Limit Lazanda® use to ≤4 episodes of breakthrough pain per day. If response to maintenance dose changes (increase in adverse reactions or alterations in pain relief), dose readjustment may be necessary. If patient is experiencing >4 breakthrough pain episodes/day, consider increasing the around-the-clock, long-acting opioid therapy; if long-acting opioid therapy dose is altered, re-evaluate and retitrate Lazanda® dose as needed.

Sublingual spray (Subsys®):

Initial dose: 100 mcg for all patients. If pain is unrelieved, 1 additional 100 mcg dose may be given 30 minutes after administration of the first dose. A maximum of 2 doses can be given per breakthrough pain episode; must wait at least 4 hours before treating another episode. **Note:** Patients must remain on around-the-clock opioids during use. Patients previously using other fentanyl products should be initiated at a dose of 100 mcg; do not convert patients from any other fentanyl product (transmucosal, transdermal, or parenteral) to Subsys® on a mcg-per-mcg basis.

Dose titration: If pain is relieved within 30 minutes, that same dose should be used to treat subsequent episodes and no titration is necessary. If pain is unrelieved, may increase to a higher dose using the recommended titration steps. Goal is to determine the dose that provides adequate analgesia (with tolerable side effects) using a single dose per breakthrough pain episode. For each breakthrough pain episode, if pain unrelieved after 30 minutes only 1 additional dose using the same strength may be given (maximum: 2 doses per breakthrough pain episode). **Must wait at least 4 hours before treating another episode with Subsys®.**

Dose titration steps: If no relief with 100 mcg dose, increase to 200 mcg dose per episode (one 200 mcg unit); if no relief with 200 mcg dose, increase to 400 mcg per episode (one 400 mcg unit); if no relief with 400 mcg dose, increase to 600 mcg dose per episode (one 600 mcg unit); if no relief with 600 mcg dose, increase to 800 mcg dose per episode (one 800 mcg unit); if no relief with 800 mcg dose, increase to 1200 mcg dose per episode (two 600 mcg units); if no relief with 1200 mcg dose, increase to 1600 mcg per episode (two 800 mcg units).

Maintenance dose: Once maintenance dose for breakthrough pain episode has been determined, use that dose for subsequent episodes. If occasional episodes of unrelieved breakthrough pain occur following 30 minutes of Subsys® administration, 1 additional dose using the same strength may be administered (maximum: 2 doses per breakthrough pain episode); patient must wait 4 hours before treating another breakthrough pain episode with Subsys®. Once maintenance dose is determined, limit Susbsys™ use to ≤4 episodes of breakthrough pain per day. If response to maintenance dose changes (increase in adverse reactions or alterations in pain relief), dose readjustment may be necessary. If patient is experiencing >4 breakthrough pain episodes/day, consider increasing the around-the-clock, long-acting opioid therapy.

Sublingual tablet (Abstral®):

Initial dose:

U.S. labeling: 100 mcg for all patients; if pain is unrelieved, a second dose may be given 30 minutes after administration of the first dose. A maximum of 2 doses can be given per breakthrough pain episode; must wait at least 2 hours before treating another episode.

Canadian labeling: 100 mcg for all patients; if pain is unrelieved 30 minutes after administration of Abstral™, an alternative rescue medication (other than Abstral™) may be given. Administer only 1 dose of Abstral™ per breakthrough pain episode; must wait at least 2 hours before treating another episode.

Note: Patients previously using another fentanyl product should be initiated at a dose of 100 mcg; do not convert patients from other fentanyl products to Abstral® on a mcg-per-mcg basis.

Dose titration: If titration required, increase in 100 mcg increments (up to 400 mcg) over consecutive breakthrough episodes. If titration requires >400 mcg/dose, increase in increments of 200 mcg, starting with 600 mcg dose. During titration, patients may use multiples of 100 mcg and/or 200 mcg tablets for any single dose; do not exceed 4 tablets at one time; safety and efficacy of doses >800 mcg have not been evaluated.

Maintenance dose: Once maintenance dose for breakthrough pain episode has been determined, use only 1 tablet in the appropriate strength per episode; if pain is unrelieved with maintenance dose:

U.S. labeling recommendations: A second dose may be given after 30 minutes; maximum of 2 doses/episode of breakthrough pain; separate treatment of subsequent episodes by ≥2 hours; limit treatment to ≤4 breakthrough episodes/day.

Canadian labeling recommendations: Administer alternative rescue medication after 30 minutes; maximum of 1 Abstral™ dose/episode of breakthrough pain; separate treatment of subsequent episodes by ≥2 hours; limit treatment to ≤4 breakthrough episodes/day.

Consider increasing the around-the-clock long-acting opioid therapy in patients experiencing >4 breakthrough pain episodes/day; if long-acting opioid therapy dose altered, re-evaluate and retitrate Abstral® dose as needed.

Chronic pain management: Adults (opioid-tolerant patients): Transdermal patch (Duragesic®):

Initial: To convert patients from oral or parenteral opioids to transdermal patch, a 24-hour analgesic requirement should be calculated (based on prior opiate use). Using the tables, the appropriate initial dose can be determined. The initial fentanyl dosage may be approximated from the 24-hour morphine dosage equivalent and titrated to minimize adverse effects and provide analgesia. With the initial application, the absorption of transdermal fentanyl requires several hours to reach plateau; therefore transdermal fentanyl is inappropriate for management of acute pain. Change patch every 72 hours.

Conversion from continuous infusion of fentanyl: In patients who have adequate pain relief with a fentanyl infusion, fentanyl may be converted to transdermal dosing at a rate equivalent to the intravenous rate. A two-step taper of the infusion to be completed over 12 hours has been recommended (Kornick, 2001) after the patch is applied. The infusion is decreased to 50% of the original rate six hours after the application of the first patch, and subsequently discontinued twelve hours after application.

Titration: Short-acting agents may be required until analgesic efficacy is established and/or as supplements for "breakthrough" pain. The amount of supplemental doses should be closely monitored. Appropriate dosage increases may be based on daily supplemental dosage using the ratio of 45 mg/24 hours of oral morphine to a 12.5 mcg/hour increase in fentanyl dosage.

Frequency of adjustment: The dosage should not be titrated more frequently than every 3 days after the initial dose or every 6 days thereafter. Patients should wear a consistent fentanyl dosage through two applications (6 days) before dosage increase based on supplemental opiate dosages can be estimated. **Note:** Upon discontinuation, ~17 hours are required for a 50% decrease in fentanyl levels.

Frequency of application: The majority of patients may be controlled on every 72-hour administration; however, a small number of patients require every 48-hour administration.

Dose conversion guidelines for transdermal fentanyl (see tables below and on following pages).

Note: U.S. and Canadian dose conversion guidelines differ. Consult appropriate table.

U.S. Labeling: Dose Conversion Guidelines: Recommended Initial Duragesic® Dose Based Upon Daily Oral Morphine Dose[1,2]

Oral 24-Hour Morphine (mg/day)	Duragesic® Dose (mcg/h)
60-134	25
135-224	50
225-314	75
315-404	100
405-494	125
495-584	150
585-674	175
675-764	200
765-854	225
855-944	250
945-1034	275
1035-1124	300

[1]The table should NOT be used to convert from transdermal fentanyl (Duragesic®) to other opioid analgesics. Rather, following removal of the patch, titrate the dose of the new opioid until adequate analgesia is achieved.

[2]Recommendations are based on U.S. product labeling for Duragesic®.

U.S. Labeling: Dose Conversion Guidelines[1,2]

Current Analgesic	Daily Dosage (mg/day)			
Morphine (I.M./I.V.)	10-22	23-37	38-52	53-67
Oxycodone (oral)	30-67	67.5-112	112.5-157	157.5-202
Oxycodone (I.M./I.V.)	15-33	33.1-56	56.1-78	78.1-101
Codeine (oral)	150-447	448-747	748-1047	1048-1347
Hydromorphone (oral)	8-17	17.1-28	28.1-39	39.1-51
Hydromorphone (I.V.)	1.5-3.4	3.5-5.6	5.7-7.9	8-10
Meperidine (I.M.)	75-165	166-278	279-390	391-503
Methadone (oral)	20-44	45-74	75-104	105-134
Methadone (I.M.)	10-22	23-37	38-52	53-67
Fentanyl transdermal recommended dose (mcg/h)	25 mcg/h	50 mcg/h	75 mcg/h	100 mcg/h

[1]The table should NOT be used to convert from transdermal fentanyl (Duragesic®) to other opioid analgesics. Rather, following removal of the patch, titrate the dose of the new opioid until adequate analgesia is achieved.

[2]Recommendations are based on U.S. product labeling for Duragesic®.

Transdermal patch (Duragesic® MAT [Canada; not available in U.S.]): Adults:

Canadian Labeling: Dose Conversion Guidelines (Adults): Recommended Initial Duragesic® MAT Dose Based Upon Daily Oral Morphine Dose[1,2]

Oral 24-Hour Morphine (Current Dose in mg/day)	Duragesic® MAT Dose (Initial Dose in mcg/h)
45-59	12
60-134	25
135-179	37
180-224	50
225-269	62
270-314	75
315-359	87
360-404	100
405-494	125
495-584	150
585-674	175
675-764	200
765-854	225
855-944	250
945-1034	275
1035-1124	300

[1]The table should NOT be used to convert from transdermal fentanyl (Duragesic® MAT) to other opioid analgesics. Rather, following removal of the patch, titrate the dose of the new opioid until adequate analgesia is achieved.

[2]Recommendations are based on Canadian product labeling for Duragesic® MAT.

Note: The 12 mcg/hour dose included in this table is to be used for incremental dose adjustment and is generally not recommended for initial dosing, except for patients in whom lower starting doses are deemed clinically appropriate.

Canadian Labeling: Dosing Conversion Guidelines (Adults)[1,2]

Current Analgesic	Daily Dosage (mg/day)						
Morphine[3] (I.M./I.V.)	20-44	45-60	61-75	76-90	n/a[4]	n/a[4]	n/a[4]
Oxycodone (oral)	30-66	67-90	91-112	113-134	135-157	158-179	180-202
Codeine (oral)	150-447	448-597	598-747	748-897	898-1047	1048-1197	1198-1347
Hydromorphone (oral)	8-16	17-22	23-28	29-33	34-39	40-45	46-51
Hydromorphone (I.V.)	4-8.4	8.5-11.4	11.5-14.4	14.5-16.5	16.6-19.5	19.6-22.5	22.6-25.5
Fentanyl transdermal recommended dose (mcg/h)	25 mcg/h	37 mcg/h	50 mcg/h	62 mcg/h	75 mcg/h	87 mcg/h	100 mcg/h

[1]The table should NOT be used to convert from transdermal fentanyl (Duragesic® MAT) to other opioid analgesics. Rather, following removal of the patch, titrate the dose of the new opioid until adequate analgesia is achieved.

[2]Recommendations are based on Canadian product labeling for Duragesic® MAT.

[3]Morphine dose conversion based upon I.M to oral dose ratio of 1:3.

[4]Insufficient data available to provide specific dosing recommendations. Use caution; adjust dose conservatively.

Renal Impairment
Transdermal (patch): Degree of impairment (ie, Cl_{cr}) not defined in manufacturer's labeling.
  Mild-to-moderate impairment: Initial: Reduce dose by 50%.
  Severe impairment: Use not recommended.
Transmucosal (buccal film/tablet, sublingual spray/tablet, lozenge) and nasal spray: Although fentanyl pharmacokinetics may be altered in renal disease, fentanyl can be used successfully in the management of breakthrough cancer pain. Doses should be titrated to reach clinical effect with careful monitoring of patients with severe renal disease.

Hepatic Impairment
Transdermal (patch):
  Mild-to-moderate impairment: Initial: Reduce dose by 50%.
  Severe impairment: Use not recommended.
Transmucosal (buccal film/tablet, sublingual spray/tablet, lozenge) and nasal spray: Although fentanyl pharmacokinetics may be altered in hepatic disease, fentanyl can be used successfully in the management of breakthrough cancer pain. Doses should be titrated to reach clinical effect with careful monitoring of patients with severe hepatic disease.

Administration
I.V.: Administer as slow I.V. infusion over 1-2 minutes. May also be administered as continuous infusion or PCA (unlabeled use) routes. Muscular rigidity may occur with rapid I.V. administration.
Transdermal patch (eg, Duragesic®): Apply to nonirritated and nonirradiated skin, such as chest, back, flank, or upper arm. Do not shave skin; hair at application site should be clipped. Prior to application, clean site with clear water and allow to dry completely. Do not use damaged, cut or leaking patches; patch may be less effective. Skin exposure from fentanyl gel leaking from patch may lead to serious adverse effects; thoroughly wash affected skin surfaces with water (do not use soap). Firmly press in place and hold for 30 seconds. Change patch every 72 hours. Do **not** use soap, alcohol, or other solvents to remove transdermal gel if it accidentally touches skin; use copious amounts of water. Avoid exposing application site to external heat sources (eg, heating pad, electric blanket, heat lamp, hot tub). If there is difficulty with patch adhesion, the edges of the system may be taped in place with first-aid tape. If there is continued difficulty with adhesion, an adhesive film dressing (eg, Bioclusive®, Tegaderm®) may be applied over the system.
Lozenge: Foil overwrap should be removed just prior to administration. Place the unit in mouth between the cheek and gum and allow it to dissolve. Do not chew. Lozenge may be moved from one side of the mouth to the other. The unit should be consumed over a period of 15 minutes. Handle should be removed after the lozenge is consumed; early removal should be considered if the patient has achieved an adequate response and/or shows signs of respiratory depression.
Buccal film: Foil overwrap should be removed just prior to administration. Prior to placing film, wet inside of cheek using tongue or by rinsing with water. Place film inside mouth with the

pink side of the unit against the inside of the moistened cheek. With finger, press the film against cheek and hold for 5 seconds. The film should stick to the inside of cheek after 5 seconds. The film should be left in place until it dissolves (usually within 15-30 minutes after application). Liquids may be consumed after 5 minutes of application. Food can be eaten after film dissolves. If using more than 1 film simultaneously (during titration period), apply films on either side of mouth (do not apply on top of each other). Do not chew or swallow film. Do not cut or tear the film. All patients must initiate therapy using the 200 mcg film.

Buccal tablet: Patient should not open blister until ready to administer. The blister backing should be peeled back to expose the tablet; tablet should not be pushed out through the blister. Immediately use tablet once removed from blister. Place entire tablet in the buccal cavity (above a rear molar, between the upper cheek and gum). Tablet should not be broken, sucked, chewed, or swallowed. Should dissolve in about 14-25 minutes when left between the cheek and the gum. If remnants remain they may be swallowed with water.

Nasal spray: Prior to initial use, prime device by spraying 4 sprays into the provided pouch (the counting window will show a green bar when the bottle is ready for use). Insert nozzle a short distance into the nose (~$\frac{1}{2}$ inch or 1 cm) and point towards the bridge of the nose (while closing off the other nostril using 1 finger). Press on finger grips until a "click" sound is heard and the number in the counting window advances by one. The "click" sound and dose counter are the only reliable methods for ensuring a dose has been administered (spray is not always felt on the nasal mucosa) following administration. Patient should remain seated for at least 1 minute following administration. Do not blow nose for ≥30 minutes after administration. Wash hands before and after use. There are 8 full therapeutic sprays in each bottle; do not continue to use bottle after "8" sprays have been used. Dispose of bottle and contents if ≥5 days have passed since last use or if it has been ≥4 days since bottle was primed. Spray the remaining contents into the provided pouch, seal in the child-resistant container, and dispose of in the trash.

Sublingual spray: Open sealed blister unit with scissors immediately prior to administration. Contents of unit should be sprayed into mouth under the tongue.

Sublingual tablet: Remove from the blister unit immediately prior to administration. Place tablet directly under the tongue on the floor of the mouth and allow to completely dissolve; do not chew, suck, or swallow. Do not eat or drink anything until tablet is completely dissolved. In patients with a dry mouth, water may be used to moisten the buccal mucosa just before administration. All patients must initiate therapy using the 100 mcg tablet.

Monitoring Parameters Respiratory and cardiovascular status, blood pressure, heart rate; signs of misuse, abuse, or addiction

Transdermal patch: Monitor for 24 hours after application of first dose

Pharmacotherapy Pearls Fentanyl is 50-100 times as potent as morphine; morphine 10 mg I.M. is equivalent to fentanyl 0.1-0.2 mg I.M.; fentanyl has less hypotensive effects than morphine due to lack of histamine release. However, fentanyl may cause rigidity with high doses. If the patient has required high-dose analgesia or has used for a prolonged period (~7 days), taper dose to prevent withdrawal; monitor for signs and symptoms of withdrawal.

Transmucosal (nasal spray, Lazanda®): Disposal of nasal spray: Before disposal, all unopened or partially used bottles must be completely emptied by spraying the contents into the provided pouch. After "8" therapeutic sprays has been reached on the counter, patients should continue to spray an additional four sprays into the pouch to ensure that any residual fentanyl has been expelled (an audible click will no longer be heard and the counter will not advance beyond "8"). The empty bottle and the sealed pouch must be put into the child-resistant container before placing in the trash. Wash hands with soap and water immediately after handling the pouch. If the pouch is lost, another one can be ordered by the patient or caregiver by calling 1-866-435-6775.

Transmucosal (oral lozenge, Actiq®): Disposal of lozenge units: After consumption of a complete unit, the handle may be disposed of in a trash container that is out of the reach of children. For a partially-consumed unit, or a unit that still has any drug matrix remaining on the handle, the handle should be placed under hot running tap water until the drug matrix has dissolved. Special child-resistant containers are available to temporarily store partially consumed units that cannot be disposed of immediately.

Transmucosal (buccal film, Onsolis®): Disposal of film: Remove foil overwrap from any unused, unneeded films and dispose by flushing in the toilet.

Transmucosal (sublingual spray, Subsys®): Disposal of spray: Dispose of each unit dose immediately after use; place used unit into one of the provided small disposal bags. After sealing appropriately, discard in the trash. Also dispose of any unused unit as soon as no longer needed. Prior to disposal, empty all the medicine into the provided disposal bottle. The disposal bottle should then be placed into the large disposal bag (provided), seal appropriately, and discard in the trash.

Transmucosal (sublingual tablet, Abstral®): Disposal of tablets: Remove any unused tablets from the blister cards and dispose by flushing in the toilet.

Transdermal patch (Duragesic®): Upon removal of the patch, ~17 hours are required before serum concentrations fall to 50% of their original values. Opioid withdrawal symptoms are possible. Gradual downward titration (potentially by the sequential use of lower-dose patches) is recommended. Keep transdermal patch (both used and unused) out of the reach of children. Do **not** use soap, alcohol, or other solvents to remove transdermal gel if it accidentally touches skin as they may increase transdermal absorption, use copious amounts of water. Avoid exposure of direct external heat sources (eg, heating pads, electric blankets, heat lamps, saunas, hot tubs, heated water beds) to application site.

Special Geriatric Considerations The elderly may be particularly susceptible to the CNS depressant and constipating effects of narcotics; therefore, use with caution. The effect of age on the pharmacokinetics of Fentora® (oral transmucosal buccal tablets) has not been studied. Instruct patients on proper use of the transdermal patch.

Controlled Substance C-II

Dosage Forms Excipient information presented when available (limited, particularly for generics); consult specific product labeling.

Film, for buccal application, as citrate [strength expressed as base]:
  Onsolis®: 200 mcg (30s); 400 mcg (30s); 600 mcg (30s); 800 mcg (30s); 1200 mcg (30s)
Injection, solution, as citrate [strength expressed as base, preservative free]: 0.05 mg/mL (2 mL, 5 mL, 10 mL, 20 mL, 50 mL)
Liquid, sublingual, as base [spray]:
  Subsys®: 100 mcg (30s); 200 mcg (30s); 400 mcg (30s); 600 mcg (30s); 800 mcg (30s) [contains dehydrated ethanol 63.6%, propylene glycol]
Lozenge, oral, as citrate [strength expressed as base, transmucosal]: 200 mcg (30s); 400 mcg (30s); 600 mcg (30s); 800 mcg (30s); 1200 mcg (30s); 1600 mcg (30s)
  Actiq®: 200 mcg (30s); 400 mcg (30s); 600 mcg (30s); 800 mcg (30s); 1200 mcg (30s); 1600 mcg (30s) [contains sugar 2 g/lozenge; berry flavor]
Patch, transdermal, as base: 12 [delivers 12.5 mcg/hr] (5s); 25 [delivers 25 mcg/hr] (5s); 50 [delivers 50 mcg/hr] (5s); 75 [delivers 75 mcg/hr] (5s); 100 [delivers 100 mcg/hr] (5s)
  Duragesic®: 12 [delivers 12.5 mcg/hr] (5s) [contains ethanol 0.1mL/10 cm^2; 5 cm^2]
  Duragesic®: 25 [delivers 25 mcg/hr] (5s) [contains ethanol 0.1 mL/10 cm^2; 10 cm^2]
  Duragesic®: 50 [delivers 50 mcg/hr] (5s) [contains ethanol 0.1 mL/10 cm^2; 20 cm^2]
  Duragesic®: 75 [delivers 75 mcg/hr] (5s) [contains ethanol 0.1 mL/10 cm^2; 30 cm^2]
  Duragesic®: 100 [delivers 100 mcg/hr] (5s) [contains ethanol 0.1 mL/10 cm^2; 40 cm^2]
Powder, for prescription compounding, as citrate: USP: 100% (1 g)
Solution, intranasal, as citrate [strength expressed as base, spray]:
  Lazanda®: 100 mcg/spray (5 mL); 400 mcg/spray (5 mL) [delivers 8 metered sprays]
Tablet, for buccal application, as citrate [strength expressed as base]:
  Fentora®: 100 mcg (28s); 200 mcg (28s); 400 mcg (28s); 600 mcg (28s); 800 mcg (28s)
Tablet, sublingual, as citrate [strength expressed as base]:
  Abstral®: 100 mcg (12s, 32s); 200 mcg (12s, 32s); 300 mcg (12s, 32s); 400 mcg (12s, 32s); 600 mcg (32s); 800 mcg (32s)

Dosage Forms: Canada Excipient information presented when available (limited, particularly for generics); consult specific product labeling.

Patch, transdermal, as base: 12 mcg/hr (5s); 25 mcg/hr (5s); 50 mcg/hr (5s); 75 mcg/hr (5s); 100 mcg/hr (5s)
  Duragesic® MAT: 12 mcg/hr (5s) [contains ethanol 0.1 mL/10 cm^2; 5 cm^2]
  Duragesic® MAT: 25 mcg/hr (5s) [contains ethanol 0.1 mL/10 cm^2; 10 cm^2]
  Duragesic® MAT: 50 mcg/hr (5s) [contains ethanol 0.1 mL/10 cm^2; 20 cm^2]
  Duragesic® MAT: 75 mcg/hr (5s) [contains ethanol 0.1 mL/10 cm^2; 30 cm^2]
  Duragesic® MAT: 100 mcg/hr (5s) [contains ethanol 0.1 mL/10 cm^2; 40 cm^2]

◆ **Ferrex™ 150 Forte Plus** *see* Polysaccharide-Iron Complex, Vitamin B12, and Folic Acid on page 1566

Ferric Gluconate (FER ik GLOO koe nate)

Medication Safety Issues
Sound-alike/look-alike issues:
Ferric gluconate may be confused with ferumoxytol

Brand Names: U.S. Ferrlecit®; Nulecit™ [DSC]

Brand Names: Canada Ferrlecit®

Index Terms Sodium Ferric Gluconate

Generic Availability (U.S.) Yes

Pharmacologic Category Iron Salt

Use Treatment of iron-deficiency anemia in patients undergoing hemodialysis in conjunction with erythropoietin therapy

Unlabeled Use Cancer-/chemotherapy-associated anemia

Contraindications Hypersensitivity to ferric gluconate or any component of the formulation

Warnings/Precautions Potentially serious hypersensitivity reactions may occur. Fatal immediate hypersensitivity reactions have occurred with other iron carbohydrate complexes. Avoid rapid administration. Flushing and transient hypotension may occur. May augment hemodialysis-induced hypotension. Use with caution in elderly patients. Use only in patients with documented iron deficiency; caution with hemoglobinopathies or other refractory anemias.

Adverse Reactions (Reflective of adult population; not specific for elderly) Percentages reported in adults unless otherwise noted:

>10%:
Cardiovascular: Hypotension (children 35%; adults 29%), hypertension (children 23%; adults 13%), tachycardia (children 17%; adults 5%)
Central nervous system: Headache (children 24%; adults 7%), dizziness (13%)
Gastrointestinal: Vomiting (adults ≤35%; children 11%), nausea (adults ≤35%; children 9%), diarrhea (adults ≤35%; children 8%)
Hematologic: Erythrocytes abnormal (11% [changes in morphology, color, or number])
Local: Injection site reaction (33%)
Neuromuscular & skeletal: Cramps (25%)
Respiratory: Dyspnea (11%)

1% to 10%:
Cardiovascular: Chest pain (10%), syncope (6%), edema (5%), angina pectoris, bradycardia, hypervolemia, MI, peripheral edema, vasodilation
Central nervous system: Pain (10%), fever (children 9%; adults 5%), fatigue (6%), agitation, chills, consciousness decreased, lightheadedness, malaise, rigors, somnolence
Dermatologic: Pruritus (6%), rash
Endocrine & metabolic: Hyperkalemia (6%), hypoglycemia, hypokalemia
Gastrointestinal: Abdominal pain (children 9%; adults 6%), anorexia, dyspepsia, eructation, flatulence, GI disorder, melena, rectal disorder
Genitourinary: Menorrhagia, UTI
Hematologic: Thrombosis (children 6%), anemia, leukocytosis, lymphadenopathy
Neuromuscular & skeletal: Leg cramps (10%), weakness (7%), paresthesias (6%), arm pain, arthralgia, back pain, leg edema, myalgia
Ocular: Arcus senilis, conjunctivitis, diplopia, puffy eyelids, redness of eyes, rolling of eyes, watery eyes
Otic: Deafness
Respiratory: Pharyngitis (children 9%), cough (6%), rhinitis (children 6%), upper respiratory infections (6%), pneumonia, pulmonary edema
Miscellaneous: Abscess, carcinoma, diaphoresis, flu-like symptoms, infection, sepsis

Drug Interactions
Metabolism/Transport Effects None known.
Avoid Concomitant Use
Avoid concomitant use of Ferric Gluconate with any of the following: Dimercaprol
Increased Effect/Toxicity
The levels/effects of Ferric Gluconate may be increased by: ACE Inhibitors; Dimercaprol
Decreased Effect
Ferric Gluconate may decrease the levels/effects of: Cefdinir; Eltrombopag; Levothyroxine; Phosphate Supplements; Trientine

The levels/effects of Ferric Gluconate may be decreased by: Pancrelipase; Trientine

Stability Store at 20°C to 25°C (68°F to 77°F). Do not freeze. For I.V. infusion, dilute 10 mL ferric gluconate in 0.9% sodium chloride (100 mL NS); use immediately after dilution.

Mechanism of Action Supplies a source to elemental iron necessary to the function of hemoglobin, myoglobin and specific enzyme systems; allows transport of oxygen via hemoglobin

Pharmacodynamics/Kinetics Half-life elimination: Bound iron: 1 hour

Dosage

Geriatric & Adult

Iron-deficiency anemia, hemodialysis patients: I.V.: 125 mg elemental iron per dialysis session. Most patients will require a cumulative dose of 1 g elemental iron over approximately 8 sequential dialysis treatments to achieve a favorable response.

Note: A test dose of 2 mL diluted in NS 50 mL administered over 60 minutes was previously recommended (not in current manufacturer's labeling). Doses >125 mg are associated with increased adverse events.

Cancer-/chemotherapy-associated anemia (unlabeled use): I.V. infusion: 125 mg over 1 hour; maximum: 250 mg/infusion. Repeat dose every week for 8 doses. Test doses (25 mg slow I.V. push or infusion) are recommended in patients with iron dextran hypersensitivity or those with other drug allergies (NCCN guidelines, v.2.2010)

Renal Impairment No dosage adjustment necessary.

Hepatic Impairment No dosage adjustment necessary.

Administration I.V.: Monitor patient for hypotension or hypersensitivity reactions during infusion.

Adults: May be diluted prior to administration; avoid rapid administration. Infusion rate should not exceed 2.1 mg/minute. If administered undiluted, infuse slowly at a rate of up to 12.5 mg/minute.

Monitoring Parameters Hemoglobin and hematocrit, serum ferritin, iron saturation; vital signs; signs and symptoms of hypersensitivity (monitor for ≥30 minutes following the end of administration and until clinically stable)

NKF K/DOQI guidelines recommend that iron status should be monitored monthly during initiation through the percent transferrin saturation (TSAT) and serum ferritin.

Reference Range CKD patients should have sufficient iron to achieve and maintain hemoglobin of 11-12 g/dL. To achieve and maintain this target Hgb, sufficient iron should be administered to maintain a TSAT of 20%, and a serum ferritin level >100 ng/mL (non-dialysis chronic kidney disease and peritoneal dialysis chronic kidney disease) or serum ferritin level >200 ng/mL (hemodialysis chronic kidney disease).

Test Interactions Serum or transferrin bound iron levels may be falsely elevated if assessed within 24 hours of ferric gluconate administration. Serum ferritin levels may be falsely elevated for 5 days after ferric gluconate administration.

Special Geriatric Considerations Anemia in the elderly is often caused by "anemia of chronic disease," a result of aging changes in the bone marrow, or associated with inflammation rather than blood loss. Iron stores are usually normal or increased, with a serum ferritin >50 ng/mL and a decreased total iron binding capacity; hence, the anemia is not secondary to iron deficiency but the inability of the reticuloendothelial system to use available iron stores. Timed release iron preparations should be avoided due to their erratic absorption. Products combined with a laxative or stool softener should not be used unless the need for the combination is demonstrated.

Dosage Forms Excipient information presented when available (limited, particularly for generics); consult specific product labeling. [DSC] = Discontinued product

Injection, solution: Elemental iron 12.5 mg/mL (5 mL)

Ferrlecit®: Elemental iron 12.5 mg/mL (5 mL) [contains benzyl alcohol, sucrose 20%]

Nulecit™: Elemental iron 12.5 mg/mL (5 mL) [DSC] [contains benzyl alcohol, sucrose ~20%]

◆ **Ferriprox®** see Deferiprone on page 497
◆ **Ferrlecit®** see Ferric Gluconate on page 774
◆ **Ferrocite™ [OTC]** see Ferrous Fumarate on page 775
◆ **Ferro-Sequels® [OTC]** see Ferrous Fumarate on page 775

Ferrous Fumarate (FER us FYOO ma rate)

Brand Names: U.S. Femiron® [OTC]; Ferretts® [OTC]; Ferro-Sequels® [OTC]; Ferrocite™ [OTC]; Hemocyte® [OTC]; Ircon® [OTC]

Brand Names: Canada Palafer®

Index Terms Iron Fumarate

Generic Availability (U.S.) Yes: Tablet

Pharmacologic Category Iron Salt

Use Prevention and treatment of iron-deficiency anemias

Contraindications Hypersensitivity to iron salts or any component of the formulation; hemochromatosis, hemolytic anemia

FERROUS FUMARATE

Warnings/Precautions Avoid in patients with peptic ulcer, enteritis, or ulcerative colitis. Administration of iron for >6 months should be avoided except in patients with continuous bleeding or menorrhagia. Anemia in the elderly is often caused by "anemia of chronic disease" or associated with inflammation rather than blood loss. Iron stores are usually normal or increased, with a serum ferritin >50 ng/mL and a decreased total iron binding capacity. Hence, the "anemia of chronic disease" is not secondary to iron deficiency but the inability of the reticuloendothelial system to reclaim available iron stores. Avoid in patients receiving frequent blood transfusions. **[U.S. Boxed Warning]: Severe iron toxicity may occur in overdose, particularly when ingested by children; iron is a leading cause of fatal poisoning in children; store out of children's reach and in child-resistant containers.**

Adverse Reactions (Reflective of adult population; not specific for elderly)

>10%: Gastrointestinal: Constipation, dark stools, nausea, stomach cramping, vomiting

1% to 10%:

Gastrointestinal: Diarrhea, heartburn, staining of teeth

Genitourinary: Discoloration of urine

Drug Interactions

Metabolism/Transport Effects None known.

Avoid Concomitant Use

Avoid concomitant use of Ferrous Fumarate with any of the following: Dimercaprol

Increased Effect/Toxicity

The levels/effects of Ferrous Fumarate may be increased by: Dimercaprol

Decreased Effect

Ferrous Fumarate may decrease the levels/effects of: Bisphosphonate Derivatives; Cefdinir; Deferiprone; Eltrombopag; Levodopa; Levothyroxine; Methyldopa; PenicillAMINE; Phosphate Supplements; Quinolone Antibiotics; Tetracycline Derivatives; Trientine

The levels/effects of Ferrous Fumarate may be decreased by: Antacids; H2-Antagonists; Pancrelipase; Proton Pump Inhibitors; Trientine

Ethanol/Nutrition/Herb Interactions Food: Cereals, dietary fiber, tea, coffee, eggs, and milk may decrease absorption.

Stability Iron is a leading cause of fatal poisoning in children. Store out of children's reach and in child-resistant containers.

Mechanism of Action Replaces iron found in hemoglobin, myoglobin, and enzymes; allows the transportation of oxygen via hemoglobin

Pharmacodynamics/Kinetics

Absorption: Iron is absorbed in the duodenum and upper jejunum; in persons with normal iron stores 10% of an oral dose is absorbed, this is increased to 20% to 30% in persons with inadequate iron stores. Food and achlorhydria will decrease absorption; aging has not been shown to affect absorption, but the percent uptake by red cells decreases from 91.2% in healthy young adults to 60% in healthy older adults.

Elimination: Iron is largely bound to serum transferrin and excreted in the urine, sweat, and sloughing of intestinal mucosa.

Dosage

Geriatric Lower doses (15-50 mg elemental iron/day) may have similar efficacy and less GI adverse events (eg, nausea,constipation) as compared to higher doses (eg, 150 mg elemental iron/day) (Rimon, 2005).

Adult

Dietary Reference Intake: Dose is RDA presented as elemental iron unless otherwise noted:

19-50 years: Male: 8 mg/day; Female: 18 mg/day

≥50 years: 8 mg/day

Doses expressed in terms of elemental iron; elemental iron content of ferrous fumarate is 33%.

Treatment of iron deficiency: Oral: Usual range: 150-200 mg elemental iron/day in divided doses; 60-100 mg elemental iron twice daily, up to 60 mg elemental iron 4 times/day

Prophylaxis of iron deficiency: Oral: 60-100 mg elemental iron/day

Note: To avoid GI upset, start with a single daily dose and increase by 1 tablet/day each week or as tolerated until desired daily dose is achieved

Administration Should be administered with water or juice on an empty stomach. Administer 2 hours prior to or 4 hours after antacids.

Monitoring Parameters Hemoglobin, hematocrit, ferritin, reticulocyte count

Reference Range

Serum iron:

Males: 75-175 mcg/dL (SI: 13.4-31.3 micromole/L)

Females: 65-165 mcg/dL (SI: 11.6-29.5 micromole/L)

Total iron binding capacity: 230-430 mcg/dL
Transferrin: 204-360 mg/dL
Percent transferrin saturation: 20% to 50%
Iron levels >300 mcg/dL can be considered toxic, should be treated as an overdose

Pharmacotherapy Pearls The elemental iron content in ferrous fumarate is 33% (ie, 200 mg ferrous fumarate is equivalent to 66 mg ferrous iron). Administration of iron for longer than 6 months should be avoided except in patients with continuous bleeding or menorrhagia.

Special Geriatric Considerations Anemia in the elderly is often caused by "anemia of chronic disease," a result of aging changes in the bone marrow, or associated with inflammation rather than blood loss. Iron stores are usually normal or increased, with a serum ferritin >50 ng/mL and a decreased total iron binding capacity. Hence, the anemia is not secondary to iron deficiency but the inability of the reticuloendothelial system to use available iron stores. Timed release iron preparations should be avoided due to their erratic absorption. Products combined with a laxative or stool softener should not be used unless the need for the combination is demonstrated.

Dosage Forms Excipient information presented when available (limited, particularly for generics); consult specific product labeling.
Tablet, oral: 324 mg [elemental iron 106 mg]
Femiron®: 63 mg [elemental iron 20 mg]
Ferretts®: 325 mg [scored; elemental iron 106 mg]
Ferrocite™: 324 mg [contains tartrazine; elemental iron 106 mg]
Hemocyte®: 324 mg [elemental iron 106 mg]
Ircon®: 200 mg [elemental iron 66 mg]
Tablet, timed release, oral:
Ferro-Sequels®: 150 mg [contains sodium benzoate; elemental iron 50 mg; with docusate sodium]

Ferrous Gluconate (FER us GLOO koe nate)

Brand Names: U.S. Ferate [OTC]; Fergon® [OTC]
Brand Names: Canada Apo-Ferrous Gluconate®; Novo-Ferrogluc
Index Terms Iron Gluconate
Generic Availability (U.S.) Yes
Pharmacologic Category Iron Salt
Use Prevention and treatment of iron-deficiency anemias
Contraindications Hypersensitivity to iron salts or any component of the formulation; hemochromatosis, hemolytic anemia
Warnings/Precautions Avoid in patients with peptic ulcer, enteritis, or ulcerative colitis. Administration of iron for >6 months should be avoided except in patients with continuous bleeding or menorrhagia. Anemia in the elderly is often caused by "anemia of chronic disease" or associated with inflammation rather than blood loss. Iron stores are usually normal or increased, with a serum ferritin >50 ng/mL and a decreased total iron binding capacity. Hence, the "anemia of chronic disease" is not secondary to iron deficiency but the inability of the reticuloendothelial system to reclaim available iron stores. Avoid in patients receiving frequent blood transfusions. **[U.S. Boxed Warning]: Severe iron toxicity may occur in overdose, particularly when ingested by children; iron is a leading cause of fatal poisoning in children; store out of children's reach and in child-resistant containers.**
Adverse Reactions (Reflective of adult population; not specific for elderly)
>10%: Gastrointestinal: Constipation, dark stools, nausea, stomach cramping, vomiting
1% to 10%:
Gastrointestinal: Diarrhea, heartburn, staining of teeth
Genitourinary: Discoloration of urine
Drug Interactions
Metabolism/Transport Effects None known.
Avoid Concomitant Use
Avoid concomitant use of Ferrous Gluconate with any of the following: Dimercaprol
Increased Effect/Toxicity
The levels/effects of Ferrous Gluconate may be increased by: Dimercaprol
Decreased Effect
Ferrous Gluconate may decrease the levels/effects of: Bisphosphonate Derivatives; Cefdinir; Deferiprone; Eltrombopag; Levodopa; Levothyroxine; Methyldopa; PenicillAMINE; Phosphate Supplements; Quinolone Antibiotics; Tetracycline Derivatives; Trientine

The levels/effects of Ferrous Gluconate may be decreased by: Antacids; H2-Antagonists; Pancrelipase; Proton Pump Inhibitors; Trientine
Ethanol/Nutrition/Herb Interactions Food: Cereals, dietary fiber, tea, coffee, eggs, and milk may decrease absorption.

FERROUS GLUCONATE

Stability Iron is a leading cause of fatal poisoning in children. Store out of children's reach and in child-resistant containers.

Mechanism of Action Replaces iron found in hemoglobin, myoglobin, and enzymes; allows the transportation of oxygen via hemoglobin

Pharmacodynamics/Kinetics

Absorption: Iron is absorbed in the duodenum and upper jejunum; in persons with normal iron stores 10% of an oral dose is absorbed, this is increased to 20% to 30% in persons with inadequate iron stores. Food and achlorhydria will decrease absorption; aging has not been shown to affect absorption, but the percent uptake by red cells decreases from 91.2% in healthy young adults to 60% in healthy older adults.

Elimination: Iron is largely bound to serum transferrin and excreted in the urine, sweat, and sloughing of intestinal mucosa

Dosage

Geriatric Lower doses (15-50 mg elemental iron/day) may have similar efficacy and less GI adverse events (eg, nausea, constipation) as compared to higher doses (eg, 150 mg elemental iron/day) (Rimon, 2005).

Adult

Dietary Reference Intake: Dose is RDA presented as elemental iron unless otherwise noted:
19-50 years: Male: 8 mg/day; Female: 18 mg/day
≥50 years: 8 mg/day

Dose expressed in terms of elemental iron:
Treatment of iron deficiency anemia: Oral: 60 mg twice daily up to 60 mg 4 times/day
Prophylaxis of iron deficiency: Oral: 60 mg/day

Administration Administer 2 hours before or 4 hours after antacids

Monitoring Parameters Serum iron, total iron binding capacity, reticulocyte count, hemoglobin

Reference Range Therapeutic: Males: 75-175 mcg/dL (SI: 13.4-31.3 micromole/L); Females: 65-165 mcg/dL (SI: 11.6-29.5 micromole/L); serum iron level >300 mcg/dL usually requires treatment of overdose due to severe toxicity

Test Interactions False-positive for blood in stool by the guaiac test

Pharmacotherapy Pearls Gluconate contains 12% elemental iron (ie, 300 mg ferrous gluconate is equivalent to 34 mg ferrous iron); administration of iron for longer than 6 months should be avoided except in patients with continued bleeding or menorrhagia

Special Geriatric Considerations Anemia in the elderly is often caused by "anemia of chronic disease," a result of aging changes in the bone marrow, or associated with inflammation rather than blood loss. Iron stores are usually normal or increased, with a serum ferritin >50 ng/mL and a decreased total iron binding capacity. Hence, the anemia is not secondary to iron deficiency but the inability of the reticuloendothelial system to use available iron stores. Timed release iron preparations should be avoided due to their erratic absorption. Products combined with a laxative or stool softener should not be used unless the need for the combination is demonstrated.

Dosage Forms Excipient information presented when available (limited, particularly for generics); consult specific product labeling.
Tablet, oral: 246 mg [elemental iron 28 mg], 324 mg [elemental iron 38 mg], 325 mg [elemental iron 36 mg]
Ferate: 240 mg [elemental iron 27 mg]
Fergon®: 240 mg [elemental iron 27 mg]

Ferrous Sulfate (FER us SUL fate)

Medication Safety Issues

Sound-alike/look-alike issues:
Feosol® may be confused with Fer-In-Sol®
Fer-In-Sol® may be confused with Feosol®
Slow FE® may be confused with Slow-K®

Administration issues:
Fer-In-Sol® (manufactured by Mead Johnson) and a limited number of generic products are available at a concentration of 15 mg/mL. However, many other generics and brand name products of ferrous sulfate oral liquid drops are available at a concentration of 15 mg/0.6 mL. Check concentration closely prior to dispensing. Prescriptions written in milliliters (mL) should be clarified.

Brand Names: U.S. Feosol® [OTC]; Fer-In-Sol® [OTC]; Fer-iron [OTC]; MyKidz Iron 10™ [OTC]; Slow FE® [OTC]; Slow Release [OTC]

Brand Names: Canada Apo-Ferrous Sulfate®; Fer-In-Sol®; Ferodan™

Index Terms FeSO₄; Iron Sulfate

Generic Availability (U.S.) Yes

Pharmacologic Category Iron Salt

Use Prevention and treatment of iron-deficiency anemias

Contraindications Hypersensitivity to iron salts or any component of the formulation; hemochromatosis, hemolytic anemia

Warnings/Precautions Avoid in patients with peptic ulcer, enteritis, or ulcerative colitis. Administration of iron for >6 months should be avoided except in patients with continuous bleeding or menorrhagia. Anemia in the elderly is often caused by "anemia of chronic disease" or associated with inflammation rather than blood loss. Iron stores are usually normal or increased, with a serum ferritin >50 ng/mL and a decreased total iron binding capacity. Hence, the "anemia of chronic disease" is not secondary to iron deficiency but the inability of the reticuloendothelial system to reclaim available iron stores. Avoid in patients receiving frequent blood transfusions.

Adverse Reactions (Reflective of adult population; not specific for elderly)

>10%: Gastrointestinal: Constipation, dark stools, epigastric pain, GI irritation, nausea, stomach cramping, vomiting

1% to 10%:

Gastrointestinal: Diarrhea, heartburn

Genitourinary: Discoloration of urine

Miscellaneous: Liquid preparations may temporarily stain the teeth

Drug Interactions

Metabolism/Transport Effects None known.

Avoid Concomitant Use

Avoid concomitant use of Ferrous Sulfate with any of the following: Dimercaprol

Increased Effect/Toxicity

The levels/effects of Ferrous Sulfate may be increased by: Dimercaprol

Decreased Effect

Ferrous Sulfate may decrease the levels/effects of: Bisphosphonate Derivatives; Cefdinir; Deferiprone; Eltrombopag; Levodopa; Levothyroxine; Methyldopa; PenicillAMINE; Phosphate Supplements; Quinolone Antibiotics; Tetracycline Derivatives; Trientine

The levels/effects of Ferrous Sulfate may be decreased by: Antacids; H2-Antagonists; Pancrelipase; Proton Pump Inhibitors; Trientine

Ethanol/Nutrition/Herb Interactions Food: Cereals, dietary fiber, tea, coffee, eggs, and milk may decrease absorption.

Stability Iron is a leading cause of fatal poisoning in children. Store out of children's reach and in child-resistant containers.

Mechanism of Action Replaces iron, found in hemoglobin, myoglobin, and other enzymes; allows the transportation of oxygen via hemoglobin

Pharmacodynamics/Kinetics

Onset of action: Hematologic response: Oral: ~3-10 days

Peak effect: Reticulocytosis: 5-10 days; hemoglobin increases within 2-4 weeks

Absorption: Iron is absorbed in the duodenum and upper jejunum; in persons with normal serum iron stores, 10% of an oral dose is absorbed; this is increased to 20% to 30% in persons with inadequate iron stores. Food and achlorhydria will decrease absorption

Protein binding: To transferrin

Excretion: Urine, sweat, sloughing of the intestinal mucosa, and menses

Dosage

Geriatric Lower doses (15-50 mg elemental iron/day) may have similar efficacy and less GI adverse events (eg, nausea, constipation) as compared to higher doses (eg, 150 mg elemental iron/day) (Rimon, 2005).

Adult Note: Multiple concentrations of ferrous sulfate oral liquid exist; close attention must be paid to the concentration when ordering and administering ferrous sulfate; incorrect selection or substitution of one ferrous sulfate liquid for another without proper dosage volume adjustment may result in serious over- or underdosing.

Dietary Reference Intake: Dose is RDA presented as elemental iron unless otherwise noted:

19-50 years: Male: 8 mg/day; Female: 18 mg/day

≥50 years: 8 mg/day

Dose expressed in terms of ferrous sulfate:

Treatment of iron deficiency anemia: Oral: 300 mg twice daily up to 300 mg 4 times/day or 250 mg (extended release) 1-2 times/day

Prophylaxis of iron deficiency: Oral: 300 mg/day

Administration Should be taken with water or juice on an empty stomach; administer ferrous sulfate 2 hours prior to, or 4 hours after antacids

◀ **Monitoring Parameters** Serum iron, total iron binding capacity, reticulocyte count, hemoglobin

Reference Range

Serum iron:

Males: 75-175 mcg/dL (SI: 13.4-31.3 micromole/L)

Females: 65-165 mcg/dL (SI: 11.6-29.5 micromole/L)

Total iron binding capacity: 230-430 mcg/dL

Transferrin: 204-360 mg/dL

Percent transferrin saturation: 20% to 50%

Test Interactions False-positive for blood in stool by the guaiac test

Special Geriatric Considerations Anemia in the elderly is often caused by "anemia of chronic disease," a result of aging changes in the bone marrow, or associated with inflammation rather than blood loss. Iron stores are usually normal or increased, with a serum ferritin >50 ng/mL and a decreased total iron binding capacity. Hence, the anemia is not secondary to iron deficiency but the inability of the reticuloendothelial system to use available iron stores. Timed release iron preparations should be avoided due to their erratic absorption. Products combined with a laxative or stool softener should not be used unless the need for the combination is demonstrated.

Dosage Forms Excipient information presented when available (limited, particularly for generics); consult specific product labeling.

Elixir, oral: 220 mg/5 mL (473 mL, 480 mL) [elemental iron 44 mg/5 mL]

Liquid, oral: 300 mg/5 mL (5 mL) [elemental iron ~60 mg/5 mL]

Liquid, oral [drops]: 75 mg/mL (50 mL) [elemental iron 15 mg/mL]

Fer-In-Sol®: 75 mg/mL (50 mL) [gluten free; contains ethanol 0.2%, sodium bisulfite; elemental iron 15 mg/mL]

Fer-iron: 75 mg/mL (50 mL) [contains ethanol 0.2%, sodium bisulfite; lemon flavor; elemental iron 15 mg/mL]

Suspension, oral [drops]:

MyKidz Iron 10™: 75 mg/1.5 mL (118 mL) [dye free, ethanol free; contains propylene glycol, sodium 12 mg/1.5 mL; strawberry-banana flavor; elemental iron 15 mg/1.5 mL]

Tablet, oral: 324 mg [elemental iron 65 mg], 325 mg [elemental iron 65 mg]

Tablet, oral [exsiccated]:

Feosol®: 200 mg [elemental iron 65 mg]

Tablet, enteric coated, oral: 324 mg [elemental iron 65 mg], 325 mg [elemental iron 65 mg]

Tablet, extended release, oral: 140 mg [elemental iron 45 mg]

Tablet, slow release, oral: 160 mg [elemental iron 50 mg]

Slow FE®: 142 mg [elemental iron 45 mg]

Slow Release: 140 mg [elemental iron 45 mg]

Ferumoxytol (fer ue MOX i tol)

Medication Safety Issues

Sound-alike/look-alike issues:

Ferumoxytol may be confused with ferric gluconate, iron dextran complex, iron sucrose

Brand Names: U.S. Feraheme®

Brand Names: Canada Feraheme®

Generic Availability (U.S.) No

Pharmacologic Category Iron Salt

Use Treatment of iron-deficiency anemia in chronic kidney disease

Contraindications Hypersensitivity to ferumoxytol or any component of the formulation

Canadian labeling: Additional contraindications (not in U.S. labeling): Evidence of iron overload; anemia not caused by iron deficiency

Warnings/Precautions Serious hypersensitivity reactions, including rare anaphylactic and anaphylactoid reactions, may occur, presenting with cardiac/cardiorespiratory arrest, clinically significant hypotension, syncope, or unresponsiveness; equipment for resuscitation and trained personnel experienced in handling emergencies should be immediately available during use. Monitor patients for signs/symptoms of hypersensitivity reactions for ≥30 minutes and until clinically stable following administration.

Do not administer in the presence of tissue iron overload; periodic monitoring of hemoglobin, serum ferritin, serum iron, and transferrin saturation is recommended. Serum iron and transferrin-bound iron may be overestimated in laboratory assays if level is drawn during the first 24 hours following administration. Administration may alter magnetic resonance (MR) imaging; conduct anticipated MRI studies prior to use. MR imaging alterations may persist for ≤3 months following use, with peak alterations anticipated in the first 2 days following administration. If MR imaging is required within 3 months after administration, use T1- or proton density-weighted MR pulse sequences to decrease effect on imagining. Do not use T2-weighted sequence MR imaging prior to 4 weeks following ferumoxytol administration. Ferumoxytol does not interfere with X-ray, computed tomography (CT), positron emission tomography (PET), single photon emission computed tomography (SPECT), ultrasound or nuclear medicine imaging.

Adverse Reactions (Reflective of adult population; not specific for elderly) 1% to 10%:

Cardiovascular: Hypotension (≤3%), edema (2%), peripheral edema (2%), chest pain (1%), hypertension (1%)

Central nervous system: Dizziness (3%), headache (2%), fever (1%)

Dermatologic: Pruritus (1%), rash (1%)

Gastrointestinal: Diarrhea (4%), nausea (3%), constipation (2%), vomiting (2%), abdominal pain (1%)

Neuromuscular & skeletal: Back pain (1%), muscle spasms (1%)

Respiratory: Cough (1%), dyspnea (1%)

Miscellaneous: Hypersensitivity reactions (≤4%; serious reactions: <1%)

Drug Interactions

Metabolism/Transport Effects None known.

Avoid Concomitant Use

Avoid concomitant use of Ferumoxytol with any of the following: Dimercaprol

Increased Effect/Toxicity

The levels/effects of Ferumoxytol may be increased by: Dimercaprol

Decreased Effect There are no known significant interactions involving a decrease in effect.

Stability Store vials at controlled room temperature of 20°C to 25°C (68°F to 77°F); excursions permitted to 15°C to 30°C (59°F to 86°F). Do not freeze.

Mechanism of Action Superparamagnetic iron oxide coated with a low molecular weight semisynthetic carbohydrate; iron-carbohydrate complex enters the reticuloendothelial system macrophages of the liver, spleen, and bone marrow where the iron is released from the complex. The released iron is either transported into storage pools or is transported via plasma transferrin for incorporation into hemoglobin.

Pharmacodynamics/Kinetics

Distribution: V_d: 3.16 L

Metabolism: Iron released from iron-carbohydrate complex after uptake in the reticuloendo-thelial system macrophages of the liver, spleen, and bone marrow

Half-life elimination: ~15 hours

Dialysis: Ferumoxytol is not removed by hemodialysis

Dosage

Geriatric & Adult Doses expressed in mg of **elemental** iron. **Note:** Test dose: Product labeling does not indicate need for a test dose.

Iron-deficiency anemia in chronic kidney disease: I.V.: 510 mg (17 mL) as a single dose, followed by a second 510 mg dose 3-8 days (U.S. labeling) or 2-8 days (Canadian labeling) after initial dose. Assess response at least 30 days following the second dose. U.S. manufacturer's labeling states the recommended dose may be readministered in patients with persistent or recurrent iron-deficiency anemia.

Renal Impairment No dosage adjustment necessary.

Hepatic Impairment No dosage adjustment provided in manufacturer's labeling.

Administration Administer intravenously as an undiluted injection at a rate ≤1 mL/second (30 mg of elemental iron/second). Do not administer if solution has particulate matter or is discolored (solution is black to reddish-brown).

Hemodialysis patients should receive injection after at least 1 hour of hemodialysis has been completed and once blood pressure has stabilized.

Monitoring Parameters Hemoglobin, serum ferritin, serum iron, transferrin saturation (for at least 1 month following second injection and periodically); signs/symptoms of hypotension following administration; signs/symptoms of hypersensitivity reactions (≥30 minutes following administration)

Reference Range

Hemoglobin: Adults:

Males: 13.5-16.5 g/dL

Females: 12.0-15.0 g/dL

Serum iron: 40-160 mcg/dL

Total iron-binding capacity: 230-430 mcg/dL

Transferrin: 204-360 mg/dL

Percent transferrin saturation: 20% to 50%

◀ **Test Interactions** May interfere with MR imaging; alterations may persist for ≤3 months following use, with peak alterations anticipated in the first 2 days following administration. If MR imaging is required within 3 months after administration, use T1- or proton density-weighted MR pulse sequences to decrease effect on imaging. Do not use T2-weighted sequence MR imaging prior to 4 weeks following administration.

Serum iron and transferrin-bound iron may be overestimated in laboratory assays if level is drawn during the first 24 hours following administration (due to contribution of iron in ferumoxytol).

Special Geriatric Considerations The manufacturer states that in clinical trials, ferumoxytol was reportedly as safe and effective in patients 65 years and older as younger patients. Anemia in the elderly is most often caused by "anemia of chronic disease", a result of aging effect in bone marrow, or associated with inflammation rather than blood loss. Iron stores are usually normal or increased, with a serum ferritin >50 ng/mL and a decreased total iron binding capacity. Hence, the anemia is not secondary to iron deficiency but the inability of the reticuloendothelial system to use available iron stores. I.V. administration of iron is often preferred over I.M. in the elderly with a decreased muscle mass and the need for daily injections.

Dosage Forms Excipient information presented when available (limited, particularly for generics); consult specific product labeling.
Injection, solution:
Feraheme®: Elemental iron 30 mg/mL (17 mL)

◆ **FESO** see Fesoterodine on page 782
◆ **FeSO₄** see Ferrous Sulfate on page 778

Fesoterodine (fes oh TER oh deen)

Related Information
Beers Criteria – Potentially Inappropriate Medications for Geriatrics on page 2183
Pharmacotherapy of Urinary Incontinence on page 2141

Medication Safety Issues
Sound-alike/look-alike issues:
Fesoterodine may be confused with fexofenadine, tolterodine
BEERS Criteria medication:
This drug may be potentially inappropriate for use in geriatric patients (Quality of evidence - varies based on comorbidity; Strength of recommendation - varies based on comorbidity)

Brand Names: U.S. Toviaz™
Index Terms FESO; Fesoterodine Fumarate
Generic Availability (U.S.) No
Pharmacologic Category Anticholinergic Agent
Use Treatment of patients with an overactive bladder with symptoms of urinary frequency, urgency, or urge incontinence.
Contraindications Hypersensitivity to fesoterodine or tolterodine (both are metabolized to 5-hydroxymethyl tolterodine) or any component of the formulation; urinary retention; gastric retention; uncontrolled narrow-angle glaucoma
Warnings/Precautions Cases of angioedema involving the face, lips, tongue, and/or larynx have been reported. Immediately discontinue if tongue, hypopharynx, or larynx are involved. May cause drowsiness and/or blurred vision, which may impair physical or mental abilities; patients must be cautioned about performing tasks which require mental alertness (eg, operating machinery or driving). Patients may experience decreased sweating; caution use in hot weather or during exercise. Use is not recommended in patients with severe hepatic impairment (Child-Pugh class C). Doses >4 mg are not recommended for patients with severe renal impairment (Cl$_{cr}$ <30 mL/minute) or patients receiving concurrent therapy with strong CYP3A4 inhibitors. Use caution in patients with bladder flow obstruction, gastrointestinal obstructive disorders, myasthenia gravis, and treated narrow-angle glaucoma. This medication is associated with potent anticholinergic properties which may be inappropriate in older adults depending on comorbidities (eg, dementia, delirium) (Beers Criteria). In addition, risk of adverse effects may be increased in elderly patients.
Adverse Reactions (Reflective of adult population; not specific for elderly)
>10%: Gastrointestinal: Xerostomia (19% to 35%; dose related)
1% to 10%:
Central nervous system: Insomnia (1%)
Dermatological: Rash (1%)
Gastrointestinal: Constipation (4% to 6%), dyspepsia (2%), nausea (1% to 2%), abdominal pain (1%)
Genitourinary: Urinary tract infection (3% to 4%), dysuria (1% to 2%), urinary retention (1%)

Hepatic: ALT increased (1%), GGT increased (1%)

Neuromuscular & skeletal: Back pain (1% to 2%)

Ocular: Dry eyes (1% to 4%)

Respiratory: Upper respiratory tract infection (2% to 3%), cough (1% to 2%), dry throat (1% to 2%)

Miscellaneous: Peripheral edema (1%)

Drug Interactions

Metabolism/Transport Effects Substrate of CYP2D6 (minor), CYP3A4 (major); **Note:** Assignment of Major/Minor substrate status based on clinically relevant drug interaction potential

Avoid Concomitant Use There are no known interactions where it is recommended to avoid concomitant use.

Increased Effect/Toxicity

Fesoterodine may increase the levels/effects of: AbobotulinumtoxinA; Anticholinergics; Cannabinoids; OnabotulinumtoxinA; Potassium Chloride; RimabotulinumtoxinB

The levels/effects of Fesoterodine may be increased by: CYP2D6 Inhibitors; CYP3A4 Inhibitors (Moderate); CYP3A4 Inhibitors (Strong); Dasatinib; Ivacaftor; Mifepristone; Pramlintide

Decreased Effect

Fesoterodine may decrease the levels/effects of: Acetylcholinesterase Inhibitors (Central); Secretin

The levels/effects of Fesoterodine may be decreased by: Acetylcholinesterase Inhibitors (Central); CYP3A4 Inducers (Strong); Deferasirox; Herbs (CYP3A4 Inducers); Peginterferon Alfa-2b; Tocilizumab

Ethanol/Nutrition/Herb Interactions Ethanol: Ethanol may potentiate adverse effects. Management: Avoid alcohol.

Stability Store at 20°C to 25°C (68°F to 77°F); excursions permitted between 15°C to 30°C (59°F to 86°F). Protect from moisture.

Mechanism of Action Fesoterodine acts as a prodrug and is converted to an active metabolite, 5-hydroxymethyl tolterodine (5-HMT); 5-HMT is responsible for fesoterodine's antimuscarinic activity and acts as a competitive antagonist of muscarinic receptors.

Urinary bladder contractions are mediated by muscarinic receptors; fesoterodine inhibits the receptors in the bladder preventing symptoms of urgency and frequency.

Pharmacodynamics/Kinetics

Absorption: Well absorbed

Distribution: I.V.: 5-HMT: V_d: 169 L

Protein binding: ~50% (primarily to albumin and alpha$_1$-acid glycoprotein)

Metabolism: Fesoterodine is rapidly and extensively metabolized to its active metabolite (5-hydroxymethyl tolterodine; 5-HMT) by nonspecific esterases; 5-HMT is further metabolized via CYP2D6 and CYP3A4 to inactive metabolites.

Bioavailability: 5-HMT: 52%

Half-life elimination: ~7 hours

Time to peak, plasma: 5-HMT: ~5 hours; C_{max} higher in poor CYP2D6 metabolizers

Excretion: Urine (~70%; 16% as 5-HMT, ~53% as inactive metabolites); feces (7%)

Dosage

Geriatric & Adult Overactive bladder: Oral: 4 mg once daily; may be increased to 8 mg once daily based on individual response and tolerability

Dosing adjustment for concomitant strong CYP3A4 inhibitors (eg, ketoconazole, itraconazole, clarithromycin): 4 mg once daily; maximum dose: 4 mg once daily

Renal Impairment

Cl_{cr} ≥30 mL/minute: No dosage adjustment necessary.

Cl_{cr} <30 mL/minute: 4 mg once daily; maximum dose: 4 mg once daily

Hepatic Impairment

Mild-to-moderate impairment (Child-Pugh class A or B): No dosage adjustment necessary.

Severe impairment (Child-Pugh class C): Use is not recommended; has not been studied.

Administration May be administered with or without food. Swallow whole; do not chew, crush, or divide.

Special Geriatric Considerations See Dosage: Renal Impairment. In clinical trials, patients >75 years of age experienced more anticholinergic side effects than younger patients.

This medication is considered to be potentially inappropriate in this patient population (Beers Criteria: Quality of evidence - varies based on comorbidity; Strength of recommendation - varies based on comorbidity)

◄ **Dosage Forms** Excipient information presented when available (limited, particularly for generics); consult specific product labeling.
Tablet, extended release, oral, as fumarate:
Toviaz™: 4 mg, 8 mg [contains soya lecithin]

♦ **Fesoterodine Fumarate** see Fesoterodine on page 782
♦ **Feverall® [OTC]** see Acetaminophen on page 31
♦ **Fexmid®** see Cyclobenzaprine on page 454

Fexofenadine (feks oh FEN a deen)

Medication Safety Issues
Sound-alike/look-alike issues:
Fexofenadine may be confused with fesoterodine
Allegra® may be confused with Viagra®
International issues:
Allegra [U.S, Canada, and multiple international markets] may be confused with Allegro brand name for fluticasone [Israel] and frovatriptan [Germany]
Brand Names: U.S. Allegra®; Allegra® Allergy 12 Hour [OTC]; Allegra® Allergy 24 Hour [OTC]; Allegra® Children's Allergy ODT [OTC]; Allegra® Children's Allergy [OTC]
Brand Names: Canada Allegra®
Index Terms Fexofenadine Hydrochloride
Generic Availability (U.S.) Yes: Excludes orally disintegrating tablet and suspension
Pharmacologic Category Histamine H_1 Antagonist; Histamine H_1 Antagonist, Second Generation; Piperidine Derivative
Use Relief of symptoms associated with seasonal allergic rhinitis; treatment of chronic idiopathic urticaria
OTC labeling: Relief of symptoms associated with allergic rhinitis
Contraindications Hypersensitivity to fexofenadine or any component of the formulation
Warnings/Precautions Use with caution in patients with renal impairment; dosage adjustment recommended. Orally disintegrating tablet contains phenylalanine.
Adverse Reactions (Reflective of adult population; not specific for elderly)
>10%:
Central nervous system: Headache (5% to 11%)
Gastrointestinal: Vomiting (children 6 months to 5 years: 4% to 12%)
1% to 10%:
Central nervous system: Fatigue (1% to 3%), somnolence (1% to 3%), dizziness (2%), fever (2%), pain (2%), drowsiness (1%)
Endocrine & metabolic: Dysmenorrhea (2%)
Gastrointestinal: Diarrhea (3% to 4%), nausea (2%), dyspepsia (1% to 2%)
Neuromuscular & skeletal: Myalgia (3%), back pain (2% to 3%), pain in extremities (2%)
Otic: Otitis media (2% to 4%)
Respiratory: Upper respiratory tract infection (3% to 4%), cough (2% to 4%), rhinorrhea (1% to 2%)
Miscellaneous: Viral infection (3%)
Drug Interactions
Metabolism/Transport Effects Substrate of CYP3A4 (minor), P-glycoprotein, SLCO1B1; **Note:** Assignment of Major/Minor substrate status based on clinically relevant drug interaction potential; **Inhibits** CYP2D6 (weak)
Avoid Concomitant Use
Avoid concomitant use of Fexofenadine with any of the following: Azelastine; Azelastine (Nasal); Methadone; Mirtazapine; Paraldehyde
Increased Effect/Toxicity
Fexofenadine may increase the levels/effects of: Alcohol (Ethyl); Anticholinergics; ARIPiprazole; Azelastine; Azelastine (Nasal); Buprenorphine; CNS Depressants; Methadone; Methotrimeprazine; Metyrosine; Mirtazapine; Paraldehyde; Selective Serotonin Reuptake Inhibitors; Zolpidem

The levels/effects of Fexofenadine may be increased by: Droperidol; Eltrombopag; Erythromycin; Erythromycin (Systemic); HydrOXYzine; Itraconazole; Ketoconazole; Ketoconazole (Systemic); Methotrimeprazine; P-glycoprotein/ABCB1 Inhibitors; Pramlintide; Verapamil
Decreased Effect
Fexofenadine may decrease the levels/effects of: Acetylcholinesterase Inhibitors (Central); Benzylpenicilloyl Polylysine; Betahistine; Hyaluronidase

The levels/effects of Fexofenadine may be decreased by: Acetylcholinesterase Inhibitors (Central); Amphetamines; Antacids; Grapefruit Juice; P-glycoprotein/ABCB1 Inducers; Rifampin; Tocilizumab

Ethanol/Nutrition/Herb Interactions

Ethanol: Ethanol may increase CNS depression. Management: Avoid ethanol.

Food: Fruit juice (apple, grapefruit, orange) may decrease bioavailability of fexofenadine by ~36%. Management: Administer with water only, avoid fruit juice.

Herb/Nutraceutical: St John's wort may decrease fexofenadine levels.

Stability Store at controlled room temperature of 20°C to 25°C (68°F to 77°F). Protect from excessive moisture.

Mechanism of Action Fexofenadine is an active metabolite of terfenadine and like terfenadine it competes with histamine for H_1-receptor sites on effector cells in the gastrointestinal tract, blood vessels and respiratory tract; it appears that fexofenadine does not cross the blood-brain barrier to any appreciable degree, resulting in a reduced potential for sedation

Pharmacodynamics/Kinetics

Onset of action: 60 minutes

Duration: Antihistaminic effect: ≥12 hours

Absorption: Rapid

Protein binding: 60% to 70%, primarily albumin and alpha$_1$-acid glycoprotein

Metabolism: Minimal (Hepatic ~5%)

Half-life elimination: 14.4 hours (31% to 72% longer in renal impairment)

Time to peak, serum: ODT: 2 hours (4 hours with high-fat meal); Tablet: ~2.6 hours; Suspension: ~1 hour

Excretion: Feces (~80%) and urine (~11%) as unchanged drug

Dosage

Geriatric Chronic idiopathic urticaria, seasonal allergic rhinitis: Oral: Use caution; adjust dose for renal impairment.

Adult

Seasonal allergic rhinitis, idiopathic urticaria, allergic rhinitis (OTC labeling): Oral: 60 mg twice daily **or** 180 mg once daily

Renal Impairment Cl$_{cr}$ <80 mL/minute: Initial: 60 mg once daily

Not effectively removed by hemodialysis

Administration

Suspension, tablet: Administer with water only; do not administer with fruit juices. Shake suspension well before use.

Orally disintegrating tablet: Take on an empty stomach. Do not remove from blister pack until administered. Using dry hands, place immediately on tongue. Tablet will dissolve within seconds, and may be swallowed with or without liquid (do not administer with fruit juices). Do not split or chew.

Monitoring Parameters Relief of symptoms

Test Interactions May suppress the wheal and flare reactions to skin test antigens.

Special Geriatric Considerations Plasma levels in the elderly are generally higher than those observed in other age groups. Once daily dosing is recommended when starting therapy in elderly patients or patients with decreased renal function.

Dosage Forms Excipient information presented when available (limited, particularly for generics); consult specific product labeling.

Suspension, oral, as hydrochloride:

Allegra®: 6 mg/mL (300 mL) [contains propylene glycol; raspberry cream flavor]

Allegra® Children's Allergy: 6 mg/mL (120 mL) [contains propylene glycol, sodium 18 mg/5 mL; berry flavor]

Tablet, oral, as hydrochloride: 30 mg, 60 mg, 180 mg

Allegra® Allergy 12 Hour: 60 mg

Allegra® Allergy 24 Hour: 180 mg

Allegra® Children's Allergy: 30 mg

Tablet, orally disintegrating, oral, as hydrochloride:

Allegra® Children's Allergy ODT: 30 mg [contains phenylalanine 5.3 mg/tablet, sodium 5 mg/tablet; orange cream flavor]

Fidaxomicin (fye DAX oh mye sin)

Brand Names: U.S. Dificid™
Brand Names: Canada Dificid™
Index Terms Difimicin; Lipiarrmycin; OPT-80; PAR-101; Tiacumicin B
Generic Availability (U.S.) No
Pharmacologic Category Antibiotic, Macrolide
Use Treatment of *Clostridium difficile*-associated diarrhea (CDAD)
Contraindications There are no contraindications listed in the manufacturer's labeling.
Warnings/Precautions Do not use for systemic infections; fidaxomicin systemic absorption is negligible. Use only in patients with proven or strongly suspected *Clostridium difficile (C. difficile)* infections.
Adverse Reactions (Reflective of adult population; not specific for elderly)
>10%: Gastrointestinal: Nausea (11%)
2% to 10%:
  Gastrointestinal: Gastrointestinal hemorrhage (4%), abdominal pain, vomiting
  Hematologic: Anemia (2%), neutropenia (2%)
Drug Interactions
Metabolism/Transport Effects None known.
Avoid Concomitant Use There are no known interactions where it is recommended to avoid concomitant use.
Increased Effect/Toxicity There are no known significant interactions involving an increase in effect.
Decreased Effect There are no known significant interactions involving a decrease in effect.
Stability Store at 20°C to 25°C (68°F to 77°F); excursions permitted to 15°C to 30°C (59°F to 86°F).
Mechanism of Action Inhibits RNA polymerase sigma subunit resulting in inhibition of protein synthesis and cell death in susceptible organisms including *C. difficile*; bactericidal
Pharmacodynamics/Kinetics
Absorption: Oral: Minimal systemic absorption
Distribution: Largely confined to the gastrointestinal tract; in single- and multiple-dose studies, fecal concentrations of fidaxomicin and its active metabolite (OP-1118) are very high while serum concentrations are minimally detectable to undetectable
Metabolism: Intestinal hydrolysis to less active metabolite (OP-1118)
Excretion: Feces (>92% as unchanged drug and metabolites); urine (<1% as metabolite)
Dosage
Geriatric & Adult Treatment of diarrhea due to *Clostridium difficile* (CDAD): Oral: 200 mg twice daily for 10 days
Renal Impairment Minimal systemic absorption; no dosage adjustment needed
Hepatic Impairment Not studied; minimally absorbed, so no dosage adjustment predicted
Administration May be administered with or without food.
Pharmacotherapy Pearls Fidaxomicin is bactericidal against gram-positive anaerobes (including *C. difficile* NAP1/B1/027 strain) and gram-positive aerobes. Fidaxomicin spectrum does **not** include gram-negative aerobes or gram-negative anaerobes (eg, *Bacteroides spp*). At the approved dose, concentrations in feces substantially exceed the 90% MIC of *C. difficile*. Postantibiotic effects against *C. difficile* in clinical studies range from 6-10 hours. Clinical studies excluded patients with a history of >1 recurrent *C. difficile*-associated diarrhea (CDAD) episode within 3 months.
Special Geriatric Considerations Fifty percent of subjects in fidaxomicin's pivotal trial were ≥65 years; 31% were ≥75 years. No difference in safety or efficacy vs vancomycin was noted between younger and older subjects. Clinical studies excluded patients with life-threatening or fulminant *C. difficile* infections or a history of more than one recurrent *C. difficile*-associated diarrhea episode in the preceding 3 months; hence, its efficacy in these patients has not been established.
Dosage Forms Excipient information presented when available (limited, particularly for generics); consult specific product labeling.
Tablet, oral:
  Dificid™: 200 mg [contains soy lecithin]

Filgrastim (fil GRA stim)

Medication Safety Issues

Sound-alike/look-alike issues:
Neupogen® may be confused with Epogen®, Neulasta®, Neumega®, Nutramigen®

International issues:
Neupogen [U.S., Canada, and multiple international markets] may be confused with Neupro brand name for rotigotine [multiple international markets]

Brand Names: U.S. Neupogen®

Brand Names: Canada Neupogen®

Index Terms G-CSF; Granulocyte Colony Stimulating Factor

Generic Availability (U.S.) No

Pharmacologic Category Colony Stimulating Factor

Use

Cancer patients (nonmyeloid malignancies) receiving myelosuppressive chemotherapy to decrease the incidence of infection (febrile neutropenia) in regimens associated with a high incidence of neutropenia with fever

Acute myelogenous leukemia (AML) following induction or consolidation chemotherapy to shorten time to neutrophil recovery and reduce the duration of fever

Cancer patients (nonmyeloid malignancies) receiving bone marrow transplant to shorten the duration of neutropenia and neutropenia-related events (eg, neutropenic fever)

Peripheral stem cell transplantation to mobilize hematopoietic progenitor cells for apheresis collection

Severe chronic neutropenia (SCN; chronic administration) to reduce the incidence and duration of neutropenic complications (fever, infections, oropharyngeal ulcers) in symptomatic patients with congenital, cyclic, or idiopathic neutropenia

Unlabeled Use Treatment of anemia in myelodysplastic syndrome (in combination with epoetin); mobilization of hematopoietic stem cells (HSC) for collection and subsequent autologous transplantation (in combination with plerixafor) in patients with non-Hodgkin's lymphoma (NHL) and multiple myeloma (MM); treatment of neutropenia in HIV-infected patients receiving zidovudine; hepatitis C treatment-associated neutropenia

Contraindications Hypersensitivity to filgrastim, E. coli-derived proteins, or any component of the formulation

Warnings/Precautions Do not use filgrastim in the period 24 hours before to 24 hours after administration of cytotoxic chemotherapy because of the potential sensitivity of rapidly dividing myeloid cells to cytotoxic chemotherapy. May potentially act as a growth factor for any tumor type, particularly myeloid malignancies; caution should be exercised in the usage of filgrastim in any malignancy with myeloid characteristics. Increases circulating leukocytes when used in conjunction with plerixafor for stem cell mobilization; monitor WBC; use with caution in patients with neutrophil count >50,000/mm^3; tumor cells released from marrow could be collected in leukapheresis product; potential effect of tumor cell reinfusion is unknown. Reports of alveolar hemorrhage, manifested as pulmonary infiltrates and hemoptysis, have occurred in healthy donors undergoing PBPC collection (not FDA approved for use in healthy donors); hemoptysis resolved upon discontinuation. Safety and efficacy have not been established with patients receiving radiation therapy (avoid concurrent radiation therapy with filgrastim), or chemotherapy associated with delayed myelosuppression (eg, nitrosoureas, mitomycin).

Allergic-type reactions (rash, urticaria, facial edema, wheezing, dyspnea, tachycardia, and/or hypotension) have occurred with first or subsequent doses. Reactions tended to involve ≥2 body systems and occur more frequently with intravenous administration and generally within 30 minutes of administration; may recur with rechallenge. Rare cases of acute respiratory distress syndrome (ARDS) have been reported (possibly due to influx of neutrophils to sites of lung inflammation); withhold or discontinue filgrastim if ARDS occurs; patients must be instructed to report respiratory distress; monitor for fever, infiltrates, or respiratory distress. Rare cases of splenic rupture have been reported (may be fatal); patients must be instructed to report left upper quadrant pain or shoulder tip pain. Cutaneous vasculitis has been reported, generally occurring in severe chronic neutropenia (SCN) patients on long-term therapy; symptoms generally developed with increasing absolute neutrophil count (ANC) and subsided when the ANC decreased; dose reductions may improve symptoms to allow for continued therapy. Use caution in patients with sickle cell disorders; severe sickle cell crises (sometimes resulting in fatalities) have been reported following filgrastim therapy. Filgrastim use prior to appropriate diagnosis of SCN may impair proper evaluation and treatment for neutropenia not due to SCN. Cytogenetic abnormalities, transformation to myelodysplastic syndrome (MDS) and acute myeloid leukemia (AML) have been observed in patients treated with filgrastim for congenital neutropenia; a longer duration of treatment and poorer ANC response appear to increase the risk. Carefully consider the risk of continuing filgrastim in patients who develop abnormal cytogenetics or MDS. The packaging of some forms may contain latex.

Adverse Reactions (Reflective of adult population; not specific for elderly)

>10%:

Central nervous system: Fever (12%)

Dermatologic: Petechiae (≤17%), rash (≤12%)

Endocrine & metabolic: LDH increased, uric acid increased

Gastrointestinal: Splenomegaly (severe chronic neutropenia: 30%; rare in other patients)

Hepatic: Alkaline phosphatase increased (21%)

Neuromuscular & skeletal: Bone/skeletal pain (22% to 33%; dose related), commonly in the lower back, posterior iliac crest, and sternum

Respiratory: Epistaxis (9% to 15%)

1% to 10%:

Cardiovascular: Hyper-/hypotension (4%), myocardial infarction/arrhythmias (3%)

Central nervous system: Headache (7%)

Gastrointestinal: Nausea (10%), vomiting (7%), peritonitis (≤2%)

Hematologic: Leukocytosis (2%)

Miscellaneous: Transfusion reaction (≤10%)

Drug Interactions

Metabolism/Transport Effects None known.

Avoid Concomitant Use There are no known interactions where it is recommended to avoid concomitant use.

Increased Effect/Toxicity

Filgrastim may increase the levels/effects of: Bleomycin; Topotecan

Decreased Effect There are no known significant interactions involving a decrease in effect.

Stability Intact vials and prefilled syringes should be stored under refrigeration at 2°C to 8°C (36°F to 46°F) and protected from direct sunlight. Filgrastim should be protected from freezing and temperatures >30°C to avoid aggregation. Do not shake.

Filgrastim vials and prefilled syringes are stable for 24 hours at 9°C to 30°C (47°F to 86°F).

Undiluted filgrastim is stable for 24 hours at 15°C to 30°C (59°F to 86°F) and for up to 14 days at 2°C to 8°C (36°F to 46°F) (data on file, Amgen Medical Information) in BD tuberculin syringes; however, sterility has only been assessed and maintained for up to 7 days when prepared under strict aseptic conditions (Jacobson, 1996; Singh, 1994). The manufacturer recommends using syringes within 24 hours due to the potential for bacterial contamination.

Do not dilute with saline at any time; product may precipitate. Filgrastim may be diluted with D_5W for I.V. infusion administration (5-15 mcg/mL; minimum concentration is 5 mcg/mL). This diluted solution is stable for 7 days at 2°C to 8°C (36°F to 46°F), however, should be used within 24 hours due to the possibility for bacterial contamination. Concentrations 5-15 mcg/mL require addition of albumin (final albumin concentration of 2 mg/mL) to prevent adsorption to plastics. Dilution to <5 mcg/mL is not recommended.

Mechanism of Action Stimulates the production, maturation, and activation of neutrophils; filgrastim activates neutrophils to increase both their migration and cytotoxicity.

Pharmacodynamics/Kinetics

Onset of action: ~24 hours; plateaus in 3-5 days

Duration: Neutrophil counts generally return to baseline within 4 days

Absorption: SubQ: 100%

Distribution: V_d: 150 mL/kg; no evidence of drug accumulation over a 11- to 20-day period

Metabolism: Systemically degraded

Half-life elimination: 1.8-3.5 hours

Time to peak, serum: SubQ: 2-8 hours

Dosage

Geriatric & Adult Details concerning dosing in combination regimens and institution protocols should also be consulted. Rounding doses to the nearest vial size may enhance patient convenience and reduce costs without compromising clinical response.

Chemotherapy-induced neutropenia SubQ, I.V.: 5 mcg/kg/day; doses may be increased by 5 mcg/kg (for each chemotherapy cycle) according to the duration and severity of the neutropenia; continue for up to 14 days or until the ANC reaches 10,000/mm³

Bone marrow transplantation (in patients with cancer; to shorten the duration of neutropenia and neutropenia-related events): SubQ, I.V.: 10 mcg/kg/day (administer ≥24 hours after chemotherapy and ≥24 hours after bone marrow infusion); adjust the dose according to the duration and severity of neutropenia; recommended steps based on neutrophil response:

When ANC >1000/mm³ for 3 consecutive days: Reduce filgrastim dose to 5 mcg/kg/day

If ANC remains >1000/mm³ for 3 more consecutive days: Discontinue filgrastim

If ANC decreases to <1000/mm³: Resume at 5 mcg/kg/day.

If ANC decreases to <1000/mm^3 during the 5 mcg/kg/day dose: Increase filgrastim to 10 mcg/kg/day and follow the above steps.

Peripheral blood progenitor cell (PBPC) collection: SubQ: 10 mcg/kg daily, usually for 6-7 days. Begin at least 4 days before the first apheresis and continue until the last apheresis; consider dose adjustment for WBC >100,000/mm^3

Severe chronic neutropenia: SubQ:

Congenital: Initial: 6 mcg/kg twice daily; adjust the dose based on ANC and clinical response

Idiopathic/cyclic: Initial: 5 mcg/kg/day; adjust the dose based on ANC and clinical response

Anemia in myelodysplastic syndrome (unlabeled use; in combination with epoetin): SubQ: 30 mcg, 75 mcg, or 150 mcg once daily (Hellstrom-Lindberg, 1998) **or** 1 mcg/kg once daily (Greenberg, 2009) **or** 75 mcg, 150 mcg or 300 mcg/dose 3 times/week (Hellstrom-Lindberg, 2003) **or** 1-2 mcg/kg/dose 1-3 times/week (NCCN MDS guidelines v.2.2011)

Hematopoietic stem cell mobilization in autologous transplantation in patients with non-Hodgkin's lymphoma or multiple myeloma (in combination with plerixafor; unlabeled use): SubQ: 10 mcg/kg once daily; begin 4 days before initiation of plerixafor; continue G-CSF on each day prior to apheresis for up to 8 days (DiPersio, *JCO* 2009; DiPersio, *Blood* 2009)

Hepatitis C treatment-associated neutropenia (unlabeled use): SubQ: 150 mcg once weekly to 300 mcg 3 times/week; titrate to maintain ANC between 750-10,000/mm^3 (Younossi, 2008)

Administration May be administered by SubQ injection, either as a bolus injection (chemotherapy-induced neutropenia) or as a continuous infusion (chemotherapy-induced neutropenia, bone marrow transplantation, and peripheral blood progenitor cell collection). May also be administered I.V. as a short infusion over 15-30 minutes (chemotherapy-induced neutropenia) or by continuous infusion (chemotherapy-induced neutropenia) or as a 4- or 24-hour infusion (bone marrow transplantation). Do not administer earlier than 24 hours after or in the 24 hours prior to cytotoxic chemotherapy.

Monitoring Parameters CBC with differential and platelets prior to treatment and twice weekly during filgrastim treatment for chemotherapy-induced neutropenia (3 times/week following marrow transplantation). For severe chronic neutropenia, monitor CBC with differential and platelets twice weekly during the first month of therapy and for 2 weeks following dose adjustments; once clinically stable, monthly for 1 year and quarterly thereafter; for congenital neutropenia also monitor bone marrow and karyotype prior to treatment; and monitor marrow and cytogenetics annually throughout treatment. Monitor temperature.

Reference Range No additional clinical benefit seen when filgrastim is used with ANC >10,000/mm^3

Test Interactions May interfere with bone imaging studies; increased hematopoietic activity of the bone marrow may appear as transient positive bone imaging changes

Special Geriatric Considerations Out of 855 participants in randomized, placebo-controlled clinical trials who had received myelosuppressive chemotherapy, a total of 232 subjects were ≥65 years and 22 subjects were ≥75 years. No overall differences in safety or effectiveness were observed between these older and younger subjects; other clinical experience has not identified differences in the responses between elderly and younger patients.

Product Availability

Tbo-filgrastim: FDA approved August 2012; availability anticipated November 2013.

Tbo-filgrastim is a short-acting recombinant form of G-CSF (biologically similar to Neupogen®), indicated to reduce the duration of severe neutropenia in patients with nonmyeloid malignancies.

Dosage Forms Excipient information presented when available (limited, particularly for generics); consult specific product labeling.

Injection, solution [preservative free]:

Neupogen®: 300 mcg/mL (1 mL, 1.6 mL) [contains polysorbate 80, sodium 0.035 mg/mL, sorbitol; vial]

Neupogen®: 600 mcg/mL (0.5 mL, 0.8 mL) [contains natural rubber/natural latex in packaging, polysorbate 80, sodium 0.035 mg/mL, sorbitol; prefilled syringe]

Finasteride (fi NAS teer ide)

Medication Safety Issues

Sound-alike/look-alike issues:

Finasteride may be confused with furosemide

Proscar® may be confused with ProSom, Provera®, PROzac®

Brand Names: U.S. Propecia®; Proscar®

Brand Names: Canada CO Finasteride; JAMP-Finasteride; Mylan-Finasteride; Novo-Finasteride; PMS-Finasteride; Propecia®; Proscar®; ratio-Finasteride; Sandoz-Finasteride; Teva-Finasteride

Generic Availability (U.S.) Yes

Pharmacologic Category 5 Alpha-Reductase Inhibitor

Use

Propecia®: Treatment of male pattern hair loss in **men only**. Safety and efficacy were demonstrated in men between 18-41 years of age.

Proscar®: Treatment of symptomatic benign prostatic hyperplasia (BPH); can be used in combination with an alpha-blocker, doxazosin

Unlabeled Use Adjuvant monotherapy after radical prostatectomy in the treatment of prostatic cancer; treatment of female hirsutism

Contraindications Hypersensitivity to finasteride or any component of the formulation

Warnings/Precautions Hazardous agent - use appropriate precautions for handling and disposal. Other urological diseases (including prostate cancer) should be ruled out before initiating. For BPH, a minimum of 6 months of treatment may be necessary to determine whether an individual will respond to finasteride; for male pattern hair loss, daily use for 3 months or longer may be required before benefit is observed. Reduces prostate specific antigen (PSA) by ~50%; in patients treated for ≥6 months the PSA value should be doubled when comparing to normal ranges in untreated patients (for interpretation of serial PSAs, a new PSA baseline should be established ≥6 months after treatment initiation and PSA monitored periodically thereafter). Failure to demonstrate a meaningful PSA decrease (<50%) or a PSA increase while on this medication may be associated with an increased risk for prostate cancer (NCCN prostate cancer early detection guidelines, v.1.2011). Patients on a 5-alpha-reductase inhibitor (5-ARI) with any increase in PSA levels, even if within normal limits, should be evaluated; may indicate presence of prostate cancer. Use with caution in patients with hepatic dysfunction; finasteride is extensively metabolized in the liver. When compared with placebo, 5-ARIs have been shown to reduce the overall incidence of prostate cancer, although an increase in the incidence of high-grade prostate cancers has been observed; 5-ARIs are not FDA-approved for the prevention of prostate cancer. Carefully monitor patients with a large residual urinary volume or severely diminished urinary flow for obstructive uropathy; these patients may not be candidates for finasteride therapy. Patients should promptly report any breast changes, including lumps, pain, or nipple discharge. Active ingredient can be absorbed through the skin; women should always use caution whenever handling. Pregnant women or women trying to conceive should not handle the product; finasteride may negatively impact fetal development.

Adverse Reactions (Reflective of adult population; not specific for elderly) Note: "Combination therapy" refers to finasteride and doxazosin.

>10%:

Endocrine & metabolic: Impotence (5% to 19%; combination therapy 23%), libido decreased (2% to 10%; combination therapy 12%)

Neuromuscular & skeletal: Weakness (5%; combination therapy 17%)

1% to 10%:

Cardiovascular: Orthostatic hypotension (9%; combination therapy 18%), edema (1%; combination therapy 3%)

Central nervous system: Dizziness (7%; combination therapy 23%), somnolence (2%; combination therapy 3%)

Dermatologic: Rash (1%)

Genitourinary: Ejaculation disturbances (<1% to 7%; combination therapy 14%), decreased volume of ejaculate (2% to 4%)

Endocrine & metabolic: Gynecomastia (1% to 2%), breast tenderness (≤1%)

Respiratory: Dyspnea (1%; combination therapy 2%), rhinitis (1%; combination therapy 2%)

Drug Interactions

Metabolism/Transport Effects Substrate of CYP3A4 (minor); **Note:** Assignment of Major/Minor substrate status based on clinically relevant drug interaction potential

Avoid Concomitant Use There are no known interactions where it is recommended to avoid concomitant use.

Increased Effect/Toxicity There are no known significant interactions involving an increase in effect.

Decreased Effect

The levels/effects of Finasteride may be decreased by: Tocilizumab

Ethanol/Nutrition/Herb Interactions Herb/Nutraceutical: St John's wort may decrease finasteride levels. Avoid saw palmetto (concurrent use has not been adequately studied).

Stability

Propecia®: Store at 15°C to 30°C (59°F to 86°F). Protect from moisture.

Proscar®: Store below 30°C (86°F). Protect from light.

Mechanism of Action Finasteride is a competitive inhibitor of both tissue and hepatic 5-alpha reductase. This results in inhibition of the conversion of testosterone to dihydrotestosterone and markedly suppresses serum dihydrotestosterone levels

Pharmacodynamics/Kinetics

Onset of action: BPH: 6 months; Male pattern hair loss: ≥3 months of daily use

Duration:

After a single oral dose as small as 0.5 mg: 65% depression of plasma dihydrotestosterone levels persists 5-7 days

After 6 months of treatment with 5 mg/day: Circulating dihydrotestosterone levels are reduced to castrate levels without significant effects on circulating testosterone; levels return to normal within 14 days of discontinuation of treatment

Distribution: V_{dss}: 76 L

Protein binding: ~90%

Metabolism: Hepatic via CYP3A4; two active metabolites (<20% activity of finasteride)

Bioavailability: Mean: 65%

Half-life elimination, serum: 6 hours (range: 3-16 hours); Elderly: 8 hours (range: 6-15 hours)

Time to peak, serum: 1-2 hours

Excretion: Feces (57%) and urine (39%) as metabolites

Dosage

Geriatric & Adult

Benign prostatic hyperplasia (Proscar®): Oral: 5 mg once daily as a single dose; clinical responses occur within 12 weeks to 6 months of initiation of therapy; long-term administration is recommended for maximal response

Male pattern baldness (Propecia®): Oral: 1 mg daily

Renal Impairment No adjustment is necessary.

Hepatic Impairment Use with caution in patients with liver function abnormalities because finasteride is metabolized extensively in the liver

Administration May be administered without regard to meals. Women of childbearing age should not touch or handle broken tablets.

Monitoring Parameters Objective and subjective signs of relief of benign prostatic hyperplasia, including improvement in urinary flow, reduction in symptoms of urgency, and relief of difficulty in micturition; for interpretation of serial PSAs, establish a new PSA baseline ≥6 months after treatment initiation and monitor PSA periodically thereafter.

Test Interactions PSA levels decrease in treated patients. After 6 months of therapy, PSA levels stabilize to a new baseline that is ~50% of pretreatment values. If following serial PSAs in a patient, re-establish a new baseline after ≥6 months of use.

Special Geriatric Considerations Clearance of finasteride is decreased in the elderly, but no dosage reductions are necessary.

Dosage Forms Excipient information presented when available (limited, particularly for generics); consult specific product labeling.

Tablet, oral: 5 mg

Propecia®: 1 mg

Proscar®: 5 mg

FlavoxATE (fla VOKS ate)

Related Information
  Beers Criteria – Potentially Inappropriate Medications for Geriatrics *on page 2183*
Medication Safety Issues
  Sound-alike/look-alike issues:
    FlavoxATE may be confused with fluvoxaMINE
  BEERS Criteria medication:
    This drug may be potentially inappropriate for use in geriatric patients (Quality of evidence - varies based on comorbidity; Strength of recommendation - varies based on comorbidity)
Brand Names: Canada Apo-Flavoxate®; Urispas®
Index Terms Flavoxate Hydrochloride; Urispas
Generic Availability (U.S.) Yes
Pharmacologic Category Antispasmodic Agent, Urinary
Use Antispasmodic to provide symptomatic relief of dysuria, nocturia, suprapubic pain, urgency, and incontinence due to detrusor instability and hyper-reflexia in elderly with cystitis, urethritis, urethrocystitis, urethrotrigonitis, and prostatitis
Contraindications Hypersensitivity to flavoxate; pyloric or duodenal obstruction; GI hemorrhage; GI obstruction; ileus; achalasia; obstructive uropathies of lower urinary tract (BPH)
Warnings/Precautions May cause drowsiness, vertigo, and ocular disturbances. Give cautiously in patients with suspected glaucoma. This medication is associated with potent anticholinergic properties which may be inappropriate in older adults depending on comorbidities (eg, dementia, delirium) (Beers Criteria).
Adverse Reactions (Reflective of adult population; not specific for elderly) Frequency not defined.
  Cardiovascular: Palpitations, tachycardia
  Central nervous system: Confusion (especially in the elderly), drowsiness, fatigue, headache, hyperpyrexia, nervousness, vertigo
  Dermatologic: Rash, urticaria
  Gastrointestinal: Constipation, dry throat, nausea, vomiting, xerostomia
  Genitourinary: Dysuria
  Hematologic: Leukopenia
  Ocular: Blurred vision, intraocular pressure increased
Drug Interactions
  Metabolism/Transport Effects None known.
  Avoid Concomitant Use There are no known interactions where it is recommended to avoid concomitant use.
  Increased Effect/Toxicity
    FlavoxATE may increase the levels/effects of: AbobotulinumtoxinA; Anticholinergics; Cannabinoids; OnabotulinumtoxinA; Potassium Chloride; RimabotulinumtoxinB

    The levels/effects of FlavoxATE may be increased by: Pramlintide
  Decreased Effect
    FlavoxATE may decrease the levels/effects of: Acetylcholinesterase Inhibitors (Central); Secretin

    The levels/effects of FlavoxATE may be decreased by: Acetylcholinesterase Inhibitors (Central)
Ethanol/Nutrition/Herb Interactions Ethanol: Avoid ethanol (may increase CNS depression).
Mechanism of Action Synthetic antispasmotic with similar actions to that of propantheline; it exerts a direct relaxant effect on smooth muscles via phosphodiesterase inhibition, providing relief to a variety of smooth muscle spasms; it is especially useful for the treatment of bladder spasticity, whereby it produces an increase in urinary capacity
Pharmacodynamics/Kinetics
  Onset of action: 55-60 minutes
  Metabolism: To methyl; flavone carboxylic acid active
  Excretion: Urine (10% to 30%) within 6 hours
Dosage
  Geriatric & Adult Urinary spasms: Oral: 100-200 mg 3-4 times/day; reduce the dose when symptoms improve.
Administration Should be administered with water on an empty stomach.
Monitoring Parameters Monitor I & O closely
Special Geriatric Considerations Caution should be used in the elderly due to anticholinergic activity (eg, confusion, constipation, blurred vision, and tachycardia).

This medication is considered to be potentially inappropriate in this patient population (Beers Criteria: Quality of evidence - varies based on comorbidity; Strength of recommendation - varies based on comorbidity)

Dosage Forms Excipient information presented when available (limited, particularly for generics); consult specific product labeling.

Tablet, oral, as hydrochloride: 100 mg

♦ **Flavoxate Hydrochloride** *see* FlavoxATE *on page* 792
♦ **Flebogamma® DIF** *see* Immune Globulin *on page* 982

Flecainide (fle KAY nide)

Related Information

Beers Criteria – Potentially Inappropriate Medications for Geriatrics *on page* 2183

Medication Safety Issues

Sound-alike/look-alike issues:

Flecainide may be confused with fluconazole

Tambocor™ may be confused with Pamelor™, Temodar®, tamoxifen, Tamiflu®

BEERS Criteria medication:

This drug may be potentially inappropriate for use in geriatric patients (Quality of evidence - high; Strength of recommendation - strong).

Brand Names: U.S. Tambocor™

Brand Names: Canada Apo-Flecainide®; Tambocor™

Index Terms Flecainide Acetate

Generic Availability (U.S.) Yes

Pharmacologic Category Antiarrhythmic Agent, Class Ic

Use Prevention and suppression of documented life-threatening ventricular arrhythmias (eg, sustained ventricular tachycardia); controlling symptomatic, disabling supraventricular tachycardias in patients without structural heart disease in whom other agents fail

Contraindications Hypersensitivity to flecainide or any component of the formulation; pre-existing second- or third-degree AV block or with right bundle branch block when associated with a left hemiblock (bifascicular block) (except in patients with a functioning artificial pacemaker); cardiogenic shock; coronary artery disease (based on CAST study results); concurrent use of ritonavir or amprenavir

Warnings/Precautions [U.S. Boxed Warning]: In the Cardiac Arrhythmia Suppression Trial (CAST), recent (>6 days but <2 years ago) myocardial infarction patients with asymptomatic, non-life-threatening ventricular arrhythmias did not benefit and may have been harmed by attempts to suppress the arrhythmia with flecainide or encainide. An increased mortality or nonfatal cardiac arrest rate (7.7%) was seen in the active treatment group compared with patients in the placebo group (3%). The applicability of the CAST results to other populations is unknown. The risks of class 1C agents and the lack of improved survival make use in patients without life-threatening arrhythmias generally unacceptable. **[U.S. Boxed Warning]: Watch for proarrhythmic effects;** monitor and adjust dose to prevent QT$_c$ prolongation. Not recommended for patients with chronic atrial fibrillation. In the treatment of atrial fibrillation in the elderly, avoid antiarrhythmics as first-line treatment. In older adults, data suggests rate control may provide more benefits than risks compared to rhythm control for most patients (Beers Criteria). **[U.S. Boxed Warning]: When treating atrial flutter, 1:1 atrioventricular conduction may occur; pre-emptive negative chronotropic therapy (eg, digoxin, beta-blockers) may lower the risk.** Pre-existing hypokalemia or hyperkalemia should be corrected before initiation (can alter drug's effect). A worsening or new arrhythmia may occur (proarrhythmic effect). Use caution in heart failure (may precipitate or exacerbate HF). Dose-related increases in PR, QRS, and QT intervals occur. Use with caution in sick sinus syndrome with permanent pacemakers or temporary pacing wires (can increase endocardial pacing thresholds). Cautious use in significant hepatic impairment.

Adverse Reactions (Reflective of adult population; not specific for elderly)

>10%:

Central nervous system: Dizziness (19% to 30%)

Ocular: Visual disturbances (16%)

Respiratory: Dyspnea (~10%)

1% to 10%:

Cardiovascular: Palpitation (6%), chest pain (5%), edema (3.5%), tachycardia (1% to 3%), proarrhythmic (4% to 12%), sinus node dysfunction (1.2%)

Central nervous system: Headache (4% to 10%), fatigue (8%), nervousness (5%) additional symptoms occurring at a frequency between 1% and 3%: fever, malaise, hypoesthesia, paresis, ataxia, vertigo, syncope, somnolence, tinnitus, anxiety, insomnia, depression

Dermatologic: Rash (1% to 3%)

Gastrointestinal: Nausea (9%), constipation (1%), abdominal pain (3%), anorexia (1% to 3%), diarrhea (0.7% to 3%)

Neuromuscular & skeletal: Tremor (5%), weakness (5%), paresthesia (1%)

Ocular: Diplopia (1% to 3%), blurred vision

Drug Interactions

Metabolism/Transport Effects Substrate of CYP1A2 (minor), CYP2D6 (major); **Note:** Assignment of Major/Minor substrate status based on clinically relevant drug interaction potential; **Inhibits** CYP2D6 (weak)

Avoid Concomitant Use

Avoid concomitant use of Flecainide with any of the following: Fosamprenavir; Highest Risk QTc-Prolonging Agents; Mifepristone; Ritonavir; Saquinavir; Tipranavir

Increased Effect/Toxicity

Flecainide may increase the levels/effects of: ARIPiprazole; Highest Risk QTc-Prolonging Agents; Moderate Risk QTc-Prolonging Agents

The levels/effects of Flecainide may be increased by: Abiraterone Acetate; Amiodarone; Boceprevir; Carbonic Anhydrase Inhibitors; CYP2D6 Inhibitors (Moderate); CYP2D6 Inhibitors (Strong); Darunavir; Fosamprenavir; Mifepristone; QTc-Prolonging Agents (Indeterminate Risk and Risk Modifying); Ritonavir; Saquinavir; Sodium Bicarbonate; Sodium Lactate; Telaprevir; Tipranavir; Tromethamine; Verapamil

Decreased Effect

The levels/effects of Flecainide may be decreased by: Etravirine; Peginterferon Alfa-2b; Sodium Bicarbonate

Ethanol/Nutrition/Herb Interactions Food: Clearance may be decreased in patients following strict vegetarian diets due to urinary pH ≥8.

Mechanism of Action Class Ic antiarrhythmic; slows conduction in cardiac tissue by altering transport of ions across cell membranes; causes slight prolongation of refractory periods; decreases the rate of rise of the action potential without affecting its duration; increases electrical stimulation threshold of ventricle, His-Purkinje system; possesses local anesthetic and moderate negative inotropic effects

Pharmacodynamics/Kinetics

Absorption: Oral: Rapid

Distribution: Adults: V_d: 5-13.4 L/kg

Protein binding: Alpha$_1$ acid glycoprotein: 40% to 50%

Metabolism: Hepatic

Bioavailability: 85% to 90%

Half-life elimination: Adults: 7-22 hours, increased with congestive heart failure or renal dysfunction; End-stage renal disease: 19-26 hours

Time to peak, serum: ~1.5-3 hours

Excretion: Urine (80% to 90%, 10% to 50% as unchanged drug and metabolites)

Dosage

Geriatric & Adult

Life-threatening ventricular arrhythmias: Oral:

Initial: 100 mg every 12 hours; increase by 50-100 mg/day (given in 2 doses/day) every 4 days; maximum: 400 mg/day

For patients receiving 400 mg/day who are not controlled and have trough concentrations <0.6 mcg/mL, dosage may be increased to 600 mg/day.

Prevention of paroxysmal supraventricular arrhythmias: Oral: (**Note:** In patients with disabling symptoms but no structural heart disease): Initial: 50 mg every 12 hours; increase by 50 mg twice daily at 4-day intervals; maximum: 300 mg/day

Paroxysmal atrial fibrillation: Outpatient: "Pill-in-the-pocket" dose (unlabeled dose): Oral: 200 mg (weight <70 kg), 300 mg (weight ≥70 kg). May not repeat in ≤24 hours. **Note:** An initial inpatient conversion trial should have been successful before sending patient home on this approach. Patient must be taking an AV nodal-blocking agent (eg, beta-blocker, nondihydropyridine calcium channel blocker) prior to initiation of antiarrhythmic.

Renal Impairment GFR ≤50 mL/minute: Decrease dose by 50%; dose increases should be made cautiously at intervals >4 days and serum levels monitored frequently.

Hemodialysis: No supplemental dose recommended.

Peritoneal dialysis: No supplemental dose recommended.

Hepatic Impairment Monitoring of plasma levels is recommended because half-life is significantly increased. When transferring from another antiarrhythmic agent, allow for 2-4 half-lives of the agent to pass before initiating flecainide therapy.

Administration Administer around-the-clock to promote less variation in peak and trough serum levels

Monitoring Parameters ECG, blood pressure, pulse, periodic serum concentrations, especially in patients with renal or hepatic impairment

Reference Range Therapeutic: 0.2-1 mcg/mL

Special Geriatric Considerations Decreased clearance and, therefore, prolonged half-life is possible; however, studies have shown no difference in response to usual doses in the elderly despite slight decrease in clearance; calculate or measure GFR since elderly patients may have GFR ≤50 mL/minute.

This medication is considered to be potentially inappropriate in this patient population (Beers Criteria: Quality of evidence - high; Strength of recommendation - strong).

Dosage Forms Excipient information presented when available (limited, particularly for generics); consult specific product labeling.

Tablet, oral, as acetate: 50 mg, 100 mg, 150 mg

Tambocor™: 50 mg

Tambocor™: 100 mg, 150 mg [scored]

♦ **Flecainide Acetate** see Flecainide on page 793
♦ **Flector®** see Diclofenac (Topical) on page 536
♦ **Fleet® Bisacodyl [OTC]** see Bisacodyl on page 214
♦ **Fleet® Enema [OTC]** see Sodium Phosphates on page 1791
♦ **Fleet® Enema Extra® [OTC]** see Sodium Phosphates on page 1791
♦ **Fleet® Glycerin Suppositories [OTC]** see Glycerin on page 891
♦ **Fleet® Liquid Glycerin [OTC]** see Glycerin on page 891
♦ **Fleet® Mineral Oil Enema [OTC]** see Mineral Oil on page 1288
♦ **Fleet® Pedia-Lax™ Chewable Tablet [OTC]** see Magnesium Hydroxide on page 1177
♦ **Fleet® Pedia-Lax™ Enema [OTC]** see Sodium Phosphates on page 1791
♦ **Fleet® Pedia-Lax™ Glycerin Suppositories [OTC]** see Glycerin on page 891
♦ **Fleet® Pedia-Lax™ Liquid Glycerin Suppositories [OTC]** see Glycerin on page 891
♦ **Fleet® Pedia-Lax™ Liquid Stool Softener [OTC]** see Docusate on page 583
♦ **Fleet® Pedia-Lax™ Quick Dissolve [OTC]** see Senna on page 1764
♦ **Fleet® Sof-Lax® [OTC]** see Docusate on page 583
♦ **Fleet® Stimulant Laxative [OTC]** see Bisacodyl on page 214
♦ **Fletcher's® [OTC]** see Senna on page 1764
♦ **Flexeril®** see Cyclobenzaprine on page 454
♦ **Flomax®** see Tamsulosin on page 1834
♦ **Flonase®** see Fluticasone (Nasal) on page 826
♦ **Flo-Pred™** see PrednisoLONE (Systemic) on page 1591
♦ **Floranex™ [OTC]** see Lactobacillus on page 1084
♦ **Flora-Q™ [OTC]** see Lactobacillus on page 1084
♦ **Florastor® [OTC]** see Saccharomyces boulardii on page 1741
♦ **Florastor® Kids [OTC]** see Saccharomyces boulardii on page 1741
♦ **Florical® [OTC]** see Calcium Carbonate on page 262
♦ **Florinef** see Fludrocortisone on page 801
♦ **Flovent** see Fluticasone (Oral Inhalation) on page 822
♦ **Flovent® Diskus®** see Fluticasone (Oral Inhalation) on page 822
♦ **Flovent® HFA** see Fluticasone (Oral Inhalation) on page 822
♦ **Floxin Otic Singles** see Ofloxacin (Otic) on page 1403
♦ **Fluarix®** see Influenza Virus Vaccine (Inactivated) on page 997
♦ **Flubenisolone** see Betamethasone on page 204

Fluconazole (floo KOE na zole)

Medication Safety Issues

Sound-alike/look-alike issues:

Fluconazole may be confused with flecainide, FLUoxetine, furosemide, itraconazole, voriconazole

Diflucan® may be confused with diclofenac, Diprivan®, disulfiram

International issues:

Canesten (oral capsules) [Great Britain] may be confused with Canesten brand name for clotrimazole (various dosage forms) [multiple international markets]; Cenestin brand name estrogens (conjugated A/synthetic) [U.S., Canada]

Brand Names: U.S. Diflucan®

Brand Names: Canada Apo-Fluconazole®; CanesOral®; CO Fluconazole; Diflucan®; Dom-Fluconazole; Fluconazole Injection; Fluconazole Omega; Monicure; Mylan-Fluconazole; Novo-Fluconazole; PHL-Fluconazole; PMS-Fluconazole; PRO-Fluconazole; Riva-Fluconazole; Taro-Fluconazole; ZYM-Fluconazole

Generic Availability (U.S.) Yes

Pharmacologic Category Antifungal Agent, Oral; Antifungal Agent, Parenteral

FLUCONAZOLE

Use Treatment of candidiasis (esophageal, oropharyngeal, peritoneal, urinary tract, vaginal); systemic candida infections (eg, candidemia, disseminated candidiasis, and pneumonia); cryptococcal meningitis; antifungal prophylaxis in allogeneic bone marrow transplant recipients

Unlabeled Use Cryptococcal pneumonia; candidal intertrigo

Contraindications Hypersensitivity to fluconazole or any component of the formulation (cross-reaction with other azole antifungal agents may occur, but has not been established; use caution); coadministration of CYP3A4 substrates which may lead to QT$_c$ prolongation (eg, cisapride, pimozide, or quinidine)

Warnings/Precautions Should be used with caution in patients with renal and hepatic dysfunction or previous hepatotoxicity from other azole derivatives. Patients who develop abnormal liver function tests during fluconazole therapy should be monitored closely and discontinued if symptoms consistent with liver disease develop. Rare exfoliative skin disorders have been observed; monitor closely if rash develops and discontinue if lesions progress. Cases of QT$_c$ prolongation and torsade de pointes associated with fluconazole use have been reported (usually high dose or in combination with agents known to prolong the QT interval); use caution in patients with concomitant medications or conditions which are arrhythmogenic. Use caution in patients treated with medications having a narrow therapeutic window and which are metabolized via CYP2C9 or CYP3A4 (monitor). Use with erythromycin should be avoided (may increase risk of cardiotoxicity). May occasionally cause dizziness or seizures; use caution driving or operating machines. Powder for oral suspension contains sucrose; use caution with fructose intolerance, sucrose-isomaltase deficiency, or glucose-galactose malabsorption.

Adverse Reactions (Reflective of adult population; not specific for elderly) Frequency not always defined.

Cardiovascular: Angioedema (rare)

Central nervous system: Headache (2% to 13%), dizziness (1%)

Dermatologic: Rash (2%)

Gastrointestinal: Nausea (2% to 7%), abdominal pain (2% to 6%), vomiting (2% to 5%), diarrhea (2% to 3%), dysgeusia (1%), dyspepsia (1%)

Hepatic: Alkaline phosphatase increased, ALT increased, AST increased, hepatic failure (rare), hepatitis, jaundice

Miscellaneous: Anaphylactic reactions (rare)

Drug Interactions

Metabolism/Transport Effects Inhibits CYP1A2 (weak), CYP2C19 (strong), CYP2C9 (strong), CYP3A4 (moderate)

Avoid Concomitant Use

Avoid concomitant use of Fluconazole with any of the following: Cisapride; Clopidogrel; Conivaptan; Dofetilide; Pimozide; QuiNIDine; Ranolazine; Tolvaptan; Voriconazole

Increased Effect/Toxicity

Fluconazole may increase the levels/effects of: Alfentanil; Aprepitant; ARIPiprazole; AtorvaSTATin; Avanafil; Benzodiazepines (metabolized by oxidation); Bosentan; Budesonide (Systemic, Oral Inhalation); BusPIRone; Busulfan; Calcium Channel Blockers; CarBAMazepine; Carvedilol; Cilostazol; Cinacalcet; Cisapride; Citalopram; Colchicine; Conivaptan; Corticosteroids (Systemic); CycloSPORINE; CycloSPORINE (Systemic); CYP2C19 Substrates; CYP2C9 Substrates; CYP3A4 Substrates; Diclofenac; DOCEtaxel; Dofetilide; Eletriptan; Eplerenone; Erlotinib; Eszopiclone; Etravirine; Everolimus; FentaNYL; Fluvastatin; Fosaprepitant; Fosphenytoin; Gefitinib; Highest Risk QTc-Prolonging Agents; Imatinib; Irbesartan; Irinotecan; Ivacaftor; Losartan; Lovastatin; Lurasidone; Macrolide Antibiotics; Methadone; Moderate Risk QTc-Prolonging Agents; Nevirapine; Phenytoin; Pimecrolimus; Pimozide; Protease Inhibitors; Proton Pump Inhibitors; QuiNIDine; Ramelteon; Ranolazine; Red Yeast Rice; Repaglinide; Rifamycin Derivatives; Salmeterol; Saxagliptin; Sildenafil; Simvastatin; Sirolimus; Solifenacin; Sulfonylureas; SUNItinib; Tacrolimus; Tacrolimus (Systemic); Tacrolimus (Topical); Tadalafil; Temsirolimus; Tolterodine; Tolvaptan; Vardenafil; Vilazodone; Vitamin K Antagonists; Voriconazole; Zidovudine; Ziprasidone; Zolpidem

The levels/effects of Fluconazole may be increased by: Etravirine; Grapefruit Juice; Macrolide Antibiotics; Mifepristone; Protease Inhibitors

Decreased Effect

Fluconazole may decrease the levels/effects of: Amphotericin B; Clopidogrel; Ifosfamide; Saccharomyces boulardii

The levels/effects of Fluconazole may be decreased by: Didanosine; Etravirine; Fosphenytoin; Phenytoin; Rifamycin Derivatives; Sucralfate

Stability

Tablet: Store at <30°C (86°F).

Powder for oral suspension: Store dry powder at <30°C (86°F). Following reconstitution, store at 5°C to 30°C (41°F to 86°F). Discard unused portion after 2 weeks. Do not freeze.

Injection: Store injection in glass at 5°C to 30°C (41°F to 86°F). Store injection in Viaflex® at 5°C to 25°C (41°F to 77°F). Do not freeze. Do not unwrap unit until ready for use.

Mechanism of Action Interferes with fungal cytochrome P450 activity (lanosterol 14-α-demethylase), decreasing ergosterol synthesis (principal sterol in fungal cell membrane) and inhibiting cell membrane formation

Pharmacodynamics/Kinetics

Distribution: V_d: ~0.6 L/kg; widely throughout body with good penetration into CSF, eye, peritoneal fluid, sputum, skin, and urine

Relative diffusion blood into CSF: Adequate with or without inflammation (exceeds usual MICs)

CSF:blood level ratio: Normal meninges: 50% to 90%; Inflamed meninges: ~80%

Protein binding, plasma: 11% to 12%

Bioavailability: Oral: >90%

Half-life elimination: Normal renal function: ~30 hours (range: 20-50 hours); Elderly: ~46 hours

Time to peak, serum: Oral: 1-2 hours

Excretion: Urine (80% as unchanged drug)

Dosage

Geriatric & Adult The daily dose of fluconazole is the same for both oral and I.V. administration

Usual dosage range: Oral, I.V: 150 mg once **or** Loading dose: 200-800 mg; maintenance: 200-800 mg once daily; duration and dosage depend on location and severity of infection

Indication-specific dosing:

Blastomycosis (unlabeled use): Oral: *CNS disease:* Consolidation: 800 mg daily for ≥12 months and until resolution of CSF abnormalities (Chapman, 2008)

Candidiasis: Oral, I.V.:

Candidemia (neutropenic and non-neutropenic): Loading dose: 800 mg (12 mg/kg) on day 1, then 400 mg daily (6 mg/kg/day) for 14 days after first negative blood culture and resolution of signs/symptoms. **Note:** Not recommended for patients with recent azole exposure, critical illness, or if *C. krusei* or *C. glabrata* are suspected (Pappas, 2009).

Chronic, disseminated: 400 mg daily (6 mg/kg/day) until calcification or lesion resolution (Pappas, 2009)

CNS candidiasis (alternative therapy): 400-800 mg daily (6-12 mg/kg/day) until CSF/radiological abnormalities resolved. **Note:** Recommended as alternative therapy in patients intolerant of amphotericin B (Pappas, 2009).

Endocarditis, prosthetic valve (unlabeled use): 400-800 mg daily (6-12 mg/kg/day) for 6 weeks after valve replacement (as step-down in stable, culture-negative patients); long-term suppression in absence of valve replacement: 400-800 mg daily (Pappas, 2009)

Endophthalmitis (unlabeled use): 400-800 mg daily (6-12 mg/kg/day) for 4-6 weeks until examination indicates resolution (Pappas, 2009)

Esophageal:

Manufacturer's recommendation: Loading dose: 200 mg on day 1, then maintenance dose of 100-400 mg daily for 21 days and for at least 2 weeks following resolution of symptoms

Alternative dosing: 200-400 mg daily for 14-21 days; suppressive therapy of 100-200 mg 3 times weekly may be used for recurrent infections (Pappas, 2009)

Intertrigo (unlabeled use): 50 mg daily or 150 mg once weekly (Coldiron, 1991; Nozickova, 1998; Stengel, 1994)

Oropharyngeal:

Manufacturer's recommendation: Loading dose: 200 mg on day 1; maintenance dose 100 mg daily for ≥2 weeks. **Note:** Therapy with 100 mg daily is associated with resistance development (Rex, 1995).

Alternative dosing: 100-200 mg daily for 7-14 days for uncomplicated, moderate-to-severe disease; chronic therapy of 100 mg 3 times weekly is recommended in immunocompromised patients with history of oropharyngeal candidiasis (OPC) (Pappas, 2009)

Osteoarticular: 400 mg daily for 6-12 months (osteomyelitis) or 6 weeks (septic arthritis) (Pappas, 2009)

Pacemaker (or ICD, VAD) infection (unlabeled use): 400-800 mg daily (6-12 mg/kg/day) for 4- 6 weeks after device removal (as step-down in stable, culture-negative patients); long-term suppression when VAD cannot be removed: 400-800 mg daily (Pappas, 2009)

Pericarditis or myocarditis: 400-800 mg daily for several months (Pappas, 2009)

Peritonitis: 50-200 mg daily. **Note:** Some clinicians do not recommend using <200 mg daily (Chen, 2004).

Prophylaxis:
Bone marrow transplant: 400 mg once daily. Patients anticipated to have severe granulocytopenia should start therapy several days prior to the anticipated onset of neutropenia and continue for 7 days after the neutrophil count is >1000 mm^3.
High-risk ICU patients in units with high incidence of invasive candidiasis: 400 mg once daily (Pappas, 2009)
Neutropenic patients: 400 mg once daily for duration of neutropenia (Pappas, 2009)
Peritoneal dialysis associated infection (concurrently treated with antibiotics), prevention of secondary fungal infection: 200 mg every 48 hours (Restrepo, 2010)
Solid organ transplant: 200-400 mg once daily for at least 7-14 days (Pappas, 2009)
Thrombophlebitis, suppurative (unlabeled use): 400-800 mg daily (6-12 mg/kg/day) and as step-down in stable patients for ≥2 weeks (Pappas, 2009)
Urinary tract:
Cystitis:
Manufacturer's recommendation: UTI: 50-200 mg once daily
Asymptomatic, patient undergoing urologic procedure: 200-400 mg once daily several days before and after the procedure (Pappas, 2009)
Symptomatic: 200 mg once daily for 2 weeks (Pappas, 2009)
Fungus balls: 200-400 mg once daily (Pappas, 2009)
Pyelonephritis: 200-400 mg once daily for 2 weeks (Pappas, 2009)
Vaginal:
Uncomplicated: Manufacturer's recommendation: 150 mg as a single oral dose
Complicated: 150 mg every 72 hours for 3 doses (Pappas, 2009)
Recurrent: 150 mg once daily for 10-14 days, followed by 150 mg once weekly for 6 months (Pappas, 2009), **or** fluconazole (oral) 100 mg, 150 mg, or 200 mg every third day for a total of 3 doses (day 1, 4, and 7), then 100 mg, 150 mg, or 200 mg dose weekly for 6 months (CDC, 2010)
Coccidioidomycosis, treatment: Oral, I.V.:
HIV-infected (unlabeled use):
Meningitis: 400-800 mg once daily continued indefinitely (CDC, 2009)
Pneumonia, focal, mild or positive serology alone: 400 mg once daily continued indefinitely (CDC, 2009)
Pneumonia, diffuse or severe extrathoracic disseminated disease (after clinical improvement noted with amphotericin B): 400 mg once daily (CDC, 2009)
Non-HIV infected (unlabeled use):
Disseminated, extrapulmonary: 400 mg once daily (some experts use 2000 mg daily [Galgiani, 2005])
Meningitis: 400 mg once daily (some experts use initial doses of 800-1000 mg daily), lifelong duration (Galgiani, 2005)
Pneumonia, acute, uncomplicated: 200-400 mg daily for 3-6 months (Catanzaro, 1995; Galgiani, 2000)
Pneumonia, chronic progressive, fibrocavitary: 200-400 mg daily for 12 months (Catanzaro, 1995; Galgiani, 2000)
Pneumonia, diffuse: Consolidation after amphotericin B induction: 400 mg daily for 12 months (lifelong in chronically immunosuppressed) (Galgiani, 2005)
Coccidioidomycosis, prophylaxis: Oral:
HIV-infected, positive serology, CD4+ count <250 cells/microL (unlabeled use): 400 mg once daily (CDC, 2009)
Solid organ transplant (unlabeled use): **Note:** Prophylaxis regimens in this setting have not been established; the following regimen has been proposed for transplant recipients who maintain residence in a *Coccidioides* spp endemic area.
Previous history >12 months prior to transplant: 200 mg once daily for 6-12 months (Vikram, 2009; Vucicevic, 2011)
Previous history ≤12 months prior to transplant: 400 mg once daily, lifelong treatment (Vikram, 2009; Vucicevic, 2011)
Positive serology before or at transplant: 400 mg once daily, lifelong treatment; if serology is negative at 12 months, consider a dose reduction to 200 mg daily (Vikram, 2009; Vucicevic, 2011)
No history (at risk for *de novo* post-transplant disease): some clinicians treat with 200 mg daily for 6-12 months (Vucicevic, 2011)
Cryptococcosis: Oral, I.V.:
Meningitis: Manufacturer's recommendation: 400 mg for 1 dose, then 200-400 mg once daily for 10-12 weeks following negative CSF culture
HIV-infected:
Meningitis (in patients amphotericin B resistant or intolerant): Induction: 400-800 mg once daily for 4-6 weeks with concomitant flucytosine (CDC, 2009) **or** 800-1200 mg once daily with concomitant flucytosine for 6 weeks (Perfect, 2010)
Consolidation: 400 mg once daily for 8 weeks (CDC, 2009)

Maintenance (suppression): 200 mg once daily lifelong or until CD4+ count >200 (CDC, 2009)

Pulmonary (immunocompetent) (unlabeled use): 400 mg once daily for 6-12 months (Perfect, 2010)

Renal Impairment
Manufacturer's recommendation: **Note:** Renal function estimated using the Cockcroft-Gault formula

No adjustment for vaginal candidiasis single-dose therapy

For multiple dosing in adults, administer loading dose of 50-400 mg, then adjust daily doses as follows: Cl_{cr} ≤50 mL/minute (no dialysis): Administer 50% of recommended dose daily

Intermittent hemodialysis (IHD): Dialyzable (50%): May administer 100% of daily dose (according to indication) after each dialysis session. Alternatively, doses of 200-400 mg every 48-72 hours **or** 100- 200 mg every 24 hours have been recommended. **Note:** Dosing dependent on the assumption of 3 times/week, complete IHD sessions (Heintz, 2009).

Continuous renal replacement therapy (CRRT) (Heintz, 2009; Trotman, 2005): Drug clearance is highly dependent on the method of renal replacement, filter type, and flow rate. Appropriate dosing requires close monitoring of pharmacologic response, signs of adverse reactions due to drug accumulation, as well as drug concentrations in relation to target trough (if appropriate). The following are general recommendations only (based on dialysate flow/ultrafiltration rates of 1-2 L/hour and minimal residual renal function) and should not supersede clinical judgment:

CVVH: Loading dose of 400-800 mg followed by 200-400 mg every 24 hours

CVVHD/CVVHDF: Loading dose of 400-800 mg followed by 400-800 mg every 24 hours (CVVHD or CVVHDF) **or** 800 mg every 24 hours (CVVHDF)

Note: Higher maintenance doses of 400 mg every 24 hours (CVVH), 800 mg every 24 hours (CVVHD), and 500-600 mg every 12 hours (CVVHDF) may be considered when treating resistant organisms and/or when employing combined ultrafiltration and dialysis flow rates of ≥2 L/hour for CVVHD/CVVHDF (Heintz, 2009; Trotman, 2005).

Administration
I.V.: Do not use if cloudy or precipitated. Infuse over ~1-2 hours; do not exceed 200 mg/hour. Oral: May be administered without regard to meals.

Monitoring Parameters Periodic liver function tests (AST, ALT, alkaline phosphatase) and renal function tests, potassium

Special Geriatric Considerations Has not been specifically studied in the elderly.

Dosage Forms Excipient information presented when available (limited, particularly for generics); consult specific product labeling. [DSC] = Discontinued product

Infusion, premixed iso-osmotic dextrose solution: 200 mg (100 mL); 400 mg (200 mL)

Infusion, premixed iso-osmotic sodium chloride solution: 100 mg (50 mL); 200 mg (100 mL); 400 mg (200 mL)

Diflucan®: 200 mg (100 mL [DSC]); 400 mg (200 mL [DSC])

Infusion, premixed iso-osmotic sodium chloride solution [preservative free]: 200 mg (100 mL); 400 mg (200 mL)

Powder for suspension, oral: 10 mg/mL (35 mL); 40 mg/mL (35 mL)

Diflucan®: 10 mg/mL (35 mL); 40 mg/mL (35 mL) [contains sodium benzoate, sucrose; orange flavor]

Tablet, oral: 50 mg, 100 mg, 150 mg, 200 mg

Diflucan®: 50 mg, 100 mg, 150 mg, 200 mg

Flucytosine (floo SYE toe seen)

Medication Safety Issues
Sound-alike/look-alike issues:
Flucytosine may be confused with fluorouracil
Ancobon® may be confused with Oncovin

High alert medication:
The Institute for Safe Medication Practices (ISMP) includes this medication among its list of drugs which have a heightened risk of causing significant patient harm when used in error.

Brand Names: U.S. Ancobon®

Brand Names: Canada Ancobon®

Index Terms 5-FC; 5-Fluorocytosine; 5-Flurocytosine

Generic Availability (U.S.) Yes

Pharmacologic Category Antifungal Agent, Oral

Use Adjunctive treatment of systemic fungal infections (eg, septicemia, endocarditis, UTI, meningitis, or pulmonary) caused by susceptible strains of *Candida* or *Cryptococcus*

Contraindications Hypersensitivity to flucytosine or any component of the formulation

FLUCYTOSINE

Warnings/Precautions [U.S. Boxed Warning]: Use with extreme caution in patients with renal dysfunction; dosage adjustment required. Avoid use as monotherapy; resistance rapidly develops. Use with caution in patients with bone marrow depression; patients with hematologic disease or who have been treated with radiation or drugs that suppress the bone marrow may be at greatest risk. Bone marrow toxicity can be irreversible. **[U.S. Boxed Warning]: Closely monitor hematologic, renal, and hepatic status.** Hepatotoxicity and bone marrow toxicity appear to be dose related; monitor levels closely and adjust dose accordingly.

Adverse Reactions (Reflective of adult population; not specific for elderly) Frequency not defined.

Cardiovascular: Cardiac arrest, myocardial toxicity, ventricular dysfunction, chest pain

Central nervous system: Ataxia, confusion, dizziness, drowsiness, fatigue, hallucinations, headache, parkinsonism, psychosis, pyrexia, sedation, seizure, vertigo

Dermatologic: Rash, photosensitivity, pruritus, toxic epidermal necrolysis, urticaria

Endocrine & metabolic: Hypoglycemia, hypokalemia

Gastrointestinal: Abdominal pain, diarrhea, dry mouth, duodenal ulcer, hemorrhage, loss of appetite, nausea, ulcerative colitis, vomiting

Hematologic: Agranulocytosis, anemia, aplastic anemia, eosinophilia, leukopenia, pancytopenia, thrombocytopenia

Hepatic: Acute hepatic injury, bilirubin increased, hepatic dysfunction, jaundice, liver enzymes increased

Neuromuscular & skeletal: Paresthesia, peripheral neuropathy, weakness

Otic: Hearing loss

Renal: Azotemia, BUN increased, crystalluria, renal failure, serum creatinine increased

Respiratory: Dyspnea, respiratory arrest

Miscellaneous: Allergic reaction

Drug Interactions

Metabolism/Transport Effects None known.

Avoid Concomitant Use

Avoid concomitant use of Flucytosine with any of the following: CloZAPine

Increased Effect/Toxicity

Flucytosine may increase the levels/effects of: CloZAPine

The levels/effects of Flucytosine may be increased by: Amphotericin B

Decreased Effect

Flucytosine may decrease the levels/effects of: Saccharomyces boulardii

The levels/effects of Flucytosine may be decreased by: Cytarabine (Conventional)

Ethanol/Nutrition/Herb Interactions Food: Food decreases the rate, but not the extent of absorption.

Stability Store at room temperature of 15°C to 30°C (59°F to 86°F). Protect from light.

Mechanism of Action Penetrates fungal cells and is converted to fluorouracil which competes with uracil interfering with fungal RNA and protein synthesis

Pharmacodynamics/Kinetics

Absorption: 76% to 89%

Distribution: Into CSF, aqueous humor, joints, peritoneal fluid, and bronchial secretions; V_d: 0.6 L/kg

Protein binding: 3% to 4%

Metabolism: Minimally hepatic; deaminated, possibly via gut bacteria, to 5-fluorouracil

Half-life elimination:

Normal renal function: 2-5 hours

Anuria: 85 hours (range: 30-250)

End stage renal disease: 75-200 hours

Time to peak, serum: ~1-2 hours

Excretion: Urine (>90% as unchanged drug)

Dosage

Geriatric & Adult

Endocarditis: Oral: 25-37.5 mg/kg every 6 hours (with amphotericin B) for at least 6 weeks after valve replacement

Meningoencephalitis, cryptococcal: Induction: Oral: 25 mg/kg/dose (with amphotericin B) every 6 hours for 2 weeks; if clinical improvement, may discontinue both amphotericin and flucytosine and follow with an extended course of fluconazole (400 mg/day); alternatively, may continue flucytosine for 6-10 weeks (with amphotericin B) without conversion to fluconazole treatment

Renal Impairment

Use lower initial dose:

Cl_{cr} 20-40 mL/minute: Administer 37.5 mg/kg every 12 hours

Cl_{cr} 10-20 mL/minute: Administer 37.5 mg/kg every 24 hours

Cl_{cr} <10 mL/minute: Administer 37.5 mg/kg every 24-48 hours, but monitor drug concentrations frequently

Hemodialysis: Dialyzable (50% to 100%); administer dose posthemodialysis

Peritoneal dialysis: Adults: Administer 0.5-1 g every 24 hours

Continuous arteriovenous or venovenous hemodiafiltration effects: Change dosing frequency to every 12-24 hours (monitor serum concentrations and adjust)

Administration Administer around-the-clock to promote less variation in peak and trough serum levels. To avoid nausea and vomiting, administer a few capsules at a time over 15 minutes until full dose is taken.

Monitoring Parameters

Pretreatment: Electrolytes (especially potassium), CBC with differential, BUN, renal function, blood culture

During treatment: CBC with differential, and LFTs (eg, alkaline phosphatase, AST/ALT) frequently, serum flucytosine concentration, renal function

Reference Range

Therapeutic: Trough: 25-50 mcg/mL; peak: 50-100 mcg/mL; peak levels should not exceed 100 mcg/mL to avoid toxic bone marrow depressive and hepatic effects

Trough: Draw just prior to dose administration

Peak: Draw 2 hours after an oral dose administration

Test Interactions Flucytosine causes markedly false elevations in serum creatinine values when the Ektachem® analyzer is used. The Jaffé reaction is recommended for determining serum creatinine.

Special Geriatric Considerations Adjust for renal function.

Dosage Forms Excipient information presented when available (limited, particularly for generics); consult specific product labeling.

Capsule, oral: 250 mg, 500 mg

Ancobon®: 250 mg, 500 mg

Fludrocortisone (floo droe KOR ti sone)

Related Information

Corticosteroids Systemic Equivalencies *on page 2112*

Medication Safety Issues

Sound-alike/look-alike issues:

Florinef® may be confused with Fioricet®, Fiorinal®

Brand Names: Canada Florinef®

Index Terms 9α-Fluorohydrocortisone Acetate; Florinef; Fludrocortisone Acetate; Fluohydrisone Acetate; Fluohydrocortisone Acetate

Generic Availability (U.S.) Yes

Pharmacologic Category Corticosteroid, Systemic

Use Partial replacement therapy for primary and secondary adrenocortical insufficiency in Addison's disease; treatment of salt-losing adrenogenital syndrome

Contraindications Hypersensitivity to fludrocortisone or any component of the formulation; systemic fungal infections

Warnings/Precautions May cause hypercorticism or suppression of hypothalamic-pituitary-adrenal (HPA) axis, particularly in patients receiving high doses for prolonged periods. HPA axis suppression may lead to adrenal crisis. Withdrawal and discontinuation of a corticosteroid should be done slowly and carefully. Fludrocortisone is primarily a mineralocorticoid agonist, but may also inhibit the HPA axis. May increase risk of infection and/or limit response to vaccinations; close observation is required in patients with latent tuberculosis and/or TB reactivity. Restrict use in active TB (only in conjunction with antituberculosis treatment). Use with caution in patients with sodium retention and potassium loss, hepatic impairment, myocardial infarction, osteoporosis, and/or renal impairment. Use with caution in the elderly. Withdraw therapy with gradual tapering of dose.

Adverse Reactions (Reflective of adult population; not specific for elderly) Frequency not defined.

Cardiovascular: CHF, edema, hypertension

Central nervous system: Dizziness, headache, seizures

Dermatologic: Acne, bruising, rash

Endocrine & metabolic: HPA axis suppression, hyperglycemia, hypokalemic alkalosis, suppression of growth

Gastrointestinal: Peptic ulcer

Neuromuscular & skeletal: Muscle weakness

Ocular: Cataracts

Miscellaneous: Anaphylaxis (generalized), diaphoresis

FLUDROCORTISONE

Drug Interactions
Metabolism/Transport Effects None known.
Avoid Concomitant Use
Avoid concomitant use of Fludrocortisone with any of the following: Aldesleukin; BCG; Mifepristone; Natalizumab; Pimecrolimus; Tacrolimus (Topical)

Increased Effect/Toxicity
Fludrocortisone may increase the levels/effects of: Acetylcholinesterase Inhibitors; Amphotericin B; Deferasirox; Leflunomide; Loop Diuretics; Natalizumab; NSAID (COX-2 Inhibitor); NSAID (Nonselective); Thiazide Diuretics; Vaccines (Live); Warfarin

The levels/effects of Fludrocortisone may be increased by: Antifungal Agents (Azole Derivatives, Systemic); Aprepitant; Calcium Channel Blockers (Nondihydropyridine); Denosumab; Estrogen Derivatives; Fluconazole; Fosaprepitant; Indacaterol; Macrolide Antibiotics; Mifepristone; Neuromuscular-Blocking Agents (Nondepolarizing); Pimecrolimus; Quinolone Antibiotics; Roflumilast; Salicylates; Tacrolimus (Topical); Telaprevir; Trastuzumab

Decreased Effect
Fludrocortisone may decrease the levels/effects of: Aldesleukin; Antidiabetic Agents; BCG; Calcitriol; Coccidioidin Skin Test; Corticorelin; Hyaluronidase; Isoniazid; Salicylates; Sipuleucel-T; Telaprevir; Vaccines (Inactivated)

The levels/effects of Fludrocortisone may be decreased by: Aminoglutethimide; Antacids; Barbiturates; Bile Acid Sequestrants; Echinacea; Mifepristone; Mitotane; Primidone; Rifamycin Derivatives

Mechanism of Action Promotes increased reabsorption of sodium and loss of potassium from renal distal tubules

Pharmacodynamics/Kinetics
Absorption: Rapid and complete
Protein binding: 42%
Metabolism: Hepatic
Half-life elimination, plasma: 30-35 minutes; Biological: 18-36 hours
Time to peak, serum: ~1.7 hours

Dosage
Geriatric & Adult Mineralocorticoid deficiency: Oral: 0.05-0.2 mg/day with ranges of 0.1 mg 3 times/week to 0.2 mg/day

Administration Administration in conjunction with a glucocorticoid is preferable

Monitoring Parameters Monitor blood pressure and signs of edema when patient is on chronic therapy; very potent mineralocorticoid with high glucocorticoid activity; monitor serum electrolytes, serum renin activity, and blood pressure; monitor for evidence of infection; stop treatment if a significant increase in weight or blood pressure, edema, or cardiac enlargement occurs

Pharmacotherapy Pearls Very potent mineralocorticoid with high glucocorticoid activity

Special Geriatric Considerations The most common use of fludrocortisone in the elderly is orthostatic hypotension that is unresponsive to more conservative measures. Attempt non-pharmacologic measures (hydration, support stockings etc) before starting drug therapy.

Dosage Forms Excipient information presented when available (limited, particularly for generics); consult specific product labeling.
Tablet, oral, as acetate: 0.1 mg

◆ **Fludrocortisone Acetate** see Fludrocortisone on page 801
◆ **FluLaval®** see Influenza Virus Vaccine (Inactivated) on page 997
◆ **Flumadine®** see Rimantadine on page 1705
◆ **FluMist®** see Influenza Virus Vaccine (Live/Attenuated) on page 1001

Flunisolide (Nasal) (floo NISS oh lide)

Medication Safety Issues
Sound-alike/look-alike issues:
Flunisolide may be confused with Flumadine®, fluocinonide
Brand Names: Canada Apo-Flunisolide®; Nasalide®; Rhinalar®
Generic Availability (U.S.) Yes
Pharmacologic Category Corticosteroid, Nasal
Use Seasonal or perennial rhinitis
Unlabeled Use Adjunct to antibiotics in empiric treatment of acute bacterial rhinosinusitis (ABRS) (Chow, 2012)

Dosage
  Geriatric & Adult Seasonal allergic rhinitis: Intranasal: 2 sprays each nostril twice daily (morning and evening); may increase to 2 sprays 3 times daily; maximum dose: 8 sprays/day in each nostril (400 mcg/day)
Special Geriatric Considerations Evaluate the patient's or caregiver's ability to safely administer the correct dose of nasal medication.
Dosage Forms Excipient information presented when available (limited, particularly for generics); consult specific product labeling.
  Solution, intranasal [spray]: 25 mcg/actuation (25 mL); 29 mcg/actuation (25 mL)

Fluocinolone (Ophthalmic) (floo oh SIN oh lone)

Medication Safety Issues
  Sound-alike/look-alike issues:
    Fluocinolone may be confused with fluocinonide
Brand Names: U.S. Retisert®
Index Terms Fluocinolone Acetonide
Generic Availability (U.S.) No
Pharmacologic Category Corticosteroid, Ophthalmic
Use Treatment of chronic, noninfectious uveitis affecting the posterior segment of the eye
Dosage
  Geriatric & Adult Chronic uveitis: Ocular implant: One silicone-encased tablet (0.59 mg) surgically implanted into the posterior segment of the eye is designed to initially release 0.6 mcg/day, decreasing over 30 days to a steady-state release rate of 0.3-0.4 mcg/day for 30 months. Recurrence of uveitis denotes depletion of tablet, requiring reimplantation.
Special Geriatric Considerations Evaluate the patient's or caregiver's ability to safely administer the correct dose of ophthalmic medication.
Dosage Forms Excipient information presented when available (limited, particularly for generics); consult specific product labeling.
  Implant, intravitreal, as acetonide:
    Retisert®: 0.59 mg (1s) [enclosed in silicone elastomer]

Fluocinolone (Otic) (floo oh SIN oh lone)

Medication Safety Issues
  Sound-alike/look-alike issues:
    Fluocinolone may be confused with fluocinonide
Brand Names: U.S. DermOtic®
Index Terms Fluocinolone Acetonide
Generic Availability (U.S.) Yes
Pharmacologic Category Corticosteroid, Otic
Use Relief of chronic eczematous external otitis
Dosage
  Geriatric & Adult Chronic eczematous external otitis: Otic: 5 drops into the affected ear twice daily for 1-2 weeks
Special Geriatric Considerations Evaluate the patient's or caregiver's ability to safely administer the correct dose of otic medication.
Dosage Forms Excipient information presented when available (limited, particularly for generics); consult specific product labeling.
  Oil, otic, as acetonide [drops]: 0.01% (20 mL)
    DermOtic®: 0.01% (20 mL) [contains peanut oil]

Fluocinolone (Topical) (floo oh SIN oh lone)

Related Information
  Topical Corticosteroids on page 2113
Medication Safety Issues
  Sound-alike/look-alike issues:
    Fluocinolone may be confused with fluocinonide
Brand Names: U.S. Capex®; Derma-Smoothe/FS®
Brand Names: Canada Capex®; Derma-Smoothe/FS®; Synalar®
Index Terms Fluocinolone Acetonide
Generic Availability (U.S.) Yes: Excludes shampoo
Pharmacologic Category Corticosteroid, Topical

Use Relief of susceptible inflammatory dermatosis [low, medium corticosteroid]; dermatitis or psoriasis of the scalp; atopic dermatitis

Dosage

Geriatric & Adult

Atopic dermatitis (Derma-Smoothe/FS® body oil): Apply thin film to affected area 3 times/day

Corticosteroid-responsive dermatoses: Topical: Cream, ointment, solution: Apply a thin layer to affected area 2-4 times/day; may use occlusive dressings to manage psoriasis or recalcitrant conditions

Inflammatory and pruritic manifestations (dental use): Topical: Apply to oral lesion 4 times/day, after meals and at bedtime

Scalp psoriasis (Derma-Smoothe/FS® scalp oil): Topical: Massage thoroughly into wet or dampened hair/scalp; cover with shower cap. Leave on overnight (or for at least 4 hours). Remove by washing hair with shampoo and rinsing thoroughly.

Seborrheic dermatitis of the scalp (Capex®): Topical: Apply no more than 1 ounce to scalp once daily; work into lather and allow to remain on scalp for ~5 minutes. Remove from hair and scalp by rinsing thoroughly with water.

Special Geriatric Considerations Due to age-related changes in skin, limit use of topical corticosteroids.

Dosage Forms Excipient information presented when available (limited, particularly for generics); consult specific product labeling.

Cream, topical, as acetonide: 0.01% (15 g, 60 g); 0.025% (15 g, 60 g)

Oil, topical, as acetonide [body oil]: 0.01% (118 mL)

Derma-Smoothe/FS®: 0.01% (120 mL) [contains isopropyl alcohol, peanut oil]

Oil, topical, as acetonide [scalp oil]: 0.01% (118 mL)

Derma-Smoothe/FS®: 0.01% (120 mL) [contains isopropyl alcohol, peanut oil]

Ointment, topical, as acetonide: 0.025% (15 g, 60 g)

Shampoo, topical, as acetonide:

Capex®: 0.01% (120 mL)

Solution, topical, as acetonide: 0.01% (60 mL)

◆ **Fluocinolone Acetonide** see Fluocinolone (Ophthalmic) on page 803
◆ **Fluocinolone Acetonide** see Fluocinolone (Otic) on page 803
◆ **Fluocinolone Acetonide** see Fluocinolone (Topical) on page 803

Fluocinonide (floo oh SIN oh nide)

Related Information

Topical Corticosteroids on page 2113

Medication Safety Issues

Sound-alike/look-alike issues:

Fluocinonide may be confused with flunisolide, fluocinolone

Lidex® may be confused with Lasix®, Videx®

Brand Names: U.S. Vanos®

Brand Names: Canada Lidemol®; Lidex®; Lyderm®; Tiamol®; Topactin; Topsyn®

Index Terms Lidex

Generic Availability (U.S.) Yes

Pharmacologic Category Corticosteroid, Topical

Use Anti-inflammatory, antipruritic; treatment of plaque-type psoriasis (up to 10% of body surface area) [high-potency topical corticosteroid]

Contraindications Hypersensitivity to fluocinonide or any component of the formulation; viral, fungal, or tubercular skin lesions, herpes simplex

Warnings/Precautions Systemic absorption of topical corticosteroids may cause hypothalamic-pituitary-adrenal (HPA) axis suppression (reversible). HPA axis suppression may lead to adrenal crisis. Risk is increased when used over large surface areas, for prolonged periods, or with occlusive dressings. Allergic contact dermatitis can occur, it is usually diagnosed by failure to heal rather than clinical exacerbation. Prolonged treatment with corticosteroids has been associated with the development of Kaposi's sarcoma (case reports); if noted, discontinuation of therapy should be considered. Adverse systemic effects including hyperglycemia, glycosuria, fluid and electrolyte changes, and HPA suppression may occur when used on large surface areas, for prolonged periods, or with an occlusive dressing. Lower-strength cream (0.05%) may be used cautiously on face or opposing skin surfaces that may rub or touch (eg, skin folds of the groin, axilla, and breasts); higher-strength (0.1%) should not be used on the face, groin, or axillae. Use of the 0.1% cream for >2 weeks is not recommended.

Adverse Reactions (Reflective of adult population; not specific for elderly) Frequency not defined.

Cardiovascular: Intracranial hypertension

Dermatologic: Acne, allergic dermatitis, contact dermatitis, dry skin, folliculitis, hypertrichosis, hypopigmentation, maceration of the skin, miliaria, perioral dermatitis, pruritus, skin atrophy, striae, telangiectasia

Endocrine & metabolic: Cushing's syndrome, growth retardation, HPA axis suppression, hyperglycemia

Local: Burning, irritation

Renal: Glycosuria

Miscellaneous: Secondary infection

Drug Interactions

Metabolism/Transport Effects None known.

Avoid Concomitant Use

Avoid concomitant use of Fluocinonide with any of the following: Aldesleukin

Increased Effect/Toxicity

Fluocinonide may increase the levels/effects of: Deferasirox

The levels/effects of Fluocinonide may be increased by: Telaprevir

Decreased Effect

Fluocinonide may decrease the levels/effects of: Aldesleukin; Corticorelin; Hyaluronidase; Telaprevir

Mechanism of Action Fluorinated topical corticosteroid considered to be of high potency. The mechanism of action for all topical corticosteroids is not well defined, however, is felt to be a combination of three important properties: anti-inflammatory activity, immunosuppressive properties, and antiproliferative actions.

Pharmacodynamics/Kinetics

Absorption: Dependent on strength of product, amount applied, and nature of skin at application site; ranges from ~1% in areas of thick stratum corneum (palms, soles, elbows, etc) to 36% in areas of thin stratum corneum (face, eyelids, etc); increased in areas of skin damage, inflammation, or occlusion

Distribution: Throughout local skin; absorbed drug into muscle, liver, skin, intestines, and kidneys

Metabolism: Primarily in skin; small amount absorbed into systemic circulation is primarily hepatic to inactive compounds

Excretion: Urine (primarily as glucuronide and sulfate, also as unconjugated products); feces (small amounts as metabolites)

Dosage

Geriatric & Adult

Pruritus and inflammation: Topical (0.05% cream): Apply thin layer to affected area 2-4 times/day depending on the severity of the condition. Therapy should be discontinued when control is achieved; if no improvement is seen, reassessment of diagnosis may be necessary.

Plaque-type psoriasis (Vanos™): Topical (0.1% cream): Apply a thin layer once or twice daily to affected areas (limited to <10% of body surface area). **Note:** Not recommended for use >2 consecutive weeks or >60 g/week total exposure. Discontinue when control is achieved.

Monitoring Parameters Relief of symptoms

Pharmacotherapy Pearls Considered a high potency steroid; avoid prolonged use on the face; may cause atrophic changes

Special Geriatric Considerations Due to age-related changes in skin, limit use of topical corticosteroids.

Dosage Forms Excipient information presented when available (limited, particularly for generics); consult specific product labeling.

Cream, topical:

Vanos®: 0.1% (30 g, 60 g, 120 g)

Cream, anhydrous, emollient, topical: 0.05% (15 g, 30 g, 60 g, 120 g)

Cream, aqueous, emollient, topical: 0.05% (15 g, 30 g, 60 g)

Gel, topical: 0.05% (15 g, 30 g, 60 g)

Ointment, topical: 0.05% (15 g, 30 g, 60 g)

Solution, topical: 0.05% (20 mL, 60 mL)

◆ **Fluohydrisone Acetate** *see* Fludrocortisone *on page 801*
◆ **Fluohydrocortisone Acetate** *see* Fludrocortisone *on page 801*
◆ **Fluorabon™** *see* Fluoride *on page 806*
◆ **Fluor-A-Day®** *see* Fluoride *on page 806*

Fluoride (FLOR ide)

Medication Safety Issues
Sound-alike/look-alike issues:
Phos-Flur® may be confused with PhosLo®
International issues:
Fluorex [France] may be confused with Flarex brand name for fluorometholone [U.S., Canada, and multiple international markets] and Fluarix brand name for influenza virus vaccine (inactivated) [U.S., and multiple international markets]

Brand Names: U.S. Act® Kids [OTC]; Act® Restoring™ [OTC]; Act® Total Care™ [OTC]; Act® [OTC]; CaviRinse™; Clinpro™ 5000; ControlRx™; ControlRx™ Multi; Denta 5000 Plus™; DentaGel™; Epiflur™; Fluor-A-Day®; Fluorabon™; Fluorinse®; Fluoritab; Flura-Drops®; Gel-Kam® Rinse; Gel-Kam® [OTC]; Just For Kids™ [OTC]; Lozi-Flur™; Neutra-Care®; NeutraGard® Advanced; Omni Gel™ [OTC]; OrthoWash™; PerioMed™; Phos-Flur®; Phos-Flur® Rinse [OTC]; PreviDent®; PreviDent® 5000 Booster; PreviDent® 5000 Dry Mouth; PreviDent® 5000 Plus®; PreviDent® 5000 Sensitive; StanGard® Perio; Stop®

Brand Names: Canada Fluor-A-Day

Index Terms Acidulated Phosphate Fluoride; Sodium Fluoride; Stannous Fluoride

Generic Availability (U.S.) Yes: Excludes lozenge, gel drops

Pharmacologic Category Nutritional Supplement

Use Prevention of dental caries

Contraindications Hypersensitivity to fluoride, tartrazine, or any component of the formulation; when fluoride content of drinking water exceeds 0.7 ppm; low sodium or sodium-free diets

Warnings/Precautions Prolonged ingestion with excessive doses may result in dental fluorosis and osseous changes; do **not** exceed recommended dosage. Some products contain tartrazine.

Drug Interactions
Metabolism/Transport Effects None known.
Avoid Concomitant Use There are no known interactions where it is recommended to avoid concomitant use.
Increased Effect/Toxicity There are no known significant interactions involving an increase in effect.
Decreased Effect There are no known significant interactions involving a decrease in effect.

Stability Store in tight plastic containers (not glass).

Mechanism of Action Promotes remineralization of decalcified enamel; inhibits the cariogenic microbial process in dental plaque; increases tooth resistance to acid dissolution

Pharmacodynamics/Kinetics
Absorption: Oral: Rapid and complete; sodium fluoride; other soluble fluoride salts; calcium, iron, or magnesium may delay absorption
Distribution: 50% of fluoride is deposited in teeth and bone after ingestion; topical application works superficially on enamel and plaque
Excretion: Urine and feces

Dosage
Geriatric & Adult Prevention of dental caries: Oral:
Dental rinse or gel: 10 mL rinse or apply to teeth and spit daily after brushing
Product-specific dosing:
PreviDent® rinse: Once weekly, rinse 10 mL vigorously around and between teeth for 1 minute, then spit; this should be done preferably at bedtime, after thoroughly brushing teeth; for maximum benefit, do not eat, drink, or rinse mouth for at least 30 minutes after treatment; do not swallow
Fluorinse®: Once weekly, vigorously swish 5-10 mL in mouth for 1 minute, then spit

Pharmacotherapy Pearls 2.2 mg of sodium fluoride is equivalent to 1 mg of fluoride ion

Special Geriatric Considerations Postmenopausal women taking high doses of sodium fluoride have increased their bone density in the lumbar spine by 35% with a smaller increase in the femoral neck. In spite of these increases, the overall rate of vertebral fracture did not decline significantly while the rate of hip fracture increased. The results of a randomized, placebo-controlled trial using an investigational slow-release fluoride formulation at a lower dose (50 mg/day) are encouraging. Patients who received fluoride for 1 year or more had a lower vertebral fracture rate and substantial increase in L2-L4 bone mass and femoral neck bone density compared to placebo. Both groups took calcium.

Dosage Forms Excipient information presented when available (limited, particularly for generics); consult specific product labeling. [DSC] = Discontinued product
Cream, oral, as sodium [toothpaste]: 1.1% (51 g) [equivalent to fluoride 2.5 mg/dose]
Denta 5000 Plus™: 1.1% (51 g) [spearmint flavor; equivalent to fluoride 2.5 mg/dose]

PreviDent® 5000 Plus®: 1.1% (51 g) [contains sodium benzoate; fruitastic™ flavor; equivalent to fluoride 2.5 mg/dose]
PreviDent® 5000 Plus®: 1.1% (51 g) [contains sodium benzoate; spearmint flavor; equivalent to fluoride 2.5 mg/dose]
Gel, topical, as acidulated phosphate:
Phos-Flur®: 1.1% (51 g) [contains propylene glycol, sodium benzoate; mint flavor; equivalent to fluoride 0.5%]
Gel, oral, as sodium [toothpaste]:
PreviDent® 5000 Booster: 1.1% (100 mL, 106 mL) [contains sodium benzoate; fruitastic™ flavor; equivalent to fluoride 2.5 mg/dose]
PreviDent® 5000 Booster: 1.1% (100 mL, 106 mL) [contains sodium benzoate; spearmint flavor; equivalent to fluoride 2.5 mg/dose]
PreviDent® 5000 Dry Mouth: 1.1% (100 mL) [mint flavor; equivalent to fluoride 2.5 mg/dose]
PreviDent® 5000 Sensitive: 1.1% (100 mL) [mild mint flavor; equivalent to fluoride 2.5 mg/dose]
Gel, topical, as sodium: 1.1% (56 g) [equivalent to fluoride 2 mg/dose]
DentaGel™: 1.1% (56 g) [fresh mint flavor; neutral pH; equivalent to fluoride 2 mg/dose]
NeutraCare®: 1.1% (60 g) [grape flavor; neutral pH]
NeutraCare®: 1.1% (60 g) [mint flavor; neutral pH]
NeutraGard® Advanced: 1.1% (60 g) [mint flavor; neutral pH]
NeutraGard® Advanced: 1.1% (60 g) [mixed berry flavor; neutral pH]
PreviDent®: 1.1% (56 g) [mint flavor; equivalent to fluoride 2 mg/dose]
PreviDent®: 1.1% (56 g) [very berry flavor; equivalent to fluoride 2 mg/dose]
Gel, topical, as stannous flouride:
Gel-Kam®: 0.4% (129 g) [cinnamon flavor]
Gel-Kam®: 0.4% (129 g) [fruit & berry flavor]
Gel-Kam®: 0.4% (129 g) [mint flavor]
Just For Kids™: 0.4% (122 g) [bubblegum flavor]
Just For Kids™: 0.4% (122 g) [fruit-punch flavor]
Just For Kids™: 0.4% (122 g) [grapey grape flavor]
Omni Gel™: 0.4% (122 g) [cinnamon flavor]
Omni Gel™: 0.4% (122 g) [grape flavor]
Omni Gel™: 0.4% (122 g) [mint flavor]
Omni Gel™: 0.4% (122 g) [natural flavor]
Omni Gel™: 0.4% (122 g) [raspberry flavor]
Stop®: 0.4% (120 g) [bubblegum flavor]
Stop®: 0.4% (120 g [DSC]) [cinnamon flavor]
Stop®: 0.4% (120 g [DSC]) [grape flavor]
Stop®: 0.4% (120 g) [mint flavor]
Liquid, oral, as base:
Fluoritab: 0.125 mg/drop [dye free]
Lozenge, oral, as sodium:
Lozi-Flur™: 2.21 mg (90s) [sugar free; cherry flavor; equivalent to fluoride 1 mg]
Paste, oral, as sodium [toothpaste]:
Clinpro™ 5000: 1.1% (113 g) [vanilla-mint flavor]
ControlRx™: 1.1% (57 g) [berry flavor]
ControlRx™: 1.1% (57 g) [vanilla-mint flavor]
ControlRx™ Multi: 1.1% (57 g) [vanilla-mint flavor]
Solution, oral, as fluoride [rinse]:
Act® Total Care™: 0.02% (1000 mL) [ethanol free; contains menthol, propylene glycol, sodium benzoate, tartrazine; fresh mint flavor; equivalent to fluoride 0.009%]
Solution, oral, as sodium [drops]: 1.1 mg/mL (50 mL) [equivalent to fluoride 0.5 mg/mL]
Fluor-A-Day®: 0.278 mg/drop (30 mL) [equivalent to fluoride 0.125 mg/drop]
Fluorabon™: 0.55 mg/0.6 mL (60 mL) [dye free, sugar free; equivalent to fluoride 0.25 mg/0.6 mL]
Flura-Drops®: 0.55 mg/drop (24 mL) [dye free, sugar free; equivalent to fluoride 0.25 mg/drop]
Solution, oral, as sodium [rinse]: 0.2% (473 mL)
Act®: 0.05% (532 mL) [contains benzyl alcohol, propylene glycol, sodium benzoate, tartrazine; cinnamon flavor; equivalent to fluoride 0.02%]
Act®: 0.05% (532 mL) [contains propylene glycol, sodium benzoate, tartrazine; mint flavor; equivalent to fluoride 0.02%]
Act® Kids: 0.05% (532 mL) [ethanol free; contains benzyl alcohol, propylene glycol, sodium benzoate; bubblegum flavor; equivalent to fluoride 0.02%]
Act® Kids: 0.05% (500 mL) [ethanol free; contains benzyl alcohol, propylene glycol, sodium benzoate; ocean berry flavor; equivalent to fluoride 0.02%]
Act® Restoring™: 0.02% (1000 mL) [contains ethanol 11%, propylene glycol, sodium benzoate; Cool Splash™ mint flavor; equivalent to fluoride 0.009%]

◄ Act® Restoring™: 0.02% (1000 mL) [contains ethanol 11%, propylene glycol, sodium benzoate; Cool Splash™ spearmint flavor; equivalent to fluoride 0.009%]

Act® Restoring™: 0.05% (532 mL) [contains ethanol 11%, propylene glycol, sodium benzoate; Cool Splash™ mint flavor; equivalent to fluoride 0.02%]

Act® Restoring™: 0.05% (532 mL) [contains ethanol 11%, propylene glycol, sodium benzoate; Cool Splash™ spearmint flavor; equivalent to fluoride 0.02%]

Act® Restoring™: 0.05% (532 mL) [contains ethanol 11%, propylene glycol, sodium benzoate; Cool Splash™ vanilla-mint flavor; equivalent to fluoride 0.02%]

Act® Total Care™: 0.02% (1000 mL) [contains ethanol 11%, propylene glycol, sodium benzoate; icy clean mint flavor; equivalent to fluoride 0.009%]

Act® Total Care™: 0.05% (88 mL, 532 mL) [contains ethanol 11%, propylene glycol, sodium benzoate; icy clean mint flavor; equivalent to fluoride 0.02%]

Act® Total Care™: 0.05% (88 mL, 532 mL) [ethanol free; contains menthol, propylene glycol, sodium benzoate, tartrazine; fresh mint flavor; equivalent to fluoride 0.02%]

CaviRinse™: 0.2% (240 mL) [mint flavor]

Fluorinse®: 0.2% (480 mL) [ethanol free; cinnamon flavor]

Fluorinse®: 0.2% (480 mL) [ethanol free; mint flavor]

OrthoWash™: 0.044% (480 mL) [contains sodium benzoate; grape flavor]

OrthoWash™: 0.044% (480 mL) [contains sodium benzoate; strawberry flavor]

Phos-Flur® Rinse: 0.044% (473 mL) [ethanol free, sugar free; bubblegum flavor]

Phos-Flur® Rinse: 0.044% (473 mL) [ethanol free, sugar free; gushing grape flavor]

Phos-Flur® Rinse: 0.044% (500 mL) [sugar free; cool mint flavor]

PreviDent®: 0.2% (473 mL) [contains benzoic acid, ethanol 6%, sodium benzoate; cool mint flavor]

Solution, oral, as stannous flouride [concentrated rinse]: 0.63% (300 mL) [equivalent to fluoride 7 mg/30 mL dose]

Gel-Kam® Rinse: 0.63% (300 mL) [mint flavor; equivalent to fluoride 7 mg/30 mL dose]

PerioMed™: 0.63% (284 mL) [ethanol free; cinnamon flavor; equivalent to fluoride 7 mg/30 mL dose]

PerioMed™: 0.63% (284 mL) [ethanol free; mint flavor; equivalent to fluoride 7 mg/30 mL dose]

PerioMed™: 0.63% (284 mL) [ethanol free; tropical fruit flavor; equivalent to fluoride 7 mg/30 mL dose]

StanGard® Perio: 0.63% (284 mL) [mint flavor]

Tablet, chewable, oral, as sodium: 0.55 mg [equivalent to fluoride 0.25 mg], 1.1 mg [equivalent to fluoride 0.5 mg], 2.2 mg [equivalent to fluoride 1 mg]

Epiflur™: 0.55 mg [sugar free; vanilla flavor; equivalent to fluoride 0.25 mg]

Epiflur™: 1.1 mg [sugar free; vanilla flavor; equivalent to fluoride 0.5 mg]

Epiflur™: 2.2 mg [sugar free; vanilla flavor; equivalent to fluoride 1 mg]

Fluor-A-Day®: 0.55 mg [raspberry flavor; equivalent to fluoride 0.25 mg]

Fluor-A-Day®: 1.1 mg [raspberry flavor; equivalent to fluoride 0.5 mg]

Fluor-A-Day®: 2.2 mg [raspberry flavor; equivalent to fluoride 1 mg]

Fluoritab: 2.2 mg [cherry flavor; equivalent to fluoride 1 mg]

Fluoritab: 1.1 mg [dye free; cherry flavor; equivalent to fluoride 0.5 mg]

◆ **Fluorinse®** *see* Fluoride *on page 806*
◆ **Fluoritab** *see* Fluoride *on page 806*
◆ **5-Fluorocytosine** *see* Flucytosine *on page 799*
◆ **9α-Fluorohydrocortisone Acetate** *see* Fludrocortisone *on page 801*

FLUoxetine (floo OKS e teen)

Related Information

Antidepressant Agents *on page 2097*

Medication Safety Issues

Sound-alike/look-alike issues:

FLUoxetine may be confused with DULoxetine, famotidine, Feldene®, fluconazole, fluvastatin, fluvoxaMINE, fosinopril, furosemide, PARoxetine, thiothixene

PROzac® may be confused with Paxil®, Prelone®, PriLOSEC®, Prograf®, Proscar®, ProSom, Provera®

Sarafem® may be confused with Serophene®

BEERS Criteria medication:

This drug may be potentially inappropriate for use in geriatric patients (Quality of evidence - moderate; Strength of recommendation - strong).

International issues:

Reneuron [Spain] may be confused with Remeron brand name for mirtazapine [U.S., Canada, and multiple international markets]

Brand Names: U.S. PROzac®; PROzac® Weekly™; Sarafem®

Brand Names: Canada Apo-Fluoxetine®; Ava-Fluoxetine; CO Fluoxetine; Dom-Fluoxetine; Fluoxetine Capsules BP; FXT 40; Gen-Fluoxetine; JAMP-Fluoxetine; Mint-Fluoxetine; Mylan-Fluoxetine; Novo-Fluoxetine; Nu-Fluoxetine; PHL-Fluoxetine; PMS-Fluoxetine; PRO-Fluoxetine; Prozac®; Q-Fluoxetine; ratio-Fluoxetine; Riva-Fluoxetine; Sandoz-Fluoxetine; Teva-Fluoxetine; ZYM-Fluoxetine

Index Terms Fluoxetine Hydrochloride

Generic Availability (U.S.) Yes

Pharmacologic Category Antidepressant, Selective Serotonin Reuptake Inhibitor

Use Treatment of major depressive disorder (MDD); treatment of binge-eating and vomiting in patients with moderate-to-severe bulimia nervosa; obsessive-compulsive disorder (OCD); premenstrual dysphoric disorder (PMDD); panic disorder with or without agoraphobia; in combination with olanzapine for treatment-resistant or bipolar I depression

Unlabeled Use Selective mutism; treatment of mild dementia-associated agitation in non-psychotic patients; post-traumatic stress disorder (PTSD); social anxiety disorder; fibromyalgia; Raynaud's phenomenon

Medication Guide Available Yes

Contraindications Hypersensitivity to fluoxetine or any component of the formulation; patients currently receiving MAO inhibitors, pimozide, or thioridazine

> **Note:** MAO inhibitor therapy must be stopped for 14 days before fluoxetine is initiated. Treatment with MAO inhibitors or thioridazine should not be initiated until 5 weeks after the discontinuation of fluoxetine.

Warnings/Precautions [U.S. Boxed Warning]: Antidepressants increase the risk of suicidal thinking and behavior in children, adolescents, and young adults (18-24 years of age) with major depressive disorder (MDD) and other psychiatric disorders; consider risk prior to prescribing. Short-term studies did not show an increased risk in patients >24 years of age and showed a decreased risk in patients ≥65 years. Closely monitor patients for clinical worsening, suicidality, or unusual changes in behavior, particularly during the initial 1-2 months of therapy or during periods of dosage adjustments (increases or decreases); the patient's family or caregiver should be instructed to closely observe the patient and communicate condition with healthcare provider. A medication guide concerning the use of antidepressants should be dispensed with each prescription.

The possibility of a suicide attempt is inherent in major depression and may persist until remission occurs. Use caution in high-risk patients. Worsening depression and severe abrupt suicidality that are not part of the presenting symptoms may require discontinuation or modification of drug therapy. The patient's family or caregiver should be alerted to monitor patients for the emergence of suicidality and associated behaviors (such as agitation, irritability, hostility, impulsivity, and hypomania) and call healthcare provider.

May worsen psychosis in some patients or precipitate a shift to mania or hypomania in patients with bipolar disorder. Patients presenting with depressive symptoms should be screened for bipolar disorder. Monotherapy in patients with bipolar disorder should be avoided. **Fluoxetine monotherapy is not FDA approved for the treatment of bipolar depression.** May cause insomnia, anxiety, nervousness, or anorexia. Use with caution in patients where weight loss is undesirable. May impair cognitive or motor performance; caution operating hazardous machinery or driving.

Serotonin syndrome and neuroleptic malignant syndrome (NMS)-like reactions have occurred with serotonin/norepinephrine reuptake inhibitors (SNRIs) and selective serotonin reuptake inhibitors (SSRIs) when used alone, and particularly when used in combination with serotonergic agents (eg, triptans) or antidopaminergic agents (eg, antipsychotics). Concurrent use with MAO inhibitors is contraindicated. Fluoxetine may elevate plasma levels of thioridazine or pimozide and increase the risk of QT_c interval prolongation. This may lead to serious ventricular arrhythmias, such as torsade de pointes-type arrhythmias, and sudden death. Fluoxetine use has been associated with occurrences of significant rash and allergic events, including vasculitis, lupus-like syndrome, laryngospasm, anaphylactoid reactions, and pulmonary inflammatory disease. Discontinue if underlying cause of rash cannot be identified.

Use caution in patients with a previous seizure disorder or condition predisposing to seizures such as brain damage, alcoholism, or concurrent therapy with other drugs which lower the seizure threshold. Use with caution in patients with hepatic or severe renal dysfunction and in elderly patients. Use caution in elderly patients; may cause or exacerbate syndrome of inappropriate antidiuretic hormone secretion or hyponatremia; monitor sodium closely with initiation or dosage adjustments in older adults (Beers Criteria). May also cause agitation, sleep disturbances, and excessive CNS stimulation. May cause hyponatremia/SIADH (elderly at increased risk); volume depletion (diuretics may increase risk). May increase the risks associated with electroconvulsive treatment. Use caution with concomitant use of NSAIDs, ASA, or other drugs that affect coagulation; the risk of bleeding may be potentiated. Use caution with history of MI or unstable heart disease; use in these patients is limited. May alter glycemic control in patients with diabetes. Due to the long half-life of fluoxetine and its metabolites, the effects and interactions noted may persist for prolonged periods following discontinuation. May cause or exacerbate sexual dysfunction. May cause mydriasis; use caution in patients at risk of acute narrow-angle glaucoma or with increased intraocular pressure. Discontinuation symptoms (eg, dysphoric mood, irritability, agitation, confusion, anxiety, insomnia, hypomania) may occur upon abrupt discontinuation. Taper dose when discontinuing therapy.

Adverse Reactions (Reflective of adult population; not specific for elderly) Percentages listed for adverse effects as reported in placebo-controlled trials and were generally similar in adults and children; actual frequency may be dependent upon diagnosis and in some cases the range presented may be lower than or equal to placebo for a particular disorder.

>10%:
  Central nervous system: Insomnia (10% to 33%), headache (21%), somnolence (5% to 17%), anxiety (6% to 15%), nervousness (8% to 14%)
  Endocrine & metabolic: Libido decreased (1% to 11%)
  Gastrointestinal: Nausea (12% to 29%), diarrhea (8% to 18%), anorexia (4% to 17%), xerostomia (4% to 12%)
  Neuromuscular & skeletal: Weakness (7% to 21%), tremor (3% to 13%)
  Respiratory: Pharyngitis (3% to 11%), yawn (≤11%)

1% to 10%:
  Cardiovascular: Vasodilation (1% to 5%), chest pain, hemorrhage, hypertension, palpitation
  Central nervous system: Dizziness (9%), abnormal dreams (1% to 5%), abnormal thinking (2%), agitation, amnesia, chills, confusion, emotional lability, sleep disorder
  Dermatologic: Rash (2% to 6%), pruritus (4%)
  Endocrine & metabolic: Ejaculation abnormal (≤7%), impotence (≤7%), menorrhagia (≥2%)
  Gastrointestinal: Dyspepsia (6% to 10%), constipation (5%), flatulence (3%), vomiting (3%), thirst (≥2%), weight loss (2%), appetite increased, taste perversion, weight gain
  Genitourinary: Urinary frequency
  Neuromuscular & skeletal: Hyperkinesia (≥2%)
  Ocular: Vision abnormal (2%)
  Otic: Ear pain, tinnitus
  Respiratory: Sinusitis (1% to 6%)
  Miscellaneous: Flu-like syndrome (3% to 10%), diaphoresis (2% to 8%), epistaxis (≥2%)

Drug Interactions
  Metabolism/Transport Effects Substrate of CYP1A2 (minor), CYP2B6 (minor), CYP2C19 (minor), CYP2C9 (major), CYP2D6 (major), CYP2E1 (minor), CYP3A4 (minor); **Note:** Assignment of Major/Minor substrate status based on clinically relevant drug interaction potential; **Inhibits** CYP1A2 (moderate), CYP2B6 (weak), CYP2C19 (moderate), CYP2C9 (weak), CYP2D6 (strong)

  Avoid Concomitant Use
  Avoid concomitant use of FLUoxetine with any of the following: Clopidogrel; Iobenguane I 123; MAO Inhibitors; Methylene Blue; Pimozide; Tryptophan

  Increased Effect/Toxicity
  FLUoxetine may increase the levels/effects of: Alpha-/Beta-Blockers; Anticoagulants; Antidepressants (Serotonin Reuptake Inhibitor/Antagonist); Antiplatelet Agents; ARIPiprazole; Aspirin; AtoMOXetine; Benzodiazepines (metabolized by oxidation); Beta-Blockers; BusPIRone; CarBAMazepine; CloZAPine; Collagenase (Systemic); CYP1A2 Substrates; CYP2C19 Substrates; CYP2D6 Substrates; Dabigatran Etexilate; Desmopressin; Dextromethorphan; Drotrecogin Alfa (Activated); Fesoterodine; Fosphenytoin; Galantamine; Haloperidol; Highest Risk QTc-Prolonging Agents; Hypoglycemic Agents; Ibritumomab; Lithium; Methadone; Methylene Blue; Metoclopramide; Mexiletine; Moderate Risk QTc-Prolonging Agents; NIFEdipine; NiMODipine; NSAID (COX-2 Inhibitor); NSAID (Nonselective); Phenytoin; Pimozide; Propafenone; QuiNIDine; RisperiDONE; Rivaroxaban; Salicylates; Serotonin Modulators; Thrombolytic Agents; Tositumomab and Iodine I 131 Tositumomab; TraMADol; Tricyclic Antidepressants; Vitamin K Antagonists

  The levels/effects of FLUoxetine may be increased by: Abiraterone Acetate; Alcohol (Ethyl); Analgesics (Opioid); Antipsychotics; ARIPiprazole; BusPIRone; Cimetidine; CNS Depressants; CYP2C9 Inhibitors (Moderate); CYP2C9 Inhibitors (Strong); CYP2D6 Inhibitors (Moderate); CYP2D6 Inhibitors (Strong); Darunavir; Glucosamine; Herbs (Anticoagulant/Antiplatelet Properties); Linezolid; Macrolide Antibiotics; MAO Inhibitors; Metoclopramide; Metyrosine; Mifepristone; Omega-3-Acid Ethyl Esters; Pentosan Polysulfate Sodium; Pentoxifylline; Prostacyclin Analogues; Tipranavir; TraMADol; Tryptophan; Vitamin E

  Decreased Effect
  FLUoxetine may decrease the levels/effects of: Clopidogrel; Iobenguane I 123; Ioflupane I 123

The levels/effects of FLUoxetine may be decreased by: CarBAMazepine; CYP2C9 Inducers (Strong); Cyproheptadine; NSAID (COX-2 Inhibitor); NSAID (Nonselective); Peginterferon Alfa-2b; Tocilizumab

Ethanol/Nutrition/Herb Interactions

Ethanol: May increase CNS depression; monitor for increased effects with coadministration. Caution patients about effects.

Herb/Nutraceutical: Avoid valerian, St John's wort, kava kava, gotu kola (may increase CNS depression).

Stability All dosage forms should be stored at controlled room temperature. Protect from light.

Mechanism of Action Inhibits CNS neuron serotonin reuptake; minimal or no effect on reuptake of norepinephrine or dopamine; does not significantly bind to alpha-adrenergic, histamine, or cholinergic receptors

Pharmacodynamics/Kinetics

Onset of action: Depression: The onset of action is within a week; however, individual response varies greatly and full response may not be seen until 8-12 weeks after initiation of treatment.

Absorption: Well absorbed; delayed 1-2 hours with weekly formulation

Distribution: V_d: 12-43 L/kg

Protein binding: 95% to albumin and alpha$_1$ glycoprotein

Metabolism: Hepatic, via CYP2C19 and 2D6, to norfluoxetine (activity equal to fluoxetine)

Half-life elimination: Adults:

Parent drug: 1-3 days (acute), 4-6 days (chronic), 7.6 days (cirrhosis)

Metabolite (norfluoxetine): 9.3 days (range: 4-16 days), 12 days (cirrhosis)

Time to peak, serum: 6-8 hours

Excretion: Urine (10% as norfluoxetine, 2.5% to 5% as fluoxetine)

Note: Weekly formulation results in greater fluctuations between peak and trough concentrations of fluoxetine and norfluoxetine compared to once-daily dosing (24% daily/164% weekly; 17% daily/43% weekly, respectively). Trough concentrations are 76% lower for fluoxetine and 47% lower for norfluoxetine than the concentrations maintained by 20 mg once-daily dosing. Steady-state fluoxetine concentrations are ~50% lower following the once-weekly regimen compared to 20 mg once daily. Average steady-state concentrations of once-daily dosing were considered to be within the ranges reported in adults (fluoxetine 91-302 ng/mL; norfluoxetine 72-258 ng/mL).

Dosage

Geriatric Oral: Some patients may require an initial dose of 10 mg/day with dosage increases of 10 mg and 20 mg every several weeks as tolerated; should not be taken at night unless patient experiences sedation.

Adult

Depression, obsessive-compulsive disorder, premenstrual dysphoric disorder, bulimia: Oral: 20 mg/day in the morning; may increase after several weeks by 20 mg/day increments; maximum: 80 mg/day; doses >20 mg may be given once daily or divided twice daily. **Note:** Lower doses of 5-10 mg/day have been used for initial treatment.

Usual dosage range:

Bulimia nervosa: Oral: 60 mg/day

Depression: Oral: Initial: 20 mg/day; may increase after several weeks if inadequate response (maximum: 80 mg/day). Patients maintained on Prozac® 20 mg/day may be changed to Prozac® Weekly™ 90 mg/week, starting dose 7 days after the last 20 mg/day dose

Depression associated with bipolar disorder (in combination with olanzapine): Oral: Initial: 20 mg in the evening; adjust as tolerated to usual range of 20-50 mg/day. See **"Note"**.

Fibromyalgia (unlabeled use): Oral: Range: 20-80 mg/day (Arnold, 2002)

Obsessive-compulsive disorder: Oral: Initial: 20 mg/day; may increase after several weeks if inadequate response; recommended range: 20-60 mg/day (maximum: 80 mg/day)

Panic disorder: Oral: Initial: 10 mg/day; after 1 week, increase to 20 mg/day; may increase after several weeks; doses >60 mg/day have not been evaluated

Post-traumatic stress disorder (PTSD) (unlabeled use): Oral: 20-40 mg/day

Premenstrual dysphoric disorder (Sarafem®): Oral: 20 mg/day continuously, **or** 20 mg/day starting 14 days prior to menstruation and through first full day of menses (repeat with each cycle)

Raynaud's phenomena (unlabeled use): Oral: 20 mg/day (Coleiro, 2001)

Social anxiety disorder (unlabeled use): Oral: Target dose: 40 mg/day; range 30-60 mg/day (Davidson, 2004)

Treatment-resistant depression (in combination with olanzapine): Oral: Initial: 20 mg in the evening; adjust as tolerated to usual range of 20-50 mg/day. See **"Note."**

Note: When using individual components of fluoxetine with olanzapine rather than fixed dose combination product (Symbyax®), approximate dosage correspondence is as follows:

Olanzapine 2.5 mg + fluoxetine 20 mg = Symbyax® 3/25
Olanzapine 5 mg + fluoxetine 20 mg = Symbyax® 6/25
Olanzapine 12.5 mg + fluoxetine 20 mg = Symbyax® 12/25
Olanzapine 5 mg + fluoxetine 50 mg = Symbyax® 6/50
Olanzapine 12.5 mg + fluoxetine 50 mg = Symbyax® 12/50

Note: Upon discontinuation of fluoxetine therapy, gradually taper dose. If intolerable symptoms occur following a dose reduction, consider resuming the previously prescribed dose and/or decrease dose at a more gradual rate.

Renal Impairment
Single dose studies: Pharmacokinetics of fluoxetine and norfluoxetine were similar among subjects with all levels of impaired renal function, including anephric patients on chronic hemodialysis.

Chronic administration: Additional accumulation of fluoxetine or norfluoxetine may occur in patients with severely impaired renal function.

Not removed by hemodialysis; use of lower dose or less frequent dosing is not usually necessary.

Hepatic Impairment Elimination half-life of fluoxetine is prolonged in patients with hepatic impairment. A lower dose or less frequent dosing of fluoxetine should be used in these patients.

Cirrhosis patient: Administer a lower dose or less frequent dosing interval.

Compensated cirrhosis without ascites: Administer 50% of normal dose.

Administration Administer without regard to meals.

Bipolar I disorder and treatment-resistant depression: Take once daily in the evening.

Major depressive disorder and obsessive compulsive disorder: Once daily doses should be taken in the morning, or twice daily (morning and noon).

Bulimia: Take once daily in the morning.

Monitoring Parameters Mental status for depression, suicidal ideation (especially at the beginning of therapy or when doses are increased or decreased), anxiety, social functioning, mania, panic attacks; akathisia, sleep status; blood glucose (for diabetic patients), baseline liver function

Reference Range Therapeutic levels have not been well established

Therapeutic: Fluoxetine: 100-800 ng/mL (SI: 289-2314 nmol/L); Norfluoxetine: 100-600 ng/mL (SI: 289-1735 nmol/L)

Toxic: Fluoxetine plus norfluoxetine: >2000 ng/mL

Pharmacotherapy Pearls ECG may reveal S-T segment depression. Not shown to be teratogenic in rodents; 15-60 mg/day, buspirone and cyproheptadine, may be useful in treatment of sexual dysfunction during treatment with a selective serotonin reuptake inhibitor.

Weekly capsules are a delayed release formulation containing enteric-coated pellets of fluoxetine hydrochloride, equivalent to 90 mg fluoxetine. Therapeutic equivalence of weekly formulation with daily formulation for delaying time to relapse has not been established.

Special Geriatric Considerations Fluoxetine's potential stimulating and anorexic effects may be bothersome to some patients and has not been shown to be superior in efficacy to other SSRIs. The long half-life in the elderly makes it less attractive compared to other SSRIs. The elderly are more prone to SSRI/SNRI-induced hyponatremia.

A systematic review and meta-analysis of antidepressant placebo-controlled trials in persons with depression and dementia found evidence "suggestive" of efficacy but not of sufficient strength to "confirm" efficacy. Antidepressant trials in this patient population are small and underpowered. Older patients with depression being treated with an antidepressant should be closely monitored for response and adverse effects. Treatment should be switched or augmented when response is inadequate with a therapeutic dose. Antidepressants that are not tolerated should be discontinued and an alternative agent should be started.

This medication is considered to be potentially inappropriate in this patient population (Beers Criteria: Quality of evidence - moderate; Strength of recommendation - strong).

Dosage Forms Excipient information presented when available (limited, particularly for generics); consult specific product labeling.

Capsule, oral: 10 mg, 20 mg, 40 mg
PROzac®: 10 mg, 20 mg, 40 mg
Capsule, delayed release, enteric coated pellets, oral: 90 mg
PROzac® Weekly™: 90 mg
Solution, oral: 20 mg/5 mL (5 mL, 120 mL)
Tablet, oral: 10 mg, 20 mg, 60 mg
Sarafem®: 10 mg, 15 mg, 20 mg

Extemporaneously Prepared A 20 mg capsule may be mixed with 4 oz of water, apple juice, or Gatorade® to provide a solution that is stable for 14 days under refrigeration

◆ **Fluoxetine and Olanzapine** see Olanzapine and Fluoxetine on page 1408
◆ **Fluoxetine Hydrochloride** see FLUoxetine on page 808

FluPHENAZine (floo FEN a zeen)

Related Information

Antipsychotic Agents on page 2103
Beers Criteria – Potentially Inappropriate Medications for Geriatrics on page 2183

Medication Safety Issues

Sound-alike/look-alike issues:

FluPHENAZine may be confused with fluvoxaMINE

BEERS Criteria medication:

This drug may be potentially inappropriate for use in geriatric patients (Quality of evidence - moderate; Strength of recommendation - strong).

International issues:

Prolixin [Turkey] may be confused with Prolixan brand name for azapropazone [Greece]

Brand Names: Canada Apo-Fluphenazine Decanoate®; Apo-Fluphenazine®; Modecate®; Modecate® Concentrate; PMS-Fluphenazine Decanoate

Index Terms Fluphenazine Decanoate; Fluphenazine Hydrochloride

Generic Availability (U.S.) Yes

Pharmacologic Category Antipsychotic Agent, Typical, Phenothiazine

Use Management of manifestations of psychotic disorders and schizophrenia; depot formulation may offer improved outcome in individuals with psychosis who are nonadherent with oral antipsychotics

Unlabeled Use Psychosis/agitation related to Alzheimer's dementia

Contraindications Hypersensitivity to fluphenazine or any component of the formulation (cross-reactivity between phenothiazines may occur); severe CNS depression; coma; subcortical brain damage; in patients receiving large doses of hypnotics; blood dyscrasias; hepatic disease

Warnings/Precautions [U.S. Boxed Warning]: Elderly patients with dementia-related psychosis treated with antipsychotics are at an increased risk of death compared to placebo. Most deaths appeared to be either cardiovascular (eg, heart failure, sudden death) or infectious (eg, pneumonia) in nature. Fluphenazine is not approved for the treatment of dementia-related psychosis. May be sedating; use with caution in disorders where CNS depression is a feature. Use with caution in Parkinson's disease. Caution in patients with hemodynamic instability; predisposition to seizures; or severe cardiac disease. Use caution in renal impairment; discontinue therapy if BUN abnormal. Use caution in hepatic impairment; use contraindicated in patients with liver damage. Esophageal dysmotility and aspiration have been associated with antipsychotic use; use with caution in patients at risk of pneumonia (ie, Alzheimer's disease). May alter temperature regulation or mask toxicity of other drugs due to antiemetic effects. May alter cardiac conduction; life-threatening arrhythmias have occurred with therapeutic doses of phenothiazines. Hypotension may occur, particularly with I.M. administration. May cause orthostatic hypotension; use with caution in patients at risk of this effect or those who would not tolerate transient hypotensive episodes (cerebrovascular disease, cardiovascular disease, or other medications which may predispose). Adverse effects of depot injections may be prolonged. Use associated with increased prolactin levels; clinical significance of hyperprolactinemia in patients with breast cancer or other prolactin-dependent tumors is unknown. May cause pigmentary retinopathy, and lenticular and corneal deposits, particularly with prolonged therapy.

Leukopenia, neutropenia, and agranulocytosis (sometimes fatal) have been reported in clinical trials and postmarketing reports with antipsychotic use; presence of risk factors (eg, pre-existing low WBC or history of drug-induced leuko-/neutropenia) should prompt periodic blood count assessment. Discontinue therapy at first signs of blood dyscrasias or if absolute neutrophil count <1000/mm^3.

Due to anticholinergic effects, use caution in patients with decreased gastrointestinal motility, urinary retention, BPH, xerostomia, visual problems, narrow-angle glaucoma, and myasthenia gravis. Relative to other antipsychotics, fluphenazine has a low potency of cholinergic blockade.

May cause extrapyramidal symptoms, including pseudoparkinsonism, acute dystonic reactions, akathisia, and tardive dyskinesia (risk of these reactions is high relative to other antipsychotics). Risk of dystonia (and possibly other EPS) may be greater with increased doses, use of conventional antipsychotics, males, and younger patients. May also be associated with neuroleptic malignant syndrome (NMS).

Use in elderly patients with dementia is associated with an increased risk of mortality and cerebrovascular accidents; avoid antipsychotic use for behavioral problems associated with dementia unless alternative nonpharmacologic therapies have failed and patient may harm self or others. In addition, use may cause or exacerbate syndrome of inappropriate antidiuretic hormone secretion or hyponatremia; monitor sodium closely with initiation or dosage adjustments in older adults May also be inappropriate in older adults depending on comorbidities (eg, dementia, delirium) due to its potent anticholinergic effects (Beers Criteria). Increased risk for developing tardive dyskinesia, particularly elderly women.

Adverse Reactions (Reflective of adult population; not specific for elderly) Frequency not defined.

Cardiovascular: Hyper-/hypotension, tachycardia, fluctuations in blood pressure, arrhythmia, edema

Central nervous system: Parkinsonian symptoms, akathisia, dystonias, tardive dyskinesia, dizziness, hyper-reflexia, headache, cerebral edema, drowsiness, lethargy, restlessness, excitement, bizarre dreams, EEG changes, depression, seizure, NMS, altered central temperature regulation

Dermatologic: Dermatitis, eczema, erythema, itching, photosensitivity, rash, seborrhea, skin pigmentation, urticaria

Endocrine & metabolic: Menstrual cycle changes, breast pain, amenorrhea, galactorrhea, gynecomastia, libido changes, prolactin increased, SIADH

Gastrointestinal: Weight gain, appetite loss, salivation, xerostomia, constipation, paralytic ileus, laryngeal edema

Genitourinary: Ejaculatory disturbances, impotence, polyuria, bladder paralysis, enuresis

Hematologic: Agranulocytosis, leukopenia, thrombocytopenia, nonthrombocytopenic purpura, eosinophilia, pancytopenia

Hepatic: Cholestatic jaundice, hepatotoxicity

Neuromuscular & skeletal: Trembling of fingers, SLE, facial hemispasm

Ocular: Pigmentary retinopathy, cornea and lens changes, blurred vision, glaucoma

Respiratory: Nasal congestion, asthma

Drug Interactions

Metabolism/Transport Effects Substrate of CYP2D6 (major); **Note:** Assignment of Major/Minor substrate status based on clinically relevant drug interaction potential; **Inhibits** CYP1A2 (weak), CYP2C9 (weak), CYP2D6 (weak), CYP2E1 (weak)

Avoid Concomitant Use

Avoid concomitant use of FluPHENAZine with any of the following: Azelastine; Azelastine (Nasal); Metoclopramide; Paraldehyde

Increased Effect/Toxicity

FluPHENAZine may increase the levels/effects of: Alcohol (Ethyl); Analgesics (Opioid); Anticholinergics; Antidepressants (Serotonin Reuptake Inhibitor/Antagonist); ARIPiprazole; Azelastine; Azelastine (Nasal); Beta-Blockers; CNS Depressants; Methotrimeprazine; Methylphenidate; Paraldehyde; Porfimer; Serotonin Modulators; Zolpidem

The levels/effects of FluPHENAZine may be increased by: Abiraterone Acetate; Acetylcholinesterase Inhibitors (Central); Antidepressants (Serotonin Reuptake Inhibitor/Antagonist); Antimalarial Agents; Beta-Blockers; CYP2D6 Inhibitors (Moderate); CYP2D6 Inhibitors (Strong); Darunavir; Droperidol; HydrOXYzine; Lithium formulations; Methotrimeprazine; Methylphenidate; Metoclopramide; Metyrosine; Pramlintide; Tetrabenazine

Decreased Effect

FluPHENAZine may decrease the levels/effects of: Amphetamines; Anti-Parkinson's Agents (Dopamine Agonist); Quinagolide

The levels/effects of FluPHENAZine may be decreased by: Antacids; Anti-Parkinson's Agents (Dopamine Agonist); Lithium formulations; Peginterferon Alfa-2b

Ethanol/Nutrition/Herb Interactions

Ethanol: May increase CNS depression; monitor for increased effects with coadministration. Caution patients about effects.

Herb/Nutraceutical: Avoid dong quai, St John's wort (may also cause photosensitization). Avoid kava kava, gotu kola, valerian, St John's wort (may increase CNS depression).

Stability Store at room temperature; avoid freezing and excessive heat. Protect all dosage forms from light. Clear or slightly yellow solutions may be used. Should be dispensed in amber or opaque vials/bottles. Solutions may be diluted or mixed with fruit juices or other liquids, but must be administered immediately after mixing. Do not prepare bulk dilutions or store bulk dilutions.

Mechanism of Action Fluphenazine is a piperazine phenothiazine antipsychotic which blocks postsynaptic mesolimbic dopaminergic D_1 and D_2 receptors in the brain; depresses the release of hypothalamic and hypophyseal hormones; believed to depress the reticular activating system, thus affecting basal metabolism, body temperature, wakefulness, vasomotor tone, and emesis

Pharmacodynamics/Kinetics
Onset of action: Decanoate: 24-72 hours;
Peak effect: Neuroleptic: Decanoate: 48-96 hours
Duration: Hydrochloride salt: 6-8 hours; Decanoate: ~4 weeks
Absorption: Oral: Erratic and variable
Half-life elimination (derivative dependent): Hydrochloride: ~14-16.4 hours; Decanoate: ~14 days
Time to peak, serum: Hydrochloride: Oral: 2 hours; Decanoate: 8-10 hours

Dosage
Geriatric Oral: Initial: 1-2.5 mg daily; titrated gradually based on patient response.
Adult
Psychosis:
Oral: Initial: 2.5-10 mg/day in divided doses at 6- to 8-hour intervals; Maintenance: 1-5 mg/day; **Note:** Some patients may require up to 40 mg/day for symptom control (long-term safety of higher doses not established)
PORT guidelines: Acute therapy: 6-20 mg/day for up to 6 weeks; Maintenance: 6-12 mg/day (Buchanan, 2009)
I.M. (hydrochloride): Initial: 1.25 mg as a single dose; depending on severity and duration, may need 2.5-10 mg/day in divided doses at 6- to 8-hour intervals (4 mg I.M. fluphenazine HCl is approximately equivalent to 10 mg oral fluphenazine HCl); use caution with doses >10 mg/day; once symptoms stabilized, transition to oral maintenance therapy
Long-acting maintenance injections (decanoate):
I.M., SubQ (decanoate): Initial: 12.5-25 mg every 2-4 weeks; response may last up to 6 weeks in some patients; titrate dose cautiously, if doses >50 mg are needed, increase in 12.5 mg increments (maximum dose: 100 mg)
Conversion from hydrochloride dosage forms to decanoate I.M.: 12.5 mg of decanoate every 2-4 weeks is approximately equivalent to 10 mg of oral hydrochloride/day; **Note:** Clinically, an every-2-week interval is frequently utilized
PORT guidelines: 6.25-25 mg every 2 weeks (Buchanan, 2009)
Renal Impairment Use with caution; not dialyzable (0% to 5%).
Hepatic Impairment Use with caution.

Administration
I.M., SubQ: The hydrochloride or decanoate formulation may be administered intramuscularly. Watch for hypotension when administering I.M. Only the decanoate formulation may be administered subcutaneously. When administering fluphenazine decanoate, use a dry syringe and needle of ≥21 gauge to administer the fluphenazine decanoate; a wet needle/syringe may cause the solution to become cloudy.
Oral: Avoid contact of oral solution or injection with skin (contact dermatitis). Oral liquid should be diluted into at least 60 mL (2 fl oz) of the following **only**: Water, saline, homogenized milk, carbonated orange beverages, pineapple, apricot, prune, orange, tomato, and grapefruit juices. Do **not** dilute in beverages containing caffeine, tannics (eg, tea), or pectinate (eg, apple juice).

Monitoring Parameters Vital signs; lipid profile, fasting blood glucose/Hgb A_{1c}; BMI; mental status, abnormal involuntary movement scale (AIMS), extrapyramidal symptoms (EPS)

Reference Range Therapeutic: 0.3-3 ng/mL (SI: 0.6-6.0 nmol/L); correlation of serum concentrations and efficacy is controversial; most often dosed to best response

Pharmacotherapy Pearls Less sedative and hypotensive effects than chlorpromazine.

Special Geriatric Considerations Any changes in disease status in any organ system can result in behavior changes.

Many elderly patients receive antipsychotic medications for inappropriate nonpsychotic behavior. Before initiating antipsychotic medication, the clinician should investigate any possible reversible cause; any stress or stress from any disease can cause acute "confusion" or worsening of baseline nonpsychotic behavior. Most commonly, acute changes in behavior are due to increases in drug dose or addition of a new drug to regimen, fluid electrolyte loss, infections, and changes in environment.

In the treatment of agitated, demented, and elderly patients, authors of meta-analysis of controlled trials of the response to the traditional antipsychotics (phenothiazines, butyrophenones) in controlling agitation have concluded that the use of neuroleptics results in a response rate of 18%. Clearly, neuroleptic therapy for behavior control should be limited with frequent attempts to withdraw the agent given for behavior control.

This medication is considered to be potentially inappropriate in this patient population (Beers Criteria: Quality of evidence - moderate; Strength of recommendation - strong).

Dosage Forms Excipient information presented when available (limited, particularly for generics); consult specific product labeling.
Elixir, oral, as hydrochloride: 2.5 mg/5 mL (60 mL, 473 mL)
Injection, oil, as decanoate: 25 mg/mL (5 mL)
Injection, solution, as hydrochloride: 2.5 mg/mL (10 mL)
Solution, oral, as hydrochloride [concentrate]: 5 mg/mL (118 mL)
Tablet, oral, as hydrochloride: 1 mg, 2.5 mg, 5 mg, 10 mg

◆ **Fluphenazine Decanoate** see FluPHENAZine on page 813
◆ **Fluphenazine Hydrochloride** see FluPHENAZine on page 813
◆ **Flura-Drops®** see Fluoride on page 806

Flurazepam (flure AZ e pam)

Related Information
Anxiolytic, Sedative/Hypnotic, and Miscellaneous Benzodiazepines on page 2106
Beers Criteria – Potentially Inappropriate Medications for Geriatrics on page 2183
Medication Safety Issues
Sound-alike/look-alike issues:
Flurazepam may be confused with temazepam
Dalmane® may be confused with Demulen®
BEERS Criteria medication:
This drug may be potentially inappropriate for use in geriatric patients (Quality of evidence - high; Strength of recommendation - strong).
Brand Names: Canada Apo-Flurazepam®; Dalmane®; Som Pam
Index Terms Flurazepam Hydrochloride
Generic Availability (U.S.) Yes
Pharmacologic Category Hypnotic, Benzodiazepine
Use Short-term treatment of insomnia
Medication Guide Available Yes
Contraindications Hypersensitivity to flurazepam or any component of the formulation (cross-sensitivity with other benzodiazepines may exist); narrow-angle glaucoma
Warnings/Precautions Use with caution in elderly or debilitated patients, patients with hepatic disease (including alcoholics), or renal impairment. Use with caution in patients with respiratory disease or impaired gag reflex. Avoid use in patients with sleep apnea.

Causes CNS depression (dose related); patients must be cautioned about performing tasks which require mental alertness (eg, operating machinery or driving). Use with caution in patients receiving other CNS depressants or psychoactive agents. Benzodiazepines have been associated with falls and traumatic injury and should be used with extreme caution in patients who are at risk of these events. In older adults, benzodiazepines increase the risk of impaired cognition, delirium, falls, fractures, and motor vehicle accidents. Due to increased sensitivity in this age group and slower metabolism of long-acting agents (such as flurazepam), avoid use for treatment of insomnia, agitation, or delirium (Beers Criteria).

Use caution in patients with depression, particularly if suicidal risk may be present. Use with caution in patients with a history of drug dependence. Benzodiazepines have been associated with dependence and acute withdrawal symptoms on discontinuation or reduction in dose (may occur after as little as 10 days of use).

As a hypnotic, should be used only after evaluation of potential causes of sleep disturbance. Failure of sleep disturbance to resolve after 7-10 days may indicate psychiatric or medical illness. A worsening of insomnia or the emergence of new abnormalities of thought or behavior may represent unrecognized psychiatric or medical illness and requires immediate and careful evaluation. Postmarketing studies have indicated that the use of hypnotic/sedative agents for sleep has been associated with hypersensitivity reactions including anaphylaxis as well as angioedema. An increased risk for hazardous sleep-related activities such as sleep-driving; cooking and eating food, and making phone calls while asleep have also been noted.

Benzodiazepines have been associated with anterograde amnesia. Paradoxical reactions have been reported, particularly in psychiatric patients. Does not have analgesic, antidepressant, or antipsychotic properties.

Adverse Reactions (Reflective of adult population; not specific for elderly) Frequency not defined.

Cardiovascular: Chest pain, flushing, hypotension, palpitation

Central nervous system: Apprehension, ataxia, confusion, depression, dizziness, drowsiness, euphoria, faintness, falling, hallucinations, hangover effect, headache, irritability, lightheadedness, memory impairment, nervousness, paradoxical reactions, restlessness, slurred speech, staggering, talkativeness

Dermatologic: Pruritus, rash

Gastrointestinal: Appetite increased/decreased, bitter taste, constipation, diarrhea, GI pain, heartburn, nausea, salivation increased/excessive, upset stomach, vomiting, weight gain/loss, xerostomia

Hematologic: Granulocytopenia, leukopenia

Hepatic: Alkaline phosphatase increased, ALT increased, AST increased, cholestatic jaundice, total bilirubin increased

Neuromuscular & skeletal: Body/joint pain, dysarthria, reflex slowing, weakness

Ocular: Blurred vision, burning eyes, difficulty focusing

Respiratory: Apnea, dyspnea

Miscellaneous: Diaphoresis, drug dependence

Postmarketing and/or case reports: Anaphylaxis, angioedema, complex sleep-related behavior (sleep-driving, cooking or eating food, making phone calls)

Drug Interactions

Metabolism/Transport Effects Substrate of CYP3A4 (major); **Note:** Assignment of Major/Minor substrate status based on clinically relevant drug interaction potential; **Inhibits** CYP2E1 (weak)

Avoid Concomitant Use

Avoid concomitant use of Flurazepam with any of the following: Azelastine; Azelastine (Nasal); Conivaptan; Methadone; Mirtazapine; OLANZapine; Paraldehyde

Increased Effect/Toxicity

Flurazepam may increase the levels/effects of: Alcohol (Ethyl); Azelastine; Azelastine (Nasal); Buprenorphine; CloZAPine; CNS Depressants; Fosphenytoin; Methadone; Methotrimeprazine; Metyrosine; Mirtazapine; Paraldehyde; Phenytoin; Selective Serotonin Reuptake Inhibitors; Zolpidem

The levels/effects of Flurazepam may be increased by: Antifungal Agents (Azole Derivatives, Systemic); Aprepitant; Calcium Channel Blockers (Nondihydropyridine); Cimetidine; Conivaptan; Contraceptives (Estrogens); Contraceptives (Progestins); CYP3A4 Inhibitors (Moderate); CYP3A4 Inhibitors (Strong); Dasatinib; Droperidol; Fosamprenavir; Fosaprepitant; Grapefruit Juice; HydrOXYzine; Isoniazid; Ivacaftor; Macrolide Antibiotics; Methotrimeprazine; Mifepristone; OLANZapine; Proton Pump Inhibitors; Ritonavir; Saquinavir; Selective Serotonin Reuptake Inhibitors

Decreased Effect

The levels/effects of Flurazepam may be decreased by: CarBAMazepine; CYP3A4 Inducers (Strong); Deferasirox; Rifamycin Derivatives; St Johns Wort; Theophylline Derivatives; Tocilizumab; Yohimbine

Ethanol/Nutrition/Herb Interactions

Ethanol: May increase CNS depression; monitor for increased effects with coadministration. Caution patients about effects.

Food: Serum levels and response to flurazepam may be increased by grapefruit juice, but unlikely because of flurazepam's high oral bioavailability.

Herb/Nutraceutical: Avoid valerian, St John's wort, kava kava, gotu kola (may increase CNS depression).

Stability Store at 15°C to 30°C (59°F to 86°F).

Mechanism of Action Binds to stereospecific benzodiazepine receptors on the postsynaptic GABA neuron at several sites within the central nervous system, including the limbic system, reticular formation. Enhancement of the inhibitory effect of GABA on neuronal excitability results by increased neuronal membrane permeability to chloride ions. This shift in chloride ions results in hyperpolarization (a less excitable state) and stabilization.

Pharmacodynamics/Kinetics

Onset of action: Hypnotic: 15-20 minutes

Peak effect: 3-6 hours

Duration: 7-8 hours

Distribution: V_d: 3.4 L/kg

Protein binding: ~97%

Metabolism: Hepatic to N-desalkylflurazepam (active) and N-hydroxyethylflurazepam

Half-life elimination:
Flurazepam: 2.3 hours
N-desalkylflurazepam:
Adults: Single dose: 74-90 hours; Multiple doses: 111-113 hours
Elderly (61-85 years): Single dose: 120-160 hours; Multiple doses: 126-158 hours
Time to peak, serum:
N-desalkylflurazepam: 10.6 hours (range: 7.6-13.6 hours)
N-hydroxyethylflurazepam: ~1 hour
Excretion: Urine: N-hydroxyethylflurazepam (22% to 55%); N-desalkylflurazepam (<1%)

Dosage
Geriatric Oral: 15 mg at bedtime. Avoid use if possible.
Adult Insomnia (short-term treatment): Oral: 15-30 mg at bedtime
Monitoring Parameters Respiratory and cardiovascular status
Reference Range Therapeutic: 0-4 ng/mL (SI: 0-9 nmol/L); Metabolite N-desalkylflurazepam: 20-110 ng/mL (SI: 43-240 nmol/L); Toxic: >0.12 mcg/mL
Special Geriatric Considerations Due to its long-acting metabolite, flurazepam is not considered a drug of choice in the elderly. Long-acting benzodiazepines have been associated with falls in the elderly. Guidelines from the Centers for Medicare and Medicaid Services (CMS) discourage the use of this agent in residents of long-term care facilities.

This medication is considered to be potentially inappropriate in this patient population (Beers Criteria: Quality of evidence - high; Strength of recommendation - strong).
Controlled Substance C-IV
Dosage Forms Excipient information presented when available (limited, particularly for generics); consult specific product labeling.
Capsule, oral, as hydrochloride: 15 mg, 30 mg

◆ **Flurazepam Hydrochloride** see Flurazepam on page 816

Flurbiprofen (Systemic) (flure BI proe fen)

Medication Safety Issues
Sound-alike/look-alike issues:
Flurbiprofen may be confused with fenoprofen
Ansaid® may be confused with Asacol®, Axid®
Brand Names: Canada Alti-Flurbiprofen; Ansaid®; Apo-Flurbiprofen®; Froben-SR®; Froben®; Novo-Flurprofen; Nu-Flurprofen
Index Terms Flurbiprofen Sodium
Generic Availability (U.S.) Yes
Pharmacologic Category Nonsteroidal Anti-inflammatory Drug (NSAID), Oral
Use Treatment of rheumatoid arthritis and osteoarthritis
Unlabeled Use Management of postoperative pain
Medication Guide Available Yes
Contraindications Hypersensitivity to flurbiprofen, aspirin, other NSAIDs, or any component of the formulation; perioperative pain in the setting of coronary artery bypass (CABG) surgery
Warnings/Precautions [U.S. Boxed Warning]: NSAIDs are associated with an increased risk of adverse cardiovascular thrombotic events, including MI and stroke. Risk may be increased with duration of use or pre-existing cardiovascular risk factors or disease. Carefully evaluate individual cardiovascular risk profiles prior to prescribing. May cause new-onset hypertension or worsening of existing hypertension. Use caution with fluid retention. Avoid use in heart failure. Concurrent administration of ibuprofen, and potentially other nonselective NSAIDs, may interfere with aspirin's cardioprotective effect. **[U.S. Boxed Warning]: Use is contraindicated for treatment of perioperative pain in the setting of coronary artery bypass graft (CABG) surgery.** Risk of MI and stroke may be increased with use following CABG surgery.

Platelet adhesion and aggregation may be decreased; may prolong bleeding time; patients with coagulation disorders or who are receiving anticoagulants should be monitored closely. Anemia may occur; patients on long-term NSAID therapy should be monitored for anemia. NSAID use may compromise existing renal function; dose-dependent decreases in prostaglandin synthesis may result from NSAID use, reducing renal blood flow which may cause renal decompensation. Patients with impaired renal function, dehydration, heart failure, liver dysfunction, those taking diuretics, and ACE inhibitors, and the elderly are at greater risk of renal toxicity. Rehydrate patient before starting therapy; monitor renal function closely. Not recommended for use in patients with advanced renal disease. Long-term NSAID use may result in renal papillary necrosis.

[U.S. Boxed Warning]: NSAIDs may increase risk of gastrointestinal irritation, inflammation, ulceration, bleeding, and perforation. These events may occur at any time during therapy and without warning. Use caution with a history of GI disease (bleeding or ulcers), concurrent therapy with aspirin, anticoagulants and/or corticosteroids, smoking, use of alcohol, the elderly, or debilitated patients. When used concomitantly with ≤325 mg of aspirin, a substantial increase in the risk of gastrointestinal complications (eg, ulcer) occurs; concomitant gastroprotective therapy (eg, proton pump inhibitors) is recommended (Bhatt, 2008).

Use the lowest effective dose for the shortest duration of time, consistent with individual patient goals, to reduce risk of cardiovascular or GI adverse events. Alternate therapies should be considered for patients at high risk.

NSAIDs may cause serious skin adverse events including exfoliative dermatitis, Stevens-Johnson syndrome (SJS), and toxic epidermal necrolysis (TEN); discontinue use at first sign of skin rash or hypersensitivity. Anaphylactoid reactions may occur, even without prior exposure; patients with "aspirin triad" (bronchial asthma, aspirin intolerance, rhinitis) may be at increased risk. Do not use in patients who experience bronchospasm, asthma, rhinitis, or urticaria with NSAID or aspirin therapy. Use caution in other forms of asthma.

Use with caution in patients with decreased hepatic function. Closely monitor patients with any abnormal LFT. Severe hepatic reactions (eg, fulminant hepatitis, liver failure) have occurred with NSAID use, rarely; discontinue if signs or symptoms of liver disease develop, or if systemic manifestations occur.

The elderly are at increased risk for adverse effects (especially peptic ulceration, CNS effects, renal toxicity) from NSAIDs even at low doses.

Withhold for at least 4-6 half-lives prior to surgical or dental procedures.

Adverse Reactions (Reflective of adult population; not specific for elderly) >1%:
Cardiovascular: Edema
Central nervous system: Amnesia, anxiety, depression, dizziness, headache, insomnia, malaise, nervousness, somnolence, vertigo
Dermatologic: Rash
Gastrointestinal: Abdominal pain, constipation, diarrhea, dyspepsia, flatulence, GI bleeding, nausea, vomiting, weight changes
Hepatic: Liver enzymes increased
Neuromuscular & skeletal: Reflexes increased, tremor, weakness
Ocular: Vision changes
Otic: Tinnitus
Respiratory: Rhinitis

Drug Interactions

Metabolism/Transport Effects Substrate of CYP2C9 (minor); **Note:** Assignment of Major/Minor substrate status based on clinically relevant drug interaction potential; **Inhibits** CYP2C9 (weak)

Avoid Concomitant Use
Avoid concomitant use of Flurbiprofen (Systemic) with any of the following: Floctafenine; Ketorolac; Ketorolac (Nasal); Ketorolac (Systemic)

Increased Effect/Toxicity
Flurbiprofen (Systemic) may increase the levels/effects of: Aliskiren; Aminoglycosides; Anticoagulants; Antiplatelet Agents; Bisphosphonate Derivatives; Collagenase (Systemic); CycloSPORINE; CycloSPORINE (Systemic); Dabigatran Etexilate; Deferasirox; Desmopressin; Digoxin; Drotrecogin Alfa (Activated); Eplerenone; Haloperidol; Ibritumomab; Lithium; Methotrexate; Nonsteroidal Anti-Inflammatory Agents; PEMEtrexed; Porfimer; Potassium-Sparing Diuretics; PRALAtrexate; Quinolone Antibiotics; Rivaroxaban; Salicylates; Thrombolytic Agents; Tositumomab and Iodine I 131 Tositumomab; Vancomycin; Vitamin K Antagonists

The levels/effects of Flurbiprofen (Systemic) may be increased by: ACE Inhibitors; Angiotensin II Receptor Blockers; Antidepressants (Tricyclic, Tertiary Amine); Corticosteroids (Systemic); CycloSPORINE; CycloSPORINE (Systemic); Glucosamine; Herbs (Anticoagulant/Antiplatelet Properties); Ketorolac; Ketorolac (Nasal); Ketorolac (Systemic); Nonsteroidal Anti-Inflammatory Agents; Omega-3-Acid Ethyl Esters; Pentosan Polysulfate Sodium; Pentoxifylline; Probenecid; Prostacyclin Analogues; Selective Serotonin Reuptake Inhibitors; Serotonin/Norepinephrine Reuptake Inhibitors; Sodium Phosphates; Tipranavir; Treprostinil; Vitamin E

Decreased Effect
Flurbiprofen (Systemic) may decrease the levels/effects of: ACE Inhibitors; Aliskiren; Angiotensin II Receptor Blockers; Antiplatelet Agents; Beta-Blockers; Eplerenone; HydrALAZINE; Loop Diuretics; Potassium-Sparing Diuretics; Salicylates; Selective Serotonin Reuptake Inhibitors; Thiazide Diuretics

The levels/effects of Flurbiprofen (Systemic) may be decreased by: Bile Acid Sequestrants; Nonsteroidal Anti-Inflammatory Agents; Salicylates

Ethanol/Nutrition/Herb Interactions

Ethanol: Avoid ethanol (may enhance gastric mucosal irritation).

Food: Food may decrease the rate but not the extent of absorption.

Herb/Nutraceutical: Avoid alfalfa, anise, bilberry, bladderwrack, bromelain, cat's claw, celery, chamomile, coleus, cordyceps, dong quai, evening primrose, fenugreek, feverfew, garlic, ginger, ginkgo biloba, ginseng (American, Panax, Siberian), grapeseed, green tea, guggul, horse chestnut seed, horseradish, licorice, prickly ash, red clover, reishi, SAMe (S-adenosylmethionine), sweet clover, turmeric, white willow (all have additional antiplatelet activity).

Mechanism of Action Reversibly inhibits cyclooxygenase-1 and 2 (COX-1 and 2) enzymes, which results in decreased formation of prostaglandin precursors; has antipyretic, analgesic, and anti-inflammatory properties

Other proposed mechanisms not fully elucidated (and possibly contributing to the anti-inflammatory effect to varying degrees), include inhibiting chemotaxis, altering lymphocyte activity, inhibiting neutrophil aggregation/activation, and decreasing proinflammatory cytokine levels.

Pharmacodynamics/Kinetics

Onset of action: ~1-2 hours

Distribution: V_d: 0.12 L/kg

Protein binding: 99%, primarily albumin

Metabolism: Hepatic via CYP2C9; forms metabolites such as 4-hydroxy-flurbiprofen (inactive)

Half-life elimination: 5.7 hours

Time to peak: 1.5 hours

Excretion: Urine (primarily as metabolites)

Dosage

Geriatric & Adult

Rheumatoid arthritis and osteoarthritis: Oral: 200-300 mg/day in 2, 3, or 4 divided doses; do not administer more than 100 mg for any single dose; maximum: 300 mg/day

Management of postoperative dental pain (unlabeled use): Oral: 100 mg every 12 hours

Renal Impairment Not recommended in patients with advanced renal disease.

Administration Administer with a full glass of water.

Monitoring Parameters Monitor response (pain, range of motion, grip strength, mobility, ADL function), inflammation; observe for weight gain, edema; monitor renal function; observe for bleeding, bruising; evaluate gastrointestinal effects (abdominal pain, bleeding, dyspepsia); mental confusion, disorientation, CBC, serum creatinine, BUN, liver function tests

Pharmacotherapy Pearls There are no clinical guidelines to predict which NSAID will give response in a particular patient. Trials with each must be initiated until response is determined. Consider dose, patient convenience, and cost.

Special Geriatric Considerations Elderly are a high-risk population for adverse effects from NSAIDs. As much as 60% of the elderly can develop peptic ulceration and/or hemorrhage asymptomatically. The concomitant use of H_2 blockers, omeprazole, and sucralfate is not effective as prophylaxis with the exception of NSAID-induced duodenal ulcers which may be prevented by the use of ranitidine. Misoprostol and proton pump inhibitors are the only agents proven to help prevent the development of NSAID-induced ulcers. Also, concomitant disease and drug use contribute to the risk for GI adverse effects. Use lowest effective dose for shortest period possible. Consider renal function decline with age. Use of NSAIDs can compromise existing renal function, especially when Cl_{cr} is ≤30 mL/minute. Tinnitus may be a difficult and unreliable indication of toxicity due to age-related hearing loss or eighth cranial nerve damage. CNS adverse effects, such as confusion, agitation, and hallucinations, are generally seen in overdose or high-dose situations, but elderly may demonstrate these adverse effects at lower doses than younger adults.

Dosage Forms Excipient information presented when available (limited, particularly for generics); consult specific product labeling.

Tablet, oral: 50 mg, 100 mg

Flurbiprofen (Ophthalmic) (flure BI proe fen)

Medication Safety Issues

Sound-alike/look-alike issues:

Flurbiprofen may be confused with fenoprofen

Ocufen® may be confused with Ocuflox®

International issues:

Ocufen [U.S., Canada, and multiple international markets] may be confused with Ocupres brand name for timolol [India]; Ocupress brand name for dorzolamide [Brazil]

Brand Names: U.S. Ocufen®
Brand Names: Canada Ocufen®
Index Terms Flurbiprofen Sodium
Generic Availability (U.S.) Yes
Pharmacologic Category Nonsteroidal Anti-inflammatory Drug (NSAID), Ophthalmic
Use Inhibition of intraoperative miosis
Dosage
  Geriatric & Adult Ophthalmic anti-inflammatory/surgical aid: Ophthalmic: Instill 1 drop every 30 minutes, beginning 2 hours prior to surgery (total of 4 drops in each affected eye)
  Special Geriatric Considerations Evaluate the patient's or caregiver's ability to safely administer the correct dose of ophthalmic medication.
Dosage Forms Excipient information presented when available (limited, particularly for generics); consult specific product labeling.
  Solution, ophthalmic, as sodium [drops]: 0.03% (2.5 mL)
    Ocufen®: 0.03% (2.5 mL)

♦ **Flurbiprofen Sodium** see Flurbiprofen (Ophthalmic) on page 820
♦ **Flurbiprofen Sodium** see Flurbiprofen (Systemic) on page 818
♦ **5-Flurocytosine** see Flucytosine on page 799

Flutamide (FLOO ta mide)

Medication Safety Issues
  Sound-alike/look-alike issues:
    Flutamide may be confused with Flumadine®, thalidomide
    Eulexin® may be confused with Edecrin®, Eurax®
Brand Names: Canada Apo-Flutamide®; Euflex®; Eulexin®; Novo-Flutamide; PMS-Flutamide; Teva-Flutamide
Index Terms 4'-Nitro-3'-Trifluoromethylisobutyrantide; Eulexin; Niftolid; NSC-147834; SCH 13521
Generic Availability (U.S.) Yes
Pharmacologic Category Antineoplastic Agent, Antiandrogen
Use Treatment of metastatic prostatic carcinoma in combination therapy with LHRH agonist analogues
Unlabeled Use Treatment of female hirsutism
Contraindications Hypersensitivity to flutamide or any component of the formulation; severe hepatic impairment
Warnings/Precautions Hazardous agent - use appropriate precautions for handling and disposal. **[U.S. Boxed Warning]: Hospitalization and, rarely, death due to liver failure have been reported in patients taking flutamide.** Elevated serum transaminase levels, jaundice, hepatic encephalopathy, and acute hepatic failure have been reported. Androgen-deprivation therapy may increase the risk for cardiovascular disease (Levine, 2010). Product labeling states flutamide is not for use in women, particularly for non-life-threatening conditions. In some patients, the toxicity reverses after discontinuation of therapy. About 50% of the cases occur within the first 3 months of treatment. Serum transaminase levels should be measured prior to starting treatment, monthly for 4 months, and periodically thereafter. Liver function tests should be obtained at the first suggestion of liver dysfunction (nausea, vomiting, abdominal pain, fatigue, anorexia, "flu-like" symptoms, hyperbilirubinuria, jaundice, or right upper quadrant tenderness). Flutamide should be immediately discontinued any time a patient has jaundice, and/or an ALT level greater than twice the upper limit of normal. Flutamide should not be used in patients whose ALT values are greater than twice the upper limit of normal.

Patients with glucose-6 phosphate dehydrogenase deficiency or hemoglobin M disease or smokers are at risk of toxicities associated with aniline exposure, including methemoglobinemia, hemolytic anemia, and cholestatic jaundice. Monitor methemoglobin levels.
Adverse Reactions (Reflective of adult population; not specific for elderly)
  >10%:
    Endocrine & metabolic: Gynecomastia, hot flashes, breast tenderness, galactorrhea (9% to 42%), impotence, libido decreased, tumor flare
    Gastrointestinal: Nausea, vomiting (11% to 12%)
    Hepatic: AST increased (transient; mild), LDH increased (transient; mild)
  1% to 10%:
    Cardiovascular: Hypertension (1%), edema
    Central nervous system: Drowsiness, confusion, depression, anxiety, nervousness, headache, dizziness, insomnia
    Dermatologic: Ecchymosis, photosensitivity, pruritus

Gastrointestinal: Anorexia, appetite increased, constipation, indigestion, upset stomach (4% to 6%); diarrhea

Hematologic: Anemia (6%), leukopenia (3%), thrombocytopenia (1%)

Neuromuscular & skeletal: Weakness (1%)

Miscellaneous: Herpes zoster

Drug Interactions

Metabolism/Transport Effects Substrate of CYP1A2 (major), CYP3A4 (major); **Note:** Assignment of Major/Minor substrate status based on clinically relevant drug interaction potential; **Inhibits** CYP1A2 (weak)

Avoid Concomitant Use

Avoid concomitant use of Flutamide with any of the following: Conivaptan

Increased Effect/Toxicity

Flutamide may increase the levels/effects of: Prilocaine

The levels/effects of Flutamide may be increased by: Abiraterone Acetate; Conivaptan; CYP1A2 Inhibitors (Moderate); CYP1A2 Inhibitors (Strong); CYP3A4 Inhibitors (Moderate); CYP3A4 Inhibitors (Strong); Dasatinib; Deferasirox; Ivacaftor; Mifepristone

Decreased Effect

The levels/effects of Flutamide may be decreased by: CYP1A2 Inducers (Strong); CYP3A4 Inducers (Strong); Cyproterone; Deferasirox; Herbs (CYP3A4 Inducers); Tocilizumab

Ethanol/Nutrition/Herb Interactions

Food: No effect on bioavailability of flutamide.

Herb/Nutraceutical: St John's wort may decrease flutamide levels.

Stability Store at room temperature.

Mechanism of Action Nonsteroidal antiandrogen that inhibits androgen uptake or inhibits binding of androgen in target tissues

Pharmacodynamics/Kinetics

Absorption: Oral: Rapid and complete

Protein binding: Parent drug: 94% to 96%; 2-hydroxyflutamide: 92% to 94%

Metabolism: Extensively hepatic to more than 10 metabolites, primarily 2-hydroxyflutamide (active)

Half-life elimination: 5-6 hours (2-hydroxyflutamide)

Excretion: Primarily urine (as metabolites)

Dosage

Geriatric & Adult Refer to individual protocols.

Prostate carcinoma: Oral: 250 mg 3 times/day; alternatively, once-daily doses of 0.5-1.5 g have been used (unlabeled dosing)

Female hirsutism (unlabeled use): Oral: 250 mg daily (Moghetti, 2000)

Administration Usually administered orally in 3 divided doses; contents of capsule may be opened and mixed with applesauce, pudding, or other soft foods; mixing with a beverage is not recommended

Monitoring Parameters Serum transaminase levels should be measured prior to starting treatment and should be repeated monthly for the first 4 months of therapy, and periodically thereafter. LFTs should be checked at the first sign or symptom of liver dysfunction (eg, nausea, vomiting, abdominal pain, fatigue, anorexia, flu-like symptoms, hyperbilirubinuria, jaundice, or right upper quadrant tenderness). Other parameters include tumor reduction, testosterone/estrogen, and phosphatase serum levels.

Special Geriatric Considerations No specific dose alterations are necessary in the elderly.

Dosage Forms Excipient information presented when available (limited, particularly for generics); consult specific product labeling.

Capsule, oral: 125 mg

Fluticasone (Oral Inhalation) (floo TIK a sone)

Related Information

Asthma on page 2125

Inhalant Agents on page 2117

Medication Safety Issues

Sound-alike/look-alike issues:

Flovent® may be confused with Flonase®

International issues:

Allegro: Brand name for fluticasone [Israel], but also the brand name for frovatriptan [Germany]

Allegro [Israel] may be confused with Allegra and Allegra-D brand names for fexofenadine and fexofenadine/pseudoephedrine, respectively [U.S., Canada, and multiple international markets]

Flovent [U.S., Canada] may be confused with Flogen brand name for naproxen [Mexico]; Flogene brand name for piroxicam [Brazil]

Brand Names: U.S. Flovent® Diskus®; Flovent® HFA

Brand Names: Canada Flovent® Diskus®; Flovent® HFA

Index Terms Flovent; Fluticasone Propionate

Generic Availability (U.S.) No

Pharmacologic Category Corticosteroid, Inhalant (Oral)

Use Maintenance treatment of asthma as prophylactic therapy; also indicated for patients requiring oral corticosteroid therapy for asthma to assist in total discontinuation or reduction of total oral dose

Contraindications Hypersensitivity to fluticasone or any component of the formulation; severe hypersensitivity to milk proteins or lactose (Flovent® Diskus®); primary treatment of status asthmaticus or other acute episodes of asthma requiring intensive measures

Canadian labeling: Additional contraindications (not in U.S. labeling): Moderate-to-severe bronchiectasis; untreated fungal, bacterial or tubercular infections of the respiratory tract

Warnings/Precautions May cause hypercorticism or suppression of hypothalamic-pituitary-adrenal (HPA) axis, particularly in patients receiving high doses for prolonged periods. HPA axis suppression may lead to adrenal crisis. Withdrawal and discontinuation of a corticosteroid should be done slowly and carefully. Particular care is required when patients are transferred from systemic corticosteroids to inhaled products due to possible adrenal insufficiency or withdrawal from steroids, including an increase in allergic symptoms. Patients receiving ≥20 mg per day of prednisone (or equivalent) may be most susceptible. Concurrent use of ritonavir (and potentially other strong inhibitors of CYP3A4) may increase fluticasone levels and effects on HPA suppression. Fatalities have occurred due to adrenal insufficiency in asthmatic patients during and after transfer from systemic corticosteroids to aerosol steroids; aerosol steroids do **not** provide the systemic steroid needed to treat patients having trauma, surgery, or infections.

Bronchospasm may occur with wheezing after inhalation; if this occurs, stop steroid and treat with a fast-acting bronchodilator. Supplemental steroids (oral or parenteral) may be needed during stress or severe asthma attacks. Corticosteroid use may cause psychiatric disturbances, including depression, euphoria, insomnia, mood swings, and personality changes. Pre-existing psychiatric conditions may be exacerbated by corticosteroid use. Prolonged use of corticosteroids may also increase the incidence of secondary infection, mask acute infection (including fungal infections), prolong or exacerbate viral infections, or limit response to vaccines. Exposure to chickenpox should be avoided; corticosteroids should not be used to treat ocular herpes simplex. Corticosteroids should not be used for cerebral malaria. Close observation is required in patients with latent tuberculosis and/or TB reactivity; restrict use in active TB (only in conjunction with antituberculosis treatment). Rare cases of vasculitis (Churg-Strauss syndrome) or other eosinophilic conditions can occur. Prolonged treatment with corticosteroids has been associated with the development of Kaposi's sarcoma (case reports); if noted, discontinuation of therapy should be considered.

Use with caution in patients with thyroid disease, hepatic impairment, renal impairment, cardiovascular disease, diabetes, glaucoma, cataracts, myasthenia gravis, patients at risk for osteoporosis, patients at risk for seizures, or GI diseases (diverticulitis, peptic ulcer, ulcerative colitis) due to perforation risk. Use caution following acute MI (corticosteroids have been associated with myocardial rupture). Because of the risk of adverse effects, systemic corticosteroids should be used cautiously in the elderly in the smallest possible effective dose for the shortest duration.

Not to be used in status asthmaticus or for the relief of acute bronchospasm. Flovent® Diskus® contains lactose; very rare anaphylactic reactions have been reported in patients with severe milk protein allergy. There have been reports of systemic corticosteroid withdrawal symptoms (eg, joint/muscle pain, lassitude, depression) when withdrawing oral inhalation therapy. Local yeast infections (eg, oral pharyngeal candidiasis) may occur. Lower respiratory tract infections, including pneumonia, have been reported in patients with COPD with an even higher incidence in the elderly.

Adverse Reactions (Reflective of adult population; not specific for elderly)
>10%:
Central nervous system: Malaise/fatigue (16%), headache (2% to 14%)
Gastrointestinal: Oral candidiasis (≤31%)
Neuromuscular & skeletal: Arthralgia/articular rheumatism (17%), musculoskeletal pain (2% to 12%)
Respiratory: Sinusitis/sinus infection (≤33%), upper respiratory tract infection (≤31%), throat irritation (3% to 22%), nasal congestion/blockage (16%), rhinitis (≤13%)
1% to 10%:
Central nervous system: Pain (10%), fever (1% to 7%)

Dermatologic: Rash (8%), pruritus (6%)

Gastrointestinal: Nausea/vomiting (1% to 9%), gastrointestinal infection (including viral; 1% to 5%), gastrointestinal discomfort/pain (1% to 4%)

Neuromuscular & skeletal: Muscle injury (≤5%)

Respiratory: Hoarseness/dysphonia (2% to 9%), cough (1% to 9%), viral respiratory infection (1% to 9%), bronchitis (≤8%), upper respiratory tract inflammation (≤5%)

Miscellaneous: Viral infection (≤5%)

Drug Interactions

Metabolism/Transport Effects Substrate of CYP3A4 (major); **Note:** Assignment of Major/ Minor substrate status based on clinically relevant drug interaction potential

Avoid Concomitant Use

Avoid concomitant use of Fluticasone (Oral Inhalation) with any of the following: Aldesleukin; BCG; CYP3A4 Inhibitors (Strong); Natalizumab; Pimecrolimus; Tacrolimus (Topical)

Increased Effect/Toxicity

Fluticasone (Oral Inhalation) may increase the levels/effects of: Amphotericin B; Deferasirox; Leflunomide; Loop Diuretics; Natalizumab; Thiazide Diuretics

The levels/effects of Fluticasone (Oral Inhalation) may be increased by: CYP3A4 Inhibitors (Moderate); CYP3A4 Inhibitors (Strong); Dasatinib; Denosumab; Ivacaftor; Mifepristone; Pimecrolimus; Tacrolimus (Topical); Telaprevir; Trastuzumab

Decreased Effect

Fluticasone (Oral Inhalation) may decrease the levels/effects of: Aldesleukin; Antidiabetic Agents; BCG; Coccidioidin Skin Test; Corticorelin; Hyaluronidase; Sipuleucel-T; Telaprevir; Vaccines (Inactivated)

The levels/effects of Fluticasone (Oral Inhalation) may be decreased by: Echinacea; Tocilizumab

Ethanol/Nutrition/Herb Interactions Herb/Nutraceutical: In theory, St John's wort may decrease serum levels of fluticasone by inducing CYP3A4 isoenzymes.

Stability

Flovent® HFA: Store at 15°C to 30°C (59°F to 86°F). Discard device when the dose counter reads "000". Store with mouthpiece down.

Flovent® Diskus®: Store at 20°C to 25°C (68°F to 77°F) in a dry place away from direct heat or sunlight. Discard after 6 weeks (50 mcg diskus) or after 2 months (100 mcg and 250 mcg diskus) from removal from protective foil pouch or when the dose counter reads "0" (whichever comes first); device is not reusable.

Mechanism of Action Fluticasone belongs to a group of corticosteroids which utilizes a fluorocarbothioate ester linkage at the 17 carbon position; extremely potent vasoconstrictive and anti-inflammatory activity. The effectiveness of inhaled fluticasone is due to its direct local effect.

Pharmacodynamics/Kinetics

Onset of action: Maximal benefit may take 1-2 weeks or longer

Absorption: Absorbed systemically (Flovent® Diskus®: ~8%) primarily via lungs, minimal GI absorption (<1%) due to presystemic metabolism

Distribution: 4.2 L/kg

Protein binding: 99%

Metabolism: Hepatic via CYP3A4 to 17β-carboxylic acid (negligible activity)

Half-life elimination: ~11-12 hours (Thorsson, 2001)

Excretion: Feces (as parent drug and metabolites); urine (<5% as metabolites)

Dosage

Geriatric & Adult Asthma: Inhalation, oral: **Note:** Titrate to the lowest effective dose once asthma stability is achieved

Flovent® HFA:

U.S. labeling: Dosing based on previous asthma therapy: **Note:** May increase dose after 2 weeks of therapy in patients who are not adequately controlled.

Bronchodilator alone: Initial: 88 mcg twice daily; maximum: 440 mcg twice daily

Inhaled corticosteroids: Initial: 88-220 mcg twice daily (initial dose >88 mcg twice daily may be considered in patients previously requiring higher doses of inhaled cortico- steroids); maximum: 440 mcg twice daily

Oral corticosteroids (OCS): Initial: 440 mcg twice daily; maximum: 880 mcg twice daily. *NIH Asthma Guidelines (NIH, 2007)* (administer in divided doses twice daily):

"Low" dose: 88-264 mcg/day

"Medium" dose: >264-440 mcg/day

"High" dose: >440 mcg/day

Canadian labeling: **Note:** May increase dose after ~1 week of therapy in patients who are not adequately controlled.

Mild asthma: 100-250 mcg twice daily

Moderate asthma: 250-500 mcg twice daily

Severe asthma: 500 mcg twice daily; may increase up to 1000 mcg twice daily in very severe patients (eg, patients using oral corticosteroids [OCS])

Flovent® Diskus®:

U.S. labeling: **Note:** May increase dose after 2 weeks of therapy in patients who are not adequately controlled.

Dosing based on previous asthma therapy:

Bronchodilator alone: Initial: 100 mcg twice daily; maximum: 500 mcg twice daily

Inhaled corticosteroids: Initial: 100-250 mcg twice daily; maximum: 500 mcg twice daily; initial dose >100 mcg twice daily may be considered in patients with poorer asthma control or those previously requiring high ranges of inhaled corticosteroids

Oral corticosteroids (OCS): Initial: 500-1000 mcg twice daily; maximum: 1000 mcg twice daily

NIH Asthma Guidelines (NIH, 2007) (administer in divided doses twice daily):

"Low" dose: 100-300 mcg/day

"Medium" dose: >300-500 mcg/day

"High" dose: >500 mcg/day

Canadian labeling: **Note:** May increase dose after ~1 week of therapy in patients who are not adequately controlled.

Mild asthma: 100-250 mcg twice daily

Moderate asthma: 250-500 mcg twice daily

Severe asthma: 500 mcg twice daily; may increase up to 1000 mcg twice daily in very severe patients (eg, patients using oral corticosteroids [OCS])

Conversion from oral systemic corticosteroids to orally inhaled corticosteroids: When converting from oral corticosteroids (OCS) to orally inhaled corticosteroids, initiate oral inhalation therapy in patients whose asthma is previously stabilized on OCS. Gradual OCS dose reductions should begin ~7 days after starting inhaled therapy. U.S. labeling recommends reducing prednisone dose no more rapidly than 2.5-5 mg/day (or equivalent of other OCS) weekly. The Canadian labeling recommends decreasing the daily dose of prednisone by 1 mg (or equivalent of other OCS) no more rapidly than weekly in adults who are closely monitored or every 10 days if not closely monitored. If adrenal insufficiency occurs, resume OCS therapy; initiate a more gradual withdrawal. When transitioning from systemic to inhaled corticosteroids, supplemental systemic corticosteroid therapy may be necessary during periods of stress or during severe asthma attacks.

Renal Impairment No dosage adjustment provided in manufacturer's labeling (has not been studied).

Hepatic Impairment No dosage adjustment provided in manufacturer's labeling (has not been studied); however, fluticasone is primarily cleared in the liver and plasma levels may be increased in patients with hepatic impairment. Use with caution; monitor.

Administration

Aerosol inhalation: Flovent® HFA: Shake container thoroughly before using. Take 3-5 deep breaths. Use inhaler on inspiration. Allow 1 full minute between inhalations. Rinse mouth with water after use to reduce aftertaste and incidence of candidiasis; do not swallow. Inhaler must be primed before first use, when not used for 7 days, or if dropped. To prime the first time, release 4 sprays into air; shake well before each spray and spray away from face. If dropped or not used for 7 days, prime by releasing a single test spray. Patient should contact pharmacy for refill when the dose counter reads "020". Discard device when the dose counter reads "000". Do not use "float" test to determine contents.

Powder for oral inhalation: Flovent® Diskus®: Do not use with a spacer device. Do not exhale into Diskus®. Do not wash or take apart. Use in horizontal position. Mouth should be rinsed with water after use (do not swallow). Discard after 6 weeks (50 mcg diskus) or after 2 months (100 mcg and 250 mcg diskus) once removed from protective pouch or when the dose counter reads "0", whichever comes first (device is not reusable).

Monitoring Parameters Signs/symptoms of HPA axis suppression/adrenal insufficiency; possible eosinophilic conditions (including Churg-Strauss syndrome); FEV_1, peak flow, and/or other pulmonary function tests; asthma symptoms

Pharmacotherapy Pearls In the United States, dosage for the metered dose inhaler (Flovent® HFA) is expressed as the amount of drug which leaves the actuater and is delivered to the patient. This differs from other countries, which express the dosage as the amount of drug which leaves the valve.

Special Geriatric Considerations No specific geriatric information is available. No differences in safety have been observed in the elderly when compared to younger patients. Based on current data, no dosage adjustment is needed based on age.

Dosage Forms Excipient information presented when available (limited, particularly for generics); consult specific product labeling.

FLUTICASONE (ORAL INHALATION)

Aerosol, for oral inhalation, as propionate:
Flovent® HFA: 44 mcg/inhalation (10.6 g); 110 mcg/inhalation (12 g); 220 mcg/inhalation (12 g) [chlorofluorocarbon free; 120 metered actuations]
Powder, for oral inhalation, as propionate:
Flovent® Diskus®: 50 mcg (60s); 100 mcg (60s); 250 mcg (60s) [contains lactose]
Dosage Forms: Canada Excipient information presented when available (limited, particularly for generics); consult specific product labeling.
Aerosol, for oral inhalation, as propionate:
Flovent® HFA: 50 mcg/inhalation (120 actuations); 125 mcg/inhalation (60 or 120 actuations); 250 mcg/inhalation (60 or 120 actuations)
Powder, for oral inhalation, as propionate:
Flovent® Diskus®: 50 mcg (60s) [contains lactose; prefilled blister pack]
Flovent® Diskus®: 100 mcg (60s) [contains lactose; prefilled blister pack]
Flovent® Diskus®: 250 mcg (60s) [contains lactose; prefilled blister pack]
Flovent® Diskus®: 500 mcg (60s) [contains lactose; prefilled blister pack]

Fluticasone (Nasal) (floo TIK a sone)

Medication Safety Issues
Sound-alike/look-alike issues:
Flonase® may be confused with Flovent®
International issues:
Allegro: Brand name for fluticasone [Israel], but also the brand name for frovatriptan [Germany]
Allegro [Israel] may be confused with Allegra and Allegra-D brand names for fexofenadine and fexofenadine/pseudoephedrine, respectively, [U.S., Canada, and multiple international markets]
Brand Names: U.S. Flonase®; Veramyst®
Brand Names: Canada Apo-Fluticasone®; Avamys®; Flonase®; ratio-Fluticasone
Index Terms Fluticasone Furoate; Fluticasone Propionate
Generic Availability (U.S.) Yes: Propionate spray
Pharmacologic Category Corticosteroid, Nasal
Use
Flonase®: Management of seasonal and perennial allergic rhinitis and nonallergic rhinitis
Veramyst®, Avamys® [CAN]: Management of seasonal and perennial allergic rhinitis
Unlabeled Use Adjunct to antibiotics in empiric treatment of acute bacterial rhinosinusitis (ABRS) (Chow, 2012)
Dosage
Geriatric & Adult Rhinitis: Intranasal:
Flonase® (fluticasone propionate): Initial: 2 sprays (50 mcg/spray) per nostril once daily (200 mcg/day); alternatively, the same total daily dosage may be divided and given as 1 spray per nostril twice daily (200 mcg/day). After the first few days, dosage may be reduced to 1 spray per nostril once daily for maintenance therapy (100 mcg/day).
Veramyst® (fluticasone furoate): Initial: 2 sprays (27.5 mcg/spray) per nostril once daily (110 mcg/day); once symptoms are controlled, may reduce dosage to 1 spray per nostril once daily (55 mcg/day) for maintenance therapy.
Avamys® [CAN] (fluticasone furoate): 2 sprays (27.5 mcg/spray) in each nostril once daily (110 mcg/day). Total daily dosage should not exceed 2 sprays in each nostril (110 mcg)/day.
Special Geriatric Considerations No differences in safety have been observed in the elderly when compared to younger patients. Based on current data, no dosage adjustment is needed based on age. Evaluate the patient's or caregiver's ability to safely administer the correct dose of nasal medication.
Dosage Forms Excipient information presented when available (limited, particularly for generics); consult specific product labeling.
Suspension, intranasal, as furoate [spray]:
Veramyst®: 27.5 mcg/inhalation (10 g) [contains benzalkonium chloride; 120 metered actuations]
Suspension, intranasal, as propionate [spray]: 50 mcg/inhalation (16 g)
Flonase®: 50 mcg/inhalation (16 g) [contains benzalkonium chloride; 120 metered actuations]
Dosage Forms: Canada Excipient information presented when available (limited, particularly for generics); consult specific product labeling.
Suspension, intranasal, as furoate [spray]:
Avamys®: 27.5 mcg/inhalation (4.5 g) [30 metered actuations; contains benzalkonium chloride]; (10 g) [120 metered actuations; contains benzalkonium chloride]

Fluticasone (Topical) (floo TIK a sone)

Related Information
Topical Corticosteroids *on page 2113*
Medication Safety Issues
Sound-alike/look-alike issues:
Cutivate® may be confused with Ultravate®
International issues:
Allegro: Brand name for fluticasone [Israel], but also the brand name for frovatriptan [Germany]
Allegro [Israel] may be confused with Allegra and Allegra-D brand names for fexofenadine and fexofenadine/pseudoephedrine, respectively, [U.S., Canada, and multiple international markets]
Brand Names: U.S. Cutivate®
Brand Names: Canada Cutivate™
Index Terms Fluticasone Propionate
Generic Availability (U.S.) Yes
Pharmacologic Category Corticosteroid, Topical
Use Relief of inflammation and pruritus associated with corticosteroid-responsive dermatoses; atopic dermatitis
Dosage
Geriatric & Adult
Corticosteroid-responsive dermatoses: Topical: Cream, lotion, ointment: Apply sparingly to affected area twice daily. If no improvement is seen within 2 weeks, reassessment of diagnosis may be necessary.
Atopic dermatitis: Topical: Cream, lotion: Apply sparingly to affected area once or twice daily. If no improvement is seen within 2 weeks, reassessment of diagnosis may be necessary.
Dosage Forms Excipient information presented when available (limited, particularly for generics); consult specific product labeling.
Cream, topical, as propionate: 0.05% (15 g, 30 g, 60 g)
Cutivate®: 0.05% (30 g, 60 g)
Lotion, topical, as propionate: 0.05% (60 mL)
Cutivate®: 0.05% (120 mL)
Ointment, topical, as propionate: 0.005% (15 g, 30 g, 60 g)
Cutivate®: 0.005% (30 g, 60 g)

Fluticasone and Salmeterol (floo TIK a sone & sal ME te role)

Related Information
Fluticasone (Oral Inhalation) *on page 822*
Salmeterol *on page 1749*
Medication Safety Issues
Sound-alike/look-alike issues:
Advair® may be confused with Adcirca®, Advicor®
Brand Names: U.S. Advair Diskus®; Advair® HFA
Brand Names: Canada Advair Diskus®; Advair®
Index Terms Fluticasone Propionate and Salmeterol Xinafoate; Salmeterol and Fluticasone
Generic Availability (U.S.) No
Pharmacologic Category Beta$_2$ Agonist; Beta$_2$-Adrenergic Agonist, Long-Acting; Corticosteroid, Inhalant (Oral)
Use Maintenance treatment of asthma; maintenance treatment of COPD
Medication Guide Available Yes
Contraindications Hypersensitivity to fluticasone, salmeterol, or any component of the formulation; status asthmaticus; acute episodes of asthma or COPD; severe hypersensitivity to milk proteins (Advair Diskus®)
Warnings/Precautions See individual agents.
Adverse Reactions (Reflective of adult population; not specific for elderly) Percentages reported in patients with asthma; also see individual agents:
>10%:
Central nervous system: Headache (12% to 21%)
Respiratory: Upper respiratory tract infection (16% to 27%), pharyngitis (9% to 13%)
>3% to 10%:
Central nervous system: Dizziness (1% to 4%)
Endocrine & metabolic: Menstruation symptoms (3% to 5%)

Gastrointestinal: Nausea/vomiting (3% to 6%), diarrhea (2% to 4%), pain/discomfort (1% to 4%), oral candidiasis (1% to 4%), gastrointestinal infections (including viral, ≤4%)

Neuromuscular & skeletal: Musculoskeletal pain (2% to 7%), muscle pain (≤4%)

Respiratory: Throat irritation (7% to 9%), bronchitis (2% to 8%), upper respiratory tract inflammation (4% to 7%), lower respiratory tract infections/pneumonia (1% to 7%; COPD diagnosis and age >65 years increase risk), cough (3% to 6%), sinusitis (4% to 5%), hoarseness/dysphonia (1% to 5%), viral respiratory tract infection (3% to 5%)

1% to 3%:

Cardiovascular: Arrhythmia, chest symptoms, fluid retention, MI, palpitation, syncope, tachycardia

Central nervous system: Compressed nerve syndromes, hypnagogic effects, migraine, pain, sleep disorders, tremor

Dermatologic: Dermatitis, dermatosis, eczema, hives, skin flakiness, urticaria, viral skin infection

Endocrine & metabolic: Hypothyroidism

Gastrointestinal: Constipation, dental discomfort/pain, gastrointestinal infection, hemorrhoids, oral discomfort/pain, oral erythema/rash, oral ulcerations, unusual taste, weight gain

Genitourinary: Urinary tract infection

Hematologic: Contusions/hematomas

Hepatic: Abnormal liver function tests

Neuromuscular & skeletal: Arthralgia, articular rheumatism, bone/cartilage disorders, bone pain, cramps, fractures, muscle injuries (≤3%), muscle spasm, muscle stiffness, tightness/rigidity

Ocular: Conjunctivitis, edema, eye redness, keratitis, xerophthalmia

Respiratory: Blood in nasal mucosa, congestion, ear/nose/throat infection, epistaxis, laryngitis, lower respiratory hemorrhage, nasal irritation, rhinitis, rhinorrhea/postnasal drip, sneezing

Miscellaneous: Allergies/allergic reactions, bacterial infection, burns, candidiasis (≤3%), diaphoresis, sweat/sebum disorders, viral infection, wounds and lacerations

Drug Interactions

Metabolism/Transport Effects Refer to individual components.

Avoid Concomitant Use

Avoid concomitant use of Fluticasone and Salmeterol with any of the following: Aldesleukin; BCG; Beta-Blockers (Nonselective); CYP3A4 Inhibitors (Strong); Iobenguane I 123; Natalizumab; Pimecrolimus; Tacrolimus (Topical); Telaprevir

Increased Effect/Toxicity

Fluticasone and Salmeterol may increase the levels/effects of: Amphotericin B; Deferasirox; Leflunomide; Loop Diuretics; Natalizumab; Sympathomimetics; Thiazide Diuretics

The levels/effects of Fluticasone and Salmeterol may be increased by: AtoMOXetine; Cannabinoids; CYP3A4 Inhibitors (Moderate); CYP3A4 Inhibitors (Strong); Dasatinib; Denosumab; Ivacaftor; MAO Inhibitors; Mifepristone; Pimecrolimus; Roflumilast; Tacrolimus (Topical); Telaprevir; Trastuzumab; Tricyclic Antidepressants

Decreased Effect

Fluticasone and Salmeterol may decrease the levels/effects of: Aldesleukin; Antidiabetic Agents; BCG; Coccidioidin Skin Test; Corticorelin; Hyaluronidase; Iobenguane I 123; Sipuleucel-T; Telaprevir; Vaccines (Inactivated)

The levels/effects of Fluticasone and Salmeterol may be decreased by: Alpha-/Beta-Blockers; Beta-Blockers (Beta1 Selective); Beta-Blockers (Nonselective); Betahistine; Echinacea; Tocilizumab

Stability

Advair Diskus®: Store at controlled room temperature of 20°C to 25°C (68°F to 77°F). Store in a dry place out of direct heat or sunlight. Diskus® device should be discarded 1 month after removal from foil pouch, or when dosing indicator reads "0" (whichever comes first); device is not reusable.

Advair® HFA: Store at controlled room temperature of 25°C (77°F). Store with mouthpiece down. Discard after 120 inhalations. Discard device when the dose counter reads "000". Device is not reusable.

Mechanism of Action Combination of fluticasone (corticosteroid) and salmeterol (long-acting beta$_2$-agonist) designed to improve pulmonary function and control over what is produced by either agent when used alone. Because fluticasone and salmeterol act locally in the lung, plasma levels do not predict therapeutic effect.

Fluticasone: The mechanism of action for all topical corticosteroids is believed to be a combination of three important properties: Anti-inflammatory activity, immunosuppressive properties, and antiproliferative actions. Fluticasone has extremely potent vasoconstrictive and anti-inflammatory activity.

Salmeterol: Relaxes bronchial smooth muscle by selective action on beta$_2$-receptors with little effect on heart rate

Pharmacodynamics/Kinetics See individual agents.

Dosage

Geriatric & Adult Do not use to transfer patients from systemic corticosteroid therapy.

COPD: Oral Inhalation:

Advair Diskus®: Fluticasone 250 mcg/salmeterol 50 mcg twice daily, 12 hours apart. **Note:** This is the maximum dose.

Advair Diskus® [Canadian labeling; not in approved U.S. labeling]: Fluticasone 250 mcg/ salmeterol 50 mcg **or** fluticasone 500 mcg/salmeterol 50 mcg twice daily, 12 hours apart. Maximum dose: Fluticasone 500 mcg/salmeterol 50 mcg per inhalation (2 inhalations/day)

Asthma (maintenance): Oral inhalation:

Advair Diskus®: One inhalation twice daily, morning and evening, 12 hours apart

Maximum dose: Fluticasone 500 mcg/salmeterol 50 mcg per inhalation (2 inhalations/day)

Advair® HFA: Two inhalations twice daily, morning and evening, 12 hours apart

Maximum dose: Fluticasone 230 mcg/salmeterol 21 mcg per inhalation (4 inhalations/day)

Advair® 125 or Advair® 250 [Canadian labeling; not in approved U.S. labeling]: Two inhalations twice daily, morning and evening, 12 hours apart

Maximum dose: Fluticasone 250 mcg/salmeterol 25 mcg per inhalation (4 inhalations/day)

Note: Initial dose prescribed should be based upon previous dose of inhaled-steroid asthma therapy. Dose should be increased after 2 weeks if adequate response is not achieved. Patients should be titrated to lowest effective dose once stable. Each suggestion below specifies the product strength to use; remember to **use 1 inhalation for Diskus® and 2 inhalations for HFA.**

Patients not currently on inhaled corticosteroids:

Advair Diskus®: Fluticasone 100 mcg/salmeterol 50 mcg **or** fluticasone 250 mcg/ salmeterol 50 mcg

Advair® HFA: Fluticasone 45 mcg/salmeterol 21 mcg **or** fluticasone 115 mcg/salmeterol 21 mcg

Patients currently using inhaled beclomethasone dipropionate:

≤160 mcg/day: Fluticasone 100 mcg/salmeterol 50 mcg **or** Advair® HFA: Fluticasone 45 mcg/salmeterol 21 mcg

320 mcg/day: Fluticasone 250 mcg/salmeterol 50 mcg **or** Advair® HFA: Fluticasone 115 mcg/salmeterol 21 mcg

640 mcg/day: Fluticasone 500 mcg/salmeterol 50 mcg **or** Advair® HFA: Fluticasone 230 mcg/salmeterol 21 mcg

Patients currently using inhaled budesonide:

≤400 mcg/day: Fluticasone 100 mcg/salmeterol 50 mcg **or** Advair® HFA: Fluticasone 45 mcg/salmeterol 21 mcg

800-1200 mcg/day: Fluticasone 250 mcg/salmeterol 50 mcg **or** Advair® HFA: Fluticasone 115 mcg/salmeterol 21mcg

1600 mcg/day: Fluticasone 500 mcg/salmeterol 50 mcg **or** Advair® HFA: Fluticasone 230 mcg/salmeterol 21 mcg

Patients currently using inhaled flunisolide CFC aerosol:

≤1000 mcg/day: Fluticasone 100 mcg/salmeterol 50 mcg **or** Advair® HFA: Fluticasone 45 mcg/salmeterol 21 mcg

1250-2000 mcg/day: Fluticasone 250 mcg/salmeterol 50 mcg **or** Advair® HFA: Fluticasone 115 mcg/salmeterol 21 mcg

Patients currently using inhaled flunisolide HFA inhalation aerosol:

≤320 mcg/day: Fluticasone 100 mcg/salmeterol 50 mcg **or** Advair® HFA: Fluticasone 45 mcg/salmeterol 21 mcg

640 mcg/day: Fluticasone 250 mcg/salmeterol 50 mcg **or** Advair® HFA: Fluticasone 115 mcg/salmeterol 21 mcg

Patients currently using inhaled fluticasone HFA aerosol:

≤176 mcg/day: Fluticasone 100 mcg/salmeterol 50 mcg **or** Advair® HFA: Fluticasone 45 mcg/salmeterol 21 mcg

440 mcg/day: Fluticasone 250 mcg/salmeterol 50 mcg **or** Advair® HFA: Fluticasone 115 mcg/salmeterol 21 mcg

660-880 mcg/day: Fluticasone 500 mcg/salmeterol 50 mcg **or** Advair® HFA: Fluticasone 230 mcg/salmeterol 21 mcg

Patients currently using inhaled fluticasone propionate powder:

≤200 mcg/day: Fluticasone 100 mcg/salmeterol 50 mcg **or** Advair® HFA: Fluticasone 45 mcg/salmeterol 21 mcg

500 mcg/day: Fluticasone 250 mcg/salmeterol 50 mcg or Advair® HFA: Fluticasone 115 mcg/salmeterol 21 mcg

1000 mcg/day: Fluticasone 500 mcg/salmeterol 50 mcg or Advair® HFA: Fluticasone 230 mcg/salmeterol 21 mcg

Patients currently using inhaled mometasone furoate powder:

220 mcg/day: Fluticasone 100 mcg/salmeterol 50 mcg or Advair® HFA: Fluticasone 45 mcg/salmeterol 21 mcg

440 mcg/day: Fluticasone 250 mcg/salmeterol 50 mcg or Advair® HFA: Fluticasone 115 mcg/salmeterol 21 mcg

880 mcg/day: Fluticasone 500 mcg/salmeterol 50 mcg or Advair® HFA: Fluticasone 230 mcg/salmeterol 21 mcg

Patients currently using inhaled triamcinolone acetonide:

≤1000 mcg/day: Fluticasone 100 mcg/salmeterol 50 mcg or Advair® HFA: Fluticasone 45 mcg/salmeterol 21 mcg

1100-1600 mcg/day: Fluticasone 250 mcg/salmeterol 50 mcg or Advair® HFA: Fluticasone 115 mcg/salmeterol 21 mcg

Hepatic Impairment No dosage adjustment required; manufacturer suggests close monitoring of patients with hepatic impairment.

Administration

Advair Diskus®: After removing from box and foil pouch, write the "Pouch opened" and "Use by" dates on the label on top of the Diskus®. The "Use by" date is 1 month from date of opening the pouch. Every time the lever is pushed back, a dose is ready to be inhaled. Do not close or tilt the Diskus® after the lever is pushed back. Do not play with the lever or move the lever more than once. The dose indicator tells you how many doses are left. When the numbers 5 to 0 appear in red, only a few doses remain. Discard device 1 month after you remove it from the foil pouch or when the dose counter reads "0" (whichever comes first). Rinse mouth with water after use and spit to reduce risk of oral candidiasis.

Advair® HFA: Shake well for 5 seconds before each spray. Prime with 4 test sprays (into air and away from face) before using for the first time. If canister is dropped or not used for >4 weeks, prime with 2 sprays. Patient should contact pharmacy for refill when the dose counter reads "020". Discard device when the dose counter reads "000". Do not spray in eyes. Rinse mouth with water after use and spit to reduce risk of oral candidiasis.

Monitoring Parameters FEV_1, peak flow, and/or other pulmonary function tests; blood pressure, heart rate; CNS stimulation. Monitor for increased use of short-acting beta$_2$-agonist inhalers; may be marker of a deteriorating asthma condition.

Pharmacotherapy Pearls Advair® HFA: Salmeterol (base) 21 mcg is equivalent to 30.45 mcg of salmeterol xinafoate.

Special Geriatric Considerations No differences in safety or effectiveness have been seen in studies of patients ≥65 years of age. However, increased sensitivity may be seen in the elderly. Use with caution in patients with concomitant cardiovascular disease.

Dosage Forms Excipient information presented when available (limited, particularly for generics); consult specific product labeling. [DSC] = Discontinued product

Aerosol, for oral inhalation:

Advair® HFA:

45/21: Fluticasone propionate 45 mcg and salmeterol 21 mcg per inhalation (8 g) [chlorofluorocarbon free; 60 metered actuations]

45/21: Fluticasone propionate 45 mcg and salmeterol 21 mcg per inhalation (12 g) [chlorofluorocarbon free; 120 metered actuations]

115/21: Fluticasone propionate 115 mcg and salmeterol 21 mcg per inhalation (8 g) [chlorofluorocarbon free; 60 metered actuations]

115/21: Fluticasone propionate 115 mcg and salmeterol 21 mcg per inhalation (12 g) [chlorofluorocarbon free; 120 metered actuations]

230/21: Fluticasone propionate 230 mcg and salmeterol 21 mcg per inhalation (8 g) [chlorofluorocarbon free; 60 metered actuations]

230/21: Fluticasone propionate 230 mcg and salmeterol 21 mcg per inhalation (12 g) [chlorofluorocarbon free; 120 metered actuations]

Powder, for oral inhalation:

Advair Diskus®:

100/50: Fluticasone propionate 100 mcg and salmeterol 50 mcg (14s, 28s [DSC], 60s) [contains lactose]

250/50: Fluticasone propionate 250 mcg and salmeterol 50 mcg (14s [DSC], 60s) [contains lactose]

500/50: Fluticasone propionate 500 mcg and salmeterol 50 mcg (14s [DSC], 60s) [contains lactose]

Dosage Forms: Canada Excipient information presented when available (limited, particularly for generics); consult specific product labeling.

Aerosol, for oral inhalation:
Advair®;
125/25: Fluticasone propionate 125 mcg and salmeterol 25 mcg per inhalation (12 g) [120 metered actuations]
250/25: Fluticasone propionate 250 mcg and salmeterol 25 mcg per inhalation (12 g) [120 metered actuations]

◆ **Fluticasone Furoate** *see* Fluticasone (Nasal) *on page 826*
◆ **Fluticasone Propionate** *see* Fluticasone (Nasal) *on page 826*
◆ **Fluticasone Propionate** *see* Fluticasone (Oral Inhalation) *on page 822*
◆ **Fluticasone Propionate** *see* Fluticasone (Topical) *on page 827*
◆ **Fluticasone Propionate and Salmeterol Xinafoate** *see* Fluticasone and Salmeterol *on page 827*

Fluvastatin (FLOO va sta tin)

Related Information
Hyperlipidemia Management *on page 2130*
Medication Safety Issues
Sound-alike/look-alike issues:
Fluvastatin may be confused with fluoxetine, nystatin, pitavastatin
Brand Names: U.S. Lescol®; Lescol® XL
Brand Names: Canada Lescol®; Lescol® XL
Generic Availability (U.S.) Yes: Capsules
Pharmacologic Category Antilipemic Agent, HMG-CoA Reductase Inhibitor
Use To be used as a component of multiple risk factor intervention in patients at risk for atherosclerosis vascular disease due to hypercholesterolemia

Adjunct to dietary therapy to reduce elevated total cholesterol (total-C), LDL-C, triglyceride, and apolipoprotein B (apo-B) levels and to increase HDL-C in primary hypercholesterolemia and mixed dyslipidemia (Fredrickson types IIa and IIb); to slow the progression of coronary atherosclerosis in patients with coronary heart disease; reduce risk of coronary revascularization procedures in patients with coronary heart disease
Contraindications Hypersensitivity to fluvastatin or any component of the formulation; active liver disease; unexplained persistent elevations of serum transaminases
Warnings/Precautions Secondary causes of hyperlipidemia should be ruled out prior to therapy. Liver function must be monitored by periodic laboratory assessment. Rhabdomyolysis with acute renal failure has occurred with fluvastatin and other HMG-CoA reductase inhibitors. Risk may be increased with concurrent use of other drugs which may cause rhabdomyolysis (including colchicine, cyclosporine, erythromycin, fibric acid derivatives, or niacin at doses ≥1 g/day). The manufacturer recommends temporary discontinuation for elective major surgery, acute medical or surgical conditions, or in any patient experiencing an acute or serious condition predisposing to renal failure (eg, sepsis, hypotension, trauma, uncontrolled seizures). However, based upon current evidence, HMG-CoA reductase inhibitor therapy should be continued in the perioperative period unless risk outweighs cardioprotective benefit. Use with caution in patients with advanced age; these patients are predisposed to myopathy. Use caution in patients with previous liver disease or heavy ethanol use.

If serious hepatotoxicity with clinical symptoms and/or hyperbilirubinemia or jaundice occurs during treatment, interrupt therapy. If an alternate etiology is not identified, do not restart fluvastatin. Liver enzyme tests should be obtained at baseline and as clinically indicated; routine periodic monitoring of liver enzymes is not necessary. Increases in Hb A_{1c} and fasting blood glucose have been reported with HMG-CoA reductase inhibitors; however, the benefits of statin therapy far outweigh the risk of dysglycemia. Use caution in patients with concurrent medications or conditions which reduce steroidogenesis.
Adverse Reactions (Reflective of adult population; not specific for elderly) As reported with fluvastatin capsules; in general, adverse reactions reported with fluvastatin extended release tablet were similar, but the incidence was less.

1% to 10%:
Central nervous system: Headache (9%), fatigue (3%), insomnia (3%)
Gastrointestinal: Dyspepsia (8%), diarrhea (5%), abdominal pain (5%), nausea (3%)
Genitourinary: Urinary tract infection (2%)
Neuromuscular & skeletal: Myalgia (5%)
Respiratory: Sinusitis (3%), bronchitis (2%)

FLUVASTATIN

Drug Interactions

Metabolism/Transport Effects Substrate of CYP2C9 (minor), CYP2D6 (minor), CYP3A4 (minor), SLCO1B1; **Note:** Assignment of Major/Minor substrate status based on clinically relevant drug interaction potential; **Inhibits** CYP1A2 (weak), CYP2C8 (weak), CYP2C9 (moderate), CYP2D6 (weak), CYP3A4 (weak)

Avoid Concomitant Use

Avoid concomitant use of Fluvastatin with any of the following: Gemfibrozil; Pimozide; Red Yeast Rice

Increased Effect/Toxicity

Fluvastatin may increase the levels/effects of: ARIPiprazole; Carvedilol; CYP2C9 Substrates; DAPTOmycin; Pazopanib; Pimozide; Trabectedin; Vitamin K Antagonists

The levels/effects of Fluvastatin may be increased by: Amiodarone; Colchicine; Cyclo-SPORINE; CycloSPORINE (Systemic); Cyproterone; Eltrombopag; Fenofibrate; Fenofibric Acid; Fluconazole; Gemfibrozil; Mifepristone; Niacin; Niacinamide; Red Yeast Rice

Decreased Effect

Fluvastatin may decrease the levels/effects of: Lanthanum

The levels/effects of Fluvastatin may be decreased by: Antacids; Cholestyramine Resin; Etravirine; Fosphenytoin; Peginterferon Alfa-2b; Phenytoin; Rifamycin Derivatives; Tocilizumab

Ethanol/Nutrition/Herb Interactions

Ethanol: Avoid excessive ethanol consumption (due to potential hepatic effects).

Food: Reduces rate but not the extent of absorption. Red yeast rice contains an estimated 2.4 mg lovastatin per 600 mg rice.

Stability Store at 15°C to 30°C (59°F to 86°F). Protect from light.

Mechanism of Action Acts by competitively inhibiting 3-hydroxyl-3-methylglutaryl-coenzyme A (HMG-CoA) reductase, the enzyme that catalyzes the reduction of HMG-CoA to mevalonate; this is an early rate-limiting step in cholesterol biosynthesis. HDL is increased while total, LDL, and VLDL cholesterols; apolipoprotein B; and plasma triglycerides are decreased.

Pharmacodynamics/Kinetics

Onset of action: Peak effect: Maximal LDL-C reductions achieved within 4 weeks

Distribution: V_d: 0.35 L/kg

Protein binding: >98%

Metabolism: To inactive and active metabolites (oxidative metabolism via CYP2C9 [75%], 2C8 [~5%], and 3A4 [~20%] isoenzymes); active forms do not circulate systemically; extensive (saturable) first-pass hepatic extraction

Bioavailability: Absolute: Capsule: 24%; Extended release tablet: 29%

Half-life elimination: Capsule: <3 hours; Extended release tablet: 9 hours

Time to peak: Capsule: 1 hour; Extended release tablet: 3 hours

Excretion: Feces (90%): urine (5%)

Dosage

Geriatric & Adult Dyslipidemia (also delay in progression of CAD): Oral:

Patients requiring ≥25% decrease in LDL-C: 40 mg capsule once daily in the evening, 80 mg extended release tablet once daily (anytime), or 40 mg capsule twice daily

Patients requiring <25% decrease in LDL-C: Initial: 20 mg capsule once daily in the evening; may increase based on tolerability and response to a maximum recommended dose of 80 mg/day, given in 2 divided doses (immediate release capsule) or as a single daily dose (extended release tablet)

Concomitant use with cyclosporine or fluconazole: Do not exceed fluvastatin 20 mg twice daily

Renal Impairment Note: Less than 6% excreted renally

Mild-to-moderate renal impairment: No dosage adjustment necessary.

Severe renal impairment: Use with caution (particularly at doses >40 mg/day; has not been studied).

Hepatic Impairment Manufacturer's labeling does not provide specific dosing recommendations; however, systemic exposure may be increased in patients with liver disease (increased AUC and C_{max}); use is contraindicated in active liver disease or unexplained transaminase elevations.

Administration Patient should be placed on a standard cholesterol-lowering diet before and during treatment. Fluvastatin may be taken without regard to meals. Adjust dosage as needed in response to periodic lipid determinations during the first 4 weeks after a dosage change; lipid-lowering effects are additive when fluvastatin is combined with a bile-acid binding resin or niacin, however, it must be administered at least 2 hours following these drugs. Do not break, chew, or crush extended release tablets; do not open capsules.

Monitoring Parameters Baseline CPK (recheck CPK in any patient with symptoms suggestive of myopathy; discontinue therapy if markedly elevated); baseline liver function tests (LFTs) and repeat when clinically indicated thereafter. Patients with elevated transaminase levels should have a second (confirmatory) test and frequent monitoring until values normalize; discontinue if increase in ALT/AST is persistently >3 times ULN (NCEP, 2002).

Lipid panel (total cholesterol, HDL, LDL, triglycerides):
ATP III recommendations (NCEP, 2002): Baseline; 6-8 weeks after initiation of drug therapy; if dose increased, then at 6-8 weeks until final dose determined. Once treatment goal achieved, follow up intervals may be reduced to every 4-6 months. Lipid panel should be assessed at least annually, and preferably at each clinic visit.
Manufacturer recommendation: Upon initiation or titration, lipid panel should be analyzed at 4 weeks.

Special Geriatric Considerations The definition of and, therefore, when to treat hyperlipidemia in the elderly is a controversial issue. The National Cholesterol Education Program recommends that all adults maintain a plasma cholesterol <160 mg/dL. In elderly patients with one additional risk factor, goal LDL would decrease to <130 mg/dL. Pharmacologic treatment should be reserved for those who are unable to obtain a desirable plasma cholesterol concentration by diet alone and for whom the benefits of treatment are believed to outweigh the potential adverse effects, drug interactions, and cost of treatment. Age ≥65 years is a risk factor for myopathy.

Dosage Forms Excipient information presented when available (limited, particularly for generics); consult specific product labeling.
Capsule, oral: 20 mg, 40 mg
  Lescol®: 20 mg, 40 mg
Tablet, extended release, oral:
  Lescol® XL: 80 mg

◆ **Fluvirin®** *see* Influenza Virus Vaccine (Inactivated) *on page* 997

FluvoxaMINE (floo VOKS a meen)

Related Information
Antidepressant Agents *on page* 2097
Medication Safety Issues
Sound-alike/look-alike issues:
FluvoxaMINE may be confused with flavoxATE, FLUoxetine, fluPHENAZine
Luvox may be confused with Lasix®, Levoxyl®, Lovenox®
BEERS Criteria medication:
This drug may be potentially inappropriate for use in geriatric patients (Quality of evidence - moderate; Strength of recommendation - strong).
Brand Names: U.S. Luvox® CR
Brand Names: Canada Alti-Fluvoxamine; Apo-Fluvoxamine®; Luvox®; Novo-Fluvoxamine; Nu-Fluvoxamine; PMS-Fluvoxamine; Rhoxal-fluvoxamine; Riva-Fluvox; Sandoz-Fluvoxamine
Index Terms Luvox
Generic Availability (U.S.) Yes: Excludes extended release capsule
Pharmacologic Category Antidepressant, Selective Serotonin Reuptake Inhibitor
Use Treatment of obsessive-compulsive disorder (OCD)
Unlabeled Use Treatment of major depression; panic disorder; treatment of mild dementia-associated agitation in nonpsychotic patients; post-traumatic stress disorder (PTSD); social anxiety disorder (SAD)
Medication Guide Available Yes
Contraindications Hypersensitivity to fluvoxamine or any component of the formulation; concurrent use with alosetron, pimozide, ramelteon, thioridazine, or tizanidine; use with or within 14 days of MAO inhibitors
Warnings/Precautions [U.S. Boxed Warning]: Antidepressants increase the risk of suicidal thinking and behavior in children, adolescents, and young adults (18-24 years of age) with major depressive disorder (MDD) and other psychiatric disorders; consider risk prior to prescribing. Short-term studies did not show an increased risk in patients >24 years of age and showed a decreased risk in patients ≥65 years. Closely monitor patients for clinical worsening, suicidality, or unusual changes in behavior, particularly during the initial 1-2 months of therapy or during periods of dosage adjustments (increases or decreases); the patient's family or caregiver should be instructed to closely observe the patient and communicate condition with healthcare provider. A medication guide concerning the use of antidepressants should be dispensed with each prescription.

The possibility of a suicide attempt is inherent in major depression and may persist until remission occurs. Use caution in high-risk patients. Worsening depression and severe abrupt suicidality that are not part of the presenting symptoms may require discontinuation or modification of drug therapy. The patient's family or caregiver should be alerted to monitor patients for the emergence of suicidality and associated behaviors (such as agitation, irritability, hostility, impulsivity, and hypomania) and call healthcare provider.

May worsen psychosis in some patients or precipitate a shift to mania or hypomania in patients with bipolar disorder. Patients presenting with depressive symptoms should be screened for bipolar disorder. Monotherapy in patients with bipolar disorder should be avoided. **Fluvoxamine is not FDA approved for the treatment of bipolar depression.**

Serotonin syndrome and neuroleptic malignant syndrome (NMS)-like reactions have occurred with serotonin/norepinephrine reuptake inhibitors (SNRIs) and selective serotonin reuptake inhibitors (SSRIs) when used alone, and particularly when used in combination with serotonergic agents (eg, triptans) or antidopaminergic agents (eg, antipsychotics). Concurrent use with MAO inhibitors is contraindicated. Fluvoxamine has a low potential to impair cognitive or motor performance; caution operating hazardous machinery or driving. Use caution in patients with a previous seizure disorder or condition predisposing to seizures such as brain damage, alcoholism, or concurrent therapy with other drugs which lower the seizure threshold. Fluvoxamine may significantly increase alosetron concentrations; concurrent use **contraindicated.** Potential for QT_c prolongation and arrhythmia with thioridazine and pimozide; concurrent use of fluvoxamine with either of these agents is **contraindicated.** Concomitant use with tizanidine may cause a significant decrease in blood pressure and increase in drowsiness; concurrent use is **contraindicated.** Fluvoxamine levels may be lower in patients who smoke.

May increase the risks associated with electroconvulsive therapy. Use with caution in patients with hepatic dysfunction and in elderly patients. May cause hyponatremia/SIADH (elderly at increased risk); volume depletion (diuretics may increase risk). Use with caution in patients at risk of bleeding or receiving concurrent anticoagulant therapy, although not consistently noted, fluvoxamine may cause impairment in platelet function. May cause or exacerbate sexual dysfunction. Use caution in elderly patients; monitor sodium closely with initiation or dosage adjustments in older adults (Beers Criteria).

Adverse Reactions (Reflective of adult population; not specific for elderly)
Frequency varies by dosage form and indication. Adverse reactions reported as a composite of all indications.

>10%:

Central nervous system: Headache (22% to 35%), insomnia (21% to 35%), somnolence (22% to 27%), dizziness (11% to 15%), nervousness (10% to 12%)

Gastrointestinal: Nausea (34% to 40%), diarrhea (11% to 18%), xerostomia (10% to 14%), anorexia (6% to 14%)

Genitourinary: Ejaculation abnormal (8% to 11%)

Neuromuscular & skeletal: Weakness (14% to 26%)

1% to 10%:

Cardiovascular: Chest pain (3%), palpitation (3%), vasodilation (2% to 3%), hypertension (1% to 2%), edema (≤1%), hypotension (≤1%), syncope (≤1%), tachycardia (≤1%)

Central nervous system: Pain (10%), anxiety (5% to 8%), abnormal dreams (3%), abnormal thinking (3%), agitation (2% to 3%), apathy (≥1% to 3%), chills (2%), CNS stimulation (2%), depression (2%), neurosis (2%), amnesia, malaise, manic reaction, psychotic reaction

Dermatologic: Bruising (4%), acne (2%)

Endocrine & metabolic: Libido decreased (2% to 10%; incidence higher in males), anorgasmia (2% to 5%), sexual function abnormal (2% to 4%), menorrhagia (3%)

Gastrointestinal: Dyspepsia (8% to 10%), constipation (4% to 10%), vomiting (4% to 6%), abdominal pain (5%), flatulence (4%), taste perversion (2% to 3%), toothache and dental caries (2% to 3%), dysphagia (2%), gingivitis (2%), weight loss (≤1% to 2%), weight gain

Genitourinary: Polyuria (2% to 3%), impotence (2%), urinary tract infection (2%), urinary retention (1%)

Hepatic: Liver function tests abnormal (≥1% to 2%)

Neuromuscular & skeletal: Tremor (5% to 8%), myalgia (5%), paresthesia (3%), hypertonia (2%), twitching (2%), hyper-/hypokinesia, myoclonus

Ocular: Amblyopia (2% to 3%)

Respiratory: Upper respiratory infection (9%), pharyngitis (6%), yawn (2% to 5%), laryngitis (3%), bronchitis (2%), dyspnea (2%), epistaxis (2%), cough increased, sinusitis

Miscellaneous: Diaphoresis (6% to 7%), flu-like syndrome (3%), viral infection (2%)

Drug Interactions

Metabolism/Transport Effects Substrate of CYP1A2 (major), CYP2D6 (major); **Note:** Assignment of Major/Minor substrate status based on clinically relevant drug interaction potential; **Inhibits** CYP1A2 (strong), CYP2B6 (weak), CYP2C19 (strong), CYP2C9 (weak), CYP2D6 (weak), CYP3A4 (weak)

Avoid Concomitant Use

Avoid concomitant use of FluvoxaMINE with any of the following: Alosetron; Clopidogrel; Iobenguane I 123; MAO Inhibitors; Methylene Blue; Pimozide; Ramelteon; Thioridazine; TiZANidine; Tryptophan

Increased Effect/Toxicity

FluvoxaMINE may increase the levels/effects of: Alosetron; Anticoagulants; Antidepressants (Serotonin Reuptake Inhibitor/Antagonist); Antiplatelet Agents; Asenapine; Aspirin; Bendamustine; Benzodiazepines (metabolized by oxidation); Bromazepam; BusPIRone; CarBAMazepine; CloZAPine; Collagenase (Systemic); CYP1A2 Substrates; CYP2C19 Substrates; Dabigatran Etexilate; Desmopressin; Drotrecogin Alfa (Activated); DULoxetine; Erlotinib; Fosphenytoin; Haloperidol; Hypoglycemic Agents; Ibritumomab; Lithium; Methadone; Methylene Blue; Metoclopramide; Mexiletine; NSAID (COX-2 Inhibitor); NSAID (Nonselective); OLANZapine; Phenytoin; Pimozide; Propafenone; Propranolol; QuiNIDine; Ramelteon; Rivaroxaban; Roflumilast; Ropivacaine; Salicylates; Serotonin Modulators; Theophylline Derivatives; Thioridazine; Thrombolytic Agents; TiZANidine; Tositumomab and Iodine I 131 Tositumomab; TraMADol; Tricyclic Antidepressants; Vitamin K Antagonists; Zolpidem

The levels/effects of FluvoxaMINE may be increased by: Abiraterone Acetate; Alcohol (Ethyl); Analgesics (Opioid); Antipsychotics; BusPIRone; CNS Depressants; CYP1A2 Inhibitors (Moderate); CYP1A2 Inhibitors (Strong); CYP2D6 Inhibitors (Moderate); CYP2D6 Inhibitors (Strong); Darunavir; Dasatinib; Deferasirox; Glucosamine; Herbs (Anticoagulant/Antiplatelet Properties); Linezolid; MAO Inhibitors; Metoclopramide; Metyrosine; Omega-3-Acid Ethyl Esters; Pentosan Polysulfate Sodium; Pentoxifylline; Prostacyclin Analogues; Tipranavir; TraMADol; Tryptophan; Vitamin E

Decreased Effect

FluvoxaMINE may decrease the levels/effects of: Clopidogrel; Iobenguane I 123; Ioflupane I 123

The levels/effects of FluvoxaMINE may be decreased by: CarBAMazepine; CYP1A2 Inducers (Strong); Cyproheptadine; Cyproterone; NSAID (COX-2 Inhibitor); NSAID (Nonselective); Peginterferon Alfa-2b

Ethanol/Nutrition/Herb Interactions

Ethanol: May increase CNS depression; monitor for increased effects with coadministration. Caution patients about effects.

Food: The bioavailability of melatonin has been reported to be increased by fluvoxamine.

Herb/Nutraceutical: Avoid valerian, St John's wort, SAMe, kava kava (may increase risk of serotonin syndrome and/or excessive sedation). Avoid alfalfa, anise, bilberry, bladderwrack, bromelain, cat's claw, celery, chamomile, coleus, cordyceps, dong quai, evening primrose, fenugreek, feverfew, garlic, ginger, ginkgo biloba, ginseng (American), ginseng (Panax), ginseng (Siberian), grape seed, green tea, guggul, horse chestnuts, horseradish, licorice, prickly ash, red clover, reishi, SAMe (S-adenosylmethionine), sweet clover, turmeric, white willow (all have additional antiplatelet activity).

Stability Protect from high humidity and store at controlled room temperature 25°C (77°F).

Mechanism of Action Inhibits CNS neuron serotonin uptake; minimal or no effect on reuptake of norepinephrine or dopamine; does not significantly bind to alpha-adrenergic, histamine or cholinergic receptors

Pharmacodynamics/Kinetics

Onset of action: Depression: The onset of action is within a week; however, individual response varies greatly and full response may not be seen until 8-12 weeks after initiation of treatment.

Distribution: V_d: ~25 L/kg

Protein binding: ~80%, primarily to albumin

Metabolism: Extensively hepatic via oxidative demethylation and deamination

Bioavailability: Immediate release: 53%; not significantly affected by food

Half-life elimination: 15-16 hours; 17-26 hours in the elderly

Time to peak, plasma: 3-8 hours

Excretion: Urine (~85% as metabolites; ~2% as unchanged drug)

Dosage

Geriatric Reduce dose; titrate slowly.

Adult

Obsessive-compulsive disorder: Oral:

Immediate release: Initial: 50 mg once daily at bedtime; may be increased in 50 mg increments at 4- to 7-day intervals, as tolerated; usual dose range: 100-300 mg/day; maximum dose: 300 mg/day. **Note:** When total daily dose exceeds 100 mg, the dose should be given in 2 divided doses with larger portion administered at bedtime.

Extended release: Initial: 100 mg once daily at bedtime; may be increased in 50 mg increments at intervals of at least 1 week; usual dosage range: 100-300 mg/day; maximum dose: 300 mg/day

Social anxiety disorder (unlabeled use): Oral: Extended release: Initial: 100 mg once daily at bedtime; may be increased in 50 mg increments at intervals of at least 1 week; usual dosage range: 100-300 mg/day; maximum dose: 300 mg/day (Davidson, 2004; Stein, 2003; Westenberg, 2004)

Post-traumatic stress disorder (PTSD) (unlabeled use): Immediate release: Oral: 75 mg twice daily (Spivak, 2006)

Hepatic Impairment Reduce dose; titrate slowly.

Administration May be administered with or without food. Do not crush, open, or chew extended release capsules.

Monitoring Parameters Mental status for depression, suicide ideation (especially at the beginning of therapy or when doses are increased or decreased), anxiety, social functioning, mania, panic attacks; akathisia, weight gain or loss, nutritional intake, sleep; liver function assessment prior to beginning drug therapy

Special Geriatric Considerations Given fluvoxamine's approved indication (OCD), the number of drug interactions, and the limited information available on its use in the elderly, it may be best to select a different agent when treating depression. The elderly are more prone to SSRI/SNRI-induced hyponatremia.

A systematic review and meta-analysis of antidepressant placebo-controlled trials in persons with depression and dementia found evidence "suggestive" of efficacy but not of sufficient strength to "confirm" efficacy. Antidepressant trials in this patient population are small and underpowered. Older patients with depression being treated with an antidepressant should be closely monitored for response and adverse effects. Treatment should be switched or augmented when response is inadequate with a therapeutic dose. Antidepressants that are not tolerated should be discontinued and an alternative agent should be started.

This medication is considered to be potentially inappropriate in this patient population (Beers Criteria: Quality of evidence - moderate; Strength of recommendation - strong).

Dosage Forms Excipient information presented when available (limited, particularly for generics); consult specific product labeling.

Capsule, extended release, oral, as maleate:
Luvox® CR: 100 mg, 150 mg [gluten free]
Tablet, oral, as maleate: 25 mg, 50 mg, 100 mg

- ♦ **Fluzone®** see Influenza Virus Vaccine (Inactivated) on page 997
- ♦ **Fluzone® High-Dose** see Influenza Virus Vaccine (Inactivated) on page 997
- ♦ **Fluzone® Intradermal** see Influenza Virus Vaccine (Inactivated) on page 997
- ♦ **Folacin** see Folic Acid on page 836
- ♦ **Folacin-800 [OTC]** see Folic Acid on page 836
- ♦ **Folate** see Folic Acid on page 836

Folic Acid (FOE lik AS id)

Medication Safety Issues

Sound-alike/look-alike issues:

Folic acid may be confused with folinic acid

Brand Names: U.S. Folacin-800 [OTC]

Brand Names: Canada Apo-Folic®

Index Terms Folacin; Folate; Pteroylglutamic Acid

Generic Availability (U.S.) Yes

Pharmacologic Category Vitamin, Water Soluble

Use Treatment of megaloblastic and macrocytic anemias due to folate deficiency; dietary supplement

Unlabeled Use Adjunctive cofactor therapy in methanol toxicity (alternative to leucovorin calcium)

Contraindications Hypersensitivity to folic acid or any component of the formulation

Warnings/Precautions Not appropriate for monotherapy with pernicious, aplastic, or normocytic anemias when anemia is present with vitamin B_{12} deficiency. Doses >0.1 mg/day may obscure pernicious anemia with continuing irreversible nerve damage progression. Resistance to treatment may occur with depressed hematopoiesis, alcoholism, and deficiencies of other vitamins. Injection contains benzyl alcohol (1.5%) as preservative.

Adverse Reactions (Reflective of adult population; not specific for elderly) Frequency not defined.

Cardiovascular: Flushing (slight)
Central nervous system: Malaise (general)
Dermatologic: Erythema, pruritus, rash
Respiratory: Bronchospasm
Miscellaneous: Allergic reaction

Drug Interactions

Metabolism/Transport Effects None known.

Avoid Concomitant Use

Avoid concomitant use of Folic Acid with any of the following: Raltitrexed

Increased Effect/Toxicity There are no known significant interactions involving an increase in effect.

Decreased Effect

Folic Acid may decrease the levels/effects of: Fosphenytoin; PHENobarbital; Phenytoin; Primidone; Raltitrexed

The levels/effects of Folic Acid may be decreased by: Green Tea

Stability Do not use with oxidizing and reducing agents or heavy metal ions.

Mechanism of Action Folic acid is necessary for formation of a number of coenzymes in many metabolic systems, particularly for purine and pyrimidine synthesis; required for nucleoprotein synthesis and maintenance in erythropoiesis; stimulates WBC and platelet production in folate deficiency anemia. Folic acid enhances the metabolism of formic acid, the toxic metabolite of methanol, to nontoxic metabolites (unlabeled use).

Pharmacodynamics/Kinetics

Onset of action: Peak effect: Oral: 0.5-1 hour

Absorption: Proximal part of small intestine

Metabolism: Hepatic

Excretion: Urine

Dosage

Geriatric Refer to adult dosing. Vitamin B_{12} deficiency must be ruled out before initiating folate therapy due to frequency of combined nutritional deficiencies: RDA requirements (1999): 400 mcg/day (0.4 mg) minimum.

Adult

Anemia: Oral, I.M., I.V., SubQ: 0.4 mg/day

RDA: Expressed as dietary folate equivalents: 400 mcg/day

Administration Oral preferred, but may also be administered by deep I.M., SubQ, or I.V. injection.

I.V. administration: May administer ≤5 mg dose undiluted over ≥1 minute **or** may dilute ≤5 mg in 50 mL of NS or D_5W and infuse over 30 minutes. May also be added to I.V. maintenance solutions and given as an infusion.

Reference Range Therapeutic: 0.005-0.015 mcg/mL

Test Interactions Falsely low serum concentrations may occur with the *Lactobacillus casei* assay method in patients on anti-infectives (eg, tetracycline)

Pharmacotherapy Pearls The RDA for folic acid is presented as dietary folate equivalents (DFE). DFE adjusts for the difference in bioavailability of folic acid from food as compared to dietary supplements.

Special Geriatric Considerations Elderly frequently have combined nutritional deficiencies. Must rule out vitamin B_{12} deficiency before initiating folate therapy. Elderly, due to decreased nutrient intake, may benefit from daily intake of a multiple vitamin with minerals.

Dosage Forms Excipient information presented when available (limited, particularly for generics); consult specific product labeling.

Injection, solution, as sodium folate: 5 mg/mL (10 mL)

Tablet, oral: 0.4 mg, 0.8 mg, 1 mg

Folacin-800: 0.8 mg [scored; gluten free, sugar free]

Fondaparinux (fon da PARE i nuks)

Related Information

Injectable Heparins/Heparinoids Comparison Table *on page 2119*

Medication Safety Issues

Sound-alike/look-alike issues:

Arixtra® may be confused with Arista® AH (hemostatic device)

High alert medication:

The Institute for Safe Medication Practices (ISMP) includes this medication among its list of drugs which have a heightened risk of causing significant patient harm when used in error.

Brand Names: U.S. Arixtra®

Brand Names: Canada Arixtra®

Index Terms Fondaparinux Sodium

Generic Availability (U.S.) Yes

Pharmacologic Category Factor Xa Inhibitor

Use Prophylaxis of deep vein thrombosis (DVT) in patients undergoing surgery for hip replacement, knee replacement, hip fracture (including extended prophylaxis following hip fracture surgery), or abdominal surgery (in patients at risk for thromboembolic complications); treatment of acute pulmonary embolism (PE); treatment of acute DVT without PE

Canadian labeling: Additional uses (not approved in U.S.): Unstable angina or non-ST segment elevation myocardial infarction (UA/NSTEMI) for the prevention of death and subsequent MI; ST segment elevation MI (STEMI) for the prevention of death and myocardial reinfarction

Unlabeled Use Prophylaxis of DVT in patients with a history of heparin-induced thrombocytopenia (HIT); treatment of acute thrombosis (unrelated to HIT) in patients with a past history of HIT; acute symptomatic superficial vein thrombosis (≥5 cm in length) of the legs

Contraindications Hypersensitivity to fondaparinux or any component of the formulation; severe renal impairment (Cl_{cr} <30 mL/minute); body weight <50 kg (prophylaxis); active major bleeding; bacterial endocarditis; thrombocytopenia associated with a positive *in vitro* test for antiplatelet antibody in the presence of fondaparinux

Warnings/Precautions **[U.S. Boxed Warning]: Spinal or epidural hematomas, including subsequent paralysis, may occur with recent or anticipated neuraxial anesthesia (epidural or spinal anesthesia) or spinal puncture in patients anticoagulated with LMWH, heparinoids, or fondaparinux.** Consider risk versus benefit prior to spinal procedures; risk is increased by the use of concomitant agents which may alter hemostasis, the use of indwelling epidural catheters for analgesia, a history of spinal deformity or spinal surgery, as well as a history of traumatic or repeated epidural or spinal punctures. Patient should be observed closely for bleeding and signs and symptoms of neurological impairment if therapy is administered during or immediately following diagnostic lumbar puncture, epidural anesthesia, or spinal anesthesia.

Discontinue use 24 hours prior to CABG and dose with unfractionated heparin per institutional practice (Jneid, 2012). Use caution in patients with moderate renal dysfunction (Cl_{cr} 30-50 mL/minute); contraindicated in patients with Cl_{cr} <30 mL/minute. Discontinue if severe dysfunction or labile function develops.

Use caution in congenital or acquired bleeding disorders; bacterial endocarditis; renal impairment; hepatic impairment; active ulcerative or angiodysplastic gastrointestinal disease; hemorrhagic stroke; shortly after brain, spinal, or ophthalmologic surgery; or in patients taking platelet inhibitors. Risk of major bleeding may be increased if initial dose is administered earlier than recommended (initiation recommended at 6-8 hours following surgery). Discontinue agents that may enhance the risk of hemorrhage if possible. Although considered an insensitive measure of fondaparinux activity, there have been postmarketing reports of bleeding associated with elevated aPTT. Thrombocytopenia has occurred with administration, including reports of thrombocytopenia with thrombosis similar to heparin-induced thrombocytopenia. Monitor patients closely and discontinue therapy if platelets fall to <100,000/mm^3.

For subcutaneous administration; not for I.M. administration. Do not use interchangeably (unit for unit) with low molecular weight heparins, heparin, or heparinoids. Use caution in patients <50 kg who are being treated for DVT/PE; dosage reduction recommended. Contraindicated in patients <50 kg when used for prophylactic therapy. Use with caution in the elderly. The needle guard contains natural latex rubber.

The administration of fondaparinux as the sole anticoagulant is **not recommended** during PCI due to an increased risk for guiding-catheter thrombosis. Use of an anticoagulant with antithrombin activity (eg, unfractionated heparin) is recommended as adjunctive therapy to PCI even if prior treatment with fondaparinux (must take into account whether GP IIb/IIIa antagonists have been administered) (Levine, 2011). Do not administer with other agents that increase the risk of hemorrhage unless they are essential for the management of the underlying condition (eg, warfarin for treatment of VTE).

Adverse Reactions (Reflective of adult population; not specific for elderly) As with all anticoagulants, bleeding is the major adverse effect. Hemorrhage may occur at any site. Risk appears increased by a number of factors including renal dysfunction, age (>75 years), and weight (<50 kg).
>10%:
  Central nervous system: Fever (4% to 14%)
  Gastrointestinal: Nausea (11%)
  Hematologic: Anemia (20%)
1% to 10%:
  Cardiovascular: Edema (9%), hypotension (4%), thrombosis PCI catheter (without heparin 1%)
  Central nervous system: Insomnia (5%), dizziness (4%), headache (2% to 5%), confusion (3%), pain (2%)
  Dermatologic: Rash (8%), purpura (4%), bullous eruption (3%)
  Endocrine & metabolic: Hypokalemia (1% to 4%)

Gastrointestinal: Constipation (5% to 9%), nausea (3%), vomiting (6%), diarrhea (3%), dyspepsia (2%)

Genitourinary: Urinary tract infection (4%), urinary retention (3%)

Hematologic: Moderate thrombocytopenia (50,000-100,000/mm^3: 3%), major bleeding (1% to 3%), minor bleeding (2% to 4%), hematoma (3%); risk of major bleeding increased as high as 5% in patients receiving initial dose <6 hours following surgery

Hepatic: ALT increased (≤3%), AST increased (≤2%)

Local: Injection site reaction (bleeding, rash, pruritus)

Miscellaneous: Wound drainage increased (5%)

Drug Interactions

Metabolism/Transport Effects None known.

Avoid Concomitant Use

Avoid concomitant use of Fondaparinux with any of the following: Rivaroxaban

Increased Effect/Toxicity

Fondaparinux may increase the levels/effects of: Anticoagulants; Collagenase (Systemic); Dabigatran Etexilate; Deferasirox; Ibritumomab; Rivaroxaban; Tositumomab and Iodine I 131 Tositumomab

The levels/effects of Fondaparinux may be increased by: Antiplatelet Agents; Dasatinib; Drotrecogin Alfa (Activated); Herbs (Anticoagulant/Antiplatelet Properties); Nonsteroidal Anti-Inflammatory Agents; Pentosan Polysulfate Sodium; Prostacyclin Analogues; Salicylates; Thrombolytic Agents; Tipranavir

Decreased Effect There are no known significant interactions involving a decrease in effect.

Ethanol/Nutrition/Herb Interactions Herb/Nutraceutical: Avoid alfalfa, anise, bilberry, bladderwrack, bromelain, cat's claw, celery, coleus, cordyceps, dong quai, evening primrose oil, fenugreek, feverfew, garlic, ginger, ginkgo biloba, ginseng (American/Panax/Siberian), grapeseed, green tea, guggul, horse chestnut seed, horseradish, licorice, prickly ash, red clover, reishi, sweet clover, turmeric, white willow (all possess anticoagulant or antiplatelet activity and as such, may enhance the anticoagulant effects of fondaparinux).

Stability Store at 25°C (77°F); excursions permitted to 15°C to 30°C (59°F to 86°F).

Canadian labeling: For I.V. administration: May mix with 25 mL or 50 mL NS; manufacturer recommends immediate use once diluted in NS, but is stable for up to 24 hours at 15°C to 30°C (59°F to 86°F).

Mechanism of Action Fondaparinux is a synthetic pentasaccharide that causes an antithrombin III-mediated selective inhibition of factor Xa. Neutralization of factor Xa interrupts the blood coagulation cascade and inhibits thrombin formation and thrombus development.

Pharmacodynamics/Kinetics

Absorption: SubQ: Rapid and complete

Distribution: V_d: 7-11 L; mainly in blood

Protein binding: ≥94% to antithrombin III

Bioavailability: SubQ: 100%

Half-life elimination: 17-21 hours; prolonged with renal impairment

Time to peak: SubQ: 2-3 hours

Excretion: Urine (~77%, unchanged drug)

Dosage

Geriatric & Adult

DVT prophylaxis: SubQ: Adults ≥50 kg: 2.5 mg once daily. **Note:** Prophylactic use contraindicated in patients <50 kg. Initiate dose after hemostasis has been established, 6-8 hours postoperatively.

DVT prophylaxis with history of HIT (unlabeled use): SubQ: 2.5 mg once daily (Blackmer, 2009; Harenberg, 2004; Parody, 2003)

Usual duration: 5-9 days (up to 10 days following abdominal surgery or up to 11 days following hip replacement or knee replacement). The American College of Chest Physicians recommends a minimum of 10-14 days for patients undergoing total hip arthroplasty, total knee arthroplasty, or hip fracture surgery; extended duration of up to 35 days suggested (Guyatt, 2012).

Acute DVT/PE treatment: SubQ: **Note:** Start warfarin on the first or second treatment day and continue fondaparinux until INR is ≥2 for at least 24 hours (usually 5-7 days) (Guyatt, 2012):

<50 kg: 5 mg once daily

50-100 kg: 7.5 mg once daily

>100 kg: 10 mg once daily

Usual duration: 5-9 days (has been administered up to 26 days)

Acute coronary syndrome (Canadian labeling; unlabeled use in U.S.):

UA/NSTEMI: SubQ: 2.5 mg once daily; initiate as soon as possible after presentation; treat for up to 8 days or until hospital discharge (Anderson, 2007; Yusuf 2006a)

STEMI: I.V.: 2.5 mg once; subsequent doses: SubQ: 2.5 mg once daily; treat for up to 8 days or until hospital discharge (Antman, 2007; Yusuf, 2006b)

Note: Discontinue fondaparinux 24 hours prior to coronary artery bypass graft (CABG) surgery; instead, administer unfractionated heparin per institutional practice (Anderson, 2007).

Acute symptomatic superficial vein thrombosis (≥5 cm in length) of the legs (unlabeled use): SubQ: 2.5 mg once daily for 45 days (Decousus, 2010; Guyatt, 2012)

Acute thrombosis (unrelated to HIT) in patients with a past history of HIT (unlabeled use; Guyatt, 2012; Warkentin, 2011): SubQ:

<50 kg: 5 mg once daily

50-100 kg: 7.5 mg once daily

>100 kg: 10 mg once daily

Renal Impairment

Cl_{cr} 30-50 mL/minute: Use caution; total clearance ~40% lower compared to patients with normal renal function. When used for thromboprophylaxis, the American College of Chest Physicians suggests a 50% reduction in dose or use of low-dose heparin instead of fondaparinux (Garcia, 2012).

Cl_{cr} <30 mL/minute: Use is contraindicated.

Hepatic Impairment

Mild-to-moderate impairment: Dosage adjustment not required; monitor for signs of bleeding.

Severe impairment: No dosage adjustment provided in manufacturer's labeling (has not been studied).

Administration Do **not** administer I.M.; intended for SubQ administration. Do not mix with other injections or infusions. Do not expel air bubble from syringe before injection. Administer according to recommended regimen; when used for DVT prophylaxis, early initiation (before 6 hours after orthopedic surgery) has been associated with increased bleeding. For STEMI patients (Canadian labeling; unlabeled use in U.S.) may administer initial dose as I.V. push or mix in 25-50 mL of NS (do not mix with other agents) and infuse over 2 minutes; flush tubing with NS after infusion to ensure complete administration for fondaparinux.

To convert from I.V. unfractionated heparin (UFH) infusion to SubQ fondaparinux (Nutescu, 2007): Calculate specific dose for fondaparinux based on indication, discontinue UFH, and begin fondaparinux within 1 hour

To convert from SubQ fondaparinux to I.V. UFH infusion (Nutescu, 2007): Discontinue fondaparinux; calculate specific dose for I.V. UFH infusion based on indication; omit heparin bolus/loading dose

For subQ fondaparinux dosed every 24 hours: Start I.V. UFH infusion 22-23 hours after last dose of fondaparinux

Monitoring Parameters Periodic monitoring of CBC, serum creatinine, occult blood testing of stools recommended. Anti-Xa activity of fondaparinux can be measured by the assay if fondaparinux is used as the calibrator. PT and aPTT are insensitive measures of fondaparinux activity. If unexpected changes in coagulation parameters or major bleeding occur, discontinue fondaparinux (elevated aPTT associated with bleeding events have been reported in postmarketing data).

Reference Range Note: Routine monitoring is not recommended; the following fondaparinux-specific anti-Xa concentrations have been reported (Garcia, 2012):

Thromboprophylaxis dose: Anti-Xa activity at 3 hours post dose: ~0.39-0.5 mg/L

Therapeutic dosing (eg, 7.5 mg once daily): Anti-Xa activity at 3 hours post dose: 1.2-1.26 mg/L

Test Interactions International standards of heparin or LMWH are not the appropriate calibrators for antifactor Xa activity of fondaparinux.

Special Geriatric Considerations Use with caution in patients with estimated or actual creatinine clearance between 30-50 mL/minute. Contraindicated in patients with Cl_{cr} <30 mL/minute.

Dosage Forms Excipient information presented when available (limited, particularly for generics); consult specific product labeling.

Injection, solution, as sodium [preservative free]: 2.5 mg/0.5 mL (0.5 mL); 5 mg/0.4 mL (0.4 mL); 7.5 mg/0.6 mL (0.6 mL); 10 mg/0.8 mL (0.8 mL)

Arixtra®: 2.5 mg/0.5 mL (0.5 mL); 5 mg/0.4 mL (0.4 mL); 7.5 mg/0.6 mL (0.6 mL); 10 mg/0.8 mL (0.8 mL)

◆ **Fondaparinux Sodium** *see* Fondaparinux *on page 837*
◆ **Foradil® Aerolizer®** *see* Formoterol *on page 841*

Formoterol (for MOH te rol)

Related Information
Inhalant Agents *on page 2117*

Medication Safety Issues
Sound-alike/look-alike issues:
Foradil® may be confused with Toradol®

Administration issues:
Foradil® capsules for inhalation are for administration via Aerolizer™ inhaler and are **not** for oral use.

International issues:
Foradil [U.S., Canada, and multiple international markets] may be confused with Theradol brand name for tramadol [Netherlands]

Brand Names: U.S. Foradil® Aerolizer®; Performoist®

Brand Names: Canada Foradil®; Oxeze® Turbuhaler®

Index Terms Formoterol Fumarate; Formoterol Fumarate Dihydrate

Generic Availability (U.S.) No

Pharmacologic Category Beta$_2$ Agonist; Beta$_2$-Adrenergic Agonist, Long-Acting

Use Maintenance treatment of asthma and prevention of bronchospasm (as concomitant therapy) in patients ≥5 years of age with reversible obstructive airway disease, including patients with symptoms of nocturnal asthma; maintenance treatment of bronchoconstriction in patients with COPD; prevention of exercise-induced bronchospasm in patients ≥5 years of age (monotherapy may be indicated in patients without persistent asthma)

Canadian labeling: Oxeze®: Also approved for acute relief of symptoms ("on demand" treatment) in patients ≥6 years of age

Medication Guide Available Yes

Contraindications Hypersensitivity to formoterol or any component of the formulation (Foradil® only); monotherapy in the treatment of asthma (ie, use without a concomitant long-term asthma control medication, such as an inhaled corticosteroid)

Canadian labeling: Oxeze®: Hypersensitivity to formoterol, inhaled lactose, or any component of the formulation; presence of tachyarrhythmias

Warnings/Precautions [U.S. Boxed Warning]: Long-acting beta$_2$-agonists (LABAs) increase the risk of asthma-related deaths. Formoterol should only be used in asthma patients as adjunvant therapy in patients who are currently receiving but are not adequately controlled on a long-term asthma control medication (ie, an inhaled cortico-steroid). Monotherapy with an LABA is contraindicated in the treatment of asthma. In a large, randomized, placebo-controlled U.S. clinical trial (SMART, 2006), salmeterol was associated with an increase in asthma-related deaths (when added to usual asthma therapy); risk is considered a class effect among all LABAs. Data are not available to determine if the addition of an inhaled corticosteroid lessens this increased risk of death associated with LABA use. Assess patients at regular intervals once asthma control is maintained on combination therapy to determine if step-down therapy is appropriate and the LABA can be discontinued (without loss of asthma control), and the patient can be maintained on an inhaled corticosteroid. LABAs are not appropriate in patients whose asthma is adequately controlled on low- or medium-dose inhaled corticosteroids. Do **not** use for acute bronchospasm. Short-acting beta$_2$-agonist (eg, albuterol) should be used for acute symptoms and symptoms occurring between treatments. Do **not** initiate in patients with significantly worsening or acutely deteriorating asthma; reports of severe (sometimes fatal) respiratory events have been reported when formoterol has been initiated in this situation. Corticosteroids should not be stopped or reduced when formoterol is initiated. Formoterol is not a substitute for inhaled or systemic corticosteroids and should not be used as monotherapy. During initiation, watch for signs of worsening asthma.

Because LABAs may disguise poorly controlled persistent asthma, frequent or chronic use of LABAs for exercise-induced bronchospasm is discouraged by the NIH Asthma Guidelines (NIH, 2007). The safety and efficacy of Performoist™ in the treatment of asthma have not been established. Oxeze® is a formulation of formoterol (available outside the U.S. [eg, Canada]) approved for acute treatment of asthmatic symptoms. The labelings for U.S. approved formulations (Foradil®, Performoist™) state that formoterol is not meant to relieve acute asthmatic symptoms.

Do **not** use for acute episodes of COPD. Do **not** initiate in patients with significantly worsening or acutely deteriorating COPD. Data are not available to determine if LABA use increases the risk of death in patients with COPD. Increased use and/or ineffectiveness of short-acting beta$_2$-agonists may indicate rapidly deteriorating disease and should prompt re-evaluation of the patient's condition.

Immediate hypersensitivity reactions (urticaria, angioedema, rash, bronchospasm) have been reported. Do not exceed recommended dose or frequency; serious adverse events (including serious asthma exacerbations and fatalities) have been associated with excessive use of inhaled sympathomimetics. Beta$_2$-agonists may increase risk of arrhythmias, decrease serum potassium, prolong QT_c interval, or increase serum glucose. These effects may be exacerbated in hypoxemia. Use caution in patients with cardiovascular disease (arrhythmia, coronary insufficiency, hypertension, or HF), seizures, diabetes, hyperthyroidism, or hypokalemia. Beta-agonists may cause elevation in blood pressure and heart rate, and result in CNS stimulation/excitation. Tolerance to the bronchodilator effect, measured by FEV_1, has been observed in studies.

Powder for oral inhalation contains lactose; very rare anaphylactic reactions have been reported in patients with severe milk protein allergy. The contents of the Foradil® capsules are for inhalation via the Aerolizer™ device. There have been reports of incorrect administration (swallowing of the capsules).

Adverse Reactions (Reflective of adult population; not specific for elderly)
1% to 10%:
  Cardiovascular: Chest pain (2% to 3%), palpitation
  Central nervous system: Anxiety (2%), dizziness (2%), fever (2%), insomnia (2%), dysphonia (1%), headache
  Dermatologic: Pruritus (2%), rash (1%)
  Gastrointestinal: Diarrhea (5%), nausea (5%), xerostomia (1% to 3%), vomiting (2%), abdominal pain, dyspepsia, gastroenteritis
  Neuromuscular & skeletal: Muscle cramps (2%), tremor
  Respiratory: Infection (3% to 7%), asthma exacerbation (age 5-12 years: 5% to 6%; age >12 years: <4%), bronchitis (5%), pharyngitis (3% to 4%), sinusitis (3%), dyspnea (2%), tonsillitis (1%)

Drug Interactions
  Metabolism/Transport Effects Substrate of CYP2C9 (minor); **Note:** Assignment of Major/Minor substrate status based on clinically relevant drug interaction potential
  Avoid Concomitant Use
  Avoid concomitant use of Formoterol with any of the following: Beta-Blockers (Nonselective); Iobenguane I 123
  Increased Effect/Toxicity
  Formoterol may increase the levels/effects of: Loop Diuretics; Sympathomimetics; Thiazide Diuretics

  The levels/effects of Formoterol may be increased by: AtoMOXetine; Caffeine; Cannabinoids; MAO Inhibitors; Theophylline Derivatives; Tricyclic Antidepressants
  Decreased Effect
  Formoterol may decrease the levels/effects of: Iobenguane I 123

  The levels/effects of Formoterol may be decreased by: Alpha-/Beta-Blockers; Beta-Blockers (Beta1 Selective); Beta-Blockers (Nonselective); Betahistine

Stability
  Foradil®: Prior to dispensing, store in refrigerator at 2°C to 8°C (36°F to 46°F). After dispensing, store at room temperature at 20°C to 25°C (68°F to 77°F). Protect from heat and moisture. Capsules should always be stored in the blister and only removed immediately before use. Always check expiration date. Use within 4 months of purchase date or product expiration date, whichever comes first.
  Perforomist™: Prior to dispensing, store in refrigerator at 2°C to 8°C (36°F to 46°F). After dispensing, store at 2°C to 25°C (36°F to 77°F) for up to 3 months. Protect from heat. Unit-dose vials should always be stored in the foil pouch and only removed immediately before use.

Mechanism of Action
Relaxes bronchial smooth muscle by selective action on beta$_2$ receptors with little effect on heart rate. Formoterol has a long-acting effect.

Pharmacodynamics/Kinetics
  Onset of action: Powder for inhalation: Within 3 minutes
  Peak effect: Powder for inhalation: 80% of peak effect within 15 minutes; Solution for nebulization: 2 hours
  Duration: Improvement in FEV_1 observed for 12 hours in most patients
  Absorption: Rapidly into plasma
  Protein binding: 61% to 64% *in vitro* at higher concentrations than achieved with usual dosing
  Metabolism: Hepatic via direct glucuronidation and O-demethylation; CYP2D6, CYP2C8/9, CYP2C19, CYP2A6 involved in O-demethylation
  Half-life elimination: Powder: ~10-14 hours; Nebulized solution: ~7 hours
  Time to peak: Maximum improvement in FEV_1 in 1-3 hours

Excretion: Urine (15% to 18% as direct glucuronide metabolites, 2% to 10% as unchanged drug)

Dosage

Geriatric & Adult

Asthma, maintenance: Inhalation: **Note:** For asthma control, long-acting beta$_2$-agonists (LABAs) should be used in combination with inhaled corticosteroids and **not** as monotherapy

Foradil®: 12 mcg capsule inhaled every 12 hours via Aerolizer™ device (maximum: 24 mcg/day)

Oxeze® (CAN): **Note:** Not labeled for use in the U.S.: Inhalation: 6 mcg or 12 mcg every 12 hours (maximum dose: 48 mcg/day)

Exercise-induced bronchospasm: Inhalation:

Foradil®: 12 mcg capsule inhaled via Aerolizer™ device at least 15 minutes before exercise on an "as needed" basis; additional doses should not be used for another 12 hours. **Note:** If already using for asthma maintenance then should not use additional doses for exercise-induced bronchospasm. Because LABAs may disguise poorly controlled persistent asthma, frequent or chronic use of LABAs for exercise-induced bronchospasm is discouraged by the NIH Asthma Guidelines (NIH, 2007).

Oxeze® (CAN): **Note:** Not labeled for use in the U.S.: Inhalation: 6 mcg or 12 mcg at least 15 minutes before exercise.

COPD (maintenance): Inhalation:

Foradil®: 12 mcg capsule inhaled every 12 hours via Aerolizer™ device (maximum: 24 mcg/day)

Performist™: 20 mcg twice daily (maximum dose: 40 mcg/day)

Acute ("on demand") relief of bronchoconstriction: *Indication for Oxeze® approved in Canada:* 6 mcg or 12 mcg as a single dose (maximum dose: 72 mcg/24-hour period). The prolonged use of high dosages (48 mcg/day for ≥3 consecutive days) may be a sign of suboptimal control, and should prompt the re-evaluation of therapy.

Renal Impairment Not studied

Administration

Foradil®: Remove capsule from foil blister **immediately** before use. Place capsule in the capsule-chamber in the base of the Aerolizer™ Inhaler. Must only use the Aerolizer™ Inhaler. Press both buttons **once only** and then release. Keep inhaler in a level, horizontal position. Exhale fully. Do not exhale into inhaler. Tilt head slightly back and inhale (rapidly, steadily, and deeply). Hold breath as long as possible. If any powder remains in capsule, exhale and inhale again. Repeat until capsule is empty. Throw away empty capsule; do not leave in inhaler. Do not use a spacer with the Aerolizer™ Inhaler. Always keep capsules and inhaler dry.

Performist™: Remove unit-dose vial from foil pouch **immediately** before use. Solution does not require dilution prior to administration; do not mix other medications with formoterol solution. Place contents of unit-dose vial into the reservoir of a standard jet nebulizer connected to an air compressor; assemble nebulizer based on the manufacturer's instructions and turn nebulizer on; breathe deeply and evenly until all of the medication has been inhaled. Discard any unused medication immediately; do not ingest contents of vial. Clean nebulizer after use.

Oxeze® Turbuhaler® [CAN; not available in U.S.]: Hold inhaler upright. Turn colored grip as far as it will go in one direction and then turn back to original position; a clicking sound should be heard which means the inhaler is ready for use. Exhale fully. Do not exhale into mouthpiece of inhaler. Place mouthpiece to lips and inhale forcefully and deeply. Do not chew or bite on mouthpiece. Clean outside of mouthpiece once weekly with a dry tissue. Avoid getting inhaler wet.

Monitoring Parameters FEV$_1$, peak flow, and/or other pulmonary function tests; blood pressure, heart rate; CNS stimulation; serum glucose, serum potassium

Special Geriatric Considerations Elderly patients should be specifically counseled about the proper use of this inhaler/spacing of doses and/or the proper use of a nebulizer system. No significant difference in both safety and effectiveness was seen between elderly and younger patients.

Dosage Forms Excipient information presented when available (limited, particularly for generics); consult specific product labeling.

Powder, for oral inhalation, as fumarate:

Foradil® Aerolizer®: 12 mcg/capsule (12s, 60s) [contains lactose 25 mg/capsule]

Solution, for nebulization, as fumarate dihydrate:

Performist®: 20 mcg/2 mL (60s)

Dosage Forms: Canada Excipient information presented when available (limited, particularly for generics); consult specific product labeling.

Powder for oral inhalation, as fumarate:

Oxeze® Turbuhaler®: 6 mcg/inhalation [delivers 60 metered doses; contains lactose 600 mcg/dose]; 12 mcg/inhalation [delivers 60 metered doses; contains lactose 600 mcg/dose]

Fosaprepitant (fos a PRE pi tant)

Medication Safety Issues
Sound-alike/look-alike issues:
Fosaprepitant may be confused with aprepitant, fosamprenavir, fospropofol
Emend® for Injection (fosaprepitant) may be confused with Emend® (aprepitant) which is an oral capsule formulation.

Brand Names: U.S. Emend® for Injection
Brand Names: Canada Emend® IV
Index Terms Aprepitant Injection; Fosaprepitant Dimeglumine; L-758,298; MK 0517
Generic Availability (U.S.) No
Pharmacologic Category Antiemetic; Substance P/Neurokinin 1 Receptor Antagonist
Use Prevention of acute and delayed nausea and vomiting associated with moderately- and highly-emetogenic chemotherapy (in combination with other antiemetics)
Contraindications Hypersensitivity to fosaprepitant, aprepitant, polysorbate 80, or any component of the formulation; concurrent use with pimozide or cisapride

Canadian labeling: Additional contraindications (not in U.S. labeling): Concurrent use with astemizole or terfenadine
Warnings/Precautions Fosaprepitant is rapidly converted to aprepitant, which has a high potential for drug interactions. Use caution with agents primarily metabolized via CYP3A4; aprepitant is a 3A4 inhibitor. Effect on orally administered 3A4 substrates is greater than those administered intravenously. Immediate hypersensitivity has been reported (rarely) with fosaprepitant; stop infusion with hypersensitivity symptoms (dyspnea, erythema, flushing, or anaphylaxis); do not reinitiate. Use caution with hepatic impairment; has not been studied in patients with severe hepatic impairment (Child-Pugh class C). Not studied for treatment of existing nausea and vomiting. Chronic continuous administration of fosaprepitant is not recommended.
Adverse Reactions (Reflective of adult population; not specific for elderly) Adverse reactions reported with aprepitant and fosaprepitant (as part of a combination chemotherapy regimen) occurring at a higher frequency than standard antiemetic therapy:

1% to 10%:
Central nervous system: Fatigue (1% to 3%), headache (2%)
Gastrointestinal: Anorexia (2%), constipation 2%), dyspepsia (2%), diarrhea (1%), eructation (1%)
Hepatic: ALT increased (1% to 3%), AST increased (1%)
Local: Injection site reactions (3%; includes erythema, induration, pain, pruritus, or thrombophlebitis)
Neuromuscular & skeletal: Weakness (3%)
Miscellaneous: Hiccups (5%)
Drug Interactions
Metabolism/Transport Effects Substrate of CYP1A2 (minor), CYP2C19 (minor), CYP3A4 (major); **Note:** Assignment of Major/Minor substrate status based on clinically relevant drug

interaction potential; **Inhibits** CYP2C19 (weak), CYP2C9 (weak), CYP3A4 (moderate); **Induces** CYP2C9 (weak/moderate), CYP3A4 (weak/moderate)

Avoid Concomitant Use

Avoid concomitant use of Fosaprepitant with any of the following: Astemizole; Axitinib; Cisapride; Conivaptan; Pimozide; Terfenadine; Tolvaptan

Increased Effect/Toxicity

Fosaprepitant may increase the levels/effects of: ARIPiprazole; Astemizole; Avanafil; Benzodiazepines (metabolized by oxidation); Budesonide (Systemic, Oral Inhalation); Cisapride; Colchicine; Corticosteroids (Systemic); CYP3A4 Substrates; Diltiazem; Eplerenone; Everolimus; FentaNYL; Halofantrine; Ivacaftor; Lurasidone; Pimecrolimus; Pimozide; Propafenone; Ranolazine; Salmeterol; Saxagliptin; Terfenadine; Tolvaptan; Vilazodone; Zuclopenthixol

The levels/effects of Fosaprepitant may be increased by: Antifungal Agents (Azole Derivatives, Systemic); Conivaptan; CYP3A4 Inhibitors (Moderate); CYP3A4 Inhibitors (Strong); Dasatinib; Diltiazem; Ivacaftor; Mifepristone

Decreased Effect

Fosaprepitant may decrease the levels/effects of: ARIPiprazole; Axitinib; Contraceptives (Estrogens); Contraceptives (Progestins); Ifosfamide; PARoxetine; Saxagliptin; TOLBUTamide; Warfarin

The levels/effects of Fosaprepitant may be decreased by: CYP3A4 Inducers (Strong); Deferasirox; Herbs (CYP3A4 Inducers); PARoxetine; Rifampin; Tocilizumab

Ethanol/Nutrition/Herb Interactions

Food: Aprepitant serum concentration may be increased when taken with grapefruit juice; avoid concurrent use.

Herb/Nutraceutical: Avoid St John's wort (may decrease aprepitant levels).

Stability Store intact vials at 2°C to 8°C (36°F to 46°F). Reconstitute either vial size with 5 mL of sodium chloride 0.9%, directing diluent down side of vial to avoid foaming; swirl gently. Add reconstituted contents of the 150 mg vial to 145 mL sodium chloride 0.9% (add 115 mg vial to 110 mL), resulting in a final concentration of 1 mg/mL; gently invert bag to mix. Solutions diluted for infusion are stable for 24 hours at room temperature of ≤25°C (≤77°F).

Mechanism of Action Fosaprepitant is a prodrug of aprepitant, a substance P/neurokinin 1 (NK1) receptor antagonist. It is rapidly converted to aprepitant which prevents acute and delayed vomiting by inhibiting the substance P/neurokinin 1 (NK1) receptor; augments the antiemetic activity of the 5-HT$_3$ receptor antagonist and corticosteroid activity and inhibits chemotherapy-induced emesis.

Pharmacodynamics/Kinetics

Distribution: Fosaprepitant: ~5 L; Aprepitant: V$_d$: ~70 L; crosses the blood-brain barrier

Protein binding: Aprepitant: >95%

Metabolism:

Fosaprepitant: Hepatic and extrahepatic; rapidly (within 30 minutes after the end of infusion) converted to aprepitant (nearly complete conversion)

Aprepitant: Hepatic via CYP3A4 (major); CYP1A2 and CYP2C19 (minor); forms 7 weakly-active metabolites

Half-life elimination: Fosaprepitant: ~2 minutes; Aprepitant: ~9-13 hours

Time to peak, plasma: Fosaprepitant is converted to aprepitant within 30 minutes after the end of infusion

Excretion: Urine (57%); feces (45%)

Dosage

Geriatric & Adult Prevention of chemotherapy-induced nausea/vomiting: I.V.:

Single-dose regimen (for highly-emetogenic chemotherapy): 150 mg over 20-30 minutes ~30 minutes prior to chemotherapy on day 1 only (in combination with a 5-HT$_3$ antagonist on day 1 and dexamethasone on days 1 to 4)

3-day regimen (for highly-emetogenic chemotherapy): 115 mg over 15 minutes 30 minutes prior to chemotherapy on day 1, followed by aprepitant 80 mg orally on days 2 and 3 (in combination with a 5-HT$_3$ antagonist on day 1 and dexamethasone on days 1 to 4)

3-day regimen (for moderately-emetogenic chemotherapy): 115 mg over 15 minutes 30 minutes prior to chemotherapy on day 1, followed by aprepitant 80 mg orally on days 2 and 3 (in combination with a 5-HT$_3$ antagonist and dexamethasone on day 1)

Renal Impairment

Mild, moderate, or severe impairment: No adjustment required.

Dialysis-dependent end-stage renal disease (ESRD): No adjustment required.

Hepatic Impairment

Child-Pugh class A or B: No adjustment required.

Child-Pugh class C: Has not been evaluated; use with caution.

Administration

115 mg: Infuse over 15 minutes 30 minutes prior to chemotherapy

150 mg: Infuse over 20-30 minutes ~30 minutes prior to chemotherapy

FOSAPREPITANT

Pharmacotherapy Pearls Oncology Comment: Fosaprepitant is recommended in the National Comprehensive Cancer Network® (NCCN) Clinical Practice Guidelines in Oncology for Antiemesis (version 1.2011) for use on day 1 in combination with a serotonin receptor antagonist and dexamethasone for chemotherapy with high emetic risk and for select moderately emetogenic regimens (carboplatin, cisplatin, doxorubicin, epirubicin, ifosfamide, irinotecan, or methotrexate). Either fosaprepitant 115 mg or aprepitant (125 mg orally) are administered on day 1; for day 2 and 3, patients should receive aprepitant 80 mg orally. The 1-day regimen (fosaprepitant 150 mg on day 1 only) is listed in the guidelines for highly emetogenic treatments.

Special Geriatric Considerations Prior studies with aprepitant by the manufacturer were demonstrated in a total of 544 patients, 31% were >65 years of age, while 5% were >75 years. No differences in safety and efficacy were noted between elderly subjects and younger adults. No dosing adjustment is necessary.

Dosage Forms Excipient information presented when available (limited, particularly for generics); consult specific product labeling. [DSC] = Discontinued product

Injection, powder for reconstitution:
Emend® for Injection: 115 mg [DSC] [contains edetate disodium, lactose 287.5 mg, polysorbate 80]
Emend® for Injection: 150 mg [contains edetate disodium, lactose 375 mg, polysorbate 80]

◆ **Fosaprepitant Dimeglumine** see Fosaprepitant on page 844

Fosinopril (foe SIN oh pril)

Related Information
Angiotensin Agents on page 2093
Heart Failure (Systolic) on page 2203
Medication Safety Issues
Sound-alike/look-alike issues:
Fosinopril may be confused with FLUoxetine, Fosamax®, furosemide, lisinopril
Monopril may be confused with Accupril®, minoxidil, moexipril, Monoket®, Monurol®, ramipril
Brand Names: Canada Apo-Fosinopril®; Jamp-Fosinopril; Monopril®; Mylan-Fosinopril; PMS-Fosinopril; RAN™-Fosinopril; Riva-Fosinopril; Teva-Fosinopril
Index Terms Fosinopril Sodium; Monopril
Generic Availability (U.S.) Yes
Pharmacologic Category Angiotensin-Converting Enzyme (ACE) Inhibitor
Use Treatment of hypertension, either alone or in combination with other antihypertensive agents; treatment of heart failure (HF)
Contraindications Hypersensitivity to fosinopril, any other ACE inhibitor, or any component of the formulation; angioedema related to previous treatment with an ACE inhibitor
Warnings/Precautions Anaphylactic reactions may occur rarely with ACE inhibitors. At any time during treatment (especially following first dose), angioedema may occur rarely with ACE inhibitors; it may involve the head and neck (potentially compromising airway) or the intestine (presenting with abdominal pain). African-Americans may be at an increased risk and patients with idiopathic or hereditary angioedema may be at an increased risk. Prolonged frequent monitoring may be required especially if tongue, glottis, or larynx are involved as they are associated with airway obstruction. Patients with a history of airway surgery may have a higher risk of airway obstruction. Aggressive early and appropriate management is critical. Use in patients with previous angioedema associated with ACE inhibitor therapy is contraindicated. Severe anaphylactoid reactions may be seen during hemodialysis (eg, CVVHD) with high-flux dialysis membranes (eg, AN69), and rarely, during low density lipoprotein apheresis with dextran sulfate cellulose. Rare cases of anaphylactoid reactions have been reported in patients undergoing sensitization treatment with hymenoptera (bee, wasp) venom while receiving ACE inhibitors.

Symptomatic hypotension with or without syncope can occur with ACE inhibitors (usually with the first several doses); effects are most often observed in volume-depleted patients; correct volume depletion prior to initiation; close monitoring of patient is required especially with initial dosing and dosing increases; blood pressure must be lowered at a rate appropriate for the patient's clinical condition. Initiation of therapy in patients with ischemic heart disease or cerebrovascular disease warrants close observation due to the potential consequences posed by falling blood pressure (eg, MI, stroke). Use with caution in hypertrophic cardiomyopathy with outflow tract obstruction, severe aortic stenosis, or before, during, or immediately after major surgery.

Hyperkalemia may occur with ACE inhibitors; risk factors include renal dysfunction, diabetes mellitus, concomitant use of potassium-sparing diuretics, potassium supplements, and/or potassium-containing salts. Use cautiously, if at all, with these agents and monitor potassium closely. Cough may occur with ACE inhibitors. Other causes of cough should be considered (eg, pulmonary congestion in patients with heart failure) and excluded prior to discontinuation.

May be associated with deterioration of renal function and/or increases in serum creatinine, particularly in patients with low renal blood flow (eg, renal artery stenosis, heart failure) whose glomerular filtration rate (GFR) is dependent on efferent arteriolar vasoconstriction by angiotensin II; deterioration may result in oliguria, acute renal failure, and progressive azotemia. Small increases in serum creatinine may occur following initiation; consider discontinuation only in patients with progressive and/or significant deterioration in renal function. Use with caution in patients with unstented unilateral/bilateral renal artery stenosis. When unstented bilateral renal artery stenosis is present, use is generally avoided due to the elevated risk of deterioration in renal function unless possible benefits outweigh risks. Concurrent use of angiotensin receptor blockers may increase the risk of clinically-significant adverse events (eg, renal dysfunction, hyperkalemia).

Rare toxicities associated with ACE inhibitors include cholestatic jaundice (which may progress to fulminant hepatic necrosis), agranulocytosis, neutropenia or leukopenia with myeloid hypoplasia. Patients with collagen vascular diseases (especially with concomitant renal impairment) or renal impairment alone may be at increased risk for hematologic toxicity; periodically monitor CBC with differential in these patients.

Adverse Reactions (Reflective of adult population; not specific for elderly) Note: Frequency ranges include data from hypertension and heart failure trials. Higher rates of adverse reactions have generally been noted in patients with CHF. However, the frequency of adverse effects associated with placebo is also increased in this population.

>10%: Central nervous system: Dizziness (2% to 12%)
1% to 10%:
  Cardiovascular: Orthostatic hypotension (1% to 2%), palpitation (1%)
  Central nervous system: Dizziness (1% to 2%; up to 12% in CHF patients), headache (3%), fatigue (1% to 2%)
  Endocrine & metabolic: Hyperkalemia (2.6%)
  Gastrointestinal: Diarrhea (2%), nausea/vomiting (1.2% to 2.2%)
  Hepatic: Transaminases increased
  Neuromuscular & skeletal: Musculoskeletal pain (<1% to 3%), noncardiac chest pain (<1% to 2%), weakness (1%)
  Renal: Serum creatinine increased, renal function worsening (in patients with bilateral renal artery stenosis or hypovolemia)
  Respiratory: Cough (2% to 10%)
  Miscellaneous: Upper respiratory infection (2%)
>1% but ≤ frequency in patients receiving placebo: Sexual dysfunction, fever, flu-like syndrome, dyspnea, rash, headache, insomnia
Other events reported with ACE inhibitors: Neutropenia, agranulocytosis, eosinophilic pneumonitis, cardiac arrest, pancytopenia, hemolytic anemia, anemia, aplastic anemia, thrombocytopenia, acute renal failure, hepatic failure, jaundice, symptomatic hyponatremia, bullous pemphigus, exfoliative dermatitis, Stevens-Johnson syndrome. In addition, a syndrome which may include fever, myalgia, arthralgia, interstitial nephritis, vasculitis, rash, eosinophilia and positive ANA, and elevated ESR has been reported for other ACE inhibitors.

Drug Interactions
Metabolism/Transport Effects None known.
Avoid Concomitant Use There are no known interactions where it is recommended to avoid concomitant use.
Increased Effect/Toxicity
  Fosinopril may increase the levels/effects of: Allopurinol; Amifostine; Antihypertensives; AzaTHIOprine; CycloSPORINE; CycloSPORINE (Systemic); Ferric Gluconate; Gold Sodium Thiomalate; Hypotensive Agents; Iron Dextran Complex; Lithium; Nonsteroidal Anti-Inflammatory Agents; RiTUXimab; Sodium Phosphates

  The levels/effects of Fosinopril may be increased by: Alfuzosin; Aliskiren; Angiotensin II Receptor Blockers; Diazoxide; DPP-IV Inhibitors; Eplerenone; Everolimus; Herbs (Hypotensive Properties); Loop Diuretics; MAO Inhibitors; Pentoxifylline; Phosphodiesterase 5 Inhibitors; Potassium Salts; Potassium-Sparing Diuretics; Prostacyclin Analogues; Sirolimus; Temsirolimus; Thiazide Diuretics; TIZANidine; Tolvaptan; Trimethoprim
Decreased Effect
  The levels/effects of Fosinopril may be decreased by: Antacids; Aprotinin; Herbs (Hypertensive Properties); Icatibant; Lanthanum; Methylphenidate; Nonsteroidal Anti-Inflammatory Agents; Salicylates; Yohimbine

FOSINOPRIL

Ethanol/Nutrition/Herb Interactions
Food: Potassium supplements and/or potassium-containing salts may cause or worsen hyperkalemia. Management: Consult prescriber before consuming a potassium-rich diet, potassium supplements, or salt substitutes.

Herb/Nutraceutical: Some herbal medications may worsen hypertension (eg, licorice); others may increase the antihypertensive effect of fosinopril (eg, shepherd's purse). Management: Avoid bayberry, blue cohosh, cayenne, ephedra, ginger, ginseng (American), kola, licorice, and yohimbe. Avoid black cohosh, california poppy, coleus, golden seal, hawthorn, mistletoe, periwinkle, quinine, and shepherd's purse.

Stability Store at 25°C (77°F); excursions permitted to 15°C to 30°C (59°F to 86°F). Protect from moisture by keeping bottle tightly closed.

Mechanism of Action Competitive inhibitor of angiotensin-converting enzyme (ACE); prevents conversion of angiotensin I to angiotensin II, a potent vasoconstrictor; results in lower levels of angiotensin II which causes an increase in plasma renin activity and a reduction in aldosterone secretion; a CNS mechanism may also be involved in hypotensive effect as angiotensin II increases adrenergic outflow from CNS; vasoactive kallikreins may be decreased in conversion to active hormones by ACE inhibitors, thus reducing blood pressure

Pharmacodynamics/Kinetics
Onset of action: 1 hour
Duration: 24 hours
Absorption: 36%
Protein binding: 95%
Metabolism: Prodrug, hydrolyzed to its active metabolite fosinoprilat by intestinal wall and hepatic esterases
Bioavailability: 36%
Half-life elimination, serum (fosinoprilat): 12 hours
Time to peak, serum: ~3 hours
Excretion: Urine and feces (as fosinoprilat and other metabolites in roughly equal proportions, 45% to 50%)

Dosage
Geriatric & Adult
Heart failure: Oral: Initial: 10 mg/day (5 mg if renal dysfunction present) and increase, as needed, to a maximum of 40 mg once daily over several weeks. Usual dose: 20-40 mg/day. If hypotension, orthostasis, or azotemia occurs during titration, consider decreasing concomitant diuretic dose, if any.

Hypertension: Oral: Initial: 10 mg/day; increase to a maximum dose of 80 mg/day. Most patients are maintained on 20-40 mg/day. May need to divide the dose into two if trough effect is inadequate. Discontinue the diuretic, if possible 2-3 days before initiation of therapy. Resume diuretic therapy carefully, if needed.

Renal Impairment None needed since hepatobiliary elimination compensates adequately diminished renal elimination.
Hemodialysis: Moderately dialyzable (20% to 50%)

Hepatic Impairment Decrease dose and monitor effects

Monitoring Parameters Blood pressure; serum creatinine and potassium; if patient has collagen vascular disease and/or renal impairment, periodically monitor CBC with differential

Test Interactions May cause false low serum digoxin levels with the Digi-Tab RIA kit for digoxin.

Pharmacotherapy Pearls Watch for hypotensive effect within 1-3 hours of first dose or new higher dose. Some patients may have a decreased hypotensive effect between 12-16 hours; consider dividing total daily dose into 2 doses 12 hours apart; if patient is receiving a diuretic, a potential for first-dose hypotension is increased; to decrease this potential, stop diuretic for 2-3 days prior to initiating fosinopril if possible; continue diuretic if needed to control blood pressure

Special Geriatric Considerations Due to frequent decreases in glomerular filtration (also creatinine clearance) with aging, elderly patients may have exaggerated responses to ACE inhibitors. Differences in clinical response due to hepatic changes are not observed. ACE inhibitors may be preferred agents in elderly patients with congestive heart failure and diabetes mellitus. Diabetic proteinuria is reduced and insulin sensitivity is enhanced. In general, the side effect profile is favorable in the elderly and causes little or no CNS confusion; use lowest dose recommendations initially. Many elderly may be volume depleted due to diuretic use and/or blunted thirst reflex resulting in inadequate fluid intake.

Dosage Forms Excipient information presented when available (limited, particularly for generics); consult specific product labeling.
Tablet, oral, as sodium: 10 mg, 20 mg, 40 mg

◆ **Fosinopril Sodium** see Fosinopril on page 846

Fosphenytoin (FOS fen i toyn)

Medication Safety Issues
Sound-alike/look-alike issues:
Cerebyx® may be confused with CeleBREX®, CeleXA®, Cerezyme®, Cervarix®
Fosphenytoin may be confused with fospropofol

Administration issues:
Overdoses have occurred due to confusion between the **mg per mL concentration** of fosphenytoin (50 mg PE/mL) and **total drug content per vial** (either 100 mg PE/2 mL vial or 500 mg PE/10 mL vial). ISMP recommends that the total drug content per container is identified instead of the concentration in mg per mL to avoid confusion and potential overdosages. Additionally, since most errors have occurred with overdoses in children, they recommend that pediatric hospitals should consider stocking only the 2 mL vial.

Brand Names: U.S. Cerebyx®

Brand Names: Canada Cerebyx®

Index Terms Fosphenytoin Sodium

Generic Availability (U.S.) Yes

Pharmacologic Category Anticonvulsant, Hydantoin

Use Used for the control of generalized convulsive status epilepticus and prevention and treatment of seizures occurring during neurosurgery; indicated for short-term parenteral administration when other means of phenytoin administration are unavailable, inappropriate, or deemed less advantageous (the safety and effectiveness of fosphenytoin use for more than 5 days has not been systematically evaluated)

Contraindications Hypersensitivity to phenytoin, other hydantoins, or any component of the formulation; patients with sinus bradycardia, sinoatrial block, second- and third-degree AV block, or Adams-Stokes syndrome; occurrence of rash during treatment (should not be resumed if rash is exfoliative, purpuric, or bullous); treatment of absence seizures

Warnings/Precautions Doses of fosphenytoin are expressed as their phenytoin sodium equivalent (PE). Antiepileptic drugs should not be abruptly discontinued. Hypotension may occur, especially after I.V. administration at high doses and high rates of administration. Administration of phenytoin has been associated with atrial and ventricular conduction depression and ventricular fibrillation. Careful cardiac monitoring is needed when administering I.V. loading doses of fosphenytoin. Acute hepatotoxicity associated with a hypersensitivity syndrome characterized by fever, skin eruptions, and lymphadenopathy has been reported to occur within the first 2 months of treatment. Discontinue if skin rash or lymphadenopathy occurs. A spectrum of hematologic effects have been reported with use (eg, neutropenia, leukopenia, thrombocytopenia, pancytopenia, and anemias). Use with caution in patients with hypotension, severe myocardial insufficiency, diabetes mellitus, porphyria, hypoalbuminemia, hypothyroidism, fever, or hepatic or renal dysfunction. Effects with other sedative drugs or ethanol may be potentiated. Severe reactions, including toxic epidermal necrolysis and Stevens-Johnson syndromes, although rarely reported, have resulted in fatalities; drug should be discontinued if there are any signs of rash. Patients of Asian descent with the variant *HLA-B*1502* may be at an increased risk of developing Stevens-Johnson syndrome and/or toxic epidermal necrolysis.

Adverse Reactions (Reflective of adult population; not specific for elderly) The more important adverse clinical events caused by the I.V. use of fosphenytoin or phenytoin are cardiovascular collapse and/or central nervous system depression. Hypotension can occur when either drug is administered rapidly by the I.V. route.

The adverse clinical events most commonly observed with the use of fosphenytoin in clinical trials were nystagmus, dizziness, pruritus, paresthesia, headache, somnolence, and ataxia. Paresthesia and pruritus were seen more often following fosphenytoin (versus phenytoin) administration and occurred more often with I.V. fosphenytoin than with I.M. administration. These events were dose and rate related (adult doses ≥15 mg/kg at a rate of 150 mg/minute). These sensations, generally described as itching, burning, or tingling are usually not at the infusion site. The location of the discomfort varied with the groin mentioned most frequently. The paresthesia and pruritus were transient events that occurred within several minutes of the start of infusion and generally resolved within 10 minutes after completion of infusion.

Transient pruritus, tinnitus, nystagmus, somnolence, and ataxia occurred 2-3 times more often at adult doses ≥15 mg/kg and rates ≥150 mg/minute.

I.V. administration (maximum dose/rate):
>10%:
  Central nervous system: Nystagmus, dizziness, somnolence, ataxia
  Dermatologic: Pruritus
1% to 10%:
  Cardiovascular: Hypotension, vasodilation, tachycardia

◄

Central nervous system: Stupor, incoordination, paresthesia, extrapyramidal syndrome, tremor, agitation, hypoesthesia, dysarthria, vertigo, brain edema, headache
Gastrointestinal: Nausea, tongue disorder, dry mouth, vomiting
Neuromuscular & skeletal: Pelvic pain, muscle weakness, back pain
Ocular: Diplopia, amblyopia
Otic: Tinnitus, deafness
Miscellaneous: Taste perversion

I.M. administration (substitute for oral phenytoin):

1% to 10%:
Central nervous system: Nystagmus, tremor, ataxia, headache, incoordination, somnolence, dizziness, paresthesia, reflexes decreased
Dermatologic: Pruritus
Gastrointestinal: Nausea, vomiting
Hematologic/lymphatic: Ecchymosis
Neuromuscular & skeletal: Muscle weakness

Drug Interactions

Metabolism/Transport Effects Substrate of CYP2C19 (major), CYP2C9 (major), CYP3A4 (minor); **Note:** Assignment of Major/Minor substrate status based on clinically relevant drug interaction potential; **Induces** CYP2B6 (strong), CYP2C19 (strong), CYP2C8 (strong), CYP2C9 (strong), CYP3A4 (strong)

Avoid Concomitant Use
Avoid concomitant use of Fosphenytoin with any of the following: Axitinib; Azelastine; Azelastine (Nasal); Boceprevir; Bortezomib; Darunavir; Delavirdine; Etravirine; Everolimus; Lurasidone; Mirtazapine; Paraldehyde; Praziquantel; Rilpivirine; Rivaroxaban; Roflumilast; SORAfenib; Telaprevir; Ticagrelor; Tolvaptan

Increased Effect/Toxicity
Fosphenytoin may increase the levels/effects of: Azelastine; Azelastine (Nasal); Barbiturates; Buprenorphine; CNS Depressants; Fosamprenavir; Highest Risk QTc-Prolonging Agents; Ifosfamide; Lithium; Metyrosine; Mirtazapine; Moderate Risk QTc-Prolonging Agents; Paraldehyde; Selective Serotonin Reuptake Inhibitors; Vecuronium; Vitamin K Antagonists; Zolpidem

The levels/effects of Fosphenytoin may be increased by: Alcohol (Ethyl); Allopurinol; Amiodarone; Antifungal Agents (Azole Derivatives, Systemic); Barbiturates; Benzodiazepines; Calcium Channel Blockers; Capecitabine; CarBAMazepine; Carbonic Anhydrase Inhibitors; CeFAZolin; Chloramphenicol; Cimetidine; CYP2C19 Inhibitors (Moderate); CYP2C19 Inhibitors (Strong); CYP2C9 Inhibitors (Moderate); CYP2C9 Inhibitors (Strong); Delavirdine; Dexmethylphenidate; Disulfiram; Efavirenz; Ethosuximide; Felbamate; Floxuridine; Fluconazole; Fluorouracil; Fluorouracil (Systemic); Fluorouracil (Topical); FLUoxetine; FluvoxaMINE; Halothane; HydrOXYzine; Isoniazid; Methylphenidate; MetroNIDAZOLE; MetroNIDAZOLE (Systemic); Mifepristone; OXcarbazepine; Proton Pump Inhibitors; Rufinamide; Sertraline; Sulfonamide Derivatives; Tacrolimus; Tacrolimus (Systemic); Telaprevir; Ticlopidine; Topiramate; TraZODone; Trimethoprim; Vitamin K Antagonists

Decreased Effect
Fosphenytoin may decrease the levels/effects of: Acetaminophen; Amiodarone; Antifungal Agents (Azole Derivatives, Systemic); Apixaban; ARIPiprazole; Axitinib; Boceprevir; Bortezomib; Brentuximab Vedotin; Busulfan; CarBAMazepine; Chloramphenicol; CloZAPine; Contraceptives (Estrogens); Contraceptives (Progestins); CycloSPORINE; CycloSPORINE (Systemic); CYP2B6 Substrates; CYP2C19 Substrates; CYP2C8 Substrates; CYP2C9 Substrates; CYP3A4 Substrates; Darunavir; Deferasirox; Delavirdine; Diclofenac; Disopyramide; Divalproex; Doxycycline; Efavirenz; Ethosuximide; Etoposide; Etoposide Phosphate; Etravirine; Everolimus; Exemestane; Felbamate; Flunarizine; Gefitinib; GuanFACINE; HMG-CoA Reductase Inhibitors; Imatinib; Irinotecan; Ixabepilone; Lacosamide; LamoTRIgine; Levodopa; Linagliptin; Loop Diuretics; Lopinavir; Lurasidone; Maraviroc; Mebendazole; Meperidine; Methadone; MethylPREDNISolone; MetroNIDAZOLE; MetroNIDAZOLE (Systemic); Metyrapone; Mexiletine; Nelfinavir; OXcarbazepine; Praziquantel; PredenisoLONE; PrednisoLONE (Systemic); PredniSONE; Primidone; QUEtiapine; QuiNIDine; QuiNINE; Rilpivirine; Ritonavir; Rivaroxaban; Roflumilast; Rufinamide; Saxagliptin; Sertraline; Sirolimus; SORAfenib; Tacrolimus; Tacrolimus (Systemic); Tadalafil; Telaprevir; Temsirolimus; Teniposide; Theophylline Derivatives; Thyroid Products; Ticagrelor; Tipranavir; Tolvaptan; Topiramate; TraZODone; Treprostinil; Ulipristal; Valproic Acid; Vecuronium; Zonisamide

The levels/effects of Fosphenytoin may be decreased by: Alcohol (Ethyl); Antacids; Barbiturates; CarBAMazepine; Ciprofloxacin; Ciprofloxacin (Systemic); CISplatin; CYP2C19 Inducers (Strong); CYP2C9 Inducers (Strong); Diazoxide; Divalproex; Folic Acid; Fosamprenavir; Ketorolac; Ketorolac (Nasal); Ketorolac (Systemic); Leucovorin Calcium-Levoleucovorin; Levomefolate; Lopinavir; Mefloquine; Methylfolate; Peginterferon Alfa-2b;

Pyridoxine; Rifamycin Derivatives; Ritonavir; Telaprevir; Theophylline Derivatives; Tiprana-vir; Tocilizumab; Valproic Acid; Vigabatrin

Ethanol/Nutrition/Herb Interactions Ethanol:

Acute use: Avoid or limit ethanol (inhibits metabolism of phenytoin). Ethanol may also increase CNS depression; monitor for increased effects with coadministration. Caution patients about effects.

Chronic use: Avoid or limit ethanol (stimulates metabolism of phenytoin).

Stability Refrigerate at 2°C to 8°C (36°F to 46°F). Do not store at room temperature for more than 48 hours. Do not use vials that develop particulate matter. Must be diluted to concentrations of 1.5-25 mg PE/mL, in normal saline or D_5W, for I.V. infusion.

Mechanism of Action Diphosphate ester salt of phenytoin which acts as a water soluble prodrug of phenytoin; after administration, plasma esterases convert fosphenytoin to phosphate, formaldehyde, and phenytoin as the active moiety; phenytoin works by stabilizing neuronal membranes and decreasing seizure activity by increasing efflux or decreasing influx of sodium ions across cell membranes in the motor cortex during generation of nerve impulses

Pharmacodynamics/Kinetics Also refer to Phenytoin monograph on page 1527 for additional information.

Protein binding: Fosphenytoin: 95% to 99% to albumin; can displace phenytoin and increase free fraction (up to 30% unbound) during the period required for conversion of fosphenytoin to phenytoin

Metabolism: Fosphenytoin is rapidly converted via hydrolysis to phenytoin; phenytoin is metabolized in the liver and forms metabolites

Bioavailability: I.M.: Fosphenytoin: 100%

Half-life elimination:

Fosphenytoin: 15 minutes

Phenytoin: Variable (mean: 12-29 hours); kinetics of phenytoin are saturable

Time to peak: Conversion to phenytoin: Following I.V. administration (maximum rate of administration): 15 minutes; following I.M. administration, peak phenytoin levels are reached in 3 hours

Excretion: Phenytoin: Urine (as inactive metabolites)

Dosage

Geriatric Phenytoin clearance is decreased in geriatric patients; lower doses may be required. In addition, older adults may have lower serum albumin which may increase the free fraction and, therefore, pharmacologic response. Refer to adult dosing.

Adult

Note: The dose, concentration in solutions, and infusion rates for fosphenytoin are expressed as phenytoin sodium equivalents (PE); fosphenytoin should always be prescribed and dispensed in phenytoin sodium equivalents (PE)

Status epilepticus: I.V.: Loading dose: 15-20 mg PE/kg I.V. administered at 100-150 mg PE/minute

Nonemergent loading and maintenance dosing: I.V. or I.M.:

Loading dose: 10-20 mg PE/kg (I.V. rate: Infuse over 30 minutes; maximum rate: 150 mg PE/minute)

Initial daily maintenance dose: 4-6 mg PE/kg/day

Substitution for oral phenytoin therapy: I.M. or I.V.: May be substituted for oral phenytoin sodium at the same total daily dose; however, Dilantin® capsules are ~90% bioavailable by the oral route; phenytoin, supplied as fosphenytoin, is 100% bioavailable by both the I.M. and I.V. routes; for this reason, plasma phenytoin concentrations may increase when I.M. or I.V. fosphenytoin is substituted for oral phenytoin sodium therapy; in clinical trials, I.M. fosphenytoin was administered as a single daily dose utilizing either 1 or 2 injection sites; some patients may require more frequent dosing

Renal Impairment Free phenytoin levels should be monitored closely in patients with renal disease or in those with hypoalbuminemia; furthermore, fosphenytoin clearance to phenytoin may be increased without a similar increase in phenytoin clearance in these patients leading to increase frequency and severity of adverse events.

Hepatic Impairment Phenytoin clearance may be substantially reduced in cirrhosis and plasma level monitoring with dose adjustment advisable. Free phenytoin levels should be monitored closely in patients with hepatic disease or in those with hypoalbuminemia; furthermore, fosphenytoin clearance to phenytoin may be increased without a similar increase in phenytoin clearance in these patients leading to increased frequency and severity of adverse events.

Administration Since there is no precipitation problem with fosphenytoin, no I.V. filter is required; I.V. administration rate should not exceed 150 mg/minute

Monitoring Parameters Continuous blood pressure, ECG, and respiratory function monitoring with loading dose and for 10-20 minutes following infusion; vital signs, CBC, liver function tests, plasma level monitoring (plasma levels should not be measured until conversion to phenytoin is complete, ~2 hours after an I.V. infusion or ~4 hours after an I.M. injection)

FOSPHENYTOIN

Reference Range
Therapeutic: 10-20 mcg/mL (SI: 40-79 micromole/L); toxicity is measured clinically, and some patients require levels outside the suggested therapeutic range
Toxic: 30-50 mcg/mL (SI: 120-200 micromole/L)
Lethal: >100 mcg/mL (SI: >400 micromole/L)

Manifestations of toxicity:
Nystagmus: 20 mcg/mL (SI: 79 micromole/L)
Ataxia: 30 mcg/mL (SI: 118.9 micromole/L)
Decreased mental status: 40 mcg/mL (SI: 159 micromole/L)
Coma: 50 mcg/mL (SI: 200 micromole/L)
Peak serum phenytoin level after a 375 mg I.M. fosphenytoin dose in healthy males: 5.7 mcg/mL
Peak serum fosphenytoin levels and phenytoin levels after a 1.2 g infusion (I.V.) in healthy subjects over 30 minutes were 129 mcg/mL and 17.2 mcg/mL, respectively

Test Interactions Falsely high plasma phenytoin concentrations (due to cross-reactivity with fosphenytoin) when measured by immunoanalytical techniques (eg, TD_X®, TD_XFL_X™, Emit® 2000) prior to complete conversion of fosphenytoin to phenytoin. Phenytoin may produce falsely low results for dexamethasone or metyrapone tests.

Pharmacotherapy Pearls 1.5 mg fosphenytoin is approximately equivalent to 1 mg phenytoin; equimolar fosphenytoin dose is 375 mg (75 mg/mL solution) to phenytoin 250 mg (50 mg/mL); 0.0037 mmol phosphate/mg PE fosphenytoin

Water solubility: 142 mg/mL at pH of 9

Antiarrhythmic effects may be similar to phenytoin; parenteral product contains no propylene sterol; this should allow for rapid intravenous bolus dosing without cardiovascular complications; formaldehyde production is not expected to be clinically consequential (about 200 mg) if used for one week

Special Geriatric Considerations No significant changes in fosphenytoin pharmacokinetics with age have been noted. Phenytoin clearance is decreased in the elderly and lower doses may be needed. Elderly may have reduced hepatic clearance due to age decline in Phase I metabolism. Elderly may have low albumin which will increase free fraction and, therefore, pharmacologic response. Monitor closely in those who are hypoalbuminemic. Free fraction measurements advised, also elderly may display a higher incidence of adverse effects (cardiovascular) when using the I.V. loading regimen; therefore, it is recommended to decrease loading I.V. dose to 25 mg/minute.

Dosage Forms Excipient information presented when available (limited, particularly for generics); consult specific product labeling.
Injection, solution, as sodium: 75 mg/mL (2 mL, 10 mL) [equivalent to phenytoin sodium 50 mg/mL]
Cerebyx®: 75 mg/mL (2 mL) [equivalent to phenytoin sodium 50 mg/mL]

◆ **Fosphenytoin Sodium** see Fosphenytoin on page 849
◆ **Fosrenol®** see Lanthanum on page 1096
◆ **Fragmin®** see Dalteparin on page 476
◆ **Freezone® [OTC]** see Salicylic Acid on page 1743
◆ **Frova®** see Frovatriptan on page 852

Frovatriptan (froe va TRIP tan)

Medication Safety Issues
International issues:
Allegro: Brand name for frovatriptan [Germany], but also the brand name for fluticasone [Israel]
Allegro [Germany] may be confused with Allegra and Allegra-D brand names for fexofenadine and fexofenadine/pseudoehedrine, respectively, in the [U.S., Canada, and multiple international markets]
Brand Names: U.S. Frova®
Brand Names: Canada Frova®
Index Terms Frovatriptan Succinate
Generic Availability (U.S.) No
Pharmacologic Category Antimigraine Agent; Serotonin 5-HT$_{1B, 1D}$ Receptor Agonist
Use Acute treatment of migraine with or without aura
Unlabeled Use Short-term prevention of menstrually-associated migraines (MAMs)

Contraindications Hypersensitivity to frovatriptan or any component of the formulation; patients with ischemic heart disease or signs or symptoms of ischemic heart disease (including Prinzmetal's angina, angina pectoris, myocardial infarction, silent myocardial ischemia); cerebrovascular syndromes (including strokes, transient ischemic attacks); peripheral vascular syndromes (including ischemic bowel disease); uncontrolled hypertension; use within 24 hours of ergotamine derivatives; use within 24 hours of another 5-HT$_1$ agonist; management of hemiplegic or basilar migraine

Canadian labeling: Additional contraindications (not in U.S. labeling): Cardiac arrhythmias, valvular heart disease, congenital heart disease, atherosclerotic disease; management of ophthalmoplegic migraine; severe hepatic impairment

Warnings/Precautions Not intended for migraine prophylaxis, or treatment of cluster headaches, hemiplegic or basilar migraines. Rule out underlying neurologic disease in patients with atypical headache, migraine (with no prior history of migraine) or inadequate clinical response to initial dosing. Cardiac events (coronary artery vasospasm, transient ischemia, MI, ventricular tachycardia/fibrillation, cardiac arrest, and death), cerebral/subarachnoid hemorrhage, stroke, peripheral vascular ischemia, and colonic ischemia have been reported with 5-HT$_1$ agonist administration. May cause vasospastic reactions resulting in colonic, peripheral, or coronary ischemia. Do not give to patients with risk factors for CAD until a cardiovascular evaluation has been performed; if evaluation is satisfactory, the healthcare provider should administer the first dose and cardiovascular status should be periodically evaluated. Significant elevation in blood pressure, including hypertensive crisis, has also been reported on rare occasions in patients using other 5-HT$_{1D}$ agonists with and without a history of hypertension. May lower seizure threshold, use caution in epilepsy or structural brain lesions. Symptoms of agitation, confusion, hallucinations, hyper-reflexia, myoclonus, shivering, and tachycardia (serotonin syndrome) may occur with concomitant proserotonergic drugs (ie, SSRIs/SNRIs or triptans) or agents which reduce frovatriptan's metabolism.

Adverse Reactions (Reflective of adult population; not specific for elderly) 1% to 10%:

Cardiovascular: Flushing (4%), chest pain (2%), palpitation (1%)

Central nervous system: Dizziness (8%), fatigue (5%), headache (4%), hot or cold sensation (3%), somnolence (≥2%), anxiety (1%), dysesthesia (1%), hypoesthesia (1%), insomnia (1%), pain (1%)

Gastrointestinal: Xerostomia (3%), nausea (≥2%), dyspepsia (2%), abdominal pain (1%), diarrhea (1%), vomiting (1%)

Neuromuscular & skeletal: Paresthesia (4%), skeletal pain (3%)

Ocular: Vision abnormal (1%)

Otic: Tinnitus (1%)

Respiratory: Rhinitis (1%), sinusitis (1%)

Miscellaneous: Diaphoresis (1%)

Drug Interactions

Metabolism/Transport Effects Substrate of CYP1A2 (minor); **Note:** Assignment of Major/Minor substrate status based on clinically relevant drug interaction potential

Avoid Concomitant Use

Avoid concomitant use of Frovatriptan with any of the following: Ergot Derivatives

Increased Effect/Toxicity

Frovatriptan may increase the levels/effects of: Ergot Derivatives; Metoclopramide; Serotonin Modulators

The levels/effects of Frovatriptan may be increased by: Antipsychotics; Ergot Derivatives

Decreased Effect There are no known significant interactions involving a decrease in effect.

Ethanol/Nutrition/Herb Interactions Food: Food does not affect frovatriptan bioavailability.

Stability Store at controlled room temperature of 25°C (77°F); excursions permitted to 15°C to 30°C (59°F to 86°F). Protect from moisture.

Mechanism of Action Selective agonist for serotonin (5-HT$_{1B}$ and 5-HT$_{1D}$ receptors) in cranial arteries; causes vasoconstriction and reduces sterile inflammation associated with antidromic neuronal transmission correlating with relief of migraine.

Pharmacodynamics/Kinetics

Distribution: Male: 4.2 L/kg; Female: 3.0 L/kg

Protein binding: ~15%

Metabolism: Primarily hepatic via CYP1A2

Bioavailability: Male: ~20%; Female: ~30%

Half-life elimination: ~26 hours

Time to peak: 2-4 hours

Excretion: Feces (62%); urine (32%; <10% as unchanged drug)

◀ **Dosage**
Geriatric & Adult Migraine: Oral:
U.S. labeling: 2.5 mg; if headache recurs, a second dose may be given if first dose provided relief and at least 2 hours have elapsed since the first dose (maximum daily dose: 7.5 mg)
Canadian labeling: 2.5 mg; if headache recurs, a second dose may be given if first dose provided relief and at least 4 hours have elapsed since the first dose (maximum daily dose: 5 mg)
Note: The safety of treating more than 4 migraines/month has not been established.
Renal Impairment No adjustment necessary.
Hepatic Impairment No adjustment necessary in mild-to-moderate hepatic impairment; use with caution in severe impairment (has not been studied in severe impairment).
Canadian labeling (not in U.S. labeling): Use is contraindicated in severe hepatic impairment.
Administration Administer with fluids.
Pharmacotherapy Pearls Blocks 5-HT$_{1B}$ and 5-HT$_{1D}$ receptors. Relieves symptoms of migraine by blocking vasoconstrictive and other effects of serotonin.
Special Geriatric Considerations Migraine headaches occur infrequently in elderly; however, since elderly often have cardiovascular disease, careful evaluation of the use of 5-HT agonists is needed to avoid complications with the use of these agents. The pharmacokinetic disposition of these agents is similar to that seen in younger adults.
Dosage Forms Excipient information presented when available (limited, particularly for generics); consult specific product labeling.
Tablet, oral:
Frova®: 2.5 mg

◆ **Frovatriptan Succinate** *see Frovatriptan on page 852*
◆ **Frusemide** *see Furosemide on page 855*

Fulvestrant (fool VES trant)

Brand Names: U.S. Faslodex®
Brand Names: Canada Faslodex®
Index Terms ICI-182,780; ZD9238
Generic Availability (U.S.) No
Pharmacologic Category Antineoplastic Agent, Estrogen Receptor Antagonist
Use Treatment of hormone receptor positive metastatic breast cancer in postmenopausal women with disease progression following antiestrogen therapy
Contraindications Hypersensitivity to fulvestrant or any component of the formulation
Warnings/Precautions Hazardous agent - use appropriate precautions for handling and disposal. Use caution in hepatic impairment; dosage adjustment is recommended in patients with moderate hepatic impairment. Safety and efficacy have not been established in severe hepatic impairment. Use with caution in patients with a history of bleeding disorders (including thrombocytopenia) and/or patients on anticoagulant therapy; bleeding/hematoma may occur from I.M. administration.
Adverse Reactions (Reflective of adult population; not specific for elderly) Adverse reactions reported with 500 mg dose.
>10%:
Endocrine & metabolic: Hot flushes (7% to 13%)
Hepatic: Alkaline phosphatase increased (>15%; grades 3/4: 1% to 2%), transaminases increased (>15%; grades 3/4: 1% to 2%)
Local: Injection site pain (12% to 14%)
Neuromuscular & skeletal: Joint disorders (14% to 19%)
1% to 10%:
Cardiovascular: Ischemic disorder (1%)
Central nervous system: Fatigue (8%), headache (8%)
Gastrointestinal: Nausea (10%), anorexia (6%), vomiting (6%), constipation (5%), weight gain (≤1%)
Genitourinary: Urinary tract infection (2% to 4%)
Neuromuscular & skeletal: Bone pain (9%), arthralgia (8%), back pain (8%), extremity pain (7%), musculoskeletal pain (6%), weakness (6%)
Respiratory: Cough (5%), dyspnea (4%)
Drug Interactions
Metabolism/Transport Effects Substrate of CYP3A4 (minor); **Note:** Assignment of Major/Minor substrate status based on clinically relevant drug interaction potential
Avoid Concomitant Use There are no known interactions where it is recommended to avoid concomitant use.

Increased Effect/Toxicity There are no known significant interactions involving an increase in effect.

Decreased Effect

The levels/effects of Fulvestrant may be decreased by: Tocilizumab

Stability Store in original carton under refrigeration at 2°C to 8°C (36°F to 46°F). Protect from light.

Mechanism of Action Estrogen receptor antagonist; competitively binds to estrogen receptors on tumors and other tissue targets, producing a nuclear complex that causes a dose-related down-regulation of estrogen receptors and inhibits tumor growth.

Pharmacodynamics/Kinetics

Duration: I.M.: Steady state concentrations reached within first month, when administered with additional dose given 2 weeks following the initial dose; plasma levels maintained for at least 1 month

Distribution: V_d: ~3-5 L/kg

Protein binding: 99%; to plasma proteins (VLDL, LDL and HDL lipoprotein fractions)

Metabolism: Hepatic via multiple biotransformation pathways (CYP3A4 substrate involved in oxidation pathway, although relative contribution to metabolism unknown); metabolites formed are either less active or have similar activity to parent compound

Half-life elimination: 250 mg: ~40 days

Excretion: Feces (~90%); urine (<1%)

Dosage

Geriatric & Adult Breast cancer, metastatic (postmenopausal women): I.M.: Initial: 500 mg on days 1, 15, and 29; Maintenance: 500 mg once monthly

Hepatic Impairment

Moderate impairment (Child-Pugh class B): Decrease initial and maintenance dose to 250 mg

Severe impairment (Child-Pugh class C): Use has not been evaluated.

Administration For I.M. administration only; do not administer I.V., SubQ, or intra-arterially. Administer 500 mg dose as two 5 mL injections (one in each buttocks) slowly over 1-2 minutes per injection.

Special Geriatric Considerations Pharmacokinetic studies in patients with breast cancer did not show age-related differences in older adults compared to younger adults.

Dosage Forms Excipient information presented when available (limited, particularly for generics); consult specific product labeling.

Injection, solution:

Faslodex®: 50 mg/mL (5 mL) [contains benzyl alcohol, benzyl benzoate, castor oil, ethanol 10% w/v]

◆ **Fung-O® [OTC]** see Salicylic Acid on page 1743
◆ **Fungoid® [OTC]** see Miconazole (Topical) on page 1276
◆ **Furadantin®** see Nitrofurantoin on page 1384
◆ **Furazosin** see Prazosin on page 1589

Furosemide (fyoor OH se mide)

Medication Safety Issues

Sound-alike/look-alike issues:

Furosemide may be confused with famotidine, finasteride, fluconazole, FLUoxetine, fosinopril, loperamide, torsemide

Lasix® may be confused with Lanoxin®, Lidex®, Lomotil®, Lovenox®, Luvox®, Luxiq®

International issues:

Lasix [U.S., Canada, and multiple international markets] may be confused with Esidrex brand name for hydrochlorothiazide [multiple international markets]; Esidrix brand name for hydrochlorothiazide [Germany]

Urex [Australia, Hong Kong, Turkey] may be confused with Eurax brand name for crotamiton [U.S., Canada, and multiple international markets]

Brand Names: U.S. Lasix®

Brand Names: Canada Apo-Furosemide®; Bio-Furosemide; Dom-Furosemide; Furosemide Injection, USP; Furosemide Special Injection; Lasix®; Lasix® Special; Novo-Semide; Nu-Furosemide; PMS-Furosemide

Index Terms Frusemide

Generic Availability (U.S.) Yes

Pharmacologic Category Diuretic, Loop

Use Management of edema associated with heart failure and hepatic or renal disease; acute pulmonary edema; treatment of hypertension (alone or in combination with other antihypertensives)

FUROSEMIDE

Canadian labeling: Additional use: Furosemide Special Injection and Lasix® Special (products not available in the U.S.): Adjunctive treatment of oliguria in patients with severe renal impairment

Contraindications Hypersensitivity to furosemide or any component of the formulation; anuria

Canadian labeling: Additional contraindications (not in U.S. labeling): Hypersensitivity to sulfonamide-derived drugs; complete renal shutdown; hepatic coma and precoma; uncorrected states of electrolyte depletion, hypovolemia, or hypotension. **Note:** Manufacturer's labeling for Lasix® Special and Furosemide Special Injection also includes: GFR <5 mL/ minute or GFR >20 mL/minute; hepatic cirrhosis; renal failure accompanied by hepatic coma and precoma; renal failure due to poisoning with nephrotoxic or hepatotoxic substances.

Warnings/Precautions [U.S. Boxed Warning]: If given in excessive amounts, furosemide, similar to other loop diuretics, can lead to profound diuresis, resulting in fluid and electrolyte depletion; close medical supervision and dose evaluation are required. Watch for and correct electrolyte disturbances; adjust dose to avoid dehydration. When electrolyte depletion is present, therapy should not be initiated unless serum electrolytes, especially potassium, are normalized. In cirrhosis, avoid electrolyte and acid/base imbalances that might lead to hepatic encephalopathy; correct electrolyte and acid/base imbalances prior to initiation when hepatic coma is present. Coadministration of antihypertensives may increase the risk of hypotension.

Monitor fluid status and renal function in an attempt to prevent oliguria, azotemia, and reversible increases in BUN and creatinine; close medical supervision of aggressive diuresis is required. May increase risk of contrast-induced nephropathy. Rapid I.V. administration, renal impairment, excessive doses, hypoproteinemia, and concurrent use of other ototoxins is associated with ototoxicity. Asymptomatic hyperuricemia has been reported with use; rarely, gout may precipitate. Photosensitization may occur.

Use with caution in patients with prediabetes or diabetes mellitus; may see a change in glucose control. Use with caution in patients with systemic lupus erythematosus (SLE); may cause SLE exacerbation or activation. Use with caution in patients with prostatic hyperplasia/ urinary stricture; may cause urinary retention. Chemical similarities are present among sulfonamides, sulfonylureas, carbonic anhydrase inhibitors, thiazides, and loop diuretics (except ethacrynic acid). A risk of cross-reaction exists in patients with allergy to any of these compounds; avoid use when previous reaction has been severe. Discontinue if signs of hypersensitivity are noted.

Adverse Reactions (Reflective of adult population; not specific for elderly) Frequency not defined.

Cardiovascular: Acute hypotension, chronic aortitis, necrotizing angiitis, orthostatic hypotension, vasculitis

Central nervous system: Dizziness, fever, headache, hepatic encephalopathy, lightheadedness, restlessness, vertigo

Dermatologic: Bullous pemphigoid, cutaneous vasculitis, drug rash with eosinophilia and systemic symptoms (DRESS), erythema multiforme, exanthematous pustulosis (generalized), exfoliative dermatitis, photosensitivity, pruritus, purpura, rash, Stevens-Johnson syndrome, toxic epidermal necrolysis, urticaria

Endocrine & metabolic: Cholesterol and triglycerides increased, glucose tolerance test altered, gout, hyperglycemia, hyperuricemia, hypocalcemia, hypochloremia, hypokalemia, hypomagnesemia, hyponatremia, metabolic alkalosis

Gastrointestinal: Anorexia, constipation, cramping, diarrhea, nausea, oral and gastric irritation, pancreatitis, vomiting

Genitourinary: Urinary bladder spasm, urinary frequency

Hematological: Agranulocytosis (rare), anemia, aplastic anemia (rare), eosinophilia, hemolytic anemia, leukopenia, thrombocytopenia

Hepatic: Intrahepatic cholestatic jaundice, ischemic hepatitis, liver enzymes increased

Local: Injection site pain (following I.M. injection), thrombophlebitis

Neuromuscular & skeletal: Muscle spasm, paresthesia, weakness

Ocular: Blurred vision, xanthopsia

Otic: Hearing impairment (reversible or permanent with rapid I.V. or I.M. administration), tinnitus

Renal: Allergic interstitial nephritis, fall in glomerular filtration rate and renal blood flow (due to overdiuresis), glycosuria, transient rise in BUN

Miscellaneous: Anaphylaxis (rare), exacerbate or activate systemic lupus erythematosus

Drug Interactions

Metabolism/Transport Effects None known.

Avoid Concomitant Use

Avoid concomitant use of Furosemide with any of the following: Chloral Hydrate; Ethacrynic Acid

Increased Effect/Toxicity

Furosemide may increase the levels/effects of: ACE Inhibitors; Allopurinol; Amifostine; Aminoglycosides; Antihypertensives; Cardiac Glycosides; Chloral Hydrate; CISplatin; Dofetilide; Ethacrynic Acid; Hypotensive Agents; Lithium; Methotrexate; Neuromuscular-Blocking Agents; RisperiDONE; RiTUXimab; Salicylates; Sodium Phosphates

The levels/effects of Furosemide may be increased by: Alfuzosin; Beta2-Agonists; Corticosteroids (Orally Inhaled); Corticosteroids (Systemic); CycloSPORINE (Systemic); Diazoxide; Herbs (Hypotensive Properties); Licorice; MAO Inhibitors; Methotrexate; Pentoxifylline; Phosphodiesterase 5 Inhibitors; Probenecid; Prostacyclin Analogues

Decreased Effect

Furosemide may decrease the levels/effects of: Hypoglycemic Agents; Lithium; Neuromuscular-Blocking Agents

The levels/effects of Furosemide may be decreased by: Aliskiren; Bile Acid Sequestrants; Fosphenytoin; Herbs (Hypertensive Properties); Methotrexate; Methylphenidate; Nonsteroidal Anti-Inflammatory Agents; Phenytoin; Probenecid; Salicylates; Sucralfate; Yohimbine

Ethanol/Nutrition/Herb Interactions

Food: Furosemide serum levels may be decreased if taken with food.

Herb/Nutraceutical: Avoid bayberry, blue cohosh, cayenne, ephedra, ginger, ginseng (American), kola, licorice (may worsen hypertension). Avoid black cohosh, California poppy, coleus, golden seal, hawthorn, mistletoe, periwinkle, quinine, shepherd's purse (may increase antihypertensive effect). Licorice may also cause or worsen hypokalemia.

Stability

Injection: Store at room temperature of 15°C to 30°C (59°F to 86°F). Protect from light. Exposure to light may cause discoloration; do not use furosemide solutions if they have a yellow color. Furosemide solutions are unstable in acidic media, but very stable in basic media. Refrigeration may result in precipitation or crystallization; however, resolubilization at room temperature or warming may be performed without affecting the drug's stability.

I.V. infusion solution mixed in NS or D₅W solution is stable for 24 hours at room temperature. May also be diluted for infusion to 1-2 mg/mL (maximum: 10 mg/mL).

Tablet: Store at 25°C (77°F); excursions permitted to 15°C to 30°C (59°F to 89°F). Protect from light.

Mechanism of Action Inhibits reabsorption of sodium and chloride in the ascending loop of Henle and distal renal tubule, interfering with the chloride-binding cotransport system, thus causing increased excretion of water, sodium, chloride, magnesium, and calcium

Pharmacodynamics/Kinetics

Onset of action: Diuresis: Oral, S.L.: 30-60 minutes; I.M.: 30 minutes; I.V.: ~5 minutes

Symptomatic improvement with acute pulmonary edema: Within 15-20 minutes; occurs prior to diuretic effect

Peak effect: Oral, S.L.: 1-2 hours

Duration: Oral, S.L.: 6-8 hours; I.V.: 2 hours

Protein binding: 91% to 99%; primarily to albumin

Metabolism: Minimally hepatic

Bioavailability: Oral tablet: 47% to 64%; Oral solution: 50%; S.L. administration of oral tablet: ~60%; results of a small comparative study (n=11) showed bioavailability of S.L. administration of tablet was ~12% higher than oral administration of tablet (Haegeli, 2007)

Half-life elimination: Normal renal function: 0.5-2 hours; End-stage renal disease: 9 hours

Excretion: Urine (Oral: 50%, I.V.: 80%) within 24 hours; feces (as unchanged drug); nonrenal clearance prolonged in renal impairment

Dosage

Geriatric Oral, I.M., I.V.: Initial: 20 mg/day; increase slowly to desired response.

Adult

Edema, heart failure:

Oral: Initial: 20-80 mg/dose; if response is not adequate, may repeat the same dose or increase dose in increments of 20-40 mg/dose at intervals of 6-8 hours; may be titrated up to 600 mg/day with severe edematous states; usual maintenance dose interval is once or twice daily. **Note:** Dosing frequency may be adjusted based on patient-specific diuretic needs.

I.M., I.V.: Initial: 20-40 mg/dose; if response is not adequate, may repeat the same dose or increase dose in increments of 20 mg/dose and administer 1-2 hours after previous dose (maximum dose: 200 mg/dose). Individually determined dose should then be given once or twice daily although some patients may initially require dosing as frequent as every 6 hours. **Note:** ACC/AHA 2009 guidelines for heart failure recommend a maximum single dose of 160-200 mg.

Continuous I.V. infusion (Howard, 2001; Hunt, 2009): Initial: I.V. bolus dose 20-40 mg over 1-2 minutes, followed by continuous I.V. infusion doses of 10-40 mg/hour. If urine output is <1 mL/kg/hour, double as necessary to a maximum of 80-160 mg/hour. The risk

◀ associated with higher infusion rates (80-160 mg/hour) must be weighed against alternative strategies. **Note:** ACC/AHA 2009 guidelines for heart failure recommend 40 mg I.V. load, then 10-40 mg/hour infusion.

Acute pulmonary edema: *I.V.:* 40 mg over 1-2 minutes. If response not adequate within 1 hour, may increase dose to 80 mg. **Note:** ACC/AHA 2009 guidelines for heart failure recommend a maximum single dose of 160-200 mg.

Hypertension, resistant (Chobanian, 2003; JNC 7): *Oral:* 20-80 mg/day in 2 divided doses

Refractory heart failure: *Oral, I.V.:* Doses up to 8 g/day have been used.

Renal Impairment

Acute renal failure: Doses up to 1-3 g/day may be necessary to initiate desired response; avoid use in oliguric states.

Not removed by hemo- or peritoneal dialysis; supplemental dose is not necessary.

Hepatic Impairment Diminished natriuretic effect with increased sensitivity to hypokalemia and volume depletion in cirrhosis. Monitor effects, particularly with high doses.

Administration

I.V.: I.V. injections should be given slowly. Undiluted direct I.V. injections may be administered at a rate of 20-40 mg per minute; maximum rate of administration for short-term intermittent infusion is 4 mg/minute; exceeding this rate increases the risk of ototoxicity.

Oral: Administer on an empty stomach (Bard, 2004). May be administered with food or milk if GI distress occurs; however, this may reduce diuretic efficacy.

Note: When I.V. or oral administration is not possible, the sublingual route may be used. Place 1 tablet under tongue for at least 5 minutes to allow for maximal absorption. Patients should be advised not to swallow during disintegration time (Haegeli, 2007).

Monitoring Parameters Monitor weight and I & O daily; blood pressure, orthostasis; serum electrolytes, renal function; monitor hearing with high doses or rapid I.V. administration

Special Geriatric Considerations Loop diuretics are potent diuretics; excess amounts can lead to profound diuresis with fluid and electrolyte loss; close medical supervision and dose evaluation is required, particularly in the elderly. Severe loss of sodium and/or increase in BUN can cause confusion. For any change in mental status in patients on furosemide, monitor electrolytes and renal function.

Dosage Forms Excipient information presented when available (limited, particularly for generics); consult specific product labeling.

Injection, solution [preservative free]: 10 mg/mL (2 mL, 4 mL, 10 mL)

Solution, oral: 40 mg/5 mL (5 mL, 500 mL); 10 mg/mL (4 mL, 60 mL, 120 mL)

Tablet, oral: 20 mg, 40 mg, 80 mg

Lasix®: 20 mg

Lasix®: 40 mg, 80 mg [scored]

Dosage Forms: Canada Excipient information presented when available (limited, particularly for generics); consult specific product labeling.

Injection, solution [preservative free]:

Furosemide Special Injection: 10 mg/mL (25 mL)

Tablet, oral:

Lasix® Special: 500 mg [scored]

Gabapentin (GA ba pen tin)

Medication Safety Issues

Sound-alike/look-alike issues:

Neurontin® may be confused with Motrin®, Neoral®, nitrofurantoin, Noroxin®, Zarontin®

Brand Names: U.S. Gralise™; Neurontin®

Brand Names: Canada Apo-Gabapentin®; CO Gabapentin; Dom-Gabapentin; Mylan-Gabapentin; Neurontin®; PHL-Gabapentin; PMS-Gabapentin; PRO-Gabapentin; RAN™-Gabapentin; ratio-Gabapentin; Riva-Gabapentin; Teva-Gabapentin

Generic Availability (U.S.) Yes

Pharmacologic Category Anticonvulsant, Miscellaneous; GABA Analog

Use Adjunct for treatment of partial seizures with and without secondary generalized seizures in patients with epilepsy; management of postherpetic neuralgia (PHN)

Unlabeled Use Neuropathic pain, diabetic peripheral neuropathy, fibromyalgia, postoperative pain, restless legs syndrome (RLS), vasomotor symptoms

Medication Guide Available Yes

Contraindications Hypersensitivity to gabapentin or any component of the formulation

Warnings/Precautions Antiepileptics are associated with an increased risk of suicidal behavior/thoughts with use (regardless of indication); patients should be monitored for signs/symptoms of depression, suicidal tendencies, and other unusual behavior changes during therapy and instructed to inform their healthcare provider immediately if symptoms occur. Avoid abrupt withdrawal, may precipitate seizures; Gralise™ should be withdrawn over

≥1 week. Use cautiously in patients with severe renal dysfunction; male rat studies demonstrated an association with pancreatic adenocarcinoma (clinical implication unknown). May cause CNS depression, which may impair physical or mental abilities. Patients must be cautioned about performing tasks which require mental alertness (eg, operating machinery or driving). Effects with other sedative drugs or ethanol may be potentiated. Gabapentin immediate release and extended release (Gralise™) products are not interchangeable with each other **or** with gabapentin encarbil (Horizant™). The safety and efficacy of extended release gabapentin (Gralise™) has not been studied in patients with epilepsy. Potentially serious, sometimes fatal multiorgan hypersensitivity (also known as drug reaction with eosinophilia and systemic symptoms [DRESS]) has been reported with some antiepileptic drugs, including gabapentin; may affect lymphatic, hepatic, renal, cardiac, and/or hematologic systems; fever, rash, and eosinophilia may also be present. Discontinue immediately if suspected.

Adverse Reactions (Reflective of adult population; not specific for elderly) As reported for immediate release (IR) formulations in patients >12 years of age, unless otherwise noted with use of extended release (ER) formulation

>10%:

Central nervous system: Dizziness (IR: 17% to 28%; ER: 11%), somnolence (IR: 19% to 21%; ER: 5%), ataxia (3% to 13%), fatigue (11%)

Miscellaneous: Viral infection

1% to 10%:

Cardiovascular: Peripheral edema (2% to 8%), vasodilatation (1%)

Central nervous system: Fever, hostility, emotional lability, headache (IR: 3%; ER: 4%), abnormal thinking (2% to 3%), amnesia (2%), depression (2%), nervousness (2%), abnormal coordination (1% to 2%), pain (ER: 1% to 2%), hyperesthesia (1%), lethargy (ER: 1%), twitching (1%), vertigo (ER: 1%)

Dermatologic: Pruritus (1%), rash (1%)

Endocrine & metabolic: Hyperglycemia (1%)

Gastrointestinal: Diarrhea (IR: 6%; ER: 3%), nausea/vomiting (3% to 4%), abdominal pain (3%), xerostomia (2% to 5%), constipation (1% to 4%), weight gain (adults and children 2% to 3%), dyspepsia (IR: 2%; ER: 1%), flatulence (2%), dry throat (2%), dental abnormalities (2%), appetite stimulation (1%)

Genitourinary: Impotence (2%), urinary tract infection (ER: 2%)

Hematologic: Decreased WBC (1%), leukopenia (1%)

Neuromuscular & skeletal: Tremor (7%), weakness (6%), hyperkinesia, abnormal gait (2%), back pain (2%), dysarthria (2%), myalgia (2%), fracture (1%)

Ocular: Nystagmus (8%), diplopia (1% to 6%), blurred vision (3% to 4%), conjunctivitis (1%)

Otic: Otitis media (1%)

Respiratory: Rhinitis (4%), bronchitis, respiratory infection, pharyngitis (1% to 3%), cough (2%)

Miscellaneous: Infection (5%)

Drug Interactions

Metabolism/Transport Effects None known.

Avoid Concomitant Use

Avoid concomitant use of Gabapentin with any of the following: Azelastine; Azelastine (Nasal); Methadone; Mirtazapine; Paraldehyde

Increased Effect/Toxicity

Gabapentin may increase the levels/effects of: Alcohol (Ethyl); Azelastine; Azelastine (Nasal); Buprenorphine; CNS Depressants; Methadone; Methotrimeprazine; Metyrosine; Mirtazapine; Paraldehyde; Selective Serotonin Reuptake Inhibitors; Zolpidem

The levels/effects of Gabapentin may be increased by: Droperidol; HydrOXYzine; Methotrimeprazine

Decreased Effect

The levels/effects of Gabapentin may be decreased by: Antacids; Ketorolac; Ketorolac (Nasal); Ketorolac (Systemic); Mefloquine

Ethanol/Nutrition/Herb Interactions

Ethanol: May increase CNS depression; monitor for increased effects with coadministration. Caution patients about effects.

Food: Tablet, solution (immediate release): No significant effect on rate or extent of absorption; tablet (extended release): Increases rate and extent of absorption.

Herb/Nutraceutical: Avoid evening primrose (seizure threshold decreased). Avoid valerian, St John's wort, kava kava, gotu kola (may increase CNS depression).

Stability

Capsules and tablets: Store at 25°C (77°F); excursions permitted to 15°C to 30°C (59°F to 86°F).

Oral solution: Store refrigerated at 2°C to 8°C (36°F to 46°F).

◀ **Mechanism of Action** Gabapentin is structurally related to GABA. However, it does not bind to GABA$_A$ or GABA$_B$ receptors, and it does not appear to influence synthesis or uptake of GABA. High affinity gabapentin binding sites have been located throughout the brain; these sites correspond to the presence of voltage-gated calcium channels specifically possessing the alpha-2-delta-1 subunit. This channel appears to be located presynaptically, and may modulate the release of excitatory neurotransmitters which participate in epileptogenesis and nociception.

Pharmacodynamics/Kinetics

Absorption: Variable, from proximal small bowel by L-amino transport system

Distribution: V_d: 58 ± 6 L

Protein binding: <3%

Bioavailability: Inversely proportional to dose due to saturable absorption:

Immediate release:
900 mg/day: 60%
1200 mg/day: 47%
2400 mg/day: 34%
3600 mg/day: 33%
4800 mg/day: 27%

Extended release: Variable; increased with higher fat content meal

Half-life elimination: 5-7 hours; anuria 132 hours; during dialysis 3.8 hours

Time to peak: Immediate release: 2-4 hours; extended release: 8 hours

Excretion: Proportional to renal function; urine (as unchanged drug)

Dosage

Geriatric Studies in elderly patients have shown a decrease in clearance as age increases. This is most likely due to age-related decreases in renal function; dose reductions may be needed.

Adult

Anticonvulsant: Oral: Immediate release:
Initial: 300 mg 3 times/day, if necessary the dose may be increased up to 1800 mg/day
Maintenance: 900-1800 mg/day administered in 3 divided doses; doses of up to 2400 mg/day have been tolerated in long-term clinical studies; up to 3600 mg/day has been tolerated in short-term studies
Note: If gabapentin is discontinued or if another anticonvulsant is added to therapy, it should be done slowly over a minimum of 1 week.

Diabetic neuropathy (unlabeled use): Oral: Immediate release: 900-3600 mg/day (Bril, 2011)

Neuropathic pain (unlabeled use): Oral: Immediate release: 300-3600 mg/day (Attal, 2010; Dworkin, 2010)

Postherpetic neuralgia: Oral:
Immediate release: Day 1: 300 mg, Day 2: 300 mg twice daily, Day 3: 300 mg 3 times/day; dose may be titrated as needed for pain relief (range: 1800-3600 mg/day in divided doses, daily doses >1800 mg do not generally show greater benefit)
Extended release (Gralise™): Day 1: 300 mg, Day 2: 600 mg, Days 3-6: 900 mg once daily, Days 7-10: 1200 mg once daily, Days 11-14: 1500 mg once daily, Days ≥15: 1800 mg once daily

Postoperative pain (unlabeled use): Oral: Immediate release: Usual dose: 300-1200 mg given 1-2 hours prior to surgery (Dauri, 2009)

Restless legs syndrome (RLS) (unlabeled use): Oral: Initial: 300 mg once daily 2 hours before bedtime. Doses ≥600 mg/day have been given in 2 divided doses (late afternoon and 2 hours before bedtime). Dose may be titrated every 2 weeks until symptom relief achieved (range: 300-1800 mg/day). Suggested maintenance dosing schedule: One-third of total daily dose given at 12 pm, remaining two-thirds total daily dose given at 8 pm. (Garcia-Borreguero, 2002; Happe, 2003; Saletu, 2010; Vignatelli, 2006)

Vasomotor symptoms associated with menopause (unlabeled use): Oral: Day 1: 300 mg at bedtime, Day 2: 300 mg twice daily, followed by 300 mg 3 times/day for 4 weeks and then tapered off (Butt, 2008)

Renal Impairment Note: Renal function may be estimated using the Cockcroft-Gault formula for dosage adjustment purposes

Immediate release:
Cl_{cr} ≥60 mL/minute: 300-1200 mg 3 times/day
Cl_{cr} >30-59 mL/minute: 200-700 mg twice daily
Cl_{cr} >15-29 mL/minute: 200-700 mg once daily
Cl_{cr} 15 mL/minute: 100-300 mg once daily
Cl_{cr} <15 mL/minute: Reduce daily dose in proportion to creatinine clearance based on dose for creatinine clearance of 15 mL/minute (eg, reduce dose by one-half [range: 50-150 mg/day] for Cl_{cr} 7.5 mL/minute)

ESRD requiring hemodialysis: Dose for Cl$_{cr}$ <15 mL/minute plus single supplemental dose of 125-350 mg (given after each 4 hours of hemodialysis)

Extended release: **Note:** Follow initial dose titration schedule if treatment-naive.

Cl$_{cr}$ ≥60 mL/minute: 1800 mg once daily

Cl$_{cr}$ >30-59 mL/minute: 600-1800 mg once daily; dependent on tolerability and clinical response

Cl$_{cr}$ <30 mL/minute: Use is not recommended.

ESRD requiring hemodialysis: Use is not recommended.

Hepatic Impairment There are no dosage adjustments provided in the manufacturer's labeling; however, gabapentin is not hepatically metabolized.

Administration

Tablet, solution (immediate release): Administer first dose on first day at bedtime to avoid somnolence and dizziness. Dosage must be adjusted for renal function; when given 3 times daily, the maximum time between doses should not exceed 12 hours.

Tablet (extended release): Take with evening meal. Swallow whole; do not chew, crush, or split.

Monitoring Parameters Monitor serum levels of concomitant anticonvulsant therapy; suicidality (eg, suicidal thoughts, depression, behavioral changes)

Test Interactions False positives have been reported with the Ames N-Multistix SG® dipstick test for urine protein

Special Geriatric Considerations Studies in the elderly have shown a decrease in clearance as age increases. This is most likely due to age-related decreases in renal function; calculations of Cl$_{cr}$ recommended since dose reductions may be needed.

Dosage Forms Excipient information presented when available (limited, particularly for generics); consult specific product labeling.

Capsule, oral: 100 mg, 300 mg, 400 mg

Neurontin®: 100 mg, 300 mg, 400 mg

Solution, oral: 250 mg/5 mL (470 mL)

Neurontin®: 250 mg/5 mL (470 mL) [cool strawberry-anise flavor]

Tablet, oral: 600 mg, 800 mg

Gralise™: 300 mg [contains soybean lecithin]

Gralise™: 600 mg

Neurontin®: 600 mg, 800 mg [scored]

Tablet, oral [combination package (each unit-dose starter kit contains)]:

Gralise™: 300 mg (9s) [white tablets; contains soybean lecithin] and 600 mg (69s) [beige tablets]

Gabapentin Enacarbil (gab a PEN tin en a KAR bil)

Brand Names: U.S. Horizant™

Index Terms GSK 1838262; Horizant™; Solzira; XP13512

Generic Availability (U.S.) No

Pharmacologic Category Anticonvulsant, Miscellaneous

Use Treatment of moderate-to-severe restless leg syndrome (RLS); management of post-herpetic neuralgia (PHN)

Medication Guide Available Yes

Contraindications There are no contraindications listed within the manufacturer's labeling.

Warnings/Precautions Potentially serious, sometimes fatal multiorgan hypersensitivity (also known as drug reaction with eosinophilia and systemic symptoms [DRESS]) has been reported with some antiepileptic drugs, including gabapentin. Monitor for signs and symptoms of possible disparate manifestations associated with lymphatic, hepatic, renal, cardiac, and/or hematologic systems; fever, rash, and eosinophilia may also be present. Discontinue immediately if suspected. Gabapentin and other antiepileptics are associated with an increased risk of suicidal behavior/thoughts with use (regardless of indication); gabapentin enacarbil is a prodrug of gabapentin and may also increase patient's risk. Patients should be monitored for signs/symptoms of depression, suicidal tendencies, and other unusual behavior changes during therapy and instructed to inform their healthcare provider immediately if symptoms occur. Doses >600 mg daily should be reduced to 600 mg daily for 1 week prior to stopping. Rat studies demonstrated an association with pancreatic adenocarcinoma (clinical implication unknown). May cause CNS depression, which may impair physical or mental abilities. Patients must be cautioned about performing tasks which require mental alertness (eg, operating machinery or driving). Effects with other sedative drugs or ethanol may be potentiated. Use with caution in patients with renal impairment; dose adjustment is needed. Gabapentin enacarbil (Horizant™) and other gabapentin products are not interchangeable due to differences in formulation, indications, and pharmacokinetics.

Restless legs syndrome (RLS): Not recommended for use in patients who are required to sleep during the day and remain awake during the night.

Adverse Reactions (Reflective of adult population; not specific for elderly) Percentages reported are for restless leg syndrome (RLS) 600 mg daily and postherpetic neuralgia (PHN) 1200 mg daily.

>10%: Central nervous system: Sedation/somnolence (PHN 10%; RLS 20%), dizziness (13% to 17%), headache (10% to 12%)

1% to 10%:

Cardiovascular: Peripheral edema (PHN 6%; RLS <1%)

Central nervous system: Fatigue (6%), irritability (≤4%), insomnia (PHN 3%), balance disorder (<2%), depression (<2%), disorientation (<2%), lethargy (<2%), drunk feeling (<2%), vertigo (<2%)

Gastrointestinal: Nausea (6% to 8%), flatulence (≤3%), xerostomia (≤3%), weight gain (2% to 3%), appetite increased (≤2%)

Ocular: Blurred vision (≤2%)

Drug Interactions

Metabolism/Transport Effects None known.

Avoid Concomitant Use

Avoid concomitant use of Gabapentin Enacarbil with any of the following: Azelastine; Azelastine (Nasal); Methadone; Mirtazapine; Paraldehyde

Increased Effect/Toxicity

Gabapentin Enacarbil may increase the levels/effects of: Alcohol (Ethyl); Azelastine; Azelastine (Nasal); Buprenorphine; CNS Depressants; Methadone; Methotrimeprazine; Metyrosine; Mirtazapine; Paraldehyde; Selective Serotonin Reuptake Inhibitors; Zolpidem

The levels/effects of Gabapentin Enacarbil may be increased by: Droperidol; HydrOXYzine; Methotrimeprazine

Decreased Effect

The levels/effects of Gabapentin Enacarbil may be decreased by: Ketorolac; Ketorolac (Nasal); Ketorolac (Systemic); Mefloquine

Ethanol/Nutrition/Herb Interactions

Ethanol: Avoid ethanol (may increase CNS depression).

Herb/Nutraceutical: Avoid evening primrose (seizure threshold decreased). Avoid valerian, St John's wort, kava kava, gotu kola (may increase CNS depression).

Stability Store at 25°C (77°F); excursions permitted to 15°C to 30°C (59°F to 86°F). Protect from moisture. Do not remove from original container.

Mechanism of Action Gabapentin enacarbil is a prodrug of gabapentin. Gabapentin is structurally related to GABA. However, it does not bind to $GABA_A$ or $GABA_B$ receptors, and it does not appear to influence synthesis or uptake of GABA. High affinity gabapentin binding sites have been located throughout the brain; these sites correspond to the presence of voltage-gated calcium channels specifically possessing the alpha-2-delta-1 subunit. This channel appears to be located presynaptically, and may modulate the release of excitatory neurotransmitters. These effects on RLS are unknown.

Pharmacodynamics/Kinetics

Absorption: Mediated by active transport via proton-linked monocarboxylate transporter, MCT-1

Distribution: V_d: 76 L

Protein binding: <3%

Bioavailability: With food: ~75%; Fasting: 42% to 65%

Metabolism: Prodrug hydrolyzed primarily in the intestines to gabapentin (active metabolite)

Time to peak, plasma: With food: 7.3 hours; Fasting: 5 hours

Half-life elimination: 5-6 hours

Excretion: Urine (94%); feces (5%)

Dosage

Geriatric & Adult

Postherpetic neuralgia (PHN): Oral: Initial: 600 mg once daily in the morning for 3 days, then increase to 600 mg twice daily; increasing to >1200 mg daily provided no additional benefit and increased side effects

Restless legs syndrome (RLS): Oral: 600 mg once daily (at ~5:00 pm); increasing to 1200 mg daily provided no additional benefit and increased side effects

Renal Impairment Note: Estimation of renal function for the purpose of drug dosing should be done using the Cockcroft-Gault formula.

PHN:

Cl_{cr} 30-59 mL/minute: Initial: 300 mg every morning for 3 days, then increase to 300 mg twice daily. May increase to 600 mg twice daily as needed based on tolerability and efficacy. When discontinuing, reduce current dose to once daily in the morning for 1 week.

Cl_{cr} 15-29: Initial: 300 mg in the morning on day 1 and on day 3; then increase to 300 mg once daily. May increase to 300 mg twice daily if needed based on tolerability and efficacy. When discontinuing, if current dose is 300 mg twice daily, reduce to 300 mg once daily for 1 week. If current dose is 300 mg once daily, no taper is needed.

Cl_{cr} <15: 300 mg every other day in the morning; may increase dose to 300 mg once daily if needed based on tolerability and efficacy. When discontinuing, no taper is needed.

Cl_{cr} <15 and on hemodialysis: 300 mg following every dialysis. May increase to 600 mg following every dialysis if needed based on tolerability and efficacy. When discontinuing, no taper is needed.

RLS:
Cl_{cr} 30-59 mL/minute: Initial dose: 300 mg daily; increase to 600 mg daily as needed
Cl_{cr} 15-29: 300 mg daily
Cl_{cr} <15: 300 mg every other day
Cl_{cr} <15 and on hemodialysis: Use is not recommended.

Administration Tablet should be swallowed whole; do not break, chew, cut, or crush. Administer with food.

Restless leg syndrome: Administer at ~5:00 pm daily.

Monitoring Parameters Suicidality (eg, suicidal thoughts, depression, behavioral changes)

Special Geriatric Considerations Since many elderly may have a creatinine clearance of <60 mL/minute due to age-related renal function decline, it is advised to estimate (calculate) the creatinine clearance before initiating gabapentin enacarbil.

Dosage Forms Excipient information presented when available (limited, particularly for generics); consult specific product labeling.
Tablet, extended release, oral:
Horizant™: 600 mg

♦ **Gabitril®** see TiaGABine on page 1886
♦ **Gablofen®** see Baclofen on page 186

Galantamine (ga LAN ta meen)

Medication Safety Issues
Sound-alike/look-alike issues:
Razadyne® may be confused with Rozerem®
International issues:
Reminyl [Canada and multiple international markets] may be confused with Amarel brand name for glimepiride [France]; Amaryl brand name for glimepiride [U.S., Canada, and multiple international markets]; Robinul brand name for glycopyrrolate [U.S. and multiple international markets]

Brand Names: U.S. Razadyne®; Razadyne® ER
Brand Names: Canada Mylan-Galantamine ER; PAT-Galantamine ER; Reminyl®; Reminyl® ER
Index Terms Galantamine Hydrobromide
Generic Availability (U.S.) Yes
Pharmacologic Category Acetylcholinesterase Inhibitor (Central)
Use Treatment of mild-to-moderate dementia of Alzheimer's disease
Unlabeled Use Severe dementia associated with Alzheimer's disease; mild-to-moderate dementia associated with Parkinson's disease; Lewy body dementia
Contraindications Hypersensitivity to galantamine or any component of the formulation
Warnings/Precautions Use caution in patients with supraventricular conduction delays (without a functional pacemaker in place); Alzheimer's treatment guidelines consider brady-cardia to be a relative contraindication for use of centrally-active cholinesterase inhibitors. Use caution in patients taking medicines that slow conduction through SA or AV node. Use caution in peptic ulcer disease (or in patients at risk); seizure disorder; asthma; COPD; mild-to-moderate liver dysfunction; moderate renal dysfunction. May cause bladder outflow obstruc-tion. May exaggerate neuromuscular blockade effects of succinylcholine and like agents.
Adverse Reactions (Reflective of adult population; not specific for elderly)
>10%: Gastrointestinal: Nausea (13% to 24%), vomiting (6% to 13%), diarrhea (6% to 12%)
1% to 10%:
Cardiovascular: Bradycardia (2% to 3%), hypertension (≥2%), peripheral edema (≥2%), syncope (0.4% to 2.2%: dose related), chest pain (≥1% to 2%)
Central nervous system: Dizziness (9%), headache (8%), depression (7%), fatigue (5%), insomnia (5%), somnolence (4%), agitation (≥2%), anxiety (≥2%), confusion (≥2%), hallucination (≥2%), fever (≥1%), malaise (≥1%)
Dermatologic: Purpura (≥2%)
Gastrointestinal: Anorexia (7% to 9%), weight loss (5% to 7%), abdominal pain (5%), dyspepsia (5%), constipation (≥2%), flatulence (≥1%)

Genitourinary: Urinary tract infection (8%), hematuria (<1% to 3%), incontinence (≥1% to 2%)

Hematologic: Anemia (3%)

Neuromuscular & skeletal: Tremor (3%), back pain (≥2%), fall (≥2%), weakness (≥1% to 2%)

Respiratory: Rhinitis (4%), bronchitis (≥2%), cough (≥2%), upper respiratory tract infection (≥2%)

Drug Interactions

Metabolism/Transport Effects Substrate of CYP2D6 (minor), CYP3A4 (minor); **Note:** Assignment of Major/Minor substrate status based on clinically relevant drug interaction potential

Avoid Concomitant Use There are no known interactions where it is recommended to avoid concomitant use.

Increased Effect/Toxicity

Galantamine may increase the levels/effects of: Antipsychotics; Beta-Blockers; Cholinergic Agonists; Highest Risk QTc-Prolonging Agents; Moderate Risk QTc-Prolonging Agents; Succinylcholine

The levels/effects of Galantamine may be increased by: Corticosteroids (Systemic); Mifepristone; Selective Serotonin Reuptake Inhibitors

Decreased Effect

Galantamine may decrease the levels/effects of: Anticholinergics; Neuromuscular-Blocking Agents (Nondepolarizing)

The levels/effects of Galantamine may be decreased by: Anticholinergics; Dipyridamole; Peginterferon Alfa-2b; Tocilizumab

Ethanol/Nutrition/Herb Interactions

Ethanol: Avoid ethanol (may increase CNS adverse events).

Herb/Nutraceutical: St John's wort may decrease galantamine serum levels; avoid concurrent use.

Stability Store at 25°C (77°F); excursions permitted to 15°C to 30°C (59°F to 86°F). Do not freeze oral solution.

Mechanism of Action Centrally-acting cholinesterase inhibitor (competitive and reversible). It elevates acetylcholine in cerebral cortex by slowing the degradation of acetylcholine. Modulates nicotinic acetylcholine receptor to increase acetylcholine from surviving presynaptic nerve terminals. May increase glutamate and serotonin levels.

Pharmacodynamics/Kinetics

Duration: 3 hours; maximum inhibition of erythrocyte acetylcholinesterase ~40% at 1 hour post 8 mg oral dose; levels return to baseline at 30 hours

Absorption: Rapid and complete

Distribution: 175 L; levels in the brain are 2-3 times higher than in plasma

Protein binding: 18%

Metabolism: Hepatic; linear, CYP2D6 and 3A4; metabolized to epigalanthaminone and galanthaminone both of which have acetylcholinesterase inhibitory activity 130 times less than galantamine

Bioavailability: ~90%

Half-life elimination: ~7 hours

Time to peak: Immediate release: 1 hour (2.5 hours with food); extended release: 4.5-5 hours

Excretion: Urine (20%)

Dosage

Geriatric & Adult Alzheimer's dementia (mild-to-moderate): Oral:

Immediate release tablet or solution: Initial: 4 mg twice a day for 4 weeks; if tolerated, increase to 8 mg twice daily for ≥4 weeks; if tolerated, increase to 12 mg twice daily. Range: 16-24 mg/day in 2 divided doses

Extended-release capsule: Initial: 8 mg once daily for 4 weeks; if tolerated, increase to 16 mg once daily for ≥4 weeks; if tolerated, increase to 24 mg once daily. Range: 16-24 mg once daily

Note: If therapy is interrupted for ≥3 days, restart at the lowest dose and increase to current dose.

Conversion from immediate release to extended release formulation: Patients may be switched from the immediate release formulation to the extended release formulation by taking the last immediate release dose in the evening and beginning the extended release dose the following morning; the same total daily dose should be used.

Conversion to galantamine from other cholinesterase inhibitors: Patients experiencing poor tolerability with donepezil or rivastigmine should wait until side effects subside or allow a 7-day washout period prior to beginning galantamine. Patients not experiencing side effects with donepezil or rivastigmine may begin galantamine therapy the day immediately following discontinuation of previous therapy (Morris, 2001).

Renal Impairment
Moderate renal impairment: Maximum dose: 16 mg/day.
Severe renal dysfunction (Cl_{cr} <9 mL/minute): Use is not recommended
Hepatic Impairment
Moderate liver dysfunction (Child-Pugh score 7-9): Maximum dose: 16 mg/day
Severe liver dysfunction (Child-Pugh score 10-15): Use is not recommended
Administration Oral: Administer solution or tablet with breakfast and dinner; administer extended release capsule with breakfast. If therapy is interrupted for ≥3 days, restart at the lowest dose and increase to current dose. If using oral solution, mix dose with 3-4 ounces of any nonalcoholic beverage; mix well and drink immediately.
Monitoring Parameters Mental status
Special Geriatric Considerations No dosage adjustment needed.
Dosage Forms Excipient information presented when available (limited, particularly for generics); consult specific product labeling.
Capsule, extended release, oral, as hydrobromide [strength expressed as base]: 8 mg, 16 mg, 24 mg
Razadyne® ER: 8 mg, 16 mg, 24 mg
Solution, oral, as hydrobromide: 4 mg/mL (100 mL)
Razadyne®: 4 mg/mL (100 mL)
Tablet, oral, as hydrobromide [strength expressed as base]: 4 mg, 8 mg, 12 mg
Razadyne®: 4 mg, 8 mg, 12 mg

- ◆ **Galantamine Hydrobromide** *see* Galantamine *on page 863*
- ◆ **GamaSTAN™ S/D** *see* Immune Globulin *on page 982*
- ◆ **Gamma Benzene Hexachloride** *see* Lindane *on page 1135*
- ◆ **Gamma E-Gems® [OTC]** *see* Vitamin E *on page 2027*
- ◆ **Gamma-E PLUS [OTC]** *see* Vitamin E *on page 2027*
- ◆ **Gammagard® Liquid** *see* Immune Globulin *on page 982*
- ◆ **Gammagard S/D®** *see* Immune Globulin *on page 982*
- ◆ **Gamma Globulin** *see* Immune Globulin *on page 982*
- ◆ **Gammaked™** *see* Immune Globulin *on page 982*
- ◆ **Gammaplex®** *see* Immune Globulin *on page 982*
- ◆ **Gamunex® [DSC]** *see* Immune Globulin *on page 982*
- ◆ **Gamunex®-C** *see* Immune Globulin *on page 982*

Ganciclovir (Systemic) (gan SYE kloe veer)

Medication Safety Issues
Sound-alike/look-alike issues:
Cytovene® may be confused with Cytosar®, Cytosar-U
Ganciclovir may be confused with acyclovir
Brand Names: U.S. Cytovene®-IV
Brand Names: Canada Cytovene®
Index Terms DHPG Sodium; GCV Sodium; Nordeoxyguanosine
Generic Availability (U.S.) Yes
Pharmacologic Category Antiviral Agent
Use Treatment of CMV retinitis in immunocompromised individuals, including patients with acquired immunodeficiency syndrome; prophylaxis of CMV infection in transplant patients
Unlabeled Use CMV retinitis: May be given in combination with foscarnet in patients who relapse after monotherapy with either drug
Contraindications Hypersensitivity to ganciclovir, acyclovir, or any component of the formulation
Warnings/Precautions Hazardous agent - use appropriate precautions for handling and disposal. **[U.S. Boxed Warning]: Granulocytopenia (neutropenia), anemia, and thrombocytopenia may occur.** Dosage adjustment or interruption of ganciclovir therapy may be necessary in patients with neutropenia and/or thrombocytopenia and patients with impaired renal function. **[U.S. Boxed Warning]: Animal studies have demonstrated carcinogenic and teratogenic effects, and inhibition of spermatogenesis;** contraceptive precautions for female and male patients need to be followed during and for at least 90 days after therapy with the drug; take care to administer only into veins with good blood flow. **[U.S. Boxed Warning]: Indicated only for treatment of CMV retinitis in the immunocompromised patient and CMV prevention in transplant patients at risk.**

◀ **Adverse Reactions (Reflective of adult population; not specific for elderly)**

>10%:

Central nervous system: Fever (48%)

Gastrointestinal: Diarrhea (44%), anorexia (14%), vomiting (13%)

Hematologic: Thrombocytopenia (57%), leukopenia (41%), anemia (16% to 26%), neutropenia with ANC <500/mm^3 (12% to 14%)

Ocular: Retinal detachment (11%; relationship to ganciclovir not established)

Renal: Serum creatinine increased (2% to 14%)

Miscellaneous: Sepsis (15%), diaphoresis (12%)

1% to 10%:

Central nervous system: Chills (10%), neuropathy (9%)

Dermatologic: Pruritus (5%)

<1%, postmarketing, and/or case reports (limited to important or life-threatening): Allergic reaction (including anaphylaxis), alopecia, arrhythmia, bronchospasm, cardiac arrest, cataracts, cholestasis, coma, dyspnea, edema, encephalopathy, exfoliative dermatitis, extrapyramidal symptoms, hepatitis, hepatic failure, pancreatitis, pancytopenia, pulmonary fibrosis, psychosis, rhabdomyolysis, seizure, alopecia, urticaria, eosinophilia, hemorrhage, Stevens-Johnson syndrome, torsade de pointes, renal failure, SIADH, visual loss

Drug Interactions

Metabolism/Transport Effects None known.

Avoid Concomitant Use

Avoid concomitant use of Ganciclovir (Systemic) with any of the following: Imipenem

Increased Effect/Toxicity

Ganciclovir (Systemic) may increase the levels/effects of: Imipenem; Mycophenolate; Reverse Transcriptase Inhibitors (Nucleoside); Tenofovir

The levels/effects of Ganciclovir (Systemic) may be increased by: Mycophenolate; Probenecid; Tenofovir

Decreased Effect There are no known significant interactions involving a decrease in effect.

Stability Intact vials should be stored at room temperature and protected from temperatures >40°C Reconstitute powder with unpreserved sterile water **not** bacteriostatic water because parabens may cause precipitation; dilute in 250-1000 mL D$_5$W or NS to a concentration ≤10 mg/mL for infusion.

Reconstituted solution is stable for 12 hours at room temperature, however, conflicting data indicates that reconstituted solution is stable for 60 days under refrigeration (4°C). Stability of parenteral admixture at room temperature (25°C) and at refrigeration temperature (4°C) is 5 days.

Mechanism of Action Ganciclovir is phosphorylated to a substrate which competitively inhibits the binding of deoxyguanosine triphosphate to DNA polymerase resulting in inhibition of viral DNA synthesis

Pharmacodynamics/Kinetics

Distribution: V$_d$: 15.26 L/1.73 m^2; widely to all tissues including CSF and ocular tissue

Protein binding: 1% to 2%

Half-life elimination: 1.7-5.8 hours; prolonged with renal impairment; End-stage renal disease: 5-28 hours

Excretion: Urine (80% to 99% as unchanged drug)

Dosage

Geriatric Refer to adult dosing. In general, dose selection should be cautious, reflecting greater frequency of organ impairment.

Adult

CMV CNS infection in HIV-exposed/-infected patients (unlabeled use; CDC, 2009): I.V.: 5 mg/kg/dose every 12 hours plus foscarnet until symptoms improve followed by chronic suppression

CMV retinitis: I.V. (slow infusion):

Induction therapy: 5 mg/kg/dose every 12 hours for 14-21 days followed by maintenance therapy

Maintenance therapy: 5 mg/kg/day as a single daily dose for 7 days/week or 6 mg/kg/day for 5 days/week

Prevention (secondary) of CMV disease in HIV-exposed/-infected patients (unlabeled use; CDC, 2009): I.V.: 5 mg/kg/dose daily

Prevention (secondary) of CMV disease in transplant patients: I.V. (slow infusion): 5 mg/kg/dose every 12 hours for 7-14 days, duration of maintenance therapy is dependent on clinical condition and degree of immunosuppression

Varicella zoster: Progressive outer retinal necrosis in HIV-exposed/-infected patients (unlabeled use; CDC, 2009): I.V.: 5 mg/kg/dose every 12 hours plus systemic foscarnet and intravitreal ganciclovir or intravitreal foscarnet

Renal Impairment

I.V. (Induction):
Cl_{cr} 50-69 mL/minute: Administer 2.5 mg/kg/dose every 12 hours.
Cl_{cr} 25-49 mL/minute: Administer 2.5 mg/kg/dose every 24 hours.
Cl_{cr} 10-24 mL/minute: Administer 1.25 mg/kg/dose every 24 hours.
Cl_{cr} <10 mL/minute: Administer 1.25 mg/kg/dose 3 times/week following hemodialysis.

I.V. (Maintenance):
Cl_{cr} 50-69 mL/minute: Administer 2.5 mg/kg/dose every 24 hours.
Cl_{cr} 25-49 mL/minute: Administer 1.25 mg/kg/dose every 24 hours.
Cl_{cr} 10-24 mL/minute: Administer 0.625 mg/kg/dose every 24 hours
Cl_{cr} <10 mL/minute: Administer 0.625 mg/kg/dose 3 times/week following hemodialysis.

Intermittent hemodialysis (IHD) (administer after hemodialysis on dialysis days): Dialyzable (50%): CMV Infection: I.V.: Induction: 1.25 mg/kg every 48-72 hours; Maintenance: 0.625 mg/kg every 48-72 hours. **Note:** Dosing dependent on the assumption of 3 times/week, complete IHD sessions.

Peritoneal dialysis (PD): Dose as for Cl_{cr} <10 mL/minute.

Continuous renal replacement therapy (CRRT) (Heintz, 2009; Trotman, 2005): Drug clearance is highly dependent on the method of renal replacement, filter type, and flow rate. Appropriate dosing requires close monitoring of pharmacologic response, signs of adverse reactions due to drug accumulation, as well as drug concentrations in relation to target trough (if appropriate). The following are general recommendations only (based on dialysate flow/ultrafiltration rates of 1-2 L/hour and minimal residual renal function) and should not supersede clinical judgment: CMV Infection:
CVVH: I.V.: Induction: 2.5 mg/kg every 24 hours; Maintenance: 1.25 mg/kg every 24 hours
CVVHD/CVVHDF: I.V.: Induction: 2.5 mg/kg every 12 hours; Maintenance: 2.5 mg/kg every 24 hours

Administration Should not be administered by I.M., SubQ, or rapid IVP; administer by slow I.V. infusion over at least 1 hour. Too rapid infusion can cause increased toxicity and excessive plasma levels.

Monitoring Parameters CBC with differential and platelet count, serum creatinine

Pharmacotherapy Pearls Sodium content of 500 mg vial: 46 mg

Special Geriatric Considerations Adjust dose based upon renal function.

Dosage Forms Excipient information presented when available (limited, particularly for generics); consult specific product labeling.
Injection, powder for reconstitution: 500 mg
Cytovene®-IV: 500 mg

Ganciclovir (Ophthalmic) (gan SYE kloe veer)

Medication Safety Issues
Sound-alike/look-alike issues:
Ganciclovir may be confused with acyclovir

Brand Names: U.S. Vitrasert®; Zirgan®

Index Terms Nordeoxyguanosine

Generic Availability (U.S.) No

Pharmacologic Category Antiviral Agent, Ophthalmic

Use
Intravitreal implant: Treatment of CMV retinitis in patients with acquired immunodeficiency syndrome
Ophthalmic gel: Treatment of acute herpetic keratitis (dendritic ulcers)

Dosage
Geriatric & Adult
CMV retinitis: *Intravitreal implant:* One implant for 5- to 8-month period; following depletion of ganciclovir, as evidenced by progression of retinitis, implant may be removed and replaced
Herpetic keratitis: *Ophthalmic gel:* Apply 1 drop in affected eye 5 times/day (approximately every 3 hours while awake) until corneal ulcer heals, then 1 drop 3 times/day for 7 days

Special Geriatric Considerations Evaluate the patient's or caregiver's ability to safely administer the correct dose of ophthalmic medication.

Dosage Forms Excipient information presented when available (limited, particularly for generics); consult specific product labeling.
Gel, ophthalmic [drops]:
Zirgan®: 0.15% (5 g) [contains benzalkonium chloride]
Implant, intravitreal:
Vitrasert®: 4.5 mg (1s) [released gradually over 5-8 months]

◆ GAR-936 see Tigecycline on page 1896

Gatifloxacin (gat i FLOKS a sin)

Brand Names: U.S. Zymaxid™
Brand Names: Canada Zymar™
Generic Availability (U.S.) No
Pharmacologic Category Antibiotic, Ophthalmic; Antibiotic, Quinolone
Use Treatment of bacterial conjunctivitis
Contraindications
Zymaxid™: There are no contraindications listed in the manufacturer's labeling.
Zymar™: Hypersensitivity to gatifloxacin, other quinolones, or any component of the formulation
Warnings/Precautions Severe hypersensitivity reactions, including anaphylaxis, have occurred with systemic quinolone therapy. Reactions may present as typical allergic symptoms after a single dose, or may manifest as severe idiosyncratic dermatologic, vascular, pulmonary, renal, hepatic, and/or hematologic events, usually after multiple doses. Prompt discontinuation of drug should occur if skin rash or other symptoms arise. Prolonged use may result in fungal or bacterial superinfection. For topical ophthalmic use only. Do not inject ophthalmic solution subconjunctivally or introduce directly into the anterior chamber of the eye. Contact lenses should not be worn during treatment of ophthalmic infections.
Adverse Reactions (Reflective of adult population; not specific for elderly) 1% to 10%:
Cardiovascular: Edema
Dermatologic: Contact dermatitis, erythema
Gastrointestinal: Taste disturbance
Ocular: Conjunctival irritation, discharge, dry eye, edema, irritation, keratitis, lacrimation increased, pain, papillary conjunctivitis, visual acuity decreased
Respiratory: Rhinorrhea
Drug Interactions
  Metabolism/Transport Effects None known.
  Avoid Concomitant Use There are no known interactions where it is recommended to avoid concomitant use.
  Increased Effect/Toxicity There are no known significant interactions involving an increase in effect.
  Decreased Effect There are no known significant interactions involving a decrease in effect.
Stability Store between 15°C to 25°C (59°F to 77°F); do not freeze.
Mechanism of Action Gatifloxacin is a DNA gyrase inhibitor, and also inhibits topoisomerase IV. DNA gyrase (topoisomerase II) is an essential bacterial enzyme that maintains the superhelical structure of DNA. DNA gyrase is required for DNA replication and transcription, DNA repair, recombination, and transposition; inhibition is bactericidal.
Pharmacodynamics/Kinetics Absorption: Ophthalmic: Not measurable
Dosage
  Geriatric & Adult Bacterial conjunctivitis: Ophthalmic:
    Zymar™:
      Days 1 and 2: Instill 1 drop into affected eye(s) every 2 hours while awake (maximum: 8 times/day)
      Days 3-7: Instill 1 drop into affected eye(s) 4 times/day while awake
    Zymaxid™:
      Day 1: Instill 1 drop into affected eye(s) every 2 hours while awake (maximum: 8 times/day)
      Days 2-7: Instill 1 drop into affected eye(s) 2-4 times/day while awake
Administration Concentrated injection (10 mg/mL) must be diluted to 2 mg/mL prior to administration. No further dilution is required for premixed 100 mL and 200 mL solutions. Suspension may be administered through a gastric feeding tube.
Monitoring Parameters Signs of infection

Test Interactions Some quinolones may produce a false-positive urine screening result for opiates using commercially-available immunoassay kits. This has been demonstrated most consistently for levofloxacin and ofloxacin, but other quinolones have shown cross-reactivity in certain assay kits. Confirmation of positive opiate screens by more specific methods should be considered.

Special Geriatric Considerations Evaluate the patient's or caregiver's ability to safely administer the correct dose of ophthalmic medication.

Dosage Forms Excipient information presented when available (limited, particularly for generics); consult specific product labeling.

Solution, ophthalmic [drops]:
Zymaxid™: 0.5% (2.5 mL) [contains benzalkonium chloride]

Dosage Forms: Canada Excipient information presented when available (limited, particularly for generics); consult specific product labeling.

Solution, ophthalmic [drops]:
Zymar™: 0.3% (1 mL, 2.5 mL, 5 mL) [contains benzalkonium chloride]

- ◆ **Gaviscon® Extra Strength [OTC]** see Aluminum Hydroxide and Magnesium Carbonate on page 79
- ◆ **Gaviscon® Liquid [OTC]** see Aluminum Hydroxide and Magnesium Carbonate on page 79
- ◆ **Gaviscon® Tablet [OTC]** see Aluminum Hydroxide and Magnesium Trisilicate on page 81
- ◆ **Gax-X® Infant [OTC]** see Simethicone on page 1776
- ◆ **G-CSF** see Filgrastim on page 787
- ◆ **G-CSF (PEG Conjugate)** see Pegfilgrastim on page 1481
- ◆ **GCV Sodium** see Ganciclovir (Systemic) on page 865
- ◆ **Gelclair®** see Mucosal Barrier Gel, Oral on page 1323
- ◆ **Gel-Kam® [OTC]** see Fluoride on page 806
- ◆ **Gel-Kam® Rinse** see Fluoride on page 806
- ◆ **Gelnique®** see Oxybutynin on page 1443
- ◆ **Gelnique 3%™** see Oxybutynin on page 1443
- ◆ **Gelusil® [OTC]** see Aluminum Hydroxide, Magnesium Hydroxide, and Simethicone on page 82

Gemfibrozil (jem FI broe zil)

Related Information
Hyperlipidemia Management on page 2130

Medication Safety Issues
Sound-alike/look-alike issues:
Lopid® may be confused with Levbid®, Lipitor®, Lodine

Brand Names: U.S. Lopid®

Brand Names: Canada Apo-Gemfibrozil®; Gen-Gemfibrozil; GMD-Gemfibrozil; Lopid®; Mylan-Gemfibrozil; Novo-Gemfibrozil; Nu-Gemfibrozil; PMS-Gemfibrozil

Index Terms CI-719

Generic Availability (U.S.) Yes

Pharmacologic Category Antilipemic Agent, Fibric Acid

Use Treatment of hypertriglyceridemia in Fredrickson types IV and V hyperlipidemia for patients who are at greater risk for pancreatitis and who have not responded to dietary intervention; to reduce the risk of CHD development in Fredrickson type IIb patients without a history or symptoms of existing CHD who have not responded to dietary and other interventions (including pharmacologic treatment) and who have decreased HDL, increased LDL, and increased triglycerides

Contraindications Hypersensitivity to gemfibrozil or any component of the formulation; hepatic or severe renal dysfunction; primary biliary cirrhosis; pre-existing gallbladder disease; concurrent use with repaglinide

Warnings/Precautions Secondary causes of hyperlipidemia should be ruled out prior to therapy. Possible increased risk of malignancy and cholelithiasis. Anemia, leukopenia, thrombocytopenia, and bone marrow hypoplasia have rarely been reported. Periodic monitoring recommended during the first year of therapy. Elevations in serum transaminases can be seen. Discontinue if lipid response not seen. Be careful in patient selection; this is not a first- or second-line choice. Other agents may be more suitable. Adjustments in warfarin therapy may be required with concurrent use. Has been associated with rare myositis or rhabdomyolysis; patients should be monitored closely. Patients should be instructed to report unexplained muscle pain, tenderness, weakness, or brown urine. Use caution when combining gemfibrozil with HMG-CoA reductase inhibitors (may lead to myopathy, rhabdomyolysis). Use with caution in patients with mild-to-moderate renal impairment; contraindicated in patients with severe impairment. Renal function deterioration has been seen when used in patients with a serum creatinine >2 mg/dL.

◄ **Adverse Reactions (Reflective of adult population; not specific for elderly)**
>10%: Gastrointestinal: Dyspepsia (20%)
1% to 10%:
  Cardiovascular: Atrial fibrillation (1%)
  Central nervous system: Fatigue (4%), vertigo (2%)
  Dermatologic: Eczema (2%), rash (2%)
  Gastrointestinal: Abdominal pain (10%), nausea/vomiting (3%)

Reports where causal relationship has not been established: Alopecia, anaphylaxis, cataracts, colitis, confusion, decreased fertility (male), drug-induced lupus-like syndrome, extrasystoles, hepatoma, intracranial hemorrhage, pancreatitis, peripheral vascular disease, photosensitivity, positive ANA, renal dysfunction, retinal edema, seizure, syncope, thrombocytopenia, vasculitis, weight loss

Drug Interactions
  Metabolism/Transport Effects Substrate of CYP3A4 (minor); **Note:** Assignment of Major/Minor substrate status based on clinically relevant drug interaction potential; **Inhibits** CYP1A2 (moderate), CYP2C19 (strong), CYP2C8 (strong), CYP2C9 (strong)

Avoid Concomitant Use
  Avoid concomitant use of Gemfibrozil with any of the following: AtorvaSTATin; Bexarotene; Bexarotene (Systemic); Clopidogrel; Fluvastatin; Lovastatin; Pitavastatin; Pravastatin; Repaglinide; Rosuvastatin; Simvastatin

Increased Effect/Toxicity
  Gemfibrozil may increase the levels/effects of: Antidiabetic Agents (Thiazolidinedione); AtorvaSTATin; Bexarotene; Bexarotene (Systemic); Carvedilol; Citalopram; Colchicine; CYP1A2 Substrates; CYP2C19 Substrates; CYP2C8 Substrates; CYP2C9 Substrates; Diclofenac; Ezetimibe; Fluvastatin; Lovastatin; Pitavastatin; Pravastatin; Repaglinide; Rosuvastatin; Simvastatin; Sulfonylureas; Treprostinil; Vitamin K Antagonists

  The levels/effects of Gemfibrozil may be increased by: CycloSPORINE; CycloSPORINE (Systemic)

Decreased Effect
  Gemfibrozil may decrease the levels/effects of: Chenodiol; Clopidogrel; CycloSPORINE; CycloSPORINE (Systemic); Ursodiol

  The levels/effects of Gemfibrozil may be decreased by: Bile Acid Sequestrants; Tocilizumab

Ethanol/Nutrition/Herb Interactions
  Ethanol: Avoid ethanol to decrease triglycerides.
  Food: When given after meals, the AUC of gemfibrozil is decreased.

Stability Store at controlled room temperature of 20°C to 25°C (68°F to 77°F). Protect from light and moisture.

Mechanism of Action The exact mechanism of action of gemfibrozil is unknown, however, several theories exist regarding the VLDL effect; it can inhibit lipolysis and decrease subsequent hepatic fatty acid uptake as well as inhibit hepatic secretion of VLDL; together these actions decrease serum VLDL levels; increases HDL-cholesterol; the mechanism behind HDL elevation is currently unknown

Pharmacodynamics/Kinetics
  Onset of action: May require several days
  Absorption: Well absorbed
  Protein binding: 99%
  Metabolism: Hepatic via oxidation to two inactive metabolites; undergoes enterohepatic recycling
  Half-life elimination: 1.5 hours
  Time to peak, serum: 1-2 hours
  Excretion: Urine (~70% primarily as conjugated drug); feces (6%)

Dosage
  Geriatric & Adult Hyperlipidemia/hypertriglyceridemia: Oral: 600 mg twice daily; administer 30 minutes before breakfast and dinner
  Renal Impairment
    Mild-to-moderate impairment: Use caution; deterioration of renal function has been reported in patients with baseline serum creatinine >2 mg/dL
    Severe impairment: Use is contraindicated
    Hemodialysis: Not removed by hemodialysis; supplemental dose is not necessary
  Hepatic Impairment Use is contraindicated.

Administration Administer 30 minutes prior to breakfast and dinner.

Monitoring Parameters Serum cholesterol, LFTs periodically, CBC periodically (first year)

Pharmacotherapy Pearls If no appreciable triglyceride or cholesterol lowering effect occurs after 3 months, the drug should be discontinued

Special Geriatric Considerations Gemfibrozil is the drug of choice for the treatment of hypertriglyceridemia and hypoalphaproteinemia in the elderly; it is usually well tolerated; myositis may be more common in patients with poor renal function. The definition of and, therefore, when to treat hyperlipidemia in the elderly is a controversial issue. The National Cholesterol Education Program recommends that all adults maintain a plasma cholesterol <160 mg/dL. Older adults with one additional risk factor, goal LDL would be <130 mg/dL. It is the authors' belief that pharmacologic treatment be reserved for those who are unable to obtain a desirable plasma cholesterol concentration by diet alone and for whom the benefits of treatment are believed to outweigh the potential adverse effects, drug interactions, and cost of treatment.

Dosage Forms Excipient information presented when available (limited, particularly for generics); consult specific product labeling.
Tablet, oral: 600 mg
  Lopid®: 600 mg [scored]

Gemifloxacin (je mi FLOKS a sin)

Related Information

Antimicrobial Drugs of Choice *on page 2163*
Community-Acquired Pneumonia in Adults *on page 2171*

Brand Names: U.S. Factive®

Brand Names: Canada Factive®

Index Terms DW286; Gemifloxacin Mesylate; LA 20304a; SB-265805

Generic Availability (U.S.) No

Pharmacologic Category Antibiotic, Quinolone; Respiratory Fluoroquinolone

Use Treatment of acute exacerbation of chronic bronchitis; treatment of community-acquired pneumonia (CAP), including pneumonia caused by multidrug-resistant strains of *S. pneumoniae* (MDRSP)

Unlabeled Use Acute sinusitis

Medication Guide Available Yes

Contraindications Hypersensitivity to gemifloxacin, other fluoroquinolones, or any component of the formulation

Warnings/Precautions [U.S. Boxed Warning]: There have been reports of tendon inflammation and/or rupture with quinolone antibiotics; risk may be increased with concurrent corticosteroids, organ transplant recipients, and in patients >60 years of age. Rupture of the Achilles tendon sometimes requiring surgical repair has been reported most frequently; but other tendon sites (eg, rotator cuff, biceps) have also been reported. Strenuous physical activity, rheumatoid arthritis, and renal impairment may be an independent risk factor for tendonitis. Discontinue at first sign of tendon inflammation or pain. May occur even after discontinuation of therapy. Use with caution in patients with rheumatoid arthritis; may increase risk of tendon rupture. Fluoroquinolones may prolong QT_c interval; avoid use of gemifloxacin in patients with a history of QT_c prolongation, uncorrected hypokalemia, hypomagnesemia, or concurrent administration of other medications known to prolong the QT interval (including Class Ia and Class III antiarrhythmics, cisapride, erythromycin, antipsychotics, and tricyclic antidepressants). Use with caution in patients with significant bradycardia or acute myocardial ischemia. CNS effects may occur (tremor, restlessness, confusion, and very rarely hallucinations, increased intracranial pressure [including pseudotumor cerebri] or seizures). Use with caution in patients with known or suspected CNS disorder. Potential for seizures, although very rare, may be increased with concomitant NSAID therapy. Use with caution in individuals at risk of seizures. Use caution in renal dysfunction; dosage adjustment required for Cl_{cr} ≤40 mL/minute.

Fluoroquinolones have been associated with the development of serious, and sometimes fatal, hypoglycemia, most often in elderly diabetics, but also in patients without diabetes. This occurred most frequently with gatifloxacin (no longer available systemically) but may occur at a lower frequency with other quinolones.

Severe hypersensitivity reactions, including anaphylaxis, have occurred with quinolone therapy. Reactions may present as typical allergic symptoms after a single dose, or may manifest as severe idiosyncratic dermatologic, vascular, pulmonary, renal, hepatic, and/or hematologic events, usually after multiple doses. May cause maculopapular rash, usually 8-10 days after treatment initiation; risk factors may include age <40 years, female gender (including postmenopausal women on HRT), and treatment duration >7 days. Prompt discontinuation of drug should occur if skin rash or other symptoms arise. **[U.S. Boxed Warning]: Quinolones may exacerbate myasthenia gravis; avoid use (rare, potentially life-threatening weakness of respiratory muscles may occur).** Avoid excessive sunlight and take precautions to limit exposure (eg, loose fitting clothing, sunscreen); may cause moderate-to-severe phototoxicity reactions. Discontinue use if photosensitivity occurs. Prolonged use may result in fungal or bacterial superinfection, including *C. difficile*-associated diarrhea (CDAD) and pseudomembranous colitis; CDAD has been observed >2 months postantibiotic treatment. Peripheral neuropathy has been linked to the use of quinolones; these cases were rare. Hemolytic reactions may (rarely) occur with quinolone use in patients with latent or actual G6PD deficiency.

Adverse Reactions (Reflective of adult population; not specific for elderly) 1% to 10%:

Central nervous system: Headache (4%), dizziness (2%)

Dermatologic: Rash (4%)

Gastrointestinal: Diarrhea (5%), nausea (4%), abdominal pain (2%), vomiting (2%)

Hepatic: Transaminases increased (1% to 4%)

Important adverse effects reported with other agents in this drug class include (not reported for gemifloxacin): Allergic reactions, CNS stimulation, hepatitis, jaundice, peripheral neuropathy, pneumonitis (eosinophilic), seizure; sensorimotor-axonal neuropathy (paresthesia, hypoesthesias, dysesthesias, weakness); severe dermatologic reactions (toxic epidermal necrolysis, Stevens-Johnson syndrome); torsade de pointes, vasculitis

Drug Interactions

Metabolism/Transport Effects None known.

Avoid Concomitant Use

Avoid concomitant use of Gemifloxacin with any of the following: BCG; Highest Risk QTc-Prolonging Agents; Mifepristone

Increased Effect/Toxicity

Gemifloxacin may increase the levels/effects of: Corticosteroids (Systemic); Highest Risk QTc-Prolonging Agents; Moderate Risk QTc-Prolonging Agents; Porfimer; Sulfonylureas; Varenicline; Vitamin K Antagonists

The levels/effects of Gemifloxacin may be increased by: Insulin; Mifepristone; Nonsteroidal Anti-Inflammatory Agents; Probenecid; QTc-Prolonging Agents (Indeterminate Risk and Risk Modifying)

Decreased Effect

Gemifloxacin may decrease the levels/effects of: BCG; Mycophenolate; Sulfonylureas; Typhoid Vaccine

The levels/effects of Gemifloxacin may be decreased by: Antacids; Calcium Salts; Didanosine; Iron Salts; Magnesium Salts; Quinapril; Sevelamer; Sucralfate; Zinc Salts

Ethanol/Nutrition/Herb Interactions Herb/Nutraceutical: Avoid dong quai, St John's wort (may also cause photosensitization).

Stability Store at 25°C (77°F). Protect from light.

Mechanism of Action Gemifloxacin is a DNA gyrase inhibitor and also inhibits topoisomerase IV. DNA gyrase (topoisomerase IV) is an essential bacterial enzyme that maintains the superhelical structure of DNA. DNA gyrase is required for DNA replication and transcription, DNA repair, recombination, and transposition; bactericidal

Pharmacodynamics/Kinetics

Absorption: Well absorbed from the GI tract

Distribution: V_{dss}: 4.2 L/kg

Protein binding: ~60% to 70%

Metabolism: Hepatic (minor); forms metabolites (CYP isoenzymes are not involved)

Bioavailability: ~71%

Half-life elimination: 7 hours (range 4-12 hours)

Time to peak, plasma: 0.5-2 hours

Excretion: Feces (61%); urine (36%)

Dosage

Geriatric & Adult

Susceptible infections: Oral: 320 mg once daily

Acute exacerbations of chronic bronchitis: Oral: 320 mg once daily for 5 days

Community-acquired pneumonia (mild-to-moderate): Oral: 320 mg once daily for 5 or 7 days (decision to use 5- or 7-day regimen should be guided by initial sputum culture; 7 days are recommended for MDRSP, *Klebsiella*, or *M. catarrhalis* infection)

Sinusitis (unlabeled use): Oral: 320 mg once daily for 10 days

Renal Impairment

Cl_{cr} >40 mL/minute: No adjustment required.

Cl_{cr} ≤40 mL/minute (or patients on hemodialysis/CAPD): 160 mg once daily (administer dose following hemodialysis).

Hepatic Impairment No adjustment required.

Administration May be administered with or without food, milk, or calcium supplements. Gemifloxacin should be taken 3 hours before or 2 hours after supplements (including multivitamins) containing iron, zinc, or magnesium.

Monitoring Parameters WBC, signs/symptoms of infection, renal function

Special Geriatric Considerations The risk of torsade de pointes and tendon inflammation and/or rupture associated with the concomitant use of corticosteroids and quinolones is increased in the elderly population. See Warnings/Precautions regarding tendon rupture in patients >60 years of age.

Dosage Forms Excipient information presented when available (limited, particularly for generics); consult specific product labeling.

Tablet, oral:

Factive®: 320 mg [scored]

◆ **Gemifloxacin Mesylate** see Gemifloxacin on page 871
◆ **Generlac** see Lactulose on page 1086
◆ **Gengraf®** see CycloSPORINE (Systemic) on page 460
◆ **Gentak®** see Gentamicin (Ophthalmic) on page 876

Gentamicin (Systemic) (jen ta MYE sin)

Related Information

Antibiotic Treatment of Adults With Infective Endocarditis on page 2157
Antimicrobial Drugs of Choice on page 2163

Medication Safety Issues

Sound-alike/look-alike issues:

Gentamicin may be confused with gentian violet, kanamycin, vancomycin

High alert medication:

The Institute for Safe Medication Practices (ISMP) includes this medication (intrathecal administration) among its list of drug classes which have a heightened risk of causing significant patient harm when used in error.

Brand Names: Canada Gentamicin Injection, USP

Index Terms Gentamicin Sulfate

Generic Availability (U.S.) Yes

Pharmacologic Category Antibiotic, Aminoglycoside

Use Treatment of susceptible bacterial infections, normally gram-negative organisms, including *Pseudomonas*, *Proteus*, *Serratia*, and gram-positive *Staphylococcus*; treatment of bone infections, respiratory tract infections, skin and soft tissue infections, as well as abdominal and urinary tract infections, and septicemia; treatment of infective endocarditis

Contraindications Hypersensitivity to gentamicin or other aminoglycosides

Warnings/Precautions [U.S. Boxed Warning]: Aminoglycosides may cause neurotoxicity and/or nephrotoxicity; usual risk factors include pre-existing renal impairment, concomitant neuro-/nephrotoxic medications, advanced age and dehydration. Ototoxicity may be directly proportional to the amount of drug given and the duration of treatment; tinnitus or vertigo are indications of vestibular injury and impending hearing loss; renal damage is usually reversible. May cause neuromuscular blockade and respiratory paralysis; especially when given soon after anesthesia or muscle relaxants.

Not intended for long-term therapy due to toxic hazards associated with extended administration; use caution in pre-existing renal insufficiency, vestibular or cochlear impairment, myasthenia gravis, hypocalcemia, conditions which depress neuromuscular transmission. Dosage modification required in patients with impaired renal function. Prolonged use may result in fungal or bacterial superinfection, including *C. difficile*-associated diarrhea (CDAD) and pseudomembranous colitis; CDAD has been observed >2 months postantibiotic treatment.

Adverse Reactions (Reflective of adult population; not specific for elderly) Frequency not defined.

Cardiovascular: Edema, hyper/hypotension

Central nervous system: Ataxia, confusion, depression, dizziness, drowsiness, encephalopathy, fever, headache, lethargy, pseudomotor cerebri, seizures, vertigo

Dermatologic: Alopecia, erythema, itching, purpura, rash, urticaria

Endocrine & metabolic: Hypocalcemia, hypokalemia, hypomagnesemia, hyponatremia

Gastrointestinal: Anorexia, appetite decreased, *C. difficile*-associated diarrhea, enterocolitis, nausea, salivation increased, splenomegaly, stomatitis, vomiting, weight loss

Hematologic: Agranulocytosis, anemia, eosinophilia, granulocytopenia, leukopenia, reticulocytes increased/decreased, thrombocytopenia

Hepatic: Hepatomegaly, LFTs increased

Local: Injection site reactions, pain at injection site, phlebitis/thrombophlebitis

◀ Neuromuscular & skeletal: Arthralgia, gait instability, muscle cramps, muscle twitching, muscle weakness, myasthenia gravis-like syndrome, numbness, paresthesia, peripheral neuropathy, tremor, weakness

Ocular: Visual disturbances

Otic: Hearing impairment, hearing loss (associated with persistently increased serum concentrations; early toxicity usually affects high-pitched sound), tinnitus

Renal: BUN increased, casts (hyaline, granular) in urine, creatinine clearance decreased, distal tubular dysfunction, Fanconi-like syndrome (high dose, prolonged course) (infants and adults), oliguria, renal failure (high trough serum concentrations), polyuria, proteinuria, serum creatinine increased, tubular necrosis, urine specific gravity decreased

Respiratory: Dyspnea, laryngeal edema, pulmonary fibrosis, respiratory depression

Miscellaneous: Allergic reaction, anaphylaxis, anaphylactoid reactions

Drug Interactions

Metabolism/Transport Effects None known.

Avoid Concomitant Use

Avoid concomitant use of Gentamicin (Systemic) with any of the following: Agalsidase Alfa; Agalsidase Beta; BCG; Gallium Nitrate

Increased Effect/Toxicity

Gentamicin (Systemic) may increase the levels/effects of: AbobotulinumtoxinA; Bisphosphonate Derivatives; CARBOplatin; Colistimethate; CycloSPORINE; CycloSPORINE (Systemic); Gallium Nitrate; Neuromuscular-Blocking Agents; OnabotulinumtoxinA; RimabotulinumtoxinB

The levels/effects of Gentamicin (Systemic) may be increased by: Amphotericin B; Capreomycin; Cephalosporins (2nd Generation); Cephalosporins (3rd Generation); Cephalosporins (4th Generation); CISplatin; Loop Diuretics; Nonsteroidal Anti-Inflammatory Agents; Vancomycin

Decreased Effect

Gentamicin (Systemic) may decrease the levels/effects of: Agalsidase Alfa; Agalsidase Beta; BCG; Typhoid Vaccine

The levels/effects of Gentamicin (Systemic) may be decreased by: Penicillins

Stability

Gentamicin is a colorless to slightly yellow solution which should be stored between 2°C to 30°C, but refrigeration is not recommended.

I.V. infusion solutions mixed in NS or D_5W solution are stable for 24 hours at room temperature and refrigeration.

Premixed bag: Manufacturer expiration date.

Out of overwrap stability: 30 days.

Mechanism of Action Interferes with bacterial protein synthesis by binding to 30S and 50S ribosomal subunits resulting in a defective bacterial cell membrane

Pharmacodynamics/Kinetics

Absorption:

Intramuscular: Rapid and complete

Oral: None

Distribution: Primarily into extracellular fluid (highly hydrophilic); high concentration in the renal cortex; minimal penetration to ocular tissues via I.V. route

V_d: Increased by edema, ascites, fluid overload; decreased with dehydration

Adults: 0.2-0.3 L/kg

Relative diffusion from blood into CSF: Minimal even with inflammation

CSF:blood level ratio: Normal meninges: Nil; Inflamed meninges: 10% to 30%

Protein binding: <30%

Half-life elimination: Adults: 1.5-3 hours; End-stage renal disease: 36-70 hours

Time to peak, serum: I.M.: 30-90 minutes; I.V.: 30 minutes after 30-minute infusion

Excretion: Urine (as unchanged drug)

Clearance: Directly related to renal function

Dosage

Geriatric & Adult Individualization is **critical** because of the low therapeutic index.

Use of ideal body weight (IBW) for determining the mg/kg/dose appears to be more accurate than dosing on the basis of total body weight (TBW). In morbid obesity, dosage requirement may best be estimated using a dosing weight of IBW + 0.4 (TBW - IBW).

Initial and periodic plasma drug levels (eg, peak and trough with conventional dosing) should be determined, particularly in critically-ill patients with serious infections or in disease states known to significantly alter aminoglycoside pharmacokinetics (eg, cystic fibrosis, burns, or major surgery).

Usual dosage ranges:
I.M., I.V.:

Conventional: 1-2.5 mg/kg/dose every 8-12 hours; to ensure adequate peak concentrations early in therapy, higher initial dosage may be considered in selected patients when extracellular water is increased (edema, septic shock, postsurgical, or trauma)

Once daily: 4-7 mg/kg/dose once daily; some clinicians recommend this approach for all patients with normal renal function; this dose is at least as efficacious with similar, if not less, toxicity than conventional dosing

Intrathecal: 4-8 mg/day

Indication-specific dosing: I.M., I.V.:

Brucellosis: 240 mg (I.M.) daily or 5 mg/kg (I.V.) daily for 7 days; either regimen recommended in combination with doxycycline

Cholangitis: 4-6 mg/kg once daily with ampicillin

Diverticulitis (complicated): 1.5-2 mg/kg every 8 hours (with ampicillin and metronidazole)

Endocarditis: Treatment: 3 mg/kg/day in 1-3 divided doses

Meningitis *Enterococcus* sp or *Pseudomonas aeruginosa:* I.V.: Loading dose 2 mg/kg, then 1.7 mg/kg/dose every 8 hours (administered with another bacteriocidal drug)

Pelvic inflammatory disease: Loading dose: 2 mg/kg, then 1.5 mg/kg every 8 hours Alternate therapy: 4.5 mg/kg once daily

Plague (*Yersinia pestis* **):** Treatment: 5 mg/kg/day, followed by postexposure prophylaxis with doxycycline

Pneumonia, hospital- or ventilator-associated: 7 mg/kg/day (with antipseudomonal beta-lactam or carbapenem)

Synergy (for gram-positive infections): 3 mg/kg/day in 1-3 divided doses (with ampicillin)

Tularemia: 5 mg/kg/day divided every 8 hours for 1-2 weeks

Urinary tract infection: 1.5 mg/kg/dose every 8 hours

Renal Impairment

Conventional dosing:

Cl_{cr} ≥60 mL/minute: Administer every 8 hours

Cl_{cr} 40-60 mL/minute: Administer every 12 hours

Cl_{cr} 20-40 mL/minute: Administer every 24 hours

Cl_{cr} <20 mL/minute: Loading dose, then monitor levels

High-dose therapy: Interval may be extended (eg, every 48 hours) in patients with moderate renal impairment (Cl_{cr} 30-59 mL/minute) and/or adjusted based on serum level determinations.

Intermittent hemodialysis (IHD) (administer after hemodialysis on dialysis days) (Heintz, 2009): Dialyzable (~50%; variable; dependent on filter, duration, and type of IHD):

Loading dose of 2-3 mg/kg loading dose followed by:

Mild UTI or synergy: 1 mg/kg every 48-72 hours; consider redosing for pre-HD or post-HD concentrations <1 mg/L

Moderate-to-severe UTI: 1-1.5 mg/kg every 48-72 hours; consider redosing for pre-HD concentrations <1.5-2 mg/L or post-HD concentrations <1 mg/L

Systemic gram-negative rod infection: 1.5-2 mg/kg every 48-72 hours; consider redosing for pre-HD concentrations <3-5 mg/L or post-HD concentrations <2 mg/L

Note: Dosing dependent on the assumption of 3 times/week, complete IHD sessions.

Peritoneal dialysis (PD):

Administration via PD fluid:

Gram-positive infection (eg, synergy): 3-4 mg/L (3-4 mcg/mL) of PD fluid

Gram-negative infection: 4-8 mg/L (4-8 mcg/mL) of PD fluid

Administration via I.V., I.M. route during PD: Dose as for Cl_{cr} <10 mL/minute and follow levels

Continuous renal replacement therapy (CRRT) (Heintz, 2009; Trotman, 2005): Drug clearance is highly dependent on the method of renal replacement, filter type, and flow rate. Appropriate dosing requires close monitoring of pharmacologic response, signs of adverse reactions due to drug accumulation, as well as drug concentrations in relation to target trough (if appropriate). The following are general recommendations only (based on dialysate flow/ultrafiltration rates of 1-2 L/hour and minimal residual renal function) and should not supersede clinical judgment:

CVVH/CVVHD/CVVHDF: Loading dose of 2-3 mg/kg followed by:

Mild UTI or synergy: 1 mg/kg every 24-36 hours (redose when concentration <1 mg/L)

Moderate-to-severe UTI: 1-1.5 mg/kg every 24-36 hours (redose when concentration <1.5-2 mg/L)

Systemic gram-negative infection: 1.5-2.5 mg/kg every 24-48 hours (redose when concentration <3-5 mg/L)

Hepatic Impairment Monitor plasma concentrations.

Administration

I.M.: Administer by deep I.M. route if possible. Slower absorption and lower peak concentrations, probably due to poor circulation in the atrophic muscle, may occur following I.M. injection; in paralyzed patients, suggest I.V. route.

Some penicillins (eg, carbenicillin, ticarcillin, and piperacillin) have been shown to inactivate aminoglycosides *in vitro*. This has been observed to a greater extent with tobramycin and gentamicin, while amikacin has shown greater stability against inactivation. Concurrent use of these agents may pose a risk of reduced antibacterial efficacy *in vivo*, particularly in the setting of profound renal impairment. However, definitive clinical evidence is lacking. If combination penicillin/aminoglycoside therapy is desired in a patient with renal dysfunction, separation of doses (if feasible), and routine monitoring of aminoglycoside levels, CBC, and clinical response should be considered.

Monitoring Parameters Urinalysis, urine output, BUN, serum creatinine; hearing should be tested before, during, and after treatment; particularly in those at risk for ototoxicity or who will be receiving prolonged therapy (>2 weeks)

Some penicillin derivatives may accelerate the degradation of aminoglycosides *in vitro*. This may be clinically-significant for certain penicillin (ticarcillin, piperacillin, carbenicillin) and aminoglycoside (gentamicin, tobramycin) combination therapy in patients with significant renal impairment. Close monitoring of aminoglycoside levels is warranted.

Reference Range

Timing of serum samples: Draw peak 30 minutes after 30-minute infusion has been completed or 1 hour after I.M. injection; draw trough immediately before next dose

Sample size: 0.5-2 mL blood (red top tube) or 0.1-1 mL serum (separated)

Therapeutic levels:

Peak:
  Serious infections: 6-8 mcg/mL (12-17 micromole/L)
  Life-threatening infections: 8-10 mcg/mL (17-21 micromole/L)
  Urinary tract infections: 4-6 mcg/mL
  Synergy against gram-positive organisms: 3-5 mcg/mL

Trough:
  Serious infections: 0.5-1 mcg/mL
  Life-threatening infections: 1-2 mcg/mL
  The American Thoracic Society (ATS) recommends trough levels of <1 mcg/mL for patients with hospital-acquired pneumonia.

Obtain drug levels after the third dose unless renal dysfunction/toxicity suspected

Test Interactions Some penicillin derivatives may accelerate the degradation of aminoglycosides *in vitro*, leading to a potential underestimation of aminoglycoside serum concentration.

Special Geriatric Considerations The aminoglycosides are important therapeutic interventions for infections due to susceptible organisms and as empiric therapy in seriously ill patients. Their use is not without risk; these risks can be minimized if initial dosing is adjusted for estimated renal function and appropriate monitoring performed. High dose, once daily aminoglycosides have been advocated as an alternative to traditional dosing regimens. Once daily or extended interval dosing is as effective and may be safer than traditional dosing. The interval must be adjusted for renal function.

Dosage Forms Excipient information presented when available (limited, particularly for generics); consult specific product labeling. [DSC] = Discontinued product

Infusion, premixed in NS: 60 mg (50 mL, 100 mL [DSC]); 80 mg (50 mL, 100 mL); 100 mg (50 mL, 100 mL); 120 mg (100 mL)

Injection, solution: 40 mg/mL (2 mL, 20 mL)

Injection, solution [pediatric]: 10 mg/mL (2 mL [DSC])

Injection, solution [pediatric, preservative free]: 10 mg/mL (2 mL)

Gentamicin (Ophthalmic) (jen ta MYE sin)

Medication Safety Issues

Sound-alike/look-alike issues:
  Gentamicin may be confused with gentian violet, kanamycin, vancomycin

Brand Names: U.S. Garamycin®; Gentak®

Brand Names: Canada Diogent®; Garamycin®; Garasone; Gentak®; Gentocin; PMS-Gentamicin

Index Terms Gentamicin Sulfate

Generic Availability (U.S.) Yes

Pharmacologic Category Antibiotic, Aminoglycoside; Antibiotic, Ophthalmic

Use Treatment of ophthalmic infections caused by susceptible bacteria

Dosage
Geriatric & Adult Ophthalmic infections: Ophthalmic:
Ointment: Instill ½" (1.25 cm) 2-3 times/day to every 3-4 hours
Solution: Instill 1-2 drops every 4 hours, up to 2 drops every hour for severe infections
Special Geriatric Considerations Evaluate the patient's or caregiver's ability to safely administer the correct dose of ophthalmic medication.
Dosage Forms Excipient information presented when available (limited, particularly for generics); consult specific product labeling.
Ointment, ophthalmic:
Gentak®: 0.3% (3.5 g)
Ointment, ophthalmic [preservative free]:
Garamycin®: 0.3% (3.5 g)
Solution, ophthalmic [drops]: 0.3% (5 mL, 15 mL)
Garamycin®: 0.3% (5 mL) [contains benzalkonium chloride]
Gentak®: 0.3% (5 mL) [contains benzalkonium chloride]

Gentamicin (Topical) (jen ta MYE sin)

Related Information
Pressure Ulcer Treatment *on page 2246*
Medication Safety Issues
Sound-alike/look-alike issues:
Gentamicin may be confused with gentian violet, kanamycin, vancomycin
Brand Names: Canada PMS-Gentamicin; ratio-Gentamicin
Generic Availability (U.S.) Yes
Pharmacologic Category Antibiotic, Aminoglycoside; Antibiotic, Topical
Use Used topically to treat superficial infections of the skin
Dosage
Geriatric & Adult Dermatologic infections: Topical: Apply 3-4 times/day to affected area
Special Geriatric Considerations Instruct patient or caregiver on appropriate use of topical gentamicin products.
Dosage Forms Excipient information presented when available (limited, particularly for generics); consult specific product labeling.
Cream, topical: 0.1% (15 g, 30 g)
Ointment, topical: 0.1% (15 g, 30 g)

♦ **Gentamicin and Prednisolone** see Prednisolone and Gentamicin *on page 1594*
♦ **Gentamicin Sulfate** see Gentamicin (Ophthalmic) *on page 876*
♦ **Gentamicin Sulfate** see Gentamicin (Systemic) *on page 873*
♦ **Geodon®** see Ziprasidone *on page 2053*
♦ **Geri-Dryl** see DiphenhydrAMINE (Systemic) *on page 556*
♦ **Geri-kot [OTC]** see Senna *on page 1764*
♦ **Geri-Stool [OTC]** see Docusate and Senna *on page 585*
♦ **Geri-Tussin [OTC]** see GuaiFENesin *on page 904*
♦ **Gets-It® [OTC]** see Salicylic Acid *on page 1743*
♦ **GF196960** see Tadalafil *on page 1826*
♦ **GG** see GuaiFENesin *on page 904*
♦ **Glargine Insulin** see Insulin Glargine *on page 1012*
♦ **Glibenclamide** see GlyBURIDE *on page 887*

Glimepiride (GLYE me pye ride)

Related Information
Diabetes Mellitus Management, Adults *on page 2193*
Medication Safety Issues
Sound-alike/look-alike issues:
Glimepiride may be confused with glipiZIDE
Amaryl® may be confused with Altace®, Amerge®
High alert medication:
The Institute for Safe Medication Practices (ISMP) includes this medication among its list of drugs which have a heightened risk of causing significant patient harm when used in error.
International issues:
Amarel [France], Amaryl [U.S., Canada, and multiple international markets] may be confused with Reminyl brand name for galantamine [multiple international markets]
Amaryl [U.S., Canada, and multiple international markets] may be confused with Almarl brand name for arotinolol [Japan]

◀ **Brand Names: U.S.** Amaryl®

Brand Names: Canada Amaryl®; Apo-Glimepiride®; CO Glimepiride; Novo-Glimepiride; PMS-Glimepiride; ratio-Glimepiride; Rhoxal-glimepiride; Sandoz-Glimepiride

Generic Availability (U.S.) Yes

Pharmacologic Category Antidiabetic Agent, Sulfonylurea

Use Management of type 2 diabetes mellitus (noninsulin dependent, NIDDM) as an adjunct to diet and exercise to lower blood glucose; may be used in combination with metformin or insulin in patients whose hyperglycemia cannot be controlled by diet and exercise in conjunction with a single oral hypoglycemic agent

Contraindications Hypersensitivity to glimepiride, any component of the formulation, or sulfonamides; diabetic ketoacidosis (with or without coma)

Warnings/Precautions All sulfonylurea drugs are capable of producing severe hypoglycemia. Hypoglycemia is more likely to occur when caloric intake is deficient, after severe or prolonged exercise, when ethanol is ingested, or when more than one glucose-lowering drug is used. It is also more likely in elderly patients, malnourished patients and in patients with impaired renal or hepatic function; use with caution. Autonomic neuropathy, advanced age, and concomitant use of beta-blockers or other sympatholytic agents may impair the patient's ability to recognize the signs and symptoms of hypoglycemia; use with caution.

Loss of efficacy may be observed following prolonged use as a result of the progression of type 2 diabetes mellitus which results in continued beta cell destruction. In patients who were previously responding to sulfonylurea therapy, consider additional factors which may be contributing to decreased efficacy (eg, inappropriate dose, nonadherence to diet and exercise regimen). If no contributing factors can be identified, consider discontinuing use of the sulfonylurea due to secondary failure of treatment. Additional antidiabetic therapy (eg, insulin) will be required. It may be necessary to discontinue therapy and administer insulin if the patient is exposed to stress (fever, trauma, infection, surgery).

Chemical similarities are present among sulfonamides, sulfonylureas, carbonic anhydrase inhibitors, thiazides, and loop diuretics (except ethacrynic acid). Use in patients with sulfonamide allergy is not specifically contraindicated in product labeling, however, a risk of cross-reaction exists in patients with allergy to any of these compounds; avoid use when previous reaction has been severe. Patients with G6PD deficiency may be at an increased risk of sulfonylurea-induced hemolytic anemia; however, cases have also been described in patients without G6PD deficiency during postmarketing surveillance. Use with caution and consider a nonsulfonylurea alternative in patients with G6PD deficiency.

Product labeling states oral hypoglycemic drugs may be associated with an increased cardiovascular mortality as compared to treatment with diet alone or diet plus insulin. Data to support this association are limited, and several studies, including a large prospective trial (UKPDS) have not supported an association.

Adverse Reactions (Reflective of adult population; not specific for elderly) 1% to 10%:

Central nervous system: Dizziness (2%), headache (2%)

Endocrine & metabolic: Hypoglycemia (1% to 2%)

Gastrointestinal: Nausea (1%)

Neuromuscular & skeletal: Weakness (2%)

Drug Interactions

Metabolism/Transport Effects Substrate of CYP2C9 (major); **Note:** Assignment of Major/Minor substrate status based on clinically relevant drug interaction potential

Avoid Concomitant Use There are no known interactions where it is recommended to avoid concomitant use.

Increased Effect/Toxicity

Glimepiride may increase the levels/effects of: Alcohol (Ethyl); Hypoglycemic Agents; Porfimer; Vitamin K Antagonists

The levels/effects of Glimepiride may be increased by: Beta-Blockers; Chloramphenicol; Cimetidine; Cyclic Antidepressants; CYP2C9 Inhibitors (Moderate); CYP2C9 Inhibitors (Strong); Fibric Acid Derivatives; Fluconazole; GLP-1 Agonists; Herbs (Hypoglycemic Properties); MAO Inhibitors; Mifepristone; Pegvisomant; Probenecid; Quinolone Antibiotics; Ranitidine; Salicylates; Selective Serotonin Reuptake Inhibitors; Sulfonamide Derivatives; Vitamin K Antagonists; Voriconazole

Decreased Effect

The levels/effects of Glimepiride may be decreased by: Colesevelam; Corticosteroids (Orally Inhaled); Corticosteroids (Systemic); CYP2C9 Inducers (Strong); Loop Diuretics; Luteinizing Hormone-Releasing Hormone Analogs; Peginterferon Alfa-2b; Quinolone Antibiotics; Rifampin; Somatropin; Thiazide Diuretics

Ethanol/Nutrition/Herb Interactions
Ethanol: Caution with ethanol (may cause hypoglycemia).
Herb/Nutraceutical: Caution with chromium, garlic, gymnema (may cause hypoglycemia).

Mechanism of Action Stimulates insulin release from the pancreatic beta cells; reduces glucose output from the liver; insulin sensitivity is increased at peripheral target sites

Pharmacodynamics/Kinetics
Onset of action: Peak effect: Blood glucose reductions: 2-3 hours
Duration: 24 hours
Absorption: 100%; delayed when given with food
Distribution: V_d: 8.8 L
Protein binding: >99.5%
Metabolism: Hepatic oxidation via CYP2C9 to M1 metabolite (~33% activity of parent compound); further oxidative metabolism to inactive M2 metabolite
Half-life elimination: 5-9 hours
Time to peak, plasma: 2-3 hours
Excretion: Urine (60%, 80% to 90% as M1 and M2); feces (40%, 70% as M1 and M2)

Dosage
Geriatric Initial: 1 mg/day; dose titration and maintenance dosing should be conservative to avoid hypoglycemia

Adult

Type 2 diabetes: Oral:
Initial: 1-2 mg once daily, administered with breakfast or the first main meal
Adjustment: Allow several days between dose titrations: usual maintenance dose: 1-4 mg once daily; after a dose of 2 mg once daily, increase in increments of 2 mg at 1- to 2-week intervals based upon the patient's blood glucose response to a maximum of 8 mg once daily. If inadequate response to maximal dose, combination therapy with metformin may be considered.

Combination with insulin therapy:
Note: Fasting glucose level for instituting combination therapy is in the range of >150 mg/dL in plasma or serum depending on the patient)
Initial: 8 mg once daily with the first main meal
Adjustment: After starting with low-dose insulin, upward adjustments of insulin can be done approximately weekly as guided by frequent measurements of fasting blood glucose. Once stable, combination-therapy patients should monitor their capillary blood glucose on an ongoing basis, preferably daily.

Conversion from therapy with long half-life agents: Observe patient carefully for 1-2 weeks when converting from a longer half-life agent (eg, chlorpropamide) to glimepiride due to overlapping hypoglycemic effects.

Renal Impairment Cl_{cr} <22 mL/minute: Initial starting dose should be 1 mg and dosage increments should be based on fasting blood glucose levels.

Administration Administer once daily with breakfast or first main meal of the day. Patients that are NPO or require decreased caloric intake may need doses held to avoid hypoglycemia.

Monitoring Parameters Monitor for signs and symptoms of hypoglycemia (fatigue, excessive hunger, profuse sweating, numbness of extremities), fasting blood glucose, hemoglobin A_{1c}

Reference Range
Recommendations for glycemic control in adults with diabetes:
Hb A_{1c}: <7%
Preprandial capillary plasma glucose: 70-130 mg/dL
Peak postprandial capillary blood glucose: <180 mg/dL
Blood pressure: <130/80 mm Hg
Recommendations for glycemic control in older adults with diabetes:
Relatively healthy, cognitively intact, and with a ≥5-year life expectancy: See Adults
Frail, life expectancy <5-years or those for whom the risks of intensive glucose control outweigh the benefits:
Hb A_{1c}: <8% to 9%
Blood pressure: <140/80 mm Hg or <130/80 mm Hg if tolerated

Special Geriatric Considerations Rapid and prolonged hypoglycemia (>12 hours) despite hypertonic glucose injections have been reported with glimepiride. Age, hepatic impairment, and renal impairment are independent risk factors for hypoglycemia; dosage titration should be made at weekly intervals. Intensive glucose control (Hb A_{1c} <6.5%) has been linked to increased all-cause and cardiovascular mortality, hypoglycemia requiring assistance, and weight gain in adult type 2 diabetes. How "tightly" to control a geriatric patient's blood glucose needs to be individualized. Such a decision should be based on several factors, including the patient's functional and cognitive status, how well he/she recognizes hypoglycemic or hyperglycemic symptoms, and how to respond to them and other disease states. An Hb A_{1c} <7.5% is an acceptable endpoint for a healthy older adult, while <8% is acceptable for frail elderly patients, those with a duration of illness >10 years, or those with comorbid conditions and requiring combination diabetes medications. For elderly patients with diabetes who are relatively healthy, attaining target goals for aspirin use, blood pressure, lipids, smoking cessation, and diet and exercise may be more important than normalized glycemic control.

Dosage Forms Excipient information presented when available (limited, particularly for generics); consult specific product labeling.

Tablet, oral: 1 mg, 2 mg, 4 mg
  Amaryl®: 1 mg, 2 mg, 4 mg [scored]

◆ **Glimepiride and Pioglitazone** see Pioglitazone and Glimepiride on page 1544
◆ **Glimepiride and Pioglitazone Hydrochloride** see Pioglitazone and Glimepiride on page 1544
◆ **Glimepiride and Rosiglitazone Maleate** see Rosiglitazone and Glimepiride on page 1731

GlipiZIDE (GLIP i zide)

Related Information
Diabetes Mellitus Management, Adults on page 2193

Medication Safety Issues
Sound-alike/look-alike issues:
  GlipiZIDE may be confused with glimepiride, glyBURIDE
  Glucotrol® may be confused with Glucophage®, Glucotrol® XL, glyBURIDE
High alert medication:
  The Institute for Safe Medication Practices (ISMP) includes this medication among its list of drugs which have a heightened risk of causing significant patient harm when used in error.

Brand Names: U.S. Glucotrol XL®; Glucotrol®
Index Terms Glydiazinamide
Generic Availability (U.S.) Yes
Pharmacologic Category Antidiabetic Agent, Sulfonylurea
Use Management of type 2 diabetes mellitus (noninsulin dependent, NIDDM)
Contraindications Hypersensitivity to glipizide or any component of the formulation, other sulfonamides; type 1 diabetes mellitus (insulin dependent, IDDM); diabetic ketoacidosis
Warnings/Precautions All sulfonylurea drugs are capable of producing severe hypoglycemia. Hypoglycemia is more likely to occur when caloric intake is deficient, after severe or prolonged exercise, when ethanol is ingested, or when more than one glucose-lowering drug is used. It is also more likely in elderly patients, malnourished patients and in patients with impaired renal or hepatic function; use with caution.

Use with caution in patients with severe hepatic disease. It may be necessary to discontinue therapy and administer insulin if the patient is exposed to stress (fever, trauma, infection, surgery). Loss of efficacy may be observed following prolonged use as a result of the progression of type 2 diabetes mellitus which results in continued beta cell destruction. In patients who were previously responding to sulfonylurea therapy, consider additional factors which may be contributing to decreased efficacy (eg, inappropriate dose, nonadherence to diet and exercise regimen). If no contributing factors can be identified, consider discontinuing use of the sulfonylurea due to secondary failure of treatment. Additional antidiabetic therapy (eg, insulin) will be required. Chemical similarities are present among sulfonamides, sulfonylureas, carbonic anhydrase inhibitors, thiazides, and loop diuretics (except ethacrynic acid). Use in patients with sulfonamide allergy is specifically contraindicated in product labeling, however, a risk of cross-reaction exists in patients with allergy to any of these compounds; avoid use when previous reaction has been severe. Patients with G6PD deficiency may be at an increased risk of sulfonylurea-induced hemolytic anemia; however, cases have also been described in patients without G6PD deficiency during postmarketing surveillance. Use with caution and consider a nonsulfonylurea alternative in patients with G6PD deficiency.

Product labeling states oral hypoglycemic drugs may be associated with an increased cardiovascular mortality as compared to treatment with diet alone or diet plus insulin. Data to support this association are limited, and several studies, including a large prospective trial (UKPDS) have not supported an association. Avoid use of extended release tablets (Glucotrol XL®) in patients with known stricture/narrowing of the GI tract.

Adverse Reactions (Reflective of adult population; not specific for elderly) Frequency not defined.
Cardiovascular: Edema, syncope
Central nervous system: Anxiety, depression, dizziness, drowsiness, headache, hypoesthesia, insomnia, nervousness, pain
Dermatologic: Eczema, erythema, maculopapular eruptions, morbilliform eruptions, photosensitivity, pruritus, rash, urticaria
Endocrine & metabolic: Disulfiram-like reaction, hypoglycemia, hyponatremia, SIADH (rare)

Gastrointestinal: Anorexia, constipation, diarrhea, epigastric fullness, flatulence, gastralgia, heartburn, nausea, vomiting

Hematologic: Agranulocytopenia, aplastic anemia, blood dyscrasias, hemolytic anemia, leukopenia, pancytopenia, porphyria cutanea tarda, thrombocytopenia

Hepatic: Hepatic porphyria

Neuromuscular & skeletal: Arthralgia, leg cramps, myalgia, paresthesia, tremor

Ocular: Blurred vision

Renal: Diuretic effect (minor)

Respiratory: Rhinitis

Miscellaneous: Diaphoresis

Drug Interactions

Metabolism/Transport Effects Substrate of CYP2C9 (major); **Note:** Assignment of Major/Minor substrate status based on clinically relevant drug interaction potential

Avoid Concomitant Use There are no known interactions where it is recommended to avoid concomitant use.

Increased Effect/Toxicity

GlipiZIDE may increase the levels/effects of: Alcohol (Ethyl); Hypoglycemic Agents; Porfimer; Vitamin K Antagonists

The levels/effects of GlipiZIDE may be increased by: Beta-Blockers; Chloramphenicol; Cimetidine; Clarithromycin; Cyclic Antidepressants; CYP2C9 Inhibitors (Moderate); CYP2C9 Inhibitors (Strong); Fibric Acid Derivatives; Fluconazole; GLP-1 Agonists; Herbs (Hypoglycemic Properties); MAO Inhibitors; Mifepristone; Pegvisomant; Posaconazole; Probenecid; Quinolone Antibiotics; Ranitidine; Salicylates; Selective Serotonin Reuptake Inhibitors; Sulfonamide Derivatives; Vitamin K Antagonists; Voriconazole

Decreased Effect

The levels/effects of GlipiZIDE may be decreased by: Colesevelam; Corticosteroids (Orally Inhaled); Corticosteroids (Systemic); CYP2C9 Inducers (Strong); Loop Diuretics; Luteinizing Hormone-Releasing Hormone Analogs; Peginterferon Alfa-2b; Quinolone Antibiotics; Rifampin; Somatropin; Thiazide Diuretics

Ethanol/Nutrition/Herb Interactions

Ethanol: Caution with ethanol (may cause hypoglycemia or rare disulfiram reaction).

Food: A delayed release of insulin may occur if glipizide is taken with food. Immediate release tablets should be administered 30 minutes before meals to avoid erratic absorption.

Herb/Nutraceutical: Herbs with hypoglycemic properties may enhance the hypoglycemic effect of glipizide. This includes alfalfa, aloe, bilberry, bitter melon, burdock, celery, damiana, fenugreek, garcinia, garlic, ginger, ginseng (American), gymnema, marshmallow, stinging nettle

Mechanism of Action Stimulates insulin release from the pancreatic beta cells; reduces glucose output from the liver; insulin sensitivity is increased at peripheral target sites

Pharmacodynamics/Kinetics

Duration: 12-24 hours

Absorption: Rapid and complete; delayed with food

Distribution: 10-11 L

Protein binding: 98% to 99%; primarily to albumin

Bioavailability: 90% to 100%

Metabolism: Hepatic via CYP2C9; forms metabolites (inactive)

Half-life elimination: 2-5 hours

Time to peak: 1-3 hours; extended release tablets: 6-12 hours

Excretion: Urine (60% to 80%, 91% to 97% as metabolites); feces (11%)

Dosage

Geriatric & Adult

Type 2 diabetes: Oral:

Immediate release tablet: Initial: 5 mg once daily; titrate in 2.5-5 mg increments no more frequently than every few days based on blood glucose response; if once-daily dose is ineffective, may divide the dose; doses >15 mg/day should be administered in divided doses. Maximum recommended once-daily dose: 15 mg; maximum recommended total daily dose: 40 mg (some clinicians recommend a maximum total daily dose of 20 mg [Defronzo, 1999]).

Extended release tablet (Glucotrol XL®): Initial: 5 mg once daily; usual dose: 5-10 mg once daily; maximum recommended dose: 20 mg/day; preferred method for monitoring response to therapy and adjusting dosage is hemoglobin A_{1c} level at initiation and at ~3-month intervals; alternatively, dosage adjustments based on blood glucose monitoring should be made no more frequently than every 7 days

When transferring from immediate release to extended release glipizide: May switch the total daily dose of immediate release to the nearest equivalent daily dose of the extended release tablet and administer once daily; alternatively, may initiate extended release at 5 mg once daily and titrate accordingly.

When transferring from insulin to glipizide immediate release or extended release tablet:

Current insulin requirement ≤20 units: Discontinue insulin and initiate glipizide at usual dose

Current insulin requirement >20 units: Decrease insulin by 50% and initiate glipizide at usual dose; gradually decrease insulin dose based on patient response.

Renal Impairment The FDA-approved labeling recommends that caution should be used with initial and maintenance dosing in patients with renal impairment; however, no specific dosage adjustment guidelines are provided. The following guidelines have been used by some clinicians (Aronoff, 2007): GFR ≤50 mL/minute: Decrease dose by 50%.

Hepatic Impairment

Immediate release tablet: Initial: 2.5 mg/day

Extended release tablet: There are no dosage adjustments provided in manufacturer's labeling; use of a lower initial and maintenance dose should be considered.

Administration Administer immediate release tablets 30 minutes before a meal to achieve greatest reduction in postprandial hyperglycemia. Extended release tablets should be given with breakfast. Patients that are NPO or require decreased caloric intake may need doses held to avoid hypoglycemia.

Monitoring Parameters Signs and symptoms of hypoglycemia (fatigue, excessive hunger, profuse sweating, numbness of extremities), blood glucose, hemoglobin A_{1c}

Reference Range

Recommendations for glycemic control in adults with diabetes:

Hb A_{1c}: <7%

Preprandial capillary plasma glucose: 70-130 mg/dL

Peak postprandial capillary blood glucose: <180 mg/dL

Blood pressure: <130/80 mm Hg

Recommendations for glycemic control in older adults with diabetes:

Relatively healthy, cognitively intact, and with a ≥5-year life expectancy: See Adults

Frail, life expectancy <5-years or those for whom the risks of intensive glucose control outweigh the benefits:

Hb A_{1c}: <8% to 9%

Blood pressure: <140/80 mm Hg or <130/80 mm Hg if tolerated

Special Geriatric Considerations Glipizide is a useful agent since there are few drug-to-drug interactions and elimination of the active drug is not dependent upon renal function. Intensive glucose control (Hb A_{1c} <6.5%) has been linked to increased all-cause and cardiovascular mortality, hypoglycemia requiring assistance, and weight gain in adult type 2 diabetes. How "tightly" to control a geriatric patient's blood glucose needs to be individualized. Such a decision should be based on several factors, including the patient's functional and cognitive status, how well he/she recognizes hypoglycemic or hyperglycemic symptoms, and how to respond to them and other disease states. An Hb A_{1c} <7.5% is an acceptable endpoint for a healthy older adult, while <8% is acceptable for frail elderly patients, those with a duration of illness >10 years, or those with comorbid conditions and requiring combination diabetes medications. For elderly patients with diabetes who are relatively healthy, attaining target goals for aspirin use, blood pressure, lipids, smoking cessation, and diet and exercise may be more important than normalized glycemic control.

Dosage Forms Excipient information presented when available (limited, particularly for generics); consult specific product labeling.

Tablet, oral: 5 mg, 10 mg

Glucotrol®: 5 mg, 10 mg [scored; dye free]

Tablet, extended release, oral: 2.5 mg, 5 mg, 10 mg

Glucotrol XL®: 2.5 mg, 5 mg, 10 mg

Glipizide and Metformin (GLIP i zide & met FOR min)

Related Information

GlipiZIDE *on page 880*

MetFORMIN *on page 1222*

Medication Safety Issues

High alert medication:

The Institute for Safe Medication Practices (ISMP) includes this medication among its list of drugs which have a heightened risk of causing significant patient harm when used in error.

Brand Names: U.S. Metaglip™

Index Terms Glipizide and Metformin Hydrochloride; Metformin and Glipizide

Generic Availability (U.S.) Yes

Pharmacologic Category Antidiabetic Agent, Biguanide; Antidiabetic Agent, Sulfonylurea

Use Indicated as an adjunct to diet and exercise to improve glycemic control in adults with type 2 diabetes mellitus (noninsulin dependent, NIDDM)

Dosage

Geriatric Conservative doses are recommended in the elderly due to potentially decreased renal function; **do not titrate to maximum dose**; should not be used in patients ≥80 years unless renal function is verified as normal

Adult Type 2 diabetes:

Patients inadequately controlled on diet and exercise alone: Initial dose: Glipizide 2.5 mg/metformin 250 mg once daily with a meal. In patients with fasting plasma glucose (FPG) 280-320 mg/dL, initiate therapy with glipizide 2.5 mg/metformin 500 mg twice daily.

Note: Increase dose by 1 tablet/day every 2 weeks (maximum daily dose: Glipizide 10 mg/metformin 2000 mg in divided doses)

Patients inadequately controlled on a sulfonylurea and/or metformin: Initial dose: Glipizide 2.5 mg/metformin 500 mg or glipizide 5 mg/metformin 500 mg twice daily with morning and evening meals; starting dose should not exceed current daily dose of glipizide (or sulfonylurea equivalent) and/or metformin.

Note: Increase dose in increments of no more than glipizide 5 mg/metformin 500 mg (maximum daily dose: Glipizide 20 mg/metformin 2000 mg)

Renal Impairment Contraindicated in the presence of renal disease or renal dysfunction (serum creatinine ≥1.5 mg/dL [males], ≥1.4 mg/dL [females], or abnormal creatinine clearance).

Hepatic Impairment Avoid use in patients with impaired liver function.

Special Geriatric Considerations See individual agents. Combination products are not recommended as first-line treatment. Use only if doses of individual agents correspond to the combination available.

Dosage Forms Excipient information presented when available (limited, particularly for generics); consult specific product labeling. [DSC] = Discontinued product

Tablet, oral: 2.5/250: Glipizide 2.5 mg and metformin hydrochloride 250 mg; 2.5/500: Glipizide 2.5 mg and metformin hydrochloride 500 mg; 5/500: Glipizide 5 mg and metformin hydrochloride 500 mg

Metaglip™ 2.5/250: Glipizide 2.5 mg and metformin hydrochloride 250 mg [DSC]

Metaglip™ 2.5/500: Glipizide 2.5 mg and metformin hydrochloride 500 mg

Metaglip™ 5/500: Glipizide 5 mg and metformin hydrochloride 500 mg

◆ **Glipizide and Metformin Hydrochloride** see Glipizide and Metformin on page 882
◆ **GlucaGen®** see Glucagon on page 883
◆ **GlucaGen® Diagnostic Kit** see Glucagon on page 883
◆ **GlucaGen® HypoKit®** see Glucagon on page 883

Glucagon (GLOO ka gon)

Brand Names: U.S. GlucaGen®; GlucaGen® Diagnostic Kit; GlucaGen® HypoKit®; Glucagon Emergency Kit

Brand Names: Canada GlucaGen®; GlucaGen® HypoKit®

Index Terms Glucagon Hydrochloride

Generic Availability (U.S.) No

Pharmacologic Category Antidote; Antidote, Hypoglycemia; Diagnostic Agent

Use Management of hypoglycemia; diagnostic aid in radiologic examinations to temporarily inhibit GI tract movement

Unlabeled Use Beta-blocker- or calcium channel blocker-induced myocardial depression (with or without hypotension) unresponsive to standard measures; suspected or documented hypoglycemia secondary to insulin or sulfonylurea overdose (as adjunct to dextrose)

Contraindications Hypersensitivity to glucagon or any component of the formulation; insulinoma; pheochromocytoma

Warnings/Precautions Use of glucagon is contraindicated in insulinoma; exogenous glucagon may cause an initial rise in blood glucose followed by rebound hypoglycemia. Use of glucagon is contraindicated in pheochromocytoma; exogenous glucagon may cause the release of catecholamines, resulting in an increase in blood pressure. Use caution with prolonged fasting, starvation, adrenal insufficiency or chronic hypoglycemia; levels of glucose stores in liver may be decreased. Supplemental carbohydrates should be given to patients who respond to glucagon for severe hypoglycemia to prevent secondary hypoglycemia. Monitor blood glucose levels closely.

In patients with hypoglycemia secondary to insulin or sulfonylurea overdose, dextrose should be immediately administered; if I.V. access cannot be established or if dextrose is not available, glucagon may be considered as alternative acute treatment until dextrose can be administered.

May contain lactose; avoid administration in hereditary galactose intolerance, Lapp lactase deficiency, or glucose-galactose malabsorption.

Adverse Reactions (Reflective of adult population; not specific for elderly) Frequency not defined.

Cardiovascular: Hypotension (up to 2 hours after GI procedures), hypertension, tachycardia

Gastrointestinal: Nausea, vomiting (high incidence with rapid administration of high doses)

Miscellaneous: Hypersensitivity reactions, anaphylaxis

Drug Interactions

Metabolism/Transport Effects None known.

Avoid Concomitant Use There are no known interactions where it is recommended to avoid concomitant use.

Increased Effect/Toxicity

Glucagon may increase the levels/effects of: Vitamin K Antagonists

Decreased Effect There are no known significant interactions involving a decrease in effect.

Ethanol/Nutrition/Herb Interactions Glucagon depletes glycogen stores.

Stability Prior to reconstitution, store at controlled room temperature of 20°C to 25°C (69°F to 77°F); do not freeze. Reconstitute powder for injection by adding 1 mL of sterile diluent to a vial containing 1 unit of the drug, to provide solutions containing 1 mg of glucagon/mL. Gently roll vial to dissolve. Use immediately after reconstitution. May be kept at 5°C for up to 48 hours if necessary. Solution for infusion may be prepared by reconstitution with and further dilution in NS or D_5W (Love, 1998).

Mechanism of Action Stimulates adenylate cyclase to produce increased cyclic AMP, which promotes hepatic glycogenolysis and gluconeogenesis, causing a raise in blood glucose levels

Pharmacodynamics/Kinetics

Onset of action: Peak effect: Blood glucose levels: Parenteral:

I.V.: 5-20 minutes

I.M.: 30 minutes

SubQ: 30-45 minutes

Duration: Glucose elevation:

SubQ: 60-90 minutes

I.V.: 30 minutes

Metabolism: Primarily hepatic; some inactivation occurring renally and in plasma

Half-life elimination, plasma: 8-18 minutes

Dosage

Geriatric & Adult

Hypoglycemia: I.M., I.V., SubQ: 1 mg; may repeat in 20 minutes as needed

Note: I.V. dextrose should be administered as soon as it is available; if patient fails to respond to glucagon, I.V. dextrose must be given.

Beta-blocker- or calcium channel blocker-induced myocardial depression (with or without hypotension) unresponsive to standard measures (unlabeled use): I.V.: 3-10 mg (or 0.05-0.15 mg/kg) bolus followed by an infusion of 3-5 mg/hour (or 0.05-0.1 mg/kg/hour); titrate infusion rate to achieve adequate hemodynamic response (ACLS, 2010)

Diagnostic aid:

I.M.: 1-2 mg 10 minutes prior to gastrointestinal procedure

I.V.: 0.25-2 mg 10 minutes prior to gastrointestinal procedure

Administration I.V.: Bolus may be associated with nausea and vomiting.

Beta-blocker/calcium channel blocker toxicity: Administer bolus over 3-5 minutes; continuous infusions may be used. Ensure adequate supply available to continue therapy.

Monitoring Parameters Blood pressure, blood glucose, ECG, heart rate, mentation

Pharmacotherapy Pearls 1 unit = 1 mg

Special Geriatric Considerations No specific recommendations needed.

Dosage Forms Excipient information presented when available (limited, particularly for generics); consult specific product labeling.

Injection, powder for reconstitution:

Glucagon Emergency Kit: 1 mg [contains glycerin (in diluent), lactose 49 mg; equivalent to 1 unit]

Injection, powder for reconstitution, as hydrochloride:

GlucaGen®: 1 mg [contains lactose 107 mg; equivalent to 1 unit]

GlucaGen® Diagnostic Kit: 1 mg [contains lactose 107 mg; equivalent to 1 unit]

GlucaGen® HypoKit®: 1 mg [contains lactose 107 mg; equivalent to 1 unit]

◆ **Glucagon Emergency Kit** *see* Glucagon *on page 883*
◆ **Glucagon Hydrochloride** *see* Glucagon *on page 883*

Glucarpidase (gloo KAR pid ase)

Brand Names: U.S. Voraxaze®
Index Terms Carboxypeptidase-G2; CPDG2; CPG2; Voraxaze
Generic Availability (U.S.) No
Pharmacologic Category Antidote; Enzyme
Use Treatment of toxic plasma methotrexate concentrations (>1 micromole/L) in patients with delayed clearance due to renal impairment

Note: Due to the risk of subtherapeutic methotrexate exposure, glucarpidase is **NOT** indicated when methotrexate clearance is within expected range (plasma methotrexate concentration ≤2 standard deviations of mean methotrexate excretion curve specific for dose administered) **or** with normal renal function or mild renal impairment.

Unlabeled Use Rescue agent to reduce methotrexate toxicity in patients with accidental intrathecal methotrexate overdose

Prescribing and Access Restrictions
Voraxaze® is distributed through ASD Healthcare; procurement information is available (24 hours a day; 365 days a year) at 1-855-7-VORAXAZE (1-855-786-7292).

Contraindications There are no contraindications listed in the manufacturer's labeling.

Warnings/Precautions Serious allergic reactions have been reported.

Leucovorin calcium administration should be continued after glucarpidase; the same dose as was given prior to glucarpidase should be continued for the first 48 hours after glucarpidase; after 48 hours, leucovorin doses should be based on methotrexate concentrations. A single methotrexate concentration should not determine when leucovorin should be discontinued; continue leucovorin until the methotrexate concentration remains below the threshold for leucovorin treatment for ≥3 days. Leucovorin calcium is a substrate for glucarpidase and may compete with methotrexate for binding sites; **do not administer leucovorin calcium within 2 hours before or after glucarpidase.** In addition to leucovorin, glucarpidase use should be accompanied with adequate hydration and urinary alkalinization. During the first 48 hours following glucarpidase administration, the only reliable method of measuring methotrexate concentrations is the chromatographic method. DAMPA, an inactive methotrexate metabolite with a half-life of 9 hours, may interfere with immunoassay and result in the overestimation of the methotrexate concentration (when collected within 48 hours of glucarpidase administration). Glucarpidase use for intrathecal methotrexate overdose (unlabeled route/use) should be used in conjunction with immediate lumbar drainage; concurrent dexamethasone (4 mg I.V. every 6 hours for 4 doses) may minimize methotrexate-induced chemical arachnoiditis; leucovorin calcium (100 mg I.V. every 6 hours for 4 doses) may prevent systemic methotrexate toxicity (Widemann, 2004).

Adverse Reactions (Reflective of adult population; not specific for elderly)
>10%: Miscellaneous: Antiglucarpidase antibody development (17%)
1% to 10%:
  Cardiovascular: Flushing (2%), hypotension (1%)
  Central nervous system: Headache (1%)
  Gastrointestinal: Nausea/vomiting (2%)
  Neuromuscular & skeletal: Paresthesia (2%)

Drug Interactions
Metabolism/Transport Effects None known.
Avoid Concomitant Use There are no known interactions where it is recommended to avoid concomitant use.
Increased Effect/Toxicity There are no known significant interactions involving an increase in effect.
Decreased Effect
Glucarpidase may decrease the levels/effects of: Leucovorin Calcium-Levoleucovorin

Stability Store intact vials refrigerated at 2°C to 8°C (36°F to 46°F); do not freeze. Reconstituted solutions should be used immediately or may be stored for up to 4 hours under refrigeration.
I.V.: Reconstitute each vial (1000 units/vial) with 1 mL normal saline. Mix gently by rolling or tilting vial; do not shake. Upon reconstitution, solution should be clear, colorless and free of particulate matter.
Intrathecal (unlabeled route/use): Reconstitute 2000 units with 12 mL preservative-free normal saline (Widemann, 2004)

GLUCARPIDASE

Mechanism of Action Recombinant enzyme which rapidly hydrolyzes the carboxyl-terminal glutamate residue from extracellular methotrexate into inactive metabolites (DAMPA and glutamate), resulting in a rapid reduction of methotrexate concentrations independent of renal function

Pharmacodynamics/Kinetics

Onset of action: Methotrexate toxicity: Reduces methotrexate concentrations by ≥97% within 15 minutes of I.V. administration

Duration: Methotrexate toxicity: Maintains a >95% reduction of methotrexate concentrations for up to 8 days

Distribution: V_d: I.V.: 3.6 L; distribution restricted to plasma volume

Half-life elimination: I.V.: Normal renal function: 6-9 hours; impaired renal function (Cl_{cr} <30 mL/minute): 8-10 hours (Phillips, 2008)

Dosage

Geriatric & Adult

Methotrexate toxicity: I.V.: 50 units/kg (Buchen, 2005; Widemann, 1997; Widemann, 2010)

Intrathecal methotrexate overdose (unlabeled route/use): Intrathecal: 2000 units as soon as possible after accidental overdose (Widemann, 2004)

Renal Impairment No dosage adjustment necessary.

Hepatic Impairment No dosage adjustment provided in the manufacturer's labeling; has not been studied.

Administration

I.V.: Infuse over 5 minutes; flush I.V. line before and after glucarpidase administration

Intrathecal (for intrathecal methotrexate overdose; unlabeled route/use): Glucarpidase was administered within 3-9 hours of accidental intrathecal methotrexate overdose in conjunction with lumbar drainage or ventriculolumbar perfusion (Widemann, 2004). Administered over 5 minutes via lumbar route, ventriculostomy, Ommaya reservoir, or lumbar and ventriculostomy (O'Marcaigh, 1996; Widemann, 2004). In one case report, 1000 units was administered through the ventricular catheter over 5 minutes and another 1000 units was administered through the lumbar catheter (O'Marcaigh, 1996).

Monitoring Parameters

Serum methotrexate levels: Use chromatographic method if <48 hours from glucarpidase administration (DAMPA interferes with immunoassay results until >48 hours)

CBC with differential, bilirubin, ALT, AST, serum creatinine; evaluate for signs/symptoms of methotrexate toxicity

Test Interactions Methotrexate levels: During the first 48 hours following glucarpidase administration, the only reliable method of measuring methotrexate concentrations is the chromatographic method. DAMPA, an inactive methotrexate metabolite with a half-life of 9 hours, may interfere with immunoassay and result in the overestimation of the methotrexate concentration (when collected within 48 hours of glucarpidase administration).

Pharmacotherapy Pearls The utility of more than one glucarpidase dose in reducing plasma methotrexate levels was evaluated in a study of 100 patients with high-dose methotrexate-induced nephrotoxicity (Widemann, 2010). Glucarpidase 50 units/kg I.V. was administered either as a single dose (n=65), 2 doses given 24 hours apart (n=28), or 3 doses given at 4 hour intervals (n=7). Six of the 65 patients randomized to a single dose also received a second delayed glucarpidase dose (>24 hours later) due to persistent methotrexate concentrations ≥1 micromole/L in spite of a ≥90% decrease in the plasma methotrexate concentration after the initial dose. The use of scheduled second and third glucarpidase doses did not result in additional methotrexate concentration decreases; and only 2 of the 6 patients who received a second delayed glucarpidase dose (>24 hours later) experienced a ≥50% methotrexate concentration reduction.

Special Geriatric Considerations Studies with elderly patients demonstrate that the elderly tolerate glucarpidase as well as younger adults. No dosage adjustment necessary for age or renal function.

Dosage Forms Excipient information presented when available (limited, particularly for generics); consult specific product labeling.

Injection, powder for reconstitution:

Voraxaze®: 1000 units [contains lactose 10 mg/vial]

GlyBURIDE (GLYE byoor ide)

Related Information
Beers Criteria – Potentially Inappropriate Medications for Geriatrics *on page 2183*
Diabetes Mellitus Management, Adults *on page 2193*

Medication Safety Issues
Sound-alike/look-alike issues:
GlyBURIDE may be confused with glipiZIDE, Glucotrol®
Diaβeta® may be confused with Zebeta®
Micronase may be confused with microK®, miconazole, Micronor®, Microzide®

High alert medication:
The Institute for Safe Medication Practices (ISMP) includes this medication among its list of drugs which have a heightened risk of causing significant patient harm when used in error.

BEERS Criteria medication:
This drug may be potentially inappropriate for use in geriatric patients (Quality of evidence - high; Strength of recommendation - strong).

Brand Names: U.S. DiaBeta®; Glynase® PresTab®

Brand Names: Canada Apo-Glyburide®; DiaBeta®; Dom-Glyburide; Euglucon®; Med-Glybe; Mylan-Glybe; Novo-Glyburide; Nu-Glyburide; PMS-Glyburide; PRO-Glyburide; ratio-Glyburide; Riva-Glyburide; Sandoz-Glyburide; Teva-Glyburide

Index Terms Diabeta; Glibenclamide; Glybenclamide; Glybenzcyclamide; Micronase

Generic Availability (U.S.) Yes

Pharmacologic Category Antidiabetic Agent, Sulfonylurea

Use Adjunct to diet and exercise for the management of type 2 diabetes mellitus (noninsulin dependent, NIDDM)

Unlabeled Use Alternative to insulin in women for the treatment of gestational diabetes mellitus (GDM) (11-33 weeks gestation)

Contraindications Hypersensitivity to glyburide or any component of the formulation; type 1 diabetes mellitus (insulin dependent, IDDM), diabetic ketoacidosis; concomitant use with bosentan

Warnings/Precautions All sulfonylurea drugs are capable of producing severe hypoglycemia. Hypoglycemia is more likely to occur when caloric intake is deficient, after severe or prolonged exercise, when ethanol is ingested, or when more than one glucose-lowering drug is used. It is also more likely in elderly patients, malnourished patients and in patients with impaired renal or hepatic function; use with caution.

It may be necessary to discontinue therapy and administer insulin if the patient is exposed to stress (fever, trauma, infection, surgery). Loss of efficacy may be observed following prolonged use as a result of the progression of type 2 diabetes mellitus which results in continued beta cell destruction. In patients who were previously responding to sulfonylurea therapy, consider additional factors which may be contributing to decreased efficacy (eg, inappropriate dose, nonadherence to diet and exercise regimen). If no contributing factors can be identified, consider discontinuing use of the sulfonylurea due to secondary failure of treatment. Additional antidiabetic therapy (eg, insulin) will be required.

Elderly: Avoid use in older adults due to increased risk of prolonged hypoglycemia (Beers Criteria). Rapid and prolonged hypoglycemia (>12 hours) despite hypertonic glucose injections have been reported; age and hepatic and renal impairment are independent risk factors for hypoglycemia; dosage titration should be made at weekly intervals.

Chemical similarities are present among sulfonamides, sulfonylureas, carbonic anhydrase inhibitors, thiazides, and loop diuretics (except ethacrynic acid). Use in patients with sulfonamide allergy is not specifically contraindicated in product labeling, however, a risk of cross-reaction exists in patients with allergy to any of these compounds; avoid use when previous reaction has been severe.

Product labeling states oral hypoglycemic drugs may be associated with an increased cardiovascular mortality as compared to treatment with diet alone or diet plus insulin. Data to support this association are limited, and several studies, including a large prospective trial (UKPDS) have not supported an association.

Patients with G6PD deficiency may be at an increased risk of sulfonylurea-induced hemolytic anemia; however, cases have also been described in patients without G6PD deficiency during postmarketing surveillance. Use with caution and consider a nonsulfonylurea alternative in patients with G6PD deficiency.

Micronized glyburide tablets are **not** bioequivalent to *conventional* glyburide tablets; retitration should occur if patients are being transferred to a different glyburide formulation (eg, micronized-to-conventional or vice versa) or from other hypoglycemic agents.

Adverse Reactions (Reflective of adult population; not specific for elderly) Frequency not defined.

Cardiovascular: Vasculitis

Central nervous system: Dizziness, headache

Dermatologic: Angioedema, erythema, maculopapular eruptions, morbilliform eruptions, photosensitivity reaction, pruritus, purpura, rash, urticaria

Endocrine & metabolic: Disulfiram-like reaction, hypoglycemia, hyponatremia (SIADH reported with other sulfonylureas)

Gastrointestinal: Anorexia, constipation, diarrhea, epigastric fullness, heartburn, nausea

Genitourinary: Nocturia

Hematologic: Agranulocytosis, aplastic anemia, hemolytic anemia, leukopenia, pancytopenia, porphyria cutanea tarda, thrombocytopenia

Hepatic: Cholestatic jaundice, hepatitis, liver failure, transaminase increased

Neuromuscular & skeletal: Arthralgia, myalgia, paresthesia

Ocular: Blurred vision

Renal: Diuretic effect (minor)

Miscellaneous: Allergic reaction

Drug Interactions

Metabolism/Transport Effects Substrate of CYP2C9 (major); **Note:** Assignment of Major/Minor substrate status based on clinically relevant drug interaction potential; **Inhibits** CYP2C8 (weak), CYP3A4 (weak)

Avoid Concomitant Use

Avoid concomitant use of GlyBURIDE with any of the following: Bosentan; Pimozide

Increased Effect/Toxicity

GlyBURIDE may increase the levels/effects of: Alcohol (Ethyl); ARIPiprazole; Bosentan; CycloSPORINE; CycloSPORINE (Systemic); Hypoglycemic Agents; Pimozide; Porfimer; Vitamin K Antagonists

The levels/effects of GlyBURIDE may be increased by: Beta-Blockers; Chloramphenicol; Cimetidine; Clarithromycin; Cyclic Antidepressants; CYP2C9 Inhibitors (Moderate); CYP2C9 Inhibitors (Strong); Fibric Acid Derivatives; Fluconazole; GLP-1 Agonists; Herbs (Hypoglycemic Properties); MAO Inhibitors; Mifepristone; Pegvisomant; Probenecid; Quinolone Antibiotics; Ranitidine; Salicylates; Selective Serotonin Reuptake Inhibitors; Sulfonamide Derivatives; Vitamin K Antagonists; Voriconazole

Decreased Effect

GlyBURIDE may decrease the levels/effects of: Bosentan

The levels/effects of GlyBURIDE may be decreased by: Bosentan; Colesevelam; Corticosteroids (Orally Inhaled); Corticosteroids (Systemic); CycloSPORINE; CycloSPORINE (Systemic); CYP2C9 Inducers (Strong); Loop Diuretics; Luteinizing Hormone-Releasing Hormone Analogs; Peginterferon Alfa-2b; Quinolone Antibiotics; Rifampin; Somatropin; Thiazide Diuretics

Ethanol/Nutrition/Herb Interactions

Ethanol: Caution with ethanol (may cause hypoglycemia).

Herb/Nutraceutical: Herbs with hypoglycemic properties may enhance the hypoglycemic effect of glyburide. This includes alfalfa, aloe, bilberry, bitter melon, burdock, celery, damiana, fenugreek, garcinia, garlic, ginger, ginseng (American), gymnema, marshmallow, stinging nettle

Mechanism of Action Stimulates insulin release from the pancreatic beta cells; reduces glucose output from the liver; insulin sensitivity is increased at peripheral target sites

Pharmacodynamics/Kinetics

Onset of action: Serum insulin levels begin to increase 15-60 minutes after a single dose

Duration: ≤24 hours

Absorption: Significant within 1 hour

Distribution: 9-10 L

Protein binding, plasma: >99% primarily to albumin

Metabolism: Hepatic; forms metabolites (weakly active)

Bioavailability: Variable among oral dosage forms

Half-life elimination: Diaβeta®: 10 hours; Glynase® PresTab®: ~4 hours; may be prolonged with renal or hepatic impairment

Time to peak, serum: Adults: 2-4 hours

Excretion: Feces (50%) and urine (50%) as metabolites

Dosage

Geriatric Regular tablets (Diaβeta®): Oral: Initial: 1.25-2.5 mg/day, increase by 1.25-2.5 mg/day every 1-3 weeks. Refer to adult dosing.

Adult Micronized glyburide tablets are **not** bioequivalent to conventional glyburide tablets; retitration should occur if patients are being transferred to a different glyburide formulation (eg, micronized-to-conventional or vice versa) or from other hypoglycemic agents.

Type 2 diabetes: Oral:
Note: Regular tablets cannot be used interchangeably with micronized tablet formulations

Regular tablets (Diaβeta®):
Initial: 2.5-5 mg/day, administered with breakfast or the first main meal of the day. In patients who are more sensitive to hypoglycemic drugs, start at 1.25 mg/day.
Adjustment: Increase in increments of no more than 2.5 mg/day at weekly intervals based on the patient's blood glucose response
Maintenance: 1.25-20 mg/day given as single or divided doses. Some patients (especially those receiving >10 mg/day) may have a more satisfactory response with twice-daily dosing. Maximum: 20 mg/day
Micronized tablets (Glynase® PresTab®):
Initial: 1.5-3 mg/day, administered with breakfast or the first main meal of the day in patients who are more sensitive to hypoglycemic drugs, start at 0.75 mg/day. Increase in increments of no more than 1.5 mg/day in weekly intervals based on the patient's blood glucose response.
Maintenance: 0.75-12 mg/day given as a single dose or in divided doses. Some patients (especially those receiving >6 mg/day) may have a more satisfactory response with twice-daily dosing. Maximum: 12 mg/day

Management of noninsulin-dependent diabetes mellitus in patients previously maintained on insulin: Oral: Initial dosage dependent upon previous insulin dosage, see table.

Dose Conversion: Insulin to Glyburide

Previous Daily Insulin Dosage (units/day)	Initial Glyburide Dosage Conventional Formulation (mg/day)	Initial Glyburide Dosage Micronized Formulation (mg/day)	Insulin Dosage Change (after glyburide started)
<20	2.5-5	1.5-3	Discontinue
20-40	5	3	Discontinue
>40	5 (increase in increments of 1.25-2.5 mg every 2-10 days)	3 (increase in increments of 0.75-1.5 mg every 2-10 days)	Reduce insulin dosage by 50% (gradually taper off insulin as glyburide dosage increased)

Renal Impairment Cl_{cr} <50 mL/minute: Not recommended
Hepatic Impairment Use conservative initial and maintenance doses and avoid use in severe disease.
Administration Administer with meals at the same time each day (twice-daily dosing may be beneficial if conventional glyburide doses are >10 mg or micronized glyburide doses are >6 mg). Patients that are NPO or require decreased caloric intake may need doses held to avoid hypoglycemia.
Monitoring Parameters Signs and symptoms of hypoglycemia, fasting blood glucose, hemoglobin A_{1c}
Reference Range Recommendations for glycemic control in adults with diabetes:
Hb A_{1c}: <7%
Preprandial capillary plasma glucose: 70-130 mg/dL
Peak postprandial capillary blood glucose: <180 mg/dL
Blood pressure: <130/80 mm Hg
Special Geriatric Considerations Glyburide is not a drug of choice for the elderly because of its association with severe hypoglycemia. Rapid and prolonged hypoglycemia (>12 hours) despite hypertonic glucose injections has been reported; age, hepatic, and renal impairment are independent risk factors for hypoglycemia; dosage titration should be made at weekly intervals. **Do not titrate to maximum dose.** Intensive glucose control (Hb A_{1c} <6.5%) has been linked to increased all-cause and cardiovascular mortality, hypoglycemia requiring assistance, and weight gain in adult type 2 diabetes. How "tightly" to control a geriatric patient's blood glucose needs to be individualized. Such a decision should be based on several factors, including the patient's functional and cognitive status, how well he/she recognizes hypoglycemic or hyperglycemic symptoms, and how to respond to them and other disease states. An Hb A_{1c} <7.5% is an acceptable endpoint for a healthy older adult, while <8% is acceptable for frail elderly patients, those with a duration of illness >10 years, or those with comorbid conditions and requiring combination diabetes medications. For elderly patients with diabetes who are relatively healthy, attaining target goals for aspirin use, blood pressure, lipids, smoking cessation, and diet and exercise may be more important than normalized glycemic control.

◀ This medication is considered to be potentially inappropriate in this patient population (Beers Criteria: Quality of evidence - high; Strength of recommendation - strong).

Dosage Forms Excipient information presented when available (limited, particularly for generics); consult specific product labeling.

Tablet, oral: 1.25 mg, 2.5 mg, 5 mg
DiaBeta®: 1.25 mg, 2.5 mg, 5 mg [scored]

Tablet, oral [micronized]: 1.5 mg, 3 mg, 5 mg, 6 mg
Glynase® PresTab®: 1.5 mg, 3 mg, 6 mg [scored]

Glyburide and Metformin (GLYE byoor ide & met FOR min)

Related Information
GlyBURIDE *on page 887*
MetFORMIN *on page 1222*

Medication Safety Issues
Sound-alike/look-alike issues:
Glucovance® may be confused with Vyvanse®

High alert medication:
The Institute for Safe Medication Practices (ISMP) includes this medication among its list of drugs which have a heightened risk of causing significant patient harm when used in error.

Brand Names: U.S. Glucovance®

Index Terms Glyburide and Metformin Hydrochloride; Metformin and Glyburide

Generic Availability (U.S.) Yes

Pharmacologic Category Antidiabetic Agent, Biguanide; Antidiabetic Agent, Sulfonylurea

Use Adjunct to diet and exercise for the management of type 2 diabetes mellitus (noninsulin dependent, NIDDM)

Dosage
Geriatric Refer to adult dosing. Adjust carefully to renal function. Should not be used in patients ≥80 years of age unless renal function is verified as normal. Do not titrate to maximum dose.

Adult Note: Dose must be individualized. All doses should be taken with a meal. Twice daily dosage should be taken with the morning and evening meals. Dosages expressed as glyburide/metformin components.

Type 2 diabetes: Oral:

No prior treatment with sulfonylurea or metformin: Initial: 1.25 mg/250 mg once daily with a meal; patients with Hb A_{1c} >9% or fasting plasma glucose (FPG) >200 mg/dL may start with 1.25 mg/250 mg twice daily with meals. Adjustment: Dosage may be increased in increments of 1.25 mg/250 mg, at intervals of not less than 2 weeks; maximum daily dose: 10 mg/2000 mg (limited experience with higher doses); **Note:** Doses of 5 mg/500 mg should not be used as initial therapy, due to risk of hypoglycemia.

Previously treated with a sulfonylurea or metformin alone: Initial: 2.5 mg/500 mg or 5 mg/500 mg twice daily with meals; increase in increments no greater than 5 mg/500 mg; maximum daily dose: 20 mg/2000 mg

Note: When switching patients previously on a sulfonylurea and metformin together, do not exceed the daily dose of glyburide (or glyburide equivalent) or metformin. When adding thiazolidinedione, continue glyburide and metformin at current dose and initiate thiazolidinedione at recommended starting dose.

Combination with thiazolidinedione: May be combined with a thiazolidinedione in patients with an inadequate response to glyburide/metformin therapy, however the risk of hypoglycemia may be increased.

Special Geriatric Considerations See individual agents. Combination products are not recommended as first-line treatment. Use only if doses of individual agents correspond to the combination available.

Dosage Forms Excipient information presented when available (limited, particularly for generics); consult specific product labeling. [DSC] = Discontinued product

Tablet: 1.25 mg/250 mg: Glyburide 1.25 mg and metformin hydrochloride 250 mg; 2.5 mg/500 mg: Glyburide 2.5 mg and metformin hydrochloride 500 mg; 5 mg/500 mg: Glyburide 5 mg and metformin hydrochloride 500 mg
Glucovance®: 1.25 mg/250 mg: Glyburide 1.25 mg and metformin hydrochloride 250 mg [DSC]
Glucovance®: 2.5 mg/500 mg: Glyburide 2.5 mg and metformin hydrochloride 500 mg
Glucovance®: 5 mg/500 mg: Glyburide 5 mg and metformin hydrochloride 500 mg

◆ **Glyburide and Metformin Hydrochloride** *see* Glyburide and Metformin *on page 890*

Glycerin (GLIS er in)

Related Information

Laxatives, Classification and Properties *on page 2121*

Treatment Options for Constipation *on page 2142*

Brand Names: U.S. Fleet® Glycerin Suppositories [OTC]; Fleet® Liquid Glycerin [OTC]; Fleet® Pedia-Lax™ Glycerin Suppositories [OTC]; Fleet® Pedia-Lax™ Liquid Glycerin Suppositories [OTC]; Orajel® Dry Mouth [OTC]; Sani-Supp® [OTC]

Index Terms Glycerol

Generic Availability (U.S.) Yes: Suppositories

Pharmacologic Category Laxative, Osmotic; Ophthalmic Agent, Miscellaneous

Use Constipation; reduction of intraocular pressure; reduction of corneal edema; glycerin has been administered orally to reduce intracranial pressure

Adverse Reactions (Reflective of adult population; not specific for elderly) Frequency not defined.

Oral:

Cardiovascular: Arrhythmias

Central nervous system: Confusion, dizziness, headache, hyperosmolar nonketotic coma

Endocrine & metabolic: Dehydration, hyperglycemia, polydipsia

Gastrointestinal: Diarrhea, dry mouth, nausea, vomiting

Rectal: Gastrointestinal: Cramping pain, rectal irritation, tenesmus

Drug Interactions

Metabolism/Transport Effects None known.

Avoid Concomitant Use There are no known interactions where it is recommended to avoid concomitant use.

Increased Effect/Toxicity There are no known significant interactions involving an increase in effect.

Decreased Effect There are no known significant interactions involving a decrease in effect.

Stability

Refrigerate suppositories; avoid freezing. Protect from heat.

Ophthalmic: Store at room temperature. Keep bottle tightly closed. Discard 6 months after dropper is first placed in the solution.

Mechanism of Action Osmotic dehydrating agent which increases osmotic pressure; draws fluid into colon and thus stimulates evacuation

Pharmacodynamics/Kinetics

Onset of action:

Decrease in intraocular pressure: Oral: 10-30 minutes

Reduction of intracranial pressure: Oral: 10-60 minutes

Constipation: Suppository: 15-30 minutes

Peak effect:

Decrease in intraocular pressure: Oral: 60-90 minutes

Reduction of intracranial pressure: Oral: 60-90 minutes

Duration:

Decrease in intraocular pressure: Oral: 4-8 hours

Reduction of intracranial pressure: Oral: ~2-3 hours

Absorption: Oral: Well absorbed; Rectal: Poorly absorbed

Half-life elimination, serum: 30-45 minutes

Dosage

Geriatric & Adult

Constipation: Rectal: 1 adult suppository 1-2 times/day as needed or 5-15 mL as an enema

Reduction of intracranial pressure: Oral: 1.5 g/kg/day divided every 4 hours; 1 g/kg/dose every 6 hours has also been used

Reduction of corneal edema: Ophthalmic solution: Instill 1-2 drops in eye(s) prior to examination OR for lubricant effect, instill 1-2 drops in eye(s) every 3-4 hours

Reduction of intraocular pressure: Oral: 1-1.8 g/kg 1-1½ hours preoperatively; additional doses may be administered at 5-hour intervals

Administration Apply topical anesthetic before instilling ophthalmic drops

Pharmacotherapy Pearls Suppository needs to melt to provide laxative effect

Special Geriatric Considerations The primary use of glycerin in the elderly is as a laxative, although it is not recommended as a first-line treatment

Dosage Forms Excipient information presented when available (limited, particularly for generics); consult specific product labeling. [DSC] = Discontinued product

Gel, oral:

Orajel® Dry Mouth: 18% (42 g) [contains benzalkonium chloride]

Liquid, for prescription compounding: USP: 100% (3840 mL)

GLYCERIN

Liquid, topical: USP: 100% (120 mL, 180 mL, 480 mL, 3840 mL)
Solution, rectal:
  Fleet® Liquid Glycerin: 5.6 g/5.5 mL (7.5 mL) [4 units per box]
  Fleet® Pedia-Lax™ Liquid Glycerin Suppositories: 2.3 g/2.3 mL (4 mL) [6 units per box]
Suppository, rectal [adult]: 80.7% (25s [DSC], 100s [DSC]); 82.5% (12s, 25s, 50s, 100s)
  Fleet® Glycerin Suppositories: 2 g (12s, 50s)
  Sani-Supp®: 82.5% (10s, 25s)
Suppository, rectal [pediatric]: 1.5 g (12s [DSC], 25s [DSC]); 82.5% (12s, 25s)
  Fleet® Pedia-Lax™ Glycerin Suppositories: 1 g (12s)
  Sani-Supp®: 82.5% (10s, 25s)

◆ **Glycerol** see Glycerin on page 891
◆ **Glycerol Guaiacolate** see GuaiFENesin on page 904
◆ **Glyceryl Trinitrate** see Nitroglycerin on page 1386

Glycopyrrolate (glye koe PYE roe late)

Medication Safety Issues
International issues:
  Robinul [U.S. and multiple international markets] may be confused with Reminyl brand name for galantamine [Canada and multiple international markets]
Brand Names: U.S. Cuvposa™; Robinul®; Robinul® Forte
Brand Names: Canada Glycopyrrolate Injection, USP
Index Terms Glycopyrronium Bromide
Generic Availability (U.S.) Yes: Excludes oral solution
Pharmacologic Category Anticholinergic Agent
Use Inhibit salivation and excessive secretions of the respiratory tract preoperatively; control of upper airway secretions; intraoperatively to counteract drug-induced or vagal mediated bradyarrhythmias; adjunct in treatment of peptic ulcer (indication listed in product labeling but currently has no place in management of peptic ulcer disease)

Cuvposa™: Reduce chronic, severe drooling in those with neurologic conditions (eg, cerebral palsy) associated with drooling
Unlabeled Use Adjunct with acetylcholinesterase inhibitors (eg, neostigmine, edrophonium, pyridostigmine) to antagonize cholinergic effects
Contraindications Hypersensitivity to glycopyrrolate or any component of the formulation; medical conditions that preclude use of anticholinergic medication; severe ulcerative colitis, toxic megacolon complicating ulcerative colitis, paralytic ileus, obstructive disease of GI tract (eg, pyloric stenosis), intestinal atony in the elderly or debilitated patient; unstable cardiovascular status in acute hemorrhage; narrow-angle glaucoma; acute hemorrhage; tachycardia; obstructive uropathy; myasthenia gravis

Oral solution: Additional contraindication: Concomitant use of potassium chloride in a solid oral dosage form
Warnings/Precautions Diarrhea may be a sign of incomplete intestinal obstruction, treatment should be discontinued if this occurs. Use caution in elderly and in patients with autonomic neuropathy, hepatic or renal disease, or ulcerative colitis; may precipitate/aggravate toxic megacolon, hyperthyroidism, CAD, CHF, arrhythmias, tachycardia, BPH, or hiatal hernia with reflux. Use of anticholinergics in gastric ulcer treatment may cause a delay in gastric emptying due to antral statis. Caution should be used in individuals demonstrating decreased pigmentation (skin and iris coloration, dark versus light) since there has been some evidence that these individuals have an enhanced sensitivity to the anticholinergic response. May cause drowsiness, eye sensitivity to light, or blurred vision; caution should be used when performing tasks which require mental alertness, such as driving. Thr risk of heat stroke with this medication may be increased during exercise or hot weather.
Adverse Reactions (Reflective of adult population; not specific for elderly)
>10% (as reported with Cuvposa™):
  Cardiovascular: Flushing (30%)
  Central nervous system: Headache (15%)
  Gastrointestinal: Vomiting (40%), xerostomia (40%), constipation (35%)
  Genitourinary: Urinary retention (15%)
  Respiratory: Nasal congestion (30%), sinusitis (15%), upper respiratory tract infection (15%)

<10% (frequency not always defined):
  Cardiovascular: Pallor (≤2%), arrhythmias, cardiac arrest, heart block, hyper-/hypotension, malignant hyperthermia, palpitation, QT_c-interval prolongation, tachycardia

Central nervous system: Aggressiveness (≤2%), agitation (≤2%), crying (abnormal; ≤2%), irritability (≤2%), mood changes (≤2%), pain (≤2%), restlessness (≤2%), confusion, dizziness, drowsiness, excitement, insomnia, nervousness, seizure

Dermatologic: Dry skin (≤2%), pruritus (≤2%), rash (≤2%), urticaria

Endocrine & metabolic: Dehydration (≤2%), lactation suppression

Gastrointestinal: Abdominal distention (≤2%), abdominal pain (≤2%), flatulence (≤2%), retching (≤2%), bloated feeling, intestinal obstruction, loss of taste, nausea, pseudo-obstruction

Genitourinary: Urinary tract infection (≤2%), impotence, urinary hesitancy

Local: Injection site reactions (edema, erythema, pain)

Neuromuscular & skeletal: Weakness

Ocular: Nystagmus (≤2%), blurred vision, cycloplegia, mydriasis, ocular tension increased, photophobia, sensitivity to light increased

Respiratory: Bronchial secretion (thickening; ≤2%), nasal dryness (≤2%), pneumonia (≤2%), respiratory depression

Miscellaneous: Anaphylactoid reactions, diaphoresis decreased, hypersensitivity reactions

Drug Interactions

Metabolism/Transport Effects None known.

Avoid Concomitant Use

Avoid concomitant use of Glycopyrrolate with any of the following: Potassium Chloride

Increased Effect/Toxicity

Glycopyrrolate may increase the levels/effects of: AbobotulinumtoxinA; Anticholinergics; Atenolol; Cannabinoids; Digoxin; MetFORMIN; OnabotulinumtoxinA; Potassium Chloride; RimabotulinumtoxinB

The levels/effects of Glycopyrrolate may be increased by: Amantadine; MAO Inhibitors; Pramlintide

Decreased Effect

Glycopyrrolate may decrease the levels/effects of: Acetylcholinesterase Inhibitors (Central); Haloperidol; Levodopa; Secretin

The levels/effects of Glycopyrrolate may be decreased by: Acetylcholinesterase Inhibitors (Central)

Ethanol/Nutrition/Herb Interactions Food: Administration with a high-fat meal significantly reduced absorption; administer on an empty stomach.

Stability Store at 20°C to 25°C (68°F to 77°F).

Mechanism of Action Blocks the action of acetylcholine at parasympathetic sites in smooth muscle, secretory glands, and the CNS; indirectly reduces the rate of salivation by preventing the stimulation of acetylcholine receptors

Pharmacodynamics/Kinetics

Onset of action: Oral: 50 minutes; I.M.: 15-30 minutes; I.V.: ~1 minute

Peak effect: Oral: ~1 hour; I.M.: 30-45 minutes

Duration: Vagal effect: 2-3 hours; Inhibition of salivation: Up to 7 hours; Anticholinergic: Oral: 8-12 hours

Absorption: Oral tablet: Poor and erratic; Oral solution: 23% lower compared to tablet

Distribution: V_d: Adults: 0.2-0.62 L/kg

Metabolism: Hepatic (minimal)

Bioavailability: Tablet: ~1% to 13%

Half-life elimination: Adults: ~60-75 minutes; Oral solution: Adults: 3 hours

Excretion: Urine (as unchanged drug, I.M.: 80%, I.V.: 85%); bile (as unchanged drug)

Dosage

Geriatric & Adult

Reduction of secretions:

Preoperative: I.M.: 4 mcg/kg 30-60 minutes before procedure

Intraoperative: I.V.: 0.1 mg repeated as needed at 2- to 3-minute intervals

Reversal of neuromuscular blockade: I.V.: 0.2 mg for each 1 mg of neostigmine or 5 mg of pyridostigmine administered or 5-15 mcg/kg glycopyrrolate with 25-70 mcg/kg of neostigmine or 0.1-0.3 mg/kg of pyridostigmine (agents usually administered simultaneously, but glycopyrrolate may be administered first if bradycardia is present)

Administration

I.V.: Administer I.V. at a rate of 0.2 mg over 1-2 minutes. May be administered I.M. or I.V. without dilution. May also be administered via the tubing of a running I.V. infusion of a compatible solution. May be administered I.V. in the same syringe with neostigmine or pyridostigmine.

Oral: Administer oral solution on an empty stomach, 1 hour before or 2 hours after meals

Monitoring Parameters Heart rate; anticholinergic effects; bowel sounds; bowel movements; effects on drooling

Special Geriatric Considerations Anticholinergic agents are generally not well tolerated in the elderly and their use should be avoided when possible.

Dosage Forms Excipient information presented when available (limited, particularly for generics); consult specific product labeling.

Injection, solution: 0.2 mg/mL (1 mL, 2 mL, 5 mL, 20 mL)
  Robinul®: 0.2 mg/mL (1 mL, 2 mL, 5 mL, 20 mL) [contains benzyl alcohol]

Solution, oral:
  Cuvposa™: 1 mg/5 mL (473 mL) [contains propylene glycol; cherry flavor]

Tablet, oral: 1 mg, 2 mg
  Robinul®: 1 mg [scored]
  Robinul® Forte: 2 mg [scored]

◆ **Glycopyrronium Bromide** see Glycopyrrolate on page 892
◆ **Glydiazinamide** see GlipiZIDE on page 880
◆ **Glynase® PresTab®** see GlyBURIDE on page 887
◆ **Gly-Oxide® [OTC]** see Carbamide Peroxide on page 291
◆ **Glyset®** see Miglitol on page 1284

Gold Sodium Thiomalate (gold SOW dee um thye oh MAL ate)

Brand Names: U.S. Myochrysine® [DSC]
Brand Names: Canada Myochrysine®
Index Terms Sodium Aurothiomalate
Generic Availability (U.S.) No
Pharmacologic Category Gold Compound
Use Adjunctive treatment of active rheumatoid arthritis
Contraindications Hypersensitivity to gold compounds or any component of the formulation; history of severe toxicity to gold compounds or heavy metals; systemic lupus erythematosus; severe debilitation
Warnings/Precautions Frequent monitoring of patients for signs and symptoms of toxicity will prevent/limit serious adverse reactions. Must not be administered by I.V. injection. In patients with hematologic abnormalities (blood dyscrasias, hemorrhagic diathesis), renal impairment, hepatic impairment, SLE or dermatitis: Consider alternative therapy (these conditions may be considered relative contraindications); may increase risk and/or symptoms of gold toxicity may be more difficult to detect.

[U.S. Boxed Warning]: **May cause significant toxicity involving dermatologic, gastro-intestinal, hematologic, pulmonary, renal and hepatic systems; patient education is required.** Dermatitis and lesions of the mucous membranes are common and may be serious; pruritus may precede the early development of a skin reaction. Signs of toxicity include hematologic depression (depressed hemoglobin, leukocytes, granulocytes, or platelets); stomatitis, persistent diarrhea, enterocolitis, cholestatic jaundice; proteinuria (nephritic syndrome), and interstitial pulmonary fibrosis. Use caution in patients with HF, hypertension, or cerebrovascular disease. Avoid use in patients with prior inflammatory bowel disease. Injection contains benzyl alcohol.

In general, NSAIDS and corticosteroids may be discontinued after initiation of therapy (corticosteroid tapering may be required). Concurrent ACE inhibitors may be associated with a higher risk of nitritoid reactions.

Adverse Reactions (Reflective of adult population; not specific for elderly) Frequency not defined.

Cardiovascular: Bradycardia, syncope
Central nervous system: Confusion, fever, Guillain-Barré syndrome, hallucinations, seizure
Dermatologic: Alopecia, angioedema, dermatitis, nail shedding, pruritus, rash, urticaria
Gastrointestinal: Anorexia, abdominal cramps, diarrhea, dysphagia, enterocolitis (ulcerative), gingivitis, glossitis, nausea, stomatitis, taste disturbance (metallic), thick tongue, vomiting
Hematologic: Agranulocytosis, aplastic anemia, eosinophilia, leukopenia, purpura, thrombo-cytopenia
Hepatic: Cholestasis, hepatitis, hepatotoxicity, jaundice
Neuromuscular & skeletal: Arthralgia, peripheral neuropathy
Ocular: Conjunctivitis, corneal ulcers, gold deposits in ocular tissues, iritis
Respiratory: Dyspnea, gold bronchitis, interstitial pneumonitis, pulmonary fibrosis
Renal: Glomerulitis, hematuria, nephrotic syndrome, proteinuria
Miscellaneous: Anaphylactoid reaction, anaphylaxis, nitritoid reaction

Drug Interactions
Metabolism/Transport Effects None known.
Avoid Concomitant Use There are no known interactions where it is recommended to avoid concomitant use.

Increased Effect/Toxicity
The levels/effects of Gold Sodium Thiomalate may be increased by: ACE Inhibitors

Decreased Effect There are no known significant interactions involving a decrease in effect.

Stability Should not be used if solution is darker than pale yellow.

Mechanism of Action Unknown, may decrease prostaglandin synthesis or may alter cellular mechanisms by inhibiting sulfhydryl systems

Pharmacodynamics/Kinetics
Onset of action: Delayed; may require up to 3 months
Half-life elimination: 5 days; may be prolonged with multiple doses
Time to peak, serum: 4-6 hours
Excretion: Urine (60% to 90%); feces (10% to 40%)

Dosage
Geriatric & Adult Rheumatoid arthritis: I.M.: 10 mg first week; 25 mg second week; then 25-50 mg/week until development of toxicity or 1 g cumulative dose has been given; if improvement occurs without adverse reactions, the dose may be decreased or the dosing interval increased; Maintenance: 25-50 mg every other week for 2-20 weeks, then every 3-4 weeks indefinitely

Note: Failure to improve during initial therapy may warrant continuation of 25-50 mg for additional 10 weeks or a dose increase in increments of 10 mg every 1-4 weeks (maximum: 100 mg/injection). Discontinue therapy if no improvement or toxicity develops.

Renal Impairment Aronoff, 2007:
Cl_{cr} 50-80 mL/minute: Administer 50% of normal dose.
Cl_{cr} <50 mL/minute: Avoid use.

Administration Deep I.M. injection into the upper outer quadrant of the gluteal region addition of 0.1 mL of 1% lidocaine to each injection may reduce the discomfort associated with I.M. administration

Monitoring Parameters Patients should have a CBC with differential, platelet count, hemoglobin determination and urinalysis for protein, white cells, red cells and casts; at baseline and prior to each injection. Skin and oral mucosa should be inspected for skin rash, bruising or oral ulceration/stomatitis. Specific questioning for symptoms such as pruritus, rash, stomatitis or metallic taste should be included. Dosing should be withheld in patients with significant gastrointestinal, renal, dermatologic, or hematologic effects (platelet count falls to <100,000/mm^3, WBC <4000, granulocytes <1500/mm^3

Reference Range Gold: Normal: 0-0.1 mcg/mL (SI: 0-0.0064 micromole/L); Therapeutic: 1-3 mcg/mL (SI: 0.06-0.18 micromole/L); Urine: <0.1 mcg/24 hour

Pharmacotherapy Pearls Approximately 50% gold

Special Geriatric Considerations Tolerance to gold decreases with advanced age; use cautiously only after traditional therapy and other disease-modifying antirheumatic drugs (DMARDs) have been attempted. Since elderly frequently have Cl_{cr} <50 mL/minute, it is advisable to measure or calculate creatinine clearance before use.

Dosage Forms Excipient information presented when available (limited, particularly for generics); consult specific product labeling. [DSC] = Discontinued product
Injection, solution:
Myochrysine®: 50 mg/mL (1 mL [DSC], 10 mL [DSC]) [contains benzyl alcohol]

Golimumab (goe LIM ue mab)

Brand Names: U.S. Simponi®
Brand Names: Canada Simponi®
Index Terms CNTO-148
Generic Availability (U.S.) No
Pharmacologic Category Antipsoriatic Agent; Antirheumatic, Disease Modifying; Monoclonal Antibody; Tumor Necrosis Factor (TNF) Blocking Agent
Use Treatment of active rheumatoid arthritis (moderate-to-severe), active psoriatic arthritis, and active ankylosing spondylitis
Medication Guide Available Yes
Contraindications There are no contraindications listed in the FDA-approved manufacturer's labeling.

Canadian labeling: Hypersensitivity to golimumab, latex, or any other component of formulation or packaging; patients with severe infections (eg, sepsis, tuberculosis, opportunistic infections)

Warnings/Precautions [U.S. Boxed Warning]: Patients receiving golimumab are at increased risk for serious infections which may result in hospitalization and/or fatality; infections usually developed in patients receiving concomitant immunosuppressive agents (eg, methotrexate or corticosteroids) and may present as disseminated (rather ▶

than local) disease. **Active tuberculosis (or reactivation of latent tuberculosis), invasive fungal (including aspergillosis, blastomycosis, candidiasis, coccidioidomycosis, histoplasmosis, and pneumocystosis) and bacterial, viral or other opportunistic infections (including legionellosis and listeriosis) have been reported in patients receiving TNF-blocking agents, including golimumab. Monitor closely for signs/symptoms of infection. Discontinue for serious infection or sepsis. Consider risks versus benefits prior to use in patients with a history of chronic or recurrent infection. Consider empiric antifungal therapy in patients who are at risk for invasive fungal infection and develop severe systemic illness.** Caution should be exercised when considering use in the elderly or in patients with conditions that predispose them to infections (eg, diabetes) or residence/travel from areas of endemic mycoses (blastomycosis, coccidioidomycosis, histoplasmosis), or with latent or localized infections. Do not initiate golimumab therapy with clinically important active infection. Patients who develop a new infection while undergoing treatment should be monitored closely.

[U.S. Boxed Warning]: Tuberculosis (disseminated or extrapulmonary) has been reported in patients receiving golimumab; both reactivation of latent infection and new infections have been reported. Patients should be evaluated for tuberculosis risk factors and latent tuberculosis infection (with a tuberculin skin test) prior to therapy. Treatment of latent tuberculosis should be initiated before use. Patients with initial negative tuberculin skin tests should receive continued monitoring for tuberculosis throughout treatment; active tuberculosis has developed in this population during treatment with TNF-blocking agents. Use with caution in patients who have resided in regions where tuberculosis is endemic. Consider antituberculosis therapy if an adequate course of treatment cannot be confirmed in patients with a history of latent or active tuberculosis or for patients with risk factors despite negative skin test.

Rare reactivation of hepatitis B virus (HBV) has occurred in chronic virus carriers; use with caution; evaluate prior to initiation and during treatment. Patients should be brought up to date with all immunizations before initiating therapy. Live vaccines should not be given concurrently. In clinical trials, humoral response to pneumococcal vaccine was not suppressed in psoriatic arthritis patients.

[U.S. Boxed Warning]: Lymphoma and other malignancies have been reported in children and adolescent patients receiving TNF-blocking agents. Half of the malignancies reported in children were lymphomas (Hodgkin's and non-Hodgkin's) while other cases varied and included malignancies not typically observed in this population. The impact of golimumab on the development and course of malignancy is not fully defined. Compared to the general population, an increased risk of lymphoma has been noted in clinical trials; however, rheumatoid arthritis alone has been previously associated with an increased rate of lymphoma. Lymphomas and other malignancies were also observed (at rates higher than expected for the general population) in adult patients receiving TNF-blocking agents. Hepatosplenic T-cell lymphoma (HSTCL), a rare T-cell lymphoma, has also been associated with TNF-blocking agents, primarily reported in adolescent and young adult males with Crohn's disease or ulcerative colitis. Treatment may result in the formation of autoimmune antibodies; cases of autoimmune disease have not been described. Neutralizing antibodies to golimumab may also be formed. Rarely, a reversible lupus-like syndrome has occurred with use of TNF blockers.

Use with caution in patients with peripheral or central nervous system demyelinating disorders; rare cases of new onset or exacerbation of demyelinating disorders (eg, multiple sclerosis, Guillain-Barré syndrome) have occurred with use of TNF-blockers, including golimumab. Consider discontinuing use in patients who develop peripheral or central nervous system demyelinating disorders during treatment. Optic neuritis, transverse myelitis, multiple sclerosis, and new onset or exacerbation of seizures has been reported. Use with caution in patients with heart failure or decreased left ventricular function and discontinue use with new onset or worsening of symptoms. Use caution in patients with a history of significant hematologic abnormalities (cytopenias).

Avoid concomitant use with abatacept (increased incidence of serious infections) or anakinra (increased incidence of neutropenia and serious infection). Use caution when switching between biological disease-modifying antirheumatic drugs (DMARDs); overlapping of biological activity may increase the risk for infection. Use with caution in the elderly (general incidence of infection is higher). Packaging (prefilled syringe and needle cover) contains dry natural rubber (latex). Some dosage forms may contain dry natural rubber (latex) and/or polysorbate 80.

Adverse Reactions (Reflective of adult population; not specific for elderly)

>10%:

Respiratory: Upper respiratory tract infection (16%; includes laryngitis, nasopharyngitis, pharyngitis, and rhinitis)

Miscellaneous: Infection (28%)

1% to 10%:

Cardiovascular: Hypertension (3%)

Central nervous system: Dizziness (2%), fever (1%)

Gastrointestinal: Constipation (1%)

Hepatic: ALT increased (4%), AST increased (3%)

Local: Injection site reactions (6%)

Neuromuscular & skeletal: Paresthesia (2%)

Respiratory: Bronchitis (2%), sinusitis (2%)

Miscellaneous: Viral infection (5%; includes herpes and influenza), antibody formation (4%), fungal infection (superficial; 2%)

Drug Interactions

Metabolism/Transport Effects None known.

Avoid Concomitant Use

Avoid concomitant use of Golimumab with any of the following: Abatacept; Anakinra; BCG; Belimumab; Canakinumab; Certolizumab Pegol; Natalizumab; Pimecrolimus; Rilonacept; Tacrolimus (Topical); Vaccines (Live)

Increased Effect/Toxicity

Golimumab may increase the levels/effects of: Abatacept; Anakinra; Belimumab; Canakinumab; Certolizumab Pegol; Leflunomide; Natalizumab; Rilonacept; Vaccines (Live)

The levels/effects of Golimumab may be increased by: Abciximab; Denosumab; Pimecrolimus; Roflumilast; Tacrolimus (Topical); Trastuzumab

Decreased Effect

Golimumab may decrease the levels/effects of: BCG; Coccidioidin Skin Test; Sipuleucel-T; Vaccines (Inactivated); Vaccines (Live)

The levels/effects of Golimumab may be decreased by: Echinacea

Stability Store under refrigeration at 2°C to 8°C (36°F to 46°F); do not freeze. Do not shake. Protect from light.

Mechanism of Action Human monoclonal antibody that binds to human tumor necrosis factor alpha (TNFα), thereby interfering with endogenous TNFα activity. Biological activities of TNFα include the induction of proinflammatory cytokines (interleukin [IL]-6, IL-8, Granulocyte-colony stimulating factor, granulocyte-macrophage colony stimulating factor), expression of adhesion molecules (E-selectin, vascular cell adhesion molecule [VCAM]-1, intercellular adhesion molecule [ICAM]-1) necessary for leukocyte infiltration, activation of neutrophils and eosinophils.

Pharmacodynamics/Kinetics

Distribution: V_d: I.V.: 0.058-0.126 L/kg

Bioavailability: SubQ: ~53%

Half-life elimination: ~2 weeks

Time to peak, serum: SubQ: 2-6 days

Dosage

Geriatric & Adult Note: Should be administered in conjunction with methotrexate in rheumatoid arthritis; may administer with or without methotrexate or other nonbiologic disease-modifying antirheumatic drugs (DMARDs) in psoriatic arthritis or ankylosing spondylitis.

Rheumatoid arthritis, psoriatic arthritis, ankylosing spondylitis: SubQ: 50 mg once per month

Administration Subcutaneous injection: Prior to administration, allow syringe to sit at room temperature for 30 minutes. Solution should be clear to slightly opalescent and colorless to light yellow. Discard if solution is cloudy, discolored, or has foreign particles. Hold autoinjector firmly against skin and inject subcutaneously into thigh, lower abdomen (below navel), or upper arm. A loud click is heard when injection has begun. Continue to hold autoinjector against skin until second click is heard (may take 3-15 seconds). Following second click, lift autoinjector from injection site. Discard any unused portion. Rotate injection sites and avoid injecting into tender, red, hard, or bruised skin.

Monitoring Parameters Monitor improvement of symptoms and physical function assessments. Latent TB screening prior to initiating and during therapy; signs/symptoms of infection (prior to, during, and following therapy); CBC with differential; signs/symptoms/worsening of heart failure; HBV screening prior to initiating (all patients), HBV carriers (during and for several months following therapy); signs and symptoms of hypersensitivity reaction;

GOLIMUMAB

symptoms of lupus-like syndrome; signs/symptoms of malignancy (eg, splenomegaly, hepatomegaly, abdominal pain, persistent fever, night sweats, weight loss).

Special Geriatric Considerations Phase three trials did not demonstrate any significant differences in adverse drug reactions, infections, or in the side effects profile in elderly compared to younger adults. However, since elderly experience a higher incidence of infections, use with caution and close monitoring in the elderly patient.

Dosage Forms Excipient information presented when available (limited, particularly for generics); consult specific product labeling.

Injection, solution [preservative free]:
Simponi®: 50 mg/0.5 mL (0.5 mL) [contains natural rubber/natural latex in packaging, polysorbate 80; autoinjector]
Simponi®: 50 mg/0.5 mL (0.5 mL) [contains natural rubber/natural latex in packaging, polysorbate 80; prefilled syringe]

♦ **Gordofilm [OTC]** see Salicylic Acid on page 1743
♦ **Gordon Boro-Packs [OTC]** see Aluminum Sulfate and Calcium Acetate on page 84

Goserelin (GOE se rel in)

Brand Names: U.S. Zoladex®
Brand Names: Canada Zoladex®; Zoladex® LA
Index Terms Goserelin Acetate; ICI-118630; ZDX
Generic Availability (U.S.) No
Pharmacologic Category Antineoplastic Agent, Gonadotropin-Releasing Hormone Agonist; Gonadotropin Releasing Hormone Agonist
Use Treatment of locally confined prostate cancer; palliative treatment of advanced prostate cancer; palliative treatment of advanced breast cancer in pre- and perimenopausal women; treatment of endometriosis, including pain relief and reduction of endometriotic lesions; endometrial thinning agent as part of treatment for dysfunctional uterine bleeding
Contraindications Hypersensitivity to goserelin, GnRH, GnRH agonist analogues, or any component of the formulation
Warnings/Precautions Hazardous agent - use appropriate precautions for handling and disposal. Allergic hypersensitivity reactions (including anaphylaxis) and antibody formation may occur; monitor. Androgen-deprivation therapy may increase the risk for cardiovascular disease (Levine, 2010). Transient increases in serum testosterone (in men with prostate cancer) and estrogen (in women with breast cancer) may result in a worsening of disease signs and symptoms (tumor flare) during the first few weeks of treatment. Urinary tract obstruction or spinal cord compression have been reported when used for prostate cancer; closely observe patients for weakness, paresthesias, and urinary tract obstruction in first few weeks of therapy. Decreased bone density has been reported in women and may be irreversible; use caution if other risk factors are present; evaluate and institute preventative treatment if necessary. Cervical resistance may be increased; use caution when dilating the cervix. The 3-month implant currently has no approved indications for use in women. Rare cases of pituitary apoplexy (frequently secondary to pituitary adenoma) have been observed with leuprolide administration (onset from 1 hour to usually <2 weeks); may present as sudden headache, vomiting, visual or mental status changes, and infrequently cardiovascular collapse; immediate medical attention required. Hyperglycemia has been reported in males and may manifest as diabetes or worsening of pre-existing diabetes. Decreased bioavailability may be observed when using the 3-month implant in obese patients. Monitor testosterone levels if desired clinical response is not observed.

Adverse Reactions (Reflective of adult population; not specific for elderly) Percentages reported with the 1-month implant:
>10%:
Cardiovascular: Peripheral edema (female 21%)
Central nervous system: Headache (female 32% to 75%; male 1% to 5%), emotional lability (female 60%), depression (female 54%; male 1% to 5%), pain (female 17%; male 8%), insomnia (female 11%; male 5%)
Dermatologic: Acne (female 42%), seborrhea (female 26%)
Endocrine & metabolic: Hot flashes (female 57% to 96%; male 62%), libido decreased (female 48% to 61%), sexual dysfunction (male 21%), breast atrophy (female 33%), breast enlargement (female 18%), erections decreased (18%), libido increased (female 12%)
Gastrointestinal: Nausea (female 8% to 11%; male 5%), abdominal pain (female 7% to 11%)
Genitourinary: Vaginitis (75%), pelvic symptoms (female 9% to 18%), dyspareunia (female 14%), lower urinary symptoms (male 13%)
Neuromuscular & skeletal: Bone mineral density decreased (female 23%; ~4% decrease from baseline in 6 months; postmarketing reports in males), weakness (female 11%)

Miscellaneous: Diaphoresis (female 16% to 45%; male 6%), tumor flare (female: 23%), infection (female 13%)

1% to 10%:

Cardiovascular: Arrhythmia, cerebrovascular accident, chest pain, edema, heart failure, hypertension, MI, palpitation, peripheral vascular disorder, tachycardia

Central nervous system: Abnormal thinking, anxiety, chills, dizziness, fever, lethargy, malaise, migraine, nervousness, somnolence

Dermatologic: Alopecia, bruising, dry skin, hair disorder, hirsutism, pruritus, rash, skin discoloration

Endocrine & metabolic: Breast pain, breast swelling/tenderness, dysmenorrhea, gout, hyperglycemia

Gastrointestinal: Anorexia, appetite increased, constipation, diarrhea, dyspepsia, flatulence, ulcer, vomiting, weight gain/loss, xerostomia

Genitourinary: Urinary frequency, urinary obstruction, urinary tract infection, vaginal hemorrhage, vulvovaginitis

Hematologic: Anemia, hemorrhage

Local: Application site reaction

Neuromuscular & skeletal: Arthralgia, back pain, hypertonia, joint disorder, leg cramps, myalgia, paresthesia

Ocular: Amblyopia, dry eyes

Renal: Renal insufficiency

Respiratory: Bronchitis, COPD, cough, epistaxis, pharyngitis, rhinitis, sinusitis, upper respiratory tract infection

Miscellaneous: Allergic reaction, flu-like syndrome, voice alteration

Drug Interactions

Metabolism/Transport Effects None known.

Avoid Concomitant Use There are no known interactions where it is recommended to avoid concomitant use.

Increased Effect/Toxicity There are no known significant interactions involving an increase in effect.

Decreased Effect

Goserelin may decrease the levels/effects of: Antidiabetic Agents

Stability Zoladex® should be stored at room temperature not to exceed 25°C or 77°F. Protect from light.

Mechanism of Action Goserelin (a gonadotropin-releasing hormone [GnRH] analog) causes an initial increase in luteinizing hormone (LH) and follicle stimulating hormone (FSH), chronic administration of goserelin results in a sustained suppression of pituitary gonadotropins. Serum testosterone falls to levels comparable to surgical castration. The exact mechanism of this effect is unknown, but may be related to changes in the control of LH or down-regulation of LH receptors.

Pharmacodynamics/Kinetics

Onset:

Females: Estradiol suppression reaches postmenopausal levels within 3 weeks and FSH and LH are suppressed to follicular phase levels within 4 weeks of initiation

Males: Testosterone suppression reaches castrate levels within 2-4 weeks after initiation

Duration:

Females: Estradiol, LH and FSH generally return to baseline levels within 12 weeks following the last monthly implant.

Males: Testosterone levels maintained at castrate levels throughout the duration of therapy.

Absorption: SubQ: Rapid and can be detected in serum in 30-60 minutes; 3.6 mg: released slowly in first 8 days, then rapid and continuous release for 28 days

Distribution: V_d: Male: 44.1 L; Female: 20.3 L

Protein binding: 27%

Time to peak, serum: SubQ: Male: 12-15 days, Female: 8-22 days

Half-life elimination: SubQ: Male: ~4 hours, Female: ~2 hours; Renal impairment: Male: 12 hours

Excretion: Urine (>90%; 20% as unchanged drug)

Dosage

Geriatric & Adult

Prostate cancer, advanced: SubQ:

28-day implant: 3.6 mg every 28 days

12-week implant: 10.8 mg every 12 weeks

Prostate cancer, locally confined (in combination with an antiandrogen and radiotherapy; begin 8 weeks prior to radiotherapy): SubQ:

Combination 28-day/12-week implant: 3.6 mg implant, followed in 28 days by 10.8 mg implant

28-day implant (alternate dosing): 3.6 mg; repeated every 28 days for a total of 4 doses

◄

Breast cancer, advanced: SubQ: 3.6 mg every 28 days
Endometriosis: SubQ: 3.6 mg every 28 days for 6 months
Endometrial thinning: SubQ: 3.6 mg every 28 days for 1 or 2 doses

Renal Impairment No adjustment is necessary.

Hepatic Impairment No adjustment is necessary.

Administration SubQ: Administer implant by inserting needle at a 30-45 degree angle into the anterior abdominal wall below the navel line. Goserelin is an implant; therefore, do not attempt to eliminate air bubbles prior to injection (may displace implant). Do not attempt to aspirate prior to injection; if a large vessel is penetrated, blood will be visualized in the syringe chamber (if vessel is penetrated, withdraw needle and inject elsewhere with a new syringe). Do not penetrate into muscle or peritoneum. Implant may be detected by ultrasound if removal is required.

Monitoring Parameters Bone mineral density, serum calcium, cholesterol/lipids

Prostate cancer: Weakness, paresthesias, and urinary tract obstruction in first few weeks of therapy; screen for diabetes

Test Interactions Interferes with pituitary gonadotropic and gonadal function tests during and for up to 12 weeks after discontinued

Pharmacotherapy Pearls If removal is necessary, implant may be located by ultrasound.

Special Geriatric Considerations No dosage adjustments are needed in the elderly. Monitoring for bone density changes, serum lipid, hemoglobin A_{1c}, blood pressure, and serum calcium changes is recommended.

Dosage Forms Excipient information presented when available (limited, particularly for generics); consult specific product labeling.

Implant, subcutaneous:
Zoladex®: 3.6 mg (1s) [1 month implant]
Zoladex®: 10.8 mg (1s) [3 month implant]

◆ **Goserelin Acetate** see Goserelin on page 898
◆ **GP 47680** see OXcarbazepine on page 1440
◆ **GR38032R** see Ondansetron on page 1425
◆ **Gralise™** see Gabapentin on page 858
◆ **Gramicidin, Neomycin, and Polymyxin B** see Neomycin, Polymyxin B, and Gramicidin on page 1357

Granisetron (gra NI se tron)

Medication Safety Issues

Sound-alike/look-alike issues:
Granisetron may be confused with dolasetron, ondansetron, palonosetron

Brand Names: U.S. Granisol™; Sancuso®

Brand Names: Canada Granisetron Hydrochloride Injection; Kytril®

Index Terms BRL 43694; Kytril

Generic Availability (U.S.) Yes: Injection, tablet

Pharmacologic Category Antiemetic; Selective 5-HT$_3$ Receptor Antagonist

Use Prophylaxis of nausea and vomiting associated with emetogenic chemotherapy and radiation therapy; prophylaxis and treatment of postoperative nausea and vomiting (PONV)

Unlabeled Use Breakthrough treatment of nausea and vomiting associated with chemotherapy

Contraindications Hypersensitivity to granisetron or any component of the formulation

Warnings/Precautions Use with caution in patients with congenital long QT syndrome or other risk factors for QT prolongation (eg, medications known to prolong QT interval, electrolyte abnormalities, and cumulative high-dose anthracycline therapy). 5-HT$_3$ antagonists have been associated with a number of dose-dependent increases in ECG intervals (eg, PR, QRS duration, QT/QT$_c$, JT), usually occurring 1-2 hours after I.V. administration. In general, these changes are not clinically relevant, however, when used in conjunction with other agents that prolong these intervals, arrhythmia may occur. When used with agents that prolong the QT interval (eg, Class I and III antiarrhythmics), clinically relevant QT interval prolongation may occur resulting in torsade de pointes. I.V. formulations of 5-HT$_3$ antagonists have more association with ECG interval changes, compared to oral formulations.

For chemotherapy-related emesis, **granisetron should be used on a scheduled basis, not on an "as needed" (PRN) basis**, since data support the use of this drug in the prevention of nausea and vomiting and not in the rescue of nausea and vomiting. Granisetron should be used only in the first 24-48 hours of receiving chemotherapy or radiation. Data do not support any increased efficacy of granisetron in delayed nausea and vomiting.

Use with caution in patients allergic to other 5-HT$_3$ receptor antagonists; cross-reactivity has been reported. Routine prophylaxis for PONV is not recommended in patients where there is little expectation of nausea and vomiting postoperatively. In patients where nausea and vomiting must be avoided postoperatively, administer to all patients even when expected incidence of nausea and vomiting is low. Use caution following abdominal surgery or in chemotherapy-induced nausea and vomiting; may mask progressive ileus or gastric distention. Application site reactions, generally mild, have occurred with transdermal patch use; if skin reaction is severe or generalized, remove patch. Cover patch application site with clothing to protect from natural or artificial sunlight exposure while patch is applied and for 10 days following removal; granisetron may potentially be affected by natural or artificial sunlight. Do not apply patch to red, irritated, or damaged skin.

Adverse Reactions (Reflective of adult population; not specific for elderly)
>10%:
  Central nervous system: Headache (3% to 21%; transdermal patch: 1%)
  Gastrointestinal: Constipation (3% to 18%)
  Neuromuscular & skeletal: Weakness (5% to 18%)
1% to 10%:
  Cardiovascular: QT$_c$ prolongation (1% to 3%), hypertension (1% to 2%)
  Central nervous system: Pain (10%), fever (3% to 9%), dizziness (4% to 5%), insomnia (<2% to 5%), somnolence (1% to 4%), anxiety (2%), agitation (<2%), CNS stimulation (<2%)
  Dermatologic: Rash (1%)
  Gastrointestinal: Diarrhea (3% to 9%), abdominal pain (4% to 6%), dyspepsia (3% to 6%), taste perversion (2%)
  Hepatic: Liver enzymes increased (5% to 6%)
  Renal: Oliguria (2%)
  Respiratory: Cough (2%)
  Miscellaneous: Infection (3%)

Drug Interactions
Metabolism/Transport Effects Substrate of CYP3A4 (minor); **Note:** Assignment of Major/Minor substrate status based on clinically relevant drug interaction potential

Avoid Concomitant Use
  Avoid concomitant use of Granisetron with any of the following: Apomorphine; Highest Risk QTc-Prolonging Agents; Mifepristone

Increased Effect/Toxicity
  Granisetron may increase the levels/effects of: Apomorphine; Highest Risk QTc-Prolonging Agents; Moderate Risk QTc-Prolonging Agents

  The levels/effects of Granisetron may be increased by: Mifepristone; QTc-Prolonging Agents (Indeterminate Risk and Risk Modifying)

Decreased Effect
  Granisetron may decrease the levels/effects of: Tapentadol; TraMADol

  The levels/effects of Granisetron may be decreased by: Tocilizumab

Stability
I.V.: Store at 15°C to 30°C (59°F to 86°F). Stable when mixed in NS or D$_5$W for 7 days under refrigeration and for 3 days at room temperature. Protect from light. Do not freeze vials.
Oral: Store tablet or oral solution at 15°C to 30°C (59°F to 86°F). Protect from light.
Transdermal patch: Store at 20°C to 25°C (68°F to 77°F). Keep patch in original packaging until immediately prior to use.

Mechanism of Action Selective 5-HT$_3$-receptor antagonist, blocking serotonin, both peripherally on vagal nerve terminals and centrally in the chemoreceptor trigger zone

Pharmacodynamics/Kinetics
Duration: Oral, I.V.: Generally up to 24 hours
Absorption: Oral: Tablets and oral solution are bioequivalent; Transdermal patch: ~66% over 7 days
Distribution: V$_d$: 2-4 L/kg; widely throughout body
Protein binding: 65%
Metabolism: Hepatic via N-demethylation, oxidation, and conjugation; some metabolites may have 5-HT$_3$ antagonist activity
Half-life elimination: Oral: 6 hours; I.V.: 9 hours
Time to peak, plasma: Transdermal patch: Maximum systemic concentrations: ~48 hours after application (range: 24-168 hours)
Excretion: Urine (12% as unchanged drug, 48% to 49% as metabolites); feces (34% to 38% as metabolites)

Dosage

Geriatric & Adult

Prophylaxis of chemotherapy-related emesis:

Oral: 2 mg once daily up to 1 hour before chemotherapy or 1 mg twice daily; the first 1 mg dose should be given up to 1 hour before chemotherapy.

I.V.:

Within U.S.: 10 mcg/kg/dose (maximum: 1 mg/dose) given 30 minutes prior to chemotherapy; for some drugs (eg, carboplatin, cyclophosphamide) with a later onset of emetic action, 10 mcg/kg every 12 hours may be necessary.

Outside U.S.: 40 mcg/kg/dose (or 3 mg/dose); maximum: 9 mg/24 hours

Breakthrough: Granisetron has not been shown to be effective in terminating nausea or vomiting once it occurs and should not be used for this purpose.

Transdermal patch: Prophylaxis of chemotherapy-related emesis: Apply 1 patch at least 24 hours prior to chemotherapy; do not apply ≥48 hours before chemotherapy. Remove patch a minimum of 24 hours after chemotherapy completion. Maximum duration: Patch may be worn up to 7 days, depending on chemotherapy regimen duration.

Prophylaxis of radiation therapy-associated emesis: Oral: 2 mg once daily given 1 hour before radiation therapy.

Postoperative nausea and vomiting (PONV): I.V.:

Prevention: 1 mg given undiluted over 30 seconds; the manufacturer recommends administration before induction of anesthesia or immediately before reversal of anesthesia. **Note:** The Society for Ambulatory Anesthesia (SAMBA) Guidelines recommend a dosage range of 0.35-1.5 mg administered at the end of surgery (Gan, 2007). However, doses ≤1 mg are generally used since doses >1 mg are not more effective. Of note, 5 mcg/kg (~0.35 mg in a 70 kg adult) has been shown to be effective; doses >5 mcg/kg were not more effective (Mikawa, 1997).

Treatment: 1 mg given undiluted over 30 seconds

Renal Impairment No dosage adjustment required.

Hepatic Impairment Kinetic studies in patients with hepatic impairment showed that total clearance was approximately halved; however, standard doses were very well tolerated, and dose adjustments are not necessary.

Administration

Oral: Doses should be given up to 1 hour prior to initiation of chemotherapy/radiation

I.V.: Administer I.V. push over 30 seconds or as a 5-10 minute-infusion

Prevention of PONV: Administer before induction of anesthesia or immediately before reversal of anesthesia.

Treatment of PONV: Administer undiluted over 30 seconds.

Transdermal (Sancuso®): Apply patch to clean, dry, intact skin on upper outer arm. Do not use on red, irritated or damaged skin. Remove patch from pouch immediately before application. Do not cut patch.

Monitoring Parameters Monitor for control of nausea and vomiting

Special Geriatric Considerations Clinical trials with patients older than 65 years of age are limited; however, the data indicates that safety and efficacy are similar to that observed in younger adults. No adjustment in dose necessary for elderly.

Dosage Forms Excipient information presented when available (limited, particularly for generics); consult specific product labeling.

Injection, solution: 1 mg/mL (1 mL, 4 mL)

Injection, solution [preservative free]: 0.1 mg/mL (1 mL); 1 mg/mL (1 mL)

Patch, transdermal:

Sancuso®: 3.1 mg/24 hours (1s) [52 cm^2, total granisetron 34.3 mg]

Solution, oral:

Granisol™: 2 mg/10 mL (30 mL) [contains sodium benzoate; orange flavor]

Tablet, oral: 1 mg

Extemporaneously Prepared A 0.2 mg/mL oral suspension may be prepared by crushing twelve (12) 1 mg tablets and mixing with 30 mL water and enough cherry syrup to provide a final volume of 60 mL; this preparation is stable for 14 days at room temperature or when refrigerated

Quercia RA, Zhang JH, Fan C, et al, "Stability of Granisetron (Kytril®) in an Extemporaneously Prepared Oral Liquid," *International Pharmaceutical Abstracts*, 1996, May 15, Vol 33.

◆ **Granisol™** *see* Granisetron *on page 900*

◆ **Granulex®** *see* Trypsin, Balsam Peru, and Castor Oil *on page 1979*

◆ **Granulocyte Colony Stimulating Factor** *see* Filgrastim *on page 787*

◆ **Granulocyte Colony Stimulating Factor (PEG Conjugate)** *see* Pegfilgrastim *on page 1481*

◆ **Grifulvin V®** *see* Griseofulvin *on page 903*

Griseofulvin (gri see oh FUL vin)

Brand Names: U.S. Grifulvin V®; Gris-PEG®

Index Terms Griseofulvin Microsize; Griseofulvin Ultramicrosize

Generic Availability (U.S.) Yes: Suspension, ultramicrosized product

Pharmacologic Category Antifungal Agent, Oral

Use Treatment of susceptible tinea infections of the skin, hair, and nails

Contraindications Hypersensitivity to griseofulvin or any component of the formulation; severe liver disease; porphyria (interferes with porphyrin metabolism)

Warnings/Precautions During long-term therapy, periodic assessment of hepatic, renal, and hematopoietic functions should be performed; avoid exposure to intense sunlight to prevent photosensitivity reactions; hypersensitivity cross reaction between penicillins and griseofulvin is possible

Adverse Reactions (Reflective of adult population; not specific for elderly) Frequency not defined.

Central nervous system: Dizziness, fatigue, headache, insomnia, mental confusion

Dermatologic: Angioneurotic edema (rare), erythema multiforme-like drug reaction, photosensitivity, rash (most common), urticaria (most common),

Gastrointestinal: Diarrhea, epigastric distress, GI bleeding, nausea, vomiting

Genitourinary: Menstrual irregularities (rare)

Hematologic: Granulocytopenia, leukopenia

Hepatic: Hepatotoxicity

Neuromuscular & skeletal: Paresthesia (rare)

Renal: Nephrosis, proteinuria

Miscellaneous: Drug-induced lupus-like syndrome (rare), oral thrush

Drug Interactions

Metabolism/Transport Effects Induces CYP1A2 (weak/moderate), CYP2C9 (weak/moderate), CYP3A4 (weak/moderate)

Avoid Concomitant Use

Avoid concomitant use of Griseofulvin with any of the following: Axitinib; Contraceptives (Progestins)

Increased Effect/Toxicity

Griseofulvin may increase the levels/effects of: Alcohol (Ethyl); Porfimer

Decreased Effect

Griseofulvin may decrease the levels/effects of: ARIPiprazole; Axitinib; Contraceptives (Estrogens); Contraceptives (Progestins); CycloSPORINE; CycloSPORINE (Systemic); Saccharomyces boulardii; Saxagliptin; Vitamin K Antagonists

The levels/effects of Griseofulvin may be decreased by: Barbiturates

Ethanol/Nutrition/Herb Interactions

Ethanol: Ethanol may increase CNS depression. Concomitant use will also cause a "disulfiram"-type reaction consisting of tachycardia, flushing, headache, nausea, and in some patients, vomiting and chest and/or abdominal pain. Management: Avoid ethanol.

Food: Griseofulvin concentrations may be increased if taken with food, especially with high-fat meals. Management: Take with a fatty meal (peanuts or ice cream) to increase absorption, or with food or milk to avoid GI upset.

Mechanism of Action Inhibits fungal cell mitosis at metaphase; binds to human keratin making it resistant to fungal invasion

Pharmacodynamics/Kinetics

Absorption: Ultramicrosize griseofulvin is almost complete; absorption of microsize griseofulvin is variable (25% to 70% of an oral dose); absorption is enhanced by ingestion of a fatty meal

Distribution: Deposited in varying concentrations in the keratin layer of the skin, hair, and nails; only a very small fraction is distributed in the body fluids and tissues

Metabolism: Extensive in the liver

Half-life: 9-22 hours

Time to peak serum concentration: ~4 hours

Elimination: <1% excreted unchanged in urine; also excreted in feces and perspiration

Dosage

Geriatric & Adult

Tinea infections: Oral:

Microsize: 500-1000 mg/day in single or divided doses

Ultramicrosize: 375 mg/day in single or divided doses; doses up to 750 mg/day have been used for infections more difficult to eradicate such as tinea unguium and tinea pedis.

Note: Duration of therapy depends on the site of infection:
Tinea corporis: 2-4 weeks
Tinea capitis: 4-6 weeks or longer (up to 8-12 weeks)
Tinea pedis: 4-8 weeks
Tinea unguium: 4-6 months

Administration Oral: Administer with a fatty meal (peanuts or ice cream) to increase absorption, or with food or milk to avoid GI upset

Gris-PEG® tablets: May be swallowed whole or crushed and sprinkled onto 1 tablespoonful of applesauce and swallowed immediately without chewing.

Monitoring Parameters Periodic renal, hepatic, and hematopoietic function tests

Test Interactions False-positive urinary VMA levels

Special Geriatric Considerations No specific changes in dosing are needed.

Dosage Forms Excipient information presented when available (limited, particularly for generics); consult specific product labeling.

Suspension, oral [microsize]: 125 mg/5 mL (118 mL, 120 mL)

Tablet, oral [microsize]:
Grifulvin V®: 500 mg [scored]

Tablet, oral [ultramicrosize]:
Gris-PEG®: 125 mg, 250 mg [scored]

♦ **Griseofulvin Microsize** *see* Griseofulvin *on page 903*
♦ **Griseofulvin Ultramicrosize** *see* Griseofulvin *on page 903*
♦ **Gris-PEG®** *see* Griseofulvin *on page 903*
♦ **GSK 1838262** *see* Gabapentin Enacarbil *on page 861*
♦ **Guaiatussin AC** *see* Guaifenesin and Codeine *on page 906*
♦ **Guaicon DMS [OTC]** *see* Guaifenesin and Dextromethorphan *on page 906*

GuaiFENesin (gwye FEN e sin)

Medication Safety Issues
Sound-alike/look-alike issues:
GuaiFENesin may be confused with guanFACINE
Mucinex® may be confused with Mucomyst®

Brand Names: U.S. Allfen [OTC]; Bidex®-400 [OTC]; Diabetic Siltussin DAS-Na [OTC]; Diabetic Tussin® EX [OTC]; Fenesin IR [OTC]; Geri-Tussin [OTC]; Humibid® Maximum Strength [OTC]; Iophen NR [OTC]; Liquituss GG [OTC]; Mucinex® Kid's Mini-Melts™ [OTC]; Mucinex® Kid's [OTC]; Mucinex® Maximum Strength [OTC]; Mucinex® [OTC]; Mucus Relief [OTC] [DSC]; Organ-I NR [OTC]; Q-Tussin [OTC]; Refenesen™ 400 [OTC]; Refenesen™ [OTC]; Robafen [OTC]; Scot-Tussin® Expectorant [OTC]; Siltussin SA [OTC]; Vicks® Casero™ Chest Congestion Relief [OTC]; Vicks® DayQuil® Mucus Control [OTC]; Xpect™ [OTC]

Brand Names: Canada Balminil Expectorant; Benylin® E Extra Strength; Koffex Expectorant; Robitussin®

Index Terms Cheratussin; GG; Glycerol Guaiacolate

Generic Availability (U.S.) Yes: Excludes extended release tablet and granules

Pharmacologic Category Expectorant

Use Help loosen phlegm and thin bronchial secretions to make coughs more productive

Contraindications Hypersensitivity to guaifenesin or any component of the formulation

Warnings/Precautions When used for self medication (OTC) notify healthcare provider if symptoms do not improve within 7 days, or are accompanied by fever, rash, or persistent headache. Do not use for persistent or chronic cough (as with smoking, asthma, chronic bronchitis, emphysema) or if cough is accompanied by excessive phlegm unless directed to do so by healthcare provider. Some products may contain phenylalanine.

Adverse Reactions (Reflective of adult population; not specific for elderly) Frequency not defined.
Central nervous system: Dizziness, drowsiness, headache
Dermatologic: Rash
Endocrine & metabolic: Uric acid levels decreased
Gastrointestinal: Nausea, stomach pain, vomiting

Drug Interactions
Metabolism/Transport Effects None known.
Avoid Concomitant Use There are no known interactions where it is recommended to avoid concomitant use.
Increased Effect/Toxicity There are no known significant interactions involving an increase in effect.
Decreased Effect There are no known significant interactions involving a decrease in effect.

Mechanism of Action Thought to act as an expectorant by irritating the gastric mucosa and stimulating respiratory tract secretions, thereby increasing respiratory fluid volumes and decreasing mucous viscosity

Pharmacodynamics/Kinetics
Absorption: Well absorbed
Half-life elimination: ~1 hour
Excretion: Urine (as unchanged drug and metabolites)

Dosage
Geriatric & Adult
Cough (expectorant): Oral: 200-400 mg every 4 hours to a maximum of 2.4 g/day
Extended release tablet: 600-1200 mg every 12 hours, not to exceed 2.4 g/day

Administration Do not crush, chew, or break extended release tablets. Administer with a full glass of water.

Monitoring Parameters Cough, sputum consistency and volume

Test Interactions Possible color interference with determination of 5-HIAA and VMA; discontinue for 48 hours prior to test

Pharmacotherapy Pearls Should not be used for persistent or chronic cough such as that occurring with smoking, asthma, chronic bronchitis, or emphysema or for cough associated with excessive phlegm; there is lack of convincing studies to document the efficacy of guaifenesin.

Special Geriatric Considerations No specific information for use in elderly.

Dosage Forms Excipient information presented when available (limited, particularly for generics); consult specific product labeling. [DSC] = Discontinued product
Caplet, oral:
Fenesin IR: 400 mg
Refenesen™ 400: 400 mg [dye free]
Granules, oral:
Mucinex® Kid's Mini-Melts™: 50 mg/packet (12s) [contains magnesium 6 mg/packet, phenylalanine 0.6 mg/packet, sodium 2 mg/packet; grape flavor]
Mucinex® Kid's Mini-Melts™: 100 mg/packet (12s) [contains magnesium 6 mg/packet, phenylalanine 1 mg/packet, sodium 3 mg/packet; bubblegum flavor]
Liquid, oral:
Diabetic Tussin® EX: 100 mg/5 mL (118 mL) [dye free, ethanol free, sugar free; contains phenylalanine 8.4 mg/5 mL]
Iophen NR: 100 mg/5 mL (480 mL) [contains propylene glycol, sodium 2 mg/5 mL, sodium benzoate; raspberry flavor]
Liquituss GG: 200 mg/5 mL (118 mL, 473 mL) [ethanol free, sugar free; contains potassium 30 mg/5 mL, propylene glycol, sodium 2 mg/5 mL; raspberry flavor]
Mucinex® Kid's: 100 mg/5 mL (118 mL) [contains propylene glycol, sodium 3 mg/5 mL; grape flavor]
Q-Tussin: 100 mg/5 mL (118 mL, 237 mL, 473 mL) [ethanol free; contains sodium 2 mg/5 mL, sodium benzoate; cherry flavor]
Scot-Tussin® Expectorant: 100 mg/5 mL (120 mL) [dye free, ethanol free, sugar free; contains benzoic acid; grape flavor]
Vicks® Casero™ Chest Congestion Relief: 100 mg/6.25 mL (120 mL, 240 mL) [contains phenylalanine 5.5 mg/12.5 mL, sodium 32 mg/12.5 mL, sodium benzoate; honey-menthol flavor]
Vicks® DayQuil® Mucus Control: 200 mg/15 mL (295 mL) [contains propylene glycol, sodium 25 mg/15 mL, sodium benzoate; citrus blend flavor]
Syrup, oral: 100 mg/5 mL (5 mL, 10 mL, 15 mL, 118 mL, 120 mL, 240 mL, 473 mL, 480 mL)
Diabetic Siltussin DAS-Na: 100 mg/5 mL (118 mL) [ethanol free, sugar free; contains benzoic acid, phenylalanine 3 mg/5 mL, propylene glycol; strawberry flavor]
Geri-Tussin: 100 mg/5 mL (480 mL) [ethanol free, sugar free; contains sodium benzoate]
Robafen: 100 mg/5 mL (120 mL, 240 mL, 480 mL) [ethanol free; contains sodium benzoate; cherry flavor]
Siltussin SA: 100 mg/5 mL (120 mL, 240 mL, 480 mL) [ethanol free, sugar free; strawberry flavor]
Tablet, oral: 200 mg, 400 mg
Allfen: 400 mg [scored]
Bidex®-400: 400 mg
Mucus Relief: 400 mg [DSC]
Organ-I NR: 200 mg
Refenesen™: 200 mg
Xpect™: 400 mg [sugar free]
Tablet, extended release, oral:
Humibid® Maximum Strength: 1200 mg
Mucinex®: 600 mg
Mucinex® Maximum Strength: 1200 mg

Guaifenesin and Codeine (gwye FEN e sin & KOE deen)

Related Information
Codeine *on page 433*
GuaiFENesin *on page 904*
Brand Names: U.S. Allfen CD; Allfen CDX; Codar® GF; Dex-Tuss; Guaiatussin AC; Iophen C-NR; M-Clear; M-Clear WC; Mar-Cof® CG; Robafen AC
Index Terms Codeine and Guaifenesin; Robitussin AC
Generic Availability (U.S.) Yes: Oral solution, syrup
Pharmacologic Category Antitussive; Cough Preparation; Expectorant
Use Temporary control of cough due to minor throat and bronchial irritation
Dosage
  Geriatric & Adult Cough (antitussive/expectorant): Oral:
    Capsule: Guaifenesin 200 mg and codeine 9 mg: Two capsules every 4 hours (maximum: 12 capsules/24 hours)
    Liquid:
      Guaifenesin 100 mg and codeine 6.33 mg per 5 mL: 15 mL every 4-6 hours (maximum: 45 mL/24 hours)
      Guaifenesin 100-200 mg and codeine 8-10 mg per 5 mL: 10 mL every 4 hours (maximum: 60 mL/24 hours)
      Guaifenesin 300 mg and codeine 10 mg per 5 mL: 5 mL every 4-6 hours (maximum: 40 mL/24 hours)
    Tablet: Guaifenesin 400 mg and codeine 10-20 mg: One tablet every 4-6 hours (maximum: 6 tablets/24 hours)
Special Geriatric Considerations Elderly may be more sensitive to the CNS depressant effects of codeine; monitor closely for excessive sedation.
Controlled Substance Capsule: C-V; Liquid products: C-V; Tablet: C-III
Dosage Forms Excipient information presented when available (limited, particularly for generics); consult specific product labeling.
  Capsule, oral:
    M-Clear: Guaifenesin 200 mg and codeine phosphate 9 mg [contains tartrazine]
  Liquid, oral:
    Codar® GF: Guaifenesin 200 mg and codeine phosphate 8 mg per 5 mL (473 mL) [contains propylene glycol; cotton candy flavor]
    Dex-Tuss: Guaifenesin 300 mg and codeine phosphate 10 mg per 5 mL (473 mL) [ethanol free, gluten free, sugar free; contains propylene glycol; grape flavor]
    Iophen C-NR: Guaifenesin 100 mg and codeine phosphate 10 mg per 5 mL (473 mL) [contains propylene glycol, sodium benzoate; raspberry flavor]
    M-Clear WC: Guaifenesin 100 mg and codeine phosphate 6.33 mg per 5 mL (473 mL) [contains propylene glycol; cotton candy flavor]
  Solution, oral: Guaifenesin 100 mg and codeine phosphate 10 mg per 5 mL (5 mL, 10 mL, 118 mL, 473 mL)
    Mar-Cof® CG: Guaifenesin 225 mg and codeine phosphate 7.5 mg per 5 mL (473 ml) [ethanol free, sugar free; contains propylene glycol, sodium benzoate, sodium 6 mg/5 mL]
  Syrup, oral: Guaifenesin 100 mg and codeine phosphate 10 mg per 5 mL (473 mL)
    Guaiatussin AC: Guaifenesin 100 mg and codeine phosphate 10 mg per 5 mL (118 mL, 473 mL) [contains ethanol 3.5%, sodium 1 mg/5 mL, sodium benzoate; cherry flavor]
    Robafen AC: Guaifenesin 100 mg and codeine phosphate 10 mg per 5 mL (120 mL, 480 mL) [contains ethanol 3.5%, sodium 4 mg/5 mL, sodium benzoate; cherry flavor]
  Tablet, oral:
    Allfen CD: Guaifenesin 400 mg and codeine phosphate 10 mg
    Allfen CDX: Guaifenesin 400 mg and codeine phosphate 20 mg

Guaifenesin and Dextromethorphan (gwye FEN e sin & deks troe meth OR fan)

Related Information
Dextromethorphan *on page 525*
GuaiFENesin *on page 904*
Medication Safety Issues
  Sound-alike/look-alike issues:
    Benylin® may be confused with Benadryl®, Ventolin®
Brand Names: U.S. Cheracol® D [OTC]; Cheracol® Plus [OTC]; Coricidin HBP® Chest Congestion and Cough [OTC]; Diabetic Siltussin-DM DAS-Na Maximum Strength [OTC]; Diabetic Siltussin-DM DAS-Na [OTC]; Diabetic Tussin® DM Maximum Strength [OTC];

Diabetic Tussin® DM [OTC]; Double Tussin DM [OTC]; Fenesin DM IR [OTC]; Guaicon DMS [OTC]; Iophen DM-NR [OTC]; Kolephrin® GG/DM [OTC]; Mucinex® DM Maximum Strength [OTC]; Mucinex® DM [OTC]; Mucinex® Kid's Cough Mini-Melts™ [OTC]; Mucinex® Kid's Cough [OTC]; Q-Tussin DM [OTC]; Refenesen™ DM [OTC]; Robafen DM Clear [OTC]; Robafen DM [OTC]; Robitussin® Peak Cold Cough + Chest Congestion DM [OTC]; Robitussin® Peak Cold Maximum Strength Cough + Chest Congestion DM [OTC]; Robitussin® Peak Cold Sugar-Free Cough + Chest Congestion DM [OTC]; Safe Tussin® DM [OTC]; Scot-Tussin® Senior [OTC]; Silexin [OTC]; Siltussin DM DAS [OTC]; Siltussin DM [OTC]; Tussi-Bid® [OTC] [DSC]; Vicks® 44E [OTC]; Vicks® DayQuil® Mucus Control DM [OTC]; Vicks® Nature Fusion™ Cough & Chest Congestion [OTC]; Vicks® Pediatric Formula 44E [OTC]

Brand Names: Canada Balminil DM E; Benylin® DM-E

Index Terms Dextromethorphan and Guaifenesin

Generic Availability (U.S.) Yes: Excludes extended release tablet, sustained release tablet

Pharmacologic Category Antitussive; Cough Preparation; Expectorant

Use Temporary control of cough due to minor throat and bronchial irritation

Dosage

Geriatric & Adult Cough (antitussive/expectorant): Oral:

General dosing guidelines: Guaifenesin 200-400 mg and dextromethorphan 10-20 mg every 4 hours (maximum dose: Guaifenesin 2400 mg and dextromethorphan 120 mg per day)

Product-specific labeling:

Mucinex® DM: 1-2 tablets every 12 hours (maximum: 4 tablets/24 hours)

Vicks® 44E: 15 mL every 4 hours (maximum: 6 doses/24 hours)

Vicks® Pediatric Formula 44E: 30 mL every 4 hours (maximum: 6 doses/24 hours)

Special Geriatric Considerations See individual agents.

Dosage Forms Excipient information presented when available (limited, particularly for generics); consult specific product labeling. [DSC] = Discontinued product

Caplet, oral:

Fenesin DM IR: Guaifenesin 400 mg and dextromethorphan hydrobromide 15 mg

Refenesen™ DM: Guaifenesin 400 mg and dextromethorphan hydrobromide 20 mg

Capsule, softgel, oral:

Coricidin HBP® Chest Congestion and Cough: Guaifenesin 200 mg and dextromethorphan hydrobromide 10 mg

Granules, oral:

Mucinex® Kid's Cough Mini-Melts™: Guaifenesin 100 mg and dextromethorphan hydrobromide 5 mg per packet (12s) [contains magnesium 6 mg/pack, phenylalanine 2 mg/packet, sodium 3 mg/packet; orange crème flavor]

Liquid, oral: Guaifenesin 100 mg and dextromethorphan hydrobromide 10 mg per 5 mL (480 mL)

Diabetic Tussin® DM: Guaifenesin 100 mg and dextromethorphan hydrobromide 10 mg per 5 mL (120 mL) [dye free, ethanol free, sugar free; contains phenylalanine 8.4 mg/5 mL]

Diabetic Tussin® DM Maximum Strength: Guaifenesin 200 mg and dextromethorphan hydrobromide 10 mg per 5 mL (120 mL) [dye free, ethanol free, sugar free; contains phenylalanine 8.4 mg/5 mL]

Double Tussin DM: Guaifenesin 300 mg and dextromethorphan hydrobromide 20 mg per 5 mL (120 mL, 480 mL) [dye free, ethanol free, sugar free]

Iophen DM-NR: Guaifenesin 100 mg and dextromethorphan hydrobromide 10 mg per 5 mL (480 mL) [contains propylene glycol, sodium benzoate; raspberry flavor]

Kolephrin® GG/DM: Guaifenesin 150 mg and dextromethorphan hydrobromide 10 mg per 5 mL (120 mL) [ethanol free; cherry flavor]

Mucinex® Kid's Cough: Guaifenesin 100 mg and dextromethorphan hydrobromide 5 mg per 5 mL (120 mL) [contains propylene glycol, sodium 3 mg/5 mL; cherry flavor]

Safe Tussin® DM: Guaifenesin 100 mg and dextromethorphan hydrobromide 15 mg per 5 mL (120 mL) [contains benzoic acid, phenylalanine 4.2 mg/5 mL, and propylene glycol; orange and mint flavors]

Scot-Tussin® Senior: Guaifenesin 200 mg and dextromethorphan hydrobromide 15 mg per 5 mL (120 mL) [ethanol free, sodium free, sugar free]

Vicks® 44E: Guaifenesin 200 mg and dextromethorphan hydrobromide 20 mg per 15 mL (120 mL, 235 mL) [contains ethanol, sodium 31 mg/15 mL, sodium benzoate]

Vicks® DayQuil® Mucus Control DM: Guaifenesin 200 mg and dextromethorphan hydrobromide 10 mg per 15 mL (295 mL) [contains propylene glycol, sodium 25 mg/15 mL, sodium benzoate; citrus blend flavor]

Vicks® Nature Fusion™ Cough & Chest Congestion: Guaifenesin 200 mg and dextromethorphan hydrobromide 20 mg per 30 mL (236 mL) [dye free, ethanol free, gluten free; contains propylene glycol, sodium 36 mg/30 mL; honey flavor]

Vicks® Pediatric Formula 44E: Guaifenesin 100 mg and dextromethorphan hydrobromide 10 mg per 15 mL (120 mL) [ethanol free; contains sodium 30 mg/15 mL, sodium benzoate; cherry flavor]
Syrup, oral: Guaifenesin 100 mg and dextromethorphan hydrobromide 10 mg per 5 mL (5 mL, 10 mL, 120 mL, 480 mL)
Cheracol® D: Guaifenesin 100 mg and dextromethorphan hydrobromide 10 mg per 5 mL (120 mL, 180 mL) [contains benzoic acid, ethanol 4.75%]
Cheracol® Plus: Guaifenesin 100 mg and dextromethorphan hydrobromide 10 mg per 5 mL (120 mL) [contains benzoic acid, ethanol 4.75%]
Diabetic Siltussin-DM DAS-Na: Guaifenesin 100 mg and dextromethorphan hydrobromide 10 mg per 5 mL (118 mL) [ethanol free, sugar free; contains benzoic acid, phenylalanine 3 mg/5 mL, propylene glycol; strawberry flavor]
Diabetic Siltussin-DM DAS-Na Maximum Strength: Guaifenesin 200 mg and dextromethorphan hydrobromide 10 mg per 5 mL (118 mL) [ethanol free, sugar free; contains benzoic acid, phenylalanine 3 mg/5 mL, propylene glycol; strawberry flavor]
Guaicon DMS: Guaifenesin 100 mg and dextromethorphan hydrobromide 10 mg per 5 mL (10 mL) [ethanol free, sugar free]
Q-Tussin DM: Guaifenesin 100 mg and dextromethorphan hydrobromide 10 mg per 5 mL (118 mL, 237 mL, 473 mL) [ethanol free, contains sodium benzoate; cherry flavor]
Robafen DM: Guaifenesin 100 mg and dextromethorphan hydrobromide 10 mg per 5 mL (120 mL, 240 mL, 480 mL) [cherry flavor]
Robafen DM Clear: Guaifenesin 100 mg and dextromethorphan hydrobromide 10 mg per 5 mL (120 mL)
Robitussin® Peak Cold Cough + Chest Congestion DM: Guaifenesin 100 mg and dextromethorphan hydrobromide 10 mg per 5 mL (120 mL, 240 mL) [contains menthol, propylene glycol, sodium 7 mg/5 mL, sodium benzoate]
Robitussin® Peak Cold Sugar-Free Cough + Chest Congestion DM: Guaifenesin 100 mg and dextromethorphan hydrobromide 10 mg per 5 mL (120 mL) [sugar free; contains propylene glycol, sodium 3 mg/5 mL, sodium benzoate]
Robitussin® Peak Cold Maximum Strength Cough + Chest Congestion DM: Guaifenesin 200 mg and dextromethorphan hydrobromide 10 mg per 5 mL (120 mL, 240 mL) [contains menthol, propylene glycol, sodium 5 mg/5 mL, sodium benzoate]
Silexin: Guaifenesin 100 mg and dextromethorphan hydrobromide 10 mg per 5 mL (45 mL) [ethanol free, sugar free)]
Siltussin DM: Guaifenesin 100 mg and dextromethorphan hydrobromide 10 mg per 5 mL (120 mL, 240 mL, 480 mL) [strawberry flavor]
Siltussin DM DAS: Guaifenesin 100 mg and dextromethorphan hydrobromide 10 mg per 5 mL (120 mL) [dye free, ethanol free, sugar free; strawberry flavor]
Tablet, oral: Guaifenesin 1000 mg and dextromethorphan hydrobromide 60 mg; guaifenesin 1200 mg and dextromethorphan hydrobromide 60 mg
Silexin: Guaifenesin 100 mg and dextromethorphan hydrobromide 10 mg
Tablet, extended release, oral:
Mucinex® DM: Guaifenesin 600 mg and dextromethorphan hydrobromide 30 mg
Mucinex® DM Maximum Strength: Guaifenesin 1200 mg and dextromethorphan hydrobromide 60 mg
Tablet, sustained release, oral
Tussi-Bid®: Guaifenesin 1200 mg and dextromethorphan hydrobromide 60 mg [DSC]
Tablet, timed release, oral [scored]: Guaifenesin 1200 mg and dextromethorphan hydrobromide 60 mg

GuanFACINE (GWAHN fa seen)

Related Information
Beers Criteria – Potentially Inappropriate Medications for Geriatrics on page 2183
Medication Safety Issues
Sound-alike/look-alike issues:
GuanFACINE may be confused with guaiFENesin, guanabenz, guanidine
Tenex® may be confused with Entex®, Xanax®
BEERS Criteria medication:
This drug may be potentially inappropriate for use in geriatric patients (Quality of evidence - low; Strength of recommendation - strong).
International issues:
Tenex [U.S., Canada] may be confused with Kinex brand name for biperiden [Mexico]
Brand Names: U.S. Intuniv®; Tenex®
Index Terms Guanfacine Hydrochloride
Generic Availability (U.S.) Yes: Excludes extended release tablet
Pharmacologic Category Alpha$_2$-Adrenergic Agonist

Use
Tablet, immediate release: Management of hypertension
Tablet, extended release: Treatment of attention-deficit/hyperactivity disorder (ADHD) as monotherapy or adjunctive therapy to stimulants
Unlabeled Use Tic disorder; Tourette's syndrome
Dosage
Geriatric
Refer to adult dosing. In the management of hypertension, consider lower initial doses and titrate to response (Aronow, 2011).
Adult Hypertension: Oral: Immediate release: 1 mg usually at bedtime, may increase if needed at 3- to 4-week intervals; usual dose range (JNC 7): 0.5-2 mg once daily
Renal Impairment
No specific dosage adjustments are recommended by the manufacturer; consider using the lower end of the dosing range in patients with renal impairment.
Hemodialysis: Dialysis clearance is ~15% of total clearance; usual doses are recommended.
Hepatic Impairment
No specific dosage adjustments are recommended by the manufacturer; however, dosage adjustments may be required.
Special Geriatric Considerations Because of adverse effects such as CNS depression, dry mouth, and constipation, guanfacine is not considered a drug of choice in the elderly.

This medication is considered to be potentially inappropriate in this patient population (Beers Criteria: Quality of evidence - low; Strength of recommendation - strong).
Dosage Forms Excipient information presented when available (limited, particularly for generics); consult specific product labeling.
Tablet, oral: 1 mg, 2 mg
  Tenex®: 1 mg, 2 mg
Tablet, extended release, oral:
  Intuniv®: 1 mg, 2 mg, 3 mg, 4 mg

◆ **Guanfacine Hydrochloride** see GuanFACINE on page 908
◆ **Gyne-Lotrimin® 3 [OTC]** see Clotrimazole (Topical) on page 426
◆ **Gyne-Lotrimin® 7 [OTC]** see Clotrimazole (Topical) on page 426
◆ **H1N1 Influenza Vaccine** see Influenza Virus Vaccine (Inactivated) on page 997
◆ **H1N1 Influenza Vaccine** see Influenza Virus Vaccine (Live/Attenuated) on page 1001
◆ **H5N1 Influenza Vaccine** see Influenza Virus Vaccine (H5N1) on page 996
◆ **HA** see Typhoid and Hepatitis A Vaccine on page 1983
◆ **Habitrol** see Nicotine on page 1372

Halcinonide (hal SIN oh nide)

Related Information
Topical Corticosteroids on page 2113
Medication Safety Issues
Sound-alike/look-alike issues:
Halcinonide may be confused with Halcion®
Halog® may be confused with Haldol®
Brand Names: U.S. Halog®
Brand Names: Canada Halog®
Generic Availability (U.S.) No
Pharmacologic Category Corticosteroid, Topical
Use Inflammation of corticosteroid-responsive dermatoses [high potency topical corticosteroid]
Dosage
Geriatric & Adult Steroid-responsive dermatoses: Topical: Apply sparingly 1-3 times/day, occlusive dressing may be used for severe or resistant dermatoses; a thin film is effective; do not overuse. Therapy should be discontinued when control is achieved; if no improvement is seen, reassessment of diagnosis may be necessary.
Special Geriatric Considerations Due to age-related changes in skin, limit use of topical corticosteroids.
Dosage Forms Excipient information presented when available (limited, particularly for generics); consult specific product labeling.
Cream, topical:
  Halog®: 0.1% (30 g, 60 g, 216 g)
Ointment, topical:
  Halog®: 0.1% (30 g, 60 g)

◆ **Halcion®** see Triazolam on page 1963
◆ **Haldol®** see Haloperidol on page 910

- ◆ **Haldol® Decanoate** see Haloperidol on page 910
- ◆ **Haley's M-O** see Magnesium Hydroxide and Mineral Oil on page 1179
- ◆ **HalfLytely® and Bisacodyl** see Polyethylene Glycol-Electrolyte Solution and Bisacodyl on page 1565
- ◆ **Halfprin® [OTC]** see Aspirin on page 154

Halobetasol (hal oh BAY ta sol)

Related Information
Topical Corticosteroids on page 2113
Medication Safety Issues
Sound-alike/look-alike issues:
Ultravate® may be confused with Cutivate®
Brand Names: U.S. Halonate™; Ultravate®
Brand Names: Canada Ultravate®
Index Terms Halobetasol Propionate
Generic Availability (U.S.) Yes
Pharmacologic Category Corticosteroid, Topical
Use Relief of inflammatory and pruritic manifestations of corticosteroid-response dermatoses [super high potency topical corticosteroid]
Dosage
Geriatric & Adult Steroid-responsive dermatoses: Topical: Apply sparingly to skin once or twice daily, rub in gently and completely; treatment should not exceed 2 consecutive weeks and total dosage should not exceed 50 g/week. Therapy should be discontinued when control is achieved; if no improvement is seen, reassessment of diagnosis may be necessary.
Special Geriatric Considerations Due to age-related changes in skin, limit use of topical corticosteroids.
Dosage Forms Excipient information presented when available (limited, particularly for generics); consult specific product labeling. [DSC] = Discontinued product
Cream, topical, as propionate: 0.05% (15 g, 50 g)
Ultravate®: 0.05% (15 g [DSC], 50 g)
Ointment, topical, as propionate: 0.05% (15 g, 50 g)
Halonate™: 0.05% (50 g)
Ultravate®: 0.05% (15 g [DSC], 50 g)

- ◆ **Halobetasol Propionate** see Halobetasol on page 910
- ◆ **Halog®** see Halcinonide on page 909
- ◆ **Halonate™** see Halobetasol on page 910

Haloperidol (ha loe PER i dole)

Related Information
Antipsychotic Agents on page 2103
Beers Criteria – Potentially Inappropriate Medications for Geriatrics on page 2183
Medication Safety Issues
Sound-alike/look-alike issues:
Haldol® may be confused with Halcion®, Halog®, Stadol
BEERS Criteria medication:
This drug may be potentially inappropriate for use in geriatric patients (Quality of evidence - moderate; Strength of recommendation - strong).
International issues:
Haldol [U.S. and multiple international markets] may be confused with Halotestin brand name for fluoxymesterone [Great Britain]
Brand Names: U.S. Haldol®; Haldol® Decanoate
Brand Names: Canada Apo-Haloperidol LA®; Apo-Haloperidol®; Haloperidol Injection, USP; Haloperidol Long Acting; Haloperidol-LA; Haloperidol-LA Omega; Novo-Peridol; PMS-Haloperidol; PMS-Haloperidol LA
Index Terms Haloperidol Decanoate; Haloperidol Lactate
Generic Availability (U.S.) Yes
Pharmacologic Category Antipsychotic Agent, Typical
Use Management of schizophrenia; control of tics and vocal utterances of Tourette's disorder in adults

Unlabeled Use Treatment of nonschizophrenia psychosis; may be used for the emergency sedation of severely-agitated or delirious patients; adjunctive treatment of ethanol dependence; postoperative nausea and vomiting (alternative therapy); psychosis/agitation related to Alzheimer's dementia

Contraindications Hypersensitivity to haloperidol or any component of the formulation; Parkinson's disease; severe CNS depression; coma

Warnings/Precautions [U.S. Boxed Warning]: Elderly patients with dementia-related psychosis treated with antipsychotics are at an increased risk of death compared to placebo. Most deaths appeared to be either cardiovascular (eg, heart failure, sudden death) or infectious (eg, pneumonia) in nature. Haloperidol is not approved for the treatment of dementia-related psychosis. Hypotension may occur, particularly with parenteral administration. Although the short-acting form (lactate) is used clinically, the I.V. use of the injection is not an FDA-approved route of administration; the decanoate form should never be administered intravenously.

May alter cardiac conduction and prolong QT interval; life-threatening arrhythmias have occurred with therapeutic doses of antipsychotics but risk may be increased with doses exceeding recommendations and/or intravenous administration (unlabeled route). Use caution or avoid use in patients with electrolyte abnormalities (eg, hypokalemia, hypomagnesemia), hypothyroidism, familial long QT syndrome, concomitant medications which may augment QT prolongation, or any underlying cardiac abnormality which may also potentiate risk. Monitor ECG closely for dose-related QT effects. Adverse effects of decanoate may be prolonged. Avoid in thyrotoxicosis.

Leukopenia, neutropenia, and agranulocytosis (sometimes fatal) have been reported in clinical trials and postmarketing reports with antipsychotic use; presence of risk factors (eg, pre-existing low WBC or history of drug-induced leuko-/neutropenia) should prompt periodic blood count assessment. Discontinue therapy at first signs of blood dyscrasias or if absolute neutrophil count <1000/mm^3.

May be sedating, use with caution in disorders where CNS depression is a feature. Effects may be potentiated when used with other sedative drugs or ethanol. Caution in patients with severe cardiovascular disease, predisposition to seizures, subcortical brain damage, or renal disease. Esophageal dysmotility and aspiration have been associated with antipsychotic use - use with caution in patients at risk of pneumonia (eg, Alzheimer's disease). Use associated with increased prolactin levels; clinical significance of hyperprolactinemia in patients with breast cancer or other prolactin-dependent tumors is unknown. May alter temperature regulation or mask toxicity of other drugs due to antiemetic effects. May cause orthostatic hypotension; use with caution in patients at risk of this effect or those who would tolerate transient hypotensive episodes (cerebrovascular disease, cardiovascular disease, or other medications which may predispose). Some tablets contain tartrazine. Antipsychotics have been associated with pigmentary retinopathy.

May cause anticholinergic effects (confusion, agitation, constipation, xerostomia, blurred vision, urinary retention). Therefore, they should be used with caution in patients with decreased gastrointestinal motility, urinary retention, BPH, xerostomia, or visual problems. Conditions which also may be exacerbated by cholinergic blockade include narrow-angle glaucoma and worsening of myasthenia gravis. Relative to other neuroleptics, haloperidol has a low potency of cholinergic blockade.

May cause extrapyramidal symptoms (EPS), including pseudoparkinsonism, acute dystonic reactions, akathisia, and tardive dyskinesia. Risk of dystonia (and possibly other EPS) may be greater with increased doses, use of conventional antipsychotics, males, and younger patients. May be associated with neuroleptic malignant syndrome (NMS). Use in elderly patients with dementia is associated with an increased risk of mortality and cerebrovascular accidents; avoid antipsychotic use for behavioral problems associated with dementia unless alternative nonpharmacologic therapies have failed and patient may harm self or others. In addition, use may cause or exacerbate syndrome of inappropriate antidiuretic hormone secretion or hyponatremia; monitor sodium closely with initiation or dosage adjustments in older adults (Beers Criteria). Increased risk for developing tardive dyskinesia, particularly elderly women.

Adverse Reactions (Reflective of adult population; not specific for elderly) Frequency not defined.
   Cardiovascular: Abnormal T waves with prolonged ventricular repolarization, arrhythmia, hyper-/hypotension, QT prolongation, sudden death, tachycardia, torsade de pointes
   Central nervous system: Agitation, akathisia, altered central temperature regulation, anxiety, confusion, depression, drowsiness, dystonic reactions, euphoria, extrapyramidal reactions, headache, insomnia, lethargy, neuroleptic malignant syndrome (NMS), pseudoparkinsonian signs and symptoms, restlessness, seizure, tardive dyskinesia, tardive dystonia, vertigo

◀

Dermatologic: Alopecia, contact dermatitis, hyperpigmentation, photosensitivity (rare), pruritus, rash

Endocrine & metabolic: Amenorrhea, breast engorgement, galactorrhea, gynecomastia, hyper-/hypoglycemia, hyponatremia, lactation, mastalgia, menstrual irregularities, sexual dysfunction

Gastrointestinal: Anorexia, constipation, diarrhea, dyspepsia, hypersalivation, nausea, vomiting, xerostomia

Genitourinary: Priapism, urinary retention

Hematologic: Agranulocytosis (rare), leukopenia, leukocytosis, neutropenia, anemia, lymphomonocytosis

Hepatic: Cholestatic jaundice, obstructive jaundice

Ocular: Blurred vision

Respiratory: Bronchospasm, laryngospasm

Miscellaneous: Diaphoresis, heat stroke

Drug Interactions

Metabolism/Transport Effects Substrate of CYP1A2 (minor), CYP2D6 (major), CYP3A4 (major); **Note:** Assignment of Major/Minor substrate status based on clinically relevant drug interaction potential; **Inhibits** CYP2D6 (moderate), CYP3A4 (moderate)

Avoid Concomitant Use

Avoid concomitant use of Haloperidol with any of the following: Azelastine; Azelastine (Nasal); Conivaptan; Highest Risk QTc-Prolonging Agents; Metoclopramide; Mifepristone; Paraldehyde; Tolvaptan

Increased Effect/Toxicity

Haloperidol may increase the levels/effects of: Alcohol (Ethyl); Anticholinergics; ARIPiprazole; Avanafil; Azelastine; Azelastine (Nasal); Budesonide (Systemic, Oral Inhalation); Buprenorphine; ChlorproMAZINE; CNS Depressants; Colchicine; CYP2D6 Substrates; CYP3A4 Substrates; Eplerenone; Everolimus; FentaNYL; Fesoterodine; Highest Risk QTc-Prolonging Agents; Ivacaftor; Lurasidone; Methylphenidate; Moderate Risk QTc-Prolonging Agents; Nebivolol; Paraldehyde; Pimecrolimus; QuiNIDine; Salmeterol; Saxagliptin; Serotonin Modulators; Tolvaptan; Zolpidem

The levels/effects of Haloperidol may be increased by: Abiraterone Acetate; Acetylcholinesterase Inhibitors (Central); ChlorproMAZINE; Conivaptan; CYP2D6 Inhibitors (Moderate); CYP2D6 Inhibitors (Strong); CYP3A4 Inhibitors (Moderate); CYP3A4 Inhibitors (Strong); Darunavir; FLUoxetine; FluvoxaMINE; HydrOXYzine; Ivacaftor; Lithium formulations; Methylphenidate; Metoclopramide; Metyrosine; Mifepristone; Nonsteroidal Anti-Inflammatory Agents; Pramlintide; QTc-Prolonging Agents (Indeterminate Risk and Risk Modifying); QuiNIDine; Tetrabenazine

Decreased Effect

Haloperidol may decrease the levels/effects of: Amphetamines; Anti-Parkinson's Agents (Dopamine Agonist); Codeine; Ifosfamide; Quinagolide

The levels/effects of Haloperidol may be decreased by: Anti-Parkinson's Agents (Dopamine Agonist); CarBAMazepine; CYP3A4 Inducers (Strong); Deferasirox; Glycopyrrolate; Lithium formulations; Peginterferon Alfa-2b; Tocilizumab

Ethanol/Nutrition/Herb Interactions

Ethanol: May increase CNS depression; monitor for increased effects with coadministration. Caution patients about effects.

Herb/Nutraceutical: Avoid valerian, St John's wort, kava kava, gotu kola (may increase CNS depression).

Stability

Protect oral dosage forms from light.

Haloperidol lactate injection should be stored at controlled room temperature; do not freeze or expose to temperatures >40°C. Protect from light; exposure to light may cause discoloration and the development of a grayish-red precipitate over several weeks.

Haloperidol lactate may be administered IVPB or I.V. infusion in D_5W solutions. NS solutions should not be used due to reports of decreased stability and incompatibility.

Standardized dose: 0.5-100 mg/50-100 mL D_5W.

Stability of standardized solutions is 38 days at room temperature (24°C).

Mechanism of Action Haloperidol is a butyrophenone antipsychotic which blocks postsynaptic mesolimbic dopaminergic D_1 and D_2 receptors in the brain; depresses the release of hypothalamic and hypophyseal hormones; believed to depress the reticular activating system thus affecting basal metabolism, body temperature, wakefulness, vasomotor tone, and emesis

Pharmacodynamics/Kinetics

Onset of action: Sedation: I.M., I.V.: 30-60 minutes

Duration: Decanoate: 2-4 weeks

Distribution: V_d: 8-18 L/kg

Protein binding: 90%

Metabolism: Hepatic: 50% to 60% glucuronidation (inactive); 23% CYP3A4-mediated reduction to inactive metabolites (some back-oxidation to haloperidol); and 20% to 30% CYP3A4-mediated N-dealkylation, including minor oxidation pathway to toxic pyridinium derivative (Kudo, 1999)

Bioavailability: Oral: 60% to 70%

Half-life elimination: 18 hours; Decanoate: 21 days

Time to peak, serum: Oral: 2-6 hours; I.M.: 20 minutes; Decanoate: 7 days

Excretion: Urine (30%, 1% as unchanged drug); feces (15%)

Dosage

Geriatric Nonpsychotic patient, dementia behavior (unlabeled use): Initial: Oral: 0.25-0.5 mg 1-2 times/day; increase dose at 4- to 7-day intervals by 0.25-0.5 mg/day. Increase dosing intervals (twice daily, 3 times/day, etc) as necessary to control response or side effects.

Adult

Psychosis:
Oral: 0.5-5 mg 2-3 times/day; usual maximum: 30 mg/day

I.M. (as lactate): 2-5 mg every 4-8 hours as needed

I.M. (as decanoate): Initial: 10-20 times the daily oral dose administered at 4-week intervals. Maintenance dose: 10-15 times initial oral dose; used to stabilize psychiatric symptoms

Delirium in the intensive care unit (unlabeled use, unlabeled route; Jacobi, 2002): I.V.: Initial: 2-10 mg depending on degree of agitation; if inadequate response, may repeat bolus dose (with sequential doubling of initial bolus dose) every 15-30 minutes until calm achieved, then administer 25% of the last bolus dose every 6 hours; monitor ECG and QT_c interval. After the patient is controlled, haloperidol therapy should be tapered over several days. **Note:** QT_c prolongation may occur with cumulative doses ≥35 mg and torsade de pointes has been reported with single doses of ≥20 mg. The optimal dose and regimen of haloperidol for the treatment of severe agitation and/or delirium has not been established.

Rapid tranquilization of severely-agitated patient (unlabeled use; administer every 30-60 minutes):
Oral: 5-10 mg

I.M. (as lactate): 5 mg

Average total dose (oral or I.M.) for tranquilization: 10-20 mg

Postoperative nausea and vomiting (PONV) (unlabeled use): I.M., I.V.: 0.5-2 mg (Gan, 2007)

Renal Impairment Hemodialysis/peritoneal dialysis: Supplemental dose is not necessary.

Administration

Injection oil (decanoate): The decanoate injectable formulation should be administered I.M. only, **do not administer decanoate I.V.**

Injection solution (lactate): The lactate injectable formulation may be administered I.V. (unlabeled route) or I.M.

Oral solution (lactate): Dilute the oral concentrate with water or juice before administration. Avoid skin contact with oral solution; may cause contact dermatitis.

Monitoring Parameters Vital signs; lipid profile, fasting blood glucose/Hgb A_{1c}; BMI; mental status, abnormal involuntary movement scale (AIMS), extrapyramidal symptoms (EPS); ECG (with off-label intravenous administration)

Reference Range

Therapeutic: 5-20 ng/mL (SI: 10-40 nmol/L) (psychotic disorders - less for Tourette's and mania)

Toxic: >42 ng/mL (SI: >84 nmol/L)

Special Geriatric Considerations Many elderly patients receive antipsychotic medications for inappropriate nonpsychotic behavior. Before initiating antipsychotic medication, the clinician should investigate any possible reversible cause; any stress or stress from any disease can cause acute "confusion" or worsening of baseline nonpsychotic behavior. Most commonly acute changes in behavior are due to increases in drug dose or addition of new drug to regimen; fluid electrolyte loss; infections; and changes in environment.

Any changes in disease status in any organ system can result in behavior changes.

In the treatment of agitated, demented, elderly patients, authors of meta-analysis of controlled trials of the response to the traditional antipsychotics (phenothiazines, butyrophenones) in controlling agitation have concluded that the use of neuroleptics results in a response rate of 18%. Clearly neuroleptic therapy for behavior control should be limited with frequent attempts to withdraw the agent given for behavior control.

Clinical studies of haloperidol did not include sufficient numbers of subjects ≥65 years of age to determine whether they respond differently from younger subjects. Other reported clinical experience has not consistently identified differences between the elderly and younger patients. However, the prevalence of tardive dyskinesia appears to be highest among the elderly, especially elderly women. Also, the pharmacokinetics of haloperidol in geriatric patients generally warrants the use of lower doses.

This medication is considered to be potentially inappropriate in this patient population (Beers Criteria: Quality of evidence - moderate; Strength of recommendation - strong).

Dosage Forms Excipient information presented when available (limited, particularly for generics); consult specific product labeling.

Injection, oil, as decanoate [strength expressed as base]: 50 mg/mL (1 mL, 5 mL); 100 mg/mL (1 mL, 5 mL)

Haldol® Decanoate: 50 mg/mL (1 mL); 100 mg/mL (1 mL) [contains benzyl alcohol, sesame oil]

Injection, solution, as lactate [strength expressed as base]: 5 mg/mL (1 mL, 10 mL)

Haldol®: 5 mg/mL (1 mL)

Solution, oral, as lactate [strength expressed as base, concentrate]: 2 mg/mL (5 mL, 15 mL, 120 mL)

Tablet, oral: 0.5 mg, 1 mg, 2 mg, 5 mg, 10 mg, 20 mg

Heparin (HEP a rin)

Related Information

Injectable Heparins/Heparinoids Comparison Table on page 2119

Medication Safety Issues

Sound-alike/look-alike issues:

Heparin may be confused with Hespan®

High alert medication:

The Institute for Safe Medication Practices (ISMP) includes this medication among its list of drugs which have a heightened risk of causing significant patient harm when used in error.

National Patient Safety Goals:

The Joint Commission (TJC) requires healthcare organizations that provide anticoagulant therapy to have a process in place to reduce the risk of anticoagulant-associated patient harm. Patients receiving anticoagulants should receive individualized care through a defined process that includes standardized ordering, dispensing, administration, monitoring and education. This does not apply to routine short-term use of anticoagulants for prevention of venous thromboembolism when the expectation is that the patient's laboratory values will remain within or close to normal values (NPSG.03.05.01).

Other safety concerns:

Heparin sodium injection 10,000 units/mL and Hep-Lock U/P 10 units/mL have been confused with each other. Fatal medication errors have occurred between the two whose labels are both blue. **Never rely on color as a sole indicator to differentiate product identity.**

Heparin lock flush solution is intended only to maintain patency of I.V. devices and is **not** to be used for anticoagulant therapy.

Brand Names: U.S. Hep-Lock; HepFlush®-10

Brand Names: Canada Hepalean®; Hepalean® Leo; Hepalean®-LOK

Index Terms Heparin Calcium; Heparin Lock Flush; Heparin Sodium

Generic Availability (U.S.) Yes

Pharmacologic Category Anticoagulant

Use Prophylaxis and treatment of thromboembolic disorders; as an anticoagulant for extracorporeal and dialysis procedures

Note: Heparin lock flush solution is intended only to maintain patency of I.V. devices and is **not** to be used for systemic anticoagulant therapy.

Unlabeled Use ST-elevation myocardial infarction (STEMI) as an adjunct to thrombolysis; unstable angina/non-STEMI (UA/NSTEMI); anticoagulant used during percutaneous coronary intervention (PCI)

Contraindications Hypersensitivity to heparin or any component of the formulation (unless a life-threatening situation necessitates use and use of an alternative anticoagulant is not possible); severe thrombocytopenia; uncontrolled active bleeding except when due to disseminated intravascular coagulation (DIC); not for use when appropriate blood coagulation tests cannot be obtained at appropriate intervals (applies to full-dose heparin only)

Warnings/Precautions Hypersensitivity reactions can occur. Only in life-threatening situations when use of an alternative anticoagulant is not possible should heparin be cautiously used in patients with a documented hypersensitivity reaction. Hemorrhage is the most common complication. Monitor for signs and symptoms of bleeding. Certain patients are at increased risk of bleeding. Risk factors for bleeding include bacterial endocarditis; congenital or acquired bleeding disorders; active ulcerative or angiodysplastic GI diseases; continuous GI tube drainage; severe uncontrolled hypertension; history of hemorrhagic stroke; or use shortly after brain, spinal, or ophthalmology surgery; patient treated concomitantly with platelet inhibitors; conditions associated with increased bleeding tendencies (hemophilia, vascular purpura); recent GI bleeding; thrombocytopenia or platelet defects; severe liver disease; hypertensive or diabetic retinopathy; renal failure; or in patients undergoing invasive procedures including spinal tap or spinal anesthesia. Many concentrations of heparin are available ranging from 1 unit/mL to 20,000 units/mL. Clinicians **must** carefully examine each prefilled syringe or vial prior to use ensuring that the correct concentration is chosen; fatal hemorrhages have occurred related to heparin overdose. A higher incidence of bleeding has been reported in patients >60 years of age, particularly women. They are also more sensitive to the dose. Discontinue heparin if hemorrhage occurs; severe hemorrhage or overdosage may require protamine.

May cause thrombocytopenia; monitor platelet count closely. Patients who develop HIT may be at risk of developing a new thrombus (heparin-induced thrombocytopenia and thrombosis [HITT]). Discontinue therapy and consider alternatives if platelets are <100,000/mm^3 and/or thrombosis develops. HIT or HITT may be delayed and can occur up to several weeks after discontinuation of heparin. Osteoporosis may occur with prolonged use (>6 months) due to a reduction in bone mineral density. Monitor for hyperkalemia; can cause hyperkalemia by suppressing aldosterone production. Patients >60 years of age may require lower doses of heparin.

Some preparations contain sulfite which may cause allergic reactions.

Heparin resistance may occur in patients with antithrombin deficiency, increased heparin clearance, elevations in heparin-binding proteins, elevations in factor VIII and/or fibrinogen; frequently encountered in patients with fever, thrombosis, thrombophlebitis, infections with thrombosing tendencies, MI, cancer, and in postsurgical patients; measurement of anticoagulant effects using antifactor Xa levels may be of benefit.

Adverse Reactions (Reflective of adult population; not specific for elderly) Note: Thrombocytopenia has been reported to occur at an incidence between 0% and 30%. It is often of no clinical significance. However, immunologically mediated heparin-induced thrombocytopenia (HIT) has been estimated to occur in 1% to 2% of patients, and is marked by a progressive fall in platelet counts and, in some cases, thromboembolic complications (skin necrosis, pulmonary embolism, gangrene of the extremities, stroke, or MI).

Frequency not defined.

Cardiovascular: Allergic vasospastic reaction (possibly related to thrombosis), chest pain, hemorrhagic shock, shock, thrombosis

Central nervous system: Chills, fever, headache

Dermatologic: Alopecia (delayed, transient), bruising (unexplained), cutaneous necrosis, dysesthesia pedis, erythematous plaques (case reports), eczema, urticaria, purpura

Endocrine & metabolic: Adrenal hemorrhage, hyperkalemia (suppression of aldosterone synthesis), ovarian hemorrhage, rebound hyperlipidemia on discontinuation

Gastrointestinal: Constipation, hematemesis, nausea, tarry stools, vomiting

Genitourinary: Frequent or persistent erection

Hematologic: Bleeding from gums, epistaxis, hemorrhage, ovarian hemorrhage, retroperitoneal hemorrhage, thrombocytopenia (see note)

Hepatic: Liver enzymes increased

Local: Irritation, erythema, pain, hematoma, and ulceration have been rarely reported with deep SubQ injections; I.M. injection (not recommended) is associated with a high incidence of these effects

Neuromuscular & skeletal: Peripheral neuropathy, osteoporosis (chronic therapy effect)

Ocular: Conjunctivitis (allergic reaction), lacrimation

Renal: Hematuria

Respiratory: Asthma, bronchospasm (case reports), hemoptysis, pulmonary hemorrhage, rhinitis

Miscellaneous: Allergic reactions, anaphylactoid reactions, heparin resistance, hypersensitivity (including chills, fever, and urticaria)

Drug Interactions

Metabolism/Transport Effects None known.

Avoid Concomitant Use

Avoid concomitant use of Heparin with any of the following: Corticorelin; Palifermin; Rivaroxaban

Increased Effect/Toxicity

Heparin may increase the levels/effects of: Anticoagulants; Collagenase (Systemic); Corticorelin; Dabigatran Etexilate; Deferasirox; Drotrecogin Alfa (Activated); Ibritumomab; Palifermin; Rivaroxaban; Tositumomab and Iodine I 131 Tositumomab

The levels/effects of Heparin may be increased by: 5-ASA Derivatives; Antiplatelet Agents; Aspirin; Dasatinib; Herbs (Anticoagulant/Antiplatelet Properties); Nonsteroidal Anti-Inflammatory Agents; Pentosan Polysulfate Sodium; Pentoxifylline; Prostacyclin Analogues; Salicylates; Thrombolytic Agents; Tipranavir

Decreased Effect

The levels/effects of Heparin may be decreased by: Nitroglycerin

Ethanol/Nutrition/Herb Interactions Herb/Nutraceutical: Avoid cat's claw, dong quai, evening primrose, feverfew, red clover, horse chestnut, garlic, green tea, ginseng, ginkgo (all have additional antiplatelet activity).

Stability

Heparin solutions are colorless to slightly yellow; minor color variations do not affect therapeutic efficacy.

Heparin should be stored at controlled room temperature. Protect from freezing and temperatures >40°C.

Stability at room temperature and refrigeration:

Prepared bag: 24-72 hours (specific to solution, concentration, and/or study conditions)

Premixed bag: After seal is broken, 4 days.

Out of overwrap stability: 30 days.

Mechanism of Action Potentiates the action of antithrombin III and thereby inactivates thrombin (as well as activated coagulation factors IX, X, XI, XII, and plasmin) and prevents the conversion of fibrinogen to fibrin; heparin also stimulates release of lipoprotein lipase (lipoprotein lipase hydrolyzes triglycerides to glycerol and free fatty acids)

Pharmacodynamics/Kinetics

Onset of action: Anticoagulation: I.V.: Immediate; SubQ: ~20-30 minutes

Absorption: Oral, rectal: Erratic at best from these routes of administration; SubQ absorption is also erratic, but considered acceptable for prophylactic use

Metabolism: Hepatic; may be partially metabolized in the reticuloendothelial system

Half-life elimination:

Dose-dependent: I.V. bolus: 25 units/kg: 30 minutes; 100 units/kg: 60 minutes; 400 units/kg: 150 minutes (Hirsh, 2008)

Mean: 1.5 hours; Range: 1-2 hours; affected by obesity, renal function, malignancy, presence of pulmonary embolism, and infections

Note: At therapeutic doses, elimination occurs rapidly via nonrenal mechanisms. With very high doses, renal elimination may play more of a role; however, dosage adjustment remains unnecessary for patients with renal impairment (Hirsh, 2008).

Excretion: Urine (small amounts as unchanged drug)

Dosage

Geriatric Patients >60 years of age may have higher serum levels and clinical response (longer aPTTs) as compared to younger patients receiving similar dosages. Lower dosages may be required.

Adult Note: Many concentrations of heparin are available ranging from 1 unit/mL to 20,000 units/mL. Carefully examine each prefilled syringe or vial prior to use ensuring that the correct concentration is chosen. Heparin lock flush solution is intended only to maintain patency of I.V. devices and is not to be used for anticoagulant therapy.

Acute coronary syndromes: I.V. infusion (weight-based dosing per institutional nomogram recommended):

STEMI: Adjunct to fibrinolysis (full-dose alteplase, reteplase, or tenecteplase) (Antman, 2008): Initial bolus of 60 units/kg (maximum: 4000 units), then 12 units/kg/hour (maximum: 1000 units/hour) as continuous infusion. Check aPTT every 4-6 hours; adjust to target of 1.5-2 times the upper limit of control (50-70 seconds). Duration of heparin therapy depends on concurrent therapy and the specific patient risks for systemic or venous thromboembolism.

Unstable angina (UA)/non-ST-elevation myocardial infarction (NSTEMI) (Anderson, 2007): Initial bolus of 60 units/kg (maximum: 4000 units), followed by an initial infusion of 12 units/kg/hour (maximum: 1000 units/hour). Check aPTT every 4-6 hours; adjust to target of 1.5-2 times the upper limit of control (50-70 seconds). Continue for 48 hours in low risk patients managed with a conservative strategy (ie, no diagnostic angiography or PCI) (Jneid, 2012).

Percutaneous coronary intervention (Levine, 2011):

No prior anticoagulant therapy:

If no GPIIb/IIIa inhibitor use planned: Initial bolus of 70-100 units/kg (target ACT 250-300 seconds for HemoTec®, 300-350 seconds for Hemochron®)

or

If planning GPIIb/IIIa inhibitor use: Initial bolus of 50-70 units/kg (target ACT 200-250 seconds regardless of device)

Prior anticoagulant therapy:

If no GPIIb/IIIa inhibitor use planned: Additional heparin as needed (eg, 2000-5000 units) (target ACT 250-300 seconds for HemoTec®, 300-350 seconds for Hemochron®)

or

If planning GPIIb/IIIa inhibitor use: Additional heparin as needed (eg, 2000-5000 units) (target ACT 200-250 seconds regardless of device)

Thromboprophylaxis (low-dose heparin): SubQ: 5000 units every 8-12 hours. **Note:** The American College of Chest Physicians recommends a minimum of 10-14 days for patients undergoing total hip arthroplasty, total knee arthroplasty, or hip fracture surgery (Guyatt, 2012).

Treatment of venous thromboembolism: Note: Start warfarin on the first or second treatment day and continue heparin until INR is ≥2 for at least 24 hours (usually 5-7 days) (Guyatt, 2012).

DVT/PE (unlabeled dosing): I.V.: 80 units/kg (or alternatively 5000 units) I.V. push followed by continuous infusion of 18 units/kg/hour (or alternatively 1000 units/hour) (Guyatt, 2012)

or

DVT/PE (unlabeled dosing): SubQ: *Unmonitored dosing regimen:* Initial: 333 units/kg then 250 units/kg every 12 hours (Guyatt, 2012; Kearon, 2006)

Intermittent I.V. Anticoagulation: Intermittent I.V.: Initial: 10,000 units, then 50-70 units/kg (5000-10,000 units) every 4-6 hours

Maintenance of line patency (line flushing): When using daily flushes of heparin to maintain patency of single and double lumen central catheters, 10 units/mL is commonly used for younger infants (eg, <10 kg) while 100 units/mL is used for older infants, children, and adults. Capped PVC catheters and peripheral heparin locks require flushing more frequently (eg, every 6-8 hours). Volume of heparin flush is usually similar to volume of catheter (or slightly greater). Additional flushes should be given when stagnant blood is observed in catheter, after catheter is used for drug or blood administration, and after blood withdrawal from catheter.

Parenteral nutrition: Addition of heparin (0.5-3 unit/mL) to peripheral and central parenteral nutrition has not been shown to decrease catheter-related thrombosis.

Renal Impairment No dosage adjustment required; adjust therapeutic heparin according to aPTT or anti-Xa activity.

Hepatic Impairment No dosage adjustment required; adjust therapeutic heparin according to aPTT or anti-Xa activity.

Administration

SubQ: Inject in subcutaneous tissue only (not muscle tissue). Injection sites should be rotated (usually left and right portions of the abdomen, above iliac crest).

I.M.: Do not administer I.M. due to pain, irritation, and hematoma formation; central venous catheters must be flushed with heparin solution when newly inserted, daily (at the time of tubing change), after blood withdrawal or transfusion, and after an intermittent infusion through an injectable cap. A volume of at least 10 mL of blood should be removed and discarded from a heparinized line before blood samples are sent for coagulation testing.

Continuous I.V. infusion: Infuse via infusion pump. If preparing solution, mix thoroughly prior to administration.

Heparin lock: Inject via injection cap using positive pressure flushing technique. Heparin lock flush solution is intended only to maintain patency of I.V. devices and is **not** to be used for anticoagulant therapy.

Monitoring Parameters Hemoglobin, hematocrit, signs of bleeding; fecal occult blood test; aPTT (or antifactor Xa activity levels) or ACT depending upon indication

Platelet counts should be routinely monitored (eg, every 2-3 days on days 4-14 of heparin therapy) when the risk of HIT is >1% (eg, receiving therapeutic dose heparin, postoperative antithrombotic prophylaxis), if the patient has received heparin or low molecular weight heparin (eg, enoxaparin) within the past 100 days, if pre-exposure history is uncertain, or if anaphylactoid reaction to heparin occurs. When the risk of HIT is <1% (eg, medical/obstetrical patients receiving heparin flushes), routine platelet count monitoring is not recommended (Guyatt, 2012).

For intermittent I.V. injections, aPTT is measured 3.5-4 hours after I.V. injection.

Note: Continuous I.V. infusion is preferred over I.V. intermittent injections. For full-dose heparin (ie, nonlow-dose), the dose should be titrated according to aPTT results. For anticoagulation, an aPTT 1.5-2.5 times normal is usually desired. Because of variation among hospitals in the control aPTT values, nomograms should be established at each institution, designed to achieve aPTT values in the target range (eg, for a control aPTT of 30 seconds, the target range [1.5-2.5 times control] would be 45-75 seconds). Measurements should be made prior to heparin therapy, 6 hours after initiation, and 6 hours after any dosage change, and should be used to adjust the heparin infusion until the aPTT exhibits a therapeutic level. When two consecutive aPTT values are therapeutic, subsequent measurements may be made every 24 hours, and if necessary, dose adjustment carried out. In addition, a significant change in the patient's clinical condition (eg, recurrent ischemia, bleeding, hypotension) should prompt an immediate aPTT determination, followed by dose adjustment if necessary. In general, may increase or decrease infusion by 2-4 units/kg/hour dependent upon aPTT.

Heparin infusion dose adjustment: A number of dose-adjustment nomograms have been developed which target an aPTT range of 1.5-2.5 times control (Cruickshank, 1991; Flaker, 1994; Hull, 1992; Raschke, 1993). However, institution-specific and indication-specific nomograms should be consulted for dose adjustment. **Note:** aPTT values vary throughout the day with maximum values occurring during the night (Decousus, 1985).

Reference Range Venous thromboembolism: Heparin: 0.3-0.7 unit/mL anti-Xa activity (by chromogenic assay) or 0.2-0.4 unit/mL (by protamine titration); aPTT: 1.5-2.5 times control (usually reflects an aPTT of 60-85 seconds) (Garcia, 2012; Monagle, 2012)

When used with thrombolytic therapy in patients with acute MI, a lower therapeutic range corresponding to an aPTT of 1.5-2 times control (or approximately an aPTT of 50-70 seconds) is recommended (Antman, 2004).

Test Interactions Increased thyroxine (competitive protein binding methods); increased PT

Aprotinin significantly increases aPTT and celite Activated Clotting Time (ACT) which may not reflect the actual degree of anticoagulation by heparin. Kaolin-based ACTs are not affected by aprotinin to the same degree as celite ACTs. While institutional protocols may vary, a minimal celite ACT of 750 seconds or kaolin-ACT of 480 seconds is recommended in the presence of aprotinin. Consult the manufacturer's information on specific ACT test interpretation in the presence of aprotinin.

Special Geriatric Considerations In the clinical setting, age has not been shown to be a reliable predictor of a patient's anticoagulant response to heparin. However, it is common for the elderly to have a "standard" response for the first 24-48 hours after a loading dose (5000 units) and a maintenance infusion of 800-1000 units/hour. After this period, they then have an exaggerated response (ie, elevated aPTT), requiring a lower infusion rate. Hence, monitor closely during this period of therapy. Elderly women are more likely to have bleeding complications and osteoporosis may be a problem when used >3 months or total daily dose exceeds 30,000 units.

Dosage Forms Excipient information presented when available (limited, particularly for generics); consult specific product labeling.

Infusion, premixed in ½ NS, as sodium [porcine intestinal mucosa source]: 25,000 units (250 mL, 500 mL)

Infusion, premixed in D5W, as sodium [porcine intestinal mucosa source]: 10,000 units (250 mL); 12,500 units (250 mL); 20,000 units (500 mL); 25,000 units (250 mL, 500 mL)

Infusion, premixed in NS, as sodium [porcine intestinal mucosa source]: 1000 units (500 mL); 2000 units (1000 mL)

Infusion, premixed in NS, as sodium [porcine intestinal mucosa source, preservative free]: 1000 units (500 mL); 2000 units (1000 mL)

Injection, solution, as sodium [lock flush preparation; porcine intestinal mucosa source]: 10 units/mL (1 mL, 2 mL, 3 mL, 5 mL, 10 mL); 100 units/mL (1 mL, 2 mL, 3 mL, 5 mL, 10 mL, 30 mL)

Hep-Lock: 100 units/mL (1 mL) [contains benzyl alcohol]

Injection, solution, as sodium [lock flush preparation; porcine intestinal mucosa source, preservative free]: 1 units/mL (2 mL, 3 mL, 5 mL); 2 units/mL (3 mL); 10 units/mL (1 mL, 2 mL, 2.5 mL, 3 mL, 5 mL, 6 mL, 10 mL); 100 units/mL (1 mL, 2 mL, 2.5 mL, 3 mL, 5 mL, 10 mL)

HepFlush®-10: 10 units/mL (10 mL)

Injection, solution, as sodium [porcine intestinal mucosa source]: 1000 units/mL (1 mL, 10 mL, 30 mL); 5000 units/mL (1 mL, 10 mL); 10,000 units/mL (1 mL, 4 mL, 5 mL); 20,000 units/mL (1 mL)

Injection, solution, as sodium [porcine intestinal mucosa source, preservative free]: 1000 units/mL (2 mL); 5000 units/mL (0.5 mL); 10,000 units/mL (0.5 mL)

♦ **Heparin Calcium** see Heparin on page 914
♦ **Heparin Lock Flush** see Heparin on page 914
♦ **Heparin Sodium** see Heparin on page 914

Hepatitis A and Hepatitis B Recombinant Vaccine
(hep a TYE tis aye & hep a TYE tis bee ree KOM be nant vak SEEN)

Related Information
Hepatitis A Vaccine on page 921
Hepatitis B Vaccine (Recombinant) on page 926
Immunization Administration Recommendations on page 2144
Immunization Recommendations on page 2149

Brand Names: U.S. Twinrix®
Brand Names: Canada Twinrix®; Twinrix® Junior
Index Terms Engerix-B® and Havrix®; Havrix® and Engerix-B®; HepA-HepB; Hepatitis B and Hepatitis A Vaccine
Generic Availability (U.S.) No
Pharmacologic Category Vaccine, Inactivated (Viral)
Use Active immunization against disease caused by hepatitis A virus and hepatitis B virus (all known subtypes) in populations desiring protection against or at high risk of exposure to these viruses.

Populations include travelers or people living in or relocating to areas of intermediate/high endemicity for **both** HAV and HBV and are at increased risk of HBV infection due to behavioral or occupational factors; patients with chronic liver disease; laboratory workers who handle live HAV and HBV; healthcare workers, police, and other personnel who render first-aid or medical assistance; workers who come in contact with sewage; employees of day care centers and correctional facilities; patients/staff of hemodialysis units; men who have sex with men; patients frequently receiving blood products; military personnel; users of injectable illicit drugs; close household contacts of patients with hepatitis A and hepatitis B infection; residents of drug and alcohol treatment centers

Contraindications Hypersensitivity to hepatitis A vaccine, hepatitis B vaccine, or any component of the formulation

Warnings/Precautions Use caution in patients on anticoagulants, with thrombocytopenia, or bleeding disorders (bleeding may occur following intramuscular injection). Treatment for anaphylactic reactions should be immediately available. Postpone vaccination in moderate-to-severe acute illness (minor illness is not a contraindication). Use with caution in severely immunocompromised patients (eg, patients receiving chemo/radiation therapy or other immunosuppressive therapy (including high-dose corticosteroids)); may have a reduced response to vaccination. In general, household and close contacts of persons with altered immunocompetence may receive all age appropriate vaccines. Syncope has been reported with use of injectable vaccines and may be accompanied by transient visual disturbances, weakness, or tonic-clonic movements. Procedures should be in place to avoid injuries from falling and to restore cerebral perfusion if syncope occurs.

May contain yeast, aluminum, and trace amounts of neomycin; packaging may contain latex. In order to maximize vaccination rates, the ACIP recommends simultaneous administration of all age-appropriate vaccines (live or inactivated) for which a person is eligible at a single clinic visit, unless contraindications exist. The use of combination vaccines is generally preferred over separate injections, taking into consideration provider assessment, patient preference, and potential adverse events. When using combination vaccines, the minimum age for administration is the oldest minimum age for any individual component; the minimum interval between dosing is the greatest minimum interval between any individual component.

Vaccination may not result in effective immunity in all patients. Response depends upon multiple factors (eg, type of vaccine, age of patient) and is improved by administering the vaccine at the recommended dose, route, and interval. Vaccines may not be effective if administered during periods of altered immune competence (CDC, 2011). Due to the long incubation periods for hepatitis, unrecognized hepatitis A or B infection may be present; immunization may not prevent infection in these patients. Use hepatitis B vaccine with caution in patients with decreased cardiopulmonary function. Patients >65 years may have lower response rates to hepatitis B vaccine.

Adverse Reactions (Reflective of adult population; not specific for elderly) In the U.S., all serious adverse reactions must be reported to the U.S. Department of Health and Human Services (DHHS) Vaccine Adverse Event Reporting System (VAERS) 1-800-822-7967 or online at https://vaers.hhs.gov/esub/index.

Incidence of adverse effects of the combination product were similar to those occurring after administration of hepatitis A vaccine and hepatitis B vaccine alone. (Incidence reported is not versus placebo.)

Adults:
>10%:
  Central nervous system: Headache (13% to 22%), fatigue (11% to 14%)
  Local: Injection site reaction: Soreness (35% to 41%), redness (8% to 11%)
1% to 10%:
  Central nervous system: Fever (2% to 4%)
  Gastrointestinal: Diarrhea (4% to 6%), nausea (2% to 4%), vomiting (≤1%)
  Local: Injection site reaction: Swelling (4% to 6%), induration
  Respiratory: Upper respiratory tract infection

Children (as reported in Canadian labeling):
>10%: Local: Injection site pain/redness
1% to 10%:
  Central nervous system: Fever (≥37.5°C), drowsiness, fatigue, headache, irritability, malaise
  Gastrointestinal: Appetite decreased, diarrhea, nausea, vomiting
  Local: Injection site edema

Drug Interactions
  Metabolism/Transport Effects None known.
  Avoid Concomitant Use There are no known interactions where it is recommended to avoid concomitant use.
  Increased Effect/Toxicity There are no known significant interactions involving an increase in effect.
  Decreased Effect There are no known significant interactions involving a decrease in effect.
  Stability Store in refrigerator at 2°C to 8°C (36°F to 46°F); do not freeze (discard if frozen).

Mechanism of Action
  Hepatitis A vaccine, an inactivated virus vaccine, offers active immunization against hepatitis A virus infection at an effective immune response rate in up to 99% of subjects.
  Recombinant hepatitis B vaccine is a noninfectious subunit viral vaccine. The vaccine is derived from hepatitis B surface antigen (HB_sAg) produced through recombinant DNA techniques from yeast cells. The portion of the hepatitis B gene which codes for HB_sAg is cloned into yeast which is then cultured to produce hepatitis B vaccine.

  In immunocompetent people, Twinrix® provides active immunization against hepatitis A virus infection (at an effective immune response rate >99% of subjects) and against hepatitis B virus infection (at an effective immune response rate of 93% to 97%) 30 days after completion of the 3-dose series. This is comparable to using hepatitis A vaccine and hepatitis B vaccine concomitantly.

Pharmacodynamics/Kinetics
  Onset of action: Seroconversion for antibodies against HAV and HBV were detected 1 month after completion of the 3-dose series.
  Duration: Patients remained seropositive for at least 4 years during clinical studies.

Dosage
  Geriatric & Adult Primary immunization: I.M.: Three doses (1 mL each) given on a 0-, 1-, and 6-month schedule
    Alternative regimen: Accelerated regimen: Four doses (1 mL each) on day 0, 7, and 21-30, followed by a booster at 12 months
  Administration I.M.: Shake well prior to use. Do not dilute prior to administration. Discard if the suspension is discolored or does not appear homogenous after shaking or if there are cracks in the vial or syringe. Administer in the deltoid region; do not administer in the gluteal region (may give suboptimal response). Do not administer at the same site, or using the same syringe, as additional vaccines or immunoglobulins.

For patients at risk of hemorrhage following intramuscular injection, the ACIP recommends "it should be administered intramuscularly if, in the opinion of the physician familiar with the patients bleeding risk, the vaccine can be administered by this route with reasonable safety. If the patient receives antihemophilia or other similar therapy, intramuscular vaccination can be scheduled shortly after such therapy is administered. A fine needle (23 gauge or smaller) can be used for the vaccination and firm pressure applied to the site (without rubbing) for at least 2 minutes. The patient should be instructed concerning the risk of hematoma from the injection." Patients on anticoagulant therapy should be considered to have the same bleeding risks and treated as those with clotting factor disorders (CDC, 2011).

Simultaneous administration of vaccines helps ensure the patients will be fully vaccinated by the appropriate age. Simultaneous administration of vaccines is defined as administering >1 vaccine on the same day at different anatomic sites. The use of licensed combination vaccines is generally preferred over separate injections of the equivalent components. Separate vaccines should not be combined in the same syringe unless indicated by product specific labeling. Separate needles and syringes should be used for each injection. The ACIP prefers each dose of a specific vaccine in a series come from the same manufacturer when possible. Adolescents and adults should be vaccinated while seated or lying down. In general, preterm infants should be vaccinated at the same chronological age as full-term infants (CDC, 2011).

Antipyretics have not been shown to prevent febrile seizures. Antipyretics may be used to treat fever or discomfort following vaccination (CDC, 2011). One study reported that routine prophylactic administration of acetaminophen to prevent fever prior to vaccination decreased the immune response of some vaccines; the clinical significance of this reduction in immune response has not been established (Prymula, 2009).

Monitoring Parameters Monitor for syncope for 15 minutes following administration. If seizure-like activity associated with syncope occurs, maintain patient in supine or Trendelenburg position to reestablish adequate cerebral perfusion.

Pharmacotherapy Pearls U.S. federal law requires that the name of medication, date of administration, the vaccine manufacturer, lot number of vaccine, and the administering person's name, title, and address be entered into the patient's permanent medical record.

Special Geriatric Considerations No adjustment for age is necessary. Some studies with HBV demonstrate a lower antibody titer in the elderly as compared to younger adults.

Dosage Forms Excipient information presented when available (limited, particularly for generics); consult specific product labeling.

Injection, suspension [preservative free]:

Twinrix®: Hepatitis A virus antigen 720 ELISA units and hepatitis B surface antigen 20 mcg per mL (1 mL) [contains aluminum, yeast protein, and trace amounts of neomycin; may contain natural rubber/natural latex in prefilled syringe]

Dosage Forms: Canada Excipient information presented when available (limited, particularly for generics); consult specific product labeling.

Injection, suspension [preservative free]:

Twinrix® Junior: Hepatitis A virus antigen 360 ELISA units and hepatitis B surface antigen 10 mcg per 0.5 mL (0.5 mL) [contains aluminum and trace amounts of neomycin]

◆ **Hepatitis A and Typhoid Vaccine** see Typhoid and Hepatitis A Vaccine on page 1983

Hepatitis A Vaccine (hep a TYE tis aye vak SEEN)

Related Information

Immunization Administration Recommendations on page 2144
Immunization Recommendations on page 2149

Medication Safety Issues

International issues:

Avaxim [Canada and multiple international markets] may be confused with Avastin brand name for bevacizumab [U.S., Canada, and multiple international markets]

Brand Names: U.S. Havrix®; VAQTA®

Brand Names: Canada Avaxim®; Avaxim®-Pediatric; HAVRIX®; VAQTA®

Index Terms HepA

Generic Availability (U.S.) No

Pharmacologic Category Vaccine, Inactivated (Viral)

Use

Active immunization against disease caused by hepatitis A virus (HAV)

The Advisory Committee on Immunization Practices (ACIP) recommends routine vaccination for:

- All children ≥12 months of age
- All unvaccinated adults requesting protection from HAV infection

- All unvaccinated adults at risk for HAV infection, such as:
  Behavioral risks: Men who have sex with men; injection drug users
  Occupational risks: Persons who work with HAV-infected primates or with HAV in a research laboratory setting
  Medical risks: Persons with chronic liver disease; patients who receive clotting-factor concentrates
- Other risks: International travelers to regions with high or intermediate levels of endemic HAV infection (a list of countries is available at http://wwwn.cdc.gov/travel/contentdiseases.aspx)
- Unvaccinated persons who anticipate close personal contact with international adoptee from a country of intermediate to high endemicity of HAV, during their first 60 days of arrival into the United States (eg, household contacts, babysitters)

Contraindications Hypersensitivity to hepatitis A vaccine or any component of the formulation

Warnings/Precautions Use caution in patients on anticoagulants, with thrombocytopenia, or bleeding disorders (bleeding may occur following intramuscular injection). Treatment for anaphylactic reactions should be immediately available. Postpone vaccination with acute infection or febrile illness. Use with caution in severely immunocompromised patients (eg, patients receiving chemo/radiation therapy or other immunosuppressive therapy (including high dose corticosteroids)); may have a reduced response to vaccination. In general, household and close contacts of persons with altered immunocompetence may receive all age appropriate vaccines. Vaccination may not result in effective immunity in all patients. Response depends upon multiple factors (eg, type of vaccine, age of patient) and is improved by administering the vaccine at the recommended dose, route, and interval. Vaccines may not be effective if administered during periods of altered immune competence (CDC, 2011). Due to the long incubation period for hepatitis A (15-50 days), unrecognized hepatitis A infection may be present; immunization may not prevent infection in these patients. Patients with chronic liver disease may have decreased antibody response. Syncope has been reported with use of injectable vaccines and may be accompanied by transient visual disturbances, weakness, or tonic-clonic movements. Procedures should be in place to avoid injuries from falling and to restore cerebral perfusion if syncope occurs. Packaging may contain natural latex rubber; some products may contain neomycin. In order to maximize vaccination rates, the ACIP recommends simultaneous administration of all age-appropriate vaccines (live or inactivated) for which a person is eligible at a single clinic visit, unless contraindications exist. The use of combination vaccines is generally preferred over separate injections, taking into consideration provider assessment, patient preference, and adverse events.

Adverse Reactions (Reflective of adult population; not specific for elderly) All serious adverse reactions must be reported to the U.S. Department of Health and Human Services (DHHS) Vaccine Adverse Event Reporting System (VAERS) at 1-800-822-7967 or online at https://vaers.hhs.gov/esub/index.

Frequency dependent upon age, product used, and concomitant vaccine administration. In general, headache and injection site reactions were less common in younger children.

>10%:
  Central nervous system: Drowsiness, fever ≥100.4°F (1-5 days post vaccination), fever >98.6°C (1-14 days post vaccination), headache, irritability
  Gastrointestinal: Appetite decreased
  Local: Injection site: Erythema, pain, soreness, swelling, tenderness, warmth

1% to 10%:
  Central nervous system: Chills, fatigue, fever ≥102°F (1-5 days postvaccination), insomnia, malaise
  Dermatologic: Rash
  Endocrine & metabolic: Menstrual disorder
  Gastrointestinal: Abdominal pain, anorexia, constipation, diarrhea, gastroenteritis, nausea, vomiting
  Local: Injection site bruising, induration
  Neuromuscular & skeletal: Arm pain, back pain, myalgia, stiffness, weakness/fatigue
  Ocular: Conjunctivitis
  Otic: Otitis media
  Respiratory: Asthma, cough, nasopharyngitis, nasal congestion, pharyngitis, rhinorrhea, rhinitis, upper respiratory tract infection
  Miscellaneous: Crying

Drug Interactions
  Metabolism/Transport Effects None known.
  Avoid Concomitant Use There are no known interactions where it is recommended to avoid concomitant use.
  Increased Effect/Toxicity There are no known significant interactions involving an increase in effect.

Decreased Effect
The levels/effects of Hepatitis A Vaccine may be decreased by: Belimumab; Fingolimod; Immunosuppressants

Stability Store under refrigeration at 2°C to 8°C (36°F to 46°F); do not freeze. The following stability information has also been reported for Havrix®: May be stored at room temperature for up to 72 hours (Cohen, 2007).

Mechanism of Action As an inactivated virus vaccine, hepatitis A vaccine offers active immunization against hepatitis A virus infection at an effective immune response rate in up to 99% of subjects

Pharmacodynamics/Kinetics

Onset of action (protection): 2-4 weeks after a single dose; 2 weeks after vaccine administration, 54% to 62% of patients develop neutralizing antibodies; this percentage increases to 94% to 100% at 1 month postvaccination (CDC, 2006)

Duration: Neutralizing antibodies have persisted for up to 8 years; based on kinetic models, antibodies may be present ≥14-20 years in children and ≥25 years in adults who receive the complete vaccination series (CDC, 2006; Van Damme, 2003).

Dosage

Geriatric & Adult Immunization: I.M.: **Note:** When used for primary immunization, the vaccine should be given at least 2 weeks prior to expected HAV exposure. When used prior to an international adoption, the vaccination series should begin when adoption is being planned, but ideally ≥2 weeks prior to expected arrival of adoptee. When used for postexposure prophylaxis, the vaccine should be given as soon as possible.

HAVRIX®: 1440 ELISA units (1 mL) with a booster dose of 1440 ELISA units to be given 6-12 months following primary immunization

VAQTA®: 50 units (1 mL) with a booster dose of 50 units (1 mL) to be given 6-18 months after primary immunization (6-12 months if initial dose was with HAVRIX®)

Administration Administer as an I.M. injection. The deltoid muscle is the preferred site for injection for adults. Do not administer to the gluteal region; may decrease efficacy. Do not administer intravenously, intradermally, or subcutaneously. Shake well prior to use; discard if the suspension is discolored or does not appear homogenous after shaking, or if there are cracks in the vial or syringe. When used for primary immunization, the vaccine should be given at least 2 weeks prior to expected HAV exposure. When used for postexposure prophylaxis, the vaccine should be given as soon as possible. For patients at risk of hemorrhage following intramuscular injection, the ACIP recommends "it should be administered intramuscularly if, in the opinion of the physician familiar with the patient's bleeding risk, the vaccine can be administered by this route with reasonable safety. If the patient receives antihemophilia or other similar therapy, intramuscular vaccination can be scheduled shortly after such therapy is administered. A fine needle (23 gauge or smaller) can be used for the vaccination and firm pressure applied to the site (without rubbing) for at least 2 minutes. The patient should be instructed concerning the risk of hematoma from the injection." Patients on anticoagulant therapy should be considered to have the same bleeding risks and treated as those with clotting factor disorders (CDC, 2011).

Simultaneous administration of vaccines helps ensure the patients will be fully vaccinated by the appropriate age. Simultaneous administration of vaccines is defined as administering >1 vaccine on the same day at different anatomic sites. The use of licensed combination vaccines is generally preferred over separate injections of the equivalent components. Separate vaccines should not be combined in the same syringe unless indicated by product specific labeling. Separate needles and syringes should be used for each injection. The ACIP prefers each dose of a specific vaccine in a series come from the same manufacturer when possible. Adults should be vaccinated while seated or lying down (CDC, 2011).

Antipyretics have not been shown to prevent febrile seizures. Antipyretics may be used to treat fever or discomfort following vaccination (CDC, 2011). One study reported that routine prophylactic administration of acetaminophen to prevent fever prior to vaccination decreased the immune response of some vaccines; the clinical significance of this reduction in immune response has not been established (Prymula, 2009).

Monitoring Parameters Liver function tests; monitor for syncope for 15 minutes following administration. If seizure-like activity associated with syncope occurs, maintain patient in supine or Trendelenburg position to reestablish adequate cerebral perfusion.

Pharmacotherapy Pearls The ACIP currently recommends that older adults, the immunocompromised, or persons with underlying medical conditions (including chronic liver disease) that are vaccinated <2 weeks from departure to an area with a high or intermediate risk of hepatitis A infection also receive immune globulin (CDC, 2007).

U.S. federal law requires that the name of medication, date of administration, the vaccine manufacturer, lot number of vaccine, and the administering person's name, title, and address be entered into the patient's permanent medical record.

◀ **Special Geriatric Considerations** There is no specific data to suggest dosing is different than it is for younger adults.

Dosage Forms Excipient information presented when available (limited, particularly for generics); consult specific product labeling. [DSC] = Discontinued product

Injection, suspension [adult, preservative free]:

Havrix®: Hepatitis A virus antigen 1440 ELISA units/mL (1 mL) [contains aluminum, neomycin (may have trace amounts); may contain natural rubber/natural latex in prefilled syringe]

VAQTA®: Hepatitis A virus antigen 50 units/mL (1 mL) [contains aluminum, natural rubber/natural latex in packaging]

Injection, suspension [pediatric, preservative free]:

Havrix®: Hepatitis A virus antigen 720 ELISA units/0.5 mL (0.5 mL) [contains aluminum, neomycin (may have trace amounts); may contain natural rubber/natural latex in prefilled syringe]

Injection, suspension [pediatric/adolescent, preservative free]:

VAQTA®: Hepatitis A virus antigen 25 units/0.5 mL (0.5 mL) [contains aluminum, natural rubber/natural latex in packaging]

◆ **Hepatitis B and Hepatitis A Vaccine** see Hepatitis A and Hepatitis B Recombinant Vaccine on page 919

Hepatitis B Immune Globulin (Human)
(hep a TYE tis bee i MYUN GLOB yoo lin YU man)

Related Information
Immunization Administration Recommendations on page 2144
Immunization Recommendations on page 2149

Medication Safety Issues
Sound-alike/look-alike issues:
HBIG may be confused with BabyBIG

Brand Names: U.S. HepaGam B®; HyperHEP B™ S/D; Nabi-HB®

Brand Names: Canada HepaGam B®; HyperHEP B™ S/D

Index Terms HBIG

Generic Availability (U.S.) No

Pharmacologic Category Blood Product Derivative; Immune Globulin

Use
Passive prophylactic immunity to hepatitis B following: Acute exposure to blood containing hepatitis B surface antigen (HBsAg); sexual exposure to HBsAg-positive persons; household exposure to persons with acute HBV infection

Prevention of hepatitis B virus recurrence after liver transplantation in HBsAg-positive transplant patients

Note: Hepatitis B immune globulin is not indicated for treatment of active hepatitis B infection and is ineffective in the treatment of chronic active hepatitis B infection.

Contraindications
HepaGam B®: Anaphylactic or severe systemic reaction to human globulin preparations; postexposure prophylaxis in patients with severe thrombocytopenia or other coagulation disorders which would contraindicate I.M. injections (administer only if benefit outweighs the risk)

HyperHEP B™ S/D: No contraindications listed in manufacturer's labeling

Nabi-HB®: Anaphylactic or severe systemic reaction to human globulin preparations

Warnings/Precautions Hypersensitivity and anaphylactic reactions can occur; immediate treatment (including epinephrine 1:1000) should be available. Use with caution in patients with previous systemic hypersensitivity to human immunoglobulins. Use with caution in patients with thrombocytopenia or coagulation disorders; I.M. injections may be contraindicated. Use with caution in patients with IgA deficiency. When administered I.V., do not exceed recommended infusion rates; may increase risk of adverse events. Patients should be monitored for adverse events during and after the infusion. Thrombotic events have been reported with administration of intravenous immune globulin; use with caution in patients of advanced age, with a history of atherosclerosis or cardiovascular and/or thrombotic risk factors, patients with impaired cardiac output, coagulation disorders, prolonged immobilization, or patients with known/suspected hyperviscosity. Consider a baseline assessment of blood viscosity in patients at risk for hyperviscosity. Product of human plasma; may potentially contain infectious agents which could transmit disease. Screening of donors, as well as testing and/or inactivation or removal of certain viruses, reduces the risk. Infections thought to be transmitted by this product should be reported to the manufacturer. Some products may contain maltose, which may result in falsely-elevated blood glucose readings.

Adverse Reactions (Reflective of adult population; not specific for elderly)

Reported with postexposure prophylaxis; frequency not defined. Adverse events reported in liver transplant patients included tremor and hypotension, were associated with a single infusion during the first week of treatment, and did not recur with additional infusions.

Central nervous system: Dizziness, fainting, headache, lightheadedness, malaise
Dermatologic: Angioedema, bruising, urticaria
Gastrointestinal: Nausea, vomiting
Hematologic: WBC decreased
Hepatic: Alkaline phosphatase increased, AST increased
Local: Ache, erythema, pain, and/or tenderness at injection site
Neuromuscular & skeletal: Arthralgia, joint stiffness, myalgia
Renal: Creatinine increased
Respiratory: Cold symptoms
Miscellaneous: Anaphylaxis, flu-like syndrome

Drug Interactions

Metabolism/Transport Effects None known.

Avoid Concomitant Use There are no known interactions where it is recommended to avoid concomitant use.

Increased Effect/Toxicity There are no known significant interactions involving an increase in effect.

Decreased Effect

Hepatitis B Immune Globulin (Human) may decrease the levels/effects of: Vaccines (Live)

Stability Refrigerate at 2°C to 8°C (36°F to 46°F); do not freeze. Do not shake vial; avoid foaming.

HepaGamB®: May dilute with NS prior to I.V. administration if preferred; do not dilute with D$_5$W. Use within 6 hours of entering vial.

HyperHEP B™ S/D: May be exposed to room temperature for a cumulative 7 days (Cohen, 2007).

Nabi-HB®: Use within 6 hours of entering vial.

Mechanism of Action Hepatitis B immune globulin (HBIG) is a nonpyrogenic sterile solution containing immunoglobulin G (IgG) specific to hepatitis B surface antigen (HB$_s$Ag). HBIG differs from immune globulin in the amount of anti-HB$_s$. Immune globulin is prepared from plasma that is not preselected for anti-HB$_s$ content. HBIG is prepared from plasma preselected for high titer anti-HB$_s$. In the U.S., HBIG has an anti-HB$_s$ high titer >1:100,000 by IRA.

Pharmacodynamics/Kinetics

Duration: Postexposure prophylaxis: 3-6 months
Absorption: I.M.: Slow
Half-life: 17-25 days
Distribution: V$_d$: 7-15 L
Time to peak, serum: I.M.: 2-10 days

Dosage

Geriatric & Adult

Postexposure prophylaxis: I.M.: 0.06 mL/kg as soon as possible after exposure (ie, within 24 hours of needlestick, ocular, or mucosal exposure or within 14 days of sexual exposure); repeat at 28-30 days after exposure in nonresponders to hepatitis B vaccine or in patients who refuse vaccination

Note: HBIG may be administered at the same time (but at a different site) or up to 1 month preceding hepatitis B vaccination without impairing the active immune response

Prevention of hepatitis B virus recurrence after liver transplantation (HepaGam B™):
I.V.: 20,000 units/dose according to the following schedule:
Anhepatic phase (Initial dose): One dose given with the liver transplant
Week 1 postop: One dose daily for 7 days (days 1-7)
Weeks 2-12 postop: One dose every 2 weeks starting day 14
Month 4 onward: One dose monthly starting on month 4
Dose adjustment: Adjust dose to reach anti-HBs levels of 500 units/L within the first week after transplantation. In patients with surgical bleeding, abdominal fluid drainage >500 mL or those undergoing plasmapheresis, administer 10,000 units/dose every 6 hours until target anti-HBs levels are reached.

Administration

I.M.: Postexposure prophylaxis: I.M. injection only in anterolateral aspect of upper thigh and deltoid muscle of upper arm; to prevent injury from injection, care should be taken when giving to patients with thrombocytopenia or bleeding disorders

I.V.:
HepaGam B™: Liver transplant: Administer at 2 mL/minute. Decrease infusion to ≤1 mL/minute for patient discomfort or infusion-related adverse events. Actual volume of infusion is dependent upon potency labeled on each individual vial.

Nabi-HB®: Although not FDA-approved for this purpose, Nabi-HB® has been administered intravenously in hepatitis B-positive liver transplant patients (Dickson, 2006)

Monitoring Parameters Liver transplant: Serum HBsAg; infusion-related adverse events

Test Interactions

Glucose testing: HepaGam B™ contains maltose. Falsely-elevated blood glucose levels may occur when glucose monitoring devices and test strips utilizing the glucose dehydrogenase pyrroloquinolinequinone (GDH-PQQ) based methods are used.

Serological testing: Antibodies transferred following administration of immune globulins may provide misleading positive test results (eg, Coombs' test)

Pharmacotherapy Pearls Each vial contains anti-HB$_s$ antibody equivalent to or exceeding the potency of anti-HB$_s$ in a U.S. reference standard hepatitis B immune globulin (FDA). The U.S. reference standard has been tested against the WHO standard hepatitis B immune globulin with listed values between 207 units/mL and 220 units/mL (included in individual product information).

Special Geriatric Considerations No data available to suggest different dosing in the elderly than in younger adults.

Dosage Forms Excipient information presented when available (limited, particularly for generics); consult specific product labeling.

Injection, solution [preservative free]:

HepaGam B®: Anti-HBs >312 units/mL (1 mL, 5 mL) [contains maltose, polysorbate 80]

HyperHEP B™ S/D: Anti-HBs ≥220 units/mL (0.5 mL, 1 mL, 5 mL)

Nabi-HB®: Anti-HBs >312 units/mL (1 mL, 5 mL) [contains polysorbate 80]

◆ **Hepatitis B Inactivated Virus Vaccine (recombinant DNA)** *see* Hepatitis B Vaccine (Recombinant) *on page 926*

Hepatitis B Vaccine (Recombinant)
(hep a TYE tis bee vak SEEN ree KOM be nant)

Related Information

Immunization Administration Recommendations *on page 2144*

Immunization Recommendations *on page 2149*

Medication Safety Issues

Sound-alike/look-alike issues:

Engerix-B® adult may be confused with Engerix-B® pediatric/adolescent

Recombivax HB® may be confused with Comvax®

Brand Names: U.S. Engerix-B®; Recombivax HB®

Brand Names: Canada Engerix-B®; Recombivax HB®

Index Terms Hepatitis B Inactivated Virus Vaccine (recombinant DNA); HepB

Generic Availability (U.S.) No

Pharmacologic Category Vaccine, Inactivated (Viral)

Use Immunization against infection caused by all known subtypes of hepatitis B virus (HBV)

The Advisory Committee on Immunization Practices (ACIP) recommends routine vaccination for the following (CDC, 2005; CDC, 2006; CDC, 2011):

- All unvaccinated adults requesting protection from HBV infection

- All unvaccinated adults at risk for HBV infection such as those with:

Behavioral risks: Sexually-active persons with >1 partner in a 6-month period; persons seeking evaluation or treatment for a sexually-transmitted disease; men who have sex with men; injection drug users

Occupational risks: Healthcare and public safety workers with reasonably anticipated risk for exposure to blood or blood contaminated body fluids

Medical risks: Persons with end-stage renal disease (including predialysis, hemodialysis, peritoneal dialysis, and home dialysis); persons with HIV infection; persons with chronic liver disease. Adults (19 through 59 years of age) with diabetes mellitus type 1 or type 2 should be vaccinated as soon as possible following diagnosis. Adults ≥60 years with diabetes mellitus may also be vaccinated at the discretion of their treating clinician.

Other risks: Household contacts and sex partners of persons with chronic HBV infection; residents and staff of facilities for developmentally disabled persons; international travelers to regions with high or intermediate levels of endemic HBV infection

In addition, the ACIP recommends vaccination for any persons who are wounded in bombings or similar mass casualty events who have penetrating injuries or nonintact skin exposure, or who have contact with mucous membranes (exception - superficial contact with intact skin), and who cannot confirm receipt of a hepatitis B vaccination (CDC, 2008).

Contraindications Hypersensitivity to yeast, hepatitis B vaccine, or any component of the formulation

Warnings/Precautions Immediate treatment for anaphylactic/anaphylactoid reaction should be available during vaccine use. Defer administration in patients with moderate or severe acute illness (with or without fever). Use caution with decreased cardiopulmonary function. Vaccination may not result in effective immunity in all patients. Response depends upon multiple factors (eg, type of vaccine, age of patient) and is improved by administering the vaccine at the recommended dose, route, and interval. Vaccines may not be effective if administered during periods of altered immune competence (CDC 60[2], 2011). Due to the long incubation period for hepatitis, unrecognized hepatitis B infection may be present prior to vaccination; immunization may not prevent infection in these patients. Patients >65 years of age may have lower response rates. Use with caution in severely immunocompromised patients (eg, patients receiving chemo/radiation therapy or other immunosuppressive therapy [including high-dose corticosteroids]); may have a reduced response to vaccination. In general, household and close contacts of persons with altered immunocompetence may receive all age appropriate vaccines. Use caution in multiple sclerosis patients; rare exacerbations of symptoms have been observed.

Syncope has been reported with use of injectable vaccines and may be accompanied by transient visual disturbances, weakness, or tonic-clonic movements. Procedures should be in place to avoid injuries from falling and to restore cerebral perfusion if syncope occurs. Some dosage forms contain dry natural latex rubber. In order to maximize vaccination rates, the ACIP recommends simultaneous administration of all age-appropriate vaccines (live or inactivated) for which a person is eligible at a single clinic visit, unless contraindications exist. The use of combination vaccines is generally preferred over separate injections, taking into consideration provider assessment, patient preference, and adverse events.

Adverse Reactions (Reflective of adult population; not specific for elderly) All serious adverse reactions must be reported to the U.S. Department of Health and Human Services (DHHS) Vaccine Adverse Event Reporting System (VAERS) at 1-800-822-7967 or online at https://vaers.hhs.gov/esub/index.

Frequency not defined. The most common adverse effects reported with both products included injection site reactions (>10%).

Cardiovascular: Flushing, hypotension

Central nervous system: Agitation, chills, dizziness, fatigue, fever (≥37.5°C/100°F), headache, insomnia, irritability, lightheadedness, malaise, somnolence, vertigo

Dermatologic: Angioedema, petechiae, pruritus, rash, urticaria

Gastrointestinal: Abdominal pain, anorexia, appetite decreased, constipation, cramps, diarrhea, dyspepsia, nausea, vomiting

Genitourinary: Dysuria

Local: Injection site reactions: Ecchymosis, erythema, induration, pain, nodule formation, soreness, swelling, tenderness, warmth

Neuromuscular & skeletal: Achiness, arthralgia, back pain, myalgia, neck pain, neck stiffness, paresthesia, shoulder pain, tingling, weakness

Otic: Earache

Respiratory: Cough, pharyngitis, rhinitis, upper respiratory tract infection

Miscellaneous: Diaphoresis, lymphadenopathy, flu-like syndrome

Drug Interactions

Metabolism/Transport Effects None known.

Avoid Concomitant Use There are no known interactions where it is recommended to avoid concomitant use.

Increased Effect/Toxicity There are no known significant interactions involving an increase in effect.

Decreased Effect

The levels/effects of Hepatitis B Vaccine (Recombinant) may be decreased by: Belimumab; Fingolimod; Immunosuppressants

Stability Refrigerate at 2°C to 8°C (36°F to 46°F); do not freeze. The following stability information has also been reported for Engerix-B®: May be stored at room temperature for up to 72 hours (Cohen, 2007).

Mechanism of Action Recombinant hepatitis B vaccine is a noninfectious subunit viral vaccine, which confers active immunity via formation of antihepatitis B antibodies. The vaccine is derived from hepatitis B surface antigen (HB$_s$Ag) produced through recombinant DNA techniques from yeast cells. The portion of the hepatitis B gene which codes for HB$_s$Ag is cloned into yeast which is then cultured to produce hepatitis B vaccine.

Pharmacodynamics/Kinetics Duration: Following a 3-dose series in children, up to 50% of patients will have low or undetectable anti-HB antibody 5-15 years postvaccination. However, anamnestic increases in anti-HB have been shown up to 23 years later suggesting a lifelong immune memory response.

◄ **Dosage**

Geriatric & Adult

Primary immunization: I.M.: 1 mL/dose (adult formulation) for 3 total doses administered at 0, 1, and 6 months

Note: Adult formulations of hepatitis B vaccine products differ by concentration (mcg/mL) but when dosed in terms of volume (mL), the dose of Engerix-B® and Recombivax HB® are the same (both 1 mL).

Alternate dosing schedules (selection of schedule should optimize compliance with vaccination): All regimens use the adult formulation administered as one dose at the following intervals (three schedules presented):

0, 1, and 4 months (CDC, 2005)

0, 2, and 4 months (CDC, 2005)

0, 12, and 24 months (CDC, 2005)

Bombings or similar mass casualty events: I.M.: In persons without a reliable history of vaccination against HepB and who have no known contraindications to the vaccine, vaccination should begin within 24 hours (but no later than 7 days) following the event (CDC, 2008).

Renal Impairment Adults on dialysis:

Engerix-B® 20 mcg/mL: Administer 2 mL per dose at 0, 1, 2, and 6 months

Recombivax HB® 40 mcg/mL: Administer 1 mL per dose at 0, 1, and 6 months

Note: Serologic testing is recommended 1-2 months after the final dose of the primary vaccine series and annually to determine the need for booster doses. Persons with anti-HB$_s$ concentrations of <10 mIU/mL should be revaccinated with 3 doses of the vaccine (CDC, 2006).

Administration Adult formulations of hepatitis B vaccine products differ by concentration (mcg/mL), but when dosed in terms of volume (mL), the dose of Engerix-B® and Recombivax HB® are the same (both 1 mL). It is possible to interchange the vaccines for completion of a series or for booster doses; the antibody produced in response to each type of vaccine is comparable, however, the quantity of the vaccine will vary.

I.M. injection only; in adults, the deltoid muscle is the preferred site. Not for gluteal administration. Shake well prior to withdrawal and use.

For patients at risk of hemorrhage following intramuscular injection, hepatitis B vaccine may be administered subcutaneously although lower titers and/or increased incidence of local reactions may result. The ACIP recommends "it should be administered intramuscularly if, in the opinion of the physician familiar with the patients bleeding risk, the vaccine can be administered by this route with reasonable safety. If the patient receives antihemophilia or other similar therapy, intramuscular vaccination can be scheduled shortly after such therapy is administered. A fine needle (23 gauge or smaller) can be used for the vaccination and firm pressure applied to the site (without rubbing) for at least 2 minutes. The patient should be instructed concerning the risk of hematoma from the injection." Patients on anticoagulant therapy should be considered to have the same bleeding risks and treated as those with clotting factor disorders (CDC, 2011).

Simultaneous administration of vaccines helps ensure the patients will be fully vaccinated by the appropriate age. Simultaneous administration of vaccines is defined as administering >1 vaccine on the same day at different anatomic sites. The use of licensed combination vaccines is generally preferred over separate injections of the equivalent components. Separate vaccines should not be combined in the same syringe unless indicated by product specific labeling. Separate needles and syringes should be used for each injection. The ACIP prefers each dose of a specific vaccine in a series come from the same manufacturer when possible. Adults should be vaccinated while seated or lying down.

Antipyretics have not been shown to prevent febrile seizures. Antipyretics may be used to treat fever or discomfort following vaccination (CDC, 2011). One study reported that routine prophylactic administration of acetaminophen to prevent fever prior to vaccination decreased the immune response of some vaccines; the clinical significance of this reduction in immune response has not been established (Prymula, 2009).

Vaccination at the time of HB$_s$Ag testing: For persons in whom vaccination is recommended, the first dose of hepatitis B vaccine can be given after blood is drawn to test for HB$_s$Ag.

Monitoring Parameters Monitor for syncope for 15 minutes following administration. If seizure-like activity associated with syncope occurs, maintain patient in supine or Trendelenburg position to reestablish adequate cerebral perfusion.

Pharmacotherapy Pearls U.S. federal law requires that the name of medication, date of administration, the vaccine manufacturer, lot number of vaccine, and the administering person's name, title, and address be entered into the patient's permanent medical record.

Special Geriatric Considerations No dose adjustments required based on age. Some studies demonstrate a lower antibody titer in the elderly as compared to young adults. The decision to vaccinate adults ≥60 years of age with diabetes should take into consideration the patients risk of acquiring HBV infection, including the need for blood-glucose monitoring in long-term care facilities, the likelihood of long-term effects if an HBV infection is acquired, and the declining immune response to vaccines associated with aging.

Dosage Forms Excipient information presented when available (limited, particularly for generics); consult specific product labeling. [DSC] = Discontinued product

Injection, suspension [adult, preservative free]:

Engerix-B®: Hepatitis B surface antigen 20 mcg/mL (1 mL) [contains aluminum, yeast protein, may contain natural rubber/natural latex in prefilled syringe]

Engerix-B®: Hepatitis B surface antigen 20 mcg/mL (1 mL) [contains aluminum, yeast protein; vial]

Recombivax HB®: Hepatitis B surface antigen 10 mcg/mL (1 mL) [contains aluminum, natural rubber/natural latex in packaging, yeast protein]

Injection, suspension [dialysis formulation, preservative free]:

Recombivax HB®: Hepatitis B surface antigen 40 mcg/mL (1 mL) [contains aluminum, natural rubber/natural latex in packaging, yeast protein]

Injection, suspension [pediatric/adolescent, preservative free]:

Engerix-B®: Hepatitis B surface antigen 10 mcg/0.5 mL (0.5 mL) [contains aluminum, yeast protein, may contain natural rubber/natural latex in prefilled syringe]

Recombivax HB®: Hepatitis B surface antigen 5 mcg/0.5 mL (0.5 mL) [contains aluminum, natural rubber/natural latex in packaging, yeast protein]

◆ **HepB** see Hepatitis B Vaccine (Recombinant) on page 926
◆ **HepFlush®-10** see Heparin on page 914
◆ **Hep-Lock** see Heparin on page 914
◆ **Hexachlorocyclohexane** see Lindane on page 1135
◆ **Hexamethylenetetramine** see Methenamine on page 1231
◆ **High Gamma Vitamin E Complete™ [OTC]** see Vitamin E on page 2027
◆ **High-Molecular-Weight Iron Dextran (DexFerrum®)** see Iron Dextran Complex on page 1039
◆ **Hiprex®** see Methenamine on page 1231
◆ **Histaprin [OTC]** see DiphenhydrAMINE (Systemic) on page 556
◆ **Hizentra®** see Immune Globulin on page 982
◆ **HMR 3647** see Telithromycin on page 1845
◆ **HOE 140** see Icatibant on page 971
◆ **Hold® DM [OTC]** see Dextromethorphan on page 525
◆ **Homatropaire** see Homatropine on page 929

Homatropine (hoe MA troe peen)

Related Information

Beers Criteria – Potentially Inappropriate Medications for Geriatrics on page 2183

Medication Safety Issues

Sound-alike/look-alike issues:

Homatropine may be confused with Humatrope®, somatropin

Brand Names: U.S. Homatropaire; Isopto® Homatropine

Index Terms Homatropine Hydrobromide

Generic Availability (U.S.) Yes

Pharmacologic Category Anticholinergic Agent, Ophthalmic; Ophthalmic Agent, Mydriatic

Use Producing cycloplegia and mydriasis for refraction; treatment of acute inflammatory conditions of the uveal tract; optical aid in axial lens opacities

Contraindications Hypersensitivity to homatropine or any component of the formulation; primary glaucoma or predisposition to glaucoma (eg, narrow-angle glaucoma)

Warnings/Precautions Excessive use may cause CNS disturbances, including confusion, delirium, agitation and coma (rare); may occur with any age group, although children and the elderly are more susceptible. May cause an increase in intraocular pressure. Use with caution in patients with keratoconus; may result in fixed pupil dilation. Use with caution in the elderly. May cause sensitivity to light; appropriate eye protection should be used. Some strengths may contain benzalkonium chloride which may be adsorbed by contact lenses; remove contacts prior to administration and wait 15 minutes before reinserting. To minimize systemic absorption, apply pressure over the nasolacrimal sac for 2-3 minutes after instillation. To avoid contamination, do not touch dropper tip to any surface. For topical ophthalmic use only.

Adverse Reactions (Reflective of adult population; not specific for elderly)
>10%: Ocular: Blurred vision, photophobia
1% to 10%:
Local: Stinging, local irritation
Ocular: Increased intraocular pressure
Respiratory: Congestion

Drug Interactions
Metabolism/Transport Effects None known.
Avoid Concomitant Use There are no known interactions where it is recommended to avoid concomitant use.
Increased Effect/Toxicity
Homatropine may increase the levels/effects of: AbobotulinumtoxinA; Anticholinergics; Cannabinoids; OnabotulinumtoxinA; Potassium Chloride; RimabotulinumtoxinB

The levels/effects of Homatropine may be increased by: Pramlintide
Decreased Effect
Homatropine may decrease the levels/effects of: Acetylcholinesterase Inhibitors (Central); Secretin

The levels/effects of Homatropine may be decreased by: Acetylcholinesterase Inhibitors (Central)
Stability Store at 8°C to 24°C (46°F to 75°F). Protect from light.
Mechanism of Action Blocks response of iris sphincter muscle and the accommodative muscle of the ciliary body to cholinergic stimulation resulting in dilation and loss of accommodation
Pharmacodynamics/Kinetics
Onset of action: Accommodation and pupil effect: Ophthalmic:
Maximum mydriatic effect: Within 10-30 minutes
Maximum cycloplegic effect: Within 30-90 minutes
Duration:
Mydriasis: 6 hours to 4 days
Cycloplegia: 10-48 hours

Dosage
Geriatric & Adult
Mydriasis and cycloplegia for refraction: Ophthalmic: Instill 1-2 drops of 2% solution or 1 drop of 5% solution before the procedure; repeat at 5- to 10-minute intervals as needed; maximum of 3 doses for refraction
Uveitis: Ophthalmic: Instill 1-2 drops of 2% or 5% 2-3 times/day up to every 3-4 hours as needed
Administration Finger pressure should be applied to lacrimal sac for 1-2 minutes after instillation to decrease risk of absorption and systemic reactions
Special Geriatric Considerations Use with caution due to susceptibility to systemic effects. Evaluate the patient's or caregiver's ability to safely administer the correct dose of ophthalmic medication.
Dosage Forms Excipient information presented when available (limited, particularly for generics); consult specific product labeling.
Solution, ophthalmic, as hydrobromide [drops]: 5% (5 mL)
Homatropaire: 5% (5 mL) [contains benzalkonium chloride]
Isopto® Homatropine: 2% (5 mL); 5% (5 mL) [contains benzalkonium chloride]

◆ **HuMist® [OTC]** *see* Sodium Chloride *on page 1787*
◆ **HumuLIN® 70/30** *see* Insulin NPH and Insulin Regular *on page 1023*
◆ **HumuLIN® N** *see* Insulin NPH *on page 1020*
◆ **HumuLIN® R** *see* Insulin Regular *on page 1025*
◆ **HumuLIN® R U-500** *see* Insulin Regular *on page 1025*

Hyaluronidase (hye al yoor ON i dase)

Brand Names: U.S. Amphadase™; Hylenex [DSC]; Vitrase®
Generic Availability (U.S.) No
Pharmacologic Category Enzyme
Use Increase the dispersion and absorption of other injected drugs; increase rate of absorption of parenteral fluids given by subcutaneous administration (hypodermoclysis)
Unlabeled Use Management of drug extravasations; local anesthetic adjuvant in bupivacaine-lidocaine mixture for retrobulbar/peribulbar block
Dosage
Geriatric & Adult
Skin test: Intradermal: 0.02 mL (3 units) of a 150 units/mL solution. Positive reaction consists of a wheal with pseudopods appearing within 5 minutes and persisting for 20-30 minutes with localized itching.
Dehydration: Hypodermoclysis: SubQ: Add 15 units to each 100 mL of replacement fluid to be administered **or** 150 units followed by subcutaneous isotonic fluid administration ≥1000 mL; rate and volume of a single clysis should not exceed those used for infusion of I.V. fluids
Extravasation (unlabeled use): SubQ: Inject 1 mL of a 150 unit/mL solution (as 5-10 injections of 0.1-0.2 mL) into affected area; doses of 15-250 units have been reported.
Note: Do not use for extravasation of pressor agents (eg, dopamine, norepinephrine).
Special Geriatric Considerations The most common use of hyaluronidase in the elderly is in hypodermoclysis. Hypodermoclysis is very useful in dehydrated patients in whom oral intake is minimal and I.V. access is a problem.
Dosage Forms Excipient information presented when available (limited, particularly for generics); consult specific product labeling. [DSC] = Discontinued product
Injection, solution [preservative free]:
Hylenex: 150 units/mL (1 mL [DSC]) [contains albumin (human), edetate disodium; recombinant]
Injection, solution [bovine derived]:
Amphadase™: 150 units/mL (1 mL) [contains edetate disodium, thimerosal]
Injection, solution [ovine derived, preservative free]:
Vitrase®: 200 units/mL (1.2 mL) [contains lactose 0.93 mg/mL]

◆ **hycet®** *see* Hydrocodone and Acetaminophen *on page 937*
◆ **Hydergine [DSC]** *see* Ergoloid Mesylates *on page 659*

HydrALAZINE (hye DRAL a zeen)

Medication Safety Issues
Sound-alike/look-alike issues:
HydrALAZINE may be confused with hydrOXYzine
Brand Names: Canada Apo-Hydralazine®; Apresoline®; Novo-Hylazin; Nu-Hydral
Index Terms Apresoline [DSC]; Hydralazine Hydrochloride
Generic Availability (U.S.) Yes
Pharmacologic Category Vasodilator
Use Management of moderate-to-severe hypertension
Unlabeled Use Heart failure
Contraindications Hypersensitivity to hydralazine or any component of the formulation; mitral valve rheumatic heart disease
Warnings/Precautions May cause peripheral neuritis or a drug-induced lupus-like syndrome (more likely on larger doses, longer duration). Discontinue hydralazine in patients who develop SLE-like syndrome or positive ANA. Use with caution in patients with severe renal disease or cerebral vascular accidents or with known or suspected coronary artery disease; monitor blood pressure closely with I.V. use. Slow acetylators, patients with decreased renal function, and patients receiving >200 mg/day (chronically) are at higher risk for SLE. Titrate dosage cautiously to patient's response. Hypotensive effect after I.V. administration may be delayed and unpredictable in some patients. Usually administered with diuretic and a beta-blocker to counteract side effects of sodium and water retention and reflex tachycardia.

◀ Adjust dose in severe renal dysfunction. Use with caution in CAD (increase in tachycardia may increase myocardial oxygen demand). Use with caution in pulmonary hypertension (may cause hypotension). Patients may be poorly compliant because of frequent dosing. Hydralazine-induced fluid and sodium retention may require addition or increased dosage of a diuretic.

Adverse Reactions (Reflective of adult population; not specific for elderly) Frequency not defined.

Cardiovascular: Angina pectoris, flushing, orthostatic hypotension, palpitations, paradoxical hypertension, peripheral edema, tachycardia, vascular collapse

Central nervous system: Anxiety, chills, depression, disorientation, dizziness, fever, headache, increased intracranial pressure (I.V.; in patient with pre-existing increased intracranial pressure), psychotic reaction

Dermatologic: Pruritus, rash, urticaria

Gastrointestinal: Anorexia, constipation, diarrhea, nausea, paralytic ileus, vomiting

Genitourinary: Dysuria, impotence

Hematologic: Agranulocytosis, eosinophilia, erythrocyte count reduced, hemoglobin decreased, hemolytic anemia, leukopenia, thrombocytopenia (rare)

Neuromuscular & skeletal: Muscle cramps, peripheral neuritis, rheumatoid arthritis, tremor, weakness

Ocular: Conjunctivitis, lacrimation

Respiratory: Dyspnea, nasal congestion

Miscellaneous: Diaphoresis, drug-induced lupus-like syndrome (dose related; fever, arthralgia, splenomegaly, lymphadenopathy, asthenia, myalgia, malaise, pleuritic chest pain, edema, positive ANA, positive LE cells, maculopapular facial rash, positive direct Coombs' test, pericarditis, pericardial tamponade)

Drug Interactions

Metabolism/Transport Effects Inhibits CYP3A4 (weak)

Avoid Concomitant Use

Avoid concomitant use of HydrALAZINE with any of the following: Pimozide

Increased Effect/Toxicity

HydrALAZINE may increase the levels/effects of: Amifostine; Antihypertensives; ARIPiprazole; Hypotensive Agents; Pimozide; RiTUXimab

The levels/effects of HydrALAZINE may be increased by: Alfuzosin; Diazoxide; Herbs (Hypotensive Properties); MAO Inhibitors; Pentoxifylline; Phosphodiesterase 5 Inhibitors; Prostacyclin Analogues

Decreased Effect

The levels/effects of HydrALAZINE may be decreased by: Herbs (Hypertensive Properties); Methylphenidate; Nonsteroidal Anti-Inflammatory Agents; Yohimbine

Ethanol/Nutrition/Herb Interactions

Ethanol: Avoid ethanol (may increase CNS depression).

Food: Food enhances bioavailability of hydralazine.

Herb/Nutraceutical: Avoid dong quai if using for hypertension (has estrogenic activity). Avoid ephedra, yohimbe, ginseng (may worsen hypertension). Avoid garlic (may have increased antihypertensive effect).

Stability Intact ampuls/vials of hydralazine should not be stored under refrigeration because of possible precipitation or crystallization. Hydralazine should be diluted in NS for IVPB administration due to decreased stability in D_5W. Stability of IVPB solution in NS is 4 days at room temperature.

Mechanism of Action Direct vasodilation of arterioles (with little effect on veins) with decreased systemic resistance

Pharmacodynamics/Kinetics

Onset of action: Oral: 20-30 minutes; I.V.: 5-20 minutes

Duration: Oral: Up to 8 hours; I.V.: 1-4 hours; **Note:** May vary depending on acetylator status of patient

Protein binding: 85% to 90%

Metabolism: Hepatically acetylated; extensive first-pass effect (oral)

Bioavailability: 30% to 50%; increased with food

Half-life elimination: Normal renal function: 2-8 hours; End-stage renal disease: 7-16 hours

Excretion: Urine (14% as unchanged drug)

Dosage

Geriatric Oral: Initial: 10 mg 2-3 times/day; increase by 10-25 mg/day every 2-5 days.

Adult

Hypertension: Oral:

Initial: 10 mg 4 times/day; increase by 10-25 mg/dose every 2-5 days (maximum: 300 mg/day); usual dose range (JNC 7): 25-100 mg/day in 2 divided doses

Acute hypertension: I.M., I.V.: Initial: 10-20 mg/dose every 4-6 hours as needed, may increase to 40 mg/dose; change to oral therapy as soon as possible.

Congestive heart failure: Oral:

Initial dose: 10-25 mg 3-4 times/day

Adjustment: Dosage must be adjusted based on individual response

Target dose: 225-300 mg/day in divided doses; use in combination with isosorbide dinitrate

Renal Impairment

Cl_{cr} 10-50 mL/minute: Administer every 8 hours.

Cl_{cr} <10 mL/minute: Administer every 8-16 hours in fast acetylators and every 12-24 hours in slow acetylators.

Hemodialysis effects: Supplemental dose is not necessary.

Peritoneal dialysis effects: Supplemental dose is not necessary.

Administration Solution for injection: Administer as a slow I.V. push; maximum rate: 5 mg/minute

Monitoring Parameters Blood pressure (monitor closely with I.V. use), standing and sitting/supine, heart rate, ANA titer

Pharmacotherapy Pearls Slow acetylators, patients with decreased renal function and patients receiving >200 mg/day (chronically) are at higher risk for SLE. Titrate dosage to patient's response. Usually administered with diuretic and a beta-blocker to counteract side effects of sodium and water retention and reflex tachycardia although the beta-blocker may not be necessary in older adults. For the treatment of CHF where hydralazine is used in place of an ACE inhibitor, it is necessary to use a combination of hydralazine and isosorbide.

Special Geriatric Considerations Due to the vasodilating effects, lower initial doses within the recommended dosage range should be used in elderly patients.

Dosage Forms Excipient information presented when available (limited, particularly for generics); consult specific product labeling.

Injection, solution, as hydrochloride: 20 mg/mL (1 mL)

Tablet, oral, as hydrochloride: 10 mg, 25 mg, 50 mg, 100 mg

◆ **Hydralazine and Isosorbide Dinitrate** *see* Isosorbide Dinitrate and Hydralazine *on page 1052*

◆ **Hydralazine Hydrochloride** *see* HydrALAZINE *on page 931*

◆ **Hydrated Chloral** *see* Chloral Hydrate *on page 349*

◆ **Hydrea®** *see* Hydroxyurea *on page 955*

◆ **Hydrisalic® [OTC]** *see* Salicylic Acid *on page 1743*

Hydrochlorothiazide (hye droe klor oh THYE a zide)

Medication Safety Issues

Sound-alike/look-alike issues:

HCTZ is an error-prone abbreviation (mistaken as hydrocortisone)

Hydrochlorothiazide may be confused with hydrocortisone, Viskazide®

Microzide™ may be confused with Maxzide®, Micronase®

International issues:

Esidrex [multiple international markets] may be confused with Lasix brand name for furosemide [U.S., Canada, and multiple international markets]

Esidrix [Germany] may be confused with Lasix brand name for furosemide [U.S., Canada, and multiple international markets]

Brand Names: U.S. Microzide®

Brand Names: Canada Apo-Hydro®; Bio-Hydrochlorothiazide; Dom-Hydrochlorothiazide; Novo-Hydrazide; Nu-Hydro; PMS-Hydrochlorothiazide

Index Terms HCTZ (error-prone abbreviation); Hydrodiuril

Generic Availability (U.S.) Yes

Pharmacologic Category Diuretic, Thiazide

Use Management of mild-to-moderate hypertension; treatment of edema in heart failure and nephrotic syndrome

Unlabeled Use Treatment of lithium-induced diabetes insipidus

Contraindications Hypersensitivity to hydrochlorothiazide or any component of the formulation, thiazides, or sulfonamide-derived drugs; anuria; renal decompensation

Warnings/Precautions Hypersensitivity reactions may occur with hydrochlorothiazide. Risk is increased in patients with a history of allergy or bronchial asthma. Avoid in severe renal disease (ineffective as a diuretic). Electrolyte disturbances (hypokalemia, hypochloremic alkalosis, hyponatremia) can occur. Use with caution in severe hepatic dysfunction; hepatic encephalopathy can be caused by electrolyte disturbances. Gout may be precipitated in certain patients with a history of gout, a familial predisposition to gout, or chronic renal failure. Thiazide diuretics reduce calcium excretion; pathologic changes in the parathyroid glands with hypercalcemia and hypophosphatemia have been observed with prolonged use. Use with caution in patients with prediabetes and diabetes; may alter glucose control. May cause SLE exacerbation or activation. Use with caution in patients with moderate or high cholesterol concentrations. Photosensitization may occur. Correct hypokalemia before initiating therapy. Thiazide diuretics may decrease renal calcium excretion; consider avoiding use in patients with hypercalcemia. May cause acute transient myopia and acute angle-closure glaucoma, typically occurring within hours to weeks following initiation; discontinue therapy immediately in patients with acute decreases in visual acuity or ocular pain. Risk factors may include a history of sulfonamide or penicillin allergy.

Chemical similarities are present among sulfonamides, sulfonylureas, carbonic anhydrase inhibitors, thiazides, and loop diuretics (except ethacrynic acid). Use in patients with sulfonamide allergy is specifically contraindicated in product labeling, however, a risk of cross-reaction exists in patients with allergy to any of these compounds; avoid use when previous reaction has been severe. Discontinue if signs of hypersensitivity are noted.

Adverse Reactions (Reflective of adult population; not specific for elderly) Frequency not defined; adverse events reported were observed at doses ≥25 mg:

Cardiovascular: Hypotension, orthostatic hypotension

Central nervous system: Dizziness, fever, headache, vertigo

Dermatologic: Alopecia, erythema multiforme, exfoliative dermatitis, photosensitivity, purpura, rash, Stevens-Johnson syndrome, toxic epidermal necrolysis, urticaria

Endocrine & metabolic: Hyperglycemia, hypokalemia, hyperuricemia

Gastrointestinal: Anorexia, constipation, cramping, diarrhea, epigastric distress, gastric irritation, nausea, pancreatitis, sialadenitis, vomiting

Genitourinary: Glycosuria, impotence

Hematologic: Agranulocytosis, aplastic anemia, hemolytic anemia, leukopenia, thrombocytopenia

Hepatic: Jaundice

Neuromuscular & skeletal: Muscle spasm, paresthesia, restlessness, weakness

Ocular: Blurred vision (transient), xanthopsia

Renal: Interstitial nephritis, renal dysfunction, renal failure

Respiratory: Respiratory distress, pneumonitis, pulmonary edema

Miscellaneous: Anaphylactic reactions, necrotizing angiitis

Drug Interactions

Metabolism/Transport Effects None known.

Avoid Concomitant Use

Avoid concomitant use of Hydrochlorothiazide with any of the following: Dofetilide

Increased Effect/Toxicity

Hydrochlorothiazide may increase the levels/effects of: ACE Inhibitors; Allopurinol; Amifostine; Antihypertensives; Benazepril; Calcium Salts; CarBAMazepine; Dofetilide; Hypotensive Agents; Lithium; OXcarbazepine; Porfimer; RiTUXimab; Sodium Phosphates; Topiramate; Toremifene; Valsartan; Vitamin D Analogs

The levels/effects of Hydrochlorothiazide may be increased by: Alcohol (Ethyl); Alfuzosin; Analgesics (Opioid); Barbiturates; Beta2-Agonists; Corticosteroids (Orally Inhaled); Corticosteroids (Systemic); Herbs (Hypotensive Properties); Licorice; MAO Inhibitors; Pentoxifylline; Phosphodiesterase 5 Inhibitors; Prostacyclin Analogues; Valsartan

Decreased Effect

Hydrochlorothiazide may decrease the levels/effects of: Antidiabetic Agents

The levels/effects of Hydrochlorothiazide may be decreased by: Benazepril; Bile Acid Sequestrants; Herbs (Hypertensive Properties); Methylphenidate; Nonsteroidal Anti-Inflammatory Agents; Yohimbine

Ethanol/Nutrition/Herb Interactions

Food: Hydrochlorothiazide peak serum levels may be decreased if taken with food. This product may deplete potassium, sodium, and magnesium.

Herb/Nutraceutical: Avoid herbs with *hypertensive* properties (bayberry, blue cohosh, cayenne, ephedra, ginger, ginseng [American], kola, licorice); may diminish the antihypertensive effect of hydrochlorothiazide. Avoid herbs with *hypotensive* properties (black cohosh, California poppy, coleus, golden seal, hawthorn, mistletoe, periwinkle, quinine, shepherd's purse); may enhance the hypotensive effect of hydrochlorothiazide.

Mechanism of Action Inhibits sodium reabsorption in the distal tubules causing increased excretion of sodium and water as well as potassium and hydrogen ions

Pharmacodynamics/Kinetics

Onset of action: Diuresis: ~2 hours

Peak effect: 4-6 hours

Duration: 6-12 hours

Absorption: ~50% to 80%

Distribution: 3.6-7.8 L/kg

Protein binding: 68%
Metabolism: Not metabolized
Bioavailability: 50% to 80%
Half-life elimination: 5.6-14.8 hours
Time to peak: 1-2.5 hours
Excretion: Urine (as unchanged drug)

Dosage

Geriatric Oral: 12.5-25 mg once daily; minimal increase in response and more electrolyte disturbances are seen with doses >50 mg/day.

Adult

Edema (diuresis): Oral: 25-100 mg/day in 1-2 doses; maximum: 200 mg/day

Hypertension: Oral: 12.5-50 mg/day; minimal increase in response and more electrolyte disturbances are seen with doses >50 mg/day

Renal Impairment Cl$_{cr}$ <10 mL/minute: Avoid use. Usually ineffective with GFR <30 mL/minute. Effective at lower GFR in combination with a loop diuretic.

Note: ACC/AHA 2009 Heart Failure guidelines suggest that thiazides lose their efficacy when Cl$_{cr}$ <40 mL/minute.

Administration May be administered with food or milk. Take early in day to avoid nocturia. Take the last dose of multiple doses no later than 6 PM unless instructed otherwise.

Monitoring Parameters Assess weight, I & O reports daily to determine fluid loss; blood pressure, serum electrolytes, BUN, creatinine

Test Interactions May interfere with parathyroid function tests and may decrease serum iodine (protein bound) without signs of thyroid disturbance.

Pharmacotherapy Pearls If given the morning of surgery, hydrochlorothiazide may render the patient volume depleted and blood pressure may be labile during general anesthesia. Effect of drug may be decreased when used every day.

Special Geriatric Considerations Hydrochlorothiazide is not effective in patients with a Cl$_{cr}$ <30 mL/minute, therefore, it may not be a useful agent in many elderly patients.

Dosage Forms Excipient information presented when available (limited, particularly for generics); consult specific product labeling.

Capsule, oral: 12.5 mg

Microzide®: 12.5 mg

Tablet, oral: 12.5 mg, 25 mg, 50 mg

Hydrochlorothiazide and Spironolactone
(hye droe klor oh THYE a zide & speer on oh LAK tone)

Related Information
Hydrochlorothiazide *on page 933*
Spironolactone *on page 1805*
Medication Safety Issues
Sound-alike/look-alike issues:
Aldactazide® may be confused with Aldactone®
Brand Names: U.S. Aldactazide®
Brand Names: Canada Aldactazide 25®; Aldactazide 50®; Novo-Spirozine
Index Terms Spironolactone and Hydrochlorothiazide
Generic Availability (U.S.) Yes
Pharmacologic Category Diuretic, Thiazide; Selective Aldosterone Blocker
Use Management of mild-to-moderate hypertension; treatment of edema in congestive heart failure and nephrotic syndrome, and cirrhosis of the liver accompanied by edema and/or ascites
Dosage
Geriatric Oral: Consider initiating therapy with the lowest available dose (usual initial doses of hydrochlorothiazide are 12.5-25 mg once daily); increase as necessary.
Adult Hypertension, edema: Oral: Hydrochlorothiazide 12.5-50 mg/day and spironolactone 12.5-50 mg/day; manufacturer's labeling states hydrochlorothiazide maximum 200 mg/day, however, usual dose in JNC-7 is 12.5-50 mg/day
Renal Impairment Efficacy of hydrochlorothiazide is limited in patients with Cl_{cr} <30 mL/minute; contraindicated in patients with anuria
Special Geriatric Considerations See individual agents. Combination products are not recommended as first-line treatment. Use only if doses of individual agents correspond to the combination available.

The efficacy of hydrochlorothiazide is limited in patients with a Cl_{cr} <30 mL/minute; monitor serum potassium.
Dosage Forms Excipient information presented when available (limited, particularly for generics); consult specific product labeling.
Tablet: Hydrochlorothiazide 25 mg and spironolactone 25 mg
Aldactazide®:
25/25: Hydrochlorothiazide 25 mg and spironolactone 25 mg
50/50: Hydrochlorothiazide 50 mg and spironolactone 50 mg

◆ **Hydrochlorothiazide and Telmisartan** see Telmisartan and Hydrochlorothiazide *on page 1849*

Hydrochlorothiazide and Triamterene
(hye droe klor oh THYE a zide & trye AM ter een)

Related Information
Hydrochlorothiazide *on page 933*
Triamterene *on page 1962*
Medication Safety Issues
Sound-alike/look-alike issues:
Dyazide® may be confused with diazoxide, Dynacin®
Maxzide® may be confused with Maxidex®, Microzide®
Brand Names: U.S. Dyazide®; Maxzide®; Maxzide®-25
Brand Names: Canada Apo-Triazide®; Nu-Triazide; Pro-Triazide; Riva-Zide; Teva-Triamterene HCTZ
Index Terms Triamterene and Hydrochlorothiazide
Generic Availability (U.S.) Yes
Pharmacologic Category Diuretic, Potassium-Sparing; Diuretic, Thiazide
Use Treatment of hypertension or edema (not recommended for initial treatment) when hypokalemia has developed on hydrochlorothiazide alone or when the development of hypokalemia must be avoided
Dosage
Geriatric & Adult Hypertension, edema: Oral:
Hydrochlorothiazide 25 mg and triamterene 37.5 mg: 1-2 tablets/capsules once daily
Hydrochlorothiazide 50 mg and triamterene 75 mg: 1/2-1 tablet daily

Special Geriatric Considerations See individual agents. Combination products are not recommended as first-line treatment. Use only if doses of individual agents correspond to the combination available.

The efficacy of hydrochlorothiazide is limited in patients with a Cl_{cr} <30 mL/minute; monitor serum potassium.

Dosage Forms Excipient information presented when available (limited, particularly for generics); consult specific product labeling.

Capsule, oral: Hydrochlorothiazide 25 mg and triamterene 37.5 mg; hydrochlorothiazide 25 mg and triamterene 50 mg

Dyazide®: Hydrochlorothiazide 25 mg and triamterene 37.5 mg

Tablet: Hydrochlorothiazide 25 mg and triamterene 37.5 mg; hydrochlorothiazide 50 mg and triamterene 75 mg

Maxzide®: Hydrochlorothiazide 50 mg and triamterene 75 mg [scored]

Maxzide®-25: Hydrochlorothiazide 25 mg and triamterene 37.5 mg [scored]

◆ **Hydrochlorothiazide and Valsartan** see Valsartan and Hydrochlorothiazide on page 1998
◆ **Hydrochlorothiazide, Olmesartan, and Amlodipine** see Olmesartan, Amlodipine, and Hydrochlorothiazide on page 1412
◆ **Hydrocil® Instant [OTC]** see Psyllium on page 1635

Hydrocodone and Acetaminophen (hye droe KOE done & a seet a MIN oh fen)

Related Information
Acetaminophen on page 31
Medication Safety Issues
Sound-alike/look-alike issues:
Lorcet® may be confused with Fioricet®
Lortab® may be confused with Cortef®
Vicodin® may be confused with Hycodan, Indocin®
Zydone® may be confused with Vytone
High alert medication:
The Institute for Safe Medication Practices (ISMP) includes this medication among its list of drug classes which have a heightened risk of causing significant patient harm when used in error.
Other safety concerns:
Duplicate therapy issues: This product contains acetaminophen, which may be a component of other combination products. Do not exceed the maximum recommended daily dose of acetaminophen.

Brand Names: U.S. hycet®; Lorcet® 10/650; Lorcet® Plus; Lortab®; Margesic® H; Maxidone®; Norco®; Stagesic™; Vicodin®; Vicodin® ES; Vicodin® HP; Xodol® 10/300; Xodol® 5/300; Xodol® 7.5/300; Zamicet™; Zolvit®; Zydone®
Index Terms Acetaminophen and Hydrocodone
Generic Availability (U.S.) Yes: Oral solution, tablet
Pharmacologic Category Analgesic Combination (Opioid)
Use Relief of moderate-to-severe pain
Contraindications Hypersensitivity to hydrocodone, acetaminophen, or any component of the formulation; CNS depression; severe respiratory depression
Warnings/Precautions Use with caution in patients with hypersensitivity reactions to other phenanthrene derivative opioid agonists (morphine, hydromorphone, levorphanol, oxycodone, oxymorphone); tolerance or drug dependence may result from extended use. Concurrent use of agonist/antagonist analgesics may precipitate withdrawal symptoms and/or reduced analgesic efficacy in patients following prolonged therapy with mu opioid agonists. Abrupt discontinuation following prolonged use may also lead to withdrawal symptoms.

Respiratory depressant effects may be increased with head injuries. Use caution with acute abdominal conditions; clinical course may be obscured. Use caution with adrenal insufficiency, biliary tract impairment, morbidly obese patients, toxic psychosis, thyroid dysfunction, prostatic hyperplasia, respiratory disease, hepatic or renal disease, and in the debilitated or elderly. Causes sedation; caution must be used in performing tasks which require alertness (eg, operating machinery or driving). Effects may be potentiated when used with other sedative drugs or ethanol. May cause hypotension.

Due to the role of CYP2D6 in the metabolism of hydrocodone to hydromorphone (an active metabolite with higher binding affinity to mu-opioid receptors compared to hydrocodone), patients with genetic variations of CYP2D6, including "poor metabolizers" or "extensive metabolizers," may have decreased or increased hydromorphone formation, respectively. Variable effects in positive and negative opioid effects have been reported in these patients;

however, limited data exists to determine if clinically significant differences of analgesia and toxicity can be predicted based on CYP2D6 phenotype (Hutchinson, 2004; Otton, 1993; Zhou, 2009).

[U.S. Boxed Warning]: Acetaminophen may cause severe hepatotoxicity, potentially requiring liver transplant or resulting in death; hepatotoxicity is usually associated with excessive acetaminophen intake (>4 g/day). Risk is increased with alcohol use, pre-existing liver disease, and intake of more than one source of acetaminophen-containing medications. Chronic daily dosing in adults has also resulted in liver damage in some patients. Hypersensitivity and anaphylactic reactions have been reported with acetaminophen use; discontinue immediately if symptoms of allergic or hypersensitivity reactions occur. Use caution in patients with known G6PD deficiency.

Adverse Reactions (Reflective of adult population; not specific for elderly) Frequency not defined.

Cardiovascular: Bradycardia, cardiac arrest, circulatory collapse, coma, hypotension

Central nervous system: Anxiety, dizziness, drowsiness, dysphoria, euphoria, fear, lethargy, lightheadedness, malaise, mental clouding, mental impairment, mood changes, physiological dependence, sedation, somnolence, stupor

Dermatologic: Pruritus, rash

Endocrine & metabolic: Hypoglycemic coma

Gastrointestinal: Abdominal pain, constipation, gastric distress, heartburn, nausea, peptic ulcer, vomiting, xerostomia

Genitourinary: Ureteral spasm, urinary retention, vesical sphincter spasm

Hematologic: Agranulocytosis, bleeding time prolonged, hemolytic anemia, iron deficiency anemia, occult blood loss, thrombocytopenia

Hepatic: Hepatic necrosis, hepatitis

Neuromuscular & skeletal: Skeletal muscle rigidity

Otic: Hearing impairment or loss (chronic overdose)

Renal: Renal toxicity, renal tubular necrosis

Respiratory: Acute airway obstruction, apnea, dyspnea, respiratory depression (dose related)

Miscellaneous: Allergic reactions, clamminess, diaphoresis

Drug Interactions

Metabolism/Transport Effects Refer to individual components.

Avoid Concomitant Use

Avoid concomitant use of Hydrocodone and Acetaminophen with any of the following: Azelastine; Azelastine (Nasal); Methadone; Mirtazapine; Paraldehyde; Pimozide

Increased Effect/Toxicity

Hydrocodone and Acetaminophen may increase the levels/effects of: Alcohol (Ethyl); Alvimopan; ARIPiprazole; Azelastine; Azelastine (Nasal); Busulfan; CNS Depressants; Dasatinib; Desmopressin; Imatinib; Methadone; Metyrosine; Mirtazapine; Paraldehyde; Pimozide; Prilocaine; Selective Serotonin Reuptake Inhibitors; SORAfenib; Thiazide Diuretics; Vitamin K Antagonists; Zolpidem

The levels/effects of Hydrocodone and Acetaminophen may be increased by: Amphetamines; Antipsychotic Agents (Phenothiazines); Dasatinib; Droperidol; HydrOXYzine; Imatinib; Isoniazid; MAO Inhibitors; Metyrapone; Probenecid; SORAfenib; Succinylcholine

Decreased Effect

Hydrocodone and Acetaminophen may decrease the levels/effects of: Pegvisomant

The levels/effects of Hydrocodone and Acetaminophen may be decreased by: Ammonium Chloride; Anticonvulsants (Hydantoin); Barbiturates; CarBAMazepine; Cholestyramine Resin; Mixed Agonist / Antagonist Opioids; Peginterferon Alfa-2b; QuiNIDine; Tocilizumab

Ethanol/Nutrition/Herb Interactions

Ethanol: Consuming ≥3 alcoholic drinks/day may increase the risk of liver damage. Ethanol may also increase CNS depression; monitor for increased effects with coadministration. Caution patients about effects.

Herb/Nutraceutical: Avoid valerian, St John's wort, SAMe, kava kava (may increase risk of excessive sedation).

Mechanism of Action Hydrocodone, as with other narcotic (opiate) analgesics, blocks pain perception in the cerebral cortex by binding to specific receptor molecules (opiate receptors) within the neuronal membranes of synapses. This binding results in a decreased synaptic chemical transmission throughout the CNS thus inhibiting the flow of pain sensations into the higher centers. Mu and kappa are the two subtypes of the opiate receptor which hydrocodone binds to cause analgesia.

Acetaminophen inhibits the synthesis of prostaglandins in the CNS and peripherally blocks pain impulse generation; produces antipyresis from inhibition of hypothalamic heat-regulating center.

Pharmacodynamics/Kinetics

Acetaminophen: See Acetaminophen monograph.

Hydrocodone:

Onset of action: Narcotic analgesic: 10-20 minutes

Duration: 4-8 hours

Metabolism: Hepatic; O-demethylation via primarily CYP2D6 to hydromorphone (major, active metabolite with ~10- to 33-fold higher or as much as a >100-fold higher binding affinity for the mu-opioid receptor than hydrocodone); N-demethylation via CYP3A4 to norhydrocodone (major metabolite); and ~40% of metabolism/clearance occurs via other non-CYP pathways, including 6-ketosteroid reduction to 6-alpha-hydrocol and 6-beta-hydrocol, and other elimination pathways (eg, fecal, biliary, intestinal, renal) (Hutchinson, 2004; Volpe, 2011; Zhou, 2009)

Half-life elimination: 3.3-4.4 hours

Excretion: Urine (26% of single dose in 72 hours, with ~12% as unchanged drug, 5% as norhydrocodone, 4% as conjugated hydrocodone, 3% as 6-hydrocodol, and 0.21% as conjugated 6-hydromorphol (Zhou, 2009)

Dosage

Geriatric Doses should be titrated to appropriate analgesic effect; 2.5-5 mg of the hydrocodone component every 4-6 hours. Do not exceed 4 g/day of acetaminophen.

Adult Pain management (analgesic): Oral (doses should be titrated to appropriate analgesic effect): Average starting dose in opioid naive patients: Hydrocodone 5-10 mg 4 times/day; the dosage of acetaminophen should be limited to ≤4 g/day (and possibly less in patients with hepatic impairment or ethanol use).

Dosage ranges (based on specific product labeling): Hydrocodone 2.5-10 mg every 4-6 hours (maximum dose of hydrocodone may be limited by the acetaminophen content of specific product)

Hepatic Impairment Use with caution. Limited, low-dose therapy usually well tolerated in hepatic disease/cirrhosis; however, cases of hepatotoxicity at daily acetaminophen dosages <4 g/day have been reported. Avoid chronic use in hepatic impairment.

Monitoring Parameters Pain relief, respiratory and mental status, blood pressure

Test Interactions Acetaminophen may cause false-positive urinary 5-hydroxyindoleacetic acid.

Special Geriatric Considerations Elderly may be particularly susceptible to the CNS depressant action (sedation, confusion) and constipating effects of narcotics.

Controlled Substance C-III

Dosage Forms Excipient information presented when available (limited, particularly for generics); consult specific product labeling.

Capsule, oral:

Margesic® H, Stagesic™: Hydrocodone bitartrate 5 mg and acetaminophen 500 mg

Elixir, oral:

Lortab®: Hydrocodone bitartrate 7.5 mg and acetaminophen 500 mg per 15 mL (480 mL) [contains ethanol 7%, propylene glycol; tropical fruit punch flavor]

Solution, oral: Hydrocodone bitartrate 7.5 mg and acetaminophen 325 mg per 15 mL; hydrocodone bitartrate 7.5 mg and acetaminophen 500 mg per 15 mL (5 mL, 10 mL, 15 mL, 118 mL, 473 mL); hydrocodone bitartrate 10 mg and acetaminophen 325 mg per 15 mL (7.5 mL, 15 mL)

hycet®: Hydrocodone bitartrate 7.5 mg and acetaminophen 325 mg per 15 mL (473 mL) [contains ethanol 7%, propylene glycol; tropical fruit punch flavor]

Zamicet™: Hydrocodone bitartrate 10 mg and acetaminophen 325 mg per 15 mL (473 mL) [contains ethanol 6.7%, propylene glycol; fruit flavor]

Zolvit®: Hydrocodone bitartrate 10 mg and acetaminophen 300 mg per 15 mL (480 mL) [contains ethanol 7%, propylene glycol; tropical fruit punch flavor]

Tablet, oral:

Hydrocodone bitartrate 2.5 mg and acetaminophen 500 mg

Hydrocodone bitartrate 5 mg and acetaminophen 300 mg

Hydrocodone bitartrate 5 mg and acetaminophen 325 mg

Hydrocodone bitartrate 5 mg and acetaminophen 500 mg

Hydrocodone bitartrate 7.5 mg and acetaminophen 300 mg

Hydrocodone bitartrate 7.5 mg and acetaminophen 325 mg

Hydrocodone bitartrate 7.5 mg and acetaminophen 500 mg

Hydrocodone bitartrate 7.5 mg and acetaminophen 650 mg

Hydrocodone bitartrate 7.5 mg and acetaminophen 750 mg

Hydrocodone bitartrate 10 mg and acetaminophen 300 mg

Hydrocodone bitartrate 10 mg and acetaminophen 325 mg

Hydrocodone bitartrate 10 mg and acetaminophen 500 mg

Hydrocodone bitartrate 10 mg and acetaminophen 650 mg

Hydrocodone bitartrate 10 mg and acetaminophen 660 mg

◀

Hydrocodone bitartrate 10 mg and acetaminophen 750 mg
Lorcet® 10/650: Hydrocodone bitartrate 10 mg and acetaminophen 650 mg
Lorcet® Plus: Hydrocodone bitartrate 7.5 mg and acetaminophen 650 mg
Lortab®:
  5/500: Hydrocodone bitartrate 5 mg and acetaminophen 500 mg
  7.5/500: Hydrocodone bitartrate 7.5 mg and acetaminophen 500 mg
  10/500: Hydrocodone bitartrate 10 mg and acetaminophen 500 mg
Maxidone®: Hydrocodone bitartrate 10 mg and acetaminophen 750 mg
Norco®:
  Hydrocodone bitartrate 5 mg and acetaminophen 325 mg
  Hydrocodone bitartrate 7.5 mg and acetaminophen 325 mg
  Hydrocodone bitartrate 10 mg and acetaminophen 325 mg
Vicodin®: Hydrocodone bitartrate 5 mg and acetaminophen 500 mg
Vicodin® ES: Hydrocodone bitartrate 7.5 mg and acetaminophen 750 mg
Vicodin® HP: Hydrocodone bitartrate 10 mg and acetaminophen 660 mg
Xodol®:
  5/300: Hydrocodone bitartrate 5 mg and acetaminophen 300 mg
  7.5/300: Hydrocodone bitartrate 7.5 mg and acetaminophen 300 mg
  10/300: Hydrocodone bitartrate 10 mg and acetaminophen 300 mg
Zydone®:
  Hydrocodone bitartrate 5 mg and acetaminophen 400 mg
  Hydrocodone bitartrate 7.5 mg and acetaminophen 400 mg
  Hydrocodone bitartrate 10 mg and acetaminophen 400 mg

Hydrocortisone (Systemic) (hye droe KOR ti sone)

Related Information
  Corticosteroids Systemic Equivalencies *on page 2112*
Medication Safety Issues
  Sound-alike/look-alike issues:
  Hydrocortisone may be confused with hydrocodone, hydroxychloroquine, hydrochlorothiazide
  Cortef® may be confused with Coreg®, Lortab®
  HCT (occasional abbreviation for hydrocortisone) is an error-prone abbreviation (mistaken as hydrochlorothiazide)
  Solu-CORTEF® may be confused with Solu-MEDROL®
Brand Names: U.S. A-Hydrocort®; Cortef®; Solu-CORTEF®
Brand Names: Canada Cortef®; Solu-Cortef®
Index Terms A-hydroCort; Compound F; Cortisol; Hydrocortisone Sodium Succinate
Generic Availability (U.S.) Yes: Tablet
Pharmacologic Category Corticosteroid, Systemic
Use Management of adrenocortical insufficiency; anti-inflammatory or immunosuppressive
Unlabeled Use Management of septic shock when blood pressure is poorly responsive to fluid resuscitation and vasopressor therapy; treatment of thyroid storm
Contraindications Hypersensitivity to hydrocortisone or any component of the formulation; serious infections, except septic shock or tuberculous meningitis; viral, fungal, or tubercular skin lesions; I.M. administration contraindicated in idiopathic thrombocytopenia purpura; intrathecal administration of injection
Warnings/Precautions Use with caution in patients with thyroid disease, hepatic impairment, renal impairment, heart failure, hypertension, diabetes, glaucoma, cataracts, myasthenia gravis, patients at risk for osteoporosis, patients at risk for seizures, or GI diseases (diverticulitis, peptic ulcer, ulcerative colitis) due to perforation risk. Use caution following acute MI (corticosteroids have been associated with myocardial rupture). Because of the risk of adverse effects, systemic corticosteroids should be used cautiously in the elderly in the smallest possible effective dose for the shortest duration. Withdraw therapy with gradual tapering of dose.

May cause hypercorticism or suppression of hypothalamic-pituitary-adrenal (HPA) axis, particularly in patients receiving high doses for prolonged periods. HPA axis suppression may lead to adrenal crisis. Withdrawal and discontinuation of a corticosteroid should be done slowly and carefully. Particular care is required when patients are transferred from systemic corticosteroids to inhaled products due to possible adrenal insufficiency or withdrawal from steroids, including an increase in allergic symptoms. Patients receiving >20 mg per day of prednisone (or equivalent) may be most susceptible. Fatalities have occurred due to adrenal insufficiency in asthmatic patients during and after transfer from systemic corticosteroids to aerosol steroids; aerosol steroids do not provide the systemic steroid needed to treat patients having trauma, surgery, or infections.

Acute myopathy has been reported with high dose corticosteroids, usually in patients with neuromuscular transmission disorders; may involve ocular and/or respiratory muscles; monitor creatine kinase; recovery may be delayed. Corticosteroid use may cause psychiatric disturbances, including depression, euphoria, insomnia, mood swings, and personality changes. Pre-existing psychiatric conditions may be exacerbated by corticosteroid use. Prolonged use of corticosteroids may also increase the incidence of secondary infection, mask acute infection (including fungal infections), prolong or exacerbate viral infections, or limit response to vaccines. Exposure to chickenpox should be avoided; corticosteroids should not be used to treat ocular herpes simplex. Corticosteroids should not be used for cerebral malaria or viral hepatitis. Oral steroid treatment is not recommended for the treatment of acute optic neuritis. Close observation is required in patients with latent tuberculosis and/or TB reactivity; restrict use in active TB (only in conjunction with antituberculosis treatment). Prolonged treatment with corticosteroids has been associated with the development of Kaposi's sarcoma (case reports); if noted, discontinuation of therapy should be considered. High-dose corticosteroids should not be used to manage acute head injury. Some dosage forms contain benzyl alcohol.

Adverse Reactions (Reflective of adult population; not specific for elderly) Frequency not defined.

Cardiovascular: Arrhythmias, bradycardia, cardiac arrest, cardiomegaly, circulatory collapse, congestive heart failure, edema, fat embolism, hypertension, hypertrophic cardiomyopathy (premature infants), myocardial rupture (post MI), syncope, tachycardia, thromboembolism, vasculitis

Central nervous system: Delirium, depression, emotional instability, euphoria, hallucinations, headache, insomnia, intracranial pressure increased, malaise, mood swings, nervousness, neuritis, neuropathy, personality changes, pseudotumor cerebri, psychic disorders, psychoses, seizure, vertigo

Dermatologic: Acne, allergic dermatitis, alopecia, bruising, burning/tingling, dry scaly skin, edema, erythema, hirsutism, hyper-/hypopigmentation, impaired wound healing, petechiae, rash, skin atrophy, skin test reaction impaired, sterile abscess, striae, urticaria

Endocrine & metabolic: Adrenal suppression, alkalosis, amenorrhea, carbohydrate intolerance increased, Cushing's syndrome, diabetes mellitus, glucose intolerance, growth suppression, hyperglycemia, hyperlipidemia, hypokalemia, hypokalemic alkalosis, menstrual irregularities, negative nitrogen balance, pituitary-adrenal axis suppression, potassium loss, protein catabolism, sodium and water retention, sperm motility increased/decreased, spermatogenesis increased/decreased

Gastrointestinal: Abdominal distention, appetite increased, bowel dysfunction (intrathecal administration), indigestion, nausea, pancreatitis, peptic ulcer, gastrointestinal perforation, ulcerative esophagitis, vomiting, weight gain

Genitourinary: Bladder dysfunction (intrathecal administration)

Hematologic: Leukocytosis (transient)

Hepatic: Hepatomegaly, transaminases increased

Local: Atrophy (at injection site), postinjection flare (intra-articular use), thrombophlebitis

Neuromuscular & skeletal: Arthralgia, necrosis (femoral and humoral heads), Charcot-like arthropathy, fractures, muscle mass loss, muscle weakness, myopathy, osteoporosis, tendon rupture, vertebral compression fractures

Ocular: Cataracts, exophthalmoses, glaucoma, intraocular pressure increased

Miscellaneous: Abnormal fat deposits, anaphylaxis, avascular necrosis, diaphoresis, hiccups, hypersensitivity reactions, infection, secondary malignancy

Drug Interactions

Metabolism/Transport Effects Substrate of CYP3A4 (minor), P-glycoprotein; **Note:** Assignment of Major/Minor substrate status based on clinically relevant drug interaction potential; **Induces** CYP3A4 (weak/moderate)

Avoid Concomitant Use

Avoid concomitant use of Hydrocortisone (Systemic) with any of the following: Aldesleukin; Axitinib; BCG; Mifepristone; Natalizumab; Pimecrolimus; Tacrolimus (Topical)

Increased Effect/Toxicity

Hydrocortisone (Systemic) may increase the levels/effects of: Acetylcholinesterase Inhibitors; Amphotericin B; Deferasirox; Leflunomide; Loop Diuretics; Natalizumab; NSAID (COX-2 Inhibitor); NSAID (Nonselective); Thiazide Diuretics; Vaccines (Live); Warfarin

The levels/effects of Hydrocortisone (Systemic) may be increased by: Antifungal Agents (Azole Derivatives, Systemic); Aprepitant; Calcium Channel Blockers (Nondihydropyridine); Denosumab; Estrogen Derivatives; Fluconazole; Fosaprepitant; Indacaterol; Macrolide Antibiotics; Mifepristone; Neuromuscular-Blocking Agents (Nondepolarizing); P-glycoprotein/ABCB1 Inhibitors; Pimecrolimus; Quinolone Antibiotics; Roflumilast; Salicylates; Tacrolimus (Topical); Telaprevir; Trastuzumab

Decreased Effect

Hydrocortisone (Systemic) may decrease the levels/effects of: Aldesleukin; Antidiabetic Agents; ARIPiprazole; Axitinib; BCG; Calcitriol; Coccidioidin Skin Test; Corticorelin; Hyaluronidase; Isoniazid; Salicylates; Sipuleucel-T; Telaprevir; Vaccines (Inactivated)

The levels/effects of Hydrocortisone (Systemic) may be decreased by: Aminoglutethimide; Antacids; Barbiturates; Bile Acid Sequestrants; Echinacea; Mifepristone; Mitotane; P-glycoprotein/ABCB1 Inducers; Primidone; Rifamycin Derivatives; Tocilizumab

Ethanol/Nutrition/Herb Interactions

Ethanol: Avoid ethanol (may enhance gastric mucosal irritation).

Food: Hydrocortisone interferes with calcium absorption.

Herb/Nutraceutical: St John's wort may decrease hydrocortisone levels. Avoid cat's claw, echinacea (have immunostimulant properties).

Stability Store at controlled room temperature 20°C to 25°C (68°F to 77°F). Protect from light. Hydrocortisone sodium phosphate and hydrocortisone sodium succinate are clear, light yellow solutions which are heat labile.

Sodium succinate: Reconstitute 100 mg vials with bacteriostatic water (not >2 mL). Act-O-Vial (self-contained powder for injection plus diluent) may be reconstituted by pressing the activator to force diluent into the powder compartment. Following gentle agitation, solution may be withdrawn via syringe through a needle inserted into the center of the stopper. May be administered (I.V. or I.M.) without further dilution. After initial reconstitution, hydrocortisone sodium succinate solutions are stable for 3 days at room temperature or under refrigeration when protected from light. Stability of parenteral admixture (Solu-Cortef®) at room temperature (25°C) and at refrigeration temperature (4°C) is concentration-dependent: Stability of concentration 1 mg/mL: 24 hours.

Stability of concentration 2 mg/mL to 60 mg/mL: At least 4 hours.

Solutions for I.V. infusion: Reconstituted solutions may be added to an appropriate volume of compatible solution for infusion. Concentration should generally not exceed 1 mg/mL. However, in cases where administration of a small volume of fluid is desirable, 100-3000 mg may be added to 50 mL of D_5W or NS (stability limited to 4 hours).

Mechanism of Action Decreases inflammation by suppression of migration of polymorphonuclear leukocytes and reversal of increased capillary permeability

Pharmacodynamics/Kinetics

Onset of action: Hydrocortisone sodium succinate (water soluble): Rapid

Absorption: Rapid

Metabolism: Hepatic

Half-life elimination: Biologic: 8-12 hours

Excretion: Urine (primarily as 17-hydroxysteroids and 17-ketosteroids)

Dosage

Geriatric & Adult Dose should be based on severity of disease and patient response.

Adrenal insufficiency (acute): I.M., I.V.: 100 mg I.V. bolus, then 300 mg/day in divided doses every 8 hours or as a continuous infusion for 48 hours. Once patient is stable change to oral, 50 mg every 8 hours for 6 doses, then taper to 30-50 mg/day in divided doses.

Adrenal insufficiency (chronic), physiologic replacement (unlabeled dosing): Oral: 15-25 mg/day in 2-3 divided doses. **Note:** Studies suggest administering one-half to two-thirds of the daily dose in the morning in order to mimic the physiological cortisol secretion pattern. If the twice-daily regimen is utilized, the second dose should be administered 6-8 hours following the first dose (Arlt, 2003).

Anti-inflammatory or immunosuppressive: Oral, I.M., I.V.: 15-240 mg every 12 hours

Congenital adrenal hyperplasia (unlabeled dosing): Oral: 15-25 mg/day in 2-3 divided doses (Speiser, 2010)

Status asthmaticus: I.V.: 1-2 mg/kg/dose every 6 hours for 24 hours, then maintenance of 0.5-1 mg/kg every 6 hours

Stress dosing (surgery) in patients known to be adrenally-suppressed or on chronic systemic steroids: I.V.:

Minor stress (ie, inguinal herniorrhaphy): 25 mg/day for 1 day

Moderate stress (ie, joint replacement, cholecystectomy): 50-75 mg/day (25 mg every 8-12 hours) for 1-2 days

Major stress (pancreatoduodenectomy, esophagogastrectomy, cardiac surgery): 100-150 mg/day (50 mg every 8-12 hours) for 2-3 days

Septic shock (unlabeled use): I.V.: 50 mg every 6 hours (Annane, 2002; Marik, 2008); not to exceed 300 mg/day (Dellinger, 2008). Practice guidelines also recommend alternative dosing of 100 mg bolus, followed by continuous infusion of 10 mg/hour (240 mg/day). Taper slowly (for total of 11 days) and do not stop abruptly. **Note:** Fludrocortisone is optional with use of hydrocortisone.

Thyroid storm (unlabeled use): I.V.: 300 mg loading dose, followed by 100 mg every 8 hours (Bahn, 2011)

Administration

Oral: Administer with food or milk to decrease GI upset

Parenteral: Hydrocortisone sodium succinate may be administered by I.M. or I.V. routes. Dermal and/or subdermal skin depression may occur at the site of injection. Avoid injection into deltoid muscle (high incidence of subcutaneous atrophy).

I.V. bolus: Dilute to 50 mg/mL and administer over 30 seconds or over 10 minutes for doses ≥500 mg

I.V. intermittent infusion: Dilute to 1 mg/mL and administer over 20-30 minutes

Monitoring Parameters Serum glucose, electrolytes; blood pressure, weight, presence of infection; monitor IOP with therapy >6 weeks; bone mineral density

Reference Range Therapeutic: AM: 5-25 mcg/dL (SI: 138-690 nmol/L), PM: 2-9 mcg/dL (SI: 55-248 nmol/L) depending on test, assay

Test Interactions Interferes with skin tests

Special Geriatric Considerations Because of the risk of adverse effects, systemic cortico-steroids should be used cautiously in the elderly, in the smallest possible dose, and for the shortest possible time.

Dosage Forms Excipient information presented when available (limited, particularly for generics); consult specific product labeling.

Injection, powder for reconstitution, as sodium succinate [strength expressed as base]:
A-Hydrocort®: 100 mg
Solu-CORTEF®: 100 mg

Injection, powder for reconstitution, as sodium succinate [strength expressed as base, preservative free]:
Solu-CORTEF®: 100 mg, 250 mg, 500 mg, 1000 mg [supplied with diluent]

Tablet, oral, as base: 5 mg, 10 mg, 20 mg
Cortef®: 5 mg, 10 mg, 20 mg [scored]

Hydrocortisone (Topical) (hye droe KOR ti sone)

Related Information

Topical Corticosteroids on page 2113

Medication Safety Issues

Sound-alike/look-alike issues:

Hydrocortisone may be confused with hydrocodone, hydroxychloroquine, hydrochlorothia-zide

Anusol® may be confused with Anusol-HC®, Aplisol®, Aquasol®

Cortizone® may be confused with cortisone

HCT (occasional abbreviation for hydrocortisone) is an error-prone abbreviation (mistaken as hydrochlorothiazide)

Hytone® may be confused with Vytone®

Proctocort® may be confused with ProctoCream®

International issues:

Nutracort [multiple international markets] may be confused with Nitrocor brand name of nitroglycerin [Italy, Russia, and Venezuela]

Brand Names: U.S. Ala-Cort; Ala-Scalp; Anu-med HC; Anucort-HC™; Anusol-HC®; Aquanil HC® [OTC]; Beta-HC® [OTC]; Caldecort® [OTC]; Colocort®; Cortaid® Advanced [OTC]; Cortaid® Intensive Therapy [OTC]; Cortaid® Maximum Strength [OTC]; Cortenema®; Corti-Cool® [OTC]; Cortifoam®; Cortizone-10® Hydratensive Healing [OTC]; Cortizone-10® Hydra-tensive Soothing [OTC]; Cortizone-10® Intensive Healing Eczema [OTC]; Cortizone-10® Maximum Strength Cooling Relief [OTC]; Cortizone-10® Maximum Strength Easy Relief [OTC]; Cortizone-10® Maximum Strength Intensive Healing Formula [OTC]; Cortizone-10® Maximum Strength [OTC]; Cortizone-10® Plus Maximum Strength [OTC]; Dermarest® Eczema Medicated [OTC]; Hemril® -30; Hydrocortisone Plus [OTC]; Hydroskin® [OTC]; Locoid Lipocream® [OTC]; Locoid®; Pandel®; Pediaderm™ HC; Preparation H® Hydrocortisone [OTC]; Procto-Pak™; Proctocort®; ProctoCream®-HC; Proctosol-HC®; Proctozone-HC 2.5%™; Recort [OTC]; Scalpana [OTC]; Texacort™; U-Cort®; Westcort®

Brand Names: Canada Aquacort®; Cortamed®; Cortenema®; Cortifoam™; Emo-Cort®; Hycort™; Hyderm; HydroVal®; Locoid®; Prevex® HC; Sarna® HC; Westcort®

Index Terms A-hydroCort; Compound F; Cortisol; Hemorrhoidal HC; Hydrocortisone Acetate; Hydrocortisone Butyrate; Hydrocortisone Probutate; Hydrocortisone Valerate; Nutracort

Generic Availability (U.S.) Yes: Excludes foam (acetate), cream (probutate), gel (base), liquid (base), lotion (base), lotion (butyrate), solution (base)

Pharmacologic Category Corticosteroid, Rectal; Corticosteroid, Topical

HYDROCORTISONE (TOPICAL)

Use Relief of inflammation of corticosteroid-responsive dermatoses (low and medium potency topical corticosteroid); adjunctive treatment of ulcerative colitis; mild-to-moderate atopic dermatitis; inflamed hemorrhoids, postirradiation (factitial) proctitis, and other inflammatory conditions of anorectum and pruritus ani

Dosage

Geriatric & Adult

Dermatosis: Topical: Apply thin film to affected area 2-4 times/day.

Hydrocortisone probutate (Pandel®): Topical: Apply thin film to affected area 1-2 times/day

Hydrocortisone valerate (Westcort®): Topical: Apply thin film to affected area 2-3 times/day

External anal and genital itching: Topical (OTC labeling): Apply to clean dry skin up to 3-4 times/day

Hemorrhoids: Rectal: One suppository (30 mg) twice daily for 2 weeks. For severe cases of proctitis, 1 suppository 3 times/day or 2 suppositories twice daily may be needed. For factitial proctitis, duration of treatment may be up to 6-8 weeks.

Ulcerative colitis: Rectal:

Foam: One applicatorful (80 mg) 1-2 times/day for 2-3 weeks, and then every other day thereafter; use lowest dose to maintain clinical response; taper dose to discontinue long-term therapy

Suspension: One enema (100 mg) every night for 21 days or until remission (clinical improvement may precede improvement of mucosal integrity); 2-3 months of therapy may be required; taper dose to discontinue long-term therapy

Special Geriatric Considerations Instruct patient or caregiver on appropriate use of topical hydrocortisone products.

Dosage Forms Excipient information presented when available (limited, particularly for generics); consult specific product labeling. [DSC] = Discontinued product

Aerosol, foam, rectal, as acetate:

Cortifoam®: 10% (15 g) [90 mg/applicator]

Cream, topical, as acetate: 1% (28.4 g, 454 g); 2% (43 g)

U-Cort®: 1% (28 g) [contains sodium metabisulfite]

Cream, topical, as acetate [strength expressed as base]: 1% (30 g)

Cream, topical, as base: 0.5% (28.4 g, 30 g); 1% (1 g, 1.5 g, 15 g, 28.4 g, 30 g, 114 g, 454 g); 2.5% (20 g, 28 g, 28.35 g, 30 g, 454 g)

Ala-Cort: 1% (28.4 g, 85.2 g)

Anusol-HC®: 2.5% (30 g) [contains benzyl alcohol]

Caldecort®: 1% (28.4 g) [contains aloe]

Cortaid® Advanced: 1% (42 g) [contains aloe]

Cortaid® Intensive Therapy: 1% (37 g, 56 g)

Cortaid® Maximum Strength: 1% (14 g, 28 g, 37 g, 56 g) [contains aloe]

Cortizone-10® Maximum Strength: 1% (15 g, 28 g, 56 g) [contains aloe]

Cortizone-10® Maximum Strength Intensive Healing Formula: 1% (28 g, 56 g) [contains aloe, benzyl alcohol]

Cortizone-10® Plus Maximum Strength: 1% (28 g, 56 g) [contains aloe, vitamin A, vitamin E]

Hydrocortisone Plus: 1% (28.4 g) [contains aloe, vitamin A, vitamin D, vitamin E]

Hydroskin®: 1% (28 g)

Preparation H® Hydrocortisone: 1% (26 g) [contains sodium benzoate]

Procto-Pak™: 1% (28.4 g)

Proctocort®: 1% (28.35 g)

ProctoCream®-HC: 2.5% (30 g) [contains benzyl alcohol]

Proctosol-HC®: 2.5% (28.35 g)

Proctozone-HC 2.5%™: 2.5% (30 g)

Recort: 1% (30 g)

Cream, topical, as butyrate: 0.1% (15 g, 45 g)

Locoid Lipocream®: 0.1% (15 g [DSC], 45 g, 60 g)

Locoid®: 0.1% (15 g, 45 g)

Cream, topical, as probutate:

Pandel®: 0.1% (15 g, 45 g, 80 g)

Cream, topical, as valerate: 0.2% (15 g, 45 g, 60 g)

Gel, topical, as base:

CortiCool®: 1% (0.9 g, 42.5 g) [contains ethanol 20%]

Cortizone-10® Maximum Strength Cooling Relief: 1% (28 g) [contains aloe, ethanol 15%]

Liquid, topical, as base:

Cortizone-10® Maximum Strength Easy Relief: 1% (36 mL) [contains aloe, ethanol 45%]

Scalpana: 1% (85.5 mL)

Lotion, topical, as base: 1% (114 g, 118 mL); 2.5% (59 mL, 60 mL, 118 mL)

Ala-Scalp: 2% (29.6 mL)

Aquanil HC®: 1% (120 mL) [contains benzyl alcohol]

Beta-HC®: 1% (60 mL)

Cortaid® Intensive Therapy: 1% (98 g)
Cortizone-10® Hydratensive Healing: 1% (113 g) [contains aloe]
Cortizone-10® Hydratensive Soothing: 1% (113 g) [contains aloe]
Cortizone-10® Intensive Healing Eczema: 1% (99 g) [contains aloe, vitamin A, vitamin C, vitamin E]
Dermarest® Eczema Medicated: 1% (118 mL)
Hydroskin®: 1% (118 mL)
Lotion, topical, as base [kit]:
Pediaderm™ HC: 2% (29.6 mL) [contains benzalkonium chloride, isopropyl alcohol; packaged with protective emollient]
Lotion, topical, as butyrate:
Locoid®: 0.1% (60 mL)
Ointment, topical, as acetate [strength expressed as base]: 1% (30 g)
Ointment, topical, as base: 0.5% (30 g); 1% (25 g, 30 g, 110 g, 430 g, 454 g); 2.5% (20 g, 30 g, 454 g)
Cortaid® Maximum Strength: 1% (28 g, 37 g)
Cortizone-10® Maximum Strength: 1% (28 g, 56 g)
Ointment, topical, as butyrate: 0.1% (15 g, 45 g)
Locoid®: 0.1% (15 g, 45 g)
Ointment, topical, as valerate: 0.2% (15 g, 45 g, 60 g)
Westcort®: 0.2% (15 g [DSC], 45 g, 60 g)
Powder, for prescription compounding, as acetate [micronized]: USP: 100% (10 g, 25 g, 100 g)
Solution, topical, as base:
Texacort™: 2.5% (30 mL) [contains ethanol 48.8%]
Solution, topical, as base [spray]:
Cortaid® Intensive Therapy: 1% (59 mL) [contains ethanol 45%]
Solution, topical, as butyrate: 0.1% (20 mL, 60 mL)
Locoid®: 0.1% (20 mL, 60 mL) [contains isopropyl alcohol 50%]
Suppository, rectal, as acetate: 25 mg (12s); 30 mg (12s)
Anu-med HC: 25 mg (12s)
Anucort-HC™: 25 mg (12s, 24s, 100s)
Anusol-HC®: 25 mg (12s, 24s)
Hemril® -30: 30 mg (12s, 24s)
Proctocort®: 30 mg (12s, 24s)
Suspension, rectal, as base: 100 mg/60 mL (60 mL)
Colocort®: 100 mg/60 mL (60 mL)
Cortenema®: 100 mg/60 mL (60 mL)

♦ **Hydrocortisone Acetate** see Hydrocortisone (Topical) on page 943
♦ **Hydrocortisone and Ciprofloxacin** see Ciprofloxacin and Hydrocortisone on page 387
♦ **Hydrocortisone Butyrate** see Hydrocortisone (Topical) on page 943
♦ **Hydrocortisone, Neomycin, Colistin, and Thonzonium** see Neomycin, Colistin, Hydrocortisone, and Thonzonium on page 1355
♦ **Hydrocortisone Plus [OTC]** see Hydrocortisone (Topical) on page 943
♦ **Hydrocortisone Probutate** see Hydrocortisone (Topical) on page 943
♦ **Hydrocortisone Sodium Succinate** see Hydrocortisone (Systemic) on page 940
♦ **Hydrocortisone Valerate** see Hydrocortisone (Topical) on page 943
♦ **Hydrodiuril** see Hydrochlorothiazide on page 933

HYDROmorphone (hye droe MOR fone)

Related Information
Opioid Analgesics on page 2122
Patient Information for Disposal of Unused Medications on page 2244
Medication Safety Issues
Sound-alike/look-alike issues:
Dilaudid® may be confused with Demerol®, Dilantin®
HYDROmorphone may be confused with morphine; significant overdoses have occurred when hydromorphone products have been inadvertently administered instead of morphine sulfate. Commercially available prefilled syringes of both products looks similar and are often stored in close proximity to each other. **Note:** Hydromorphone 1 mg oral is

approximately equal to morphine 4 mg oral; hydromorphone 1 mg I.V. is approximately equal to morphine 5 mg I.V.

High alert medication:
The Institute for Safe Medication Practices (ISMP) includes this medication among its list of drug classes which have a heightened risk of causing significant patient harm when used in error.

Administration issues:
Dilaudid®, Dilaudid-HP®: Extreme caution should be taken to avoid confusing the highly-concentrated (Dilaudid-HP®) injection with the less-concentrated (Dilaudid®) injectable product.

Exalgo™: Extreme caution should be taken to avoid confusing the extended release Exalgo™ 8 mg tablets with immediate release hydromorphone 8 mg tablets.

Significant differences exist between oral and I.V. dosing. Use caution when converting from one route of administration to another.

Brand Names: U.S. Dilaudid-HP®; Dilaudid®; Exalgo™

Brand Names: Canada Dilaudid-HP-Plus®; Dilaudid-HP®; Dilaudid-XP®; Dilaudid®; Dilaudid® Sterile Powder; Hydromorph Contin®; Hydromorph-IR®; Hydromorphone HP; Hydromorphone HP® 10; Hydromorphone HP® 20; Hydromorphone HP® 50; Hydromorphone HP® Forte; Hydromorphone Hydrochloride Injection, USP; Jurnista™; PMS-Hydromorphone

Index Terms Dihydromorphinone; Hydromorphone Hydrochloride

Generic Availability (U.S.) Yes: Excludes extended release tablet, powder for injection

Pharmacologic Category Analgesic, Opioid

Use Management of moderate-to-severe pain

Exalgo™: Management of moderate-to-severe pain in opioid-tolerant patients (requiring around-the-clock analgesia for an extended period of time)

Prescribing and Access Restrictions Exalgo™: As a requirement of the REMS program, healthcare providers who prescribe Exalgo™ need to receive training on the proper use and potential risks of Exalgo™. For training, please refer to http://www.exalgorems.com. Prescribers will need retraining every 2 years or following any significant changes to the Exalgo™ REMS program.

Medication Guide Available Yes

Contraindications Hypersensitivity to hydromorphone, any component of the formulation; acute or severe asthma, severe respiratory depression (in absence of resuscitative equipment or ventilatory support); severe CNS depression; obstetrical analgesia

Warnings/Precautions Use with caution in patients with hypersensitivity reactions to other phenanthrene derivative opioid agonists (codeine, hydrocodone, levorphanol, oxycodone, oxymorphone). Hydromorphone shares toxic potential of opiate agonists, including CNS depression and respiratory depression. Precautions associated with opiate agonist therapy should be observed. May cause CNS depression, which may impair physical or mental abilities; patients must be cautioned about performing tasks which require mental alertness (eg, operating machinery or driving). Myoclonus and seizures have been reported with high doses. Critical respiratory depression may occur, even at therapeutic dosages, particularly in elderly or debilitated patients or in patients with pre-existing respiratory compromise (hypoxia and/or hypercapnia). Use caution in COPD or other obstructive pulmonary disease. Use with caution in patients with hypersensitivity to other phenanthrene opiates, kyphoscoliosis, cardiovascular disease, morbid obesity, adrenocortical insufficiency, hypothyroidism, acute alcoholism, delirium tremens, toxic psychoses, prostatic hyperplasia and/or urinary stricture, or severe liver or renal failure. Use with caution in patients with biliary tract dysfunction. Hydromorphone may increase biliary tract pressure following spasm in sphincter of Oddi. Use caution in patients with inflammatory or obstructive bowel disorder, acute pancreatitis secondary to biliary tract disease, and patients undergoing biliary surgery. Use extreme caution in patients with head injury, intracranial lesions, or elevated intracranial pressure; exaggerated elevation of ICP may occur (in addition, hydromorphone may complicate neurologic evaluation due to pupillary dilation and CNS depressant effects). Use with caution in patients with depleted blood volume or drugs which may exaggerate hypotensive effects (including phenothiazines or general anesthetics). May obscure diagnosis or clinical course of patients with acute abdominal conditions.

[U.S. Boxed Warning]: Hydromorphone has a high potential for abuse. Those at risk for opioid abuse include patients with a history of substance abuse or mental illness. Tolerance or drug dependence may result from extended use; however, concerns for abuse should not prevent effective management of pain. In general, abrupt discontinuation of therapy in dependent patients should be avoided.

An opioid-containing analgesic regimen should be tailored to each patient's needs and based upon the type of pain being treated (acute versus chronic), the route of administration, degree of tolerance for opioids (naive versus chronic user), age, weight, and medical condition. The optimal analgesic dose varies widely among patients. Doses should be titrated to pain relief/prevention. I.M. use may result in variable absorption and a lag time to peak effect.

Dosage form specific warnings:

[U.S. Boxed Warning]: Dilaudid-HP®: Extreme caution should be taken to avoid confusing the highly-concentrated (Dilaudid-HP®) injection with the less-concentrated (Dilaudid®) injectable product. Dilaudid-HP® should only be used in patients who are opioid-tolerant.

Controlled release: Capsules should only be used when continuous analgesia is required over an extended period of time. Controlled release products are not to be used on an "as needed" (PRN) basis.

Extended release tablets (Exalgo™): [U.S. Boxed Warning]: For use in opioid tolerant patients only; fatal respiratory depression may occur in patient who are not opioid tolerant. Indicated for the management of moderate-to-severe pain when around the clock pain control is needed for an extended time period. Not for use as an as-needed analgesic or for the management of acute or postoperative pain. Tablets should be swallowed whole; do not crush, break, chew, dissolve or inject; doing so may lead to rapid release and absorption of a potentially fatal dose of hydromorphone. Accidental consumption may lead to fatal overdose, especially in children. Exalgo™ tablets are nondeformable; do not administer to patients with preexisting severe gastrointestinal narrowing (eg, esophageal stricture, small bowel inflammatory disease, short gut syndrome, history of peritonitis, cystic fibrosis, chronic intestinal pseudo-obstruction, Meckel's diverticulum); obstruction may occur. Exalgo™ is not recommended for use within 14 days of MAO inhibitors; severe and unpredictable potentiation by MAO inhibitors has been reported with opioid analgesics

Some dosage forms contain trace amounts of sodium metabisulfite which may cause allergic reactions in susceptible individuals.

Adverse Reactions (Reflective of adult population; not specific for elderly) Frequency not defined.

Cardiovascular: Bradycardia, extrasystoles, flushing of face, hyper-/hypotension, palpitation, peripheral edema, peripheral vasodilation, syncope, tachycardia

Central nervous system: Abnormal dreams, abnormal feelings, agitation, aggression, apprehension, attention disturbances, chills, coordination impaired, CNS depression, confusion, cognitive disorder, crying, dizziness, drowsiness, dysphoria, encephalopathy, euphoria, fatigue, hallucinations, headache, hyper-reflexia, hypo/hyperesthesia, hypothermia, increased intracranial pressure, insomnia, lightheadedness, listlessness, malaise, memory impairment, mental depression, mood alterations, nervousness, panic attacks, paranoia, psychomotor hyperactivity, restlessness, sedation, seizure, somnolence, suicide ideation, vertigo

Dermatologic: Hyperhidrosis, pruritus, rash, urticaria

Endocrine & metabolic: Amylase decreased, dehydration, erectile dysfunction, fluid retention, hyperuricemia, hypogonadism, hypokalemia, libido decreased, sexual dysfunction, testosterone decreased

Gastrointestinal: Abdominal distention, anal fissure, anorexia, appetite increased, bezoar (Exalgo™), biliary tract spasm, constipation, diarrhea, diverticulum, diverticulitis, duodenitis, dysgeusia, dysphagia, eructation, flatulence, gastric emptying impaired, gastrointestinal motility disorder (Exalgo™), gastroenteritis, hematochezia, ileus, intestinal obstruction (Exalgo™), large intestine perforation (Exalgo™), nausea, painful defecation, paralytic ileus, stomach cramps, taste perversion, vomiting, weight loss, xerostomia

Genitourinary: Dysuria, micturition disorder, ureteral spasm, urinary frequency, urinary hesitation, urinary retention, urinary tract spasm, urination decreased

Hepatic: LFTs increased

Local: Pain at injection site (I.M.), wheal/flare over vein (I.V.)

Neuromuscular & skeletal: Arthralgia, dysarthria, dyskinesia, muscle rigidity, muscle spasms, myalgia, myoclonus, paresthesia, trembling, tremor, uncoordinated muscle movements, weakness

Ocular: Blurred vision, diplopia, dry eyes, miosis, nystagmus

Otic: Tinnitus

Respiratory: Apnea, bronchospasm, dyspnea, hyperventilation, hypoxia, laryngospasm, oxygen saturation decreased, respiratory depression/distress, rhinorrhea

Miscellaneous: Antidiuretic effects, balance disorder, diaphoresis, difficulty walking, histamine release, physical and psychological dependence

Drug Interactions

Metabolism/Transport Effects None known.

Avoid Concomitant Use

Avoid concomitant use of HYDROmorphone with any of the following: Azelastine; Azelastine (Nasal); MAO Inhibitors; Methadone; Mirtazapine; Paraldehyde

Increased Effect/Toxicity

HYDROmorphone may increase the levels/effects of: Alcohol (Ethyl); Alvimopan; Azelastine; Azelastine (Nasal); CNS Depressants; Desmopressin; Methadone; Metyrosine; Mirtazapine; Paraldehyde; Selective Serotonin Reuptake Inhibitors; Thiazide Diuretics; Zolpidem

The levels/effects of HYDROmorphone may be increased by: Amphetamines; Antipsychotic Agents (Phenothiazines); Droperidol; HydrOXYzine; MAO Inhibitors; Succinylcholine

Decreased Effect

HYDROmorphone may decrease the levels/effects of: Pegvisomant

The levels/effects of HYDROmorphone may be decreased by: Ammonium Chloride; Mixed Agonist / Antagonist Opioids

Ethanol/Nutrition/Herb Interactions

Ethanol: Ethanol may increase CNS depression. Management: Monitor for increased effects with coadministration. Caution patients about effects.

Herb/Nutraceutical: Gotu kola, valerian, and kava kava may increase CNS depression. Management: Avoid gotu kola, valerian, and kava kava.

Stability Store injection and oral dosage forms at 15°C to 30°C (59°F to 86°F). Protect tablets from light. A slightly yellowish discoloration has not been associated with a loss of potency.

Mechanism of Action Binds to opiate receptors in the CNS, causing inhibition of ascending pain pathways, altering the perception of and response to pain; causes cough supression by direct central action in the medulla; produces generalized CNS depression

Pharmacodynamics/Kinetics

Onset of action: Analgesic: Immediate release formulations:

Oral: 15-30 minutes; Peak effect: 30-60 minutes

I.V.: 5 minutes; Peak effect: 10-20 minutes

Duration: Immediate release formulations: Oral, I.V.: 4-5 hours

Absorption: I.M.: Variable and delayed

Distribution: V_d: 4 L/kg

Protein binding: ~8% to 19%

Metabolism: Hepatic via glucuronidation; to inactive metabolites

Bioavailability: 62%

Half-life elimination:

Immediate release formulations: 2-3 hours

Extended release tablets (Exalgo™): ~11 hours

Excretion: Urine (primarily as glucuronide conjugates)

Dosage

Geriatric Doses should be titrated to appropriate analgesic effects. When changing routes of administration, oral doses and parenteral doses are **NOT** equivalent; parenteral doses are up to 5 times more potent. Therefore, when administered parenterally, one-fifth of the oral dose will provide similar analgesia.

Pain: Oral: 1-2 mg every 4-6 hours

Adult

Acute pain (moderate-to-severe): Note: These are guidelines and do not represent the maximum doses that may be required in all patients. Doses should be titrated to provide adequate pain relief. When changing routes of administration, oral doses and parenteral doses are **NOT** equivalent; parenteral doses are up to 5 times more potent. Therefore, when administered parenterally, one-fifth of the oral dose will provide similar analgesia.

Oral: Initial: Opiate-naive: 2-4 mg every 3-4 hours as needed; elderly/debilitated patients may require lower doses; patients with prior opiate exposure may require higher initial doses. **Note:** In adults with severe pain, the American Pain Society recommends an initial dose of 4-8 mg.

I.V.: Initial: Opiate-naive: 0.2-0.6 mg every 2-3 hours as needed; patients with prior opiate exposure may require higher initial doses.

Mechanically ventilated/critically ill patients (unlabeled use): 0.7-4 mg (based on 70 kg patient) every 4 hours as needed. **Note:** More frequent dosing may be needed (eg, every 1-2 hours); dose should be adjusted based on patient response; elderly patients may be more sensitive (Jacobi, 2002).

Continuous infusion: Usual dosage range: 0.5-1 mg/hour (based on 70 kg patient) or 7-15 mcg/kg/**hour**

Patient-controlled analgesia (PCA): **Note:** Opiate-naive: Consider lower end of dosing range:
- Usual concentration: 0.2 mg/mL
- Demand dose: Usual: 0.1-0.2 mg; range: 0.05-0.4 mg
- Lockout interval: 5-10 minutes

Epidural PCA (de Leon-Casasola, 1996; Liu, 2010; Smith, 2009):
- Bolus dose: 0.4-1 mg
- Infusion rate: 0.03-0.3 mg/**hour**
- Demand dose: 0.02-0.05 mg
- Lockout interval: 10-15 minutes

I.M., SubQ: **Note:** I.M. use may result in variable absorption and lag time to peak effect.
- Initial: Opiate-naive: 0.8-1 mg every 4-6 hours as needed; patients with prior opiate exposure may require higher initial doses
- Usual dosage range: 1-2 mg every 4-6 hours as needed

Rectal: 3 mg every 6-8 hours as needed

Chronic pain: Note: Patients taking opioids chronically may become tolerant and require doses higher than the usual dosage range to maintain the desired effect. Tolerance can be managed by appropriate dose titration. There is no optimal or maximal dose for hydromorphone in chronic pain. The appropriate dose is one that relieves pain throughout its dosing interval without causing unmanageable side effects.

Controlled release formulation (Hydromorph Contin®, not available in U.S.): Oral: 3-30 mg every 12 hours. **Note:** A patient's hydromorphone requirement should be established using prompt release formulations; conversion to long acting products may be considered when chronic, continuous treatment is required. Higher dosages should be reserved for use only in opioid-tolerant patients.

Extended release formulation (Exalgo™): Dosing range: 8-64 mg every 24 hours. For use in opioid-tolerant patients only; discontinue all other extended release opioids when starting therapy. Suggested recommendations for converting to Exalgo™ from other analgesics are presented, but when selecting the initial dose, other characteristics (eg, patient status, degree of opioid tolerance, concurrent medications, type of pain, risk factors for addiction or diversion, etc) should also be considered.

Individualization of dose: Pain relief and adverse events should be assessed frequently. Dose increases may occur not more often than every 3-4 days; consider titrating with increases of 25% to 50% of the current daily dose. If more than 2 doses of rescue medications are needed within 24 hours for 2 consecutive days, consider increasing the dose of Exalgo™. Do not administer more frequently than every 24 hours.

Discontinuing Exalgo™: Taper by gradually decreasing the dose by 25% to 50% every 2-3 days to a dose of 8 mg every 24 hours before discontinuing therapy.

Conversion from other oral hydromorphone formulations to Exalgo™: Start with the equivalent total daily dose of hydromorphone administered once daily. May titrate every 3-4 days until adequate pain relief with tolerable side effects have been achieved.

Conversion from other opioids to Exalgo™: In general, start Exalgo™ at 50% of the calculated total daily dose every 24 hours. Titrate until adequate pain relief with tolerable side effects has been achieved. The following conversion ratios may be used to convert from **oral** opioid therapy to Exalgo™.

Conversion ratios to Exalgo™ (see table): Select the opioid, sum the total daily dose, then multiply by the conversion ratio to calculate the *approximate* oral hydromorphone equivalent; start Exalgo™ at 50% of the calculated total daily dose every 24 hours. (**Note:** The conversion ratios and approximate equivalent doses in this conversion table are only to be used for the conversion from current opioid therapy to Exalgo™).

Conversion Ratios to Exalgo™[1]

Previous Opioid	Approximate Equivalent Oral Dose	Oral Conversion Ratio[2]
Hydromorphone	12 mg	1
Codeine	200 mg	0.06
Hydrocodone	30 mg	0.4
Methadone[3]	20 mg	0.6
Morphine	60 mg	0.2
Oxycodone	30 mg	0.4
Oxymorphone	20 mg	0.6

[1] *Approximate* equivalent doses for conversion from current opioid therapy to Exalgo™.

[2] Ratio for converting oral opioid dose to approximate hydromorphone equivalent dose.

[3] Monitor closely; ratio between methadone and other opioid agonists may vary widely as a function of previous drug exposure. Methadone has a long half-life and may accumulate in the plasma.

◀ *Conversion from transdermal fentanyl to Exalgo™:* Treatment with Exalgo™ can be started 18 hours after the removal of the transdermal fentanyl patch. For every fentanyl 25 mcg/hour transdermal dose, the equianalgesic dose of Exalgo™ is 12 mg every 24 hours. An appropriate starting dose is 50% of the calculated total daily dose given every 24 hours.

Renal Impairment Exalgo™:
Moderate impairment: Start with a reduced dose and monitor closely.
Severe impairment: Consider use of an alternate analgesic with better dosing flexibility.

Hepatic Impairment Dose adjustment should be considered.
Exalgo™: In patients with moderate and severe hepatic impairment, start with a reduced dose and monitor closely. Consider use of an alternate analgesic with better dosing flexibility.

Administration
Parenteral: May be given SubQ or I.M.; vial stopper contains latex
I.V.: For IVP, must be given slowly over 2-3 minutes (rapid IVP has been associated with an increase in side effects, especially respiratory depression and hypotension)
Oral: Hydromorph Contin®: Capsule should be swallowed whole; do not crush or chew; contents may be sprinkled on soft food and swallowed

Monitoring Parameters Pain relief, respiratory and mental status, blood pressure

Test Interactions Some quinolones may produce a false-positive urine screening result for opiates using commercially-available immunoassay kits. This has been demonstrated most consistently for levofloxacin and ofloxacin, but other quinolones have shown cross-reactivity in certain assay kits. Confirmation of positive opiate screens by more specific methods should be considered.

Pharmacotherapy Pearls Equianalgesic doses: Morphine 10 mg I.M. = hydromorphone 1.5 mg I.M.
Exalgo™ is indicated for the management of moderate-to-severe pain in opioid-tolerant patients (requiring around-the-clock analgesia for an extended period of time). Patients are considered to be opioid tolerant if they have been taking oral morphine ≥60 mg/day, fentanyl transdermal ≥25 mcg/hour, oral oxycodone ≥30 mg/day, oral hydromorphone ≥8 mg/day, oral oxymorphone ≥25 mg/day, or an equianalgesic dose of another opioid for ≥1 week.

Special Geriatric Considerations Elderly may be particularly susceptible to the CNS depressant and constipating effects of narcotics.

Controlled Substance C-II

Dosage Forms Excipient information presented when available (limited, particularly for generics); consult specific product labeling.
Injection, powder for reconstitution, as hydrochloride:
Dilaudid-HP®: 250 mg [contains natural rubber/natural latex in packaging, sodium metabisulfite]
Injection, solution, as hydrochloride: 1 mg/mL (1 mL); 2 mg/mL (1 mL, 20 mL); 4 mg/mL (1 mL); 10 mg/mL (1 mL, 5 mL, 50 mL)
Dilaudid-HP®: 10 mg/mL (50 mL) [contains natural rubber/natural latex in packaging, sodium metabisulfite]
Dilaudid-HP®: 10 mg/mL (1 mL, 5 mL) [contains sodium metabisulfite]
Dilaudid®: 1 mg/mL (1 mL); 2 mg/mL (1 mL); 4 mg/mL (1 mL) [contains sodium metabisulfite]
Injection, solution, as hydrochloride [preservative free]: 10 mg/mL (1 mL, 5 mL, 50 mL)
Liquid, oral, as hydrochloride: 1 mg/mL (473 mL)
Dilaudid®: 1 mg/mL (473 mL) [contains sodium metabisulfite (may have trace amounts)]
Powder, for prescription compounding, as hydrochloride: USP: 100% (972 mg)
Suppository, rectal, as hydrochloride: 3 mg (6s)
Tablet, oral, as hydrochloride: 2 mg, 4 mg, 8 mg
Dilaudid®: 2 mg, 4 mg [contains sodium metabisulfite (may have trace amounts)]
Dilaudid®: 8 mg [scored; contains sodium metabisulfite (may have trace amounts)]
Tablet, extended release, oral, as hydrochloride:
Exalgo™: 8 mg, 12 mg, 16 mg [contains sodium metabisulfite]

Dosage Forms: Canada Excipient information presented when available (limited, particularly for generics); consult specific product labeling.
Capsule, controlled release:
Hydromorph Contin®: 3 mg, 6 mg, 12 mg, 18 mg, 24 mg, 30 mg

◆ **Hydromorphone Hydrochloride** see HYDROmorphone *on page 945*

◆ **Hydroskin® [OTC]** see Hydrocortisone (Topical) *on page 943*

Hydroxocobalamin (hye droks oh koe BAL a min)

Brand Names: U.S. Cyanokit®
Brand Names: Canada Cyanokit®
Index Terms Vitamin B_{12a}
Generic Availability (U.S.) Yes: Excludes powder for injection
Pharmacologic Category Antidote; Vitamin, Water Soluble
Use

I.M. injection: Treatment of pernicious anemia; treatment of vitamin B_{12} deficiency due to dietary deficiencies or malabsorption diseases, inadequate secretion of intrinsic factor, competition for vitamin B_{12} by intestinal parasites/bacteria, or inadequate utilization of B_{12} (eg, during neoplastic treatment); diagnostic agent for Schilling test

I.V. infusion (Cyanokit®): Treatment of cyanide poisoning (known or suspected)

Contraindications

I.M.: Hypersensitivity to hydroxocobalamin or any component of the formulation

I.V. (Cyanokit®): There are no contraindications listed in the manufacturer's labeling.

Warnings/Precautions

Solution for I.M. injection: Treatment of severe vitamin B_{12} megaloblastic anemia may result in thrombocytosis and severe hypokalemia, sometimes fatal, due to intracellular potassium shift upon anemia resolution. Use caution in folic acid deficient megaloblastic anemia; administration of vitamin B_{12} alone is not a substitute for folic acid and might mask true diagnosis. Vitamin B_{12} deficiency masks signs of polycythemia vera; vitamin B_{12} administration may unmask this condition. Neurologic manifestations of vitamin B_{12} deficiency will not be prevented with folic acid unless vitamin B_{12} is also given; spinal cord degeneration might also occur when folic acid is used as a substitute for vitamin B_{12} in anemia prevention. Blunted therapeutic response to vitamin B_{12} may occur in certain conditions (eg, infection, uremia, concurrent iron or folic acid deficiency) or in patients on medications with bone marrow suppressant properties (eg, chloramphenicol). Approved for use as I.M. injection only.

Cyanokit®: Use caution or consider alternatives in patients known to be allergic to, or who have experienced anaphylaxis,with hydroxocobalamin or cyanocobalamin. Increased blood pressure (≥180 mm Hg systolic or ≥110 mm Hg diastolic) may occur with infusion; elevations usually noted at the beginning of the infusion, peak toward the end of the infusion and return to baseline within 4 hours of the infusion. May offset hypotension induced by nitrite administration or cyanide. Collection of pretreatment blood cyanide concentrations does not preclude administration and should not delay administration in the emergency management of suspected or confirmed cyanide toxicity. Pretreatment cyanide concentrations may be useful as post infusion concentrations may be inaccurate. Treatment of cyanide poisoning should include decontamination and supportive therapy. Fire victims may present with both cyanide and carbon monoxide poisoning. In this scenario, hydroxocobalamin is the agent of choice for cyanide intoxication. Hydroxocobalamin can discolor the skin and exudates, complicating the assessment of burn severity. Use caution with concurrent use of other cyanide antidotes; safety has not been established. Hydroxocobalamin may interfere with and/or trip alarms in patients who use hemodialysis machines that rely on colorimetric technology. Photosensitivity is a potential concern; avoid direct sunlight while skin remains discolored.

Adverse Reactions (Reflective of adult population; not specific for elderly)

I.M. injection: Frequency not defined:
Dermatologic: Exanthema (transient), itching
Gastrointestinal: Diarrhea (mild, transient)
Local: Injection site pain
Miscellaneous: Anaphylaxis, feeling of swelling of the entire body

I.V. infusion (Cyanokit®):
>10%:
Cardiovascular: Blood pressure increased (18% to 28%)
Central nervous system: Headache (6% to 33%)
Dermatologic: Erythema (94% to 100%; may last up to 2 weeks), rash (predominantly acneiform; 20% to 44%; can appear 7-28 days after administration and usually resolves within a few weeks)
Gastrointestinal: Nausea (6% to 11%)
Genitourinary: Chromaturia (100%; may last up to 5 weeks after administration)
Hematologic: Lymphocytes decreased (8% to 17%)
Local: Infusion site reaction (6% to 39%)

HYDROXOCOBALAMIN

Frequency not defined:
Cardiovascular: Chest discomfort, hot flashes, peripheral edema
Central nervous system: Dizziness, memory impairment, restlessness
Dermatologic: Pruritus, urticaria
Gastrointestinal: Abdominal discomfort, diarrhea, dyspepsia, dysphagia, hematochezia, vomiting
Ocular: Irritation, redness, swelling
Respiratory: Dry throat, dyspnea, throat tightness
Miscellaneous: Allergic reaction (including anaphylaxis)

Drug Interactions

Metabolism/Transport Effects None known.

Avoid Concomitant Use There are no known interactions where it is recommended to avoid concomitant use.

Increased Effect/Toxicity There are no known significant interactions involving an increase in effect.

Decreased Effect There are no known significant interactions involving a decrease in effect.

Stability

Solution for I.M. injection: Store at 20°C to 25°C (68°F to 77°F). Protect from light.

I.V. infusion (Cyanokit®): Prior to reconstitution, store at 25°C (77°F): excursions permitted to 15°C to 30°C (59°F to 86°F).

Temperature variation exposure allowed for transport of lyophilized form:
Usual transport: ≤15 days at 5°C to 40°C (41°F to 104°F)
Desert transport: ≤4 days at 5°C to 60°C (41°F to 140°F)
Freezing/defrosting cycles: ≤15 days at -20°C to 40°C (-4°F to 104°F)

Reconstitute each 5 g vial with 200 mL of NS using provided sterile transfer spike. If NS is unavailable, may use LR or D_5W. Invert or rock each vial for 60 seconds prior to infusion; do not shake. Discard if solution is **not** dark red. Following reconstitution, store up to 6 hours at ≤40°C (104°F); do not freeze. Discard any remaining solution after 6 hours.

Mechanism of Action Hydroxocobalamin (vitamin B_{12a}) is a precursor to cyanocobalamin (vitamin B_{12}). Cyanocobalamin acts as a coenzyme for various metabolic functions, including fat and carbohydrate metabolism and protein synthesis, used in cell replication and hematopoiesis. In the presence of cyanide, each hydroxocobalamin molecule can bind one cyanide ion by displacing it for the hydroxo ligand linked to the trivalent cobalt ion, forming cyanocobalamin, which is then excreted in the urine.

Pharmacodynamics/Kinetics Following I.V. administration of Cyanokit®:
Protein binding: Significant; forms various cobalamin-(III) complexes
Half-life elimination: 26-31 hours
Excretion: Urine (50% to 60% within initial 72 hours)

Dosage

Geriatric & Adult

Cyanide poisoning: I.V.: **Note:** If cyanide poisoning is suspected, antidotal therapy must be given immediately. Initial: 5 **g** as single infusion; may repeat a second 5 **g** dose depending on the severity of poisoning and clinical response. Maximum cumulative dose: 10 **g**.

Schilling test: I.M.: 1000 mcg

Vitamin B_{12} deficiency: I.M.: Initial: 30 mcg once daily for 5-10 days; maintenance: 100-200 mcg once per month. **Note:** Larger doses may be required in critically-ill patients or if patient has neurologic disease, an infectious disease, or hyperthyroidism.

Renal Impairment No dosage adjustments provided in manufacturer's labeling (has not been studied).

Hepatic Impairment No dosage adjustments provided in manufacturer's labeling (has not been studied).

Administration

I.M.: Administer 1000 mcg/mL solution I.M. only

I.V.: Cyanokit®: Administer initial dose by I.V. infusion over 15 minutes; if a second dose is needed, administer the second dose over 15 minutes to 2 hours; hydroxocobalamin is chemically incompatible with sodium thiosulfate and sodium nitrite and separate I.V. lines must be used if concomitant administration is desired **(the safety of coadministration is not established)**

Monitoring Parameters Vitamin B_{12}, hematocrit, hemoglobin, reticulocyte count, red blood cell counts, folate and iron levels should be obtained prior to treatment and periodically during treatment.

Cyanide poisoning: Blood pressure and heart rate during and after infusion, serum lactate levels, venous-arterial PO_2 gradient. Pretreatment cyanide levels may be useful as post infusion levels may be inaccurate.

Megaloblastic anemia: In addition to normal hematological parameters, serum potassium and platelet counts should be monitored during therapy, particularly in the first 48 hours of treatment.

Test Interactions The following values may be affected, *in vitro*, following hydroxocobalamin 5 g dose. Interference following hydroxocobalamin 10 g dose can be expected to last up to an additional 24 hours. **Note:** Extent and duration of interference dependent on analyzer used and patient variability.

Falsely elevated:
Basophils, hemoglobin, MCH, and MCHC [duration: 12-16 hours]
Albumin, alkaline phosphatase, cholesterol, creatinine, glucose, total protein, and triglycerides [duration: 24 hours]
Bilirubin [duration: up to 4 days]
Urinalysis: Glucose, protein, erythrocytes, leukocytes, ketones, bilirubin, urobilinogen, nitrite [duration: 2-8 days]

Falsely decreased: ALT and amylase [duration: 24 hours]

Unpredictable:
AST, CK, CKMB, LDH, phosphate, and uric acid [duration: 24 hours]
PT (quick or INR) and aPTT [duration: 24-48 hours]
Urine pH [duration: 2-8 days]

May also interfere with colorimetric tests and cause hemodialysis machines to shut down due to false detection of a blood leak from the blood-like appearance of the solution.

Special Geriatric Considerations Evidence exists that people, particularly elderly, whose serum cobalamin concentrations are <500 pg/mL, should receive replacement parenteral therapy. This recommendation is based upon neuropsychiatric disorders and cardiovascular disorders associated with lower serum cobalamin concentrations.

Dosage Forms Excipient information presented when available (limited, particularly for generics); consult specific product labeling. [DSC] = Discontinued product
Injection, powder for reconstitution:
Cyanokit®: 2.5 g [DSC], 5 g
Injection, solution: 1000 mcg/mL (30 mL)

◆ **Hydroxycarbamide** *see* Hydroxyurea *on page 955*

Hydroxychloroquine (hye droks ee KLOR oh kwin)

Medication Safety Issues
Sound-alike/look-alike issues:
Hydroxychloroquine may be confused with hydrocortisone
Plaquenil® may be confused with Platinol
Brand Names: U.S. Plaquenil®
Brand Names: Canada Apo-Hydroxyquine®; Gen-Hydroxychloroquine; Mylan-Hydroxychloroquine; Plaquenil®; PRO-Hydroxyquine
Index Terms Hydroxychloroquine Sulfate
Generic Availability (U.S.) Yes
Pharmacologic Category Aminoquinoline (Antimalarial)
Use Suppression and treatment of acute attacks of malaria; treatment of systemic lupus erythematosus (SLE) and rheumatoid arthritis
Unlabeled Use Treatment of porphyria cutanea tarda, polymorphous light eruptions
Contraindications Hypersensitivity to hydroxychloroquine, 4-aminoquinoline derivatives, or any component of the formulation; retinal or visual field changes attributable to 4-aminoquinolines
Warnings/Precautions May cause ophthalmic adverse effects (risk factors include daily doses >6.5 mg/kg lean body weight) or neuromyopathy; perform baseline and periodic (every 3 months) ophthalmologic examinations; test periodically for muscle weakness. Rare cardiomyopathy has been associated with long-term use of hydroxychloroquine. Aminoquinolines have been associated with rare hematologic reactions, including agranulocytosis, aplastic anemia, and thrombocytopenia; monitoring (CBC) is recommended in prolonged therapy. Use with caution in patients with hepatic disease, G6PD deficiency, psoriasis, and porphyria. Not effective in the treatment of malaria caused by chloroquine resistant *P. falciparum*. **[U.S. Boxed Warning]: Should be prescribed by physicians familiar with its use.**
Adverse Reactions (Reflective of adult population; not specific for elderly) Frequency not defined.
Cardiovascular: Cardiomyopathy (rare, relationship to hydroxychloroquine unclear)
Central nervous system: Ataxia, dizziness, emotional changes, headache, irritability, lassitude, nervousness, nightmares, psychosis, seizure, vertigo

Dermatologic: Alopecia, angioedema, bleaching of hair, pigmentation changes (skin and mucosal; black-blue color), rash (acute generalized exanthematous pustulosis, erythema annulare centrifugum, exfoliative dermatitis, lichenoid, maculopapular, morbilliform, purpuric, Stevens-Johnson syndrome, urticarial), urticaria

Gastrointestinal: Abdominal cramping, anorexia, diarrhea, nausea, vomiting, weight loss

Hematologic: Agranulocytosis, aplastic anemia, hemolysis (in patients with glucose-6-phosphate deficiency), leukopenia, thrombocytopenia

Hepatic: Abnormal liver function/hepatic failure (isolated cases)

Neuromuscular & skeletal: Myopathy, palsy, or neuromyopathy leading to progressive weakness and atrophy of proximal muscle groups (may be associated with mild sensory changes, loss of deep tendon reflexes, and abnormal nerve conduction)

Ocular: Abnormal color vision, abnormal retinal pigmentation, atrophy, attenuation of retinal arterioles, corneal changes/deposits (visual disturbances, blurred vision, photophobia [reversible on discontinuation]), decreased visual acuity, disturbance in accommodation, keratopathy, macular edema, nystagmus, optic disc pallor/atrophy, pigmentary retinopathy, retinopathy (early changes reversible [may progress despite discontinuation if advanced]), scotoma

Otic: Deafness, tinnitus

Miscellaneous: Exacerbation of porphyria and nonlight sensitive psoriasis

Respiratory: Bronchospasm, respiratory failure (myopathy-related)

Drug Interactions

Metabolism/Transport Effects None known.

Avoid Concomitant Use

Avoid concomitant use of Hydroxychloroquine with any of the following: Artemether; BCG; Lumefantrine; Mefloquine; Natalizumab; Pimecrolimus; Tacrolimus (Topical)

Increased Effect/Toxicity

Hydroxychloroquine may increase the levels/effects of: Antipsychotic Agents (Phenothiazines); Beta-Blockers; Cardiac Glycosides; Dapsone; Dapsone (Systemic); Dapsone (Topical); Leflunomide; Lumefantrine; Mefloquine; Natalizumab; Vaccines (Live)

The levels/effects of Hydroxychloroquine may be increased by: Artemether; Dapsone; Dapsone (Systemic); Denosumab; Mefloquine; Pimecrolimus; Roflumilast; Tacrolimus (Topical); Trastuzumab

Decreased Effect

Hydroxychloroquine may decrease the levels/effects of: Anthelmintics; BCG; Coccidioidin Skin Test; Sipuleucel-T; Vaccines (Inactivated)

The levels/effects of Hydroxychloroquine may be decreased by: Echinacea

Ethanol/Nutrition/Herb Interactions Ethanol: Avoid ethanol (due to GI irritation).

Mechanism of Action Interferes with digestive vacuole function within sensitive malarial parasites by increasing the pH and interfering with lysosomal degradation of hemoglobin; inhibits locomotion of neutrophils and chemotaxis of eosinophils; impairs complement-dependent antigen-antibody reactions

Pharmacodynamics/Kinetics

Onset of action: Rheumatic disease: May require 4-6 weeks to respond

Absorption: Rapid and complete

Protein binding: 55%

Metabolism: Hepatic; metabolites include desethylhydroxychloroquine and desethylchloroquine

Half-life elimination: 32-50 days

Time to peak: Rheumatic disease: Several months

Excretion: Urine (as metabolites and unchanged drug [up to 60%]); may be enhanced by urinary acidification

Dosage

Geriatric & Adult Note: Hydroxychloroquine sulfate 200 mg is equivalent to 155 mg hydroxychloroquine base and 250 mg chloroquine phosphate. All doses below expressed as hydroxychloroquine sulfate. Second-line alternative treatment for malaria (chloroquine is preferred).

Malaria, chemoprophylaxis: Oral: 400 mg weekly on same day each week; begin 2 weeks before exposure; continue for 4 weeks (per CDC guidelines) after leaving endemic area; if suppressive therapy is not begun prior to the exposure, double the initial dose and give in 2 doses, 6 hours apart and continue treatment for 8 weeks

Malaria, acute attack: Oral: 800 mg initially, followed by 400 mg at 6, 24, and 48 hours

Rheumatoid arthritis: Oral: Initial: 400-600 mg/day taken with food or milk; increase dose gradually until optimum response level is reached; usually after 4-12 weeks dose should be reduced by 1/2 to a maintenance dose of 200-400 mg/day

Lupus erythematosus: Oral: 400 mg every day or twice daily for several weeks-months depending on response; 200-400 mg/day for prolonged maintenance therapy

Renal Impairment Use with caution; dosage adjustment may be necessary in severe dysfunction (Bernstein, 1992); specific guidelines not available.

Hepatic Impairment Use with caution; dosage adjustment may be necessary.

Administration Administer with food or milk.

Monitoring Parameters Ophthalmologic exam at baseline and every 3 months during prolonged therapy (including visual acuity, slit-lamp, fundoscopic, and visual field exam); CBC at baseline and periodically; muscle strength (especially proximal, as a symptom of neuromyopathy) during long-term therapy

Special Geriatric Considerations No specific recommendations for dosing.

Dosage Forms Excipient information presented when available (limited, particularly for generics); consult specific product labeling.

Tablet, oral, as sulfate: 200 mg [equivalent to 155 mg base]

    Plaquenil®: 200 mg [equivalent to 155 mg base]

- ◆ **Hydroxychloroquine Sulfate** see Hydroxychloroquine on page 953
- ◆ **Hydroxyethylcellulose** see Artificial Tears on page 148
- ◆ **9-hydroxy-risperidone** see Paliperidone on page 1457

Hydroxyurea (hye droks ee yoor EE a)

Medication Safety Issues
Sound-alike/look-alike issues:

Hydroxyurea may be confused with hydrOXYzine

High alert medication:

This medication is in a class the Institute for Safe Medication Practices (ISMP) includes among its list of drugs which have a heightened risk of causing significant patient harm when used in error.

International issues:

Hydrea [U.S., Canada, and multiple international markets] may be confused with Hydra brand name for isoniazid [Japan]

Brand Names: U.S. Droxia®; Hydrea®

Brand Names: Canada Apo-Hydroxyurea®; Gen-Hydroxyurea; Hydrea®; Mylan-Hydroxyurea

Index Terms Hydroxycarbamide; Hydurea

Generic Availability (U.S.) Yes

Pharmacologic Category Antineoplastic Agent, Antimetabolite

Use Treatment of melanoma, refractory chronic myelocytic leukemia (CML); recurrent, metastatic, or inoperable ovarian cancer; radiosensitizing agent in the treatment of squamous cell head and neck cancer (excluding lip cancer); adjunct in the management of sickle cell patients who have had at least three painful crises in the previous 12 months (to reduce frequency of these crises and the need for blood transfusions)

Unlabeled Use Treatment of HIV; treatment of psoriasis, treatment of hematologic conditions such as essential thrombocythemia, polycythemia vera, hypereosinophilia, and hyperleukocytosis due to acute leukemia; treatment of uterine, cervix and nonsmall cell lung cancers; radiosensitizing agent in the treatment of primary brain tumors; has shown activity against renal cell cancer and prostate cancer

Contraindications Hypersensitivity to hydroxyurea or any component of the formulation; severe anemia; severe bone marrow suppression; WBC <2500/mm^3 or platelet count <100,000/mm^3 (neutrophils <2000/mm^3, platelets <80,000/mm^3, and hemoglobin <4.5 g/dL for sickle cell anemia)

Warnings/Precautions Hazardous agent - use appropriate precautions for handling and disposal; to decrease risk of exposure, wear gloves when handling and wash hands before and after contact. Leukopenia may commonly occur (thrombocytopenia and anemia are less common; reversible with treatment interruption). Use with caution in patients with a history of prior chemotherapy or radiation therapy; myelosuppression is more common. Correct severe anemia prior to initiating treatment. Patients with a history of radiation therapy are also at risk for exacerbation of post irradiation erythema. Self-limiting megaloblastic erythropoiesis may be seen early in treatment (may resemble pernicious anemia, but is unrelated to vitamin B$_{12}$ or folic acid deficiency). Plasma iron clearance may be delayed and iron utilization rate (by erythrocytes) may be reduced. When treated concurrently with hydroxyurea and antiretroviral agents (including didanosine), HIV-infected patients are at higher risk for potentially fatal pancreatitis, hepatotoxicity, hepatic failure, and severe peripheral neuropathy. Hyperuricemia may occur with treatment; adequate hydration and initiation or dosage adjustment of uricosuric agents (eg, allopurinol) may be necessary.

HYDROXYUREA

In patients with sickle cell anemia, use is not recommended if neutrophils <2000/mm^3, platelets <80,000/mm^3, hemoglobin <4.5 g/dL, or reticulocytes <80,000/mm^3 when hemoglobin <9 g/dL. May cause macrocytosis, which can mask folic acid deficiency; prophylactic fold acid supplementation is recommended. **[U.S. Boxed Warning]: Hydroxyurea is mutagenic and clastogenic. Treatment of myeloproliferative disorders (eg, polycythemia vera, thrombocythemia) with long-term hydroxyurea is associated with secondary leukemia;** it is unknown if this is drug-related or disease-related. Cutaneous vasculitic toxicities (vasculitic ulceration and gangrene) have been reported with hydroxyurea treatment, most often in patients with a history of or receiving concurrent interferon therapy; discontinue hydroxyurea and consider alternate cytoreductive therapy if cutaneous vasculitic toxicity develops. Use caution with renal dysfunction; may require dose reductions. Elderly patients may be more sensitive to the effects of hydroxyurea; may require lower doses. **[U.S. Boxed Warning]: Should be administered under the supervision of a physician experienced in the treatment of sickle cell anemia** or in cancer chemotherapy.

Adverse Reactions (Reflective of adult population; not specific for elderly) Frequency not defined.

Cardiovascular: Edema

Central nervous system: Chills, disorientation, dizziness, drowsiness (dose-related), fever, hallucinations, headache, malaise, seizure

Dermatologic: Alopecia, cutaneous vasculitic toxicities, dermatomyositis-like skin changes, facial erythema, gangrene, hyperpigmentation, maculopapular rash, nail atrophy, nail discoloration, peripheral erythema, scaling, skin atrophy, skin cancer, skin ulcer, vasculitis ulcerations, violet papules

Endocrine & metabolic: Hyperuricemia

Gastrointestinal: Anorexia, constipation, diarrhea, gastrointestinal irritation and mucositis, (potentiated with radiation therapy), nausea, pancreatitis, stomatitis, vomiting

Genitourinary: Dysuria

Hematologic: Myelosuppression (anemia, leukopenia [common; reversal of WBC count occurs rapidly], thrombocytopenia); macrocytosis, megaloblastic erythropoiesis, secondary leukemias (long-term use)

Hepatic: Hepatic enzymes increased, hepatotoxicity

Neuromuscular & skeletal: Peripheral neuropathy, weakness

Renal: BUN increased, creatinine increased

Respiratory: Acute diffuse pulmonary infiltrates (rare), dyspnea, pulmonary fibrosis (rare)

Drug Interactions

Metabolism/Transport Effects None known.

Avoid Concomitant Use
Avoid concomitant use of Hydroxyurea with any of the following: BCG; CloZAPine; Didanosine; Natalizumab; Pimecrolimus; Stavudine; Tacrolimus (Topical); Vaccines (Live)

Increased Effect/Toxicity
Hydroxyurea may increase the levels/effects of: CloZAPine; Didanosine; Leflunomide; Natalizumab; Stavudine; Vaccines (Live)

The levels/effects of Hydroxyurea may be increased by: Denosumab; Didanosine; Pimecrolimus; Roflumilast; Stavudine; Tacrolimus (Topical); Trastuzumab

Decreased Effect
Hydroxyurea may decrease the levels/effects of: BCG; Coccidioidin Skin Test; Sipuleucel-T; Vaccines (Inactivated); Vaccines (Live)

The levels/effects of Hydroxyurea may be decreased by: Echinacea

Stability Store at room temperature of 25°C (77°F); excursions permitted between 15°C and 30°C (59°F and 86°F).

Mechanism of Action Antimetabolite which selectively inhibits ribonucleoside diphosphate reductase, preventing the conversion of ribonucleotides to deoxyribonucleotides, halting the cell cycle at the G1/S phase and therefore has radiation sensitizing activity by maintaining cells in the G$_1$ phase and interfering with DNA repair. In sickle cell anemia, hydroxyurea increases red blood cell (RBC) hemoglobin F levels, RBC water content, deformability of sickled cells, and alters adhesion of RBCs to endothelium.

Pharmacodynamics/Kinetics

Onset: Sickle cell anemia: Fetal hemoglobin increase: 4-12 weeks

Absorption: Readily (≥80%)

Distribution: Readily crosses blood-brain barrier; distributes into intestine, brain, lung, kidney tissues, effusions and ascites

Metabolism: 60% via hepatic and GI tract

Half-life elimination: 3-4 hours

Time to peak: 1-4 hours

Excretion: Urine (sickle cell anemia: 40% of administered dose)

Dosage

Geriatric & Adult

Antineoplastic uses: Titrate dose to patient response; if WBC count falls to <2500/mm^3, or the platelet count to <100,000/mm^3, therapy should be stopped for at least 3 days and resumed when values rise toward normal

Chronic myeloid leukemia (resistant): Oral: Continuous therapy: 20-30 mg/kg once daily

Solid tumors: Oral:

Intermittent therapy: 80 mg/kg as a single dose every third day

Continuous therapy: 20-30 mg/kg once daily

Concomitant therapy with irradiation (head and neck cancer): 80 mg/kg as a single dose every third day starting at least 7 days before initiation of irradiation

Sickle cell anemia: Oral: Initial: 15 mg/kg/day; if blood counts are in an acceptable range, may increase by 5 mg/kg every 12 weeks until the maximum tolerated dose of 35 mg/kg/day is achieved or the dose that does not produce toxic effects (do not increase dose if blood counts are between acceptable and toxic ranges). Monitor for toxicity every 2 weeks; if toxicity occurs, withhold treatment until the bone marrow recovers, then restart with a dose reduction of 2.5 mg/kg/day; if no toxicity occurs over the next 12 weeks, then the subsequent dose may be increased by 2.5 mg/kg/day every 12 weeks to a maximum tolerated dose (dose which does not produce hematologic toxicity for 24 consecutive weeks). If hematologic toxicity recurs a second time at a specific dose, do not retry that dose.

Acceptable hematologic ranges: Neutrophils ≥2500/mm^3; platelets ≥95,000/mm^3; hemoglobin >5.3 g/dL, and reticulocytes ≥95,000/mm^3 if the hemoglobin concentration is <9 g/dL

Toxic hematologic ranges: Neutrophils <2000/mm^3; platelets <80,000/mm^3; hemoglobin <4.5 g/dL; and reticulocytes <80,000/mm^3 if the hemoglobin concentration is <9 g/dL

Cervical cancer (unlabeled use; with concurrent radiation therapy, cisplatin and fluorouracil): Oral: 2000 mg/m^2 (2 hours prior to radiation treatment) twice a week for 6 weeks (Rose, 2007)

Essential thrombocythemia, high-risk (unlabeled use): Oral: 500-1000 mg daily; adjust dose to maintain platelets <400,000/mm^3 (Harrison, 2005)

Head and neck cancer (unlabeled dosing; with concurrent radiation therapy and fluorouracil): Oral: 1000 mg every 12 hours for 11 doses (Garden, 2004)

Hypereosinophilic syndrome (unlabeled use): Oral: 1000-3000 mg/day (Klion, 2006)

Meningioma (unlabeled use): Oral: 20 mg/kg once daily (Newton, 2000; Rosenthal, 2002)

Polycythemia vera, high-risk (unlabeled use): Oral: 15-20 mg/kg/day (Finazzi, 2007)

Renal Impairment

The FDA-approved labeling recommends the following adjustment:

Sickle cell anemia:

Cl_{cr} ≥60 mL/minute: No adjustment (of initial dose) required.

Cl_{cr} <60 mL/minute: Reduce initial dose to 7.5 mg/kg/day; titrate to response/avoidance of toxicity (refer to Dosage: Geriatric & Adult).

ESRD: Reduce initial dose to 7.5 mg/kg/dose (administer after dialysis on dialysis days); titrate to response/avoidance of toxicity.

Other approved indications: It is recommended to reduce the initial dose; however, no specific guidelines are available.

The following guidelines have been used by some clinicians:

Aronoff, 2007: Adults:

Cl_{cr} 10-50 mL/minute: Administer 50% of dose.

Cl_{cr} <10 mL/minute: Administer 20% of dose.

Hemodialysis: Administer dose after dialysis on dialysis days; supplemental dose is not necessary. Hydroxyurea is a low molecular weight compound with high aqueous solubility that may be freely dialyzable, however, clinical studies confirming this hypothesis have not been performed.

Continuous renal replacement therapy (CRRT): Administer 50% of dose.

Kintzel, 1995:

Cl_{cr} 46-60 mL/minute: Administer 85% of dose.

Cl_{cr} 31-45 mL/minute: Administer 80% of dose.

Cl_{cr} <30 mL/minute: Administer 75% of dose.

Hepatic Impairment Specific guidelines are not available for dosage adjustment in hepatic impairment. The FDA-approved labeling recommends closely monitoring for bone marrow toxicity in patients with hepatic impairment.

Administration Capsules may be opened and emptied into water (will not dissolve completely); observe proper handling procedures

Monitoring Parameters CBC with differential and platelets, renal function and liver function tests, serum uric acid

Sickle cell disease: Monitor for toxicity every 2 weeks. If toxicity occurs, stop treatment until the bone marrow recovers; restart at 2.5 mg/kg/day less than the dose at which toxicity occurs. If no toxicity occurs over the next 12 weeks, then the subsequent dose should be increased by 2.5 mg/kg/day. Reduced dosage of hydroxyurea alternating with erythropoietin may decrease myelotoxicity and increase levels of fetal hemoglobin in patients who have not been helped by hydroxyurea alone.

Acceptable range: Neutrophils ≥2500 cells/mm^3, platelets ≥95,000/mm^3, hemoglobin >5.3 g/dL, and reticulocytes ≥95,000/mm^3 if the hemoglobin concentration is <9 g/dL

Toxic range: Neutrophils <2000 cells/mm^3, platelets <80,000/mm^3, hemoglobin <4.5 g/dL, and reticulocytes <80,000/mm^3 if the hemoglobin concentration is <9 g/dL

Test Interactions False-negative triglyceride measurement by a glycerol oxidase method

Pharmacotherapy Pearls Although I.V. use is reported, no parenteral product is commercially available in the U.S.

If WBC decreases to <2500/mm^3 or platelet count to <100,000/mm^3, interrupt therapy until values rise significantly toward normal. Treat anemia with whole blood replacement; do not interrupt therapy. Adequate trial period to determine the antineoplastic effectiveness is 6 weeks. Almost all patients receiving hydroxyurea in clinical trials needed to have their medication stopped for a time to allow their low blood count to return to acceptable levels.

Special Geriatric Considerations Elderly may be more sensitive to the effects of this drug and may require a lower dosage regimen; advance dose slowly and adjust dose for renal function with careful monitoring.

Dosage Forms Excipient information presented when available (limited, particularly for generics); consult specific product labeling.

Capsule, oral: 500 mg
Droxia®: 200 mg, 300 mg, 400 mg
Hydrea®: 500 mg

HydrOXYzine (hye DROKS i zeen)

Related Information
Beers Criteria − Potentially Inappropriate Medications for Geriatrics *on page 2183*

Medication Safety Issues
Sound-alike/look-alike issues:
HydrOXYzine may be confused with hydrALAZINE, hydroxyurea
Atarax® may be confused with Ativan®
Vistaril® may be confused with Restoril™, Versed, Zestril®

BEERS Criteria medication:
This drug may be potentially inappropriate for use in geriatric patients (Quality of evidence - high; Strength of recommendation - strong).

International issues:
Vistaril [U.S. and Turkey] may be confused with Vastarel brand name for trimetazidine [multiple international markets]

Brand Names: U.S. Vistaril®

Brand Names: Canada Apo-Hydroxyzine®; Atarax®; Hydroxyzine Hydrochloride Injection, USP; Novo-Hydroxyzin; Nu-Hydroxyzine; PMS-Hydroxyzine; Riva-Hydroxyzine

Index Terms Hydroxyzine Hydrochloride; Hydroxyzine Pamoate

Generic Availability (U.S.) Yes

Pharmacologic Category Antiemetic; Histamine H$_1$ Antagonist; Histamine H$_1$ Antagonist, First Generation; Piperazine Derivative

Use Treatment of anxiety/agitation (including adjunctive therapy in alcoholism); adjunct to pre- and postoperative analgesia and anesthesia; antipruritic; antiemetic

Contraindications Hypersensitivity to hydroxyzine or any component of the formulation; SubQ, intra-arterial, or I.V. injection

Warnings/Precautions Causes sedation, caution must be used in performing tasks which require alertness (eg, operating machinery or driving). Sedative effects of CNS depressants or ethanol are potentiated. SubQ, I.V., and intra-arterial administration are contraindicated since tissue damage, intravascular hemolysis, thrombosis, and digital gangrene can occur. Use with caution with narrow-angle glaucoma, prostatic hyperplasia, bladder neck obstruction, asthma, or COPD. In the elderly, avoid use of this potent anticholinergic agent due to increased risk of confusion, dry mouth, constipation, and other anticholinergic effects; clearance decreases in patients of advanced age (Beers Criteria).

Adverse Reactions (Reflective of adult population; not specific for elderly) Frequency not defined.
Central nervous system: Dizziness, drowsiness, fatigue, hallucination, headache, nervousness, seizure
Dermatologic: Pruritus, rash, urticaria

Gastrointestinal: Xerostomia
Neuromuscular & skeletal: Involuntary movements, paresthesia, tremor
Ocular: Blurred vision
Respiratory: Respiratory depression (at higher than recommended doses)
Miscellaneous: Allergic reaction

Drug Interactions
Metabolism/Transport Effects Inhibits CYP2D6 (weak)
Avoid Concomitant Use
Avoid concomitant use of HydrOXYzine with any of the following: Azelastine; Azelastine (Nasal); Methadone; Mirtazapine; Paraldehyde
Increased Effect/Toxicity
HydrOXYzine may increase the levels/effects of: Alcohol (Ethyl); Anticholinergics; ARIPiprazole; Azelastine; Azelastine (Nasal); Barbiturates; Buprenorphine; CNS Depressants; Meperidine; Methadone; Methotrimeprazine; Metyrosine; Mirtazapine; Paraldehyde; Selective Serotonin Reuptake Inhibitors; Zolpidem

The levels/effects of HydrOXYzine may be increased by: Droperidol; Methotrimeprazine; Pramlintide
Decreased Effect
HydrOXYzine may decrease the levels/effects of: Acetylcholinesterase Inhibitors (Central); Benzylpenicilloyl Polylysine; Betahistine; Hyaluronidase

The levels/effects of HydrOXYzine may be decreased by: Acetylcholinesterase Inhibitors (Central); Amphetamines

Ethanol/Nutrition/Herb Interactions
Ethanol: May increase CNS depression; monitor for increased effects with coadministration. Caution patients about effects.
Herb/Nutraceutical: Avoid valerian, St John's wort, kava kava, gotu kola (may increase CNS depression).

Stability
Injection: Store at 20°C to 25°C (68°F to 77°F); excursions permitted to 15°C to 30°C (59°F to 86°F). Protect from light.
Tablets: Store at 20°C to 25°C (68°F to 77°F).

Mechanism of Action Competes with histamine for H_1-receptor sites on effector cells in the gastrointestinal tract, blood vessels, and respiratory tract. Possesses skeletal muscle relaxing, bronchodilator, antihistamine, antiemetic, and analgesic properties.

Pharmacodynamics/Kinetics
Onset of action: Oral: 15-30 minutes; Injection: Rapid
Duration: Decreased histamine-induced wheal and flare areas: 2 to ≥36 hours; Suppression of pruritus: 1-12 hours (Simons, 1984)
Absorption: Oral: Rapid
Distribution: Adults: V_d ~16 L/kg (Simons, 1984); Elderly: ~23 L/kg (Simons K, 1989); Hepatic dysfunction: ~23 L/kg (Simons F, 1989)
Metabolism: Hepatic to multiple metabolites, including cetirizine (active) (Simons F, 1989)
Half-life elimination: Adults: ~20 hours (Simons, 1984); Elderly: ~29 hours (Simons K, 1989); Hepatic dysfunction: ~37 hours (Simons F, 1989)
Time to peak: Oral administration: Serum: ~2 hours; Peak suppression of antihistamine-induced wheal and flare: 4-12 hours (Simons, 1984)
Excretion: Urine

Dosage
Geriatric Initiate dosing using the lower end of the recommended dosage range due to an increased potential for anticholinergic side effects. Refer to adult dosing.
Adult
Note: Adjust dose based on patient response.
Antiemetic: I.M.: 25-100 mg/dose
Anxiety:
Oral: 50-100 mg 4 times/day
I.M.: Initial: 50-100 mg, then every 4-6 hours as needed
Preoperative sedation:
Oral: 50-100 mg
I.M.: 25-100 mg
Pruritus: Oral: 25 mg 3-4 times/day
Renal Impairment No dosage adjustment provided in the manufacturer's labeling; however, the following guidelines have been used by some clinicians (Aronoff, 2007): Adults:
GFR >50 mL/minute: No adjustment recommended.
GFR ≤50 mL/minute: Administer 50% of normal dose.
Continuous renal replacement therapy (CRRT), hemodialysis, peritoneal dialysis: Administer 50% of the normal dose.

◀ **Hepatic Impairment** Change dosing interval to every 24 hours in patients with primary biliary cirrhosis (Simons F, 1989)

Administration

Injection: For I. M. use only. Do not administer I.V., SubQ, or intra-arterially. Administer I.M. deep in large muscle. In adults, the preferred site is the upper outer quadrant of the buttock or midlateral thigh. The upper outer quadrant of the gluteal region should be used only when necessary to minimize potential damage to the sciatic nerve. With I.V. administration, extravasation can result in sterile abscess and marked tissue induration.

Oral: Shake suspension vigorously prior to use.

Monitoring Parameters Relief of symptoms, mental status, blood pressure

Test Interactions May cause false-positive serum TCA screen.

Special Geriatric Considerations Anticholinergic effects are not well tolerated in the elderly and frequently result in bowel, bladder, and mental status changes (ie, constipation, confusion, and urinary retention). Hydroxyzine may be useful as a short-term antipruritic, but it is not recommended for use as a sedative or anxiolytic in the elderly.

This medication is considered to be potentially inappropriate in this patient population (Beers Criteria: Quality of evidence - high; Strength of recommendation - strong).

Dosage Forms Excipient information presented when available (limited, particularly for generics); consult specific product labeling.

Capsule, oral, as pamoate: 25 mg, 50 mg, 100 mg
  Vistaril®: 25 mg, 50 mg
Injection, solution, as hydrochloride: 25 mg/mL (1 mL); 50 mg/mL (1 mL, 2 mL, 10 mL)
Solution, oral, as hydrochloride: 10 mg/5 mL (473 mL)
Syrup, oral, as hydrochloride: 10 mg/5 mL (118 mL, 473 mL)
Tablet, oral, as hydrochloride: 10 mg, 25 mg, 50 mg

◆ **Hydroxyzine Hydrochloride** see HydrOXYzine on page 958
◆ **Hydroxyzine Pamoate** see HydrOXYzine on page 958
◆ **Hydurea** see Hydroxyurea on page 955
◆ **Hygroton** see Chlorthalidone on page 364
◆ **Hylenex [DSC]** see Hyaluronidase on page 931
◆ **HyoMax™-DT** see Hyoscyamine on page 960
◆ **HyoMax™-FT** see Hyoscyamine on page 960
◆ **HyoMax®-SL** see Hyoscyamine on page 960
◆ **HyoMax® -SR** see Hyoscyamine on page 960
◆ **Hyonatol** see Hyoscyamine, Atropine, Scopolamine, and Phenobarbital on page 963
◆ **Hyoscine Butylbromide** see Scopolamine (Systemic) on page 1756
◆ **Hyoscine Hydrobromide** see Scopolamine (Ophthalmic) on page 1759

Hyoscyamine (hye oh SYE a meen)

Related Information
  Beers Criteria - Potentially Inappropriate Medications for Geriatrics on page 2183
Medication Safety Issues
  Sound-alike/look-alike issues:
    Anaspaz® may be confused with Anaprox®, Antispas®
    Levbid® may be confused with Enbrel®, Lithobid®, Lopid®, Lorabid®
    Levsinex® may be confused with Lanoxin®
    Levsin/SL® maybe confused with Levaquin®
  BEERS Criteria medication:
    This drug may be potentially inappropriate for use in geriatric patients (Quality of evidence - moderate; Strength of recommendation - strong).
Brand Names: U.S. Anaspaz®; ED-SPAZ; HyoMax® -SR; HyoMax®-SL; HyoMax™-DT; HyoMax™-FT; Hyosyne; Levbid®; Levsin®; Levsin®/SL; NuLev®; Oscimin; Symax® DuoTab; Symax® FasTab; Symax® SL; Symax® SR
Brand Names: Canada Levsin®
Index Terms l-Hyoscyamine Sulfate; Hyoscyamine Sulfate
Generic Availability (U.S.) Yes: Excludes chewable/disintegrating, dispersible, and variable release tablets, and injection
Pharmacologic Category Anticholinergic Agent
Use
  Oral: Adjunctive therapy for peptic ulcers, irritable bowel, neurogenic bladder/bowel; GI tract disorders caused by spasm; to reduce rigidity, tremors, sialorrhea, and hyperhidrosis associated with parkinsonism; as a drying agent in acute rhinitis
  Injection: Preoperative antimuscarinic to reduce secretions and block cardiac vagal inhibitory reflexes; to improve radiologic visibility of the kidneys; symptomatic relief of biliary and renal

colic; reduce GI motility to facilitate diagnostic procedures (ie, endoscopy, hypotonic duodenography); reduce pain and hypersecretion in pancreatitis, certain cases of partial heart block associated with vagal activity; reversal of neuromuscular blockade

Contraindications Hypersensitivity to belladonna alkaloids or any component of the formulation; glaucoma; obstructive uropathy; myasthenia gravis; obstructive GI tract disease, paralytic ileus, intestinal atony of elderly or debilitated patients, severe ulcerative colitis, toxic megacolon complicating ulcerative colitis; unstable cardiovascular status in acute hemorrhage, myocardial ischemia

Warnings/Precautions Heat prostration may occur in hot weather. Diarrhea may be a sign of incomplete intestinal obstruction, treatment should be discontinued if this occurs. May produce side effects as seen with other anticholinergic medications including drowsiness, dizziness, blurred vision, or psychosis. Elderly may be more susceptible to these effects. Use with caution in patients with autonomic neuropathy, coronary heart disease, CHF, cardiac arrhythmias, prostatic hyperplasia, hyperthyroidism, hypertension, renal disease, and hiatal hernia associated with reflux esophagitis. Avoid use in the elderly due to potent anticholinergic adverse effects and uncertain effectiveness (Beers Criteria). NuLev™ contains phenylalanine.

Adverse Reactions (Reflective of adult population; not specific for elderly) Frequency not defined.

Cardiovascular: Palpitation, tachycardia

Central nervous system: Ataxia, dizziness, drowsiness, headache, insomnia, mental confusion/excitement, nervousness, speech disorder

Dermatologic: Urticaria

Endocrine & metabolic: Lactation suppression

Gastrointestinal: Bloating, constipation, dry mouth, loss of taste, nausea, vomiting

Genitourinary: Impotence, urinary hesitancy, urinary retention

Neuromuscular & skeletal: Weakness

Ocular: Blurred vision, cycloplegia, increased ocular tension, mydriasis

Miscellaneous: Allergic reactions, sweating decreased

Drug Interactions

Metabolism/Transport Effects None known.

Avoid Concomitant Use There are no known interactions where it is recommended to avoid concomitant use.

Increased Effect/Toxicity

Hyoscyamine may increase the levels/effects of: AbobotulinumtoxinA; Anticholinergics; Cannabinoids; OnabotulinumtoxinA; Potassium Chloride; RimabotulinumtoxinB

The levels/effects of Hyoscyamine may be increased by: Pramlintide

Decreased Effect

Hyoscyamine may decrease the levels/effects of: Acetylcholinesterase Inhibitors (Central); Secretin

The levels/effects of Hyoscyamine may be decreased by: Acetylcholinesterase Inhibitors (Central)

Stability Store at controlled room temperature.

Mechanism of Action Blocks the action of acetylcholine at parasympathetic sites in smooth muscle, secretory glands, and the CNS; increases cardiac output, dries secretions, antagonizes histamine and serotonin

Pharmacodynamics/Kinetics

Onset of action: 2-3 minutes

Duration: 4-6 hours

Absorption: Well absorbed

Protein binding: 50%

Metabolism: Hepatic

Half-life elimination: 3-5 hours

Excretion: Urine

Dosage

Geriatric & Adult

Gastrointestinal spasms:

Oral or S.L.: 0.125-0.25 mg every 4 hours or as needed (before meals or food); maximum: 1.5 mg/24 hours

Oral, timed release: 0.375-0.75 mg every 12 hours; maximum: 1.5 mg/24 hours

I.M., I.V., SubQ: 0.25-0.5 mg; may repeat as needed up to 4 times/day, at 4-hour intervals

Diagnostic procedures: I.V.: 0.25-0.5 mg given 5-10 minutes prior to procedure

Preanesthesia: I.V.: 5 mcg/kg given 30-60 minutes prior to induction of anesthesia or at the time preoperative narcotics or sedatives are administered

To reduce drug-induced bradycardia during surgery: I.V.: 0.125 mg; repeat as needed

Reverse neuromuscular blockade: I.V.: 0.2 mg for every 1 mg neostigmine (or the physostigmine/pyridostigmine equivalent)

◀ **Administration**
Oral: Tablets should be administered before meals or food.
Levbid®: Tablets are scored and may be broken in half for dose titration; do not crush or chew.
Levsin/SL®: Tablets may be used sublingually, chewed, or swallowed whole.
Symax® SL: Tablets may be used sublingually or swallowed whole.
I.M.: May be administered without dilution.
I.V.: Inject over at least 1 minute. May be administered without dilution.

Special Geriatric Considerations Avoid long-term use; the potential for toxic reactions is higher than the potential benefit, elderly are particularly prone to CNS side effects of anticholinergics (eg, confusion, delirium, hallucinations). Side effects often occur before clinical response is obtained.

This medication is considered to be potentially inappropriate in this patient population (Beers Criteria: Quality of evidence - moderate; Strength of recommendation - strong).

Dosage Forms Excipient information presented when available (limited, particularly for generics); consult specific product labeling.
Elixir, oral, as sulfate: 0.125 mg/5 mL (473 mL)
Hyosyne: 0.125 mg/5 mL (473 mL) [contains ethanol 20%, sodium benzoate; orange-lemon flavor]
Injection, solution, as sulfate:
Levsin®: 0.5 mg/mL (1 mL)
Solution, oral, as sulfate [drops]: 0.125 mg/mL (15 mL)
Hyosyne: 0.125 mg/mL (15 mL) [contains ethanol 5%, sodium benzoate; orange-lemon flavor]
Tablet, oral, as sulfate: 0.125 mg
Levsin®: 0.125 mg
Tablet, sublingual, as sulfate: 0.125 mg
HyoMax®-SL: 0.125 mg [peppermint flavor]
Levsin®/SL: 0.125 mg
Oscimin: 0.125 mg [peppermint flavor]
Symax® SL: 0.125 mg
Tablet, chewable/disintegrating, oral, as sulfate:
HyoMax™-FT: 0.125 mg [mint flavor]
NuLev®: 0.125 mg [peppermint flavor]
Oscimin: 0.125 mg [peppermint flavor]
Symax® FasTab: 0.125 mg [mint flavor]
Tablet, dispersible, oral, as sulfate:
Oscimin: 0.125 mg [peppermint flavor]
Tablet, extended release, oral, as sulfate: 0.375 mg
Levbid®: 0.375 mg
Oscimin: 0.375 mg
Tablet, orally disintegrating, oral, as sulfate: 0.125 mg
Anaspaz®: 0.125 mg [scored]
ED-SPAZ: 0.125 mg [scored]
Tablet, sustained release, oral, as sulfate: 0.375 mg
HyoMax® -SR: 0.375 mg [scored]
Symax® SR: 0.375 mg
Tablet, variable release, oral:
HyoMax™-DT: Hyoscyamine sulfate 0.125 mg [immediate release] and hyoscyamine sulfate 0.25 mg [sustained release]
Symax® DuoTab: Hyoscyamine sulfate 0.125 mg [immediate release] and hyoscyamine sulfate 0.25 mg [sustained release]

Hyoscyamine, Atropine, Scopolamine, and Phenobarbital
(hye oh SYE a meen, A troe peen, skoe POL a meen, & fee noe BAR bi tal)

Related Information
Atropine *on page 166*
Hyoscyamine *on page 960*
PHENobarbital *on page 1520*
Scopolamine (Systemic) *on page 1756*

Medication Safety Issues
Sound-alike/look-alike issues:
Donnatal® may be confused with Donnagel, Donnatal Extentabs®
BEERS Criteria medication:
This drug may be potentially inappropriate for use in geriatric patients (Quality of evidence - moderate; Strength of recommendation - strong).

Brand Names: U.S. Donnatal Extentabs®; Donnatal®; Hyonatol

Index Terms Atropine, Hyoscyamine, Phenobarbital, and Scopolamine; Belladonna Alkaloids With Phenobarbital; Phenobarbital, Hyoscyamine, Atropine, and Scopolamine; Scopolamine, Hyoscyamine, Atropine, and Phenobarbital

Generic Availability (U.S.) Yes: Elixir, tablet

Pharmacologic Category Anticholinergic Agent; Antispasmodic Agent, Gastrointestinal

Use Adjunct in treatment of irritable bowel syndrome, acute enterocolitis, duodenal ulcer

Dosage
Geriatric & Adult Spasmolytic: Oral:
Immediate release: 1-2 tablets or 5-10 mL of elixir 3-4 times/day
Extended release: One tablet every 12 hours; may increase to 1 tablet every 8 hours if needed

Special Geriatric Considerations Because of the anticholinergic effects of this product, it is not recommended for use in the elderly.

This medication is considered to be potentially inappropriate in this patient population (Beers Criteria: Quality of evidence - moderate; Strength of recommendation - strong).

Dosage Forms Excipient information presented when available (limited, particularly for generics); consult specific product labeling. [DSC] = Discontinued product

Elixir: Hyoscyamine sulfate 0.1037 mg, atropine sulfate 0.0194 mg, scopolamine hydrobromide 0.0065 mg, and phenobarbital 16.2 mg per 5 mL (473 mL)
Donnatal®: Hyoscyamine sulfate 0.1037 mg, atropine sulfate 0.0194 mg, scopolamine hydrobromide 0.0065 mg, and phenobarbital 16.2 mg per 5 mL (120 mL, 480 mL) [contains ethanol <23.8%; citrus flavor] [DSC]
Donnatal®: Hyoscyamine sulfate 0.1037 mg, atropine sulfate 0.0194 mg, scopolamine hydrobromide 0.0065 mg, and phenobarbital 16.2 mg per 5 mL (120 mL, 480 mL) [contains ethanol <23.8%; grape flavor]

Tablet: Hyoscyamine sulfate 0.1037 mg, atropine sulfate 0.0194 mg, scopolamine hydrobromide 0.0065 mg, and phenobarbital 16.2 mg
Donnatal®: Hyoscyamine sulfate 0.1037 mg, atropine sulfate 0.0194 mg, scopolamine hydrobromide 0.0065 mg, and phenobarbital 16.2 mg
Hyonatol: Hyoscyamine sulfate 0.1037 mg, atropine sulfate 0.0194 mg, scopolamine hydrobromide 0.0065 mg, and phenobarbital 16.2 mg

Tablet, extended release:
Donnatal Extentabs®: Hyoscyamine sulfate 0.3111 mg, atropine sulfate 0.0582 mg, scopolamine hydrobromide 0.0195 mg, and phenobarbital 48.6 mg

Ibandronate (eye BAN droh nate)

Related Information
  Osteoporosis Management *on page* 2136
Brand Names: U.S. Boniva®
Index Terms Ibandronate Sodium; Ibandronic Acid
Generic Availability (U.S.) Yes: Tablet
Pharmacologic Category Bisphosphonate Derivative
Use Treatment and prevention of osteoporosis in postmenopausal females
Unlabeled Use Hypercalcemia of malignancy; reduce bone pain and skeletal complications from metastatic bone disease due to breast cancer
Medication Guide Available Yes
Contraindications Hypersensitivity to ibandronate or any component of the formulation; hypocalcemia; oral tablets are also contraindicated in patients unable to stand or sit upright for at least 60 minutes and in patients with abnormalities of the esophagus which delay esophageal emptying, such as stricture or achalasia
Warnings/Precautions Hypocalcemia must be corrected before therapy initiation. Ensure adequate calcium and vitamin D intake. Osteonecrosis of the jaw (ONJ) has been reported in patients receiving bisphosphonates. Risk factors include invasive dental procedures (eg, tooth extraction, dental implants, boney surgery); a diagnosis of cancer, with concomitant chemotherapy or corticosteroids; poor oral hygiene, ill-fitting dentures; and comorbid disorders (anemia, coagulopathy, infection, pre-existing dental disease). Most reported cases occurred after I.V. bisphosphonate therapy; however, cases have been reported following oral therapy. A dental exam and preventative dentistry should be performed prior to placing patients with risk factors on chronic bisphosphonate therapy. The manufacturer's labeling states that discontinuing bisphosphonates in patients requiring invasive dental procedures may reduce the risk of ONJ. However, other experts suggest that there is no evidence that discontinuing therapy reduces the risk of developing ONJ (Assael, 2009). The benefit/risk must be assessed by the treating physician and/or dentist/surgeon prior to any invasive dental procedure. Patients developing ONJ while on bisphosphonates should receive care by an oral surgeon.

Atypical femur fractures have been reported in patients receiving bisphosphonates for treatment/prevention of osteoporosis. The fractures include subtrochanteric femur (bone just below the hip joint) and diaphyseal femur (long segment of the thigh bone). Some patients experience prodromal pain weeks or months before the fracture occurs. It is unclear if bisphosphonate therapy is the cause for these fractures, although the majority have been reported in patients taking bisphosphonates. Patients receiving long-term (>3-5 years) therapy may be at an increased risk. Discontinue bisphosphonate therapy in patients who develop a femoral shaft fracture.

Infrequently, severe (and occasionally debilitating) bone, joint, and/or muscle pain have been reported during bisphosphonate treatment. The onset of pain ranged from a single day to several months. Consider discontinuing therapy in patients who experience severe symptoms; symptoms usually resolve upon discontinuation. Some patients experienced recurrence when rechallenged with same drug or another bisphosphonate; avoid use in patients with a history of these symptoms in association with bisphosphonate therapy.

Oral bisphosphonates may cause dysphagia, esophagitis, esophageal or gastric ulcer; risk may increase in patients unable to comply with dosing instructions; discontinue use if new or worsening symptoms develop. Intravenous bisphosphonates may cause transient decreases in serum calcium and have also been associated with renal toxicity.

Use not recommended with severe renal impairment (Cl_{cr} <30 mL/minute).
Adverse Reactions (Reflective of adult population; not specific for elderly) Percentages vary based on frequency of administration (daily vs monthly). Unless specified, percentages are reported with oral use.
  >10%:
    Gastrointestinal: Dyspepsia (6% to 12%)
    Neuromuscular & skeletal: Back pain (4% to 14%)
  1% to 10%:
    Cardiovascular: Hypertension (6% to 7%)
    Central nervous system: Headache (3% to 7%), dizziness (1% to 4%), insomnia (1% to 2%)
    Dermatologic: Rash (1% to 2%)
    Endocrine & metabolic: Hypercholesterolemia (5%)
    Gastrointestinal: Abdominal pain (5% to 8%), diarrhea (4% to 7%), nausea (5%), constipation (3% to 4%), vomiting (3%)
    Genitourinary: Urinary tract infection (2% to 6%)
    Hepatic: Alkaline phosphatase decreased (frequency not defined)

Local: Injection site reaction (<2%)

Neuromuscular & skeletal: Pain in extremity (1% to 8%), arthralgia (4% to 6%), myalgia (1% to 6%), joint disorder (4%), osteonecrosis of the jaw (4%), weakness (4%), osteoarthritis (localized; 1% to 3%), muscle cramp (2%)

Respiratory: Bronchitis (3% to 10%), pneumonia (6%), pharyngitis/nasopharyngitis (3% to 4%), upper respiratory infection (2%)

Miscellaneous: Acute phase reaction (I.V. 10%; oral 3% to 9%), infection (4%), flu-like syndrome (1% to 4%), allergic reaction (3%)

Drug Interactions

Metabolism/Transport Effects None known.

Avoid Concomitant Use There are no known interactions where it is recommended to avoid concomitant use.

Increased Effect/Toxicity

Ibandronate may increase the levels/effects of: Deferasirox; Phosphate Supplements; SUNItinib

The levels/effects of Ibandronate may be increased by: Aminoglycosides; Nonsteroidal Anti-Inflammatory Agents

Decreased Effect

The levels/effects of Ibandronate may be decreased by: Antacids; Calcium Salts; Iron Salts; Magnesium Salts; Proton Pump Inhibitors

Ethanol/Nutrition/Herb Interactions

Ethanol: Ethanol may increase risk of osteoporosis. Management: Avoid ethanol.

Food: May reduce absorption; mean oral bioavailability is decreased up to 90% when given with food. Management: Take with a full glass (6-8 oz) of plain water, at least 60 minutes prior to any food, beverages, or medications. Mineral water with a high calcium content should be avoided. Wait at least 60 minutes after taking ibandronate before taking anything else.

Stability Store at controlled room temperature of 25°C (77°F); excursions permitted to 15°C to 30°C (59°F to 86°F).

Mechanism of Action A bisphosphonate which inhibits bone resorption via actions on osteoclasts or on osteoclast precursors; decreases the rate of bone resorption, leading to an indirect increase in bone mineral density.

Pharmacodynamics/Kinetics

Distribution: Terminal V_d: 90 L; 40% to 50% of circulating ibandronate binds to bone

Protein binding: 85.7% to 99.5%

Metabolism: Not metabolized

Bioavailability: Oral: Minimal; reduced ~90% following standard breakfast

Half-life elimination:
  Oral: 150 mg dose: Terminal: 37-157 hours
  I.V.: Terminal: ~5-25 hours

Time to peak, plasma: Oral: 0.5-2 hours

Excretion: Urine (50% to 60% of absorbed dose, excreted as unchanged drug); feces (unabsorbed drug)

Dosage

Geriatric & Adult

Postmenopausal osteoporosis (treatment): Patients should receive supplemental calcium and vitamin D if dietary intake is inadequate
  Oral: 150 mg once a month
  I.V.: 3 mg every 3 months

Postmenopausal osteoporosis (prevention): Patients should receive supplemental calcium and vitamin D if dietary intake is inadequate: Oral: 150 mg once a month

Hypercalcemia of malignancy (unlabeled use): I.V.: 2-6 mg over 1-2 hours (Pecherstorfer, 2003; Ralston, 1997)

Metastatic bone disease due to breast cancer (unlabeled use): I.V.: 6 mg every 3-4 weeks (Diel, 2004)

Renal Impairment

Osteoporosis: Oral, I.V.:
  Cl_{cr} ≥30 mL/minute: No dosage adjustment necessary.
  Cl_{cr} <30 mL/minute: Use not recommended.

Oncologic uses (unlabeled): I.V.: Cl_{cr} <30 mL/minute: 2 mg every 3-4 weeks (von Moos, 2005)

Hepatic Impairment No dosage adjustment necessary.

Administration

Oral: Administer 60 minutes before the first food or drink of the day (other than water) and prior to taking any oral medications or supplements (eg, calcium, antacids, vitamins). Ibandronate should be taken in an upright position with a full glass (6-8 oz) of plain water and the patient should avoid lying down for 60 minutes to minimize the possibility of GI side effects. Mineral water with a high calcium content should be avoided. The tablet should be swallowed whole; do not chew or suck. Do not eat or drink anything (except water) for 60 minutes following administration of ibandronate.

Take on the same date each month. In case of a missed dose, do not take two 150 mg tablets within the same week. If the next scheduled dose is 1-7 days away, wait until the next scheduled dose to take the tablet. If the next scheduled dose is >7 days away, take the dose the morning it is remembered, and then resume taking the once-monthly dose on the originally scheduled day.

I.V.: Administer as a 15-30 second bolus. Do not mix with calcium-containing solutions or other drugs. For osteoporosis, do not administer more frequently than every 3 months. Infuse over 1 hour for metastatic bone disease due to breast cancer (Diel, 2004) and over 1-2 hours for hypercalcemia of malignancy (Pecherstorfer, 2003; Ralston, 1997).

Monitoring Parameters

Osteoporosis: Bone mineral density as measured by central dual-energy x-ray absorptiometry (DXA) of the hip or spine (prior to initiation of therapy and at least every 2 years); annual measurements of height and weight, assessment of chronic back pain; serum calcium and 25(OH)D; may consider measuring biochemical markers of bone turnover

Serum creatinine prior to each I.V. dose

Test Interactions Bisphosphonates may interfere with diagnostic imaging agents such as technetium-99m-diphosphonate in bone scans.

Special Geriatric Considerations The elderly are frequently treated long-term for osteoporosis. Elderly patients should be advised to report any lower extremity, jaw (osteonecrosis), or muscle pain that cannot be explained or lasts longer than 2 weeks. Additionally, the elderly often receive concomitant diuretic therapy and therefore their electrolyte status (eg, calcium, phosphate) should be periodically evaluated. Since the elderly may have creatinine clearances <30 mL/minute, creatinine clearance should be measured or calculated before initiating therapy with ibandronate.

Due to the reports of atypical femur fractures and osteonecrosis of the jaw, recommendations for duration of bisphosphonate use in osteoporosis have been modified. Based on available data, consider discontinuing bisphosphonates after 5 years of use in low-risk patients, since the risk of nonvertebral fracture is the same as those patients taking bisphosphonates for 10 years. Those patients with high risk (fracture history) may be continued for a longer period, taking into consideration the risks vs benefits associated with continued therapy.

Dosage Forms Excipient information presented when available (limited, particularly for generics); consult specific product labeling.

Injection, solution:
  Boniva®: 1 mg/mL (3 mL)
Tablet, oral: 150 mg
  Boniva®: 150 mg [once-monthly formulation]

◆ **Ibandronate Sodium** see Ibandronate on page 964
◆ **Ibandronic Acid** see Ibandronate on page 964
◆ **Ibidomide Hydrochloride** see Labetalol on page 1078
◆ **Ibu®** see Ibuprofen on page 966
◆ **Ibu-200 [OTC]** see Ibuprofen on page 966

Ibuprofen (eye byoo PROE fen)

Related Information

Beers Criteria – Potentially Inappropriate Medications for Geriatrics on page 2183

Medication Safety Issues

Sound-alike/look-alike issues:
  Haltran® may be confused with Halfprin®
  Motrin® may be confused with Neurontin®

BEERS Criteria medication:
  This drug may be potentially inappropriate for use in geriatric patients (Quality of evidence - moderate; Strength of recommendation - strong).

Administration issues:
  Injectable formulations: Both ibuprofen and ibuprofen lysine are available for parenteral use. Ibuprofen lysine is **only** indicated for closure of a clinically-significant patent ductus arteriosus.

Brand Names: U.S. Addaprin [OTC]; Advil® Children's [OTC]; Advil® Infants' [OTC]; Advil® Migraine [OTC]; Advil® [OTC]; Caldolor™; I-Prin [OTC]; Ibu-200 [OTC]; Ibu®; Midol® Cramps & Body Aches [OTC]; Motrin® Children's [OTC]; Motrin® IB [OTC]; Motrin® Infants' [OTC]; Motrin® Junior [OTC]; Proprinal® [OTC]; TopCare® Junior Strength [OTC]; Ultraprin [OTC]

Brand Names: Canada Advil®; Apo-Ibuprofen®; Motrin® (Children's); Motrin® IB; Novo-Profen; Nu-Ibuprofen

Index Terms *p*-Isobutylhydratropic Acid

Generic Availability (U.S.) Yes: Caplet, liquid-filled capsule, softgel capsule, suspension, tablet

Pharmacologic Category Nonsteroidal Anti-inflammatory Drug (NSAID), Oral

Use

Oral: Inflammatory diseases and rheumatoid disorders including juvenile idiopathic arthritis (JIA), mild-to-moderate pain, fever, dysmenorrhea, osteoarthritis

Ibuprofen injection (Caldolor™): Management of mild-to-moderate pain; management moderate-to-severe pain when used concurrently with an opioid analgesic; reduction of fever

Unlabeled Use Cystic fibrosis, gout, ankylosing spondylitis, acute migraine headache, migraine prophylaxis

Medication Guide Available Yes

Contraindications Hypersensitivity to ibuprofen; history of asthma, urticaria, or allergic-type reaction to aspirin or other NSAIDs; aspirin triad (eg, bronchial asthma, aspirin intolerance, rhinitis); perioperative pain in the setting of coronary artery bypass graft (CABG) surgery

Warnings/Precautions [U.S. Boxed Warning]: NSAIDs are associated with an increased risk of adverse cardiovascular thrombotic events, including fatal MI and stroke. Risk may be increased with duration of use or pre-existing cardiovascular risk factors or disease. Carefully evaluate individual cardiovascular risk profiles prior to prescribing. May cause new-onset hypertension or worsening of existing hypertension. Response to ACE inhibitors, thiazides, or loop diuretics may be impaired with concurrent use of NSAIDs. Use caution with fluid retention. Avoid use in heart failure. Concurrent administration of ibuprofen, and potentially other nonselective NSAIDs, may interfere with aspirin's cardioprotective effect. **[U.S. Boxed Warning]: Use is contraindicated for treatment of perioperative pain in the setting of coronary artery bypass graft (CABG) surgery.** Risk of MI and stroke may be increased with use following CABG surgery.

May increase the risk of aseptic meningitis, especially in patients with systemic lupus erythematosus (SLE) and mixed connective tissue disorders. Platelet adhesion and aggregation may be decreased; may prolong bleeding time; patients with coagulation disorders or who are receiving anticoagulants should be monitored closely. Anemia may occur; patients on long-term NSAID therapy should be monitored for anemia. Rarely, NSAID use may cause severe blood dyscrasias (eg, agranulocytosis, aplastic anemia, thrombocytopenia).

NSAID use may compromise existing renal function; dose-dependent decreases in prostaglandin synthesis may result from NSAID use, reducing renal blood flow which may cause renal decompensation. NSAID use may increase the risk for hyperkalemia. Patients with impaired renal function, dehydration, heart failure, liver dysfunction, those taking diuretics, and ACE inhibitors, and the elderly are at greater risk of renal toxicity and hyperkalemia. Rehydrate patient before starting therapy; monitor renal function closely. Not recommended for use in patients with advanced renal disease. Long-term NSAID use may result in renal papillary necrosis.

NSAIDs may increase risk of gastrointestinal irritation, inflammation, ulceration, bleeding, and perforation. These events can be fatal and may occur at any time during therapy and without warning. Use caution with a history of GI disease (bleeding or ulcers), concurrent therapy with aspirin, anticoagulants and/or corticosteroids, smoking, use of ethanol, the elderly or debilitated patients. When used concomitantly with ≤325 mg of aspirin, a substantial increase in the risk of gastrointestinal complications (eg, ulcer) occurs; concomitant gastroprotective therapy (eg, proton pump inhibitors) is recommended (Bhatt, 2008).

Use the lowest effective dose for the shortest duration of time, consistent with individual patient goals, to reduce risk of cardiovascular or GI adverse events. Alternate therapies should be considered for patients at high risk.

NSAIDs may cause serious skin adverse events including exfoliative dermatitis, Stevens-Johnson Syndrome (SJS) and toxic epidermal necrolysis (TEN); discontinue use at first sign of skin rash or hypersensitivity. Anaphylactoid reactions may occur, even without prior exposure; patients with "aspirin triad" (bronchial asthma, aspirin intolerance, rhinitis) may be at increased risk. Do not use in patients who experience bronchospasm, asthma, rhinitis, or urticaria with NSAID or aspirin therapy. Use caution in other forms of asthma.

NSAIDS may cause drowsiness, dizziness, blurred vision and other neurologic effects which may impair physical or mental abilities; patients must be cautioned about performing tasks which require mental alertness (eg, operating machinery or driving). Monitor vision with long-term therapy. Blurred/diminished vision, scotomata, and changes in color vision have been reported. Discontinue use with altered vision and perform ophthalmologic exam.

◄

Use with caution in patients with decreased hepatic function. Closely monitor patients with any abnormal LFT. Severe hepatic reactions (eg, fulminant hepatitis, liver failure) have occurred with NSAID use, rarely; discontinue if signs or symptoms of liver disease develop, or if systemic manifestations occur.

In the elderly, avoid chronic use (unless alternative agents ineffective and patient can receive concomitant gastroprotective agent); nonselective oral NSAID use is associated with an increased risk of GI bleeding and peptic ulcer disease in older adults in high risk category (eg, >75 years or age or receiving concomitant oral/parenteral corticosteroids, anticoagulants, or antiplatelet agents) (Beers Criteria).

Withhold for at least 4-6 half-lives prior to surgical or dental procedures. Some products may contain phenylalanine. Ibuprofen injection (Caldolor™) must be diluted prior to administration; hemolysis can occur if not diluted.

Self medication (OTC use): Prior to self-medication, patients should contact healthcare provider if they have had recurring stomach pain or upset, ulcers, bleeding problems, high blood pressure, heart or kidney disease, other serious medical problems, are currently taking a diuretic, aspirin, anticoagulant, or are ≥60 years of age. If patients are using for migraines, they should also contact healthcare provider if they have not had a migraine diagnosis by healthcare provider, a headache that is different from usual migraine, worst headache of life, fever and neck stiffness, headache from head injury or coughing, first headache at ≥50 years of age, daily headache, or migraine requiring bed rest. Recommended dosages should not be exceeded, due to an increased risk of GI bleeding. Stop use and consult a healthcare provider if symptoms get worse, newly appear, fever lasts for >10 days (adults). Do not give for >10 days unless instructed by healthcare provider. Consuming ≥3 alcoholic beverages/day or taking longer than recommended may increase the risk of GI bleeding.

Adverse Reactions (Reflective of adult population; not specific for elderly)
Oral:
1% to 10%:
Cardiovascular: Edema (1% to 3%)
Central nervous system: Dizziness (3% to 9%), headache (1% to 3%), nervousness (1% to 3%)
Dermatologic: Rash (3% to 9%), itching (1% to 3%)
Endocrine & metabolic: Fluid retention (1% to 3%)
Gastrointestinal: Epigastric pain (3% to 9%), heartburn (3% to 9%), nausea (3% to 9%), abdominal pain/cramps/distress (1% to 3%), appetite decreased (1% to 3%), constipation (1% to 3%), diarrhea (1% to 3%), dyspepsia (1% to 3%), flatulence (1% to 3%), vomiting (1% to 3%)
Otic: Tinnitus (3% to 9%)

Injection: Ibuprofen (Caldolor™):
Cardiovascular: Edema, hypertension
Central nervous system: Dizziness, headache
Dermatologic: Pruritus
Endocrine & metabolic: Hypernatremia, hypokalemia
Gastrointestinal: Abdominal pain, dyspepsia, flatulence, nausea, vomiting
Genitourinary: Urinary retention
Hematologic: Anemia, hemorrhage, neutropenia
Renal: BUN increased
Respiratory: Cough

Drug Interactions
Metabolism/Transport Effects Substrate of CYP2C19 (minor), CYP2C9 (minor); **Note:** Assignment of Major/Minor substrate status based on clinically relevant drug interaction potential; **Inhibits** CYP2C9 (weak)

Avoid Concomitant Use
Avoid concomitant use of Ibuprofen with any of the following: Floctafenine; Ketorolac; Ketorolac (Nasal); Ketorolac (Systemic)

Increased Effect/Toxicity
Ibuprofen may increase the levels/effects of: Aliskiren; Aminoglycosides; Anticoagulants; Antiplatelet Agents; Bisphosphonate Derivatives; Collagenase (Systemic); CycloSPORINE; CycloSPORINE (Systemic); Dabigatran Etexilate; Deferasirox; Desmopressin; Digoxin; Drotrecogin Alfa (Activated); Eplerenone; Haloperidol; Ibritumomab; Lithium; Methotrexate; Nonsteroidal Anti-Inflammatory Agents; PEMEtrexed; Porfimer; Potassium-Sparing Diuretics; PRALAtrexate; Quinolone Antibiotics; Rivaroxaban; Salicylates; Thrombolytic Agents; Tositumomab and Iodine I 131 Tositumomab; Vancomycin; Vitamin K Antagonists

The levels/effects of Ibuprofen may be increased by: ACE Inhibitors; Angiotensin II Receptor Blockers; Antidepressants (Tricyclic, Tertiary Amine); Corticosteroids (Systemic); Cyclo-SPORINE; CycloSPORINE (Systemic); Dasatinib; Floctafenine; Glucosamine; Herbs (Anti-coagulant/Antiplatelet Properties); Ketorolac; Ketorolac (Nasal); Ketorolac (Systemic); Nonsteroidal Anti-Inflammatory Agents; Omega-3-Acid Ethyl Esters; Pentosan Polysulfate Sodium; Pentoxifylline; Probenecid; Prostacyclin Analogues; Selective Serotonin Reuptake Inhibitors; Serotonin/Norepinephrine Reuptake Inhibitors; Sodium Phosphates; Tipranavir; Treprostinil; Vitamin E; Voriconazole

Decreased Effect

Ibuprofen may decrease the levels/effects of: ACE Inhibitors; Aliskiren; Angiotensin II Receptor Blockers; Antiplatelet Agents; Beta-Blockers; Eplerenone; HydrALAZINE; Imatinib; Loop Diuretics; Potassium-Sparing Diuretics; Salicylates; Selective Serotonin Reuptake Inhibitors; Thiazide Diuretics

The levels/effects of Ibuprofen may be decreased by: Bile Acid Sequestrants; Nonsteroidal Anti-Inflammatory Agents; Salicylates

Ethanol/Nutrition/Herb Interactions

Ethanol: Avoid ethanol (may enhance gastric mucosal irritation).

Food: Ibuprofen peak serum levels may be decreased if taken with food.

Herb/Nutraceutical: Avoid alfalfa, anise, bilberry, bladderwrack, bromelain, cat's claw, celery, chamomile, coleus, cordyceps, dong quai, evening primrose, fenugreek, feverfew, garlic, ginger, ginkgo biloba, ginseng (American, Panax, Siberian), grapeseed, green tea, guggul, horse chestnut seed, horseradish, licorice, prickly ash, red clover, reishi, SAMe (S-adenosylmethionine), sweet clover, turmeric, white willow (all have additional antiplatelet activity).

Stability

Ibuprofen injection (Caldolor™): Store intact vials at room temperature of 20°C to 25°C (68°F to 77°F). Must be diluted prior to use. Dilute with D_5W, NS or LR to a final concentration ≤4 mg/mL. Diluted solutions stable for 24 hours at room temperature.

Suspension, tablet: Store at room temperature of 20°C to 25°C (68°F to 77°F).

Mechanism of Action Reversibly inhibits cyclooxygenase-1 and 2 (COX-1 and 2) enzymes, which results in decreased formation of prostaglandin precursors; has antipyretic, analgesic, and anti-inflammatory properties

Other proposed mechanisms not fully elucidated (and possibly contributing to the anti-inflammatory effect to varying degrees), include inhibiting chemotaxis, altering lymphocyte activity, inhibiting neutrophil aggregation/activation, and decreasing proinflammatory cytokine levels.

Pharmacodynamics/Kinetics

Onset of action: Oral: Analgesic: 30-60 minutes; Anti-inflammatory: ≤7 days

Duration: Oral: 4-6 hours

Absorption: Oral: Rapid (85%)

Distribution: V_d: 6.35 L

Protein binding: 90% to 99%

Metabolism: Hepatic via oxidation

Half-life elimination: Adults: 2-4 hours; End-stage renal disease: Unchanged

Time to peak: Oral: ~1-2 hours

Excretion: Urine (primarily as metabolites; 1% as unchanged drug); some feces

Dosage

Geriatric & Adult

Inflammatory disease: Oral: 400-800 mg/dose 3-4 times/day (maximum: 3.2 g/day)

Analgesia/pain/fever/dysmenorrhea: Oral: 200-400 mg/dose every 4-6 hours (maximum daily dose: 1.2 g, unless directed by physician; under physician supervision daily doses ≤2.4 g may be used)

Analgesic: I.V. (Caldolor®): 400-800 mg every 6 hours as needed (maximum: 3.2 g/day). **Note:** Patients should be well hydrated prior to administration.

Antipyretic: I.V. (Caldolor®): Initial: 400 mg, then every 4-6 hours or 100-200 mg every 4 hours as needed (maximum: 3.2 g/day). **Note:** Patients should be well hydrated prior to administration.

OTC labeling (analgesic, antipyretic): Oral: 200 mg every 4-6 hours as needed (maximum: 1200 mg/24 hours); treatment for >10 days is not recommended unless directed by healthcare provider.

Migraine: 2 capsules at onset of symptoms (maximum: 400 mg/24 hours unless directed by healthcare provider)

Renal Impairment If anuria or oliguria evident, hold dose until renal function returns to normal.

Hepatic Impairment Avoid use in severe hepatic impairment.

Administration
Oral: Administer with food
I.V.:
Caldolor™: For I.V. administration only; must be diluted to a final concentration of ≤4 mg/mL prior to administration; infuse over at least 30 minutes

Monitoring Parameters CBC, chemistry profile, occult blood loss and periodic liver function tests; monitor response (pain, range of motion, grip strength, mobility, ADL function), inflammation; observe for weight gain, edema; monitor renal function (urine output, serum BUN and creatinine); observe for bleeding, bruising; evaluate gastrointestinal effects (abdominal pain, bleeding, dyspepsia); mental confusion, disorientation; with long-term therapy, periodic ophthalmic exams

Reference Range Plasma concentrations >200 mcg/mL may be associated with severe toxicity
PDA: Minimum effective concentration: 10-12 mg/L

Test Interactions May interfere with urine detection of PCP, cannabinoids, and barbiturates (false-positives)

Special Geriatric Considerations Elderly are a high-risk population for adverse effects from NSAIDs. As much as 60% of elderly can develop peptic ulceration and/or hemorrhage asymptomatically. The concomitant use of H_2 blockers and sucralfate is not effective as prophylaxis with the exception of NSAID-induced duodenal ulcers which may be prevented by the use of ranitidine. Misoprostol and proton pump inhibitors are the only agents proven to help prevent the development of NSAID-induced ulcers. Also, concomitant disease and drug use contribute to the risk for GI adverse effects. Use lowest effective dose for shortest period possible. Consider renal function decline with age. Use of NSAIDs can compromise existing renal function especially when Cl_{cr} is ≤30 mL/minute. Tinnitus may be a difficult and unreliable indication of toxicity due to age-related hearing loss or eighth cranial nerve damage. CNS adverse effects such as confusion, agitation, and hallucination are generally seen in overdose or high dose situations, but the elderly may demonstrate these adverse effects at lower doses than younger adults.

This medication is considered to be potentially inappropriate in this patient population (Beers Criteria: Quality of evidence - moderate; Strength of recommendation - strong).

Dosage Forms Excipient information presented when available (limited, particularly for generics); consult specific product labeling.
Caplet, oral: 200 mg
Advil®: 200 mg
Motrin® IB: 200 mg
Motrin® Junior: 100 mg [scored]
Capsule, liquid filled, oral: 200 mg
Advil®: 200 mg [contains potassium 20 mg/capsule; solubilized ibuprofen]
Advil® Migraine: 200 mg [contains potassium 20 mg/capsule; solubilized ibuprofen]
Capsule, softgel, oral: 200 mg
Gelcap, oral:
Advil®: 200 mg [contains coconut oil]
Injection, solution:
Caldolor™: 100 mg/mL (4 mL, 8 mL)
Suspension, oral: 100 mg/5 mL (5 mL, 10 mL, 120 mL, 480 mL)
Advil® Children's: 100 mg/5 mL (120 mL) [contains propylene glycol, sodium 10 mg/5 mL, sodium benzoate; blue raspberry flavor]
Advil® Children's: 100 mg/5 mL (120 mL) [contains propylene glycol, sodium 3 mg/5 mL, sodium benzoate; grape flavor]
Advil® Children's: 100 mg/5 mL (120 mL) [contains sodium 3 mg/5 mL, sodium benzoate; fruit flavor]
Motrin® Children's: 100 mg/5 mL (120 mL) [dye free, ethanol free; contains sodium 2 mg/5 mL, sodium benzoate; berry flavor]
Motrin® Children's: 100 mg/5 mL (60 mL, 120 mL) [ethanol free; contains sodium 2 mg/5 mL, sodium benzoate; berry flavor]
Motrin® Children's: 100 mg/5 mL (120 mL) [ethanol free; contains sodium 2 mg/5 mL, sodium benzoate; bubblegum flavor]
Motrin® Children's: 100 mg/5 mL (120 mL) [ethanol free; contains sodium 2 mg/5 mL, sodium benzoate; grape flavor]
Motrin® Children's: 100 mg/5 mL (120 mL) [ethanol free; contains sodium 2 mg/5 mL, sodium benzoate; tropical punch flavor]
Suspension, oral [concentrate/drops]: 40 mg/mL (15 mL)
Advil® Infants': 40 mg/mL (15 mL) [contains sodium benzoate; grape flavor]
Advil® Infants': 40 mg/mL (15 mL) [dye free; contains propylene glycol, sodium benzoate; white grape flavor]

Motrin® Infants': 40 mg/mL (15 mL) [dye free, ethanol free; contains sodium benzoate; berry flavor]

Motrin® Infants': 40 mg/mL (15 mL) [ethanol free; contains sodium benzoate; berry flavor]

Tablet, oral: 200 mg, 400 mg, 600 mg, 800 mg

Addaprin: 200 mg

Advil®: 200 mg [contains sodium benzoate]

I-Prin: 200 mg

Ibu-200: 200 mg

Ibu®: 400 mg, 600 mg, 800 mg

Midol® Cramps & Body Aches: 200 mg

Motrin® IB: 200 mg

Proprinal®: 200 mg [contains sodium benzoate]

Ultraprin: 200 mg [sugar free]

Tablet, chewable, oral:

Motrin® Junior: 100 mg [contains phenylalanine 2.8 mg/tablet; grape flavor]

Motrin® Junior: 100 mg [contains phenylalanine 2.8 mg/tablet; orange flavor]

TopCare® Junior Strength: 100 mg [scored; orange flavor]

Ibuprofen and Famotidine (eye byoo PROE fen & fa MOE ti deen)

Brand Names: U.S. Duexis®

Index Terms Famotidine and Ibuprofen; HZT-501

Generic Availability (U.S.) No

Pharmacologic Category Histamine H_2 Antagonist; Nonsteroidal Anti-inflammatory Drug (NSAID), Oral

Use Reduction of the risk of NSAID-associated gastric ulcers in patients who require an NSAID for the treatment of rheumatoid arthritis or osteoarthritis

Medication Guide Available Yes

Dosage

Geriatric & Adult NSAID-associated ulcer prophylaxis during treatment for osteo-arthritis/rheumatoid arthritis: Oral: One tablet (800 mg ibuprofen/26.6 mg famotidine) 3 times daily

Renal Impairment Cl_{cr} <50 mL/minute: Use not recommended.

Special Geriatric Considerations See individual agents.

Dosage Forms Excipient information presented when available (limited, particularly for generics); consult specific product labeling.

Tablet, oral:

Duexis®: Ibuprofen 800 mg and famotidine 26.6 mg

Icatibant (eye KAT i bant)

Brand Names: U.S. Firazyr®

Index Terms HOE 140; Icatibant Acetate

Pharmacologic Category Selective Bradykinin B2 Receptor Antagonist

Use Treatment of acute attacks of hereditary angioedema (HAE)

Contraindications There are no contraindications listed in the manufacturer's labeling.

Warnings/Precautions Airway obstruction may occur during acute laryngeal attacks of HAE. Patients with laryngeal attacks should be instructed to seek medical attention immediately in addition to treatment with icatibant. Icatibant may potentially attenuate the antihypertensive effect of ACE inhibitors; patients taking ACE inhibitors were excluded from initial clinical trials.

Adverse Reactions (Reflective of adult population; not specific for elderly)

>10%: Local: Injection site reaction (97%)

1% to 10%:

Central nervous system: Pyrexia (4%), dizziness (3%)

Hepatic: Transaminase increased (4%)

Drug Interactions

Metabolism/Transport Effects None known.

Avoid Concomitant Use There are no known interactions where it is recommended to avoid concomitant use.

Increased Effect/Toxicity There are no known significant interactions involving an increase in effect.

Decreased Effect

Icatibant may decrease the levels/effects of: ACE Inhibitors

Stability Store between 2°C to 25°C (36°F to 77°F); do not freeze. Store in original container until time of administration.

Mechanism of Action Icatibant is a selective competitive antagonist for the bradykinin B_2 receptor. Patients with HAE have an absence or dysfunction of C1-esterase-inhibitor which leads to the production of bradykinin. The presence of bradykinin may cause symptoms of localized swelling, inflammation, and pain. Icatibant inhibits bradykinin from binding at the B_2 receptor, thereby treating the symptoms associated with acute attack.

Pharmacodynamics/Kinetics
Onset: Median time to 50% decrease of symptoms: ~2 hours
Duration: Inhibits symptoms caused by bradykinin for ~6 hours
Distribution: V_{dss}: 20.3-37.7 L
Metabolism: Metabolized by proteolytic enzymes to metabolites (inactive)
Bioavailability: ~97%
Half-life elimination: 1-1.8 hours
Time to peak: 0.75 hours
Excretion: Urine (<10% unchanged)

Dosage
Geriatric Refer to adult dosing. Systemic exposure may be increased; however, no dosage adjustments are recommended.
Adult Hereditary angioedema (HAE): SubQ: 30 mg/dose; may repeat one dose every 6 hours if response is inadequate or symptoms recur (maximum: 3 doses/24 hours)
Renal Impairment No dosage adjustments are recommended.
Hepatic Impairment No dosage adjustments are recommended.

Administration For SubQ injection only. Inject into the abdomen over ≥30 seconds, using the 25 gauge needle provided. Inject 2-4 inches below belly button and away from any scars; do not inject into an area that is bruised, swollen, or painful.

Monitoring Parameters Symptom relief; laryngeal symptoms or airway obstruction (immediate medical attention required in addition to icatibant therapy)

Special Geriatric Considerations Data suggests icatibant's pharmacokinetics are not affected by liver or renal impairment; however, clearance is reduced in the elderly, resulting in an AUC ~50% to 60% higher in 75- to 80-year-old patients compared to 40-year-old patients. Despite an increased AUC, no difference in safety and efficacy has been noted between elderly and younger adults and dosage adjustments are not recommended.

Dosage Forms Excipient information presented when available (limited, particularly for generics); consult specific product labeling.
Injection, solution [preservative free]:
Firazyr®: 10 mg/mL (3 mL)

Iloperidone (eye loe PER i done)

Related Information
Medication Safety Issues
Sound-alike/look-alike issues:
Fanapt® may be confused with Xanax®
Iloperidone may be confused with domperidone
BEERS Criteria medication:
This drug may be potentially inappropriate for use in geriatric patients (Quality of evidence - moderate; Strength of recommendation - strong).
Brand Names: U.S. Fanapt®
Generic Availability (U.S.) No
Pharmacologic Category Antipsychotic Agent, Atypical
Use Acute treatment of schizophrenia
Contraindications Hypersensitivity to iloperidone or any component of the formulation

Warnings/Precautions [U.S. Boxed Warning]: Elderly patients with dementia-related psychosis treated with antipsychotics are at an increased risk of death compared to placebo. Most deaths appeared to be either cardiovascular (eg, heart failure, sudden death) or infectious (eg, pneumonia) in nature. In addition, an increased incidence of cerebrovascular effects (eg, transient ischemic attack, cerebrovascular accidents) has been reported in studies of placebo-controlled trials of antipsychotics in elderly patients with dementia-related psychosis. Iloperidone is not approved for the treatment of dementia-related psychosis.

May be sedating; use with caution in disorders where CNS depression is a feature. Caution in patients with predisposition to seizures. Use is not recommended in patients with hepatic impairment. Esophageal dysmotility and aspiration have been associated with antipsychotic use; use with caution in patients at risk of aspiration pneumonia (ie, Alzheimer's disease). Use is associated with increased prolactin levels; clinical significance of hyperprolactinemia in patients with breast cancer or other prolactin-dependent tumors is unknown. May alter temperature regulation. Leukopenia, neutropenia, and agranulocytosis (sometimes fatal) have been reported in clinical trials and postmarketing reports; presence of risk factors (eg, pre-existing low WBC or history of drug-induced leuko-/neutropenia) should prompt periodic blood count assessment and discontinuation at first signs of blood dyscrasias.

May alter cardiac conduction and prolong the QT_c interval; life-threatening arrhythmias have occurred with therapeutic doses of antipsychotics. Risks may be increased by conditions or concomitant medications which cause bradycardia, hypokalemia, and/or hypomagnesemia. Avoid use in combination with QT_c-prolonging drugs and in patients with congenital long QT syndrome, history of cardiac arrhythmia, recent MI, or uncompensated heart failure. Discontinue treatment in patients found to have persistent QT_c intervals >500 msec. Further cardiac evaluation is warranted in patients with symptoms of dizziness, palpitations, or syncope. May cause orthostatic hypotension; use with caution in patients at risk of this effect (eg, concurrent medication use which may predispose to hypotension/bradycardia or presence of hypovolemia) or in those who would not tolerate transient hypotensive episodes. Use with caution in patients with cardiovascular diseases (eg, heart failure, history of myocardial infarction or ischemia, cerebrovascular disease, conduction abnormalities).

May cause anticholinergic effects (confusion, agitation, constipation, xerostomia, blurred vision, urinary retention); therefore, use with caution in patients with decreased gastrointestinal motility, urinary retention, BPH, xerostomia, or visual problems (including narrow-angle glaucoma). May cause extrapyramidal symptoms (EPS), including pseudoparkinsonism, acute dystonic reactions, akathisia, and tardive dyskinesia. Risk of dystonia (and probably other EPS) may be greater with increased doses, use of conventional antipsychotics, males, and younger patients. Risk of neuroleptic malignant syndrome (NMS) may be increased in patients with Parkinson's disease or Lewy body dementia. May cause hyperglycemia; in some cases may be extreme and associated with ketoacidosis, hyperosmolar coma, or death. Use with caution in patients with diabetes or other disorders of glucose regulation; monitor for worsening of glucose control. Dyslipidemia has been reported with atypical antipsychotics; risk profile may differ between agents. In clinical trials, changes in triglyceride and total cholesterol levels observed with iloperidone were similar to those observed with placebo or were clinically insignificant.

Significant weight gain has been observed with antipsychotic therapy; incidence varies with product. Monitor waist circumference and BMI. Rare cases of priapism have been reported.

Use in elderly patients with dementia is associated with an increased risk of mortality and cerebrovascular accidents; avoid antipsychotic use for behavioral problems associated with dementia unless alternative nonpharmacologic therapies have failed and patient may harm self or others. In addition, use may cause or exacerbate syndrome of inappropriate antidiuretic hormone secretion or hyponatremia; monitor sodium closely with initiation or dosage adjustments in older adults (Beers Criteria).

Dosage adjustments are recommended for iloperidone when given concomitantly with strong CYP2D6 or CYP3A4 inhibitors or in poor metabolizers of CYP2D6. The possibility of a suicide attempt is inherent in psychotic illness; use caution in high-risk patients during initiation of therapy. Prescriptions should be written for the smallest quantity consistent with good patient care. Continued use for >6 weeks has not been evaluated.

Adverse Reactions (Reflective of adult population; not specific for elderly)
>10%:
  Cardiovascular: Tachycardia (3% to 12%; dose related)
  Central nervous system: Dizziness (10% to 20%; dose related), somnolence (9% to 15%)
1% to 10%:
  Cardiovascular: Orthostatic hypotension (3% to 5%), hypotension (<1% to 3%; dose related), palpitations (≥1%)

Central nervous system: Fatigue (4% to 6%), extrapyramidal symptoms (4% to 5%), tremor (3%), lethargy (1% to 3%), akathisia (2%), aggression (≥1%), delusion (≥1%), restless- ness (≥1%)

Dermatologic: Rash (2% to 3%)

Gastrointestinal: Nausea (≤10%), xerostomia (8% to 10%), weight gain (1% to 9%; dose related), diarrhea (5% to 7%), abdominal discomfort (≤3%; dose related), weight loss (≥1%)

Genitourinary: Ejaculation failure (2%), erectile dysfunction (≥1%), urinary inconti- nence (≥1%)

Neuromuscular & skeletal: Arthralgia (3%), stiffness (1% to 3%; dose related), dyskinesia (<2%), muscle spasm (≥1%), myalgia (≥1%)

Ocular: Blurred vision (≤3%), conjunctivitis (≥1%)

Respiratory: Nasal congestion (5% to 8%), nasopharyngitis (≤4%), upper respiratory tract infection (2% to 3%), dyspnea (2%)

Drug Interactions

Metabolism/Transport Effects Substrate of CYP2D6 (major), CYP3A4 (minor); **Note:** Assignment of Major/Minor substrate status based on clinically relevant drug interaction potential

Avoid Concomitant Use

Avoid concomitant use of Iloperidone with any of the following: Azelastine; Azelastine (Nasal); Highest Risk QTc-Prolonging Agents; Metoclopramide; Mifepristone; Moderate Risk QTc-Prolonging Agents; Paraldehyde

Increased Effect/Toxicity

Iloperidone may increase the levels/effects of: Alcohol (Ethyl); Azelastine; Azelastine (Nasal); Buprenorphine; CNS Depressants; Highest Risk QTc-Prolonging Agents; Methyl- phenidate; Paraldehyde; Serotonin Modulators; Zolpidem

The levels/effects of Iloperidone may be increased by: Abiraterone Acetate; Acetylcholines- terase Inhibitors (Central); CYP2D6 Inhibitors (Moderate); CYP2D6 Inhibitors (Strong); CYP3A4 Inhibitors (Strong); HydrOXYzine; Lithium formulations; MAO Inhibitors; Methyl- phenidate; Metoclopramide; Metyrosine; Mifepristone; Moderate Risk QTc-Prolonging Agents; QTc-Prolonging Agents (Indeterminate Risk and Risk Modifying); Tetrabenazine

Decreased Effect

Iloperidone may decrease the levels/effects of: Amphetamines; Anti-Parkinson's Agents (Dopamine Agonist); Quinagolide

The levels/effects of Iloperidone may be decreased by: CYP2D6 Inhibitors (Strong); Lithium formulations; Peginterferon Alfa-2b; Tocilizumab

Ethanol/Nutrition/Herb Interactions

Ethanol: May increase CNS depression; monitor for increased effects with coadministration. Caution patients about effects.

Herb/Nutraceutical: Avoid St John's wort (may decrease serum levels of iloperidone). Avoid kava kava, gotu kola, valerian, St John's wort (may increase CNS depression).

Stability Store at 25°C (77°F); excursions permitted at 15°C to 30°C (59°F to 86°F). Protect from light and moisture.

Mechanism of Action Iloperidone is a piperidinyl-benzisoxazole atypical antipsychotic with mixed D_2/5-HT$_2$ antagonist activity. It exhibits high affinity for 5-HT$_{2A}$, D_2, and D_3 receptors, low to moderate affinity for D_1, D_4, H_1, 5-HT$_{1A}$, 5-HT$_6$, 5HT$_7$, and NE$_{\alpha 1}$ receptors, and no affinity for muscarinic receptors. The addition of serotonin antagonism to dopamine antago- nism (classic neuroleptic mechanism) is thought to improve negative symptoms of psychoses and reduce the incidence of extrapyramidal side effects. Iloperidone's low affinity for histamine H_1 receptors may decrease the risk for weight gain and somnolence while its affinity for NE$_{\alpha 1/\alpha 2C}$ may provide antidepressant and anxiolytic activity and improved cognitive function.

Pharmacodynamics/Kinetics

Absorption: Well absorbed

Distribution: V_d: 1340-2800 L

Protein binding: ~95% (iloperidone and active metabolites)

Metabolism: Hepatic via carbonyl reduction, hydroxylation (CYP2D6) and O-demethylation (CYP3A4); forms active metabolites (P88 and P95)

Bioavailability: Oral: Tablet (relative to solution): 96%

Half-life elimination:

Extensive metabolizers: Iloperidone: 18 hours; P88: 26 hours; P95: 23 hours

Poor metabolizers: Iloperidone: 33 hours; P88: 37 hours; P95: 31 hours

Time to peak, plasma: 2-4 hours

Excretion: Urine (58% extensive metabolizers, 45% poor metabolizers); feces (20% extensive metabolizers, 22% poor metabolizers)

Dosage
  Geriatric & Adult Schizophrenia: Oral: Initial: 1 mg twice daily; recommended dosage range: 6-12 mg twice daily (maximum: 24 mg/day)

  Recommended titration schedule: Increase in 2 mg increments every 24 hours on days 2-7 (eg, Day 2: 2 mg twice daily; Day 3: 4 mg twice daily; Day 4: 6 mg twice daily; Day 5: 8 mg twice daily; Day 6: 10 mg twice daily; Day 7: 12 mg twice daily)

  Note: Titrate dose to effect (to avoid orthostatic hypotensive effects); treatment >6 weeks has not been evaluated; when reinitiating treatment after discontinuation (>3 days), the initial titration schedule should be followed.

  Dosage adjustment in patients receiving strong CYP2D6 inhibitors (eg, paroxetine, fluoxetine, quinidine): Decrease iloperidone dose by 50%; when the CYP2D6 inhibitor is discontinued, return to previous dose.

  Dosage adjustment in patients receiving strong CYP3A4 inhibitors (eg, ketoconazole, clarithromycin): Decrease iloperidone dose by 50%; when the CYP3A4 inhibitor is discontinued, return to previous dose.

  Dosage adjustment in poor metabolizers of CYP2D6: Decrease iloperidone dose by 50%.

  Hepatic Impairment Not recommended in patients with hepatic impairment due to lack of data.

Administration May be administered with or without food.

Monitoring Parameters Vital signs; fasting blood glucose/Hgb A$_{1c}$ (prior to treatment and periodically during treatment); signs and symptoms of hyperglycemia; signs and symptoms of cardiac arrhythmia; CBC (frequently during first few months of therapy); serum potassium and magnesium levels (prior to treatment and periodically during treatment); orthostatic blood pressure changes; assess weight prior to and periodically during treatment;

Special Geriatric Considerations Any change in disease status in any organ system may result in behavior changes. EPS appears significantly less than with the other agents in this class. Many elderly patients receive antipsychotic medications for inappropriate nonpsychotic behavior. Before initiating antipsychotic medication, the clinician should investigate any reversible cause; any stress or stress from any disease can cause acute "confusion" or worsening of baseline nonpsychotic behavior. Most commonly, acute changes in behavior are due to increases in drug dose or addition of a new medication to the regimen, fluid and electrolyte loss, infection, or changes in their environment.

Studies of elderly patients with psychosis associated with Alzheimer's disease, treated with antipsychotics, have demonstrated an increased risk of mortality and cardiovascular events as compared to younger patient populations.

This medication is considered to be potentially inappropriate in this patient population (Beers Criteria: Quality of evidence - moderate; Strength of recommendation - strong).

Dosage Forms Excipient information presented when available (limited, particularly for generics); consult specific product labeling.
  Tablet, oral:
    Fanapt®: 1 mg, 2 mg, 4 mg, 6 mg, 8 mg, 10 mg, 12 mg
  Tablet, oral [combination package (each titration pack contains)]:
    Fanapt®: 1 mg (2s), 2 mg (2s), 4 mg (2s), and 6 mg (2s)

◆ **Imdur®** *see* Isosorbide Mononitrate *on page 1052*
◆ **Imferon** *see* Iron Dextran Complex *on page 1039*
◆ **Imipemide** *see* Imipenem and Cilastatin *on page 975*

Imipenem and Cilastatin (i mi PEN em & sye la STAT in)

Related Information
  Antibiotic Treatment of Adults With Infective Endocarditis *on page 2157*
  Community-Acquired Pneumonia in Adults *on page 2171*
Medication Safety Issues
  Sound-alike/look-alike issues:
    Imipenem may be confused with ertapenem, meropenem
    Primaxin® may be confused with Premarin®, Primacor®
Brand Names: U.S. Primaxin® I.V.
Brand Names: Canada Imipenem and Cilastatin for Injection; Primaxin® I.V. Infusion; RAN™-Imipenem-Cilastatin
Index Terms Imipemide; Primaxin® I.M. [DSC]
Generic Availability (U.S.) Yes
Pharmacologic Category Antibiotic, Carbapenem

IMIPENEM AND CILASTATIN

Use Treatment of lower respiratory tract, urinary tract, intra-abdominal, gynecologic, bone and joint, skin and skin structure, endocarditis (caused by *Staphylococcus aureus*) and polymicrobic infections as well as bacterial septicemia. Antibacterial activity includes gram-positive bacteria (methicillin-sensitive *S. aureus* and *Streptococcus* spp), resistant gram-negative bacilli (including extended spectrum beta-lactamase-producing *Escherichia coli* and *Klebsiella* spp, *Enterobacter* spp, and *Pseudomonas aeruginosa*), and anaerobes.

Unlabeled Use Hepatic abscess; neutropenic fever; melioidosis

Contraindications Hypersensitivity to imipenem/cilastatin or any component of the formulation

Warnings/Precautions Dosage adjustment required in patients with impaired renal function; elderly patients often require lower doses (adjust carefully to renal function). Prolonged use may result in fungal or bacterial superinfection, including *C. difficile*-associated diarrhea (CDAD) and pseudomembranous colitis; CDAD has been observed >2 months postantibiotic treatment. Has been associated with CNS adverse effects, including confusional states and seizures (myoclonic); use with caution in patients with a history of seizures or hypersensitivity to beta-lactams (including penicillins and cephalosporins); patients with impaired renal function are at increased risk of seizures if not properly dose adjusted. May decrease divalproex sodium/valproic acid concentrations leading to breakthrough seizures; concomitant use not recommended. Serious hypersensitivity reactions, including anaphylaxis, have been reported (some without a history of previous allergic reactions to beta-lactams). Doses for I.M. administration are mixed with lidocaine; consult information on lidocaine for associated warnings/precautions. Two different imipenem/cilastatin products are available; due to differences in formulation, the I.V. and I.M. preparations **cannot** be interchanged.

Adverse Reactions (Reflective of adult population; not specific for elderly)
1% to 10%:
  Cardiovascular: Tachycardia (infants 2%; adults <1%)
  Central nervous system: Seizure (infants 6%; adults <1%)
  Dermatologic: Rash (≤1%, children 2%)
  Gastrointestinal: Nausea (1% to 2%), diarrhea (children 3% to 4%; adults 1% to 2%), vomiting (≤2%)
  Genitourinary: Oliguria/anuria (infants 2%; adults <1%)
  Local: Phlebitis/thrombophlebitis (3%)

Drug Interactions

Metabolism/Transport Effects None known.

Avoid Concomitant Use
  Avoid concomitant use of Imipenem and Cilastatin with any of the following: BCG; Ganciclovir (Systemic); Ganciclovir-Valganciclovir

Increased Effect/Toxicity
  Imipenem and Cilastatin may increase the levels/effects of: CycloSPORINE; CycloSPORINE (Systemic)

  The levels/effects of Imipenem and Cilastatin may be increased by: CycloSPORINE; CycloSPORINE (Systemic); Ganciclovir (Systemic); Ganciclovir-Valganciclovir; Probenecid

Decreased Effect
  Imipenem and Cilastatin may decrease the levels/effects of: BCG; CycloSPORINE; CycloSPORINE (Systemic); Divalproex; Typhoid Vaccine; Valproic Acid

Stability Imipenem/cilastatin powder for injection should be stored at <25°C (77°F).
  I.V.: Prior to use, dilute dose into 100-250 mL of an appropriate solution. Imipenem is inactivated at acidic or alkaline pH. Final concentration should not exceed 5 mg/mL. The I.M. formulation is not buffered and cannot be used to prepare I.V. solutions. Reconstituted I.V. solutions are stable for 4 hours at room temperature and 24 hours when refrigerated. Do not freeze.

Mechanism of Action Inhibits bacterial cell wall synthesis by binding to one or more of the penicillin-binding proteins (PBPs); which in turn inhibits the final transpeptidation step of peptidoglycan synthesis in bacterial cell walls, thus inhibiting cell wall biosynthesis. Bacteria eventually lyse due to ongoing activity of cell wall autolytic enzymes (autolysins and murein hydrolases) while cell wall assembly is arrested. Cilastatin prevents renal metabolism of imipenem by competitive inhibition of dehydropeptidase along the brush border of the renal tubules.

Pharmacodynamics/Kinetics

  Distribution: Rapidly and widely to most tissues and fluids including sputum, pleural fluid, peritoneal fluid, interstitial fluid, bile, aqueous humor, and bone; highest concentrations in pleural fluid, interstitial fluid, and peritoneal fluid; low concentrations in CSF
  Protein binding: Imipenem: 20%; cilastatin: 40%
  Metabolism: Imipenem is metabolized in the kidney by dehydropeptidase I; cilastatin prevents imipenem metabolism by this enzyme; cilastatin is partially metabolized renally
  Half-life elimination: I.V.: Both drugs: 60 minutes; prolonged with renal impairment
  Excretion: Both drugs: Urine (~70% as unchanged drug)

Dosage

Geriatric & Adult Doses based on **imipenem** content.

Usual dosage range: Weight ≥70 kg: 250-1000 mg every 6-8 hours; maximum: 4 g/day.
Note: For adults weighing <70 kg, refer to Dosage: Renal Impairment.

Indication-specific dosing:

Burkholderia pseudomallei **(melioidosis) (unlabeled use):** I.V.: Initial: 20 mg/kg every 8 hours for at least 10 days (White, 2003) **or** 25 mg/kg (up to 1 g) every 6 hours for at least 10 days (Currie, 2003); continue parenteral therapy until clinical improvement then switch to oral therapy if tolerated and/or appropriate.

Intra-abdominal infections: I.V.:

Mild infection: 250-500 mg every 6 hours

Severe infection: 500 mg every 6 hours **or** 1 g every 8 hours for 4-7 days (provided source controlled). **Note:** Not recommended for mild-to-moderate, community-acquired intra-abdominal infections due to risk of toxicity and the development of resistant organisms (Solomkin, 2010)

Liver abscess (unlabeled use): I.V.: 500 mg every 6 hours for 4-6 weeks (Ulug, 2010)

Moderate infections: I.V.:

Fully-susceptible organisms: 500 mg every 6-8 hours

Moderately-susceptible organisms: 500 mg every 6 hours or 1 g every 8 hours

Neutropenic fever (unlabeled use): I.V.: 500 mg every 6 hours (Paul, 2006)

Pseudomonas **infections:** I.V.: 500 mg every 6 hours; **Note:** Higher doses may be required based on organism sensitivity.

Severe infections: I.V.:

Fully-susceptible organisms: 500 mg every 6 hours

Moderately-susceptible organisms: 1 g every 6-8 hours

Maximum daily dose should not exceed 50 mg/kg or 4 g/day, whichever is lower

Urinary tract infection, uncomplicated: I.V.: 250 mg every 6 hours

Urinary tract infection, complicated: I.V.: 500 mg every 6 hours

Mild infections: Note: Rarely a suitable option in mild infections; normally reserved for moderate-severe cases: I.V.:

Fully-susceptible organisms: 250 mg every 6 hours

Moderately-susceptible organisms: 500 mg every 6 hours

Renal Impairment I.V.:

Patients with a Cl_{cr} ≤5 mL/minute/1.73 m^2 should not receive imipenem/cilastatin unless hemodialysis is instituted within 48 hours.

Patients weighing <30 kg with impaired renal function should not receive imipenem/cilastatin.

Reduced I.V. dosage regimen based on creatinine clearance and/or body weight: See table.

Intermittent hemodialysis (IHD) (administer after hemodialysis on dialysis days): Use the dosing recommendation for patients with a Cl_{cr} 6-20 mL/minute; administer dose after dialysis session and every 12 hours thereafter **or** 250-500 mg every 12 hours (Heintz, 2009). **Note:** Dosing dependent on the assumption of 3 times/week, complete IHD sessions.

Peritoneal dialysis (unlabeled dosing): Dose as for Cl_{cr} 6-20 mL/minute (Somani, 1988)

Continuous renal replacement therapy (CRRT) (Heintz, 2009; Trotman, 2005): Drug clearance is highly dependent on the method of renal replacement, filter type, and flow rate. Appropriate dosing requires close monitoring of pharmacologic response, signs of adverse reactions due to drug accumulation, as well as drug concentrations in relation to target trough (if appropriate). The following are general recommendations only (based on dialysate flow/ultrafiltration rates of 1-2 L/hour and minimal residual renal function) and should not supersede clinical judgment:

CVVH: Loading dose of 1 g followed by either 250 mg every 6 hours **or** 500 mg every 8 hours

CVVHD: Loading dose of 1 g followed by either 250 mg every 6 hours **or** 500 mg every 6-8 hours

CVVHDF: Loading dose of 1 g followed by either 250 mg every 6 hours **or** 500 mg every 6 hours

Note: Data suggest that 500 mg every 8-12 hours may provide sufficient time above MIC to cover organisms with MIC values ≤2 mg/L; however, a higher dose of 500 mg every 6 hours is recommended for resistant organisms (particularly *Pseudomonas* spp) with MIC ≥4 mg/L or deep-seated infections (Fish, 2005).

◄ Reduced I.V. dosage regimen based on creatinine clearance and/or body weight:
U.S. labeling: See table.

Imipenem and Cilastatin Dosage in Renal Impairment

Reduced I.V. Dosage Regimen Based on Creatinine Clearance (mL/minute/1.73 m^2) and/or Body Weight <70 kg				
Body Weight (kg)				
≥70	60	50	40	30
Total daily dose for normal renal function: 1 g/day				
Cl$_{cr}$ ≥71	250 mg q6h	250 mg q8h	125 mg q6h	125 mg q6h	125 mg q8h
Cl$_{cr}$ 41-70	250 mg q8h	125 mg q6h	125 mg q6h	125 mg q8h	125 mg q8h
Cl$_{cr}$ 21-40	250 mg q12h	250 mg q12h	125 mg q8h	125 mg q12h	125 mg q12h
Cl$_{cr}$ 6-20	250 mg q12h	125 mg q12h	125 mg q12h	125 mg q12h	125 mg q12h
Total daily dose for normal renal function: 1.5 g/day				
Cl$_{cr}$ ≥71	500 mg q8h	250 mg q6h	250 mg q6h	250 mg q8h	125 mg q6h
Cl$_{cr}$ 41-70	250 mg q6h	250 mg q8h	250 mg q8h	125 mg q6h	125 mg q8h
Cl$_{cr}$ 21-40	250 mg q8h	250 mg q8h	250 mg q12h	125 mg q8h	125 mg q8h
Cl$_{cr}$ 6-20	250 mg q12h	250 mg q12h	250 mg q12h	125 mg q12h	125 mg q12h
Total daily dose for normal renal function: 2 g/day				
Cl$_{cr}$ ≥71	500 mg q6h	500 mg q8h	250 mg q6h	250 mg q6h	250 mg q8h
Cl$_{cr}$ 41-70	500 mg q8h	250 mg q6h	250 mg q6h	250 mg q8h	125 mg q6h
Cl$_{cr}$ 21-40	250 mg q6h	250 mg q8h	250 mg q8h	250 mg q12h	125 mg q8h
Cl$_{cr}$ 6-20	250 mg q12h	250 mg q12h	250 mg q12h	250 mg q12h	125 mg q12h
Total daily dose for normal renal function: 3 g/day				
Cl$_{cr}$ ≥71	1000 mg q8h	750 mg q8h	500 mg q6h	500 mg q8h	250 mg q6h
Cl$_{cr}$ 41-70	500 mg q6h	500 mg q8h	500 mg q8h	250 mg q6h	250 mg q8h
Cl$_{cr}$ 21-40	500 mg q8h	500 mg q8h	250 mg q6h	250 mg q8h	250 mg q8h
Cl$_{cr}$ 6-20	500 mg q12h	500 mg q12h	250 mg q12h	250 mg q12h	250 mg q12h
Total daily dose for normal renal function: 4 g/day				
Cl$_{cr}$ ≥71	1000 mg q6h	1000 mg q8h	750 mg q8h	500 mg q6h	500 mg q8h
Cl$_{cr}$ 41-70	750 mg q8h	750 mg q8h	500 mg q6h	500 mg q8h	250 mg q6h
Cl$_{cr}$ 21-40	500 mg q6h	500 mg q8h	500 mg q8h	250 mg q6h	250 mg q8h
Cl$_{cr}$ 6-20	500 mg q12h	500 mg q12h	500 mg q12h	250 mg q12h	250 mg q12h

Canadian labeling: Reduced I.V. dosage regimen based on creatinine clearance (mL/minute/1.73 m^2) and body weight ≥70 kg (**Note:** The manufacturer's labeling recommends further proportionate dose reductions for patients <70 kg, but does not provide specific dosing recommendations):

Mild renal impairment (Cl$_{cr}$ 31-70 mL/minute/1.73 m^2):
  Fully-susceptible organisms: Maximum dosage: 500 mg every 8 hours
  Less susceptible organisms (primarily some *Pseudomonas* strains): Maximum dosage: 500 mg every 6 hours

Moderate renal impairment (Cl$_{cr}$ 21-30 mL/minute/1.73 m^2):
  Fully-susceptible organisms: Maximum dosage: 500 mg every 12 hours
  Less susceptible organisms (primarily some *Pseudomonas* strains): Maximum dosage: 500 mg every 8 hours

Severe renal impairment (Cl$_{cr}$ 0-20 mL/minute/1.73 m^2):
  Fully-susceptible organisms: Maximum dosage: 250 mg every 12 hours
  Less susceptible organisms (primarily some *Pseudomonas* strains): Maximum dosage: 500 mg every 12 hours

  Note: Patients with Cl$_{cr}$ 6-20 mL/minute/1.73 m^2 should receive 250 mg every 12 hours or 3.5 mg/kg (whichever is lower) every 12 hours for most pathogens; seizure risk may increase with higher dosing.

Hepatic Impairment Hepatic dysfunction may further impair cilastatin clearance in patients receiving chronic renal replacement therapy; consider decreasing the dosing frequency.

Administration I.V.: Do not administer I.V. push. Infuse doses ≤500 mg over 20-30 minutes; infuse doses ≥750 mg over 40-60 minutes.

Monitoring Parameters Periodic renal, hepatic, and hematologic function tests; monitor for signs of anaphylaxis during first dose

Test Interactions Interferes with urinary glucose determination using Clinitest®; positive Coombs' [direct]

Special Geriatric Considerations Imipenem/cilastatin's role is limited to the treatment of infections caused by susceptible multiresistant organism(s) and in patients whose bacterial infection(s) have failed to respond to other appropriate antimicrobials; many of the seizures attributed to imipenem/cilastatin were in elderly patients; dose must be adjusted for creatinine clearance and body weight.

Dosage Forms Excipient information presented when available (limited, particularly for generics); consult specific product labeling.

Injection, powder for reconstitution: Imipenem 250 mg and cilastatin 250 mg; imipenem 500 mg and cilastatin 500 mg

Primaxin® I.V.: Imipenem 250 mg and cilastatin 250 mg [contains sodium 18.8 mg (0.8 mEq)]; imipenem 500 mg and cilastatin 500 mg [contains sodium 37.5 mg (1.6 mEq)]

Imipramine (im IP ra meen)

Related Information
Antidepressant Agents *on page* 2097
Beers Criteria – Potentially Inappropriate Medications for Geriatrics *on page* 2183
Pharmacotherapy of Urinary Incontinence *on page* 2141

Medication Safety Issues
Sound-alike/look-alike issues:
Imipramine may be confused with amitriptyline, desipramine, Norpramin®
BEERS Criteria medication:
This drug may be potentially inappropriate for use in geriatric patients (Quality of evidence - high [moderate for SIADH]; Strength of recommendation - strong).

Brand Names: U.S. Tofranil-PM®; Tofranil®

Brand Names: Canada Apo-Imipramine®; Novo-Pramine; Tofranil®

Index Terms Imipramine Hydrochloride; Imipramine Pamoate

Generic Availability (U.S.) Yes

Pharmacologic Category Antidepressant, Tricyclic (Tertiary Amine)

Use Treatment of depression

Unlabeled Use Analgesic for certain chronic and neuropathic pain (including diabetic neuropathy); panic disorder; attention-deficit/hyperactivity disorder (ADHD); post-traumatic stress disorder (PTSD)

Medication Guide Available Yes

Contraindications Hypersensitivity to imipramine (cross-reactivity with other dibenzodiazepines may occur) or any component of the formulation; concurrent use of MAO inhibitors (within 14 days); in a patient during acute recovery phase of MI

Warnings/Precautions [U.S. Boxed Warning]: Antidepressants increase the risk of suicidal thinking and behavior in children, adolescents, and young adults (18-24 years of age) with major depressive disorder (MDD) and other psychiatric disorders; consider risk prior to prescribing. Short-term studies did not show an increased risk in patients >24 years of age and showed a decreased risk in patients ≥65 years. Closely monitor for clinical worsening, suicidality, or unusual changes in behavior; the patient's family or caregiver should be instructed to closely observe the patient and communicate condition with healthcare provider. A medication guide should be dispensed with each prescription.

The possibility of a suicide attempt is inherent in major depression and may persist until remission occurs. Monitor for worsening of depression or suicidality, especially during initiation of therapy (generally first 1-2 months) or with dose increases or decreases. Use caution in high-risk patients. Worsening depression and severe abrupt suicidality that are not part of the presenting symptoms may require discontinuation or modification of drug therapy. The patient's family or caregiver should be alerted to monitor patients for the emergence of suicidality and associated behaviors (such as agitation, irritability, hostility, impulsivity, and hypomania) and notify healthcare provider.

May worsen psychosis in some patients or precipitate a shift to mania or hypomania in patients with bipolar disorder. Patients presenting with depressive symptoms should be screened for bipolar disorder. Monotherapy in patients with bipolar disorder should be avoided. **Imipramine is not FDA approved for the treatment of bipolar depression.**

TCAs may rarely cause bone marrow suppression; monitor for any signs of infection and obtain CBC if symptoms (eg, fever, sore throat) evident. The degree of sedation, anticholinergic effects, orthostasis, and conduction abnormalities are high relative to other antidepressants. Imipramine often causes drowsiness/sedation, resulting in impaired performance of tasks requiring alertness (eg, operating machinery or driving). Sedative effects may be additive with other CNS depressants and/or ethanol. Use with caution in patients with a history of cardiovascular disease (including previous MI, stroke, tachycardia, or conduction abnormalities). Use with caution in patients with urinary retention, benign prostatic hyperplasia, narrow-angle glaucoma, xerostomia, visual problems, constipation, or a history of bowel obstruction.

Consider discontinuing, when possible, prior to elective surgery. Therapy should not be abruptly discontinued in patients receiving high doses for prolonged periods. May lower seizure threshold - use caution in patients with a previous seizure disorder or condition predisposing to seizures such as brain damage, alcoholism, or concurrent therapy with other drugs which lower the seizure threshold. May increase the risks associated with electroconvulsive therapy. Use with caution in hyperthyroid patients or those receiving thyroid supplementation. Use with caution in patients with diabetes mellitus; may alter glucose regulation. Use with caution in patients with hepatic or renal dysfunction and in elderly patients. Has been associated with photosensitization.

Avoid use in the elderly due to its potent anticholinergic and sedative properties, and potential to cause orthostatic hypotension.In addition, may also cause or exacerbate syndrome of inappropriate antidiuretic hormone secretion or hyponatremia; monitor sodium closely with initiation or dosage adjustments in older adults (Beers Criteria).

Adverse Reactions (Reflective of adult population; not specific for elderly)
Reported for tricyclic antidepressants in general. Frequency not defined.

Cardiovascular: Arrhythmia, CHF, ECG changes, heart block, hypertension, MI, orthostatic hypotension, palpitation, stroke, tachycardia

Central nervous system: Agitation, anxiety, confusion, delusions, disorientation, dizziness, drowsiness, fatigue, hallucination, headache, hypomania, insomnia, nightmares, psychosis, restlessness, seizure

Dermatologic: Alopecia, itching, petechiae, photosensitivity, purpura, rash, urticaria

Endocrine & metabolic: Breast enlargement, galactorrhea, gynecomastia, increase or decrease in blood sugar, increase or decrease in libido, SIADH

Gastrointestinal: Abdominal cramps, anorexia, black tongue, constipation, diarrhea, epigastric disorders, ileus, nausea, stomatitis, taste disturbance, vomiting, weight gain/loss, xerostomia

Genitourinary: Impotence, testicular swelling, urinary retention

Hematologic: Agranulocytosis, eosinophilia, thrombocytopenia

Hepatic: Cholestatic jaundice, transaminases increased

Neuromuscular & skeletal: Ataxia, extrapyramidal symptoms, incoordination, numbness, paresthesia, peripheral neuropathy, tingling, tremor, weakness

Ocular: Blurred vision, disturbances of accommodation, mydriasis

Otic: Tinnitus

Miscellaneous: Diaphoresis, falling, hypersensitivity (eg, drug fever, edema)

Drug Interactions
Metabolism/Transport Effects Substrate of CYP1A2 (minor), CYP2B6 (minor), CYP2C19 (major), CYP2D6 (major), CYP3A4 (minor); **Note:** Assignment of Major/Minor substrate status based on clinically relevant drug interaction potential; **Inhibits** CYP1A2 (weak), CYP2C19 (weak), CYP2D6 (moderate), CYP2E1 (weak)

Avoid Concomitant Use
Avoid concomitant use of Imipramine with any of the following: Iobenguane I 123; MAO Inhibitors; Methylene Blue

Increased Effect/Toxicity
Imipramine may increase the levels/effects of: Alpha-/Beta-Agonists (Direct-Acting); Alpha1-Agonists; Amphetamines; Anticholinergics; Aspirin; Beta2-Agonists; CYP2D6 Substrates; Desmopressin; Fesoterodine; Highest Risk QTc-Prolonging Agents; Methylene Blue; Metoclopramide; Moderate Risk QTc-Prolonging Agents; Nebivolol; NSAID (COX-2 Inhibitor); NSAID (Nonselective); QuiNIDine; Serotonin Modulators; Sodium Phosphates; Sulfonylureas; TraMADol; Vitamin K Antagonists; Yohimbine

The levels/effects of Imipramine may be increased by: Abiraterone Acetate; Altretamine; Antipsychotics; BuPROPion; Cimetidine; Cinacalcet; CYP2C19 Inhibitors (Moderate); CYP2C19 Inhibitors (Strong); CYP2D6 Inhibitors (Moderate); CYP2D6 Inhibitors (Strong); Dexmethylphenidate; Divalproex; DULoxetine; Linezolid; Lithium; MAO Inhibitors; Methylphenidate; Metoclopramide; Metyrosine; Mifepristone; Pramlintide; Protease Inhibitors; QuiNIDine; Selective Serotonin Reuptake Inhibitors; Terbinafine; Terbinafine (Systemic); Valproic Acid

Decreased Effect
Imipramine may decrease the levels/effects of: Acetylcholinesterase Inhibitors (Central); Alpha2-Agonists; Codeine; Iobenguane I 123

The levels/effects of Imipramine may be decreased by: Acetylcholinesterase Inhibitors (Central); Barbiturates; CarBAMazepine; CYP2C19 Inducers (Strong); Peginterferon Alfa-2b; St Johns Wort; Tocilizumab

Ethanol/Nutrition/Herb Interactions

Ethanol: May increase CNS depression; monitor for increased effects with coadministration. Caution patients about effects.

Herb/Nutraceutical: St John's wort may decrease imipramine levels. Avoid valerian, St John's wort, SAMe, kava kava (may increase risk of serotonin syndrome and/or excessive sedation).

Mechanism of Action Traditionally believed to increase the synaptic concentration of serotonin and/or norepinephrine in the central nervous system by inhibition of their reuptake by the presynaptic neuronal membrane. However, additional receptor effects have been found including desensitization of adenyl cyclase, down regulation of beta-adrenergic receptors, and down regulation of serotonin receptors.

Pharmacodynamics/Kinetics

Onset of action: Peak antidepressant effect: Usually after ≥2 weeks

Absorption: Well absorbed

Metabolism: Hepatic, primarily via CYP2D6 to desipramine (active) and other metabolites; significant first-pass effect

Half-life elimination: 6-18 hours

Excretion: Urine (as metabolites)

Dosage

Geriatric

Depression: Initial: 25-50 mg at bedtime; may increase every 3 days for inpatients and weekly for outpatients if tolerated to a recommended maximum of 100 mg/day.

Adult

Depression:

Outpatients: Initial: 75 mg/day; may increase gradually to 150 mg/day. May be given in divided doses or as a single bedtime dose; maximum: 200 mg/day

Inpatients: Initial: 100-150 mg/day; may increase gradually to 200 mg/day; if no response after 2 weeks, may further increase to 250-300 mg/day. May be given in divided doses or as a single bedtime dose; maximum: 300 mg/day.

Note: Maximum antidepressant effect may not be seen for 2 or more weeks after initiation of therapy.

Post-traumatic stress disorder (PTSD) (unlabeled use): Oral: 75-200 mg/day

Monitoring Parameters Monitor blood pressure and pulse rate prior to and during initial therapy; ECG in older adults, with high doses, and/or in patients with pre-existing cardiovascular disease; evaluate mental status, suicide ideation (especially at the beginning of therapy or when doses are increased or decreased); blood levels are useful for therapeutic monitoring

Reference Range Therapeutic: Imipramine and desipramine: 150-250 ng/mL (SI: 530-890 nmol/L); desipramine: 150-300 ng/mL (SI: 560-1125 nmol/L); Toxic: >500 ng/mL (SI: 446-893 nmol/L); utility of serum level monitoring controversial

Special Geriatric Considerations Avoid in the elderly. Orthostatic hypotension is a concern with this agent, especially in patients taking other medications that may affect blood pressure. May precipitate arrhythmias in predisposed patients; may aggravate seizures. Strong anticholinergic properties; a less anticholinergic antidepressant may be a better choice.

A systematic review and meta-analysis of antidepressant placebo-controlled trials in persons with depression and dementia found evidence "suggestive" of efficacy but not of sufficient strength to "confirm" efficacy. Antidepressant trials in this patient population are small and underpowered. Older patients with depression being treated with an antidepressant should be closely monitored for response and adverse effects. Treatment should be switched or augmented when response is inadequate with a therapeutic dose. Antidepressants that are not tolerated should be discontinued and an alternative agent should be started.

This medication is considered to be potentially inappropriate in this patient population (Beers Criteria: Quality of evidence - high [moderate for SIADH]; Strength of recommendation - strong).

Dosage Forms Excipient information presented when available (limited, particularly for generics); consult specific product labeling.

Capsule, oral, as pamoate: 75 mg, 100 mg, 125 mg, 150 mg

Tofranil-PM®: 75 mg, 100 mg, 125 mg, 150 mg

Tablet, oral, as hydrochloride: 10 mg, 25 mg, 50 mg

Tofranil®: 10 mg, 25 mg, 50 mg

◆ **Imipramine Hydrochloride** *see* Imipramine *on page* 979
◆ **Imipramine Pamoate** *see* Imipramine *on page* 979
◆ **Imitrex®** *see* SUMAtriptan *on page* 1822

Immune Globulin (i MYUN GLOB yoo lin)

Related Information
Immunization Administration Recommendations *on page 2144*
Immunization Recommendations *on page 2149*
Medication Safety Issues
Sound-alike/look-alike issues:
Gamimune® N may be confused with CytoGam®
Immune globulin (intravenous) may be confused with hepatitis B immune globulin
Brand Names: U.S. Carimune® NF; Flebogamma® DIF; GamaSTAN™ S/D; Gammagard S/D®; Gammagard® Liquid; Gammaked™; Gammaplex®; Gamunex® [DSC]; Gamunex®-C; Hizentra®; Octagam®; Privigen®; Vivaglobin® [DSC]
Brand Names: Canada Gamastan S/D; Gamimune® N; Gammagard Liquid; Gammagard S/D; Gamunex®; Hizentra®; IGIVnex®; Privigen®; Vivaglobin®
Index Terms Gamma Globulin; IG; IGIM; IGIV; Immune Globulin Subcutaneous (Human); Immune Serum Globulin; ISG; IV Immune Globulin; IVIG; Panglobulin; SCIG
Generic Availability (U.S.) No
Pharmacologic Category Blood Product Derivative; Immune Globulin
Use
Treatment of primary humoral immunodeficiency syndromes (congenital agammaglobuline-mia, severe combined immunodeficiency syndromes [SCIDS], common variable immuno-deficiency, X-linked immunodeficiency, Wiskott-Aldrich syndrome) (Carimune® NF, Flebogamma® DIF, Gammagard® Liquid, Gammagard S/D®, Gammaked™, Gammaplex®, Gamunex®, Gamunex®-C, Hizentra®, Octagam®, Privigen®, Vivaglobin®)
Treatment of acute and chronic immune (idiopathic) thrombocytopenic purpura (ITP) (Carimune® NF, Gammagard S/D®, Gammaked™, Gamunex®, Gamunex®-C, Privigen® [chronic only])
Treatment of chronic inflammatory demyelinating polyneuropathy (CIDP) (Gammaked™, Gamunex®, Gamunex®-C)
Prevention of coronary artery aneurysms associated with Kawasaki syndrome (in combination with aspirin) (Gammagard S/D®)
Prevention of bacterial infection in patients with hypogammaglobulinemia and/or recurrent bacterial infections with B-cell chronic lymphocytic leukemia (CLL) (Gammagard S/D®)
Prevention of serious infection in immunoglobulin deficiency (select agammaglobulinemias) (GamaSTAN™ S/D)
Provision of passive immunity in the following susceptible individuals (GamaSTAN™ S/D):
Hepatitis A: Pre-exposure prophylaxis; postexposure: within 14 days and/or prior to manifestation of disease
Measles: For use within 6 days of exposure in an unvaccinated person, who has not previously had measles
Varicella: For immunosuppressed patients when varicella zoster immune globulin is not available
Unlabeled Use Acquired hypogammaglobulinemia secondary to malignancy; Guillain-Barré syndrome; hematopoietic stem cell transplantation (HSCT), to prevent bacterial infections among allogeneic recipients with severe hypogammaglobulinemia (IgG <400 mg/dL) at <100 days post transplant (CDC guidelines); HIV-associated thrombocytopenia; multiple sclerosis (relapsing, remitting when other therapies cannot be used); Lambert-Eaton myasthenic syndrome (LEMS); multifocal motor neuropathy; myasthenia gravis; refractory dermatomyo-sitis/polymyositis
Contraindications Hypersensitivity to immune globulin or any component of the formulation; selective IgA deficiency; hyperprolinemia (Hizentra®, Privigen®); severe thrombocytopenia or coagulation disorders; severe thrombocytopenia or coagulation disorders where IM injections are contraindicated
Warnings/Precautions [U.S. Boxed Warning]: I.V. formulation only: Acute renal dysfunction (increased serum creatinine, oliguria, acute renal failure, osmotic nephrosis) can rarely occur; usually within 7 days of use (more likely with products stabilized with sucrose). Use with caution in the elderly, patients with renal disease, diabetes mellitus, volume depletion, sepsis, paraproteinemia, and nephrotoxic medications due to risk of renal dysfunction. In patients at risk of renal dysfunction, the rate of infusion and concentration of solution should be minimized. Discontinue if renal function deteriorates. High-dose regimens (1 g/kg for 1-2 days) are not recommended for individuals with fluid overload or where fluid volume may be of concern. Hypersensitivity and anaphylactic reactions can occur; a severe fall in blood pressure may rarely occur with anaphylactic reaction; immediate treatment (including epinephrine 1:1000) should be available. Product of human plasma; may potentially contain infectious agents which could transmit disease. Screening of donors, as well as testing and/or inactivation or removal of certain viruses, reduces the risk. Infections

thought to be transmitted by this product should be reported to the manufacturer. Aseptic meningitis may occur with high doses (≥1-2 g/kg [product-dependent]) and/or rapid infusion; syndrome usually appears within several hours to 2 days following treatment; usually resolves within several days after product is discontinued; patients with a migraine history may be at higher risk for AMS. Increased risk of hypersensitivity, especially in patients with anti-IgA antibodies. Increased risk of hematoma formation when administered subcutaneously for the treatment of ITP.

Intravenous immune globulin has been associated with antiglobulin hemolysis; monitor for signs of hemolytic anemia. Patients should be adequately hydrated prior to initiation of therapy. Hyperproteinemia, increased serum viscosity and hyponatremia may occur; distinguish hyponatremia from pseudohyponatremia to prevent volume depletion, a further increase in serum viscosity, and a higher risk of thrombotic events. Use caution in patients with a history of thrombotic events or a history of atherosclerosis or cardiovascular disease or patients with known/suspected hyperviscosity; there is clinical evidence of a possible association between thrombotic events and administration of intravenous immune globulin and subcutaneous immune globulin. Consider a baseline assessment of blood viscosity in patients at risk for hyperviscosity. Patients should be monitored for adverse events during and after the infusion. Stop administration with signs of infusion reaction (fever, chills, nausea, vomiting, and rarely shock). Risk may be increased with initial treatment, when switching brands of immune globulin, and with treatment interruptions of >8 weeks. Monitor for transfusion-related acute lung injury (TRALI); noncardiogenic pulmonary edema has been reported with intravenous immune globulin use. TRALI is characterized by severe respiratory distress, pulmonary edema, hypoxemia, and fever (in the presence of normal left ventricular function) and usually occurs within 1-6 hours after infusion. Response to live vaccinations may be impaired. Some clinicians may administer intravenous immune globulin products as a subcutaneous infusion based on patient tolerability and clinical judgment. SubQ infusion should begin 1 week after the last I.V. dose; dose should be individualized based on clinical response and serum IgG trough concentrations; consider premedicating with acetaminophen and diphenhydramine.

Some products may contain maltose, which may result in falsely-elevated blood glucose readings; maltose-containing products are contraindicated in patients with an allergy to corn. Some products may contain polysorbate 80, sodium, and/or sucrose. Some products may contain sorbitol; do not use in patients with fructose intolerance. Hizentra® and Privigen® contain the stabilizer L-proline and are contraindicated in patients with hyperprolinemia. Packaging of some products may contain natural latex/natural rubber; skin testing should not be performed with GamaSTAN™ S/D as local irritation can occur and be misinterpreted as a positive reaction.

Adverse Reactions (Reflective of adult population; not specific for elderly) Frequency not defined.

Cardiovascular: Angioedema, chest tightness, edema, flushing of the face, hyper-/hypotension, palpitation, tachycardia

Central nervous system: Anxiety, aseptic meningitis syndrome, chills, dizziness, drowsiness, fatigue, fever, headache, irritability, lethargy, lightheadedness, malaise, migraine, pain

Dermatologic: Bruising, contact dermatitis, eczema, erythema, hyperhidrosis, petechiae, pruritus, purpura, rash, urticaria

Gastrointestinal: Abdominal cramps, abdominal pain, diarrhea, discomfort, dyspepsia, gastroenteritis, nausea, sore throat, toothache, vomiting

Hematologic: Anemia, autoimmune hemolytic anemia, hematocrit decreased, hematoma, hemolysis (mild), hemorrhage, thrombocytopenia

Hepatic: Bilirubin increased, LDH increased, liver function test increased

Local: Muscle stiffness at I.M. site; pain, swelling, redness or irritation at the infusion site

Neuromuscular & skeletal: Arthralgia, back or hip pain, leg cramps, muscle cramps, myalgia, neck pain, rigors, weakness

Ocular: Conjunctivitis

Otic: Ear pain

Renal: Acute renal failure, acute tubular necrosis, anuria, BUN increased, creatinine increased, oliguria, proximal tubular nephropathy, osmotic nephrosis

Respiratory: Asthma aggravated, bronchitis, cough, dyspnea, epistaxis, nasal congestion, oropharyngeal pain, pharyngeal pain, pharyngitis, rhinitis, rhinorrhea, sinus headache, sinusitis, upper respiratory infection, wheezing

Miscellaneous: Anaphylaxis, diaphoresis, flu-like syndrome, hypersensitivity reactions, infusion reaction, thermal burn

◄ **Drug Interactions**
Metabolism/Transport Effects None known.
Avoid Concomitant Use There are no known interactions where it is recommended to avoid concomitant use.
Increased Effect/Toxicity There are no known significant interactions involving an increase in effect.
Decreased Effect
Immune Globulin may decrease the levels/effects of: Vaccines (Live)
Stability Stability is dependent upon the manufacturer and brand. Do not freeze. Dilution is dependent upon the manufacturer and brand. Gently swirl; do not shake; avoid foaming. Do not mix products from different manufacturers together. Discard unused portion of vials.

Carimune® NF: Prior to reconstitution, store at or below 30°C (86°F). Reconstitute with NS, D_5W, or SWFI. Following reconstitution in a sterile laminar air flow environment, store under refrigeration. Begin infusion within 24 hours.

Flebogamma® DIF: Store at 2°C to 25°C (36°F to 77°F); do not freeze. Dilution is not recommended.

GamaSTAN™ S/D: Store under refrigeration at 2°C to 8°C (36°F to 46°F). The following stability information has also been reported for GamaSTAN™ S/D: May be exposed to room temperature for a cumulative 7 days (Cohen, 2007).

Gammagard® Liquid: May dilute in D_5W only. Prior to use, store at 2°C to 8°C (36°F to 46°F); do not freeze. May store at room temperature of 25°C (77°F) within the first 24 months of manufacturing. Storage time at room temperature varies with length of time previously refrigerated; refer to product labeling for details.

Gammagard S/D®: Store at ≤25°C (≤77°F). Reconstitute with SWFI; may store diluted solution under refrigeration at 2°C to 8°C (36°F to 46°F) for up to 24 hours if originally prepared in a sterile laminar air flow environment.

Gammaked™: Store at 2°C to 8°C (36°F to 46°F); may be stored at ≤25°C (≤77°F) for up to 6 months. Dilute in D_5W only.

Gammaplex®: Store at 2°C to 25°C (36°F to 77°F); do not freeze. Protect from light.

Gamunex®, Gamunex®-C: Store at 2°C to 8°C (36°F to 46°F); may be stored at ≤25°C (≤77°F) for up to 6 months. Dilute in D_5W only.

Hizentra®: Store at ≤25°C (≤77°F); do not freeze or use product if previously frozen. Do not shake.

Octagam®: Store at 2°C to 25°C (36°F to 77°F).

Privigen®: Store at ≤25°C (≤77°F); do not freeze (do not use if previously frozen). Protect from light. If necessary to further dilute, D_5W may be used.

Vivaglobin®: Store at 2°C to 8°C (36°F to 46°F); do not freeze or use product if previously frozen. Do not shake.

Mechanism of Action Replacement therapy for primary and secondary immunodeficiencies, and IgG antibodies against bacteria, viral, parasitic and mycoplasma antigens; interference with F_c receptors on the cells of the reticuloendothelial system for autoimmune cytopenias and ITP; provides passive immunity by increasing the antibody titer and antigen-antibody reaction potential

Pharmacodynamics/Kinetics
Onset of action: I.V.: Provides immediate antibody levels
Duration: I.M., I.V.: Immune effect: 3-4 weeks (variable)
Distribution: V_d: 0.09-0.13 L/kg
  Intravascular portion (primarily): Healthy subjects: 41% to 57%; Patients with congenital humoral immunodeficiencies: ~70%
Bioavailability: SubQ: Vivaglobin®: 73%
Half-life elimination: I.M.: ~23 days; I.V.: IgG (variable among patients): Healthy subjects: 14-24 days; Patients with congenital humoral immunodeficiencies: 26-40 days; hypermetabolism associated with fever and infection have coincided with a shortened half-life
Time to peak:
  Plasma: SubQ: Gammagard® Liquid: 2.9 days; Hizentra®: 2.9 days; Vivaglobin®: 2.5 days
  Serum: I.M.: ~48 hours

Dosage
Geriatric & Adult According to manufacturer product labeling, intravenous formulations are for intravenous administration only. However, some clinicians may administer intravenous formulations as a subcutaneous infusion based on clinical judgment and patient tolerability. Some clinicians dose IVIG on ideal body weight or an adjusted ideal body weight in morbidly-obese patients (Siegel, 2010).
B-cell chronic lymphocytic leukemia (CLL) (Gammagard S/D®): I.V.: 400 mg/kg every 3-4 weeks

Chronic inflammatory demyelinating polyneuropathy (CIDP) (Gamunex®, Gamunex-C®): I.V.: Loading dose: 2000 mg/kg (given in divided doses over 2-4 consecutive days); Maintenance: 1000 mg/kg every 3 weeks. Alternatively, administer 500 mg/kg/day for 2 consecutive days every 3 weeks.

Hepatitis A (GamaSTAN™ S/D): I.M.:

Pre-exposure prophylaxis upon travel into endemic areas (hepatitis A vaccine preferred):
0.02 mL/kg for anticipated risk of exposure <3 months
0.06 mL/kg for anticipated risk of exposure ≥3 months; repeat every 4-6 months.

Postexposure prophylaxis: 0.02 mL/kg given within 14 days of exposure and/or prior to manifestation of disease; not needed if at least 1 dose of hepatitis A vaccine was given at ≥1 month before exposure

Immunoglobulin deficiency (GamaSTAN™ S/D): I.M.: 0.66 mL/kg (minimum dose should be 100 mg/kg) every 3-4 weeks. Administer a double dose at onset of therapy; some patients may require more frequent injections.

Immune (idiopathic) thrombocytopenic purpura (ITP):
Carimune® NF: I.V.: Initial: 400 mg/kg/day for 2-5 days; Maintenance: 400 mg/kg as needed to maintain platelet count ≥30,000/mm^3 and/or to control significant bleeding; may increase dose if needed (range: 800-1000 mg/kg)

Gammagard S/D®: I.V.: 1000 mg/kg; up to 3 additional doses may be given based on patient response and/or platelet count. **Note:** Additional doses should be given on alternate days.

Gamunex®, Gamunex-C®: I.V.: 1000 mg/kg/day for 2 consecutive days (second dose may be withheld if adequate platelet response in 24 hours) **or** 400 mg/kg once daily for 5 consecutive days

Privigen®: I.V.: 1000 mg/kg/day for 2 consecutive days

Kawasaki syndrome (Gammagard S/D®): I.V.:
Gammagard S/D®: 1000 mg/kg as a single dose **or** 400 mg/kg/day for 4 consecutive days. Begin within 7 days of onset of fever.

AHA guidelines (2004): 2000 mg/kg as a single dose within 10 days of disease onset

Note: Must be used in combination with aspirin: 80-100 mg/kg/day orally, divided every 6 hours for up to 14 days (until fever resolves for at least 48 hours); then decrease dose to 3-5 mg/kg/day once daily. In patients without coronary artery abnormalities, give lower dose for 6-8 weeks. In patients with coronary artery abnormalities, low-dose aspirin should be continued indefinitely.

Measles:
GamaSTAN™ S/D: I.M.: Immunocompetent: 0.25 mL/kg given within 6 days of exposure followed by live attenuated measles vaccine in 5-6 months when indicated (Watson, 1998)

Gamunex-C®, Octagam®: I.V.:
Prophylaxis in patients with primary humoral immunodeficiency (**ONLY** if routine dose is <400 mg/kg): ≥400 mg/kg immediately before expected exposure
Treatment in patients with primary immunodeficiency: 400 mg/kg administered as soon as possible after exposure

Hizentra®: SubQ infusion: Measles exposure in patients with primary humoral immunodeficiency: Weekly dose: ≥200 mg/kg for 2 consecutive weeks for patients at risk of measles exposure (eg, during an outbreak; travel to endemic area). In patients who have been exposed to measles, administer the minimum dose as soon as possible following exposure.

Primary humoral immunodeficiency disorders:
Carimune® NF: I.V.: 400-800 mg/kg every 3-4 weeks
Flebogamma® DIF, Gammagard® Liquid, Gammagard S/D®, Gamunex®, Gamunex-C®, Octagam®: I.V.: 300-600 mg/kg every 3-4 weeks; adjusted based on dosage and interval in conjunction with monitored serum IgG concentrations and clinical response
Gammaplex®: I.V.: 300-800 mg/kg every 3-4 weeks
Gamunex-C®: SubQ infusion: Begin 1 week after last I.V. dose. Use the following equation to calculate initial dose:
Initial weekly dose (grams) = [1.37 x IGIV dose (grams)] divided by [I.V. dose interval (weeks)]
Note: For subsequent dose adjustments, refer to product labeling.
Hizentra®: SubQ infusion: Begin 1 week after last I.V. dose. Use the following equation to calculate initial dose:
Initial weekly dose (grams) = [1.53 x IGIV dose (grams)] divided by [I.V. dose interval (weeks)]
Note: For subsequent dose adjustments, refer to product labeling.
Privigen®: I.V.: 200-800 mg/kg every 3-4 weeks; adjusted based on dosage and interval in conjunction with monitored serum IgG concentrations and clinical response

◀

Vivaglobin®: SubQ infusion: Begin 1 week after last I.V. dose; **Note:** Patient should have received an I.V. immune globulin routinely for at least 3 months before switching to SubQ. Use the following equation to calculate initial dose:

Initial weekly dose (grams) = [1.37 x IGIV dose (grams)] divided by [I.V. dose interval (weeks)]

Note: For subsequent dose adjustments, refer to product labeling.

Varicella (GamaSTAN™ S/D): I.M.: Prophylaxis: 0.6-1.2 mL/kg (varicella zoster immune globulin preferred) within 72 hours of exposure

Unlabeled uses: I.V.:

Acquired hypogammaglobulinemia secondary to malignancy (unlabeled use): Adults: 400 mg/kg/dose every 3 weeks; reevaluate every 4-6 months (Anderson, 2007)

Guillain-Barré syndrome (unlabeled use): Adults: Various regimens have been used, including:

400 mg/kg/day for 5 days (Hughes, 2003)

or

2000 mg/kg in divided doses administered over 2-5 days (Feasby, 2007)

Hematopoietic stem cell transplantation with hypogammaglobulinemia (CDC guidelines, 2000; unlabeled use): Adults: 500 mg/kg/week

HIV-associated thrombocytopenia (unlabeled use): Adults: 1000 mg/kg/day for 2 days (Anderson, 2007)

Multiple sclerosis (relapsing-remitting, when other therapies cannot be used) (unlabeled use): Adults: 1000 mg/kg per month, with or without an induction of 400 mg/kg/day for 5 days (Feasby, 2007)

Myasthenia gravis (severe exacerbation) (unlabeled use): Adults: Total dose of 2000 mg/kg over 2-5 days (Feasby, 2007)

Refractory dermatomyositis/polymyositis (unlabeled uses): Adults: 2000 mg/kg per treatment course administered over 2-5 days (Feasby, 2007)

Dosing adjustment/comments in renal impairment: Cl$_{cr}$ <10 mL/minute: Avoid use; in patients at risk of renal dysfunction, consider infusion at a rate less than maximum.

Renal Impairment I.V.: Cl$_{cr}$ <10 mL/minute: Avoid use; in patients at risk of renal dysfunction, consider infusion at a rate less than maximum.

Administration Note: If plasmapheresis employed for treatment of condition, administer immune globulin **after** completion of plasmapheresis session.

I.M.: Administer I.M. in the anterolateral aspects of the upper thigh or deltoid muscle of the upper arm. Avoid gluteal region due to risk of injury to sciatic nerve. Divide doses >10 mL and inject in multiple sites.

GamaSTAN™ S/D is for I.M. administration only.

I.V. infusion: Infuse over 2-24 hours; administer in separate infusion line from other medications; if using primary line, flush with saline prior to administration. Decrease dose, rate and/or concentration of infusion in patients who may be at risk of renal failure. Decreasing the rate or stopping the infusion may help relieve some adverse effects (flushing, changes in pulse rate, changes in blood pressure). Epinephrine should be available during administration. For initial treatment or in the elderly, a lower concentration and/or a slower rate of infusion should be used. Initial rate of administration and titration is specific to each IVIG product. Consult specific product prescribing information for detailed recommendations. Refrigerated product should be warmed to room temperature prior to infusion. Some products require filtration; refer to individual product labeling. Antecubital veins should be used, especially with concentrations ≥10% to prevent injection site discomfort.

SubQ infusion: Initial dose should be administered in a healthcare setting capable of providing monitoring and treatment in the event of hypersensitivity. Using aseptic technique, follow the infusion device manufacturer's instructions for filling the reservoir and preparing the pump. Remove air from administration set and needle by priming. Appropriate injection sites include the abdomen, thigh, upper arm, and/or lateral hip; dose may be infused into multiple sites (spaced ≥2 inches apart) simultaneously. After the sites are clean and dry, insert subcutaneous needle and prime administration set. Attach sterile needle to administration set, gently pull back on the syringe to assure a blood vessel has not been inadvertently accessed (do not use needle and tubing if blood present). Repeat for each injection site; deliver the dose following instructions for the infusion device. Rotate the site(s) weekly. Treatment may be transitioned to the home/home care setting in the absence of adverse reactions.

Gamunex-C®:

Injection sites: ≤8 simultaneous injection sites

Recommended infusion rate: 20 mL/hour per injection site

Hizentra®:

Injection sites: ≤4 simultaneous injection sites

Maximum infusion rate: First infusion: 15 mL/hour per injection site; subsequent infusions: 25 mL/hour per injection site (maximum: 50 mL/hour for all simultaneous sites combined)

Maximum infusion volume: First 4 infusions: 15 mL per injection site; subsequent infusions: 20 mL per injection site (maximum: 25 mL per site as tolerated)

Vivaglobin®:

Injection sites: Adults ≤65 years: ≤6 simultaneous injection sites; Adults >65 years: ≤4 simultaneous injection sites

Maximum infusion rate: 20 mL/hour per injection site (maximum: 3 mg/kg/minute [1.13 mL/kg/hour] for all simultaneous sites combined)

Maximum infusion volume: 15 mL per injection site

Monitoring Parameters Renal function, urine output, IgG concentrations, hemoglobin and hematocrit, platelets (in patients with ITP); infusion- or injection-related adverse reactions, anaphylaxis, signs and symptoms of hemolysis; blood viscosity (in patients at risk for hyperviscosity); presence of antineutrophil antibodies (if TRALI is suspected); volume status; neurologic symptoms (if AMS suspected); clinical response

SubQ infusion: Monitor IgG trough levels every 2-3 months before/after conversion from I.V.; subcutaneous infusions provide more constant IgG levels than usual I.V. immune globulin treatments.

Test Interactions Octagam® contains maltose. Falsely-elevated blood glucose levels may occur when glucose monitoring devices and test strips utilizing the glucose dehydrogenase pyrroloquinolinequinone (GDH-PQQ) based methods are used. Glucose monitoring devices and test strips which utilize the glucose-specific method are recommended. Passively-transferred antibodies may yield false-positive serologic testing results; may yield false-positive direct and indirect Coombs' test. Skin testing should not be performed with GamaSTAN™ S/D as local irritation can occur and be misinterpreted as a positive reaction.

Pharmacotherapy Pearls I.M.: When administering immune globulin for hepatitis A prophylaxis, use should be considered for the following close contacts of persons with confirmed hepatitis A: unvaccinated household and sexual contacts, persons who have shared illicit drugs, regular babysitters, staff and attendees of child care centers, food handlers within the same establishment (CDC, 2006).

All household contacts of measles patients should be evaluated to receive immune globulin unless the measles vaccine has been given on or after the first birthday, unless immunocompromised (CDC, 1998).

For travelers, immune globulin is not an alternative to careful selection of foods and water; immune globulin can interfere with the antibody response to parenterally administered live virus vaccines. Frequent travelers should be tested for hepatitis A antibody, immune hemolytic anemia, and neutropenia (with ITP, I.V. route is usually used).

IgA content:

Carimune® NF: 720 mcg/mL

Flebogamma® 5% DIF: 2.9 ± 0.1 mcg/mL

Flebogamma® 10% DIF: <100 mcg/mL

Gammagard® Liquid: 37 mcg/mL

Gammagard S/D® 5% solution: <1 mcg/mL or <2.2 mcg/mL(product dependent)

Gammaked™: 46 mcg/mL

Gammaplex®: <10 mcg/mL

Gamunex-C®: 46 mcg/mL

Hizentra®: ≤50 mcg/mL

Octagam®: ≤200 mcg/mL

Privigen®: ≤25 mcg/mL

Vivaglobin®: ≤1700 mcg/mL

Dosage Forms Excipient information presented when available (limited, particularly for generics); consult specific product labeling. [DSC] = Discontinued product

Injection, powder for reconstitution [preservative free]:

Carimune® NF: 3 g, 6 g, 12 g [contains sucrose]

Gammagard S/D®: 2.5 g [contains albumin (human), glucose, glycine, natural rubber/natural latex in packaging, polyethylene glycol, polysorbate 80; IgA <2.2 mcg/mL]

Gammagard S/D®: 5 g [contains albumin (human), glucose, glycine, natural rubber/natural latex in packaging, polyethylene glycol, polysorbate 80; IgA <1 mcg/mL]

Gammagard S/D®: 5 g [contains albumin (human), glucose, glycine, natural rubber/natural latex in packaging, polyethylene glycol, polysorbate 80; IgA <2.2 mcg/mL]

Gammagard S/D®: 10 g [contains albumin (human), glucose, glycine, natural rubber/natural latex in packaging, polyethylene glycol, polysorbate 80; IgA <1 mcg/mL]

Gammagard S/D®: 10 g [contains albumin (human), glucose, glycine, natural rubber/natural latex in packaging, polyethylene glycol, polysorbate 80; IgA <2.2 mcg/mL]

◀ Injection, solution [preservative free]:
   Flebogamma® DIF: 5% [50 mg/mL] (10 mL, 50 mL, 100 mL, 200 mL, 400 mL); 10%
      [100 mg/mL] (100 mL, 200 mL) [contains polyethylene glycol, sorbitol]
   GamaSTAN™ S/D: 15% to 18% [150 to 180 mg/mL] (2 mL, 10 mL)
   Gammagard® Liquid: 10% [100 mg/mL] (10 mL, 25 mL, 50 mL, 100 mL, 200 mL) [sucrose
      free; contains glycine]
   Gammaked™: 10% [100 mg/mL] (10 mL, 25 mL, 50 mL, 100 mL, 200 mL) [sucrose free;
      contains glycine]
   Gammaplex®: 5% [50 mg/mL] (50 mL, 100 mL, 200 mL) [sucrose free; contains glycine,
      natural rubber/natural latex in packaging, polysorbate 80, sorbitol]
   Gamunex®: 10% [100 mg/mL] (10 mL [DSC], 25 mL [DSC], 50 mL [DSC], 100 mL [DSC],
      200 mL [DSC]) [contains glycine]
   Gamunex®-C: 10% [100 mg/mL] (10 mL, 25 mL, 50 mL, 100 mL, 200 mL) [contains glycine]
   Hizentra®: 200 mg/mL (5 mL, 10 mL, 20 mL) [contains L-proline, polysorbate 80]
   Octagam®: 5% [50 mg/mL] (20 mL, 50 mL, 100 mL, 200 mL) [sucrose free; contains
      maltose, sodium 30 mmol/L]
   Privigen®: 10% [100 mg/mL] (50 mL, 100 mL, 200 mL) [sucrose free; contains L-proline]
   Vivaglobin®: 160 mg/mL (3 mL [DSC], 10 mL [DSC], 20 mL [DSC])

◆ **Immune Globulin Subcutaneous (Human)** *see* Immune Globulin *on page* 982
◆ **Immune Serum Globulin** *see* Immune Globulin *on page* 982
◆ **Imodium® A-D [OTC]** *see* Loperamide *on page* 1153
◆ **Imodium® A-D EZ Chews [OTC]** *see* Loperamide *on page* 1153
◆ **Imodium® A-D for children [OTC]** *see* Loperamide *on page* 1153
◆ **Imodium® Multi-Symptom Relief [OTC]** *see* Loperamide and Simethicone *on page* 1154
◆ **Imogam® Rabies-HT** *see* Rabies Immune Globulin (Human) *on page* 1662
◆ **Imovax® Rabies** *see* Rabies Vaccine *on page* 1663
◆ **Imuran®** *see* AzaTHIOprine *on page* 174

IncobotulinumtoxinA (in kuh BOT yoo lin num TOKS in aye)

Medication Safety Issues
Other safety concerns:
   Botulinum products are not interchangeable; potency differences may exist between the
   products.

Brand Names: U.S. Xeomin®
Brand Names: Canada Xeomin®
Index Terms Botulinum Toxin Type A
Generic Availability (U.S.) No
Pharmacologic Category Neuromuscular Blocker Agent, Toxin; Ophthalmic Agent, Toxin
Use Treatment of blepharospasm in patients previously treated with onabotulinumtoxinA
(Botox®); treatment of cervical dystonia in botulinum toxin-naïve and previously treated
patients; temporary improvement in the appearance of moderate-to-severe glabellar lines
associated with corrugator and/or procerus muscle activity

Canadian labeling: Treatment of hypertonicity disorders of the seventh nerve (eg, blephar-
ospasm, hemifacial spasm); treatment of poststroke spasticity of upper limb(s); treatment of
cervical dystonia (spasmodic torticollis)
Medication Guide Available Yes
Dosage
   Geriatric Refer to adult dosing. Initiate therapy at lowest recommended dose.
   Adult
      Blepharospasm: I.M.:
         U.S. labeling: Initial: Total dose should be the same as previously administered onabotu-
            linumtoxinA dose. If prior onabotulinumtoxinA dose is not known: 1.25-2.5 units/injection
            site (maximum initial dose: 35 units/eye or 70 units/both eyes). Number and location of
            injection sites based on disease severity and previous dose/response to onabotulinum-
            toxinA (in clinical trials, a mean number of 6 injections per eye were administered).
            Cumulative dose should not exceed 35 units/eye or 70 units/both eyes administered no
            more frequently than every 3 months.
         Canadian labeling: Initial: 1.25-2.5 units/injection site (maximum initial dose: 25 units/eye).
            Dose may be increased up to twice the previous dose if the response from the initial dose
            lasted ≤2 months; maximum dose per site: 5 units. Cumulative dose should not exceed
            35 units/eye or 70 units/both eyes administered no more frequently than every 3 months.
      Cervical dystonia: I.M.:
         U.S. labeling: Initial total dose: 120 units (in clinical trials, similar efficacy was noted with
            initial total doses of 120 and 240 units and between treatment experienced and treatment
            naïve patients). Dose and number of injection sites should be individualized based on

prior treatment, response, duration of effect, adverse events, number/location of muscle(s) to be treated and disease severity. In clinical trials most patients received a total of 2-10 injections into treated muscles. Administer no more frequently than every 3 months
Canadian labeling: Usual total dose: 200 units (maximum: 300 units; maximum dose per injection site: 50 units); administer no more frequently than every 3 months

Reduction of glabellar lines: I.M.: Inject 4 units into each of the 5 sites (2 injections in each corrugator muscle and 1 injection in the procerus muscle) for a total dose of 20 units per treatment session. Administer no more frequently than every 3 months.

Spasticity of upper limb (poststroke): *Canadian labeling (not in U.S. labeling):* I.M.: Individualize dose based on patient size, extent, and location of muscle involvement, degree of spasticity, local muscle weakness, and response to prior treatment. In clinical trials, total doses up to 400 units were administered as separate injections typically divided among selected muscles; may repeat therapy at ≥3 months with appropriate dosage based upon the clinical condition of patient at time of retreatment.

Suggested guidelines for the treatment of stroke-related upper limb spasticity: Note: The lowest recommended starting dose should be used. Dosage and number of injection sites should be individualized. Multiple injections may minimize adverse effects. Dose listed is total dose administered to site:

Biceps: 80 units
Brachialis: 50 units
Brachioradialis: 60 units
Flexor carpi radialis: 50 units
Flexor carpi ulnaris: 40 units
Flexor digitorum profundus: 40 units
Flexor digitorum superficialis: 40 units
Adductor pollicis: 10 units
Flexor pollicis brevis: 10 units
Flexor pollicis longus: 20 units
Pronator quadratus 25 units
Pronator teres: 40 units

Renal Impairment There are no dosage adjustments provided in manufacturer's labeling.
Hepatic Impairment There are no dosage adjustments provided in manufacturer's labeling.
Special Geriatric Considerations No specific information for use in elderly.
Dosage Forms Excipient information presented when available (limited, particularly for generics); consult specific product labeling.
Injection, powder for reconstitution:
Xeomin®: 50 units, 100 units [contains albumin (human), sucrose 4.7 mg]

Indacaterol (in da KA ter ol)

Brand Names: U.S. Arcapta™ Neohaler™
Brand Names: Canada Onbrez® Breezhaler®
Index Terms Indacaterol Maleate; QAB149
Generic Availability (U.S.) No
Pharmacologic Category Beta$_2$ Agonist; Beta$_2$-Adrenergic Agonist, Long-Acting
Use Long-term maintenance treatment of airflow obstruction in chronic obstructive pulmonary disease (COPD) including chronic bronchitis and/or emphysema
Medication Guide Available Yes
Contraindications Monotherapy in the treatment of asthma (ie, use without a concomitant long-term asthma control medication, such as an inhaled corticosteroid). **Note:** Indacaterol is not FDA approved for treatment of asthma.

Canadian labeling: Additional contraindications (not in U.S. labeling): Hypersensitivity to indacaterol or any component of the formulation

Warnings/Precautions Asthma-related deaths: **[U.S. Boxed Warning]: Long-acting beta$_2$-agonists (LABAs) increase the risk of asthma-related deaths. Indacaterol is not indicated for treatment of asthma and should not be used.** In a large, randomized, placebo-controlled U.S. clinical trial (SMART, 2006), salmeterol was associated with an increase in asthma-related deaths (when added to usual asthma therapy); risk is considered a class effect among all LABAs. It is unknown if indacaterol increases asthma-related deaths. Do not use for acutely deteriorating COPD or as rescue therapy in acute episodes. Short-acting beta$_2$-agonists (eg, albuterol) should be used for acute symptoms and symptoms occurring between treatments. If deterioration develops, prompt evaluation of the COPD regimen is warranted. Do not increase the dose or frequency of indacaterol. Data are not available to determine if LABA use increases the risk of death in patients with COPD. Do not use more than once daily or at a higher dose than indicated; do not combine use with other long-acting beta$_2$-agonists. Deaths and significant cardiovascular effects have been reported with excessive sympathomimetic use. Rarely, paradoxical bronchospasm may occur with use of inhaled bronchodilators; this should be distinguished from inadequate response.

Use caution in patients with cardiovascular disease (eg, arrhythmias, coronary insufficiency, hypertension), diabetes mellitus, hyperthyroidism, seizure disorders, or hypokalemia. Beta-agonists may cause elevation in blood pressure, heart rate, CNS stimulation/excitation, increased risk of arrhythmia, increase serum glucose, or decrease serum potassium.

Adverse Reactions (Reflective of adult population; not specific for elderly)
>10%: Respiratory: Cough (post inhalation 7% to 24%)
1% to 10%:
Central nervous system: Headache (5%)
Gastrointestinal: Nausea (2%)
Respiratory: Nasopharyngitis (5%), oropharyngeal pain (2%)

Drug Interactions
Metabolism/Transport Effects Substrate of CYP2D6 (minor), CYP3A4 (minor), P-glyco-protein, UGT1A1; **Note:** Assignment of Major/Minor substrate status based on clinically relevant drug interaction potential

Avoid Concomitant Use
Avoid concomitant use of Indacaterol with any of the following: Beta-Blockers (Nonselective); Highest Risk QTc-Prolonging Agents; Iobenguane I 123; Mifepristone

Increased Effect/Toxicity
Indacaterol may increase the levels/effects of: Corticosteroids (Systemic); Highest Risk QTc-Prolonging Agents; Loop Diuretics; Moderate Risk QTc-Prolonging Agents; Sympathomimetics; Thiazide Diuretics

The levels/effects of Indacaterol may be increased by: AtoMOXetine; Caffeine; Cannabinoids; MAO Inhibitors; Mifepristone; QTc-Prolonging Agents (Indeterminate Risk and Risk Modifying); Theophylline Derivatives; Tricyclic Antidepressants

Decreased Effect
Indacaterol may decrease the levels/effects of: Iobenguane I 123

The levels/effects of Indacaterol may be decreased by: Alpha-/Beta-Blockers; Beta-Blockers (Beta1 Selective); Beta-Blockers (Nonselective); Betahistine; Peginterferon Alfa-2b; Tocilizumab

Stability Store capsules at controlled room temperature of 25°C (77°F); excursions permitted to 15°C to 30°C (59°F to 86°F). Protect from direct sunlight and moisture. Remove from blister pack immediately before use; discard capsule if not used immediately.

Mechanism of Action Relaxes bronchial smooth muscle by selective action on beta₂-receptors with little effect on heart rate; acts locally in the lung.

Pharmacodynamics/Kinetics
Onset of action: 5 minutes
Peak effect: 1-4 hours
Duration: 24 hours
Absorption: Systemic: Inhalation: 43% to 45% bioavailable
Protein binding: ~95%
Metabolism: Hepatic; hydroxylated via CYP3A4, CYP2D6, and CYP1A1
Half-life elimination: 40-56 hours
Time to peak, serum: ~15 minutes
Excretion: Feces (>90%; 54% as unchanged drug [after oral administration]); urine (<2% as unchanged drug)

Dosage
Geriatric & Adult COPD (maintenance): Inhalation: One inhalation (75 mcg/inhalation) once daily; maximum: 1 inhalation once daily. **Note:** A dose of 150-300 mcg once daily is recommended by the 2010 Updated GOLD Guidelines; the 2010 update was published prior to the FDA approval of the 75 mcg dose.

Renal Impairment No dosage adjustment necessary.

Hepatic Impairment
Mild-to-moderate impairment: No dosage adjustment necessary.
Severe impairment: No dosage adjustment provided in manufacturer's labeling.

Administration Inhalation: **For inhalation using Neohaler™ inhaler (U.S.) or Onbrez® Breezhaler® (Canada) only.** Do **not** swallow indacaterol capsules. Use the new inhaler included with each prescription. Do not remove capsules from blister until immediately before use. Use at the same time each day. Not to be used for the relief of acute attacks. Not for use with a spacer device. Do not wash mouthpiece; inhalation device should be kept dry. Discard any capsules that are exposed to air and not used immediately.

Monitoring Parameters FEV_1, FVC, and/or other pulmonary function tests; serum potassium, serum glucose; blood pressure, heart rate; CNS stimulation. Monitor for increased use of short-acting beta$_2$-agonist inhalers; may be marker of a deteriorating condition. Monitor for changes in risk factors (eg, environmental exposure, smoking status).

Pharmacotherapy Pearls In November 2009, the European Medicines Agency approved indacaterol (Onbrez® Breezhaler®) at a dose of 150-300 mcg/day. Indacaterol at this dose, along with other long acting bronchodilators, is recommended by the 2010 Updated GOLD guidelines for maintenance treatment of moderate to very severe COPD. In reviewing the available data, the FDA concluded that the benefit of higher dosing (ie, >75 mcg/day) was not justified due to lack of additional benefit seen at the end of 2 weeks and a higher incidence of adverse reactions.

Special Geriatric Considerations No differences in adverse effects were seen in elderly patients compared to younger adults. No dosage adjustment needed.

Dosage Forms Excipient information presented when available (limited, particularly for generics); consult specific product labeling.

Powder, for oral inhalation:

Arcapta™ Neohaler™: 75 mcg/capsule (30s) [contains contains lactose~25 mg/capsule]

◆ **Indacaterol Maleate** see Indacaterol on page 989

Indapamide (in DAP a mide)

Medication Safety Issues
Sound-alike/look-alike issues:
Indapamide may be confused with Iopidine®
International issues:
Pretanix [Hungary] may be confused with Protonix brand name for pantoprazole [U.S., Canada]

Brand Names: Canada Apo-Indapamide®; Dom-Indapamide; Indapamide Hemihydrate; JAMP-Indapamide; Lozide®; Mylan-Indapamide; Novo-Indapamide; Nu-Indapamide; PHL-Indapamide; PMS-Indapamide; PRO-Indapamide; Riva-Indapamide

Generic Availability (U.S.) Yes

Pharmacologic Category Diuretic, Thiazide-Related

Use Management of mild-to-moderate hypertension; treatment of edema in heart failure

Unlabeled Use Nephrotic syndrome (Tanaka, 2005)

Contraindications Hypersensitivity to indapamide or any component of the formulation or sulfonamide-derived drugs; anuria

Canadian labeling: Additional contraindications (not in U.S. labeling): Severe renal failure (Cl_{cr} <30 mL/minute); hepatic encephalopathy; severe hepatic impairment; hypokalemia; concomitant use with nonantiarrhythmic agents causing torsade de pointes

Warnings/Precautions Use with caution in severe renal disease; Canadian labeling contraindicates use in severe renal failure (Cl_{cr} <30 mL/minute). Electrolyte disturbances including severe hyponatremia (with hypokalemia, hypochloremic alkalosis, hypomagnesemia, or hypercalcemia) can occur; risk may be dose dependent. Correct hypokalemia before initiating therapy (Canadian labeling contraindicates use in hypokalemia). Use with caution in severe hepatic dysfunction; hepatic encephalopathy can be caused by electrolyte disturbances (Canadian labeling contraindicates use in severe hepatic impairment or hepatic encephalopathy). Gout may be precipitated in certain patients with a history of gout, a familial predisposition to gout, or chronic renal failure. Use caution in patients with prediabetes or diabetes; may alter glucose control. May cause SLE exacerbation or activation. Use with caution in patients with moderate or high cholesterol concentrations. Photosensitization may occur.

Chemical similarities are present among sulfonamides, sulfonylureas, carbonic anhydrase inhibitors, thiazides, and loop diuretics (except ethacrynic acid). Use in patients with sulfonamide allergy is specifically contraindicated in product labeling, however, a risk of cross-reaction exists in patients with allergy to any of these compounds; avoid use when previous reaction has been severe. Discontinue if signs of hypersensitivity are noted. Formulation may contain lactose; Canadian labeling recommends avoiding use in patients with hereditary conditions of galactose intolerance, glucose-galactose malabsorption, or lactase deficiency.

Adverse Reactions (Reflective of adult population; not specific for elderly)
≥5%:
Central nervous system: Agitation, anxiety, dizziness, fatigue, headache, irritability, lethargy, malaise, nervousness (dose dependent), pain, tension, tiredness
Endocrine & metabolic: Hypokalemia (<3.5 mEq/L: 20% to 72%, dose dependent)
Neuromuscular & skeletal: Back pain, muscle cramps/spasm, paresthesia, weakness

Respiratory: Rhinitis

Miscellaneous: Infection

≥1% to <5%:

Cardiovascular: Arrhythmia, chest pain, flushing, orthostatic hypotension, palpitation, peripheral edema, PVC, vasculitis

Central nervous system: Depression, drowsiness, insomnia, lightheadedness, vertigo

Dermatologic: Hives, pruritus, rash

Endocrine & metabolic: Hyperglycemia, hyperuricemia, hypochloremia, hyponatremia, libido decreased

Gastrointestinal: Abdominal pain, anorexia, constipation, cramping, diarrhea, dyspepsia, gastric irritation, nausea, vomiting, weight loss, xerostomia

Genitourinary: Nocturia, polyuria

Neuromuscular & skeletal: Hypertonia

Ocular: Blurred vision, conjunctivitis

Renal: BUN increased, creatinine increased, glycosuria

Respiratory: Cough, pharyngitis, rhinorrhea, sinusitis

Miscellaneous: Flu-like syndrome

Drug Interactions

Metabolism/Transport Effects None known.

Avoid Concomitant Use

Avoid concomitant use of Indapamide with any of the following: Dofetilide

Increased Effect/Toxicity

Indapamide may increase the levels/effects of: ACE Inhibitors; Allopurinol; Amifostine; Antihypertensives; Calcium Salts; CarBAMazepine; Dofetilide; Highest Risk QTc-Prolonging Agents; Hypotensive Agents; Lithium; Moderate Risk QTc-Prolonging Agents; OXcarbazepine; Porfimer; RiTUXimab; Sodium Phosphates; Topiramate; Toremifene; Vitamin D Analogs

The levels/effects of Indapamide may be increased by: Alcohol (Ethyl); Analgesics (Opioid); Barbiturates; Beta2-Agonists; Corticosteroids (Orally Inhaled); Corticosteroids (Systemic); Herbs (Hypotensive Properties); Licorice; MAO Inhibitors; Mifepristone; Pentoxifylline; Phosphodiesterase 5 Inhibitors; Prostacyclin Analogues

Decreased Effect

Indapamide may decrease the levels/effects of: Antidiabetic Agents

The levels/effects of Indapamide may be decreased by: Bile Acid Sequestrants; Herbs (Hypertensive Properties); Methylphenidate; Nonsteroidal Anti-Inflammatory Agents; Yohimbine

Ethanol/Nutrition/Herb Interactions Herb/Nutraceutical: Avoid herbs with *hypertensive* properties (bayberry, blue cohosh, cayenne, ephedra, ginger, ginseng [American], kola, licorice); may diminish the antihypertensive effect of indapamide. Avoid herbs with *hypotensive* properties (black cohosh, California poppy, coleus, golden seal, hawthorn, mistletoe, periwinkle, quinine, shepherd's purse); may enhance the hypotensive effect of indapamide.

Stability Store at 20°C to 25°C (68°F to 77°F).

Mechanism of Action Diuretic effect is localized at the proximal segment of the distal tubule of the nephron; it does not appear to have significant effect on glomerular filtration rate nor renal blood flow; like other diuretics, it enhances sodium, chloride, and water excretion by interfering with the transport of sodium ions across the renal tubular epithelium

Pharmacodynamics/Kinetics

Absorption: Rapid and complete

Distribution: V_d: 25 L (Grebow, 1982)

Protein binding, plasma: 71% to 79%

Metabolism: Extensively hepatic

Bioavailability: 93% (Ernst, 2009)

Half-life elimination: Biphasic: 14 and 25 hours

Time to peak: 2 hours

Excretion: Urine (~70%; 7% as unchanged drug within 48 hours); feces (23%)

Dosage

Geriatric & Adult

Edema: Oral: Initial: 2.5 mg/day; if inadequate response after 1 week, may increase dose to 5 mg/day. **Note:** There is little therapeutic benefit to increasing the dose >5 mg/day; there is, however, an increased risk of electrolyte disturbances

Hypertension: Oral: Initial: 1.25 mg/day; if inadequate response, may increase dose once every 4 weeks to 2.5 mg/day and then to 5 mg/day if needed. Consider adding another antihypertensive and decreasing the dose if response is not adequate. **Note:** Canadian labeling recommends a maximum dose of 2.5 mg/day.

Administration May be administered without regard to meals (Caruso, 1983); however, administration with food or milk may decrease GI adverse effects. Administer early in day to avoid nocturia.

Monitoring Parameters Blood pressure (both standing and sitting/supine); serum electrolytes, hepatic function, renal function, uric acid; assess weight, I & O reports daily to determine fluid loss

Special Geriatric Considerations Indapamide has the advantage over other related thiazide diuretics in that it may be effective when Cl_{cr} is <30 mL/minute.

Dosage Forms Excipient information presented when available (limited, particularly for generics); consult specific product labeling.
Tablet, oral: 1.25 mg, 2.5 mg

◆ **Inderal® LA** *see* Propranolol *on page 1622*
◆ **Inderide** *see* Propranolol and Hydrochlorothiazide *on page 1626*
◆ **Indocin®** *see* Indomethacin *on page 993*
◆ **Indocin® I.V.** *see* Indomethacin *on page 993*
◆ **Indometacin** *see* Indomethacin *on page 993*

Indomethacin (in doe METH a sin)

Related Information
Beers Criteria − Potentially Inappropriate Medications for Geriatrics *on page 2183*

Medication Safety Issues
Sound-alike/look-alike issues:
Indocin® may be confused with Imodium®, Lincocin®, Minocin®, Vicodin®

BEERS Criteria medication:
This drug may be potentially inappropriate for use in geriatric patients (Quality of evidence - moderate; Strength of recommendation - strong).

Brand Names: U.S. Indocin®; Indocin® I.V.

Brand Names: Canada Apo-Indomethacin®; Indocid® P.D.A.; Novo-Methacin; Nu-Indo; Pro-Indo; ratio-Indomethacin; Sandoz-Indomethacin

Index Terms Indometacin; Indomethacin Sodium Trihydrate

Generic Availability (U.S.) Yes: Excludes oral suspension, suppository

Pharmacologic Category Nonsteroidal Anti-inflammatory Drug (NSAID), Oral; Nonsteroidal Anti-inflammatory Drug (NSAID), Parenteral

Use Acute gouty arthritis, acute bursitis/tendonitis, moderate-to-severe osteoarthritis, rheumatoid arthritis, ankylosing spondylitis

Medication Guide Available Yes

Contraindications Hypersensitivity to indomethacin, aspirin, other NSAIDs, or any component of the formulation; perioperative pain in the setting of coronary artery bypass graft (CABG) surgery; patients with a history of proctitis or recent rectal bleeding (suppositories)

Warnings/Precautions [U.S. Boxed Warning]: NSAIDs are associated with an increased risk of adverse cardiovascular thrombotic events, including MI and stroke. Risk may be increased with duration of use or pre-existing cardiovascular risk factors or disease. May cause new-onset hypertension or worsening of existing hypertension. Use caution with fluid retention. Avoid use in heart failure. Concurrent administration of ibuprofen, and potentially other nonselective NSAIDs, may interfere with aspirin's cardioprotective effect. **[U.S. Boxed Warning]: Use is contraindicated for treatment of perioperative pain in the setting of coronary artery bypass graft (CABG) surgery.** Risk of MI and stroke may be increased with use following CABG surgery.

Platelet adhesion and aggregation may be decreased; may prolong bleeding time; patients with coagulation disorders or who are receiving anticoagulants should be monitored closely. Anemia may occur; patients on long-term NSAID therapy should be monitored for anemia. Rarely, NSAID use may cause severe blood dyscrasias (eg, agranulocytosis, aplastic anemia, thrombocytopenia).

NSAID use may compromise existing renal function; dose-dependent decreases in prostaglandin synthesis may result from NSAID use, reducing renal blood flow which may cause renal decompensation. NSAID use may increase the risk for hyperkalemia. Patients with impaired renal function, dehydration, heart failure, liver dysfunction, those taking diuretics, and ACE inhibitors are at greater risk of renal toxicity and hyperkalemia. Rehydrate patient before starting therapy; monitor renal function closely. Not recommended for use in patients with advanced renal disease. Long-term NSAID use may result in renal papillary necrosis.

[U.S. Boxed Warning]: NSAIDs may increase risk of gastrointestinal irritation, inflammation, ulceration, bleeding, and perforation. Use caution with a history of GI disease (bleeding or ulcers), concurrent therapy with aspirin, anticoagulants and/or corticosteroids, smoking, use of alcohol, the elderly or debilitated patients. When used concomitantly with ≤325 mg of aspirin, a substantial increase in the risk of gastrointestinal complications (eg, ulcer) occurs; concomitant gastroprotective therapy (eg, proton pump inhibitors) is recommended (Bhatt, 2008).

Use the lowest effective dose for the shortest duration of time, consistent with individual patient goals, to reduce risk of cardiovascular or GI adverse events. Alternate therapies should be considered for patients at high risk.

NSAIDS may cause drowsiness, dizziness, blurred vision and other neurologic effects which may impair physical or mental abilities; patients must be cautioned about performing tasks which require mental alertness (eg, operating machinery or driving). Discontinue use with blurred or diminished vision and perform ophthalmologic exam. Monitor vision with long-term therapy.

NSAIDs may cause serious skin adverse events including exfoliative dermatitis, Stevens-Johnson syndrome (SJS) and toxic epidermal necrolysis (TEN); discontinue use at first sign of skin rash or hypersensitivity. Anaphylactoid reactions may occur, even without prior exposure; patients with "aspirin triad" (bronchial asthma, aspirin intolerance, rhinitis) may be at increased risk. Do not use in patients who experience bronchospasm, asthma, rhinitis, or urticaria with NSAID or aspirin therapy. Use caution in other forms of asthma.

Use with caution in patients with decreased hepatic function. Closely monitor patients with any abnormal LFT. Severe hepatic reactions (eg, fulminant hepatitis, liver failure) have occurred with NSAID use, rarely; discontinue if signs or symptoms of liver disease develop, or if systemic manifestations occur. The elderly are at increased risk for adverse effects (especially peptic ulceration, CNS effects, renal toxicity) from NSAIDs even at low doses. Prolonged use may cause corneal deposits and retinal disturbances; discontinue if visual changes are observed. Use caution with depression, epilepsy, or Parkinson's disease.

Withhold for at least 4-6 half-lives prior to surgical or dental procedures.

Elderly: Nonselective oral NSAID use is associated with an increased risk of GI bleeding and peptic ulcer disease in older adults in high risk category (eg, >75 years or age or receiving concomitant oral/parenteral corticosteroids, anticoagulants, or antiplatelet agents). Risk of adverse events may be higher with indomethacin compared to other NSAIDs; avoid use in this age group (Beers Criteria).

Adverse Reactions (Reflective of adult population; not specific for elderly)

>10%: Central nervous system: Headache (12%)

1% to 10%:

Central nervous system: Dizziness (3% to 9%), depression (<3%), fatigue (<3%), malaise (<3%), somnolence (<3%), vertigo (<3%)

Gastrointestinal: Dyspepsia (3% to 9%), epigastric pain (3% to 9%), heartburn (3% to 9%), indigestion (3% to 9%), nausea (3% to 9%), abdominal pain/cramps/distress (<3%), constipation (<3%), diarrhea (<3%), rectal irritation (suppository), tenesmus (suppository), vomiting

Otic: Tinnitus (<3%)

Drug Interactions

Metabolism/Transport Effects Substrate of CYP2C19 (minor), CYP2C9 (minor); **Note:** Assignment of Major/Minor substrate status based on clinically relevant drug interaction potential; **Inhibits** CYP2C19 (weak), CYP2C9 (weak)

Avoid Concomitant Use

Avoid concomitant use of Indomethacin with any of the following: Floctafenine; Ketorolac; Ketorolac (Nasal); Ketorolac (Systemic)

Increased Effect/Toxicity

Indomethacin may increase the levels/effects of: Aliskiren; Aminoglycosides; Anticoagulants; Antiplatelet Agents; Bisphosphonate Derivatives; Collagenase (Systemic); CycloSPORINE; CycloSPORINE (Systemic); Dabigatran Etexilate; Deferasirox; Desmopressin; Digoxin; Drotrecogin Alfa (Activated); Eplerenone; Haloperidol; Ibritumomab; Lithium; Methotrexate; Nonsteroidal Anti-Inflammatory Agents; PEMEtrexed; Porfimer; Potassium-Sparing Diuretics; PRALAtrexate; Quinolone Antibiotics; Rivaroxaban; Salicylates; Thrombolytic Agents; Tiludronate; Tositumomab and Iodine I 131 Tositumomab; Triamterene; Vancomycin; Vitamin K Antagonists

The levels/effects of Indomethacin may be increased by: ACE Inhibitors; Angiotensin II Receptor Blockers; Antidepressants (Tricyclic, Tertiary Amine); Corticosteroids (Systemic); CycloSPORINE; CycloSPORINE (Systemic); Dasatinib; Floctafenine; Glucosamine; Herbs (Anticoagulant/Antiplatelet Properties); Ketorolac; Ketorolac (Nasal); Ketorolac (Systemic); Nonsteroidal Anti-Inflammatory Agents; Omega-3-Acid Ethyl Esters; Pentosan Polysulfate Sodium; Pentoxifylline; Probenecid; Prostacyclin Analogues; Selective Serotonin Reuptake

Inhibitors; Serotonin/Norepinephrine Reuptake Inhibitors; Sodium Phosphates; Tipranavir; Treprostinil; Vitamin E

Decreased Effect

Indomethacin may decrease the levels/effects of: ACE Inhibitors; Aliskiren; Angiotensin II Receptor Blockers; Antiplatelet Agents; Beta-Blockers; Eplerenone; HydrALAZINE; Loop Diuretics; Potassium-Sparing Diuretics; Salicylates; Selective Serotonin Reuptake Inhibitors; Thiazide Diuretics

The levels/effects of Indomethacin may be decreased by: Bile Acid Sequestrants; Non-steroidal Anti-Inflammatory Agents; Salicylates

Ethanol/Nutrition/Herb Interactions

Ethanol: Avoid ethanol (may enhance gastric mucosal irritation).

Food: Food may decrease the rate but not the extent of absorption. Indomethacin peak serum levels may be delayed if taken with food.

Herb/Nutraceutical: Avoid alfalfa, anise, bilberry, bladderwrack, bromelain, cat's claw, celery, chamomile, coleus, cordyceps, dong quai, evening primrose, fenugreek, feverfew, garlic, ginger, ginkgo biloba, ginseng (American, Panax, Siberian), grapeseed, green tea, guggul, horse chestnut seed, horseradish, licorice, prickly ash, red clover, reishi, SAMe (S-adeno-sylmethionine), sweet clover, turmeric, white willow (all have additional antiplatelet activity).

Stability

Capsules: Store at controlled room temperature.

I.V.: Store below 30°C (86°F). Protect from light. Not stable in alkaline solution. Reconstitute with 1-2 mL preservative free NS or SWFI just prior to administration. Discard any unused portion. Do not use preservative-containing diluents for reconstitution.

Suppositories: Store refrigerated at 2°C to 8°C (36°F to 46°F).

Suspension: Store at controlled room temperature.

Mechanism of Action Reversibly inhibits cyclooxygenase-1 and 2 (COX-1 and 2) enzymes, which results in decreased formation of prostaglandin precursors; has antipyretic, analgesic, and anti-inflammatory properties

Other proposed mechanisms not fully elucidated (and possibly contributing to the anti-inflammatory effect to varying degrees), include inhibiting chemotaxis, altering lymphocyte activity, inhibiting neutrophil aggregation/activation, and decreasing proinflammatory cytokine levels.

Pharmacodynamics/Kinetics

Onset of action: ~30 minutes

Duration: 4-6 hours

Absorption: Oral: Immediate release: Prompt and extensive; Extended release: 90% over 12 hours

Distribution: V_d: 0.34-1.57 L/kg; crosses blood-brain barrier

Protein binding: 99%

Metabolism: Hepatic; significant enterohepatic recirculation

Bioavailability: 100%

Half-life elimination: 4.5 hours

Time to peak: Oral: Immediate release: 2 hours

Excretion: Urine (60%, primarily as glucuronide conjugates); feces (33%, primarily as metabolites)

Dosage

Geriatric Refer to adult dosing. Use lowest recommended dose and frequency in elderly to initiate therapy for indications listed in adult dosing.

Adult

Inflammatory/rheumatoid disorders (use lowest effective dose): Oral, rectal: 25-50 mg/dose 2-3 times/day; maximum dose: 200 mg/day; extended release capsule should be given on a 1-2 times/day schedule (maximum dose for extended release: 150 mg/day). In patients with arthritis and persistent night pain and/or morning stiffness, may give the larger portion (up to 100 mg) of the total daily dose at bedtime.

Bursitis/tendonitis: Oral, rectal: Initial dose: 75-150 mg/day in 3-4 divided doses **or** 1-2 divided doses for extended release; usual treatment is 7-14 days

Acute gouty arthritis: Oral, rectal: 50 mg 3 times daily until pain is tolerable then reduce dose; usual treatment <3-5 days

Renal Impairment No dosage adjustment provided in the manufacturer's labeling; not recommended in patients with advanced renal disease.

Hepatic Impairment No dosage adjustment provided in the manufacturer's labeling; use with caution.

Administration

Oral: Administer with food, milk, or antacids to decrease GI adverse effects. Extended release capsules must be swallowed whole; do not crush.

I.V.: Administer over 20-30 minutes. Reconstitute I.V. formulation just prior to administration; discard any unused portion; avoid I.V. bolus administration or infusion via an umbilical catheter into vessels near the superior mesenteric artery as these may cause vaso-constriction and can compromise blood flow to the intestines. Do not administer intra-arterially.

Monitoring Parameters Monitor response (pain, range of motion, grip strength, mobility, ADL function), inflammation; observe for weight gain, edema; monitor renal function (serum creatinine, BUN); observe for bleeding, bruising; evaluate gastrointestinal effects (abdominal pain, bleeding, dyspepsia); mental confusion, disorientation, CBC, liver function tests; ophthalmologic exams with prolonged therapy

Test Interactions False-negative dexamethasone suppression test

Special Geriatric Considerations Elderly are a high-risk population for adverse effects from NSAIDs. As much as 60% of elderly can develop peptic ulceration and/or hemorrhage asymptomatically. The concomitant use of H_2 blockers and sucralfate is not effective as prophylaxis with the exception of NSAID-induced duodenal ulcers which may be prevented by the use of ranitidine. Misoprostol and proton pump inhibitors are the only agents proven to help prevent the development of NSAID-induced ulcers. Also, concomitant disease and drug use contribute to the risk for GI adverse effects. Use lowest effective dose for shortest period possible. Consider renal function decline with age. Use of NSAIDs may compromise existing renal function especially when Cl_{cr} is ≤30 mL/minute. Tinnitus may be a difficult and unreliable indication of toxicity due to age-related hearing loss or eighth cranial nerve damage. CNS adverse effects such as confusion, agitation, and hallucination are generally seen in overdose or high-dose situations, but the elderly may demonstrate these adverse effects at lower doses than younger adults. Indomethacin frequently causes confusion at recommended doses in the elderly.

This medication is considered to be potentially inappropriate in this patient population (Beers Criteria: Quality of evidence - moderate; Strength of recommendation - strong).

Dosage Forms Excipient information presented when available (limited, particularly for generics); consult specific product labeling.
Capsule, oral: 25 mg, 50 mg
Capsule, extended release, oral: 75 mg
Injection, powder for reconstitution: 1 mg
  Indocin® I.V.: 1 mg
Suppository, rectal:
  Indocin®: 50 mg (30s)
Suspension, oral:
  Indocin®: 25 mg/5 mL (237 mL) [contains ethanol 1%; pineapple-coconut-mint flavor]

◆ **Indomethacin Sodium Trihydrate** *see* Indomethacin *on page 993*
◆ **Infanrix®** *see* Diphtheria and Tetanus Toxoids, and Acellular Pertussis Vaccine *on page 567*
◆ **Infantaire [OTC]** *see* Acetaminophen *on page 31*
◆ **Infantaire Gas [OTC]** *see* Simethicone *on page 1776*
◆ **Infants Gas Relief Drops [OTC] [DSC]** *see* Simethicone *on page 1776*
◆ **INFeD®** *see* Iron Dextran Complex *on page 1039*
◆ **Influenza Vaccine** *see* Influenza Virus Vaccine (Inactivated) *on page 997*
◆ **Influenza Vaccine** *see* Influenza Virus Vaccine (Live/Attenuated) *on page 1001*

Influenza Virus Vaccine (H5N1) (in floo EN za VYE rus vak SEEN H5N1)

Related Information
  Immunization Administration Recommendations *on page 2144*
  Immunization Recommendations *on page 2149*
Medication Safety Issues
  Sound-alike/look-alike issues:
    Influenza virus vaccine (H5N1) may be confused with the nonavian strain of influenza virus vaccine
Index Terms Avian Influenza Virus Vaccine; Bird Flu Vaccine; H5N1 Influenza Vaccine; Influenza Virus Vaccine (Monovalent)
Generic Availability (U.S.) No
Pharmacologic Category Vaccine, Inactivated (Viral)
Use Active immunization of adults at increased risk of exposure to the H5N1 viral subtype of influenza
Prescribing and Access Restrictions Commercial distribution is not planned. The vaccine will be included as part of the U.S. Strategic National Stockpile. It will be distributed by public health officials if needed.

Dosage

Adult Immunization: Adults 18-64 years: I.M.: 1 mL, followed by second 1 mL dose given 28 days later (acceptable range: 21-35 days)

Special Geriatric Considerations No clinical studies in elderly have been done to date. Differences in immune response may be different than the titer response seen in younger adults.

Dosage Forms Excipient information presented when available (limited, particularly for generics); consult specific product labeling.

Injection, suspension [monovalent]: Hemagglutinin (H5N1strain) 90 mcg/mL (5 mL) [contains chicken, egg, and porcine protein, and thimerosal]

Influenza Virus Vaccine (Inactivated)

(in floo EN za VYE rus vak SEEN, in ak ti VAY ted)

Related Information

Immunization Administration Recommendations *on page 2144*
Immunization Recommendations *on page 2149*

Medication Safety Issues

Sound-alike/look-alike issues:

Fluarix® may be confused with Flarex®

Influenza virus vaccine may be confused with flumazenil

Influenza virus vaccine may be confused with tetanus toxoid and tuberculin products. Medication errors have occurred when tuberculin skin tests (PPD) have been inadvertently administered instead of tetanus toxoid products and influenza virus vaccine. These products are refrigerated and often stored in close proximity to each other.

International issues:

Fluarix [U.S., Canada, and multiple international markets] may be confused with Flarex brand name for fluorometholone [U.S. and multiple international markets] and Fluorex brand name for fluoride [France]

Brand Names: U.S. Afluria®; Fluarix®; FluLaval®; Fluvirin®; Fluzone®; Fluzone® High-Dose; Fluzone® Intradermal

Brand Names: Canada Agriflu™; Fluad™; Fluviral®; Influvac®; Intanza®; Vaxigrip®

Index Terms H1N1 Influenza Vaccine; Influenza Vaccine; Influenza Virus Vaccine (Purified Surface Antigen); Influenza Virus Vaccine (Split-Virus); TIV; Trivalent Inactivated Influenza Vaccine

Generic Availability (U.S.) No

Pharmacologic Category Vaccine, Inactivated (Viral)

Use Provide active immunity to influenza virus strains contained in the vaccine

The Advisory Committee on Immunization Practices (ACIP) recommends annual vaccination with the seasonal trivalent inactivated influenza vaccine (TIV) (injection) for all persons ≥6 months of age.

When vaccine supply is limited, target groups for vaccination (those at higher risk of complications from influenza infection and their close contacts) include the following:

- Persons ≥50 years of age
- Residents of nursing homes and other chronic-care facilities that house persons of any age with chronic medical conditions
- Adults with chronic disorders of the pulmonary or cardiovascular systems (except hypertension), including asthma
- Adults who have chronic metabolic diseases (including diabetes mellitus), hepatic disease, renal dysfunction, hematologic disorders, or immunosuppression (including immunosuppression caused by medications or HIV)
- Adults with cognitive or neurologic/neuromuscular conditions (including conditions such as spinal cord injuries or seizure disorders) which may compromise respiratory function, the handling of respiratory secretions, or that can increase the risk of aspiration
- Healthcare personnel
- Household contacts and caregivers of children <5 years (particularly children <6 months) and adults ≥50 years
- Household contacts and caregivers of persons with medical conditions which put them at high risk of complications from influenza infection
- American Indians/Alaska Natives
- Morbidly obese (BMI ≥40)

Contraindications Prior life-threatening reaction to previous influenza vaccination; hypersensitivity to any component of the formulation

Fluviral® (not available in U.S.): Canadian labeling: Additional contraindications: Presence of acute respiratory infection, other active infections, or serious febrile illness

▶

Warnings/Precautions Anaphylactoid/hypersensitivity reactions: Immediate treatment (including epinephrine 1:1000) for anaphylactoid and/or hypersensitivity reactions should be available during vaccine use. Influenza vaccines from previous seasons must not be used. May consider deferring administration in patients with moderate or severe acute illness (with or without fever); may administer to patients with mild acute illness (with or without fever). Use with caution in patients with a history of bleeding disorders (including thrombocytopenia) and/or patients on anticoagulant therapy; bleeding/hematoma may occur from I.M. administration. Use with caution in patients with history of Guillain-Barré syndrome (GBS); patients with history of GBS have a greater likelihood of developing GBS than those without. As a precaution, the ACIP recommends that patients with a history of GBS and who are at low risk for severe influenza complications, and patients known to have experienced GBS within 6 weeks following previous vaccination should generally not be vaccinated (consider influenza antiviral chemoprophylaxis in these patients). The benefits of vaccination may outweigh the potential risks in persons with a history of GBS who are also at high risk for complications of influenza.

Use with caution in severely immunocompromised patients (eg, patients receiving chemo/radiation therapy or other immunosuppressive therapy [including high-dose corticosteroids]); may have a reduced response to vaccination. Inactivated vaccine is preferred over live virus vaccine for household members, healthcare workers and others coming in close contact with severely-immunosuppressed persons requiring care in a protected environment. Antigenic response may not be as great as expected in HIV-infected persons with CD4 cells <100/mm³ and viral copies of HIV type 1 >30,000/mL. In order to maximize vaccination rates, the ACIP recommends simultaneous administration of all age-appropriate vaccines (live or inactivated) for which a person is eligible at a single clinic visit, unless contraindications exist. Some products are manufactured with gentamicin, neomycin, polymyxin, and/or thimerosal. Packaging may contain natural latex rubber. All products are manufactured with chicken egg protein (expressed as ovalbumin content). The ovalbumin content may vary from season to season and lot to lot of vaccine. Allergy to eggs must be distinguished from allergy to the vaccine. Recommendations are available from the CDC regarding influenza vaccination to persons who report egg allergies; however, a prior severe allergic reaction to influenza vaccine, regardless of the component suspected, is a contraindication to vaccination (CDC, 2011).

Adverse Reactions (Reflective of adult population; not specific for elderly) All serious adverse reactions must be reported to the U.S. Department of Health and Human Services (DHHS) Vaccine Adverse Event Reporting System (VAERS) 1-800-822-7967 or online at https://vaers.hhs.gov/esub/index. In Canada, adverse reactions may be reported to local provincial/territorial health agencies or to the Vaccine Safety Section at Public Health Agency of Canada (1-866-844-0018).

Frequency not defined. Adverse reactions in adults ≥65 years of age may be greater using the high-dose vaccine, but are typically mild and transient.

Cardiovascular: Chest tightness, facial edema

Central nervous system: Chills, drowsiness, fatigue, fever, headache, irritability, malaise, migraine, shivering

Endocrine & metabolic: Dysmenorrhea

Gastrointestinal: Appetite decreased, diarrhea, nausea, sore throat, upper abdominal pain, vomiting

Local: Injection site reactions (including bruising, erythema, induration, inflammation, pain, soreness [≤64%; may last up to 2 days], pruritus, swelling, tenderness)

Neuromuscular & skeletal: Arthralgia, back pain, myalgia (may start within 6-12 hours and last 1-2 days; incidence equal to placebo in adults; occurs more frequently than placebo in children)

Ocular: Red eyes

Otic: Earache

Respiratory: Cough, nasal congestion, nasopharyngitis, pharyngolaryngeal pain, rhinitis, upper respiratory tract infection, wheezing

Miscellaneous: Diaphoresis

Drug Interactions

Metabolism/Transport Effects None known.

Avoid Concomitant Use There are no known interactions where it is recommended to avoid concomitant use.

Increased Effect/Toxicity There are no known significant interactions involving an increase in effect.

Decreased Effect

Influenza Virus Vaccine (Inactivated) may decrease the levels/effects of: Pneumococcal Conjugate Vaccine (13-Valent)

The levels/effects of Influenza Virus Vaccine (Inactivated) may be decreased by: Belimumab; Fingolimod; Immunosuppressants; Pneumococcal Conjugate Vaccine (13-Valent)

Stability Store all products between 2°C to 8°C (36°F to 46°F). Potency is destroyed by freezing; do not use if product has been frozen.

Agriflu™, Fluad™, Fluarix®: Protect from light.

Afluria®, FluLaval®, Fluviral®: Discard 28 days after initial entry. Protect from light.

Fluvirin®, Fluzone®, Fluzone® High Dose: Between uses, the multiple dose vial should be stored at 2°C to 8°C (36°F to 46°F).

Vaxigrip®: Between uses, the multiple dose vial should be stored at 2°C to 8°C (36°F to 46°F). Discard 7 days after initial entry. Protect from light.

Mechanism of Action Promotes immunity to seasonal influenza virus by inducing specific antibody production. Each year the formulation is standardized according to the U.S. Public Health Service. Preparations from previous seasons must not be used.

Pharmacodynamics/Kinetics

Onset of action: Protective antibody titers achieved ~3 weeks after vaccination

Duration: Protective antibody titers persist approximately ≥6 months. Elderly: Protective antibody titers may fall ≤4 months after vaccination.

Dosage

Geriatric It is important to note that influenza seasons vary in their timing and duration from year to year. In general, vaccination should begin soon after the vaccine becomes available and prior to onset of influenza activity in the community. However, vaccination should continue throughout the influenza season as long as vaccine is available.

Immunization: Adults ≥65 years:

Afluria®, Fluarix®, FluLaval®, Fluvirin®, Fluzone®, Fluzone® High-Dose: I.M.: 0.5 mL/dose (1 dose per season). The ACIP does not have a preference for any given TIV formulation when used within their specified age indications.

Canadian labeling (product not available in U.S.):

Fluad™: I.M.: 0.5 mL/dose (1 dose per season)

Intanza® 15 mcg/strain: Intradermal: Refer to adult dosing

Adult It is important to note that influenza seasons vary in their timing and duration from year to year. In general, vaccination should begin soon after the vaccine becomes available and prior to onset of influenza activity in the community. However, vaccination should continue throughout the influenza season as long as vaccine is available. Unless noted, the ACIP does not have a preference for any given TIV formulation when used within their specified age indications.

Immunization:

I.M.: *Afluria®, Fluarix®, FluLaval®, Fluvirin®, Fluzone®:* 0.5 mL/dose (1 dose per season)

Intradermal: Adults 18-64 years: *Fluzone® Intradermal:* 0.1 mL/dose (1 dose per season)

Canadian labeling (products not available in U.S.):

I.M.: *Agriflu™, Fluviral®, Vaxigrip®:* 0.5 mL/dose (1 dose per season)

I.M., SubQ: *Influvac®:* 0.5 mL/dose (1 per season)

Intradermal:

Intanza® 9 mcg/strain: Adults 18-59 years: 0.1 mL/dose (1 dose per season)

Intanza® 15 mcg/strain: Adults ≥60 years: 0.1 mL/dose (1 dose per season)

Administration

Fluzone® Intradermal: For intradermal administration over the deltoid muscle only. Shake gently prior to use. Hold system using the thumb and middle finger (do not place fingers on windows). Insert needle perpendicular to the skin; inject using index finger to push on plunger. Do not aspirate.

Afluria®, Fluarix®, FluLaval®, Fluvirin®, Fluzone®, Fluzone® High-Dose: For I.M. administration only. Inspect for particulate matter and discoloration prior to administration. Adults should be vaccinated in the deltoid muscle using a ≥1 inch needle length. Do not inject into the gluteal region or areas where there may be a major nerve trunk. Suspensions should be shaken well prior to use.

If a pediatric vaccine (0.25 mL) is inadvertently administered to an adult, an additional 0.25 mL should be administered to provide the full adult dose (0.5 mL). If the error is discovered after the patient has left, an adult dose should be given as soon as the patient can return.

Note: For patients at risk of hemorrhage following intramuscular injection, the ACIP recommends "it should be administered intramuscularly if, in the opinion of the physician familiar with the patients bleeding risk, the vaccine can be administered by this route with reasonable safety. If the patient receives antihemophilia or other similar therapy, intramuscular vaccination can be scheduled shortly after such therapy is administered. A fine needle (23 gauge or smaller) can be used for the vaccination and firm pressure applied to the site (without rubbing) for at least 2 minutes. The patient should be instructed concerning the risk of hematoma from the injection." Patients on anticoagulant therapy should be considered to have the same bleeding risks and treated as those with clotting factor disorders (CDC, 2011).

Simultaneous administration of vaccines helps ensure the patients will be fully vaccinated by the appropriate age. Simultaneous administration of vaccines is defined as administering >1 vaccine on the same day at different anatomic sites. Separate vaccines should not be combined in the same syringe unless indicated by product specific labeling. Separate needles and syringes should be used for each injection. However, in general, vaccination should not be deferred if the brand name or route of the previous dose is not available or not known (CDC, 2011). Adolescents and adults should be vaccinated while seated or lying down.

Antipyretics have not been shown to prevent febrile seizures. Antipyretics may be used to treat fever or discomfort following vaccination (CDC, 2011). One study reported that routine prophylactic administration of acetaminophen to prevent fever prior to vaccination decreased the immune response of some vaccines; the clinical significance of this reduction in immune response has not been established (Prymula, 2009).

Monitoring Parameters Monitor for syncope for 15 minutes following administration. If seizure-like activity associated with syncope occurs, maintain patient in supine or Trendelenburg position to reestablish adequate cerebral perfusion. For those individuals who report a history of egg allergy but it is determined that the inactivated vaccine can be used, observe vaccine recipient for at least 30 minutes after receipt of vaccine.

Pharmacotherapy Pearls Pharmacies will stock the formulations(s) standardized according to the USPHS requirements for the season. Influenza vaccines from previous seasons must not be used. U.S. federal law requires that the name of medication, date of administration, the vaccine manufacturer, lot number of vaccine, and the administering person's name, title, and address be entered into the patient's permanent medical record.

It is important to note that influenza seasons vary in their timing and duration from year to year. In general, vaccination should begin soon after the vaccine becomes available and if possible, prior to October. However, vaccination should continue throughout the influenza season as long as vaccine is available.

When vaccine supply is limited, administration should focus on the ACIP target groups. When TIV vaccine is in short supply, administering LAIV to eligible persons is encouraged to increase available TIV to those patients in whom LAIV cannot be used. During periods of inactivated influenza vaccine (TIV) shortage, the CDC and ACIP have recommended vaccination be prioritized based on the following three tiers. The grouping is based on influenza associated mortality and hospitalization rates. Those listed in group 1 should be vaccinated first, followed by persons in group 2, and then group 3. If the vaccine supply is extremely limited, group 1 has also been subdivided in three tiers, where those in group 1A should be vaccinated first, followed by 1B, then 1C.

Priority groups for vaccination with inactivated seasonal influenza vaccine during periods of vaccine shortage:
Tier 1A:
  Persons ≥65 years with comorbid conditions
  Residents of long-term-care facilities
Tier 1B:
  Persons 2-64 years with comorbid conditions
  Persons ≥65 years without comorbid conditions
  Children 6-23 months
  Pregnant women
Tier 1C:
  Healthcare personnel
  Household contacts and out-of-home caregivers of children <6 months
Tier 2:
  Household contacts of children and adults at increased risk of influenza-associated complications
  Healthy persons 50-64 years
Tier 3:
  Persons 2-49 years without high-risk conditions
Further information available at http://www.cdc.gov/mmwr/preview/mmwrhtml/mm5430a4.htm

Special Geriatric Considerations Limited data on the elderly exists due to ethical considerations precluding use of placebo and differences in studies and vaccines; 80% develop a 1:40 HA titer, 70% are completely protected, 90% protected from death.

Dosage Forms Excipient information presented when available (limited, particularly for generics); consult specific product labeling.

Injection, suspension [purified split-virus]:
  Afluria®: Hemagglutinin 45 mcg/0.5 mL (5 mL) [contains chicken egg protein, neomycin (may have trace amounts), polymyxin B (may have trace amounts), thimerosal]
  FluLaval®: Hemagglutinin 45 mcg/0.5 mL (5 mL) [contains chicken egg protein, thimerosal]
  Fluvirin®: Hemagglutinin 45 mcg/0.5 mL (5 mL) [contains chicken egg protein, neomycin (may have trace amounts), polymyxin B (may have trace amounts), thimerosal]
  Fluzone®: Hemagglutinin 45 mcg/0.5 mL (5 mL) [contains chicken egg protein, thimerosal]
Injection, suspension [purified split-virus, preservative free]:
  Afluria®: Hemagglutinin 45 mcg/0.5 mL (0.5 mL) [contains chicken egg protein, neomycin (may have trace amounts), polymyxin B (may have trace amounts)]
  Fluarix®: Hemagglutinin 45 mcg/0.5 mL (0.5 mL) [contains chicken egg protein, gentamicin (may have trace amounts), hydrocortisone (may have trace amounts), may contain natural rubber/natural latex in prefilled syringe, polysorbate 80]
  Fluvirin®: Hemagglutinin 45 mcg/0.5 mL (0.5 mL) [contains chicken egg protein, may contain natural rubber/natural latex in prefilled syringe, neomycin (may have trace amounts), polymyxin B (may have trace amounts)]
  Fluzone®: Hemagglutinin 22.5 mcg/0.25 mL (0.25 mL); Hemagglutinin 45 mcg/0.5 mL (0.5 mL) [contains chicken egg protein]
  Fluzone® High-Dose: Hemagglutinin 180 mcg/0.5 mL (0.5 mL) [contains chicken egg protein]
  Fluzone® Intradermal: Hemagglutinin 27 mcg/0.1 mL (0.1 mL) [contains chicken egg protein]

Dosage Forms: Canada Excipient information presented when available (limited, particularly for generics); consult specific product labeling.
Injection, suspension [purified split-virus]:
  Fluviral®: Hemagglutinin 45 mcg/0.5 mL (5 mL) [contains chicken egg protein, thimerosal]
  Vaxigrip®: Hemagglutinin 45 mcg/0.5 mL (5 mL) [contains chicken egg protein, neomycin (may have trace amounts), thimerosal]
Injection, suspension [purified split-virus, preservative free]:
  Agriflu™: Hemagglutinin 45 mcg/0.5 mL (0.5 mL) [contains chicken egg protein, neomycin (may have trace amounts), kanamycin (may have trace amounts), polysorbate 80]
  Fluad™: Hemagglutinin 45 mcg/0.5 mL (0.5 mL) [contains chicken egg protein, neomycin (may have trace amounts), kanamycin (may have trace amounts), polysorbate 80]
  Influvac®: Hemagglutinin 45 mcg/0.5 mL (0.5 mL) [contains chicken egg protein, gentamicin (may have trace amounts), polysorbate 80]
  Intanza®: Hemagglutinin 27 mcg/0.1 mL (0.1 mL) [contains chicken egg protein, neomycin (may have trace amounts)]
  Intanza®: Hemagglutinin 45 mcg/0.1 mL (0.1 mL) [contains chicken egg protein, neomycin (may have trace amounts)]
  Vaxigrip®: Hemagglutinin 45 mcg/0.5 mL (0.25 mL, 0.5 mL) [contains chicken egg protein, neomycin (may have trace amounts)]

Influenza Virus Vaccine (Live/Attenuated)
(in floo EN za VYE rus vak SEEN live ah TEN yoo aye ted)

Related Information
Immunization Administration Recommendations *on page 2144*
Immunization Recommendations *on page 2149*
Medication Safety Issues
Sound-alike/look-alike issues:
Influenza virus vaccine may be confused with flumazenil
Brand Names: U.S. FluMist®
Brand Names: Canada FluMist®
Index Terms H1N1 Influenza Vaccine; Influenza Vaccine; Influenza Virus Vaccine (Trivalent, Live); LAIV; Live Attenuated Influenza Vaccine
Generic Availability (U.S.) No
Pharmacologic Category Vaccine, Live (Viral)
Use Provide active immunity to influenza virus strains contained in the vaccine

The Advisory Committee on Immunization Practices (ACIP) states that healthy, nonpregnant persons aged 2-49 years may receive vaccination with either the seasonal live, attenuated influenza vaccine (LAIV) (nasal spray) or the seasonal trivalent inactivated influenza vaccine (TIV) (injection).
Contraindications Prior life-threatening reaction to previous influenza vaccination; hypersensitivity to any component of the formulation
Warnings/Precautions Immediate treatment (including epinephrine 1:1000) for anaphylactoid and/or hypersensitivity reactions should be available during vaccine use. Influenza

vaccines from previous seasons must not be used. May consider deferring administration in patients with moderate or severe acute illness (with or without fever); may administer to patients with mild acute illness (with or without fever). Defer immunization if nasal congestion is present which may impede delivery of vaccine. Use with caution in patients with history of Guillain-Barré syndrome (GBS); patients with history of GBS have a greater likelihood of developing GBS than those without. As a precaution, the ACIP recommends that patients with a history of GBS and who are at low risk for severe influenza complications, and patients known to have experienced GBS within 6 weeks following previous vaccination should generally not be vaccinated (consider influenza antiviral chemoprophylaxis in these patients). Based on limited data, the benefits of vaccinating persons with a history of GBS who are also at high risk for complications of influenza, may outweigh the risks. The nasal spray should not be used in patients with asthma; risk of wheezing following vaccination is increased. Patients with severe asthma or active wheezing were not included in clinical trials. Because safety and efficacy information is limited, the ACIP does not recommend the use of LAIV in patients with chronic pulmonary disorders including asthma.

Because safety and efficacy information is limited, the ACIP does not recommend the use of LAIV in patients with chronic disorders of the cardiovascular system (except isolated hypertension), diabetes, with hematologic disorders and hemoglobinopathies, hepatic disease, neurologic or neuromuscular disorders, or renal disease. Data on the use of the nasal spray in immunocompromised patients is limited. **Avoid contact with severely immunocompromised individuals for at least 7 days following vaccination (at least 14 days per Canadian labeling).** Because safety and efficacy information is limited, the ACIP does not recommend the use of LAIV in immunosuppressed patients including patients with HIV. In order to maximize vaccination rates, the ACIP recommends simultaneous administration of all age-appropriate vaccines (live or inactivated) for which a person is eligible at a single clinic visit, unless contraindications exist. The U.S. labeling states that safety and efficacy of the nasal spray have not been established in adults ≥50 years of age; use in adults <60 years is approved in the Canadian labeling. Manufactured using arginine, chicken egg protein, gelatin, and gentamicin. Allergy to eggs must be distinguished from allergy to the vaccine. Recommendations are available from the CDC regarding influenza vaccination to persons who report egg allergies; however, a prior severe allergic reaction to influenza vaccine, regardless of the component suspected, is a contraindication to vaccination. Use of TIV is preferred over LAIV when considering vaccination in persons reporting an egg allergy (CDC, 2011).

Adverse Reactions (Reflective of adult population; not specific for elderly) All serious adverse reactions must be reported to the U.S. Department of Health and Human Services (DHHS) Vaccine Adverse Event Reporting System (VAERS) 1-800-822-7967 or online at https://vaers.hhs.gov/esub/index. In Canada, adverse reactions may be reported to local provincial/territorial health agencies or to the Vaccine Safety Section at Public Health Agency of Canada (1-866-844-0018).

Frequency of events reported within 10 days.
>10%:
  Central nervous system: Headache (children 3% to 9%; adults 40%), irritability (children 12% to 21%), lethargy (children 7% to 14%)
  Gastrointestinal: Appetite decreased (children 13% to 21%), abdominal pain (children 2% to 12%)
  Neuromuscular & skeletal: Tiredness/weakness (adults 26%), muscle aches (children 2% to 6%; adults 17%)
  Respiratory: Cough (adults 14%), nasal congestion/ runny nose (children 51% to 58%; adults 9% to 44%), sore throat (children 5% to 11%; adults 28%)
1% to 10%:
  Central nervous system: Chills (children 2% to 4%, adults 9%), fever (100°F to 101°F: children 6% to 9%; >101°F: children 1% to 4%)
  Otic: Otitis media (children 3%)
  Respiratory: Sinusitis (adults 4%), sneezing (children 2%), wheezing (children 6-23 months 6%; children 24-59 months 2%)

Drug Interactions
  Metabolism/Transport Effects None known.
  Avoid Concomitant Use
    Avoid concomitant use of Influenza Virus Vaccine (Live/Attenuated) with any of the following: Belimumab; Fingolimod; Immunosuppressants; Salicylates
  Increased Effect/Toxicity
    Influenza Virus Vaccine (Live/Attenuated) may increase the levels/effects of: Salicylates

    The levels/effects of Influenza Virus Vaccine (Live/Attenuated) may be increased by: AzaTHIOprine; Belimumab; Corticosteroids (Systemic); Fingolimod; Hydroxychloroquine; Immunosuppressants; Leflunomide; Mercaptopurine; Methotrexate

Decreased Effect

Influenza Virus Vaccine (Live/Attenuated) may decrease the levels/effects of: Tuberculin Tests

The levels/effects of Influenza Virus Vaccine (Live/Attenuated) may be decreased by: Antiviral Agents (Influenza A and B); Fingolimod; Immune Globulins; Immunosuppressants

Stability Store in refrigerator at 2°C to 8°C (36°F to 46°F). **Do not freeze.**

Mechanism of Action Promotes immunity to seasonal influenza virus by inducing specific antibody production. Each year the formulation is standardized according to the U.S. Public Health Service. Preparations from previous seasons must not be used.

Pharmacodynamics/Kinetics

Onset of action: Protective antibody titers achieved ~3 weeks after vaccination

Duration: Protective antibody titers persist approximately ≥6 months. Elderly: Protective antibody titers may fall ≤4 months after vaccination.

Distribution: Following nasal administration, vaccine is distributed in the nasal cavity (~90%), stomach (~3%), brain (~2%), and lung (0.4%)

Dosage

Geriatric Not indicated for use in patients ≥50 years (U.S. labeling) or ≥60 years (Canadian labeling).

Adult It is important to note that influenza seasons vary in their timing and duration from year to year. In general, vaccination should begin soon after the vaccine becomes available and prior to onset of influenza activity in the community. However, vaccination should continue throughout the influenza season as long as vaccine is available.

Immunization: Intranasal (FluMist®):

U.S. labeling: Adults ≤49 years: 0.2 mL/dose (1 dose per season)

Canadian labeling: Adults ≤59 years: 0.2 mL/dose (1 dose per season)

Administration LAIV: Intranasal: Half the dose (0.1 mL) is administered to each nostril; patient should be in upright position. A dose divider clip is provided. Severely immunocompromised persons should not administer the live vaccine. If recipient sneezes following administration, the dose should not be repeated.

Simultaneous administration of vaccines helps ensure the patients will be fully vaccinated by the appropriate age. Simultaneous administration of vaccines is defined as administering >1 vaccine on the same day at different anatomic sites. The ACIP prefers each dose of a specific vaccine in a series come from the same manufacturer when possible. However, in general, vaccination should not be deferred if the brand name or route of the previous dose is not available or not known (CDC, 2011).

Antipyretics have not been shown to prevent febrile seizures. Antipyretics may be used to treat fever or discomfort following vaccination (CDC, 2011). One study reported that routine prophylactic administration of acetaminophen to prevent fever prior to vaccination decreased the immune response of some vaccines; the clinical significance of this reduction in immune response has not been established (Prymula, 2009).

Vaccine administration with oral influenza antiviral medications: Live influenza virus vaccine (LAIV) should not be given until 48 hours after the completion of influenza antiviral therapy (influenza A and B). Influenza antiviral therapy (influenza A and B) should not be administered for 2 weeks after receiving LAIV. If influenza antiviral therapy (influenza A and B) and LAIV are administered concomitantly, revaccination should be considered.

Test Interactions Administration of the intranasal influenza virus vaccine (live, LAIV) may cause a positive result on the rapid influenza diagnostic test for the 7 days after vaccine administration; for a person with influenza-like illness during this time, the positive test could be caused by either the live attenuated vaccine or wild-type influenza virus.

Pharmacotherapy Pearls Pharmacies will stock the formulations(s) standardized according to the USPHS requirements for the season. Influenza vaccines from previous seasons must not be used. U.S. federal law requires that the name of medication, date of administration, the vaccine manufacturer, lot number of vaccine, and the administering person's name, title, and address, and documentation of the vaccine information statement (VIS; date on VIS and date given to patient) be entered into the patient's permanent medical record.

It is important to note that influenza seasons vary in their timing and duration from year to year. In general, vaccination should begin soon after the vaccine becomes available and prior to onset of influenza activity in the community. However, vaccination should continue throughout the influenza season as long as vaccine is available.

When vaccine supply is not limited, either TIV or LAIV can be used in healthy, nonpregnant persons aged 2-49 years of age.

◀ When vaccine supply is limited, administration should focus on the ACIP target groups. When TIV vaccine is in short supply, administering LAIV to eligible persons is encouraged to increase available TIV to those patients in whom LAIV cannot be used. During periods of inactivated influenza vaccine (TIV) shortage, the CDC and ACIP have recommended vaccination be prioritized based on the following three tiers. The grouping is based on influenza-associated mortality and hospitalization rates. Those listed in group 1 should be vaccinated first, followed by persons in group 2, and then group 3. If the vaccine supply is extremely limited, group 1 has also been subdivided in three tiers, where those in group 1A should be vaccinated first, followed by 1B, then 1C.

Priority groups for vaccination with inactivated seasonal influenza vaccine during periods of vaccine shortage:
Tier 1A:
  Persons ≥65 years with comorbid conditions
  Residents of long-term-care facilities
Tier 1B:
  Persons 2-64 years with comorbid conditions
  Persons ≥65 years without comorbid conditions
  Children 6-23 months
  Pregnant women
Tier 1C:
  Healthcare personnel
  Household contacts and out-of-home caregivers of children <6 months
Tier 2:
  Household contacts of children and adults at increased risk of influenza-associated complications
  Healthy persons 50-64 years
Tier 3:
  Persons 2-49 years without high-risk conditions
Further information available at http://www.cdc.gov/mmwr/preview/mmwrhtml/mm5430a4.htm

Special Geriatric Considerations Limited data on the elderly exists due to ethical considerations precluding use of placebo and differences in studies and vaccines; 80% develop a 1:40 HA titer, 70% are completely protected, 90% protected from death.

Product Availability FluMist® Quadrivalent Vaccine: FDA approved February 2012; availability anticipated for the 2013-2014 flu season. Consult prescribing information for additional information.

Dosage Forms Excipient information presented when available (limited, particularly for generics); consult specific product labeling.
Solution, intranasal [spray, preservative free]:
  FluMist®: (0.2 mL) [contains arginine, chicken egg protein, gelatin, gentamicin (may have trace amounts)]

◆ **Influenza Virus Vaccine (Monovalent)** see Influenza Virus Vaccine (H5N1) on page 996
◆ **Influenza Virus Vaccine (Purified Surface Antigen)** see Influenza Virus Vaccine (Inactivated) on page 997
◆ **Influenza Virus Vaccine (Split-Virus)** see Influenza Virus Vaccine (Inactivated) on page 997
◆ **Influenza Virus Vaccine (Trivalent, Live)** see Influenza Virus Vaccine (Live/Attenuated) on page 1001
◆ **Infumorph 200** see Morphine (Systemic) on page 1312
◆ **Infumorph 500** see Morphine (Systemic) on page 1312

Ingenol Mebutate (IN je nol MEB u tate)

Brand Names: U.S. Picato®
Index Terms Euphorbia peplus Derivative; PEP005
Generic Availability (U.S.) No
Pharmacologic Category Topical Skin Product
Use Topical treatment of actinic keratosis
Contraindications There are no contraindications listed in the manufacturer's labeling.
Warnings/Precautions Severe dermatologic reactions including erythema, crusting, swelling, vesiculation/pustulation, and erosion/ulceration can occur. Severe eye pain, eyelid edema, eyelid ptosis, and periorbital edema can occur after exposure; avoid contact with the periocular area (patients should wash hands immediately after applying and avoid transferring to the eye area).

Apply to intact and nonirritated skin only. Instruct patients to wash hands well after applying and to avoid contact with the periocular area during and after application. Avoid touching the treated area for 6 hours after application. If inadvertent exposure to other area(s) occurs, flush the area with water and seek medical care as soon as possible. Avoid inadvertent transfer to other individuals. Administration of ingenol mebutate gel is not recommended until the skin is healed from any previous drug or surgical treatment. For topical use only; not for oral, ophthalmic, or intravaginal use.

Adverse Reactions (Reflective of adult population; not specific for elderly)

>10%: Dermatologic: Erythema (92% to 94%), flaking/scaling (85% to 90%), crusting (74% to 80%), swelling (64% to 79%), vesiculation/pustulation (44% to 56%), erosion/ulceration (26% to 32%), application site pain (2% to 15%)

1% to 10%:

Central nervous system: Headache (2%)

Dermatologic: Application site pruritus (8%), application site irritation (4%), application site infection (3%)

Ocular: Periorbital edema (3%)

Respiratory: Nasopharyngitis (2%)

Drug Interactions

Metabolism/Transport Effects None known.

Avoid Concomitant Use There are no known interactions where it is recommended to avoid concomitant use.

Increased Effect/Toxicity There are no known significant interactions involving an increase in effect.

Decreased Effect There are no known significant interactions involving a decrease in effect.

Stability Store in a refrigerator at 2°C to 8°C (36°F to 46°F); excursions are permitted to 0°C to 15°C (32°F to 59°F); do not freeze. Discard tubes after single use.

Mechanism of Action Ingenol mebutate appears to induce primary necrosis of actinic keratosis with a subsequent neutrophil-mediated inflammatory response with antibody-dependent cytotoxicity of residual disease cells; killing residual disease cells may prevent future relapse.

Pharmacodynamics/Kinetics Absorption: Absorption through the skin is minimal (with proper use); expected systemic exposure is <0.1 ng/mL.

Dosage

Geriatric & Adult Actinic keratoses: Topical:

Face and scalp: Apply 0.015% gel once daily to affected area for 3 consecutive days

Trunk/extremities: Apply 0.05% gel once daily to affected area for 2 consecutive days

Administration Apply to one contiguous affected area of skin using one unit-dose tube; one unit-dose tube will cover ~5 cm x 5 cm (~25 cm^2 or ~2 inch x 2 inch). Spread evenly then allow gel to dry for 15 minutes. Do not cover with bandages or occlusive dressings. Wash hands immediately after applying and avoid transferring gel to any other areas. Avoid washing or touching the treatment area for at least 6 hours, and following this period of time, patients may wash the area with a mild soap. Not for oral, ophthalmic, or intravaginal use.

Special Geriatric Considerations

In clinical trials, there was no significant difference in efficacy or safety when comparing older and younger patients.

Dosage Forms Excipient information presented when available (limited, particularly for generics); consult specific product labeling.

Gel, topical:

Picato®: 0.015% (3s); 0.05% (2s) [contains benzyl alcohol, isopropyl alcohol]

♦ **INH** see Isoniazid on page 1047
♦ **InnoPran XL®** see Propranolol on page 1622
♦ **Inspra™** see Eplerenone on page 649

Insulin Aspart (IN soo lin AS part)

Related Information

Diabetes Mellitus Management, Adults on page 2193
Insulin Regular on page 1025

Medication Safety Issues

Sound-alike/look-alike issues:

NovoLOG® may be confused with HumaLOG®, HumuLIN® R, NovoLIN® N, NovoLIN® R, NovoLOG® Mix 70/30

High alert medication:

The Institute for Safe Medication Practices (ISMP) includes this medication among its list of drugs which have a heightened risk of causing significant patient harm when used in error. ▶

◀ *Due to the number of insulin preparations, it is essential to identify/clarify the type of insulin to be used.*

Other safety concerns:
Cross-contamination may occur if insulin pens are shared among multiple patients. Steps should be taken to prohibit sharing of insulin pens.

Brand Names: U.S. NovoLOG®; NovoLOG® FlexPen®; NovoLOG® Penfill®

Brand Names: Canada NovoRapid®

Index Terms Aspart Insulin

Generic Availability (U.S.) No

Pharmacologic Category Insulin, Rapid-Acting

Use Treatment of type 1 diabetes mellitus (insulin dependent, IDDM) and type 2 diabetes mellitus (noninsulin dependent, NIDDM) to improve glycemic control

Unlabeled Use Mild-to-moderate diabetic ketoacidosis (DKA); mild-to-moderate hyperosmolar hyperglycemic state (HHS)

Contraindications Hypersensitivity to insulin aspart or any component of the formulation; during episodes of hypoglycemia

Warnings/Precautions Refer to Insulin Regular on page 1025.

Due to the short duration of action of insulin aspart, a longer acting insulin or CSII via an external insulin pump is needed to maintain adequate glucose control in patients with type 1 diabetes mellitus. In both type 1 and type 2 diabetes, preprandial administration of insulin aspart should be immediately followed by a meal within 5-10 minutes. May also be administered via CSII; do not dilute or mix with other insulin formulations when using an external insulin pump. Rule out pump failure if unexplained hyperglycemia or ketosis occurs; temporary SubQ insulin administration may be required until the problem is identified and corrected. Insulin aspart may also be administered I.V. in selected clinical situations to control hyperglycemia; close monitoring of blood glucose and serum potassium as well as medical supervision is required.

Drug Interactions

Metabolism/Transport Effects None known.

Avoid Concomitant Use There are no known interactions where it is recommended to avoid concomitant use.

Increased Effect/Toxicity
Insulin Aspart may increase the levels/effects of: Antidiabetic Agents (Thiazolidinedione); Hypoglycemic Agents; Quinolone Antibiotics

The levels/effects of Insulin Aspart may be increased by: Beta-Blockers; Edetate CALCIUM Disodium; Edetate Disodium; Herbs (Hypoglycemic Properties); MAO Inhibitors; Pegvisomant; Salicylates; Selective Serotonin Reuptake Inhibitors

Decreased Effect
The levels/effects of Insulin Aspart may be decreased by: Corticosteroids (Orally Inhaled); Corticosteroids (Systemic); Loop Diuretics; Luteinizing Hormone-Releasing Hormone Analogs; Somatropin; Thiazide Diuretics

Ethanol/Nutrition/Herb Interactions Refer to Insulin Regular on page 1025.

Stability Unopened vials, cartridges, and prefilled pens may be stored under refrigeration between 2°C and 8°C (36°F to 46°F) until the expiration date or at room temperature <30°C (<86°F) for 28 days; do not freeze; keep away from heat and sunlight. Once punctured (in use), vials may be stored under refrigeration or at room temperature <30°C (<86°F); use within 28 days. Cartridges and prefilled pens that have been punctured (in use) should be stored at temperatures <30°C (<86°F) and used within 28 days; do not freeze or refrigerate. When used for CSII, insulin aspart contained within an external insulin pump reservoir should be replaced at least every 6 days; discard if exposed to temperatures >37°C (>98.6°F).
For SubQ administration: *NovoLog® vials:* May be diluted with Insulin Diluting Medium for NovoLog® to a concentration of 10 units/mL (U-10) or 50 units/mL (U-50). According to the manufacturer, diluted insulin should be stored at temperatures <30°C (<86°F) and used within 28 days; do not dilute insulin contained in a cartridge, prefilled pen, or external insulin pump.
For I.V. infusion: May be diluted in NS, D_5W, or $D_{10}W$ to concentrations of 0.05-1 unit/mL. Stable for 24 hours at room temperature.

Mechanism of Action Insulin aspart is a rapid-acting insulin analog.
Refer to Insulin Regular on page 1025.

Pharmacodynamics/Kinetics Note: Rate of absorption, onset, and duration of activity may be affected by site of injection, exercise, presence of lipodystrophy, local blood supply, and/or temperature.
Onset of action: 0.2-0.3 hours
Peak effect: 1-3 hours
Duration: 3-5 hours

Protein binding: <10%
Half-life elimination: SubQ: 81 minutes
Time to peak, plasma: 40-50 minutes
Excretion: Urine

Dosage

Geriatric & Adult Note: When compared to insulin regular, insulin aspart has a more rapid onset and shorter duration of activity.

Diabetes mellitus, type 1 and type 2: SubQ: Refer to Insulin Regular on page 1025.

Glycemic control in selected clinical situations and under appropriate medical supervision: I.V.: Refer to Insulin Regular on page 1025.

Diabetic ketoacidosis (DKA), mild-to-moderate (unlabeled use): SubQ: Refer to Insulin Regular on page 1025.

Hyperosmolar hyperglycemic state (HHS), mild-to-moderate (unlabeled use): SubQ: Refer to Insulin Regular on page 1025.

Renal Impairment Refer to Insulin Regular on page 1025.

Hepatic Impairment Refer to Insulin Regular on page 1025.

Administration

SubQ administration: Do not use if solution is viscous or cloudy; use only if clear and colorless. Insulin aspart should be administered immediately (within 5-10 minutes) before a meal. Cold injections should be avoided. SubQ administration is usually made into the thighs, arms, buttocks, or abdomen; rotate injection sites. When mixing insulin aspart with other preparations of insulin (eg, insulin NPH), insulin aspart should be drawn into syringe first. Do not dilute or mix other insulin formulations with insulin aspart contained in a cartridge or prefilled pen.

CSII administration: Do not use if solution is viscous or cloudy; use only if clear and colorless. Patients should be trained in the proper use of their external insulin pump and in intensive insulin therapy. Infusion sets and infusion set insertion sites should be changed at least every 3 days; rotate infusion sites. Do not dilute or mix other insulin formulations with insulin aspart that is to be used in an external insulin pump.

I.V. administration: Do not use if solution is viscous or cloudy; use only if clear and colorless. May be administered I.V. with close monitoring of blood glucose and serum potassium; appropriate medical supervision is required. **Do not administer insulin mixtures intravenously.**

I.V. infusions: To minimize adsorption to I.V. solution bag: **Note:** Refer to institution-specific protocols where appropriate.

*If new tubing is **not** needed:* Wait a minimum of 30 minutes between the preparation of the solution and the initiation of the infusion

If new tubing is needed: After receiving the insulin drip solution, the administration set should be attached to the I.V. container and the entire line should be flushed with a priming infusion of 20-50 mL of the insulin solution (Goldberg, 2006; Hirsch, 2006). Wait 30 minutes, and then flush the line again with the insulin solution prior to initiating the infusion.

Because of adsorption, the actual amount of insulin being administered via I.V. infusion could be substantially less than the apparent amount. Therefore, adjustment of the I.V. infusion rate should be based on effect and not solely on the apparent insulin dose. The apparent dose may be used as a starting point for determining the subsequent SubQ dosing regimen (Moghissi, 2009); however, the transition to SubQ administration requires continuous medical supervision, frequent monitoring of blood glucose, and careful adjustment of therapy. In addition, SubQ insulin should be given 1-4 hours prior to the discontinuation of I.V. insulin to prevent hyperglycemia (Moghissi, 2009).

Monitoring Parameters

Diabetes mellitus: Plasma glucose, electrolytes, Hb A_{1c}

I.V. administration: Close monitoring of blood glucose and serum potassium

Reference Range Refer to Insulin Regular on page 1025.

Pharmacotherapy Pearls Refer to Insulin Regular on page 1025.

Special Geriatric Considerations Intensive glucose control (Hb A_{1c} <6.5%) has been linked to increased all-cause and cardiovascular mortality, hypoglycemia requiring assistance, and weight gain in adult type 2 diabetes. How "tightly" to control a geriatric patient's blood glucose needs to be individualized. Such a decision should be based on several factors, including the patient's functional and cognitive status, how well he/she recognizes hypoglycemic or hyperglycemic symptoms, and how to respond to them and other disease states. An Hb A_{1c} <7.5% is an acceptable endpoint for a healthy older adult, while <8% is acceptable for frail elderly patients, those with a duration of illness >10 years, or those with comorbid conditions and requiring combination diabetes medications. Patients who are unable to accurately draw up their dose will need assistance, such as prefilled syringes. Initial doses may require considerations for renal function in the elderly with dosing adjusted subsequently based on blood glucose monitoring. For elderly patients with diabetes who are relatively

◀ healthy, attaining target goals for aspirin use, blood pressure, lipids, smoking cessation, and diet and exercise may be more important than normalized glycemic control.

Dosage Forms Excipient information presented when available (limited, particularly for generics); consult specific product labeling.

Injection, solution:
NovoLOG®: 100 units/mL (10 mL) [vial]
NovoLOG® FlexPen®: 100 units/mL (3 mL)
NovoLOG® Penfill®: 100 units/mL (3 mL) [cartridge]

◆ **Insulin Aspart and Insulin Aspart Protamine** see Insulin Aspart Protamine and Insulin Aspart on page 1008

Insulin Aspart Protamine and Insulin Aspart
(IN soo lin AS part PROE ta meen & IN soo lin AS part)

Related Information
Diabetes Mellitus Management, Adults on page 2193
Insulin Regular on page 1025

Medication Safety Issues
Sound-alike/look-alike issues:
NovoLOG® Mix 70/30 may be confused with HumaLOG® Mix 75/25™, HumuLIN® 70/30, NovoLIN® 70/30, NovoLOG®

High alert medication:
The Institute for Safe Medication Practices (ISMP) includes this medication among its list of drugs which have a heightened risk of causing significant patient harm when used in error. *Due to the number of insulin preparations, it is essential to identify/clarify the type of insulin to be used.*

Other safety concerns:
Cross-contamination may occur if insulin pens are shared among multiple patients. Steps should be taken to prohibit sharing of insulin pens.

Brand Names: U.S. NovoLOG® Mix 70/30; NovoLOG® Mix 70/30 FlexPen®

Brand Names: Canada NovoMix® 30

Index Terms Insulin Aspart and Insulin Aspart Protamine; NovoLog 70/30

Generic Availability (U.S.) No

Pharmacologic Category Insulin, Combination

Use Treatment of type 1 diabetes mellitus (insulin dependent, IDDM) and type 2 diabetes mellitus (noninsulin dependent, NIDDM) to improve glycemic control

Contraindications Hypersensitivity to any component of the formulation; during episodes of hypoglycemia

Warnings/Precautions Refer to Insulin Regular on page 1025. Insulin aspart protamine and insulin aspart premixed combination products are **NOT** intended for I.V. or I.M. administration.

Adverse Reactions (Reflective of adult population; not specific for elderly) Refer to Insulin Regular on page 1025.

Drug Interactions
Metabolism/Transport Effects None known.
Avoid Concomitant Use There are no known interactions where it is recommended to avoid concomitant use.

Increased Effect/Toxicity
Insulin Aspart Protamine and Insulin Aspart may increase the levels/effects of: Antidiabetic Agents (Thiazolidinedione); Hypoglycemic Agents; Quinolone Antibiotics

The levels/effects of Insulin Aspart Protamine and Insulin Aspart may be increased by: Beta-Blockers; Edetate CALCIUM Disodium; Edetate Disodium; Herbs (Hypoglycemic Properties); MAO Inhibitors; Pegvisomant; Salicylates; Selective Serotonin Reuptake Inhibitors

Decreased Effect
The levels/effects of Insulin Aspart Protamine and Insulin Aspart may be decreased by: Corticosteroids (Orally Inhaled); Corticosteroids (Systemic); Loop Diuretics; Luteinizing Hormone-Releasing Hormone Analogs; Somatropin; Thiazide Diuretics

Ethanol/Nutrition/Herb Interactions Refer to Insulin Regular on page 1025.

Stability Unopened vials and prefilled pens may be stored under refrigeration between 2°C and 8°C (36°F to 46°F) until the expiration date or at room temperature <30°C (<86°F) for 14 days (prefilled pens) or 28 days (vials); do not freeze; keep away from heat and sunlight. Once punctured (in use), vials may be stored under refrigeration or at room temperature <30°C (<86°F); use within 28 days. Prefilled pens that have been punctured (in use) should be stored at room temperature <30°C (<86°F) and used within 14 days; do not freeze or refrigerate.

Mechanism of Action Insulin aspart protamine and insulin aspart is an intermediate-acting combination insulin product with a more rapid onset and similar duration of action as compared to that of insulin NPH and insulin regular combination products. Refer to Insulin Regular on page 1025.

Pharmacodynamics/Kinetics Note: Rate of absorption, onset, and duration of activity may be affected by site of injection, exercise, presence of lipodystrophy, local blood supply, and/or temperature.

Onset of action: 10-20 minutes

Peak effect: 1-4 hours

Duration: 18-24 hours

Protein binding: ≤9%

Half-life elimination: ~8-9 hours

Time to peak, plasma: 1-1.5 hours

Excretion: Urine

Dosage

Geriatric & Adult Note: Insulin aspart protamine and insulin aspart combination products are approximately equipotent to insulin NPH and insulin regular combination products but with a more rapid onset and similar duration of activity. The proportion of rapid-acting to long-acting insulin is fixed in the combination products; basal versus prandial dose adjustments cannot be made.

Diabetes mellitus, type 1 and type 2: SubQ: Refer to Insulin Regular on page 1025.

Renal Impairment Refer to Insulin Regular on page 1025.

Hepatic Impairment Refer to Insulin Regular on page 1025.

Administration SubQ administration: In order to properly resuspend the insulin, vials and prefilled pens should be gently rolled between the palms ten times; in addition, prefilled pens should be inverted 180° ten times. Properly resuspended insulin should look uniformly cloudy or milky; do not use if any white insulin substance remains at the bottom of the container, if any clumps are present, if the insulin remains clear after adequate mixing, or if white particles are stuck to the bottom or wall of the container. Cold injections should be avoided. Insulin aspart protamine and insulin aspart combination products should be administered within 15 minutes before a meal (type 1 diabetes) or 15 minutes before or after a meal (type 2 diabetes); typically given twice daily. SubQ administration is usually made into the thighs, arms, buttocks, or abdomen; rotate injection sites. Do not dilute or mix with any other insulin formulation or solution; not recommended for use in external SubQ insulin infusion pump.

Monitoring Parameters Diabetes mellitus: Plasma glucose, electrolytes, Hb A_{1c}

Reference Range Refer to Insulin Regular on page 1025.

Pharmacotherapy Pearls Refer to Insulin Regular on page 1025.

Special Geriatric Considerations Intensive glucose control (Hb A_{1c} <6.5%) has been linked to increased all-cause and cardiovascular mortality, hypoglycemia requiring assistance, and weight gain in adult type 2 diabetes. How "tightly" to control a geriatric patient's blood glucose needs to be individualized. Such a decision should be based on several factors, including the patient's functional and cognitive status, how well he/she recognizes hypoglycemic or hyperglycemic symptoms, and how to respond to them and other disease states. An Hb A_{1c} <7.5% is an acceptable endpoint for a healthy older adult, while <8% is acceptable for frail elderly patients, those with a duration of illness >10 years, or those with comorbid conditions and requiring combination diabetes medications. Patients who are unable to accurately draw up their dose will need assistance, such as prefilled syringes. Initial doses may require considerations for renal function in the elderly with dosing adjusted subsequently based on blood glucose monitoring. For elderly patients with diabetes who are relatively healthy, attaining target goals for aspirin use, blood pressure, lipids, smoking cessation, and diet and exercise may be more important than normalized glycemic control.

Dosage Forms Excipient information presented when available (limited, particularly for generics); consult specific product labeling.

Injection, suspension:

NovoLOG® Mix 70/30: Insulin aspart protamine suspension 70% [intermediate acting] and insulin aspart solution 30% [rapid acting]: 100 units/mL (10 mL)

NovoLOG® Mix 70/30 FlexPen®: Insulin aspart protamine suspension 70% [intermediate acting] and insulin aspart solution 30% [rapid acting]: 100 units/mL (3 mL)

Insulin Detemir (IN soo lin DE te mir)

Related Information
Diabetes Mellitus Management, Adults *on page 2193*
Insulin Regular *on page 1025*

Medication Safety Issues
High alert medication:
The Institute for Safe Medication Practices (ISMP) includes this medication among its list of drugs which have a heightened risk of causing significant patient harm when used in error. ***Due to the number of insulin preparations, it is essential to identify/clarify the type of insulin to be used.***

Administration issues:
Insulin detemir is a clear solution, but it is NOT intended for I.V. or I.M. administration.

Other safety concerns:
Cross-contamination may occur if insulin pens are shared among multiple patients. Steps should be taken to prohibit sharing of insulin pens.

Brand Names: U.S. Levemir®; Levemir® FlexPen®
Brand Names: Canada Levemir®
Index Terms Detemir Insulin
Generic Availability (U.S.) No
Pharmacologic Category Insulin, Intermediate- to Long-Acting
Use Treatment of type 1 diabetes mellitus (insulin dependent, IDDM) and type 2 diabetes mellitus (noninsulin dependent, NIDDM) to improve glycemic control
Contraindications Hypersensitivity to insulin detemir or any component of the formulation
Warnings/Precautions Refer to Insulin Regular on page 1025.

The duration of action of insulin detemir is dose-dependent; consider this factor during dosage adjustment and titration. Insulin detemir, although a clear solution, is **NOT** intended for I.V. or I.M. administration

Adverse Reactions (Reflective of adult population; not specific for elderly) Primarily symptoms of hypoglycemia
Cardiovascular: Pallor, palpitation, tachycardia
Central nervous system: Fatigue, headache, hypothermia, loss of consciousness, mental confusion
Dermatologic: Redness, urticaria
Endocrine & metabolic: Hypoglycemia, hypokalemia
Gastrointestinal: Hunger, nausea, numbness of mouth
Local: Atrophy or hypertrophy of SubQ fat tissue; edema, itching, pain or warmth at injection site; stinging
Neuromuscular & skeletal: Muscle weakness, paresthesia, tremor
Ocular: Transient presbyopia or blurred vision
Miscellaneous: Anaphylaxis, diaphoresis, local and/or systemic hypersensitivity reactions

Drug Interactions
Metabolism/Transport Effects None known.
Avoid Concomitant Use There are no known interactions where it is recommended to avoid concomitant use.
Increased Effect/Toxicity
Insulin Detemir may increase the levels/effects of: Antidiabetic Agents (Thiazolidinedione); Hypoglycemic Agents; Quinolone Antibiotics

The levels/effects of Insulin Detemir may be increased by: Beta-Blockers; Edetate CALCIUM Disodium; Edetate Disodium; Herbs (Hypoglycemic Properties); MAO Inhibitors; Pegvisomant; Salicylates; Selective Serotonin Reuptake Inhibitors
Decreased Effect
The levels/effects of Insulin Detemir may be decreased by: Corticosteroids (Orally Inhaled); Corticosteroids (Systemic); Loop Diuretics; Luteinizing Hormone-Releasing Hormone Analogs; Somatropin; Thiazide Diuretics
Ethanol/Nutrition/Herb Interactions Refer to Insulin Regular on page 1025.
Stability Unopened vials, cartridges, and prefilled pens may be stored under refrigeration between 2°C and 8°C (36°F to 46°F) until the expiration date or at room temperature <30°C (<86°F) for 42 days; do not freeze; keep away from heat and sunlight. Once punctured (in use), vials may be stored under refrigeration or at room temperature <30°C (<86°F); use within 42 days. Cartridges and prefilled pens that have been punctured (in use) should be stored at temperatures <30°C (<86°F) and used within 42 days; do not freeze or refrigerate.
Mechanism of Action Insulin detemir is an intermediate- to long-acting insulin analog. Refer to Insulin Regular on page 1025.

Pharmacodynamics/Kinetics Note: Rate of absorption, onset, and duration of activity may be affected by site of injection, exercise, presence of lipodystrophy, local blood supply, and/or temperature.

Onset of action: 3-4 hours

Peak effect: 3-9 hours (Plank, 2005)

Duration: Dose dependent: 6-23 hours; **Note:** Duration is dose-dependent. At lower dosages (0.1-0.2 units/kg), mean duration is variable (5.7-12.1 hours). At 0.4 units/kg, the mean duration was 19.9 hours. At high dosages (≥0.8 units/kg) the duration is longer and less variable (mean of 22-23 hours) (Plank, 2005).

Distribution: V_d: 0.1 L/kg

Protein binding: >98% (albumin)

Bioavailability: 60%

Half-life elimination: 5-7 hours (dose-dependent)

Time to peak, plasma: 6-8 hours

Excretion: Urine

Dosage

Geriatric & Adult Note: When compared to insulin NPH, insulin detemir has a slower, more prolonged absorption; duration is dose-dependent. Insulin detemir may be given once or twice daily when used as the basal insulin component of therapy. Changing the basal insulin component from another insulin to insulin detemir can be done on a unit-to-unit basis.

Diabetes mellitus:

Type 1: SubQ: Refer to Insulin Regular on page 1025; the recommended starting dose should be approximately one-third of the total daily insulin requirement; a rapid acting or short acting insulin should also be used.

Type 2: SubQ: Refer to Insulin Regular on page 1025.

Initial basal insulin dose: Manufacturer recommendations: 10 units (**or** 0.1-0.2 units/kg) once daily in the evening; may also administer total daily dose in 2 divided doses

Renal Impairment Refer to Insulin Regular on page 1025.

Hepatic Impairment Refer to Insulin Regular on page 1025.

Administration Do **not** administer I.M or I.V.; for SubQ administration only: Do not use if solution is viscous or cloudy; use only if clear and colorless with no visible particles. Insulin detemir should be administered once or twice daily. When given once daily, administer with the evening meal or at bedtime. When given twice daily, administer the evening dose within the evening meal, at bedtime, or 12 hours following the morning dose. Cold injections should be avoided. SubQ administration is usually made into the thighs, arms, or abdomen; rotate injection sites. Do not dilute or mix insulin detemir with any other insulin formulation or solution; **not** recommended for use in external SubQ insulin infusion pump.

Monitoring Parameters Diabetes mellitus: Plasma glucose, electrolytes, Hb A_{1c}, lipid profile, renal function

Reference Range Refer to Insulin Regular on page 1025.

Pharmacotherapy Pearls Insulin detemir differs from human insulin by a single amino acid omission (threonine at B30) and the addition of a 14-carbon fatty acid chain attached at the B29 position. On injection, the fatty acid chain facilitates self-association between the molecules as well as binding to albumin. The delayed release of insulin from the injection site and albumin binding sites result in more prolonged action and limits variability in the amount of free insulin at steady-state. Insulin detemir has a duration of action which is dose-dependent. The FDA-approved product labeling identifies this product as a long-acting insulin analog; however, at lower dosages (<0.4 units/kg) published data regarding its duration of action is consistent with an intermediate insulin form (12-20 hours) (Plank, 2005). In clinical trials it has been compared primarily with NPH insulin and dosed in a similar manner. In some patients, or at higher dosages, it may have a duration of action up to 24 hours, which is consistent with a long-acting insulin (Le Floch, 2009; Plank, 2005; Porcellati, 2007).

Refer to Insulin Regular on page 1025

Special Geriatric Considerations Intensive glucose control (Hb A_{1c} <6.5%) has been linked to increased all-cause and cardiovascular mortality, hypoglycemia requiring assistance, and weight gain in adult type 2 diabetes. How "tightly" to control a geriatric patient's blood glucose needs to be individualized. Such a decision should be based on several factors, including the patient's functional and cognitive status, how well he/she recognizes hypoglycemic or hyperglycemic symptoms, and how to respond to them and other disease states. An Hb A_{1c} <7.5% is an acceptable endpoint for a healthy older adult, while <8% is acceptable for frail elderly patients, those with a duration of illness >10 years, or those with comorbid conditions and requiring combination diabetes medications. Patients who are unable to accurately draw up their dose will need assistance, such as prefilled syringes. Initial doses may require considerations for renal function in the elderly with dosing adjusted subsequently based on blood glucose monitoring. For elderly patients with diabetes who are relatively healthy, attaining target goals for aspirin use, blood pressure, lipids, smoking cessation, and diet and exercise may be more important than normalized glycemic control.

◄ **Dosage Forms** Excipient information presented when available (limited, particularly for generics); consult specific product labeling.
Injection, solution:
Levemir®: 100 units/mL (10 mL)
Levemir® FlexPen®: 100 units/mL (3 mL)

Insulin Glargine (IN soo lin GLAR jeen)

Related Information
Diabetes Mellitus Management, Adults *on page 2193*
Insulin Regular *on page 1025*
Medication Safety Issues
Sound-alike/look-alike issues:
Insulin glargine may be confused with insulin glulisine
Lantus® may be confused with latanoprost, Latuda®, Xalatan®
High alert medication:
The Institute for Safe Medication Practices (ISMP) includes this medication among its list of drugs which have a heightened risk of causing significant patient harm when used in error. *Due to the number of insulin preparations, it is essential to identify/clarify the type of insulin to be used.*
Administration issues:
Insulin glargine is a clear solution, but it is NOT intended for I.V. or I.M. administration.
Other safety concerns:
Cross-contamination may occur if insulin pens are shared among multiple patients. Steps should be taken to prohibit sharing of insulin pens.
International issues:
Lantus [U.S., Canada, and multiple international markets] may be confused with Lanvis brand name for thioguanine [Canada and multiple international markets]
Brand Names: U.S. Lantus®; Lantus® Solostar®
Brand Names: Canada Lantus®; Lantus® OptiSet®
Index Terms Glargine Insulin
Generic Availability (U.S.) No
Pharmacologic Category Insulin, Long-Acting
Use Treatment of type 1 diabetes mellitus (insulin dependent, IDDM) and type 2 diabetes mellitus (noninsulin dependent, NIDDM) to improve glycemic control
Contraindications Hypersensitivity to insulin glargine or any component of the formulation
Warnings/Precautions Refer to Insulin Regular on page 1025. Insulin glargine is a clear solution, but it is **NOT** intended for I.V. or I.M. administration.
Adverse Reactions (Reflective of adult population; not specific for elderly) Refer to Insulin Regular on page 1025.
Drug Interactions
Metabolism/Transport Effects None known.
Avoid Concomitant Use There are no known interactions where it is recommended to avoid concomitant use.
Increased Effect/Toxicity
Insulin Glargine may increase the levels/effects of: Antidiabetic Agents (Thiazolidinedione); Hypoglycemic Agents; Quinolone Antibiotics

The levels/effects of Insulin Glargine may be increased by: Beta-Blockers; Edetate CALCIUM Disodium; Edetate Disodium; Herbs (Hypoglycemic Properties); MAO Inhibitors; Pegvisomant; Salicylates; Selective Serotonin Reuptake Inhibitors
Decreased Effect
The levels/effects of Insulin Glargine may be decreased by: Corticosteroids (Orally Inhaled); Corticosteroids (Systemic); Loop Diuretics; Luteinizing Hormone-Releasing Hormone Analogs; Somatropin; Thiazide Diuretics
Ethanol/Nutrition/Herb Interactions Refer to Insulin Regular on page 1025.
Stability Unopened vials, cartridges, and prefilled pens may be stored under refrigeration between 2°C and 8°C (36°F to 46°F) until the expiration date or at room temperature <30°C (<86°F) for 28 days; do not freeze; keep away from heat and sunlight. Once punctured (in use), vials may be stored under refrigeration or at room temperature <30°C (<86°F); use within 28 days. Cartridges used in the OptiClik® system and prefilled pens (SoloStar®) that have been punctured (in use) should be stored at temperatures <30°C (<86°F) and used within 28 days; do not freeze or refrigerate.
Mechanism of Action Insulin glargine is a long-acting insulin analog.
Refer to Insulin Regular on page 1025.

Pharmacodynamics/Kinetics Note: Rate of absorption, onset, and duration of activity may be affected by site of injection, exercise, presence of lipodystrophy, local blood supply, and/or temperature.

Onset of action: 3-4 hours

Peak effect: No pronounced peak

Duration: Generally 24 hours or longer; reported range: 10.8 to >24 hours (up to 32 hours documented in some studies)

Absorption: Slow; upon injection into the subcutaneous tissue, microprecipitates form which allow small amounts of insulin glargine to release over time

Metabolism: Partially metabolized in the skin to form two active metabolites

Time to peak, plasma: No pronounced peak

Excretion: Urine

Dosage

Geriatric & Adult Note: Insulin glargine is approximately equipotent to human insulin, but has a slower onset, no pronounced peak, and a longer duration of activity. Changing the basal insulin component from another insulin to insulin glargine can be done on a unit-to-unit basis.

Diabetes mellitus, type 1 and type 2: SubQ: Refer to Insulin Regular on page 1025.

Renal Impairment Refer to Insulin Regular on page 1025.

Hepatic Impairment Refer to Insulin Regular on page 1025.

Administration SubQ administration: Do not use if solution is viscous or cloudy; use only if clear and colorless with no visible particles. Insulin glargine should be administered once daily, at any time of day; however, administer at the same time each day. Cold injections should be avoided. SubQ administration is usually made into the thighs, arms, buttocks, or abdomen; rotate injection sites. Do not dilute or mix insulin glargine with any other insulin formulation or solution.

Monitoring Parameters Diabetes mellitus: Plasma glucose, electrolytes, Hb A_{1c}

Reference Range Refer to Insulin Regular on page 1025.

Pharmacotherapy Pearls The duration of action of insulin glargine is generally 24 hours or longer with a relatively flat action profile throughout this interval. Many pharmacokinetic and pharmacodynamic studies were terminated at 24 hours despite the fact that insulin glargine continued to exhibit hypoglycemic activity beyond 24 hours; therefore, it is difficult to determine the absolute duration of action.

Clinicians should be aware that, in rare cases, patients may exhibit hypoglycemic activity beyond 24 hours and that accumulation of insulin glargine is possible. Adequate monitoring and subsequent dosage adjustments should be made in patients who are requiring less insulin to maintain euglycemia after several days of therapy.

On the other hand, insulin glargine has a reported duration of action that ranges from 10.8 to >24 hours. On rare occasions, patients may require twice-daily injections of insulin glargine to deliver adequate basal insulin coverage over 24 hours. Some clinicians may also switch to twice-daily dosing in patients who require >100 units of insulin glargine per day to allow for complete absorption. Dosing insulin glargine 3 times daily is not recommended.

Also, refer to Insulin Regular on page 1025.

Special Geriatric Considerations Intensive glucose control (Hb A_{1c} <6.5%) has been linked to increased all-cause and cardiovascular mortality, hypoglycemia requiring assistance, and weight gain in adult type 2 diabetes. How "tightly" to control a geriatric patient's blood glucose needs to be individualized. Such a decision should be based on several factors, including the patient's functional and cognitive status, how well he/she recognizes hypoglycemic or hyperglycemic symptoms, and how to respond to them and other disease states. An Hb A_{1c} <7.5% is an acceptable endpoint for a healthy older adult, while <8% is acceptable for frail elderly patients, those with a duration of illness >10 years, or those with comorbid conditions and requiring combination diabetes medications. Patients who are unable to accurately draw up their dose will need assistance, such as prefilled syringes. Initial doses may require considerations for renal function in the elderly with dosing adjusted subsequently based on blood glucose monitoring. For elderly patients with diabetes who are relatively healthy, attaining target goals for aspirin use, blood pressure, lipids, smoking cessation, and diet and exercise may be more important than normalized glycemic control.

Dosage Forms Excipient information presented when available (limited, particularly for generics); consult specific product labeling.

Injection, solution:

Lantus®: 100 units/mL (3 mL) [cartridge]

Lantus®: 100 units/mL (10 mL) [vial]

Lantus® Solostar®: 100 units/mL (3 mL) [prefilled pen]

Insulin Glulisine (IN soo lin gloo LIS een)

Related Information
Diabetes Mellitus Management, Adults *on page 2193*
Insulin Regular *on page 1025*

Medication Safety Issues
Sound-alike/look-alike issues:
Insulin glulisine may be confused with insulin glargine

High alert medication:
The Institute for Safe Medication Practices (ISMP) includes this medication among its list of drugs which have a heightened risk of causing significant patient harm when used in error. *Due to the number of insulin preparations, it is essential to identify/clarify the type of insulin to be used.*

Other safety concerns:
Cross-contamination may occur if insulin pens are shared among multiple patients. Steps should be taken to prohibit sharing of insulin pens.

Brand Names: U.S. Apidra®; Apidra® SoloStar®
Brand Names: Canada Apidra®
Index Terms Glulisine Insulin
Generic Availability (U.S.) No
Pharmacologic Category Insulin, Rapid-Acting

Use Treatment of type 1 diabetes mellitus (insulin dependent, IDDM) and type 2 diabetes mellitus (noninsulin dependent, NIDDM) to improve glycemic control

Contraindications Hypersensitivity to insulin glulisine or any component of the formulation; during episodes of hypoglycemia

Warnings/Precautions Refer to Insulin Regular on page 1025.

Due to the short duration of action of insulin glulisine, a longer acting insulin or CSII via an external insulin pump is needed to maintain adequate glucose control in patients with type 1 diabetes mellitus. In both type 1 and type 2 diabetes, preprandial administration of insulin glulisine should be immediately followed by a meal within 15 minutes. May also be administered via CSII; do not dilute or mix with other insulin formulations when using an external insulin pump. Rule out pump failure if unexplained hyperglycemia or ketosis occurs; temporary SubQ insulin administration may be required until the problem is identified and corrected. Insulin glulisine may also be administered I.V. in selected clinical situations to control hyperglycemia; close monitoring of blood glucose and serum potassium as well as medical supervision is required.

Adverse Reactions (Reflective of adult population; not specific for elderly) Refer to Insulin Regular on page 1025.

Drug Interactions
Metabolism/Transport Effects None known.

Avoid Concomitant Use There are no known interactions where it is recommended to avoid concomitant use.

Increased Effect/Toxicity
Insulin Glulisine may increase the levels/effects of: Antidiabetic Agents (Thiazolidinedione); Hypoglycemic Agents; Quinolone Antibiotics

The levels/effects of Insulin Glulisine may be increased by: Beta-Blockers; Edetate CALCIUM Disodium; Edetate Disodium; Herbs (Hypoglycemic Properties); MAO Inhibitors; Pegvisomant; Salicylates; Selective Serotonin Reuptake Inhibitors

Decreased Effect
The levels/effects of Insulin Glulisine may be decreased by: Corticosteroids (Orally Inhaled); Corticosteroids (Systemic); Loop Diuretics; Luteinizing Hormone-Releasing Hormone Analogs; Somatropin; Thiazide Diuretics

Ethanol/Nutrition/Herb Interactions Refer to Insulin Regular on page 1025.

Stability Unopened vials, cartridges, and prefilled pens may be stored under refrigeration between 2°C and 8°C (36°F to 46°F) until the expiration date or at room temperature for 28 days; do not freeze; keep away from heat and sunlight. Once punctured (in use), vials may be stored under refrigeration or at room temperature ≤25°C (≤77°F); use within 28 days. Cartridges and prefilled pens that have been punctured (in use) should be stored at temperatures ≤25°C (≤77°F) and used within 28 days; do not freeze or refrigerate. When used for CSII, insulin glulisine contained within an external insulin pump reservoir should be replaced every 48 hours; discard if exposed to temperatures >37°C (>98.6°F).

For I.V. infusion: May be diluted in NS to concentrations of 0.05-1 unit/mL. Stable for 48 hours at room temperature.

Mechanism of Action Insulin glulisine is a rapid-acting insulin analog.
Refer to Insulin Regular on page 1025.

Pharmacodynamics/Kinetics Note: Rate of absorption, onset, and duration of activity may be affected by site of injection, exercise, presence of lipodystrophy, local blood supply, and/or temperature.

Onset of action: 0.2-0.5 hours
Peak effect: 1.6-2.8 hours
Duration: 3-4 hours
Distribution: I.V.: 13 L
Bioavailability: SubQ: ~70%
Half-life elimination:
I.V.: 13 minutes
SubQ: 42 minutes
Time to peak, plasma: 0.6-2 hours
Excretion: Urine

Dosage

Geriatric & Adult Note: Insulin glulisine is equipotent to insulin regular, but has a more rapid onset and shorter duration of activity.

Diabetes mellitus, type 1 and type 2: SubQ: Refer to Insulin Regular on page 1025.

Glycemic control in selected clinical situations and under appropriate medical supervision: I.V.: Refer to Insulin Regular on page 1025.

Renal Impairment Refer to Insulin Regular on page 1025.

Hepatic Impairment Refer to Insulin Regular on page 1025.

Administration

SubQ administration: Do not use if solution is viscous or cloudy; use only if clear and colorless. Insulin glulisine should be administered within 15 minutes before or within 20 minutes after starting a meal. Cold injections should be avoided. SubQ administration is usually made into the thighs, arms, buttocks, or abdomen; rotate injection sites. When mixing insulin glulisine with other preparations of insulin (eg, insulin NPH), insulin glulisine should be drawn into syringe first. Do not mix other insulin formulations with insulin glulisine contained in a cartridge or prefilled pen.

CSII administration: Do not use if solution is viscous or cloudy; use only if clear and colorless. Patients should be trained in the proper use of their external insulin pump and in intensive insulin therapy. Infusion sets, reservoirs, and infusion set insertion sites should be changed every 48 hours; rotate infusion sites. Do not dilute or mix other insulin formulations with insulin glulisine that is to be used in an external insulin pump.

I.V. administration: Do not use if solution is viscous or cloudy; use only if clear and colorless. May be administered I.V. with close monitoring of blood glucose and serum potassium; appropriate medical supervision is required. **Do not administer insulin mixtures intravenously.**

I.V. infusions: To minimize adsorption to I.V. solution bag: **Note:** Refer to institution-specific protocols where appropriate.

If new tubing is **not** *needed:* Wait a minimum of 30 minutes between the preparation of the solution and the initiation of the infusion.

If new tubing is needed: After receiving the insulin drip solution, the administration set should be attached to the I.V. container and the entire line should be flushed with a priming infusion of 20-50 mL of the insulin solution (Goldberg, 2006; Hirsch, 2006). Wait 30 minutes, and then flush the line again with the insulin solution prior to initiating the infusion.

Because of adsorption, the actual amount of insulin being administered via I.V. infusion could be substantially less than the apparent amount. Therefore, adjustment of the I.V. infusion rate should be based on effect and not solely on the apparent insulin dose. The apparent dose may be used as a starting point for determining the subsequent SubQ dosing regimen (Moghissi, 2009); however, the transition to SubQ administration requires continuous medical supervision, frequent monitoring of blood glucose, and careful adjustment of therapy. In addition, SubQ insulin should be given 1-4 hours prior to the discontinuation of I.V. insulin to prevent hyperglycemia (Moghissi, 2009).

Monitoring Parameters

Diabetes mellitus: Plasma glucose, electrolytes, Hb A_{1c}
I.V. administration: Close monitoring of blood glucose and serum potassium

Reference Range Refer to Insulin Regular on page 1025.

Pharmacotherapy Pearls Refer to Insulin Regular on page 1025.

Special Geriatric Considerations Intensive glucose control (Hb A_{1c} <6.5%) has been linked to increased all-cause and cardiovascular mortality, hypoglycemia requiring assistance, and weight gain in adult type 2 diabetes. How "tightly" to control a geriatric patient's blood glucose needs to be individualized. Such a decision should be based on several factors, including the patient's functional and cognitive status, how well he/she recognizes hypoglycemic or hyperglycemic symptoms, and how to respond to them and other disease states. An

◀ Hb A_{1c} <7.5% is an acceptable endpoint for a healthy older adult, while <8% is acceptable for frail elderly patients, those with a duration of illness >10 years, or those with comorbid conditions and requiring combination diabetes medications. Patients who are unable to accurately draw up their dose will need assistance, such as prefilled syringes. Initial doses may require considerations for renal function in the elderly with dosing adjusted subsequently based on blood glucose monitoring. For elderly patients with diabetes who are relatively healthy, attaining target goals for aspirin use, blood pressure, lipids, smoking cessation, and diet and exercise may be more important than normalized glycemic control.

Dosage Forms Excipient information presented when available (limited, particularly for generics); consult specific product labeling.

Injection, solution:

Apidra®: 100 units/mL (3 mL) [cartridge]

Apidra®: 100 units/mL (10 mL) [vial]

Apidra® SoloStar®: 100 units/mL (3 mL) [prefilled pen]

Insulin Lispro (IN soo lin LYE sproe)

Related Information

Diabetes Mellitus Management, Adults on page 2193

Insulin Regular on page 1025

Medication Safety Issues

Sound-alike/look-alike issues:

HumaLOG® may be confused with HumaLOG® Mix 50/50, Humira®, HumuLIN® N, HumuLIN® R, NovoLOG®

High alert medication:

The Institute for Safe Medication Practices (ISMP) includes this medication among its list of drugs which have a heightened risk of causing significant patient harm when used in error. *Due to the number of insulin preparations, it is essential to identify/clarify the type of insulin to be used.*

Other safety concerns:

Cross-contamination may occur if insulin pens are shared among multiple patients. Steps should be taken to prohibit sharing of insulin pens.

Brand Names: U.S. HumaLOG®; HumaLOG® KwikPen™

Brand Names: Canada Humalog®

Index Terms Lispro Insulin

Generic Availability (U.S.) No

Pharmacologic Category Insulin, Rapid-Acting

Use Treatment of type 1 diabetes mellitus (insulin dependent, IDDM) and type 2 diabetes mellitus (noninsulin dependent, NIDDM) to improve glycemic control

Unlabeled Use Mild-to-moderate diabetic ketoacidosis (DKA); mild-to-moderate hyperosmolar hyperglycemic state (HHS)

Contraindications Hypersensitivity to insulin lispro or any component of the formulation; during episodes of hypoglycemia

Warnings/Precautions Refer to Insulin Regular on page 1025.

Due to the short duration of action of insulin lispro, a longer acting insulin or CSII via an external insulin pump is needed to maintain adequate glucose control in patients with type 1 diabetes mellitus. In both type 1 and type 2 diabetes, preprandial administration of insulin lispro should be immediately followed by a meal within 15 minutes. May also be administered via CSII; do not dilute or mix with other insulin formulations when using an external insulin pump. Rule out pump failure if unexplained hyperglycemia or ketosis occurs; temporary SubQ insulin administration may be required until the problem is identified and corrected. Insulin lispro may also be administered I.V. in selected clinical situations to control hyperglycemia; close monitoring of blood glucose and serum potassium as well as medical supervision is required.

Adverse Reactions (Reflective of adult population; not specific for elderly) Primarily symptoms of hypoglycemia

Cardiovascular: Pallor, palpitation, tachycardia

Central nervous system: Fatigue, headache, hypothermia, loss of consciousness, mental confusion

Dermatologic: Redness, urticaria

Endocrine & metabolic: Hypoglycemia, hypokalemia

Gastrointestinal: Hunger, nausea, numbness of mouth

Local: Atrophy or hypertrophy of SubQ fat tissue; edema, itching, pain or warmth at injection site; stinging

Neuromuscular & skeletal: Muscle weakness, paresthesia, tremor

Ocular: Transient presbyopia or blurred vision

Miscellaneous: Anaphylaxis, diaphoresis, local and/or systemic hypersensitivity reactions

Drug Interactions

Metabolism/Transport Effects None known.

Avoid Concomitant Use There are no known interactions where it is recommended to avoid concomitant use.

Increased Effect/Toxicity

Insulin Lispro may increase the levels/effects of: Antidiabetic Agents (Thiazolidinedione); Hypoglycemic Agents; Quinolone Antibiotics

The levels/effects of Insulin Lispro may be increased by: Beta-Blockers; Edetate CALCIUM Disodium; Edetate Disodium; Herbs (Hypoglycemic Properties); MAO Inhibitors; Pegvisomant; Salicylates; Selective Serotonin Reuptake Inhibitors

Decreased Effect

The levels/effects of Insulin Lispro may be decreased by: Corticosteroids (Orally Inhaled); Corticosteroids (Systemic); Loop Diuretics; Luteinizing Hormone-Releasing Hormone Analogs; Somatropin; Thiazide Diuretics

Ethanol/Nutrition/Herb Interactions Refer to Insulin Regular on page 1025.

Stability Unopened vials, cartridges, and prefilled pens may be stored under refrigeration between 2°C and 8°C (36°F to 46°F) until the expiration date or at room temperature <30°C (<86°F) for 28 days; do not freeze; keep away from heat and sunlight. Once punctured (in use), vials may be stored under refrigeration or at room temperature <30°C (<86°F); use within 28 days. Cartridges and prefilled pens that have been punctured (in use) should be stored at temperatures <30°C (<86°F) and used within 28 days; do not freeze or refrigerate. When used for CSII, insulin lispro contained within an external insulin pump reservoir should be changed every 7 days and insulin lispro contained within a 3 mL cartridge should be discarded after 7 days; discard if exposed to temperatures >37°C (>98.6°F).

For SubQ administration: *Humalog® vials:* May be diluted with the universal diluent, Sterile Diluent for Humalog®, Humulin® N, Humulin® R, Humulin® 70/30, and Humulin® R U-500, to a concentration of 10 units/mL (U-10) or 50 units/mL (U-50). According to the manufacturer, diluted insulin should be stored at 30°C (86°F) and used within 14 days or 5°C (41°F) and used within 28 days; do not dilute insulin contained in a cartridge, prefilled pen, or external insulin pump.

For I.V. infusion (unlabeled use): May be diluted in NS or D_5W to concentrations of 0.025-2 units/mL. Stable for 48 hours at room temperature.

Mechanism of Action Insulin lispro is a rapid-acting insulin analog. Refer to Insulin Regular on page 1025.

Pharmacodynamics/Kinetics Note: Rate of absorption, onset, and duration of activity may be affected by site of injection, exercise, presence of lipodystrophy, local blood supply, and/or temperature.

Onset of action: 0.25-0.5 hours

Peak effect: 0.5-2.5 hours

Duration: ≤5 hours

Distribution: V_d: 0.26-0.36 L/kg

Bioavailability: 55% to 77%

Half-life elimination:

I.V.: ~0.5-1 hour (dose-dependent)

SubQ: 1 hour

Time to peak, plasma: 0.5-1.5 hours

Excretion: Urine

Dosage

Geriatric & Adult Note: When compared to insulin regular, insulin lispro has a more rapid onset and shorter duration of activity.

Diabetes mellitus, type 1 and type 2: SubQ: Refer to Insulin Regular on page 1025.

Diabetic ketoacidosis (DKA), mild-to-moderate (unlabeled use): SubQ: Refer to Insulin Regular on page 1025.

Gestational diabetes mellitus (unlabeled use): Refer to Insulin Regular on page 1025.

Glycemic control in selected clinical situations and under appropriate medical supervision (unlabeled use): I.V.: Refer to Insulin Regular on page 1025.

Hyperosmolar hyperglycemic state (HHS), mild-to-moderate (unlabeled use): SubQ: Refer to Insulin Regular on page 1025.

Renal Impairment Refer to Insulin Regular on page 1025.

Hepatic Impairment Refer to Insulin Regular on page 1025.

Administration

SubQ administration: Do not use if solution is viscous or cloudy; use only if clear and colorless. Insulin lispro should be administered within 15 minutes before or immediately after a meal. Cold injections should be avoided. SubQ administration is usually made into the thighs, arms, buttocks, or abdomen; rotate injection sites. When mixing insulin lispro with other preparations of insulin (eg, insulin NPH), insulin lispro should be drawn into syringe first. Do not dilute or mix other insulin formulations with insulin lispro contained in a cartridge or prefilled pen.

CSII administration: Do not use if solution is viscous or cloudy; use only if clear and colorless. Patients should be trained in the proper use of their external insulin pump and in intensive insulin therapy. Infusion sets and infusion set insertion sites should be changed every 3 days; rotate infusion sites. Insulin in reservoir should be changed every 7 days. Do not dilute or mix other insulin formulations with insulin lispro contained in an external insulin pump.

I.V. administration (unlabeled use): Do not use if solution is viscous or cloudy; use only if clear and colorless. May be administered I.V. with close monitoring of blood glucose and serum potassium; appropriate medical supervision is required. **Do not administer insulin mixtures intravenously.**

I.V. infusions: To minimize adsorption to I.V. solution bag: **Note:** Refer to institution-specific protocols where appropriate.

*If new tubing is **not** needed:* Wait a minimum of 30 minutes between the preparation of the solution and the initiation of the infusion. Wait a minimum of 30 minutes between the preparation of the solution and the initiation of the infusion.

If new tubing is needed: After receiving the insulin drip solution, the administration set should be attached to the I.V. container and the entire line should be flushed with a priming infusion of 20-50 mL of the insulin solution (Goldberg, 2006; Hirsch, 2006). Wait 30 minutes, and then flush the line again with the insulin solution prior to initiating the infusion.

Because of adsorption, the actual amount of insulin being administered via I.V. infusion could be substantially less than the apparent amount. Therefore, adjustment of the I.V. infusion rate should be based on effect and not solely on the apparent insulin dose. The apparent dose may be used as a starting point for determining the subsequent SubQ dosing regimen (Moghissi, 2009); however, the transition to SubQ administration requires continuous medical supervision, frequent monitoring of blood glucose, and careful adjustment of therapy. In addition, SubQ insulin should be given 1-4 hours prior to the discontinuation of I.V. insulin to prevent hyperglycemia (Moghissi, 2009).

Monitoring Parameters

Diabetes mellitus: Plasma glucose, electrolytes, Hb A_{1c}

I.V. administration (unlabeled use): Close monitoring of blood glucose and serum potassium

Reference Range Refer to Insulin Regular on page 1025.

Pharmacotherapy Pearls Refer to Insulin Regular on page 1025.

Special Geriatric Considerations Intensive glucose control (Hb A_{1c} <6.5%) has been linked to increased all-cause and cardiovascular mortality, hypoglycemia requiring assistance, and weight gain in adult type 2 diabetes. How "tightly" to control a geriatric patient's blood glucose needs to be individualized. Such a decision should be based on several factors, including the patient's functional and cognitive status, how well he/she recognizes hypoglycemic or hyperglycemic symptoms, and how to respond to them and other disease states. An Hb A_{1c} <7.5% is an acceptable endpoint for a healthy older adult, while <8% is acceptable for frail elderly patients, those with a duration of illness >10 years, or those with comorbid conditions and requiring combination diabetes medications. Patients who are unable to accurately draw up their dose will need assistance, such as prefilled syringes. Initial doses may require considerations for renal function in the elderly with dosing adjusted subsequently based on blood glucose monitoring. For elderly patients with diabetes who are relatively healthy, attaining target goals for aspirin use, blood pressure, lipids, smoking cessation, and diet and exercise may be more important than normalized glycemic control.

Dosage Forms Excipient information presented when available (limited, particularly for generics); consult specific product labeling.

Injection, solution:

HumaLOG®: 100 units/mL (3 mL) [cartridge]

HumaLOG®: 100 units/mL (3 mL, 10 mL) [vial]

HumaLOG® KwikPen™: 100 units/mL (3 mL)

♦ **Insulin Lispro and Insulin Lispro Protamine** *see* Insulin Lispro Protamine and Insulin Lispro *on page 1019*

Insulin Lispro Protamine and Insulin Lispro
(IN soo lin LYE sproe PROE ta meen & IN soo lin LYE sproe)

Related Information
- Diabetes Mellitus Management, Adults *on page 2193*
- Insulin Regular *on page 1025*

Medication Safety Issues
Sound-alike/look-alike issues:
HumaLOG® Mix 50/50™ may be confused with HumaLOG®
HumaLOG® Mix 75/25™ may be confused with HumuLIN® 70/30, NovoLIN® 70/30, and NovoLOG® Mix 70/30

High alert medication:
The Institute for Safe Medication Practices (ISMP) includes this medication among its list of drugs which have a heightened risk of causing significant patient harm when used in error. *Due to the number of insulin preparations, it is essential to identify/clarify the type of insulin to be used.*

Other safety concerns:
Cross-contamination may occur if insulin pens are shared among multiple patients. Steps should be taken to prohibit sharing of insulin pens.

Brand Names: U.S. HumaLOG® Mix 50/50™; HumaLOG® Mix 50/50™ KwikPen™; HumaLOG® Mix 75/25™; HumaLOG® Mix 75/25™ KwikPen™

Brand Names: Canada Humalog® Mix 25

Index Terms Insulin Lispro and Insulin Lispro Protamine

Generic Availability (U.S.) No

Pharmacologic Category Insulin, Combination

Use Treatment of type 1 diabetes mellitus (insulin dependent, IDDM) and type 2 diabetes mellitus (noninsulin dependent, NIDDM) to improve glycemic control

Contraindications Hypersensitivity to any component of the formulation; during episodes of hypoglycemia

Warnings/Precautions Refer to Insulin Regular on page 1025. Insulin lispro protamine and insulin lispro premixed combination products are **NOT** intended for I.V. or I.M. administration.

Adverse Reactions (Reflective of adult population; not specific for elderly) Refer to Insulin Regular on page 1025.

Drug Interactions
Metabolism/Transport Effects None known.
Avoid Concomitant Use There are no known interactions where it is recommended to avoid concomitant use.
Increased Effect/Toxicity
Insulin Lispro Protamine and Insulin Lispro may increase the levels/effects of: Antidiabetic Agents (Thiazolidinedione); Hypoglycemic Agents; Quinolone Antibiotics

The levels/effects of Insulin Lispro Protamine and Insulin Lispro may be increased by: Beta-Blockers; Edetate CALCIUM Disodium; Edetate Disodium; Herbs (Hypoglycemic Properties); MAO Inhibitors; Pegvisomant; Salicylates; Selective Serotonin Reuptake Inhibitors

Decreased Effect
The levels/effects of Insulin Lispro Protamine and Insulin Lispro may be decreased by: Corticosteroids (Orally Inhaled); Corticosteroids (Systemic); Loop Diuretics; Luteinizing Hormone-Releasing Hormone Analogs; Somatropin; Thiazide Diuretics

Ethanol/Nutrition/Herb Interactions Refer to Insulin Regular on page 1025.

Stability Unopened vials and prefilled pens may be stored under refrigeration between 2°C and 8°C (36°F to 46°F) until the expiration date or at room temperature <30°C (<86°F) for 10 days (prefilled pens) or 28 days (vials); do not freeze; keep away from heat and sunlight. Once punctured (in use), vials may be stored under refrigeration or at room temperature <30°C (<86°F); use within 28 days. Prefilled pens that have been punctured (in use) should be stored at room temperature <30°C (<86°F) and used within 10 days; do not freeze or refrigerate.

Mechanism of Action Insulin lispro protamine and insulin lispro is an intermediate-acting combination product with a more rapid onset and similar duration of action as compared to that of insulin NPH and insulin regular combination products. Refer to Insulin Regular on page 1025.

Pharmacodynamics/Kinetics Note: Rate of absorption, onset, and duration of activity may be affected by site of injection, exercise, presence of lipodystrophy, local blood supply, and/or temperature.
Onset of action: 0.25-0.5 hours
Peak effect:
Humalog® Mix 50/50™: 0.8-4.8 hours
Humalog® Mix 75/25™: 1-6.5 hours

Duration: 14-24 hours
Time to peak, plasma:
Humalog® Mix 50/50™: 0.75-13.5 hours
Humalog® Mix 75/25™: 0.5-4 hours
Excretion: Urine

Dosage

Geriatric & Adult Note: Insulin lispro protamine and insulin lispro combination products are approximately equipotent to insulin NPH and insulin regular combination products but with a more rapid onset and similar duration of activity.

Diabetes mellitus, type 1 and type 2: SubQ: Refer to Insulin Regular on page 1025

Renal Impairment Refer to Insulin Regular on page 1025.

Hepatic Impairment Refer to Insulin Regular on page 1025.

Administration SubQ administration: In order to properly resuspend the insulin, vials should be carefully shaken or rolled several times and prefilled pens should be rolled between the palms ten times and inverted 180° ten times. Properly resuspended insulin should look uniformly cloudy or milky; do not use if any white insulin substance remains at the bottom of the container, if any clumps are present, if the insulin remains clear after adequate mixing, or if white particles are stuck to the bottom or wall of the container. Cold injections should be avoided. Insulin lispro protamine and insulin lispro combination products should be administered within 15 minutes before a meal; typically given once- or twice daily. SubQ administration is usually made into the thighs, arms, buttocks, or abdomen; rotate injection sites. Do not dilute or mix with any other insulin formulation or solution; **not** recommended for use in external SubQ insulin infusion pump.

Monitoring Parameters Diabetes mellitus: Plasma glucose, electrolytes, Hb A_{1c}

Reference Range Refer to Insulin Regular on page 1025.

Pharmacotherapy Pearls Refer to Insulin Regular on page 1025.

Special Geriatric Considerations Intensive glucose control (Hb A_{1c} <6.5%) has been linked to increased all-cause and cardiovascular mortality, hypoglycemia requiring assistance, and weight gain in adult type 2 diabetes. How "tightly" to control a geriatric patient's blood glucose needs to be individualized. Such a decision should be based on several factors, including the patient's functional and cognitive status, how well he/she recognizes hypoglycemic or hyperglycemic symptoms, and how to respond to them and other disease states. An Hb A_{1c} <7.5% is an acceptable endpoint for a healthy older adult, while <8% is acceptable for frail elderly patients, those with a duration of illness >10 years, or those with comorbid conditions and requiring combination diabetes medications. Patients who are unable to accurately draw up their dose will need assistance, such as prefilled syringes. Initial doses may require considerations for renal function in the elderly with dosing adjusted subsequently based on blood glucose monitoring. For elderly patients with diabetes who are relatively healthy, attaining target goals for aspirin use, blood pressure, lipids, smoking cessation, and diet and exercise may be more important than normalized glycemic control.

Dosage Forms Excipient information presented when available (limited, particularly for generics); consult specific product labeling.
Injection, suspension:
HumaLOG® Mix 50/50™: Insulin lispro protamine suspension 50% [intermediate acting] and insulin lispro solution 50% [rapid acting]: 100 units/mL (10 mL)
HumaLOG® Mix 50/50™ KwikPen™: Insulin lispro protamine suspension 50% [intermediate acting] and insulin lispro solution 50% [rapid acting]: 100 units/mL (3 mL)
HumaLOG® Mix 75/25™: Insulin lispro protamine suspension 75% [intermediate acting] and insulin lispro solution 25% [rapid acting]: 100 units/mL (10 mL)
HumaLOG® Mix 75/25™ KwikPen™: Insulin lispro protamine suspension 75% [intermediate acting] and insulin lispro solution 25% [rapid acting]: 100 units/mL (3 mL)

Insulin NPH (IN soo lin N P H)

Related Information
Diabetes Mellitus Management, Adults *on page* 2193
Insulin Regular *on page* 1025

Medication Safety Issues
Sound-alike/look-alike issues:
HumuLIN® N may be confused with HumuLIN® R, HumaLOG®, Humira®
NovoLIN® N may be confused with NovoLIN® R, NovoLOG®

High alert medication:
The Institute for Safe Medication Practices (ISMP) includes this medication among its list of drugs which have a heightened risk of causing significant patient harm when used in error.

Due to the number of insulin preparations, it is essential to identify/clarify the type of insulin to be used.

Other safety concerns:

Cross-contamination may occur if insulin pens are shared among multiple patients. Steps should be taken to prohibit sharing of insulin pens.

Brand Names: U.S. HumuLIN® N; NovoLIN® N

Brand Names: Canada Humulin® N; Novolin® ge NPH

Index Terms Isophane Insulin; NPH Insulin

Generic Availability (U.S.) No

Pharmacologic Category Insulin, Intermediate-Acting

Use Treatment of type 1 diabetes mellitus (insulin dependent, IDDM) and type 2 diabetes mellitus (noninsulin dependent, NIDDM) to improve glycemic control

Unlabeled Use No geriatric-specific information.

Contraindications Hypersensitivity to insulin NPH or any component of the formulation

Warnings/Precautions Refer to Insulin Regular on page 1025. Insulin NPH is **NOT** intended for I.V. or I.M. administration.

Adverse Reactions (Reflective of adult population; not specific for elderly) Primarily symptoms of hypoglycemia

Cardiovascular: Pallor, palpitation, tachycardia

Central nervous system: Fatigue, headache, hypothermia, loss of consciousness, mental confusion

Dermatologic: Redness, urticaria

Endocrine & metabolic: Hypoglycemia, hypokalemia

Gastrointestinal: Hunger, nausea, numbness of mouth

Local: Atrophy or hypertrophy of SubQ fat tissue; edema, itching, pain or warmth at injection site; stinging

Neuromuscular & skeletal: Muscle weakness, paresthesia, tremor

Ocular: Transient presbyopia or blurred vision

Miscellaneous: Anaphylaxis, diaphoresis, local and/or systemic hypersensitivity reactions

Drug Interactions

Metabolism/Transport Effects None known.

Avoid Concomitant Use There are no known interactions where it is recommended to avoid concomitant use.

Increased Effect/Toxicity

Insulin NPH may increase the levels/effects of: Antidiabetic Agents (Thiazolidinedione); Hypoglycemic Agents; Quinolone Antibiotics

The levels/effects of Insulin NPH may be increased by: Beta-Blockers; Edetate CALCIUM Disodium; Edetate Disodium; Herbs (Hypoglycemic Properties); MAO Inhibitors; Pegvisomant; Salicylates; Selective Serotonin Reuptake Inhibitors

Decreased Effect

The levels/effects of Insulin NPH may be decreased by: Corticosteroids (Orally Inhaled); Corticosteroids (Systemic); Loop Diuretics; Luteinizing Hormone-Releasing Hormone Analogs; Somatropin; Thiazide Diuretics

Ethanol/Nutrition/Herb Interactions Refer to Insulin Regular on page 1025.

Stability

Humulin® N vials: Store unopened vials in refrigerator between 2°C and 8°C (36°F to 46°F; do not freeze; keep away from heat and sunlight. Once punctured (in use), vials may be stored for up to 31 days in the refrigerator between 2°C and 8°C (36°F to 46°F) or at room temperature ≤30°C (≤86°F)

Humulin® N pens and cartridges: Store unopened pens and unused cartridges in the refrigerator between 2°C and 8°C (36°F to 46°F); do not freeze; keep away from heat and sunlight. Once punctured (in use), cartridge/pen should be stored at room temperature 15°C to 30°C (59°F to 86°F) for up to 14 days.

Novolin® N vials: Store unopened vials in refrigerator between 2°C and 8°C (36°F to 46°F) until product expiration date or at room temperature ≤25°C (≤77°F) for up to 42 days; do not freeze; keep away from heat and sunlight. Once punctured (in use), store vials at room temperature ≤25°C (≤77°F) for up to 42 days (this includes any days stored at room temperature prior to opening vial); refrigeration of in-use vials is not recommended.

Canadian labeling (not in U.S. labeling): All products: Unopened vials, cartridges, and pens should be stored under refrigeration between 2°C and 8°C (36°F to 46°F) until the expiration date; do not freeze; keep away from heat and sunlight. Once punctured (in use), Humulin® vials, cartridges and pens should be stored at room temperature <25°C (<77°F) for up to 4 weeks. Once punctured (in use), Novolin® ge vials, cartridges, and pens may be stored for up to 1 month at room temperature <25°C (<77°F) for vials or <30°C (<86°F) for pens/cartridges; do not refrigerate.

For SubQ administration:

Humulin® N vials: May be diluted with the universal diluent, Sterile Diluent for Humalog®, Humulin® N, Humulin® R, Humulin® 70/30, and Humulin® R U-500. According to the manufacturer, storage and stability information are not available for diluted Humulin® N; do not dilute insulin contained in a cartridge or prefilled pen.

Novolin® N: Insulin Diluting Medium for NovoLog® is not intended for use with Novolin® N or any insulin product other than insulin aspart.

Mechanism of Action Insulin NPH, an isophane suspension of human insulin, is an intermediate-acting insulin.

Refer to Insulin Regular on page 1025.

Pharmacodynamics/Kinetics Note: Rate of absorption, onset, and duration of activity may be affected by site of injection, exercise, presence of lipodystrophy, local blood supply, and/or temperature.

Onset of action: 1-2 hours

Peak effect: 4-12 hours

Duration: 14-24 hours

Time to peak, plasma: 6-10 hours

Excretion: Urine

Dosage

Geriatric & Adult Note: When compared to insulin regular, insulin NPH has a slower onset and longer duration of activity.

Diabetes mellitus, type 1 and type 2: SubQ: Refer to Insulin Regular on page 1025.

Renal Impairment Refer to Insulin Regular on page 1025.

Hepatic Impairment Refer to Insulin Regular on page 1025.

Administration SubQ administration: In order to properly resuspend the insulin, vials should be carefully shaken or rolled several times, prefilled pens should be rolled between the palms ten times and inverted 180° ten times, and cartridges should be inverted 180° at least ten times. Properly resuspended insulin NPH should look uniformly cloudy or milky; do not use if any white insulin substance remains at the bottom of the container, if any clumps are present, or if white particles are stuck to the bottom or wall of the container. Cold injections should be avoided. SubQ administration is usually made into the thighs, arms, buttocks, or abdomen; rotate injection sites. When mixing insulin NPH with other preparations of insulin (eg, insulin aspart, insulin glulisine, insulin lispro, insulin regular), insulin NPH should be drawn into the syringe **after** the other insulin preparations. Do not dilute or mix other insulin formulations with insulin NPH contained in a cartridge or prefilled pen. Insulin NPH is **not** recommended for use in external SubQ insulin infusion pump.

Monitoring Parameters Diabetes mellitus: Plasma glucose, electrolytes, Hb A_{1c}

Reference Range Refer to Insulin Regular on page 1025.

Pharmacotherapy Pearls Refer to Insulin Regular on page 1025.

Special Geriatric Considerations Intensive glucose control (Hb A_{1c} <6.5%) has been linked to increased all-cause and cardiovascular mortality, hypoglycemia requiring assistance, and weight gain in adult type 2 diabetes. How "tightly" to control a geriatric patient's blood glucose needs to be individualized. Such a decision should be based on several factors, including the patient's functional and cognitive status, how well he/she recognizes hypoglycemic or hyperglycemic symptoms, and how to respond to them and other disease states. An Hb A_{1c} <7.5% is an acceptable endpoint for a healthy older adult, while <8% is acceptable for frail elderly patients, those with a duration of illness >10 years, or those with comorbid conditions and requiring combination diabetes medications. Patients who are unable to accurately draw up their dose will need assistance, such as prefilled syringes. Initial doses may require considerations for renal function in the elderly with dosing adjusted subsequently based on blood glucose monitoring. For elderly patients with diabetes who are relatively healthy, attaining target goals for aspirin use, blood pressure, lipids, smoking cessation, and diet and exercise may be more important than normalized glycemic control.

Dosage Forms Excipient information presented when available (limited, particularly for generics); consult specific product labeling.

Injection, suspension:

HumuLIN® N: 100 units/mL (3 mL) [prefilled pen]

HumuLIN® N: 100 units/mL (3 mL, 10 mL) [vial]

NovoLIN® N: 100 units/mL (10 mL) [vial]

Dosage Forms: Canada Excipient information presented when available (limited, particularly for generics); consult specific product labeling.

Injection, suspension:

Novolin® ge NPH: 100 units/mL (3 mL) [NovolinSet® prefilled syringe or PenFill® prefilled cartridge]; 10 mL [vial]

Insulin NPH and Insulin Regular (IN soo lin N P H & IN soo lin REG yoo ler)

Related Information

Diabetes Mellitus Management, Adults *on page 2193*

Insulin Regular *on page 1025*

Medication Safety Issues

Sound-alike/look-alike issues:

HumuLIN® 70/30 may be confused with HumaLOG® Mix 75/25, HumuLIN® R, NovoLIN® 70/30, NovoLOG® Mix 70/30

NovoLIN® 70/30 may be confused with HumaLOG® Mix 75/25, HumuLIN® 70/30, HumuLIN® R, NovoLIN® R, and NovoLOG® Mix 70/30

High alert medication:

The Institute for Safe Medication Practices (ISMP) includes this medication among its list of drugs which have a heightened risk of causing significant patient harm when used in error. *Due to the number of insulin preparations, it is essential to identify/clarify the type of insulin to be used.*

Other safety concerns:

Cross-contamination may occur if insulin pens are shared among multiple patients. Steps should be taken to prohibit sharing of insulin pens.

Brand Names: U.S. HumuLIN® 70/30; NovoLIN® 70/30

Brand Names: Canada Humulin® 20/80; Humulin® 70/30; Novolin® ge 30/70; Novolin® ge 40/60; Novolin® ge 50/50

Index Terms Insulin Regular and Insulin NPH; Isophane Insulin and Regular Insulin; NPH Insulin and Regular Insulin

Generic Availability (U.S.) No

Pharmacologic Category Insulin, Combination

Use Treatment of type 1 diabetes mellitus (insulin dependent, IDDM) and type 2 diabetes mellitus (noninsulin dependent, NIDDM) to improve glycemic control

Unlabeled Use No geriatric-specific information.

Contraindications Hypersensitivity to any component of the formulation; during episodes of hypoglycemia

Warnings/Precautions Refer to Insulin Regular on page 1025. Insulin NPH and insulin regular combination products are **NOT** intended for I.V. or I.M. administration

Adverse Reactions (Reflective of adult population; not specific for elderly) Primarily symptoms of hypoglycemia

Cardiovascular: Pallor, palpitation, tachycardia

Central nervous system: Fatigue, headache, hypothermia, loss of consciousness, mental confusion

Dermatologic: Redness, urticaria

Endocrine & metabolic: Hypoglycemia, hypokalemia

Gastrointestinal: Hunger, nausea, numbness of mouth

Local: Atrophy or hypertrophy of SubQ fat tissue; edema, itching, pain or warmth at injection site; stinging

Neuromuscular & skeletal: Muscle weakness, paresthesia, tremor

Ocular: Transient presbyopia or blurred vision

Miscellaneous: Anaphylaxis, diaphoresis, local and/or systemic hypersensitivity reactions

Drug Interactions

Metabolism/Transport Effects None known.

Avoid Concomitant Use There are no known interactions where it is recommended to avoid concomitant use.

Increased Effect/Toxicity

Insulin NPH and Insulin Regular may increase the levels/effects of: Antidiabetic Agents (Thiazolidinedione); Hypoglycemic Agents; Quinolone Antibiotics

The levels/effects of Insulin NPH and Insulin Regular may be increased by: Beta-Blockers; Edetate CALCIUM Disodium; Edetate Disodium; Herbs (Hypoglycemic Properties); MAO Inhibitors; Pegvisomant; Salicylates; Selective Serotonin Reuptake Inhibitors

Decreased Effect

The levels/effects of Insulin NPH and Insulin Regular may be decreased by: Corticosteroids (Orally Inhaled); Corticosteroids (Systemic); Loop Diuretics; Luteinizing Hormone-Releasing Hormone Analogs; Somatropin; Thiazide Diuretics

Ethanol/Nutrition/Herb Interactions Refer to Insulin Regular on page 1025.

Stability

Humulin® 70/30 vials: Store unopened vials in refrigerator between 2°C and 8°C (36°F to 46°F); do not freeze; keep away from heat and sunlight. Once punctured (in use), vials may be stored for up to 31 days in the refrigerator between 2°C and 8°C (36°F to 46°F) or at room temperature ≤30°C (≤86°F).

Humulin® 70/30 pens and cartridges: Store unopened pen and unused cartridges in refrigerator between 2°C and 8°C (36°F to 46°F); do not freeze; keep away from heat and sunlight. Once punctured (in use), cartridge/pen should be stored at room temperature 15°C to 30°C (59°F to 86°F) for up to 10 days.

Novolin® 70/30 vials: Store unopened vials in refrigerator between 2°C and 8°C (36°F to 46°F) until product expiration date or at room temperature ≤25°C (≤77°F) for up to 42 days; do not freeze; keep away from heat and sunlight. Once punctured (in use), store vials at room temperature ≤25°C (≤77°F) for up to 42 days (this includes any days stored at room temperature prior to opening vial); refrigeration of in-use vials is not recommended.

Canadian labeling (not in U.S. labeling): All products: Unopened vials, cartridges, and pens should be stored under refrigeration between 2°C and 8°C (36°F to 46°F) until the expiration date; do not freeze; keep away from heat and sunlight. Once punctured (in use), Humulin® vials, cartridges, and pens should be stored at room temperature <25°C (<77°F) for up to 4 weeks. Once punctured (in use), Novolin® ge vials, cartridges, and pens may be stored for up to 1 month at room temperature <25°C (<77°F) for vials or <30°C (<86°F) for pens/cartridges; do not refrigerate.

For SubQ administration:

Humulin® 70/30: May be diluted with the universal diluent, Sterile Diluent for Humalog®, Humulin® N, Humulin® R, Humulin® 70/30, and Humulin® R U-500. According to the manufacturer, storage and stability information are not available for diluted Humulin® 70/30; do not dilute insulin contained in a cartridge or prefilled pen.

Novolin® 70/30: Insulin Diluting Medium for NovoLog® is not intended for use with Novolin® 70/30 or any insulin product other than insulin aspart.

Mechanism of Action Insulin NPH and insulin regular is an intermediate-acting combination insulin product with a more rapid onset than that of insulin NPH alone. Refer to Insulin Regular on page 1025.

Pharmacodynamics/Kinetics Note: Rate of absorption, onset, and duration of activity may be affected by site of injection, exercise, presence of lipodystrophy, local blood supply, and/or temperature.

Onset of action: 0.5 hours

Peak effect: 2-12 hours

Duration: 18-24 hours

Time to peak, plasma: Based on individual components:

Insulin regular: 0.8-2 hours

Insulin NPH: 6-10 hours

Excretion: Urine

Dosage

Geriatric & Adult Note: When compared to insulin NPH, the combination product (insulin NPH and insulin regular) has a more rapid onset of action and a similar duration of action.

Diabetes mellitus, type 1 and type 2: SubQ: Refer to Insulin Regular on page 1025.

Renal Impairment Refer to Insulin Regular on page 1025.

Hepatic Impairment Refer to Insulin Regular on page 1025.

Administration SubQ administration: In order to properly resuspend the insulin, vials should be carefully shaken or rolled several times, prefilled pens should be rolled between the palms ten times and inverted 180° ten times, and cartridges should be inverted 180° at least ten times. Properly resuspended insulin should look uniformly cloudy or milky; do not use if any white insulin substance remains at the bottom of the container, if any clumps are present, if the insulin remains clear after adequate mixing, or if white particles are stuck to the bottom or wall of the container. Cold injections should be avoided. Insulin NPH and insulin regular combination products should be administered within 30 minutes before a meal; typically given once- or twice daily. SubQ administration is usually made into the thighs, arms, buttocks, or abdomen; rotate injection sites. Do not mix with any other insulin formulation. Do not dilute combination product (insulin NPH and insulin regular) contained in a cartridge or prefilled pen. Combination insulin products are not recommended for use in an external SubQ insulin infusion pump.

Monitoring Parameters Diabetes mellitus: Plasma glucose, electrolytes, Hb A_{1c}

Reference Range Refer to Insulin Regular on page 1025.

Pharmacotherapy Pearls Refer to Insulin Regular on page 1025.

Special Geriatric Considerations Intensive glucose control (Hb A_{1c} <6.5%) has been linked to increased all cause and cardiovascular mortality, hypoglycemia requiring assistance, and weight gain in adult type 2 diabetes. For elderly patients with diabetes who are relatively healthy, attaining target goals for aspirin use, blood pressure, lipids, smoking cessation, and diet and exercise may be more important than normalized glycemic control.

Dosage Forms Excipient information presented when available (limited, particularly for generics); consult specific product labeling.

Injection, suspension:

HumuLIN® 70/30: Insulin NPH suspension 70% [intermediate acting] and insulin regular solution 30% [short acting]: 100 units/mL (3 mL) [prefilled pen, vial]

HumuLIN® 70/30: Insulin NPH suspension 70% [intermediate acting] and insulin regular solution 30% [short acting]: 100 units/mL (10 mL) [vial]

NovoLIN® 70/30: Insulin NPH suspension 70% [intermediate acting] and insulin regular solution 30% [short acting]: 100 units/mL (10 mL) [vial]

Dosage Forms: Canada Excipient information presented when available (limited, particularly for generics); consult specific product labeling.

Injection, suspension:

Humulin® 20/80: Insulin regular solution 20% [short acting] and insulin NPH suspension 80% [intermediate acting]: 100 units/mL (3 mL) [PenFill® prefilled cartridge]

Novolin® ge 30/70: Insulin regular solution 30% [short acting] and insulin NPH suspension 70% [intermediate acting]: 100 units/mL (3 mL) [prefilled syringe or PenFill® prefilled cartridge]; (10 mL) [vial]

Novolin® ge 40/60: Insulin regular solution 40% [short acting] and insulin NPH suspension 60% [intermediate acting]: 100 units/mL (3 mL) [PenFill® prefilled cartridge]

Novolin® ge 50/50: Insulin regular solution 50% [short acting] and insulin NPH suspension 50% [intermediate acting]: 100 units/mL (3 mL) [PenFill® prefilled cartridge]

Insulin Regular (IN soo lin REG yoo ler)

Related Information

Beers Criteria – Potentially Inappropriate Medications for Geriatrics *on page 2183*
Diabetes Mellitus Management, Adults *on page 2193*
Insulin Aspart *on page 1005*
Insulin Aspart Protamine and Insulin Aspart *on page 1008*
Insulin Detemir *on page 1010*
Insulin Glargine *on page 1012*
Insulin Glulisine *on page 1014*
Insulin Lispro *on page 1016*
Insulin Lispro Protamine and Insulin Lispro *on page 1019*
Insulin NPH *on page 1020*
Insulin NPH and Insulin Regular *on page 1023*

Medication Safety Issues

Sound-alike/look-alike issues:

HumuLIN® R may be confused with HumaLOG®, Humira®, HumuLIN® 70/30, HumuLIN® N, NovoLIN® 70/30, NovoLIN® R, NovoLOG®

NovoLIN® R may be confused with HumuLIN® R, NovoLIN® 70/30, NovoLIN® N, NovoLOG®

High alert medication:

The Institute for Safe Medication Practices (ISMP) includes this medication among its list of drugs which have a heightened risk of causing significant patient harm when used in error. ***Due to the number of insulin preparations, it is essential to identify/clarify the type of insulin to be used.***

BEERS Criteria medication:

This drug may be potentially inappropriate for use in geriatric patients (Quality of evidence - moderate; Strength of recommendation - strong).

Administration issues:

Concentrated solutions (eg, U-500) should not be available in patient care areas. U-500 regular insulin should be stored, dispensed, and administered separately from U-100 regular insulin. For patients who receive U-500 insulin in the hospital setting, highlighting the strength prominently on the patient's medical chart and medication record may help to reduce dispensing errors.

Other safety concerns:

Cross-contamination may occur if insulin pens are shared among multiple patients. Steps should be taken to prohibit sharing of insulin pens.

Brand Names: U.S. HumuLIN® R; HumuLIN® R U-500; NovoLIN® R

Brand Names: Canada Humulin® R; Novolin® ge Toronto

Index Terms Regular Insulin

Generic Availability (U.S.) No

Pharmacologic Category Insulin, Short-Acting

INSULIN REGULAR

Use Treatment of type 1 diabetes mellitus (insulin dependent, IDDM) and type 2 diabetes mellitus (noninsulin dependent, NIDDM) to improve glycemic control

Unlabeled Use Hyperkalemia; gestational diabetes mellitus (GDM), diabetic ketoacidosis (DKA); hyperosmolar hyperglycemic state (HHS); adjunct of parenteral nutrition

Contraindications Hypersensitivity to regular insulin or any component of the formulation; during episodes of hypoglycemia

Warnings/Precautions Hypoglycemia is the most common adverse effect of insulin. The timing of hypoglycemia differs among various insulin formulations. Hypoglycemia may result from increased work or exercise without eating; use of long-acting insulin preparations (eg, insulin detemir, insulin glargine) may delay recovery from hypoglycemia. Profound and prolonged episodes of hypoglycemia may result in convulsions, unconsciousness, temporary or permanent brain damage or even death. Insulin requirements may be altered during illness, emotional disturbances or other stressors. Insulin may produce hypokalemia which, if left untreated, may result in respiratory paralysis, ventricular arrhythmia and even death. Use with caution in patients at risk for hypokalemia (eg, I.V. insulin use). Use with caution in renal or hepatic impairment. In the elderly, avoid use of sliding scale insulin in this population due to increased risk of hypoglycemia without benefits in management of hyperglycemia regardless of care setting (Beers Criteria).

Human insulin differs from animal-source insulin. Any change of insulin should be made cautiously; changing manufacturers, type, and/or method of manufacture may result in the need for a change of dosage. U-500 regular insulin is a concentrated insulin formulation which contains 500 units of insulin per mL; for SubQ administration only using a U-100 insulin syringe or tuberculin syringe; **not for I.V. administration**. To avoid dosing errors when using a U-100 insulin syringe, the prescribed dose should be written in actual insulin units and as unit markings on the U-100 insulin syringe (eg, 50 units [10 units on a U-100 insulin syringe]). To avoid dosing errors when using a tuberculin syringe, the prescribed dose should be written in actual insulin units and as a volume (eg, 50 units [0.1 mL]). Mixing U-500 regular insulin with other insulin formulations is not recommended.

Regular insulin may be administered I.V. or I.M. in selected clinical situations; close monitoring of blood glucose and serum potassium, as well as medical supervision, is required.

The general objective of exogenous insulin therapy is to approximate the physiologic pattern of insulin secretion which is characterized by two distinct phases. Phase 1 insulin secretion suppresses hepatic glucose production and phase 2 insulin secretion occurs in response to carbohydrate ingestion; therefore, exogenous insulin therapy may consist of basal insulin (eg, intermediate- or long-acting insulin or via continuous subcutaneous insulin infusion [CSII]) and/or preprandial insulin (eg, short- or rapid-acting insulin) (see Related Information: Insulin Products). Patients with type 1 diabetes do not produce endogenous insulin; therefore, these patients require both basal and preprandial insulin administration. Patients with type 2 diabetes retain some beta-cell function in the early stages of their disease; however, as the disease progresses, phase 1 insulin secretion may become completely impaired and phase 2 insulin secretion becomes delayed and/or inadequate in response to meals. Therefore, patients with type 2 diabetes may be treated with oral antidiabetic agents, basal insulin, and/or preprandial insulin depending on the stage of disease and current glycemic control. Since treatment regimens often consist of multiple agents, dosage adjustments must address the specific phase of insulin release that is primarily contributing to the patient's impaired glycemic control. Diabetes self-management education (DSME) is essential to maximize the effectiveness of therapy. Treatment and monitoring regimens must be individualized.

Adverse Reactions (Reflective of adult population; not specific for elderly) Primarily symptoms of hypoglycemia

Cardiovascular: Pallor, palpitation, tachycardia

Central nervous system: Fatigue, headache, hypothermia, loss of consciousness, mental confusion

Dermatologic: Redness, urticaria

Endocrine & metabolic: Hypoglycemia, hypokalemia

Gastrointestinal: Hunger, nausea, numbness of mouth

Local: Atrophy or hypertrophy of SubQ fat tissue; edema, itching, pain or warmth at injection site; stinging

Neuromuscular & skeletal: Muscle weakness, paresthesia, tremor

Ocular: Transient presbyopia or blurred vision

Miscellaneous: Anaphylaxis, diaphoresis, local and/or systemic hypersensitivity reactions

Drug Interactions

Metabolism/Transport Effects None known.

Avoid Concomitant Use There are no known interactions where it is recommended to avoid concomitant use.

Increased Effect/Toxicity

Insulin Regular may increase the levels/effects of: Antidiabetic Agents (Thiazolidinedione); Hypoglycemic Agents; Quinolone Antibiotics

The levels/effects of Insulin Regular may be increased by: Beta-Blockers; Edetate CALCIUM Disodium; Edetate Disodium; Herbs (Hypoglycemic Properties); MAO Inhibitors; Pegvisomant; Salicylates; Selective Serotonin Reuptake Inhibitors

Decreased Effect

The levels/effects of Insulin Regular may be decreased by: Corticosteroids (Orally Inhaled); Corticosteroids (Systemic); Loop Diuretics; Luteinizing Hormone-Releasing Hormone Analogs; Somatropin; Thiazide Diuretics

Ethanol/Nutrition/Herb Interactions

Ethanol: Use caution with ethanol; may increase risk of hypoglycemia.

Herb/Nutraceutical: Use caution with alfalfa, aloe, bilberry, bitter melon, burdock, celery, damiana, fenugreek, garcinia, garlic, ginger, ginseng (American), gymnema, marshmallow, stinging nettle; may increase risk of hypoglycemia.

Stability

Humulin® R, Humulin® R U-500: Store unopened vials in refrigerator between 2°C and 8°C (36°F to 46°F); do not freeze; keep away from heat and sunlight. Once punctured (in use), vials may be stored for up to 31 days in the refrigerator between 2°C and 8°C (36°F to 46°F) or at room temperature of ≤30°C (≤86°F).

Novolin® R: Store unopened vials in refrigerator between 2°C and 8°C (36°F to 46°F) until product expiration date or at room temperature ≤25°C (≤77°F) for up to 42 days; do not freeze; keep away from heat and sunlight. Once punctured (in use), store vials at room temperature ≤25°C (≤77°F) for up to 42 days (this includes any days stored at room temperature prior to opening vial); refrigeration of in-use vials is not recommended.

Canadian labeling (not in U.S. labeling): All products: Unopened vials, cartridges, and pens should be stored under refrigeration between 2°C and 8°C (36°F to 46°F) until the expiration date; do not freeze; keep away from heat and sunlight. Once punctured (in use), Humulin® vials, cartridges, and pens should be stored at room temperature <25°C (<77°F) for up to 4 weeks. Once punctured (in use), Novolin® ge vials, cartridges, and pens may be stored for up to 1 month at room temperature <25°C (<77°F) for vials or <30°C (<86°F) for pens/cartridges; do not refrigerate.

For SubQ administration:

Humulin® R: May be diluted with the universal diluent, Sterile Diluent for Humalog®, Humulin® N, Humulin® R, Humulin® 70/30, and Humulin® R U-500, to a concentration of 10 units/mL (U-10) or 50 units/mL (U-50). According to the manufacturer, diluted insulin should be stored at 30°C (86°F) and used within 14 days **or** at 5°C (41°F) and used within 28 days.

Novolin® R: Insulin Diluting Medium for NovoLog® is **not** intended for use with Novolin® R or any insulin product other than insulin aspart.

For I.V. infusion:

Humulin® R: May be diluted in NS or D_5W to concentrations of 0.1-1 unit/mL. Stable for 48 hours at room temperature or for 48 hours under refrigeration followed by 48 hours at room temperature.

Novolin® R: May be diluted in NS, D_5W, or $D_{10}W$ with 40 mEq/L potassium chloride at concentrations of 0.05-1 unit/mL. Stable for 24 hours at room temperature

Mechanism of Action Insulin acts via specific membrane-bound receptors on target tissues to regulate metabolism of carbohydrate, protein, and fats. Target organs for insulin include the liver, skeletal muscle, and adipose tissue.

Within the liver, insulin stimulates hepatic glycogen synthesis. Insulin promotes hepatic synthesis of fatty acids, which are released into the circulation as lipoproteins. Skeletal muscle effects of insulin include increased protein synthesis and increased glycogen synthesis. Within adipose tissue, insulin stimulates the processing of circulating lipoproteins to provide free fatty acids, facilitating triglyceride synthesis and storage by adipocytes; also directly inhibits the hydrolysis of triglycerides. In addition, insulin stimulates the cellular uptake of amino acids and increases cellular permeability to several ions, including potassium, magnesium, and phosphate. By activating sodium-potassium ATPases, insulin promotes the intracellular movement of potassium.

Normally secreted by the pancreas, insulin products are manufactured for pharmacologic use through recombinant DNA technology using either *E. coli* or *Saccharomyces cerevisiae*. Insulins are categorized based on the onset, peak, and duration of effect (eg, rapid-, short-, intermediate-, and long-acting insulin).

Pharmacodynamics/Kinetics Note: Rate of absorption, onset, and duration of activity may be affected by site of injection, exercise, presence of lipodystrophy, local blood supply, and/or temperature.

INSULIN REGULAR

Onset of action: SubQ: 0.5 hours
  Peak effect: SubQ: 2.5-5 hours
Duration: SubQ:
  U-100: 4-12 hours (may increase with dose)
  U-500: Up to 24 hours
Distribution: V_d: 0.26-0.36 L/kg
Bioavailability: SubQ: 55% to 77%
Half-life elimination: I.V.: ~0.5-1 hour (dose-dependent); SubQ: 1.5 hours
Time to peak, plasma: SubQ: 0.8-2 hours
Excretion: Urine

Dosage

Geriatric & Adult

Diabetes mellitus: SubQ: **Note:** Insulin requirements vary dramatically between patients and therapy requires dosage adjustments with careful medical supervision. Specific formulations may require distinct administration procedures; please see individual agents.

Type 1: **Note:** Multiple daily injections (MDI) guided by blood glucose monitoring or the use of continuous subcutaneous insulin infusions (CSII) is the standard of care for patients with type 1 diabetes. Combinations of insulin formulations are commonly used.

Initial dose: 0.5-1.0 units/kg/day in divided doses. Conservative initial doses of 0.2-0.4 units/kg/day may be recommended to avoid the potential for hypoglycemia.

Division of daily insulin requirement: Generally, 50% to 75% of the total daily dose (TDD) is given as an intermediate- or long-acting form of insulin (in 1-2 daily injections). The remaining portion of the TDD is then divided and administered before or at mealtimes (depending on the formulation) as a rapid-acting or short-acting form of insulin. Premixed combinations are available that deliver the rapid- or short-acting component at the same time as the intermediate- or long-acting component. Some patients may benefit from the use of CSII which delivers rapid-acting insulin as a continuous infusion throughout the day and as boluses at mealtimes via an external pump device.

Adjustment of dose: Dosage must be titrated to achieve glucose control and avoid hypoglycemia. Adjust dose to maintain preprandial plasma glucose between 70-130 mg/dL for most patients. Since treatment regimens often consist of multiple formulations, dosage adjustments must address the specific phase of insulin release that is primarily contributing to the patient's impaired glycemic control. Treatment and monitoring regimens must be individualized. Also see Pharmacotherapy Pearls.

Usual maintenance range: 0.5-1.2 units/kg/day in divided doses. Insulin requirements are patient-specific and may vary based on age, body weight, and/or activity factors.

Type 2: The goal of therapy is to achieve an Hb A_{1c} <7% as quickly as possible using the safe titration of medications. According to a consensus statement by the ADA and European Association for the Study of Diabetes (EASD), basal insulin therapy (eg, intermediate- or long-acting insulin) should be considered in patients with type 2 diabetes who fail to achieve glycemic goals with lifestyle interventions and metformin ± a sulfonylurea. Pioglitazone or a GLP-1 agonist may also be considered prior to initiation of basal insulin therapy. In patients who continue to fail to achieve glycemic goals despite the addition of basal insulin, intensification of insulin therapy should be considered; this generally consists of multiple daily injections with a combination of insulin formulations (Nathan, 2009).

Initial basal insulin dose: 0.2 units/kg or 10 units/day (Nathan, 2009). **Note:** Current guidelines recommend that insulin therapy begin with intermediate- or long-acting insulin given at bedtime or long-acting insulin given in the morning (Nathan, 2009).

Adjustment of basal insulin dose: Increase dose by 2 units/day every 3 days until fasting glucose levels are consistently within target range (70-130 mg/dL); may increase dose in larger increments (eg, 4 units/day) if fasting glucose levels are >180 mg/dL (Nathan, 2009)

Note: If the patient experiences hypoglycemia following adjustment, reduce dose by 4 units/day or 10% of total daily dose, whichever is greater (Nathan, 2009). Additional algorithms, such as the "1-1-100", "2-4-6-8", "3-0-3", and "3-2-1" algorithms, exist to aid in the titration of basal insulin (Davies, 2005; Gerstein, 2006; Meneghini, 2007; Riddle, 2003); therapy should be individualized and based on patient-specific details.

Intensification of therapy: Add a second injection of a short-, rapid-, or intermediate-acting insulin as needed based on blood glucose monitoring; the timing of administration and type of insulin added for intensification of therapy depends on the blood glucose level that is consistently out of the target range (eg, preprandial glucose levels before lunch or dinner, postprandial glucose levels, and/or bedtime glucose levels). Additional injections and subsequent dosage adjustments must address the specific phase of insulin release that is primarily contributing to the patient's impaired glycemic control. Intensification of therapy can usually begin with a second injection of ~4 units/day followed by adjustments of ~2 units/day every 3 days until the targeted blood glucose is within range (Nathan, 2009).

In the setting of glucose toxicity (loss of beta-cell sensitivity to glucose concentrations), insulin therapy may be used for short-term management to restore sensitivity of beta-cells; in these cases, the dose may need to be rapidly reduced/withdrawn when sensitivity is re-established.

Diabetic ketoacidosis (DKA) (unlabeled use): Only I.V. regular insulin should be used for severe DKA; use of SubQ rapid-acting insulin analogs (eg, aspart, lispro) may be appropriate for mild-moderate DKA (Kitabchi, 2009). Treatment should continue until reversal of acid-base derangement/ketonemia. Serum glucose is not a direct indicator of these abnormalities, and may decrease more rapidly than correction of the metabolic abnormalities. Also, refer to institution-specific protocols where appropriate.

Adults <20 years (Kitabchi, 2004):

I.V. infusion: 0.1 units/kg/hour

Adjustment: If serum glucose does not fall by 50 mg/dL in the first hour, check hydration status; if acceptable, double insulin dose hourly until glucose levels fall at rate of 50-75 mg/dL per hour. Once serum glucose reaches 250 mg/dL, decrease dose to 0.05-0.1 units/kg/hour; dextrose-containing I.V. fluids should be administered to maintain serum glucose between 150-250 mg/dL until the acidosis clears. After resolution of DKA, supplement I.V. insulin with SubQ insulin as needed until the patient is able to eat and transition fully to a SubQ insulin regimen. An overlap of ~1-2 hours between discontinuation of I.V. insulin and administration of SubQ insulin is recommended to ensure adequate plasma insulin levels.

SubQ, I.M. (**Note:** Only use the SubQ and I.M route if I.V. infusion access is unavailable): 0.1-0.3 units/kg SubQ bolus, followed by 0.1 units/kg given every hour SubQ or I.M. or 0.15-0.2 units/kg every 2 hours SubQ; continue until acidosis clears, then decrease to 0.05 units/kg given every hour until SubQ replacement dosing can be initiated (Kitabchi, 2004; Wolfsdorf, 2007)

Adults ≥20 years (Kitabchi, 2009):

I.V.:

Bolus: 0.1 units/kg (optional)

Infusion: 0.1-0.14 units/kg/hour. **Note:** If no I.V. bolus was administered, patients should receive a continuous infusion of 0.14 units/kg/hour; lower doses may not achieve adequate insulin concentrations to suppress hepatic ketone body production.

Adjustment: If serum glucose does not fall by at least 10% in the first hour, give an I.V. bolus of 0.14 units/kg and continue previous regimen. In addition, if serum glucose does not fall by 50-70 mg/dL in the first hour, the insulin infusion dose should be increased hourly until a steady glucose decline is achieved Once serum glucose reaches 200 mg/dL, decrease infusion dose to 0.02-0.05 units/kg/hour or switch to SubQ rapid-acting insulin (eg, aspart, lispro) at 0.1 units/kg every 2 hours; dextrose-containing I.V. fluids should be administered to maintain serum glucose between 150-250 mg/dL until the acidosis clears. After resolution of DKA, supplement I.V. insulin with SubQ insulin as needed until the patient is able to eat and transition fully to a SubQ insulin regimen. An overlap of ~1-2 hours between discontinuation of I.V. insulin and administration of SubQ insulin is recommended to ensure adequate plasma insulin levels.

SubQ, I.M.: According to the 2009 ADA consensus statement on hyperglycemic crises, a rapid-acting insulin analog (eg, aspart, lispro) given every 1-2 hours via the SubQ route may be appropriate for mild-moderate DKA; however, specific dosing recommendations are not provided (Kitabchi, 2009). If using the I.V. route for severe DKA, consider switching to SubQ rapid-acting insulin once serum glucose reaches 200 mg/dL (Kitabchi, 2009). The following dosing regimen from the 2004 ADA position statement recommends regular insulin (Kitabchi, 2004):

Bolus: 0.4 units/kg; **Note:** Give half of the dose (0.2 units/kg) as an I.V. bolus and half of the dose (0.2 units/kg) as SubQ or I.M.

Intermittent: 0.1 units/kg given every hour SubQ or I.M.

Adjustment: If serum glucose does not fall by 50-70 mg/dL in the first hour, administer 10 units hourly by I.V. bolus until glucose levels fall at a rate of 50-70 mg/dL per hour. Once serum glucose reaches 250 mg/dL, decrease dose to 5-10 units SubQ every 2 hours; dextrose-containing I.V. fluids should be administered to maintain serum glucose between 150-250 mg/dL until the acidosis clears.

Gestational diabetes mellitus (unlabeled use): Insulin therapy should be considered when medical nutrition therapy has not achieved GDM glycemic goals (fasting plasma glucose: <95 mg/dL; 1-hour postprandial levels: <130-140 mg/dL; 2-hour postprandial levels: <120 mg/dL); dose and timing of administration should be based on frequent monitoring of plasma glucose levels (ACOG, 2001; ADA, 2004). Human insulin may be preferred (ADA, 2004); however, rapid-acting insulin analogues may also be considered (ACOG, 2001).

Hyperkalemia, moderate-to-severe (unlabeled use): I.V.: 10 units regular insulin mixed with 25 g dextrose (50 mL $D_{50}W$) given over 15-30 minutes (ACLS, 2010); alternatively, 50 mL $D_{50}W$ over 5 minutes followed by 10 units regular insulin I.V. push over seconds may be administered in the setting of imminent cardiac arrest. In patients with ongoing cardiac arrest (eg, PEA with presumed hyperkalemia), administration of $D_{50}W$ over <5 minutes is routine. Effects on potassium are temporary. As appropriate, consider methods of enhancing potassium removal/excretion.

Hyperosmolar hyperglycemic state (HHS) (unlabeled use): Only regular insulin should be used. Infusion should continue until reversal of mental status changes and hyperosmolality. Serum glucose is not a direct indicator of these abnormalities, and may decrease more rapidly than correction of the metabolic abnormalities. Also, refer to institution-specific protocols where appropriate.

Adults <20 years (Kitabchi, 2004):

I.V.:

Infusion: 0.1 units/kg/hour

Adjustment: If serum glucose does not fall by 50 mg/dL in the first hour, check hydration status; if acceptable, double insulin dose hourly until glucose levels fall at rate of 50-75 mg/dL per hour. Once serum glucose reaches 300 mg/dL, decrease dose to 0.05-0.1 units/kg/hour; dextrose-containing I.V. fluids should be administered to maintain serum glucose between 250-300 mg/dL until hyperosmolality clears and mental status returns to normal. After resolution of HHS, supplement I.V. insulin with SubQ insulin as needed until the patient is able to eat and transition fully to a SubQ insulin regimen. An overlap of ~1-2 hours between discontinuation of I.V. insulin and administration of SubQ insulin is recommended to ensure adequate plasma insulin levels.

SubQ, I.M. (**Note:** Only use the SubQ and I.M route if I.V. infusion access is unavailable): 0.1-0.3 units/kg SubQ bolus, followed by 0.1 units/kg given every hour SubQ or I.M. or 0.15-0.2 units/kg every 2 hours SubQ; continue until resolution of hyperosmolality, then decrease to 0.05 units/kg given every hour until SubQ replacement dosing can be initiated (Kitabchi, 2004; Wolfsdorf, 2007)

Adults ≥20 years (Kitabchi, 2009):

I.V.:

Bolus: 0.1 units/kg bolus (optional)

Infusion: 0.1-0.14 units/kg/hour. **Note:** If no I.V. bolus was administered, patients should receive a continuous infusion of 0.14 units/kg/hour.

Adjustment: If serum glucose does not fall by at least 10% in the first hour, give an I.V. bolus of 0.14 units/kg and continue previous regimen. In addition, if serum glucose does not fall by 50-70 mg/dL in the first hour, the insulin infusion dose should be increased hourly until a steady glucose decline is achieved. Once serum glucose reaches 300 mg/dL, decrease dose to 0.02-0.05 units/kg/hour; dextrose-containing I.V. fluids should be administered to maintain serum glucose between 200-300 mg/dL until the patient is mentally alert. After resolution of HHS, supplement I.V. insulin with SubQ insulin as needed until the patient is able to eat and transition fully to a SubQ insulin regimen. An overlap of ~1-2 hours between discontinuation of I.V. insulin and administration of SubQ insulin is recommended to ensure adequate plasma insulin levels.

Renal Impairment Insulin requirements are reduced due to changes in insulin clearance or metabolism. Close monitoring of blood glucose and adjustment of therapy is required in renal impairment.

Cl_{cr} 10-50 mL/minute: Administer at 75% of normal dose and monitor glucose closely

Cl_{cr} <10 mL/minute: Administer at 25% to 50% of normal dose and monitor glucose closely

Hemodialysis: Because of a large molecular weight (6000 daltons), insulin is not significantly removed by hemodialysis; supplemental dose is not necessary.

Peritoneal dialysis: Because of a large molecular weight (6000 daltons), insulin is not significantly removed by peritoneal dialysis; supplemental dose is not necessary.

Continuous renal replacement therapy: Administer 75% of normal dose and monitor glucose closely; supplemental dose is not necessary.

Hepatic Impairment Insulin requirements may be reduced. Close monitoring of blood glucose and adjustment of therapy is required in hepatic impairment.

Administration

SubQ administration: Do not use if solution is viscous or cloudy; use only if clear and colorless. Regular insulin should be administered within 30-60 minutes before a meal. Cold injections should be avoided. SubQ administration is usually made into the thighs, arms, buttocks, or abdomen; rotate injection sites. When mixing regular insulin with other preparations of insulin, regular insulin should be drawn into syringe first. Regular insulin is not recommended for use in external SubQ insulin infusion pump.

I.M. administration: Do not use if solution is viscous or cloudy; use only if clear and colorless. May be administered I.M. in selected clinical situations; close monitoring of blood glucose and serum potassium as well as medical supervision is required.

I.V. administration: Do not use if solution is viscous or cloudy; use only if clear and colorless. May be administered I.V. with close monitoring of blood glucose and serum potassium; appropriate medical supervision is required. **Do not administer mixtures of insulin formulations intravenously.** I.V. administration of U-500 regular insulin is not recommended.

I.V. infusions: To minimize adsorption to I.V. solution bag (**Note:** Refer to institution-specific protocols where appropriate):

*If new tubing is **not** needed:* Wait a minimum of 30 minutes between the preparation of the solution and the initiation of the infusion.

If new tubing is needed: After receiving the insulin drip solution, the administration set should be attached to the I.V. container and the entire line should be flushed with a priming infusion of 20-50 mL of the insulin solution (Goldberg, 2006; Hirsch, 2006). Wait 30 minutes, then flush the line again with the insulin solution prior to initiating the infusion.

If insulin is required prior to the availability of the insulin drip, regular insulin should be administered by I.V. push injection.

Because of adsorption, the actual amount of insulin being administered via I.V. infusion could be substantially less than the apparent amount. Therefore, adjustment of the I.V. infusion rate should be based on effect and not solely on the apparent insulin dose. The apparent dose may be used as a starting point for determining the subsequent SubQ dosing regimen (Moghissi, 2009); however, the transition to SubQ administration requires continuous medical supervision, frequent monitoring of blood glucose, and careful adjustment of therapy. In addition, SubQ insulin should be given 1-4 hours prior to the discontinuation of I.V. insulin to prevent hyperglycemia (Moghissi, 2009).

Monitoring Parameters

Diabetes mellitus: Plasma glucose, electrolytes, Hb A_{1c}

DKA/HHS: Serum electrolytes, glucose, BUN, creatinine, osmolality, venous pH (repeat arterial blood gases are generally unnecessary), anion gap, urine output, urinalysis, mental status

Hyperkalemia: Serum potassium and glucose must be closely monitored to avoid hypokalemia, rebound hyperkalemia, and hypoglycemia.

Reference Range

Therapeutic, serum insulin (fasting): 5-20 µIU/mL (SI: 35-145 pmol/L)

Glucose, fasting:

Adults: 60-110 mg/dL

Elderly: 100-180 mg/dL

Recommendations for glycemic control in adults with diabetes mellitus:

Hb A_{1c}: <7%

Preprandial capillary plasma glucose: 70-130 mg/dL

Peak postprandial capillary plasma glucose: <180 mg/dL

Pharmacotherapy Pearls

Split-mixed or basal-bolus regimens: Combination regimens which optimize differences in the onset and duration of different insulin products are commonly used to approximate physiologic secretion. In split-mixed regimens, an intermediate-acting insulin (eg, NPH insulin) is administered once or twice daily and supplemented by short-acting (regular) or rapid-acting (lispro, aspart, or glulisine) insulin. Blood glucose measurements are completed several times daily. Dosages are adjusted emphasizing the individual component of the regimen which most directly influences the blood sugar in question (either the intermediate-acting component or the shorter-acting component). Fixed-ratio formulations (eg, 70/30 mix) may be used as twice daily injections in this scenario; however, the ability to titrate the dosage of an individual component is limited. An example of a "split-mixed" regimen would be 21 units of NPH plus 9 units of regular insulin in the morning and an evening meal dose consisting of 14 units of NPH plus 6 units of regular insulin.

Basal-bolus regimens are designed to more closely mimic physiologic secretion. These regimens employ a long-acting insulin (eg, glargine) to simulate basal insulin secretion. The basal component is frequently administered at bedtime or in the early morning. This is supplemented by multiple daily injections of rapid-acting products (lispro, aspart, or glulisine) immediately prior to a meal, which provides insulin at the time when nutrients are absorbed. An example of a basal-bolus regimen would be 30 units of glargine at bedtime and 12 units of lispro insulin prior to each meal.

Estimation of the effect per unit: A "Rule of 1500" has been frequently used as a means to estimate the change in blood sugar relative to each unit of insulin administered. In fact, the recommended values used in these calculations may vary from 1500-2200 (a value of 1500 is generally recommended for regular insulin while 1800 is recommended for "rapid-acting insulins"). The higher values lead to more conservative estimates of the effect per unit of insulin, and therefore lead to more cautious adjustments. The effect per unit of insulin is approximated by dividing the selected numerical value (eg, 1500-2200) by the number of units/day received by the patient. This may be used as a crude approximation of the patient's insulin sensitivity as adjustments to individual components of the regimen are made. Each additional unit of insulin added to the corresponding insulin dose may be expected to lower the blood glucose by this amount.

To illustrate, in the "basal-bolus" regimen example presented above, the rule of 1800 would indicate an expected change of 27 mg/dL per unit of lispro insulin (the total daily insulin dose is 66 units; using the formula: 1800/66 = 27). A patient may be instructed to add additional insulin if the preprandial glucose is >125 mg/dL. For a prelunch glucose of 195 mg/dL, this would mean the patient would administer the scheduled 12 units of lispro along with an additional "correctional" 3 units for a total of 15 units prior to the meal. If correctional doses are required on a consistent basis, an adjustment of the patients diet and/or scheduled insulin dose may be necessary.

Special Geriatric Considerations Intensive glucose control (Hb A$_{1c}$ <6.5%) has been linked to increased all-cause and cardiovascular mortality, hypoglycemia requiring assistance, and weight gain in adult type 2 diabetes. How "tightly" to control a geriatric patient's blood glucose needs to be individualized. Such a decision should be based on several factors, including the patient's functional and cognitive status, how well he/she recognizes hypoglycemic or hyperglycemic symptoms, and how to respond to them and other disease states. An Hb A$_{1c}$ <7.5% is an acceptable endpoint for a healthy older adult, while <8% is acceptable for frail elderly patients, those with a duration of illness >10 years, or those with comorbid conditions and requiring combination diabetes medications. Patients who are unable to accurately draw up their dose will need assistance, such as prefilled syringes. Initial doses may require considerations for renal function in the elderly with dosing adjusted subsequently based on blood glucose monitoring. For elderly patients with diabetes who are relatively healthy, attaining target goals for aspirin use, blood pressure, lipids, smoking cessation, and diet and exercise may be more important than normalized glycemic control.

This medication is considered to be potentially inappropriate when used in a sliding scale regimen in this patient population (Beers Criteria: Quality of evidence - moderate; Strength of recommendation - strong).

Dosage Forms Excipient information presented when available (limited, particularly for generics); consult specific product labeling.

Injection, solution:
HumuLIN® R: 100 units/mL (3 mL, 10 mL)
NovoLIN® R: 100 units/mL (10 mL)
Injection, solution [concentrate]:
HumuLIN® R U-500: 500 units/mL (20 mL)

◆ **Insulin Regular and Insulin NPH** *see* Insulin NPH and Insulin Regular *on page* 1023
◆ **Interferon Alfa-2b (PEG Conjugate)** *see* Peginterferon Alfa-2b *on page* 1485

Interferon Beta-1b (in ter FEER on BAY ta won bee)

Brand Names: U.S. Betaseron®; Extavia®
Brand Names: Canada Betaseron®; Extavia®
Index Terms rIFN beta-1b
Generic Availability (U.S.) No
Pharmacologic Category Interferon
Use Treatment of relapsing forms of multiple sclerosis (MS); treatment of first clinical episode with MRI features consistent with MS

Canadian labeling: Additional use (not in U.S. labeling): Treatment of secondary-progressive MS

Medication Guide Available Yes
Contraindications Hypersensitivity to *E. coli*-derived products, natural or recombinant interferon beta, albumin human or any other component of the formulation
Warnings/Precautions Anaphylaxis has been reported rarely with use. Associated with a high incidence of flu-like adverse effects; improvement in symptoms occurs over time. Hepatotoxicity has been reported with beta interferons, including rare reports of hepatitis (autoimmune) and hepatic failure requiring transplant. Interferons have been associated with severe psychiatric adverse events (psychosis, mania, depression, suicidal behavior/ideation) in patients with and without previous psychiatric symptoms, avoid use in severe psychiatric disorders and use caution in patients with a history of depression; patients exhibiting symptoms of depression should be closely monitored and discontinuation of therapy should be considered. Use caution in patients with pre-existing cardiovascular disease, pulmonary disease, seizure disorders, renal impairment or hepatic impairment. Use caution in myelosuppression; routine monitoring for leukopenia is recommended; dose reduction may be

required. Thyroid dysfunction has rarely been reported with use. Severe injection site reactions (necrosis) may occur, which may or may not heal with continued therapy; patient and/or caregiver competency in injection technique should be confirmed and periodically re-evaluated. Contains albumin, which may carry a remote risk of transmitting viral diseases.

Adverse Reactions (Reflective of adult population; not specific for elderly) Note: Flu-like syndrome (including at least two of the following - headache, fever, chills, malaise, diaphoresis, and myalgia) are reported in the majority of patients (60%) and decrease over time (average duration ~1 week).

>10%:
 Cardiovascular: Peripheral edema (15%), chest pain (11%)
 Central nervous system: Headache (57%), fever (36%), pain (51%), chills (25%), dizziness (24%), insomnia (24%)
 Dermatologic: Rash (24%), skin disorder (12%)
 Endocrine & metabolic: Metrorrhagia (11%)
 Gastrointestinal: Nausea (27%), diarrhea (19%), abdominal pain (19%), constipation (20%), dyspepsia (14%)
 Genitourinary: Urinary urgency (13%)
 Hematologic: Lymphopenia (88%), neutropenia (14%), leukopenia (14%)
 Local: Injection site reaction (85%), inflammation (53%), pain (18%)
 Neuromuscular & skeletal: Weakness (61%), myalgia (27%), hypertonia (50%), myasthenia (46%), arthralgia (31%), incoordination (21%)
 Miscellaneous: Flu-like syndrome (decreases over treatment course; 60%), neutralizing antibodies (≤45%; significance not known)
1% to 10%:
 Cardiovascular: Palpitation (4%), vasodilation (8%), hypertension (7%), tachycardia (4%), peripheral vascular disorder (6%)
 Central nervous system: Anxiety (10%), malaise (8%), nervousness (7%)
 Dermatologic: Alopecia (4%)
 Endocrine & metabolic: Menorrhagia (8%), dysmenorrhea (7%)
 Gastrointestinal: Weight gain (7%)
 Genitourinary: Impotence (9%), pelvic pain (6%), cystitis (8%), urinary frequency (7%), prostatic disorder (3%)
 Hematologic: Lymphadenopathy (8%)
 Hepatic: ALT increased >5x baseline (10%), AST increased >5x baseline (3%)
 Local: Injection site necrosis (4% to 5%), edema (3%), mass (2%)
 Neuromuscular & skeletal: Leg cramps (4%)
 Respiratory: Dyspnea (7%)
 Miscellaneous: Diaphoresis (8%), hypersensitivity (3%)

Drug Interactions
 Metabolism/Transport Effects None known.
 Avoid Concomitant Use There are no known interactions where it is recommended to avoid concomitant use.
 Increased Effect/Toxicity
  Interferon Beta-1b may increase the levels/effects of: Theophylline Derivatives; Zidovudine
  Decreased Effect There are no known significant interactions involving a decrease in effect.

Stability Store at room temperature of 25°C (77°F); excursions permitted to 15°C to 30°C (59°F to 86°F). To reconstitute solution, inject 1.2 mL of diluent (provided); gently swirl to dissolve, do not shake. Reconstituted solution provides 0.25 mg/mL (8 million units). If not used immediately following reconstitution, refrigerate solution at 2°C to 8°C (36°F to 46°F) and use within 3 hours; do not freeze or shake solution. Discard unused portion of vial.

Mechanism of Action Interferon beta-1b differs from naturally occurring human protein by a single amino acid substitution and the lack of carbohydrate side chains; mechanism in the treatment of MS is unknown; however, immunomodulatory effects attributed to interferon beta-1b include enhancement of suppressor T cell activity, reduction of proinflammatory cytokines, down-regulation of antigen presentation, and reduced trafficking of lymphocytes into the central nervous system. Improves MRI lesions, decreases relapse rate, and disease severity in patients with secondary progressive MS.

Pharmacodynamics/Kinetics Limited data due to small doses used
 Half-life elimination: 8 minutes to 4.3 hours
 Time to peak, serum: 1-8 hours

Dosage
 Geriatric & Adult Note: Gradual dose-titration, analgesics, and/or antipyretics may help decrease flu-like symptoms on treatment days.
  Multiple sclerosis (relapsing): Initial: 0.0625 mg (2 million units [0.25 mL]) every other day; gradually increase dose by 0.0625 every 2 weeks
   Target dose: 0.25 mg (8 million units [1 mL]) every other day

INTERFERON BETA-1B

Multiple sclerosis (secondary-progressive) [Canadian labeling; not in U.S. labeling]:
Initial: 0.125 mg (4 million units [0.5 mL]) every other day for 2 weeks
Target dose: 0.25 mg (8 million units [1 mL]) every other day

Administration Withdraw dose of reconstituted solution from the vial into a sterile syringe fitted with a 27-gauge needle and inject the solution subcutaneously; sites for self-injection include outer surface of the arms, abdomen, hips, and thighs. Rotate SubQ injection site. Patient should be well hydrated.

Monitoring Parameters Complete blood chemistries (including platelet count) and liver function tests are recommended at 1, 3, and 6 months following initiation of therapy and periodically thereafter. Thyroid function should be assessed every 6 months in patients with history of thyroid dysfunction.

Pharmacotherapy Pearls American Academy of Neurology and MS Council guidelines suggest that, based upon published data, 6 million units of Avonex® (interferon beta-1a) (30 mcg) is equivalent to approximately 7-9 million units of Betaseron® (220-280 mcg).

Special Geriatric Considerations No specific recommendations necessary for use in the elderly. Monitor for CNS adverse effects which may be significant in the elderly.

Dosage Forms Excipient information presented when available (limited, particularly for generics); consult specific product labeling.
Injection, powder for reconstitution [preservative free]:
Betaseron®: 0.3 mg [~9.6 million units] [contains albumin (human); supplied with diluent]
Extavia®: 0.3 mg [~9.6 million units] [contains albumin (human); supplied with diluent]

- ◆ **Interleukin-1 Receptor Antagonist** *see* Anakinra *on page* 132
- ◆ **Intermezzo®** *see* Zolpidem *on page* 2064
- ◆ **Intropin** *see* DOPamine *on page* 593
- ◆ **Intuniv®** *see* GuanFACINE *on page* 908
- ◆ **INVanz®** *see* Ertapenem *on page* 662
- ◆ **Invega®** *see* Paliperidone *on page* 1457
- ◆ **Invega® Sustenna®** *see* Paliperidone *on page* 1457
- ◆ **Iodine and Potassium Iodide** *see* Potassium Iodide and Iodine *on page* 1575

Iodoquinol (eye oh doe KWIN ole)

Brand Names: U.S. Yodoxin®
Brand Names: Canada Diodoquin®
Index Terms Diiodohydroxyquin
Generic Availability (U.S.) No
Pharmacologic Category Amebicide
Use Treatment of acute and chronic intestinal amebiasis; asymptomatic cyst passers; *Blastocystis hominis* infections; ineffective for amebic hepatitis or hepatic abscess
Dosage
Geriatric This agent is no longer a drug of choice; use only if other therapy is contraindicated or has failed. Due to optic nerve damage, use cautiously in the elderly.
Adult Treatment of susceptible infections: Oral: 650 mg 3 times/day after meals for 20 days; not to exceed 2 g/day

Special Geriatric Considerations This agent is no longer a drug of choice; use only if other therapy is contraindicated or has failed. Due to optic nerve damage, use cautiously in the elderly.

Dosage Forms Excipient information presented when available (limited, particularly for generics); consult specific product labeling.
Tablet, oral:
Yodoxin®: 210 mg, 650 mg

- ◆ **Ionil® [OTC]** *see* Salicylic Acid *on page* 1743
- ◆ **Ionil Plus® [OTC]** *see* Salicylic Acid *on page* 1743
- ◆ **Iophen C-NR** *see* Guaifenesin and Codeine *on page* 906
- ◆ **Iophen DM-NR [OTC]** *see* Guaifenesin and Dextromethorphan *on page* 906
- ◆ **Iophen NR [OTC]** *see* GuaiFENesin *on page* 904
- ◆ **Iopidine®** *see* Apraclonidine *on page* 138
- ◆ **IPOL®** *see* Poliovirus Vaccine (Inactivated) *on page* 1561

Ipratropium (Oral Inhalation) (i pra TROE pee um)

Related Information
Inhalant Agents *on page 2117*
Medication Safety Issues
Sound-alike/look-alike issues:
Atrovent® may be confused with Alupent, Serevent®
Ipratropium may be confused with tiotropium
Brand Names: U.S. Atrovent® HFA
Brand Names: Canada Atrovent® HFA; Gen-Ipratropium; Mylan-Ipratropium Sterinebs; Novo-Ipramide; Nu-Ipratropium; PMS-Ipratropium
Index Terms Ipratropium Bromide
Generic Availability (U.S.) Yes: Solution for nebulization
Pharmacologic Category Anticholinergic Agent
Use Anticholinergic bronchodilator used in bronchospasm associated with COPD, bronchitis, and emphysema
Contraindications Hypersensitivity to ipratropium, atropine (and its derivatives), or any component of the formulation
Warnings/Precautions Immediate hypersensitivity reactions (urticaria, angioedema, rash, bronchospasm) have been reported. Rarely, paradoxical bronchospasm may occur with use of inhaled bronchodilating agents; this should be distinguished from inadequate response. Not indicated for the initial treatment of acute episodes of bronchospasm where rescue therapy is required for rapid response. Should only be used in acute exacerbations of asthma in conjunction with short-acting beta-adrenergic agonists for acute episodes. Use with caution in patients with myasthenia gravis, narrow-angle glaucoma, benign prostatic hyperplasia (BPH), or bladder neck obstruction
Adverse Reactions (Reflective of adult population; not specific for elderly)
>10%: Respiratory: Upper respiratory tract infection (9% to 34%), bronchitis (10% to 23%), sinusitis (1% to 11%)
1% to 10%:
Cardiovascular: Chest pain (3%), palpitation
Central nervous system: Headache (6% to 7%), dizziness (2% to 3%)
Gastrointestinal: Dyspepsia (1% to 5%), nausea (4%), xerostomia (2% to 4%)
Genitourinary: Urinary tract infection (2% to 10%)
Neuromuscular & skeletal: Back pain (2% to 7%)
Respiratory: Dyspnea (7% to 10%), rhinitis (2% to 6%), cough (3% to 5%), pharyngitis (4%), bronchospasm (2%), sputum increased (1%)
Miscellaneous: Flu-like syndrome (4% to 8%)
Drug Interactions
Metabolism/Transport Effects None known.
Avoid Concomitant Use There are no known interactions where it is recommended to avoid concomitant use.
Increased Effect/Toxicity
Ipratropium (Oral Inhalation) may increase the levels/effects of: AbobotulinumtoxinA; Anticholinergics; Cannabinoids; OnabotulinumtoxinA; Potassium Chloride; RimabotulinumtoxinB

The levels/effects of Ipratropium (Oral Inhalation) may be increased by: Pramlintide
Decreased Effect
Ipratropium (Oral Inhalation) may decrease the levels/effects of: Acetylcholinesterase Inhibitors (Central); Secretin

The levels/effects of Ipratropium (Oral Inhalation) may be decreased by: Acetylcholinesterase Inhibitors (Central)
Stability
Aerosol: Store at controlled room temperature of 25°C (77°F). Do not store near heat or open flame.
Solution: Store at 15°C to 30°C (59°F to 86°F). Protect from light.
Mechanism of Action Blocks the action of acetylcholine at parasympathetic sites in bronchial smooth muscle causing bronchodilation; local application to nasal mucosa inhibits serous and seromucous gland secretions.
Pharmacodynamics/Kinetics
Onset of action: Bronchodilation: Within 15 minutes
Peak effect: 1-2 hours
Duration: 2-5 hours
Absorption: Negligible

◀ Distribution: 15% of dose reaches lower airways
Protein Binding: ≤9%
Half-life elimination: 2 hours
Excretion: Urine

Dosage
Geriatric & Adult
Asthma exacerbation, acute (*NIH Asthma Guidelines, 2007*):
  Nebulization: 500 mcg every 20 minutes for 3 doses, then as needed. **Note:** Should be given in combination with a short-acting beta-adrenergic agonist.
  Metered-dose inhaler: 8 inhalations every 20 minutes as needed for up to 3 hours. **Note:** Should be given in combination with a short-acting beta-adrenergic agonist.
Bronchospasm associated with COPD:
  Nebulization: 500 mcg (one unit-dose vial) 3-4 times/day with doses 6-8 hours apart
  Metered-dose inhaler: 2 inhalations 4 times/day, up to 12 inhalations/24 hours

Administration Avoid spraying into the eyes.
Atrovent® HFA: Prior to initial use, prime inhaler by releasing 2 test sprays into the air. If the inhaler has not been used for >3 days, reprime.

Monitoring Parameters Pulmonary function tests

Special Geriatric Considerations The elderly may find it difficult to use the metered dose inhaler. A spacer device may be useful. Monitor urinary function in elderly men with benign prostatic hyperplasia while on this medication.

Dosage Forms Excipient information presented when available (limited, particularly for generics); consult specific product labeling.
Aerosol, for oral inhalation, as bromide:
  Atrovent® HFA: 17 mcg/actuation (12.9 g) [chlorofluorocarbon free; 200 metered actuations]
  Solution, for nebulization, as bromide: 0.02% [500 mcg/2.5 mL] (25s, 30s, 60s)
  Solution, for nebulization, as bromide [preservative free]: 0.02% [500 mcg/2.5 mL] (25s, 30s, 60s)

Ipratropium (Nasal) (i pra TROE pee um)

Related Information
Inhalant Agents *on page 2117*

Medication Safety Issues
Sound-alike/look-alike issues:
  Atrovent® may be confused with Alupent, Serevent®
  Ipratropium may be confused with tiotropium

Brand Names: U.S. Atrovent®

Brand Names: Canada Alti-Ipratropium; Apo-Ipravent®; Atrovent®; Mylan-Ipratropium Solution

Index Terms Ipratropium Bromide

Generic Availability (U.S.) Yes

Pharmacologic Category Anticholinergic Agent

Use Symptomatic relief of rhinorrhea associated with the common cold and allergic and nonallergic rhinitis

Dosage
Geriatric & Adult
Colds (symptomatic relief of rhinorrhea): Safety and efficacy of use beyond 4 days not established: *Intranasal:* Nasal spray (0.06%): 2 sprays in each nostril 3-4 times/day
Allergic/nonallergic rhinitis: *Intranasal:* Nasal spray (0.03%): 2 sprays in each nostril 2-3 times/day
Seasonal allergic rhinitis (safety and efficacy of use beyond 3 weeks in patients with seasonal allergic rhinitis has not been established): *Intranasal:* Nasal spray (0.06%): 2 sprays in each nostril 4 times/day

Special Geriatric Considerations Evaluate the patient's or caregiver's ability to safely administer the correct dose of nasal medication.

Ipratropium nasal has not been specifically studied in the elderly.

Dosage Forms Excipient information presented when available (limited, particularly for generics); consult specific product labeling.
Solution, intranasal, as bromide [spray]: 0.03% (30 mL); 0.06% (15 mL) [delivers 42 mcg/spray; 165 sprays]; 0.06% (15 mL)
  Atrovent®: 0.03% (30 mL) [contains benzalkonium chloride; delivers 21 mcg/spray; 345 sprays]
  Atrovent®: 0.06% (15 mL) [contains benzalkonium chloride; delivers 42 mcg/spray; 165 sprays]

Ipratropium and Albuterol (i pra TROE pee um & al BYOO ter ole)

Related Information
Albuterol *on page 49*
Ipratropium (Oral Inhalation) *on page 1035*
Medication Safety Issues
Sound-alike/look-alike issues:
Combivent® may be confused with Combivir®, Serevent®
DuoNeb® may be confused with DuoTrav™, Duovent® UDV
Brand Names: U.S. Combivent®; DuoNeb®
Brand Names: Canada CO Ipra-Sal; Combivent UDV; Gen-Combo Sterinebs; ratio-Ipra Sal UDV
Index Terms Albuterol and Ipratropium; Salbutamol and Ipratropium
Generic Availability (U.S.) Yes: Solution for nebulization
Pharmacologic Category Anticholinergic Agent; Beta$_2$-Adrenergic Agonist
Use Treatment of COPD in those patients who are currently on a regular bronchodilator who continue to have bronchospasms and require a second bronchodilator
Dosage
Geriatric & Adult
COPD:
Aerosol for inhalation: 2 metered-dose inhalations 4 times/day; may receive additional doses as necessary, but total number of doses in 24 hours should not exceed 12 inhalations.
Solution for nebulization: Initial: 3 mL every 6 hours (maximum: 3 mL every 4 hours)
Special Geriatric Considerations See individual agents.
Product Availability
Combivent® Respimat®: FDA approved October 2011; availability expected mid-2012
Combivent® Respimat® spray is a non-CFC ipratropium and albuterol inhalation formulation approved for the treatment of COPD and will replace Combivent® inhalation aerosol, which is being phased out in accordance with the Montreal Protocol on Substances that Deplete the Ozone Layer.
Dosage Forms Excipient information presented when available (limited, particularly for generics); consult specific product labeling.
Aerosol, for oral inhalation:
Combivent®: Ipratropium bromide 18 mcg and albuterol (base) 90 mcg per inhalation (14.7 g) [contains chlorofluorocarbon, soya lecithin; 200 metered actuations]
Solution, for nebulization: Ipratropium bromide 0.5 mg and albuterol (base) 2.5 mg per 3 mL (30s, 60s)
DuoNeb®: Ipratropium bromide 0.5 mg and albuterol (base) 2.5 mg per 3 mL (30s, 60s)

Irbesartan (ir be SAR tan)

Related Information
Angiotensin Agents *on page 2093*
Medication Safety Issues
Sound-alike/look-alike issues:
Avapro® may be confused with Anaprox®
Brand Names: U.S. Avapro®
Brand Names: Canada Avapro®; CO Irbesartan; PMS-Irbesartan; ratio-Irbesartan; Sandoz-Irbesartan; Teva-Irbesartan
Generic Availability (U.S.) Yes
Pharmacologic Category Angiotensin II Receptor Blocker
Use Treatment of hypertension alone or in combination with other antihypertensives; treatment of diabetic nephropathy in patients with type 2 diabetes mellitus (noninsulin dependent, NIDDM) and hypertension
Contraindications Hypersensitivity to irbesartan or any component of the formulation

Warnings/Precautions May cause hyperkalemia; avoid potassium supplementation unless specifically required by healthcare provider. May be associated with deterioration of renal function and/or increases in serum creatinine, particularly in patients with low renal blood flow (eg, renal artery stenosis, heart failure) whose glomerular filtration rate (GFR) is dependent on efferent arteriolar vasoconstriction by angiotensin II. Avoid use or use a much smaller dose in patients who are intravascularly volume-depleted; use caution in patients with unstented unilateral or bilateral renal artery stenosis. When unstented bilateral renal artery stenosis is present, use is generally avoided due to the elevated risk of deterioration in renal function unless possible benefits outweigh risks. AUCs of irbesartan (not the active metabolite) are about 50% greater in patients with Cl_{cr} <30 mL/minute and are doubled in hemodialysis patients. Concurrent use of ACE inhibitors may increase the risk of clinically-significant adverse events (eg, renal dysfunction, hyperkalemia).

Adverse Reactions (Reflective of adult population; not specific for elderly) Unless otherwise indicated, percentage of incidence is reported for patients with hypertension.

>10%: Endocrine & metabolic: Hyperkalemia (19%, diabetic nephropathy; rarely seen in HTN)

1% to 10%:
  Cardiovascular: Orthostatic hypotension (5%, diabetic nephropathy)
  Central nervous system: Fatigue (4%), dizziness (10%, diabetic nephropathy)
  Gastrointestinal: Diarrhea (3%), dyspepsia (2%)
  Respiratory: Upper respiratory infection (9%), cough (2.8% versus 2.7% in placebo)

Drug Interactions

Metabolism/Transport Effects Substrate of CYP2C9 (minor); **Note:** Assignment of Major/Minor substrate status based on clinically relevant drug interaction potential; **Inhibits** CYP2C8 (moderate), CYP2C9 (moderate), CYP2D6 (weak), CYP3A4 (weak)

Avoid Concomitant Use

Avoid concomitant use of Irbesartan with any of the following: Pimozide

Increased Effect/Toxicity

Irbesartan may increase the levels/effects of: ACE Inhibitors; Amifostine; Antihypertensives; ARIPiprazole; Carvedilol; CYP2C8 Substrates; CYP2C9 Substrates; Hypotensive Agents; Lithium; Nonsteroidal Anti-Inflammatory Agents; Pimozide; Potassium-Sparing Diuretics; RiTUXimab; Sodium Phosphates

The levels/effects of Irbesartan may be increased by: Alfuzosin; Aliskiren; Diazoxide; Eplerenone; Fluconazole; Herbs (Hypotensive Properties); MAO Inhibitors; Pentoxifylline; Phosphodiesterase 5 Inhibitors; Potassium Salts; Prostacyclin Analogues; Tolvaptan; Trimethoprim

Decreased Effect

The levels/effects of Irbesartan may be decreased by: Herbs (Hypertensive Properties); Methylphenidate; Nonsteroidal Anti-Inflammatory Agents; Rifamycin Derivatives; Yohimbine

Ethanol/Nutrition/Herb Interactions Herb/Nutraceutical: Dong quai has estrogenic activity. Some herbal medications may worsen hypertension (eg, ephedra); garlic may have additional antihypertensive effects. Management: Avoid dong quai if using for hypertension. Avoid ephedra, yohimbe, ginseng, and garlic.

Stability Store at room temperature of 15°C to 30°C (59°F to 86°F).

Mechanism of Action Irbesartan is an angiotensin receptor antagonist. Angiotensin II acts as a vasoconstrictor. In addition to causing direct vasoconstriction, angiotensin II also stimulates the release of aldosterone. Once aldosterone is released, sodium as well as water are reabsorbed. The end result is an elevation in blood pressure. Irbesartan binds to the AT1 angiotensin II receptor. This binding prevents angiotensin II from binding to the receptor thereby blocking the vasoconstriction and the aldosterone secreting effects of angiotensin II.

Pharmacodynamics/Kinetics

Onset of action: Peak effect: 1-2 hours
Duration: >24 hours
Distribution: V_d: 53-93 L
Protein binding, plasma: 90%
Metabolism: Hepatic, primarily CYP2C9
Bioavailability: 60% to 80%
Half-life elimination: Terminal: 11-15 hours
Time to peak, serum: 1.5-2 hours
Excretion: Feces (80%); urine (20%)

Dosage

Geriatric & Adult

Hypertension: Oral: 150 mg once daily; patients may be titrated to 300 mg once daily. **Note:** Starting dose in volume-depleted patients should be 75 mg.

Nephropathy in patients with type 2 diabetes and hypertension: Oral: Target dose: 300 mg once daily

Renal Impairment No dosage adjustment necessary with mild to severe impairment unless the patient is also volume depleted.

Monitoring Parameters Electrolytes, serum creatinine, BUN, urinalysis

Special Geriatric Considerations No dosage adjustment is necessary when initiating angiotensin II receptor antagonists in the elderly. In clinical studies, no differences between younger adults and the elderly were demonstrated. Many elderly may be volume depleted due to diuretic use and/or blunted thirst reflex resulting in inadequate fluid intake.

Dosage Forms Excipient information presented when available (limited, particularly for generics); consult specific product labeling.

Tablet, oral: 75 mg, 150 mg, 300 mg

Avapro®: 75 mg, 150 mg, 300 mg

Irbesartan and Hydrochlorothiazide
(ir be SAR tan & hye droe klor oh THYE a zide)

Related Information
Hydrochlorothiazide *on page 933*
Irbesartan *on page 1037*

Medication Safety Issues
Sound-alike/look-alike issues:
Avalide® may be confused with Avandia®

Brand Names: U.S. Avalide®

Brand Names: Canada Avalide®; CO Irbesartan HCT; Irbesartan-HCTZ; PMS-Irbesartan HCTZ; Ran™-Irbesartan HCTZ; ratio-Irbesartan HCTZ; Sandoz-Irbesartan HCT; Teva-Irbesartan HCTZ

Index Terms Avapro® HCT; Hydrochlorothiazide and Irbesartan

Generic Availability (U.S.) Yes

Pharmacologic Category Angiotensin II Receptor Blocker; Diuretic, Thiazide

Use Combination therapy for the management of hypertension; may be used as initial therapy in patients likely to need multiple drugs to achieve blood pressure goals

Dosage
Geriatric & Adult Dose must be individualized.

Hypertension: Oral: **Note:** Maximum antihypertensive effects are attained within 2-4 weeks after initiation or a change in dose; however, if necessary, may carefully titrate dose as soon as after 1 week of treatment.

Add-on therapy: A patient who is not controlled with either agent alone may be switched to the combination product. The lowest dosage available is irbesartan 150 mg/hydrochlorothiazide 12.5 mg.

Initial therapy: Irbesartan 150 mg/hydrochlorothiazide 12.5 mg once daily. If initial response is inadequate, may titrate dose after 1-2 weeks, to a maximum dose of irbesartan 300 mg/hydrochlorothiazide 25 mg once daily.

Renal Impairment Not recommended in patients with Cl_{cr} ≤30 mL/minute.

Hepatic Impairment Use with caution.

Special Geriatric Considerations See individual agents. Combination products are not recommended as first-line treatment. Use only if doses of individual agents correspond to the combination available.

Dosage Forms Excipient information presented when available (limited, particularly for generics); consult specific product labeling. [DSC] = Discontinued product

Tablet: 150/12.5: Irbesartan 150 mg and hydrochlorothiazide 12.5 mg; 300/12.5: Irbesartan 300 mg and hydrochlorothiazide 12.5 mg

Avalide® 150/12.5: Irbesartan 150 mg and hydrochlorothiazide 12.5 mg

Avalide® 300/12.5: Irbesartan 300 mg and hydrochlorothiazide 12.5 mg [DSC]

Avalide® 300/25: Irbesartan 300 mg and hydrochlorothiazide 25 mg [DSC]

♦ **Ircon® [OTC]** *see* Ferrous Fumarate *on page 775*
♦ **Iron Dextran** *see* Iron Dextran Complex *on page 1039*

Iron Dextran Complex (EYE ern DEKS tran KOM pleks)

Medication Safety Issues
Sound-alike/look-alike issues:
Dexferrum® may be confused with Desferal®
Iron dextran complex may be confused with ferumoxytol

Brand Names: U.S. Dexferrum®; INFeD®

Brand Names: Canada Dexiron™; Infufer®

Index Terms High-Molecular-Weight Iron Dextran (DexFerrum®); Imferon; Iron Dextran; Low-Molecular-Weight Iron Dextran (INFeD®)

Generic Availability (U.S.) No

Pharmacologic Category Iron Salt

Use Treatment of iron deficiency in patients in whom oral administration is infeasible or ineffective

Unlabeled Use Cancer-/chemotherapy-associated anemia

Contraindications Hypersensitivity to iron dextran or any component of the formulation; any anemia not associated with iron deficiency

Warnings/Precautions [U.S. Boxed Warning]: Deaths associated with parenteral administration following anaphylactic-type reactions have been reported (use only where resuscitation equipment and personnel are available). A test dose should be administered to all patients prior to the first therapeutic dose. Fatal reactions have occurred even in patients who tolerated the test dose. Monitor patients for signs/symptoms of anaphylactic reactions during any iron dextran administration. A history of drug allergy (including multiple drug allergies) and/or the concomitant use of an ACE inhibitor may increase the risk of anaphylactic-type reactions. Adverse events (including life-threatening) associated with iron dextran usually occur with the high-molecular-weight formulation (Dexferrum®), compared to low-molecular-weight (INFeD®) (Chertow, 2006). Delayed (1-2 days) infusion reaction (including arthralgia, back pain, chills, dizziness, and fever) may occur with large doses (eg, total dose infusion) of I.V. iron dextran; usually subsides within 3-4 days. Delayed reaction may also occur (less commonly) with I.M. administration; subsiding within 3-7 days. Use with caution in patients with a history of significant allergies, asthma, serious hepatic impairment, pre-existing cardiac disease (may exacerbate cardiovascular complications), and rheumatoid arthritis (may exacerbate joint pain and swelling). Avoid use during acute kidney infection.

In patients with chronic kidney disease (CKD) requiring iron supplementation, the I.V. route is preferred for hemodialysis patients; either oral iron or I.V. iron may be used for nondialysis and peritoneal dialysis CKD patients. In patients with cancer-related anemia (either due to cancer or chemotherapy-induced) requiring iron supplementation, the I.V. route is superior to oral therapy; I.M. administration is not recommended for parenteral iron supplementation.

[U.S. Boxed Warning]: Use only in patients where the iron deficient state is not amenable to oral iron therapy. Discontinue oral iron prior to initiating parenteral iron therapy. Exogenous hemosiderosis may result from excess iron stores; patients with refractory anemias and/or hemoglobinopathies may be prone to iron overload with unwarranted iron supplementation. Anemia in the elderly is often caused by "anemia of chronic disease" or associated with inflammation rather than blood loss. Iron stores are usually normal or increased, with a serum ferritin >50 ng/mL and a decreased total iron binding capacity. I.V. administration of iron dextran is often preferred over I.M. in the elderly secondary to a decreased muscle mass and the need for daily injections. Intramuscular injections of iron-carbohydrate complexes may have a risk of delayed injection site tumor development. Iron dextran products differ in chemical characteristics. The high-molecular-weight formulation (Dexferrum®) and the low-molecular-weight formulation (INFeD®) are not clinically interchangeable.

Adverse Reactions (Reflective of adult population; not specific for elderly) Frequency not defined. **Note:** Adverse event risk is reported to be higher with the high-molecular-weight iron dextran formulation.

Cardiovascular: Arrhythmia, bradycardia, cardiac arrest, chest pain, chest tightness, cyanosis, flushing, hyper-/hypotension, shock, syncope, tachycardia

Central nervous system: Chills, disorientation, dizziness, fever, headache, malaise, seizure, unconsciousness, unresponsiveness

Dermatologic: Pruritus, purpura, rash, urticaria

Gastrointestinal: Abdominal pain, diarrhea, nausea, taste alteration, vomiting

Genitourinary: Discoloration of urine

Hematologic: Leukocytosis, lymphadenopathy

Local: Injection site reactions (cellulitis, inflammation, pain, phlebitis, soreness, swelling), muscle atrophy/fibrosis (with I.M. injection), skin/tissue staining (at the site of I.M. injection), sterile abscess

Neuromuscular & skeletal: Arthralgia, arthritis/arthritis exacerbation, back pain, myalgia, paresthesia, weakness

Respiratory: Bronchospasm, dyspnea, respiratory arrest, wheezing

Renal: Hematuria

Miscellaneous: Anaphylactic reactions (sudden respiratory difficulty, cardiovascular collapse), diaphoresis

Drug Interactions

Metabolism/Transport Effects None known.

Avoid Concomitant Use

Avoid concomitant use of Iron Dextran Complex with any of the following: Dimercaprol

Increased Effect/Toxicity

The levels/effects of Iron Dextran Complex may be increased by: ACE Inhibitors; Dimercaprol

Decreased Effect There are no known significant interactions involving a decrease in effect.

Stability Store at controlled room temperature. Solutions for infusion should be diluted in 250-1000 mL NS.

Mechanism of Action The released iron, from the plasma, eventually replenishes the depleted iron stores in the bone marrow where it is incorporated into hemoglobin

Pharmacodynamics/Kinetics

Onset of action: I.V.: Serum ferritin peak: 7-9 days after dose

Absorption:

I.M.: 50% to 90% is promptly absorbed, balance is slowly absorbed over month

I.V.: Uptake of iron by the reticuloendothelial system appears to be constant at about 10-20 mg/hour

Excretion: Urine and feces via reticuloendothelial system

Dosage

Geriatric & Adult

Note: A 0.5 mL test dose should be given prior to starting iron dextran therapy.

Iron-deficiency anemia: I.M. (INFeD®), I.V. (Dexferrum®, INFeD®):

Dose (mL) = 0.0442 (desired Hgb - observed Hgb) x LBW + (0.26 x LBW)

Desired hemoglobin: Usually 14.8 g/dL

LBW = Lean body weight in kg

Iron replacement therapy for blood loss: (INFeD®), I.V. (Dexferrum®, INFeD®): Replacement iron (mg) = blood loss (mL) x Hct

Maximum daily dosage: Manufacturer's labeling: **Note:** Replacement of larger estimated iron deficits may be achieved by serial administration of smaller incremental dosages. Daily dosages should be limited to 100 mg iron (2 mL)

Total dose infusion (unlabeled): The entire dose (estimated iron deficit) may be diluted and administered as a one-time I.V. infusion.

Cancer-/chemotherapy-associated anemia (NCCN guidelines v.2.2010) (unlabeled use): I.V.: Test dose: 25 mg slow I.V. slow push, followed 1 hour later by 100 mg over 5 minutes; larger doses (unlabeled), up to total dose infusion (over several hours) may be administered. Low-molecular-weight iron dextran preferred.

Administration Note: Test dose: A test dose should be given on the first day of therapy; patient should be observed for 1 hour for hypersensitivity reaction, then the remaining dose (dose minus test dose) should be given. Epinephrine should be available.

I.M. (INFeD®): Use Z-track technique (displacement of the skin laterally prior to injection); injection should be deep into the upper outer quadrant of buttock; alternate buttocks with subsequent injections. Administer test dose at same recommended site using the same technique.

I.V.: Test dose should be given gradually over at least 30 seconds (INFeD®) or 5 minutes (Dexferrum®). Subsequent dose(s) may be administered by I.V. bolus undiluted at a rate not to exceed 50 mg/minute or diluted in 250-1000 mL NS and infused over 1-6 hours (initial 25 mL should be given slowly and patient should be observed for allergic reactions); avoid dilutions with dextrose (increased incidence of local pain and phlebitis)

Monitoring Parameters Hemoglobin, hematocrit, reticulocyte count, serum ferritin, serum iron, TIBC; monitor for anaphylaxis/hypersensitivity reaction (during test dose and therapeutic dose)

Reference Range

Hemoglobin: Adults:

Males: 13.5-16.5 g/dL

Females: 12.0-15.0 g/dL

Serum iron: 40-160 mcg/dL

Total iron binding capacity: 230-430 mcg/dL

Transferrin: 204-360 mg/dL

Percent transferrin saturation: 20% to 50%

Test Interactions May cause falsely elevated values of serum bilirubin and falsely decreased values of serum calcium. Residual iron dextran may remain in reticuloendothelial cells; may affect accuracy of examination of bone marrow iron stores. Bone scans with 99m Tc-labeled bone seeking agents may show reduced bony uptake, marked renal activity, and excess blood pooling and soft tissue accumulation following I.V. iron dextran infusion or with high serum ferritin levels. Following I.M. iron dextran, bone scans with 99m Tc-diphosphonate may show dense activity in the buttocks.

◄ **Pharmacotherapy Pearls** Avoid iron injection if oral intake is feasible; a test dose of 0.5 mL I.V. or I.M. should be given to observe for adverse reactions

Special Geriatric Considerations Anemia in the elderly is most often caused by "anemia of chronic disease," a result of aging effect in bone marrow, or associated with inflammation rather than blood loss. Iron stores are usually normal or increased, with a serum ferritin >50 ng/mL and a decreased total iron binding capacity. Hence, the anemia is not secondary to iron deficiency but the inability of the reticuloendothelial system to use available iron stores. I.V. administration of iron is often preferred over I.M. in the elderly secondary to a decreased muscle mass and the need for daily injections.

Dosage Forms Excipient information presented when available (limited, particularly for generics); consult specific product labeling.

Injection, solution:

Dexferrum®: Elemental iron 50 mg/mL (1 mL, 2 mL) [high-molecular-weight iron dextran]

INFeD®: Elemental iron 50 mg/mL (2 mL) [low-molecular-weight iron dextran]

◆ **Iron Fumarate** see Ferrous Fumarate on page 775
◆ **Iron Gluconate** see Ferrous Gluconate on page 777
◆ **Iron-Polysaccharide Complex, Vitamin B12, and Folic Acid** see Polysaccharide-Iron Complex, Vitamin B12, and Folic Acid on page 1566

Iron Sucrose (EYE ern SOO krose)

Medication Safety Issues

Sound-alike/look-alike issues:

Iron sucrose may be confused with ferumoxytol

Brand Names: U.S. Venofer®

Brand Names: Canada Venofer®

Generic Availability (U.S.) No

Pharmacologic Category Iron Salt

Use Treatment of iron-deficiency anemia in chronic renal failure, including nondialysis-dependent patients (with or without erythropoietin therapy) and dialysis-dependent patients receiving erythropoietin therapy

Unlabeled Use Cancer-/chemotherapy-associated anemia

Contraindications Hypersensitivity to iron sucrose or any component of the formulation; evidence of iron overload; anemia not caused by iron deficiency

Warnings/Precautions Hypersensitivity reactions, including rare postmarketing anaphylactic and anaphylactoid reactions, have been reported. Hypotension has been reported frequently in hemodialysis-dependent patients. Hypotension has also been reported in peritoneal dialysis and nondialysis patients. Hypotension may be related to total dose or rate of administration (avoid rapid I.V. injection), follow recommended guidelines. Withhold iron in the presence of tissue iron overload; periodic monitoring of hemoglobin, hematocrit, serum ferritin, and transferrin saturation is recommended.

Adverse Reactions (Reflective of adult population; not specific for elderly)

>10%:

Cardiovascular: Hypotension (1% to 7%; 39% in hemodialysis patients; may be related to total dose or rate of administration), peripheral edema (2% to 17%)

Central nervous system: Headache (3% to 13%)

Gastrointestinal: Diarrhea (1% to 17%), nausea (1% to 15%), vomiting (3% to 12%)

Neuromuscular & skeletal: Muscle cramps (1% to 3%; 29% in hemodialysis patients)

1% to 10%:

Cardiovascular: Hypertension (6% to 8%), edema (1% to 7%), chest pain (1% to 6%), murmur (<1% to 3%), heart failure (2%), myocardial infarction (1%)

Central nervous system: Dizziness (1% to 10%), fatigue (2% to 5%), fever (1% to 3%), stroke (1%)

Dermatologic: Pruritus (1% to 7%), rash (≤1%)

Endocrine & metabolic: Gout (2% to 7%), hypoglycemia (<1% to 4%), hyperglycemia (3% to 4%), fluid overload (1% to 3%)

Gastrointestinal: Taste perversion (1% to 9%), peritoneal infection (≤8%), constipation (1% to 7%), abdominal pain (1% to 4%), positive fecal occult blood (1% to 3%)

Genitourinary: Urinary tract infection (≤1%)

Local: Injection site reaction (2% to 6%), catheter site infection (≤4%)

Neuromuscular & skeletal: Arthralgia (1% to 8%), back pain (1% to 8%), muscle pain (1% to 7%), extremity pain (3% to 6%), weakness (1% to 3%)

Ocular: Conjunctivitis (<1% to 3%)

Otic: Ear pain (1% to 7%)

Respiratory: Dyspnea (1% to 10%), pharyngitis (<1% to 7%), cough (1% to 7%), sinusitis (1% to 4%), nasopharyngitis (≤3%), upper respiratory infection (1% to 3%), nasal congestion (1%), pneumonia (1%), pulmonary edema (1%), rhinitis (≤1%)

Miscellaneous: Graft complication (1% to 10%), sepsis (2%)

Drug Interactions

Metabolism/Transport Effects None known.

Avoid Concomitant Use

Avoid concomitant use of Iron Sucrose with any of the following: Dimercaprol

Increased Effect/Toxicity

The levels/effects of Iron Sucrose may be increased by: Dimercaprol

Decreased Effect There are no known significant interactions involving a decrease in effect.

Stability Store vials at controlled room temperature of 25°C (77°F); do not freeze. May be administered via the dialysis line as an undiluted solution or by diluting 100 mg (5 mL) in a maximum of 100 mL normal saline. Doses ≥200 mg should be diluted in a maximum of 250 mL normal saline. Iron sucrose is stable for 7 days at room temperature or under refrigeration when undiluted in a plastic syringe or following dilution in normal saline in a plastic syringe (2-10 mg/mL) or I.V. bag (1-2 mg/mL) (data on file [American Regent, Inc, 2010]).

Mechanism of Action Iron sucrose is dissociated by the reticuloendothelial system into iron and sucrose. The released iron increases serum iron concentrations and is incorporated into hemoglobin.

Pharmacodynamics/Kinetics

Distribution: V_{dss}: Healthy adults: 7.9 L

Metabolism: Dissociated into iron and sucrose by the reticuloendothelial system

Half-life elimination: Healthy adults: 6 hours

Excretion: Healthy adults: Urine (5%) within 24 hours

Dosage

Geriatric Insufficient data to identify differences between elderly and other adults; use caution.

Adult Doses expressed in mg of **elemental** iron. **Note:** Test dose: Product labeling does not indicate need for a test dose in product-naive patients.

Iron-deficiency anemia in chronic renal disease: I.V.:

Hemodialysis-dependent patient: 100 mg over 2-5 minutes administered 1-3 times/week during dialysis; administer no more than 3 times/week to a cumulative total dose of 1000 mg (10 doses); may continue to administer at lowest dose necessary to maintain target hemoglobin, hematocrit, and iron storage parameters

Peritoneal dialysis-dependent patient: Two infusions of 300 mg each over 1.5 hours 14 days apart, followed by a single 400 mg infusion over 2.5 hours 14 days later (total cumulative dose of 1000 mg in 3 divided doses)

Nondialysis-dependent patient: 200 mg slow injection (over 2-5 minutes) on 5 different occasions within a 14-day period. Total cumulative dose: 1000 mg in 14-day period. **Note:** Dosage has also been administered as two infusions of 500 mg in a maximum of 250 mL normal saline infused over 3.5-4 hours on day 1 and day 14 (limited experience)

Cancer-/chemotherapy-associated anemia (unlabeled use): I.V. infusion: 200 mg over 1 hour; maximum 300-400 mg/infusion. Repeat dose every 2-3 weeks. Test doses (25 mg slow I.V. push) are recommended in patients with iron dextran hypersensitivity or those with other drug allergies (NCCN guidelines, v.2.2010)

Administration Not for rapid I.V. injection; inject slowly over 2-5 minutes. Can be administered through dialysis line. Do not mix with other medications or parenteral nutrient solutions.

Slow I.V. injection: May administer undiluted by slow I.V. injection (100 mg over 2-5 minutes in hemodialysis-dependent patients **or** 200 mg over 2-5 minutes in nondialysis-dependent patients)

Infusion: Dilute 100 mg in maximum of 100 mL normal saline; infuse over at least 15 minutes; 300 mg/250 mL should be infused over at least 1.5 hours; 400 mg/250 mL should be infused over at least 2.5 hours; 500 mg/250 mL should be infused over at least 3.5 hours

Monitoring Parameters Hematocrit, hemoglobin, serum ferritin, transferrin, percent transferrin saturation, TIBC; takes about 4 weeks of treatment to see increased serum iron and ferritin, and decreased TIBC. Serum iron concentrations should be drawn 48 hours after last dose.

Reference Range

Hemoglobin: Adults:

Males: 13.5-16.5 g/dL

Females: 12.0-15.0 g/dL

Serum iron: 40-160 mcg/dL

Total iron binding capacity: 230-430 mcg/dL

Transferrin: 204-360 mg/dL

Percent transferrin saturation: 20% to 50%

◀ **Test Interactions** May cause falsely elevated values of serum bilirubin and falsely decreased values of serum calcium.

Special Geriatric Considerations Anemia in the elderly is most often caused by "anemia of chronic disease," a result of aging effect in bone marrow, or associated with inflammation rather than blood loss. Iron stores are usually normal or increased, with a serum ferritin >50 ng/mL and a decreased total iron binding capacity. Hence, the anemia is not secondary to iron deficiency but the inability of the reticuloendothelial system to use available iron stores. I.V. administration of iron is often preferred over I.M. in the elderly secondary to a decreased muscle mass and the need for daily injections.

Dosage Forms Excipient information presented when available (limited, particularly for generics); consult specific product labeling.

Injection, solution [preservative free]:

Venofer®: Elemental iron 20 mg/mL (2.5 mL, 5 mL, 10 mL)

- ◆ **Iron Sulfate** see Ferrous Sulfate on page 778
- ◆ **ISD** see Isosorbide Dinitrate on page 1050
- ◆ **ISDN** see Isosorbide Dinitrate on page 1050
- ◆ **ISG** see Immune Globulin on page 982
- ◆ **ISMN** see Isosorbide Mononitrate on page 1052
- ◆ **Ismo®** see Isosorbide Mononitrate on page 1052
- ◆ **Isobamate** see Carisoprodol on page 298

Isocarboxazid (eye soe kar BOKS a zid)

Related Information
Antidepressant Agents on page 2097
Brand Names: U.S. Marplan®
Generic Availability (U.S.) No
Pharmacologic Category Antidepressant, Monoamine Oxidase Inhibitor
Use Treatment of depression
Medication Guide Available Yes
Contraindications

Hypersensitivity to isocarboxazid or any component of the formulation; cardiovascular disease (including CHF, or HTN); cerebrovascular disease; history of hepatic disease or abnormal liver function tests; pheochromocytoma; renal disease or severe renal impairment

Concurrent use of sympathomimetics (including amphetamines, cocaine, dopamine, epinephrine, methylphenidate, norepinephrine, or phenylephrine) and related compounds (methyldopa, levodopa, phenylalanine, tryptophan, or tyrosine), as well as ophthalmic alpha$_2$-agonists (apraclonidine, brimonidine); may result in behavioral and neurologic symptoms

CNS depressants, cyclobenzaprine, dextromethorphan, ethanol, meperidine, bupropion, buspirone; may result in delirium, excitation, hyper-/hypotension, hyperpyrexia, seizures, and coma

Isocarboxazid **initiation**: At least 2 weeks should elapse between the discontinuation of serotoninergic agents (including SSRIs and tricyclics) and the initiation of isocarboxazid; at least 5 weeks should elapse between the discontinuation of fluoxetine and the initiation of isocarboxazid; at least 1 week should elapse between the discontinuation of other monoamine oxidase (MAO) inhibitors and the initiation of isocarboxazid (using half the normal starting dose). In all cases, a sufficient amount of time must be allowed for the clearance of the serotoninergic agent and any active metabolites prior to the initiation of isocarboxazid.

Isocarboxazid **discontinuation**: At least 2 weeks should elapse between the discontinuation of isocarboxazid and the initiation of the following agents: Serotoninergic agents (including SSRIs, fluoxetine, and tricyclics), bupropion, and other antidepressants. Two to 3 weeks should elapse between the discontinuation of isocarboxazid and the initiation of meperidine. At least 10 days should elapse between the discontinuation of isocarboxazid and initiation of buspirone. At least 1 week should elapse between the discontinuation of isocarboxazid and the initiation of other MAO inhibitors (see specific agent for details).

Antihypertensive agents (including thiazide diuretics): may result in potentiation of antihypertensive effects.

General anesthesia, spinal anesthesia (hypotension may be exaggerated). Use caution with local anesthetics containing sympathomimetic agents. Discontinue drug 10 days prior to elective surgery.

Foods high in tyramine or dopamine content; foods and/or supplements containing tyrosine, phenylalanine, tryptophan, or caffeine; may result in hypertensive reactions.

Warnings/Precautions [U.S. Boxed Warning]: Antidepressants increase the risk of suicidal thinking and behavior in children, adolescents, and young adults (18-24 years of age) with major depressive disorder (MDD) and other psychiatric disorders; consider risk prior to prescribing. Short-term studies did not show an increased risk in patients >24 years of age and showed a decreased risk in patients ≥65 years. Closely monitor for clinical worsening, suicidality, or unusual changes in behavior; the patient's family or caregiver should be instructed to closely observe the patient and communicate condition with healthcare provider. A medication guide should be dispensed with each prescription.

The possibility of a suicide attempt is inherent in major depression and may persist until remission occurs. Monitor for worsening of depression or suicidality, especially during initiation of therapy (generally first 1-2 months) or with dose increases or decreases. Use caution in high-risk patients. Worsening depression and severe abrupt suicidality that are not part of the presenting symptoms may require discontinuation or modification of drug therapy. The patient's family or caregiver should be alerted to monitor patients for the emergence of suicidality and associated behaviors (such as agitation, irritability, hostility, impulsivity, and hypomania) and notify healthcare provider.

May worsen psychosis in some patients or precipitate a shift to mania or hypomania in patients with bipolar disorder. Patients presenting with depressive symptoms should be screened for bipolar disorder. Monotherapy in patients with bipolar disorder should be avoided. Isocarboxazid is not FDA approved for the treatment of bipolar depression. Isocarboxazid should not be used for initial therapy but reserved for patients who have not responded to other antidepressants.

Use with caution in patients who are hyperactive, hyperexcitable, have a seizure disorder, or who have glaucoma, hyperthyroidism, or diabetes, or renal impairment; avoid use in hepatic impairment or severe renal impairment. High potential for interactions; do not use with other MAO inhibitors or antidepressants. Avoid products containing sympathomimetic stimulants, dextromethorphan, disulfiram, and meperidine. Concurrent use with antihypertensive agents may lead to exaggeration of hypotensive effects. May cause orthostatic hypotension (especially at dosages >30 mg/day). Use with caution in patients with hypotension or patients who would not tolerate transient hypotensive episodes; effects may be additive when used with other agents known to cause orthostasis (phenothiazines). Hypertensive crisis may occur with foods/supplements high in tyramine, tryptophan, phenylalanine, or tyrosine content.

Discontinue at least 48 hours prior to myelography. May increase the risks associated with electroconvulsive therapy. Consider discontinuing, when possible, prior to elective surgery. Use with caution in patients receiving disulfiram.

Adverse Reactions (Reflective of adult population; not specific for elderly)
>10%: Central nervous system: Dizziness (29%), headache (15%)
1% to 10%:
Cardiovascular: Orthostatic hypotension (4%), syncope (2%), palpitation (2%)
Central nervous system: Sleep disturbance (5%), drowsiness (4%), anxiety (2%), chills (2%), forgetfulness (2%), hyperactivity (2%), lethargy (2%), sedation (2%)
Gastrointestinal: Xerostomia (9%), constipation (7%), nausea (6%), diarrhea (2%)
Genitourinary: Urinary frequency (2%), impotence (2%), urinary hesitancy (1%)
Neuromuscular & skeletal: Tremor (4%), myoclonus (2%), paresthesia (2%)
Miscellaneous: Diaphoresis (2%), heavy feeling (2%)

Drug Interactions
Metabolism/Transport Effects Inhibits Monoamine Oxidase
Avoid Concomitant Use
Avoid concomitant use of Isocarboxazid with any of the following: Alpha-/Beta-Agonists (Indirect-Acting); Alpha1-Agonists; Alpha2-Agonists (Ophthalmic); Amphetamines; Anilidopiperidine Opioids; Antidepressants (Serotonin Reuptake Inhibitor/Antagonist); AtoMOXetine; Bezafibrate; Buprenorphine; BuPROPion; BusPIRone; CarBAMazepine; Cyclobenzaprine; Dexmethylphenidate; Dextromethorphan; Diethylpropion; HYDROmorphone; Linezolid; Maprotiline; Meperidine; Methyldopa; Methylene Blue; Methylphenidate; Mirtazapine; Oxymorphone; Pizotifen; Selective Serotonin Reuptake Inhibitors; Serotonin 5-HT1D Receptor Agonists; Serotonin/Norepinephrine Reuptake Inhibitors; Tapentadol; Tetrabenazine; Tetrahydrozoline; Tetrahydrozoline (Nasal); Tricyclic Antidepressants; Tryptophan
Increased Effect/Toxicity
Isocarboxazid may increase the levels/effects of: Alpha-/Beta-Agonists (Direct-Acting); Alpha-/Beta-Agonists (Indirect-Acting); Alpha1-Agonists; Alpha2-Agonists (Ophthalmic); Amphetamines; Anticholinergics; Antidepressants (Serotonin Reuptake Inhibitor/Antagonist); Antihypertensives; AtoMOXetine; Beta2-Agonists; Bezafibrate; BuPROPion; Dexmethylphenidate; Dextromethorphan; Diethylpropion; Doxapram; HYDROmorphone; Hypoglycemic Agents; Linezolid; Lithium; Meperidine; Methadone; Methyldopa; Methylene Blue; Methylphenidate; Metoclopramide; Mirtazapine; Orthostatic Hypotension Producing Agents; Pizotifen; Reserpine; Selective Serotonin Reuptake Inhibitors; Serotonin 5-HT1D

Receptor Agonists; Serotonin Modulators; Serotonin/Norepinephrine Reuptake Inhibitors; Tetrahydrozoline; Tetrahydrozoline (Nasal); Tricyclic Antidepressants

The levels/effects of Isocarboxazid may be increased by: Altretamine; Anilidopiperidine Opioids; Antipsychotics; Buprenorphine; BusPIRone; CarBAMazepine; COMT Inhibitors; Cyclobenzaprine; Levodopa; MAO Inhibitors; Maprotiline; Oxymorphone; Pramlintide; Tapentadol; Tetrabenazine; TraMADol; Tryptophan

Decreased Effect

Isocarboxazid may decrease the levels/effects of: Acetylcholinesterase Inhibitors (Central)

The levels/effects of Isocarboxazid may be decreased by: Acetylcholinesterase Inhibitors (Central)

Ethanol/Nutrition/Herb Interactions

Ethanol: Ethanol may increase CNS depression. Management: Monitor for increased effects with coadministration; caution patients about effects. Avoid beverages containing tyramine (eg, hearty red wine and beer).

Food: Concurrent ingestion of foods rich in tyramine, dopamine, tyrosine, phenylalanine, tryptophan, or caffeine may cause sudden and severe high blood pressure (hypertensive crisis or serotonin syndrome). Management: Avoid tyramine-containing foods (aged or matured cheese, air-dried or cured meats including sausages and salamis; fava or broad bean pods, tap/draft beers, Marmite concentrate, sauerkraut, soy sauce, and other soybean condiments). Food's freshness is also an important concern; improperly stored or spoiled food can create an environment in which tyramine concentrations may increase. Avoid foods containing dopamine, tyrosine, phenylalanine, tryptophan, or caffeine.

Herb/Nutraceutical: Kava kava, valerian, St John's wort, and SAMe may increase the risk of serotonin syndrome and/or excessive sedation. Supplements containing caffeine, tyrosine, tryptophan, or phenylalanine may increase the risk of severe side effects like hypertensive reactions or serotonin syndrome. Management: Avoid kava kava, valerian, St John's wort, SAMe, and supplements containing caffeine, tyrosine, tryptophan, or phenylalanine.

Mechanism of Action Thought to act by increasing endogenous concentrations of epinephrine, norepinephrine, dopamine, and serotonin through inhibition of the enzyme (monoamine oxidase) responsible for the breakdown of these neurotransmitters

Pharmacodynamics/Kinetics

Absorption: Oral: Well absorbed; undergoes acetylation in the liver; older patients have been reported to have higher blood concentrations than younger adults after 2 weeks of continuous treatment

Elimination: In urine primarily as metabolites and unchanged drug

Dosage

Geriatric & Adult Depression: Oral: Initial: 10 mg 2-4 times/day; may increase by 10 mg/day every 2-4 days to 40 mg/day by the end of the first week (divided into 2-4 doses). After first week, may increase by up to 20 mg/week to a maximum of 60 mg/day. May take 3-6 weeks to see effects. Dose should be reduced once maximum clinical effect is seen. If no response obtained within 6 weeks, additional titration is unlikely to be beneficial. **Note:** Use caution in patients on >40 mg/day; experience is limited.

Monitoring Parameters Blood pressure, heart rate; mood, suicidal ideation (especially at the beginning of therapy or when doses are increased or decreased)

Special Geriatric Considerations The MAO inhibitors are effective and generally well tolerated by elderly patients. It is their potential interactions with tyramine-containing foods and other drugs and their effects on blood pressure that have limited their use. The MAO inhibitors are usually reserved for patients who do not tolerate or respond to the traditional "cyclic" or "second generation" antidepressants. Information on the use of isocarboxazid in the elderly is limited.

A systematic review and meta-analysis of antidepressant placebo-controlled trials in persons with depression and dementia found evidence "suggestive" of efficacy but not of sufficient strength to "confirm" efficacy. Antidepressant trials in this patient population are small and underpowered. Older patients with depression being treated with an antidepressant should be closely monitored for response and adverse effects. Treatment should be switched or augmented when response is inadequate with a therapeutic dose. Antidepressants that are not tolerated should be discontinued and an alternative agent should be started.

Dosage Forms Excipient information presented when available (limited, particularly for generics); consult specific product labeling.

Tablet, oral:

Marplan®: 10 mg [scored]

Isoniazid (eye soe NYE a zid)

Related Information
Antimicrobial Drugs of Choice *on page 2163*
Medication Safety Issues
International issues:
Hydra [Japan] may be confused with Hydrea brand name for hydroxyurea [U.S., Canada, and multiple international markets]
Brand Names: Canada Isotamine®; PMS-Isoniazid
Index Terms INH; Isonicotinic Acid Hydrazide
Generic Availability (U.S.) Yes
Pharmacologic Category Antitubercular Agent
Use Treatment of susceptible tuberculosis infections; treatment of latent tuberculosis infection (LTBI)
Contraindications Hypersensitivity to isoniazid or any component of the formulation; acute liver disease; previous history of hepatic damage during isoniazid therapy; previous severe adverse reaction (drug fever, chills, arthritis) to isoniazid
Warnings/Precautions Use with caution in patients with severe renal impairment and liver disease. **[U.S. Boxed Warning]: Severe and sometimes fatal hepatitis may occur; usually occurs within the first 3 months of treatment, although may develop even after many months of treatment.** The risk of developing hepatitis is age-related; daily ethanol consumption may also increase the risk. Patients must report any prodromal symptoms of hepatitis, such as fatigue, weakness, malaise, anorexia, nausea, abdominal pain, jaundice, or vomiting. Patients should be instructed to immediately discontinue therapy if any of these symptoms occur, even if a clinical evaluation has yet to be conducted. Treatment with isoniazid for latent tuberculosis infection should be deferred in patients with acute hepatic diseases. Periodic ophthalmic examinations are recommended even when usual symptoms do not occur. Pyridoxine (10-50 mg/day) is recommended in individuals at risk for development of peripheral neuropathies (eg, HIV infection, nutritional deficiency, diabetes). Multidrug regimens should be utilized for the treatment of active tuberculosis to prevent the emergence of drug resistance.
Adverse Reactions (Reflective of adult population; not specific for elderly) Frequency not defined.
Cardiovascular: Hypertension, palpitation, tachycardia, vasculitis
Central nervous system: Depression, dizziness, encephalopathy, fever, lethargy, memory impairment, psychosis, seizure, slurred speech, toxic encephalopathy
Dermatologic: Flushing, rash (morbilliform, maculopapular, pruritic, or exfoliative)
Endocrine & metabolic: Gynecomastia, hyperglycemia, metabolic acidosis, pellagra, pyridoxine deficiency
Gastrointestinal: Anorexia, epigastric distress, nausea, stomach pain, vomiting
Hematologic: Agranulocytosis, anemia (sideroblastic, hemolytic, or aplastic), eosinophilia, thrombocytopenia
Hepatic: LFTs mildly increased (10% to 20%), hyperbilirubinemia, bilirubinuria, jaundice, hepatic dysfunction, hepatitis (may involve progressive liver damage; risk increases with age; 2.3% in patients >50 years)
Neuromuscular & skeletal: Arthralgia, hyper-reflexia, paresthesia, peripheral neuropathy (dose-related incidence, 10% to 20% incidence with 10 mg/kg/day), weakness
Ocular: Blurred vision, loss of vision, optic neuritis and atrophy
Miscellaneous: Lupus-like syndrome, lymphadenopathy, rheumatic syndrome
Drug Interactions
Metabolism/Transport Effects Substrate of CYP2E1 (major); **Note:** Assignment of Major/Minor substrate status based on clinically relevant drug interaction potential; **Inhibits** CYP1A2 (weak), CYP2A6 (moderate), CYP2C19 (strong), CYP2C9 (weak), CYP2D6 (moderate), CYP2E1 (moderate), CYP3A4 (weak); **Induces** CYP2E1 (weak/moderate)
Avoid Concomitant Use
Avoid concomitant use of Isoniazid with any of the following: Clopidogrel; Pimozide; Thioridazine
Increased Effect/Toxicity
Isoniazid may increase the levels/effects of: Acetaminophen; ARIPiprazole; Benzodiazepines (metabolized by oxidation); CarBAMazepine; Chlorzoxazone; Citalopram; CycloSERINE; CYP2A6 Substrates; CYP2C19 Substrates; CYP2D6 Substrates; CYP2E1 Substrates; Fesoterodine; Fosphenytoin; Nebivolol; Phenytoin; Pimozide; Theophylline Derivatives; Thioridazine

The levels/effects of Isoniazid may be increased by: Disulfiram; Ethionamide; Propafenone; Rifamycin Derivatives

◀ **Decreased Effect**

Isoniazid may decrease the levels/effects of: Clopidogrel; Codeine; Itraconazole; Ketoco-nazole; Ketoconazole (Systemic); Tamoxifen; TraMADol

The levels/effects of Isoniazid may be decreased by: Antacids; Corticosteroids (Systemic); Cyproterone

Ethanol/Nutrition/Herb Interactions

Ethanol: Ethanol increases the risk of hepatitis. Management: Avoid ethanol.

Food: Serum levels may be decreased if taken with food. Has some ability to inhibit tyramine metabolism; several case reports of mild reactions (flushing, palpitations) after ingestion of cheese (with or without wine). Reactions resembling allergic symptoms following ingestion of fish high in histamine content have been reported. Isoniazid decreases folic acid absorption. Isoniazid alters pyridoxine metabolism. Management: Take on an empty stomach 1 hour before or 2 hours after a meal, increase dietary intake of folate, niacin, and magnesium. Avoid tyramine-containing foods (eg, aged or matured cheese, air-dried or cured meats including sausages and salamis; fava or broad bean pods, tap/draft beers, Marmite concentrate, sauerkraut, soy sauce, and other soybean condiments). Food's freshness is also an important concern; improperly stored or spoiled food can create an environment in which tyramine concentrations may increase. Avoid histamine-containing foods.

Stability

Tablet: Store at 20°C to 25°C (68°F to 77°F). Protect from light.

Oral solution; Store at 15°C to 30°C (59°F to 86°F). Protect from light.

Mechanism of Action Unknown, but may include the inhibition of mycolic acid synthesis resulting in disruption of the bacterial cell wall

Pharmacodynamics/Kinetics

Absorption: Rapid and complete; rate can be slowed with food

Distribution: All body tissues and fluids including CSF

Protein binding: 10% to 15%

Metabolism: Hepatic with decay rate determined genetically by acetylation phenotype

Half-life elimination: Fast acetylators: 30-100 minutes; Slow acetylators: 2-5 hours; may be prolonged with hepatic or severe renal impairment

Time to peak, serum: 1-2 hours

Excretion: Urine (75% to 95%); feces; saliva

Dosage

Geriatric & Adult Recommendations often change due to resistant strains and newly-developed information; consult *MMWR* for current CDC recommendations. Intramuscular injection is available for patients who are unable to either take or absorb oral therapy.

Nontuberculous mycobacterium (*M. kansasii*) (unlabeled use): Oral, I.M.: 5 mg/kg/day (maximum: 300 mg/day) for duration to include 12 months of culture-negative sputum; typically used in combination with ethambutol and rifampin

Treatment of latent tuberculosis infection (LTBI): Oral, I.M.: CDC recommendations: 5 mg/kg (maximum: 300 mg/dose) once daily or 15 mg/kg (maximum: 900 mg/dose) twice weekly by directly observed therapy (DOT) for 6-9 months in patients who do not have HIV infection (9 months is optimal, 6 months may be considered to reduce costs of therapy) and 9 months in patients who have HIV infection. Extend to 12 months of therapy if interruptions in treatment occur (*MMWR*, 2000).

Treatment of active TB infection (drug susceptible): Oral, I.M.:

Daily therapy: CDC recommendations: 5 mg/kg/day once daily (usual dose: 300 mg/day) (*MMWR*, 2003)

Directly observed therapy (DOT): CDC recommendations: 15 mg/kg (maximum: 900 mg/dose) twice weekly or 3 times/week; **Note:** CDC guidelines state that once-weekly therapy (15 mg/kg/dose) may be considered, but only after the first 2 months of initial therapy in HIV-negative patients, and only in combination with rifapentine (*MMWR*, 2003).

Note: Treatment may be defined by the number of doses administered (eg, "six-month" therapy involves 182 doses of INH and rifampin, and 56 doses of pyrazinamide). Six months is the shortest interval of time over which these doses may be administered, assuming no interruption of therapy.

Note: Concomitant administration of 10-50 mg/day pyridoxine is recommended in malnour-ished patients or those prone to neuropathy (eg, alcoholics, patients with diabetes)

Renal Impairment No adjustment necessary

Hemodialysis: Dialyzable (50% to 100%); administer dose postdialysis

Hepatic Impairment No adjustment required, however, use with caution, may accumulate and additional liver damage may occur in patients with pre-existing liver disease. For ALT or AST >3 times the ULN: discontinue or temporarily withhold treatment. Treatment with isoniazid for latent tuberculosis infection should be deferred in patients with acute hepatic diseases.

Administration Should be administered 1 hour before or 2 hours after meals on an empty stomach.

Monitoring Parameters Baseline and periodic (more frequently in patients with higher risk for hepatitis) liver function tests (ALT and AST); sputum cultures monthly (until 2 consecutive negative cultures reported); monitoring for prodromal signs of hepatitis

LTBI therapy: American Thoracic Society/Centers for Disease Control (ATS/CDC) recommendations: Monthly clinical evaluation, including brief physical exam for adverse events. Baseline serum AST or ALT and bilirubin should be considered for patients at higher risk for adverse events (eg, history of liver disease, chronic ethanol use, HIV-infected patients, older adults with concomitant medications or diseases). Routine, periodic monitoring is recommended for any patient with an abnormal baseline or at increased risk for hepatotoxicity.

Test Interactions False-positive urinary glucose with Clinitest®

Pharmacotherapy Pearls Pyridoxine should be given concomitantly in persons with conditions in which neuropathy is common (eg, diabetes, alcoholism, malnutrition)

Special Geriatric Considerations Age has not been shown to affect the pharmacokinetics of INH since acetylation phenotype determines clearance and half-life, acetylation rate does not change significantly with age. Most strains of *M. tuberculosis* found the elderly should be susceptible to INH since most acquired their initial infection prior to INH's introduction.

Dosage Forms Excipient information presented when available (limited, particularly for generics); consult specific product labeling.
Injection, solution: 100 mg/mL (10 mL)
Solution, oral: 50 mg/5 mL (473 mL)
Tablet, oral: 100 mg, 300 mg

♦ **Isonicotinic Acid Hydrazide** see Isoniazid *on page 1047*
♦ **Isonipecaine Hydrochloride** see Meperidine *on page 1208*
♦ **Isophane Insulin** see Insulin NPH *on page 1020*
♦ **Isophane Insulin and Regular Insulin** see Insulin NPH and Insulin Regular *on page 1023*

Isoproterenol (eye soe proe TER e nole)

Medication Safety Issues
Sound-alike/look-alike issues:
Isuprel® may be confused with Disophrol®, Isordil®
Brand Names: U.S. Isuprel®
Index Terms Isoproterenol Hydrochloride
Generic Availability (U.S.) No
Pharmacologic Category Beta$_1$- & Beta$_2$-Adrenergic Agonist Agent
Use Manufacturer's labeled indications (see **"Note"**): Mild or transient episodes of heart block that do not require electric shock or pacemaker therapy; serious episodes of heart block and Adams-Stokes attacks (except when caused by ventricular tachycardia or fibrillation); cardiac arrest until electric shock or pacemaker therapy is available; bronchospasm during anesthesia; adjunct to fluid and electrolyte replacement therapy and other drugs and procedures in the treatment of hypovolemic or septic shock and low cardiac output states (eg, decompensated heart failure, cardiogenic shock)

Note: The use of isoproterenol in advanced cardiac life support (ACLS) has largely been supplanted by the use of other adrenergic agents (eg, epinephrine and dopamine). The use of isoproterenol for bronchospasm during anesthesia and cardiogenic, hypovolemic, or septic shock is no longer recommended. See *Unlabeled Use* for more appropriate, yet unlabeled, uses.

Unlabeled Use Pharmacologic overdrive pacing for refractory torsade de pointes; pharmacologic provocation during tilt table testing for syncope; temporary control of bradycardia in denervated heart transplant patients unresponsive to atropine; ventricular arrhythmias due to AV nodal block; beta-blocker overdose

Dosage
Geriatric & Adult Note: Patients may exhibit dose-dependent vasodilation due to unopposed beta$_2$-agonism elicited by isoproterenol.

Bradyarrhythmias, AV nodal block, or refractory torsade de pointes: Continuous I.V. infusion: Usual range: 2-10 mcg/minute; titrate to patient response.

Brugada syndrome with electrical storm (unlabeled use): I.V. bolus: Initial: 1-2 mcg, followed by a continuous infusion of 0.15-0.3 mcg/minute for 1 day; may repeat sequence if ventricular tachycardia/fibrillation recurs (Watanabe, 2006; Zipes, 2006).

Tilt table testing for syncope (Benditt, 1996; Brignole, 2004): Continuous I.V infusion: Initial: 1 mcg/minute; increase as necessary based on response; maximum dose: 5 mcg/minute. **Note:** Timing of initiation and dose adjustment during test may be institution-specific.

◀ **Special Geriatric Considerations** No specific information for use in elderly. Use caution and initiate therapy on the lower end of the recommended dosage range.

Dosage Forms Excipient information presented when available (limited, particularly for generics); consult specific product labeling.
Injection, solution, as hydrochloride:
Isuprel®: 0.2 mg/mL (1 mL, 5 mL) [contains sodium metabisulfite; 1:5000]

◆ **Isoproterenol Hydrochloride** see Isoproterenol on page 1049
◆ **Isoptin® SR** see Verapamil on page 2014
◆ **Isopto® Atropine** see Atropine on page 166
◆ **Isopto® Carbachol** see Carbachol on page 285
◆ **Isopto® Carpine** see Pilocarpine (Ophthalmic) on page 1536
◆ **Isopto® Homatropine** see Homatropine on page 929
◆ **Isopto® Hyoscine** see Scopolamine (Ophthalmic) on page 1759
◆ **Isordil® Titradose™** see Isosorbide Dinitrate on page 1050

Isosorbide Dinitrate (eye soe SOR bide dye NYE trate)

Medication Safety Issues
Sound-alike/look-alike issues:
Isordil® may be confused with Inderal®, Isuprel®, Plendil®
Brand Names: U.S. Dilatrate®-SR; Isordil® Titradose™
Brand Names: Canada ISDN; Isosorbide; Novo-Sorbide; PMS-Isosorbide
Index Terms ISD; ISDN
Generic Availability (U.S.) Yes: Excludes capsule
Pharmacologic Category Antianginal Agent; Vasodilator
Use Prevention and treatment of angina pectoris

Note: Due to slower onset of action, not the drug of choice to abort an acute anginal episode.

Unlabeled Use Patients with heart failure (HF) who do not tolerate an ACE inhibitor or an angiotensin receptor blocker (ARB); African-American (self-identified) patients with HF remaining symptomatic despite optimal standard therapy; esophageal spastic disorders

Contraindications Hypersensitivity to isosorbide dinitrate or any component of the formulation; hypersensitivity to organic nitrates; concurrent use with phosphodiesterase-5 (PDE-5) inhibitors (sildenafil, tadalafil, or vardenafil)

Warnings/Precautions Severe hypotension can occur; paradoxical bradycardia and increased angina pectoris can accompany hypotension. Postural hypotension can also occur; ethanol may potentiate this effect. Use with caution in volume depletion and moderate hypotension, and use with extreme caution with inferior wall MI and suspected right ventricular infarctions. Nitrates may reduce preload, exacerbating obstruction and cause hypotension or syncope and/or worsening of heart failure (Gibbons, 2003). Avoid use in patients with hypertrophic cardiomyopathy (HCM).

Use of isosorbide dinitrate sublingual tablets to treat acute angina attacks is recommended only in patients unresponsive to sublingual nitroglycerin; however, current clinical practice guidelines do not recommend use during an acute anginal episode. Avoid use of extended release formulations in acute MI or acute HF; cannot easily reverse effects if adverse events develop. Nitrates may precipitate or aggravate increased intracranial pressure and subsequently may worsen clinical outcomes in patients with neurologic injury (eg, intracranial hemorrhage, traumatic brain injury). Appropriate dosing intervals are needed to minimize tolerance development. Tolerance can only be overcome by short periods of nitrate absence from the body. Dose escalation does not overcome this effect. When used for HF in combination with hydralazine, tolerance is less of a concern (Gogia, 1995).

Avoid concurrent use with PDE-5 inhibitors (eg, sildenafil, tadalafil, vardenafil). When nitrate administration becomes medically necessary, may administer nitrates only if 24 hours have elapsed after use of sildenafil or vardenafil (48 hours after tadalafil use) (Trujillo, 2007).

Adverse Reactions (Reflective of adult population; not specific for elderly) Frequency not defined.
Cardiovascular: Crescendo angina (uncommon), hypotension, orthostatic hypotension, rebound hypertension (uncommon), syncope (uncommon)
Central nervous system: Headache (most common), lightheadedness (related to blood pressure changes)
Hematologic: Methemoglobinemia (rare, overdose)

Drug Interactions
Metabolism/Transport Effects Substrate of CYP3A4 (major); **Note:** Assignment of Major/Minor substrate status based on clinically relevant drug interaction potential

Avoid Concomitant Use
Avoid concomitant use of Isosorbide Dinitrate with any of the following: Conivaptan; Phosphodiesterase 5 Inhibitors
Increased Effect/Toxicity
Isosorbide Dinitrate may increase the levels/effects of: Hypotensive Agents; Prilocaine; Rosiglitazone

The levels/effects of Isosorbide Dinitrate may be increased by: Conivaptan; CYP3A4 Inhibitors (Moderate); CYP3A4 Inhibitors (Strong); Dasatinib; Ivacaftor; Mifepristone; Phosphodiesterase 5 Inhibitors
Decreased Effect
The levels/effects of Isosorbide Dinitrate may be decreased by: CYP3A4 Inducers (Strong); Deferasirox; Herbs (CYP3A4 Inducers); Tocilizumab
Ethanol/Nutrition/Herb Interactions
Ethanol: Caution with ethanol (may increase risk of hypotension).
Herb/Nutraceutical: Avoid black cohosh, California poppy, coleus, golden seal, hawthorn, mistletoe, periwinkle, quinine, shepherd's purse (may cause hypotension).
Mechanism of Action Stimulation of intracellular cyclic-GMP results in vascular smooth muscle relaxation of both arterial and venous vasculature with more prominent effects on the veins. Primarily reduces cardiac oxygen demand by decreasing preload (left ventricular end-diastolic pressure); may modestly reduce afterload. Additionally, coronary artery dilation improves collateral flow to ischemic regions.
Pharmacodynamics/Kinetics
Onset of action: Sublingual tablet: ~3 minutes; Oral tablet and capsule (includes extended-release formulations): ~1 hour
Duration: Sublingual tablet: 1-2 hours; Oral tablet and capsule (includes extended-release formulations): Up to 8 hours
Distribution: V_d: 2-4 L/kg
Metabolism: Extensively hepatic to conjugated metabolites, including isosorbide 5-mononitrate (active) and 2-mononitrate (active)
Bioavailability: Sublingual tablet: 40% to 50%; Oral immediate release formulations: Highly variable (10% to 90%); increases with chronic therapy
Half-life elimination: Parent drug: ~1 hour; Metabolites (5-mononitrate: 5 hours; 2-mononitrate: 2 hours)
Excretion: Urine and feces
Dosage
Geriatric Elderly patients should be given lowest recommended adult daily doses initially and titrate upward.
Adult
Angina:
Oral:
Immediate release: Initial: 5-20 mg 2-3 times/day; Maintenance: 10-40 mg 2-3 times/day **or** 5-80 mg 2-3 times/day (Anderson, 2007; Gibbons, 2002)
Sustained release: 40-160 mg/day has been used in clinical trials (a nitrate free interval of at least 18 hours is recommended; however, a clinically efficacious dosage interval has not been clearly established) **or** 40 mg 1-2 times/day (Anderson, 2007; Gibbons, 2002)
Sublingual:
Prophylactic use: 2.5-5 mg administered 15 minutes prior to activities which may provoke an anginal episode
Treatment of acute anginal episode (use only if patient has failed sublingual nitroglycerin): 2.5-5 mg every 5-10 minutes for maximum of 3 doses in 15-30 minutes
Heart failure (unlabeled use; Cohn, 1991; HFSA, 2010; Hunt, 2009): *Oral:*
Immediate release (**Note:** Use in combination with hydralazine):
Initial dose: 20 mg 3-4 times per day
Target dose: 160 mg/day in 4 divided doses
Esophageal spastic disorders (unlabeled use; Goyal, 1998): *Oral, sublingual:* Immediate release: 10-30 mg before meals
Renal Impairment
Hemodialysis: Supplemental dose is not necessary
Peritoneal dialysis: Supplemental dose is not necessary
Administration May consider administration of first dose in physician office; observe for maximal cardiovascular dynamic effects and adverse effects (orthostatic hypotension, headache). Do not administer around the clock; allow nitrate-free interval ≥14 hours (immediate release products) and >18 hours (sustained release products). Do not crush sublingual tablets or extended release formulations.

Immediate release products: When prescribed twice daily, consider administering at 8 AM and 1 PM. For 3 times/day dosing, consider 8 AM, 1 PM, and 6 PM.

Sustained release products: Consider once daily in morning or twice-daily dosing at 8 AM and between 1-2 PM.

Monitoring Parameters Blood pressure, heart rate

Special Geriatric Considerations The first dose of nitrates (sublingual, chewable, oral) should be taken in a physician's office to observe for maximal cardiovascular dynamic effects and adverse effects (eg, orthostatic blood pressure drop, headache). The use of nitrates for angina may occasionally promote reflux esophagitis. This may require dose adjustments or changing therapeutic agents to correct this adverse effect.

Dosage Forms Excipient information presented when available (limited, particularly for generics); consult specific product labeling.

Capsule, sustained release, oral:
    Dilatrate®-SR: 40 mg
Tablet, oral: 5 mg, 10 mg, 20 mg, 30 mg
    Isordil® Titradose™: 5 mg, 40 mg [scored]
Tablet, sublingual: 2.5 mg, 5 mg
Tablet, extended release, oral: 40 mg

Isosorbide Dinitrate and Hydralazine
(eye soe SOR bide dye NYE trate & hye DRAL a zeen)

Related Information
    HydrALAZINE *on page 931*
    Isosorbide Dinitrate *on page 1050*
Brand Names: U.S. BiDil®
Index Terms Hydralazine and Isosorbide Dinitrate
Generic Availability (U.S.) No
Pharmacologic Category Vasodilator
Use Treatment of heart failure, adjunct to standard therapy, in self-identified African-Americans
Dosage
    Geriatric & Adult Heart failure: Oral: Initial: 1 tablet 3 times/day; may titrate to a maximum dose of 2 tablets 3 times/day
Special Geriatric Considerations The pharmacokinetics of hydralazine and isosorbide dinitrate alone or in combination have not been studied. As with all antihypertensives and nitrate products, caution should be used on initiation of therapy, as hypotension may be encountered. Since many elderly are volume depleted, secondary to their blunted thirst reflex and/or use of diuretics, doses used initially should be at lowest recommended dose. The use of nitrates may occasionally promote reflux esophagitis. Monitor for these effects at start of therapy.
Dosage Forms
    Tablet, oral:
        BiDil®: Isosorbide dinitrate 20 mg and hydralazine 37.5 mg

Isosorbide Mononitrate (eye soe SOR bide mon oh NYE trate)

Medication Safety Issues
    Sound-alike/look-alike issues:
        Imdur® may be confused with Imuran®, Inderal® LA, K-Dur®
        Monoket® may be confused with Monopril®
Brand Names: U.S. Imdur®; Ismo®; Monoket® [DSC]
Brand Names: Canada Apo-ISMN®; Imdur®; PMS-ISMN; PRO-ISMN
Index Terms ISMN
Generic Availability (U.S.) Yes
Pharmacologic Category Antianginal Agent; Vasodilator
Use Prevention of angina pectoris
Contraindications Hypersensitivity to isosorbide mononitrate or any component of the formulation; hypersensitivity to organic nitrates; concurrent use with phosphodiesterase-5 (PDE-5) inhibitors (sildenafil, tadalafil, or vardenafil)
Warnings/Precautions Avoid use in hypertrophic cardiomyopathy. Use with caution in volume depletion, moderate hypotension, and extreme caution with inferior wall MI and suspected right ventricular infarctions. Nitrates may precipitate or aggravate increased intra-cranial pressure and subsequently may worsen clinical outcomes in patients with neurologic injury (eg, intracranial hemorrhage, traumatic brain injury). Postural hypotension, transient episodes of weakness, dizziness, or syncope may occur even with small doses; ethanol

accentuates these effects; tolerance and cross-tolerance to nitrate antianginal and hemodynamic effects may occur during prolonged isosorbide mononitrate therapy; (minimized by using the smallest effective dose, by alternating coronary vasodilators or offering drug-free intervals of as little as 12 hours). Excessive doses may result in severe headache, blurred vision, or xerostomia; increased anginal symptoms may be a result of dosage increases. Avoid concurrent use with PDE-5 inhibitors (eg, sildenafil, tadalafil, vardenafil). When nitrate administration becomes medically necessary, may administer nitrates only if 24 hours have elapsed after use of sildenafil or vardenafil (48 hours after tadalafil use) (O'Connor, 2010).

Adverse Reactions (Reflective of adult population; not specific for elderly)
>10%: Central nervous system: Headache (13% to 35%)
1% to 10%:
  Cardiovascular: Angina (≤2%), flushing (≤2%)
  Central nervous system: Dizziness (≤4%), fatigue (≤4%), pain (≤4%), emotional lability (≤2%)
  Dermatologic: Pruritus (≤2%), rash (≤2%)
  Gastrointestinal: Nausea (≤3%), abdominal pain (≤2%), diarrhea (≤2%)
  Respiratory: Upper respiratory infection (≤4%), cough increased (≤2%)
  Miscellaneous: Allergic reaction (≤2%)

Drug Interactions
  Metabolism/Transport Effects Substrate of CYP3A4 (major); **Note:** Assignment of Major/Minor substrate status based on clinically relevant drug interaction potential
  Avoid Concomitant Use
  Avoid concomitant use of Isosorbide Mononitrate with any of the following: Conivaptan; Phosphodiesterase 5 Inhibitors
  Increased Effect/Toxicity
  Isosorbide Mononitrate may increase the levels/effects of: Hypotensive Agents; Prilocaine; Rosiglitazone

  The levels/effects of Isosorbide Mononitrate may be increased by: Conivaptan; CYP3A4 Inhibitors (Moderate); CYP3A4 Inhibitors (Strong); Dasatinib; Ivacaftor; Mifepristone; Phosphodiesterase 5 Inhibitors
  Decreased Effect
  The levels/effects of Isosorbide Mononitrate may be decreased by: CYP3A4 Inducers (Strong); Deferasirox; Herbs (CYP3A4 Inducers); Tocilizumab

Ethanol/Nutrition/Herb Interactions Ethanol: Caution with ethanol (may increase risk of hypotension).

Stability Tablets should be stored in a tight container at room temperature of 15°C to 30°C (59°F to 86°F).

Mechanism of Action Nitroglycerin and other nitrates form free radical nitric oxide. In smooth muscle, nitric oxide activates guanylate cyclase which increases guanosine 3'5' monophosphate (cGMP) leading to dephosphorylation of myosin light chains and smooth muscle relaxation. Produces a vasodilator effect on the peripheral veins and arteries with more prominent effects on the veins. Primarily reduces cardiac oxygen demand by decreasing preload (left ventricular end-diastolic pressure); may modestly reduce afterload; dilates coronary arteries and improves collateral flow to ischemic regions.

Pharmacodynamics/Kinetics
Onset of action: 30-60 minutes
Duration: Immediate release: ≥6 hours (Thadani, 1987); Extended release: ≥12-24 hours (Anderson, 2007)
Absorption: Nearly complete and low intersubject variability in its pharmacokinetic parameters and plasma concentrations
Distribution: V_d: ~0.6 L/kg
Protein binding: <5%
Metabolism: Hepatic
Bioavailability: ~100%
Half-life elimination: Mononitrate: ~5-6 hours
Excretion: Predominantly urine (2% as unchanged drug); feces (1% of dose)

Dosage
  Geriatric Start with lowest recommended adult dose.
  Adult
    Angina: Oral:
      Regular release tablet: Initial: 5-20 mg twice daily with the 2 doses given 7 hours apart (eg, 8 AM and 3 PM) to decrease tolerance development; patients initiating therapy with 5 mg twice daily (eg, small stature) should be titrated up to 10 mg twice daily in first 2-3 days.
      Extended release tablet: Initial: 30-60 mg given once daily in the morning; titrate upward as needed, giving at least 3 days between increases; maximum daily single dose: 240 mg

Note: Tolerance to nitrate effects develops with chronic exposure. Dose escalation does not overcome this effect. Tolerance can only be overcome by short periods of nitrate absence from the body. Short periods of nitrate withdrawal may help minimize tolerance. Recommended twice daily dosage regimens incorporate this interval. Administer sustained release tablet once daily in the morning.

Renal Impairment Dose adjustment not necessary.

Hemodialysis: Dose supplementation is not necessary.

Peritoneal dialysis: Dose supplementation is not necessary.

Hepatic Impairment Dose adjustment not necessary.

Administration Do not administer around-the-clock. Immediate release tablet should be scheduled twice daily with doses 7 hours apart (8 AM and 3 PM); extended release tablet may be administered once daily in the morning upon rising with a half-glassful of fluid and should not be chewed or crushed.

Monitoring Parameters Monitor for orthostasis, increased hypotension

Special Geriatric Considerations The first dose of nitrates (sublingual, chewable, oral) should be taken in a physician's office to observe for maximal cardiovascular dynamic effects and adverse effects (eg, orthostatic blood pressure drop, headache). The use of nitrates for angina may occasionally promote reflux esophagitis. This may require dose adjustments or changing therapeutic agents to correct this adverse effect.

Dosage Forms Excipient information presented when available (limited, particularly for generics); consult specific product labeling. [DSC] = Discontinued product

Tablet, oral: 10 mg, 20 mg

Ismo®: 20 mg [scored]

Monoket®: 10 mg [DSC], 20 mg [DSC] [scored]

Tablet, extended release, oral: 30 mg, 60 mg, 120 mg

Imdur®: 30 mg, 60 mg [scored]

Imdur®: 120 mg

Isoxsuprine (eye SOKS syoo preen)

Related Information

Beers Criteria – Potentially Inappropriate Medications for Geriatrics *on page 2183*

Medication Safety Issues

Sound-alike/look-alike issues:

Vasodilan may be confused with Vasocidin®

BEERS Criteria medication:

This drug may be potentially inappropriate for use in geriatric patients (Quality of evidence - high; Strength of recommendation - strong).

Index Terms Isoxsuprine Hydrochloride; Vasodilan

Generic Availability (U.S.) Yes

Pharmacologic Category Vasodilator

Use Treatment of peripheral vascular diseases, such as arteriosclerosis obliterans, thromboangiitis obliterans (Buerger's disease), and Raynaud's disease; relief of symptoms associated with cerebrovascular insufficiency

Note: More appropriate therapies (medical or surgical) should be considered; efficacy of isoxsuprine in the treatment of these conditions has not been well established.

Dosage

Geriatric Refer to adult dosing. Start with lower dose due to potential hypotension.

Adult Peripheral vascular disease or symptoms of cerebrovascular insufficiency: Oral: 10-20 mg 3-4 times/day

Special Geriatric Considerations The use of vasodilators for cognitive dysfunction is not recommended or proven by appropriate scientific study.

This medication is considered to be potentially inappropriate in this patient population (Beers Criteria: Quality of evidence - high; Strength of recommendation - strong).

Dosage Forms Excipient information presented when available (limited, particularly for generics); consult specific product labeling.

Tablet, oral, as hydrochloride: 10 mg, 20 mg

◆ **Isoxsuprine Hydrochloride** *see* Isoxsuprine *on page 1054*

Isradipine (iz RA di peen)

Related Information
Calcium Channel Blockers – Comparative Pharmacokinetics *on page 2111*
Medication Safety Issues
Sound-alike/look-alike issues:
DynaCirc® may be confused with Dynacin®
Brand Names: U.S. DynaCirc CR®
Generic Availability (U.S.) Yes: Capsule
Pharmacologic Category Calcium Channel Blocker; Calcium Channel Blocker, Dihydropyridine
Use Treatment of hypertension
Contraindications Hypersensitivity to isradipine or any component of the formulation; hypotension (<90 mm Hg systolic)
Warnings/Precautions Increased angina and/or MI has occurred with initiation or dosage titration of calcium channel blockers. The most common side effect is peripheral edema; occurs within 2-3 weeks of starting therapy. Reflex tachycardia may occur with use. Symptomatic hypotension with or without syncope can rarely occur; blood pressure must be lowered at a rate appropriate for the patient's clinical condition. Use cautiously in HF, hypertrophic cardiomyopathy (IHSS), and in hepatic dysfunction. Use controlled release tablets with caution in patients with severe GI narrowing. Adjust doses at 2- to 4-week intervals.

Adverse Reactions (Reflective of adult population; not specific for elderly) Percentages reported with capsule formulation.
>10%: Central nervous system: Headache (dose related 2% to 22%)
1% to 10%:
  Cardiovascular: Edema (dose related 1% to 9%), palpitation (dose related 1% to 5%), flushing (dose related 1% to 5%), tachycardia (1% to 3%), chest pain (2% to 3%)
  Central nervous system: Dizziness (2% to 8%), fatigue (dose related 1% to 9%)
  Dermatologic: Rash (2%)
  Gastrointestinal: Nausea (1% to 5%), abdominal discomfort (≤3%), vomiting (≤1%), diarrhea (≤3%)
  Neuromuscular & skeletal: Weakness (≤1%)
  Renal: Urinary frequency (1% to 3%)
  Respiratory: Dyspnea (1% to 3%)

Drug Interactions
Metabolism/Transport Effects Substrate of CYP3A4 (major); **Note:** Assignment of Major/Minor substrate status based on clinically relevant drug interaction potential; **Inhibits** CYP3A4 (weak)
Avoid Concomitant Use
Avoid concomitant use of Isradipine with any of the following: Conivaptan
Increased Effect/Toxicity
Isradipine may increase the levels/effects of: Amifostine; Antihypertensives; ARIPiprazole; Beta-Blockers; Calcium Channel Blockers (Nondihydropyridine); Fosphenytoin; Highest Risk QTc-Prolonging Agents; Hypotensive Agents; Magnesium Salts; Moderate Risk QTc-Prolonging Agents; Neuromuscular-Blocking Agents (Nondepolarizing); Nitroprusside; Phenytoin; QuiNIDine; RiTUXimab; Tacrolimus; Tacrolimus (Systemic)

The levels/effects of Isradipine may be increased by: Alpha1-Blockers; Antifungal Agents (Azole Derivatives, Systemic); Calcium Channel Blockers (Nondihydropyridine); Cimetidine; Conivaptan; CycloSPORINE; CycloSPORINE (Systemic); CYP3A4 Inhibitors (Moderate); CYP3A4 Inhibitors (Strong); Diazoxide; Fluconazole; Herbs (Hypotensive Properties); Ivacaftor; Macrolide Antibiotics; Magnesium Salts; MAO Inhibitors; Mifepristone; Pentoxifylline; Phosphodiesterase 5 Inhibitors; Prostacyclin Analogues; Protease Inhibitors; QuiNIDine
Decreased Effect
Isradipine may decrease the levels/effects of: Clopidogrel; QuiNIDine

The levels/effects of Isradipine may be decreased by: Barbiturates; Calcium Salts; CarBAMazepine; CYP3A4 Inducers (Strong); Deferasirox; Herbs (CYP3A4 Inducers); Herbs (Hypertensive Properties); Methylphenidate; Nafcillin; Rifamycin Derivatives; Tocilizumab; Yohimbine
Ethanol/Nutrition/Herb Interactions
Food: Administration with food delays absorption, but does not affect availability
Herb/Nutraceutical: St John's wort may decrease isradipine levels; dong quai has estrogenic effects. Some herbal medications may worsen hypertension (eg, licorice); garlic may have additional antihypertensive effects. Management: Avoid dong quai and St John's wort. Avoid

bayberry, blue cohosh, cayenne, ephedra, ginger, ginseng (American), gotu kola, licorice, yohimbe, and garlic.

Mechanism of Action Inhibits calcium ion from entering the "slow channels" or select voltage-sensitive areas of vascular smooth muscle and myocardium during depolarization, producing a relaxation of coronary vascular smooth muscle and coronary vasodilation; increases myocardial oxygen delivery in patients with vasospastic angina

Pharmacodynamics/Kinetics

Onset of action: Immediate release: 2-3 hours

Duration: Immediate release: >12 hours

Absorption: 90% to 95%

Distribution: V_d: 3 L/kg

Protein binding: 95%

Metabolism: Hepatic; CYP3A4 substrate (major); extensive first-pass effect; forms metabolites (inactive)

Bioavailability: 15% to 24%

Half-life elimination: Terminal: 8 hours

Time to peak, serum: 1-1.5 hours

Excretion: Urine (60% to 65% as metabolites); feces (25% to 30%)

Dosage

Geriatric

Capsule: Refer to adult dosing.

Controlled release tablet: Initial dose: 5 mg once daily

Adult Hypertension: Oral:

Capsule: 2.5 mg twice daily; antihypertensive response occurs in 2-3 hours; maximal response in 2-4 weeks; increase dose at 2- to 4-week intervals at 2.5-5 mg increments; usual dose range (JNC 7): 2.5-10 mg/day in 2 divided doses. **Note:** Most patients show no improvement with doses >10 mg/day except adverse reaction rate increases; therefore, maximal dose in older adults should be 10 mg/day.

Controlled release tablet: 5 mg once daily; antihypertensive response occurs in 2 hours. Adjust dose in increments of 5 mg at 2-4 week intervals. Maximum dose: 20 mg/day; adverse events are increased at doses >10 mg/day.

Renal Impairment

Cl_{cr} 30-80 mL/minute: Bioavailability increased by 45%

Cl_{cr} <10 mL/minute on hemodialysis: Bioavailability decreased by 20% to 50%

Capsule: Refer to adult dosing.

Controlled release tablet: Initial dose: 5 mg once daily

Hepatic Impairment

Peak serum concentrations are increased by 32% and bioavailability is increased by 52%.

Capsule: Refer to adult dosing.

Controlled release tablet: Initial dose: 5 mg once daily

Administration Controlled release tablets should be swallowed whole; do not divide or chew

Monitoring Parameters Blood pressure; renal, hepatic dysfunction

Special Geriatric Considerations Elderly may experience a greater hypotensive response. Constipation may be more of a problem in the elderly. Calcium channel blockers are no more effective in the elderly than other therapies; however, they do not cause significant CNS effects which is an advantage over some antihypertensive agents.

Dosage Forms Excipient information presented when available (limited, particularly for generics); consult specific product labeling.

Capsule, oral: 2.5 mg, 5 mg

Tablet, controlled release, oral:

DynaCirc CR®: 5 mg, 10 mg

◆ **Istalol®** see Timolol (Ophthalmic) *on page 1902*
◆ **Isuprel®** see Isoproterenol *on page 1049*

Itraconazole (i tra KOE na zole)

Medication Safety Issues

Sound-alike/look-alike issues:

Itraconazole may be confused with fluconazole

Sporanox® may be confused with Suprax®, Topamax®

Brand Names: U.S. Sporanox®

Brand Names: Canada Sporanox®

Generic Availability (U.S.) Yes: Capsule

Pharmacologic Category Antifungal Agent, Oral

Use

Oral capsules: Treatment of susceptible fungal infections in immunocompromised and immunocompetent patients including blastomycosis and histoplasmosis; indicated for aspergillosis (in patients intolerant/refractory to amphotericin B), and onychomycosis of the toenail and fingernail (in nonimmunocompromised patients)

Oral solution: Treatment of oral and esophageal candidiasis

Contraindications Hypersensitivity to itraconazole (use caution in patients with a history of hypersensitivity to other azoles), any component of the formulation; concurrent administration with cisapride, dofetilide, ergot derivatives, felodipine, levomethadyl, lovastatin, methadone, midazolam (oral), nisoldipine, pimozide, quinidine, simvastatin, or triazolam; treatment of onychomycosis (or other non-life-threatening indications) in patients with evidence of ventricular dysfunction, heart failure (HF) or a history of HF

Warnings/Precautions [U.S. Boxed Warning]: Negative inotropic effects have been observed following intravenous administration. Discontinue or reassess use if signs or symptoms of HF (heart failure) occur during treatment. [U.S. Boxed Warning]: Use is contraindicated for treatment of onychomycosis in patients with ventricular dysfunction or a history of HF. HF has been reported, particularly in patients receiving a total daily oral dose of 400 mg. Use with caution in patients with risk factors for HF (COPD, renal failure, edematous disorders, ischemic or valvular disease). Discontinue if signs or symptoms of HF or neuropathy occur during treatment. Due to potential toxicity, the manufacturer recommends confirmation of diagnosis testing of nail specimens prior to treatment of onychomycosis.

[U.S. Boxed Warning]: Serious cardiovascular adverse events including, QT prolongation, ventricular tachycardia, torsade de pointes, cardiac arrest and/or sudden death have been observed due to itraconazole-induced increased serum concentrations of the following: cisapride, dofetilide, ergot alkaloids (dihydroergotamine, ergonovine, ergotamine, methylergonovine), felodipine, levomethadyl, lovastatin, methadone, midazolam (oral), nisoldipine, pimozide, simvastatin, quinidine, or triazolam; concurrent use contraindicated.

Calcium channel blockers (CCBs) may cause additive negative inotropic effects when used concurrently with itraconazole. Itraconazole may also inhibit the metabolism of CCBs. Use caution with concurrent use of itraconazole and CCBs due to an increased risk of HF. Concurrent use of itraconazole and nisoldipine is contraindicated.

Use with caution in patients with renal impairment. Rare cases of serious hepatotoxicity (including liver failure and death) have been reported (including some cases occurring within the first week of therapy); hepatotoxicity was reported in some patients without pre-existing liver disease or risk factors. Use with caution in patients with pre-existing hepatic impairment; monitor liver function closely and dosage adjustment may be warranted. Not recommended for use in patients with active liver disease, elevated liver enzymes, or prior hepatotoxic reactions to other drugs unless the expected benefit exceeds the risk of hepatotoxicity. Transient or permanent hearing loss has been reported. Quinidine (a contraindicated drug) was used concurrently in several of these cases. Hearing loss usually resolves after discontinuation, but may persist in some patients.

Large differences in itraconazole pharmacokinetic parameters have been observed in cystic fibrosis patients receiving the solution; if a patient with cystic fibrosis does not respond to therapy, alternate therapies should be considered. Due to differences in bioavailability, oral capsules and oral solution cannot be used interchangeably. Only the oral solution has proven efficacy for oral and esophageal candidiasis. Initiation of treatment with oral solution is not recommended in patients at immediate risk for systemic candidiasis (eg, patients with severe neutropenia).

Adverse Reactions (Reflective of adult population; not specific for elderly)

>10%: Gastrointestinal: Nausea (3% to 11%), diarrhea (3% to 11%)

1% to 10%:

Cardiovascular: Edema (4%), hypertension (3%), chest pain (3%)

Central nervous system: Headache (4% to 10%), fever (2% to 7%), dizziness (2% to 4%), anxiety (3%), depression (2% to 3%), fatigue (2% to 3%), pain (2% to 3%), malaise (1% to 3%), dreams abnormal (2%)

Dermatologic: Rash (3% to 9%), pruritus (≤5%)

Endocrine & metabolic: Hypertriglyceridemia (≤3%), hypokalemia (2%)

Gastrointestinal: Vomiting (5% to 7%), abdominal pain (2% to 6%), dyspepsia (≤4%), flatulence (≤4%), gingivitis (3%), stomatitis (ulcerative) (≤3%), constipation (2% to 3%), appetite increased (2%), gastritis (2%), gastroenteritis (2%)

Hepatic: LFTs abnormal (≤4%)

Neuromuscular & skeletal: Bursitis (3%), myalgia (≤3%), tremor (2%), weakness (≤2%)

Renal: Cystitis (3%), urinary tract infection (3%)

Respiratory: Rhinitis (5% to 9%), upper respiratory tract infection (8%), sinusitis (2% to 7%), cough (4%), dyspnea (2%), pharyngitis (≤2%), pneumonia (2%), sputum increased (2%)

Miscellaneous: Diaphoresis increased (3%), herpes zoster (2%)

Drug Interactions

Metabolism/Transport Effects Substrate of CYP3A4 (major); **Note:** Assignment of Major/Minor substrate status based on clinically relevant drug interaction potential; **Inhibits** CYP3A4 (strong), P-glycoprotein

Avoid Concomitant Use

Avoid concomitant use of Itraconazole with any of the following: Alfuzosin; Aliskiren; Apixaban; Avanafil; Axitinib; Cisapride; Conivaptan; Crizotinib; CYP3A4 Inducers (Strong); Dihydroergotamine; Dofetilide; Dronedarone; Eplerenone; Ergoloid Mesylates; Ergonovine; Ergotamine; Everolimus; Fluticasone (Oral Inhalation); Halofantrine; Lapatinib; Lovastatin; Lurasidone; Methadone; Methylergonovine; Nevirapine; Nilotinib; Nisoldipine; Pimozide; QuiNIDine; Ranolazine; Red Yeast Rice; Rivaroxaban; RomiDEPsin; Salmeterol; Silodosin; Simvastatin; Tamsulosin; Ticagrelor; Tolvaptan; Topotecan; Toremifene

Increased Effect/Toxicity

Itraconazole may increase the levels/effects of: Alfentanil; Alfuzosin; Aliskiren; Almotriptan; Alosetron; Apixaban; Aprepitant; ARIPiprazole; AtorvaSTATin; Avanafil; Axitinib; Benzodiazepines (metabolized by oxidation); Boceprevir; Bortezomib; Bosentan; Brentuximab Vedotin; Brinzolamide; Budesonide (Nasal); Budesonide (Systemic, Oral Inhalation); BusPIRone; Busulfan; Calcium Channel Blockers; CarBAMazepine; Cardiac Glycosides; Ciclesonide; Cilostazol; Cisapride; Colchicine; Conivaptan; Corticosteroids (Orally Inhaled); Corticosteroids (Systemic); Crizotinib; CycloSPORINE; CycloSPORINE (Systemic); CYP3A4 Substrates; Dabigatran Etexilate; Dienogest; Dihydroergotamine; DOCEtaxel; Dofetilide; Dronedarone; Dutasteride; Eletriptan; Eplerenone; Ergoloid Mesylates; Ergonovine; Ergotamine; Erlotinib; Eszopiclone; Etravirine; Everolimus; FentaNYL; Fesoterodine; Fexofenadine; Fluticasone (Nasal); Fluticasone (Oral Inhalation); Fosaprepitant; Fosphenytoin; Gefitinib; GuanFACINE; Halofantrine; Highest Risk QTc-Prolonging Agents; Iloperidone; Imatinib; Irinotecan; Ivacaftor; Ixabepilone; Lapatinib; Losartan; Lovastatin; Lumefantrine; Lurasidone; Macrolide Antibiotics; Maraviroc; Methadone; Methylergonovine; MethylPREDNISolone; Mifepristone; Moderate Risk QTc-Prolonging Agents; Nilotinib; Nisoldipine; Paliperidone; Paricalcitol; Pazopanib; P-glycoprotein/ABCB1 Substrates; Phenytoin; Pimecrolimus; Pimozide; Pravastatin; Propafenone; Protease Inhibitors; Prucalopride; QuiNIDine; Ramelteon; Ranolazine; Red Yeast Rice; Repaglinide; Rifamycin Derivatives; Rivaroxaban; RomiDEPsin; Ruxolitinib; Salmeterol; Saxagliptin; Sildenafil; Silodosin; Simvastatin; Sirolimus; Solifenacin; SORAfenib; SUNItinib; Tacrolimus; Tacrolimus (Systemic); Tacrolimus (Topical); Tadalafil; Tamsulosin; Telaprevir; Temsirolimus; Ticagrelor; Tolterodine; Tolvaptan; Topotecan; Toremifene; Vardenafil; Vemurafenib; Vilazodone; VinBLAStine; VinCRIStine; Vinorelbine; Vitamin K Antagonists; Ziprasidone; Zolpidem; Zuclopenthixol

The levels/effects of Itraconazole may be increased by: Boceprevir; Etravirine; Grapefruit Juice; Macrolide Antibiotics; Mifepristone; Protease Inhibitors; Telaprevir

Decreased Effect

Itraconazole may decrease the levels/effects of: Amphotericin B; Ifosfamide; Prasugrel; Saccharomyces boulardii; Ticagrelor

The levels/effects of Itraconazole may be decreased by: Antacids; CYP3A4 Inducers (Strong); Deferasirox; Didanosine; Efavirenz; Etravirine; Fosphenytoin; H2-Antagonists; Herbs (CYP3A4 Inducers); Isoniazid; Nevirapine; Phenytoin; Proton Pump Inhibitors; Rifamycin Derivatives; Sucralfate; Tocilizumab

Ethanol/Nutrition/Herb Interactions

Food:

Capsules: Absorption enhanced by food and possibly by gastric acidity. Cola drinks have been shown to increase the absorption of the capsules in patients with achlorhydria or those taking H2-receptor antagonists or other gastric acid suppressors. Grapefruit/grapefruit juice may increase serum levels. Management: Take capsules immediately after meals. Avoid grapefruit juice.

Solution: Food decreases the bioavailability and increases the time to peak concentration. Management: Take solution on an empty stomach 1 hour before or 2 hours after meals.

Herb/Nutraceutical: St John's wort may decrease itraconazole levels.

Stability

Capsule: Store at room temperature, 15°C to 25°C (59°F to 77°F). Protect from light and moisture.

Oral solution: Store at ≤25°C (77°F); do not freeze.

Mechanism of Action Interferes with cytochrome P450 activity, decreasing ergosterol synthesis (principal sterol in fungal cell membrane) and inhibiting cell membrane formation

Pharmacodynamics/Kinetics

Absorption: Requires gastric acidity; capsule better absorbed with food, solution better absorbed on empty stomach

Distribution: V_d (average): 796 ± 185 L or 10 L/kg; highly lipophilic and tissue concentrations are higher than plasma concentrations. The highest concentrations: adipose, omentum, endometrium, cervical and vaginal mucus, and skin/nails. Aqueous fluids (eg, CSF and urine) contain negligible amounts.

Protein binding, plasma: 99.8%; metabolite hydroxy-itraconazole: 99.5%

Metabolism: Extensively hepatic via CYP3A4 into >30 metabolites including hydroxy-itraconazole (major metabolite); appears to have *in vitro* antifungal activity. Main metabolic pathway is oxidation; may undergo saturation metabolism with multiple dosing.

Bioavailability: Variable, ~55% (oral solution) in 1 small study; **Note:** Oral solution has a higher degree of bioavailability (149% ± 68%) relative to oral capsules; should not be interchanged

Half-life elimination: Oral: Single dose: ~21 hours, steady state: 64 hours; Cirrhosis (single dose): 37 hours (range: 20-54 hours)

Time to peak, plasma: Capsules: 3-5 hours; Oral solution: 2-3 hours

Excretion: Urine (<0.03% active drug, 40% as inactive metabolites); feces (~3% to 18%)

Dosage

Geriatric & Adult

Usual dosage ranges: Adults: 100-400 mg/day; doses >200 mg/day are given in 2 divided doses; length of therapy varies from 1 day to >6 months depending on the condition and mycological response

Aspergillosis, invasive (salvage therapy): Duration of therapy should be a minimum of 6-12 weeks or throughout period of immunosuppression: Oral: 200-400 mg/day; **Note:** 2008 IDSA guidelines recommend 600 mg/day for 3 days, followed by 400 mg/day (Walsh, 2008).

Appropriate use: Itraconazole should **NOT** be used for voriconazole-refractory aspergillosis since the same antifungal and/or resistance mechanism(s) may be shared by both agents. Itraconazole oral solution and capsule formulations are not bioequivalent or interchangeable. Due to variable bioavailability of oral preparations, therapeutic drug monitoring is advisable (Walsh, 2008).

Aspergillosis, allergic (ABPA, sinusitis): Oral: 200 mg/day; may be used in conjunction with corticosteroids (Walsh, 2008)

Blastomycosis: Oral: 200 mg 3 times/day for 3 days, then 200 mg twice daily for 6-12 months; in moderately-severe to severe infection, therapy should be initiated with ~2 weeks of amphotericin B (Chapman, 2008)

Candidiasis: Oral:

Oropharyngeal: Oral solution: 200 mg once daily for 1-2 weeks; in patients unresponsive or refractory to fluconazole: 100 mg twice daily (clinical response expected in 2-4 weeks)

Esophageal: Oral solution: 100-200 mg once daily for a minimum of 3 weeks; continue dosing for 2 weeks after resolution of symptoms

Coccidioidomycosis (nonprogressive, nondisseminated disease): 200 mg twice daily or 3 times/day (Galgiani, 2005)

Histoplasmosis: Oral: 200 mg 3 times/day for 3 days, then 200 mg twice daily (or once daily in mild-moderate disease) for 6-12 weeks in mild-moderate disease or ≥12 months in progressive disseminated or chronic cavitary pulmonary histoplasmosis; in moderately-severe to severe infection, therapy should be initiated with ~2 weeks of a lipid formation of amphotericin B (Wheat, 2007)

Long-term suppression therapy: 200 mg/day (CDC, 2009b)

Meningitis: Oral:

Coccidioides: 400-600 mg/day (Galgiani, 2005)

Coccidioides, HIV-positive (unlabeled use): 200 mg 3 times/day for 3 days, then 200 mg twice daily; maintenance: 200 mg twice daily life-long (CDC, 2009b)

Appropriate use: Fluconazole is preferred for meningeal infections (CDC, 2009b; Galgiani, 2005).

Onychomycosis: Oral: 200 mg once daily for 12 consecutive weeks; alternative "pulse-dosing" may be considering for fingernail involvement only: 200 mg twice daily for 1 week; repeat 1-week course after 3-week off-time

Penicilliosis, HIV-positive (unlabeled use): Oral: 400 mg daily for 8 weeks (mild disease) or 10 weeks (severe infections). In severely ill patients, initiate therapy with 2 weeks of amphotericin B. Maintenance: 200 mg/day (CDC, 2009b)

Pneumonia: Oral:

Coccidioides: Mild-to-moderate: 200 mg twice daily

Coccidioides, HIV-positive (focal pneumonia): 200 mg 3 times/day for 3 days, then 200 mg twice daily (CDC, 2009b)

Sporotrichosis: Oral:

Lymphocutaneous: 100-200 mg/day for 3-6 months (Kauffman, 2007)

◄

Osteoarticular and pulmonary: 200 mg twice daily for ≥1 years (may use amphotericin B initially for stabilization) (Kauffman, 2007)

Renal Impairment The FDA-approved labeling states to use with caution in patients with renal impairment; wide variations observed in plasma concentrations versus time profiles in patients with uremia, or receiving hemodialysis or continuous ambulatory peritoneal dialysis. The following guidelines have been used by some clinicians:

Aronoff, 2007:

Cl_{cr} >10 mL/minute: No adjustment recommended.

Cl_{cr} <10 mL/minute: Administer 50% of normal dose.

Poorly dialyzed; no supplemental dose or dosage adjustment necessary, including patients on intermittent hemodialysis, peritoneal dialysis, or continuous renal replacement therapy (eg, CVVHD).

Hepatic Impairment No dosage adjustment provided in manufacturer's labeling; however, use caution and monitor closely for signs/symptoms of toxicity.

Administration Doses >200 mg/day are given in 2 divided doses; do not administer with antacids. Capsule and oral solution formulations are not bioequivalent and thus are not interchangeable. Capsule absorption is best if taken with food, therefore, it is best to administer itraconazole after meals; solution should be taken on an empty stomach. When treating oropharyngeal and esophageal candidiasis, solution should be swished vigorously in mouth (10 mL at a time), then swallowed.

Monitoring Parameters Liver function in patients with pre-existing hepatic dysfunction, and in all patients being treated for longer than 1 month; serum concentrations particularly for oral therapy (due to erratic bioavailability with capsule formulation); renal function

Reference Range Serum concentrations may be performed to assure therapeutic levels. Itraconazole plus the metabolite hydroxyitraconazole concentrations should be >1 mcg/mL (not to exceed 10 mcg/mL).

Timing of serum samples: Obtain level after ~2 weeks of therapy, level may be drawn anytime during the dosing interval.

Special Geriatric Considerations No specific data for the elderly. Transient or permanent hearing loss reported in the elderly; several reports include concurrent administration of quinidine.

Dosage Forms Excipient information presented when available (limited, particularly for generics); consult specific product labeling.

Capsule, oral: 100 mg

Sporanox®: 100 mg

Solution, oral:

Sporanox®: 10 mg/mL (150 mL) [contains propylene glycol; cherry-caramel flavor]

Ivermectin (Topical) (eye ver MEK tin)

Brand Names: U.S. Sklice™

Generic Availability (U.S.) No

Pharmacologic Category Antiparasitic Agent, Topical; Pediculocide

Use Topical treatment of head lice (*Pediculus capitis*) infestation

Contraindications There are no contraindications listed in the manufacturer's labeling.

Warnings/Precautions For topical use on scalp and scalp hair only; avoid contact with eyes. Wash hands after application.

Stability Store at 20°C to 25°C (68°F to 77°F); excursions permitted between 15°C to 30°C (59°F to 86°F); do not freeze.

Mechanism of Action Ivermectin is a semisynthetic anthelminthic agent; it binds selectively and with strong affinity to glutamate-gated chloride ion channels which occur in invertebrate nerve and muscle cells. This leads to increased permeability of cell membranes to chloride ions then hyperpolarization of the nerve or muscle cell, and death of the parasite.

Dosage

Geriatric & Adult Head lice: Topical: Apply sufficient amount (up to 1 tube) to completely cover dry scalp and hair; for single-dose use only

Administration Topical lotion. For external use only. Apply to dry scalp and hair closest to scalp first, then apply outward towards ends of hair; completely covering scalp and hair. Leave on for 10 minutes (start timing treatment after the scalp and hair have been completely covered). The hair should then be rinsed thoroughly with warm water. Avoid contact with the eyes. Nit combing is not required, although a fine-tooth comb may be used to remove treated lice and nits. Lotion is for one-time use; discard any unused portion.

Ivermectin should be a portion of a whole lice removal program, which should include washing or dry cleaning all clothing, hats, bedding, and towels recently worn or used by the patient and washing combs, brushes, and hair accessories in hot soapy water.

Monitoring Parameters Monitor scalp for live lice.

Special Geriatric Considerations Specific information on the safety and efficacy of ivermectin in persons ≥65 years of age is not available, as this age group was not sufficiently represented in clinical trials.

Dosage Forms Excipient information presented when available (limited, particularly for generics); consult specific product labeling.
Lotion, topical:
Sklice™: 0.5% (117 g) [contains shea butter]

Kanamycin (kan a MYE sin)

Related Information
Antimicrobial Drugs of Choice *on page 2163*
Medication Safety Issues
Sound-alike/look-alike issues:
Kanamycin may be confused with Garamycin®, gentamicin
Index Terms Kanamycin Sulfate
Generic Availability (U.S.) Yes
Pharmacologic Category Antibiotic, Aminoglycoside
Use Treatment of serious infections caused by susceptible strains of *E. coli*, *Proteus* species, *Enterobacter aerogenes*, *Klebsiella pneumoniae*, *Serratia marcescens*, and *Acinetobacter* species; second-line treatment of *Mycobacterium tuberculosis*
Contraindications Hypersensitivity to kanamycin, any component of the formulation, or other aminoglycosides
Warnings/Precautions [U.S. Boxed Warning]: Aminoglycosides may cause neurotoxicity and/or nephrotoxicity; usual risk factors include pre-existing renal impairment, concomitant neuro-/nephrotoxic medications, advanced age, and dehydration. Ototoxicity may be directly proportional to the amount of drug given and the duration of treatment. Tinnitus or vertigo are indications of vestibular injury and impending hearing loss. Renal damage is usually reversible. May cause neuromuscular blockade and respiratory paralysis; especially when given soon after anesthesia or muscle relaxants.

Not intended for long-term therapy due to toxic hazards associated with extended administration. Use caution in pre-existing renal insufficiency, vestibular or cochlear impairment, myasthenia gravis, hypocalcemia, and conditions which depress neuromuscular transmission. Dosage modification required in patients with impaired renal function. Prolonged use may result in fungal or bacterial superinfection, including *C. difficile*-associated diarrhea (CDAD) and pseudomembranous colitis; CDAD has been observed >2 months postantibiotic treatment.

Adverse Reactions (Reflective of adult population; not specific for elderly) Frequency not defined.
Cardiovascular: Edema
Central nervous system: Neurotoxicity, drowsiness, headache, pseudomotor cerebri
Dermatologic: Skin itching, redness, rash, photosensitivity, erythema
Gastrointestinal: Nausea, vomiting, diarrhea, malabsorption syndrome (with prolonged and high-dose therapy of hepatic coma), anorexia, weight loss, salivation increased, enterocolitis
Hematologic: Granulocytopenia, agranulocytosis, thrombocytopenia
Local: Burning, stinging
Neuromuscular & skeletal: Weakness, tremor, muscle cramps
Otic: Ototoxicity (auditory), ototoxicity (vestibular)
Renal: Nephrotoxicity
Respiratory: Dyspnea

Drug Interactions

Metabolism/Transport Effects None known.

Avoid Concomitant Use

Avoid concomitant use of Kanamycin with any of the following: BCG; Gallium Nitrate

Increased Effect/Toxicity

Kanamycin may increase the levels/effects of: AbobotulinumtoxinA; Bisphosphonate Derivatives; CARBOplatin; Colistimethate; CycloSPORINE; CycloSPORINE (Systemic); Gallium Nitrate; Neuromuscular-Blocking Agents; OnabotulinumtoxinA; RimabotulinumtoxinB

The levels/effects of Kanamycin may be increased by: Amphotericin B; Capreomycin; Cephalosporins (2nd Generation); Cephalosporins (3rd Generation); Cephalosporins (4th Generation); CISplatin; Loop Diuretics; Nonsteroidal Anti-Inflammatory Agents; Vancomycin

Decreased Effect

Kanamycin may decrease the levels/effects of: BCG; Cardiac Glycosides; Typhoid Vaccine

The levels/effects of Kanamycin may be decreased by: Penicillins

Stability Store vial at controlled room temperature. Darkening of vials does not indicate loss of potency.

I.V.: Must be further diluted prior to I.V. infusion. For adults, dilute 500 mg in 100-200 mL of appropriate solution or 1 g in 200-400 mL.

Intraperitoneal: Dilute dose in 20 mL sterile distilled water.

Aerosol: Dilute 250 mg in 3 mL normal saline.

Mechanism of Action Interferes with protein synthesis in bacterial cell by binding to ribosomal subunit

Pharmacodynamics/Kinetics

Absorption:

I.M.: Rapid

Oral: Minimal

Distribution: V_d: ~0.3 L/kg:

Relative diffusion from blood into CSF: Good only with inflammation (exceeds usual MICs)

CSF:blood level ratio: Normal meninges: Nil; Inflamed meninges: 43%

Protein binding: 0%

Half-life elimination: 2-4 hours; Anuria: 80 hours; End-stage renal disease: 40-96 hours

Time to peak, serum: I.M.: 1-2 hours (decreased in burn patients)

Excretion: Urine (as unchanged drug)

Dosage

Geriatric I.M., I.V.: Initial dose should be 5-7.5 mg/kg based on ideal body weight (except in obese patients); maintenance dose and interval should be adjusted for estimated renal function; dosing interval in most older patients is every 12-24 hours (see Dosage: Renal Impairment).

Adult Note: Dosing should be based on ideal body weight

Susceptible systemic infections: I.M., I.V.: 5-7.5 mg/kg/dose in divided doses every 8-12 hours (<15 mg/kg/day)

Following surgical contamination, peritonitis: Intraperitoneal: 500 mg

Irrigating solution: 0.25%; maximum 1.5 g/day (via all administration routes)

Aerosol: 250 mg 2-4 times/day

Renal Impairment

Cl_{cr} 50-80 mL/minute: Administer 60% to 90% of dose or administer every 8-12 hours.

Cl_{cr} 10-50 mL/minute: Administer 30% to 70% of dose or administer every 12 hours.

Cl_{cr} <10 mL/minute: Administer 20% to 30% of dose or administer every 24-48 hours.

Administration Dilute to 100-200 mL and infuse over 30 minutes; I.M. doses should be given in a large muscle mass (ie, gluteus maximus)

Monitoring Parameters Serum creatinine and BUN every 2-3 days; peak and trough concentrations; hearing

Some penicillin derivatives may accelerate the degradation of aminoglycosides *in vitro*. This may be clinically-significant for certain penicillin (ticarcillin, piperacillin, carbenicillin) and aminoglycoside (gentamicin, tobramycin) combination therapy in patients with significant renal impairment. Close monitoring of aminoglycoside levels is warranted.

Reference Range Therapeutic: Peak: 15-30 mcg/mL; Trough: 5-10 mcg/mL; Toxic: Peak: >35 mcg/mL; Trough: >10 mcg/mL

Test Interactions Some penicillin derivatives may accelerate the degradation of aminoglycosides *in vitro*, leading to a potential underestimation of aminoglycoside serum concentration.

Pharmacotherapy Pearls Aminoglycoside levels in blood taken from silastic central catheters can sometime give falsely high readings.

Special Geriatric Considerations This is not a drug of choice since elderly may have increased adverse effects (renal).

Dosage Forms Excipient information presented when available (limited, particularly for generics); consult specific product labeling.
Injection, solution, as sulfate: 1 g/3 mL (3 mL)

- **Kanamycin Sulfate** *see Kanamycin on page 1061*
- **Kaon-CL® 10** *see Potassium Chloride on page 1571*
- **Kaopectate® [OTC]** *see Bismuth on page 216*
- **Kaopectate® Extra Strength [OTC]** *see Bismuth on page 216*
- **Kaopectate® Stool Softener [OTC]** *see Docusate on page 583*
- **Kao-Tin [OTC]** *see Bismuth on page 216*
- **Kao-Tin [OTC]** *see Docusate on page 583*
- **Kapidex** *see Dexlansoprazole on page 523*
- **Kapvay®** *see CloNIDine on page 413*
- **Kayexalate®** *see Sodium Polystyrene Sulfonate on page 1794*
- **KCl** *see Potassium Chloride on page 1571*
- **Kdur** *see Potassium Chloride on page 1571*
- **Keflex®** *see Cephalexin on page 341*
- **Kenalog®** *see Triamcinolone (Topical) on page 1961*
- **Kenalog®-10** *see Triamcinolone (Systemic) on page 1957*
- **Kenalog®-40** *see Triamcinolone (Systemic) on page 1957*
- **Keoxifene Hydrochloride** *see Raloxifene on page 1666*
- **Keppra®** *see LevETIRAcetam on page 1109*
- **Keppra XR®** *see LevETIRAcetam on page 1109*
- **Keralyt®** *see Salicylic Acid on page 1743*
- **Kerlone®** *see Betaxolol (Systemic) on page 207*
- **Ketek®** *see Telithromycin on page 1845*

Ketoconazole (Systemic) (kee toe KOE na zole)

Medication Safety Issues
Sound-alike/look-alike issues:
Nizoral® may be confused with Nasarel, Neoral®, Nitrol®
Brand Names: Canada Apo-Ketoconazole®; Novo-Ketoconazole
Generic Availability (U.S.) Yes
Pharmacologic Category Antifungal Agent, Oral

Use Treatment of susceptible fungal infections, including candidiasis, oral thrush, blastomycosis, histoplasmosis, paracoccidioidomycosis, coccidioidomycosis, chromomycosis, candiduria, chronic mucocutaneous candidiasis, as well as certain recalcitrant cutaneous dermatophytoses

Unlabeled Use Treatment of prostate cancer (androgen synthesis inhibitor)

Contraindications Hypersensitivity to ketoconazole or any component of the formulation; CNS fungal infections (due to poor CNS penetration); coadministration with ergot derivatives, cisapride, or triazolam is contraindicated due to risk of potentially fatal cardiac arrhythmias

Warnings/Precautions [U.S. Boxed Warning]: Ketoconazole has been associated with hepatotoxicity, including some fatalities; use with caution in patients with impaired hepatic function and perform periodic liver function tests. **[U.S. Boxed Warning]: Concomitant use with cisapride is contraindicated due to the occurrence of ventricular arrhythmias.** High doses of ketoconazole may depress adrenocortical function.

Adverse Reactions (Reflective of adult population; not specific for elderly) 1% to 10%:
Dermatologic: Pruritus (2%)
Gastrointestinal: Nausea/vomiting (3% to 10%), abdominal pain (1%)

Drug Interactions
Metabolism/Transport Effects Substrate of CYP3A4 (major); **Note:** Assignment of Major/Minor substrate status based on clinically relevant drug interaction potential; **Inhibits** CYP1A2 (strong), CYP2A6 (moderate), CYP2B6 (weak), CYP2C19 (moderate), CYP2C8 (weak), CYP2C9 (strong), CYP2D6 (moderate), CYP3A4 (strong), P-glycoprotein

Avoid Concomitant Use
Avoid concomitant use of Ketoconazole (Systemic) with any of the following: Alfuzosin; Apixaban; Avanafil; Axitinib; Cisapride; Clopidogrel; Conivaptan; Crizotinib; Dihydroergotamine; Dofetilide; Dronedarone; Eplerenone; Ergoloid Mesylates; Ergonovine; Ergotamine; Everolimus; Fluticasone (Oral Inhalation); Halofantrine; Lapatinib; Lovastatin; Lurasidone; Methylergonovine; Nevirapine; Nilotinib; Nisoldipine; Pimozide; QuiNIDine; Ranolazine; Red Yeast Rice; Rivaroxaban; RomiDEPsin; Salmeterol; Silodosin; Simvastatin; Tamsulosin; Ticagrelor; Tolvaptan; Topotecan; Toremifene

Increased Effect/Toxicity

Ketoconazole (Systemic) may increase the levels/effects of: Alfentanil; Alfuzosin; Aliskiren; Almotriptan; Alosetron; Apixaban; Aprepitant; ARIPiprazole; AtorvaSTATin; Avanafil; Axitinib; Bendamustine; Benzodiazepines (metabolized by oxidation); Boceprevir; Bortezomib; Bosentan; Brentuximab Vedotin; Brinzolamide; Budesonide (Nasal); Budesonide (Systemic, Oral Inhalation); BusPIRone; Busulfan; Calcium Channel Blockers; CarBAMazepine; Carvedilol; Ciclesonide; Cilostazol; Cinacalcet; Cisapride; Colchicine; Conivaptan; Corticosteroids (Orally Inhaled); Corticosteroids (Systemic); Crizotinib; CycloSPORINE; CycloSPORINE (Systemic); CYP1A2 Substrates; CYP2A6 Substrates; CYP2C19 Substrates; CYP2C9 Substrates; CYP2D6 Substrates; CYP3A4 Substrates; Dabigatran Etexilate; Diclofenac; Dienogest; Dihydroergotamine; DOCEtaxel; Dofetilide; Dronedarone; Dutasteride; Eletriptan; Eplerenone; Ergoloid Mesylates; Ergonovine; Ergotamine; Erlotinib; Eszopiclone; Etravirine; Everolimus; FentaNYL; Fesoterodine; Fexofenadine; Fluticasone (Nasal); Fluticasone (Oral Inhalation); Fosaprepitant; Fosphenytoin; Gefitinib; GuanFACINE; Halofantrine; Highest Risk QTc-Prolonging Agents; Iloperidone; Imatinib; Irinotecan; Ivacaftor; Ixabepilone; Lapatinib; Losartan; Lovastatin; Lumefantrine; Lurasidone; Macrolide Antibiotics; Maraviroc; Methadone; Methylergonovine; MethylPREDNISolone; Mifepristone; Moderate Risk QTc-Prolonging Agents; Nebivolol; Nilotinib; Nisoldipine; Paricalcitol; Pazopanib; P-glycoprotein/ABCB1 Substrates; Phenytoin; Pimecrolimus; Pimozide; Praziquantel; Propafenone; Protease Inhibitors; Proton Pump Inhibitors; Prucalopride; QuiNIDine; Ramelteon; Ranolazine; Red Yeast Rice; Repaglinide; Rifamycin Derivatives; Rilpivirine; Rivaroxaban; RomiDEPsin; Ruxolitinib; Salmeterol; Saxagliptin; Sildenafil; Silodosin; Simvastatin; Sirolimus; Solifenacin; SORAfenib; SUNItinib; Tacrolimus; Tacrolimus (Systemic); Tacrolimus (Topical); Tadalafil; Tamsulosin; Telaprevir; Temsirolimus; Ticagrelor; Tolterodine; Tolvaptan; Topotecan; Toremifene; Vardenafil; Vemurafenib; Vilazodone; Vitamin K Antagonists; Ziprasidone; Zolpidem; Zuclopenthixol

The levels/effects of Ketoconazole (Systemic) may be increased by: AtorvaSTATin; Boceprevir; Etravirine; Grapefruit Juice; Macrolide Antibiotics; Mifepristone; Protease Inhibitors; Telaprevir

Decreased Effect

Ketoconazole (Systemic) may decrease the levels/effects of: Amphotericin B; Clopidogrel; Codeine; Ifosfamide; Prasugrel; Saccharomyces boulardii; Ticagrelor; TraMADol

The levels/effects of Ketoconazole (Systemic) may be decreased by: Antacids; CYP3A4 Inducers (Strong); Deferasirox; Didanosine; Etravirine; Fosphenytoin; H2-Antagonists; Herbs (CYP3A4 Inducers); Isoniazid; Nevirapine; Phenytoin; Proton Pump Inhibitors; Rifamycin Derivatives; Rilpivirine; Sucralfate; Tocilizumab

Ethanol/Nutrition/Herb Interactions

Food: Ketoconazole peak serum levels may be prolonged if taken with food.

Herb/Nutraceutical: St John's wort may decrease ketoconazole levels.

Stability Store at 15°C to 25°C (59°F to 77°F).

Mechanism of Action Alters the permeability of the cell wall by blocking fungal cytochrome P450; inhibits biosynthesis of triglycerides and phospholipids by fungi; inhibits several fungal enzymes that results in a build-up of toxic concentrations of hydrogen peroxide; also inhibits androgen synthesis

Pharmacodynamics/Kinetics

Absorption: Rapid (~75%)

Distribution: Well into inflamed joint fluid, saliva, bile, urine, sebum, cerumen, feces, tendons, skin and soft tissue, and testes; crosses blood-brain barrier poorly; only negligible amounts reach CSF

Protein binding: 93% to 96%

Metabolism: Partially hepatic via CYP3A4 to inactive compounds

Bioavailability: Decreases as gastric pH increases

Half-life elimination: Biphasic: Initial: 2 hours; Terminal: 8 hours

Time to peak, serum: 1-2 hours

Excretion: Feces (57%); urine (13%)

Dosage

Geriatric & Adult

Fungal infections: Oral: 200-400 mg/day as a single daily dose

Prostate cancer (unlabeled use): Oral: 400 mg 3 times/day

Renal Impairment Hemodialysis: Not dialyzable (0% to 5%)

Hepatic Impairment Dose reductions should be considered in patients with severe liver disease.

Administration Administer oral tablets 2 hours prior to antacids to prevent decreased absorption due to the high pH of gastric contents.

Monitoring Parameters Liver function tests

Special Geriatric Considerations No specific recommendations.

Dosage Forms Excipient information presented when available (limited, particularly for generics); consult specific product labeling.
Tablet, oral: 200 mg

Ketoconazole (Topical) (kee toe KOE na zole)

Medication Safety Issues
Sound-alike/look-alike issues:
Nizoral® may be confused with Nasarel, Neoral®, Nitrol®
Brand Names: U.S. Extina®; Nizoral®; Nizoral® A-D [OTC]; Xolegel®
Brand Names: Canada Ketoderm®; Xolegel®
Generic Availability (U.S.) Yes: Aerosol, cream, shampoo
Pharmacologic Category Antifungal Agent, Topical
Use
Cream: Treatment of tinea corporis, tinea cruris, tinea versicolor, cutaneous candidiasis, seborrheic dermatitis
Foam, gel: Treatment of seborrheic dermatitis
Shampoo: Treatment of dandruff, seborrheic dermatitis, tinea versicolor
Unlabeled Use Cream: Treatment of susceptible fungal infections in the oral cavity including candidiasis, oral thrush, and chronic mucocutaneous candidiasis
Dosage
Geriatric & Adult
Fungal infections: *Topical:*
Cream: Tinea infections: Rub gently into the affected area once daily. Duration of treatment: Tinea corporis, cruris: 2 weeks; tinea pedis: 6 weeks
Shampoo (ketoconazole 2%): Tinea versicolor: Apply to damp skin, lather, leave on 5 minutes, and rinse (one application should be sufficient)
Seborrheic dermatitis: *Topical:*
Cream: Rub gently into the affected area twice daily for 4 weeks or until clinical response is noted.
Foam: Apply to affected area twice daily for 4 weeks
Gel: Rub gently into the affected area once daily for 2 weeks.
Shampoo (ketoconazole 1%): Apply twice weekly for up to 8 weeks with at least 3 days between each shampoo
Susceptible fungal infections in the oral cavity (candidiasis, oral thrush, and chronic mucocutaneous candidiasis) (unlabeled use): *Topical:* Cream: Apply locally as directed with a thin coat to inner surface of denture and affected areas after meals
Special Geriatric Considerations Instruct patient or caregiver on appropriate use of topical ketoconazole products.
Dosage Forms Excipient information presented when available (limited, particularly for generics); consult specific product labeling. [DSC] = Discontinued product
Aerosol, foam, topical: 2% (50 g, 100 g)
Extina®: 2% (50 g, 100 g)
Cream, topical: 2% (15 g, 30 g, 60 g)
Gel, topical:
Xolegel®: 2% (15 g [DSC], 45 g) [contains dehydrated ethanol 34%]
Shampoo, topical: 2% (120 mL)
Nizoral®: 2% (120 mL)
Nizoral® A-D: 1% (120 mL, 210 mL)

Ketoprofen (kee toe PROE fen)

Related Information
Beers Criteria – Potentially Inappropriate Medications for Geriatrics *on page 2183*
Medication Safety Issues
Sound-alike/look-alike issues:
Ketoprofen may be confused with ketotifen
BEERS Criteria medication:
This drug may be potentially inappropriate for use in geriatric patients (Quality of evidence - moderate; Strength of recommendation - strong).
Brand Names: Canada Apo-Keto SR®; Apo-Keto-E®; Apo-Keto®; Ketoprofen SR; Keto-profen-E; Nu-Ketoprofen; Nu-Ketoprofen-E; PMS-Ketoprofen; PMS-Ketoprofen-E
Generic Availability (U.S.) Yes
Pharmacologic Category Nonsteroidal Anti-inflammatory Drug (NSAID), Oral
Use Acute and long-term treatment of rheumatoid arthritis and osteoarthritis; primary dysmenorrhea; mild-to-moderate pain

◀ **Unlabeled Use** Migraine prophylaxis

Medication Guide Available Yes

Contraindications Hypersensitivity to ketoprofen, aspirin, other NSAIDs, or any component of the formulation; perioperative pain in the setting of coronary artery bypass graft (CABG) surgery

Warnings/Precautions [U.S. Boxed Warning]: NSAIDs are associated with an increased risk of adverse cardiovascular thrombotic events, including MI and stroke Risk may be increased with duration of use or pre-existing cardiovascular risk factors or disease. Carefully evaluate individual cardiovascular risk profiles prior to prescribing. May cause new-onset hypertension or worsening of existing hypertension. Use caution with fluid retention. Avoid use in heart failure. Concurrent administration of ibuprofen, and potentially other nonselective NSAIDs, may interfere with aspirin's cardioprotective effect. **[U.S. Boxed Warning]: Use is contraindicated for treatment of perioperative pain in the setting of coronary artery bypass graft (CABG) surgery.** Risk of MI and stroke may be increased with use following CABG surgery.

NSAID use may compromise existing renal function; dose-dependent decreases in prosta-glandin synthesis may result from NSAID use, reducing renal blood flow which may cause renal decompensation. NSAID use may increase the risk for hyperkalemia. Patients with impaired renal function, dehydration, heart failure, liver dysfunction, those taking diuretics, and ACE inhibitors, and the elderly are at greater risk of renal toxicity and hyperkalemia. Rehydrate patient before starting therapy; monitor renal function closely. Not recommended for use in patients with advanced renal disease. Long-term NSAID use may result in renal papillary necrosis.

[U.S. Boxed Warning]: NSAIDs may increase risk of gastrointestinal irritation, inflam-mation, ulceration, bleeding, and perforation. These events may occur at any time during therapy and without warning. Use caution with a history of GI disease (bleeding or ulcers), concurrent therapy with aspirin, anticoagulants and/or corticosteroids, smoking, use of alcohol, the elderly or debilitated patients. When used concomitantly with ≤325 mg of aspirin, a substantial increase in the risk of gastrointestinal complications (eg, ulcer) occurs; con-comitant gastroprotective therapy (eg, proton pump inhibitors) is recommended (Bhatt, 2008). Platelet adhesion and aggregation may be decreased; may prolong bleeding time; patients with coagulation disorders or who are receiving anticoagulants should be monitored closely. Anemia may occur; patients on long-term NSAID therapy should be monitored for anemia. Rarely, NSAID use may cause severe blood dyscrasias (eg, agranulocytosis, aplastic anemia, thrombocytopenia).

In the elderly, avoid chronic use (unless alternative agents ineffective and patient can receive concomitant gastroprotective agent); nonselective oral NSAID use is associated with an increased risk of GI bleeding and peptic ulcer disease in older adults in high risk category (eg, >75 years or age or receiving concomitant oral/parenteral corticosteroids, anticoagulants, or antiplatelet agents) (Beers Criteria).

Use the lowest effective dose for the shortest duration of time, consistent with individual patient goals, to reduce risk of cardiovascular or GI adverse events. Alternate therapies should be considered for patients at high risk.

NSAIDS may cause drowsiness, dizziness, blurred vision and other neurologic effects which may impair physical or mental abilities; patients must be cautioned about performing tasks which require mental alertness (eg, operating machinery or driving). Discontinue use with blurred or diminished vision and perform ophthalmologic exam. Monitor vision with long-term therapy.

NSAIDs may cause serious skin adverse events including exfoliative dermatitis, Stevens-Johnson syndrome (SJS), and toxic epidermal necrolysis (TEN); discontinue use at first sign of skin rash or hypersensitivity. Anaphylactoid reactions may occur, even without prior exposure; patients with "aspirin triad" (bronchial asthma, aspirin intolerance, rhinitis) may be at increased risk. Do not use in patients who experience bronchospasm, asthma, rhinitis, or urticaria with NSAID or aspirin therapy. Use caution in other forms of asthma.

Use with caution in patients with decreased hepatic function. Closely monitor patients with any abnormal LFT. Severe hepatic reactions (eg, fulminant hepatitis, liver failure) have occurred with NSAID use, rarely; discontinue if signs or symptoms of liver disease develop, or if systemic manifestations occur. The elderly are at increased risk for adverse effects (especially peptic ulceration, CNS effects, renal toxicity) from NSAIDs, even at low doses.

Withhold for at least 4-6 half-lives prior to surgical or dental procedures.

Adverse Reactions (Reflective of adult population; not specific for elderly)

>10%:
  Gastrointestinal: Dyspepsia (11%)
  Hepatic: Liver function test abnormal (≤15%)
1% to 10%:
  Cardiovascular: Peripheral edema (2%)
  Central nervous system: Headache (3% to 9%), depression, dizziness (>1%), dreams, insomnia, malaise, nervousness, somnolence
  Dermatologic: Rash (>1%)
  Gastrointestinal: Abdominal pain (3% to 9%), constipation (3% to 9%), diarrhea (3% to 9%), flatulence (3% to 9%), nausea (3% to 9%), gastrointestinal bleeding (>2%), peptic ulcer (>2%), anorexia (>1%), stomatitis (>1%), vomiting (>1%)
  Genitourinary: Urinary tract irritation (>1%)
  Ocular: Visual disturbances (>1%)
  Otic: Tinnitus (>1%)
  Renal: Renal dysfunction (3% to 9%)

Drug Interactions

Metabolism/Transport Effects Inhibits CYP2C9 (weak)

Avoid Concomitant Use

Avoid concomitant use of Ketoprofen with any of the following: Floctafenine; Ketorolac; Ketorolac (Nasal); Ketorolac (Systemic)

Increased Effect/Toxicity

Ketoprofen may increase the levels/effects of: Aliskiren; Aminoglycosides; Anticoagulants; Antiplatelet Agents; Bisphosphonate Derivatives; Collagenase (Systemic); CycloSPORINE; CycloSPORINE (Systemic); Dabigatran Etexilate; Deferasirox; Desmopressin; Digoxin; Drotrecogin Alfa (Activated); Eplerenone; Haloperidol; Ibritumomab; Lithium; Methotrexate; Nonsteroidal Anti-Inflammatory Agents; PEMEtrexed; Porfimer; Potassium-Sparing Diuretics; PRALAtrexate; Quinolone Antibiotics; Rivaroxaban; Salicylates; Thrombolytic Agents; Tositumomab and Iodine I 131 Tositumomab; Vancomycin; Vitamin K Antagonists

The levels/effects of Ketoprofen may be increased by: ACE Inhibitors; Angiotensin II Receptor Blockers; Antidepressants (Tricyclic, Tertiary Amine); Corticosteroids (Systemic); CycloSPORINE; CycloSPORINE (Systemic); Dasatinib; Floctafenine; Glucosamine; Herbs (Anticoagulant/Antiplatelet Properties); Ketorolac; Ketorolac (Nasal); Ketorolac (Systemic); Nonsteroidal Anti-Inflammatory Agents; Omega-3-Acid Ethyl Esters; Pentosan Polysulfate Sodium; Pentoxifylline; Probenecid; Prostacyclin Analogues; Selective Serotonin Reuptake Inhibitors; Serotonin/Norepinephrine Reuptake Inhibitors; Sodium Phosphates; Tipranavir; Treprostinil; Vitamin E

Decreased Effect

Ketoprofen may decrease the levels/effects of: ACE Inhibitors; Aliskiren; Angiotensin II Receptor Blockers; Antiplatelet Agents; Beta-Blockers; Eplerenone; HydrALAZINE; Loop Diuretics; Potassium-Sparing Diuretics; Salicylates; Selective Serotonin Reuptake Inhibitors; Thiazide Diuretics

The levels/effects of Ketoprofen may be decreased by: Bile Acid Sequestrants; Nonsteroidal Anti-Inflammatory Agents; Salicylates

Ethanol/Nutrition/Herb Interactions

Ethanol: Avoid ethanol (due to GI irritation).
Food: Food slows rate of absorption resulting in delayed and reduced peak serum concentrations; total bioavailability is not affected by food.
Herb/Nutraceutical: Avoid alfalfa, anise, bilberry, bladderwrack, bromelain, cat's claw, celery, chamomile, coleus, cordyceps, dong quai, evening primrose, fenugreek, feverfew, garlic, ginger, ginkgo biloba, ginseng (American, Panax, Siberian), grapeseed, green tea, guggul, horse chestnut seed, horseradish, licorice, prickly ash, red clover, reishi, SAMe (S-adenosylmethionine), sweet clover, turmeric, and white willow (all have additional antiplatelet activity).

Stability Store at room temperature of 25°C (77°F). Protect from light; avoid excessive heat and humidity.

Mechanism of Action Reversibly inhibits cyclooxygenase-1 and 2 (COX-1 and 2) enzymes, which results in decreased formation of prostaglandin precursors; has antipyretic, analgesic, and anti-inflammatory properties

Other proposed mechanisms not fully elucidated (and possibly contributing to the anti-inflammatory effect to varying degrees), include inhibiting chemotaxis, altering lymphocyte activity, inhibiting neutrophil aggregation/activation, and decreasing proinflammatory cytokine levels.

Pharmacodynamics/Kinetics

Onset of action: Regular release: <30 minutes

Duration: Regular release: Up to 6 hours

Absorption: Almost complete

Distribution: 0.1 L/kg

Protein binding: >99%, primarily to albumin; Hepatic impairment: Unbound fraction is approximately doubled

Metabolism: Hepatic via glucuronidation; metabolite (inactive) can be converted back to parent compound; may have enterohepatic recirculation

Bioavailability: ~90%

Half-life elimination:

Regular release: 2-4 hours; Renal impairment: Mild: 3 hours; moderate-to-severe: 5-9 hours

Extended release: ~3-7.5 hours

Time to peak, serum:

Regular release: 0.5-2 hours

Extended release: 6-7 hours

Excretion: Urine (~80%, primarily as glucuronide conjugates)

Dosage

Geriatric Initial: 25-50 mg 3-4 times/day; increase up to 150-300 mg/day (maximum daily dose: 300 mg)

Adult Note: The extended release formulation is not recommended for the treatment of acute pain.

Rheumatoid arthritis or osteoarthritis: Oral:

Regular release: 50 mg 4 times/day **or** 75 mg 3 times/day; up to a maximum of 300 mg/day

Extended release: 200 mg once daily

Note: Lower doses may be used in small patients or in the elderly, or debilitated.

Dysmenorrhea, mild-to-moderate pain: Oral: Regular release: 25-50 mg every 6-8 hours up to a maximum of 300 mg/day

Renal Impairment In general, NSAIDs are not recommended for use in patients with advanced renal disease, but the manufacturer of ketoprofen does provide some guidelines for adjustment in renal dysfunction:

Mild impairment: Maximum dose: 150 mg/day

Severe impairment: Cl_{cr} <25 mL/minute: Maximum dose: 100 mg/day

Hepatic Impairment Hepatic impairment and serum albumin <3.5 g/dL: Maximum dose: 100 mg/day

Administration May take with food to reduce GI upset. Do not crush or break extended release capsules.

Monitoring Parameters CBC, chemistry profile, occult blood loss, periodic liver function; renal function (urine output, serum BUN, creatinine)

Special Geriatric Considerations Elderly are a high-risk population for adverse effects from NSAIDs. As much as 60% of the elderly can develop peptic ulceration and/or hemorrhage asymptomatically. The concomitant use of H_2 blockers and sucralfate is not effective as prophylaxis with the exception of NSAID-induced duodenal ulcers which may be prevented by the use of ranitidine. Misoprostol and proton pump inhibitors are the only agents proven to help prevent the development of NSAID-induced ulcers. Also, concomitant disease and drug use contribute to the risk for GI adverse effects. Use lowest effective dose for shortest period possible. Consider renal function decline with age. Use of NSAIDs can compromise existing renal function especially when Cl_{cr} is ≤30 mL/minute. Tinnitus may be a difficult and unreliable indication of toxicity due to age-related hearing loss or eighth cranial nerve damage. CNS adverse effects such as confusion, agitation, and hallucination are generally seen in overdose or high dose situations, but elderly may demonstrate these adverse effects at lower doses than younger adults.

This medication is considered to be potentially inappropriate in this patient population (Beers Criteria: Quality of evidence - moderate; Strength of recommendation - strong).

Dosage Forms Excipient information presented when available (limited, particularly for generics); consult specific product labeling.

Capsule, oral: 50 mg, 75 mg

Capsule, extended release, oral: 200 mg

Ketorolac (Systemic) (KEE toe role ak)

Related Information
Beers Criteria – Potentially Inappropriate Medications for Geriatrics *on page 2183*
Medication Safety Issues
Sound-alike/look-alike issues:
Ketorolac may be confused with Ketalar®
Toradol® may be confused with Foradil®, Inderal®, TEGretol®, traMADol, tromethamine
BEERS Criteria medication:
This drug may be potentially inappropriate for use in geriatric patients (Quality of evidence - high; Strength of recommendation - strong).
International issues:
Toradol [Canada and multiple international markets] may be confused with Theradol brand name for tramadol [Netherlands]
Brand Names: Canada Apo-Ketorolac Injectable®; Apo-Ketorolac®; Ketorolac Tromethamine Injection, USP; Novo-Ketorolac; Nu-Ketorolac; Toradol®; Toradol® IM
Index Terms Ketorolac Tromethamine; Toradol
Generic Availability (U.S.) Yes
Pharmacologic Category Nonsteroidal Anti-inflammatory Drug (NSAID), Oral; Nonsteroidal Anti-inflammatory Drug (NSAID), Parenteral
Use Short-term (≤5 days) management of moderate-to-severe acute pain requiring analgesia at the opioid level
Medication Guide Available Yes
Contraindications Hypersensitivity to ketorolac, aspirin, other NSAIDs, or any component of the formulation; active or history of peptic ulcer disease; recent or history of GI bleeding or perforation; patients with advanced renal disease or risk of renal failure (due to volume depletion); prophylaxis before major surgery; suspected or confirmed cerebrovascular bleeding; hemorrhagic diathesis, incomplete hemostasis, or high risk of bleeding; concurrent ASA or other NSAIDs; concomitant probenecid or pentoxifylline; epidural or intrathecal administration; perioperative pain in the setting of coronary artery bypass graft (CABG) surgery
Warnings/Precautions [U.S. Boxed Warning]: May inhibit platelet function; contraindicated in patients with cerebrovascular bleeding (suspected or confirmed), hemorrhagic diathesis, incomplete hemostasis and patients at high risk for bleeding. Effects on platelet adhesion and aggregation may prolong bleeding time. Anemia may occur; patients on long-term NSAID therapy should be monitored for anemia. Rarely, NSAID use has been associated with potentially severe blood dyscrasias (eg, agranulocytosis, thrombocytopenia, aplastic anemia).

[U.S. Boxed Warning]: NSAIDs are associated with an increased risk of adverse cardiovascular thrombotic events, including MI and stroke. Risk may be increased with duration of use or pre-existing cardiovascular risk factors or disease. Carefully evaluate individual cardiovascular risk profiles prior to prescribing. May cause new-onset hypertension or worsening of existing hypertension. Use caution with fluid retention. Avoid use in heart failure. Concurrent administration of ibuprofen, and potentially other nonselective NSAIDs, may interfere with aspirin's cardioprotective effect. **[U.S. Boxed Warning]: Use is contraindicated as prophylactic analgesic before any major surgery and is contraindicated for treatment of perioperative pain in the setting of coronary artery bypass graft (CABG) surgery.** Risk of MI and stroke may be increased with use following CABG surgery. Wound bleeding and postoperative hematomas have been associated with ketorolac use in the perioperative setting. Withhold for at least 4-6 half-lives prior to surgical or dental procedures.

[U.S. Boxed Warning]: Ketorolac is contraindicated in patients with advanced renal impairment and in patients at risk for renal failure due to volume depletion. NSAID use may compromise existing renal function; dose-dependent decreases in prostaglandin synthesis may result from NSAID use, reducing renal blood flow which may cause renal decompensation. NSAID use may increase the risk for hyperkalemia. Patients with impaired renal function, dehydration, heart failure, liver dysfunction, those taking diuretics and ACE inhibitors, and the elderly are at greater risk of renal toxicity. Use with caution in patients with impaired renal function or history of kidney disease; dosage adjustment is required in patients with moderate elevation in serum creatinine. Monitor renal function closely. Acute renal failure, interstitial nephritis, and nephrotic syndrome have been reported with ketorolac use; papillary necrosis and renal injury have been reported with the use of NSAIDs. Use of NSAIDs can compromise existing renal function. Rehydrate patient before starting therapy.

[U.S. Boxed Warning]: NSAIDs may increase risk of gastrointestinal irritation, inflammation, ulceration, bleeding, and perforation. These events may occur at any time during therapy and without warning. Use caution with a history of GI disease (bleeding, ulcers, inflammatory bowel disease), concurrent therapy with aspirin, anticoagulants and/or cortico-steroids, smoking, use of alcohol, the elderly, or debilitated patients. When used concomitantly with ≤325 mg of aspirin, a substantial increase in the risk of gastrointestinal complications (eg, ulcer) occurs; concomitant gastroprotective therapy (eg, proton pump inhibitors) is recommended (Bhatt, 2008).

NSAIDs may cause serious skin adverse events including exfoliative dermatitis, Stevens-Johnson syndrome (SJS), and toxic epidermal necrolysis (TEN); discontinue use at first sign of skin rash or hypersensitivity. Hypersensitivity or anaphylactoid reactions may occur, even without prior exposure; patients with "aspirin triad" (bronchial asthma, aspirin intolerance, rhinitis) may be at increased risk. Do not use in patients who experience bronchospasm, asthma, rhinitis, or urticaria with NSAID or aspirin therapy. **[U.S. Boxed Warning]: Ketorolac injection is contraindicated in patients with prior hypersensitivity reaction to aspirin or NSAIDs**. Use caution in other forms of asthma.

Use with caution in patients with hepatic impairment or a history of liver disease. Closely monitor patients with any abnormal LFT. Rarely, severe hepatic reactions (eg, fulminant hepatitis, hepatic necrosis, liver failure) have occurred with NSAID use; discontinue if signs or symptoms of liver disease develop, or if systemic manifestations occur.

[U.S. Boxed Warning]: Dosage adjustment is required for patients ≥65 years of age. Avoid use in older adults; use is associated with an increased risk of GI bleeding and peptic ulcer disease in older adults in high risk category (eg, >75 years or age or receiving concomitant oral/parenteral corticosteroids, anticoagulants, or antiplatelet agents) (Beers Criteria). **[U.S. Boxed Warning]: Dosage adjustment is required for patients weighing <50 kg (<110 pounds). [U.S. Boxed Warning]: Concurrent use of ketorolac with aspirin or other NSAIDs is contraindicated due to the increased risk of adverse reactions.**

[U.S. Boxed Warning]: Contraindicated for epidural or intrathecal administration. [U.S. Boxed Warning]: Systemic ketorolac is indicated for short term (≤5 days) use in adults for treatment of moderately severe acute pain requiring opioid-level analgesia. Low doses of narcotics may be needed for breakthrough pain. **[U.S. Boxed Warning]: Oral therapy is only indicated for use as continuation treatment, following parenteral ketorolac and is not indicated for minor or chronic painful conditions. The maximum daily oral dose is 40 mg (adults); doses above 40 mg/day do not improve efficacy but may increase the risk of serious adverse effects.** The combined therapy duration (oral and parenteral) should not exceed 5 days. Use the lowest effective dose for the shortest duration of time, consistent with individual patient goals, to reduce risk of cardiovascular or GI adverse events. Alternate therapies should be considered for patients at high risk.

NSAIDS may cause drowsiness, dizziness, blurred vision and other neurologic effects which may impair physical or mental abilities; patients must be cautioned about performing tasks which require mental alertness (eg, operating machinery or driving). Discontinue use with blurred or diminished vision and perform ophthalmologic exam. Monitor vision with long-term therapy.

Adverse Reactions (Reflective of adult population; not specific for elderly)
Frequencies noted for parenteral administration:

>10%:
Central nervous system: Headache (17%)
Gastrointestinal: Gastrointestinal pain (13%), dyspepsia (12%), nausea (12%)

>1% to 10%:
Cardiovascular: Edema (4%), hypertension
Central nervous system: Dizziness (7%), drowsiness (6%)
Dermatologic: Pruritus, purpura, rash
Gastrointestinal: Diarrhea (7%), constipation, flatulence, GI bleeding, GI fullness, GI perfo-ration, GI ulcer, heartburn, stomatitis, vomiting
Hematologic: Anemia, bleeding time increased
Hepatic: Liver enzymes increased
Local: Injection site pain (2%)
Otic: Tinnitus
Renal: Renal function abnormal
Miscellaneous: Diaphoresis

Drug Interactions
Metabolism/Transport Effects None known.
Avoid Concomitant Use
Avoid concomitant use of Ketorolac (Systemic) with any of the following: Aspirin; Floctafe-nine; Ketorolac; Ketorolac (Nasal); Nonsteroidal Anti-Inflammatory Agents; Pentoxifylline; Probenecid

Increased Effect/Toxicity

Ketorolac (Systemic) may increase the levels/effects of: Aliskiren; Aminoglycosides; Anticoagulants; Antiplatelet Agents; Aspirin; Bisphosphonate Derivatives; Collagenase (Systemic); CycloSPORINE; CycloSPORINE (Systemic); Dabigatran Etexilate; Deferasirox; Desmopressin; Digoxin; Drotrecogin Alfa (Activated); Eplerenone; Haloperidol; Ibritumomab; Lithium; Methotrexate; Neuromuscular-Blocking Agents (Nondepolarizing); Nonsteroidal Anti-Inflammatory Agents; PEMEtrexed; Pentoxifylline; Porfimer; Potassium-Sparing Diuretics; PRALAtrexate; Quinolone Antibiotics; Rivaroxaban; Salicylates; Thrombolytic Agents; Tositumomab and Iodine I 131 Tositumomab; Vancomycin; Vitamin K Antagonists

The levels/effects of Ketorolac (Systemic) may be increased by: ACE Inhibitors; Angiotensin II Receptor Blockers; Antidepressants (Tricyclic, Tertiary Amine); Corticosteroids (Systemic); CycloSPORINE; CycloSPORINE (Systemic); Dasatinib; Floctafenine; Glucosamine; Herbs (Anticoagulant/Antiplatelet Properties); Ketorolac; Ketorolac (Nasal); Omega-3-Acid Ethyl Esters; Pentosan Polysulfate Sodium; Probenecid; Prostacyclin Analogues; Selective Serotonin Reuptake Inhibitors; Serotonin/Norepinephrine Reuptake Inhibitors; Sodium Phosphates; Tipranavir; Treprostinil; Vitamin E

Decreased Effect

Ketorolac (Systemic) may decrease the levels/effects of: ACE Inhibitors; Aliskiren; Angiotensin II Receptor Blockers; Anticonvulsants; Antiplatelet Agents; Beta-Blockers; Eplerenone; HydrALAZINE; Loop Diuretics; Potassium-Sparing Diuretics; Salicylates; Selective Serotonin Reuptake Inhibitors; Thiazide Diuretics

The levels/effects of Ketorolac (Systemic) may be decreased by: Bile Acid Sequestrants; Salicylates

Ethanol/Nutrition/Herb Interactions

Ethanol: Avoid ethanol (may enhance gastric mucosal irritation).

Food: Oral: High-fat meals may delay time to peak (by ~1 hour) and decrease peak concentrations.

Herb/Nutraceutical: Avoid alfalfa, anise, bilberry, bladderwrack, bromelain, cat's claw, celery, chamomile, coleus, cordyceps, dong quai, evening primrose, fenugreek, feverfew, garlic, ginger, ginkgo biloba, ginseng (American, Panax, Siberian), grapeseed, green tea, guggul, horse chestnut seed, horseradish, licorice, prickly ash, red clover, reishi, SAMe (S-adenosylmethionine), sweet clover, turmeric, and white willow (all have additional antiplatelet activity).

Stability

Injection: Store at room temperature of 15°C to 30°C (59°F to 86°F). Protect from light. Injection is clear and has a slight yellow color. Precipitation may occur at relatively low pH values.

Tablet: Store at room temperature of 15°C to 30°C (59°F to 86°F).

Mechanism of Action

Reversibly inhibits cyclooxygenase-1 and 2 (COX-1 and 2) enzymes, which results in decreased formation of prostaglandin precursors; has antipyretic, analgesic, and anti-inflammatory properties

Other proposed mechanisms not fully elucidated (and possibly contributing to the anti-inflammatory effect to varying degrees), include inhibiting chemotaxis, altering lymphocyte activity, inhibiting neutrophil aggregation/activation, and decreasing proinflammatory cytokine levels.

Pharmacodynamics/Kinetics

Onset of action: Analgesic: I.M.: ~10 minutes

Peak effect: Analgesic: 2-3 hours

Duration: Analgesic: 6-8 hours

Absorption: Oral: Well absorbed (100%)

Distribution: ~13 L; poor penetration into CSF

Protein binding: 99%

Metabolism: Hepatic

Half-life elimination: 2-6 hours; prolonged 30% to 50% in elderly; up to 19 hours in renal impairment

Time to peak, serum: I.M.: 30-60 minutes

Excretion: Urine (92%, ~60% as unchanged drug); feces ~6%

Dosage

Geriatric Dosage adjustments in elderly (≥65 years), renal insufficiency, or low body weight (<50 kg): **Note:** These groups have an increased incidence of GI bleeding, ulceration, and perforation. The maximum combined duration of treatment (for parenteral and oral) is 5 days.

I.M.: 30 mg as a single dose or 15 mg every 6 hours (maximum daily dose: 60 mg)

I.V.: 15 mg as a single dose or 15 mg every 6 hours (maximum daily dose: 60 mg)

Oral: 10 mg, followed by 10 mg every 4-6 hours; do not exceed 40 mg/day; oral dosing is intended to be a continuation of I.M. or I.V. therapy only

◄ **Adult Pain management (acute; moderately-severe): Note:** The maximum combined duration of treatment (for parenteral and oral) is 5 days; do not increase dose or frequency; supplement with low dose opioids if needed for breakthrough pain. For patients <50 kg and/or ≥65 years of age, see Dosage: Geriatric.

I.M.: 60 mg as a single dose or 30 mg every 6 hours (maximum daily dose: 120 mg)

I.V.: 30 mg as a single dose or 30 mg every 6 hours (maximum daily dose: 120 mg)

Oral: 20 mg, followed by 10 mg every 4-6 hours; do not exceed 40 mg/day; oral dosing is intended to be a continuation of I.M. or I.V. therapy only

Renal Impairment Contraindicated in patients with advanced renal impairment. Patients with moderately-elevated serum creatinine should use half the recommended dose, not to exceed 60 mg/day I.M./I.V.

Hepatic Impairment Use with caution, may cause elevation of liver enzymes; discontinue if clinical signs and symptoms of liver disease develop.

Administration

Oral: May take with food to reduce GI upset.

I.M.: Administer slowly and deeply into the muscle. Analgesia begins in 30 minutes and maximum effect within 2 hours.

I.V.: Administer I.V. bolus over a minimum of 15 seconds; onset within 30 minutes; peak analgesia within 2 hours.

Monitoring Parameters Monitor response (pain, range of motion, grip strength, mobility, ADL function), inflammation; observe for weight gain, edema; monitor renal function (serum creatinine, BUN, urine output); CBC and platelets, liver function tests; observe for bleeding, bruising; evaluate gastrointestinal effects (abdominal pain, bleeding, dyspepsia); mental confusion, disorientation

Reference Range Serum concentration: Therapeutic: 0.3-5 mcg/mL; Toxic: >5 mcg/mL

Pharmacotherapy Pearls First parenteral NSAID for analgesia; 30 mg provides the analgesia comparable to 12 mg of morphine or 100 mg of meperidine.

Special Geriatric Considerations Ketorolac is cleared more slowly in the elderly. It is recommended to use lower doses in the elderly. Elderly are a high-risk population for adverse effects from NSAIDs. As much as 60% of elderly can develop peptic ulceration and/or hemorrhage asymptomatically. The concomitant use of H_2 blockers and sucralfate is not effective as prophylaxis with the exception of NSAID-induced duodenal ulcers which may be prevented by the use of ranitidine. Misoprostol and proton pump inhibitors are the only agents proven to help prevent the development of NSAID-induced ulcers. Also, concomitant disease and drug use contribute to the risk for GI adverse effects. Use lowest effective dose for shortest period possible. Consider renal function decline with age. Use of NSAIDs can compromise existing renal function especially when Cl_{cr} is ≤30 mL/minute or weight <50 kg. Tinnitus may be a difficult and unreliable indication of toxicity due to age-related hearing loss or eighth cranial nerve damage. CNS adverse effects such as confusion, agitation, and hallucination are generally seen in overdose or high dose situations, but elderly may demonstrate these adverse effects at lower doses than younger adults.

This medication is considered to be potentially inappropriate in this patient population (Beers Criteria: Quality of evidence - high; Strength of recommendation - strong).

Dosage Forms Excipient information presented when available (limited, particularly for generics); consult specific product labeling.

Injection, solution, as tromethamine: 15 mg/mL (1 mL, 2 mL); 30 mg/mL (1 mL, 2 mL, 10 mL)

Tablet, oral, as tromethamine: 10 mg

Ketorolac (Nasal) (KEE toe role ak)

Medication Safety Issues

Sound-alike/look-alike issues:

Ketorolac may be confused with Ketalar®

BEERS Criteria medication:

This drug may be potentially inappropriate for use in geriatric patients (Quality of evidence - high; Strength of recommendation - strong).

Brand Names: U.S. Sprix®

Index Terms Ketorolac Tromethamine

Generic Availability (U.S.) No

Pharmacologic Category Nonsteroidal Anti-inflammatory Drug (NSAID), Nasal

Use Short-term (≤5 days) management of moderate-to-moderately-severe acute pain requiring analgesia at the opioid level

Medication Guide Available Yes

Contraindications Hypersensitivity to ketorolac, aspirin, other NSAIDs, or any component of the formulation; history of asthma, urticaria, or other allergic-type reactions following aspirin or other NSAID use; active or history of peptic ulcer disease; recent or history of GI bleeding or perforation; patients with advanced renal disease or risk of renal failure (due to volume depletion); prophylaxis before major surgery; suspected or confirmed cerebrovascular bleeding; hemorrhagic diathesis, incomplete hemostasis, or high risk of bleeding; concomitant probenecid or pentoxifylline; perioperative pain in the setting of coronary artery bypass graft (CABG) surgery

Warnings/Precautions **[U.S. Boxed Warning]: May inhibit platelet function; contraindicated in patients with cerebrovascular bleeding (suspected or confirmed), hemorrhagic diathesis, incomplete hemostasis and patients at high risk for bleeding.** Effects on platelet adhesion and aggregation may prolong bleeding time. Anemia may occur; patients on long-term NSAID therapy should be monitored for anemia. Rarely, NSAID use has been associated with potentially severe blood dyscrasias (eg, agranulocytosis, thrombocytopenia, aplastic anemia).

[U.S. Boxed Warning]: NSAIDs are associated with an increased risk of adverse cardiovascular thrombotic events, including MI and stroke. Risk may be increased with duration of use or pre-existing cardiovascular risk factors or disease. Carefully evaluate individual cardiovascular risk profiles prior to prescribing. Use caution with fluid retention. Avoid use in heart failure. Use may cause new-onset hypertension or worsening of existing hypertension. Concurrent administration of ibuprofen, and potentially other nonselective NSAIDs, may interfere with aspirin's cardioprotective effect. **[U.S. Boxed Warning]: Use is contraindicated for treatment of perioperative pain in the setting of coronary artery bypass graft (CABG) surgery.** Risk of MI and stroke may be increased with use following CABG surgery. Use is also contraindicated as prophylactic analgesic before any major surgery. Wound bleeding and postoperative hematomas have been associated with ketorolac use in the perioperative setting. Withhold for at least 4-6 half-lives prior to surgical or dental procedures.

[U.S. Boxed Warning]: Ketorolac is contraindicated in patients with advanced renal impairment and in patients at risk for renal failure due to volume depletion. NSAID use may compromise existing renal function; dose-dependent decreases in prostaglandin synthesis may result from NSAID use, reducing renal blood flow which may cause renal decompensation. NSAID use may increase the risk of hyperkalemia. Patients with impaired renal function, dehydration, heart failure, liver dysfunction, those taking diuretics and ACE inhibitors, and the elderly are at greater risk of renal toxicity. Use with caution in patients with impaired renal function or history of kidney disease. Dosage adjustment is required in patients with moderate elevation in serum creatinine. Acute renal failure, interstitial nephritis, and nephrotic syndrome have been reported with ketorolac use; papillary necrosis and renal injury have been reported with the use of NSAIDs. Rehydrate patient before starting therapy; monitor renal function closely.

[U.S. Boxed Warning]: NSAIDs may increase risk of gastrointestinal irritation, inflammation, ulceration, bleeding, and perforation. These events may occur at any time during therapy and without warning. Use caution with a history of GI disease (bleeding, ulcers, inflammatory bowel disease), concurrent therapy with aspirin, anticoagulants and/or corticosteroids, smoking, use of alcohol, the elderly, or debilitated patients.

NSAIDs may cause serious skin adverse events including exfoliative dermatitis, Stevens-Johnson syndrome (SJS), and toxic epidermal necrolysis (TEN); discontinue use at first sign of skin rash or hypersensitivity. Hypersensitivity or anaphylactoid reactions may occur, even without prior exposure. Ketorolac nasal spray is contraindicated in patients with prior hypersensitivity reaction to aspirin or NSAIDs. Use caution in patients with other forms of asthma.

Use with caution in patients with hepatic impairment or a history of liver disease. Closely monitor patients with any abnormal LFT. Rarely, severe hepatic reactions (eg, fulminant hepatitis, hepatic necrosis, liver failure) have occurred with NSAID use; discontinue if signs or symptoms of liver disease develop, or if systemic manifestations occur.

[U.S. Boxed Warning]: Ketorolac nasal spray is indicated for short term (≤5 days) use in adults for treatment of moderate to moderately severe acute pain requiring opioid-level analgesia. The combined therapy duration (nasal and other ketorolac formulations) should not exceed 5 days. Therapy is not appropriate for minor or chronic pain therapy. Use the lowest effective dose for the shortest duration of time, consistent with individual patient goals, to reduce risk of cardiovascular or GI adverse events. Alternate therapies should be considered for patients at high risk.

Dosage adjustment is required for adults weighing <50 kg (<110 pounds) and/or for patients ≥65 years of age. Avoid use in older adults; nonselective oral NSAID use is associated with an increased risk of GI bleeding and peptic ulcer disease in older adults in high risk category (eg, >75 years or age or receiving concomitant oral/parenteral corticosteroids, anticoagulants, or antiplatelet agents) (Beers Criteria). Avoid contact with the eyes; if eye exposure occurs, wash eye with water or saline; consult physician if irritation continues >1 hour. Preparation contains edetate sodium (EDTA); do not use in patients with hypersensitivity to EDTA.

Adverse Reactions (Reflective of adult population; not specific for elderly) Events reported with intranasal use; refer to Ketorolac (Systemic) monograph on page 1069 for other potential ketorolac-related adverse events.

>10%: Respiratory: Nasal discomfort (15%), rhinalgia (13%)

>1% to 10%:
  Cardiovascular: Bradycardia (2%), hypertension (2%)
  Dermatologic: Rash (3%)
  Gastrointestinal: Throat irritation (4%)
  Genitourinary: Urine output decreased (2%)
  Hepatic: ALT/AST increased (2%)
  Ocular: Lacrimation increased (5%)
  Respiratory: Rhinitis (2%)
  Renal: Oliguria (3%)

Drug Interactions

Metabolism/Transport Effects None known.

Avoid Concomitant Use

Avoid concomitant use of Ketorolac (Nasal) with any of the following: Aspirin; Floctafenine; Ketorolac; Ketorolac (Systemic); Nonsteroidal Anti-Inflammatory Agents; Pentoxifylline; Probenecid

Increased Effect/Toxicity

Ketorolac (Nasal) may increase the levels/effects of: Aliskiren; Aminoglycosides; Anticoagulants; Antiplatelet Agents; Aspirin; Bisphosphonate Derivatives; Collagenase (Systemic); CycloSPORINE; CycloSPORINE (Systemic); Dabigatran Etexilate; Deferasirox; Desmopressin; Digoxin; Drotrecogin Alfa (Activated); Eplerenone; Haloperidol; Ibritumomab; Lithium; Methotrexate; Neuromuscular-Blocking Agents (Nondepolarizing); Nonsteroidal Anti-Inflammatory Agents; PEMEtrexed; Pentoxifylline; Porfimer; Potassium-Sparing Diuretics; PRALAtrexate; Quinolone Antibiotics; Rivaroxaban; Salicylates; Thrombolytic Agents; Tositumomab and Iodine I 131 Tositumomab; Vancomycin; Vitamin K Antagonists

The levels/effects of Ketorolac (Nasal) may be increased by: ACE Inhibitors; Angiotensin II Receptor Blockers; Antidepressants (Tricyclic, Tertiary Amine); Corticosteroids (Systemic); CycloSPORINE; CycloSPORINE (Systemic); Dasatinib; Floctafenine; Glucosamine; Herbs (Anticoagulant/Antiplatelet Properties); Ketorolac; Ketorolac (Systemic); Omega-3-Acid Ethyl Esters; Pentosan Polysulfate Sodium; Probenecid; Prostacyclin Analogues; Selective Serotonin Reuptake Inhibitors; Serotonin/Norepinephrine Reuptake Inhibitors; Sodium Phosphates; Tipranavir; Treprostinil; Vitamin E

Decreased Effect

Ketorolac (Nasal) may decrease the levels/effects of: ACE Inhibitors; Aliskiren; Angiotensin II Receptor Blockers; Anticonvulsants; Antiplatelet Agents; Beta-Blockers; Eplerenone; HydrALAZINE; Loop Diuretics; Potassium-Sparing Diuretics; Salicylates; Selective Serotonin Reuptake Inhibitors; Thiazide Diuretics

The levels/effects of Ketorolac (Nasal) may be decreased by: Bile Acid Sequestrants; Salicylates

Ethanol/Nutrition/Herb Interactions Herb/Nutraceutical: Avoid alfalfa, anise, bilberry, bladderwrack, bromelain, cat's claw, celery, chamomile, coleus, cordyceps, dong quai, evening primrose, fenugreek, feverfew, garlic, ginger, ginkgo biloba, ginseng (American, Panax, Siberian), grapeseed, green tea, guggul, horse chestnut seed, horseradish, licorice, prickly ash, red clover, reishi, SAMe (S-adenosylmethionine), sweet clover, turmeric, and white willow (all have additional antiplatelet activity).

Stability Store unopened nasal spray refrigerated at 2°C to 8°C (36°F to 46°F); protect from freezing. Protect from light. During use, store at room temperature of 15°C to 30°C (59°F to 86°F) and out of direct sunlight. Discard each nasal spray bottle within 24 hours of priming.

Mechanism of Action Reversibly inhibits cyclooxygenase-1 and 2 (COX-1 and 2) enzymes, which results in decreased formation of prostaglandin precursors; has antipyretic, analgesic, and anti-inflammatory properties

Other proposed mechanisms not fully elucidated (and possibly contributing to the anti-inflammatory effect to varying degrees), include inhibiting chemotaxis, altering lymphocyte activity, inhibiting neutrophil aggregation/activation, and decreasing proinflammatory cytokine levels.

Pharmacodynamics/Kinetics
Onset of analgesia: Within 20 minutes

Absorption: Rapid and well absorbed; C_{max}, t_{max} and AUC values were similar following multiple administrations for 5 days compared to the single-dose study in healthy volunteers.

Distribution: ~13 L following complete distribution; following intranasal administration, ketorolac is deposited primarily in the nasal cavity and pharynx; <20% deposited in the esophagus and stomach; <0.5% in the lungs

Protein binding: 99%

Metabolism: Hepatic to hydroxylated and conjugated forms

Bioavailability: ~60% to 70% relative to I.M. administration

Half-life elimination: ~5-6 hours (similar to I.M. administration); prolonged ~35% in elderly; up to 19 hours in renal impairment

Time to peak: 0.5-0.75 hours

Excretion: Urine (~92%, ~60% as unchanged drug); feces ~6%

Dosage
Geriatric Elderly (≥65 years): Intranasal: One spray (15.75 mg) in 1 nostril (total dose: 15.75 mg) every 6-8 hours; maximum dose: 4 doses (63 mg)/day

Adult Pain management (acute; moderate-to-moderately-severe): Note: The maximum combined duration of treatment (for nasal spray or other ketorolac formulations) is 5 days.

Intranasal: Adults<65 years and ≥50 kg: One spray (15.75 mg) in each nostril (total dose: 31.5 mg) every 6-8 hours; maximum dose: 4 doses (126 mg)/day

Dosage adjustments in adults with low body weight (<50 kg): One spray (15.75 mg) in 1 nostril (total dose: 15.75 mg) every 6-8 hours; maximum dose: 4 doses (63 mg)/day

Renal Impairment

Renal insufficiency: Intranasal: One spray (15.75 mg) in 1 nostril (total dose: 15.75 mg) every 6-8 hours; maximum dose: 4 doses (63 mg)/day

Advanced renal impairment (or at risk for renal failure due to volume depletion): Use is contraindicated

Hepatic Impairment Use with caution with hepatic impairment or history of hepatic disease; use may cause elevation of liver enzymes; discontinue if clinical signs and symptoms of liver disease develop.

Administration Each nasal spray contains medication for 1 day of therapy. Before first use of a nasal spray container, prime by pressing pump 5 times. There is no need to prime the pump again if more doses are administered during the next 24 hours using the same nasal container. Repeat priming each day prior to first use of each new nasal spray. Blow nose to clear nostrils. Sit up straight or stand; tilt head slightly forward. Insert tip of container into nostril, keeping bottle upright, and point container away from the center of nose. Spray once, pressing down evenly on both sides of container.

Discard container within 24 hours of priming even if there is unused medication.

Monitoring Parameters Monitor for weight gain/edema; renal function (serum creatinine, BUN, urine output); observe for bleeding, bruising; evaluate gastrointestinal effects (abdominal pain, bleeding, dyspepsia); CBC and platelets, liver function tests

Reference Range Serum concentration: Therapeutic: 0.3-5 mcg/mL; Toxic: >5 mcg/mL

Special Geriatric Considerations Ketorolac is cleared more slowly in the elderly. It is recommended to use lower doses in the elderly. Elderly are a high-risk population for adverse effects from NSAIDs. As much as 60% of elderly can develop peptic ulceration and/or hemorrhage asymptomatically. The concomitant use of H_2 blockers and sucralfate is not effective as prophylaxis with the exception of NSAID-induced duodenal ulcers which may be prevented by the use of ranitidine. Misoprostol and proton pump inhibitors are the only agents proven to help prevent the development of NSAID-induced ulcers. Also, concomitant disease and drug use contribute to the risk for GI adverse effects. Use lowest effective dose for shortest period possible. Consider renal function decline with age. Use of NSAIDs can compromise existing renal function especially when Cl_{cr} is ≤30 mL/minute or weight <50 kg. Tinnitus may be a difficult and unreliable indication of toxicity due to age-related hearing loss or eighth cranial nerve damage. CNS adverse effects such as confusion, agitation, and hallucination are generally seen in overdose or high dose situations, but elderly may demonstrate these adverse effects at lower doses than younger adults.

This medication is considered to be potentially inappropriate in this patient population (Beers Criteria: Quality of evidence - high; Strength of recommendation - strong).

Dosage Forms Excipient information presented when available (limited, particularly for generics); consult specific product labeling.

Solution, intranasal, as tromethamine [spray, preservative free]:
Sprix®: 15.75 mg/spray (1.7 g) [delivers 8 metered sprays]

Ketorolac (Ophthalmic) (KEE toe role ak)

Medication Safety Issues
  Sound-alike/look-alike issues:
    Acular® may be confused with Acthar®, Ocular
    Ketorolac may be confused with Ketalar®
Brand Names: U.S. Acular LS®; Acular®; Acuvail®
Brand Names: Canada Acular LS®; Acular®; ratio-Ketorolac
Index Terms Ketorolac Tromethamine
Generic Availability (U.S.) Yes
Pharmacologic Category Nonsteroidal Anti-inflammatory Drug (NSAID), Ophthalmic
Use Temporary relief of ocular itching due to seasonal allergic conjunctivitis; postoperative inflammation following cataract extraction; reduction of ocular pain and photophobia following incisional refractive surgery; reduction of ocular pain, burning, and stinging following corneal refractive surgery
Dosage
  Adult
    Seasonal allergic conjunctivitis (relief of ocular itching) (Acular®): *Ophthalmic:* Instill 1 drop (0.25 mg) 4 times/day
    Inflammation following cataract extraction (Acular®): *Ophthalmic:* Instill 1 drop (0.25 mg) to affected eye(s) 4 times/day beginning 24 hours after surgery; continue for 2 weeks
    Pain following corneal refractive surgery (Acular LS®): *Ophthalmic:* Instill 1 drop 4 times/day as needed to affected eye for up to 4 days
Special Geriatric Considerations Evaluate the patient's or caregiver's ability to safely administer the correct dose of ophthalmic medication.
Dosage Forms Excipient information presented when available (limited, particularly for generics); consult specific product labeling. [DSC] = Discontinued product
  Solution, ophthalmic, as tromethamine [drops]: 0.4% (5 mL); 0.5% (3 mL, 5 mL, 10 mL)
    Acular LS®: 0.4% (5 mL) [contains benzalkonium chloride]
    Acular®: 0.5% (5 mL, 10 mL [DSC]) [contains benzalkonium chloride]
  Solution, ophthalmic, as tromethamine [drops, preservative free]:
    Acuvail®: 0.45% (0.4 mL)

◆ **Ketorolac Tromethamine** *see* Ketorolac (Nasal) *on page 1072*
◆ **Ketorolac Tromethamine** *see* Ketorolac (Ophthalmic) *on page 1076*
◆ **Ketorolac Tromethamine** *see* Ketorolac (Systemic) *on page 1069*

Ketotifen (Ophthalmic) (kee toe TYE fen)

Medication Safety Issues
  Sound-alike/look-alike issues:
    Claritin™ Eye (ketotifen) may be confused with Claritin® (loratadine)
    Ketotifen may be confused with ketoprofen
    ZyrTEC® Itchy Eye (ketotifen) may be confused with ZyrTEC® (cetirizine)
Brand Names: U.S. Alaway™ [OTC]; Claritin™ Eye [OTC]; Zaditor® [OTC]; ZyrTEC® Itchy Eye [OTC]
Brand Names: Canada Zaditor®
Index Terms Ketotifen Fumarate
Generic Availability (U.S.) Yes
Pharmacologic Category Histamine H_1 Antagonist; Histamine H_1 Antagonist, Second Generation; Mast Cell Stabilizer; Piperidine Derivative
Use Ophthalmic: Temporary relief of eye itching due to allergic conjunctivitis
Contraindications Hypersensitivity to ketotifen or any component of the formulation
Warnings/Precautions Do not use to treat acute asthmatic attacks. Therapy for acute symptoms of asthma (eg, corticosteroids, beta$_2$-agonists, xanthine derivatives) should be maintained and gradually reduced. Several weeks of oral ketotifen therapy may be needed to observe clinical response while full therapeutic response is usually observed after 10 weeks of treatment. Patients with inadequate response to therapy should be maintained on therapy 2-3 months; then if no response, gradually discontinue therapy over 2-4 weeks. Oral dosage forms may cause sedation early in therapy. Sedative effects may be reduced by initiating therapy at one-half the recommended daily dose with gradual increase over 5 days to maintenance dose. Caution patients about performing tasks which require mental alertness (eg, driving or operating machinery). Thrombocytopenia has occurred rarely when used concomitantly with oral antidiabetic agents. Use caution in diabetics and individuals with benzoate allergies as the syrup preparation contains carbohydrates and benzoate

compounds. Ophthalmic solution should not be used to treat contact lens-related irritation. After ketotifen use, soft contact lens wearers should wait at least 10 minutes before reinserting contact lenses. Do not wear contact lenses if eyes are red. Do not contaminate dropper tip or solution when placing drops in eyes.

When using ophthalmic solution for self-medication (OTC), notify healthcare provider if symptoms worsen or do not improve within 3 days. Contact healthcare provider if change in vision, eye pain, or redness occur. Do not use if solution is cloudy or changes color.

Adverse Reactions (Reflective of adult population; not specific for elderly) 1% to 10%:

Ocular: Allergic reactions, burning or stinging, conjunctivitis, discharge, dry eyes, eye pain, eyelid disorder, itching, keratitis, lacrimation disorder, mydriasis, photophobia, rash

Respiratory: Pharyngitis

Miscellaneous: Flu syndrome

Drug Interactions

Metabolism/Transport Effects None known.

Avoid Concomitant Use

Avoid concomitant use of Ketotifen (Ophthalmic) with any of the following: Azelastine; Azelastine (Nasal); Methadone; Mirtazapine; Paraldehyde

Increased Effect/Toxicity

Ketotifen (Ophthalmic) may increase the levels/effects of: Alcohol (Ethyl); Anticholinergics; Azelastine; Azelastine (Nasal); Buprenorphine; CNS Depressants; Methadone; Methotrimeprazine; Metyrosine; Mirtazapine; Paraldehyde; Selective Serotonin Reuptake Inhibitors; Zolpidem

The levels/effects of Ketotifen (Ophthalmic) may be increased by: Droperidol; HydrOXYzine; Methotrimeprazine; Pramlintide

Decreased Effect

Ketotifen (Ophthalmic) may decrease the levels/effects of: Acetylcholinesterase Inhibitors (Central); Benzylpenicilloyl Polylysine; Betahistine; Hyaluronidase

The levels/effects of Ketotifen (Ophthalmic) may be decreased by: Acetylcholinesterase Inhibitors (Central); Amphetamines

Stability Store at 4°C to 25°C (39°F to 77°F).

Mechanism of Action Exhibits noncompetitive H_1-receptor antagonist and mast cell stabilizer properties. Efficacy in conjunctivitis likely results from a combination of anti-inflammatory and antihistaminergic actions including interference with chemokine-induced migration of eosinophils into inflamed conjunctiva.

Pharmacodynamics/Kinetics

Ophthalmic:

Onset of action: Minutes

Duration: 8-12 hours

Absorption: Minimally systemic

Oral:

Absorption: Rapid, ≥60%

Protein binding: 75%

Metabolism: Hepatic via N-glucuronidation to inactive metabolite ketotifen-N-glucoronide; N-demethylation to active metabolite nor-ketotifen; and keto-reduction to hydroxyl derivative

Bioavailability: ~50%

Half-life elimination: ~9-9.5 hours

Time to peak, plasma: 2-4 hours

Excretion: Urine (60% to 70% as metabolites, 1% as unchanged drug)

Dosage

Geriatric & Adult Allergic conjunctivitis: Ophthalmic: Instill 1 drop into the affected eye(s) twice daily, every 8-12 hours

Administration For use in eyes only. Wash hands before use. Do not let tip of applicator touch eye; do not contaminate tip of applicator. Remove contact lenses prior to administration. Wait 10 minutes before reinserting if using products containing benzalkonium chloride. Do not wear contact lenses if eyes are red. Allow at least 5 minutes between applications with other eye drops.

Special Geriatric Considerations Instruct the patient on proper instillation of ophthalmic solution.

Dosage Forms Excipient information presented when available (limited, particularly for generics); consult specific product labeling.

Solution, ophthalmic [drops]: 0.025% (5 mL)

Alaway™: 0.025% (10 mL) [contains benzalkonium chloride]

Claritin™ Eye: 0.025% (5 mL) [contains benzalkonium chloride]

Zaditor®: 0.025% (5 mL) [contains benzalkonium chloride]

ZyrTEC® Itchy Eye: 0.025% (5 mL) [contains benzalkonium chloride]

Dosage Forms: Canada Excipient information presented when available (limited, particularly for generics); consult specific product labeling.

Solution, ophthalmic [drops]:
  Zaditor®: 0.025% (5 mL) [contains benzalkonium chloride]

Solution, ophthalmic [drops], preservative free:
  Zaditor®: 0.025% (0.4 mL) (30s)

- ◆ **Ketotifen Fumarate** *see* Ketotifen (Ophthalmic) *on page 1076*
- ◆ **Key-E® [OTC]** *see* Vitamin E *on page 2027*
- ◆ **Key-E® Kaps [OTC]** *see* Vitamin E *on page 2027*
- ◆ **Key-E® Powder [OTC]** *see* Vitamin E *on page 2027*
- ◆ **Kineret®** *see* Anakinra *on page 132*
- ◆ **Kinrix®** *see* Diphtheria and Tetanus Toxoids, Acellular Pertussis, and Poliovirus Vaccine *on page 565*
- ◆ **Kionex®** *see* Sodium Polystyrene Sulfonate *on page 1794*
- ◆ **Klaron®** *see* Sulfacetamide (Topical) *on page 1812*
- ◆ **KlonoPIN®** *see* ClonazePAM *on page 411*
- ◆ **Klor-Con®** *see* Potassium Chloride *on page 1571*
- ◆ **Klor-Con® 8** *see* Potassium Chloride *on page 1571*
- ◆ **Klor-Con® 10** *see* Potassium Chloride *on page 1571*
- ◆ **Klor-Con®/25** *see* Potassium Chloride *on page 1571*
- ◆ **Klor-Con® M10** *see* Potassium Chloride *on page 1571*
- ◆ **Klor-Con® M15** *see* Potassium Chloride *on page 1571*
- ◆ **Klor-Con® M20** *see* Potassium Chloride *on page 1571*
- ◆ **KMD 3213** *see* Silodosin *on page 1773*
- ◆ **Kolephrin® GG/DM [OTC]** *see* Guaifenesin and Dextromethorphan *on page 906*
- ◆ **Kombiglyze™ XR** *see* Saxagliptin and Metformin *on page 1755*
- ◆ **Kondremul® [OTC]** *see* Mineral Oil *on page 1288*
- ◆ **Konsyl® [OTC]** *see* Psyllium *on page 1635*
- ◆ **Konsyl-D™ [OTC]** *see* Psyllium *on page 1635*
- ◆ **Konsyl® Easy Mix™ [OTC]** *see* Psyllium *on page 1635*
- ◆ **Konsyl® Fiber [OTC]** *see* Polycarbophil *on page 1563*
- ◆ **Konsyl® Orange [OTC]** *see* Psyllium *on page 1635*
- ◆ **Konsyl® Original [OTC]** *see* Psyllium *on page 1635*
- ◆ **K-Phos® MF** *see* Potassium Phosphate and Sodium Phosphate *on page 1578*
- ◆ **K-Phos® Neutral** *see* Potassium Phosphate and Sodium Phosphate *on page 1578*
- ◆ **K-Phos® No. 2** *see* Potassium Phosphate and Sodium Phosphate *on page 1578*
- ◆ **K-Phos® Original** *see* Potassium Phosphate Acid Phosphate *on page 1570*
- ◆ **Kristalose®** *see* Lactulose *on page 1086*
- ◆ **Krystexxa™** *see* Pegloticase *on page 1490*
- ◆ **K-Tab®** *see* Potassium Chloride *on page 1571*
- ◆ **Kytril** *see* Granisetron *on page 900*
- ◆ **L-749,345** *see* Ertapenem *on page 662*
- ◆ **L-758,298** *see* Fosaprepitant *on page 844*
- ◆ **L-M-X® 4 [OTC]** *see* Lidocaine (Topical) *on page 1128*
- ◆ **L-M-X® 5 [OTC]** *see* Lidocaine (Topical) *on page 1128*
- ◆ **L 754030** *see* Aprepitant *on page 139*
- ◆ **LA 20304a** *see* Gemifloxacin *on page 871*

Labetalol (la BET a lole)

Related Information
Beta-Blockers *on page 2108*

Medication Safety Issues
Sound-alike/look-alike issues:
  Labetalol may be confused with betaxolol, lamoTRIgine, Lipitor®
  Normodyne® may be confused with Norpramin®
  Trandate® may be confused with traMADol, TRENtal®

High alert medication:
  The Institute for Safe Medication Practices (ISMP) includes this medication among its list of drugs which have a heightened risk of causing significant patient harm when used in error.

Administration issues:
  Significant differences exist between oral and I.V. dosing. Use caution when converting from one route of administration to another.

Brand Names: U.S. Trandate®

Brand Names: Canada Apo-Labetalol®; Labetalol Hydrochloride Injection, USP; Normodyne®; Trandate®

Index Terms Ibidomide Hydrochloride; Labetalol Hydrochloride

Generic Availability (U.S.) Yes

Pharmacologic Category Beta-Blocker With Alpha-Blocking Activity

Use Treatment of mild-to-severe hypertension; I.V. for severe hypertension (eg, hypertensive emergencies)

Unlabeled Use Hypertension during acute ischemic stroke

Contraindications Hypersensitivity to labetalol or any component of the formulation; severe bradycardia; heart block greater than first degree (except in patients with a functioning artificial pacemaker); cardiogenic shock; bronchial asthma; uncompensated cardiac failure; conditions associated with severe and prolonged hypotension

Warnings/Precautions Consider pre-existing conditions such as sick sinus syndrome before initiating. Symptomatic hypotension with or without syncope may occur with labetalol; close monitoring of patient is required especially with initial dosing and dosing increases; blood pressure must be lowered at a rate appropriate for the patient's clinical condition. Initiation with a low dose and gradual up-titration may help to decrease the occurrence of hypotension or syncope. Patients should be advised to avoid driving or other hazardous tasks during initiation of therapy due to the risk of syncope. Orthostatic hypotension may occur with I.V. administration; patient should remain supine during and for up to 3 hours after I.V. administration. Use with caution in impaired hepatic function; bioavailability is increased due to decreased first-pass metabolism. Severe hepatic injury including some fatalities have also been rarely reported with use: periodically monitor LFTs with prolonged use. Use with caution in patients with diabetes mellitus; may potentiate hypoglycemia and/or mask signs and symptoms. Bradycardia may be observed more frequently in elderly patients (>65 years of age); dosage reductions may be necessary. May also reduce release of insulin in response to hyperglycemia; dosage of antidiabetic agents may need to be adjusted. May mask signs of hyperthyroidism (eg, tachycardia); if hyperthyroidism is suspected, carefully manage and monitor; abrupt withdrawal may exacerbate symptoms of hyperthyroidism or precipitate thyroid storm. Elimination of labetalol is reduced in elderly patients; lower maintenance doses may be required.

Use only with extreme caution in compensated heart failure and monitor for a worsening of the condition. Beta-blocker therapy should not be withdrawn abruptly (particularly in patients with CAD), but gradually tapered to avoid acute tachycardia, hypertension, and/or ischemia. Chronic beta-blocker therapy should not be routinely withdrawn prior to major surgery. Use caution with concurrent use of digoxin, verapamil, or diltiazem; bradycardia or heart block can occur. Use with caution in patients receiving inhaled anesthetic agents known to depress myocardial contractility. Patients with bronchospastic disease should not receive beta-blockers; if used at all, should be used cautiously with close monitoring. Use with caution in patients with myasthenia gravis or psychiatric disease (may cause or exacerbate CNS depression). Can precipitate or aggravate symptoms of arterial insufficiency in patients with PVD and Raynaud's disease; use with caution and monitor for progression of arterial obstruction. If possible, obtain diagnostic tests for pheochromocytoma prior to use. May induce or exacerbate psoriasis. Labetalol has been shown to be effective in lowering blood pressure and relieving symptoms in patients with pheochromocytoma. However, some patients have experienced paradoxical hypertensive responses; use with caution in patients with pheochromocytoma. Additional alpha-blockade may be required during use of labetalol. Use caution with history of severe anaphylaxis to allergens; patients taking beta-blockers may become more sensitive to repeated challenges. Treatment of anaphylaxis (eg, epinephrine) in patients taking beta-blockers may be ineffective or promote undesirable effects.

Intraoperative floppy iris syndrome has been observed in cataract surgery patients who were on or were previously treated with alpha$_1$-blockers; causality has not been established and there appears to be no benefit in discontinuing alpha-blocker therapy prior to surgery. Instruct patients to inform ophthalmologist of labetalol use when considering eye surgery.

Adverse Reactions (Reflective of adult population; not specific for elderly)

>10%:

　Cardiovascular: Orthostatic hypotension (I.V. use; ≤58%)

　Central nervous system: Dizziness (1% to 20%), fatigue (1% to 11%)

　Gastrointestinal: Nausea (≤19%)

1% to 10%:

　Cardiovascular: Hypotension (1% to 5%), edema (≤2%), flushing (1%), ventricular arrhythmia (I.V. use; 1%)

　Central nervous system: Somnolence (3%), headache (2%), vertigo (1% to 2%)

　Dermatologic: Scalp tingling (≤7%), pruritus (1%), rash (1%)

　Gastrointestinal: Dyspepsia (≤4%), vomiting (≤3%), taste disturbance (1%)

　Genitourinary: Ejaculatory failure (≤5%), impotence (1% to 4%)

　Hepatic: Transaminases increased (4%)

　Neuromuscular & skeletal: Paresthesia (≤5%), weakness (1%)

Ocular: Vision abnormal (1%)
Renal: BUN increased (≤8%)
Respiratory: Nasal congestion (1% to 6%), dyspnea (2%)
Miscellaneous: Diaphoresis (≤4%)
Other adverse reactions noted with beta-adrenergic blocking agents include mental depression, catatonia, disorientation, short-term memory loss, emotional lability, clouded sensorium, intensification of pre-existing AV block, laryngospasm, respiratory distress, agranulocytosis, thrombocytopenic purpura, nonthrombocytopenic purpura, mesenteric artery thrombosis, and ischemic colitis.

Drug Interactions

Metabolism/Transport Effects None known.

Avoid Concomitant Use
Avoid concomitant use of Labetalol with any of the following: Beta2-Agonists; Floctafenine; Methacholine

Increased Effect/Toxicity
Labetalol may increase the levels/effects of: Alpha-/Beta-Agonists (Direct-Acting); Alpha1-Blockers; Alpha2-Agonists; Amifostine; Antihypertensives; Antipsychotic Agents (Phenothiazines); Bupivacaine; Cardiac Glycosides; Cholinergic Agonists; Fingolimod; Hypotensive Agents; Insulin; Lidocaine; Lidocaine (Systemic); Lidocaine (Topical); Mepivacaine; Methacholine; Midodrine; RiTUXimab; Sulfonylureas

The levels/effects of Labetalol may be increased by: Acetylcholinesterase Inhibitors; Aminoquinolines (Antimalarial); Amiodarone; Anilidopiperidine Opioids; Antipsychotic Agents (Phenothiazines); Calcium Channel Blockers (Dihydropyridine); Calcium Channel Blockers (Nondihydropyridine); Diazoxide; Dipyridamole; Disopyramide; Dronedarone; Floctafenine; Herbs (Hypotensive Properties); MAO Inhibitors; Pentoxifylline; Phosphodiesterase 5 Inhibitors; Propafenone; Prostacyclin Analogues; QuiNIDine; Reserpine; Selective Serotonin Reuptake Inhibitors

Decreased Effect
Labetalol may decrease the levels/effects of: Beta2-Agonists; Theophylline Derivatives

The levels/effects of Labetalol may be decreased by: Barbiturates; Herbs (Hypertensive Properties); Methylphenidate; Nonsteroidal Anti-Inflammatory Agents; Rifamycin Derivatives; Yohimbine

Ethanol/Nutrition/Herb Interactions

Food: Labetalol serum concentrations may be increased if taken with food.
Herb/Nutraceutical: Avoid dong quai if using for hypertension (has estrogenic activity). Avoid ephedra, yohimbe, ginseng (may worsen hypertension). Avoid natural licorice (causes sodium and water retention and increases potassium loss). Avoid garlic (may have increased antihypertensive effect).

Stability

Tablets: Store at room temperature (refer to manufacturer's labeling for detailed storage requirements). Protect from light and excessive moisture.
Injectable: Store at room temperature (refer to manufacturer's labeling for detailed storage requirements); do not freeze. Protect from light. The solution is clear to slightly yellow.
Parenteral admixture: Stability of parenteral admixture at room temperature (25°C) and refrigeration temperature (4°C): 3 days.

Mechanism of Action Blocks alpha-, beta$_1$-, and beta$_2$-adrenergic receptor sites; elevated renins are reduced. The ratios of alpha- to beta-blockade differ depending on the route of administration: 1:3 (oral) and 1:7 (I.V.).

Pharmacodynamics/Kinetics

Onset of action: Oral: 20 minutes to 2 hours; I.V.: 2-5 minutes
Peak effect: Oral: 1-4 hours; I.V.: 5-15 minutes
Duration: Blood pressure response:
  Oral: 8-12 hours (dose dependent)
  I.V.: 2-18 hours (dose dependent; based on single and multiple sequential doses of 0.25-0.5 mg/kg with cumulative dosing up to 3.25 mg/kg)
Absorption: Complete
Distribution: V$_d$: Adults: 3-16 L/kg; mean: <9.4 L/kg; moderately lipid soluble, therefore, can enter CNS
Protein binding: 50%
Metabolism: Hepatic, primarily via glucuronide conjugation; extensive first-pass effect
Bioavailability: Oral: 25%; increased with liver disease, elderly, and concurrent cimetidine
Half-life elimination: Oral: 6-8 hours; I.V.: ~5.5 hours
Time to peak, plasma: Oral: 1-2 hours
Excretion: Urine (55% to 60% as glucuronide conjugates, <5% as unchanged drug)

Dosage

Geriatric & Adult

Hypertension: Oral: Initial: 100 mg twice daily, may increase as needed every 2-3 days by 100 mg twice daily (titration increments not to exceed 200 mg twice daily) until desired response is obtained; usual dose: 100-400 mg twice daily (JNC 7); may require up to 2.4 g/day.

Acute hypertension (hypertensive emergency/urgency):

I.V. bolus: Per the manufacturer: Initial: 20 mg I.V. push over 2 minutes; may administer 40-80 mg at 10-minute intervals, up to 300 mg total cumulative dose; as appropriate, follow with oral antihypertensive regimen

I.V. infusion (acute loading): Per the manufacturer: Initial: 2 mg/minute; titrate to response up to 300 mg total cumulative dose (eg, discontinue after 2.5 hours of 2 mg/minute); usual total dose required: 50-200 mg; as appropriate, follow with oral antihypertensive regimen

Note: Although loading infusions are well described in the product labeling, the labeling is silent in specific clinical situations, such as in the patient who has an initial response to labetalol infusions but cannot be converted to an oral route for subsequent dosing. There is limited documentation of prolonged continuous infusions (ie, >300 mg/day). In rare clinical situations, higher continuous infusion doses up to 6 mg/minute have been used in the critical care setting (eg, aortic dissection) and up to 8 mg/minute (eg, hypertension with ongoing acute ischemic stroke). At these doses, it may be best to consider an alternative agent if the labetalol infusion is not meeting the goals of therapy. At the other extreme, continuous infusions at relatively low doses (0.03-0.1 mg/minute) have been used in some settings (following loading infusion in patients who are unable to be converted to oral regimens or in some cases as a continuation of outpatient oral regimens). These prolonged infusions should not be confused with loading infusions. Because of wide variation in the use of infusions, an awareness of institutional policies and practices is extremely important. Careful clarification of orders and specific infusion rates/units is required to avoid confusion. Due to the prolonged duration of action, careful monitoring should be extended for the duration of the infusion and for several hours after the infusion. Excessive administration may result in prolonged hypotension and/or bradycardia.

Arterial hypertension in acute ischemic stroke (unlabeled use [Adams, 2007; Jauch, 2010]): I.V.:

Patient otherwise eligible for reperfusion treatment (eg, alteplase): Blood pressure (BP): Systolic >185 mm Hg or diastolic >110 mm Hg: 10-20 mg over 1-2 minutes; may repeat once. If BP does not decline and remains >185/110 mm Hg, alteplase should not be administered.

Management of BP during and after reperfusion treatment (eg, alteplase): BP: Systolic ≥180 mm Hg or diastolic ≥105 mm Hg: 10 mg over 1-2 minutes; may repeat every 10-20 minutes (maximum dose: 300 mg) **or** 10 mg followed by an infusion of 2-8 mg/minute. If hypertension is refractory, consider other I.V. antihypertensives (eg, nitroprusside).

I.V. to oral conversion: Upon discontinuation of I.V. infusion, may initiate oral dose of 200 mg followed in 6-12 hours with an additional dose of 200-400 mg. Thereafter, dose patients with 400-2400 mg/day in divided doses depending on blood pressure response.

Renal Impairment Not removed by hemo- or peritoneal dialysis; supplemental dose is not necessary.

Hepatic Impairment Dosage reduction may be necessary.

Administration Bolus dose may be administered I.V. push at a rate of 10 mg/minute; may follow with continuous I.V. infusion

Monitoring Parameters Blood pressure, standing and sitting/supine, pulse, cardiac monitor and blood pressure monitor required for I.V. administration

Test Interactions False-positive urine catecholamines, vanillylmandelic acid (VMA) if measured by fluorometric or photometric methods; use HPLC or specific catecholamine radioenzymatic technique; false-positive amphetamine if measured by thin-layer chromatography or radioenzymatic assay (gas chromatographic-mass spectrometer technique should be used)

Special Geriatric Considerations Due to alterations in the beta-adrenergic autonomic nervous system, beta-adrenergic blockade may result in less hemodynamic response than seen in younger adults. Studies indicate that despite decreased sensitivity to the chronotropic effects of beta-blockade with age, there appears to be an increased myocardial sensitivity to the negative inotropic effect during stress (ie, exercise). Controlled trials have shown the overall response rate for propranolol to be only 20% to 50% in elderly populations. Therefore, all beta-adrenergic blocking drugs may result in a decreased response as compared to younger adults.

LABETALOL

Dosage Forms Excipient information presented when available (limited, particularly for generics); consult specific product labeling.
Injection, solution, as hydrochloride: 5 mg/mL (4 mL, 20 mL, 40 mL)
   Trandate®: 5 mg/mL (20 mL, 40 mL) [contains edetate disodium]
Tablet, oral, as hydrochloride: 100 mg, 200 mg, 300 mg
   Trandate®: 100 mg [scored]
   Trandate®: 200 mg [scored; contains sodium benzoate]
   Trandate®: 300 mg [scored]

◆ **Labetalol Hydrochloride** see Labetalol on page 1078

Lacosamide (la KOE sa mide)

Medication Safety Issues
Sound-alike/look-alike issues:
   Lacosamide may be confused with zonisamide
   Vimpat® may be confused with Vimovo™
Brand Names: U.S. Vimpat®
Brand Names: Canada Vimpat®
Index Terms ADD 234037; Harkoseride; LCM; SPM 927
Generic Availability (U.S.) No
Pharmacologic Category Anticonvulsant, Miscellaneous
Use Adjunctive therapy in the treatment of partial-onset seizures
Medication Guide Available Yes
Contraindications There are no contraindications listed in manufacturer's labeling.
Warnings/Precautions Antiepileptics are associated with an increased risk of suicidal behavior/thoughts with use (regardless of indication); patients should be monitored for signs/symptoms of depression, suicidal tendencies, and other unusual behavior changes during therapy and instructed to inform their healthcare provider immediately if symptoms occur. CNS effects may occur; patients should be cautioned about performing tasks which require alertness (eg, operating machinery or driving). Lacosamide may prolong PR interval; use caution in patients with conduction problems (eg, first/second degree atrioventricular block and sick sinus syndrome without pacemaker), myocardial ischemia, heart failure, or if concurrent use with other drugs that prolong the PR interval; ECG is recommended prior to initiating therapy and when at steady state. During investigational trials, atrial fibrillation/flutter, or syncope occurred slightly more often in patients with diabetic neuropathy and/or cardiovascular disease. Use caution with renal or hepatic impairment; dosage adjustment may be necessary. Multiorgan hypersensitivity reactions can occur (rare); monitor patient and discontinue therapy if necessary. Withdraw therapy gradually (≥1 week) to minimize the potential of increased seizure frequency. Effects with ethanol may be potentiated. Some products may contain phenylalanine.
Adverse Reactions (Reflective of adult population; not specific for elderly)
>10%:
   Central nervous system: Dizziness (31%), headache (13%)
   Gastrointestinal: Nausea (11%)
   Ocular: Diplopia (11%)
1% to 10%:
   Cardiovascular: Syncope (adults 1%; dose-related: >400 mg/day)
   Central nervous system: Fatigue (9%), ataxia (8%), somnolence (7%), coordination impaired (4%), vertigo (4%), depression (2%), memory impairment (2%)
   Dermatologic: Pruritus (2%)
   Gastrointestinal: Vomiting (9%), diarrhea (4%)
   Hepatic: ALT increased (1%)
   Local: Contusion (3%), skin laceration (3%), injection site pain/discomfort (2.5%), irritation (1%)
   Neuromuscular & skeletal: Tremor (7%), gait instability (2%), weakness (2%)
   Ocular: Blurred vision (8%), nystagmus (5%)
Drug Interactions
   Metabolism/Transport Effects Substrate of CYP2C19 (minor); **Note:** Assignment of Major/Minor substrate status based on clinically relevant drug interaction potential; **Inhibits** CYP2C19 (weak)
   Avoid Concomitant Use There are no known interactions where it is recommended to avoid concomitant use.
   Increased Effect/Toxicity There are no known significant interactions involving an increase in effect.

Decreased Effect

The levels/effects of Lacosamide may be decreased by: CarBAMazepine; Fosphenytoin; PHENobarbital; Phenytoin

Ethanol/Nutrition/Herb Interactions Ethanol: Avoid ethanol (may increase CNS depression).

Stability

Injection: Store at 20°C to 25°C (68°F to 77°F); excursions permitted between 15°C to 30°C (59°F to 86°F). Do not freeze. Can be administered without further dilution or may be mixed with compatible diluents (NS, LR, D$_5$W). Reconstituted solution is stable for ≤24 hours in glass or PVC at room temperature of 15°C to 30°C (59°F to 86°F). Any unused portion should be discarded.

Oral solution, tablets: Store at 20°C to 25°C (68°F to 77°F); excursions permitted between 15°C to 30°C (59°F to 86°F). Do not freeze oral solution. Discard any unused portion of oral solution after 7 weeks.

Mechanism of Action In vitro studies have shown that lacosamide stabilizes hyperexcitable neuronal membranes and inhibits repetitive neuronal firing by enhancing the slow inactivation of sodium channels (with no effects on fast inactivation of sodium channels).

Pharmacodynamics/Kinetics

Absorption: Oral: Completely

Distribution: V$_d$: ~0.6 L/kg

Protein binding: <15%

Metabolism: Hepatic; forms metabolite, O-desmethyl-lacosamide (inactive)

Bioavailability: ~100%

Half-life elimination: ~13 hours

Time to peak, plasma: Oral: 1-4 hours postdose

Excretion: Urine (95%; 40% as unchanged drug, 30% as inactive metabolite, 20% as uncharacterized metabolite); feces (<0.5%)

Dosage

Geriatric & Adult Partial onset seizure: Oral, I.V.:

Initial: 50 mg twice daily; may be increased at weekly intervals by 100 mg/day

Maintenance dose: 200-400 mg/day

Note: When switching from oral to I.V. formulations, the total daily dose and frequency should be the same; I.V. therapy should only be used temporarily.

Renal Impairment Use caution when titrating dose.

Mild-to-moderate renal impairment: No dose adjustment necessary.

Severe renal impairment (Cl$_{cr}$ ≤30 mL/minute): Maximum dose: 300 mg/day.

Hemodialysis: Removed by hemodialysis; after 4-hour HD treatment, a supplemental dose of up to 50% should be considered.

Hepatic Impairment Use caution when titrating dose.

Mild-to-moderate hepatic impairment: Maximum dose: 300 mg/day.

Severe hepatic impairment: Use is not recommended.

Administration

Injection: Administer over 30-60 minutes. Twice daily I.V. infusions have been used for up to 5 days.

Tablet: May be administered with or without food.

Monitoring Parameters Patients with conduction problems or severe cardiac disease should have ECG tracing prior to start of therapy and when at steady-state; suicidality (eg, suicidal thoughts, depression, behavioral changes)

Special Geriatric Considerations Elderly often have compromised renal function with creatinine clearance <30 mL/minute. Evaluate (calculate) creatinine clearance in the elderly before initiating lacosamide therapy. Monitor closely those elderly with cardiac disease and/or conduction disease. In healthy elderly patients, the AUC and C$_{max}$ pharmacokinetic parameters were 20% higher than in younger adults. The higher serum concentrations may reflect differences in total body water (lean body mass) found in the elderly, as well as reduced renal function with aging.

Controlled Substance C-V

Dosage Forms Excipient information presented when available (limited, particularly for generics); consult specific product labeling.

Injection, solution:

Vimpat®: 10 mg/mL (20 mL)

Solution, oral:

Vimpat®: 10 mg/mL (465 mL) [contains phenylalanine 0.32 mg/20 mL, propylene glycol; strawberry flavor]

Tablet, oral:

Vimpat®: 50 mg, 100 mg, 150 mg, 200 mg

◆ **LaCrosse Complete [OTC]** see Sodium Phosphates on page 1791

♦ **Lactinex™ [OTC]** *see Lactobacillus on page 1084*

Lactobacillus (lak toe ba SIL us)

Brand Names: U.S. Bacid® [OTC]; Culturelle® [OTC]; Dofus [OTC]; Flora-Q™ [OTC]; Floranex™ [OTC]; Kala® [OTC]; Lactinex™ [OTC]; Lacto-Bifidus [OTC]; Lacto-Key [OTC]; Lacto-Pectin [OTC]; Lacto-TriBlend [OTC]; Megadophilus® [OTC]; MoreDophilus® [OTC]; RisaQuad®-2 [OTC]; RisaQuad™ [OTC]; Superdophilus® [OTC]; VSL #3® [OTC]; VSL #3®-DS

Brand Names: Canada Bacid®; Fermalac

Index Terms *Lactobacillus acidophilus*; *Lactobacillus bifidus*; *Lactobacillus bulgaricus*; *Lactobacillus casei*; *Lactobacillus paracasei*; *Lactobacillus plantarum*; *Lactobacillus reuteri*; *Lactobacillus rhamnosus* GG

Generic Availability (U.S.) Yes

Pharmacologic Category Dietary Supplement; Probiotic

Use Promote normal bacterial flora of the intestinal tract

Contraindications Hypersensitivity to any component of the formulation

Warnings/Precautions *Lactobacillus* species have been studied for various gastrointestinal disorders including diarrhea, inflammatory bowel disease, gastrointestinal infection. Effectiveness may be dependent upon actual species used; studies are ongoing. Currently, there are no FDA-approved disease-prevention or therapeutic indications for these products.

Adverse Reactions (Reflective of adult population; not specific for elderly) Gastrointestinal: Bloating (intestinal), flatulence

Drug Interactions

Metabolism/Transport Effects None known.

Avoid Concomitant Use There are no known interactions where it is recommended to avoid concomitant use.

Increased Effect/Toxicity There are no known significant interactions involving an increase in effect.

Decreased Effect There are no known significant interactions involving a decrease in effect.

Stability

Bacid®: Store at room temperature.

Flora-Q™: Store at or below room temperature; do not store in bathroom.

Kala®, MoreDophilus®: Refrigeration recommended after opening.

Lactinex™, Dofus: Store in refrigerator.

VSL #3®, VSL #3®-DS: Store in refrigerator; may be stored at room temperature for up to 1 week without loss in potency

Mechanism of Action Helps re-establish normal intestinal flora; suppresses the growth of potentially pathogenic microorganisms by producing lactic acid which favors the establishment of an aciduric flora.

Pharmacodynamics/Kinetics

Absorption: Oral: None

Distribution: Local, primarily colon

Excretion: Feces

Dosage

Geriatric & Adult Dietary supplement: Oral: Dosing varies by manufacturer; consult product labeling

Bacid®: 2 caplets/day

Culturelle®: 1 capsule daily; may increase to twice daily

Flora-Q™: 1 capsule/day

Lacto-Key 100 or 600: 1-2 capsules/day

Lactinex™: 1 packet or 4 tablets 3-4 times/day

VSL #3®: 1-8 sachets or 2-32 capsules/day

VSL #3®-DS: 1-4 packets/day

Administration

Culturelle®: Capsules may be opened and mixed in a cool beverage or sprinkled onto baby food or applesauce.

Flora-Q™: May be taken with or without food.

Lactinex™: Granules may be added to or administered with cereal, food, or milk.

Megadophilus®, Superdophilus®: Administer on an empty stomach; powder should be mixed in unchilled water.

Monitoring Parameters Monitor for decrease in frequency of stool and increased mass of stool

Special Geriatric Considerations No specific recommendations due to age; keep in mind that elderly suffer significantly with fluid and electrolyte loss (lethargy, confusion, etc) and diarrhea should be aggressively treated

Dosage Forms Excipient information presented when available (limited, particularly for generics); consult specific product labeling.

Capsule:

Culturelle®: *L. rhamnosus* GG 10 billion colony-forming units [contains casein and whey]

Dofus: *L. acidophilus* and *L. bifidus* 10:1 ratio [beet root powder base]

Flora-Q™: *L. acidophilus* and *L. paracasei* ≥8 billion colony-forming units [also contains *Bifidobacterium* and *S. thermophilus*]

Lacto-Key:

100: *L. acidophilus* 1 billion colony-forming units [milk, soy, and yeast free; rice derived]

600: *L. acidophilus* 6 billion colony-forming units [milk, soy, and yeast free; rice derived]

Lacto-Bifidus:

100: *L. bifidus* 1 billion colony-forming units [milk, soy, and yeast free; rice derived]

600: *L. bifidus* 6 billion colony-forming units [milk, soy, and yeast free; rice derived]

Lacto-Pectin: *L. acidophilus* and *L. casei* ≥5 billion colony-forming units [also contains *Bifidobacterium lactis* and citrus pectin cellulose complex]

Lacto-TriBlend:

100: *L. acidophilus, L. bifidus,* and *L. bulgaricus* 1 billion colony-forming units [milk, soy and yeast free; rice derived]

600: *L. acidophilus, L. bifidus,* and *L. bulgaricus* 6 billion colony-forming units [milk, soy and yeast free; rice derived]

Megadophilus®, Superdophilus®: *L. acidophilus* 2 billion units [available in dairy based or dairy free formulations]

RisaQuad™: *L. acidophilus* and *L. paracasei* 8 billion colony-forming units [also includes *Bifidobacterium* and *Streptococcus thermophilus*]

VSL #3®: *L. acidophilus, L. plantarum, L. paracasei, L. bulgaricus* 112 billion live cells [also contains *Bifidobacterium breve, B. longum, B. infantis,* and *Streptococcus thermophilus*]

Capsule, double strength:

RisaQuad®-2: *L. acidophilus* and *L. paracasei* 16 billion colony-forming units [gluten free; also includes *Bifidobacterium* and *Streptococcus thermophilus*]

Capsule, softgel: *L. acidophilus* 100 active units

Caplet:

Bacid®: *L. acidophilus* and *L. bulgaricus* [also contains *Bifidobacterium biffidum* and *Streptococcus thermophilus*

Granules:

Floranex™: *L. acidophilus* and *L. bulgaricus* 100 million live cells per 1 g packet (12s) [contains milk, sodium 5 mg/packet, soy]

Lactinex™: *L. acidophilus* and *L. bulgaricus* 100 million live cells per 1 g packet (12s) [gluten free; contains calcium 5 mg/packet, lactose 380 mg/packet, potassium 20 mg/packet, sodium 5 mg/packet, sucrose 34 mg/packet, whey, evaporated milk, and soy peptone]

Powder:

Lacto-TriBlend: *L. acidophilus, L. bifidus,* and *L. bulgaricus* 10 billion colony-forming units per ¼ teaspoon (60 g) [milk, soy, and yeast free; rice derived]

Megadophilus®, Superdophilus®: *L. acidophilus* 2 billion units per half-teaspoon (49 g, 70 g, 84 g, 126 g) [available in dairy based or dairy free (garbanzo bean) formulations]

MoreDophilus®: *L. acidophilus* 12.4 billion units per teaspoon (30 g, 120 g) [dairy free, yeast free; soy and carrot derived]

VSL #3®: *L. acidophilus, L. plantarum, L. paracasei, L. bulgaricus* 450 billion live cells per sachet (10s, 30s) [gluten free; also contains *Bifidobacterium breve, B. longum, B. infantis,* and *Streptococcus thermophilus*; lemon cream flavor and unflavored]

VSL #3®-DS: *L. acidophilus, L. plantarum, L. paracasei, L. bulgaricus* 900 billion live cells per packet (20s,) [gluten free; also contains *Bifidobacterium breve, B. longum, B. infantis,* and *Streptococcus thermophilus*]

Tablet:

Kala®: *L. acidophilus* 200 million units [dairy free, yeast free; soy based]

Tablet, chewable: *L. reuteri* 100 million organisms

Floranex™: *L. acidophilus* and *L. bulgaricus* 1 million colony-forming units [contains lactose, nonfat dried milk, whey]

Lactinex™: *L. acidophilus* and *L. bulgaricus* 1 million live cells [gluten free; contains calcium 5.2 mg/4 tablets, lactose 960 mg/4 tablets, potassium 20 mg/4 tablets, sodium 5.6 mg/4 tablets, and sucrose 500 sucrose/4 tablets; contains whey, evaporated milk, and soy peptone]

Wafer: *L. acidophilus* 90 mg and *L. bifidus* 25 mg (100s) [provides 1 billion organisms/wafer at time of manufacture; milk free]

◆ **Lactobacillus acidophilus** see Lactobacillus on page 1084

- *Lactobacillus bifidus* see Lactobacillus on page *1084*
- *Lactobacillus bulgaricus* see Lactobacillus on page *1084*
- *Lactobacillus casei* see Lactobacillus on page *1084*
- *Lactobacillus paracasei* see Lactobacillus on page *1084*
- *Lactobacillus plantarum* see Lactobacillus on page *1084*
- *Lactobacillus reuteri* see Lactobacillus on page *1084*
- *Lactobacillus rhamnosus* GG see Lactobacillus on page *1084*
- *Lacto-Bifidus* [OTC] *see Lactobacillus on page 1084*
- *Lacto-Key* [OTC] *see Lactobacillus on page 1084*
- *Lacto-Pectin* [OTC] *see Lactobacillus on page 1084*
- *Lacto-TriBlend* [OTC] *see Lactobacillus on page 1084*

Lactulose (LAK tyoo lose)

Related Information
Laxatives, Classification and Properties *on page 2121*
Treatment Options for Constipation *on page 2142*

Medication Safety Issues
Sound-alike/look-alike issues:
Lactulose may be confused with lactose

Brand Names: U.S. Constulose; Enulose; Generlac; Kristalose®
Brand Names: Canada Acilac; Apo-Lactulose®; Laxilose; PMS-Lactulose
Generic Availability (U.S.) Yes: Excludes crystals for solution
Pharmacologic Category Ammonium Detoxicant; Laxative, Osmotic

Use Prevention and treatment of portal-systemic encephalopathy (including hepatic precoma and coma); treatment of constipation

Contraindications Use in patients requiring a low galactose diet

Warnings/Precautions Use with caution in patients with diabetes mellitus; solution contains galactose and lactose. Monitor periodically for electrolyte imbalance when lactulose is used >6 months or in patients predisposed to electrolyte abnormalities (eg, elderly). Hepatic disease may predispose patients to electrolyte imbalance. Patients receiving lactulose and an oral anti-infective agent should be monitored for possible inadequate response to lactulose. During proctoscopy or colonoscopy procedures involving electrocautery, a theoretical risk of reaction between H_2 gas accumulation and electrical spark may exist; thorough bowel cleansing with a nonfermentable solution is recommended.

Adverse Reactions (Reflective of adult population; not specific for elderly) Frequency not defined.
Endocrine & metabolic: Dehydration, hypernatremia, hypokalemia
Gastrointestinal: Abdominal discomfort, abdominal distention, belching, cramping, diarrhea (excessive dose), flatulence, nausea, vomiting

Drug Interactions
Metabolism/Transport Effects None known.
Avoid Concomitant Use There are no known interactions where it is recommended to avoid concomitant use.
Increased Effect/Toxicity There are no known significant interactions involving an increase in effect.
Decreased Effect There are no known significant interactions involving a decrease in effect.

Stability Store at room temperature; do not freeze. Protect from light. Discard solution if cloudy or very dark. Prolonged exposure to cold temperatures will cause thickening which will return to normal upon warming to room temperature.

Mechanism of Action The bacterial degradation of lactulose resulting in an acidic pH inhibits the diffusion of NH_3 into the blood by causing the conversion of NH_3 to NH_4+; also enhances the diffusion of NH_3 from the blood into the gut where conversion to NH_4+ occurs; produces an osmotic effect in the colon with resultant distention promoting peristalsis; reduces blood ammonia concentration to reduce the degree of portal systemic encephalopathy

Pharmacodynamics/Kinetics
Onset:
Constipation: Up to 24-48 hours to produce a normal bowel movement
Encephalopathy: At least 24-48 hours
Absorption: Not appreciable
Metabolism: Via colonic flora to lactic acid and acetic acid; requires colonic flora for drug activation
Excretion: Primarily feces; urine (≤3%)

Dosage

Geriatric & Adult

Constipation: Oral: 10-20 g (15-30 mL) daily; may increase to 40 g (60 mL) daily if necessary

Prevention of portal systemic encephalopathy (PSE): Oral: 20-30 g (30-45 mL) 3-4 times/day; adjust dose every 1-2 days to produce 2-3 soft stools/day

Treatment of acute PSE:

Oral: 20-30 g (30-45 mL) every 1 hour to induce rapid laxation; reduce to 20-30 g (30-45 mL) 3-4 times/day after laxation is achieved titrate to produce 2-3 soft stools/day

Rectal administration (retention enema): 200 g (300 mL) diluted with 700 mL of water or NS via rectal balloon catheter; retain for 30-60 minutes; may repeat every 4-6 hours; transition to oral treatment prior to discontinuing rectal administration

Administration

Oral solution: May mix with fruit juice, water or milk.

Crystals for oral solution: Dissolve contents of packet in 120 mL water.

Rectal: Mix with water or normal saline; administer as retention enema using a rectal balloon catheter; retain for 30-60 minutes. Transition to oral lactulose when appropriate (able to take oral medication and no longer a risk for aspiration) prior to discontinuing rectal administration

Monitoring Parameters Blood pressure, standing/supine; serum electrolytes, serum ammonia; bowel movement patterns, fluid status

Special Geriatric Considerations Elderly are more likely to show CNS signs of dehydration and electrolyte loss than younger adults. Therefore, monitor closely for fluid and electrolyte loss with chronic use. Sorbitol is equally effective as a laxative and less expensive. However, sorbitol **cannot be substituted** in the treatment of hepatic encephalopathy.

Dosage Forms Excipient information presented when available (limited, particularly for generics); consult specific product labeling. [DSC] = Discontinued product

Crystals for solution, oral:

Kristalose®: 10 g/packet (30s); 20 g/packet (30s)

Solution, oral: 10 g/15 mL (15 mL, 30 mL, 237 mL, 473 mL, 500 mL, 946 mL, 1892 mL)

Constulose: 10 g/15 mL (237 mL [DSC], 946 mL)

Enulose: 10 g/15 mL (473 mL)

Solution, oral/rectal: 10 g/15 mL (237 mL, 473 mL, 946 mL)

Generlac: 10 g/15 mL (473 mL, 1892 mL)

- ◆ **LAIV** see Influenza Virus Vaccine (Live/Attenuated) on page 1001
- ◆ **LaMICtal®** see LamoTRIgine on page 1087
- ◆ **LaMICtal® ODT™** see LamoTRIgine on page 1087
- ◆ **LaMICtal® XR™** see LamoTRIgine on page 1087
- ◆ **LamISIL®** see Terbinafine (Systemic) on page 1853
- ◆ **LamISIL AT® [OTC]** see Terbinafine (Topical) on page 1856

LamoTRIgine (la MOE tri jeen)

Medication Safety Issues

Sound-alike/look-alike issues:

LamoTRIgine may be confused with labetalol, LamISIL®, lamiVUDine, levothyroxine, Lomotil®

LaMICtal® may be confused with LamISIL®, Lomotil®

Administration issues:

Potential exists for medication errors to occur among different formulations of LaMICtal® (tablets, extended release tablets, orally disintegrating tablets, and chewable/dispersible tablets). Patients should be instructed to visually inspect tablets dispensed to verify receiving the correct medication and formulation. The medication guide includes illustrations to aid in tablet verification.

International issues:

Lamictal [U.S., Canada, and multiple international markets] may be confused with Ludiomil brand name for maprotiline [multiple international markets]

Lamotrigine [U.S., Canada, and multiple international markets] may be confused with Ludiomil brand name for maprotiline [multiple international markets]

Brand Names: U.S. LaMICtal®; LaMICtal® ODT™; LaMICtal® XR™

Brand Names: Canada Apo-Lamotrigine®; Lamictal®; Mylan-Lamotrigine; Novo-Lamotrigine; PMS-Lamotrigine; ratio-Lamotrigine; Teva-Lamotrigine

Index Terms BW-430C; LTG

Generic Availability (U.S.) Yes; excludes extended release tablet, orally disintegrating tablet

Pharmacologic Category Anticonvulsant, Miscellaneous

LAMOTRIGINE

Use Adjunctive therapy in the treatment of generalized seizures of Lennox-Gastaut syndrome, primary generalized tonic-clonic seizures, and partial seizures; conversion to monotherapy in patients with partial seizures who are receiving treatment with valproic acid or a single enzyme-inducing antiepileptic drug (specifically carbamazepine, phenytoin, phenobarbital, or primidone); maintenance treatment of bipolar I disorder

Medication Guide Available Yes

Contraindications Hypersensitivity to lamotrigine or any component of the formulation

Warnings/Precautions [U.S. Boxed Warning]: Severe and potentially life-threatening skin rashes requiring hospitalization have been reported; incidence of serious rash is higher in pediatric patients than adults; risk may be increased by coadministration with valproic acid, higher than recommended starting doses, and exceeding recommended dose titration. The majority of cases occur in the first 8 weeks; however, isolated cases may occur after prolonged treatment or in patients without these risk factors. Discontinue at first sign of rash and do not reinitiate therapy unless rash is clearly not drug related. Rare cases of Stevens-Johnson syndrome, toxic epidermal necrolysis, and angioedema have been reported.

Antiepileptics are associated with an increased risk of suicidal behavior/thoughts with use (regardless of indication); patients should be monitored for signs/symptoms of depression, suicidal tendencies, and other unusual behavior changes during therapy and instructed to inform their healthcare provider immediately if symptoms occur.

A spectrum of hematologic effects have been reported with use (eg, neutropenia, leukopenia, thrombocytopenia, pancytopenia, anemias, and rarely, aplastic anemia and pure red cell aplasia); patients with a previous history of adverse hematologic reaction to any drug may be at increased risk. Early detection of hematologic change is important; advise patients of early signs and symptoms including fever, sore throat, mouth ulcers, infections, easy bruising, petechial or purpuric hemorrhage. May be associated with hypersensitivity syndrome. Acute multiorgan failure has also been reported. Increased risk of developing aseptic meningitis has been reported; symptoms (eg, headache, nuchal rigidity, fever, nausea/vomiting, rash, photophobia) have generally occurred within 1-45 days following therapy initiation. Use caution in patients with renal or hepatic impairment. Avoid abrupt cessation, taper over at least 2 weeks if possible.

May cause CNS depression, which may impair physical or mental abilities. Patients must be cautioned about performing tasks which require mental alertness (eg, operating machinery or driving). Effects with other sedative drugs or ethanol may be potentiated. Binds to melanin and may accumulate in the eye and other melanin-rich tissues; the clinical significance of this is not known. Safety and efficacy have not been established for use as initial monotherapy, conversion to monotherapy from antiepileptic drugs (AED) other than carbamazepine, phenytoin, phenobarbital, primidone or valproic acid or conversion to monotherapy from two or more AEDs. Patients treated for bipolar disorder should be monitored closely for clinical worsening or suicidality; prescriptions should be written for the smallest quantity consistent with good patient care. Valproic acid may cause an increase in lamotrigine levels requiring dose adjustment. There is a potential for medication errors with similar-sounding medications and among different lamotrigine formulations; medication errors have occurred.

Adverse Reactions (Reflective of adult population; not specific for elderly) Percentages reported in adults on monotherapy for epilepsy or bipolar disorder.

>10%: Gastrointestinal: Nausea (7% to 14%)

1% to 10%:

Cardiovascular: Chest pain (5%), peripheral edema (2% to 5%), edema (1% to 5%)

Central nervous system: Insomnia (5% to 10%), somnolence (9%), fatigue (8%), coordination impaired (7%), dizziness (7%), anxiety (5%), pain (5%), ataxia (2% to 5%), irritability (2% to 5%), suicidal ideation (2% to 5%), agitation (1% to 5%), amnesia (1% to 5%), depression (1% to 5%), dream abnormality (1% to 5%), emotional lability (1% to 5%), fever (1% to 5%), hypoesthesia (1% to 5%), migraine (1% to 5%), thought abnormality (1% to 5%), confusion (1%)

Dermatologic: Rash (nonserious: 7%), dermatitis (2% to 5%), dry skin (2% to 5%)

Endocrine & metabolic: Dysmenorrhea (5%), libido increased (2% to 5%)

Gastrointestinal: Vomiting (5% to 9%), dyspepsia (7%), abdominal pain (6%), xerostomia (2% to 6%), constipation (5%), weight loss (5%), anorexia (2% to 5%), peptic ulcer (2% to 5%), rectal hemorrhage (2% to 5%), flatulence (1% to 5%), weight gain (2% to 5%)

Genitourinary: Urinary frequency (1% to 5%)

Neuromuscular & skeletal: Back pain (8%), weakness (2% to 5%), arthralgia (1% to 5%), myalgia (1% to 5%), neck pain (1% to 5%), paresthesia (1%)

Ocular: Nystagmus (2% to 5%), vision abnormal (2% to 5%), amblyopia (1%)

Respiratory: Rhinitis (7%), cough (5%), pharyngitis (5%), bronchitis (2% to 5%), dyspnea (2% to 5%), epistaxis (2% to 5%), sinusitis (1% to 5%)

Miscellaneous: Infection (5%), diaphoresis (2% to 5%), reflexes increased/decreased (2% to 5%), dyspraxia (1% to 5%)

Drug Interactions

Metabolism/Transport Effects None known.

Avoid Concomitant Use

Avoid concomitant use of LamoTRIgine with any of the following: Azelastine; Azelastine (Nasal); Methadone; Mirtazapine; Paraldehyde

Increased Effect/Toxicity

LamoTRIgine may increase the levels/effects of: Alcohol (Ethyl); Azelastine; Azelastine (Nasal); Buprenorphine; CarBAMazepine; CNS Depressants; Desmopressin; MetFORMIN; Methadone; Methotrimeprazine; Metyrosine; Mirtazapine; OLANZapine; Paraldehyde; Procainamide; Selective Serotonin Reuptake Inhibitors; Zolpidem

The levels/effects of LamoTRIgine may be increased by: Divalproex; Droperidol; HydrOXYzine; Methotrimeprazine; Valproic Acid

Decreased Effect

LamoTRIgine may decrease the levels/effects of: Contraceptives (Progestins)

The levels/effects of LamoTRIgine may be decreased by: Barbiturates; CarBAMazepine; Contraceptives (Estrogens); Fosphenytoin; Ketorolac; Ketorolac (Nasal); Ketorolac (Systemic); Mefloquine; Phenytoin; Primidone; Rifampin; Ritonavir

Ethanol/Nutrition/Herb Interactions

Ethanol: May increase CNS depression; monitor for increased effects with coadministration. Caution patients about effects.

Food: Has no effect on absorption.

Herb/Nutraceutical: Avoid evening primrose (seizure threshold decreased).

Stability Store at 25°C (77°F); excursions permitted to 15°C to 30°C (59°F to 86°F). Protect from light.

Mechanism of Action A triazine derivative which inhibits release of glutamate (an excitatory amino acid) and inhibits voltage-sensitive sodium channels, which stabilizes neuronal membranes. Lamotrigine has weak inhibitory effect on the 5-HT$_3$ receptor; *in vitro* inhibits dihydrofolate reductase.

Pharmacodynamics/Kinetics

Absorption: Immediate release: Rapid and complete

Distribution: V_d: 0.9-1.3 L/kg

Protein binding: ~55%

Metabolism: Hepatic and renal; metabolized primarily by glucuronic acid conjugation to inactive metabolites

Bioavailability: Immediate release: 98%; **Note:** AUCs were similar for immediate release and extended release preparations in patients receiving nonenzyme-inducing AEDs. In subjects receiving concomitant enzyme-inducing AEDs, bioavailability of extended release product was ~21% lower than immediate release product; in some of these subjects, a decrease in AUC of up to 70% was observed when switching from immediate release to extended release tablets.

Half-life elimination: Immediate release: Adults: 25-33 hours, Elderly: 25-43 hours; Extended release: Similar to immediate release

Concomitant valproic acid therapy: 48-70 hours

Concomitant phenytoin, phenobarbital, primidone, or carbamazepine therapy: 13-14 hours

Chronic renal failure: 43 hours

Hemodialysis: 13 hours during dialysis; 57 hours between dialysis (~20% of a dose is eliminated in a 4-hour dialysis session)

Hepatic impairment:

Mild: 26-66 hours

Moderate: 28-116 hours

Severe without ascites: 56-78 hours

Severe with ascites: 52-148 hours

Time to peak, plasma: Immediate release: 1-1.5 hours; Extended release: 4-11 hours (dependent on adjunct therapy)

Excretion: Urine (94%, ~90% as glucuronide conjugates and ~10% unchanged); feces (2%)

Dosage

Geriatric & Adult Note: Only whole tablets should be used for dosing, round calculated dose down to the nearest whole tablet. Enzyme-inducing regimens specifically refer to those containing carbamazepine, phenytoin, phenobarbital, or primidone.

Lennox-Gastaut (adjunctive), primary generalized tonic-clonic seizures (adjunctive) or partial seizures (adjunctive): Oral:

Immediate release formulations:

Regimens **not containing** carbamazepine, phenytoin, phenobarbital, primidone, or valproic acid: Initial: Week 1 and 2: 25 mg once daily; Week 3 and 4: 50 mg once daily; Week 5 and beyond: Increase by 50 mg/day every 1-2 weeks; Maintenance: 225-375 mg/day in 2 divided doses

Regimens **containing** valproic acid: Initial: Week 1 and 2: 25 mg every other day; Week 3 and 4: 25 mg once daily; Week 5 and beyond: Increase by 25-50 mg/day every 1-2 weeks; Maintenance: 100-200 mg/day (valproic acid alone) or 100-400 mg/day (valproic acid and other drugs that induce glucuronidation)

Regimens **containing** carbamazepine, phenytoin, phenobarbital, or primidone and without valproic acid: Initial: Week 1 and 2: 50 mg once daily; Week 3 and 4: 100 mg/day in 2 divided doses; Week 5 and beyond: Increase by 100 mg/day every 1-2 weeks; Maintenance: 300-500 mg/day in 2 divided doses; maximum daily dose: 700 mg

Partial seizures (adjunctive) and primary generalized tonic-clonic seizures (adjunctive):

Extended release formulation: **Note:** Dose increases after week 8 should not exceed 100 mg/day at weekly intervals:

Regimens **not containing** carbamazepine, phenytoin, phenobarbital, primidone, or valproic acid: Initial: Week 1 and 2: 25 mg once daily; Week 3 and 4: 50 mg once daily; Week 5: 100 mg once daily; Week 6: 150 mg once daily; Week 7: 200 mg once daily; Maintenance: 300-400 mg once daily

Regimens **containing** valproic acid: Initial: Week 1 and 2: 25 mg every other day; Week 3 and 4: 25 mg once daily; Week 5: 50 mg once daily; Week 6: 100 mg once daily; Week 7: 150 mg once daily; Maintenance: 200-250 mg once daily

Regimens **containing** carbamazepine, phenytoin, phenobarbital, or primidone and without valproic acid: Initial: Week 1 and 2: 50 mg once daily; Week 3 and 4: 100 mg once daily; Week 5: 200 mg once daily; Week 6: 300 mg once daily; Week 7: 400 mg once daily; Maintenance: 400-600 mg once daily

Conversion from adjunctive therapy with a single enzyme-inducing AED regimen for partial seizures to monotherapy with lamotrigine: **Note:** Goal is to achieve a lamotrigine monotherapy dose of 500 mg/day in 2 divided doses for immediate release formulations and a lamotrigine monotherapy dosage range of 250-300 mg once daily for the extended release formulation.

Conversion strategy from adjunctive therapy with valproic acid:

Immediate release formulations:

- Initiate and titrate as per escalation recommendations for adjunctive therapy to a lamotrigine dose of 200 mg/day.
- Then taper valproic acid dose in decrements of not >500 mg/day/week to a valproic acid dosage of 500 mg/day; this dosage should be maintained for 1 week. The lamotrigine dosage should then be increased to 300 mg/day while valproic acid is simultaneously decreased to 250 mg/day; this dosage should be maintained for 1 week.
- Valproic acid may then be discontinued, while the lamotrigine dose is increased by 100 mg/day at weekly intervals to achieve a lamotrigine maintenance dose of 500 mg/day in 2 divided doses.

Extended release formulation:

- Initiate and titrate as per escalation recommendations for adjunctive therapy to a lamotrigine dose of 150 mg/day.
- Then taper valproic acid dose in decrements of not >500 mg/day/week to a valproic acid dose of 500 mg/day; this dosage should be maintained for 1 week. The lamotrigine dosage should then be increased to 200 mg/day while valproic acid is simultaneously decreased to 250 mg/day; this dosage should be maintained for 1 week.
- Valproic acid may then be discontinued, while the lamotrigine dose is increased to achieve a maintenance dosage range of 250-300 mg once daily.

Conversion strategy from adjunctive therapy with carbamazepine, phenytoin, phenobarbital, or primidone: *Immediate release formulations and extended release formulation:*

- Initiate and titrate as per escalation recommendations for adjunctive therapy to a lamotrigine dose of 500 mg/day.
- Concomitant enzyme-inducing AED should then be withdrawn by 20% decrements each week over a 4-week period.
- Following withdrawal of the enzyme-inducing AED, the dosage of lamotrigine extended release may be tapered in decrements of not >100 mg/day at intervals of 1 week to achieve a maintenance dosage range of 250-300 mg once daily; no further dosage reduction is required for lamotrigine immediate release formulations.

Conversion strategy from adjunctive therapy with AED other than carbamazepine, pheny-toin, phenobarbital, primidone or valproic acid:

Immediate release formulations: No specific guidelines available

Extended release formulation: Initiate and titrate as per escalation recommendations for adjunctive therapy to a lamotrigine dose of 250-300 mg/day. Concomitant AED should then be withdrawn by 20% decrements each week over a 4 week period.

Bipolar disorder: *Immediate release formulations:*

Regimens **not containing** carbamazepine, phenytoin, phenobarbital, primidone, or val-proic acid: Initial: Week 1 and 2: 25 mg once daily; Week 3 and 4: 50 mg once daily; Week 5: 100 mg once daily; Week 6 and maintenance: 200 mg once daily

Regimens **containing** valproic acid: Initial: Week 1 and 2: 25 mg every other day; Week 3 and 4: 25 mg once daily; Week 5: 50 mg once daily; Week 6 and maintenance: 100 mg once daily

Regimens **containing** carbamazepine, phenytoin, phenobarbital, or primidone and without valproic acid: Initial: Week 1 and 2: 50 mg once daily; Week 3 and 4: 100 mg/day in divided doses; Week 5: 200 mg/day in divided doses; Week 6: 300 mg/day in divided doses; Maintenance: up to 400 mg/day in divided doses

Adjustment following discontinuation of psychotropic medication:

Discontinuing valproic acid with current dose of lamotrigine 100 mg/day: 150 mg/day for week 1, then increase to 200 mg/day beginning week 2

Discontinuing carbamazepine, phenytoin, phenobarbital, primidone, or rifampin with current dose of lamotrigine 400 mg/day: 400 mg/day for week 1, then decrease to 300 mg/day for week 2, then decrease to 200 mg/day beginning week 3

Conversion from immediate release to extended release (Lamictal® XR™): Initial dose of the extended release tablet should match the total daily dose of the immediate-release formulation. Adjust dose as needed within the recommended dosing guidelines.

Discontinuing therapy: Children and Adults: Decrease dose by ~50% per week, over at least 2 weeks unless safety concerns require a more rapid withdrawal. Discontinuing carbamazepine, phenytoin, phenobarbital, primidone, or rifampin should prolong the half-life of lamotrigine; discontinuing valproic acid should shorten the half-life of lamotrigine

Restarting therapy after discontinuation: If lamotrigine has been withheld for >5 half-lives, consider restarting according to initial dosing recommendations. **Note:** Concomitant medications may affect the half-life of lamotrigine; consider pharmacokinetic interactions when restarting therapy.

Dosage adjustment with estrogen-containing hormonal contraceptives: Follow initial lamotrigine dosing guidelines, maintenance dose should be adjusted as follows, based on concomitant medications:

Patients taking concomitant carbamazepine, phenytoin, phenobarbital, primidone or rifampin: No dosing adjustment required

Patients **not** taking concomitant carbamazepine, phenytoin, phenobarbital, primidone or rifampin: Lamotrigine maintenance dose may need increased by twofold over target dose. If already taking a stable dose of lamotrigine and starting contraceptive, main-tenance dose may need increased by twofold. Dose increases should start when contraceptive is started and titrated to clinical response increasing no more rapidly than 50-100 mg/day every week. Gradual increases of lamotrigine plasma levels may occur during the inactive "pill-free" week and will be greater when dose increases are made the week before. If increased adverse events consistently occur during "pill-free" week, overall maintenance dose adjustments may be required. When discontinuing estrogen-containing hormonal contraceptive, dose of lamotrigine may need decreased by as much as 50%; do not decrease by more than 25% of total daily dose over a 2-week period unless clinical response or plasma levels indicate otherwise. Dose adjustments during "pill-free" week are not recommended.

Renal Impairment Decreased maintenance dosage may be effective in patients with significant renal impairment; has not been adequately studied; use with caution.

Hepatic Impairment

Mild impairment: No adjustment required.

Moderate-to-severe impairment without ascites: Decrease initial, escalation, and mainte-nance doses by ~25%; adjust according to clinical response.

Moderate-to-severe impairment with ascites: Decrease initial, escalation, and maintenance doses by ~50%; adjust according to clinical response.

Administration Doses should be rounded down to the nearest whole tablet.

Lamictal® chewable/dispersible tablets: May be chewed, dispersed in water or diluted fruit juice, or swallowed whole. To disperse tablets, add to a small amount of liquid (just enough to cover tablet); let sit ~1 minute until dispersed; swirl solution and consume immediately. Do not administer partial amounts of liquid. If tablets are chewed, a small amount of water or diluted fruit juice should be used to aid in swallowing.

Lamictal® ODT™: Place tablets on tongue and move around in the mouth. Tablets will dissolve rapidly and can be swallowed with or without food or water.

Lamictal® XR™: Administer without regard to meals. Swallow whole; do not chew, crush, or cut.

Monitoring Parameters Seizure, frequency and duration; serum levels of concurrent anticonvulsants, hypersensitivity reactions (especially rash); suicidality (eg, suicidal thoughts, depression, behavioral changes); signs/symptoms of aseptic meningitis

Reference Range A therapeutic serum concentration range has not been established for lamotrigine. Dosing should be based on therapeutic response. Lamotrigine plasma concentrations of 0.25-29.1 mcg/mL have been reported in the literature.

Special Geriatric Considerations No pharmacokinetic differences noted between young adults and the elderly. Use with caution in the elderly with significant renal decline.

Dosage Forms Excipient information presented when available (limited, particularly for generics); consult specific product labeling.

Tablet, oral: 25 mg, 100 mg, 150 mg, 200 mg

LaMICtal®: 25 mg, 100 mg, 150 mg, 200 mg [scored]

Tablet, oral [combination package (each unit-dose starter kit contains)]:

LaMICtal®: 25 mg (84s) [white tablets] and 100 mg (14s) [peach tablets] [scored; green kit; for patients taking carbamazepine, phenytoin, phenobarbital, primidone, or rifampin and **not** taking valproic acid]

LaMICtal®: 25 mg (42s) [white tablets] and 100 mg (7s) [peach tablets] [scored; orange kit; for patients **not** taking carbamazepine, phenytoin, phenobarbital, primidone, rifampin, or valproic acid]

Tablet, oral [each unit-dose starter kit contains]:

LaMICtal®: 25 mg [scored; blue kit; for patients taking valproic acid]

Tablet, chewable/dispersible, oral: 5 mg, 25 mg

LaMICtal®: 2 mg [black currant flavor]

LaMICtal®: 5 mg [scored; black currant flavor]

LaMICtal®: 25 mg [black currant flavor]

Tablet, extended release, oral:

LaMICtal® XR™: 25 mg, 50 mg, 100 mg, 200 mg, 250 mg, 300 mg

Tablet, extended release, oral [combination package (each patient titration kit contains)]:

LaMICtal® XR™: 25 mg (21s) [yellow/white tablets] and 50 mg (7s) [green/white tablets] [blue XR kit, for patients taking valproic acid]

LaMICtal® XR™: 50 mg (14s) [green/white tablets], 100 mg (14s) [orange/white tablets], and 200 mg (7s) [blue/white tablets] [green XR kit, for patients taking carbamazepine, phenytoin, phenobarbital, primidone, and **not** taking valproic acid]

LaMICtal® XR™: 25 mg (14s) [yellow/white tablets], 50 mg (14s) [green/white tablets], and 100 mg (7s) [orange/white tablets] [orange XR kit, for patients **not** taking carbamazepine, phenytoin, phenobarbital, primidone, or valproic acid]

Tablet, orally disintegrating, oral:

LaMICtal® ODT™: 25 mg, 50 mg, 100 mg, 200 mg [cherry flavor]

Tablet, orally disintegrating, oral [combination package (each patient titration kit contains)]:

LaMICtal® ODT™: 25 mg (21s) and 50 mg (7s) [cherry flavor; blue kit, for patients taking valproic acid]

LaMICtal® ODT™: 50 mg (42s) and 100 mg (14s) [cherry flavor; green kit, for patients taking carbamazepine, phenytoin, phenobarbital, primidone, or rifampin and **not** taking valproic acid]

LaMICtal® ODT™: 25 mg (14s), 50 mg (14s), and 100 mg (7s) [cherry flavor; orange kit, for patients **not** taking carbamazepine, phenytoin, phenobarbital, primidone, rifampin, or valproic acid]

Extemporaneously Prepared A 1 mg/mL oral suspension may be compounded as follows: Crush one 100 mg immediate release tablet and reduce to a fine powder. Add small amount of Ora-Sweet® or Ora-Plus® and mix to uniform paste. Transfer to graduate and qs to 100 mL. Shake well before using and refrigerate. Suspension is stable for 91 days.

Nahata M, Morosco R, Hipple T. "Stability of Lamotrigine in Two Extemporaneously Prepared Oral Suspensions at 4 and 25°C," *Am J Health Syst Pharm,* 1999, 56:240-2.

◆ **Lanoxin®** *see* Digoxin *on page 543*

Lansoprazole (lan SOE pra zole)

Related Information
H. pylori Treatment in Adult Patients on page 2116
Medication Safety Issues
Sound-alike/look-alike issues:
Lansoprazole may be confused with aripiprazole, dexlansoprazole
Prevacid® may be confused with Pravachol®, Prevpac®, PriLOSEC®, Prinivil®
Brand Names: U.S. First®-Lansoprazole; Prevacid®; Prevacid® 24 HR [OTC]; Prevacid® SoluTab™
Brand Names: Canada Apo-Lansoprazole®; Mylan-Lansoprazole; Prevacid®; Prevacid® FasTab; Teva-Lansoprazole
Generic Availability (U.S.) Yes: Capsule
Pharmacologic Category Proton Pump Inhibitor; Substituted Benzimidazole
Use Short-term treatment of active duodenal ulcers; maintenance treatment of healed duodenal ulcers; as part of a multidrug regimen for H. pylori eradication to reduce the risk of duodenal ulcer recurrence; short-term treatment of active benign gastric ulcer; treatment of NSAID-associated gastric ulcer; to reduce the risk of NSAID-associated gastric ulcer in patients with a history of gastric ulcer who require an NSAID; short-term treatment of symptomatic GERD; short-term treatment for all grades of erosive esophagitis; to maintain healing of erosive esophagitis; long-term treatment of pathological hypersecretory conditions, including Zollinger-Ellison syndrome

OTC labeling: Relief of frequent heartburn (≥2 days/week)
Contraindications Hypersensitivity to lansoprazole or any component of the formulation
Warnings/Precautions Use of proton pump inhibitors (PPIs) may increase the risk of gastrointestinal infections (eg, Salmonella, Campylobacter). Relief of symptoms does not preclude the presence of a gastric malignancy. Atrophic gastritis (by biopsy) has been noted with long-term omeprazole therapy; this may also occur with lansoprazole. No reports of enterochromaffin-like (ECL) cell carcinoids, dysplasia, or neoplasia have occurred. Severe liver dysfunction may require dosage reductions. Decreased H. pylori eradication rates have been observed with short-term (≤7 days) combination therapy. The American College of Gastroenterology recommends 10-14 days of therapy (triple or quadruple) for eradication of H. pylori (Chey, 2007).

PPIs may diminish the therapeutic effect of clopidogrel thought to be due to reduced formation of the active metabolite of clopidogrel. The manufacturer of clopidogrel recommends either avoidance of omeprazole or use of a PPI with less potent CYP2C19 inhibition (eg, pantoprazole). Lansoprazole exhibits the most potent CYP2C19 inhibition; given the potency of lansoprazole's CYP2C19 inhibitory activity, avoidance of lansoprazole would appear prudent. Others have recommended the continued use of PPIs, regardless of the degree of inhibition, in patients with a history of GI bleeding or multiple risk factors for GI bleeding who are also receiving clopidogrel since no evidence has established clinically meaningful differences in outcome; however, a clinically-significant interaction cannot be excluded in those who are poor metabolizers of clopidogrel (Abraham, 2010; Levine, 2011). Additionally, concomitant use of lansoprazole with some drugs may require cautious use, may not be recommended, or may require dosage adjustments.

Increased incidence of osteoporosis-related bone fractures of the hip, spine, or wrist may occur with PPI therapy. Patients on high-dose or long-term therapy should be monitored. Use the lowest effective dose for the shortest duration of time, use vitamin D and calcium supplementation, and follow appropriate guidelines to reduce risk of fractures in patients at risk.

Hypomagnesemia, reported rarely, usually with prolonged PPI use of >3 months (most cases >1 year of therapy); may be symptomatic or asymptomatic; severe cases may cause tetany, seizures, and cardiac arrhythmias. Consider obtaining serum magnesium concentrations prior to beginning long-term therapy, especially if taking concomitant digoxin, diuretics, or other drugs known to cause hypomagnesemia; and periodically thereafter. Hypomagnesemia may be corrected by magnesium supplementation, although discontinuation of lansoprazole may be necessary; magnesium levels typically return to normal within 1 week of stopping.

When used for self-medication, patients should be instructed not to use if they have difficulty swallowing, are vomiting blood, or have bloody or black stools. Prior to use, patients should contact healthcare provider if they have liver disease, heartburn for >3 months, heartburn with dizziness, lightheadedness, or sweating, MI symptoms, frequent chest pain, frequent wheezing (especially with heartburn), unexplained weight loss, nausea/vomiting, stomach pain, or are taking antifungals, atazanavir, digoxin, tacrolimus, theophylline, or warfarin. Patients should stop use and consult a healthcare provider if heartburn continues or worsens, or if they need to take for >14 days or more often than every 4 months. Patients should be informed that it may take 1-4 days for full effect to be seen; should not be used for immediate relief.

Adverse Reactions (Reflective of adult population; not specific for elderly) 1% to 10%:

Central nervous system: Headache (children 1-11 years 3%, 12-17 years 7%), dizziness (children 12-17 years 3%; adults <1%)

Gastrointestinal: Diarrhea (1% to 5%; 60 mg/day: 7%), abdominal pain (children 12-17 years 5%; adults 2%), constipation (children 1-11 years 5%; adults 1%), nausea (children 12-17 years 3%; adults 1%)

Drug Interactions

Metabolism/Transport Effects Substrate of CYP2C19 (major), CYP2C9 (minor), CYP3A4 (major); **Note:** Assignment of Major/Minor substrate status based on clinically relevant drug interaction potential; **Inhibits** CYP2C19 (moderate), CYP2C9 (weak), CYP2D6 (weak), CYP3A4 (weak); **Induces** CYP1A2 (weak/moderate)

Avoid Concomitant Use

Avoid concomitant use of Lansoprazole with any of the following: Delavirdine; Erlotinib; Nelfinavir; Pimozide; Posaconazole; Rilpivirine

Increased Effect/Toxicity

Lansoprazole may increase the levels/effects of: Amphetamines; ARIPiprazole; Citalopram; CYP2C19 Substrates; Dexmethylphenidate; Imatinib; Methotrexate; Methylphenidate; Pimozide; Raltegravir; Saquinavir; Tacrolimus; Tacrolimus (Systemic); Vitamin K Antagonists; Voriconazole

The levels/effects of Lansoprazole may be increased by: Fluconazole; Ketoconazole; Ketoconazole (Systemic)

Decreased Effect

Lansoprazole may decrease the levels/effects of: Atazanavir; Bisphosphonate Derivatives; Cefditoren; Clopidogrel; Dabigatran Etexilate; Dasatinib; Delavirdine; Erlotinib; Gefitinib; Indinavir; Iron Salts; Itraconazole; Ketoconazole; Ketoconazole (Systemic); Mesalamine; Mycophenolate; Nelfinavir; Nilotinib; Posaconazole; Rilpivirine; Vismodegib

The levels/effects of Lansoprazole may be decreased by: CYP2C19 Inducers (Strong); CYP3A4 Inducers (Strong); Deferasirox; Herbs (CYP3A4 Inducers); Tipranavir; Tocilizumab

Ethanol/Nutrition/Herb Interactions

Ethanol: Avoid ethanol (may cause gastric mucosal irritation).

Food: Lansoprazole serum concentrations may be decreased if taken with food.

Herb/Nutraceutical: Avoid St John's wort (may decrease the levels/effect of lansoprazole).

Stability Store at 25°C (77°F); excursions permitted to 15°C to 30°C (59°F to 86°F).

Mechanism of Action Decreases acid secretion in gastric parietal cells through inhibition of (H+, K+)-ATPase enzyme system, blocking the final step in gastric acid production.

Pharmacodynamics/Kinetics

Onset of action: Gastric acid suppression: Oral: 1-3 hours

Duration: Gastric acid suppression: Oral: >1 day

Absorption: Rapid

Distribution: V_d: 14-18 L

Protein binding: 97%

Metabolism: Hepatic via CYP2C19 and 3A4, and in parietal cells to two active metabolites that are not present in systemic circulation

Bioavailability: ≥80%; decreased 50% to 70% if given 30 minutes after food

Half-life elimination: 1.5 ± 1 hours; Elderly: 2-3 hours; Hepatic impairment: 3-7 hours

Time to peak, plasma: 1.7 hours

Excretion: Feces (67%); urine (33%)

Dosage

Geriatric & Adult

Symptomatic GERD: Oral: Short-term treatment: 15 mg once daily for up to 8 weeks

Erosive esophagitis: Oral: Short-term treatment: 30 mg once daily for up to 8 weeks; continued treatment for an additional 8 weeks may be considered for recurrence or for patients who do not heal after the first 8 weeks of therapy; maintenance therapy: 15 mg once daily

Hypersecretory conditions: Oral: Initial: 60 mg once daily; adjust dose based upon patient response and to reduce acid secretion to <10 mEq/hour (5 mEq/hour in patients with prior gastric surgery); doses of 90 mg twice daily have been used; administer doses >120 mg/day in divided doses

Duodenal ulcer: Oral: Short-term treatment: 15 mg once daily for 4 weeks; maintenance therapy: 15 mg once daily

Helicobacter pylori **eradication:**
Manufacturer's labeling: 30 mg 3 times/day administered with amoxicillin 1000 mg 3 times/day for 14 days **or** 30 mg twice daily administered with amoxicillin 1000 mg *and* clarithromycin 500 mg twice daily for 10-14 days

American College of Gastroenterology guidelines (Chey, 2007):
Nonpenicillin allergy: 30 mg twice daily administered with amoxicillin 1000 mg *and* clarithromycin 500 mg twice daily for 10-14 days

Penicillin allergy: 30 mg twice daily administered with clarithromycin 500 mg *and* metronidazole 500 mg twice daily for 10-14 days **or** 30 mg once or twice daily administered with bismuth subsalicylate 525 mg *and* metronidazole 250 mg *plus* tetracycline 500 mg 4 times/day for 10-14 days

Gastric ulcer: Oral: Short-term treatment: 30 mg once daily for up to 8 weeks

NSAID-associated gastric ulcer (healing): Oral: 30 mg once daily for 8 weeks; controlled studies did not extend past 8 weeks

NSAID-associated gastric ulcer (to reduce risk): Oral: 15 mg once daily for up to 12 weeks; controlled studies did not extend past 12 weeks

Heartburn (OTC labeling): Oral: 15 mg once daily for 14 days; may repeat 14 days of therapy every 4 months. Do not take for >14 days or more often than every 4 months, unless instructed by healthcare provider.

Renal Impairment No adjustment is necessary.

Hepatic Impairment Severe hepatic impairment: Consider a dose reduction.

Administration

Oral: Administer before food; best if taken before breakfast. The intact granules should not be chewed or crushed; however, several options are available for those patients unable to swallow capsules:

Capsules may be opened and the intact granules sprinkled on 1 tablespoon of applesauce, Ensure® pudding, cottage cheese, yogurt, or strained pears. The granules should then be swallowed immediately.

Capsules may be opened and emptied into ~60 mL orange juice, apple juice, or tomato juice; mix and swallow immediately. Rinse the glass with additional juice and swallow to assure complete delivery of the dose.

Orally-disintegrating tablets: Should not be swallowed whole, broken, cut, or chewed. Place tablet on tongue; allow to dissolve (with or without water) until particles can be swallowed. Orally-disintegrating tablets may also be administered via an oral syringe: Place the 15 mg tablet in an oral syringe and draw up ~4 mL water, or place the 30 mg tablet in an oral syringe and draw up ~10 mL water. After tablet has dispersed, administer within 15 minutes. Refill the syringe with water (2 mL for the 15 mg tablet; 5 mL for the 30 mg tablet), shake gently, then administer any remaining contents.

Nasogastric tube administration:

Capsule: Capsule can be opened, the granules mixed (not crushed) with 40 mL of apple juice and then injected through the NG tube into the stomach, then flush tube with additional apple juice. Do not mix with other liquids.

Orally-disintegrating tablet: Nasogastric tube ≥8 French: Place a 15 mg tablet in a syringe and draw up ~4 mL water, or place the 30 mg tablet in a syringe and draw up ~10 mL water. After tablet has dispersed, administer within 15 minutes. Refill the syringe with ~5 mL water, shake gently, and then flush the nasogastric tube.

Monitoring Parameters Patients with Zollinger-Ellison syndrome should be monitored for gastric acid output, which should be maintained at ≤10 mEq/hour during the last hour before the next lansoprazole dose; lab monitoring should include CBC, liver function, renal function, and serum gastrin levels

Special Geriatric Considerations The clearance of lansoprazole is decreased in the elderly; however, the half-life is only increased by 50% to 100%, resulting in a continued short half-life with no accumulation in the elderly. No dosage adjustment is required with normal hepatic function. The rate of healing and side effects are similar to younger adults.

An increased risk of fractures of the hip, spine, or wrist has been observed in epidemiologic studies with proton pump inhibitor (PPI) use, primarily in older adults ≥50 years of age. The greatest risk was seen in patients receiving high doses or on long-term therapy (≥1 year). Calcium and vitamin D supplementation and close monitoring are recommended to reduce the risk of fracture in high-risk patients. Additionally, long-term use of proton pump inhibitors has resulted in reports of hypomagnesemia and *Clostridium difficile* infections.

Dosage Forms Excipient information presented when available (limited, particularly for generics); consult specific product labeling. [DSC] = Discontinued product

Capsule, delayed release, oral: 15 mg, 30 mg
Prevacid®: 15 mg, 30 mg
Prevacid® 24 HR: 15 mg

Powder for suspension, oral [compounding kit]:
First®-Lansoprazole: 3 mg/mL (90 mL, 150 mL, 300 mL) [contains benzyl alcohol]

◀ Tablet, delayed release, orally disintegrating, oral: 15 mg [DSC], 30 mg [DSC]
    Prevacid® SoluTab™: 15 mg [contains phenylalanine 2.5 mg/tablet; strawberry flavor]
    Prevacid® SoluTab™: 30 mg [contains phenylalanine 5.1 mg/tablet; strawberry flavor]

Lanthanum (LAN tha num)

Medication Safety Issues
Sound-alike/look-alike issues:
  Lanthanum may be confused with lithium
Brand Names: U.S. Fosrenol®
Brand Names: Canada Fosrenol®
Index Terms Lanthanum Carbonate
Generic Availability (U.S.) No
Pharmacologic Category Phosphate Binder
Use Reduction of serum phosphate in patients with stage 5 chronic kidney disease (end-stage renal disease [ESRD]; kidney failure: GFR <15 mL/minute/1.73 m² or dialysis)
Medication Guide Available Yes
Contraindications Bowel obstruction, fecal impaction, ileus
Warnings/Precautions Gastrointestinal (GI) obstruction may occur in patients with altered gastrointestinal anatomy, hypomotility disorders (including constipation, ileus, and diabetes), or concomitant medications (eg, calcium channel blockers); may also occur without history of GI disease. Use caution with active peptic ulcer, ulcerative colitis, or Crohn's disease. Abdominal x-rays may have a radiopaque appearance in patients taking lanthanum. Chew tablet thoroughly to decrease risk of adverse GI effects; do not swallow whole.
Adverse Reactions (Reflective of adult population; not specific for elderly)
Reported in short-term (4-6 weeks) trials at frequency >placebo:
>10%: Gastrointestinal: Nausea (11%)
1% to 10%: Gastrointestinal: Vomiting (9%), abdominal pain (5%)
Drug Interactions
Metabolism/Transport Effects None known.
Avoid Concomitant Use There are no known interactions where it is recommended to avoid concomitant use.
Increased Effect/Toxicity There are no known significant interactions involving an increase in effect.
Decreased Effect
Lanthanum may decrease the levels/effects of: ACE Inhibitors; Ampicillin; Chloroquine; Halofantrine; Quinolone Antibiotics; Tetracycline Derivatives; Thyroid Products

The levels/effects of Lanthanum may be decreased by: HMG-CoA Reductase Inhibitors
Stability Store at 25°C (77°F); excursions permitted to 15°C to 30°C (59°F to 86°F). Protect from moisture.
Mechanism of Action Disassociates in the upper gastrointestinal tract to lanthanum ions (La^{3+}) which bind to dietary phosphate resulting in insoluble lanthanum phosphate complexes and a net decrease in serum phosphate and calcium levels.
Pharmacodynamics/Kinetics
Absorption: <0.002%
Protein binding: >99%
Metabolism: Not metabolized
Half-life elimination: Plasma: 53 hours; Bone: 2-3.6 years
Excretion: Feces primarily; urine <2%
Dosage
Geriatric & Adult Reduction of serum phosphorous: Oral: Initial: 1500 mg/day divided and taken with meals; typical increases of 750 mg/day every 2-3 weeks are suggested as needed to reduce the serum phosphate level <6 mg/dL; usual dosage range: 1500-3000 mg; doses of up to 4500 mg have been evaluated
Administration Administer with or immediately after meals; tablet should be chewed completely prior to swallowing; do not swallow whole. Tablet may be crushed to aid in chewing.
Monitoring Parameters Serum calcium and phosphorus. Frequency of measurement may be dependent upon the presence and magnitude of abnormalities, the rate of progression of CKD, and the use of treatments for CKD-mineral and bone disorders (KDIGO, 2009): CKD stage 5 and 5D: Every 1-3 months
Reference Range
Corrected total serum calcium (K/DOQI, 2003): CKD stage 5: 8.4-9.5 mg/dL (2.1-2.37 mmol/L); KDIGO guidelines recommend maintaining normal ranges for CKD stage 5 and 5D (KDIGO, 2009)

Phosphorus (K/DOQI, 2003): CKD stage 5 (including those treated with dialysis): 3.5-5.5 mg/dL (1.13-1.78 mmol/L); KDIGO guidelines recommend maintaining normal ranges for CKD stage 5 and lowering elevated phosphorus levels toward the normal range for CKD stage 5D (KDIGO, 2009)

Serum calcium-phosphorus product (K/DOQI, 2003): CKD stage 5: <55 mg^2/dL^2

Test Interactions Abdominal x-rays may have a radiopaque appearance.

Special Geriatric Considerations In initial studies, no overall clinical differences were noted in those >65 years of age compared to younger adults.

Dosage Forms Excipient information presented when available (limited, particularly for generics); consult specific product labeling.

Tablet, chewable, oral:

Fosrenol®: 500 mg, 750 mg, 1000 mg

♦ **Lanthanum Carbonate** *see* Lanthanum *on page 1096*
♦ **Lantus®** *see* Insulin Glargine *on page 1012*
♦ **Lantus® Solostar®** *see* Insulin Glargine *on page 1012*
♦ **Lasix®** *see* Furosemide *on page 855*
♦ **Lastacaft™** *see* Alcaftadine *on page 52*

Latanoprost (la TA noe prost)

Related Information

Glaucoma Drug Therapy *on page 2115*

Medication Safety Issues

Sound-alike/look-alike issues:

Latanoprost may be confused with Lantus®

Xalatan® may be confused with Lantus®, Travatan®, Xalacom™, Zarontin®

Brand Names: U.S. Xalatan®

Brand Names: Canada Apo-Latanoprost®; CO Latanoprost; GD-Latanoprost; Xalatan®

Generic Availability (U.S.) Yes

Pharmacologic Category Ophthalmic Agent, Antiglaucoma; Prostaglandin, Ophthalmic

Use Reduction of elevated intraocular pressure in patients with open-angle glaucoma or ocular hypertension

Contraindications Hypersensitivity to latanoprost, benzalkonium chloride, or any component of the formulation

Warnings/Precautions May permanently change/increase brown pigmentation of the iris, the eyelid skin, and eyelashes. In addition, may increase the length and/or number of eyelashes (may vary between eyes); changes occur slowly and may not be noticeable for months or years. Long-term consequences and potential injury to eye are not known. Use with caution in patients with intraocular inflammation, aphakic patients, pseudophakic patients with a torn posterior lens capsule, or patients with risk factors for macular edema. Safety and efficacy have not been determined for use in patients with angle-closure-, inflammatory-, or neo-vascular glaucoma.

There have been reports of bacterial keratitis associated with the use of multiple-dose containers of topical ophthalmic products. Contains benzalkonium chloride which may be absorbed by contact lenses; remove contacts prior to administration and wait 15 minutes before reinserting.

Adverse Reactions (Reflective of adult population; not specific for elderly)

>5% to 15%: Ocular: Blurred vision, burning and stinging, conjunctival hyperemia, foreign body sensation, itching, increased pigmentation of the iris, punctate epithelial keratopathy

1% to 5%:

Cardiovascular: Angina pectoris (1% to 2%), chest pain (1% to 2%)

Dermatologic: Allergic skin reaction (1% to 2%), rash (1% to 2%)

Neuromuscular & skeletal: Arthralgia (1% to 2%), back pain (1% to 2%), myalgia (1% to 2%)

Ocular: Dry eye (1% to 4%), excessive tearing (1% to 4%), eye pain (1% to 4%), lid crusting (1% to 4%), lid edema (1% to 4%), lid erythema (1% to 4%), lid discomfort/pain (1% to 4%), photophobia (1% to 4%)

Respiratory: Cold (4%), flu (4%), upper respiratory tract infection (4%)

Miscellaneous: Flu-like syndrome (4%)

Drug Interactions

Metabolism/Transport Effects None known.

Avoid Concomitant Use There are no known interactions where it is recommended to avoid concomitant use.

Increased Effect/Toxicity

Latanoprost may increase the levels/effects of: Bimatoprost

Decreased Effect
The levels/effects of Latanoprost may be decreased by: NSAID (Ophthalmic)

Stability Store intact bottles under refrigeration (2°C to 8°C/36°F to 46°F). Protect from light. Once opened, the container may be stored at room temperature up to 25°C (77°F) for 6 weeks.

Mechanism of Action Latanoprost is a prostaglandin F_2-alpha analog believed to reduce intraocular pressure by increasing the outflow of the aqueous humor

Pharmacodynamics/Kinetics
Onset of action: 3-4 hours
Peak effect: Maximum: 8-12 hours
Absorption: Through the cornea where the isopropyl ester prodrug is hydrolyzed by esterases to the biologically active acid. Peak concentration is reached in 2 hours after topical administration in the aqueous humor.
Distribution: V_d: 0.16 L/kg
Metabolism: Primarily hepatic via fatty acid beta-oxidation
Half-life elimination: 17 minutes
Excretion: Urine (as metabolites)

Dosage
Geriatric & Adult Glaucoma: Ophthalmic: 1 drop (1.5 mcg) in the affected eye(s) once daily in the evening; do not exceed the once daily dosage because it has been shown that more frequent administration may decrease the IOP lowering effect
Note: A medication delivery device (Xal-Ease™) is available for use with Xalatan®.

Administration If more than one topical ophthalmic drug is being used, administer the drugs at least 5 minutes apart. A delivery aid, Xal-Ease™, is available for administering Xalatan®.

Special Geriatric Considerations Evaluate the patient's or caregiver's ability to safely administer the correct dose of ophthalmic medication.

Dosage Forms Excipient information presented when available (limited, particularly for generics); consult specific product labeling.
Solution, ophthalmic [drops]: 0.005% (2.5 mL)
Xalatan®: 0.005% (2.5 mL) [contains benzalkonium chloride]

◆ **Latisse®** *see* Bimatoprost *on page* 213
◆ **Latuda®** *see* Lurasidone *on page* 1172
◆ **Lazanda®** *see* FentaNYL *on page* 761
◆ ***l*-Bunolol Hydrochloride** *see* Levobunolol *on page* 1112
◆ **LCM** *see* Lacosamide *on page* 1082
◆ **L-Deoxythymidine** *see* Telbivudine *on page* 1843
◆ **L-Deprenyl** *see* Selegiline *on page* 1760
◆ **LdT** *see* Telbivudine *on page* 1843
◆ **LEA29Y** *see* Belatacept *on page* 192

Leflunomide (le FLOO noh mide)

Brand Names: U.S. Arava®
Brand Names: Canada Apo-Leflunomide®; Arava®; Mylan-Leflunomide; Novo-Leflunomide; PHL-Leflunomide; PMS-Leflunomide; Sandoz-Leflunomide
Generic Availability (U.S.) Yes
Pharmacologic Category Antirheumatic, Disease Modifying
Use Treatment of active rheumatoid arthritis; indicated to reduce signs and symptoms, and to inhibit structural damage and improve physical function
Unlabeled Use Treatment of cytomegalovirus (CMV) disease in transplant recipients resistant to standard antivirals; prevention of acute and chronic rejection in recipients of solid organ transplants
Contraindications Hypersensitivity to leflunomide or any component of the formulation
Warnings/Precautions Hazardous agent - use appropriate precautions for handling and disposal. **[U.S. Boxed Warning]: Use has been associated with rare reports of hepato-toxicity, hepatic failure, and death. Treatment should not be initiated in patients with pre-existing acute or chronic liver disease or ALT >2 x ULN. Use caution in patients with concurrent exposure to potentially hepatotoxic drugs. Monitor ALT levels during therapy; discontinue if ALT >3 x ULN occurs and, if hepatotoxicity is likely leflu-nomide-induced, start drug elimination procedures** (eg, cholestyramine, activated charcoal).

Use has been associated (rarely) with interstitial lung disease; discontinue in patients who develop new onset or worsening of pulmonary symptoms. Drug elimination procedures should be considered (eg, cholestyramine, activated charcoal) if interstitial lung disease occurs; fatal outcomes have been reported. May increase susceptibility to infection, including opportunistic pathogens. Severe infections, sepsis, and fatalities have been reported. Not recommended in patients with severe immunodeficiency, bone marrow dysplasia, or severe, uncontrolled infections. Caution should be exercised when considering the use in patients with a history of new/recurrent infections, with conditions that predispose them to infections, or with chronic, latent, or localized infections. Patients who develop a new infection while undergoing treatment should be monitored closely; consider discontinuation of therapy and drug elimination procedures if infection is serious.

Use may affect defenses against malignancies; impact on the development and course of malignancies is not fully defined. As compared to the general population, an increased risk of lymphoma has been noted in clinical trials; however, rheumatoid arthritis has been previously associated with an increased rate of lymphoma. Use with caution in patients with a prior history of significant hematologic abnormalities; avoid use with bone marrow dysplasia. Use has been associated with rare pancytopenia, agranulocytosis, and thrombocytopenia, generally when given concurrently or recently with methotrexate or other immunosuppressive agents. Monitoring of hematologic function is required; discontinue if evidence of bone marrow suppression and begin drug elimination procedures (eg, cholestyramine or activated charcoal). Rare cases of dermatologic reactions (including Stevens-Johnson syndrome and toxic epidermal necrolysis) have been reported; discontinue if evidence of severe dermatologic reaction occurs, and begin drug elimination procedures (eg, cholestyramine or activated charcoal). Cases of peripheral neuropathy have been reported; use with caution in patients >60 years of age, receiving concomitant neurotoxic medications, or patients with diabetes; discontinue if evidence of peripheral neuropathy occurs and begin drug elimination procedures (eg, cholestyramine, activated charcoal).

Safety has not been established in patients with latent tuberculosis infection. Patients should be screened for tuberculosis and if necessary, treated prior to initiating therapy. Use with caution in patients with renal impairment. Patients should be brought up to date with all immunizations before initiating therapy. Live vaccines should not be given concurrently; there is no data available concerning secondary transmission of live vaccines in patients receiving therapy. Due to variations in clearance, it may take up to 2 years to reach low levels of leflunomide metabolite serum concentrations. A drug elimination procedure using cholestyramine or activated charcoal is recommended when a more rapid elimination is needed.

Adverse Reactions (Reflective of adult population; not specific for elderly)

>10%:
  Gastrointestinal: Diarrhea (17%)
  Respiratory: Respiratory tract infection (4% to 15%)
1% to 10%:
  Cardiovascular: Hypertension (10%), chest pain (2%), edema (peripheral), palpitation, tachycardia, vasodilation, varicose vein, vasculitis
  Central nervous system: Headache (7%), dizziness (4%), pain (2%), anxiety, depression, fever, insomnia, malaise, migraine, sleep disorder, vertigo
  Dermatologic: Alopecia (10%), rash (10%), pruritus (4%), dry skin (2%), eczema (2%), acne, bruising, dermatitis, hair discoloration, hematoma, nail disorder, skin disorder/discoloration, skin ulcer, subcutaneous nodule
  Endocrine & metabolic: Hypokalemia (1%), diabetes mellitus, hyperglycemia, hyperlipidemia, hyperthyroidism, menstrual disorder
  Gastrointestinal: Nausea (9%), abdominal pain (5% to 6%), dyspepsia (5%), weight loss (4%), anorexia (3%), gastroenteritis (3%), mouth ulceration (3%), vomiting (3%), candidiasis (oral), colitis, constipation, esophagitis, flatulence, gastritis, gingivitis, melena, salivary gland enlarged, stomatitis, taste disturbance, xerostomia
  Genitourinary: Urinary tract infection (5%), albuminuria, cystitis, dysuria, prostate disorder, urinary frequency, vaginal candidiasis
  Hematologic: Anemia
  Hepatic: Abnormal LFTs (5%), cholelithiasis
  Local: Abscess
  Neuromuscular & skeletal: Back pain (5%), joint disorder (4%), weakness (3%), tenosynovitis (3%), synovitis (2%), paresthesia (2%), arthralgia (1%), leg cramps (1%), arthrosis, bone necrosis, bone pain, bursitis, CPK increased, myalgia, neck pain, neuralgia, neuritis, pelvic pain, tendon rupture
  Ocular: Blurred vision, cataract, conjunctivitis, eye disorder
  Renal: Hematuria
  Respiratory: Bronchitis (7%), cough (3%), pharyngitis (3%), pneumonia (2%), rhinitis (2%), sinusitis (2%), asthma, dyspnea, epistaxis
  Miscellaneous: Accidental injury (5%), allergic reactions (2%), flu-like syndrome (2%), cyst, diaphoresis, hernia, herpes infection

◄ **Drug Interactions**
   Metabolism/Transport Effects Inhibits CYP2C9 (moderate)
   Avoid Concomitant Use
      Avoid concomitant use of Leflunomide with any of the following: BCG; Natalizumab; Pimecrolimus; Tacrolimus (Topical)
   Increased Effect/Toxicity
      Leflunomide may increase the levels/effects of: Carvedilol; CYP2C9 Substrates; Natalizumab; TOLBUTamide; Vaccines (Live); Vitamin K Antagonists

      The levels/effects of Leflunomide may be increased by: Denosumab; Immunosuppressants; Methotrexate; Pimecrolimus; Rifampin; Roflumilast; Tacrolimus (Topical); TOLBUTamide; Trastuzumab
   Decreased Effect
      Leflunomide may decrease the levels/effects of: BCG; Coccidioidin Skin Test; Sipuleucel-T; Vaccines (Inactivated)

      The levels/effects of Leflunomide may be decreased by: Bile Acid Sequestrants; Charcoal, Activated; Echinacea
   Ethanol/Nutrition/Herb Interactions
      Food: No interactions with food have been noted. Management: Maintain adequate hydration, unless instructed to restrict fluid intake.
      Herb/Nutraceutical: Echinacea may diminish the therapeutic effect of leflunomide.
   Stability Store at 25°C (77°F); excursions permitted to 15°C to 30°C (59°F to 86°F). Protect from light.
   Mechanism of Action Leflunomide is an immunodulatory agent that inhibits pyrimidine synthesis, resulting in antiproliferative and anti-inflammatory effects. Leflunomide is a prodrug; the active metabolite is responsible for activity. For CMV, may interfere with virion assembly.
   Pharmacodynamics/Kinetics
      Distribution: V_d: M1: 0.13 L/kg
      Protein binding; M1: >99% to albumin
      Metabolism: Hepatic to an active metabolite M1 (also known as A77 1726 or teriflunomide), which accounts for nearly all pharmacologic activity; further metabolism to multiple inactive metabolites; undergoes enterohepatic recirculation
      Bioavailability: 80% (relative to oral solution)
      Half-life elimination: M1: Mean: 14-15 days; enterohepatic recycling appears to contribute to the long half-life of this agent, since activated charcoal and cholestyramine substantially reduce plasma half-life
      Time to peak: M1: 6-12 hours
      Excretion: Feces (48%); urine (43%)
   Dosage
      Geriatric & Adult
         Rheumatoid arthritis: Oral: Loading dose: 100 mg/day for 3 days, followed by 20 mg/day; **Note:** The loading dose may be omitted in patients at increased risk of hepatic or hematologic toxicity (eg, recent concomitant methotrexate). Dosage may be decreased to 10 mg/day in patients who have difficulty tolerating the 20 mg dose. Due to the long half-life of the active metabolite, serum concentrations may require a prolonged period to decline after dosage reduction.
         CMV disease, resistant to standard antivirals (unlabeled use): Oral: Some authors recommend 100-200 mg/day for 5-7 days, followed by 40-60 mg/day (Avery, 2004; Avery, 2010). Others have utilized the standard rheumatoid arthritis dosing (John, 2004). Adjust dose based on serum concentrations of metabolite and adverse events (Avery, 2008; Avery, 2010; Williams, 2002).
      Renal Impairment No specific dosage adjustment is recommended. There is no clinical experience in the use of leflunomide in patients with renal impairment. The free fraction of M1 is doubled in dialysis patients. Patients should be monitored closely for adverse effects requiring dosage adjustment.
      Hepatic Impairment Not recommended for use in patients with pre-existing liver disease or in patients with significant hepatic impairment (ALT >2 times ULN). Patients should have LFTs monitored closely. Discontinue leflunomide if ALT >3 times ULN.
   Administration Administer without regard to meals.
   Monitoring Parameters A complete blood count (WBC, platelet count, hemoglobin or hematocrit), serum phosphate, as well as serum transaminase determinations should be monitored at baseline and monthly during the initial 6 months of treatment; if stable, monitoring frequency may be decreased to every 6-8 weeks thereafter (continue monthly when used in combination with other immunosuppressive agents). ALT should be monitored at least monthly for the first 6 months of treatment, then every 6-8 weeks thereafter (discontinue if ALT >3 x ULN, treat with cholestyramine, and monitor liver function at least weekly until normal). In addition, monitor for signs/symptoms of severe infection, abnormalities in hepatic function

tests, symptoms of hepatotoxicity, and blood pressure. If coadministered with methotrexate, monthly transaminases (ALT, AST) and serum albumin levels are recommended. Screen for tuberculosis prior to therapy.

When used for CMV disease, monitor serum trough concentrations of active metabolite (also see Reference Range).

Reference Range CMV disease:

Timing of serum samples: Initial: Obtain 24 hours after last dose of loading regimen and periodically thereafter

Therapeutic concentration: Active metabolite (A77 1726, M1, or teriflunomide): Trough: 50-80 mcg/mL (Avery, 2010) or up to 100 mcg/mL (Williams, 2002)

Special Geriatric Considerations In Phase III studies, no difference in safety and effectiveness were seen between older and younger adults. No dosage reduction necessary based on age alone; monitor in renal and hepatic impairment.

Dosage Forms Excipient information presented when available (limited, particularly for generics); consult specific product labeling.

Tablet, oral: 10 mg, 20 mg

Arava®: 10 mg, 20 mg

♦ **Lescol®** see Fluvastatin on page 831
♦ **Lescol® XL** see Fluvastatin on page 831

Letrozole (LET roe zole)

Medication Safety Issues

Sound-alike/look-alike issues:

Femara® may be confused with Famvir®, femhrt®, Provera®

Letrozole may be confused with anastrozole

Brand Names: U.S. Femara®

Brand Names: Canada Femara®; JAMP-Letrozole; Letrozole Tablets, USP; MED-Letrozole; Myl-Letrozole; PMS-Letrozole; Sandoz-Letrozole

Index Terms CGS-20267

Generic Availability (U.S.) Yes

Pharmacologic Category Antineoplastic Agent, Aromatase Inhibitor

Use For use in postmenopausal women in the adjuvant treatment of hormone receptor positive early breast cancer, extended adjuvant treatment of early breast cancer after 5 years of tamoxifen, advanced breast cancer with disease progression following antiestrogen therapy, hormone receptor positive or hormone receptor unknown, locally-advanced, or first-line (or second-line) treatment of advanced or metastatic breast cancer

Unlabeled Use Treatment of ovarian (epithelial) cancer, endometrial cancer

Contraindications Canadian labeling: Additional contraindications (not in U.S. labeling): Hypersensitivity to letrozole, other aromatase inhibitors, or any component of the formulation

Warnings/Precautions Hazardous agent - use appropriate precautions for handling and disposal. Use caution with hepatic impairment; dose adjustment recommended in patients with cirrhosis or severe hepatic dysfunction. May cause dizziness, fatigue, and somnolence; patients should be cautioned before performing tasks which require mental alertness (eg, operating machinery or driving). May increase total serum cholesterol; in patients treated with adjuvant therapy and cholesterol levels within normal limits, an increase of >1.5 x ULN in total cholesterol has been demonstrated in 8.2% of letrozole-treated patients (25% requiring lipid-lowering medications) vs 3.2% of tamoxifen-treated patients (16% requiring medications); monitor cholesterol panel; may require antihyperlipidemics. May cause decreases in bone mineral density (BMD); a decrease in hip BMD by 3.8% from baseline in letrozole-treated patients vs 2% in placebo at 2 years has been demonstrated; however, there was no statistical difference in changes to the lumbar spine BMD scores; monitor BMD.

Adverse Reactions (Reflective of adult population; not specific for elderly)

>10%:

Cardiovascular: Edema (7% to 18%)

Central nervous system: Headache (4% to 20%), dizziness (3% to 14%), fatigue (8% to 13%)

Endocrine & metabolic: Hypercholesterolemia (3% to 52%), hot flashes (6% to 50%)

Gastrointestinal: Nausea (9% to 17%), weight gain (2% to 13%), constipation (2% to 11%)

Neuromuscular & skeletal: Weakness (4% to 34%), arthralgia (8% to 25%), arthritis (7% to 25%), bone pain (5% to 22%), back pain (5% to 18%), bone mineral density decreased/osteoporosis (5% to 15%), bone fracture (10% to 14%)

Respiratory: Dyspnea (6% to 18%), cough (6% to 13%)

Miscellaneous: Diaphoresis (≤24%), night sweats (15%)

◀ 1% to 10%:
Cardiovascular: Chest pain (6% to 8%), hypertension (5% to 8%), chest wall pain (6%), peripheral edema (5%); cerebrovascular accident including hemorrhagic stroke, thrombotic stroke (2% to 3%); thromboembolic event including venous thrombosis, thrombophlebitis, portal vein thrombosis, pulmonary embolism (2% to 3%); MI (1% to 2%), angina (1% to 2%), transient ischemic attack
Central nervous system: Insomnia (6% to 7%), pain (5%), anxiety (<5%), depression (<5%), vertigo (<5%), somnolence (3%)
Dermatologic: Rash (5%), alopecia (3% to 5%), pruritus (1%)
Endocrine & metabolic: Breast pain (2% to 7%), hypercalcemia (<5%)
Gastrointestinal: Diarrhea (5% to 8%), vomiting (3% to 7%), weight loss (6% to 7%), abdominal pain (6%), anorexia (1% to 5%), dyspepsia (3%)
Genitourinary: Urinary tract infection (6%), vaginal bleeding (5%), vaginal dryness (5%), vaginal hemorrhage (5%), vaginal irritation (5%)
Neuromuscular & skeletal: Limb pain (4% to 10%), myalgia (7% to 9%)
Ocular: Cataract (2%)
Renal: Renal disorder (5%)
Respiratory: Pleural effusion (<5%)
Miscellaneous: Infection (7%), influenza (6%), viral infection (6%), secondary malignancy (2% to 4%)

Drug Interactions
Metabolism/Transport Effects Substrate of CYP2A6 (minor), CYP3A4 (minor); **Note:** Assignment of Major/Minor substrate status based on clinically relevant drug interaction potential; **Inhibits** CYP2A6 (strong), CYP2C19 (weak)
Avoid Concomitant Use There are no known interactions where it is recommended to avoid concomitant use.
Increased Effect/Toxicity
Letrozole may increase the levels/effects of: CYP2A6 Substrates
Decreased Effect
The levels/effects of Letrozole may be decreased by: Tamoxifen; Tocilizumab
Stability Store at room temperature of 25°C (77°F); excursions permitted to 15°C to 30°C (59°F to 86°F).
Mechanism of Action Nonsteroidal competitive inhibitor of the aromatase enzyme system which binds to the heme group of aromatase, a cytochrome P450 enzyme which catalyzes conversion of androgens to estrogens (specifically, androstenedione to estrone and testosterone to estradiol). This leads to inhibition of the enzyme and a significant reduction in plasma estrogen (estrone, estradiol and estrone sulfate) levels. Does not affect synthesis of adrenal or thyroid hormones, aldosterone, or androgens.

Pharmacodynamics/Kinetics
Absorption: Rapid and well absorbed; not affected by food
Distribution: V_d: ~1.9 L/kg
Protein binding, plasma: Weak
Metabolism: Hepatic via CYP3A4 and 2A6 to an inactive carbinol metabolite
Half-life elimination: Terminal: ~2 days
Time to steady state, plasma: 2-6 weeks
Excretion: Urine (90%; 6% as unchanged drug, 75% as glucuronide carbinol metabolite, 9% as unidentified metabolites)

Dosage
Geriatric & Adult Females: Postmenopausal:
Breast cancer, advanced (first- or second-line treatment): Oral: 2.5 mg once daily; continue until tumor progression
Breast cancer, early (adjuvant treatment): Oral: 2.5 mg once daily; optimal duration unknown, duration in clinical trial is 5 years; discontinue at relapse
Breast cancer, early (extended adjuvant treatment): Oral: 2.5 mg once daily; optimal duration unknown, duration in clinical trials is 5 years (after 5 years of tamoxifen); discontinue at relapse
Ovarian (epithelial) cancer (unlabeled use): Oral: 2.5 mg once daily; continue until disease progression (Ramirez, 2008)
Renal Impairment No dosage adjustment is required in patients with renal impairment if Cl_{cr} is ≥10 mL/minute.
Hepatic Impairment
Mild-to-moderate impairment (Child-Pugh class A or B): No adjustment recommended.
Severe impairment (Child-Pugh class C) and cirrhosis: 2.5 mg every other day.
Administration Administer with or without food.
Monitoring Parameters Monitor periodically during therapy: Complete blood counts, thyroid function tests; serum electrolytes, cholesterol, transaminases, and creatinine; blood pressure; bone density

Pharmacotherapy Pearls Oncology Comment: The American Society of Clinical Oncology (ASCO) guidelines for adjuvant endocrine therapy in postmenopausal women with HR-positive breast cancer (Burstein, 2010) recommend considering aromatase inhibitor (AI) therapy at some point in the treatment course (primary, sequentially, or extended). Optimal duration at this time is not known; however, treatment with an AI should not exceed 5 years in primary and extended therapies, and 2-3 years if followed by tamoxifen in sequential therapy (total of 5 years). If initial therapy with AI has been discontinued before the 5 years, consideration should be taken to receive tamoxifen for a total of 5 years. The optimal time to switch to an AI is also not known, but data supports switching after 2-3 years of tamoxifen (sequential) or after 5 years of tamoxifen (extended). If patient becomes intolerant or has poor adherence, consideration should be made to switch to another AI or initiate tamoxifen.

Special Geriatric Considerations No dosage adjustment recommended.

Dosage Forms Excipient information presented when available (limited, particularly for generics); consult specific product labeling.

Tablet, oral: 2.5 mg

Femara®: 2.5 mg

◆ **Leukeran®** *see Chlorambucil on page 350*

Leuprolide (loo PROE lide)

Medication Safety Issues

Sound-alike/look-alike issues:

Lupron Depot® (1-month or 3-month formulation) may be confused with Lupron Depot-Ped® (1-month or 3-month formulation)

Lupron Depot-Ped® is available in two formulations, a 1-month formulation and a 3-month formulation. Both formulations offer an 11.25 mg strength which may further add confusion.

Brand Names: U.S. Eligard®; Lupron Depot-Ped®; Lupron Depot®

Brand Names: Canada Eligard®; Lupron®; Lupron® Depot®

Index Terms Abbott-43818; Leuprolide Acetate; Leuprorelin Acetate; TAP-144

Generic Availability (U.S.) Yes: Injection (solution)

Pharmacologic Category Antineoplastic Agent, Gonadotropin-Releasing Hormone Agonist; Gonadotropin Releasing Hormone Agonist

Use Palliative treatment of advanced prostate cancer; management of endometriosis; treatment of anemia caused by uterine leiomyomata (fibroids)

Unlabeled Use Treatment of breast cancer

Contraindications Hypersensitivity to leuprolide, GnRH, GnRH-agonist analogs, or any component of the formulation; undiagnosed abnormal vaginal bleeding

Lupron Depot® 22.5 mg, 30 mg, and 45 mg are also not indicated for use in women

Warnings/Precautions Hazardous agent - use appropriate precautions for handling and disposal. Transient increases in testosterone serum levels (~50% above baseline) occur at the start of treatment. Androgen-deprivation therapy (ADT) may increase the risk for cardiovascular disease (Levine, 2010); sudden cardiac death and stroke have been reported in men receiving GnRH agonists; long-term ADT may prolong the QT interval; consider the benefits of ADT versus the risk for QT prolongation in patients with a history of QT_c prolongation, with medications known to prolong the QT interval, or with pre-existing cardiac disease. Tumor flare, bone pain, neuropathy, urinary tract obstruction, and spinal cord compression have been reported when used for prostate cancer; closely observe patients for weakness, paresthesias, hematuria, and urinary tract obstruction in first few weeks of therapy. Observe patients with metastatic vertebral lesions or urinary obstruction closely. Exacerbation of endometriosis or uterine leiomyomata may occur initially. Decreased bone density has been reported when used for ≥6 months; use caution in patients with additional risk factors for bone loss (eg, chronic alcohol use, corticosteroid therapy). In patients with prostate cancer, androgen deprivation therapy may increase the risk for cardiovascular disease, diabetes, insulin resistance, obesity, alterations in lipids, and fractures. Use caution in patients with a history of psychiatric illness; alteration in mood, memory impairment, and depression have been associated with use. Rare cases of pituitary apoplexy (frequently secondary to pituitary adenoma) have been observed with leuprolide administration (onset from 1 hour to usually <2 weeks); may present as sudden headache, vomiting, visual or mental status changes, and infrequently cardiovascular collapse; immediate medical attention required.

Some dosage forms may contain benzyl alcohol; patients with benzyl alcohol allergy may demonstrate a hypersensitivity reaction (usually local) in the form of erythema and induration at the injection site. Vehicle used in depot injectable formulations (polylactide-co-glycolide microspheres) has rarely been associated with retinal artery occlusion in patients with abnormal arteriovenous anastomosis. Due to different release properties, combinations of dosage forms or fractions of dosage forms should not be interchanged.

Adverse Reactions (Reflective of adult population; not specific for elderly)

Adults: Note: For prostate cancer treatment, an initial rise in serum testosterone concentrations may cause "tumor flare" or worsening of symptoms, including bone pain, neuropathy, hematuria, or ureteral or bladder outlet obstruction during the first 2 weeks. Similarly, an initial increase in estradiol levels, with a temporary worsening of symptoms, may occur in women treated with leuprolide.

Delayed release formulations:

>10%:

Cardiovascular: Edema (≤14%)

Central nervous system: Headache (≤65%), pain (<2% to 33%), depression (≤31%), insomnia (≤31%), fatigue (≤17%), dizziness/vertigo (≤16%)

Dermatologic: Skin reaction (≤12%)

Endocrine & metabolic: Hot flashes (25% to 98%), testicular atrophy (≤20%), hyperlipidemia (≤12%), libido decreased (≤11%)

Gastrointestinal: Nausea/vomiting (≤25%), bowel function altered (≤14%), weight gain/loss (≤13%)

Genitourinary: Vaginitis (11% to 28%), urinary disorder (13% to 15%)

Local: Injection site burning/stinging (transient: ≤35%)

Neuromuscular & skeletal: Weakness (≤18%), joint disorder (≤12%)

Miscellaneous: Flu-like syndrome (≤12%)

1% to 10% (limited to important or life-threatening):

Cardiovascular: Angina (<5%), arrhythmia (<5%), atrial fibrillation (<5%), bradycardia (<5%), CHF (<5%), deep thrombophlebitis (<5%), hyper-/hypotension (<5%), palpitation (<5%), syncope (<5%), tachycardia (<5%)

Central nervous system: Nervousness (≤8%), anxiety (≤6%), confusion (<5%), delusions (<5%), dementia (<5%), fever (<5%), seizure (<5%)

Dermatologic: Acne (≤10%), alopecia (≤5%), bruising (≤5%), cellulitis (≤5%), pruritus (≤3%), rash (≤2%), hirsutism (<2%)

Endocrine & metabolic: Dehydration (≤8%), gynecomastia (≤7%), breast tenderness/pain (≤6%), bicarbonate decreased (≥5%), hyper-/hypocholesterolemia (≥5%), hyperglycemia (≥5%), hyperphosphatemia (≥5%), hyperuricemia (≥5%), hypoalbuminemia (≥5%), hypoproteinemia (≥5%), lactation (<5%), testicular pain (≤4%), menstrual disorder (≤2%)

Gastrointestinal: Dysphagia (<5%), gastrointestinal hemorrhage (<5%), intestinal obstruction (<5%), ulcer (<5%), constipation (≤3%), gastroenteritis/colitis (≤3%), diarrhea (≤2%)

Genitourinary: Prostatic acid phosphatase increased/decreased (≥5%), urine specific gravity increased/decreased (≥5%), impotence (≤5%), balanitis (<5%), incontinence (<5%), penile/testis disorder (<5%), urinary tract infection (<5%), nocturia (≤4%), polyuria (2% to 4%), dysuria (≤2%), bladder spasm (<2%), erectile dysfunction (<2%), hematuria (<2%), urinary retention (<2%), urinary urgency (<2%)

Hematologic: Eosinophilia (≥5%), leukopenia (≥5%), platelets increased (≥5%), anemia

Hepatic: Liver function tests abnormal (≥5%), partial thromboplastin time increased (≥5%), prothrombin time increased (≥5%), hepatomegaly (<5%)

Local: Injection site pain (2% to 5%), injection site erythema (1% to 3%)

Neuromuscular & skeletal: Myalgia (≤8%), paresthesia (≤8%), neuropathy (<5%), paralysis (<5%), pathologic fracture (<5%), bone pain (<2%), arthralgia (≤1%)

Renal: BUN increased (≥5%), creatinine increased (≥5%)

Respiratory: Emphysema (<5%), epistaxis (<5%), hemoptysis (<5%), pleural effusion (<5%), pulmonary edema (<5%), dyspnea (≤2%), cough (≤1%)

Miscellaneous: Diaphoresis (≤5%), allergic reaction (<5%), infection (5%), lymphadenopathy (<5%)

Immediate release formulation:

>10%:

Cardiovascular: ECG changes/ischemia (19%), peripheral edema (12%)

Central nervous system: Pain (13%)

Endocrine & metabolic: Hot flashes (55%)

1% to 10% (limited to important or life-threatening):

Cardiovascular: Hypertension (8%), murmur (3%), thrombosis/phlebitis (2%), CHF (1%), angina, arrhythmia, MI, syncope

Central nervous system: Headache (7%), insomnia (7%), dizziness/lightheadedness (5%), anxiety, depression, fatigue, fever, nervousness

Dermatologic: Dermatitis (5%), alopecia, bruising, itching, lesions, pigmentation

Endocrine & metabolic: Gynecomastia/breast tenderness/pain (7%), testicular size decreased (7%), diabetes, hypercalcemia, hypoglycemia, libido decreased, thyroid enlarged

Gastrointestinal: Constipation (7%), anorexia (6%), nausea/vomiting (5%), diarrhea, dysphagia, gastrointestinal bleeding, peptic ulcer, rectal polyps

Genitourinary: Urinary frequency/urgency (6%), impotence (4%), urinary tract infection (3%), bladder spasm, dysuria, incontinence, testicular pain, urinary obstruction

Hematologic: Anemia (5%)

Local: Injection site reaction

Neuromuscular & skeletal: Weakness (10%), bone pain (5%), peripheral neuropathy

Ocular: Blurred vision

Renal: Hematuria (6%), BUN increased, creatinine increased

Respiratory: Dyspnea (2%), cough, pneumonia, pulmonary embolus, pulmonary fibrosis

Miscellaneous: Infection, inflammation

Drug Interactions

Metabolism/Transport Effects None known.

Avoid Concomitant Use There are no known interactions where it is recommended to avoid concomitant use.

Increased Effect/Toxicity There are no known significant interactions involving an increase in effect.

Decreased Effect

Leuprolide may decrease the levels/effects of: Antidiabetic Agents

Stability

Eligard®: Store at 2°C to 8°C (36°F to 46°C). Allow to reach room temperature prior to using. Once mixed, must be administered within 30 minutes. Eligard® is packaged in two syringes; one contains the Atrigel® polymer system and the second contains leuprolide acetate powder. Follow package instructions for mixing.

Lupron Depot®, Lupron Depot-Ped®: Store at room temperature of 25°C (77°F); excursions permitted to 15°C to 30°C (59°F to 86°F). Upon reconstitution, the suspension does not contain a preservative and should be used immediately; discard if not used within 2 hours. Reconstitute only with diluent provided.

Leuprolide acetate 5 mg/mL solution: Store at 20°C to 25°C (68°F to 77°F); excursions permitted to 15°C to 30°C (59°F to 86°F). Protect from light and store vial in carton until use. Do not freeze.

Mechanism of Action Leuprolide, is an agonist of luteinizing hormone-releasing hormone (LHRH). Acting as a potent inhibitor of gonadotropin secretion; continuous administration results in suppression of ovarian and testicular steroidogenesis due to decreased levels of LH and FSH with subsequent decrease in testosterone (male) and estrogen (female) levels. In males, testosterone levels are reduced to below castrate levels. Leuprolide may also have a direct inhibitory effect on the testes, and act by a different mechanism not directly related to reduction in serum testosterone.

Pharmacodynamics/Kinetics

Onset of action: Following transient increase, testosterone suppression occurs in ~2-4 weeks of continued therapy

Distribution: Males: V_d: 27 L

Protein binding: 43% to 49%

Metabolism: Major metabolite, pentapeptide (M-1)

Bioavailability: SubQ: 94%

Excretion: Urine (<5% as parent and major metabolite)

Dosage

Geriatric & Adult

Advanced prostate cancer:

I.M.:

Lupron Depot® 7.5 mg (monthly): 7.5 mg every month **or**

Lupron Depot® 22.5 mg (3 month): 22.5 mg every 12 weeks **or**

Lupron Depot® 30 mg (4 month): 30 mg every 16 weeks **or**

Lupron Depot® 45 mg (6 month): 45 mg every 24 weeks

SubQ:

Eligard®: 7.5 mg monthly **or** 22.5 mg every 3 months **or** 30 mg every 4 months **or** 45 mg every 6 months

Leuprolide acetate 5 mg/mL solution: 1 mg/day

Endometriosis: I.M.: Initial therapy may be with leuprolide alone or in combination with norethindrone; if retreatment for an additional 6 months is necessary, concomitant norethindrone should be used. Retreatment is not recommended for longer than one additional 6-month course.

Lupron Depot®: 3.75 mg every month for up to 6 months **or**

Lupron Depot®-3 month: 11.25 mg every 3 months for up to 2 doses (6 months total duration of treatment)

Uterine leiomyomata (fibroids): I.M. (in combination with iron):

Lupron Depot®: 3.75 mg every month for up to 3 months **or**

Lupron Depot®-3 month: 11.25 mg as a single injection

Breast cancer, premenopausal ovarian ablation (unlabeled use): I.M.:
Lupron Depot®: 3.75 mg every 28 days for up to 24 months (Boccardo, 1999) **or**
Lupron Depot®-3 month: 11.25 mg every 3 months for up to 24 months (Boccardo, 1999; Schmid, 2007)

Administration
I.M.: Lupron Depot®, Lupron Depot-Ped®: Administer as a single injection. Vary injection site periodically

SubQ:
Eligard®: Vary injection site; choose site with adequate subcutaneous tissue (eg, upper or mid-abdomen, upper buttocks); avoid areas that may be compressed or rubbed (eg, belt or waistband)
Leuprolide acetate 5 mg/mL solution: Vary injection site; if an alternate syringe from the syringe provided is required, insulin syringes should be used

Monitoring Parameters Bone mineral density
Prostatic cancer: LH and FSH levels, serum testosterone (~4 weeks after initiation of therapy), PSA; weakness, paresthesias, and urinary tract obstruction in first few weeks of therapy. Screen for diabetes (blood glucose and Hb A_{1c}) and cardiovascular risk prior to initiating and periodically during treatment.

Test Interactions Interferes with pituitary gonadotropic and gonadal function tests during and up to 3 months after monthly administration of leuprolide therapy.

Pharmacotherapy Pearls
Eligard® Atrigel®: A nongelatin-based, biodegradable, polymer matrix

Oncology Comment: Guidelines from the American Society of Clinical Oncology (ASCO) for hormonal management of advanced prostate cancer which is androgen-sensitive (Loblaw, 2007) recommend either orchiectomy or luteinizing hormone-releasing hormone (LHRH) agonists as initial treatment for androgen deprivation.

Special Geriatric Considerations No dosage adjustments are needed in the elderly. Monitoring for bone density changes, serum lipid, hemoglobin A_{1c}, blood pressure, and serum calcium changes is recommended.

Product Availability
Lupron Depot-Ped® 3-month formulation: FDA approved August 2011; availability expected August 2011
Lupron Depot-Ped® 3-month formulation will be available in two strengths, 11.25 mg and 30 mg.

Dosage Forms Excipient information presented when available (limited, particularly for generics); consult specific product labeling.
Injection, powder for reconstitution, as acetate [depot formulation, preservative free]:
Eligard®: 7.5 mg (monthly), 22.5 mg (3 month), 30 mg (4 month), 45 mg (6 month) [contains polylactide-co-glycolide; supplied with diluent]
Lupron Depot-Ped®: 7.5 mg (monthly), 11.25 mg (3 month), 11.25 mg (monthly), 15 mg (monthly), 30 mg (3 month) [contains polylactide-co-glycolide, polysorbate 80]
Lupron Depot®: 3.75 mg (monthly), 7.5 mg (monthly), 11.25 mg (3 month), 22.5 mg (3 month), 30 mg (4 month), 45 mg (6 month) [contains polylactide-co-glycolide, polysorbate 80]
Injection, solution, as acetate: 5 mg/mL (2.8 mL)

◆ **Leuprolide Acetate** see Leuprolide on page 1103
◆ **Leuprorelin Acetate** see Leuprolide on page 1103

Levalbuterol (leve al BYOO ter ole)

Related Information
Inhalant Agents on page 2117
Medication Safety Issues
Sound-alike/look-alike issues:
Xopenex® may be confused with Xanax®
Brand Names: U.S. Xopenex HFA™; Xopenex®
Brand Names: Canada Xopenex®
Index Terms Levalbuterol Hydrochloride; Levalbuterol Tartrate; R-albuterol
Generic Availability (U.S.) Yes: Excludes aerosol
Pharmacologic Category Beta$_2$ Agonist
Use Treatment or prevention of bronchospasm in adults with reversible obstructive airway disease
Contraindications Hypersensitivity to levalbuterol, albuterol, or any component of the formulation

Warnings/Precautions Optimize anti-inflammatory treatment before initiating maintenance treatment with levalbuterol. Do not use as a component of chronic therapy without an anti-inflammatory agent. Only the mildest form of asthma (Step 1 and/or exercise-induced) would not require concurrent use based upon asthma guidelines. Patient must be instructed to seek medical attention in cases where acute symptoms are not relieved or a previous level of response is diminished. The need to increase frequency of use may indicate deterioration of asthma, and treatment must not be delayed. A spacer device or valved holding chamber is recommended when using a metered-dose inhaler.

Use caution in patients with cardiovascular disease (arrhythmia or hypertension or HF), convulsive disorders, diabetes, glaucoma, hyperthyroidism, or hypokalemia. Beta-agonists may cause elevation in blood pressure, heart rate, and result in CNS stimulation/excitation. $Beta_2$-agonists may increase risk of arrhythmia, increase serum glucose, or decrease serum potassium.

Immediate hypersensitivity reactions (urticaria, angioedema, rash, bronchospasm) have been reported. Do not exceed recommended dose; serious adverse events including fatalities, have been associated with excessive use of inhaled sympathomimetics. Rarely, paradoxical bronchospasm may occur with use of inhaled bronchodilating agents; this should be distinguished from inadequate response.

Adverse Reactions (Reflective of adult population; not specific for elderly)
>10%:
  Endocrine & metabolic: Serum glucose increased, serum potassium decreased
  Neuromuscular & skeletal: Tremor (≤7%)
  Respiratory: Rhinitis (3% to 11%)
  Miscellaneous: Viral infection (7% to 12%)
>2% to 10%:
  Central nervous system: Headache (8% to 12%), nervousness (3% to 10%), dizziness (1% to 3%), anxiety (≤3%), migraine (≤3%), weakness (3%)
  Cardiovascular: Tachycardia (~3%)
  Dermatologic: Rash (≤8%)
  Gastrointestinal: Diarrhea (2% to 6%), dyspepsia (1% to 3%)
  Neuromuscular & skeletal: Leg cramps (≤3%)
  Respiratory: Asthma (9%), pharyngitis (3% to 10%), cough (1% to 4%), sinusitis (1% to 4%), nasal edema (1% to 3%)
  Miscellaneous: Flu-like syndrome (1% to 4%), accidental injury (≤3%)
Note: Immediate hypersensitivity reactions have occurred (including angioedema, oropharyngeal edema, urticaria, and anaphylaxis).

Drug Interactions
  Metabolism/Transport Effects None known.
  Avoid Concomitant Use
    Avoid concomitant use of Levalbuterol with any of the following: Beta-Blockers (Non-selective); Iobenguane I 123
  Increased Effect/Toxicity
    Levalbuterol may increase the levels/effects of: Loop Diuretics; Sympathomimetics; Thiazide Diuretics

    The levels/effects of Levalbuterol may be increased by: AtoMOXetine; Cannabinoids; MAO Inhibitors; Tricyclic Antidepressants
  Decreased Effect
    Levalbuterol may decrease the levels/effects of: Iobenguane I 123

    The levels/effects of Levalbuterol may be decreased by: Alpha-/Beta-Blockers; Beta-Blockers (Beta1 Selective); Beta-Blockers (Nonselective); Betahistine

Stability
  Aerosol: Store at room temperature of 20°C to 25°C (68°F to 77°F); protect from freezing and direct sunlight. Store with mouthpiece down. Discard after 200 actuations.
  Solution for nebulization: Store in protective foil pouch at room temperature of 20°C to 25°C (68°F to 77°F). Protect from light and excessive heat. Vials should be used within 2 weeks after opening protective pouch. Use within 1 week and protect from light if removed from pouch. Vials of concentrated solution should be used immediately after removing from protective pouch. Concentrated solution should be diluted with 2.5 mL NS prior to use.

Mechanism of Action Relaxes bronchial smooth muscle by action on $beta_2$-receptors with little effect on heart rate

Pharmacodynamics/Kinetics

Onset of action (as measured by a 15% increase in FEV$_1$):
Aerosol: 5.5-10.2 minutes
Peak effect: ~77 minutes
Nebulization: 10-17 minutes
Peak effect: 1.5 hours
Duration (as measured by a 15% increase in FEV$_1$):
Aerosol: 3-4 hours (up to 6 hours in some patients)
Nebulization: 5-6 hours (up to 8 hours in some patients)
Absorption: A portion of inhaled dose is absorbed to systemic circulation
Half-life elimination: 3.3-4 hours
Time to peak, serum:
Aerosol: 0.5 hours
Nebulization: 0.2 hours

Dosage

Geriatric Only a small number of patients have been studied. Although greater sensitivity of some elderly patients cannot be ruled out, no overall differences in safety or effectiveness were observed. An initial dose of 0.63 mg should be used in all patients >65 years of age.

Adult

Bronchospasm:
Metered-dose inhaler: 2 puffs every 4-6 hours
Solution for nebulization: 0.63 mg 3 times/day at intervals of 6-8 hours; dosage may be increased to 1.25 mg 3 times/day with close monitoring for adverse effects

Exacerbation of asthma (acute, severe) *(NIH Guidelines, 2007):*
Metered-dose inhaler: 4-8 puffs every 20 minutes for up to 4 hours, then every 1-4 hours as needed
Solution for nebulization: 1.25-2.5 mg every 20 minutes for 3 doses, then 1.25-5 mg every 1-4 hours as needed

Administration Inhalation:

Metered-dose inhaler: Shake well before use; prime with 4 test sprays prior to first use or if inhaler has not been use of more than 3 days. Clean actuator (mouthpiece) weekly. A spacer device or valved holding chamber is recommended when using a metered-dose inhaler.

Solution for nebulization: Safety and efficacy were established when administered with the following nebulizers: PARI LC Jet™, PARI LC Plus™, as well as the following compressors: PARI Master®, Dura-Neb® 2000, and Dura-Neb® 3000. Concentrated solution should be diluted prior to use. Blow-by administration is not recommended, use a mask device if patient unable to hold mouthpiece in mouth for administration.

Monitoring Parameters Asthma symptoms; FEV$_1$, peak flow, and/or other pulmonary function tests; heart rate, blood pressure, CNS stimulation; arterial blood gases (if condition warrants); serum potassium, serum glucose (in selected patients)

Pharmacotherapy Pearls Slightly smaller increase in heart rate and slightly lower incidence of nervousness were seen with levalbuterol compared to albuterol.

Special Geriatric Considerations For aerosol formulation, start with low end of dosage range. Refer to dosing information for nebulization dosing specifics. Instruct patient on proper use of metered-dose inhaler.

Dosage Forms Excipient information presented when available (limited, particularly for generics); consult specific product labeling.

Aerosol, for oral inhalation, as tartrate [strength expressed as base]:
Xopenex HFA™: 45 mcg/actuation (15 g) [chlorofluorocarbon free; 200 actuations]
Solution, for nebulization, as hydrochloride [strength expressed as base, preservative free]:
0.31 mg/3 mL (3 mL); 0.63 mg/3 mL (3 mL); 1.25 mg/3 mL (3 mL)
Xopenex®: 0.31 mg/3 mL (24s); 0.63 mg/3 mL (24s); 1.25 mg/3 mL (24s)
Solution, for nebulization, as hydrochloride [strength expressed as base, concentrate, preservative free]: 1.25 mg/0.5 mL (30s)

LevETIRAcetam (lee va tye RA se tam)

Medication Safety Issues

Sound-alike/look-alike issues:

Keppra® may be confused with Keflex®, Keppra XR®

LevETIRAcetam may be confused with levOCARNitine, levofloxacin

Potential for dispensing errors between Keppra® and Kaletra® (lopinavir/ritonavir)

Brand Names: U.S. Keppra XR®; Keppra®

Brand Names: Canada Apo-Levetiracetam®; Ava-Levetiracetam; CO Levetiracetam; Dom-Levetiracetam; Keppra®; PHL-Levetiracetam; PMS-Levetiracetam; PRO-Levetiracetam

Generic Availability (U.S.) Yes

Pharmacologic Category Anticonvulsant, Miscellaneous

Use Adjunctive therapy in the treatment of partial onset, myoclonic, and/or primary generalized tonic-clonic seizures

Medication Guide Available Yes

Contraindications There are no contraindications listed in the U.S. manufacturer's labeling.

Canadian labeling: Hypersensitivity to levetiracetam or any component of the formulation

Warnings/Precautions Antiepileptics are associated with an increased risk of suicidal behavior/thoughts with use (regardless of indication); patients should be monitored for signs/symptoms of depression, suicidal tendencies, and other unusual behavior changes during therapy and instructed to inform their healthcare provider immediately if symptoms occur.

Severe dermatologic reactions (toxic epidermal necrolysis and Stevens-Johnson syndrome) have been reported; onset usually within ~2 weeks of treatment initiation but may be delayed (>4 months); discontinue for any signs of a hypersensitivity reaction or unspecified rash.

Psychotic symptoms (psychosis, hallucinations) and behavioral symptoms (including aggression, anger, anxiety, depersonalization, depression, personality disorder) may occur. Dose reduction or discontinuation may be required. Levetiracetam should be withdrawn gradually, when possible, to minimize the potential of increased seizure frequency. Use caution with renal impairment; dosage adjustment may be necessary. Impaired coordination, weakness, dizziness, and somnolence may occur, most commonly during the first month of therapy; use caution when driving or operating heavy machinery. Although rare, decreases in red blood cell counts, hemoglobin, hematocrit, white blood cell counts and neutrophils have been observed.

Adverse Reactions (Reflective of adult population; not specific for elderly)

>10%:

Central nervous system: Behavioral symptoms (agitation, aggression, anger, anxiety, apathy, depersonalization, depression, emotional lability, hostility, hyperkinesias, irritability, nervousness, neurosis and personality disorder: adults 5% to 13%; children 5% to 38%), somnolence (8% to 23%), headache (14%), hostility (2% to 12%)

Gastrointestinal: Vomiting (15%), anorexia (3% to 13%)

Neuromuscular & skeletal: Weakness (9% to 15%)

Respiratory: Pharyngitis (6% to 14%), rhinitis (4% to 13%), cough (2% to 11%)

Miscellaneous: Accidental injury (17%), infection (2% to 13%)

1% to 10%:

Cardiovascular: Facial edema (2%)

Central nervous system: Fatigue (10%), nervousness (4% to 10%), dizziness (5% to 9%), personality disorder (8%), pain (6% to 7%), agitation (6%), irritability (6% to 7%), emotional lability (2% to 6%), mood swings (5%), depression (3% to 5%), vertigo (3% to 5%), ataxia (3%), amnesia (2%), anxiety (2%), confusion (2%)

Dermatologic: Bruising (4%), pruritus (2%), rash (2%), skin discoloration (2%)

Endocrine & metabolic: Dehydration (2%)

Gastrointestinal: Diarrhea (8%), nausea (5%), gastroenteritis (4%), constipation (3%)

Genitourinary: Urine abnormality (2%)

Hematologic: Leukocytes decreased (2% to 3%)

Neuromuscular & skeletal: Neck pain (2% to 8%), paresthesia (2%), reflexes increased (2%)

Ocular: Conjunctivitis (3%), diplopia (2%), amblyopia (2%)

Otic: Ear pain (2%)

Renal: Albuminuria (4%)

Respiratory: Influenza (5%), asthma (2%), sinusitis (2%)

Miscellaneous: Flu-like syndrome (3% to 8%), viral infection (2%)

Drug Interactions
  Metabolism/Transport Effects None known.
  Avoid Concomitant Use
    Avoid concomitant use of LevETIRAcetam with any of the following: Azelastine; Azelastine (Nasal); Methadone; Mirtazapine; Paraldehyde
  Increased Effect/Toxicity
    LevETIRAcetam may increase the levels/effects of: Alcohol (Ethyl); Azelastine; Azelastine (Nasal); Buprenorphine; CNS Depressants; Methadone; Methotrimeprazine; Metyrosine; Mirtazapine; Paraldehyde; Selective Serotonin Reuptake Inhibitors; Zolpidem

    The levels/effects of LevETIRAcetam may be increased by: Droperidol; HydrOXYzine; Methotrimeprazine
  Decreased Effect
    The levels/effects of LevETIRAcetam may be decreased by: Ketorolac; Ketorolac (Nasal); Ketorolac (Systemic); Mefloquine
Ethanol/Nutrition/Herb Interactions
  Ethanol: May increase CNS depression; monitor for increased effects with coadministration. Caution patients about effects.
  Food: Food may delay, but does not affect the extent of absorption.
Stability
  Oral solution, tablets: Store at 25°C (77°F); excursions permitted to 15°C to 30°C (59°F to 86°F).
  Premixed solution for infusion: Store at 20°C to 25°C (68°F to 77°F).
  Vials for injection: Store at 25°C (77°F); excursions permitted to 15°C to 30°C (59°F to 86°F). Must dilute dose in 100 mL of NS, LR, or D_5W. Admixed solution is stable for 24 hours in PVC bags kept at room temperature.
Mechanism of Action The precise mechanism by which levetiracetam exerts its antiepileptic effect is unknown. However, several studies have suggested the mechanism may involve one or more of the following central pharmacologic effects: inhibition of voltage-dependent N-type calcium channels; facilitation of GABA-ergic inhibitory transmission through displacement of negative modulators; reduction of delayed rectifier potassium current; and/or binding to synaptic proteins which modulate neurotransmitter release.
Pharmacodynamics/Kinetics
  Absorption: Oral: Rapid and almost complete
  Distribution: V_d: Similar to total body water
  Protein binding: <10%
  Metabolism: Not extensive; primarily by enzymatic hydrolysis; forms metabolites (inactive)
  Bioavailability: 100%
  Half-life elimination: ~6-8 hours; extended release tablet: ~7 hours; half-life increased in renal dysfunction
  Time to peak, plasma: Oral: Immediate release: ~1 hour; Extended release: ~4 hours
  Excretion: Urine (66% as unchanged drug)
Dosage
  Geriatric & Adult Note: When switching from oral to I.V. formulations, the total daily dose should be the same.
    Myoclonic seizures:
      Oral: Immediate release: Initial: 500 mg twice daily; may increase every 2 weeks by 500 mg/dose to the recommended dose of 1500 mg twice daily. Efficacy of doses other than 3000 mg/day has not been established.
      I.V.: Initial: 500 mg twice daily; may increase every 2 weeks by 500 mg/dose to the recommended dose of 1500 mg twice daily. Efficacy of doses other than 3000 mg /day has not been established.
    Partial onset seizures:
      Oral:
        Immediate release: Initial: 500 mg twice daily; may increase every 2 weeks by 500 mg/dose to a maximum of 1500 mg twice daily. Doses >3000 mg/day have been used in trials; however, there is no evidence of increased benefit.
        Extended release: Initial: 1000 mg once daily; may increase every 2 weeks by 1000 mg/dose to a maximum of 3000 mg once daily.
      I.V.: Initial: 500 mg twice daily; may increase every 2 weeks by 500 mg/dose to a maximum of 1500 mg twice daily. Doses >3000 mg/day have been used in trials; however, there is no evidence of increased benefit.
    Tonic-clonic seizures:
      Oral: Immediate release: Initial: 500 mg twice daily; may increase every 2 weeks by 500 mg/dose to the recommended dose of 1500 mg twice daily. Efficacy of doses other than 3000 mg/day has not been established.

I.V.: Initial: 500 mg twice daily; may increase every 2 weeks by 500 mg/dose to the recommended dose of 1500 mg twice daily. Efficacy of doses other than 3000 mg/day has not been established.

Loading dose (unlabeled): Oral: Immediate release: Initial doses of 1500-2000 mg have been well-tolerated (Betts, 2000; Koubeissi, 2008), although the necessity of a loading dose has not been established

Refractory status epilepticus (unlabeled use): I.V.: 1000-3000 mg administered over 15 minutes (Meierkord, 2010); 2500 mg has been safely administered over 5 minutes in one report (Uges, 2009). **Note:** Levetiracetam has not been well studied in comparison to other agents routinely used in this setting.

Renal Impairment Adults:

Immediate release and I.V. formulations:

Cl_{cr} >80 mL/minute/1.73 m^2: 500-1500 mg every 12 hours

Cl_{cr} 50-80 mL/minute/1.73 m^2: 500-1000 mg every 12 hours

Cl_{cr} 30-50 mL/minute/1.73 m^2: 250-750 mg every 12 hours

Cl_{cr} <30 mL/minute/1.73 m^2: 250-500 mg every 12 hours

End-stage renal disease (ESRD) requiring hemodialysis: 500-1000 mg every 24 hours; supplemental dose of 250-500 mg is recommended posthemodialysis

Peritoneal dialysis (PD): 500-1000 mg every 24 hours (Aronoff, 2007)

Continuous renal replacement therapy (CRRT): 250-750 mg every 12 hours (Arnoff, 2007)

Extended release tablets:

Cl_{cr} >80 mL/minute/1.73 m^2: 1000-3000 mg every 24 hours

Cl_{cr} 50-80 mL/minute/1.73 m^2: 1000-2000 mg every 24 hours

Cl_{cr} 30-50 mL/minute/1.73 m^2: 500-1500 mg every 24 hours

Cl_{cr} <30 mL/minute/1.73 m^2: 500-1000 mg every 24 hours

End-stage renal disease (ESRD) requiring hemodialysis: Use of immediate release formulation is recommended

Hepatic Impairment

U.S. labeling: No dosage adjustment necessary

Canadian labeling:

Mild-to-moderate impairment: No dosage adjustment necessary

Severe impairment: Reduce maintenance dose by 50% in patients who **also** have Cl_{cr} <60 mL/minute/1.73 m^2

Administration

I.V.: Infuse over 15 minutes

Oral: May be administered without regard to meals.

Oral solution: Should be administered with a calibrated measuring device (not a household teaspoon or tablespoon)

Tablet (immediate release and extended release): Only administer as whole tablet; do not crush, break or chew.

Monitoring Parameters Suicidality (eg, suicidal thoughts, depression, behavioral changes)

Special Geriatric Considerations In a study of 16 older adults (61-88 years of age) receiving levetiracetam daily and with creatinine clearances ranging from 30-74 mL/minute, a decrease in creatinine clearance (38%) and a 2.5 hour longer half-life were recorded in the elderly compared to younger adults. The authors concluded that the difference was due to renal function. Other studies show no overall difference in safety and efficacy, although larger numbers in studies are needed to verify efficacy. Levetiracetam has demonstrated a low incidence of cognitive effects. When using the drug in elderly, it is essential to base the dose on estimated creatinine clearance and adjust appropriately.

Dosage Forms Excipient information presented when available (limited, particularly for generics); consult specific product labeling. [DSC] = Discontinued product

Infusion, premixed in sodium chloride 0.54%: 1500 mg (100 mL)

Infusion, premixed in sodium chloride 0.75%: 1000 mg (100 mL)

Infusion, premixed in sodium chloride 0.82%: 500 mg (100 mL)

Injection, solution: 100 mg/mL (5 mL)

Keppra®: 100 mg/mL (5 mL)

Solution, oral: 100 mg/mL (5 mL, 118 mL [DSC], 472 mL, 473 mL, 480 mL, 500 mL)

Keppra®: 100 mg/mL (480 mL) [dye free; grape flavor]

Tablet, oral: 250 mg, 500 mg, 750 mg, 1000 mg

Keppra®: 250 mg, 500 mg, 750 mg, 1000 mg [scored; gluten free]

Tablet, extended release, oral: 500 mg, 750 mg

Keppra XR®: 500 mg, 750 mg

◆ **Levitra®** *see* Vardenafil *on page 2004*

Levobunolol (lee voe BYOO noe lole)

Related Information
Glaucoma Drug Therapy *on page 2115*

Medication Safety Issues
Sound-alike/look-alike issues:
Levobunolol may be confused with levocabastine
Betagan® may be confused with Betadine®, Betoptic® S

Brand Names: U.S. Betagan®

Brand Names: Canada Apo-Levobunolol®; Betagan®; Novo-Levobunolol; Optho-Bunolol®; PMS-Levobunolol; Sandoz-Levobunolol

Index Terms *l*-Bunolol Hydrochloride; Levobunolol Hydrochloride

Generic Availability (U.S.) Yes

Pharmacologic Category Beta-Adrenergic Blocker, Nonselective; Ophthalmic Agent, Anti-glaucoma

Use To lower intraocular pressure in chronic open-angle glaucoma or ocular hypertension

Contraindications Hypersensitivity to levobunolol or any component of the formulation; bronchial asthma, severe COPD, sinus bradycardia, second- or third-degree AV block, cardiac failure, cardiogenic shock

Warnings/Precautions Consider pre-existing conditions such as sick sinus syndrome before initiating. Use with caution in patients with HF, diabetes mellitus, bronchospastic disease, myasthenia gravis, peripheral vascular disease, psychiatric disease, hyperthyroidism; contains metabisulfite. Because systemic absorption does occur with ophthalmic administration, the elderly with other disease states or syndromes that may be affected by a beta-blocker (HF, COPD, etc) should be monitored closely. Use caution with history of severe anaphylaxis to allergens; patients taking beta-blockers may become more sensitive to repeated challenges. Treatment of anaphylaxis (eg, epinephrine) in patients taking beta-blockers may be ineffective or promote undesirable effects. Product contains benzalkonium chloride which may be absorbed by soft contact lenses; do not administer while wearing soft contact lenses. Ophthalmic solutions contain metabisulfite.

Adverse Reactions (Reflective of adult population; not specific for elderly)
>10%: Ocular: Stinging/burning eyes
1% to 10%:
Cardiovascular: Bradycardia, arrhythmia, hypotension
Central nervous system: Dizziness, headache
Dermatologic: Alopecia, erythema
Local: Stinging, burning
Ocular: Blepharoconjunctivitis, conjunctivitis
Respiratory: Bronchospasm

Drug Interactions
Metabolism/Transport Effects None known.

Avoid Concomitant Use
Avoid concomitant use of Levobunolol with any of the following: Beta2-Agonists; Floctafenine; Methacholine

Increased Effect/Toxicity
Levobunolol may increase the levels/effects of: Alpha-/Beta-Agonists (Direct-Acting); Bupivacaine; Cholinergic Agonists; Fingolimod; Hypotensive Agents; Lidocaine (Systemic); Lidocaine (Topical); Mepivacaine; Methacholine; Midodrine

The levels/effects of Levobunolol may be increased by: Anilidopiperidine Opioids; Dronedarone; Floctafenine; MAO Inhibitors; QuiNIDine; Reserpine

Decreased Effect
Levobunolol may decrease the levels/effects of: Beta2-Agonists; Theophylline Derivatives

Mechanism of Action A nonselective beta-adrenergic blocking agent that lowers intraocular pressure by reducing aqueous humor production and possibly increases the outflow of aqueous humor

Pharmacodynamics/Kinetics
Onset of action: ~1 hour
Peak effect: 2-6 hours
Duration: 1 day
Excretion: Not well defined

Dosage
Geriatric & Adult Glaucoma: Ophthalmic: Instill 1 drop in the affected eye(s) 1-2 times/day

Administration Apply finger pressure over nasolacrimal duct to decrease systemic absorption.

Monitoring Parameters Intraocular pressure, heart rate, funduscopic exam, visual field testing

Special Geriatric Considerations Because systemic absorption does occur with ophthalmic administration, the elderly with other disease states or syndromes that may be affected by a beta-blocker (CHF, COPD, etc) should be monitored closely. Evaluate the patient's or caregiver's ability to safely administer the correct dose of ophthalmic medication.

Dosage Forms Excipient information presented when available (limited, particularly for generics); consult specific product labeling. [DSC] = Discontinued product

Solution, ophthalmic, as hydrochloride [drops]: 0.25% (5 mL, 10 mL); 0.5% (5 mL, 10 mL, 15 mL)

  Betagan®: 0.25% (5 mL [DSC], 10 mL [DSC]); 0.5% (2 mL [DSC], 5 mL, 10 mL, 15 mL) [contains benzalkonium chloride, sodium metabisulfite]

♦ **Levobunolol Hydrochloride** see Levobunolol on page 1112
♦ **Levocabastine Hydrochloride** see Levocabastine (Nasal) on page 1113
♦ **Levocabastine Hydrochloride** see Levocabastine (Ophthalmic) on page 1113

Levocabastine (Nasal) (LEE voe kab as teen)

Medication Safety Issues
Sound-alike/look-alike issues:
Levocabastine may be confused with levobunolol, levOCARNitine
Livostin® may be confused with lovastatin
International issues:
Livostin [Canada and multiple international markets] may be confused with Limoxin brand name for ambroxol [Indonesia] and amoxicillin [Mexico]; Lovastin brand name for lovastatin [Malaysia, Poland, Singapore]

Brand Names: Canada Livostin®
Index Terms Levocabastine Hydrochloride
Pharmacologic Category Histamine H_1 Antagonist; Histamine H_1 Antagonist, Second Generation; Piperidine Derivative
Use Symptomatic treatment of allergic rhinitis
Dosage
Adult Allergic rhinitis: Intranasal: Adults ≤65 years: Two sprays in each nostril twice daily; if necessary, may increase dose to 2 sprays 3-4 times daily; consider therapy discontinuation if no response within 3 days. Continuous treatment >10 weeks has not been evaluated.
Renal Impairment Use caution; manufacturer's labeling provides no specific dosing recommendations.
Special Geriatric Considerations Evaluate the patient's or caregiver's ability to safely administer the correct dose of nasal medication.
Product Availability Not available in U.S.
Dosage Forms: Canada Excipient information presented when available (limited, particularly for generics); consult specific product labeling.
Microsuspension, intranasal, as hydrochloride [spray]:
  Livostin®: 0.05% [50 mcg/spray] (15 mL) [contains benzalkonium chloride]

Levocabastine (Ophthalmic) (LEE voe kab as teen)

Medication Safety Issues
Sound-alike/look-alike issues:
Levocabastine may be confused with levobunolol, levOCARNitine
Livostin® may be confused with lovastatin
International issues:
Livostin [Canada and multiple international markets] may be confused with Limoxin brand name for ambroxol [Indonesia] and amoxicillin [Mexico]; Lovastin brand name for lovastatin [Malaysia, Poland, Singapore]

Brand Names: Canada Livostin® Eye Drops
Index Terms Levocabastine Hydrochloride
Pharmacologic Category Histamine H_1 Antagonist; Histamine H_1 Antagonist, Second Generation; Piperidine Derivative
Use Treatment of seasonal allergic conjunctivitis
Dosage
Adult Allergic conjunctivitis: Adults ≤65 years: Ophthalmic: Usual dose: Instill 1 drop in affected eye(s) 2 times/day; may increase to 1 drop 3-4 times/day. If no improvement within 3 days, consider discontinuation of therapy. Continuous therapy >16 weeks has not been studied.

◀ **Special Geriatric Considerations** Evaluate the patient's or caregiver's ability to safely administer the correct dose of ophthalmic medication.
Product Availability Not available in U.S.
Dosage Forms: Canada Excipient information presented when available (limited, particularly for generics); consult specific product labeling.
Suspension, ophthalmic:
Livostin®: 0.05% (5 mL, 10 mL) [contains benzalkonium chloride]

Levocetirizine (LEE vo se TI ra zeen)

Medication Safety Issues
Sound-alike/look-alike issues:
Levocetirizine may be confused with cetirizine
Brand Names: U.S. Xyzal®
Index Terms Levocetirizine Dihydrochloride
Generic Availability (U.S.) Yes
Pharmacologic Category Histamine H_1 Antagonist; Histamine H_1 Antagonist, Second Generation; Piperazine Derivative
Use Relief of symptoms of perennial and seasonal allergic rhinitis; treatment of skin manifestations (uncomplicated) of chronic idiopathic urticaria
Contraindications Hypersensitivity to levocetirizine, cetirizine, or any component of the formulation; end-stage renal disease (Cl_{cr} <10 mL/minute); hemodialysis
Warnings/Precautions Use with caution in adults with mild-to-moderate renal impairment; dosage adjustments may be needed. Use is contraindicated in end-stage renal disease (Cl_{cr} <10 mL/minute), and patients undergoing hemodialysis. Use with caution in the elderly. May cause drowsiness; use caution performing tasks which require alertness (eg, operating machinery or driving). Effects may be potentiated when used with other sedative drugs or ethanol.
Adverse Reactions (Reflective of adult population; not specific for elderly)
>10%: Gastrointestinal: Diarrhea
1% to 10%:
Central nervous system: Somnolence (2% to 6%), fever, fatigue (1% to 4%)
Gastrointestinal: Constipation, vomiting, xerostomia (2% to 3%)
Neuromuscular & skeletal: Weakness (2%)
Otic: Otitis media
Respiratory: Nasopharyngitis (4% to 6%), cough, epistaxis, pharyngitis (1% to 2%)

The following potentially-severe adverse reactions have been reported with cetirizine and, therefore, may also occur with levocetirizine: Cholestasis, glomuleronephritis, hallucination, hypotension (severe), orofacial dyskinesia, suicidal ideation
Drug Interactions
Metabolism/Transport Effects None known.
Avoid Concomitant Use
Avoid concomitant use of Levocetirizine with any of the following: Azelastine; Azelastine (Nasal); Methadone; Mirtazapine; Paraldehyde
Increased Effect/Toxicity
Levocetirizine may increase the levels/effects of: Alcohol (Ethyl); Anticholinergics; Azelastine; Azelastine (Nasal); Buprenorphine; CNS Depressants; Methadone; Methotrimeprazine; Metyrosine; Mirtazapine; Paraldehyde; Selective Serotonin Reuptake Inhibitors; Zolpidem

The levels/effects of Levocetirizine may be increased by: Droperidol; HydrOXYzine; Methotrimeprazine; Pramlintide
Decreased Effect
Levocetirizine may decrease the levels/effects of: Acetylcholinesterase Inhibitors (Central); Benzylpenicilloyl Polylysine; Betahistine; Hyaluronidase

The levels/effects of Levocetirizine may be decreased by: Acetylcholinesterase Inhibitors (Central); Amphetamines
Ethanol/Nutrition/Herb Interactions Ethanol: May increase CNS depression; monitor for increased effects with coadministration. Caution patients about effects.
Stability Store at room temperature of 20°C to 25°C (68°F to 77°F); excursions permitted to 15°C to 30°C (59°F to 86°F).
Mechanism of Action Levocetirizine is an antihistamine which selectively competes with histamine for H_1-receptor sites on effector cells in the gastrointestinal tract, blood vessels, and respiratory tract. Levocetirizine, the active enantiomer of cetirizine, has twice the binding affinity at the H_1-receptor compared to cetirizine.

LEVODOPA, CARBIDOPA, AND ENTACAPONE

Pharmacodynamics/Kinetics
Absorption: Rapid and extensive
Distribution: 0.4 L/kg
Protein binding: 91% to 92%
Metabolism: Minimal (<14%); via aromatic oxidation, N and O-dealkylation (via CYPA4), and taurine conjugation
Half-life elimination: Adults: ~8 hours; Renal impairment: 11-34 hours; End-stage renal disease: 46 hours
Time to peak, plasma: Adults: 0.9 hours
Excretion: Urine (85%); feces (13%)

Dosage
Geriatric Refer to adult dosing; dosing should begin at the lower end of the dosing range.
Adult Allergic rhinitis, chronic urticaria: Oral: 5 mg once daily (in the evening); some patients may experience relief of symptoms with 2.5 mg once daily
Renal Impairment Adults:
Cl_{cr} 50-80 mL/minute: 2.5 mg once daily
Cl_{cr} 30-50 mL/minute: 2.5 mg once every other day
Cl_{cr} 10-30 mL/minute: 2.5 mg twice weekly (every 3 or 4 days)
Cl_{cr} <10 mL/minute, hemodialysis patients: Contraindicated
Hepatic Impairment No adjustment required.
Administration Administer in the evening. May be administered without regard to meals.
Monitoring Parameters Creatinine clearance (prior to treatment for dosing adjustment)
Special Geriatric Considerations Use with caution in the elderly due to potential sedative effects. Dosage should be adjusted based on renal function.
Dosage Forms Excipient information presented when available (limited, particularly for generics); consult specific product labeling.
Solution, oral, as dihydrochloride: 0.5 mg/mL (150 mL)
Xyzal®: 0.5 mg/mL (150 mL)
Tablet, oral, as dihydrochloride: 5 mg
Xyzal®: 5 mg [scored]

♦ **Levocetirizine Dihydrochloride** *see* Levocetirizine *on page 1114*
♦ **Levodopa and Carbidopa** *see* Carbidopa and Levodopa *on page 293*

Levodopa, Carbidopa, and Entacapone
(lee voe DOE pa, kar bi DOE pa, & en TA ka pone)

Related Information
Antiparkinsonian Agents *on page 2101*
Carbidopa *on page 291*
Entacapone *on page 641*
Medication Safety Issues
Administration issues:
Strengths listed in Stalevo® brand names correspond to the **levodopa** component of the formulation only. All strengths of Stalevo® contain a levodopa/carbidopa ratio of 4:1 plus entacapone 200 mg.
Brand Names: U.S. Stalevo®
Brand Names: Canada Stalevo®
Index Terms Carbidopa, Entacapone, and Levodopa; Carbidopa, Levodopa, and Entacapone; Entacapone, Carbidopa, and Levodopa
Generic Availability (U.S.) Yes
Pharmacologic Category Anti-Parkinson's Agent, COMT Inhibitor; Anti-Parkinson's Agent, Decarboxylase Inhibitor; Anti-Parkinson's Agent, Dopamine Precursor
Use Treatment of idiopathic Parkinson's disease
Dosage
Geriatric & Adult
Note: All strengths of Stalevo® contain a carbidopa/levodopa ratio of 1:4 plus entacapone 200 mg.
Parkinson's disease: Oral: Dose should be individualized based on therapeutic response; doses may be adjusted by changing strength or adjusting interval. Fractionated doses are not recommended and only 1 tablet should be given at each dosing interval; maximum daily dose: 8 tablets of Stalevo® 50, 75, 100, 125, or 150, **or** 6 tablets of Stalevo® 200.
Patients previously treated with carbidopa/levodopa immediate release tablets (ratio of 1:4):
With current entacapone therapy: May switch directly to corresponding strength of combination tablet. No data available on transferring patients from controlled release preparations or products with a 1:10 ratio of carbidopa/levodopa.

Without entacapone therapy:
  If current levodopa dose is >600 mg/day: Levodopa dose reduction may be required when adding entacapone to therapy; therefore, titrate dose using individual products first (carbidopa/levodopa immediate release with a ratio of 1:4 plus entacapone 200 mg); then transfer to combination product once stabilized.
  If current levodopa dose is <600 mg without dyskinesias: May transfer to corresponding dose of combination product; monitor, dose reduction of levodopa may be required.

Patients previously treated with benserazide/levodopa immediate release tablets (Canadian labeling, not in U.S. labeling): *With current entacapone therapy:* Prior to switching to combination product (carbidopa/levodopa/entacapone), withhold treatment for 1 night, then initiate (carbidopa/levodopa/entacapone) therapy the following morning at a dose that provides either an equivalent amount or ~5% to 10% more levodopa.

Renal Impairment Use caution with severe renal impairment; specific dosing recommendations not available.

Hepatic Impairment Use with caution; specific dosing recommendations not available.

Special Geriatric Considerations This combination product may be convenient for elderly patients to improve adherence.

Dosage Forms Excipient information presented when available (limited, particularly for generics); consult specific product labeling.
  Tablet:
    Stalevo® 50: Levodopa 50 mg, carbidopa 12.5 mg, and entacapone 200 mg
    Stalevo® 75: Levodopa 75 mg, carbidopa 18.75 mg, and entacapone 200 mg
    Stalevo® 100: Levodopa 100 mg, carbidopa 25 mg, and entacapone 200 mg
    Stalevo® 125: Levodopa 125 mg, carbidopa 31.25 mg, and entacapone 200 mg
    Stalevo® 150: Levodopa 150 mg, carbidopa 37.5 mg, and entacapone 200 mg
    Stalevo® 200: Levodopa 200 mg, carbidopa 50 mg, and entacapone 200 mg

◆ **Levo-Dromoran** *see* Levorphanol *on page 1120*

Levofloxacin (Systemic) (lee voe FLOKS a sin)

Related Information
Antibiotic Treatment of Adults With Infective Endocarditis *on page 2157*
Antimicrobial Drugs of Choice *on page 2163*
Community-Acquired Pneumonia in Adults *on page 2171*
H. pylori Treatment in Adult Patients *on page 2116*
Medication Safety Issues
  Sound-alike/look-alike issues:
    Levaquin® may be confused with Levoxyl®, Levsin/SL®, Lovenox®
    Levofloxacin may be confused with levETIRAcetam, levodopa, Levophed®, levothyroxine
Brand Names: U.S. Levaquin®
Brand Names: Canada Levaquin®; Novo-Levofloxacin; PMS-Levofloxacin
Generic Availability (U.S.) Yes
Pharmacologic Category Antibiotic, Quinolone; Respiratory Fluoroquinolone
Use Treatment of community-acquired pneumonia, including multidrug resistant strains of *S. pneumoniae* (MDRSP); nosocomial pneumonia; chronic bronchitis (acute bacterial exacerbation); acute bacterial rhinosinusitis (ABRS); prostatitis, urinary tract infection (uncomplicated or complicated); acute pyelonephritis; skin or skin structure infections (uncomplicated or complicated); reduce incidence or disease progression of inhalational anthrax (postexposure)
Unlabeled Use Diverticulitis, enterocolitis (*Shigella* spp), epididymitis (nongonococcal), gonococcal infections, complicated intra-abdominal infections (in combination with metronidazole), Legionnaires' disease, peritonitis, PID, tuberculosis (second-line therapy)
  Note: As of April 2007, the CDC no longer recommends the use of fluoroquinolones for the treatment of gonococcal disease.
Medication Guide Available Yes
Contraindications Hypersensitivity to levofloxacin, any component of the formulation, or other quinolones

Canadian labeling: Additional contraindications (not in U.S. labeling): History of tendinitis or tendon rupture associated with use of any quinolone antimicrobial agent
Warnings/Precautions [U.S. Boxed Warning]: There have been reports of tendon inflammation and/or rupture with quinolone antibiotics; risk may be increased with concurrent corticosteroids, organ transplant recipients, and in patients >60 years of age. Rupture of the Achilles tendon sometimes requiring surgical repair has been reported most frequently; but other tendon sites (eg, rotator cuff, biceps) have also been reported. Strenuous physical activity, rheumatoid arthritis, and renal impairment may be an independent risk factor for tendonitis. Discontinue at first sign of tendon inflammation or pain. May occur

even after discontinuation of therapy. Use with caution in patients with rheumatoid arthritis; may increase risk of tendon rupture. CNS effects may occur (tremor, restlessness, confusion, and very rarely hallucinations, increased intracranial pressure [including pseudotumor cerebri] or seizures). Potential for seizures, although very rare, may be increased with concomitant NSAID therapy. Use with caution in individuals at risk of seizures, with known or suspected CNS disorders or renal dysfunction. Avoid excessive sunlight and take precautions to limit exposure (eg, loose fitting clothing, sunscreen); may cause moderate-to-severe phototoxicity reactions. Discontinue use if photosensitivity occurs.

Rare cases of torsade de pointes have been reported in patients receiving levofloxacin. Use caution in patients with known prolongation of QT interval, bradycardia, hypokalemia, hypomagnesemia, or in those receiving concurrent therapy with Class Ia or Class III antiarrhythmics.

Severe hypersensitivity reactions, including anaphylaxis, have occurred with quinolone therapy. Reactions may present as typical allergic symptoms after a single dose, or may manifest as severe idiosyncratic dermatologic, vascular, pulmonary, renal, hepatic, and/or hematologic events, usually after multiple doses. Prompt discontinuation of drug should occur if skin rash or other symptoms arise. Prolonged use may result in fungal or bacterial superinfection, including *C. difficile*-associated diarrhea (CDAD) and pseudomembranous colitis; CDAD has been observed >2 months postantibiotic treatment. Peripheral neuropathies have been linked to levofloxacin use; discontinue if numbness, tingling, or weakness develops. **[U.S. Boxed Warning]: Quinolones may exacerbate myasthenia gravis; avoid use (rare, potentially life-threatening weakness of respiratory muscles may occur).** Unrelated to hypersensitivity, severe hepatotoxicity (including acute hepatitis and fatalities) has been reported. Elderly patients may be at greater risk. Discontinue therapy immediately if signs and symptoms of hepatitis occur. Hemolytic reactions may (rarely) occur with quinolone use in patients with latent or actual G6PD deficiency.

Fluoroquinolones have been associated with the development of serious, and sometimes fatal, hypoglycemia, most often in elderly diabetics, but also in patients without diabetes. This occurred most frequently with gatifloxacin (no longer available systemically) but may occur at a lower frequency with other quinolones.

Adverse Reactions (Reflective of adult population; not specific for elderly) 1% to 10%:

Cardiovascular: Chest pain (1%), edema (1%)

Central nervous system: Headache (6%), insomnia (4%), dizziness (3%), fatigue (1%), pain (1%)

Dermatologic: Rash (2%), pruritus (1%)

Gastrointestinal: Nausea (7%), diarrhea (5%), constipation (3%), abdominal pain (2%), dyspepsia (2%), vomiting (2%)

Genitourinary: Vaginitis (1%)

Local: Injection site reaction (1%)

Respiratory: Pharyngitis (4%), dyspnea (1%)

Miscellaneous: Moniliasis (1%)

Drug Interactions

Metabolism/Transport Effects None known.

Avoid Concomitant Use

Avoid concomitant use of Levofloxacin (Systemic) with any of the following: BCG; Highest Risk QTc-Prolonging Agents; Mifepristone

Increased Effect/Toxicity

Levofloxacin (Systemic) may increase the levels/effects of: Corticosteroids (Systemic); Highest Risk QTc-Prolonging Agents; Moderate Risk QTc-Prolonging Agents; Porfimer; Sulfonylureas; Varenicline; Vitamin K Antagonists

The levels/effects of Levofloxacin (Systemic) may be increased by: Insulin; Mifepristone; Nonsteroidal Anti-Inflammatory Agents; Probenecid; QTc-Prolonging Agents (Indeterminate Risk and Risk Modifying)

Decreased Effect

Levofloxacin (Systemic) may decrease the levels/effects of: BCG; Mycophenolate; Sulfonylureas; Typhoid Vaccine

The levels/effects of Levofloxacin (Systemic) may be decreased by: Antacids; Calcium Salts; Didanosine; Iron Salts; Lanthanum; Magnesium Salts; Quinapril; Sevelamer; Sucralfate; Zinc Salts

Stability

Solution for injection:

Vial: Store at room temperature. Protect from light. When diluted to 5 mg/mL in a compatible I.V. fluid, solution is stable for 72 hours when stored at room temperature; stable for 14 days when stored under refrigeration. When frozen, stable for 6 months; do not refreeze. Do not thaw in microwave or by bath immersion.

Premixed: Store at ≤25°C (77°F); do not freeze. Brief exposure to 40°C (104°F) does not affect product. Protect from light.

Tablet, oral solution: Store at 25°C (77°F); excursions permitted to 15°C to 30°C (59°F to 86°F).

Mechanism of Action As the S(-) enantiomer of the fluoroquinolone, ofloxacin, levofloxacin, inhibits DNA-gyrase in susceptible organisms thereby inhibits relaxation of supercoiled DNA and promotes breakage of DNA strands. DNA gyrase (topoisomerase II), is an essential bacterial enzyme that maintains the superhelical structure of DNA and is required for DNA replication and transcription, DNA repair, recombination, and transposition.

Pharmacodynamics/Kinetics

Absorption: Rapid and complete

Distribution: V_d: 74-112 L; CSF concentrations ~15% of serum levels; high concentrations are achieved in prostate, lung, and gynecological tissues, sinus, saliva

Protein binding: ~24% to 38%; primarily to albumin

Metabolism: Minimally hepatic

Bioavailability: ~99%

Half-life elimination: ~6-8 hours

Time to peak, serum: Oral: 1-2 hours

Excretion: Urine (~87% as unchanged drug, <5% as metabolites); feces (<4%)

Dosage

Geriatric & Adult Note: Sequential therapy (intravenous to oral) may be instituted based on prescriber's discretion.

Acute bacterial rhinosinusitis: Oral, I.V.:

Manufacturer's recommendations: 750 mg every 24 hours for 5 days or 500 mg every 24 hours for 10-14 days

Alternate recommendations: 500 mg every 24 hours for 5-7 days (Chow, 2012)

Anthrax (inhalational): 500 mg every 24 hours for 60 days, beginning as soon as possible after exposure

Chronic bronchitis (acute bacterial exacerbation): Oral, I.V.: 500 mg every 24 hours for at least 7 days

Diverticulitis, peritonitis (unlabeled use): Oral, I.V.: 750 mg every 24 hours for 7-10 days; use adjunctive metronidazole therapy

Dysenteric enterocolitis, *Shigella spp.* (unlabeled use): Oral, I.V.: 500 mg every 24 hours for 3-5 days

Epididymitis, nongonococcal (unlabeled use): 500 mg once daily for 10 days

Gonococcal infection (unlabeled use): Oral, I.V.:

Cervicitis, urethritis: 250 mg for one dose with azithromycin or doxycycline; **Note:** As of April 2007, the CDC no longer recommends the use of fluoroquinolones for the treatment of uncomplicated gonococcal disease.

Disseminated infection: 250 mg I.V. once daily; 24 hours after symptoms improve may change to 500 mg orally every 24 hours to complete total therapy of 7 days; **Note:** As of April 2007, the CDC no longer recommends the use of fluoroquinolones for the treatment of more serious gonococcal disease, unless no other options exist and susceptibility can be confirmed via culture.

Intra-abdominal infection, complicated, community-acquired (in combination with metronidazole) (unlabeled use): I.V.: 750 mg once daily for 4-7 days (provided source controlled). **Note:** Avoid using in settings where *E. coli* susceptibility to fluoroquinolones is <90%.

Pelvic inflammatory disease (unlabeled use): 500 mg once daily for 14 days with or without adjunctive metronidazole; **Note:** The CDC recommends use only if standard cephalosporin therapy is not feasible and community prevalence of quinolone-resistant gonococcal organisms is low. Culture sensitivity must be confirmed.

Pneumonia: Oral, I.V.:

Community-acquired (CAP): 500 mg every 24 hours for 7-14 days or 750 mg every 24 hours for 5 days (efficacy of 5-day regimen for MDRSP not established)

Healthcare-associated (HAP): 750 mg every 24 hours for 7-14 days

Prostatitis (chronic bacterial): Oral, I.V.: 500 mg every 24 hours for 28 days

Skin and skin structure infections: Oral, I.V.:

Uncomplicated: 500 mg every 24 hours for 7-10 days

Complicated: 750 mg every 24 hours for 7-14 days

Traveler's diarrhea (unlabeled use): Oral, I.V.: 500 mg for one dose

Tuberculosis, drug-resistant tuberculosis, or intolerance to first-line agents (unlabeled use): Oral: 500-1000 mg every 24 hours (*MMWR*, 2003)

Urinary tract infections: Oral, I.V.:

Uncomplicated: 250 mg once daily for 3 days

Complicated, including acute pyelonephritis: 250 mg once daily for 10 days **or** 750 mg once daily for 5 days

Renal Impairment

Normal renal function dosing of 750 mg/day:

Cl_{cr} 20-49 mL/minute: Administer 750 mg every 48 hours

Cl_{cr} 10-19 mL/minute: Administer 750 mg initial dose, followed by 500 mg every 48 hours

Hemodialysis (administer after hemodialysis on dialysis days)/peritoneal dialysis (PD): Administer 750 mg initial dose, followed by 500 mg every 48 hours

Normal renal function dosing of 500 mg/day:

Cl_{cr} 20-49 mL/minute: Administer 500 mg initial dose, followed by 250 mg every 24 hours

Cl_{cr} 10-19 mL/minute: Administer 500 mg initial dose, followed by 250 mg every 48 hours

Hemodialysis (administer after hemodialysis on dialysis days)/peritoneal dialysis (PD): Administer 500 mg initial dose, followed by 250 mg every 48 hours

Normal renal function dosing of 250 mg/day:

Cl_{cr} 20-49 mL/minute: No dosage adjustment required

Cl_{cr} 10-19 mL/minute: Administer 250 mg every 48 hours (except in uncomplicated UTI, where no dosage adjustment is required)

Hemodialysis (administer after hemodialysis on dialysis days)/peritoneal dialysis (PD): No information available.

Continuous renal replacement therapy (CRRT) (Heintz, 2009; Trotman, 2005): Drug clearance is highly dependent on the method of renal replacement, filter type, and flow rate. Appropriate dosing requires close monitoring of pharmacologic response, signs of adverse reactions due to drug accumulation, as well as drug concentrations in relation to target trough (if appropriate). The following are general recommendations only (based on dialysate flow/ultrafiltration rates of 1-2 L/hour and minimal residual renal function) and should not supersede clinical judgment:

CVVH: Loading dose of 500-750 mg followed by 250 mg every 24 hours

CVVHD: Loading dose of 500-750 mg followed by 250-500 mg every 24 hours

CVVHDF: Loading dose of 500-750 mg followed by 250-750 mg every 24 hours

Administration

Oral: Tablets may be administered without regard to meals. Oral solution should be administered 1 hour before or 2 hours after meals. Maintain adequate hydration of patient to prevent crystalluria.

I.V.: Infuse 250-500 mg I.V. solution over 60 minutes; infuse 750 mg I.V. solution over 90 minutes. Too rapid of infusion can lead to hypotension. Avoid administration through an intravenous line with a solution containing multivalent cations (eg, magnesium, calcium). Maintain adequate hydration of patient to prevent crystalluria.

Monitoring Parameters Evaluation of organ system functions (renal, hepatic, and hematopoietic) is recommended periodically during therapy; the possibility of crystalluria should be assessed; WBC and signs of infection

Test Interactions Some quinolones may produce a false-positive urine screening result for opiates using commercially-available immunoassay kits. This has been demonstrated most consistently for levofloxacin and ofloxacin, but other quinolones have shown cross-reactivity in certain assay kits. Confirmation of positive opiate screens by more specific methods should be considered.

Special Geriatric Considerations The risk of torsade de pointes and tendon inflammation and/or rupture associated with the concomitant use of corticosteroids and quinolones is increased in the elderly population. See Warnings/Precautions regarding tendon rupture in patients >60 years of age. Adjust dose for renal function.

Dosage Forms Excipient information presented when available (limited, particularly for generics); consult specific product labeling. [DSC] = Discontinued product

Infusion, premixed in D_5W [preservative free]: 250 mg (50 mL); 500 mg (100 mL); 750 mg (150 mL)

Levaquin®: 250 mg (50 mL); 500 mg (100 mL); 750 mg (150 mL)

Injection, solution [preservative free]: 25 mg/mL (20 mL, 30 mL)

Levaquin®: 25 mg/mL (20 mL [DSC], 30 mL [DSC])

Solution, oral: 25 mg/mL (100 mL, 200 mL, 480 mL)

Levaquin®: 25 mg/mL (480 mL) [contains benzyl alcohol, propylene glycol]

Tablet, oral: 250 mg, 500 mg, 750 mg

Levaquin®: 250 mg, 500 mg, 750 mg

Levofloxacin (Ophthalmic) (lee voe FLOKS a sin)

Medication Safety Issues
Sound-alike/look-alike issues:
Levofloxacin may be confused with levETIRAcetam, levodopa, levothyroxine
Brand Names: U.S. Iquix®; Quixin®
Generic Availability (U.S.) Yes
Pharmacologic Category Antibiotic, Ophthalmic; Antibiotic, Quinolone
Use Treatment of bacterial conjunctivitis caused by susceptible organisms (Quixin® 0.5% ophthalmic solution); treatment of corneal ulcer caused by susceptible organisms (Iquix® 1.5% ophthalmic solution)

Dosage
Geriatric & Adult
Conjunctivitis (0.5% ophthalmic solution): Ophthalmic:
Treatment day 1 and day 2: Instill 1-2 drops into affected eye(s) every 2 hours while awake, up to 8 times/day
Treatment day 3 through day 7: Instill 1-2 drops into affected eye(s) every 4 hours while awake, up to 4 times/day
Corneal ulceration (1.5% ophthalmic solution): Ophthalmic:
Treatment day 1 through day 3: Instill 1-2 drops into affected eye(s) every 30 minutes to 2 hours while awake and 4-6 hours after retiring.
Treatment day 4 through completion: Instill 1-2 drops into affected eye(s) every 1-4 hours while awake.

Special Geriatric Considerations Evaluate the patient's or caregiver's ability to safely administer the correct dose of ophthalmic medication.
Dosage Forms Excipient information presented when available (limited, particularly for generics); consult specific product labeling.
Solution, ophthalmic [drops]: 0.5% (5 mL)
Iquix®: 1.5% (5 mL)
Quixin®: 0.5% (5 mL) [contains benzalkonium chloride]

Levorphanol (lee VOR fa nole)

Related Information
Opioid Analgesics *on page 2122*
Medication Safety Issues
High alert medication:
The Institute for Safe Medication Practices (ISMP) includes this medication among its list of drug classes which have a heightened risk of causing significant patient harm when used in error.
Index Terms Levo-Dromoran; Levorphan Tartrate; Levorphanol Tartrate
Generic Availability (U.S.) Yes: Tablet
Pharmacologic Category Analgesic, Opioid
Use Relief of moderate-to-severe pain; preoperative sedation/analgesia; management of chronic pain (eg, cancer) requiring opioid therapy
Contraindications Hypersensitivity to levorphanol or any component of the formulation
Warnings/Precautions An opioid-containing analgesic regimen should be tailored to each patient's needs and based upon the type of pain being treated (acute versus chronic), the route of administration, degree of tolerance for opioids (naive versus chronic user), age, weight, and medical condition. The optimal analgesic dose varies widely among patients. Doses should be titrated to pain relief/prevention.

May cause CNS depression, which may impair physical or mental abilities; patients must be cautioned about performing tasks which require mental alertness (eg, operating machinery or driving). Effects may be potentiated when used with other sedative drugs or ethanol. Use with caution in patients with hypersensitivity reactions to other phenanthrene derivative opioid agonists (morphine, hydrocodone, hydromorphone, oxycodone, oxymorphone); respiratory diseases including asthma, emphysema, COPD, hypothyroidism, head trauma, morbid obesity, adrenal insufficiency, prostatic hyperplasia/urinary stricture, or severe liver or renal insufficiency. Use with caution in patients with biliary tract dysfunction; acute pancreatitis may cause constriction of sphincter of Oddi. May be habit-forming. May cause hypotension; use with caution in patients with depleted blood volume or drugs which may exaggerate hypotensive effects (including phenothiazines or general anesthetics). May obscure diagnosis or clinical course of patients with acute abdominal conditions. Concurrent use of agonist/antagonist analgesics may precipitate withdrawal symptoms and/or reduced analgesic efficacy in patients following prolonged therapy with mu opioid agonists. Abrupt discontinuation following prolonged use may also lead to withdrawal symptoms. Elderly and debilitated patients may be particularly susceptible to the adverse effects of narcotics.

Adverse Reactions (Reflective of adult population; not specific for elderly) Frequency not defined.

Cardiovascular: Palpitation, hypotension, bradycardia, peripheral vasodilation, cardiac arrest, shock, tachycardia

Central nervous system: CNS depression, fatigue, drowsiness, dizziness, nervousness, headache, restlessness, anorexia, malaise, confusion, coma, convulsion, insomnia, amnesia, mental depression, hallucinations, paradoxical CNS stimulation, intracranial pressure (increased)

Dermatologic: Pruritus, urticaria, rash

Endocrine & metabolic: Antidiuretic hormone release

Gastrointestinal: Nausea, vomiting, dyspepsia, stomach cramps, xerostomia, constipation, abdominal pain, dry mouth, biliary tract spasm, paralytic ileus

Genitourinary: Decreased urination, urinary tract spasm, urinary retention

Neuromuscular & skeletal: Weakness

Ocular: Miosis, diplopia

Respiratory: Respiratory depression, apnea, hypoventilation, cyanosis

Miscellaneous: Histamine release, physical and psychological dependence

Drug Interactions

Metabolism/Transport Effects None known.

Avoid Concomitant Use

Avoid concomitant use of Levorphanol with any of the following: Azelastine; Azelastine (Nasal); Methadone; Mirtazapine; Paraldehyde

Increased Effect/Toxicity

Levorphanol may increase the levels/effects of: Alcohol (Ethyl); Alvimopan; Azelastine; Azelastine (Nasal); CNS Depressants; Desmopressin; Methadone; Metyrosine; Mirtazapine; Paraldehyde; Selective Serotonin Reuptake Inhibitors; Thiazide Diuretics; Zolpidem

The levels/effects of Levorphanol may be increased by: Amphetamines; Antipsychotic Agents (Phenothiazines); Droperidol; HydrOXYzine; Succinylcholine

Decreased Effect

Levorphanol may decrease the levels/effects of: Pegvisomant

The levels/effects of Levorphanol may be decreased by: Ammonium Chloride; Mixed Agonist / Antagonist Opioids

Ethanol/Nutrition/Herb Interactions

Ethanol: May increase CNS depression; monitor for increased effects with coadministration. Caution patients about effects.

Herb/Nutraceutical: Avoid valerian, St John's wort, kava kava, gotu kola (may increase CNS depression).

Stability Store at 25°C (77°F); excursions permitted to 15°C to 30°C (59°F to 86°F).

Mechanism of Action Levorphanol tartrate is a synthetic opioid agonist that is classified as a morphinan derivative. Opioids interact with stereospecific opioid receptors in various parts of the central nervous system and other tissues. Analgesic potency parallels the affinity for these binding sites. These drugs do not alter the threshold or responsiveness to pain, but the perception of pain.

Pharmacodynamics/Kinetics

Onset of action: Oral: 10-60 minutes

Duration: 4-8 hours

Metabolism: Hepatic

Half-life elimination: 11-16 hours

Excretion: Urine (as inactive metabolite)

Dosage

Geriatric & Adult Note: These are guidelines and do not represent the maximum doses that may be required in all patients. Doses should be titrated to pain relief/prevention.

Acute pain (moderate-to-severe): Oral: Initial: Opiate-naive: 2 mg every 6-8 hours as needed; patients with prior opiate exposure may require higher initial doses; usual dosage range: 2-4 mg every 6-8 hours as needed

Note: The American Pain Society recommends an initial dose of 4 mg for severe pain in adults (APS, 6th ed)

Chronic pain: Patients taking opioids chronically may become tolerant and require doses higher than the usual dosage range to maintain the desired effect. Tolerance can be managed by appropriate dose titration. **There is no optimal or maximal dose for levorphanol in chronic pain. The appropriate dose is one that relieves pain throughout its dosing interval without causing unmanageable side effects.**

Renal Impairment Use with caution; initial dose should be reduced in severe renal impairment.

Hepatic Impairment Use with caution; initial dose should be reduced in severe hepatic impairment.

Monitoring Parameters Pain relief, respiratory and mental status, blood pressure

Pharmacotherapy Pearls 2 mg levorphanol I.M. produces analgesia comparable to that produced by 10 mg of morphine I.M.

Special Geriatric Considerations The elderly may be particularly susceptible to the CNS depressant and constipating effects of narcotics.

Controlled Substance C-II

Dosage Forms Excipient information presented when available (limited, particularly for generics); consult specific product labeling.

Tablet, oral, as tartrate: 2 mg,

- ◆ **Levorphanol Tartrate** *see* Levorphanol *on page 1120*
- ◆ **Levorphan Tartrate** *see* Levorphanol *on page 1120*
- ◆ **Levothroid®** *see* Levothyroxine *on page 1122*

Levothyroxine (lee voe thye ROKS een)

Medication Safety Issues

Sound-alike/look-alike issues:

Levothyroxine may be confused with lamoTRIgine, Lanoxin®, levofloxacin, liothyronine

Levoxyl® may be confused with Lanoxin®, Levaquin®, Luvox®

Synthroid® may be confused with Symmetrel®

Administration issues:

Significant differences exist between oral and I.V. dosing. Use caution when converting from one route of administration to another.

Other safety concerns:

To avoid errors due to misinterpretation of a decimal point, always express dosage in mcg (**not** mg).

Brand Names: U.S. Levothroid®; Levoxyl®; Synthroid®; Tirosint®; Unithroid®

Brand Names: Canada Eltroxin®; Euthyrox; Levothyroxine Sodium; Synthroid®

Index Terms L-Thyroxine Sodium; Levothyroxine Sodium; T_4

Generic Availability (U.S.) Yes: Excludes capsule

Pharmacologic Category Thyroid Product

Use Replacement or supplemental therapy in hypothyroidism; pituitary TSH suppression

Unlabeled Use Management of hemodynamically unstable potential organ donors increasing the quantity of organs available for transplantation

Contraindications Hypersensitivity to levothyroxine sodium or any component of the formulation; acute MI; thyrotoxicosis of any etiology; uncorrected adrenal insufficiency

Capsule: Additional contraindication: Inability to swallow capsules

Warnings/Precautions [U.S. Boxed Warning]: Thyroid supplements are ineffective and potentially toxic when used for the treatment of obesity or for weight reduction, especially in euthyroid patients. High doses may produce serious or even life-threatening toxic effects particularly when used with some anorectic drugs (eg, sympathomimetic amines). Routine use of T_4 for TSH suppression is not recommended in patients with benign thyroid nodules. In patients deemed appropriate candidates, treatment should never be fully suppressive (TSH <0.1 mIU/L). Use with caution and reduce dosage in patients with angina pectoris or other cardiovascular disease; decrease initial dose. Use cautiously in the elderly since they may be more likely to have compromised cardiovascular functions. Patients with adrenal insufficiency, myxedema, diabetes mellitus and insipidus may have symptoms exaggerated or aggravated. Chronic hypothyroidism predisposes patients to coronary artery disease. Long-term therapy can decrease bone mineral density. Levoxyl® may rapidly swell and disintegrate causing choking or gagging (should be administered with a full glass of water); use caution in patients with dysphagia or other swallowing disorders.

Adverse Reactions (Reflective of adult population; not specific for elderly) Frequency not defined.

Cardiovascular: Angina, arrhythmia, cardiac arrest, flushing, heart failure, hypertension, MI, palpitation, pulse increased, tachycardia

Central nervous system: Anxiety, emotional lability, fatigue, fever, headache, hyperactivity, insomnia, irritability, nervousness, pseudotumor cerebri (children), seizure (rare)

Dermatologic: Alopecia

Endocrine & metabolic: Fertility impaired, menstrual irregularities

Gastrointestinal: Abdominal cramps, appetite increased, diarrhea, vomiting, weight loss

Hepatic: Liver function tests increased

Neuromuscular & skeletal: Bone mineral density decreased, muscle weakness, tremor, slipped capital femoral epiphysis (children)

Respiratory: Dyspnea

Miscellaneous: Diaphoresis, heat intolerance, hypersensitivity (to inactive ingredients, symptoms include urticaria, pruritus, rash, flushing, angioedema, GI symptoms, fever, arthralgia, serum sickness, wheezing)

Levoxyl®: Choking, dysphagia, gagging

Drug Interactions

Metabolism/Transport Effects None known.

Avoid Concomitant Use

Avoid concomitant use of Levothyroxine with any of the following: Sodium Iodide I131

Increased Effect/Toxicity

Levothyroxine may increase the levels/effects of: Vitamin K Antagonists

Decreased Effect

Levothyroxine may decrease the levels/effects of: Sodium Iodide I131; Theophylline Derivatives

The levels/effects of Levothyroxine may be decreased by: Aluminum Hydroxide; Bile Acid Sequestrants; Calcium Polystyrene Sulfonate; Calcium Salts; CarBAMazepine; Estrogen Derivatives; Fosphenytoin; Iron Salts; Lanthanum; Orlistat; Phenytoin; Raloxifene; Rifampin; Sevelamer; Sodium Polystyrene Sulfonate; Sucralfate

Ethanol/Nutrition/Herb Interactions Food: Taking levothyroxine with enteral nutrition may cause reduced bioavailability and may lower serum thyroxine levels leading to signs or symptoms of hypothyroidism. Soybean flour (infant formula), cottonseed meal, walnuts, and dietary fiber may decrease absorption of levothyroxine from the GI tract. Management: Take in the morning on an empty stomach at least 30 minutes before food. Consider an increase in dose if taken with enteral tube feed.

Stability

Capsules, tablets: Store at room temperature; excursions permitted to 15°C to 30°C (59°F to 86°F). Protect from light and moisture.

Injection: Store at room temperature; excursions permitted to 15°C to 30°C (59°F to 86°F). Dilute vials for injection with 5 mL normal saline. Reconstituted concentrations for the 100 mcg, 200 mcg, and 500 mcg vials are 20 mcg/mL, 40 mcg/mL, and 100 mcg/mL, respectively. Shake well and use immediately after reconstitution (manufacturer recommendation); discard any unused portions.

Additional stability data:

Stability in polypropylene syringes (100 mcg/mL in NS) at 5°C ± 1°C is 7 days (Gupta, 2000). Stability in latex-free, PVC minibags protected from light and stored at 15°C to 30°C (59°F to 86°F) was 12 hours for a 2 mcg/mL concentration or 18 hours for a 0.4 mcg/mL concentration in NS. May be exposed to light; however, stability time is significantly reduced, especially for the 2 mcg/mL concentration (Strong, 2010).

Mechanism of Action Levothyroxine (T_4) is a synthetic form of thyroxine, an endogenous hormone secreted by the thyroid gland. T_4 is converted to its active metabolite, L-triiodothyronine (T_3). Thyroid hormones (T_4 and T_3) then bind to thyroid receptor proteins in the cell nucleus and exert metabolic effects through control of DNA transcription and protein synthesis; involved in normal metabolism, growth, and development; promotes gluconeogenesis, increases utilization and mobilization of glycogen stores, and stimulates protein synthesis, increases basal metabolic rate

Pharmacodynamics/Kinetics

Onset of action: Therapeutic: Oral: 3-5 days; I.V. 6-8 hours

Peak effect: I.V.: 24 hours

Absorption: Oral: Erratic (40% to 80% [per manufacturer]); may be decreased by age and specific foods and drugs

Protein binding: >99% bound to plasma proteins including thyroxine-binding globulin, thyroxine-binding prealbumin, and albumin

Metabolism: Hepatic to triiodothyronine (T_3; active); ~80% thyroxine (T_4) deiodinated in kidney and periphery; glucuronidation/conjugation also occurs; undergoes enterohepatic recirculation

Bioavailability: Oral tablets: 64% (nonfasting state) to 79% to 81% (fasting state)

Time to peak, serum: 2-4 hours

Half-life elimination: Euthyroid: 6-7 days; Hypothyroid: 9-10 days; Hyperthyroid: 3-4 days

Excretion: Urine (major route of elimination; decreases with age); feces (~20%)

◀ **Dosage**

Geriatric Doses should be adjusted based on clinical response and laboratory parameters.
Hypothyroidism: Elderly patients may require <1 mcg/kg/day:

Oral:

>50 years without cardiac disease **or** <50 years with cardiac disease: Initial: 25-50 mcg/day; adjust dose by 12.5-25 mcg increments at 6- to 8-week intervals as needed

>50 years with cardiac disease: Initial: 12.5-25 mcg/day; adjust dose by 12.5-25 mcg increments at 4- to 6-week intervals (many clinicians prefer to adjust at 6- to 8-week intervals).

Note: Patients with combined hypothyroidism and cardiac disease should be monitored carefully for changes in stability.

I.M., I.V.: Refer to adult dosing.

Myxedema coma: *I.V.:* Refer to adult dosing; lower doses may be needed.

Adult Doses should be adjusted based on clinical response and laboratory parameters.

Hypothyroidism: Adults, healthy adults <50 years of age, and older adults who have been recently treated for hyperthyroidism or who have been hypothyroid for only a few months):

Oral: ~1.7 mcg/kg/day; usual doses are ≤200 mcg/day (range: 100-125 mcg/day [70 kg adult]); doses ≥300 mcg/day are rare (consider poor compliance, malabsorption, and/or drug interactions). Titrate dose every 6 weeks.

Patients >50 years or patients with cardiac disease: Refer to geriatric dosing.

I.M., I.V.: 50% of the oral dose; alternatively, some clinicians administer up to 80% of the oral dose. **Note:** Bioavailability of the oral formulation is highly variable, but absorption has been measured to be ~80%, when the oral tablet formulation was administered in the recommended fasting state (Dickerson, 2010; Fish, 1987).

Severe hypothyroidism: Oral: Initial: 12.5-25 mcg/day; adjust dose by 25 mcg/day every 2-4 weeks as appropriate

Subclinical hypothyroidism (if treated): Oral: 1 mcg/kg/day

TSH suppression: Oral:

Well-differentiated thyroid cancer: Highly individualized; Doses >2 mcg/kg/day may be needed to suppress TSH to <0.1 mIU/L in intermediate- to high-risk tumors. Low-risk tumors may be maintained at or slightly below the lower limit of normal (0.1-0.5 mIU/L) (Cooper, 2009).

Benign nodules and nontoxic multinodular goiter: Routine use of T_4 for TSH suppression is not recommended in patients with benign thyroid nodules. In patients deemed appropriate candidates, treatment should never be fully suppressive (TSH <0.1 mIU/L) (Cooper, 2009; Gharib, 2010). Avoid use if TSH is already suppressed.

Myxedema coma or stupor: I.V.: 200-500 mcg, then 100-300 mcg the next day if necessary; smaller doses should be considered in patients with cardiovascular disease

Administration

Oral: Administer in the morning on an empty stomach, at least 30 minutes before food.

Capsule: Must be swallowed whole; do not cut, crush, or attempt to dissolve capsules in water to prepare a suspension

Tablet: May be crushed and suspended in 5-10 mL of water; suspension should be used immediately. Levoxyl® should be administered with a full glass of water to prevent gagging (due to tablet swelling).

Nasogastric tube: Bioavailability of levothyroxine is reduced if administered with enteral tube feeds. Since holding feedings for at least 1 hour before and after levothyroxine administration may not completely resolve the interaction, an increase in dose (eg, additional 25 mcg) may be necessary (Dickerson, 2010).

Parenteral: Dilute vial with 5 mL normal saline; use immediately after reconstitution; should not be admixed with other solutions

Monitoring Parameters Thyroid function test (serum thyroxine, thyrotropin concentrations), resin triiodothyronine uptake (rT_3U), free thyroxine index (FTI), T_4, TSH, heart rate, blood pressure, clinical signs of hypo- and hyperthyroidism; TSH is the most reliable guide for evaluating adequacy of thyroid replacement dosage. TSH may be elevated during the first few months of thyroid replacement despite patients being clinically euthyroid. In cases where T_4 remains low and TSH is within normal limits, an evaluation of "free" (unbound) T_4 is needed to evaluate further increase in dosage

Adults: Monitor TSH every 6-8 weeks until normalized; 8-12 weeks after dosage changes; every 6-12 months throughout therapy

Reference Range Approximate adult normal range: 4-12 mcg/dL (SI: 51-154 nmol/L). Borderline high: 11.1-13 mcg/dL (SI: 143-167 nmol/L); high: ≥13.1 mcg/dL (SI: 169 nmol/L). TSH: 0.4-10 (for those ≥80 years) mIU/L; T_4: 4-12 mcg/dL (SI: 51-154 nmol/L); T_3 (RIA) (total T_3): 80-230 ng/dL (SI: 1.2-3.5 nmol/L); T_4 free (free T_4): 0.7-1.8 ng/dL (SI: 9-23 pmol/L).

Test Interactions Many drugs may have effects on thyroid function tests (see Pharmacotherapy Pearls). Infectious hepatitis and acute intermittent porphyria may increase TBG concentrations; nephrosis, severe hypoproteinemia, severe liver disease, and acromegaly may decrease TBG concentrations.

Pharmacotherapy Pearls Equivalent doses: The following statement on relative potency of thyroid products is included in a joint statement by American Thyroid Association (ATA), American Association of Clinical Endocrinologists (AACE) and The Endocrine Society (TES): For purposes of conversion, levothyroxine sodium (T_4) 100 mcg is usually considered equivalent to desiccated thyroid 60 mg, thyroglobulin 60 mg, or liothyronine sodium (T_3) 25 mcg. However, these are rough guidelines only and do not obviate the careful re-evaluation of a patient when switching thyroid hormone preparations, including a change from one brand of levothyroxine to another. Joint position statement is available at http://www.thyroid.org/professionals/advocacy/04_12_08_thyroxine.html.

Note: Several medications have effects on thyroid production or conversion. The impact in thyroid replacement has not been specifically evaluated, but patient response should be monitored:

Methimazole: Decreases thyroid hormone secretion, while propylthiouracil decrease thyroid hormone secretion and decreases conversion of T_4 to T_3.

Beta-adrenergic antagonists: Decrease conversion of T_4 to T_3 (dose related, propranolol ≥160 mg/day); patients may be clinically euthyroid.

Iodide, iodine-containing radiographic contrast agents may decrease thyroid hormone secretion; may also increase thyroid hormone secretion, especially in patients with Graves' disease.

Other agents reported to impact on thyroid production/conversion include aminoglutethimide, amiodarone, chloral hydrate, diazepam, ethionamide, interferon-alpha, interleukin-2, lithium, lovastatin (case report), glucocorticoids (dose-related), mercaptopurine, sulfonamides, thiazide diuretics, and tolbutamide.

In addition, a number of medications have been noted to cause transient depression in TSH secretion, which may complicate interpretation of monitoring tests for levothyroxine, including corticosteroids, octreotide, and dopamine. Metoclopramide may increase TSH secretion

Special Geriatric Considerations Elderly do not have a change in serum thyroxine associated with aging; however, plasma T_3 concentrations are decreased 25% to 40% in the elderly. There is not a compensatory rise in thyrotropin suggesting that lower T_3 is not reacted upon as a deficiency by the pituitary. This indicates a slightly lower than normal dosage of thyroid hormone replacement is usually sufficient in elderly patients than in younger adult patients. TSH must be monitored since insufficient thyroid replacement (elevated TSH) is a risk for coronary artery disease and excessive replacement (low TSH) may cause signs of hyperthyroidism and excessive bone loss. Some clinicians suggest levothyroxine is the drug of choice for replacement therapy.

Dosage Forms Excipient information presented when available (limited, particularly for generics); consult specific product labeling. [DSC] = Discontinued product

Capsule, soft gelatin, oral, as sodium:
Tirosint®: 13 mcg, 25 mcg, 50 mcg, 75 mcg, 88 mcg, 100 mcg, 112 mcg, 125 mcg, 137 mcg, 150 mcg

Injection, powder for reconstitution, as sodium: 100 mcg, 200 mcg [DSC], 500 mcg

Tablet, oral, as sodium: 25 mcg, 50 mcg, 75 mcg, 88 mcg, 100 mcg, 112 mcg, 125 mcg, 137 mcg, 150 mcg, 175 mcg, 200 mcg, 300 mcg

Levothroid®: 25 mcg, 75 mcg, 88 mcg, 100 mcg, 112 mcg, 125 mcg, 137 mcg, 150 mcg, 175 mcg, 200 mcg, 300 mcg [scored]

Levothroid®: 50 mcg [scored; dye free]

Levoxyl®: 25 mcg, 75 mcg, 88 mcg, 100 mcg, 112 mcg, 125 mcg, 137 mcg, 150 mcg, 175 mcg, 200 mcg [scored]

Levoxyl®: 50 mcg [scored; dye free]

Synthroid®: 25 mcg, 75 mcg, 88 mcg, 100 mcg, 112 mcg, 125 mcg, 137 mcg, 150 mcg, 175 mcg, 200 mcg, 300 mcg [scored]

Synthroid®: 50 mcg [scored; dye free]

Unithroid®: 25 mcg, 75 mcg, 88 mcg, 100 mcg, 112 mcg, 125 mcg, 150 mcg, 175 mcg, 200 mcg, 300 mcg [scored]

Unithroid®: 50 mcg [scored; dye free]

◆ **Levothyroxine and Liothyronine** see Liotrix on page 1142
◆ **Levothyroxine and Liothyronine** see Thyroid, Desiccated on page 1885
◆ **Levothyroxine Sodium** see Levothyroxine on page 1122
◆ **Levoxyl®** see Levothyroxine on page 1122
◆ **Levsin®** see Hyoscyamine on page 960
◆ **Levsin®/SL** see Hyoscyamine on page 960

- ◆ **Levulan® Kerastick®** *see* Aminolevulinic Acid *on page 91*
- ◆ **Lexapro®** *see* Escitalopram *on page 670*
- ◆ **Lexiscan®** *see* Regadenoson *on page 1683*
- ◆ ***l*-Hyoscyamine Sulfate** *see* Hyoscyamine *on page 960*
- ◆ **Lialda®** *see* Mesalamine *on page 1217*
- ◆ **Librax®** *see* Clidinium and Chlordiazepoxide *on page 398*
- ◆ **Librium** *see* ChlordiazePOXIDE *on page 354*
- ◆ **LidaMantle®** *see* Lidocaine (Topical) *on page 1128*
- ◆ **Lidex** *see* Fluocinonide *on page 804*

Lidocaine (Systemic) (LYE doe kane)

Medication Safety Issues
High alert medication:
The Institute for Safe Medication Practices (ISMP) includes this medication (epidural administration; I.V. formulation) among its list of drugs which have a heightened risk of causing significant patient harm when used in error.

International issues:
Lidosen [Italy] may be confused with Lincocin brand name for lincomycin [U.S., Canada, and multiple international markets]; Lodosyn brand name for carbidopa [U.S.]

Brand Names: U.S. Xylocaine®; Xylocaine® Dental; Xylocaine® MPF

Brand Names: Canada Xylocard®

Index Terms Lidocaine Hydrochloride; Lignocaine Hydrochloride

Generic Availability (U.S.) Yes

Pharmacologic Category Antiarrhythmic Agent, Class Ib; Local Anesthetic

Use Local and regional anesthesia by infiltration, nerve block, epidural, or spinal techniques; acute treatment of ventricular arrhythmias from myocardial infarction or cardiac manipulation

Unlabeled Use
ACLS guidelines: Hemodynamically stable monomorphic ventricular tachycardia (VT) (preserved ventricular function); polymorphic VT (preserved ventricular function); drug-induced monomorphic VT; when amiodarone is not available, pulseless VT or ventricular fibrillation (VF) (unresponsive to defibrillation, CPR, and vasopressor administration)

PALS guidelines: When amiodarone is not available, pulseless VT or VF (unresponsive to defibrillation, CPR, and epinephrine administration); consider in patients with cocaine overdose to prevent arrhythmias secondary to MI

I.V. infusion for chronic pain syndrome

Contraindications Hypersensitivity to lidocaine or any component of the formulation; hypersensitivity to another local anesthetic of the amide type; Adam-Stokes syndrome; severe degrees of SA, AV, or intraventricular heart block (except in patients with a functioning artificial pacemaker); premixed injection may contain corn-derived dextrose and its use is contraindicated in patients with allergy to corn-related products

Warnings/Precautions Use caution in patients with severe hepatic dysfunction or pseudocholinesterase deficiency; may have increased risk of lidocaine toxicity.

Intravenous: Constant ECG monitoring is necessary during I.V. administration. Use cautiously in hepatic impairment, any degree of heart block, Wolff-Parkinson-White syndrome, HF, marked hypoxia, severe respiratory depression, hypovolemia, history of malignant hyperthermia, or shock. Increased ventricular rate may be seen when administered to a patient with atrial fibrillation. Correct electrolyte disturbances, especially hypokalemia or hypomagnesemia, prior to use and throughout therapy. Correct any underlying causes of ventricular arrhythmias. Monitor closely for signs and symptoms of CNS toxicity. The elderly may be prone to increased CNS and cardiovascular side effects. Reduce dose in hepatic dysfunction and CHF.

Injectable anesthetic: Follow appropriate administration techniques so as not to administer any intravascularly. Solutions containing antimicrobial preservatives should not be used for epidural or spinal anesthesia. Some solutions contain a bisulfite; avoid in patients who are allergic to bisulfite. Resuscitative equipment, medicine and oxygen should be available in case of emergency. Use products containing epinephrine cautiously in patients with significant vascular disease, compromised blood flow, or during or following general anesthesia (increased risk of arrhythmias). Adjust the dose for the elderly, acutely ill, and debilitated patients.

Adverse Reactions (Reflective of adult population; not specific for elderly) Effects vary with route of administration. Many effects are dose related.
Frequency not defined.

Cardiovascular: Arrhythmia, bradycardia, arterial spasms, cardiovascular collapse, defibrillator threshold increased, edema, flushing, heart block, hypotension, sinus node supression, vascular insufficiency (periarticular injections)

Central nervous system: Agitation, anxiety, apprehension, coma, confusion, disorientation, dizziness, drowsiness, euphoria, hallucinations, headache, hyperesthesia, hypoesthesia, lethargy, lightheadedness, nervousness, psychosis, seizure, slurred speech, somnolence, unconsciousness

Gastrointestinal: Metallic taste, nausea, vomiting

Local: Thrombophlebitis

Neuromuscular & skeletal: Paresthesia, transient radicular pain (subarachnoid administration; up to 1.9%), tremor, twitching, weakness

Otic: Tinnitus

Respiratory: Bronchospasm, dyspnea, respiratory depression or arrest

Miscellaneous: Allergic reactions, anaphylactoid reaction, sensitivity to temperature extremes

Following spinal anesthesia: Positional headache (3%), shivering (2%) nausea, peripheral nerve symptoms, respiratory inadequacy and double vision (<1%), hypotension, cauda equina syndrome

Drug Interactions

Metabolism/Transport Effects Substrate of CYP1A2 (major), CYP2A6 (minor), CYP2B6 (minor), CYP2C9 (minor), CYP3A4 (major); **Note:** Assignment of Major/Minor substrate status based on clinically relevant drug interaction potential; **Inhibits** CYP1A2 (weak)

Avoid Concomitant Use

Avoid concomitant use of Lidocaine (Systemic) with any of the following: Conivaptan; Saquinavir

Increased Effect/Toxicity

Lidocaine (Systemic) may increase the levels/effects of: Prilocaine

The levels/effects of Lidocaine (Systemic) may be increased by: Abiraterone Acetate; Amiodarone; Beta-Blockers; Conivaptan; CYP1A2 Inhibitors (Moderate); CYP1A2 Inhibitors (Strong); CYP3A4 Inhibitors (Moderate); CYP3A4 Inhibitors (Strong); Darunavir; Dasatinib; Deferasirox; Disopyramide; Hyaluronidase; Ivacaftor; Mifepristone; Saquinavir; Telaprevir

Decreased Effect

The levels/effects of Lidocaine (Systemic) may be decreased by: CYP1A2 Inducers (Strong); CYP3A4 Inducers (Strong); Cyproterone; Deferasirox; Etravirine; Herbs (CYP3A4 Inducers); Tocilizumab

Ethanol/Nutrition/Herb Interactions Herb/Nutraceutical: St John's wort may decrease lidocaine levels; avoid concurrent use.

Stability Injection: Stable at room temperature. Stability of parenteral admixture at room temperature (25°C) is the expiration date on premixed bag; out of overwrap stability is 30 days.

Mechanism of Action Class Ib antiarrhythmic; suppresses automaticity of conduction tissue, by increasing electrical stimulation threshold of ventricle, His-Purkinje system, and spontaneous depolarization of the ventricles during diastole by a direct action on the tissues; blocks both the initiation and conduction of nerve impulses by decreasing the neuronal membrane's permeability to sodium ions, which results in inhibition of depolarization with resultant blockade of conduction

Pharmacodynamics/Kinetics

Onset of action: Single bolus dose: 45-90 seconds

Duration: 10-20 minutes

Distribution: V_d: 1.1-2.1 L/kg; alterable by many patient factors; decreased in CHF and liver disease; crosses blood-brain barrier

Protein binding: 60% to 80% to alpha$_1$ acid glycoprotein

Metabolism: 90% hepatic; active metabolites monoethylglycinexylidide (MEGX) and glycinexylidide (GX) can accumulate and may cause CNS toxicity

Half-life elimination: Biphasic: Prolonged with congestive heart failure, liver disease, shock, severe renal disease; Initial: 7-30 minutes; Terminal: 1.5-2 hours

Excretion: Urine (<10% as unchanged drug, ~90% as metabolites)

Dosage

Geriatric & Adult

Antiarrhythmic (ACLS, 2010):

VF or pulseless VT (after defibrillation attempts, CPR, and vasopressor administration) if amiodarone is not available: I.V., intraosseous (I.O.): Initial: 1-1.5 mg/kg. If refractory VF or pulseless VT, repeat 0.5-0.75 mg/kg bolus every 5-10 minutes (maximum cumulative dose: 3 mg/kg). Follow with continuous infusion (1-4 mg/minute) after return of perfusion. Reappearance of arrhythmia during constant infusion: 0.5 mg/kg bolus and reassessment of infusion (Zipes, 2000)

◀

Endotracheal (loading dose only): 2-3.75 mg/kg (2-2.5 times the recommended I.V. dose); dilute in 5-10 mL NS or sterile water. **Note:** Absorption is greater with sterile water and results in less impairment of PaO$_2$.

Hemodynamically stable monomorphic VT: I.V.: 1-1.5 mg/kg; repeat with 0.5-0.75 mg/kg every 5-10 minutes as necessary (maximum cumulative dose: 3 mg/kg). Follow with continuous infusion of 1-4 mg/minute (or 14-57 mcg/kg/minute).

Note: Reduce maintenance infusion in patients with CHF, shock, or hepatic disease; initiate infusion at 10 mcg/kg/minute (maximum dose: 1.5 mg/minute or 20 mcg/kg/minute).

Anesthesia, local injectable: Varies with procedure, degree of anesthesia needed, vascularity of tissue, duration of anesthesia required, and physical condition of patient; maximum: 4.5 mg/kg/dose not to exceed 300 mg; do not repeat within 2 hours.

Renal Impairment Not dialyzable (0% to 5%) by hemo- or peritoneal dialysis; supplemental dose is not necessary.

Hepatic Impairment Reduce maintenance infusion. Initial: 0.75 mg/minute or 10 mcg/kg/minute; maximum dose: 1.5 mg/minute or 20 mcg/kg/minute. Monitor lidocaine concentrations closely and adjust infusion rate as necessary; consider alternative therapy.

Administration

Local infiltration: Buffered lidocaine for injectable local anesthetic may be prepared: Add 2 mL of sodium bicarbonate 8.4% to 18 mL of lidocaine 1% (Christoph, 1988)

Endotracheal (unlabeled administration route): Dilute in NS or sterile water. Absorption is greater with sterile water and results in less impairment of PaO$_2$ (Hahnel, 1990). Stop compressions, spray drug quickly down tube. Flush with 5 mL of NS and follow immediately with several quick insufflations and continue chest compressions.

Intraosseous (I.O.; unlabeled administration route): In adults, I.O. administration is a reasonable alternative when quick I.V. access is not feasible (ACLS, 2010).

Reference Range

Therapeutic: 1.5-5.0 mcg/mL (SI: 6-21 micromole/L)

Potentially toxic: >6 mcg/mL (SI: >26 micromole/L)

Toxic: >9 mcg/mL (SI: >38 micromole/L)

Special Geriatric Considerations Due to decreases in Phase I metabolism and possibly decrease in splanchnic perfusion with age, there may be a decreased clearance or increased half-life in the elderly and increased risk for CNS side effects and cardiac effects.

Dosage Forms Excipient information presented when available (limited, particularly for generics); consult specific product labeling. [DSC] = Discontinued product

Infusion, premixed in D$_5$W, as hydrochloride: 0.4% [4 mg/mL] (250 mL, 500 mL); 0.8% [8 mg/mL] (250 mL, 500 mL [DSC])

Injection, solution, as hydrochloride: 0.5% [5 mg/mL] (50 mL [DSC]); 1% [10 mg/mL] (2 mL, 10 mL, 20 mL, 30 mL, 50 mL); 2% [20 mg/mL] (2 mL, 5 mL, 20 mL, 50 mL)

Xylocaine®: 0.5% [5 mg/mL] (50 mL); 1% [10 mg/mL] (10 mL, 20 mL, 50 mL); 2% [20 mg/mL] (10 mL, 20 mL, 50 mL) [contains methylparaben]

Injection, solution, as hydrochloride [preservative free]: 0.5% [5 mg/mL] (50 mL); 1% [10 mg/mL] (2 mL, 5 mL, 30 mL); 1.5% [15 mg/mL] (20 mL); 2% [20 mg/mL] (2 mL, 5 mL, 10 mL); 4% [40 mg/mL] (5 mL)

Xylocaine®: 2% [20 mg/mL] (5 mL)

Xylocaine® MPF: 0.5% [5 mg/mL] (50 mL); 1% [10 mg/mL] (2 mL, 5 mL, 10 mL, 30 mL); 1.5% [15 mg/mL] (10 mL, 20 mL); 2% [20 mg/mL] (2 mL, 5 mL, 10 mL); 4% [40 mg/mL] (5 mL)

Injection, solution, as hydrochloride [for dental use]:

Xylocaine® Dental: 2% [20 mg/mL] (1.8 mL)

Injection, solution, premixed in D$_{7.5}$W, as hydrochloride [preservative free]: 5% [50 mg/mL] (2 mL)

Lidocaine (Topical) (LYE doe kane)

Brand Names: U.S. AneCream™ [OTC]; Anestafoam™ [OTC]; Band-Aid® Hurt Free™ Antiseptic Wash [OTC]; Burn Jel Plus [OTC]; Burn Jel® [OTC]; L-M-X® 4 [OTC]; L-M-X® 5 [OTC]; LidaMantle®; Lidoderm®; LidoPatch™ [OTC]; LTA® 360; Premjact®; RectiCare™ [OTC]; Regenecare®; Regenecare® HA [OTC]; Solarcaine® cool aloe Burn Relief [OTC]; Topicaine® [OTC]; Unburn® [OTC]; Xylocaine®

Brand Names: Canada Betacaine®; Lidodan™; Lidoderm®; Maxilene®; Xylocaine®

Index Terms Lidocaine Hydrochloride; Lidocaine Patch; Lignocaine Hydrochloride; Viscous Lidocaine; Xylocaine Viscous

Generic Availability (U.S.) Yes: Hydrochloride cream, jelly, ointment, solution

Pharmacologic Category Analgesic, Topical; Local Anesthetic

Use

Rectal: Temporary relief of pain and itching due to anorectal disorders

Topical: Local anesthetic for oral mucous membrane; use in laser/cosmetic surgeries; minor burns, cuts, and abrasions of the skin

Oral topical solution (viscous): Topical anesthesia of irritated oral mucous membranes and pharyngeal tissue

Patch (Lidoderm®): Relief of allodynia (painful hypersensitivity) and chronic pain in post-herpetic neuralgia

Patch (LidoPatch™): Temporary relief of localized pain

Dosage

Geriatric & Adult Anesthesia, topical:

Cream:

LidaMantle®: Skin irritation: Apply a thin film to affected area 2-3 times/day as needed

L-M-X® 4: Skin irritation: Apply up to 3-4 times daily to intact skin

L-M-X® 5: Relief of anorectal pain and itching: Apply to affected area up to 6 times/day

Gel, ointment: Apply to affected area ≤4 times/day as needed (maximum dose: 4.5 mg/kg, not to exceed 300 mg)

Topical solution: Apply 1-5 mL (40-200 mg) to affected area

Jelly: Maximum dose: 30 mL (600 mg) in any 12-hour period:

Anesthesia of male urethra: 5-30 mL (100-600 mg)

Anesthesia of female urethra: 3-5 mL (60-100 mg)

Oral topical solution (viscous):

Anesthesia of the mouth: 15 mL swished in the mouth and spit out no more frequently than every 3 hours (maximum: 8 doses per 24-hour period)

Anesthesia of the pharynx: 15 mL gargled no more frequently than every 3 hours (maximum: 8 doses per 24-hour period); may be swallowed

Patch:

Lidoderm®: Postherpetic neuralgia: Apply patch to most painful area. Up to 3 patches may be applied in a single application. Patch(es) may remain in place for up to 12 hours in any 24-hour period.

LidoPatch™: Pain (localized): Apply patch to painful area. Patch may remain in place for up to 12 hours in any 24-hour period. No more than 1 patch should be used in a 24-hour period.

Special Geriatric Considerations Instruct patient or caregiver on appropriate use of topical lidocaine products.

Dosage Forms Excipient information presented when available (limited, particularly for generics); consult specific product labeling. [DSC] = Discontinued product

Aerosol, foam, topical:

Anestafoam™: 4% (30 g) [contains benzalkonium chloride, benzyl alcohol]

Aerosol, spray, topical:

Solarcaine® cool aloe Burn Relief: 0.5% (127 g) [contains aloe, vitamin E]

Cream, rectal:

L-M-X® 5: 5% (15 g, 30 g) [contains benzyl alcohol]

Cream, topical:

AneCream™: 4% (5 g, 15 g, 30 g) [contains benzyl alcohol, soybean lecithin]

L-M-X® 4: 4% (5 g, 15 g, 30 g) [contains benzyl alcohol]

RectiCare™: 5% (30 g) [contains benzyl alcohol, natural rubber/natural latex in packaging, propylene glycol]

Cream, topical, as hydrochloride: 0.5% (0.9 g)

LidaMantle®: 3% (85 g)

Gel, topical:

Topicaine®: 4% (10 g, 30 g, 113 g); 5% (10 g, 30 g, 113 g) [contains aloe, benzyl alcohol, ethanol 35%, jojoba]

Gel, topical, as hydrochloride:

Burn Jel Plus: 2.5% (118 mL) [contains vitamin E]

Burn Jel®: 2% (59 mL, 118 mL); 2% (3.5 g)

Regenecare®: 2% (14 g, 85 g) [contains aloe; contains calcium alginate]

Regenecare® HA: 2% (85 g) [contains aloe; contains hyaluronic acid]

Solarcaine® cool aloe Burn Relief: 0.5% (113 g, 226 g) [contains aloe, isopropyl alcohol, menthol, tartrazine]

Unburn®: 2.5% (59 mL) [contains vitamin E]

Jelly, topical, as hydrochloride: 2% (5 mL, 30 mL)

Xylocaine®: 2% (5 mL [DSC], 30 mL [DSC])

Jelly, topical, as hydrochloride [preservative free]: 2% (5 mL, 10 mL, 20 mL)

Lotion, topical, as hydrochloride:

LidaMantle®: 3% (177 mL)

Ointment, topical: 5% (35.4 g, 50 g)

Patch, topical:
  Lidoderm®: 5% (30s)
  LidoPatch™: 3.99% (3s) [contains menthol]
Solution, topical [spray]:
  Premjact®: 9.6% (13 mL)
Solution, topical, as hydrochloride: 4% [40 mg/mL] (50 mL)
  Band-Aid® Hurt Free™ Antiseptic Wash: 2% [20 mg/mL] (177 mL) [contains aloe, benzal-
    konium chloride]
  LTA® 360: 4% [40 mg/mL] (4 mL)
  Xylocaine®: 4% [40 mg/mL] (50 mL)
Solution, topical, as hydrochloride [preservative free]: 4% [40 mg/mL] (4 mL)
Solution, viscous, oral topical, as hydrochloride: 2% [20 mg/mL] (20 mL, 100 mL)

Lidocaine and Tetracaine (LYE doe kane & TET ra kane)

Medication Safety Issues
  Other safety concerns:
    Transdermal patch may contain conducting metal (eg, aluminum); remove patch prior to
    MRI.
Brand Names: U.S. Synera®
Index Terms Eutectic Mixture of Lidocaine and Tetracaine; Tetracaine and Lidocaine
Generic Availability (U.S.) No
Pharmacologic Category Analgesic, Topical; Local Anesthetic
Use Topical anesthetic for use on normal intact skin for minor procedures (eg, I.V. cannulation
  or venipuncture) and superficial dermatologic procedures
Dosage
  Geriatric & Adult
    Venipuncture or intravenous cannulation: Transdermal patch: Prior to procedure, apply
      to intact skin for 20-30 minutes; **Note:** Adults can use another patch at a new location to
      facilitate venous access after a failed attempt; remove previous patch.
    Superficial dermatological procedures: Transdermal patch: Prior to procedure, apply to
      intact skin for 30 minutes
  Hepatic Impairment Use caution in patients with severe hepatic dysfunction.
Special Geriatric Considerations The manufacturer reports that in clinical studies there
  were no significant differences in safety between geriatric adjustments and younger subjects.
Dosage Forms Excipient information presented when available (limited, particularly for
  generics); consult specific product labeling.
  Patch, transdermal:
    Synera®: Lidocaine 70 mg and tetracaine 70 mg (10s) [contains heating component, metal;
      each patch is ~50 cm^2]

- ◆ **Lidocaine Hydrochloride** see Lidocaine (Systemic) on page 1126
- ◆ **Lidocaine Hydrochloride** see Lidocaine (Topical) on page 1128
- ◆ **Lidocaine Patch** see Lidocaine (Topical) on page 1128
- ◆ **Lidoderm®** see Lidocaine (Topical) on page 1128
- ◆ **LidoPatch™ [OTC]** see Lidocaine (Topical) on page 1128
- ◆ **Lignocaine Hydrochloride** see Lidocaine (Systemic) on page 1126
- ◆ **Lignocaine Hydrochloride** see Lidocaine (Topical) on page 1128

Linagliptin (lin a GLIP tin)

Related Information
  Diabetes Mellitus Management, Adults on page 2193
Medication Safety Issues
  High alert medication:
    The Institute for Safe Medication Practices (ISMP) includes this medication among its list of
    drug classes which have a heightened risk of causing significant patient harm when used
    in error.
Brand Names: U.S. Tradjenta™
Brand Names: Canada Trajenta™
Index Terms BI-1356; Trajenta
Pharmacologic Category Antidiabetic Agent, Dipeptidyl Peptidase IV (DPP-IV) Inhibitor
Use Management of type 2 diabetes mellitus (noninsulin dependent, NIDDM) as an adjunct to
  diet and exercise as monotherapy or in combination with other antidiabetic agents

Contraindications Hypersensitivity to linagliptin or any component of the formulation

Canadian labeling: Additional contraindications: Use in type 1 diabetes mellitus or diabetic ketoacidosis

Warnings/Precautions Avoid use in type 1 diabetes mellitus (insulin dependent, IDDM) and diabetic ketoacidosis (DKA) due to lack of efficacy in these populations. Use caution if used in conjunction with insulin or insulin secretagogues; risk of hypoglycemia is increased. Monitor blood glucose closely; dosage adjustments of insulin or insulin secretagogues may be necessary. Diabetes self-management education (DSME) is essential to maximize the effectiveness of therapy.

Adverse Reactions (Reflective of adult population; not specific for elderly)

>10%: Endocrine & metabolic: Hypoglycemia (combined with metformin/sulfonylurea [15%], metformin [<1%], pioglitazone [<1%]; monotherapy [<1%]) (Scott, 2011)

1% to 10%:

Central nervous system: Headache (6%)

Endocrine & metabolic: Hyperuricemia (3%), lipids increased (3%), triglycerides increased (2%), weight gain (2%)

Neuromuscular & skeletal: Arthralgia (6%), back pain (6%)

Respiratory: Nasopharyngitis (6%), cough (2%)

Drug Interactions

Metabolism/Transport Effects Substrate of CYP3A4 (major), P-glycoprotein; **Note:** Assignment of Major/Minor substrate status based on clinically relevant drug interaction potential

Avoid Concomitant Use There are no known interactions where it is recommended to avoid concomitant use.

Increased Effect/Toxicity

Linagliptin may increase the levels/effects of: ACE Inhibitors; Hypoglycemic Agents

The levels/effects of Linagliptin may be increased by: Herbs (Hypoglycemic Properties); MAO Inhibitors; Pegvisomant; P-glycoprotein/ABCB1 Inhibitors; Ritonavir; Salicylates; Selective Serotonin Reuptake Inhibitors

Decreased Effect

The levels/effects of Linagliptin may be decreased by: Corticosteroids (Orally Inhaled); Corticosteroids (Systemic); CYP3A4 Inducers (Strong); Deferasirox; Herbs (CYP3A4 Inducers); Loop Diuretics; Luteinizing Hormone-Releasing Hormone Analogs; P-glycoprotein/ABCB1 Inducers; Somatropin; Thiazide Diuretics; Tocilizumab

Ethanol/Nutrition/Herb Interactions

Ethanol: Caution with ethanol (may cause hypoglycemia).

Herb/Nutraceutical: Herbs with hypoglycemic properties may enhance the hypoglycemic effect of linagliptin. This includes alfalfa, aloe, bilberry, bitter melon, burdock, celery, damiana, fenugreek, garcinia, garlic, ginger, ginseng (American), gymnema, marshmallow, stinging nettle.

Stability Store at 25°C (77°F); excursions permitted between 15°C to 30°C (59°F to 86°F).

Mechanism of Action Linagliptin inhibits dipeptidyl peptidase IV (DPP-IV) enzyme resulting in prolonged active incretin levels. Incretin hormones (eg, glucagon-like peptide-1 [GLP-1] and glucose-dependent insulinotropic polypeptide [GIP]) regulate glucose homeostasis by increasing insulin synthesis and release from pancreatic beta cells and decreasing glucagon secretion from pancreatic alpha cells. Decreased glucagon secretion results in decreased hepatic glucose production. Under normal physiologic circumstances, incretin hormones are released by the intestine throughout the day and levels are increased in response to a meal; incretin hormones are rapidly inactivated by the DPP-IV enzyme.

Pharmacodynamics/Kinetics

Absorption: Rapid

Distribution: Extensive

Protein binding: 70% to 80%; concentration dependent

Metabolism: Not extensively metabolized

Bioavailability: 30%

Half-life elimination: Effective (therapeutic): ~12 hours; Terminal (DPP-IV saturable binding): >100 hours

Time to peak: 1.5 hours

Excretion: 80% feces unchanged; 5% urine unchanged

Dosage

Geriatric & Adult Type 2 diabetes: Oral: 5 mg once daily

Concomitant use with insulin and/or insulin secretagogues (eg, sulfonylureas): Reduced dose of insulin and/or insulin secretagogues may be needed.

Renal Impairment No dosage adjustment necessary. **Note:** Canadian labeling does not recommend use in severe renal impairment.

Hepatic Impairment No dosage adjustment necessary. **Note:** Canadian labeling does not recommend use in severe hepatic impairment.

Administration May be administered with or without food.

Monitoring Parameters Hb A_{1c}, serum glucose

Reference Range Recommendations for glycemic control in adults with diabetes:

Hb A_{1c}: <7%

Preprandial capillary plasma glucose: 70-130 mg/dL

Peak postprandial capillary blood glucose: <180 mg/dL

Special Geriatric Considerations According to the manufacturer, ~26% of participants in clinical trials were ≥65 years; ~3% were ≥75 years. No difference in efficacy or safety was noted between younger and older patients. Intensive glucose control (Hb A_{1c} <6.5%) has been linked to increased all-cause and cardiovascular mortality, hypoglycemia requiring assistance, and weight gain in adult type 2 diabetes. How "tightly" to control a geriatric patient's blood glucose needs to be individualized. Such a decision should be based on several factors, including the patient's functional and cognitive status, how well he/she recognizes hypoglycemic or hyperglycemic symptoms, and how to respond to them and other disease states. An Hb A_{1c} <7.5% is an acceptable endpoint for a healthy older adult, while <8% is acceptable for frail elderly patients, those with a duration of illness >10 years, or those with comorbid conditions and requiring combination diabetes medications. For elderly patients with diabetes who are relatively healthy, attaining target goals for aspirin use, blood pressure, lipids, smoking cessation, and diet and exercise may be more important than normalized glycemic control.

Dosage Forms Excipient information presented when available (limited, particularly for generics); consult specific product labeling.

Tablet, oral:

Tradjenta™: 5 mg

Linagliptin and Metformin (lin a GLIP tin & met FOR min)

Related Information

Diabetes Mellitus Management, Adults *on page 2193*

Medication Safety Issues

Sound-alike/look-alike issues:

Linagliptin and Metformin may be confused with Sitagliptin and Metformin

High alert medication:

The Institute for Safe Medication Practices (ISMP) includes this medication among its list of drug classes which have a heightened risk of causing significant patient harm when used in error.

Brand Names: U.S. Jentadueto™

Index Terms Linagliptin and Metformin Hydrochloride; Metformin and Linagliptin; Metformin Hydrochloride and Linagliptin

Generic Availability (U.S.) No

Pharmacologic Category Antidiabetic Agent, Biguanide; Antidiabetic Agent, Dipeptidyl Peptidase IV (DPP-IV) Inhibitor

Use Management of type 2 diabetes mellitus (noninsulin dependent, NIDDM) as an adjunct to diet and exercise in patients not adequately controlled on metformin or linagliptin monotherapy

Contraindications Hypersensitivity to linagliptin, metformin, or any component of the formulation; renal disease or renal dysfunction (serum creatinine ≥1.5 mg/dL [≥136 micromole/L] in males or ≥1.4 mg/dL [≥124 micromole/L] in females), or abnormal creatinine clearance which may also result from conditions such as cardiovascular collapse, acute myocardial infarction, and septicemia; acute or chronic metabolic acidosis including diabetic ketoacidosis (with or without coma).

Warnings/Precautions [U.S. Boxed Warning]: Lactic acidosis is a rare, but potentially severe consequence of therapy with metformin. Lactic acidosis should be suspected in any patient with diabetes receiving metformin with evidence of acidosis but without evidence of ketoacidosis. Discontinue metformin in clinical situations predisposing to hypoxemia, including conditions such as cardiovascular collapse, respiratory failure, acute myocardial infarction, acute heart failure, and septicemia. Not indicated for use in patients with insulin-dependent diabetes mellitus (IDDM) (type 1). Use caution in patients with heart failure requiring pharmacologic management, particularly in patients with unstable or acute heart failure; risk of lactic acidosis may be increased secondary to hypoperfusion. Avoid use in patients with impaired liver function due to potential for lactic acidosis. Patients should be instructed to avoid excessive acute or chronic ethanol use; ethanol may potentiate metformin's effect on lactate metabolism.

Metformin is substantially excreted by the kidney; patients with renal function below the limit of normal for their age should not receive therapy. In elderly patients, renal function should be monitored regularly; should not be used in any patient ≥80 years of age unless normal renal function is confirmed. The risk of accumulation and lactic acidosis increases with the degree of impairment of renal function. Use of concomitant medications that may affect renal function (eg, affect tubular secretion) may also affect metformin disposition. Concomitant use of carbonic anhydrase inhibitors may increase risk of metformin-induced lactic acidosis; use with caution. Metformin should be withheld in patients with dehydration and/or prerenal azotemia. Metformin therapy should be temporarily discontinued prior to or at the time of intravascular administration of iodinated contrast media (potential for acute alteration in renal function). Metformin should be withheld for 48 hours after the radiologic study and restarted only after renal function has been confirmed as normal. Therapy should be suspended for any surgical procedures (resume only after normal intake resumed and normal renal function is verified). It may be necessary to discontinue metformin and administer insulin if the patient is exposed to stress (eg, fever, trauma, infection, surgery). Metformin may impair vitamin B_{12} absorption; very rarely associated with anemia. Rapid reversal of vitamin B_{12} deficiency may be observed with discontinuation of therapy or supplementation; monitor vitamin B_{12} serum concentrations periodically with long-term therapy. Use with caution in conjunction with insulin or insulin secretagogues (eg, sulfonylureas); risk of hypoglycemia is increased. Monitor blood glucose closely; dosage adjustments of insulin or the secretagogue may be necessary.

Adverse Reactions (Reflective of adult population; not specific for elderly) Reactions/percentages reported with combination product; also see individual agents.

1% to 10%:
Gastrointestinal: Diarrhea (6%)
Respiratory: Nasopharyngitis (6%)
Frequency not defined:
Dermatologic: Pruritus
Gastrointestinal: Appetite decreased, nausea, pancreatitis, vomiting
Respiratory: Cough
Miscellaneous: Hypersensitivity reactions

Drug Interactions

Metabolism/Transport Effects Refer to individual components.

Avoid Concomitant Use There are no known interactions where it is recommended to avoid concomitant use.

Increased Effect/Toxicity

Linagliptin and Metformin may increase the levels/effects of: ACE Inhibitors; Dalfampridine; Dofetilide; Hypoglycemic Agents

The levels/effects of Linagliptin and Metformin may be increased by: Carbonic Anhydrase Inhibitors; Cephalexin; Cimetidine; Dalfampridine; Glycopyrrolate; Herbs (Hypoglycemic Properties); Iodinated Contrast Agents; LamoTRIgine; MAO Inhibitors; Pegvisomant; P-glycoprotein/ABCB1 Inhibitors; Ritonavir; Salicylates; Selective Serotonin Reuptake Inhibitors

Decreased Effect

Linagliptin and Metformin may decrease the levels/effects of: Trospium

The levels/effects of Linagliptin and Metformin may be decreased by: Corticosteroids (Orally Inhaled); Corticosteroids (Systemic); CYP3A4 Inducers (Strong); Deferasirox; Herbs (CYP3A4 Inducers); Loop Diuretics; Luteinizing Hormone-Releasing Hormone Analogs; P-glycoprotein/ABCB1 Inducers; Somatropin; Thiazide Diuretics; Tocilizumab

Ethanol/Nutrition/Herb Interactions Ethanol: Excessive ethanol intake (acute or chronic) may increase risks for metformin accumulation and lactic acidosis. Management: Avoid excessive ethanol intake.

Stability Store at 25°C (77°F); excursions permitted to 15°C to 30°C (59°F to 86°F).

Mechanism of Action

Linagliptin inhibits dipeptidyl peptidase IV (DPP-IV) enzymes resulting in prolonged active incretin levels. Incretin hormones [eg, glucagon-like peptide-1 (GLP-1) and glucose-dependent insulinotropic polypeptide (GIP)] regulate glucose homeostasis by increasing insulin synthesis and release from pancreatic beta cells and decreasing glucagon secretion from pancreatic alpha cells. Decreased glucagon secretion results in decreased hepatic glucose production. Under normal physiologic circumstances, incretin hormones are released by the intestine throughout the day and levels are increased in response to a meal; incretin hormones are rapidly inactivated by DPP-IV enzymes.

Metformin decreases hepatic glucose production, decreasing intestinal absorption of glucose, and improves insulin sensitivity (increases peripheral glucose uptake and utilization).

Pharmacodynamics/Kinetics See individual agents.

◄ **Dosage**

Geriatric Refer to adult dosing. The initial and maintenance dosing should be conservative, due to the potential for decreased renal function (monitor). Do not use in patients ≥80 years of age unless normal renal function has been established.

Adult Note: Patients receiving concomitant insulin and/or insulin secretagogues (eg, sulfonylureas) may require dosage adjustments of these agents.

Type 2 diabetes mellitus: Oral: Initial doses should be based on current dose of linagliptin and metformin.

Patients inadequately controlled on metformin alone: Initial dose: Linagliptin 5 mg/day plus current daily dose of metformin given in 2 equally divided doses; maximum: linagliptin 5 mg/metformin 2000 mg daily.

Patients inadequately controlled on linagliptin alone: Initial dose: Metformin 1000 mg/day plus linagliptin 5 mg/day given in 2 equally divided doses.

Dosing adjustment: Metformin component may be gradually increased up to the maximum dose. Maximum dose: Linagliptin 5 mg/metformin 2000 mg daily

Renal Impairment Use is contraindicated in patients with renal disease or renal dysfunction (serum creatinine ≥1.5 mg/dL [≥136 micromole/L] in males or ≥1.4 mg/dL [≥124 micromole/L] in females or abnormal clearance)

Hepatic Impairment Avoid metformin; liver disease is a risk factor for the development of lactic acidosis during metformin therapy.

Administration Administer with meals, at the same time each day.

Monitoring Parameters Hb A_{1c} and serum glucose; hematologic parameters (eg, hemoglobin/hematocrit, red blood cell indices) annually; hepatic function, renal function (prior to initiation of therapy then annually or more frequent if necessary); vitamin B_{12} (periodically with long-term treatment) and folate (if megaloblastic anemia is suspected)

Reference Range

Recommendations for glycemic control in adults with diabetes mellitus (ADA, 2009):

Hb A_{1c}: <7%

Preprandial capillary plasma glucose: 70-130 mg/dL

Peak postprandial capillary blood glucose: <180 mg/dL

Recommendations for glycemic control in older adults with diabetes:

Relatively healthy, cognitively intact, and with a ≥5-year life expectancy: See Adults

Frail, life expectancy <5-years or those for whom the risks of intensive glucose control outweigh the benefits:

Hb A_{1c}: <8% to 9%

Blood pressure: <140/80 mm Hg or <130/80 mm Hg if tolerated

Special Geriatric Considerations According to the manufacturer, ~26% of participants in clinical trials with **linagliptin** were ≥65 years; ~3% were ≥75 years. No difference in efficacy or safety was noted between younger and older patients. Limited data suggest that metformin's total body clearance may be decreased and AUC and half-life increased in elderly patients; presumably due to decreased renal clearance. Metformin has been well tolerated by the elderly but lower doses and frequent monitoring are recommended. In one study of elderly subjects, its effects could not be distinguished from tolbutamide, except for weight loss. The initial and maintenance dosing should be conservative, due to the potential for decreased renal function. Generally, elderly patients should not be titrated to the maximum dose of metformin. Do not use in patients ≥80 years unless normal renal function has been established. Intensive glucose control (Hb A_{1c} <6.5%) has been linked to increased all-cause and cardiovascular mortality, hypoglycemia requiring assistance, and weight gain in adult type 2 diabetes. How "tightly" to control a geriatric patient's blood glucose needs to be individualized. Such a decision should be based on several factors, including the patient's functional and cognitive status, how well he/she recognizes hypoglycemic or hyperglycemic symptoms, and how to respond to them and other disease states. An Hb A_{1c} <7.5% is an acceptable endpoint for a healthy older adult, while <8% is acceptable for frail elderly patients, those with a duration of illness >10 years, or those with comorbid conditions and requiring combination diabetes medications. For elderly patients with diabetes who are relatively healthy, attaining target goals for aspirin use, blood pressure, lipids, smoking cessation, and diet and exercise may be more important than normalized glycemic control.

Dosage Forms Excipient information presented when available (limited, particularly for generics); consult specific product labeling.

Tablet, oral:

Jentadueto™ 2.5/500: Linagliptin 2.5 mg and metformin hydrochloride 500 mg

Jentadueto™ 2.5/850: Linagliptin 2.5 mg and metformin hydrochloride 850 mg

Jentadueto™ 2.5/1000: Linagliptin 2.5 mg and metformin hydrochloride 1000 mg

◆ **Linagliptin and Metformin Hydrochloride** see Linagliptin and Metformin on page 1132

Lindane (LIN dane)

Brand Names: Canada Hexit™; PMS-Lindane

Index Terms Benzene Hexachloride; Gamma Benzene Hexachloride; Hexachlorocyclohexane

Generic Availability (U.S.) Yes

Pharmacologic Category Antiparasitic Agent, Topical; Pediculocide; Scabicidal Agent

Use Treatment of *Sarcoptes scabiei* (scabies), *Pediculus capitis* (head lice), and *Phthirus pubis* (crab lice); FDA recommends reserving lindane as a second-line agent or with inadequate response to other therapies

Medication Guide Available Yes

Contraindications Hypersensitivity to lindane or any component of the formulation; uncontrolled seizure disorders; crusted (Norwegian) scabies, acutely-inflamed skin or raw, weeping surfaces or other skin conditions which may increase systemic absorption

Warnings/Precautions [U.S. Boxed Warning]: Not considered a drug of first choice; use only in patients who have failed first-line treatments, or in patients who cannot tolerate these agents. Because of the potential for systemic absorption and CNS side effects, lindane should be used with caution; consider permethrin or crotamiton agent first. Oil-based hair dressing may increase toxic potential.

[U.S. Boxed Warning]: May be associated with severe neurologic toxicities (contraindicated in uncontrolled seizure disorders). Seizures and death have been reported with use; use with caution in patients <50 kg, or patients with a history of seizures; use caution with conditions which may increase risk of seizures or medications which decrease seizure threshold; use caution with hepatic impairment; avoid contact with face, eyes, mucous membranes, and urethral meatus.

[U.S. Boxed Warning]: A lindane medication use guide must be given to all patients along with instructions for proper use. Patients should be informed that itching may occur following successful killing of lice and re-treatment may not be indicated. Should be used as a part of an overall lice management program.

Adverse Reactions (Reflective of adult population; not specific for elderly) Frequency not defined (includes postmarketing and/or case reports).

Cardiovascular: Cardiac arrhythmia

Central nervous system: Ataxia, dizziness, headache, restlessness, seizure, pain

Dermatologic: Alopecia, contact dermatitis, skin and adipose tissue may act as repositories, eczematous eruptions, pruritus, urticaria

Gastrointestinal: Nausea, vomiting

Hematologic: Aplastic anemia

Hepatic: Hepatitis

Local: Burning and stinging

Neuromuscular & skeletal: Paresthesia

Renal: Hematuria

Respiratory: Pulmonary edema

Drug Interactions

Metabolism/Transport Effects None known.

Avoid Concomitant Use There are no known interactions where it is recommended to avoid concomitant use.

Increased Effect/Toxicity There are no known significant interactions involving an increase in effect.

Decreased Effect There are no known significant interactions involving a decrease in effect.

Mechanism of Action Directly absorbed by parasites and ova through the exoskeleton; stimulates the nervous system resulting in seizures and death of parasitic arthropods

Pharmacodynamics/Kinetics

Absorption: ≤13% systemically

Distribution: Stored in body fat; accumulates in brain; skin and adipose tissue may act as repositories

Metabolism: Hepatic

Excretion: Urine and feces

Dosage

Geriatric & Adult

Scabies: Topical: Apply a thin layer of lotion and massage it on skin from the neck to the toes; after 8-12 hours, bathe and remove the drug

Head lice, crab lice: Topical: Apply shampoo to dry hair and massage into hair for 4 minutes; add small quantities of water to hair until lather forms, then rinse hair thoroughly and comb with a fine tooth comb to remove nits. Amount of shampoo needed is based on length and density of hair; most patients will require 30 mL (maximum: 60 mL).

Administration For topical use only; never administer orally. Caregivers should apply with gloves (avoid natural latex, may be permeable to lindane). Rinse off with warm (not hot) water.

Lotion: Apply to dry, cool skin; do not apply to face or eyes. Wait at least 1 hour after bathing or showering (wet or warm skin increases absorption). Skin should be clean and free of any other lotions, creams, or oil prior to lindane application.

Shampoo: Apply to clean, dry hair. Wait at least 1 hour after washing hair before applying lindane shampoo. Hair should be washed with a shampoo not containing a conditioner; hair and skin of head and neck should be free of any lotions, oils, or creams prior to lindane application.

Special Geriatric Considerations Because of the potential for systemic absorption and CNS side effects, lindane should be used with caution. Not considered a drug of first choice; consider permethrin or crotamiton agent first.

Dosage Forms Excipient information presented when available (limited, particularly for generics); consult specific product labeling.

Lotion, topical: 1% (60 mL)

Shampoo, topical: 1% (60 mL)

Linezolid (li NE zoh lid)

Related Information

Antibiotic Treatment of Adults With Infective Endocarditis *on page 2157*
Antimicrobial Drugs of Choice *on page 2163*
Community-Acquired Pneumonia in Adults *on page 2171*

Medication Safety Issues

Sound-alike/look-alike issues:

Zyvox® may be confused with Zosyn®, Zovirax®

Brand Names: U.S. Zyvox®

Brand Names: Canada Zyvoxam®

Generic Availability (U.S.) No

Pharmacologic Category Antibiotic, Oxazolidinone

Use Treatment of vancomycin-resistant *Enterococcus faecium* (VRE) infections, nosocomial pneumonia caused by *Staphylococcus aureus* (including MRSA) or *Streptococcus pneumoniae* (including multidrug-resistant strains [MDRSP]), complicated and uncomplicated skin and skin structure infections (including diabetic foot infections without concomitant osteomyelitis), and community-acquired pneumonia caused by susceptible gram-positive organisms

Contraindications Hypersensitivity to linezolid or any other component of the formulation; concurrent use or within 2 weeks of MAO inhibitors; patients with uncontrolled hypertension, pheochromocytoma, thyrotoxicosis, and/or taking sympathomimetics (eg, pseudoephedrine), vasopressive agents (eg, epinephrine, norepinephrine), or dopaminergic agents (eg, dopamine, dobutamine) unless closely monitored for increased blood pressure; patients with carcinoid syndrome and/or taking SSRIs, tricyclic antidepressants, serotonin $5-HT_{1B,1D}$ receptor agonists, meperidine, or buspirone unless closely monitored for sign/symptoms of serotonin syndrome

Warnings/Precautions Myelosuppression has been reported and may be dependent on duration of therapy (generally >2 weeks of treatment); use with caution in patients with pre-existing myelosuppression, in patients receiving other drugs which may cause bone marrow suppression, or in chronic infection (previous or concurrent antibiotic therapy). Weekly CBC monitoring is recommended. Consider discontinuation in patients developing myelosuppression (or in whom myelosuppression worsens during treatment).

Lactic acidosis has been reported with use. Linezolid exhibits mild MAO inhibitor properties and has the potential to have the same interactions as other MAO inhibitors; use with caution and monitor closely in patients with uncontrolled hypertension, pheochromocytoma, carcinoid syndrome, or untreated hyperthyroidism; use is contraindicated in the absence of close monitoring. Symptoms of agitation, confusion, hallucinations, hyper-reflexia, myoclonus, shivering, and tachycardia may occur with concomitant proserotonergic drugs (eg, SSRIs/SNRIs or triptans) or agents which reduce linezolid's metabolism; concurrent use with these medications is contraindicated unless patient is closely monitored for signs/symptoms of serotonin syndrome. Unnecessary use may lead to the development of resistance to linezolid; consider alternatives before initiating outpatient treatment.

Peripheral and optic neuropathy (with vision loss) has been reported and may occur primarily with extended courses of therapy >28 days; any symptoms of visual change or impairment warrant immediate ophthalmic evaluation and possible discontinuation of therapy. Seizures have been reported; use with caution in patients with a history of seizures. Prolonged use may result in fungal or bacterial superinfection, including *C. difficile*-associated diarrhea (CDAD) and pseudomembranous colitis; CDAD has been observed >2 months postantibiotic treatment.

Linezolid should not be used in the empiric treatment of catheter-related bloodstream infection (CRBSI), but may be appropriate for targeted therapy (Mermel, 2009). Oral suspension contains phenylalanine.

Adverse Reactions (Reflective of adult population; not specific for elderly) Percentages as reported in adults; frequency similar in pediatric patients

>10%:
  Central nervous system: Headache (<1% to 11%)
  Gastrointestinal: Diarrhea (3% to 11%)

1% to 10%:
  Central nervous system: Insomnia (3%), dizziness (≤2%), fever (2%)
  Dermatologic: Rash (2%)
  Gastrointestinal: Nausea (3% to 10%), lipase increased (3% to 4%), vomiting (1% to 4%), constipation (2%), taste alteration (1% to 2%), amylase increased (<1% to 2%), tongue discoloration (≤1%), oral moniliasis (≤1%), pancreatitis
  Genitourinary: Vaginal moniliasis (1% to 2%)
  Hematologic: Thrombocytopenia (<1% to 10%), hemoglobin decreased (1% to 7%), leukopenia (<1% to 2%), neutropenia (≤1%)
  Hepatic: ALT increased (2% to 10%), AST increased (2% to 5%), alkaline phosphatase increased (<1% to 4%), bilirubin increased (≤1%)
  Renal: BUN increased (≤2%)
  Miscellaneous: Fungal infection (≤1% to 2%), lactate dehydrogenase increased (<1% to 2%)

Drug Interactions

Metabolism/Transport Effects Inhibits Monoamine Oxidase

Avoid Concomitant Use

Avoid concomitant use of Linezolid with any of the following: Alpha-/Beta-Agonists (Indirect-Acting); Alpha1-Agonists; Alpha2-Agonists (Ophthalmic); Amphetamines; Anilidopiperidine Opioids; Antidepressants (Serotonin Reuptake Inhibitor/Antagonist); AtoMOXetine; Bezafibrate; Buprenorphine; BuPROPion; BusPIRone; CarBAMazepine; CloZAPine; Cyclobenzaprine; Dexmethylphenidate; Dextromethorphan; Diethylpropion; HYDROmorphone; MAO Inhibitors; Maprotiline; Meperidine; Methyldopa; Methylene Blue; Methylphenidate; Mirtazapine; Oxymorphone; Pizotifen; Selective Serotonin Reuptake Inhibitors; Serotonin 5-HT1D Receptor Agonists; Serotonin/Norepinephrine Reuptake Inhibitors; Tapentadol; Tetrabenazine; Tetrahydrozoline; Tetrahydrozoline (Nasal); Tricyclic Antidepressants; Tryptophan

Increased Effect/Toxicity

Linezolid may increase the levels/effects of: Alpha-/Beta-Agonists (Direct-Acting); Alpha-/Beta-Agonists (Indirect-Acting); Alpha1-Agonists; Alpha2-Agonists (Ophthalmic); Amphetamines; Antidepressants (Serotonin Reuptake Inhibitor/Antagonist); Antihypertensives; AtoMOXetine; Beta2-Agonists; Bezafibrate; BuPROPion; CloZAPine; Dexmethylphenidate; Dextromethorphan; Diethylpropion; Doxapram; HYDROmorphone; Hypoglycemic Agents; Lithium; Meperidine; Methadone; Methyldopa; Methylene Blue; Methylphenidate; Metoclopramide; Mirtazapine; Nefazodone; Orthostatic Hypotension Producing Agents; Pizotifen; Reserpine; Selective Serotonin Reuptake Inhibitors; Serotonin 5-HT1D Receptor Agonists; Serotonin Modulators; Serotonin/Norepinephrine Reuptake Inhibitors; Sympathomimetics; Tetrahydrozoline; Tetrahydrozoline (Nasal); TraZODone; Tricyclic Antidepressants

The levels/effects of Linezolid may be increased by: Altretamine; Anilidopiperidine Opioids; Antipsychotics; Buprenorphine; BusPIRone; CarBAMazepine; COMT Inhibitors; Cyclobenzaprine; Levodopa; MAO Inhibitors; Maprotiline; Oxymorphone; Tapentadol; Tetrabenazine; TraMADol; Tryptophan

Decreased Effect There are no known significant interactions involving a decrease in effect.

Ethanol/Nutrition/Herb Interactions

Ethanol: May cause additional CNS depressant effects and provide potential source of additional tyramine content. Management: Avoid ethanol.

Food: Concurrent ingestion of foods rich in tyramine may cause sudden and severe high blood pressure (hypertensive crisis). Food's freshness is also an important concern; improperly stored or spoiled food can create an environment where tyramine concentrations may increase. Management: Avoid tyramine-containing foods with MAOIs.

Herb/Nutraceutical: Ingestion of large quantities of supplements containing caffeine, tyrosine, tryptophan, or phenylalanine may increase the risk of severe side effects (eg, hypertensive reactions, serotonin syndrome). Management: Avoid supplements containing caffeine, tyrosine, tryptophan, or phenylalanine.

Stability

Infusion: Store at 25°C (77°F); excursions permitted to 15°C to 30°C (59°F to 86°F). Protect from light. Keep infusion bags in overwrap until ready for use. Protect infusion bags from freezing.

Oral suspension: Reconstitute with 123 mL of distilled water (in 2 portions); shake vigorously. Concentration is 100 mg/5 mL. Prior to administration mix gently by inverting bottle; do not shake. Following reconstitution, store at 25°C (77°F); excursions permitted to 15°C to 30°C (59°F to 86°F). Use reconstituted suspension within 21 days. Protect from light.

Tablet: Store at 25°C (77°F); excursions permitted to 15°C to 30°C (59°F to 86°F). Protect from light; protect from moisture.

Mechanism of Action Inhibits bacterial protein synthesis by binding to bacterial 23S ribosomal RNA of the 50S subunit. This prevents the formation of a functional 70S initiation complex that is essential for the bacterial translation process. Linezolid is bacteriostatic against enterococci and staphylococci and bactericidal against most strains of streptococci.

Pharmacodynamics/Kinetics

Absorption: Rapid and extensive

Distribution: V_{dss}: Adults: 40-50 L

Protein binding: Adults: 31%

Metabolism: Hepatic via oxidation of the morpholine ring, resulting in two inactive metabolites (aminoethoxyacetic acid, hydroxyethyl glycine); minimally metabolized, may be mediated by cytochrome P450

Bioavailability: Oral: ~100%

Half-life elimination: Adults: 4-5 hours

Time to peak: Adults: Oral: 1-2 hours

Excretion: Urine (~30% of total dose as parent drug, ~50% of total dose as metabolites); feces (~9% of total dose as metabolites)

Nonrenal clearance: Adults: ~65%

Dosage

Geriatric & Adult

Usual dosage: Oral, I.V.: 600 mg every 12 hours

Indication-specific dosing:

Pneumonia:

Community-acquired pneumonia (CAP):

Manufacturer's recommendation (includes concurrent bacteremia): Oral, I.V.: 600 mg every 12 hours for 10-14 days. **Note:** May consider 7-day treatment course (versus manufacturer recommended 10-14 days) in patients with healthcare-, hospital-, and ventilator-associated pneumonia who have demonstrated good clinical response (ATS/IDSA, 2005).

Alternate recommendation (Liu, 2011): Oral, I.V.: *S. aureus* (methicillin-resistant): 600 mg every 12 hours for 7-21 days

Healthcare-associated (HA) pneumonia:

Manufacturer's recommendation: Oral, I.V.: 600 mg every 12 hours for 10-14 days.

Note: May consider 7-day treatment course (versus manufacturer recommended 10-14 days) in patients with healthcare-, hospital-, and ventilator- associated pneumonia who have demonstrated good clinical response (ATS/IDSA, 2005).

Alternate recommendations (Liu, 2011): Oral, I.V.: *S. aureus* (methicillin-resistant): 600 mg every 12 hours for 7-21 days

Skin and skin structure infections, complicated: Oral, I.V.: 600 mg every 12 hours for 10-14 days. **Note:** For diabetic foot infections, initial treatment duration is up to 4 weeks depending on severity of infection and response to therapy (Lipsky, 2012).

Skin and skin structure infections, uncomplicated: Oral: 400 mg every 12 hours for 10-14 days. **Note:** 400 mg dose is recommended in the product labeling; however, 600 mg dose is commonly employed clinically; consider 5- to 10-day treatment course as opposed to the manufacturer recommended 10-14 days (Liu, 2011; Stevens, 2005). For diabetic foot infections, may extend treatment duration up to 4 weeks if slow to resolve (Lipsky, 2012).

VRE infections including concurrent bacteremia: Oral, I.V.: 600 mg every 12 hours for 14-28 days

Brain abscess, subdural empyema, spinal epidural abscess (*S. aureus* [methicillin-resistant]) (unlabeled use; Liu, 2011): Oral, I.V.: 600 mg every 12 hours for 4-6 weeks

Meningitis (*S. aureus* [methicillin-resistant]) (unlabeled use; Liu, 2011): Oral, I.V.: 600 mg every 12 hours for 2 weeks

Osteomyelitis (*S. aureus* [methicillin-resistant]) (unlabeled use; Liu, 2011): Oral, I.V.: 600 mg every 12 hours for a minimum of 8 weeks (some experts combine with rifampin)

Septic arthritis (*S. aureus* [methicillin-resistant]) (unlabeled use; Liu, 2011): Oral, I.V.: 600 mg every 12 hours for 3-4 weeks

Septic thrombosis of cavernous or dural venous sinus (*S. aureus* [methicillin-resistant]) (unlabeled use; Liu, 2011): Oral, I.V.: 600 mg every 12 hours for 4-6 weeks

Renal Impairment No adjustment is recommended. The two primary metabolites may accumulate in patients with renal impairment but the clinical significance is unknown. Weigh the risk of accumulation of metabolites versus the benefit of therapy. Monitor for hematopoietic (eg, anemia, leukopenia, thrombocytopenia) and neuropathic (eg, peripheral neuropathy) adverse events when administering for extended periods.

Intermittent hemodialysis (administer after hemodialysis on dialysis days): Dialyzable (~30% removed during 3-hour dialysis session): If administration time is not immediately after dialysis session, may consider administration of a supplemental dose especially early in the treatment course to maintain levels above the MIC (Brier, 2003). Others have recommended no supplemental dose or dosage adjustment for patients on intermittent hemodialysis, peritoneal dialysis, or continuous renal replacement therapy (eg, CVVHD) (Heintz, 2009; Trotman, 2005).

Hepatic Impairment

Mild-to-moderate hepatic impairment (Child-Pugh class A or B): No dosage adjustment required.

Severe hepatic impairment (Child-Pugh class C): Use has not been adequately evaluated.

Administration

I.V.: Administer intravenous infusion over 30-120 minutes. Do not mix or infuse with other medications. When the same intravenous line is used for sequential infusion of other medications, flush line with D_5W, NS, or LR before and after infusing linezolid. The yellow color of the injection may intensify over time without affecting potency.

Oral suspension: Invert gently to mix prior to administration, do not shake. Administer without regard to meals.

Monitoring Parameters Weekly CBC, particularly in patients at increased risk of bleeding, with pre-existing myelosuppression, on concomitant medications that cause bone marrow suppression, in those who require >2 weeks of therapy, or in those with chronic infection who have received previous or concomitant antibiotic therapy; visual function with extended therapy (≥3 months) or in patients with new onset visual symptoms, regardless of therapy length

Special Geriatric Considerations According to the manufacturer the pharmacokinetics of linezolid are not significantly altered in patients ≥65 years of age.

Dosage Forms Excipient information presented when available (limited, particularly for generics); consult specific product labeling.

Infusion, premixed:

Zyvox®: 200 mg (100 mL); 600 mg (300 mL) [contains sodium 0.38 mg/mL]

Powder for suspension, oral:

Zyvox®: 100 mg/5 mL (150 mL) [contains phenylalanine 20 mg/5 mL, sodium 8.52 mg (0.4 mEq)/5 mL, sodium benzoate; orange flavor]

Tablet, oral:

Zyvox®: 600 mg [contains sodium 2.92 mg (0.1 mEq)/tablet]

♦ **Lioresal®** see Baclofen on page 186

Liothyronine (lye oh THYE roe neen)

Medication Safety Issues

Sound-alike/look-alike issues:

Liothyronine may be confused with levothyroxine

Other safety concerns:

T3 is an error-prone abbreviation (mistaken as acetaminophen and codeine [ie, Tylenol® #3])

Brand Names: U.S. Cytomel®; Triostat®

Brand Names: Canada Cytomel®

Index Terms Liothyronine Sodium; Sodium L-Triiodothyronine; T_3 Sodium (error-prone abbreviation)

Generic Availability (U.S.) Yes

Pharmacologic Category Thyroid Product

Use

Oral: Replacement or supplemental therapy in hypothyroidism; management of nontoxic goiter; a diagnostic aid

I.V.: Treatment of myxedema coma/precoma

Unlabeled Use Management of hemodynamically unstable potential organ donors increasing the quantity of organs available for transplantation

Contraindications Hypersensitivity to liothyronine sodium or any component of the formulation; undocumented or uncorrected adrenal insufficiency; recent myocardial infarction or thyrotoxicosis; artificial rewarming (injection)

Warnings/Precautions [U.S. Boxed Warning]: Ineffective and potentially toxic for weight reduction. High doses may produce serious or even life-threatening toxic effects particularly when used with some anorectic drugs. Use with extreme caution in patients with angina pectoris or other cardiovascular disease (including hypertension) or coronary artery disease. Use with caution in elderly patients since they may be more likely to have compromised cardiovascular function. Patients with adrenal insufficiency, myxedema, diabetes mellitus and insipidus may have symptoms exaggerated or aggravated. Thyroid replacement requires periodic assessment of thyroid status. Chronic hypothyroidism predisposes patients to coronary artery disease.

Adverse Reactions (Reflective of adult population; not specific for elderly) 1% to 10%: Cardiovascular: Arrhythmia (6%), tachycardia (3%), cardiopulmonary arrest (2%), hypotension (2%), MI (2%)

Drug Interactions

Metabolism/Transport Effects None known.

Avoid Concomitant Use

Avoid concomitant use of Liothyronine with any of the following: Sodium Iodide I131

Increased Effect/Toxicity

Liothyronine may increase the levels/effects of: Vitamin K Antagonists

Decreased Effect

Liothyronine may decrease the levels/effects of: Sodium Iodide I131; Theophylline Derivatives

The levels/effects of Liothyronine may be decreased by: Bile Acid Sequestrants; Calcium Polystyrene Sulfonate; Calcium Salts; CarBAMazepine; Estrogen Derivatives; Fosphenytoin; Lanthanum; Phenytoin; Rifampin; Sodium Polystyrene Sulfonate

Stability Vials must be stored under refrigeration at 2°C to 8°C (36°F to 46°F). Store tablets at 15°C to 30°C (59°F to 86°F).

Mechanism of Action Exact mechanism of action is unknown; however, it is believed the thyroid hormone exerts its many metabolic effects through control of DNA transcription and protein synthesis; involved in normal metabolism, growth, and development; promotes gluconeogenesis, increases utilization and mobilization of glycogen stores, and stimulates protein synthesis, increases basal metabolic rate

Pharmacodynamics/Kinetics

Onset of action: ~3 hours

Peak response: 2-3 days

Absorption: Oral: Well absorbed (95% in 4 hours)

Half-life elimination: 2.5 days

Excretion: Urine

Dosage

Geriatric Oral: 5 mcg/day; increase by 5 mcg/day every 2 weeks

Adult

Hypothyroidism: Oral: 25 mcg/day increase by 12.5-25 mcg/day every 1-2 weeks to a maximum of 100 mcg/day; usual maintenance dose: 25-75 mcg/day

Patients with cardiovascular disease: Refer to geriatric dosing.

Suppression test: (T_3): Oral: 75-100 mcg/day for 7 days; use lowest dose for elderly

Myxedema: Oral: Initial: 5 mcg/day; increase in increments of 5-10 mcg/day every 1-2 weeks. When 25 mcg/day is reached, dosage may be increased at intervals of 5-25 mcg/day every 1-2 weeks. Usual maintenance dose: 50-100 mcg/day.

Myxedema coma: I.V.: 25-50 mcg

Patients with known or suspected cardiovascular disease: 10-20 mcg

Note: Normally, at least 4 hours should be allowed between doses to adequately assess therapeutic response and no more than 12 hours should elapse between doses to avoid fluctuations in hormone levels. Oral therapy should be resumed as soon as the clinical situation has been stabilized and the patient is able to take oral medication. If levothyroxine rather than liothyronine sodium is used in initiating oral therapy, the prescriber should bear in mind that there is a delay of several days in the onset of levothyroxine activity and that I.V. therapy should be discontinued gradually.

Simple (nontoxic) goiter: Oral: Initial: 5 mcg/day; increase by 5-10 mcg every 1-2 weeks; after 25 mcg/day is reached, may increase dose by 12.5-25 mcg. Usual maintenance dose: 75 mcg/day.

Administration I.V.: For I.V. use only; **do not administer I.M. or SubQ**

Administer doses at least 4 hours, and no more than 12 hours, apart

Resume oral therapy as soon as the clinical situation has been stabilized and the patient is able to take oral medication

When switching to tablets, discontinue the injectable, initiate oral therapy at a low dosage and increase gradually according to response

If **levothyroxine** is used for oral therapy, there is a delay of several days in the onset of activity; therefore, discontinue I.V. therapy gradually

Monitoring Parameters T_3, TSH, heart rate, blood pressure, renal function, clinical signs of hypo- and hyperthyroidism; TSH is the most reliable guide for evaluating adequacy of thyroid replacement dosage. TSH may be elevated during the first few months of thyroid replacement despite patients being clinically euthyroid. In cases where T_4 remains low and TSH is within normal limits, an evaluation of "free" (unbound) T_4 is needed to evaluate further increase in dosage.

Reference Range Free T_3, serum: 250-390 pg/dL; TSH: 0.4 and up to 10 ($\geq$80 years) mIU/L

Test Interactions Many drugs may have effects on thyroid function tests (see Pharmacotherapy Pearls). Infectious hepatitis and acute intermittent porphyria may increase TBG concentrations; nephrosis, severe hypoproteinemia, severe liver disease, and acromegaly may decrease TBG concentrations.

Pharmacotherapy Pearls Equivalent doses: The following statement on relative potency of thyroid products is included in a joint statement by American Thyroid Association (ATA), American Association of Clinical Endocrinologists (AACE) and The Endocrine Society (TES): For purposes of conversion, levothyroxine sodium (T_4) 100 mcg is usually considered equivalent to desiccated thyroid 60 mg, thyroglobulin 60 mg, or liothyronine sodium (T_3) 25 mcg. However, these are rough guidelines only and do not obviate the careful re-evaluation of a patient when switching thyroid hormone preparations, including a change from one brand of levothyroxine to another. Joint position statement is available at http://www.thyroid.org/professionals/advocacy/04_12_08_thyroxine.html.

A synthetic form of *L*-Triiodothyronine (T_3) can be used in patients allergic to products derived from pork or beef.

Note: Several medications have effects on thyroid production or conversion. The impact in thyroid replacement has not been specifically evaluated, but patient response should be monitored:

Methimazole: Decreases thyroid hormone secretion, while propylthiouracil decrease thyroid hormone secretion and decreases conversion of T_4 to T_3.

Beta-adrenergic antagonists: Decrease conversion of T_4 to T_3 (dose related, propranolol $\geq$160 mg/day); patients may be clinically euthyroid.

Iodide, iodine-containing radiographic contrast agents may decrease thyroid hormone secretion; may also increase thyroid hormone secretion, especially in patients with Graves' disease.

Other agents reported to impact on thyroid production/conversion include aminoglutethimide, amiodarone, chloral hydrate, diazepam, ethionamide, interferon-alpha, interleukin-2, lithium, lovastatin (case report), glucocorticoids (dose-related), mercaptopurine, sulfonamides, thiazide diuretics, and tolbutamide.

In addition, a number of medications have been noted to cause transient depression in TSH secretion, which may complicate interpretation of monitoring tests for thyroid hormones, including corticosteroids, octreotide, and dopamine. Metoclopramide may increase TSH secretion.

Special Geriatric Considerations Elderly do not have a change in serum thyroxine associated with aging; however, plasma T_3 concentrations are decreased 25% to 40% in the elderly. There is not a compensatory rise in thyrotropin suggesting that lower T_3 is not reacted upon as a deficiency by the pituitary. This indicates a slightly lower than normal dosage of thyroid hormone replacement is usually sufficient in elderly patients than in younger adult patients. TSH must be monitored since insufficient thyroid replacement (elevated TSH) is a risk for coronary artery disease and excessive replacement (low TSH) may cause signs of hyperthyroidism and excessive bone loss.

Dosage Forms Excipient information presented when available (limited, particularly for generics); consult specific product labeling.

Injection, solution: 10 mcg/mL (1 mL)

Triostat®: 10 mcg/mL (1 mL) [contains ethanol 6.8%]

Tablet, oral: 5 mcg, 25 mcg, 50 mcg

Cytomel®: 5 mcg

Cytomel®: 25 mcg, 50 mcg [scored]

◆ **Liothyronine and Levothyroxine** see Liotrix *on page* 1142
◆ **Liothyronine Sodium** see Liothyronine *on page* 1139

Liotrix (LYE oh triks)

Medication Safety Issues
Sound-alike/look-alike issues:
Liotrix may be confused with Klotrix®
Thyrolar® may be confused with Thyrogen®
Brand Names: U.S. Thyrolar®
Brand Names: Canada Thyrolar®
Index Terms Levothyroxine and Liothyronine; Liothyronine and Levothyroxine; T_3/T_4 Liotrix
Generic Availability (U.S.) No
Pharmacologic Category Thyroid Product
Use
Replacement or supplemental therapy in hypothyroidism (uniform mixture of T_4:T_3 in 4:1 ratio by weight)
Thyroid-stimulating hormone (TSH) suppressant therapy used in the management of thyroid cancer (levothyroxine is generally recommended for this indication); prevention or treatment of euthyroid goiters (eg, thyroid nodules, subacute or chronic lymphocytic thyroiditis [Hashimoto's], multinodular goiters)
Diagnostic agent in suppression tests to diagnose suspected mild hyperthyroidism or to demonstrate thyroid gland autonomy
Contraindications Hypersensitivity to liotrix or any component of the formulation; uncorrected adrenal insufficiency; untreated thyrotoxicosis
Warnings/Precautions [U.S. Boxed Warning]: In euthyroid patients, thyroid supplements are ineffective and potentially toxic for weight reduction (unapproved use); high doses may produce serious or even life-threatening toxic effects, particularly when used with some anorectic drugs. Use is not justified for the treatment of male or female infertility in euthyroid patients (unapproved use). Use with caution and reduce dosage in the elderly since they may be more likely to have compromised cardiovascular function and in patients with angina pectoris or other cardiovascular disease (chronic hypothyroidism predisposes patients to coronary artery disease). Suppressed TSH levels in the elderly may increase risk of atrial fibrillation and mortality secondary to cardiovascular disease (Gharib, 2010; Parle, 2001). Use with caution in patients with adrenal insufficiency, diabetes mellitus or insipidus, and myxedema; symptoms may be exaggerated or aggravated; initial dosage reduction is recommended in patients with long-standing myxedema.
Adverse Reactions (Reflective of adult population; not specific for elderly) Frequency not defined.
Cardiovascular: Blood pressure increased, cardiac arrhythmia, chest pain, palpitation, tachycardia
Central nervous system: Anxiety, ataxia, fever, headache, insomnia, nervousness
Dermatologic: Alopecia, hyperhidrosis, pruritus, urticaria
Endocrine & metabolic: Changes in menstrual cycle, increased appetite, weight loss
Gastrointestinal: Abdominal cramps, constipation, diarrhea, nausea, vomiting
Neuromuscular & skeletal: Hand tremor, myalgia, tremor
Respiratory: Dyspnea
Miscellaneous: Allergic skin reactions (rare), diaphoresis
Drug Interactions
Metabolism/Transport Effects None known.
Avoid Concomitant Use
Avoid concomitant use of Liotrix with any of the following: Sodium Iodide I131
Increased Effect/Toxicity
Liotrix may increase the levels/effects of: Vitamin K Antagonists
Decreased Effect
Liotrix may decrease the levels/effects of: Sodium Iodide I131; Theophylline Derivatives

The levels/effects of Liotrix may be decreased by: Bile Acid Sequestrants; Calcium Polystyrene Sulfonate; Calcium Salts; CarBAMazepine; Estrogen Derivatives; Fosphenytoin; Lanthanum; Phenytoin; Rifampin; Sodium Polystyrene Sulfonate
Ethanol/Nutrition/Herb Interactions Food: Management: Take once a day on an empty stomach 30-60 minutes before meals.
Stability Store at 2°C to 8°C (36°F to 46°F). Protect from light.
Mechanism of Action The primary active compound is T_3 (triiodothyronine), which may be converted from T_4 (thyroxine) and then circulates throughout the body to influence growth and maturation of various tissues. Liotrix is uniform mixture of synthetic T_4 and T_3 in 4:1 ratio; exact mechanism of action is unknown; however, it is believed the thyroid hormone exerts its many metabolic effects through control of DNA transcription and protein synthesis; involved in normal metabolism, growth, and development; promotes gluconeogenesis, increases

utilization and mobilization of glycogen stores and stimulates protein synthesis, increases basal metabolic rate

Pharmacodynamics/Kinetics

Onset of action: Liothyronine (T_3): ~3 hours

Absorption: Thyroxine (T_4): 40% to 80%; T_3: 95%

Protein binding: T_4: >99% bound to plasma proteins including thyroxine-binding globulin, thyroxine-binding prealbumin, and albumin

Metabolism: Hepatic to triiodothyronine (active); ~80% T_4 deiodinated in kidney and periphery; glucuronidation/conjugation also occurs; undergoes enterohepatic recirculation

Half-life elimination:

T_4: Euthyroid: 6-7 days; Hyperthyroid: 3-4 days; Hypothyroid: 9-10 days

T_3: 2.5 days

Time to peak, serum: T_4: 2-4 hours; T_3: 2-3 days

Excretion: Urine (major route of elimination); partially feces

Dosage

Geriatric Initial: Levothyroxine 12.5-25 mcg/Liothyronine 3.1-6.25 mcg once daily; may increase by levothyroxine 12.5 mcg/Liothyronine 3.1 mcg every 2-3 weeks

Adult Hypothyroidism: Oral: Initial: Levothyroxine 25 mcg/Liothyronine 6.25 mcg once daily; may increase by levothyroxine 12.5 mcg/Liothyronine 3.1 mcg every 2-3 weeks. A lower initial dose (levothyroxine 12.5 mcg/Liothyronine 3.1 mcg) is recommended in patients with long-standing myxedema, especially if cardiovascular impairment coexists. If angina occurs, reduce dose (usual maintenance dose: levothyroxine 50-100 mcg/Liothyronine 12.5-25 mcg)

Monitoring Parameters T_4, TSH, heart rate, blood pressure, clinical signs of hypo- and hyperthyroidism; TSH is the most reliable guide for evaluating adequacy of thyroid replacement dosage. TSH may be elevated during the first few months of thyroid replacement despite patients being clinically euthyroid. In cases where T_4 remains low and TSH is within normal limits, an evaluation of "free" (unbound) T_4 is needed to evaluate further increase in dosage.

Reference Range

TSH: Age 21-54 years: 0.4-4.2 mIU/L; Age 55-87 years: 0.5-8.9 mIU/L

T_4: 4-12 mcg/dL (SI: 51-154 nmol/L)

T_3 (RIA) (total T_3): 80-230 ng/dL (SI: 1.2-3.5 nmol/L)

T_4 free (free T_4): 0.7-1.8 ng/dL (SI: 9-23 pmol/L)

Test Interactions Many drugs may have effects on thyroid function tests: para-aminosalicylic acid, aminoglutethimide, amiodarone, barbiturates, carbamazepine, chloral hydrate, clofibrate, colestipol, corticosteroids, danazol, diazepam, estrogens, ethionamide, fluorouracil, I.V. heparin, insulin, lithium, methadone, methimazole, mitotane, nitroprusside, oxyphenbutazone, phenylbutazone, PTU, perphenazine, phenytoin, propranolol, salicylates, sulfonylureas, and thiazides

Pharmacotherapy Pearls Equivalent doses: The following statement on relative potency of thyroid products is included in a joint statement by American Thyroid Association (ATA), American Association of Clinical Endocrinologists (AACE) and The Endocrine Society (TES): For purposes of conversion, levothyroxine sodium (T_4) 100 mcg is usually considered equivalent to desiccated thyroid 60 mg, thyroglobulin 60 mg, or liothyronine sodium (T_3) 25 mcg. However, these are rough guidelines only and do not obviate the careful re-evaluation of a patient when switching thyroid hormone preparations, including a change from one brand of levothyroxine to another. Joint position statement is available at http://www.thyroid.org/professionals/advocacy/04_12_08_thyroxine.html.

Since T_3 is produced by monodeiodination of T_4 in peripheral tissues (80%) and since elderly have decreased T_3 (25% to 40%), little advantage to this product exists and cost is not justified; no advantage over synthetic levothyroxine sodium.

Special Geriatric Considerations Elderly do not have a change in serum thyroxine associated with aging; however, plasma T_3 concentrations are decreased 25% to 40% in older adults. There is not a compensatory rise in thyrotropin suggesting that lower T_3 is not reacted upon as a deficiency by the pituitary. This indicates a slightly lower than normal dosage of thyroid hormone replacement is usually sufficient in older patients than in younger adult patients. TSH must be monitored since insufficient thyroid replacement (elevated TSH) is a risk for coronary artery disease and excessive replacement (low TSH) may cause signs of hyperthyroidism and excessive bone loss.

Dosage Forms Excipient information presented when available (limited, particularly for generics); consult specific product labeling.

Tablet, oral:

Thyrolar®: 1/4 [levothyroxine sodium 12.5 mcg and liothyronine sodium 3.1 mcg]

Thyrolar®: 1/2 [levothyroxine sodium 25 mcg and liothyronine sodium 6.25 mcg]

Thyrolar®: 1 [levothyroxine sodium 50 mcg and liothyronine sodium 12.5 mcg]

Thyrolar®: 2 [levothyroxine sodium 100 mcg and liothyronine sodium 25 mcg]

Thyrolar®: 3 [levothyroxine sodium 150 mcg and liothyronine sodium 37.5 mcg]

Liraglutide (lir a GLOO tide)

Related Information
Diabetes Mellitus Management, Adults on page 2193
Medication Safety Issues
Other safety concerns:
Cross-contamination may occur if pens are shared among multiple patients. Steps should be taken to prohibit sharing of pens.
Brand Names: U.S. Victoza®
Brand Names: Canada Victoza®
Index Terms NN2211
Generic Availability (U.S.) No
Pharmacologic Category Antidiabetic Agent, Glucagon-Like Peptide-1 (GLP-1) Receptor Agonist
Use Treatment of type 2 diabetes mellitus (noninsulin dependent, NIDDM) to improve glycemic control
Medication Guide Available Yes
Contraindications Hypersensitivity to liraglutide or any component of the formulation; history of or family history of medullary thyroid carcinoma (MTC); patients with multiple endocrine neoplasia syndrome type 2 (MEN2)
Warnings/Precautions [U.S. Boxed Warning] Dose and duration dependent thyroid C-cell tumors have developed in animal studies with liraglutide therapy; relevance in humans unknown. During clinical studies a few cases of thyroid C-cell hyperplasia were reported. Due to the finding in animal studies, patients were monitored with serum calcitonin or thyroid ultrasound during clinical trials; however it us unknown if this is beneficial in decreasing the risk of thyroid tumors. Consultation with an endocrinologist is recommended in patients who develop elevated calcitonin concentrations. Patients should be counseled on the risk and symptoms of thyroid tumors. Use is contraindicated in patients with or a family history of medullary thyroid cancer and in patients with multiple endocrine neoplasia syndrome type 2 (MEN2). Serious hypersensitivity reactions, including anaphylactic reactions and angioedema, have been reported with use; discontinue therapy in the event of a hypersensitivity reaction. Use with caution in patients with a history of angioedema to other GLP-1 receptor agonists (angioedema has been reported with other GLP-1 receptor agonists); potential for cross-sensitivity is unknown. Cases of acute and chronic pancreatitis (including one case of fatal necrotizing pancreatitis) have been reported although conclusive evidence to liraglutide therapy has not been established; monitor for unexplained severe abdominal pain, and if pancreatitis is suspected, discontinue use. Do not resume unless an alternative etiology of pancreatitis is confirmed. Use with caution in patients with a history of pancreatitis, cholelithiasis, and/or alcohol abuse. Most common reactions are gastrointestinal related; these symptoms may be dose-related and may decrease in frequency/severity with gradual titration and continued use. Slows gastric emptying; has not been studied in patients with pre-existing gastroparesis. Use may be associated with weight loss (likely due to reduced intake) independent of the change in hemoglobin A_{1c}. Use with caution in patients with hepatic impairment. Use with caution in renal impairment, particularly during initiation of therapy and dose escalation; cases of acute renal failure and chronic renal failure exacerbation have been reported; some cases have been reported in patients with no known pre-existing renal disease.

Concomitant use of an insulin secretagogue (eg, sulfonylurea, meglitinide) or insulin may increase the risk of hypoglycemia; dosage reduction of secretagogues or insulin may be required. Concurrent use with prandial insulin therapy has not been evaluated. Due to its effects on gastric emptying, liraglutide may reduce the rate and extent of absorption of orally-administered drugs; use with caution in patients receiving medications with a narrow therapeutic window or require rapid absorption from the GI tract. Not recommended for first-line therapy; use as adjunct to diet and exercise. Do not use in patients with type 1 diabetes mellitus or for the treatment of diabetic ketoacidosis; not a substitute for insulin. Diabetes self-management education (DSME) is essential to maximize the effectiveness of therapy.

Adverse Reactions (Reflective of adult population; not specific for elderly) Incidence reported in monotherapy trials unless otherwise specified.

>10%: Gastrointestinal: Nausea (28%), diarrhea (17%), vomiting (11%)

1% to 10%:

Central nervous system: Headache (9%)

Gastrointestinal: Constipation (10%)

Hepatic: Hyperbilirubinemia (monotherapy and combination trials: 4%)

Local: Injection site reactions (monotherapy and combination trials: 2% [includes rash, erythema])

Miscellaneous: Antiliraglutide antibodies (low titers [concentrations not requiring dilution of serum]; monotherapy and combination trials: 9%), cross-reacting antiliraglutide antibodies to native GLP-1 (monotherapy: 7%; combination trials: 5%)

Drug Interactions

Metabolism/Transport Effects None known.

Avoid Concomitant Use There are no known interactions where it is recommended to avoid concomitant use.

Increased Effect/Toxicity

Liraglutide may increase the levels/effects of: Sulfonylureas

The levels/effects of Liraglutide may be increased by: Pegvisomant

Decreased Effect

The levels/effects of Liraglutide may be decreased by: Corticosteroids (Orally Inhaled); Corticosteroids (Systemic); Luteinizing Hormone-Releasing Hormone Analogs; Somatropin; Thiazide Diuretics

Ethanol/Nutrition/Herb Interactions Ethanol: Ethanol may cause hypoglycemia. Management: Avoid ethanol.

Stability Prior to initial use, store under refrigeration at 2°C to 8°C (36°F to 46°F); after initial use, may be stored in refrigerator or at room temperature of 15°C to 30°C (59°F to 86°F). Do not freeze (discard if freezing occurs). Protect from heat and light. Pen should be discarded 30 days after initial use.

Mechanism of Action Liraglutide is a long acting analog of human glucagon-like peptide-1 (GLP-1) (an incretin hormone) which increases glucose-dependent insulin secretion, decreases inappropriate glucagon secretion, increases B-cell growth/replication, slows gastric emptying, and decreases food intake. Liraglutide administration results in decreases in hemoglobin A_{1c} by approximately 1%.

Pharmacodynamics/Kinetics

Distribution: V_d: SubQ: ~13 L; I.V.: 0.07 L/kg

Protein binding: >98%

Metabolism: Endogenously metabolized by dipeptidyl peptidase IV (DPP-IV) and endogenous endopeptidases (Croom, 2009); metabolism occurs slower than that seen with native GLP-1

Bioavailability: SubQ: ~55%

Half-life, elimination: ~13 hours

Time to peak, plasma: 8-12 hours

Excretion: Urine (6%, as metabolites); feces (5%, as metabolites)

Dosage

Geriatric & Adult Note: Initial dose is intended to reduce GI symptoms; does not provide effective glycemic control.

Treatment of type 2 diabetes: SubQ: Initial: 0.6 mg once daily for 1 week; then increase to 1.2 mg once daily; may increase further to 1.8 mg once daily if optimal glycemic response not achieved with 1.2 mg/day

Missed doses: In the event of a missed dose, the once daily regimen can be resumed with the next scheduled dose (an extra dose or an increase in the next dose should not be attempted); if >3 days have passed since the last liraglutide dose, reinitiate therapy at 0.6 mg/day to avoid GI symptoms and titrate according to prescriber discretion.

Renal Impairment

U.S. labeling: Mild-to-severe impairment: No dosage adjustment provided in manufacturer's labeling; however, use with caution, due to limited experience and reports of acute renal failure and exacerbation of chronic renal failure.

Canadian labeling:

Mild impairment: No dosage adjustment necessary.

Moderate-to-severe impairment: Use is not recommended.

Hepatic Impairment

U.S. labeling: Mild-to-severe impairment: No dosage adjustment provided in manufacturer's labeling; use with caution, due to limited experience.

Canadian labeling: Mild-to-severe impairment: Use is not recommended.

◀ **Administration** SubQ: Use only if clear, colorless, and free of particulate matter. Administer via injection in the upper arm, thigh, or abdomen. Administer without regard to meals or time of day. Change needle with each administration. Do not share pens between patients even if needle is changed. If using concomitantly with insulin, administer as separate injections (do **not** mix); may inject in the same body region as insulin, but not adjacent to one another.

Monitoring Parameters Plasma glucose, Hb A_{1c}

Reference Range Recommendations for glycemic control in adults with diabetes (ADA, 2012):

Hb A_{1c}: <7%

Preprandial capillary plasma glucose: 70-130 mg/dL

Peak postprandial capillary blood glucose: <180 mg/dL

Special Geriatric Considerations In clinical trials liraglutide's pharmacokinetics did not differ between younger and older participants. The manufacturer reports that the safety and efficacy of liraglutide did not differ in older diabetics. Intensive glucose control (Hb A_{1c} <6.5%) has been linked to increased all-cause and cardiovascular mortality, hypoglycemia requiring assistance, and weight gain in adult type 2 diabetes. How "tightly" to control a geriatric patient's blood glucose needs to be individualized. Such a decision should be based on several factors, including the patient's functional and cognitive status, how well he/she recognizes hypoglycemic or hyperglycemic symptoms, and how to respond to them and other disease states. An Hb A_{1c} <7.5% is an acceptable endpoint for a healthy older adult, while <8% is acceptable for frail elderly patients, those with a duration of illness >10 years, or those with comorbid conditions and requiring combination diabetes medications. For elderly patients with diabetes who are relatively healthy, attaining target goals for aspirin use, blood pressure, lipids, smoking cessation, and diet and exercise may be more important than normalized glycemic control.

Dosage Forms Excipient information presented when available (limited, particularly for generics); consult specific product labeling.

Injection, solution [rDNA origin]:

Victoza®: 6 mg/mL (3 mL) [contains propylene glycol 14 mg/3 mL; prefilled pen]

Lisinopril (lyse IN oh pril)

Related Information

Angiotensin Agents *on page 2093*

Heart Failure (Systolic) *on page 2203*

Medication Safety Issues

Sound-alike/look-alike issues:

Lisinopril may be confused with fosinopril, Lioresal®, Lipitor®, RisperDAL®

Prinivil® may be confused with Plendil®, Pravachol®, Prevacid®, PriLOSEC®, Proventil®

Zestril® may be confused with Desyrel, Restoril™, Vistaril®, Zegerid®, Zerit®, Zetia®, Zostrix®, ZyPREXA®

International issues:

Acepril [Malaysia] may be confused with Accupril which is a brand name for quinapril [U.S.]

Acepril: Brand name for lisinopril [Malaysia], but also the brand name for captopril [Great Britain]; enalapril [Hungary, Switzerland]

Brand Names: U.S. Prinivil®; Zestril®

Brand Names: Canada Apo-Lisinopril®; CO Lisinopril; Dom-Lisinopril; JAMP-Lisinopril; Mint-Lisinopril; Mylan-Lisinopril; PMS-Lisinopril; Prinivil®; PRO-Lisinopril; RAN™-Lisinopril; ratio-Lisinopril; ratio-Lisinopril P; ratio-Lisinopril Z; Riva-Lisinopril; Sandoz-Lisinopril; Teva-Lisinopril (Type P); Teva-Lisinopril (Type Z); Zestril®

Generic Availability (U.S.) Yes

Pharmacologic Category Angiotensin-Converting Enzyme (ACE) Inhibitor

Use Treatment of hypertension, either alone or in combination with other antihypertensive agents; adjunctive therapy in treatment of heart failure (afterload reduction); treatment of acute myocardial infarction within 24 hours in hemodynamically-stable patients to improve survival; treatment of left ventricular dysfunction after myocardial infarction

Contraindications Hypersensitivity to lisinopril or any component of the formulation; angioedema related to previous treatment with an ACE inhibitor; patients with idiopathic or hereditary angioedema

Warnings/Precautions Anaphylactic reactions may occur rarely with ACE inhibitors. At any time during treatment (especially following first dose), angioedema may occur rarely with ACE inhibitors; it may involve the head and neck (potentially compromising airway) or the intestine (presenting with abdominal pain). African-Americans may be at an increased risk. Prolonged frequent monitoring may be required especially if tongue, glottis, or larynx are involved as they are associated with airway obstruction. Patients with a history of airway surgery may have a higher risk of airway obstruction. Aggressive early and appropriate management is critical.

Use in patients with idiopathic or hereditary angioedema or previous angioedema associated with ACE inhibitor therapy is contraindicated. Severe anaphylactoid reactions may be seen during hemodialysis (eg, CVVHD) with high-flux dialysis membranes (eg, AN69), and rarely, during low density lipoprotein apheresis with dextran sulfate cellulose. Rare cases of anaphylactoid reactions have been reported in patients undergoing sensitization treatment with hymenoptera (bee, wasp) venom while receiving ACE inhibitors.

Symptomatic hypotension with or without syncope can occur with ACE inhibitors (usually with the first several doses); effects are most often observed in volume depleted patients; correct volume depletion prior to initiation; close monitoring of patient is required especially with initial dosing and dosing increases; blood pressure must be lowered at a rate appropriate for the patient's clinical condition. Initiation of therapy in patients with ischemic heart disease or cerebrovascular disease warrants close observation due to the potential consequences posed by falling blood pressure (eg, MI, stroke). Use with caution in hypertrophic cardiomyopathy with outflow tract obstruction, severe aortic stenosis, or before, during, or immediately after major surgery.

Hyperkalemia may occur with ACE inhibitors; risk factors include renal dysfunction, diabetes mellitus, concomitant use of potassium-sparing diuretics, potassium supplements, and/or potassium-containing salts. Use cautiously, if at all, with these agents and monitor potassium closely. Cough may occur with ACE inhibitors. Other causes of cough should be considered (eg, pulmonary congestion in patients with heart failure) and excluded prior to discontinuation.

May be associated with deterioration of renal function and/or increases in serum creatinine, particularly in patients with low renal blood flow (eg, renal artery stenosis, heart failure) whose glomerular filtration rate (GFR) is dependent on efferent arteriolar vasoconstriction by angiotensin II; deterioration may result in oliguria, acute renal failure, and progressive azotemia. Small increases in serum creatinine may occur following initiation; consider discontinuation only in patients with progressive and/or significant deterioration in renal function. Use with caution in patients with unstented unilateral/bilateral renal artery stenosis. When unstented bilateral renal artery stenosis is present, use is generally avoided due to the elevated risk of deterioration in renal function unless possible benefits outweigh risks. Concurrent use of angiotensin receptor blockers may increase the risk of clinically-significant adverse events (eg, renal dysfunction, hyperkalemia).

Rare toxicities associated with ACE inhibitors include cholestatic jaundice (which may progress to fulminant hepatic necrosis), agranulocytosis, neutropenia, or leukopenia with myeloid hypoplasia. Patients with collagen vascular diseases (especially with concomitant renal impairment) or renal impairment alone may be at increased risk for hematologic toxicity; periodically monitor CBC with differential in these patients.

Adverse Reactions (Reflective of adult population; not specific for elderly) Note: Frequency ranges include data from hypertension and heart failure trials. Higher rates of adverse reactions have generally been noted in patients with heart failure. However, the frequency of adverse effects associated with placebo is also increased in this population.

1% to 10%:
Cardiovascular: Orthostatic effects (1%), hypotension (1% to 4%)
Central nervous system: Headache (4% to 6%), dizziness (5% to 12%), fatigue (3%)
Dermatologic: Rash (1% to 2%)
Endocrine & metabolic: Hyperkalemia (2% to 5%)
Gastrointestinal: Diarrhea (3% to 4%), nausea (2%), vomiting (1%), abdominal pain (2%)
Genitourinary: Impotence (1%)
Hematologic: Decreased hemoglobin (small)
Neuromuscular & skeletal: Chest pain (3%), weakness (1%)
Renal: BUN increased (2%); deterioration in renal function (in patients with bilateral renal artery stenosis or hypovolemia); serum creatinine increased (often transient)
Respiratory: Cough (4% to 9%), upper respiratory infection (1% to 2%)

Drug Interactions

Metabolism/Transport Effects None known.

Avoid Concomitant Use There are no known interactions where it is recommended to avoid concomitant use.

Increased Effect/Toxicity
Lisinopril may increase the levels/effects of: Allopurinol; Amifostine; Antihypertensives; AzaTHIOprine; CycloSPORINE; CycloSPORINE (Systemic); Ferric Gluconate; Gold Sodium Thiomalate; Hypotensive Agents; Iron Dextran Complex; Lithium; Nonsteroidal Anti-Inflammatory Agents; RiTUXimab; Sodium Phosphates

◀ *The levels/effects of Lisinopril may be increased by:* Alfuzosin; Aliskiren; Angiotensin II Receptor Blockers; Diazoxide; DPP-IV Inhibitors; Eplerenone; Everolimus; Herbs (Hypotensive Properties); Loop Diuretics; MAO Inhibitors; Pentoxifylline; Phosphodiesterase 5 Inhibitors; Potassium Salts; Potassium-Sparing Diuretics; Prostacyclin Analogues; Sirolimus; Temsirolimus; Thiazide Diuretics; TiZANidine; Tolvaptan; Trimethoprim

Decreased Effect

The levels/effects of Lisinopril may be decreased by: Antacids; Aprotinin; Herbs (Hypertensive Properties); Icatibant; Lanthanum; Methylphenidate; Nonsteroidal Anti-Inflammatory Agents; Salicylates; Yohimbine

Ethanol/Nutrition/Herb Interactions

Food: Potassium supplements and/or potassium-containing salts may cause or worsen hyperkalemia. Management: Consult prescriber before consuming a potassium-rich diet, potassium supplements, or salt substitutes.

Herb/Nutraceutical: Some herbal medications may worsen hypertension (eg, licorice); others may increase the antihypertensive effect of lisinopril (eg, shepherd's purse). Management: Avoid bayberry, blue cohosh, cayenne, ephedra, ginger, ginseng (American), kola, licorice, and yohimbe. Avoid black cohosh, California poppy, coleus, golden seal, hawthorn, mistletoe, periwinkle, quinine, and shepherd's purse.

Mechanism of Action Competitive inhibitor of angiotensin-converting enzyme (ACE); prevents conversion of angiotensin I to angiotensin II, a potent vasoconstrictor; results in lower levels of angiotensin II which causes an increase in plasma renin activity and a reduction in aldosterone secretion; a CNS mechanism may also be involved in hypotensive effect as angiotensin II increases adrenergic outflow from CNS; vasoactive kallikreins may be decreased in conversion to active hormones by ACE inhibitors, thus reducing blood pressure

Pharmacodynamics/Kinetics

Onset of action: 1 hour
 Peak effect: Hypotensive: Oral: ~6 hours
Duration: 24 hours
Absorption: Well absorbed; unaffected by food
Protein binding: 25%
Metabolism: Not metabolized
Bioavailability: Decreased with NYHA Class II-IV heart failure
Half-life elimination: 11-12 hours
Time to peak: ~7 hours
Excretion: Primarily urine (as unchanged drug)

Dosage

Geriatric Refer to adult dosing. In the management of hypertension, consider lower initial doses (eg, 2.5-5 mg/day) and titrate to response (Aronow, 2011).

Adult

Heart failure: Oral: Initial: 2.5-5 mg once daily; then increase by no more than 10 mg increments at intervals no less than 2 weeks to a maximum daily dose of 40 mg. Usual maintenance: 5-40 mg/day as a single dose. Target dose: 20-40 mg once daily (ACC/AHA 2009 Heart Failure Guidelines)
  Note: If patient has hyponatremia (serum sodium <130 mEq/L) or renal impairment (Cl_{cr} <30 mL/minute or creatinine >3 mg/dL), then initial dose should be 2.5 mg/day

Hypertension: Oral: Usual dosage range (JNC 7): 10-40 mg/day
 Not maintained on diuretic: Initial: 10 mg/day
 Maintained on diuretic: Initial: 5 mg/day
  Note: Antihypertensive effect may diminish toward the end of the dosing interval especially with doses of 10 mg/day. An increased dose may aid in extending the duration of antihypertensive effect. Doses up to 80 mg/day have been used, but do not appear to give greater effect.
  Patients taking diuretics should have them discontinued 2-3 days prior to initiating lisinopril if possible. Restart diuretic after blood pressure is stable if needed. If diuretic cannot be discontinued prior to therapy, begin with 5 mg with close supervision until stable blood pressure. In patients with hyponatremia (<130 mEq/L), start dose at 2.5 mg/day.

Acute myocardial infarction (within 24 hours in hemodynamically stable patients): Oral: 5 mg immediately, then 5 mg at 24 hours, 10 mg at 48 hours, and 10 mg every day thereafter for 6 weeks. Patients should continue to receive standard treatments such as thrombolytics, aspirin, and beta-blockers.

Renal Impairment Adults: Initial doses should be modified and upward titration should be cautious, based on response (maximum: 40 mg/day)
Cl_{cr} >30 mL/minute: Initial: 10 mg/day
Cl_{cr} 10-30 mL/minute: Initial: 5 mg/day
Hemodialysis: Initial: 2.5 mg/day; dialyzable (50%)

Administration Watch for hypotensive effects within 1-3 hours of first dose or new higher dose.

Monitoring Parameters BUN, serum creatinine, renal function, WBC, and potassium; if patient has collagen vascular disease and/or renal impairment, periodically monitor CBC with differential

Test Interactions May cause false-positive results in urine acetone determinations using sodium nitroprusside reagent

Special Geriatric Considerations Due to frequent decreases in glomerular filtration (also creatinine clearance) with aging, elderly patients may have exaggerated responses to ACE inhibitors. Differences in clinical response due to hepatic changes are not observed. ACE inhibitors may be preferred agents in elderly patients with congestive heart failure and diabetes mellitus. Diabetic proteinuria is reduced and insulin sensitivity is enhanced. In general, the side effect profile is favorable in the elderly and causes little or no CNS confusion. Use lowest dose recommendations initially. Many elderly may be volume depleted due to diuretic use and/or blunted thirst reflex resulting in inadequate fluid intake.

Dosage Forms Excipient information presented when available (limited, particularly for generics); consult specific product labeling.

Tablet, oral: 2.5 mg, 5 mg, 10 mg, 20 mg, 30 mg, 40 mg
  Prinivil®: 5 mg, 10 mg, 20 mg [scored]
  Zestril®: 2.5 mg
  Zestril®: 5 mg [scored]
  Zestril®: 10 mg, 20 mg, 30 mg, 40 mg

Lisinopril and Hydrochlorothiazide
(lyse IN oh pril & hye droe klor oh THYE a zide)

Related Information
Hydrochlorothiazide *on page 933*
Lisinopril *on page 1146*

Brand Names: U.S. Prinzide®; Zestoretic®

Brand Names: Canada Apo-Lisinopril®/Hctz; Mylan-Lisinopril/Hctz; Novo-Lisinopril/Hctz; Prinzide®; Sandoz-Lisinopril/Hctz; Teva-Lisinopril/Hctz (Type P); Teva-Lisinopril/Hctz (Type Z); Zestoretic®

Index Terms Hydrochlorothiazide and Lisinopril

Generic Availability (U.S.) Yes

Pharmacologic Category Angiotensin-Converting Enzyme (ACE) Inhibitor; Diuretic, Thiazide

Use Treatment of hypertension

Dosage

Geriatric & Adult Hypertension: Oral: Initial: Lisinopril 10 mg/hydrochlorothiazide 12.5 mg or lisinopril 20 mg/hydrochlorothiazide 12.5 mg with further increases of either or both components could depend on clinical response. Doses >80 mg/day lisinopril or >50 mg/day hydrochlorothiazide are not recommended.

Renal Impairment Dosage adjustments should be made with caution. Usual regimens of therapy need not be adjusted as long as patient's Cl_{cr} >30 mL/minute. In patients with more severe renal impairment, loop diuretics are preferred.

Special Geriatric Considerations See individual agents. Combination products are not recommended as first-line treatment. Use only if doses of individual agents correspond to the combination available.

Dosage Forms Excipient information presented when available (limited, particularly for generics); consult specific product labeling.

Tablet, oral: 10/12.5: Lisinopril 10 mg and hydrochlorothiazide 12.5 mg; 20/12.5: Lisinopril 20 mg and hydrochlorothiazide 12.5 mg; 20/25: Lisinopril 20 mg and hydrochlorothiazide 25 mg
  Prinzide®:
    10/12.5: Lisinopril 10 mg and hydrochlorothiazide 12.5 mg
    20/12.5: Lisinopril 20 mg and hydrochlorothiazide 12.5 mg
  Zestoretic®:
    10/12.5: Lisinopril 10 mg and hydrochlorothiazide 12.5 mg
    20/12.5: Lisinopril 20 mg and hydrochlorothiazide 12.5 mg
    20/25: Lisinopril 20 mg and hydrochlorothiazide 25 mg

◆ **Lispro Insulin** *see* Insulin Lispro *on page 1016*

Lithium (LITH ee um)

Medication Safety Issues

Sound-alike/look-alike issues:

Eskalith may be confused with Estratest

Lithium may be confused with lanthanum

Lithobid® may be confused with Levbid®, Lithostat®

Other safety concerns:

Do not confuse **mEq** (milliequivalent) with **mg** (milligram). **Note:** 300 mg lithium carbonate or citrate contain 8 mEq lithium. Dosage should be written in **mg** (milligrams) to avoid confusion.

Check prescriptions for unusually high volumes of the syrup for dosing errors.

Brand Names: U.S. Lithobid®

Brand Names: Canada Apo-Lithium® Carbonate; Apo-Lithium® Carbonate SR; Carbolith™; Duralith®; Euro-Lithium; Lithane™; Lithmax; PHL-Lithium Carbonate; PMS-Lithium Carbonate; PMS-Lithium Citrate

Index Terms Eskalith; Lithium Carbonate; Lithium Citrate

Generic Availability (U.S.) Yes

Pharmacologic Category Antimanic Agent

Use Management of bipolar disorders; treatment of mania in individuals with bipolar disorder (maintenance treatment prevents or diminishes intensity of subsequent episodes)

Unlabeled Use Potential augmenting agent for antidepressants; treatment of aggression, post-traumatic stress disorder

Contraindications Hypersensitivity to lithium or any component of the formulation; avoid use in patients with severe cardiovascular or renal disease, or with severe debilitation, dehydration, or sodium depletion

Warnings/Precautions [U.S. Boxed Warning]: Lithium toxicity is closely related to serum levels and can occur at therapeutic doses; serum lithium determinations are required to monitor therapy. Use with caution in patients with thyroid disease, mild-moderate renal impairment, or mild-moderate cardiovascular disease. Use caution in patients receiving medications which alter sodium excretion (eg, diuretics, ACE inhibitors, NSAIDs), or in patients with significant fluid loss (protracted sweating, diarrhea, or prolonged fever); temporary reduction or cessation of therapy may be warranted. Some elderly patients may be extremely sensitive to the effects of lithium, see Dosage and Reference Range. Chronic therapy results in diminished renal concentrating ability (nephrogenic DI); this is usually reversible when lithium is discontinued. Changes in renal function should be monitored, and re-evaluation of treatment may be necessary. Use caution in patients at risk of suicide (suicidal thoughts or behavior).

Use with caution in patients receiving neuroleptic medications - a syndrome resembling NMS has been associated with concurrent therapy. Lithium may impair the patient's alertness, affecting the ability to operate machinery or driving a vehicle. Neuromuscular-blocking agents should be administered with caution; the response may be prolonged.

Higher serum concentrations may be required and tolerated during an acute manic phase; however, the tolerance decreases when symptoms subside. Normal fluid and salt intake must be maintained during therapy.

Adverse Reactions (Reflective of adult population; not specific for elderly) Frequency not defined.

Cardiovascular: Cardiac arrhythmia, hypotension, sinus node dysfunction, flattened or inverted T waves (reversible), edema, bradycardia, syncope

Central nervous system: Blackout spells, coma, confusion, dizziness, dystonia, fatigue, headache, lethargy, pseudotumor cerebri, psychomotor retardation, restlessness, sedation, seizure, slowed intellectual functioning, slurred speech, stupor, tics, vertigo

Dermatologic: Dry or thinning of hair, folliculitis, alopecia, exacerbation of psoriasis, rash

Endocrine & metabolic: Euthyroid goiter and/or hypothyroidism, hyperthyroidism, hyperglycemia, diabetes insipidus

Gastrointestinal: Polydipsia, anorexia, nausea, vomiting, diarrhea, xerostomia, metallic taste, weight gain, salivary gland swelling, excessive salivation

Genitourinary: Incontinence, polyuria, glycosuria, oliguria, albuminuria

Hematologic: Leukocytosis

Neuromuscular & skeletal: Tremor, muscle hyperirritability, ataxia, choreoathetoid movements, hyperactive deep tendon reflexes, myasthenia gravis (rare)

Ocular: Nystagmus, blurred vision, transient scotoma

Miscellaneous: Coldness and painful discoloration of fingers and toes

Postmarketing and/or case reports: Drug-induced Brugada syndrome

Drug Interactions

Metabolism/Transport Effects None known.

Avoid Concomitant Use There are no known interactions where it is recommended to avoid concomitant use.

Increased Effect/Toxicity

Lithium may increase the levels/effects of: Antipsychotics; Highest Risk QTc-Prolonging Agents; Metoclopramide; Moderate Risk QTc-Prolonging Agents; Neuromuscular-Blocking Agents; Serotonin Modulators; Tricyclic Antidepressants

The levels/effects of Lithium may be increased by: ACE Inhibitors; Angiotensin II Receptor Blockers; Antipsychotics; Calcium Channel Blockers (Nondihydropyridine); CarBAMazepine; Desmopressin; Fosphenytoin; Loop Diuretics; MAO Inhibitors; Methyldopa; Mifepristone; Nonsteroidal Anti-Inflammatory Agents; Phenytoin; Potassium Iodide; Selective Serotonin Reuptake Inhibitors; Thiazide Diuretics; Topiramate

Decreased Effect

Lithium may decrease the levels/effects of: Amphetamines; Antipsychotics; Desmopressin

The levels/effects of Lithium may be decreased by: Calcitonin; Calcium Polystyrene Sulfonate; Carbonic Anhydrase Inhibitors; Loop Diuretics; Sodium Bicarbonate; Sodium Chloride; Sodium Polystyrene Sulfonate; Theophylline Derivatives

Ethanol/Nutrition/Herb Interactions Food: Limit caffeine.

Mechanism of Action Alters cation transport across cell membrane in nerve and muscle cells and influences reuptake of serotonin and/or norepinephrine; second messenger systems involving the phosphatidylinositol cycle are inhibited; postsynaptic D2 receptor supersensitivity is inhibited

Pharmacodynamics/Kinetics

Absorption: Rapid and complete

Distribution: V_d: Initial: 0.3-0.4 L/kg; V_{dss}: 0.7-1 L/kg; crosses placenta; enters breast milk at 35% to 50% the concentrations in serum; distribution is complete in 6-10 hours

CSF, liver concentrations: $1/3$ to $1/2$ of serum concentration

Erythrocyte concentration: ~$1/2$ of serum concentration

Heart, lung, kidney, muscle concentrations: Equivalent to serum concentration

Saliva concentration: 2-3 times serum concentration

Thyroid, bone, brain tissue concentrations: Increase 50% over serum concentrations

Protein binding: Not protein bound

Metabolism: Not metabolized

Bioavailability: Not affected by food; Capsule, immediate release tablet: 95% to 100%; Extended release tablet: 60% to 90%; Syrup: 100%

Half-life elimination: 18-24 hours; can increase to more than 36 hours in elderly or with renal impairment

Time to peak, serum: Immediate release: ~0.5-2 hours; extended release: 4-12 hours; syrup: 15-60 minutes

Excretion: Urine (90% to 98% as unchanged drug); sweat (4% to 5%); feces (1%)

Clearance: 80% of filtered lithium is reabsorbed in the proximal convoluted tubules; therefore, clearance approximates 20% of GFR or 20-40 mL/minute

Dosage

Geriatric Bipolar disorders: Oral: Initial: 300 mg twice daily; increase weekly in increments of 300 mg/day, monitoring levels; rarely need >900-1200 mg/day.

Adult

Bipolar disorders: Oral: 900-2400 mg/day in 3-4 divided doses or 900-1800 mg/day in two divided doses of extended release

Note: Monitor serum concentrations and clinical response (efficacy and toxicity) to determine proper dose

Renal Impairment

Cl_{cr} 10-50 mL/minute: Administer 50% to 75% of normal dose.

Cl_{cr} <10 mL/minute: Administer 25% to 50% of normal dose.

Dialyzable (50% to 100%); 4-7 times more efficient than peritoneal dialysis

Administration Administer with meals to decrease GI upset. Extended release tablets must be swallowed whole; do not crush or chew.

Monitoring Parameters Serum lithium every 4-5 days during initial therapy; draw lithium serum concentrations 12 hours postdose; renal, thyroid, and cardiovascular function; fluid status; serum electrolytes; CBC with differential, urinalysis; monitor for signs of toxicity

Reference Range Levels should be obtained twice weekly until both patient's clinical status and levels are stable then levels may be obtained every 1-3 months

Timing of serum samples: Draw trough just before next dose (8-12 hours after previous dose)

Therapeutic levels:
Acute mania: 0.6-1.2 mEq/L (SI: 0.6-1.2 mmol/L)
Protection against future episodes in most patients with bipolar disorder: 0.8-1 mEq/L (SI: 0.8-1.0 mmol/L); a higher rate of relapse is described in subjects who are maintained at <0.4 mEq/L (SI: 0.4 mmol/L)
Elderly patients can usually be maintained at lower end of therapeutic range (0.6-0.8 mEq/L)
Toxic concentration: >1.5 mEq/L (SI: >1.5 mmol/L)
Adverse effect levels:
GI complaints/tremor: 1.5-2 mEq/L
Confusion/somnolence: 2-2.5 mEq/L
Seizures/death: >2.5 mEq/L

Special Geriatric Considerations Some elderly patients may be extremely sensitive to the effects of lithium. Initial doses need to be adjusted for renal function in the elderly; thereafter, adjust doses based upon serum concentrations and response.

Dosage Forms Excipient information presented when available (limited, particularly for generics); consult specific product labeling.
Capsule, oral, as carbonate: 150 mg, 300 mg, 600 mg
Solution, oral, as citrate: 300 mg/5 mL (5 mL, 500 mL) [equivalent to amount of lithium in lithium carbonate]
Tablet, oral, as carbonate: 300 mg, 600 mg
Tablet, extended release, oral, as carbonate: 300 mg, 450 mg
Lithobid®: 300 mg

◆ **Lithium Carbonate** see Lithium on page 1150
◆ **Lithium Citrate** see Lithium on page 1150
◆ **Lithobid®** see Lithium on page 1150
◆ **Little Fevers™ [OTC]** see Acetaminophen on page 31
◆ **Little Noses® Decongestant [OTC]** see Phenylephrine (Nasal) on page 1526
◆ **Little Noses® Saline [OTC]** see Sodium Chloride on page 1787
◆ **Little Noses® Sterile Saline Nasal Mist [OTC]** see Sodium Chloride on page 1787
◆ **Little Noses® Stuffy Nose Kit [OTC]** see Sodium Chloride on page 1787
◆ **Little Phillips'® Milk of Magnesia [OTC]** see Magnesium Hydroxide on page 1177
◆ **Little Tummys® Gas Relief [OTC]** see Simethicone on page 1776
◆ **Little Tummys® Laxative [OTC]** see Senna on page 1764
◆ **Livalo®** see Pitavastatin on page 1556
◆ **Live Attenuated Influenza Vaccine** see Influenza Virus Vaccine (Live/Attenuated) on page 1001
◆ **L-methylfolate** see Methylfolate on page 1245
◆ **L-methylfolate, Methylcobalamin, and N-acetylcysteine** see Methylfolate, Methylcobalamin, and Acetylcysteine on page 1246
◆ **Locoid®** see Hydrocortisone (Topical) on page 943
◆ **Locoid Lipocream®** see Hydrocortisone (Topical) on page 943
◆ **Lodine** see Etodolac on page 729
◆ **Lodosyn®** see Carbidopa on page 291

Lodoxamide (loe DOKS a mide)

Medication Safety Issues
International issues:
Thilomide [Greece, Turkey] may be confused with Thalomid brand name for thalidomide [U.S., Canada]
Brand Names: U.S. Alomide®
Brand Names: Canada Alomide®
Index Terms Lodoxamide Tromethamine
Generic Availability (U.S.) No
Pharmacologic Category Mast Cell Stabilizer
Use Treatment of vernal keratoconjunctivitis, vernal conjunctivitis, and vernal keratitis
Dosage
Geriatric & Adult Vernal conjunctivitis, keratitis: Ophthalmic: Instill 1-2 drops in eye(s) 4 times/day for up to 3 months
Special Geriatric Considerations Evaluate the patient's or caregiver's ability to safely administer the correct dose of ophthalmic medication.
Dosage Forms Excipient information presented when available (limited, particularly for generics); consult specific product labeling.
Solution, ophthalmic [drops]:
Alomide®: 0.1% (10 mL) [contains benzalkonium chloride]

◆ **Lodoxamide Tromethamine** see Lodoxamide on page 1152

◆ **Lofibra®** *see* Fenofibrate *on page 752*
◆ **LoHist-12 [DSC]** *see* Brompheniramine *on page 226*
◆ **Lomotil®** *see* Diphenoxylate and Atropine *on page 560*

Loperamide (loe PER a mide)

Medication Safety Issues
Sound-alike/look-alike issues:
Imodium® A-D may be confused with Indocin®
Loperamide may be confused with furosemide, Lomotil®
International issues:
Indiaral [France] may be confused with Inderal and Inderal LA brand names for propranolol [U.S., Canada, and multiple international markets]
Lomotil: Brand name for loperamide [Mexico, Philippines], but also the brand name for diphenoxylate [U.S., Canada, and multiple international markets]
Lomotil [Mexico, Phillipines] may be confused with Ludiomil brand name for maprotiline [multiple international markets]

Brand Names: U.S. Anti-Diarrheal [OTC]; Diamode [OTC]; Imodium® A-D EZ Chews [OTC]; Imodium® A-D for children [OTC]; Imodium® A-D [OTC]

Brand Names: Canada Apo-Loperamide®; Diarr-Eze; Dom-Loperamide; Imodium®; Loperacap; Novo-Loperamide; PMS-Loperamine; Rhoxal-loperamide; Rho®-Loperamine; Riva-Loperamide; Sandoz-Loperamide

Index Terms Loperamide Hydrochloride

Generic Availability (U.S.) Yes: Excludes chewable tablet

Pharmacologic Category Antidiarrheal

Use Control and symptomatic relief of chronic diarrhea associated with inflammatory bowel disease and of acute nonspecific diarrhea; to reduce volume of ileostomy discharge
OTC labeling: Control of symptoms of diarrhea, including Traveler's diarrhea

Unlabeled Use Cancer treatment-induced diarrhea (eg, irinotecan induced); chronic diarrhea caused by bowel resection

Contraindications Hypersensitivity to loperamide or any component of the formulation; abdominal pain without diarrhea
Avoid use as primary therapy in acute dysentery, acute ulcerative colitis, bacterial enterocolitis, pseudomembranous colitis

Warnings/Precautions Rare cases of anaphylaxis and anaphylactic shock have been reported. Should not be used if diarrhea is accompanied by high fever or blood in stool. Concurrent fluid and electrolyte replacement is often necessary in all age groups depending upon severity of diarrhea. Should not be used when inhibition of peristalsis is undesirable or dangerous. Discontinue if constipation, abdominal pain, or ileus develop. Use caution in treatment of AIDS patients; stop therapy at the sign of abdominal distention. Cases of toxic megacolon have occurred in this population. Loperamide is a symptom-directed treatment; if an underlying diagnosis is made, other disease-specific treatment may be indicated; Use caution in patients with hepatic impairment because of reduced first-pass metabolism; monitor for signs of CNS toxicity.

OTC labeling: If diarrhea lasts longer than 2 days, patient should stop taking loperamide and consult healthcare provider.

Adverse Reactions (Reflective of adult population; not specific for elderly) 1% to 10%:
Central nervous system: Dizziness (1%)
Gastrointestinal: Constipation (2% to 5%), abdominal cramping (≤3%), nausea (≤3%)
Postmarketing and/or case reports: Abdominal distention, abdominal pain, allergic reactions, anaphylactic shock, anaphylactoid reactions, angioedema, bullous eruption (rare), drowsiness, dyspepsia, erythema multiforme (rare), fatigue, flatulence, hypersensitivity, paralytic ileus, megacolon, pruritus, rash, Stevens-Johnson syndrome (rare), toxic epidermal necrolysis (rare), toxic megacolon, urinary retention, urticaria, vomiting, xerostomia

Drug Interactions
Metabolism/Transport Effects Substrate of P-glycoprotein
Avoid Concomitant Use There are no known interactions where it is recommended to avoid concomitant use.
Increased Effect/Toxicity
The levels/effects of Loperamide may be increased by: P-glycoprotein/ABCB1 Inhibitors
Decreased Effect
The levels/effects of Loperamide may be decreased by: P-glycoprotein/ABCB1 Inducers
Stability Store at 20°C to 25°C (68°F to 77°F).

Mechanism of Action Acts directly on circular and longitudinal intestinal muscles, through the opioid receptor, to inhibit peristalsis and prolong transit time; reduces fecal volume, increases viscosity, and diminishes fluid and electrolyte loss; demonstrates antisecretory activity. Loperamide increases tone on the anal sphincter

Pharmacodynamics/Kinetics
Absorption: Poor
Distribution: Poor penetration into brain
Metabolism: Hepatic via oxidative N-demethylation
Half-life elimination: 9-14 hours
Time to peak, plasma: Liquid: 2.5 hours; Capsule: 5 hours

Dosage
Geriatric & Adult
Acute diarrhea: Oral: Initial: 4 mg, followed by 2 mg after each loose stool, up to 16 mg/day
Chronic diarrhea: Oral: Initial: Follow acute diarrhea; maintenance dose should be slowly titrated downward to minimum required to control symptoms (typically, 4-8 mg/day in divided doses)
Traveler's diarrhea: Oral: Initial: 4 mg after first loose stool, followed by 2 mg after each subsequent stool (maximum dose: 8 mg/day)
Cancer treatment-induced diarrhea (unlabeled use): Oral: 4 mg followed by 2 mg every 4 hours or after each unformed stool; Maximum 16 mg/day (Benson, 2004) **or** 4 mg followed by 2 mg every 2 hours (4 mg every 4 hours at night) until 12 hours have passed without a loose bowel movement (Sharma, 2005)
Irinotecan-induced delayed diarrhea (unlabeled use): Oral: 4 mg after first loose or frequent bowel movement, then 2 mg every 2 hours (4 mg every 4 hours at night) until 12 hours have passed without a bowel movement (Rothenberg, 1996)
Renal Impairment No dosage adjustment necessary.
Hepatic Impairment No dosage adjustment provided in manufacturer's labeling; use with caution.
Monitoring Parameters Monitor stool frequency and consistency; observe for toxicity with use more than 48 hours
Pharmacotherapy Pearls Therapy for chronic diarrhea should not exceed 10 days; if diarrhea persists longer than 48 hours for acute diarrhea, etiology should be examined
Special Geriatric Considerations Elderly are particularly sensitive to fluid and electrolyte loss. This generally results in lethargy, weakness, and confusion. Repletion and maintenance of electrolytes and water are essential in the treatment of diarrhea. Drug therapy must be limited in order to avoid toxicity with this agent.
Dosage Forms Excipient information presented when available (limited, particularly for generics); consult specific product labeling. [DSC] = Discontinued product
Caplet, oral, as hydrochloride: 2 mg
Anti-Diarrheal: 2 mg
Diamode: 2 mg
Imodium® A-D: 2 mg [scored]
Capsule, oral, as hydrochloride: 2 mg
Liquid, oral, as hydrochloride: 1 mg/5 mL (120 mL [DSC]); 1 mg/7.5 mL (120 mL)
Imodium® A-D: 1 mg/7.5 mL (240 mL) [creamy-mint flavor]
Imodium® A-D: 1 mg/7.5 mL (120 mL) [contains sodium 10 mg/30 mL, sodium benzoate; creamy-mint flavor]
Imodium® A-D for children: 1 mg/7.5 mL (120 mL) [contains sodium 16 mg/30 mL, sodium benzoate; creamy-mint flavor]
Solution, oral, as hydrochloride: 1 mg/5 mL (5 mL, 10 mL, 118 mL)
Anti-Diarrheal: 1 mg/5 mL (120 mL)
Tablet, chewable, oral:
Imodium® A-D EZ Chews: 2 mg [mint flavor]

Loperamide and Simethicone (loe PER a mide & sye METH i kone)

Related Information
Loperamide *on page* 1153
Simethicone *on page* 1776
Brand Names: U.S. Imodium® Multi-Symptom Relief [OTC]
Brand Names: Canada Imodium® Advanced Multi-Symptom
Index Terms Simethicone and Loperamide Hydrochloride
Generic Availability (U.S.) No
Pharmacologic Category Antidiarrheal; Antiflatulent
Use Control of symptoms of diarrhea and gas (bloating, pressure, and cramps)

Dosage

Geriatric & Adult Acute diarrhea: Oral: 1 caplet or tablet after first loose stool, followed by 1 caplet or tablet with each subsequent loose stool (maximum: 4 caplets or tablets/24 hours)

Special Geriatric Considerations See individual agents. Elderly are particularly sensitive to fluid and electrolyte loss. This generally results in lethargy, weakness, and confusion. Repletion and maintenance of electrolytes and water are essential in the treatment of diarrhea. Drug therapy must be limited in order to avoid toxicity with this agent. Before treating excess gas or pain due to gas accumulation, a thorough evaluation must be made to determine cause since many bowel diseases may present with flatulence and bloating.

Dosage Forms Excipient information presented when available (limited, particularly for generics); consult specific product labeling.

Caplet:
Imodium® Multi-Symptom Relief: Loperamide hydrochloride 2 mg and simethicone 125 mg [contains calcium 65 mg/caplet, sodium 4 mg/caplet]

Tablet, chewable:
Imodium® Multi-Symptom Relief: Loperamide hydrochloride 2 mg and simethicone 125 mg [contains calcium 50 mg/tablet; mint flavor]

◆ **Loperamide Hydrochloride** *see* Loperamide *on page 1153*
◆ **Lopid®** *see* Gemfibrozil *on page 869*
◆ **Lopressor®** *see* Metoprolol *on page 1263*
◆ **Lopressor HCT®** *see* Metoprolol and Hydrochlorothiazide *on page 1267*
◆ **Loprox®** *see* Ciclopirox *on page 373*
◆ **Loradamed [OTC]** *see* Loratadine *on page 1155*

Loratadine (lor AT a deen)

Related Information

Beers Criteria – Potentially Inappropriate Medications for Geriatrics *on page 2183*

Medication Safety Issues

Sound-alike/look-alike issues:
Claritin® may be confused with clarithromycin
Claritin® (loratadine) may be confused with Claritin™ Eye (ketotifen)

BEERS Criteria medication:
This drug may be potentially inappropriate for use in geriatric patients (Quality of evidence - varies based on comorbidity; Strength of recommendation - varies based on comorbidity)

Brand Names: U.S. Alavert® Allergy 24 Hour [OTC]; Alavert® Children's Allergy [OTC]; Claritin® 24 Hour Allergy [OTC]; Claritin® Children's Allergy [OTC]; Claritin® Liqui-Gels® 24 Hour Allergy [OTC]; Claritin® RediTabs® 24 Hour Allergy [OTC]; Loradamed [OTC]

Brand Names: Canada Apo-Loratadine®; Claritin®; Claritin® Kids

Index Terms Tavist ND

Generic Availability (U.S.) Yes: Excludes capsule, chewable tablet

Pharmacologic Category Histamine H_1 Antagonist; Histamine H_1 Antagonist, Second Generation; Piperidine Derivative

Use Relief of nasal and non-nasal symptoms of seasonal allergic rhinitis; treatment of chronic idiopathic urticaria

Contraindications Hypersensitivity to loratadine or any component of the formulation

Warnings/Precautions Use with caution in patients with liver or renal impairment; dosage adjustment recommended. Some products may contain phenylalanine. May be inappropriate in older adults depending on comorbidities (eg, dementia, delirium) due to its potent anticholinergic effects (Beers Criteria).

Adverse Reactions (Reflective of adult population; not specific for elderly)

Central nervous system: Headache (12% adults), somnolence (8% adults), nervousness (4% ages 6-12 years), fatigue (4% adults; 3% ages 6-12 years, 2% to 3% ages 2-5 years), malaise (2% ages 6-12 years)

Dermatologic: Rash (2% to 3% ages 2-5 years)

Gastrointestinal: Xerostomia (3% adults), stomatitis (2% to 3% ages 2-5 years), abdominal pain (2% ages 6-12 years)

Neuromuscular & skeletal: Hyperkinesia (3% ages 6-12 years)

Ocular: Conjunctivitis (2% ages 6-12 years)

Respiratory: Wheezing (4% ages 6-12 years), epistaxis (2% to 3% ages 2-5 years), pharyngitis (2% to 3% ages 2-5 years), dysphonia (2% ages 6-12 years), upper respiratory infection (2% ages 6-12 years)

Miscellaneous: Flu-like syndrome (2% to 3% ages 2-5 years), viral infection (2% to 3% ages 2-5 years)

Drug Interactions

Metabolism/Transport Effects Substrate of CYP2D6 (minor), CYP3A4 (minor), P-glyco-protein; **Note:** Assignment of Major/Minor substrate status based on clinically relevant drug interaction potential; **Inhibits** CYP2C19 (weak), CYP2C8 (weak), CYP2D6 (weak)

Avoid Concomitant Use

Avoid concomitant use of Loratadine with any of the following: Azelastine; Azelastine (Nasal); Methadone; Mirtazapine; Paraldehyde

Increased Effect/Toxicity

Loratadine may increase the levels/effects of: Alcohol (Ethyl); Anticholinergics; ARIPiprazole; Azelastine; Azelastine (Nasal); Buprenorphine; CNS Depressants; Methadone; Methotrimeprazine; Metyrosine; Mirtazapine; Paraldehyde; Selective Serotonin Reuptake Inhibitors; Zolpidem

The levels/effects of Loratadine may be increased by: Amiodarone; Droperidol; HydrOXYzine; Methotrimeprazine; P-glycoprotein/ABCB1 Inhibitors; Pramlintide

Decreased Effect

Loratadine may decrease the levels/effects of: Acetylcholinesterase Inhibitors (Central); Benzylpenicilloyl Polylysine; Betahistine; Hyaluronidase

The levels/effects of Loratadine may be decreased by: Acetylcholinesterase Inhibitors (Central); Amphetamines; Peginterferon Alfa-2b; P-glycoprotein/ABCB1 Inducers; Tocilizumab

Ethanol/Nutrition/Herb Interactions

Ethanol: May increase CNS depression; monitor for increased effects with coadministration. Caution patients about effects.

Food: Increases bioavailability and delays peak.

Herb/Nutraceutical: St John's wort may decrease loratadine levels.

Stability Store at 2°C to 25°C (36°F to 77°F).

Rapidly-disintegrating tablets: Use within 6 months of opening foil pouch, and immediately after opening individual tablet blister. Store in a dry place.

Mechanism of Action Long-acting tricyclic antihistamine with selective peripheral histamine H_1-receptor antagonistic properties

Pharmacodynamics/Kinetics

Onset of action: 1-3 hours

Peak effect: 8-12 hours

Duration: >24 hours

Absorption: Rapid

Metabolism: Extensively hepatic via CYP2D6 and 3A4 to active metabolite

Half-life elimination: 12-15 hours

Excretion: Urine (40%) and feces (40%) as metabolites

Dosage

Geriatric & Adult Seasonal allergic rhinitis, chronic idiopathic urticaria: Oral: 10 mg/day

Renal Impairment Cl_{cr} ≤30 mL/minute:

Adults: 10 mg every other day.

Hepatic Impairment Elimination half-life increases with severity of disease.

Adults: 10 mg every other day.

Administration May be administered without regard to meals.

Test Interactions May suppress the wheal and flare reactions to skin test antigens

Special Geriatric Considerations Loratadine is a nonsedating antihistamine. Because of its low incidence of side effects, it seems to be a good choice in the elderly; however, there is a wide variation in loratadine half-life reported in the elderly and this should be kept in mind when initiating dosing. Because of its OTC status, patients should be counseled on appropriate use.

This medication is considered to be potentially inappropriate in this patient population (Beers Criteria: Quality of evidence - varies based on comorbidity; Strength of recommendation - varies based on comorbidity).

Dosage Forms Excipient information presented when available (limited, particularly for generics); consult specific product labeling.

Capsule, liquid gel, oral:

Claritin® Liqui-Gels® 24 Hour Allergy: 10 mg

Solution, oral: 5 mg/5 mL (120 mL)

Syrup, oral: 5 mg/5 mL (120 mL, 240 mL)

Claritin® Children's Allergy: 5 mg/5 mL (60 mL, 120 mL) [dye free, ethanol free; contains propylene glycol, sodium benzoate; fruit flavor]

Claritin® Children's Allergy: 5 mg/5 mL (60 mL, 120 mL) [dye free, ethanol free, sugar free; contains propylene glycol, sodium 6 mg/5 mL, sodium benzoate; grape flavor]

Tablet, oral: 10 mg
Alavert® Allergy 24 Hour: 10 mg [dye free, gluten free, sucrose free]
Claritin® 24 Hour Allergy: 10 mg
Loradamed: 10 mg
Tablet, chewable, oral:
Claritin® Children's Allergy: 5 mg [contains phenylalanine 1.4 mg/tablet; grape flavor]
Tablet, orally disintegrating, oral: 10 mg
Alavert® Allergy 24 Hour: 10 mg [dye free, gluten free, sucrose free; contains phenylalanine 8.4 mg/tablet; Citrus Burst™ flavor]
Alavert® Allergy 24 Hour: 10 mg [dye free, gluten free, sucrose free; contains phenylalanine 8.4 mg/tablet; mint flavor]
Alavert® Children's Allergy: 10 mg [dye free, gluten free, sucrose free; contains phenylalanine 8.4 mg/tablet; Citrus Burst™ flavor]
Alavert® Children's Allergy: 10 mg [dye free, gluten free, sucrose free; contains phenylalanine 8.4 mg/tablet; bubblegum flavor]
Claritin® RediTabs® 24 Hour Allergy: 10 mg [mint flavor]

LORazepam (lor A ze pam)

Related Information
Anxiolytic, Sedative/Hypnotic, and Miscellaneous Benzodiazepines *on page 2106*
Beers Criteria – Potentially Inappropriate Medications for Geriatrics *on page 2183*

Medication Safety Issues
Sound-alike/look-alike issues:
LORazepam may be confused with ALPRAZolam, clonazePAM, diazepam, KlonoPIN®, Lovaza®, temazepam, zolpidem
Ativan® may be confused with Ambien®, Atarax®, Atgam®, Avitene®

BEERS Criteria medication:
This drug may be potentially inappropriate for use in geriatric patients (Quality of evidence - high; Strength of recommendation - strong).

Administration issues:
Injection dosage form contains propylene glycol. Monitor for toxicity when administering continuous lorazepam infusions.

Brand Names: U.S. Ativan®; Lorazepam Intensol™

Brand Names: Canada Apo-Lorazepam®; Ativan®; Dom-Lorazepam; Lorazepam Injection, USP; Novo-Lorazem; Nu-Loraz; PHL-Lorazepam; PMS-Lorazepam; PRO-Lorazepam

Generic Availability (U.S.) Yes

Pharmacologic Category Benzodiazepine

Use
Oral: Management of anxiety disorders or short-term (≤4 months) relief of the symptoms of anxiety, anxiety associated with depressive symptoms, or insomnia due to anxiety or transient stress
I.V.: Status epilepticus, amnesia, sedation

Unlabeled Use Ethanol detoxification; psychogenic catatonia; partial complex seizures; agitation (I.V.); antiemetic for chemotherapy; rapid tranquilization of the agitated patient

Contraindications Hypersensitivity to lorazepam or any component of the formulation (cross-sensitivity with other benzodiazepines may exist); acute narrow-angle glaucoma; sleep apnea (parenteral); intra-arterial injection of parenteral formulation; severe respiratory insufficiency (except during mechanical ventilation)

Warnings/Precautions Use with caution in elderly or debilitated patients, patients with hepatic disease (including alcoholics) or renal impairment. In older adults, benzodiazepines increase the risk of impaired cognition, delirium, falls, fractures, and motor vehicle accidents. Due to increased sensitivity in this age group, avoid use for treatment of insomnia, agitation, or delirium. (Beers Criteria). Use with caution in patients with respiratory disease (COPD or sleep apnea) or limited pulmonary reserve, or impaired gag reflex. Initial doses in elderly or debilitated patients should be at the lower end of the dosing range. May worsen hepatic encephalopathy.

Causes CNS depression (dose-related) resulting in sedation, dizziness, confusion, or ataxia which may impair physical and mental capabilities. Patients must be cautioned about performing tasks which require mental alertness (eg, operating machinery or driving). Use with caution in patients receiving other CNS depressants or psychoactive agents. Effects with other sedative drugs or ethanol may be potentiated. Benzodiazepines have been associated with falls and traumatic injury and should be used with extreme caution in patients who are at risk of these events.

Lorazepam may cause anterograde amnesia. Paradoxical reactions, including hyperactive or aggressive behavior have been reported with benzodiazepines, particularly in adolescent/ pediatric or psychiatric patients. Does not have analgesic, antidepressant, or antipsychotic properties.

Use caution in patients with depression, particularly if suicidal risk may be present. Pre-existing depression may worsen or emerge during therapy. Not recommended for use in primary depressive or psychotic disorders. Use with caution in patients with a history of drug dependence, alcoholism, or significant personality disorders. Benzodiazepines have been associated with dependence and acute withdrawal symptoms on discontinuation or reduction in dose. Acute withdrawal, including seizures, may be precipitated after administration of flumazenil to patients receiving long-term benzodiazepine therapy.

As a hypnotic agent, should be used only after evaluation of potential causes of sleep disturbance. Failure of sleep disturbance to resolve after 7-10 days may indicate psychiatric or medical illness. A worsening of insomnia or the emergence of new abnormalities of thought or behavior may represent unrecognized psychiatric or medical illness and requires immediate and careful evaluation.

Parenteral formulation of lorazepam contains polyethylene glycol which has resulted in toxicity during high-dose and/or longer-term infusions. Parenteral formulation also contains propylene glycol (PG); may be associated with dose-related toxicity and can occur ≥48 hours after initiation of lorazepam. Limited data suggest increased risk of PG accumulation at doses of ≥6 mg/hour for 48 hours or more (Nelson, 2008). Consider monitoring for signs of toxicity which may include acute renal failure, lactic acidosis, and/or osmol gap. In high-risk patients requiring higher doses/extended treatment durations, use of enteral delivery of lorazepam tablets may be beneficial (Jacobi, 2002). Also contains benzyl alcohol.

Adverse Reactions (Reflective of adult population; not specific for elderly)
>10%:
  Central nervous system: Sedation
  Respiratory: Respiratory depression
1% to 10%:
  Cardiovascular: Hypotension
  Central nervous system: Akathisia, amnesia, ataxia, confusion, depression, disorientation, dizziness, headache
  Dermatologic: Dermatitis, rash
  Gastrointestinal: Changes in appetite, nausea, weight gain/loss
  Neuromuscular & skeletal: Weakness
  Ocular: Visual disturbances
  Respiratory: Apnea, hyperventilation, nasal congestion

Drug Interactions
Metabolism/Transport Effects None known.
Avoid Concomitant Use
  Avoid concomitant use of LORazepam with any of the following: Azelastine; Azelastine (Nasal); Methadone; Mirtazapine; OLANZapine; Paraldehyde
Increased Effect/Toxicity
  LORazepam may increase the levels/effects of: Alcohol (Ethyl); Azelastine; Azelastine (Nasal); Buprenorphine; CloZAPine; CNS Depressants; Fosphenytoin; Methadone; Methotrimeprazine; Metyrosine; Mirtazapine; Paraldehyde; Phenytoin; Selective Serotonin Reuptake Inhibitors; Zolpidem

  The levels/effects of LORazepam may be increased by: Divalproex; Droperidol; HydrOXYzine; Loxapine; Methotrimeprazine; OLANZapine; Probenecid; Valproic Acid
Decreased Effect
  The levels/effects of LORazepam may be decreased by: Theophylline Derivatives; Yohimbine

Ethanol/Nutrition/Herb Interactions
Ethanol: May increase CNS depression; monitor for increased effects with coadministration. Caution patients about effects.
Herb/Nutraceutical: Avoid valerian, St John's wort, kava kava, gotu kola (may increase CNS depression).

Stability
I.V.: Intact vials should be refrigerated. Protect from light. Do not use discolored or precipitate-containing solutions. May be stored at room temperature for up to 3 months [data on file (Hospira Inc, 2010)]. Parenteral admixture is stable at room temperature (25°C) for 24 hours. Dilute I.V. dose with equal volume of compatible diluent (D₅W, NS, SWFI).
Infusion: Use 2 mg/mL injectable vial to prepare; there may be decreased stability when using 4 mg/mL vial. Dilute ≤1 mg/mL and mix in glass bottle. Precipitation may develop. Can also be administered undiluted via infusion.
Tablet: Store at room temperature.

Mechanism of Action Binds to stereospecific benzodiazepine receptors on the postsynaptic GABA neuron at several sites within the central nervous system, including the limbic system, reticular formation. Enhancement of the inhibitory effect of GABA on neuronal excitability results by increased neuronal membrane permeability to chloride ions. This shift in chloride ions results in hyperpolarization (a less excitable state) and stabilization.

Pharmacodynamics/Kinetics

Onset of action:
  Hypnosis: I.M.: 20-30 minutes
  Sedation: I.V.: 5-20 minutes
  Anticonvulsant: I.V.: 5 minutes, oral: 30-60 minutes
Duration: 6-8 hours
Absorption: Oral, I.M.: Prompt
Distribution: V_d: Adults: 1.3 L/kg
Protein binding: 85%; free fraction may be significantly higher in elderly
Metabolism: Hepatic to inactive compounds
Bioavailability: Oral: 90%
Half-life elimination: Adults: 12.9 hours; Elderly: 15.9 hours; End-stage renal disease: 32-70 hours
Time to peak: Oral: 2 hours
Excretion: Urine; feces (minimal)

Dosage

Geriatric

Anxiety, sedation, and procedural amnesia: Oral: Initial: 1-2 mg/day in divided doses; Beers Criteria: Avoid maintenance doses >3 mg/day

Other indications: Refer to adult dosing. Dose selection should generally be on the low end of the dosage range (ie, initial dose not to exceed 2 mg).

Adult

Antiemetic: Oral, I.V. (**Note:** May be administered sublingually; not a labeled route): 0.5-2 mg every 4-6 hours as needed

Anxiety, sedation, and procedural amnesia:
  Oral: 1-10 mg/day in 2-3 divided doses; usual dose: 2-6 mg/day in divided doses or 1-2 mg 1 hour before procedure
  I.M.: 0.05 mg/kg administered 2 hours before surgery (maximum: 4 mg/dose)
  I.V.: 0.044 mg/kg 15-20 minutes before surgery (usual dose: 2 mg; maximum: 4 mg/dose)

Insomnia: Oral: 2-4 mg at bedtime

Status epilepticus: I.V.: 4 mg/dose slow I.V. (maximum rate: 2 mg/minute); may repeat in 10-15 minutes; usual maximum dose: 8 mg. May be given I.M, but I.V. preferred.

Rapid tranquilization of agitated patient (unlabeled use): Oral, I.M.: 1-2 mg administered every 30-60 minutes; may be administered with an antipsychotic (eg, haloperidol) (Battaglia, 2005; De Fruyt, 2004)
  Average total dose for tranquilization: 4-8 mg

Agitation in the ICU patient (unlabeled):
  I.V.: 0.02-0.06 mg/kg every 2-6 hours or 0.01-0.1 mg/kg/hour (Jacobi, 2002)
  Dosage adjustment for lorazepam with concomitant medications: *Probenecid or valproic acid:* Reduce lorazepam dose by 50%

Alcohol withdrawal syndrome (unlabeled use): Oral: 2 mg every 6 hours for 4 doses, then 1 mg every 6 hours for 8 additional doses (Mayo-Smith, 1997)

Alcohol withdrawal delirium (unlabeled use) (Mayo-Smith, 2004):
  I.V.: 1-4 mg every 5-15 minutes until calm, then every hour as needed to maintain light somnolence
  I.M.: 1-4 mg every 30-60 minutes until calm, then every hour as needed to maintain light somnolence

Renal Impairment I.V.: Risk of propylene glycol toxicity. Monitor closely if using for prolonged periods or at high doses.

Hepatic Impairment No dose reduction necessary.

Administration

I.M.: Should be administered deep into the muscle mass
I.V.: Do not exceed 2 mg/minute or 0.05 mg/kg over 2-5 minutes; dilute I.V. dose with equal volume of compatible diluent (D_5W, NS, SWFI). Continuous infusion solutions should have an in-line filter and the solution should be checked frequently for possible precipitation. Avoid intra-arterial administration. Monitor I.V. site for extravasation.

Monitoring Parameters Respiratory and cardiovascular status, blood pressure, heart rate, symptoms of anxiety
Clinical signs of propylene glycol toxicity (for continuous high-dose and/or long duration intravenous use): Serum creatinine, BUN, serum lactate, osmol gap

Reference Range Therapeutic: 50-240 ng/mL (SI: 156-746 nmol/L)

◀ **Pharmacotherapy Pearls** Oral doses >0.09 mg/kg produced increased ataxia without increased sedative benefit vs lower doses; preferred anxiolytic when I.M. route needed. Abrupt discontinuation after sustained use (generally >10 days) may cause withdrawal symptoms.

Special Geriatric Considerations Because lorazepam is relatively short-acting with an inactive metabolite, it is a preferred agent to use in elderly patients when a benzodiazepine is indicated.

This medication is considered to be potentially inappropriate in this patient population (Beers Criteria: Quality of evidence - high; Strength of recommendation - strong).

Controlled Substance C-IV

Dosage Forms Excipient information presented when available (limited, particularly for generics); consult specific product labeling. [DSC] = Discontinued product

Injection, solution: 2 mg/mL (1 mL, 10 mL); 4 mg/mL (1 mL, 10 mL)

Ativan®: 2 mg/mL (1 mL [DSC], 10 mL [DSC]); 4 mg/mL (1 mL [DSC], 10 mL [DSC]) [contains benzyl alcohol, polyethylene glycol 400, propylene glycol]

Solution, oral [concentrate]: 2 mg/mL (30 mL)

Lorazepam Intensol™: 2 mg/mL (30 mL) [dye free, ethanol free, sugar free; contains propylene glycol]

Tablet, oral: 0.5 mg, 1 mg, 2 mg

Ativan®: 0.5 mg

Ativan®: 1 mg, 2 mg [scored]

♦ **Lorazepam Intensol™** see LORazepam on page 1157

♦ **Lorcet® 10/650** see Hydrocodone and Acetaminophen on page 937

♦ **Lorcet® Plus** see Hydrocodone and Acetaminophen on page 937

♦ **Lortab®** see Hydrocodone and Acetaminophen on page 937

♦ **Lorzone™** see Chlorzoxazone on page 364

Losartan (loe SAR tan)

Related Information
Angiotensin Agents on page 2093

Heart Failure (Systolic) on page 2203

Medication Safety Issues

Sound-alike/look-alike issues:

Cozaar® may be confused with Colace®, Coreg®, Hyzaar®, Zocor®

Losartan may be confused with valsartan

Brand Names: U.S. Cozaar®

Brand Names: Canada Apo-Losartan; CO Losartan; Cozaar®; Mylan-Losartan; PMS-Losartan; Teva-Losartan

Index Terms DuP 753; Losartan Potassium; MK594

Generic Availability (U.S.) Yes

Pharmacologic Category Angiotensin II Receptor Blocker

Use Treatment of hypertension (HTN); treatment of diabetic nephropathy in patients with type 2 diabetes mellitus (noninsulin dependent, NIDDM) and a history of hypertension; stroke risk reduction in patients with HTN and left ventricular hypertrophy (LVH)

Contraindications Hypersensitivity to losartan or any component of the formulation

Warnings/Precautions Avoid use or use a much smaller dose in patients who are volume-depleted; correct depletion first. Use with caution in patients with significant aortic/mitral stenosis. May cause hyperkalemia; avoid potassium supplementation unless specifically required by healthcare provider. May be associated with deterioration of renal function and/or increases in serum creatinine, particularly in patients with low renal blood flow (eg, renal artery stenosis, heart failure) whose glomerular filtration rate (GFR) is dependent on efferent arteriolar vasoconstriction by angiotensin II. Use caution in patients with unstented unilateral/bilateral renal artery stenosis. When unstented bilateral renal artery stenosis is present, use is generally avoided due to the elevated risk of deterioration in renal function unless possible benefits outweigh risks. Use with caution with pre-existing renal insufficiency. AUCs of losartan (not the active metabolite) are about 50% greater in patients with Cl_{cr} <30 mL/minute and are doubled in hemodialysis patients. Concurrent use of ACE inhibitors may increase the risk of clinically-significant adverse events (eg, renal dysfunction, hyperkalemia).

At any time during treatment (especially following first dose), angioedema may occur rarely; may involve the head and neck (potentially compromising airway) or the intestine (presenting with abdominal pain). Patients with idiopathic or hereditary angioedema or previous angioedema associated with ACE-inhibitor therapy may be at an increased risk. Prolonged frequent monitoring may be required, especially if tongue, glottis, or larynx are involved, as they are associated with airway obstruction. Patients with a history of airway surgery may have a higher risk of airway obstruction. Aggressive early management is critical; intramuscular (I.M.) administration of epinephrine may be necessary.

When used to reduce the risk of stroke in patients with HTN and LVH, may not be effective in African-American population. Use caution with hepatic dysfunction, dose adjustment may be needed.

Adverse Reactions (Reflective of adult population; not specific for elderly) Note: The incidence of some adverse reactions varied based on the underlying disease state. Notations are made, where applicable, for data derived from trials conducted in diabetic nephropathy and hypertensive patients, respectively.
>10%:
  Cardiovascular: Chest pain (12% diabetic nephropathy)
  Central nervous system: Fatigue (14% diabetic nephropathy)
  Endocrine: Hypoglycemia (14% diabetic nephropathy)
  Gastrointestinal: Diarrhea (2% hypertension to 15% diabetic nephropathy)
  Genitourinary: Urinary tract infection (13% diabetic nephropathy)
  Hematologic: Anemia (14% diabetic nephropathy)
  Neuromuscular & skeletal: Weakness (14% diabetic nephropathy), back pain (2% hypertension to 12% diabetic nephropathy)
  Respiratory: Cough (≤3% to 11%; similar to placebo; incidence higher in patients with previous cough related to ACE inhibitor therapy)
1% to 10%:
  Cardiovascular: Hypotension (7% diabetic nephropathy), orthostatic hypotension (4% hypertension to 4% diabetic nephropathy), first-dose hypotension (dose related: <1% with 50 mg, 2% with 100 mg)
  Central nervous system: Dizziness (4%), hypoesthesia (5% diabetic nephropathy), fever (4% diabetic nephropathy), insomnia (1%)
  Dermatology: Cellulitis (7% diabetic nephropathy)
  Endocrine: Hyperkalemia (<1% hypertension to 7% diabetic nephropathy)
  Gastrointestinal: Gastritis (5% diabetic nephropathy), weight gain (4% diabetic nephropathy), dyspepsia (1% to 4%), abdominal pain (2%), nausea (2%)
  Neuromuscular & skeletal: Muscular weakness (7% diabetic nephropathy), knee pain (5% diabetic nephropathy), leg pain (1% to 5%), muscle cramps (1%), myalgia (1%)
  Respiratory: Bronchitis (10% diabetic nephropathy), upper respiratory infection (8%), nasal congestion (2%), sinusitis (1% hypertension to 6% diabetic nephropathy)
  Miscellaneous: Infection (5% diabetic nephropathy), flu-like syndrome (10% diabetic nephropathy)

Drug Interactions
Metabolism/Transport Effects Substrate of CYP2C9 (major), CYP3A4 (major); **Note:** Assignment of Major/Minor substrate status based on clinically relevant drug interaction potential; **Inhibits** CYP1A2 (weak), CYP2C19 (weak), CYP2C8 (moderate), CYP2C9 (moderate), CYP3A4 (weak)

Avoid Concomitant Use
Avoid concomitant use of Losartan with any of the following: Pimozide

Increased Effect/Toxicity
Losartan may increase the levels/effects of: ACE Inhibitors; Amifostine; Antihypertensives; ARIPiprazole; Carvedilol; CYP2C8 Substrates; CYP2C9 Substrates; Hypoglycemic Agents; Hypotensive Agents; Lithium; Nonsteroidal Anti-Inflammatory Agents; Pimozide; Potassium-Sparing Diuretics; RiTUXimab; Sodium Phosphates

The levels/effects of Losartan may be increased by: Alfuzosin; Aliskiren; Antifungal Agents (Azole Derivatives, Systemic); CYP2C9 Inhibitors (Moderate); CYP2C9 Inhibitors (Strong); Diazoxide; Eplerenone; Fluconazole; Herbs (Hypoglycemic Properties); Herbs (Hypotensive Properties); MAO Inhibitors; Mifepristone; Milk Thistle; Pentoxifylline; Phosphodiesterase 5 Inhibitors; Potassium Salts; Prostacyclin Analogues; Salicylates; Selective Serotonin Reuptake Inhibitors; Tolvaptan; Trimethoprim

Decreased Effect
The levels/effects of Losartan may be decreased by: CYP2C9 Inducers (Strong); CYP3A4 Inducers (Strong); Deferasirox; Herbs (CYP3A4 Inducers); Herbs (Hypertensive Properties); Loop Diuretics; Methylphenidate; Nonsteroidal Anti-Inflammatory Agents; Peginterferon Alfa-2b; Rifamycin Derivatives; Tocilizumab; Yohimbine

Ethanol/Nutrition/Herb Interactions Herb/Nutraceutical: St John's wort may decrease levels of losartan. Some herbal medications may worsen hypertension (eg, licorice); others may increase the antihypertensive effect of losartan (eg, shepherd's purse). Some herbal medications may increase the hypoglycemic effects of losartan (eg, alfalfa). Management: Avoid St John's wort. Avoid bayberry, blue cohosh, ginseng (American), kola, licorice, and yohimbe. Avoid black cohosh, California poppy, coleus, golden seal, hawthorn, mistletoe, periwinkle, quinine, and shepherd's purse. Avoid alfalfa, aloe, bilberry, bitter melon, burdock, celery, damiana, fenugreek, garcinia, garlic, ginger, ginseng (American), gymnema, marsh-mallow, and stinging nettle.

Stability Store at 15°C to 30°C (59°F to 86°F). Protect from light.

Mechanism of Action As a selective and competitive, nonpeptide angiotensin II receptor antagonist, losartan blocks the vasoconstrictor and aldosterone-secreting effects of angiotensin II; losartan interacts reversibly at the AT1 and AT2 receptors of many tissues and has slow dissociation kinetics; its affinity for the AT1 receptor is 1000 times greater than the AT2 receptor. Angiotensin II receptor antagonists may induce a more complete inhibition of the renin-angiotensin system than ACE inhibitors, they do not affect the response to bradykinin, and are less likely to be associated with nonrenin-angiotensin effects (eg, cough and angioedema). Losartan increases urinary flow rate and in addition to being natriuretic and kaliuretic, increases excretion of chloride, magnesium, uric acid, calcium, and phosphate.

Pharmacodynamics/Kinetics
Onset of action: 6 hours
Distribution: V_d: Losartan: 34 L; E-3174: 12 L; does not cross blood-brain barrier
Protein binding, plasma: High
Metabolism: Hepatic (14%) via CYP2C9 and 3A4 to active metabolite, E-3174 (40 times more potent than losartan); extensive first-pass effect
Bioavailability: 25% to 33%; AUC of E-3174 is four times greater than that of losartan
Half-life elimination: Losartan: 1.5-2 hours; E-3174: 6-9 hours
Time to peak, serum: Losartan: 1 hour; E-3174: 3-4 hours
Excretion: Urine (4% as unchanged drug, 6% as active metabolite)
Clearance: Plasma: Losartan: 600 mL/minute; Active metabolite: 50 mL/minute

Dosage
Geriatric & Adult
Hypertension: Oral: Usual starting dose: 50 mg once daily; can be administered once or twice daily with total daily doses ranging from 25-100 mg
Usual initial doses in patients receiving diuretics or those with intravascular volume depletion: 25 mg once daily
Nephropathy in patients with type 2 diabetes and hypertension: Oral: Initial: 50 mg once daily; can be increased to 100 mg once daily based on blood pressure response
Stroke reduction (HTN with LVH): Oral: 50 mg once daily (maximum daily dose: 100 mg); may be used in combination with a thiazide diuretic
Renal Impairment Adults: No adjustment necessary.
Hepatic Impairment Adults: Reduce the initial dose to 25 mg/day
Administration May be administered without regard to meals.
Monitoring Parameters Supine blood pressure, electrolytes, serum creatinine, BUN, urinalysis, symptomatic hypotension and tachycardia, CBC
Special Geriatric Considerations Serum concentrations of losartan and its metabolites are not significantly different and no initial dose adjustment is necessary even in low creatinine clearance states (<30 mL/minute). Many elderly may be volume depleted due to diuretic use and/or blunted thirst reflex resulting in inadequate fluid intake.
Dosage Forms Excipient information presented when available (limited, particularly for generics); consult specific product labeling.
Tablet, oral, as potassium: 25 mg, 50 mg, 100 mg
Cozaar®: 25 mg [contains potassium 2.12 mg (0.054 mEq)]
Cozaar®: 50 mg [contains potassium 4.24 mg (0.108 mEq)]
Cozaar®: 100 mg [contains potassium 8.48 mg (0.216 mEq)]
Extemporaneously Prepared To prepare losartan suspension, combine 10 mL of purified water and ten (10) losartan 50 mg tablets in an 8 ounce bottle. Shake well for ≥2 minutes. Allow concentrate to stand for 1 hour then shake for 1 minute. Separately, prepare 190 mL of a 50/50 mixture of Ora-Plus™ and Ora-Sweet SF™. Add to tablet and water mixture; shake for 1 minute. Resulting 200 mL suspension will contain losartan 2.5 mg/mL. Store under refrigeration for up to 4 weeks; shake well before use.

Losartan and Hydrochlorothiazide (loe SAR tan & hye droe klor oh THYE a zide)

Related Information
Hydrochlorothiazide on page 933
Losartan on page 1160
Medication Safety Issues
Sound-alike/look-alike issues:
Hyzaar® may be confused with Cozaar®
Brand Names: U.S. Hyzaar®
Brand Names: Canada Apo-Losartan/HCTZ; Hyzaar®; Hyzaar® DS; Mylan-Losartan/HCTZ; Teva-Losartan/HCTZ

Index Terms Hydrochlorothiazide and Losartan
Generic Availability (U.S.) Yes
Pharmacologic Category Angiotensin II Receptor Blocker; Diuretic, Thiazide
Use Treatment of hypertension; stroke risk reduction in patients with HTN and left ventricular hypertrophy (LVH)
Dosage
  Geriatric Refer to dosing in individual monographs.
  Adult Note: Dose is individualized (combination substituted for individual components); dose may be titrated after 2-4 weeks of therapy
    Hypertension/stroke reduction in hypertension (with LVH): Usual recommended starting dose of losartan: 50 mg once daily when used as monotherapy in patients who are not volume depleted
  Renal Impairment Cl$_{cr}$ ≤30 mL/minute: Use of combination formulation is not recommended.
  Hepatic Impairment Use is not recommended.
Special Geriatric Considerations See individual agents. Combination products are not recommended as first-line treatment. Use only if doses of individual agents correspond to the combination available.
Dosage Forms Excipient information presented when available (limited, particularly for generics); consult specific product labeling.
  Tablet: 50/12.5: Losartan potassium 50 mg and hydrochlorothiazide 12.5 mg; 100/12.5: Losartan potassium 100 mg and hydrochlorothiazide 12.5 mg; 100/25: Losartan potassium 100 mg and hydrochlorothiazide 25 mg
    Hyzaar® 50/12.5: Losartan potassium 50 mg and hydrochlorothiazide 12.5 mg [contains potassium 4.24 mg (0.108 mEq)]
    Hyzaar® 100/12.5: Losartan potassium 100 mg and hydrochlorothiazide 12.5 mg [contains potassium 8.48 mg (0.216 mEq)]
    Hyzaar® 100/25: Losartan potassium 100 mg and hydrochlorothiazide 25 mg [contains potassium 8.48 mg (0.216 mEq)]

◆ **Losartan Potassium** *see Losartan on page 1160*
◆ **Lotemax®** *see Loteprednol on page 1163*
◆ **Lotensin®** *see Benazepril on page 197*
◆ **Lotensin HCT®** *see Benazepril and Hydrochlorothiazide on page 199*

Loteprednol (loe te PRED nol)

Brand Names: U.S. Alrex®; Lotemax®
Brand Names: Canada Alrex®; Lotemax®
Index Terms Loteprednol Etabonate
Generic Availability (U.S.) No
Pharmacologic Category Corticosteroid, Ophthalmic
Use
  Ointment, 0.5% (Lotemax®): Treatment of postoperative inflammation and pain following ocular surgery
  Suspension, 0.2% (Alrex®): Temporary relief of signs and symptoms of seasonal allergic conjunctivitis
  Suspension, 0.5% (Lotemax®): Inflammatory conditions (treatment of steroid-responsive inflammatory conditions of the palpebral and bulbar conjunctiva, cornea, and anterior segment of the globe such as allergic conjunctivitis, acne rosacea, superficial punctate keratitis, herpes zoster keratitis, iritis, cyclitis, selected infective conjunctivitis, when the inherent hazard of steroid use is accepted to obtain an advisable diminution in edema and inflammation) and treatment of postoperative inflammation following ocular surgery
Dosage
  Geriatric & Adult
    Seasonal allergic conjunctivitis: Ophthalmic: 0.2% suspension (Alrex®): Instill 1 drop into affected eye(s) 4 times/day.
    Inflammatory conditions: Ophthalmic: 0.5% suspension (Lotemax®): Apply 1-2 drops into the conjunctival sac of the affected eye(s) 4 times/day. During the initial treatment within the first week, the dosing may be increased up to 1 drop every hour. Advise patients not to discontinue therapy prematurely. If signs and symptoms fail to improve after 2 days, re-evaluate the patient.
    Postoperative inflammation: Ophthalmic:
      Ointment, 0.5% (Lotemax®): Apply ~1/2 inch ribbon into the conjunctival sac of the affected eye(s) 4 times/day beginning 24 hours after surgery and continuing throughout the first 2 weeks of the postoperative period

Suspension, 0.5% (Lotemax®): Apply 1-2 drops into the conjunctival sac of the operated eye(s) 4 times/day beginning 24 hours after surgery and continuing throughout the first 2 weeks of the postoperative period.

Special Geriatric Considerations Evaluate the patient's or caregiver's ability to safely administer the correct dose of ophthalmic medication.

Product Availability
Lotemax® 0.5% ointment: FDA approved April 2011; expected availability undetermined
Lotemax® 0.5% ointment is a topical corticosteroid approved for the treatment of postoperative inflammation and pain following ocular surgery.

Dosage Forms Excipient information presented when available (limited, particularly for generics); consult specific product labeling. [DSC] = Discontinued product
Ointment, ophthalmic, as etabonate:
Lotemax®: 0.5% (3.5 g)
Suspension, ophthalmic, as etabonate [drops]:
Alrex®: 0.2% (5 mL, 10 mL) [contains benzalkonium chloride]
Lotemax®: 0.5% (2.5 mL [DSC], 5 mL, 10 mL, 15 mL) [contains benzalkonium chloride]

Loteprednol and Tobramycin (loe te PRED nol & toe bra MYE sin)

Related Information
Loteprednol on page 1163
Brand Names: U.S. Zylet®
Index Terms Loteprednol Etabonate and Tobramycin; Tobramycin and Loteprednol Etabonate
Generic Availability (U.S.) No
Pharmacologic Category Antibiotic/Corticosteroid, Ophthalmic
Use Treatment of steroid-responsive ocular inflammatory conditions where either a superficial bacterial ocular infection or the risk of a superficial bacterial ocular infection exists
Dosage
Geriatric & Adult Ophthalmic: Instill 1-2 drops into the affected eye(s) every 4-6 hours; may increase frequency during the first 24-48 hours to every 1-2 hours. Interval should increase as signs and symptoms improve. Further evaluation should occur for use of greater than 20 mL.
Special Geriatric Considerations Evaluate the patient's or caregiver's ability to safely administer the correct dose of ophthalmic medication.
Dosage Forms Excipient information presented when available (limited, particularly for generics); consult specific product labeling.
Suspension, ophthalmic [drops]:
Zylet®: Loteprednol etabonate 0.5% and tobramycin 0.3% (2.5 mL, 5 mL, 10 mL) [contains benzalkonium chloride]

◆ **Loteprednol Etabonate** see Loteprednol on page 1163
◆ **Loteprednol Etabonate and Tobramycin** see Loteprednol and Tobramycin on page 1164
◆ **Lotrel®** see Amlodipine and Benazepril on page 106
◆ **Lotrimin AF® [OTC]** see Miconazole (Topical) on page 1276
◆ **Lotrimin® AF Athlete's Foot [OTC]** see Clotrimazole (Topical) on page 426
◆ **Lotrimin® AF for Her [OTC]** see Clotrimazole (Topical) on page 426
◆ **Lotrimin® AF Jock Itch [OTC]** see Clotrimazole (Topical) on page 426

Lovastatin (LOE va sta tin)

Related Information
Hyperlipidemia Management on page 2130
Medication Safety Issues
Sound-alike/look-alike issues:
Lovastatin may be confused with atorvaSTATin, Leustatin®, Livostin®, Lotensin®, nystatin, pitavastatin
Mevacor® may be confused with Benicar®, Lipitor®
International issues:
Lovacol [Chile and Finland] may be confused with Levatol brand name for penbutolol [U.S.]
Lovastin [Malaysia, Poland, and Singapore] may be confused with Livostin brand name for levocabastine [multiple international markets]
Mevacor [U.S., Canada, and multiple international markets} may be confused with Mivacron brand name for mivacurium [multiple international markets]
Brand Names: U.S. Altoprev®; Mevacor®

Brand Names: Canada Apo-Lovastatin®; CO Lovastatin; Dom-Lovastatin; Gen-Lovastatin; Mevacor®; Mylan-Lovastatin; Novo-Lovastatin; Nu-Lovastatin; PHL-Lovastatin; PMS-Lovastatin; PRO-Lovastatin; RAN™-Lovastatin; ratio-Lovastatin; Riva-Lovastatin; Sandoz-Lovastatin

Index Terms Mevinolin; Monacolin K

Generic Availability (U.S.) Yes: Excludes extended release tablet

Pharmacologic Category Antilipemic Agent, HMG-CoA Reductase Inhibitor

Use

Adjunct to dietary therapy to decrease elevated serum total and LDL-cholesterol concentrations in primary hypercholesterolemia

Primary prevention of coronary artery disease (patients without symptomatic disease with average to moderately elevated total and LDL-cholesterol and below average HDL-cholesterol); slow progression of coronary atherosclerosis in patients with coronary heart disease and reduce the risk of myocardial infarction, unstable angina, and coronary revascularization procedures.

Contraindications Hypersensitivity to lovastatin or any component of the formulation; active liver disease; unexplained persistent elevations of serum transaminases; concomitant use of strong CYP3A4 inhibitors (eg, clarithromycin, erythromycin, itraconazole, ketoconazole, nefazodone, posaconazole, protease inhibitors [including boceprevir and telaprevir], telithromycin)

Warnings/Precautions Secondary causes of hyperlipidemia should be ruled out prior to therapy. Liver enzyme tests should be obtained at baseline and as clinically indicated; routine periodic monitoring of liver enzymes is not necessary. Use with caution in patients who consume large amounts of ethanol or have a history of liver disease; use is contraindicated with active liver disease and with unexplained transaminase elevations. Rhabdomyolysis with or without acute renal failure has occurred. Risk of rhabdomyolysis is dose-related and increased with concurrent use of lipid-lowering agents which may also cause rhabdomyolysis (fibric acid derivatives or niacin at doses ≥1 g/day) or during concurrent use with potent CYP3A4 inhibitors. Use is contraindicated in patients taking strong CYP3A4 inhibitors. Concomitant use of lovastatin with some drugs may require cautious use, may not be recommended, may require dosage adjustments, or may be contraindicated. Increases in Hb A_{1c} and fasting blood glucose have been reported with HMG-CoA reductase inhibitors; however, the benefits of statin therapy far outweigh the risk of dysglycemia. Monitor closely if used with other drugs associated with myopathy (eg, colchicine). Patients should be instructed to report unexplained muscle pain or weakness; lovastatin should be discontinued if myopathy is suspected/confirmed. The manufacturer recommends temporary discontinuation for elective major surgery, acute medical or surgical conditions, or in any patient experiencing an acute or serious condition predisposing to renal failure (eg, sepsis, hypotension, trauma, uncontrolled seizures). However, based upon current evidence, HMG-CoA reductase inhibitor therapy should be continued in the perioperative period unless risk outweighs cardioprotective benefit. Use with caution in patients with advanced age; these patients are predisposed to myopathy.

Adverse Reactions (Reflective of adult population; not specific for elderly) Percentages as reported with immediate release tablets; similar adverse reactions seen with extended release tablets.

>10%: Neuromuscular & skeletal: CPK increased (>2x normal) (11%)

1% to 10%:

Central nervous system: Headache (2% to 3%), dizziness (≤1%)

Dermatologic: Rash (≤1%)

Gastrointestinal: Flatulence (4% to 5%), constipation (2% to 4%), abdominal pain (2% to 3%), diarrhea (2% to 3%), nausea (2% to 3%), dyspepsia (1% to 2%)

Neuromuscular & skeletal: Myalgia (2% to 3%), weakness (1% to 2%), muscle cramps (≤1%)

Ocular: Blurred vision (≤1%)

Additional class-related events or case reports (not necessarily reported with lovastatin therapy): Alkaline phosphatase increased, alteration in taste, anaphylaxis, angioedema, anorexia, anxiety, arthritis, cataracts, chills, cholestatic jaundice, cirrhosis, depression, dryness of skin/mucous membranes, dyspnea, eosinophilia, erectile dysfunction, erythema multiforme, ESR increased, facial paresis, fatty liver, fever, flushing, fulminant hepatic necrosis, GGT increased, gynecomastia, hemolytic anemia, hepatitis, hepatoma, hyperbilirubinemia, hypersensitivity reaction, impaired extraocular muscle movement, impotence, interstitial lung disease, leukopenia, libido decreased, malaise, myopathy, nail changes, nodules, ophthalmoplegia, pancreatitis, peripheral nerve palsy, peripheral neuropathy, photosensitivity, polymyalgia rheumatica, positive ANA, psychic disturbance, purpura, renal failure (secondary to rhabdomyolysis), rhabdomyolysis, skin discoloration, Stevens-Johnson syndrome, systemic lupus erythematosus-like syndrome, thrombocytopenia, thyroid dysfunction, toxic epidermal necrolysis, transaminases increased, tremor, urticaria, vasculitis, vertigo

Drug Interactions

Metabolism/Transport Effects Substrate of CYP3A4 (major), P-glycoprotein; **Note:** Assignment of Major/Minor substrate status based on clinically relevant drug interaction potential; **Inhibits** CYP2C9 (weak), CYP3A4 (weak)

Avoid Concomitant Use

Avoid concomitant use of Lovastatin with any of the following: Boceprevir; CycloSPORINE; CycloSPORINE (Systemic); CYP3A4 Inhibitors (Strong); Erythromycin; Gemfibrozil; Mifepristone; Pimozide; Protease Inhibitors; Red Yeast Rice; Telaprevir

Increased Effect/Toxicity

Lovastatin may increase the levels/effects of: ARIPiprazole; DAPTOmycin; Diltiazem; Pazopanib; Pimozide; Trabectedin; Vitamin K Antagonists

The levels/effects of Lovastatin may be increased by: Amiodarone; Boceprevir; Colchicine; CycloSPORINE; CycloSPORINE (Systemic); CYP3A4 Inhibitors (Moderate); CYP3A4 Inhibitors (Strong); Cyproterone; Danazol; Dasatinib; Diltiazem; Dronedarone; Erythromycin; Fenofibrate; Fenofibric Acid; Fluconazole; Gemfibrozil; Grapefruit Juice; Ivacaftor; Macrolide Antibiotics; Mifepristone; Niacin; Niacinamide; P-glycoprotein/ABCB1 Inhibitors; Protease Inhibitors; QuiNINE; Ranolazine; Red Yeast Rice; Sildenafil; Telaprevir; Ticagrelor; Verapamil

Decreased Effect

Lovastatin may decrease the levels/effects of: Lanthanum

The levels/effects of Lovastatin may be decreased by: Antacids; Bosentan; CYP3A4 Inducers (Strong); Deferasirox; Efavirenz; Etravirine; Fosphenytoin; P-glycoprotein/ABCB1 Inducers; Phenytoin; Rifamycin Derivatives; St Johns Wort; Tocilizumab

Ethanol/Nutrition/Herb Interactions

Ethanol: Excessive ethanol consumption may have harmful hepatic effects. Management: Avoid excessive ethanol consumption.

Food: Food decreases the bioavailability of lovastatin extended release tablets and increases the bioavailability of lovastatin immediate release tablets. Lovastatin serum concentrations may be increased if taken with grapefruit juice. Management: Avoid concurrent intake of large quantities (>1 quart/day) of grapefruit juice. Red yeast rice contains an estimated 2.4 mg lovastatin per 600 mg rice.

Herb/Nutraceutical: St John's wort may decrease lovastatin levels.

Stability

Tablet, immediate release: Store at 20°C to 25°C (68°F to 77°F). Protect from light

Tablet, extended release: Store between 20°C to 25°C (68°F to 77°F); excursions permitted between 15°C to 30°C (59°F to 86°F). Avoid excessive heat and humidity.

Mechanism of Action Lovastatin acts by competitively inhibiting 3-hydroxyl-3-methylglutaryl-coenzyme A (HMG-CoA) reductase, the enzyme that catalyzes the rate-limiting step in cholesterol biosynthesis

Pharmacodynamics/Kinetics

Onset of action: LDL-cholesterol reductions: 3 days

Absorption: 30%; increased with extended release tablets when taken in the fasting state

Protein binding: >95%

Metabolism: Hepatic; extensive first-pass effect; hydrolyzed to β-hydroxyacid (active)

Bioavailability: Increased with extended release tablets

Half-life elimination: 1.1-1.7 hours

Time to peak, serum: Immediate release: 2-4 hours; extended release: 12-14 hours

Excretion: Feces (~80% to 85%); urine (10%)

Dosage

Geriatric & Adult

Dyslipidemia and primary prevention of CAD: Oral: Initial: 20 mg with evening meal, then adjust at 4-week intervals; maximum: 80 mg/day immediate release tablet **or** 60 mg/day extended release tablet.

Note: Doses should be individualized according to the baseline LDL-cholesterol levels, the recommended goal of therapy, and patient response.

Lovastatin dose limits based on concurrent therapy:

Amiodarone: Maximum recommended lovastatin dose: 40 mg/day (immediate release) **or** 20 mg/day (extended release)

Danazol or diltiazem: Initial lovastatin (immediate release) dose: 10 mg/day; Maximum recommended lovastatin (immediate release) dose: 20 mg/day

Verapamil: Initial lovastatin (immediate release) dose: 10 mg/day; Maximum recommended lovastatin (extended release and immediate release) dose: 20 mg/day

Renal Impairment Cl_{cr} <30 mL/minute: Use with caution and carefully consider doses >20 mg/day.

Administration Administer immediate release tablet with the evening meal. Administer extended release tablet at bedtime; do not crush or chew.

Monitoring Parameters Baseline CPK (recheck CPK in any patient with symptoms suggestive of myopathy; discontinue therapy if markedly elevated); baseline liver function tests (LFTs) and repeat when clinically indicated thereafter. Patients with elevated transaminase levels should have a second (confirmatory) test and frequent monitoring until values normalize; discontinue if increase in ALT/AST is persistently >3 times ULN (NCEP, 2002).

Lipid panel (total cholesterol, HDL, LDL, triglycerides):
ATP III recommendations (NCEP, 2002): Baseline; 6-8 weeks after initiation of drug therapy; if dose increased, then at 6-8 weeks until final dose determined. Once treatment goal achieved, follow up intervals may be reduced to every 4-6 months. Lipid panel should be assessed at least annually, and preferably at each clinic visit.
Manufacturer recommendation: Analyze lipid panel at intervals of 4 weeks or more.

Test Interactions Altered thyroid function tests

Special Geriatric Considerations The definition of and, therefore, when to treat hyperlipidemia in the elderly is a controversial issue. The National Cholesterol Education Program recommends that all adults maintain a plasma cholesterol <160 mg/dL. For elderly patients with one additional risk factor, goal LDL would be <130 mg/dL. It is the authors' belief that pharmacologic treatment be reserved for those who are unable to obtain a desirable plasma cholesterol concentration by diet alone and for whom the benefits of treatment are believed to outweigh the potential adverse effects, drug interactions, and cost of treatment. Age ≥65 years is a risk factor for myopathy.

Dosage Forms Excipient information presented when available (limited, particularly for generics); consult specific product labeling.
Tablet, oral: 10 mg, 20 mg, 40 mg
  Mevacor®: 20 mg, 40 mg
Tablet, extended release, oral:
  Altoprev®: 20 mg, 40 mg, 60 mg

◆ **Lovastatin and Niacin** *see* Niacin and Lovastatin *on page 1366*
◆ **Lovaza®** *see* Omega-3-Acid Ethyl Esters *on page 1416*
◆ **Lovenox®** *see* Enoxaparin *on page 637*
◆ **Low-Molecular-Weight Iron Dextran (INFeD®)** *see* Iron Dextran Complex *on page 1039*

Loxapine (LOKS a peen)

Related Information
Antipsychotic Agents *on page 2103*
Beers Criteria – Potentially Inappropriate Medications for Geriatrics *on page 2183*
Medication Safety Issues
Sound-alike/look-alike issues:
  Loxitane® may be confused with Lexapro®, Soriatane®
BEERS Criteria medication:
  This drug may be potentially inappropriate for use in geriatric patients (Quality of evidence - moderate; Strength of recommendation - strong).
International issues:
  Loxitane [U.S.] may be confused with Lexotan which is a brand name for bromazepam [multiple international markets]
Brand Names: U.S. Loxitane®
Brand Names: Canada Apo-Loxapine®; Dom-Loxapine; Loxapac; Nu-Loxapine; PHL-Loxapine; Xylac™
Index Terms Loxapine Succinate; Oxilapine Succinate
Generic Availability (U.S.) Yes
Pharmacologic Category Antipsychotic Agent, Typical
Use Management of psychotic disorders
Unlabeled Use Psychosis/agitation related to Alzheimer's dementia
Contraindications Hypersensitivity to loxapine or any component of the formulation; severe drug-induced CNS depression; coma

Canadian labeling: Additional contraindication (not in U.S. labeling): Circulatory collapse

Warnings/Precautions [U.S. Boxed Warning]: Elderly patients with dementia-related psychosis treated with antipsychotics are at an increased risk of death compared to placebo. Most deaths appeared to be either cardiovascular (eg, heart failure, sudden death) or infectious (eg, pneumonia) in nature. Loxapine is not approved for the treatment of dementia-related psychosis.

Antipsychotic use has been associated with esophageal dysmotility and aspiration; use with caution in patients at risk of pneumonia (ie, Alzheimer's disease). May cause extrapyramidal symptoms (EPS), including pseudoparkinsonism, acute dystonic reactions, akathisia, and tardive dyskinesia. Risk of dystonia (and possibly other EPS) may be greater with increased doses, use of conventional antipsychotics, males, and younger patients. Risk of tardive dyskinesia may be increased in elderly patients; antipsychotics may also mask signs/symptoms of tardive dyskinesia. Consider therapy discontinuation with signs/symptoms of tardive dyskinesia. Increased incidence of EPS has been observed with I.M. administration compared to oral administration. Use may be associated with neuroleptic malignant syndrome (NMS); monitor for mental status changes, fever, muscle rigidity, and/or autonomic instability. Discontinue treatment immediately with onset of NMS; recurrence has been reported in patients rechallenged with antipsychotic therapy.

Use in elderly patients with dementia is associated with an increased risk of mortality and cerebrovascular accidents; avoid antipsychotic use for behavioral problems associated with dementia unless alternative nonpharmacologic therapies have failed and patient may harm self or others In addition, use may cause or exacerbate syndrome of inappropriate antidiuretic hormone secretion or hyponatremia; monitor sodium closely with initiation or dosage adjustments in older adults May also be inappropriate in older adults depending on comorbidities (eg, dementia, delirium, etc) due to its potent anticholinergic effects (Beers Criteria). Increased risk for developing tardive dyskinesia, particularly elderly women.

Use with caution in patients with cardiovascular disease. May alter cardiac conduction; life-threatening arrhythmias have occurred with therapeutic doses of antipsychotics. Avoid use in patients with underlying QT prolongation, in those taking medicines that prolong the QT interval, or cause polymorphic ventricular tachycardia; monitor ECG closely for dose-related QT effects. May cause orthostatic hypotension; use with caution in patients at risk of this effect or in those who would not tolerate transient hypotensive episodes (cerebrovascular disease, cardiovascular disease, hypovolemia, or concurrent medication use which may predispose to hypotension/bradycardia).

Leukopenia, neutropenia, and agranulocytosis (sometimes fatal) have been reported in clinical trials and postmarketing reports with antipsychotic use; presence of risk factors (eg, pre-existing low WBC or history of drug-induced leuko-/neutropenia) should prompt periodic blood count assessment. Discontinue therapy at first signs of blood dyscrasias or if absolute neutrophil count <1000/mm^3.

Use with caution in patients with narrow-angle glaucoma, myasthenia gravis, Parkinson's disease, or seizure disorder. May be sedating, use with caution in disorders where CNS depression is a feature; patients must be cautioned about performing tasks which require mental alertness (eg, operating machinery or driving). Effects may be potentiated when used with other sedative drugs or ethanol. May cause anticholinergic effects (constipation, xerostomia, blurred vision, urinary retention); use with caution in patients with decreased gastrointestinal motility, paralytic ileus, urinary retention, BPH, xerostomia, or visual problems. Impaired core body temperature regulation may occur; caution with strenuous exercise, heat exposure, dehydration, and concomitant medication possessing anticholinergic effects. Relative to other antipsychotics, loxapine has a low potency of cholinergic blockade. May mask toxicity of other drugs or conditions (eg, intestinal obstruction, Reye's syndrome, brain tumor) due to antiemetic effects. Use associated with increased prolactin levels; clinical significance of hyperprolactinemia in patients with breast cancer or other prolactin-dependent tumors is unknown. May cause pigmentary retinopathy, and lenticular and corneal deposits, particularly with prolonged therapy. Canadian labeling recommends avoiding use in severe hepatic disease. Reserve injection (Canadian availability; not available in U.S.) for patients unable to tolerate oral administration; convert to oral dosage form with symptom control and ability to tolerate oral administration.

Adverse Reactions (Reflective of adult population; not specific for elderly) Frequency not defined.

Cardiovascular: ECG changes, edema, facial flushing, hyper-/hypotension, orthostatic hypotension, tachycardia, syncope

Central nervous system: Agitation, altered central temperature regulation, confusion, dizziness, drowsiness, extrapyramidal reactions (akathisia, akinesia, dystonia, pseudoparkinsonism, tardive dyskinesia), faintness, headache, hyperpyrexia, insomnia, lightheadedness, neuroleptic malignant syndrome (NMS), sedation, seizure, slurred speech, tension

Dermatologic: Alopecia, dermatitis, photosensitivity, pruritus, rash, seborrhea

Endocrine & metabolic: Amenorrhea, galactorrhea, gynecomastia, hyperprolactinemia, impotence, menstrual irregularity, polydipsia

Gastrointestinal: Adynamic ileus, constipation, nausea, vomiting, weight gain/loss, xerostomia

Genitourinary: Priapism (rare), urinary retention

Hematologic: Agranulocytosis, leukopenia, thrombocytopenia

Hepatic: ALT increased, AST increased, hepatitis, jaundice

Neuromuscular & skeletal: Gait instability, muscle twitching, numbness, paresthesia, weakness

Ocular: Blurred vision, ptosis

Respiratory: Dyspnea, nasal congestion

Drug Interactions

Metabolism/Transport Effects None known.

Avoid Concomitant Use

Avoid concomitant use of Loxapine with any of the following: Azelastine; Azelastine (Nasal); Metoclopramide; Paraldehyde

Increased Effect/Toxicity

Loxapine may increase the levels/effects of: Alcohol (Ethyl); Anticholinergics; Azelastine; Azelastine (Nasal); Buprenorphine; CNS Depressants; Highest Risk QTc-Prolonging Agents; LORazepam; Methylphenidate; Moderate Risk QTc-Prolonging Agents; Paraldehyde; Serotonin Modulators; Zolpidem

The levels/effects of Loxapine may be increased by: Acetylcholinesterase Inhibitors (Central); HydrOXYzine; Lithium formulations; Methylphenidate; Metoclopramide; Metyrosine; Mifepristone; Pramlintide; Tetrabenazine

Decreased Effect

Loxapine may decrease the levels/effects of: Amphetamines; Anti-Parkinson's Agents (Dopamine Agonist); Quinagolide

The levels/effects of Loxapine may be decreased by: Anti-Parkinson's Agents (Dopamine Agonist); Lithium formulations

Ethanol/Nutrition/Herb Interactions

Ethanol: May increase CNS depression; monitor for increased effects with coadministration. Caution patients about effects.

Herb/Nutraceutical: Avoid kava kava, gotu kola, valerian, St John's wort (may increase CNS depression).

Stability

Capsules: Store at 20°C to 25°C (68°F to 77°F).

Canadian products (not available in U.S.): Injection solution, oral solution, tablets: Store at 15°C to 30°C (59°F to 86°F).

Mechanism of Action Loxapine is a dibenzoxazepine antipsychotic which blocks postsynaptic mesolimbic D_1 and D_2 receptors in the brain, and also possesses serotonin 5-HT$_2$ blocking activity

Pharmacodynamics/Kinetics

Onset of action: Oral, I.M.: Within 30 minutes

Peak effect: 1.5-3 hours

Duration: ~12 hours

Absorption: Oral, I.M.: Rapid and complete

Metabolism: Hepatic to glucuronide conjugates

Half-life elimination: Biphasic: Initial: 5 hours; Terminal: 19 hours

Excretion: Urine (56% to 70%, as metabolites); feces (as metabolites)

Dosage

Geriatric Reduced dosing may be indicated due to risks of adverse events associated with high-dose therapy. Refer to adult dosing.

Adult Psychosis:

Oral: Initial: 10 mg twice daily (up to 50 mg/day may be considered in severely disturbed patients), increase dose until psychotic symptoms are controlled; usual maintenance: 60-100 mg/day in divided doses 2-4 times/day; satisfactory response often observed with doses of 20-60 mg/day (maximum: 250 mg/day).Therapy should be maintained at lowest effective dose.

I.M. (Canadian availability; not available in the U.S.): 12.5-50 mg every 4-6 hours or longer; individualize dose early in therapy; some patients respond satisfactorily to twice-daily dosing

Renal Impairment There are no dosage adjustments provided in the manufacturer's labeling.

Hepatic Impairment There are no dosage adjustments provided in the manufacturer's labeling. Canadian labeling does not recommend use in severe hepatic disease.

Administration

Oral solution (Canadian availability; not available in the U.S.) should be mixed with orange or grapefruit juice prior to administration.

Injection (Canadian availability; not available in the U.S.) is administered by I.M. injection. Do **not** administer I.V.

Monitoring Parameters Vital signs, orthostatic blood pressures 3-5 days after initiation of therapy or a dose increase; liver and kidney function, CBC at baseline and then at regular ▶

intervals (in patients at risk for blood dyscrasias), lipid profile, fasting blood glucose/Hgb A$_{1c}$; BMI; mental status, abnormal involuntary movement scale (AIMS), extrapyramidal symptoms (EPS)

Test Interactions False-positives for phenylketonuria, amylase, uroporphyrins, urobilinogen

Special Geriatric Considerations Many elderly patients receive antipsychotic medications for inappropriate nonpsychotic behavior. Before initiating antipsychotic medication, the clinician should investigate any possible reversible cause; any stress or stress from any disease can cause acute "confusion" or worsening of baseline nonpsychotic behavior. Most commonly acute changes in behavior are due to increases in drug dose or addition of new drug to regimen; fluid electrolyte loss; infections; and changes in environment.

Any changes in disease status in any organ system can result in behavior changes.

In the treatment of agitated, demented, elderly patients, authors of meta-analysis of controlled trials of the response to the traditional antipsychotics (phenothiazines, butyrophenones) in controlling agitation have concluded that the use of neuroleptics results in a response rate of 18%. Clearly neuroleptic therapy for behavior control should be limited with frequent attempts to withdraw the agent given for behavior control.

This medication is considered to be potentially inappropriate in this patient population (Beers Criteria: Quality of evidence - moderate; Strength of recommendation - strong).

Dosage Forms Excipient information presented when available (limited, particularly for generics); consult specific product labeling.
Capsule, oral: 5 mg, 10 mg, 25 mg, 50 mg
    Loxitane®: 5 mg, 10 mg, 25 mg, 50 mg

Dosage Forms: Canada Excipient information presented when available (limited, particularly for generics); consult specific product labeling.
Injection, solution, as hydrochloride [strength expressed as base]:
    Loxapac: 50 mg/mL (1 mL) [contains polysorbate 80, propylene glycol]
Solution, oral, as hydrochloride [strength expressed as base; concentrate]:
    Xylac™: 25 mg/mL (100 mL) [contains propylene glycol]
Tablet, oral, as succinate [strength expressed as base]:
    Xylac™: 2.5 mg, 5 mg, 10 mg, 25 mg, 50 mg

Lubiprostone (loo bi PROS tone)

Related Information
Laxatives, Classification and Properties on page 2121
Brand Names: U.S. Amitiza®
Index Terms RU 0211; SPI 0211
Generic Availability (U.S.) No
Pharmacologic Category Chloride Channel Activator; Gastrointestinal Agent, Miscellaneous
Use Treatment of chronic idiopathic constipation; treatment of irritable bowel syndrome with constipation in adult women
Contraindications Known or suspected mechanical bowel obstruction
Warnings/Precautions Symptoms of mechanical gastrointestinal obstruction should be evaluated before prescribing this medicine; use is contraindicated in patients with bowel obstruction. Avoid use in patients with severe diarrhea. Nausea may occur; administer with food to reduce symptoms. In long-term clinical studies for chronic idiopathic constipation, patients were allowed to reduce the dose to 24 mcg once daily if nausea was severe. Dyspnea, often described as chest tightness, has been observed with use, including postmarketing reports; generally occurs following the first dose with an acute onset (within 30-60 minutes) and resolves within a few hours; however, has been frequently reported with subsequent dosing. Dose adjustment is recommended in patients with moderate-to-severe hepatic impairment (Child Pugh class B or C). Not approved for use in males with irritable bowel syndrome with constipation.

Adverse Reactions (Reflective of adult population; not specific for elderly)
>10%:
  Central nervous system: Headache (3% to 11%)
  Gastrointestinal: Nausea (7% to 29%; severe: 4%; dose related), diarrhea (7% to 12%; severe 2%)
1% to 10%:
  Cardiovascular: Edema (3%), chest discomfort/pain (2%)
  Central nervous system: Dizziness (3%), fatigue (2%)
  Gastrointestinal: Abdominal pain (1% to 8%), abdominal distention (3% to 6%), flatulence (3% to 6%), vomiting (3%), loose stools (3%), dyspepsia (2%), xerostomia (1%)
  Respiratory: Dyspnea (2% to 3%)

Drug Interactions
  Metabolism/Transport Effects None known.
  Avoid Concomitant Use There are no known interactions where it is recommended to avoid concomitant use.
  Increased Effect/Toxicity There are no known significant interactions involving an increase in effect.
  Decreased Effect There are no known significant interactions involving a decrease in effect.

Stability Store at 25°C (77°F); excursions permitted to 15°C to 30°C (59°F to 86°F).

Mechanism of Action Bicyclic fatty acid that acts locally at the apical portion of the intestine as a chloride channel activator, increasing intestinal fluid secretion and intestinal motility. Does not alter serum sodium or potassium concentrations.

Pharmacodynamics/Kinetics
  Absorption: Systemic: Parent drug: Poor (below levels of detection); Active metabolite (M3): Low
  Distribution: Gastrointestinal tissue; minimal beyond gastrointestinal tissue
  Metabolism: Rapid and extensive within stomach and jejunum by carbonyl reductase to M3 (active metabolite) and others
  Bioavailability: Minimal
  Half-life elimination: M3: 0.9-1.4 hours
  Excretion: Parent drug and M3: Feces (trace amounts)

Dosage
  Geriatric & Adult
    Chronic idiopathic constipation: Adults: 24 mcg twice daily
    Irritable bowel syndrome with constipation: Females ≥18 years: 8 mcg twice daily
  Renal Impairment No dosage adjustment required.
  Hepatic Impairment
    Moderate hepatic impairment (Child-Pugh class B):
      Chronic idiopathic constipation: 16 mcg twice daily; may increase to 24 mcg twice daily if tolerated and an adequate response has not been obtained with lower dosage
      Irritable bowel syndrome with constipation: No dosage adjustment required
    Severe hepatic impairment (Child-Pugh class C):
      Chronic idiopathic constipation: 8 mcg twice daily; may increase to 16-24 mcg twice daily if tolerated and an adequate response has not been obtained with lower dosage
      Irritable bowel syndrome with constipation: 8 mcg once daily; may increase to 8 mcg twice daily if tolerated and an adequate response has not been obtained at lower dosage

Administration Administer with food and water. Swallow whole; do not break or chew.

Special Geriatric Considerations Elderly with chronic idiopathic constipation, when studied, demonstrated consistent efficacy to that seen in younger populations. Of note, the elderly experienced less nausea than younger subjects.

Dosage Forms Excipient information presented when available (limited, particularly for generics); consult specific product labeling.
Capsule, softgel, oral:
  Amitiza®: 8 mcg, 24 mcg

Lurasidone (loo RAS i done)

Related Information
Antipsychotic Agents *on page 2103*
Atypical Antipsychotics *on page 2107*
Beers Criteria – Potentially Inappropriate Medications for Geriatrics *on page 2183*
Medication Safety Issues
Sound-alike/look-alike issues:
Latuda® may be confused with Lantus®
BEERS Criteria medication:
This drug may be potentially inappropriate for use in geriatric patients (Quality of evidence - moderate; Strength of recommendation - strong).
Brand Names: U.S. Latuda®
Index Terms Lurasidone Hydrochloride; SM-13496
Generic Availability (U.S.) No
Pharmacologic Category Antipsychotic Agent, Atypical
Use Treatment of schizophrenia
Contraindications Hypersensitivity to lurasidone or any component of the formulation; concomitant use with potent CYP3A4 inhibitors (eg, ketoconazole) and inducers (eg, rifampin)
Warnings/Precautions [U.S. Boxed Warning]: Elderly patients with dementia-related psychosis treated with antipsychotics are at an increased risk of death compared to placebo. Most deaths appeared to be either cardiovascular (eg, heart failure, sudden death) or infectious (eg, pneumonia) in nature. Lurasidone is not approved for the treatment of dementia-related psychosis. An increased incidence of cerebrovascular effects (eg, transient ischemic attack, stroke), including fatalities, has been reported in placebo-controlled trials of antipsychotics for the unapproved use in elderly patients with dementia-related psychosis.

Leukopenia, neutropenia, and agranulocytosis (sometimes fatal) have been reported in clinical trials and postmarketing reports with antipsychotic use; presence of risk factors (eg, pre-existing low WBC or history of drug-induced leuko-/neutropenia) should prompt periodic blood count assessment. Discontinue therapy at first signs of blood dyscrasias or if absolute neutrophil count <1000/mm^3.

Low to moderately sedating, use with caution in disorders where CNS depression is a feature. Use with caution in Parkinson's disease. Caution in patients with predisposition to seizures. Use with caution in renal or hepatic dysfunction; dose reduction recommended in moderate-to-severe impairment. Esophageal dysmotility and aspiration have been associated with antipsychotic use; use with caution in patients at risk of aspiration pneumonia (ie, Alzheimer's disease). Use is associated with increased prolactin levels; clinical significance of hyper-prolactinemia in patients with breast cancer or other prolactin-dependent tumors is unknown. May alter temperature regulation.

Use with caution in patients with severe cardiac disease, hemodynamic instability, prior myocardial infarction or ischemic heart disease. May cause orthostatic hypotension; use with caution in patients at risk of this effect (eg, concurrent medication use which may predispose to hypotension/bradycardia or presence of hypovolemia) or in those who would not tolerate transient hypotensive episodes. Antipsychotics may alter cardiac conduction; life-threatening arrhythmias have occurred with therapeutic doses of antipsychotics. Relative to other antipsychotics, lurasidone has minimal effects on the QT$_c$ interval and therefore, risk for arrhythmias is low. Increases in total cholesterol and triglyceride concentrations have been observed with atypical antipsychotic use; during clinical trials of lurasidone, there were no significant changes in total cholesterol or triglycerides observed. Concurrent use with strong inhibitors/inducers of CYP3A4 is contraindicated; dosage adjustment is recommended with concurrent use of moderate CYP3A4 inhibitors (eg, diltiazem).

May cause extrapyramidal symptoms (EPS), including pseudoparkinsonism, acute dystonic reactions, akathisia, and tardive dyskinesia (potentially irreversible). Risk of tardive dyskinesia may be increased in elderly patients, particularly elderly women. Risk of dystonia (and probably other EPS) may be greater with increased doses, use of conventional antipsychotics, males, and younger patients. Use may be associated with neuroleptic malignant syndrome (NMS); monitor for mental status changes, fever, muscle rigidity and/or autonomic instability (risk may be increased in patients with Parkinson's disease or Lewy body dementia). May cause hyperglycemia; in some cases may be extreme and associated with ketoacidosis, hyperosmolar coma, or death. Use with caution in patients with diabetes or other disorders of glucose regulation; monitor for worsening of glucose control. Significant weight gain has been observed with antipsychotic therapy; incidence varies with product. Monitor waist circumference and BMI.

Use in elderly patients with dementia is associated with an increased risk of mortality and cerebrovascular accidents; avoid antipsychotic use for behavioral problems associated with dementia unless alternative nonpharmacologic therapies have failed and patient may harm self or others. In addition, use may cause or exacerbate syndrome of inappropriate antidiuretic hormone secretion or hyponatremia; monitor sodium closely with initiation or dosage adjustments in older adults (Beers Criteria).

The possibility of a suicide attempt is inherent in psychotic illness or bipolar disorder; use caution in high-risk patients during initiation of therapy. Prescriptions should be written for the smallest quantity consistent with good patient care.

Adverse Reactions (Reflective of adult population; not specific for elderly)

10%:

Central nervous system: Somnolence (dose-related: 19% to 23%), akathisia (dose-related: 11% to 15%)

Endocrine & metabolic: Fasting glucose increased (10% to 14%)

Gastrointestinal: Nausea (12%)

Neuromuscular & skeletal: Extrapyramidal symptoms (24% to 26%), parkinsonism (11%)

1% to 10%:

Cardiovascular: Tachycardia

Central nervous system: Insomnia (8%), agitation (6%), anxiety (6%), dizziness (5%), dystonia (5%), fatigue (4%), restlessness (3%)

Dermatologic: Pruritus, rash

Endocrine & metabolic: Prolactin increased ($\geq$5 x ULN: females: 8%; males: 2%)

Gastrointestinal: Dyspepsia (8%), vomiting (8%), weight gain ($\geq$7% increase in baseline body weight: 6%), salivary hypersecretion (2%), abdominal pain, appetite decreased, diarrhea

Neuromuscular & skeletal: Back pain (4%), CPK increased

Ocular: Blurred vision

Renal: Creatinine increased (3%)

Drug Interactions

Metabolism/Transport Effects Substrate of CYP3A4 (major); **Note:** Assignment of Major/Minor substrate status based on clinically relevant drug interaction potential; **Inhibits** CYP3A4 (weak)

Avoid Concomitant Use

Avoid concomitant use of Lurasidone with any of the following: Azelastine; Azelastine (Nasal); CYP3A4 Inducers (Strong); CYP3A4 Inhibitors (Strong); DOPamine; EPINEPHrine; EPINEPHrine (Systemic, Oral Inhalation); Methadone; Metoclopramide; Paraldehyde; Pimozide

Increased Effect/Toxicity

Lurasidone may increase the levels/effects of: Alcohol (Ethyl); ARIPiprazole; Azelastine; Azelastine (Nasal); Buprenorphine; CNS Depressants; Disopyramide; Methadone; Methotrimeprazine; Methylphenidate; Paraldehyde; Pimozide; Procainamide; QuiNIDine; Serotonin Modulators; Zolpidem

The levels/effects of Lurasidone may be increased by: Acetylcholinesterase Inhibitors (Central); CYP3A4 Inhibitors (Moderate); CYP3A4 Inhibitors (Strong); Dasatinib; DOPamine; Droperidol; EPINEPHrine; EPINEPHrine (Systemic, Oral Inhalation); HydrOXYzine; Ivacaftor; Lithium formulations; MAO Inhibitors; Methotrimeprazine; Methylphenidate; Metoclopramide; Metyrosine; Mifepristone; Tetrabenazine

Decreased Effect

Lurasidone may decrease the levels/effects of: Amphetamines; Anti-Parkinson's Agents (Dopamine Agonist); Quinagolide

The levels/effects of Lurasidone may be decreased by: CYP3A4 Inducers (Strong); Deferasirox; Lithium formulations; Tocilizumab

Ethanol/Nutrition/Herb Interactions

Ethanol: May increase CNS depression; monitor for increased effects with coadministration. Caution patients about effects.

Food: Administration with food ($\geq$350 calories) increased C_{max} and AUC of lurasidone ~3 times and 2 times, respectively, compared to administration during fasting conditions. Lurasidone exposure was not affected by the fat content of the meal.

Stability Store at controlled room temperature of 25°C (77°F).

Mechanism of Action Lurasidone is a benzoisothiazol-derivative atypical antipsychotic with mixed serotonin-dopamine antagonist activity. It exhibits high affinity for D_2, $5-HT_{2A}$, and $5-HT_7$ receptors; moderate affinity for $alpha_{2C}$-adrenergic receptors; and is a partial agonist for $5-HT_{1A}$ receptors. Lurasidone has no significant affinity for muscarinic M_1 and histamine H_1 receptors. The addition of serotonin antagonism to dopamine antagonism (classic neuroleptic mechanism) is thought to improve negative symptoms of psychoses and reduce the incidence of extrapyramidal side effects as compared to typical antipsychotics.

Pharmacodynamics/Kinetics

Distribution: V_d: 6173 L

Protein binding: ~99%

Metabolism: Primarily via CYP3A4; two active metabolites (ID-14283 and ID-14326) and two major nonactive metabolites (ID-20219 and ID-20220) produced

Bioavailability: 9% to 19%

Half-life elimination: 18 hours; Main active metabolite, ID-14283 (exo-hydroxy metabolite), exhibits a half-life of 7.5-10 hours

Time to peak: 1-3 hours; steady state concentrations achieved within 7 days

Excretion: Urine (~9%); feces (~80%)

Dosage

Geriatric & Adult Schizophrenia: Oral: Initial: 40 mg once daily; titration is not required; maximum recommended dose: 160 mg/day

Concomitant CYP3A4 inhibitors/inducers:

CYP3A4 inhibitors: If concomitant administration with a moderate CYP3A4 inhibitor (eg, diltiazem) is necessary, do not exceed 80 mg/day of lurasidone. Concomitant administration with a strong CYP3A4 inhibitor (eg, ketoconazole) is contraindicated.

CYP3A4 inducers: Concomitant administration with a strong CYP3A4 inducer (eg, rifampin) is contraindicated.

Renal Impairment

Cl_{cr} ≥50 mL/minute: No dosage adjustment necessary

Cl_{cr} <50 mL/minute: Initial: 20 mg/day; maximum: 80 mg/day

Hepatic Impairment

Mild impairment (Child-Pugh class A): No dosage adjustment necessary

Moderate impairment (Child-Pugh class B): Initial: 20 mg/day; maximum: 80 mg/day

Severe impairment (Child-Pugh class C): Initial: 20 mg/day; maximum: 40 mg/day

Administration Administer with food (≥350 calories).

Monitoring Parameters Vital signs; fasting lipid profile and fasting blood glucose/Hgb A_{1c} (baseline and periodically); CBC frequently during first few months of therapy in patients with pre-existing low WBC or a history of drug-induced leukopenia/neutropenia; BMI, personal/family history of obesity, waist circumference; blood pressure; mental status, abnormal involuntary movement scale (AIMS), extrapyramidal symptoms; orthostatic blood pressure changes for 3-5 days after starting or increasing dose. Weight should be assessed prior to treatment and regularly throughout therapy. Consider titrating to a different antipsychotic agent for a weight gain ≥5% of the initial weight.

Special Geriatric Considerations Clinical studies of schizophrenic patients did not include sufficient numbers of elderly to determine a difference in response compared to younger adults. Elderly with psychosis had similar serum concentrations to younger adults; therefore, no dosage adjustments are recommended for elderly patients with psychosis. This drug is not recommended/indicated for use in elderly patients with dementia-related psychosis. Such patients are at an increased risk of death compared to placebo. Most deaths were cardiovascular (eg, heart failure, sudden death) or infectious (eg, pneumonia) in nature.

This medication is considered to be potentially inappropriate in this patient population (Beers Criteria: Quality of evidence - moderate; Strength of recommendation - strong).

Dosage Forms Excipient information presented when available (limited, particularly for generics); consult specific product labeling.

Tablet, oral, as hydrochloride:

Latuda®: 20 mg, 40 mg, 80 mg

◆ **Macrobid®** *see* Nitrofurantoin *on page 1384*
◆ **Macrodantin®** *see* Nitrofurantoin *on page 1384*
◆ **Macugen®** *see* Pegaptanib *on page 1480*
◆ **Mag-Al [OTC]** *see* Aluminum Hydroxide and Magnesium Hydroxide *on page 80*

Magaldrate and Simethicone (MAG al drate & sye METH i kone)

Related Information
Simethicone *on page 1776*
Medication Safety Issues
Sound-alike/look-alike issues:
Riopan Plus® may be confused with Repan®
Index Terms Riopan Plus; Simethicone and Magaldrate
Generic Availability (U.S.) Yes
Pharmacologic Category Antacid; Antiflatulent
Use Relief of hyperacidity associated with peptic ulcer, gastritis, peptic esophagitis, and hiatal hernia which are accompanied by symptoms of gas
Dosage
Geriatric & Adult Hyperacidity/gas: Oral: 5-10 mL (540-1080 mg magaldrate) between meals and at bedtime
Special Geriatric Considerations No specific information for use in elderly.
Dosage Forms Excipient information presented when available (limited, particularly for generics); consult specific product labeling.
Suspension, oral: Magaldrate 540 mg and simethicone 20 mg per 5 mL (360 mL)

◆ **Mag-Al Ultimate [OTC]** *see* Aluminum Hydroxide and Magnesium Hydroxide *on page 80*
◆ **Magan®** *see* Salicylates (Various Salts) *on page 1742*
◆ **Mag Citrate** *see* Magnesium Citrate *on page 1175*
◆ **Maginex™ [OTC]** *see* Magnesium L-aspartate Hydrochloride *on page 1180*
◆ **Maginex™ DS [OTC]** *see* Magnesium L-aspartate Hydrochloride *on page 1180*
◆ **Magnesia Magma** *see* Magnesium Hydroxide *on page 1177*
◆ **Magnesium L-lactate Dihydrate** *see* Magnesium L-lactate *on page 1180*
◆ **Magnesium Carbonate and Aluminum Hydroxide** *see* Aluminum Hydroxide and Magnesium Carbonate *on page 79*

Magnesium Citrate (mag NEE zhum SIT rate)

Related Information
Laxatives, Classification and Properties *on page 2121*
Brand Names: U.S. Citroma® [OTC]
Brand Names: Canada Citro-Mag®
Index Terms Citrate of Magnesia; Mag Citrate
Generic Availability (U.S.) Yes
Pharmacologic Category Laxative, Saline; Magnesium Salt
Use Evacuation of bowel prior to certain surgical and diagnostic procedures or overdose situations; relieves occasional constipation
Contraindications Renal failure, appendicitis, abdominal pain, intestinal impaction, obstruction or perforation, diabetes mellitus, complications in gastrointestinal tract, patients with colostomy or ileostomy, ulcerative colitis or diverticulitis
Warnings/Precautions Use with caution in patients with impaired renal function (accumulation of magnesium may lead to magnesium intoxication).

Constipation (self-medication, OTC use): For occasional use only; serious side effects may occur with prolonged use. For use only under the supervision of a healthcare provider in patients with kidney dysfunction, or with a sudden change in bowel habits which persist for >2 weeks. Do not use if abdominal pain, nausea, or vomiting are present.
Adverse Reactions (Reflective of adult population; not specific for elderly) 1% to 10%:
Cardiovascular: Hypotension
Endocrine & metabolic: Hypermagnesemia
Gastrointestinal: Abdominal cramps, diarrhea, gas formation
Respiratory: Respiratory depression

Drug Interactions

Metabolism/Transport Effects None known.

Avoid Concomitant Use

Avoid concomitant use of Magnesium Citrate with any of the following: Calcium Polystyrene Sulfonate; Sodium Polystyrene Sulfonate

Increased Effect/Toxicity

Magnesium Citrate may increase the levels/effects of: Aluminum Hydroxide; Calcium Channel Blockers; Calcium Polystyrene Sulfonate; Neuromuscular-Blocking Agents; Sodium Polystyrene Sulfonate

The levels/effects of Magnesium Citrate may be increased by: Alfacalcidol; Calcitriol; Calcium Channel Blockers

Decreased Effect

Magnesium Citrate may decrease the levels/effects of: Bisphosphonate Derivatives; Deferiprone; Eltrombopag; Mycophenolate; Phosphate Supplements; Quinolone Antibiotics; Tetracycline Derivatives; Trientine

The levels/effects of Magnesium Citrate may be decreased by: Trientine

Mechanism of Action Promotes bowel evacuation by causing osmotic retention of fluid which distends the colon with increased peristaltic activity

Pharmacodynamics/Kinetics

Absorption: Oral: 15% to 30%

Excretion: Urine

Dosage

Geriatric & Adult Cathartic: Oral: 150-300 mL

Renal Impairment Patients in severe renal failure should not receive magnesium due to toxicity from accumulation. Patients with a Cl_{cr} <25 mL/minute should be monitored by serum magnesium levels.

Administration To increase palatability, chill the solution prior to administration.

Reference Range Serum magnesium: 1.5-2.5 mg/dL; slightly different ranges are reported by different laboratories

Test Interactions Increased magnesium; decreased protein, decreased calcium (S), decreased potassium (S)

Pharmacotherapy Pearls To increase palatability, manufacturer suggests chilling the solution prior to administration.

3.85-4.71 mEq of magnesium/5 mL

Special Geriatric Considerations Elderly, due to disease or drug therapy, may be predisposed to diarrhea. Diarrhea may result in electrolyte imbalance. Decreased renal function (Cl_{cr} <30 mL/minute) may result in toxicity; monitor for toxicity and Cl_{cr} <30 mL/minute.

Dosage Forms Excipient information presented when available (limited, particularly for generics); consult specific product labeling.

Solution, oral: 290 mg/5 mL (296 mL)

Citroma®: 290 mg/5 mL (340 mL) [contains benzoic acid, magnesium 48 mg/5 mL, sodium 0.5 mg/5 mL; grape flavor]

Citroma®: 290 mg/5 mL (296 mL) [contains magnesium 48 mg/5 mL, potassium 13 mg/5 mL; cherry flavor]

Citroma®: 290 mg/5 mL (296 mL) [contains magnesium 48 mg/5 mL, potassium 13 mg/5 mL; lemon flavor]

Citroma®: 290 mg/5 mL (296 mL) [contains magnesium 48 mg/5 mL, sodium 7.5 mg/5 mL; grape flavor]

Citroma®: 290 mg/5 mL (296 mL) [contains magnesium 48 mg/5 mL, sodium 7.5 mg/5 mL; lemon flavor]

Tablet, oral: Elemental magnesium 100 mg

◆ **Magnesium Gluceptate** *see* Magnesium Glucoheptonate *on page 1176*

Magnesium Glucoheptonate (mag NEE zhum gloo koh HEP toh nate)

Brand Names: Canada Magnesium Glucoheptonate

Index Terms Magnesium Gluceptate

Pharmacologic Category Magnesium Salt

Use Dietary supplement

Dosage

Geriatric & Adult Note: Serum magnesium is poor reflection of repletional status as the majority of magnesium is intracellular; serum levels may be transiently normal for a few hours after a dose is given, therefore, aim for consistently high normal serum levels in patients with normal renal function for most efficient repletion.

RDA (elemental magnesium):
  19-30 years:
    Female: 310 mg/day
    Male: 400 mg/day
  ≥31 years:
    Female: 320 mg/day
    Male: 420 mg/day

Hypomagnesemia: Oral: 1500-3000 mg (75-150 mg elemental magnesium) 1-3 times/day

Renal Impairment
  Mild-to-moderate renal impairment: Use with caution; monitor serum magnesium levels carefully.
  Severe renal impairment: Use is contraindicated.

Special Geriatric Considerations Elderly, due to disease or drug therapy, may be predisposed to diarrhea. Diarrhea may result in electrolyte imbalance. Decreased renal function (Cl_{cr} <30 mL/minute) may result in toxicity; monitor for toxicity and Cl_{cr} <30 mL/minute.

Product Availability Not available in U.S.

Dosage Forms: Canada Excipient information presented when available (limited, particularly for generics); consult specific product labeling.
  Solution, oral: 100 mg/mL

Magnesium Hydroxide (mag NEE zhum hye DROKS ide)

Related Information
Laxatives, Classification and Properties *on page 2121*
Treatment Options for Constipation *on page 2142*

Brand Names: U.S. Fleet® Pedia-Lax™ Chewable Tablet [OTC]; Little Phillips'® Milk of Magnesia [OTC]; Milk of Magnesia [OTC]; Milk of Magnesium [OTC]; Phillips'® Milk of Magnesia [OTC]

Index Terms Magnesia Magma; Milk of Magnesia; MOM

Generic Availability (U.S.) Yes: Liquid

Pharmacologic Category Antacid; Laxative; Magnesium Salt

Use Short-term treatment of occasional constipation and symptoms of hyperacidity, laxative

Contraindications Hypersensitivity to magnesium hydroxide or any component of the formulation

Warnings/Precautions Use magnesium with caution in patients with impaired renal function (accumulation of magnesium may lead to magnesium intoxication). Use with extreme caution in patients with myasthenia gravis or other neuromuscular disease.

For self-medication (OTC use): For occasional use only; serious side effects may occur with prolonged use. For use only under the supervision of a healthcare provider in patients with kidney dysfunction, or with a sudden change in bowel habits which persist for >2 weeks. Patients should notify healthcare provider of any sudden change in bowel habits which last >14 days, stomach pain, nausea, or vomiting or if use is needed for >1 week.

Drug Interactions

Metabolism/Transport Effects None known.

Avoid Concomitant Use
  Avoid concomitant use of Magnesium Hydroxide with any of the following: Calcium Polystyrene Sulfonate; QuiNINE; Sodium Polystyrene Sulfonate

Increased Effect/Toxicity
  Magnesium Hydroxide may increase the levels/effects of: Alpha-/Beta-Agonists; Amphetamines; Calcium Channel Blockers; Calcium Polystyrene Sulfonate; Dexmethylphenidate; Methylphenidate; Misoprostol; Neuromuscular-Blocking Agents; QuiNIDine; Sodium Polystyrene Sulfonate

  The levels/effects of Magnesium Hydroxide may be increased by: Alfacalcidol; Calcitriol; Calcium Channel Blockers

Decreased Effect
  Magnesium Hydroxide may decrease the levels/effects of: ACE Inhibitors; Allopurinol; Anticonvulsants (Hydantoin); Antipsychotic Agents (Phenothiazines); Atazanavir; Bisacodyl; Bisphosphonate Derivatives; Cefditoren; Cefpodoxime; Cefuroxime; Chloroquine;

Corticosteroids (Oral); Dabigatran Etexilate; Dasatinib; Deferiprone; Delavirdine; Eltrombopag; Erlotinib; Fexofenadine; Gabapentin; HMG-CoA Reductase Inhibitors; Iron Salts; Isoniazid; Itraconazole; Ketoconazole; Ketoconazole (Systemic); Mesalamine; Methenamine; Mycophenolate; Nilotinib; PenicillAMINE; Phosphate Supplements; Protease Inhibitors; QuiNINE; Quinolone Antibiotics; Rilpivirine; Tetracycline Derivatives; Trientine; Vismodegib

The levels/effects of Magnesium Hydroxide may be decreased by: Trientine

Mechanism of Action Promotes bowel evacuation by causing osmotic retention of fluid which distends the colon with increased peristaltic activity; reacts with hydrochloric acid in stomach to form magnesium chloride

Pharmacodynamics/Kinetics

Onset of action: Laxative: 30 minutes to 6 hours

Excretion: Urine (up to 30% as absorbed magnesium ions); feces (as unabsorbed drug)

Dosage

Geriatric & Adult

Antacid: OTC labeling: Oral:

Liquid: Magnesium hydroxide 400 mg/5 mL: 5-15 mL as needed up to 4 times/day

Tablet: Magnesium hydroxide 311 mg/tablet: 2-4 tablets every 4 hours up to 4 times/day

Laxative: OTC labeling: Oral:

Liquid:

Magnesium hydroxide 400 mg/5 mL: 30-60 mL/day once daily at bedtime or in divided doses

Magnesium hydroxide 800 mg/5 mL: 15-30 mL/day once daily at bedtime or in divided doses

Tablet: Magnesium hydroxide 311 mg/tablet: 8 tablets/day once daily at bedtime or in divided doses

Renal Impairment Patients in severe renal failure should not receive magnesium due to toxicity from accumulation. Patients with a Cl_{cr} <30 mL/minute should be monitored by serum magnesium levels.

Administration Liquid doses may be diluted with a small amount of water prior to administration. All doses should be followed by 8 ounces of water.

Test Interactions Increased magnesium; decreased protein, calcium (S), decreased potassium (S)

Special Geriatric Considerations Elderly, due to disease or drug therapy, may be predisposed to diarrhea. Diarrhea may result in electrolyte imbalance. Decreased renal function (Cl_{cr} <30 mL/minute) may result in toxicity; monitor for toxicity.

Dosage Forms Excipient information presented when available (limited, particularly for generics); consult specific product labeling.

Suspension, oral: 400 mg/5 mL (30 mL, 473 mL)

Milk of Magnesia: 400 mg/5 mL (360 mL, 480 mL)

Milk of Magnesia: 400 mg/5 mL (360 mL, 480 mL) [mint flavor]

Milk of Magnesia: 400 mg/5 mL (480 mL) [ethanol free, sugar free]

Milk of Magnesium: 400 mg/5 mL (3.78 L, 473 mL) [contains magnesium 165 mg/5 mL]

Phillips'® Milk of Magnesia: 400 mg/5 mL (120 mL, 360 mL, 780 mL) [contains magnesium 167 mg/5 mL; fresh mint flavor]

Phillips'® Milk of Magnesia: 400 mg/5 mL (120 mL, 360 mL, 780 mL) [contains magnesium 167 mg/5 mL; original flavor]

Phillips'® Milk of Magnesia: 400 mg/5 mL (120 mL, 240 mL, 360 mL, 780 mL) [contains magnesium 167 mg/5 mL, sodium 2 mg/5 mL; cherry flavor]

Suspension, oral [concentrate]: 2400 mg/10 mL (10 mL)

Little Phillips'® Milk of Magnesia: 800 mg/5 mL (120 mL) [contains magnesium 333 mg/5 mL, propylene glycol; strawberry flavor]

Milk of Magnesia: 800 mg/5 mL (100 mL, 400 mL) [contains sodium 20 mg/10 mL, sucrose 0.8 g/10 mL; lemon flavor]

Phillips'® Milk of Magnesia: 800 mg/5 mL (240 mL) [contains magnesium 333 mg/5 mL, propylene glycol; strawberry flavor]

Tablet, chewable, oral:

Fleet® Pedia-Lax™ Chewable Tablet: 400 mg [contains magnesium 170 mg/tablet; watermelon flavor]

Phillips'® Milk of Magnesia: 311 mg [mint flavor]

Phillips'® Milk of Magnesia: 311 mg [contains magnesium 130 mg/tablet; mint flavor]

◆ **Magnesium Hydroxide, Aluminum Hydroxide, and Simethicone** see Aluminum Hydroxide, Magnesium Hydroxide, and Simethicone *on page 82*

◆ **Magnesium Hydroxide and Aluminum Hydroxide** see Aluminum Hydroxide and Magnesium Hydroxide *on page 80*

Magnesium Hydroxide and Mineral Oil
(mag NEE zhum hye DROKS ide & MIN er al oyl)

Related Information
Magnesium Hydroxide *on page 1177*
Mineral Oil *on page 1288*
Brand Names: U.S. Phillips'® M-O [OTC]
Index Terms Haley's M-O; MOM/Mineral Oil Emulsion
Generic Availability (U.S.) No
Pharmacologic Category Laxative
Use Short-term treatment of occasional constipation
Contraindications Hypersensitivity magnesium hydroxide, mineral oil, or any component of the formulation
Warnings/Precautions Use magnesium with caution in patients with severe renal impairment (especially when doses are >50 mEq magnesium/day); hypermagnesemia and toxicity may occur due to decreased renal clearance of absorbed magnesium. Decreased renal function (Cl_{cr} <30 mL/minute) may result in toxicity; monitor for toxicity.

For self-medication (OTC use): Patients should notify healthcare provider of any sudden change in bowel habits which last >14 days, stomach pain, nausea, vomiting, or if use is needed for >1 week. Not for OTC use in bedridden patients or patients with dysphagia. Avoid concomitant use with stool softener laxatives.

Drug Interactions
Metabolism/Transport Effects None known.
Avoid Concomitant Use
Avoid concomitant use of Magnesium Hydroxide and Mineral Oil with any of the following: Calcium Polystyrene Sulfonate; QuiNINE; Sodium Polystyrene Sulfonate
Increased Effect/Toxicity
Magnesium Hydroxide and Mineral Oil may increase the levels/effects of: Alpha-/Beta-Agonists; Amphetamines; Calcium Channel Blockers; Calcium Polystyrene Sulfonate; Dexmethylphenidate; Methylphenidate; Misoprostol; Neuromuscular-Blocking Agents; QuiNIDine; Sodium Polystyrene Sulfonate

The levels/effects of Magnesium Hydroxide and Mineral Oil may be increased by: Alfacalcidol; Calcitriol; Calcium Channel Blockers
Decreased Effect
Magnesium Hydroxide and Mineral Oil may decrease the levels/effects of: ACE Inhibitors; Allopurinol; Anticonvulsants (Hydantoin); Antipsychotic Agents (Phenothiazines); Atazanavir; Bisacodyl; Bisphosphonate Derivatives; Cefditoren; Cefpodoxime; Cefuroxime; Chloroquine; Corticosteroids (Oral); Dabigatran Etexilate; Dasatinib; Deferiprone; Delavirdine; Eltrombopag; Erlotinib; Fexofenadine; Gabapentin; HMG-CoA Reductase Inhibitors; Iron Salts; Isoniazid; Itraconazole; Ketoconazole; Ketoconazole (Systemic); Mesalamine; Methenamine; Mycophenolate; Nilotinib; PenicillAMINE; Phosphate Supplements; Phytonadione; Protease Inhibitors; QuiNINE; Quinolone Antibiotics; Rilpivirine; Tetracycline Derivatives; Trientine; Vismodegib; Vitamin D Analogs

The levels/effects of Magnesium Hydroxide and Mineral Oil may be decreased by: Trientine
Pharmacodynamics/Kinetics
Onset of action: Laxative: 30 minutes to 6 hours hours
Excretion: Magnesium: Urine (up to 30% as absorbed magnesium ions); feces (as unabsorbed drug)
Dosage
Geriatric & Adult Laxative: OTC labeling: Oral: 45-60 mL at bedtime
Renal Impairment Patients in severe renal failure should not receive magnesium due to toxicity from accumulation. Patients with a Cl_{cr} <30 mL/minute should be monitored by serum magnesium levels.
Administration Shake well; administer with full glass of water
Special Geriatric Considerations The use of mineral oil products may be hazardous in the elderly with conditions predisposing them to aspiration. Elderly, due to disease or drug therapy, may be predisposed to diarrhea. Diarrhea may result in electrolyte imbalance. Decreased renal function (Cl_{cr} <30 mL/minute) may result in toxicity from magnesium absorption; monitor for toxicity.
Dosage Forms Excipient information presented when available (limited, particularly for generics); consult specific product labeling.
Suspension, oral:
Phillips'® M-O: Magnesium hydroxide 300 mg and mineral oil 1.25 mL per 5 mL (360 mL, 780 mL) [contains magnesium 125 mg and sodium 1.5 mg per 5 mL mint flavors]

◆ **Magnesium Hydroxide, Famotidine, and Calcium Carbonate** see Famotidine, Calcium Carbonate, and Magnesium Hydroxide on page 746

Magnesium L-aspartate Hydrochloride
(mag NEE zhum el as PAR tate hye droe KLOR ide)

Brand Names: U.S. Maginex™ DS [OTC]; Maginex™ [OTC]
Index Terms MAH
Generic Availability (U.S.) No
Pharmacologic Category Electrolyte Supplement, Oral; Magnesium Salt
Use Dietary supplement
Dosage
  Geriatric & Adult
    RDA (elemental magnesium):
      19-30 years:
        Female: 310 mg/day
        Male: 400 mg/day
      ≥31 years:
        Female: 320 mg/day
        Male: 420 mg/day
    Dietary supplement: Oral: Magnesium-L-aspartate 1230 mg (magnesium 122 mg) up to 3 times/day
  Renal Impairment Cl$_{cr}$ <30 mL/minute: Use with caution; monitor for hypermagnesemia
  Special Geriatric Considerations Elderly, due to disease or drug therapy, may be predisposed to diarrhea. Diarrhea may result in electrolyte imbalance. Decreased renal function (Cl$_{cr}$ <30 mL/minute) may result in toxicity; monitor for toxicity. Monitor for signs of confusion or worsening signs of dementia.
  Dosage Forms Excipient information presented when available (limited, particularly for generics); consult specific product labeling.
    Granules for solution, oral [preservative free]:
      Maginex™ DS: 1230 mg/packet (30s) [sugar free; lemon flavor; equivalent to elemental magnesium 122 mg]
    Tablet, enteric coated, oral [preservative free]:
      Maginex™: 615 mg [sugar free; equivalent to elemental magnesium 61 mg]

Magnesium L-lactate (mag NEE zhum el LAK tate)

Brand Names: U.S. Mag-Tab® SR
Index Terms Magnesium L-lactate Dihydrate
Generic Availability (U.S.) No
Pharmacologic Category Electrolyte Supplement; Magnesium Salt
Use Dietary supplement
Dosage
  Geriatric & Adult
    Dietary supplement: Oral:1-2 caplets every 12 hours
    RDA (elemental magnesium):
      19-30 years:
        Female: 310 mg/day
        Male: 400 mg/day
      ≥31 years:
        Female: 320 mg/day
        Male: 420 mg/day
  Renal Impairment Cl$_{cr}$ <30 mL/minute: Use with caution; monitor for hypermagnesemia
  Special Geriatric Considerations Elderly, due to disease or drug therapy, may be predisposed to diarrhea. Diarrhea may result in electrolyte imbalance. Decreased renal function (Cl$_{cr}$ <30 mL/minute) may result in toxicity; monitor for toxicity and Cl$_{cr}$ <30 mL/minute.
  Dosage Forms Excipient information presented when available (limited, particularly for generics); consult specific product labeling.
    Caplet, sustained release, oral:
      Mag-Tab® SR: Elemental magnesium 84 mg [scored]

Magnesium Oxide (mag NEE zhum OKS ide)

Related Information
Calculations *on page 2087*
Brand Names: U.S. Mag-Ox® 400 [OTC]; MAGnesium-Oxide™ [OTC]; Phillips'® Laxative Dietary Supplement Cramp-Free [OTC]; Uro-Mag® [OTC]
Index Terms Mag Oxide
Generic Availability (U.S.) Yes: Excludes capsule
Pharmacologic Category Electrolyte Supplement, Oral; Magnesium Salt
Use Electrolyte replacement
Contraindications Hypersensitivity to any component of the formulation
Warnings/Precautions Use magnesium with caution in patients with impaired renal function (accumulation of magnesium may lead to magnesium intoxication). Use with extreme caution in patients with myasthenia gravis or other neuromuscular disease.

Constipation (self-medication, OTC use): For occasional use only; serious side effects may occur with prolonged use. For use only under the supervision of a healthcare provider in patients with kidney dysfunction, or with a sudden change in bowel habits which persist for >2 weeks. Do not use if abdominal pain, nausea, or vomiting are present.
Adverse Reactions (Reflective of adult population; not specific for elderly) Frequency not defined: Gastrointestinal: Diarrhea (excessive oral doses)
Drug Interactions
Metabolism/Transport Effects None known.
Avoid Concomitant Use
Avoid concomitant use of Magnesium Oxide with any of the following: Calcium Polystyrene Sulfonate; Sodium Polystyrene Sulfonate
Increased Effect/Toxicity
Magnesium Oxide may increase the levels/effects of: Calcium Channel Blockers; Calcium Polystyrene Sulfonate; Neuromuscular-Blocking Agents; Sodium Polystyrene Sulfonate

The levels/effects of Magnesium Oxide may be increased by: Alfacalcidol; Calcitriol; Calcium Channel Blockers
Decreased Effect
Magnesium Oxide may decrease the levels/effects of: Bisphosphonate Derivatives; Deferiprone; Eltrombopag; Mycophenolate; Phosphate Supplements; Quinolone Antibiotics; Tetracycline Derivatives; Trientine

The levels/effects of Magnesium Oxide may be decreased by: Trientine
Mechanism of Action Magnesium is important as a cofactor in many enzymatic reactions in the body involving protein synthesis and carbohydrate metabolism (at least 300 enzymatic reactions require magnesium). Actions on lipoprotein lipase have been found to be important in reducing serum cholesterol and on sodium/potassium ATPase in promoting polarization (eg, neuromuscular functioning).
Pharmacodynamics/Kinetics
Absorption: Oral: Inversely proportional to amount ingested; 40% to 60% under controlled dietary conditions; 15% to 36% at higher doses
Distribution: Bone (50% to 60%); extracellular fluid (1% to 2%)
Protein binding: 30%, to albumin
Excretion: Urine (as magnesium)
Dosage
Geriatric & Adult
RDA (elemental magnesium): Oral:
19-30 years:
Female: 310 mg/day
Male: 400 mg/day
≥31 years:
Female: 320 mg/day
Male: 420 mg/day

Dietary supplement: Oral:
Mag-Ox 400®: 2 tablets daily with food
Mag-Caps, Uro-Mag®: 4-5 capsules daily with food
Renal Impairment Cl_{cr} <30 mL/minute: Use with caution; monitor for hypermagnesemia
Reference Range Serum magnesium: 1.5-2.5 mg/dL; slightly different ranges are reported by different laboratories

◄ **Special Geriatric Considerations** Elderly, due to disease or drug therapy, may be predisposed to diarrhea. Diarrhea may result in electrolyte imbalance. Decreased renal function (Cl_{cr} <30 mL/minute) may result in toxicity; monitor for toxicity.

Dosage Forms Excipient information presented when available (limited, particularly for generics); consult specific product labeling.

Caplet, oral: Elemental magnesium 250 mg

Phillips'® Laxative Dietary Supplement Cramp-Free: Elemental magnesium 500 mg

Capsule, oral:

Uro-Mag®: 140 mg [equivalent to elemental magnesium 84.5 mg]

Tablet, oral: 400 mg [equivalent to elemental magnesium 240 mg], 400 mg, 420 mg, 500 mg [equivalent to elemental magnesium 500 mg]

Mag-Ox® 400: 400 mg [scored; equivalent to elemental magnesium 240 mg]

MAGnesium-Oxide™: 400 mg [equivalent to elemental magnesium 240 mg]

◆ **MAGnesium-Oxide™ [OTC]** *see* Magnesium Oxide *on page 1181*
◆ **Magnesium Salicylate** *see* Salicylates (Various Salts) *on page 1742*

Magnesium Salts (Various Salts) (mag NEE zhum salts)

Brand Names: U.S. Almora® [OTC]; Epsom Salt [OTC]; Magonate® [OTC]; Mg-plus® [OTC]; Slow-Mag® [OTC]

Generic Availability (U.S.) Yes

Stability Refrigeration of intact ampuls may result in precipitation or crystallization; stability of parenteral admixture at room temperature (25°C): 60 days

Mechanism of Action Promotes bowel evacuation by causing osmotic retention of fluid which distends the colon with increased peristaltic activity when taken orally; parenterally, decreases acetylcholine in motor nerve terminals and acts on myocardium by slowing rate of S-A node impulse formation and prolonging conduction time

Pharmacodynamics/Kinetics

Absorption: Absorbed magnesium is rapidly eliminated by the kidneys.

Elimination: Primarily excreted in feces

Test Interactions Increased magnesium; decreased protein, calcium (S), decreased potassium (S)

Pharmacotherapy Pearls 1 g magnesium = 8.3 mEq (41.1 mmol); see individual agents for magnesium content per dose

Special Geriatric Considerations Elderly, due to disease or drug therapy, may be predisposed to diarrhea. Diarrhea may result in electrolyte imbalance. Decreased renal function (Cl_{cr} <30 mL/minute) may result in toxicity; monitor for toxicity.

Dosage Forms

Granules, as sulfate: ~40 mEq magnesium/5 g (240 g)

Injection, as sulfate: 10% = 0.8 mEq/mL (2 mL, 10 mL, 20 mL, 30 mL, 50 mL); 20% = 1.97 mEq/mL (2 mL, 10 mL, 20 mL, 30 mL, 50 mL); 50% = 4 mEq/mL (2 mL, 10 mL, 20 mL, 30 mL, 50 mL)

Liquid, as sulfate: 54 mg/5 mL; gluconate: 54 mg/5 mL (gluconate has 27 mg magnesium)

Tablet, as various salts: 140 mg, 400 mg, 500 mg

◆ **Magnesium Trisilicate and Aluminum Hydroxide** *see* Aluminum Hydroxide and Magnesium Trisilicate *on page 81*
◆ **Magonate® [OTC]** *see* Magnesium Salts (Various Salts) *on page 1182*
◆ **Mag-Ox® 400 [OTC]** *see* Magnesium Oxide *on page 1181*
◆ **Mag Oxide** *see* Magnesium Oxide *on page 1181*
◆ **Mag-Tab® SR** *see* Magnesium L-lactate *on page 1180*
◆ **MAH** *see* Magnesium L-aspartate Hydrochloride *on page 1180*
◆ **Mantoux** *see* Tuberculin Tests *on page 1980*
◆ **Mapap® [OTC]** *see* Acetaminophen *on page 31*
◆ **Mapap® Arthritis Pain [OTC]** *see* Acetaminophen *on page 31*
◆ **Mapap® Children's [OTC]** *see* Acetaminophen *on page 31*
◆ **Mapap® Extra Strength [OTC]** *see* Acetaminophen *on page 31*
◆ **Mapap® Infant's [OTC]** *see* Acetaminophen *on page 31*
◆ **Mapap® Junior Rapid Tabs [OTC]** *see* Acetaminophen *on page 31*
◆ **Mapap® Sinus PE [OTC]** *see* Acetaminophen and Phenylephrine *on page 37*

Maprotiline (ma PROE ti leen)

Related Information
Antidepressant Agents on page 2097
Medication Safety Issues
International issues
Ludiomil [multiple international markets] may be confused with Lamictal brand name for lamotrigine [U.S., Canada, and multiple international markets]; lamotrigine [U.S., Canada, and multiple international markets]; Lomotil brand name for diphenoxylate [U.S, Canada, and multiple international markets] and brand name for loperamide [Mexico, Philippines]
Brand Names: Canada Novo-Maprotiline; Teva-Maprotiline
Index Terms Ludiomil; Maprotiline Hydrochloride
Generic Availability (U.S.) Yes
Pharmacologic Category Antidepressant, Tetracyclic
Use Treatment of major depressive disorder (MDD) or of anxiety associated with depression
Unlabeled Use Chronic pain; panic attacks
Medication Guide Available Yes
Dosage
Geriatric Depression/anxiety: Oral: Initial: 25 mg/day for 2 weeks; Maintenance: Increase by 25 mg as tolerated; usual dose: 50-75 mg/day, higher doses may be necessary in nonresponders
Adult
Mild-to-moderate depression/anxiety: Oral: Initial: 75 mg/day for 2 weeks (lower doses may be considered in some patients); Maintenance: Increase by 25 mg as tolerated up to 150 mg/day; given in divided doses or in a single daily dose
Severe depression: Oral: Initial: 100-150 mg/day for 2 weeks; Maintenance: Increase by 25 mg as tolerated up to 225 mg/day; given in divided doses or in a single daily dose
Special Geriatric Considerations Avoid in the elderly due to sedation and anticholinergic effects (eg, confusion, constipation, difficulty urinating, dry mouth).

A systematic review and meta-analysis of antidepressant placebo-controlled trials in persons with depression and dementia found evidence "suggestive" of efficacy but not of sufficient strength to "confirm" efficacy. Antidepressant trials in this patient population are small and underpowered. Older patients with depression being treated with an antidepressant should be closely monitored for response and adverse effects. Treatment should be switched or augmented when response is inadequate with a therapeutic dose. Antidepressants that are not tolerated should be discontinued and an alternative agent should be started.
Dosage Forms Excipient information presented when available (limited, particularly for generics); consult specific product labeling.
Tablet, oral, as hydrochloride: 25 mg, 50 mg, 75 mg

◆ **MDL 73,147EF** *see* Dolasetron *on page* 589

Measles, Mumps, and Rubella Virus Vaccine
(MEE zels, mumpz & roo BEL a VYE rus vak SEEN)

Related Information
Immunization Administration Recommendations *on page* 2144
Immunization Recommendations *on page* 2149

Medication Safety Issues
Sound-alike/look-alike issues:
MMR (measles, mumps and rubella virus vaccine) may be confused with MMRV (measles, mumps, rubella, and varicella) vaccine

Brand Names: U.S. M-M-R® II

Brand Names: Canada M-M-R® II; Priorix™

Index Terms MMR; Mumps, Measles and Rubella Vaccines; Rubella, Measles and Mumps Vaccines

Generic Availability (U.S.) No

Pharmacologic Category Vaccine, Live (Viral)

Use Measles, mumps, and rubella prophylaxis
The Advisory Committee on Immunization Practices (ACIP) recommends routine vaccination for the following:
- All children (first dose given at 12-15 months of age)
- Adults born 1957 or later (without evidence of immunity or documentation of vaccination).
- Adults at higher risk for exposure to and transmission of measles mumps and rubella should receive special consideration for vaccination, unless an acceptable evidence of immunity exists. This includes international travelers, persons attending colleges and other post-high school education, persons working in healthcare facilities.

Contraindications Hypersensitivity to measles, mumps, and/or rubella vaccine or any component of the formulation; current febrile respiratory illness or other febrile infection; patients receiving immunosuppressive therapy (does not include corticosteroids as replacement therapy); primary and acquired immunodeficiency states; individuals with blood dyscrasias, leukemia, lymphomas, or other malignant neoplasms affecting the bone marrow or lymphatic systems; family history of congenital or hereditary immunodeficiency (until immune competence in the vaccine recipient is demonstrated).

Warnings/Precautions Use caution with history of cerebral injury, seizures, or other conditions where stress due to fever should be avoided. Immediate treatment for anaphylactic/anaphylactoid reaction should be available during vaccine use. Use caution in patients with thrombocytopenia and those who develop thrombocytopenia after first dose; thrombocytopenia may worsen. Consider delaying vaccination during acute moderate or severe febrile illness; per the ACIP, patients with minor illnesses with or without fever may receive vaccine. Use is contraindicated in severely immunocompromised patients. However, leukemia patients who are in remission and who have not received chemotherapy for at least 3 months may be vaccinated; patients with HIV infection, who are asymptomatic and not severely immunosuppressed may be vaccinated. In general, household and close contacts of persons with altered immunocompetence may receive all age appropriate vaccines. Recent administration of blood or blood products may interfere with immune response.

Therapy to treat tuberculosis should be started prior to administering vaccine to patients with active tuberculosis. Patients with untreated, active tuberculosis should not receive vaccine. Exposure to measles is not a contraindication to vaccine; use within 72 hours of exposure may provide some protection. Vaccine contains trace amounts of chick embryo antigen. Use caution in patients with history of immediate hypersensitivity/anaphylactic reactions following egg ingestion. Generally, the MMR vaccine can be safely administered to persons with an egg allergy (CDC, 2011). Manufactured with neomycin. Patients with history of anaphylaxis should not receive vaccine; contact dermatitis to neomycin is not a contraindication to the vaccine. Contains gelatin; contraindicated if known hypersensitivity to gelatin. In order to maximize vaccination rates, the ACIP recommends simultaneous administration of all age-appropriate vaccines (live or inactivated) for which a person is eligible at a single clinic visit, unless contraindications exist. The use of combination vaccines is generally preferred over separate injections, taking into consideration provider assessment, patient preference, and potential adverse events. Acceptable evidence of immunity is recommended healthcare workers prior to employment, students entering institutions of higher learning, and travelers to endemic areas.

Adverse Reactions (Reflective of adult population; not specific for elderly) All serious adverse reactions must be reported to the U.S. Department of Health and Human Services (DHHS) Vaccine Adverse Event Reporting System (VAERS) 1-800-822-7967 or online at https://vaers.hhs.gov/esub/index. In Canada, adverse reactions may be reported to local provincial/territorial health agencies or to the Vaccine Safety Section at Public Health Agency of Canada (1-866-844-0018).

Frequency not defined:

Cardiovascular: Syncope, vasculitis

Central nervous system: Ataxia, dizziness, febrile seizure, fever, encephalitis, encephalopathy, Guillain-Barré syndrome, headache, irritability, malaise, measles inclusion body encephalitis, polyneuritis, polyneuropathy, seizure, subacute sclerosing panencephalitis.

Dermatologic: Angioneurotic edema, erythema multiforme, measles-like rash, pruritus, purpura, rash, Stevens-Johnson syndrome, urticaria

Endocrine & metabolic: Diabetes mellitus, parotitis

Gastrointestinal: Diarrhea, nausea, pancreatitis, sore throat, vomiting

Genitourinary: Epididymitis, orchitis

Hematologic: Leukocytosis, thrombocytopenia

Local: Injection site reactions which include burning, induration, redness, stinging, swelling, tenderness, wheal and flare, vesiculation

Neuromuscular & skeletal: Arthralgia/arthritis (variable; highest rates in women, 12% to 26% versus children, up to 3%), myalgia, paresthesia

Ocular: Conjunctivitis, ocular palsies, optic neuritis, papillitis, retinitis, retrobulbar neuritis

Otic: Nerve deafness, otitis media

Renal: Conjunctivitis, retinitis, optic neuritis, papillitis, retrobulbar neuritis

Respiratory: Bronchospasm, cough, pneumonia, pneumonitis, rhinitis

Miscellaneous: Anaphylactoid reactions, anaphylaxis, atypical measles, panniculitis, regional lymphadenopathy

Drug Interactions

Metabolism/Transport Effects None known.

Avoid Concomitant Use

Avoid concomitant use of Measles, Mumps, and Rubella Virus Vaccine with any of the following: Belimumab; Fingolimod; Immunosuppressants

Increased Effect/Toxicity

The levels/effects of Measles, Mumps, and Rubella Virus Vaccine may be increased by: AzaTHIOprine; Belimumab; Corticosteroids (Systemic); Fingolimod; Hydroxychloroquine; Immunosuppressants; Leflunomide; Mercaptopurine; Methotrexate

Decreased Effect

Measles, Mumps, and Rubella Virus Vaccine may decrease the levels/effects of: Tuberculin Tests

The levels/effects of Measles, Mumps, and Rubella Virus Vaccine may be decreased by: Fingolimod; Immune Globulins; Immunosuppressants

Stability To maintain potency, the lyophilized vaccine must be stored between -50°C to 8°C (-58°F to 46°F). Temperatures below -50°C (-58°F) may occur if stored in dry ice. Prior to reconstitution, store the powder at 2°C to 8°C (36°F to 46°F). Protect from light. Diluent may be stored in refrigerator or at room temperature. Do not freeze diluent. Use entire contents of the provided diluent to reconstitute vaccine. Gently agitate to mix thoroughly. Discard if powder does not dissolve. Use as soon as possible following reconstitution (may be stored at 2°C to 8°C/36°F to 46°F; protect from light); discard if not used within 8 hours.

Mechanism of Action As a live, attenuated vaccine, MMR vaccine offers active immunity to disease caused by the measles, mumps, and rubella viruses.

Dosage

Adult

Immunization: SubQ: 0.5 mL

Birth year in or after 1957 without evidence of immunity: 1 or 2 doses (0.5 mL/dose); minimum interval between doses is 28 days

Adults born in or after 1957 without documentation of live vaccine on or after first birthday, or without physician-diagnosed measles or mumps, or without laboratory evidence of immunity, should be vaccinated with at least one dose; a second dose, separated by no less than 1 month, is indicated for those previously vaccinated with one dose of measles vaccine, students entering institutions of higher learning, recently exposed in an outbreak setting, healthcare workers at time of employment, and for travelers to endemic areas (CDC, 1998).

Persons vaccinated between 1963 and 1967 with a killed measles vaccine, followed by live vaccine within 3 months, or with a vaccine of unknown type should be revaccinated with live measles virus vaccine (CDC, 1998).

Healthcare personnel (unvaccinated) born prior to 1957 and who are without laboratory evidence of measles, mumps, and/or rubella immunity or laboratory confirmation of disease: Consider 2 doses of MMR vaccine at the appropriate interval. Two doses of the MMR vaccine are needed for measles and mumps, one dose is needed for rubella (CDC, 2006).

Administration Administer SubQ in outer aspect of the upper arm in patients ≥12 months. **Not for I.V. administration.**

Simultaneous administration of vaccines helps ensure the patients will be fully vaccinated by the appropriate age. Simultaneous administration of vaccines is defined as administering >1 vaccine on the same day at different anatomic sites. The use of licensed combination vaccines is generally preferred over separate injections of the equivalent components. Separate vaccines should not be combined in the same syringe unless indicated by product specific labeling. Separate needles and syringes should be used for each injection. The ACIP prefers each dose of a specific vaccine in a series come from the same manufacturer when possible. Adolescents and adults should be vaccinated while seated or lying down. In general, preterm infants should be vaccinated at the same chronological age as full-term infants (CDC, 2011).

Antipyretics have not been shown to prevent febrile seizures. Antipyretics may be used to treat fever or discomfort following vaccination (CDC, 2011). One study reported that routine prophylactic administration of acetaminophen to prevent fever prior to vaccination decreased the immune response of some vaccines; the clinical significance of this reduction in immune response has not been established (Prymula, 2009).

Monitoring Parameters Monitor for syncope for 15 minutes following administration. If seizure-like activity associated with syncope occurs, maintain patient in supine or Trendelenburg position to reestablish adequate cerebral perfusion.

Test Interactions Temporary suppression of TB skin test reactivity. Tuberculin test may be given simultaneously at separate sites on the same day as measles -containing vaccine or ≥4 weeks later.

Pharmacotherapy Pearls U.S. federal law requires that the name of medication, date of administration, the vaccine manufacturer, lot number of vaccine, and the administering person's name, title, and address be entered into the patient's permanent medical record.

Acceptable presumptive evidence of immunity includes one of the following:
1. Documentation of adequate vaccination (for measles, mumps, and rubella). Adequate vaccination for mumps is defined as 1 dose of a live mumps virus vaccine for preschool children and adults not at high risk; 2 doses of a live mumps virus vaccine for school-aged children and high-risk adults. Healthcare workers, international travelers, and students in institutions of higher learning are considered high-risk adults.
2. Laboratory evidence of immunity (for measles, mumps, and rubella)
3. Birth prior to 1957 (measles and mumps); for women of childbearing potential, birth prior to 1957 is not acceptable evidence of immunity to rubella
4. Documentation of physician-diagnosed disease (for measles, mumps); exception, not acceptable evidence of immunity for healthcare workers

Special Geriatric Considerations Most adults and elderly are immune to measles (rubeola) and it is not necessary to vaccinate. If no history of measles exposure or patient is from an isolated community where measles is not endemic, vaccination may be required. Testing may be indicated; may need to test for rubella. Vaccinate those traveling into endemic areas with no evidence of immunity. No dose restriction necessary.

Dosage Forms Excipient information presented when available (limited, particularly for generics); consult specific product labeling.

Injection, powder for reconstitution [preservative free]:

M-M-R® II: Measles virus ≥1000 $TCID_{50}$, mumps virus ≥20,000 $TCID_{50}$, and rubella virus ≥1000 $TCID_{50}$ [contains albumin (human), bovine serum, chicken egg protein, gelatin, neomycin, sorbitol, and sucrose 1.9 mg/vial; supplied with diluent]

Meclizine (MEK li zeen)

Related Information
Beers Criteria – Potentially Inappropriate Medications for Geriatrics *on page 2183*

Medication Safety Issues
Sound-alike/look-alike issues:
Antivert® may be confused with Anzemet®, Axert®

BEERS Criteria medication:
This drug may be potentially inappropriate for use in geriatric patients (Quality of evidence - varies based on comorbidity; Strength of recommendation - varies based on comorbidity)

Brand Names: U.S. Antivert®; Bonine® [OTC] [DSC]; Dramamine® Less Drowsy Formula [OTC]; Medi-Meclizine [OTC]; Trav-L-Tabs® [OTC]; VertiCalm™ [OTC]

Index Terms Meclizine Hydrochloride; Meclozine Hydrochloride

Generic Availability (U.S.) Yes

Pharmacologic Category Antiemetic; Histamine H_1 Antagonist; Histamine H_1 Antagonist, First Generation; Piperazine Derivative

Use Prevention and treatment of symptoms of motion sickness; management of vertigo with diseases affecting the vestibular system

Contraindications Hypersensitivity to meclizine or any component of the formulation

Warnings/Precautions Use with caution in patients with asthma, angle-closure glaucoma, prostatic hyperplasia, pyloric or duodenal obstruction, or bladder neck obstruction. May be inappropriate in older adults depending on comorbidities (eg, dementia, delirium, etc) due to its potent anticholinergic effects (Beers Criteria). Use with caution in the elderly; may be more sensitive to adverse effects. If vertigo does not respond in 1-2 weeks, it is advised to discontinue use. May be sedating, use with caution in disorders where CNS depression is a feature; patients must be cautioned about performing tasks which require mental alertness (eg, operating machinery or driving). Effects may be potentiated when used with other sedative drugs or ethanol.

Adverse Reactions (Reflective of adult population; not specific for elderly) Frequency not defined.

Central nervous system: Drowsiness, fatigue, headache

Gastrointestinal: Vomiting, xerostomia

Ocular: Blurred vision

Miscellaneous: Anaphylactoid reaction

Drug Interactions

Metabolism/Transport Effects None known.

Avoid Concomitant Use

Avoid concomitant use of Meclizine with any of the following: Azelastine; Azelastine (Nasal); Methadone; Mirtazapine; Paraldehyde

Increased Effect/Toxicity

Meclizine may increase the levels/effects of: Alcohol (Ethyl); Anticholinergics; Azelastine; Azelastine (Nasal); Buprenorphine; CNS Depressants; Methadone; Methotrimeprazine; Metyrosine; Mirtazapine; Paraldehyde; Selective Serotonin Reuptake Inhibitors; Zolpidem

The levels/effects of Meclizine may be increased by: Droperidol; HydrOXYzine; Methotrimeprazine; Pramlintide

Decreased Effect

Meclizine may decrease the levels/effects of: Acetylcholinesterase Inhibitors (Central); Benzylpenicilloyl Polylysine; Betahistine; Hyaluronidase

The levels/effects of Meclizine may be decreased by: Acetylcholinesterase Inhibitors (Central); Amphetamines

Ethanol/Nutrition/Herb Interactions Ethanol: May increase CNS depression; monitor for increased effects with coadministration. Caution patients about effects.

Mechanism of Action Has central anticholinergic action by blocking chemoreceptor trigger zone; decreases excitability of the middle ear labyrinth and blocks conduction in the middle ear vestibular-cerebellar pathways

Pharmacodynamics/Kinetics

Onset of action: ~1 hour (Wang, 2011a)

Duration: ~24 hours (Wang, 2011a)

Distribution: V_d: 7 L/kg (Wang, 2011a)

Metabolism: Hepatic to norchlorcyclizine (Wang, 2011a)

Half-life elimination: 5 hours (Wang, 2011a; Wang, 2011b)

Time to peak, plasma: 3 hours (Wang, 2011a; Wang, 2011b)

Excretion: Urine and feces as unchanged drug and metabolites (Wang, 2011a)

Dosage

Geriatric & Adult

Motion sickness: Oral: 25-50 mg 1 hour before travel, repeat dose every 24 hours if needed

Vertigo: Oral: 25-100 mg daily in divided doses

Special Geriatric Considerations Due to anticholinergic action, use lowest dose in divided doses to avoid side effects and their inconvenience. Limit use if possible. May cause confusion or aggravate symptoms of confusion in those with dementia. If vertigo does not respond in 1-2 weeks, discontinue use.

This medication is considered to be potentially inappropriate in this patient population (Beers Criteria: Quality of evidence - varies based on comorbidity; Strength of recommendation - varies based on comorbidity).

Dosage Forms Excipient information presented when available (limited, particularly for generics); consult specific product labeling. [DSC] = Discontinued product

Caplet, oral, as hydrochloride: 12.5 mg

◀ Tablet, oral, as hydrochloride: 12.5 mg, 25 mg
    Antivert®: 12.5 mg, 25 mg
    Antivert®: 50 mg [scored]
    Dramamine® Less Drowsy Formula: 25 mg
    Medi-Meclizine: 25 mg
    Trav-L-Tabs®: 25 mg
    VertiCalm™: 25 mg
Tablet, chewable, oral, as hydrochloride: 25 mg
    Bonine®: 25 mg [DSC] [scored; raspberry flavor]

♦ **Meclizine Hydrochloride** *see* Meclizine *on page* 1186

Meclofenamate (me kloe fen AM ate)

Related Information
Beers Criteria – Potentially Inappropriate Medications for Geriatrics *on page* 2183

Medication Safety Issues
BEERS Criteria medication:
This drug may be potentially inappropriate for use in geriatric patients (Quality of evidence - moderate; Strength of recommendation - strong).

Brand Names: Canada Meclomen®

Index Terms Meclofenamate Sodium

Generic Availability (U.S.) Yes

Pharmacologic Category Nonsteroidal Anti-inflammatory Drug (NSAID), Oral

Use Treatment of inflammatory disorders, arthritis, mild-to-moderate pain, dysmenorrhea

Medication Guide Available Yes

Contraindications Hypersensitivity to meclofenamate, aspirin, other NSAIDs, or any component of the formulation; perioperative pain in the setting of coronary artery bypass graft (CABG) surgery

Warnings/Precautions NSAIDs are associated with an increased risk of adverse cardiovascular thrombotic events, including MI and stroke. Risk may be increased with duration of use or pre-existing cardiovascular risk factors or disease. Carefully evaluate individual cardiovascular risk profiles prior to prescribing. May cause new-onset hypertension or worsening of existing hypertension. Use caution with fluid retention. Avoid use in heart failure. Concurrent administration of ibuprofen, and potentially other nonselective NSAIDs, may interfere with aspirin's cardioprotective effect. Risk of MI and stroke may be increased with use following CABG surgery.

Platelet adhesion and aggregation may be decreased; may prolong bleeding time; patients with coagulation disorders or who are receiving anticoagulants should be monitored closely. Anemia may occur; patients on long-term NSAID therapy should be monitored for anemia. Rarely, NSAID use may cause severe blood dyscrasias (eg, agranulocytosis, aplastic anemia, thrombocytopenia).

NSAID use may compromise existing renal function; dose-dependent decreases in prostaglandin synthesis may result from NSAID use, reducing renal blood flow which may cause renal decompensation. NSAID use may increase the risk for hyperkalemia. Patients with impaired renal function, dehydration, heart failure, liver dysfunction, those taking diuretics, and ACE inhibitors, and the elderly are at greater risk of renal toxicity and hyperkalemia. Rehydrate patient before starting therapy; monitor renal function closely. Not recommended for use in patients with advanced renal disease. Long-term NSAID use may result in renal papillary necrosis.

NSAIDs may increase risk of gastrointestinal irritation, inflammation, ulceration, bleeding, and perforation. These events may occur at any time during therapy and without warning. Use caution with a history of GI disease (bleeding or ulcers), concurrent therapy with aspirin, anticoagulants and/or corticosteroids, smoking, use of alcohol, the elderly or debilitated patients. When used concomitantly with ≤325 mg of aspirin, a substantial increase in the risk of gastrointestinal complications (eg, ulcer) occurs; concomitant gastroprotective therapy (eg, proton pump inhibitors) is recommended (Bhatt, 2008).

Use the lowest effective dose for the shortest duration of time, consistent with individual patient goals, to reduce risk of cardiovascular or GI adverse events. Alternate therapies should be considered for patients at high risk.

NSAIDs may cause serious skin adverse events including exfoliative dermatitis, Stevens-Johnson syndrome (SJS) and toxic epidermal necrolysis (TEN); discontinue use at first sign of skin rash or hypersensitivity. Anaphylactoid reactions may occur, even without prior exposure; patients with "aspirin triad" (bronchial asthma, aspirin intolerance, rhinitis) may be at increased risk. Do not use in patients who experience bronchospasm, asthma, rhinitis, or urticaria with NSAID or aspirin therapy. Use caution in other forms of asthma.

Use with caution in patients with decreased hepatic function. Closely monitor patients with any abnormal LFT. Severe hepatic reactions (eg, fulminant hepatitis, liver failure) have occurred with NSAID use, rarely; discontinue if signs or symptoms of liver disease develop, or if systemic manifestations occur.

NSAIDS may cause drowsiness, dizziness, blurred vision and other neurologic effects which may impair physical or mental abilities; patients must be cautioned about performing tasks which require mental alertness (eg, operating machinery or driving). Discontinue use with blurred or diminished vision and perform ophthalmologic exam. Monitor vision with long-term therapy.

In the elderly, avoid chronic use (unless alternative agents ineffective and patient is able to receive concomitant gastroprotective agent); nonselective oral NSAID use is associated with an increased risk of GI bleeding and peptic ulcer disease in older adults in high risk category (eg, >75 years or age or receiving concomitant oral/parenteral corticosteroids, anticoagulants, or antiplatelet agents) (Beers Criteria).

Withhold for at least 4-6 half-lives prior to surgical or dental procedures.

Adverse Reactions (Reflective of adult population; not specific for elderly)

>10%:
Central nervous system: Dizziness
Dermatologic: Rash
Gastrointestinal: Abdominal cramps, heartburn, indigestion, nausea

1% to 10%:
Central nervous system: Headache, nervousness
Dermatologic: Itching
Endocrine & metabolic: Fluid retention
Gastrointestinal: Vomiting
Otic: Tinnitus

Drug Interactions

Metabolism/Transport Effects None known.

Avoid Concomitant Use

Avoid concomitant use of Meclofenamate with any of the following: Floctafenine; Ketorolac; Ketorolac (Nasal); Ketorolac (Systemic)

Increased Effect/Toxicity

Meclofenamate may increase the levels/effects of: Aliskiren; Aminoglycosides; Anticoagulants; Antiplatelet Agents; Bisphosphonate Derivatives; Collagenase (Systemic); CycloSPORINE; CycloSPORINE (Systemic); Dabigatran Etexilate; Deferasirox; Desmopressin; Digoxin; Drotrecogin Alfa (Activated); Eplerenone; Haloperidol; Ibritumomab; Lithium; Methotrexate; Nonsteroidal Anti-Inflammatory Agents; PEMEtrexed; Porfimer; Potassium-Sparing Diuretics; PRALAtrexate; Quinolone Antibiotics; Rivaroxaban; Salicylates; Thrombolytic Agents; Tositumomab and Iodine I 131 Tositumomab; Vancomycin; Vitamin K Antagonists

The levels/effects of Meclofenamate may be increased by: ACE Inhibitors; Angiotensin II Receptor Blockers; Antidepressants (Tricyclic, Tertiary Amine); Corticosteroids (Systemic); CycloSPORINE; CycloSPORINE (Systemic); Dasatinib; Floctafenine; Glucosamine; Herbs (Anticoagulant/Antiplatelet Properties); Ketorolac; Ketorolac (Nasal); Ketorolac (Systemic); Nonsteroidal Anti-Inflammatory Agents; Omega-3-Acid Ethyl Esters; Pentosan Polysulfate Sodium; Pentoxifylline; Probenecid; Prostacyclin Analogues; Selective Serotonin Reuptake Inhibitors; Serotonin/Norepinephrine Reuptake Inhibitors; Sodium Phosphates; Tipranavir; Treprostinil; Vitamin E

Decreased Effect

Meclofenamate may decrease the levels/effects of: ACE Inhibitors; Aliskiren; Angiotensin II Receptor Blockers; Antiplatelet Agents; Beta-Blockers; Eplerenone; HydrALAZINE; Loop Diuretics; Potassium-Sparing Diuretics; Salicylates; Selective Serotonin Reuptake Inhibitors; Thiazide Diuretics

The levels/effects of Meclofenamate may be decreased by: Bile Acid Sequestrants; Nonsteroidal Anti-Inflammatory Agents; Salicylates

◀ **Ethanol/Nutrition/Herb Interactions**
Ethanol: Avoid ethanol (may enhance gastric mucosal irritation).
Herb/Nutraceutical: Avoid alfalfa, anise, bilberry, bladderwrack, bromelain, cat's claw, celery, chamomile, coleus, cordyceps, dong quai, evening primrose, fenugreek, feverfew, garlic, ginger, ginkgo biloba, ginseng (American, Panax, Siberian), grapeseed, green tea, guggul, horse chestnut seed, horseradish, licorice, prickly ash, red clover, reishi, SAMe (S-adeno-sylmethionine), sweet clover, turmeric, white willow (all have additional antiplatelet activity).

Mechanism of Action Reversibly inhibits cyclooxygenase-1 and 2 (COX-1 and 2) enzymes, which results in decreased formation of prostaglandin precursors; has antipyretic, analgesic, and anti-inflammatory properties.

Other proposed mechanisms not fully elucidated (and possibly contributing to the anti-inflammatory effect to varying degrees) include inhibiting chemotaxis, altering lymphocyte activity, inhibiting neutrophil aggregation/activation, and decreasing proinflammatory cytokine levels.

Pharmacodynamics/Kinetics
Duration: 2-4 hours
Distribution: Meclofenamate sodium: 9.1-43.2 L/kg
Protein binding: ≥99%
Metabolism: Metabolized to metabolite I (active) and ~6 other minor metabolites
Bioavailability: 100%
Half-life elimination: Meclofenamate sodium: 0.8-2.1 hours; metabolite I 15.3 hours
Time to peak, serum: Meclofenamate sodium 0.5-1.5 hours; metabolite I 0.5-4 hours
Excretion: Primarily urine (70%; primarily as metabolites); feces (30%)

Dosage
Geriatric & Adult
Mild-to-moderate pain: Oral: 50 mg every 4-6 hours; increases to 100 mg may be required; maximum dose: 400 mg
Rheumatoid arthritis/osteoarthritis: Oral: 50 mg every 4-6 hours; increase, over weeks, to 200-400 mg/day in 3-4 divided doses; do not exceed 400 mg/day; maximal benefit for any dose may not be seen for 2-3 weeks

Test Interactions Increased chloride (S), increased sodium (S)

Special Geriatric Considerations Elderly are a high-risk population for adverse effects from NSAIDs. As much as 60% of elderly can develop peptic ulceration and/or hemorrhage asymptomatically. The concomitant use of H_2 blockers and sucralfate is not effective as prophylaxis with the exception of NSAID-induced duodenal ulcers which may be prevented by the use of ranitidine. Misoprostol and proton pump inhibitors are the only agents proven to help prevent the development of NSAID-induced ulcers. Also, concomitant disease and drug use contribute to the risk for GI adverse effects. Use lowest effective dose for shortest period possible. Consider renal function decline with age. Use of NSAIDs can compromise existing renal function especially when Cl_{cr} is ≤30 mL/minute. Tinnitus may be a difficult and unreliable indication of toxicity due to age-related hearing loss or eighth cranial nerve damage. CNS adverse effects such as confusion, agitation, and hallucination are generally seen in overdose or high dose situations, but elderly may demonstrate these adverse effects at lower doses than younger adults.

This medication is considered to be potentially inappropriate in this patient population (Beers Criteria: Quality of evidence - moderate; Strength of recommendation - strong).

Dosage Forms Excipient information presented when available (limited, particularly for generics); consult specific product labeling.
Capsule, oral, as sodium: 50 mg, 100 mg

◆ **Meclofenamate Sodium** see Meclofenamate on page 1188
◆ **Meclozine Hydrochloride** see Meclizine on page 1186
◆ **Medicone® Suppositories [OTC]** see Phenylephrine (Topical) on page 1527
◆ **Medi-First® Sinus Decongestant [OTC]** see Phenylephrine (Systemic) on page 1523
◆ **Medi-Meclizine [OTC]** see Meclizine on page 1186
◆ **Medi-Phenyl [OTC]** see Phenylephrine (Systemic) on page 1523
◆ **Mediproxen [OTC]** see Naproxen on page 1338
◆ **Medrol®** see MethylPREDNISolone on page 1252
◆ **Medrol Dose Pack** see MethylPREDNISolone on page 1252
◆ **Medrol® Dosepak™** see MethylPREDNISolone on page 1252

MedroxyPROGESTERone (me DROKS ee proe JES te rone)

Medication Safety Issues
Sound-alike/look-alike issues:
Depo-Provera® may be confused with depo-subQ provera 104™

MedroxyPROGESTERone may be confused with hydroxyprogesterone caproate, methyl-PREDNISolone, methylTESTOSTERone

Provera® may be confused with Covera®, Femara®, Parlodel®, Premarin®, Proscar®, PROzac®

Administration issues:
The injectable dosage form is available in different formulations. Carefully review prescriptions to assure the correct formulation and route of administration.

Brand Names: U.S. Depo-Provera®; Depo-Provera® Contraceptive; depo-subQ provera 104®; Provera®

Brand Names: Canada Alti-MPA; Apo-Medroxy®; Depo-Prevera®; Depo-Provera®; Dom-Medroxyprogesterone; Gen-Medroxy; Medroxy; Medroxyprogesterone Acetate Injectable Suspension USP; Novo-Medrone; PMS-Medroxyprogesterone; Provera-Pak; Provera®; Teva-Medroxyprogesterone

Index Terms Acetoxymethylprogesterone; Medroxyprogesterone Acetate; Methylacetoxyprogesterone; MPA

Generic Availability (U.S.) Yes

Pharmacologic Category Contraceptive; Progestin

Use Secondary amenorrhea or abnormal uterine bleeding due to hormonal imbalance; reduction of endometrial hyperplasia in nonhysterectomized postmenopausal women receiving conjugated estrogens; management of endometriosis-associated pain; adjunctive therapy and palliative treatment of recurrent and metastatic endometrial carcinoma

Unlabeled Use Treatment of low-grade endometrial stromal sarcoma

Contraindications Hypersensitivity to medroxyprogesterone or any component of the formulation; history of or current thrombophlebitis or venous thromboembolic disorders (including DVT, PE); cerebral vascular disease; severe hepatic dysfunction or disease; carcinoma of the breast or other estrogen- or progesterone-dependent neoplasia; undiagnosed vaginal bleeding

Warnings/Precautions [U.S. Boxed Warning]: Prolonged use of medroxyprogesterone contraceptive injection may result in a loss of bone mineral density (BMD). [U.S. Boxed Warning]: Long-term use (ie, >2 years) should be limited to situations where other birth control methods are inadequate. Consider other methods of birth control in women with (or at risk for) osteoporosis. Anaphylaxis or anaphylactoid reactions have been reported with use of the injection; medication for the treatment of hypersensitivity reactions should be available for immediate use.

[U.S. Boxed Warning]: Estrogens with or without progestin should not be used to prevent cardiovascular disease. Using data from the Women's Health Initiative (WHI) studies, an increased risk of deep vein thrombosis (DVT) and stroke has been reported with CE and an increased risk of DVT, stroke, pulmonary emboli (PE) and myocardial infarction (MI) has been reported with CE with MPA in postmenopausal women. Additional risk factors include diabetes mellitus, hypercholesterolemia, hypertension, SLE, obesity, tobacco use, and/or history of venous thromboembolism (VTE). Risk factors should be managed appropriately; discontinue use if adverse cardiovascular events occur or are suspected. If thrombosis develops with contraceptive treatment, discontinue treatment (unless no other acceptable contraceptive alternative). Whenever possible, progestins in combination with estrogens should be discontinued at least 4-6 weeks prior to and for 2 weeks following elective surgery associated with an increased risk of thromboembolism or during periods of prolonged immobilization.

[U.S. Boxed Warning]: Estrogens with or without progestin should not be used to prevent dementia. In the Women's Health Initiative Memory Study (WHIMS), an increased incidence of dementia was observed in women ≥65 years of age taking CE alone or in combination with MPA.

[U.S. Boxed Warning]: Based on data from the Women's Health Initiative (WHI) studies, an increased risk of invasive breast cancer was observed in postmenopausal women using conjugated estrogens (CE) in combination with medroxyprogesterone acetate (MPA). This risk may be associated with duration of use and declines once combined therapy is discontinued (Chlebowski, 2009). The risk of invasive breast cancer was decreased in postmenopausal women with a hysterectomy using CE only, regardless of weight. However, the risk was not significantly decreased in women at high risk for breast cancer (family history of breast cancer, personal history of benign breast disease) (Anderson, 2012). An increase in abnormal mammogram findings has also been reported with estrogen alone or in combination with progestin therapy. Use is contraindicated in patients with known or suspected breast cancer.

MPA is used to reduce the risk of endometrial hyperplasia in nonhysterectomized postmenopausal women receiving conjugated estrogens. The use of unopposed estrogen in women with an intact uterus is associated with an increased risk of endometrial cancer. The addition of a progestin to estrogen therapy may decrease the risk of endometrial hyperplasia, a precursor to endometrial cancer. Adequate diagnostic measures, including endometrial sampling if indicated, should be performed to rule out malignancy in postmenopausal women with undiagnosed abnormal vaginal bleeding. Estrogens may exacerbate endometriosis. Malignant transformation of residual endometrial implants has been reported posthysterectomy with unopposed estrogen therapy. Consider adding a progestin in women with residual endometriosis posthysterectomy. Postmenopausal estrogen therapy and combined estrogen/progesterone therapy may increase the risk of ovarian cancer; however, the absolute risk to an individual woman is small. Although results from various studies are not consistent, risk does not appear to be significantly associated with the duration, route, or dose of therapy. In one study, the risk decreased after 2 years following discontinuation of therapy (Mørch, 2009). Although the risk of ovarian cancer is rare, women who are at an increased risk (eg, family history) should be counseled about the association (NAMS, 2012).

[U.S. Boxed Warning]: Estrogens with or without progestin should be used for the shortest duration possible at the lowest effective dose consistent with treatment goals. Before prescribing estrogen therapy to postmenopausal women, the risks and benefits must be weighed for each patient. Women should be informed of these risks and benefits, as well as possible effects of progestin when added to estrogen therapy. Patients should be reevaluated as clinically appropriate to determine if treatment is still necessary. Available data related to treatment risks are from Women's Health Initiative (WHI) studies, which evaluated oral CE 0.625 mg with or without MPA 2.5 mg relative to placebo in postmenopausal women. Other combinations and dosage forms of estrogens and progestins were not studied. **Outcomes reported from clinical trials using CE with or without MPA should be assumed to be similar for other doses and other dosage forms of estrogens and progestins until comparable data becomes available.**

Discontinue pending examination in cases of sudden partial or complete vision loss, sudden onset of proptosis, diplopia, or migraine; discontinue permanently if papilledema or retinal vascular lesions are observed on examination. Use with caution in patients with diseases that may be exacerbated by fluid retention (including asthma, epilepsy, migraine, cardiac, or renal dysfunction). Contraceptive therapy with medroxyprogesterone commonly results in an average weight gain of ~2.5 kg after 1 year and ~3.7 kg after 2 years of treatment. Use caution with history of depression.

May have adverse effects on glucose tolerance; use caution in women with diabetes. MPA is extensively metabolized in the liver. Discontinue if jaundice develops or if acute or chronic hepatic disturbances occur. Use is contraindicated with severe hepatic disease. Unscheduled bleeding/spotting may occur. Presentation of irregular, unresolving vaginal bleeding following previously regular cycles warrants further evaluation including endometrial sampling, if indicated, to rule out malignancy. Not for use prior to menarche. The use of estrogens and/or progestins may change the results of some laboratory tests (eg, coagulation factors, lipids, glucose tolerance, binding proteins). The dose, route, and the specific estrogen/progestin influences these changes. In addition, personal risk factors (eg, cardiovascular disease, smoking, diabetes, age) also contribute to adverse events; use of specific products may be contraindicated in women with certain risk factors.

Adverse Reactions (Reflective of adult population; not specific for elderly) Adverse effects as reported with any dosage form; percent ranges presented are noted with the MPA I.M. contraceptive injection:

>5%:
  Central nervous system: Dizziness, headache, nervousness
  Endocrine & metabolic: Libido decreased, menstrual irregularities (includes bleeding, amenorrhea, or both)
  Gastrointestinal: Abdominal pain/discomfort, weight gain (>10 lbs at 24 months: 38%)
1% to 5%:
  Cardiovascular: Edema
  Central nervous system: Depression, fatigue, insomnia
  Dermatologic: Acne, alopecia, rash
  Endocrine & metabolic: Breast pain, hot flashes
  Gastrointestinal: Bloating, nausea
  Genitourinary: Dysmenorrhea, leukorrhea, vaginitis
  Local: Injection site reaction (SubQ administration): Atrophy, induration, pain
  Neuromuscular & skeletal: Arthralgia, backache, leg cramp, weakness

Drug Interactions

Metabolism/Transport Effects Substrate of CYP3A4 (major); **Note:** Assignment of Major/Minor substrate status based on clinically relevant drug interaction potential; **Induces** CYP3A4 (weak/moderate)

Avoid Concomitant Use

Avoid concomitant use of MedroxyPROGESTERone with any of the following: Axitinib; Griseofulvin

Increased Effect/Toxicity

MedroxyPROGESTERone may increase the levels/effects of: Benzodiazepines (metabolized by oxidation); Selegiline; Tranexamic Acid; Voriconazole

The levels/effects of MedroxyPROGESTERone may be increased by: Boceprevir; Herbs (Progestogenic Properties); Mifepristone; Voriconazole

Decreased Effect

MedroxyPROGESTERone may decrease the levels/effects of: ARIPiprazole; Axitinib; Saxagliptin; Vitamin K Antagonists

The levels/effects of MedroxyPROGESTERone may be decreased by: Acitretin; Aminoglutethimide; Aprepitant; Artemether; Barbiturates; Bexarotene; Bexarotene (Systemic); Bile Acid Sequestrants; Bosentan; CarBAMazepine; Clobazam; CYP3A4 Inducers (Strong); Deferasirox; Felbamate; Fosaprepitant; Fosphenytoin; Griseofulvin; LamoTRIgine; Mifepristone; Mycophenolate; Nevirapine; OXcarbazepine; Phenytoin; Prucalopride; Retinoic Acid Derivatives; Rifamycin Derivatives; St Johns Wort; Telaprevir; Tocilizumab; Topiramate

Ethanol/Nutrition/Herb Interactions

Ethanol: Avoid ethanol (may increase risk of osteoporosis).

Food: Bioavailability of the oral tablet is increased when taken with food; half-life is unchanged.

Herb/Nutraceutical: St John's wort may diminish the therapeutic effect of progestin contraceptives (contraceptive failure is possible).

Stability Store at controlled room temperature.

Mechanism of Action Inhibits secretion of pituitary gonadotropins, which prevents follicular maturation and ovulation; causes endometrial thinning

Pharmacodynamics/Kinetics

Absorption: Oral: Well absorbed; I.M.: Slow

Protein binding: 86% to 90% primarily to albumin; does not bind to sex hormone-binding globulin

Metabolism: Extensively hepatic via hydroxylation and conjugation; forms metabolites

Half-life elimination: Oral: 12-17 hours; I.M. (Depo-Provera® Contraceptive): ~50 days; SubQ: ~40 days

Time to peak: Oral: 2-4 hours; I.M. (Depo-Provera® Contraceptive): ~3 weeks; SubQ: ~1 week

Excretion: Urine

Dosage

Geriatric & Adult

Abnormal uterine bleeding: Oral: 5-10 mg for 5-10 days starting on day 16 or 21 of cycle

Endometriosis (depo-subQ provera 104™): SubQ: 104 mg every 3 months (every 12-14 weeks)

Endometrial carcinoma, recurrent or metastatic (adjunctive/palliative treatment) (Depo-Provera®): I.M.: 400-1000 mg/week

Accompanying cyclic estrogen therapy, postmenopausal: Oral: 5-10 mg for 12-14 consecutive days each month, starting on day 1 or day 16 of the cycle; lower doses may be used if given with estrogen continuously throughout the cycle

Hepatic Impairment Use is contraindicated with severe impairment. Discontinue with jaundice or if liver function disturbances occur. Consider lower dose or less frequent administration with mild-to-moderate impairment. Use of the contraceptive injection has not been studied in patients with hepatic impairment; consideration should be given to not readminister if jaundice develops

Administration No geriatric-specific information.

Monitoring Parameters Before starting therapy, a physical exam with reference to the breasts and pelvis are recommended, including a Papanicolaou smear. Monitor patient closely for loss of vision; sudden onset of proptosis, diplopia, or migraine; signs and symptoms of thromboembolic disorders; signs or symptoms of depression; glucose in patients with diabetes; or blood pressure. BMD with long-term use (per manufacturer).

Adequate diagnostic measures, including endometrial sampling, if indicated, should be performed to rule out malignancy in all cases of undiagnosed abnormal vaginal bleeding.

Special Geriatric Considerations No specific information for use in elderly.

MEDROXYPROGESTERONE

◀ **Dosage Forms** Excipient information presented when available (limited, particularly for generics); consult specific product labeling.
Injection, suspension, as acetate: 150 mg/mL (1 mL)
  Depo-Provera®: 400 mg/mL (2.5 mL)
  Depo-Provera® Contraceptive: 150 mg/mL (1 mL) [contains polysorbate 80]
  depo-subQ provera 104®: 104 mg/0.65 mL (0.65 mL) [contains polysorbate 80]
Tablet, oral, as acetate: 2.5 mg, 5 mg, 10 mg
  Provera®: 2.5 mg, 5 mg, 10 mg [scored]

◆ **Medroxyprogesterone Acetate** see MedroxyPROGESTERone on page 1190
◆ **Medroxyprogesterone and Estrogens (Conjugated)** see Estrogens (Conjugated/Equine) and Medroxyprogesterone on page 711

Mefenamic Acid (me fe NAM ik AS id)

Related Information
  Beers Criteria – Potentially Inappropriate Medications for Geriatrics on page 2183
Medication Safety Issues
  Sound-alike/look-alike issues:
  Ponstel® may be confused with Pronestyl
  BEERS Criteria medication:
    This drug may be potentially inappropriate for use in geriatric patients (Quality of evidence - moderate; Strength of recommendation - strong).
Brand Names: U.S. Ponstel®
Brand Names: Canada Apo-Mefenamic®; Dom-Mefenamic Acid; Mefenamic-250; Nu-Mefenamic; PMS-Mefenamic Acid; Ponstan®
Generic Availability (U.S.) Yes
Pharmacologic Category Nonsteroidal Anti-inflammatory Drug (NSAID), Oral
Use Short-term relief of mild-to-moderate pain
Medication Guide Available Yes
Dosage
  Geriatric & Adult Mild-moderate pain: Oral: Initial: 500 mg; then 250 mg every 6 hours as needed; maximum therapy: 1 week
  Renal Impairment Not recommended for use
Special Geriatric Considerations Elderly are a high-risk population for adverse effects from NSAIDs. As much as 60% of elderly can develop peptic ulceration and/or hemorrhage asymptomatically. The concomitant use of H_2 blockers, omeprazole, and sucralfate is not effective as prophylaxis with the exception of NSAID-induced duodenal ulcers which may be prevented by the use of ranitidine. Misoprostol and proton pump inhibitors are the only agents proven to help prevent the development of NSAID-induced ulcers. Also, concomitant disease and drug use contribute to the risk for GI adverse effects. Use lowest effective dose for shortest period possible. Consider renal function decline with age. Use of NSAIDs can compromise existing renal function especially when Cl_{cr} is ≤30 mL/minute. Tinnitus may be a difficult and unreliable indication of toxicity due to age-related hearing loss or eighth cranial nerve damage. CNS adverse effects such as confusion, agitation, and hallucination are generally seen in overdose or high-dose situations, but elderly may demonstrate these adverse effects at lower doses than younger adults.

This medication is considered to be potentially inappropriate in this patient population (Beers Criteria: Quality of evidence - moderate; Strength of recommendation - strong).
Dosage Forms Excipient information presented when available (limited, particularly for generics); consult specific product labeling.
Capsule, oral: 250 mg
  Ponstel®: 250 mg

◆ **Mefoxin®** see CefOXitin on page 322
◆ **Megace®** see Megestrol on page 1194
◆ **Megace® ES** see Megestrol on page 1194
◆ **Megadophilus® [OTC]** see Lactobacillus on page 1084

Megestrol (me JES trole)

Related Information
  Beers Criteria – Potentially Inappropriate Medications for Geriatrics on page 2183
Medication Safety Issues
  Sound-alike/look-alike issues:
  Megace® may be confused with Reglan®
  Megestrol may be confused with mesalamine

BEERS Criteria medication:
This drug may be potentially inappropriate for use in geriatric patients (Quality of evidence - moderate; Strength of recommendation - strong).

Brand Names: U.S. Megace®; Megace® ES

Brand Names: Canada Apo-Megestrol®; Megace®; Megace® OS; Nu-Megestrol

Index Terms 5071-1DL(6); Megestrol Acetate; NSC-71423

Generic Availability (U.S.) Yes: Excludes Megace® ES

Pharmacologic Category Antineoplastic Agent, Hormone; Appetite Stimulant; Progestin

Use Palliative treatment of breast and endometrial carcinoma; treatment of anorexia, cachexia, or unexplained significant weight loss in patients with AIDS

Contraindications Hypersensitivity to megestrol or any component of the formulation

Warnings/Precautions Hazardous agent - use appropriate precautions for handling and disposal. May suppress hypothalamic-pituitary-adrenal (HPA) axis during chronic administration; consider the possibility of adrenal suppression in any patient receiving or being withdrawn from chronic therapy when signs/symptoms suggestive of hypoadrenalism are noted (during stress or in unstressed state). Laboratory evaluation and replacement/stress doses of rapid-acting glucocorticoid should be considered. New-onset diabetes and exacerbation of pre-existing diabetes have been reported with long-term use. Use with caution in patients with a history of thromboembolic disease. Avoid use in older adults due to minimal effect on weight, and an increased risk of thrombosis and possibly death (Beers Criteria). Vaginal bleeding or discharge may occur in females. Megace® ES suspension is not equivalent to other formulations on a mg per mg basis; Megace® ES suspension 625 mg/5 mL is equivalent to megestrol acetate suspension 800 mg/20 mL.

Adverse Reactions (Reflective of adult population; not specific for elderly)
Frequency not always defined.
Cardiovascular: Hypertension (≤8%), cardiomyopathy (1% to 3%), chest pain (1% to 3%), edema (1% to 3%), palpitation (1% to 3%), peripheral edema (1% to 3%), heart failure
Central nervous system: Headache (≤10%), insomnia (≤6%), fever (1% to 6%), pain (≤6%, similar to placebo), abnormal thinking (1% to 3%), confusion (1% to 3%), depression (1% to 3%), hypoesthesia (1% to 3%), seizure (1% to 3%), mood changes, malaise, lethargy
Dermatologic: Rash (2% to 12%), alopecia (1% to 3%), pruritus (1% to 3%), vesiculobullous rash (1% to 3%)
Endocrine & metabolic: Hyperglycemia (≤6%), gynecomastia (1% to 3%), adrenal insufficiency, amenorrhea, breakthrough bleeding, cervical erosion and secretions (changes), breast tenderness increased, Cushing's syndrome, diabetes, glucose intolerance, HPA axis suppression, hot flashes, hypercalcemia, menstrual flow changes, spotting, vaginal bleeding pattern changes
Gastrointestinal: Diarrhea (6% to 15%, similar to placebo), flatulence (≤10%), vomiting (≤6%), nausea (≤5%), dyspepsia (≤4%), abdominal pain (1% to 3%), constipation (1% to 3%), salivation increased (1% to 3%), xerostomia (1% to 3%), weight gain (not attributed to edema or fluid retention)
Genitourinary: Impotence (4% to 14%), decreased libido (≤5%), urinary incontinence (1% to 3%), urinary tract infection (1% to 3%), urinary frequency (≤2%)
Hematologic: Anemia (≤5%), leukopenia (1% to 3%)
Hepatic: Hepatomegaly (1% to 3%), LDH increased (1% to 3%), cholestatic jaundice, hepatotoxicity
Neuromuscular & skeletal: Weakness (2% to 6%), neuropathy (1% to 3%), paresthesia (1% to 3%), carpal tunnel syndrome
Ocular: Amblyopia (1% to 3%)
Renal: Albuminuria (1% to 3%)
Respiratory: Dyspnea (1% to 3%), cough (1% to 3%), pharyngitis (1% to 3%), pneumonia (≤2%), hyperpnea
Miscellaneous: Diaphoresis (1% to 3%), herpes infection (1% to 3%), infection (1% to 3%), moniliasis (1% to 3%), tumor flare

Drug Interactions

Metabolism/Transport Effects None known.

Avoid Concomitant Use
Avoid concomitant use of Megestrol with any of the following: Dofetilide

Increased Effect/Toxicity
Megestrol may increase the levels/effects of: Dofetilide

The levels/effects of Megestrol may be increased by: Herbs (Progestogenic Properties)

Decreased Effect
The levels/effects of Megestrol may be decreased by: Aminoglutethimide

Ethanol/Nutrition/Herb Interactions Herb/Nutraceutical: Avoid herbs with progestogenic properties (eg, bloodroot, chasteberry, damiana, oregano, and yucca); may enhance the adverse/toxic effect of megestrol.

Stability
Suspension: Store at 15°C to 25°C (59°F to 77°F); protect from heat.
Tablet: Store at 25°C (77°F); excursions permitted to 15°C to 30°C (59°F to 86°F); protect from heat (temperatures >40°C [>104°F])

Mechanism of Action A synthetic progestin with antiestrogenic properties which disrupt the estrogen receptor cycle. Megestrol interferes with the normal estrogen cycle and results in a lower LH titer. May also have a direct effect on the endometrium. Megestrol is an antineoplastic progestin thought to act through an antileutenizing effect mediated via the pituitary. May stimulate appetite by antagonizing the metabolic effects of catabolic cytokines.

Pharmacodynamics/Kinetics
Absorption: Well absorbed orally
Metabolism: Hepatic (to free steroids and glucuronide conjugates)
Half-life elimination: 13-105 hours
Time to peak, serum: 1-3 hours
Excretion: Urine (57% to 78%; 5% to 8% as metabolites); feces (8% to 30%)

Dosage
Geriatric & Adult Note: Megace® ES suspension is not equivalent to other formulations on a mg-per-mg basis.
Breast carcinoma (females): Refer to individual protocols: Oral: Tablet: 40 mg 4 times/day
Endometrial carcinoma: Refer to individual protocols: Oral: Tablet: 40-320 mg/day in divided doses; use for 2 months to determine efficacy; maximum doses used have been up to 800 mg/day.
HIV-related cachexia (males/females): Oral: Suspension:
Megace®: Initial dose: 800 mg/day; daily doses of 400 and 800 mg/day were found to be clinically effective
Megace® ES: 625 mg/day
Renal Impairment No data available; however, the urinary excretion of megestrol acetate administered in doses of 4-90 mg ranged from 57% to 78% within 10 days.

Administration Megestrol acetate (Megace®) oral suspension is compatible with water, orange juice, apple juice, or Sustacal H.C. for immediate consumption. Shake suspension well before use.

Monitoring Parameters Observe for signs of thromboembolic events; blood pressure, weight; serum glucose

Test Interactions Altered thyroid and liver function tests

Special Geriatric Considerations Elderly females may have vaginal bleeding or discharge and need to be forewarned of this side effect and inconvenience. No specific changes in dose are required for the elderly. Megestrol has been used in the treatment of the failure to thrive syndrome in cachectic elderly in addition to proper nutrition. Data does not support the use of megestrol for weight gain. The increase in weight tends to be mostly fat instead of lean body mass. Also, this agent is associated with DVTs and increased mortality.

This medication is considered to be potentially inappropriate in this patient population (Beers Criteria: Quality of evidence - moderate; Strength of recommendation - strong).

Dosage Forms Excipient information presented when available (limited, particularly for generics); consult specific product labeling.
Suspension, oral, as acetate: 40 mg/mL (10 mL, 20 mL, 237 mL, 240 mL, 473 mL, 480 mL)
Megace®: 40 mg/mL (240 mL) [contains ethanol 0.06%, sodium benzoate; lemon-lime flavor]
Megace® ES: 125 mg/mL (150 mL) [contains ethanol 0.06%, sodium benzoate; lemon-lime flavor]
Tablet, oral, as acetate: 20 mg, 40 mg

◆ **Megestrol Acetate** see Megestrol on page 1194
◆ **Mellaril** see Thioridazine on page 1880

Meloxicam (mel OKS i kam)

Related Information
Beers Criteria – Potentially Inappropriate Medications for Geriatrics on page 2183
Medication Safety Issues
BEERS Criteria medication:
This drug may be potentially inappropriate for use in geriatric patients (Quality of evidence - moderate; Strength of recommendation - strong).
Brand Names: U.S. Mobic®

Brand Names: Canada Apo-Meloxicam®; CO Meloxicam; Dom-Meloxicam; Mobicox®; Mobic®; Mylan-Meloxicam; Novo-Meloxicam; PHL-Meloxicam; PMS-Meloxicam; ratio-Melox-icam; Teva-Meloxicam

Generic Availability (U.S.) Yes:

Pharmacologic Category Nonsteroidal Anti-inflammatory Drug (NSAID), Oral

Use Relief of signs and symptoms of osteoarthritis, rheumatoid arthritis, and juvenile idiopathic arthritis (JIA)

Medication Guide Available Yes

Contraindications Hypersensitivity (eg, asthma, urticaria, allergic-type reactions) to melox-icam, aspirin, other NSAIDs, or any component of the formulation; perioperative pain in the setting of coronary artery bypass graft (CABG) surgery

Warnings/Precautions [U.S. Boxed Warning]: NSAIDs are associated with an increased risk of adverse cardiovascular thrombotic events, including MI and stroke. Risk may be increased with duration of use or pre-existing cardiovascular risk factors or disease. Carefully evaluate individual cardiovascular risk profiles prior to prescribing. May cause new-onset hypertension or worsening of existing hypertension. Use caution with fluid retention. Avoid use in heart failure. Concurrent administration of ibuprofen, and potentially other nonselective NSAIDs, may interfere with aspirin's cardioprotective effect. **[U.S. Boxed Warning]: Use is contraindicated for treatment of perioperative pain in the setting of coronary artery bypass graft (CABG) surgery.** Risk of MI and stroke may be increased with use within the first 10-14 days following CABG surgery.

Platelet adhesion and aggregation may be decreased; may prolong bleeding time; patients with coagulation disorders or who are receiving anticoagulants should be monitored closely. Anemia may occur; patients on long-term NSAID therapy should be monitored for anemia. Rarely, NSAID use may cause severe blood dyscrasias (eg, agranulocytosis, aplastic anemia, thrombocytopenia).

NSAID use may compromise existing renal function; dose-dependent decreases in prosta-glandin synthesis may result from NSAID use, reducing renal blood flow which may cause renal decompensation. NSAID use may increase the risk for hyperkalemia. Patients with impaired renal function, dehydration, heart failure, liver dysfunction, those taking diuretics, and ACE inhibitors, and the elderly are at greater risk of renal toxicity and hyperkalemia. Rehydrate patient before starting therapy; monitor renal function closely. Not recommended for use in patients with advanced renal disease. Long-term NSAID use may result in renal papillary necrosis.

[U.S. Boxed Warning]: NSAIDs may increase risk of gastrointestinal irritation, inflam-mation, ulceration, bleeding, and perforation. These events may occur at any time during therapy and without warning. Use caution with a history of GI disease (bleeding or ulcers), concurrent therapy with aspirin, anticoagulants and/or corticosteroids, smoking, use of alcohol, the elderly or debilitated patients. When used concomitantly with ≤325 mg of aspirin, a substantial increase in the risk of gastrointestinal complications (eg, ulcer) occurs; con-comitant gastroprotective therapy (eg, proton pump inhibitors) is recommended (Bhatt, 2008).

Use the lowest effective dose for the shortest duration of time, consistent with individual patient goals, to reduce risk of cardiovascular or GI adverse events. Alternate therapies should be considered for patients at high risk.

NSAIDs may cause serious skin adverse events including exfoliative dermatitis, Stevens-Johnson syndrome (SJS) and toxic epidermal necrolysis (TEN); discontinue use at first sign of skin rash or hypersensitivity. Anaphylactoid reactions may occur, even without prior exposure; patients with "aspirin triad" (bronchial asthma, aspirin intolerance, rhinitis) may be at increased risk. Do not use in patients who experience bronchospasm, asthma, rhinitis, or urticaria with NSAID or aspirin therapy. Use caution in other forms of asthma.

Use with caution in patients with decreased hepatic function. Closely monitor patients with any abnormal LFT. Severe hepatic reactions (eg, fulminant hepatitis, liver failure) have occurred with NSAID use, rarely; discontinue if signs or symptoms of liver disease develop, or if systemic manifestations occur.

NSAIDS may cause drowsiness, dizziness, blurred vision and other neurologic effects which may impair physical or mental abilities; patients must be cautioned about performing tasks which require mental alertness (eg, operating machinery or driving). Discontinue use with blurred or diminished vision and perform ophthalmologic exam. Monitor vision with long-term therapy.

In the elderly, avoid chronic use (unless alternative agents ineffective and patient can receive concomitant gastroprotective agent); nonselective oral NSAID use is associated with an increased risk of GI bleeding and peptic ulcer disease in older adults in high risk category (eg, >75 years or age or receiving concomitant oral/parenteral corticosteroids, anticoagulants, or antiplatelet agents) (Beers Criteria).

Oral suspension formulation may contain sorbitol. Concomitant use with sodium polystyrene sulfonate (Kayexalate®) may cause intestinal necrosis (including fatal cases); combined use should be avoided. Withhold for at least 4-6 half-lives prior to surgical or dental procedures.

Adverse Reactions (Reflective of adult population; not specific for elderly) Percentages reported in adult patients; abdominal pain, diarrhea, fever, headache, pyrexia, and vomiting were reported more commonly in pediatric patients

2% to 10%:
  Cardiovascular: Edema (≤5%)
  Central nervous system: Headache (2% to 8%), pain (1% to 5%), dizziness (≤4%), insomnia (≤4%)
  Dermatologic: Pruritus (≤2%), rash (≤3%)
  Gastrointestinal: Dyspepsia (4% to 10%), diarrhea (2% to 8%), nausea (2% to 7%), abdominal pain (2% to 5%), constipation (≤3%), flatulence (≤3%), vomiting (≤3%)
  Genitourinary: Urinary tract infection (≤7%), micturition (≤2%)
  Hematologic: Anemia (≤4%)
  Neuromuscular & skeletal: Arthralgia (≤5%), back pain (≤3%)
  Respiratory: Upper respiratory infection (≤8%), cough (≤2%), pharyngitis (≤3%)
  Miscellaneous: Flu-like syndrome (2% to 6%), falls (≤3%)

Drug Interactions

  Metabolism/Transport Effects Substrate of CYP3A4 (minor); **Note:** Assignment of Major/Minor substrate status based on clinically relevant drug interaction potential; **Inhibits** CYP2C9 (weak)

  Avoid Concomitant Use
  Avoid concomitant use of Meloxicam with any of the following: Calcium Polystyrene Sulfonate; Floctafenine; Ketorolac; Ketorolac (Nasal); Ketorolac (Systemic); Sodium Polystyrene Sulfonate

  Increased Effect/Toxicity
  Meloxicam may increase the levels/effects of: Aliskiren; Aminoglycosides; Anticoagulants; Antiplatelet Agents; Bisphosphonate Derivatives; Calcium Polystyrene Sulfonate; Collagenase (Systemic); CycloSPORINE; CycloSPORINE (Systemic); Dabigatran Etexilate; Deferasirox; Desmopressin; Digoxin; Drotrecogin Alfa (Activated); Eplerenone; Haloperidol; Ibritumomab; Lithium; Methotrexate; Nonsteroidal Anti-Inflammatory Agents; PEMEtrexed; Porfimer; Potassium-Sparing Diuretics; PRALAtrexate; Quinolone Antibiotics; Rivaroxaban; Salicylates; Sodium Polystyrene Sulfonate; Thrombolytic Agents; Tositumomab and Iodine I 131 Tositumomab; Vancomycin; Vitamin K Antagonists

  The levels/effects of Meloxicam may be increased by: ACE Inhibitors; Angiotensin II Receptor Blockers; Antidepressants (Tricyclic, Tertiary Amine); Corticosteroids (Systemic); CycloSPORINE; CycloSPORINE (Systemic); Dasatinib; Floctafenine; Glucosamine; Herbs (Anticoagulant/Antiplatelet Properties); Ketorolac; Ketorolac (Nasal); Ketorolac (Systemic); Nonsteroidal Anti-Inflammatory Agents; Omega-3-Acid Ethyl Esters; Pentosan Polysulfate Sodium; Pentoxifylline; Probenecid; Prostacyclin Analogues; Selective Serotonin Reuptake Inhibitors; Serotonin/Norepinephrine Reuptake Inhibitors; Sodium Phosphates; Tipranavir; Treprostinil; Vitamin E; Voriconazole

  Decreased Effect
  Meloxicam may decrease the levels/effects of: ACE Inhibitors; Aliskiren; Angiotensin II Receptor Blockers; Antiplatelet Agents; Beta-Blockers; Eplerenone; HydrALAZINE; Loop Diuretics; Potassium-Sparing Diuretics; Salicylates; Selective Serotonin Reuptake Inhibitors; Thiazide Diuretics

  The levels/effects of Meloxicam may be decreased by: Bile Acid Sequestrants; Nonsteroidal Anti-Inflammatory Agents; Salicylates; Tocilizumab

Ethanol/Nutrition/Herb Interactions
  Ethanol: Avoid ethanol (may enhance gastric mucosal irritation).
  Herb/Nutraceutical: Avoid alfalfa, anise, bilberry, bladderwrack, bromelain, cat's claw, celery, chamomile, coleus, cordyceps, dong quai, evening primrose, fenugreek, feverfew, garlic, ginger, ginkgo biloba, ginseng (American, Panax, Siberian), grapeseed, green tea, guggul, horse chestnut seed, horseradish, licorice, prickly ash, red clover, reishi, SAMe (S-adenosylmethionine), sweet clover, turmeric, white willow (all have additional antiplatelet activity).

Stability Store at 25°C (77°F). Protect tablets from moisture.

Mechanism of Action Reversibly inhibits cyclooxygenase-1 and 2 (COX-1 and 2) enzymes, which results in decreased formation of prostaglandin precursors; has antipyretic, analgesic, and anti-inflammatory properties

Other proposed mechanisms not fully elucidated (and possibly contributing to the anti-inflammatory effect to varying degrees), include inhibiting chemotaxis, altering lymphocyte activity, inhibiting neutrophil aggregation/activation, and decreasing proinflammatory cytokine levels.

Pharmacodynamics/Kinetics
Distribution: 10 L
Protein binding: ~99%, primarily to albumin
Metabolism: Hepatic via CYP2C9 and CYP3A4 (minor); forms 4 metabolites (inactive)
Bioavailability: 89%
Half-life elimination: Adults: 15-20 hours
Time to peak: Initial: 4-5 hours; Secondary: 12-14 hours
Excretion: Urine and feces (as inactive metabolites)

Dosage
Geriatric & Adult Osteoarthritis, rheumatoid arthritis: Oral: Initial: 7.5 mg once daily; some patients may receive additional benefit from increasing dose to 15 mg once daily; maximum dose: 15 mg/day.

Renal Impairment
Mild-to-moderate impairment: No specific dosage recommendations
Significant impairment ($Cl_{cr} \leq 20$ mL/minute): Patients with severe renal impairment have not been adequately studied; use not recommended.
Hemodialysis: Maximum dose: 7.5 mg/day

Hepatic Impairment
Mild-to-moderate hepatic impairment (Child-Pugh class A or B): No dosage adjustment is necessary
Severe hepatic impairment: Patients with severe hepatic impairment have not been adequately studied

Administration May be administered with or without meals; take with food or milk to minimize gastrointestinal irritation. Oral suspension: Shake gently prior to use.

Monitoring Parameters Periodic CBC, serum chemistries, liver function, renal function (serum BUN and creatinine) with long-term use; signs and symptoms of bleeding

Special Geriatric Considerations Men ≥65 years of age exhibited steady-state plasma concentrations and pharmacokinetics similar to younger men. Elderly women (≥65 years of age) had nearly a 50% greater AUC and 32% higher C_{max} compared to younger women.

Elderly are a high-risk population for adverse effects from NSAIDs. As much as 60% of elderly can develop peptic ulceration and/or hemorrhage asymptomatically. The concomitant use of H_2 blockers and sucralfate is not effective as prophylaxis with the exception of NSAID-induced duodenal ulcers which may be prevented by the use of ranitidine. Misoprostol and proton pump inhibitors are the only agents proven to help prevent the development of NSAID-induced ulcers. Also, concomitant disease and drug use contribute to the risk for GI adverse effects. Use lowest effective dose for shortest period possible. Consider renal function decline with age. Use of NSAIDs can compromise existing renal function especially when Cl_{cr} is ≤30 mL/minute. Tinnitus may be a difficult and unreliable indication of toxicity due to age-related hearing loss or eighth cranial nerve damage. CNS adverse effects, such as confusion, agitation, and hallucination, are generally seen in overdose or high-dose situations, but the elderly may demonstrate these adverse effects at lower doses than younger adults.

This medication is considered to be potentially inappropriate in this patient population (Beers Criteria: Quality of evidence - moderate; Strength of recommendation - strong).

Dosage Forms Excipient information presented when available (limited, particularly for generics); consult specific product labeling.
Suspension, oral: 7.5 mg/5 mL (100 mL)
Mobic®: 7.5 mg/5 mL (100 mL) [contains sodium benzoate; raspberry flavor]
Tablet, oral: 7.5 mg, 15 mg
Mobic®: 7.5 mg, 15 mg

Melphalan (MEL fa lan)

Medication Safety Issues
Sound-alike/look-alike issues:
Melphalan may be confused with Mephyton®, Myleran®
Alkeran® may be confused with Alferon®, Leukeran®, Myleran®

High alert medication:
This medication is in a class the Institute for Safe Medication Practices (ISMP) includes among its list of drug classes which have a heightened risk of causing significant patient harm when used in error.

Brand Names: U.S. Alkeran®

Brand Names: Canada Alkeran®

Index Terms L-PAM; L-Phenylalanine Mustard; L-Sarcolysin; Phenylalanine Mustard

Generic Availability (U.S.) Yes: Excludes tablet

Pharmacologic Category Antineoplastic Agent, Alkylating Agent

Use Palliative treatment of multiple myeloma and nonresectable epithelial ovarian carcinoma

Unlabeled Use Treatment of Hodgkin lymphoma, light chain amyloidosis; conditioning regimen for autologous hematopoietic stem cell transplantation in adults with hematologic disorders (eg, multiple myeloma)

Contraindications Hypersensitivity to melphalan or any component of the formulation; patients whose disease was resistant to prior melphalan therapy

Warnings/Precautions [U.S. Boxed Warning: Bone marrow suppression is common; may be severe and result in infection or bleeding; has been demonstrated more with the I.V. formulation (compared to oral); myelosuppression is dose-related. Monitor blood counts; may require treatment delay or dose modification for thrombocytopenia or neutropenia. Use with caution in patients with prior bone marrow suppression, impaired renal function (consider dose reduction), or who have received prior (or concurrent) chemotherapy or irradiation. Myelotoxicity is generally reversible, although irreversible bone marrow failure has been reported. In patients who are candidates for autologous transplantation, avoid melphalan-containing regimens prior to transplant (due to the effects on stem cell reserve). Signs of infection, such as fever and WBC rise, may not occur; lethargy and confusion may be more prominent signs of infection.

[U.S. Boxed Warning]: Hypersensitivity reactions (including anaphylaxis) have occurred in ~2% of patients receiving I.V. melphalan, usually after multiple treatment cycles. Discontinue infusion and treat symptomatically. Hypersensitivity may also occur (rarely) with oral melphalan. Do not readminister (oral or I.V.) in patients who experience hypersensitivity to melphalan.

Gastrointestinal toxicities, including nausea, vomiting, diarrhea and mucositis, are common. When administering high-dose melphalan in autologous transplantation, cryotherapy is recommended to prevent mucositis (Keefe, 2007). Abnormal liver function tests may occur; hepatitis and jaundice have also been reported; hepatic sinusoidal obstruction syndrome (SOS; formerly called veno-occlusive disease) has been reported with I.V. melphalan. Pulmonary fibrosis (some fatal) and interstitial pneumonitis have been observed with treatment. Dosage reduction is recommended with I.V. melphalan in patients with renal impairment; reduced initial doses may also be recommended with oral melphalan. Closely monitor patients with azotemia.

[U.S. Boxed Warning]: Produces chromosomal changes and is leukemogenic and potentially mutagenic; secondary malignancies (including acute myeloid leukemia, myeloproliferative disease, and carcinoma) have been reported reported (some patients were receiving combination chemotherapy or radiation therapy); the risk is increased with increased treatment duration and cumulative doses. Suppresses ovarian function and produces amenorrhea; may also cause testicular suppression.

Extravasation may cause local tissue damage; administration by slow injection into a fast running I.V. solution into an injection port or via a central line is recommended; do not administer directly into a peripheral vein. **[U.S. Boxed Warning]: Should be administered under the supervision of an experienced cancer chemotherapy physician.** Avoid vaccination with live vaccines during treatment if immunocompromised. Toxicity may be increased in elderly; start with lowest recommended adult doses.

Adverse Reactions (Reflective of adult population; not specific for elderly)
>10%:
Gastrointestinal: Nausea/vomiting, diarrhea, oral ulceration
Hematologic: Myelosuppression, leukopenia (nadir: 14-21 days; recovery: 28-35 days), thrombocytopenia (nadir: 14-21 days; recovery: 28-35 days), anemia
Miscellaneous: Secondary malignancy (<2% to 20%; cumulative dose and duration dependent, includes acute myeloid leukemia, myeloproliferative syndrome, carcinoma)
1% to 10%: Miscellaneous: Hypersensitivity (I.V.: 2%; includes bronchospasm, dyspnea, edema, hypotension, pruritus, rash, tachycardia, urticaria)

Drug Interactions
Metabolism/Transport Effects None known.

Avoid Concomitant Use

Avoid concomitant use of Melphalan with any of the following: BCG; CloZAPine; Nalidixic Acid; Natalizumab; Pimecrolimus; Tacrolimus (Topical); Vaccines (Live)

Increased Effect/Toxicity

Melphalan may increase the levels/effects of: Carmustine; CloZAPine; CycloSPORINE; CycloSPORINE (Systemic); Leflunomide; Natalizumab; Vaccines (Live); Vitamin K Antagonists

The levels/effects of Melphalan may be increased by: Denosumab; Nalidixic Acid; Pimecrolimus; Roflumilast; Tacrolimus (Topical); Trastuzumab

Decreased Effect

Melphalan may decrease the levels/effects of: BCG; Cardiac Glycosides; Coccidioidin Skin Test; Sipuleucel-T; Vaccines (Inactivated); Vaccines (Live); Vitamin K Antagonists

The levels/effects of Melphalan may be decreased by: Echinacea

Ethanol/Nutrition/Herb Interactions

Ethanol: Avoid ethanol (due to GI irritation).

Food: Food interferes with oral absorption.

Stability Use appropriate precautions for handling and disposal.

Tablet: Store in refrigerator at 2°C to 8°C (36°F to 46°F). Protect from light.

Injection: Store at room temperature of 15°C to 30°C (59°F to 86°F). Protect from light. Stability is limited; must be prepared fresh. **The time between reconstitution/dilution and administration of parenteral melphalan must be kept to a minimum (manufacturer recommends <60 minutes) because reconstituted and diluted solutions are unstable.** Dissolve powder initially with 10 mL of supplied diluent to a concentration of 5 mg/mL; shake immediately and vigorously to dissolve. This solution is chemically and physically stable for ≤90 minutes when stored at room temperature, although the manufacturer recommends administration be completed within 60 minutes of reconstitution. **Immediately** dilute dose in NS to a concentration of ≤0.45 mg/mL (manufacturer recommended concentration). Do not refrigerate solution; precipitation occurs.

Mechanism of Action Alkylating agent which is a derivative of mechlorethamine that inhibits DNA and RNA synthesis via formation of carbonium ions; cross-links strands of DNA; acts on both resting and rapidly dividing tumor cells.

Pharmacodynamics/Kinetics Note: Pharmacokinetics listed are for FDA-approved doses.

Absorption: Oral: Variable and incomplete

Distribution: V_d: 0.5 L/kg; low penetration into CSF

Protein binding: 53% to 92%; primarily to albumin (40% to 60%), ~20% to α_1-acid glycoprotein

Metabolism: Hepatic; chemical hydrolysis to monohydroxymelphalan and dihydroxymelphalan

Bioavailability: Oral: Variable; 56% to 93%; exposure is reduced with a high-fat meal

Half-life elimination: Terminal: I.V.: 75 minutes; Oral: 1-2 hours

Time to peak, serum: Oral: ~1-2 hours

Excretion: Oral: Feces (20% to 50%); urine (~10% as unchanged drug)

Dosage

Geriatric Refer to adult dosing. Use caution and begin at the lower end of dosing range.

Adult

Details regarding dosing in combination regimens should also be consulted. Adjust dose based on patient response and weekly blood counts.

Multiple myeloma (palliative treatment): Note: Response is gradual; may require repeated courses to realize benefit:

Oral: Usual dose (as described in the manufacturer's labeling):

6 mg once daily for 2-3 weeks initially, followed by up to 4 weeks rest, then a maintenance dose of 2 mg daily as hematologic recovery begins **or**

10 mg daily for 7-10 days; institute 2 mg daily maintenance dose after WBC >4000 cells/mm³ and platelets >100,000 cells/mm³ (~4-8 weeks); titrate maintenance dose to hematologic response **or**

0.15 mg/kg/day for 7 days, with a 2-6 week rest, followed by a maintenance dose of ≤0.05 mg/kg/day as hematologic recovery begins **or**

0.25 mg/kg/day for 4 days (or 0.2 mg/kg/day for 5 days); repeat at 4- to 6-week intervals as ANC and platelet counts return to normal

Other dosing regimens in **combination therapy** *(unlabeled doses):*

4 mg/m²/day for 7 days every 4 weeks (in combination with prednisone **or** with prednisone and thalidomide) (Palumbo, 2006; Palumbo, 2008) **or**

6 mg/m²/day for 7 days every 4 weeks (in combination with prednisone) (Palumbo, 2004) **or**

0.25 mg/kg/day for 4 days every 6 weeks (in combination with prednisone [Facon, 2006; Facon, 2007] **or** with prednisone and thalidomide [Facon, 2007]) **or**

9 mg/m²/day for 4 days every 6 weeks (in combination with prednisone **or** with prednisone and bortezomib) (Dimopoulos, 2009; San Miguel, 2008)

◀ I.V.: 16 mg/m^2 administered at 2-week intervals for 4 doses, then administer at 4-week intervals after adequate hematologic recovery.

Ovarian carcinoma: Oral: 0.2 mg/kg/day for 5 days, repeat every 4-5 weeks **or**

Unlabeled dosing: 7 mg/m^2/day in 2 divided doses for 5 days, repeat every 28 days (Wadler, 1996)

Amyloidosis, light chain (unlabeled use): Oral: 0.22 mg/kg/day for 4 days every 28 days (in combination with oral dexamethasone) (Palladini, 2004) **or** 10 mg/m^2/day for 4 days every month (in combination with oral dexamethasone) for 12-18 treatment cycles (Jaccard, 2007)

Hodgkin lymphoma (unlabeled use): I.V.: 30 mg/m^2 on day 6 of combination chemotherapy (mini-BEAM) regimen (Colwill, 1995; Martin, 2001)

Conditioning regimen for autologous hematopoietic stem cell transplantation (unlabeled use): I.V.:

200 mg/m^2 alone 2 days prior to transplantation (Fermand, 2005; Moreau, 2002) **or**

140 mg/m^2 2 days prior to transplantation (combined with busulfan) (Fermand, 2005) **or**

140 mg/m^2 2 days prior to transplantation (combined with total body irradiation [TBI]) (Moreau, 2002) **or**

140 mg/m^2 5 days prior to transplantation (combined with TBI) (Barlogie, 2006)

Renal Impairment

The FDA-approved labeling contains the following adjustment recommendations (for approved dosing levels) based on route of administration:

Oral: Moderate-to-severe renal impairment: Consider a reduced dose initially.

I.V.: BUN ≥30 mg/dL: Reduce dose by up to 50%.

The following guidelines have been used by some clinicians:

Aronoff, 2007 (route of administration not specified): Adults (based on a 6 mg once-daily dose):

Cl$_{cr}$ 10-50 mL/minute: Administer 75% of dose.

Cl$_{cr}$ <10 mL/minute: Administer 50% of dose.

Hemodialysis: Administer dose after hemodialysis.

Continuous ambulatory peritoneal dialysis (CAPD): Administer 50% of dose.

Continuous renal replacement therapy (CRRT): Administer 75% of dose.

Carlson, 2005: Oral (for melphalan-prednisone combination therapy; based on a study evaluating toxicity with melphalan dosed at 0.25 mg/kg/day for 4 days/cycle):

Cl$_{cr}$ >10 to <30 mL/minute: Administer 75% of dose

Cl$_{cr}$ ≤10 mL/minute: Data is insufficient for a recommendation

Kintzel, 1995:

Oral: Adjust dose in the presence of hematologic toxicity

I.V.:

Cl$_{cr}$ 46-60 mL/minute: Administer 85% of normal dose.

Cl$_{cr}$ 31-45 mL/minute: Administer 75% of normal dose.

Cl$_{cr}$ <30 mL/minute: Administer 70% of normal dose.

Badros, 2001: I.V.: Autologous stem cell transplant (single-agent conditioning regimen; no busulfan or irradiation): Serum creatinine >2 mg/dL: Reduce dose from 200 mg/m^2 over 2 days (as 100 mg/m^2/day for 2 days) to 140 mg/m^2 given as a single-dose infusion

Hepatic Impairment Melphalan is hepatically metabolized; however, dosage adjustment does not appear to be necessary (King, 2001).

Administration

Oral: Administer on an empty stomach (1 hour prior to or 2 hours after meals)

Parenteral: Due to limited stability, complete administration of I.V. dose should occur within 60 minutes of reconstitution

I.V.: Infuse over 15-30 minutes. Extravasation may cause local tissue damage; administration by slow injection into a fast running I.V. solution into an injection port or via a central line is recommended; do not administer by direct injection into a peripheral vein.

Monitoring Parameters CBC with differential and platelet count, serum electrolytes, serum uric acid

Test Interactions False-positive Coombs' test [direct]

Special Geriatric Considerations Toxicity to immunosuppressives is increased in the elderly. Start with lowest recommended adult doses. Signs of infection, such as fever and WBC rise, may not occur. Lethargy and confusion may be more prominent signs of infection.

Dosage Forms Excipient information presented when available (limited, particularly for generics); consult specific product labeling.

Injection, powder for reconstitution: 50 mg

Alkeran®: 50 mg [contains ethanol (in diluent), propylene glycol (in diluent)]

Tablet, oral:

Alkeran®: 2 mg

Memantine (me MAN teen)

Medication Safety Issues
Sound-alike/look-alike issues:
Memantine may be confused with mesalamine

Brand Names: U.S. Namenda®

Brand Names: Canada Apo-Memantine; CO Memantine; Ebixa®; PMS-Memantine; ratio-Memantine; Riva-Memantine; Sandoz-Memantine

Index Terms Memantine Hydrochloride; Namenda XR

Generic Availability (U.S.) No

Pharmacologic Category N-Methyl-D-Aspartate Receptor Antagonist

Use Treatment of moderate-to-severe dementia of the Alzheimer's type

Unlabeled Use Treatment of mild-to-moderate vascular dementia

Contraindications Hypersensitivity to memantine or any component of the formulation

Warnings/Precautions Use with caution in patients with cardiovascular disease; an increased incidence of cardiac failure, angina, bradycardia, and hypertension (compared with placebo) was observed in clinical trials. Use caution with seizure disorders or severe hepatic impairment. Use with caution in severe renal impairment; dose adjustments may be required. Worsening of corneal condition has been observed in a clinical trial; periodic ophthalmic exams during use have been recommended (Canadian labeling). Clearance is significantly reduced by alkaline urine; use caution with medications, dietary changes, or patient conditions which may alter urine pH.

Adverse Reactions (Reflective of adult population; not specific for elderly) 1% to 10%:
Cardiovascular: Hypertension (4%), cardiac failure, cerebrovascular accident, syncope, transient ischemic attack
Central nervous system: Dizziness (7%), confusion (6%), headache (6%), hallucinations (3%), pain (3%), somnolence (3%), fatigue (2%), aggressive reaction, ataxia, vertigo
Dermatologic: Rash
Gastrointestinal: Constipation (5%), vomiting (3%), weight loss
Genitourinary: Micturition
Hematologic: Anemia
Hepatic: Alkaline phosphatase increased
Neuromuscular & skeletal: Back pain (3%), hypokinesia
Ocular: Cataract, conjunctivitis
Respiratory: Cough (4%), dyspnea (2%), pneumonia

Drug Interactions
Metabolism/Transport Effects None known.

Avoid Concomitant Use There are no known interactions where it is recommended to avoid concomitant use.

Increased Effect/Toxicity
Memantine may increase the levels/effects of: Trimethoprim

The levels/effects of Memantine may be increased by: Carbonic Anhydrase Inhibitors; Sodium Bicarbonate; Trimethoprim

Decreased Effect There are no known significant interactions involving a decrease in effect.

Stability Store at 25°C (77°F); excursions permitted to 15°C to 30°C (59°F to 86°F).

Mechanism of Action Glutamate, the primary excitatory amino acid in the CNS, may contribute to the pathogenesis of Alzheimer's disease (AD) by overstimulating various glutamate receptors leading to excitotoxicity and neuronal cell death. Memantine is an uncompetitive antagonist of the N-methyl-D-aspartate (NMDA) type of glutamate receptors, located ubiquitously throughout the brain. Under normal physiologic conditions, the (unstimulated) NMDA receptor ion channel is blocked by magnesium ions, which are displaced after agonist-induced depolarization. Pathologic or excessive receptor activation, as postulated to occur during AD, prevents magnesium from reentering and blocking the channel pore resulting in a chronically open state and excessive calcium influx. Memantine binds to the intra-pore magnesium site, but with longer dwell time, and thus functions as an effective receptor blocker only under conditions of excessive stimulation; memantine does not affect normal neurotransmission.

Pharmacodynamics/Kinetics
Distribution: 9-11 L/kg
Protein binding: 45%
Metabolism: Partially hepatic, primarily independent of the CYP enzyme system; forms 3 metabolites (minimal activity)
Half-life elimination: Terminal: ~60-80 hours; severe renal impairment (Cl_{cr} 5-29 mL/minute): 117-156 hours

Time to peak, serum: 3-7 hours

Excretion: Urine (74%; ~48% of the total dose as unchanged drug; undergoes active tubular secretion moderated by pH-dependent tubular reabsorption; excretion reduced by alkaline urine pH)

Dosage

Geriatric & Adult

Alzheimer's disease: Oral: Initial: 5 mg daily; increase dose by 5 mg daily to a target dose of 20 mg daily; wait ≥1 week between dosage changes. Doses >5 mg daily should be given in 2 divided doses.

Suggested titration: 5 mg daily for ≥1 week; 5 mg twice daily for ≥1 week; 15 mg daily given in 5 mg and 10 mg separated doses for ≥1 week; then 10 mg twice daily

Mild-to-moderate vascular dementia (unlabeled use): Oral: Initial: 5 mg daily, titrated by 5 mg daily weekly to a target dose of 10 mg twice daily (Orgogozo, 2002)

Renal Impairment Note: Renal function may be estimated using the Cockcroft-Gault formula for dosage adjustment purposes.

Mild impairment: No adjustment required

Moderate impairment:

U.S. labeling: No adjustment required

Canadian labeling: (Cl_{cr} 30-49 mL/minute): Initial: 5 mg once daily; after at least 1 week of therapy and if tolerated, titrate up to 5 mg twice daily; based on clinical response (and if well tolerated), may further titrate dosage upward in weekly increments to 20 mg daily according to suggested titration schedule.

Severe impairment:

U.S. labeling: Cl_{cr} 5-29 mL/minute: Initial: 5 mg once daily; after at least 1 week of therapy and if tolerated, may titrate up to a target dose of 5 mg twice daily

Canadian labeling: Cl_{cr} 15-29 mL/minute: Initial: 5 mg once daily; after at least 1 week of therapy and if tolerated, may titrate up to a target dose of 5 mg twice daily

Hepatic Impairment

Mild-to-moderate impairment: No dosage adjustment necessary.

Severe impairment:

U.S. labeling: No dosage adjustment provided in the manufacturer's labeling (has not been studied); use with caution.

Canadian labeling: No dosage adjustment provided in the manufacturer's labeling (has not been studied); avoid use.

Administration Administer without regard to meals.

Monitoring Parameters Periodic ophthalmic exam (Canadian labeling)

Special Geriatric Considerations In clinical trials, patients on memantine had less of a decline in cognitive function and activities of daily living (ADL) as compared to placebo. This was true for monotherapy with memantine, as well as combination therapy with donepezil, an acetylcholinesterase inhibitor.

Product Availability

Namenda XR™: FDA approved in June 2010; anticipated availability is currently undetermined

Namenda XR™ is an extended release capsule (once-daily administration) approved for the treatment of moderate-to-severe dementia associated with Alzheimer's disease

Dosage Forms Excipient information presented when available (limited, particularly for generics); consult specific product labeling.

Combination package, oral, as hydrochloride [titration pack contains two separate tablet formulations]:

Namenda®: Tablet: 5 mg (28s) and Tablet: 10 mg (21s)

Solution, oral, as hydrochloride:

Namenda®: 2 mg/mL (360 mL) [ethanol free, sugar free; contains propylene glycol; peppermint flavor]

Tablet, oral, as hydrochloride:

Namenda®: 5 mg, 10 mg

Meningococcal (Groups A / C / Y and W-135) Diphtheria Conjugate Vaccine

(me NIN joe kok al groops aye, see, why & dubl yoo won thur tee fyve dif THEER ee a KON joo gate vak SEEN)

Related Information

Immunization Administration Recommendations *on page 2144*
Immunization Recommendations *on page 2149*

Medication Safety Issues

Administration issue:

Menactra® (MCV4) should be administered by intramuscular (I.M.) injection only. Inadvertent subcutaneous (SubQ) administration has been reported; possibly due to confusion of this product with Menomune® (MPSV4), also a meningococcal polysaccharide vaccine, which is administered by the SubQ route.

Brand Names: U.S. Menactra®; Menveo®

Brand Names: Canada Menactra®; Menveo®

Index Terms MCV; MCV4; MenACWY-CRM (Menveo®); MenACWY-D (Menactra®); Meningococcal Conjugate Vaccine

Generic Availability (U.S.) No

Pharmacologic Category Vaccine, Inactivated (Bacterial)

Use Provide active immunization of children and adults against invasive meningococcal disease caused by *N. meningitidis* serogroups A, C, Y, and W-135.

The Advisory Committee on Immunization Practices (ACIP) recommends routine vaccination of all persons at age 11 or 12 years of age, followed by a booster at age 16 years of age (CDC, 60[3], 2011).

The ACIP also recommends vaccination for:

Children 9 through 23 months of age at increased risk for meningococcal disease (CDC, 60 [40], 2011). Children at increased risk include:
- Children traveling to or who reside in countries where *N. meningitidis* is hyperendemic or epidemic
- Children with persistent complement component deficiencies (eg, C5-C9, properdin, factor H, or factor D)

Persons 2 through 55 years of age at increased risk for meningococcal disease (CDC, 60[3], 2011). Meningococcal conjugate vaccine (MCV4) is preferred for persons aged 2-55 years; meningococcal polysaccharide vaccine (MPSV4) is preferred in adults ≥56 years of age (CDC, 2005). Persons at increased risk include:
- Previously unvaccinated college freshmen living in dormitories
- Microbiologists routinely exposed to isolates of *N. meningitidis*
- Military recruits
- Persons traveling to or who reside in countries where *N. meningitidis* is hyperendemic or epidemic, particularly if contact with local population will be prolonged
- Persons with persistent complement component deficiencies (eg, C5-C9, properdin, factor H, or factor D)
- Persons with anatomic or functional asplenia

Use is also recommended during meningococcal outbreaks caused by vaccine preventable serogroups (all recommended age groups) (CDC, 2005; CDC, 60[40], 2011).

Dosage

Adult Immunization: I.M.:

Menactra®, Menveo®: Adults ≤55 years: 0.5 mL/dose given as single dose

ACIP recommendations:

Adults ≤55 years with persistent complement component deficiency; functional or anatomic asplenia or HIV infection: Two doses, 2 months apart. A booster dose should be given every 5 years if still at risk for meningococcal disease (CDC, 60[3], 2011).

Adults ≤55 years with prolonged increased risk of exposure: One dose. A booster dose should be given every 5 years if still at risk for meningococcal disease (CDC, 60[3], 2011).

College students: Persons ≤21 years of age should have documentation of vaccination ≤5 years prior to enrollment. If the primary dose was given at <16 years of age, a booster dose should be given any time after the 16th birthday and prior to college enrollment. The minimum interval between doses is 8 weeks (CDC, 60[3], 2011).

Special Geriatric Considerations May be used though safety and efficacy have not been established in patients >55 years of age.

MENINGOCOCCAL (GROUPS A / C / Y AND W-135) DIPHTHERIA CONJUGATE VACCINE

Dosage Forms Excipient information presented when available (limited, particularly for generics); consult specific product labeling.

Injection, solution [preservative free]:

Menactra®: 4 mcg each of polysaccharide antigen groups A, C, Y, and W-135 [bound to diphtheria toxoid 48 mcg] per 0.5 mL [MCV4 or MenACWY-D]

Menveo®: MenA oligosaccharide 10 mcg, MenC oligosaccharide 5 mcg, MenY oligosaccharide 5 mcg, and MenW-135 oligosaccharide 5 mcg [bound to CRM$_{197}$ protein 32.7-64.1 mcg] per 0.5 mL (0.5 mL) [MenACWY-CRM; supplied in two vials, one containing MenA powder and one containing MenCYW-135 liquid]

◆ **Meningococcal Polysaccharide Vaccine** see Meningococcal Polysaccharide Vaccine (Groups A / C / Y and W-135) on page 1206

Meningococcal Polysaccharide Vaccine (Groups A / C / Y and W-135)

(me NIN joe kok al pol i SAK a ride vak SEEN groops aye, see, why & dubl yoo won thur tee fyve)

Related Information

Immunization Administration Recommendations on page 2144
Immunization Recommendations on page 2149

Medication Safety Issues

Administration issue:

Menomune® (MPSV4) should be administered by subcutaneous (SubQ) injection. Menactra® (MCV4), also a meningococcal polysaccharide vaccine, is to be administered by intramuscular (I.M.) injection only.

Brand Names: U.S. Menomune®-A/C/Y/W-135

Brand Names: Canada Menomune®-A/C/Y/W-135

Index Terms Meningococcal Polysaccharide Vaccine; MPSV; MPSV4

Generic Availability (U.S.) No

Pharmacologic Category Vaccine, Inactivated (Bacterial)

Use Provide active immunity to meningococcal serogroups contained in the vaccine

The Advisory Committee on Immunization Practices (ACIP) recommends routine vaccination for persons at increased risk for meningococcal disease. Meningococcal conjugate vaccine (MCV4) is preferred for persons aged 2-55 years; meningococcal polysaccharide vaccine (MPSV4) is preferred in adults ≥56 years of age (CDC, 2005).

Persons at increased risk include:

- Previously unvaccinated college freshmen living in dormitories
- Microbiologists routinely exposed to isolates of N. meningitidis
- Military recruits
- Persons traveling to or who reside in countries where N. meningitidis is hyperendemic or epidemic, particularly if contact with local population will be prolonged
- Persons with persistent complement component deficiencies (eg, C5-C9, properidin, factor H, or factor D)
- Persons with anatomic or functional asplenia
- Persons with HIV infection

Use is also recommended during meningococcal outbreaks caused by vaccine preventable serogroups.

Contraindications Hypersensitivity to any component of the formulation

Warnings/Precautions Immediate treatment (including epinephrine 1:1000) for anaphylactoid and/or hypersensitivity reactions should be available during vaccine use. Response may not be as great as desired in immunosuppressed patients. In general, household and close contacts of persons with altered immunocompetence may receive all age appropriate vaccines. Not to be used to treat meningococcal infections or to provide immunity against N. meningitidis serogroup B. May consider deferring administration in patients with moderate or severe acute illness (with or without fever); may administer to patients with mild acute illness (with or without fever). Vaccination may not result in effective immunity in all patients. Response depends upon multiple factors (eg, type of vaccine, age of patient) and may be improved by administering the vaccine at the recommended dose, route, and interval. Vaccines may not be effective if administered during periods of altered immune competence (CDC, 2011). Syncope has been reported with use of injectable vaccines and may be accompanied by transient visual disturbances, weakness, or tonic-clonic movements. Procedures should be in place to avoid injuries from falling and to restore cerebral perfusion if syncope occurs. Use with caution in patients with latex sensitivity; the stopper to the vial contains dry, natural latex rubber. Some dosage forms contain thimerosal. In order to maximize vaccination rates, the ACIP recommends simultaneous administration of all age-appropriate vaccines (live or inactivated) for which a person is eligible at a single clinic visit, unless contraindications exist.

Adverse Reactions (Reflective of adult population; not specific for elderly) All serious adverse reactions must be reported to the U.S. Department of Health and Human Services (DHHS) Vaccine Adverse Event Reporting System (VAERS) 1-800-822-7967 or online at https://vaers.hhs.gov/esub/index. In Canada, adverse reactions may be reported to local provincial/territorial health agencies or to the Vaccine Safety Section at Public Health Agency of Canada (1-866-844-0018).

>10%:

Central nervous system: Headache (29% to 42%), fatigue (25% to 32%), malaise (17% to 22%), irritability (12%), drowsiness (11%)

Gastrointestinal: Diarrhea (10% to 14%)

Local: Injection site: Pain (26% to 48%), redness (6% to 16%), induration (4% to 11%)

Neuromuscular & skeletal: Arthralgia (5% to 16%)

1% to 10%:

Central nervous system: Chills (4% to 6%), fever (≤5%)

Dermatologic: Rash (≤3%)

Gastrointestinal: Anorexia (8% to 10%), vomiting (1% to 3%)

Local: Injection site: Swelling (3% to 8%)

Drug Interactions

Metabolism/Transport Effects None known.

Avoid Concomitant Use There are no known interactions where it is recommended to avoid concomitant use.

Increased Effect/Toxicity There are no known significant interactions involving an increase in effect.

Decreased Effect

The levels/effects of Meningococcal Polysaccharide Vaccine (Groups A / C / Y and W-135) may be decreased by: Belimumab; Fingolimod; Immunosuppressants

Stability Prior to and following reconstitution, store vaccine and diluent at 2°C to 8°C (35°F to 46°F); do not freeze. Reconstitute using provided diluent; shake well. Use single-dose vial within 30 minutes of reconstitution. Use single-dose vial immediately after reconstitution. Use multidose vial within 35 days of reconstitution.

Mechanism of Action Induces the formation of bactericidal antibodies to meningococcal antigens; the presence of these antibodies is strongly correlated with immunity to meningococcal disease caused by *Neisseria meningitidis* groups A, C, Y and W-135.

Pharmacodynamics/Kinetics

Onset of action: Antibody levels: 7-10 days

Duration: Antibodies against group A and C polysaccharides decline markedly (to prevaccination levels) over the first 3 years following a single dose of vaccine, especially in children <4 years of age

Dosage

Geriatric & Adult Immunization: SubQ: 0.5 mL/dose

ACIP recommendations:

Adults ≤55 years: 0.5 mL/dose; however, use is not generally recommended; meningococcal conjugate vaccine (MCV4) is preferred (CDC, 2011); If MCV4 is unavailable, meningococcal polysaccharide vaccine (MPSV4) is an acceptable alternative (CDC, 2005). Persons at prolonged increased risk for meningococcal disease should be revaccinated with MCV4 (CDC, 2009).

Adults >55 years: 0.5 mL/dose (MPSV4 preferred in this population) (CDC, 2005)

Administration Administer by SubQ injection to the deltoid region; do not administer intradermally, I.M., or I.V.

Simultaneous administration of vaccines helps ensure the patients will be fully vaccinated by the appropriate age. Simultaneous administration of vaccines is defined as administering ≥1 vaccine on the same day at different anatomic sites. Separate vaccines should not be combined in the same syringe unless indicated by product specific labeling. Separate needles and syringes should be used for each injection. The ACIP prefers each dose of a specific vaccine in a series come from the same manufacturer when possible. Adolescents and adults should be vaccinated while seated or lying down. In general, preterm infants should be vaccinated at the same chronological age as full-term infants (CDC, 2011).

Antipyretics have not been shown to prevent febrile seizures. Antipyretics may be used to treat fever or discomfort following vaccination (CDC, 2011). One study reported that routine prophylactic administration of acetaminophen to prevent fever prior to vaccination decreased the immune response of some vaccines; the clinical significance of this reduction in immune response has not been established (Prymula, 2009).

Monitoring Parameters Monitor for syncope for 15 minutes following administration. If seizure-like activity associated with syncope occurs, maintain patient in supine or Trendelenburg position to reestablish adequate cerebral perfusion.

Pharmacotherapy Pearls U.S. federal law requires that the name of medication, date of administration, the vaccine manufacturer, lot number of vaccine, and the administering person's name, title and address be entered into the patient's permanent medical record.

Special Geriatric Considerations No specific data; only recommended when traveling to highly endemic areas.

Dosage Forms Excipient information presented when available (limited, particularly for generics); consult specific product labeling.

Injection, powder for reconstitution [MPSV4]:

Menomune®-A/C/Y/W-135: 50 mcg each of polysaccharide antigen groups A, C, Y, and W-135 per 0.5 mL dose [contains lactose 2.5-5 mg/0.5 mL, natural rubber/natural latex in packaging, thimerosal in diluent for multidose vial]

◆ **Menomune®-A/C/Y/W-135** see Meningococcal Polysaccharide Vaccine (Groups A / C / Y and W-135) on page 1206

◆ **Menostar®** see Estradiol (Systemic) on page 681

◆ **Menveo®** see Meningococcal (Groups A / C / Y and W-135) Diphtheria Conjugate Vaccine on page 1205

Meperidine (me PER i deen)

Related Information
Beers Criteria – Potentially Inappropriate Medications for Geriatrics on page 2183
Opioid Analgesics on page 2122
Patient Information for Disposal of Unused Medications on page 2244

Medication Safety Issues
Sound-alike/look-alike issues:
Meperidine may be confused with meprobamate
Demerol® may be confused with Demulen®, Desyrel, Dilaudid®, Pamelor™

High alert medication:
The Institute for Safe Medication Practices (ISMP) includes this medication among its list of drug classes which have a heightened risk of causing significant patient harm when used in error.

BEERS Criteria medication:
This drug may be potentially inappropriate for use in geriatric patients (Quality of evidence - high; Strength of recommendation - strong).

Other safety concerns:
Avoid the use of meperidine for pain control, especially in elderly and renally-compromised patients because of the risk of neurotoxicity (American Pain Society, 2008; Institute for Safe Medication Practices [ISMP], 2007)

Brand Names: U.S. Demerol®
Brand Names: Canada Demerol®
Index Terms Isonipecaine Hydrochloride; Meperidine Hydrochloride; Pethidine Hydrochloride
Generic Availability (U.S.) Yes
Pharmacologic Category Analgesic, Opioid
Use Management of moderate-to-severe pain; adjunct to anesthesia and preoperative sedation
Unlabeled Use Reduce postoperative shivering; reduce rigors from amphotericin B (conventional)
Contraindications Hypersensitivity to meperidine or any component of the formulation; use with or within 14 days of MAO inhibitors; severe respiratory insufficiency
Warnings/Precautions Oral meperidine is not recommended for acute/chronic pain management. Meperidine should not be used for acute/cancer pain because of the risk of neurotoxicity. Normeperidine (an active metabolite and CNS stimulant) may accumulate and precipitate anxiety, tremors, or seizures; risk increases with CNS or renal dysfunction, prolonged use (>48 hours), and cumulative dose (>600 mg/24 hours). The Institute for Safe Medication Practice recommends avoiding the use of meperidine for pain control, especially in the elderly and renally-impaired (ISMP, 2007). In the elderly; meperidine is not an effective oral analgesic at commonly used doses; may cause neurotoxicity; other agents are preferred in the elderly (Beers Criteria).

May cause CNS depression, which may impair physical or mental abilities; patients must be cautioned about performing tasks which require mental alertness (eg, operating machinery or driving). Effects (eg, sedation, respiratory depression, hypotension) may be potentiated when used with other sedative/hypnotic drugs, general anesthetics, phenothiazines, or ethanol; consider reduced dose of meperidine if using concomitantly. Use only with extreme caution (if at all) in patients with head injury or increased intracranial pressure (ICP). Use caution with pulmonary, hepatic, or renal disorders, supraventricular tachycardias (including atrial flutter), acute abdominal conditions, delirium tremens, hypothyroidism, myxedema, toxic psychosis, kyphoscoliosis, morbid obesity, Addison's disease, seizure disorders, pheochromocytoma, BPH, or urethral stricture. Use with caution in patients with biliary tract dysfunction; acute pancreatitis may cause constriction of sphincter of Oddi. May cause hypotension (including orthostatic hypotension); use with caution in patients with depleted blood volume or drugs which may exaggerate hypotensive effects (including phenothiazines or general anesthetics).

An opioid-containing analgesic regimen should be tailored to each patient's needs and based upon the type of pain being treated (acute versus chronic), the route of administration, degree of tolerance for opioids (naive versus chronic user), age, weight, and medical condition. The optimal analgesic dose varies widely among patients. Some preparations contain sulfites which may cause allergic reaction. Tolerance or drug dependence may result from extended use. Healthcare provider should be alert to problems of abuse, misuse, and diversion. Concurrent use of agonist/antagonist analgesics may precipitate withdrawal symptoms and/ or reduced analgesic efficacy in patients following prolonged therapy with mu opioid agonists. Abrupt discontinuation following prolonged use may also lead to withdrawal symptoms. Avoid use in the elderly.

Adverse Reactions (Reflective of adult population; not specific for elderly) Frequency not defined.

Cardiovascular: Bradycardia, cardiac arrest, circulatory depression, hypotension, palpitation, shock, syncope, tachycardia

Central nervous system: Agitation, confusion, delirium, disorientation, dizziness, drowsiness, dysphoria, euphoria, fatigue, flushing, hallucinations, headache, intracranial pressure increased, lightheadedness, malaise, mental depression, nervousness, paradoxical CNS stimulation, restlessness, sedation, seizure (associated with metabolite accumulation), serotonin syndrome

Dermatologic: Pruritus, rash, urticaria

Gastrointestinal: Abdominal cramps, anorexia, biliary spasm, constipation, nausea, paralytic ileus, sphincter of Oddi spasm, vomiting, xerostomia

Genitourinary: Ureteral spasms, urinary retention

Local: Injection site reaction (including pain, wheal, and flare)

Neuromuscular & skeletal: Muscle twitching, myoclonus, tremor, weakness

Ocular: Visual disturbances

Respiratory: Dyspnea, respiratory arrest, respiratory depression

Miscellaneous: Anaphylaxis, diaphoresis, histamine release, hypersensitivity reactions, physical and psychological dependence

Drug Interactions

Metabolism/Transport Effects None known.

Avoid Concomitant Use

Avoid concomitant use of Meperidine with any of the following: Azelastine; Azelastine (Nasal); MAO Inhibitors; Methadone; Paraldehyde

Increased Effect/Toxicity

Meperidine may increase the levels/effects of: Alcohol (Ethyl); Alvimopan; Azelastine; Azelastine (Nasal); CNS Depressants; Desmopressin; Methadone; Metoclopramide; Metyrosine; Paraldehyde; Selective Serotonin Reuptake Inhibitors; Serotonin Modulators; Thiazide Diuretics; Zolpidem

The levels/effects of Meperidine may be increased by: Amphetamines; Antipsychotic Agents (Phenothiazines); Antipsychotics; Barbiturates; HydrOXYzine; MAO Inhibitors; Protease Inhibitors; Succinylcholine

Decreased Effect

Meperidine may decrease the levels/effects of: Pegvisomant

The levels/effects of Meperidine may be decreased by: Ammonium Chloride; Fosphenytoin; Mixed Agonist / Antagonist Opioids; Phenytoin; Protease Inhibitors

Ethanol/Nutrition/Herb Interactions

Ethanol: May increase CNS depression; monitor for increased effects with coadministration. Caution patients about effects.

Herb/Nutraceutical: Avoid valerian, St John's wort, kava kava, gotu kola (may increase CNS depression).

Stability

Injection solution: Store at 20°C to 25°C (68°F to 77°F); excursions permitted to 15°C to 30°C (59°F to 86°F).

Tablets: Store at 25°C (77°F); excursions permitted to 15°C to 30°C (59°F to 86°F).

Mechanism of Action Binds to opioid receptors in the CNS, causing inhibition of ascending pain pathways, altering the perception of and response to pain; produces generalized CNS depression

Pharmacodynamics/Kinetics

Onset of action: Analgesic: Oral, SubQ: 10-15 minutes; I.V.: ~5 minutes

Peak effect: SubQ.: ~1 hour; Oral: 2 hours

Duration: Oral, SubQ.: 2-4 hours

Absorption: I.M.: Erratic and highly variable

Protein binding: 65% to 75%

Metabolism: Hepatic; hydrolyzed to meperidinic acid (inactive) or undergoes N-demethylation to normeperidine (active; has $1/2$ the analgesic effect and 2-3 times the CNS effects of meperidine)

Bioavailability: ~50% to 60%; increased with liver disease

Half-life elimination:

Parent drug: Terminal phase: Adults: 2.5-4 hours, Liver disease: 7-11 hours

Normeperidine (active metabolite): 15-30 hours; can accumulate with high doses (>600 mg/day) or with decreased renal function

Excretion: Urine (as metabolites)

Dosage

Geriatric Avoid use (American Pain Society, 2008; ISMP, 2007).

Adult Note: The American Pain Society (2008) and ISMP (2007) do not recommend meperidine's use as an analgesic. If use in acute pain (in patients without renal or CNS disease) cannot be avoided, treatment should be limited to ≤48 hours and doses should not exceed 600 mg/24 hours. Oral route is not recommended for treatment of acute or chronic pain. If I.V. route is required, consider a reduced dose. Patients with prior opioid exposure may require higher initial doses.

Pain (analgesic): Oral, I.M., SubQ: 50-150 mg every 3-4 hours as needed

Preoperatively: I.M., SubQ: 50-150 mg given 30-90 minutes before the beginning of anesthesia

Obstetrical analgesia: I.M., SubQ: 50-100 mg when pain becomes regular; may repeat at every 1-3 hours

Postoperative shivering (unlabeled use): I.V.: 25-50 mg once (Crowley, 2008; Kranke, 2002; Mercandante, 1994; Wang, 1999)

Renal Impairment Avoid use in renal impairment (American Pain Society, 2008; ISMP, 2007).

Hepatic Impairment Use with caution in severe hepatic impairment; consider a lower initial dose when initiating therapy. An increased opioid effect may be seen in patients with cirrhosis; dose reduction is more important for the oral than I.V. route.

Administration

Solution for injection: Meperidine may be administered I.M., SubQ, or I.V.; I.V. push should be administered slowly using a diluted solution, use of a 10 mg/mL concentration has been recommended.

Oral solution: Administer solution in $1/2$ glass of water; undiluted solution may exert topical anesthetic effect on mucous membranes

Monitoring Parameters Pain relief, respiratory and mental status, blood pressure; observe patient for excessive sedation, CNS depression, seizures, respiratory depression

Test Interactions Increased amylase (S), increased BSP retention, increased CPK (I.M. injections)

Special Geriatric Considerations Meperidine is not recommended as a drug of first choice for the treatment of chronic pain in the elderly due to the accumulation of its metabolite, normeperidine, which leads to serious CNS side effects (eg, tremor, seizures). If used for acute pain, its use should be limited to 1-2 doses.

This medication is considered to be potentially inappropriate in this patient population (Beers Criteria: Quality of evidence - high; Strength of recommendation - strong).

Controlled Substance C-II

Dosage Forms Excipient information presented when available (limited, particularly for generics); consult specific product labeling. [DSC] = Discontinued product

Injection, solution, as hydrochloride: 25 mg/mL (1 mL); 50 mg/mL (1 mL [DSC]); 100 mg/mL (1 mL [DSC])

Demerol®: 25 mg/mL (1 mL); 25 mg/0.5 mL (0.5 mL); 50 mg/mL (1 mL, 1.5 mL, 2 mL, 30 mL); 75 mg/mL (1 mL); 100 mg/mL (1 mL, 20 mL)

Injection, solution, as hydrochloride [for PCA pump]: 10 mg/mL (30 mL)

Solution, oral, as hydrochloride: 50 mg/5 mL (500 mL)

Tablet, oral, as hydrochloride: 50 mg, 100 mg

Demerol®: 50 mg [scored]

Demerol®: 100 mg

◆ **Meperidine Hydrochloride** *see* Meperidine *on page 1208*

◆ **Mephyton®** *see* Phytonadione *on page 1534*

Meprobamate (me proe BA mate)

Related Information
Beers Criteria – Potentially Inappropriate Medications for Geriatrics *on page 2183*
Medication Safety Issues
Sound-alike/look-alike issues:
Meprobamate may be confused with meperidine
Equanil may be confused with Elavil®
BEERS Criteria medication:
This drug may be potentially inappropriate for use in geriatric patients (Quality of evidence - moderate; Strength of recommendation - strong).
Brand Names: Canada Novo-Mepro
Index Terms Equanil
Generic Availability (U.S.) Yes
Pharmacologic Category Antianxiety Agent, Miscellaneous
Use Management of anxiety disorders
Unlabeled Use Demonstrated value for muscle contraction, headache, external sphincter spasticity, muscle rigidity, opisthotonos-associated with tetanus; treatment of muscle spasm associated with acute temporomandibular joint (TMJ) pain
Contraindications Hypersensitivity to meprobamate, related compounds (including carisoprodol), or any component of the formulation; acute intermittent porphyria
Warnings/Precautions Physical and psychological dependence and abuse may occur; abrupt cessation may precipitate withdrawal. Use with caution in patients with depression or suicidal tendencies, or in patients with a history of drug abuse. May cause CNS depression, which may impair physical or mental abilities. Patients must be cautioned about performing tasks which require mental alertness (eg, operating machinery or driving). Effects with other sedative drugs or ethanol may be potentiated. Allergic reaction may occur in patients with history of dermatological condition (usually by fourth dose). Use with caution in patients with renal or hepatic impairment, or with a history of seizures. Avoid use in older adults; use associated with excessive sedation and high rate of physical dependence (Beers Criteria).
Adverse Reactions (Reflective of adult population; not specific for elderly) Frequency not defined.
Cardiovascular: Arrhythmia EEG abnormalities, hypotensive crisis, peripheral edema, palpitation, syncope, tachycardia
Central nervous system: Ataxia, chills, dizziness, drowsiness, euphoria, fever, headache, overstimulation, paradoxical excitement, slurred speech, vertigo
Dermatologic: Angioneurotic edema, bruising, dermatitis, erythema multiforme, petechiae, purpura, rash, Stevens-Johnson syndrome
Gastrointestinal: Diarrhea, nausea, proctitis, stomatitis, vomiting
Hematologic: Agranulocytosis, aplastic anemia, eosinophilia, leukopenia, porphyria exacerbation, thrombocytopenic purpura
Neuromuscular & skeletal: Paresthesia, weakness
Ocular: Impairment of accommodation
Renal: Anuria, oliguria
Respiratory: Bronchospasm
Miscellaneous: Anaphylaxis, hypersensitivity
Drug Interactions
Metabolism/Transport Effects None known.
Avoid Concomitant Use
Avoid concomitant use of Meprobamate with any of the following: Azelastine; Azelastine (Nasal); Methadone; Mirtazapine; Paraldehyde
Increased Effect/Toxicity
Meprobamate may increase the levels/effects of: Alcohol (Ethyl); Azelastine; Azelastine (Nasal); Buprenorphine; CNS Depressants; Methadone; Methotrimeprazine; Metyrosine; Mirtazapine; Paraldehyde; Selective Serotonin Reuptake Inhibitors; Zolpidem

The levels/effects of Meprobamate may be increased by: Droperidol; HydrOXYzine; Methotrimeprazine
Decreased Effect
The levels/effects of Meprobamate may be decreased by: Yohimbine
Ethanol/Nutrition/Herb Interactions
Ethanol: May increase CNS depression; monitor for increased effects with coadministration. Caution patients about effects.
Herb/Nutraceutical: Avoid valerian, St John's wort, kava kava, gotu kola (may increase CNS depression).

Mechanism of Action Affects the thalamus and limbic system; also appears to inhibit multineuronal spinal reflexes

Pharmacodynamics/Kinetics

Onset of action: Sedation: ~1 hour

Metabolism: Hepatic

Half-life elimination: 10 hours

Excretion: Urine (8% to 20% as unchanged drug); feces (10% as metabolites)

Dosage

Adult Anxiety or muscle spasm (TMJ) pain (unlabeled use): Oral: 1200-1600 mg/day in 3-4 divided doses, up to 2400 mg/day

Renal Impairment

Cl_{cr} 10-50 mL/minute: Administer every 9-12 hours.

Cl_{cr} <10 mL/minute: Administer every 12-18 hours.

Moderately dialyzable (20% to 50%)

Hepatic Impairment Probably necessary in patients with liver disease; no specific recommendations.

Monitoring Parameters Mental status

Reference Range Therapeutic: 6-12 mcg/mL (SI: 28-55 micromole/L); Toxic: >60 mcg/mL (SI: >275 micromole/L)

Pharmacotherapy Pearls Withdrawal should be gradual over 1-2 weeks. Benzodiazepine and buspirone are better choices for treatment of anxiety disorders.

Special Geriatric Considerations Meprobamate is not considered a drug of choice in the elderly because of its potential to cause physical and psychological dependence. Guidelines from the Centers for Medicare and Medicaid Services (CMS) strongly discourage the use of meprobamate in residents of long-term care facilities.

This medication is considered to be potentially inappropriate in this patient population (Beers Criteria: Quality of evidence - moderate; Strength of recommendation - strong).

Controlled Substance C-IV

Dosage Forms Excipient information presented when available (limited, particularly for generics); consult specific product labeling.

Tablet, oral: 200 mg, 400 mg

Mercaptopurine (mer kap toe PYOOR een)

Medication Safety Issues

Sound-alike/look-alike issues:

Mercaptopurine may be confused with methotrexate

Purinethol® may be confused with propylthiouracil

High alert medication:

This medication is in a class the Institute for Safe Medication Practices (ISMP) includes among its list of drug classes which have a heightened risk of causing significant patient harm when used in error.

Other safety concerns:

To avoid potentially serious dosage errors, the terms "6-mercaptopurine" or "6-MP" should be avoided; use of these terms has been associated with sixfold overdosages.

Azathioprine is metabolized to mercaptopurine; concurrent use of these commercially-available products has resulted in profound myelosuppression.

Brand Names: U.S. Purinethol®

Brand Names: Canada Purinethol®

Index Terms 6-Mercaptopurine (error-prone abbreviation); 6-MP (error-prone abbreviation)

Generic Availability (U.S.) Yes

Pharmacologic Category Antineoplastic Agent, Antimetabolite; Antineoplastic Agent, Antimetabolite (Purine Analog); Immunosuppressant Agent

Use Maintenance treatment component of acute lymphoblastic leukemia (ALL)

Unlabeled Use Steroid-sparing agent for corticosteroid-dependent Crohn's disease (CD) and ulcerative colitis (UC); maintenance of remission in CD; fistulizing Crohn's disease; maintenance treatment in acute promyelocytic leukemia (APL); treatment component for non Hodgkin lymphoma (NHL), treatment of autoimmune hepatitis

Contraindications Hypersensitivity to mercaptopurine or any component of the formulation; patients whose disease showed prior resistance to mercaptopurine

Warnings/Precautions Hazardous agent - use appropriate precautions for handling and disposal.

Hepatotoxicity has been reported, including jaundice, ascites, hepatic necrosis (may be fatal), intrahepatic cholestasis, parenchymal cell necrosis, and/or hepatic encephalopathy; may be due to direct hepatic cell damage or hypersensitivity. While hepatotoxicity or hepatic injury may occur at any dose, dosages >2.5 mg/kg/day are associated with a higher incidence. Signs of jaundice generally appear early in treatment, after ~1-2 months (range: 1 week to 8 years) and may resolve following discontinuation; recurrence with rechallenge has been noted. Monitor liver function tests (monitor more frequently if used in combination with other hepatotoxic drugs or in patients with pre-existing hepatic impairment. Consider a reduced dose in patients with hepatic impairment. Withhold treatment for clinical signs of jaundice (hepatomegaly, anorexia, tenderness), deterioration in liver function tests, toxic hepatitis, or biliary stasis until hepatotoxicity is ruled out.

Dose-related leukopenia, thrombocytopenia, and anemia are common; however, may be indicative of disease progression. Hematologic toxicity may be delayed. Bone marrow may appear hypoplastic (could also appear normal). Monitor for bleeding (due to thrombocytopenia) or infection (due to neutropenia). Patients with homozygous genetic defect of thiopurine methyltransferase (TPMT) are more sensitive to myelosuppressive effects; generally associated with rapid myelosuppression. Significant mercaptopurine dose reductions will be necessary (possibly with continued concomitant chemotherapy at normal doses). Patients who are heterozygous for TPMT defects will have intermediate activity; may have increased toxicity (primarily myelosuppression) although will generally tolerate normal mercaptopurine doses. Consider TPMT testing for severe toxicities/excessive myelosuppression. Patients on concurrent therapy with drugs which may inhibit TPMT (eg, olsalazine) or xanthine oxidase (eg, allopurinol) may be sensitive to myelosuppressive effects.

May increase the risk for secondary malignancies; hepatic T-cell lymphoma (HTCL) has been reported with mercaptopurine when used for the treatment of irritable bowel disease (an unlabeled use). Because azathioprine is metabolized to mercaptopurine, concomitant use with azathioprine may result in profound myelosuppression and should be avoided. Mercaptopurine is immunosuppressive; the risk for infection is increased; common signs of infection, such as fever and leukocytosis may not occur; lethargy and confusion may be more prominent signs of infection. Immune response to vaccines may be diminished. Consider adjusting dosage in patients with renal impairment. To avoid potentially serious dosage errors, the terms "6-mercaptopurine" or "6-MP" should be avoided; use of these terms has been associated with sixfold overdosages.

Adverse Reactions (Reflective of adult population; not specific for elderly) Frequency not defined.

Central nervous system: Drug fever

Dermatologic: Alopecia, hyperpigmentation, rash

Endocrine & metabolic: Hyperuricemia

Gastrointestinal: Anorexia, diarrhea, intestinal ulcers, mucositis/oral lesions (rare), nausea (minimal), pancreatitis, sprue-like symptoms, stomach pain, vomiting (minimal)

Genitourinary: Oligospermia

Hematologic: Myelosuppression (onset 7-10 days; nadir 14 days; recovery: 21 days); anemia, bleeding, granulocytopenia, leukopenia, marrow hypoplasia, thrombocytopenia

Hepatic: Hepatotoxicity, ascites, biliary stasis, hepatic damage/injury, hepatic encephalopathy, hepatic necrosis, hepatomegaly, intrahepatic cholestasis, jaundice, parenchymal cell necrosis, toxic hepatitis

Renal: Hyperuricosuria, renal toxicity

Miscellaneous: Hepatosplenic T cell lymphoma, immunosuppression, infection, secondary malignancy

Drug Interactions

Metabolism/Transport Effects None known.

Avoid Concomitant Use

Avoid concomitant use of Mercaptopurine with any of the following: AzaTHIOprine; BCG; CloZAPine; Febuxostat; Natalizumab; Pimecrolimus; Tacrolimus (Topical)

Increased Effect/Toxicity

Mercaptopurine may increase the levels/effects of: CloZAPine; Leflunomide; Natalizumab; Vaccines (Live); Vitamin K Antagonists

The levels/effects of Mercaptopurine may be increased by: 5-ASA Derivatives; Allopurinol; AzaTHIOprine; Denosumab; Febuxostat; Pimecrolimus; Roflumilast; Sulfamethoxazole; Tacrolimus (Topical); Trastuzumab; Trimethoprim

Decreased Effect

Mercaptopurine may decrease the levels/effects of: BCG; Coccidioidin Skin Test; Sipuleucel-T; Vaccines (Inactivated); Vitamin K Antagonists

The levels/effects of Mercaptopurine may be decreased by: Echinacea

Ethanol/Nutrition/Herb Interactions Food: Absorption is variable with food. Management: Take on an empty stomach at the same time each day 1 hour before or 2 hours after a meal. Maintain adequate hydration, unless instructed to restrict fluid intake.

Stability Store at room temperature of 15°C to 25°C (59°F to 77°F). Protect from moisture.

MERCAPTOPURINE

Mechanism of Action Purine antagonist which inhibits DNA and RNA synthesis; acts as false metabolite and is incorporated into DNA and RNA, eventually inhibiting their synthesis; specific for the S phase of the cell cycle

Pharmacodynamics/Kinetics
Absorption: Variable and incomplete (~50%)
Distribution: V_d >total body water; CNS penetration is poor
Protein binding: ~19%
Metabolism: Hepatic and in GI mucosa; hepatically via xanthine oxidase and methylation via TPMT to sulfate conjugates, 6-thiouric acid, and other inactive compounds; first-pass effect
Half-life elimination (age dependent): Adults: 47 minutes
Time to peak, serum: ~2 hours
Excretion: Urine (46% as mercaptopurine and metabolites)

Dosage
Geriatric Due to renal decline with age, initiate treatment at the low end of recommended dose range.
Adult Also consult details concerning dosing in combination regimens.
 Acute lymphoblastic leukemia (ALL): Maintenance: Oral: 1.5-2.5 mg/kg/day **or**
 Unlabeled ALL dosing (combination chemotherapy; refer to specific reference for combinations):
  Early intensification (two 4-week courses): 60 mg/m^2/day days 1-14 (Larson, 1995; Larson, 1998)
  Interim maintenance (12-week course): 60 mg/m^2/day days 1-70 (Larson, 1995; Larson, 1998)
  Maintenance (prolonged): 50 mg 3 times/day for 2 years (Kantarjian, 2000; Thomas, 2004) **or** 60 mg/m^2/day for 2 years from diagnosis (Larson, 1995; Larson, 1998)
 Acute promyelocytic leukemia (APL) maintenance (unlabeled use): 60 mg/mm^2/day for 1 year (in combination with tretinoin and methotrexate) (Powell, 2010)
 Crohn's disease, remission maintenance or reduction of steroid use (unlabeled use): Oral: 1-1.5 mg/kg/day (Lichtenstein, 2009)
 Ulcerative colitis (unlabeled use): Oral:
  Initial: 50 mg once daily; titrate dose up if clinical remission not achieved or down if leukopenia occurs (Lobel, 2004) **or**
  Initial: 50 mg (25 mg if heterozygous for TPMT activity) once daily; titrate up to goal of 1.5 mg/kg (0.75 mg/kg if heterozygous for TPMT activity) if WBC >4000/mm^3 (and at least 50% of baseline) and LFTs and amylase are stable (Siegel, 2005) **or**
  Maintenance: 1-1.5 mg/kg/day (Carter, 2004) **or**
  Remission maintenance: 1.5 mg/kg/day (Danese, 2011)

 Dosage adjustment with concurrent allopurinol: Reduce mercaptopurine dosage to 25% to 33% of the usual dose.
 Dosage adjustment in TPMT-deficiency: Not always established; substantial reductions are generally required only in homozygous deficiency.
Renal Impairment The manufacturer's labeling recommends starting with reduced doses in patients with renal impairment to avoid accumulation; however, no specific dosage adjustment is provided.
Hepatic Impairment The manufacturer's labeling recommends considering a reduced dose in patients with hepatic impairment; however, no specific dosage adjustment is provided.
Administration Preferably on an empty stomach (1 hour before or 2 hours after meals)

For the treatment of ALL in children (Schmiegelow, 1997): Administration in the evening has demonstration superior outcome; administration with food did not significantly affect outcome.
Monitoring Parameters CBC with differential (weekly initially, although clinical status may require increased frequency), bone marrow exam (to evaluate marrow status), liver function tests (weekly initially, then monthly; monitor more frequently if on concomitant hepatotoxic agents), renal function, urinalysis; consider TPMT genotyping to identify TPMT defect (if severe toxicity occurs)

For use as immunomodulatory therapy in CD or UC, monitor CBC with differential weekly for 1 month, then biweekly for 1 month, followed by monitoring every 1-2 months throughout the course of therapy. LFTs should be assessed every 3 months. Monitor for signs/symptoms of malignancy (eg, splenomegaly, hepatomegaly, abdominal pain, persistent fever, night sweats, weight loss).
Test Interactions TPMT testing: Recent transfusions may result in a misinterpretation of the actual TPMT activity. Concomitant drugs may influence TPMT activity in the blood.
Special Geriatric Considerations Toxicity to immunosuppressives is increased in the elderly. Start with lowest recommended adult doses. Signs of infection, such as fever and WBC rise, may not occur. Lethargy and confusion may be more prominent signs of infection.

Dosage Forms Excipient information presented when available (limited, particularly for generics); consult specific product labeling.
Tablet, oral: 50 mg
Purinethol®: 50 mg [scored]

◆ **6-Mercaptopurine (error-prone abbreviation)** *see* Mercaptopurine *on page 1212*

Meropenem (mer oh PEN em)

Related Information
Antimicrobial Drugs of Choice *on page 2163*
Community-Acquired Pneumonia in Adults *on page 2171*
Medication Safety Issues
Sound-alike/look-alike issues:
Meropenem may be confused with ertapenem, imipenem, metroNIDAZOLE
Brand Names: U.S. Merrem® I.V.
Brand Names: Canada Merrem®
Generic Availability (U.S.) Yes
Pharmacologic Category Antibiotic, Carbapenem
Use
Treatment of intra-abdominal infections (complicated appendicitis and peritonitis); treatment of complicated skin and skin structure infections caused by susceptible organisms

Canadian labeling: Additional indications (not in U.S. labeling): Treatment of lower respiratory tract infections (community-acquired and nosocomial pneumonias), complicated urinary tract infections, gynecologic infections (excluding chlamydia), and septicemia; treatment of bacterial meningitis in adults caused by *S. pneumoniae*, *H. influenzae*, and *N. meningitidis* (use in adult meningitis based on pediatric data)
Unlabeled Use *Burkholderia pseudomallei* (melioidosis), febrile neutropenia, liver abscess, otitis externa
Contraindications Hypersensitivity to meropenem, any component of the formulation, or other carbapenems (eg, doripenem, ertapenem, imipenem); patients who have experienced anaphylactic reactions to other beta-lactams
Warnings/Precautions Serious hypersensitivity reactions, including anaphylaxis, have been reported (some without a history of previous allergic reactions to beta-lactams). Carbapenems have been associated with CNS adverse effects, including confusional states and seizures (myoclonic); use caution with CNS disorders (eg, brain lesions and history of seizures) and adjust dose in renal impairment to avoid drug accumulation, which may increase seizure risk. Prolonged use may result in fungal or bacterial superinfection, including *C. difficile*-associated diarrhea (CDAD) and pseudomembranous colitis; CDAD has been observed >2 months postantibiotic treatment. Use with caution in patients with renal impairment; dosage adjustment required in patients with moderate-to-severe renal dysfunction. Thrombocytopenia has been reported in patients with renal dysfunction. Lower doses (based upon renal function) are often required in the elderly. May decrease divalproex sodium/valproic acid concentrations leading to breakthrough seizures; concomitant use not recommended. Alternative antimicrobial agents should be considered; if concurrent meropenem is necessary, consider additional antiseizure medication.
Adverse Reactions (Reflective of adult population; not specific for elderly) 1% to 10%:
Central nervous system: Headache (2% to 8%), pain (≤5%)
Dermatologic: Rash (2% to 3%, includes diaper-area moniliasis in infants), pruritus (1%)
Endocrine & metabolic: Hypoglycemia
Gastrointestinal: Diarrhea (4% to 7%), nausea/vomiting (1% to 8%), constipation (1% to 7%), oral moniliasis (up to 2% in pediatric patients), glossitis (1%)
Hematologic: Anemia (≤6%)
Local: Inflammation at the injection site (2%), phlebitis/thrombophlebitis (1%), injection site reaction (1%)
Respiratory: Apnea (1%), pharyngitis, pneumonia
Miscellaneous: Sepsis (2%), shock (1%)
Drug Interactions
Metabolism/Transport Effects None known.
Avoid Concomitant Use
Avoid concomitant use of Meropenem with any of the following: BCG; Probenecid
Increased Effect/Toxicity
The levels/effects of Meropenem may be increased by: Probenecid

Decreased Effect

Meropenem may decrease the levels/effects of: BCG; Divalproex; Typhoid Vaccine; Valproic Acid

Stability Dry powder should be stored at controlled room temperature 20°C to 25°C (68°F to 77°F). Meropenem infusion vials may be reconstituted with SWFI or a compatible diluent (eg, NS). The 500 mg vials should be reconstituted with 10 mL, and 1 g vials with 20 mL. May be further diluted with compatible solutions for infusion. Consult detailed reference/product labeling for compatibility.

Injection reconstitution: Stability in vial when constituted (up to 50 mg/mL) with:

SWFI: Stable for up to 2 hours at controlled room temperature of 15°C to 25°C (59°F to 77°F) or for up to 12 hours under refrigeration.

Sodium chloride: Stable for up to 2 hours at controlled room temperature of 15°C to 25°C (59°F to 77°F) or for up to 18 hours under refrigeration.

Dextrose 5% injection: Stable for 1 hour at controlled room temperature of 15°C to 25°C (59°F to 77°F) or for 8 hours under refrigeration.

Infusion admixture (1-20 mg/mL): Solution stability when diluted in NS is 4 hours at controlled room temperature of 15°C to 25°C (59°F to 77°F) or 24 hours under refrigeration. Stability in D_5W is 1 hour at controlled room temperature of 15°C to 25°C (59°F to 77°F) or 4 hours under refrigeration. For other diluents, see prescribing information.

Mechanism of Action Inhibits bacterial cell wall synthesis by binding to several of the penicillin-binding proteins, which in turn inhibit the final transpeptidation step of peptidoglycan synthesis in bacterial cell walls, thus inhibiting cell wall biosynthesis; bacteria eventually lyse due to ongoing activity of cell wall autolytic enzymes (autolysins and murein hydrolases) while cell wall assembly is arrested

Pharmacodynamics/Kinetics

Distribution: V_d: Adults: 15-20 L; penetrates well into most body fluids and tissues; CSF concentrations approximate those of the plasma

Protein binding: ~2%

Metabolism: Hepatic; metabolized to open beta-lactam form (inactive)

Half-life elimination:

Normal renal function: 1-1.5 hours

Cl_{cr} 30-80 mL/minute: 1.9-3.3 hours

Cl_{cr} 2-30 mL/minute: 3.82-5.7 hours

Time to peak, tissue: 1 hour following infusion

Excretion: Urine (~70% as unchanged drug)

Dosage

Geriatric & Adult

Usual dosage range: I.V.: 1.5-6 g/day divided every 8 hours

Extended infusion method (unlabeled dosing): I.V.: 0.5-2 g over 3 hours every 8 hours (Crandon, 2011; Dandekar, 2003). **Note:** Dosing used at some centers and is based on pharmacokinetic/pharmacodynamic modeling and not clinical efficacy data.

Indication-specific dosing:

***Burkholderia pseudomallei* (melioidosis) (unlabeled use), *Pseudomonas*:** I.V.: 1 g every 8 hours

Cholangitis, intra-abdominal infections, complicated: I.V.: 1 g every 8 hours. **Note:** 2010 IDSA guidelines recommend treatment duration of 4-7 days (provided source controlled). Not recommended for mild-to-moderate, community-acquired intra-abdominal infections due to risk of toxicity and the development of resistant organisms (Solomkin, 2010).

Febrile neutropenia, otitis externa, pneumonia (unlabeled uses): I.V.: 1 g every 8 hours

Gynecologic and pelvic inflammatory disease: *Canadian labeling (not in U.S. labeling):* I.V.: 500 mg every 8 hours

Liver abscess (unlabeled use): I.V.: 1 g every 8 hours for 2-3 weeks, then oral therapy for duration of 4-6 weeks

Meningitis: *Canadian labeling (not in U.S. labeling):* I.V.: 2 g every 8 hours

Mild-to-moderate infection, other severe infections (unlabeled use): I.V.: 1.5-3 g/day divided every 8 hours

Pneumonia (community-acquired): *Canadian labeling (not in U.S. labeling):* I.V.: 500 mg every 8 hours

Pneumonia (nosocomial): *Canadian labeling (not in U.S. labeling):* I.V.: 1 g every 8 hours

Septicemia: *Canadian labeling (not in U.S. labeling):* I.V.: 1 g every 8 hours

Skin and skin structure infections:

Complicated: I.V.: 500 mg every 8 hours; diabetic foot: 1 g every 8 hours

Uncomplicated: *Canadian labeling (not in U.S. labeling):* I.V.: 500 mg every 8 hours

Urinary tract infections (complicated): *Canadian labeling (not in U.S. labeling):* I.V.: 500 mg every 8 hours. **Note:** Up to 1 g every 8 hours may be administered (Pallett, 2010).

Renal Impairment

Adults:

Cl$_{cr}$ 26-50 mL/minute: Administer recommended dose based on indication every 12 hours

Cl$_{cr}$ 10-25 mL/minute: Administer one-half recommended dose based on indication every 12 hours

Cl$_{cr}$ <10 mL/minute: Administer one-half recommended dose based on indication every 24 hours

Alternative dosing recommendations: (unlabeled dosing; Aronoff, 2007):

GFR 10-50 mL/minute: Administer recommended dose (based on indication) every 12 hours

GFR <10 mL/minute: Administer recommended dose (based on indication) every 24 hours

Intermittent hemodialysis (IHD) (administer after hemodialysis on dialysis days): Meropenem and its metabolite are readily dialyzable: 500 mg every 24 hours. **Note:** Dosing dependent on the assumption of 3 times/week, complete IHD sessions.

Peritoneal dialysis (unlabeled dosing): Administer recommended dose (based on indication) every 24 hours (Aronoff, 2007).

Continuous renal replacement therapy (CRRT) (Heintz, 2009; Trotman, 2005): Drug clearance is highly dependent on the method of renal replacement, filter type, and flow rate. Appropriate dosing requires close monitoring of pharmacologic response, signs of adverse reactions due to drug accumulation, as well as drug concentrations in relation to target trough (if appropriate). The following are general recommendations only (based on dialysate flow/ultrafiltration rates of 1-2 L/hour and minimal residual renal function) and should not supersede clinical judgment:

CVVH: Loading dose of 1 g followed by either 0.5 g every 8 hours **or** 1 g every 12 hours

CVVHD/CVVHDF: Loading dose of 1 g followed by either 0.5 g every 6-8 hours **or** 1 g every 8-12 hours

Note: Consider giving patients receiving CVVHDF dosages of 750 mg every 8 hours **or** 1500 mg every 12 hours (Heintz, 2009). Substantial variability exists in various published recommendations, ranging from 1-3 g/day in 2-3 divided doses. One gram every 12 hours achieves a target trough of ~4 mg/L.

Administration Administer I.V. infusion over 15-30 minutes; I.V. bolus injection (5-20 mL) over 3-5 minutes

Extended infusion administration (unlabeled dosing): Administer over 3 hours (Crandon 2011; Dandekar, 2003). **Note:** Must consider meropenem's limited room temperature stability if using extended infusions

Monitoring Parameters Perform culture and sensitivity testing prior to initiating therapy. Monitor for signs of anaphylaxis during first dose. During prolonged therapy, monitor renal function, liver function, CBC.

Test Interactions Positive Coombs' [direct]

Special Geriatric Considerations Adjust dose based on renal function.

Dosage Forms Excipient information presented when available (limited, particularly for generics); consult specific product labeling.

Injection, powder for reconstitution: 500 mg, 1 g

Merrem® I.V.: 500 mg [contains sodium 45.1 mg as sodium carbonate (1.96 mEq)]

Merrem® I.V.: 1 g [contains sodium 90.2 mg as sodium carbonate (3.92 mEq)]

◆ **Merrem® I.V.** *see* Meropenem *on page 1215*

Mesalamine (me SAL a meen)

Medication Safety Issues

Sound-alike/look-alike issues:

Mesalamine may be confused with mecamylamine, megestrol, memantine, metaxalone, methenamine

Apriso™ may be confused with Apri®

Asacol® may be confused with Ansaid®, Os-Cal®, Visicol®

Lialda® may be confused with Aldara®

Pentasa® may be confused with Pancrease®, Pangestyme®

Brand Names: U.S. Apriso™; Asacol®; Asacol® HD; Canasa®; Lialda®; Pentasa®; Rowasa®; sfRowasa™

Brand Names: Canada 5-ASA; Asacol®; Asacol® 800; Mesasal®; Mezavant®; Novo-5 ASA; Novo-5 ASA-ECT; Pentasa®; Salofalk®; Salofalk® 5-ASA

Index Terms 5-Aminosalicylic Acid; 5-ASA; Fisalamine; Mesalazine

Generic Availability (U.S.) Yes: Rectal suspension

Pharmacologic Category 5-Aminosalicylic Acid Derivative

Use

Oral:

Asacol®, Lialda®, Mezavant®, Pentasa®: Treatment and maintenance of remission of mildly- to moderately-active ulcerative colitis

Apriso™: Maintenance of remission of ulcerative colitis

Asacol® HD: Treatment of moderately-active ulcerative colitis

Rectal: Treatment of active mild-to-moderate distal ulcerative colitis, proctosigmoiditis, or proctitis

Contraindications Hypersensitivity to mesalamine, aminosalicylates, salicylates, or any component of the formulation

Canadian labeling (Mezavant®): Additional contraindications: Severe renal impairment (GFR <30 mL/minute/1.73m²); severe hepatic impairment

Warnings/Precautions May cause an acute intolerance syndrome (cramping, acute abdominal pain, bloody diarrhea; sometimes fever, headache, rash); discontinue if this occurs. Use caution in patients with active peptic ulcers. Patients with pyloric stenosis may have prolonged gastric retention of tablets, delaying the release of mesalamine in the colon. Pericarditis or myocarditis should be considered in patients with chest pain; use with caution in patients predisposed to these conditions. Pancreatitis should be considered in patients with new abdominal discomfort. Symptomatic worsening of colitis/IBD may occur following initiation of therapy. Oligospermia (rare, reversible) has been reported in males. Use caution in patients with sulfasalazine hypersensitivity. Use caution in patients with impaired hepatic function; hepatic failure has been reported. Renal impairment (including minimal change nephropathy and acute/chronic interstitial nephritis) and rarely failure have been reported; use caution in patients with renal impairment. Use of Mezavant® contraindicated in severe renal and/or hepatic impairment. Use caution with other medications converted to mesalamine. Postmarketing reports suggest an increased incidence of blood dyscrasias in patients >65 years of age. In addition, elderly may have difficulty administering and retaining rectal suppositories or may have decreased renal function; use with caution and monitor.

Apriso™ contains phenylalanine. The Asacol® HD 800 mg tablet has not been shown to be bioequivalent to 2 Asacol® 400 mg tablets. Canasa® suppositories contain saturated vegetable fatty acid esters (contraindicated in patients with allergy to these components). Rowasa® enema contains potassium metabisulfite; may cause severe hypersensitivity reactions (ie, anaphylaxis) in patients with sulfite allergies.

Adverse Reactions (Reflective of adult population; not specific for elderly) Adverse effects vary depending upon dosage form. Incidence usually on lower end with enema and suppository dosage forms.

>10%:

Central nervous system: Headache (2% to 35%), pain (≤14%)

Gastrointestinal: Abdominal pain (1% to 18%), eructation (16%), nausea (3% to 13%)

Respiratory: Pharyngitis (11%)

1% to 10%:

Cardiovascular: Chest pain (3%), peripheral edema (3%), vasodilation (≥2%)

Central nervous system: Dizziness (2% to 8%), fever (1% to 6%), chills (3%), malaise (2% to 3%), fatigue (<3%), vertigo (<3%), anxiety (≥2%), migraine (≥2%), nervousness (≥2%), insomnia (2%)

Dermatologic: Rash (1% to 6%), pruritus (1% to 3%), alopecia (<3%), acne (1% to 2%)

Endocrine & metabolic: Triglyceride increased (<3%)

Gastrointestinal: Diarrhea (2% to 8%), dyspepsia (1% to 6%), flatulence (1% to 6%), constipation (5%), vomiting (1% to 5%), colitis exacerbation (1% to 3%), rectal bleeding (<3%), abdominal distention (≥2%), gastroenteritis (≥2%), gastrointestinal bleeding (≥2%), stool abnormalities (≥2%), tenesmus (≥2%), rectal pain (1% to 2%), hemorrhoids (1%)

Genitourinary: Polyuria (≥2%)

Hematologic: Hematocrit/hemoglobin decreased (<3%)

Hepatic: Cholestatic hepatitis (<3%), transaminases increased (<3%), ALT increased (1%)

Local: Pain on insertion of enema tip (1%)

Neuromuscular & skeletal: Back pain (1% to 7%), arthralgia (≤5%), hypertonia (5%), myalgia (3%), paresthesia (≥2%), weakness (≥2%), arthritis (2%), leg/joint pain (2%)

Ocular: Vision abnormalities (≥2%), conjunctivitis (2%)

Otic: Tinnitus (<3%), ear pain (≥2%)

Renal: Creatinine clearance decreased (<3%), hematuria (<3%)

Respiratory: Nasopharyngitis (1% to 4%), dyspnea (<3%), bronchitis (≥2%), sinusitis (≥2%), cough (≤2%)

Miscellaneous: Flu-like syndrome (1% to 5%), infection (≥2%), diaphoresis (3%), intolerance syndrome (3%)

Drug Interactions

Metabolism/Transport Effects None known.

Avoid Concomitant Use There are no known interactions where it is recommended to avoid concomitant use.

Increased Effect/Toxicity

Mesalamine may increase the levels/effects of: Heparin; Heparin (Low Molecular Weight); Thiopurine Analogs; Varicella Virus-Containing Vaccines

Decreased Effect

Mesalamine may decrease the levels/effects of: Cardiac Glycosides

The levels/effects of Mesalamine may be decreased by: Antacids; H2-Antagonists; Proton Pump Inhibitors

Stability

Capsule:

Apriso™: Store at controlled room temperature of 20°C to 25°C (68°F to 77°F)

Pentasa®: Store at controlled room temperature of 15°C to 30°C (59°F to 86°F). Protect from light.

Enema: Store at controlled room temperature. Use promptly once foil wrap is removed. Contents may darken with time (do not use if dark brown).

Suppository: Store below 25°C (below 77°F). May store under refrigeration; do not freeze. Protect from direct heat, light, and humidity.

Tablet: Store at controlled room temperature:

Asacol®, Asacol® HD: 20°C to 25°C (68°F to 77°F)

Lialda®: 15°C to 30°C (59°F to 86°F)

Mezavant®: 15°C to 25°C (59°F to 77°F)

Mechanism of Action Mesalamine (5-aminosalicylic acid) is the active component of sulfasalazine; the specific mechanism of action of mesalamine is unknown; however, it is thought that it modulates local chemical mediators of the inflammatory response, especially leukotrienes, and is also postulated to be a free radical scavenger or an inhibitor of tumor necrosis factor (TNF); action appears topical rather than systemic

Pharmacodynamics/Kinetics

Absorption: Rectal: Variable and dependent upon retention time, underlying GI disease, and colonic pH; Oral: Tablet: ~20% to 28%, Capsule: ~20% to 40%

Distribution: ~18 L

Protein binding: Mesalamine (5-ASA): ~43%; N-acetyl-5-ASA: ~78%

Metabolism: Hepatic and via GI tract to N-acetyl-5-aminosalicylic acid

Half-life elimination: 5-ASA: 0.5-10 hours; N-acetyl-5-ASA: 2-15 hours

Time to peak, serum:

Capsule: Apriso™: ~4 hours; Pentasa®: 3 hours

Rectal: 4-7 hours

Tablet: Asacol®: 4-12 hours; Asacol® HD: 10-16 hours; Lialda®: 9-12 hours; Mezavant®: 8 hours

Excretion: Urine (primarily as metabolites, <8% as unchanged drug); feces (<2%)

Dosage

Geriatric & Adult

Treatment of ulcerative colitis: Oral: Usual course of therapy is 3-8 weeks:

Capsule (Pentasa®): 1 g 4 times/day; **Note:** Apriso™ capsules are approved for maintenance of remission only.

Tablet: Initial:

Asacol®: 800 mg 3 times/day for 6 weeks

Asacol® HD: 1.6 g 3 times/day for 6 weeks

Lialda®, Mezavant®: 2.4-4.8 g once daily for up to 8 weeks

Maintenance of remission of ulcerative colitis: Oral:

Capsule:

Apriso™: 1.5 g once daily in the morning

Pentasa®: 1 g 4 times/day

Tablet:

Asacol®: 1.6 g/day in divided doses

Lialda®, Mezavant®: 2.4 g once daily

Note: Asacol® HD is approved for treatment only.

Active mild-to-moderate distal ulcerative colitis, proctosigmoiditis, or proctitis: Retention enema: 60 mL (4 g) at bedtime, retained overnight, approximately 8 hours

Active ulcerative proctitis: Rectal suppository (Canasa®): Insert one 1000 mg suppository in rectum daily at bedtime; retained for at least 1-3 hours to achieve maximum benefit

Note: Duration of rectal therapy is 3-6 weeks; some patients may require rectal and oral therapy concurrently.

Renal Impairment No dosage adjustment provided in manufacturer's labeling.
Hepatic Impairment No dosage adjustment provided in manufacturer's labeling.
Administration Oral: Swallow capsules or tablets whole, do not break, chew, or crush.

Capsules:

Apriso™: Administer with or without food; do not administer with antacids. The capsule should be swallowed whole per the manufacturer's labeling; however, opening the capsule and placing the contents (delayed release granules) on food with a pH <6 is not expected to affect the release of mesalamine once ingested (data on file, Salix Pharmaceuticals Medical Information). There is no safety/efficacy information regarding this practice. The contents of the capsules should not be chewed or crushed.

Pentasa®: Administer with or without food. Although the manufacturer recommends swallowing the capsule whole, if a patient is unable to swallow the capsule, some clinicians support opening the capsules and placing the contents (controlled-release beads) on yogurt or peanut butter (Crohn's & Colitis Foundation of America). There are currently no published data evaluating the safety/efficacy of this practice. The contents of the capsules should not be chewed or crushed.

Tablets:

Asacol®: Do not break outer coating.

Asacol® HD: Do not break outer coating; administer with or without food.

Lialda®: Do not break outer coating; should be administered once daily with a meal

Mezavant®: Do not break outer coating; should be administered once daily with a meal

Rectal enema: Shake bottle well. Retain enemas for 8 hours or as long as practical.

Suppository: Remove foil wrapper; avoid excessive handling. Should be retained for at least 1-3 hours to achieve maximum benefit.

Monitoring Parameters Renal function (prior to and periodically during therapy); CBC (particularly in elderly patients)

Special Geriatric Considerations Use with caution. Elderly may have difficulty administering and retaining rectal suppositories. Given renal function decline with aging, monitor serum creatinine often during therapy.

Dosage Forms Excipient information presented when available (limited, particularly for generics); consult specific product labeling.

Capsule, controlled release, oral:

Pentasa®: 250 mg, 500 mg

Capsule, delayed and extended release, oral:

Apriso™: 0.375 g [contains phenylalanine 0.56 mg/capsule]

Suppository, rectal:

Canasa®: 1000 mg (30s, 42s) [contains saturated vegetable fatty esters]

Suspension, rectal: 4 g/60 mL (7s, 28s)

Rowasa®: 4 g/60 mL (7s) [contains potassium metabisulfite, sodium benzoate; packaged with wipes]

Rowasa®: 4 g/60 mL (28s) [contains potassium metabisulfite, sodium benzoate; packaged with wipes]

sfRowasa™: 4 g/60 mL (7s, 28s) [contains sodium benzoate]

Tablet, delayed release, enteric coated, oral:

Asacol®: 400 mg

Asacol® HD: 800 mg

Lialda®: 1.2 g

Dosage Forms: Canada Excipient information presented when available (limited, particularly for generics); consult specific product labeling.

Tablet, delayed and extended release:

Mezavant®: 1.2 g

- ◆ **Mesalazine** see Mesalamine on page 1217
- ◆ **Mestinon®** see Pyridostigmine on page 1638
- ◆ **Mestinon® Timespan®** see Pyridostigmine on page 1638
- ◆ **Metadate CD®** see Methylphenidate on page 1247
- ◆ **Metadate® ER** see Methylphenidate on page 1247
- ◆ **Metaglip™** see Glipizide and Metformin on page 882
- ◆ **Metamucil® [OTC]** see Psyllium on page 1635
- ◆ **Metamucil® Plus Calcium [OTC]** see Psyllium on page 1635
- ◆ **Metamucil® Smooth Texture [OTC]** see Psyllium on page 1635

Metaproterenol (met a proe TER e nol)

Medication Safety Issues

Sound-alike/look-alike issues:

Metaproterenol may be confused with metipranolol, metoprolol

Alupent may be confused with Atrovent®

Brand Names: Canada Apo-Orciprenaline®; ratio-Orciprenaline®; Tanta-Orciprenaline®

Index Terms Alupent; Metaproterenol Sulfate; Orciprenaline Sulfate

Generic Availability (U.S.) Yes

Pharmacologic Category Beta$_2$ Agonist

Use Bronchodilator in reversible airway obstruction due to asthma or COPD

Contraindications Hypersensitivity to metaproterenol or any component of the formulation; pre-existing cardiac arrhythmias associated with tachycardia

Warnings/Precautions Use beta$_2$-agonists with caution in patients with cardiovascular disease (arrhythmia or hypertension or HF), convulsive disorders, diabetes, glaucoma, hyperthyroidism, or hypokalemia. Beta-agonists may cause elevation in blood pressure, heart rate, and result in CNS stimulation/excitation. Beta$_2$-agonists may increase risk of arrhythmia, increase serum glucose, or decrease serum potassium. Immediate hypersensitivity reactions (urticaria, angioedema, rash, bronchospasm) have been reported.

Asthma: Appropriate use: Metaproterenol (a less selective beta$_2$-agonist) is not recommended in the management of asthma due to potential for excessive cardiac stimulation. Oral systemic agents (eg, tablets, syrup) should be avoided due to increased risk of adverse effects (eg, excessive cardiac stimulation).

Chronic obstructive lung disease (COPD): Appropriate use: Inhaled bronchodilators are preferred therapy for COPD exacerbations; oral systemic agents (eg, tablets, syrup) should be avoided due to increased risk of adverse effects (eg, excessive cardiac stimulation).

Adverse Reactions (Reflective of adult population; not specific for elderly)
>10%:
  Cardiovascular: Tachycardia (6% to 17%)
  Central nervous system: Nervousness (5% to 20%), headache (1% to 7%)
  Neuromuscular & skeletal: Tremor (2% to 17%)
1% to 10%:
  Cardiovascular: Palpitation (4%)
  Central nervous system: Dizziness (2%), insomnia (2%), fatigue (1%)
  Gastrointestinal: Nausea (1% to 4%), diarrhea (1%)
  Respiratory: Asthma exacerbation (2%)

Drug Interactions
  Metabolism/Transport Effects None known.
  Avoid Concomitant Use
    Avoid concomitant use of Metaproterenol with any of the following: Beta-Blockers (Non-selective); Iobenguane I 123
  Increased Effect/Toxicity
    Metaproterenol may increase the levels/effects of: Loop Diuretics; Sympathomimetics; Thiazide Diuretics

    The levels/effects of Metaproterenol may be increased by: AtoMOXetine; Cannabinoids; MAO Inhibitors; Tricyclic Antidepressants
  Decreased Effect
    Metaproterenol may decrease the levels/effects of: Iobenguane I 123

    The levels/effects of Metaproterenol may be decreased by: Alpha-/Beta-Blockers; Beta-Blockers (Beta1 Selective); Beta-Blockers (Nonselective); Betahistine

Stability Store at room temperature; protect from light. Protect tablets from moisture.

Mechanism of Action Stimulates beta$_2$-receptors which increases the conversion of adenosine triphosphate (ATP) to 3'-5'-cyclic adenosine monophosphate (cAMP), resulting in bronchial smooth muscle relaxation

Pharmacodynamics/Kinetics
  Onset of action: Bronchodilation: Oral: ~30 minutes
  Peak effect: Oral: ~1 hour
  Duration: ~2-6 hours

Dosage
  Geriatric & Adult Bronchoconstriction: Oral: 20 mg 3-4 times/day

Administration Administer orally without regards to food. May administer with food if GI upset occurs.

Monitoring Parameters Lung sounds, heart rate, and blood pressure; FEV$_1$, peak flow, and/or other pulmonary function tests; CNS stimulation; serum glucose, serum potassium (in selected patients)

Pharmacotherapy Pearls Use with caution perioperatively due to beta$_1$ effect of agent. Hypertension and tachycardia are increased with exogenous sympathomimetics.

Special Geriatric Considerations Oral systemic beta-agonists should be avoided due to the increased incidence of adverse effects compared to inhaled agents.

◀ **Dosage Forms** Excipient information presented when available (limited, particularly for generics); consult specific product labeling.
Syrup, oral, as sulfate: 10 mg/5 mL (473 mL)
Tablet, oral, as sulfate: 10 mg, 20 mg

♦ **Metaproterenol Sulfate** see Metaproterenol on page 1220

MetFORMIN (met FOR min)

Related Information
Diabetes Mellitus Management, Adults on page 2193
Medication Safety Issues
Sound-alike/look-alike issues:
MetFORMIN may be confused with metroNIDAZOLE
Glucophage® may be confused with Glucotrol®, Glutofac®
High alert medication:
The Institute for Safe Medication Practices (ISMP) includes this medication among its list of drug classes which have a heightened risk of causing significant patient harm when used in error.
International issues:
Dianben [Spain] may be confused with Diovan brand name for valsartan [U.S., Canada, and multiple international markets]
Brand Names: U.S. Fortamet®; Glucophage®; Glucophage® XR; Glumetza®; Riomet®
Brand Names: Canada Apo-Metformin®; Ava-Metformin; CO Metformin; Dom-Metformin; Glucophage®; Glumetza®; Glycon; JAMP-Metformin; JAMP-Metformin Blackberry; Med-Metformin; Mylan-Metformin; Novo-Metformin; Nu-Metformin; PHL-Metformin; PMS-Metformin; PRO-Metformin; Q-Metformin; RAN™-Metformin; ratio-Metformin; Riva-Metformin; Sandoz-Metformin FC
Index Terms Metformin Hydrochloride
Generic Availability (U.S.) Yes: Excludes solution
Pharmacologic Category Antidiabetic Agent, Biguanide
Use Management of type 2 diabetes mellitus (noninsulin dependent, NIDDM) when hyperglycemia cannot be managed with diet and exercise alone.
Unlabeled Use Prevention of type 2 diabetes mellitus
Contraindications Hypersensitivity to metformin or any component of the formulation; renal disease or renal dysfunction (serum creatinine ≥1.5 mg/dL in males or ≥1.4 mg/dL in females) or abnormal creatinine clearance from any cause, including shock, acute myocardial infarction, or septicemia; acute or chronic metabolic acidosis with or without coma (including diabetic ketoacidosis).

Note: Temporarily discontinue in patients undergoing radiologic studies in which intravascular iodinated contrast media are utilized.

Warnings/Precautions [U.S. Boxed Warning]: Lactic acidosis is a rare, but potentially severe consequence of therapy with metformin. Lactic acidosis should be suspected in any patient with diabetes receiving metformin with evidence of acidosis but without evidence of ketoacidosis. Discontinue metformin in clinical situations predisposing to hypoxemia, including conditions such as cardiovascular collapse, respiratory failure, acute myocardial infarction, acute congestive heart failure, and septicemia. Use caution in patients with congestive heart failure requiring pharmacologic management, particularly in patients with unstable or acute CHF; risk of lactic acidosis may be increased secondary to hypoperfusion.

Metformin is substantially excreted by the kidney. The risk of accumulation and lactic acidosis increases with the degree of impairment of renal function. Patients with renal function below the limit of normal for their age should not receive metformin. In elderly patients, renal function should be monitored regularly; should not be initiated in patients ≥80 years of age unless normal renal function is confirmed. Use of concomitant medications that may affect renal function (ie, affect tubular secretion) may also affect metformin disposition. Metformin should be withheld in patients with dehydration and/or prerenal azotemia. Therapy should be suspended for any surgical procedures (resume only after normal oral intake resumed and normal renal function is verified). Therapy should be temporarily discontinued prior to or at the time of intravascular administration of iodinated contrast media (potential for acute alteration in renal function). Metformin should be withheld for 48 hours after the radiologic study and restarted only after renal function has been confirmed as normal. It may be necessary to discontinue metformin and administer insulin if the patient is exposed to stress (fever, trauma, infection, surgery).

Avoid use in patients with impaired liver function. Patient must be instructed to avoid excessive acute or chronic ethanol use; ethanol may potentiate metformin's effect on lactate metabolism. Administration of oral antidiabetic drugs has been reported to be associated with increased cardiovascular mortality; metformin does not appear to share this risk. Insoluble tablet shell of Glumetza® 1000 mg extended release tablet may remain intact and be visible in the stool. Other extended released tablets (Fortamet®, Glucophage® XR, Glumetza® 500 mg) may appear in the stool as a soft mass resembling the tablet.

Adverse Reactions (Reflective of adult population; not specific for elderly)
>10%:
  Gastrointestinal: Diarrhea (IR tablet: 12% to 53%; ER tablet: 10% to 17%), nausea/vomiting (IR tablet: 7% to 26%; ER tablet: 7% to 9%), flatulence (12%)
  Neuromuscular & skeletal: Weakness (9%)
1% to 10%:
  Cardiovascular: Chest discomfort, flushing, palpitation
  Central nervous system: Headache (6%), chills, dizziness, lightheadedness
  Dermatologic: Rash
  Endocrine & metabolic: Hypoglycemia
  Gastrointestinal: Indigestion (7%), abdominal discomfort (6%), abdominal distention, abnormal stools, constipation, dyspepsia/ heartburn, taste disorder
  Neuromuscular & skeletal: Myalgia
  Respiratory: Dyspnea, upper respiratory tract infection
  Miscellaneous: Decreased vitamin B_{12} levels (7%), increased diaphoresis, flu-like syndrome, nail disorder

Drug Interactions
  Metabolism/Transport Effects None known.
  Avoid Concomitant Use There are no known interactions where it is recommended to avoid concomitant use.
  Increased Effect/Toxicity
    MetFORMIN may increase the levels/effects of: Dalfampridine; Dofetilide

    The levels/effects of MetFORMIN may be increased by: Carbonic Anhydrase Inhibitors; Cephalexin; Cimetidine; Dalfampridine; Glycopyrrolate; Iodinated Contrast Agents; LamoTRIgine; Pegvisomant
  Decreased Effect
    MetFORMIN may decrease the levels/effects of: Trospium

    The levels/effects of MetFORMIN may be decreased by: Corticosteroids (Orally Inhaled); Corticosteroids (Systemic); Luteinizing Hormone-Releasing Hormone Analogs; Somatropin; Thiazide Diuretics

Ethanol/Nutrition/Herb Interactions
  Ethanol: Avoid or limit ethanol (incidence of lactic acidosis may be increased; may cause hypoglycemia).
  Food: Food decreases the extent and slightly delays the absorption. May decrease absorption of vitamin B_{12} and/or folic acid.
  Herb/Nutraceutical: Caution with chromium, garlic, gymnema (may cause hypoglycemia).

Stability
  Oral solution: Store at 15°C to 30°C (59°F to 86°F).
  Tablets: Store at 20°C to 25°C (68°F to 77°F); excursion permitted to 15°C to 30°C (59°F to 86°F). Protect from light and moisture.

Mechanism of Action Decreases hepatic glucose production, decreasing intestinal absorption of glucose and improves insulin sensitivity (increases peripheral glucose uptake and utilization)

Pharmacodynamics/Kinetics
  Onset of action: Within days; maximum effects up to 2 weeks
  Distribution: V_d: 654 ± 358 L; partitions into erythrocytes
  Protein binding: Negligible
  Metabolism: Not metabolized by the liver
  Bioavailability: Absolute: Fasting: 50% to 60%
  Half-life elimination: Plasma: 4-9 hours
  Time to peak, serum: Immediate release: 2-3 hours; Extended release: 7 hours (range: 4-8 hours)
  Excretion: Urine (90% as unchanged drug; active secretion)

Dosage
  Geriatric The initial and maintenance dosing should be conservative, due to the potential for decreased renal function. Generally, elderly patients should **not** be titrated to the maximum dose of metformin. Do not use in patients ≥80 years of age unless normal renal function has been established.

◄ **Adult**

Management of type 2 diabetes mellitus: Oral: **Note:** Allow 1-2 weeks between dose titrations: Generally, clinically significant responses are not seen at doses <1500 mg daily; however, a lower recommended starting dose and gradual increased dosage is recommended to minimize gastrointestinal symptoms.

Immediate release tablet or solution: Adults ≥17 years: Initial: 500 mg twice daily **or** 850 mg once daily; titrate in increments of 500 mg weekly or 850 mg every other week; may also titrate from 500 mg twice a day to 850 mg twice a day after 2 weeks

Doses of up to 2000 mg/day may be given twice daily. If a dose >2000 mg/day is required, it may be better tolerated in three divided doses. Maximum recommended dose: 2550 mg/day.

Extended release tablet: **Note:** If glycemic control is not achieved at maximum dose, may divide dose and administer twice daily.

Fortamet®: Initial: 500-1000 mg once daily;dosage may be increased by 500 mg weekly; maximum dose: 2500 mg once daily

Glucophage® XR: Initial: 500 mg once daily; dosage may be increased by 500 mg weekly; maximum dose: 2000 mg once daily

Glumetza®: Initial: 1000 mg once daily; dosage may be increased by 500 mg weekly; maximum dose: 2000 mg once daily

Transfer from other antidiabetic agents: No transition period is generally necessary except when transferring from chlorpropamide. When transferring from chlorpropamide, care should be exercised during the first 2 weeks because of the prolonged retention of chlorpropamide in the body, leading to overlapping drug effects and possible hypoglycemia.

Concomitant metformin and oral sulfonylurea therapy: If patients have not responded to 4 weeks of the maximum dose of metformin monotherapy, consider a gradual addition of an oral sulfonylurea, even if prior primary or secondary failure to a sulfonylurea has occurred. Continue metformin at the maximum dose. If adequate response has not occurred following 3 months of metformin and sulfonylurea combination therapy, consider switching to insulin with or without metformin.

Failed sulfonylurea therapy: Patients with prior failure on glyburide may be treated by gradual addition of metformin. Initiate with glyburide 20 mg and metformin 500 mg daily. Metformin dosage may be increased by 500 mg/day at weekly intervals, up to a maximum metformin dose (dosage of glyburide maintained at 20 mg/day).

Concomitant metformin and insulin therapy: Initial: 500 mg metformin once daily, continue current insulin dose; increase by 500 mg metformin weekly until adequate glycemic control is achieved

Maximum daily dose: Immediate release and solution: 2550 mg metformin; Extended release: 2000-2500 mg (varies by product)

Decrease insulin dose 10% to 25% when FPG <120 mg/dL; monitor and make further adjustments as needed

Type 2 diabetes prevention (unlabeled use): *Immediate release tablet or solution:* Oral: Initial: 850 mg once daily; Target: 850 mg twice daily (Knowler, 2002)

Renal Impairment The plasma and blood half-life of metformin is prolonged and the renal clearance is decreased in proportion to the decrease in creatinine clearance. Per the manufacturer, metformin is contraindicated in the presence of renal dysfunction defined as a serum creatinine ≥1.5 mg/dL in males, or ≥1.4 mg/dL in females and in patients with abnormal clearance. The Canadian labeling recommends that metformin be avoided in patients with Cl_{cr} <60 mL/minute.

Hepatic Impairment Avoid metformin; liver disease is a risk factor for the development of lactic acidosis during metformin therapy.

Administration Administer with a meal (to decrease GI upset).

Extended release: Swallow whole; do not crush, break, or chew. Administer once daily doses with the evening meal. Fortamet® should also be administered with a full glass of water.

Monitoring Parameters Urine for glucose and ketones, fasting blood glucose, and hemoglobin A_{1c}. Initial and periodic monitoring of hematologic parameters (eg, hemoglobin/ hematocrit and red blood cell indices) and renal function should be performed, at least annually. Check vitamin B_{12} and folate if anemia is present.

Reference Range Recommendations for glycemic control in adults with diabetes:

Hb A_{1c}: <7%

Preprandial capillary plasma glucose: 70-130 mg/dL

Peak postprandial capillary blood glucose: <180 mg/dL

Blood pressure: <130/80 mm Hg

Special Geriatric Considerations Limited data suggest that metformin's total body clearance may be decreased and AUC and half-life increased in elderly patients; presumably due to decreased renal clearance. Metformin has been well tolerated by the elderly but lower doses and frequent monitoring are recommended. In one study of elderly subjects, its effects could not be distinguished from tolbutamide, except for weight loss. The initial and maintenance dosing should be conservative, due to the potential for decreased renal function. Generally, elderly patients should not be titrated to the maximum dose of metformin. Do not use in patients ≥80 years of age unless normal renal function has been established. Intensive glucose control (Hb A_{1c} <6.5%) has been linked to increased all-cause and cardiovascular mortality, hypoglycemia requiring assistance, and weight gain in adult type 2 diabetes. How "tightly" to control a geriatric patient's blood glucose needs to be individualized. Such a decision should be based on several factors, including the patient's functional and cognitive status, how well he/she recognizes hypoglycemic or hyperglycemic symptoms, and how to respond to them and other disease states. An Hb A_{1c} <7.5% is an acceptable endpoint for a healthy older adult, while <8% is acceptable for frail elderly patients, those with a duration of illness >10 years, or those with comorbid conditions and requiring combination diabetes medications. For elderly patients with diabetes who are relatively healthy, attaining target goals for aspirin use, blood pressure, lipids, smoking cessation, and diet and exercise may be more important than normalized glycemic control.

Dosage Forms Excipient information presented when available (limited, particularly for generics); consult specific product labeling.

Solution, oral, as hydrochloride:
Riomet®: 100 mg/mL (118 mL, 473 mL) [dye free, ethanol free, sugar free; contains saccharin; cherry flavor]

Tablet, oral, as hydrochloride: 500 mg, 850 mg, 1000 mg
Glucophage®: 500 mg, 850 mg
Glucophage®: 1000 mg [scored]

Tablet, extended release, oral, as hydrochloride: 500 mg, 750 mg, 1000 mg
Fortamet®: 500 mg, 1000 mg
Glucophage® XR: 500 mg, 750 mg
Glumetza®: 500 mg, 1000 mg

◆ **Metformin and Glipizide** see Glipizide and Metformin on page 882
◆ **Metformin and Glyburide** see Glyburide and Metformin on page 890
◆ **Metformin and Linagliptin** see Linagliptin and Metformin on page 1132
◆ **Metformin and Repaglinide** see Repaglinide and Metformin on page 1687
◆ **Metformin and Rosiglitazone** see Rosiglitazone and Metformin on page 1732
◆ **Metformin and Saxagliptin** see Saxagliptin and Metformin on page 1755
◆ **Metformin and Sitagliptin** see Sitagliptin and Metformin on page 1783
◆ **Metformin Hydrochloride** see MetFORMIN on page 1222
◆ **Metformin Hydrochloride and Linagliptin** see Linagliptin and Metformin on page 1132
◆ **Metformin Hydrochloride and Pioglitazone Hydrochloride** see Pioglitazone and Metformin on page 1545
◆ **Metformin Hydrochloride and Rosiglitazone Maleate** see Rosiglitazone and Metformin on page 1732
◆ **Metformin Hydrochloride and Saxagliptin** see Saxagliptin and Metformin on page 1755

Methadone (METH a done)

Related Information
Opioid Analgesics on page 2122
Patient Information for Disposal of Unused Medications on page 2244

Medication Safety Issues
Sound-alike/look-alike issues:
Methadone may be confused with dexmethylphenidate, Mephyton®, methylphenidate, Metadate CD®, Metadate® ER, morphine
High alert medication:
The Institute for Safe Medication Practices (ISMP) includes this medication among its list of drug classes which have a heightened risk of causing significant patient harm when used in error.

Brand Names: U.S. Dolophine®; Methadone Diskets®; Methadone Intensol™; Methadose®
Brand Names: Canada Metadol-D™; Metadol™
Index Terms Methadone Hydrochloride
Generic Availability (U.S.) Yes
Pharmacologic Category Analgesic, Opioid
Use Management of moderate-to-severe pain; detoxification and maintenance treatment of opioid addiction as part of an FDA-approved program

◄ **Prescribing and Access Restrictions** When used for treatment of opioid addiction: May only be dispensed in accordance to guidelines established by the Substance Abuse and Mental Health Services Administration's (SAMHSA) Center for Substance Abuse Treatment (CSAT). Regulations regarding methadone use may vary by state and/or country. Obtain advice from appropriate regulatory agencies and/or consult with pain management/palliative care specialists.

Note: Regulatory Exceptions to the General Requirement to Provide Opioid Agonist Treatment (per manufacturer's labeling):

1. During inpatient care, when the patient was admitted for any condition other than concurrent opioid addiction, to facilitate the treatment of the primary admitting diagnosis.
2. During an emergency period of no longer than 3 days while definitive care for the addiction is being sought in an appropriately licensed facility.

Medication Guide Available Yes

Contraindications Hypersensitivity to methadone or any component of the formulation; respiratory depression (in the absence of resuscitative equipment or in an unmonitored setting); acute bronchial asthma or hypercarbia; paralytic ileus; concurrent use of selegiline

Warnings/Precautions An opioid-containing analgesic regimen should be tailored to each patient's needs and based upon the type of pain being treated (acute versus chronic), the route of administration, degree of tolerance for opioids (naive versus chronic user), age, weight, and medical condition. The optimal analgesic dose varies widely among patients. Doses should be titrated to pain relief/prevention. Patients maintained on stable doses of methadone may need higher and/or more frequent doses in case of acute pain (eg, postoperative pain, physical trauma). Methadone is ineffective for the relief of anxiety.

[U.S. Boxed Warning]: May prolong the QT_c interval and increase risk for torsade de pointes. Patients should be informed of the potential arrhythmia risk, evaluated for any history of structural heart disease, arrhythmia, syncope, and for existence of potential drug interactions including drugs that possess QT_c interval-prolonging properties, promote hypokalemia, hypomagnesemia, or hypocalcemia, or reduce elimination of methadone (eg, CYP3A4 inhibitors). Obtain baseline ECG for all patients and risk stratify according to QT_c interval (see Monitoring Parameters). Use with caution in patients at risk for QT_c prolongation, with medications known to prolong the QT_c interval, promote electrolyte depletion, or inhibit CYP3A4, or history of conduction abnormalities. QT_c interval prolongation and torsade de pointes may be associated with doses >100 mg/day, but have also been observed with lower doses. May cause severe hypotension; use caution with severe volume depletion or other conditions which may compromise maintenance of normal blood pressure. Use caution with cardiovascular disease or patients predisposed to dysrhythmias.

[U.S. Boxed Warning]: May cause respiratory depression. Use caution in patients with respiratory disease or pre-existing respiratory conditions (eg, severe obesity, asthma, COPD, sleep apnea, CNS depression). Because the respiratory effects last longer than the analgesic effects, slow titration is required. Use extreme caution during treatment initiation, dose titration and conversion from other opioid agonists. Incomplete cross tolerance may occur; patients tolerant to other mu opioid agonists may not be tolerant to methadone. Abrupt cessation may precipitate withdrawal symptoms.

May cause CNS depression, which may impair physical or mental abilities. Patients must be cautioned about performing tasks which require mental alertness (eg, operating machinery or driving). Effects with other sedative drugs or ethanol may be potentiated. Use with caution in patients with depression or suicidal tendencies, or in patients with a history of drug abuse. Tolerance or psychological and physical dependence may occur with prolonged use.

Use with caution in patients with head injury or increased intracranial pressure. May obscure diagnosis or clinical course of patients with acute abdominal conditions. Elderly may be more susceptible to adverse effects (eg, CNS, respiratory, gastrointestinal). Decrease initial dose and use caution in the elderly or debilitated; with hyper/hypothyroidism, morbid obesity, adrenal insufficiency, prostatic hyperplasia, or urethral stricture; or with severe renal or hepatic failure. Use with caution in patients with biliary tract dysfunction; acute pancreatitis may cause constriction of sphincter of Oddi. **[U.S. Boxed Warning]: For oral administration only;** excipients to deter use by injection are contained in tablets.

[U.S. Boxed Warning]: When used for treatment of narcotic addiction: May only be dispensed by opioid treatment programs certified by the Substance Abuse and Mental Health Services Administration (SAMHSA) and certified by the designated state authority. Exceptions include inpatient treatment of other conditions and emergency period (not >3 days) while definitive substance abuse treatment is being sought.

Adverse Reactions (Reflective of adult population; not specific for elderly) Frequency not defined. During prolonged administration, adverse effects may decrease over several weeks; however, constipation and sweating may persist.

Cardiovascular: Arrhythmia, bigeminal rhythms, bradycardia, cardiac arrest, cardiomyopathy, ECG changes, edema, extrasystoles, faintness, flushing, heart failure, hypotension, palpitation, peripheral vasodilation, phlebitis, orthostatic hypotension, QT interval prolonged, shock, syncope, tachycardia, torsade de pointes, T-wave inversion, ventricular fibrillation, ventricular tachycardia,

Central nervous system: Agitation, confusion, disorientation, dizziness, drowsiness, dysphoria, euphoria, hallucination, headache, insomnia, lightheadedness, sedation, seizure

Dermatologic: Hemorrhagic urticaria, pruritus, rash, urticaria

Endocrine & metabolic: Antidiuretic effect, amenorrhea, hypokalemia, hypomagnesemia, libido decreased

Gastrointestinal: Abdominal pain, anorexia, biliary tract spasm, constipation, glossitis, nausea, stomach cramps, vomiting, weight gain, xerostomia

Genitourinary: Impotence, urinary retention or hesitancy

Hematologic: Thrombocytopenia (reversible, reported in patients with chronic hepatitis)

Neuromuscular & skeletal: Weakness

Local: I.M./SubQ injection: Erythema, pain, swelling; I.V. injection: Hemorrhagic urticaria (rare), pruritus, urticaria, rash

Ocular: Miosis, visual disturbances

Respiratory: Pulmonary edema, respiratory depression, respiratory arrest

Miscellaneous: Death, diaphoresis, physical and psychological dependence

Drug Interactions

Metabolism/Transport Effects Substrate of CYP2B6 (major), CYP2C19 (minor), CYP2C9 (minor), CYP2D6 (minor), CYP3A4 (major); **Note:** Assignment of Major/Minor substrate status based on clinically relevant drug interaction potential; **Inhibits** CYP2D6 (moderate), CYP3A4 (weak)

Avoid Concomitant Use

Avoid concomitant use of Methadone with any of the following: Alcohol (Ethyl); Azelastine; Azelastine (Nasal); CNS Depressants; Conivaptan; Highest Risk QTc-Prolonging Agents; Itraconazole; Mifepristone; Mirtazapine; Paraldehyde; Posaconazole

Increased Effect/Toxicity

Methadone may increase the levels/effects of: Alvimopan; ARIPiprazole; Azelastine; Azelastine (Nasal); CYP2D6 Substrates; Desmopressin; Fesoterodine; Highest Risk QTc-Prolonging Agents; Metyrosine; Mirtazapine; Moderate Risk QTc-Prolonging Agents; Nebivolol; Paraldehyde; Selective Serotonin Reuptake Inhibitors; Thiazide Diuretics; Zidovudine; Zolpidem

The levels/effects of Methadone may be increased by: Alcohol (Ethyl); Amphetamines; Antipsychotic Agents (Phenothiazines); Boceprevir; CNS Depressants; Conivaptan; CYP2B6 Inhibitors (Moderate); CYP2B6 Inhibitors (Strong); CYP3A4 Inhibitors (Moderate); CYP3A4 Inhibitors (Strong); Fluconazole; HydrOXYzine; Interferons (Alfa); Itraconazole; Ivacaftor; Ketoconazole; Ketoconazole (Systemic); MAO Inhibitors; Mifepristone; Posaconazole; QTc-Prolonging Agents (Indeterminate Risk and Risk Modifying); Quazepam; Selective Serotonin Reuptake Inhibitors; Succinylcholine; Voriconazole

Decreased Effect

Methadone may decrease the levels/effects of: Codeine; Didanosine; Pegvisomant; TraMADol

The levels/effects of Methadone may be decreased by: Ammonium Chloride; Boceprevir; CarBAMazepine; CYP3A4 Inducers (Strong); Deferasirox; Etravirine; Fosphenytoin; Herbs (CYP3A4 Inducers); Mixed Agonist / Antagonist Opioids; Phenytoin; Protease Inhibitors; Reverse Transcriptase Inhibitors (Non-Nucleoside); Rifamycin Derivatives; Telaprevir; Tocilizumab

Ethanol/Nutrition/Herb Interactions

Ethanol: Ethanol may increase CNS depression. Management: Avoid ethanol.

Food: Grapefruit/grapefruit juice may increase levels of methadone. Management: Avoid concurrent use of grapefruit juice.

Herb/Nutraceutical: St John's wort may decrease methadone levels and increase CNS depression; valerian, kava kava, and gotu kola may increase CNS depression. Management: Avoid St John's wort, valerian, kava kava, and gotu kola.

Stability

Injection: Store at controlled room temperature of 15°C to 30°C (59°F to 86°F). Protect from light.

Oral concentrate, oral solution, tablet: Store at controlled room temperature of 15°C to 30°C (59°F to 86°F).

Mechanism of Action Binds to opiate receptors in the CNS, causing inhibition of ascending pain pathways, altering the perception of and response to pain; produces generalized CNS depression

◀ **Pharmacodynamics/Kinetics**

Onset of action: Oral: Analgesic: 0.5-1 hour; Parenteral: 10-20 minutes

Peak effect: Parenteral: 1-2 hours; Oral: Continuous dosing: 3-5 days

Duration of analgesia: Oral: 4-8 hours, increases to 22-48 hours with repeated doses

Distribution: V_{dss}: 1-8 L/kg

Protein binding: 85% to 90%

Metabolism: Hepatic; N-demethylation primarily via CYP3A4, CYP2B6, and CYP2C19 to inactive metabolites

Bioavailability: Oral: 36% to 100%

Half-life elimination: 8-59 hours; may be prolonged with alkaline pH

Time to peak, plasma: 1-7.5 hours

Excretion: Urine (<10% as unchanged drug); increased with urine pH <6

Dosage

Geriatric Oral, I.M.: 2.5 mg every 8-12 hours; refer to adult dosing.

Adult Regulations regarding methadone use may vary by state and/or country. Obtain advice from appropriate regulatory agencies and/or consult with pain management/palliative care specialists. **Note:** These are guidelines and do not represent the maximum doses that may be required in all patients. Methadone accumulates with repeated doses and dosage may need reduction after 3-5 days to prevent CNS depressant effects. Some patients may benefit from every 8-12 hour dosing interval for chronic pain management. Doses should be titrated to appropriate effects.

Acute pain (moderate-to-severe):

Opioid-naive: *Oral:* Initial: 2.5-10 mg every 8-12 hours; more frequent administration may be required during initiation to maintain adequate analgesia. Dosage interval may range from 4-12 hours, since duration of analgesia is relatively short during the first days of therapy, but increases substantially with continued administration.

Chronic pain (opioid-tolerant): Conversion from oral morphine to oral methadone:

Daily oral morphine dose <100 mg: Estimated daily oral methadone dose: 20% to 30% of total daily morphine dose

Daily oral morphine dose 100-300 mg: Estimated daily oral methadone dose: 10% to 20% of total daily morphine dose

Daily oral morphine dose 300-600 mg: Estimated daily oral methadone dose: 8% to 12% of total daily morphine dose

Daily oral morphine dose 600-1000 mg: Estimated daily oral methadone dose: 5% to 10% of total daily morphine dose.

Daily oral morphine dose >1000 mg: Estimated daily oral methadone dose: <5% of total daily morphine dose.

Note: The total daily methadone dose should then be divided to reflect the intended dosing schedule.

I.V.: Manufacturer's labeling: Initial: 2.5-10 mg every 8-12 hours in opioid-naive patients; titrate slowly to effect; may also be administered by SubQ or I.M. injection

Conversion from oral to parenteral dose: Initial dose: Parenteral:Oral ratio: 1:2 (eg, 5 mg parenteral methadone equals 10 mg oral methadone)

Detoxification: *Oral:*

Initial: A single dose of 20-30 mg is usually sufficient to suppress symptoms. Should not exceed 30 mg; lower doses should be considered in patients with low tolerance at initiation (eg, absence of opioids ≥5 days); an additional 5-10 mg of methadone may be provided if withdrawal symptoms have not been suppressed or if symptoms reappear after 2-4 hours; total daily dose on the first day should not exceed 40 mg, unless the program physician documents in the patient's record that 40 mg did not control opiate abstinence symptoms.

Maintenance: Titrate to a dosage which prevents craving, attenuates euphoric effect of self-administered opiates, and tolerance to sedative effects of methadone. Usual range: 80-120 mg/day (titration should occur cautiously)

Withdrawal: Dose reductions should be <10% of the maintenance dose, every 10-14 days

Detoxification (short-term): *Oral:*

Initial: Titrate to ~40 mg/day in divided doses to achieve stabilization. May continue 40 mg dose for 2-3 days

Maintenance: Titrate to a dosage which prevents/attenuates euphoric effects of self-administered opioids, reduces drug craving, and withdrawal symptoms are prevented for 24 hours.

Withdrawal: Requires individualization. Decrease daily or every other day, keeping withdrawal symptoms tolerable; hospitalized patients may tolerate a 20% reduction/day; ambulatory patients may require a slower reduction

Renal Impairment Cl_{cr} <10 mL/minute: Administer 50% to 75% of normal dose.

Hepatic Impairment Avoid in severe liver disease.

Administration Oral dose for detoxification and maintenance may be administered in fruit juice or water. Dispersible tablet should not be chewed or swallowed; add to liquid and allow to dissolve before administering. May rinse if residual remains.

Monitoring Parameters Obtain baseline ECG (evaluate QT_c interval), within 30 days of initiation, and then annually for all patients receiving methadone. Increase ECG monitoring if patient receiving >100 mg/day or if unexplained syncope or seizure occurs while on methadone (Krantz, 2008).

If before or at anytime during therapy:

QT_c >450-499 msecs: Discuss potential risks and benefits; monitor QT_c more frequently

QT_c ≥500 msecs: Consider discontinuation or reducing methadone dose **or** eliminate factors promoting QT_c prolongation (eg, potassium-wasting drugs) **or** use alternative therapy (eg, buprenorphine)

Pain relief, respiratory and mental status, blood pressure

Reference Range Prevention of opiate withdrawal: Therapeutic: 100-400 ng/mL (SI: 0.32-1.29 micromole/L); Toxic: >2 mcg/mL (SI: >6.46 micromole/L)

Test Interactions Some quinolones may produce a false-positive urine screening result for opiates using commercially-available immunoassay kits. This has been demonstrated most consistently for levofloxacin and ofloxacin, but other quinolones have shown cross-reactivity in certain assay kits. Confirmation of positive opiate screens by more specific methods should be considered.

Special Geriatric Considerations Because of its long half-life and risk of accumulation, methadone is difficult to titrate and is not considered a drug of first choice. It should be prescribed only by physicians who are experienced in using it. Elderly may be particularly susceptible to the CNS depressant and constipating effects of narcotics.

Controlled Substance C-II

Dosage Forms Excipient information presented when available (limited, particularly for generics); consult specific product labeling.

Injection, solution, as hydrochloride: 10 mg/mL (20 mL)

Solution, oral, as hydrochloride: 5 mg/5 mL (500 mL); 10 mg/5 mL (500 mL)

Solution, oral, as hydrochloride [concentrate]: 10 mg/mL (946 mL, 1000 mL, 1000s)

Methadone Intensol™: 10 mg/mL (30 mL) [dye free, sugar free; contains sodium benzoate; unflavored]

Methadose®: 10 mg/mL (1000 mL) [contains propylene glycol; cherry flavor]

Methadose®: 10 mg/mL (1000 mL) [dye free, sugar free; contains sodium benzoate; unflavored]

Tablet, oral, as hydrochloride: 5 mg, 10 mg

Dolophine®: 5 mg, 10 mg [scored]

Tablet, dispersible, oral, as hydrochloride: 40 mg

Methadone Diskets®: 40 mg [scored; orange-pineapple flavor]

Methadose®: 40 mg [scored]

- ◆ **Methadone Diskets®** *see* Methadone *on page 1225*
- ◆ **Methadone Hydrochloride** *see* Methadone *on page 1225*
- ◆ **Methadone Intensol™** *see* Methadone *on page 1225*
- ◆ **Methadose®** *see* Methadone *on page 1225*
- ◆ **Methaminodiazepoxide Hydrochloride** *see* ChlordiazePOXIDE *on page 354*

Methazolamide (meth a ZOE la mide)

Related Information

Glaucoma Drug Therapy *on page 2115*

Medication Safety Issues

Sound-alike/look-alike issues:

Methazolamide may be confused with methenamine, metolazone

Neptazane™ may be confused with Nesacaine®

Brand Names: U.S. Neptazane™

Brand Names: Canada Apo-Methazolamide®

Generic Availability (U.S.) Yes

Pharmacologic Category Carbonic Anhydrase Inhibitor; Diuretic, Carbonic Anhydrase Inhibitor; Ophthalmic Agent, Antiglaucoma

Use Treatment of chronic open-angle or secondary glaucoma; short-term therapy of acute angle-closure glaucoma prior to surgery

Contraindications Marked kidney or liver dysfunction; adrenal gland failure; cirrhosis; hyperchloremic acidosis; hyponatremia; hypokalemia; long-term treatment of angle-closure glaucoma

Warnings/Precautions May impair mental alertness and/or physical coordination. Use with caution in patients with prediabetes or diabetes mellitus; may see a change in glucose control. ▶

Initially, potassium excretion may be increased; periodically monitor serum electrolytes and signs of hypokalemia in at risk patients. Use with caution in patients with respiratory disease such as emphysema or pulmonary obstruction; may precipitate or aggravate respiratory acidosis. Use with caution in patients with hepatic impairment; may precipitate hepatic encephalopathy. Use is contraindicated in patients with marked liver impairment or cirrhosis.

Chemical similarities are present among sulfonamides, sulfonylureas, carbonic anhydrase inhibitors, thiazides, and loop diuretics (except ethacrynic acid). Use in patients with sulfonylurea allergy is not specifically contraindicated in product labeling, however, a risk of cross-reaction exists in patients with allergy to any of these compounds; avoid use when previous reaction has been severe. Discontinue if signs of hypersensitivity are noted. Use with caution in patients taking high dose aspirin concurrently; may lead to severe adverse effects including death, coma, tachypnea, anorexia, and lethargy

Adverse Reactions (Reflective of adult population; not specific for elderly) Frequency not defined.
Central nervous system: Confusion, drowsiness, fatigue, fever, malaise, seizure
Dermatologic: Erythema multiforme, photosensitivity, rash, Stevens-Johnson syndrome, toxic epidermal necrolysis, urticaria
Endocrine & metabolic: Electrolyte imbalance, metabolic acidosis
Gastrointestinal: Appetite decreased, diarrhea, melena, nausea, taste alteration, vomiting
Genitourinary: Crystalluria, glycosuria, hematuria, polyuria, renal calculi
Hematologic: Agranulocytosis, aplastic anemia, bone marrow depression, hemolytic anemia, leukopenia, pancytopenia, thrombocytopenic purpura
Hepatic: Fulminant hepatic necrosis, hepatic insufficiency
Neuromuscular & skeletal: Flaccid paralysis, paresthesia
Ocular: Myopia
Otic: Hearing disturbance, tinnitus
Miscellaneous: Anaphylaxis, hypersensitivity

Drug Interactions
Metabolism/Transport Effects None known.
Avoid Concomitant Use
Avoid concomitant use of Methazolamide with any of the following: Carbonic Anhydrase Inhibitors
Increased Effect/Toxicity
Methazolamide may increase the levels/effects of: Alpha-/Beta-Agonists; Amifostine; Amphetamines; Anticonvulsants (Barbiturate); Anticonvulsants (Hydantoin); Antihypertensives; CarBAMazepine; Carbonic Anhydrase Inhibitors; Flecainide; Hypotensive Agents; Memantine; MetFORMIN; Primidone; QuiNIDine; RiTUXimab; Sodium Phosphates

The levels/effects of Methazolamide may be increased by: Alfuzosin; Diazoxide; Herbs (Hypotensive Properties); MAO Inhibitors; Pentoxifylline; Phosphodiesterase 5 Inhibitors; Prostacyclin Analogues; Salicylates
Decreased Effect
Methazolamide may decrease the levels/effects of: Lithium; Methenamine; Primidone; Trientine

The levels/effects of Methazolamide may be decreased by: Herbs (Hypertensive Properties); Methylphenidate; Yohimbine

Stability Store at 20°C to 25°C (68°F to 77°F).

Mechanism of Action Noncompetitive inhibition of the enzyme carbonic anhydrase; thought that carbonic anhydrase is located at the luminal border of cells of the proximal tubule. When the enzyme is inhibited, there is an increase in urine volume and a change to an alkaline pH with a subsequent decrease in the excretion of titratable acid and ammonia.

Pharmacodynamics/Kinetics
Onset of action: Slow in comparison with acetazolamide (2-4 hours)
Peak effect: 6-8 hours
Duration: 10-18 hours
Absorption: Slow
Distribution: V_d: 17-23 L
Protein binding: ~55%
Metabolism: Slowly from GI tract
Half-life elimination: ~14 hours
Excretion: Urine (~25% as unchanged drug)

Dosage
Geriatric & Adult Glaucoma: Oral: 50-100 mg 2-3 times/day
Monitoring Parameters Intraocular pressure, serum potassium, serum bicarbonate, serum sodium

Special Geriatric Considerations Oral carbonic anhydrase inhibitors are an alternative useful for patients who have difficulty administering ophthalmic drugs, who do not achieve sufficient lowering of intraocular pressure, or who cannot tolerate other agents. Malaise and complaints of tiredness and myalgia are signs of excessive dosing and acidosis in the elderly.

Dosage Forms Excipient information presented when available (limited, particularly for generics); consult specific product labeling.

Tablet, oral: 25 mg, 50 mg
  Neptazane™: 25 mg
  Neptazane™: 50 mg [scored]

Methenamine (meth EN a meen)

Medication Safety Issues
Sound-alike/look-alike issues:
  Hiprex® may be confused with Mirapex®
  Methenamine may be confused with mesalamine, methazolamide, methionine
  Urex may be confused with Eurax®, Serax
International issues:
  Urex: Brand name for methenamine [U.S. (discontinued)], but also the brand name for furosemide [Australia, China, Turkey]
  Urex [U.S. (discontinued)] may be confused with Eurax brand name for crotamitin [U.S., Canada, and multiple international markets]

Brand Names: U.S. Hiprex®

Brand Names: Canada Dehydral®; Hiprex®; Mandelamine®; Urasal®

Index Terms Hexamethylenetetramine; Methenamine Hippurate; Methenamine Mandelate; Urex

Generic Availability (U.S.) Yes

Pharmacologic Category Antibiotic, Miscellaneous

Use Prophylaxis or suppression of recurrent urinary tract infections; urinary tract discomfort secondary to hypermotility

Contraindications Hypersensitivity to methenamine or any component of the formulation; severe dehydration, renal insufficiency, severe hepatic insufficiency; concurrent treatment with sulfonamides

Warnings/Precautions Methenamine should not be used to treat infections outside of the lower urinary tract. Use with caution in patients with hepatic disease (contraindicated with severe impairment), gout, and the elderly; doses of 8 g/day for 3-4 weeks may cause bladder irritation. Use care to maintain an acid pH of the urine, especially when treating infections due to urea splitting organisms (eg, *Proteus* and strains of *Pseudomonas*); reversible increases in LFTs have occurred during therapy especially in patients with hepatic dysfunction. Prolonged use may result in fungal or bacterial superinfection, including *C. difficile*-associated diarrhea (CDAD) and pseudomembranous colitis; CDAD has been observed >2 months postantibiotic treatment. Hiprex® contains tartrazine dye.

Adverse Reactions (Reflective of adult population; not specific for elderly) <4%:
Dermatologic: Pruritus, rash
Gastrointestinal: Dyspepsia, nausea, vomiting
Hepatic: ALT increased (reversible; rare), AST increased (reversible; rare)
Note: Large doses (higher than recommended) have resulted in bladder irritation, frequent/painful micturition, albuminuria, and hematuria.

Drug Interactions
Metabolism/Transport Effects None known.

Avoid Concomitant Use
  Avoid concomitant use of Methenamine with any of the following: BCG; Sulfonamide Derivatives

Increased Effect/Toxicity
  Methenamine may increase the levels/effects of: Sulfonamide Derivatives

Decreased Effect
  Methenamine may decrease the levels/effects of: Amphetamines; BCG; Typhoid Vaccine

  The levels/effects of Methenamine may be decreased by: Antacids; Carbonic Anhydrase Inhibitors

Ethanol/Nutrition/Herb Interactions Food: Foods/diets which alkalinize urine (pH >5.5) decrease therapeutic effect of methenamine.

Stability Store at room temperature of 15°C to 30°C (59°F to 86°F). Protect from light.

Mechanism of Action Methenamine is hydrolyzed to formaldehyde and ammonia in acidic urine; formaldehyde has nonspecific bactericidal action. Other components, hippuric acid or mandelic acid, aid in maintaining urine acidity and may aid in suppressing bacteria.

◀ **Pharmacodynamics/Kinetics**
Absorption: Readily
Metabolism: Gastric juices: Hydrolyze 10% to 30% unless protected via enteric coating; Hepatic: ~10% to 25%
Half-life elimination: 3-6 hours
Excretion: Urine (90% as unchanged drug) within 24 hours

Dosage
Geriatric & Adult Urinary tract infection: Oral:
Hippurate: 1 g twice daily
Mandelate: 1 g 4 times/day after meals and at bedtime
Renal Impairment Cl_{cr} <50 mL/minute: Avoid use.

Administration Administer around-the-clock to promote less variation in effect.

Monitoring Parameters Urinalysis, periodic liver function tests

Test Interactions Increased urinary catecholamines, 17-hydroxycorticosteroid and vanillyl-mandelic acid (VMA) levels; decreased urinary 5-hydroxyindoleacetic acid (5HIAA) and estriol levels

Pharmacotherapy Pearls Should not be used to treat infections outside of the lower urinary tract. Methenamine has little, if any, role in the treatment or prevention of infections in patients with indwelling urinary (Foley) catheters. Furthermore, in noncatheterized patients, more effective antibiotics are available for the prevention or treatment of urinary tract infections.

Special Geriatric Considerations Methenamine has little, if any, role in the treatment or prevention of infections in patients with indwelling urinary (Foley) catheters. Furthermore, in noncatheterized patients, more effective antibiotics are available for the prevention or treatment of urinary tract infections. The influence of decreased renal function on the pharmacologic effects of methenamine results are unknown.

Dosage Forms Excipient information presented when available (limited, particularly for generics); consult specific product labeling.
Tablet, oral, as hippurate: 1 g
  Hiprex®: 1 g [scored; contains tartrazine]
Tablet, oral, as mandelate: 500 mg, 1 g

◆ **Methenamine Hippurate** *see* Methenamine *on page 1231*
◆ **Methenamine Mandelate** *see* Methenamine *on page 1231*

Methimazole (meth IM a zole)

Medication Safety Issues
Sound-alike/look-alike issues:
Methimazole may be confused with metolazone
Brand Names: U.S. Tapazole®
Brand Names: Canada Dom-Methimazole; PHL-Methimazole; Tapazole®
Index Terms Thiamazole
Generic Availability (U.S.) Yes
Pharmacologic Category Antithyroid Agent; Thioamide
Use Treatment of hyperthyroidism; improve hyperthyroidism prior to thyroidectomy or radio-active iodine therapy
Unlabeled Use
Treatment of Graves' disease
Contraindications Hypersensitivity to methimazole or any component of the formulation
Warnings/Precautions Antithyroid agents have been associated (rarely) with significant bone marrow depression. The most severe manifestation is agranulocytosis. Aplastic anemia, thrombocytopenia, and leukopenia may also occur. Use with extreme caution in patients receiving other drugs known to cause myelosuppression (particularly agranulocytosis) and in patients >40 years of age; avoid doses ≥40 mg/day (increased myelosuppression). Monitor patients closely; discontinue if significant bone marrow suppression occurs, particularly agranulocytosis or aplastic anemia.

May cause hypoprothrombinemia and bleeding. Rare, severe hepatic reactions (hepatic necrosis, hepatitis, encephalopathy) may occur; possibly fatal. Symptoms suggestive of hepatic dysfunction should prompt evaluation. Discontinue in the presence of hepatitis (transaminase >3 times upper limit of normal). In addition, other rare hypersensitivity reactions to antithyroid agents have been reported, including the development of ANCA-positive vasculitis, drug fever, exfoliative dermatitis, glomerulonephritis, leukocytoclastic vasculitis, and a lupus-like syndrome; prompt discontinuation is warranted in patients who develop symptoms consistent with a form of autoimmunity or other hypersensitivity during therapy. Minor dermatologic reactions may not require discontinuation, depending on severity.

Adverse Reactions (Reflective of adult population; not specific for elderly) Frequency not defined.

Cardiovascular: ANCA-positive vasculitis, edema, leukocytoclastic vasculitis, periarteritis

Central nervous system: Drowsiness, fever, headache, neuritis, vertigo

Dermatologic: Alopecia, exfoliative dermatitis, pruritus, skin pigmentation, skin rash, urticaria

Endocrine & metabolic: Goiter, hypoglycemic coma

Gastrointestinal: Constipation, epigastric distress, loss of taste perception, nausea, salivary gland swelling, vomiting, weight gain

Hematologic: Agranulocytosis, aplastic anemia, granulocytopenia, hypoprothrombinemia, leukopenia, thrombocytopenia

Hepatic: Hepatic necrosis, hepatitis, jaundice

Neuromuscular & skeletal: Arthralgia, myalgia, paresthesia

Renal: Nephritis

Miscellaneous: Insulin autoimmune syndrome, lymphadenopathy, SLE-like syndrome

Drug Interactions

Metabolism/Transport Effects Inhibits CYP1A2 (weak), CYP2A6 (weak), CYP2B6 (weak), CYP2C19 (weak), CYP2C9 (weak), CYP2D6 (weak), CYP2E1 (weak), CYP3A4 (weak)

Avoid Concomitant Use

Avoid concomitant use of Methimazole with any of the following: CloZAPine; Pimozide; Sodium Iodide I131

Increased Effect/Toxicity

Methimazole may increase the levels/effects of: ARIPiprazole; Cardiac Glycosides; CloZAPine; Pimozide; Theophylline Derivatives

Decreased Effect

Methimazole may decrease the levels/effects of: Sodium Iodide I131; Vitamin K Antagonists

Stability Store at 20°C to 25°C (68°F to 77°F); excursion permitted to 15°C to 30°C (59°F to 86°F). Protect from light.

Mechanism of Action Inhibits the synthesis of thyroid hormones by blocking the oxidation of iodine in the thyroid gland. As a result, methimazole inhibits the ability of iodine to combine with tyrosine to form thyroxine and triiodothyronine (T_3); does not inactivate circulating T_4 and T_3

Pharmacodynamics/Kinetics

Onset of action: Antithyroid: Oral: 12-18 hours

Duration: 36-72 hours

Distribution: Concentrated in thyroid gland

Protein binding, plasma: None

Metabolism: Hepatic

Bioavailability: ~93%

Half-life elimination: 4-6 hours

Time to peak, serum concentration: 1-2 hours

Excretion: Urine

Dosage

Geriatric & Adult

Hyperthyroidism: Oral: Initial: 15 mg/day in 3 divided doses (approximately every 8 hours) for mild hyperthyroidism; 30-40 mg/day in moderately severe hyperthyroidism; 60 mg/day in severe hyperthyroidism; maintenance: 5-15 mg/day (may be given as a single daily dose in many cases)

Adjust dosage as required to achieve and maintain serum T_3, T_4, and TSH levels in the normal range. An elevated T_3 may be the sole indicator of inadequate treatment. An elevated TSH indicates excessive antithyroid treatment.

Graves' disease (unlabeled use): Oral: Initial: 10-20 mg once daily to restore euthyroidism; maintenance: 5-10 mg once daily for a total of 12-18 months, then tapered or discontinued if TSH is normal at that time (Bahn, 2011)

Iodine-induced thyrotoxicosis (unlabeled use): Oral: 20-40 mg/day given either once or twice daily (Bahn, 2011)

Thyrotoxic crisis (unlabeled use): Oral: **Note:** Recommendations vary; use in combination with other specific agents. Dosages of 20-25 mg every 6 hours have been used; once stable, dosing frequency may be reduced to once or twice daily (Nayak, 2006). The American Thyroid Association and the American Association of Clinical Endocrinologists recommend 60-80 mg/day (Bahn, 2011). Rectal administration has also been described (Nabil, 1982).

Thyrotoxicosis (type I amiodarone-induced; unlabeled use): Oral: 40 mg once daily to restore euthyroidism (generally 3-6 months). **Note:** If high doses continue to be required, dividing the dose may be more effective (Bahn, 2011).

Administration Administer consistently in relation to meals every day. In thyrotoxic crisis, rectal administration has been described (Nabil, 1982).

◀ **Monitoring Parameters** Monitor for signs of hypothyroidism, hyperthyroidism, T_4, T_3; CBC with differential, liver function (baseline and as needed), serum thyroxine, free thyroxine index; prothrombin time

Pharmacotherapy Pearls A potency ratio of methimazole to propylthiouracil of at least 20-30:1 is recommended when changing from one drug to another (eg, 300 mg of propylthiouracil would be roughly equivalent to 10-15 mg of methimazole) (Bahn, 2011).

Special Geriatric Considerations The use of antithyroid thioamides is as effective in the elderly as they are in younger adults.

Dosage Forms Excipient information presented when available (limited, particularly for generics); consult specific product labeling.

Tablet, oral: 5 mg, 10 mg

Tapazole®: 5 mg, 10 mg [scored]

◆ **Methitest™** see MethylTESTOSTERone on page 1256

Methocarbamol (meth oh KAR ba mole)

Related Information

Beers Criteria – Potentially Inappropriate Medications for Geriatrics on page 2183

Medication Safety Issues

Sound-alike/look-alike issues:

Methocarbamol may be confused with mephobarbital

Robaxin® may be confused with ribavirin, Skelaxin®

BEERS Criteria medication:

This drug may be potentially inappropriate for use in geriatric patients (Quality of evidence - moderate; Strength of recommendation - strong).

International issues:

Robaxin [U.S., Canada, Great Britain, Greece, Spain] may be confused with Rubex brand name for ascorbic acid [Ireland]; doxorubicin [Brazil]

Brand Names: U.S. Robaxin®; Robaxin®-750

Brand Names: Canada Robaxin®

Generic Availability (U.S.) Yes: Tablet

Pharmacologic Category Skeletal Muscle Relaxant

Use Adjunctive treatment of muscle spasm associated with acute painful musculoskeletal conditions (eg, tetanus)

Contraindications Hypersensitivity to methocarbamol or any component of the formulation; renal impairment (injection formulation)

Warnings/Precautions May cause CNS depression, which may impair physical or mental abilities; patients must be cautioned about performing tasks which require mental alertness (eg, operating machinery or driving). Effects may be potentiated when used with other sedative drugs or ethanol. Plasma protein binding and clearance are decreased and the half-life is increased in patients with hepatic impairment. Muscle relaxants are poorly tolerated by the elderly due to potent anticholinergic effects, sedation, and risk of fracture. Efficacy is questionable at dosages tolerated by elderly patients; avoid use (Beers Criteria).

Injection: Contraindicated in renal impairment. Contains polyethylene glycol. Rate of injection should not exceed 3 mL/minute; solution is hypertonic; avoid extravasation. Use with caution in patients with a history of seizures. Use caution with hepatic impairment. Vial stopper contains latex. Recommended only for the treatment of tetanus in pediatric patients.

Adverse Reactions (Reflective of adult population; not specific for elderly) Frequency not defined.

Cardiovascular: Bradycardia, flushing, hypotension, syncope

Central nervous system: Amnesia, confusion, coordination impaired (mild), dizziness, drowsiness, fever, headache, insomnia, lightheadedness, sedation, seizures, vertigo

Dermatologic: Angioneurotic edema, pruritus, rash, urticaria

Gastrointestinal: Dyspepsia, metallic taste, nausea, vomiting

Hematologic: Leukopenia

Hepatic: Jaundice

Local: Pain at injection site, thrombophlebitis

Ocular: Blurred vision, conjunctivitis, diplopia, nystagmus

Respiratory: Nasal congestion

Miscellaneous: Hypersensitivity reactions including anaphylaxis

Drug Interactions

Metabolism/Transport Effects None known.

Avoid Concomitant Use

Avoid concomitant use of Methocarbamol with any of the following: Azelastine; Azelastine (Nasal); Methadone; Mirtazapine; Paraldehyde

Increased Effect/Toxicity

Methocarbamol may increase the levels/effects of: Alcohol (Ethyl); Azelastine; Azelastine (Nasal); Buprenorphine; CNS Depressants; Methadone; Methotrimeprazine; Metyrosine; Mirtazapine; Paraldehyde; Selective Serotonin Reuptake Inhibitors; Zolpidem

The levels/effects of Methocarbamol may be increased by: Droperidol; HydrOXYzine; Methotrimeprazine

Decreased Effect

Methocarbamol may decrease the levels/effects of: Pyridostigmine

Ethanol/Nutrition/Herb Interactions

Ethanol: May increase CNS depression; monitor for increased effects with coadministration. Caution patients about effects.

Herb/Nutraceutical: Avoid valerian, St John's wort, kava kava, gotu kola (may increase CNS depression).

Stability

Injection: Prior to dilution, store at controlled room temperature of 20°C to 25°C (68°F to 77°F); excursions permitted to 15°C to 30°C (59°F to 86°F).

Tablet: Store at controlled room temperature of 20°C to 25°C (68°F to 77°F).

Mechanism of Action Causes skeletal muscle relaxation by general CNS depression

Pharmacodynamics/Kinetics

Onset of action: Muscle relaxation: Oral: ~30 minutes

Protein binding: 46% to 50%

Metabolism: Hepatic via dealkylation and hydroxylation

Half-life elimination: 1-2 hours

Time to peak, serum: Oral: 1-2 hours

Excretion: Urine (primarily as metabolites)

Dosage

Adult

Muscle spasm:

Oral: 1.5 g 4 times/day for 2-3 days (up to 8 g/day may be given in severe conditions), then decrease to 4-4.5 g/day in 3-6 divided doses

I.M., I.V.: Initial: 1 g; may repeat every 8 hours if oral administration not possible; maximum dose: 3 g/day for no more than 3 consecutive days. If condition persists, may repeat course of therapy after a drug-free interval of 48 hours.

Tetanus: I.V.: Initial dose: 1-2 g by direct I.V. injection, which may be followed by an additional 1-2 g by infusion (maximum initial dose: 3 g total); may repeat initial dose every 6 hours until NG tube or oral therapy possible; total oral daily dose of up to 24 g may be needed; injection should not be used for more than 3 consecutive days

Renal Impairment Administration of the parenteral formulation is contraindicated in patients with renal dysfunction due to the presence of polyethylene glycol.

Hepatic Impairment Specific dosing guidelines are not available.

Administration

Injection:

I.M.: A maximum of 5 mL can be administered into each gluteal region.

I.V.: Maximum rate: 3 mL/minute; may be administered undiluted or mixed with 5% dextrose or 0.9% saline (1 vial/≤250 mL diluent). Monitor closely for extravasation. Administer I.V. while in recumbent position. Maintain position for at least 10-15 minutes following infusion.

Tablet: May be crushed and mixed with food or liquid if needed.

Monitoring Parameters Monitor closely for extravasation (I.V. administration).

Test Interactions May cause color interference in certain screening tests for 5-HIAA using nitrosonaphthol reagent and in screening tests for urinary VMA using the Gitlow method.

Special Geriatric Considerations Methocarbamol has a short half-life, so it may be considered one of the safer skeletal muscle relaxants.

This medication is considered to be potentially inappropriate in this patient population (Beers Criteria: Quality of evidence - moderate; Strength of recommendation - strong).

Dosage Forms Excipient information presented when available (limited, particularly for generics); consult specific product labeling.

Injection, solution:

Robaxin®: 100 mg/mL (10 mL) [contains natural rubber/natural latex in packaging, polyethylene glycol 300]

Tablet, oral: 500 mg, 750 mg

Robaxin®: 500 mg [scored]

Robaxin®-750: 750 mg

Methotrexate (meth oh TREKS ate)

Medication Safety Issues

Sound-alike/look-alike issues:
Methotrexate may be confused with mercaptopurine, methylPREDNISolone sodium succinate, metolazone, metroNIDAZOLE, mitoXANtrone, PRALAtrexate

High alert medication:
The Institute for Safe Medication Practices (ISMP) includes this medication among its list of drugs which have a heightened risk of causing significant patient harm when used in error.

Administration issues:
Errors have occurred (resulting in death) when methotrexate was administered as "daily" dose instead of the recommended "weekly" dose.

Intrathecal medication safety: The American Society of Clinical Oncology (ASCO)/Oncology Nursing Society (ONS) chemotherapy administration safety standards (Jacobson, 2009) encourage the following safety measures for intrathecal chemotherapy:
- Intrathecal medication should not be prepared during the preparation of any other agents
- After preparation, store in an isolated location or container clearly marked with a label identifying as "intrathecal" use only
- Delivery to the patient should only be with other medications intended for administration into the central nervous system

Other safety concerns:
MTX is an error-prone abbreviation (mistaken as mitoxantrone)

International issues:
Trexall [U.S.] may be confused with Trexol brand name for tamadol [Mexico]; Truxal brand name for chlorprothixene [multiple international markets]

Brand Names: U.S. Rheumatrex®; Trexall™

Brand Names: Canada Apo-Methotrexate®; ratio-Methotrexate

Index Terms Amethopterin; Methotrexate Sodium; Methotrexatum; MTX (error-prone abbreviation)

Generic Availability (U.S.) Yes

Pharmacologic Category Antineoplastic Agent, Antimetabolite (Antifolate); Antirheumatic, Disease Modifying; Immunosuppressant Agent

Use

Oncology-related uses: Treatment of trophoblastic neoplasms (gestational choriocarcinoma, chorioadenoma destruens and hydatidiform mole), acute lymphocytic leukemia (ALL), meningeal leukemia, breast cancer, head and neck cancer (epidermoid), cutaneous T-Cell lymphoma (advanced mycosis fungoides), lung cancer (squamous cell and small cell), advanced non-Hodgkin's lymphomas (NHL), osteosarcoma

Nononcology uses: Treatment of psoriasis (severe, recalcitrant, disabling) and severe rheumatoid arthritis (RA), including polyarticular-course juvenile idiopathic arthritis (JIA)

Unlabeled Use Treatment and maintenance of remission in Crohn's disease; dermatomyositis; bladder cancer, central nervous system tumors (including nonleukemic meningeal cancers), acute promyelocytic leukemia (maintenance treatment), soft tissue sarcoma (desmoid tumors)

Contraindications Hypersensitivity to methotrexate or any component of the formulation

Additional contraindications for patients with psoriasis or rheumatoid arthritis: Alcoholism, alcoholic liver disease or other chronic liver disease, immunodeficiency syndrome (overt or laboratory evidence); pre-existing blood dyscrasias (eg, bone marrow hypoplasia, leukopenia, thrombocytopenia, significant anemia)

Warnings/Precautions Hazardous agent - use appropriate precautions for handling and disposal.

[U.S. Boxed Warning]: Methotrexate has been associated with acute (elevated transaminases) and potentially fatal chronic (fibrosis, cirrhosis) hepatotoxicity. Risk is related to cumulative dose and prolonged exposure. Monitor closely (with liver function tests, including serum albumin) for liver toxicities. Liver enzyme elevations may be noted, but may not be predictive of hepatic disease in long term treatment for psoriasis (but generally is predictive in rheumatoid arthritis [RA] treatment). With long-term use, liver biopsy may show histologic changes, fibrosis, or cirrhosis; periodic liver biopsy is recommended with long-term use for psoriasis patients with risk factors for hepatotoxicity and for persistent abnormal liver function tests in psoriasis patients without risk factors for hepatotoxicity and in RA patients; discontinue methotrexate with moderate-to-severe change in liver biopsy. Risk factors for hepatotoxicity include history of above moderate ethanol consumption, persistent abnormal liver chemistries, history of chronic liver disease (including hepatitis B or C), family history of inheritable liver disease, diabetes, obesity, hyperlipidemia, lack of folate supplementation during methotrexate therapy, and history of significant exposure to hepatotoxic drugs. Use caution with preexisting liver impairment; may require dosage reduction. Use caution when used with other hepatotoxic agents (azathioprine, retinoids, sulfasalazine). **[U.S. Boxed Warning]: Methotrexate elimination is reduced in patients with ascites;** may require dose reduction or discontinuation. Monitor closely for toxicity.

[U.S. Boxed Warning]: May cause renal damage leading to acute renal failure, especially with high-dose methotrexate; monitor renal function and methotrexate levels closely, maintain adequate hydration and urinary alkalinization. Use caution in osteosarcoma patients treated with high-dose methotrexate in combination with nephrotoxic chemotherapy (eg, cisplatin). **[U.S. Boxed Warning]: Methotrexate elimination is reduced in patients with renal impairment;** may require dose reduction or discontinuation; monitor closely for toxicity. **[U.S. Boxed Warning]: Tumor lysis syndrome may occur in patients with high tumor burden;** use appropriate prevention and treatment.

[U.S. Boxed Warning]: May cause potentially life-threatening pneumonitis (may occur at any time during therapy and at any dosage); monitor closely for pulmonary symptoms, particularly dry, nonproductive cough. Other potential symptoms include fever, dyspnea, hypoxemia, or pulmonary infiltrate. **[U.S. Boxed Warning]: Methotrexate elimination is reduced in patients with pleural effusions;** may require dose reduction or discontinuation. Monitor closely for toxicity.

[U.S. Boxed Warning]: Bone marrow suppression may occur, resulting in anemia, aplastic anemia, pancytopenia, leukopenia, neutropenia, and/or thrombocytopenia. Use caution in patients with pre-existing bone marrow suppression. Discontinue therapy in RA or psoriasis if a significant decrease in hematologic components is noted. **[U.S. Boxed Warning]: Use of low dose methotrexate has been associated with the development of malignant lymphomas;** may regress upon discontinuation of therapy; treat lymphoma appropriately if regression is not induced by cessation of methotrexate.

[U.S. Boxed Warning]: Diarrhea and ulcerative stomatitis may require interruption of therapy; death from hemorrhagic enteritis or intestinal perforation has been reported. Use with caution in patients with peptic ulcer disease, ulcerative colitis.

May cause neurotoxicity including seizures (usually in pediatric ALL patients), leukoencephalopathy (usually with concurrent cranial irradiation) and stroke-like encephalopathy (usually with high-dose regimens). Chemical arachnoiditis (headache, back pain, nuchal rigidity, fever), myelopathy and chronic leukoencephalopathy may result from intrathecal administration.

[U.S. Boxed Warning]: Any dose level or route of administration may cause severe and potentially fatal dermatologic reactions, including toxic epidermal necrolysis, Stevens-Johnson syndrome, exfoliative dermatitis, skin necrosis, and erythema multiforme. Radiation dermatitis and sunburn may be precipitated by methotrexate administration. Psoriatic lesions may be worsened by concomitant exposure to ultraviolet radiation.

[U.S. Boxed Warning]: Concomitant administration with NSAIDs may cause severe bone marrow suppression, aplastic anemia, and GI toxicity. Do not administer NSAIDs prior to or during high dose methotrexate therapy; may increase and prolong serum methotrexate levels. Doses used for psoriasis may still lead to unexpected toxicities; use caution when administering NSAIDs or salicylates with lower doses of methotrexate for RA. Methotrexate may increase the levels and effects of mercaptopurine; may require dosage adjustments. Vitamins containing folate may decrease response to systemic methotrexate; folate deficiency may increase methotrexate toxicity. **[U.S. Boxed Warning]: Concomitant methotrexate administration with radiotherapy may increase the risk of soft tissue necrosis and osteonecrosis.**

[U.S. Boxed Warnings]: Should be administered under the supervision of a physician experienced in the use of antimetabolite therapy; serious and fatal toxicities have occurred at all dose levels. Immune suppression may lead to potentially fatal opportunistic infections. For rheumatoid arthritis and psoriasis, immunosuppressive therapy should only be used when disease is active and less toxic, traditional therapy is ineffective. Methotrexate formulations and/or diluents containing preservatives should not be used for intrathecal or high-dose therapy. May cause impairment of fertility, oligospermia, and menstrual dysfunction. Toxicity from methotrexate or any immunosuppressive is increased in the elderly.

When used for intrathecal administration, should not be prepared during the preparation of any other agents; after preparation, store intrathecal medications in an isolated location or container clearly marked with a label identifying as "intrathecal" use only; delivery of intrathecal medications to the patient should only be with other medications intended for administration into the central nervous system (Jacobson, 2009).

Adverse Reactions (Reflective of adult population; not specific for elderly) Note: Adverse reactions vary by route and dosage. Hematologic and/or gastrointestinal toxicities may be common at dosages used in chemotherapy; these reactions are much less frequent when used at typical dosages for rheumatic diseases.

>10%:

Central nervous system (with I.T. administration or very high-dose therapy):

Arachnoiditis: Acute reaction manifested as severe headache, nuchal rigidity, vomiting, and fever; may be alleviated by reducing the dose

Subacute toxicity: 10% of patients treated with 12-15 mg of I.T. methotrexate may develop this in the second or third week of therapy; consists of motor paralysis of extremities, cranial nerve palsy, seizure, or coma. This has also been seen in pediatric cases receiving very high-dose I.V. methotrexate.

Demyelinating encephalopathy: Seen months or years after receiving methotrexate; usually in association with cranial irradiation or other systemic chemotherapy

Dermatologic: Reddening of skin

Endocrine & metabolic: Hyperuricemia, oligospermia

Gastrointestinal: Ulcerative stomatitis, glossitis, gingivitis, nausea, vomiting, diarrhea, intestinal perforation, mucositis (dose dependent; appears in 3-7 days after therapy, resolving within 2 weeks)

Hematologic: Leukopenia, myelosuppression (nadir: 7-10 days), thrombocytopenia

Renal: Renal failure, azotemia, nephropathy

Respiratory: Pharyngitis

Miscellaneous: Immunosuppression

1% to 10%:

Cardiovascular: Vasculitis

Central nervous system: Dizziness, malaise, fever, chills

Dermatologic: Alopecia, rash, photosensitivity, depigmentation or hyperpigmentation of skin, pruritus, dermatitis

Endocrine & metabolic: Diabetes

Genitourinary: Cystitis

Hematologic: Hemorrhage

Hepatic: Cirrhosis (chronic therapy), liver function tests increased (chronic therapy), portal fibrosis (chronic therapy)

Neuromuscular & skeletal: Arthralgia

Ocular: Blurred vision

Renal: Renal dysfunction: Manifested by an abrupt rise in serum creatinine and BUN and a fall in urine output; more common with high-dose methotrexate, and may be due to precipitation of the drug.

Respiratory: Pneumonitis: Associated with fever, cough, and interstitial pulmonary infiltrates; treatment is to withhold methotrexate during the acute reaction; interstitial pneumonitis has been reported to occur with an incidence of 1% in patients with RA (dose 7.5-15 mg/week)

Miscellaneous: Infection

Drug Interactions

Metabolism/Transport Effects Substrate of P-glycoprotein, SLCO1B1

Avoid Concomitant Use

Avoid concomitant use of Methotrexate with any of the following: Acitretin; BCG; CloZAPine; Natalizumab; Pimecrolimus; Tacrolimus (Topical)

Increased Effect/Toxicity

Methotrexate may increase the levels/effects of: CloZAPine; CycloSPORINE; CycloSPORINE (Systemic); Leflunomide; Loop Diuretics; Natalizumab; Theophylline Derivatives; Vaccines (Live); Vitamin K Antagonists

The levels/effects of Methotrexate may be increased by: Acitretin; Ciprofloxacin; Ciprofloxacin (Systemic); CycloSPORINE; CycloSPORINE (Systemic); Denosumab; Eltrombopag; Loop Diuretics; Nonsteroidal Anti-Inflammatory Agents; Penicillins; P-glycoprotein/ABCB1 Inhibitors; Pimecrolimus; Probenecid; Proton Pump Inhibitors; Roflumilast; Salicylates; SulfaSALAzine; Sulfonamide Derivatives; Tacrolimus (Topical); Trastuzumab; Trimethoprim

Decreased Effect

Methotrexate may decrease the levels/effects of: BCG; Cardiac Glycosides; Coccidioidin Skin Test; Loop Diuretics; Sapropterin; Sipuleucel-T; Vaccines (Inactivated); Vitamin K Antagonists

The levels/effects of Methotrexate may be decreased by: Bile Acid Sequestrants; Echinacea; P-glycoprotein/ABCB1 Inducers

Ethanol/Nutrition/Herb Interactions

Ethanol: Ethanol may be associated with increased liver injury. Management: Avoid ethanol.

Food: Methotrexate peak serum levels may be decreased if taken with food. Milk-rich foods may decrease methotrexate absorption. Folate may decrease drug response.

Herb/Nutraceutical: Echinacea has immunostimulant properties. Management: Avoid echinacea.

Stability Store tablets and intact vials at room temperature (15°C to 25°C). Use appropriate precautions for handling and disposal. Protect from light. **Use preservative-free preparations for intrathecal or high-dose methotrexate administration.**

I.M., I.V., SubQ: Dilute powder with D_5W or NS to a concentration of ≤25 mg/mL (20 mg and 50 mg vials) and 50 mg/mL (1 g vial). Further dilution in D_5W or NS is stable for 24 hours at room temperature (21°C to 25°C). Reconstituted solutions with a preservative may be stored under refrigeration for up to 3 months, and up to 4 weeks at room temperature.

Intrathecal: Prepare intrathecal solutions with preservative-free NS, lactated Ringer's, or Elliot's B solution to a final volume of up to 12 mL (volume generally based on institution or practitioner preference). Intrathecal methotrexate concentrations may be institution specific or based on practitioner preference, generally ranging from a final concentration of 1 mg/mL (per prescribing information; Grossman, 1993; Lin, 2008) up to ~2-4 mg/mL (de Lemos, 2009; Glantz, 1999). For triple intrathecal therapy (methotrexate 12 mg/hydrocortisone 24 mg/cytarabine 36 mg), preparation to final volume of 12 mL is reported (Lin, 2008). Intrathecal dilutions are preservative-free and should be used as soon as possible after preparation. Intrathecal medications should **NOT** be prepared during the preparation of any other agents. After preparation, store intrathecal medications (until use) in an isolated location or container clearly marked with a label identifying as "intrathecal" use only.

Mechanism of Action Methotrexate is a folate antimetabolite that inhibits DNA synthesis. Methotrexate irreversibly binds to dihydrofolate reductase, inhibiting the formation of reduced folates, and thymidylate synthetase, resulting in inhibition of purine and thymidylic acid synthesis. Methotrexate is cell cycle specific for the S phase of the cycle.

The MOA in the treatment of rheumatoid arthritis is unknown, but may affect immune function. In psoriasis, methotrexate is thought to target rapidly proliferating epithelial cells in the skin.

In Crohn's disease, it may have immune modulator and anti-inflammatory activity.

Pharmacodynamics/Kinetics

Onset of action: Antirheumatic: 3-6 weeks; additional improvement may continue longer than 12 weeks

Absorption: Oral: Dose dependent; well absorbed at low doses (<30 mg/m²), incomplete after higher doses; I.M. injection: Complete

Distribution: Penetrates slowly into 3rd space fluids (eg, pleural effusions, ascites), exits slowly from these compartments (slower than from plasma); sustained concentrations retained in kidney and liver

V_d: 0.18 L/kg (initial); 0.4-0.8 L/kg (steady state)

Protein binding: ~50%

Metabolism: <10%; degraded by intestinal flora to DAMPA by carboxypeptidase; hepatic aldehyde oxidase converts methotrexate to 7-OH methotrexate; polyglutamates are produced intracellularly and are just as potent as methotrexate; their production is dose- and duration-dependent and they are slowly eliminated by the cell once formed. Polyglutamated forms can be converted back to methotrexate.

Bioavailability: Dose dependent; ~60% at low doses

Half-life elimination: Low dose: 3-10 hours; High dose: 8-15 hours

Time to peak, serum: Oral: 1-2 hours; I.M.: 30-60 minutes

Excretion: Urine (44% to 100%); feces (small amounts)

Dosage

Geriatric Refer to individual protocols; adjust for renal impairment.

Meningeal leukemia: I.T.: Consider a dose reduction (CSF volume and turnover may decrease with age)

Rheumatoid arthritis/psoriasis: Oral: Initial: 5-7.5 mg/week, not to exceed 20 mg/week

Adult Details concerning dosing in combination regimens should also be consulted.

Note: Doses between 100-500 mg/m² **may require** leucovorin rescue. Doses >500 mg/m² **require** leucovorin rescue: I.V., I.M., Oral: Leucovorin 10-15 mg/m² every 6 hours for 8 or 10 doses, starting 24 hours after the start of methotrexate infusion. Continue until the methotrexate level is ≤0.1 micromolar (10^{-7} M). Some clinicians continue leucovorin until the methotrexate level is <0.05 micromolar (5 x 10^{-8} M) or 0.01 micromolar (10^{-8} M).

If the 48-hour methotrexate level is >1 micromolar (10^{-6} M) or the 72-hour methotrexate level is >0.2 micromolar (2 x 10^{-7} M): I.V., I.M, Oral: Leucovorin 100 mg/m² every 6 hours until the methotrexate level is ≤0.1 micromolar (10^{-7} M). Some clinicians continue leucovorin until the methotrexate level is <0.05 micromolar (5 x 10^{-8} M) or 0.01 micromolar (10^{-8} M).

Antineoplastic dosage range: I.V.: Range is wide from 30-40 mg/m^2/week to 100-12,000 mg/m^2 with leucovorin rescue

Trophoblastic neoplasms:
Oral, I.M.: 15-30 mg/day for 5 days; repeat in 7 days for 3-5 courses
I.V.: 11 mg/m^2 days 1 through 5 every 3 weeks

Head and neck cancer: Oral, I.M., I.V.: 25-50 mg/m^2 once weekly

Mycosis fungoides (cutaneous T-cell lymphoma): Oral, I.M.: Initial (early stages):
5-50 mg once weekly **or**
15-37.5 mg twice weekly

Breast cancer: I.V.: 30-60 mg/m^2 Day 1 and 8 every 3-4 weeks

Lymphoma, non-Hodgkin's: I.V.:
30 mg/m^2 days 3 and 10 every 3 weeks **or**
120 mg/m^2 day 8 and 15 every 3-4 weeks **or**
200 mg/m^2 day 8 and 15 every 3 weeks **or**
400 mg/m^2 every 4 weeks for 3 cycles **or**
1 g/m^2 every 3 weeks **or**
1.5 g/m^2 every 4 weeks

Meningeal leukemia: I.T.: Usual dose: 12 mg/dose

Osteosarcoma: I.V.: 8-12 g/m^2 weekly for 2-4 weeks

Rheumatoid arthritis: Some experts recommend concomitant folic acid at a dose of least 5 mg/week (except the day of methotrexate) to reduce hematologic, gastrointestinal, and hepatic adverse events related to methotrexate.
Oral (manufacturer's labeling): 7.5 mg once weekly or 2.5 mg every 12 hours for 3 doses/week (dosage exceeding 20 mg/week may cause a higher incidence and severity of adverse events); *alternatively,* 10-15 mg once weekly, increased by 5 mg every 2-4 weeks to a maximum of 20-30 mg once weekly has been recommended by some experts (Visser, 2009)
I.M., SubQ (unlabeled route): 15 mg once weekly (dosage varies, similar to oral) (Braun, 2008)

Psoriasis: Some experts recommend concomitant folic acid 1-5 mg/day (except the day of methotrexate) to reduce hematologic, gastrointestinal, and hepatic adverse events related to methotrexate.
Oral: 2.5-5 mg/dose every 12 hours for 3 doses given weekly **or**
Oral, I.M., SubQ: 10-25 mg/dose given once weekly; titrate to lowest effective dose
Note: An initial test dose of 2.5-5 mg is recommended in patients with risk factors for hematologic toxicity or renal impairment. (Kalb, 2009).

Bladder cancer (unlabeled use): I.V.:
30 mg/m^2 day 1 and 8 every 3 weeks **or**
30 mg/m^2 day 1, 15, and 22 every 4 weeks

Nonleukemic meningeal cancer (unlabeled uses): I.T.: 10-12 mg/dose twice weekly for 4 weeks, then weekly for 4 weeks, then monthly (NCCN CNS cancer guidelines v.2.2009) **or** 12 mg/dose twice weekly for 4 weeks, then weekly for 4 doses, then monthly for 4 doses (Glantz, 1998) **or** 10 mg twice weekly for 4 weeks, then weekly for 1 month, then every 2 weeks for 2 months (Glantz, 1999)

Active Crohn's disease (unlabeled use): Induction of remission: I.M., SubQ: 15-25 mg once weekly; remission maintenance: 15 mg once weekly
Note: Oral dosing has been reported as effective but oral absorption is highly variable. If patient relapses after a switch to oral, may consider returning to injectable.

Renal Impairment The FDA-approved labeling does not contain dosage adjustment guidelines.
The following guidelines have been used by some clinicians:
Cl$_{cr}$ 61-80 mL/minute: Administer 75% of dose
Cl$_{cr}$ 51-60 mL/minute: Administer 70% of dose
Cl$_{cr}$ 10-50 mL/minute: Administer 30% to 50% of dose
Cl$_{cr}$ <10 mL/minute: Avoid use
Hemodialysis: Not dialyzable (0% to 5%); supplemental dose is not necessary
Peritoneal dialysis effects: Supplemental dose is not necessary
CAVH effects: Unknown

Aronoff, 2007:
Adults:
Cl$_{cr}$ 10-50 mL/minute: Administer 50% of dose
Cl$_{cr}$ <10 mL/minute: Avoid use
Hemodialysis: Administer 50% of dose
Continuous renal replacement therapy (CRRT): Administer 50% of dose

Kintzel, 1995:

Cl_{cr} 46-60 mL/minute: Administer 65% of normal dose

Cl_{cr} 31-45 mL/minute: Administer 50% of normal dose

Cl_{cr} <30 mL/minute: Avoid use

Hepatic Impairment The FDA-approved labeling does not contain dosage adjustment guidelines. The following guidelines have been used by some clinicians (Floyd, 2006):

Bilirubin 3.1-5 mg/dL **or** transaminases >3 times ULN: Administer 75% of dose

Bilirubin >5 mg/dL: Avoid use

Administration Methotrexate may be administered I.M., I.V., or I.T.; I.V. administration may be as slow push, short bolus infusion, or 24- to 42-hour continuous infusion. Specific dosing schemes vary, but high dose should be followed by leucovorin calcium to prevent toxicity.

Monitoring Parameters Laboratory tests should be performed on day 5 or day 6 of the weekly methotrexate cycle (eg, psoriasis, RA) to detect the leukopenia nadir and to avoid elevated LFTs 1-2 days after taking dose.

Patients with psoriasis:

CBC with differential and platelets (baseline, 7-14 days after initiating therapy or dosage increase, every 2-4 weeks for first few months, then every 1-3 months); BUN and serum creatinine (baseline and every 2-3 months); consider PPD for latent TB screening (baseline); LFTs (baseline, monthly for first 6 months, then every 1-2 months); chest x-ray (baseline if underlying lung disease)

Liver biopsy for patients **with** risk factors for hepatotoxicity: Baseline or after 2-6 months of therapy and with each 1-1.5 g cumulative dose interval

Liver biopsy for patients **without** risk factors for hepatotoxicity: If persistent elevations in 5 of 9 AST levels during a 12-month period, or decline of serum albumin below the normal range with normal nutritional status. Consider biopsy after cumulative dose of 3.5-4 g and after each additional 1.5 g.

Patients with RA:

CBC with differential and platelets, serum creatinine and LFTs (baseline then every 2-4 weeks for initial 3 months of therapy, then every 8-12 weeks for 3-6 months of therapy and then every 12 weeks after 6 months of therapy); chest x-ray (baseline); pulmonary function test (if methotrexate-induced lung disease suspected); hepatitis B or C testing (baseline)

Liver biopsy (if persistent abnormal baseline LFTs, history of alcoholism, or chronic hepatitis B or C) or during treatment if persistent LFT elevations (6 of 12 tests abnormal over 1 year or 5 of 9 results when LFTs performed at 6-week intervals)

Patients with cancer: Baseline and frequently during treatment: CBC with differential and platelets, serum creatinine, LFTs; chest x-ray (baseline); methotrexate levels and urine pH (with high-dose therapy); pulmonary function test (if methotrexate-induced lung disease suspected)

Reference Range Therapeutic levels: Variable; Toxic concentration: Variable; therapeutic range is dependent upon therapeutic approach.

High-dose regimens produce drug levels that are between 0.1-1 micromole/L 24-72 hours after drug infusion

Toxic: Low-dose therapy: >0.2 micromole/L; high-dose therapy: >1 micromole/L

Pharmacotherapy Pearls Oncology Comment: Methotrexate overexposure: The investigational rescue agent, glucarpidase, is an enzyme which rapidly hydrolyzes extracellular methotrexate into inactive metabolites, resulting in a rapid reduction of methotrexate concentrations. Glucarpidase is available for intrathecal (IT) use through an Emergency Use IND and for I.V. use under an Open-Label Treatment protocol.

Special Geriatric Considerations Toxicity to methotrexate or any immunosuppressive is increased in the elderly. Must monitor carefully. For rheumatoid arthritis and psoriasis, immunosuppressive therapy should only be used when disease is active and less toxic, traditional therapy is ineffective. Recommended doses should be reduced when initiating therapy in the elderly due to possible decreased metabolism, reduced renal function, and presence of interacting diseases and drugs. Adjust dose as needed for renal function (Cl_{cr}).

Dosage Forms Excipient information presented when available (limited, particularly for generics); consult specific product labeling.

Injection, powder for reconstitution: 1 g

Injection, solution: 25 mg/mL (2 mL, 10 mL)

Injection, solution [preservative free]: 25 mg/mL (2 mL, 4 mL, 8 mL, 10 mL, 40 mL)

Tablet, oral: 2.5 mg

Trexall™: 5 mg, 7.5 mg, 10 mg, 15 mg [scored]

Tablet, oral [dose-pack]:

Rheumatrex®: 2.5 mg [scored]

◆ **Methotrexate Sodium** see Methotrexate on page 1236

◆ **Methotrexatum** see Methotrexate on page 1236

Methsuximide (meth SUKS i mide)

Medication Safety Issues
Sound-alike/look-alike issues:
Methsuximide may be confused with ethosuximide
Brand Names: U.S. Celontin®
Brand Names: Canada Celontin®
Generic Availability (U.S.) No
Pharmacologic Category Anticonvulsant, Succinimide
Use Control of absence (petit mal) seizures that are refractory to other drugs
Unlabeled Use Treatment of partial complex (psychomotor) seizures
Medication Guide Available Yes
Contraindications History of hypersensitivity to succinimides
Warnings/Precautions Antiepileptics are associated with an increased risk of suicidal behavior/thoughts with use (regardless of indication); patients should be monitored for signs/symptoms of depression, suicidal tendencies, and other unusual behavior changes during therapy and instructed to inform their healthcare provider immediately if symptoms occur. Use with caution in patients with hepatic or renal disease. Abrupt withdrawal of the drug may precipitate absence status. Methsuximide may increase tonic-clonic seizures when used alone in patients with mixed seizure disorders. Methsuximide must be used in combination with other anticonvulsants in patients with both absence and tonic-clonic seizures. May cause CNS depression, which may impair physical or mental abilities; patients must be cautioned about performing tasks which require mental alertness (eg, operating machinery or driving). Effects with other sedative drugs or ethanol may be potentiated. Consider evaluation of blood counts in patients with signs/symptoms of infection. Succinimides have been associated with severe blood dyscrasias and cases of systemic lupus erythematosus.
Adverse Reactions (Reflective of adult population; not specific for elderly) Frequency not defined.
Cardiovascular: Hyperemia
Central nervous system: Aggressiveness, ataxia, confusion, depression, dizziness, drowsiness, hallucinations (auditory), headache, hypochondriacal behavior, insomnia, irritability, mental instability, mental slowness, nervousness, psychosis, suicidal behavior
Dermatologic: Pruritus, rash, Stevens-Johnson syndrome, urticaria
Gastrointestinal: Abdominal pain, anorexia, constipation, diarrhea, epigastric pain, nausea, vomiting, weight loss
Genitourinary: Hematuria (microscopic), proteinuria
Hematologic: Eosinophilia, leukopenia, monocytosis, pancytopenia
Ocular: Blurred vision, periorbital edema, photophobia
Miscellaneous: Hiccups, systemic lupus erythematosus
Drug Interactions
Metabolism/Transport Effects Substrate of CYP2C19 (major); **Note:** Assignment of Major/Minor substrate status based on clinically relevant drug interaction potential; **Inhibits** CYP2C19 (weak)
Avoid Concomitant Use
Avoid concomitant use of Methsuximide with any of the following: Azelastine; Azelastine (Nasal); Methadone; Mirtazapine; Paraldehyde
Increased Effect/Toxicity
Methsuximide may increase the levels/effects of: Alcohol (Ethyl); Azelastine; Azelastine (Nasal); Buprenorphine; CNS Depressants; Methadone; Methotrimeprazine; Metyrosine; Mirtazapine; Paraldehyde; Selective Serotonin Reuptake Inhibitors; Zolpidem

The levels/effects of Methsuximide may be increased by: CYP2C19 Inhibitors (Moderate); CYP2C19 Inhibitors (Strong); Droperidol; HydrOXYzine; Methotrimeprazine
Decreased Effect
The levels/effects of Methsuximide may be decreased by: CYP2C19 Inducers (Strong); Ketorolac; Ketorolac (Nasal); Ketorolac (Systemic); Mefloquine
Stability Store at 25°C (77°F); excursions permitted to 15°C to 30°C (59°F to 86°F); protect from excessive heat 40°C (104°F). Protect from light and moisture. **Note:** Methsuximide has a relatively low melting temperature (124°F); do not store in conditions that promote high temperatures (eg, in a closed vehicle).
Mechanism of Action Increases the seizure threshold and suppresses paroxysmal spike-and-wave pattern in absence seizures; depresses nerve transmission in the motor cortex

Pharmacodynamics/Kinetics
Metabolism: Hepatic; rapidly demethylated to N-desmethylmethsuximide (active metabolite)
Half-life elimination: 2-4 hours
Time to peak, serum: Within 1-3 hours
Excretion: Urine (<1% as unchanged drug)

Dosage
Geriatric & Adult Anticonvulsant: Oral: 300 mg/day for the first week; may increase by 300 mg/day at weekly intervals up to 1.2 g/day in 2-4 divided doses/day

Monitoring Parameters CBC, hepatic function tests, urinalysis; suicidality (eg, suicidal thoughts, depression, behavioral changes)

Reference Range Therapeutic: N-desmethylmethsuximide: 20-40 mcg/mL

Special Geriatric Considerations No specific data available for the elderly. This drug is rarely used in the elderly, however, if it is used for partial complex seizure control, monitor closely.

Dosage Forms Excipient information presented when available (limited, particularly for generics); consult specific product labeling.
Capsule, oral:
Celontin®: 150 mg, 300 mg

◆ **Methylacetoxyprogesterone** see MedroxyPROGESTERone on page 1190
◆ **Methylcobalamin, Acetylcysteine, and Methylfolate** see Methylfolate, Methylcobalamin, and Acetylcysteine on page 1246

Methyldopa (meth il DOE pa)

Related Information
Beers Criteria – Potentially Inappropriate Medications for Geriatrics on page 2183
Medication Safety Issues
Sound-alike/look-alike issues:
Methyldopa may be confused with L-dopa, levodopa
BEERS Criteria medication:
This drug may be potentially inappropriate for use in geriatric patients (Quality of evidence - low; Strength of recommendation - strong).
Brand Names: Canada Apo-Methyldopa®; Nu-Medopa
Index Terms Aldomet; Methyldopate Hydrochloride
Generic Availability (U.S.) Yes
Pharmacologic Category Alpha$_2$-Adrenergic Agonist
Use Management of moderate-to-severe hypertension
Contraindications Hypersensitivity to methyldopa or any component of the formulation; active hepatic disease; liver disorders previously associated with use of methyldopa; concurrent use of MAO inhibitors
Warnings/Precautions Rare cases of reversible granulocytopenia and thrombocytopenia have been reported. May rarely produce hemolytic anemia; positive Coombs' test occurs in 10% to 20% of patients (perform CBC periodically). If Coombs'-positive hemolytic anemia occurs during therapy, discontinue use and do not reinitiate; Coombs' test may not revert back to normal for weeks to months following discontinuation. Sedation (usually transient) may occur during initial therapy or whenever the dose is increased. May rarely produce liver disorders including fatal hepatic necrosis; use with caution in patients with previous liver disease or dysfunction. Periodically monitor liver function during the first 6-12 weeks of therapy or when unexplained fever occurs; discontinue use if fever, abnormal liver function tests, or jaundice is present. Patients with severe bilateral cerebrovascular disease have exhibited involuntary choreoathetotic movements (rare); discontinue use if these symptoms develop. Patients with impaired renal function may respond to smaller doses. Active metabolites of methyldopa accumulate in patients with renal impairment. Tolerance may occur usually between the second and third month of therapy; adding a diuretic or increasing the dosage of methyldopa frequently restores blood pressure control. May produce clinical edema; discontinue if edema worsens or signs of heart failure arise. Mild edema may be controlled with the concomitant use of diuretic therapy. May be inappropriate in the elderly due to a risk of bradycardia and depression (Beers Criteria); use with caution in the elderly; may experience syncope (avoid by giving smaller doses); not considered a drug of choice in this age group. Do not use injectable if bisulfite allergy.
Adverse Reactions (Reflective of adult population; not specific for elderly) Frequency not defined.
Cardiovascular: Angina pectoris aggravation, bradycardia, carotid sinus hypersensitivity prolonged, heart failure, myocarditis, orthostatic hypotension, paradoxical pressor response (I.V. use), pericarditis, peripheral edema, symptoms of cerebrovascular insufficiency, vasculitis

Central nervous system: Bell's palsy, dizziness, drug fever, headache, lightheadedness, mental acuity decreased, mental depression, nightmares, parkinsonism, sedation

Dermatologic: Rash, toxic epidermal necrolysis

Endocrine & metabolic: Amenorrhea, breast enlargement, gynecomastia, hyperprolactinemia, lactation, libido decreased

Gastrointestinal: Abdominal distension, colitis, constipation, diarrhea, flatulence, nausea, pancreatitis, sialadenitis, sore or "black" tongue, vomiting, weight gain, xerostomia

Genitourinary: Impotence

Hematologic: Bone marrow suppression, eosinophilia, granulocytopenia, hemolytic anemia; positive tests for ANA, LE cells, rheumatoid factor, Coombs test (positive); leukopenia, thrombocytopenia

Hepatic: Abnormal LFTs, liver disorders (hepatitis), jaundice

Neuromuscular & skeletal: Arthralgia, choreoathetosis, myalgia, paresthesias, weakness

Renal: BUN increased

Respiratory: Nasal congestion

Miscellaneous: SLE-like syndrome

Drug Interactions

Metabolism/Transport Effects Substrate of COMT

Avoid Concomitant Use

Avoid concomitant use of Methyldopa with any of the following: Iobenguane I 123; MAO Inhibitors

Increased Effect/Toxicity

Methyldopa may increase the levels/effects of: Amifostine; Antihypertensives; Lithium; RiTUXimab

The levels/effects of Methyldopa may be increased by: Alfuzosin; COMT Inhibitors; Diazoxide; Herbs (Hypotensive Properties); MAO Inhibitors; Pentoxifylline; Phosphodiesterase 5 Inhibitors; Prostacyclin Analogues

Decreased Effect

Methyldopa may decrease the levels/effects of: Iobenguane I 123

The levels/effects of Methyldopa may be decreased by: Herbs (Hypertensive Properties); Iron Salts; Methylphenidate; Yohimbine

Ethanol/Nutrition/Herb Interactions Herb/Nutraceutical: Avoid dong quai if using for hypertension (has estrogenic activity). Avoid ephedra, yohimbe, ginseng (may worsen hypertension). Avoid valerian, St John's wort, kava kava, gotu kola (may increase CNS depression). Avoid natural licorice (causes sodium and water retention and increases potassium loss). Avoid garlic (may have increased antihypertensive effect).

Stability

Injection: Store at controlled room temperature 20°C to 25°C (68°F to 77°F); excursions permitted to 15°C to 30°C (59°F to 86°F). Injectable dosage form is most stable at acid to neutral pH. Stability of parenteral admixture at room temperature (25°C) is 24 hours. Parenteral admixture is stable at room temperature for up to 125 hours (Newton, 1981). Standard diluent: 250-500 mg/100 mL D_5W.

Tablets: Store at controlled room temperature 20°C to 25°C (68°F to 77°F).

Mechanism of Action Stimulation of central alpha-adrenergic receptors by a false neurotransmitter (alpha-methylnorepinephrine) that results in a decreased sympathetic outflow to the heart, kidneys, and peripheral vasculature

Pharmacodynamics/Kinetics

Onset of action: Peak effect: Hypotensive: Oral, I.V.: 4-6 hours

Duration: Oral: Single-dose: 12-24, Multiple-dose: 24-48 hours; I.V.: 10-16 hours

Absorption: Oral: Incomplete due to presystemic gut metabolism (Skerjanec, 1995)

Distribution: V_d: 0.23 L/kg (Myhre, 1982)

Protein binding: 10% to 15% (Myhre, 1982)

Metabolism: Intestinal and hepatic

Bioavailability: ~42% (Skerjanec, 1995)

Half-life elimination: 1.5-2 hours; End-stage renal disease: Prolonged (Myhre, 1982)

Time to peak, plasma: Oral: 2-4 hours (Myhre, 1982)

Excretion: Urine (~70% as parent drug and metabolites); excretion complete within 36 hours

Dosage

Geriatric Refer to adult dosing. Initiate at the lower end of the dosage range.

Adult Hypertension:

Oral: Initial: 250 mg 2-3 times/day; increase every 2 days as needed (maximum dose: 3 g/day); usual dose range (JNC 7): 250-1000 mg/day in 2 divided doses. **Note:** When administered with other antihypertensives other than thiazide diuretics, limit initial daily dose of methyldopa to 500 mg/day.

I.V.: 250-1000 mg every 6-8 hours; maximum: 1 g every 6 hours

Renal Impairment
No dosage adjustment provided in manufacturer's labeling; however, the following adjustments have been recommended (Aronoff, 2007):
Cl_{cr} >50 mL/minute: Administer every 8 hours.
Cl_{cr} 10-50 mL/minute: Administer every 8-12 hours.
Cl_{cr} <10 mL/minute: Administer every 12-24 hours.
Intermittent hemodialysis (administer after hemodialysis on dialysis days): Moderately dialyzable (up to 60% with a 6-hour session) (Yeh, 1970).
Peritoneal dialysis (PD): Administer every 12-24 hours.
Continuous renal replacement therapy (CRRT): Administer every 8-12 hours. **Note:** Use of antihypertensives in patients requiring CRRT is generally not recommended since CRRT is typically employed when patient cannot tolerate intermittent hemodialysis due to hypotension.

Hepatic Impairment No dosage adjustment provided in manufacturer's labeling; however, use is contraindicated in patients with active hepatic disease (eg, acute hepatitis and cirrhosis).

Administration
I.V.: Infuse over 30-60 minutes.
Oral: Administer new dosage increases in the evening to minimize sedation.

Monitoring Parameters Blood pressure (standing and sitting/lying down), CBC, liver enzymes (periodically during the first 6-12 weeks or when unexplained fever occurs), Coombs' test (direct) (may obtain prior to initiation and at 6 and 12 months); blood pressure monitor required during I.V. administration

Test Interactions Methyldopa interferes with the following laboratory tests: urinary uric acid, serum creatinine (alkaline picrate method), AST (colorimetric method), and urinary catecholamines (falsely high levels)

Special Geriatric Considerations Because of its CNS effects, methyldopa is not considered a drug of first choice in the elderly. Adjust dose for renal function.

This medication is considered to be potentially inappropriate in this patient population (Beers Criteria: Quality of evidence - low; Strength of recommendation - strong).

Dosage Forms Excipient information presented when available (limited, particularly for generics); consult specific product labeling.
Injection, solution, as hydrochloride: 50 mg/mL (5 mL)
Tablet, oral: 250 mg, 500 mg

◆ **Methyldopate Hydrochloride** *see* Methyldopa *on page 1243*

Methylfolate (meth il FO late)

Brand Names: U.S. Deplin®
Index Terms 6(S)-5-methyltetrahydrofolate; 6(S)-5-MTHF; L-methylfolate
Generic Availability (U.S.) Yes
Pharmacologic Category Dietary Supplement
Use Medicinal food for management of patients with low plasma and/or low red blood cell folate
Contraindications Hypersensitivity to any component of the formulation
Warnings/Precautions Folate administration is not appropriate for monotherapy with pernicious or other megaloblastic anemias when anemia is present with vitamin B_{12} deficiency. Doses >0.1 mg/day may obscure pernicious anemia with continuing irreversible nerve damage progression. Product is a medicinal food for use only under the supervision of a healthcare provider.
Drug Interactions
Metabolism/Transport Effects None known.
Avoid Concomitant Use
Avoid concomitant use of Methylfolate with any of the following: Raltitrexed
Increased Effect/Toxicity There are no known significant interactions involving an increase in effect.
Decreased Effect
Methylfolate may decrease the levels/effects of: CarBAMazepine; Divalproex; Fosphenytoin; PHENobarbital; Phenytoin; Primidone; Pyrimethamine; Raltitrexed; Valproic Acid

The levels/effects of Methylfolate may be decreased by: Cholestyramine Resin; Colestipol; SulfaSALAzine
Stability Store at controlled room temperature of 15°C to 30°C (59°F to 86°F). Protect from light and moisture.
Mechanism of Action Methylfolate, or L-methylfolate, is the active form of folate in the body, which can be transported into peripheral tissues and across the blood-brain barrier. Folate is

necessary for formation of numerous coenzymes in many metabolic systems, particularly for purine, pyrimidine, and nucleoprotein synthesis, and maintenance in erythropoiesis; stimulates WBC and platelet production in folate deficiency anemia.

Dosage
Geriatric & Adult Medicinal food: Oral: One tablet (7.5 mg) daily
Pharmacotherapy Pearls Information in this monograph is currently limited to the fields presented. Consult product labeling for additional details.

The manufacturer of Deplin™ indicates a use of methylfolate in individuals who have a major depressive disorder that has not fully responded or may not fully respond to antidepressant therapy. Limited data exists of the investigational use of folate supplementation as an adjunct to the treatment of major depressive disorder. Adjunctive use in major depressive disorders requires further studies, but some studies (using various forms of folic acid) suggest a possible benefit of supplementation by augmentation of response to antidepressants, particularly in patients with low serum folate levels prior to supplementation.

Special Geriatric Considerations No special recommendations. Elderly frequently have combined nutritional deficiencies. Must rule out vitamin B_{12} deficiency before initiating folate therapy. Elderly, due to decreased nutrient intake, may benefit from daily intake of a multiple vitamin with minerals.

Dosage Forms Excipient information presented when available (limited, particularly for generics); consult specific product labeling.
Caplet, oral: L-methylfolate 15 mg
Deplin®: L-methylfolate 15 mg [gluten free, sugar free; contains tartrazine]
Tablet, oral: L-methylfolate 7.5 mg
Deplin®: L-methylfolate 7.5 mg [gluten free, sugar free]

Methylfolate, Methylcobalamin, and Acetylcysteine
(meth il FO late meth il koe BAL a min & a se teel SIS teen)

Related Information
Methylfolate *on page 1245*
Brand Names: U.S. Cerefolin® NAC
Index Terms Acetylcysteine, Methylcobalamin, and Methylfolate; Acetylcysteine, Methylfolate, and Methylcobalamin; L-methylfolate, Methylcobalamin, and N-acetylcysteine; Methylcobalamin, Acetylcysteine, and Methylfolate
Generic Availability (U.S.) No
Pharmacologic Category Dietary Supplement
Use Medicinal food for use in patients with neurovascular oxidative stress and/or hyperhomocysteinemia
Dosage
Adult Medicinal food: Oral: One caplet daily
Special Geriatric Considerations No specific information for use in elderly.
Dosage Forms Excipient information presented when available (limited, particularly for generics); consult specific product labeling.
Caplet, oral:
Cerefolin® NAC: L-methylfolate 5.6 mg, methylcobalamin 2 mg, and N-acetylcysteine 600 mg [gluten free, sugar free]

◆ **Methylin®** *see* Methylphenidate *on page 1247*
◆ **Methylin® ER [DSC]** *see* Methylphenidate *on page 1247*
◆ **Methylmorphine** *see* Codeine *on page 433*

Methylnaltrexone (meth il nal TREKS one)

Medication Safety Issues
Sound-alike/look-alike issues:
Methylnaltrexone may be confused with naltrexone
Brand Names: U.S. Relistor®
Brand Names: Canada Relistor®
Index Terms Methylnaltrexone Bromide; N-methylnaltrexone Bromide
Generic Availability (U.S.) No
Pharmacologic Category Gastrointestinal Agent, Miscellaneous; Opioid Antagonist, Peripherally-Acting
Use Treatment of opioid-induced constipation in patients with advanced illness receiving palliative care with inadequate response to conventional laxative regimens

Dosage

Geriatric & Adult Opioid-induced constipation: SubQ: Dosing is according to body weight: Administer 1 dose every other day as needed; maximum: 1 dose/24 hours

<38 kg: 0.15 mg/kg (round dose up to nearest 0.1 mL of volume)

38 to <62 kg: 8 mg

62-114 kg: 12 mg

>114 kg: 0.15 mg/kg (round dose up to nearest 0.1 mL of volume)

Renal Impairment

Mild-to-moderate renal impairment: No adjustment required.

Severe renal impairment (Cl_{cr} <30 mL/minute): Administer 50% of normal dose.

End-stage renal impairment (dialysis-dependent): Has not been studied.

Hepatic Impairment

Mild-to-moderate hepatic impairment (Child-Pugh class A or B): No adjustment required.

Severe hepatic impairment: Has not been studied.

Special Geriatric Considerations In small studies (Phase 2 and 3), no differences in safety and efficacy were noted between elderly and young adults. No dose adjustment is required in elderly.

Dosage Forms Excipient information presented when available (limited, particularly for generics); consult specific product labeling.

Injection, solution:

Relistor®: 8 mg/0.4 mL (0.4 mL); 12 mg/0.6 mL (0.6 mL) [contains edetate calcium disodium; prefilled syringe]

Relistor®: 12 mg/0.6 mL (0.6 mL) [contains edetate calcium disodium; vial]

◆ **Methylnaltrexone Bromide** see Methylnaltrexone on page 1246

Methylphenidate (meth il FEN i date)

Related Information

Patient Information for Disposal of Unused Medications on page 2244

Medication Safety Issues

Sound-alike/look-alike issues:

Metadate CD® may be confused with Metadate® ER

Metadate® ER may be confused with methadone

Methylphenidate may be confused with methadone

Ritalin® may be confused with Rifadin®, ritodrine

Ritalin LA® may be confused with Ritalin-SR®

Brand Names: U.S. Concerta®; Daytrana®; Metadate CD®; Metadate® ER; Methylin®; Methylin® ER [DSC]; Ritalin LA®; Ritalin-SR®; Ritalin®

Brand Names: Canada Apo-Methylphenidate®; Apo-Methylphenidate® SR; Biphentin®; Concerta®; PHL-Methylphenidate; PMS-Methylphenidate; ratio-Methylphenidate; Ritalin®; Ritalin® SR; Sandoz-Methylphenidate SR; Teva-Methylphenidate ER-C

Index Terms Methylphenidate Hydrochloride

Generic Availability (U.S.) Yes: Extended release capsule, extended/sustained release tablet, immediate release tablet, oral solution

Pharmacologic Category Central Nervous System Stimulant

Use Treatment of attention-deficit/hyperactivity disorder (ADHD); symptomatic management of narcolepsy

Unlabeled Use Depression (especially elderly or medically ill)

Medication Guide Available Yes

Contraindications Hypersensitivity to methylphenidate, any component of the formulation, or idiosyncratic reactions to sympathomimetic amines; marked anxiety, tension, and agitation; glaucoma; use during or within 14 days following MAO inhibitor therapy; family history or diagnosis of Tourette's syndrome or tics

Metadate CD® and Metadate® ER: Additional contraindications: Severe hypertension, heart failure, arrhythmia, hyperthyroidism, recent MI or angina; concomitant use of halogenated anesthetics

Warnings/Precautions CNS stimulant use has been associated with serious cardiovascular events (eg, sudden death in children and adolescents; sudden death, stroke, and MI in adults) in patients with pre-existing structural cardiac abnormalities or other serious heart problems. These products should be avoided in patients with known serious structural cardiac abnormalities, cardiomyopathy, serious heart rhythm abnormalities, or other serious cardiac problems that could further increase their risk of sudden death. Patients should be carefully evaluated for cardiac disease prior to initiation of therapy. Use of stimulants can cause an increase in blood pressure (average 2-4 mm Hg) and increases in heart rate (average 3-6 bpm), although some patients may have larger than average increases. Use caution with hypertension, hyperthyroidism, or other cardiovascular conditions that might be exacerbated by increases in blood pressure or heart rate. Some products are contraindicated in patients with heart failure, arrhythmias, severe hypertension, hyperthyroidism, angina, or recent MI.

Has demonstrated value as part of a comprehensive treatment program for ADHD. Use with caution in patients with bipolar disorder (may induce mixed/manic episode). May exacerbate symptoms of behavior and thought disorder in psychotic patients; new-onset psychosis or mania may occur with stimulant use; observe for symptoms of aggression and/or hostility. Use caution with seizure disorders (may reduce seizure threshold). Use caution in patients with history of ethanol or drug abuse. May exacerbate symptoms of behavior and thought disorder in psychotic patients. **[U.S. Boxed Warning]: Potential for drug dependency exists - avoid abrupt discontinuation in patients who have received for prolonged periods.** Visual disturbances have been reported (rare).

Concerta® should not be used in patients with esophageal motility disorders or pre-existing severe gastrointestinal narrowing (small bowel disease, short gut syndrome, history of peritonitis, cystic fibrosis, chronic intestinal pseudo-obstruction, Meckel's diverticulum). Metadate CD® contains sucrose; avoid administration in fructose intolerance, glucose-galactose malabsorption, or sucrase-isomaltase insufficiency. Metadate® ER contains lactose; avoid administration in hereditary galactose intolerance, Lapp lactase deficiency, or glucose-galactose malabsorption. Concomitant use with halogenated anesthetics is contraindicated; may cause sudden elevations in blood pressure; if surgery is planned, do not administer Metadate CD® or Metadate® ER on the day of surgery. Transdermal system may cause allergic contact sensitization, characterized by intense local reactions (edema, papules) that may spread beyond the patch site; sensitization may subsequently manifest systemically with other routes of methylphenidate administration; monitor closely. Avoid exposure of application site to any direct external heat sources (eg, hair dryers, heating pads, electric blankets); may increase the rate and extent of absorption and risk of overdose. Efficacy of transdermal methylphenidate therapy for >7 weeks has not been established.

Adverse Reactions (Reflective of adult population; not specific for elderly)
All dosage forms: Frequency not defined:
Cardiovascular: Angina, cardiac arrhythmia, cerebral arteritis, cerebral hemorrhage, cerebral occlusion, cerebrovascular accidents, vasculitis, hyper-/hypotension, MI, murmur, palpitation, pulse increased/decreased, Raynaud's phenomenon, tachycardia
Central nervous system: Aggression, agitation, anger, anxiety, confusional state, depression, dizziness, drowsiness, fatigue, fever, headache, hypervigilance, insomnia, irritability, lethargy, mood alterations, nervousness, neuroleptic malignant syndrome (NMS) (rare), restlessness, stroke, tension, Tourette's syndrome (rare), toxic psychosis, tremor, vertigo
Dermatologic: Alopecia, erythema multiforme, exfoliative dermatitis, hyperhidrosis, rash, urticaria
Endocrine & metabolic: Dysmenorrhea, growth retardation, libido decreased
Gastrointestinal: Abdominal pain, anorexia, appetite decreased, bruxism, constipation, diarrhea, dyspepsia, nausea, vomiting, weight loss, xerostomia
Genitourinary: Erectile dysfunction
Hematologic: Anemia, leukopenia, pancytopenia, thrombocytopenic purpura, thrombocytopenia
Hepatic: Bilirubin increased, liver function tests abnormal, hepatic coma, transaminases increased
Neuromuscular & skeletal: Arthralgia, dyskinesia, muscle tightness, paresthesia
Ocular: Blurred vision, dry eyes, mydriasis, visual accommodation disturbance
Renal: Necrotizing vasculitis
Respiratory: Cough increased, dyspnea, pharyngitis, pharyngolaryngeal pain, rhinitis, sinusitis, upper respiratory tract infection
Miscellaneous: Accidental injury, hypersensitivity reactions

Transdermal system: Frequency of adverse events as reported in trials of 7-week duration. Incidence of some events higher with extended use.
>10%:
Central nervous system: Headache (≤15%; long-term use in children: 28%), insomnia (6% to 13%; long-term use in children: 30%), irritability (7% to 11%)
Gastrointestinal: Appetite decreased (26%), nausea (10% to 12%)
Miscellaneous: Viral infection (long-term use in children: 28%)
1% to 10%:
Cardiovascular: Tachycardia (≤1%)
Central nervous system: Tic (7%), dizziness (adolescents 6%), emotional instability (6%)
Gastrointestinal: Vomiting (3% to 10%), weight loss (6% to 9%), abdominal pain (5% to 7%), anorexia (5%; long-term use in children: 46%)
Local: Application site reaction
Respiratory: Nasal congestion (6%) nasopharyngitis (5%)

Postmarketing and/or case reports (limited to important or life-threatening): Allergic contact dermatitis/sensitization, anaphylaxis, angioedema, hallucinations, seizures

Drug Interactions

Metabolism/Transport Effects Inhibits CYP2D6 (weak)

Avoid Concomitant Use

Avoid concomitant use of Methylphenidate with any of the following: Inhalational Anesthetics; Iobenguane I 123; MAO Inhibitors

Increased Effect/Toxicity

Methylphenidate may increase the levels/effects of: Anti-Parkinson's Agents (Dopamine Agonist); Antipsychotics; CloNIDine; Fosphenytoin; Inhalational Anesthetics; PHENobarbital; Phenytoin; Primidone; Sympathomimetics; Tricyclic Antidepressants; Vitamin K Antagonists

The levels/effects of Methylphenidate may be increased by: Antacids; Antipsychotics; AtoMOXetine; Cannabinoids; H2-Antagonists; MAO Inhibitors; Proton Pump Inhibitors

Decreased Effect

Methylphenidate may decrease the levels/effects of: Antihypertensives; Iobenguane I 123; Ioflupane I 123

Ethanol/Nutrition/Herb Interactions

Ethanol: Avoid ethanol (may cause CNS depression).

Food: Food may increase oral absorption; Concerta® formulation is not affected. Food delays early peak and high-fat meals increase C_{max} and AUC of Metadate CD® formulation.

Herb/Nutraceutical: Avoid ephedra (may cause hypertension or arrhythmias) and yohimbe (also has CNS stimulatory activity).

Stability

Capsule: *Extended release:* Store at 25°C (77°F); excursions permitted to 15°C to 30°C (59°F to 86°F). Protect from light.

Solution: Store at controlled room temperature of 20°C to 25°C (68°F to 77°F).

Tablet:

Chewable: Store at controlled room temperature of 20°C to 25°C (68°F to 77°F). Protect from light and moisture.

Extended and sustained release: Store at controlled room temperature of 20°C to 25°C (68°F to 77°F). Protect from light and moisture.

Immediate release: Store at controlled room temperature of 20°C to 25°C (68°F to 77°F). Protect from light and moisture.

Osmotic controlled release (Concerta®): Store at controlled room temperature of 25°C; excursions permitted to 15°C to 30°C (59°F to 86°F). Protect from humidity.

Transdermal system: Store at 25°C (77°F); excursions permitted to 15°C to 30°C (59°F to 86°F). Keep patches stored in protective pouch. Once tray is opened, use patches within 2 months; once an individual patch has been removed from the pouch and the protective liner removed, use immediately. Do not refrigerate or freeze.

Mechanism of Action Mild CNS stimulant; blocks the reuptake of norepinephrine and dopamine into presynaptic neurons; appears to stimulate the cerebral cortex and subcortical structures similar to amphetamines

Pharmacodynamics/Kinetics

Onset of action: Peak effect:

Immediate release tablet: Cerebral stimulation: ~2 hours

Extended release capsule (Metadate CD®, Ritalin LA®): Biphasic; initial peak similar to immediate release product, followed by second rising portion (corresponding to extended release portion)

Sustained release tablet: 4-7 hours

Osmotic release tablet (Concerta®): Initial: 1-2 hours

Transdermal: ~2 hours; may be expedited by the application of external heat

Duration: Immediate release tablet: 3-6 hours; Sustained release tablet: 8 hours; Extended release tablet: Methylin® ER, Metadate® ER: 8 hours, Concerta®: 12 hours

Absorption:

Oral: Readily absorbed

Transdermal: Absorption increased when applied to inflamed skin or exposed to heat. Absorption is continuous for 9 hours after application.

Distribution: V_d: *d*-methylphenidate: 2.65 ± 1.11 L/kg, *l*-methylphenidate: 1.80 ± 0.91 L/kg

Protein binding: 10% to 33%

Metabolism: Hepatic via carboxylesterase CES1A1 to minimally active metabolite

Half-life elimination: *d*-methylphenidate: 3-4 hours; *l*-methylphenidate: 1-3 hours

Time to peak: Concerta®: C_{max}: 6-8 hours; Daytrana™: 7.5-10.5 hours

Excretion: Urine (90% as metabolites and unchanged drug)

Dosage
  Geriatric & Adult
  ADHD: Oral:
  Concerta®:
  Patients not currently taking methylphenidate: Initial dose:
    U.S. labeling: 18-36 mg once every morning
    Canadian labeling: 18 mg once every morning
  Patients currently taking methylphenidate: **Note:** Initial dose: Dosing based on current regimen and clinical judgment; suggested dosing listed below:
    - Patients taking methylphenidate 5 mg 2-3 times/day **or** methylphenidate SR 20 mg/day (Canadian labeling; not in U.S. labeling): 18 mg once every morning
    - Patients taking methylphenidate 10 mg 2-3 times/day **or** methylphenidate SR 40 mg/day (Canadian labeling; not in U.S. labeling): 36 mg once every morning
    - Patients taking methylphenidate 15 mg 2-3 times/day **or** methylphenidate SR 60 mg/day (Canadian labeling; not in U.S. labeling): 54 mg once every morning
    - Patients taking methylphenidate 20 mg 2-3 times/day: 72 mg once every morning
  Dose adjustment: May increase dose in increments of 18 mg; dose may be adjusted at weekly intervals. A dosage strength of 27 mg is available for situations in which a dosage between 18-36 mg is desired. Maximum dose: 72 mg/day.
  Metadate® ER, Methylin® ER, Ritalin® SR: May be given in place of immediate release products, once the daily dose is titrated and the titrated 8-hour dosage corresponds to sustained or extended release tablet size; maximum: 60 mg/day
  Metadate CD®, Ritalin LA®: Initial: 20 mg once daily; may be adjusted in 10-20 mg increments at weekly intervals; maximum: 60 mg/day

  Narcolepsy: Oral: 10 mg 2-3 times/day, up to 60 mg/day

  Depression (unlabeled use): Oral: Initial: 2.5 mg every morning before 9 AM; dosage may be increased by 2.5-5 mg every 2-3 days as tolerated to a maximum of 20 mg/day; may be divided (ie, 7 AM and 12 noon), but should not be given after noon; do not use sustained release product
  Note: Discontinue periodically to re-evaluate or if no improvement occurs within 1 month.
Administration
  Oral: Do not crush or allow patient to chew sustained or extended release dosage form. To effectively avoid insomnia, dosing should be completed by noon.
    Concerta®: Administer dose once daily in the morning. May be taken with or without food, but must be taken with water, milk, or juice.
    Metadate CD®, Ritalin LA®: Capsules may be opened and the contents sprinkled onto a small amount (equal to 1 tablespoon) of cold applesauce. Swallow applesauce without chewing. Do not crush or chew capsule contents.
    Methylin® chewable tablet: Administer with at least 8 ounces of water or other fluid.
  Topical: Transdermal (Daytrana™): Apply to clean, dry, non-oily, intact skin to the hip area, avoiding the waistline; do not premedicate the patch site with hydrocortisone or other solutions, creams, ointments, or emollients. Apply at the same time each day to alternating hips. Press firmly for 30 seconds to ensure proper adherence. Avoid exposure of application site to external heat source, which may increase the amount of drug absorbed. If difficulty is experienced when separating the patch from the liner or if any medication (sticky substance) remains on the liner after separation; discard that patch and apply a new patch. Do not use a patch that has been damaged or torn; do not cut patch. If patch should dislodge, may replace with new patch (to different site) but total wear time should not exceed 9 hours; do not reapply with dressings, tape, or common adhesives. Patch may be removed early if a shorter duration of effect is desired or if late day side effects occur. Wash hands with soap and water after handling. Avoid touching the sticky side of the patch. If patch removal is difficult, an oil-based product (eg, petroleum jelly, olive oil) may be applied to the patch edges to aid removal; never apply acetone-based products (eg, nail polish remover) to patch. Dispose of used patch by folding adhesive side onto itself, and discard in toilet or appropriate lidded container.
Monitoring Parameters Blood pressure, heart rate, signs and symptoms of depression, aggression, or hostility; CBC, differential and platelet counts, liver function tests; signs of central nervous system stimulation

  Transdermal: Signs of worsening erythema, blistering or edema which does not improve within 48 hours of patch removal, or spreads beyond patch site.

  When used for the treatment of ADHD, thoroughly evaluate for cardiovascular risk. Monitor heart rate, blood pressure, and consider obtaining ECG prior to initiation (Vetter, 2008).

Test Interactions May interfere with urine detection of amphetamines/methamphetamines (false-positive).

Pharmacotherapy Pearls Treatment with methylphenidate may include "drug holidays" or periodic discontinuation in order to assess the patient's requirements and to decrease tolerance and limit suppression of linear growth and weight. Specific patients may require 3 doses/day for treatment of ADHD (ie, additional dose at 4 PM).

Concerta® is an osmotic controlled release formulation (OROS®) of methylphenidate. The tablet has an immediate-release overcoat that provides an initial dose of methylphenidate within 1 hour. The overcoat covers a trilayer core. The trilayer core is composed of two layers containing the drug and excipients, and one layer of osmotic components. As water from the gastrointestinal tract enters the core, the osmotic components expand and methylphenidate is released.

Metadate CD® capsules contain a mixture of immediate release and extended release beads, designed to release 30% of the dose immediately and 70% over an extended period.

Ritalin LA® uses a combination of immediate release and enteric coated, delayed release beads.

Special Geriatric Considerations Methylphenidate is often useful in treating elderly patients who are discouraged, withdrawn, apathetic, or disinterested in their activities. In particular, it is useful in patients who are starting a rehabilitation program but have resigned themselves to fail; these patients may not have a major depressive disorder; will not improve memory or cognitive function; use with caution in patients with dementia who may have increased agitation and confusion. In elderly patients with insomnia, this medication is considered potentially inappropriate (Beers Criteria, 2012).

Controlled Substance C-II

Dosage Forms Excipient information presented when available (limited, particularly for generics); consult specific product labeling. [DSC] = Discontinued product

Capsule, extended release, oral, as hydrochloride [bi-modal release]: 20 mg [generic for Ritalin LA®], 30 mg [generic for Ritalin LA®], 40 mg [generic for Ritalin LA®]

Metadate CD®: 10 mg [contains sucrose; 3 mg immediate release, 7 mg extended release]

Metadate CD®: 20 mg [contains sucrose; 6 mg immediate release, 14 mg extended release]

Metadate CD®: 30 mg [contains sucrose; 9 mg immediate release, 21 mg extended release]

Metadate CD®: 40 mg [contains sucrose; 12 mg immediate release, 28 mg extended release]

Metadate CD®: 50 mg [contains sucrose; 15 mg immediate release, 35 mg extended release]

Metadate CD®: 60 mg [contains sucrose; 18 mg immediate release, 42 mg extended release]

Ritalin LA®: 10 mg [5 mg immediate release, 5 mg extended release]

Ritalin LA®: 20 mg [10 mg immediate release, 10 mg extended release]

Ritalin LA®: 30 mg [15 mg immediate release, 15 mg extended release]

Ritalin LA®: 40 mg [20 mg immediate release, 20 mg extended release]

Patch, transdermal:

Daytrana®: 10 mg/9 hours (30s) [12.5 cm^2, total methylphenidate 27.5 mg]

Daytrana®: 15 mg/9 hours (30s) [18.75 cm^2, total methylphenidate 41.3 mg]

Daytrana®: 20 mg/9 hours (30s) [25 cm^2, total methylphenidate 55 mg]

Daytrana®: 30 mg/9 hours (30s) [37.5 cm^2, total methylphenidate 82.5 mg]

Solution, oral, as hydrochloride: 5 mg/5 mL (500 mL); 10 mg/mL (500 mL)

Methylin®: 5 mg/5 mL (500 mL); 10 mg/5 mL (500 mL) [grape flavor]

Tablet, oral, as hydrochloride: 5 mg, 10 mg, 20 mg

Methylin®: 5 mg [DSC]

Methylin®: 10 mg [DSC], 20 mg [DSC] [scored]

Ritalin®: 5 mg

Ritalin®: 10 mg, 20 mg [scored]

Tablet, chewable, oral, as hydrochloride:

Methylin®: 2.5 mg [contains phenylalanine 0.42 mg/tablet; grape flavor]

Methylin®: 5 mg [contains phenylalanine 0.84 mg/tablet; grape flavor]

Methylin®: 10 mg [scored; contains phenylalanine 1.68 mg/tablet; grape flavor]

Tablet, extended release, oral, as hydrochloride: 10 mg, 20 mg

Metadate® ER: 20 mg [contains lactose]

Methylin® ER: 10 mg [DSC], 20 mg [DSC]

Tablet, extended release, oral, as hydrochloride [bi-modal release]: 18 mg, 27 mg, 36 mg, 54 mg
Concerta®: 18 mg [4 mg immediate release, 14 mg extended release]
Concerta®: 27 mg [6 mg immediate release, 21 mg extended release]
Concerta®: 36 mg [8 mg immediate release, 28 mg extended release]
Concerta®: 54 mg [12 mg immediate release, 42 mg extended release]
Tablet, sustained release, oral, as hydrochloride: 20 mg
Ritalin-SR®: 20 mg [dye free]

- ◆ **Methylphenidate Hydrochloride** see Methylphenidate on page 1247
- ◆ **Methylphenyl Isoxazolyl Penicillin** see Oxacillin on page 1434
- ◆ **Methylphytyl Napthoquinone** see Phytonadione on page 1534

MethylPREDNISolone (meth il pred NIS oh lone)

Related Information
Corticosteroids Systemic Equivalencies on page 2112

Medication Safety Issues
Sound-alike/look-alike issues:
MethylPREDNISolone may be confused with medroxyPROGESTERone, methotrexate, methylTESTOSTERone, predniSONE
Depo-Medrol® may be confused with Solu-Medrol®
Medrol® may be confused with Mebaral®
Solu-MEDROL® may be confused with salmeterol, Solu-CORTEF®

International issues:
Medrol [U.S., Canada, and multiple international markets] may be confused with Medral brand name for omeprazole [Mexico]

Brand Names: U.S. A-Methapred®; Depo-Medrol®; Medrol®; Medrol® Dosepak™; Solu-MEDROL®

Brand Names: Canada Depo-Medrol®; Medrol®; Methylprednisolone Acetate; Solu-Medrol®

Index Terms 6-α-Methylprednisolone; A-Methapred; Medrol Dose Pack; Methylprednisolone Acetate; Methylprednisolone Sodium Succinate; Solumedrol

Generic Availability (U.S.) Yes: Excludes preservative free injection

Pharmacologic Category Corticosteroid, Systemic

Use Primarily as an anti-inflammatory or immunosuppressant agent in the treatment of a variety of diseases including those of hematologic, allergic, inflammatory, neoplastic, and autoimmune origin. Prevention and treatment of graft-versus-host disease following allogeneic bone marrow transplantation.

Unlabeled Use Acute spinal cord injury

Contraindications Hypersensitivity to methylprednisolone or any component of the formulation; systemic fungal infection (except intra-articular injection in localized joint conditions); administration of live virus vaccines. I.M. administration in idiopathic thrombocytopenia purpura; intrathecal administration

Warnings/Precautions Use with caution in patients with thyroid disease, hepatic impairment, renal impairment, cardiovascular disease, diabetes, glaucoma, cataracts, myasthenia gravis, patients at risk for osteoporosis, patients at risk for seizures, or GI diseases (diverticulitis, peptic ulcer, ulcerative colitis) due to perforation risk. Not recommended for the treatment of optic neuritis; may increase frequency of new episodes. Use caution following acute MI (corticosteroids have been associated with myocardial rupture). Cardiomegaly and congestive heart failure have been reported following concurrent use of amphotericin B and hydrocortisone for the management of fungal infections.

Because of the risk of adverse effects, systemic corticosteroids should be used cautiously in the elderly in the smallest possible effective dose for the shortest duration. Withdraw therapy with gradual tapering of dose.

May cause hypercorticism or suppression of hypothalamic-pituitary-adrenal (HPA) axis, particularly in younger children or in patients receiving high doses for prolonged periods. HPA axis suppression may lead to adrenal crisis. Withdrawal and discontinuation of a corticosteroid should be done slowly and carefully. Particular care is required when patients are transferred from systemic corticosteroids to inhaled products due to possible adrenal insufficiency or withdrawal from steroids, including an increase in allergic symptoms. Patients receiving >20 mg per day of prednisone (or equivalent) may be most susceptible. Fatalities have occurred due to adrenal insufficiency in asthmatic patients during and after transfer from systemic corticosteroids to aerosol steroids; aerosol steroids do not provide the systemic steroid needed to treat patients having trauma, surgery, or infections.

Acute myopathy has been reported with high dose corticosteroids, usually in patients with neuromuscular transmission disorders; may involve ocular and/or respiratory muscles; monitor creatine kinase; recovery may be delayed. Corticosteroid use may cause psychiatric disturbances, including depression, euphoria, insomnia, mood swings, and personality changes. Pre-existing psychiatric conditions may be exacerbated by corticosteroid use. Prolonged use of corticosteroids may also increase the incidence of secondary infection, cause activation of latent infections, mask acute infection (including fungal infections), prolong or exacerbate viral or parasitic infections, or limit response to vaccines. Exposure to chickenpox or measles should be avoided; corticosteroids should not be used to treat ocular herpes simplex. Corticosteroids should not be used for cerebral malaria or viral hepatitis. Close observation is required in patients with latent tuberculosis and/or TB reactivity; restrict use in active TB (only in conjunction with antituberculosis treatment). Amebiasis should be ruled out in any patient with recent travel to tropic climates or unexplained diarrhea prior to initiation of corticosteroids. Prolonged treatment with corticosteroids has been associated with the development of Kaposi's sarcoma (case reports); discontinuation may result in clinical improvement.

High-dose corticosteroids should not be used to manage acute head injury. Rare cases of anaphylactoid reactions have been observed in patients receiving corticosteroids. Avoid injection or leakage into the dermis; dermal and/or subdermal skin depression may occur at the site of injection. Avoid deltoid muscle injection; subcutaneous atrophy may occur.

Adverse Reactions (Reflective of adult population; not specific for elderly) Frequency not defined.

Cardiovascular: Arrhythmias, bradycardia, cardiac arrest, cardiomegaly, circulatory collapse, congestive heart failure, edema, fat embolism, hypertension, hypertrophic cardiomyopathy in premature infants, myocardial rupture (post MI), syncope, tachycardia, thromboembolism, vasculitis

Central nervous system: Delirium, depression, emotional instability, euphoria, hallucinations, headache, intracranial pressure increased, insomnia, malaise, mood swings, nervousness, neuritis, personality changes, psychic disorders, pseudotumor cerebri (usually following discontinuation), seizure, vertigo

Dermatologic: Acne, allergic dermatitis, alopecia, dry scaly skin, ecchymoses, edema, erythema, hirsutism, hyper-/hypopigmentation, hypertrichosis, impaired wound healing, petechiae, rash, skin atrophy, sterile abscess, skin test reaction impaired, striae, urticaria

Endocrine & metabolic: Adrenal suppression, amenorrhea, carbohydrate intolerance increased, Cushing's syndrome, diabetes mellitus, fluid retention, glucose intolerance, growth suppression (children), hyperglycemia, hyperlipidemia, hypokalemia, hypokalemic alkalosis, menstrual irregularities, negative nitrogen balance, pituitary-adrenal axis suppression, protein catabolism, sodium and water retention

Gastrointestinal: Abdominal distention, appetite increased, bowel/bladder dysfunction (after intrathecal administration), gastrointestinal hemorrhage, gastrointestinal perforation, nausea, pancreatitis, peptic ulcer, perforation of the small and large intestine, ulcerative esophagitis, vomiting, weight gain

Hematologic: Leukocytosis (transient)

Hepatic: Hepatomegaly, transaminases increased

Local: Postinjection flare (intra-articular use), thrombophlebitis

Neuromuscular & skeletal: Arthralgia, arthropathy, aseptic necrosis (femoral and humoral heads), fractures, muscle mass loss, muscle weakness, myopathy (particularly in conjunction with neuromuscular disease or neuromuscular-blocking agents), neuropathy, osteoporosis, parasthesia, tendon rupture, vertebral compression fractures, weakness

Ocular: Cataracts, exophthalmoses, glaucoma, intraocular pressure increased

Renal: Glycosuria

Respiratory: Pulmonary edema

Miscellaneous: Abnormal fat disposition, anaphylactoid reaction, anaphylaxis, angioedema, avascular necrosis, diaphoresis, hiccups, hypersensitivity reactions, infections, secondary malignancy

Drug Interactions

Metabolism/Transport Effects Substrate of CYP3A4 (minor); **Note:** Assignment of Major/Minor substrate status based on clinically relevant drug interaction potential; **Inhibits** CYP2C8 (weak), CYP3A4 (weak)

Avoid Concomitant Use

Avoid concomitant use of MethylPREDNISolone with any of the following: Aldesleukin; BCG; Mifepristone; Natalizumab; Pimecrolimus; Pimozide; Tacrolimus (Topical)

Increased Effect/Toxicity

MethylPREDNISolone may increase the levels/effects of: Acetylcholinesterase Inhibitors; Amphotericin B; ARIPiprazole; CycloSPORINE; CycloSPORINE (Systemic); Deferasirox; Leflunomide; Loop Diuretics; Natalizumab; NSAID (COX-2 Inhibitor); NSAID (Nonselective); Pimozide; Thiazide Diuretics; Vaccines (Live); Warfarin

METHYLPREDNISOLONE

The levels/effects of MethylPREDNISolone may be increased by: Antifungal Agents (Azole Derivatives, Systemic); Aprepitant; Calcium Channel Blockers (Nondihydropyridine); Cyclo-SPORINE; CycloSPORINE (Systemic); CYP3A4 Inhibitors (Strong); Denosumab; Estrogen Derivatives; Fluconazole; Fosaprepitant; Indacaterol; Macrolide Antibiotics; Mifepristone; Neuromuscular-Blocking Agents (Nondepolarizing); Pimecrolimus; Quinolone Antibiotics; Roflumilast; Salicylates; Tacrolimus (Topical); Telaprevir; Trastuzumab

Decreased Effect

MethylPREDNISolone may decrease the levels/effects of: Aldesleukin; Antidiabetic Agents; BCG; Calcitriol; Coccidioidin Skin Test; Corticorelin; CycloSPORINE; CycloSPORINE (Systemic); Hyaluronidase; Isoniazid; Salicylates; Sipuleucel-T; Telaprevir; Vaccines (Inactivated)

The levels/effects of MethylPREDNISolone may be decreased by: Aminoglutethimide; Antacids; Barbiturates; Bile Acid Sequestrants; CarBAMazepine; Echinacea; Fosphenytoin; Mifepristone; Mitotane; Phenytoin; Primidone; Rifamycin Derivatives; Tocilizumab

Ethanol/Nutrition/Herb Interactions

Ethanol: Ethanol may increase gastric mucosal irritation. Management: Avoid ethanol.

Food: Methylprednisolone interferes with calcium absorption. May cause GI upset. Management: Administer with food. Limit caffeine.

Herb/Nutraceutical: St John's wort may decrease methylprednisolone levels. Cat's claw and echinacea have immunostimulant properties. Management: Avoid St John's wort, cat's claw, and echinacea.

Stability

Intact vials of methylprednisolone sodium succinate should be stored at controlled room temperature of 20°C to 25°C (68°F to 77°F). Protect from light.

Reconstituted solutions of methylprednisolone sodium succinate should be stored at room temperature of 20°C to 25°C (68°F to 77°F), and used within 48 hours.

Stability of parenteral admixture at room temperature (25°C) and at refrigeration temperature (4°C) is 48 hours.

Standard diluent (Solu-Medrol®): 40 mg/50 mL D_5W; 125 mg/50 mL D_5W.

Minimum volume (Solu-Medrol®): 50 mL D_5W.

Mechanism of Action In a tissue-specific manner, corticosteroids regulate gene expression subsequent to binding specific intracellular receptors and translocation into the nucleus. Corticosteroids exert a wide array of physiologic effects including modulation of carbohydrate, protein, and lipid metabolism and maintenance of fluid and electrolyte homeostasis. Moreover cardiovascular, immunologic, musculoskeletal, endocrine, and neurologic physiology are influenced by corticosteroids. Decreases inflammation by suppression of migration of poly-morphonuclear leukocytes and reversal of increased capillary permeability.

Pharmacodynamics/Kinetics

Onset of action: Peak effect (route dependent): Oral: 1-2 hours; I.M.: 4-8 days; Intra-articular: 1 week; methylprednisolone sodium succinate is highly soluble and has a rapid effect by I.M. and I.V. routes

Duration (route dependent): Oral: 30-36 hours; I.M.: 1-4 weeks; Intra-articular: 1-5 weeks; methylprednisolone acetate has a low solubility and has a sustained I.M. effect

Distribution: V_d: 0.7-1.5 L/kg

Half-life elimination: 3-3.5 hours; reduced in obese

Excretion: Clearance: Reduced in obese

Dosage

Geriatric & Adult Only sodium succinate may be given I.V.; methylprednisolone sodium succinate is highly soluble and has a rapid effect by I.M. and I.V. routes. Methylprednisolone acetate has a low solubility and has a sustained I.M. effect.

Acute spinal cord injury (unlabeled use): I.V. (sodium succinate): 30 mg/kg over 15 minutes, followed in 45 minutes by a continuous infusion of 5.4 mg/kg/hour for 23 hours. **Note:** Due to insufficient evidence of clinical efficacy (ie, preserving or improving spinal cord function), the routine use of methylprednisolone in the treatment of acute spinal cord injury is no longer recommended. If used in this setting, methylprednisolone should not be initiated >8 hours after the injury; not effective in penetrating trauma (eg, gunshot) (Consortium for Spinal Cord Medicine, 2008).

Allergic conditions: Oral: Tapered-dosage schedule (eg, dose-pack containing 21 x 4 mg tablets):

Day 1: 24 mg on day 1 administered as 8 mg (2 tablets) before breakfast, 4 mg (1 tablet) after lunch, 4 mg (1 tablet) after supper, and 8 mg (2 tablets) at bedtime **OR** 24 mg (6 tablets) as a single dose or divided into 2 or 3 doses upon initiation (regardless of time of day)

Day 2: 20 mg on day 2 administered as 4 mg (1 tablet) before breakfast, 4 mg (1 tablet) after lunch, 4 mg (1 tablet) after supper, and 8 mg (2 tablets) at bedtime

Day 3: 16 mg on day 3 administered as 4 mg (1 tablet) before breakfast, 4 mg (1 tablet) after lunch, 4 mg (1 tablet) after supper, and 4 mg (1 tablet) at bedtime

Day 4: 12 mg on day 4 administered as 4 mg (1 tablet) before breakfast, 4 mg (1 tablet) after lunch, and 4 mg (1 tablet) at bedtime

Day 5: 8 mg on day 5 administered as 4 mg (1 tablet) before breakfast and 4 mg (1 tablet) at bedtime

Day 6: 4 mg on day 6 administered as 4 mg (1 tablet) before breakfast

Anti-inflammatory or immunosuppressive:

Oral: 2-60 mg/day in 1-4 divided doses to start, followed by gradual reduction in dosage to the lowest possible level consistent with maintaining an adequate clinical response.

I.M. (sodium succinate): 10-80 mg/day once daily

I.M. (acetate): 10-80 mg every 1-2 weeks

I.V. (sodium succinate): 10-40 mg over a period of several minutes and repeated I.V. or I.M. at intervals depending on clinical response; when high dosages are needed, give 30 mg/kg over a period ≥30 minutes and may be repeated every 4-6 hours for 48 hours.

Arthritis: Intra-articular (acetate): Administer every 1-5 weeks.

Large joints (eg, knee, ankle): 20-80 mg

Medium joints (eg, elbow, wrist): 10-40 mg

Small joints: 4-10 mg

Asthma exacerbations, including status asthmaticus (emergency medical care or hospital doses): Oral, I.V.: 40-80 mg/day in 1- 2 divided doses until peak expiratory flow is 70% of predicted or personal best (NIH Asthma Guidelines, NAEPP, 2007)

Asthma, severe persistent, long-term control: Oral: 7.5-60 mg/day (or on alternate days) (NIH Asthma Guidelines, NAEPP, 2007)

Dermatitis, acute severe: I.M. (acetate): 80-120 mg as a single dose

Dermatitis, chronic: I.M. (acetate): 40-120 mg every 5-10 days

Dermatologic conditions (eg, keloids, lichen planus): Intralesional (acetate): 20-60 mg

Dermatomyositis/polymyositis: I.V. (sodium succinate): 1 g/day for 3-5 days for severe muscle weakness, followed by conversion to oral prednisone (Drake, 1996)

Lupus nephritis: High-dose "pulse" therapy: I.V. (sodium succinate): 0.5-1 g/day for 3 days (Ponticelli, 2010)

***Pneumocystis* pneumonia in AIDS patients:** I.V.: 30 mg twice daily for 5 days, then 30 mg once daily for 5 days, then 15 mg once daily for 11 days

Renal Impairment

Hemodialysis effects: Slightly dialyzable (5% to 20%)

Administer dose posthemodialysis.

Administration Administer with meals to decrease GI upset.

Parenteral: Methylprednisolone sodium succinate may be administered I.M. or I.V.; I.V. administration may be IVP over one to several minutes or IVPB or continuous I.V. infusion. **Acetate salt should not be given I.V.** Avoid injection into the deltoid muscle due to a high incidence of subcutaneous atrophy. Avoid injection or leakage into the dermis; dermal and/or subdermal skin depression may occur at the site of injection.

I.V.: Succinate:

Low dose: ≤1.8 mg/kg or ≤125 mg/dose: I.V. push over 3-15 minutes

Moderate dose: ≥2 mg/kg or 250 mg/dose: I.V. over 15-30 minutes

High dose: 15 mg/kg or ≥500 mg/dose: I.V. over ≥30 minutes

Doses >15 mg/kg or ≥1 g: Administer over 1 hour

Do **not** administer high-dose I.V. push; hypotension, cardiac arrhythmia, and sudden death have been reported in patients given high-dose methylprednisolone I.V. push (>0.5 g over <10 minutes); intermittent infusion over 15-60 minutes; maximum concentration: I.V. push 125 mg/mL

I.M.: Avoid injection into the deltoid muscle due to a high incidence of subcutaneous atrophy. Avoid injection or leakage into the dermis; dermal and/or subdermal skin depression may occur at the site of injection. Do not inject into areas that have evidence of acute local infection.

Monitoring Parameters Blood pressure, blood glucose, electrolytes

Test Interactions Interferes with skin tests

Pharmacotherapy Pearls Sodium content of 1 g sodium succinate injection: 2.01 mEq; 53 mg of sodium succinate salt is equivalent to 40 mg of methylprednisolone base

Methylprednisolone acetate: Depo-Medrol®

Methylprednisolone sodium succinate: Solu-Medrol®

Special Geriatric Considerations Because of the risk of adverse effects, systemic corticosteroids should be used cautiously in the elderly, in the smallest possible dose, and for the shortest possible time.

Dosage Forms Excipient information presented when available (limited, particularly for generics); consult specific product labeling.

Injection, powder for reconstitution, as sodium succinate [strength expressed as base]: 40 mg, 125 mg, 500 mg, 1 g

A-Methapred®: 40 mg [contains benzyl alcohol (in diluent), lactose 25 mg/vial]

A-Methapred®: 40 mg [contains lactose 25 mg/vial]

A-Methapred®: 125 mg

A-Methapred®: 125 mg [contains benzyl alcohol (in diluent)]

Solu-MEDROL®: 500 mg, 1 g

Solu-MEDROL®: 2 g [contains benzyl alcohol (in diluent)]

Injection, powder for reconstitution, as sodium succinate [strength expressed as base, preservative free]:

Solu-MEDROL®: 40 mg [contains lactose 25 mg/vial; supplied with diluent]

Solu-MEDROL®: 125 mg, 500 mg, 1 g [supplied with diluent]

Injection, suspension, as acetate: 40 mg/mL (1 mL, 5 mL, 10 mL); 80 mg/mL (1 mL, 5 mL)

Depo-Medrol®: 20 mg/mL (5 mL) [contains benzyl alcohol, polysorbate 80]

Depo-Medrol®: 40 mg/mL (1 mL)

Depo-Medrol®: 40 mg/mL (5 mL, 10 mL); 80 mg/mL (5 mL) [contains benzyl alcohol, polysorbate 80]

Injection, suspension, as acetate [preservative free]:

Depo-Medrol®: 80 mg/mL (1 mL)

Tablet, oral: 4 mg, 8 mg, 16 mg, 32 mg

Medrol®: 2 mg, 4 mg, 8 mg, 16 mg, 32 mg [scored]

Tablet, oral [dose-pack]: 4 mg [21s]

Medrol® Dosepak™: 4 mg [scored; 21s]

♦ **6-α-Methylprednisolone** *see* MethylPREDNISolone *on page 1252*

♦ **Methylprednisolone Acetate** *see* MethylPREDNISolone *on page 1252*

♦ **Methylprednisolone Sodium Succinate** *see* MethylPREDNISolone *on page 1252*

MethylTESTOSTERone (meth il tes TOS te rone)

Related Information

Beers Criteria – Potentially Inappropriate Medications for Geriatrics *on page 2183*

Medication Safety Issues

Sound-alike/look-alike issues:

MethylTESTOSTERone may be confused with medroxyPROGESTERone, methylPREDNISolone

BEERS Criteria medication:

This drug may be potentially inappropriate for use in geriatric patients (Quality of evidence - moderate; Strength of recommendation - weak).

Brand Names: U.S. Android®; Methitest™; Testred®

Generic Availability (U.S.) No

Pharmacologic Category Androgen

Use

Male: Hypogonadism; impotence and climacteric symptoms

Female: Palliative treatment of metastatic breast cancer

Unlabeled Use Hypogonadism (male); delayed puberty (male)

Contraindications Males with carcinoma of the breast or the prostate (known or suspected)

Warnings/Precautions Prolonged use and/or high doses may cause peliosis hepatis or liver cell tumors which may not be apparent until liver failure or intra-abdominal hemorrhage develops. Discontinue in case of cholestatic hepatitis with jaundice or abnormal liver function tests. Use with caution in patients with breast cancer; may cause hypercalcemia by stimulating osteolysis. Use with caution in patients with diabetes mellitus; monitor carefully. Use with caution in patients with conditions influenced by edema (e.g, cardiovascular disease, migraine, seizure disorder, renal impairment); may cause fluid retention. Discontinue with evidence of mild virilization in women. Use with caution in hepatic impairment. May be inappropriate for use in the elderly due to potential risk of cardiac problems and contraindication for use in men with prostate cancer; in general, avoid use in older adults except in the setting of moderate-to-severe hypogonadism (Beers Criteria). In addition, elderly patients may be at greater risk for fluid retention and transaminase elevations. Product may contain tartrazine.

Adverse Reactions (Reflective of adult population; not specific for elderly) Frequency not defined.

Male: Gynecomastia, impotence, oligospermia (at high doses), priapism, prostatic carcinoma, prostatic hyperplasia, testicular atrophy, virilism

Female: Atrophy, breast soreness, hirsutism, menstrual problems (amenorrhea), virilism

Cardiovascular: Edema

Central nervous system: Anxiety, depression, headache

Dermatologic: Acne, "male pattern" baldness

Endocrine & metabolic: Hypercalcemia, hypercholesterolemia, libido (changes in)

Gastrointestinal: Nausea, vomiting

Hematologic: Polycythemia, suppression of clotting factors
Hepatic: Cholestatic hepatitis, hepatic dysfunction, hepatic necrosis, hepatocellular neoplasm (rare), jaundice, liver function tests (abnormal), peliosis hepatitis
Neuromuscular & skeletal: Paresthesia
Miscellaneous: Anaphylactoid reactions (rare)

Drug Interactions

Metabolism/Transport Effects None known.

Avoid Concomitant Use There are no known interactions where it is recommended to avoid concomitant use.

Increased Effect/Toxicity
MethylTESTOSTERone may increase the levels/effects of: CycloSPORINE; CycloSPORINE (Systemic); Vitamin K Antagonists

Decreased Effect There are no known significant interactions involving a decrease in effect.

Mechanism of Action Stimulates receptors in organs and tissues to promote growth and development of male sex organs and maintains secondary sex characteristics in androgen-deficient males

Pharmacodynamics/Kinetics
Metabolism: Hepatic
Excretion: Urine

Dosage
Geriatric & Adult
Hypogonadism (male), delayed puberty (males): Oral: Individualize dose based on response and tolerability.
Androgen deficiency (males): Oral: 10-50 mg/day
Breast cancer (females): Oral: 50-200 mg/day

Monitoring Parameters Cholesterol, PSA, electrolyte changes

Special Geriatric Considerations Testosterone should be reserved for men with moderate to severe testosterone deficiency. Retention of sodium and water could be a problem in patients with CHF and hypertension.

This medication is considered to be potentially inappropriate in this patient population (Beers Criteria: Quality of evidence - moderate; Strength of recommendation - weak).

Controlled Substance C-III

Dosage Forms Excipient information presented when available (limited, particularly for generics); consult specific product labeling.
Capsule, oral:
Android®: 10 mg
Testred®: 10 mg
Tablet, oral:
Methitest™: 10 mg [scored]

Metipranolol (met i PRAN oh lol)

Related Information
Glaucoma Drug Therapy *on page 2115*

Medication Safety Issues
Sound-alike/look-alike issues:
Metipranolol may be confused with metaproterenol
International issues:
Betanol [Monaco] may be confused with Beta-Val brand name for betamethasone [U.S.]; Betimol brand name for timolol [U.S.]; Patanol brand name for olopatadine [U.S., Canada, and multiple international markets]

Brand Names: U.S. OptiPranolol®
Brand Names: Canada OptiPranolol®
Index Terms Metipranolol Hydrochloride
Generic Availability (U.S.) Yes
Pharmacologic Category Beta-Blocker, Nonselective; Ophthalmic Agent, Antiglaucoma
Use Treatment of chronic open-angle glaucoma or ocular hypertension
Contraindications Hypersensitivity to metipranolol or any component of the formulation; bronchial asthma, severe COPD, sinus bradycardia, second- and third-degree AV block, cardiac failure, cardiogenic shock
Warnings/Precautions Consider pre-existing conditions such as sick sinus syndrome before initiating. Use with caution in patients with bronchospastic disease, cardiac failure, diabetes mellitus, myasthenia gravis, peripheral vascular disease, or psychiatric disease. Systemic absorption and adverse effects may occur with ophthalmic use, including bradycardia and/or hypotension. Beta-blocker therapy should not be withdrawn abruptly (particularly in patients

with CAD), but gradually tapered to avoid acute tachycardia, hypertension, and/or ischemia. Use caution with history of severe anaphylaxis to allergens; patients taking beta-blockers may become more sensitive to repeated challenges. Treatment of anaphylaxis (eg, epinephrine) in patients taking beta-blockers may be ineffective or promote undesirable effects. Some products may contain benzalkonium chloride which may be absorbed by soft contact lenses; do not administer while wearing soft contact lenses.

Adverse Reactions (Reflective of adult population; not specific for elderly) Frequency not defined.

Cardiovascular: Angina, atrial fibrillation, bradycardia, hypertension, MI, palpitation

Central nervous system: Anxiety, depression, dizziness, headache, nervousness, somnolence

Dermatologic: Rash

Gastrointestinal: Nausea

Neuromuscular & skeletal: Arthritis, myalgia, weakness

Ocular: Abnormal vision, blepharitis, blurred vision, browache, conjunctivitis, discomfort, edema, eyelid dermatitis, photophobia, tearing, uveitis

Respiratory: Bronchitis, cough, dyspnea, epistaxis, rhinitis

Miscellaneous: Allergic reaction

Drug Interactions

Metabolism/Transport Effects None known.

Avoid Concomitant Use

Avoid concomitant use of Metipranolol with any of the following: Beta2-Agonists; Floctafenine; Methacholine

Increased Effect/Toxicity

Metipranolol may increase the levels/effects of: Alpha-/Beta-Agonists (Direct-Acting); Bupivacaine; Cholinergic Agonists; Fingolimod; Hypotensive Agents; Lidocaine (Systemic); Lidocaine (Topical); Mepivacaine; Methacholine; Midodrine

The levels/effects of Metipranolol may be increased by: Anilidopiperidine Opioids; Dronedarone; Floctafenine; MAO Inhibitors; QuiNIDine; Reserpine

Decreased Effect

Metipranolol may decrease the levels/effects of: Beta2-Agonists; Theophylline Derivatives

Mechanism of Action Beta-adrenoceptor-blocking agent; lacks intrinsic sympathomimetic activity and membrane-stabilizing effects and possesses only slight local anesthetic activity; mechanism of action of metipranolol in reducing intraocular pressure appears to be via reduced production of aqueous humor. This effect may be related to a reduction in blood flow to the iris root-ciliary body. It remains unclear if the reduction in intraocular pressure observed with beta-blockers is actually secondary to beta-adrenoceptor blockade.

Pharmacodynamics/Kinetics

Onset of action: ≤30 minutes

Peak effect: Maximum: ~2 hours

Duration: Intraocular pressure reduction: Up to 24 hours

Metabolism: Rapid and complete to deacetyl metipranolol, an active metabolite

Half-life elimination: ~3 hours

Dosage

Geriatric & Adult Glaucoma: Ophthalmic: Instill 1 drop in the affected eye(s) twice daily

Administration Do not allow the dispenser tip to touch the eye. Remove contact lenses prior to administration and wait 15 minutes before reinserting.

Monitoring Parameters Intraocular pressure, funduscopic exam, visual field testing

Special Geriatric Considerations Because systemic absorption occurs with ophthalmic administration, elderly patients with other disease states or syndromes that may be affected by a beta-blocker (ie, CHF, COPD, etc) should be closely monitored. Evaluate the patient's or caregiver's ability to safely administer the correct dose of ophthalmic medication.

Dosage Forms Excipient information presented when available (limited, particularly for generics); consult specific product labeling.

Solution, ophthalmic [drops]: 0.3% (5 mL, 10 mL)

OptiPranolol®: 0.3% (5 mL, 10 mL) [contains benzalkonium chloride]

◆ **Metipranolol Hydrochloride** *see* Metipranolol *on page 1257*

Metoclopramide (met oh KLOE pra mide)

Related Information

Beers Criteria − Potentially Inappropriate Medications for Geriatrics *on page 2183*

Medication Safety Issues

Sound-alike/look-alike issues:

Metoclopramide may be confused with metolazone, metoprolol, metroNIDAZOLE

Reglan® may be confused with Megace®, Regonol®, Renagel®

BEERS Criteria medication:
This drug may be potentially inappropriate for use in geriatric patients (Quality of evidence - moderate; Strength of recommendation - strong).

Brand Names: U.S. Metozolv™ ODT; Reglan®

Brand Names: Canada Apo-Metoclop®; Metoclopramide Hydrochloride Injection; Metoclopramide Omega; Nu-Metoclopramide; PMS-Metoclopramide

Generic Availability (U.S.) Yes: Excludes oral-disintegrating tablet

Pharmacologic Category Antiemetic; Gastrointestinal Agent, Prokinetic

Use
Oral: Symptomatic treatment of diabetic gastroparesis; gastroesophageal reflux

I.V., I.M.: Symptomatic treatment of diabetic gastroparesis; postpyloric placement of enteral feeding tubes; prevention and/or treatment of nausea and vomiting associated with chemotherapy, or postsurgery; to stimulate gastric emptying and intestinal transit of barium during radiological examination of the stomach/small intestine

Medication Guide Available Yes

Contraindications Hypersensitivity to metoclopramide or any component of the formulation; GI obstruction, perforation or hemorrhage; pheochromocytoma; history of seizures or concomitant use of other agents likely to increase extrapyramidal reactions

Warnings/Precautions [U.S. Boxed Warning]: May cause tardive dyskinesia, which is often irreversible; duration of treatment and total cumulative dose are associated with an increased risk. Therapy durations >12 weeks should be avoided (except in rare cases following risk:benefit assessment). Risk appears to be increased in the elderly, women, and diabetics; however, it is not possible to predict which patients will develop tardive dyskinesia. Therapy should be discontinued in any patient if signs/symptoms of tardive dyskinesia appear.

May cause extrapyramidal symptoms, generally manifested as acute dystonic reactions within the initial 24-48 hours of use. Risk of these reactions is increased at higher doses. Pseudoparkinsonism (eg, bradykinesia, tremor, rigidity) may also occur (usually within first 6 months of therapy) and is generally reversible following discontinuation. Use with caution or avoid in patients with Parkinson's disease. Avoid use in older adults (except for gastroparesis) due to risk of extrapyramidal effects, including tardive dyskinesia; risk potentially even greater in frail older adults (Beers Criteria). In addition, risk of tardive dyskinesia may be increased in older women. Neuroleptic malignant syndrome (NMS) has been reported (rarely) with metoclopramide.

May cause transient increase in serum aldosterone; use caution in patients who are at risk of fluid overload (HF, cirrhosis). Use caution in patients with hypertension or following surgical anastomosis/closure. Use caution with a history of mental illness; has been associated with depression. Abrupt discontinuation may (rarely) result in withdrawal symptoms (dizziness, headache, nervousness). Use caution and adjust dose in renal impairment. Patients with NADH-cytochrome b5 reductase deficiency are at increased risk of methemoglobinemia and/or sulfhemoglobinemia.

Adverse Reactions (Reflective of adult population; not specific for elderly) Frequency not always defined.
Cardiovascular: AV block, bradycardia, HF, fluid retention, flushing (following high I.V. doses), hyper-/hypotension, supraventricular tachycardia

Central nervous system: Drowsiness (~10% to 70%; dose related), acute dystonic reactions (<1% to 25%; dose and age related), fatigue (2% to 10%), lassitude (~10%), restlessness (~10%), headache (4% to 5%), dizziness (1% to 4%), somnolence (2% to 3%), akathisia, confusion, depression, hallucinations (rare), insomnia, neuroleptic malignant syndrome (rare), Parkinsonian-like symptoms, suicidal ideation, seizure, tardive dyskinesia

Dermatologic: Angioneurotic edema (rare), rash, urticaria

Endocrine & metabolic: Amenorrhea, galactorrhea, gynecomastia, hyperprolactinemia, impotence

Gastrointestinal: Nausea (4% to 6%), vomiting (1% to 2%), diarrhea

Hematologic: Agranulocytosis, leukopenia, neutropenia, porphyria

Hepatic: Hepatotoxicity (rare)

Ocular: Visual disturbance

Respiratory: Bronchospasm, laryngeal edema (rare), laryngospasm (rare)

Miscellaneous: Allergic reactions, methemoglobinemia, sulfhemoglobinemia

Drug Interactions
Metabolism/Transport Effects Substrate of CYP1A2 (minor), CYP2D6 (minor); **Note:** Assignment of Major/Minor substrate status based on clinically relevant drug interaction potential; **Inhibits** CYP2D6 (weak)

Avoid Concomitant Use
Avoid concomitant use of Metoclopramide with any of the following: Antipsychotics; Droperidol; Promethazine; Tetrabenazine

Increased Effect/Toxicity
Metoclopramide may increase the levels/effects of: Antipsychotics; CycloSPORINE; Cyclo-SPORINE (Systemic); Prilocaine; Promethazine; Selective Serotonin Reuptake Inhibitors; Tetrabenazine; Tricyclic Antidepressants; Venlafaxine

The levels/effects of Metoclopramide may be increased by: Droperidol; Metyrosine; Serotonin Modulators

Decreased Effect
Metoclopramide may decrease the levels/effects of: Anti-Parkinson's Agents (Dopamine Agonist); Posaconazole; Quinagolide

The levels/effects of Metoclopramide may be decreased by: Peginterferon Alfa-2b

Ethanol/Nutrition/Herb Interactions Ethanol: Avoid ethanol (may increase CNS depression).

Stability
Injection: Store intact vial at controlled room temperature. Injection is photosensitive and should be protected from light during storage. Parenteral admixtures in D_5W or NS are stable for at least 24 hours and do not require light protection if used within 24 hours.

Tablet: Store at controlled room temperature of 20°C to 25°C (68°F to 77°F).

Mechanism of Action Blocks dopamine receptors and (when given in higher doses) also blocks serotonin receptors in chemoreceptor trigger zone of the CNS; enhances the response to acetylcholine of tissue in upper GI tract causing enhanced motility and accelerated gastric emptying without stimulating gastric, biliary, or pancreatic secretions; increases lower esophageal sphincter tone

Pharmacodynamics/Kinetics
Onset of action: Oral: 30-60 minutes; I.V.: 1-3 minutes; I.M.: 10-15 minutes

Duration: Therapeutic: 1-2 hours, regardless of route

Absorption: Oral: Rapid

Distribution: V_d: ~3.5 L/kg

Protein binding: ~30%

Bioavailability: Oral: Range: 65% to 95%

Half-life elimination: Normal renal function: Adults: 5-6 hours (may be dose dependent)

Time to peak, serum: Oral: 1-2 hours

Excretion: Urine (~85%)

Dosage
Geriatric Initial: Dose at the lower end of the recommended range. Refer to adult dosing.

Adult

Gastroesophageal reflux: Oral: 10-15 mg/dose up to 4 times/day 30 minutes before meals or food and at bedtime; single doses of 20 mg are occasionally needed prior to provoking situations. Treatment >12 weeks is not recommended.

Diabetic gastroparesis:
Oral: 10 mg/dose up to 4 times/day 30 minutes before meals or food and at bedtime for 2-8 weeks

I.M., I.V. (for severe symptoms): 10 mg over 1-2 minutes; 10 days of I.V. therapy may be necessary before symptoms are controlled to allow transition to oral administration

Chemotherapy-induced emesis prophylaxis: I.V.: 1-2 mg/kg 30 minutes before chemotherapy and repeated every 2 hours for 2 doses, then every 3 hours for 3 doses (manufacturer's labeling); pretreatment with diphenhydramine will decrease risk of extrapyramidal reactions

Alternate dosing: **Note:** Metoclopramide is considered an antiemetic with a low therapeutic index; use is generally reserved for agents with low emetogenic potential or in patients intolerant/refractory to first line antiemetics.

Low-risk chemotherapy (unlabeled): I.V., Oral: 10-40 mg prior to dose, then every 4-6 hours as needed (NCCN Antiemesis guidelines, v.4.2009)

Breakthrough treatment (unlabeled): I.V., Oral: 10-40 mg every 4-6 hours (NCCN Antiemesis guidelines, v.4.2009)

Delayed-emesis prophylaxis (unlabeled): Oral: 20-40 mg/dose (or 0.5 mg/kg/dose) 2-4 times/day for 3-4 days (in combination with dexamethasone [ASCO guidelines, 2006])

Refractory or intolerant to antiemetics with a higher therapeutic index (unlabeled; Hesketh, 2008):

I.V.: 1-2 mg/kg/dose before chemotherapy and repeat 2 hours after chemotherapy

Oral: 0.5 mg/kg every 6 hours on days 2-4

Postoperative nausea and vomiting prophylaxis: I.M., I.V. (unlabeled route): 10-20 mg near end of surgery. **Note:** Guidelines discourage use of 10 mg metoclopramide as being ineffective (Gan, 2007); comparative study indicates higher dose (20 mg) may be efficacious (Quaynor, 2002).

Postpyloric feeding tube placement, radiological exam: I.V.: 10 mg as a single dose

Renal Impairment

Cl$_{cr}$ <40 mL/minute: Administer 50% of normal dose.

Not dialyzable (0% to 5%); supplemental dose is not necessary.

Administration

Injection solution: May be given I.M., direct I.V. push, short infusion (15-30 minutes), or continuous infusion; lower doses (≤10 mg) of metoclopramide can be given I.V. push undiluted over 1-2 minutes; higher doses (>10 mg) to be diluted in 50 mL of compatible solution (preferably NS) and given IVPB over at least 15 minutes; continuous SubQ infusion and rectal administration have been reported. **Note:** Rapid I.V. administration may be associated with a transient (but intense) feeling of anxiety and restlessness, followed by drowsiness.

Orally-disintegrating tablets: Administer on an empty stomach at least 30 minutes prior to food. Do not remove from packaging until time of administration. If tablet breaks or crumbles while handling, discard and remove new tablet. Using dry hands, place tablet on tongue and allow to dissolve. Swallow with saliva.

Monitoring Parameters Dystonic reactions; signs of hypoglycemia in patients using insulin and those being treated for gastroparesis; agitation, and confusion

Test Interactions Increased aminotransferase [ALT/AST] (S), increased amylase (S)

Special Geriatric Considerations Elderly are more likely to develop tardive dyskinesia syndrome (especially elderly females) reactions than younger adults. Use lowest recommended doses initially. Must consider renal function (estimate creatinine clearance). It is recommended to do involuntary movement assessments on elderly using this medication at high doses and for long-term therapy.

This medication is considered to be potentially inappropriate in this patient population (Beers Criteria: Quality of evidence - moderate; Strength of recommendation - strong).

Dosage Forms Excipient information presented when available (limited, particularly for generics); consult specific product labeling. [DSC] = Discontinued product

Injection, solution [preservative free]: 5 mg/mL (2 mL)

Reglan®: 5 mg/mL (2 mL [DSC], 10 mL [DSC], 30 mL [DSC])

Solution, oral: 5 mg/5 mL (0.9 mL, 10 mL, 473 mL)

Tablet, oral: 5 mg, 10 mg

Reglan®: 5 mg

Reglan®: 10 mg [scored]

Tablet, orally disintegrating, oral:

Metozolv™ ODT: 5 mg, 10 mg [mint flavor]

Extemporaneously Prepared

Reglan® suppository: 5 pulverized tablets in polyethylene glycol; administer 1 suppository 30-60 minutes before meals and at bedtime; use ¹/₂ for older adults.

Metoclophen nausea suppository:

Metoclopramide powder (USP) 40 mg

Haloperidol powder (USP) 1 mg

Dexamethasone powder (USP) 10 mg

Diphenhydramine HCl (USP) 25 mg

Benztropine mesylate (USP) 1 mg

Silica gel powder 200 mg

Fatty base (emulsifying type) qs 2.2 g

Metoclophen-modified nausea suppository:

Metoclopramide powder (USP) 40 mg

Haloperidol powder (USP) 1 mg

Lorazepam (USP) 1 mg

Benztropine mesylate (USP) 1 mg

Fatty base (emulsifying type) qs 2.2 g

Grind all powders (and/or tablets) into a fine uniform powder. Melt the fatty base on low temperature, then add the powder. Stir the mixture until uniform. With continuous stirring, draw up part of the mixture and instill into calibrated suppository molds. Refrigerate.

Francom M, "Compounding Nausea Aid," *Am Pharm*, 1991, NS31(7):7.

Metolazone (me TOLE a zone)

Medication Safety Issues

Sound-alike/look-alike issues:

Metolazone may be confused with metaxalone, methazolamide, methimazole, methotrexate, metoclopramide, metoprolol, minoxidil

Zaroxolyn® may be confused with Zarontin®

Brand Names: U.S. Zaroxolyn®

Brand Names: Canada Zaroxolyn®

METOLAZONE

Generic Availability (U.S.) Yes

Pharmacologic Category Diuretic, Thiazide-Related

Use Management of mild-to-moderate hypertension; treatment of edema in heart failure and nephrotic syndrome, impaired renal function

Contraindications Hypersensitivity to metolazone, any component of the formulation, other thiazides, and sulfonamide derivatives; anuria; hepatic coma

Warnings/Precautions Electrolyte disturbances (hypokalemia, hypochloremic alkalosis, hyponatremia) can occur. Large or prolonged fluid and electrolyte losses may occur with concomitant furosemide administration. Use with caution in severe hepatic dysfunction; hepatic encephalopathy can be caused by electrolyte disturbances. Gout can be precipitate in certain patients with a history of gout, a familial predisposition to gout, or chronic renal failure. Cautious use in patients with prediabetes or diabetes; may see a change in glucose control. Can cause SLE exacerbation or activation. Use caution in severe renal impairment. Use with caution in patients with moderate or high cholesterol concentrations. Photosensitization may occur.

Chemical similarities are present among sulfonamides, sulfonylureas, carbonic anhydrase inhibitors, thiazides, and loop diuretics (except ethacrynic acid). Use in patients with thiazide or sulfonamide allergy is specifically contraindicated in product labeling, however, a risk of cross-reaction exists in patients with allergy to any of these compounds; avoid use when previous reaction has been severe. Discontinue if signs of hypersensitivity are noted.

Adverse Reactions (Reflective of adult population; not specific for elderly) Frequency not defined.

Cardiovascular: Chest pain/discomfort, necrotizing angiitis, orthostatic hypotension, palpitation, syncope, venous thrombosis, vertigo, volume depletion

Central nervous system: Chills, depression, dizziness, drowsiness, fatigue, headache, lightheadedness, restlessness

Dermatologic: Petechiae, photosensitivity, pruritus, purpura, rash, skin necrosis, Stevens-Johnson syndrome, toxic epidermal necrolysis, urticaria

Endocrine & metabolic: Gout attacks, hypercalcemia, hyperglycemia, hyperuricemia, hypochloremia, hypochloremic alkalosis, hypokalemia, hypomagnesemia, hyponatremia, hypophosphatemia

Gastrointestinal: Abdominal bloating, abdominal pain, anorexia, constipation, diarrhea, epigastric distress, nausea, pancreatitis, vomiting, xerostomia

Genitourinary: Impotence

Hematologic: Agranulocytosis, aplastic/hypoplastic anemia, hemoconcentration, leukopenia, thrombocytopenia

Hepatic: Cholestatic jaundice, hepatitis

Neuromuscular & skeletal: Joint pain, muscle cramps/spasm, neuropathy, paresthesia, weakness

Ocular: Blurred vision (transient)

Renal: BUN increased, glucosuria

Drug Interactions

Metabolism/Transport Effects None known.

Avoid Concomitant Use

Avoid concomitant use of Metolazone with any of the following: Dofetilide

Increased Effect/Toxicity

Metolazone may increase the levels/effects of: ACE Inhibitors; Allopurinol; Amifostine; Antihypertensives; Calcium Salts; CarBAMazepine; Dofetilide; Hypotensive Agents; Lithium; OXcarbazepine; Porfimer; RiTUXimab; Sodium Phosphates; Topiramate; Toremifene; Vitamin D Analogs

The levels/effects of Metolazone may be increased by: Alcohol (Ethyl); Alfuzosin; Analgesics (Opioid); Barbiturates; Beta2-Agonists; Corticosteroids (Orally Inhaled); Corticosteroids (Systemic); Herbs (Hypotensive Properties); Licorice; MAO Inhibitors; Pentoxifylline; Phosphodiesterase 5 Inhibitors; Prostacyclin Analogues

Decreased Effect

Metolazone may decrease the levels/effects of: Antidiabetic Agents

The levels/effects of Metolazone may be decreased by: Bile Acid Sequestrants; Herbs (Hypertensive Properties); Methylphenidate; Nonsteroidal Anti-Inflammatory Agents; Yohimbine

Ethanol/Nutrition/Herb Interactions

Ethanol: May potentiate hypotensive effect of metazolone.

Herb/Nutraceutical: Avoid herbs with *hypertensive* properties (bayberry, blue cohosh, cayenne, ephedra, ginger, ginseng [American], kola, licorice); may diminish the antihypertensive effect of metolazone. Avoid herbs with *hypotensive* properties (black cohosh, California poppy, coleus, golden seal, hawthorn, mistletoe, periwinkle, quinine, shepherd's purse); may enhance the hypotensive effect of metolazone.

Mechanism of Action Inhibits sodium reabsorption in the distal tubules causing increased excretion of sodium and water, as well as, potassium and hydrogen ions

Pharmacodynamics/Kinetics

Onset of action: Diuresis: ~60 minutes

Duration: ≥24 hours

Absorption: Incomplete

Protein binding: 95%

Half-life elimination: 20 hours

Excretion: Urine (80%); bile (10%)

Dosage

Geriatric Oral: Initial: 2.5 mg/day or every other day

Adult

Edema: Oral: Initial: 2.5-10 mg once daily; may increase as necessary to 20 mg once daily (ACC/AHA 2009 Heart Failure Guidelines); **Note:** Dosing frequency may be adjusted based on patient-specific diuretic needs (eg, administration every other day or weekly) (Lindenfeld, 2010).

Hypertension: Oral: 2.5-5 mg/dose every 24 hours

Renal Impairment Not dialyzable (0% to 5%) via hemo- or peritoneal dialysis; supplemental dose is not necessary

Administration May be taken with food or milk. Take early in day to avoid nocturia. Take the last dose of multiple doses no later than 6 PM unless instructed otherwise.

Monitoring Parameters Serum electrolytes (potassium, sodium, chloride, bicarbonate), renal function, blood pressure (standing, sitting/supine)

Pharmacotherapy Pearls 5 mg is approximately equivalent to 50 mg of hydrochlorothiazide; may be effective in patients with glomerular filtration rate <20 mL/minute; metolazone is often used in combination with a loop diuretic in patients who are unresponsive to the loop diuretic alone

Special Geriatric Considerations When metolazone is used in combination with other diuretics, there is an increased risk of azotemia and electrolyte depletion, particularly in the elderly; therefore, monitor closely. May be effective in patients with glomerular filtration rate <20 mL/minute. Metolazone is often used in combination with a loop diuretic in patients who are unresponsive to the loop diuretic alone.

Dosage Forms Excipient information presented when available (limited, particularly for generics); consult specific product labeling.

Tablet, oral: 2.5 mg, 5 mg, 10 mg

Zaroxolyn®: 2.5 mg, 5 mg

Metoprolol (me toe PROE lole)

Related Information

Beta-Blockers *on page 2108*

Heart Failure (Systolic) *on page 2203*

Medication Safety Issues

Sound-alike/look-alike issues:

Lopressor® may be confused with Lyrica®

Metoprolol may be confused with metaproterenol, metoclopramide, metolazone, misoprostol

Metoprolol succinate may be confused with metoprolol tartrate

Toprol-XL® may be confused with TEGretol®, TEGretol®-XR, Topamax®

High alert medication:

The Institute for Safe Medication Practices (ISMP) includes this medication among its list of drugs which have a heightened risk of causing significant patient harm when used in error.

Administration issues:

Significant differences exist between oral and I.V. dosing. Use caution when converting from one route of administration to another.

Brand Names: U.S. Lopressor®; Toprol-XL®

Brand Names: Canada Apo-Metoprolol (Type L®); Apo-Metoprolol SR®; Apo-Metoprolol®; Ava-Metoprolol; Ava-Metoprolol (Type L); Betaloc®; Dom-Metoprolol-B; Dom-Metoprolol-L; JAMP-Metoprolol-L; Lopresor SR®; Lopresor®; Metoprolol Tartrate Injection, USP; Metopro-lol-25; Metoprolol-L; Mylan-Metoprolol (Type L); Nu-Metop; PMS-Metoprolol-B; PMS-Meto-prolol-L; Riva-Metoprolol-L; Sandoz-Metoprolol (Type L); Sandoz-Metoprolol SR; Teva-Metoprolol

Index Terms Metoprolol Succinate; Metoprolol Tartrate

Generic Availability (U.S.) Yes

Pharmacologic Category Antianginal Agent; Beta-Blocker, Beta-1 Selective

METOPROLOL

Use Treatment of angina pectoris, hypertension, or hemodynamically-stable acute myocardial infarction

Extended release: Treatment of angina pectoris or hypertension; to reduce mortality/hospitalization in patients with heart failure (stable NYHA Class II or III) already receiving ACE inhibitors, diuretics, and/or digoxin

Unlabeled Use Treatment of ventricular arrhythmias, atrial ectopy; migraine prophylaxis, essential tremor; prevention of reinfarction and sudden death after myocardial infarction; prevention and treatment of atrial fibrillation and atrial flutter; multifocal atrial tachycardia; symptomatic treatment of hypertrophic obstructive cardiomyopathy; management of thyrotoxicosis

Contraindications

Hypersensitivity to metoprolol, any component of the formulation, or other beta-blockers
Note: Additional contraindications are formulation and/or indication specific.
Immediate release tablets/injectable formulation:
Hypertension and angina: Sinus bradycardia; second- and third-degree heart block; cardiogenic shock; overt heart failure; sick sinus syndrome (except in patients with a functioning artificial pacemaker); severe peripheral arterial disease; pheochromocytoma (without alpha blockade)
Myocardial infarction: Severe sinus bradycardia (heart rate <45 beats/minute); significant first-degree heart block (P-R interval ≥0.24 seconds); second- and third-degree heart block; systolic blood pressure <100 mm Hg; moderate-to-severe cardiac failure
Extended release tablet: Severe bradycardia, second- and third degree heart block; cardiogenic shock; decompensated heart failure; sick sinus syndrome (except in patients with a functioning artificial pacemaker)

Warnings/Precautions [U.S. Boxed Warning]: Beta-blocker therapy should not be withdrawn abruptly (particularly in patients with CAD), but gradually tapered over 1-2 weeks to avoid acute tachycardia, hypertension, and/or ischemia. Consider pre-existing conditions such as sick sinus syndrome before initiating. Metoprolol commonly produces mild first-degree heart block (P-R interval >0.2-0.24 sec). May also produce severe first- (P-R interval ≥0.26 sec), second-, or third-degree heart block. Patients with acute MI (especially right ventricular MI) have a high risk of developing heart block of varying degrees. If severe heart block occurs, metoprolol should be discontinued and measures to increase heart rate should be employed. Symptomatic hypotension may occur with use. May precipitate or aggravate symptoms of arterial insufficiency in patients with PVD and Raynaud's disease; use with caution and monitor for progression of arterial obstruction. Use caution with concurrent use of digoxin, verapamil, or diltiazem; bradycardia or heart block can occur; avoid concurrent I.V. use of both agents. Use with caution in patients receiving inhaled anesthetic agents known to depress myocardial contractility. Use with caution in patients receiving CYP2D6 inhibitors (eg, bupropion, chlorpromazine, cimetidine, diphenhydramine, hydroxychloroquine, fluoxetine, paroxetine, propafenone, propoxyphene, quinidine, ritonavir, terbinafine, thioridazine); concurrent use may increase metoprolol plasma concentrations.

In general, beta-blockers should be avoided in patients with bronchospastic disease. Metoprolol, with B$_1$ selectivity, should be used cautiously in bronchospastic disease with close monitoring. Use cautiously in patients with diabetes because it can mask prominent hypoglycemic symptoms. May mask signs of hyperthyroidism (eg, tachycardia); if hyperthyroidism is suspected, carefully manage and monitor; abrupt withdrawal may exacerbate symptoms of hyperthyroidism or precipitate thyroid storm. Alterations in thyroid function tests may be observed. Use caution with hepatic dysfunction. Use with caution in patients with myasthenia gravis or psychiatric disease (may cause CNS depression). Although perioperative beta-blocker therapy is recommended prior to elective surgery in selected patients, use of high-dose extended release metoprolol in patients naïve to beta-blocker therapy undergoing noncardiac surgery has been associated with bradycardia, hypotension, stroke, and death. Chronic beta-blocker therapy should not be routinely withdrawn prior to major surgery. Use of beta-blockers may unmask cardiac failure in patients without a history of dysfunction. Adequate alpha-blockade is required prior to use of any beta-blocker for patients with untreated pheochromocytoma. May induce or exacerbate psoriasis. Use caution with history of severe anaphylaxis to allergens; patients taking beta-blockers may become more sensitive to repeated allergen challenges. Treatment of anaphylaxis (eg, epinephrine) in patients taking beta-blockers may be ineffective or promote undesirable effects. Bradycardia may be observed more frequently in elderly patients (>65 years of age); dosage reductions may be necessary.

Extended release: Use with caution in patients with compensated heart failure; monitor for a worsening of heart failure.

Adverse Reactions (Reflective of adult population; not specific for elderly) Frequency may not be defined.

Cardiovascular: Hypotension (1% to 27%), bradycardia (2% to 16%), first-degree heart block (P-R interval ≥0.26 sec; 5%), arterial insufficiency (usually Raynaud type; 1%), chest pain (1%), CHF (1%), edema (peripheral; 1%), palpitation (1%), syncope (1%)

Central nervous system: Dizziness (2% to 10%), fatigue (1% to 10%), depression (5%), confusion, hallucinations, headache, insomnia, memory loss (short-term), nightmares, sleep disturbances, somnolence, vertigo

Dermatology: Pruritus (5%), rash (5%), photosensitivity, psoriasis exacerbated

Endocrine & metabolic: Libido decreased, Peyronie's disease (<1%), diabetes exacerbated

Gastrointestinal: Diarrhea (5%), constipation (1%), flatulence (1%), gastrointestinal pain (1%), heartburn (1%), nausea (1%), xerostomia (1%), vomiting

Hematologic: Claudication

Neuromuscular & skeletal: Musculoskeletal pain

Ocular: Blurred vision, visual disturbances

Otic: Tinnitus

Respiratory: Dyspnea (1% to 3%), bronchospasm (1%), wheezing (1%), rhinitis, shortness of breath

Miscellaneous: Cold extremities (1%)

Other events reported with beta-blockers: Catatonia, emotional lability, fever, hypersensitivity reactions, laryngospasm, nonthrombocytopenic purpura, respiratory distress, thrombocytopenic purpura

Drug Interactions

Metabolism/Transport Effects Substrate of CYP2C19 (minor), CYP2D6 (major); **Note:** Assignment of Major/Minor substrate status based on clinically relevant drug interaction potential; **Inhibits** CYP2D6 (weak)

Avoid Concomitant Use

Avoid concomitant use of Metoprolol with any of the following: Floctafenine; Methacholine

Increased Effect/Toxicity

Metoprolol may increase the levels/effects of: Alpha-/Beta-Agonists (Direct-Acting); Alpha1-Blockers; Alpha2-Agonists; Amifostine; Antihypertensives; Antipsychotic Agents (Phenothiazines); ARIPiprazole; Bupivacaine; Cardiac Glycosides; Cholinergic Agonists; Fingolimod; Hypotensive Agents; Insulin; Lidocaine; Lidocaine (Systemic); Lidocaine (Topical); Mepivacaine; Methacholine; Midodrine; RiTUXimab; Sulfonylureas

The levels/effects of Metoprolol may be increased by: Abiraterone Acetate; Acetylcholinesterase Inhibitors; Aminoquinolines (Antimalarial); Amiodarone; Anilidopiperidine Opioids; Antipsychotic Agents (Phenothiazines); Calcium Channel Blockers (Dihydropyridine); Calcium Channel Blockers (Nondihydropyridine); CYP2D6 Inhibitors (Moderate); CYP2D6 Inhibitors (Strong); Darunavir; Diazoxide; Dipyridamole; Disopyramide; Dronedarone; Floctafenine; Herbs (Hypotensive Properties); MAO Inhibitors; Pentoxifylline; Phosphodiesterase 5 Inhibitors; Propafenone; Prostacyclin Analogues; QuiNIDine; Reserpine; Selective Serotonin Reuptake Inhibitors

Decreased Effect

Metoprolol may decrease the levels/effects of: Beta2-Agonists; Theophylline Derivatives

The levels/effects of Metoprolol may be decreased by: Barbiturates; Herbs (Hypertensive Properties); Methylphenidate; Nonsteroidal Anti-Inflammatory Agents; Peginterferon Alfa-2b; Rifamycin Derivatives; Yohimbine

Ethanol/Nutrition/Herb Interactions

Food: Food increases absorption. Metoprolol serum levels may be increased if taken with food. Management: Take immediate release tartrate tablets with food; succinate can be taken with or without food.

Herb/Nutraceutical: Some herbal medications may worsen hypertension (eg, licorice); others may increase the antihypertensive effect of metoprolol (eg, shepherd's purse). Management: Avoid bayberry, blue cohosh, cayenne, ephedra, ginger, ginseng (American), gotu kola, licorice, and yohimbe. Avoid black cohosh, California poppy, coleus, golden seal, hawthorn, mistletoe, periwinkle, quinine, and shepherd's purse.

Stability

Injection: Store at 25°C (77°F); excursions permitted to 15°C to 30°C (59°F to 86°F). Protect from light.

Tablet: Store at 25°C (77°F); excursions permitted to 15°C to 30°C (59°F to 86°F). Protect from moisture.

Mechanism of Action Selective inhibitor of beta1-adrenergic receptors; competitively blocks beta1-receptors, with little or no effect on beta2-receptors at doses <100 mg; does not exhibit any membrane stabilizing or intrinsic sympathomimetic activity

◄ **Pharmacodynamics/Kinetics**
Onset of action: Peak effect: Oral: 1.5-4 hours; I.V.: 20 minutes (when infused over 10 minutes)
Duration: Oral: Immediate release: 10-20 hours, Extended release: ~24 hours; I.V.: 5-8 hours
Absorption: 95%, rapid and complete
Distribution: V_d: 5.5 L/kg
Protein binding: 12% to albumin
Metabolism: Extensively hepatic via CYP2D6; significant first-pass effect (~50%)
Bioavailability: Oral: ~50%
Half-life elimination: 3-8 hours (dependent on rate of CYP2D6 metabolism)
Excretion: Urine (<5% to 10% as unchanged drug)

Dosage

Geriatric Refer to adult dosing. In the management of hypertension, consider lower initial doses and titrate to response (Aronow, 2011).

Adult

Angina: Oral:
Immediate release: Initial: 50 mg twice daily; usual dosage range: 50-200 mg twice daily; maximum: 400 mg/day; increase dose at weekly intervals to desired effect
Extended release: Initial: 100 mg/day (maximum: 400 mg/day)

Atrial fibrillation/flutter (ventricular rate control), supraventricular tachycardia (SVT) (acute treatment; unlabeled use; Antman, 2004; Fuster, 2006; Neumar, 2010): I.V.: 2.5-5 mg every 2-5 minutes (maximum total dose: 15 mg over a 10-15 minute period). **Note:** Initiate cautiously in patients with concomitant heart failure; avoid in patients with decompensated heart failure.
Maintenance: Oral (immediate release): 25-100 mg twice daily

Heart failure: Oral: *Extended release:* Initial: 25 mg once daily (reduce to 12.5 mg once daily in NYHA class higher than class II); may double dosage every 2 weeks as tolerated (target dose: 200 mg/day)

Hypertension: Oral:
Immediate release: Initial: 50 mg twice daily; effective dosage range: 100-450 mg/day in 2-3 divided doses; increase dose at weekly intervals to desired effect; maximum: 450 mg/day; usual dosage range (JNC 7): 50-100 mg/day
Extended release: Initial: 25-100 mg once daily; increase doses at weekly (or longer) intervals to desired effect; maximum: 400 mg/day; usual dosage range (JNC 7): 50-100 mg/day

Hypertension/ventricular rate control: I.V. (in patients having nonfunctioning GI tract): Initial: 1.25-5 mg every 6-12 hours; titrate initial dose to response. Initially, low doses may be appropriate to establish response; however, although not routine, up to 15 mg administered as frequently as every 3 hours has been employed in patients with refractory tachycardia.

Myocardial infarction:
Acute: I.V.: 5 mg every 2 minutes for 3 doses in early treatment of myocardial infarction; thereafter, give 50 mg orally every 6 hours beginning 15 minutes after last I.V. dose and continue for 48 hours; then administer a maintenance dose of 100 mg twice daily. **Note:** Do not initiate this regimen in those with signs of heart failure, a low output state, increased risk of cardiogenic shock, or other contraindications (eg, second- or third-degree heart block). If initial I.V. dosing is not tolerated, may give 25-50 mg orally (depending on degree of intolerance) every 6 hours beginning 15 minutes after the last I.V. dose or as soon as clinical condition permits.
Secondary prevention (unlabeled use; Olsson, 1992): Oral: Immediate release: 25-100 mg twice daily; optimize dose based on heart rate and blood pressure; continue indefinitely.

Thyrotoxicosis (unlabeled use): Oral: Immediate release: 25-50 mg every 6 hours; may also consider administering extended release formulation (Bahn, 2011)

Note: Switching dosage forms:
When switching from immediate release metoprolol to extended release, the same total daily dose of metoprolol should be used.
When switching between oral and intravenous dosage forms, equivalent beta-blocking effect is achieved when doses in a 2.5:1 (Oral:I.V.) ratio is used. For example, if the patient is receiving an oral dose of 25 mg twice daily (50 mg/day), this would translate to 5 mg I.V. every 6 hours; consider reducing initial I.V. dose to evaluate patient response.

Renal Impairment No adjustment required.

Hepatic Impairment Reduced dose may be necessary.

Administration

Oral: Extended release tablets may be divided in half; do not crush or chew.

I.V.: I.V. dose is much smaller than oral dose. When administered acutely for cardiac treatment, monitor ECG and blood pressure; may administer by rapid infusion (I.V. push) over 1 minute. May also be administered by slow infusion (ie, 5-10 mg of metoprolol in 50 mL of fluid) over ~30-60 minutes during less urgent situations (eg, substitution for oral metoprolol).

Monitoring Parameters Acute cardiac treatment: Monitor ECG and blood pressure with I.V. administration; heart rate and blood pressure with oral administration. I.V. use in a non-emergency situation: Necessary monitoring for surgical patients who are unable to take oral beta-blockers (because of prolonged ileus) has not been defined. Some institutions require monitoring of baseline and postinfusion heart rate and blood pressure when a patient's response to beta-blockade has not been characterized (ie, the patient's initial dose or following a change in dose). Consult individual institutional policies and procedures.

Special Geriatric Considerations Due to alterations in the beta-adrenergic autonomic nervous system, beta-adrenergic blockade may result in less hemodynamic response than seen in younger adults. Studies indicate that despite decreased sensitivity to the chronotropic effects of beta-blockade with age, there appears to be an increased myocardial sensitivity to the negative inotropic effect during stress (ie, exercise). Controlled trials have shown the overall response rate for propranolol to be only 20% to 50% in the elderly populations. Therefore, all beta-adrenergic blocking drugs may result in a decreased response as compared to younger adults.

Dosage Forms Excipient information presented when available (limited, particularly for generics); consult specific product labeling.

Injection, solution, as tartrate: 1 mg/mL (5 mL)
    Lopressor®: 1 mg/mL (5 mL)
Injection, solution, as tartrate [preservative free]: 1 mg/mL (5 mL)
Tablet, oral, as tartrate: 25 mg, 50 mg, 100 mg
    Lopressor®: 50 mg, 100 mg [scored]
Tablet, extended release, oral, as succinate: 25 mg [expressed as mg equivalent to tartrate], 50 mg [expressed as mg equivalent to tartrate], 100 mg [expressed as mg equivalent to tartrate], 200 mg [expressed as mg equivalent to tartrate]
    Toprol-XL®: 25 mg, 50 mg, 100 mg, 200 mg [scored; expressed as mg equivalent to tartrate]

Extemporaneously Prepared To prepare a metoprolol 10 mg/mL liquid, crush 12 metoprolol tartrate 100 mg tablets into a fine powder. Add ~20 mL of either Ora-Sweet® and Ora-Plus® (1:1 preparation), or Ora-Sweet® SF and Ora-Plus® (1:1 preparation), or cherry syrup. Mix to a uniform paste. Continue to add the vehicle to bring the final volume to 120 mL. The preparation is stable for 60 days; shake well before using and protect from light.

Allen LV and Erickson III MA, "Stability of Labetalol Hydrochloride, Metoprolol Tartrate, Verapamil Hydrochloride, and Spironolactone With Hydrochlorothiazide in Extemporaneously Compounded Oral Liquids," *Am J Health Syst Pharm*, 1996, 53:2304-9.

Metoprolol and Hydrochlorothiazide
(me toe PROE lole & hye droe klor oh THYE a zide)

Related Information

Hydrochlorothiazide *on page 933*
Metoprolol *on page 1263*

Brand Names: U.S. Dutoprol™; Lopressor HCT®

Index Terms Hydrochlorothiazide and Metoprolol; Hydrochlorothiazide and Metoprolol Succinate; Hydrochlorothiazide and Metoprolol Tartrate; Metoprolol Succinate and Hydrochlorothiazide; Metoprolol Tartrate and Hydrochlorothiazide

Generic Availability (U.S.) Yes: Excludes extended release tablet

Pharmacologic Category Beta-Blocker, Beta-1 Selective; Diuretic, Thiazide

Use Treatment of hypertension (not recommended for initial treatment)

Dosage

Geriatric & Adult Hypertension: Oral: Dosage should be determined by titration of the individual agents and the combination product substituted based upon the daily requirements. **Note:** Hydrochlorothiazide >50 mg/day is not recommended.

Metoprolol **tartrate** (immediate release) and hydrochlorothiazide:
    Dosage range: Metoprolol tartrate 100-200 mg and hydrochlorothiazide 25-50 mg once daily **or** metoprolol tartrate 50-100 mg and hydrochlorothiazide 12.5-25 mg twice daily
Metoprolol **succinate** (extended release) and hydrochlorothiazide:
    Dosage range: Metoprolol succinate 25-200 mg and hydrochlorothiazide 12.5-25 mg once daily; titration may occur once every 2 weeks to the maximum daily dose of metoprolol succinate 200 mg/hydrochlorothiazide 25 mg

Note: Metoprolol **succinate** 50 mg and hydrochlorothiazide 6.25 mg dose may be achieved by splitting the metoprolol succinate 100 mg/hydrochlorothiazide 12.5 mg tablet.

Concomitant therapy: It is recommended that if an additional antihypertensive agent is required, gradual titration should occur using ½ the usual starting dose of the other agent to avoid hypotension.

Renal Impairment

Cl_{cr} >30 mL/minute: No dosage adjustment necessary.

Cl_{cr} ≤30 mL/minute: Loop diuretics preferred; the use of hydrochlorothiazide may not be effective.

Anuria: Use is contraindicated.

Hepatic Impairment

Mild impairment: No adjustment necessary.

Moderate impairment: Initial: Consider lower hydrochlorothiazide doses.

Special Geriatric Considerations See individual agents. Combination products are not recommended as first-line treatment. Use only if doses of individual agents correspond to the combination available.

Dosage Forms Excipient information presented when available (limited, particularly for generics); consult specific product labeling.

Tablet, oral: 50/25: Metoprolol tartrate 50 mg and hydrochlorothiazide 25 mg; 100/25: Metoprolol tartrate 100 mg and hydrochlorothiazide 25 mg; 100/50: Metoprolol tartrate 100 mg and hydrochlorothiazide 50 mg

Lopressor HCT® 50/25: Metoprolol tartrate 50 mg and hydrochlorothiazide 25 mg

Lopressor HCT® 100/25: Metoprolol tartrate 100 mg and hydrochlorothiazide 25 mg

Tablet, extended release, oral:

Dutoprol™: 25/12.5: Metoprolol succinate 25 mg [extended release, expressed as mg equivalent to tartrate] and hydrochlorothiazide 12.5 mg

Dutoprol™: 50/12.5: Metoprolol succinate 50 mg [extended release, expressed as mg equivalent to tartrate] and hydrochlorothiazide 12.5 mg

Dutoprol™: 100/12.5: Metoprolol succinate 100 mg [extended release, expressed as mg equivalent to tartrate] and hydrochlorothiazide 12.5 mg [scored]

◆ **Metoprolol Succinate** *see* Metoprolol *on page 1263*
◆ **Metoprolol Succinate and Hydrochlorothiazide** *see* Metoprolol and Hydrochlorothiazide *on page 1267*
◆ **Metoprolol Tartrate** *see* Metoprolol *on page 1263*
◆ **Metoprolol Tartrate and Hydrochlorothiazide** *see* Metoprolol and Hydrochlorothiazide *on page 1267*
◆ **Metozolv™ ODT** *see* Metoclopramide *on page 1258*
◆ **MetroCream®** *see* MetroNIDAZOLE (Topical) *on page 1271*
◆ **MetroGel®** *see* MetroNIDAZOLE (Topical) *on page 1271*
◆ **MetroGel® 1% Kit [DSC]** *see* MetroNIDAZOLE (Topical) *on page 1271*
◆ **MetroGel-Vaginal®** *see* MetroNIDAZOLE (Topical) *on page 1271*
◆ **MetroLotion®** *see* MetroNIDAZOLE (Topical) *on page 1271*

MetroNIDAZOLE (Systemic) (met roe NYE da zole)

Related Information

Antimicrobial Drugs of Choice *on page 2163*

H. pylori Treatment in Adult Patients *on page 2116*

Medication Safety Issues

Sound-alike/look-alike issues:

MetroNIDAZOLE may be confused with mebendazole, meropenem, metFORMIN, methotrexate, metoclopramide, miconazole

Brand Names: U.S. Flagyl®; Flagyl® 375; Flagyl® ER

Brand Names: Canada Apo-Metronidazole®; Flagyl®; Florazole® ER

Index Terms Metronidazole Hydrochloride

Generic Availability (U.S.) Yes: Excludes extended release tablet

Pharmacologic Category Amebicide; Antibiotic, Miscellaneous; Antiprotozoal, Nitroimidazole

Use Treatment of susceptible anaerobic bacterial and protozoal infections in the following conditions: Amebiasis, symptomatic and asymptomatic trichomoniasis; skin and skin structure infections, bone and joint infections, CNS infections, endocarditis, gynecologic infections, intra-abdominal infections (as part of combination regimen), respiratory tract infections (lower), systemic anaerobic infections; treatment of antibiotic-associated pseudomembranous colitis (AAPC); as part of a multidrug regimen for *H. pylori* eradication to reduce the risk of duodenal ulcer recurrence; surgical prophylaxis (colorectal); useful as single agent or in combination with amoxicillin, amoxicillin/clavulanic acid, or ciprofloxacin in the treatment of periodontitis associated with the presence of *Actinobacillus actinomycetemcomitans* (AA).

Unlabeled Use Crohn's disease

Contraindications Hypersensitivity to metronidazole, nitroimidazole derivatives, or any component of the formulation

Warnings/Precautions Use with caution in patients with severe liver impairment due to potential accumulation, blood dyscrasias; history of seizures, CHF or other sodium-retaining states; reduce dosage in patients with severe liver impairment, CNS disease, and consider dosage reduction in longer-term therapy with severe renal failure (Cl_{cr} <10 mL/minute); if *H. pylori* is not eradicated in patients being treated with metronidazole in a regimen, it should be assumed that metronidazole-resistance has occurred and it should not again be used; aseptic meningitis, encephalopathy, seizures, and neuropathies have been reported especially with increased doses and chronic treatment; monitor and consider discontinuation of therapy if symptoms occur. **[U.S. Boxed Warning]: Possibly carcinogenic based on animal data.** Prolonged use may result in fungal or bacterial superinfection, including *C. difficile*-associated diarrhea (CDAD) and pseudomembranous colitis; CDAD has been observed >2 months postantibiotic treatment. The Infectious Disease Society of America (IDSA) recommends the use of oral metronidazole for initial treatment of mild-to-moderate *C. difficile* infection and the use of oral vancomycin for initial treatment of severe *C. difficile* infection with or without I.V. metronidazole depending on the presence of complications. May treat recurrent mild-to-moderate infection once with oral metronidazole; avoid use beyond first reoccurrence due to potential cumulative neurotoxicity (Cohen, 2010). Candidiasis infection (known or unknown) maybe more prominent during metronidazole treatment, antifungal treatment required. Disulfiram-like reactions to ethanol have been reported with oral metronidazole; avoid alcoholic beverages during therapy

Adverse Reactions (Reflective of adult population; not specific for elderly) Frequency not always defined.

Cardiovascular: Flattening of the T-wave, flushing, syncope

Central nervous system: Aseptic meningitis, ataxia, confusion, coordination impaired, depression, dizziness, encephalopathy, fever, headache, insomnia, irritability, seizure, vertigo

Dermatologic: Erythematous rash, pruritus, Stevens-Johnson syndrome, toxic epidermal necrolysis, urticaria

Endocrine & metabolic: Disulfiram-like reaction, dysmenorrhea

Gastrointestinal: Nausea (~12%), anorexia, abdominal cramping, constipation, diarrhea, epigastric distress, furry tongue, glossitis, pancreatitis (rare), proctitis, stomatitis, unusual/metallic taste, vomiting, xerostomia

Genitourinary: Cystitis, darkened urine (rare), dyspareunia, dysuria, incontinence, libido decreased, pelvic pressure, polyuria, vaginal dryness, vaginitis

Hematologic: Neutropenia (reversible), thrombocytopenia (reversible, rare)

Local: Thrombophlebitis

Neuromuscular & skeletal: Dysarthria, peripheral neuropathy, weakness

Ocular: Optic neuropathy

Respiratory: Nasal congestion, pharyngitis, rhinitis, sinusitis, pharyngitis

Miscellaneous: Flu-like syndrome, joint pains resembling serum sickness, moniliasis

Drug Interactions

Metabolism/Transport Effects Inhibits CYP2C9 (weak), CYP3A4 (moderate)

Avoid Concomitant Use

Avoid concomitant use of MetroNIDAZOLE (Systemic) with any of the following: BCG; Disulfiram; Pimozide; Tolvaptan

Increased Effect/Toxicity

MetroNIDAZOLE (Systemic) may increase the levels/effects of: Alcohol (Ethyl); ARIPiprazole; Avanafil; Budesonide (Systemic, Oral Inhalation); Busulfan; Calcineurin Inhibitors; Colchicine; CYP3A4 Substrates; Eplerenone; Everolimus; FentaNYL; Fluorouracil; Fluorouracil (Systemic); Fosphenytoin; Halofantrine; Ivacaftor; Lurasidone; Phenytoin; Pimecrolimus; Pimozide; Propafenone; Ranolazine; Salmeterol; Saxagliptin; Tipranavir; Tolvaptan; Vilazodone; Vitamin K Antagonists; Zuclopenthixol

The levels/effects of MetroNIDAZOLE (Systemic) may be increased by: Disulfiram; Mebendazole

Decreased Effect

MetroNIDAZOLE (Systemic) may decrease the levels/effects of: BCG; Ifosfamide; Mycophenolate; Typhoid Vaccine

The levels/effects of MetroNIDAZOLE (Systemic) may be decreased by: Fosphenytoin; PHENobarbital; Phenytoin

Ethanol/Nutrition/Herb Interactions

Ethanol: The manufacturer recommends to avoid all ethanol or any ethanol-containing drugs (may cause disulfiram-like reaction characterized by flushing, headache, nausea, vomiting, sweating, or tachycardia).

Food: Peak antibiotic serum concentration lowered and delayed, but total drug absorbed not affected.

Stability

Injection: Store at controlled room temperature of 15°C to 30°C (59°F to 86°F). Protect from light. Keep in overwrap until ready to use. Product may be refrigerated but crystals may form. Crystals redissolve on warming to room temperature. Prolonged exposure to light will cause a darkening of the product. However, short-term exposure to normal room light does not adversely affect metronidazole stability. Direct sunlight should be avoided. Stability of parenteral admixture at room temperature (25°C); Out of overwrap stability: 30 days. Standard diluent: 500 mg/100 mL NS.

Tablets: Store at room temperature. Protect from light and moisture.

Mechanism of Action After diffusing into the organism, interacts with DNA to cause a loss of helical DNA structure and strand breakage resulting in inhibition of protein synthesis and cell death in susceptible organisms

Pharmacodynamics/Kinetics

Absorption: Oral: Well absorbed

Distribution: To saliva, bile, seminal fluid, bone, liver, and liver abscesses, lung and vaginal secretions; crosses blood-brain barrier

CSF:blood level ratio: Normal meninges: 16% to 43%; Inflamed meninges: 100%

Protein binding: <20%

Metabolism: Hepatic (30% to 60%)

Half-life elimination: 6-8 hours, prolonged with hepatic impairment; End-stage renal disease: 21 hours

Time to peak, serum: Oral: Immediate release: 1-2 hours

Excretion: Urine (60% to 80% as unchanged drug); feces (6% to 15%)

Dosage

Geriatric Refer to adult dosing. Use the lower end of the dosing recommendations for adults; do not administer as single dose as efficacy has not been established.

Adult

Anaerobic infections (diverticulitis, intra-abdominal, peritonitis, cholangitis, or abscess): Oral, I.V.: 500 mg every 6-8 hours, not to exceed 4 g/day; **Note:** Initial: 1 g I.V. loading dose may be administered

Amebiasis: Oral: 500-750 mg every 8 hours for 5-10 days

Antibiotic-associated pseudomembranous colitis: IDSA Guidelines (Cohen, 2010):

Mild-to-moderate infection: Oral: 500 mg 3 times/day for 10-14 days

Severe complicated infection: I.V.: 500 mg 3 times/day with oral vancomycin (recommended agent) for 10-14 days

Note: Due to the emergence of a new strain of *C. difficile*, some clinicians recommend converting to oral vancomycin therapy if the patient does not show a clear clinical response after 2 days of metronidazole therapy.

Giardiasis: 500 mg twice daily for 5-7 days

Intra-abdominal infection, complicated, community-acquired, mild-to-moderate (in combination with cephalosporin or fluoroquinolone): I.V.: 500 mg every 8-12 hours or 1.5 g every 24 hours for for 4-7 days (provided source controlled)

Peptic ulcer disease: *Helicobacter pylori* eradication: Oral: 250-500 mg with meals and at bedtime for 14 days; requires combination therapy with at least one other antibiotic and an acid-suppressing agent (proton pump inhibitor or H₂ blocker)

Bacterial vaginosis or vaginitis due to *Gardnerella, Mobiluncus*: Oral: 500 mg twice daily (regular release) or 750 mg once daily (extended release tablet) for 7 days

Pelvic inflammatory disease (unlabeled use): Oral: 500 mg twice daily for 14 days (in combination with a cephalosporin and doxycycline) (CDC, 2010)

Periodontitis treatment (monotherapy or combination) associated with presence of *Actinobacillus actinomycetemcomitans* **(AA):** Oral: 250-500 mg every 8 hours for 8-10 days used in addition to scaling and root planing (Varela, 2011)

Trichomoniasis: Oral: 250 mg every 8 hours for 7 days **or** 375 mg twice daily for 7 days **or** 2 g as a single dose **or** 1 g twice daily for 2 doses (on same day)

Urethritis (unlabeled use): Oral: 2 g as a single dose with azithromycin (CDC, 2010)

Surgical prophylaxis (colorectal): I.V. 15 mg/kg 1 hour prior to surgery; followed by 7.5 mg/kg 6 and 12 hours after initial dose

Renal Impairment Cl_{cr} <10 mL/minute (not on dialysis): Recommendations vary: To reduce possible accumulation in patients receiving multiple doses, consider reduction to 50% of dose or administer normal dose every 12 hours; **Note:** Dosage reduction is unnecessary in short courses of therapy. Some references do not recommend reduction at any level of renal impairment (Lamp, 1999).

Intermittent hemodialysis (IHD) (administer after hemodialysis on dialysis days): Dialyzable (50% to 100%): 500 mg every 8-12 hours. **Note:** Dosing regimen highly dependent on clinical indication (trichomoniasis vs *C. difficile* colitis) (Heintz, 2009). **Note:** Dosing dependent on the assumption of thrice weekly, complete IHD sessions.

Peritoneal dialysis (PD): Dose as for Cl_{cr} <10 mL/minute

Continuous renal replacement therapy (CRRT) (Heintz, 2009; Trotman, 2005): Drug clearance is highly dependent on the method of renal replacement, filter type, and flow rate. Appropriate dosing requires close monitoring of pharmacologic response, signs of adverse reactions due to drug accumulation, as well as drug concentrations in relation to target trough (if appropriate). The following are general recommendations only (based on dialysate flow/ultrafiltration rates of 1-2 L/hour and minimal residual renal function) and should not supersede clinical judgment:

CVVH/CVVHD/CVVHDF: 500 mg every 6-12 hours (or per clinical indication; dosage reduction generally not necessary)

Hepatic Impairment Unchanged in mild liver disease; reduce dosage in severe liver disease.

Administration

I.V.: Infuse intravenously over 30-60 minutes. Avoid contact of drug solution with equipment containing aluminum.

Oral: May be taken with food to minimize stomach upset. Extended release tablets should be taken on an empty stomach (1 hour before or 2 hours after meals).

Test Interactions May interfere with AST, ALT, triglycerides, glucose, and LDH testing

Special Geriatric Considerations Adjust dose based on renal function.

Dosage Forms Excipient information presented when available (limited, particularly for generics); consult specific product labeling.

Capsule, oral: 375 mg
Flagyl® 375: 375 mg

Infusion, premixed iso-osmotic sodium chloride solution: 500 mg (100 mL)

Tablet, oral: 250 mg, 500 mg
Flagyl®: 250 mg, 500 mg

Tablet, extended release, oral:
Flagyl® ER: 750 mg

MetroNIDAZOLE (Topical) (met roe NYE da zole)

Related Information

Antimicrobial Drugs of Choice *on page 2163*
Pressure Ulcer Treatment *on page 2246*

Brand Names: U.S. MetroCream®; MetroGel-Vaginal®; MetroGel®; MetroGel® 1% Kit [DSC]; MetroLotion®; Noritate®; Rosadan™; Vandazole®

Brand Names: Canada MetroCream®; Metrogel®; MetroLotion®; Nidagel™; Noritate®; Rosasol®

Index Terms Metronidazole Hydrochloride

Generic Availability (U.S.) Yes

Pharmacologic Category Antibiotic, Topical

Use

Topical: Treatment of inflammatory lesions and erythema of rosacea
Vaginal gel: Bacterial vaginosis

Dosage

Geriatric Use the lower end of the dosing recommendations for adults

Adult

Acne rosacea: Topical:
0.75%: Apply and rub a thin film twice daily, morning and evening, to entire affected areas after washing.
1%: Apply thin film to affected area once daily

Bacterial vaginosis or vaginitis due to *Gardnerella, Mobiluncus*: Vaginal: One applicatorful (~37.5 mg metronidazole) intravaginally once or twice daily for 5 days; apply once in morning and evening if using twice daily, if daily, use at bedtime

Special Geriatric Considerations Instruct patient or caregiver on appropriate use of topical metronidazole products.

◀ **Dosage Forms** Excipient information presented when available (limited, particularly for generics); consult specific product labeling. [DSC] = Discontinued product

Cream, topical: 0.75% (45 g)
MetroCream®: 0.75% (45 g) [contains benzyl alcohol]
Noritate®: 1% (60 g)
Rosadan™: 0.75% (45 g) [contains benzyl alcohol]

Gel, topical: 0.75% (45 g)
MetroGel®: 1% (55 g, 60 g)
MetroGel® 1% Kit: 1% (60 g [DSC])

Gel, vaginal: 0.75% (70 g)
MetroGel-Vaginal®: 0.75% (70 g)
Vandazole®: 0.75% (70 g)

Lotion, topical: 0.75% (59 mL, 60 mL)
MetroLotion®: 0.75% (59 mL) [contains benzyl alcohol]

◆ **Metronidazole Hydrochloride** *see* MetroNIDAZOLE (Systemic) *on page 1268*
◆ **Metronidazole Hydrochloride** *see* MetroNIDAZOLE (Topical) *on page 1271*
◆ **Mevacor®** *see* Lovastatin *on page 1164*
◆ **Mevinolin** *see* Lovastatin *on page 1164*

Mexiletine (meks IL e teen)

Brand Names: Canada Novo-Mexiletine
Generic Availability (U.S.) Yes
Pharmacologic Category Antiarrhythmic Agent, Class Ib
Use Management of serious ventricular arrhythmias; suppression of PVCs
Unlabeled Use Treatment of diabetic neuropathy
Contraindications Hypersensitivity to mexiletine or any component of the formulation; cardiogenic shock; second- or third-degree AV block (except in patients with a functioning artificial pacemaker)
Warnings/Precautions [U.S. Boxed Warning]: In the Cardiac Arrhythmia Suppression Trial (CAST), recent (>6 days but <2 years ago) myocardial infarction patients with asymptomatic, non-life-threatening ventricular arrhythmias did not benefit and may have been harmed by attempts to suppress the arrhythmia with flecainide or encainide. An increased mortality or non-fatal cardiac arrest rate (7.7%) was seen in the active treatment group compared with patients in the placebo group (3%). The applicability of the CAST results to other populations is unknown. Antiarrhythmic agents should be reserved for patients with life-threatening ventricular arrhythmias. Can be proarrhythmic. Electrolyte disturbances alter response; should be corrected before initiating therapy. Use cautiously in patients with first-degree block, pre-existing sinus node dysfunction, intraventricular conduction delays, significant hepatic dysfunction, hypotension, or severe HF. Alterations in urinary pH may change urinary excretion. Rare hepatic toxicity may occur; may cause acute hepatic injury.
Adverse Reactions (Reflective of adult population; not specific for elderly)
>10%:
Central nervous system: Lightheadedness (11% to 25%), dizziness (20% to 25%), nervousness (5% to 10%), incoordination (10%)
Gastrointestinal: GI distress (41%), nausea/vomiting (40%)
Neuromuscular & skeletal: Trembling, unsteady gait, tremor (13%), ataxia (10% to 20%)
1% to 10%:
Cardiovascular: Chest pain (3% to 8%), premature ventricular contractions (1% to 2%), palpitation (4% to 8%), angina (2%), proarrhythmia (10% to 15% in patients with malignant arrhythmia)
Central nervous system: Confusion, headache, insomnia (5% to 7%), depression (2%)
Dermatologic: Rash (4%)
Gastrointestinal: Constipation or diarrhea (4% to 5%), xerostomia (3%), abdominal pain (1%)
Neuromuscular & skeletal: Weakness (5%), numbness of fingers or toes (2% to 4%), paresthesia (2%), arthralgia (1%)
Ocular: Blurred vision (5% to 7%), nystagmus (6%)
Otic: Tinnitus (2% to 3%)
Respiratory: Dyspnea (3%)
Drug Interactions
Metabolism/Transport Effects Substrate of CYP1A2 (major), CYP2D6 (major); **Note:** Assignment of Major/Minor substrate status based on clinically relevant drug interaction potential; **Inhibits** CYP1A2 (strong).
Avoid Concomitant Use There are no known interactions where it is recommended to avoid concomitant use.

Increased Effect/Toxicity

Mexiletine may increase the levels/effects of: Bendamustine; CYP1A2 Substrates; Theophylline Derivatives

The levels/effects of Mexiletine may be increased by: Abiraterone Acetate; CYP1A2 Inhibitors (Moderate); CYP1A2 Inhibitors (Strong); CYP2D6 Inhibitors (Moderate); CYP2D6 Inhibitors (Strong); Darunavir; Deferasirox; Selective Serotonin Reuptake Inhibitors

Decreased Effect

The levels/effects of Mexiletine may be decreased by: CYP1A2 Inducers (Strong); Cyproterone; Etravirine; Fosphenytoin; Peginterferon Alfa-2b; Phenytoin

Ethanol/Nutrition/Herb Interactions Food: Food may decrease the rate, but not the extent of oral absorption; diets which affect urine pH can increase or decrease excretion of mexiletine. Avoid dietary changes that alter urine pH.

Mechanism of Action Class IB antiarrhythmic, structurally related to lidocaine, which inhibits inward sodium current, decreases rate of rise of phase 0, increases effective refractory period/action potential duration ratio

Pharmacodynamics/Kinetics

Absorption: Well absorbed; elderly have a slightly slower rate, but extent of absorption is the same as young adults

Distribution: V_d: 5-7 L/kg

Protein binding: 50% to 60%

Metabolism: Hepatic; low first-pass effect

Bioavailability: 80% to 95%

Half-life elimination: Adults: 10-14 hours (average: elderly: 14.4 hours, younger adults: 12 hours); prolonged with hepatic impairment or heart failure

Time to peak, serum: 2-3 hours

Excretion: Urine (10% to 15% as unchanged drug); urinary acidification increases excretion, alkalinization decreases excretion

Dosage

Geriatric & Adult Arrhythmias: Oral: Initial: 200 mg every 8 hours (may load with 400 mg if necessary); adjust dose every 2-3 days; usual dose: 200-300 mg every 8 hours; maximum: 1.2 g/day (some patients respond to every 12-hour dosing). When switching from another antiarrhythmic, initiate a 200 mg dose 6-12 hours after stopping former agents, 3-6 hours after stopping procainamide.

Hepatic Impairment Patients with hepatic impairment or CHF may require dose reduction; reduce dose to 25% to 30% of usual dose

Administration Administer with food, around-the-clock rather than 3 times/day to promote less variation in peak and trough serum levels.

Monitoring Parameters ECG, blood pressure, pulse, serum concentrations

Reference Range Therapeutic range: 0.5-2 mcg/mL; potentially toxic: >2 mcg/mL

Test Interactions Abnormal liver function test, positive ANA, thrombocytopenia

Special Geriatric Considerations No specific changes in dose are necessary.

Dosage Forms Excipient information presented when available (limited, particularly for generics); consult specific product labeling.

Capsule, oral, as hydrochloride: 150 mg, 200 mg, 250 mg

- ◆ **MG217® Sal-Acid [OTC]** *see* Salicylic Acid *on page 1743*
- ◆ **Mg-plus® [OTC]** *see* Magnesium Salts (Various Salts) *on page 1182*
- ◆ **Miacalcin®** *see* Calcitonin *on page 254*
- ◆ **Mi-Acid [OTC]** *see* Aluminum Hydroxide, Magnesium Hydroxide, and Simethicone *on page 82*
- ◆ **Mi-Acid Gas Relief [OTC]** *see* Simethicone *on page 1776*
- ◆ **Mi-Acid Maximum Strength [OTC] [DSC]** *see* Aluminum Hydroxide, Magnesium Hydroxide, and Simethicone *on page 82*
- ◆ **Micaderm® [OTC]** *see* Miconazole (Topical) *on page 1276*

Micafungin (mi ka FUN gin)

Brand Names: U.S. Mycamine®

Brand Names: Canada Mycamine®

Index Terms Micafungin Sodium

Generic Availability (U.S.) No

Pharmacologic Category Antifungal Agent, Parenteral; Echinocandin

Use Treatment of esophageal candidiasis; *Candida* prophylaxis in patients undergoing hematopoietic stem cell transplant (HSCT); treatment of candidemia, acute disseminated candidiasis, and other *Candida* infections (peritonitis and abscesses)

Unlabeled Use Treatment of infections due to *Aspergillus* spp; prophylaxis of HIV-related esophageal candidiasis

Contraindications Hypersensitivity to micafungin, other echinocandins, or any component of the formulation

Warnings/Precautions Anaphylactic reactions, including shock, have been reported. New onset or worsening hepatic failure has been reported; use caution in pre-existing mild-moderate hepatic impairment; safety in severe liver failure has not been evaluated. Hemolytic anemia and hemoglobinuria have been reported. Increased BUN, serum creatinine, renal dysfunction, and/or acute renal failure has been reported; use with caution in patients with pre-existing renal impairment and monitor closely.

Adverse Reactions (Reflective of adult population; not specific for elderly)

>10%:

Central nervous system: Fever (7% to 20%), headache (2% to 16%), dizziness (13%)

Endocrine & metabolic: Hypokalemia (14% to 18%), hypomagnesemia (6% to 13%)

Gastrointestinal: Diarrhea (8% to 23%), nausea (7% to 22%), vomiting (7% to 22%), mucosal inflammation (14%), constipation (11%)

Hematologic: Thrombocytopenia (4% to 15%), neutropenia (14%)

Local: Phlebitis (with peripheral administration; 5% to 19%)

1% to 10%:

Cardiovascular: Hypotension (6% to 10%), tachycardia (3% to 8%), hypertension (3% to 5%), peripheral edema (7%), edema (5%), bradycardia (3% to 5%), atrial fibrillation (3% to 5%)

Central nervous system: Insomnia (4% to 10%), anxiety (6%), fatigue (6%)

Dermatologic: Rash (2% to 9%), pruritus (6%)

Endocrine & metabolic: Hypocalcemia (7%), hypoglycemia (6% to 7%), hyperglycemia (6%), hypernatremia (4% to 6%), hyperkalemia (4% to 5%), fluid overload (5%)

Gastrointestinal: Abdominal pain (2% to 10%), anorexia (6%), dyspepsia (6%)

Hematologic: Anemia (3% to 10%), febrile neutropenia (6%)

Hepatic: AST increased (6%), ALT increased (5%), serum alkaline phosphatase increased (6% to 8%)

Neuromuscular & skeletal: Rigors (9%), back pain (5%)

Respiratory: Cough (8%), dyspnea (6%), epistaxis (6%)

Miscellaneous: Bacteremia (5% to 9%), sepsis (5% to 6%)

Drug Interactions

Metabolism/Transport Effects Substrate of CYP3A4 (minor); **Note:** Assignment of Major/Minor substrate status based on clinically relevant drug interaction potential; **Inhibits** CYP3A4 (weak)

Avoid Concomitant Use

Avoid concomitant use of Micafungin with any of the following: Pimozide

Increased Effect/Toxicity

Micafungin may increase the levels/effects of: ARIPiprazole; Pimozide

Decreased Effect

Micafungin may decrease the levels/effects of: Saccharomyces boulardii

The levels/effects of Micafungin may be decreased by: Tocilizumab

Stability Store at controlled room temperature of 25°C (77°F). Reconstituted and diluted solutions are stable for 24 hours at room temperature. Protect from light. Aseptically add 5 mL of NS (preservative-free) to each 50 or 100 mg vial. Swirl to dissolve; do not shake. Further dilute 50-150 mg in 100 mL NS. Protect from light. Alternatively, D₅W may be used for reconstitution and dilution.

Mechanism of Action Concentration-dependent inhibition of 1,3-beta-D-glucan synthase resulting in reduced formation of 1,3-beta-D-glucan, an essential polysaccharide comprising 30% to 60% of *Candida* cell walls (absent in mammalian cells); decreased glucan content leads to osmotic instability and cellular lysis

Pharmacodynamics/Kinetics

Distribution: 0.28-0.5 L/kg

Protein binding: >99%; primarily to albumin

Metabolism: Hepatic; forms M-1 (catechol) and M-2 (methoxy) metabolites (activity unknown)

Half-life elimination: 11-21 hours

Excretion: Primarily feces (71%); urine (<15%)

Dosage

Geriatric & Adult

Candidemia, acute disseminated candidiasis, and *Candida* peritonitis and abscesses: I.V.: 100 mg daily; mean duration of therapy (from clinical trials) was 15 days (range: 10-47 days)

Esophageal candidiasis: I.V.: 150 mg daily; mean duration of therapy (from clinical trials) was 15 days (range: 10-30 days)

Prophylaxis of *Candida* infection in hematopoietic stem cell transplantation: 50 mg daily

Renal Impairment No dosage adjustment required in renal impairment.

Poorly dialyzed; no supplemental dose or dosage adjustment necessary, including patients on intermittent hemodialysis, peritoneal dialysis, or continuous renal replacement therapy (eg, CVVHD).

Hepatic Impairment No dosage adjustment required for moderate hepatic impairment (Child-Pugh score 7-9). Patients with severe hepatic dysfunction have not been studied.

Administration For intravenous use only; infuse over 1 hour. Flush line with NS prior to administration.

Monitoring Parameters Liver function tests

Special Geriatric Considerations No specific data for the elderly; does not require alteration in dose or dose intervals.

Dosage Forms Excipient information presented when available (limited, particularly for generics); consult specific product labeling.

Injection, powder for reconstitution, as sodium:
  Mycamine®: 50 mg, 100 mg [contains lactose 200 mg]

◆ **Micafungin Sodium** *see* Micafungin *on page 1273*
◆ **Micardis®** *see* Telmisartan *on page 1847*
◆ **Micardis® HCT** *see* Telmisartan and Hydrochlorothiazide *on page 1849*
◆ **Micatin® [OTC]** *see* Miconazole (Topical) *on page 1276*

Miconazole (Oral) (mi KON a zole)

Medication Safety Issues
  Sound-alike/look-alike issues:
  Miconazole may be confused with metroNIDAZOLE, Micronase, Micronor®

Brand Names: U.S. Oravig® [DSC]
Index Terms Miconazole Nitrate
Generic Availability (U.S.) No
Pharmacologic Category Antifungal Agent, Oral Nonabsorbed
Use Treatment of oropharyngeal candidiasis
Contraindications Hypersensitivity to miconazole, milk protein concentrate, or any component of the formulation

Warnings/Precautions Hypersensitivity reactions have been reported. Monitor patients who have a history of azole hypersensitivity for reactions; risk of cross-reactivity is unknown. Use with caution in patients with hepatic impairment.

Adverse Reactions (Reflective of adult population; not specific for elderly)
>10%: Local: Application site reaction (10% to 12%; including burning, discomfort, edema, glossodynia, pain, pruritus, toothache, ulceration)
1% to 10%:
  Central nervous system: Headache (5% to 8%), fatigue (3%), pain (1%)
  Dermatologic: Pruritus (2%)
  Gastrointestinal: Diarrhea (6% to 9%), nausea (1% to 7%), vomiting (1% to 4%), abnormal taste (3% to 4%), oral discomfort (3%), xerostomia (3%), abdominal pain (1% to 3%), ageusia (2%), gastroenteritis (1%)
  Hematologic: Anemia (3%), lymphopenia (2%), neutropenia (1%)
  Hepatic: GGT increased (1%)
  Respiratory: Cough (3%), upper respiratory infection (2%), pharyngeal pain (1%)

Drug Interactions
  Metabolism/Transport Effects Inhibits CYP2C19 (moderate), CYP2C9 (moderate), CYP2D6 (moderate), CYP3A4 (moderate)
  Avoid Concomitant Use
  Avoid concomitant use of Miconazole (Oral) with any of the following: Clopidogrel; Gliclazide; Pimozide; Thioridazine; Tolvaptan
  Increased Effect/Toxicity
  Miconazole (Oral) may increase the levels/effects of: ARIPiprazole; Avanafil; Budesonide (Systemic, Oral Inhalation); Carvedilol; Citalopram; Colchicine; CYP2C19 Substrates; CYP2C9 Substrates; CYP2D6 Substrates; CYP3A4 Substrates; Eplerenone; Everolimus; FentaNYL; Fesoterodine; Gliclazide; Halofantrine; Ivacaftor; Lurasidone; Nebivolol; Pimecrolimus; Pimozide; Propafenone; Ranolazine; Salmeterol; Saxagliptin; Thioridazine; Tolvaptan; Vilazodone; Warfarin; Zuclopenthixol

  The levels/effects of Miconazole (Oral) may be increased by: Propafenone

◄ **Decreased Effect**
Miconazole (Oral) may decrease the levels/effects of: Clopidogrel; Codeine; Ifosfamide; Tamoxifen; TraMADol

Stability Store at 20°C to 25°C (68°F to 77°F); excursions permitted to15°C to 30°C (59°F to 86°F). Protect from moisture.

Mechanism of Action Inhibits biosynthesis of ergosterol, damaging the fungal cell wall membrane, which increases permeability causing leaking of nutrients

Pharmacodynamics/Kinetics
Duration: Buccal adhesion: 15 hours
Absorption: Minimal

Dosage
Geriatric & Adult Oropharyngeal candidiasis: Buccal tablet: 50 mg (1 tablet) applied to the upper gum region once daily for 14 days
Renal Impairment No dosing adjustment is required.
Hepatic Impairment Use with caution in patients with hepatic impairment.

Administration Apply in the morning after brushing teeth. With dry hands, place either side of the tablet against the upper gum above the incisor tooth; hold with slight pressure over the upper lip for 30 seconds. Placing the rounded side of the tablet against the gum may be more comfortable. Alternate sides of the mouth with each application; do not crush, chew, or swallow. Avoid chewing gum while in place.

If the tablet does not adhere to the gum or falls off within 6 hours of application, the same tablet should be repositioned immediately. If the tablet does not adhere, use a new tablet. If the tablet is swallowed within 6 hours of application, the patient should drink a glass of water and apply a new tablet (only once). If the tablet falls off or is swallowed >6 hours after application, a new tablet should not be applied until the next regularly scheduled dose.

Special Geriatric Considerations No specific data for the elderly; does not require alteration in dose or dose intervals. Assess patient's ability to self-administer.

Dosage Forms Excipient information presented when available (limited, particularly for generics); consult specific product labeling. [DSC] = Discontinued product
Tablet, for buccal application:
Oravig®: 50 mg [DSC]

Miconazole (Topical) (mi KON a zole)

Medication Safety Issues
Sound-alike/look-alike issues:
Miconazole may be confused with metroNIDAZOLE, Micronase, Micronor®
Lotrimin® may be confused with Lotrisone®, Otrivin®
Micatin® may be confused with Miacalcin®

Brand Names: U.S. 3M™ Cavilon™ Antifungal [OTC]; Aloe Vesta® Antifungal [OTC]; Baza® Antifungal [OTC]; Carrington® Antifungal [OTC]; Critic-Aid® Clear AF [OTC]; DermaFungal [OTC]; Dermagran® AF [OTC]; DiabetAid® Antifungal Foot Bath [OTC]; Fungoid® [OTC]; Lotrimin AF® [OTC]; Micaderm® [OTC]; Micatin® [OTC]; Micro-Guard® [OTC]; Miranel AF™ [OTC]; Mitrazol® [OTC]; Monistat® 1 Day or Night [OTC]; Monistat® 1 [OTC]; Monistat® 3 [OTC]; Monistat® 7 [OTC]; Neosporin® AF [OTC]; Podactin Cream [OTC]; Secura® Antifungal Extra Thick [OTC]; Secura® Antifungal Greaseless [OTC]; Ting® Spray Powder [OTC]; Zeasorb®-AF [OTC]

Brand Names: Canada Dermazole; Micatin®; Micozole; Monistat®; Monistat® 3

Index Terms Miconazole Nitrate

Generic Availability (U.S.) Yes: Cream (topical and vaginal), vaginal suppository

Pharmacologic Category Antifungal Agent, Topical; Antifungal Agent, Vaginal

Use Treatment of vulvovaginal candidiasis and a variety of skin and mucous membrane fungal infections

Contraindications Hypersensitivity to miconazole or any component of the formulation

Warnings/Precautions For topical use only; avoid contact with eyes. Discontinue if sensitivity or irritation develop. Petrolatum-based vaginal products may damage rubber or latex condoms or diaphragms. Separate use by 3 days. Consult with healthcare provider prior to self-medication (OTC use) of vaginal products if experiencing vaginal itching/discomfort, lower abdominal pain, back or shoulder pain, chills, nausea, vomiting, foul-smelling discharge, if this is the first vaginal yeast infection, or if exposed to HIV. Contact healthcare provider if symptoms do not begin to improve after 3 days or last longer than 7 days.

Fungoid® tincture: Patients with diabetes, circulatory problems, renal or hepatic dysfunction should contact healthcare provider prior to self-medication (OTC use).

Adverse Reactions (Reflective of adult population; not specific for elderly) Frequency not defined.

Topical: Allergic contact dermatitis, burning, maceration

Vaginal: Abdominal cramps, burning, irritation, itching

Drug Interactions

Metabolism/Transport Effects None known.

Avoid Concomitant Use There are no known interactions where it is recommended to avoid concomitant use.

Increased Effect/Toxicity

Miconazole (Topical) may increase the levels/effects of: Vitamin K Antagonists

Decreased Effect There are no known significant interactions involving a decrease in effect.

Ethanol/Nutrition/Herb Interactions Herb/Nutraceutical: St John's wort may decrease miconazole levels.

Mechanism of Action Inhibits biosynthesis of ergosterol, damaging the fungal cell wall membrane, which increases permeability causing leaking of nutrients

Pharmacodynamics/Kinetics

Absorption: Topical: Negligible

Excretion: Feces; urine

Dosage

Geriatric & Adult

Tinea corporis: Topical: Apply twice daily for 4 weeks

Tinea pedis: Topical: Apply twice daily for 4 weeks

Effervescent tablet: Dissolve 1 tablet in ~1 gallon of water; soak feet for 15-30 minutes; pat dry

Tinea cruris: Topical: Apply twice daily for 2 weeks

Vulvovaginal candidiasis: Vaginal:

Cream, 2%: Insert 1 applicatorful at bedtime for 7 days

Cream, 4%: Insert 1 applicatorful at bedtime for 3 days

Suppository, 100 mg: Insert 1 suppository at bedtime for 7 days

Suppository, 200 mg: Insert 1 suppository at bedtime for 3 days

Suppository, 1200 mg: Insert 1 suppository (a one-time dose); may be used at bedtime or during the day

Note: Many products are available as a combination pack, with a suppository for vaginal instillation and cream to relieve external symptoms. External cream may be used twice daily, as needed, for up to 7 days.

Special Geriatric Considerations Instruct patient or caregiver on appropriate use of topical miconazole products.

Dosage Forms Excipient information presented when available (limited, particularly for generics); consult specific product labeling. [DSC] = Discontinued product

Aerosol, powder, topical, as nitrate:

Lotrimin AF®: 2% (133 g)

Lotrimin AF®: 2% (133 g) [deodorant formulation]

Micatin®: 2% (90 g)

Neosporin® AF: 2% (85 g)

Ting® Spray Powder: 2% (128 g) [contains aloe, ethanol 10% w/w]

Aerosol, spray, topical, as nitrate:

Micatin®: 2% (90 g)

Micatin®: 2% (105 mL) [contains benzyl alcohol]

Neosporin® AF: 2% (105 mL)

Combination package, topical/vaginal, as nitrate: Cream, topical: 2% (9 g) and Suppository, vaginal: 200 mg (3s)

Monistat® 3: Cream, topical: 2% (9 g) and Insert, vaginal: 200 mg (3s)

Monistat® 7: Cream, topical: 2% (9 g) and Cream, vaginal: 2% (45 g), Cream, topical: 2% (9 g) and Cream, vaginal: 2% (7 x 5 g) [contains benzoic acid]

Monistat® 3: Cream, topical: 2% (9 g) and Cream, vaginal: 4% (25 g), Cream, topical: 2% (9 g) and Cream, vaginal: 4% (3 x 5 g) [contains benzoic acid; vaginal cream 200 mg/ applicator]

Monistat® 7: Cream, topical: 2% (9 g) and Suppository, vaginal: 100 mg (7s) [contains benzoic acid (in cream)]

Monistat® 1: Cream, topical: 2% (9 g) and Insert, vaginal: 1200 mg (1) [contains benzoic acid (in cream), soya lecithin (in insert)]

Monistat® 1 Day or Night: Cream, topical: 2% (9 g) and Insert, vaginal: 1200 mg (1) [contains benzoic acid (in cream), mineral oil (in insert), soya lecithin (in insert)]

Cream, topical, as nitrate: 2% (15 g, 30 g, 45 g)
  Baza® Antifungal: 2% (4 g, 57 g, 142 g) [zinc oxide based formula]
  Carrington® Antifungal: 2% (150 g)
  Micaderm®: 2% (30 g)
  Micatin®: 2% (14 g) [contains benzoic acid]
  Micro-Guard®: 2% (60 g [DSC])
  Miranel AF™: 2% (28 g) [contains ethanol]
  3M™ Cavilon™ Antifungal: 2% (56 g, 141 g) [contains castor oil]
  Neosporin® AF: 2% (14 g, 15 g) [contains benzoic acid]
  Podactin Cream: 2% (30 g)
  Secura® Antifungal Extra Thick: 2% (97.5 g) [contains zinc oxide]
  Secura® Antifungal Greaseless: 2% (60 g)
Cream, vaginal, as nitrate: 2% (45 g); 4% (25 g [DSC])
  Monistat® 7: 2% (45 g) [contains benzoic acid; 100 mg/applicator]
  Monistat® 3: 4% (15 g, 25 g) [contains benzoic acid; 200 mg/applicator]
Liquid, topical, as nitrate [spray]:
  Lotrimin AF®: 2% (150 g)
Ointment, topical, as nitrate:
  Aloe Vesta® Antifungal: 2% (60 g, 150 g) [contains aloe]
  Critic-Aid® Clear AF: 2% (57 g, 142 g, 300s)
  DermaFungal: 2% (120 g)
  Dermagran® AF: 2% (120 g) [zinc oxide based formula]
Powder, topical, as nitrate:
  Lotrimin AF®: 2% (90 g)
  Micro-Guard®: 2% (90 g)
  Mitrazol®: 2% (30 g)
  Zeasorb®-AF: 2% (70 g)
Suppository, vaginal, as nitrate: 100 mg (7s); 200 mg (3s)
Tablet for solution, topical, as nitrate [effervescent]:
  DiabetAid® Antifungal Foot Bath: 2% (10s)
Tincture, topical, as nitrate:
  Fungoid®: 2% (7.39 mL, 30 mL) [contains isopropyl alcohol 30%]

◆ **Miconazole Nitrate** see Miconazole (Oral) on page 1275
◆ **Miconazole Nitrate** see Miconazole (Topical) on page 1276
◆ **Micro-Guard® [OTC]** see Miconazole (Topical) on page 1276
◆ **microK®** see Potassium Chloride on page 1571
◆ **microK® 10** see Potassium Chloride on page 1571
◆ **Micronase** see GlyBURIDE on page 887
◆ **Microzide®** see Hydrochlorothiazide on page 933

Midazolam (MID aye zoe lam)

Related Information
Anxiolytic, Sedative/Hypnotic, and Miscellaneous Benzodiazepines on page 2106
Medication Safety Issues
Sound-alike/look-alike issues:
Versed may be confused with VePesid, Vistaril®
High alert medication:
The Institute for Safe Medication Practices (ISMP) includes this medication among its list of drugs which have a heightened risk of causing significant patient harm when used in error.
Brand Names: Canada Apo-Midazolam®; Midazolam Injection
Index Terms Midazolam Hydrochloride; Versed
Generic Availability (U.S.) Yes
Pharmacologic Category Benzodiazepine
Use Preoperative sedation; moderate sedation prior to diagnostic or radiographic procedures; ICU sedation (continuous infusion); induction and maintenance of general anesthesia
Unlabeled Use Anxiety, status epilepticus, conscious sedation (intranasal route)
Contraindications Hypersensitivity to midazolam or any component of the formulation; intrathecal or epidural injection of parenteral forms containing preservatives (ie, benzyl alcohol); acute narrow-angle glaucoma; concurrent use of potent inhibitors of CYP3A4 (amprenavir, atazanavir, or ritonavir)

Per respective protease inhibitor manufacturer's labeling: Concurrent use of oral midazolam with amprenavir, atazanavir, darunavir, indinavir, lopinavir-ritonavir, nelfinavir, ritonavir, saquinavir, tipranavir and concurrent use of oral or injectable midazolam with fosamprenavir

Warnings/Precautions [U.S. Boxed Warning]: **May cause severe respiratory depression, respiratory arrest, or apnea. Use with extreme caution, particularly in noncritical care settings.** Appropriate resuscitative equipment and qualified personnel must be available for administration and monitoring. Initial dosing must be cautiously titrated and individualized, particularly in elderly or debilitated patients, patients with hepatic impairment (including alcoholics), or in renal impairment, particularly if other CNS depressants (including opiates) are used concurrently. [U.S. Boxed Warning]: **Initial doses in elderly or debilitated patients should be conservative; as little as 1 mg, but not to exceed 2.5 mg.** Use with caution in patients with respiratory disease or impaired gag reflex. Use during upper airway procedures may increase risk of hypoventilation. Prolonged responses have been noted following extended administration by continuous infusion (possibly due to metabolite accumulation) or in the presence of drugs which inhibit midazolam metabolism.

Causes CNS depression (dose-related) resulting in sedation, dizziness, confusion, or ataxia which may impair physical and mental capabilities. Patients must be cautioned about performing tasks which require mental alertness (eg, operating machinery or driving). A minimum of 1 day should elapse after midazolam administration before attempting these tasks. Use with caution in patients receiving other CNS depressants or psychoactive agents. Effects with other sedative drugs or ethanol may be potentiated. Benzodiazepines have been associated with falls and traumatic injury and should be used with extreme caution in patients who are at risk of these events (especially the elderly).

May cause hypotension - hemodynamic events are more common in pediatric patients or patients with hemodynamic instability. Hypotension and/or respiratory depression may occur more frequently in patients who have received opioid analgesics. Use with caution in obese patients, chronic renal failure, and HF. Does not protect against increases in heart rate or blood pressure during intubation. Should not be used in shock, coma, or acute alcohol intoxication.

Avoid intra-arterial administration or extravasation of parenteral formulation. Some parenteral dosage forms may contain benzyl alcohol. Some formulations may contain cherry flavoring.

Midazolam causes anterograde amnesia. Paradoxical reactions, including hyperactive or aggressive behavior have been reported with benzodiazepines, particularly in psychiatric patients. Does not have analgesic, antidepressant, or antipsychotic properties.

Benzodiazepines have been associated with dependence and acute withdrawal symptoms on discontinuation or reduction in dose. Acute withdrawal, including seizures, may be precipitated after administration of flumazenil to patients receiving long-term benzodiazepine therapy.

Adverse Reactions (Reflective of adult population; not specific for elderly) As reported in adults unless otherwise noted:

>10%: Respiratory: Decreased tidal volume and/or respiratory rate decrease, apnea

1% to 10%:

Cardiovascular: Hypotension

Central nervous system: Drowsiness (1%), oversedation, headache (1%), seizure-like activity

Gastrointestinal: Nausea (3%), vomiting (3%)

Local: Pain and local reactions at injection site (4% I.M., 5% I.V.; severity less than diazepam)

Ocular: Nystagmus

Respiratory: Cough (1%)

Miscellaneous: Physical and psychological dependence with prolonged use, hiccups (4%), paradoxical reaction

Drug Interactions

Metabolism/Transport Effects Substrate of CYP2B6 (minor), CYP3A4 (major); **Note:** Assignment of Major/Minor substrate status based on clinically relevant drug interaction potential; **Inhibits** CYP2C8 (weak), CYP2C9 (weak), CYP3A4 (weak)

Avoid Concomitant Use

Avoid concomitant use of Midazolam with any of the following: Azelastine; Azelastine (Nasal); Boceprevir; Conivaptan; Efavirenz; Methadone; Mirtazapine; OLANZapine; Paraldehyde; Pimozide; Protease Inhibitors; Telaprevir

Increased Effect/Toxicity

Midazolam may increase the levels/effects of: Alcohol (Ethyl); ARIPiprazole; Azelastine; Azelastine (Nasal); Buprenorphine; CloZAPine; CNS Depressants; Fosphenytoin; Methadone; Methotrimeprazine; Metyrosine; Mirtazapine; Paraldehyde; Phenytoin; Pimozide; Propofol; Selective Serotonin Reuptake Inhibitors; Zolpidem

The levels/effects of Midazolam may be increased by: Antifungal Agents (Azole Derivatives, Systemic); Aprepitant; AtorvaSTATin; Boceprevir; Calcium Channel Blockers (Nondihydro-pyridine); Cimetidine; Conivaptan; Contraceptives (Estrogens); Contraceptives (Progestins); CYP3A4 Inhibitors (Moderate); CYP3A4 Inhibitors (Strong); Dasatinib; Droperidol; Efavir-enz; Fosaprepitant; Grapefruit Juice; HydrOXYzine; Isoniazid; Ivacaftor; Macrolide Anti-biotics; Methotrimeprazine; Mifepristone; OLANZapine; Propofol; Protease Inhibitors; Proton Pump Inhibitors; Selective Serotonin Reuptake Inhibitors; Telaprevir

Decreased Effect

The levels/effects of Midazolam may be decreased by: CarBAMazepine; CYP3A4 Inducers (Strong); Deferasirox; Ginkgo Biloba; Rifamycin Derivatives; St Johns Wort; Theophylline Derivatives; Tocilizumab; Yohimbine

Ethanol/Nutrition/Herb Interactions

Ethanol: Ethanol may increase CNS depression. Management: Avoid ethanol.

Food: Grapefruit juice may increase serum concentrations of midazolam. Management: Avoid concurrent use of grapefruit juice with oral midazolam.

Herb/Nutraceutical: St John's wort may decrease midazolam levels and increase CNS depression; valerian, kava kava, and gotu kola may increase CNS depression. Manage-ment: Avoid concurrent use with St John's wort, valerian, kava kava, and gotu kola.

Stability The manufacturer states that midazolam, at a final concentration of 0.5 mg/mL, is stable for up to 24 hours when diluted with D_5W or NS. A final concentration of 1 mg/mL in NS has been documented to be stable for up to 10 days (McMullen, 1995). Admixtures do not require protection from light for short-term storage.

Mechanism of Action Binds to stereospecific benzodiazepine receptors on the postsynaptic GABA neuron at several sites within the central nervous system, including the limbic system, reticular formation. Enhancement of the inhibitory effect of GABA on neuronal excitability results by increased neuronal membrane permeability to chloride ions. This shift in chloride ions results in hyperpolarization (a less excitable state) and stabilization.

Pharmacodynamics/Kinetics

Onset of action: I.M.: Sedation: ~15 minutes; I.V.: 3-5 minutes; Oral: 10-20 minutes
Peak effect: I.M.: 0.5-1 hour

Duration: I.M.: Up to 6 hours; Mean: 2 hours; I.V.: Single dose: <2 hours (dose-dependent) (Fragen, 1997); Cirrhosis: Up to 6 hours (MacGilcrhist, 1986)

Absorption: Oral: Rapid

Distribution: V_d: 1-3.1 L/kg; increased in females, elderly, and obesity

Protein binding: ~97%; in patients with cirrhosis, protein binding is reduced with a free fraction of ~5% (Trouvin, 1988)

Metabolism: Extensively hepatic CYP3A4; 60% to 70% of biotransformed midazolam is the active metabolite 1-hydroxy-midazolam (or alpha-hydroxymidazolam)

Bioavailability: Oral: 40% to 50% (Kanto, 1985); I.M.: >90%

Half-life elimination: 2-6 hours; prolonged in cirrhosis, congestive heart failure, obesity, renal failure, and elderly. **Note:** In patients with renal failure, reduced elimination of active hydroxylated metabolites leads to drug accumulation and prolonged sedation.

Excretion: I.V.: Urine (primarily as glucuronide conjugates of the hydroxylated metabolites); Oral: Urine (~90% within 24 hours; primarily [60% to 70%] as glucuronide conjugates of the hydroxylated metabolites; <0.03% as unchanged drug); feces (~2% to 10% over 5 days) (Kanto, 1985; Smith, 1981)

Dosage

Geriatric The dose of midazolam needs to be individualized based on the patient's age, underlying diseases, and concurrent medications. Consider reducing dose by 20% to 50% in elderly, chronically ill, or debilitated patients and those receiving opioids or other CNS depressants.

Anesthesia: I.V.:
Induction: Adults >55 years:
Unpremedicated patients: Initial dose: 0.3 mg/kg
Premedicated patients: Reduce dose by at least 20% (Miller, 2010).
Maintenance: Refer to adult dosing.

Conscious sedation: I.V.: Initial: 0.5 mg slow I.V.; give no more than 1.5 mg in a 2-minute period; if additional titration is needed, give no more than 1 mg over 2 minutes, waiting another 2 or more minutes to evaluate sedative effect; a total dose of >3.5 mg is rarely necessary

Preoperative/preprocedural sedation: Adults >60 years (without concomitant opioid administration): I.M.: 2-3 mg (or 0.02-0.05 mg/kg) 30-60 minutes prior to surgery/proce-dure; some may only require 1 mg (or 0.01 mg/kg) if anticipated intensity and duration of sedation is less critical.

Adult The dose of midazolam needs to be individualized based on the patient's age, underlying diseases, and concurrent medications. Consider reducing dose by 20% to 50% in elderly, chronically ill, or debilitated patients and those receiving opioids or other CNS depressants.

Preoperative/preprocedural sedation: Healthy adults <60 years:
I.M.: 0.07-0.08 mg/kg 30-60 minutes prior to surgery/procedure; usual dose: 5 mg
I.V.: 0.02-0.04 mg/kg; repeat every 5 minutes as needed to desired effect or up to 0.1-0.2 mg/kg
Intranasal (unlabeled route): 0.1 mg/kg; administer 10-20 minutes prior to surgery/proce- dure (Uygur-Bayramiçli, 2002). **Note:** Use 5 mg/mL injectable concentrated solution to deliver dose. Due to the low pH of the solution, burning upon administration is likely to occur.

Conscious sedation: I.V.:
Manufacturer's labeling:
Healthy adults <60 years:
Initial: Some patients respond to doses as low as 1 mg; no more than 2.5 mg should be administered over a period of 2 minutes. Additional doses of midazolam may be administered after a 2-minute waiting period and evaluation of sedation after each dose increment. A total dose >5 mg is generally not needed.
Maintenance: 25% of dose used to reach sedative effect
Adults ≥60 years, debilitated, or chronically ill: Refer to geriatric dosing.
Alternate recommendations: American Society for Gastrointestinal Endoscopy: Initial: 0.5-2 mg slow I.V. over at least 2 minutes; slowly titrate to effect by repeating doses every 2-3 minutes if needed; usual total dose: 2.5-5 mg (Waring, 2003)

Anesthesia: I.V.:
Induction: Adults <55 years:
Unpremedicated patients: 0.3-0.35 mg/kg over 20-30 seconds; after 2 minutes, may repeat if necessary at 25% of initial dose every 2 minutes, up to a total dose of 0.6 mg/kg in resistant cases
Premedicated patients: Usual dosage range: 0.05-0.2 mg/kg (Barash, 2009; Miller, 2010). Use of 0.2 mg/kg administered over 5-10 seconds has been shown to safely produce anesthesia within 30 seconds (Samuelson, 1981) and is recommended for ASA physical status P1 and P2 patients. When used with other anesthetic drugs (ie, co- induction), the dose is <0.1 mg/kg (Miller, 2010).
ASA physical status >P3 or debilitation: Reduce dose by at least 20% (Miller, 2010).
Maintenance: 0.05 mg/kg as needed (Miller, 2010), or continuous infusion 0.015-0.06 mg/kg/**hour** (0.25-1 **mcg**/kg/minute) (Barash, 2009; Miller, 2010)

Sedation in mechanically ventilated patients: I.V.:
Manufacturer's labeling: Initial dose: 0.01-0.05 mg/kg (~0.5-4 mg); may repeat at 5- to 15-minute intervals until adequate sedation achieved; maintenance infusion: 0.02-0.1 mg/kg/**hour** (0.3-1.7 **mcg**/kg/minute). Titrate to reach desired level of sedation. Consider a trial of daily awakening; if agitated after discontinuation of drip, then restart at 50% of the previous dose (Kress, 2000).
or
Initial dose: 0.02-0.08 mg/kg (~1-5 mg in 70 kg adult); may repeat at 5- to 15-minute intervals until adequate sedation achieved; maintenance infusion: 0.04-0.2 mg/kg/**hour** (0.67-3.3 **mcg**/kg/minute). Titrate to reach desired level of sedation (Jacobi, 2002).

Status epilepticus refractory to standard therapy (unlabeled use): I.V.: **Note:** Intubation required; adjust dose based on hemodynamics, seizure activity, and EEG. 0.15-0.3 mg/kg (usual dose: 5-15 mg); may repeat every 10-15 minutes as needed **or** 0.2 mg/kg bolus followed by a continuous infusion of 0.05-0.6 mg/kg/**hour** (0.83-10 **mcg**/kg/minute) (Low- enstein, 2005; Meierkord, 2010)

Status epilepticus, prehospital treatment (unlabeled use): I.V.: **Note:**Administered by paramedics when convulsions last >5 minutes **or** if convulsions are occurring after having intermittent seizures without regaining consciousness for >5 minutes: 10 mg once (Silber- gleit, 2012)

Renal Impairment There are no dosage adjustments provided in manufacturer's labeling; however, patients with renal failure receiving a continuous infusion cannot adequately eliminate the active hydroxylated metabolites (eg, 1-hydroxymidazolam) contributing to prolonged sedation sometimes for days after discontinuation (Spina, 2007).
Intermittent hemodialysis: Supplemental dose is not necessary.
Continuous venovenous hemofiltration (CVVH): Unconjugated 1-hydroxymidazolam not effectively removed; 1-hydroxymidazolamglucuronide effectively removed; sieving coeffi- cient = 0.45 (Swart, 2005).
Peritoneal dialysis: Significant drug removal is unlikely based on physiochemical character- istics.

◄

Hepatic Impairment

Severe hepatic impairment (eg, cirrhosis): **Note:** Use with caution in patients with any degree of hepatic impairment; patients with hepatic encephalopathy likely to be more sensitive to midazolam.

Single dose (eg, induction): No dosage adjustment recommended; patients with hepatic impairment may be more sensitive compared to patients without hepatic impairment; anticipate longer duration of action (MacGilchrist, 1986; Trouvin, 1988).

Multiple dosing or continuous infusion: Expect longer duration of action and accumulation; based on patient response, dosage reduction likely to be necessary (Trouvin, 1988).

Administration

Intranasal: **Note:** Due to the low pH of the solution, burning upon administration is likely to occur. Use of an atomizer, such as the MAD 300 Mucosal Atomizer which attaches to a tuberculin syringe, can reduce irritation. If possible, based upon dose to be administered, use higher concentration injectable solution to minimize volume administered intranasal. Smaller volume will reduce irritation and swallowing of administered dose. The maximum recommended dose volume per nare is 1 mL.

Using the 5 mg/mL injectable solution, draw up desired dose with a 1-3 mL needleless syringe; may attach a nasal mucosal atomization device prior to delivering dose. Deliver half of the total dose volume (of the 5 mg/mL concentration) into the first nare using the atomizer device or by dripping slowly into nostril, then deliver the other half of the dose into the second nare.

Oral: Do not mix with any liquid (such as grapefruit juice) prior to administration

Parenteral:

I.M.: Administer deep I.M. into large muscle.

I.V.: Administer by slow I.V. injection over at least 2-5 minutes at a concentration of 1-5 mg/mL or by I.V. infusion. For induction of anesthesia, administer I.V. bolus over 5-30 seconds. Continuous infusions should be administered via an infusion pump.

Monitoring Parameters Respiratory and cardiovascular status, blood pressure, blood pressure monitor required during I.V. administration

Pharmacotherapy Pearls Abrupt discontinuation after sustained use (generally >10 days) may cause withdrawal symptoms. With continuous infusion, midazolam may accumulate in peripheral tissues; use lowest effective infusion rate to reduce accumulation effects; midazolam is 3-4 times as potent as diazepam.

Special Geriatric Considerations In the elderly if concomitant CNS depressant medications are used, the midazolam dose will be at least 50% less than doses used in healthy, young, unpremedicated patients.

Controlled Substance C-IV

Dosage Forms Excipient information presented when available (limited, particularly for generics); consult specific product labeling.

Injection, solution: 1 mg/mL (2 mL, 5 mL, 10 mL); 5 mg/mL (1 mL, 2 mL, 5 mL, 10 mL)

Injection, solution [preservative free]: 1 mg/mL (2 mL, 5 mL); 5 mg/mL (1 mL, 2 mL)

Syrup, oral: 2 mg/mL (118 mL)

◆ **Midazolam Hydrochloride** see Midazolam on page 1278

Midodrine (MI doe dreen)

Medication Safety Issues

Sound-alike/look-alike issues:

Midodrine may be confused with Midrin®, minoxidil

ProAmatine may be confused with protamine

Brand Names: Canada Amatine®; Apo-Midodrine®

Index Terms Midodrine Hydrochloride; ProAmatine

Generic Availability (U.S.) Yes

Pharmacologic Category Alpha$_1$ Agonist

Use Orphan drug: Treatment of symptomatic orthostatic hypotension

Unlabeled Use Investigational: Management of urinary incontinence

Contraindications Hypersensitivity to midodrine or any component of the formulation; severe organic heart disease; acute renal failure; urinary retention; pheochromocytoma; thyrotoxicosis; persistent and significant supine hypertension

Warnings/Precautions [U.S. Boxed Warning]: Indicated for patients for whom orthostatic hypotension significantly impairs their daily life despite standard clinical care. May cause hypertension. Use is not recommended with supine hypertension. May slow heart rate primarily due to vagal reflex. Use caution when administered concurrently with negative chronotropes (eg, digoxin, beta blockers). Use is not recommended with supine hypertension. Use cautiously in patients with renal impairment and initiate with a reduced dose; contraindicated in patients with acute renal failure. Caution should be exercised in patients with diabetes, visual problems (especially if receiving fludrocortisone), urinary retention (reduce initial dose), or hepatic dysfunction; monitor renal and hepatic function prior to and periodically during therapy.

Adverse Reactions (Reflective of adult population; not specific for elderly)
>10%:
- Cardiovascular: Supine hypertension (7% to 13%)
- Dermatologic: Piloerection (13%), pruritus (12%)
- Genitourinary: Urinary urgency, retention, or polyuria, dysuria (up to 13%)
- Neuromuscular & skeletal: Paresthesia (18%)

1% to 10%:
- Central nervous system: Chills (5%), pain (5%)
- Dermatologic: Rash (2%)
- Gastrointestinal: Abdominal pain

Drug Interactions
Metabolism/Transport Effects None known.

Avoid Concomitant Use
Avoid concomitant use of Midodrine with any of the following: Ergot Derivatives; Iobenguane I 123; MAO Inhibitors

Increased Effect/Toxicity
Midodrine may increase the levels/effects of: Sympathomimetics

The levels/effects of Midodrine may be increased by: AtoMOXetine; Beta-Blockers; Calcium Channel Blockers (Nondihydropyridine); Cannabinoids; Cardiac Glycosides; Ergot Derivatives; MAO Inhibitors; Tricyclic Antidepressants

Decreased Effect
Midodrine may decrease the levels/effects of: Benzylpenicilloyl Polylysine; Iobenguane I 123

Mechanism of Action Midodrine forms an active metabolite, desglymidodrine, which is an alpha$_1$-agonist. This agent increases arteriolar and venous tone resulting in a rise in standing, sitting, and supine systolic and diastolic blood pressure in patients with orthostatic hypotension.

Pharmacodynamics/Kinetics
Onset of action: ~1 hour

Duration: 2-3 hours

Absorption: Rapid

Distribution: V_d (desglymidodrine): <1.6 L/kg; poorly across membrane (eg, blood-brain barrier)

Protein binding: Minimal

Metabolism: Hepatic and many other tissues; midodrine is a prodrug which undergoes rapid deglycination to desglymidodrine (active metabolite)

Bioavailability: Desglymidodrine: 93%

Half-life elimination: Desglymidodrine: ~3-4 hours; Midodrine: 25 minutes

Time to peak, serum: Desglymidodrine: 1-2 hours; Midodrine: 30 minutes

Excretion: Urine (Midodrine: Insignificant; Desglymidodrine: 80% by active renal secretion)

Dosage
Geriatric & Adult
Orthostatic hypotension: Oral: 10 mg 3 times/day during daytime hours (every 3-4 hours) when patient is upright (maximum: 40 mg/day)

Prevention of hemodialysis-induced hypotension (unlabeled use): Oral: 2.5-10 mg given 15-30 minutes prior to dialysis session (Cruz, 1998; KDOQI, 2005; Prakash, 2004)

Vasovagal syncope (unlabeled use): Oral: Initial: 5 mg 3 times/day during daytime hours (every 6 hours) increased up to 15 mg/dose if necessary (Perez-Lugones, 2001; Ward, 1998)

Renal Impairment Orthostatic hypotension: 2.5 mg 3 times/day; gradually increase as tolerated.

Hemodialysis: Dialyzable; dose after hemodialysis unless used for prevention of hemodialysis-induced hypotension.

Administration Doses may be given in approximately 3- to 4-hour intervals (eg, shortly before or upon rising in the morning, at midday, in the late afternoon not later than 6 PM). Avoid dosing after the evening meal or within 4 hours of bedtime. Continue therapy only in patients who appear to attain symptomatic improvement during initial treatment. Standing systolic blood pressure may be elevated 15-30 mm Hg at 1 hour after a 10 mg dose. Some effect may persist for 2-3 hours.

Monitoring Parameters Blood pressure (standing and sitting), renal and hepatic parameters, symptoms of orthostasis

Special Geriatric Considerations Adjust dosage for renal impairment.

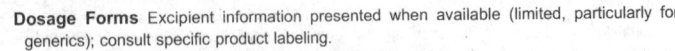

Dosage Forms Excipient information presented when available (limited, particularly for generics); consult specific product labeling.

Tablet, oral, as hydrochloride: 2.5 mg, 5 mg, 10 mg

◆ **Midodrine Hydrochloride** see Midodrine on page 1282
◆ **Midol® Cramps & Body Aches [OTC]** see Ibuprofen on page 966
◆ **Midol® Extended Relief [OTC]** see Naproxen on page 1338
◆ **Migergot®** see Ergotamine and Caffeine on page 662

Miglitol (MIG li tol)

Related Information
Diabetes Mellitus Management, Adults on page 2193

Medication Safety Issues
Sound-alike/look-alike issues:
Glyset® may be confused with Cycloset®

Brand Names: U.S. Glyset®

Generic Availability (U.S.) No

Pharmacologic Category Antidiabetic Agent, Alpha-Glucosidase Inhibitor

Use Type 2 diabetes mellitus (noninsulin-dependent, NIDDM):

Monotherapy as an adjunct to diet to improve glycemic control in patients with type 2 diabetes mellitus (noninsulin-dependent, NIDDM) whose hyperglycemia cannot be managed with diet alone

Combination therapy with a sulfonylurea when diet plus either miglitol or a sulfonylurea alone do not result in adequate glycemic control. The effect of miglitol to enhance glycemic control is additive to that of sulfonylureas when used in combination.

Contraindications Hypersensitivity to miglitol or any of component of the formulation; diabetic ketoacidosis; inflammatory bowel disease; colonic ulceration; partial intestinal obstruction or predisposition to intestinal obstruction; chronic intestinal diseases associated with marked disorders of digestion or absorption or with conditions that may deteriorate as a result of increased gas formation in the intestine

Warnings/Precautions GI symptoms are the most common reactions. The incidence of abdominal pain and diarrhea tend to diminish considerably with continued treatment. Use with caution in patients with mild-to-moderate renal impairment; not recommended in severe impairment (serum creatinine >2 mg/dL); studies have not been conducted. In combination with a sulfonylurea will cause a further lowering of blood glucose and may increase the hypoglycemic potential of the sulfonylurea. It may be necessary to discontinue miglitol and administer insulin if the patient is exposed to stress (ie, fever, trauma, infection, surgery).

Adverse Reactions (Reflective of adult population; not specific for elderly)
>10%: Gastrointestinal: Flatulence (42%), diarrhea (29%), abdominal pain (12%)
1% to 10%: Dermatologic: Rash (4%)

Drug Interactions
Metabolism/Transport Effects None known.

Avoid Concomitant Use There are no known interactions where it is recommended to avoid concomitant use.

Increased Effect/Toxicity
Miglitol may increase the levels/effects of: Hypoglycemic Agents

The levels/effects of Miglitol may be increased by: Herbs (Hypoglycemic Properties); MAO Inhibitors; Pegvisomant; Salicylates; Selective Serotonin Reuptake Inhibitors

Decreased Effect
The levels/effects of Miglitol may be decreased by: Corticosteroids (Orally Inhaled); Corticosteroids (Systemic); Loop Diuretics; Luteinizing Hormone-Releasing Hormone Analogs; Somatropin; Thiazide Diuretics

Stability Store at 25°C (77°F); excursions permitted to 15°C to 30°C (59°F to 86°F).

Mechanism of Action In contrast to sulfonylureas, miglitol does not enhance insulin secretion; the antihyperglycemic action of miglitol results from a reversible inhibition of membrane-bound intestinal alpha-glucosidases which hydrolyze oligosaccharides and disaccharides to glucose and other monosaccharides in the brush border of the small intestine. In patients with diabetes, this enzyme inhibition results in delayed glucose absorption and lowering of postprandial hyperglycemia.

Pharmacodynamics/Kinetics
Absorption: Saturable at high doses: 25 mg dose: Completely absorbed; 100 mg dose: 50% to 70% absorbed
Distribution: V_d: 0.18 L/kg
Protein binding: <4%
Metabolism: None
Half-life elimination: ~2 hours
Time to peak: 2-3 hours
Excretion: Urine (as unchanged drug)

Dosage
Geriatric & Adult Type 2 diabetes (noninsulin dependent, NIDDM): Oral: Initial: 25 mg 3 times/day with the first bite of food at each meal; the dose may be increased to 50 mg 3 times/day after 4-8 weeks; maximum recommended dose: 100 mg 3 times/day

Renal Impairment Miglitol is primarily excreted by the kidneys; no dosage adjustment recommended in mild-moderate impairment. Not recommended in patients with a S_{cr} >2 mg/dL; studies have not been conducted.

Hepatic Impairment No adjustment necessary.

Administration Should be taken orally at the start (with the first bite) of each main meal

Monitoring Parameters Monitor therapeutic response by periodic blood glucose tests; measurement of glycosylated hemoglobin is recommended for the monitoring of long-term glycemic control

Reference Range
Recommendations for glycemic control in adults with diabetes:
Hb A_{1c}: <7%
Preprandial capillary plasma glucose: 70-130 mg/dL
Peak postprandial capillary blood glucose: <180 mg/dL
Blood pressure: <130/80 mm Hg
Recommendations for glycemic control in older adults with diabetes:
Relatively healthy, cognitively intact, and with a ≥5-year life expectancy: See Adults
Frail, life expectancy <5-years or those for whom the risks of intensive glucose control outweigh the benefits:
Hb A_{1c}: <8% to 9%
Blood pressure: <140/80 mm Hg or <130/80 mm Hg if tolerated

Special Geriatric Considerations In a double-blind randomized, placebo-controlled trial, glyburide caused significantly greater reductions in hemoglobin A_{1c} compared to miglitol 25 mg or 50 mg three times per day, but was associated with more weight gain. Diarrhea, soft stools, and flatulence were more common with miglitol. Intensive glucose control (Hb A_{1c} <6.5%) has been linked to increased all-cause and cardiovascular mortality, hypoglycemia requiring assistance, and weight gain in adult type 2 diabetes. How "tightly" to control a geriatric patient's blood glucose needs to be individualized. Such a decision should be based on several factors, including the patient's functional and cognitive status, how well he/she recognizes hypoglycemic or hyperglycemic symptoms, and how to respond to them and other disease states. An Hb A_{1c} <7.5% is an acceptable endpoint for a healthy older adult, while <8% is acceptable for frail elderly patients, those with a duration of illness >10 years, or those with comorbid conditions and requiring combination diabetes medications. For elderly patients with diabetes who are relatively healthy, attaining target goals for aspirin use, blood pressure, lipids, smoking cessation, and diet and exercise may be more important than normalized glycemic control.

Dosage Forms Excipient information presented when available (limited, particularly for generics); consult specific product labeling.
Tablet, oral:
Glyset®: 25 mg, 50 mg, 100 mg

◆ **Migranal®** see Dihydroergotamine on page 548
◆ **Mild-C® [OTC]** see Ascorbic Acid on page 149
◆ **Milk of Magnesia** see Magnesium Hydroxide on page 1177
◆ **Milk of Magnesia [OTC]** see Magnesium Hydroxide on page 1177
◆ **Milk of Magnesium [OTC]** see Magnesium Hydroxide on page 1177
◆ **Millipred™** see PrednisoLONE (Systemic) on page 1591
◆ **Millipred™ DP** see PrednisoLONE (Systemic) on page 1591

Milnacipran (mil NAY ci pran)

Related Information
Antidepressant Agents *on page 2097*
Medication Safety Issues
Sound-alike/look-alike issues:
Savella® may be confused with cevimeline, sevelamer
Brand Names: U.S. Savella®
Generic Availability (U.S.) No
Pharmacologic Category Antidepressant, Serotonin/Norepinephrine Reuptake Inhibitor
Use Management of fibromyalgia
Medication Guide Available Yes
Contraindications Concomitant use or within 2 weeks of MAO inhibitors; uncontrolled narrow-angle glaucoma
Warnings/Precautions [U.S. Boxed Warning]: Milnacipran is a serotonin/norepinephrine reuptake inhibitor (SNRI) similar to SNRIs used to treat depression and other psychiatric disorders. **Antidepressants increase the risk of suicidal thinking and behavior in children, adolescents, and young adults (18-24 years of age) with major depressive disorder (MDD) and other psychiatric disorders**; consider risk prior to prescribing. Short-term studies did not show an increased risk in patients >24 years of age and showed a decreased risk in patients ≥65 years. Closely monitor for clinical worsening, suicidality, or unusual changes in behavior; the patient's family or caregiver should be instructed to closely observe the patient and communicate condition with healthcare provider. A medication guide should be dispensed with each prescription.

Suicide risks should be monitored in patients treated with SNRIs regardless of the indication. The possibility of a suicide attempt is inherent in major depression and may persist until remission occurs. Monitor for worsening of depression or suicidality, especially during initiation of therapy (generally first 1-2 months) or with dose increases or decreases. Use caution in high-risk patients. Worsening depression and severe abrupt suicidality that are not part of the presenting symptoms may require discontinuation or modification of drug therapy. The patient's family or caregiver should be alerted to monitor patients for the emergence of suicidality and associated behaviors (such as agitation, irritability, hostility, impulsivity, and hypomania) and call healthcare provider.

Patients with major depressive disorder were excluded from clinical trials evaluating milnacipran for fibromyalgia; however, mania has been reported in patients with mood disorders taking similar medications. May worsen psychosis in some patients or precipitate a shift to mania or hypomania in patients with bipolar disorder. Patients presenting with depressive symptoms should be screened for bipolar disorder. Monotherapy in patients with bipolar disorder should be avoided. **Milnacipran is not FDA approved for the treatment of bipolar depression.**

Serotonin syndrome and neuroleptic malignant syndrome (NMS)-like reactions have occurred with serotonin/norepinephrine reuptake inhibitors (SNRIs) and selective serotonin reuptake inhibitors (SSRIs) when used alone, and particularly when used in combination with serotonergic agents (eg, triptans) or antidopaminergic agents (eg, antipsychotics). Concurrent use with MAO inhibitors is contraindicated. May cause sustained increase in blood pressure or heart rate. Control pre-existing hypertension and cardiovascular disease prior to initiation of milnacipran. Use caution in patients with renal impairment; dose reduction required in severe renal impairment. Use caution in patients with hepatic impairment. Avoid ethanol use. Use cautiously in patients with a history of seizures. May impair platelet aggregation, resulting in bleeding. May cause increased urinary resistance. Use caution in patients with controlled narrow-angle glaucoma; use is contraindicated with uncontrolled narrow-angle glaucoma.

Abrupt discontinuation or dosage reduction after extended therapy may lead to agitation, dysphoria, anxiety, and other symptoms. When discontinuing therapy, dosage should be tapered gradually. If intolerable symptoms occur following a decrease in dosage or upon discontinuation of therapy, then resuming the previous dose with a more gradual taper should be considered.
Adverse Reactions (Reflective of adult population; not specific for elderly)
>10%:
Central nervous system: Headache (18%), insomnia (12%)
Endocrine & metabolic: Hot flashes (12%)
Gastrointestinal: Nausea (37%), constipation (16%)

1% to 10%:
Cardiovascular: Palpitation (7%), heart rate increased (6%), hypertension (5%), flushing (3%), blood pressure increased (3%), tachycardia (2%), peripheral edema (≥1%)
Central nervous system: Dizziness (10%), migraine (5%), chills (2%), tremor (2%), depression (≥1%), fatigue (≥1%), fever (≥1%), irritability (≥1%), somnolence (≥1%)
Dermatologic: Hyperhidrosis (9%), rash (3%)
Endocrine & metabolic: Hypercholesterolemia (≥1%)
Gastrointestinal: Vomiting (7%), xerostomia (5%), abdominal pain (3%), appetite decreased (2%), abdominal distension (≥1%), abnormal taste (≥1%), diarrhea (≥1%), dyspepsia (≥1%), flatulence (≥1%), gastroesophageal reflux disease (≥1%), weight changes (≥1%)
Genitourinary: Dysuria (≥2%), ejaculation disorder/failure (≥2%), erectile dysfunction (≥2%), libido decreased (≥2%), prostatitis (≥2%), scrotal pain (≥2%), testicular pain (≥2%), testicular swelling (≥2%), urethral pain (≥2%), urinary hesitation (≥2%), urinary retention (≥2%), urine flow decreased (≥2%), cystitis (≥1%), urinary tract infection (≥1%)
Neuromuscular & skeletal: Falling (≥1%)
Ocular: Blurred vision (2%)
Respiratory: Dyspnea (2%)
Miscellaneous: Night sweats (≥1%)

Drug Interactions
Metabolism/Transport Effects None known.
Avoid Concomitant Use
Avoid concomitant use of Milnacipran with any of the following: Iobenguane I 123; MAO Inhibitors; Methylene Blue
Increased Effect/Toxicity
Milnacipran may increase the levels/effects of: Alpha-/Beta-Agonists; Aspirin; Digoxin; Methylene Blue; Metoclopramide; NSAID (Nonselective); Serotonin Modulators; Vitamin K Antagonists

The levels/effects of Milnacipran may be increased by: Alcohol (Ethyl); Antipsychotics; ClomiPRAMINE; Linezolid; MAO Inhibitors
Decreased Effect
Milnacipran may decrease the levels/effects of: Alpha2-Agonists; Iobenguane I 123; Ioflupane I 123

Ethanol/Nutrition/Herb Interactions
Ethanol: Ethanol may increase CNS depression. Management: Avoid ethanol.
Herb/Nutraceutical: Some herbal medications may increase risk of serotonin syndrome and/or excessive sedation. Management: Avoid valerian, St John's wort, SAMe, kava kava, and tryptophan.

Stability Store at 25°C (77°F); excursions permitted between 15°C to 30°C (59°F to 86°F).

Mechanism of Action Potent inhibitor of norepinephrine and serotonin reuptake (3:1). Milnacipran has no significant activity for serotonergic, alpha- and beta-adrenergic, muscarinic, histaminergic, dopaminergic, opiate, benzodiazepine, and GABA receptors. It does not possess MAO-inhibitory activity.

Pharmacodynamics/Kinetics
Absorption: Well absorbed
Distribution: I.V: V_d: ~400 L
Protein binding: 13%
Metabolism: Hepatic to inactive metabolites
Bioavailability: 85% to 90%
Half-life elimination: 6-8 hours
Time to peak, plasma: Oral: 2-4 hours
Excretion: Urine (55% as unchanged drug)

Dosage
Geriatric & Adult Fibromyalgia: Oral: 50 mg twice daily (maximum dose: 200 mg/day).
Titration schedule: 12.5 mg once on day 1, then 12.5 mg twice daily on days 2-3, 25 mg twice daily on days 4-7, then 50 mg twice daily thereafter. Dose may be increased to 100 mg twice daily, based on individual response. Doses >200 mg/day have not been studied.
Discontinuation of therapy: Gradually taper dose. If intolerable symptoms occur following a dose reduction, consider resuming the previously prescribed dose and/or decrease dose at a more gradual rate.
Renal Impairment
Mild renal impairment: No dose adjustment is recommended.
Moderate renal impairment: Use with caution.
Severe renal impairment (Cl_{cr} ≤29 mL/minute): Reduce maintenance dose to 25 mg twice daily; dose may be increased to 50 mg twice daily, based on individual tolerance.
End-stage renal disease (ESRD): Use not recommended.

Hepatic Impairment
Mild-to-moderate hepatic impairment: No dose adjustment is recommended.
Severe hepatic impairment: Use with caution.

Administration May be administered with or without food; food may improve tolerability.

Monitoring Parameters Blood pressure and heart rate should be regularly monitored; renal function should be monitored for dosing purposes; mental status for suicidal ideation (especially at the beginning of therapy or when doses are increased or decreased); intraocular pressure should be monitored in those with baseline elevations or a history of glaucoma

Special Geriatric Considerations According to the manufacturer of milnacipran, 402 participants in the clinical trials were age 60 years and older; no difference in efficacy or safety were reported compared to younger participants. Milnacipran should be used cautiously in patients with moderate renal impairment and its dose reduced in patients with Cl_{cr} 5-29 mL/minute. The risk of hyponatremia may be greater in the elderly.

Dosage Forms Excipient information presented when available (limited, particularly for generics); consult specific product labeling.
Combination package, oral [titration pack contains three separate tablet formulations]:
Savella®: Tablet: 12.5 mg (5s), Tablet: 25 mg (8s), and Tablet: 50 mg (42s)
Tablet, oral:
Savella®: 12.5 mg, 25 mg, 50 mg, 100 mg

Mineral Oil (MIN er al oyl)

Related Information
Beers Criteria – Potentially Inappropriate Medications for Geriatrics *on page 2183*
Laxatives, Classification and Properties *on page 2121*
Treatment Options for Constipation *on page 2142*

Medication Safety Issues
BEERS Criteria medication:
This drug may be potentially inappropriate for use in geriatric patients (Quality of evidence - moderate; Strength of recommendation - strong).

Brand Names: U.S. Fleet® Mineral Oil Enema [OTC]; Kondremul® [OTC]

Index Terms Heavy Mineral Oil; Liquid Paraffin; White Mineral Oil

Generic Availability (U.S.) Yes: Oral oil

Pharmacologic Category Laxative, Lubricant

Use Temporary relief of occasional constipation, relief of fecal impaction; removal of barium sulfate residues following barium administration

Contraindications Patients with colostomy or an ileostomy, appendicitis, ulcerative colitis, diverticulitis

Warnings/Precautions Lipid pneumonitis results from aspiration of mineral oil. Aspiration risk increased in patients in prolonged supine position or conditions which interfere with swallowing or epiglottal function (eg, stroke, Parkinson's disease, Alzheimer's disease, esophageal dysmotility). Due to potential for aspiration and other adverse effects, use in the elderly should be avoided (Beers Criteria).

When used for self-medication (OTC): Healthcare provider should be contacted in case of sudden changes in bowel habits which last over 2 weeks or if abdominal pain, nausea, vomiting, or rectal bleeding occur following use; do not use for >1 week, unless otherwise directed by healthcare provider.

Adverse Reactions (Reflective of adult population; not specific for elderly) Frequency not defined.
Gastrointestinal: Abdominal cramps, diarrhea, nausea, vomiting
Respiratory: Lipid pneumonitis with aspiration
Miscellaneous: Large doses may cause anal leakage causing anal itching, irritation, hemorrhoids, perianal discomfort, soiling of clothes

Drug Interactions
Metabolism/Transport Effects None known.
Avoid Concomitant Use There are no known interactions where it is recommended to avoid concomitant use.
Increased Effect/Toxicity There are no known significant interactions involving an increase in effect.
Decreased Effect
Mineral Oil may decrease the levels/effects of: Phytonadione; Vitamin D Analogs

Mechanism of Action Eases passage of stool by decreasing water absorption and lubricating the intestine; retards colonic absorption of water

Pharmacodynamics/Kinetics
Onset of action: Oral: 6-8 hours; Rectal: 2-15 minutes
Distribution: Site of action is the colon
Excretion: Feces

Dosage
Geriatric & Adult
Constipation:
Oral: 15-45 mL/day
   Kondremul®: 30-75 mL/day
   Liqui-Doss®: 15-45 mL at bedtime
   Rectal (Fleet® Mineral Oil): 118 mL as a single dose
Fecal impaction or following barium studies: Rectal (Fleet® Mineral Oil): 118 mL as a single dose

Administration
Oral: Mineral oil may be more palatable if refrigerated. Administer on an empty stomach in an upright position.
Kondremul®: Shake well before use.
Liqui-Doss®: Shake well before use. Prior to use, mix with 120 mL of any beverage; administer only at bedtime.
Rectal (Fleet® Mineral Oil): Gently insert enema rectally with patient lying on left side and left knee slightly bent, right knee drawn to chest.

Monitoring Parameters Monitor for response (stool frequency, consistency). Avoid use in patients who may aspirate.

Special Geriatric Considerations Other therapies should be attempted before using mineral oil to relieve constipation to avoid complications with mineral oil; doses, if used, should begin low and should be used as infrequently as possible.

This medication is considered to be potentially inappropriate in this patient population (Beers Criteria: Quality of evidence - moderate; Strength of recommendation - strong).

Dosage Forms Excipient information presented when available (limited, particularly for generics); consult specific product labeling.
Microemulsion, oral:
   Kondremul®: 2.5 mL/5 mL (480 mL) [sugar free; mint flavor]
Oil, oral: 100% (30 mL, 480 mL)
Oil, oral [heavy]: 100% (480 mL, 3840 mL)
Oil, rectal [enema]:
   Fleet® Mineral Oil Enema: 100% per 118 mL delivered dose (133 mL)
Oil, topical: 100% (480 mL)
Oil, topical [light]: 100% (3840 mL)

♦ **Minipress®** see Prazosin on page 1589
♦ **Minitran™** see Nitroglycerin on page 1386
♦ **Minocin®** see Minocycline on page 1289
♦ **Minocin® PAC** see Minocycline on page 1289

Minocycline (mi noe SYE kleen)

Related Information
Antimicrobial Drugs of Choice on page 2163
Medication Safety Issues
Sound-alike/look-alike issues:
Dynacin® may be confused with Dyazide®, DynaCirc®, Dynapen
Minocin® may be confused with Indocin®, Lincocin®, Minizide®, niacin
Brand Names: U.S. Dynacin®; Minocin®; Minocin® PAC; Solodyn®
Brand Names: Canada Apo-Minocycline®; Arestin Microspheres; Dom-Minocycline; Minocin®; Mylan-Minocycline; Novo-Minocycline; PHL-Minocycline; PMS-Minocycline; ratio-Minocycline; Riva-Minocycline; Sandoz-Minocycline
Index Terms Minocycline Hydrochloride
Generic Availability (U.S.) Yes: Excludes injection, pellet-filled capsule
Pharmacologic Category Antibiotic, Tetracycline Derivative
Use Treatment of susceptible bacterial infections of both gram-negative and gram-positive organisms; treatment of anthrax (inhalational, cutaneous, and gastrointestinal); moderate-to-severe acne; meningococcal (asymptomatic) carrier state; Rickettsial diseases (including Rocky Mountain spotted fever, Q fever); nongonococcal urethritis, gonorrhea; acute intestinal amebiasis; respiratory tract infection; skin/soft tissue infections; chlamydial infections
Extended release (Solodyn®): Only indicated for treatment of inflammatory lesions of non-nodular moderate-to-severe acne

◄ **Unlabeled Use** Rheumatoid arthritis (patients with low disease activity of short duration); nocardiosis; alternative treatment for community-acquired MRSA infection

Contraindications Hypersensitivity to minocycline, other tetracyclines, or any component of the formulation

Warnings/Precautions May be associated with increases in BUN secondary to antianabolic effects; use caution in patients with renal impairment (Cl_{cr} <80 mL/minute). Hepatotoxicity has been reported; use caution in patients with hepatic insufficiency. Autoimmune syndromes (eg, lupus-like, hepatitis, and vasculitis) have been reported; discontinue if symptoms occur. CNS effects (lightheadedness, vertigo) may occur; patients must be cautioned about performing tasks which require mental alertness (eg, operating machinery or driving). Pseudotumor cerebri has been (rarely) reported with tetracycline use; usually resolves with discontinuation. May cause photosensitivity; discontinue if skin erythema occurs. Prolonged use may result in fungal or bacterial superinfection, including *C. difficile*-associated diarrhea (CDAD) and pseudomembranous colitis; CDAD has been observed >2 months postantibiotic treatment. Rash, along with eosinophilia, fever, and organ failure (Drug Rash with Eosinophilia and Systemic Symptoms [DRESS] syndrome) has been reported; discontinue treatment immediately if DRESS syndrome is suspected.

Adverse Reactions (Reflective of adult population; not specific for elderly) Frequency not defined.

Cardiovascular: Myocarditis, pericarditis, vasculitis

Central nervous system: Bulging fontanels, dizziness, fatigue, fever, headache, hypoesthesia, malaise, mood changes, paresthesia, pseudotumor cerebri, sedation, seizure, somnolence, vertigo

Dermatologic: Alopecia, angioedema, drug rash with eosinophilia and systemic symptoms (DRESS), erythema multiforme, erythema nodosum, erythematous rash, exfoliative dermatitis, hyperpigmentation of nails, maculopapular rash, photosensitivity, pigmentation of the skin and mucous membranes, pruritus, Stevens-Johnson syndrome, toxic epidermal necrolysis, urticaria

Endocrine & metabolic: Thyroid cancer, thyroid discoloration, thyroid dysfunction

Gastrointestinal: Anorexia, diarrhea, dyspepsia, dysphagia, enamel hypoplasia, enterocolitis, esophageal ulcerations, esophagitis, glossitis, inflammatory lesions (oral/anogenital), moniliasis, nausea, oral cavity discoloration, pancreatitis, pseudomembranous colitis, stomatitis, tooth discoloration, vomiting, xerostomia

Genitourinary: Balanitis, vulvovaginitis

Hematologic: Agranulocytosis, eosinophilia, hemolytic anemia, leukopenia, neutropenia, pancytopenia, thrombocytopenia

Hepatic: Autoimmune hepatitis, hepatic cholestasis, hepatic failure, hepatitis, hyperbilirubinemia, jaundice, liver enzyme increases

Local: Injection site reaction (I.V. administration)

Neuromuscular & skeletal: Arthralgia, arthritis, bone discoloration, joint stiffness, joint swelling, myalgia

Otic: Hearing loss, tinnitus

Renal: Acute renal failure, BUN increased, interstitial nephritis

Respiratory: Asthma, bronchospasm, cough, dyspnea, pneumonitis, pulmonary infiltrate (with eosinophilia)

Miscellaneous: Anaphylaxis, hypersensitivity, lupus erythematosus, lupus-like syndrome, serum sickness

Drug Interactions

Metabolism/Transport Effects None known.

Avoid Concomitant Use

Avoid concomitant use of Minocycline with any of the following: BCG; Retinoic Acid Derivatives

Increased Effect/Toxicity

Minocycline may increase the levels/effects of: Neuromuscular-Blocking Agents; Porfimer; Retinoic Acid Derivatives; Vitamin K Antagonists

Decreased Effect

Minocycline may decrease the levels/effects of: Atazanavir; BCG; Penicillins; Typhoid Vaccine

The levels/effects of Minocycline may be decreased by: Antacids; Bile Acid Sequestrants; Bismuth; Bismuth Subsalicylate; Calcium Salts; Iron Salts; Lanthanum; Magnesium Salts; Quinapril; Sucralfate; Zinc Salts

Ethanol/Nutrition/Herb Interactions

Food: Minocycline serum concentrations are not significantly altered if taken with food or dairy products.

Herb/Nutraceutical: Avoid dong quai, St John's wort (may also cause photosensitization).

Stability

Capsule (including pellet-filled), tablet: Store at 20°C to 25°C (68°F to 77°F); protect from heat. Protect from light and moisture.

Extended release tablet: Store at 15°C to 30°C (59°F to 86°F); protect from heat. Protect from light and moisture.

Injection: Store vials at 20°C to 25°C (68°F to 77°F) prior to reconstitution. Reconstitute with 5 mL of sterile water for injection, and further dilute in 500-1000 mL of NS, D_5W, D_5NS, Ringer's injection, or LR. Reconstituted solution is stable at room temperature for 24 hours. Final dilutions should be administered immediately.

Mechanism of Action Inhibits bacterial protein synthesis by binding with the 30S and possibly the 50S ribosomal subunit(s) of susceptible bacteria; cell wall synthesis is not affected

Rheumatoid arthritis: The mechanism of action of minocycline in rheumatoid arthritis is not completely understood. It is thought to have antimicrobial, anti-inflammatory, immunomodulatory, and chondroprotective effects. More specifically, it is thought to be a potent inhibitor of metalloproteinases, which are active in rheumatoid arthritis joint destruction.

Pharmacodynamics/Kinetics

Absorption: Oral: Well absorbed

Protein binding: 70% to 75%

Metabolism: Hepatic to inactive metabolites

Half-life elimination: I.V.: 15-23 hours; Oral: 16 hours (range: 11-22 hours)

Time to peak: Capsule, pellet filled: 1-4 hours; Extended release tablet: 3.5-4 hours

Excretion: Urine, feces

Dosage

Geriatric & Adult

Usual dosage range:

I.V.: Initial: 200 mg, followed by 100 mg every 12 hours (maximum: 400 mg/day)

Oral: Initial: 200 mg, followed by 100 mg every 12 hours; more frequent dosing intervals may be used (100-200 mg initially, followed by 50 mg 4 times daily)

Acne: Oral: Capsule or immediate-release tablet: 50-100 mg twice daily

Inflammatory, non-nodular, moderate-to-severe acne (Solodyn®):

45-54 kg: 45 mg once daily

55-77 kg: 65 mg once daily

78-102 kg: 90 mg once daily

103-125 kg: 115 mg once daily

126-136 kg: 135 mg once daily

Note: Therapy should be continued for 12 weeks. Higher doses do not confer greater efficacy and may be associated with more acute vestibular side effects. Safety of use beyond 12 weeks has not been established.

Cellulitis (purulent) due to community-acquired MRSA (unlabeled use): Oral: Initial: 200 mg; Maintenance: 100 mg twice daily for 5-10 days (Liu, 2011)

Chlamydial or *Ureaplasma urealyticum* infection, uncomplicated: Oral, I.V.: Urethral, endocervical, or rectal: Oral: 100 mg every 12 hours for at least 7 days

Gonococcal infection, uncomplicated (males): Oral, I.V.:

Without urethritis or anorectal infection: Initial: 200 mg, followed by 100 mg every 12 hours for at least 4 days (cultures 2-3 days post-therapy)

Urethritis: 100 mg every 12 hours for 5 days

Meningococcal carrier state (manufacturer's labeling): Oral: 100 mg every 12 hours for 5 days. **Note:** CDC recommendations do not mention use of minocycline for eradicating nasopharyngeal carriage of meningococcal

Mycobacterium marinum: Oral: 100 mg every 12 hours for 6-8 weeks

Nocardiosis, cutaneous (non-CNS) (unlabeled use): Oral: 100-200 mg every 12 hours

Rheumatoid arthritis (unlabeled use): Oral: 100 mg twice daily (O'Dell, 2001)

Syphilis: Oral, I.V.: Initial: 200 mg, followed by 100 mg every 12 hours for 10-15 days

Renal Impairment Use with caution; monitor BUN and creatinine clearance. Consider decreasing dose or increasing dosing interval (extended release).

Cl_{cr} <80 mL/minute: Do not exceed 200 mg/day

Administration

I.V.: Infuse slowly; avoid rapid administration. The manufacturer's labeling does not provide a recommended administration rate. The injectable route should be used only if the oral route is not feasible or adequate. Prolonged intravenous therapy may be associated with thrombophlebitis.

Oral: May be administered with or without food. Administer with adequate fluid to decrease the risk of esophageal irritation and ulceration. Swallow pellet-filled capsule and extended release tablet whole; do not chew, crush, or split.

Monitoring Parameters LFTs, BUN, renal function with long-term treatment; if symptomatic for autoimmune disorder, include ANA, CBC

◀ **Test Interactions** May cause interference with fluorescence test for urinary catecholamines (false elevations)

Special Geriatric Considerations Minocycline has not been studied in the elderly but its CNS effects may limit its use. Dose reduction for renal function not necessary.

Dosage Forms Excipient information presented when available (limited, particularly for generics); consult specific product labeling.

Capsule, oral: 50 mg, 75 mg, 100 mg

Capsule, pellet filled, oral:
  Minocin®: 50 mg, 100 mg
  Minocin® PAC: 50 mg, 100 mg

Injection, powder for reconstitution:
  Minocin®: 100 mg

Tablet, oral: 50 mg, 75 mg, 100 mg
  Dynacin®: 50 mg, 75 mg, 100 mg

Tablet, extended release, oral: 45 mg, 90 mg, 135 mg
  Solodyn®: 45 mg, 65 mg, 90 mg, 115 mg, 135 mg

◆ **Minocycline Hydrochloride** see Minocycline on page 1289

Minoxidil (Systemic) (mi NOKS i dil)

Medication Safety Issues

Sound-alike/look-alike issues:
  Loniten® may be confused with Lipitor®
  Minoxidil may be confused with metolazone, midodrine, Minipress®, Minocin®, Monopril®, Noxafil®

International issues:
  Noxidil [Thailand] may be confused with Noxafil brand name for posaconazole [U.S. and multiple international markets]

Brand Names: Canada Loniten®

Generic Availability (U.S.) Yes

Pharmacologic Category Vasodilator, Direct-Acting

Use Management of severe hypertension (usually in combination with a diuretic and beta-blocker)

Contraindications Hypersensitivity to minoxidil or any component of the formulation; pheochromocytoma

Warnings/Precautions [U.S. Boxed Warning]: Minoxidil may cause pericarditis and pericardial effusion that may progress to tamponade; patients with renal impairment not on dialysis may be at higher risk. Observe patients closely. **[U.S. Boxed Warning]: May increase oxygen demand and exacerbate angina pectoris;** concomitant use with a beta-blocker (if no contraindication exists may help reduce the effect. Use with caution in patients with pulmonary hypertension, significant renal failure, or HF; use with caution in patients with coronary artery disease or recent myocardial infarction; renal failure or dialysis patients may require smaller doses; usually used with a beta-blocker (to treat minoxidil-induced tachycardia) and a diuretic (for treatment of water retention/edema. Compared to placebo minoxidil increased the frequency of clinical events, including increased need for diuretics, angina, ventricular arrhythmias, worsening heart failure and death (Franciosa, 1984). Use with caution in the elderly; initiate at the low end of the dosage range and monitor closely.

[U.S. Boxed Warning]: Maximum therapeutic doses of a diuretic and two antihypertensives should be used before this drug is ever added. Should be given with a diuretic to minimize fluid gain and a beta-blocker (if no contraindications) to prevent tachycardia. Anyone with malignant hypertension should be hospitalized with close medical supervision to ensure blood pressure is reducing and to prevent too rapid of a reduction in blood pressure. Inform patients of excessive hair growth before initiating therapy; may take 1-6 months for hypertrichosis to reverse itself after discontinuation of the drug.

Adverse Reactions (Reflective of adult population; not specific for elderly) Frequency not always reported.

Cardiovascular: ECG changes (T-wave changes 60%), peripheral edema (7%), pericardial effusion with tamponade (3%), pericardial effusion without tamponade (3%), angina pectoris, heart failure, pericarditis, rebound hypertension (in children after a gradual withdrawal), sodium and water retention, tachycardia

Dermatologic: Hypertrichosis (common; 80%), bullous eruption (rare), rash, Stevens-Johnson syndrome (rare)

Endocrine & metabolic: Breast tenderness (rare; <1%)

Gastrointestinal: Nausea, vomiting, weight gain

Hematologic: Leukopenia (rare), thrombocytopenia (rare), transient decreased erythrocyte count (hemodilution), transient decreased hematocrit/hemoglobin (hemodilution)

Hepatic: Increased alkaline phosphatase

Renal: Transient increase in serum BUN and creatinine

Respiratory: Pulmonary edema

Drug Interactions

Metabolism/Transport Effects None known.

Avoid Concomitant Use There are no known interactions where it is recommended to avoid concomitant use.

Increased Effect/Toxicity

Minoxidil (Systemic) may increase the levels/effects of: Amifostine; Antihypertensives; Hypotensive Agents; RiTUXimab

The levels/effects of Minoxidil (Systemic) may be increased by: Alfuzosin; CycloSPORINE; CycloSPORINE (Systemic); Diazoxide; Herbs (Hypotensive Properties); MAO Inhibitors; Pentoxifylline; Phosphodiesterase 5 Inhibitors; Prostacyclin Analogues

Decreased Effect

The levels/effects of Minoxidil (Systemic) may be decreased by: Herbs (Hypertensive Properties); Methylphenidate; Yohimbine

Ethanol/Nutrition/Herb Interactions Herb/Nutraceutical: Bayberry, blue cohosh, cayenne, ephedra, ginger, ginseng (American), kola, licorice may diminish the antihypertensive effects of minoxidil. Black cohosh, California poppy, coleus, golden seal, hawthorn, mistletoe, periwinkle, quinine, shepherd's purse may enhance the hypotensive effects of minoxidil.

Stability Store at controlled room temperature of 15°C to 30°C (59°F to 86°F).

Mechanism of Action Produces vasodilation by directly relaxing arteriolar smooth muscle, with little effect on veins; effects may be mediated by cyclic AMP; stimulation of hair growth is secondary to vasodilation, increased cutaneous blood flow and stimulation of resting hair follicles

Pharmacodynamics/Kinetics

Onset of action: Hypotensive: ~30 minutes

Peak effect: 2-8 hours

Duration: 2-5 days

Protein binding: None

Metabolism: 88%, primarily via glucuronidation

Bioavailability: 90%

Half-life elimination: Adults: 3.5-4.2 hours

Excretion: Urine (12% as unchanged drug)

Dosage

Geriatric Hypertension: Initial: 2.5 mg once daily; increase gradually.

Adult Hypertension: Oral: Initial: 5 mg once daily, increase gradually every 3 days (maximum: 100 mg/day); usual dosage range (JNC 7): 2.5-80 mg/day in 1-2 divided doses

Note: Dosage adjustment is needed when added to concomitant therapy.

Renal Impairment Patient with renal failure and/or receiving dialysis may require dosage reduction.

Supplemental dose is not necessary after hemo- or peritoneal dialysis.

Monitoring Parameters Blood pressure, standing and sitting/supine; fluid and electrolyte balance and body weight should be monitored. Any tests that are abnormal at the time of initiation (including, renal function tests, ECG, echocardiogram, chest x-ray) should be repeated initially every 1-3 months then every 6-12 months once stable.

Special Geriatric Considerations Use caution when initiating therapy in elderly patients. In general, select lower initial doses within the recommended dosage range.

Dosage Forms Excipient information presented when available (limited, particularly for generics); consult specific product labeling.

Tablet, oral: 2.5 mg, 10 mg

◆ **Mintox Plus [OTC]** *see* Aluminum Hydroxide, Magnesium Hydroxide, and Simethicone *on page 82*

◆ **Miostat®** *see* Carbachol *on page 285*

◆ **MiraLAX® [OTC]** *see* Polyethylene Glycol 3350 *on page 1564*

◆ **Miranel AF™ [OTC]** *see* Miconazole (Topical) *on page 1276*

◆ **Mirapex®** *see* Pramipexole *on page 1579*

◆ **Mirapex® ER®** *see* Pramipexole *on page 1579*

Mirtazapine (mir TAZ a peen)

Related Information
Antidepressant Agents *on page 2097*
Beers Criteria – Potentially Inappropriate Medications for Geriatrics *on page 2183*

Medication Safety Issues
Sound-alike/look-alike issues:
Remeron® may be confused with Premarin®, ramelteon, Rozerem®, Zemuron®

BEERS Criteria medication:
This drug may be potentially inappropriate for use in geriatric patients (SIADH: Quality of evidence - moderate; Strength of recommendation - strong).

International issues:
Avanza [Australia] may be confused with Albenza brand name for albendazole [U.S.]; Avandia brand name for rosiglitazone [U.S., Canada, and multiple international markets]
Remeron [U.S., Canada, and multiple international markets] may be confused with Reneuron which is a brand name for fluoxetine [Spain]

Brand Names: U.S. Remeron SolTab®; Remeron®

Brand Names: Canada Apo-Mirtazapine®; Auro-Mirtazapine; Ava-Mirtazapine; CO Mirtazapine; Dom-Mirtazapine; GD-Mirtazapine; Jamp-Mirtazapine; Mylan-Mirtazapine; Novo-Mirtazapine; PMS-Mirtazapine; PRO-Mirtazapine; ratio-Mirtazapine; Remeron®; Remeron® RD; Riva-Mirtazapine; Sandoz-Mirtazapine; Sandoz-Mirtazapine FC; ZYM-Mirtazapine

Generic Availability (U.S.) Yes

Pharmacologic Category Antidepressant, Alpha-2 Antagonist

Use Treatment of depression

Unlabeled Use Alzheimer's dementia-related depression; post-traumatic stress disorder (PTSD)

Medication Guide Available Yes

Contraindications Hypersensitivity to mirtazapine or any component of the formulation; use with or within 14 days of MAO inhibitors

Warnings/Precautions [U.S. Boxed Warning]: Antidepressants increase the risk of suicidal thinking and behavior in children, adolescents, and young adults (18-24 years of age) with major depressive disorder (MDD) and other psychiatric disorders; consider risk prior to prescribing. Short-term studies did not show an increased risk in patients >24 years of age and showed a decreased risk in patients ≥65 years. Closely monitor for clinical worsening, suicidality, or unusual changes in behavior; the patient's family or caregiver should be instructed to closely observe the patient and communicate condition with healthcare provider. A medication guide should be dispensed with each prescription.

The possibility of a suicide attempt is inherent in major depression and may persist until remission occurs. Monitor for worsening of depression or suicidality, especially during initiation of therapy (generally first 1-2 months) or with dose increases or decreases. Use caution in high-risk patients. Worsening depression and severe abrupt suicidality that are not part of the presenting symptoms may require discontinuation or modification of drug therapy. The patient's family or caregiver should be alerted to monitor patients for the emergence of suicidality and associated behaviors (such as agitation, irritability, hostility, impulsivity, and hypomania) and call healthcare provider.

May worsen psychosis in some patients or precipitate a shift to mania or hypomania in patients with bipolar disorder. Patients presenting with depressive symptoms should be screened for bipolar disorder. Monotherapy in patients with bipolar disorder should be avoided. **Mirtazapine is not FDA approved for the treatment of bipolar depression.**

Patients should not discontinue treatment abruptly, unless significant life-threatening event, due to risk of withdrawal symptoms. A gradual reduction in the dose over several weeks is recommended.

Discontinue immediately if signs and symptoms of neutropenia/agranulocytosis occur. May cause sedation, resulting in impaired performance of tasks requiring alertness (eg, operating machinery or driving). Sedative effects may be additive with other CNS depressants and/or ethanol. The degree of sedation is moderate-high relative to other antidepressants. Conversely, may increase psychomotor restlessness within first few weeks of therapy. The risks of orthostatic hypotension or anticholinergic effects are low relative to other antidepressants. The incidence of sexual dysfunction with mirtazapine is generally lower than with selective serotonin reuptake inhibitors (SSRIs). Serotonin syndrome (SS) and neuroleptic malignant syndrome (NMS)-like reactions have occurred with serotonin/norepinephrine reuptake inhibitors (SNRIs), SSRIs, MAOIs, and other serotonergic medications, including mirtazapine, when used alone, and particularly when used in combination with serotonergic agents (eg, triptans) or antidopaminergic agents (eg, antipsychotics). Discontinue treatment (and any concomitant serotonergic and/or antidopaminergic agents) immediately if signs/symptoms arise. Concurrent use of serotonin precursors (eg, tryptophan) is not recommended. Concurrent use with or within 14 days of MAO inhibitors is contraindicated. May increase appetite and stimulate weight gain. In clinical trials, an increased incidence of weight gain in adults and children was observed with mirtazapine compared to placebo; up to 8% of patients discontinued therapy due to weight gain. May increase serum cholesterol and triglyceride levels.

Use caution in patients with a previous seizure disorder or condition predisposing to seizures such as brain damage, alcoholism, or concurrent therapy with other drugs which lower the seizure threshold. Use with caution in patients with hepatic or renal dysfunction. Use caution in elderly patients; may cause or exacerbate syndrome of inappropriate antidiuretic hormone secretion or hyponatremia; monitor sodium closely with initiation or dosage adjustments in older adults (Beers Criteria). Clinically significant transaminase elevations have been observed. SolTab® formulation contains phenylalanine.

Adverse Reactions (Reflective of adult population; not specific for elderly)
>10%:
Central nervous system: Somnolence (54%)
Endocrine & metabolic: Cholesterol increased
Gastrointestinal: Xerostomia (25%), appetite increased (17%), constipation (13%), weight gain (12%; weight gain of >7% reported in 8% of adults, ≤49% of pediatric patients)
1% to 10%:
Cardiovascular: Peripheral edema (2%), edema (1%), hypertension, vasodilatation
Central nervous system: Dizziness (7%), abnormal dreams (4%), abnormal thoughts (3%), confusion (2%), agitation, amnesia, anxiety, apathy, depression, hyper/hypokinesia, hypoesthesia, malaise, vertigo
Dermatologic: Pruritus, rash
Endocrine & metabolic: Triglycerides increased
Gastrointestinal: Abdominal pain, anorexia, vomiting
Genitourinary: Urinary frequency (2%), urinary tract infection
Hepatic: SGPT increased (≥3 times ULN: 2%)
Neuromuscular & skeletal: Weakness (8%), back pain (2%), myalgia (2%), tremor (2%), arthralgia, myasthenia, paresthesia, twitching
Respiratory: Dyspnea (1%), cough increased, sinusitis
Miscellaneous: Flu-like syndrome (5%), thirst

Drug Interactions
Metabolism/Transport Effects Substrate of CYP1A2 (major), CYP2C9 (minor), CYP2D6 (major), CYP3A4 (major); **Note:** Assignment of Major/Minor substrate status based on clinically relevant drug interaction potential; **Inhibits** CYP1A2 (weak), CYP3A4 (weak)

Avoid Concomitant Use
Avoid concomitant use of Mirtazapine with any of the following: Alcohol (Ethyl); Azelastine; Azelastine (Nasal); CNS Depressants; Conivaptan; MAO Inhibitors; Methadone; Methylene Blue; Paraldehyde; Tryptophan

Increased Effect/Toxicity
Mirtazapine may increase the levels/effects of: Azelastine; Azelastine (Nasal); Buprenorphine; Methadone; Methylene Blue; Metoclopramide; Metyrosine; Paraldehyde; Serotonin Modulators; Warfarin; Zolpidem

The levels/effects of Mirtazapine may be increased by: Abiraterone Acetate; Alcohol (Ethyl); Antipsychotics; CNS Depressants; Conivaptan; CYP1A2 Inhibitors (Moderate); CYP1A2 Inhibitors (Strong); CYP2D6 Inhibitors (Moderate); CYP2D6 Inhibitors (Strong); CYP3A4 Inhibitors (Moderate); CYP3A4 Inhibitors (Strong); Darunavir; Dasatinib; Deferasirox; HydrOXYzine; Ivacaftor; Linezolid; MAO Inhibitors; Mifepristone; Tryptophan

Decreased Effect
Mirtazapine may decrease the levels/effects of: Alpha2-Agonists

The levels/effects of Mirtazapine may be decreased by: CYP1A2 Inducers (Strong); CYP3A4 Inducers (Strong); Cyproterone; Deferasirox; Peginterferon Alfa-2b; Tocilizumab

Ethanol/Nutrition/Herb Interactions
Ethanol: May increase CNS depression; monitor for increased effects with coadministration. Caution patients about effects.
Herb/Nutraceutical: Avoid St John's wort (may decrease mirtazapine levels). Avoid valerian, St John's wort, SAMe, kava kava (may increase CNS depression).

Stability
Orally disintegrating tablet: Store at controlled room temperature of 25°C (77°F); excursions permitted to 15°C to 30°C (59°F to 86°F). Protect from light and moisture. Use immediately upon opening tablet blister.
Tablet: Store at controlled room temperature of 25°C (77°F); excursions permitted to 15°C to 30°C (59°F to 86°F). Protect from light and moisture.

Mechanism of Action Mirtazapine is a tetracyclic antidepressant that works by its central presynaptic alpha$_2$-adrenergic antagonist effects, which results in increased release of norepinephrine and serotonin. It is also a potent antagonist of 5-HT$_2$ and 5-HT$_3$ serotonin receptors and H1 histamine receptors and a moderate peripheral alpha$_1$-adrenergic and muscarinic antagonist; it does not inhibit the reuptake of norepinephrine or serotonin.

Pharmacodynamics/Kinetics

Absorption: Rapid and complete

Distribution: 4.5 L/kg

Protein binding: ~85%

Metabolism: Extensively hepatic via CYP1A2, 2C9, 2D6, 3A4 and via demethylation (forms demethylmirtazapine, an active metabolite) and hydroxylation (forms inactive metabolites)

Bioavailability: ~50%

Half-life elimination: 20-40 hours; increased with renal or hepatic impairment

Time to peak, serum: ~2 hours

Excretion: Urine (75%) and feces (15%) as metabolites

Dosage

Geriatric Refer to adult dosing. Use with caution. Compared to younger adults, clearance is decreased 40% in elderly males and 10% in elderly females; manufacturer's labeling does not include specific dosage adjustment

Alzheimer's dementia-related depression (unlabeled use): Initial: 7.5 mg at bedtime; may increase at 7.5-15 mg increments to 45-60 mg daily (Rabins, 2007)

Adult

Depression: Oral: Initial: 15 mg nightly, may titrate dose up no more frequently than every 1-2 weeks to a maximum of 45 mg daily; dosage range: 15-45 mg daily; there is an inverse relationship between dose and sedation

Post-traumatic stress disorder (PTSD) (unlabeled use): Oral: 30-60 mg daily (Bandelow, 2008; Benedek, 2009)

Renal Impairment No dosage adjustment provided in manufacturer's labeling; clearance is decreased 30% in moderate (Cl$_{cr}$ 11-39 mL/minute/1.73 m^2) impairment and is decreased 50% in severe (Cl$_{cr}$ <10 mL/minute/1.73 m^2) impairment. Use with caution.

Hepatic Impairment No dosage adjustment is provided in manufacturer's labeling; a decrease in clearance by 30% has been observed in hepatic impairment. Use with caution.

Administration

Orally disintegrating tablet: Administer without regard to meals. Open blister pack and place tablet on the tongue; tablet is formulated to dissolve on the tongue without water; do not split tablet.

Tablet: Administer without regard to meals. Canadian labeling does not recommend chewing tablet.

Monitoring Parameters Patients should be monitored for signs of agranulocytosis or severe neutropenia such as sore throat, stomatitis or other signs of infection or a low WBC; renal and hepatic function; mental status for depression, suicide ideation (especially at the beginning of therapy or when doses are increased or decreased), anxiety, social functioning, mania, panic attacks; signs/symptoms of serotonin syndrome or NMS-like reactions; lipid profile; weight gain

Special Geriatric Considerations Limited published data specifically in the elderly or addressing *in vivo* drug interactions.

A systematic review and meta-analysis of antidepressant placebo-controlled trials in persons with depression and dementia found evidence "suggestive" of efficacy but not of sufficient strength to "confirm" efficacy. Antidepressant trials in this patient population are small and underpowered. Older patients with depression being treated with an antidepressant should be closely monitored for response and adverse effects. Treatment should be switched or augmented when response is inadequate with a therapeutic dose. Antidepressants that are not tolerated should be discontinued and an alternative agent should be started.

This medication is considered to be potentially inappropriate in this patient population (Beers Criteria: SIADH: Quality of evidence - moderate; Strength of recommendation - strong).

Dosage Forms Excipient information presented when available (limited, particularly for generics); consult specific product labeling.

Tablet, oral: 7.5 mg, 15 mg, 30 mg, 45 mg

Remeron®: 15 mg, 30 mg [scored]

Remeron®: 45 mg

Tablet, orally disintegrating, oral: 15 mg, 30 mg, 45 mg

Remeron SolTab®: 15 mg [contains phenylalanine 2.6 mg/tablet; orange flavor]

Remeron SolTab®: 30 mg [contains phenylalanine 5.2 mg/tablet; orange flavor]

Remeron SolTab®: 45 mg [contains phenylalanine 7.8 mg/tablet; orange flavor]

Misoprostol (mye soe PROST ole)

Medication Safety Issues
  Sound-alike/look-alike issues:
    Cytotec® may be confused with Cytoxan
    Misoprostol may be confused with metoprolol, mifepristone
Brand Names: U.S. Cytotec®
Brand Names: Canada Apo-Misoprostol®; Novo-Misoprostol; PMS-Misoprostol
Generic Availability (U.S.) Yes
Pharmacologic Category Prostaglandin
Use Prevention of NSAID-induced gastric ulcers
Unlabeled Use Fat malabsorption in cystic fibrosis
Contraindications Hypersensitivity to prostaglandins
Warnings/Precautions [U.S. Boxed Warning]: Due to the abortifacient property of this medication, patients must be warned not to give this drug to others. Use with caution in patients with renal impairment, cardiovascular disease and the elderly.
Adverse Reactions (Reflective of adult population; not specific for elderly)
  >10%: Gastrointestinal: Diarrhea, abdominal pain
  1% to 10%:
    Central nervous system: Headache
    Gastrointestinal: Constipation, dyspepsia, flatulence, nausea, vomiting
Drug Interactions
  Metabolism/Transport Effects None known.
  Avoid Concomitant Use
    Avoid concomitant use of Misoprostol with any of the following: Carbetocin
  Increased Effect/Toxicity
    Misoprostol may increase the levels/effects of: Carbetocin; Oxytocin

    The levels/effects of Misoprostol may be increased by: Antacids
  Decreased Effect There are no known significant interactions involving a decrease in effect.
Ethanol/Nutrition/Herb Interactions Food: Misoprostol peak serum concentrations may be decreased if taken with food (not clinically significant).
Stability Store at or below 25°C (77°F).
Mechanism of Action Misoprostol is a synthetic prostaglandin E_1 analog that replaces the protective prostaglandins consumed with prostaglandin-inhibiting therapies (eg, NSAIDs); has been shown to induce uterine contractions
Pharmacodynamics/Kinetics
  Absorption: Oral: Rapid
  Half-life (parent and metabolite combined): 1.5 hours; metabolite: 20-40 minutes
  Time to peak serum concentration (active metabolite): Within 15-30 minutes
  Rapidly de-esterified to misoprostol acid
  Elimination: In urine (64% to 73% in 24 hours) and feces (15% in 24 hours)
  Since older adults have decreased clearance (increased AUC), it may be necessary to reduce dose to 100 mcg 4 times/day
Dosage
  Geriatric Oral: 100-200 mcg 4 times/day with food; if 200 mcg 4 times/day not tolerated, reduce to 100 mcg 4 times/day. **Note:** To avoid the diarrhea potential, doses can be initiated at 100 mcg/day and increased 100 mcg/day at 3-day intervals until desired dose is achieved; also, recommend administering with food to decrease diarrhea incidence.
  Adult
    Prevention of NSAID-induced ulcers: Oral: 200 mcg 4 times/day with food; if not tolerated, may decrease dose to 100 mcg 4 times/day with food. Last dose of the day should be taken at bedtime.
  Renal Impairment Half-life, maximum plasma concentration, and bioavailability may be increased; however, a correlation has not been observed with degree of dysfunction. Decrease dose if recommended dose is not tolerated. It is not known if misoprostol is removed by dialysis.
Administration Incidence of diarrhea may be lessened by having patient take dose right after meals and avoiding magnesium-containing antacids.
Monitoring Parameters Adequate diagnostic measures in all cases of undiagnosed abnormal vaginal bleeding
Special Geriatric Considerations Elderly, due to extensive use of NSAIDs and the high percentage of asymptomatic hemorrhage and perforation from NSAIDs, are at risk for NSAID-induced ulcers and may be candidates for misoprostol use. However, routine use for prophylaxis is not justified. Patients must be selected upon demonstration that they are at

◄ risk for NSAID-induced lesions. Misoprostol should not be used as a first-line therapy for gastric or duodenal ulcers.

Dosage Forms Excipient information presented when available (limited, particularly for generics); consult specific product labeling.

Tablet, oral: 100 mcg, 200 mcg
  Cytotec®: 100 mcg
  Cytotec®: 200 mcg [scored]

♦ **Misoprostol and Diclofenac** *see* Diclofenac and Misoprostol *on page* 537
♦ **Mitomycin-C** *see* MitoMYcin (Ophthalmic) *on page* 1298

MitoMYcin (Ophthalmic) (mye toe MYE sin)

Medication Safety Issues

Sound-alike/look-alike issues:
MitoMYcin (Ophthalmic) may be confused with MitoMYcin (Systemic), mitotane, mitoXANtrone

High alert medication:
This medication is in a class the Institute for Safe Medication Practices (ISMP) includes among its list of drug classes which have a heightened risk of causing significant patient harm when used in error.

Administration issues:
Mitosol® is not intended for intraocular administration; intraocular administration may result in cell death and lead to corneal and retinal infarction, and ciliary body atrophy.
Mitosol® is only intended for topical application to the surgical site of glaucoma filtration surgery.

Brand Names: U.S. Mitosol®

Index Terms Mitomycin-C; MMC

Generic Availability (U.S.) No

Pharmacologic Category Antineoplastic Agent, Antibiotic; Ophthalmic Agent, Miscellaneous

Use Adjunct to *ab externo* glaucoma surgery

Contraindications Hypersensitivity to mitomycin or any component of the formulation

Warnings/Precautions Solution should **not** be administered intraocularly; intraocular administration may result in cell death, potentially causing corneal and retinal infarction, and ciliary body atrophy. Therapy is only intended for topical application to the surgical site of glaucoma filtration surgery. Increased incidence of postoperative hypotony has been observed with use. Increased incidence of lenticular change and cataract formation has been correlated with use in phakic patients. Inadvertent corneal and/or scleral damage, including thinning or perforation, may occur with use of mitomycin solution in concentrations >0.2 mg/mL or for time periods >2 minutes. In addition, direct contact of the solution with the corneal endothelium will cause cell death. Use appropriate precautions for handling and disposal.

Adverse Reactions (Reflective of adult population; not specific for elderly) Frequency not defined: Ocular: Astigmatism induced, bleb (encapsulated/cystic/thin-walled), bleb leak (chronic), bleb ulceration, bleb-related infection, blebitis, capsule opacification, capsular constriction, capsulotomy rupture, cataract development, cataract progression, choroidal detachment, choroidal effusion, ciliary block, conjunctival necrosis, corneal endothelial damage, corneal vascularization, cystic conjunctival degeneration, Descemet's detachment, disk hemorrhage, disk swelling, endophthalmitis, epithelial defect, fibrin reaction, glaucoma (malignant), hemiretinal vein occlusion, hyphema, hypotony, hypotony maculopathy, implants dislocated, intraocular lens capture, iritis, lacrimal drainage system obstruction, loss of vision (severe), macular edema, retinal detachment (serious and rhegatogenous), retinal hemorrhage, retinal pigment epithelial tear, retinal vein occlusion, sclera thinning/ulceration, subconjunctival hemorrhage, superficial punctuate keratitis, suprachoroidal effusion (including hypoechogenic), suprachoroidal hemorrhage, supraciliochoroidal fluid present, synechiae (anterior and posterior), upper eyelid retraction, visual acuity decreased, vitreal hemorrhage/clot, wound dehiscence (associated with blebitis and scleritis)

Drug Interactions

Metabolism/Transport Effects None known.

Avoid Concomitant Use There are no known interactions where it is recommended to avoid concomitant use.

Increased Effect/Toxicity There are no known significant interactions involving an increase in effect.

Decreased Effect There are no known significant interactions involving a decrease in effect.

Stability Store at 20°C to 25°C (68°F to 77°F). Protect from light.
Kit should only be opened and reconstituted by sterile surgical scrub technician. To reconstitute, add 1 mL of SWFI; shake/swirl to dissolve (detailed instructions are available in the kit). If powder does not dissolve immediately, allow to stand at room temperature until it dissolves completely into solution. Reconstituted solution is stable for 1 hour at room temperature. Use appropriate precautions for handling and disposal.

Mechanism of Action Acts like an alkylating agent and produces DNA cross-linking (primarily with guanine and cytosine pairs); cell-cycle nonspecific; inhibits DNA and RNA synthesis; degrades preformed DNA, causes nuclear lysis and formation of giant cells. While not phase-specific per se, mitomycin has its maximum effect against cells in late G and early S phases.

During use in trabeculectomy (filtration surgery) for glaucoma, mitomycin topical application is believed to alter conjunctival vascular endothelium and inhibit fibroblast proliferation.

Pharmacodynamics/Kinetics
Absorption: Systemic absorption following ocular administration is unknown; however, systemic concentrations are expected to be of multiple orders of magnitude lower than concentrations produced following parenteral administration.
Metabolism: Cleared from ophthalmic tissue following topical administration and irrigation; systemic metabolism primarily occurs in the liver

Dosage
Geriatric & Adult Glaucoma surgery, adjunctive therapy: Topical ophthalmic: 0.2 mg solution is aseptically applied via saturated sponges to surgical site of glaucoma filtration surgery for 2 minutes

Administration The inner tray and the contents of the kit are sterile and should only be handled, opened and assembled by a sterile surgical scrub technician. Use within 1 hour of reconstitution. Technician should fully saturate sponges provided in the kit with the entire reconstituted solution (0.2 mg). Allow saturated sponges to remain undisturbed in kit for 60 seconds. Saturated sponges should be applied aseptically with the use of surgical forceps in a single layer to a treatment area ~10 mm x 6 mm (± 2 mm); sponges should be removed from the treatment area after 2 minutes. Following removal of sponges from eye, the surgical site should be copiously irrigated. Saturated sponges should be returned to the provided tray for ultimate disposal into chemotherapy waste bag. Consult product labeling for additional details. Solution is **not** intended for intraocular administration.

Special Geriatric Considerations The manufacturer reports no overall differences in safety and effectiveness have been observed between elderly and younger patients.

Dosage Forms Excipient information presented when available (limited, particularly for generics); consult specific product labeling.
Powder for solution, ophthalmic [kit]:
Mitosol®: 0.2 mg [supplied with diluent]

◆ **Mitosol®** see MitoMYcin (Ophthalmic) on page 1298
◆ **Mitrazol® [OTC]** see Miconazole (Topical) on page 1276
◆ **MK-217** see Alendronate on page 53
◆ **MK383** see Tirofiban on page 1909
◆ **MK-0431** see SitaGLIPtin on page 1781
◆ **MK462** see Rizatriptan on page 1722
◆ **MK 0517** see Fosaprepitant on page 844
◆ **MK594** see Losartan on page 1160
◆ **MK0826** see Ertapenem on page 662
◆ **MK 869** see Aprepitant on page 139
◆ **MMC** see MitoMYcin (Ophthalmic) on page 1298
◆ **MMR** see Measles, Mumps, and Rubella Virus Vaccine on page 1184
◆ **M-M-R® II** see Measles, Mumps, and Rubella Virus Vaccine on page 1184
◆ **Mobic®** see Meloxicam on page 1196
◆ **Mobidin®** see Salicylates (Various Salts) on page 1742

Modafinil (moe DAF i nil)

Brand Names: U.S. Provigil®
Brand Names: Canada Alertec®; Apo-Modafinil®
Generic Availability (U.S.) Yes
Pharmacologic Category Stimulant
Use Improve wakefulness in patients with excessive daytime sleepiness associated with narcolepsy and shift work sleep disorder (SWSD); adjunctive therapy for obstructive sleep apnea/hypopnea syndrome (OSAHS)

Unlabeled Use Attention-deficit/hyperactivity disorder (ADHD); treatment of fatigue in MS and other disorders

Medication Guide Available Yes

Contraindications Hypersensitivity to modafinil, armodafinil, or any component of the formulation

Warnings/Precautions For use following complete evaluation of sleepiness and in conjunction with other standard treatments (eg, CPAP). The degree of sleepiness should be reassessed frequently; some patients may not return to a normal level of wakefulness. Use is not recommended with a history of angina, cardiac ischemia, recent history of myocardial infarction, left ventricular hypertrophy, or patients with mitral valve prolapse who have developed mitral valve prolapse syndrome with previous CNS stimulant use.

Serious and life-threatening rashes (including Stevens-Johnson syndrome and toxic epidermal necrolysis) have been reported with modafinil. Most cases have occurred within the first 5 weeks of therapy; however, rare cases have occurred after long-term use. No risk factors have been identified to predict occurrence or severity. Patients should be advised to discontinue at first sign of rash.

In addition, rare cases of multiorgan hypersensitivity reactions in association with modafinil use, and lone cases of angioedema and anaphylactoid reactions with armodafinil, have been reported. Signs and symptoms are diverse, reflecting the involvement of specific organs. Patients typically present with fever and rash associated with organ-system dysfunction. Patients should be advised to report any signs and symptoms related to these effects; discontinuation of therapy is recommended.

Caution should be exercised when modafinil is given to patients with a history of psychosis; may impair the ability to engage in potentially hazardous activities. Stimulants may unmask tics in individuals with coexisting Tourette's syndrome. Use caution with renal or hepatic impairment (dosage adjustment in hepatic dysfunction is recommended).

Adverse Reactions (Reflective of adult population; not specific for elderly)
>10%:
  Central nervous system: Headache (adults 34%; children 20%; dose related)
  Gastrointestinal: Appetite decreased (children 16%), abdominal pain (children 12%), nausea (11%)
1% to 10%:
  Cardiovascular: Chest pain (3%), hypertension (3%), palpitation (2%), tachycardia (2%), vasodilation (2%), edema (1%)
  Central nervous system: Nervousness (7%), dizziness (5%), anxiety (5%; dose related), insomnia (5%), depression (2%), somnolence (2%), chills (1%), agitation (1%), confusion (1%), emotional lability (1%), vertigo (1%)
  Dermatologic: Rash (1%; includes some severe cases requiring hospitalization)
  Gastrointestinal: Diarrhea (6%), dyspepsia (5%), weight loss (children 5%), xerostomia (4%), anorexia (4%), constipation (2%), flatulence (1%), mouth ulceration (1%), taste perversion (1%)
  Genitourinary: Abnormal urine (1%), hematuria (1%), pyuria (1%)
  Hematologic: Eosinophilia (1%)
  Hepatic: LFTs abnormal (2%)
  Neuromuscular & skeletal: Back pain (6%), paresthesia (2%), dyskinesia (1%), hyperkinesia (1%), hypertonia (1%), neck rigidity (1%), tremor (1%)
  Ocular: Amblyopia (1%), eye pain (1%), vision abnormal (1%)
  Respiratory: Rhinitis (7%), pharyngitis (4%), lung disorder (2%), asthma (1%), epistaxis (1%)
  Miscellaneous: Flu-like syndrome (4%), thirst (1%), diaphoresis (1%), herpes simplex infection (1%)

Drug Interactions
  Metabolism/Transport Effects Substrate of CYP3A4 (major); **Inhibits** CYP1A2 (weak), 2A6 (weak), 2C8/9 (weak), 2C19 (strong), 2E1 (weak), 3A4 (weak); **Induces** CYP1A2 (weak), 2B6 (weak), 3A4 (weak)

Avoid Concomitant Use
  Avoid concomitant use of Modafinil with any of the following: Axitinib; Clopidogrel; Conivaptan; Iobenguane I 123; Pimozide

Increased Effect/Toxicity Modafinil may increase the levels/effects of citalopram, diazepam, methsuximide, phenytoin, propranolol, sertraline, or other CYP2C19 substrates. Modafinil may increase levels of warfarin. In populations deficient in the CYP2D6 isoenzyme, where CYP2C19 acts as a secondary metabolic pathway, concentrations of tricyclic antidepressants and selective serotonin reuptake inhibitors may be increased during coadministration. The levels/effects of modafinil may be increased by azole antifungals, ciprofloxacin, clarithromycin, diclofenac, doxycycline, erythromycin, imatinib, isoniazid, nefazodone, nicardipine, propofol, protease inhibitors, quinidine, telithromycin, verapamil, or other CYP3A4 inhibitors.

Decreased Effect Modafinil may decrease serum concentrations of oral contraceptives, cyclosporine, and to a lesser degree, theophylline. The levels/effects of modafinil may be decreased by aminoglutethimide, carbamazepine, nafcillin, nevirapine, phenobarbital, phenytoin, rifamycins, and other CYP3A4 inducers. There is also evidence to suggest that modafinil may induce its own metabolism.

Ethanol/Nutrition/Herb Interactions
Ethanol: Avoid or limit ethanol.
Food: Delays absorption, but does not affect bioavailability.

Stability Store at 20°C to 25°C (68°F to 77°F).

Mechanism of Action The exact mechanism of action is unclear, it does not appear to alter the release of dopamine or norepinephrine, it may exert its stimulant effects by decreasing GABA-mediated neurotransmission, although this theory has not yet been fully evaluated; several studies also suggest that an intact central alpha-adrenergic system is required for modafinil's activity; the drug increases high-frequency alpha waves while decreasing both delta and theta wave activity, and these effects are consistent with generalized increases in mental alertness

Pharmacodynamics/Kinetics Modafinil is a racemic compound (10% *d*-isomer and 90% *l*-isomer at steady state) whose enantiomers have different pharmacokinetics

Distribution: V_d: 0.9 L/kg
Protein binding: ~60%, primarily to albumin
Metabolism: Hepatic; multiple pathways including CYP3A4
Half-life elimination: Effective half-life: 15 hours
Time to peak, serum: 2-4 hours
Excretion: Urine (as metabolites, <10% as unchanged drug)

Dosage

Geriatric Elimination of modafinil and its metabolites may be reduced as a consequence of aging and as a result, consider initiating at lower doses in this patient population.

Adult
ADHD (unlabeled use): Oral: 100-400 mg/day (Taylor, 2000)
Narcolepsy, obstructive sleep apnea/hypopnea syndrome (OSAHS): Oral: Initial: 200 mg as a single daily dose in the morning.
Shift work sleep disorder (SWSD): Oral: Initial: 200 mg as a single dose taken ~1 hour prior to start of work shift.
Note: Doses of 400 mg/day, given as a single dose, have been well tolerated, but there is no consistent evidence that this dose confers additional benefit.

Renal Impairment Safety and efficacy have not been established in severe renal impairment.

Hepatic Impairment Severe hepatic impairment: Dose should be reduced to one-half of that recommended for patients with normal liver function.

Administration For the treatment of narcolepsy and obstructive sleep apnea/hypopnea syndrome (OSAHS), administer dose in the morning. For the treatment of shift work sleep disorder (SWSD), administer dose ~1 hour prior to start of work shift.

Monitoring Parameters Levels of sleepiness; blood pressure in patients with hypertension

Special Geriatric Considerations Clearance of modafinil may be reduced in the elderly. Safety and effectiveness in persons >65 years of age have not been established. In the limited number of elderly patients studied, the incidence of adverse events was similar to younger patients.

Controlled Substance C-IV

Dosage Forms Excipient information presented when available (limited, particularly for generics); consult specific product labeling.
Tablet, oral: 100 mg, 200 mg
Provigil®: 100 mg
Provigil®: 200 mg [scored]

◆ **Modified Shohl's Solution** see Sodium Citrate and Citric Acid on page 1790

Moexipril (mo EKS i pril)

Related Information
Angiotensin Agents on page 2093
Medication Safety Issues
Sound-alike/look-alike issues:
Moexipril may be confused with Monopril®
Brand Names: U.S. Univasc®

Index Terms Moexipril Hydrochloride

Generic Availability (U.S.) Yes

Pharmacologic Category Angiotensin-Converting Enzyme (ACE) Inhibitor

Use Treatment of hypertension, alone or in combination with thiazide diuretics

Contraindications Hypersensitivity to moexipril or any component of the formulation; angioedema related to previous treatment with an ACE inhibitor

Warnings/Precautions Anaphylactic reactions may occur rarely with ACE inhibitors. At any time during treatment (especially following first dose) angioedema may occur rarely with ACE inhibitors; it may involve the head and neck (potentially compromising airway) or the intestine (presenting with abdominal pain). African-Americans and patients with idiopathic or hereditary angioedema may be at an increased risk. Prolonged frequent monitoring may be required especially if tongue, glottis, or larynx are involved as they are associated with airway obstruction. Patients with a history of airway surgery may have a higher risk of airway obstruction. Aggressive early and appropriate management is critical. Use in patients with previous angioedema associated with ACE inhibitor therapy is contraindicated. Severe anaphylactoid reactions may be seen during hemodialysis (eg, CVVHD) with high-flux dialysis membranes (eg, AN69), and rarely, during low density lipoprotein apheresis with dextran sulfate cellulose. Rare cases of anaphylactoid reactions have been reported in patients undergoing sensitization treatment with hymenoptera (bee, wasp) venom while receiving ACE inhibitors.

Symptomatic hypotension with or without syncope can occur with ACE inhibitors (usually with the first several doses); effects are most often observed in volume depleted patients; correct volume depletion prior to initiation; close monitoring of patient is required especially with initial dosing and dosing increases; blood pressure must be lowered at a rate appropriate for the patient's clinical condition. Initiation of therapy in patients with ischemic heart disease or cerebrovascular disease warrants close observation due to the potential consequences posed by falling blood pressure (eg, MI, stroke). Use with caution in hypertrophic cardiomyopathy with outflow tract obstruction, severe aortic stenosis, or before, during, or immediately after major surgery.

Hyperkalemia may occur with ACE inhibitors; risk factors include renal dysfunction, diabetes mellitus, concomitant use of potassium-sparing diuretics, potassium supplements, and/or potassium-containing salts. Use cautiously, if at all, with these agents and monitor potassium closely. Cough may occur with ACE inhibitors. Other causes of cough should be considered (eg, pulmonary congestion in patients with heart failure) and excluded prior to discontinuation.

May be associated with deterioration of renal function and/or increases in serum creatinine, particularly in patients with low renal blood flow (eg, renal artery stenosis, heart failure) whose glomerular filtration rate (GFR) is dependent on efferent arteriolar vasoconstriction by angiotensin II; deterioration may result in oliguria, acute renal failure, and progressive azotemia. Small increases in serum creatinine may occur following initiation; consider discontinuation only in patients with progressive and/or significant deterioration in renal function. Use with caution in patients with unstented unilateral/bilateral renal artery stenosis. When unstented bilateral renal artery stenosis is present, use is generally avoided due to the elevated risk of deterioration in renal function unless possible benefits outweigh risks. Concurrent use of angiotensin receptor blockers may increase the risk of clinically-significant adverse events (eg, renal dysfunction, hyperkalemia).

Rare toxicities associated with ACE inhibitors include cholestatic jaundice (which may progress to fulminant hepatic necrosis), agranulocytosis, neutropenia, or leukopenia with myeloid hypoplasia. Patients with collagen vascular diseases (especially with concomitant renal impairment) or renal impairment alone may be at increased risk for hematologic toxicity; periodically monitor CBC with differential in these patients.

Adverse Reactions (Reflective of adult population; not specific for elderly) 1% to 10%:

Cardiovascular: Hypotension, peripheral edema

Central nervous system: Headache, dizziness, fatigue

Dermatologic: Flushing, rash

Endocrine & metabolic: Hyperkalemia, hyponatremia

Gastrointestinal: Diarrhea, nausea, heartburn

Genitourinary: Polyuria

Neuromuscular & skeletal: Myalgia

Renal: Reversible increases in creatinine or BUN

Respiratory: Cough, pharyngitis, upper respiratory infection, sinusitis

Drug Interactions

Metabolism/Transport Effects None known.

Avoid Concomitant Use There are no known interactions where it is recommended to avoid concomitant use.

Increased Effect/Toxicity

Moexipril may increase the levels/effects of: Allopurinol; Amifostine; Antihypertensives; AzaTHIOprine; CycloSPORINE; CycloSPORINE (Systemic); Ferric Gluconate; Gold Sodium Thiomalate; Highest Risk QTc-Prolonging Agents; Hypotensive Agents; Iron Dextran Complex; Lithium; Moderate Risk QTc-Prolonging Agents; Nonsteroidal Anti-Inflammatory Agents; RiTUXimab; Sodium Phosphates

The levels/effects of Moexipril may be increased by: Aliskiren; Angiotensin II Receptor Blockers; Diazoxide; DPP-IV Inhibitors; Eplerenone; Everolimus; Herbs (Hypotensive Properties); Loop Diuretics; MAO Inhibitors; Mifepristone; Pentoxifylline; Phosphodiesterase 5 Inhibitors; Potassium Salts; Potassium-Sparing Diuretics; Prostacyclin Analogues; Sirolimus; Temsirolimus; Thiazide Diuretics; TiZANidine; Tolvaptan; Trimethoprim

Decreased Effect

The levels/effects of Moexipril may be decreased by: Antacids; Aprotinin; Herbs (Hypertensive Properties); Icatibant; Lanthanum; Methylphenidate; Nonsteroidal Anti-Inflammatory Agents; Salicylates; Yohimbine

Ethanol/Nutrition/Herb Interactions

Food: Food may delay and reduce peak serum levels. Potassium supplements and/or potassium-containing salts may cause or worsen hyperkalemia. Management: Take on an empty stomach 1 hour before or 2 hours after a meal. Consult prescriber before consuming a potassium-rich diet, potassium supplements, or salt substitutes.

Herb/Nutraceutical: Some herbal medications may worsen hypertension (eg, licorice); others may increase the antihypertensive effect of moexipril (eg, shepherd's purse). Management: Avoid bayberry, blue cohosh, cayenne, ephedra, ginger, ginseng (American), kola, licorice, and yohimbe. Avoid black cohosh, California poppy, coleus, golden seal, hawthorn, mistletoe, periwinkle, quinine, and shepherd's purse.

Mechanism of Action Competitive inhibitor of angiotensin-converting enzyme (ACE); prevents conversion of angiotensin I to angiotensin II, a potent vasoconstrictor; results in lower levels of angiotensin II which causes an increase in plasma renin activity and a reduction in aldosterone secretion

Pharmacodynamics/Kinetics

Onset of action: Peak effect: 1-2 hours

Duration: >24 hours

Absorption: Incomplete

Distribution: V_d (moexiprilat): 180 L

Protein binding, plasma: Moexipril: 90%; Moexiprilat: 50% to 70%

Metabolism: Parent drug: Hepatic and via GI tract to moexiprilat, 1000 times more potent than parent

Bioavailability: Moexiprilat: 13%; reduced with food (AUC decreased by ~40%)

Half-life elimination: Moexipril: 1 hour; Moexiprilat: 2-9 hours

Time to peak: 1.5 hours

Excretion: Feces (50%)

Dosage

Geriatric Dose the same as adults; adjust for renal impairment. Tablet may be cut in half (3.75 mg) for starting therapy (see Dosage: Renal Impairment).

Adult Hypertension: Oral: Initial: 7.5 mg once daily (in patients **not** receiving diuretics), 1 hour prior to a meal **or** 3.75 mg once daily (when combined with thiazide diuretics); maintenance dose: 7.5-30 mg/day in 1 or 2 divided doses 1 hour before meals

Renal Impairment Cl_{cr} ≤40 mL/minute: Patients may be cautiously placed on 3.75 mg once daily, then upwardly titrated to a maximum of 15 mg/day.

Administration Administer on an empty stomach.

Monitoring Parameters Blood pressure; serum creatinine and potassium; if patient has collagen vascular disease and/or renal impairment, periodically monitor CBC with differential

Test Interactions Increases BUN, creatinine, potassium, positive Coombs' [direct]; decreases cholesterol (S); may cause false-positive results in urine acetone determinations using sodium nitroprusside reagent

Special Geriatric Considerations Due to frequent decreases in glomerular filtration (also creatinine clearance) with aging, elderly patients may have exaggerated responses to ACE inhibitors; differences in clinical response due to hepatic changes are not observed. ACE inhibitors may be preferred agents in elderly patients with congestive heart failure and diabetes mellitus. Diabetic proteinuria is reduced and insulin sensitivity is enhanced. In general, the side effect profile is favorable in the elderly and causes little or no CNS confusion; use lowest dose recommendations initially; adjust dose for renal impairment in the elderly. The elderly may be volume depleted due to diuretic use and/or blunted thirst reflex resulting in inadequate fluid intake.

◀ **Dosage Forms** Excipient information presented when available (limited, particularly for generics); consult specific product labeling.

Tablet, oral, as hydrochloride: 7.5 mg, 15 mg

Univasc®: 7.5 mg, 15 mg [scored]

♦ **Moexipril Hydrochloride** see Moexipril on page 1301

♦ **Moi-Stir® [OTC]** see Saliva Substitute on page 1748

♦ **MOM** see Magnesium Hydroxide on page 1177

Mometasone (Oral Inhalation) (moe MET a sone)

Related Information

Asthma on page 2125

Inhalant Agents on page 2117

Brand Names: U.S. Asmanex® Twisthaler®

Brand Names: Canada Asmanex® Twisthaler®

Index Terms Mometasone Furoate

Generic Availability (U.S.) No

Pharmacologic Category Corticosteroid, Inhalant (Oral)

Use Maintenance treatment of asthma as prophylactic therapy

Contraindications Hypersensitivity to mometasone or any component of the formulation; hypersensitivity to milk proteins; primary treatment of status asthmaticus or acute bronchospasm

Canadian labeling: Additional contraindications (not in U.S. labeling): Untreated systemic fungal, bacterial, viral, or parasitic infections; active or quiet tuberculosis infection of the respiratory tract; ocular herpes simplex

Warnings/Precautions May cause hypercorticism or suppression of hypothalamic-pituitary-adrenal (HPA) axis, particularly in patients receiving high doses for prolonged periods. HPA axis suppression may lead to adrenal crisis. Withdrawal and discontinuation of a corticosteroid should be done slowly and carefully. Particular care is required when patients are transferred from systemic corticosteroids to inhaled products due to possible adrenal insufficiency or withdrawal from steroids, including an increase in allergic symptoms. Patients receiving >20 mg per day of prednisone (or equivalent) may be most susceptible. Fatalities have occurred due to adrenal insufficiency in asthmatic patients during and after transfer from systemic corticosteroids to aerosol steroids; aerosol steroids do not provide the systemic steroid needed to treat patients having trauma, surgery, or infections. When transferring to oral inhaler, previously-suppressed allergic conditions (rhinitis, conjunctivitis, eczema) may be unmasked.

Bronchospasm may occur with wheezing after inhalation; if this occurs stop steroid and treat with a fast-acting bronchodilator. Supplemental steroids (oral or parenteral) may be needed during stress or severe asthma attacks. Not to be used in status asthmaticus or for the relief of acute bronchospasm. Corticosteroid use may cause psychiatric disturbances, including depression, euphoria, insomnia, mood swings, and personality changes. Pre-existing psychiatric conditions may be exacerbated by corticosteroid use. Prolonged use of corticosteroids may also increase the incidence of secondary infection, mask acute infection (including fungal infections), prolong or exacerbate viral infections, or limit response to vaccines. Exposure to chickenpox should be avoided; corticosteroids should not be used to treat ocular herpes simplex. Corticosteroids should not be used for cerebral malaria or viral hepatitis. Close observation is required in patients with latent tuberculosis and/or TB reactivity; restrict use in active TB (only in conjunction with antituberculosis treatment). Prolonged treatment with corticosteroids has been associated with the development of Kaposi's sarcoma (case reports); if noted, discontinuation of therapy should be considered.

Use with caution in patients with thyroid disease, hepatic impairment, renal impairment, cardiovascular disease, diabetes, glaucoma, cataracts, myasthenia gravis, patients with or who are at risk for osteoporosis, patients at risk for seizures, or GI diseases (diverticulitis, peptic ulcer, ulcerative colitis) due to perforation risk. Use caution following acute MI (corticosteroids have been associated with myocardial rupture). Because of the risk of adverse effects, systemic corticosteroids should be used cautiously in the elderly in the smallest possible effective dose for the shortest duration.

Adverse Reactions (Reflective of adult population; not specific for elderly)
>10%:
Central nervous system: Headache (17% to 22%), fatigue (1% to 13%), depression (11%)
Neuromuscular & skeletal: Musculoskeletal pain (4% to 22%), arthralgia (13%)
Respiratory: Sinusitis (5% to 22%), rhinitis (4% to 20%), upper respiratory infection (8% to 15%), pharyngitis (8% to 13%)
Miscellaneous: Oral candidiasis (4% to 22%)
1% to 10%:
Central nervous system: Fever (children 7%), pain (1% to <3%)
Dermatologic: Bruising (children 2%)
Gastrointestinal: Abdominal pain (2% to 6%), dyspepsia (3% to 5%), nausea (1% to 3%), vomiting (1% to ≤3%), anorexia (1% to <3%), dry throat (1% to <3%), gastroenteritis (1% to <3%)
Genitourinary: Dysmenorrhea (4% to 9%), urinary tract infection (children 2%)
Neuromuscular & skeletal: Back pain (3% to 6%), myalgia (2% to 3%)
Ocular: Ocular pressure increased (3%), cataracts (1%)
Otic: Earache (1% to <3%)
Respiratory: Sinus congestion (9%), dysphonia (1% to <3%), epistaxis (1% to <3%), nasal irritation (1% to <3%)
Miscellaneous: Flu-like syndrome (1% to <3%), infection (1% to <3%)

Drug Interactions
Metabolism/Transport Effects Substrate of CYP3A4 (minor); **Note:** Assignment of Major/Minor substrate status based on clinically relevant drug interaction potential
Avoid Concomitant Use
Avoid concomitant use of Mometasone (Oral Inhalation) with any of the following: Aldesleukin
Increased Effect/Toxicity
Mometasone (Oral Inhalation) may increase the levels/effects of: Amphotericin B; Deferasirox; Loop Diuretics; Thiazide Diuretics

The levels/effects of Mometasone (Oral Inhalation) may be increased by: CYP3A4 Inhibitors (Strong); Telaprevir
Decreased Effect
Mometasone (Oral Inhalation) may decrease the levels/effects of: Aldesleukin; Antidiabetic Agents; Corticorelin; Hyaluronidase; Telaprevir

The levels/effects of Mometasone (Oral Inhalation) may be decreased by: Tocilizumab
Stability Store at 25°C (77°F); excursions permitted to 15°C to 30°C (59°F to 86°F). Discard when oral dose counter reads "00" (or 45 days [U.S. labeling] or 60 days [Canadian labeling] after opening the foil pouch).
Mechanism of Action May depress the formation, release, and activity of endogenous chemical mediators of inflammation (kinins, histamine, liposomal enzymes, prostaglandins). Leukocytes and macrophages may have to be present for the initiation of responses mediated by the above substances. Inhibits the margination and subsequent cell migration to the area of injury, and also reverses the dilatation and increased vessel permeability in the area resulting in decreased access of cells to the sites of injury.
Pharmacodynamics/Kinetics
Absorption: <1%
Protein binding: 98% to 99%
Metabolism: Hepatic via CYP3A4; forms metabolite
Half-life elimination: 5 hours
Excretion: Feces, bile, urine
Dosage
Geriatric & Adult Asthma: Oral inhalation: **Note:** Dosage forms available in the U.S. (110 mcg and 220 mcg Twisthaler®) deliver 100 and 200 mcg mometasone furoate per actuation respectively.
U.S. labeling: Adults: Previous therapy:
Bronchodilators or inhaled corticosteroids: Initial: 1 inhalation (220 mcg) daily (maximum: 2 inhalations or 440 mcg/day); may be given in the evening or in divided doses twice daily
Oral corticosteroids: Initial: 440 mcg twice daily (maximum: 880 mcg/day); prednisone should be reduced no faster than 2.5 mg/day on a weekly basis, beginning after at least 1 week of mometasone furoate use
Canadian labeling: Adults:
Usual dose: 400 mcg once daily in the morning; maintenance: 200-400 mcg once daily in the morning. **Note:** Some patients (eg, previously receiving high-dose inhaled corticosteroids) may respond more favorably to 400 mcg daily administered in 2 divided doses.

Severe asthma and requiring oral corticosteroids: Initial: 400 mcg twice daily; taper off oral corticosteroid gradually by decreasing daily prednisone dose by 1 mg/day (or equivalent of other corticosteroid) on a weekly basis, beginning after at least 1 week of mometasone furoate use; upon successful taper off of oral steroids, titrate mometasone to lowest effective dose.

NIH Asthma Guidelines (NIH, 2007): Adults:
"Low" dose: 200 mcg/day
"Medium" dose: 400 mcg/day
"High" dose: >400 mcg/day
Note: Maximum effects may not be evident for 1-2 weeks or longer; dose should be titrated to effect, using the lowest possible dose

Administration Exhale fully prior to bringing the Twisthaler® up to the mouth. Place between lips and inhale quickly and deeply. Do not breathe out through the inhaler. Remove inhaler and hold breath for 10 seconds if possible. Rinse mouth after use.

Monitoring Parameters HPA axis suppression
Asthma: FEV_1, peak flow, and/or other pulmonary function tests

Special Geriatric Considerations Instruct patient on proper use of inhaler.

Dosage Forms Excipient information presented when available (limited, particularly for generics); consult specific product labeling.
Powder, for oral inhalation, as furoate:
Asmanex® Twisthaler®: 110 mcg (7 units, 30 units) [contains lactose; delivers 100 mcg/actuation]
Asmanex® Twisthaler®: 220 mcg (14 units, 30 units, 60 units, 120 units) [contains lactose; delivers 200 mcg/actuation]

Dosage Forms: Canada Excipient information presented when available (limited, particularly for generics); consult specific product labeling.
Powder, for oral inhalation, as furoate:
Asmanex® Twisthaler®: 200 mcg (30 doses, 60 doses) [contains lactose; delivers 200 mcg/actuation]
Asmanex® Twisthaler®: 400 mcg (30 doses, 60 doses) [contains lactose; delivers 400 mcg/actuation]

Mometasone (Nasal) (moe MET a sone)

Brand Names: U.S. Nasonex®
Brand Names: Canada Nasonex®
Index Terms Mometasone Furoate
Generic Availability (U.S.) No
Pharmacologic Category Corticosteroid, Nasal
Use Treatment of nasal symptoms of seasonal and perennial allergic rhinitis; prevention of nasal symptoms associated with seasonal allergic rhinitis; treatment of nasal polyps in adults

Canadian labeling: Additional use (not in U.S. labeling): Treatment of mild-to-moderate uncomplicated rhinosinusitis or as adjunctive treatment (with antimicrobials) in acute rhinosinusitis

Unlabeled Use Adjunct to antibiotics in empiric treatment of acute bacterial rhinosinusitis (ABRS) (Chow, 2012)

Dosage

Geriatric & Adult

Seasonal and perennial allergic rhinitis: Intranasal:
U.S. labeling:
Treatment: 2 sprays (100 mcg) in each nostril once daily
Prevention: 2 sprays (100 mcg) in each nostril once daily beginning 2-4 weeks prior to pollen season
Canadian labeling (not in U.S. labeling): Initial: 2 sprays (100 mcg) in each nostril once daily; upon symptom control, may consider dose reduction to 1 spray (50 mcg) in each nostril once daily as maintenance therapy. **Note:** If adequate symptom control is not achieved with initial dosing, may increase dose to 4 sprays (200 mcg) in each nostril once daily (total daily dose: 400 mcg). Dose reduction is recommended upon symptom control.

Treatment of nasal polyps: Intranasal: 2 sprays (100 mcg) in each nostril twice daily; 2 sprays (100 mcg) once daily may be effective in some patients

Rhinosinusitis, adjunctive treatment (acute): Intranasal: Canadian labeling (not in U.S. labeling): 2 sprays (100 mcg) in each nostril twice daily; if inadequate symptom control, may increase to 4 sprays (200 mcg) in each nostril twice daily (total daily dose: 800 mcg)

Rhinosinusitis treatment (acute, mild-to-moderate, uncomplicated): Intranasal: Canadian labeling (not in U.S. labeling): 2 sprays (100 mcg) in each nostril twice daily; use beyond 15 days has not been studied.

Special Geriatric Considerations Evaluate the patient's or caregiver's ability to safely administer the correct dose of nasal medication.

Dosage Forms Excipient information presented when available (limited, particularly for generics); consult specific product labeling.

Suspension, intranasal, as furoate [spray]:
Nasonex®: 50 mcg/spray (17 g) [contains benzalkonium chloride; delivers 120 sprays]

Dosage Forms: Canada Excipient information presented when available (limited, particularly for generics); consult specific product labeling.

Suspension, intranasal, as furoate [spray]:
Nasonex®: 50 mcg/spray [contains benzalkonium chloride; delivers 140 sprays]

Mometasone (Topical) (moe MET a sone)

Related Information
Topical Corticosteroids *on page 2113*

Medication Safety Issues
Sound-alike/look-alike issues:
Elocon® lotion may be confused with ophthalmic solutions. Manufacturer's labeling emphasizes the product is **NOT** for use in the eyes.

Brand Names: U.S. Elocon®

Brand Names: Canada Elocom®; PMS-Mometasone; ratio-Mometasone; Taro-Mometasone

Index Terms Mometasone Furoate

Generic Availability (U.S.) Yes

Pharmacologic Category Corticosteroid, Topical

Use Relief of the inflammatory and pruritic manifestations of corticosteroid-responsive dermatoses (medium potency topical corticosteroid)

Dosage
Geriatric & Adult Treatment of corticosteroid-responsive dermatoses: Topical: Apply sparingly, do not use occlusive dressings. Therapy should be discontinued when control is achieved; if no improvement is seen in 2 weeks, reassessment of diagnosis may be necessary.
Cream, ointment: Apply a thin film to affected area once daily
Lotion: Apply a few drops to affected area once daily

Special Geriatric Considerations Due to age-related changes in skin, limit use of topical corticosteroids.

Dosage Forms Excipient information presented when available (limited, particularly for generics); consult specific product labeling.

Cream, topical, as furoate: 0.1% (15 g, 45 g)
Elocon®: 0.1% (15 g, 45 g)
Lotion, topical, as furoate: 0.1% (30 mL, 60 mL)
Elocon®: 0.1% (30 mL, 60 mL) [contains isopropyl alcohol 40%]
Ointment, topical, as furoate: 0.1% (15 g, 45 g)
Elocon®: 0.1% (15 g, 45 g)

Mometasone and Formoterol (moe MET a sone & for MOH te rol)

Related Information
Formoterol *on page 841*
Mometasone (Oral Inhalation) *on page 1304*

Brand Names: U.S. Dulera®

Brand Names: Canada Zenhale™

Index Terms Formoterol and Mometasone; Formoterol and Mometasone Furoate; Formoterol Fumarate Dihydrate and Mometasone

Generic Availability (U.S.) No

Pharmacologic Category Beta$_2$ Agonist, Long-Acting; Beta$_2$-Adrenergic Agonist, Long-Acting; Corticosteroid, Inhalant (Oral)

Use Maintenance treatment of asthma where combination therapy is indicated

Medication Guide Available Yes

Contraindications Hypersensitivity to mometasone, formoterol, or any component of the formulation; need for acute bronchodilation (including status asthmaticus)

Warnings/Precautions [U.S. Boxed Warning]: Long-acting beta$_2$-agonists (LABAs), such as formoterol, increase the risk of asthma-related deaths; mometasone and formoterol should only be used in patients not adequately controlled on a long-term

◀ **asthma control medication (ie, inhaled corticosteroid) or whose disease severity requires initiation of two maintenance therapies.** In a large, randomized, placebo-controlled U.S. clinical trial (SMART, 2006), salmeterol was associated with an increase in asthma-related deaths (when added to usual asthma therapy); risk is considered a class effect among all LABAs. Data are not available to determine if the addition of an inhaled corticosteroid lessens this increased risk of death associated with LABA use. Assess patients at regular intervals once asthma control is maintained on combination therapy to determine if step-down therapy is appropriate (without loss of asthma control), and the patient can be maintained on an inhaled corticosteroid only. LABAs are not appropriate in patients whose asthma is adequately controlled on low- or medium-dose inhaled corticosteroids.

Do **not** use for acute bronchospasm. Short-acting beta$_2$-agonist (eg, albuterol) should be used for acute symptoms and symptoms occurring between treatments. Do **not** initiate in patients with significantly worsening or acutely deteriorating asthma. Patients must be instructed to seek medical attention in cases where acute symptoms are not relieved by short-acting beta-agonist (not formoterol) or a previous level of response is diminished. Medical evaluation must not be delayed. Patients using inhaled, short-acting beta$_2$-agonists should be instructed to discontinue routine use of these medications prior to beginning treatment with Dulera®; short-acting agents should be reserved for symptomatic relief of acute symptoms. Patients should not use additional long-acting beta$_2$-adrenergic agonists.

Immediate hypersensitivity reactions (urticaria, angioedema, rash, bronchospasm) have been reported. Do not exceed recommended dose; serious adverse events, including fatalities, have been associated with excessive use of inhaled sympathomimetics. Rarely, paradoxical bronchospasm may occur with use of inhaled bronchodilating agents; this should be distinguished from inadequate response.

Use caution in patients with cardiovascular disease (arrhythmia or hypertension or HF), seizure disorders, diabetes, osteoporosis, ocular disease, thyroid disease, or hypokalemia. Beta agonists may cause elevation in blood pressure, heart rate, and result in CNS stimulation/excitation. Beta$_2$-agonists may increase risk of arrhythmia, increase serum glucose, or decrease serum potassium. Long-term use may affect bone mineral density in adults. Infections with *Candida albicans* in the mouth and throat (thrush) have been reported with use. Use with caution in patients taking strong CYP3A4 inhibitors (see Drug Interactions); consider alternative agents that avoid or lessen the potential for CYP-mediated interactions.

Mometasone may cause hypercorticism and/or suppression of hypothalamic-pituitary-adrenal (HPA) axis, particularly in patients receiving high doses for prolonged periods. Caution is required when patients are transferred from systemic corticosteroids to products with lower systemic bioavailability (ie, inhalation). May lead to possible adrenal insufficiency or withdrawal symptoms, including an increase in allergic symptoms. Patients receiving prolonged therapy ≥20 mg per day of prednisone (or equivalent) may be most susceptible. Aerosol steroids do not provide the systemic steroid needed to treat patients having trauma, surgery, or infections.

Prolonged use of corticosteroids may also increase the incidence of secondary infection, mask acute infection (including fungal infections), prolong or exacerbate viral infections, or limit response to vaccines. Exposure to chickenpox should be avoided; corticosteroids should not be used to treat ocular herpes simplex. Corticosteroids should not be used for cerebral malaria. Close observation is required in patients with latent tuberculosis and/or TB reactivity restrict use in active TB (only in conjunction with antituberculosis treatment).

Withdraw systemic therapy with gradual tapering of dose. There have been reports of systemic corticosteroid withdrawal symptoms (eg, joint/muscle pain, lassitude, depression) when withdrawing oral inhalation therapy.

Adverse Reactions (Reflective of adult population; not specific for elderly) Also see individual agents.
1% to 10%:
Central nervous system: Headache (up to 5%)
Respiratory: Nasopharyngitis (5%), dysphonia (4% to 5%), sinusitis (2% to 3%)

Drug Interactions
Metabolism/Transport Effects Refer to individual components.
Avoid Concomitant Use
Avoid concomitant use of Mometasone and Formoterol with any of the following: Aldesleukin; BCG; Beta-Blockers (Nonselective); Iobenguane I 123; Mifepristone; Natalizumab; Pimecrolimus; Tacrolimus (Topical)

Increased Effect/Toxicity

Mometasone and Formoterol may increase the levels/effects of: Acetylcholinesterase Inhibitors; Amphotericin B; Deferasirox; Leflunomide; Loop Diuretics; Natalizumab; NSAID (COX-2 Inhibitor); NSAID (Nonselective); Sympathomimetics; Thiazide Diuretics; Vaccines (Live); Warfarin

The levels/effects of Mometasone and Formoterol may be increased by: Antifungal Agents (Azole Derivatives, Systemic); Aprepitant; AtoMOXetine; Caffeine; Calcium Channel Blockers (Nondihydropyridine); Cannabinoids; CYP3A4 Inhibitors (Strong); Denosumab; Estrogen Derivatives; Fluconazole; Fosaprepitant; Indacaterol; Macrolide Antibiotics; MAO Inhibitors; Mifepristone; Neuromuscular-Blocking Agents (Nondepolarizing); Pimecrolimus; Quinolone Antibiotics; Roflumilast; Salicylates; Tacrolimus (Topical); Telaprevir; Theophylline Derivatives; Trastuzumab; Tricyclic Antidepressants

Decreased Effect

Mometasone and Formoterol may decrease the levels/effects of: Aldesleukin; Antidiabetic Agents; BCG; Calcitriol; Coccidioidin Skin Test; Corticorelin; Hyaluronidase; Iobenguane I 123; Isoniazid; Salicylates; Sipuleucel-T; Telaprevir; Vaccines (Inactivated)

The levels/effects of Mometasone and Formoterol may be decreased by: Alpha-/Beta-Blockers; Aminoglutethimide; Barbiturates; Beta-Blockers (Beta1 Selective); Beta-Blockers (Nonselective); Betahistine; Echinacea; Mifepristone; Mitotane; Primidone; Rifamycin Derivatives; Tocilizumab

Stability Store at room temperature of 20°C to 25°C (68°F to 77°F). Do not puncture, incinerate, or store near heat or open flame. Discard inhaler after the labeled number of inhalations have been used.

Mechanism of Action Formoterol relaxes bronchial smooth muscle by selective action on $beta_2$ receptors with little effect on heart rate. Formoterol has a long-acting effect. Mometasone is a corticosteroid which controls the rate of protein synthesis, depresses the migration of polymorphonuclear leukocytes/fibroblasts, and reverses capillary permeability and lysosomal stabilization at the cellular level to prevent or control inflammation.

Pharmacodynamics/Kinetics See individual agents.

Dosage

Geriatric & Adult Asthma: Oral inhalation:

Previous therapy included inhaled low-dose corticosteroids: Canadian labeling (not in U.S. labeling): Mometasone 50 mcg/formoterol 5 mcg: Two inhalations twice daily. Maximum daily dose: 4 inhalations

Previous therapy included inhaled medium-dose corticosteroids: Mometasone 100 mcg/formoterol 5 mcg: Two inhalations twice daily. Consider the higher dose combination for patients not adequately controlled on the lower combination following 1-2 weeks of therapy. Maximum daily dose: 4 inhalations

Previous therapy included inhaled high-dose corticosteroids: Mometasone 200 mcg/formoterol 5 mcg: Two inhalations twice daily. Maximum daily dose: 4 inhalations

Hepatic Impairment Mometasone systemic exposure appears to increase with increasing extent of impairment; however, there is no dosage adjustment recommended in the manufacturer's labeling.

Administration Prior to first use, inhaler must be primed by releasing 4 test sprays into the air; shake well before each spray. Inhaler must be reprimed if not used for >5 days. Shake well before each use. Discard inhaler after the labeled number of inhalations have been used.

Delivery of dose: Instruct patient to place mouthpiece gently between teeth, closing lips around inhaler. Instruct patient to inhale deeply and hold breath held for 5-10 seconds. The amount of drug delivered is small, and the individual will not sense the medication as it is inhaled. Remove mouthpiece from mouth prior to exhalation. Patient should not breathe out through the mouthpiece. After use of the inhaler, patient should rinse mouth/oropharynx with water and spit out rinse solution.

Monitoring Parameters FEV$_1$, peak flow meter, and/or other pulmonary function tests; monitor symptom relief, monitor for increased use if short-acting beta$_2$-adrenergic agonists (may be a sign of asthma deterioration)

Special Geriatric Considerations No significant difference in both safety and effectiveness was seen between elderly and young patients. Elderly patients should be specifically counseled about the proper use of metered-dose inhalers.

Dosage Forms Excipient information presented when available (limited, particularly for generics); consult specific product labeling.

Aerosol, for oral inhalation:

Dulera®: Mometasone furoate 100 mcg and formoterol fumarate dihydrate 5 mcg per inhalation (13 g) [120 metered actuations]

Dulera®: Mometasone furoate 200 mcg and formoterol fumarate dihydrate 5 mcg per inhalation (13 g) [120 metered actuations]

Dosage Forms: Canada Excipient information presented when available (limited, particularly for generics); consult specific product labeling.

Aerosol, for oral inhalation:

Zenhale™: Mometasone furoate 50 mcg and formoterol fumarate dihydrate 5 mcg per inhalation [120 metered actuations]

Montelukast (mon te LOO kast)

Medication Safety Issues
Sound-alike/look-alike issues:
Singulair® may be confused with SINEquan®
Brand Names: U.S. Singulair®
Brand Names: Canada Apo-Montelukast; Montelukast Sodium Tablets; Mylan-Montelukast; PMS-Montelukast; PMS-Montelukast FC; Sandoz-Montelukast; Sandoz-Montelukast Granules; Singulair®; Teva-Montelukast
Index Terms Montelukast Sodium
Generic Availability (U.S.) Yes: Excludes granules
Pharmacologic Category Leukotriene-Receptor Antagonist
Use Prophylaxis and chronic treatment of asthma; relief of symptoms of seasonal allergic rhinitis and perennial allergic rhinitis; prevention of exercise-induced bronchoconstriction
Unlabeled Use Acute asthma
Contraindications Hypersensitivity to montelukast or any component of the formulation
Warnings/Precautions Montelukast is not FDA approved for use in the reversal of bronchospasm in acute asthma attacks, including status asthmaticus; some clinicians, however, support its use as adjunctive therapy (Camargo, 2003; Cylly, 2003; Ferreira, 2001; Harmancik 2006). Appropriate rescue medication should be available. Appropriate rescue medication should be available. Appropriate clinical monitoring and a gradual dose reduction are recommended when systemic corticosteroid reduction is considered in patients initiating or receiving montelukast. Patients should be instructed to notify prescriber if behavioral changes occur. Inform phenylketonuric patients that the chewable tablet contains phenylalanine.

In rare cases, patients on therapy with montelukast may present with systemic eosinophilia, sometimes presenting with clinical features of vasculitis consistent with Churg-Strauss syndrome, a condition which is often treated with systemic corticosteroid therapy. Healthcare providers should be alert to eosinophilia, vasculitic rash, worsening pulmonary symptoms, cardiac complications, and/or neuropathy presenting in their patients. A causal association between montelukast and these underlying conditions has not been established. Montelukast will not interrupt bronchoconstrictor response to aspirin or other NSAIDs; aspirin sensitive asthmatics should continue to avoid these agents. Postmarketing reports of behavior changes (agitation, aggression, depression, insomnia) have been noted in children and adults.

Adverse Reactions (Reflective of adult population; not specific for elderly) 1% to 10%:
Central nervous system: Dizziness (2%), fatigue (2%), fever (2%)
Dermatologic: Rash (2%)
Gastrointestinal: Abdominal pain (3%), dyspepsia (2%), dental pain (2%), gastroenteritis (2%)
Hepatic: AST increased (2%)
Neuromuscular & skeletal: Weakness (2%)
Respiratory: Cough (3%), nasal congestion (2%)

Drug Interactions
Metabolism/Transport Effects Substrate of CYP2C9 (major), CYP3A4 (major); **Note:** Assignment of Major/Minor substrate status based on clinically relevant drug interaction potential; **Inhibits** CYP2C8 (weak), CYP2C9 (weak)
Avoid Concomitant Use There are no known interactions where it is recommended to avoid concomitant use.

Increased Effect/Toxicity

The levels/effects of Montelukast may be increased by: CYP2C9 Inhibitors (Moderate); CYP2C9 Inhibitors (Strong); Mifepristone

Decreased Effect

The levels/effects of Montelukast may be decreased by: CYP2C9 Inducers (Strong); CYP3A4 Inducers (Strong); Deferasirox; Herbs (CYP3A4 Inducers); Peginterferon Alfa-2b; Tocilizumab

Ethanol/Nutrition/Herb Interactions Herb/Nutraceutical: St John's wort may decrease montelukast levels.

Stability Store at room temperature of 25°C (77°F); excursions permitted to 15°C to 30°C (59°F to 86°F). Store in original package. Protect from moisture and light. Granules must be used within 15 minutes of opening packet.

Mechanism of Action Selective leukotriene receptor antagonist that inhibits the cysteinyl leukotriene receptor. Cysteinyl leukotrienes and leukotriene receptor occupation have been correlated with the pathophysiology of asthma, including airway edema, smooth muscle contraction, and altered cellular activity associated with the inflammatory process, which contribute to the signs and symptoms of asthma. Cysteinyl leukotrienes are also released from the nasal mucosa following allergen exposure leading to symptoms associated with allergic rhinitis.

Pharmacodynamics/Kinetics

Duration: >24 hours

Absorption: Rapid

Distribution: V_d: 8-11 L

Protein binding, plasma: >99%

Metabolism: Extensively hepatic via CYP3A4 and 2C9

Bioavailability: Tablet: 10 mg, Mean: 64%; Chewable tablet: 5 mg: 73% (63% when administered with a standard meal)

Half-life elimination, plasma: Mean: 2.7-5.5 hours; Prolonged in mild-to-moderate hepatic impairment: Mean: 7.4 hours

Time to peak, serum: Tablet: 10 mg: 3-4 hours; Chewable tablet: 2-2.5 hours; granules: 1-3 hours (fasting) and 3.5 to ~9 hours (with high-fat meal)

Excretion: Feces (86%); urine (<0.2%)

Dosage

Geriatric & Adult

Asthma, allergic seasonal or perennial rhinitis: Oral: 10 mg once daily

Asthma, acute (unlabeled use): Oral: 10 mg as a single dose administered with first-line therapy (Camargo, 2003; Cylly, 2003)

Bronchoconstriction, exercise-induced (prevention): Oral: 10 mg at least 2 hours prior to exercise; additional doses should not be administered within 24 hours. Daily administration to prevent exercise-induced bronchoconstriction has not been evaluated. Patients receiving montelukast for another indication should not take an additional dose to prevent exercise-induced bronchoconstriction.

Renal Impairment No dosage adjustment necessary.

Hepatic Impairment

Mild-to-moderate impairment: No dosage adjustment necessary.

Severe impairment: No dosage adjustment provided in manufacturer's labeling; has not been studied.

Administration When treating asthma, administer dose in the evening. Patients with allergic rhinitis may individualize administration time (morning or evening). Patients with both asthma and allergic rhinitis should take their dose in the evening. Granules may be administered directly in the mouth or mixed with a spoonful of applesauce, carrots, rice, ice cream, baby formula, or breast milk; do not add to any other liquids or foods. Administer within 15 minutes of opening packet. May administer without regard to meals.

Monitoring Parameters Mood or behavior changes, including suicidal thinking/behavior

Special Geriatric Considerations The pharmacokinetic profile in the elderly is similar to younger adults except the half-life is slightly longer in the elderly. Despite this difference, no adjustment in dose is necessary in the elderly. Elimination is mostly fecal and bile with insignificant amounts from renal elimination, which is an advantage for the elderly.

Dosage Forms Excipient information presented when available (limited, particularly for generics); consult specific product labeling.

Granules, oral:

Singulair®: 4 mg/packet (30s)

Tablet, oral: 10 mg

Singulair®: 10 mg [contains lactose 89.3 mg/tablet]

Tablet, chewable, oral: 4 mg, 5 mg

Singulair®: 4 mg [contains phenylalanine 0.67 mg/tablet; cherry flavor]

Singulair®: 5 mg [contains phenylalanine 0.84 mg/tablet; cherry flavor]

◆ **Montelukast Sodium** see Montelukast on page 1310
◆ **MoreDophilus® [OTC]** see Lactobacillus on page 1084

Morphine (Systemic) (MOR feen)

Related Information
Opioid Analgesics on page 2122
Patient Information for Disposal of Unused Medications on page 2244

Medication Safety Issues

Sound-alike/look-alike issues:
Morphine may be confused with HYDROmorphone, methadone
Morphine sulfate may be confused with magnesium sulfate
Kadian® may be confused with Kapidex [DSC]
MS Contin® may be confused with OxyCONTIN®
MSO_4 and MS are error-prone abbreviations (mistaken as magnesium sulfate)
AVINza® may be confused with Evista®, INVanz®
Roxanol may be confused with OxyFast®, Roxicet™, Roxicodone®

High alert medication:
The Institute for Safe Medication Practices (ISMP) includes this medication (I.V. formulation) among its list of drug classes which have a heightened risk of causing significant patient harm when used in error.

Other safety concerns:
Use care when prescribing and/or administering morphine solutions. These products are available in different concentrations. Always prescribe dosage in mg; **not** by volume (mL).
Use caution when selecting a morphine formulation for use in neurologic infusion pumps (eg, Medtronic delivery systems). The product should be appropriately labeled as "preservative-free" and suitable for intraspinal use via continuous infusion. In addition, the product should be formulated in a pH range that is compatible with the device operation specifications.
Significant differences exist between oral and I.V. dosing. Use caution when converting from one route of administration to another.

Brand Names: U.S. Astramorph®/PF; AVINza®; Duramorph; Infumorph 200; Infumorph 500; Kadian®; MS Contin®; Oramorph® SR

Brand Names: Canada Doloral; Kadian®; M-Eslon®; M.O.S.-SR®; M.O.S.-Sulfate®; M.O.S.® 10; M.O.S.® 20; M.O.S.® 30; Morphine Extra Forte Injection; Morphine Forte Injection; Morphine HP®; Morphine LP® Epidural; Morphine SR; Morphine-EPD; MS Contin SRT; MS Contin®; MS-IR®; Novo-Morphine SR; PMS-Morphine Sulfate SR; ratio-Morphine; ratio-Morphine SR; Sandoz-Morphine SR; Statex®; Teva-Morphine SR

Index Terms MS (error-prone abbreviation and should not be used); MSO_4 (error-prone abbreviation and should not be used); Roxanol

Generic Availability (U.S.) Yes: Excludes controlled release tablet, sustained release tablet

Pharmacologic Category Analgesic, Opioid

Use Relief of moderate-to-severe acute and chronic pain; relief of pain of myocardial infarction; relief of dyspnea of acute left ventricular failure and pulmonary edema; preanesthetic medication
Infumorph®: Used in continuous microinfusion devices for intrathecal or epidural administration in treatment of intractable chronic pain
Controlled, extended, or sustained release products: Only intended/indicated for use when repeated doses for an extended period of time are required. The 100 mg and 200 mg tablets or capsules of Kadian®, MS Contin®, and morphine sulfate controlled-release tablets and the 60 mg, 90 mg, and 120 mg capsules of Avinza® should only be used in opioid-tolerant patients.

Medication Guide Available Yes

Contraindications Note: Some contraindications are product specific. For details, please see detailed product prescribing information.

Hypersensitivity to morphine sulfate or any component of the formulation; severe respiratory depression (without resuscitative equipment); acute or severe asthma; known or suspected paralytic ileus; sustained release products are not recommended with gastrointestinal obstruction or in acute/postoperative pain. Oral solutions contraindicated in patients with heart failure due to chronic lung disease, cardiac arrhythmias, head injuries, brain tumors, acute alcoholism, deliriums tremens, seizure disorders, Injectable solution contraindicated during labor when a premature birth is anticipated. Some products contraindicated in patients with head injuries or increased intracranial pressure. MS Contin® and Kadian® contraindicated in patients with hypercarbia. Some immediate release formulations (tablets and solution) contraindicated in post biliary tract surgery, suspected surgical abdomen, surgical anastomosis, MAO inhibitor use (concurrent or within 14 days), general CNS depression.

Warnings/Precautions An opioid-containing analgesic regimen should be tailored to each patient's needs and based upon the type of pain being treated (acute versus chronic), the route of administration, degree of tolerance for opioids (naive versus chronic user), age, weight, and medical condition. The optimal analgesic dose varies widely among patients. Doses should be titrated to pain relief/prevention. When used as an epidural injection, monitor for delayed sedation. **[U.S. Boxed Warning]: Healthcare provider should be alert to problems of abuse, misuse, and diversion.**

May cause respiratory depression; use with caution in patients (particularly elderly or debilitated) with impaired respiratory function, morbid obesity, adrenal insufficiency, prostatic hyperplasia, urinary stricture, renal impairment, or severe hepatic dysfunction and in patients with hypersensitivity reactions to other phenanthrene derivative opioid agonists (codeine, hydrocodone, hydromorphone, levorphanol, oxycodone, oxymorphone). Use with caution in patients with biliary tract dysfunction; acute pancreatitis may cause constriction of sphincter of Oddi. Some preparations contain sulfites which may cause allergic reactions.

May cause CNS depression, which may impair physical or mental abilities; patients must be cautioned about performing tasks which require mental alertness (eg, operating machinery or driving). Effects may be potentiated when used with other sedative drugs or ethanol. May cause hypotension in patients with acute myocardial infarction, volume depletion, or concurrent drug therapy which may exaggerate vasodilation. Use with extreme caution in patients with head injury, intracranial lesions, or elevated intracranial pressure; exaggerated elevation of ICP may occur. May cause seizures if high doses are used; use with caution in patients with seizure disorders. Tolerance or drug dependence may result from extended use. Concurrent use of agonist/antagonist analgesics may precipitate withdrawal symptoms and/or reduced analgesic efficacy in patients following prolonged therapy with mu opioid agonists. Abrupt discontinuation following prolonged use may also lead to withdrawal symptoms. Elderly may be particularly susceptible to adverse effects of narcotics. May obscure diagnosis or clinical course of patients with acute abdominal conditions.

Extended or sustained-release formulations:

[U.S. Boxed Warning]: Extended or sustained release dosage forms should not be crushed or chewed. Controlled-, extended-, or sustained-release products are not intended for "as needed (PRN)" use. **MS Contin® 100 or 200 mg tablets and Kadian® 100 mg or 200 mg capsules are for use only in opioid-tolerant patients.** Avinza®, Kadian®, MS Contin®: **[U.S. Boxed Warning]: Indicated for the management of moderate-to-severe pain when around the clock pain control is needed for an extended time period.**

[U.S. Boxed Warning]: Avinza®: Do not administer with alcoholic beverages or ethanol-containing products, which may disrupt extended-release characteristic of product.

Highly concentrated oral solutions: [U.S. Boxed Warning]: Check doses carefully when using highly concentrated oral solutions.

Injections: Note: Products are designed for administration by specific routes (I.V., intrathecal, epidural). Use caution when prescribing, dispensing, or administering to use formulations only by intended route(s).

[U.S. Boxed Warning]: Duramorph®: Due to the risk of severe and/or sustained cardiopulmonary depressant effects of Duramorph® must be administered in a fully equipped and staffed environment. Naloxone injection should be immediately available. Patient should remain in this environment for at least 24 hours following the initial dose.

[U.S. Boxed Warning]: Intrathecal dosage is usually $^1/_{10}$ that of epidural dosage.

Infumorph® solutions are **for use in microinfusion devices only**; not for I.V., I.M., or SubQ administration, or for single-dose administration.

When used as an epidural injection, monitor for delayed sedation.

Adverse Reactions (Reflective of adult population; not specific for elderly) Note: Individual patient differences are unpredictable, and percentage may differ in acute pain (surgical) treatment. Reactions may be dose, formulation, and/or route dependent.

Frequency not defined:
   Cardiovascular: Circulatory depression, flushing, shock
   Central nervous system: Dysphonia, physical and psychological dependence, sedation
   Endocrine & metabolic: Antidiuretic hormone release, hypogonadism
   Neuromuscular & skeletal: Bone mineral density decreased

>10%:

Cardiovascular: Bradycardia, hypotension

Central nervous system: Drowsiness (9% to 48%; tolerance usually develops to drowsiness with regular dosing for 1-2 weeks), dizziness (6% to 20%), fever (<3% to >10%), confusion, headache (following epidural or intrathecal use)

Dermatologic: Pruritus (may be dose related)

Gastrointestinal: Xerostomia (78%), constipation (9% to 40%; tolerance develops very slowly if at all), nausea (7% to 28%; tolerance usually develops to nausea and vomiting with chronic use), vomiting

Genitourinary: Urinary retention (16%; may be prolonged, up to 20 hours, following epidural or intrathecal use)

Hematologic: Anemia (following intrathecal use)

Local: Pain at injection site

Neuromuscular & skeletal: Weakness

Respiratory: Oxygen saturation decreased

Miscellaneous: Histamine release

1% to 10%:

Cardiovascular: Atrial fibrillation (<3%), chest pain (<3%), edema, hypertension, palpitation, peripheral edema, syncope, tachycardia, vasodilation

Central nervous system: Amnesia, agitation, anxiety, apathy, apprehension, ataxia, chills, coma, delirium, depression, dream abnormalities, euphoria, false sense of well being, hallucination, hypoesthesia, insomnia, lethargy, malaise, nervousness, restlessness, seizure, slurred speech, somnolence, vertigo

Dermatologic: Dry skin, rash, urticaria

Endocrine & metabolic: Gynecomastia (<3%), hypokalemia, hyponatremia, libido decreased

Gastrointestinal: Abdominal distension, abdominal pain, anorexia, biliary colic, diarrhea, dyspepsia, dysphagia, flatulence, gastroenteritis, GERD, GI irritation, paralytic ileus, rectal disorder, taste perversion, weight loss

Genitourinary: Bladder spasm, dysuria, ejaculation abnormal, impotence, urination decreased

Hematologic: Leukopenia (<3%), thrombocytopenia (<3%), hematocrit decreased

Hepatic: Liver function tests increased

Neuromuscular & skeletal: Arthralgia, back pain, bone pain, foot drop, gait abnormalities, paresthesia, rigors, skeletal muscle rigidity, tremor

Ocular: Amblyopia, conjunctivitis, eye pain, vision problems/disturbance

Renal: Oliguria

Respiratory: Asthma, atelectasis, dyspnea, hiccups, hypercapnia, hypoxia, pulmonary edema (noncardiogenic), respiratory depression, rhinitis

Miscellaneous: Diaphoresis, flu-like syndrome, infection, thirst, voice alteration, withdrawal syndrome

Drug Interactions

Metabolism/Transport Effects Substrate of CYP2D6 (minor); **Note:** Assignment of Major/Minor substrate status based on clinically relevant drug interaction potential

Avoid Concomitant Use

Avoid concomitant use of Morphine (Systemic) with any of the following: Azelastine; Azelastine (Nasal); Methadone; Mirtazapine; Paraldehyde

Increased Effect/Toxicity

Morphine (Systemic) may increase the levels/effects of: Alcohol (Ethyl); Alvimopan; Azelastine; Azelastine (Nasal); CNS Depressants; Desmopressin; Methadone; Metyrosine; Mirtazapine; Paraldehyde; Selective Serotonin Reuptake Inhibitors; Thiazide Diuretics; Zolpidem

The levels/effects of Morphine (Systemic) may be increased by: Amphetamines; Antipsychotic Agents (Phenothiazines); Droperidol; HydrOXYzine; Succinylcholine

Decreased Effect

Morphine (Systemic) may decrease the levels/effects of: Pegvisomant

The levels/effects of Morphine (Systemic) may be decreased by: Ammonium Chloride; Mixed Agonist / Antagonist Opioids; Peginterferon Alfa-2b; Rifamycin Derivatives

Ethanol/Nutrition/Herb Interactions

Ethanol: Alcoholic beverages or ethanol-containing products may disrupt extended-release formulation resulting in rapid release of entire morphine dose. Ethanol may also increase CNS depression. Management: Avoid alcohol.

Food: Administration of oral morphine solution with food may increase bioavailability (ie, a report of 34% increase in morphine AUC when morphine oral solution followed a high-fat meal). The bioavailability of Avinza®, Oramorph SR®, or Kadian® does not appear to be affected by food. Management: Take consistently with or without meals.

Herb/Nutraceutical: Gotu kola, valerian, and kava kava may increase CNS depression. Management: Avoid gotu kola, valerian, and kava kava.

Stability

Capsule, sustained release (Avinza®, Kadian®): Store at 25°C (77°F); excursions permitted to 15°C to 30°C (59°F to 86°F). Protect from light and moisture.

Injection: Store at controlled room temperature of 20°C to 25°C (68°F to 77°F); do not freeze. Protect from light. Degradation depends on pH and presence of oxygen; relatively stable in pH ≤4; darkening of solutions indicate degradation. Usual concentration for continuous I.V. infusion: 0.1-1 mg/mL in D_5W.

Oral solution: Store at controlled room temperature of 25°C (68°F to 77°F); do not freeze.

Suppositories: Store at controlled room temperature 25°C (77°F). Protect from light.

Tablet, extended release: Store at controlled room temperature of 25°C (77°F).

Tablet, immediate release: Store at controlled room temperature of 25°C (77°F). Protect from moisture.

Mechanism of Action Binds to opiate receptors in the CNS, causing inhibition of ascending pain pathways, altering the perception of and response to pain; produces generalized CNS depression

Pharmacodynamics/Kinetics

Onset of action (patient dependent; dosing must be individualized): Oral (immediate release): ~30 minutes; I.V.: 5-10 minutes

Duration (patient dependent; dosing must be individualized): Pain relief:
  Immediate release formulations: 4 hours
  Extended release capsule and tablet: 8-24 hours (formulation dependent)

Absorption: Variable

Distribution: V_d: 3-4 L/kg; binds to opioid receptors in the CNS and periphery (eg, GI tract)

Protein binding: 30% to 35%

Metabolism: Hepatic via conjugation with glucuronic acid primarily to morphine-6-glucuronide (active analgesic) morphine-3-glucuronide (inactive as analgesic); minor metabolites include morphine-3-6-diglucuronide; other minor metabolites include normorphine (active) and morphine 3-ethereal sulfate

Bioavailability: Oral: 17% to 33% (first-pass effect limits oral bioavailability; oral:parenteral effectiveness reportedly varies from 1:6 in opioid naive patients to 1:3 with chronic use)

Half-life elimination: Adults: 2-4 hours (immediate release forms)

Time to peak, plasma: Avinza®: 30 minutes (maintained for 24 hours); Kadian®: ~10 hours; Oramorph® SR: ~4 hours

Excretion: Urine (primarily as morphine-3-glucuronide, ~2% to 12% excreted unchanged); feces (~7% to 10%). It has been suggested that accumulation of morphine-6-glucuronide might cause toxicity with renal insufficiency. All of the metabolites (ie, morphine-3-glucuronide, morphine-6-glucuronide, and normorphine) have been suggested as possible causes of neurotoxicity (eg, myoclonus).

Dosage

Geriatric Refer to adult dosing. Use with caution; may require reduced dosage in the elderly and debilitated patients.

Adult These are guidelines and do not represent the doses that may be required in all patients. Doses and dosage intervals should be titrated to pain relief/prevention.

Acute pain (moderate-to-severe):

Oral (immediate release formulations): Opiate-naive: Initial: 10 mg every 4 hours as needed; patients with prior opiate exposure may require higher initial doses: usual dosage range: 10-30 mg every 4 hours as needed

I.M., SubQ: **Note:** Repeated SubQ administration causes local tissue irritation, pain, and induration.
  Initial: Opiate-naive: 5-10 mg every 4 hours as needed; patients with prior opiate exposure may require higher initial doses; usual dosage range: 5-20 mg every 4 hours as needed

Rectal: 10-20 mg every 3-4 hours

I.V.: Initial: Opiate-naive: 2.5-5 mg every 3-4 hours; patients with prior opiate exposure may require higher initial doses. **Note:** Repeated doses (up to every 5 minutes if needed) in small increments (eg, 1-4 mg) may be preferred to larger and less frequent doses.
  Acute myocardial infarction, analgesia (ACC/AHA 2004 Guidelines): Initial management: 2-4 mg, give 2-8 mg every 5-15 minutes as needed
  Critically-ill patients (unlabeled dose): 0.7-10 mg (based on 70 kg patient) **or** 0.01-0.15 mg/kg every 1-2 hours as needed. **Note:** More frequent dosing may be needed (eg, mechanically-ventilated patients).

I.V., SubQ continuous infusion: 0.8-10 mg/hour; usual range: Up to 80 mg/hour
  Continuous infusion: Usual dosage range: 5-35 mg/hour (based on 70 kg patient) **or** 0.07-0.5 mg/kg/hour

Patient-controlled analgesia (PCA): (Opiate-naive: Consider lower end of dosing range):
Usual concentration: 1 mg/mL
Demand dose: Usual: 1 mg; range: 0.5-2.5 mg
Lockout interval: 5-10 minutes

Intrathecal (I.T.): **Note: Must be preservative-free.** Administer with extreme caution and in reduced dosage to geriatric or debilitated patients. I.T. dose is usually $^1/_{10}$ that of epidural dosage.

Opioid-naive: 0.2-1 mg/dose (may provide adequate relief for up to 24 hours); repeat doses are **not** recommended. **Note:** The American Pain Society recommends 0.1-0.3 mg/dose; adjust dose for age, injection site, and patient's medical condition and degree of opioid tolerance.
Continuous microinfusion (Infumorph®): Initial: 0.2-1 mg/day

Opioid-tolerant: 1-10 mg/day
Continuous microinfusion (Infumorph®): Initial: 1-10 mg/day, titrate to effect; usual maximum is ~20 mg/day

Epidural: Pain management: **Note: Must be preservative-free.** Administer with extreme caution and in reduced dosage to geriatric or debilitated patients. Vigilant monitoring is particularly important in these patients.

Single-dose (Astromorph/PF™, Duramorph®): Initial: 5 mg, if pain relief not achieved in 1 hour, careful administration of 1-2 mg at intervals sufficient to assess effectiveness may be given; maximum: 10 mg/24 hours (single doses may provide adequate relief for up to 24 hours)
Infusion: Bolus dose: 1-6 mg; infusion rate: 0.1-0.2 mg/hour; maximum dose: 10 mg/24 hours.
Note: The American Pain Society recommends 1-6 mg/dose as a single dose or an infusion of 0.1-1 mg/hour; adjust dose for age, injection site, and patient's medical condition and degree of opioid tolerance.
Continuous microinfusion (Infumorph®):
Opioid-naive: Initial: 0.2-1 mg/day
Opioid-tolerant: Initial: 1-10 mg/day, titrate to effect; usual maximum is ~20 mg/day

Chronic pain: Note: Patients taking opioids chronically may become tolerant and require doses higher than the usual dosage range to maintain the desired effect. Tolerance can be managed by appropriate dose titration. There is no optimal or maximal dose for morphine in chronic pain. The appropriate dose is one that relieves pain throughout its dosing interval without causing unmanageable side effects.

Oral: Controlled-, extended-, or sustained-release formulations: A patient's morphine requirement should be established using prompt-release formulations. Conversion to long-acting products may be considered when chronic, continuous treatment is required. Higher dosages should be reserved for use only in opioid-tolerant patients.

Capsules, extended release (Avinza®): Daily dose administered once daily (for best results, administer at same time each day)
Capsules, sustained release (Kadian®): Daily dose administered once daily or in 2 divided doses daily (every 12 hours)
Tablets, controlled release (MS Contin®), sustained release (Oramorph SR®), or extended release: Daily dose divided and administered every 8 or every 12 hours

Renal Impairment
Cl_{cr} 10-50 mL/minute: Administer at 75% of normal dose
Cl_{cr} <10 mL/minute: Administer at 50% of normal dose
Intermittent HD: Adults: No dosage adjustment necessary
CRRT: Administer 75% of normal dose, titrate

Hepatic Impairment Unchanged in mild liver disease; substantial extrahepatic metabolism may occur. Excessive sedation may occur in cirrhosis.

Administration
Oral: Do not crush controlled release drug product, swallow whole. Kadian® and Avinza® can be opened and sprinkled on applesauce; do not crush or chew the beads. Contents of Kadian® capsules may be opened and sprinkled over 10 mL water and flushed through prewetted 16F gastrostomy tube; do not administer Kadian® through nasogastric tube.
I.V.: When giving morphine I.V. push, it is best to first dilute with sterile water or NS for a final concentration of 1-2 mg/mL and then administer slowly.
Epidural: Use preservative-free solutions for intrathecal or epidural use.

Monitoring Parameters Pain relief, respiratory and mental status, blood pressure
Astromorph/PF™, Duramorph®, Infumorph®: Patients should be observed in a fully-equipped and staffed environment for at least 24 hours following initiation, and as appropriate for the first several days after catheter implantation.

Test Interactions Some quinolones may produce a false-positive urine screening result for opiates using commercially-available immunoassay kits. This has been demonstrated most consistently for levofloxacin and ofloxacin, but other quinolones have shown cross-reactivity in certain assay kits. Confirmation of positive opiate screens by more specific methods should be considered.

Special Geriatric Considerations The elderly may be particularly susceptible to the CNS depressant and constipating effects of narcotics. For chronic administration of narcotic analgesics, morphine is preferable in the elderly due to its pharmacokinetics and side effect profile as compared to meperidine and methadone.

Controlled Substance C-II

Dosage Forms Excipient information presented when available (limited, particularly for generics); consult specific product labeling.

Capsule, extended release, oral, as sulfate: 10 mg, 20 mg, 30 mg, 50 mg, 60 mg, 80 mg, 100 mg, 200 mg

AVINza®: 30 mg, 45 mg, 60 mg, 75 mg, 90 mg, 120 mg

Kadian®: 10 mg, 20 mg, 30 mg, 50 mg, 60 mg, 80 mg, 100 mg, 200 mg

Injection, solution, as sulfate: 1 mg/mL (10 mL); 2 mg/mL (1 mL); 4 mg/mL (1 mL); 5 mg/mL (1 mL); 8 mg/mL (1 mL); 10 mg/mL (1 mL, 10 mL); 10 mg/0.7 mL (0.7 mL); 15 mg/mL (1 mL, 20 mL); 25 mg/mL (4 mL, 10 mL); 50 mg/mL (20 mL, 50 mL)

Injection, solution, as sulfate [preservative free]: 0.5 mg/mL (10 mL); 1 mg/mL (10 mL); 25 mg/mL (10 mL)

Injection, solution, as sulfate [epidural or intrathecal infusion via microinfusion device, preservative free]:

Infumorph 200: 10 mg/mL (20 mL)

Infumorph 500: 25 mg/mL (20 mL)

Injection, solution, as sulfate [epidural, intrathecal, or I.V. infusion, preservative free]:

Astramorph®/PF: 0.5 mg/mL (2 mL, 10 mL); 1 mg/mL (2 mL, 10 mL)

Duramorph: 0.5 mg/mL (10 mL); 1 mg/mL (10 mL)

Injection, solution, as sulfate [for PCA pump]: 1 mg/mL (30 mL)

Injection, solution, as sulfate [for PCA pump, preservative free]: 1 mg/mL (30 mL); 5 mg/mL (30 mL)

Solution, oral, as sulfate: 10 mg/5 mL (5 mL, 100 mL, 500 mL); 20 mg/5 mL (100 mL, 500 mL)

Solution, oral, as sulfate [concentrate]: 100 mg/5 mL (15 mL, 30 mL, 120 mL, 240 mL)

Suppository, rectal, as sulfate: 5 mg (12s); 10 mg (12s); 20 mg (12s); 30 mg (12s)

Tablet, oral, as sulfate: 15 mg, 30 mg

Tablet, controlled release, oral, as sulfate:

MS Contin®: 15 mg, 30 mg, 60 mg, 100 mg, 200 mg

Tablet, extended release, oral, as sulfate: 15 mg, 30 mg, 60 mg, 100 mg, 200 mg

Tablet, sustained release, oral, as sulfate:

Oramorph® SR: 15 mg, 30 mg, 60 mg, 100 mg

Dosage Forms: Canada Excipient information presented when available (limited, particularly for generics); consult specific product labeling.

Solution, oral, as sulfate:

Doloral: 1 mg/mL (10 mL, 250 mL, 500 mL); 5 mg/mL (10 mL, 250 mL, 500 mL)

Morphine (Liposomal) (MOR feen)

Related Information

Opioid Analgesics *on page 2122*

Medication Safety Issues

Sound-alike/look-alike issues:

Morphine may be confused with HYDROmorphone

Morphine sulfate may be confused with magnesium sulfate

MSO$_4$ and MS are error-prone abbreviations (mistaken as magnesium sulfate)

High alert medication:

The Institute for Safe Medication Practices (ISMP) includes this medication among its list of drug classes which have a heightened risk of causing significant patient harm when used in error.

Brand Names: U.S. DepoDur®

Index Terms Extended Release Epidural Morphine; MS (error-prone abbreviation and should not be used); MSO$_4$ (error-prone abbreviation and should not be used)

Generic Availability (U.S.) No

Pharmacologic Category Analgesic, Opioid

Use Epidural (lumbar) single-dose management of surgical pain

Contraindications Hypersensitivity to morphine sulfate or any component of the formulation; severe respiratory depression (without resuscitative equipment); acute or severe asthma; known or suspected paralytic ileus; patients with head injuries or increased intracranial pressure; circulatory shock; upper airway obstruction.

Warnings/Precautions May cause respiratory depression. Risk increased in elderly patients, debilitated patients, and patients with conditions associated with hypoxia or hypercapnia. Prolonged, serious respiratory depression has been associated with nonapproved routes of administration (subarachnoid puncture and intrathecal). Although respiratory depression is reversible with naloxone, patients must be monitored for at least 48 hours due to the duration of action of the liposomal formulation and the potential for rebound sedation. Use with caution in patients with pre-existing respiratory compromise (hypoxia and/or hypercapnia), COPD or other obstructive pulmonary disease, and kyphoscoliosis or other skeletal disorder which may alter respiratory function.

May cause CNS depression and/or hypotension; use with caution in patients with hypovolemia, cardiovascular disease (including acute MI), circulatory shock, or drugs which may exaggerate hypotensive effects (including phenothiazines or general anesthetics). Use with caution in patients with CNS depression or coma. May cause orthostatic hypotension and syncope in ambulatory patients.

Use with caution in patients with hypersensitivity reactions to other phenanthrene derivative opioid agonists (codeine, hydrocodone, hydromorphone, levorphanol, oxycodone, oxymorphone). Use with caution in patients with biliary tract dysfunction and acute pancreatitis. Use may cause constriction of sphincter of Oddi diminishing biliary and pancreatic secretions. May obscure diagnosis or clinical course of patients with acute abdominal conditions. May worsen gastrointestinal ileus due to the effects on GI motility. Use with caution in patients with adrenal insufficiency, including Addison's disease. Use with caution in patients with severe hepatic impairment, renal impairment, prostatic hyperplasia, and/or urinary stricture. Use with caution in patients with seizure disorders or thyroid disease.

Use with caution in the elderly; may be more sensitive to adverse effects.

For lumbar administration only. Monitor for delayed sedation. Physician should evaluate patient for contraindications for epidural injection (eg, anticoagulant therapy, bleeding, diathesis). Intrathecal administration has resulted in prolonged respiratory depression. Freezing may adversely affect modified-release mechanism of drug; check freeze indicator within carton prior to administration. To minimize the pharmacokinetic interaction resulting in higher peak serum concentrations of morphine, administer the test dose of the local anesthetic at least 15 minutes prior to administration. Use of DepoDur® with epidural local anesthetics has not been studied. Other medications should not be administered into the epidural space for at least 48 hours after administration.

Adverse Reactions (Reflective of adult population; not specific for elderly)
>10%:
Cardiovascular: Hypotension
Central nervous system: Dizziness, fever, headache
Dermatologic: Pruritus
Gastrointestinal: Constipation, nausea, vomiting
Genitourinary: Urinary retention (may be prolonged)
Hematologic: Anemia
Local: Pain at injection site
Neuromuscular & skeletal: Weakness
Respiratory: Oxygen saturation decreased
2% to 10%:
Cardiovascular: Bradycardia, hypertension, tachycardia
Central nervous system: Anxiety, insomnia, somnolence
Gastrointestinal: Abdominal distension, dyspepsia, flatulence, paralytic ileus
Genitourinary: Bladder spasm, oliguria
Hematologic: Hematocrit decreased
Neuromuscular & skeletal: Back pain, hypoesthesia, paresthesia, rigors
Respiratory: Dyspnea, hypercapnea, hypoxia, respiratory depression
Miscellaneous: Sweating increased

Drug Interactions
Metabolism/Transport Effects Substrate of CYP2D6 (minor); **Note:** Assignment of Major/Minor substrate status based on clinically relevant drug interaction potential
Avoid Concomitant Use
Avoid concomitant use of Morphine (Liposomal) with any of the following: Azelastine; Azelastine (Nasal); Methadone; Mirtazapine; Paraldehyde

Increased Effect/Toxicity

Morphine (Liposomal) may increase the levels/effects of: Alcohol (Ethyl); Alvimopan; Azelastine; Azelastine (Nasal); CNS Depressants; Desmopressin; Methadone; Metyrosine; Mirtazapine; Paraldehyde; Selective Serotonin Reuptake Inhibitors; Thiazide Diuretics; Zolpidem

The levels/effects of Morphine (Liposomal) may be increased by: Amphetamines; Antipsychotic Agents (Phenothiazines); Droperidol; HydrOXYzine; Succinylcholine

Decreased Effect

Morphine (Liposomal) may decrease the levels/effects of: Pegvisomant

The levels/effects of Morphine (Liposomal) may be decreased by: Ammonium Chloride; Mixed Agonist / Antagonist Opioids; Peginterferon Alfa-2b

Stability DepoDur®: Store under refrigeration at 2°C to 8°C (36°F to 46°F); keep vials in carton during refrigeration; do not freeze. Check freeze indicator before administration; do not administer if bulb is pink or purple. May store at room temperature for up to 30 days in sealed, unopened vials. DepoDur® may be diluted in preservative-free NS to a volume of 5 mL. Gently invert to suspend particles prior to removal from vial. Once vial is opened, use within 4 hours.

Mechanism of Action Binds to opiate receptors in the CNS, causing inhibition of ascending pain pathways, altering the perception of and response to pain; produces generalized CNS depression

Pharmacodynamics/Kinetics

Duration (patient dependent; dosing must be individualized): >48 hours

Distribution: V_d: 3-4 L/kg; binds to opioid receptors in the CNS and periphery (eg, GI tract)

Protein binding: 30% to 35%

Metabolism: Hepatic via conjugation with glucuronic acid primarily to morphine-6-glucuronide (active analgesic) morphine-3-glucuronide (inactive as analgesic); minor metabolites include morphine-3-6-diglucuronide; other minor metabolites include normorphine (active) and morphine 3-ethereal sulfate

Excretion: Urine (primarily as morphine-3-glucuronide, ~2% to 12% excreted unchanged); feces (~7% to 10%). It has been suggested that accumulation of morphine-6-glucuronide might cause toxicity with renal insufficiency. All of the metabolites (ie, morphine-3-glucuronide, morphine-6-glucuronide, and normorphine) have been suggested as possible causes of neurotoxicity (eg, myoclonus).

Dosage

Geriatric Refer to adult dosing. Use with caution; may require reduced dosage in the elderly and debilitated patients.

Adult Surgical anesthesia: Epidural: Single-dose (extended release, DepoDur®): Lumbar epidural only; not recommended in patients <18 years of age:

Cesarean section: 10 mg (after clamping umbilical cord)

Lower abdominal/pelvic surgery: 10-15 mg

Major orthopedic surgery of lower extremity: 15 mg; **Note:** Some patients may benefit from a 20 mg dose; however, the incidence of adverse effects may be increased.

To minimize the pharmacokinetic interaction resulting in higher peak serum concentrations of morphine, administer the test dose of the local anesthetic at least 15 minutes prior to administration. Use with epidural local anesthetics has not been studied. Other medications should not be administered into the epidural space for at least 48 hours after administration.

Renal Impairment Dosing adjustment is not required.

Hepatic Impairment Dosing adjustment is not required.

Administration Epidural: Intended for lumbar administration only. Thoracic administration has not been studied. May be administered undiluted or diluted up to 5 mL total volume in preservative-free NS. Do not use an in-line filter during administration. Not for I.V., I.M., or intrathecal administration.

Resedation may occur following epidural administration; this may be delayed ≥48 hours in patients receiving extended-release epidural injections.

Administration of an epidural test dose (lidocaine 1.5% and epinephrine 1:200,000) may affect the release of morphine from the liposomal preparation. Delaying the dose for an interval of at least 15 minutes following the test dose minimizes this pharmacokinetic interaction. Except for a test dose, other epidural local anesthetics or medications should not be administered epidurally before or after this product for a minimum of 48 hours.

Monitoring Parameters Pain relief, respiratory and mental status, blood pressure; patient should be monitored for at least 48 hours following administration.

Special Geriatric Considerations Elderly patients may be more sensitive to the adverse effects of opiates. In general, dosage should be on the lower end of the dosage range when administering opiates to elderly patients.

Controlled Substance C-II

◀ **Dosage Forms** Excipient information presented when available (limited, particularly for generics); consult specific product labeling.

Injection, extended release liposomal suspension, as sulfate [lumbar epidural injection, preservative free]:

DepoDur®: 10 mg/mL (1 mL, 1.5 mL)

♦ **Mosco® Callus & Corn Remover [OTC]** see Salicylic Acid on page 1743
♦ **Mosco® One Step Corn Remover [OTC]** see Salicylic Acid on page 1743
♦ **Motrin® Children's [OTC]** see Ibuprofen on page 966
♦ **Motrin® IB [OTC]** see Ibuprofen on page 966
♦ **Motrin® Infants' [OTC]** see Ibuprofen on page 966
♦ **Motrin® Junior [OTC]** see Ibuprofen on page 966
♦ **Mouth Kote® [OTC]** see Saliva Substitute on page 1748
♦ **Moxatag™** see Amoxicillin on page 112
♦ **Moxeza™** see Moxifloxacin (Ophthalmic) on page 1323

Moxifloxacin (Systemic) (moxs i FLOKS a sin)

Related Information
Antibiotic Treatment of Adults With Infective Endocarditis on page 2157
Antimicrobial Drugs of Choice on page 2163
Community-Acquired Pneumonia in Adults on page 2171

Medication Safety Issues
Sound-alike/look-alike issues:
Avelox® may be confused with Avonex®

Brand Names: U.S. Avelox®; Avelox® ABC Pack; Avelox® I.V.

Brand Names: Canada Avelox®; Avelox® I.V.

Index Terms Moxifloxacin Hydrochloride

Generic Availability (U.S.) No

Pharmacologic Category Antibiotic, Quinolone; Respiratory Fluoroquinolone

Use Treatment of mild-to-moderate community-acquired pneumonia, including multidrug-resistant *Streptococcus pneumoniae* (MDRSP); acute bacterial exacerbation of chronic bronchitis; acute bacterial rhinosinusitis (ABRS); complicated and uncomplicated skin and skin structure infections; complicated intra-abdominal infections

Unlabeled Use Treatment of *Legionella* pneumonia; treatment of mild-to-moderate community-acquired pneumonia (CAP), including multidrug-resistant *Streptococcus pneumoniae* (MDRSP); tuberculosis (second-line therapy)

Medication Guide Available Yes

Contraindications Hypersensitivity to moxifloxacin, other quinolone antibiotics, or any component of the formulation

Warnings/Precautions [U.S. Boxed Warning]: There have been reports of tendon inflammation and/or rupture with quinolone antibiotics; risk may be increased with concurrent corticosteroids, organ transplant recipients, and in patients >60 years of age. Rupture of the Achilles tendon sometimes requiring surgical repair has been reported most frequently; but other tendon sites (eg, rotator cuff, biceps) have also been reported. Strenuous physical activity, rheumatoid arthritis, and renal impairment may be an independent risk factor for tendonitis. Discontinue at first sign of tendon inflammation or pain. Tendon rupture may occur even after discontinuation of therapy. Use with caution in patients with rheumatoid arthritis or renal impairment; may increase risk of tendon rupture.

Use with caution in patients with significant bradycardia or acute myocardial ischemia. Moxifloxacin causes a concentration-dependent QT prolongation. Do not exceed recommended dose or infusion rate. Avoid use with uncorrected hypokalemia, with other drugs that prolong the QT interval or induce bradycardia, or with class Ia or III antiarrhythmic agents. CNS effects may occur (tremor, restlessness, confusion, and very rarely hallucinations, increased intracranial pressure [including pseudotumor cerebri] or seizures). Use with caution in patients with known or suspected CNS disorder. Potential for seizures, although very rare, may be increased with concomitant NSAID therapy. Use with caution in individuals at risk of seizures. Use with caution in patients with mild, moderate, or severe hepatic impairment or liver cirrhosis; may increase the risk of QT prolongation. Fulminant hepatitis potentially leading to liver failure (including fatalities) has been reported with use. Use with caution in diabetes; glucose regulation may be altered.

Fluoroquinolones have been associated with the development of serious, and sometimes fatal, hypoglycemia, most often in elderly diabetics, but also in patients without diabetes. This occurred most frequently with gatifloxacin (no longer available systemically) but may occur at a lower frequency with other quinolones.

Severe hypersensitivity reactions, including anaphylaxis, have occurred with quinolone therapy. Reactions may present as typical allergic symptoms after a single dose, or may manifest as severe idiosyncratic dermatologic, vascular, pulmonary, renal, hepatic, and/or hematologic events, usually after multiple doses. Prompt discontinuation of drug should occur if skin rash or other symptoms arise. Avoid excessive sunlight and take precautions to limit exposure (eg, loose fitting clothing, sunscreen); may cause moderate-to-severe phototoxicity reactions. Discontinue use if photosensitivity occurs. Prolonged use may result in fungal or bacterial superinfection, including *C. difficile*-associated diarrhea (CDAD) and pseudomembranous colitis; CDAD has been observed >2 months postantibiotic treatment. **[U.S. Boxed Warning]: Quinolones may exacerbate myasthenia gravis; avoid use (rare, potentially life-threatening weakness of respiratory muscles may occur).** Peripheral neuropathy may rarely occur. Hemolytic reactions may (rarely) occur with quinolone use in patients with latent or actual G6PD deficiency. Adverse effects (eg, tendon rupture, QT changes) may be increased in the elderly. Some quinolones may exacerbate myasthenia gravis, use with caution (rare, potentially life-threatening weakness of respiratory muscles may occur).

Adverse Reactions (Reflective of adult population; not specific for elderly)

2% to 10%:

Central nervous system: Dizziness (2%)

Endocrine & metabolic: Serum chloride increased (≥2%), serum ionized calcium increased (≥2%), serum glucose decreased (≥2%)

Gastrointestinal: Nausea (6%), diarrhea (5%), amylase decreased (≥2%)

Hematologic: Decreased serum levels of the following (≥2%): Basophils, eosinophils, hemoglobin, RBC, neutrophils; increased serum levels of the following (≥2%): MCH, neutrophils, WBC

Hepatic: Bilirubin decreased/increased (≥2%)

Renal: Serum albumin increased (≥2%)

Respiratory: PO_2 decreased (≥2%)

0.1% to <2%:

Cardiovascular: Cardiac arrhythmias, palpitation, QT_c prolongation, tachycardia, vasodilation

Central nervous system: Anxiety, headache, insomnia, malaise, nervousness, pain, somnolence, vertigo

Dermatologic: Pruritus, rash (maculopapular, purpuric, pustular), urticaria

Gastrointestinal: Abdominal pain, amylase increased, anorexia, constipation, dyspepsia, flatulence, glossitis, lactic dehydrogenase increased, stomatitis, taste perversion, vomiting, xerostomia

Genitourinary: Vaginal moniliasis, vaginitis

Hematologic: Eosinophilia, leukopenia, prothrombin time prolonged, increased INR, thrombocythemia

Hepatic: GGTP increased, liver function test abnormal

Local: Injection site reaction

Neuromuscular & skeletal: Arthralgia, myalgia, tremor, weakness

Respiratory: Pharyngitis, pneumonia, rhinitis, sinusitis

Miscellaneous: Allergic reaction, infection, diaphoresis, oral moniliasis

Drug Interactions

Metabolism/Transport Effects None known.

Avoid Concomitant Use

Avoid concomitant use of Moxifloxacin (Systemic) with any of the following: BCG; Highest Risk QTc-Prolonging Agents; Mifepristone

Increased Effect/Toxicity

Moxifloxacin (Systemic) may increase the levels/effects of: Corticosteroids (Systemic); Highest Risk QTc-Prolonging Agents; Moderate Risk QTc-Prolonging Agents; Porfimer; Sulfonylureas; Varenicline; Vitamin K Antagonists

The levels/effects of Moxifloxacin (Systemic) may be increased by: Insulin; Mifepristone; Nonsteroidal Anti-Inflammatory Agents; Probenecid; QTc-Prolonging Agents (Indeterminate Risk and Risk Modifying)

Decreased Effect

Moxifloxacin (Systemic) may decrease the levels/effects of: BCG; Mycophenolate; Sulfonylureas; Typhoid Vaccine

The levels/effects of Moxifloxacin (Systemic) may be decreased by: Antacids; Didanosine; Iron Salts; Lanthanum; Magnesium Salts; Quinapril; Sevelamer; Sucralfate; Zinc Salts

Ethanol/Nutrition/Herb Interactions Food: Absorption is not affected by administration with a high-fat meal or yogurt.

Stability Store at controlled room temperature of 25°C (77°F). Do not refrigerate infusion solution.

Mechanism of Action Moxifloxacin is a DNA gyrase inhibitor, and also inhibits topoisomerase IV. DNA gyrase (topoisomerase II) is an essential bacterial enzyme that maintains the superhelical structure of DNA. DNA gyrase is required for DNA replication and transcription, DNA repair, recombination, and transposition; inhibition is bactericidal.

Pharmacodynamics/Kinetics

Absorption: Well absorbed; not affected by high-fat meal or yogurt

Distribution: V_d: 1.7 to 2.7 L/kg; tissue concentrations often exceed plasma concentrations in respiratory tissues, alveolar macrophages, abdominal tissues/fluids, uterine tissue (endometrium, myometrium), and sinus tissues

Protein binding: ~30% to 50%

Metabolism: Hepatic (~52% of dose) via glucuronide (~14%) and sulfate (~38%) conjugation

Bioavailability: ~90%

Half-life elimination: Single dose: Oral: 12-16 hours; I.V.: 8-15 hours

Excretion: Urine (as unchanged drug [20%] and glucuronide conjugates); feces (as unchanged drug [25%] and sulfate conjugates)

Dosage

Geriatric & Adult

Acute bacterial rhinosinusitis: Oral, I.V.: 400 mg every 24 hours for 10 days or 5-7 days (Chow, 2012). **Note:** Recommended in patients with beta-lactam allergy; may also be used if initial therapy fails, in areas with high endemic rates of penicillin nonsusceptible *S. pneumoniae*, those with severe infections, age >65 years, recent hospitalization, antibiotic use within the past month, or who are immunocompromised.

Chronic bronchitis, acute bacterial exacerbation: Oral, I.V.: 400 mg every 24 hours for 5 days

Community-acquired pneumonia (CAP) (including MDRSP): Oral, I.V.: 400 mg every 24 hours for 7-14 days

Intra-abdominal infections, complicated: 400 mg every 24 hours for 5-14 days (initiate with I.V.); **Note:** 2010 IDSA guidelines recommend a treatment duration of 4-7 days (provided source controlled) for community-acquired, mild-to-moderate IAI

M. genitalium infections (including confirmed cases or clinically significant persistent cervicitis, pelvic inflammatory disease or urethritis in patients who previously received azithromycin or doxycycline; unlabeled use): Oral, I.V.: 400 mg every 24 hours for 7-10 days (Manhart, 2011)

Skin and skin structure infections: Oral, I.V.:
Complicated: 400 mg every 24 hours for 7-21 days
Uncomplicated: 400 mg every 24 hours for 7 days

Tuberculosis, drug-resistant tuberculosis, or intolerance to first-line agents (unlabeled use): Oral: 400 mg every 24 hours (*MMWR*, 2003)

Renal Impairment No dosage adjustment required in renal impairment.

Poorly dialyzed; no supplemental dose or dosage adjustment necessary, including patients on intermittent hemodialysis, peritoneal dialysis, or continuous renal replacement therapy (eg, CVVHD).

Hepatic Impairment No dosage adjustment is required in mild, moderate, or severe hepatic insufficiency (Child-Pugh class A, B, or C); however, use with caution in this patient population secondary to the risk of QT prolongation.

Administration Administer without regard to meals.

I.V.: Infuse over 60 minutes; do not infuse by rapid or bolus intravenous infusion

Monitoring Parameters WBC, signs of infection

Test Interactions Some quinolones may produce a false-positive urine screening result for opiates using commercially-available immunoassay kits. This has been demonstrated most consistently for levofloxacin and ofloxacin, but other quinolones have shown cross-reactivity in certain assay kits. Confirmation of positive opiate screens by more specific methods should be considered.

Special Geriatric Considerations The risk of torsade de pointes and tendon inflammation and/or rupture associated with the concomitant use of corticosteroids and quinolones is increased in the elderly population. See Warnings/Precautions regarding tendon rupture in patients >60 years of age. No dosage adjustments are required based on age.

Dosage Forms Excipient information presented when available (limited, particularly for generics); consult specific product labeling.

Infusion, premixed in sodium chloride 0.8% [preservative free]:
Avelox® I.V.: 400 mg (250 mL) [contains sodium ~787 mg (34.2 mEq)/250 mL]
Tablet, oral:
Avelox®: 400 mg
Avelox® ABC Pack: 400 mg

Moxifloxacin (Ophthalmic) (moxs i FLOKS a sin)

Medication Safety Issues
International issues:
Vigamox [U.S., Canada, and multiple international markets] may be confused with Fisamox brand name for amoxicillin [Australia]
Brand Names: U.S. Moxeza™; Vigamox®
Brand Names: Canada Vigamox®
Index Terms Moxifloxacin Hydrochloride
Generic Availability (U.S.) No
Pharmacologic Category Antibiotic, Ophthalmic; Antibiotic, Quinolone
Use Treatment of bacterial conjunctivitis caused by susceptible organisms
Dosage
Geriatric & Adult Bacterial conjunctivitis: Ophthalmic:
Moxeza™: Instill 1 drop into affected eye(s) 2 times/day for 7 days
Vigamox®: Instill 1 drop into affected eye(s) 3 times/day for 7 days
Special Geriatric Considerations Evaluate the patient's or caregiver's ability to safely administer the correct dose of ophthalmic medication.
Dosage Forms Excipient information presented when available (limited, particularly for generics); consult specific product labeling.
Solution, ophthalmic [drops]:
Moxeza™: 0.5% (3 mL)
Vigamox®: 0.5% (3 mL)

◆ **Moxifloxacin Hydrochloride** *see* Moxifloxacin (Ophthalmic) *on page 1323*
◆ **Moxifloxacin Hydrochloride** *see* Moxifloxacin (Systemic) *on page 1320*
◆ **MPA** *see* MedroxyPROGESTERone *on page 1190*
◆ **MPA and Estrogens (Conjugated)** *see* Estrogens (Conjugated/Equine) and Medroxyprogesterone *on page 711*
◆ **6-MP (error-prone abbreviation)** *see* Mercaptopurine *on page 1212*
◆ **MPSV** *see* Meningococcal Polysaccharide Vaccine (Groups A / C / Y and W-135) *on page 1206*
◆ **MPSV4** *see* Meningococcal Polysaccharide Vaccine (Groups A / C / Y and W-135) *on page 1206*
◆ **MRA** *see* Tocilizumab *on page 1918*
◆ **MS Contin®** *see* Morphine (Systemic) *on page 1312*
◆ **MS (error-prone abbreviation and should not be used)** *see* Morphine (Liposomal) *on page 1317*
◆ **MS (error-prone abbreviation and should not be used)** *see* Morphine (Systemic) *on page 1312*
◆ **MSO₄ (error-prone abbreviation and should not be used)** *see* Morphine (Liposomal) *on page 1317*
◆ **MSO₄ (error-prone abbreviation and should not be used)** *see* Morphine (Systemic) *on page 1312*
◆ **MTX (error-prone abbreviation)** *see* Methotrexate *on page 1236*
◆ **Mucinex® [OTC]** *see* GuaiFENesin *on page 904*
◆ **Mucinex® DM [OTC]** *see* Guaifenesin and Dextromethorphan *on page 906*
◆ **Mucinex® DM Maximum Strength [OTC]** *see* Guaifenesin and Dextromethorphan *on page 906*
◆ **Mucinex® Kid's [OTC]** *see* GuaiFENesin *on page 904*
◆ **Mucinex® Kid's Mini-Melts™ [OTC]** *see* GuaiFENesin *on page 904*
◆ **Mucinex® Kid's Cough [OTC]** *see* Guaifenesin and Dextromethorphan *on page 904*
◆ **Mucinex® Kid's Cough Mini-Melts™ [OTC]** *see* Guaifenesin and Dextromethorphan *on page 906*
◆ **Mucinex® Maximum Strength [OTC]** *see* GuaiFENesin *on page 904*

Mucosal Barrier Gel, Oral (myoo KOH sul BAR ee er GEL, OR al)

Brand Names: U.S. Gelclair®
Index Terms Mucosal Bioadherent Gel
Pharmacologic Category Gastrointestinal Agent, Miscellaneous
Use Management of oral mucosal pain caused by oral mucositis/stomatitis (resulting from chemotherapy or radiation therapy), irritation due to oral surgery, traumatic ulcers caused by braces/ill-fitting dentures or disease, diffuse aphthous ulcers (canker sores)

Dosage

Geriatric & Adult Mucosal protection: Oral: Gargle and spit the mixture of 1 single-use packet (15 mL) and water 3 times daily, or as needed. May be used undiluted if water is unavailable.

Special Geriatric Considerations No specific data for elderly patients available. No dosage adjustment necessary.

Dosage Forms Excipient information presented when available (limited, particularly for generics); consult specific product labeling.

Gel, oral [concentrate]:

Gelclair®: 15 mL/packet (15s) [contains benzalkonium chloride, castor oil, propylene glycol, sodium benzoate]

◆ **Mucosal Bioadherent Gel** *see* Mucosal Barrier Gel, Oral *on page 1323*
◆ **Mucus Relief [OTC] [DSC]** *see* GuaiFENesin *on page 904*
◆ **Multaq®** *see* Dronedarone *on page 612*
◆ **Mumps, Measles and Rubella Vaccines** *see* Measles, Mumps, and Rubella Virus Vaccine *on page 1184*

Mupirocin (myoo PEER oh sin)

Related Information

Pressure Ulcer Treatment *on page 2246*

Medication Safety Issues

Sound-alike/look-alike issues:

Bactroban® may be confused with bacitracin, baclofen, Bactrim™

Brand Names: U.S. Bactroban Cream®; Bactroban Nasal®; Bactroban®; Centany®; Centany® AT

Brand Names: Canada Bactroban®

Index Terms Mupirocin Calcium; Pseudomonic Acid A

Generic Availability (U.S.) Yes: Topical ointment

Pharmacologic Category Antibiotic, Topical

Use

Intranasal: Eradication of nasal colonization with MRSA in adult patients and healthcare workers

Topical: Treatment of impetigo or secondary infected traumatic skin lesions due to *S. aureus* and *S. pyogenes*

Unlabeled Use Intranasal: Surgical prophylaxis to prevent wound infections

Contraindications Hypersensitivity to mupirocin or any component of the formulation

Warnings/Precautions Potentially toxic amounts of polyethylene glycol contained in some topical products may be absorbed percutaneously in patients with extensive burns or open wounds; use caution with renal impairment. Prolonged use may result in over growth of nonsusceptible organisms. For external use only; avoid contact with eyes. Not for treatment of pressure sores. If skin irritation occurs, discontinue use.

Adverse Reactions (Reflective of adult population; not specific for elderly) Frequency not defined.

Central nervous system: Dizziness, headache

Dermatologic: Cellulitis, dermatitis, dry skin, erythema, hives, pruritus, rash

Gastrointestinal: Abdominal pain, diarrhea, nausea, taste perversion, ulcerative stomatitis, xerostomia

Local: Burning, edema, pain, stinging, tenderness

Ocular: Blepharitis

Otic: Ear pain

Respiratory: Cough, pharyngitis, rhinitis, upper respiratory tract congestion

Miscellaneous: Secondary wound infection

Drug Interactions

Metabolism/Transport Effects None known.

Avoid Concomitant Use

Avoid concomitant use of Mupirocin with any of the following: BCG

Increased Effect/Toxicity There are no known significant interactions involving an increase in effect.

Decreased Effect

Mupirocin may decrease the levels/effects of: BCG; Typhoid Vaccine

Mechanism of Action Binds to bacterial isoleucyl transfer-RNA synthetase resulting in the inhibition of protein synthesis

Pharmacodynamics/Kinetics

Absorption: Topical: Penetrates outer layers of skin; systemic absorption minimal through intact skin

Metabolism: Skin: 3% to monic acid (inactive)

Excretion: Urine

Dosage

Geriatric & Adult

Impetigo: Topical: Ointment: Apply to affected area 3 times/day; re-evaluate after 3-5 days if no clinical response

Secondary skin infections: Topical: Cream: Apply to affected area 3 times/day for 10 days; re-evaluate after 3-5 days if no clinical response

Elimination of MRSA colonization: Intranasal: Approximately one-half of the ointment from the single-use tube should be applied into one nostril and the other half into the other nostril twice daily for 5 days

Administration

Intranasal ointment: After application into nostrils, press sides of nose together and gently massage to spread ointment throughout the insides of the nostrils; discard tube after use

Topical cream, ointment: For external use only; area may be covered with gauze if desired

Monitoring Parameters If no clinical response in 3-5 days, re-evaluate use

Pharmacotherapy Pearls Contains polyethylene glycol vehicle

Special Geriatric Considerations Not for treatment of pressure sores.

Dosage Forms Excipient information presented when available (limited, particularly for generics); consult specific product labeling.

Cream, topical, as calcium [strength expressed as base]:

Bactroban Cream®: 2% (15 g, 30 g) [contains benzyl alcohol]

Ointment, topical: 2% (22 g)

Bactroban®: 2% (22 g) [contains polyethylene glycol]

Centany®: 2% (30 g)

Centany® AT: 2% (1s) [kit includes Centany® ointment (30 g),12 gauze pads, and 24 cloth tape strips]

Ointment, intranasal, as calcium [strength expressed as base]:

Bactroban Nasal®: 2% (1 g)

Nabumetone (na BYOO me tone)

Related Information
Beers Criteria – Potentially Inappropriate Medications for Geriatrics *on page 2183*

Medication Safety Issues
BEERS Criteria medication:
This drug may be potentially inappropriate for use in geriatric patients (Quality of evidence - moderate; Strength of recommendation - strong).

Brand Names: Canada Apo-Nabumetone®; Gen-Nabumetone; Mylan-Nabumetone; Novo-Nabumetone; Relafen®; Rhoxal-nabumetone; Sandoz-Nabumetone

Index Terms Relafen

Generic Availability (U.S.) Yes

Pharmacologic Category Nonsteroidal Anti-inflammatory Drug (NSAID), Oral

Use Management of osteoarthritis and rheumatoid arthritis

Unlabeled Use Moderate pain

Medication Guide Available Yes

Contraindications Hypersensitivity to nabumetone, aspirin, other NSAIDs, or any component of the formulation; perioperative pain in the setting of coronary artery bypass graft (CABG) surgery

Warnings/Precautions [U.S. Boxed Warning]: NSAIDs are associated with an increased risk of adverse cardiovascular thrombotic events, including MI and stroke. Risk may be increased with duration of use or pre-existing cardiovascular risk factors or disease. Carefully evaluate individual cardiovascular risk profiles prior to prescribing. May cause new-onset hypertension or worsening of existing hypertension. Use caution with fluid retention. Avoid use in heart failure. Concurrent administration of ibuprofen, and potentially other nonselective NSAIDs, may interfere with aspirin's cardioprotective effect. **[U.S. Boxed Warning]: Use is contraindicated for treatment of perioperative pain in the setting of coronary artery bypass graft (CABG) surgery.** Risk of MI and stroke may be increased with use following CABG surgery.

Platelet adhesion and aggregation may be decreased; may prolong bleeding time; patients with coagulation disorders or who are receiving anticoagulants should be monitored closely. Anemia may occur; patients on long-term NSAID therapy should be monitored for anemia. Rarely, NSAID use may cause severe blood dyscrasias (eg, agranulocytosis, aplastic anemia, thrombocytopenia).

NSAID use may compromise existing renal function; dose-dependent decreases in prostaglandin synthesis may result from NSAID use, reducing renal blood flow which may cause renal decompensation. NSAID use may increase the risk for hyperkalemia. Patients with impaired renal function, dehydration, heart failure, liver dysfunction, those taking diuretics, and ACE inhibitors, and the elderly are at greater risk of renal toxicity and hyperkalemia. Rehydrate patient before starting therapy; monitor renal function closely. Not recommended for use in patients with advanced renal disease. Long-term NSAID use may result in renal papillary necrosis.

[U.S. Boxed Warning]: NSAIDs may increase risk of gastrointestinal irritation, inflammation, ulceration, bleeding, and perforation. These events may occur at any time during therapy and without warning. Use caution with a history of GI disease (bleeding or ulcers), concurrent therapy with aspirin, anticoagulants and/or corticosteroids, smoking, use of alcohol, the elderly or debilitated patients. When used concomitantly with ≤325 mg of aspirin, a substantial increase in the risk of gastrointestinal complications (eg, ulcer) occurs; concomitant gastroprotective therapy (eg, proton pump inhibitors) is recommended (Bhatt, 2008).

Use the lowest effective dose for the shortest duration of time, consistent with individual patient goals, to reduce risk of cardiovascular or GI adverse events. Alternate therapies should be considered for patients at high risk.

NSAIDs may cause serious skin adverse events including exfoliative dermatitis, Stevens-Johnson syndrome (SJS) and toxic epidermal necrolysis (TEN); discontinue use at first sign of skin rash or hypersensitivity. Anaphylactoid reactions may occur, even without prior exposure; patients with "aspirin triad" (bronchial asthma, aspirin intolerance, rhinitis) may be at increased risk. Do not use in patients who experience bronchospasm, asthma, rhinitis, or urticaria with NSAID or aspirin therapy. Use caution in other forms of asthma.

Use with caution in patients with decreased hepatic function. Closely monitor patients with any abnormal LFT. Severe hepatic reactions (eg, fulminant hepatitis, liver failure) have occurred with NSAID use, rarely; discontinue if signs or symptoms of liver disease develop, or if systemic manifestations occur.

NSAIDS may cause drowsiness, dizziness, blurred vision and other neurologic effects which may impair physical or mental abilities; patients must be cautioned about performing tasks which require mental alertness (eg, operating machinery or driving). Discontinue use with blurred or diminished vision and perform ophthalmologic exam. Monitor vision with long-term therapy.

In the elderly, avoid chronic use (unless alternative agents ineffective and patient can receive concomitant gastroprotective agent); nonselective oral NSAID use is associated with an increased risk of GI bleeding and peptic ulcer disease in older adults in high risk category (eg, >75 years or age or receiving concomitant oral/parenteral corticosteroids, anticoagulants, or antiplatelet agents) (Beers Criteria).

Withhold for at least 4-6 half-lives prior to surgical or dental procedures. May cause photo-sensitivity reactions.

Adverse Reactions (Reflective of adult population; not specific for elderly)
>10%: Gastrointestinal: Diarrhea (14%), dyspepsia (13%), abdominal pain (12%)
1% to 10%:
  Cardiovascular: Edema (3% to 9%)
  Central nervous system: Dizziness (3% to 9%), headache (3% to 9%), fatigue (1% to 3%), insomnia (1% to 3%), nervousness (1% to 3%), somnolence (1% to 3%)
  Dermatologic: Pruritus (3% to 9%), rash (3% to 9%)
  Gastrointestinal: Constipation (3% to 9%), flatulence (3% to 9%), guaiac positive (3% to 9%), nausea (3% to 9%), gastritis (1% to 3%), stomatitis (1% to 3%), vomiting (1% to 3%), xerostomia (1% to 3%)
  Otic: Tinnitus
  Miscellaneous: Diaphoresis (1% to 3%)

Drug Interactions
Metabolism/Transport Effects None known.
Avoid Concomitant Use
Avoid concomitant use of Nabumetone with any of the following: Floctafenine; Ketorolac; Ketorolac (Nasal); Ketorolac (Systemic)
Increased Effect/Toxicity
Nabumetone may increase the levels/effects of: Aliskiren; Aminoglycosides; Anticoagulants; Antiplatelet Agents; Bisphosphonate Derivatives; Collagenase (Systemic); CycloSPORINE; CycloSPORINE (Systemic); Dabigatran Etexilate; Deferasirox; Desmopressin; Digoxin; Drotrecogin Alfa (Activated); Eplerenone; Haloperidol; Ibritumomab; Lithium; Methotrexate; Nonsteroidal Anti-Inflammatory Agents; PEMEtrexed; Porfimer; Potassium-Sparing Diuretics; PRALAtrexate; Quinolone Antibiotics; Rivaroxaban; Salicylates; Thrombolytic Agents; Tositumomab and Iodine I 131 Tositumomab; Vancomycin; Vitamin K Antagonists

The levels/effects of Nabumetone may be increased by: ACE Inhibitors; Angiotensin II Receptor Blockers; Antidepressants (Tricyclic, Tertiary Amine); Corticosteroids (Systemic); CycloSPORINE; CycloSPORINE (Systemic); Dasatinib; Floctafenine; Glucosamine; Herbs (Anticoagulant/Antiplatelet Properties); Ketorolac; Ketorolac (Nasal); Ketorolac (Systemic); Nonsteroidal Anti-Inflammatory Agents; Omega-3-Acid Ethyl Esters; Pentosan Polysulfate Sodium; Pentoxifylline; Probenecid; Prostacyclin Analogues; Selective Serotonin Reuptake Inhibitors; Serotonin/Norepinephrine Reuptake Inhibitors; Sodium Phosphates; Tipranavir; Treprostinil; Vitamin E
Decreased Effect
Nabumetone may decrease the levels/effects of: ACE Inhibitors; Aliskiren; Angiotensin II Receptor Blockers; Antiplatelet Agents; Beta-Blockers; Eplerenone; HydrALAZINE; Loop Diuretics; Potassium-Sparing Diuretics; Salicylates; Selective Serotonin Reuptake Inhibitors; Thiazide Diuretics

The levels/effects of Nabumetone may be decreased by: Bile Acid Sequestrants; Non-steroidal Anti-Inflammatory Agents; Salicylates

Ethanol/Nutrition/Herb Interactions
Ethanol: Avoid ethanol (may enhance gastric mucosal irritation).
Food: Nabumetone peak serum concentrations may be increased if taken with food or dairy products.
Herb/Nutraceutical: Avoid alfalfa, anise, bilberry, bladderwrack, bromelain, cat's claw, celery, chamomile, coleus, cordyceps, dong quai, evening primrose, fenugreek, feverfew, garlic, ginger, ginkgo biloba, ginseng (American, Panax, Siberian), grapeseed, green tea, guggul, horse chestnut seed, horseradish, licorice, prickly ash, red clover, reishi, SAMe (S-adenosylmethionine), sweet clover, turmeric, white willow (all have additional antiplatelet activity).

Mechanism of Action
Reversibly inhibits cyclooxygenase-1 and 2 (COX-1 and 2) enzymes, which results in decreased formation of prostaglandin precursors; has antipyretic, analgesic, and anti-inflammatory properties

Other proposed mechanisms not fully elucidated (and possibly contributing to the anti-inflammatory effect to varying degrees), include inhibiting chemotaxis, altering lymphocyte activity, inhibiting neutrophil aggregation/activation, and decreasing proinflammatory cytokine levels.

Pharmacodynamics/Kinetics
Onset of action: Several days
Distribution: Diffusion occurs readily into synovial fluid
V_d: 6MNA: 29-82 L
Protein binding: 6MNA: >99%
Metabolism: Prodrug, rapidly metabolized in the liver to an active metabolite [6-methoxy-2-naphthylacetic acid (6MNA)] and inactive metabolites; extensive first-pass effect
Half-life elimination: 6MNA: ~24 hours
Time to peak, serum: 6MNA: Oral: 2.5-4 hours; Synovial fluid: 4-12 hours
Excretion: 6MNA: Urine (80%) and feces (9%)

Dosage
Geriatric Refer to adult dosing; do not exceed 2000 mg/day.
Adult Osteoarthritis, rheumatoid arthritis: Oral: 1000 mg/day; an additional 500-1000 mg may be needed in some patients to obtain more symptomatic relief; may be administered once or twice daily; maximum dose: 2000 mg/day
Note: Patients <50 kg are less likely to require doses >1000 mg/day.
Renal Impairment In general, NSAIDs are not recommended for use in patients with advanced renal disease, but the manufacturer of nabumetone does provide some guidelines for adjustment in renal dysfunction:
Moderate impairment (Cl_{cr} 30-49 mL/minute): Initial dose: 750 mg/day; maximum dose: 1500 mg/day
Severe impairment (Cl_{cr} <30 mL/minute): Initial dose: 500 mg/day; maximum dose: 1000 mg/day

Monitoring Parameters Patients with renal insufficiency: Baseline renal function followed by repeat test within weeks (to determine if renal function has deteriorated)
Special Geriatric Considerations In trials with nabumetone, no significant differences were noted between young and the elderly in regards to efficacy and safety. However, the elderly are a high-risk population for adverse effects from NSAIDs. As much as 60% of elderly can develop peptic ulceration and/or hemorrhage asymptomatically. The concomitant use of H_2 blockers and sucralfate is not effective as prophylaxis with the exception of NSAID-induced duodenal ulcers which may be prevented by the use of ranitidine. Misoprostol and proton pump inhibitors are the only agents proven to help prevent the development of NSAID-induced ulcers. Also, concomitant disease and drug use contribute to the risk for GI adverse effects. Use lowest effective dose for shortest period possible. Consider renal function decline with age. Use of NSAIDs can compromise existing renal function especially when Cl_{cr} is ≤30 mL/minute. Tinnitus may be a difficult and unreliable indication of toxicity due to age-related hearing loss or eighth cranial nerve damage. CNS adverse effects such as confusion, agitation, and hallucination are generally seen in overdose or high dose situations, but the elderly may demonstrate these adverse effects at lower doses than younger adults.

This medication is considered to be potentially inappropriate in this patient population (Beers Criteria: Quality of evidence - moderate; Strength of recommendation - strong).
Dosage Forms Excipient information presented when available (limited, particularly for generics); consult specific product labeling.
Tablet, oral: 500 mg, 750 mg

♦ **N-Acetyl-P-Aminophenol** see Acetaminophen on page 31
♦ **NaCl** see Sodium Chloride on page 1787

Nadolol (NAY doe lol)

Related Information
Beta-Blockers on page 2108
Medication Safety Issues
Sound-alike/look-alike issues:
Corgard® may be confused with Cognex®, Coreg®
International issues:
Nadolol may be confused with Mandol brand name for cefamandole [Belgium, Netherlands, New Zealand, Russia]
Brand Names: U.S. Corgard®
Brand Names: Canada Alti-Nadolol; Apo-Nadol®; Corgard®; Novo-Nadolol; Teva-Nadolol
Generic Availability (U.S.) Yes
Pharmacologic Category Antianginal Agent; Beta-Blocker, Nonselective

Use Treatment of hypertension and angina pectoris; prophylaxis of migraine headaches

Unlabeled Use Primary and secondary prophylaxis of variceal hemorrhage; management of thyrotoxicosis

Contraindications Hypersensitivity to nadolol or any component of the formulation; bronchial asthma; sinus bradycardia; sinus node dysfunction; heart block greater than first degree (except in patients with a functioning artificial pacemaker); cardiogenic shock; uncompensated cardiac failure

Warnings/Precautions Consider pre-existing conditions such as sick sinus syndrome before initiating. Administer only with extreme caution in patients with compensated heart failure, monitor for a worsening of the condition. Efficacy in heart failure has not been established for nadolol. **[U.S. Boxed Warning]: Beta-blocker therapy should not be withdrawn abruptly (particularly in patients with CAD), but gradually tapered to avoid acute tachycardia, hypertension, and/or ischemia.** Chronic beta-blocker therapy should not be routinely withdrawn prior to major surgery. Use with caution in patients on concurrent digoxin, verapamil or diltiazem; bradycardia or heart block can occur. Use with caution in patients receiving inhaled anesthetic agents known to depress myocardial contractility. In general, patients with bronchospastic disease should not receive beta-blockers. Nadolol, if used at all, should be used cautiously in bronchospastic disease with close monitoring. Use cautiously in diabetics because it can mask prominent hypoglycemic symptoms. May mask signs of hyperthyroidism (eg, tachycardia); if hyperthyroidism is suspected, carefully manage and monitor; abrupt withdrawal may exacerbate symptoms of hyperthyroidism or precipitate thyroid storm. Use cautiously in the renally impaired (dosage adjustments are required). Use with caution in patients with myasthenia gravis, peripheral vascular disease, or psychiatric disease (may cause CNS depression). Bradycardia may be observed more frequently in elderly patients (>65 years of age); dosage reductions may be necessary. Adequate alpha-blockade is required prior to use of any beta-blocker for patients with untreated pheochromocytoma. May induce or exacerbate psoriasis. Use caution with history of severe anaphylaxis to allergens; patients taking beta-blockers may become more sensitive to repeated challenges. Treatment of anaphylaxis (eg, epinephrine) in patients taking beta-blockers may be ineffective or promote undesirable effects.

Adverse Reactions (Reflective of adult population; not specific for elderly)
>10%:
Central nervous system: Drowsiness, insomnia
Endocrine & metabolic: Decreased sexual ability
1% to 10%:
Cardiovascular: Bradycardia, palpitation, edema, CHF, reduced peripheral circulation
Central nervous system: Mental depression
Gastrointestinal: Diarrhea or constipation, nausea, vomiting, stomach discomfort
Respiratory: Bronchospasm
Miscellaneous: Cold extremities

Drug Interactions

Metabolism/Transport Effects Substrate of P-glycoprotein

Avoid Concomitant Use
Avoid concomitant use of Nadolol with any of the following: Beta2-Agonists; Floctafenine; Methacholine

Increased Effect/Toxicity
Nadolol may increase the levels/effects of: Alpha-/Beta-Agonists (Direct-Acting); Alpha1-Blockers; Alpha2-Agonists; Amifostine; Antihypertensives; Bupivacaine; Cardiac Glycosides; Cholinergic Agonists; Fingolimod; Hypotensive Agents; Insulin; Lidocaine; Lidocaine (Systemic); Lidocaine (Topical); Mepivacaine; Methacholine; Midodrine; RiTUXimab; Sulfonylureas

The levels/effects of Nadolol may be increased by: Acetylcholinesterase Inhibitors; Amiodarone; Anilidopiperidine Opioids; Calcium Channel Blockers (Dihydropyridine); Calcium Channel Blockers (Nondihydropyridine); Diazoxide; Dipyridamole; Disopyramide; Dronedarone; Floctafenine; Herbs (Hypotensive Properties); MAO Inhibitors; Pentoxifylline; P-glycoprotein/ABCB1 Inhibitors; Phosphodiesterase 5 Inhibitors; Prostacyclin Analogues; Reserpine

Decreased Effect
Nadolol may decrease the levels/effects of: Beta2-Agonists; Theophylline Derivatives

The levels/effects of Nadolol may be decreased by: Herbs (Hypertensive Properties); Methylphenidate; Nonsteroidal Anti-Inflammatory Agents; P-glycoprotein/ABCB1 Inducers; Yohimbine

Ethanol/Nutrition/Herb Interactions Herb/Nutraceutical: Avoid dong quai if using for hypertension (has estrogenic activity). Avoid ephedra, garlic, yohimbe, ginseng (may worsen hypertension). Avoid natural licorice (causes sodium and water retention and increases potassium loss).

NADOLOL

Mechanism of Action Competitively blocks response to beta$_1$- and beta$_2$-adrenergic stimulation; does not exhibit any membrane stabilizing or intrinsic sympathomimetic activity. Nonselective beta-adrenergic blockers (propranolol, nadolol) reduce portal pressure by producing splanchnic vasoconstriction (beta$_2$ effect) thereby reducing portal blood flow.

Pharmacodynamics/Kinetics

Duration: 17-24 hours

Absorption: 30% to 40%

Distribution: V_d: 1.9 L/kg

Protein binding: 30%

Metabolism: Not metabolized

Half-life elimination: Adults: 10-24 hours; prolonged with renal impairment; End-stage renal disease: 45 hours

Time to peak, serum: 2-4 hours

Excretion: Urine (as unchanged drug)

Dosage

Geriatric Refer to adult dosing. In the management of hypertension, consider lower initial doses (eg, 20 mg/day) and titrate to response (Aronow, 2011).

Adult

Angina: Oral: Initial: 40 mg/day, increase dosage gradually by 40-80 mg increments at 3- to 7-day intervals until optimum clinical response is obtained with profound slowing of heart rate; doses up to 160-240 mg/day in angina

Hypertension: Oral: Initial: 40 mg/day, increase dosage gradually by 40-80 mg increments until optimum blood pressure reduction achieved. Usual dosage range (JNC 7): 40-120 mg once daily; doses up to 240-320 mg/day in hypertension may be necessary

Variceal hemorrhage prophylaxis (unlabeled use) (Garcia-Tsao, 2007): Oral:

Primary prophylaxis: Initial: 40 mg once daily; adjust to maximal tolerated dose. **Note:** Risk factors for hemorrhage include Child-Pugh class B/C or variceal red wale markings on endoscopy.

Secondary prophylaxis: Initial: 40 mg once daily; adjust to maximal tolerated dose

Thyrotoxicosis (unlabeled use): Oral: 40-160 mg once daily (Bahn, 2011)

Renal Impairment

Cl_{cr} >50 mL/minute/1.73 m^2: Administer every 24 hours

Cl_{cr} 31-50 mL/minute/1.73 m^2: Administer every 24-36 hours

Cl_{cr} 10-30 mL/minute/1.73 m^2: Administer every 24-48 hours

Cl_{cr} <10 mL/minute/1.73 m^2: Administer every 40-60 hours

Dosage adjustments for dialysis are not provided in the manufacturer's labeling; however, the following guidelines have been used by some clinicians (Aronoff, 2007):

ESRD requiring hemodialysis: Administer dose postdialysis.

Peritoneal dialysis: Supplemental dose is not necessary.

Hepatic Impairment There are no dosage adjustments provided in the manufacturer's labeling.

Administration May be administered without regard to meals.

Special Geriatric Considerations Due to alterations in the beta-adrenergic autonomic nervous system, beta-adrenergic blockade may result in less hemodynamic response than seen in younger adults. Studies indicate that despite decreased sensitivity to the chronotropic effects of beta-blockade with age, there appears to be an increased myocardial sensitivity to the negative inotropic effect during stress (ie, exercise). Controlled trials have shown the overall response rate for propranolol to be only 20% to 50% in elderly populations. Therefore, all beta-adrenergic blocking drugs may result in a decreased response as compared to younger adults. Must adjust dose for renal function.

Dosage Forms Excipient information presented when available (limited, particularly for generics); consult specific product labeling.

Tablet, oral: 20 mg, 40 mg, 80 mg

Corgard®: 20 mg, 40 mg, 80 mg [scored]

Nafcillin (naf SIL in)

Related Information

Antibiotic Treatment of Adults With Infective Endocarditis *on page 2157*

Brand Names: Canada Nallpen®; Unipen®

Index Terms Ethoxynaphthamido Penicillin Sodium; Nafcillin Sodium; Nallpen; Sodium Nafcillin

Generic Availability (U.S.) Yes

Pharmacologic Category Antibiotic, Penicillin

Use Treatment of infections such as osteomyelitis, septicemia, endocarditis, and CNS infections caused by susceptible strains of staphylococci species

Contraindications Hypersensitivity to nafcillin, or any component of the formulation, or penicillins; premixed injection may contain corn-derived dextrose and its use is contraindicated in patients with allergy to corn-related products

Warnings/Precautions Serious and occasionally severe or fatal hypersensitivity (anaphylactoid) reactions have been reported in patients on penicillin therapy, especially with a history of beta-lactam hypersensitivity, history of sensitivity to multiple allergens, or previous IgE-mediated reactions (eg, anaphylaxis, angioedema, urticaria). Use with caution in asthmatic patients. Extravasation of I.V. infusions should be avoided. Modification of dosage is necessary in patients with both severe renal and hepatic impairment. Prolonged use may result in fungal or bacterial superinfection, including *C. difficile*-associated diarrhea (CDAD) and pseudomembranous colitis; CDAD has been observed >2 months postantibiotic treatment.

Adverse Reactions (Reflective of adult population; not specific for elderly) Frequency not defined.

Central nervous system: Neurotoxicity (high doses)

Gastrointestinal: Pseudomembranous colitis

Hematologic: Agranulocytosis, bone marrow depression, neutropenia

Local: Inflammation, pain, phlebitis, skin sloughing, swelling, and thrombophlebitis at the injection site; tissue necrosis with sloughing (SubQ extravasation)

Renal: Interstitial nephritis (rare), renal tubular damage (rare)

Miscellaneous: Anaphylaxis, hypersensitivity reactions (immediate and delayed; general incidence of 1% to 10% for penicillins), serum sickness

Drug Interactions

Metabolism/Transport Effects Induces CYP3A4 (strong)

Avoid Concomitant Use

Avoid concomitant use of Nafcillin with any of the following: Axitinib; BCG; Bortezomib; Crizotinib; Dienogest; Dronedarone; Everolimus; Itraconazole; Lapatinib; Lurasidone; Mifepristone; Nilotinib; Pazopanib; Praziquantel; Ranolazine; Rivaroxaban; Roflumilast; RomiDEPsin; SORAfenib; Ticagrelor; Tolvaptan; Toremifene; Vandetanib

Increased Effect/Toxicity

Nafcillin may increase the levels/effects of: Clarithromycin; Ifosfamide; Methotrexate; Vitamin K Antagonists

The levels/effects of Nafcillin may be increased by: Clarithromycin; Probenecid

Decreased Effect

Nafcillin may decrease the levels/effects of: Apixaban; ARIPiprazole; Axitinib; BCG; Boceprevir; Bortezomib; Brentuximab Vedotin; Calcium Channel Blockers; Clarithromycin; Contraceptives (Estrogens); Crizotinib; CycloSPORINE; CycloSPORINE (Systemic); CYP3A4 Substrates; Dasatinib; Dienogest; Dronedarone; Everolimus; Exemestane; Gefitinib; GuanFACINE; Imatinib; Itraconazole; Ixabepilone; Lapatinib; Linagliptin; Lurasidone; Maraviroc; Mifepristone; Mycophenolate; Nilotinib; Pazopanib; Praziquantel; Ranolazine; Rivaroxaban; Roflumilast; RomiDEPsin; Saxagliptin; SORAfenib; SUNItinib; Tadalafil; Ticagrelor; Tolvaptan; Toremifene; Typhoid Vaccine; Ulipristal; Vandetanib; Vemurafenib; Vitamin K Antagonists; Zuclopenthixol

The levels/effects of Nafcillin may be decreased by: Fusidic Acid; Tetracycline Derivatives

Stability

Premixed infusions: Store in a freezer at -20°C (4°F). Thaw at room temperature or under refrigeration only. Thawed bags are stable for 21 days under refrigeration or 72 hours at room temperature. Do not refreeze.

Vials: Reconstituted parenteral solution is stable for 3 days at room temperature and 7 days when refrigerated or 12 weeks when frozen. For I.V. infusion in NS or D$_5$W, solution is stable for 24 hours at room temperature and 96 hours when refrigerated.

Mechanism of Action Interferes with bacterial cell wall synthesis during active multiplication, causing cell wall death and resultant bactericidal activity against susceptible bacteria

Pharmacodynamics/Kinetics

Distribution: Widely distributed; CSF penetration is poor but enhanced by meningeal inflammation

Protein binding: ~90%; primarily to albumin

Metabolism: Primarily hepatic; undergoes enterohepatic recirculation

Half-life elimination: Normal renal/hepatic function: 30-60 minutes

Time to peak, serum: I.M.: 30-60 minutes

Excretion: Primarily feces; urine (10% to 30% as unchanged drug)

Dosage

Geriatric & Adult

Susceptible infections:

I.M.: 500 mg every 4-6 hours

I.V.: 500-2000 mg every 4-6 hours

Endocarditis: MSSA:
Native valve: I.V.: 12 g/24 hours in 4-6 divided doses for 6 weeks
Prosthetic valve: I.V.: 12 g/24 hours in 6 divided doses for ≥6 weeks (use with rifampin and gentamicin)
Joint:
Bursitis, septic: I.V.: 2 g every 4 hours
Prosthetic: I.V.: 2 g every 4-6 hours with rifampin for 6 weeks
***Staphylococcus aureus,* methicillin-susceptible infections, including brain abscess, empyema, erysipelas, mastitis, myositis, orbital cellulitis, osteomyelitis, pneumonia, splenic abscess, toxic shock, urinary tract (perinephric abscess):** I.V.: 2 g every 4 hours
Renal Impairment Not necessary unless renal impairment is in the setting of concomitant hepatic impairment.
Poorly dialyzed; no supplemental dose or dosage adjustment necessary, including patients on intermittent hemodialysis, peritoneal dialysis, or continuous renal replacement therapy (eg, CVVHD).
Hepatic Impairment In patients with both hepatic and renal impairment, modification of dosage may be necessary; no data available.
Administration Administer around-the-clock rather than 4 times/day, 3 times/day, etc (ie, 12-6-12-6, not 9-1-5-9) to promote less variation in peak and trough serum concentrations; burning on I.V. administration may be decreased by further diluting the preparation to 250 mL NS or D₅W
Monitoring Parameters Baseline and periodic CBC with differential; periodic urinalysis, BUN, serum creatinine, AST and ALT; observe for signs and symptoms of anaphylaxis during first dose
Test Interactions Positive Coombs' test (direct), false-positive urinary and serum proteins; may inactivate aminoglycosides *in vitro*
Pharmacotherapy Pearls Sodium content of 1 g: 66.7 mg (2.9 mEq)
Special Geriatric Considerations Nafcillin has not been studied exclusively in the elderly, however, given its route of elimination, dosage adjustments based upon age and renal function is not necessary
Dosage Forms Excipient information presented when available (limited, particularly for generics); consult specific product labeling.
Infusion, premixed iso-osmotic dextrose solution: 1 g (50 mL); 2 g (100 mL)
Injection, powder for reconstitution: 1 g, 2 g, 10 g

♦ **Nafcillin Sodium** *see* Nafcillin *on page 1330*

Naftifine (NAF ti feen)

Brand Names: U.S. Naftin®
Index Terms Naftifine Hydrochloride
Generic Availability (U.S.) No
Pharmacologic Category Antifungal Agent, Topical
Use Topical treatment of tinea cruris (jock itch), tinea corporis (ringworm), and tinea pedis (athlete's foot)
Contraindications Hypersensitivity to naftifine or any component of the formulation
Warnings/Precautions For topical use only; not intended for oral, ophthalmic, or vaginal use. Avoid use of occlusive dressings and contact with eyes, nose, mouth, or mucous membranes. Discontinue if sensitivity or irritation occurs.
Adverse Reactions (Reflective of adult population; not specific for elderly) 1% to 10%:
Dermatologic: Burning/stinging (5% to 6%), erythema (≤2%), pruritus (1% to 2%)
Local: Dryness (3%), irritation (2%)
Drug Interactions
Metabolism/Transport Effects None known.
Avoid Concomitant Use There are no known interactions where it is recommended to avoid concomitant use.
Increased Effect/Toxicity There are no known significant interactions involving an increase in effect.
Decreased Effect There are no known significant interactions involving a decrease in effect.
Stability Store at 25°C (77°F); excursions permitted to 15°C to 30°C (59°F to 86°F).
Mechanism of Action Synthetic, broad-spectrum antifungal agent in the allylamine class; appears to have both fungistatic and fungicidal activity. Exhibits antifungal activity by selectively inhibiting the enzyme squalene epoxidase in a dose-dependent manner which results in a reduced synthesis of ergosterol, the primary sterol within the fungal membrane, and increased squalene in cells.

Pharmacodynamics/Kinetics
Absorption: Systemic: Cream: 6%; Gel: 4%
Half-life elimination: 2-3 days
Excretion: Urine and feces (as unchanged drug and/or metabolites)

Dosage
Geriatric & Adult **Tinea corporis, tinea cruris, tinea pedis:** Topical:
Cream: Apply once daily to affected area and surrounding skin for up to 2 weeks (1%) or up to 4 weeks (2%)
Gel: Apply twice daily (morning and evening) to affected area and surrounding skin for up to 4 weeks

Administration Topical: Wash hands before and after use. Apply to clean, dry skin. Avoid occlusive dressings.

Monitoring Parameters Culture and KOH exam; re-evaluate if no improvement after 4 weeks of therapy

Special Geriatric Considerations No specific recommendations for use in the elderly.

Dosage Forms Excipient information presented when available (limited, particularly for generics); consult specific product labeling.
Cream, topical, as hydrochloride:
Naftin®: 1% (30 g, 60 g, 90 g); 2% (45 g) [contains benzyl alcohol]
Gel, topical, as hydrochloride:
Naftin®: 1% (40 g, 60 g, 90 g) [contains ethanol 52%]

◆ **Naftifine Hydrochloride** *see* Naftifine *on page 1332*
◆ **Naftin®** *see* Naftifine *on page 1332*
◆ **NaHCO₃** *see* Sodium Bicarbonate *on page 1785*

Nalbuphine (NAL byoo feen)

Related Information
Opioid Analgesics *on page 2122*

Medication Safety Issues
Sound-alike/look-alike issues:
Nubain may be confused with Navane®, Nebcin
High alert medication:
The Institute for Safe Medication Practices (ISMP) includes this medication among its list of drug classes which have a heightened risk of causing significant patient harm when used in error.

Index Terms Nalbuphine Hydrochloride; Nubain

Generic Availability (U.S.) Yes

Pharmacologic Category Analgesic, Opioid; Analgesic, Opioid Partial Agonist

Use Relief of moderate-to-severe pain; preoperative analgesia, postoperative and surgical anesthesia, and obstetrical analgesia during labor and delivery

Unlabeled Use Opioid-induced pruritus

Contraindications Hypersensitivity to nalbuphine or any component of the formulation

Warnings/Precautions Use caution in CNS depression. Sedation and psychomotor impairment are likely, and are additive with other CNS depressants or ethanol. May cause respiratory depression. Ambulatory patients must be cautioned about performing tasks which require mental alertness (eg, operating machinery or driving). Effects may be potentiated when used with other sedative drugs or ethanol. Use with caution in patients with recent myocardial infarction, biliary tract impairment, morbid obesity, thyroid dysfunction, head trauma, or increased intracranial pressure. Use caution in patients with prostatic hyperplasia and/or urinary stricture, adrenal insufficiency, decreased hepatic or renal function. Use with caution in patients with pre-existing respiratory compromise (hypoxia and/or hypercapnia), COPD or other obstructive pulmonary disease; critical respiratory depression may occur, even at therapeutic dosages. May cause hypotension; use with caution in patients with hypovolemia, cardiovascular disease (including acute MI), or drugs which may exaggerate hypotensive effects (including phenothiazines or general anesthetics). May obscure diagnosis or clinical course of patients with acute abdominal conditions. May result in tolerance and/or drug dependence with chronic use; use with caution in patients with a history of drug dependence. Abrupt discontinuation following prolonged use may lead to withdrawal symptoms. May precipitate withdrawal symptoms in patients following prolonged therapy with mu opioid agonists. Use with caution in the elderly and debilitated patients; may be more sensitive to adverse effects.

Adverse Reactions (Reflective of adult population; not specific for elderly)
>10%: Central nervous system: Sedation (36%)
1% to 10%:
Central nervous system: Dizziness (5%), headache (3%)
Gastrointestinal: Nausea/vomiting (6%), xerostomia (4%)
Miscellaneous: Clamminess (9%)

Drug Interactions
Metabolism/Transport Effects None known.
Avoid Concomitant Use
Avoid concomitant use of Nalbuphine with any of the following: Azelastine; Azelastine (Nasal); Mirtazapine; Paraldehyde
Increased Effect/Toxicity
Nalbuphine may increase the levels/effects of: Alcohol (Ethyl); Alvimopan; Azelastine; Azelastine (Nasal); CNS Depressants; Desmopressin; Metyrosine; Mirtazapine; Paraldehyde; Selective Serotonin Reuptake Inhibitors; Thiazide Diuretics; Zolpidem

The levels/effects of Nalbuphine may be increased by: Amphetamines; Antipsychotic Agents (Phenothiazines); Droperidol; HydrOXYzine; Succinylcholine
Decreased Effect
Nalbuphine may decrease the levels/effects of: Analgesics (Opioid); Pegvisomant

The levels/effects of Nalbuphine may be decreased by: Ammonium Chloride; Mixed Agonist/ Antagonist Opioids
Ethanol/Nutrition/Herb Interactions
Ethanol: May increase CNS depression; monitor for increased effects with coadministration. Caution patients about effects.
Herb/Nutraceutical: Avoid valerian, St John's wort, kava kava, gotu kola (may increase CNS depression).
Stability Store at room temperature of 15°C to 30°C (59°F to 86°F). Protect from light.
Mechanism of Action Agonist of kappa opiate receptors and partial antagonist of mu opiate receptors in the CNS, causing inhibition of ascending pain pathways, altering the perception of and response to pain; produces generalized CNS depression
Pharmacodynamics/Kinetics
Onset of action: Peak effect: SubQ, I.M.: <15 minutes; I.V.: 2-3 minutes
Metabolism: Hepatic
Half-life elimination: 5 hours
Excretion: Feces; urine (~7% as metabolites)
Dosage
Geriatric Refer to adult dosing; use with caution.
Adult
Pain management: I.M., I.V., SubQ: 10 mg/70 kg every 3-6 hours; maximum single dose in nonopioid-tolerant patients: 20 mg; maximum daily dose: 160 mg
Surgical anesthesia supplement: I.V.: Induction: 0.3-3 mg/kg over 10-15 minutes; maintenance doses of 0.25-0.5 mg/kg may be given as required
Opioid-induced pruritus (unlabeled use): I.V. 2.5-5 mg; may repeat dose
Renal Impairment Use with caution and reduce dose. Monitor.
Hepatic Impairment Use with caution and reduce dose.
Administration Administer I.M., SubQ, or I.V.
Monitoring Parameters Relief of pain, respiratory and mental status, blood pressure
Test Interactions May interfere with certain enzymatic methods used to detect opioids, depending on sensitivity and specificity of the test (refer to test manufacturer for details)
Special Geriatric Considerations The elderly may be particularly susceptible to CNS effects; monitor closely.
Dosage Forms Excipient information presented when available (limited, particularly for generics); consult specific product labeling.
Injection, solution, as hydrochloride: 10 mg/mL (10 mL); 20 mg/mL (10 mL)
Injection, solution, as hydrochloride [preservative free]: 10 mg/mL (1 mL); 20 mg/mL (1 mL)

◆ **Nalbuphine Hydrochloride** *see* Nalbuphine *on page 1333*
◆ **Nalfon®** *see* Fenoprofen *on page 758*
◆ **Nallpen** *see* Nafcillin *on page 1330*
◆ **N-allylnoroxymorphine Hydrochloride** *see* Naloxone *on page 1335*

Naloxone (nal OKS one)

Medication Safety Issues
Sound-alike/look-alike issues:
Naloxone may be confused with Lanoxin®, naltrexone
Narcan may be confused with Marcaine®, Norcuron®
International issues:
Narcan [multiple international markets] may be confused with Marcen brand name for ketazolam [Spain]
Brand Names: Canada Naloxone Hydrochloride Injection®; Naloxone Hydrochloride Injection® USP
Index Terms N-allylnoroxymorphine Hydrochloride; Naloxone Hydrochloride; Narcan
Generic Availability (U.S.) Yes
Pharmacologic Category Antidote; Opioid Antagonist
Use Complete or partial reversal of opioid drug effects, including respiratory depression; management of known or suspected opioid overdose; diagnosis of suspected opioid dependence or acute opioid overdose
Unlabeled Use Opioid-induced pruritus
Contraindications Hypersensitivity to naloxone or any component of the formulation
Warnings/Precautions Due to an association between naloxone and acute pulmonary edema, use with caution in patients with cardiovascular disease or in patients receiving medications with potential adverse cardiovascular effects (eg, hypotension, pulmonary edema, or arrhythmias). Administration of naloxone causes the release of catecholamines; may precipitate acute withdrawal or unmask pain in those who regularly take opioids. Excessive dosages should be avoided after use of opiates in surgery. Abrupt postoperative reversal may result in nausea, vomiting, sweating, tachycardia, hypertension, seizures, and other cardiovascular events (including pulmonary edema and arrhythmias). May precipitate withdrawal symptoms in patients addicted to opiates, including pain, hypertension, sweating, agitation, irritability; carefully titrate dose to reverse hypoventilation; do not fully awaken patient or reverse analgesic effect (postoperative patient). Use caution in patients with history of seizures; avoid use in treatment of meperidine-induced seizures. Recurrence of respiratory depression is possible if the opioid involved is long-acting; observe patients until there is no reasonable risk of recurrent respiratory depression.
Adverse Reactions (Reflective of adult population; not specific for elderly) Adverse reactions are related to reversing dependency and precipitating withdrawal. Withdrawal symptoms are the result of sympathetic excess. Adverse events occur secondarily to reversal (withdrawal) of narcotic analgesia and sedation.
Cardiovascular: Cardiac arrest, fever, flushing, hypertension, hypotension, tachycardia, ventricular fibrillation ventricular tachycardia
Central nervous system: Agitation, coma, crying (excessive [neonates]), encephalopathy, hallucination, irritability, nervousness, restlessness, seizure (neonates), tremulousness
Gastrointestinal: Abdominal cramps, diarrhea, nausea, vomiting
Local: Injection site reaction
Neuromuscular & skeletal: Ache, hyperreflexia (neonates), paresthesia, piloerection, tremor, weakness
Respiratory: Dyspnea, hypoxia, pulmonary edema, respiratory depression, rhinorrhea, sneezing
Miscellaneous: Diaphoresis, hot flashes, shivering, yawning
Drug Interactions
Metabolism/Transport Effects None known.
Avoid Concomitant Use There are no known interactions where it is recommended to avoid concomitant use.
Increased Effect/Toxicity There are no known significant interactions involving an increase in effect.
Decreased Effect There are no known significant interactions involving a decrease in effect.
Stability Store at 20°C to 25°C (68°F to 77°F). Protect from light.
I.V. push: Dilute naloxone 0.4 mg (1 mL ampul) with 9 mL of NS for a total volume of 10 mL to achieve a concentration of 0.04 mg/mL (APS, 2008)
I.V. infusion: Dilute naloxone 2 mg in 500 mL of NS or D$_5$W to make a final concentration of 4 **mcg**/mL; use within 24 hours
Inhalation via nebulization (unlabeled route): Dilute 2 mg of naloxone with 3 mL of normal saline (Mycyk, 2003; Weber, 2012)
Mechanism of Action Pure opioid antagonist that competes and displaces narcotics at opioid receptor sites

Pharmacodynamics/Kinetics
Onset of action: Endotracheal, I.M., SubQ: 2-5 minutes; I.V.: ~2 minutes
Duration: ~30-120 minutes depending on route of administration; I.V. has a shorter duration of action than I.M. administration; since naloxone's action is shorter than that of most opioids, repeated doses are usually needed
Metabolism: Primarily hepatic via glucuronidation
Half-life elimination: 0.5-1.5 hours
Excretion: Urine (as metabolites)

Dosage
Geriatric & Adult Note: Available routes of administration include I.V. (preferred), I.M., and SubQ; other available routes (unlabeled) include inhalation via nebulization (adults only), intranasal (adults only), and intraosseous (I.O.). Endotracheal administration is the least desirable and is supported by only anecdotal evidence (case report) (Neumar, 2010); nebulized naloxone has been shown to be an effective alternative to parenteral administration when needleless administration is desired (Weber, 2012):

Opioid overdose (with standard ACLS protocols):
I.V., I.M., SubQ: Initial: 0.4-2 mg; may need to repeat doses every 2-3 minutes; after reversal, may need to readminister dose(s) at a later interval (ie, 20-60 minutes) depending on type/duration of opioid. If no response is observed after 10 mg total, consider other causes of respiratory depression.
Continuous infusion (unlabeled dosing): I.V.: **Note:** For use with exposures to long-acting opioids (eg, methadone), sustained release product, and symptomatic body packers after initial naloxone response. Calculate dosage/hour based on effective intermittent dose used and duration of adequate response seen (Tenenbein, 1984) **or** use two-thirds ($2/3$) of the initial effective naloxone bolus on an hourly basis (typically 0.25-6.25 mg/hour); one-half ($1/2$) of the initial bolus dose should be readministered 15 minutes after initiation of the continuous infusion to prevent a drop in naloxone levels; adjust infusion rate as needed to assure adequate ventilation and prevent withdrawal symptoms (Goldfrank, 1986).
Endotracheal (unlabeled route): 0.08-5 mg (dose is 2-2.5 times I.V. dose); may repeat (Neumar, 2010)
Inhalation via nebulization (unlabeled route): 2 mg; may repeat. Switch to I.V. or I.M. administration when possible (Weber, 2012).
Intranasal administration (unlabeled route): 2 mg (1 mg per nostril); may repeat in 5 minutes if respiratory depression persists. **Note:** Onset of action is slightly delayed compared to I.M. or I.V. routes (Kelly, 2005; Robertson, 2009; Vanden Hoek, 2010).

Reversal of respiratory depression with therapeutic opioid doses: I.V., I.M., SubQ.: Initial: 0.04-0.4 mg; may repeat until desired response achieved. If desired response is not observed after 0.8 mg total, consider other causes of respiratory depression.
Continuous infusion (unlabeled dosing): I.V.: **Note:** For use with exposures to long-acting opioids (eg, methadone) or sustained release products. Calculate dosage/hour based on effective intermittent dose used and duration of adequate response seen (Tenenbein, 1984) **or** use two-thirds ($2/3$) of the initial effective naloxone bolus on an hourly basis (typically 0.2-0.6 mg/hour); one-half ($1/2$) of the initial bolus dose should be readministered 15 minutes after initiation of the continuous infusion to prevent a drop in naloxone levels; adjust infusion rate as needed to assure adequate ventilation and prevent withdrawal symptoms (Goldfrank, 1986).
Opioid-dependent patients being treated for cancer pain (NCCN guidelines, v.2.2011): I.V.: 0.04-0.08 mg (40-80 **mcg**) slow I.V. push; administer every 30-60 seconds until improvement in symptoms; if no response is observed after total naloxone dose 1 mg, consider other causes of respiratory depression. **Note:** May dilute 0.4 mg (1 mL) ampul into 9 mL of normal saline for a total volume of 10 mL to achieve a 0.04 mg/mL (40 **mcg**/mL) concentration.
Postoperative reversal: I.V.: 0.1-0.2 mg every 2-3 minutes until desired response (adequate ventilation and alertness without significant pain). **Note:** Repeat doses may be needed within 1-2 hour intervals depending on type, dose, and timing of the last dose of opioid administered.
Opioid-induced pruritus (unlabeled use): I.V. infusion: 0.25 mcg/kg/hour; **Note:** Monitor pain control; verify that the naloxone is not reversing analgesia (Gan, 1997)

Administration
Endotracheal: There is only anecdotal support for this route of administration. May require a slightly higher dose than used in other routes. Dilute to 1-2 mL with normal saline; flush with 5 cc of saline and then administer 5 ventilations
Intratracheal: Dilute to 1-2 mL with normal saline
I.V. push: Administer over 30 seconds as undiluted preparation **or** (unlabeled) administer as diluted preparation slow I.V. push by diluting 0.4 mg (1 mL) ampul with 9 mL of normal saline for a total volume of 10 mL to achieve a concentration of 0.04 mg/mL
I.V. continuous infusion: Dilute to 4 mcg/mL in D_5W or normal saline

Monitoring Parameters Respiratory rate, heart rate, blood pressure, temperature, level of consciousness, ABGs or pulse oximetry

Pharmacotherapy Pearls Too rapid a reversal of narcotic depression may result in nausea, vomiting, sweating, tachycardia, increased blood pressure, and tremulousness

Special Geriatric Considerations No specific information for use in elderly.

Dosage Forms Excipient information presented when available (limited, particularly for generics); consult specific product labeling. [DSC] = Discontinued product

Injection, solution, as hydrochloride: 0.4 mg/mL (10 mL)

Injection, solution, as hydrochloride [preservative free]: 0.4 mg/mL (1 mL); 1 mg/mL (2 mL [DSC])

♦ **Naloxone Hydrochloride** *see* Naloxone *on page 1335*

♦ **Namenda®** *see* Memantine *on page 1203*

♦ **Namenda XR** *see* Memantine *on page 1203*

Naphazoline (Nasal) (naf AZ oh leen)

Brand Names: U.S. Privine® [OTC]

Index Terms Naphazoline Hydrochloride

Pharmacologic Category Alpha$_1$ Agonist

Use Temporary relief of nasal congestion associated with the common cold, upper respiratory allergies, or sinusitis

Dosage

Geriatric & Adult Nasal congestion (decongestant): Intranasal: 0.05%, instill 1-2 drops or sprays every 6 hours if needed; therapy should not exceed 3 days

Special Geriatric Considerations Evaluate the patient's or caregiver's ability to safely administer the correct dose of nasal medication. Use cautiously in patients with cardiovascular disease.

Dosage Forms Excipient information presented when available (limited, particularly for generics); consult specific product labeling.

Solution, intranasal, as hydrochloride [drops]:

Privine®: 0.05% (25 mL) [contains benzalkonium chloride]

Solution, intranasal, as hydrochloride [spray]:

Privine®: 0.05% (20 mL) [contains benzalkonium chloride]

Naphazoline (Ophthalmic) (naf AZ oh leen)

Brand Names: U.S. AK-Con™; Clear eyes® for Dry Eyes Plus ACR Relief [OTC]; Clear eyes® for Dry Eyes plus Redness Relief [OTC]; Clear eyes® Redness Relief [OTC]; Clear eyes® Seasonal Relief [OTC]

Brand Names: Canada Naphcon Forte®; Vasocon®

Index Terms Naphazoline Hydrochloride

Generic Availability (U.S.) No

Pharmacologic Category Alpha$_1$ Agonist; Ophthalmic Agent, Vasoconstrictor

Use Topical ocular vasoconstrictor; relief of redness of the eye due to minor irritation

Dosage

Geriatric & Adult Decrease in eye redness (vasoconstrictor): Ophthalmic:

0.1% solution (prescription): 1-2 drops into conjuctival sac every 3-4 hours as needed

0.012% or 0.025% solution (OTC): 1-2 drops into affected eye(s) up to 4 times/day; therapy should not exceed 3 days

Special Geriatric Considerations Evaluate the patient's or caregiver's ability to safely administer the correct dose of ophthalmic medication. Use cautiously in patients with cardiovascular disease.

Dosage Forms Excipient information presented when available (limited, particularly for generics); consult specific product labeling.

Solution, ophthalmic, as hydrochloride [drops]:

AK-Con™: 0.1% (15 mL) [contains benzalkonium chloride]

Clear eyes® for Dry Eyes Plus ACR Relief: 0.025% (15 mL) [contains hypromellose, zinc sulfate]

Clear eyes® for Dry Eyes plus Redness Relief: 0.012% (15 mL) [contains benzalkonium chloride, glycerin, hypromellose]

Clear eyes® Redness Relief: 0.012% (6 mL, 15 mL, 30 mL) [contains benzalkonium chloride, glycerin]

Clear eyes® Seasonal Relief: 0.012% (15 mL, 30 mL) [contains benzalkonium chloride, glycerin, zinc sulfate]

Naphazoline and Pheniramine (naf AZ oh leen & fen NIR a meen)

Related Information
Naphazoline (Ophthalmic) *on page 1337*
Medication Safety Issues
Sound-alike/look-alike issues:
Visine® may be confused with Visken®
Brand Names: U.S. Naphcon-A® [OTC]; Opcon-A® [OTC]; Visine-A® [OTC]
Brand Names: Canada Naphcon-A®; Visine® Advanced Allergy
Index Terms Pheniramine and Naphazoline
Generic Availability (U.S.) No
Pharmacologic Category Alkylamine Derivative; Alpha$_1$ Agonist; Histamine H$_1$ Antagonist; Histamine H$_1$ Antagonist, First Generation; Imidazoline Derivative; Ophthalmic Agent, Vasoconstrictor
Use Treatment of ocular congestion, irritation, and itching
Dosage
Geriatric & Adult Ophthalmic: 1-2 drops into the affected eye(s) up to 4 times/day
Special Geriatric Considerations Evaluate the patient's or caregiver's ability to safely administer the correct dose of ophthalmic medication. Use cautiously in patients with cardiovascular disease.
Dosage Forms Excipient information presented when available (limited, particularly for generics); consult specific product labeling.
Solution, ophthalmic:
Naphcon-A®: Naphazoline hydrochloride 0.025% and pheniramine maleate 0.3% (5 mL) [contains benzalkonium chloride; 2 bottles/box], (15 mL) [contains benzalkonium chloride]
Opcon-A®: Naphazoline hydrochloride 0.027% and pheniramine maleate 0.3% (15 mL) [contains benzalkonium chloride]
Visine-A®: Naphazoline hydrochloride 0.025% and pheniramine maleate 0.3% (15 mL) [contains benzalkonium chloride]

- ◆ **Naphazoline Hydrochloride** *see* Naphazoline (Nasal) *on page 1337*
- ◆ **Naphazoline Hydrochloride** *see* Naphazoline (Ophthalmic) *on page 1337*
- ◆ **Naphcon-A® [OTC]** *see* Naphazoline and Pheniramine *on page 1338*
- ◆ **Naprelan®** *see* Naproxen *on page 1338*
- ◆ **Naprosyn®** *see* Naproxen *on page 1338*

Naproxen (na PROKS en)

Related Information
Beers Criteria – Potentially Inappropriate Medications for Geriatrics *on page 2183*
Medication Safety Issues
Sound-alike/look-alike issues:
Naproxen may be confused with Natacyn®, Nebcin
Anaprox® may be confused with Anaspaz®, Avapro®
Naprelan® may be confused with Naprosyn®
Naprosyn® may be confused with Natacyn®, Nebcin
BEERS Criteria medication:
This drug may be potentially inappropriate for use in geriatric patients (Quality of evidence - moderate; Strength of recommendation - strong).
International issues:
Flogen [Mexico] may be confused with Flovent brand name for fluticasone [U.S., Canada]
Flogen [Mexico] may be confused with Floxin brand name for flunarizine [Thailand], norfloxacin [South Africa], ofloxacin [U.S., Canada], and perfloxacin [Philippines]
Brand Names: U.S. Aleve® [OTC]; All Day Relief [OTC]; Anaprox®; Anaprox® DS; EC-Naprosyn®; Mediproxen [OTC]; Midol® Extended Relief [OTC]; Naprelan®; Naprosyn®; Pamprin® Maximum Strength All Day Relief [OTC]
Brand Names: Canada Anaprox®; Anaprox® DS; Apo-Napro-Na DS®; Apo-Napro-Na®; Apo-Naproxen®; Apo-Naproxen EC®; Apo-Naproxen SR®; Apo-Naproxen®; Mylan-Naproxen EC; Naprelan™; Naprosyn®; Naprosyn® E; Naprosyn® SR; Naproxen Sodium DS; Naproxen-NA; Naproxen-NA DF; PMS-Naproxen; PMS-Naproxen EC; PRO-Naproxen EC; Riva-Naproxen; Riva-Naproxen Sodium; Riva-Naproxen Sodium DS; Teva-Naproxen; Teva-Naproxen EC; Teva-Naproxen Sodium; Teva-Naproxen Sodium DS; Teva-Naproxen SR
Index Terms Naproxen Sodium
Generic Availability (U.S.) Yes: Caplet, suspension, tablet
Pharmacologic Category Nonsteroidal Anti-inflammatory Drug (NSAID), Oral

Use Management of ankylosing spondylitis, osteoarthritis, and rheumatoid disorders; acute gout; mild-to-moderate pain; tendonitis, bursitis; fever

Unlabeled Use Migraine prophylaxis

Medication Guide Available Yes

Contraindications Hypersensitivity to naproxen, aspirin, other NSAIDs, or any component of the formulation; perioperative pain in the setting of coronary artery bypass graft (CABG) surgery

Warnings/Precautions [U.S. Boxed Warning]: NSAIDs are associated with an increased risk of adverse cardiovascular thrombotic events, including MI and stroke. Risk may be increased with duration of use or pre-existing cardiovascular risk factors or disease. Carefully evaluate individual cardiovascular risk profiles prior to prescribing. May cause new-onset hypertension or worsening of existing hypertension. Use caution with fluid retention. Avoid use in heart failure. Use the lowest effective dose for the shortest duration of time, consistent with individual patient goals, to reduce risk of cardiovascular or GI adverse events. Alternate therapies should be considered for patients at high risk. Concurrent administration of ibuprofen, and potentially other nonselective NSAIDs, may interfere with aspirin's cardioprotective effect. **[U.S. Boxed Warning]: Use is contraindicated for treatment of perioperative pain in the setting of coronary artery bypass graft (CABG) surgery.** Risk of MI and stroke may be increased with use following CABG surgery.

[U.S. Boxed Warning]: NSAIDs may increase risk of gastrointestinal irritation, inflammation, ulceration, bleeding, and perforation. These events may occur at any time during therapy and without warning. Use caution with a history of GI disease (bleeding or ulcers), concurrent therapy with aspirin, anticoagulants and/or corticosteroids, smoking, use of alcohol, the elderly or debilitated patients. When used concomitantly with ≤325 mg of aspirin, a substantial increase in the risk of gastrointestinal complications (eg, ulcer) occurs; concomitant gastroprotective therapy (eg, proton pump inhibitors) is recommended (Bhatt, 2008).

May increase the risk of aseptic meningitis, especially in patients with systemic lupus erythematosus (SLE) and mixed connective tissue disorders. Platelet adhesion and aggregation may be decreased; may prolong bleeding time; patients with coagulation disorders or who are receiving anticoagulants should be monitored closely. Anemia may occur; patients on long-term NSAID therapy should be monitored for anemia. Rarely, NSAID use may cause severe blood dyscrasias (eg, agranulocytosis, aplastic anemia, thrombocytopenia).

NSAID use may compromise existing renal function; dose-dependent decreases in prostaglandin synthesis may result from NSAID use, reducing renal blood flow which may cause renal decompensation. NSAID use may increase the risk for hyperkalemia. Patients with impaired renal function, dehydration, heart failure, liver dysfunction, those taking diuretics, and ACE inhibitors, and the elderly are at greater risk of renal toxicity and hyperkalemia. Rehydrate patient before starting therapy; monitor renal function closely. Not recommended for use in patients with advanced renal disease. Long-term NSAID use may result in renal papillary necrosis.

NSAIDs may cause serious skin adverse events including exfoliative dermatitis, Stevens-Johnson Syndrome (SJS) and toxic epidermal necrolysis (TEN); discontinue use at first sign of skin rash or hypersensitivity. Anaphylactoid reactions may occur, even without prior exposure; patients with "aspirin triad" (bronchial asthma, aspirin intolerance, rhinitis) may be at increased risk. Do not use in patients who experience bronchospasm, asthma, rhinitis, or urticaria with NSAID or aspirin therapy. Use caution in other forms of asthma.

Use with caution in patients with decreased hepatic function. Closely monitor patients with any abnormal LFT. Severe hepatic reactions (eg, fulminant hepatitis, liver failure) have occurred with NSAID use, rarely; discontinue if signs or symptoms of liver disease develop, or if systemic manifestations occur.

NSAIDS may cause drowsiness, dizziness, blurred vision and other neurologic effects which may impair physical or mental abilities; patients must be cautioned about performing tasks which require mental alertness (eg, operating machinery or driving). Discontinue use with blurred or diminished vision and perform ophthalmologic exam. Monitor vision with long-term therapy.

In the elderly, avoid chronic use (unless alternative agents ineffective and patient can receive concomitant gastroprotective agent); nonselective oral NSAID use is associated with an increased risk of GI bleeding and peptic ulcer disease in older adults in high risk category (eg, >75 years or age or receiving concomitant oral/parenteral corticosteroids, anticoagulants, or antiplatelet agents) (Beers Criteria).

Withhold for at least 4-6 half-lives prior to surgical or dental procedures.

◀ **OTC labeling:** Prior to self-medication, patients should contact healthcare provider if they have had recurring stomach pain or upset, ulcers, bleeding problems, asthma, high blood pressure, heart or kidney disease, other serious medical problems, are currently taking a diuretic, anticoagulant, other NSAIDs, or are ≥60 years of age. Recommended dosages and duration should not be exceeded, due to an increased risk of GI bleeding, MI, and stroke. Patients should stop use and consult a healthcare provider if symptoms get worse, newly appear, or continue; if an allergic reaction occurs; if feeling faint, vomit blood or have bloody/ black stools; if having difficulty swallowing or heartburn, or if fever lasts for >3 days or pain >10 days. Consuming ≥3 alcoholic beverages/day or taking longer than recommended may increase the risk of GI bleeding.

Adverse Reactions (Reflective of adult population; not specific for elderly) 1% to 10%:

Cardiovascular: Edema (3% to 9%), palpitations (<3%)

Central nervous system: Dizziness (3% to 9%), drowsiness (3% to 9%), headache (3% to 9%), lightheadedness (<3%), vertigo (<3%)

Dermatologic: Pruritus (3% to 9%), skin eruption (3% to 9%), ecchymosis (3% to 9%), purpura (<3%), rash

Endocrine & metabolic: Fluid retention (3% to 9%)

Gastrointestinal: Abdominal pain (3% to 9%), constipation (3% to 9%), nausea (3% to 9%), heartburn (3% to 9%), diarrhea (<3%), dyspepsia (<3%), stomatitis (<3%), flatulence, gross bleeding/perforation, indigestion, ulcers, vomiting

Genitourinary: Abnormal renal function

Hematologic: Hemolysis (3% to 9%), ecchymosis (3% to 9%), anemia, bleeding time increased

Hepatic: LFTs increased

Ocular: Visual disturbances (<3%)

Otic: Tinnitus (3% to 9%), hearing disturbances (<3%)

Respiratory: Dyspnea (3% to 9%)

Miscellaneous: Diaphoresis (<3%), thirst (<3%)

Drug Interactions

Metabolism/Transport Effects Substrate of CYP1A2 (minor), CYP2C9 (minor); **Note:** Assignment of Major/Minor substrate status based on clinically relevant drug interaction potential

Avoid Concomitant Use

Avoid concomitant use of Naproxen with any of the following: Floctafenine; Ketorolac; Ketorolac (Nasal); Ketorolac (Systemic)

Increased Effect/Toxicity

Naproxen may increase the levels/effects of: Aliskiren; Aminoglycosides; Anticoagulants; Antiplatelet Agents; Bisphosphonate Derivatives; Collagenase (Systemic); CycloSPORINE; CycloSPORINE (Systemic); Dabigatran Etexilate; Deferasirox; Desmopressin; Digoxin; Drotrecogin Alfa (Activated); Eplerenone; Haloperidol; Ibritumomab; Lithium; Methotrexate; Nonsteroidal Anti-Inflammatory Agents; PEMEtrexed; Porfimer; Potassium-Sparing Diuretics; PRALAtrexate; Quinolone Antibiotics; Rivaroxaban; Salicylates; Thrombolytic Agents; Tositumomab and Iodine I 131 Tositumomab; Vancomycin; Vitamin K Antagonists

The levels/effects of Naproxen may be increased by: ACE Inhibitors; Angiotensin II Receptor Blockers; Antidepressants (Tricyclic, Tertiary Amine); Corticosteroids (Systemic); Cyclo-SPORINE; CycloSPORINE (Systemic); Dasatinib; Floctafenine; Glucosamine; Herbs (Anti-coagulant/Antiplatelet Properties); Ketorolac; Ketorolac (Nasal); Ketorolac (Systemic); Nonsteroidal Anti-Inflammatory Agents; Omega-3-Acid Ethyl Esters; Pentosan Polysulfate Sodium; Pentoxifylline; Probenecid; Prostacyclin Analogues; Selective Serotonin Reuptake Inhibitors; Serotonin/Norepinephrine Reuptake Inhibitors; Sodium Phosphates; Tipranavir; Treprostinil; Vitamin E

Decreased Effect

Naproxen may decrease the levels/effects of: ACE Inhibitors; Aliskiren; Angiotensin II Receptor Blockers; Antiplatelet Agents; Beta-Blockers; Eplerenone; HydrALAZINE; Loop Diuretics; Potassium-Sparing Diuretics; Salicylates; Selective Serotonin Reuptake Inhibitors; Thiazide Diuretics

The levels/effects of Naproxen may be decreased by: Bile Acid Sequestrants; Nonsteroidal Anti-Inflammatory Agents; Salicylates

Ethanol/Nutrition/Herb Interactions

Ethanol: Avoid ethanol (may enhance gastric mucosal irritation).

Food: Naproxen absorption rate/levels may be decreased if taken with food.

Herb/Nutraceutical: Avoid alfalfa, anise, bilberry, bladderwrack, bromelain, cat's claw, celery, chamomile, coleus, cordyceps, dong quai, evening primrose, fenugreek, feverfew, garlic, ginger, ginkgo biloba, ginseng (American, Panax, Siberian), grapeseed, green tea, guggul, horse chestnut seed, horseradish, licorice, prickly ash, red clover, reishi, SAMe (S-adenosylmethionine), sweet clover, turmeric, white willow (all have additional antiplatelet activity).

Stability Store oral suspension and tablet at 15°C to 30°C (59°F to 86°F).

Mechanism of Action Reversibly inhibits cyclooxygenase-1 and 2 (COX-1 and 2) enzymes, which results in decreased formation of prostaglandin precursors; has antipyretic, analgesic, and anti-inflammatory properties

Other proposed mechanisms not fully elucidated (and possibly contributing to the anti-inflammatory effect to varying degrees), include inhibiting chemotaxis, altering lymphocyte activity, inhibiting neutrophil aggregation/activation, and decreasing proinflammatory cytokine levels.

Pharmacodynamics/Kinetics
Onset of action: Analgesic: 1 hour; Anti-inflammatory: ~2 weeks
  Peak effect: Anti-inflammatory: 2-4 weeks
Duration: Analgesic: ≤7 hours; Anti-inflammatory: ≤12 hours
Absorption: Almost 100%
Distribution: 0.16 L/kg
Protein binding: >99% to albumin; increased free fraction in elderly
Metabolism: Hepatic to metabolites
Bioavailability: 95%
Half-life elimination: Normal renal function: 12-17 hours; End-stage renal disease: No change
Time to peak, serum: 1-4 hours
Excretion: Urine (95%; primarily as metabolites); feces (≤3%)

Dosage
Geriatric & Adult Note: Dosage expressed as naproxen base; 200 mg naproxen base is equivalent to 220 mg naproxen sodium.
  Gout, acute: Oral: Initial: 750 mg, followed by 250 mg every 8 hours until attack subsides. **Note:** EC-Naprosyn® is not recommended.
  Migraine, acute (unlabeled use): Initial: 500-750 mg; an additional 250-500 mg may be given if needed (maximum: 1250 mg in 24 hours). **Note:** EC-Naprosyn® is not recommended.
  Pain (mild-to-moderate), dysmenorrhea, acute tendonitis, bursitis: Oral: Initial: 500 mg, then 250 mg every 6-8 hours; maximum: 1250 mg/day naproxen base
  Rheumatoid arthritis, osteoarthritis, and ankylosing spondylitis: 500-1000 mg/day in 2 divided doses; may increase to 1.5 g/day of naproxen base for limited time period
  OTC labeling: Pain/fever: 200 mg naproxen base every 8-12 hours; if needed, may take 400 mg naproxen base for the initial dose; maximum: 400 mg naproxen base in any 8- to 12-hour period or 600 mg naproxen base/24 hours
Renal Impairment Cl$_{cr}$ <30 mL/minute: use is not recommended.

Administration Administer with food, milk, or antacids to decrease GI adverse effects
Suspension: Shake suspension well before administration.
Tablet, extended release: Swallow tablet whole; do not break, crush, or chew.

Monitoring Parameters Occult blood loss, periodic liver function test, CBC, BUN, serum creatinine; urine output

Test Interactions Naproxen may interfere with 5-HIAA urinary assays; due to an interaction with m-dinitrobenzene, naproxen should be discontinued 72 hours before adrenal function testing if the Porter-Silber test is used. May interfere with urine detection of cannabinoids and barbiturates (false-positives).

Special Geriatric Considerations Elderly are a high-risk population for adverse effects from NSAIDs. As much as 60% of the elderly can develop peptic ulceration and/or hemorrhage asymptomatically. The concomitant use of H$_2$ blockers and sucralfate is not effective as prophylaxis with the exception of NSAID-induced duodenal ulcers which may be prevented by the use of ranitidine. Misoprostol and proton pump inhibitors are the only agents proven to help prevent the development of NSAID-induced ulcers. Also, concomitant disease and drug use contribute to the risk for GI adverse effects. Use lowest effective dose for shortest period possible. Consider renal function decline with age. Use of NSAIDs can compromise existing renal function especially when Cl$_{cr}$ is ≤30 mL/minute. Tinnitus may be a difficult and unreliable indication of toxicity due to age-related hearing loss or eighth cranial nerve damage. CNS adverse effects such as confusion, agitation, and hallucination are generally seen in overdose or high-dose situations, but elderly may demonstrate these adverse effects at lower doses than younger adults.

This medication is considered to be potentially inappropriate in this patient population (Beers Criteria: Quality of evidence - moderate; Strength of recommendation - strong).

Dosage Forms Excipient information presented when available (limited, particularly for generics); consult specific product labeling.

Caplet, oral, as sodium: 220 mg [equivalent to naproxen base 200 mg]
  Aleve®: 220 mg [contains sodium 20 mg; equivalent to naproxen base 200 mg]
  All Day Relief: 220 mg [contains sodium 20 mg; equivalent to naproxen base 200 mg]
  Midol® Extended Relief: 220 mg [contains sodium 20 mg; equivalent to naproxen base 200 mg]
  Pamprin® Maximum Strength All Day Relief: 220 mg [contains sodium 20 mg; equivalent to naproxen base 200 mg]

Capsule, liquid gel, oral, as sodium:
  Aleve®: 220 mg [contains sodium 20 mg; equivalent to naproxen base 200 mg]

Combination package, oral, as sodium [dose-pack/each package contains]:
  Naprelan®: Day 1-3: Tablet, controlled release: 825 mg [equivalent to naproxen base 750 mg] (6s) [contains sodium 75 mg] and Day 4-10: Tablet, controlled release: 550 mg [equivalent to naproxen base 500 mg] (14s) [contains sodium 50 mg]

Gelcap, oral, as sodium:
  Aleve®: 220 mg [contains sodium 20 mg; equivalent to naproxen base 200 mg]

Suspension, oral: 125 mg/5 mL (500 mL)
  Naprosyn®: 125 mg/5 mL (473 mL) [contains sodium 39 mg (1.5 mEq)/5 mL; orange-pineapple flavor]

Tablet, oral: 250 mg, 375 mg, 500 mg
  Naprosyn®: 250 mg [scored]
  Naprosyn®: 375 mg
  Naprosyn®: 500 mg [scored]

Tablet, oral, as sodium: 220 mg [equivalent to naproxen base 200 mg], 275 mg [equivalent to naproxen base 250 mg], 550 mg [equivalent to naproxen base 500 mg]
  Aleve®: 220 mg [contains sodium 20 mg; equivalent to naproxen base 200 mg]
  Anaprox®: 275 mg [contains sodium 25 mg; equivalent to naproxen base 250 mg]
  Anaprox® DS: 550 mg [scored; contains sodium 50 mg; equivalent to naproxen base 500 mg]
  Mediproxen: 220 mg [contains sodium 20 mg; equivalent to naproxen base 200 mg]

Tablet, controlled release, oral, as sodium:
  Naprelan®: 412.5 mg [contains sodium 37.5 mg; equivalent to naproxen base 375 mg]
  Naprelan®: 550 mg [contains sodium 50 mg; equivalent to naproxen base 500 mg]
  Naprelan®: 825 mg [contains sodium 75 mg; equivalent to naproxen base 750 mg]

Tablet, delayed release, enteric coated, oral: 375 mg, 500 mg
  EC-Naprosyn®: 375 mg, 500 mg

Naproxen and Esomeprazole (na PROKS en & es oh ME pray zol)

Related Information
  Esomeprazole *on page 676*
  Naproxen *on page 1338*

Medication Safety Issues
  Sound-alike/look-alike issues:
    Vimovo™ may be confused with Vimpat®

Brand Names: U.S. Vimovo™

Brand Names: Canada Vimovo™

Index Terms Esomeprazole and Naproxen

Generic Availability (U.S.) No

Pharmacologic Category Nonsteroidal Anti-inflammatory Drug (NSAID), Oral; Proton Pump Inhibitor; Substituted Benzimidazole

Use Reduction of the risk of NSAID-associated gastric ulcers in patients at risk of developing gastric ulcers who require an NSAID for the treatment of rheumatoid arthritis, osteoarthritis, and ankylosing spondylitis

Medication Guide Available Yes

Contraindications Hypersensitivity to esomeprazole, substituted benzimidazoles (ie, esomeprazole, omeprazole, pantoprazole, rabeprazole), naproxen, aspirin, other NSAIDs, or any component of the formulation; perioperative pain in the setting of coronary artery bypass graft (CABG) surgery

Warnings/Precautions See individual agents.

Adverse Reactions (Reflective of adult population; not specific for elderly) See individual agents.

Drug Interactions
  Metabolism/Transport Effects Refer to individual components.

Avoid Concomitant Use

Avoid concomitant use of Naproxen and Esomeprazole with any of the following: Delavirdine; Erlotinib; Floctafenine; Ketorolac; Ketorolac (Nasal); Ketorolac (Systemic); Nelfinavir; Posaconazole; Rifampin; Rilpivirine; St Johns Wort

Increased Effect/Toxicity

Naproxen and Esomeprazole may increase the levels/effects of: Aliskiren; Aminoglycosides; Amphetamines; Anticoagulants; Antiplatelet Agents; Benzodiazepines (metabolized by oxidation); Cilostazol; Collagenase (Systemic); CycloSPORINE; CycloSPORINE (Systemic); CYP2C19 Substrates; Deferasirox; Desmopressin; Dexmethylphenidate; Drotrecogin Alfa (Activated); Eplerenone; Haloperidol; Ibritumomab; Lithium; Methotrexate; Methylphenidate; Nonsteroidal Anti-Inflammatory Agents; PEMEtrexed; Porfimer; Potassium-Sparing Diuretics; PRALAtrexate; Quinolone Antibiotics; Raltegravir; Rivaroxaban; Salicylates; Saquinavir; Tacrolimus; Tacrolimus (Systemic); Thrombolytic Agents; Tositumomab and Iodine I 131 Tositumomab; Vancomycin; Vitamin K Antagonists; Voriconazole

The levels/effects of Naproxen and Esomeprazole may be increased by: ACE Inhibitors; Angiotensin II Receptor Blockers; Antidepressants (Tricyclic, Tertiary Amine); Corticosteroids (Systemic); CycloSPORINE; CycloSPORINE (Systemic); Floctafenine; Fluconazole; Glucosamine; Herbs (Anticoagulant/Antiplatelet Properties); Ketoconazole; Ketoconazole (Systemic); Ketorolac; Ketorolac (Nasal); Ketorolac (Systemic); Nonsteroidal Anti-Inflammatory Agents; Omega-3-Acid Ethyl Esters; Pentosan Polysulfate Sodium; Pentoxifylline; Probenecid; Prostacyclin Analogues; Selective Serotonin Reuptake Inhibitors; Serotonin/Norepinephrine Reuptake Inhibitors; Sodium Phosphates; Treprostinil; Vitamin E

Decreased Effect

Naproxen and Esomeprazole may decrease the levels/effects of: ACE Inhibitors; Aliskiren; Angiotensin II Receptor Blockers; Antiplatelet Agents; Atazanavir; Beta-Blockers; Bisphosphonate Derivatives; Cefditoren; Clopidogrel; Dabigatran Etexilate; Dasatinib; Delavirdine; Eplerenone; Erlotinib; Gefitinib; HydrALAZINE; Indinavir; Iron Salts; Itraconazole; Ketoconazole; Ketoconazole (Systemic); Loop Diuretics; Mesalamine; Mycophenolate; Nelfinavir; Nilotinib; Posaconazole; Potassium-Sparing Diuretics; Rilpivirine; Salicylates; Selective Serotonin Reuptake Inhibitors; Thiazide Diuretics; Vismodegib

The levels/effects of Naproxen and Esomeprazole may be decreased by: Bile Acid Sequestrants; CYP2C19 Inducers (Strong); Nonsteroidal Anti-Inflammatory Agents; Rifampin; Salicylates; St Johns Wort; Tipranavir; Tocilizumab

Stability Store at 25°C (77°F); excursions permitted to 15°C to 30°C (59°F to 86°F). Protect from moisture.

Mechanism of Action

Naproxen: Reversibly inhibits cyclooxygenase-1 and 2 (COX-1 and 2) enzymes, which result in decreased formation of prostaglandin precursors; has antipyretic, analgesic, and anti-inflammatory properties

Esomeprazole: Proton pump inhibitor which decreases acid secretion in gastric parietal cells

Pharmacodynamics/Kinetics See individual agents.

Dosage

Geriatric Naproxen: Dosing adjustment should be considered; use lowest effective dose. Refer to adult dosing.

Adult Reduce NSAID-associated gastric ulcers during treatment for arthritis: Oral: One tablet (375 mg naproxen/20 mg esomeprazole or 500 mg naproxen/20 mg esomeprazole) twice daily; maximum daily esomeprazole dose: 40 mg.

Note: If a daily dose of esomeprazole <40 mg/day is necessary, alternate treatment should be considered.

Renal Impairment Moderate-to-severe renal impairment (Cl_{cr} <30 mL/minute): Use is not recommended.

Hepatic Impairment Severe liver disease: Use of this combination product not recommended since esomeprazole dose will exceed 20 mg/day.

Administration Administer dose at least 30 minutes prior to meals. Tablets should be swallowed whole; do not chew, crush, dissolve, or split tablet.

Monitoring Parameters Occult blood loss; periodic liver function test, CBC, BUN, serum creatinine

Test Interactions See individual agents.

Special Geriatric Considerations See individual agents.

An increased risk of fractures of the hip, spine, or wrist has been observed in epidemiologic studies with proton pump inhibitor (PPI) use, primarily in older adults ≥50 years of age. The greatest risk was seen in patients receiving high doses or on long-term therapy (≥1 year). Calcium and vitamin D supplementation and close monitoring are recommended to reduce the risk of fracture in high-risk patients. Additionally, long-term use of proton pump inhibitors has resulted in reports of hypomagnesemia and Clostridium difficile infections.

NAPROXEN AND ESOMEPRAZOLE

Dosage Forms Excipient information presented when available (limited, particularly in generics); consult specific product labeling.
Tablet, variable release, oral:
  Vimovo™: Naproxen [delayed release] 375 mg and esomeprazole [immediate release] 20 mg, Naproxen [delayed release] 500 mg and esomeprazole [immediate release] 20 mg

- ◆ **Naproxen and Sumatriptan** *see* Sumatriptan and Naproxen *on page 1825*
- ◆ **Naproxen Sodium** *see* Naproxen *on page 1338*
- ◆ **Naproxen Sodium and Sumatriptan** *see* Sumatriptan and Naproxen *on page 1825*
- ◆ **Naproxen Sodium and Sumatriptan Succinate** *see* Sumatriptan and Naproxen *on page 1825*

Naratriptan (NAR a trip tan)

Medication Safety Issues
Sound-alike/look-alike issues:
  Amerge® may be confused with Altace®, Amaryl®
Brand Names: U.S. Amerge®
Brand Names: Canada Amerge®; Sandoz-Naratriptan; Teva-Naratriptan
Index Terms Naratriptan Hydrochloride
Generic Availability (U.S.) Yes
Pharmacologic Category Antimigraine Agent; Serotonin 5-HT$_{1B, 1D}$ Receptor Agonist
Use Treatment of acute migraine headache with or without aura
Unlabeled Use Short-term prevention of menstrually-associated migraines (MAMs)
Contraindications Hypersensitivity to naratriptan or any component of the formulation; cerebrovascular, peripheral vascular disease (ischemic bowel disease), ischemic heart disease (angina pectoris, history of myocardial infarction, or proven silent ischemia); or in patients with symptoms consistent with ischemic heart disease, coronary artery vasospasm, or Prinzmetal's angina; uncontrolled hypertension or patients who have received within 24 hours another 5-HT agonist (sumatriptan, zolmitriptan) or ergotamine-containing product; patients with known risk factors associated with coronary artery disease; patients with severe hepatic (Child-Pugh grade C) or renal disease (Cl$_{cr}$ <15 mL/minute); do not administer naratriptan to patients with hemiplegic or basilar migraine
Warnings/Precautions Use only if there is a clear diagnosis of migraine. Dosage reduction is required in mild-to-moderate hepatic impairment and moderate renal impairment; use is contraindicated in patients with severe hepatic or renal impairment. Do not give to patients with risk factors for CAD until a cardiovascular evaluation has been performed; if evaluation is satisfactory, the healthcare provider should administer the first dose (consider ECG monitoring) and cardiovascular status should be periodically re-evaluated. Cardiac events (coronary artery vasospasm, transient ischemia, myocardial infarction, ventricular tachycardia/fibrillation, cardiac arrest, and death), cerebral/subarachnoid hemorrhage, stroke, peripheral vascular ischemia, and colonic ischemia have been reported with 5-HT$_1$ agonist administration. Patients who experience sensations of chest pain/pressure/tightness or symptoms suggestive of angina following dosing should be evaluated for coronary artery disease or Prinzmetal's angina before receiving additional doses; if dosing is resumed and similar symptoms recur, monitor with ECG. Significant elevation in blood pressure, including hypertensive crisis, has also been reported on rare occasions in patients with and without a history of hypertension. Only indicated for the acute treatment of migraine; not indicated for migraine prophylaxis, or for the treatment of cluster headache, hemiplegic or basilar migraine. If a patient does not respond to the first dose, the diagnosis of migraine should be reconsidered; rule out underlying neurologic disease in patients with atypical headache and in patients with no prior history of migraine.

Symptoms of agitation, confusion, hallucinations, hyper-reflexia, myoclonus, shivering, and tachycardia may occur with concomitant proserotonergic drugs (ie, SSRIs/SNRIs or triptans) or agents which reduce naratriptan's metabolism. Concurrent use of serotonin precursors (eg, tryptophan) is not recommended. If concomitant administration with SSRIs is warranted, monitor closely, especially at initiation and with dose increases.
Adverse Reactions (Reflective of adult population; not specific for elderly) 1% to 10%:
  Central nervous system: Pain/pressure (2% to 4%), malaise/fatigue (2%), dizziness (1% to 2%), drowsiness (1% to 2%), vertigo (1%)
  Gastrointestinal: Nausea (4% to 5%), hyposalivation (1%), vomiting (1%)
  Neuromuscular & skeletal: Paresthesia (1% to 2%)
  Ocular: Photophobia (1%)
  Miscellaneous: Ear/nose/throat infection (1%), pressure/tightness/heaviness sensations (1%), warm/cold temperature sensations (1%)

Drug Interactions
 Metabolism/Transport Effects None known.
 Avoid Concomitant Use
  Avoid concomitant use of Naratriptan with any of the following: Ergot Derivatives
 Increased Effect/Toxicity
  Naratriptan may increase the levels/effects of: Ergot Derivatives; Metoclopramide; Serotonin Modulators

  The levels/effects of Naratriptan may be increased by: Antipsychotics; Ergot Derivatives
 Decreased Effect There are no known significant interactions involving a decrease in effect.
Stability Store at 20°C to 25°C (68°F to 77°F).
Mechanism of Action Selective agonist for serotonin (5-HT$_{1B}$ and 5-HT$_{1D}$ receptors) in cranial arteries; causes vasoconstriction and reduces sterile inflammation associated with antidromic neuronal transmission correlating with relief of migraine
Pharmacodynamics/Kinetics
 Onset of action: ~1-2 hours (Bomhof, 1999; Tfelt-Hansen, 2000)
 Absorption: Well absorbed
 Distribution: V$_{dss}$: 170 L
 Protein binding, plasma: 28% to 31%
 Metabolism: Hepatic via CYP
 Bioavailability: ~70%
 Half-life, elimination: 6 hours; increased in renal impairment (moderate impairment; mean: 11 hours; range 7-20 hours); increased in hepatic impairment (moderate impairment: 8-16 hours)
 Time to peak: 2-3 hours
 Excretion: Urine (50% of total dose as unchanged drug; 30% of total dose as metabolites)
Dosage
 Geriatric Not recommended for use in the elderly.
 Adult Migraine: Oral: 1 mg to 2.5 mg at the onset of headache. It is recommended to use the lowest possible dose to minimize adverse effects. If headache returns or does not fully resolve, the dose may be repeated after 4 hours. Do not exceed 5 mg in 24 hours.
 Renal Impairment
  Mild-to-moderate renal impairment: Initial: 1 mg; do not exceed 2.5 mg in 24 hours.
  Severe renal impairment (Cl$_{cr}$ <15 mL/minute): Use is contraindicated.
 Hepatic Impairment
  Mild-to-moderate hepatic impairment (Child-Pugh grade A or B): Initial: 1 mg; do not exceed 2.5 mg in 24 hours
  Severe hepatic impairment (Child-Pugh grade C): Use is contraindicated.
Administration Do **not** crush or chew tablet; swallow whole with water.
Special Geriatric Considerations Naratriptan was not studied in patients >65 years of age. Use in elderly patients is not recommended because of the presence of risk factors associated with adverse effects. These include the presence of coronary artery disease, decreased liver or renal function, and the risk of pronounced blood pressure increases.
Dosage Forms Excipient information presented when available (limited, particularly for generics); consult specific product labeling.
 Tablet, oral: 1 mg, 2.5 mg
 Amerge®: 1 mg, 2.5 mg

- **Naratriptan Hydrochloride** *see* Naratriptan *on page 1344*
- **Narcan** *see* Naloxone *on page 1335*
- **Nardil®** *see* Phenelzine *on page 1517*
- **Nasacort® AQ** *see* Triamcinolone (Nasal) *on page 1960*
- **NasalCrom® [OTC]** *see* Cromolyn (Nasal) *on page 450*
- **Nascobal®** *see* Cyanocobalamin *on page 452*
- **Nasonex®** *see* Mometasone (Nasal) *on page 1306*
- **Natacyn®** *see* Natamycin *on page 1345*

Natamycin (na ta MYE sin)

Medication Safety Issues
 Sound-alike/look-alike issues:
  Natacyn® may be confused with Naprosyn®
Brand Names: U.S. Natacyn®
Brand Names: Canada Natacyn®
Index Terms Pimaricin
Generic Availability (U.S.) No
Pharmacologic Category Antifungal Agent, Ophthalmic

NATAMYCIN

Use Treatment of blepharitis, conjunctivitis, and keratitis caused by susceptible fungi (*Aspergillus*, *Candida*, *Cephalosporium*, *Fusarium*, and *Penicillium*)

Contraindications Hypersensitivity to natamycin or any component of the formulation

Warnings/Precautions For topical eye use only. Failure to improve (keratitis) after 7-10 days of administration suggests infection caused by a microorganism not susceptible to natamycin; efficacy as a single agent in fungal endophthalmitis has not been established. Suspension may adhere to epithelial ulcers; retention of the suspension in the fornices occurs regularly. Contains benzalkonium chloride which may be absorbed by contact lenses; remove contact lens prior to administration and wait 15 minutes before reinserting. Contact lens should not be worn if signs/symptoms of fungal blepharitis, conjunctivitis, and/or keratitis are present.

Adverse Reactions (Reflective of adult population; not specific for elderly) Post-marketing and/or case reports: Allergic reaction, chest pain, corneal opacity, dyspnea, eye discomfort, edema, hyperemia, irritation and/or pain, foreign body sensation, parasthesia, tearing, vision changes

Drug Interactions

Metabolism/Transport Effects None known.

Avoid Concomitant Use There are no known interactions where it is recommended to avoid concomitant use.

Increased Effect/Toxicity There are no known significant interactions involving an increase in effect.

Decreased Effect There are no known significant interactions involving a decrease in effect.

Stability Store at 2°C to 24°C (36°F to 75°F); do not freeze. Protect from excessive heat and light.

Mechanism of Action Increases cell membrane permeability in susceptible fungi

Pharmacodynamics/Kinetics

Absorption: Ophthalmic: Systemic, <2%; Gastrointestinal: Poor

Distribution: Adheres to cornea, retained in conjunctival fornices; does not produce effective intraocular fluid concentrations

Dosage

Geriatric & Adult

Fungal keratitis: Ophthalmic: Instill 1 drop in conjunctival sac every 1-2 hours, after 3-4 days reduce to one drop 6-8 times/day; usual course of therapy is 2-3 weeks or until resolution of active fungal keratitis (may be useful to gradually reduce dosage at 4-7 day intervals to assure elimination of organism)

Fungal blepharitis or conjunctivitis: Ophthalmic: Instill 1 drop in conjunctival sac every 4-6 hours

Administration Ophthalmic: Shake well before using, do not touch dropper to eye.

Monitoring Parameters Monitor tolerance to the drug at least twice weekly

Special Geriatric Considerations Evaluate the patient's or caregiver's ability to safely administer the correct dose of ophthalmic medication.

Dosage Forms Excipient information presented when available (limited, particularly for generics); consult specific product labeling.

Suspension, ophthalmic [drops]:

Natacyn® 5% (15 mL) [contains benzalkonium chloride]

Nateglinide (na te GLYE nide)

Related Information

Diabetes Mellitus Management, Adults *on page 2193*

Medication Safety Issues

High alert medication:

The Institute for Safe Medication Practices (ISMP) includes this medication among its list of drug classes which have a heightened risk of causing significant patient harm when used in error.

Brand Names: U.S. Starlix®

Brand Names: Canada Starlix®

Generic Availability (U.S.) Yes

Pharmacologic Category Antidiabetic Agent, Meglitinide Derivative

Use Management of type 2 diabetes mellitus (noninsulin dependent, NIDDM) as monotherapy when hyperglycemia cannot be managed by diet and exercise alone; in combination with metformin or a thiazolidinedione to lower blood glucose in patients whose hyperglycemia cannot be controlled by exercise, diet, or a single agent alone

Contraindications Hypersensitivity to nateglinide or any component of the formulation; diabetic ketoacidosis, with or without coma (treat with insulin); type 1 diabetes mellitus (insulin dependent, IDDM)

Warnings/Precautions Use with caution in patients with moderate-to-severe hepatic impairment. Use caution in severe renal dysfunction, elderly, malnourished, or patients with adrenal/pituitary dysfunction; may be more susceptible to glucose-lowering effects. All oral hypoglycemic agents are capable of producing hypoglycemia. Proper patient selection, dosage, and instructions to the patients are important to avoid hypoglycemic episodes. It may be necessary to discontinue nateglinide and administer insulin if the patient is exposed to stress (ie, fever, trauma, infection, surgery). Indicated for adjunctive therapy with metformin; not to be used as a substitute for metformin monotherapy. Combination treatment with sulfonylureas is not recommended (no additional benefit). Patients not adequately controlled on oral agents which stimulate insulin release (eg, glyburide) should not be switched to nateglinide or have nateglinide added to therapy.

Adverse Reactions (Reflective of adult population; not specific for elderly) As reported with nateglinide monotherapy:

>10%: Respiratory: Upper respiratory infection (11%)

1% to 10%:

Central nervous system: Dizziness (4%)

Endocrine & metabolic: Hypoglycemia (2%), uric acid increased

Gastrointestinal: Diarrhea (3%), weight gain

Neuromuscular & skeletal: Back pain, (4%), arthropathy (3%)

Respiratory: Bronchitis (3%), cough (2%)

Miscellaneous: Flu-like syndrome (4%)

Drug Interactions

Metabolism/Transport Effects Substrate of CYP2C9 (major), CYP3A4 (major), SLCO1B1; **Note:** Assignment of Major/Minor substrate status based on clinically relevant drug interaction potential; **Inhibits** CYP2C9 (weak)

Avoid Concomitant Use

Avoid concomitant use of Nateglinide with any of the following: Conivaptan

Increased Effect/Toxicity

Nateglinide may increase the levels/effects of: Hypoglycemic Agents

The levels/effects of Nateglinide may be increased by: Conivaptan; CYP2C9 Inhibitors (Moderate); CYP2C9 Inhibitors (Strong); CYP3A4 Inhibitors (Moderate); CYP3A4 Inhibitors (Strong); Dasatinib; Eltrombopag; Herbs (Hypoglycemic Properties); Ivacaftor; MAO Inhibitors; Mifepristone; Pegvisomant; Salicylates; Selective Serotonin Reuptake Inhibitors

Decreased Effect

The levels/effects of Nateglinide may be decreased by: Corticosteroids (Orally Inhaled); Corticosteroids (Systemic); CYP2C9 Inducers (Strong); CYP3A4 Inducers (Strong); Deferasirox; Herbs (CYP3A4 Inducers); Loop Diuretics; Luteinizing Hormone-Releasing Hormone Analogs; Peginterferon Alfa-2b; Somatropin; Thiazide Diuretics; Tocilizumab

Ethanol/Nutrition/Herb Interactions

Ethanol: Avoid ethanol (increased risk of hypoglycemia).

Food: Rate of absorption is decreased and time to T_{max} is delayed when taken with food. Food does not affect AUC. Multiple peak plasma concentrations may be observed if fasting. Not affected by composition of meal.

Herb/Nutraceutical: Avoid alfalfa, aloe, bilberry, bitter melon, burdock, celery, damiana, fenugreek, garcinia, garlic, ginger, ginseng (American), gymnema, marshmallow, and stinging nettle (may enhance the hypoglycemic effects of antidiabetic agents). St. John's wort may decrease the levels/effect of nateglinide.

Stability Store at 25°C (77°F).

Mechanism of Action A phenylalanine derivative, nonsulfonylurea hypoglycemic agent used in the management of type 2 diabetes mellitus (noninsulin dependent, NIDDM); stimulates insulin release from the pancreatic beta cells to reduce postprandial hyperglycemia; amount of insulin release is dependent upon existing glucose levels

Pharmacodynamics/Kinetics

Onset of action: Insulin secretion: ~20 minutes

Peak effect: 1 hour

Duration: 4 hours

Absorption: Rapid

Distribution: 10 L

Protein binding: 98%, primarily to albumin

Metabolism: Hepatic via hydroxylation followed by glucuronide conjugation via CYP2C9 (70%) and CYP3A4 (30%) to metabolites

Bioavailability: 73%

Half-life elimination: 1.5 hours

Time to peak: ≤1 hour

Excretion: Urine (83%, 16% as unchanged drug); feces (10%)

Dosage

Geriatric & Adult Management of type 2 diabetes mellitus: Oral: Initial and maintenance dose: 120 mg 3 times/day, 1-30 minutes before meals; may be given alone or in combination with metformin or a thiazolidinedione; patients close to Hb A_{1c} goal may be started at 60 mg 3 times/day

Renal Impairment No specific dosage adjustment is recommended for patients with mild-to-severe renal disease. Patients on dialysis showed reduced medication exposure and plasma protein binding. Patients with severe renal dysfunction are more susceptible to glucose-lowering effect; use with caution.

Hepatic Impairment Increased serum levels are seen with mild hepatic insufficiency; no dosage adjustment is needed. Has not been studied in patients with moderate-to-severe liver disease; use with caution.

Administration Patients who are anorexic or NPO will need to have their dose held to avoid hypoglycemia.

Monitoring Parameters Glucose and Hb A_{1c} levels, weight, lipid profile

Reference Range
Recommendations for glycemic control in adults with diabetes:
Hb A_{1c}: <7%
Preprandial capillary plasma glucose: 70-130 mg/dL
Peak postprandial capillary blood glucose: <180 mg/dL
Blood pressure: <130/80 mm Hg
Recommendations for glycemic control in older adults with diabetes:
Relatively healthy, cognitively intact, and with a ≥5-year life expectancy: See Adults
Frail, life expectancy <5-years or those for whom the risks of intensive glucose control outweigh the benefits:
Hb A_{1c}: <8% to 9%
Blood pressure: <140/80 mm Hg or <130/80 mm Hg if tolerated

Pharmacotherapy Pearls An increase in weight was seen in nateglinide monotherapy, which was not seen when used in combination with metformin.

Special Geriatric Considerations No changes in safety and efficacy were seen in patients ≥65 years; however, some older adults may show increased sensitivity to dosing. Intensive glucose control (Hb A_{1c} <6.5%) has been linked to increased all-cause and cardiovascular mortality, hypoglycemia requiring assistance, and weight gain in adult type 2 diabetes. How "tightly" to control a geriatric patient's blood glucose needs to be individualized. Such a decision should be based on several factors, including the patient's functional and cognitive status, how well he/she recognizes hypoglycemic or hyperglycemic symptoms, and how to respond to them and other disease states. An Hb A_{1c} <7.5% is an acceptable endpoint for a healthy older adult, while <8% is acceptable for frail elderly patients, those with a duration of illness >10 years, or those with comorbid conditions and requiring combination diabetes medications. Patients who are unable to accurately draw up their dose will need assistance, such as prefilled syringes. Initial doses may require considerations for renal function in the elderly with dosing adjusted subsequently based on blood glucose monitoring. For elderly patients with diabetes who are relatively healthy, attaining target goals for aspirin use, blood pressure, lipids, smoking cessation, and diet and exercise may be more important than normalized glycemic control.

Dosage Forms Excipient information presented when available (limited, particularly for generics); consult specific product labeling.
Tablet, oral: 60 mg, 120 mg
Starlix®: 60 mg, 120 mg

Nebivolol (ne BIV oh lole)

Related Information
Beta-Blockers on page 2108
Brand Names: U.S. Bystolic®
Index Terms Nebivolol Hydrochloride
Generic Availability (U.S.) No

Pharmacologic Category Beta-Blocker, Beta-1 Selective

Use Treatment of hypertension, alone or in combination with other agents

Unlabeled Use Heart failure

Contraindications Hypersensitivity to nebivolol or any component of the formulation; severe bradycardia; heart block greater than first-degree (except in patients with a functioning artificial pacemaker); cardiogenic shock; decompensated cardiac failure; sick sinus syndrome (unless a permanent pacemaker is in place); severe hepatic impairment (Child-Pugh class C)

Warnings/Precautions Use caution in patients with heart failure (HF); use gradual and careful titration; monitor for symptoms of congestive heart failure. Patients should be stabilized on HF regimen prior to initiation of beta-blocker; adjustment of other medications (ACE inhibitors and/or diuretics) may be required. **Note:** Nebivolol has not been shown to reduce morbidity or mortality in the general HF population. Use with caution in patients with myasthenia gravis, psychiatric disease (may cause CNS depression), bronchospastic disease, undergoing anesthesia; and in those with impaired hepatic function. Bradycardia may be observed more frequently in elderly patients (>65 years of age); dosage reductions may be necessary. Nebivolol should not be withdrawn abruptly (particularly in patients with CAD), but gradually tapered over 1-2 weeks to avoid acute tachycardia, hypertension, and/or ischemia. Chronic beta-blocker therapy should not be routinely withdrawn prior to major surgery. Can precipitate or aggravate symptoms of arterial insufficiency in patients with PVD and Raynaud's disease. Use with caution and monitor for progression of arterial obstruction. Use caution with concurrent use of digoxin, verapamil, or diltiazem; bradycardia or heart block may occur. Use caution with concurrent use of CYP2D6 inhibitors. Use with caution in patients receiving inhaled anesthetic agents known to depress myocardial contractility.

Nebivolol, with beta$_1$-selectivity, may be used cautiously in bronchospastic disease with close monitoring. Use cautiously in patients with diabetes because it can mask prominent hypoglycemic symptoms. May mask signs of hyperthyroidism (eg, tachycardia); if hyperthyroidism is suspected, carefully manage and monitor; abrupt withdrawal may exacerbate symptoms of hyperthyroidism or precipitate thyroid storm. Dosage adjustment is required in patients with moderate hepatic or severe renal impairment. Adequate alpha-blockade is required prior to use of any beta-blocker for patients with untreated pheochromocytoma. May induce or exacerbate psoriasis. Use caution with history of severe anaphylaxis to allergens; patients taking beta-blockers may become more sensitive to repeated challenges. Treatment of anaphylaxis (eg, epinephrine) in patients taking beta-blockers may be ineffective or promote undesirable effects.

Adverse Reactions (Reflective of adult population; not specific for elderly) 1% to 10%:

Cardiovascular: Peripheral edema (1%), bradycardia (≤1%), chest pain (≤1%)

Central nervous system: Headache (6% to 9%), fatigue (dose related; 2% to 5%), dizziness (2% to 4%), insomnia (1%)

Dermatologic: Rash (≤1%)

Endocrine & metabolic: HDL levels decreased, hypercholesterolemia, triglyceride levels increased, uric acid levels increased

Gastrointestinal: Diarrhea (dose related; 2% to 3%), nausea (1% to 3%), abdominal pain

Hematologic: Platelet count decreased

Neuromuscular & skeletal: Paresthesia, weakness

Renal: BUN increased

Respiratory: Dyspnea (≤1%)

Drug Interactions

Metabolism/Transport Effects Substrate of CYP2D6 (minor); **Note:** Assignment of Major/Minor substrate status based on clinically relevant drug interaction potential

Avoid Concomitant Use

Avoid concomitant use of Nebivolol with any of the following: Floctafenine; Methacholine

Increased Effect/Toxicity

Nebivolol may increase the levels/effects of: Alpha-/Beta-Agonists (Direct-Acting); Alpha1-Blockers; Alpha2-Agonists; Amifostine; Antihypertensives; Antipsychotic Agents (Phenothiazines); Bupivacaine; Cardiac Glycosides; Cholinergic Agonists; Fingolimod; Hypotensive Agents; Insulin; Lidocaine; Lidocaine (Systemic); Lidocaine (Topical); Mepivacaine; Methacholine; Midodrine; RiTUXimab; Sulfonylureas

The levels/effects of Nebivolol may be increased by: Acetylcholinesterase Inhibitors; Aminoquinolines (Antimalarial); Amiodarone; Anilidopiperidine Opioids; Antipsychotic Agents (Phenothiazines); Calcium Channel Blockers (Dihydropyridine); Calcium Channel Blockers (Nondihydropyridine); CYP2D6 Inhibitors (Moderate); CYP2D6 Inhibitors (Strong); Diazoxide; Dipyridamole; Disopyramide; Dronedarone; Floctafenine; Herbs (Hypotensive Properties); MAO Inhibitors; Pentoxifylline; Phosphodiesterase 5 Inhibitors; Propafenone; Prostacyclin Analogues; QuiNIDine; Reserpine; Selective Serotonin Reuptake Inhibitors

Decreased Effect
Nebivolol may decrease the levels/effects of: Beta2-Agonists; Theophylline Derivatives

The levels/effects of Nebivolol may be decreased by: Barbiturates; Herbs (Hypertensive Properties); Methylphenidate; Nonsteroidal Anti-Inflammatory Agents; Peginterferon Alfa-2b; Rifamycin Derivatives; Yohimbine

Ethanol/Nutrition/Herb Interactions Herb/Nutraceutical: Avoid bayberry, blue cohosh, cayenne, ephedra, ginger, ginseng (American), kola, licorice (may worsen hypertension). Avoid black cohosh, California poppy, coleus, golden seal, hawthorn, mistletoe, periwinkle, quinine, shepherd's purse (may increase antihypertensive effect).

Stability Store at 20°C to 25°C (68°F to 77°F). Protect from light.

Mechanism of Action Highly-selective inhibitor of beta$_1$-adrenergic receptors; at doses ≤10 mg nebivolol preferentially blocks beta$_1$-receptors. Nebivolol, unlike other beta-blockers, also produces an endothelium-derived nitric oxide-dependent vasodilation resulting in a reduction of systemic vascular resistance.

Pharmacodynamics/Kinetics
Absorption: Rapid
Distribution: V_d: 8-12 L/kg
Protein binding: ~98%, primarily to albumin
Metabolism: Hepatic; via glucuronidation and CYP2D6; extensive first-pass metabolism to multiple active metabolites with variable activity
Bioavailability: ~12% (extensive metabolizers); 96% (poor metabolizers)
Half-life elimination: Terminal: 10-12 hours (extensive metabolizers); 19-32 hours in poor metabolizers
Time to peak, plasma: 1.5-4 hours
Excretion: Urine (extensive metabolizers: 38%; poor metabolizers: 67%; <0.5% of total dose as unchanged drug); feces (extensive metabolizers: 44%; poor metabolizers: 13%; <0.5% of total dose as unchanged drug)

Dosage
Geriatric & Adult
Hypertension: Oral: Initial: 5 mg once daily; if initial response is inadequate, may be increased at 2-week intervals to a maximum dose of 40 mg once daily
Heart failure (unlabeled use): Adults ≥70 years: Oral: Initial: 1.25 mg once daily; if tolerated, may increase by 2.5 mg at 1- to 2-week intervals to a maximum dose of 10 mg once daily (Flather, 2005). **Note:** Nebivolol has not been shown to reduce morbidity or mortality in the general HF population.

Renal Impairment Severe impairment (Cl_{cr} <30 mL/minute): Initial: 2.5 mg/day; increase cautiously.

Hepatic Impairment Moderate impairment (Child-Pugh class B): Initial: 2.5 mg/day; increase cautiously.

Administration May be administered with or without food.

Monitoring Parameters Blood pressure, ECG; serum glucose (in diabetic patients)

Special Geriatric Considerations Due to alterations in the beta-adrenergic autonomic nervous system, beta-adrenergic blockade may result in less hemodynamic response than seen in younger adults. Studies indicate that despite decreased sensitivity to the chronotropic effects of beta-blockade with age, there appears to be an increased myocardial sensitivity to the negative inotropic effect during stress (eg, exercise). Controlled trials have shown the overall response rate for propranolol to be only 20% to 50% in elderly populations. Therefore, all beta-adrenergic blocking drugs may result in a decreased response as compared to younger adults.

Dosage Forms Excipient information presented when available (limited, particularly for generics); consult specific product labeling.
Tablet, oral:
Bystolic®: 2.5 mg, 5 mg, 10 mg, 20 mg

◆ **Nebivolol Hydrochloride** *see* Nebivolol *on page* 1348
◆ **NebuSal™** *see* Sodium Chloride *on page* 1787

Nedocromil (ne doe KROE mil)

Related Information
Inhalant Agents *on page* 2117
Brand Names: U.S. Alocril®
Brand Names: Canada Alocril®
Index Terms Nedocromil Sodium
Generic Availability (U.S.) No
Pharmacologic Category Mast Cell Stabilizer

Use Treatment of itching associated with allergic conjunctivitis

Contraindications Hypersensitivity to nedocromil or any component of the formulation

Warnings/Precautions Ophthalmic solution contains benzalkonium chloride, which may be absorbed by contact lenses; users of contact lenses should not wear them during periods of symptomatic allergic conjunctivitis.

Adverse Reactions (Reflective of adult population; not specific for elderly)
>10%:
Central nervous system: Headache (40%)
Gastrointestinal: Unpleasant taste
Ocular: Burning, irritation, stinging
Respiratory: Nasal congestion
1% to 10%:
Ocular: Conjunctivitis, eye redness, photophobia
Respiratory: Asthma, rhinitis

Drug Interactions
Metabolism/Transport Effects None known.
Avoid Concomitant Use There are no known interactions where it is recommended to avoid concomitant use.
Increased Effect/Toxicity There are no known significant interactions involving an increase in effect.
Decreased Effect There are no known significant interactions involving a decrease in effect.

Stability Store at 2°C to 25°C (36°F to 77°F).

Mechanism of Action Inhibits the activation of and mediator release from a variety of inflammatory cell types associated with hypersensitivity reactions including eosinophils, neutrophils, macrophages, mast cells, monocytes, and platelets; it inhibits the release of histamine, leukotrienes, and slow-reacting substance of anaphylaxis.

Pharmacodynamics/Kinetics
Absorption: Low (<4%)
Excretion: Urine 70% (as unchanged drug); feces 30% (as unchanged drug)

Dosage
Geriatric & Adult Allergic conjunctivitis: Ophthalmic: 1-2 drops in each eye twice daily throughout the period of exposure to allergen

Administration For ophthalmic use only; do not allow tip of container to touch eye, surrounding structures, fingers, or other surfaces to avoid bacterial contamination.

Special Geriatric Considerations Evaluate the patient's or caregiver's ability to safely administer the correct dose of ophthalmic medication.

Dosage Forms Excipient information presented when available (limited, particularly for generics); consult specific product labeling.
Solution, ophthalmic, as sodium [drops]:
Alocril®: 2% (5 mL) [contains benzalkonium chloride]

◆ **Nedocromil Sodium** see Nedocromil on page 1350

Nefazodone (nef AY zoe done)

Related Information
Antidepressant Agents on page 2097
Medication Safety Issues
Sound-alike/look-alike issues:
Serzone® may be confused with selegiline, SEROquel®, sertraline
Index Terms Nefazodone Hydrochloride; Serzone
Generic Availability (U.S.) Yes
Pharmacologic Category Antidepressant, Serotonin Reuptake Inhibitor/Antagonist
Use Treatment of depression
Unlabeled Use Treatment of post-traumatic stress disorder
Medication Guide Available Yes
Contraindications Hypersensitivity to nefazodone, related compounds (phenylpiperazines), or any component of the formulation; liver injury due to previous nefazodone treatment, active liver disease, or elevated serum transaminases; concurrent use or use of MAO inhibitors within previous 14 days; use in a patient during the acute recovery phase of MI; concurrent use with carbamazepine, cisapride, or pimozide; concurrent therapy with triazolam or alprazolam is generally contraindicated (dosage must be reduced by 75% for triazolam and 50% for alprazolam; such reductions may not be possible with available dosage forms).
Warnings/Precautions [U.S. Boxed Warning]: Antidepressants increase the risk of suicidal thinking and behavior in children, adolescents, and young adults (18-24 years of age) with major depressive disorder (MDD) and other psychiatric disorders; consider ▶

risk prior to prescribing. Short-term studies did not show an increased risk in patients >24 years of age and showed a decreased risk in patients ≥65 years. Closely monitor for clinical worsening, suicidality, or unusual changes in behavior; the patient's family or caregiver should be instructed to closely observe the patient and communicate condition with healthcare provider. A medication guide should be dispensed with each prescription.

The possibility of a suicide attempt is inherent in major depression and may persist until remission occurs. Monitor for worsening of depression or suicidality, especially during initiation of therapy (generally first 1-2 months) or with dose increases or decreases. Use caution in high-risk patients. Worsening depression and severe abrupt suicidality that are not part of the presenting symptoms may require discontinuation or modification of drug therapy. The patient's family or caregiver should be alerted to monitor patients for the emergence of suicidality and associated behaviors (such as agitation, irritability, hostility, impulsivity, and hypomania) and call healthcare provider.

May worsen psychosis in some patients or precipitate a shift to mania or hypomania in patients with bipolar disorder. Patients presenting with depressive symptoms should be screened for bipolar disorder. Monotherapy in patients with bipolar disorder should be avoided. **Nefazodone is not FDA approved for the treatment of bipolar depression.**

Cases of life-threatening hepatic failure have been reported (risk should be considered when choosing an agent for the treatment of depression); discontinue if clinical signs or symptoms suggest liver failure. May cause sedation, resulting in impaired performance of tasks requiring alertness (eg, operating machinery or driving). May increase the risks associated with electroconvulsive therapy. Consider discontinuing, when possible, prior to elective surgery. Therapy should not be abruptly discontinued in patients receiving high doses for prolonged periods. Rare reports of priapism have occurred. The incidence of sexual dysfunction with nefazodone is generally lower than with SSRIs.

The risk of sedation, conduction disturbances, orthostatic hypotension, or anticholinergic effects are very low relative to other antidepressants. Use with caution in patients with a history of cardiovascular disease (including previous MI, stroke, tachycardia, or conduction abnormalities). Use with caution in patients with urinary retention, benign prostatic hyperplasia, narrow-angle glaucoma, xerostomia, visual problems, constipation, or history of bowel obstruction (due to anticholinergic effects).

Use caution in patients with a previous seizure disorder or condition predisposing to seizures such as brain damage, alcoholism, or concurrent therapy with other drugs which lower the seizure threshold. Use with caution in patients with renal dysfunction and in elderly patients.

Adverse Reactions (Reflective of adult population; not specific for elderly)

>10%:
Central nervous system: Headache, drowsiness, insomnia, agitation, dizziness
Gastrointestinal: Xerostomia, nausea, constipation
Neuromuscular & skeletal: Weakness

1% to 10%:
Cardiovascular: Bradycardia, hypotension, orthostatic hypotension, peripheral edema, vasodilation
Central nervous system: Chills, fever, incoordination, lightheadedness, confusion, memory impairment, abnormal dreams, decreased concentration, ataxia, psychomotor retardation, tremor
Dermatologic: Pruritus, rash
Endocrine & metabolic: Breast pain, impotence, libido decreased
Gastrointestinal: Gastroenteritis, vomiting, dyspepsia, diarrhea, increased appetite, thirst, taste perversion
Genitourinary: Urinary frequency, urinary retention
Hematologic: Hematocrit decreased
Neuromuscular & skeletal: Arthralgia, hypertonia, paresthesia, neck rigidity, tremor
Ocular: Blurred vision (9%), abnormal vision (7%), eye pain, visual field defect
Otic: Tinnitus
Respiratory: Bronchitis, cough, dyspnea, pharyngitis
Miscellaneous: Flu syndrome, infection

Drug Interactions

Metabolism/Transport Effects Substrate of CYP2D6 (major), CYP3A4 (major); **Note:** Assignment of Major/Minor substrate status based on clinically relevant drug interaction potential; **Inhibits** CYP1A2 (weak), CYP2B6 (weak), CYP2C8 (weak), CYP2D6 (weak), CYP3A4 (strong); **Induces** P-glycoprotein

Avoid Concomitant Use

Avoid concomitant use of Nefazodone with any of the following: Alfuzosin; Avanafil; Axitinib; CarBAMazepine; Cisapride; Conivaptan; Crizotinib; Dabigatran Etexilate; Dronedarone; Eplerenone; Everolimus; Fluticasone (Oral Inhalation); Halofantrine; Lapatinib; Lovastatin;

Lurasidone; MAO Inhibitors; Methylene Blue; Nilotinib; Nisoldipine; Pimozide; Ranolazine; Red Yeast Rice; Rivaroxaban; RomiDEPsin; Salmeterol; Silodosin; Simvastatin; Tamsulosin; Ticagrelor; Tolvaptan; Toremifene

Increased Effect/Toxicity

Nefazodone may increase the levels/effects of: Alfuzosin; Almotriptan; Alosetron; Antipsychotic Agents (Phenothiazines); ARIPiprazole; Avanafil; Axitinib; Bortezomib; Brentuximab Vedotin; Brinzolamide; Budesonide (Nasal); Budesonide (Systemic, Oral Inhalation); CarBAMazepine; Cardiac Glycosides; Ciclesonide; Cisapride; CloZAPine; Colchicine; Conivaptan; Corticosteroids (Orally Inhaled); Crizotinib; CYP3A4 Substrates; Dienogest; Dronedarone; Dutasteride; Eplerenone; Everolimus; FentaNYL; Fesoterodine; Fluticasone (Nasal); Fluticasone (Oral Inhalation); GuanFACINE; Halofantrine; Iloperidone; Ivacaftor; Ixabepilone; Lapatinib; Lovastatin; Lumefantrine; Lurasidone; Maraviroc; Methylene Blue; MethylPREDNISolone; Metoclopramide; Mifepristone; Nilotinib; Nisoldipine; Paricalcitol; Pazopanib; Pimecrolimus; Pimozide; Propafenone; Ranolazine; Red Yeast Rice; Rivaroxaban; RomiDEPsin; Ruxolitinib; Salmeterol; Saxagliptin; Serotonin Modulators; Sildenafil; Silodosin; Simvastatin; SORAfenib; Tacrolimus; Tacrolimus (Systemic); Tacrolimus (Topical); Tadalafil; Tamsulosin; Ticagrelor; Tolterodine; Tolvaptan; Toremifene; Vardenafil; Vemurafenib; Vilazodone; Zuclopenthixol

The levels/effects of Nefazodone may be increased by: Abiraterone Acetate; Antipsychotic Agents (Phenothiazines); Antipsychotics; BusPIRone; CYP2D6 Inhibitors (Moderate); CYP2D6 Inhibitors (Strong); CYP3A4 Inhibitors (Moderate); CYP3A4 Inhibitors (Strong); Dasatinib; Linezolid; MAO Inhibitors; Protease Inhibitors; Selective Serotonin Reuptake Inhibitors

Decreased Effect

Nefazodone may decrease the levels/effects of: Dabigatran Etexilate; Ifosfamide; Linagliptin; P-glycoprotein/ABCB1 Substrates; Prasugrel; Ticagrelor

The levels/effects of Nefazodone may be decreased by: CarBAMazepine; CYP3A4 Inducers (Strong); Deferasirox; Peginterferon Alfa-2b; Tocilizumab

Ethanol/Nutrition/Herb Interactions

Ethanol: May increase CNS depression; monitor for increased effects with coadministration. Caution patients about effects.

Food: Nefazodone absorption may be delayed and bioavailability may be decreased if taken with food.

Herb/Nutraceutical: Avoid valerian, St John's wort, SAMe, kava kava (may increase risk of serotonin syndrome and/or excessive sedation).

Stability Store at room temperature, below 40°C (104°F) in a tight container.

Mechanism of Action Inhibits neuronal reuptake of serotonin and norepinephrine; also blocks $5-HT_2$ and alpha$_1$ receptors; has no significant affinity for alpha$_2$, beta-adrenergic, $5-HT_{1A}$, cholinergic, dopaminergic, or benzodiazepine receptors

Pharmacodynamics/Kinetics

Onset of action: Therapeutic: Up to 6 weeks

Distribution: V_d: 0.22-0.87 L/kg

Protein binding: >99%

Metabolism: Hepatic to three active metabolites: Triazoledione, hydroxynefazodone, and m-chlorophenylpiperazine (mCPP)

Bioavailability: 20% (variable)

Half-life elimination: Parent drug: 2-4 hours; active metabolites persist longer

Time to peak, serum: 1 hour, prolonged in presence of food

Excretion: Primarily urine (as metabolites); feces

Dosage

Geriatric Oral: Initial: 50 mg twice daily; increase dose to 100 mg twice daily in 2 weeks; usual maintenance dose: 200-400 mg/day

Adult

Depression: Oral: 200 mg/day, administered in two divided doses initially, with a range of 300-600 mg/day in 2 divided doses thereafter.

Post-traumatic stress disorder (PTSD) (unlabeled use): Oral: Initial: 100 mg twice daily; target dose: 600 mg/day (average daily dose: 463 mg).

Administration Dosing after meals may decrease lightheadedness and postural hypotension, but may also decrease absorption and therefore effectiveness.

Monitoring Parameters If AST/ALT increase >3 times ULN, the drug should be discontinued and not reintroduced; mental status for depression, suicide ideation (especially at the beginning of therapy or when doses are increased or decreased), anxiety, social functioning, mania, panic attacks

Reference Range Therapeutic plasma levels have not yet been defined

Pharmacotherapy Pearls May cause less sexual dysfunction than other antidepressants. Women and elderly receiving single doses attain significant higher peak concentrations than male volunteers.

Special Geriatric Considerations Data on nefazodone in the elderly are limited, specifically regarding efficacy; clinical trials in adult patients have found it superior to placebo and similar to imipramine. Nefazodone's C_{max} and AUC have been reported to be increased twofold in the elderly and women after a single dose compared to younger patients; however, these differences were markedly reduced with multiple dosing with women having AUC values of nefazodone and its hydroxy metabolite remaining approximately 50% higher

A systematic review and meta-analysis of antidepressant placebo-controlled trials in persons with depression and dementia found evidence "suggestive" of efficacy but not of sufficient strength to "confirm" efficacy. Antidepressant trials in this patient population are small and underpowered. Older patients with depression being treated with an antidepressant should be closely monitored for response and adverse effects. Treatment should be switched or augmented when response is inadequate with a therapeutic dose. Antidepressants that are not tolerated should be discontinued and an alternative agent should be started.

Dosage Forms Excipient information presented when available (limited, particularly for generics); consult specific product labeling.
Tablet, oral, as hydrochloride: 50 mg, 100 mg, 150 mg, 200 mg, 250 mg

◆ **Nefazodone Hydrochloride** *see* Nefazodone *on page 1351*
◆ **Neofrin** *see* Phenylephrine (Ophthalmic) *on page 1526*

Neomycin and Polymyxin B (nee oh MYE sin & pol i MIKS in bee)

Brand Names: U.S. Neosporin® G.U. Irrigant
Brand Names: Canada Neosporin® Irrigating Solution
Index Terms Polymyxin B and Neomycin
Generic Availability (U.S.) Yes
Pharmacologic Category Antibiotic, Topical; Genitourinary Irrigant
Use Short-term as a continuous irrigant or rinse in the urinary bladder to prevent bacteriuria and gram-negative rod septicemia associated with the use of indwelling catheters
Contraindications Hypersensitivity to neomycin, polymyxin B, or any component of the formulation
Adverse Reactions (Reflective of adult population; not specific for elderly) Frequency not defined.
Dermatologic: Contact dermatitis, erythema, rash, urticaria
Genitourinary: Bladder irritation
Local: Burning
Neuromuscular & skeletal: Neuromuscular blockade
Otic: Ototoxicity
Renal: Nephrotoxicity
Drug Interactions
Metabolism/Transport Effects None known.
Avoid Concomitant Use
Avoid concomitant use of Neomycin and Polymyxin B with any of the following: BCG; Gallium Nitrate
Increased Effect/Toxicity
Neomycin and Polymyxin B may increase the levels/effects of: AbobotulinumtoxinA; Acarbose; Bisphosphonate Derivatives; CARBOplatin; Colistimethate; CycloSPORINE; CycloSPORINE (Systemic); Gallium Nitrate; Neuromuscular-Blocking Agents; OnabotulinumtoxinA; RimabotulinumtoxinB; Vitamin K Antagonists

The levels/effects of Neomycin and Polymyxin B may be increased by: Amphotericin B; Capreomycin; Cephalosporins (2nd Generation); Cephalosporins (3rd Generation); Cephalosporins (4th Generation); CISplatin; Loop Diuretics; Nonsteroidal Anti-Inflammatory Agents; Vancomycin
Decreased Effect
Neomycin and Polymyxin B may decrease the levels/effects of: BCG; Cardiac Glycosides; SORAfenib

The levels/effects of Neomycin and Polymyxin B may be decreased by: Penicillins
Stability Store irrigation solution in refrigerator. The following stability information has also been reported: May be stored at room temperature for up to 6 months if undiluted (Cohen, 2007). Aseptically prepared dilutions (1 mL/1 L) should be stored in the refrigerator and discarded after 48 hours.

Mechanism of Action Neomycin: Interferes with bacterial protein synthesis by binding to 30S ribosomal subunits

Polymyxin B: Binds to phospholipids, alters permeability, and damages the bacterial cytoplasmic membrane permitting leakage of intracellular constituents

Pharmacodynamics/Kinetics Absorption: Topical: Clinically insignificant amounts of neomycin and polymyxin B are absorbed following irrigation of an intact urinary bladder. Systemic absorption may occur from a denuded bladder.

Dosage
  Geriatric & Adult Bladder irrigation: **Not for I.V. injection**; add 1 mL irrigant to 1 L isotonic saline solution and connect container to the inflow of lumen of 3-way catheter. Continuous irrigant or rinse in the urinary bladder for up to a maximum of 10 days with administration rate adjusted to patient's urine output; usually no more than 1 L of irrigant is used per day.
  Administration Bladder irrigant: Do not inject irrigant solution; concentrated irrigant solution must be diluted in 1 L normal saline before administration; connect irrigation container to the inflow lumen of a 3-way catheter to permit continuous irrigation of the urinary bladder

Special Geriatric Considerations No specific information for use in elderly.

Dosage Forms Excipient information presented when available (limited, particularly for generics); consult specific product labeling.
  Solution, irrigation: Neomycin 40 mg and polymyxin B sulfate 200,000 units per 1 mL (1 mL, 20 mL)
    Neosporin® G.U. Irrigant: Neomycin 40 mg and polymyxin sulfate B 200,000 units per 1 mL (1 mL, 20 mL)

Neomycin, Colistin, Hydrocortisone, and Thonzonium
(nee oh MYE sin, koe LIS tin, hye droe KOR ti sone, & thon ZOE nee um)

Brand Names: U.S. Coly-Mycin® S; Cortisporin®-TC
Index Terms Colistin, Hydrocortisone, Neomycin, and Thonzonium; Hydrocortisone, Neomycin, Colistin, and Thonzonium; Thonzonium, Neomycin, Colistin, and Hydrocortisone
Generic Availability (U.S.) No
Pharmacologic Category Antibiotic, Otic; Antibiotic/Corticosteroid, Otic; Corticosteroid, Otic
Use Treatment of superficial and susceptible bacterial infections of the external auditory canal; for treatment of susceptible bacterial infections of mastoidectomy and fenestration cavities
Dosage
  Geriatric & Adult Ear inflammation/infection: Otic:
  Calibrated dropper: 5 drops in affected ear 3-4 times/day
  Dropper bottle: 4 drops in affected ear 3-4 times/day
    Note: Alternatively, a cotton wick may be inserted in the ear canal and saturated with suspension every 4 hours; wick should be replaced at least every 24 hours
Special Geriatric Considerations No specific information in the elderly.
Dosage Forms Excipient information presented when available (limited, particularly for generics); consult specific product labeling.
  Suspension, otic [drops]:
  Coly-Mycin® S: Neomycin 0.33%, colistin 0.3%, hydrocortisone acetate 1%, and thonzonium bromide 0.05% (5 mL) [contains thimerosal]
  Cortisporin®-TC: Neomycin 0.33%, colistin 0.3%, hydrocortisone acetate 1%, and thonzonium bromide 0.05% (10 mL) [contains thimerosal]

Neomycin, Polymyxin B, and Dexamethasone
(nee oh MYE sin, pol i MIKS in bee, & deks a METH a sone)

Related Information
  Dexamethasone (Ophthalmic) *on page 521*
Brand Names: U.S. Maxitrol®
Brand Names: Canada Dioptrol®; Maxitrol®
Index Terms Dexamethasone, Neomycin, and Polymyxin B; Polymyxin B, Neomycin, and Dexamethasone
Generic Availability (U.S.) Yes
Pharmacologic Category Antibiotic/Corticosteroid, Ophthalmic
Use Steroid-responsive inflammatory ocular conditions in which a corticosteroid is indicated and where bacterial infection or a risk of bacterial infection exists
Contraindications Hypersensitivity to neomycin, polymyxin B, dexamethasone, or any component of the formulation; viral disease of the cornea and conjunctiva (including epithelial herpes simplex keratitis [dendritic keratitis], vaccinia, varicella); mycobacterial or fungal infection of the eye

Warnings/Precautions For ophthalmic use only; not for injection. Steroids may mask infection or enhance existing ocular infection; prolonged use may result in secondary bacterial or fungal superinfection due to immunosuppression. Prolonged use of corticosteroids may result in glaucoma; damage to the optic nerve, defects in visual acuity and fields of vision, corneal and scleral thinning (leading to perforation) and posterior subcapsular cataract formation may occur. Sensitivity to neomycin may develop; discontinue if sensitivity reaction occurs. Use following cataract surgery may delay healing or increase the incidence of bleb formation. Some products contain benzalkonium chloride which may be absorbed by soft contact lenses; contact lenses should not be worn during treatment of ophthalmologic infections. A maximum of 8 g of ointment or 20 mL of suspension should be prescribed initially; patients should be re-evaluated (eg, intraocular pressure and exams using magnification and fluorescein staining, where appropriate) prior to additional refills. Use >10 days should include routine monitoring of intraocular pressure. Inadvertent contamination of multiple-dose ophthalmic solutions has caused bacterial keratitis.

Adverse Reactions (Reflective of adult population; not specific for elderly) See individual agents.

Drug Interactions

Metabolism/Transport Effects Refer to individual components.

Avoid Concomitant Use

Avoid concomitant use of Neomycin, Polymyxin B, and Dexamethasone with any of the following: Aldesleukin; Axitinib; BCG; Conivaptan; Crizotinib; Dabigatran Etexilate; Dronedarone; Everolimus; Gallium Nitrate; Lapatinib; Lurasidone; Mifepristone; Natalizumab; Nilotinib; Nisoldipine; Pazopanib; Pimecrolimus; Praziquantel; Ranolazine; Rilpivirine; Rivaroxaban; RomiDEPsin; Tacrolimus (Topical); Ticagrelor; Tolvaptan; Toremifene; Vandetanib

Increased Effect/Toxicity

Neomycin, Polymyxin B, and Dexamethasone may increase the levels/effects of: AbobotulinumtoxinA; Acarbose; Acetylcholinesterase Inhibitors; Amphotericin B; Bisphosphonate Derivatives; CARBOplatin; Colistimethate; CycloSPORINE; CycloSPORINE (Systemic); Deferasirox; Gallium Nitrate; Ifosfamide; Leflunomide; Lenalidomide; Loop Diuretics; Natalizumab; Neuromuscular-Blocking Agents; NSAID (COX-2 Inhibitor); NSAID (Nonselective); OnabotulinumtoxinA; RimabotulinumtoxinB; Thalidomide; Thiazide Diuretics; Vaccines (Live); Vitamin K Antagonists; Warfarin

The levels/effects of Neomycin, Polymyxin B, and Dexamethasone may be increased by: Amphotericin B; Antifungal Agents (Azole Derivatives, Systemic); Aprepitant; Asparaginase (E. coli); Asparaginase (Erwinia); Calcium Channel Blockers (Nondihydropyridine); Capreomycin; Cephalosporins (2nd Generation); Cephalosporins (3rd Generation); Cephalosporins (4th Generation); CISplatin; Conivaptan; CycloSPORINE; CycloSPORINE (Systemic); CYP3A4 Inhibitors (Moderate); CYP3A4 Inhibitors (Strong); Dasatinib; Denosumab; Estrogen Derivatives; Fluconazole; Fosaprepitant; Indacaterol; Ivacaftor; Loop Diuretics; Macrolide Antibiotics; Mifepristone; Neuromuscular-Blocking Agents (Nondepolarizing); P-glycoprotein/ABCB1 Inhibitors; Pimecrolimus; Quinolone Antibiotics; Roflumilast; Salicylates; Tacrolimus (Topical); Telaprevir; Trastuzumab; Vancomycin

Decreased Effect

Neomycin, Polymyxin B, and Dexamethasone may decrease the levels/effects of: Aldesleukin; Antidiabetic Agents; Apixaban; ARIPiprazole; Axitinib; BCG; Boceprevir; Brentuximab Vedotin; Calcitriol; Cardiac Glycosides; Caspofungin; Coccidioidin Skin Test; Corticorelin; Crizotinib; CycloSPORINE; CycloSPORINE (Systemic); CYP3A4 Substrates; Dabigatran Etexilate; Dasatinib; Dronedarone; Everolimus; Exemestane; Gefitinib; GuanFACINE; Hyaluronidase; Imatinib; Isoniazid; Ixabepilone; Lapatinib; Lurasidone; Maraviroc; NIFEdipine; Nilotinib; Nisoldipine; Pazopanib; P-glycoprotein/ABCB1 Substrates; Praziquantel; Ranolazine; Rivaroxaban; RomiDEPsin; Salicylates; Sipuleucel-T; SORAfenib; SUNItinib; Tadalafil; Telaprevir; Ticagrelor; Tolvaptan; Toremifene; Ulipristal; Vaccines (Inactivated); Vandetanib; Vemurafenib; Zuclopenthixol

The levels/effects of Neomycin, Polymyxin B, and Dexamethasone may be decreased by: Aminoglutethimide; Antacids; Barbiturates; Bile Acid Sequestrants; CYP3A4 Inducers (Strong); Echinacea; Herbs (CYP3A4 Inducers); Mifepristone; Mitotane; Penicillins; P-glycoprotein/ABCB1 Inducers; Primidone; Rifamycin Derivatives; Rilpivirine; Tocilizumab

Stability

Ointment: Store between 15°C to 30°C (59°F to 86°F).

Suspension: Store between 8°C to 27°C (46°F to 80°F).

Mechanism of Action

Neomycin: Interferes with bacterial protein synthesis by binding to 30S ribosomal subunits

Polymyxin B: Binds to phospholipids, alters permeability, and damages the bacterial cytoplasmic membrane permitting leakage of intracellular constituents

Dexamethasone: Decreases inflammation by suppression of neutrophil migration, decreased production of inflammatory mediators, and reversal of increased capillary permeability; suppresses normal immune response. Dexamethasone's mechanism of antiemetic activity is unknown.

Pharmacodynamics/Kinetics See individual agents.

Dosage

Geriatric & Adult Ocular inflammation/infection: Ophthalmic:

Suspension: Instill 1-2 drops into the conjunctival sac of the affected eye(s) 4-6 times/day; in severe disease, drops may be used hourly and tapered to discontinuation

Ointment: Place ~1/2" ribbon in the conjunctival sac of the affected eye(s) 3-4 times/day or apply at bedtime as an adjunct with suspension

Note: If signs and symptoms do not improve after 2 days of treatment, the patient should be re-evaluated.

Administration Ophthalmic: **Note:** Contact lenses should not be worn during therapy.

Ointment: Apply into pocket between eyeball and lower lid; patient should look downward before closing eye. Do not touch tip of tube to eye.

Suspension: Shake well before using. Tilt head back, instill suspension into the conjunctival sac and close eye(s). Apply light finger pressure on lacrimal sac for 1 minute following instillation. Do not touch dropper to eye.

Monitoring Parameters Monitor intraocular pressure with use longer than 10 days

Special Geriatric Considerations Evaluate the patient's or caregiver's ability to safely administer the correct dose of ophthalmic medication.

Dosage Forms Excipient information presented when available (limited, particularly for generics); consult specific product labeling.

Ointment, ophthalmic: Neomycin 3.5 mg, polymyxin B sulfate 10,000 units, and dexamethasone 0.1% per g (3.5 g)

Maxitrol®: Neomycin 3.5 mg, polymyxin B sulfate 10,000 units, and dexamethasone 0.1% per g (3.5 g)

Suspension, ophthalmic [drops]: Neomycin 3.5 mg, polymyxin B sulfate 10,000 units, and dexamethasone 0.1% per 1 mL (5 mL)

Maxitrol®: Neomycin 3.5 mg, polymyxin B sulfate 10,000 units, and dexamethasone 0.1% per 1 mL (5 mL) [contains benzalkonium chloride]

Neomycin, Polymyxin B, and Gramicidin
(nee oh MYE sin, pol i MIKS in bee, & gram i SYE din)

Brand Names: U.S. Neosporin® Ophthalmic Solution

Brand Names: Canada Neosporin®; Optimyxin Plus®

Index Terms Gramicidin, Neomycin, and Polymyxin B; Polymyxin B, Neomycin, and Gramicidin

Generic Availability (U.S.) Yes

Pharmacologic Category Antibiotic, Ophthalmic

Use Treatment of superficial ocular infection

Contraindications Hypersensitivity to neomycin, polymyxin B, gramicidin or any component of the formulation

Warnings/Precautions Symptoms of neomycin sensitization include itching, reddening, edema, failure to heal; prolonged use may result in glaucoma, defects in visual acuity, posterior subcapsular cataract formation, and secondary ocular infections

Adverse Reactions (Reflective of adult population; not specific for elderly) Frequency not defined: Ocular: Transient irritation, burning, stinging, itching, inflammation, angioneurotic edema, urticaria, vesicular and maculopapular dermatitis

Drug Interactions

Metabolism/Transport Effects None known.

Avoid Concomitant Use

Avoid concomitant use of Neomycin, Polymyxin B, and Gramicidin with any of the following: BCG; Gallium Nitrate

Increased Effect/Toxicity

Neomycin, Polymyxin B, and Gramicidin may increase the levels/effects of: AbobotulinumtoxinA; Acarbose; Bisphosphonate Derivatives; CARBOplatin; Colistimethate; CycloSPORINE; CycloSPORINE (Systemic); Gallium Nitrate; Neuromuscular-Blocking Agents; OnabotulinumtoxinA; RimabotulinumtoxinB; Vitamin K Antagonists

The levels/effects of Neomycin, Polymyxin B, and Gramicidin may be increased by: Amphotericin B; Capreomycin; Cephalosporins (2nd Generation); Cephalosporins (3rd Generation); Cephalosporins (4th Generation); CISplatin; Loop Diuretics; Nonsteroidal Anti-Inflammatory Agents; Vancomycin

Decreased Effect

Neomycin, Polymyxin B, and Gramicidin may decrease the levels/effects of: BCG; Cardiac Glycosides; SORAfenib

The levels/effects of Neomycin, Polymyxin B, and Gramicidin may be decreased by: Penicillins

Mechanism of Action Interferes with bacterial protein synthesis by binding to 30S ribosomal subunits; binds to phospholipids, alters permeability, and damages the bacterial cytoplasmic membrane permitting leakage of intracellular constituents

Dosage

Geriatric & Adult Ophthalmic: Instill 1-2 drops 4-6 times/day or more frequently as required for severe infections

Special Geriatric Considerations Evaluate the patient's or caregiver's ability to safely administer the correct dose of ophthalmic medication.

Dosage Forms Excipient information presented when available (limited, particularly for generics); consult specific product labeling.

Solution, ophthalmic [drops]: Neomycin 1.75 mg, polymyxin B 10,000 units, and gramicidin 0.025 mg per 1 mL (10 mL)

Neosporin® Ophthalmic Solution: Neomycin 1.75 mg, polymyxin B 10,000 units, and gramicidin 0.025 mg per 1 mL (10 mL)

- **Neoral®** *see* CycloSPORINE (Systemic) *on page 460*
- **Neosar** *see* Cyclophosphamide *on page 456*
- **Neosporin® AF [OTC]** *see* Miconazole (Topical) *on page 1276*
- **Neosporin® G.U. Irrigant** *see* Neomycin and Polymyxin B *on page 1354*
- **Neosporin® Ophthalmic Solution** *see* Neomycin, Polymyxin B, and Gramicidin *on page 1357*

Neostigmine (nee oh STIG meen)

Medication Safety Issues

Sound-alike/look-alike issues:

Prostigmin® may be confused with physostigmine

Brand Names: U.S. Prostigmin®

Brand Names: Canada Prostigmin®

Index Terms Neostigmine Bromide; Neostigmine Methylsulfate

Generic Availability (U.S.) Yes: Injection

Pharmacologic Category Acetylcholinesterase Inhibitor

Use Reversal of the effects of nondepolarizing neuromuscular-blocking agents; treatment of myasthenia gravis; prevention and treatment of postoperative bladder distention and urinary retention

Contraindications Hypersensitivity to neostigmine, bromides, or any component of the formulation; GI or GU obstruction

Warnings/Precautions Does **not** antagonize and may prolong the Phase I block of depolarizing muscle relaxants (eg, succinylcholine). Use with caution in patients with epilepsy, asthma, bradycardia, hyperthyroidism, cardiac arrhythmias, or peptic ulcer; not generally recommended for use in patients with vagotonia. Adequate facilities should be available for cardiopulmonary resuscitation when testing and adjusting dose for myasthenia gravis. Have atropine and epinephrine ready to treat hypersensitivity reactions. Overdosage may result in cholinergic crisis, this must be distinguished from myasthenic crisis. Anticholinesterase insensitivity can develop for brief or prolonged periods.

Adverse Reactions (Reflective of adult population; not specific for elderly) Frequency not defined.

Cardiovascular: Arrhythmias (especially bradycardia), AV block, cardiac arrest, flushing, hypotension, nodal rhythm, nonspecific ECG changes, syncope, tachycardia

Central nervous system: Convulsions, dizziness, drowsiness, dysarthria, dysphonia, headache, loss of consciousness

Dermatologic: Skin rash, thrombophlebitis (I.V.), urticaria

Gastrointestinal: Diarrhea, dysphagia, flatulence, hyperperistalsis, nausea, salivation, stomach cramps, vomiting

Genitourinary: Urinary urgency

Neuromuscular & skeletal: Arthralgias, fasciculations, muscle cramps, spasms, weakness

Ocular: Lacrimation, small pupils

Respiratory: Bronchiolar constriction, bronchospasm, dyspnea, increased bronchial secretions, laryngospasm, respiratory arrest, respiratory depression, respiratory muscle paralysis

Miscellaneous: Allergic reactions, anaphylaxis, diaphoresis increased

Drug Interactions

Metabolism/Transport Effects None known.

Avoid Concomitant Use There are no known interactions where it is recommended to avoid concomitant use.

Increased Effect/Toxicity

Neostigmine may increase the levels/effects of: Beta-Blockers; Cholinergic Agonists; Succinylcholine

The levels/effects of Neostigmine may be increased by: Corticosteroids (Systemic)

Decreased Effect

Neostigmine may decrease the levels/effects of: Neuromuscular-Blocking Agents (Non-depolarizing)

The levels/effects of Neostigmine may be decreased by: Dipyridamole

Mechanism of Action Inhibits destruction of acetylcholine by acetylcholinesterase which facilitates transmission of impulses across myoneural junction

Pharmacodynamics/Kinetics

Onset of action: I.M.: 20-30 minutes; I.V.: 1-20 minutes

Duration: I.M.: 2.5-4 hours; I.V.: 1-2 hours

Absorption: Oral: Poor, <2%

Metabolism: Hepatic

Half-life elimination: Normal renal function: 0.5-2.1 hours; End-stage renal disease: Prolonged

Excretion: Urine (50% as unchanged drug)

Dosage

Geriatric & Adult

Myasthenia gravis, diagnosis: I.M.: 0.02 mg/kg as a single dose; **Note:** In the diagnosis of myasthenia gravis, all anticholinesterase medications should be discontinued for at least 8 hours before administering neostigmine.

Myasthenia gravis, treatment:

Oral: 15 mg/dose every 3-4 hours up to 375 mg/day maximum; interval between doses must be individualized to maximal response

I.M., I.V., SubQ: 0.5-2.5 mg every 1-3 hours up to 10 mg/24 hours maximum

Reversal of nondepolarizing neuromuscular blockade after surgery in conjunction with atropine: I.V.: 0.5-2.5 mg; total dose not to exceed 5 mg; must administer atropine several minutes prior to neostigmine

Bladder atony: I.M., SubQ:

Prevention: 0.25 mg every 4-6 hours for 2-3 days

Treatment: 0.5-1 mg every 3 hours for 5 doses after bladder has emptied

Renal Impairment

Cl_{cr} 10-50 mL/minute: Administer 50% of normal dose.

Cl_{cr} <10 mL/minute: Administer 25% of normal dose.

Administration May be administered undiluted by slow I.V. injection over several minutes

Monitoring Parameters Respiratory rate, pulse, blood pressure, signs of cholinergic crisis.

Pharmacotherapy Pearls In the diagnosis of myasthenia gravis, all anticholinesterase medications should be discontinued for at least 8 hours before administering neostigmine.

Special Geriatric Considerations Many elderly will have diseases which may influence the use of neostigmine. Also, many elderly will need doses reduced by 50% due to creatinine clearances in the 10-50 mL/minute range. Side effects or concomitant disease may warrant use of pyridostigmine.

Dosage Forms Excipient information presented when available (limited, particularly for generics); consult specific product labeling.

Injection, solution, as methylsulfate: 0.5 mg/mL (10 mL); 1 mg/mL (10 mL)

Tablet, oral, as bromide:

Prostigmin®: 15 mg [scored]

- ◆ **Neostigmine Bromide** *see* Neostigmine *on page 1358*
- ◆ **Neostigmine Methylsulfate** *see* Neostigmine *on page 1358*
- ◆ **Neo-Synephrine® Extra Strength [OTC]** *see* Phenylephrine (Nasal) *on page 1526*
- ◆ **Neo-Synephrine® Mild Formula [OTC]** *see* Phenylephrine (Nasal) *on page 1526*
- ◆ **Neo-Synephrine® Nighttime12-Hour [OTC]** *see* Oxymetazoline (Nasal) *on page 1452*
- ◆ **Neo-Synephrine® Regular Strength [OTC]** *see* Phenylephrine (Nasal) *on page 1526*

Nepafenac (ne pa FEN ak)

Brand Names: U.S. Nevanac®

Brand Names: Canada Nevanac®

Generic Availability (U.S.) No

◀

Pharmacologic Category Nonsteroidal Anti-inflammatory Drug (NSAID), Ophthalmic

Use Treatment of pain and inflammation associated with cataract surgery

Contraindications Hypersensitivity to nepafenac, other NSAIDs, or any component of the formulation

Warnings/Precautions Use caution in patients with previous sensitivity to acetylsalicylic acid and phenylacetic acid derivatives, including patients who experience bronchospasm, asthma, rhinitis, or urticaria following NSAID or aspirin. May slow/delay healing or prolong bleeding time following surgery. Use caution in patients with a predisposition to bleeding (bleeding tendencies or medications which interfere with coagulation).

May cause keratitis; continued use of nepafenac in a patient with keratitis may cause severe corneal adverse reactions, potentially resulting in loss of vision. Immediately discontinue use in patients with evidence of corneal epithelial damage.

Use caution in patients with complicated ocular surgeries, corneal denervation, corneal epithelial defects, diabetes mellitus, ocular surface disease, rheumatoid arthritis, or repeat ocular surgeries (within a short timeframe); may be at risk of corneal adverse events, potentially resulting in loss of vision. Use more than 1 day prior to surgery or for 14 days beyond surgery may increase risk and severity of corneal adverse events. Patients using ophthalmic drops should not wear soft contact lenses.

Adverse Reactions (Reflective of adult population; not specific for elderly) 1% to 10%:

Cardiovascular: Hypertension (1% to 4%)

Central nervous system: Headache (1% to 4%)

Gastrointestinal: Nausea (1% to 4%), vomiting (1% to 4%)

Ocular: Capsular opacity (5% to 10%), foreign body sensation (5% to 10%), intraocular pressure increased (5% to 10%), sticky sensation (5% to 10%), visual acuity decreased (5% to 10%), conjunctival edema (1% to 5%), corneal edema (1% to 5%), dry eye (1% to 5%), lid margin crusting (1% to 5%), ocular discomfort (1% to 5%), ocular hyperemia (1% to 5%), ocular pain (1% to 5%), ocular pruritus (1% to 5%), photophobia (1% to 5%), tearing (1% to 5%), vitreous detachment (1% to 5%)

Respiratory: Sinusitis (1% to 4%)

Drug Interactions

Metabolism/Transport Effects None known.

Avoid Concomitant Use There are no known interactions where it is recommended to avoid concomitant use.

Increased Effect/Toxicity There are no known significant interactions involving an increase in effect.

Decreased Effect

Nepafenac may decrease the levels/effects of: Latanoprost

Stability Store at 2°C to 25°C (36°F to 77°F).

Mechanism of Action Nepafenac is a prodrug which once converted to amfenac inhibits prostaglandin synthesis by decreasing the activity of the enzyme, cyclooxygenase, which results in decreased formation of prostaglandin precursors.

Pharmacodynamics/Kinetics

Absorption: Low levels (0.2-0.5 ng/mL) of nepafenac and amfenac are detected in the plasma following ophthalmic administration

Metabolism: Hydrolyzed in ocular tissue to amfenac (active)

Dosage

Geriatric & Adult Pain, inflammation associated with cataract surgery: Ophthalmic: Instill 1 drop into affected eye(s) 3 times/day, beginning 1 day prior to surgery, the day of surgery, and through the first 2 weeks of the postoperative period

Administration Shake well prior to use. May be used with other eye drops; wait at least 5 minutes between application of each medication. For topical ophthalmic use only; avoid touching tip of applicator to eye, fingers, or other surfaces.

Special Geriatric Considerations No differences in safety and efficacy noted between elderly and younger adults. No dosage adjustment necessary. Elderly may be taking other medications that will increase bleeding.

Dosage Forms Excipient information presented when available (limited, particularly for generics); consult specific product labeling.

Suspension, ophthalmic [drops]:

Nevanac®: 0.1% (3 mL) [contains benzalkonium chloride]

◆ **Nephro-Calci® [OTC]** *see* Calcium Carbonate *on page* 262

◆ **Neptazane™** *see* Methazolamide *on page* 1229

Nesiritide (ni SIR i tide)

Medication Safety Issues
High alert medication:
The Institute for Safe Medication Practices (ISMP) includes this medication among its list of drugs which have a heightened risk of causing significant patient harm when used in error.
International issues:
Natrecor [U.S., Canada, Argentina, Venezuela] may be confused with Nitrocor brand name for nitroglycerin [Italy, Russia, Venezuela]

Brand Names: U.S. Natrecor®

Brand Names: Canada Natrecor®

Index Terms B-type Natriuretic Peptide (Human); hBNP; Natriuretic Peptide

Generic Availability (U.S.) No

Pharmacologic Category Natriuretic Peptide, B-Type, Human

Use Treatment of acutely decompensated heart failure (HF) with dyspnea at rest or with minimal activity

Contraindications Hypersensitivity to natriuretic peptide or any component of the formulation; cardiogenic shock (when used as primary therapy); hypotension (systolic blood pressure <90 mm Hg)

Warnings/Precautions May cause hypotension; administer in clinical situations when blood pressure may be closely monitored. Use caution in patients systolic blood pressure <100 mm Hg (contraindicated if <90 mm Hg); more likely to experience hypotension. Effects may be additive with other agents capable of causing hypotension. Hypotensive effects may last for several hours.

Should not be used in patients with low cardiac filling pressures, or in patients with conditions which depend on venous return including significant valvular stenosis, restrictive or obstructive cardiomyopathy, constrictive pericarditis, and pericardial tamponade. May be associated with development of azotemia; use caution in patients with renal impairment or in patients where renal perfusion is dependent on renin-angiotensin-aldosterone system; avoid initiation at doses higher than recommended.

Monitor for allergic or anaphylactic reactions. Use caution with prolonged infusions; limited experience with infusions >48 hours.

Adverse Reactions (Reflective of adult population; not specific for elderly) Note: Frequencies cited below were recorded in VMAC trial at dosages similar to approved labeling. Higher frequencies have been observed in trials using higher dosages of nesiritide. The percentages marked with an asterisk (*) indicate frequency less than or equal to placebo or other standard therapy.

>10%:
Cardiovascular: Hypotension (total: 11%; symptomatic: 4% at recommended dose, up to 17% at higher doses)
Renal: Increased serum creatinine (28% with >0.5 mg/dL increase over baseline)
1% to 10%:
Cardiovascular: Ventricular tachycardia (3%)*, ventricular extrasystoles (3%)*, angina (2%)*, bradycardia (1%), tachycardia, atrial fibrillation, AV node conduction abnormalities
Central nervous system: Headache (8%)*, dizziness (3%), insomnia (2%)*, anxiety (3%), confusion, fever, paresthesia, somnolence, tremor
Dermatologic: Pruritus, rash
Gastrointestinal: Nausea (4%)*, abdominal pain (1%)*, vomiting (1%)*
Hematologic: Anemia
Local: Injection site reaction, catheter pain
Neuromuscular & skeletal: Back pain (4%), leg cramps
Ocular: Amblyopia
Respiratory: Apnea, cough increased, hemoptysis
Miscellaneous: Diaphoresis
Postmarketing and/or case reports: Hypersensitivity reactions (rare)

Drug Interactions
Metabolism/Transport Effects None known.

Avoid Concomitant Use There are no known interactions where it is recommended to avoid concomitant use.

Increased Effect/Toxicity
Nesiritide may increase the levels/effects of: Hypotensive Agents

Decreased Effect There are no known significant interactions involving a decrease in effect. ▶

Ethanol/Nutrition/Herb Interactions Herb/Nutraceutical: Avoid bayberry, blue cohosh, cayenne, ephedra, ginger, ginseng (American), kola, and licorice (may increase blood pressure). Avoid black cohosh, California poppy, coleus, golden seal, hawthorn, mistletoe, periwinkle, quinine, and shepherd's purse (may enhance decreased blood pressure).

Stability Vials may be stored below 25°C (77°F); do not freeze. Protect from light. Following reconstitution, vials are stable at 2°C to 25°C (36°F to 77°F) for up to 24 hours. Use reconstituted solution within 24 hours.

Reconstitute 1.5 mg vial with 5 mL of diluent removed from a prefilled 250 mL plastic I.V. bag (compatible with D_5W, $D_5^{1/2}NS$, $D_5^{1/4}NS$, NS). Do not shake vial to dissolve (roll gently). Withdraw entire contents of vial and add to 250 mL I.V. bag. Invert several times to mix. Resultant concentration of solution is ~6 mcg/mL.

Mechanism of Action Binds to guanylate cyclase receptor on vascular smooth muscle and endothelial cells, increasing intracellular cyclic GMP, resulting in smooth muscle cell relaxation. Has been shown to produce dose-dependent reductions in pulmonary capillary wedge pressure (PCWP) and systemic arterial pressure.

Pharmacodynamics/Kinetics

Onset of action: 15 minutes (60% of 3-hour effect achieved)

Duration: >60 minutes (up to several hours) for systolic blood pressure; hemodynamic effects persist longer than serum half-life would predict

Distribution: V_{ss}: 0.19 L/kg

Metabolism: Proteolytic cleavage by vascular endopeptidases and proteolysis following binding to the membrane bound natriuretic peptide (NPR-C) and cellular internalization

Half-life elimination: Initial (distribution) 2 minutes; Terminal: 18 minutes

Time to peak: 1 hour

Excretion: Primarily eliminated by metabolism; also excreted in the urine

Dosage

Geriatric & Adult

Acute decompensated heart failure: I.V.: Initial: 2 mcg/kg (bolus optional); followed by continuous infusion at 0.01 mcg/kg/minute. **Note:** Should not be initiated at a dosage higher than initial recommended dose. There is limited experience with increasing the dose >0.01 mcg/kg/minute; in one trial, a limited number of patients received higher doses that were increased no faster than every 3 hours by 0.005 mcg/kg/minute (preceded by a bolus of 1 mcg/kg), up to a maximum of 0.03 mcg/kg/minute. Increases beyond the initial infusion rate should be limited to selected patients and accompanied by close hemodynamic and renal function monitoring.

Patients experiencing hypotension during the infusion: Infusion dose should be reduced or discontinued. Other measures to support blood pressure should be initiated (eg, I.V. fluids, Trendelenburg position). May attempt to restart at a lower dose (reduce previous infusion dose by 30% and omit bolus).

Maximum dosing weight: According to the manufacturer, the PRECEDENT Trial capped dosing weight at 160 kg and the VMAC Trial capped dosing weight at 175 kg. There are no specific guidelines on maximum dosing weight and clinical judgment should be used.

Renal Impairment No adjustment required but use cautiously in patients with renal impairment or those patients who rely on the renin-angiotensin-aldosterone system for renal perfusion. Monitor renal function closely.

Hepatic Impairment No dosage adjustment recommended.

Administration Do not administer through a heparin-coated catheter (concurrent administration of heparin via a separate catheter is acceptable, per manufacturer).

Prime I.V. tubing with 5 mL of infusion prior to connection with vascular access port and prior to administering bolus or starting the infusion. Withdraw bolus from the prepared infusion bag and administer over 60 seconds. Begin infusion immediately following administration of the bolus.

Monitoring Parameters Blood pressure, hemodynamic responses (PCWP, RAP, CI), BUN, creatinine; urine output

Pharmacotherapy Pearls The duration of symptomatic improvement with nesiritide following discontinuation of the infusion has been limited (generally lasting several days). Atrial natriuretic peptide, which is related to nesiritide, has been associated with increased vascular permeability. This has not been observed in clinical trials with nesiritide, but patients should be monitored for this effect.

Special Geriatric Considerations No specific data to date; elderly are liable to have hypotension, see Warnings/Precautions for blood pressure criteria. Elderly with reduced renal function should be monitored closely.

Dosage Forms Excipient information presented when available (limited, particularly for generics); consult specific product labeling.

Injection, powder for reconstitution:

Natrecor®: 1.5 mg

- ◆ **NESP** *see* Darbepoetin Alfa *on page 488*
- ◆ **Neulasta®** *see* Pegfilgrastim *on page 1481*
- ◆ **Neupogen®** *see* Filgrastim *on page 787*
- ◆ **Neupro®** *see* Rotigotine *on page 1736*
- ◆ **Neurontin®** *see* Gabapentin *on page 858*
- ◆ **Neut®** *see* Sodium Bicarbonate *on page 1785*
- ◆ **NeutraCare®** *see* Fluoride *on page 806*
- ◆ **NeutraGard® Advanced** *see* Fluoride *on page 806*
- ◆ **Neutra-Phos** *see* Potassium Phosphate and Sodium Phosphate *on page 1578*
- ◆ **Neutra-Phos®-K [OTC] [DSC]** *see* Potassium Phosphate *on page 1575*
- ◆ **NeutraSal®** *see* Saliva Substitute *on page 1748*
- ◆ **Neutrogena® Acne Stress Control [OTC]** *see* Salicylic Acid *on page 1743*
- ◆ **Neutrogena® Advanced Solutions™ [OTC]** *see* Salicylic Acid *on page 1743*
- ◆ **Neutrogena® Blackhead Eliminating™ [OTC]** *see* Salicylic Acid *on page 1743*
- ◆ **Neutrogena® Blackhead Eliminating™ 2-in-1 Foaming Pads [OTC]** *see* Salicylic Acid *on page 1743*
- ◆ **Neutrogena® Blackhead Eliminating™ Daily Scrub [OTC]** *see* Salicylic Acid *on page 1743*
- ◆ **Neutrogena® Body Clear® [OTC]** *see* Salicylic Acid *on page 1743*
- ◆ **Neutrogena® Clear Pore™ Oil-Controlling Astringent [OTC]** *see* Salicylic Acid *on page 1743*
- ◆ **Neutrogena® Maximum Strength T/Sal® [OTC]** *see* Salicylic Acid *on page 1743*
- ◆ **Neutrogena® Oil-Free Acne [OTC]** *see* Salicylic Acid *on page 1743*
- ◆ **Neutrogena® Oil-Free Acne Stress Control [OTC]** *see* Salicylic Acid *on page 1743*
- ◆ **Neutrogena® Oil-Free Acne Wash [OTC]** *see* Salicylic Acid *on page 1743*
- ◆ **Neutrogena® Oil-Free Acne Wash 60 Second Mask Scrub [OTC]** *see* Salicylic Acid *on page 1743*
- ◆ **Neutrogena® Oil-Free Acne Wash Cream Cleanser [OTC]** *see* Salicylic Acid *on page 1743*
- ◆ **Neutrogena® Oil-Free Acne Wash Foam Cleanser [OTC]** *see* Salicylic Acid *on page 1743*
- ◆ **Neutrogena® Oil-Free Anti-Acne [OTC]** *see* Salicylic Acid *on page 1743*
- ◆ **Neutrogena® Rapid Clear® [OTC]** *see* Salicylic Acid *on page 1743*
- ◆ **Neutrogena® Rapid Clear® Acne Defense [OTC]** *see* Salicylic Acid *on page 1743*
- ◆ **Neutrogena® Rapid Clear® Acne Eliminating [OTC]** *see* Salicylic Acid *on page 1743*
- ◆ **Nevanac®** *see* Nepafenac *on page 1359*
- ◆ **Nexiclon™ XR** *see* CloNIDine *on page 413*
- ◆ **NexIUM®** *see* Esomeprazole *on page 676*
- ◆ **NexIUM® I.V.** *see* Esomeprazole *on page 676*
- ◆ **Nexterone®** *see* Amiodarone *on page 96*
- ◆ **NGX-4010** *see* Capsaicin *on page 280*

Niacin (NYE a sin)

Related Information
Hyperlipidemia Management *on page 2130*
Medication Safety Issues
Sound-alike/look-alike issues:
Niacin may be confused with Minocin®, niacinamide, Niaspan®
Brand Names: U.S. Niacin-Time® [OTC]; Niacor®; Niaspan®; Slo-Niacin® [OTC]
Brand Names: Canada Niaspan®; Niaspan® FCT; Niodan
Index Terms Nicotinic Acid; Vitamin B_3
Generic Availability (U.S.) Yes
Pharmacologic Category Antilipemic Agent, Miscellaneous; Vitamin, Water Soluble
Use Treatment of dyslipidemias (Fredrickson types IIa and IIb or primary hypercholesterolemia) as mono- or adjunctive therapy; to lower the risk of recurrent MI in patients with a history of MI and hyperlipidemia; to slow progression or promote regression of coronary artery disease; treatment of hypertriglyceridemia in patients at risk of pancreatitis; dietary supplement
Unlabeled Use Treatment of pellagra
Contraindications Hypersensitivity to niacin, niacinamide, or any component of the formulation; active hepatic disease or significant or unexplained persistent elevations in hepatic transaminases; active peptic ulcer; arterial hemorrhage
Warnings/Precautions Use with caution in patients with unstable angina or MI, diabetes (may interfere with glucose control), renal disease, active gallbladder disease (can exacerbate), gout, or with anticoagulants (may slightly increase prothrombin time). Use with caution in patients with a past history of hepatic impairment and/or who consume substantial amounts of ethanol; contraindicated with active liver disease or unexplained persistent transaminase elevation. Rare cases of rhabdomyolysis have occurred during concomitant use with

HMG-CoA reductase inhibitors. With concurrent use or if symptoms suggestive of myopathy occur, monitor creatine phosphokinase (CPK) and potassium; use with caution in patients with renal impairment, inadequately treated hypothyroidism, patients with diabetes or the elderly; risk for myopathy and rhabdomyolysis may be increased.

Immediate and extended or sustained release products are not interchangeable. Cases of severe hepatotoxicity have occurred when immediate release (crystalline) niacin products have been substituted with sustained-release (modified release, timed-release) niacin products at equivalent doses. Patients should be initiated with low doses (eg, 500 mg at bedtime) with titration to achieve desired response. Flushing and pruritus, common adverse effects of niacin, may be attenuated with a gradual increase in dose, and/or by taking aspirin (adults: 325 mg) or an NSAID 30-60 minutes before dosing. Compliance is enhanced with twice-daily dosing (extended-release product excluded). Prior to initiation, secondary causes for hypercholesterolemia (eg, poorly controlled diabetes mellitus, hypothyroidism) should be excluded; management with diet and other nonpharmacologic measures (eg, exercise or weight reduction) should be attempted prior to initiation. Use has not been evaluated in Fredrickson type I or III dyslipidemias.

Adverse Reactions (Reflective of adult population; not specific for elderly) Frequency not defined.

Cardiovascular: Arrhythmias, atrial fibrillation, edema, flushing, hypotension, orthostasis, palpitation, syncope (rare), tachycardia

Central nervous system: Chills, dizziness, headache, insomnia, migraine, nervousness, pain

Dermatologic: Acanthosis nigricans, burning skin, dry skin, hyperpigmentation, maculopapular rash, pruritus, rash, skin discoloration, urticaria

Endocrine & metabolic: Glucose tolerance decreased, gout, phosphorous levels decreased, hyperuricemia

Gastrointestinal: Abdominal pain, amylase increased, diarrhea, dyspepsia, eructation, flatulence, nausea, peptic ulcers, vomiting

Hematologic: Platelet counts decreased

Hepatic: Hepatic necrosis (rare), hepatitis, jaundice, transaminases increased (dose-related), prothrombin time increased, total bilirubin increased

Neuromuscular & skeletal: CPK increased, leg cramps, myalgia, myasthenia, myopathy (with concurrent HMG-CoA reductase inhibitor), paresthesia, rhabdomyolysis (with concurrent HMG-CoA reductase inhibitor; rare), weakness

Ocular: Blurred vision, cystoid macular edema, toxic amblyopia

Respiratory: Cough, dyspnea

Miscellaneous: Diaphoresis, hypersensitivity reactions (rare; includes anaphylaxis, angioedema, laryngismus, vesiculobullous rash), LDH increased

Drug Interactions

Metabolism/Transport Effects None known.

Avoid Concomitant Use There are no known interactions where it is recommended to avoid concomitant use.

Increased Effect/Toxicity

Niacin may increase the levels/effects of: HMG-CoA Reductase Inhibitors

Decreased Effect

The levels/effects of Niacin may be decreased by: Bile Acid Sequestrants

Ethanol/Nutrition/Herb Interactions Ethanol: Avoid heavy use; avoid use around niacin dose.

Stability

Niaspan®: Store at room temperature of 20°C to 25°C (68°F to 77°F).

Niacor®: Store at controlled room temperature of 15°C to 30°C (59°F to 86°F).

Mechanism of Action Component of two coenzymes which is necessary for tissue respiration, lipid metabolism, and glycogenolysis; inhibits the synthesis of very low density lipoproteins (VLDL) and low density lipoproteins (LDL); may also increase the rate of chylomicron triglyceride removal from plasma.

Pharmacodynamics/Kinetics

Absorption: Rapid and extensive (60% to 76%)

Distribution: Mainly to hepatic, renal, and adipose tissue

Metabolism: Extensive first-pass effects; converted to nicotinamide adenine dinucleotide, nicotinuric acid, and other metabolites

Half-life elimination: 20-45 minutes

Time to peak, serum: Immediate release formulation: 30-60 minutes; extended release formulation: 4-5 hours

Excretion: Urine 60% to 88% (unchanged drug [up to 12% recovered after multiple dosing] and metabolites)

Dosage

Geriatric & Adult Note: Formulations of niacin (regular release versus extended release) are not interchangeable.

Recommended daily allowances (National Academy of Sciences, 1998): Oral:
≥19 years: Female: 14 mg/day; Male: 16 mg/day

Dietary supplement (OTC labeling): Oral: 50 mg twice daily or 100 mg once daily. **Note:** Many over-the-counter formulations exist.

Hyperlipidemia: Oral:

Regular release formulation (Niacor®): Initial: 250 mg once daily (with evening meal); increase frequency and/or dose every 4-7 days to desired response or first-level therapeutic dose (1.5-2 g/day in 2-3 divided doses); after 2 months, may increase at 2- to 4-week intervals to 3 g/day in 3 divided doses (maximum dose: 6 g/day [NCEP recommends 4.5 g/day] in 3 divided doses). Usual daily dose after titration (NCEP, 2002): 1.5-3 g/day. **Note:** Many over-the-counter formulations exist.

Sustained release (or controlled release) formulations: **Note:** Several over-the-counter formulations exist. Usual daily dose after titration (NCEP, 2002): 1-2 g/day

Extended release formulation (Niaspan®): Initial: 500 mg at bedtime for 4 weeks, then 1 g at bedtime for 4 weeks; adjust dose to response and tolerance; may increase dose every 4 weeks by 500 mg/day to a maximum of 2 g/day. Usual daily dose after titration (NCEP, 2002): 1-2 g once daily

If additional LDL-lowering is necessary with lovastatin or simvastatin: Recommended initial lovastatin or simvastatin dose: 20 mg/day (maximum lovastatin or simvastatin dose: 40 mg/day); **Note:** Lovastatin prescribing information recommends a maximum dose of 20 mg/day with concurrent use of niacin (>1 g/day).

Pellagra (unlabeled use): Oral: 50-100 mg 3-4 times/day; maximum: 500 mg/day (some experts prefer niacinamide for treatment due to more favorable side effect profile)

Renal Impairment No dosage adjustment recommended; use with caution.

Hepatic Impairment Contraindicated in patients with significant or unexplained hepatic dysfunction, active liver disease or unexplained persistent transaminase elevations.

Administration Administer with food.

Niaspan®: Administer at bedtime. Tablet strengths are not interchangeable. When switching from immediate release tablet, initiate Niaspan® at lower dose and titrate. If therapy is interrupted for an extended period, dose should be retitrated. Long-acting forms should not be crushed, broken, or chewed. Do not substitute long-acting forms for immediate release ones.

Monitoring Parameters Blood glucose (in diabetic patients); CPK and serum potassium (if on concurrent HMG-CoA reductase inhibitor); liver function tests pretreatment, every 6-12 weeks for first year, then periodically (approximately every 6 months), monitor liver function more frequently if history of transaminase elevation with prior use; lipid profile; platelets; PT (if on anticoagulants); uric acid (if predisposed to gout); phosphorus (if predisposed to hypophosphatemia)

Test Interactions False elevations in some fluorometric determinations of plasma or urinary catecholamines; false-positive urine glucose (Benedict's reagent)

Pharmacotherapy Pearls If flushing is bothersome or persistent, 325 mg of aspirin 30 minutes before each dose or increasing the dose slowly with weekly increase may minimize this reaction; for explicit guidelines on the risk factors for CHD and when to treat high blood cholesterol. Due to liver function test abnormalities induced by sustained release niacin, these dosage forms are not currently recommended

Special Geriatric Considerations The definition of and, therefore, when to treat hyperlipidemia in the elderly is a controversial issue. The National Cholesterol Education Program recommends that all adults maintain a plasma cholesterol <160 mg/dL. Elderly with one additional risk factor, goal LDL would be <130 mg/dL. It is the authors' belief that pharmacologic treatment be reserved for those who are unable to obtain a desirable plasma cholesterol concentration by diet alone and for whom the benefits of treatment are believed to outweigh the potential adverse effects, drug interactions, and cost of treatment.

Dosage Forms Excipient information presented when available (limited, particularly for generics); consult specific product labeling.

Caplet, timed release, oral: 500 mg

Capsule, oral: 50 mg, 250 mg

Capsule, extended release, oral: 250 mg, 500 mg

Capsule, timed release, oral: 250 mg, 400 mg, 500 mg

Tablet, oral: 50 mg, 100 mg, 250 mg, 500 mg
  Niacor®: 500 mg [scored]

Tablet, controlled release, oral:
  Slo-Niacin®: 250 mg, 500 mg, 750 mg [scored]

Tablet, extended release, oral:
  Niaspan®: 500 mg, 750 mg, 1000 mg

Tablet, timed release, oral: 250 mg, 500 mg, 750 mg, 1000 mg
  Niacin-Time®: 500 mg

Niacinamide (nye a SIN a mide)

Medication Safety Issues
  Sound-alike/look-alike issues:
    Niacinamide may be confused with niacin, niCARdipine
Index Terms Nicomide-T; Nicotinamide; Nicotinic Acid Amide; Vitamin B_3
Generic Availability (U.S.) Yes
Pharmacologic Category Vitamin, Water Soluble
Use Dietary supplement
Unlabeled Use Prophylaxis and treatment of pellagra
Contraindications Hypersensitivity to niacin, niacinamide, or any component of the formulation
Drug Interactions
  Metabolism/Transport Effects None known.
  Avoid Concomitant Use There are no known interactions where it is recommended to avoid concomitant use.
  Increased Effect/Toxicity
    Niacinamide may increase the levels/effects of: HMG-CoA Reductase Inhibitors
  Decreased Effect There are no known significant interactions involving a decrease in effect.
Mechanism of Action Used by the body as a source of niacin; is a component of two coenzymes which is necessary for tissue respiration, lipid metabolism, and glycogenolysis; does not have hypolipidemia or vasodilating effects.
Pharmacodynamics/Kinetics
  Absorption: Oral: Rapid
  Metabolism: Hepatic
  Half-life elimination: 45 minutes
  Time to peak, serum: 20-70 minutes
  Excretion: Urine (as metabolites)
Dosage
  Geriatric & Adult Pellagra (unlabeled use): Oral: 100 mg every 6 hours for several days (or until resolution of major signs and symptoms), followed by 50 mg every 8-12 hours until skin lesions heal (Hegyi, 2004)
Test Interactions False elevations of urinary catecholamines in some fluorometric determinations
Special Geriatric Considerations No specific information for use in elderly.
Dosage Forms Excipient information presented when available (limited, particularly for generics); consult specific product labeling.
  Tablet, oral: 100 mg, 250 mg, 500 mg

Niacin and Lovastatin (NYE a sin & LOE va sta tin)

Related Information
  Hyperlipidemia Management *on page 2130*
  Lovastatin *on page 1164*
  Niacin *on page 1363*
Medication Safety Issues
  Sound-alike/look-alike issues:
    Advicor® may be confused with Adcirca®, Advair®
Brand Names: U.S. Advicor®
Brand Names: Canada Advicor®
Index Terms Lovastatin and Niacin
Generic Availability (U.S.) No
Pharmacologic Category Antilipemic Agent, HMG-CoA Reductase Inhibitor; Antilipemic Agent, Miscellaneous
Use For use when treatment with both extended-release niacin and lovastatin is appropriate in combination with a standard cholesterol-lowering diet:
    Extended-release niacin: Adjunctive treatment of dyslipidemias (types IIa and IIb or primary hypercholesterolemia) to lower the risk of recurrent MI and/or slow progression of coronary artery disease, including combination therapy with other antidyslipidemic agents when additional triglyceride-lowering or HDL-increasing effects are desired; treatment of hypertriglyceridemia in patients at risk of pancreatitis

Lovastatin: Treatment of primary hypercholesterolemia (Frederickson types IIa and IIb); primary and secondary prevention of cardiovascular disease

Dosage

Geriatric & Adult Dosage forms are a fixed combination of niacin and lovastatin.

Dyslipidemia: Oral: Lowest dose: Niacin 500 mg/lovastatin 20 mg; may increase by not more than 500 mg (niacin) at 4-week intervals (maximum dose: niacin 2000 mg/lovastatin 40 mg daily); should be taken at bedtime with a low-fat snack. **Note:** If therapy is interrupted for >7 days, reinstitution of therapy should begin with the lowest dose followed by retitration as needed.

Not for use as initial therapy of dyslipidemias. May be substituted for equivalent dose of Niaspan®; however, manufacturer does not recommend direct substitution with other niacin products.

Dosage adjustment for lovastatin component with concomitant medications:

Amiodarone: Maximum recommended lovastatin dose: 40 mg/day

Danazol, diltiazem, or verapamil: Initial lovastatin dose: 10 mg/day; Maximum recommended lovastatin dose: 20 mg/day

Renal Impairment

Mild-to-moderate impairment: No dosage adjustment required

Cl_{cr} <30 mL/minute: Use doses of lovastatin >20 mg/day with caution

Hepatic Impairment Do not use in active liver disease or unexplained persistent elevations of serum transaminases.

Special Geriatric Considerations See individual agents.

The definition of and, therefore, when to treat hyperlipidemia in the elderly is a controversial issue. The National Cholesterol Education Program recommends that all adults maintain a plasma cholesterol <160 mg/dL. For elderly patients with one additional risk factor, the goal LDL cholesterol is <130 mg/dL. It is the authors' belief that pharmacologic treatment be reserved for those who are unable to obtain a desirable plasma cholesterol concentration by diet alone and for whom the benefits of treatment are believed to outweigh the potential adverse effects, drug interactions, and cost of treatment. Patients ≥65 years of age are at risk for myopathy.

Dosage Forms Excipient information presented when available (limited, particularly for generics); consult specific product labeling.

Tablet, variable release, oral (Advicor®):

500/20: Niacin 500 mg [extended release] and lovastatin 20 mg [immediate release]

750/20: Niacin 750 mg [extended release] and lovastatin 20 mg [immediate release]

1000/20: Niacin 1000 mg [extended release] and lovastatin 20 mg [immediate release]

1000/40: Niacin 1000 mg [extended release] and lovastatin 40 mg [immediate release]

Niacin and Simvastatin (NYE a sin & sim va STAT in)

Related Information

Hyperlipidemia Management *on page 2130*
Niacin *on page 1363*
Simvastatin *on page 1777*

Brand Names: U.S. Simcor®

Index Terms Simvastatin and Niacin

Generic Availability (U.S.) No

Pharmacologic Category Antilipemic Agent, HMG-CoA Reductase Inhibitor; Antilipemic Agent, Miscellaneous

Use Reduce total cholesterol, LDL, Apo B, non-HDL, TG, and/or increase HDL in patients with primary hypercholesterolemia, mixed dyslipidemia, or hypertriglyceridemia in combination with standard cholesterol-lowering diet when simvastatin or niacin monotherapy is inadequate

Dosage

Adult Dosage forms are a fixed combination of niacin extended-release and simvastatin.

Dyslipidemia: Oral:

Initial dose:

Patients naïve to niacin therapy: Niacin 500 mg/simvastatin 20 mg once daily at bedtime; increase dose every 4 weeks as needed in increments of not more than 500 mg of niacin

Patients currently on immediate-release niacin products: Niacin 500 mg/simvastatin 20 mg once daily at bedtime; increase dose every 4 weeks as needed in increments of not more than 500 mg of niacin

Patients currently on simvastatin (20-40 mg/day): Niacin 500 mg/simvastatin 40 mg once daily at bedtime; increase dose every 4 weeks as needed in increments of not more than 500 mg of niacin

◀ Maintenance dose: Niacin 1000-2000 mg/ simvastatin 20-40 mg once daily (maximum daily dose: niacin 2000 mg/simvastatin 40 mg)

Note: If therapy is interrupted for >7 days, reinstitution of therapy should begin with the lowest dose followed by retitration as tolerated. Not for use as initial therapy of dyslipidemias. May be substituted for equivalent dose of niacin extended-release, however, manufacturer does not recommend direct substitution with immediate-release preparations.

Dosage adjustment for simvastatin component with concomitant medications: *Amlodipine, amiodarone, or ranolazine:* Dose should **not** exceed niacin 1000 mg/simvastatin 20 mg once daily

Renal Impairment

Mild-to-moderate impairment: No dosage adjustment required; use caution.

Severe renal impairment: Use with extreme caution or avoid unless patient already tolerating simvastatin doses ≥10 mg.

Hepatic Impairment Contraindicated in active liver disease or unexplained persistent elevations of serum transaminases.

Special Geriatric Considerations See individual agents.

The definition of and, therefore, when to treat hyperlipidemia in the elderly is a controversial issue. The National Cholesterol Education Program recommends that all adults maintain a plasma cholesterol <160 mg/dL. For elderly patients with one additional risk factor, the goal LDL would be <130 mg/dL. It is the authors' belief that pharmacologic treatment be reserved for those who are unable to obtain a desirable plasma cholesterol concentration by diet alone and for whom the benefits of treatment are believed to outweigh the potential adverse effects, drug interactions, and cost of treatment. Patients ≥65 years of age are at risk for myopathy.

Dosage Forms Excipient information presented when available (limited, particularly for generics); consult specific product labeling.

Tablet, variable release, oral:

Simcor®:

500/20: Niacin 500 mg [extended release] and simvastatin 20 mg [immediate release]
500/40: Niacin 500 mg [extended release] and simvastatin 40 mg [immediate release]
750/20: Niacin 750 mg [extended release] and simvastatin 20 mg [immediate release]
1000/20: Niacin 1000 mg [extended release] and simvastatin 20 mg [immediate release]
1000/40: Niacin 1000 mg [extended release] and simvastatin 40 mg [immediate release]

◆ **Niacin-Time® [OTC]** *see* Niacin *on page 1363*
◆ **Niacor®** *see* Niacin *on page 1363*
◆ **Niaspan®** *see* Niacin *on page 1363*

NiCARdipine (nye KAR de peen)

Related Information

Calcium Channel Blockers – Comparative Pharmacokinetics *on page 2111*

Medication Safety Issues

Sound-alike/look-alike issues:

NiCARdipine may be confused with niacinamide, NIFEdipine, niMODipine

Cardene® may be confused with Cardizem®, Cardura®, codeine

Administration issues:

Significant differences exist between oral and I.V. dosing. Use caution when converting from one route of administration to another.

International issues:

Cardene [U.S., Great Britain, Netherlands] may be confused with Cardem brand name for celiprolol [Spain]; Cardin brand name for simvastatin [Poland]

Brand Names: U.S. Cardene® I.V.; Cardene® SR

Index Terms Nicardipine Hydrochloride

Generic Availability (U.S.) Yes: Capsule, injection

Pharmacologic Category Antianginal Agent; Calcium Channel Blocker; Calcium Channel Blocker, Dihydropyridine

Use Chronic stable angina (immediate-release product only); management of hypertension (immediate and sustained release products); parenteral only for short-term use when oral treatment is not feasible

Unlabeled Use Congestive heart failure, control of blood pressure in acute ischemic stroke and spontaneous intracranial hemorrhage, postoperative hypertension associated with carotid endarterectomy, perioperative hypertension, prevention of migraine headaches, subarachnoid hemorrhage associated cerebral vasospasm

Contraindications Hypersensitivity to nicardipine or any component of the formulation; advanced aortic stenosis

Warnings/Precautions Symptomatic hypotension with or without syncope can rarely occur; blood pressure must be lowered at a rate appropriate for the patient's clinical condition. Close monitoring of blood pressure and heart rate is required. Reflex tachycardia may occur resulting in angina and/or MI in patients with obstructive coronary disease especially in the absence of concurrent beta blockade. The most common side effect is peripheral edema (dose-dependent); occurs within 2-3 weeks of starting therapy. Use with caution in CAD (can cause increase in angina), HF (can worsen heart failure symptoms), aortic stenosis (may reduce coronary perfusion resulting in ischemia; use is contraindicated in patients with advanced aortic stenosis), and hypertrophic cardiomyopathy with outflow tract obstruction. To minimize infusion site reactions, peripheral infusion sites (for I.V. therapy) should be changed every 12 hours; use of small peripheral veins should be avoided. Titrate I.V. dose cautiously in patients with HF, renal or hepatic dysfunction. Use the I.V. form cautiously in patients with portal hypertension (can cause increase in hepatic pressure gradient). Initiate at the low end of the dosage range in the elderly.

Adverse Reactions (Reflective of adult population; not specific for elderly) 1% to 10%:

Cardiovascular: Cardiovascular: Flushing (6% to 10%), peripheral edema (dose related; 6% to 8%), hypotension (I.V. 6%), increased angina (dose related; 6%), palpitation (3% to 4%), tachycardia (1% to 4%), vasodilation (1% to 5%), chest pain (I.V. 1%), ECG abnormal (I.V. 1%), extrasystoles (I.V. 1%), hemopericardium (I.V. 1%), hypertension (I.V. 1%), orthostasis (1%), supraventricular tachycardia (I.V. 1%), syncope (1%), ventricular extrasystoles (I.V. 1%), ventricular tachycardia (I.V. 1%)

Central nervous system: Headache (6% to 15%), dizziness (1% to 7%), hypoesthesia (1%), intracranial hemorrhage (1%) pain (1%), somnolence (1%)

Dermatologic: Rash (1%)

Endocrine & metabolic: Hypokalemia (I.V. 1%)

Gastrointestinal: Nausea (2% to 5%), vomiting (I.V. 5%), dyspepsia (oral 2%), abdominal pain (I.V. 1%), dry mouth (1%)

Genitourinary: Polyuria (1%)

Local: Injection site pain (I.V. 1%), injection site reaction (I.V. 1%)

Neuromuscular & skeletal: Weakness (1% to 6%), myalgia (1%), paresthesia (1%)

Renal: Hematuria (1%)

Respiratory: Dyspnea (1%)

Miscellaneous: Diaphoresis (1%)

Drug Interactions

Metabolism/Transport Effects Substrate of CYP1A2 (minor), CYP2C9 (minor), CYP2D6 (minor), CYP2E1 (minor), CYP3A4 (major), P-glycoprotein; **Note:** Assignment of Major/Minor substrate status based on clinically relevant drug interaction potential; **Inhibits** CYP2C19 (moderate), CYP2C9 (strong), CYP2D6 (moderate), CYP3A4 (strong), P-glycoprotein

Avoid Concomitant Use

Avoid concomitant use of NiCARdipine with any of the following: Alfuzosin; Avanafil; Axitinib; Conivaptan; Crizotinib; Dronedarone; Eplerenone; Everolimus; Fluticasone (Oral Inhalation); Halofantrine; Lapatinib; Lovastatin; Lurasidone; Nilotinib; Nisoldipine; Pimozide; Ranolazine; Red Yeast Rice; Rivaroxaban; RomiDEPsin; Salmeterol; Silodosin; Simvastatin; Tamsulosin; Ticagrelor; Tolvaptan; Topotecan; Toremifene

Increased Effect/Toxicity

NiCARdipine may increase the levels/effects of: Alfuzosin; Almotriptan; Alosetron; Amifostine; Antihypertensives; ARIPiprazole; Avanafil; Axitinib; Beta-Blockers; Bortezomib; Brentuximab Vedotin; Brinzolamide; Budesonide (Nasal); Budesonide (Systemic, Oral Inhalation); Calcium Channel Blockers (Nondihydropyridine); Ciclesonide; Colchicine; Conivaptan; Corticosteroids (Orally Inhaled); Crizotinib; CYP2C19 Substrates; CYP2C9 Substrates; CYP2D6 Substrates; CYP3A4 Substrates; Dabigatran Etexilate; Diclofenac; Dienogest; Dronedarone; Dutasteride; Eplerenone; Everolimus; FentaNYL; Fesoterodine; Fluticasone (Nasal); Fluticasone (Oral Inhalation); Fosphenytoin; GuanFACINE; Halofantrine; Highest Risk QTc-Prolonging Agents; Hypotensive Agents; Iloperidone; Ivacaftor; Ixabepilone; Lapatinib; Lovastatin; Lumefantrine; Lurasidone; Magnesium Salts; Maraviroc; MethylPREDNISolone; Mifepristone; Moderate Risk QTc-Prolonging Agents; Neuromuscular-Blocking Agents (Nondepolarizing); Nilotinib; Nisoldipine; Nitroprusside; Paricalcitol; Pazopanib; P-glycoprotein/ABCB1 Substrates; Phenytoin; Pimecrolimus; Pimozide; Propafenone; Prucalopride; QuiNIDine; Ranolazine; Red Yeast Rice; RiTUXimab; Rivaroxaban; RomiDEPsin; Ruxolitinib; Salmeterol; Saxagliptin; Sildenafil; Silodosin; Simvastatin; SORAfenib; Tacrolimus; Tacrolimus (Systemic); Tadalafil; Tamsulosin; Ticagrelor; Tolterodine; Tolvaptan; Topotecan; Toremifene; Vardenafil; Vemurafenib; Vilazodone; Zuclopenthixol

◀ *The levels/effects of NiCARdipine may be increased by:* Alpha1-Blockers; Antifungal Agents (Azole Derivatives, Systemic); Calcium Channel Blockers (Nondihydropyridine); Cyclo-SPORINE; CycloSPORINE (Systemic); CYP3A4 Inhibitors (Moderate); CYP3A4 Inhibitors (Strong); Diazoxide; Fluconazole; Grapefruit Juice; Herbs (Hypotensive Properties); Macro-lide Antibiotics; Magnesium Salts; MAO Inhibitors; Mifepristone; Pentoxifylline; P-glycopro-tein/ABCB1 Inhibitors; Prostacyclin Analogues; Protease Inhibitors; QuiNIDine

Decreased Effect

NiCARdipine may decrease the levels/effects of: Clopidogrel; Codeine; Ifosfamide; Prasu-grel; QuiNIDine; Ticagrelor; TraMADol

The levels/effects of NiCARdipine may be decreased by: Barbiturates; Calcium Salts; CarBAMazepine; CYP3A4 Inducers (Strong); Deferasirox; Herbs (CYP3A4 Inducers); Herbs (Hypertensive Properties); Methylphenidate; Nafcillin; Peginterferon Alfa-2b; P-glycoprotein/ABCB1 Inducers; Rifamycin Derivatives; Tocilizumab; Yohimbine

Ethanol/Nutrition/Herb Interactions

Ethanol: Ethanol may increase CNS depression. Management: Avoid ethanol.

Food: Nicardipine average peak concentrations may be decreased if taken with food. Serum concentrations/toxicity of nicardipine may be increased by grapefruit juice. Management: Avoid grapefruit juice.

Herb/Nutraceutical: St John's wort may decrease levels. Some herbal medications may worsen hypertension (eg, licorice); others may increase the antihypertensive effect of nicardipine (eg, shepherd's purse). Management: Avoid St John's wort. Avoid bayberry, blue cohosh, cayenne, ephedra, ginger, ginseng (American), kola, licorice, and yohimbe. Avoid black cohosh, California poppy, coleus, golden seal, hawthorn, mistletoe, periwinkle, quinine, and shepherd's purse.

Stability

I.V.:

Premixed bags: Store at controlled room temperature of 20°C to 25°C (68°F to 77°F). Protect from light and excessive heat. Do not freeze.

Vials: Store at controlled room temperature of 20°C to 25°C (68°F to 77°F). Protect from light. Dilute 25 mg vial with 240 mL of compatible solution to provide a 250 mL total volume solution and a final concentration of 0.1 mg/mL. Diluted solution (0.1 mg/mL) is stable at room temperature for 24 hours in glass or PVC containers. Stability has also been demonstrated at room temperature at concentrations up to 0.5 mg/mL in PVC containers for 24 hours or in glass containers for up to 7 days (Baaske, 1996).

Oral (Cardene®, Cardene SR®): Store at 15°C to 30°C (59°F to 86°F). Protect from light. Freezing does not affect stability.

Mechanism of Action Inhibits calcium ion from entering the "slow channels" or select voltage-sensitive areas of vascular smooth muscle and myocardium during depolarization, producing a relaxation of coronary vascular smooth muscle and coronary vasodilation; increases myocardial oxygen delivery in patients with vasospastic angina

Pharmacodynamics/Kinetics

Onset of action: Oral: 0.5-2 hours; I.V.: 10 minutes; Hypotension: ~20 minutes

Duration:

I.V.: ≤8 hours

Oral: Immediate release capsules: ≤8 hours; Sustained release capsules: 8-12 hours

Absorption: Oral: ~100%

Protein binding: >95%

Metabolism: Hepatic; CYP3A4 substrate (major); extensive first-pass effect (saturable)

Bioavailability: 35%

Half-life elimination: 2-4 hours

Time to peak, serum: Oral: Immediate release: 30-120 minutes; Sustained release: 60-240 minutes

Excretion: Urine (49% to 60% as metabolites); feces (43% as metabolites)

Dosage

Geriatric Initiate at the low end of the dosage range. Specific guidelines for adjustment of nicardipine are not available, but careful monitoring is warranted and adjustment may be necessary.

Adult

Angina: Immediate release: Oral: 20 mg 3 times/day; usual range: 60-120 mg/day; increase dose at 3-day intervals

Hypertension: Oral:

Immediate release: Initial: 20 mg 3 times/day; usual: 20-40 mg 3 times/day (allow 3 days between dose increases)

Sustained release: Initial: 30 mg twice daily, titrate up to 60 mg twice daily

Note: The total daily dose of immediate-release product may not automatically be equivalent to the daily sustained-release dose; use caution in converting.

Acute hypertension: I.V.: Initial: Initial: 5 mg/hour increased by 2.5 mg/hour every 5 minutes (for rapid titration) to every 15 minutes (for gradual titration) up to a maximum of 15 mg/hour; rapidly titrated patients, consider reduction to 3 mg/hour after response is achieved.

Arterial hypertension in acute ischemic stroke (unlabeled use [Adams, 2007; Jauch, 2010]): I.V.:

Patient otherwise eligible for reperfusion treatment (eg, alteplase): Blood pressure (BP): Systolic >185 mm Hg or diastolic >110 mm Hg: 5 mg/hour; titrate by 2.5 mg/hour at 5-15 minute intervals (maximum dose: 15 mg/hour). When goal BP obtained, reduce dose to 3 mg/hour. If BP does not decline and remains >185/110 mm Hg, alteplase should not be administered.

Management of BP during and after reperfusion treatment (eg, alteplase): BP: Systolic >230 mm Hg or diastolic >121-140 mm Hg: 5 mg/hour; titrate by 2.5 mg/hour at 5-minute intervals (maximum dose: 15 mg/hour). If hypertension is refractory, consider other I.V. antihypertensives (eg, nitroprusside).

Substitution for oral therapy (approximate equivalents):
20 mg every 8 hours oral, equivalent to 0.5 mg/hour I.V. infusion
30 mg every 8 hours oral, equivalent to 1.2 mg/hour I.V. infusion
40 mg every 8 hours oral, equivalent to 2.2 mg/hour I.V. infusion

Conversion to oral antihypertensive agent: Initiate oral antihypertensive at the same time that I.V. nicardipine is discontinued, if transitioning to oral nicardipine, start oral nicardipine 1 hour prior to I.V. discontinuation.

Renal Impairment

Oral: Per the manufacturer: Titrate dose beginning with 20 mg 3 times/day (immediate release) or 30 mg twice daily (sustained release capsule).

I.V.: Specific guidelines for adjustment of nicardipine are not available, but careful monitoring is warranted and adjustment may be necessary.

Hepatic Impairment

Oral: Per the manufacturer: Starting dose: 20 mg twice daily (immediate release) with titration. Refer to **"Note"** in adult dosing.

I.V.: Specific guidelines for adjustment of nicardipine are not available, but careful monitoring is warranted and adjustment may be necessary.

Administration

Oral: The total daily dose of immediate-release product may not automatically be equivalent to the daily sustained-release dose; use caution in converting. Do not chew or crush the sustained release formulation, swallow whole. Do not open or cut capsules.

I.V.:

Vials must be diluted before use. Administer as a slow continuous infusion at a concentration of 0.1 mg/mL or 0.2 mg/mL. Concentrations of 0.5 mg/mL may be administered via a central line only.

Premixed bags: No further dilution needed. For single use only, discard any unused portion. Use only if solution is clear; the manufacturer recommends not to admix or run in the same line as other medications.

Monitoring Parameters Blood pressure, heart rate

Special Geriatric Considerations Elderly may experience a greater hypotensive response. Constipation may be more of a problem in the elderly. Calcium channel blockers are no more effective in the elderly than other therapies; however, they do not cause significant CNS effects which is an advantage over some antihypertensive agents.

Dosage Forms Excipient information presented when available (limited, particularly for generics); consult specific product labeling.

Capsule, oral, as hydrochloride: 20 mg, 30 mg

Capsule, sustained release, oral, as hydrochloride:
Cardene® SR: 30 mg, 45 mg, 60 mg

Infusion, premixed iso-osmotic dextrose solution, as hydrochloride:
Cardene® I.V.: 20 mg (200 mL); 40 mg (200 mL)

Infusion, premixed iso-osmotic sodium chloride solution, as hydrochloride:
Cardene® I.V.: 20 mg (200 mL); 40 mg (200 mL)

Injection, solution, as hydrochloride: 2.5 mg/mL (10 mL)
Cardene® I.V.: 2.5 mg/mL (10 mL)

◆ **Nicardipine Hydrochloride** *see* NiCARdipine *on page 1368*
◆ **NicoDerm® CQ® [OTC]** *see* Nicotine *on page 1372*
◆ **Nicomide-T** *see* Niacinamide *on page 1366*
◆ **Nicorelief [OTC]** *see* Nicotine *on page 1372*
◆ **Nicorette® [OTC]** *see* Nicotine *on page 1372*
◆ **Nicotinamide** *see* Niacinamide *on page 1366*

Nicotine (nik oh TEEN)

Medication Safety Issues
Sound-alike/look-alike issues:
NicoDerm® may be confused with Nitroderm
Nicorette® may be confused with Nordette®

Other safety concerns:
Transdermal patch may contain conducting metal (eg, aluminum); remove patch prior to MRI.

Brand Names: U.S. Commit® [OTC]; NicoDerm® CQ® [OTC]; Nicorelief [OTC]; Nicorette® [OTC]; Nicotrol® Inhaler; Nicotrol® NS; Thrive™ [OTC]

Brand Names: Canada Habitrol®; Nicoderm®; Nicorette®; Nicorette® Plus; Nicotrol®

Index Terms Habitrol; Nicotine Patch

Generic Availability (U.S.) Yes: Transdermal patch and gum

Pharmacologic Category Smoking Cessation Aid

Use Treatment to aid smoking cessation for the relief of nicotine withdrawal symptoms (including nicotine craving)

Unlabeled Use Management of ulcerative colitis (transdermal)

Contraindications Hypersensitivity to nicotine or any component of the formulation; patients who are smoking during the postmyocardial infarction period; patients with life-threatening arrhythmias, or severe or worsening angina pectoris; active temporomandibular joint disease (gum); not for use in nonsmokers

Warnings/Precautions Hazardous agent - use appropriate precautions for handling and disposal. Use caution in patients with hyperthyroidism, pheochromocytoma, or insulin-dependent diabetes. Use with caution in oropharyngeal inflammation and in patients with history of esophagitis, peptic ulcer, coronary artery disease, recent MI, serious cardiac arrhythmias, vasospastic disease, angina, hypertension, hyperthyroidism, pheochromocytoma, diabetes, severe renal dysfunction, and hepatic dysfunction. The oral inhaler and nasal spray should be used with caution in patients with bronchospastic disease (other forms of nicotine replacement may be preferred). Use of nasal product is not recommended with chronic nasal disorders (eg, allergy, rhinitis, nasal polyps, and sinusitis). Transdermal patch may contain conducting metal (eg, aluminum); remove patch prior to MRI. Cautious use of topical nicotine in patients with certain skin diseases. Hypersensitivity to the topical products can occur. Dental problems may be worsened by chewing the gum. Urge patients to stop smoking completely when initiating therapy.

Adverse Reactions (Reflective of adult population; not specific for elderly)
Nasal spray/inhaler:
>10%:
Central nervous system: Headache (18% to 26%)
Gastrointestinal: Inhaler: Mouth/throat irritation (66%), dyspepsia (18%)
Respiratory: Inhaler: Cough (32%), rhinitis (23%)
1% to 10%:
Dermatologic: Acne (3%)
Endocrine & metabolic: Dysmenorrhea (3%)
Gastrointestinal: Flatulence (4%), gum problems (4%), diarrhea, hiccup, nausea, taste disturbance, tooth abrasions
Neuromuscular & skeletal: Back pain (6%), arthralgia (5%), jaw/neck pain
Respiratory: Nasal burning (nasal spray), sinusitis
Miscellaneous: Withdrawal symptoms

Adverse events previously reported in prescription labeling for chewing gum, lozenge and/or transdermal systems. Frequency not defined; may be product or dose specific:
Central nervous system: Concentration impaired, depression, dizziness, headache, insomnia, nervousness, pain
Gastrointestinal: Aphthous stomatitis, constipation, cough, diarrhea, dyspepsia, flatulence, gingival bleeding, glossitis, hiccups, jaw pain, nausea, salivation increased, stomatitis, taste perversion, tooth abrasions, ulcerative stomatitis, xerostomia
Dermatologic: Rash
Local: Application site reaction, local edema, local erythema
Neuromuscular & skeletal: Arthralgia, myalgia, paresthesia
Respiratory: Cough, sinusitis
Miscellaneous: Allergic reaction, diaphoresis

Drug Interactions
Metabolism/Transport Effects Substrate of CYP1A2 (minor), CYP2A6 (minor), CYP2B6 (minor), CYP2C19 (minor), CYP2C9 (minor), CYP2D6 (minor), CYP2E1 (minor), CYP3A4 (minor); **Note:** Assignment of Major/Minor substrate status based on clinically relevant drug interaction potential; **Inhibits** CYP2A6 (weak), CYP2E1 (weak)

Avoid Concomitant Use There are no known interactions where it is recommended to avoid concomitant use.

Increased Effect/Toxicity

Nicotine may increase the levels/effects of: Adenosine

The levels/effects of Nicotine may be increased by: Cimetidine

Decreased Effect

The levels/effects of Nicotine may be decreased by: Peginterferon Alfa-2b; Tocilizumab

Ethanol/Nutrition/Herb Interactions Food: Lozenge: Acidic foods/beverages decrease absorption of nicotine.

Stability

Nicotrol®: Store inhaler cartridge at room temperature not to exceed 30°C (86°F). Protect cartridges from light.

Nicotrol® NS: Store at room temperature not to exceed 30°C (86°F).

Mechanism of Action Nicotine is one of two naturally-occurring alkaloids which exhibit their primary effects via autonomic ganglia stimulation. The other alkaloid is lobeline which has many actions similar to those of nicotine but is less potent. Nicotine is a potent ganglionic and central nervous system stimulant, the actions of which are mediated via nicotine-specific receptors. Biphasic actions are observed depending upon the dose administered. The main effect of nicotine in small doses is stimulation of all autonomic ganglia; with larger doses, initial stimulation is followed by blockade of transmission. Biphasic effects are also evident in the adrenal medulla; discharge of catecholamines occurs with small doses, whereas prevention of catecholamines release is seen with higher doses as a response to splanchnic nerve stimulation. Stimulation of the central nervous system (CNS) is characterized by tremors and respiratory excitation. However, convulsions may occur with higher doses, along with respiratory failure secondary to both central paralysis and peripheral blockade to respiratory muscles.

Pharmacodynamics/Kinetics

Onset of action: Intranasal: More closely approximate the time course of plasma nicotine levels observed after cigarette smoking than other dosage forms

Duration: Transdermal: 24 hours

Absorption: Transdermal: Slow

Metabolism: Hepatic, primarily to cotinine (1/5 as active)

Half-life elimination: 4 hours; Nasal spray: 1-2 hours

Time to peak, serum: Transdermal: 8-9 hours; Nasal spray: 10-20 minutes

Excretion: Urine

Clearance: Renal: pH dependent

Dosage

Geriatric & Adult

Tobacco cessation (patients should be advised to completely stop smoking upon initiation of therapy):

Gum: Chew 1 piece of gum when urge to smoke, up to 24 pieces/day. Patients who smoke <25 cigarettes/day should start with 2-mg strength; patients smoking ≥25 cigarettes/day should start with the 4-mg strength. Use according to the following 12-week dosing schedule:

Weeks 1-6: Chew 1 piece of gum every 1-2 hours; to increase chances of quitting, chew at least 9 pieces/day during the first 6 weeks

Weeks 7-9: Chew 1 piece of gum every 2-4 hours

Weeks 10-12: Chew 1 piece of gum every 4-8 hours

Inhaler: Oral: Usually 6-16 cartridges per day; best effect was achieved by frequent continuous puffing (20 minutes); recommended duration of treatment is 3 months, after which patients may be weaned from the inhaler by gradual reduction of the daily dose over 6-12 weeks

Lozenge: Oral: Patients who smoke their first cigarette within 30 minutes of waking should use the 4-mg strength; otherwise the 2-mg strength is recommended. Use according to the following 12-week dosing schedule:

Weeks 1-6: One lozenge every 1-2 hours

Weeks 7-9: One lozenge every 2-4 hours

Weeks 10-12: One lozenge every 4-8 hours

Note: Use at least 9 lozenges/day during first 6 weeks to improve chances of quitting; do not use more than one lozenge at a time (maximum: 5 lozenges every 6 hours, 20 lozenges/day)

Spray: Nasal: 1-2 sprays/hour; do not exceed more than 5 doses (10 sprays) per hour [maximum: 40 doses/day (80 sprays); each dose (2 sprays) contains 1 mg of nicotine]

Transdermal patch: Topical: Apply new patch every 24 hours to nonhairy, clean, dry skin on the upper body or upper outer arm; each patch should be applied to a different site. **Note:** Adjustment may be required during initial treatment (move to higher dose if experiencing withdrawal symptoms; lower dose if side effects are experienced).

NicoDerm CQ®:

Patients smoking >10 cigarettes/day: Begin with step 1 (21 mg/day) for 6 weeks, **followed by** step 2 (14 mg/day) for 2 weeks; **finish with** step 3 (7 mg/day) for 2 weeks

Patients smoking ≤10 cigarettes/day: Begin with step 2 (14 mg/day) for 6 weeks, **followed by** step 3 (7 mg/day) for 2 weeks

Note: Patients who are receiving >600 mg/day of cimetidine: Decrease to the next lower patch size

Benefits of use of nicotine transdermal patches beyond 3 months have not been demonstrated

Administration

Gum: Should be chewed slowly to avoid jaw ache and to maximize benefit. Chew slowly until it tingles, then park gum between cheek and gum until tingle is gone; repeat process until most of tingle is gone (~30 minutes).

Lozenge: Should not be chewed or swallowed; allow to dissolve slowly (~20-30 minutes)

Nasal spray: Prime pump prior to first use (pump 6-8 times until fine spray appears) or if it has not been used for 24 hours (pump 1-2 times). Blow nose prior to use. Tilt head back slightly and insert tip of bottle into nostril. Breathe through mouth and spray once in each nostril. Do not sniff, swallow, or inhale through the nose during administration. After administration, wait 2-3 minutes before blowing nose.

Oral Inhalant: Insert cartridge into inhaler and push hard until it pops into place. Replace mouthpiece and twist the top and bottom so that markings do not line up. Inhale deeply into the back of the throat or puff in short breaths. Nicotine in cartridge is used up after about 20 minutes of active puffing.

Transdermal patch: Do not cut patch; causes rapid evaporation, rendering the patch useless

Monitoring Parameters Heart rate and blood pressure periodically during therapy; discontinue therapy if signs of nicotine toxicity occur (eg, severe headache, dizziness, mental confusion, disturbed hearing and vision, abdominal pain; rapid, weak and irregular pulse; salivation, nausea, vomiting, diarrhea, cold sweat, weakness); therapy should be discontinued if rash develops; discontinuation may be considered if other adverse effects of patch occur such as myalgia, arthralgia, abnormal dreams, insomnia, nervousness, dry mouth, sweating

Pharmacotherapy Pearls A cigarette has 10-25 mg nicotine.

Special Geriatric Considerations Must evaluate benefit in the elderly who may have chronic diseases mentioned in Warning and Contraindications. The transdermal systems are as effective in the elderly as they are in younger adults; however, complaints of body aches, dizziness, and asthenia were reported more often in the elderly.

Dosage Forms Excipient information presented when available (limited, particularly for generics); consult specific product labeling.

Gum, chewing, oral, as polacrilex: 2 mg (20s, 40s, 50s, 100s, 110s); 4 mg (20s, 40s, 50s, 100s, 110s)

Nicorelief: 2 mg (50s, 110s)

Nicorelief: 2 mg (50s, 110s) [mint flavor]

Nicorelief: 4 mg (50s, 110s)

Nicorelief: 4 mg (50s, 110s) [mint flavor]

Nicorette®: 2 mg (40s, 100s) [fresh mint flavor]

Nicorette®: 2 mg (48s, 50s, 108s, 110s, 168s, 170s, 192s, 200s, 216s) [mint flavor]

Nicorette®: 2 mg (48s, 108s) [orange flavor]

Nicorette®: 2 mg (48s, 50s, 108s, 110s, 168s, 170s, 192s, 200s, 216s) [original flavor]

Nicorette®: 2 mg (40s, 100s) [contains calcium 94 mg/gum, sodium 11 mg/gum; fruit chill flavor]

Nicorette®: 4 mg (40s, 100s) [fresh mint flavor]

Nicorette®: 4 mg (48s, 108s, 110s, 168s, 170s, 192s, 200s, 216s) [mint flavor]

Nicorette®: 4 mg (48s, 108s, 110s) [orange flavor]

Nicorette®: 4 mg (48s, 50s, 108s, 110s, 168s, 170s, 192s, 200s, 216s) [original flavor]

Nicorette®: 4 mg (40s, 100s) [contains calcium 94 mg/gum, sodium 13 mg/gum; fruit chill flavor]

Thrive™: 2 mg (40s); 4 mg (40s) [gluten free, sucrose free; mint flavor]

Lozenge, oral, as polacrilex:

Commit®: 2 mg (48s, 72s); 4 mg (48s, 72s) [gluten free, sugar free; contains phenylalanine 3.4 mg/lozenge, sodium 18 mg/lozenge; mint flavor]

Nicorette®: 4 mg (50s) [mint flavor]

Oral inhalation system, for oral inhalation:

Nicotrol® Inhaler: 10 mg (10 mL) [contains menthol; delivering 4 mg nicotine]

Patch, transdermal: 7 mg/24 hours (7s, 14s); 14 mg/24 hours (7s, 14s); 21 mg/24 hours (7s, 14s)

NicoDerm® CQ®: 7 mg/24 hours (14s) [contains metal; step 3; clear patch]

NicoDerm® CQ®: 7 mg/24 hours (14s) [contains metal; step 3; tan patch]

NicoDerm® CQ®: 14 mg/24 hours (14s) [contains metal; step 2; clear patch]
NicoDerm® CQ®: 14 mg/24 hours (14s) [contains metal; step 2; tan patch]
NicoDerm® CQ®: 21 mg/24 hours (7s, 14s) [contains metal; step 1; clear patch]
NicoDerm® CQ®: 21 mg/24 hours (7s, 14s) [contains metal; step 1; tan patch]
Solution, intranasal [spray]:
Nicotrol® NS: 10 mg/mL (10 mL) [chlorofluorocarbon free; delivers ~0.5 mg/spray; ~200 sprays]

◆ **Nicotine Patch** *see* Nicotine *on page 1372*
◆ **Nicotinic Acid** *see* Niacin *on page 1363*
◆ **Nicotinic Acid Amide** *see* Niacinamide *on page 1366*
◆ **Nicotrol® Inhaler** *see* Nicotine *on page 1372*
◆ **Nicotrol® NS** *see* Nicotine *on page 1372*
◆ **Nifediac CC®** *see* NIFEdipine *on page 1375*
◆ **Nifedical XL®** *see* NIFEdipine *on page 1375*

NIFEdipine (nye FED i peen)

Related Information
Beers Criteria – Potentially Inappropriate Medications for Geriatrics *on page 2183*
Calcium Channel Blockers – Comparative Pharmacokinetics *on page 2111*
Medication Safety Issues
Sound-alike/look-alike issues:
NIFEdipine may be confused with niCARdipine, niMODipine, nisoldipine
Procardia XL® may be confused with Cartia XT®
BEERS Criteria medication:
This drug may be potentially inappropriate for use in geriatric patients (Quality of evidence - high; Strength of recommendation - strong).
International issues:
Depin [India] may be confused with Depen brand name for penicillamine [U.S.]; Depon brand name for acetaminophen [Greece]; Dipen brand name for diltiazem [Greece]
Nipin [Italy and Singapore] may be confused with Nipent brand name for pentostatin [U.S., Canada, and multiple international markets]
Brand Names: U.S. Adalat® CC; Afeditab® CR; Nifediac CC®; Nifedical XL®; Procardia XL®; Procardia®
Brand Names: Canada Adalat® XL®; Apo-Nifed PA®; Mylan-Nifedipine Extended Release; Nu-Nifed; Nu-Nifedipine-PA; PMS-Nifedipine
Generic Availability (U.S.) Yes
Pharmacologic Category Antianginal Agent; Calcium Channel Blocker; Calcium Channel Blocker, Dihydropyridine
Use Management of chronic stable or vasospastic angina; treatment of hypertension (sustained release products only)
Unlabeled Use Management of pulmonary hypertension and Raynaud's phenomenon; prevention and treatment of high altitude pulmonary edema
Contraindications Hypersensitivity to nifedipine or any component of the formulation; concomitant use with strong CYP3A4 inducers (eg, rifampin); cardiogenic shock; immediate release preparation for treatment of urgent or emergent hypertension (Chobanian, 2003); acute MI (Antman, 2004)
Warnings/Precautions Symptomatic hypotension with or without syncope can rarely occur; blood pressure must be lowered at a rate appropriate for the patient's clinical condition. **The use of immediate release nifedipine (sublingually or orally) in hypertensive emergencies and urgencies is neither safe nor effective.** Serious adverse events (eg, death, cerebrovascular ischemia, syncope, stroke, acute myocardial infarction, and fetal distress) have been reported. **Immediate release nifedipine should not be used for acute blood pressure reduction.**

Blood pressure lowering should be done at a rate appropriate for the patient's condition. Rapid drops in blood pressure can lead to arterial insufficiency. Increased angina and/or MI have occurred with initiation or dosage titration of dihydropyridine calcium channel blockers; use with caution in patients with obstructive coronary disease especially in the absence of concurrent beta-blockade. Use with caution before major surgery. Cardiopulmonary bypass, intraoperative blood loss or vasodilating anesthesia may result in severe hypotension and/or increased fluid requirements. Consider withdrawing nifedipine (>36 hours) before surgery if possible.

The most common side effect is peripheral edema; occurs within 2-3 weeks of starting therapy. Reflex tachycardia may occur with use. Use with caution in HF or severe aortic stenosis (especially with concomitant beta-adrenergic blocker), severe left ventricular dysfunction, renal impairment, hypertrophic cardiomyopathy (especially obstructive), concomitant therapy with beta-blockers or digoxin, and edema. Use caution in patients with severe hepatic impairment. Clearance of nifedipine is reduced in cirrhotic patients leading to increased systemic exposure; monitor closely for adverse effects/toxicity and consider dose adjustments. Mild and transient elevations in liver function enzymes may be apparent within 8 weeks of therapy initiation. Abrupt withdrawal may cause rebound angina in patients with CAD. In the elderly, immediate release nifedipine should be avoided in due to potential to cause hypotension and risk of precipitating myocardial ischemia (Beers Criteria). Immediate release formulations should not be used to manage essential hypertension, adequate studies to evaluate outcomes have not been conducted. Avoid use of extended release tablets (Procardia XL®) in patients with known stricture/narrowing of the GI tract. Adalat® CC tablets contain lactose; do not use with galactose intolerance, Lapp lactase deficiency, or glucose-galactose malabsorption syndromes.

Use with caution in patients taking CYP3A4 inhibitors; may result in increased nifedipine concentrations; monitor for adverse effects/toxicity and consider dose adjustments. Use with strong CYP3A4 inducers (eg, rifampin, rifabutin, phenobarbital, phenytoin, carbamazepine, St John's wort) is contraindicated due to reduced bioavailability and efficacy.

Adverse Reactions (Reflective of adult population; not specific for elderly)
>10%:
  Cardiovascular: Flushing (10% to 25%; extended release products 3% to 4%), peripheral edema (dose related 7% to 30%)
  Central nervous system: Dizziness/lightheadedness/giddiness (10% to 27%), headache (10% to 23%)
  Gastrointestinal: Nausea/heartburn (10% to 11%)
≥1% to 10%:
  Cardiovascular: Palpitation (≤2% to 7%), transient hypotension (dose related 5%), CHF (2%)
  Central nervous system: Nervousness/mood changes (≤2% to 7%), fatigue (6%), shakiness (≤2%), jitteriness (≤2%), sleep disturbances (≤2%), difficulties in balance (≤2%), fever (≤2%), chills (≤2%)
  Dermatologic: Dermatitis (≤2%), pruritus (≤2%), urticaria (≤2%)
  Endocrine & metabolic: Sexual difficulties (≤2%)
  Gastrointestinal: Diarrhea (≤2%), constipation (≤2%), cramps (≤2%), flatulence (≤2%), gingival hyperplasia (≤10%)
  Neuromuscular & skeletal: Muscle cramps/tremor (≤2% to 8%), weakness (<3%), inflammation (≤2%), joint stiffness (≤2%)
  Ocular: Blurred vision (≤2%)
  Respiratory: Cough/wheezing (6%), nasal congestion/sore throat (≤2% to 6%), chest congestion (≤2%), dyspnea (≤2%)
  Miscellaneous: Diaphoresis (≤2%)

Drug Interactions
Metabolism/Transport Effects Substrate of CYP2D6 (minor), CYP3A4 (major); **Note:** Assignment of Major/Minor substrate status based on clinically relevant drug interaction potential; **Inhibits** CYP1A2 (moderate), CYP2C9 (weak), CYP2D6 (weak), CYP3A4 (weak)

Avoid Concomitant Use
  Avoid concomitant use of NIFEdipine with any of the following: Conivaptan; Grapefruit Juice; Pimozide

Increased Effect/Toxicity
  NIFEdipine may increase the levels/effects of: Amifostine; Antihypertensives; ARIPiprazole; Beta-Blockers; Calcium Channel Blockers (Nondihydropyridine); Calcium Channel Blockers; Digoxin; Fosphenytoin; Hypotensive Agents; Magnesium Salts; Neuromuscular-Blocking Agents (Nondepolarizing); Nitroprusside; Phenytoin; Pimozide; QuiNIDine; RiTUXimab; Tacrolimus; Tacrolimus (Systemic); VinCRIStine

  The levels/effects of NIFEdipine may be increased by: Alcohol (Ethyl); Alpha1-Blockers; Antifungal Agents (Azole Derivatives, Systemic); Calcium Channel Blockers (Nondihydropyridine); Cimetidine; Cisapride; Conivaptan; CycloSPORINE; CycloSPORINE (Systemic); CYP3A4 Inhibitors (Moderate); CYP3A4 Inhibitors (Strong); Dasatinib; Diazoxide; Fluconazole; FLUoxetine; Grapefruit Juice; Herbs (Hypotensive Properties); Ivacaftor; Macrolide Antibiotics; Magnesium Salts; MAO Inhibitors; Mifepristone; Pentoxifylline; Phosphodiesterase 5 Inhibitors; Prostacyclin Analogues; Protease Inhibitors; QuiNIDine

Decreased Effect
  NIFEdipine may decrease the levels/effects of: Clopidogrel; QuiNIDine

  The levels/effects of NIFEdipine may be decreased by: Barbiturates; Calcium Salts; CarBAMazepine; CYP3A4 Inducers (Strong); Deferasirox; Herbs (CYP3A4 Inducers); Herbs (Hypertensive Properties); Methylphenidate; Nafcillin; Peginterferon Alfa-2b; Rifamycin Derivatives; Tocilizumab; Yohimbine

Ethanol/Nutrition/Herb Interactions

Ethanol: Ethanol may increase CNS depression and may increase the effects of nifedipine. Management: Avoid ethanol.

Food: Nifedipine serum levels may be decreased if taken with food. Food may decrease the rate but not the extent of absorption of Procardia XL®. Increased nifedipine concentrations resulting in therapeutic and vasodilator side effects, including severe hypotension and myocardial ischemia, may occur if nifedipine is taken by patients ingesting grapefruit. Management: Avoid grapefruit/grapefruit juice. Avoid caffeine.

Herb/Nutraceutical: St John's wort may decrease nifedipine levels. Some herbal medications (eg, licorice) may worsen hypertension; others may increase the antihypertensive effect of nifedipine (eg, shepherd's purse). Management: Avoid bayberry, blue cohosh, cayenne, ephedra, ginger, ginseng (American), kola, licorice, and yohimbe. Avoid black cohosh, California poppy, coleus, golden seal, hawthorn, mistletoe, periwinkle, quinine, and shepherd's purse.

Mechanism of Action Inhibits calcium ion from entering the "slow channels" or select voltage-sensitive areas of vascular smooth muscle and myocardium during depolarization, producing a relaxation of coronary vascular smooth muscle and coronary vasodilation; increases myocardial oxygen delivery in patients with vasospastic angina; also reduces peripheral vascular resistance, producing a reduction in arterial blood pressure.

Pharmacodynamics/Kinetics

Onset of action: Immediate release: ~20 minutes

Protein binding (concentration dependent): 92% to 98%

Metabolism: Hepatic via CYP3A4 to inactive metabolites

Bioavailability: Capsule: 40% to 77%; Sustained release: 65% to 89% relative to immediate release capsules; bioavailability increased with significant hepatic disease

Half-life elimination: Adults: Healthy: 2-5 hours; Cirrhosis: 7 hours; Elderly: 7 hours (extended release tablet)

Excretion: Urine (60% to 80% as inactive metabolites); feces

Dosage

Geriatric Refer to adult dosing. In the management of hypertension, consider lower initial doses and titrate to response (Aronow, 2011).

Adult Dosage adjustments should occur at 7- to 14-day intervals, to allow for adequate assessment of new dose; when switching from immediate release to sustained release formulations, use same total daily dose.

Chronic stable or vasospastic angina: Oral:

Immediate release: Initial: 10 mg 3 times/day; usual dose: 10-20 mg 3 times/day; coronary artery spasm may require up to 20-30 mg 3-4 times/day; single doses >30 mg and total daily doses >120 mg are rarely needed; maximum: 180 mg/day; **Note:** Do not use for acute anginal episodes; may precipitate myocardial infarction

Extended release: Initial: 30 or 60 mg once daily; maximum: 120-180 mg/day

Hypertension: Oral: Extended release: Initial: 30 or 60 mg once daily; maximum: 90-120 mg/day

High altitude pulmonary edema (unlabeled use; Luks, 2010): Oral:

Prevention: Extended release: 30 mg every 12 hours starting the day before ascent and may be discontinued after staying at the same elevation for 5 days or if descent initiated

Treatment: Extended release: 30 mg every 12 hours

Pulmonary hypertension (unlabeled use; Galie, 2004): Oral: Extended release: Initial: 30 mg twice daily; may increase cautiously to 120-240 mg/day

Raynaud's phenomenon (unlabeled use; Wigley, 2002): Oral: Extended release: Dosage range: 30-120 mg once daily

Renal Impairment

Hemodialysis: Supplemental dose is not necessary.

Peritoneal dialysis effects: Supplemental dose is not necessary.

Hepatic Impairment Clearance of nifedipine is reduced in cirrhotic patients leading to increased systemic exposure; monitor closely for adverse effects/toxicity and consider dose adjustments.

Administration

Immediate release: In general, may be administered with or without food.

Extended release: Tablets should be swallowed whole; do not crush, split, or chew.

Adalat® CC, Afeditab® CR, Nifediac CC®: Administer on an empty stomach (per manufacturer). Other extended release products may not have this recommendation; consult product labeling.

Monitoring Parameters Heart rate, blood pressure, signs and symptoms of CHF, peripheral edema

Pharmacotherapy Pearls When measuring smaller doses from the liquid-filled capsules, consider the following concentrations (for Procardia®) 10 mg capsule = 10 mg/0.34 mL; 20 mg capsule = 20 mg/0.45 mL; may be used preoperative to treat hypertensive urgency.

Considerable attention has been directed to potential increases in mortality and morbidity when short-acting nifedipine is used in treating hypertension. The rapid reduction in blood pressure may precipitate adverse cardiovascular events.

Short-acting nifedipine should not be used for acute anginal episodes since this may precipitate myocardial infarction. Extended-release formulations are preferred for the management of chronic or vasospastic angina (Poole-Wilson, 2004).

Equivalency of extended release formulation (Adalat® CC): The manufacturer states that it is acceptable to interchange two 30 mg tablets with one 60 mg tablet to effectively deliver a 60 mg dose. However, it is not recommended to substitute one 90 mg tablet with three 30 mg tablets, since the resulting C_{max} is 29% higher compared to giving the single 90 mg tablet.

Special Geriatric Considerations Elderly may experience a greater hypotensive response. Theoretically, constipation may be more of a problem in elderly patients. The half-life of nifedipine is extended in elderly patients (6.7 hours) as compared to younger subjects (3.8 hours).

This medication is considered to be potentially inappropriate in this patient population (Beers Criteria: Quality of evidence - high; Strength of recommendation - strong).

Dosage Forms Excipient information presented when available (limited, particularly for generics); consult specific product labeling.

Capsule, softgel, oral: 10 mg, 20 mg
  Procardia®: 10 mg
Tablet, extended release, oral: 30 mg, 60 mg, 90 mg
  Adalat® CC: 30 mg, 60 mg, 90 mg
  Afeditab® CR: 30 mg, 60 mg
  Nifediac CC®: 30 mg, 60 mg
  Nifediac CC®: 90 mg [contains tartrazine]
  Nifedical XL®: 30 mg, 60 mg
  Procardia XL®: 30 mg, 60 mg, 90 mg

- ◆ **Niftolid** see Flutamide on page 821
- ◆ **Nilandron®** see Nilutamide on page 1378

Nilutamide (ni LOO ta mide)

Medication Safety Issues
  Sound-alike/look-alike issues:
    Nilutamide may be confused with nilotinib
Brand Names: U.S. Nilandron®
Brand Names: Canada Anandron®
Index Terms RU-23908
Generic Availability (U.S.) No
Pharmacologic Category Antiandrogen; Antineoplastic Agent, Antiandrogen
Use Treatment of metastatic prostate cancer (in combination with surgical castration)
Contraindications Hypersensitivity to nilutamide or any component of the formulation; severe hepatic impairment; severe respiratory insufficiency
Warnings/Precautions Hazardous agent - use appropriate precautions for handling and disposal. **[U.S. Boxed Warning]: Interstitial pneumonitis has been reported in 2% of patients exposed to nilutamide.** Symptoms typically include exertional dyspnea, cough, chest pain and fever; interstitial changes (including pulmonary fibrosis) leading to hospitalization and fatalities have been reported (rarely). The suggestive signs of pneumonitis most often occurred within the first 3 months of treatment. X-rays showed interstitial or alveolo-interstitial changes; pulmonary function tests revealed a restrictive pattern with decreased DLco. Consider baseline pulmonary function testing. Discontinue if signs and/or symptoms of interstitial pneumonitis are noted.

Hepatitis or marked increases in liver enzymes leading to drug discontinuation occurred in 1% of nilutamide patients; rare cases of hospitalization or deaths due to severe liver injury have been reported. Discontinue treatment for jaundice or ALT >2 times the upper limit of normal (ULN).

A delay in adaptation to dark has been reported; in clinical studies, this was reported by 13% to 57% of patients; the delay ranged from seconds to a few minutes after passing from a light to a dark area (this may not abate with continued treatment although may be alleviated by wearing tinted sunglasses); caution patients who experience adaptation delay about driving at night or through tunnels. Not indicated for use in women. Patients with disease progression while receiving antiandrogen therapy may experience clinical improvement with discontinuation of the antiandrogen.

Adverse Reactions (Reflective of adult population; not specific for elderly)
>10%:
Central nervous system: Insomnia (16%), headache (14%)
Endocrine & metabolic: Hot flashes (28% to 67%)
Gastrointestinal: Nausea (10% to 24%), constipation (7% to 20%), anorexia (11%), abdominal pain (10%)
Genitourinary: Testicular atrophy (16%), libido decreased (11%)
Hepatic: AST increased (8% to 13%), ALT increased (8% to 9%)
Ocular: Impaired dark adaptation (13% to 57%)
Respiratory: Dyspnea (6% to 11%)
1% to 10%:
Cardiovascular: Hypertension (5% to 9%), chest pain (7%), heart failure (3%), angina (2%), edema (2%), syncope (2%)
Central nervous system: Dizziness (7% to 10%), depression (9%), hypoesthesia (5%), malaise (2%), nervousness (2%)
Dermatologic: Alopecia (6%), dry skin (5%), rash (5%), pruritus (2%)
Endocrine & metabolic: Alcohol intolerance (5%), hyperglycemia (4%)
Gastrointestinal: Vomiting (6%), diarrhea (2%), GI hemorrhage (2%), melena (2%), weight loss (2%), xerostomia (2%), dyspepsia
Genitourinary: Nocturia (7%)
Hematologic: Anemia (7%), haptoglobin increased (2%), leukopenia (2%)
Hepatic: Alkaline phosphatase increased (3%)
Neuromuscular & skeletal: Bone pain (6%), arthritis (2%), paresthesia (2%)
Ocular: Chromatopsia (9%), impaired light adaptation (8%), abnormal vision (6% to 7%), cataract (2%), photophobia (2%)
Renal: Hematuria (8%), BUN increased (2%), creatinine increased (2%)
Respiratory: Pneumonia (5%), cough (2%), interstitial pneumonitis (2%), rhinitis (2%)
Miscellaneous: Flu-like syndrome (7%), diaphoresis (6%)

Drug Interactions
Metabolism/Transport Effects Substrate of CYP2C19 (major); **Note:** Assignment of Major/Minor substrate status based on clinically relevant drug interaction potential; **Inhibits** CYP2C19 (weak)
Avoid Concomitant Use There are no known interactions where it is recommended to avoid concomitant use.
Increased Effect/Toxicity
The levels/effects of Nilutamide may be increased by: CYP2C19 Inhibitors (Moderate); CYP2C19 Inhibitors (Strong)
Decreased Effect
The levels/effects of Nilutamide may be decreased by: CYP2C19 Inducers (Strong)
Ethanol/Nutrition/Herb Interactions Ethanol: Approximately 5% of patients experience an intolerance (facial flushing, hypotension, malaise) when ethanol is combined with nilutamide. Management: Avoid ethanol.
Stability Store at room temperature of 25°C (77°F); excursions permitted between 15°C to 30°C (59°F to 86°F). Protect from light.
Mechanism of Action Nonsteroidal antiandrogen which blocks testosterone effects at the androgen receptor level, preventing androgen response.
Pharmacodynamics/Kinetics
Absorption: Rapid and complete
Metabolism: Hepatic (extensive), forms active metabolites
Half-life elimination: Terminal: 38-59 hours; Metabolites: 59-126 hours
Excretion: Urine (62%; <2% as unchanged drug); feces (1% to 7%)
Dosage
Geriatric & Adult Prostate cancer, metastatic: Oral: 300 mg once daily (starting the same day or day after surgical castration) for 30 days, followed by 150 mg once daily
Hepatic Impairment
Prior to treatment initiation: Severe hepatic impairment: Use is contraindicated.
During treatment: ALT >2 times ULN or jaundice: Discontinue treatment.
Administration Administer without regard to meals.
Monitoring Parameters Hepatic enzymes (at baseline, regularly during the first 4 months of treatment, periodically thereafter); chest x-ray (at baseline); consider pulmonary function testing (at baseline)
Special Geriatric Considerations Eyes may be slow to adapt to darkness, tinted glasses may help; patients should be careful when driving at night.
Dosage Forms Excipient information presented when available (limited, particularly for generics); consult specific product labeling.
Tablet, oral:
Nilandron®: 150 mg

NiMODipine (nye MOE di peen)

Related Information
Calcium Channel Blockers – Comparative Pharmacokinetics *on page 2111*

Medication Safety Issues
Sound-alike/look-alike issues:
NiMODipine may be confused with niCARdipine, NIFEdipine, nisoldipine
Administration issues:
For oral administration only. For patients unable to swallow a capsule, the drug should be dispensed in an oral syringe (preferably amber in color) labeled **"WARNING: For ORAL use only"** or **"Not for I.V. use."** Nimodipine has inadvertently been administered I.V. when withdrawn from capsules into a syringe for subsequent nasogastric tube administration. Severe cardiovascular adverse events, including fatalities, have resulted. Employ precautions against such an event.

Brand Names: Canada Nimotop®
Generic Availability (U.S.) Yes
Pharmacologic Category Calcium Channel Blocker; Calcium Channel Blocker, Dihydropyridine

Use Vasospasm following subarachnoid hemorrhage from ruptured intracranial aneurysms
Contraindications Hypersensitivity to nimodipine or any component of the formulation
Warnings/Precautions Increased angina and/or MI has occurred with initiation or dosage titration of calcium channel blockers. The most common side effect is peripheral edema; occurs within 2-3 weeks of starting therapy. Reflex tachycardia may occur with use. Symptomatic hypotension with or without syncope can rarely occur; blood pressure must be lowered at a rate appropriate for the patient's clinical condition. Use caution in hepatic impairment. Intestinal pseudo-obstruction and ileus have been reported during the use of nimodipine. Use caution in patients with decreased GI motility of a history of bowel obstruction. Use caution when treating patients with hypertrophic cardiomyopathy.

[U.S. Boxed Warning]: Nimodipine has inadvertently been administered I.V. when withdrawn from capsules into a syringe for subsequent nasogastric administration. Severe cardiovascular adverse events, including fatalities, have resulted; precautions (eg, adequate labeling, use of oral syringes) should be employed against such an event.
Adverse Reactions (Reflective of adult population; not specific for elderly) 1% to 10%:
Cardiovascular: Reductions in systemic blood pressure (1% to 8%)
Central nervous system: Headache (1% to 4%)
Dermatologic: Rash (1% to 2%)
Gastrointestinal: Diarrhea (2% to 4%), abdominal discomfort (2%)

Drug Interactions
Metabolism/Transport Effects Substrate of CYP3A4 (major); **Note:** Assignment of Major/Minor substrate status based on clinically relevant drug interaction potential
Avoid Concomitant Use
Avoid concomitant use of NiMODipine with any of the following: Conivaptan; Grapefruit Juice
Increased Effect/Toxicity
NiMODipine may increase the levels/effects of: Amifostine; Antihypertensives; Beta-Blockers; Calcium Channel Blockers (Nondihydropyridine); Fosphenytoin; Hypotensive Agents; Magnesium Salts; Neuromuscular-Blocking Agents (Nondepolarizing); Nitroprusside; Phenytoin; QuiNIDine; RiTUXimab; Tacrolimus; Tacrolimus (Systemic)

The levels/effects of NiMODipine may be increased by: Alpha1-Blockers; Antifungal Agents (Azole Derivatives, Systemic); Calcium Channel Blockers (Nondihydropyridine); Cimetidine; Conivaptan; CycloSPORINE; CycloSPORINE (Systemic); CYP3A4 Inhibitors (Moderate); CYP3A4 Inhibitors (Strong); Dasatinib; Diazoxide; Fluconazole; FLUoxetine; Grapefruit Juice; Herbs (Hypotensive Properties); Ivacaftor; Macrolide Antibiotics; Magnesium Salts; MAO Inhibitors; Mifepristone; Pentoxifylline; Phosphodiesterase 5 Inhibitors; Prostacyclin Analogues; Protease Inhibitors; QuiNIDine
Decreased Effect
NiMODipine may decrease the levels/effects of: Clopidogrel; QuiNIDine

The levels/effects of NiMODipine may be decreased by: Barbiturates; Calcium Salts; CarBAMazepine; CYP3A4 Inducers (Strong); Deferasirox; Herbs (CYP3A4 Inducers); Herbs (Hypertensive Properties); Methylphenidate; Nafcillin; Rifamycin Derivatives; Tocilizumab; Yohimbine
Ethanol/Nutrition/Herb Interactions
Food: Nimodipine has shown a 1.5-fold increase in bioavailability when taken with grapefruit juice. Management: Avoid concurrent use of grapefruit juice and nimodipine.

Herb/Nutraceutical: St John's wort may decrease levels. Dong quai has estrogenic activity. Some herbal medications may worsen hypertension (eg, ephedra); garlic may increase antihypertensive effects of nimodipine. Management: Avoid dong quai if using for hypertension. Avoid St John's wort, ephedra, yohimbe, ginseng, and garlic.

Mechanism of Action Nimodipine shares the pharmacology of other calcium channel blockers; animal studies indicate that nimodipine has a greater effect on cerebral arterials than other arterials; this increased specificity may be due to the drug's increased lipophilicity and cerebral distribution as compared to nifedipine; inhibits calcium ion from entering the "slow channels" or select voltage sensitive areas of vascular smooth muscle and myocardium during depolarization

Pharmacodynamics/Kinetics
Protein binding: >95%
Metabolism: Extensively hepatic
Bioavailability: 13%
Half-life elimination: 1-2 hours; prolonged with renal impairment
Time to peak, serum: ~1 hour
Excretion: Urine (50%) and feces (32%) within 4 days

Dosage
Geriatric & Adult Note: Capsules and contents are for oral/NG tube administration **ONLY.**
Subarachnoid hemorrhage: Oral: 60 mg every 4 hours for 21 days, start therapy within 96 hours after subarachnoid hemorrhage.
Renal Impairment Not removed by hemo- or peritoneal dialysis; supplemental dose is not necessary.
Hepatic Impairment Reduce dosage to 30 mg every 4 hours in patients with liver failure.

Administration For oral administration ONLY. Life-threatening adverse events have occurred when administered parenterally. Administer on an empty stomach.

Nasogastric (NG) tube administration: If the capsules cannot be swallowed, the liquid may be removed by making a hole in each end of the capsule with an 18-gauge needle and extracting the contents into a syringe; transfer these contents into an oral syringe (amber-colored oral syringe preferred). It is strongly recommended that preparation be done in the pharmacy. Label oral syringe with **"WARNING: For ORAL use only"** or **"Not for I.V. use."** Follow with a flush of 30 mL NS.

Monitoring Parameters CNS response, heart rate, blood pressure, signs and symptoms of congestive heart failure

Special Geriatric Considerations Elderly may experience a greater hypotensive response. Constipation may be more of a problem in the elderly. Studies in the treatment of Alzheimer's disease have not demonstrated clear clinical effect.

Dosage Forms Excipient information presented when available (limited, particularly for generics); consult specific product labeling.
Capsule, liquid filled, oral: 30 mg
Capsule, softgel, oral: 30 mg

♦ **Niravam™** see ALPRAZolam on page 67

Nisoldipine (nye SOL di peen)

Related Information
Calcium Channel Blockers – Comparative Pharmacokinetics on page 2111
Medication Safety Issues
Sound-alike/look-alike issues:
Nisoldipine may be confused with NIFEdipine, niMODipine
Brand Names: U.S. Sular®
Generic Availability (U.S.) Yes
Pharmacologic Category Calcium Channel Blocker; Calcium Channel Blocker, Dihydropyridine
Use Management of hypertension, alone or in combination with other antihypertensive agents
Contraindications Hypersensitivity to nisoldipine, any component of the formulation, or other dihydropyridine calcium channel blockers
Warnings/Precautions With initiation or dosage titration of dihydropyridine calcium channel blockers, reflex tachycardia may occur resulting in angina and/or MI in patients with obstructive coronary disease especially in the absence of concurrent beta-blockade. Use with caution in patients with severe aortic stenosis, HF, and hypertrophic cardiomyopathy with outflow tract obstruction. Use with caution in hepatic impairment; lower starting dose required. The most common side effect is peripheral edema; occurs within 2-3 weeks of starting therapy. Symptomatic hypotension with or without syncope can rarely occur; blood pressure must be lowered at a rate appropriate for the patient's clinical condition. Some dosage forms

contain tartrazine, which may cause allergic reactions in certain individuals (eg, aspirin hypersensitivity). Use with caution in patients >65 years of age; lower starting dose recommended.

Adverse Reactions (Reflective of adult population; not specific for elderly)
>10%:
  Cardiovascular: Peripheral edema (dose related; 7% to 29%)
  Central nervous system: Headache (22%)
1% to 10%:
  Cardiovascular: Vasodilation (4%), palpitation (3%), angina exacerbation (2%), chest pain (2%)
  Central nervous system: Dizziness (3% to 10%)
  Dermatologic: Rash (2%)
  Gastrointestinal: Nausea (2%)
  Respiratory: Pharyngitis (5%), sinusitis (3%)

Drug Interactions
  Metabolism/Transport Effects Substrate of CYP3A4 (major); **Note:** Assignment of Major/ Minor substrate status based on clinically relevant drug interaction potential; **Inhibits** CYP1A2 (weak), CYP3A4 (weak)
  Avoid Concomitant Use
    Avoid concomitant use of Nisoldipine with any of the following: CYP3A4 Inducers (Strong); CYP3A4 Inhibitors (Strong); Grapefruit Juice; Pimozide
  Increased Effect/Toxicity
    Nisoldipine may increase the levels/effects of: Amifostine; Antihypertensives; ARIPiprazole; Beta-Blockers; Calcium Channel Blockers (Nondihydropyridine); Fosphenytoin; Hypotensive Agents; Magnesium Salts; Neuromuscular-Blocking Agents (Nondepolarizing); Nitroprusside; Phenytoin; Pimozide; RiTUXimab; Tacrolimus; Tacrolimus (Systemic)

    The levels/effects of Nisoldipine may be increased by: Alpha1-Blockers; Antifungal Agents (Azole Derivatives, Systemic); Calcium Channel Blockers (Nondihydropyridine); Cimetidine; CycloSPORINE; CycloSPORINE (Systemic); CYP3A4 Inhibitors (Moderate); CYP3A4 Inhibitors (Strong); Dasatinib; Diazoxide; Fluconazole; Grapefruit Juice; Herbs (Hypotensive Properties); Ivacaftor; Macrolide Antibiotics; Magnesium Salts; MAO Inhibitors; Mifepristone; Pentoxifylline; Phosphodiesterase 5 Inhibitors; Prostacyclin Analogues; Protease Inhibitors
  Decreased Effect
    Nisoldipine may decrease the levels/effects of: Clopidogrel

    The levels/effects of Nisoldipine may be decreased by: Barbiturates; Calcium Salts; CarBAMazepine; CYP3A4 Inducers (Strong); Deferasirox; Herbs (CYP3A4 Inducers); Herbs (Hypertensive Properties); Methylphenidate; Nafcillin; Rifamycin Derivatives; Tocilizumab; Yohimbine

Ethanol/Nutrition/Herb Interactions
  Food: Peak concentrations of nisoldipine may be significantly increased if taken with high-lipid foods; however, total exposure (AUC) may be reduced. Grapefruit juice has been shown to significantly increase the bioavailability of nisoldipine. Management: Take on an empty stomach 1 hour before or 2 hours after a meal. Avoid a high-fat diet. Avoid grapefruit products before and after dosing.
  Herb/Nutraceutical: St John's wort may decrease nisoldipine levels. Some herbal medications may worsen hypertension (eg, licorice); others may increase the antihypertensive effect of nisoldipine (eg, shepherd's purse). Management: Avoid St John's wort. Avoid bayberry, blue cohosh, cayenne, ephedra, ginger, ginseng (American), kola, licorice, and yohimbe. Avoid black cohosh, California poppy, coleus, golden seal, hawthorn, mistletoe, periwinkle, quinine, and shepherd's purse.

Stability Store at controlled room temperature of 20°C to 25°C (68°F to 77°F). Protect from light; protect from moisture.

Mechanism of Action As a dihydropyridine calcium channel blocker, structurally similar to nifedipine, nisoldipine impedes the movement of calcium ions into vascular smooth muscle and cardiac muscle. Dihydropyridines are potent vasodilators and are not as likely to suppress cardiac contractility and slow cardiac conduction as other calcium antagonists such as verapamil and diltiazem; nisoldipine is 5-10 times as potent a vasodilator as nifedipine.

Pharmacodynamics/Kinetics
  Duration: >24 hours
  Absorption: Well absorbed. Peak concentrations significantly increased with high-lipid meals; however, AUC is reduced.
  Protein binding: >99%
  Metabolism: Extensively hepatic; 1 active metabolite (10% of activity of parent); first-pass effect
  Bioavailability: ~5%
  Half-life elimination: 9-18 hours

Time to peak: 4-14 hours

Excretion: Urine (60% to 80% as inactive metabolites); feces

Dosage

Geriatric Hypertension: Oral:

Sular® (Geomatrix® delivery system): Initial dose: 8.5 mg once daily; increase by 8.5 mg/week (or longer intervals) to attain adequate blood pressure control

Nisoldipine extended-release (original formulation): Initial dose: 10 mg once daily; increase by 10 mg/week (or longer intervals) to attain adequate blood pressure control.

Conversion from nisoldipine extended-release (original formulation) to Sular® Geomatrix® delivery system: Refer to adult dosing.

Adult Hypertension: Oral:

Sular® (Geomatrix® delivery system): Oral: Initial: 17 mg once daily, then increase by 8.5 mg/week (or longer intervals) to attain adequate control of blood pressure
Usual dose range: 17-34 mg once daily; doses >34 mg once daily are not recommended

Nisoldipine extended-release tablet (original formulation): Initial: 20 mg once daily, then increase by 10 mg/week (or longer intervals) to attain adequate control of blood pressure
Usual dose range (JNC 7): 10-40 mg once daily; doses >60 mg once daily are not recommended

Conversion from nisoldipine extended-release (original formulation) to Sular® Geomatrix® delivery system:

Nisoldipine Extended Release Dosing Equivalency

Original Extended Release Formulation	Sular® Extended Release (Geomatrix® delivery system)
10 mg	8.5 mg
20 mg	17 mg
30 mg	25.5 mg
40 mg	34 mg

Hepatic Impairment

Sular® (Geomatrix® delivery system): An initial dose exceeding 8.5 mg once daily is not recommended for patients with hepatic impairment.

Nisoldipine extended-release (original formulation): An initial dose exceeding 10 mg once daily is not recommended for patients with hepatic impairment.

Administration Administer at the same time each day to ensure minimal fluctuation of serum levels. Avoid high-fat diet. Administer on an empty stomach (1 hour before or 2 hours after a meal). Swallow whole; do not crush, break, split, or chew.

Monitoring Parameters Heart rate, blood pressure, signs and symptoms of CHF, peripheral edema

Special Geriatric Considerations Elderly have been found to have two- to threefold greater serum concentrations than younger adults. Therefore, begin therapy at lowest recommended doses. Elderly may experience a greater hypotensive response. Constipation may be more of a problem in the elderly. Calcium channel blockers are no more effective in the elderly than other therapies; however, they do not cause significant CNS effects which is an advantage over some antihypertensive agents.

Dosage Forms Excipient information presented when available (limited, particularly for generics); consult specific product labeling. [DSC] = Discontinued product

Tablet, extended release, oral: 8.5 mg, 17 mg, 25.5 mg, 34 mg

Sular®: 8.5 mg

Sular®: 17 mg [contains tartrazine]

Sular®: 25.5 mg [DSC], 34 mg

Tablet, extended release, oral [original formula]: 20 mg, 30 mg, 40 mg

◆ **Nitalapram** *see* Citalopram *on page 387*

◆ **Nitro-Bid®** *see* Nitroglycerin *on page 1386*

◆ **Nitro-Dur®** *see* Nitroglycerin *on page 1386*

Nitrofurantoin (nye troe fyoor AN toyn)

Related Information
Antimicrobial Drugs of Choice *on page 2163*
Beers Criteria – Potentially Inappropriate Medications for Geriatrics *on page 2183*

Medication Safety Issues
Sound alike/look alike issues:
Macrobid® may be confused with microK®, Nitro-Bid®
Nitrofurantoin may be confused with Neurontin®, nitroglycerin

BEERS Criteria medication:
This drug may be potentially inappropriate for use in geriatric patients (Quality of evidence - moderate; Strength of recommendation - strong).

Brand Names: U.S. Furadantin®; Macrobid®; Macrodantin®

Brand Names: Canada Apo-Nitrofurantoin®; Macrobid®; Macrodantin®; Novo-Furantoin; Teva-Nitrofurantoin

Generic Availability (U.S.) Yes

Pharmacologic Category Antibiotic, Miscellaneous

Use Prevention and treatment of urinary tract infections caused by susceptible strains of *E. coli, S. aureus, Enterococcus, Klebsiella,* and *Enterobacter*

Contraindications Hypersensitivity to nitrofurantoin or any component of the formulation; significant renal impairment (anuria, oliguria, significantly elevated serum creatinine, or Cl_{cr} <60 mL/minute); use in patients with a history of cholestatic jaundice or hepatic impairment with previous nitrofurantoin therapy

Warnings/Precautions Use with caution in patients with G6PD deficiency (increased risk of hemolytic anemia). Therapeutic concentrations of nitrofurantoin are not attained in urine of patients with Cl_{cr} <60 mL/minute, therefore, use contraindicated in these patients. Use with caution if prolonged therapy is anticipated due to possible pulmonary toxicity. Acute, subacute, or chronic (usually after 6 months of therapy) pulmonary reactions (possibly fatal) have been observed in patients treated with nitrofurantoin; if these occur, discontinue therapy immediately; monitor closely for malaise, dyspnea, cough, fever, radiologic evidence of diffuse interstitial pneumonitis or fibrosis. Rare, but severe and sometimes fatal hepatic reactions (eg, cholestatic jaundice, hepatitis, hepatic necrosis) have been associated with nitrofurantoin (onset may be insidious); discontinue immediately if hepatitis occurs. Monitor liver function test periodically. Has been associated with peripheral neuropathy (rare); risk may be increased in patients with anemia, renal impairment, diabetes, vitamin B deficiency, debilitating disease, or electrolyte imbalance; use caution. Use in the elderly, particularly females receiving long-term prophylaxis for recurrent UTIs, has been associated with an increased risk of hepatic and pulmonary toxicity, and peripheral neuropathy. In the elderly, avoid use for long-term suppression or in patients with decreased renal function (contraindicated in Cl_{cr} <60 mL/minute) due to potential for pulmonary toxicity and availability of safer alternative agents (Beers Criteria). Use in the elderly, particularly females receiving long-term prophylaxis for recurrent UTIs, has also been associated with an increased risk of hepatic toxicity and peripheral neuropathy; monitor closely for toxicities during use. Prolonged use may result in fungal or bacterial superinfection, including *C. difficile*-associated diarrhea (CDAD) and pseudomembranous colitis; CDAD has been observed >2 months postantibiotic treatment. Not indicated for the treatment of pyelonephritis or perinephric abscesses.

Adverse Reactions (Reflective of adult population; not specific for elderly) Frequency not defined.
Cardiovascular: Cyanosis, ECG changes (nonspecific ST/T wave changes, bundle branch block)
Central nervous system: Bulging fontanels (infants), chills, confusion, depression, dizziness, drowsiness, fever, headache, malaise, pseudotumor cerebri, psychotic reaction, vertigo
Dermatologic: Alopecia, angioedema, erythema multiforme, exfoliative dermatitis, pruritus, rash (eczematous, erythematous, maculopapular), Stevens-Johnson syndrome, urticaria
Endocrine & metabolic: Hyperphosphatemia
Gastrointestinal: Abdominal pain, anorexia, *C. difficile* colitis, constipation, diarrhea, dyspepsia, flatulence, nausea, pancreatitis, pseudomembranous colitis, sialadenitis, vomiting
Genitourinary: Urine discoloration (brown)
Hematologic: Agranulocytosis, aplastic anemia, eosinophilia, glucose-6-phosphate dehydrogenase deficiency anemia, granulocytopenia, hemoglobin decreased, hemolytic anemia, leukopenia, megaloblastic anemia, thrombocytopenia
Hepatic: Hepatitis, hepatic necrosis, transaminases increased, jaundice (cholestatic)
Neuromuscular & skeletal: Arthralgia, myalgia, numbness, paresthesia, peripheral neuropathy, weakness
Ocular: Amblyopia, nystagmus, optic neuritis

Respiratory: Cough, dyspnea, pneumonitis, pulmonary fibrosis (with long-term use), pulmonary infiltration

Miscellaneous: Acute pulmonary reaction (symptoms include chills, chest pain, cough, dyspnea, fever, and eosinophilia), anaphylaxis, hypersensitivity (including acute pulmonary hypersensitivity), lupus-like syndrome, superinfections (eg, *Pseudomonas* or *Candida*)

Drug Interactions

Metabolism/Transport Effects None known.

Avoid Concomitant Use

Avoid concomitant use of Nitrofurantoin with any of the following: BCG; Magnesium Trisilicate; Norfloxacin

Increased Effect/Toxicity

Nitrofurantoin may increase the levels/effects of: Eplerenone; Prilocaine; Spironolactone

The levels/effects of Nitrofurantoin may be increased by: Probenecid

Decreased Effect

Nitrofurantoin may decrease the levels/effects of: BCG; Norfloxacin; Typhoid Vaccine

The levels/effects of Nitrofurantoin may be decreased by: Magnesium Trisilicate

Ethanol/Nutrition/Herb Interactions

Ethanol: Avoid ethanol (may increase CNS depression).

Food: Nitrofurantoin serum concentrations may be increased if taken with food.

Stability Store at 20°C to 25°C (68°F to 77°F); excursions permitted to 15°C to 30°C (59°F to 86°F). Protect oral suspension from light.

Mechanism of Action Inhibits several bacterial enzyme systems including acetyl coenzyme A interfering with metabolism and possibly cell wall synthesis

Pharmacodynamics/Kinetics

Absorption: Well absorbed; macrocrystalline form absorbed more slowly due to slower dissolution (causes less GI distress)

Distribution: V_d: 0.8 L/kg

Protein binding: 60% to 90%

Metabolism: Body tissues (except plasma) metabolize 60% of drug to inactive metabolites

Bioavailability: Increased with food

Half-life elimination: 20-60 minutes; prolonged with renal impairment

Excretion:

Suspension: Urine (~40%) and feces (small amounts) as metabolites and unchanged drug

Macrocrystals: Urine (20% to 25% as unchanged drug)

Dosage

Geriatric Avoid use; alternative agents preferred. Refer to adult dosing

Adult

UTI treatment:

Furadantin®, Macrodantin®: Oral: 50-100 mg/dose every 6 hours; administer for 7 days or at least 3 days after obtaining sterile urine

Macrobid®: Oral: 100 mg twice daily for 7 days

UTI prophylaxis (Furadantin®, Macrodantin®): Oral: 50-100 mg/dose at bedtime

Renal Impairment

Cl_{cr} <60 mL/minute: Contraindicated

Contraindicated in hemo- and peritoneal dialysis and continuous arteriovenous or venovenous hemofiltration.

Administration Administer with meals to improve absorption and decrease adverse effects; suspension may be mixed with water, milk, or fruit juice. Shake suspension well before use.

Monitoring Parameters Signs of pulmonary reaction; signs of numbness or tingling of the extremities; CBC, periodic liver function tests, periodic renal function tests with long-term use

Test Interactions False-positive urine glucose (Benedict's and Fehling's methods); no false positives with enzymatic tests

Special Geriatric Considerations Because of nitrofurantoin's decreased efficacy in patients with a Cl_{cr} <60 mL/minute and its side effect profile, it is not an antibiotic of choice for acute or prophylactic treatment of urinary tract infections in the elderly. An increased rate of severe hepatic toxicity has been suggested by postmarketing reports.

This medication is considered to be potentially inappropriate in this patient population (Beers Criteria: Quality of evidence - moderate; Strength of recommendation - strong).

Dosage Forms Excipient information presented when available (limited, particularly for generics); consult specific product labeling.

Capsule, oral [macrocrystal]: 50 mg, 100 mg

Macrodantin®: 25 mg, 50 mg, 100 mg

Capsule, oral [macrocrystal/monohydrate]: 100 mg

Macrobid®: 100 mg [nitrofurantoin macrocrystal 25% and nitrofurantoin monohydrate 75%]

Suspension, oral: 25 mg/5 mL (230 mL)

Furadantin®: 25 mg/5 mL (230 mL)

Nitroglycerin (nye troe GLI ser in)

Medication Safety Issues
Sound-alike/look-alike issues:
Nitroglycerin may be confused with nitrofurantoin, nitroprusside
Nitro-Bid® may be confused with Macrobid®
Nitroderm may be confused with NicoDerm®
Nitrol may be confused with Nizoral®
Nitrostat® may be confused with Nilstat, nystatin

Other safety concerns:
Transdermal patch may contain conducting metal (eg, aluminum); remove patch prior to MRI.

International issues:
Nitrocor [Italy, Russia, and Venezuela] may be confused with Natrecor brand name for nesiritide [U.S., Canada, and multiple international markets]; Nutracort brand name for hydrocortisone in the [U.S. and multiple international markets]; Nitro-Dur [U.S., Canada, and multiple international markets]

Brand Names: U.S. Minitran™; Nitro-Bid®; Nitro-Dur®; Nitro-Time®; Nitrolingual®; Nitro-Mist®; Nitrostat®; Rectiv™

Brand Names: Canada Minitran™; Mylan-Nitro Sublingual Spray; Nitro-Dur®; Nitroglycerin Injection, USP; Nitrol®; Nitrostat®; Rho®-Nitro Pump Spray; Transderm-Nitro®; Trinipatch®

Index Terms Glyceryl Trinitrate; Nitroglycerol; NTG; Tridil

Generic Availability (U.S.) Yes: Capsule, infusion, injection, patch, solution

Pharmacologic Category Antianginal Agent; Vasodilator

Use Treatment or prevention of angina pectoris
Intravenous (I.V.) administration: Treatment or prevention of angina pectoris; acute decompensated heart failure (especially when associated with acute myocardial infarction); perioperative hypertension (especially during cardiovascular surgery); induction of intraoperative hypotension
Intra-anal administration (Rectiv™ ointment): Treatment of moderate-to-severe pain associated with chronic anal fissure

Unlabeled Use Short-term management of pulmonary hypertension (I.V.); esophageal spastic disorders; uterine relaxation

Contraindications Hypersensitivity to organic nitrates or any component of the formulation (includes adhesives for transdermal product); concurrent use with phosphodiesterase-5 (PDE-5) inhibitors (sildenafil, tadalafil, or vardenafil); increased intracranial pressure; severe anemia

Additional contraindications for I.V. product: Constrictive pericarditis; pericardial tamponade; restrictive cardiomyopathy

Note: According to the 2010 American Heart Association guidelines for the treatment of acute coronary syndromes, nitrates are considered contraindicated in the following conditions: Hypotension (SBP <90 mm Hg or ≥30 mm Hg below baseline), extreme bradycardia (<50 bpm), tachycardia in the absence of heart failure (>100 bpm), and right ventricular infarction (O'Connor, 2010).

Warnings/Precautions Severe hypotension can occur. Use with caution in volume depletion, moderate hypotension, and extreme caution with inferior wall MI and suspected right ventricular involvement. Use considered contraindicated in patients with severe hypotension (SBP <90 mm Hg or ≥30 mm Hg below baseline), extreme bradycardia (<50 bpm), and right ventricular MI (O'Connor, 2010).

Paradoxical bradycardia and increased angina pectoris can accompany hypotension. Orthostatic hypotension can also occur. Ethanol can accentuate this. Tolerance does develop to nitrates and appropriate dosing is needed to minimize this (drug-free interval). Avoid use of long-acting agents in acute MI or acute HF; cannot easily reverse effects. Nitrates may aggravate angina caused by hypertrophic cardiomyopathy. Nitroglycerin may precipitate or aggravate increased intracranial pressure and subsequently may worsen clinical outcomes in patients with neurologic injury (eg, intracranial hemorrhage, traumatic brain injury). Nitroglycerin transdermal patches may contain conducting metal (eg, aluminum); remove patch prior to MRI. Avoid concurrent use with PDE-5 inhibitors. When nitrate administration becomes medically necessary, may administer nitrates only if 24 hours have elapsed after use of sildenafil or vardenafil (48 hours after tadalafil use) (Trujillo, 2007).

Use caution when treating rectal anal fissures with nitroglycerin ointment formulation in patients with suspected or known significant cardiovascular disorders (eg, cardiomyopathies, heart failure, acute MI); intra-anal nitroglycerin administration may decrease systolic blood pressure and decrease arterial vascular resistance.

Adverse Reactions (Reflective of adult population; not specific for elderly) Frequency not defined.

Cardiovascular: Flushing, hypotension, orthostatic hypotension, peripheral edema, syncope, tachycardia

Central nervous system: Headache (common), dizziness, lightheadedness

Gastrointestinal: Nausea, vomiting, xerostomia

Neuromuscular & skeletal: Paresthesia, weakness

Respiratory: Dyspnea, pharyngitis, rhinitis

Miscellaneous: Diaphoresis

Drug Interactions

Metabolism/Transport Effects None known.

Avoid Concomitant Use

Avoid concomitant use of Nitroglycerin with any of the following: Ergot Derivatives; Phosphodiesterase 5 Inhibitors

Increased Effect/Toxicity

Nitroglycerin may increase the levels/effects of: Ergot Derivatives; Hypotensive Agents; Prilocaine; Rosiglitazone

The levels/effects of Nitroglycerin may be increased by: Alfuzosin; Phosphodiesterase 5 Inhibitors

Decreased Effect

Nitroglycerin may decrease the levels/effects of: Alteplase; Heparin

The levels/effects of Nitroglycerin may be decreased by: Ergot Derivatives

Ethanol/Nutrition/Herb Interactions

Ethanol: Avoid ethanol (may increase the hypotensive effects of nitroglycerin). Monitor.

Herb/Nutraceutical: Avoid bayberry, blue cohosh, cayenne, ephedra, ginger, ginseng (American), kola, licorice (may worsen hypertension). Avoid black cohosh, California poppy, coleus, golden seal, hawthorn, mistletoe, periwinkle, quinine, shepherd's purse (may cause hypotension).

Stability

I.V. solution: Doses should be made in glass bottles, EXCEL® or PAB® containers. Adsorption occurs to soft plastic (eg, PVC). Nitroglycerin diluted in D_5W or NS in glass containers is physically and chemically stable for 48 hours at room temperature and 7 days under refrigeration. In D_5W or NS in EXCEL®/PAB® containers it is physically and chemically stable for 24 hours at room temperature.

Store sublingual tablets, topical ointment, and rectal ointment in tightly closed containers at 20°C to 25°C (68°F to 77°F); slow release capsules at 20°C to 25°C (68°F to 77°F); translingual spray and transdermal patch at 15°C to 30°C (59°F to 86°F).

Mechanism of Action Nitroglycerin forms free radical nitric oxide. In smooth muscle, nitric oxide activates guanylate cyclase which increases guanosine 3'5' monophosphate (cGMP) leading to dephosphorylation of myosin light chains and smooth muscle relaxation. Produces a vasodilator effect on the peripheral veins and arteries with more prominent effects on the veins. Primarily reduces cardiac oxygen demand by decreasing preload (left ventricular end-diastolic pressure); may modestly reduce afterload; dilates coronary arteries and improves collateral flow to ischemic regions. For use in rectal fissures, intra-anal administration results in decreased sphincter tone and intra-anal pressure.

Pharmacodynamics/Kinetics

Onset of action: Sublingual tablet: 1-3 minutes; Translingual spray: Similar to sublingual tablet; Extended release: ~60 minutes; Topical: 15-30 minutes; Transdermal: ~30 minutes; I.V.: Immediate

Peak effect: Sublingual tablet: 5 minutes; Translingual spray: 4-10 minutes; Extended release: 2.5-4 hours; Topical: ~60 minutes; Transdermal: 120 minutes; I.V.: Immediate

Duration: Sublingual tablet: At least 25 minutes; Translingual spray: Similar to sublingual tablet; Extended release: 4-8 hours (Gibbons, 2002); Topical: 7 hours; Transdermal: 10-12 hours; I.V.: 3-5 minutes

Distribution: V_d: ~3 L/kg

Protein binding: 60%

Metabolism: Extensive first-pass effect; metabolized hepatically to glycerol di- and mono-nitrate metabolites via liver reductase enzyme; subsequent metabolism to glycerol and organic nitrate; nonhepatic metabolism via red blood cells and vascular walls also occurs

Half-life elimination: ~1-4 minutes

Excretion: Urine (as inactive metabolites)

◀ **Dosage**

Geriatric & Adult Note: Hemodynamic and antianginal tolerance often develop within 24-48 hours of continuous nitrate administration. Nitrate-free interval (10-12 hours/day) is recommended to avoid tolerance development; gradually decrease dose in patients receiving NTG for prolonged period to avoid withdrawal reaction.

Angina/coronary artery disease:

Oral: 2.5-6.5 mg 3-4 times/day (maximum dose: 26 mg 4 times/day)

I.V.: 5 mcg/minute, increase by 5 mcg/minute every 3-5 minutes to 20 mcg/minute. If no response at 20 mcg/minute, may increase by 10-20 mcg/minute every 3-5 minutes (generally accepted maximum dose: 400 mcg/minute)

Topical ointment: 1/2" upon rising and 1/2" 6 hours later; if necessary, the dose may be doubled to 1" and subsequently doubled again to 2" if response is inadequate. Doses of 1/2" to 2" were used in clinical trials. Recommended maximum: 2 doses/day; include a nitrate free-interval ~10-12 hours/day.

Topical patch, transdermal: 0.2-0.4 mg/hour initially and titrate to doses of 0.4-0.8 mg/hour. Tolerance is minimized by using a patch-on period of 12-14 hours/day and patch-off period of 10-12 hours/day.

Sublingual: 0.3-0.6 mg every 5 minutes for maximum of 3 doses in 15 minutes; may also use prophylactically 5-10 minutes prior to activities which may provoke an attack.

Translingual: 1-2 sprays onto or under tongue every 3-5 minutes for maximum of 3 doses in 15 minutes, may also be used prophylactically 5-10 minutes prior to activities which may provoke an angina attack

Anal fissure, chronic (0.4% ointment): Intra-anal: 1 inch (equals 1.5 mg of nitroglycerin) every 12 hours for up to 3 weeks

Esophageal spastic disorders (unlabeled use): Sublingual: 0.3-0.6 mg (Swamy, 1977)

Uterine relaxation (unlabeled use): I.V. bolus: 100-200 mcg; may repeat dose every 2 minutes as necessary (Axemo, 1998; Chandraharan, 2005)

Administration

I.V.: Prepare in glass bottles, EXCEL® or PAB® containers. Adsorption occurs to soft plastic (eg, PVC); use administration sets intended for nitroglycerin

Intra-anal ointment: Using a finger covering (eg, plastic wrap, surgical glove, finger cot), place finger beside 1 inch measuring guide on the box and squeeze ointment the length of the measuring line directly onto covered finger. Insert ointment into the anal canal using the covered finger up to first finger joint (do not insert further than the first finger joint) and apply ointment around the side of the anal canal. If intra-anal application is too painful, may apply the ointment to the outside of the anus. Wash hands following application.

Oral (extended release capsule): Swallow whole. Do not chew, break, or crush. Take with a full glass of water.

Sublingual: Do not crush sublingual product (tablet). Place under tongue and allow to dissolve.

Topical ointment: Wash hands prior to and after use. Application site should be clean, dry, and hair-free. Apply to chest or back with the applicator or dose-measuring paper. Spread in a thin layer over a 2.25 x 3.5 inch area. Do not rub into skin. Tape applicator into place.

Topical patch, transdermal: Application site should be clean, dry and hair-free. Remove patch after 12-14 hours. Rotate patch sites.

Translingual spray: Do not shake container. Prior to initial use, the pump must be primed by spraying 5 times (Nitrolingual®) or 10 times (Nitromist®) into the air. Priming sprays should be directed away from patient and others. Release spray onto or under tongue. Close mouth after administration. Do not rinse the mouth for at least 5-10 minutes. The end of the pump should be covered by the fluid in the bottle. If pump is unused for 6 weeks, a single priming spray (Nitrolingual®) or 2 priming sprays (Nitromist®) should be completed.

Monitoring Parameters Blood pressure, heart rate

Test Interactions I.V. formulation: Due to propylene glycol content, triglyceride assays dependent on glycerol oxidase may be falsely elevated.

Pharmacotherapy Pearls I.V. preparations contain alcohol and/or propylene glycol; may need to use nitrate-free interval (10-12 hours/day) to avoid tolerance development. Tolerance may possibly be reversed with acetylcysteine; gradually decrease dose in patients receiving NTG for prolonged period to avoid withdrawal reaction.

Concomitant use of sildenafil (Viagra®) or other phosphodiesterase-5 enzyme inhibitors (PDE-5) may precipitate acute hypotension, myocardial infarction, or death. Nitrates used in right ventricular infarction may induce acute hypotension. Nitrate use in severe pericardial effusion may reduce cardiac filling pressure and precipitate cardiac tamponade. In the management of heart failure, the combination of isosorbide dinitrate and hydralazine confers beneficial effects on disease progression and cardiac outcomes.

Special Geriatric Considerations Caution should be used when using nitrate therapy in the elderly due to hypotension. Hypotension is enhanced in the elderly due to decreased baroreceptor response, decreased venous tone, and often hypovolemia (dehydration) or other hypotensive drugs.

Dosage Forms Excipient information presented when available (limited, particularly for generics); consult specific product labeling.

Aerosol, spray, translingual:
NitroMist®: 0.4 mg/spray (8.5 g) [230 metered sprays]

Capsule, extended release, oral: 2.5 mg, 6.5 mg, 9 mg
Nitro-Time®: 2.5 mg, 6.5 mg, 9 mg

Infusion, premixed in D5W: 25 mg (250 mL) [100 mcg/mL]; 50 mg (250 mL, 500 mL) [100 mcg/mL]; 50 mg (250 mL, 500 mL) [200 mcg/mL]; 100 mg (250 mL) [400 mcg/mL]

Injection, solution: 5 mg/mL (10 mL)

Ointment, rectal:
Rectiv™: 0.4% (30 g) [contains propylene glycol; ~1.5 mg/inch]

Ointment, topical:
Nitro-Bid®: 2% (1 g, 30 g, 60 g) [~15 mg/inch]

Patch, transdermal: 0.1 mg/hr (30s); 0.2 mg/hr (30s); 0.4 mg/hr (30s); 0.6 mg/hr (30s)
Minitran™: 0.1 mg/hr (30s); 0.2 mg/hr (30s); 0.4 mg/hr (30s); 0.6 mg/hr (30s)
Nitro-Dur®: 0.1 mg/hr (30s); 0.2 mg/hr (30s); 0.3 mg/hr (30s); 0.4 mg/hr (30s); 0.6 mg/hr (30s); 0.8 mg/hr (30s)

Solution, translingual [spray]: 0.4 mg/spray (4.9 g, 12 g)
Nitrolingual®: 0.4 mg/spray (12 g) [contains ethanol 20%; 200 metered sprays]
Nitrolingual®: 0.4 mg/spray (4.9 g) [contains ethanol 20%; 60 metered sprays]

Tablet, sublingual:
Nitrostat®: 0.3 mg, 0.4 mg, 0.6 mg

◆ **Nitroglycerol** see Nitroglycerin on page 1386
◆ **Nitrolingual®** see Nitroglycerin on page 1386
◆ **NitroMist®** see Nitroglycerin on page 1386
◆ **Nitropress®** see Nitroprusside on page 1389

Nitroprusside (nye troe PRUS ide)

Medication Safety Issues
Sound-alike/look-alike issues:
Nitroprusside may be confused with nitroglycerin
High alert medication:
The Institute for Safe Medication Practices (ISMP) includes this medication among its list of drugs which have a heightened risk of causing significant patient harm when used in error.

Brand Names: U.S. Nitropress®
Brand Names: Canada Nipride®
Index Terms Nitroprusside Sodium; Sodium Nitroferricyanide; Sodium Nitroprusside
Generic Availability (U.S.) Yes
Pharmacologic Category Vasodilator
Use Management of hypertensive crises; acute decompensated heart failure (HF); used for controlled hypotension to reduce bleeding during surgery
Contraindications Treatment of compensatory hypertension (aortic coarctation, arteriovenous shunting); to produce controlled hypotension during surgery in patients with known inadequate cerebral circulation or in moribund patients requiring emergency surgery; high output heart failure associated with reduced systemic vascular resistance (eg, septic shock); congenital optic atrophy or tobacco amblyopia
Warnings/Precautions [U.S. Boxed Warning] **Excessive hypotension resulting in compromised perfusion of vital organs may occur; continuous blood pressure monitoring by experienced personnel is required. Except when used briefly or at low (<2 mcg/kg/minute) infusion rates, nitroprusside gives rise to large cyanide quantities. Do not use the maximum dose for more than 10 minutes; if blood pressure is not controlled by the maximum rate after 10 minutes, discontinue infusion. Monitor for cyanide toxicity via acid-base balance and venous oxygen concentration; however, clinicians should note that these indicators may not always reliably indicate cyanide toxicity.** When nitroprusside is used for controlled hypotension during surgery, correct pre-existing anemia and hypovolemia prior to use when possible. Use with extreme caution in patients with elevated intracranial pressure (head trauma, cerebral hemorrhage), severe renal impairment, hepatic failure, hypothyroidism. Use the lowest end of the dosage range with renal impairment. Cyanide toxicity may occur in patients with decreased liver function. Thiocyanate toxicity occurs in patients with renal impairment or those on prolonged infusions. **[U.S. Boxed Warning]: Solution must be further diluted with 5% dextrose in water. Do not administer by direct injection.**

◀ **Adverse Reactions (Reflective of adult population; not specific for elderly)** Frequency not defined.

Cardiovascular: Bradycardia, ECG changes, flushing, hypotension (excessive), palpitation, substernal distress, tachycardia

Central nervous system: Apprehension, dizziness, headache, intracranial pressure increased, restlessness

Dermatologic: Rash

Endocrine & metabolic: Metabolic acidosis (secondary to cyanide toxicity), hypothyroidism

Gastrointestinal: Abdominal pain, ileus, nausea, retching, vomiting

Hematologic: Methemoglobinemia, platelet aggregation decreased

Local: Injection site irritation

Neuromuscular & skeletal: Hyperreflexia (secondary to thiocyanate toxicity), muscle twitching

Ocular: Miosis (secondary to thiocyanate toxicity)

Otic: Tinnitus (secondary to thiocyanate toxicity)

Respiratory: Hyperoxemia (secondary to cyanide toxicity)

Miscellaneous: Cyanide toxicity, diaphoresis, thiocyanate toxicity

Drug Interactions

Metabolism/Transport Effects None known.

Avoid Concomitant Use There are no known interactions where it is recommended to avoid concomitant use.

Increased Effect/Toxicity

Nitroprusside may increase the levels/effects of: Amifostine; Antihypertensives; Hypotensive Agents; Prilocaine; RiTUXimab

The levels/effects of Nitroprusside may be increased by: Alfuzosin; Calcium Channel Blockers; Diazoxide; Herbs (Hypotensive Properties); MAO Inhibitors; Pentoxifylline; Phosphodiesterase 5 Inhibitors; Prostacyclin Analogues

Decreased Effect

The levels/effects of Nitroprusside may be decreased by: Herbs (Hypertensive Properties); Methylphenidate; Yohimbine

Stability Store the intact vial at 20°C to 25°C (68°F to 77°F). Protect from light.

Prior to administration, nitroprusside sodium should be further diluted by diluting 50 mg in 250-1000 mL of D_5W.

Use only clear solutions; solutions of nitroprusside exhibit a color described as brownish, brown, brownish-pink, light orange, and straw. Solutions are highly sensitive to light. Exposure to light causes decomposition, resulting in a highly colored solution of orange, dark brown or blue. **A blue color indicates almost complete decomposition.** Do not use discolored solutions (eg, blue, green, red) or solutions in which particulate matter is visible. **Prepared solutions should be wrapped with aluminum foil or other opaque material to protect from light (do as soon as possible).**

Stability of parenteral admixture at room temperature (25°C) and at refrigeration temperature (4°C) is 24 hours.

Mechanism of Action Causes peripheral vasodilation by direct action on venous and arteriolar smooth muscle, thus reducing peripheral resistance; will increase cardiac output by decreasing afterload; reduces aortal and left ventricular impedance

Pharmacodynamics/Kinetics

Onset of action: Hypotensive effect: <2 minutes

Duration: Hypotensive effect: 1-10 minutes

Metabolism: Nitroprusside combines with hemoglobin to produce cyanide and cyanmethemoglobin. Cyanide detoxification occurs via rhodanase-mediated conversion of cyanide to thiocyanate; rhodanase couples cyanide molecules to sulfane sulfur groups from a sulfur donor (eg, thiosulfate, cystine, cysteine). This process has limited capacity and may become overwhelmed with large exposures once sulfur donor supplies are exhausted resulting in toxicity.

Half-life elimination: Nitroprusside, circulatory: ~2 minutes; Thiocyanate, elimination: ~3 days (may be doubled or tripled in renal failure)

Excretion: Urine (as thiocyanate)

Dosage

Geriatric & Adult

Acute hypertension: I.V.: Initial: 0.25-0.3 mcg/kg/minute; may be titrated by 0.5 mcg/kg/minute every few minutes to achieve desired hemodynamic effect (JNC 7; Rhoney, 2009); usual dose: 3 mcg/kg/minute; maximum dose: 10 mcg/kg/minute. When administered in doses >3 mcg/kg/minute for prolonged periods of time (eg, 3-4 days), thiocyanate levels should be monitored daily.

Acute decompensated heart failure: I.V.: Initial: 5-10 **mcg/minute**; may be titrated rapidly (eg, up to every 5 minutes) to achieve desired hemodynamic effect; usual dosage range: 5-300 **mcg/minute**. Doses >400 **mcg/minute** are not recommended due to minimal added benefit and increased risk for thiocyanate toxicity (HFSA, 2010).

Renal Impairment There are no dosage adjustments provided in manufacturer's labeling. However, use in patients with renal impairment may lead to the accumulation of thiocyanate and subsequent toxicity; limit use.

Hepatic Impairment There are no dosage adjustments provided in manufacturer's labeling; due to the risk of cyanide toxicity, use with caution.

Administration I.V. infusion only; infusion pump required. Must be diluted with D_5W (preferred), LR, or NS prior to administration; not for direct injection. Due to potential for excessive hypotension, continuously monitor patient's blood pressure during therapy.

Monitoring Parameters Blood pressure, heart rate; monitor for cyanide and thiocyanate toxicity; monitor acid-base status as acidosis can be the earliest sign of cyanide toxicity; monitor thiocyanate levels if requiring prolonged infusion (>3 days) or dose >3 mcg/kg/minute or patient has renal dysfunction; monitor cyanide blood levels in patients with decreased hepatic function; cardiac monitor and blood pressure monitor required

Reference Range Serum thiocyanate levels are not helpful in detecting toxicity. A level may be confirmatory if a patient is exhibiting signs and symptoms of thiocyanate toxicity. Initial signs of toxicity (eg, tinnitus) may be observed at levels >35 mcg/mL (manufacturer suggests 60 mcg/mL), but serious toxicity typically may not occur with levels <100 mcg/mL.

Special Geriatric Considerations Elderly patients may have an increased sensitivity to nitroprusside possibly due to a decreased baroreceptor reflex, altered sensitivity to vaso-dilating effects or a resistance of cardiac adrenergic receptors to stimulation by catecholamines.

Dosage Forms Excipient information presented when available (limited, particularly for generics); consult specific product labeling.
Injection, solution, as sodium:
    Nitropress®: 25 mg/mL (2 mL)

◆ **Nitroprusside Sodium** *see* Nitroprusside *on page 1389*
◆ **Nitrostat®** *see* Nitroglycerin *on page 1386*
◆ **Nitro-Time®** *see* Nitroglycerin *on page 1386*
◆ **4'-Nitro-3'-Trifluoromethylisobutyrantide** *see* Flutamide *on page 821*
◆ **Nix® Complete Lice Treatment System [OTC]** *see* Permethrin *on page 1512*
◆ **Nix® Creme Rinse [OTC]** *see* Permethrin *on page 1512*
◆ **Nix® Creme Rinse Lice Treatment [OTC]** *see* Permethrin *on page 1512*
◆ **Nix® Lice Control Spray [OTC]** *see* Permethrin *on page 1512*

Nizatidine (ni ZA ti deen)

Medication Safety Issues
Sound-alike/look-alike issues:
Axid® may be confused with Ansaid®
International issues:
Tazac [Australia] may be confused with Tazact brand name for piperacillin/tazobactam [India]; Tiazac brand name for diltiazem [U.S., Canada]
Brand Names: U.S. Axid®
Brand Names: Canada Apo-Nizatidine®; Axid®; Gen-Nizatidine; Novo-Nizatidine; Nu-Nizatidine; PMS-Nizatidine
Generic Availability (U.S.) Yes
Pharmacologic Category Histamine H_2 Antagonist
Use Treatment and maintenance of duodenal ulcer; treatment of benign gastric ulcer; treatment of gastroesophageal reflux disease (GERD)
Unlabeled Use Part of a multidrug regimen for *H. pylori* eradication to reduce the risk of duodenal ulcer recurrence
Contraindications Hypersensitivity to nizatidine or any component of the formulation; hypersensitivity to other H_2 antagonists (cross-sensitivity has been observed)
Warnings/Precautions Relief of symptoms does not preclude the presence of a gastric malignancy. Use with caution in patients with liver and renal impairment. Dosage modification required in patients with renal impairment
Adverse Reactions (Reflective of adult population; not specific for elderly)
>10%: Central nervous system: Headache (16%)
1% to 10%:
    Central nervous system: Anxiety, dizziness, fever (reported in children), insomnia, irritability (reported in children), somnolence, nervousness
    Dermatologic: Pruritus, rash

Gastrointestinal: Abdominal pain, anorexia, constipation, diarrhea, dry mouth, flatulence, heartburn, nausea, vomiting

Respiratory: Reported in children: Cough, nasal congestion, nasopharyngitis

Drug Interactions

Metabolism/Transport Effects Inhibits CYP3A4 (weak)

Avoid Concomitant Use

Avoid concomitant use of Nizatidine with any of the following: Delavirdine; Pimozide

Increased Effect/Toxicity

Nizatidine may increase the levels/effects of: ARIPiprazole; Dexmethylphenidate; Methylphenidate; Pimozide; Saquinavir; Varenicline

Decreased Effect

Nizatidine may decrease the levels/effects of: Atazanavir; Cefditoren; Cefpodoxime; Cefuroxime; Dasatinib; Delavirdine; Erlotinib; Fosamprenavir; Gefitinib; Indinavir; Iron Salts; Itraconazole; Ketoconazole; Ketoconazole (Systemic); Mesalamine; Nelfinavir; Nilotinib; Posaconazole; Rilpivirine; Vismodegib

Ethanol/Nutrition/Herb Interactions

Ethanol: Avoid ethanol (may cause gastric mucosal irritation).

Food: Administration with apple juice may decrease absorption.

Mechanism of Action Competitive inhibition of histamine at H_2-receptors of the gastric parietal cells resulting in reduced gastric acid secretion, gastric volume and hydrogen ion concentration reduced. In healthy volunteers, nizatidine suppresses gastric acid secretion induced by pentagastrin infusion or food.

Pharmacodynamics/Kinetics

Distribution: V_d: 0.8-1.5 L/kg

Protein binding: 35% to α_1-acid glycoprotein

Metabolism: Partially hepatic; forms metabolites

Bioavailability: >70%

Half-life elimination: 1-2 hours; prolonged with renal impairment

Time to peak, plasma: 0.5-3.0 hours

Excretion: Urine (90%; ~60% as unchanged drug); feces (<6%)

Dosage

Geriatric & Adult

Duodenal ulcer: Oral:

Treatment of active ulcer: 300 mg at bedtime or 150 mg twice daily

Maintenance of healed ulcer: 150 mg/day at bedtime

Gastric ulcer: Oral: 150 mg twice daily or 300 mg at bedtime

GERD: Oral: 150 mg twice daily

Eradication of *Helicobacter pylori* (unlabeled use): Oral: 150 mg twice daily; requires combination therapy

Renal Impairment

Active treatment:

Cl_{cr} 20-50 mL/minute: 150 mg/day

Cl_{cr} <20 mL/minute: 150 mg every other day

Maintenance treatment:

Cl_{cr} 20-50 mL/minute: 150 mg every other day

Cl_{cr} <20 mL/minute: 150 mg every 3 days

Test Interactions False-positive urine protein using Multistix®, gastric acid secretion test, skin tests allergen extracts, serum creatinine and serum transaminase concentrations, urine protein test

Pharmacotherapy Pearls Giving dose at 6 PM (rather than 10 PM) may better suppress nocturnal acid secretion

Special Geriatric Considerations H_2 blockers are the preferred drugs for treating peptic ulcer disorder (PUD) in the elderly due to cost and ease of administration. These agents are no less or more effective than any other therapy. The preferred agents (due to side effects and drug interaction profile and pharmacokinetics) are ranitidine, famotidine, and nizatidine. Treatment for PUD in the elderly is recommended for 12 weeks since their lesions are larger, and therefore, take longer to heal. Always adjust dose based upon creatinine clearance.

Dosage Forms Excipient information presented when available (limited, particularly for generics); consult specific product labeling.

Capsule, oral: 150 mg, 300 mg

Solution, oral: 15 mg/mL (473 mL)

Axid®: 15 mg/mL (480 mL) [bubblegum flavor]

◆ **Nizoral®** *see* Ketoconazole (Topical) *on page 1065*

◆ **Nizoral® A-D [OTC]** *see* Ketoconazole (Topical) *on page 1065*

◆ **N-methylnaltrexone Bromide** *see* Methylnaltrexone *on page 1246*

◆ **NN2211** *see* Liraglutide *on page 1144*

♦ **Nolvadex** *see* Tamoxifen *on page 1831*
♦ **Non-Aspirin Pain Reliever [OTC]** *see* Acetaminophen *on page 31*
♦ **Norco®** *see* Hydrocodone and Acetaminophen *on page 937*
♦ **Nordeoxyguanosine** *see* Ganciclovir (Ophthalmic) *on page 867*
♦ **Nordeoxyguanosine** *see* Ganciclovir (Systemic) *on page 865*
♦ **Norflex™** *see* Orphenadrine *on page 1429*

Norfloxacin (nor FLOKS a sin)

Medication Safety Issues
Sound-alike/look-alike issues:
Norfloxacin may be confused with Norflex™, Noroxin®
Noroxin® may be confused with Neurontin®, Norflex™
Brand Names: U.S. Noroxin®
Brand Names: Canada Apo-Norflox®; CO Norfloxacin; Norfloxacine®; Novo-Norfloxacin; PMS-Norfloxacin; Riva-Norfloxacin
Generic Availability (U.S.) No
Pharmacologic Category Antibiotic, Quinolone
Use Uncomplicated and complicated urinary tract infections caused by susceptible gram-negative and gram-positive bacteria; sexually-transmitted disease (eg, uncomplicated urethral and cervical gonorrhea) caused by *N. gonorrhoeae*; prostatitis due to *E. coli*
Note: As of April 2007, the CDC no longer recommends the use of fluoroquinolones for the treatment of gonococcal disease.
Medication Guide Available Yes
Contraindications Hypersensitivity to norfloxacin, quinolones, or any component of the formulation; history of tendonitis or tendon rupture associated with quinolone use
Warnings/Precautions [U.S. Boxed Warning]: There have been reports of tendon inflammation and/or rupture with quinolone antibiotics; risk may be increased with concurrent corticosteroids, organ transplant recipients, and in patients >60 years of age. Rupture of the Achilles tendon sometimes requiring surgical repair has been reported most frequently; but other tendon sites (eg, rotator cuff, biceps) have also been reported. Strenuous physical activity, rheumatoid arthritis, and renal impairment may be an independent risk factor for tendonitis. Discontinue at first sign of tendon inflammation or pain. May occur even after discontinuation of therapy. Use with caution in patients with rheumatoid arthritis; may increase risk of tendon rupture. Use with caution in patients with known or suspected CNS disorders. CNS stimulation may occur which may lead to tremor, restlessness, confusion, and very rarely to hallucinations or convulsive seizures. Potential for seizures, although very rare, may be increased with concomitant NSAID therapy. Use with caution in individuals at risk of seizures. Use may be associated (rarely) with prolongation of QT$_c$ interval; avoid concurrent use with class Ia and class III antiarrhythmics; use caution with other drugs may cause QT$_c$ prolongation.

Fluoroquinolones have been associated with the development of serious, and sometimes fatal, hypoglycemia, most often in elderly diabetics, but also in patients without diabetes. This occurred most frequently with gatifloxacin (no longer available systemically) but may occur at a lower frequency with other quinolones.

Severe hypersensitivity reactions, including anaphylaxis, have occurred with quinolone therapy. Reactions may present as typical allergic symptoms after a single dose, or may manifest as severe idiosyncratic dermatologic, vascular, pulmonary, renal, hepatic, and/or hematologic events, usually after multiple doses. Prompt discontinuation of drug should occur if skin rash or other symptoms arise. Prolonged use may result in fungal or bacterial superinfection, including *C. difficile*-associated diarrhea (CDAD) and pseudomembranous colitis; CDAD has been observed >2 months postantibiotic treatment. Avoid excessive sunlight and take precautions to limit exposure (eg, loose fitting clothing, sunscreen); may cause moderate-to-severe phototoxicity reactions. Discontinue use if photosensitivity occurs. May be associated with the development of peripheral neuropathy and/or paresthesias; discontinue in patients who develop symptoms consistent with neuropathy. **[U.S. Boxed Warning]: Quinolones may exacerbate myasthenia gravis; avoid use (rare, potentially life-threatening weakness of respiratory muscles may occur).** Use caution with renal impairment. Since norfloxacin is ineffective in the treatment of syphilis and may mask symptoms, all patients should be tested for syphilis at the time of gonorrheal diagnosis and 3 months later. Hemolytic reactions may (rarely) occur with quinolone use in patients with latent or actual G6PD deficiency.
Adverse Reactions (Reflective of adult population; not specific for elderly)
>1% to 10%:
Central nervous system: Dizziness (2% to 3%), headache (2% to 3%)
Gastrointestinal: Nausea (3% to 4%), abdominal cramping (2%)

Hematologic: Eosinophilia (1% to 2%)
Hepatic: Liver enzymes increased (1% to 2%)
≥0.3% to 1%:
Central nervous system: Fever, somnolence
Dermatologic: Hyperhidrosis, pruritus, rash
Gastrointestinal: Abdominal pain, anorectal pain, anorexia, constipation, diarrhea, dyspepsia, flatulence, loose stools, vomiting, xerostomia
Hematologic: Hematocrit/hemoglobin decreased (1%), leukopenia (1%), thrombocytopenia (1%)
Neuromuscular & skeletal: Back pain, paresthesia, weakness
Renal: Proteinuria (1%)

Drug Interactions

Metabolism/Transport Effects Inhibits CYP1A2 (strong), CYP3A4 (moderate)

Avoid Concomitant Use

Avoid concomitant use of Norfloxacin with any of the following: BCG; Nitrofurantoin; Tolvaptan

Increased Effect/Toxicity

Norfloxacin may increase the levels/effects of: ARIPiprazole; Avanafil; Bendamustine; Caffeine; Colchicine; Corticosteroids (Systemic); CycloSPORINE; CycloSPORINE (Systemic); CYP1A2 Substrates; CYP3A4 Substrates; Eplerenone; Everolimus; FentaNYL; Highest Risk QTc-Prolonging Agents; Ivacaftor; Lurasidone; Moderate Risk QTc-Prolonging Agents; Pimecrolimus; Porfimer; Salmeterol; Saxagliptin; Sulfonylureas; Theophylline Derivatives; Tolvaptan; Varenicline; Vilazodone; Vitamin K Antagonists

The levels/effects of Norfloxacin may be increased by: Insulin; Mifepristone; Nonsteroidal Anti-Inflammatory Agents; Probenecid

Decreased Effect

Norfloxacin may decrease the levels/effects of: BCG; Ifosfamide; Mycophenolate; Sulfonylureas; Typhoid Vaccine

The levels/effects of Norfloxacin may be decreased by: Antacids; Calcium Salts; Didanosine; Iron Salts; Lanthanum; Magnesium Salts; Nitrofurantoin; Quinapril; Sevelamer; Sucralfate; Zinc Salts

Ethanol/Nutrition/Herb Interactions

Food: Norfloxacin average peak serum concentrations may be decreased if taken with dairy products or other polyvalent cations. Norfloxacin may increase blood levels of caffeine. Management: Best taken on an empty stomach with water 1 hour before or 2 hours after meals, milk, or other dairy products. Hold antacids, sucralfate, or multivitamins/supplements containing iron, zinc, magnesium, or aluminum for 2 hours after giving norfloxacin; do not administer together. Use caution with caffeine-containing beverages/foods.

Herb/Nutraceutical: Dong quai and St John's wort may cause photosensitization. Management: Avoid dong quai and St John's wort.

Stability Store at 25°C (77°F). Keep container tightly closed.

Mechanism of Action Norfloxacin is a DNA gyrase inhibitor. DNA gyrase is an essential bacterial enzyme that maintains the superhelical structure of DNA. DNA gyrase is required for DNA replication and transcription, DNA repair, recombination, and transposition; bactericidal

Pharmacodynamics/Kinetics

Absorption: Oral: Rapid, up to 40%
Protein binding: 10% to 15%
Metabolism: Hepatic
Half-life elimination: 3-4 hours; Renal impairment (Cl$_{cr}$ ≤30 mL/minute): 6.5 hours; Elderly: 4 hours
Time to peak, serum: 1-2 hours
Excretion: Urine (26% to 32% as unchanged drug; 5% to 8% as metabolites); feces (39%)

Dosage

Geriatric & Adult

Dysenteric enterocolitis *(Shigella* unlabeled use): Oral: 400 mg twice daily for 5 days
Prostatitis: Oral: 400 mg every 12 hours for 4-6 weeks
Traveler's diarrhea (unlabeled use): Oral: 400 mg twice daily for 3 days, single dose may also be effective
Uncomplicated gonorrhea: Oral: 800 mg as a single dose. **Note:** As of April 2007, the CDC no longer recommends the use of fluoroquinolones for the treatment of uncomplicated gonococcal disease.
Urinary tract infections: Oral:
Uncomplicated due to *E. coli, K. pneumoniae, P. mirabilis*: 400 mg twice daily for 3 days
Uncomplicated due to other organisms: 400 mg twice daily for 7-10 days
Complicated: 400 mg twice daily for 10-21 days
Renal Impairment Cl$_{cr}$ ≤30 mL/minute/1.73 m^2: Administer 400 mg every 24 hours

Administration Hold antacids, sucralfate, or multivitamins/supplements containing iron, zinc, magnesium, or aluminum for 2 hours after giving norfloxacin; do not administer together. Best taken on an empty stomach with water (1 hour before or 2 hours after meals, milk, or other dairy products).

Special Geriatric Considerations The risk of torsade de pointes and tendon inflammation and/or rupture associated with the concomitant use of corticosteroids and quinolones is increased in the elderly population. See Warnings/Precautions regarding tendon rupture in patients >60 years of age. Adjust dose for renal function.

Dosage Forms Excipient information presented when available (limited, particularly for generics); consult specific product labeling.
Tablet, oral:
Noroxin®: 400 mg

♦ **Norgestimate and Estradiol** see Estradiol and Norgestimate on page 692
♦ **Noritate®** see MetroNIDAZOLE (Topical) on page 1271
♦ **Normal Saline** see Sodium Chloride on page 1787
♦ **Noroxin®** see Norfloxacin on page 1393
♦ **Norpace®** see Disopyramide on page 574
♦ **Norpace® CR** see Disopyramide on page 574
♦ **Norpramin®** see Desipramine on page 505
♦ **Nortemp Children's [OTC]** see Acetaminophen on page 31

Nortriptyline (nor TRIP ti leen)

Related Information
Antidepressant Agents on page 2097
Beers Criteria – Potentially Inappropriate Medications for Geriatrics on page 2183
Medication Safety Issues
Sound-alike/look-alike issues:
Aventyl® HCl may be confused with Bentyl®
Nortriptyline may be confused with amitriptyline, desipramine, Norpramin®
Pamelor™ may be confused with Demerol®, Tambocor™
BEERS Criteria medication:
This drug may be potentially inappropriate for use in geriatric patients (SIADH: Quality of evidence - moderate; Strength of recommendation - strong).
Brand Names: U.S. Pamelor™
Brand Names: Canada Apo-Nortriptyline®; Ava-Nortriptyline; Aventyl®; Dom-Nortriptyline; Norventyl; Nu-Nortriptyline; PMS-Nortriptyline; Teva-Nortriptyline
Index Terms Nortriptyline Hydrochloride
Generic Availability (U.S.) Yes
Pharmacologic Category Antidepressant, Tricyclic (Secondary Amine)
Use Treatment of symptoms of depression
Unlabeled Use Chronic pain (including neuropathic pain), myofascial pain, burning mouth sydrome, anxiety disorders, attention-deficit/hyperactivity disorder (ADHD); enuresis; adjunctive therapy for smoking cessation
Medication Guide Available Yes
Contraindications Hypersensitivity to nortriptyline and similar chemical class, or any component of the formulation; use of MAO inhibitors within 14 days; use in a patient during the acute recovery phase of MI
Warnings/Precautions [U.S. Boxed Warning]: Antidepressants increase the risk of suicidal thinking and behavior in children, adolescents, and young adults (18-24 years of age) with major depressive disorder (MDD) and other psychiatric disorders; consider risk prior to prescribing. Short-term studies did not show an increased risk in patients >24 years of age and showed a decreased risk in patients ≥65 years. Closely monitor for clinical worsening, suicidality, or unusual changes in behavior; the patient's family or caregiver should be instructed to closely observe the patient and communicate condition with healthcare provider. A medication guide should be dispensed with each prescription.

The possibility of a suicide attempt is inherent in major depression and may persist until remission occurs. Monitor for worsening of depression or suicidality, especially during initiation of therapy (generally first 1-2 months) or with dose increases or decreases. Use caution in high-risk patients. Worsening depression and severe abrupt suicidality that are not part of the presenting symptoms may require discontinuation or modification of drug therapy. The patient's family or caregiver should be alerted to monitor patients for the emergence of suicidality and associated behaviors (such as agitation, irritability, hostility, impulsivity, and hypomania) and call healthcare provider.

May worsen psychosis in some patients or precipitate a shift to mania or hypomania in patients with bipolar disorder. Patients presenting with depressive symptoms should be screened for bipolar disorder. Monotherapy in patients with bipolar disorder should be avoided. **Nortriptyline is not FDA approved for the treatment of bipolar depression.**

TCAs may rarely cause bone marrow suppression; monitor for any signs of infection and obtain CBC if symptoms (eg, fever, sore throat) evident. The risk of sedation and orthostatic effects are low relative to other antidepressants. However, nortriptyline may result in impaired performance of tasks requiring alertness (eg, operating machinery or driving). Sedative effects may be additive with other CNS depressants and/or ethanol. The degree of anticholinergic blockade produced by this agent is moderate relative to other cyclic antidepressants, however, caution should still be used in patients with urinary retention, benign prostatic hyperplasia, narrow-angle glaucoma, xerostomia, visual problems, constipation, or history of bowel obstruction. May cause orthostatic hypotension (risk is low relative to other antidepressants) or conduction disturbances. Use with caution in patients with a history of cardiovascular disease (including previous MI, stroke, tachycardia, or conduction abnormalities). The risk conduction abnormalities with this agent is moderate relative to other antidepressants.

Consider discontinuing, when possible, prior to elective surgery. Therapy should not be abruptly discontinued in patients receiving high doses for prolonged periods. May alter glucose regulation - use caution in patients with diabetes. Use caution in patients with a previous seizure disorder or condition predisposing to seizures such as brain damage, alcoholism, or concurrent therapy with other drugs which lower the seizure threshold. May increase the risks associated with electroconvulsive therapy. Use with caution in hyperthyroid patients or those receiving thyroid supplementation. Use with caution in patients with hepatic or renal dysfunction.

Use caution in elderly patients; may cause or exacerbate syndrome of inappropriate antidiuretic hormone secretion or hyponatremia; monitor sodium closely with initiation or dosage adjustments in older adults. May be inappropriate in older adults depending on comorbidities (eg, dementia, delirium) due to its potent anticholinergic effects (Beers Criteria).

Adverse Reactions (Reflective of adult population; not specific for elderly) Frequency not defined.

Cardiovascular: Arrhythmia, flushing, heart block, hypertension, MI, orthostatic hypotension, palpitation, tachycardia

Central nervous system: Agitation, anxiety, ataxia, confusion, delirium, delusions, disorientation, dizziness, drowsiness, EEG changes, exacerbation of psychosis, extrapyramidal symptoms, fatigue, hallucinations, headache, hypomania, incoordination, insomnia, nightmares, panic, restlessness, seizure

Dermatologic: Alopecia, itching, petechiae, photosensitivity, rash, urticaria

Endocrine & metabolic: Blood sugar increased/decreased, breast enlargement, galactorrhea, gynecomastia, libido increased/decreased, sexual dysfunction, SIADH

Gastrointestinal: Abdominal cramps, anorexia, black tongue, constipation, diarrhea, epigastric distress, nausea, paralytic ileus, stomatitis, taste disturbance, vomiting, weight gain/loss, xerostomia

Genitourinary: Delayed micturition, impotence, nocturia, polyuria, testicular edema, urinary retention

Hematologic: Agranulocytosis (rare), eosinophilia, purpura, thrombocytopenia

Hepatic: Cholestatic jaundice, transaminases increased

Neuromuscular & skeletal: Numbness, paresthesia, peripheral neuropathy, tingling, tremor, weakness

Ocular: Blurred vision, disturbances in accommodation, eye pain, mydriasis

Otic: Tinnitus

Miscellaneous: Allergic reactions (eg, general edema or of the face/tongue), diaphoresis (excessive), withdrawal symptoms

Drug Interactions

Metabolism/Transport Effects Substrate of CYP1A2 (minor), CYP2C19 (minor), CYP2D6 (major), CYP3A4 (minor); **Note:** Assignment of Major/Minor substrate status based on clinically relevant drug interaction potential; **Inhibits** CYP2D6 (weak), CYP2E1 (weak)

Avoid Concomitant Use

Avoid concomitant use of Nortriptyline with any of the following: Iobenguane I 123; MAO Inhibitors; Methylene Blue

Increased Effect/Toxicity

Nortriptyline may increase the levels/effects of: Alpha-/Beta-Agonists (Direct-Acting); Alpha1-Agonists; Amphetamines; Anticholinergics; Beta2-Agonists; Desmopressin; Highest Risk QTc-Prolonging Agents; Methylene Blue; Metoclopramide; Moderate Risk QTc-Prolonging Agents; QuiNIDine; Serotonin Modulators; Sodium Phosphates; Sulfonylureas; TraMADol; Vitamin K Antagonists; Yohimbine

The levels/effects of Nortriptyline may be increased by: Abiraterone Acetate; Altretamine; Antipsychotics; BuPROPion; Cimetidine; Cinacalcet; CYP2D6 Inhibitors (Moderate); CYP2D6 Inhibitors (Strong); Dexmethylphenidate; Divalproex; DULoxetine; Linezolid; Lithium; MAO Inhibitors; Methylphenidate; Metoclopramide; Metyrosine; Mifepristone; Pramlintide; Protease Inhibitors; QuiNIDine; Selective Serotonin Reuptake Inhibitors; Terbinafine; Terbinafine (Systemic); Valproic Acid

Decreased Effect

Nortriptyline may decrease the levels/effects of: Acetylcholinesterase Inhibitors (Central); Alpha2-Agonists; Iobenguane I 123

The levels/effects of Nortriptyline may be decreased by: Acetylcholinesterase Inhibitors (Central); Barbiturates; CarBAMazepine; Peginterferon Alfa-2b; St Johns Wort; Tocilizumab

Ethanol/Nutrition/Herb Interactions

Ethanol: May increase CNS depression; monitor for increased effects with coadministration. Caution patients about effects.

Herb/Nutraceutical: Avoid valerian, St John's wort, SAMe, kava kava (may increase risk of serotonin syndrome and/or excessive sedation).

Stability Store at 20°C to 25°C (68°F to 77°F). Protect from light.

Mechanism of Action Traditionally believed to increase the synaptic concentration of serotonin and/or norepinephrine in the central nervous system by inhibition of their reuptake by the presynaptic neuronal membrane. However, additional receptor effects have been found including desensitization of adenyl cyclase, down regulation of beta-adrenergic receptors, and down regulation of serotonin receptors.

Pharmacodynamics/Kinetics

Onset of action: Therapeutic: 1-3 weeks

Distribution: V_d: 21 L/kg

Protein binding: 93% to 95%

Metabolism: Primarily hepatic; extensive first-pass effect

Half-life elimination: 28-31 hours

Time to peak, serum: 7-8.5 hours

Excretion: Urine (as metabolites and small amounts of unchanged drug); feces (small amounts)

Dosage

Geriatric: Initial: 30-50 mg/day, given as a single daily dose or in divided doses. **Note:** Nortriptyline is one of the best tolerated TCAs in the elderly.

Adult

Depression: Oral: 25 mg 3-4 times/day up to 150 mg/day; doses may be given once daily.

Chronic urticaria, angioedema, nocturnal pruritus (unlabeled use): Oral: 75 mg/day

Myofascial pain, neuralgia, burning mouth syndrome (unlabeled uses): Initial: 10-25 mg at bedtime; dosage may be increased by 25 mg/day weekly, if tolerated; usual maintenance dose: 75 mg as a single bedtime dose or 2 divided doses

Smoking cessation (unlabeled use; Fiore, 2008): Oral: Initial: 25 mg/day; titrate dose to 75-100 mg/day 10-28 days prior to selected "quit" date; continue therapy for ≥12 weeks after "quit" day

Hepatic Impairment Lower doses and slower titration are recommended dependent on individualization of dosage.

Monitoring Parameters Blood pressure and pulse rate (ECG, cardiac monitoring) prior to and during initial therapy in older adults; weight; blood levels are useful for therapeutic monitoring; suicide ideation (especially at the beginning of therapy or when doses are increased or decreased)

Reference Range Plasma levels do not always correlate with clinical effectiveness

Therapeutic: 50-150 ng/mL (SI: 190-570 nmol/L)

Toxic: >500 ng/mL (SI: >1900 nmol/L)

Pharmacotherapy Pearls The maximum antidepressant effect of nortriptyline may not be seen for ≥2 weeks after initiation of therapy.

Special Geriatric Considerations Nortriptyline is the least likely of the tricyclic antidepressants (TCAs) to cause orthostatic hypotension and one of the least anticholinergic and sedating TCAs, it is a preferred agent when a TCA is indicated.

A systematic review and meta-analysis of antidepressant placebo-controlled trials in persons with depression and dementia found evidence "suggestive" of efficacy but not of sufficient strength to "confirm" efficacy. Antidepressant trials in this patient population are small and underpowered. Older patients with depression being treated with an antidepressant should be closely monitored for response and adverse effects. Treatment should be switched or augmented when response is inadequate with a therapeutic dose. Antidepressants that are not tolerated should be discontinued and an alternative agent should be started.

This medication is considered to be potentially inappropriate in this patient population (Beers Criteria: SIADH: Quality of evidence - moderate; Strength of recommendation - strong).

Dosage Forms Excipient information presented when available (limited, particularly for generics); consult specific product labeling. [DSC] = Discontinued product

Capsule, oral: 10 mg, 25 mg, 50 mg, 75 mg
  Pamelor™: 10 mg, 25 mg, 50 mg, 75 mg
Solution, oral: 10 mg/5 mL (473 mL, 480 mL [DSC])
  Pamelor™: 10 mg/5 mL (480 mL [DSC]) [contains benzoic acid, ethanol 4%]

◆ **Nortriptyline Hydrochloride** *see* Nortriptyline *on page* 1395
◆ **Norvasc®** *see* AmLODIPine *on page* 104
◆ **Nostrilla® [OTC]** *see* Oxymetazoline (Nasal) *on page* 1452
◆ **Novel Erythropoiesis-Stimulating Protein** *see* Darbepoetin Alfa *on page* 488
◆ **NovoLIN® 70/30** *see* Insulin NPH and Insulin Regular *on page* 1023
◆ **NovoLIN® N** *see* Insulin NPH *on page* 1020
◆ **NovoLIN® R** *see* Insulin Regular *on page* 1025
◆ **NovoLOG®** *see* Insulin Aspart *on page* 1005
◆ **NovoLog 70/30** *see* Insulin Aspart Protamine and Insulin Aspart *on page* 1008
◆ **NovoLOG® FlexPen®** *see* Insulin Aspart *on page* 1005
◆ **NovoLOG® Mix 70/30** *see* Insulin Aspart Protamine and Insulin Aspart *on page* 1008
◆ **NovoLOG® Mix 70/30 FlexPen®** *see* Insulin Aspart Protamine and Insulin Aspart *on page* 1008
◆ **NovoLOG® Penfill®** *see* Insulin Aspart *on page* 1005
◆ **Noxafil®** *see* Posaconazole *on page* 1567
◆ **NPH Insulin** *see* Insulin NPH *on page* 1020
◆ **NPH Insulin and Regular Insulin** *see* Insulin NPH and Insulin Regular *on page* 1023
◆ **NRS® [OTC]** *see* Oxymetazoline (Nasal) *on page* 1452
◆ **NSC-71423** *see* Megestrol *on page* 1194
◆ **NSC-147834** *see* Flutamide *on page* 821
◆ **NTG** *see* Nitroglycerin *on page* 1386
◆ **Nubain** *see* Nalbuphine *on page* 1333
◆ **Nucynta®** *see* Tapentadol *on page* 1836
◆ **Nucynta® ER** *see* Tapentadol *on page* 1836
◆ **Nulecit™ [DSC]** *see* Ferric Gluconate *on page* 774
◆ **NuLev®** *see* Hyoscyamine *on page* 960
◆ **Nulojix®** *see* Belatacept *on page* 192
◆ **Numoisyn™** *see* Saliva Substitute *on page* 1748
◆ **Nutracort** *see* Hydrocortisone (Topical) *on page* 943
◆ **Nutralox® [OTC]** *see* Calcium Carbonate *on page* 262
◆ **Nuvigil®** *see* Armodafinil *on page* 147
◆ **Nyamyc®** *see* Nystatin (Topical) *on page* 1399
◆ **Nycoff [OTC]** *see* Dextromethorphan *on page* 525

Nystatin (Oral) (nye STAT in)

Medication Safety Issues

Sound-alike/look-alike issues:
Nystatin may be confused with HMG-CoA reductase inhibitors (also known as "statins"; eg, atorvaSTATin, fluvastatin, lovastatin, pitavastatin, pravastatin, rosuvastatin, simvastatin), Nitrostat®

Brand Names: Canada PMS-Nystatin

Generic Availability (U.S.) Yes

Pharmacologic Category Antifungal Agent, Oral Nonabsorbed

Use Treatment of susceptible cutaneous, mucocutaneous, and oral cavity fungal infections normally caused by the *Candida* species

Contraindications Hypersensitivity to nystatin or any component of the formulation

Adverse Reactions (Reflective of adult population; not specific for elderly) 1% to 10%: Gastrointestinal: Diarrhea, nausea, stomach pain, vomiting

Drug Interactions

Metabolism/Transport Effects None known.

Avoid Concomitant Use There are no known interactions where it is recommended to avoid concomitant use.

Increased Effect/Toxicity There are no known significant interactions involving an increase in effect.

Decreased Effect
Nystatin (Oral) may decrease the levels/effects of: Saccharomyces boulardii

Stability

Tablet and suspension: Store at controlled room temperature of 15°C to 25°C (59°F to 77°F). Powder for suspension: Store under refrigeration at 2°C to 8°C (36°F to 46°F).

Mechanism of Action Binds to sterols in fungal cell membrane, changing the cell wall permeability allowing for leakage of cellular contents

Pharmacodynamics/Kinetics

Onset of action: Symptomatic relief from candidiasis: 24-72 hours

Absorption: Poorly absorbed

Excretion: Feces (as unchanged drug)

Dosage

Geriatric & Adult

Oral candidiasis: Suspension (swish and swallow): 400,000-600,000 units 4 times/day; swish in the mouth and retain for as long as possible (several minutes) before swallowing

Intestinal infections: Oral tablets: 500,000-1,000,000 units every 8 hours

Note: Powder for compounding: 1/8 teaspoon (500,000 units) to equal approximately 1/2 cup of water; give 4 times/day

Administration Suspension: Shake well before using. Should be swished about the mouth and retained in the mouth for as long as possible (several minutes) before swallowing.

Special Geriatric Considerations For oral infections, patients who wear dentures must have them removed and cleaned in order to eliminate source of reinfection.

Dosage Forms Excipient information presented when available (limited, particularly for generics); consult specific product labeling.

Powder, for prescription compounding: 50 million units (10 g); 150 million units (30 g); 500 million units (100 g)

Suspension, oral: 100,000 units/mL (5 mL, 60 mL, 473 mL, 480 mL)

Tablet, oral: 500,000 units

Nystatin (Topical) (nye STAT in)

Medication Safety Issues

Sound-alike/look-alike issues:

Nystatin may be confused with HMG-CoA reductase inhibitors (also known as "statins"; eg, atorvaSTATin, fluvastatin, lovastatin, pitavastatin, pravastatin, rosuvastatin, simvastatin), Nitrostat®

Brand Names: U.S. Nyamyc®; Nystop®; Pedi-Dri®; Pediaderm™ AF

Brand Names: Canada Candistatin®; Nyaderm

Generic Availability (U.S.) Yes

Pharmacologic Category Antifungal Agent, Topical; Antifungal Agent, Vaginal

Use Treatment of susceptible cutaneous and mucocutaneous fungal infections normally caused by the *Candida* species

Dosage

Geriatric & Adult

Mucocutaneous infections: Topical: Apply 2-3 times/day to affected areas; very moist topical lesions are treated best with powder.

Vaginal infections: Vaginal tablets: Insert 1 tablet/day at bedtime for 2 weeks. (May also be given orally.)

Special Geriatric Considerations Instruct patient or caregiver on appropriate use of topical nystatin products.

Dosage Forms Excipient information presented when available (limited, particularly for generics); consult specific product labeling.

Cream, topical: 100,000 units/g (15 g, 30 g)

Cream, topical [kit]:

Pediaderm™ AF: 100,000 units/g (30 g) [packaged with protective emollient]

Ointment, topical: 100,000 units/g (15 g, 30 g)

Powder, topical: 100,000 units/g (15 g, 30 g, 60 g)

Nyamyc®: 100,000 units/g (15 g, 30 g, 60 g) [contains talc]

Nystop®: 100,000 units/g (15 g, 30 g, 60 g) [contains talc]

Pedi-Dri®: 100,000 units/g (56.7 g) [contains talc]

Tablet, vaginal: 100,000 units

Nystatin and Triamcinolone (nye STAT in & trye am SIN oh lone)

Related Information
Nystatin (Topical) *on page 1399*
Triamcinolone (Topical) *on page 1961*
Index Terms Triamcinolone and Nystatin
Generic Availability (U.S.) Yes
Pharmacologic Category Antifungal Agent, Topical; Corticosteroid, Topical
Use Treatment of cutaneous candidiasis
Dosage
  Geriatric & Adult Cutaneous *Candida*: Topical: Apply sparingly 2-4 times/day
Special Geriatric Considerations Instruct patient or caregiver on appropriate use of topical nystatin and triamcinolone products.
Dosage Forms Excipient information presented when available (limited, particularly for generics); consult specific product labeling.
  Cream: Nystatin 100,000 units and triamcinolone acetonide 0.1% (15 g, 30 g, 60 g)
  Ointment: Nystatin 100,000 units and triamcinolone acetonide 0.1% (15 g, 30 g, 60 g)

- ◆ **Nystop®** *see* Nystatin (Topical) *on page 1399*
- ◆ **Nytol® Quick Caps [OTC]** *see* DiphenhydrAMINE (Systemic) *on page 556*
- ◆ **Nytol® Quick Gels [OTC]** *see* DiphenhydrAMINE (Systemic) *on page 556*
- ◆ **Oasis®** *see* Saliva Substitute *on page 1748*
- ◆ **OCBZ** *see* OXcarbazepine *on page 1440*
- ◆ **Ocean® [OTC]** *see* Sodium Chloride *on page 1787*
- ◆ **Ocean® for Kids [OTC]** *see* Sodium Chloride *on page 1787*
- ◆ **Octagam®** *see* Immune Globulin *on page 982*
- ◆ **Ocudox™** *see* Doxycycline *on page 606*
- ◆ **Ocufen®** *see* Flurbiprofen (Ophthalmic) *on page 820*
- ◆ **Ocuflox®** *see* Ofloxacin (Ophthalmic) *on page 1402*
- ◆ **O-desmethylvenlafaxine** *see* Desvenlafaxine *on page 514*
- ◆ **ODV** *see* Desvenlafaxine *on page 514*
- ◆ **Ofirmev™** *see* Acetaminophen *on page 31*

Ofloxacin (Systemic) (oh FLOKS a sin)

Related Information
Antimicrobial Drugs of Choice *on page 2163*
Brand Names: Canada Apo-Oflox®; Novo-Ofloxacin
Generic Availability (U.S.) Yes
Pharmacologic Category Antibiotic, Quinolone
Use Quinolone antibiotic for the treatment of acute exacerbations of chronic bronchitis, community-acquired pneumonia, skin and skin structure infections (uncomplicated), urethral and cervical gonorrhea (acute, uncomplicated), urethritis and cervicitis (nongonococcal), mixed infections of the urethra and cervix, pelvic inflammatory disease (acute), cystitis (uncomplicated), urinary tract infections (complicated), prostatitis
  Note: As of April 2007, the CDC no longer recommends the use of fluoroquinolones for the treatment of gonococcal disease.
Unlabeled Use Epididymitis (nongonococcal), leprosy, Traveler's diarrhea
Medication Guide Available Yes
Contraindications Hypersensitivity to ofloxacin or other members of the quinolone group, such as oxolinic acid, cinoxacin, norfloxacin, and ciprofloxacin; hypersensitivity to any component of the formulation
Warnings/Precautions [U.S. Boxed Warning]: There have been reports of tendon inflammation and/or rupture with quinolone antibiotics; risk may be increased with concurrent corticosteroids, organ transplant recipients, and in patients >60 years of age. Rupture of the Achilles tendon sometimes requiring surgical repair has been reported most frequently; but other tendon sites (eg, rotator cuff, biceps) have also been reported. Strenuous physical activity, rheumatoid arthritis, and renal impairment may be an independent risk factor for tendonitis. Discontinue at first sign of tendon inflammation or pain. May occur even after discontinuation of therapy. Use with caution in patients with rheumatoid arthritis; may increase risk of tendon rupture. Use with caution in patients with epilepsy or other CNS diseases which could predispose seizures; potential for seizures, although very rare, may be increased with concomitant NSAID therapy. Tremor, restlessness, confusion, and very rarely hallucinations or seizures may occur; use with caution in patients with known or suspected CNS disorder. Discontinue in patients who experience significant CNS adverse effects (eg, dizziness, hallucinations, suicidal ideations or actions). Use with caution in patients with renal

or hepatic impairment. Peripheral neuropathies have been linked to ofloxacin use; discontinue if numbness, tingling, or weakness develops.

Fluoroquinolones have been associated with the development of serious, and sometimes fatal, hypoglycemia, most often in elderly diabetics, but also in patients without diabetes. This occurred most frequently with gatifloxacin (no longer available systemically) but may occur at a lower frequency with other quinolones.

Rare cases of torsade de pointes have been reported in patients receiving ofloxacin and other quinolones. Risk may be minimized by avoiding use in patients with known prolongation of the QT interval, bradycardia, hypokalemia, hypomagnesemia, cardiomyopathy, or in those receiving concurrent therapy with Class Ia or Class III antiarrhythmics.

Severe hypersensitivity reactions, including anaphylaxis, have occurred with quinolone therapy. Reactions may present as typical allergic symptoms after a single dose, or may manifest as severe idiosyncratic dermatologic, vascular, pulmonary, renal, hepatic, and/or hematologic events, usually after multiple doses. Prompt discontinuation of drug should occur if skin rash or other symptoms arise. Prolonged use may result in fungal or bacterial superinfection, including *C. difficile*-associated diarrhea (CDAD) and pseudomembranous colitis; CDAD has been observed >2 months postantibiotic treatment. **[U.S. Boxed Warning]: Quinolones may exacerbate myasthenia gravis; avoid use (rare, potentially life-threatening weakness of respiratory muscles may occur).** Avoid excessive sunlight and take precautions to limit exposure (eg, loose fitting clothing, sunscreen); may cause moderate-to-severe phototoxicity reactions. Discontinue use if photosensitivity occurs. Since ofloxacin is ineffective in the treatment of syphilis and may mask symptoms, all patients should be tested for syphilis at the time of gonorrheal diagnosis and 3 months later. Hemolytic reactions may (rarely) occur with quinolone use in patients with latent or actual G6PD deficiency.

Adverse Reactions (Reflective of adult population; not specific for elderly) 1% to 10%:

Cardiovascular: Chest pain (1% to 3%)

Central nervous system: Headache (1% to 9%), insomnia (3% to 7%), dizziness (1% to 5%), fatigue (1% to 3%), somnolence (1% to 3%), sleep disorders (1% to 3%), nervousness (1% to 3%), pyrexia (1% to 3%)

Dermatologic: Rash/pruritus (1% to 3%)

Gastrointestinal: Diarrhea (1% to 4%), vomiting (1% to 4%), GI distress (1% to 3%), abdominal cramps (1% to 3%), flatulence (1% to 3%), abnormal taste (1% to 3%), xerostomia (1% to 3%), appetite decreased (1% to 3%), nausea (3% to 10%), constipation (1% to 3%)

Genitourinary: Vaginitis (1% to 5%), external genital pruritus in women (1% to 3%)

Ocular: Visual disturbances (1% to 3%)

Respiratory: Pharyngitis (1% to 3%)

Miscellaneous: Trunk pain

Drug Interactions

Metabolism/Transport Effects Inhibits CYP1A2 (strong)

Avoid Concomitant Use

Avoid concomitant use of Ofloxacin (Systemic) with any of the following: BCG; Highest Risk QTc-Prolonging Agents; Mifepristone

Increased Effect/Toxicity

Ofloxacin (Systemic) may increase the levels/effects of: Bendamustine; Corticosteroids (Systemic); CYP1A2 Substrates; Highest Risk QTc-Prolonging Agents; Moderate Risk QTc-Prolonging Agents; Porfimer; Sulfonylureas; Theophylline Derivatives; Varenicline; Vitamin K Antagonists

The levels/effects of Ofloxacin (Systemic) may be increased by: Insulin; Mifepristone; Nonsteroidal Anti-Inflammatory Agents; Probenecid; QTc-Prolonging Agents (Indeterminate Risk and Risk Modifying)

Decreased Effect

Ofloxacin (Systemic) may decrease the levels/effects of: BCG; Mycophenolate; Sulfonylureas; Typhoid Vaccine

The levels/effects of Ofloxacin (Systemic) may be decreased by: Antacids; Calcium Salts; Didanosine; Iron Salts; Lanthanum; Magnesium Salts; Quinapril; Sevelamer; Sucralfate; Zinc Salts

Ethanol/Nutrition/Herb Interactions

Food: Ofloxacin average peak serum concentrations may be decreased by 20% if taken with food.

Herb/Nutraceutical: Avoid dong quai, St John's wort (may also cause photosensitization).

Stability Store at 25°C (77°F); excursions permitted to 15°C to 30°C (59°F to 86°F).

OFLOXACIN (SYSTEMIC)

Mechanism of Action Ofloxacin is a DNA gyrase inhibitor. DNA gyrase is an essential bacterial enzyme that maintains the superhelical structure of DNA. DNA gyrase is required for DNA replication and transcription, DNA repair, recombination, and transposition; bactericidal

Pharmacodynamics/Kinetics

Absorption: Well absorbed; food causes only minor alterations

Distribution: V_d: 2.4-3.5 L/kg

Protein binding: 32%

Bioavailability: 98%

Half-life elimination: Biphasic: 4-5 hours and 20-25 hours (accounts for <5%); prolonged with renal impairment

Excretion: Primarily urine (as unchanged drug)

Dosage

Geriatric Oral: 200-400 mg every 12-24 hours (based on estimated renal function) for 7 days to 6 weeks depending on indication.

Adult

Cervicitis/urethritis (nongonococcal): Oral:

Nongonococcal: 300 mg every 12 hours for 7 days

Gonococcal (acute, uncomplicated): 400 mg as a single dose; **Note:** As of April 2007, the CDC no longer recommends the use of fluoroquinolones for the treatment of uncomplicated gonococcal disease.

Chronic bronchitis (acute exacerbation), community-acquired pneumonia, skin and skin structure infections (uncomplicated): Oral: 400 mg every 12 hours for 10 days

Epididymitis, nongonococcal (unlabeled use): Oral: 300 mg twice daily for 10 days (CDC, 2010); 200 mg twice daily for 14 days (Canadian STI Guidelines, 2008)

Leprosy (unlabeled use): Oral: 400 mg once daily

Pelvic inflammatory disease (acute): Oral: 400 mg every 12 hours for 10-14 days; **Note:** The CDC recommends use only if standard cephalosporin therapy is not feasible and community prevalence of quinolone-resistant gonococcal organisms is low. Culture sensitivity must be confirmed.

Prostatitis: Oral:

Acute: 400 mg for 1 dose, then 300 mg twice daily for 10 days

Chronic: 200 mg every 12 hours for 6 weeks

Traveler's diarrhea (unlabeled use): Oral: 300 mg twice daily for 3 days

UTI: Oral:

Uncomplicated: 200 mg every 12 hours for 3-7 days

Complicated: 200 mg every 12 hours for 10 days

Renal Impairment Adults: Oral: After a normal initial dose, adjust as follows:

Cl_{cr} 20-50 mL/minute: Administer usual dose every 24 hours

Cl_{cr} <20 mL/minute: Administer half the usual dose every 24 hours

Continuous arteriovenous or venovenous hemodiafiltration effects: Administer 300 mg every 24 hours

Hepatic Impairment Severe impairment: Maximum dose: 400 mg/day

Administration Do not take within 2 hours of food or any antacids which contain zinc, magnesium, or aluminum.

Test Interactions Some quinolones may produce a false-positive urine screening result for opiates using commercially-available immunoassay kits. This has been demonstrated most consistently for levofloxacin and ofloxacin, but other quinolones have shown cross-reactivity in certain assay kits. Confirmation of positive opiate screens by more specific methods should be considered.

Special Geriatric Considerations Adjust dose for renal function. The half-life of ofloxacin may be prolonged and serum concentrations are elevated in elderly patients even in the absence of overt renal impairment. The risk of torsade de pointes and tendon inflammation and/or rupture associated with the concomitant use of corticosteroids and quinolones is increased in the elderly population. See Warnings/Precautions regarding tendon rupture in patients >60 years of age.

Dosage Forms Excipient information presented when available (limited, particularly for generics); consult specific product labeling.

Tablet, oral: 200 mg, 300 mg, 400 mg

Ofloxacin (Ophthalmic) (oh FLOKS a sin)

Medication Safety Issues

Sound-alike/look-alike issues:

Ocuflox® may be confused with Occlusal™-HP, Ocufen®

Brand Names: U.S. Ocuflox®

Brand Names: Canada Ocuflox®

Generic Availability (U.S.) Yes
Pharmacologic Category Antibiotic, Ophthalmic; Antibiotic, Quinolone
Use Treatment of superficial ocular infections involving the conjunctiva or cornea due to strains of susceptible organisms
Dosage
Adult
Conjunctivitis: Ophthalmic: Instill 1-2 drops in affected eye(s) every 2-4 hours for the first 2 days, then use 4 times/day for an additional 5 days.
Corneal ulcer: Ophthalmic: Instill 1-2 drops every 30 minutes while awake and every 4-6 hours after retiring for the first 2 days; beginning on day 3, instill 1-2 drops every hour while awake for 4-6 additional days; thereafter, 1-2 drops 4 times/day until clinical cure.
Special Geriatric Considerations Evaluate the patient's or caregiver's ability to safely administer the correct dose of ophthalmic medication.
Dosage Forms Excipient information presented when available (limited, particularly for generics); consult specific product labeling.
Solution, ophthalmic [drops]: 0.3% (5 mL, 10 mL)
Ocuflox®: 0.3% (5 mL) [contains benzalkonium chloride]

Ofloxacin (Otic) (oh FLOKS a sin)

Medication Safety Issues
Sound-alike/look-alike issues:
Floxin may be confused with Flexeril®
International issues:
Floxin: Brand name for ofloxacin [U.S., Canada], but also the brand name for flunarizine [Thailand], norfloxacin [South Africa], and perfloxacin [Philippines]
Floxin [U.S., Canada] may be confused with Flexin brand name for diclofenac [Argentina], cyclobenzaprine [Chile], and orphenadrine [Israel]; Flogen brand name for naproxen [Mexico]
Index Terms Floxin Otic Singles
Generic Availability (U.S.) Yes
Pharmacologic Category Antibiotic, Quinolone
Use Otitis externa, chronic suppurative otitis media, acute otitis media
Dosage
Adult
Otitis media, chronic suppurative with perforated tympanic membranes: Otic: Instill 10 drops (or the contents of 2 single-dose containers) into affected ear twice daily for 14 days
Otitis externa: Otic: Instill 10 drops (or the contents of 2 single-dose containers) into affected ear(s) once daily for 7 days
Special Geriatric Considerations Evaluate the patient's or caregiver's ability to safely administer the correct dose of otic medication.
Dosage Forms Excipient information presented when available (limited, particularly for generics); consult specific product labeling.
Solution, otic [drops]: 0.3% (5 mL, 10 mL)

◆ **9-OH-risperidone** see Paliperidone on page 1457

OLANZapine (oh LAN za peen)

Related Information
Antipsychotic Agents on page 2103
Atypical Antipsychotics on page 2107
Beers Criteria – Potentially Inappropriate Medications for Geriatrics on page 2183
Medication Safety Issues
Sound-alike/look-alike issues:
OLANZapine may be confused with olsalazine, QUEtiapine
ZyPREXA® may be confused with CeleXA®, Reprexain™, Zestril®, ZyrTEC®
ZyPREXA® Zydis® may be confused with Zelapar®, zolpidem
ZyPREXA® Relprevv™ may be confused with ZyPREXA® IntraMuscular
BEERS Criteria medication:
This drug may be potentially inappropriate for use in geriatric patients (Quality of evidence - moderate; Strength of recommendation - strong).
Brand Names: U.S. ZyPREXA®; ZyPREXA® IntraMuscular; ZyPREXA® Relprevv™; ZyPREXA® Zydis®

OLANZAPINE

Brand Names: Canada Apo-Olanzapine ODT®; Apo-Olanzapine®; Ava-Olanzapine; CO Olanzapine; CO Olanzapine ODT; Mylan-Olanzapine; Olanzapine ODT; PHL-Olanzapine; PHL-Olanzapine ODT; PMS-Olanzapine; PMS-Olanzapine ODT; Riva-Olanzapine; Riva-Olanzapine ODT; Sandoz-Olanzapine; Sandoz-Olanzapine ODT; Teva-Olanzapine; Teva-Olanzapine OD; Zyprexa®; Zyprexa® Intramuscular; Zyprexa® Zydis®

Index Terms LY170053; Olanzapine Pamoate; Zyprexa Zydis

Generic Availability (U.S.) Yes: Excludes Injection (powder for suspension, extended release)

Pharmacologic Category Antimanic Agent; Antipsychotic Agent, Atypical

Use

Oral: Treatment of the manifestations of schizophrenia; treatment of acute or mixed mania episodes associated with bipolar I disorder (as monotherapy or in combination with lithium or valproate); maintenance treatment of bipolar disorder; in combination with fluoxetine for treatment-resistant or bipolar I depression

I.M., extended-release (Zyprexa® Relprevv™): Treatment of schizophrenia

I.M., short-acting (Zyprexa® IntraMuscular): Treatment of acute agitation associated with schizophrenia and bipolar I mania

Unlabeled Use Chronic pain; prevention of chemotherapy-associated delayed nausea or vomiting; psychosis/agitation related to Alzheimer's dementia; acute treatment of delirium

Prescribing and Access Restrictions As a requirement of the REMS program, only prescribers, healthcare facilities, and pharmacies registered with the Zyprexa® Relprevv™ Patient Care Program are able to prescribe, distribute, or dispense Zyprexa® Relprevv™ for patients who are enrolled in and meet all conditions of the program. Zyprexa® Relprevv™ must be administered at a registered healthcare facility. Prescribers will need to be recertified every 3 years. Contact the Zyprexa® Relprevv™ Patient Care Program at 1-877-772-9390.

Medication Guide Available Yes

Contraindications There are no contraindications listed in the manufacturer's labeling.

Canadian labeling: Hypersensitivity to olanzapine or any component of the formulation

Warnings/Precautions [U.S. Boxed Warning]: Elderly patients with dementia-related psychosis treated with antipsychotics are at an increased risk of death compared to placebo. Most deaths appeared to be either cardiovascular (eg, heart failure, sudden death) or infectious (eg, pneumonia) in nature. In addition, an increased incidence of cerebrovascular effects (eg, transient ischemic attack, stroke) has been reported in studies of placebo-controlled trials of olanzapine in elderly patients with dementia-related psychosis. Olanzapine is not approved for the treatment of dementia-related psychosis.

Moderate to highly sedating, use with caution in disorders where CNS depression is a feature; patients must be cautioned about performing tasks which require mental alertness (eg, operating machinery or driving). Use caution in patients with cardiac disease. Use with caution in Parkinson's disease, predisposition to seizures, or severe hepatic or renal disease. Life-threatening arrhythmias have occurred with therapeutic doses of some neuroleptics. May induce orthostatic hypotension; use caution with history of cardiovascular disease, hemodynamic instability, prior myocardial infarction, or ischemic heart disease. Increases in cholesterol and triglycerides have been noted. Use with caution in patients with pre-existing abnormal lipid profile. Esophageal dysmotility and aspiration have been associated with antipsychotic use; use with caution in patients at risk of aspiration pneumonia. May increase prolactin levels; clinical significance of hyperprolactinemia in patients with breast cancer or other prolactin-dependent tumors is unknown. Significant weight gain (>7% of baseline weight) may occur; monitor waist circumference and BMI. Impaired core body temperature regulation may occur; caution with strenuous exercise, heat exposure, dehydration, and concomitant medication possessing anticholinergic effects.

Leukopenia, neutropenia, and agranulocytosis (sometimes fatal) have been reported in clinical trials and postmarketing reports with antipsychotic use; presence of risk factors (eg, pre-existing low WBC or history of drug-induced leuko-/neutropenia) should prompt periodic blood count assessment. Discontinue therapy at first signs of blood dyscrasias or if absolute neutrophil count <1000/mm^3.

May cause anticholinergic effects; use with caution in patients with decreased gastrointestinal motility, urinary retention, BPH, xerostomia, or narrow-angle glaucoma. Relative to other neuroleptics, olanzapine has a moderate potency of cholinergic blockade. May cause extrapyramidal symptoms (EPS), although risk of these reactions is lower relative to other neuroleptics. Risk of dystonia (and probably other EPS) may be greater with increased doses, use of conventional antipsychotics, and males. May be associated with neuroleptic malignant syndrome (NMS). May cause extreme and life-threatening hyperglycemia; use with caution in patients with diabetes or other disorders of glucose regulation; monitor. Olanzapine levels may be lower in patients who smoke; the manufacturer does not require dosage adjustments, although dosage adjustments may be considered.

Use in elderly patients with dementia is associated with an increased risk of mortality and cerebrovascular accidents; avoid antipsychotic use for behavioral problems associated with dementia unless alternative nonpharmacologic therapies have failed and patient may harm self or others. In addition, use may cause or exacerbate syndrome of inappropriate antidiuretic hormone secretion or hyponatremia; monitor sodium closely with initiation or dosage adjustments in older adults. May also be inappropriate in older adults depending on comorbidities (eg, dementia, delirium) due to its potent anticholinergic effects (Beers Criteria).

The possibility of a suicide attempt is inherent in psychotic illness or bipolar disorder; use caution in high-risk patients during initiation of therapy. Prescriptions should be written for the smallest quantity consistent with good patient care.

There are two Zyprexa® formulations for intramuscular injection: Zyprexa® Relprevv™ is an extended-release formulation and Zyprexa® Intramuscular is short-acting:
  Extended-release I.M. injection (Zyprexa® Relprevv™): Monitor for post injection delirium/sedation syndrome; patients should be continuously watched (≥3 hours) for symptoms of olanzapine overdose. Only available through a restricted drug distribution program.
  Short-acting I.M. injection (Zyprexa® IntraMuscular): Patients should remain recumbent if drowsy/dizzy until hypotension, bradycardia, and/or hypoventilation have been ruled out. Concurrent use of I.M./I.V. benzodiazepines is not recommended (fatalities have been reported, though causality not determined).

Adverse Reactions (Reflective of adult population; not specific for elderly)
  Oral: Unless otherwise noted, adverse events are reported for placebo-controlled trials in adult patients on monotherapy:
  >10%:
    Central nervous system: Somnolence (dose dependent; 20% to 39%; adolescents 39% to 48%), extrapyramidal symptoms (dose dependent; ≤32%), dizziness (11% to 18%), headache (adolescents 17%), fatigue (adolescents 3% to 14%), insomnia (12%)
    Endocrine & metabolic: Prolactin increased (30%; adolescents 47%)
    Gastrointestinal: Weight gain (5% to 6%, has been reported as high as 40%; adolescents 29% to 31%), appetite increased (3% to 6%; adolescents 17% to 29%), xerostomia (dose dependent; 3% to 22%), constipation (9% to 11%), dyspepsia (7% to 11%)
    Hepatic: ALT increased ≥3 x ULN (adolescents 12%; adults 5%)
    Neuromuscular & skeletal: Weakness (dose dependent; 8% to 20%)
    Miscellaneous: Accidental injury (12%)
  1% to 10%:
    Cardiovascular: Chest pain, hypertension, orthostatic hypotension, peripheral edema, tachycardia
    Central nervous system: Fever, personality changes, restlessness (adolescents)
    Dermatologic: Bruising
    Endocrine & metabolic: Breast-related events ([adolescents] discharge, enlargement, galactorrhea, gynecomastia, lactation disorder); menstrual-related events (amenorrhea, hypomenorrhea, menstruation delayed, oligomenorrhea); sexual function-related events (anorgasmia, ejaculation delayed, erectile dysfunction, changes in libido, abnormal orgasm, sexual dysfunction)
    Gastrointestinal: Abdominal pain (adolescents), diarrhea (adolescents), flatulence, nausea (dose dependent), vomiting
    Genitourinary: Incontinence, UTI
    Hepatic: Hepatic enzymes increased
    Neuromuscular & skeletal: Abnormal gait, akathisia, articulation impairment, back pain, falling, hypertonia, joint/extremity pain, muscle stiffness (adolescents), tremor (dose dependent)
    Ocular: Amblyopia
    Respiratory: Cough, epistaxis (adolescents), pharyngitis, respiratory tract infection (adolescents), rhinitis, sinusitis (adolescents)

  Injection: Unless otherwise noted, adverse events are reported for placebo-controlled trials in adult patients on extended-release I.M. injection (Zyprexa® Relprevv™). Also refer to adverse reactions noted with oral therapy.
  >10%: Central nervous system: Headache (13% to 18%), sedation (8% to 13%)
  1% to 10%:
    Cardiovascular: Hypertension, hypotension (short-acting), orthostatic hypotension (short-acting), QT prolongation
    Central nervous system: Abnormal dreams, abnormal thinking, auditory hallucination, dizziness, dysarthria, extrapyramidal symptoms, fatigue, fever, pain, restlessness, somnolence
    Dermatologic: Acne
    Gastrointestinal: Abdominal pain, appetite increased, diarrhea, flatulence, nausea, vomiting, weight gain, xerostomia

Genitourinary: Vaginal discharge

Hepatic: Liver enzymes increased

Local: Injection site pain

Neuromuscular & skeletal: Arthralgia, back pain, muscle spasms, stiffness, tremor, weakness (short-acting)

Otic: Ear pain

Respiratory: Cough, nasal congestion, nasopharyngitis, pharyngolaryngeal pain, sneezing, upper respiratory tract infection

Miscellaneous: Toothache, tooth infection, viral infection

<1%, postmarketing, and/or case reports (limited to important or life-threatening): CPK increased, post-injection delirium/sedation syndrome, syncope (short-acting)

Drug Interactions

Metabolism/Transport Effects Substrate of CYP1A2 (major), CYP2D6 (minor); **Note:** Assignment of Major/Minor substrate status based on clinically relevant drug interaction potential; **Inhibits** CYP1A2 (weak), CYP2C19 (weak), CYP2C9 (weak), CYP2D6 (weak), CYP3A4 (weak)

Avoid Concomitant Use

Avoid concomitant use of OLANZapine with any of the following: Azelastine; Azelastine (Nasal); Benzodiazepines; Methadone; Metoclopramide; Paraldehyde; Pimozide

Increased Effect/Toxicity

OLANZapine may increase the levels/effects of: Alcohol (Ethyl); Anticholinergics; ARIPiprazole; Azelastine; Azelastine (Nasal); Benzodiazepines; Buprenorphine; CNS Depressants; Methadone; Methotrimeprazine; Methylphenidate; Paraldehyde; Pimozide; Serotonin Modulators; Zolpidem

The levels/effects of OLANZapine may be increased by: Abiraterone Acetate; Acetylcholinesterase Inhibitors (Central); CYP1A2 Inhibitors (Moderate); CYP1A2 Inhibitors (Strong); Deferasirox; Droperidol; FluvoxaMINE; HydrOXYzine; LamoTRIgine; Lithium formulations; Methotrimeprazine; Methylphenidate; Metoclopramide; Metyrosine; Pramlintide; Tetrabenazine

Decreased Effect

OLANZapine may decrease the levels/effects of: Amphetamines; Anti-Parkinson's Agents (Dopamine Agonist); Quinagolide

The levels/effects of OLANZapine may be decreased by: CYP1A2 Inducers (Strong); Cyproterone; Lithium formulations; Peginterferon Alfa-2b

Ethanol/Nutrition/Herb Interactions

Ethanol: May increase CNS depression; monitor for increased effects with coadministration. Caution patients about effects.

Herb/Nutraceutical: Avoid dong quai, St John's wort (may also cause photosensitization). Avoid kava kava, gotu kola, valerian, St John's wort (may increase CNS depression).

Stability

Injection, extended-release: Store at 20°C to 25°C (68°F to 77°F); excursions permitted to 15°C to 30°C (59°F to 86°F). Dilute as directed to final concentration of 150 mg/mL. Shake vigorously to mix; will form yellow, opaque suspension. Following reconstitution, suspension may be stored at room temperature and used within 24 hours. Shake vigorously to resuspend prior to administration. Use immediately once suspension is in syringe. Suspension may be irritating to skin; wear gloves during reconstitution.

Injection, short-acting: Store at 20°C to 25°C (68°F to 77°F); excursions permitted to 15°C to 30°C (59°F to 86°F); do not freeze. Protect from light. Reconstitute 10 mg vial with 2.1 mL SWFI. Resulting solution is ~5 mg/mL. Use immediately (within 1 hour) following reconstitution. Discard any unused portion.

Tablet and orally-disintegrating tablet: Store at 20°C to 25°C (68°F to 77°F); excursions permitted to 15°C to 30°C (59°F to 86°F). Protect from light and moisture.

Mechanism of Action Olanzapine is a second generation thienobenzodiazepine antipsychotic which displays potent antagonism of serotonin 5-HT$_{2A}$ and 5-HT$_{2C}$, dopamine D$_{1-4}$, histamine H$_1$ and alpha$_1$-adrenergic receptors. Olanzapine shows moderate antagonism of 5-HT$_3$ and muscarinic M$_{1-5}$ receptors, and weak binding to GABA-A, BZD, and beta-adrenergic receptors. Although the precise mechanism of action in schizophrenia and bipolar disorder is not known, the efficacy of olanzapine is thought to be mediated through combined antagonism of dopamine and serotonin type 2 receptor sites.

Pharmacodynamics/Kinetics

Absorption:

Oral: Well absorbed; not affected by food; tablets and orally-disintegrating tablets are bioequivalent

Short-acting injection: Rapidly absorbed

Distribution: V$_d$: Extensive, 1000 L

Protein binding, plasma: 93% bound to albumin and alpha$_1$-glycoprotein

Metabolism: Highly metabolized via direct glucuronidation and cytochrome P450 mediated oxidation (CYP1A2, CYP2D6); 40% removed via first pass metabolism

Half-life elimination: 21-54 hours; ~1.5 times greater in elderly; Extended-release injection: ~30 days

Time to peak, plasma: Maximum plasma concentrations after I.M. administration are 5 times higher than maximum plasma concentrations produced by an oral dose.

Extended-release injection: ~7 days

Short-acting injection: 15-45 minutes

Oral: ~6 hours

Excretion: Urine (57%, 7% as unchanged drug); feces (30%)

Clearance: 40% increase in olanzapine clearance in smokers; 30% decrease in females

Dosage

Geriatric & Adult

Schizophrenia:

Oral: Initial: 5-10 mg once daily (increase to 10 mg once daily within 5-7 days); thereafter, adjust by 5 mg/day at 1-week intervals, up to a recommended maximum of 20 mg/day. Maintenance: 10-20 mg once daily. Doses of 30-50 mg/day have been used; however, doses >10 mg/day have not demonstrated better efficacy, and safety and efficacy of doses >20 mg/day have not been evaluated.

Extended-release I.M. injection: **Note:** Establish tolerance to oral olanzapine prior to changing to extended-release I.M. injection. Maximum dose: 300 mg/2 weeks or 405 mg/4 weeks

Patients established on oral olanzapine 10 mg/day: Initial dose: 210 mg every 2 weeks for 4 doses or 405 mg every 4 weeks for 2 doses; Maintenance dose: 150 mg every 2 weeks or 300 mg every 4 weeks

Patients established on oral olanzapine 15 mg/day: Initial dose: 300 mg every 2 weeks for 4 doses; Maintenance dose: 210 mg every 2 weeks or 405 mg every 4 weeks

Patients established on oral olanzapine 20 mg/day: Initial and maintenance dose: 300 mg every 2 weeks

Acute mania associated with bipolar disorder: Oral:

Monotherapy: Initial: 10-15 mg once daily; increase by 5 mg/day at intervals of not less than 24 hours. Maintenance: 5-20 mg/day; recommended maximum dose: 20 mg/day.

Combination therapy (with lithium or valproate): Initial: 10 mg once daily; dosing range: 5-20 mg/day

Agitation (acute, associated with bipolar disorder or schizophrenia): Short-acting I.M. injection: Initial dose: 10 mg (a lower dose of 5-7.5 mg may be considered when clinical factors warrant); additional doses (up to 10 mg) may be considered; however, 2-4 hours should be allowed between doses to evaluate response (maximum total daily dose: 30 mg, per manufacturer's recommendation)

Depression:

Depression associated with bipolar disorder (in combination with fluoxetine): Oral: Initial: 5 mg in the evening; adjust as tolerated to usual range of 5-12.5 mg/day. See **"Note."**

Treatment-resistant depression (in combination with fluoxetine): Oral: Initial: 5 mg in the evening; adjust as tolerated to range of 5-20 mg/day. See **"Note."**

Note: When using individual components of fluoxetine with olanzapine rather than fixed dose combination product (Symbyax®), approximate dosage correspondence is as follows:

Olanzapine 2.5 mg + fluoxetine 20 mg = Symbyax® 3/25

Olanzapine 5 mg + fluoxetine 20 mg = Symbyax® 6/25

Olanzapine 12.5 mg + fluoxetine 20 mg = Symbyax® 12/25

Olanzapine 5 mg + fluoxetine 50 mg = Symbyax® 6/50

Olanzapine 12.5 mg + fluoxetine 50 mg = Symbyax® 12/50

Delirium (unlabeled use): Oral: 5 mg once daily for up to 5 days (NICE, 2010)

Prevention of chemotherapy-associated delayed nausea or vomiting (unlabeled use; in combination with a corticosteroid and serotonin [5HT$_3$] antagonist): Oral: 10 mg once daily for 3-5 days, beginning on day 1 of chemotherapy **or** 5 mg once daily for 2 days before chemotherapy, followed by 10 mg once daily (beginning on the day of chemotherapy) for 3-8 days

Renal Impairment No dosage adjustment required. Not removed by dialysis.

Hepatic Impairment Dosage adjustment may be necessary; however, there are no specific recommendations. Monitor closely.

Administration

Short-acting I.M. injection: **For I.M. administration only**; do not administer injection intravenously or subcutaneously; inject slowly, deep into muscle. If dizziness and/or drowsiness are noted, patient should remain recumbent until examination indicates postural hypotension and/or bradycardia are not a problem.

Extended-release I.M. injection: **For I.M. gluteal injection only**; do not administer I.V. or subcutaneously. After needle insertion into muscle, aspirate to verify that no blood appears. Do not massage injection site. Use diluent, syringes, and needles provided in convenience kit; obtain a new kit if aspiration of blood occurs.

Tablet: May be administered without regard to meals.

Orally-disintegrating: Remove from foil blister by peeling back (do not push tablet through the foil); place tablet in mouth immediately upon removal; tablet dissolves rapidly in saliva and may be swallowed with or without liquid. May be administered with or without food/meals.

Monitoring Parameters Vital signs; fasting lipid profile and fasting blood glucose/Hgb A$_{1c}$ (prior to treatment, at 3 months, then annually); periodic assessment of hepatic transaminases (in patients with hepatic disease); BMI, waist circumference; orthostatic blood pressure; mental status, abnormal involuntary movement scale (AIMS), extrapyramidal symptoms (EPS). Weight should be assessed prior to treatment, at 4 weeks, 8 weeks, 12 weeks, and then at quarterly intervals. Consider titrating to a different antipsychotic agent for a weight gain ≥5% of the initial weight.

Extended-release I.M. injection: Sedation/delirium for 3 hours after each dose

Special Geriatric Considerations Elderly patients have an increased risk of adverse response to side effects or adverse reactions to antipsychotics. A higher incidence of falls has been reported in elderly patients, particularly in debilitated patients. Olanzapine half-life that was 1.5 times that of younger (<65 years of age) adults; therefore, lower initial doses are recommended. Olanzapine is not indicated in dementia-related psychosis.

Studies with patients ≥65 years of age with schizophrenia showed no difference in tolerability compared to younger adults. Studies in the elderly with dementia-related psychosis suggested a different tolerability compared to younger patients with schizophrenia. In light of significant risks and adverse effects in the elderly population (compared with limited data demonstrating efficacy in the treatment of dementia-related psychosis, aggression, and agitation), an extensive risk:benefit analysis should be performed prior to use. Therefore, use with caution and at lower recommended doses.

This medication is considered to be potentially inappropriate in this patient population (Beers Criteria: Quality of evidence - moderate; Strength of recommendation - strong).

Dosage Forms Excipient information presented when available (limited, particularly for generics); consult specific product labeling.

Injection, powder for reconstitution: 10 mg
    ZyPREXA® IntraMuscular: 10 mg [contains lactose 50 mg]
Injection, powder for suspension, extended release:
    ZyPREXA® Relprevv™: 210 mg, 300 mg, 405 mg [contains polysorbate 80 (in diluent); supplied with diluent]
Tablet, oral: 2.5 mg, 5 mg, 7.5 mg, 10 mg, 15 mg, 20 mg
    ZyPREXA®: 2.5 mg, 5 mg, 7.5 mg, 10 mg, 15 mg, 20 mg
Tablet, orally disintegrating, oral: 5 mg, 10 mg, 15 mg, 20 mg
    ZyPREXA® Zydis®: 5 mg [contains phenylalanine 0.34 mg/tablet]
    ZyPREXA® Zydis®: 10 mg [contains phenylalanine 0.45 mg/tablet]
    ZyPREXA® Zydis®: 15 mg [contains phenylalanine 0.67 mg/tablet]
    ZyPREXA® Zydis®: 20 mg [contains phenylalanine 0.9 mg/tablet]

Olanzapine and Fluoxetine (oh LAN za peen & floo OKS e teen)

Medication Safety Issues
    Sound-alike/look-alike issues:
        Symbyax® may be confused with Cymbalta®
    BEERS Criteria medication:
        This drug may be potentially inappropriate for use in geriatric patients (Quality of evidence - moderate; Strength of recommendation - strong).
Brand Names: U.S. Symbyax®
Index Terms Fluoxetine and Olanzapine; Olanzapine and Fluoxetine Hydrochloride
Generic Availability (U.S.) Yes
Pharmacologic Category Antidepressant, Selective Serotonin Reuptake Inhibitor; Antipsychotic Agent, Atypical
Use Treatment of depressive episodes associated with bipolar I disorder; treatment-resistant depression (unresponsive to 2 trials of different antidepressants in the current episode)
Medication Guide Available Yes
Contraindications Hypersensitivity to olanzapine, fluoxetine, or any component of the formulation; patients currently receiving MAO inhibitors, thioridazine, pimozide, or mesoridazine; treatment within 14 days of MAO therapy
Warnings/Precautions See individual agents.

Adverse Reactions (Reflective of adult population; not specific for elderly) As reported with combination product (also see individual agents):

>10%:

Central nervous system: Somnolence (14%), fatigue (12%)

Endocrine & metabolic: Hyperprolactinemia (28%), bicarbonate decreased (14%)

Gastrointestinal: Weight gain (25%), appetite increased (20%), xerostomia (15%)

Hepatic: Hyperbilirubinemia (15%)

1% to 10%:

Cardiovascular: Peripheral edema (9%), edema (3%), vasodilation (≥1%)

Central nervous system: Sedation (8%), attention disturbance (5%), hypersomnia (5%), restlessness (4%), lethargy (3%), pain in extremity (3%), fever (2%), nervousness (2%), pain (2%), thinking abnormal (2%), chills (≥1%), amnesia (≥1%)

Dermatologic: Photosensitivity (≥1%), ecchymosis (≥1%)

Endocrine & metabolic: Hypoalbuminemia (3%), uric acid levels increased (3%), hypophosphatemia (2%), breast pain (≥1%), menorrhagia (≥1%)

Gastrointestinal: Flatulence (3%), abdominal distension (2%), diarrhea (≥1%), taste perversion (≥1%), weight loss (≥1%)

Genitourinary: Erectile dysfunction (2%), urinary frequency (≥1%), urinary incontinence (≥1%)

Hematologic: Hemoglobin decreased (3%), lymphocytopenia (2%)

Hepatic: ALT increased (3%)

Neuromuscular & skeletal: Tremor (9%), arthralgia (4%), weakness (3%), stiffness (2%), neck rigidity (≥1%)

Ocular: Blurred vision (5%)

Renal: Glucosuria (4%)

Respiratory: Sinusitis (2%)

Frequency not defined: Alkaline phosphate increased, AST increased, cholesterol increased, GGT increased, hyperglycemia, hyponatremia, orthostatic hypotension, triglycerides increased

Drug Interactions

Metabolism/Transport Effects Refer to individual components.

Avoid Concomitant Use

Avoid concomitant use of Olanzapine and Fluoxetine with any of the following: Azelastine; Azelastine (Nasal); Benzodiazepines; Clopidogrel; Iobenguane I 123; MAO Inhibitors; Methylene Blue; Metoclopramide; Paraldehyde; Pimozide; Tryptophan

Increased Effect/Toxicity

Olanzapine and Fluoxetine may increase the levels/effects of: Alpha-/Beta-Blockers; Anticholinergics; Anticoagulants; Antidepressants (Serotonin Reuptake Inhibitor/Antagonist); Antiplatelet Agents; ARIPiprazole; Aspirin; AtoMOXetine; Azelastine; Azelastine (Nasal); Benzodiazepines; Benzodiazepines (metabolized by oxidation); Beta-Blockers; BusPIRone; CarBAMazepine; CloZAPine; Collagenase (Systemic); CYP1A2 Substrates; CYP2C19 Substrates; CYP2D6 Substrates; Dabigatran Etexilate; Desmopressin; Dextromethorphan; Drotrecogin Alfa (Activated); Fesoterodine; Fosphenytoin; Galantamine; Haloperidol; Highest Risk QTc-Prolonging Agents; Hypoglycemic Agents; Ibritumomab; Lithium; Methadone; Methylene Blue; Methylphenidate; Metoclopramide; Mexiletine; Moderate Risk QTc-Prolonging Agents; NIFEdipine; NiMODipine; NSAID (COX-2 Inhibitor); NSAID (Nonselective); Paraldehyde; Phenytoin; Pimozide; Propafenone; QuiNIDine; RisperiDONE; Rivaroxaban; Salicylates; Serotonin Modulators; Thrombolytic Agents; Tositumomab and Iodine I 131 Tositumomab; TraMADol; Tricyclic Antidepressants; Vitamin K Antagonists; Zolpidem

The levels/effects of Olanzapine and Fluoxetine may be increased by: Abiraterone Acetate; Acetylcholinesterase Inhibitors (Central); Alcohol (Ethyl); Analgesics (Opioid); Antipsychotics; ARIPiprazole; BusPIRone; Cimetidine; CNS Depressants; CYP1A2 Inhibitors (Moderate); CYP1A2 Inhibitors (Strong); CYP2C9 Inhibitors (Moderate); CYP2C9 Inhibitors (Strong); CYP2D6 Inhibitors (Moderate); CYP2D6 Inhibitors (Strong); Darunavir; Deferasirox; FluvoxaMINE; Glucosamine; Herbs (Anticoagulant/Antiplatelet Properties); HydrOXYzine; LamoTRIgine; Linezolid; Lithium formulations; Macrolide Antibiotics; MAO Inhibitors; Methylphenidate; Metoclopramide; Metyrosine; Mifepristone; Omega-3-Acid Ethyl Esters; Pentosan Polysulfate Sodium; Pentoxifylline; Pramlintide; Prostacyclin Analogues; Tetrabenazine; Tipranavir; TraMADol; Tryptophan; Vitamin E

Decreased Effect

Olanzapine and Fluoxetine may decrease the levels/effects of: Amphetamines; Anti-Parkinson's Agents (Dopamine Agonist); Clopidogrel; Iobenguane I 123; Ioflupane I 123; Quinagolide

OLANZAPINE AND FLUOXETINE

The levels/effects of Olanzapine and Fluoxetine may be decreased by: CarBAMazepine; CYP1A2 Inducers (Strong); CYP2C9 Inducers (Strong); Cyproheptadine; Cyproterone; Lithium formulations; NSAID (COX-2 Inhibitor); NSAID (Nonselective); Peginterferon Alfa-2b; Tocilizumab

Ethanol/Nutrition/Herb Interactions See individual agents.

Stability Store at controlled room temperature of 15°C to 30°C (59°F to 86°F). Protect from moisture.

Mechanism of Action Olanzapine is a second generation thienobenzodiazepine antipsychotic which displays potent antagonism of serotonin 5-HT$_{2A}$ and 5-HT$_{2C}$, dopamine D$_{1-4}$, histamine H$_1$ and alpha$_1$-adrenergic receptors. Olanzapine shows moderate antagonism of 5-HT$_3$ and muscarinic M$_{1-5}$ receptors, and weak binding to GABA-A, BZD, and beta-adrenergic receptors. Fluoxetine inhibits CNS neuron serotonin reuptake; minimal or no effect on reuptake of norepinephrine or dopamine; does not significantly bind to alpha-adrenergic, histamine, or cholinergic receptors. The enhanced antidepressant effect of the combination may be due to synergistic increases in serotonin, norepinephrine, and dopamine.

Pharmacodynamics/Kinetics See individual agents.

Dosage

Geriatric Oral: Initial: Olanzapine 3-6 mg/fluoxetine 25 mg once daily in the evening; use caution adjusting dose (metabolism may be decreased). Safety and efficacy have not been established in patients >65 years of age.

Adult Lower doses (olanzapine 3-6 mg/fluoxetine 25 mg) should be used in patients predisposed to hypotension, with hepatic impairment, with combined factors for reduced metabolism (females, the elderly, nonsmokers), or enhanced sensitivity to olanzapine; dose adjustments should be made with caution in this patient population.

Depression associated with bipolar I disorder: Initial: Olanzapine 6 mg/fluoxetine 25 mg once daily in the evening. Dosing range: Olanzapine 6-12 mg/fluoxetine 25-50 mg. Safety of daily doses of olanzapine >18 mg/fluoxetine >75 mg have not been evaluated.

Treatment-resistant depression: Initial: Olanzapine 6 mg/fluoxetine 25 mg once daily in the evening. Dosing range: Olanzapine 6-18 mg/fluoxetine 25-50 mg. Safety of daily doses of olanzapine >18 mg/fluoxetine >75 mg have not been evaluated.

Note: When using individual components of fluoxetine with olanzapine rather than fixed dose combination product (Symbyax®), approximate dosage correspondence is as follows:

Olanzapine 2.5 mg + fluoxetine 20 mg = Symbyax® 3/25
Olanzapine 5 mg + fluoxetine 20 mg = Symbyax® 6/25
Olanzapine 12.5 mg + fluoxetine 20 mg = Symbyax® 12/25
Olanzapine 5 mg + fluoxetine 50 mg = Symbyax® 6/50
Olanzapine 12.5 mg + fluoxetine 50 mg = Symbyax® 12/50

Hepatic Impairment Initial: Olanzapine 3-6 mg/fluoxetine 25 mg once daily in the evening; use caution adjusting dose (metabolism may be decreased).

Administration Capsules should be taken once daily in the evening; may be taken without regard to meals.

Monitoring Parameters Vital signs; lipid profile, fasting blood glucose/Hgb A$_{1c}$; BMI; mental status; abnormal involuntary movement scale (AIMS), extrapyramidal symptoms (EPS); signs and symptoms of depression, anxiety, suicidal ideation (especially at the beginning of therapy or when doses are increased or decreased); sleep; liver function tests in patients with hepatic disease; complete blood count in patients at risk for neutropenia

Special Geriatric Considerations This medication is considered to be potentially inappropriate in this patient population (Beers Criteria: Quality of evidence - moderate; Strength of recommendation - strong).

Dosage Forms Excipient information presented when available (limited, particularly for generics); consult specific product labeling.

Capsule, oral: 6/25: Olanzapine 6 mg and fluoxetine 25 mg; 6/50: Olanzapine 6 mg and fluoxetine 50 mg; 12/25: Olanzapine 12 mg and fluoxetine 25 mg; 12/50: Olanzapine 12 mg and fluoxetine 50 mg

Symbyax® 3/25: Olanzapine 3 mg and fluoxetine 25 mg
Symbyax® 6/25: Olanzapine 6 mg and fluoxetine 25 mg
Symbyax® 6/50: Olanzapine 6 mg and fluoxetine 50 mg
Symbyax® 12/25: Olanzapine 12 mg and fluoxetine 25 mg
Symbyax® 12/50: Olanzapine 12 mg and fluoxetine 50 mg

◆ **Olanzapine and Fluoxetine Hydrochloride** *see* Olanzapine and Fluoxetine *on page 1408*
◆ **Olanzapine Pamoate** *see* OLANZapine *on page 1403*
◆ **Oleptro™** *see* TraZODone *on page 1953*
◆ **Oleum Ricini** *see* Castor Oil *on page 305*

Olmesartan (ole me SAR tan)

Related Information
Angiotensin Agents on page 2093
Medication Safety Issues
Sound-alike/look-alike issues:
Benicar® may be confused with Mevacor®
Brand Names: U.S. Benicar®
Brand Names: Canada Olmetec®
Index Terms Olmesartan Medoxomil
Generic Availability (U.S.) No
Pharmacologic Category Angiotensin II Receptor Blocker
Use Treatment of hypertension with or without concurrent use of other antihypertensive agents
Contraindications There are no contraindications listed in the manufacturer's labeling.
Warnings/Precautions May cause hyperkalemia; avoid potassium supplementation unless specifically required by healthcare provider. Avoid use or use a smaller dose in patients who are volume depleted; correct depletion first. May be associated with deterioration of renal function and/or increases in serum creatinine, particularly in patients with low renal blood flow (eg, renal artery stenosis, heart failure) whose glomerular filtration rate (GFR) is dependent on efferent arteriolar vasoconstriction by angiotensin II. Use with caution in unstented unilateral/bilateral renal artery stenosis. When unstented bilateral renal artery stenosis is present, use is generally avoided due to the elevated risk of deterioration in renal function unless possible benefits outweigh risks. Use with caution with pre-existing renal insufficiency; significant aortic/mitral stenosis. Concurrent use of ACE inhibitors may increase the risk of clinically-significant adverse events (eg, renal dysfunction, hyperkalemia).
Adverse Reactions (Reflective of adult population; not specific for elderly) 1% to 10%:
Central nervous system: Dizziness (3%), headache
Endocrine & metabolic: Hyperglycemia, hypertriglyceridemia
Gastrointestinal: Diarrhea
Neuromuscular & skeletal: Back pain, CPK increased
Renal: Hematuria
Respiratory: Bronchitis, pharyngitis, rhinitis, sinusitis
Miscellaneous: Flu-like syndrome
Drug Interactions
Metabolism/Transport Effects Substrate of SLCO1B1
Avoid Concomitant Use There are no known interactions where it is recommended to avoid concomitant use.
Increased Effect/Toxicity
Olmesartan may increase the levels/effects of: ACE Inhibitors; Amifostine; Antihypertensives; Hypotensive Agents; Lithium; Nonsteroidal Anti-Inflammatory Agents; Potassium-Sparing Diuretics; RiTUXimab; Sodium Phosphates

The levels/effects of Olmesartan may be increased by: Alfuzosin; Aliskiren; Diazoxide; Eltrombopag; Eplerenone; Herbs (Hypotensive Properties); MAO Inhibitors; Pentoxifylline; Phosphodiesterase 5 Inhibitors; Potassium Salts; Prostacyclin Analogues; Tolvaptan; Trimethoprim
Decreased Effect
The levels/effects of Olmesartan may be decreased by: Colesevelam; Herbs (Hypertensive Properties); Methylphenidate; Nonsteroidal Anti-Inflammatory Agents; Yohimbine
Ethanol/Nutrition/Herb Interactions
Food: Does not affect olmesartan bioavailability. Potassium supplements and/or potassium-containing salts may cause or worsen hyperkalemia. Management: Consult prescriber before consuming a potassium-rich diet, potassium supplements, or salt substitutes.
Herb/Nutraceutical: Some herbal medications may worsen hypertension (eg, licorice); others may increase the antihypertensive effect of olmesartan (eg, shepherd's purse). Management: Avoid bayberry, blue cohosh, cayenne, ephedra, ginger, ginseng (American), kola, licorice, and yohimbe. Avoid black cohosh, California poppy, coleus, golden seal, hawthorn, mistletoe, periwinkle, quinine, and shepherd's purse.
Stability Store at 20°C to 25°C (68°F to 77°F).
Mechanism of Action As a selective and competitive, nonpeptide angiotensin II receptor antagonist, olmesartan blocks the vasoconstrictor and aldosterone-secreting effects of angiotensin II; olmesartan interacts reversibly at the AT1 and AT2 receptors of many tissues and has slow dissociation kinetics; its affinity for the AT1 receptor is 12,500 times greater than the AT2 receptor. Angiotensin II receptor antagonists may induce a more complete inhibition of the renin-angiotensin system than ACE inhibitors, they do not affect the response to

bradykinin, and are less likely to be associated with nonrenin-angiotensin effects (eg, cough and angioedema). Olmesartan increases urinary flow rate and, in addition to being natriuretic and kaliuretic, increases excretion of chloride, magnesium, uric acid, calcium, and phosphate.

Pharmacodynamics/Kinetics
Distribution: 17 L; does not cross the blood-brain barrier (animal studies)
Protein binding: 99%
Metabolism: Olmesartan medoxomil is hydrolyzed in the GI tract to active olmesartan. No further metabolism occurs.
Bioavailability: 26%
Half-life elimination: Terminal: 13 hours
Time to peak: 1-2 hours
Excretion: All as unchanged drug: Feces (50% to 65%); urine (35% to 50%)

Dosage
Geriatric No initial dosage adjustment necessary per labeling; however, may consider starting at 5-10 mg/day (due to concomitant disease or age changes).
Adult Hypertension: Oral: Initial: Usual starting dose is 20 mg once daily; if initial response is inadequate, may be increased to 40 mg once daily after 2 weeks. May administer with other antihypertensive agents if blood pressure inadequately controlled with olmesartan. Consider lower starting dose in patients with possible depletion of intravascular volume (eg, patients receiving diuretics).
Renal Impairment No specific guidelines for dosage adjustment; patients undergoing hemodialysis have not been studied.
Hepatic Impairment No initial dosage adjustment necessary.
Administration May be administered with or without food.
Monitoring Parameters Blood pressure, serum potassium
Special Geriatric Considerations No dosage adjustment is necessary when initiating angiotensin II receptor antagonists in the elderly. In clinical studies, no differences between younger adults and the elderly were demonstrated.

For age alone, consider hydration status to avoid hypotension; many elderly are volume depleted due to age-related blunting of the thirst reflex and diuretic use. May consider starting this medication at 5-10 mg once daily.
Dosage Forms Excipient information presented when available (limited, particularly for generics); consult specific product labeling.
Tablet, oral, as medoxomil:
Benicar®: 5 mg, 20 mg, 40 mg

Olmesartan, Amlodipine, and Hydrochlorothiazide
(ole me SAR tan, am LOE di peen, & hye droe klor oh THYE a zide)

Related Information
AmLODIPine on page 104
Hydrochlorothiazide on page 933
Olmesartan on page 1411
Brand Names: U.S. Tribenzor™
Index Terms Amlodipine Besylate, Olmesartan Medoxomil, and Hydrochlorothiazide; Amlodipine, Hydrochlorothiazide, and Olmesartan; Hydrochlorothiazide, Olmesartan, and Amlodipine; Olmesartan, Hydrochlorothiazide, and Amlodipine
Generic Availability (U.S.) No
Pharmacologic Category Angiotensin II Receptor Blocker; Antianginal Agent; Calcium Channel Blocker; Calcium Channel Blocker, Dihydropyridine; Diuretic, Thiazide
Use Treatment of hypertension (not for initial therapy)
Dosage
Geriatric Patients ≥75 years of age should start amlodipine at 2.5 mg (combination product dosage form not available in this strength).
Adult Note: Not for initial therapy. Dose is individualized; combination product may be substituted for individual components in patients currently maintained on all 3 agents separately or in patients not adequately controlled with any 2 of the following antihypertensive classes: Calcium channel blockers, angiotensin II receptor blockers, and diuretics.
Hypertension: Oral: Add-on/switch/replacement therapy: Amlodipine 5-10 mg, olmesartan 20-40 mg, and hydrochlorothiazide 12.5-25 mg once daily; dose may be titrated after 2 weeks of therapy. Maximum recommended daily dose: Amlodipine 10 mg/olmesartan 40 mg/hydrochlorothiazide 25 mg

Renal Impairment
Cl_{cr} >30 mL/minute: No adjustment needed.
Cl_{cr} ≤30 mL/minute: Use of combination not recommended; contraindicated in patients with anuria

Hepatic Impairment
Mild-to-moderate hepatic impairment: Use with caution; specific dosing recommendations are not provided in manufacturer's labeling.
Severe hepatic impairment: Patients with severe hepatic impairment should start amlodipine at 2.5 mg (combination product dosage form not available).

Special Geriatric Considerations See individual agents. Combination products are not recommended as first-line treatment. Use only if doses of individual agents correspond to the combination available.

Dosage Forms Excipient information presented when available (limited, particularly for generics); consult specific product labeling.
Tablet, oral:
Tribenzor™: Olmesartan medoxomil 20 mg, amlodipine 5 mg, and hydrochlorothiazide 12.5 mg
Tribenzor™: Olmesartan medoxomil 40 mg, amlodipine 5 mg, and hydrochlorothiazide 12.5 mg
Tribenzor™: Olmesartan medoxomil 40 mg, amlodipine 5 mg, and hydrochlorothiazide 25 mg
Tribenzor™: Olmesartan medoxomil 40 mg, amlodipine 10 mg, and hydrochlorothiazide 12.5 mg
Tribenzor™: Olmesartan medoxomil 40 mg, amlodipine 10 mg, and hydrochlorothiazide 25 mg

◆ **Olmesartan and Amlodipine** see Amlodipine and Olmesartan on page 106

Olmesartan and Hydrochlorothiazide
(ole me SAR tan & hye droe klor oh THYE a zide)

Related Information
Hydrochlorothiazide on page 933
Olmesartan on page 1411
Brand Names: U.S. Benicar HCT®
Brand Names: Canada Olmetec Plus®
Index Terms Hydrochlorothiazide and Olmesartan Medoxomil; Olmesartan Medoxomil and Hydrochlorothiazide
Generic Availability (U.S.) No
Pharmacologic Category Angiotensin II Receptor Blocker; Diuretic, Thiazide
Use Treatment of hypertension (not recommended for initial treatment)
Dosage
Geriatric & Adult
Hypertension: Oral: Dosage must be individualized; may be titrated at 2- to 4-week intervals.
Replacement therapy: May be substituted for previously titrated dosages of the individual components.
Patients not controlled with single-agent therapy: Initiate by adding the lowest available dose of the alternative component (hydrochlorothiazide 12.5 mg or olmesartan 20 mg). Titrate to effect (maximum hydrochlorothiazide dose: 25 mg, maximum olmesartan dose: 40 mg).

Renal Impairment Cl_{cr} ≤30 mL/minute: Use not recommended.
Hepatic Impairment No dosage adjustment necessary.
Special Geriatric Considerations See individual agents. Combination products are not recommended as first-line treatment. Use only if doses of individual agents correspond to the combination available.

Dosage Forms Excipient information presented when available (limited, particularly for generics); consult specific product labeling.
Tablet:
20/12.5: Olmesartan medoxomil 20 mg and hydrochlorothiazide 12.5 mg
40/12.5: Olmesartan medoxomil 40 mg and hydrochlorothiazide 12.5 mg
40/25: Olmesartan medoxomil 40 mg and hydrochlorothiazide 25 mg

◆ **Olmesartan, Hydrochlorothiazide, and Amlodipine** see Olmesartan, Amlodipine, and Hydrochlorothiazide on page 1412
◆ **Olmesartan Medoxomil** see Olmesartan on page 1411

◆ **Olmesartan Medoxomil and Hydrochlorothiazide** *see* Olmesartan and Hydrochlorothiazide *on page 1413*

Olopatadine (Nasal) (oh la PAT a deen)

Brand Names: U.S. Patanase®
Index Terms Olopatadine Hydrochloride
Generic Availability (U.S.) No
Pharmacologic Category Histamine H_1 Antagonist; Histamine H_1 Antagonist, Second Generation; Piperidine Derivative
Use Treatment of the symptoms of seasonal allergic rhinitis
Dosage
  Geriatric & Adult Seasonal allergic rhinitis: Intranasal: 2 sprays into each nostril twice daily
Special Geriatric Considerations Evaluate the patient's or caregiver's ability to safely administer the correct dose of nasal medication.

No specific information in the elderly.
Dosage Forms Excipient information presented when available (limited, particularly for generics); consult specific product labeling.
  Solution, intranasal [spray]:
    Patanase®: 0.6% (30.5 g) [contains benzalkonium chloride; equivalent to olopatadine hydrochloride 665 mcg/100 microliters; 240 metered sprays]

Olopatadine (Ophthalmic) (oh la PAT a deen)

Medication Safety Issues
  Sound-alike/look-alike issues:
    Patanol® may be confused with Platinol
  International issues:
    Patanol [U.S., Canada, and multiple international markets] may be confused with Bétanol brand name for metipranolol [Monaco]
Brand Names: U.S. Pataday™; Patanol®
Brand Names: Canada Pataday™; Patanol®
Index Terms Olopatadine Hydrochloride
Generic Availability (U.S.) No
Pharmacologic Category Histamine H_1 Antagonist; Histamine H_1 Antagonist, Second Generation; Piperidine Derivative
Use Treatment of the signs and symptoms of allergic conjunctivitis
Dosage
  Geriatric & Adult Allergic conjunctivitis: Ophthalmic:
    Patanol®: Instill 1 drop into each affected eye twice daily (allowing 6-8 hours between doses); results from an environmental study demonstrated that olopatadine was effective when dosed twice daily for up to 6 weeks
    Pataday™: Instill 1 drop into each affected eye once daily
Special Geriatric Considerations Evaluate the patient's or caregiver's ability to safely administer the correct dose of ophthalmic medication.

No specific information in the elderly.
Dosage Forms Excipient information presented when available (limited, particularly for generics); consult specific product labeling.
  Solution, ophthalmic [drops]:
    Pataday™: 0.2% (2.5 mL) [contains benzalkonium chloride]
    Patanol®: 0.1% (5 mL) [contains benzalkonium chloride]

◆ **Olopatadine Hydrochloride** *see* Olopatadine (Nasal) *on page 1414*
◆ **Olopatadine Hydrochloride** *see* Olopatadine (Ophthalmic) *on page 1414*

Olsalazine (ole SAL a zeen)

Medication Safety Issues
  Sound-alike/look-alike issues:
    Olsalazine may be confused with OLANZapine
    Dipentum® may be confused with Dilantin®
Brand Names: U.S. Dipentum®
Brand Names: Canada Dipentum®

Index Terms Olsalazine Sodium

Generic Availability (U.S.) No

Pharmacologic Category 5-Aminosalicylic Acid Derivative

Use Maintenance of remission of ulcerative colitis in patients intolerant to sulfasalazine

Contraindications Hypersensitivity to olsalazine, salicylates, or any component of the formulation

Warnings/Precautions Diarrhea is a common adverse effect of olsalazine. May exacerbate symptoms of colitis. Use with caution in patients with renal or hepatic impairment. Use with caution in elderly patients. Use with caution in patients with severe allergies or asthma.

Adverse Reactions (Reflective of adult population; not specific for elderly)

>10%: Gastrointestinal: Diarrhea (11% to 17%; dose related)

1% to 10%:

Central nervous system: Depression (2%), dizziness/vertigo (1%)

Dermatologic: Rash (2%), pruritus (1%)

Gastrointestinal: Abdominal pain/cramps (10%), nausea (5%), bloating (2%), stomatitis (1%), vomiting (1%)

Neuromuscular & skeletal: Arthralgia (4%)

Respiratory: Upper respiratory infection (2%)

Drug Interactions

Metabolism/Transport Effects None known.

Avoid Concomitant Use There are no known interactions where it is recommended to avoid concomitant use.

Increased Effect/Toxicity

Olsalazine may increase the levels/effects of: Heparin; Heparin (Low Molecular Weight); Thiopurine Analogs; Varicella Virus-Containing Vaccines

Decreased Effect

Olsalazine may decrease the levels/effects of: Cardiac Glycosides

Stability Store at 20°C to 25°C (77°F); excursions permitted to 15°C to 30°C (59°F to 86°F).

Mechanism of Action Mesalamine (5-aminosalicylic acid) is the active component of olsalazine; the specific mechanism of action of mesalamine is unknown; however, it is thought that it modulates local chemical mediators of the inflammatory response, especially leukotrienes, and is also postulated to be a free radical scavenger or an inhibitor of tumor necrosis factor (TNF); action appears topical rather than systemic.

Pharmacodynamics/Kinetics

Absorption: <3%; very little intact olsalazine is systemically absorbed

Protein binding, plasma: >99%

Metabolism: Primarily via colonic bacteria to active drug, 5-aminosalicylic acid (5-ASA)

Half-life elimination: 54 minutes

Time to peak: ~1 hour

Excretion: Primarily feces; urine (<1%)

Dosage

Geriatric & Adult Ulcerative colitis: Oral: 1 g/day in 2 divided doses

Administration Take with food in evenly divided doses.

Monitoring Parameters CBC, hepatic function, renal function; stool frequency

Special Geriatric Considerations No specific data is available on elderly to suggest the drug needs alterations in dose. Since so little is absorbed, dosing should not be changed for reasons of age. Diarrhea may pose a serious problem for elderly in that it may cause dehydration, electrolyte imbalance, hypotension, and confusion.

Dosage Forms Excipient information presented when available (limited, particularly for generics); consult specific product labeling.

Capsule, oral, as sodium:

Dipentum®: 250 mg

◆ **Olsalazine Sodium** *see* Olsalazine *on page 1414*

◆ **Olux®** *see* Clobetasol *on page 406*

◆ **Olux-E™** *see* Clobetasol *on page 406*

◆ **Omega 3** *see* Omega-3-Acid Ethyl Esters *on page 1416*

Omega-3-Acid Ethyl Esters (oh MEG a three AS id ETH il ES ters)

Medication Safety Issues
Sound-alike/look-alike issues:
Lovaza® may be confused with LORazepam
International issues:
Omacor [multiple international markets] may be confused with Amicar brand name for aminocaproic acid [U.S.]
Other safety concerns:
The Institute for Safe Medication Practices (ISMP) reported a case of a foam plastic cup dissolving after contact with the liquid contents from a Lovaza® capsule. ISMP is requesting the manufacturer to add warnings to its labeling and that healthcare providers add Lovaza® to their list of medications to not crush.

Brand Names: U.S. Lovaza®
Index Terms Ethyl Esters of Omega-3 Fatty Acids; Fish Oil; Omega 3; P-OM3
Pharmacologic Category Antilipemic Agent, Miscellaneous
Use Lovaza®: Adjunct to diet therapy in the treatment of hypertriglyceridemia (≥500 mg/dL)
Note: A number of OTC formulations containing omega-3 fatty acids are marketed as nutritional supplements; these do not have FDA-approved indications and may not contain the same amounts of the active ingredient.
Unlabeled Use Omacor®: Treatment of IgA nephropathy
Contraindications Hypersensitivity to omega-3-acid ethyl esters or any component of the formulation
Warnings/Precautions Use with caution in patients with known allergy or sensitivity to fish. Should be used as an adjunct to diet therapy and exercise and only in those with very high triglyceride levels (≥500 mg/dL). Treatment of primary metabolic disorders (eg, diabetes, thyroid disease) and/or evaluation of the patient's medication regimen for possible etiologic agents should be completed prior to a decision to initiate therapy. Secondary causes of hyperlipidemia should be ruled out prior to therapy. If triglyceride levels do not adequately respond after 2 months of treatment with omega-3-acid ethyl esters, discontinue treatment. ALT may be increased without ALT increasing. May increase LDL levels; periodically monitor LDL levels. Prolongation of bleeding time has been observed in some clinical studies; use with caution in patients with coagulopathy or in those receiving therapeutic anticoagulation; monitor INR.
Adverse Reactions (Reflective of adult population; not specific for elderly)
Cardiovascular: Angina (1%)
Central nervous system: Pain (2%)
Dermatologic: Rash (2%)
Gastrointestinal: Eructation (5%), dyspepsia (3%), taste perversion (3%)
Neuromuscular & skeletal: Back pain (2%)
Miscellaneous: Flu-like syndrome (4%), infection (4%)
Drug Interactions
Metabolism/Transport Effects None known.
Avoid Concomitant Use There are no known interactions where it is recommended to avoid concomitant use.
Increased Effect/Toxicity
Omega-3-Acid Ethyl Esters may increase the levels/effects of: Antiplatelet Agents; Warfarin
Decreased Effect There are no known significant interactions involving a decrease in effect.
Ethanol/Nutrition/Herb Interactions
Ethanol: Monitor ethanol use (alcohol use may increase triglycerides).
Stability Store at controlled room temperature of 25°C (77°F); do not freeze.
Mechanism of Action Mechanism has not been completely defined. Possible mechanisms include inhibition of acyl CoA:1,2 diacylglycerol acyltransferase, increased hepatic beta-oxidation, a reduction in the hepatic synthesis of triglycerides, or an increase in plasma lipoprotein lipase activity.
Dosage
Geriatric & Adult
Hypertriglyceridemia: Oral: 4 g/day as a single daily dose or in 2 divided doses.
Treatment of IgA nephropathy (unlabeled use): Oral: 4 g/day
Renal Impairment No dosage adjustment required.
Administration May be administered with meals.
Monitoring Parameters Triglycerides and other lipids (LDL-C) should be monitored at baseline and periodically. Hepatic transaminase levels, particularly ALT, should be monitored periodically.

Pharmacotherapy Pearls Due to reports of prescribing errors associated with the similarity between Omacor® and Amicar,® (aminocaproic acid) the name Omacor® has been changed to Lovaza®. The size, strength, ingredients, and dose all remain the same

Special Geriatric Considerations Specific information about the safety and efficacy of omega-3-acid ethyl esters is limited. The manufacturer states there were no apparent differences between persons <60 and >60 years of age.

Dosage Forms Excipient information presented when available (limited, particularly for generics); consult specific product labeling.

Capsule, liquid gel, oral:

Lovaza®: 1 g [contains DHA ~375 mg/capsule, EPA ~465 mg/capsule, soybean oil]

Omeprazole (oh MEP ra zole)

Related Information

H. pylori Treatment in Adult Patients *on page 2116*

Medication Safety Issues

Sound-alike/look-alike issues:

Omeprazole may be confused with aripiprazole, fomepizole

PriLOSEC® may be confused with Plendil®, Prevacid®, predniSONE, prilocaine, Prinivil®, Proventil®, PROzac®

International issues:

Losec [multiple international markets] may be confused with Lasix brand name for furosemide [U.S., Canada, and multiple international markets]

Medral [Mexico] may be confused with Medrol brand name for methylprednisolone [U.S., Canada, and multiple international markets]

Norpramin: Brand name for omeprazole [Spain], but also the brand name for desipramine [U.S., Canada] and enalapril/hydrochlorothiazide [Portugal]

Brand Names: U.S. First®-Omeprazole; PriLOSEC OTC® [OTC]; PriLOSEC®

Brand Names: Canada Apo-Omeprazole®; Losec®; Mylan-Omeprazole; PMS-Omeprazole; PMS-Omeprazole DR; ratio-Omeprazole; Sandoz-Omeprazole

Index Terms Omeprazole Magnesium

Generic Availability (U.S.) Yes: Excludes granules for suspension

Pharmacologic Category Proton Pump Inhibitor; Substituted Benzimidazole

Use Short-term (4-8 weeks) treatment of active duodenal ulcer disease or active benign gastric ulcer; treatment of heartburn and other symptoms associated with gastroesophageal reflux disease (GERD); short-term (4-8 weeks) treatment of endoscopically-diagnosed erosive esophagitis; maintenance healing of erosive esophagitis; long-term treatment of pathological hypersecretory conditions; as part of a multidrug regimen for *H. pylori* eradication to reduce the risk of duodenal ulcer recurrence

OTC labeling: Short-term treatment of frequent, uncomplicated heartburn occurring ≥2 days/week

Unlabeled Use Healing NSAID-induced ulcers; prevention of NSAID-induced ulcer; stress-ulcer prophylaxis in the critically-ill

Contraindications Hypersensitivity to omeprazole, substituted benzimidazoles (eg, esomeprazole, lansoprazole), or any component of the formulation

Warnings/Precautions Use of proton pump inhibitors (PPIs) may increase the risk of gastrointestinal infections (eg, *Salmonella*, *Campylobacter*). Relief of symptoms does not preclude the presence of a gastric malignancy. Atrophic gastritis (by biopsy) has been noted with long-term omeprazole therapy. In long-term (2-year) studies in rats, omeprazole produced a dose-related increase in gastric carcinoid tumors. While available endoscopic evaluations and histologic examinations of biopsy specimens from human stomachs have not detected a risk from short-term exposure to omeprazole, further human data on the effect of sustained hypochlorhydria and hypergastrinemia are needed to rule out the possibility of an increased risk for the development of tumors in humans receiving long-term therapy.

PPIs may diminish the therapeutic effect of clopidogrel, thought to be due to reduced formation of the active metabolite of clopidogrel. The manufacturer of clopidogrel recommends either avoidance of omeprazole (even when scheduled 12 hours apart) or use of a PPI with less potent CYP2C19 inhibition (eg, pantoprazole). Others have recommended the continued use of PPIs, regardless of the degree of inhibition, in patients with a history of GI bleeding or multiple risk factors for GI bleeding who are also receiving clopidogrel since no evidence has established clinically meaningful differences in outcome; however, a clinically-significant interaction cannot be excluded in those who are poor metabolizers of clopidogrel (Abraham, 2010; Levine, 2011). Additionally, concomitant use of omeprazole with some drugs may require cautious use, may not be recommended, or may require dosage adjustments.

Increased incidence of osteoporosis-related bone fractures of the hip, spine, or wrist may occur with PPI therapy. Patients on high-dose (multiple daily doses)or long-term (≥1 year) therapy should be monitored. Use the lowest effective dose for the shortest duration of time, use vitamin D and calcium supplementation, and follow appropriate guidelines to reduce risk of fractures in patients at risk.

Hypomagnesemia, reported rarely, usually with prolonged PPI use of >3 months (most cases >1 year of therapy); may be symptomatic or asymptomatic; severe cases may cause tetany, seizures, and cardiac arrhythmias. Consider obtaining serum magnesium concentrations prior to beginning long-term therapy, especially if taking concomitant digoxin, diuretics, or other drugs known to cause hypomagnesemia; and periodically thereafter. Hypomagnesemia may be corrected by magnesium supplementation, although discontinuation of omeprazole may be necessary; magnesium levels typically return to normal within 1 week of stopping. Serum chromogranin A levels may be increased if assessed while patient on omeprazole; may lead to diagnostic errors related to neuroendocrine tumors.

Decreased *H. pylori* eradication rates have been observed with short-term (≤7 days) combination therapy. The American College of Gastroenterology recommends 10-14 days of therapy (triple or quadruple) for eradication of *H. pylori* (Chey, 2007). Bioavailability may be increased in Asian populations and patients with hepatic dysfunction; consider dosage reductions, especially for maintenance healing of erosive esophagitis. Bioavailability may be increased in the elderly. When used for self-medication (OTC), do not use for >14 days.

Adverse Reactions (Reflective of adult population; not specific for elderly) 1% to 10%:
Central nervous system: Headache (7%), dizziness (2%)
Dermatologic: Rash (2%)
Gastrointestinal: Abdominal pain (5%), diarrhea (4%), nausea (4%), vomiting (3%), flatulence (3%), acid regurgitation (2%), constipation (2%)
Neuromuscular & skeletal: Back pain (1%), weakness (1%)
Respiratory: Upper respiratory infection (2%), cough (1%)

Drug Interactions
Metabolism/Transport Effects Substrate of CYP2A6 (minor), CYP2C19 (major), CYP2C9 (minor), CYP2D6 (minor), CYP3A4 (minor); **Note:** Assignment of Major/Minor substrate status based on clinically relevant drug interaction potential; **Inhibits** CYP1A2 (weak), CYP2C19 (moderate), CYP2C9 (moderate), CYP2D6 (weak), CYP3A4 (weak); **Induces** CYP1A2 (weak/moderate)

Avoid Concomitant Use
Avoid concomitant use of Omeprazole with any of the following: Clopidogrel; Delavirdine; Erlotinib; Nelfinavir; Pimozide; Posaconazole; Rifampin; Rilpivirine; St Johns Wort

Increased Effect/Toxicity
Omeprazole may increase the levels/effects of: Amphetamines; ARIPiprazole; Benzodiazepines (metabolized by oxidation); Carvedilol; Cilostazol; Citalopram; CloZAPine; CycloSPORINE; CycloSPORINE (Systemic); CYP2C19 Substrates; CYP2C9 Substrates; Dexmethylphenidate; Escitalopram; Fosphenytoin; Methotrexate; Methylphenidate; Phenytoin; Pimozide; Raltegravir; Saquinavir; Tacrolimus; Tacrolimus (Systemic); Vitamin K Antagonists; Voriconazole

The levels/effects of Omeprazole may be increased by: Fluconazole; Ketoconazole; Ketoconazole (Systemic)

Decreased Effect
Omeprazole may decrease the levels/effects of: Atazanavir; Bisphosphonate Derivatives; Cefditoren; Clopidogrel; CloZAPine; Dabigatran Etexilate; Dasatinib; Delavirdine; Erlotinib; Gefitinib; Indinavir; Iron Salts; Itraconazole; Ketoconazole; Ketoconazole (Systemic); Mesalamine; Mycophenolate; Nelfinavir; Nilotinib; Posaconazole; Rilpivirine; Vismodegib

The levels/effects of Omeprazole may be decreased by: CYP2C19 Inducers (Strong); Peginterferon Alfa-2b; Rifampin; St Johns Wort; Tipranavir; Tocilizumab

Ethanol/Nutrition/Herb Interactions
Ethanol: Avoid ethanol (may cause gastric mucosal irritation).
Food: Food delays absorption.
Herb/Nutraceutical: Avoid use of St John's wort (may decrease efficacy of omeprazole).

Stability
Capsules, tablets: Store at 15°C to 30°C (59°F to 86°F). Protect from light and moisture.
Granules for oral suspension: Store at 25°C (77°F); excursions permitted to 15°C to 30°C (59°F to 86°F). For oral administration, empty the contents of the 2.5 mg packet into 5 mL of water (10 mg packet into 15 mL of water); stir. For NG administration, add 5 mL of water into a catheter-tipped syringe, and then add the contents of a 2.5 mg packet (15 mL water for the 10 mg packet); shake. **Note:** Regardless of the route of administration, the suspension should be left to thicken for 2-3 minutes prior to administration.

Mechanism of Action Proton pump inhibitor; suppresses gastric basal and stimulated acid secretion by inhibiting the parietal cell H+/K+ ATP pump

Pharmacodynamics/Kinetics

Onset of action: Antisecretory: ~1 hour

Peak effect: Within 2 hours

Duration: Up to 72 hours; 50% of maximum effect at 24 hours; after stopping treatment, secretory activity gradually returns over 3-5 days

Absorption: Rapid

Protein binding: ~95%

Metabolism: Hepatic via CYP2C19 primarily and (to a lesser extent) via 3A4 to hydroxy, desmethyl, and sulfone metabolites (all inactive); saturable first-pass effect

Bioavailability: Oral: ~30% to 40%; increased in Asian patients, elderly patients, and patients with hepatic dysfunction

Half-life elimination: 0.5-1 hour; hepatic impairment: ~3 hours

Time to peak, plasma: 0.5-3.5 hours

Excretion: Urine (~77% as metabolites, very small amount as unchanged drug); feces

Dosage

Geriatric & Adult

Active duodenal ulcer: Oral: 20 mg once daily for 4-8 weeks

Gastric ulcers: Oral: 40 mg once daily for 4-8 weeks

Symptomatic GERD (without esophageal lesions): Oral: 20 mg once daily for up to 4 weeks

Erosive esophagitis: Oral: 20 mg once daily for 4-8 weeks; maintenance of healing: 20 mg once daily for up to 12 months total therapy (including treatment period of 4-8 weeks)

Helicobacter pylori **eradication:** Oral: Dose varies with regimen:

Manufacturer's labeling: 40 mg once daily administered with clarithromycin 500 mg 3 times/day for 14 days **or** 20 mg twice daily administered with amoxicillin 1000 mg *and* clarithromycin 500 mg twice daily for 10 days. **Note:** Presence of ulcer at time of therapy initiation may necessitate an additional 14-18 days of omeprazole 20 mg/day (monotherapy) after completion of combination therapy.

American College of Gastroenterology guidelines (Chey, 2007):

Nonpenicillin allergy: 20 mg twice daily administered with amoxicillin 1000 mg *and* clarithromycin 500 mg twice daily for 10-14 days

Penicillin allergy: 20 mg twice daily administered with clarithromycin 500 mg *and* metronidazole 500 mg twice daily for 10-14 days **or** 20 mg once or twice daily administered with bismuth subsalicylate 525 mg *and* metronidazole 250 mg *plus* tetracycline 500 mg 4 times/day for 10-14 days

Pathological hypersecretory conditions: Oral: Initial: 60 mg once daily; doses up to 120 mg 3 times/day have been administered; administer daily doses >80 mg in divided doses

Stress-ulcer prophylaxis (ICU patients; unlabeled use): Oral: 40 mg once daily; periodically evaluate patient for continued need (Levy, 1997)

Frequent heartburn (OTC labeling): Oral: 20 mg once daily for 14 days; treatment may be repeated after 4 months if needed

Renal Impairment No adjustment is necessary.

Hepatic Impairment Bioavailability is increased with chronic liver disease. Consider dosage adjustment, especially for maintenance of erosive esophagitis. Specific guidelines are not available.

Administration

Oral: Best if administered before breakfast.

Capsule: Should be swallowed whole; do not chew or crush. Delayed release capsule may be opened and contents added to 1 tablespoon of applesauce (use immediately after adding to applesauce); mixture should not be chewed or warmed.

Oral suspension: Following reconstitution, the suspension should be left to thicken for 2-3 minutes and administered within 30 minutes. If any material remains after administration, add more water, stir, and administer immediately.

Tablet: Should be swallowed whole; do not crush or chew.

Nasogastric/orogastric (NG/OG) tube administration:

Capsule: When using capsules to extemporaneously prepare a solution for NG administration, the manufacturers of Prilosec® recommend the use of an acidic juice for preparation and administration. Alternative methods have been described as follows:

NG/OG tube administration for the prevention of stress-related mucosal damage in ventilated, critically-ill patients:

Study 1 (Phillips, 1996): Pour the contents of one or two 20 mg omeprazole delayed release capsules (depending on the dose) into a syringe (after removing plunger); withdraw 10-20 mL of an 8.4% sodium bicarbonate solution into the syringe; allow 30 minutes for the enteric-coated omeprazole granules to break down. Shake the resulting milky substance prior to administration. Flush the NG tube with 5-10 mL of water and clamp for at least 1 hour.

Study 2 (Balaban, 1997): Open the omeprazole delayed release capsule (20 mg or 40 mg), then pour the intact granules into a container holding 30 mL of water. Pour one-third to one-half of the granules into a 30 mL syringe (with the plunger removed) attached to a nasogastric tube (NG). Replace the plunger with 1 cm of air between the granules and the plunger top while the plunger is depressed. Repeat this process until all the granules are flushed, then flush a final 15 mL of water through the tube.

Oral suspension: Following reconstitution in a catheter-tipped syringe, shake the suspension well and leave to thicken for 2-3 minutes. Administer within 30 minutes of reconstitution. Use an NG tube or gastric tube that is a size 6 French or larger; flush the syringe and tube with water.

Monitoring Parameters Susceptibility testing is recommended in patients who fail *H. pylori* eradication regimen.

Test Interactions Omeprazole may falsely elevate serum chromogranin A (CgA) levels. The increased CgA level may cause false-positive results in the diagnosis of a neuroendocrine tumor. Temporarily stop omeprazole if assessing CgA level; repeat level if initially elevated; use the same laboratory for all testing of CgA levels.

Special Geriatric Considerations In clinical trials, the incidence of side effects in the elderly is no different than that of younger adults (≤65 years) despite slight decrease in elimination and increase in bioavailability. Bioavailability may be increased in the elderly (≥65 years of age), however, dosage adjustments are not necessary.

An increased risk of fractures of the hip, spine, or wrist has been observed in epidemiologic studies with proton pump inhibitor (PPI) use, primarily in older adults ≥50 years of age. The greatest risk was seen in patients receiving high doses or on long-term therapy (≥1 year). Calcium and vitamin D supplementation and close monitoring are recommended to reduce the risk of fracture in high-risk patients. Additionally, long-term use of proton pump inhibitors has resulted in reports of hypomagnesemia and *Clostridium difficile* infections.

Dosage Forms Excipient information presented when available (limited, particularly for generics); consult specific product labeling.

Capsule, delayed release, oral: 10 mg, 20 mg, 40 mg
  PriLOSEC®: 10 mg, 20 mg, 40 mg
Granules for suspension, delayed release, oral:
  PriLOSEC®: 2.5 mg/packet (30s); 10 mg/packet (30s)
Powder for suspension, oral [compounding kit]:
  First®-Omeprazole: 2 mg/mL (90 mL, 150 mL, 300 mL) [contains benzyl alcohol]
Tablet, delayed release, oral: 20 mg
  PriLOSEC OTC®: 20 mg

Omeprazole and Sodium Bicarbonate
(oh MEP ra zole & SOW dee um bye KAR bun ate)

Related Information
  Omeprazole *on page 1417*
  Sodium Bicarbonate *on page 1785*
Medication Safety Issues
  Sound-alike/look-alike issues:
    Zegerid® may be confused with Zestril®
Brand Names: U.S. Zegerid OTC™ [OTC]; Zegerid®
Index Terms Sodium Bicarbonate and Omeprazole
Generic Availability (U.S.) Yes: Capsule
Pharmacologic Category Proton Pump Inhibitor; Substituted Benzimidazole
Use Short-term (4-8 weeks) treatment of active duodenal ulcer or active benign gastric ulcer; treatment of heartburn and other symptoms associated with gastroesophageal reflux disease (GERD); short-term (4-8 weeks) treatment of endoscopically-diagnosed erosive esophagitis; maintenance healing of erosive esophagitis; reduction of risk of upper gastrointestinal bleeding in critically-ill patients

OTC labeling: Short-term (2 weeks) treatment of frequent (2 days/week), uncomplicated heartburn

Contraindications Hypersensitivity to omeprazole, sodium bicarbonate, or any component of the formulation
Warnings/Precautions See individual agents.

Adverse Reactions (Reflective of adult population; not specific for elderly)

Percentages of adverse events reported from a controlled clinical trial of 359 critically-ill patients receiving the oral powder for suspension

>10%:
Central nervous system: Pyrexia (20%)
Endocrine & metabolic: Hypokalemia (12%), hyperglycemia (11%)
Respiratory: Nosocomial pneumonia (11%)

1% to 10%:
Cardiovascular: Hypotension (10%), hypertension (8%), atrial fibrillation (6%), ventricular tachycardia (5%), bradycardia (4%), tachycardia (3%), supraventricular tachycardia (3%), edema (3%)
Central nervous system: Hyperpyrexia (5%), agitation (3%)
Dermatological: Rash (6%), decubitus ulcer (3%)
Endocrine & metabolic: Hypomagnesemia (10%), hypocalcemia (6%), hypophosphatemia (6%), fluid overload (5%), hypoglycemia (3%), hyponatremia (4%), hypernatremia (2%), hyperkalemia (2%)
Gastrointestinal: Constipation (5%), diarrhea (4%), hypomotility (2%)
Genitourinary: Urinary tract infection (2%)
Hematological: Thrombocytopenia (10%), anemia (8%), anemia increased (2%)
Hepatic: LFTs increased (2%)
Respiratory: ARDS (3%), respiratory failure (2%), pneumothorax (1%)
Miscellaneous: Sepsis (5%), oral candidiasis (4%), candidal infection (2%)

Drug Interactions

Metabolism/Transport Effects Refer to individual components.

Avoid Concomitant Use

Avoid concomitant use of Omeprazole and Sodium Bicarbonate with any of the following: Clopidogrel; Delavirdine; Erlotinib; Nelfinavir; Pimozide; Posaconazole; Rifampin; Rilpivirine; St Johns Wort

Increased Effect/Toxicity

Omeprazole and Sodium Bicarbonate may increase the levels/effects of: Alpha-/Beta-Agonists; Amphetamines; ARIPiprazole; Benzodiazepines (metabolized by oxidation); Calcium Polystyrene Sulfonate; Cilostazol; CloZAPine; CycloSPORINE; CycloSPORINE (Systemic); CYP2C19 Substrates; CYP2C9 Substrates; Dexmethylphenidate; Escitalopram; Flecainide; Fosphenytoin; Memantine; Methotrexate; Methylphenidate; Phenytoin; Pimozide; QuiNIDine; QuiNINE; Raltegravir; Saquinavir; Tacrolimus; Tacrolimus (Systemic); Vitamin K Antagonists; Voriconazole

The levels/effects of Omeprazole and Sodium Bicarbonate may be increased by: AcetaZOLAMIDE; Fluconazole; Ketoconazole; Ketoconazole (Systemic)

Decreased Effect

Omeprazole and Sodium Bicarbonate may decrease the levels/effects of: ACE Inhibitors; Anticonvulsants (Hydantoin); Antipsychotic Agents (Phenothiazines); Atazanavir; Bisacodyl; Bisphosphonate Derivatives; Cefditoren; Cefpodoxime; Cefuroxime; Chloroquine; Clopidogrel; CloZAPine; Corticosteroids (Oral); Dabigatran Etexilate; Dasatinib; Delavirdine; Erlotinib; Flecainide; Gabapentin; Gefitinib; HMG-CoA Reductase Inhibitors; Indinavir; Iron Salts; Isoniazid; Itraconazole; Ketoconazole; Ketoconazole (Systemic); Lithium; Mesalamine; Methenamine; Mycophenolate; Nelfinavir; Nilotinib; PenicillAMINE; Phosphate Supplements; Posaconazole; Protease Inhibitors; Rilpivirine; Tetracycline Derivatives; Trientine; Vismodegib

The levels/effects of Omeprazole and Sodium Bicarbonate may be decreased by: CYP2C19 Inducers (Strong); Peginterferon Alfa-2b; Rifampin; St Johns Wort; Tipranavir; Tocilizumab

Ethanol/Nutrition/Herb Interactions

Ethanol: Avoid ethanol (may cause gastric mucosal irritation).
Food: Food delays absorption. When given 1 hour after a meal, absorption is reduced.
Herb/Nutraceutical: St John's wort may decrease omeprazole levels.

Stability

Capsules, powder for oral suspension: Store at 25°C (77°F); excursions permitted to 15°C to 30°C (59°F to 86°F). Protect from light.
OTC capsules: Store at 20°C to 25°C (68°F to 77°F).

Mechanism of Action Suppresses gastric basal and stimulated acid secretion by inhibiting the parietal cell H+/K+ ATP pump

Pharmacodynamics/Kinetics

Onset of action: Antisecretory: ~1 hour; Peak antisecretory effect: 2 hours; Full therapeutic effect: 1-4 days
Duration: 72 hours
Absorption: Rapid
Protein binding: ~95%

Metabolism: Extensively hepatic to inactive metabolites

Bioavailability: Oral: ~30% to 40%; increased in Asian patients and patients with hepatic dysfunction

Half-life elimination: ~1 hour (range: 0.4-3.2 hours)

Time to peak, serum: ~30 minutes

Excretion: Urine (77% as metabolites, very small amount as unchanged drug); feces

Dosage

Geriatric & Adult Note: Both strengths of Zegerid® capsule and powder for oral suspension have identical sodium bicarbonate content, respectively. Do not substitute two 20 mg capsules/packets for one 40 mg dose.

Active duodenal ulcer: Oral: 20 mg/day for 4-8 weeks

Gastric ulcers: Oral: 40 mg/day for 4-8 weeks

Heartburn (OTC labeling): Oral: 20 mg once daily for 14 days. Do not take for >14 days or more often than every 4 months, unless instructed by healthcare provider.

Symptomatic GERD: Oral: 20 mg/day for up to 4 weeks

Erosive esophagitis: Oral: 20 mg/day for 4-8 weeks; maintenance of healing: 20 mg/day for up to 12 months total therapy (including treatment period of 4-8 weeks)

Risk reduction of upper GI bleeding in critically-ill patients (Zegerid® powder for oral suspension): Oral:

Loading dose: Day 1: 40 mg every 6-8 hours for two doses

Maintenance dose: 40 mg/day for up to 14 days; therapy >14 days has not been evaluated

Renal Impairment No adjustment is necessary.

Hepatic Impairment Bioavailability is increased with chronic liver disease. Consider dosage adjustment, especially for maintenance of healing of erosive esophagitis. Specific guidelines are not available.

Administration Note: Both strengths of Zegerid® capsule and powder for oral suspension have identical sodium bicarbonate content, respectively. Do not substitute two 20 mg capsules/packets for one 40 mg dose.

Capsule: Should be swallowed whole with water (do not use other liquids); do not chew or crush. Capsules should **not** be opened, sprinkled on food, or administered via NG. Best if taken at least 1 hour before breakfast.

Powder for oral suspension:

Oral: Administer 1 hour before a meal. Mix with 15-30 mL of water; stir well and drink immediately. Rinse cup with water and drink. Do not use other liquids or sprinkle on food.

Nasogastric/orogastric tube: Mix well with 20 mL of water (do not use other liquids) and administer immediately; flush tube with an additional 20 mL of water. Suspend enteral feeding for 3 hours before and 1 hour after administering.

Special Geriatric Considerations The incidence of side effects in the elderly is no different than that of younger adults (≤65 years of age) despite slight decrease in elimination and increase in bioavailability. Dosage adjustments are not necessary. Use cautiously in patients requiring sodium restriction, hypertension, or congestive heart failure.

An increased risk of fractures of the hip, spine, or wrist has been observed in epidemiologic studies with proton pump inhibitor (PPI) use, primarily in older adults ≥50 years of age. The greatest risk was seen in patients receiving high doses or on long-term therapy (≥1 year). Calcium and vitamin D supplementation and close monitoring are recommended to reduce the risk of fracture in high-risk patients. Additionally, long-term use of proton pump inhibitors has resulted in reports of hypomagnesemia and *Clostridium difficile* infections.

Dosage Forms Excipient information presented when available (limited, particularly for generics); consult specific product labeling.

Capsule, oral: Omeprazole 20 mg [immediate release] and sodium bicarbonate 1100 mg; omeprazole 40 mg [immediate release] and sodium bicarbonate 1100 mg

Zegerid®: Omeprazole 20 mg [immediate release] and sodium bicarbonate 1100 mg [contains sodium 304 mg (13 mEq) per capsule]

Zegerid®: Omeprazole 40 mg [immediate release] and sodium bicarbonate 1100 mg [contains sodium 304 mg (13 mEq) per capsule]

Zegerid OTC™: Omeprazole 20 mg [immediate release] and sodium bicarbonate 1100 mg [contains sodium 303 mg (13 mEq) per capsule]

Powder for suspension, oral:

Zegerid®: Omeprazole 20 mg and sodium bicarbonate 1680 mg per packet (30s) [contains sodium 460 mg (20 mEq) per packet]

Zegerid®: Omeprazole 40 mg and sodium bicarbonate 1680 mg per packet (30s) [contains sodium 460 mg (20 mEq) per packet]

◆ **Omeprazole Magnesium** see Omeprazole on page 1417

◆ **Omnaris®** see Ciclesonide (Nasal) on page 373

◆ **Omnicef® [DSC]** see Cefdinir on page 311

◆ **Omni Gel™ [OTC]** see Fluoride on page 806

♦ **Omnipred™** *see* PrednisoLONE (Ophthalmic) *on page 1594*
♦ **Omontys®** *see* Peginesatide *on page 1483*

OnabotulinumtoxinA (oh nuh BOT yoo lin num TOKS in aye)

Medication Safety Issues
Other safety concerns:
Botulinum products are not interchangeable; potency differences may exist between the products.
Brand Names: U.S. Botox®; Botox® Cosmetic
Brand Names: Canada Botox®; Botox® Cosmetic
Index Terms Botulinum Toxin Type A; BTX-A
Generic Availability (U.S.) No
Pharmacologic Category Neuromuscular Blocker Agent, Toxin; Ophthalmic Agent, Toxin
Use Treatment of strabismus and blepharospasm associated with dystonia (including benign essential blepharospasm or VII nerve disorders) in patients ≥12 years of age; treatment of cervical dystonia (spasmodic torticollis) in patients ≥16 years of age; temporary improvement in the appearance of lines/wrinkles of the face (moderate-to-severe glabellar lines associated with corrugator and/or procerus muscle activity) in adult patients ≤65 years of age; treatment of severe primary axillary hyperhidrosis in adults not adequately controlled with topical treatments; treatment of focal spasticity (specifically upper limb spasticity) in adults; prophylaxis of chronic migraine headache (≥15 days/month with ≥4 hours/day headache duration) in adults

Canadian labeling: Additional use (not in U.S. labeling): Treatment of forehead, lateral canthus, and glabellar lines in adults >65 years of age
Unlabeled Use Treatment of oromandibular dystonia, spasmodic dysphonia (laryngeal dystonia) and other dystonias (ie, writer's cramp, focal task-specific dystonias)
Medication Guide Available Yes
Dosage
Geriatric Initiate therapy at lowest recommended dose. Refer to adult dosing.
Adult Note: In adults treated for more than one indication, the maximum cumulative dose should be ≤360 units/3 months. Canadian labeling recommends a maximum cumulative dose of 6 units/kg (up to 360 units) over 3 months in adult patients receiving additional treatment for noncosmetic indications.

Blepharospasm: I.M.:
Botox®: Initial dose: 1.25-2.5 units injected into the medial and lateral pretarsal orbicularis oculi of the upper lid and lateral pretarsal orbicularis oculi of lower lid
Dose may be increased up to twice the previous dose if the response from the initial dose lasted ≤2 months; maximum dose per site: 5 units. Tolerance may occur if treatments are given more often than every 3 months, but the effect is not usually permanent. Cumulative dose:
U.S. labeling: ≤200 units in 30-day period
Canadian labeling (not in U.S. labeling): Botox®: ≤200 units in 2-month period
Cervical dystonia: I.M.: For dosing guidance, the mean dose is 236 units (25th to 75th percentile range 198-300 units) divided among the affected muscles in patients previously treated with botulinum toxin (maximum: ≤50 units/site). Initial dose in previously untreated patients should be lower. Sequential dosing should be based on the patient's head and neck position, localization of pain, muscle hypertrophy, patient response, and previous adverse reactions. The total dose injected into the sternocleidomastoid muscles should be ≤100 units to decrease the occurrence of dysphagia.
Canadian labeling (not in U.S. labeling): I.M.: Botox®: Effective range of 200-360 units has been used in clinical practice; administer no more frequently than every 2 months
Chronic migraine: I.M.: Administer 5 units/0.1 mL per site. Recommended total dose is 155 units once every 12 weeks. Each 155 unit dose should be equally divided and administered bilaterally, into 31 total sites as described below (refer to prescribing information for specific diagrams of recommended injection sites):
Corrugator: 5 units to each side (2 sites)
Procerus: 5 units (1 site only)
Frontalis: 10 units to each side (divided into 2 sites/side)
Temporalis: 20 units to each side (divided into 4 sites/side)
Occipitalis: 15 units to each side (divided into 3 sites/side)
Cervical paraspinal: 10 units to each side (divided into 2 sites/side)
Trapezius: 15 units to each side (divided into 3 sites/side)

Detrusor overactivity associated with neurologic condition: Intradetrusor: 30 injections of ~6.7 units/mL for a total dose of 200 units/30 mL; may consider retreatment with diminishing effect but no sooner than 12 weeks from previous administration.

Spasticity (focal): I.M.: Individualize dose based on patient size, extent, and location of muscle involvement, degree of spasticity, local muscle weakness, and response to prior treatment. In clinical trials, total doses up to 360 units (Botox®) were administered as separate injections typically divided among selected muscles; may repeat therapy at ≥3 months with appropriate dosage based upon the clinical condition of patient at time of retreatment.

Suggested guidelines for the treatment of upper limb spasticity. The lowest recommended starting dose should be used and ≤50 units/site should be administered. **Note:** Dose listed is total dose administered as individual or separate intramuscular injection(s):

Biceps brachii: 100-200 units (divided into 4 sites)
Flexor digitorum profundus: 30-50 units (1 site)
Flexor digitorum sublimes: 30-50 units (1 site)
Flexor carpi radialis: 12.5-50 units (1 site)
Flexor carpi ulnaris: 12.5-50 units (1 site)

Suggested guidelines for the treatment of stroke-related upper limb spasticity: *Canadian labeling:* **Note:** Dose listed is total dose administered as individual or separate intramuscular injection(s):

Biceps brachii: 100-200 units (up to 4 sites)
Flexor digitorum profundus: 15-50 units (1-2 sites)
Flexor digitorum sublimes: 15-50 units (1-2 sites)
Flexor carpi radialis: 15-60 units (1-2 sites)
Flexor carpi ulnaris: 10-50 units (1-2 sites)
Adductor pollicis: 20 units (1-2 sites)
Flexor pollicis longus: 20 units (1-2 sites)

Strabismus: I.M.: **Note:** Several minutes prior to injection, administration of local anesthetic and ocular decongestant drops are recommended.

Initial dose:

Vertical muscles and for horizontal strabismus <20 prism diopters: 1.25-2.5 units in any one muscle

Horizontal strabismus of 20-50 prism diopters: 2.5-5 units in any one muscle

Persistent VI nerve palsy ≥1 month: 1.25-2.5 units in the medial rectus muscle

Re-examine patients 7-14 days after each injection to assess the effect of that dose. Subsequent doses for patients experiencing incomplete paralysis of the target may be increased up to twice the previous administered dose. The maximum recommended dose as a single injection for any one muscle is 25 units. Do not administer subsequent injections until the effects of the previous dose are gone.

Primary axillary hyperhidrosis: Intradermal: 50 units/axilla. Injection area should be defined by standard staining techniques. Injections should be evenly distributed into multiple sites (10-15), administered in 0.1-0.2 mL aliquots, ~1-2 cm apart. May repeat when clinical effect diminishes.

Cosmetic uses:

Reduction of glabellar lines: Adults ≤65 years: I.M.: An effective dose is determined by gross observation of the patient's ability to activate the superficial muscles injected. The location, size, and use of muscles may vary markedly among individuals. Inject 0.1 mL (4 units) dose into each of five sites, two in each corrugator muscle and one in the procerus muscle for a total dose 0.5 mL (20 units) administered no more frequently than every 3-4 months. **Note:** Treatment of adults >65 years is approved in the Canadian labeling.

Reduction of forehead lines *(Canadian labeling; not in U.S. labeling):* I.M.: Inject 2-6 units into each of four sites in the frontalis muscle every 1-2 cm along either side of forehead crease and 2-3 cm above eyebrows for total dose of 24 units.

Reduction of lateral canthus lines; *(Canadian labeling; not in U.S. labeling):* I.M.: Inject 2-6 units into each of 1-3 injection sites, lateral to the lateral orbital rim.

Special Geriatric Considerations No specific dosing adjustment recommended.

Dosage Forms Excipient information presented when available (limited, particularly for generics); consult specific product labeling.

Injection, powder for reconstitution [preservative free]:

Botox®: *Clostridium botulinum* type A neurotoxin complex 100 units, *Clostridium botulinum* type A neurotoxin complex 200 units [contains albumin (human)]

Botox® Cosmetic: *Clostridium botulinum* type A neurotoxin complex 100 units, *Clostridium botulinum* type A neurotoxin complex 50 units [contains albumin (human)]

Dosage Forms: Canada Excipient information presented when available (limited, particularly for generics); consult specific product labeling.

Injection, powder for reconstitution [preservative free]:

Botox®: Botulinum toxin A 50 units [contains albumin (human)], 100 units [contains albumin (human)], 200 units [contains albumin (human)]

Botox Cosmetic®: Botulinum toxin A 50 units [contains albumin (human)], 100 units [contains albumin (human)], 200 units [contains albumin (human)]

Ondansetron (on DAN se tron)

Medication Safety Issues
Sound-alike/look-alike issues:

Ondansetron may be confused with dolasetron, granisetron, palonosetron

Zofran® may be confused with Zantac®, Zosyn®

Brand Names: U.S. Zofran®; Zofran® ODT; Zuplenz®

Brand Names: Canada Apo-Ondansetron®; CO Ondansetron; Dom-Ondansetron; JAMP-Ondansetron; Mint-Ondansetron; Mylan-Ondansetron; Ondansetron Injection; Ondansetron Injection USP; Ondansetron-Odan; Ondansetron-Omega; PHL-Ondansetron; PMS-Ondansetron; RAN™-Ondansetron; ratio-Ondansetron; Sandoz-Ondansetron; Teva-Ondansetron; Zofran®; Zofran® ODT; ZYM-Ondansetron

Index Terms GR38032R; Ondansetron Hydrochloride; Zuplenz®

Generic Availability (U.S.) Yes: Excludes oral soluble film

Pharmacologic Category Antiemetic; Selective 5-HT$_3$ Receptor Antagonist

Use

I.V.: Prevention of nausea and vomiting associated with initial and repeat courses of emetogenic cancer chemotherapy (including high-dose cisplatin); prevention of postoperative nausea and/or vomiting (PONV); treatment of PONV if no prophylactic dose of ondansetron received

Oral: Prevention of nausea and vomiting associated with highly emetogenic cancer chemotherapy (including high-dose cisplatin); prevention of nausea and vomiting associated with initial and repeat courses of moderately emetogenic cancer chemotherapy; prevention of nausea and vomiting associated with radiotherapy (either total body irradiation, single high-dose fraction to the abdomen, or daily fractions to the abdomen); prevention of PONV

Unlabeled Use Hyperemesis gravidarum (severe or refractory); breakthrough treatment of nausea and vomiting associated with chemotherapy

Contraindications Hypersensitivity to ondansetron or any component of the formulation; concomitant use of apomorphine

Warnings/Precautions Ondansetron should be used on a scheduled basis, not on an "as needed" (PRN) basis, since data support the use of this drug only in the prevention of nausea and vomiting (due to antineoplastic therapy) and not in the rescue of nausea and vomiting. Ondansetron should only be used in the first 24-48 hours of chemotherapy. Data do not support any increased efficacy of ondansetron in delayed nausea and vomiting. Does not stimulate gastric or intestinal peristalsis; may mask progressive ileus and/or gastric distension. Use with caution in patients allergic to other 5-HT$_3$ receptor antagonists; cross-reactivity has been reported.

Dose-dependent QT interval prolongation occurs with ondansetron use. Cases of torsade de pointes have also been reported to the manufacturer. Selective 5-HT$_3$ antagonists, including ondansetron, have been associated with a number of dose-dependent increases in ECG intervals (eg, PR, QRS duration, QT/QT$_c$, JT), usually occurring 1-2 hours after I.V. administration. Single doses >16 mg ondansetron I.V. are no longer recommended due to the potential for an increased risk of QT prolongation. In most patients, these changes are not clinically relevant; however, when used in conjunction with other agents that prolong these intervals or in those at risk for QT prolongation, arrhythmia may occur. When used with agents that prolong the QT interval (eg, Class I and III antiarrhythmics) or in patients with cardiovascular disease, clinically relevant QT interval prolongation may occur resulting in torsade de pointes. Avoid ondansetron use in patients with congenital long QT syndrome. Use caution and monitor ECG in patients with other risk factors for QT prolongation (eg, medications known to prolong QT interval, electrolyte abnormalities [hypokalemia or hypomagnesemia], heart failure, bradyarrhythmias, and cumulative high-dose anthracycline therapy). I.V. formulations of 5-HT$_3$ antagonists have more association with ECG interval changes, compared to oral formulations. Dose limitations are recommended for patients with severe hepatic impairment (Child-Pugh class C); use with caution in mild-moderate hepatic impairment; clearance is decreased and half-life increased in hepatic impairment.

Orally-disintegrating tablets contain phenylalanine.

Adverse Reactions (Reflective of adult population; not specific for elderly) Note: Percentages reported in adult patients.

>10%:
  Central nervous system: Headache (9% to 27%), malaise/fatigue (9% to 13%)
  Gastrointestinal: Constipation (6% to 11%)

1% to 10%:
  Central nervous system: Drowsiness (8%), fever (2% to 8%), dizziness (7%), anxiety (6%), cold sensation (2%)
  Dermatologic: Pruritus (2% to 5%), rash (1%)
  Gastrointestinal: Diarrhea (2% to 7%)
  Genitourinary: Gynecological disorder (7%), urinary retention (5%)
  Hepatic: ALT increased (>2 times ULN: 1% to 5%), AST increased (>2 times ULN: 1% to 5%)
  Local: Injection site reaction (4%; pain, redness, burning)
  Neuromuscular & skeletal: Paresthesia (2%)
  Respiratory: Hypoxia (9%)

Drug Interactions

  Metabolism/Transport Effects Substrate of CYP1A2 (minor), CYP2C9 (minor), CYP2D6 (minor), CYP2E1 (minor), CYP3A4 (major), P-glycoprotein; **Note:** Assignment of Major/Minor substrate status based on clinically relevant drug interaction potential; **Inhibits** CYP1A2 (weak), CYP2C9 (weak), CYP2D6 (weak)

  Avoid Concomitant Use
  Avoid concomitant use of Ondansetron with any of the following: Apomorphine; Highest Risk QTc-Prolonging Agents; Mifepristone

  Increased Effect/Toxicity
  Ondansetron may increase the levels/effects of: Apomorphine; ARIPiprazole; Highest Risk QTc-Prolonging Agents; Moderate Risk QTc-Prolonging Agents

  The levels/effects of Ondansetron may be increased by: Mifepristone; P-glycoprotein/ABCB1 Inhibitors; QTc-Prolonging Agents (Indeterminate Risk and Risk Modifying)

  Decreased Effect
  Ondansetron may decrease the levels/effects of: Tapentadol; TraMADol

  The levels/effects of Ondansetron may be decreased by: CYP3A4 Inducers (Strong); Deferasirox; Herbs (CYP3A4 Inducers); Peginterferon Alfa-2b; P-glycoprotein/ABCB1 Inducers; Rifamycin Derivatives; Tocilizumab

Ethanol/Nutrition/Herb Interactions
  Food: Tablet: Food slightly increases the extent of absorption.
  Herb/Nutraceutical: St John's wort may decrease ondansetron levels.

Stability
  Oral soluble film: Store between 20°C and 25°C (68°F and 77°F). Store pouches in cartons; keep film in individual pouch until ready to use.
  Oral solution: Store between 15°C and 30°C (59°F and 86°F). Protect from light.
  Tablet: Store between 2°C and 30°C (36°F and 86°F).
  Vial: Store between 2°C and 30°C (36°F and 86°F). Protect from light. Prior to I.V. infusion, dilute in 50 mL D_5W or NS. Solution is stable for 48 hours at room temperature.

Mechanism of Action Selective 5-HT$_3$-receptor antagonist, blocking serotonin, both peripherally on vagal nerve terminals and centrally in the chemoreceptor trigger zone

Pharmacodynamics/Kinetics
  Onset of action: ~30 minutes
  Absorption: Oral: Well absorbed from GI tract
  Distribution: V_d: Adults: 2.2-2.5 L/kg
  Protein binding, plasma: 70% to 76%
  Metabolism: Extensively hepatic via hydroxylation, followed by glucuronide or sulfate conjugation; CYP1A2, CYP2D6, and CYP3A4 substrate; some demethylation occurs
  Bioavailability: Oral: 56% to 71% (some first pass metabolism); Rectal: 58% to 74%
  Half-life elimination: Adults: 3-6 hours
    Mild-to-moderate hepatic impairment (Child-Pugh classes A and B): Adults: 12 hours
    Severe hepatic impairment (Child-Pugh class C): Adults: 20 hours
  Time to peak: Oral: ~2 hours; Oral soluble film: ~1 hour
  Excretion: Urine (44% to 60% as metabolites, ~5% as unchanged drug); feces (~25%)

Dosage
  Geriatric & Adult
    Prevention of nausea and vomiting associated with emetogenic chemotherapy:
      Manufacturer's labeling:
        I.V.: 0.15 mg/kg/dose (maximum: 16 mg/dose) over 15 minutes for 3 doses, beginning 30 minutes prior to chemotherapy, followed by subsequent doses 4 and 8 hours after the first dose

Highly-emetogenic agents/single-day therapy: Oral: 24 mg given as three 8 mg tablets 30 minutes prior to the start of therapy

Moderately-emetogenic agents: Oral: 8 mg beginning 30 minutes before chemotherapy; repeat dose 8 hours after initial dose, then 8 mg every 12 hours for 1-2 days after chemotherapy completed

Alternate recommendations (unlabeled dose): American Society of Clinical Oncology Antiemetic Guidelines (Basch, 2011): High emetic risk: Day(s) of chemotherapy:

I.V.: 8 mg or 0.15 mg/kg. **Note:** Single I.V. doses >16 mg are no longer recommended by the manufacturer due to the potential for QT prolongation.

Oral: 8 mg twice daily

Prevention of nausea and vomiting associated with radiation therapy:

Manufacturer's labeling:

Total body irradiation: Oral: 8 mg 1-2 hours before each daily fraction of radiotherapy

Single high-dose fraction radiotherapy to abdomen: Oral: 8 mg 1-2 hours before irradiation, then 8 mg every 8 hours after first dose for 1-2 days after completion of radiotherapy

Daily fractionated radiotherapy to abdomen: Oral: 8 mg 1-2 hours before irradiation, then 8 mg every 8 hours after first dose for each day of radiotherapy

Alternate recommendations: American Society of Clinical Oncology Antiemetic Guidelines (Basch, 2011): Give before each fraction throughout radiation therapy (for high emetic risk, continue for at least 24 hours after completion; for low emetic risk, may give either as prevention or rescue; for minimal emetic risk, give as rescue; if rescue used for either low or minimal emetic risk, then prophylaxis should be given until the end of radiation therapy):

I.V. (unlabeled route): 8 mg or 0.15 mg/kg. **Note:** Single I.V. doses >16 mg are no longer recommended by the manufacturer due to the potential for QT prolongation.

Oral (unlabeled regimen): 8 mg twice daily

Postoperative nausea and vomiting (PONV):

Oral: 16 mg given 1 hour prior to induction of anesthesia

I.M., I.V.: 4 mg as a single dose (over 2-5 minutes if giving I.V.) administered ~30 minutes before the end of anesthesia (see Note) or as treatment if vomiting occurs after surgery (Gan, 2007).

Note: The manufacturer recommends administration immediately before induction of anesthesia; however, this has been shown not to be as effective as administration at the end of surgery (Sun, 1997). Repeat doses given in response to inadequate control of nausea/vomiting from preoperative doses are generally ineffective.

Treatment of severe or refractory hyperemesis gravidum (unlabeled use):

Oral: 8 mg every 12 hours (Levichek, 2002)

I.V.: 8 mg administered over 15 minutes every 12 hours (ACOG, 2004)

Renal Impairment No dosage adjustment necessary (there is no experience for oral ondansetron beyond day 1)

Hepatic Impairment Severe impairment (Child-Pugh C):

I.V.: Day 1: Maximum dose: 8 mg (there is no experience beyond day 1)

Oral: Maximum daily dose: 8 mg

Administration

Oral: Oral dosage forms should be administered 30 minutes prior to chemotherapy; 1-2 hours before radiotherapy; 1 hour prior to the induction of anesthesia.

Orally-disintegrating tablets: Do not remove from blister until needed. Peel backing off the blister, do not push tablet through. Using dry hands, place tablet on tongue and allow to dissolve. Swallow with saliva.

Oral soluble film: Do not remove from pouch until immediately before use. Using dry hands, place film on top of tongue and allow to dissolve (4-20 seconds). Swallow with or without liquid. If using more than one film, each film should be allowed to dissolve completely before administering the next film.

I.M.: Should be administered undiluted.

I.V.:

IVPB: Dilute in 50 mL D_5W or NS. Infuse over 15-30 minutes; 24-hour continuous infusions have been reported, but are rarely used.

Chemotherapy-induced nausea and vomiting: Give first dose 30 minutes prior to beginning chemotherapy.

I.V. push: Prevention of postoperative nausea and vomiting: Single doses may be administered I.V. injection over 2-5 minutes as undiluted solution.

Monitoring Parameters Emetic episodes, diarrhea, headache

Special Geriatric Considerations Elderly have a slightly decreased hepatic clearance rate. This does not, however, require a dose adjustment.

Dosage Forms Excipient information presented when available (limited, particularly for generics); consult specific product labeling. [DSC] = Discontinued product

Film, soluble, oral:
  Zuplenz®: 4 mg (10s); 8 mg (10s) [peppermint flavor]
Infusion, premixed in D₅W [preservative free]: 32 mg (50 mL)
  Zofran®: 32 mg (50 mL [DSC])
Infusion, premixed in NS [preservative free]: 32 mg (50 mL)
Injection, solution: 2 mg/mL (2 mL, 20 mL)
  Zofran®: 2 mg/mL (20 mL)
Injection, solution [preservative free]: 2 mg/mL (2 mL)
Solution, oral: 4 mg/5 mL (5 mL, 50 mL)
  Zofran®: 4 mg/5 mL (50 mL) [contains sodium benzoate; strawberry flavor]
Tablet, oral: 4 mg, 8 mg
  Zofran®: 4 mg, 8 mg
Tablet, orally disintegrating, oral: 4 mg, 8 mg
  Zofran® ODT: 4 mg, 8 mg [contains phenylalanine <0.03 mg/tablet; strawberry flavor]

Extemporaneously Prepared A 0.8 mg/mL syrup may be made by crushing ten 8 mg tablets; flaking of the tablet coating occurs. Mix thoroughly with 50 mL of the suspending vehicle, Ora-Plus® (Paddock), in 5 mL increments. Add sufficient volume of any of the following syrups: Cherry syrup USP, Syrpalta® (Humco), Ora-Sweet® (Paddock), or Ora-Sweet® Sugar-Free (Paddock) to make a final volume of 100 mL. Stability is 42 days refrigerated.

Trissel LA, "Trissel's Stability of Compounded Formulations," American Pharmaceutical Association, 1996

Rectal suppositories: Calibrate a suppository mold for the base being used. Determine the displacement factor (DF) for ondansetron for the base being used (Fattibase® = 1.1; Polybase® = 0.6). Weigh the ondansetron tablet. Divide the tablet weight by the DF. Subtract the weight of base displaced from the calculated weight of base required for each suppository. Grind the ondansetron tablets to a fine powder in a mortar. Weigh out the appropriate weight of suppository base. Melt the base over a water bath (<55°C). Add the ondansetron powder to the suppository base and mix well. Pour the mixture into the suppository mold and cool. Stable for at least 30 days under refrigeration.

Allen LV, "Ondansetron Suppositories," US Pharm, 20(7):84-6.

Orlistat (OR li stat)

Medication Safety Issues
Sound-alike/look-alike issues:
Xenical® may be confused with Xeloda®
Brand Names: U.S. Alli® [OTC]; Xenical®
Brand Names: Canada Xenical®
Generic Availability (U.S.) No
Pharmacologic Category Lipase Inhibitor
Use Management of obesity, including weight loss and weight management, when used in conjunction with a reduced-calorie and low-fat diet; reduce the risk of weight regain after prior weight loss; indicated for obese patients with an initial body mass index (BMI) ≥30 kg/m^2 or ≥27 kg/m^2 in the presence of other risk factors (eg, diabetes, dyslipidemia, hypertension)
Dosage
Geriatric & Adult Obesity: Oral:
Xenical®: 120 mg 3 times/day with each main meal containing fat (during or up to 1 hour after the meal); omit dose if meal is occasionally missed or contains no fat.
Alli™: OTC labeling: 60 mg 3 times/day with each main meal containing fat
Special Geriatric Considerations There is no specific geriatric information since there were not enough elderly subjects in clinical trials.
Dosage Forms Excipient information presented when available (limited, particularly for generics); consult specific product labeling.
Capsule, oral:
Alli®: 60 mg
Xenical®: 120 mg

Orphenadrine (or FEN a dreen)

Related Information
Beers Criteria – Potentially Inappropriate Medications for Geriatrics *on page 2183*
Medication Safety Issues
Sound-alike/look-alike issues:
Norflex™ may be confused with norfloxacin, Noroxin®
BEERS Criteria medication:
This drug may be potentially inappropriate for use in geriatric patients (Quality of evidence - moderate; Strength of recommendation - strong).
International issues:
Flexin: Brand name for orphenadrine [Israel] but is also the brand name for cyclobenzaprine [Chile] and diclofenac [Argentina]
Flexin [Israel] may be confused with Floxin which is a brand name for flunarizine [Thailand], norfloxacin [South Africa], ofloxacin [U.S., Canada], and perfloxacin [Philippines]
Brand Names: U.S. Norflex™
Brand Names: Canada Norflex™; Orphenace®; Rhoxal-orphendrine
Index Terms Orphenadrine Citrate
Generic Availability (U.S.) Yes
Pharmacologic Category Skeletal Muscle Relaxant
Use Treatment of muscle spasm associated with acute painful musculoskeletal conditions
Contraindications Hypersensitivity to orphenadrine or any component of the formulation; glaucoma; GI obstruction, stenosing peptic ulcer; prostatic hypertrophy, bladder neck obstruction; cardiospasm; myasthenia gravis
Warnings/Precautions Use with caution in patients with HF, cardiac decompensation, coronary insufficiency, tachycardia or cardiac arrhythmias. May cause CNS depression, which may impair physical or mental abilities. Muscle relaxants are poorly tolerated by the elderly due to potent anticholinergic effects, sedation, and risk of fracture. Efficacy is questionable at dosages tolerated by elderly patients; avoid use (Beers Criteria). Potential for abuse; use with caution in patients with history of drug abuse. Solution for injection contains sodium bisulfite which may cause allergic reaction in some individuals. Has not been evaluated for continuous long-term use; monitor closely.
Adverse Reactions (Reflective of adult population; not specific for elderly) Frequency not defined.
Cardiovascular: Palpitation, tachycardia
Central nervous system: Agitation, dizziness, drowsiness, euphoria, hallucination, headache, mental confusion
Dermatologic: Pruritus, urticaria
Gastrointestinal: Constipation, gastric irritation, nausea, vomiting, xerostomia

Genitourinary: Urination hesitancy, urinary retention

Hematologic: Aplastic anemia (rare)

Neuromuscular & skeletal: Tremor, weakness

Ocular: Blurred vision, intraocular pressure increased, nystagmus, pupil dilation

Respiratory: Nasal congestion

Miscellaneous: Anaphylactic reaction (injection, rare), hypersensitivity

Drug Interactions

Metabolism/Transport Effects Substrate of CYP1A2 (minor), CYP2B6 (minor), CYP2D6 (minor), CYP3A4 (minor); **Note:** Assignment of Major/Minor substrate status based on clinically relevant drug interaction potential; **Inhibits** CYP1A2 (weak), CYP2A6 (weak), CYP2B6 (weak), CYP2C19 (weak), CYP2C9 (weak), CYP2D6 (weak), CYP2E1 (weak), CYP3A4 (weak)

Avoid Concomitant Use

Avoid concomitant use of Orphenadrine with any of the following: Azelastine; Azelastine (Nasal); Methadone; Mirtazapine; Paraldehyde; Pimozide

Increased Effect/Toxicity

Orphenadrine may increase the levels/effects of: AbobotulinumtoxinA; Alcohol (Ethyl); Anticholinergics; ARIPiprazole; Azelastine; Azelastine (Nasal); Buprenorphine; Cannabinoids; CNS Depressants; Methadone; Methotrimeprazine; Metyrosine; Mirtazapine; OnabotulinumtoxinA; Paraldehyde; Pimozide; Potassium Chloride; RimabotulinumtoxinB; Selective Serotonin Reuptake Inhibitors; Zolpidem

The levels/effects of Orphenadrine may be increased by: Droperidol; HydrOXYzine; Methotrimeprazine; Pramlintide

Decreased Effect

Orphenadrine may decrease the levels/effects of: Acetylcholinesterase Inhibitors (Central); Secretin

The levels/effects of Orphenadrine may be decreased by: Acetylcholinesterase Inhibitors (Central); Peginterferon Alfa-2b; Tocilizumab

Ethanol/Nutrition/Herb Interactions

Ethanol: Avoid ethanol (may increase CNS depression).

Herb/Nutraceutical: Avoid valerian, St John's wort, kava kava, gotu kola (may increase CNS depression).

Stability Store at controlled room temperature. Protect injection solution from light.

Mechanism of Action Indirect skeletal muscle relaxant thought to work by central atropine-like effects; has some euphorigenic and analgesic properties

Pharmacodynamics/Kinetics

Onset of effect: Peak effect: Oral: 2-4 hours

Duration: 4-6 hours

Protein binding: 20%

Metabolism: Extensively hepatic

Half-life elimination: 14-16 hours

Excretion: Primarily urine (8% as unchanged drug)

Dosage

Geriatric Use caution; generally not recommended for use in the elderly.

Adult Muscle spasms:

Oral: 100 mg twice daily

I.M., I.V.: 60 mg every 12 hours

Administration Do not crush sustained release drug product.

Special Geriatric Considerations Because of its anticholinergic side effects (eg, constipation, urinary retention, confusion), orphenadrine is not a drug of choice in the elderly.

This medication is considered to be potentially inappropriate in this patient population (Beers Criteria: Quality of evidence - moderate; Strength of recommendation - strong).

Dosage Forms Excipient information presented when available (limited, particularly for generics); consult specific product labeling.

Injection, solution, as citrate: 30 mg/mL (2 mL)

Norflex™: 30 mg/mL (2 mL) [contains sodium bisulfite]

Injection, solution, as citrate [preservative free]: 30 mg/mL (2 mL)

Tablet, extended release, oral, as citrate: 100 mg

Oseltamivir (oh sel TAM i vir)

Related Information
Community-Acquired Pneumonia in Adults *on page 2171*
Medication Safety Issues
Sound-alike/look-alike issues:
Tamiflu® may be confused with Tambocor™, Thera-Flu®
Other safety concerns:
Oseltamivir (Tamiflu®) oral suspension is packaged with an oral syringe. When dispensing commercially prepared oseltamivir oral suspension, verify the intended concentration to be dispensed and the correct dose, dosing instructions, and oral dosing device provided for the patient. Oseltamivir oral suspension is available in a 6 mg/mL concentration. The previous concentration (12 mg/mL) has been discontinued, but may be still be on the market until product expires. The 6 mg/mL concentration is packaged with an oral syringe calibrated in **milliliters** up to a total of 10 mL. The previous, discontinued concentration (12 mg/mL) was packaged with an oral syringe calibrated in mg (30 mg, 45 mg, and 60 mg graduations). **When the oral syringe is dispensed, instructions to the patient should be provided based on these units of measure (ie, mL or mg).** Patients should always be provided with a measuring device calibrated the same way as their labeled instructions.

When commercially-prepared oseltamivir oral suspension is not available, an extemporaneously prepared suspension may be compounded to provide a 6 mg/mL concentration (to match the preferred, currently manufactured commercially available oral suspension concentration).

Brand Names: U.S. Tamiflu®
Brand Names: Canada Tamiflu®
Generic Availability (U.S.) No
Pharmacologic Category Antiviral Agent; Neuraminidase Inhibitor
Use Treatment of uncomplicated acute illness due to influenza (A or B) infection in adults who have been symptomatic for no more than 2 days; prophylaxis against influenza (A or B) infection in adults

The Advisory Committee on Immunization Practices (ACIP) recommends that **treatment** be considered for the following:
• Persons with severe, complicated or progressive illness
• Hospitalized persons
• Persons at higher risk for influenza complications:
  - Adults ≥65 years of age
  - Persons with chronic disorders of the pulmonary (including asthma) or cardiovascular systems (except hypertension)
  - Persons with chronic metabolic diseases (including diabetes mellitus), hepatic disease, renal dysfunction, hematologic disorders (including sickle cell disease), or immunosuppression (including immunosuppression caused by medications or HIV)
  - Persons with neurologic/neuromuscular conditions (including conditions such as spinal cord injuries, seizure disorders, cerebral palsy, stroke, mental retardation, moderate to severe developmental delay, or muscular dystrophy) which may compromise respiratory function, the handling of respiratory secretions, or that can increase the risk of aspiration
  - American Indians and Alaskan Natives
  - Persons who are morbidly obese (BMI ≥40)
  - Residents of nursing homes or other chronic care facilities
• Use may also be considered for previously healthy, nonhigh-risk outpatients with confirmed or suspected influenza based on clinical judgment when treatment can be started within 48 hours of illness onset.

The ACIP recommends that **prophylaxis** be considered for the following:
• Postexposure prophylaxis may be considered for family or close contacts of suspected or confirmed cases, who are at higher risk of influenza complications, and who have not been vaccinated against the circulating strain at the time of the exposure.
• Postexposure prophylaxis may be considered for unvaccinated healthcare workers who had occupational exposure without protective equipment.
• Pre-exposure prophylaxis should only be used for persons at very high risk of influenza complications who cannot be otherwise protected at times of high risk for exposure.
• Prophylaxis should also be administered to all eligible residents of institutions that house patients at high risk when needed to control outbreaks.
Contraindications Hypersensitivity to oseltamivir or any component of the formulation

Warnings/Precautions Oseltamivir is not a substitute for the influenza virus vaccine. It has not been shown to prevent primary or concomitant bacterial infections that may occur with influenza virus. Use caution with renal impairment; dosage adjustment is required for creatinine clearance <30 mL/minute. Safety and efficacy for use in patients with chronic cardiac and/or kidney disease, severe hepatic impairment, or for treatment or prophylaxis in immunocompromised patients have not been established. Rare but severe hypersensitivity reactions (anaphylaxis, severe dermatologic reactions) have been associated with use. Rare occurrences of neuropsychiatric events (including confusion, delirium, hallucinations, and/or self-injury) have been reported from postmarketing surveillance (primarily in pediatric patients); direct causation is difficult to establish (influenza infection may also be associated with behavioral and neurologic changes). Monitor closely for signs of any unusual behavior.

Antiviral treatment should begin within 48 hours of symptom onset. However, the CDC recommends that treatment may still be beneficial and should be started in hospitalized patients with severe, complicated or progressive illness if >48 hours. Nonhospitalized persons who are not at high risk for developing severe or complicated illness and who have a mild disease are not likely to benefit if treatment is started >48 hours after symptom onset. Nonhospitalized persons who are already beginning to recover do not need treatment.

Adverse Reactions (Reflective of adult population; not specific for elderly)
>10%: Gastrointestinal: Vomiting (2% to 15%)
1% to 10%:
  Gastrointestinal: Nausea (4% to 10%), abdominal pain (2% to 5%), diarrhea (1% to 3%)
  Ocular: Conjunctivitis (1%)
  Respiratory: Epistaxis (1%)

Drug Interactions
  Metabolism/Transport Effects None known.
  Avoid Concomitant Use There are no known interactions where it is recommended to avoid concomitant use.
  Increased Effect/Toxicity
    The levels/effects of Oseltamivir may be increased by: Probenecid
  Decreased Effect
    Oseltamivir may decrease the levels/effects of: Influenza Virus Vaccine (Live/Attenuated)

Stability
  Capsules: Store at 25°C (77°F); excursions permitted to 15°C to 30°C (59°F to 86°F).
  Oral suspension: Store powder for suspension at 25°C (77°F); excursions permitted to 15°C to 30°C (59°F to 86°F). Once reconstituted, store suspension under refrigeration at 2°C to 8°C (36°F to 46°F); do not freeze. Use within 10 days of preparation if stored at room temperature or within 17 days of preparation if stored under refrigeration.
    New concentration (6 mg/mL): Reconstitute with 55 mL of water to a final concentration of 6 mg/mL (to make 60 mL total suspension).
    Discontinued concentration (12 mg/mL): Reconstitute with 23 mL of water to a final concentration of 12 mg/mL (to make 25 mL total suspension).

Mechanism of Action Oseltamivir, a prodrug, is hydrolyzed to the active form, oseltamivir carboxylate (OC). OC inhibits influenza virus neuraminidase, an enzyme known to cleave the budding viral progeny from its cellular envelope attachment point (neuraminic acid) just prior to release.

Pharmacodynamics/Kinetics
  Absorption: Well absorbed
  Distribution: V_d: 23-26 L (oseltamivir carboxylate)
  Protein binding, plasma: Oseltamivir carboxylate: 3%; Oseltamivir: 42%
  Metabolism: Hepatic (90%) to oseltamivir carboxylate; neither the parent drug nor active metabolite has any effect on the cytochrome P450 system
  Bioavailability: 75% as oseltamivir carboxylate
  Half-life elimination: Oseltamivir: 1-3 hours; Oseltamivir carboxylate: 6-10 hours
  Excretion: Urine (>90% as oseltamivir carboxylate); feces

Dosage
  Geriatric & Adult
    Influenza prophylaxis: Oral: 75 mg once daily; initiate prophylaxis within 48 hours of contact with an infected individual; duration of prophylaxis: 10 days. During community outbreaks, duration of protection lasts for length of dosing period; safety and efficacy have been demonstrated for use up to 6 weeks in immunocompetent patients and safety has been demonstrated for use up to 12 weeks in patients who are immunocompromised.
    Prophylaxis (institutional outbreak; CDC, 2011): Continue for ≥2 weeks and until ~10 days after identification of illness onset in the last patient
    Influenza treatment: Oral: 75 mg twice daily initiated within 48 hours of onset of symptoms; duration of treatment: 5 days

Note: Hospitalized patients with severe influenza infection may require longer (eg, ≥10 days) treatment courses. Some experts also recommend empirically doubling the treatment dose. Initiate as early as possible in any hospitalized patient with suspected/confirmed influenza (CDC, 2011); may be administered via naso- or orogastric tube in mechanically-ventilated patients (Taylor, 2008).

Renal Impairment

Treatment: Adults:

U.S. labeling: Cl_{cr} 10-30 mL/minute: 75 mg once daily for 5 days

Canadian labeling:

Cl_{cr} >30-60 mL/minute: 30 mg twice daily for 5 days

Cl_{cr} 10-30 mL/minute: 30 mg once daily for 5 days

High-dose treatment (unlabeled [eg, severely-ill hospitalized patients with 2009 H1N1 influenza]): Currently no data are available; consider 150 mg once daily

Prophylaxis: Adults:

U.S. labeling: Cl_{cr} 10-30 mL/minute: 75 mg every other day or 30 mg once daily

Canadian labeling:

Cl_{cr} >30-60 mL/minute: 30 mg once daily for 10-14 days

Cl_{cr} 10-30 mL/minute: 30 mg every other day for 10-14 days

CAPD: Adults:

Unlabeled dose: 30 mg once weekly (Robson, 2006)

Canadian labeling (not in U.S. labeling):

Treatment: 30 mg prior to start of dialysis

Prophylaxis: 30 mg prior to start of dialysis, then 30 mg every 7 days for 10-14 days

Hemodialysis: Adults:

Unlabeled dose: 30 mg after every other session (Robson, 2006)

Canadian labeling (not in U.S. labeling):

Treatment: 30 mg prior to dialysis; if symptomatic between dialysis sessions, then administer 30 mg after each dialysis session over period of 5 days

Prophylaxis: 30 mg prior to dialysis, then 30 mg after every other dialysis session for period of 10-14 days

Hepatic Impairment

Mild-to-moderate impairment: No adjustment necessary

Severe impairment: Pharmacokinetics and safety have not been evaluated

Administration May be administered without regard to meals; take with food to improve tolerance.

Capsules may be opened and mixed with sweetened liquid (eg, chocolate syrup).

Mechanically-ventilated critically-ill patients: May administer via naso- or orogastric (NG/OG) tube. For a 150 mg dose, dissolve powder from two 75 mg capsules in 20 mL of sterile water and inject down the NG/OG tube; follow with a 10 mL sterile water flush (Taylor, 2008).

Monitoring Parameters Signs or symptoms of unusual behavior, including attempts at self-injury, confusion, and/or delirium

Critically-ill patients: Repeat rRT-PCR or viral culture may help to determine on-going viral replication

Pharmacotherapy Pearls In clinical studies of the influenza virus, 1.3% of post-treatment isolates in adults had decreased neuraminidase susceptibility *in vitro* to oseltamivir carboxylate.

The absence of symptoms does not rule out viral influenza infection and clinical judgment should guide the decision for therapy. Treatment should not be delayed while waiting for the results of diagnostic tests. Treatment should be considered for high-risk patients with symptoms despite a negative rapid influenza test when the illness cannot be contributed to another cause. Use of oseltamivir is not a substitute for vaccination (when available); susceptibility to influenza infection returns once therapy is discontinued.

Special Geriatric Considerations Preferred influenza antiviral because of its ease of use compared to zanamivir and resistance associated with amantadine and rimantadine.

Dosage Forms Excipient information presented when available (limited, particularly for generics); consult specific product labeling. [DSC] = Discontinued product

Capsule, oral, as phosphate:

Tamiflu®: 30 mg, 45 mg, 75 mg

Powder for suspension, oral:

Tamiflu®: 6 mg/mL (60 mL); 12 mg/mL (25 mL [DSC]) [contains sodium benzoate; tutti frutti flavor]

Extemporaneously Prepared

If the commercially prepared oral suspension is not available, the manufacturer provides the following compounding information to prepare a **15 mg/mL** suspension in emergency situations. **Note:** The strength and dosing instructions differ from that of the commercially prepared product (see chart on next page).

1. Calculate the total volume needed by patient weight (refer to chart).
2. Calculate the number of capsules and required volume of vehicle (refer to chart). **Note:** Acceptable vehicles are cherry syrup or Ora-Sweet® SF.
3. Transfer contents of capsules into mortar and triturate granules into a fine powder.
4. Add ~1/3 of vehicle and triturate into a uniform suspension.
5. Add another 1/3 of vehicle and triturate, transfer to amber prescription bottle.
6. Add remaining vehicle to prescription bottle; shake well.

Suspension is stable for 35 days under refrigeration at 2°C to 8°C (36°F to 46°F) or 5 days at room temperature of 25°C (77°F). Shake gently prior to use. Do **not** dispense with dosing device provided with commercially-available product.

Preparation of Oseltamivir 15 mg/mL Suspension

Body Weight	Total Volume per Patient[1]	# of 75 mg Capsules[2]	Required Volume of Vehicle[2,3]	Treatment Dose (wt based)[4]	Prophylactic Dose (wt based)[4]
24-40 kg	50 mL	10	48 mL	4 mL (60 mg) twice daily for 5 days	4 mL (60 mg) once daily for 10 days
≥41 kg	60 mL	12	57 mL	5 mL (75 mg) twice daily for 5 days	5 mL (75 mg) once daily for 10 days

[1]Entire course of therapy.

[2]Based on total volume per patient.

[3]Acceptable vehicles are cherry syrup or Ora-Sweet® SF.

[4]Using 15 mg/mL suspension.

- ◆ **OsmoPrep®** *see* Sodium Phosphates *on page 1791*
- ◆ **OTFC (Oral Transmucosal Fentanyl Citrate)** *see* FentaNYL *on page 761*
- ◆ **Otix® [OTC]** *see* Carbamide Peroxide *on page 291*
- ◆ **Ovace®** *see* Sulfacetamide (Topical) *on page 1812*
- ◆ **Ovace® Plus** *see* Sulfacetamide (Topical) *on page 1812*

Oxacillin (oks a SIL in)

Related Information
Antibiotic Treatment of Adults With Infective Endocarditis *on page 2157*
Index Terms Methylphenyl Isoxazolyl Penicillin; Oxacillin Sodium
Generic Availability (U.S.) Yes
Pharmacologic Category Antibiotic, Penicillin
Use Treatment of infections such as osteomyelitis, septicemia, endocarditis, and CNS infections caused by susceptible strains of *Staphylococcus*
Contraindications Hypersensitivity to oxacillin or other penicillins or any component of the formulation
Warnings/Precautions Modify dosage in patients with renal impairment and in the elderly. Serious and occasionally severe or fatal hypersensitivity (anaphylactoid) reactions have been reported in patients on penicillin therapy, especially with a history of beta-lactam hypersensitivity, history of sensitivity to multiple allergens, or previous IgE-mediated reactions (eg, anaphylaxis, angioedema, urticaria). Use with caution in asthmatic patients. Prolonged use may result in fungal or bacterial superinfection, including *C. difficile*-associated diarrhea (CDAD) and pseudomembranous colitis; CDAD has been observed >2 months postantibiotic treatment.
Adverse Reactions (Reflective of adult population; not specific for elderly) Frequency not defined.
Central nervous system: Fever
Dermatologic: Rash
Gastrointestinal: Nausea, diarrhea, vomiting
Hematologic: Eosinophilia, leukopenia, neutropenia, thrombocytopenia, agranulocytosis
Hepatic: Hepatotoxicity, AST increased
Renal: Acute interstitial nephritis, hematuria
Miscellaneous: Serum sickness-like reactions
Drug Interactions
Metabolism/Transport Effects None known.
Avoid Concomitant Use
Avoid concomitant use of Oxacillin with any of the following: BCG

Increased Effect/Toxicity

Oxacillin may increase the levels/effects of: Methotrexate; Vitamin K Antagonists

The levels/effects of Oxacillin may be increased by: Probenecid

Decreased Effect

Oxacillin may decrease the levels/effects of: BCG; Mycophenolate; Typhoid Vaccine

The levels/effects of Oxacillin may be decreased by: Fusidic Acid; Tetracycline Derivatives

Stability Reconstituted parenteral solution is stable for 3 days at room temperature and 7 days when refrigerated. For I.V. infusion in NS or D_5W, solution is stable for 24 hours at room temperature.

Mechanism of Action Inhibits bacterial cell wall synthesis by binding to one or more of the penicillin-binding proteins (PBPs); which in turn inhibits the final transpeptidation step of peptidoglycan synthesis in bacterial cell walls, thus inhibiting cell wall biosynthesis. Bacteria eventually lyse due to ongoing activity of cell wall autolytic enzymes (autolysins and murein hydrolases) while cell wall assembly is arrested.

Pharmacodynamics/Kinetics

Distribution: Into bile, synovial and pleural fluids, bronchial secretions; also distributes to peritoneal and pericardial fluids; penetrates the blood-brain barrier only when meninges are inflamed

Protein binding: ~94%

Metabolism: Hepatic to active metabolites

Half-life elimination: Adults: 23-60 minutes

Time to peak, serum: I.M.: 30-60 minutes

Excretion: Urine and feces (small amounts as unchanged drug and metabolites)

Dosage

Geriatric & Adult

Endocarditis: I.V.: 2 g every 4 hours with gentamicin

Mild-to-moderate infections: I.M., I.V.: 250-500 mg every 4-6 hours

Prosthetic joint infection: I.V.: 2 g every 4 hours with rifampin

Severe infections: I.M., I.V.: 1-2 g every 4-6 hours

***Staphylococcus aureus,* methicillin-susceptible infections, including brain abscess, bursitis, erysipelas, mastitis, mastoiditis, osteomyelitis, perinephric abscess, pneumonia, pyomyositis, scalded skin syndrome, toxic shock syndrome:** I.V.: 2 g every 4 hours

Renal Impairment

Cl_{cr} <10 mL/minute: Clinical practice varies; some clinicians recommend adjustment to the lower range of the usual dosage as based on severity of infection.

Not dialyzable (0% to 5%)

Administration Administer around-the-clock to promote less variation in peak and trough serum levels. Administer IVP over 10 minutes. Administer IVPB over 30 minutes.

Monitoring Parameters Observe for signs and symptoms of anaphylaxis during first dose; monitor periodic CBC, urinalysis, BUN, serum creatinine, AST and ALT

Test Interactions May interfere with urinary glucose tests using cupric sulfate (Benedict's solution, Clinitest®); may inactivate aminoglycosides *in vitro*; false-positive urinary and serum proteins

Special Geriatric Considerations Oxacillin has not been studied in the elderly. Dosing adjustments are not necessary except in renal failure (eg, Cl_{cr} <10 mL/minute). Consider sodium content in patients who may be sensitive to volume expansion (ie, CHF).

Dosage Forms Excipient information presented when available (limited, particularly for generics); consult specific product labeling.

Infusion, premixed iso-osmotic solution: 1 g (50 mL); 2 g (50 mL)

Injection, powder for reconstitution: 1 g, 2 g, 10 g

♦ **Oxacillin Sodium** *see* Oxacillin *on page 1434*

Oxaprozin (oks a PROE zin)

Related Information

Beers Criteria − Potentially Inappropriate Medications for Geriatrics *on page 2183*

Medication Safety Issues

Sound-alike/look-alike issues:

Oxaprozin may be confused with oxazepam

BEERS Criteria medication:

This drug may be potentially inappropriate for use in geriatric patients (Quality of evidence - moderate; Strength of recommendation - strong).

Brand Names: U.S. Daypro®

Brand Names: Canada Apo-Oxaprozin®; Daypro®

Generic Availability (U.S.) Yes

Pharmacologic Category Nonsteroidal Anti-inflammatory Drug (NSAID), Oral

Use Management of signs and symptoms of osteoarthritis, rheumatoid arthritis, and juvenile idiopathic arthritis (JIA)

Medication Guide Available Yes

Contraindications Hypersensitivity to oxaprozin, aspirin, other NSAIDs, or any component of the formulation; perioperative pain in the setting of coronary artery bypass graft (CABG) surgery

Warnings/Precautions [U.S. Boxed Warning]: NSAIDs are associated with an increased risk of adverse cardiovascular thrombotic events, including MI and stroke. Risk may be increased with duration of use or pre-existing cardiovascular risk factors or disease. Carefully evaluate individual cardiovascular risk profiles prior to prescribing. May cause new onset hypertension or worsening of existing hypertension. Use caution with fluid retention. Avoid use in heart failure. Concurrent administration of ibuprofen, and potentially other nonselective NSAIDs, may interfere with aspirin's cardioprotective effect. **[U.S. Boxed Warning]: Use is contraindicated for treatment of perioperative pain in the setting of coronary artery bypass graft (CABG) surgery.** Risk of MI and stroke may be increased with use following CABG surgery.

Platelet adhesion and aggregation may be decreased; may prolong bleeding time; patients with coagulation disorders or who are receiving anticoagulants should be monitored closely. Anemia may occur; patients on long-term NSAID therapy should be monitored for anemia. Rarely, NSAID use may cause severe blood dyscrasias (eg, agranulocytosis, aplastic anemia, thrombocytopenia).

NSAID use may compromise existing renal function; dose-dependent decreases in prosta-glandin synthesis may result from NSAID use, reducing renal blood flow which may cause renal decompensation. NSAID use may increase the risk for hyperkalemia. Patients with impaired renal function, dehydration, heart failure, liver dysfunction, those taking diuretics, and ACE inhibitors, and the elderly are at greater risk of renal toxicity and hyperkalemia. In the elderly, may be inappropriate for long-term use due to potential for GI bleeding, hypertension, heart failure, and renal failure (Beers Criteria). Rehydrate patient before starting therapy; monitor renal function closely. Not recommended for use in patients with advanced renal disease. Long-term NSAID use may result in renal papillary necrosis.

[U.S. Boxed Warning]: NSAIDs may increase risk of gastrointestinal irritation, inflammation, ulceration, bleeding, and perforation. These events may occur at any time during therapy and without warning. Use caution with a history of GI disease (bleeding or ulcers); concurrent therapy with aspirin, anticoagulants, and/or corticosteroids; smoking; use of alcohol; and the elderly or debilitated patients. When used concomitantly with ≤325 mg of aspirin, a substantial increase in the risk of gastrointestinal complications (eg, ulcer) occurs; concomitant gastroprotective therapy (eg, proton pump inhibitors) is recommended (Bhatt, 2008).

Use the lowest effective dose for the shortest duration of time, consistent with individual patient goals, to reduce risk of cardiovascular or GI adverse events. Alternate therapies should be considered for patients at high risk.

NSAIDs may cause serious skin adverse events including exfoliative dermatitis, Stevens-Johnson syndrome (SJS), and toxic epidermal necrolysis (TEN); discontinue use at first sign of skin rash or hypersensitivity. Anaphylactoid reactions may occur, even without prior exposure; patients with "aspirin triad" (bronchial asthma, aspirin intolerance, rhinitis) may be at increased risk. Do not use in patients who experience bronchospasm, asthma, rhinitis, or urticaria with NSAID or aspirin therapy. Use caution in other forms of asthma.

Use with caution in patients with decreased hepatic function. Closely monitor patients with any abnormal LFT. Severe hepatic reactions (eg, fulminant hepatitis, liver failure) have occurred with NSAID use, rarely; discontinue if signs or symptoms of liver disease develop, or if systemic manifestations occur.

NSAIDS may cause drowsiness, dizziness, blurred vision and other neurologic effects which may impair physical or mental abilities; patients must be cautioned about performing tasks which require mental alertness (eg, operating machinery or driving). Discontinue use with blurred or diminished vision and perform ophthalmologic exam. Monitor vision with long-term therapy.

In the elderly, avoid chronic use (unless alternative agents ineffective and patient can receive concomitant gastroprotective agent); nonselective oral NSAID use is associated with an increased risk of GI bleeding and peptic ulcer disease in older adults in high risk category (eg, >75 years or age or receiving concomitant oral/parenteral corticosteroids, anticoagulants, or antiplatelet agents) (Beers Criteria).

Withhold for at least 4-6 half-lives prior to surgical or dental procedures. May cause mild photosensitivity reactions.

Adverse Reactions (Reflective of adult population; not specific for elderly)
1% to 10%:
Cardiovascular: Edema
Central nervous system: Confusion, depression, dizziness, headache, sedation, sleep disturbance, somnolence
Dermatologic: Pruritus, rash
Gastrointestinal: Abdominal distress, abdominal pain, anorexia, constipation, diarrhea, dyspepsia, flatulence, gastrointestinal ulcer, gross bleeding with perforation, heartburn, nausea, vomiting
Hematologic: Anemia, bleeding time increased
Hepatic: Liver enzymes increased
Otic: Tinnitus
Renal: Dysuria, renal function abnormal, urinary frequency

Drug Interactions
Metabolism/Transport Effects None known.
Avoid Concomitant Use
Avoid concomitant use of Oxaprozin with any of the following: Floctafenine; Ketorolac; Ketorolac (Nasal); Ketorolac (Systemic)

Increased Effect/Toxicity
Oxaprozin may increase the levels/effects of: Aliskiren; Aminoglycosides; Anticoagulants; Antiplatelet Agents; Bisphosphonate Derivatives; Collagenase (Systemic); CycloSPORINE; CycloSPORINE (Systemic); Dabigatran Etexilate; Deferasirox; Desmopressin; Digoxin; Drotrecogin Alfa (Activated); Eplerenone; Haloperidol; Ibritumomab; Lithium; Methotrexate; Nonsteroidal Anti-Inflammatory Agents; PEMEtrexed; Porfimer; Potassium-Sparing Diuretics; PRALAtrexate; Quinolone Antibiotics; Rivaroxaban; Salicylates; Thrombolytic Agents; Tositumomab and Iodine I 131 Tositumomab; Vancomycin; Vitamin K Antagonists

The levels/effects of Oxaprozin may be increased by: ACE Inhibitors; Angiotensin II Receptor Blockers; Antidepressants (Tricyclic, Tertiary Amine); Corticosteroids (Systemic); CycloSPORINE; CycloSPORINE (Systemic); Dasatinib; Floctafenine; Glucosamine; Herbs (Anticoagulant/Antiplatelet Properties); Ketorolac; Ketorolac (Nasal); Ketorolac (Systemic); Nonsteroidal Anti-Inflammatory Agents; Omega-3-Acid Ethyl Esters; Pentosan Polysulfate Sodium; Pentoxifylline; Probenecid; Prostacyclin Analogues; Selective Serotonin Reuptake Inhibitors; Serotonin/Norepinephrine Reuptake Inhibitors; Sodium Phosphates; Tipranavir; Treprostinil; Vitamin E

Decreased Effect
Oxaprozin may decrease the levels/effects of: ACE Inhibitors; Aliskiren; Angiotensin II Receptor Blockers; Antiplatelet Agents; Beta-Blockers; Eplerenone; HydrALAZINE; Loop Diuretics; Potassium-Sparing Diuretics; Salicylates; Selective Serotonin Reuptake Inhibitors; Thiazide Diuretics

The levels/effects of Oxaprozin may be decreased by: Bile Acid Sequestrants; Nonsteroidal Anti-Inflammatory Agents; Salicylates

Ethanol/Nutrition/Herb Interactions
Ethanol: Avoid ethanol (may enhance gastric mucosal irritation).
Herb/Nutraceutical: Avoid alfalfa, anise, bilberry, bladderwrack, bromelain, cat's claw, celery, chamomile, coleus, cordyceps, dong quai, evening primrose, fenugreek, feverfew, garlic, ginger, ginkgo biloba, ginseng (American, Panax, Siberian), grapeseed, green tea, guggul, horse chestnut seed, horseradish, licorice, prickly ash, red clover, reishi, SAMe (S-adenosylmethionine), sweet clover, turmeric, white willow (all have additional antiplatelet activity).

Stability Store at 25°C (77°F); excursions permitted to 15°C to 30°C (59°F to 86°F). Protect from light; keep bottle tightly closed.

Mechanism of Action Reversibly inhibits cyclooxygenase-1 and 2 (COX-1 and 2) enzymes, which results in decreased formation of prostaglandin precursors; has antipyretic, analgesic, and anti-inflammatory properties.

Other proposed mechanisms not fully elucidated (and possibly contributing to the anti-inflammatory effect to varying degrees) include inhibiting chemotaxis, altering lymphocyte activity, inhibiting neutrophil aggregation/activation, and decreasing proinflammatory cytokine levels.

Pharmacodynamics/Kinetics
Absorption: Oral: 95%
Distribution: V_d: 11-17 L/70 kg
Protein binding: 99% primarily to albumin
Metabolism: Hepatic via oxidation and glucuronidation; no active metabolites

Half-life elimination: 41-55 hours

Time to peak: 2-3 hours

Excretion: Urine (5% unchanged, 65% as metabolites); feces (35% as metabolites)

Dosage

Geriatric & Adult Note: Individualize dosage to lowest effective dose for the shortest duration to minimize adverse effects.

Osteoarthritis, rheumatoid arthritis: Oral: 1200 mg once daily. **Note:** Patients with low body weight should start with 600 mg daily. A one-time loading dose of 1200-1800 mg (≤26 mg/kg) may be used when a quick onset of action is desired.

Maximum doses:

Patient <50 kg: Maximum: 1200 mg daily

Patient >50 kg with normal renal/hepatic function and low risk of peptic ulcer: Maximum: 1800 mg daily or 26 mg/kg/day (whichever is lower) in divided doses

Renal Impairment In general, NSAIDs are not recommended for use in patients with advanced renal disease but the manufacturer of oxaprozin does provide some guidelines for adjustment in renal dysfunction.

Severe renal impairment or on dialysis: 600 mg once daily; may increase cautiously to 1200 mg daily with close monitoring.

Hepatic Impairment Use caution in patients with severe hepatic impairment.

Monitoring Parameters Blood pressure; CBC; signs/symptoms of GI bleeding; hepatic and renal function

Test Interactions False-positive urine immunoassay screening tests for benzodiazepines have been reported and may occur several days after discontinuing oxaprozin.

Special Geriatric Considerations Elderly are a high-risk population for adverse effects from NSAIDs. As much as 60% of the elderly can develop peptic ulceration and/or hemorrhage asymptomatically. The concomitant use of H_2 blockers and sucralfate is not generally effective as prophylaxis with the exception of NSAID-induced duodenal ulcers which may be prevented by the use of ranitidine. Misoprostol and proton pump inhibitors are the only agents proven to help prevent the development of NSAID-induced ulcers. Also, concomitant disease and drug use contribute to the risk for GI adverse effects. Use lowest effective dose for shortest period possible. Consider renal function decline with age. Use of NSAIDs can compromise existing renal function especially when Cl_{cr} is ≤30 mL/minute. Tinnitus may be a difficult and unreliable indication of toxicity due to age-related hearing loss or eighth cranial nerve damage. CNS adverse effects, such as confusion, agitation, and hallucination, are generally seen in overdose or high dose situations, but the elderly may demonstrate these adverse effects at lower doses than younger adults.

This medication is considered to be potentially inappropriate in this patient population (Beers Criteria: Quality of evidence - moderate; Strength of recommendation - strong).

Dosage Forms Excipient information presented when available (limited, particularly for generics); consult specific product labeling.

Caplet, oral:

Daypro®: 600 mg [scored]

Tablet, oral: 600 mg

Oxazepam (oks A ze pam)

Related Information

Anxiolytic, Sedative/Hypnotic, and Miscellaneous Benzodiazepines *on page 2106*

Beers Criteria – Potentially Inappropriate Medications for Geriatrics *on page 2183*

Medication Safety Issues

Sound-alike/look-alike issues:

Oxazepam may be confused with oxaprozin, quazepam

Serax may be confused with Eurax®, Urex, ZyrTEC®

BEERS Criteria medication:

This drug may be potentially inappropriate for use in geriatric patients (Quality of evidence - high; Strength of recommendation - strong).

International issues:

Murelax [Australia] may be confused with MiraLax brand name for polyethylene glycol 3350 [U.S.]

Brand Names: Canada Apo-Oxazepam®; Bio-Oxazepam; Novoxapram®; Oxpam®; Oxpram®; PMS-Oxazepam; Riva-Oxazepam

Index Terms Serax

Generic Availability (U.S.) Yes

Pharmacologic Category Benzodiazepine

Use Treatment of anxiety; management of ethanol withdrawal

Unlabeled Use Anticonvulsant in management of simple partial seizures; hypnotic

Contraindications Hypersensitivity to oxazepam or any component of the formulation (cross-sensitivity with other benzodiazepines may exist); narrow-angle glaucoma (not in product labeling, however, benzodiazepines are contraindicated); not indicated for use in the treatment of psychosis

Warnings/Precautions May cause hypotension (rare) - use with caution in patients with cardiovascular or cerebrovascular disease, or in patients who would not tolerate transient decreases in blood pressure.

Use with caution in elderly or debilitated patients, patients with hepatic disease (including alcoholics), or renal impairment. In older adults, benzodiazepines increase the risk of impaired cognition, delirium, falls, fractures, and motor vehicle accidents. Due to increased sensitivity in this age group, avoid use for treatment of insomnia, agitation, or delirium. (Beers Criteria). Use with caution in patients with respiratory disease or impaired gag reflex. Avoid use in patients with sleep apnea.

Causes CNS depression (dose-related) resulting in sedation, dizziness, confusion, or ataxia which may impair physical and mental capabilities. Patients must be cautioned about performing tasks which require mental alertness (eg, operating machinery or driving). Use with caution in patients receiving other CNS depressants or psychoactive agents. Benzodiazepines have been associated with falls and traumatic injury and should be used with extreme caution in patients who are at risk of these events.

Use caution in patients with depression, particularly if suicidal risk may be present. Use with caution in patients with a history of drug dependence. Benzodiazepines have been associated with dependence and acute withdrawal symptoms on discontinuation or reduction in dose. Acute withdrawal, including seizures, may be precipitated after administration of flumazenil to patients receiving long-term benzodiazepine therapy.

Benzodiazepines have been associated with anterograde amnesia. Paradoxical reactions, including hyperactive or aggressive behavior have been reported with benzodiazepines, particularly in psychiatric patients. Does not have analgesic, antidepressant, or antipsychotic properties.

Adverse Reactions (Reflective of adult population; not specific for elderly) Frequency not defined.
Cardiovascular: Syncope (rare), edema
Central nervous system: Drowsiness, ataxia, dizziness, vertigo, memory impairment, headache, paradoxical reactions (excitement, stimulation of effect), lethargy, amnesia, euphoria
Dermatologic: Rash
Endocrine & metabolic: Decreased libido, menstrual irregularities
Genitourinary: Incontinence
Hematologic: Leukopenia, blood dyscrasias
Hepatic: Jaundice
Neuromuscular & skeletal: Dysarthria, tremor, reflex slowing
Ocular: Blurred vision, diplopia
Miscellaneous: Drug dependence
Drug Interactions
Metabolism/Transport Effects None known.
Avoid Concomitant Use
Avoid concomitant use of Oxazepam with any of the following: Azelastine; Azelastine (Nasal); Methadone; Mirtazapine; OLANZapine; Paraldehyde
Increased Effect/Toxicity
Oxazepam may increase the levels/effects of: Alcohol (Ethyl); Azelastine; Azelastine (Nasal); Buprenorphine; CloZAPine; CNS Depressants; Fosphenytoin; Methadone; Methotrimeprazine; Metyrosine; Mirtazapine; Paraldehyde; Phenytoin; Selective Serotonin Reuptake Inhibitors; Zolpidem

The levels/effects of Oxazepam may be increased by: Droperidol; HydrOXYzine; Methotrimeprazine; OLANZapine
Decreased Effect
The levels/effects of Oxazepam may be decreased by: Theophylline Derivatives; Yohimbine
Ethanol/Nutrition/Herb Interactions
Ethanol: May increase CNS depression; monitor for increased effects with coadministration. Caution patients about effects.
Herb/Nutraceutical: Avoid valerian, St John's wort, kava kava, gotu kola (may increase CNS depression).

◄ **Mechanism of Action** Binds to stereospecific benzodiazepine receptors on the postsynaptic GABA neuron at several sites within the central nervous system, including the limbic system, reticular formation. Enhancement of the inhibitory effect of GABA on neuronal excitability results by increased neuronal membrane permeability to chloride ions. This shift in chloride ions results in hyperpolarization (a less excitable state) and stabilization.

Pharmacodynamics/Kinetics
Absorption: Almost complete
Protein binding: 86% to 99%
Metabolism: Hepatic to inactive compounds (primarily as glucuronides)
Half-life elimination: 2.8-5.7 hours
Time to peak, serum: 2-4 hours
Excretion: Urine (as unchanged drug [50%] and metabolites)

Dosage
Geriatric Oral: Anxiety: 10 mg 2-3 times/day; increase gradually as needed to a total of 30-45 mg/day. Dose titration should be slow to evaluate sensitivity.
Adult
Anxiety: Oral: 10-30 mg 3-4 times/day
Ethanol withdrawal: Oral: 15-30 mg 3-4 times/day
Hypnotic: Oral: 15-30 mg
Renal Impairment Not dialyzable (0% to 5%)

Administration Administer orally in divided doses.

Monitoring Parameters Respiratory and cardiovascular status

Reference Range Therapeutic: 0.2-1.4 mcg/mL (SI: 0.7-4.9 micromole/L)

Pharmacotherapy Pearls Not intended for management of anxieties and minor distresses associated with everyday life. Treatment longer than 4 months should be re-evaluated to determine the patient's need for the drug. Abrupt discontinuation after sustained use (generally >10 days) may cause withdrawal symptoms.

Special Geriatric Considerations Because of its relatively short half-life and its lack of active metabolites, oxazepam could be considered for use in the elderly when a benzodiazepine is indicated.

This medication is considered to be potentially inappropriate in this patient population (Beers Criteria: Quality of evidence - high; Strength of recommendation - strong).

Controlled Substance C-IV

Dosage Forms Excipient information presented when available (limited, particularly for generics); consult specific product labeling.
Capsule, oral: 10 mg, 15 mg, 30 mg

OXcarbazepine (ox car BAZ e peen)

Medication Safety Issues
Sound-alike/look-alike issues:
OXcarbazepine may be confused with carBAMazepine
Trileptal® may be confused with TriLipix®

Brand Names: U.S. Trileptal®
Brand Names: Canada Apo-Oxcarbazepine®; Trileptal®
Index Terms GP 47680; OCBZ
Generic Availability (U.S.) Yes
Pharmacologic Category Anticonvulsant, Miscellaneous
Use Monotherapy or adjunctive therapy in the treatment of partial seizures
Unlabeled Use Bipolar disorder; treatment of neuropathic pain
Medication Guide Available Yes
Contraindications Hypersensitivity to oxcarbazepine or any component of the formulation
Warnings/Precautions Hazardous agent - use appropriate precautions for handling and disposal. Antiepileptics are associated with an increased risk of suicidal behavior/thoughts with use (regardless of indication); patients should be monitored for signs/symptoms of depression, suicidal tendencies, and other unusual behavior changes during therapy and instructed to inform their healthcare provider immediately if symptoms occur.

Clinically-significant hyponatremia (serum sodium <125 mmol/L) may develop during oxcarbazepine use. Rare cases of anaphylaxis and angioedema have been reported, even after initial dosing; permanently discontinue should symptoms occur. Use caution in patients with previous hypersensitivity to carbamazepine (cross-sensitivity occurs in 25% to 30%). Potentially serious, sometimes fatal, dermatologic reactions (eg, Stevens-Johnson, toxic epidermal necrolysis) and multiorgan hypersensitivity reactions have been reported in adults and children; monitor for signs and symptoms of skin reactions and possible disparate manifestations associated with lymphatic, hepatic, renal, and/or hematologic organ systems;

discontinuation and conversion to alternate therapy may be required. As with all antiepileptic drugs, oxcarbazepine should be withdrawn gradually to minimize the potential of increased seizure frequency. Use of oxcarbazepine has been associated with CNS-related adverse events, most significant of these were cognitive symptoms including psychomotor slowing, difficulty with concentration, speech or language problems, somnolence or fatigue, and coordination abnormalities, including ataxia and gait disturbances. Effects with other sedative drugs or ethanol may be potentiated. Single-dose studies show that half-life of the primary active metabolite is prolonged three- to fourfold and AUC is doubled in patients with Cl_{cr} <30 mL/minute; dose adjustment required in these patients. May reduce the efficacy of oral contraceptives (nonhormonal contraceptive measures are recommended). Agranulocytosis, leukopenia, and pancytopenia have been reported with use (rare). Discontinuation and conversion to alternate therapy may be required.

Adverse Reactions (Reflective of adult population; not specific for elderly) As reported in adults with doses of up to 2400 mg/day (includes patients on monotherapy, adjunctive therapy, and those not previously on AEDs); incidence in children was similar.

>10%:
   Central nervous system: Dizziness (22% to 49%), somnolence (20% to 36%), headache (13% to 32%), ataxia (5% to 31%), fatigue (12% to 15%), vertigo (6% to 15%)
   Gastrointestinal: Vomiting (7% to 36%), nausea (15% to 29%), abdominal pain (10% to 13%)
   Neuromuscular & skeletal: Abnormal gait (5% to 17%), tremor (3% to 16%)
   Ocular: Diplopia (14% to 40%), nystagmus (7% to 26%), abnormal vision (4% to 14%)
1% to 10%:
   Cardiovascular: Hypotension (≤2%), leg edema (1% to 2%)
   Central nervous system: Nervousness (2% to 5%), amnesia (4%), abnormal thinking (≤4%), insomnia (2% to 4%), fever (3%), speech disorder (1% to 3%), abnormal feelings (≤2%), EEG abnormalities (≤2%), agitation (1% to 2%), confusion (1% to 2%)
   Dermatologic: Rash (4%), acne (1% to 2%)
   Endocrine & metabolic: Hyponatremia (1% to 3%)
   Gastrointestinal: Diarrhea (5% to 7%), dyspepsia (5% to 6%), constipation (2% to 6%), taste perversion (5%), xerostomia (3%), gastritis (1% to 2%), weight gain (1% to 2%)
   Genitourinary: Micturition (2%)
   Neuromuscular & skeletal: Weakness (3% to 6%), back pain (4%), falling down (4%), abnormal coordination (1% to 4%), dysmetria (1% to 3%), sprains/strains (≤2%), muscle weakness (1% to 2%)
   Ocular: Abnormal accommodation (≤2%)
   Respiratory: Upper respiratory tract infection (7%), rhinitis (2% to 5%), chest infection (4%), epistaxis (4%), sinusitis (4%)

Drug Interactions

Metabolism/Transport Effects Induces CYP3A4 (strong)

Avoid Concomitant Use
   Avoid concomitant use of OXcarbazepine with any of the following: Axitinib; Bortezomib; Crizotinib; Dronedarone; Everolimus; Itraconazole; Lapatinib; Lurasidone; Mifepristone; Nilotinib; Nisoldipine; Pazopanib; Praziquantel; Ranolazine; Rilpivirine; Rivaroxaban; Roflumilast; RomiDEPsin; Selegiline; SORAfenib; Ticagrelor; Tolvaptan; Toremifene; Vandetanib

Increased Effect/Toxicity
   OXcarbazepine may increase the levels/effects of: Clarithromycin; Fosphenytoin; Ifosfamide; Phenytoin; Selegiline

   The levels/effects of OXcarbazepine may be increased by: Clarithromycin; Thiazide Diuretics

Decreased Effect
   OXcarbazepine may decrease the levels/effects of: Apixaban; ARIPiprazole; Axitinib; Boceprevir; Bortezomib; Brentuximab Vedotin; Clarithromycin; Contraceptives (Estrogens); Contraceptives (Progestins); Crizotinib; CYP3A4 Substrates; Dasatinib; Dronedarone; Everolimus; Exemestane; Gefitinib; GuanFACINE; Imatinib; Ixabepilone; Lapatinib; Linagliptin; Lurasidone; Maraviroc; Mifepristone; NIFEdipine; Nilotinib; Nisoldipine; Pazopanib; Praziquantel; Ranolazine; Rilpivirine; Rivaroxaban; Roflumilast; RomiDEPsin; Saxagliptin; SORAfenib; SUNItinib; Tadalafil; Ticagrelor; Tolvaptan; Toremifene; Ulipristal; Vandetanib; Vemurafenib; Zuclopenthixol

   The levels/effects of OXcarbazepine may be decreased by: Divalproex; Fosphenytoin; PHENobarbital; Phenytoin; Valproic Acid

Ethanol/Nutrition/Herb Interactions
   Ethanol: Avoid ethanol (may increase CNS depression).
   Herb/Nutraceutical: St John's wort may decrease oxcarbazepine levels. Avoid evening primrose (seizure threshold decreased). Avoid valerian, St John's wort, kava kava, gotu kola.

Stability Store tablets and suspension at 25°C (77°F). Use suspension within 7 weeks of first opening container.

Mechanism of Action Pharmacological activity results from both oxcarbazepine and its monohydroxy metabolite (MHD). Precise mechanism of anticonvulsant effect has not been defined. Oxcarbazepine and MHD block voltage-sensitive sodium channels, stabilizing hyper-excited neuronal membranes, inhibiting repetitive firing, and decreasing the propagation of synaptic impulses. These actions are believed to prevent the spread of seizures. Oxcarba-zepine and MHD also increase potassium conductance and modulate the activity of high-voltage activated calcium channels.

Pharmacodynamics/Kinetics

Absorption: Complete; food has no affect on rate or extent

Distribution: MHD: V_d: 49 L

Protein binding, serum: MHD: 40%

Metabolism: Hepatic to 10-monohydroxy metabolite (MHD; active); MHD is further glucur-onidated or oxidized to a 10,11-dihydroxy metabolite (DHD; inactive)

Bioavailability: Increased in elderly >60 years

Half-life elimination: Parent drug: 2 hours; MHD: 9 hours; renal impairment (Cl_{cr} 30 mL/minute): MHD: 19 hours

Time to peak, serum (median): Tablets: 4.5 hours; oral suspension: 6 hours

Excretion: Urine (95%, <1% as unchanged oxcarbazepine, 27% as unchanged MHD, 49% as MHD glucuronides); feces (<4%)

Dosage

Geriatric & Adult

Adjunctive therapy, partial seizures (epilepsy): Oral: Initial: 600 mg/day in 2 divided doses; dosage may be increased by 600 mg/day at approximate weekly intervals. Recommended daily dose is 1200 mg/day in 2 divided doses. Although daily doses >1200 mg/day were somewhat more efficacious, most patients were unable to tolerate 2400 mg/day (due to CNS effects).

Conversion to monotherapy, partial seizures (epilepsy): Oral: Patients receiving con-comitant antiepileptic drugs (AEDs): Initial: 600 mg/day in 2 divided doses while simulta-neously reducing the dose of concomitant AEDs. Withdraw concomitant AEDs completely over 3-6 weeks, while increasing the oxcarbazine dose in increments of 600 mg/day at weekly intervals, reaching the maximum oxcarbazine dose (2400 mg/day) in about 2-4 weeks (lower doses have been effective in patients in whom monotherapy has been initiated).

Initiation of monotherapy, partial seizures (epilepsy): Oral: Patients not receiving prior AEDs: Initial: 600 mg/day in 2 divided doses. Increase dose by 300 mg/day every third day to a dose of 1200 mg/day. Higher dosages (2400 mg/day) have been shown to be effective in patients converted to monotherapy from other AEDs.

Renal Impairment Cl_{cr} <30 mL/minute: Therapy should be initiated at one-half the usual starting dose (300 mg/day in adults) and increased slowly to achieve the desired clinical response

Hepatic Impairment Adjustment not needed for mild-to-moderate impairment. No data in patients with severe impairment.

Administration All dosing should be administered twice daily.

Suspension: Prior to using for the first time, firmly insert the plastic adapter provided with the bottle. Cover adapter with child-resistant cap when not in use. Shake bottle for at least 10 seconds, remove child-resistant cap, and insert the oral dosing syringe provided to withdraw appropriate dose. Dose may be taken directly from oral syringe or may be mixed in a small glass of water immediately prior to swallowing. Rinse syringe with warm water after use and allow to dry thoroughly. Discard any unused portion after 7 weeks of first opening bottle.

Monitoring Parameters Seizure frequency, serum sodium as deemed necessary (particu-larly during first 3 months of therapy), symptoms of CNS depression (dizziness, headache, somnolence). Additional serum sodium monitoring recommended during maintenance treat-ment in patients receiving other medications known to decrease sodium levels, in patients with signs/symptoms of hyponatremia, and in patients with an increase in seizure frequency or severity. Monitor for suicidality (eg, suicidal thoughts, depression, behavioral changes). Serum levels of concomitant antiepileptic drugs during titration as necessary.

Test Interactions Thyroid function tests; may depress serum T_4 without affecting T_3 levels or TSH

Special Geriatric Considerations The elderly frequently use diuretics which theoretically may increase the risk of hyponatremia associated with oxcarbazepine use. Serum sodium should be monitored closely for the first 3 months when oxcarbazepine therapy is initiated.

Dosage Forms Excipient information presented when available (limited, particularly for generics); consult specific product labeling.

Suspension, oral: 300 mg/5 mL (250 mL)

Trileptal®: 300 mg/5 mL (250 mL) [contains ethanol, propylene glycol]

Tablet, oral: 150 mg, 300 mg, 600 mg

Trileptal®: 150 mg, 300 mg, 600 mg [scored]

♦ **Oxecta™** see OxyCODONE on page 1446
♦ **Oxilapine Succinate** see Loxapine on page 1167
♦ **Oxpentifylline** see Pentoxifylline on page 1507
♦ **OXY® [OTC]** see Salicylic Acid on page 1743
♦ **OXY® Body Wash [OTC]** see Salicylic Acid on page 1743

Oxybutynin (oks i BYOO ti nin)

Related Information

Beers Criteria – Potentially Inappropriate Medications for Geriatrics on page 2183
Pharmacotherapy of Urinary Incontinence on page 2141

Medication Safety Issues

Sound-alike/look-alike issues:

Oxybutynin may be confused with OxyCONTIN®

Ditropan may be confused with Detrol®, diazepam, Diprivan®, dithranol

BEERS Criteria medication:

This drug may be potentially inappropriate for use in geriatric patients (Quality of evidence - varies based on comorbidity; Strength of recommendation - varies based on comorbidity)

Other safety concerns:

Transdermal patch may contain conducting metal (eg, aluminum); remove patch prior to MRI.

Brand Names: U.S. Ditropan XL®; Gelnique 3%™; Gelnique®; Oxytrol®

Brand Names: Canada Apo-Oxybutynin®; Ditropan XL®; Dom-Oxybutynin; Gelnique®; Mylan-Oxybutynin; Novo-Oxybutynin; Nu-Oxybutyn; Oxybutynin; Oxybutynine; Oxytrol®; PHL-Oxybutynin; PMS-Oxybutynin; Riva-Oxybutynin; Uromax®

Index Terms Ditropan; Oxybutynin Chloride

Generic Availability (U.S.) Yes: Excludes gel, transdermal patch

Pharmacologic Category Antispasmodic Agent, Urinary

Use Antispasmodic for neurogenic bladder (urgency, frequency, leakage, urge incontinence, dysuria); extended release formulation also indicated for treatment of symptoms associated with detrusor overactivity due to a neurological condition (eg, spina bifida)

Contraindications Hypersensitivity to oxybutynin or any component of the formulation; patients with or at risk for uncontrolled narrow-angle glaucoma, urinary retention, gastric retention or conditions with severely decreased GI motility

Warnings/Precautions Cases of angioedema have been reported with oral oxybutynin; some cases have occurred after a single dose. Discontinue immediately if develops. Use with caution in patients with bladder outflow obstruction, angle-closure glaucoma (treated), hyperthyroidism, reflux esophagitis (including concurrent therapy with oral bisphosphonates or drugs which may increase the risk of esophagitis), heart disease, hepatic or renal disease, prostatic hyperplasia, autonomic neuropathy, ulcerative colitis (may cause ileus and toxic megacolon), hypertension, hiatal hernia, myasthenia gravis, dementia, ulcerative colitis, or intestinal atony. May increase the risk of heat prostration. May cause anticholinergic effects (agitation, confusion, hallucinations, somnolence) which may require dose reduction or discontinuation of therapy. May cause CNS depression, which may impair physical or mental abilities; patients must be cautioned about performing tasks which require mental alertness (eg, operating machinery or driving).

This medication is associated with potent anticholinergic properties which may be inappropriate in older adults depending on comorbidities (eg, dementia, delirium) (Beers Criteria).

The extended release formulation consists of drug within a nondeformable matrix; following drug release/absorption, the matrix/shell is expelled in the stool. The use of nondeformable products in patients with known stricture/narrowing of the GI tract has been associated with symptoms of obstruction. Transdermal patch may contain conducting metal (eg, aluminum); remove patch prior to MRI. When using the topical gel, cover treatment area with clothing after gel has dried to minimize transferring medication to others. Discontinue gel if skin irritation occurs. Gel contains ethanol; do not expose to open flame or smoking until gel has dried.

Adverse Reactions (Reflective of adult population; not specific for elderly)

Oral:

>10%:

Central nervous system: Dizziness (4% to 17%), somnolence (2% to 14%)

Gastrointestinal: Xerostomia (29% to 71%; dose related), constipation (7% to 15%), nausea (2% to 12%)

1% to 10%:

Cardiovascular: Arrhythmia (sinus; 1% to <5%), blood pressure change (increased/decreased; 1% to <5%), chest pain (1% to <5%), edema (1% to <5%), flushing (1% to <5%), palpitation (1% to <5%), peripheral edema (1% to <5%)

Central nervous system: Headache (6% to 10%), pain (1% to 7%), nervousness (1% to 7%), insomnia (1% to 6%), confusion (1% to <5%), depression (1% to <5%), fatigue (1% to <5%)

Dermatologic: Dry skin (1% to <5%), pruritus (1% to <5%)

Endocrine & metabolic: Fluid retention (1% to <5%), hyperglycemia (1% to <5%)

Gastrointestinal: Diarrhea (1% to 9%), dyspepsia (5% to 7%), abdominal pain (1% to <5%), abnormal taste (1% to <5%), dry throat (1% to <5%), dysphagia (1% to <5%), eructation (1% to <5%), flatulence (1% to <5%), gastrointestinal reflux disease (1% to <5%), vomiting (1% to <5%)

Genitourinary: Urinary hesitation (9%), urinary tract infection (5% to 7%), urinary retention (6%), cystitis (1% to <5%), dysuria (1% to <5%), pollakiuria (1% to <5%)

Neuromuscular & skeletal: Weakness (1% to 7%), arthralgia (1% to <5%), back pain (1% to <5%), extremity pain (1% to <5%), flank pain (1% to <5%)

Ocular: Blurred vision (1% to 10%), dry eyes (3% to 6%), eye irritation (1% to <5%), keratoconjunctivitis sicca (1% to <5%)

Respiratory: Rhinitis (2% to 6%), asthma (1% to <5%), bronchitis (1% to <5%), cough (1% to <5%), hoarseness (1% to <5%), nasal congestion (1% to <5%), nasal dryness (1% to <5%), nasopharyngitis (1% to <5%), pharyngolaryngeal pain (1% to <5%), sinus congestion (1% to <5%), sinusitis (1% to <5%), upper respiratory tract infection (1% to <5%)

Miscellaneous: Fungal infection (1% to <5%), thirst (1% to <5%)

Postmarketing and/or case reports: Agitation, anaphylaxis, angioedema, cycloplegia, GI motility decreased, glaucoma, hallucinations, hypersensitivity reactions, impotence, lactation suppression, memory impairment, mydriasis, psychotic disorder, QT_c prolongation, rash, seizures, sweating decreased, tachycardia

Topical gel:

>10%:

Gastrointestinal: Xerostomia (7% to 12%)

Local: Application site reaction (4% to 14%; includes dermatitis, erythema, irritation, pain, papules, pruritus, rash)

1% to 10%:

Central nervous system: Dizziness (2% to 3%), fatigue (2%), headache (2%)

Dermatologic: Pruritus (1%)

Gastrointestinal: Gastroenteritis (2%), constipation (1%)

Genitourinary: Urinary tract infection (5% to 7%)

Ocular: Conjunctivitis (4%), blurred vision (<2%), dry eyes (<2%)

Respiratory: Nasopharyngitis (3% to 5%)

Transdermal:

>10%: Local: Application site reaction (17%), pruritus (14%)

1% to 10%:

Gastrointestinal: Xerostomia (4% to 10%), diarrhea (3%), constipation (3%)

Genitourinary: Dysuria (2%)

Local: Erythema (6% to 8%), vesicles (3%), rash (3%)

Ocular: Vision changes (3%)

Drug Interactions

Metabolism/Transport Effects Substrate of CYP3A4 (minor); **Note:** Assignment of Major/Minor substrate status based on clinically relevant drug interaction potential; **Inhibits** CYP2C8 (weak), CYP2D6 (weak), CYP3A4 (weak)

Avoid Concomitant Use

Avoid concomitant use of Oxybutynin with any of the following: Pimozide

Increased Effect/Toxicity

Oxybutynin may increase the levels/effects of: AbobotulinumtoxinA; Anticholinergics; ARIPiprazole; Cannabinoids; OnabotulinumtoxinA; Pimozide; Potassium Chloride; RimabotulinumtoxinB

The levels/effects of Oxybutynin may be increased by: Pramlintide

Decreased Effect

Oxybutynin may decrease the levels/effects of: Acetylcholinesterase Inhibitors (Central); Secretin

The levels/effects of Oxybutynin may be decreased by: Acetylcholinesterase Inhibitors (Central); Tocilizumab

Ethanol/Nutrition/Herb Interactions Ethanol: Use ethanol with caution (may increase CNS depression and toxicity). Watch for sedation.

Stability

Immediate release: Store at controlled room temperature of 15°C to 30°C (59°F to 86°F). Protect syrup from light.

Extended release: Store at 25°C (77°F); excursions permitted to 15°C to 30°C (59°F to 86°F). Protect from moisture and humidity.

Gel (pump or sachet), transdermal patch: Store at 25°C (77°F); excursions permitted to 15°C to 30°C (59°F to 86°F). Protect from moisture and humidity. Keel gel away from open flame. Keep patch in sealed pouch. Throw away used sachets or patches where children and pets cannot reach.

Mechanism of Action Direct antispasmodic effect on smooth muscle, also inhibits the action of acetylcholine on smooth muscle (exhibits $1/5$ the anticholinergic activity of atropine, but is 4-10 times the antispasmodic activity); does not block effects at skeletal muscle or at autonomic ganglia; increases bladder capacity, decreases uninhibited contractions, and delays desire to void, therefore, decreases urgency and frequency

Pharmacodynamics/Kinetics

Onset of action: Oral: 30-60 minutes

Peak effect: 3-6 hours

Duration: 6-10 hours (up to 24 hours for extended release oral formulation)

Absorption: Oral: Rapid and well absorbed; Transdermal: High

Distribution: I.V.: V_d: 193 L

Protein binding: >99% primarily to alpha$_1$-acid glycoprotein

Metabolism: Hepatic via CYP3A4; Oral: High first-pass metabolism; forms active and inactive metabolites

Bioavailability: Oral: ~6%

Half-life elimination: I.V.: ~2 hours (parent drug), 7-8 hours (metabolites); Oral: Immediate release: ~2-3 hours; Extended release: ~13 hours; Transdermal: 30-64 hours

Time to peak, serum: Oral: Immediate release: ~60 minutes; Extended release: 4-6 hours; Transdermal: 24-48 hours

Excretion: Urine, as metabolites and unchanged drug (<0.1%)

Dosage

Geriatric

Oral: Immediate release: Initial: 2.5 mg 2-3 times/day; increase cautiously

Topical gel, transdermal patch: Refer to adult dosing.

Adult Bladder spasms:

Oral:

Immediate release: 5 mg 2-3 times/day; maximum: 5 mg 4 times/day

Extended release: Initial: 5-10 mg once daily, adjust dose in 5 mg increments at weekly intervals; maximum: 30 mg daily

Topical gel:

Gelnique 3%™: Apply 3 pumps (84 mg) once daily

Gelnique® 10%: Apply contents of 1 sachet (100 mg/g) once daily

Transdermal: Apply one 3.9 mg/day patch twice weekly (every 3-4 days)

Renal Impairment No dosage adjustment provided in the manufacturer's labeling (not studied); use with caution.

Hepatic Impairment No dosage adjustment provided in the manufacturer's labeling (not studied); use with caution.

Administration

Oral: Administer without regard to meals. Extended release tablets must be swallowed whole with liquid; do not crush, divide, or chew; take at approximately the same time each day.

Topical gel: For topical use only. Apply to clean, dry, intact skin on abdomen, thighs, or upper arms/shoulders. Wash hands after use. Cover treated area with clothing after gel has dried to prevent transfer of medication to others. Do not bathe, shower, or swim until 1 hour after gel applied. Do not apply to recently shaved skin.

Gelnique 3%™: Prior to initial use, press pump 4 times to prime pump; discard any gel dispensed from pump during priming. Rotate application sites to avoid skin irritation.

Gelnique® 10%: Rotate site; do not apply to same site on consecutive days.

Transdermal: Apply to clean, dry skin on abdomen, hip, or buttock. Select a new site for each new system (avoid reapplication to same site within 7 days).

Monitoring Parameters Incontinence episodes, postvoid residual (PVR)

Test Interactions May suppress the wheal and flare reactions to skin test antigens.

Special Geriatric Considerations Caution should be used in the elderly due to anticholinergic activity (eg, confusion, constipation, blurred vision, and tachycardia). Start with lower doses. Transdermal dosage form may have less potential for these effects. Oxybutynin may cause memory problems in the elderly. A study of 12 healthy volunteers with an average age of 69 showed cognitive decline while taking the drug (Katz, 1998). Studies using transdermal dosage form did not reveal any differences in safety or efficacy between elderly and younger adults.

This medication is considered to be potentially inappropriate in this patient population (Beers Criteria: Quality of evidence - varies based on comorbidity; Strength of recommendation - varies based on comorbidity)

Dosage Forms Excipient information presented when available (limited, particularly for generics); consult specific product labeling.

Gel, topical:
  Gelnique 3%™: 3% (92 g) [contains ethanol; delivers oxybutynin 28 mg/pump actuation]
Gel, topical, as chloride:
  Gelnique®: 10% (1 g) [contains ethanol; oxybutynin chloride 100 mg/1 g sachet]
Patch, transdermal:
  Oxytrol®: 3.9 mg/24 hours (8s) [39 cm^2; total oxybutynin 36 mg]
Syrup, oral, as chloride: 5 mg/5 mL (5 mL, 473 mL)
Tablet, oral, as chloride: 5 mg
Tablet, extended release, oral, as chloride: 5 mg, 10 mg, 15 mg
  Ditropan XL®: 5 mg, 10 mg, 15 mg

◆ **Oxybutynin Chloride** see Oxybutynin on page 1443
◆ **OXY® Chill Factor® [OTC]** see Salicylic Acid on page 1743

OxyCODONE (oks i KOE done)

Related Information
Opioid Analgesics on page 2122
Patient Information for Disposal of Unused Medications on page 2244

Medication Safety Issues
Sound-alike/look-alike issues:
OxyCODONE may be confused with HYDROcodone, OxyCONTIN®, oxymorphone
OxyCONTIN® may be confused with MS Contin®, oxybutynin
OxyFast® may be confused with Roxanol
Roxicodone® may be confused with Roxanol

High alert medication:
The Institute for Safe Medication Practices (ISMP) includes this medication among its list of drug classes which have a heightened risk of causing significant patient harm when used in error.

Brand Names: U.S. Oxecta™; OxyCONTIN®; Roxicodone®

Brand Names: Canada Oxy.IR®; OxyContin®; OxyNEO™; PMS-Oxycodone; Supeudol®

Index Terms Dihydrohydroxycodeinone; Oxecta™; Oxycodone Hydrochloride

Generic Availability (U.S.) Yes: Excludes controlled release tablet

Pharmacologic Category Analgesic, Opioid

Use Management of moderate-to-severe pain, normally used in combination with nonopioid analgesics

OxyContin® is indicated for around-the-clock management of moderate-to-severe pain when an analgesic is needed for an extended period of time.

Prescribing and Access Restrictions As a requirement of the REMS program, healthcare providers who prescribe OxyContin® need to receive training on the proper use and potential risks of OxyContin®. For training, please refer to http://www.oxycontinrems.com. Prescribers will need retraining every 2 years or following any significant changes to the OxyContin® REMS program.

Medication Guide Available Yes

Contraindications Hypersensitivity to oxycodone or any component of the formulation; significant respiratory depression; hypercarbia; acute or severe bronchial asthma; paralytic ileus (known or suspected)

Warnings/Precautions May cause CNS depression, which may impair physical or mental abilities; patients must be cautioned about performing tasks which require mental alertness (eg, operating machinery or driving). Effects may be potentiated when used with other sedative drugs or ethanol. Use with caution in patients with hypersensitivity reactions to other phenanthrene derivative opioid agonists (morphine, hydrocodone, hydromorphone, levorphanol, oxymorphone), respiratory diseases including asthma, emphysema, or COPD. Use with caution in pancreatitis or biliary tract disease, acute alcoholism (including delirium tremens), morbid obesity, adrenocortical insufficiency, history of seizure disorders, CNS depression/coma, kyphoscoliosis (or other skeletal disorder which may alter respiratory function), hypothyroidism (including myxedema), prostatic hyperplasia, urethral stricture, and toxic psychosis. May obscure diagnosis or clinical course of patients with acute abdominal conditions.

Use with caution in the elderly, debilitated, and hepatic or renal function. Hemodynamic effects (hypotension, orthostasis) may be exaggerated in patients with hypovolemia, concurrent vasodilating drugs, or in patients with head injury. Respiratory depressant effects and capacity to elevate CSF pressure may be exaggerated in presence of head injury, other intracranial lesion, or pre-existing intracranial pressure.

[U.S. Boxed Warning]: Concomitant use with CYP3A4 inhibitors may result in increased effects and potentially fatal respiratory depression. Concurrent use of agonist/antagonist analgesics may precipitate withdrawal symptoms and/or reduced analgesic efficacy in patients following prolonged therapy with mu opioid agonists. Abrupt discontinuation following prolonged use may also lead to withdrawal symptoms. **[U.S. Boxed Warning]: Healthcare provider should be alert to problems of abuse, misuse, and diversion.** Tolerance or drug dependence may result from extended use. Patients should be assessed for risk of abuse or addition prior to therapy and all patients should be monitored for signs of misuse, abuse, and addiction.

Controlled-release formulations: **[U.S. Boxed Warning]: OxyContin® is not intended for use as an "as needed" analgesic or for immediately-postoperative pain management** (should be used postoperatively only if the patient has received it prior to surgery or if severe, persistent pain is anticipated). **[U.S. Boxed Warning]: Do NOT crush, break, or chew controlled-release tablets**; 60 mg and 80 mg strengths, a single dose >40 mg, or a total dose of >80 mg/day are for use only in opioid-tolerant patients. Tablets may be difficult to swallow and could become lodged in throat; patients with swallowing difficulties may be at increased risk. Cases of intestinal obstruction or diverticulitis exacerbation have also been reported, including cases requiring medical intervention to remove the tablet; patients with an underlying GI disease (eg, esophageal cancer, colon cancer) may be at increased risk.

Highly-concentrated oral solutions: **[U.S. Boxed Warning]: Concentrated oral solutions (20 mg/mL) should only be used in opioid tolerant patients (taking ≥30 mg/day of oxycodone or equivalent for ≥1 week); orders should be clearly written to include the intended dose (in mg vs mL) and the intended product concentration to be dispensed.**

Adverse Reactions (Reflective of adult population; not specific for elderly) Note: Percentages as reported with OxyContin®

>10%:
  Central nervous system: Somnolence (23%), dizziness (13%)
  Dermatologic: Pruritus (13%)
  Gastrointestinal: Constipation (23%), nausea (23%), vomiting (12%)
1% to 10%:
  Cardiovascular: Orthostatic hypotension (1% to 5%)
  Central nervous system: Headache (7%), abnormal dreams (1% to 5%), anxiety (1% to 5%), chills (1% to 5%), confusion (1% to 5%), dysphoria (1% to 5%), euphoria (1% to 5%), fever (1% to 5%), insomnia (1% to 5%), nervousness (1% to 5%), thought abnormalities (1% to 5%)
  Dermatologic: Rash (1% to 5%)
  Gastrointestinal: Xerostomia (6%), abdominal pain (1% to 5%), anorexia (1% to 5%), diarrhea (1% to 5%), dyspepsia (1% to 5%), gastritis (1% to 5%)
  Neuromuscular & skeletal: Weakness (6%), twitching (1% to 5%)
  Respiratory: Dyspnea (1% to 5%), hiccups (1% to 5%)
  Miscellaneous: Diaphoresis (5%)

Drug Interactions

Metabolism/Transport Effects Substrate of CYP2D6 (minor), CYP3A4 (major); **Note:** Assignment of Major/Minor substrate status based on clinically relevant drug interaction potential

Avoid Concomitant Use

  Avoid concomitant use of OxyCODONE with any of the following: Azelastine; Azelastine (Nasal); Conivaptan; Methadone; Mirtazapine; Paraldehyde

Increased Effect/Toxicity

  OxyCODONE may increase the levels/effects of: Alcohol (Ethyl); Alvimopan; Azelastine; Azelastine (Nasal); CNS Depressants; Desmopressin; Methadone; Metyrosine; Mirtazapine; Paraldehyde; Selective Serotonin Reuptake Inhibitors; Thiazide Diuretics; Zolpidem

The levels/effects of OxyCODONE may be increased by: Amphetamines; Antipsychotic Agents (Phenothiazines); Conivaptan; CYP3A4 Inhibitors (Moderate); CYP3A4 Inhibitors (Strong); Dasatinib; Droperidol; HydrOXYzine; Ivacaftor; Mifepristone; Succinylcholine; Voriconazole

Decreased Effect

OxyCODONE may decrease the levels/effects of: Pegvisomant

The levels/effects of OxyCODONE may be decreased by: Ammonium Chloride; CYP3A4 Inducers (Strong); Deferasirox; Mixed Agonist / Antagonist Opioids; Rifampin; St Johns Wort; Tocilizumab

Ethanol/Nutrition/Herb Interactions

Ethanol: May increase CNS depression; monitor for increased effects with coadministration. Caution patients about effects.

Herb/Nutraceutical: Avoid valerian, St John's wort, kava kava, gotu kola (may increase CNS depression).

Stability Store at 25°C (77°F); excursions permitted between 15°C to 30°C (59°F to 86°F). Protect from light.

Mechanism of Action Binds to opiate receptors in the CNS, causing inhibition of ascending pain pathways, altering the perception of and response to pain; produces generalized CNS depression

Pharmacodynamics/Kinetics

Onset of action: Pain relief: Immediate release: 10-15 minutes

Peak effect: Immediate release: 0.5-1 hour

Duration: Immediate release: 3-6 hours; Controlled release: ≤12 hours

Distribution: V_d: 2.6 L/kg; distributed to skeletal muscle, liver, intestinal tract, lungs, spleen, and brain

Protein binding: ~45%

Metabolism: Hepatically via CYP3A4 to noroxycodone (has weak analgesic), noroxymorphone, and alpha- and beta-noroxycodol. CYP2D6 mediated metabolism produces oxymorphone (has analgesic activity; low plasma concentrations), alpha- and beta-oxymorphol.

Bioavailability: Controlled release, immediate release: 60% to 87%

Half-life elimination: Immediate release: 2-4 hours; controlled release: ~5 hours

Time to peak, plasma: Immediate release: 1.2-1.9 hours; Controlled release: 4-5 hours

Excretion: Urine (~19% as parent; >64% as metabolites)

Dosage

Geriatric & Adult Management of pain: Oral:

Regular or immediate release formulations: Initial: 5-15 mg every 4-6 hours as needed; dosing range: 5-20 mg/dose (APS 6th edition). For severe chronic pain, administer on a regularly scheduled basis, every 4-6 hours, at the lowest dose that will achieve adequate analgesia.

Controlled release:

Opioid-naïve: 10 mg every 12 hours

Concurrent CNS depressants: Reduce usual dose by $1/3$ to $1/2$

Conversion from transdermal fentanyl: For each 25 mcg/hour transdermal dose, substitute 10 mg controlled release oxycodone every 12 hours; should be initiated 18 hours after the removal of the transdermal fentanyl patch

Currently on opioids: Use standard conversion chart to convert daily dose to oxycodone equivalent. Divide daily dose in 2 (for twice-daily dosing, usually every 12 hours) and round down to nearest dosage form.

Dose adjustment: Doses may be adjusted by changing the total daily dose (not by changing the dosing interval). Doses may be adjusted every 1-2 days and may be increased by 25% to 50%. Dose should be gradually tapered when no longer required in order to prevent withdrawal.

Note: 60 mg and 80 mg strengths, a single dose >40 mg, or a total dose of >80 mg/day are for use only in opioid-tolerant patients.

Multiplication factors for converting the daily dose of current oral opioid to the daily dose of oral oxycodone:

Current opioid mg/day dose x factor = Oxycodone mg/day dose

Codeine mg/day oral dose **x** 0.15 = Oxycodone mg/day dose

Hydrocodone mg/day oral dose **x** 0.9 = Oxycodone mg/day dose

Hydromorphone mg/day oral dose **x** 4 = Oxycodone mg/day dose

Levorphanol mg/day oral dose **x** 7.5 = Oxycodone mg/day dose

Meperidine mg/day oral dose **x** 0.1 = Oxycodone mg/day dose

Methadone mg/day oral dose **x** 1.5 = Oxycodone mg/day dose

Morphine mg/day oral dose **x** 0.5 = Oxycodone mg/day dose

Note: Divide the oxycodone mg/day dose into the appropriate dosing interval for the specific form being used.

Renal Impairment Serum concentrations are increased ~50% in patients with Cl$_{cr}$ <60 mL/minute; adjust dose based on clinical situation.

Hepatic Impairment Reduce dosage in patients with liver disease. Decrease the dose of controlled release tablets to $^1/_3$ to $^1/_2$ the usual starting dose; titrate carefully.

Administration

Controlled release: Do not moisten, crush, break, or chew controlled release tablets. Controlled release tablets are not indicated for rectal administration; increased risk of adverse events due to better rectal absorption. Controlled release tablets should be administered one at a time and each followed with water immediately after placing in the mouth.

Immediate release (Oxecta™): Must be swallowed whole with enough water to ensure complete swallowing immediately after placing in the mouth. The tablet should not be wet prior to placing in the mouth. Do not crush, chew, or dissolve the tablets. Do not administer via feeding tubes (eg, gastric, NG) due to potential for obstruction. The formulation uses technology designed to discourage common methods of tampering to prevent misuse/abuse.

Appropriate laxatives should be administered to avoid the constipating side effects associated with use. Antiemetics may be needed for persistent nausea.

Monitoring Parameters Pain relief, respiratory and mental status, blood pressure; signs of misuse, abuse, and addiction

Reference Range Blood level of 5 mg/L associated with fatality

Test Interactions Some quinolones may produce a false-positive urine screening result for opiates using commercially-available immunoassay kits. This has been demonstrated most consistently for levofloxacin and ofloxacin, but other quinolones have shown cross-reactivity in certain assay kits. Confirmation of positive opiate screens by more specific methods should be considered.

Pharmacotherapy Pearls Oxecta™ utilizes Acura Pharmaceutical's Aversion® technology which may help discourage misuse and abuse potential. Reduced abuse potential of Oxecta™ compared to other immediate-release oxycodone tablet formulations has not been proven; the FDA is requiring Pfizer to complete a post-approval epidemiological study to determine whether the formulation actually results in a decrease of misuse/abuse. In one clinical trial in nondependent recreational opioid users, the "drug-liking" responses and safety of crushed Oxecta™ tablets were compared to crushed immediate-release oxycodone tablets following the self-administered intranasal use. A small difference in "drug-liking" scores was observed, with lower scores reported in the crushed Oxecta™ group. In regards to safety, there was an increased incidence of nasopharyngeal and facial adverse events in the Oxecta™ group. In addition, there was decreased ability in the Oxecta™ group to completely administer the two crushed Oxecta™ tablets intranasally within a set time period. However, whether these differences translate into a significant clinical difference is unknown. Of note, pharmacokinetic studies showed that Oxecta™ is bioequivalent with oxycodone immediate-release tablets with no differences in T$_{max}$ and half-life when administered in the fasted state.

Special Geriatric Considerations The elderly may be particularly susceptible to the CNS depressant and constipating effects of narcotics. Prophylactic use of a laxative should be considered. Serum concentrations at a given dose may also be increased relative to concentrations in younger patients.

Controlled Substance C-II

Dosage Forms Excipient information presented when available (limited, particularly for generics); consult specific product labeling.

Capsule, oral, as hydrochloride: 5 mg

Solution, oral, as hydrochloride: 5 mg/5 mL (5 mL, 500 mL)

Solution, oral, as hydrochloride [concentrate]: 20 mg/mL (30 mL)

Tablet, oral, as hydrochloride: 5 mg, 10 mg, 15 mg, 20 mg, 30 mg
  Oxecta™: 5 mg, 7.5 mg
  Roxicodone®: 5 mg, 15 mg, 30 mg [scored]

Tablet, controlled release, oral, as hydrochloride:
  OxyCONTIN®: 10 mg, 15 mg, 20 mg, 30 mg, 40 mg, 60 mg, 80 mg

---

Oxycodone and Acetaminophen (oks i KOE done & a seet a MIN oh fen)

Related Information

Acetaminophen on page 31

OxyCODONE on page 1446

Medication Safety Issues

Sound-alike/look-alike issues:

Endocet® may be confused with Indocid®

Percocet® may be confused with Fioricet®, Percodan®

Roxicet™ may be confused with Roxanol

Tylox® may be confused with Trimox, Tylenol®, Xanax®

High alert medication:

The Institute for Safe Medication Practices (ISMP) includes this medication among its list of drug classes which have a heightened risk of causing significant patient harm when used in error.

Other safety concerns:

Duplicate therapy issues: This product contains acetaminophen, which may be a component of other combination products. Do not exceed the maximum recommended daily dose of acetaminophen.

Brand Names: U.S. Endocet®; Percocet®; Primlev™; Roxicet™; Roxicet™ 5/500; Tylox®

Brand Names: Canada Endocet®; Novo-Oxycodone Acet; Oxycocet®; Percocet®; Percocet®-Demi; PMS-Oxycodone-Acetaminophen

Index Terms Acetaminophen and Oxycodone

Generic Availability (U.S.) Yes: Excludes caplet and solution

Pharmacologic Category Analgesic Combination (Opioid)

Use Management of moderate-to-severe pain

Contraindications Hypersensitivity to oxycodone, acetaminophen, or any component of the formulation; severe respiratory depression (in absence of resuscitative equipment or ventilatory support)

Warnings/Precautions Use with caution in patients with hypersensitivity reactions to other phenanthrene-derivative opioid agonists (morphine, codeine, hydrocodone, hydromorphone, levorphanol, oxymorphone); respiratory diseases including asthma, emphysema, COPD; severe liver or renal insufficiency; hypothyroidism; Addison's disease; seizure disorder; toxic psychosis; morbid obesity; CNS depression/coma; biliary tract impairment; prostatic hyperplasia; or urethral stricture. May obscure diagnosis or clinical course of patients with acute abdominal conditions. Some preparations contain sulfites which may cause allergic reactions. May be habit-forming. Causes sedation; caution must be used in performing tasks which require alertness (eg, operating machinery or driving). Effects may be potentiated when used with other sedative drugs or ethanol. May cause hypotension. Concurrent use of agonist/antagonist analgesics may precipitate withdrawal symptoms and/or reduced analgesic efficacy in patients following prolonged therapy with mu opioid agonists. Abrupt discontinuation following prolonged use may also lead to withdrawal symptoms.

Use with caution in patients with head injury and increased intracranial pressure (respiratory depressant effects increased and may also elevate CSF pressure).

Enhanced analgesia has been seen in elderly and debilitated patients on therapeutic doses of narcotics. Duration of action may be increased in the elderly. The elderly may be particularly susceptible to the CNS depressant and constipating effects of narcotics.

[U.S. Boxed Warning]: Acetaminophen may cause severe hepatotoxicity, potentially requiring liver transplant or resulting in death; hepatotoxicity is usually associated with excessive acetaminophen intake (>4 g/day). Risk is increased with alcohol use, preexisting liver disease, and intake of more than one source of acetaminophen-containing medications. Chronic daily dosing in adults has also resulted in liver damage in some patients. Hypersensitivity and anaphylactic reactions have been reported with acetaminophen use; discontinue immediately if symptoms of allergic or hypersensitivity reactions occur. Use with caution in patients with known G6PD deficiency.

Adverse Reactions (Reflective of adult population; not specific for elderly) Frequency not defined (also see individual agents): Allergic reaction, constipation, dizziness, dysphoria, euphoria, lightheadedness, nausea, pruritus, respiratory depression, sedation, skin rash, vomiting

Drug Interactions

Metabolism/Transport Effects Refer to individual components.

Avoid Concomitant Use

Avoid concomitant use of Oxycodone and Acetaminophen with any of the following: Azelastine; Azelastine (Nasal); Conivaptan; Methadone; Mirtazapine; Paraldehyde; Pimozide

Increased Effect/Toxicity

Oxycodone and Acetaminophen may increase the levels/effects of: Alcohol (Ethyl); Alvimopan; ARIPiprazole; Azelastine; Azelastine (Nasal); Busulfan; CNS Depressants; Dasatinib; Desmopressin; Imatinib; Methadone; Metyrosine; Mirtazapine; Paraldehyde; Pimozide; Prilocaine; Selective Serotonin Reuptake Inhibitors; SORAfenib; Thiazide Diuretics; Vitamin K Antagonists; Zolpidem

The levels/effects of Oxycodone and Acetaminophen may be increased by: Amphetamines; Antipsychotic Agents (Phenothiazines); Conivaptan; CYP3A4 Inhibitors (Moderate);

CYP3A4 Inhibitors (Strong); Dasatinib; Droperidol; HydrOXYzine; Imatinib; Isoniazid; Ivacaftor; Metyrapone; Mifepristone; Probenecid; SORAfenib; Succinylcholine; Voriconazole

Decreased Effect

Oxycodone and Acetaminophen may decrease the levels/effects of: Pegvisomant

The levels/effects of Oxycodone and Acetaminophen may be decreased by: Ammonium Chloride; Anticonvulsants (Hydantoin); Barbiturates; CarBAMazepine; Cholestyramine Resin; CYP3A4 Inducers (Strong); Deferasirox; Mixed Agonist / Antagonist Opioids; Peginterferon Alfa-2b; Rifampin; St Johns Wort; Tocilizumab

Ethanol/Nutrition/Herb Interactions Ethanol: Excessive intake of ethanol may increase the risk of acetaminophen-induced hepatotoxicity. Avoid ethanol or limit to <3 drinks/day. Ethanol may also increase CNS depression; monitor for increased effects with co-administration. Caution patients about effects.

Stability Store at controlled room temperature of 20°C to 25°C (68°F to 77°F). Protect from moisture.

Mechanism of Action

Oxycodone, as with other narcotic (opiate) analgesics, blocks pain perception in the cerebral cortex by binding to specific receptor molecules (opiate receptors) within the neuronal membranes of synapses. This binding results in a decreased synaptic chemical transmission throughout the CNS thus inhibiting the flow of pain sensations into the higher centers. Mu and kappa are the two subtypes of the opiate receptor to which oxycodone binds to cause analgesia.

Acetaminophen inhibits the synthesis of prostaglandins in the CNS and peripherally blocks pain impulse generation; produces antipyresis from inhibition of hypothalamic heat-regulating center.

Pharmacodynamics/Kinetics See individual agents.

Dosage

Geriatric Doses should be titrated to appropriate analgesic effects: Oral: Initial dose, **based on oxycodone content:** 2.5-5 mg every 6 hours. Do not exceed 4 g/day of acetaminophen.

Adult

Note: Initial dose is based on the **oxycodone** content; however, the maximum daily dose is based on the **acetaminophen** content.

Management of pain: Doses should be given every 4-6 hours as needed and titrated to appropriate analgesic effects.

Maximum daily dose, based on acetaminophen content: Oral: 4 g/day.

Mild-to-moderate pain: Oral: Initial dose, **based on oxycodone content:** 2.5-5 mg

Severe pain: Oral: Initial dose, **based on oxycodone content:** 10-30 mg

Hepatic Impairment Dose should be reduced in patients with severe liver disease.

Monitoring Parameters Monitor for pain relief, respiratory and mental status, blood pressure, constipation

Test Interactions See individual agents.

Special Geriatric Considerations The elderly may be particularly susceptible to the CNS depressant and constipating effects of narcotics. Prophylactic use of a laxative should be considered.

Controlled Substance C-II

Dosage Forms Excipient information presented when available (limited, particularly for generics); consult specific product labeling.

Caplet:

Roxicet™ 5/500: Oxycodone hydrochloride 5 mg and acetaminophen 500 mg

Capsule: 5/500: Oxycodone hydrochloride 5 mg and acetaminophen 500 mg

Tylox®: 5/500: Oxycodone hydrochloride 5 mg and acetaminophen 500 mg [contains sodium benzoate and sodium metabisulfite]

Solution, oral:

Roxicet™: Oxycodone hydrochloride 5 mg and acetaminophen 325 mg per 5 mL (5 mL, 500 mL) [contains ethanol <0.5%; mint flavor]

Tablet: 2.5/325: Oxycodone hydrochloride 2.5 mg and acetaminophen 325 mg; 5/325: Oxycodone hydrochloride 5 mg and acetaminophen 325 mg; 7.5/325: Oxycodone hydrochloride 7.5 mg and acetaminophen 325 mg; 7.5/500: Oxycodone hydrochloride 7.5 mg and acetaminophen 500 mg; 10/325: Oxycodone hydrochloride 10 mg and acetaminophen 325 mg; 10/650: Oxycodone hydrochloride 10 mg and acetaminophen 650 mg

Endocet® 5/325 [scored]: Oxycodone hydrochloride 5 mg and acetaminophen 325 mg

Endocet® 7.5/325: Oxycodone hydrochloride 7.5 mg and acetaminophen 325 mg

Endocet® 7.5/500: Oxycodone hydrochloride 7.5 mg and acetaminophen 500 mg

Endocet® 10/325: Oxycodone hydrochloride 10 mg and acetaminophen 325 mg

Endocet® 10/650: Oxycodone hydrochloride 10 mg and acetaminophen 650 mg

Percocet® 2.5/325: Oxycodone hydrochloride 2.5 mg and acetaminophen 325 mg

Percocet® 5/325 [scored]: Oxycodone hydrochloride 5 mg and acetaminophen 325 mg

Percocet® 7.5/325: Oxycodone hydrochloride 7.5 mg and acetaminophen 325 mg
Percocet® 7.5/500: Oxycodone hydrochloride 7.5 mg and acetaminophen 500 mg
Percocet® 10/325: Oxycodone hydrochloride 10 mg and acetaminophen 325 mg
Percocet® 10/650: Oxycodone hydrochloride 10 mg and acetaminophen 650 mg
Primlev™ 5/300: Oxycodone hydrochloride 5 mg and acetaminophen 300 mg
Primlev™ 7.5/300: Oxycodone hydrochloride 7.5 mg and acetaminophen 300 mg
Primlev™ 10/300: Oxycodone hydrochloride 10 mg and acetaminophen 300 mg
Roxicet™ [scored]: Oxycodone hydrochloride 5 mg and acetaminophen 325 mg

Oxycodone and Aspirin (oks i KOE done & AS pir in)

Related Information
Aspirin on page 154
OxyCODONE on page 1446
Medication Safety Issues
Sound-alike/look-alike issues:
Percodan® may be confused with Decadron, Percocet®, Percogesic®, Periactin
High alert medication:
The Institute for Safe Medication Practices (ISMP) includes this medication among its list of drug classes which have a heightened risk of causing significant patient harm when used in error.
Brand Names: U.S. Endodan®; Percodan®
Brand Names: Canada Endodan®; Oxycodan®; Percodan®
Index Terms Aspirin and Oxycodone
Generic Availability (U.S.) Yes
Pharmacologic Category Analgesic Combination (Opioid)
Use Management of moderate- to moderately-severe pain
Dosage
Geriatric & Adult Analgesic: Oral: One tablet every 6 hours as needed for pain; maximum aspirin dose should not exceed 4 g/day.
Renal Impairment Use with caution. Avoid use of aspirin in patients with Cl_{cr} <10 mL/minute.
Hepatic Impairment Use with caution. Avoid use of aspirin-containing products in severe impairment.
Special Geriatric Considerations See individual agents.
Controlled Substance C-II
Dosage Forms Excipient information presented when available (limited, particularly for generics); consult specific product labeling.
Tablet: Oxycodone hydrochloride 4.8355 mg and aspirin 325 mg
Endodan®, Percodan®: Oxycodone hydrochloride 4.8355 mg and aspirin 325 mg

♦ **Oxycodone Hydrochloride** see OxyCODONE on page 1446
♦ **OxyCONTIN®** see OxyCODONE on page 1446
♦ **OXY® Daily [OTC]** see Salicylic Acid on page 1743
♦ **OXY® Daily Cleansing [OTC]** see Salicylic Acid on page 1743
♦ **OXY® Face Wash [OTC]** see Salicylic Acid on page 1743
♦ **OXY® Maximum [OTC]** see Salicylic Acid on page 1743
♦ **OXY® Maximum Daily Cleansing [OTC]** see Salicylic Acid on page 1743

Oxymetazoline (Nasal) (oks i met AZ oh leen)

Medication Safety Issues
Sound-alike/look-alike issues:
Oxymetazoline may be confused with oxymetholone
Afrin® may be confused with aspirin
Afrin® (oxymetazoline) may be confused with Afrin® (saline)
Neo-Synephrine® (oxymetazoline) may be confused with Neo-Synephrine® (phenylephrine, nasal)
Brand Names: U.S. 12 Hour Nasal Relief [OTC]; 4-Way® 12 Hour [OTC]; Afrin® Extra Moisturizing [OTC]; Afrin® Original [OTC]; Afrin® Severe Congestion [OTC]; Afrin® Sinus [OTC]; Dristan® [OTC]; Duramist Plus [OTC]; Neo-Synephrine® Nighttime12-Hour [OTC]; Nostrilla® [OTC]; NRS® [OTC]; Vicks® Sinex® VapoSpray 12-Hour; Vicks® Sinex® VapoSpray 12-Hour UltraFine Mist [OTC]; Vicks® Sinex® VapoSpray Moisturizing 12-Hour UltraFine Mist [OTC]
Brand Names: Canada Claritin® Allergic Decongestant; Dristan® Long Lasting Nasal; Drixoral® Nasal

Index Terms Oxymetazoline Hydrochloride

Generic Availability (U.S.) Yes: Intranasal solution (spray)

Pharmacologic Category Adrenergic Agonist Agent; Decongestant; Imidazoline Derivative

Use Adjunctive therapy for nasal congestion, associated with acute or chronic rhinitis, the common cold, sinusitis, hay fever, or other allergies

Dosage

Geriatric & Adult Nasal congestion: Intranasal: Instill 2-3 sprays into each nostril twice daily for ≤3 days

Special Geriatric Considerations Evaluate the patient's or caregiver's ability to safely administer the correct dose of nasal medication. Use with caution in patients with cardiovascular disease.

Dosage Forms Excipient information presented when available (limited, particularly for generics); consult specific product labeling.

Solution, intranasal, as hydrochloride [mist]:

Afrin® Original: 0.05% (15 mL) [contains benzalkonium chloride]

Vicks® Sinex® VapoSpray 12-Hour UltraFine Mist: 0.05% (15 mL) [contains benzalkonium chloride, menthol]

Vicks® Sinex® VapoSpray Moisturizing 12-Hour UltraFine Mist: 0.05% (15 mL) [contains aloe, benzalkonium chloride]

Solution, intranasal, as hydrochloride [mist/no drip formula]:

Afrin® Extra Moisturizing: 0.05% (15 mL) [contains benzyl alcohol, glycerin]

Afrin® Original: 0.05% (15 mL) [contains benzalkonium chloride, benzyl alcohol]

Afrin® Severe Congestion: 0.05% (15 mL) [contains benzalkonium chloride, benzyl alcohol, camphor, menthol]

Afrin® Sinus: 0.05% (15 mL) [contains benzalkonium chloride, benzyl alcohol, camphor, menthol]

Solution, intranasal, as hydrochloride [spray]: 0.05% (15 mL, 30 mL)

12 Hour Nasal Relief: 0.05% (15 mL, 30 mL)

4-Way® 12 Hour: 0.05% (15 mL) [contains benzalkonium chloride]

Afrin® Extra Moisturizing: 0.05% (15 mL) [contains benzalkonium chloride, glycerin]

Afrin® Original: 0.05% (15 mL, 30 mL) [contains benzalkonium chloride]

Afrin® Severe Congestion: 0.05% (15 mL) [contains benzalkonium chloride, benzyl alcohol, camphor, menthol]

Afrin® Sinus: 0.05% (15 mL) [contains benzalkonium chloride, benzyl alcohol, camphor, menthol]

Dristan®: 0.05% (15 mL) [contains benzalkonium chloride, benzyl alcohol]

Duramist Plus: 0.05% (15 mL) [contains benzalkonium chloride]

Neo-Synephrine® Nighttime12-Hour: 0.05% (15 mL) [contains benzalkonium chloride, glycerin]

Nostrilla®: 0.05% (15 mL) [contains benzalkonium chloride]

NRS®: 0.05% (15 mL, 30 mL) [contains benzalkonium chloride]

Vicks® Sinex® VapoSpray 12-Hour: 0.05% (15 mL) [contains benzalkonium chloride]

Oxymetazoline (Ophthalmic) (oks i met AZ oh leen)

Medication Safety Issues

Sound-alike/look-alike issues:

Oxymetazoline may be confused with oxymetholone

Visine® may be confused with Visken®

Brand Names: U.S. Visine® L.R.® [OTC]

Index Terms Oxymetazoline Hydrochloride

Pharmacologic Category Vasoconstrictor

Use Relief of redness of eye due to minor eye irritations

Dosage

Geriatric & Adult Relief of eye redness: Ophthalmic: Instill 1-2 drops in affected eye(s) every 6 hours as needed or as directed by healthcare provider for ≤72 hours

Special Geriatric Considerations Evaluate the patient's or caregiver's ability to safely administer the correct dose of ophthalmic medication.

Dosage Forms Excipient information presented when available (limited, particularly for generics); consult specific product labeling.

Solution, ophthalmic, as hydrochloride [drops]:

Visine® L.R.®: 0.025% (15 mL, 30 mL) [contains benzalkonium chloride]

◆ **Oxymetazoline Hydrochloride** see Oxymetazoline (Nasal) *on page 1452*

◆ **Oxymetazoline Hydrochloride** see Oxymetazoline (Ophthalmic) *on page 1453*

Oxymorphone (oks i MOR fone)

Related Information
Opioid Analgesics *on page* 2122
Patient Information for Disposal of Unused Medications *on page* 2244

Medication Safety Issues
Sound-alike/look-alike issues:
Oxymorphone may be confused with oxycodone, oxymetholone

High alert medication:
The Institute for Safe Medication Practices (ISMP) includes this medication among its list of drug classes which have a heightened risk of causing significant patient harm when used in error.

Brand Names: U.S. Opana®; Opana® ER

Index Terms Oxymorphone Hydrochloride

Generic Availability (U.S.) Yes: Excludes injection solution

Pharmacologic Category Analgesic, Opioid

Use
Parenteral: Management of moderate-to-severe acute pain; relief of anxiety in patients with dyspnea associated with pulmonary edema secondary to acute left ventricular failure
Oral, regular release: Management of moderate-to-severe acute pain
Oral, extended release: Management of moderate-to-severe pain in patients requiring around-the-clock opioid treatment for an extended period of time

Medication Guide Available Yes

Contraindications Hypersensitivity to oxymorphone, other morphine analogs (phenanthrene derivatives), or any component of the formulation; paralytic ileus (known or suspected); moderate-to-severe hepatic impairment; severe respiratory depression (unless in monitored setting with resuscitative equipment); acute/severe bronchial asthma; hypercarbia
Note: Injection formulation is also contraindicated in the treatment of upper airway obstruction and pulmonary edema due to a chemical respiratory irritant.

Warnings/Precautions An opioid-containing analgesic regimen should be tailored to each patient's needs and based upon the type of pain being treated (acute versus chronic), the route of administration, degree of tolerance for opioids (naive versus chronic user), age, weight, and patient comorbidities. The optimal analgesic dose varies widely among patients. Doses should be titrated to pain relief/prevention.

May cause CNS depression, which may impair physical or mental abilities; patients must be cautioned about performing tasks which require mental alertness (eg, operating machinery or driving). Effects may be potentiated when used with other sedative drugs or ethanol. Use not recommended within 14 days of MAO inhibitors. Use with caution in patients with hypersensitivity reactions to other phenanthrene-derivative opioid agonists (codeine, hydrocodone, hydromorphone, levorphanol, oxycodone). May cause respiratory depression. Use extreme caution in patients with COPD or other chronic respiratory conditions characterized by hypoxia, hypercapnia, or diminished respiratory reserve (myxedema, cor pulmonale, kypho-scoliosis, obstructive sleep apnea, severe obesity). Use with caution in patients (particularly elderly or debilitated) with impaired respiratory function, adrenal disease, morbid obesity, seizure disorders, toxic psychosis, thyroid dysfunction, prostatic hyperplasia, or renal impairment. Use caution in mild hepatic dysfunction; use is contraindicated in moderate-to-severe hepatic impairment. Use only with extreme caution (if at all) in patients with head injury or increased intracranial pressure (ICP); potential to elevate ICP and/or blunt papillary response may be greatly exaggerated in these patients. Use with caution in biliary tract disease or acute pancreatitis (may cause constriction of sphincter of Oddi). May obscure diagnosis or clinical course of patients with acute abdominal conditions.

Oxymorphone shares the toxic potential of opiate agonists and usual precautions of opiate agonist therapy should be observed; may cause hypotension in patients with acute myocardial infarction, volume depletion, or concurrent drug therapy which may exaggerate vasodilation. The elderly may be particularly susceptible to adverse effects of narcotics.

[U.S. Boxed Warning]: Healthcare provider should be alert to problems of abuse, misuse, and diversion. Tolerance or drug dependence may result from extended use. Use caution in patients with a history of drug dependence or abuse. Abrupt discontinuation may precipitate withdrawal syndrome.

Extended release formulation:

[U.S. Boxed Warnings]: Opana® ER is an extended release oral formulation of oxy-morphone and is not suitable for use as an "as needed" analgesic. Tablets should not be broken, chewed, dissolved, or crushed; tablets should be swallowed whole. Opana® ER is intended for use in long-term, continuous management of moderate-to-severe chronic pain. It is not indicated for use in the immediate postoperative period (12-24 hours). [U.S. Boxed Warning: The coingestion of ethanol or ethanol-containing medications with Opana® ER may result in accelerated release of drug from the dosage form, abruptly increasing plasma levels, which may have fatal consequences.

Adverse Reactions (Reflective of adult population; not specific for elderly) Inci-dence usually on higher end with extended release tablet.

>10%:

Central nervous system: Somnolence (9% to 19%), dizziness (7% to 18%), fever (1% to 14%), headache (7% to 12%)

Dermatologic: Pruritus (8% to 15%)

Gastrointestinal: Nausea (19% to 33%), constipation (4% to 28%), vomiting (9% to 16%)

1% to 10%:

Cardiovascular: Hypotension (<10%), tachycardia (<10%), edema (<10%), flushing (<10%), hypertension (<10%)

Central nervous system: Anxiety (1% to <10%), sedation (1% to <10%), depression (<10%), disorientation (<10%), lethargy (<10%), nervousness (<10%), restlessness (<10%), fatigue (≤4%), insomnia (≤4%), confusion (3%)

Endocrine & metabolic: Dehydration (<10%)

Gastrointestinal: Abdominal distension (<10%), flatulence (1% to <10%), xerostomia (1% to <10%), dyspepsia (<10%), weight loss (<10%), diarrhea (≤4%), abdominal pain (≤3%), appetite decreased (≤3%)

Neuromuscular & skeletal: Weakness (<10%)

Ocular: Blurred vision (<10%)

Respiratory: Hypoxia (<10%), dyspnea (<10%)

Miscellaneous: Diaphoresis (1% to <10%)

Drug Interactions

Metabolism/Transport Effects None known.

Avoid Concomitant Use

Avoid concomitant use of Oxymorphone with any of the following: Azelastine; Azelastine (Nasal); MAO Inhibitors; Methadone; Mirtazapine; Paraldehyde

Increased Effect/Toxicity

Oxymorphone may increase the levels/effects of: Alcohol (Ethyl); Alvimopan; Azelastine; Azelastine (Nasal); CNS Depressants; Desmopressin; MAO Inhibitors; Methadone; Metyr-osine; Mirtazapine; Paraldehyde; Selective Serotonin Reuptake Inhibitors; Thiazide Diu-retics; Zolpidem

The levels/effects of Oxymorphone may be increased by: Amphetamines; Antipsychotic Agents (Phenothiazines); Droperidol; HydrOXYzine; Succinylcholine

Decreased Effect

Oxymorphone may decrease the levels/effects of: Pegvisomant

The levels/effects of Oxymorphone may be decreased by: Ammonium Chloride; Mixed Agonist / Antagonist Opioids

Ethanol/Nutrition/Herb Interactions

Ethanol: Ethanol ingestion with extended-release tablets is specifically contraindicated due to possible accelerated release and potentially fatal overdose. Ethanol may also increase CNS depression; monitor for increased effects with coadministration. Caution patients about effects.

Food: When taken orally with a high-fat meal, peak concentration is 38% to 50% greater. Both immediate-release and extended-release tablets should be taken 1 hour before or 2 hours after eating.

Herb/Nutraceutical: Avoid valerian, St John's wort, kava kava, gotu kola (may increase CNS depression).

Stability Injection solution, tablet: Store at 25°C (77°F); excursions permitted to 15°C to 30°C (59°F to 86°F). Protect injection from light.

Mechanism of Action Oxymorphone hydrochloride is a potent narcotic analgesic with uses similar to those of morphine. The drug is a semisynthetic derivative of morphine (phenan-threne derivative) and is closely related to hydromorphone chemically (Dilaudid®).

Pharmacodynamics/Kinetics

Onset of action: Parenteral: 5-10 minutes

Duration: Analgesic: Parenteral: 3-6 hours

Distribution: V_d: I.V.: 1.94-4.22 L/kg

Protein binding: 10% to 12%

Metabolism: Hepatic via glucuronidation to active and inactive metabolites

Bioavailability: Oral: ~10%

Half-life elimination: Oral: Immediate release: 7-9 hours; Extended release: 9-11 hours

Excretion: Urine (<1% as unchanged drug); feces

Dosage

Geriatric Refer to adult dosing. **Note:** Initiate dosing at the lower end of the dosage range.

Adult Analgesia: **Note:** Dosage must be individualized.

I.M., SubQ: Initial: 1-1.5 mg; may repeat every 4-6 hours as needed

I.V.: Initial: 0.5 mg

Oral:

Immediate release:

Opioid-naive: 10-20 mg every 4-6 hours as needed. Initial dosages as low as 5 mg may be considered in selected patients and/or patients with renal impairment. Dosage adjustment should be based on level of analgesia, side effects, pain intensity, and patient comorbidities. Initiation of therapy with initial dose >20 mg is **not** recommended. **Note:** The American Pain Society recommends an initial dose of 5-10 mg for adult patients with severe pain.

Currently on stable dose of parenteral oxymorphone: ~10 times the daily parenteral requirement. The calculated amount should be divided and given in 4-6 equal doses.

Currently on other opioids: Use standard conversion chart to convert daily dose to oxymorphone equivalent. Generally start with 1/2 the calculated daily oxymorphone dosage and administered in divided doses every 4-6 hours.

Extended release (Opana® ER):

Opioid-naive: Initial: 5 mg every 12 hours. Supplemental doses of immediate-release oxymorphone may be used as "rescue" medication as dosage is titrated.

Note: Continued requirement for supplemental dosing may be used to titrate the dose of extended-release continuous therapy. Adjust therapy incrementally, by 5-10 mg every 12 hours at intervals of every 3-7 days. Ideally, scheduled (basal) dosage may be titrated to generally mild pain or no pain with the regular use of fewer than 2 supplemental doses per 24 hours.

Currently on stable dose of parenteral oxymorphone: Approximately 10 times the daily parenteral requirement. The calculated amount should be given in 2 divided doses (for every 12-hour oxymorphone extended release dosing).

Currently on opioids: Use conversion chart (see **"Note"**) to convert daily dose of current opioid to oxymorphone equivalent. Generally start with 1/2 the calculated daily oxymorphone dosage. Divide daily dose in 2 (for every 12-hour oxymorphone extended release dosing) and round down to nearest dosage strength. **Note:** Per manufacturer, the following approximate oral dosages are equivalent to a daily dose of oxymorphone 10 mg:

Hydrocodone 20 mg

Oxycodone 20 mg

Methadone 20 mg (methadone has a long half-life and accumulates; ratio can vary widely)

Morphine 30 mg

Conversion of stable dose of immediate-release oxymorphone to extended-release oxymorphone (Opana®): Administer 1/2 of the daily dose of immediate-release oxymorphone (Opana®) as the extended-release formulation (Opana® ER) every 12 hours

Renal Impairment Cl$_{cr}$ <50 mL/minute: Reduce initial dosage of oral formulations (bioavailability increased 57% to 65%). Begin therapy at lowest dose and titrate carefully.

Hepatic Impairment Generally, contraindicated for use in patients with moderate-to-severe liver disease. Initiate with lowest possible dose and titrate slowly in mild impairment.

Administration Administer immediate release and extended release tablets 1 hour before or 2 hours after eating. Opana® ER tablet should be swallowed; do not break, crush, or chew.

Monitoring Parameters Respiratory rate, heart rate, blood pressure, CNS activity

Test Interactions Some quinolones may produce a false-positive urine screening result for opiates using commercially-available immunoassay kits. This has been demonstrated most consistently for levofloxacin and ofloxacin, but other quinolones have shown cross-reactivity in certain assay kits. Confirmation of positive opiate screens by more specific methods should be considered. May cause elevation in amylase (due to constriction of the sphincter of Oddi).

Special Geriatric Considerations Elderly may be particularly susceptible to the CNS depressant and constipating effects of narcotics. Plasma levels of oxymorphone were about 40% higher in elderly patients as compared to younger patients.

Controlled Substance C-II

Dosage Forms Excipient information presented when available (limited, particularly for generics); consult specific product labeling.

Injection, solution, as hydrochloride:
Opana®: 1 mg/mL (1 mL)
Tablet, oral, as hydrochloride: 5 mg, 10 mg
Opana®: 5 mg, 10 mg
Tablet, extended release, oral, as hydrochloride: 7.5 mg, 15 mg
Opana® ER: 5 mg, 10 mg, 20 mg, 30 mg, 40 mg

♦ **Oxymorphone Hydrochloride** *see* Oxymorphone *on page 1454*
♦ **OXY® Post-Shave [OTC]** *see* Salicylic Acid *on page 1743*
♦ **OXY® Spot Treatment [OTC]** *see* Salicylic Acid *on page 1743*
♦ **Oxytrol®** *see* Oxybutynin *on page 1443*
♦ **Oysco D [OTC]** *see* Calcium and Vitamin D *on page 261*
♦ **Oysco 500 [OTC]** *see* Calcium Carbonate *on page 262*
♦ **Oysco 500+D [OTC]** *see* Calcium and Vitamin D *on page 261*
♦ **Oyst-Cal-D 500 [OTC]** *see* Calcium and Vitamin D *on page 261*
♦ **Oystercal™ 500 [OTC]** *see* Calcium Carbonate *on page 262*
♦ **Ozurdex®** *see* Dexamethasone (Ophthalmic) *on page 521*
♦ **P-071** *see* Cetirizine *on page 346*
♦ **Pacerone®** *see* Amiodarone *on page 96*
♦ **Pain Eze [OTC]** *see* Acetaminophen *on page 31*
♦ **Pain & Fever Children's [OTC]** *see* Acetaminophen *on page 31*

Paliperidone (pal ee PER i done)

Related Information
Antipsychotic Agents *on page 2103*
Atypical Antipsychotics *on page 2107*
Beers Criteria – Potentially Inappropriate Medications for Geriatrics *on page 2183*
Medication Safety Issues
BEERS Criteria medication:
This drug may be potentially inappropriate for use in geriatric patients (Quality of evidence - moderate; Strength of recommendation - strong).
Brand Names: U.S. Invega®; Invega® Sustenna®
Brand Names: Canada Invega®; Invega® Sustenna®
Index Terms 9-hydroxy-risperidone; 9-OH-risperidone; Paliperidone Palmitate
Generic Availability (U.S.) No
Pharmacologic Category Antipsychotic Agent, Atypical
Use
Oral: Acute and maintenance treatment of schizophrenia; acute treatment of schizoaffective disorder (monotherapy or adjunctive therapy to mood stabilizers and/or antidepressants)
Injection: Acute and maintenance treatment of schizophrenia
Unlabeled Use Psychosis/agitation related to Alzheimer's dementia
Contraindications Hypersensitivity to paliperidone, risperidone, or any component of the formulation
Warnings/Precautions [U.S. Boxed Warning]: Elderly patients with dementia-related psychosis treated with antipsychotics are at an increased risk of death compared to placebo. Most deaths appeared to be either cardiovascular (eg, heart failure, sudden death) or infectious (eg, pneumonia) in nature. In addition, an increased incidence of cerebrovascular adverse effects (eg, transient ischemic attack, cerebrovascular accidents) has been reported in studies of placebo-controlled trials of risperidone (paliperidone is the primary active metabolite of risperidone) in elderly patients with dementia-related psychosis. Paliperidone is not approved for the treatment of dementia-related psychosis.

Compared with risperidone, paliperidone is low to moderately sedating; use with caution in disorders where CNS depression is a feature. Use caution in patients with predisposition to seizures. Use with caution in renal dysfunction; dose reduction recommended. Esophageal dysmotility and aspiration have been associated with antipsychotic use; use with caution in patients at risk of aspiration pneumonia (eg, Alzheimer's disease).

Leukopenia, neutropenia, and agranulocytosis (sometimes fatal) have been reported in clinical trials and postmarketing reports with antipsychotic use; presence of risk factors (eg, pre-existing low WBC or history of drug-induced leuko-/neutropenia) should prompt periodic blood count assessment. Discontinue therapy at first signs of blood dyscrasias or if absolute neutrophil count <1000/mm^3.

Paliperidone is associated with increased prolactin levels; clinical significance of hyperprolactinemia in patients with breast cancer or other prolactin-dependent tumors is unknown. May alter temperature regulation. May mask toxicity of other drugs or conditions (eg intestinal obstruction, Reye's syndrome, brain tumor) due to antiemetic effects. Priapism has been reported rarely with use.

May cause orthostasis and syncope. Use with caution in patients with cardiovascular diseases (eg, heart failure, history of myocardial infarction or ischemia, cerebrovascular disease, conduction abnormalities). Use caution in patients receiving medications for hypertension (orthostatic effects may be exacerbated) or in patients with hypovolemia or dehydration. May alter cardiac conduction; life-threatening arrhythmias have occurred with therapeutic doses of neuroleptics. Avoid use in combination with QT_c-prolonging drugs. Avoid use in patients with congenital long QT syndrome and in patients with history of cardiac arrhythmia.

May cause extrapyramidal symptoms (EPS), including pseudoparkinsonism, acute dystonic reactions, akathisia, and tardive dyskinesia (risk of these reactions is low relative to other neuroleptics, and is dose dependent). Risk of dystonia (and probably other EPS) may be greater with increased doses, use of conventional antipsychotics, males, and younger patients. Risk of neuroleptic malignant syndrome (NMS) may be increased in patients with Parkinson's disease or Lewy body dementia; monitor for symptoms of confusion, obtundation, postural instability and extrapyramidal symptoms. May cause hyperglycemia; in some cases may be extreme and associated with ketoacidosis, hyperosmolar coma, or death. Use with caution in patients with diabetes (or risk factors) or other disorders of glucose regulation; monitor for worsening of glucose control. Significant weight gain has been observed with antipsychotic therapy; incidence varies with product. Monitor waist circumference and BMI. May cause lipid abnormalities (LDL and triglycerides increased; HDL decreased).

The possibility of a suicide attempt is inherent in psychotic illness or bipolar disorder; use caution in high-risk patients during initiation of therapy. Prescriptions should be written for the smallest quantity consistent with good patient care.

Use in elderly patients with dementia is associated with an increased risk of mortality and cerebrovascular accidents; avoid antipsychotic use for behavioral problems associated with dementia unless alternative nonpharmacologic therapies have failed and patient may harm self or others. In addition, use may cause or exacerbate syndrome of inappropriate antidiuretic hormone secretion or hyponatremia; monitor sodium closely with initiation or dosage adjustments in older adults (Beers Criteria).

The tablet formulation consists of drug within a nonabsorbable shell that is expelled and may be visible in the stool. Use is not recommended in patients with pre-existing severe gastrointestinal narrowing disorders. Patients with upper GI tract alterations in transit time may have increased or decreased bioavailability of paliperidone. Do not use in patients unable to swallow the tablet whole.

Adverse Reactions (Reflective of adult population; not specific for elderly) Unless otherwise noted, frequency of adverse effects is reported for the oral/I.M. formulation in adults.

>10%:

Cardiovascular: Tachycardia (1% to 14%)

Central nervous system: EPS (≤26%; dose dependent), insomnia (10% to 15%), headache (6% to 15%), parkinsonism (3% to 14%; dose dependent), somnolence (adolescents 9% to 26%; adults 1% to 12%; dose dependent)

Neuromuscular & skeletal: Tremor (2% to 12%)

3% to 10%:

Cardiovascular: Orthostatic hypotension (1% to 4%; dose dependent), bundle branch block (≤3%)

Central nervous system: Agitation (4% to 10%), akathisia (adolescents 4% to 17%; adults 1% to 10%; dose dependent), anxiety (adolescents ≤9%; adults 3% to 8%), dizziness (1% to 6%), dystonia (1% to 5%; dose dependent), dysarthria (1% to 4%; dose dependent), fatigue (adolescents ≤4%), sleep disorder (≤3%), lethargy (adolescents ≤3%)

Endocrine & metabolic: Amenorrhea (adolescents ≤6%), galactorrhea (adolescents ≤4%), gynecomastia (adolescents ≤3%)

Gastrointestinal: Weight gain (1% to 9%; dose dependent), nausea (2% to 8%), dyspepsia (5% to 6%), vomiting (adolescents ≤11%; adults 2% to 5%), constipation (1% to 5%), salivation increased (adolescents ≤6%; adults ≤4%; dose dependent), appetite increased (2% to 3%), toothache (1% to 3%), abdominal pain (≤3%), diarrhea (≤3%), xerostomia (≤3%); tongue swelling (adolescents ≤3%), tongue paralysis (adolescents ≤3%)

Local: I.M. formulation: Injection site reaction (≤10%)

Neuromuscular & skeletal: Hyperkinesia (2% to 10% dose dependent), dyskinesia (1% to 9%), weakness (≤4%), myalgia (≤4% dose dependent), back pain (1% to 3%), extremity pain (≤3%)

Ocular: Blurred vision (adolescents ≤3%)

Respiratory: Nasopharyngitis (≤5%; dose dependent), upper respiratory tract infection (1% to 4%), cough (≤3%; dose dependent), rhinitis (1% to 3%; dose dependent)

Drug Interactions

Metabolism/Transport Effects Substrate of P-glycoprotein

Avoid Concomitant Use

Avoid concomitant use of Paliperidone with any of the following: Azelastine; Azelastine (Nasal); Highest Risk QTc-Prolonging Agents; Metoclopramide; Mifepristone; Moderate Risk QTc-Prolonging Agents; Paraldehyde

Increased Effect/Toxicity

Paliperidone may increase the levels/effects of: Alcohol (Ethyl); Azelastine; Azelastine (Nasal); Buprenorphine; CNS Depressants; Highest Risk QTc-Prolonging Agents; Methylphenidate; Paraldehyde; Serotonin Modulators; Zolpidem

The levels/effects of Paliperidone may be increased by: Acetylcholinesterase Inhibitors (Central); Divalproex; HydrOXYzine; Itraconazole; Lithium formulations; Methylphenidate; Metoclopramide; Metyrosine; Mifepristone; Moderate Risk QTc-Prolonging Agents; P-glycoprotein/ABCB1 Inhibitors; QTc-Prolonging Agents (Indeterminate Risk and Risk Modifying); RisperiDONE; Tetrabenazine; Valproic Acid

Decreased Effect

Paliperidone may decrease the levels/effects of: Amphetamines; Anti-Parkinson's Agents (Dopamine Agonist); Quinagolide

The levels/effects of Paliperidone may be decreased by: CarBAMazepine; Lithium formulations; P-glycoprotein/ABCB1 Inducers

Ethanol/Nutrition/Herb Interactions

Ethanol: May increase CNS depression; monitor for increased effects with coadministration. Caution patients about effects.

Herb/Nutraceutical: Avoid kava kava, gotu kola, valerian, St John's wort (may increase CNS depression).

Stability Store at controlled room temperature of ≤25°C (77°F); excursions permitted to 15°C to 30°C (59°F to 86°F). Protect tablets from moisture.

Mechanism of Action Paliperidone is considered a benzisoxazole atypical antipsychotic as it is the primary active metabolite of risperidone. As with other atypical antipsychotics, its therapeutic efficacy is believed to result from mixed central serotonergic and dopaminergic antagonism. The addition of serotonin antagonism to dopamine antagonism (classic neuroleptic mechanism) is thought to improve negative symptoms of psychoses and reduce the incidence of extrapyramidal side effects. Similar to risperidone, paliperidone demonstrates high affinity to α_1, D_2, H_1, and 5-HT$_{2C}$ receptors, and low affinity for muscarinic and 5-HT$_{1A}$ receptors. In contrast to risperidone, paliperidone displays nearly 10-fold lower affinity for α_2 and 5-HT$_{2A}$ receptors, and nearly three- to fivefold less affinity for 5-HT$_{1A}$ and 5-HT$_{1D}$, respectively.

Pharmacodynamics/Kinetics

Absorption: I.M.: Slow release (begins on day 1 and continues up to 126 days)

Distribution: V_d: 391-487 L

Protein binding: 74%

Metabolism: Hepatic via CYP2D6 and 3A4 (limited role in elimination); minor metabolism (<10% each) via dealkylation, hydroxylation, dehydrogenation, and benzisoxazole scission

Bioavailability: 28%

Half-life elimination:

Oral: 23 hours; 24-51 hours with renal impairment (Cl$_{cr}$ <80 mL/minute)

I.M. (following a single-dose administration): Range: 25-49 days

Time to peak, plasma: Oral: ~24 hours; I.M.: 13 days

Excretion: Urine (80%); feces (11%)

Dosage

Geriatric Refer to adult dosing. Additional monitoring of renal function and orthostatic blood pressure may be warranted.

Adult

U.S. labeling:

Schizoaffective disorder, schizophrenia: Oral: Usual: 6 mg once daily in the morning; titration not required, though some may benefit from higher or lower doses. If exceeding 6 mg/day, increases of 3 mg/day are recommended no more frequently than every 4 days in schizoaffective disorder or every 5 days in schizophrenia, up to a maximum of 12 mg/day. Some patients may require only 3 mg/day.

Schizophrenia: I.M.: **Note:** Prior to initiation of I.M therapy, tolerability should be established with oral paliperidone or oral risperidone. Previous oral antipsychotics can be discontinued at the time of initiation of I.M. therapy. **Dosing based on paliperidone palmitate.**

Initiation of therapy:

Initial: 234 mg on treatment day 1 followed by 156 mg 1 week later. The second dose may be administered 2 days before or after the weekly timepoint.

Maintenance: Following the 1-week initiation regimen, begin a maintenance dose of 117 mg every month. Some patients may benefit from higher or lower monthly maintenance doses (monthly maintenance dosage range: 39-234 mg). The monthly maintenance dose may be administered 7 days before or after the monthly timepoint.

Conversion from oral paliperidone to I.M paliperidone: Initiate I.M. therapy as described using the 1-week initiation regimen. Patients previously stabilized on oral doses can expect similar steady state exposure during maintenance treatment with I.M. therapy using the following conversion:

Oral extended release dose of 12 mg, then I.M. maintenance dose of 234 mg

Oral extended release dose of 6 mg, then I.M. maintenance dose of 117 mg

Oral extended release dose of 3 mg, then I.M. maintenance dose of 39-78 mg

Switching from other long-acting injectable antipsychotics to I.M. paliperidone: Initiate I.M. paliperidone in the place of the next scheduled injection and continue at monthly intervals. The 1-week initiation regimen is not required in these patients.

Dosage adjustments: Adjustments may be made monthly (full effect from adjustments may not be seen for several months)

Missed doses:

If <6 weeks has elapsed since the last monthly injection: Administer the missed dose as soon as possible and continue therapy at monthly intervals.

If >6 weeks and ≤6 months has elapsed since the last monthly injection:

If the maintenance dose was <234 mg: Administer the same dose the patient was previously stabilized on as soon as possible, followed by a second equivalent dose 1 week later, then resume maintenance dose at monthly intervals.

If the maintenance dose was 234 mg: Administer a 156 mg dose as soon as possible, followed by a second dose of 156 mg 1 week later, then resume maintenance dose at monthly intervals.

If >6 months has elapsed since last monthly maintenance injection: Therapy must be reinitiated following dosing recommendations for initiation of therapy.

Canadian labeling:

Schizophrenia: Oral: Usual: 6 mg once daily in the morning; titration not required, though some may benefit from higher or lower doses. If exceeding 6 mg/day, increases of 3 mg/day are recommended no more frequently than every 5 days in schizophrenia, up to a maximum of 12 mg/day. Some patients may require only 3 mg/day.

Schizophrenia: I.M.: **Note:** Prior to initiation of I.M therapy, tolerability should be established with oral paliperidone or oral risperidone. Previous oral antipsychotics can be discontinued at the time of initiation of I.M. therapy. **Dosing based on paliperidone.**

Initiation of therapy:

Initial: 150 mg on treatment day 1 followed by 100 mg 1 week later (day 8). The second dose may be administered 2 days before or after the weekly timepoint.

Maintenance: Following the 1-week initiation regimen, begin a maintenance dose of 75 mg every month. Some patients may benefit from higher or lower monthly maintenance doses (monthly maintenance dosage range: 25-150 mg). The monthly maintenance dose may be administered 7 days before or after the monthly timepoint.

Conversion from oral paliperidone to I.M paliperidone: Initiate I.M. therapy as described using the 1-week initiation regimen. Patients previously stabilized on oral doses can expect similar steady state exposure during maintenance treatment with I.M. therapy using the following conversion:

Oral extended release dose of 12 mg, then I.M. maintenance dose of 150 mg

Oral extended release dose of 6 mg, then I.M. maintenance dose of 75 mg

Oral extended release dose of 3 mg, then I.M. maintenance dose of 25-50 mg

Switching from injectable risperidone (Risperdal® Consta®) to I.M. paliperidone:

Risperdal® Consta® dose of 25 mg every 2 weeks, then I.M. paliperidone maintenance dose of 50 mg

Risperdal® Consta® dose of 37.5 mg every 2 weeks, then I.M. paliperidone maintenance dose of 75 mg

Risperdal® Consta® dose of 50 mg every 2 weeks, then I.M. paliperidone maintenance dose of 100 mg

Switching from other long-acting injectable antipsychotics to I.M. paliperidone: Initiate I.M. paliperidone in the place of the next scheduled injection and continue at monthly intervals. The 1-week initiation regimen is not required in these patients.

Dosage adjustments: Adjustments may be made monthly (full effect from adjustments may not be seen for several months)

Missed doses:

If <6 weeks has elapsed since the last monthly injection: Administer the missed dose as soon as possible and continue therapy at monthly intervals.

If >6 weeks and ≤6 months has elapsed since the last monthly injection: Therapy may be resumed at same dose (25-100 mg) the patient was previously stabilized on and then repeated 1 week later (day 8). Resume usual monthly maintenance dosing cycle thereafter. If the dose was 150 mg, administer a 100 mg dose as soon as possible and repeat 1 week later (day 8), then resume usual monthly maintenance dosing cycle 25-150 mg.

If >6 months has elapsed since last monthly maintenance injection: Therapy must be reinitiated following dosing recommendations for initiation of therapy.

Renal Impairment Clearance is decreased in renal impairment; adjust dose according to renal function:

Oral:

Mild impairment (Cl_{cr} 50-79 mL/minute): Initial dose: 3 mg once daily; maximum dose: 6 mg once daily

Moderate-to-severe impairment (Cl_{cr} 10-49 mL/minute): Initial dose: 1.5 mg once daily; maximum dose: 3 mg once daily

Severe impairment (Cl_{cr} <10 mL/minute): Use not recommended; not studied in this population

I.M., U.S. labeling:

Mild impairment (Cl_{cr} 50-79 mL/minute): Initiation of therapy: 156 mg on treatment day 1, followed by 117 mg 1 week later, followed by a maintenance dose of 78 mg every month

Moderate-to-severe impairment (Cl_{cr} <50 mL/minute): Use not recommended

I.M., Canadian labeling:

Mild impairment (Cl_{cr} 50-79 mL/minute): Initiation of therapy: 100 mg on treatment day 1, followed by 75 mg 1 week later followed by a maintenance dose of 50 mg every month

Moderate-to-severe impairment (Cl_{cr} <50 mL/minute): Use not recommended

Hepatic Impairment Oral, I.M.: No adjustment necessary for mild-to-moderate (Child-Pugh class A or B) impairment. Not studied in severe impairment.

Administration

Oral: Administer in the morning without regard to meals. Extended release tablets should be swallowed whole with liquids; do not crush, chew, or divide.

Injection: Invega® Sustenna™ should be administered by I.M. route only as a single injection (do not divide); do not administer I.V. or subcutaneously. Avoid inadvertent injection into vasculature. Prior to injection, shake syringe for at least 10 seconds to ensure a homogenous suspension. The 2 initial injections should be administered in the deltoid muscle using a 1½ inch, 22-gauge needle for patients ≥90 kg, and a 1 inch, 23-gauge needle for patients <90 kg. The 2 initial deltoid intramuscular injections help attain therapeutic concentrations rapidly. Alternate deltoid injections (right and left deltoid muscle). The second dose may be administered 2 days before or after the weekly timepoint. Monthly maintenance doses can be administered in either the deltoid or gluteal muscle. Administer injections in the gluteal muscle using a 1½ inch, 22-gauge needle in the upper-outer quadrant of the gluteal area. Alternate gluteal injections (right and left gluteal muscle). The monthly maintenance dose may be administered 7 days before or after the monthly timepoint.

Monitoring Parameters Vital signs; fasting lipid profile and fasting blood glucose/Hgb A_{1c} (prior to treatment, at 3 months, then annually), prolactin levels, CBC frequently during first few months of therapy in patients with pre-existing low WBC or a history of drug-induced leukopenia/neutropenia; BMI, personal/family history of obesity, diabetes, waist circumference; blood pressure; mental status, abnormal involuntary movement scale (AIMS), extrapyramidal symptoms; orthostatic blood pressure changes for 3-5 days after starting or increasing dose. Weight should be assessed prior to treatment, at 4 weeks, 8 weeks, 12 weeks, and then at quarterly intervals. Consider titrating to a different antipsychotic agent for a weight gain ≥5% of the initial weight.

Pharmacotherapy Pearls Invega® is an extended release tablet based on the OROS® osmotic delivery system. Water from the GI tract enters through a semipermeable membrane coating the tablet, solubilizing the drug into a gelatinous form which, through hydrophilic expansion, is then expelled through laser-drilled holes in the coating.

Special Geriatric Considerations Any changes in disease status in any organ system can result in behavior changes. Extrapyramidal syndrome symptoms occur less with this agent when total daily dose remains ≤6 mg as compared with phenothiazines and butyrophenone classes of antipsychotics.

In the treatment of agitated, demented, elderly patients, authors of meta-analysis of controlled trials of the response to the traditional antipsychotics (phenothiazines, butyrophenones) in controlling agitation have concluded that the use of neuroleptics results in a response rate of 18%. Clearly neuroleptic therapy for behavior control should be limited with frequent attempts to withdraw the agent given for behavior control. In light of significant risks and adverse effects in elderly population compared with limited data demonstrating efficacy in the treatment of dementia related psychosis, aggression, and agitation, an extensive risk:benefit analysis should be performed prior to use.

This medication is considered to be potentially inappropriate in this patient population (Beers Criteria: Quality of evidence - moderate; Strength of recommendation - strong).

Dosage Forms Excipient information presented when available (limited, particularly for generics); consult specific product labeling.

Injection, suspension, extended release, as palmitate:

Invega® Sustenna®: 39 mg/0.25 mL (0.25 mL); 78 mg/0.5 mL (0.5 mL); 117 mg/0.75 mL (0.75 mL); 156 mg/mL (1 mL); 234 mg/1.5 mL (1.5 mL)

Tablet, extended release, oral:

Invega®: 1.5 mg, 3 mg, 6 mg, 9 mg [osmotic controlled release]

Dosage Forms: Canada Excipient information presented when available (limited, particularly for generics); consult specific product labeling.

Injection, suspension, extended release:

Invega® Sustenna™: 25 mg/0.25 mL (0.25 mL), 50 mg/0.5 mL (0.5 mL), 75 mg/0.75 mL (0.75 mL), 100 mg/1 mL (1 mL), 150 mg/1.5 mL (1.5 mL)

♦ **Paliperidone Palmitate** see Paliperidone on page 1457
♦ **Palmer's® Skin Success Acne Cleanser [OTC]** see Salicylic Acid on page 1743
♦ **Pamelor™** see Nortriptyline on page 1395

Pamidronate (pa mi DROE nate)

Medication Safety Issues
Sound-alike/look-alike issues:
Aredia® may be confused with Adriamycin®
Pamidronate may be confused with papaverine

Brand Names: U.S. Aredia®

Brand Names: Canada Aredia®; Pamidronate Disodium Omega; Pamidronate Disodium®; PMS-Pamidronate

Index Terms Pamidronate Disodium

Generic Availability (U.S.) Yes

Pharmacologic Category Antidote; Bisphosphonate Derivative

Use Treatment of moderate or severe hypercalcemia associated with malignancy (in conjunction with adequate hydration) with or without bone metastases; treatment of osteolytic bone lesions associated with multiple myeloma or metastatic breast cancer; moderate-to-severe Paget's disease of bone

Unlabeled Use Treatment of osteogenesis imperfecta; treatment of symptomatic bone metastases of thyroid cancer; prevention of bone loss associated with androgen deprivation treatment in prostate cancer

Contraindications Hypersensitivity to pamidronate, other bisphosphonates, or any component of the formulation

Warnings/Precautions Osteonecrosis of the jaw (ONJ) has been reported in patients receiving bisphosphonates. Risk factors include invasive dental procedures (eg, tooth extraction, dental implants, boney surgery); a diagnosis of cancer, with concomitant chemotherapy, radiotherapy, or corticosteroids; poor oral hygiene, ill-fitting dentures; and comorbid disorders (anemia, coagulopathy, infection, pre-existing dental disease). Most reported cases occurred after I.V. bisphosphonate therapy; however, cases have been reported following oral therapy. A dental exam and preventative dentistry should be performed prior to placing patients with risk factors on chronic bisphosphonate therapy. The manufacturer's labeling states that discontinuing bisphosphonates in patients requiring invasive dental procedures reduces the risk of ONJ. However, other experts suggest that there is no evidence that discontinuing therapy reduces the risk of developing ONJ (Assael, 2009). The benefit/risk must be assessed by the treating physician and/or dentist/surgeon prior to any invasive dental procedure. Patients developing ONJ while on bisphosphonates should receive care by an oral surgeon.

Infrequently, severe (and occasionally debilitating) musculoskeletal (bone, joint, and/or muscle) pain have been reported during bisphosphonate treatment. The onset of pain ranged from a single day to several months. Consider discontinuing therapy in patients who experience severe symptoms; symptoms usually resolve upon discontinuation. Some patients experienced recurrence when rechallenged with same drug or another bisphosphonate; avoid use in patients with a history of these symptoms in association with bisphosphonate therapy.

Initial or single doses have been associated with renal deterioration, progressing to renal failure and dialysis. Withhold pamidronate treatment (until renal function returns to baseline) in patients with evidence of renal deterioration. Glomerulosclerosis (focal segmental) with or without nephrotic syndrome has also been reported. Longer infusion times (>2 hours) may reduce the risk for renal toxicity, especially in patients with pre-existing renal insufficiency. Single pamidronate doses should not exceed 90 mg. Patients with serum creatinine >3 mg/dL were not studied in clinical trials; limited data are available in patients with Cl_{cr} <30 mL/minute. Evaluate serum creatinine prior to each treatment. For the treatment of bone metastases, use is not recommended in patients with severe renal impairment; for renal impairment in indications other than bone metastases, use clinical judgment to determine if benefits outweigh potential risks.

Use has been associated with asymptomatic electrolyte abnormalities (including hypophosphatemia, hypokalemia, hypomagnesemia, and hypocalcemia). Rare cases of symptomatic hypocalcemia, including tetany have been reported. Patients with a history of thyroid surgery may have relative hypoparathyroidism; predisposing them to pamidronate-related hypocalcemia. Patients with pre-existing anemia, leukopenia, or thrombocytopenia should be closely monitored during the first 2 weeks of treatment.

According to the American Society of Clinical Oncology (ASCO) guidelines for bisphosphonates in multiple myeloma, treatment with pamidronate is not recommended for asymptomatic (smoldering) or indolent myeloma or with solitary plasmacytoma (Kyle, 2007). The National Comprehensive Cancer Network® (NCCN) multiple myeloma guidelines (v.1.2011) also do not recommend pamidronate use in stage 1 or smoldering disease, unless part of a clinical trial.

Adequate hydration is required during treatment (urine output ~2 L/day); avoid overhydration, especially in patients with heart failure. Vein irritation and thrombophlebitis may occur with infusions.

Adverse Reactions (Reflective of adult population; not specific for elderly) Note: Actual percentages may vary by indication; treatment for multiple myeloma is associated with higher percentage.

>10%:
  Central nervous system: Fever (18% to 39%; transient), fatigue (≤37%), headache (≤26%), insomnia (≤22%)
  Endocrine & metabolic: Hypophosphatemia (≤18%), hypokalemia (4% to 18%), hypomagnesemia (4% to 12%), hypocalcemia (≤12%)
  Gastrointestinal: Nausea (≤54%), vomiting (≤36%), anorexia (≤26%), abdominal pain (≤23%), dyspepsia (≤23%)
  Genitourinary: Urinary tract infection (≤19%)
  Hematologic: Anemia (≤43%), granulocytopenia (≤20%)
  Local: Infusion site reaction (≤18%; includes induration, pain, redness and swelling)
  Neuromuscular & skeletal: Myalgia (≤26%), weakness (≤22%), arthralgia (≤14%), osteonecrosis of the jaw (cancer patients: 1% to 11%)
  Renal: Serum creatinine increased (≤19%)
  Respiratory: Dyspnea (≤30%), cough (≤26%), upper respiratory tract infection (≤24%), sinusitis (≤16%), pleural effusion (≤11%)
1% to 10%:
  Cardiovascular: Atrial fibrillation (≤6%), hypertension (≤6%), syncope (≤6%), tachycardia (≤6%), atrial flutter (≤1%), cardiac failure (≤1%), edema (≤1%)
  Central nervous system: Somnolence (≤6%), psychosis (≤4%), seizure (≤2%)
  Endocrine & metabolic: Hypothyroidism (≤6%)
  Gastrointestinal: Constipation (≤6%), gastrointestinal hemorrhage (≤6%), diarrhea (≤1%), stomatitis (≤1%)
  Hematologic: Leukopenia (≤4%), neutropenia (≤1%), thrombocytopenia (≤1%)
  Neuromuscular & skeletal: Back pain, bone pain
  Renal: Uremia (≤4%)
  Respiratory: Rales (≤6%), rhinitis (≤6%)
  Miscellaneous: Moniliasis (≤6%)

Drug Interactions

Metabolism/Transport Effects None known.

Avoid Concomitant Use There are no known interactions where it is recommended to avoid concomitant use.

Increased Effect/Toxicity

Pamidronate may increase the levels/effects of: Deferasirox; Phosphate Supplements; SUNItinib

The levels/effects of Pamidronate may be increased by: Aminoglycosides; Nonsteroidal Anti-Inflammatory Agents; Thalidomide

Decreased Effect

The levels/effects of Pamidronate may be decreased by: Proton Pump Inhibitors

Stability

Powder for injection: Store below 30°C (86°F). Reconstitute by adding 10 mL of SWFI to each vial of lyophilized pamidronate disodium powder; the resulting solution will be 30 mg/10 mL or 90 mg/10 mL. The reconstituted solution is stable for 24 hours stored under refrigeration at 2°C to 8°C (36°F to 46°F).

Solution for injection: Store at 20°C to 25°C (68°F to 77°F).

Pamidronate may be further diluted in 250-1000 mL of 0.45% or 0.9% sodium chloride or 5% dextrose. (The manufacturer recommends dilution in 1000 mL for hypercalcemia of malignancy, 500 mL for Paget's disease and bone metastases of myeloma, and 250 mL for bone metastases of breast cancer.) Pamidronate solution for infusion is stable at room temperature for up to 24 hours.

Mechanism of Action Nitrogen-containing bisphosphonate; inhibits bone resorption and decreases mineralization by disrupting osteoclast activity (Gralow, 2009; Rogers, 2011)

Pharmacodynamics/Kinetics

Onset of action:

Hypercalcemia of malignancy (HCM): ≤24 hours for decrease in albumin-corrected serum calcium; maximum effect: ≤7 days

Paget's disease: ~1 month for ≥50% decrease in serum alkaline phosphatase

Duration: HCM: 7-14 days; Paget's disease: 1-372 days

Absorption: Oral: Poor

Metabolism: Not metabolized

Half-life elimination: 21-35 hours

Excretion: Biphasic; urine (30% to 62% as unchanged drug; lower in patients with renal dysfunction) within 120 hours

Dosage

Geriatric Refer to adult dosing. Begin at lower end of adult dosing range.

Adult Note: Single doses should not exceed 90 mg.

Hypercalcemia of malignancy: I.V.:

Moderate cancer-related hypercalcemia (corrected serum calcium: 12-13.5 mg/dL): 60-90 mg, as a single dose over 2-24 hours

Severe cancer-related hypercalcemia (corrected serum calcium: >13.5 mg/dL): 90 mg, as a single dose over 2-24 hours

Retreatment in patients who show an initial complete or partial response (allow at least 7 days to elapse prior to retreatment): May retreat at the same dose if serum calcium does not return to normal or does not remain normal after initial treatment.

Multiple myeloma, osteolytic bone lesions: I.V.: 90 mg over 4 hours monthly

Lytic disease: American Society of Clinical Oncology (ASCO) guidelines: 90 mg over at least 2 hours every 3-4 weeks for 2 years; discontinue after 2 years in patients with responsive and/or stable disease; resume therapy with new-onset skeletal-related events (Kyle, 2007)

Newly-diagnosed, symptomatic (unlabeled dose): 30 mg over 2.5 hours monthly for at least 3 years (Gimsing, 2010)

Breast cancer, osteolytic bone metastases: I.V.: 90 mg over 2 hours every 3-4 weeks

Paget's disease (moderate-to-severe): I.V.: 30 mg over 4 hours daily for 3 consecutive days (total dose = 90 mg); may retreat at initial dose if clinically indicated

Prevention of androgen deprivation-induced osteoporosis (unlabeled use): I.V.: 60 mg over 2 hours every 3 months (Smith, 2001)

Renal Impairment Patients with serum creatinine >3 mg/dL were excluded from clinical trials; there are only limited pharmacokinetic data in patients with Cl_{cr} <30 mL/minute.

Manufacturer recommends the following guidelines:

Treatment of bone metastases: Use is not recommended in patients with severe renal impairment.

Renal impairment in indications other than bone metastases: Use clinical judgment to determine if benefits outweigh potential risks.

Multiple myeloma: American Society of Clinical Oncology (ASCO) guidelines (Kyle, 2007):

Severe renal impairment (serum creatinine >3 mg/dL or Cl_{cr} <30 mL/minute) and extensive bone disease: 90 mg over 4-6 hours. However, a reduced initial dose should be considered if renal impairment was pre-existing.

Albuminuria >500 mg/24 hours (unexplained): Withhold dose until returns to baseline, then recheck every 3-4 weeks; consider reinitiating at a dose not to exceed 90 mg every 4 weeks and with a longer infusion time of at least 4 hours

Dosing adjustment in renal toxicity: In patients with bone metastases, treatment should be withheld for deterioration in renal function (increase of serum creatinine ≥0.5 mg/dL in patients with normal baseline or ≥1.0 mg/dL in patients with abnormal baseline). Resumption of therapy may be considered when serum creatinine returns to within 10% of baseline.

Hepatic Impairment No dosage adjustment necessary in patients with mild-to-moderate hepatic impairment; not studied in patients with severe hepatic impairment.

Administration I.V.: Infusion rate varies by indication. Longer infusion times (>2 hours) may reduce the risk for renal toxicity, especially in patients with pre-existing renal insufficiency. The manufacturer recommends infusing over 2-24 hours for hypercalcemia of malignancy; over 2 hours for osteolytic bone lesions with metastatic breast cancer; and over 4 hours for Paget's disease and for osteolytic bone lesions with multiple myeloma. The ASCO guidelines for bisphosphonate use in multiple myeloma recommend infusing pamidronate over at least 2 hours; if therapy is withheld due to renal toxicity, infuse over at least 4 hours upon reintroduction of treatment after renal recovery (Kyle, 2007).

Monitoring Parameters Serum creatinine (prior to each treatment); serum electrolytes, including calcium, phosphate, magnesium, and potassium; CBC with differential; monitor for hypocalcemia for at least 2 weeks after therapy; dental exam and preventative dentistry prior to therapy for patients at risk of osteonecrosis, including all cancer patients; patients with pre-existing anemia, leukopenia, or thrombocytopenia should be closely monitored during the first 2 weeks of treatment; in addition, monitor urine albumin every 3-6 months in multiple myeloma patients

Reference Range Calcium (total): Adults: 9.0-11.0 mg/dL (SI: 2.05-2.54 mmol/L), may slightly decrease with aging; Phosphorus: 2.5-4.5 mg/dL (SI: 0.81-1.45 mmol/L)

Test Interactions Bisphosphonates may interfere with diagnostic imaging agents such as technetium-99m-diphosphonate in bone scans.

Pharmacotherapy Pearls

Oncology Comment:

Metastatic breast cancer: The American Society of Clinical Oncology (ASCO) updated guidelines on the role of bone-modifying agents (BMAs) in the prevention and treatment of skeletal-related events for metastatic breast cancer patients (Van Poznak, 2011). The guidelines recommend initiating a BMA (denosumab, pamidronate, zoledronic acid) in patients with metastatic breast cancer to the bone. There is currently no literature indicating the superiority of one particular BMA. Optimal duration is not defined; however, the guidelines recommend continuing therapy until substantial decline in patient's performance status. In patients with normal Cl_{cr} (>60 mL/minute), no dosage/interval/infusion rate changes for pamidronate or zoledronic acid are necessary. For patients with Cl_{cr} <30 mL/minute, pamidronate and zoledronic acid are not recommended. While no renal dose adjustments are recommended for denosumab, close monitoring is advised for risk of hypocalcemia in patients with Cl_{cr} <30 mL/minute or on dialysis. The ASCO guidelines are in alignment with package insert guidelines for dosing, renal dose adjustments, infusion times, prevention and management of osteonecrosis of the jaw, and monitoring of laboratory parameter recommendations. BMAs are not the first-line therapy for pain. BMAs are to be used as adjunctive therapy for cancer-related bone pain associated with bone metastasis, demonstrating a modest pain control benefit. BMAs should be used in conjunction with agents such as NSAIDs, opioid and nonopioid analgesics, corticosteroids, radiation/surgery, and interventional procedures.

Multiple myeloma: The American Society of Clinical Oncology (ASCO) has also published guidelines on the use of bisphosphonates for prevention and treatment of bone disease in multiple myeloma (Kyle, 2007). Pamidronate or zoledronic acid use is recommended in multiple myeloma patients with lytic bone destruction or compression spine fracture from osteopenia. Clodronate (not available in the U.S.; available in Canada), administered orally or I.V., is an alternative treatment. The use of the bisphosphonates pamidronate and zoledronic acid may be considered in patients with pain secondary to osteolytic disease, adjunct therapy to stabilize fractures or impending fractures, and I.V. bisphosphonates for multiple myeloma patients with osteopenia but no radiographic evidence of lytic bone disease. Bisphosphonates are not recommended in patients with solitary plasmacytoma, smoldering (asymptomatic) or indolent myeloma, or monoclonal gammopathy of undetermined significance. The guidelines recommend monthly treatment for a period of 2 years. At that time, physicians need to consider discontinuing in responsive and stable patients, and reinitiate if a new-onset skeletal-related event occurs. The ASCO guidelines are in alignment with package insert guidelines for dosing, renal dose adjustments, infusion times, prevention and management of osteonecrosis of the jaw, and monitoring of laboratory parameter recommendations. The guidelines also recommend in patients with extensive bone disease with existing severe renal disease (a serum creatinine >3 mg/dL or Cl_{cr} <30 mL/minute) pamidronate at a dose of 90 mg over 4-6 hours (unless pre-existing renal disease in which a reduced initial dose should be considered). ASCO also recommends monitoring for albuminuria every 3-6 months. In patients with unexplained albuminuria >500 mg/24 hours, withhold the dose until level returns to baseline, then recheck every 3-4 weeks. Pamidronate may be reinitiated at a dose not to exceed 90 mg every 4 weeks with a longer infusion time of at least 4 hours. Also consider increasing the infusion time of zoledronic acid to at least 30 minutes; although one study demonstrated that extending the infusion to 30 minutes did not change the safety profile (Berenson, 2011).

◀ **Special Geriatric Considerations** Elderly patients should be advised to report any lower extremity, jaw (osteonecrosis), or muscle pain that cannot be explained or lasts longer than 2 weeks. Additionally, elderly often receive concomitant diuretic therapy and therefore their electrolyte status (eg, calcium, phosphate) should be periodically evaluated.

Dosage Forms Excipient information presented when available (limited, particularly for generics); consult specific product labeling. [DSC] = Discontinued product

Injection, powder for reconstitution, as disodium: 30 mg, 90 mg
  Aredia®: 30 mg, 90 mg [DSC]
Injection, solution, as disodium: 3 mg/mL (10 mL); 6 mg/mL (10 mL); 9 mg/mL (10 mL)
Injection, solution, as disodium [preservative free]: 3 mg/mL (10 mL); 9 mg/mL (10 mL)

- ◆ **Pamidronate Disodium** *see* Pamidronate *on page 1462*
- ◆ **p-amino-benzenesulfonamide** *see* Sulfanilamide *on page 1817*
- ◆ **p-Aminoclonidine** *see* Apraclonidine *on page 138*
- ◆ **Pamprin® Maximum Strength All Day Relief [OTC]** *see* Naproxen *on page 1338*
- ◆ **Pancreatic Enzymes** *see* Pancrelipase *on page 1466*
- ◆ **Pancreaze™** *see* Pancrelipase *on page 1466*

Pancrelipase (pan kre LYE pase)

Medication Safety Issues
Sound-alike/look-alike issues:
Pancrelipase may be confused with pancreatin

Brand Names: U.S. Creon®; Pancreaze™; Pancrelipase™; Viokace™; Zenpep®
Brand Names: Canada Cotazym®; Creon®; Pancrease® MT; Ultrase®; Ultrase® MT; Viokase®
Index Terms Amylase, Lipase, and Protease; Lipancreatin; Lipase, Protease, and Amylase; Pancreatic Enzymes; Protease, Lipase, and Amylase; Ultresa™; Viokace™
Generic Availability (U.S.) Yes
Pharmacologic Category Enzyme
Use Treatment of exocrine pancreatic insufficiency (EPI) due to conditions such as cystic fibrosis (Creon®, Pancreaze™, Zenpep®); chronic pancreatitis (Creon®); or pancreatectomy (Creon®)
Medication Guide Available Yes
Contraindications There are no contraindications listed in the manufacturer's labeling.
Warnings/Precautions Fibrosing colonopathy advancing to colonic strictures have been reported with doses of lipase >6000 units/kg/meal over long periods of time in children <12 years of age. Patients taking doses of lipase >6000 units/kg/meal should be examined and the dose decreased. Doses of lipase >2500 units/kg/meal (or lipase >10,000 units/kg/day) should be used with caution and only with documentation of 3-day fecal fat measures. Crushing or chewing the contents of the capsules, or mixing the contents with foods outside of product labeling, may cause early release of the enzymes, causing irritation of the oral mucosa and/or loss of enzyme activity. When mixing the contents of capsules with food, the mixture should be swallowed immediately and followed with water or juice to ensure complete ingestion. Use caution in patients with gout, hyperuricemia, or renal impairment; products contain purines which may increase uric acid concentrations. Products are derived from porcine pancreatic glands. Severe, allergic reactions (rare) have been observed; use with caution in patients hypersensitive to pork proteins. Transmission of porcine viruses is theoretically a risk; however, testing and/or inactivation or removal of certain viruses, reduces the risk. There have been no cases of transmission of an infectious illness reported. Available brand products are **not** interchangeable.
Adverse Reactions (Reflective of adult population; not specific for elderly) The following adverse reactions were reported in a short-term safety studies; actual frequency varies with different products; adverse events, particularly gastrointestinal events, were often greater with placebo:
10%:
  Central nervous system: Headache (6% to 15%)
  Gastrointestinal: Abdominal pain (4% to 18%)
1% to 10%:
  Central nervous system: Dizziness (4% to 6%)
  Endocrine & metabolic: Diabetes mellitus exacerbation (4%), hyperglycemia (4% to 8%), hypoglycemia (4%)
  Gastrointestinal: Flatulence (4% to 9%), early satiety (6%), weight loss (3% to 6%), vomiting (6%), upper abdominal pain (≤5%), diarrhea (≤4%), feces abnormal (≤4%)
  Respiratory: Cough (4% to 6%), nasopharyngitis (4%)
Drug Interactions
  Metabolism/Transport Effects None known.

Avoid Concomitant Use There are no known interactions where it is recommended to avoid concomitant use.

Increased Effect/Toxicity There are no known significant interactions involving an increase in effect.

Decreased Effect

Pancrelipase may decrease the levels/effects of: Iron Salts

Ethanol/Nutrition/Herb Interactions Food: Avoid placing contents of opened capsules on alkaline food; pancrelipase may impair absorption of oral iron.

Stability

Creon®: Store at room temperature of 25°C (77°F); excursions permitted between 25°C to 40°C (77°F to 104°F) for ≤30 days. Protect from moisture, and discard if moisture conditions are >70%. Keep bottle tightly closed.

Pancreaze™: Store at ≤25°C (77°F). Protect from moisture; keep bottle tightly closed.

Zenpep®: Store at room temperature 20°C to 25°C (68°F to 77°F). Protect from moisture; keep bottle tightly closed after opening.

Mechanism of Action Pancrelipase is a natural product harvested from the porcine pancreatic glands. It contains a combination of lipase, amylase, and protease. Products are formulated to dissolve in the more basic pH of the duodenum so that they may act locally to break down fats, protein, and starch.

Pharmacodynamics/Kinetics

Absorption: None; acts locally in GI tract

Excretion: Feces

Dosage

Geriatric & Adult Note: Adjust dose based on body weight, clinical symptoms, and stool fat content. Allow several days between dose adjustments. Total daily dose reflects ~3 meals/day and 2-3 snacks/day, with half the mealtime dose given with a snack. Doses of lipase >2500 units/kg/meal (or lipase >10,000 units/kg/day) should be used with caution and only with documentation of 3-day fecal fat measures. Doses of lipase >6000 units/kg/meal are associated with colonic stricture and should be decreased.

Pancreatic insufficiency: Oral: Initial: Lipase 500 units/kg/meal. Dosage range: Lipase 500-2500 units/kg/meal. Maximum dose: Lipase 10,000 units/kg/day **or** lipase 4000 units/g of fat per day

Pancreatic insufficiency due to chronic pancreatitis or pancreatectomy (Creon®): Oral: Lipase 72,000 units/meal while consuming ≥100 g of fat per day; alternatively, lower initial doses of lipase 500 units/kg/meal with individualized dosage titrations have also been used

Administration Oral: Administer with meals or snacks and swallow whole with a generous amount of liquid. Do not crush or chew; retention in the mouth before swallowing may cause mucosal irritation and stomatitis. If necessary, capsules may also be opened and contents added to a small amount of an acidic food (pH ≤4.5), such as applesauce. The food should be at room temperature and swallowed immediately after mixing. The contents of the capsule should not be crushed or chewed. Follow with water or juice to ensure complete ingestion and that no medication remains in the mouth.

Creon®: Capsules contain enteric coated spheres which are 0.71-1.6 mm in diameter

Pancreaze™: Capsules contain enteric coated microtablets which are ~2 mm in diameter

Zenpep®: Capsules contain enteric coated beads which are 1.8-2.5 mm in diameter

Administration via gastrostomy (G) tube: An *in vitro* study demonstrated that Creon® delayed-release capsules sprinkled onto a small amount of baby food (pH <4.5; applesauce or bananas manufactured by both Gerber and Beech-Nut) stirred gently and after 15 minutes was administered through the following G-tubes without significant loss of lipase activity: Kimberly-Clark MIC Bolus® size 18 Fr, Kimberly-Clark MIC-KEY® size 16 Fr, Bard® Tri-Funnel size 18 Fr, and Bard® Button size 18 Fr (Shlieout, 2011).

Monitoring Parameters Abdominal symptoms, nutritional intake, weight, stool character, fecal fat

Pharmacotherapy Pearls Unapproved PEPs are no longer allowed to be distributed in the U.S. There are three PEPs with FDA approval commercially available in the U.S.: Creon®, Pancreaze™, and Zenpep®. PEPs are **not** interchangeable, and patients will require new prescriptions when changing from one product to another. However, Pancrelipase™ lipase 5000 units strength (manufactured by Eurand Pharmaceuticals and distributed by X-Gen Pharmaceuticals) is an authorized generic which may be used interchangeably with the Zenpep® lipase 5000 units product (manufactured by Eurand Pharmaceuticals).

Special Geriatric Considerations No special considerations are necessary since drug is dosed to response; however, drug-induced diarrhea can result in unwanted side effects (eg, confusion, hypotension, lethargy, fluid and electrolyte loss).

◄ **Product Availability**
  Pertzye™: FDA approved May 2012; anticipated availability currently undetermined. Consult prescribing information for additional information.
  Ultresa™: FDA approved March 2012; anticipated availability currently undetermined. Consult prescribing information for additional information.
Dosage Forms Excipient information presented when available (limited, particularly for generics); consult specific product labeling.
  Capsule, delayed release, enteric coated beads, oral [porcine derived]:
    Pancrelipase™: Lipase 5000 units, protease 17,000 units, amylase 27,000 units
    Zenpep®: Lipase 3000 units, protease 10,000 units, and amylase 16,000 units
    Zenpep®: Lipase 5000 units, protease 17,000 units, and amylase 27,000 units
    Zenpep®: Lipase 10,000 units, protease 34,000 units, and amylase 55,000 units
    Zenpep®: Lipase 15,000 units, protease 51,000 units, and amylase 82,000 units
    Zenpep®: Lipase 20,000 units, protease 68,000 units, and amylase 109,000 units
    Zenpep®: Lipase 25,000 units, protease 85,000 units, and amylase 136,000 units
  Capsule, delayed release, enteric coated microspheres, oral [new formulation; porcine derived]:
    Creon®: Lipase 3000 units, protease 9500 units, and amylase 15,000 units
    Creon®: Lipase 6000 units, protease 19,000 units, and amylase 30,000 units
    Creon®: Lipase 12000 units, protease 38,000 units, and amylase 60,000 units
    Creon®: Lipase 24,000 units, protease 76,000 units, and amylase 120,000 units
  Capsule, delayed release, enteric coated microtablets, oral [porcine derived]:
    Pancreaze™: Lipase 4200 units, protease 10,000 units, and amylase 17,500 units
    Pancreaze™: Lipase 10,500 units, protease 25,000 units, and amylase 43,750 units
    Pancreaze™: Lipase 16,800 units, protease 40,000 units, and amylase 70,000 units
    Pancreaze™: Lipase 21,000 units, protease 37,000 units, and amylase 61,000 units

◆ **Pancrelipase™** *see* Pancrelipase *on page 1466*
◆ **Pandel®** *see* Hydrocortisone (Topical) *on page 943*
◆ **Panglobulin** *see* Immune Globulin *on page 982*

Pantoprazole (pan TOE pra zole)

Medication Safety Issues
  Sound-alike/look-alike issues:
    Pantoprazole may be confused with ARIPiprazole
    Protonix® may be confused with Lotronex®, Lovenox®, protamine
  Administration issues:
    Vials containing Protonix® I.V. for injection are not recommended for use with spiked I.V. system adaptors. Nurses and pharmacists have reported breakage of the glass vials during attempts to connect spiked I.V. system adaptors, which may potentially result in injury to healthcare professionals.
  International issues:
    Protonix [U.S., Canada] may be confused with Pretanix brand name for indapamide [Hungary]
Brand Names: U.S. Protonix®; Protonix® I.V.
Brand Names: Canada Apo-Pantoprazole®; Ava-Pantoprazole; CO Pantoprazole; Mylan-Pantoprazole; Pantoloc®; Pantoprazole for Injection; Panto™ I.V.; PMS-Pantoprazole; Q-Pantoprazole; RAN™-Pantoprazole; ratio-Pantoprazole; Riva-Pantoprazole; Sandoz-Pantoprazole; Tecta®; Teva-Pantoprazole
Index Terms Pantoprazole Magnesium; Pantoprazole Sodium
Generic Availability (U.S.) Yes: Delayed release tablet
Pharmacologic Category Proton Pump Inhibitor; Substituted Benzimidazole
Use
  Oral: Treatment and maintenance of healing of erosive esophagitis associated with GERD; reduction in relapse rates of daytime and nighttime heartburn symptoms in GERD; hypersecretory disorders associated with Zollinger-Ellison syndrome or other GI hypersecretory disorders
  I.V.: Short-term treatment (7-10 days) of patients with gastroesophageal reflux disease (GERD) and a history of erosive esophagitis; hypersecretory disorders associated with Zollinger-Ellison syndrome or other neoplastic disorders

  Canadian labeling: Additional use (not in U.S. labeling): Oral: Peptic ulcer disease (eg, duodenal or gastric ulcer); adjunct treatment with antibiotics for *Helicobacter pylori* eradication; prevention of GI lesions in patients receiving prolonged NSAID therapy
Unlabeled Use Peptic ulcer disease, active ulcer bleeding (parenteral formulation); adjunct treatment with antibiotics for *Helicobacter pylori* eradication; stress-ulcer prophylaxis in the critically-ill

Contraindications Hypersensitivity to pantoprazole, substituted benzamidazoles (eg, esomeprazole, lansoprazole, omeprazole, rabeprazole), or any component of the formulation

Warnings/Precautions Use of proton pump inhibitors (PPIs) may increase the risk of gastrointestinal infections (eg, *Salmonella, Campylobacter*). Relief of symptoms does not preclude the presence of a gastric malignancy. Long-term pantoprazole therapy (especially in patients who were *H. pylori* positive) has caused biopsy-proven atrophic gastritis. Benign and malignant neoplasia has been observed in long-term rodent studies; while not reported in humans, the relevance of these findings in regards to tumorigenicity in humans is not known. Not indicated for maintenance therapy; safety and efficacy for use beyond 16 weeks have not been established. Prolonged treatment (typically >3 years) may lead to vitamin B_{12} malabsorption and subsequent deficiency. Intravenous preparation contains edetate sodium (EDTA); use caution in patients who are at risk for zinc deficiency if other EDTA-containing solutions are coadministered. Decreased *H. pylori* eradication rates have been observed with short-term (≤7 days) combination therapy. The American College of Gastroenterology recommends 10-14 days of therapy (triple or quadruple) for eradication of *H. pylori* (Chey, 2007).

PPIs may diminish the therapeutic effect of clopidogrel, thought to be due to reduced formation of the active metabolite of clopidogrel. Of the PPIs, pantoprazole has the lowest degree of CYP2C19 inhibition. Therefore, the manufacturer of clopidogrel prefers pantoprazole if concomitant use of a PPI is necessary. Others have recommended the continued use of PPIs, regardless of the degree of inhibition, in patients with a history of GI bleeding or multiple risk factors for GI bleeding who are also receiving clopidogrel since no evidence has established clinically meaningful differences in outcome; however, a clinically-significant interaction cannot be excluded in those who are poor metabolizers of clopidogrel (Abraham, 2010; Levine, 2011). Concomitant use of pantoprazole with some drugs may require cautious use, may not be recommended, or may require dosage adjustments.

Increased incidence of osteoporosis-related bone fractures of the hip, spine, or wrist may occur with PPI therapy. Patients on high-dose or long-term therapy (≥1 year) should be monitored. Use the lowest effective dose for the shortest duration of time, use vitamin D and calcium supplementation, and follow appropriate guidelines to reduce risk of fractures in patients at risk. Thrombophlebitis and hypersensitivity reactions including anaphylaxis, Stevens-Johnson syndrome, and toxic epidermal necrolysis have been reported with IV administration.

Hypomagnesemia, reported rarely, usually with prolonged PPI use of >3 months (most cases >1 year of therapy); may be symptomatic or asymptomatic; severe cases may cause tetany, seizures, and cardiac arrhythmias. Consider obtaining serum magnesium concentrations prior to beginning long-term therapy, especially if taking concomitant digoxin, diuretics, or other drugs known to cause hypomagnesemia; and periodically thereafter. Hypomagnesemia may be corrected by magnesium supplementation, although discontinuation of pantoprazole may be necessary; magnesium levels typically return to normal within 2 weeks of stopping.

Adverse Reactions (Reflective of adult population; not specific for elderly)

>10%: Central nervous system: Headache (adults 12%; children >4%)

1% to 10%:

Cardiovascular: Facial edema (≤4%), generalized edema (≤2%)

Central nervous system: Dizziness (≤4%), vertigo (≤4%), depression (≤2%), fever (adults ≤2%; children >4%)

Dermatologic: Rash (adults ≤2%; children >4%), urticaria (≤4%), photosensitivity (≤2%), pruritus (≤2%)

Endocrine & metabolic: Triglycerides increased (≤4%)

Gastrointestinal: Diarrhea (≤9%), abdominal pain (children >4%), vomiting (≥4%), constipation (≤4%), flatulence (children ≤4%), nausea (children ≤4%), xerostomia (≤2%)

Hematologic: Leukopenia (≤2%), thrombocytopenia (≤2%)

Hepatic: Liver function tests abnormal (≤2%), hepatitis (≤2%)

Local: Injection site reaction (thrombophlebitis ≤2%)

Neuromuscular & skeletal: Arthralgia (≤4%), myalgia (≤4%), CPK increased (≤4%)

Ocular: Blurred vision (≤2%)

Respiratory: Upper respiratory tract infection (children >4%)

Miscellaneous: Allergic reaction (≤4%)

Drug Interactions

Metabolism/Transport Effects Substrate of CYP2C19 (major), CYP2D6 (minor), CYP3A4 (minor); **Note:** Assignment of Major/Minor substrate status based on clinically relevant drug interaction potential; **Inhibits** BCRP, CYP2C19 (moderate); **Induces** CYP1A2 (weak/moderate)

Avoid Concomitant Use

Avoid concomitant use of Pantoprazole with any of the following: Delavirdine; Erlotinib; Nelfinavir; Posaconazole; Rilpivirine

Increased Effect/Toxicity

Pantoprazole may increase the levels/effects of: Amphetamines; Citalopram; CYP2C19 Substrates; Dexmethylphenidate; Methotrexate; Methylphenidate; Raltegravir; Saquinavir; Topotecan; Voriconazole

The levels/effects of Pantoprazole may be increased by: Fluconazole; Ketoconazole; Ketoconazole (Systemic)

Decreased Effect

Pantoprazole may decrease the levels/effects of: Atazanavir; Bisphosphonate Derivatives; Cefditoren; Clopidogrel; Dabigatran Etexilate; Dasatinib; Delavirdine; Erlotinib; Gefitinib; Indinavir; Iron Salts; Itraconazole; Ketoconazole; Ketoconazole (Systemic); Mesalamine; Mycophenolate; Nelfinavir; Nilotinib; Posaconazole; Rilpivirine; Vismodegib

The levels/effects of Pantoprazole may be decreased by: CYP2C19 Inducers (Strong); Peginterferon Alfa-2b; Tipranavir; Tocilizumab

Ethanol/Nutrition/Herb Interactions

Ethanol: Avoid ethanol (may cause gastric mucosal irritation).

Herb/Nutraceutical: Prolonged treatment (typically >3 years) may lead to vitamin B_{12} malabsorption and subsequent deficiency.

Stability

Oral: Store tablet and oral suspension at controlled room temperature of 20°C to 25°C (68°F to 77°F); excursions permitted to 15°C to 30°C (59°F to 86°F).

I.V.: Prior to reconstitution, store at controlled room temperature of 20°C to 25°C (68°F to 77°F); excursions permitted to 15°C to 30°C (59°F to 86°F). Do not freeze. Protect from light prior to reconstitution; upon reconstitution, protection from light is not required. Reconstitute with 10 mL NS (final concentration 4 mg/mL). Reconstituted solution may be given intravenously (over 2 minutes) or may be added to 100 mL D_5W, NS, or LR (for 15-minute infusion). Per manufacturer's labeling, reconstituted solution is stable at room temperature for 6 hours; further diluted (admixed) solution should be stored at room temperature and used within 24 hours from the time of initial reconstitution. However, studies have shown that reconstituted solution (4 mg/mL) in polypropylene syringes is stable up to 96 hours at room temperature (Johnson, 2005). Upon further dilution, the admixed solution should be used within 96 hours from the time of initial reconstitution. The preparation should be stored at 3°C to 5°C (37°F to 41°F) if it is stored beyond 48 hours to minimize discoloration.

Mechanism of Action Suppresses gastric acid secretion by inhibiting the parietal cell H^+/K^+ ATP pump

Pharmacodynamics/Kinetics

Absorption: Rapid, well absorbed

Distribution: V_d: 11-24 L

Protein binding: 98%, primarily to albumin

Metabolism: Extensively hepatic; CYP2C19 (demethylation), CYP3A4; no evidence that metabolites have pharmacologic activity

Bioavailability: ~77%

Half-life elimination: 1 hour; increased to 3.5-10 hours with CYP2C19 deficiency

Time to peak: Oral: 2.5 hours

Excretion: Urine (71%); feces (18%)

Dosage

Geriatric & Adult

Erosive esophagitis associated with GERD:

Oral:

Treatment: 40 mg once daily for up to 8 weeks; an additional 8 weeks may be used in patients who have not healed after an 8-week course. **Note:** Canadian labeling recommends initial treatment for up to 4 weeks and an additional 4 weeks in patients who have not healed after the initial 4-week course. Lower doses (20 mg once daily) have been used successfully in mild GERD treatment (Dettmer, 1998).

Maintenance of healing: 40 mg once daily (U.S. labeling) or 20-40 mg once daily (Canadian labeling); 20 mg once daily has been used successfully in maintenance of healing (Escourrou, 1999)

I.V.: 40 mg once daily for 7-10 days

Hypersecretory disorders (including Zollinger-Ellison):

Oral: Initial: 40 mg twice daily; adjust dose based on patient needs; doses up to 240 mg/day have been administered

I.V.: 80 mg twice daily; adjust dose based on acid output measurements; 160-240 mg/day in divided doses has been used for a limited period (up to 7 days)

Prevention of rebleeding in peptic ulcer bleed (unlabeled use): I.V.: 80 mg, followed by 8 mg/hour infusion for 72 hours. **Note:** A daily infusion of 40 mg does not raise gastric pH sufficiently to enhance coagulation in active GI bleeds.

Helicobacter pylori eradication (unlabeled use in U.S.): *Oral:*
American College of Gastroenterology guidelines (Chey, 2007):
Nonpenicillin allergy: 40 mg twice daily administered with amoxicillin 1000 mg *and* clarithromycin 500 mg twice daily for 10-14 days
Penicillin allergy: 40 mg twice daily administered with clarithromycin 500 mg *and* metronidazole 500 mg twice daily for 10-14 days **or** 40 mg once or twice daily administered with bismuth subsalicylate 525 mg *and* metronidazole 250 mg *plus* tetracycline 500 mg 4 times/day for 10-14 days
Canadian labeling: 40 mg twice daily administered with clarithromycin 500 mg twice daily *and* either metronidazole 500 mg **or** amoxicillin 1000 mg twice daily for 7 days
Peptic ulcer disease (Canadian labeling): Oral: Treatment: 40 mg once daily for 2 weeks (duodenal ulcer) or 4 weeks (gastric ulcer); may extend therapy for an additional 2 or 4 weeks (based on indication) for inadequate healing
Prevention of GI lesions associated with NSAID use (Canadian labeling): Oral: 20 mg once daily
Symptomatic GERD (Canadian labeling): Oral: Treatment: 40 mg once daily for up to 4 weeks; failure to achieve adequate symptom relief after the initial 4 weeks of therapy warrants further evaluation
Renal Impairment No dosage adjustment necessary; pantoprazole is not removed by hemodialysis.
Hepatic Impairment
U.S. labeling: No dosage adjustment necessary.
Canadian labeling:
Mild-moderate impairment: No dosage adjustment necessary.
Severe impairment: I.V., Oral: Manufacturer's labeling suggests a maximum dose of 20 mg/day.

Administration

I.V.: Flush I.V. line before and after administration. In-line filter not required.
2-minute infusion: The volume of reconstituted solution (4 mg/mL) to be injected may be administered intravenously over at least 2 minutes.
15-minute infusion: Infuse over 15 minutes at a rate not to exceed 7 mL/minute (3 mg/minute).
Oral:
Tablet: Should be swallowed whole, do not crush or chew. Best if taken before breakfast.
Delayed-release oral suspension: Should only be administered in apple juice or applesauce and taken ~30 minutes before a meal. Do not administer with any other liquid (eg, water) or foods.
Oral administration in **applesauce**: Sprinkle intact granules on 1 tablespoon of applesauce and swallow within 10 minutes of preparation.
Oral administration in **apple juice**: Empty intact granules into 5 mL of apple juice, stir for 5 seconds, and swallow immediately after preparation. Rinse container once or twice with apple juice and swallow immediately.
Nasogastric tube administration: Separate the plunger from the barrel of a 60 mL catheter tip syringe and connect to a ≥16 French nasogastric tube. Holding the syringe attached to the tubing as high as possible, empty the contents of the packet into barrel of the syringe, add 10 mL of apple juice and gently tap/shake the barrel of the syringe to help empty the syringe. Add an additional 10 mL of apple juice and gently tap/shake the barrel to help rinse. Repeat rinse with at least 2-10 mL aliquots of apple juice. No granules should remain in the syringe.
Monitoring Parameters Hypersecretory disorders: Acid output measurements, target level <10 mEq/hour (<5 mEq/hour if prior gastric acid-reducing surgery)
Test Interactions False-positive urine screening tests for tetrahydrocannabinol (THC) have been noted in patients receiving proton pump inhibitors, including pantoprazole.
Special Geriatric Considerations Dosage adjustment not required.

An increased risk of fractures of the hip, spine, or wrist has been observed in epidemiologic studies with proton pump inhibitor (PPI) use, primarily in older adults ≥50 years of age. The greatest risk was seen in patients receiving high doses or on long-term therapy (≥1 year). Calcium and vitamin D supplementation and close monitoring are recommended to reduce the risk of fracture in high-risk patients. Additionally, long-term use of proton pump inhibitors has resulted in reports of hypomagnesemia and *Clostridium difficile* infections.
Dosage Forms Excipient information presented when available (limited, particularly for generics); consult specific product labeling.
Granules for suspension, delayed release, enteric coated, oral:
Protonix®: 40 mg/packet (30s)
Injection, powder for reconstitution:
Protonix® I.V.: 40 mg [contains edetate disodium]
Tablet, delayed release, oral: 20 mg, 40 mg
Protonix®: 20 mg, 40 mg

Dosage Forms: Canada Excipient information presented when available (limited, particularly for generics); consult specific product labeling.
Note: Strength expressed as base
Tablet, enteric coated, as magnesium:
Tecta®: 40 mg

♦ **Pantoprazole Magnesium** see Pantoprazole on page 1468
♦ **Pantoprazole Sodium** see Pantoprazole on page 1468

Papaverine (pa PAV er een)

Medication Safety Issues
Sound-alike/look-alike issues:
Papaverine may be confused with pamidronate
Index Terms Papaverine Hydrochloride; Pavabid
Generic Availability (U.S.) Yes
Pharmacologic Category Vasodilator
Use Oral: Relief of peripheral and cerebral ischemia associated with arterial spasm and myocardial ischemia complicated by arrhythmias
Unlabeled Use Investigational: Parenteral: Various vascular spasms associated with muscle spasms as in myocardial infarction, angina, peripheral and pulmonary embolism, peripheral vascular disease, angiospastic states, and visceral spasm (ureteral, biliary, and GI colic); testing for impotence

Papaverine has been used for many conditions where vasodilatation is felt to be of some benefit; however, to date, insufficient scientific evidence exists for any therapeutic value to its use except in testing for impotence.
Dosage
Geriatric & Adult Arterial spasm:
Oral, sustained release: 150-300 mg every 12 hours; in difficult cases: 150 mg every 8 hours
I.M., I.V.: 30-65 mg (rarely up to 120 mg); may repeat every 3 hours
Special Geriatric Considerations The use of vasodilators for cognitive dysfunction is not recommended or proven by appropriate scientific study.
Dosage Forms Excipient information presented when available (limited, particularly for generics); consult specific product labeling. [DSC] = Discontinued product
Capsule, sustained release, oral, as hydrochloride: 150 mg [DSC]
Injection, solution, as hydrochloride: 30 mg/mL (2 mL, 10 mL)

♦ **Papaverine Hydrochloride** see Papaverine on page 1472
♦ **PAR-101** see Fidaxomicin on page 786
♦ **Para-Aminosalicylate Sodium** see Aminosalicylic Acid on page 95
♦ **Paracetamol** see Acetaminophen on page 31
♦ **Parafon Forte® DSC** see Chlorzoxazone on page 364
♦ **Parathyroid Hormone (1-34)** see Teriparatide on page 1859
♦ **Parcopa®** see Carbidopa and Levodopa on page 293

Paricalcitol (pah ri KAL si tole)

Medication Safety Issues
Sound alike/look alike issues:
Paricalcitol may be confused with calcitriol
Zemplar® may be confused with zaleplon, Zelapar®, zolpidem, ZyPREXA® Zydis®
Brand Names: U.S. Zemplar®
Brand Names: Canada Zemplar®
Generic Availability (U.S.) No
Pharmacologic Category Vitamin D Analog
Use
I.V.: Prevention and treatment of secondary hyperparathyroidism associated with stage 5 chronic kidney disease (CKD)
Oral: Prevention and treatment of secondary hyperparathyroidism associated with stage 3 and 4 CKD and stage 5 CKD patients on hemodialysis or peritoneal dialysis
Contraindications Hypersensitivity to paricalcitol or any component of the formulation; patients with evidence of vitamin D toxicity; hypercalcemia
Warnings/Precautions Excessive administration may lead to over suppression of PTH, hypercalcemia, hypercalciuria, hyperphosphatemia and adynamic bone disease. Acute hypercalcemia may increase risk of cardiac arrhythmias and seizures; use caution with

cardiac glycosides as digitalis toxicity may be increased. Chronic hypercalcemia may lead to generalized vascular and other soft-tissue calcification. Phosphate and vitamin D (and its derivatives) should be withheld during therapy to avoid hypercalcemia. Risk of hypercalcemia may be increased by concomitant use of calcium-containing supplements and/or medications that increase serum calcium (eg, thiazide diuretics). Avoid regular administration to prevent aluminum overload and toxicity. Dialysate concentration of aluminum should be maintained at <10 mcg/L.

Adverse Reactions (Reflective of adult population; not specific for elderly)
>10%:
Gastrointestinal: Nausea (5% to 13%), diarrhea (7% to 12%)
Miscellaneous: Infection (bacterial, fungal, viral: 3% to 15%)
2% to 10%:
Cardiovascular: Edema (7%), hypertension (7%), hypervolemia (5%), hypotension (5%), palpitation (3%), chest pain (3%), peripheral edema (3%), syncope (3%)
Central nervous system: Pain (8%), dizziness (5% to 7%), chills (5%), insomnia (5%), lightheadedness (5%), vertigo (5%), fever (3% to 5%), headache (3% to 5%), anxiety (3%), depression (3%)
Dermatologic: Rash (6%), bruising (3%), skin ulcer (3%)
Endocrine & metabolic: Dehydration (3%), hypoglycemia (3%)
Gastrointestinal: Vomiting (5% to 8%), GI bleeding (5%), constipation (4% to 5%), abdominal pain (4%), dyspepsia (3%), xerostomia (3%)
Genitourinary: Urinary tract infection (3%)
Neuromuscular & skeletal: Arthritis (5%), weakness (3% to 5%), back pain (4%), leg cramps (3%)
Renal: Uremia (3%)
Respiratory: Pneumonia (5%), rhinitis (5%), oropharyngeal pain (4%), bronchitis (3%), cough (3%), sinusitis (3%)
Miscellaneous: Allergic reaction (6%), flu-like syndrome (5%), peritonitis (5%), sepsis (5%)

Drug Interactions
Metabolism/Transport Effects Substrate of CYP3A4 (minor); **Note:** Assignment of Major/Minor substrate status based on clinically relevant drug interaction potential
Avoid Concomitant Use
Avoid concomitant use of Paricalcitol with any of the following: Aluminum Hydroxide; Sucralfate; Vitamin D Analogs
Increased Effect/Toxicity
Paricalcitol may increase the levels/effects of: Aluminum Hydroxide; Cardiac Glycosides; Digoxin; Sucralfate; Vitamin D Analogs

The levels/effects of Paricalcitol may be increased by: Calcium Salts; CYP3A4 Inhibitors (Strong); Danazol; Thiazide Diuretics
Decreased Effect
The levels/effects of Paricalcitol may be decreased by: Bile Acid Sequestrants; Mineral Oil; Orlistat; Tocilizumab
Stability Store at 25°C (77°F); excursions permitted between 15°C to 30°C (59°F to 86°F).
Mechanism of Action Decreased renal conversion of vitamin D to its primary active metabolite (1,25-hydroxyvitamin D) in chronic renal failure leads to reduced activation of vitamin D receptor (VDR), which subsequently removes inhibitory suppression of parathyroid hormone (PTH) release; increased serum PTH (secondary hyperparathyroidism) reduces calcium excretion and enhances bone resorption. Paricalcitol is a synthetic vitamin D analog which binds to and activates the VDR in kidney, parathyroid gland, intestine and bone, thus reducing PTH levels and improving calcium and phosphate homeostasis.

Pharmacodynamics/Kinetics
Distribution: V_d:
Healthy subjects: Oral: 34 L; I.V.: 24 L
Stage 3 and 4 CKD: Oral: 44-46 L
Stage 5 CKD: Oral: 38-49 L; I.V.: 31-35 L
Protein binding: >99%
Metabolism: Hydroxylation and glucuronidation via hepatic and nonhepatic enzymes, including CYP24, CYP3A4, UGT1A4; forms metabolites (at least one active)
Bioavailability: Oral: 72% to 86% in healthy subjects
Half-life elimination:
Healthy subjects: Oral: 4-6 hours; I.V.: 5-7 hours
Stage 3 and 4 CKD: Oral: 14-20 hours
Stage 5 CKD: Oral: 14-20 hours; I.V.: 14-15 hours
Time to peak, plasma: 3 hours: Delayed by food
Excretion: Healthy subjects: Feces (oral: 70%; I.V.: 63%); urine (oral: 18%, I.V.: 19%)

Dosage

Geriatric & Adult Note: In stage 3-5 CKD maintain Ca x P <55 mg^2/dL^2, reduce or interrupt dosing if recommended calcium phosphorus product (Ca x P) is exceeded or hypercalcemia is observed (K/DOQI Clinical Practice Guidelines, 2003).

Secondary hyperparathyroidism associated with chronic renal failure (stage 5 CKD):
I.V.: 0.04-0.1 mcg/kg (2.8-7 mcg) given as a bolus dose no more frequently than every other day at any time during dialysis; dose may be increased by 2-4 mcg every 2-4 weeks; doses as high as 0.24 mcg/kg (16.8 mcg) have been administered safely; the dose of paricalcitol should be adjusted based on serum intact PTH (iPTH) levels, as follows:

Same or increasing iPTH level: Increase paricalcitol dose

iPTH level decreased by <30%: Increase paricalcitol dose

iPTH level decreased by >30% and <60%: Maintain paricalcitol dose

iPTH level decrease by >60%: Decrease paricalcitol dose

iPTH level 1.5-3 times upper limit of normal: Maintain paricalcitol dose

Oral: Initial dose, in mcg, based on baseline iPTH level divided by 80. Administered 3 times weekly, no more frequently than every other day. **Note:** To reduce the risk of hypercalcemia initiate only after baseline serum calcium has been adjusted to ≤9.5 mg/dL.

Dose titration:

Titration dose (mcg) = Most recent iPTH level (pg/mL) divided by 80

Note: In situations where monitoring of iPTH, calcium, and phosphorus occurs less frequently than once per week, a more modest initial and dose titration rate may be warranted:

Modest titration dose (mcg) = Most recent iPTH level (pg/mL) divided by 100

Dosage adjustment for hypercalcemia or elevated Ca x P: Decrease calculated dose by 2-4 mcg. If further adjustment is required, dose should be reduced or interrupted until these parameters are normalized. If applicable, phosphate binder dosing may also be adjusted or withheld, or switch to a noncalcium-based phosphate binder

Secondary hyperparathyroidism associated with stage 3 and 4 CKD: Adults: Oral: Initial dose based on baseline serum iPTH:

iPTH ≤500 pg/mL: 1 mcg/day or 2 mcg 3 times/week

iPTH >500 pg/mL: 2 mcg/day or 4 mcg 3 times/week

Dosage adjustment based on iPTH level relative to baseline, adjust dose at 2-4 week intervals:

iPTH same or increased: Increase paricalcitol dose by 1 mcg/day or 2 mcg 3 times/week

iPTH decreased by <30%: Increase paricalcitol dose by 1 mcg/day or 2 mcg 3 times/week

iPTH decreased by ≥30% and ≤60%: Maintain paricalcitol dose

iPTH decreased by >60%: Decrease paricalcitol dose by 1 mcg/day* or 2 mcg 3 times/week

iPTH <60 pg/mL: Decrease paricalcitol dose by 1 mcg/day* or 2 mcg 3 times/week

*If patient is taking the lowest dose on a once-daily regimen, but further dose reduction is needed, decrease dose to 1 mcg 3 times/week. If further dose reduction is required, withhold drug as needed and restart at a lower dose. If applicable, calcium-phosphate binder dosing may also be adjusted or withheld, or switch to noncalcium-based binder.

Renal Impairment Refer to Dosage: Geriatric & Adult.

Hepatic Impairment

Mild-to-moderate hepatic impairment: No dosage adjustment required.

Severe hepatic impairment: Use has not been evaluated.

Administration

Oral: May be administered with or without food. With the 3 times/week dosing schedule, doses should not be given more frequently than every other day.

I.V.: Administered as a bolus dose at anytime during dialysis. Doses should not be administered more often than every other day.

Monitoring Parameters

Signs and symptoms of vitamin D intoxication

Serum calcium and phosphorus (closely monitor levels during dosage titration and after initiation of a strong CYP3A4 inhibitor):

I.V.: Twice weekly during initial phase, then at least monthly once dose established

Oral: At least every 2 weeks for 3 months or following dose adjustment, then monthly for 3 months, then every 3 months

Serum or plasma intact PTH (iPTH):

I.V.: Every 3 months

Oral: At least every 2 weeks for 3 months or following dose adjustment, then monthly for 3 months, then every 3 months

Reference Range

Corrected total serum calcium (K/DOQI, 2003): CKD stages 3 and 4: 8.4-10.2 mg/dL (2.1-2.6 mmol/L); CKD stage 5: 8.4-9.5 mg/dL (2.1-2.37 mmol/L); KDIGO guidelines recommend maintaining normal ranges for all stages of CKD (3-5D) (KDIGO, 2009)

Phosphorus (K/DOQI, 2003):

CKD stages 3 and 4: 2.7-4.6 mg/dL (0.87-1.48 mmol/L) (adults)

CKD stage 5 (including those treated with dialysis): 3.5-5.5 mg/dL (1.13-1.78 mmol/L) (adults)

KDIGO guidelines recommend maintaining normal ranges for CKD stages 3-5 and lowering elevated phosphorus levels toward the normal range for CKD stage 5D (KDIGO, 2009)

Serum calcium-phosphorus product (K/DOQI, 2003): CKD stage 3-5: <55 mg^2/dL^2 (adults)

PTH: Whole molecule, immunochemiluminometric assay (ICMA): 1.0-5.2 pmol/L; whole molecule, radioimmunoassay (RIA): 10.0-65.0 pg/mL; whole molecule, immunoradiometric, double antibody (IRMA): 1.0-6.0 pmol/L

Target ranges by stage of chronic kidney disease (KDIGO, 2009): CKD stage 3-5: Optimal iPTH is unknown; maintain normal range (assay-dependent); CKD stage 5D: Maintain iPTH within 2-9 times the upper limit of normal for the assay used

Special Geriatric Considerations No specific dose changes necessary. Monitor closely. It may be advised to obtain baseline electrolytes, calcium, phosphorous, and digoxin serum concentrations, if applicable.

Dosage Forms Excipient information presented when available (limited, particularly for generics); consult specific product labeling.

Capsule, soft gelatin, oral:

Zemplar®: 1 mcg, 2 mcg, 4 mcg [contains coconut oil (may have trace amounts), ethanol, palm kernel oil (may have trace amounts)]

Injection, solution:

Zemplar®: 2 mcg/mL (1 mL); 5 mcg/mL (1 mL, 2 mL) [contains ethanol 20%, propylene glycol 30%]

◆ **Pariprazole** see RABEprazole on page 1659
◆ **Parlodel®** see Bromocriptine on page 223
◆ **Parlodel® SnapTabs®** see Bromocriptine on page 223
◆ **Parnate®** see Tranylcypromine on page 1949

PARoxetine (pa ROKS e teen)

Related Information

Antidepressant Agents on page 2097

Beers Criteria – Potentially Inappropriate Medications for Geriatrics on page 2183

Medication Safety Issues

Sound-alike/look-alike issues:

PARoxetine may be confused with FLUoxetine, PACLitaxel, piroxicam, pyridoxine

Paxil® may be confused with Doxil®, PACLitaxel, Plavix®, PROzac®, Taxol®

BEERS Criteria medication:

This drug may be potentially inappropriate for use in geriatric patients (SIADH: Quality of evidence - moderate; Strength of recommendation - strong).

Brand Names: U.S. Paxil CR®; Paxil®; Pexeva®

Brand Names: Canada Apo-Paroxetine®; CO Paroxetine; Dom-Paroxetine; Mylan-Paroxetine; Novo-Paroxetine; Paxil CR®; Paxil®; PHL-Paroxetine; PMS-Paroxetine; ratio-Paroxetine; Riva-Paroxetine; Sandoz-Paroxetine; Teva-Paroxetine

Index Terms Paroxetine Hydrochloride; Paroxetine Mesylate

Generic Availability (U.S.) Yes: Excludes suspension, tablet (mesylate)

Pharmacologic Category Antidepressant, Selective Serotonin Reuptake Inhibitor

Use Treatment of major depressive disorder (MDD); treatment of panic disorder with or without agoraphobia; obsessive-compulsive disorder (OCD); social anxiety disorder (social phobia); generalized anxiety disorder (GAD); post-traumatic stress disorder (PTSD)

Unlabeled Use May be useful in eating disorders, impulse control disorders; vasomotor symptoms of menopause; treatment of mild dementia-associated agitation in nonpsychotic patients

Medication Guide Available Yes

Contraindications Hypersensitivity to paroxetine or any component of the formulation; use with or within 14 days of MAO inhibitors intended to treat depression; concurrent use with reversible MAO inhibitors (eg, linezolid, methylene blue); concurrent use with thioridazine or pimozide

Warnings/Precautions Hazardous agent - use appropriate precautions for handling and disposal. Short-term studies did not show an increased risk in patients >24 years of age and showed a decreased risk in patients ≥65 years. Closely monitor patients for clinical worsening, suicidality, or unusual changes in behavior, particularly during the initial 1-2 months of therapy or during periods of dosage adjustments (increases or decreases); the patient's family or caregiver should be instructed to closely observe the patient and communicate condition with healthcare provider. A medication guide concerning the use of antidepressants should be dispensed with each prescription.

The possibility of a suicide attempt is inherent in major depression and may persist until remission occurs. Patients treated with antidepressants (for any indication) should be observed for clinical worsening and suicidality, especially during the initial few months of a course of drug therapy, or at times of dose changes, either increases or decreases. Use caution in high-risk patients. Worsening depression and severe abrupt suicidality that are not part of the presenting symptoms may require discontinuation or modification of drug therapy. The patient's family or caregiver should be alerted to monitor patients for the emergence of suicidality and associated behaviors (such as agitation, irritability, hostility, impulsivity, and hypomania) and call healthcare provider.

May worsen psychosis in some patients or precipitate a shift to mania or hypomania in patients with bipolar disorder. Patients presenting with depressive symptoms should be screened for bipolar disorder. Monotherapy in patients with bipolar disorder should be avoided. **Paroxetine is not FDA approved for the treatment of bipolar depression.**

Serotonin syndrome and neuroleptic malignant syndrome (NMS)-like reactions have occurred with serotonin/norepinephrine reuptake inhibitors (SNRIs) and selective serotonin reuptake inhibitors (SSRIs) when used alone, and particularly when used in combination with serotonergic agents (eg, triptans) or antidopaminergic agents (eg, antipsychotics). Concurrent use with MAO inhibitors, including reversible MAO inhibitors (eg, linezolid, methylene blue) is contraindicated. If the administration of linezolid or methylene blue cannot be avoided, paroxetine should be discontinued prior to administration of the reversible MAO inhibitor. Monitor for symptoms of serotonin syndrome/NMS-like reactions for 2 weeks or 24 hours after the last dose of the reversible MAO inhibitor (whichever comes first). Paroxetine may then be resumed 24 hours after the last dose of linezolid or methylene blue.

Paroxetine may increase the risks associated with electroconvulsive therapy. Has a low potential to impair cognitive or motor performance - use caution when operating hazardous machinery or driving. Symptoms of agitation and/or restlessness may occur during initial few weeks of therapy. Low potential for sedation or anticholinergic effects relative to cyclic antidepressants.

Use caution in elderly patients; may cause or exacerbate syndrome of inappropriate antidiuretic hormone secretion or hyponatremia; monitor sodium closely with initiation or dosage adjustments in older adults. Medication associated with potent anticholinergic properties which may be inappropriate in older adults depending on comorbidities (eg, dementia, delirium) (Beers Criteria).

Use caution in patients with a previous seizure disorder or condition predisposing to seizures such as brain damage, alcoholism, or concurrent therapy with other drugs which lower the seizure threshold. Use with caution in patients with hepatic dysfunction. May cause volume depletion (diuretics may increase risk). Use with caution with concomitant use of NSAIDs, ASA, or other drugs that affect coagulation; the risk of bleeding may be potentiated. Concurrent use with tamoxifen may decrease the efficacy of tamoxifen; consider an alternative antidepressant with little or no CYP2D6 inhibition when using tamoxifen for the treatment or prevention of breast cancer. Use with caution in patients with renal insufficiency or other concurrent illness (due to limited experience); dose reduction recommended with severe renal impairment. May cause or exacerbate sexual dysfunction. Use caution in patients with narrow-angle glaucoma.

Upon discontinuation of paroxetine therapy, gradually taper dose and monitor for discontinuation symptoms (eg, dizziness, dysphoric mood, irritability, agitation, confusion, paresthesias). If intolerable symptoms occur following a decrease in dosage or upon discontinuation of therapy, then resuming the previous dose with a more gradual taper should be considered.

Adverse Reactions (Reflective of adult population; not specific for elderly) Frequency varies by dose and indication. Adverse reactions reported as a composite of all indications.

>10%:
- Central nervous system: Somnolence (15% to 24%), insomnia (11% to 24%), headache (17% to 18%), dizziness (6% to 14%)
- Endocrine & metabolic: Libido decreased (3% to 15%)
- Gastrointestinal: Nausea (19% to 26%), xerostomia (9% to 18%), constipation (5% to 16%), diarrhea (9% to 12%)
- Genitourinary: Ejaculatory disturbances (13% to 28%)
- Neuromuscular & skeletal: Weakness (12% to 22%), tremor (4% to 11%)
- Miscellaneous: Diaphoresis (5% to 14%)

1% to 10%:
Cardiovascular: Vasodilation (2% to 4%), chest pain (3%), palpitation (2% to 3%), hypertension (≥1%), tachycardia (≥1%)
Central nervous system: Nervousness (4% to 9%), anxiety (5%), agitation (3% to 5%), abnormal dreams (3% to 4%), concentration impaired (3% to 4%), yawning (2% to 4%), depersonalization (≤3%), amnesia (2%), chills (2%), emotional lability (≥1%), vertigo (≥1%), confusion (1%)
Dermatologic: Rash (2% to 3%), pruritus (≥1%)
Endocrine & metabolic: Orgasmic disturbance (2% to 9%), dysmenorrhea (5%)
Gastrointestinal: Appetite decreased (5% to 9%), dyspepsia (2% to 5%), flatulence (4%), abdominal pain (4%), appetite increased (2% to 4%), vomiting (2% to 3%), taste perversion (2%), weight gain (≥1%)
Genitourinary: Genital disorder (male 10%; female 2% to 9%), impotence (2% to 9%), urinary frequency (2% to 3%), urinary tract infection (2%)
Neuromuscular & skeletal: Paresthesia (4%), myalgia (2% to 4%), back pain (3%), myoclonus (2% to 3%), myopathy (2%), myasthenia (1%), arthralgia (≥1%)
Ocular: Blurred vision (4%), abnormal vision (2% to 4%)
Otic: Tinnitus (≥1%)
Respiratory: Respiratory disorder (≤7%), pharyngitis (4%), sinusitis (≤4%), rhinitis (3%)
Miscellaneous: Infection (5% to 6%)

Drug Interactions

Metabolism/Transport Effects Substrate of CYP2D6 (major); **Note:** Assignment of Major/Minor substrate status based on clinically relevant drug interaction potential; **Inhibits** CYP1A2 (weak), CYP2B6 (moderate), CYP2C19 (weak), CYP2C9 (weak), CYP2D6 (strong), CYP3A4 (weak)

Avoid Concomitant Use

Avoid concomitant use of PARoxetine with any of the following: Iobenguane I 123; MAO Inhibitors; Methylene Blue; Pimozide; Tryptophan

Increased Effect/Toxicity

PARoxetine may increase the levels/effects of: Alpha-/Beta-Blockers; Anticoagulants; Antidepressants (Serotonin Reuptake Inhibitor/Antagonist); Antiplatelet Agents; ARIPiprazole; Aspirin; AtoMOXetine; Beta-Blockers; BusPIRone; CarBAMazepine; CloZAPine; Collagenase (Systemic); CYP2B6 Substrates; CYP2D6 Substrates; Dabigatran Etexilate; Desmopressin; Dextromethorphan; Drotrecogin Alfa (Activated); DULoxetine; Fesoterodine; Galantamine; Highest Risk QTc-Prolonging Agents; Hypoglycemic Agents; Ibritumomab; Lithium; Methadone; Methylene Blue; Metoclopramide; Mexiletine; Moderate Risk QTc-Prolonging Agents; NSAID (COX-2 Inhibitor); NSAID (Nonselective); Pimozide; Propafenone; RisperiDONE; Rivaroxaban; Salicylates; Serotonin Modulators; Thrombolytic Agents; Tositumomab and Iodine I 131 Tositumomab; TraMADol; Tricyclic Antidepressants; Vitamin K Antagonists

The levels/effects of PARoxetine may be increased by: Abiraterone Acetate; Alcohol (Ethyl); Analgesics (Opioid); Antipsychotics; ARIPiprazole; Asenapine; BusPIRone; Cimetidine; CNS Depressants; CYP2D6 Inhibitors (Moderate); CYP2D6 Inhibitors (Strong); Glucosamine; Herbs (Anticoagulant/Antiplatelet Properties); Linezolid; MAO Inhibitors; Metoclopramide; Metyrosine; Mifepristone; Omega-3-Acid Ethyl Esters; Pentosan Polysulfate Sodium; Pentoxifylline; Pravastatin; Prostacyclin Analogues; Tipranavir; TraMADol; Tryptophan; Vitamin E

Decreased Effect

PARoxetine may decrease the levels/effects of: Aprepitant; Fosaprepitant; Iobenguane I 123; Ioflupane I 123

The levels/effects of PARoxetine may be decreased by: Aprepitant; CarBAMazepine; Cyproheptadine; Darunavir; Fosamprenavir; Fosaprepitant; NSAID (COX-2 Inhibitor); NSAID (Nonselective); Peginterferon Alfa-2b

Ethanol/Nutrition/Herb Interactions

Ethanol: May increase CNS depression; monitor for increased effects with coadministration. Caution patients about effects.
Food: Peak concentration is increased, but bioavailability is not significantly altered by food.
Herb/Nutraceutical: Avoid valerian, St John's wort, SAMe, kava kava.

Stability

Suspension: Store at ≤25°C (≤77°F).
Tablets:
Paxil®: Store at 15°C to 30°C (59°F to 86°F).
Paxil CR®: Store at ≤25°C (≤77°F).
Pexeva®: Store at 25°C (77°F); excursions permitted to 15°C to 30°C (59°F to 86°F).

◄ **Mechanism of Action** Paroxetine is a selective serotonin reuptake inhibitor, chemically unrelated to tricyclic, tetracyclic, or other antidepressants; presumably, the inhibition of serotonin reuptake from brain synapse stimulated serotonin activity in the brain

Pharmacodynamics/Kinetics

Onset of action: Depression: The onset of action is within a week; however, individual response varies greatly and full response may not be seen until 8-12 weeks after initiation of treatment.

Absorption: Completely absorbed following oral administration

Distribution: V_d: 8.7 L/kg (3-28 L/kg)

Protein binding: 93% to 95%

Metabolism: Extensively hepatic via CYP2D6 enzymes; primary metabolites are formed via oxidation and methylation of parent drug, with subsequent glucuronide/sulfate conjugation; nonlinear pharmacokinetics (via 2D6 saturation) may be seen with higher doses and longer duration of therapy. Metabolites exhibit ~2% potency of parent compound. C_{min} concentrations are 70% to 80% greater in the elderly compared to nonelderly patients; clearance is also decreased.

Half-life elimination: 21 hours (3-65 hours)

Time to peak: Immediate release: 5.2-8.1 hours; controlled release: 6-10 hours

Excretion: Urine (64%, 2% as unchanged drug); feces (36% primarily via bile, <1% as unchanged drug)

Dosage

Geriatric

Major depressive disorder, obsessive compulsive disorder, panic attack, social anxiety disorder:

Paxil®, Pexeva®: Oral: Initial: 10 mg/day; increase if needed by 10 mg/day increments at intervals of at least 1 week; maximum dose: 40 mg/day

Paxil CR®: Initial: 12.5 mg/day; increase if needed by 12.5 mg/day increments at intervals of at least 1 week; maximum dose: 50 mg/day

Note: Upon discontinuation of paroxetine therapy, gradually taper dose:

Paxil®, Pexeva®: 10 mg/day at weekly intervals; when 20 mg/day dose is reached, continue for 1 week before treatment is discontinued. Some patients may need to be titrated to 10 mg/day for 1 week before discontinuation.

Paxil CR®: Patients receiving 37.5 mg/day in clinical trials had their dose decreased by 12.5 mg/day to a dose of 25 mg/day and remained at a dose of 25 mg/day for 1 week before treatment was discontinued.

Adult

Major depressive disorder: Oral:

Paxil®, Pexeva®: Initial: 20 mg once daily, preferably in the morning; increase if needed by 10 mg/day increments at intervals of at least 1 week; maximum dose: 50 mg/day

Paxil CR®: Initial: 25 mg once daily; increase if needed by 12.5 mg/day increments at intervals of at least 1 week; maximum dose: 62.5 mg/day

Generalized anxiety disorder (Paxil®, Pexeva®): Oral: Initial: 20 mg once daily, preferably in the morning (if dose is increased, adjust in increments of 10 mg/day at 1-week intervals); doses of 20-50 mg/day were used in clinical trials, however, no greater benefit was seen with doses >20 mg.

Obsessive-compulsive disorder (Paxil®, Pexeva®): Oral: Initial: 20 mg once daily, preferably in the morning; increase if needed by 10 mg/day increments at intervals of at least 1 week; recommended dose: 40 mg/day; range: 20-60 mg/day; maximum dose: 60 mg/day

Panic disorder: Oral:

Paxil®, Pexeva®: Initial: 10 mg once daily, preferably in the morning; increase if needed by 10 mg/day increments at intervals of at least 1 week; recommended dose: 40 mg/day; range: 10-60 mg/day; maximum dose: 60 mg/day

Paxil CR®: Initial: 12.5 mg once daily; increase if needed by 12.5 mg/day at intervals of at least 1 week; maximum dose: 75 mg/day

Post-traumatic stress disorder (Paxil®): Oral: Initial: 20 mg once daily, preferably in the morning; increase if needed by 10 mg/day increments at intervals of at least 1 week; range: 20-50 mg. Limited data suggest doses of 40 mg/day were not more efficacious than 20 mg/day.

Social anxiety disorder: Oral:

Paxil®: Initial: 20 mg once daily, preferably in the morning; recommended dose: 20 mg/day; range: 20-60 mg/day; doses >20 mg may not have additional benefit

Paxil CR®: Initial: 12.5 mg once daily, preferably in the morning; may be increased by 12.5 mg/day at intervals of at least 1 week; maximum dose: 37.5 mg/day

Menopause-associated vasomotor symptoms (unlabeled use, Paxil CR®): Oral: 12.5-25 mg/day

Note: Upon discontinuation of paroxetine therapy, gradually taper dose:

Paxil®, Pexeva®: 10 mg/day at weekly intervals; when 20 mg/day dose is reached, continue for 1 week before treatment is discontinued. Some patients may need to be titrated to 10 mg/day for 1 week before discontinuation.

Paxil CR®: Patients receiving 37.5 mg/day in clinical trials had their dose decreased by 12.5 mg/day to a dose of 25 mg/day and remained at a dose of 25 mg/day for 1 week before treatment was discontinued.

Renal Impairment Adults:

Cl_{cr} 30-60 mL/minute: Plasma concentration is 2 times that seen in normal function. There are no dosage adjustments provided in manufacturer's labeling.

Severe impairment (Cl_{cr} <30 mL/minute): Mean plasma concentration is ~4 times that seen in normal function.

Paxil®, Pexeva®: Initial: 10 mg/day; increase if needed by 10 mg/day increments at intervals of at least 1 week; maximum dose: 40 mg/day

Paxil CR®: Initial: 12.5 mg/day; increase if needed by 12.5 mg/day increments at intervals of at least 1 week; maximum dose: 50 mg/day

Hepatic Impairment Adults: In hepatic dysfunction, plasma concentration is 2 times that seen in normal function.

Mild-to-moderate impairment: There are no dosage adjustments provided in manufacturer's labeling.

Severe impairment:

Paxil®, Pexeva®: Initial: 10 mg/day; increase if needed by 10 mg/day increments at intervals of at least 1 week; maximum dose: 40 mg/day

Paxil CR®: Initial: 12.5 mg/day; increase if needed by 12.5 mg/day increments at intervals of at least 1 week; maximum dose: 50 mg/day

Administration May be administered without regard to meals, preferably in the morning. Do not crush, break, or chew controlled release tablets.

Monitoring Parameters Mental status for depression, suicide ideation (especially at the beginning of therapy or when doses are increased or decreased), anxiety, social functioning, mania, panic attacks; akathisia

Pharmacotherapy Pearls Paxil CR® incorporates a degradable polymeric matrix (Geomatrix™) to control dissolution rate over a period of 4-5 hours. An enteric coating delays the start of drug release until tablets have left the stomach.

Special Geriatric Considerations Paroxetine is the most sedating and anticholinergic of the selective serotonin reuptake inhibitors. The elderly are more prone to SSRI/SNRI-induced hyponatremia.

A systematic review and meta-analysis of antidepressant placebo-controlled trials in persons with depression and dementia found evidence "suggestive" of efficacy but not of sufficient strength to "confirm" efficacy. Antidepressant trials in this patient population are small and underpowered. Older patients with depression being treated with an antidepressant should be closely monitored for response and adverse effects. Treatment should be switched or augmented when response is inadequate with a therapeutic dose. Antidepressants that are not tolerated should be discontinued and an alternative agent should be started.

This medication is considered to be potentially inappropriate in this patient population (Beers Criteria: SIADH: Quality of evidence - moderate; Strength of recommendation - strong).

Dosage Forms Excipient information presented when available (limited, particularly for generics); consult specific product labeling.

Suspension, oral, as hydrochloride [strength expressed as base]:

Paxil®: 10 mg/5 mL (250 mL) [contains propylene glycol; orange flavor]

Tablet, oral, as hydrochloride [strength expressed as base]: 10 mg, 20 mg, 30 mg, 40 mg

Paxil®: 10 mg, 20 mg [scored]

Paxil®: 30 mg, 40 mg

Tablet, oral, as mesylate [strength expressed as base]:

Pexeva®: 10 mg

Pexeva®: 20 mg [scored]

Pexeva®: 30 mg, 40 mg

Tablet, controlled release, enteric coated, oral, as hydrochloride [strength expressed as base]: 12.5 mg, 25 mg, 37.5 mg

Paxil CR®: 12.5 mg, 25 mg, 37.5 mg

Tablet, extended release, enteric coated, oral, as hydrochloride [strength expressed as base]: 12.5 mg, 25 mg

◆ **Paroxetine Hydrochloride** *see* PARoxetine *on page 1475*

◆ **Paroxetine Mesylate** *see* PARoxetine *on page 1475*

◆ **PAS** *see* Aminosalicylic Acid *on page 95*

◆ **Paser®** *see* Aminosalicylic Acid *on page 95*

◆ **Pataday™** *see* Olopatadine (Ophthalmic) *on page 1414*

- **Patanase®** see Olopatadine (Nasal) on page 1414
- **Patanol®** see Olopatadine (Ophthalmic) on page 1414
- **Pavabid** see Papaverine on page 1472
- **Paxil®** see PARoxetine on page 1475
- **Paxil CR®** see PARoxetine on page 1475
- **PCA (error-prone abbreviation)** see Procainamide on page 1605
- **PCE®** see Erythromycin (Systemic) on page 665
- **PCEC** see Rabies Vaccine on page 1663
- **PediaCare® Children's Allergy [OTC]** see DiphenhydrAMINE (Systemic) on page 556
- **PediaCare® Children's Decongestant [OTC]** see Phenylephrine (Systemic) on page 1523
- **PediaCare® Children's Long-Acting Cough [OTC]** see Dextromethorphan on page 525
- **PediaCare® Children's NightTime Cough [OTC]** see DiphenhydrAMINE (Systemic) on page 556
- **Pediaderm™ AF** see Nystatin (Topical) on page 1399
- **Pediaderm™ HC** see Hydrocortisone (Topical) on page 943
- **Pediaderm™ TA** see Triamcinolone (Topical) on page 1961
- **Pediapred®** see PrednisoLONE (Systemic) on page 1591
- **Pediatex® TD** see Triprolidine and Pseudoephedrine on page 1975
- **Pedi-Boro® [OTC]** see Aluminum Sulfate and Calcium Acetate on page 84
- **Pedi-Dri®** see Nystatin (Topical) on page 1399
- **Pedipirox™ -4 Kit** see Ciclopirox on page 373
- **PEG** see Polyethylene Glycol 3350 on page 1564

Pegaptanib (peg AP ta nib)

Medication Safety Issues
Sound-alike/look-alike issues:
Pegaptanib may be confused with peginesatide, pegaspargase, pegfilgrastim, peginterferon, pegvisomant

Brand Names: U.S. Macugen®

Brand Names: Canada Macugen®

Index Terms EYE001; Pegaptanib Sodium

Generic Availability (U.S.) No

Pharmacologic Category Ophthalmic Agent; Vascular Endothelial Growth Factor (VEGF) Inhibitor

Use Treatment of neovascular (wet) age-related macular degeneration (AMD)

Contraindications Hypersensitivity to pegaptanib or any component of the formulation; ocular or periocular infection

Warnings/Precautions Intravitreous injections may be associated with endophthalmitis and retinal detachments. Proper aseptic injection techniques should be used and patients should be instructed to report any signs of infection immediately. Intraocular pressure may increase following injection. Safety and efficacy for administration into both eyes concurrently have not been studied. Safety and efficacy have not been established with hepatic impairment, or in patients requiring hemodialysis. Rare hypersensitivity reactions (including anaphylaxis) have been associated with pegaptanib, occurring within several hours of use; monitor closely. Equipment and appropriate personnel should be available for monitoring and treatment of anaphylaxis. Thromboembolic events (eg, nonfatal stroke/MI, vascular death) have been reported following intravitreal administration of other VEGF inhibitors.

Adverse Reactions (Reflective of adult population; not specific for elderly)
10% to 40%:
Cardiovascular: Hypertension
Ocular: Anterior chamber inflammation, blurred vision, cataract, conjunctival hemorrhage, corneal edema, eye discharge, eye irritation, eye pain, intraocular pressure increased, ocular discomfort, punctate keratitis, visual acuity decreased, visual disturbance, vitreous floaters, vitreous opacities
1% to 10%:
Cardiovascular: Carotid artery occlusion (1% to 5%), cerebrovascular accident (1% to 5%), chest pain (1% to 5%), transient ischemic attack (1% to 5%)
Central nervous system: Dizziness (6% to 10%), headache (6% to 10%), vertigo (1% to 5%)
Dermatologic: Contact dermatitis (1% to 5%)
Endocrine & metabolic: Diabetes mellitus (1% to 5%)
Gastrointestinal: Diarrhea (6% to 10%), nausea (6% to 10%), dyspepsia (1% to 5%), vomiting (1% to 5%)
Genitourinary: Urinary retention (1% to 5%)
Neuromuscular & skeletal: Arthritis (1% to 5%), bone spur (1% to 5%)
Ocular: Blepharitis (6% to 10%), conjunctivitis (6% to 10%), photopsia (6% to 10%), vitreous disorder (6% to 10%), allergic conjunctivitis (1% to 5%), conjunctival edema (1% to 5%),

corneal abrasion (1% to 5%), corneal deposits (1% to 5%), corneal epithelium disorder (1% to 5%), endophthalmitis (1% to 5%), eye inflammation (1% to 5%), eye swelling (1% to 5%), eyelid irritation (1% to 5%), meibomianitis (1% to 5%), mydriasis (1% to 5%), periorbital hematoma (1% to 5%), retinal edema (1% to 5%), vitreous hemorrhage (1% to 5%)

Otic: Hearing loss (1% to 5%)

Renal: Urinary tract infection (6% to 10%)

Respiratory: Bronchitis (6% to 10%), pleural effusion (1% to 5%)

Miscellaneous: Contusion (1% to 5%)

Drug Interactions

Metabolism/Transport Effects None known.

Avoid Concomitant Use There are no known interactions where it is recommended to avoid concomitant use.

Increased Effect/Toxicity There are no known significant interactions involving an increase in effect.

Decreased Effect

The levels/effects of Pegaptanib may be decreased by: Pegloticase

Stability Store under refrigeration at 2°C to 8°C (36°F to 46°F); do not freeze. Do not shake vigorously.

Mechanism of Action Pegaptanib is an apatamer, an oligonucleotide covalently bound to polyethylene glycol, which can adopt a three-dimensional shape and bind to vascular endothelial growth factor (VEGF). Pegaptanib binds to extracellular VEGF, inhibiting VEGF from binding to its receptors and thereby suppressing neovascularization and slowing vision loss.

Pharmacodynamics/Kinetics

Absorption: Slow systemic absorption following intravitreous injection

Metabolism: Metabolized by endo- and exonucleases

Half-life elimination: Plasma: 6-14 days

Dosage

Geriatric & Adult AMD: Intravitreal injection: 0.3 mg into affected eye every 6 weeks

Renal Impairment Adjustment not required with renal impairment; information not available for patients requiring hemodialysis.

Administration For ophthalmic intravitreal injection only. Attach a 30 gauge $1/2$ inch needle to the medication syringe. Depress plunger to expel excess air and medication (refer to product labeling for detailed instructions). Adequate anesthesia and a broad spectrum antibiotic should be administered prior to the procedure.

Monitoring Parameters Intraocular pressure (within 30 minutes and 2-7 days after injection); signs of infection/inflammation (for first week following injection); retinal perfusion, endophthalmitis, visual acuity

Special Geriatric Considerations In studies, 94% of patients treated with pegaptanib were ≥65 years of age. No difference in efficacy was seen as compared to younger adults.

Dosage Forms Excipient information presented when available (limited, particularly for generics); consult specific product labeling.

Injection, solution [preservative free]:

Macugen®: 0.3 mg/0.09 mL (0.09 mL)

◆ **Pegaptanib Sodium** see Pegaptanib on page 1480

Pegfilgrastim (peg fil GRA stim)

Medication Safety Issues

Sound-alike/look-alike issues:

Neulasta® may be confused with Neumega®, Neupogen®, and Lunesta®

Brand Names: U.S. Neulasta®

Brand Names: Canada Neulasta®

Index Terms G-CSF (PEG Conjugate); Granulocyte Colony Stimulating Factor (PEG Conjugate); Pegylated G-CSF; SD/01

Generic Availability (U.S.) No

Pharmacologic Category Colony Stimulating Factor

Use To decrease the incidence of infection, by stimulation of granulocyte production, in patients with nonmyeloid malignancies receiving myelosuppressive therapy associated with a significant risk of febrile neutropenia

Contraindications Hypersensitivity to pegfilgrastim, filgrastim, or any component of the formulation

Warnings/Precautions Do not use pegfilgrastim in the period 14 days before to 24 hours after administration of cytotoxic chemotherapy because of the potential sensitivity of rapidly dividing myeloid cells to cytotoxic chemotherapy. Benefit has not been demonstrated with regimens under a two-week duration. Administration on the same day as chemotherapy is not recommended (NCCN Myeloid Growth Factor Guidelines, v.1.2009). Pegfilgrastim can potentially act as a growth factor for any tumor type, particularly myeloid malignancies. Caution should be exercised in the usage of pegfilgrastim in any malignancy with myeloid characteristics. Tumors of nonhematopoietic origin may have surface receptors for pegfilgrastim. Pegfilgrastim has not been evaluated with patients receiving radiation therapy, or with chemotherapy associated with delayed myelosuppression (nitrosoureas, mitomycin C). Safety and efficacy have not been evaluated for peripheral blood progenitor cell (PBPC) mobilization.

Allergic-type reactions (anaphylaxis, angioedema, erythema, skin rash, urticaria) have occurred primarily with the initial dose and may recur (possibly delayed) after discontinuation; close follow up for several days and permanent discontinuation are recommended for severe reactions. Rare cases of splenic rupture have been reported; patients must be instructed to report left upper quadrant pain or shoulder tip pain. Acute respiratory distress syndrome (ARDS) has been associated with use; evaluate patients with pulmonary symptoms such as fever, lung infiltrates, or respiratory distress; discontinue or withhold pegfilgrastim if ARDS occurs. May precipitate sickle cell crises in patients with sickle cell disease; carefully evaluate potential risks and benefits. The packaging (needle cover) contains latex.

Adverse Reactions (Reflective of adult population; not specific for elderly)
>10%:
Cardiovascular: Peripheral edema (12%)
Central nervous system: Headache (16%)
Gastrointestinal: Vomiting (13%)
Neuromuscular & skeletal: Bone pain (31% to 57%), myalgia (21%), arthralgia (16%), weakness (13%)
1% to 10%:
Gastrointestinal: Constipation (10%)
Miscellaneous: Antibody formation (1% to 6%)

Drug Interactions
Metabolism/Transport Effects None known.
Avoid Concomitant Use There are no known interactions where it is recommended to avoid concomitant use.
Increased Effect/Toxicity There are no known significant interactions involving an increase in effect.
Decreased Effect
The levels/effects of Pegfilgrastim may be decreased by: Pegloticase

Stability Store under refrigeration 2°C to 8°C (36°F to 46°F); do not freeze. If inadvertently frozen, allow to thaw in refrigerator; discard if frozen more than one time. Protect from light. Do not shake. Allow to reach room temperature prior to injection. May be kept at room temperature for up to 48 hours.
Mechanism of Action Stimulates the production, maturation, and activation of neutrophils, pegfilgrastim activates neutrophils to increase both their migration and cytotoxicity. Pegfilgrastim has a prolonged duration of effect relative to filgrastim and a reduced renal clearance.
Pharmacodynamics/Kinetics Half-life elimination: SubQ: Adults: 15-80 hours

Dosage
Geriatric & Adult Do not administer in the period between 14 days before and 24 hours after administration of cytotoxic chemotherapy. According to the NCCN guidelines, efficacy has been demonstrated with every-2-week chemotherapy regimens, however, benefit has not been demonstrated with regimens under a two-week duration (NCCN Myeloid Growth Factor Guidelines, v.1.2011)
Prevention of chemotherapy-induced neutropenia: SubQ: 6 mg once per chemotherapy cycle, beginning 24-72 hours after completion of chemotherapy
Renal Impairment No adjustment necessary.
Administration Administer subcutaneously. Engage/activate needle guard following use to prevent accidental needlesticks.
Monitoring Parameters Complete blood count (with differential) and platelet count should be obtained prior to chemotherapy. Leukocytosis (white blood cell counts 100,000/mm³) has been observed in <1% of patients receiving pegfilgrastim. Monitor platelets and hematocrit regularly. Evaluate fever, pulmonary infiltrates, and respiratory distress; evaluate for left upper abdominal pain, shoulder tip pain, or splenomegaly. Monitor for sickle cell crisis (in patients with sickle cell anemia).
Test Interactions May interfere with bone imaging studies; increased hematopoietic activity of the bone marrow may appear as transient positive bone imaging changes
Special Geriatric Considerations Do not use in patients <45 kg.
Dosage Forms Excipient information presented when available (limited, particularly for generics); consult specific product labeling.

Injection, solution [preservative free]:
Neulasta®: 6 mg/0.6 mL (0.6 mL) [contains natural rubber/natural latex in packaging]

♦ **PEG-IFN Alfa-2b** *see* Peginterferon Alfa-2b *on page 1485*

Peginesatide (peg in ESS a tide)

Medication Safety Issues
Sound-alike/look-alike issues:
Peginesatide may be confused with pegaptanib, pegaspargase, pegfilgrastim, peginterferon, pegvisomant

Brand Names: U.S. Omontys®
Index Terms Erythropoiesis-Stimulating Agent (ESA); Hematide; Omontys®
Generic Availability (U.S.) No
Pharmacologic Category Colony Stimulating Factor; Erythropoiesis-Stimulating Agent (ESA); Growth Factor
Use Treatment of anemia due to chronic kidney disease (CKD) in patients receiving dialysis
Note: Peginesatide is **not** indicated for use under the following conditions:
  • CKD patients not receiving dialysis
  • Cancer patients with anemia that is not due to CKD
  • As a substitute for RBC transfusion in patients requiring immediate correction of anemia
Note: Peginesatide has not demonstrated improved symptoms, physical functioning, or health-related quality of life.
Medication Guide Available Yes
Contraindications Uncontrolled hypertension
Warnings/Precautions [U.S. Boxed Warning]: An increased risk of death, serious cardiovascular events, and stroke was reported in chronic kidney disease (CKD) patients administered ESAs to target hemoglobin levels >11 g/dL; use the lowest dose sufficient to reduce the need for RBC transfusions. An optimal target hemoglobin level, dose, or dosing strategy to reduce these risks have not been identified in clinical trials. Hemoglobin rising >1 g/dL in a 2-week period may contribute to the risk (dosage reduction recommended). CKD patients who exhibit an inadequate hemoglobin response to ESA therapy may be at a higher risk for cardiovascular events and mortality compared to other patients. Adjustments in dialysis parameters may be needed after initiation of peginesatide. Patients treated with peginesatide may require increased heparinization during dialysis to prevent clotting of the extracorporeal circuit. Therapy is not appropriate for anemia treatment in CKD patients *not* receiving dialysis.

Use with caution in patients with a history of hypertension (contraindicated in uncontrolled hypertension) or cardiovascular disease (history or active) and stroke. Blood pressure should be controlled prior to start of (and during) therapy; monitor closely throughout treatment and reduce or withhold peginesatide if blood pressure becomes difficult to control. In clinical trials involving ESAs, an increased risk of death was observed in patients undergoing coronary artery bypass surgery (CABG) and an increased risk of deep vein thrombosis (DVT) was seen in those undergoing orthopedic procedures. Clinical trials involving ESAs in cancer patients have shown an increased risk of death, MI, and stroke. Peginesatide is not indicated in cancer patients with anemia who do not have chronic kidney disease. Due to the delayed onset of erythropoiesis, peginesatide is not recommended for acute correction of severe anemia or as a substitute for emergency transfusion.

Allergic reactions have been reported (rarely). Discontinue and treat symptoms appropriately in patients who experience serious allergic/anaphylactic reactions. Seizures have been observed in clinical studies with use; use with caution in patients with a history of seizures. Monitor closely for neurologic symptoms during the first several months of therapy. Prior to and periodically during therapy, iron stores must be evaluated. Supplemental iron is recommended if serum ferritin <100 mcg/L or serum transferrin saturation <20%. Most patients with CKD will require iron supplementation.

Prior to treatment, correct or exclude deficiencies of iron, vitamin B_{12}, and/or folate, as well as other factors which may impair erythropoiesis (inflammatory conditions, infections, bleeding). Patients with a sudden loss of hemoglobin response should also be evaluated for potential causes of decreased response. If common causes are excluded, patient should be evaluated for the presence of peginesatide antibodies. During trials, peginesatide-specific binding antibodies were detected rarely (with a higher incidence noted in patients receiving subcutaneous compared to I.V. administration); however, no cases of pure red cell aplasia (PRCA) were observed in studies. Peginesatide is a synthetic, peptide-based ESA agent and cross-reactivity of the immune response against either endogenous or recombinant protein-based erythropoietin agents (eg, epoetin, darbepoetin) to peginesatide is unlikely due to the difference in amino acid sequence (Macdougall, 2011).

Adverse Reactions (Reflective of adult population; not specific for elderly)
>10%:
Cardiovascular: Hypotension (14%), hypertension (13%), procedural hypotension (11%)
Central nervous system: Headache (15%), fever (12%)
Endocrine & metabolic: Hyperkalemia (11%)
Gastrointestinal: Diarrhea (18%), nausea (17%), vomiting (15%)
Neuromuscular & skeletal: Muscle spasms (15%), arthralgia (11%), back pain (11%), extremity pain (11%)
Respiratory: Dyspnea (18%), cough (16%), upper respiratory tract infection (11%)
Miscellaneous: Arteriovenous fistula site complication (16%)
1% to 10%: Miscellaneous: Peginesatide-specific binding antibodies (1%)

Drug Interactions
Metabolism/Transport Effects None known.
Avoid Concomitant Use There are no known interactions where it is recommended to avoid concomitant use.
Increased Effect/Toxicity There are no known significant interactions involving an increase in effect.
Decreased Effect There are no known significant interactions involving a decrease in effect.

Stability Store refrigerated at 2°C to 8°C (36°F to 46°F). Protect from light. If necessary, may store at temperatures ≤25°C (77°F) for ≤30 days. After initial entry, store multidose vials at 2°C to 8°C (36°F to 46°F); discard after 28 days. Do not dilute prior to administration.

Mechanism of Action Peginesatide, a pegylated synthetic peptide, binds to the human erythropoietin receptor to induce erythropoiesis by stimulating the division and differentiation of committed erythroid progenitor cells; induces the release of reticulocytes from the bone marrow into the bloodstream, where they mature to erythrocytes. There is a dose response relationship with this effect. This results in an increase in reticulocyte counts followed by a rise in hemoglobin levels.

Pharmacodynamics/Kinetics
Distribution: I.V.: Dialysis patients: V_d: 34.9 mL/kg
Bioavailability: SubQ: ~46%
Half-life elimination: I.V.: Healthy subjects: 25 hours, Dialysis patients: 47.9 hours; SubQ: Healthy patients: 53 hours
Time to peak: SubQ: ~48 hours

Dosage
Geriatric & Adult Anemia associated with chronic kidney disease in patients receiving dialysis: I.V., SubQ: Individualize dosing and use the lowest dose necessary to reduce the need for RBC transfusions.
Patients not currently receiving an erythropoiesis-stimulating agent (ESA) (initiate when hemoglobin is <10 g/dL): I.V., SubQ: Initial dose: 0.04 mg/kg once monthly
Conversion from another ESA (epoetin or darbepoetin) to peginesatide: **Note:** The initial monthly peginesatide dose can be estimated based on the weekly dose of epoetin or darbepoetin at the time of substitution (see table); the same route of administration (SubQ or I.V.) of the previous ESA should be maintained after conversion to peginesatide. If previous ESA was epoetin, the first dose of peginesatide should be 1 week after the last epoetin dose. If previous ESA was darbepoetin, the first dose of peginesatide should be given in the place of darbepoetin at the next scheduled dose.

Conversion from Another ESA (Epoetin or Darbepoetin) to Peginesatide

Previous Epoetin Alfa Total WEEKLY Dose (units/wk)	Previous Darbepoetin Alfa WEEKLY Dose (mcg/wk)	Initial Peginesatide MONTHLY Dose (mg/mo)
<2500	<12	2
2500 to <4300	12 to <18	3
4300 to <6500	18 to <25	4
6500 to <8900	25 to <35	5
8900 to <13,000	35 to <45	6
13,000 to <19,000	45 to <60	8
19,000 to <33,000	60 to <95	10
33,000 to <68,000	95 to <175	15
≥68,000	≥175	20

Dosage adjustments:

If hemoglobin does not increase by >1 g/dL after 4 weeks: Increase dose by 25%; do not increase the dose more frequently than once every 4 weeks

If hemoglobin increases >1 g/dL in the 2-week period prior to the dose or >2 g/dL in 4 weeks: Reduce dose by 25% (or more) as needed to reduce rapid response

If hemoglobin approaches or exceeds 11 g/dL: Reduce or interrupt dose; after dose has been withheld and once the hemoglobin begins to decrease, may resume dose at ~25% below the previous dose

Inadequate or lack of response over a 12-week escalation period: Further increases are unlikely to improve response and may increase risks; use the minimum effective dose that will maintain a Hgb level sufficient to avoid RBC transfusions and evaluate patient for other causes of anemia. Discontinue therapy if responsiveness does not improve.

Missed doses: Administer a missed dose as soon as possible and restart peginesatide at the prescribed once monthly dosing frequency.

Renal Impairment No dosage adjustment provided in manufacturer's labeling.

Hepatic Impairment No dosage adjustment provided in manufacturer's labeling (has not been studied).

Administration May be administered as an I.V. injection or SubQ injection. The I.V. route is generally used for hemodialysis patients; medication is injected via a special access port on the dialysis tubing during the dialysis procedure. Peritoneal dialysis patients should only administer therapy via the SubQ route. For SubQ injections, may inject in either the outer area of the upper arms, the front of the middle thighs, the abdomen (excluding the 2-inch area around the navel), or the upper outer buttocks area. Do not inject in skin that is tender, red, hard, scarred, or bruised.

Monitoring Parameters Transferrin saturation and serum ferritin (prior to initiation and during therapy); hemoglobin (every 2 weeks after initiation and following dose adjustments until stable and sufficient to minimize need for RBC transfusion, then at least monthly following hemoglobin stability); blood pressure; seizures (following initiation for first few months, includes new-onset or change in seizure frequency or premonitory symptoms); allergic reaction; presence of antibodies (if common causes of lack or loss of response are ruled out)

Pharmacotherapy Pearls For information regarding evaluating patients for the presence of binding and neutralizing antibodies to peginesatide, contact Affymax, Inc (1-855-466-6689).

Special Geriatric Considerations In Phase 3 clinical trials, 32.5% of dialysis patients were ≥65 years and 13% were ≥75 years. No differences in safety or efficacy were reported between younger and older patients.

Dosage Forms Excipient information presented when available (limited, particularly for generics); consult specific product labeling.

Injection, solution:

Omontys®: 10 mg/mL (1 mL, 2 mL)

Peginterferon Alfa-2b (peg in ter FEER on AL fa too bee)

Medication Safety Issues

Sound-alike/look-alike issues:

Peginterferon alfa-2b may be confused with interferon alfa-2a, interferon alfa-2b, interferon alfa-n3, peginterferon alfa-2a

PegIntron® may be confused with Intron® A

International issues:

Peginterferon alfa-2b may be confused with interferon alpha multi-subtype which is available in international markets

Brand Names: U.S. PegIntron®; PegIntron™ Redipen®; Sylatron™

Brand Names: Canada PegIntron®

Index Terms Interferon Alfa-2b (PEG Conjugate); PEG-IFN Alfa-2b; Pegylated Interferon Alfa-2b; Polyethylene Glycol Interferon Alfa-2b; Sylatron™

Generic Availability (U.S.) No

Pharmacologic Category Interferon

Use

PegIntron®: Treatment of chronic hepatitis C (CHC; in combination with ribavirin) in patients who have compensated liver disease; treatment of chronic hepatitis C (as monotherapy) in adult patients with compensated liver disease who have never received alfa interferons

Sylatron™: Adjuvant treatment of melanoma (with microscopic or gross nodal involvement within 84 days of definitive surgical resection, including lymphadenectomy)

Medication Guide Available Yes

◀ **Contraindications** Hypersensitivity (including urticaria, angioedema, bronchoconstriction, anaphylaxis, Stevens Johnson syndrome and toxic epidermal necrolysis) to peginterferon alfa-2b, interferon alfa-2b, other alfa interferons, or any component of the formulation); autoimmune hepatitis; decompensated liver disease (Child-Pugh score >6, classes B and C)

Combination therapy with peginterferon alfa-2b and ribavirin is also contraindicated in males with pregnant partners; hemoglobinopathies (eg, thalassemia major, sickle-cell anemia); renal dysfunction (Cl_{cr} <50 mL/minute)

Warnings/Precautions Hazardous agent - use appropriate precautions for handling and disposal.

[U.S. Boxed Warnings]: May cause or aggravate severe depression or other neuropsychiatric adverse events (including suicide and suicidal ideation) in patients with and without a history of psychiatric disorder; may be irreversible; discontinue treatment permanently with worsening or persistently severe signs/symptoms of neuropsychiatric disorders (eg, depression, encephalopathy, psychosis). May cause or aggravate fatal or life-threatening autoimmune disorders, infectious disorders, ischemic disorders, and/or hemorrhagic cerebrovascular events; discontinue treatment for persistent severe or worsening symptoms.

Neuropsychiatric disorders: Neuropsychiatric effects may occur in patients with and without a history of psychiatric disorder; addiction relapse, aggression, depression, homicidal ideation and suicidal behavior/ideation have been observed with peginterferon alfa-2b; bipolar disorder, encephalopathy, hallucinations, mania, and psychosis have been observed with other alfa interferons. Onset may be delayed (up to 6 months after discontinuation). Higher doses may be associated with the development of encephalopathy (higher risk in elderly patients). Use with extreme caution in patients with a history of psychiatric disorders, including depression. Monitor all patients for evidence of depression; patients being treated for melanoma should be monitored for depression and psychiatric symptoms every 3 weeks during the first eight weeks of treatment and every 6 months thereafter; discontinue treatment if psychiatric symptoms persist, worsen or if suicidal behavior develops. All patients should continue to be monitored for 6 months after completion of therapy.

Bone marrow suppression: Causes bone marrow suppression, including potentially severe cytopenias; alfa interferons may (rarely) cause aplastic anemia. Use with caution in patients who are chronically immunosuppressed, with low peripheral blood counts or myelosuppression, including concurrent use of myelosuppressive therapy. Use with caution in patients with an increased risk for severe anemia (eg, spherocytosis, history of GI bleeding). Dosage modification may be necessary for hematologic toxicity. Combination therapy with ribavirin may potentiate the neutropenic effects of alfa interferons. When used in combination with ribavirin, an increased incidence of anemia was observed when using ribavirin weight-based dosing, as compared to flat-dose ribavirin.

Hepatic disease: Use is contraindicated in patients with hepatic decompensation. Discontinue treatment immediately with hepatic decompensation (Child Pugh score >6). Patients with chronic hepatitis C (CHC) with cirrhosis receiving peginterferon alfa-2b are at risk for hepatic decompensation. CHC patients coinfected with human immunodeficiency virus (HIV) are at increased risk for hepatic decompensation when receiving highly active antiretroviral therapy (HAART); monitor closely. A transient increase in ALT (2-5 times above baseline) which is not associated with deterioration of liver function may occur with peginterferon alfa-2b use (for the treatment of chronic hepatitis C); therapy generally may continue with monitoring.

Gastrointestinal disorders: Pancreatitis has been observed with alfa interferon therapy; discontinue therapy if known or suspected pancreatitis develops. Ulcerative or hemorrhagic/ischemic colitis has been observed with alfa interferons; withhold treatment for suspected pancreatitis; discontinue therapy for known pancreatitis. Ulcerative or hemorrhagic/ischemic colitis has been observed with alfa interferons; discontinue therapy if signs of colitis (abdominal pain, bloody diarrhea, fever) develop; symptoms typically resolve within 1-3 weeks.

Autoimmune disorders: Thyroiditis, thrombotic thrombocytopenic purpura, idiopathic thrombocytopenic purpura, rheumatoid arthritis, interstitial nephritis, systemic lupus erythematosus, and psoriasis have been reported with therapy; use with caution in patients with autoimmune disorders.

Cardiovascular disease: Use with caution in patients with cardiovascular disease or a history of cardiovascular disease; hypotension, arrhythmia, bundle branch block, tachycardia, cardiomyopathy, angina pectoris and MI have been observed with treatment. Patients with pre-existing cardiac abnormalities should have baseline ECGs prior to combination treatment with ribavirin; closely monitor patients with a history of MI or arrhythmia. Patients with a history of significant or unstable cardiac disease should not receive combination treatment with ribavirin.

Discontinue treatment (permanently) for new-onset ventricular arrhythmia or cardiovascular decompensation.

Endocrine disorders: Diabetes mellitus (including new-onset type I diabetes), hyperglycemia, and thyroid disorders have been reported; discontinue peginterferon alfa-2b if cannot be effectively managed with medication. Use caution in patients with a history of diabetes mellitus, particularly if prone to DKA. Use with caution in patients with thyroid disorders; may cause or aggravate hyper- or hypothyroidism.

Pulmonary disease: May cause or aggravate dyspnea, pulmonary infiltrates, pneumonia, bronchiolitis obliterans, interstitial pneumonitis, pulmonary hypertension, and sarcoidosis which may result in respiratory failure; may recur upon rechallenge with treatment; monitor closely. Use with caution in patients with existing pulmonary disease (eg, chronic obstructive pulmonary disease). Withhold combination therapy with ribavirin for development of pulmonary infiltrate or pulmonary function impairment.

Ophthalmic disorders: Ophthalmologic disorders (including decreased visual acuity, blindness, macular edema, retinal hemorrhages, optic neuritis, papilledema, cotton wool spots, retinal detachment [serous], and retinal artery or vein thrombosis) have occurred with peginterferon alfa-2b and/or with other alfa interferons. Prior to start of therapy, ophthalmic exams are recommended for all patients; patients with diabetic or hypertensive retinopathy should have periodic ophthalmic exams during treatment; a complete eye exam should be done promptly in patients who develop ocular symptoms. Permanently discontinue treatment with new or worsening ophthalmic disorder.

[U.S. Boxed Warning]: Combination treatment with ribavirin may cause birth defects and/or fetal mortality (avoid pregnancy in females and female partners of male patients); hemolytic anemia (which may worsen cardiac disease), genotoxicity, mutagenicity, and may possibly be carcinogenic. Interferon therapy is commonly associated with flu-like symptoms, including fever; rule out other causes/infection with persistent or high fever. Acute hypersensitivity reactions and cutaneous reactions (eg, Stevens-Johnson syndrome, toxic epidermal necrolysis) have been reported (rarely) with alfa interferons; prompt discontinuation is recommended; transient rashes do not require interruption of therapy. Hypertriglyceridemia has been reported with use; discontinue if persistent and severe (triglycerides >1000 mg/dL), particularly if combined with symptoms of pancreatitis. Use with caution in patients with renal impairment (Cl_{cr} <50 mL/minute); monitor closely. For the treatment of chronic hepatitis C, dosage adjustments are recommended with monotherapy in patients with moderate-to-severe impairment; do not use combination therapy with ribavirin in adult patients renal dysfunction (Cl_{cr} <50 mL/minute). Has not been studied in melanoma patients with renal impairment. Serum creatinine increases have been reported in patients with renal insufficiency. Use with caution in the elderly; the potential adverse effects may be more pronounced in the elderly. Elderly patients generally do not respond to interferon treatment as well as younger patients. Dental/periodontal disorders have been reported with combination therapy; dry mouth may affect teeth and mucous membranes; instruct patients to brush teeth twice daily; encourage regular dental exams.

Combination therapy with ribavirin is preferred over monotherapy for the treatment of chronic hepatitis C (combination therapy provides a better response). Safety and efficacy have not been established in patients who have received organ transplants, are coinfected with HIV or hepatitis B, or received treatment for >1 year. Patients with significant bridging fibrosis or cirrhosis, genotype 1 infection or who have not responded to prior therapy, including previous pegylated interferon treatment are less likely to benefit from combination therapy with peginterferon alfa-2b and ribavirin. Due to differences in dosage, patients should not change brands of interferon.

Adverse Reactions (Reflective of adult population; not specific for elderly) Note: Percentages reported for adults receiving monotherapy unless noted:

>10%:

    Central nervous system: Fatigue (52% to 94%), fever (22% to 75%), headache (56% to 70%), chills (≤63%), depression (29% to 59%; may be severe), dizziness (12% to 35%), anxiety/emotional liability/irritability (28%), insomnia (23%), olfactory nerve disorder (≤23%)

    Dermatologic: Rash (6% to 36%), alopecia (22% to 34%), pruritus (12%), dry skin (11%)

    Gastrointestinal: Anorexia (20% to 69%), nausea (26% to 64%), taste perversion (≤38%), diarrhea (18% to 37%), vomiting (7% to 26%), abdominal pain (15%), weight loss (11%)

    Hematologic: Neutropenia (6% to 70%; grade 4: 1%), thrombocytopenia (7% to 20%; grades 3/4: <4%), anemia (6%; in combination with ribavirin: 12% to 47%)

    Hepatic: Transaminases increased (10% to 77%), alkaline phosphatase increased (≤23%)

    Local: Injection site inflammation/reaction (23% to 62%)

    Neuromuscular & skeletal: Myalgia (54% to 68%), weakness (52%), arthralgia (23% to 51%), musculoskeletal pain (28%), rigors (23%), paresthesia (21%)

    Miscellaneous: Viral infection (11%)

>1% to 10%:
Cardiovascular: Chest pain (6%), flushing (6%)
Central nervous system: Concentration impaired (10%), malaise (7%), nervousness (4%), agitation (2%), suicidal behavior (ideation/attempt/suicide ≤2%)
Endocrine & metabolic: Hypothyroidism (5%), menstrual disorder (4%), hyperthyroidism (3%)
Gastrointestinal: Dyspepsia (6%), xerostomia (6%), constipation (1%)
Hepatic: GGT increased (8%), hepatomegaly (6%)
Local: Injection site pain (2% to 3%)
Ocular: Conjunctivitis (4%), blurred vision (2%)
Renal: Proteinuria (≤7%)
Respiratory: Pharyngitis (10%), cough (5% to 8%), sinusitis (7%), dyspnea (4% to 6%), rhinitis (2%)
Miscellaneous: Diaphoresis (6%), neutralizing antibodies (2%)

Drug Interactions
Metabolism/Transport Effects Inhibits CYP1A2 (weak)
Avoid Concomitant Use
Avoid concomitant use of Peginterferon Alfa-2b with any of the following: CloZAPine; Telbivudine
Increased Effect/Toxicity
Peginterferon Alfa-2b may increase the levels/effects of: Aldesleukin; CloZAPine; Methadone; Ribavirin; Telbivudine; Theophylline Derivatives; Zidovudine
Decreased Effect
Peginterferon Alfa-2b may decrease the levels/effects of: CYP2C9 Substrates; CYP2D6 Substrates; FLUoxetine

The levels/effects of Peginterferon Alfa-2b may be decreased by: Pegloticase
Ethanol/Nutrition/Herb Interactions Ethanol: Avoid use in patients with hepatitis C virus.
Stability Prior to reconstitution, store Redipen® at 2°C to 8°C (36°F to 46°F). Store intact vials at 25°C (77°F); excursions permitted to 15°C to 30°C (59°F to 86°F). Do not freeze.
Redipen®: Hold cartridge upright and press the two halves together until there is a "click". Gently invert to mix; do not shake. Single-use pen.
Pegintron® (vial): Add 0.7 mL sterile water for injection, USP (supplied single-use diluent) to the vial. Gently swirl. Do not re-enter vial after dose removed.
Sylatron™ (vial): Add 0.7 mL sterile water for injection and swirl gently, resulting in the following concentrations:
296 mcg vial: 40 mcg/0.1 mL
444 mcg vial: 60 mcg/0.1 mL
888 mcg vial: 120 mcg/0.1 mL
Once reconstituted each product should be used immediately or may be stored for ≤24 hours at 2°C to 8°C (36°F to 46°F); do not freeze. Do not shake. Products do not contain preservative.
Mechanism of Action Alpha interferons are a family of proteins, produced by nucleated cells, that have antiviral, antiproliferative, and immune-regulating activity. There are 16 known subtypes of alpha interferons. Interferons interact with cells through high affinity cell surface receptors. Following activation, multiple effects can be detected including induction of gene transcription. Inhibits cellular growth, alters the state of cellular differentiation, interferes with oncogene expression, alters cell surface antigen expression, increases phagocytic activity of macrophages, and augments cytotoxicity of lymphocytes for target cells.
Pharmacodynamics/Kinetics
Bioavailability: Increases with chronic dosing
Half-life elimination: CHC: ~40 hours (range: 22-60 hours); Melanoma: ~43-51 hours
Time to peak: CHC: 15-44 hours
Excretion: Urine (~30%)
Dosage
Geriatric May require dosage reduction based upon renal dysfunction; however, no established guidelines are available.
Adult
Melanoma: SubQ: 6 mcg/kg/week for 8 doses, followed by 3 mcg/kg/week for up to 5 years.
Note: Premedicate with acetaminophen (500-1000 mg orally) 30 minutes prior to the first dose and as needed thereafter.
Chronic hepatitis C (CHC): SubQ: Administer dose once weekly; **Note:** Treatment duration is 48 weeks for genotype 1, 24 weeks for genotypes 2 and 3, or 48 weeks for patients who previously failed therapy (regardless of genotype). Discontinue after 12 weeks in patients with HCV (genotype 1) if HCV RNA decreases <2 log (compared to pretreatment) or if detectable HCV RNA at 24.

Monotherapy: Initial (based on average weekly dose of 1 mcg/kg):
≤45 kg: 40 mcg once weekly
46-56 kg: 50 mcg once weekly
57-72 kg: 64 mcg once weekly
73-88 kg: 80 mcg once weekly
89-106 kg: 96 mcg once weekly
107-136 kg: 120 mcg once weekly
137-160 kg: 150 mcg once weekly
Combination therapy with ribavirin: Initial (based on average weekly dose of 1.5 mcg/kg):
<40 kg: 50 mcg once weekly (with ribavirin 800 mg/day)
40-50 kg: 64 mcg once weekly (with ribavirin 800 mg/day)
51-60 kg: 80 mcg once weekly (with ribavirin 800 mg/day)
61-65 kg: 96 mcg once weekly (with ribavirin 800 mg/day)
66-75 kg: 96 mcg once weekly (with ribavirin 1000 mg/day)
76-80 kg: 120 mcg once weekly (with ribavirin 1000 mg/day)
81-85 kg: 120 mcg once weekly (with ribavirin 1200 mg/day)
86-105 kg: 150 mcg once weekly (with ribavirin 1200 mg/day)
>105 kg: 1.5 mcg/kg once weekly (with ribavirin 1400 mg/day)

Note: *American Association for the Study of Liver Diseases (AASLD) guidelines recommendation:* Adults with chronic HCV infection: Treatment of choice: Ribavirin plus **peginterferon**; clinical condition and ability of patient to tolerate therapy should be evaluated to determine length and/or likely benefit of therapy. Recommended treatment duration (AASLD guidelines; Ghany, 2009): Genotypes 1,4: 48 weeks; Genotypes 2,3: 24 weeks; Coinfection with HIV: 48 weeks.

Renal Impairment Chronic hepatitis C:
Peginterferon alfa-2b monotherapy:
Cl$_{cr}$ 30-50 mL/minute: Reduce dose by 25%
Cl$_{cr}$ 10-29 mL/minute: Reduce dose by 50%
Hemodialysis: Reduce dose by 50%
Discontinue use if renal function declines during treatment.
Peginterferon alfa-2b combination with ribavirin: Cl$_{cr}$ <50 mL/minute: Combination therapy with ribavirin is not recommended.

Hepatic Impairment Contraindicated in decompensated liver disease

Administration For SubQ administration; rotate injection site; thigh, outer surface of upper arm, and abdomen are preferred injection sites; do not inject near navel or waistline; patients who are thin should only use thigh or upper arm. Do not inject into bruised, infected, irritated, red, or scarred skin. The weekly dose may be administered at bedtime to reduce flu-like symptoms.

Monitoring Parameters Baseline and periodic TSH (for patients being treated for melanoma, obtain baseline within 4 weeks prior to treatment initiation, and then at 3 and 6 months, and every 6 months thereafter during treatment); hematology (including hemoglobin, CBC with differential, platelets); chemistry (including LFTs) testing, renal function, triglycerides. Clinical studies (for combination therapy) tested as follows: CBC (including hemoglobin, WBC, and platelets) and chemistries (including liver function tests and uric acid) measured at weeks 2, 4, 8, and 12, and then every 6 weeks; TSH measured every 12 weeks during treatment.

Serum HCV RNA levels (pretreatment, 12 and 24 weeks after therapy initiation, 24 weeks after completion of therapy). **Note:** Discontinuation of therapy may be considered after 12 weeks in patients with HCV (genotype 1) who fail to achieve an early virologic response (EVR) (defined as ≥2-log decrease in HCV RNA compared to pretreatment) or after 24 weeks with detectable HCV RNA. Treat patients with HCV (genotypes 2,3) for 24 weeks (if tolerated) and then evaluate HCV RNA levels (Ghany, 2009).

Evaluate for depression and other psychiatric symptoms before and after initiation of therapy; patients being treated for melanoma should be monitored for depression and psychiatric symptoms every 3 weeks during the first eight weeks of treatment and every 6 months thereafter; baseline ophthalmic eye examination; periodic ophthalmic exam in patients with diabetic or hypertensive retinopathy; baseline ECG in patients with cardiac disease; serum glucose or Hb A$_{1c}$ (for patients with diabetes mellitus). In combination therapy with ribavirin, pregnancy tests (for women of childbearing age who are receiving treatment or who have male partners who are receiving treatment), continue monthly up to 6 months after discontinuation of therapy.

Reference Range Chronic hepatitis C:
Early viral response (EVR): ≥2 log decrease in HCV RNA after 12 weeks of treatment
End of treatment response (ETR): Absence of detectable HCV RNA at end of the recommended treatment period
Sustained treatment response (STR): Absence of HCV RNA in the serum 6 months following completion of full treatment course

Special Geriatric Considerations May require dosage reduction based upon renal dysfunction, but no established guidelines are available. Geriatric patients often have Cl_{cr} <50 mL/minute, as well as, many diseases that put them at risk for adverse effects with this agent. Calculation and measuring creatinine clearance must be done prior to initiating this drug.

Dosage Forms Excipient information presented when available (limited, particularly for generics); consult specific product labeling.

Injection, powder for reconstitution:

Sylatron™: 296 mcg [contains polysorbate 80, sucrose 59.2 mg; supplied with diluent]

Sylatron™: 444 mcg [contains polysorbate 80, sucrose 59.2 mg; supplied with diluent]

Sylatron™: 888 mcg [contains polysorbate 80, sucrose 59.2 mg; supplied with diluent]

Injection, powder for reconstitution [preservative free]:

PegIntron®: 50 mcg, 80 mcg, 120 mcg, 150 mcg [contains polysorbate 80, sucrose 59.2 mg; supplied with diluent]

PegIntron™ Redipen®: 50 mcg, 80 mcg, 120 mcg, 150 mcg [contains polysorbate 80, sucrose 54 mg; supplied with diluent]

◆ **PegIntron®** *see* Peginterferon Alfa-2b *on page 1485*

◆ **PegIntron™ Redipen®** *see* Peginterferon Alfa-2b *on page 1485*

Pegloticase (peg LOE ti kase)

Brand Names: U.S. Krystexxa™

Index Terms PEG-Uricase; Pegylated Urate Oxidase; Polyethylene Glycol-Conjugated Uricase; Recombinant Urate Oxidase, Pegylated; Urate Oxidase, Pegylated

Generic Availability (U.S.) No

Pharmacologic Category Enzyme; Enzyme, Urate-Oxidase (Recombinant)

Use Treatment of chronic gout refractory to conventional therapy

Medication Guide Available Yes

Contraindications Glucose-6-phosphate dehydrogenase (G6PD) deficiency

Warnings/Precautions [U.S. Boxed Warning]: Anaphylaxis and infusion reactions have been reported during and after administration; patients should be closely monitored during infusion and for an appropriate period of time after the infusion. Therapy should be administered in a healthcare facility by skilled medical personnel prepared for the immediate treatment of anaphylaxis. All patients should be premedicated with antihistamines and corticosteroids. Anaphylaxis may occur at any time during treatment (including the initial dose). **Reactions generally occur within 2 hours of administration; however, delayed hypersensitivity reactions have also been reported.** Infusion reactions are varied; symptoms range from chest pain, pruritus/urticaria, or dyspnea to a clinical presentation of anaphylaxis (eg, hemodynamic instability, perioral or lingual edema). If a less severe (non-anaphylactic) infusion reaction occurs, the infusion may be slowed, or stopped and restarted at a slower rate, at the physician's discretion. **Risk of an infusion reaction is increased in patients whose uric acid is >6 mg/dL; therefore, monitor serum uric acid concentrations prior to infusion and consider discontinuing treatment if concentrations exceed 6 mg/dL, particularly in the event of 2 consecutive concentrations >6 mg/dL.**

Therapy with antihyperuricemic agents commonly results in gout flare, particularly upon initiation due to rapid lowering of urate concentrations; gout flare-ups during treatment do not warrant discontinuation of therapy. Gout flare prophylaxis is recommended, using non-steroidal anti-inflammatory agents (NSAID) or colchicines, unless contraindicated, beginning ≥1 week before initiation of pegloticase and continuing for at least 6 months. Exacerbation of heart failure has been observed in clinical trials; use caution in patients with pre-existing heart failure. Due to the risk for hemolysis and methemoglobinemia, pegloticase is contraindicated in patients with G6PD deficiency. Patients at higher risk for G6PD deficiency (eg, African, Mediterranean) should be screened prior to therapy. Therapy is not appropriate for the treatment of asymptomatic hyperuricemia. Potential for immunogenicity exists with the use of therapeutic proteins. Antipegloticase antibodies and antiPEG antibodies commonly occurred during clinical trials in pegloticase-treated patients. High antipegloticase antibody titers were associated with failure to maintain uric acid normalization and were also associated with a higher incidence of infusion reactions. Due to potential for immunogenicity, closely monitor patients who reinitiate therapy after discontinuing treatment for >4 weeks; patients may be at increased risk for anaphylaxis and infusion reactions.

Adverse Reactions (Reflective of adult population; not specific for elderly)

>10%:

Dermatologic: Bruising (11%), urticaria (11%)

Gastrointestinal: Nausea (12%)

Miscellaneous: Antibody formation (antipegloticase antibodies: 92%; antiPEG antibodies: 42%), gout flare (74% within the first 3 months), infusion reactions (26%)

1% to 10%:
Cardiovascular: Chest pain (6% to 10%)
Dermatologic: Erythema (10%), pruritus (10%)
Gastrointestinal: Constipation (6%), vomiting (5%)
Respiratory: Dyspnea (7%), nasopharyngitis (7%)
Miscellaneous: Anaphylaxis (≤7%)
Frequency not defined: Anemia, diarrhea, headache, muscle spasms, nephrolithiasis

Drug Interactions

Metabolism/Transport Effects None known.

Avoid Concomitant Use There are no known interactions where it is recommended to avoid concomitant use.

Increased Effect/Toxicity There are no known significant interactions involving an increase in effect.

Decreased Effect

Pegloticase may decrease the levels/effects of: Certolizumab Pegol; Pegademase Bovine; Pegaptanib; Pegaspargase; Pegfilgrastim; Peginterferon Alfa-2a; Peginterferon Alfa-2b; Pegvisomant

Stability Prior to use, vials must be stored in the carton to protect from light and kept under refrigeration between 2°C to 8°C (36°F to 46°F) at all times. Do **not** shake or freeze.

To prepare solution for administration, withdraw 1 mL (8 mg) and add to a 250 mL bag of NS or ½NS; invert bag several times to mix thoroughly (do **not** shake). Do not use vial if particulate matter is present or if solution is discolored (solution should be a clear and colorless). After withdrawal, discard any unused portion of the product remaining in the vial. Diluted solution may be stored up to 4 hours at 2°C to 8°C (36°F to 46°F). Diluted solution is also stable for 4 hours at room temperature of 20°C to 25°C (68°F to 77°F); however, refrigeration is preferred. The diluted solution should be protected from light, not frozen, and used within 4 hours of dilution. Prior to administration, allow the diluted solution to reach room temperature; do not warm to room temperature using any form of artificial heating such as a microwave or warm water bath.

Mechanism of Action Pegloticase is a pegylated recombinant form of urate-oxidase enzyme, also known as uricase (an enzyme normally absent in humans and high primates), which converts uric acid to allantoin (an inactive and water soluble metabolite of uric acid); it does not inhibit the formation of uric acid.

Pharmacodynamics/Kinetics

Onset of action: ~24 hours following the first dose, serum uric acid concentrations decreased
Duration: >300 hours (12.5 days)
Half-life elimination: Median: ~14 days

Dosage

Geriatric & Adult Refractory gout: I.V.: 8 mg every 2 weeks

Note: Premedicate with antihistamines and corticosteroids. Gout flare prophylaxis with either NSAIDs or colchicine is also recommended, beginning at least 1 week prior to initiation and continuing for at least 6 months.

Renal Impairment Creatinine clearance did not alter the pharmacokinetics; dosage adjustments are not needed.

Administration Administer diluted solution by I.V. infusion over ≥120 minutes via gravity feed or an infusion pump or syringe-type pump. Do **not** administer by I.V. push or bolus. Administer in a healthcare setting by healthcare providers prepared to manage potential anaphylaxis. Monitor closely for infusion reactions during infusion and for an appropriate period of time after the infusion (anaphylaxis has been reported within 2 hours of the infusion). In the event or a less severe infusion reaction, infusion may be slowed, or stopped and restarted at a slower rate, based on the discretion of the physician.

Reference Range

Adults:
Males: 3.4-7 mg/dL or slightly more
Females: 2.4-6 mg/dL or slightly more
Values >7 mg/dL are sometimes arbitrarily regarded as hyperuricemia, but there is no sharp line between normals on the one hand, and the serum uric acid of those with clinical gout. Normal ranges cannot be adjusted for purine ingestion, but high purine diet increases uric acid. Uric acid may be increased with body size, exercise, and stress.

Special Geriatric Considerations Age did not influence pharmacokinetics. In clinical trials, there was no significant difference in safety or efficacy in older versus younger patients.

Dosage Forms Excipient information presented when available (limited, particularly for generics); consult specific product labeling.

Injection, solution:
Krystexxa™: Uricase protein 8 mg/mL (2 mL)

♦ **PEG-Uricase** *see* Pegloticase *on page 1490*

◆ **Pegylated G-CSF** see Pegfilgrastim on page 1481
◆ **Pegylated Interferon Alfa-2b** see Peginterferon Alfa-2b on page 1485
◆ **Pegylated Urate Oxidase** see Pegloticase on page 1490

Penbutolol (pen BYOO toe lole)

Related Information
Beta-Blockers on page 2108
Medication Safety Issues
Sound-alike/look-alike issues:
Levatol® may be confused with Lipitor®
International issues:
Levatol [U.S.] may be confused with Lovacol brand name for lovastatin [Chile and Finland]
Brand Names: U.S. Levatol®
Brand Names: Canada Levatol®
Index Terms Penbutolol Sulfate
Generic Availability (U.S.) No
Pharmacologic Category Beta-Blocker With Intrinsic Sympathomimetic Activity
Use Treatment of mild-to-moderate arterial hypertension
Contraindications Hypersensitivity to penbutolol or any component of the formulation; uncompensated congestive heart failure; cardiogenic shock; bradycardia or heart block (except in patients with a functioning artificial pacemaker); sinus node dysfunction; asthma; bronchospastic disease; COPD; pulmonary edema
Warnings/Precautions Consider pre-existing conditions such as sick sinus syndrome before initiating. Beta-blocker therapy should not be withdrawn abruptly (particularly in patients with CAD), but gradually tapered to avoid acute tachycardia, hypertension, and/or ischemia. Chronic beta-blocker therapy should not be routinely withdrawn prior to major surgery. In general, patients with bronchospastic disease should not receive beta-blockers; if used at all, should be used cautiously with close monitoring. Bradycardia may be observed more frequently in elderly patients (>65 years of age); dosage reductions may be necessary. Use caution with concurrent use of digoxin, verapamil, or diltiazem; bradycardia or heart block can occur. Use with caution in patients receiving inhaled anesthetic agents known to depress myocardial contractility. Can precipitate or aggravate symptoms of arterial insufficiency in patients with PVD and Raynaud's disease. Use with caution and monitor for progression of arterial obstruction.

Use with caution in patients with psychiatric disease (may cause CNS depression) or myasthenia gravis. Use cautiously in patients with diabetes because it can mask prominent hypoglycemic symptoms. May mask signs of hyperthyroidism (eg, tachycardia); if hyperthyroidism is suspected, carefully manage and monitor; abrupt withdrawal may exacerbate symptoms of hyperthyroidism or precipitate thyroid storm. Beta-blockers with intrinsic sympathomimetic activity (including penbutolol) do not appear to be of benefit in HF. Adequate alpha-blockade is required prior to use of any beta-blocker for patients with untreated pheochromocytoma. Use caution with history of severe anaphylaxis to allergens; patients taking beta-blockers may become more sensitive to repeated challenges. Treatment of anaphylaxis (eg, epinephrine) in patients taking beta-blockers may be ineffective or promote undesirable effects.
Adverse Reactions (Reflective of adult population; not specific for elderly) 1% to 10%:
Cardiovascular: CHF, arrhythmia
Central nervous system: Mental depression, headache, dizziness, fatigue
Gastrointestinal: Nausea, diarrhea, dyspepsia
Neuromuscular & skeletal: Arthralgia
Drug Interactions
Metabolism/Transport Effects None known.
Avoid Concomitant Use
Avoid concomitant use of Penbutolol with any of the following: Beta2-Agonists; Floctafenine; Methacholine
Increased Effect/Toxicity
Penbutolol may increase the levels/effects of: Alpha-/Beta-Agonists (Direct-Acting); Alpha1-Blockers; Alpha2-Agonists; Amifostine; Antihypertensives; Antipsychotic Agents (Phenothiazines); Bupivacaine; Cardiac Glycosides; Cholinergic Agonists; Fingolimod; Hypotensive Agents; Insulin; Lidocaine; Lidocaine (Systemic); Lidocaine (Topical); Mepivacaine; Methacholine; Midodrine; RiTUXimab; Sulfonylureas

The levels/effects of Penbutolol may be increased by: Acetylcholinesterase Inhibitors; Aminoquinolines (Antimalarial); Amiodarone; Anilidopiperidine Opioids; Antipsychotic Agents (Phenothiazines); Calcium Channel Blockers (Dihydropyridine); Calcium Channel Blockers (Nondihydropyridine); Diazoxide; Dipyridamole; Disopyramide; Dronedarone; Floctafenine; Herbs (Hypotensive Properties); MAO Inhibitors; Pentoxifylline; Phosphodiesterase 5 Inhibitors; Propafenone; Prostacyclin Analogues; QuiNIDine; Reserpine

Decreased Effect

Penbutolol may decrease the levels/effects of: Beta2-Agonists; Theophylline Derivatives

The levels/effects of Penbutolol may be decreased by: Barbiturates; Herbs (Hypertensive Properties); Methylphenidate; Nonsteroidal Anti-Inflammatory Agents; Rifamycin Derivatives; Yohimbine

Mechanism of Action Blocks both beta$_1$- and beta$_2$-receptors and has mild intrinsic sympathomimetic activity; has negative inotropic and chronotropic effects and can significantly slow AV nodal conduction

Pharmacodynamics/Kinetics

Onset of action: Peak effect: 1.3-3 hours

Duration: >20 hours

Absorption: ~100%

Protein binding: 80% to 98%

Metabolism: Extensively hepatic (oxidation and conjugation)

Bioavailability: ~100%

Half-life elimination: Penbutolol: 5 hours; Conjugated metabolite: ~20 hours with normal renal function, 100 hours with end-stage renal disease

Time to peak, plasma: 2-3 hours

Excretion: Urine

Dosage

Geriatric & Adult Hypertension: Oral: Initial: 20 mg once daily, full effect of a 20 or 40 mg dose is seen by the end of a 2-week period, doses of 40-80 mg have been tolerated but have shown little additional antihypertensive effects; usual dose range (JNC 7): 10-40 mg once daily

Monitoring Parameters Blood pressure, orthostatic hypotension, heart rate, CNS effects

Special Geriatric Considerations Due to alterations in the beta-adrenergic autonomic nervous system, beta-adrenergic blockade may result in less hemodynamic response than seen in younger adults. Studies indicate that despite decreased sensitivity to the chronotropic effects of beta-blockade with age, there appears to be an increased myocardial sensitivity to the negative inotropic effect during stress (ie, exercise). Controlled trials have shown the overall response rate for propranolol to be only 20% to 50% in elderly populations. Therefore, all beta-adrenergic blocking drugs may result in a decreased response as compared to younger adults.

Dosage Forms Excipient information presented when available (limited, particularly for generics); consult specific product labeling.

Tablet, oral, as sulfate:

Levatol®: 20 mg [scored]

◆ **Penbutolol Sulfate** *see* Penbutolol *on page 1492*

PenicillAMINE (pen i SIL a meen)

Medication Safety Issues

Sound-alike/look-alike issues:

Penicillamine may be confused with penicillin

International issues:

Depen [U.S.] may be confused with Depin brand name for nifedipine [India]; Depon brand name for acetaminophen [Greece]; Dipen brand name for diltiazem [Greece]

Pemine [Italy] may be confused with Pamine brand name for methscopolamine [U.S., Canada]

Brand Names: U.S. Cuprimine®; Depen®

Brand Names: Canada Cuprimine®

Index Terms D-3-Mercaptovaline; D-Penicillamine; β,β-Dimethylcysteine

Generic Availability (U.S.) No

Pharmacologic Category Chelating Agent

Use Treatment of Wilson's disease, cystinuria; adjunctive treatment of severe, active rheumatoid arthritis

Canadian labeling: Additional use (not in U.S. labeling): Treatment of chronic lead poisoning ▶

Contraindications Renal insufficiency (in patients with rheumatoid arthritis); patients with previous penicillamine-related aplastic anemia or agranulocytosis

Canadian labeling: Additional contraindications (not in U.S. labeling): Hypersensitivity to penicillamine or any component of the formulation; use in patients with chronic lead poisoning who have radiographic evidence of lead-containing substances in the GI tract; concomitant use with gold therapy, antimalarial or cytotoxic drugs, oxyphenbutazone or phenylbutazone

Warnings/Precautions Approximately 33% of patients will experience an allergic reaction; toxicity may be dose related; use caution in the elderly. Once instituted for Wilson's disease or cystinuria, continue treatment on a daily basis; interruptions of even a few days have been followed by hypersensitivity with reinstitution of therapy. Rash may occur early (more commonly) or late in therapy; early-onset rash typically resolves within days of discontinuation of therapy and does not recur upon rechallenge with reduced dose; discontinue therapy for late-onset rash (eg, after >6 months) and do not rechallenge; rash typically recurs with rechallenge. Drug fever sometimes in conjunction with macular cutaneous eruptions may be observed usually 2-3 weeks after therapy initiation. Discontinue use in patients with rheumatoid arthritis, Wilson's disease or cystinuria who develop a marked febrile response. Consider alternative therapy for patients with rheumatoid arthritis due to high incidence of fever reoccurrence with penicillamine rechallenge. May resume therapy at a reduced dose in Wilson's disease or cystinuria upon resolution of fever. Discontinue therapy for skin reactions accompanied by lymphadenopathy, fever, arthralgia, or other allergic reactions. Patients with a penicillin allergy may theoretically have cross-sensitivity to penicillamine; however, the possibility has been eliminated now that penicillamine is produced synthetically and no longer contains trace amounts of penicillin.

[U.S. Boxed Warning]: Patients should be warned to report promptly any symptoms suggesting toxicity (fever, sore throat, chills, bruising, or bleeding); penicillamine has been associated with fatalities due to agranulocytosis, aplastic anemia, and thrombocytopenia. Use caution with other hematopoietic-depressant drugs (eg, gold, immunosuppressants, antimalarials, phenylbutazone; Canadian labeling contraindicates concomitant use with these agents). Discontinue therapy for WBC <3500/mm^3. Withhold therapy at least temporarily for platelet counts <100,000/mm^3 or a progressive fall in WBC or platelets in 3 successive determinations, even though values may remain within the normal range. Proteinuria or hematuria may develop; monitor for membranous glomerulopathy which can lead to nephrotic syndrome. In rheumatoid arthritis patients, discontinue if gross hematuria or persistent microscopic hematuria develop and discontinue therapy or reduce dose for proteinuria that is either >1 g/day or progressively increasing. Dose reduction may lead to resolution of proteinuria.

[U.S. Boxed Warning]: Should be administered under the close supervision of a physician familiar with the toxicity and dosage considerations. Monitor liver function tests periodically due to rare reports of intrahepatic cholestasis or toxic hepatitis. Has been associated with myasthenic syndrome which in some cases progressed to myasthenia gravis. Resolution of symptoms has been observed in most cases following discontinuation of therapy. Bronchiolitis obliterans has been reported rarely with use. Pemphigus may occur early or late in therapy; discontinue use with suspicion of pemphigus. Lupus erythematosus-like syndrome may be observed in some patients; Taste alteration may occur (rare in Wilson's disease); usually self-limited with continued therapy, however may last ≥2 months and result in total loss of taste. Oral ulceration (eg, stomatitis) may occur; typically recurs on rechallenge, but often resolves with dose reduction. Other dose-related lesions (eg, glossitis, gingivostomatitis) have been observed with use and may require therapy discontinuation. Pyridoxine supplementation (25-50 mg/day) is recommended in Wilson's disease (Roberts, 2008) or 25 mg/day in cystinuria or in rheumatoid arthritis patients with impaired nutrition.

Penicillamine increases the amount of soluble collagen; may increase skin friability, particularly at sites subject to pressure or trauma (eg, knees, elbows shoulders). Purpuric areas with localized bleeding (if skin is broken) or vesicles with dark blood may be observed. Effects are considered localized and do not necessitate discontinuation of therapy; may not recur with dose reduction. Dose reduction may be considered prior to surgical procedures. May resume normal recommended dosing postoperatively once wound healing is complete.

Lead poisoning: Investigate, identify, and remove sources of lead exposure and confirm lead-containing substances are absent from the GI tract prior to initiating therapy. Do not permit patients to re-enter the contaminated environment until lead abatement has been completed. Penicillamine should only be used when unacceptable reactions have occurred with edetate CALCIUM disodium and succimer. Primary care providers should consult experts in the chemotherapy of lead toxicity before using chelation drug therapy.

Adverse Reactions (Reflective of adult population; not specific for elderly) Frequency not always defined and may vary by indication.

Cardiovascular: Vasculitis

Central nervous system: Anxiety, agitation, fever, Guillain-Barré syndrome, hyperpyrexia, psychiatric disturbances, worsening neurologic symptoms

Dermatologic: Alopecia, cheilosis, dermatomyositis, drug eruptions, exfoliative dermatitis, lichen planus, pemphigus, pruritus, rash (early and late: 5%), skin friability increased, toxic epidermal necrolysis, urticaria, wrinkling (excessive), yellow nail syndrome

Endocrine & metabolic: Hypoglycemia, thyroiditis

Gastrointestinal: Diarrhea (17%), taste alteration (12%), anorexia, epigastric pain, gingivostomatitis, glossitis, nausea, oral ulcerations, pancreatitis, peptic ulcer reactivation, vomiting

Hematologic: Thrombocytopenia (4%), leukopenia (2%), agranulocytosis, aplastic anemia, eosinophilia, hemolytic anemia, leukocytosis, monocytosis, red cell aplasia, sideroblastic anemia, thrombotic thrombocytopenia purpura, thrombocytosis

Hepatic: Alkaline phosphatase increased, hepatic failure, intrahepatic cholestasis, toxic hepatitis

Local: Thrombophlebitis, white papules at venipuncture and surgical sites

Neuromuscular & skeletal: Arthralgia, dystonia, myasthenia gravis, muscle weakness, neuropathies, polyarthralgia (migratory, often with objective synovitis), polymyositis

Ocular: Diplopia, extraocular muscle weakness, optic neuritis, ptosis, visual disturbances

Otic: Tinnitus

Renal: Proteinuria (6%), Goodpasture's syndrome, hematuria, nephrotic syndrome, renal failure, renal vasculitis

Respiratory: Asthma, interstitial pneumonitis, pulmonary fibrosis, obliterative bronchiolitis

Miscellaneous: Allergic alveolitis, anetoderma, elastosis perforans serpiginosa, lupus-like syndrome, lactic dehydrogenase increased, lymphadenopathy, mammary hyperplasia, positive ANA test

Drug Interactions

Metabolism/Transport Effects None known.

Avoid Concomitant Use There are no known interactions where it is recommended to avoid concomitant use.

Increased Effect/Toxicity There are no known significant interactions involving an increase in effect.

Decreased Effect

PenicillAMINE may decrease the levels/effects of: Digoxin

The levels/effects of PenicillAMINE may be decreased by: Antacids; Iron Salts

Ethanol/Nutrition/Herb Interactions

Ethanol: Management: Avoid or limit ethanol.

Food: Penicillamine serum levels may be decreased if taken with food. Management: Administer on an empty stomach 1 hour before or 2 hours after meals and at least 1 hour apart from other drugs, milk, antacids, and zinc- or iron-containing products. Certain disease states require further diet adjustment. Limit intake of vitamin A.

Stability Store in tight, well-closed containers.

Mechanism of Action Chelates with lead, copper, mercury and other heavy metals to form stable, soluble complexes that are excreted in urine; depresses circulating IgM rheumatoid factor, depresses T-cell but not B-cell activity; combines with cystine to form a compound which is more soluble, thus cystine calculi are prevented

Pharmacodynamics/Kinetics

Onset of action: Rheumatoid arthritis: 2-3 months; Wilson's disease: 1-3 months

Absorption: Rapid but incomplete

Protein binding: >80% to albumin and ceruloplasmin

Metabolism: Hepatic (small amounts metabolized to s-methyl-d-penicillamine)

Bioavailability: 40% to 70%; reduced by food, antacids, and iron

Half-life elimination: 1.7-7 hours (Roberts, 2008)

Time to peak, serum: 1-3 hours

Excretion: Urine (primarily as disulfides)

Dosage

Geriatric Therapy should be initiated at low end of dosing range and titrated upward cautiously. Refer to adult dosing.

Adult Note: Dose reduction to 250 mg/day may be considered prior to surgical procedures. May resume normal recommended dosing post-operatively once wound healing is complete.

Cystinuria: Oral: 1-4 g/day in 4 divided doses; usual dose: 2 g/day; initiation of therapy at 250 mg/day with gradual upward titration may reduce the risk of unwanted effects. **Note:** Adjust dose to limit cystine excretion to 100-200 mg/day (<100 mg/day with history of stone formation).

Lead poisoning: Oral: *Canadian labeling:* 900-1500 mg/day in 3 divided doses for 1-2 weeks, then 750 mg/day in divided doses until blood lead concentrations <60 mcg/dL or urinary lead excretion <500 mcg/L for 2 consecutive months.

Rheumatoid arthritis: Oral: Initial: 125-250 mg/day, may increase dose by 125-250 mg/day at 1- to 3-month intervals up to 1-1.5 g/day; discontinue in patients failing to improve after 3-4 months at these doses

Wilson's disease: Oral: **Note:** Dose that results in an initial 24-hour urinary copper excretion >2 mg/day should be continued for ~3 months; maintenance dose defined by amount resulting in <10 mcg serum free copper/dL.

Manufacturer's labeling recommendations: 750-1500 mg/day in divided doses; maximum dose: 2000 mg/day.

Alternate recommendations (unlabeled dosing): To increase tolerability, therapy may be initiated at 250-500 mg/day then titrated upward in 250 mg increments every 4-7 days; usual maintenance dose: 750-1000 mg/day in 2 divided doses; maximum: 1000-1500 mg/day in 2-4 divided doses. (American Association for the Study of Liver Diseases [AASLD] guidelines) (Roberts, 2008).

Renal Impairment *Manufacturer's labeling recommendations:* No dosage adjustment provided in manufacturer's labeling; however, the manufacturer's labeling does suggest a cautious approach to dosing as this drug undergoes mainly renal elimination.

Alternate recommendations:

Cl_{cr} <50 mL/minute: Avoid use (Aronoff, 2007

Hemodialysis: Dialyzable; Administer 33% of usual dose (Aronoff, 2007); a dosing decrease from 250 mg/day to 250 mg 3 times/week after dialysis has been suggested in the treatment of rheumatoid arthritis (Swarup, 2004).

Hepatic Impairment No dosage adjustment provided in manufacturer's labeling; however, only a small fraction is metabolized hepatically.

Administration Doses ≤500 mg may be administered as single dose; doses >500 mg should be administered in divided doses. For patients who cannot swallow, contents of capsules may be administered in 15-30 mL of chilled puréed fruit or fruit juice within 5 minutes of administration. Administer on an empty stomach (1 hour before or 2 hours after meals) and at least 1 hour apart from other drugs, milk, antacids, and zinc or iron-containing products. Canadian labeling recommends administering at least 2 hours before meals in patients with lead poisoning.

Cystinuria: If administering 4 equal doses is not feasible, administer the larger dose at bedtime.

Monitoring Parameters Urinalysis, CBC with differential, platelet count, skin, lymph nodes, and body temperature twice weekly during the first month of therapy, then every 2 weeks for 5 months, then monthly; LFTs every 6 months; signs/symptoms of hypersensitivity

Cystinuria: Urinary cystine, annual X-ray for renal stones

Lead poisoning: Serum lead concentration (baseline and 7-21 days after completing chelation therapy); hemoglobin or hematocrit, iron status, free erythrocyte protoporphyrin or zinc protoporphyrin; neurodevelopmental changes

Wilson's disease: Serum non-ceruloplasmin bound copper, 24-hour urinary copper excretion, LFTs every 3 months (at least) during the first year of treatment; periodic ophthalmic exam

Urinalysis: Monitor for proteinuria and hematuria. A quantitative 24-hour urine protein at 1- to 2-week intervals initially (first 2-3 months) is recommended if proteinuria develops.

Reference Range Wilson's disease: 24-hour urinary copper excretion: 200-500 mcg (3-8 micromoles)/day

Special Geriatric Considerations Close monitoring of elderly is necessary; since steady-state serum/tissue concentrations rise slowly, "go slow" with dose increase intervals; steady-state concentrations decline slowly after discontinuation suggesting extensive tissue distribution. Skin rashes and taste abnormalities occur more frequently in the elderly than in young adults; leukopenia, thrombocytopenia, and proteinuria occur with equal frequency in both younger adults and elderly. Since toxicity may be dose related, it is recommended not to exceed 750 mg/day in the elderly.

Dosage Forms Excipient information presented when available (limited, particularly for generics); consult specific product labeling.

Capsule, oral:

Cuprimine®: 250 mg

Tablet, oral:

Depen®: 250 mg [scored]

Penicillin G Benzathine (pen i SIL in jee BENZ a theen)

Medication Safety Issues

Sound-alike/look-alike issues:

Penicillin may be confused with penicillamine

Bicillin® may be confused with Wycillin®

Administration issues:

Penicillin G benzathine may only be administered by deep intramuscular injection; intravenous administration of penicillin G benzathine has been associated with cardiopulmonary arrest and death.

Other safety concerns:

Bicillin® C-R (penicillin G benzathine and penicillin G procaine) may be confused with Bicillin® L-A (penicillin G benzathine). Penicillin G benzathine is the only product currently approved for the treatment of syphilis. Administration of penicillin G benzathine and penicillin G procaine combination instead of Bicillin® L-A may result in inadequate treatment response.

Brand Names: U.S. Bicillin® L-A

Brand Names: Canada Bicillin® L-A

Index Terms Benzathine Benzylpenicillin; Benzathine Penicillin G; Benzylpenicillin Benzathine

Generic Availability (U.S.) No

Pharmacologic Category Antibiotic, Penicillin

Use Active against some gram-positive organisms, few gram-negative organisms such as *Neisseria gonorrhoeae*, and some anaerobes and spirochetes; used in the treatment of syphilis; used only for the treatment of mild to moderately-severe upper respiratory tract infections caused by organisms susceptible to low concentrations of penicillin G or for prophylaxis of infections caused by these organisms; primary and secondary prevention of rheumatic fever

Contraindications Hypersensitivity to penicillin(s) or any component of the formulation

Warnings/Precautions Use with caution in patients with impaired renal function, seizure disorder, or history of hypersensitivity to other beta-lactams; CDC and AAP do not currently recommend the use of penicillin G benzathine to treat congenital syphilis or neurosyphilis due to reported treatment failures and lack of published clinical data on its efficacy. Prolonged use may result in fungal or bacterial superinfection, including *C. difficile*-associated diarrhea (CDAD) and pseudomembranous colitis; CDAD has been observed >2 months postantibiotic treatment. **[U.S. Boxed Warning]: Not for intravenous use; cardiopulmonary arrest and death have occurred from inadvertent I.V. administration;** administer by deep I.M. injection only; injection into or near an artery or nerve could result in severe neurovascular damage or permanent neurological damage. Extended duration of therapy or use associated with high serum concentrations may be associated with an increased risk for some adverse reactions.

Adverse Reactions (Reflective of adult population; not specific for elderly) Frequency not defined.

Cardiovascular: Cardiac arrest, cerebral vascular accident, cyanosis, gangrene, hypotension, pallor, palpitations, syncope, tachycardia, vasodilation, vasospasm, vasovagal reaction

Central nervous system: Anxiety, coma, confusion, dizziness, euphoria, fatigue, headache, nervousness, pain, seizure, somnolence

In addition, a syndrome of CNS symptoms has been reported which includes: Severe agitation with confusion, hallucinations (auditory and visual), and fear of death (Hoigne's syndrome); other symptoms include cyanosis, dizziness, palpitations, psychosis, seizures, tachycardia, taste disturbance, tinnitus

Gastrointestinal: Bloody stool, intestinal necrosis, nausea, vomiting

Genitourinary: Impotence, priapism

Hepatic: AST increased

Local: Injection site reactions: Abscess, atrophy, bruising, cellulitis, edema, hemorrhage, inflammation, lump, necrosis, pain, skin ulcer

Neuromuscular & skeletal: Arthritis exacerbation, joint disorder, neurovascular damage, numbness, periostitis, rhabdomyolysis, transverse myelitis, tremor, weakness

Ocular: Blindness, blurred vision

Renal: BUN increased, creatinine increased, hematuria, myoglobinuria, neurogenic bladder, proteinuria, renal failure

Miscellaneous: Diaphoresis, hypersensitivity reactions, Jarisch-Herxheimer reaction, lymphadenopathy, mottling, warmth

Drug Interactions

Metabolism/Transport Effects None known.

Avoid Concomitant Use
Avoid concomitant use of Penicillin G Benzathine with any of the following: BCG

Increased Effect/Toxicity
Penicillin G Benzathine may increase the levels/effects of: Methotrexate; Vitamin K Antagonists

The levels/effects of Penicillin G Benzathine may be increased by: Probenecid

Decreased Effect
Penicillin G Benzathine may decrease the levels/effects of: BCG; Mycophenolate; Typhoid Vaccine

The levels/effects of Penicillin G Benzathine may be decreased by: Fusidic Acid; Tetracycline Derivatives

Stability Refrigerate at 2°C to 8°C (36°F to 46°F); do not freeze. The following stability information has also been reported: May be stored at 25°C (77°F) for 7 days (Cohen, 2007).

Mechanism of Action Interferes with bacterial cell wall synthesis during active multiplication, causing cell wall death and resultant bactericidal activity against susceptible bacteria

Pharmacodynamics/Kinetics
Duration: 1-4 weeks (dose dependent); larger doses result in more sustained levels
Distribution: Highest levels in the kidney; lesser amounts in liver, skin, intestines
Protein Binding: ~60%
Absorption: I.M.: Slow
Time to peak, serum: 12-24 hours

Dosage
Geriatric & Adult
Usual dosage range: I.M.: 1.2-2.4 million units as a single dose
Group A streptococcal upper respiratory infection: 1.2 million units as a single dose
Secondary prevention of glomerulonephritis: 1.2 million units every 4 weeks or 600,000 units twice monthly
Secondary prevention of rheumatic fever: 1.2 million units every 3-4 weeks or 600,000 units twice monthly
Syphilis (CDC, 2010):
Primary, Secondary, Early Latent (<1 year duration): 2.4 million units as a single dose in 2 injection sites
Late Latent, Latent with unknown duration: 2.4 million units in 2 injection sites once weekly for 3 doses
Neurosyphilis: Not indicated as single-drug therapy, but may be given once weekly for 3 weeks following I.V. treatment; refer to Penicillin G Parenteral/Aqueous monograph on page 1500 for dosing

Administration I.M. Administer undiluted injection by deep injection in the upper outer quadrant of the buttock do **not** administer I.V., intra-arterially, or SubQ

Monitoring Parameters Observe for signs and symptoms of anaphylaxis during first dose

Test Interactions Positive Coombs' [direct], false-positive urinary and/or serum proteins; false-positive or negative urinary glucose using Clinitest®

Special Geriatric Considerations Not indicated as single drug therapy for neurosyphilis, but may be given 1 time/week for 3 weeks following I.V. treatment with Penicillin G (Parenteral/Aqueous). No adjustment for renal function or age is necessary.

Dosage Forms Excipient information presented when available (limited, particularly for generics); consult specific product labeling.
Injection, suspension:
Bicillin® L-A: 600,000 units/mL (1 mL, 2 mL, 4 mL)

Penicillin G Benzathine and Penicillin G Procaine
(pen i SIL in jee BENZ a theen & pen i SIL in jee PROE kane)

Related Information
Penicillin G Benzathine on page 1497
Penicillin G Procaine on page 1502

Medication Safety Issues
Sound-alike/look-alike issues:
Penicillin may be confused with penicillamine
Bicillin® may be confused with Wycillin®

Administration issues:
Penicillin G benzathine may only be administered by deep intramuscular injection; intravenous administration of penicillin G benzathine has been associated with cardiopulmonary arrest and death.

Other safety concerns:
Bicillin® C-R (penicillin G benzathine and penicillin G procaine) may be confused with Bicillin® L-A (penicillin G benzathine). Penicillin G benzathine is the only product currently approved for the treatment of syphilis. Administration of penicillin G benzathine and penicillin G procaine combination instead of Bicillin® L-A may result in inadequate treatment response.

Brand Names: U.S. Bicillin® C-R; Bicillin® C-R 900/300

Index Terms Penicillin G Procaine and Benzathine Combined

Generic Availability (U.S.) No

Pharmacologic Category Antibiotic, Penicillin

Use May be used in specific situations in the treatment of streptococcal infections; primary prevention of rheumatic fever

Contraindications Hypersensitivity to penicillin(s), procaine, or any component of the formulation

Warnings/Precautions Use with caution in patients with impaired renal function. Serious and occasionally severe or fatal hypersensitivity (anaphylactoid) reactions have been reported in patients on penicillin therapy, especially with a history of beta-lactam hypersensitivity, history of sensitivity to multiple allergens, or previous IgE-mediated reactions (eg, anaphylaxis, angioedema, urticaria). Use with caution in asthmatic patients. Prolonged use may result in fungal or bacterial superinfection, including *C. difficile*-associated diarrhea (CDAD) and pseudomembranous colitis; CDAD has been observed >2 months postantibiotic treatment. **[U.S. Boxed Warning]: Not for intravenous use; cardiopulmonary arrest and death have occurred from inadvertent I.V. administration;** administer by deep I.M. injection only; injection into or near an artery or nerve could result in severe neurovascular damage or permanent neurological damage. Extended duration of therapy or use associated with high serum concentrations may be associated with an increased risk for some adverse reactions.

Adverse Reactions (Reflective of adult population; not specific for elderly) See individual agents.

Drug Interactions
Metabolism/Transport Effects None known.
Avoid Concomitant Use
Avoid concomitant use of Penicillin G Benzathine and Penicillin G Procaine with any of the following: BCG
Increased Effect/Toxicity
Penicillin G Benzathine and Penicillin G Procaine may increase the levels/effects of: Methotrexate; Vitamin K Antagonists

The levels/effects of Penicillin G Benzathine and Penicillin G Procaine may be increased by: Probenecid
Decreased Effect
Penicillin G Benzathine and Penicillin G Procaine may decrease the levels/effects of: BCG; Mycophenolate; Typhoid Vaccine

The levels/effects of Penicillin G Benzathine and Penicillin G Procaine may be decreased by: Fusidic Acid; Tetracycline Derivatives

Stability Refrigerate at 2°C to 8°C (36°F to 46°F); do not freeze. The following stability information has also been reported: May be stored at 25°C (77°F) for 7 days (Cohen, 2007).

Mechanism of Action Inhibits bacterial cell wall synthesis by binding to one or more of the penicillin-binding proteins (PBPs); which in turn inhibits the final transpeptidation step of peptidoglycan synthesis in bacterial cell walls, thus inhibiting cell wall biosynthesis. Bacteria eventually lyse due to ongoing activity of cell wall autolytic enzymes (autolysins and murein hydrolases) while cell wall assembly is arrested.

Pharmacodynamics/Kinetics
Absorption: I.M.: Released slowly
Distribution: Highest levels in the kidney; lesser amounts in liver, skin, intestines
Protein binding: ~60%
Time to peak, serum: I.M.: Within 3 hours

Dosage
Geriatric & Adult Streptococcal infections: I.M.: 2.4 million units in a single dose

Administration Administer by deep I.M. injection in the upper outer quadrant of the buttock do **not** administer I.V., intravascularly, or intra-arterially

Monitoring Parameters Observe for signs and symptoms of anaphylaxis during first dose ▶

◄ **Test Interactions** May interfere with urinary glucose tests using cupric sulfate (Benedict's solution, Clinitest®); may inactivate aminoglycosides *in vitro*; positive Coombs' [direct], increased protein

Special Geriatric Considerations No adjustment for renal function or age is necessary.

Dosage Forms Excipient information presented when available (limited, particularly for generics); consult specific product labeling. [DSC] = Discontinued product

Injection, suspension [prefilled syringe]:

Bicillin® C-R:

600,000 units: Penicillin G benzathine 300,000 units and penicillin G procaine 300,000 units per 1 mL (1 mL) [DSC]

1,200,000 units: Penicillin G benzathine 600,000 units and penicillin G procaine 600,000 units per 2 mL (2 mL)

2,400,000 units: Penicillin G benzathine 1,200,000 units and penicillin G procaine 1,200,000 units per 4 mL (4 mL) [DSC]

Bicillin® C-R 900/300: 1,200,000 units: Penicillin G benzathine 900,000 units and penicillin G procaine 300,000 units per 2 mL (2 mL)

Penicillin G (Parenteral/Aqueous) (pen i SIL in jee, pa REN ter al, AYE kwee us)

Related Information

Antibiotic Treatment of Adults With Infective Endocarditis *on page 2157*

Antimicrobial Drugs of Choice *on page 2163*

Medication Safety Issues

Sound-alike/look-alike issues:

Penicillin may be confused with penicillamine

Brand Names: U.S. Pfizerpen®

Brand Names: Canada Crystapen®

Index Terms Benzylpenicillin Potassium; Benzylpenicillin Sodium; Crystalline Penicillin; Penicillin G Potassium; Penicillin G Sodium

Generic Availability (U.S.) Yes

Pharmacologic Category Antibiotic, Penicillin

Use Treatment of infections (including sepsis, pneumonia, pericarditis, endocarditis, meningitis, anthrax) caused by susceptible organisms; active against some gram-positive organisms, generally not *Staphylococcus aureus*; some gram-negative organisms such as *Neisseria gonorrhoeae*, and some anaerobes and spirochetes

Contraindications Hypersensitivity to penicillin or any component of the formulation

Warnings/Precautions Avoid intra-arterial administration or injection into or near major peripheral nerves or blood vessels since such injections may cause severe and/or permanent neurovascular damage; use with caution in patients with renal impairment (dosage reduction required), concomitant renal and hepatic impairment (further dosage adjustment may be required), pre-existing seizure disorders, or with a history of hypersensitivity to cephalosporins. Prolonged use may result in fungal or bacterial superinfection, including *C. difficile*-associated diarrhea (CDAD) and pseudomembranous colitis; CDAD has been observed >2 months postantibiotic treatment. Serious and occasionally severe or fatal hypersensitivity (anaphylactoid) reactions have been reported in patients on penicillin therapy, especially with a history of beta-lactam hypersensitivity, history of sensitivity to multiple allergens, or previous IgE-mediated reactions (eg, anaphylaxis, angioedema, urticaria). Use with caution in asthmatic patients. Extended duration of therapy or use associated with high serum concentrations may be associated with an increased risk for some adverse reactions. Product contains sodium and potassium; high doses of I.V. therapy may alter serum levels.

Adverse Reactions (Reflective of adult population; not specific for elderly) Frequency not defined.

Central nervous system: Coma (high doses), hyper-reflexia (high doses), seizures (high doses)

Dermatologic: Contact dermatitis, rash

Endocrine & metabolic: Electrolyte imbalance (high doses)

Gastrointestinal: Pseudomembranous colitis

Hematologic: Neutropenia, positive Coombs' hemolytic anemia (rare, high doses)

Local: Injection site reaction, phlebitis, thrombophlebitis

Neuromuscular & skeletal: Myoclonus (high doses)

Renal: Acute interstitial nephritis (high doses), renal tubular damage (high doses)

Miscellaneous: Anaphylaxis, hypersensitivity reactions (immediate and delayed), Jarisch-Herxheimer reaction, serum sickness

Drug Interactions

Metabolism/Transport Effects None known.

Avoid Concomitant Use

Avoid concomitant use of Penicillin G (Parenteral/Aqueous) with any of the following: BCG

Increased Effect/Toxicity

Penicillin G (Parenteral/Aqueous) may increase the levels/effects of: Methotrexate; Vitamin K Antagonists

The levels/effects of Penicillin G (Parenteral/Aqueous) may be increased by: Probenecid

Decreased Effect

Penicillin G (Parenteral/Aqueous) may decrease the levels/effects of: BCG; Mycophenolate; Typhoid Vaccine

The levels/effects of Penicillin G (Parenteral/Aqueous) may be decreased by: Fusidic Acid; Tetracycline Derivatives

Stability

Penicillin G potassium powder for injection should be stored below 86°F (30°C). Following reconstitution, solution may be stored for up to 7 days under refrigeration. Premixed bags for infusion should be stored in the freezer (-20°C to -4°F); frozen bags may be thawed at room temperature or in refrigerator. Once thawed, solution is stable for 14 days if stored in refrigerator or for 24 hours when stored at room temperature. Do not refreeze once thawed. Penicillin G sodium powder for injection should be stored at controlled room temperature. Reconstituted solution may be stored under refrigeration for up to 3 days.

Reconstitution:

Intermittent I.V.: 5 million unit vial: Add 8.2 mL for a final concentration of 500,000 units/mL; add 3.2 mL for a final concentration of 1,000,000 units/mL. Dilute further to 50,000-145,000 units/mL prior to infusion.

Continuous I.V. infusion: 20 million unit vial: Add 11.5 mL for a final concentration of 1,000,000 units/mL. Dilute further in 1-2 L of infusion solution and administer over a 24-hour period.

Mechanism of Action Interferes with bacterial cell wall synthesis during active multiplication, causing cell wall death and resultant bactericidal activity against susceptible bacteria

Pharmacodynamics/Kinetics

Distribution: Poor penetration across blood-brain barrier, despite inflamed meninges

Relative diffusion from blood into CSF: Poor unless meninges inflamed (exceeds usual MICs)

CSF:blood level ratio: Normal meninges: <1%; Inflamed meninges: 2% to 6%

Protein binding: 65%

Metabolism: Hepatic (30%) to penicilloic acid

Half-life elimination:

Adults: Normal renal function: 30-50 minutes

End-stage renal disease: 3.3-5.1 hours

Time to peak, serum: I.M.: ~30 minutes; I.V.: ~1 hour

Excretion: Urine (58% to 85% as unchanged drug)

Dosage

Geriatric & Adult

Actinomyces species: I.V.: 10-20 million units/day divided every 4-6 hours for 4-6 weeks

Clostridium perfringens: I.V.: 24 million units/day divided every 4-6 hours with clindamycin

Corynebacterium diphtheriae: I.V.: 2-3 million units/day in divided doses every 4-6 hours for 10-12 days

Erysipelas: I.V.: 1-2 million units every 4-6 hours

Erysipelothrix: I.V.: 2-4 million units every 4 hours

Fascial space infections: I.V.: 2-4 million units every 4-6 hours with metronidazole

Leptospirosis: I.V.: 1.5 million units every 6 hours for 7 days

Listeria: I.V.: 15-20 million units/day in divided doses every 4-6 hours for 2 weeks (meningitis) or 4 weeks (endocarditis)

Lyme disease (meningitis): I.V.: 20 million units/day in divided doses

Neurosyphilis: I.V.: 18-24 million units/day in divided doses every 4 hours (or by continuous infusion) for 10-14 days (CDC, 2006; CDC, 2009; CDC, 2010)

Streptococcus:

Brain abscess: I.V.: 18-24 million units/day in divided doses every 4 hours with metronidazole

Endocarditis or osteomyelitis: I.V.: 3-4 million units every 4 hours for at least 4 weeks

Skin and soft tissue: I.V.: 3-4 million units every 4 hours for 10 days

Toxic shock: I.V.: 24 million units/day in divided doses with clindamycin

Streptococcal pneumonia: I.V.: 2-3 million units every 4 hours

Whipple's disease: I.V.: 2 million units every 4 hours for 2 weeks, followed by oral trimethoprim/sulfamethoxazole or doxycycline for 1 year

Relapse or CNS involvement: 4 million units every 4 hours for 4 weeks

Renal Impairment

Uremic patients with Cl_{cr} >10 mL/minute/1.73 m²: Administer full loading dose followed by ½ of the loading dose given every 4-5 hours

Cl_{cr} <10 mL/minute/1.73 m²: Administer full loading dose followed by ½ of the loading dose given every 8-10 hours

Intermittent hemodialysis (IHD) (administer after hemodialysis on dialysis days): Administer normal loading dose followed by either 25% to 50% of normal dose every 4-6 hours **or** 50% to 100% of normal dose every 8-12 hours. For mild-to-moderate infections, administer 0.5-1 million units every 4-6 hours **or** 1-2 million units every 8-12 hours. For neurosyphilis, endocarditis, or serious infections, administer up to 2 million units every 4-6 hours; administer after dialysis on dialysis days **or** supplement with 500,000 units after dialysis (Heintz, 2009). **Note:** Dosing dependent on the assumption of 3 times/week, complete IHD sessions.

Continuous renal replacement therapy (CRRT) (Heintz, 2009; Trotman, 2005): Drug clearance is highly dependent on the method of renal replacement, filter type, and flow rate. Appropriate dosing requires close monitoring of pharmacologic response, signs of adverse reactions due to drug accumulation, as well as drug concentrations in relation to target trough (if appropriate). The following are general recommendations only (based on dialysate flow/ultrafiltration rates of 1-2 L/hour and minimal residual renal function) and should not supersede clinical judgment:

CVVH: Loading dose of 4 million units, followed by 2 million units every 4-6 hours

CVVHD: Loading dose of 4 million units, followed by 2-3 million units every 4-6 hours

CVVHDF: Loading dose of 4 million units, followed by 2-4 million units every 4-6 hours

Administration

I.M.; Administer I.M. by deep injection in the upper outer quadrant of the buttock

I.V.: **Note:** The 20 million unit dosage form may be administered by continuous I.V. infusion only.

Intermittent I.V.: May be dissolved in small amounts of SWFI, NS, D₅W and administered peripherally as a 50,000-100,000 unit/mL solution. In fluid-restricted patients, 146,000 units/mL in SW results in a maximum recommended osmolality for peripheral infusion. Infuse over 15-30 minutes.

Continuous I.V. infusion: Determine the volume of fluid and rate of its administration required by the patient in a 24-hour period. Add the appropriate daily dosage of penicillin to this fluid. For example, if the daily dose is 10 million units and 2 L of fluid/day is required, add 5 million units to 1 L and adjust the rate of flow so the liter will be infused over 12 hours (83 mL/hour). Repeat steps (5 million units/L at 83 mL/hour) for the remaining 12 hours.

Monitoring Parameters Periodic electrolyte, hepatic, renal, cardiac and hematologic function tests during prolonged/high-dose therapy; observe for signs and symptoms of anaphylaxis during first dose

Test Interactions False-positive or negative urinary glucose determination using Clinitest®; positive Coombs' [direct]; false-positive urinary and/or serum proteins

Pharmacotherapy Pearls 1 million units is approximately equal to 625 mg.

Special Geriatric Considerations Despite a reported prolonged half-life, it is usually not necessary to adjust the dose of penicillin G or VK in elderly to account for renal function changes with age, however, it is advised to calculate an estimated creatinine clearance and adjust dose accordingly.

Dosage Forms Excipient information presented when available (limited, particularly for generics); consult specific product labeling.

Infusion, premixed iso-osmotic dextrose solution, as potassium: 1 million units (50 mL); 2 million units (50 mL); 3 million units (50 mL)

Injection, powder for reconstitution, as potassium: 5 million units, 20 million units

Pfizerpen®: 5 million units, 20 million units [contains potassium 65.6 mg (1.68 mEq) per 1 million units, sodium 6.8 mg (0.3 mEq) per 1 million units]

Injection, powder for reconstitution, as sodium: 5 million units

♦ **Penicillin G Potassium** *see* Penicillin G (Parenteral/Aqueous) *on page 1500*

Penicillin G Procaine (pen i SIL in jee PROE kane)

Medication Safety Issues

Sound-alike/look-alike issues:

Penicillin G procaine may be confused with penicillin V potassium

Wycillin® may be confused with Bicillin®

Brand Names: Canada Pfizerpen-AS®; Wycillin®

Index Terms APPG; Aqueous Procaine Penicillin G; Procaine Benzylpenicillin; Procaine Penicillin G; Wycillin [DSC]

Generic Availability (U.S.) Yes

Pharmacologic Category Antibiotic, Penicillin

Use Treatment of moderately-severe infections due to *Treponema pallidum* and other penicillin G-sensitive microorganisms that are susceptible to low, but prolonged serum penicillin concentrations; anthrax due to *Bacillus anthracis* (postexposure) to reduce the incidence or progression of disease following exposure to aerolized *Bacillus anthracis*

Contraindications Hypersensitivity to penicillin, procaine, or any component of the formulation

Warnings/Precautions May need to modify dosage in patients with severe renal impairment or seizure disorders; avoid I.V., intravascular, or intra-arterial administration of penicillin G procaine since severe and/or permanent neurovascular damage may occur. Serious and occasionally severe or fatal hypersensitivity (anaphylactoid) reactions have been reported in patients on penicillin therapy, especially with a history of beta-lactam hypersensitivity, history of sensitivity to multiple allergens, or previous IgE-mediated reactions (eg, anaphylaxis, angioedema, urticaria). Use with caution in asthmatic patients. Extended duration of therapy or use associated with high serum concentrations may be associated with an increased risk for some adverse reactions. Prolonged use may result in fungal or bacterial superinfection, including *C. difficile*-associated diarrhea (CDAD) and pseudomembranous colitis; CDAD has been observed >2 months postantibiotic treatment.

Adverse Reactions (Reflective of adult population; not specific for elderly) Frequency not defined.
Cardiovascular: Conduction disturbances, myocardial depression, vasodilation
Central nervous system: CNS stimulation, confusion, drowsiness, myoclonus, seizure
Hematologic: Hemolytic anemia, neutropenia, positive Coombs' reaction
Local: Pain at injection site, sterile abscess at injection site, thrombophlebitis
Renal: Interstitial nephritis
Miscellaneous: Hypersensitivity reactions, Jarisch-Herxheimer reaction, pseudoanaphylactic reactions, serum sickness

Drug Interactions
  Metabolism/Transport Effects None known.
  Avoid Concomitant Use
  Avoid concomitant use of Penicillin G Procaine with any of the following: BCG
  Increased Effect/Toxicity
  Penicillin G Procaine may increase the levels/effects of: Methotrexate; Vitamin K Antagonists

  The levels/effects of Penicillin G Procaine may be increased by: Probenecid
  Decreased Effect
  Penicillin G Procaine may decrease the levels/effects of: BCG; Mycophenolate; Typhoid Vaccine

  The levels/effects of Penicillin G Procaine may be decreased by: Fusidic Acid; Tetracycline Derivatives

Stability Refrigerate

Mechanism of Action Inhibits bacterial cell wall synthesis by binding to one or more of the penicillin-binding proteins (PBPs); which in turn inhibits the final transpeptidation step of peptidoglycan synthesis in bacterial cell walls, thus inhibiting cell wall biosynthesis. Bacteria eventually lyse due to ongoing activity of cell wall autolytic enzymes (autolysins and murein hydrolases) while cell wall assembly is arrested.

Pharmacodynamics/Kinetics
Absorption: I.M.: Slow
Distribution: Penetration across the blood-brain barrier is poor, despite inflamed meninges
Protein binding: 65%
Half-life: 20-50 minutes
Time to peak serum concentration: Within 1-4 hours and can persist within the therapeutic range for 15-24 hours
Elimination: 60% to 90% of drug is excreted unchanged via renal tubular excretion; ~30% of dose inactivated in the liver
Renal clearance is delayed in patients with impaired renal function

Dosage
  Geriatric & Adult
    Anthrax:
      Inhalational (postexposure prophylaxis): I.M.: 1,200,000 units every 12 hours
        Note: Overall treatment duration should be 60 days. Available safety data suggest continued administration of penicillin G procaine for longer than 2 weeks may incur additional risk of adverse reactions. Clinicians may consider switching to effective alternative treatment for completion of therapy beyond 2 weeks.
      Cutaneous (treatment): I.M.: 600,000-1,200,000 units/day; alternative therapy is recommended in severe cutaneous or other forms of anthrax infection

Endocarditis caused by susceptible viridans *Streptococcus* **(when used in conjunction with an aminoglycoside):** I.M.: 1.2 million units every 6 hours for 2-4 weeks

Gonorrhea (uncomplicated): 4.8 million units as a single dose divided in 2 sites given 30 minutes after probenecid 1 g orally

Neurosyphilis: I.M.: 2.4 million units/day with 500 mg probenecid by mouth 4 times/day for 10-14 days; **Note: penicillin G aqueous I.V. is the preferred agent**

Whipple's disease: I.M.: 1.2 million units/day (with streptomycin) for 10-14 days, followed by oral trimethoprim/sulfamethoxazole or doxycycline for 1 year

Renal Impairment

Cl_{cr} 10-30 mL/minute: Administer every 8-12 hours.

Cl_{cr} <10 mL/minute: Administer every 12-18 hours.

Moderately dialyzable (20% to 50%)

Administration Procaine suspension for deep I.M. injection only; administer around-the-clock rather than 4 times/day, 3 times/day, etc (ie, 12-6-12-6, not 9-1-5-9) to promote less variation in peak and trough serum concentrations; when doses are repeated, rotate the injection site; avoid I.V., intravascular, or intra-arterial administration of penicillin G procaine since severe and/or permanent neurovascular damage may occur; renal and hematologic systems should be evaluated periodically during prolonged therapy

Monitoring Parameters Periodic renal and hematologic function tests with prolonged therapy; fever, mental status, WBC count

Test Interactions Positive Coombs' [direct], false-positive urinary and/or serum proteins

Special Geriatric Considerations Dosage does not usually need to be adjusted in the elderly, however, if multiple doses are to be given, adjust dose for renal function.

Dosage Forms Excipient information presented when available (limited, particularly for generics); consult specific product labeling.

Injection, suspension: 600,000 units/mL (1 mL, 2 mL)

♦ **Penicillin G Procaine and Benzathine Combined** *see* Penicillin G Benzathine and Penicillin G Procaine *on page 1498*

♦ **Penicillin G Sodium** *see* Penicillin G (Parenteral/Aqueous) *on page 1500*

Penicillin V Potassium (pen i SIL in vee poe TASS ee um)

Related Information

Antimicrobial Drugs of Choice *on page 2163*

Medication Safety Issues

Sound-alike/look-alike issues:

Penicillin V procaine may be confused with penicillin G potassium

Brand Names: Canada Apo-Pen VK®; Novo-Pen-VK; Nu-Pen-VK

Index Terms Pen VK; Phenoxymethyl Penicillin

Generic Availability (U.S.) Yes

Pharmacologic Category Antibiotic, Penicillin

Use Treatment of infections caused by susceptible organisms involving the respiratory tract, otitis media, sinusitis, skin, and urinary tract; prophylaxis in rheumatic fever

Contraindications Hypersensitivity to penicillin or any component of the formulation

Warnings/Precautions Use with caution in patients with severe renal impairment (modify dosage) or history of seizures. Serious and occasionally severe or fatal hypersensitivity (anaphylactoid) reactions have been reported in patients on penicillin therapy, especially with a history of beta-lactam hypersensitivity, history of sensitivity to multiple allergens, or previous IgE-mediated reactions (eg, anaphylaxis, angioedema, urticaria). Use with caution in asthmatic patients. Extended duration of therapy or use associated with high serum concentrations may be associated with an increased risk for some adverse reactions. Prolonged use may result in fungal or bacterial superinfection, including *C. difficile*-associated diarrhea (CDAD) and pseudomembranous colitis; CDAD has been observed >2 months postantibiotic treatment.

Adverse Reactions (Reflective of adult population; not specific for elderly) >10%:

Gastrointestinal: Mild diarrhea, vomiting, nausea, oral candidiasis

Drug Interactions

Metabolism/Transport Effects None known.

Avoid Concomitant Use

Avoid concomitant use of Penicillin V Potassium with any of the following: BCG

Increased Effect/Toxicity

Penicillin V Potassium may increase the levels/effects of: Methotrexate; Vitamin K Antagonists

The levels/effects of Penicillin V Potassium may be increased by: Probenecid

Decreased Effect

Penicillin V Potassium may decrease the levels/effects of: BCG; Mycophenolate; Typhoid Vaccine

The levels/effects of Penicillin V Potassium may be decreased by: Fusidic Acid; Tetracycline Derivatives

Ethanol/Nutrition/Herb Interactions Food: Decreases drug absorption rate; decreases drug serum concentration. Management: Take on an empty stomach 1 hour before or 2 hours after meals around-the-clock to promote less variation in peak and trough serum levels.

Stability Refrigerate suspension after reconstitution; discard after 14 days

Mechanism of Action Inhibits bacterial cell wall synthesis by binding to one or more of the penicillin-binding proteins (PBPs); which in turn inhibits the final transpeptidation step of peptidoglycan synthesis in bacterial cell walls, thus inhibiting cell wall biosynthesis. Bacteria eventually lyse due to ongoing activity of cell wall autolytic enzymes (autolysins and murein hydrolases) while cell wall assembly is arrested.

Pharmacodynamics/Kinetics

Absorption: 60% to 73%

Distribution: Widely distributed to kidneys, liver, skin, tonsils, and into synovial, pleural, and pericardial fluids

Protein binding, plasma: 80%

Half-life elimination: 30 minutes; prolonged with renal impairment

Time to peak, serum: 0.5-1 hour

Excretion: Urine (as unchanged drug and metabolites)

Dosage

Geriatric & Adult

Actinomycosis:

Mild: 2-4 g/day in 4 divided doses for 8 weeks

Surgical: 2-4 g/day in 4 divided doses for 6-12 months (after I.V. penicillin G therapy of 4-6 weeks)

Erysipelas: 500 mg 4 times/day

Pharyngitis (streptococcal): 500 mg 3-4 times/day for 10 days

Prophylaxis of pneumococcal or recurrent rheumatic fever infections: 250 mg twice daily

Renal Impairment

Cl_{cr} 10-50 mL/minute: Administer every 8-12 hours.

Cl_{cr} <10 mL/minute: Administer every 12-16 hours.

Administration Administer on an empty stomach to increase oral absorption

Monitoring Parameters Periodic renal and hematologic function tests during prolonged therapy; monitor for signs of anaphylaxis during first dose

Test Interactions False-positive or negative urinary glucose determination using Clinitest®; positive Coombs' [direct]; false-positive urinary and/or serum proteins

Pharmacotherapy Pearls 0.7 mEq of potassium per 250 mg penicillin V; 250 mg equals 400,000 units of penicillin

Special Geriatric Considerations Dosage adjustment in the elderly is usually not necessary.

Dosage Forms Excipient information presented when available (limited, particularly for generics); consult specific product labeling.

Powder for solution, oral: 125 mg/5 mL (100 mL, 200 mL); 250 mg/5 mL (100 mL, 200 mL)

Tablet, oral: 250 mg, 500 mg

◆ **Penlac®** *see Ciclopirox on page 373*
◆ **Pennsaid®** *see Diclofenac (Topical) on page 536*
◆ **Pentasa®** *see Mesalamine on page 1217*

Pentazocine (pen TAZ oh seen)

Related Information

Beers Criteria – Potentially Inappropriate Medications for Geriatrics on page 2183
Opioid Analgesics on page 2122

Medication Safety Issues

High alert medication:

The Institute for Safe Medication Practices (ISMP) includes this medication among its list of drug classes which have a heightened risk of causing significant patient harm when used in error.

BEERS Criteria medication:

This drug may be potentially inappropriate for use in geriatric patients (Quality of evidence - low; Strength of recommendation - strong).

PENTAZOCINE

Brand Names: U.S. Talwin®
Brand Names: Canada Talwin®
Index Terms Pentazocine Lactate
Generic Availability (U.S.) No
Pharmacologic Category Analgesic, Opioid; Analgesic, Opioid Partial Agonist
Use Relief of moderate-to-severe pain; has also been used as a sedative prior to surgery and as a supplement to surgical anesthesia
Contraindications Hypersensitivity to pentazocine or any component of the formulation
Warnings/Precautions May increase systemic and pulmonary arterial pressure and systemic vascular resistance; use with caution in patients who may not tolerate these alterations in hemodynamics (eg, heart failure). May cause CNS depression, which may impair physical or mental abilities; patients must be cautioned about performing tasks which require mental alertness (eg, operating machinery or driving). Effects may be potentiated when used with other sedative drugs or ethanol. Use with caution in seizure-prone patients, acute myocardial infarction, patients undergoing biliary tract impairment, thyroid dysfunction, prostatic hyperplasia/urinary stricture, patients with respiratory, adrenal insufficiency, morbid obesity, renal and hepatic dysfunction, head trauma, increased intracranial pressure, and patients with a history of prior opioid dependence or abuse; pentazocine may precipitate opiate withdrawal symptoms in patients who have been receiving opiates regularly; injection contains sulfites which may cause allergic reaction; tolerance or drug dependence may result from extended use. May cause hypotension; use with caution in patients with hypovolemia, cardiovascular disease (including acute MI), or drugs which may exaggerate hypotensive effects (including phenothiazines or general anesthetics). May obscure diagnosis or clinical course of patients with acute abdominal conditions. Abrupt discontinuation may result in withdrawal symptoms; taper dose to decrease risk of withdrawal symptoms. Severe sclerosis has occurred at the injection-site following multiple injections; rotate sites of injection. Use with caution in the elderly and debilitated patients; may be more sensitive to adverse effects.

Avoid use in the elderly due to increased risk of CNS effects (confusion and hallucinations) compared to other narcotics; safer alternative agents preferred (Beers Criteria). If used, use lower initial doses.

Adverse Reactions (Reflective of adult population; not specific for elderly) Frequency not defined.
Cardiovascular: Circulatory depression, facial edema, flushing, hyper-/hypotension, shock, syncope, systemic vascular resistance increased, tachycardia
Central nervous system: Chills, CNS depression, confusion, disorientation, dizziness, drowsiness, euphoria, excitement, hallucinations, headache, insomnia, irritability, lightheadedness, malaise, nightmares, sedation
Dermatologic: Dermatitis, erythema multiforme, pruritus, rash, Stevens-Johnson syndrome, toxic epidermal necrolysis, urticaria
Gastrointestinal: Abdominal distress, anorexia, constipation, diarrhea, nausea, taste alteration, vomiting, xerostomia
Genitourinary: Urinary retention
Hematologic: Agranulocytosis (rare), eosinophilia, WBCs decreased
Local: Injection site reaction (tissue damage and irritation)
Neuromuscular & skeletal: Paresthesia, tremor, weakness
Ocular: Blurred vision, diplopia, miosis, nystagmus
Otic: Tinnitus
Respiratory: Dyspnea, respiratory depression (rare)
Miscellaneous: Anaphylaxis, diaphoresis, physical and psychological dependence
Drug Interactions
Metabolism/Transport Effects None known.
Avoid Concomitant Use
Avoid concomitant use of Pentazocine with any of the following: Azelastine; Azelastine (Nasal); Mirtazapine; Paraldehyde
Increased Effect/Toxicity
Pentazocine may increase the levels/effects of: Alcohol (Ethyl); Alvimopan; Azelastine; Azelastine (Nasal); CNS Depressants; Desmopressin; Metyrosine; Mirtazapine; Paraldehyde; Selective Serotonin Reuptake Inhibitors; Thiazide Diuretics; Zolpidem

The levels/effects of Pentazocine may be increased by: Amphetamines; Antipsychotic Agents (Phenothiazines); Droperidol; HydrOXYzine; Succinylcholine
Decreased Effect
Pentazocine may decrease the levels/effects of: Analgesics (Opioid); Pegvisomant

The levels/effects of Pentazocine may be decreased by: Ammonium Chloride
Stability Store at 20°C to 25°C (68°F to 77°F).

Mechanism of Action Agonist of kappa opiate receptors and partial agonist of mu opiate receptors in the CNS, causing inhibition of ascending pain pathways, altering the perception of and response to pain; produces analgesia, respiratory depression and sedation similar to opioids

Pharmacodynamics/Kinetics

Onset of action: I.M., SubQ: 15-20 minutes; I.V.: 2-3 minutes

Duration: 2-3 hours

Protein binding: 60%

Metabolism: Hepatic via oxidative and glucuronide conjugation pathways; extensive first-pass effect

Half-life elimination: 2-3 hours; prolonged with hepatic impairment

Excretion: Urine (small amounts as unchanged drug)

Dosage

Geriatric Use with caution; may be more sensitive to analgesic and sedative effects; decrease initial dose and monitor closely

Adult

Analgesic:

I.M., SubQ: 30-60 mg every 3-4 hours; do **not** exceed 60 mg/dose (maximum: 360 mg/day)

I.V.: 30 mg every 3-4 hours; do **not** exceed 30 mg/dose (maximum: 360 mg/day)

Renal Impairment

Cl_{cr} 10-50 mL/minute: Administer 75% of normal dose.

Cl_{cr} <10 mL/minute: Administer 50% of normal dose.

Hepatic Impairment Reduce dose or avoid use in patients with liver disease.

Administration Rotate injection site for I.M.; avoid intra-arterial injection; avoid SubQ use unless absolutely necessary (may cause tissue damage)

Monitoring Parameters Relief of pain, respiratory and mental status, blood pressure

Special Geriatric Considerations Pentazocine is not recommended for use in the elderly because of its propensity to cause delirium and agitation. If pentazocine must be used, adjust dose for renal function.

This medication is considered to be potentially inappropriate in this patient population (Beers Criteria: Quality of evidence - low; Strength of recommendation - strong).

Controlled Substance C-IV

Dosage Forms Excipient information presented when available (limited, particularly for generics); consult specific product labeling.

Injection, solution:

Talwin®: 30 mg/mL (1 mL)

Talwin®: 30 mg/mL (10 mL) [contains sodium bisulfite]

◆ **Pentazocine Lactate** see Pentazocine on page 1505

Pentoxifylline (pen toks IF i lin)

Medication Safety Issues

Sound-alike/look-alike issues:

Pentoxifylline may be confused with tamoxifen

TRENtal® may be confused with Bentyl®, TEGretol®, Trandate®

Brand Names: U.S. TRENtal®

Brand Names: Canada Albert® Pentoxifylline; Apo-Pentoxifylline SR®; Nu-Pentoxifylline SR; ratio-Pentoxifylline; Trental®

Index Terms Oxpentifylline

Generic Availability (U.S.) Yes

Pharmacologic Category Blood Viscosity Reducer Agent

Use Treatment of intermittent claudication on the basis of chronic occlusive arterial disease of the limbs; may improve function and symptoms, but not intended to replace more definitive therapy

Note: The American College of Chest Physicians (ACCP) discourages the use of pentoxifyl-line for the treatment of intermittent claudication refractory to exercise therapy (and smoking cessation) (Guyatt, 2012).

Unlabeled Use Severe alcoholic hepatitis; venous leg ulcers (with compression therapy)

Contraindications Hypersensitivity to pentoxifylline, xanthines (eg, caffeine, theophylline), or any component of the formulation; recent cerebral and/or retinal hemorrhage

Warnings/Precautions Use with caution in renal impairment; active metabolite may accumulate in renal impairment leading to increased risk of adverse effects. Use caution in the elderly and assess renal function before initiating.

Adverse Reactions (Reflective of adult population; not specific for elderly) 1% to 10%: Gastrointestinal: Nausea (2%), vomiting (1%)

Drug Interactions

Metabolism/Transport Effects Inhibits CYP1A2 (weak)

Avoid Concomitant Use

Avoid concomitant use of Pentoxifylline with any of the following: Ketorolac; Ketorolac (Nasal); Ketorolac (Systemic)

Increased Effect/Toxicity

Pentoxifylline may increase the levels/effects of: Antihypertensives; Antiplatelet Agents; Heparin; Heparin (Low Molecular Weight); Theophylline Derivatives; Vitamin K Antagonists

The levels/effects of Pentoxifylline may be increased by: Cimetidine; Ciprofloxacin; Ciprofloxacin (Systemic); Ketorolac; Ketorolac (Nasal); Ketorolac (Systemic)

Decreased Effect There are no known significant interactions involving a decrease in effect.

Ethanol/Nutrition/Herb Interactions Food: Food may decrease rate but not extent of absorption. Pentoxifylline peak serum levels may be decreased if taken with food.

Stability Store between 15°C to 30°C (59°F to 86°F).

Mechanism of Action Reduces blood viscosity via increased leukocyte and erythrocyte deformability and decreased neutrophil adhesion/activation; improves peripheral tissue oxygenation presumably through enhanced blood flow.

Pharmacodynamics/Kinetics

Absorption: Well absorbed

Metabolism: Hepatic to 3-carboxybutyl (M-IV, inactive) and 3-carboxypropyl (M-V, active) and via erythrocytes to 5-hydroxyhexyl (M-I, active); extensive first-pass effect; M-I is further metabolized in the liver

Half-life elimination: Parent drug: 24-48 minutes; Metabolites: 60-96 minutes

Time to peak, serum: 2-4 hours

Excretion: Primarily urine (50% to 80% as M-V, 20% as other metabolites); feces (<4%)

Dosage

Geriatric Refer to adult dosing. Dosage adjustment based on creatinine clearance can be considered (see Dosage: Renal Impairment).

Adult

Intermittent claudication: Oral: 400 mg 3 times/day; maximal therapeutic benefit may take 2-4 weeks to develop; recommended to maintain therapy for at least 8 weeks. May reduce to 400 mg twice daily if GI or CNS side effects occur.

Note: Use for the treatment of intermittent claudication refractory to exercise therapy (and smoking cessation) has been discouraged by The American College of Chest Physicians (ACCP) (Guyatt, 2012).

Severe alcoholic hepatitis (Maddrey Discriminant Function [MDF] score ≥32, especially when corticosteroids contraindicated) (unlabeled use): Oral: 400 mg 3 times/day for 4 weeks (O'Shea, 2010)

Venous leg ulcer (unlabeled use): Oral: 400 mg 3 times/day (with compression therapy) (Jull, 2002; Robson, 2006)

Renal Impairment Dosage adjustment in renal impairment: No dosage adjustments provided in the manufacturer's labeling; however, the following guidelines have been used by some clinicians:

Aronoff, 2007: Adults:

Cl_{cr} >50 mL/minute: 400 mg every 8-12 hours

Cl_{cr} 10-50 mL/minute: 400 mg every 12-24 hours

Cl_{cr} <10 mL minute: 400 mg every 24 hours

Hemodialysis: supplemental postdialysis dose is not necessary.

Peritoneal dialysis: 400 mg every 24 hours

Paap, 1996: Adults:

Moderate renal impairment (Cl_{cr} ~60 mL/minute): 400 mg twice daily.

Severe renal impairment (Cl_{cr} ~20 mL/minute): 400 mg once daily; further reduction may be required; Paap suggests 200 mg once daily, but with current products (extended or controlled release; unscored) may require adaptation to 400 mg once every other day.

Administration Tablets should be swallowed whole; do not chew, break, or crush. May be administered with food.

Test Interactions False-positive theophylline levels

Special Geriatric Considerations Pentoxifylline's value in the treatment of intermittent claudication is controversial. Walking distance improved statistically in some clinical trials, but the actual distance was minimal when applied to improving physical activity. Dose adjustment in moderate and severe kidney impairment has been recommended based on accumulation of two active metabolites. However, these doses have not been studied for clinical or safety outcomes.

Dosage Forms Excipient information presented when available (limited, particularly for generics); consult specific product labeling.
Tablet, controlled release, oral:
  TRENtal®: 400 mg
Tablet, extended release, oral: 400 mg

- ◆ **Pen VK** see Penicillin V Potassium on page 1504
- ◆ **PEP005** see Ingenol Mebutate on page 1004
- ◆ **Pepcid®** see Famotidine on page 744
- ◆ **Pepcid® AC [OTC]** see Famotidine on page 744
- ◆ **Pepcid® AC Maximum Strength [OTC]** see Famotidine on page 744
- ◆ **Pepcid® Complete® [OTC]** see Famotidine, Calcium Carbonate, and Magnesium Hydroxide on page 746
- ◆ **Peptic Relief [OTC]** see Bismuth on page 216
- ◆ **Pepto-Bismol® [OTC]** see Bismuth on page 216
- ◆ **Pepto-Bismol® Maximum Strength [OTC]** see Bismuth on page 216
- ◆ **Pepto Relief [OTC]** see Bismuth on page 216
- ◆ **Percocet®** see Oxycodone and Acetaminophen on page 1449
- ◆ **Percodan®** see Oxycodone and Aspirin on page 1452
- ◆ **Perdiem® Overnight Relief [OTC]** see Senna on page 1764
- ◆ **Perforomist®** see Formoterol on page 841
- ◆ **Periactin** see Cyproheptadine on page 467
- ◆ **Peri-Colace® [OTC]** see Docusate and Senna on page 585

Perindopril Erbumine (per IN doe pril er BYOO meen)

Related Information
  Angiotensin Agents on page 2093
  Heart Failure (Systolic) on page 2203
Brand Names: U.S. Aceon®
Brand Names: Canada Apo-Perindopril®; Coversyl®
Generic Availability (U.S.) Yes
Pharmacologic Category Angiotensin-Converting Enzyme (ACE) Inhibitor
Use Treatment of hypertension; reduction of cardiovascular mortality or nonfatal myocardial infarction in patients with stable coronary artery disease

  Canadian labeling: Additional use (unlabeled use in U.S.): Treatment of mild-moderate (NYHA I-III) heart failure
Unlabeled Use To delay the progression of nephropathy and reduce risks of cardiovascular events in hypertensive patients with type 1 or 2 diabetes mellitus
Contraindications Hypersensitivity to perindopril, any other ACE inhibitor, or any component of the formulation; angioedema related to previous treatment with an ACE inhibitor

  Canadian labeling: Additional contraindications (not in U.S. labeling): History of hereditary/idiopathic angioedema
Warnings/Precautions Anaphylactic reactions may occur rarely with ACE inhibitors. At any time during treatment (especially following first dose), angioedema may occur rarely with ACE inhibitors; it may involve the head and neck (potentially compromising airway) or the intestine (presenting with abdominal pain). African-Americans and patients with idiopathic or hereditary angioedema may be at an increased risk. Prolonged frequent monitoring may be required especially if tongue, glottis, or larynx are involved as they are associated with airway obstruction. Patients with a history of airway surgery may have a higher risk of airway obstruction. Aggressive early and appropriate management is critical. Use in patients with previous angioedema associated with ACE inhibitor therapy is contraindicated. Severe anaphylactoid reactions may be seen during hemodialysis (eg, CVVHD) with high-flux dialysis membranes (eg, AN69), and rarely, during low density lipoprotein apheresis with dextran sulfate cellulose. Rare cases of anaphylactoid reactions have been reported in patients undergoing sensitization treatment with hymenoptera (bee, wasp) venom while receiving ACE inhibitors.

  Symptomatic hypotension with or without syncope can occur with ACE inhibitors (usually with the first several doses); effects are most often observed in volume-depleted patients; correct volume depletion prior to initiation; close monitoring of patient is required especially with initial dosing and dosing increases; blood pressure must be lowered at a rate appropriate for the patient's clinical condition. Initiation of therapy in patients with ischemic heart disease or cerebrovascular disease warrants close observation due to the potential consequences posed by falling blood pressure (eg, MI, stroke). Use with caution in hypertrophic cardiomyopathy ▶

with outflow tract obstruction, severe aortic stenosis, or before, during, or immediately after major surgery.

Hyperkalemia may occur with ACE inhibitors; risk factors include renal dysfunction, diabetes mellitus, concomitant use of potassium-sparing diuretics, potassium supplements, and/or potassium-containing salts. Use cautiously, if at all, with these agents and monitor potassium closely. Cough may occur with ACE inhibitors. Other causes of cough should be considered (eg, pulmonary congestion in patients with heart failure) and excluded prior to discontinuation.

May be associated with deterioration of renal function and/or increases in serum creatinine, particularly in patients with low renal blood flow (eg, renal artery stenosis, heart failure) whose glomerular filtration rate (GFR) is dependent on efferent arteriolar vasoconstriction by angiotensin II; deterioration may result in oliguria, acute renal failure, and progressive azotemia. Small increases in serum creatinine may occur following initiation; consider discontinuation only in patients with progressive and/or significant deterioration in renal function. Use with caution in patients with unstented unilateral/bilateral renal artery stenosis. When unstented bilateral renal artery stenosis is present, use is generally avoided due to the elevated risk of deterioration in renal function unless possible benefits outweigh risks. Concurrent use of angiotensin receptor blockers may increase the risk of clinically-significant adverse events (eg, renal dysfunction, hyperkalemia).

Rare toxicities associated with ACE inhibitors include cholestatic jaundice (which may progress to fulminant hepatic necrosis), agranulocytosis, neutropenia or leukopenia with myeloid hypoplasia. Patients with collagen vascular diseases (especially with concomitant renal impairment) or renal impairment alone may be at increased risk for hematologic toxicity; periodically monitor CBC with differential in these patients.

Adverse Reactions (Reflective of adult population; not specific for elderly)

>10%:
Central nervous system: Headache (24%)
Respiratory: Cough (incidence is higher in women, 3:1) (12%)

1% to 10%:
Cardiovascular: Edema (4%), chest pain (2%), ECG abnormal (2%), palpitation (1%)
Central nervous system: Dizziness (8%, less than placebo), sleep disorders (3%), depression (2%), fever (2%), nervousness (1%), somnolence (1%)
Dermatologic: Rash (2%)
Endocrine & metabolic: Hyperkalemia (1%, less than placebo), triglycerides increased (1%), menstrual disorder (1%)
Gastrointestinal: Diarrhea (4%), abdominal pain (3%), nausea (2%), vomiting (2%), dyspepsia (2%), flatulence (1%)
Genitourinary: Urinary tract infection (3%), sexual dysfunction (male 1%)
Hepatic: ALT increased (2%)
Neuromuscular & skeletal: Weakness (8%), back pain (6%), lower extremity pain (5%), upper extremity pain (3%), hypertonia (3%), paresthesia (2%), joint pain (1%), myalgia (1%), arthritis (1%), neck pain (1%)
Renal: Proteinuria (2%)
Respiratory: Upper respiratory tract infection (9%), sinusitis (5%), rhinitis (5%), pharyngitis (3%)
Otic: Tinnitus (2%), ear infection (1%)
Miscellaneous: Viral infection (3%), seasonal allergy (2%)
Note: Some reactions occurred at an incidence >1% but ≤ placebo.

Additional adverse effects that have been reported with **ACE inhibitors** include agranulocytosis (especially in patients with renal impairment or collagen vascular disease), neutropenia, anemia, bullous pemphigoid, cardiac arrest, eosinophilic pneumonitis, exfoliative dermatitis, falls, hepatic failure, hyponatremia, jaundice, pancreatitis (acute), pancytopenia, pemphigus, psoriasis, thrombocytopenia; decreases in creatinine clearance in some elderly hypertensive patients or those with chronic renal failure, and worsening of renal function in patients with bilateral renal artery stenosis or hypovolemic patients (diuretic therapy). In addition, a syndrome which may include fever, myalgia, arthralgia, interstitial nephritis, vasculitis, rash, eosinophilia and positive ANA, and elevated ESR has been reported with ACE inhibitors.

Drug Interactions

Metabolism/Transport Effects None known.

Avoid Concomitant Use There are no known interactions where it is recommended to avoid concomitant use.

Increased Effect/Toxicity
Perindopril Erbumine may increase the levels/effects of: Allopurinol; Amifostine; Antihypertensives; AzaTHIOprine; CycloSPORINE; CycloSPORINE (Systemic); Ferric Gluconate; Gold Sodium Thiomalate; Hypotensive Agents; Iron Dextran Complex; Lithium; Nonsteroidal Anti-Inflammatory Agents; RiTUXimab; Sodium Phosphates

The levels/effects of Perindopril Erbumine may be increased by: Alfuzosin; Aliskiren; Angiotensin II Receptor Blockers; Diazoxide; DPP-IV Inhibitors; Eplerenone; Everolimus; Herbs (Hypotensive Properties); Loop Diuretics; MAO Inhibitors; Pentoxifylline; Phosphodiesterase 5 Inhibitors; Potassium Salts; Potassium-Sparing Diuretics; Prostacyclin Analogues; Sirolimus; Temsirolimus; Thiazide Diuretics; TiZANidine; Tolvaptan; Trimethoprim

Decreased Effect

The levels/effects of Perindopril Erbumine may be decreased by: Antacids; Aprotinin; Herbs (Hypertensive Properties); Icatibant; Lanthanum; Methylphenidate; Nonsteroidal Anti-Inflammatory Agents; Salicylates; Yohimbine

Ethanol/Nutrition/Herb Interactions

Food: Perindopril active metabolite concentrations may be lowered if taken with food. Potassium supplements and/or potassium-containing salts may cause or worsen hyperkalemia. Management: Consult prescriber before consuming a potassium-rich diet, potassium supplements, or salt substitutes.

Herb/Nutraceutical: Some herbal medications may worsen hypertension (eg, licorice); others may increase the antihypertensive effect of perindopril (eg, shepherd's purse). Avoid bayberry, blue cohosh, cayenne, ephedra, ginger, ginseng (American), kola, licorice, and yohimbe. Avoid black cohosh, California poppy, coleus, golden seal, hawthorn, mistletoe, periwinkle, quinine, and shepherd's purse.

Stability Store at room temperature of 20°C to 25°C (68°F to 77°F). Protect from moisture.

Mechanism of Action Perindopril is a prodrug for perindoprilat, which acts as a competitive inhibitor of angiotensin-converting enzyme (ACE); prevents conversion of angiotensin I to angiotensin II, a potent vasoconstrictor; results in lower levels of angiotensin II which, in turn, causes an increase in plasma renin activity and a reduction in aldosterone secretion

Pharmacodynamics/Kinetics

Onset of action: Peak effect: 1-2 hours

Protein binding: Perindopril: 60%; Perindoprilat: 10% to 20%

Metabolism: Hepatically hydrolyzed to active metabolite, perindoprilat (~17% to 20% of a dose) and other inactive metabolites

Bioavailability: Perindopril: 75%; Perindoprilat ~25% (~16% with food)

Half-life elimination: Parent drug: 1.5-3 hours; Metabolite: Effective: 3-10 hours, Terminal: 30-120 hours

Time to peak: Chronic therapy: Perindopril: 1 hour; Perindoprilat: 3-7 hours (maximum perindoprilat serum levels are 2-3 times higher and T_{max} is shorter following chronic therapy); CHF: Perindoprilat: 6 hours

Excretion: Urine (75%, 4% to 12% as unchanged drug)

Dosage

Geriatric

Hypertension: >65 years: Oral:

U.S. labeling: Initial: 4 mg/day; maintenance: 8 mg/day; experience with doses >8 mg/day is limited; may be given in 1-2 divided doses

Canadian labeling: Initial: 2 mg/day; if necessary may increase dose after 4 weeks to 4 mg/day; then to 8 mg/day (based on renal function); may be given in 1 or 2 divided doses.

ACCF/AHA Expert Consensus recommendations: Consider lower initial doses and titrating to response (Aronow, 2011)

Stable coronary artery disease: >70 years: Oral: Initial: 2 mg/day for 1 week; then increase as tolerated to 4 mg/day for 1 week; then increase as tolerated to 8 mg/day.

Adult

Heart failure (Canadian labeling; unlabeled use in U.S.): Initial: 2 mg once daily; if necessary, may titrate over 2-4 weeks to 4 mg once daily. The American College of Cardiology/ American Heart Association (ACC/AHA) 2009 Heart Failure Guidelines recommend an initial dose of 2 mg once daily with dose titration at 1- to 2- week intervals to a target dose of 8-16 mg once daily.

Hypertension: Oral: Initial: 4 mg/day but may be titrated to response; usual range: 4-8 mg/day (may be given in 2 divided doses); increase at 1- to 2-week intervals (maximum: 16 mg/day). **Note:** The Canadian labeling recommended maximum dose is 8 mg/day.

Concomitant therapy with diuretics: To reduce the risk of hypotension, discontinue diuretic, if possible, 2-3 days prior to initiating perindopril. If unable to stop diuretic, initiate perindopril at 2-4 mg/day (given in 1-2 divided doses) and monitor blood pressure closely for the first 2 weeks of therapy, and after any dose adjustment of perindopril or diuretic.

Stable coronary artery disease: Oral: Initial: 4 mg once daily for 2 weeks; then increase as tolerated to 8 mg once daily.

Renal Impairment

U.S. labeling:

Cl_{cr} >30 mL/minute: Initial: 2 mg/day; maintenance dosing not to exceed 8 mg/day

Cl_{cr} <30 mL/minute: Safety and efficacy not established.

Hemodialysis: Perindopril and its metabolites are dialyzable

Canadian labeling:

Cl_{cr} ≥60 mL/minute: Initial: 4 mg/day; maintenance dosing not to exceed 8 mg/day

Cl_{cr} 30-60 mL/minute: 2 mg/day

Cl_{cr} 15-30 mL/minute: 2 mg every other day

Hemodialysis (Cl_{cr} <15 mL/minute): 2 mg on dialysis days (given after dialysis)

Hepatic Impairment No adjustment necessary.

Administration Administer prior to a meal.

Monitoring Parameters Blood pressure; serum creatinine and potassium; if patient has collagen vascular disease and/or renal impairment, periodically monitor CBC with differential

Special Geriatric Considerations Due to frequent decreases in glomerular filtration (also creatinine clearance) with aging, elderly patients may have exaggerated responses to ACE inhibitors; differences in clinical response due to hepatic changes are not observed. ACE inhibitors may be preferred agents in elderly patients with congestive heart failure and diabetes mellitus. Diabetic proteinuria is reduced and insulin sensitivity is enhanced. In general, the side effect profile is favorable in elderly and causes little or no CNS confusion; use lowest dose recommendations initially. Many elderly may be volume depleted due to diuretic use and/or blunted thirst reflex resulting in inadequate fluid intake.

Dosage Forms Excipient information presented when available (limited, particularly for generics); consult specific product labeling.

Tablet, oral: 2 mg, 4 mg, 8 mg

Aceon® : 2 mg, 4 mg, 8 mg [scored]

♦ **PerioMed™** see Fluoride on page 806
♦ **Periostat®** see Doxycycline on page 606

Permethrin (per METH rin)

Brand Names: U.S. A200® Lice [OTC]; Nix® Complete Lice Treatment System [OTC]; Nix® Creme Rinse Lice Treatment [OTC]; Nix® Creme Rinse [OTC]; Nix® Lice Control Spray [OTC]; Rid® [OTC]

Brand Names: Canada Kwellada-P™; Nix®

Index Terms Elimite

Generic Availability (U.S.) Yes: Excludes liquid spray

Pharmacologic Category Antiparasitic Agent, Topical; Pediculocide; Scabicidal Agent

Use Single-application treatment of infestation with *Pediculus humanus capitis* (head louse) and its nits or *Sarcoptes scabiei* (scabies); indicated for prophylactic use during epidemics of lice

Contraindications Hypersensitivity to pyrethroid, pyrethrin, chrysanthemums, or any component of the formulation

Warnings/Precautions Treatment may temporarily exacerbate the symptoms of itching, redness, swelling; for external use only.

Adverse Reactions (Reflective of adult population; not specific for elderly) 1% to 10%:

Dermatologic: Pruritus, erythema, rash of the scalp

Local: Burning, stinging, tingling, numbness or scalp discomfort, edema

Drug Interactions

Metabolism/Transport Effects None known.

Avoid Concomitant Use There are no known interactions where it is recommended to avoid concomitant use.

Increased Effect/Toxicity There are no known significant interactions involving an increase in effect.

Decreased Effect There are no known significant interactions involving a decrease in effect.

Mechanism of Action Inhibits sodium ion influx through nerve cell membrane channels in parasites resulting in delayed repolarization and thus paralysis and death of the pest

Pharmacodynamics/Kinetics

Absorption: <2%

Metabolism: Hepatic via ester hydrolysis to inactive metabolites

Excretion: Urine

Dosage

Geriatric & Adult

Head lice: Topical: After hair has been washed with shampoo, rinsed with water and towel dried, apply a sufficient volume of creme rinse to saturate the hair and scalp; also apply behind the ears and at the base of the neck; leave on hair for 10 minutes before rinsing off with water; remove remaining nits. May repeat in 1 week if lice or nits still present; in areas of head lice resistance to 1% permethrin, 5% permethrin has been applied to clean, dry hair and left on overnight (8-14 hours) under a shower cap.

Scabies: Topical: Apply cream from head to toe; leave on for 8-14 hours before washing off with water; may reapply in 1 week if live mites appear. Time of application was limited to 6 hours before rinsing with soap and water.

Administration Because scabies and lice are so contagious, use caution to avoid spreading or infecting oneself; wear gloves when applying. See Dosage.

Special Geriatric Considerations Because of its minimal absorption, permethrin is a drug of choice and is preferred over lindane.

Dosage Forms Excipient information presented when available (limited, particularly for generics); consult specific product labeling.

Cream, topical: 5% (60 g)

Liquid, topical [creme rinse formulation]:

Nix® Complete Lice Treatment System: 1% (1s) [contains isopropyl alcohol 20%]

Nix® Creme Rinse: 1% (60 mL) [contains isopropyl alcohol 20%]

Nix® Creme Rinse Lice Treatment: 1% (60 mL) [contains isopropyl alcohol 20%]

Liquid, topical [for bedding, furniture and garments/spray]:

Nix® Lice Control Spray: 0.25% (150 mL)

Lotion, topical: 1% (60 mL)

Solution, topical [for bedding, furniture and garments/spray]:

A200® Lice: 0.5% (170.1 g)

Rid®: 0.5% (150 mL)

Perphenazine (per FEN a zeen)

Related Information

Antipsychotic Agents *on page 2103*

Beers Criteria – Potentially Inappropriate Medications for Geriatrics *on page 2183*

Medication Safety Issues

Sound-alike/look-alike issues:

Trilafon may be confused with Tri-Levlen®

BEERS Criteria medication:

This drug may be potentially inappropriate for use in geriatric patients (Quality of evidence - moderate; Strength of recommendation - strong).

Brand Names: Canada Apo-Perphenazine®

Index Terms Trilafon

Generic Availability (U.S.) Yes

Pharmacologic Category Antiemetic; Antipsychotic Agent, Typical, Phenothiazine

Use Treatment of schizophrenia; severe nausea and vomiting

Unlabeled Use Psychosis; psychosis/agitation related to Alzheimer's dementia (risks vs benefits)

Contraindications Hypersensitivity to perphenazine or any component of the formulation (cross-reactivity between phenothiazines may occur); severe CNS depression (comatose or patients receiving large doses of CNS depressants); subcortical brain damage (with or without hypothalamic damage); bone marrow suppression; blood dyscrasias; liver damage

Warnings/Precautions [U.S. Boxed Warning]: Elderly patients with dementia-related psychosis treated with antipsychotics are at an increased risk of death compared to placebo. Most deaths appeared to be either cardiovascular (eg, heart failure, sudden death) or infectious (eg, pneumonia) in nature. Perphenazine is not approved for the treatment of dementia-related psychosis.

Leukopenia, neutropenia, and agranulocytosis (sometimes fatal) have been reported in clinical trials and postmarketing reports with antipsychotic use; presence of risk factors (eg, pre-existing low WBC or history of drug-induced leuko-/neutropenia) should prompt periodic blood count assessment. Discontinue therapy at first signs of blood dyscrasias or if absolute neutrophil count <1000/mm^3.

May cause hypotension. May be sedating, use with caution in disorders where CNS depression is a feature. Use with caution in depressed patients. Use with caution in Parkinson's disease. Caution in patients with hemodynamic instability; predisposition to seizures; severe cardiac, renal, or respiratory disease. Monitor hepatic and renal function during use; contraindicated in patients with liver damage. Esophageal dysmotility and aspiration have been associated with antipsychotic use; use with caution in patients at risk of pneumonia (eg, Alzheimer's disease). Use associated with increased prolactin levels; clinical significance of hyperprolactinemia in patients with breast cancer or other prolactin-dependent tumors is unknown. May alter temperature regulation or mask toxicity of other drugs due to antiemetic effects. May alter cardiac conduction; life-threatening arrhythmias have occurred with therapeutic doses of phenothiazines. May cause orthostatic hypotension; use with caution in patients at risk of this effect or those who would tolerate transient hypotensive episodes (cerebrovascular disease, cardiovascular disease, or other medications which may predispose).

Phenothiazines may cause anticholinergic effects (confusion, agitation, constipation, xerostomia, blurred vision, urinary retention); therefore, they should be used with caution in patients with decreased gastrointestinal motility, urinary retention, BPH, xerostomia, or visual problems. Conditions which also may be exacerbated by cholinergic blockade include narrow-angle glaucoma and worsening of myasthenia gravis. Relative to other neuroleptics, perphenazine has a low potency of cholinergic blockade. Use with caution in patients with reduced functional alleles of CYP2D6. Poor metabolizers may have higher plasma concentrations at usual doses, increasing risk for adverse reactions.

May cause extrapyramidal reactions (EPS), including pseudoparkinsonism, acute dystonic reactions, akathisia, and tardive dyskinesia. Risk of dystonia (and possibly other EPS) may be greater with increased doses, use of conventional antipsychotics, males, and younger patients. Risk of tardive dyskinesia and potential for irreversibility often associated with total cumulative dose and therapy duration and may also be increased in elderly patients (particularly elderly women); antipsychotics may also mask signs/symptoms of tardive dyskinesia. May be associated with neuroleptic malignant syndrome (NMS). May cause pigmentary retinopathy, and lenticular and corneal deposits, particularly with prolonged therapy. May cause photosensitization. Use with caution in the elderly.

Use in elderly patients with dementia is associated with an increased risk of mortality and cerebrovascular accidents; avoid antipsychotic use for behavioral problems associated with dementia unless alternative nonpharmacologic therapies have failed and patient may harm self or others. In addition, use may cause or exacerbate syndrome of inappropriate antidiuretic hormone secretion or hyponatremia; monitor sodium closely with initiation or dosage adjustments in older adults. May also be inappropriate in older adults depending on comorbidities (eg, dementia, delirium) due to its potent anticholinergic effects (Beers Criteria). Potential for an increased risk of adverse events (eg, sedation, orthostatic hypotension, anticholinergic effects) and an increased risk for developing tardive dyskinesia, particularly in elderly women.

Adverse Reactions (Reflective of adult population; not specific for elderly) Frequency not defined.

Cardiovascular: Bradycardia, cardiac arrest, ECG changes, hyper-/hypotension, orthostatic hypotension, pallor, peripheral edema, sudden death, tachycardia

Central nervous system: Bizarre dreams, catatonic-like states, cerebral edema, dizziness, drowsiness, extrapyramidal symptoms (pseudoparkinsonism, akathisia, dystonias, tardive dyskinesia), faintness, headache, hyperactivity, hyperpyrexia, impairment of temperature regulation, insomnia, lethargy, neuroleptic malignant syndrome (NMS), nocturnal confusion, paradoxical excitement, paranoid reactions, restlessness, seizure

Dermatologic: Discoloration of skin (blue-gray), photosensitivity

Endocrine & metabolic: Amenorrhea, breast enlargement, hyper-/hypoglycemia, galactorrhea, lactation, libido changes, gynecomastia, menstrual irregularity, parotid swelling (rare), SIADH

Gastrointestinal: Adynamic ileus, anorexia, appetite increased, constipation, diarrhea, fecal impaction, obstipation, nausea, salivation, vomiting, weight gain, xerostomia

Genitourinary: Bladder paralysis, ejaculatory disturbances, incontinence, polyuria, urinary retention

Hematologic: Agranulocytosis, eosinophilia, hemolytic anemia, leukopenia, pancytopenia, thrombocytopenic purpura

Hepatic: Hepatotoxicity, jaundice

Neuromuscular & skeletal: Muscle weakness

Ocular: Blurred vision, cornea and lens changes, epithelial keratopathies, glaucoma, mydriasis, myosis, photophobia, pigmentary retinopathy

Renal: Glycosuria

Respiratory: Nasal congestion

Miscellaneous: Allergic reactions, diaphoresis, systemic lupus erythematosus-like syndrome

Drug Interactions

Metabolism/Transport Effects Substrate of CYP1A2 (minor), CYP2C19 (minor), CYP2C9 (minor), CYP2D6 (major), CYP3A4 (minor); **Note:** Assignment of Major/Minor substrate status based on clinically relevant drug interaction potential; **Inhibits** CYP1A2 (weak), CYP2D6 (weak)

Avoid Concomitant Use

Avoid concomitant use of Perphenazine with any of the following: Azelastine; Azelastine (Nasal); Metoclopramide; Paraldehyde

Increased Effect/Toxicity

Perphenazine may increase the levels/effects of: Alcohol (Ethyl); Analgesics (Opioid); Anticholinergics; Antidepressants (Serotonin Reuptake Inhibitor/Antagonist); ARIPiprazole; Azelastine; Azelastine (Nasal); Beta-Blockers; CNS Depressants; Methotrimeprazine; Methylphenidate; Paraldehyde; Porfimer; Serotonin Modulators; Zolpidem

The levels/effects of Perphenazine may be increased by: Abiraterone Acetate; Acetylcholinesterase Inhibitors (Central); Antidepressants (Serotonin Reuptake Inhibitor/Antagonist); Antimalarial Agents; Beta-Blockers; CYP2D6 Inhibitors (Moderate); CYP2D6 Inhibitors (Strong); Darunavir; Droperidol; HydrOXYzine; Lithium formulations; Methotrimeprazine; Methylphenidate; Metoclopramide; Metyrosine; Pramlintide; Tetrabenazine

Decreased Effect

Perphenazine may decrease the levels/effects of: Amphetamines; Anti-Parkinson's Agents (Dopamine Agonist); Quinagolide

The levels/effects of Perphenazine may be decreased by: Antacids; Anti-Parkinson's Agents (Dopamine Agonist); Lithium formulations; Peginterferon Alfa-2b; Tocilizumab

Ethanol/Nutrition/Herb Interactions

Ethanol: May increase CNS depression; monitor for increased effects with coadministration. Caution patients about effects.

Herb/Nutraceutical: Avoid kava kava, gotu kola, valerian, St John's wort (may increase CNS depression).

Stability Store at controlled room temperature of 20°C to 25°C (68°F to 77°F). Protect from light.

Mechanism of Action Perphenazine is a piperazine phenothiazine antipsychotic which blocks postsynaptic mesolimbic dopaminergic receptors in the brain; exhibits alpha-adrenergic blocking effect and depresses the release of hypothalamic and hypophyseal hormones

Pharmacodynamics/Kinetics

Absorption: Oral: Well absorbed

Metabolism: Extensively hepatic to metabolites via sulfoxidation, hydroxylation, dealkylation, and glucuronidation; primarily metabolized by CYP2D6 to N-dealkylated perphenazine, perphenazine sulfoxide, and 7-hydroxyperphenazine (active metabolite with 70% of the activity of perphenazine)

Half-life elimination: Perphenazine: 9-12 hours; 7-hydroxyperphenazine: 10-19 hours

Time to peak, serum: Perphenazine: 1-3 hours; 7-hydroxyperphenazine: 2-4 hours

Excretion: Urine and feces

Dosage

Geriatric No dosage adjustment provided in manufacturer's labeling; however, initiate dosing at the lower end of the dosing range. Refer to adult dosing.

Adult

Schizophrenia: Oral:

Nonhospitalized: Initial: 4-8 mg 3 times/day; reduce dose as soon as possible to minimum effective dosage (maximum: 24 mg/day)

Hospitalized: 8-16 mg 2-4 times/day (maximum: 64 mg/day)

Nausea/vomiting: Oral: 8-16 mg/day in divided doses; reduce dose as soon as possible to minimum effective dosage (maximum: 24 mg/day)

Renal Impairment 0% to 5% removed by hemodialysis (HD); no dosage adjustment provided in manufacturer's labeling.

Hepatic Impairment No dosage adjustment provided in manufacturer's labeling.

Administration May be administered without regard to meals.

Monitoring Parameters Vital signs; lipid profile, fasting blood glucose/Hgb A_{1c}, liver and kidney function (periodically during therapy), CBC (prior to and periodically during therapy); BMI; mental status, abnormal involuntary movement scale (AIMS), extrapyramidal symptoms (EPS)

Reference Range 2-6 nmol/L

Special Geriatric Considerations Any changes in disease status in any organ system can result in behavior changes.

◀ Many elderly patients receive antipsychotic medications for inappropriate nonpsychotic behavior. Before initiating antipsychotic medication, the clinician should investigate any possible reversible cause; any stress or stress from any disease can cause acute "confusion" or worsening of baseline nonpsychotic behavior. Most commonly acute changes in behavior are due to increases in drug dose or addition of new drug to regimen; fluid electrolyte loss; infections; and changes in environment.

In the treatment of agitated, demented, elderly patients, authors of meta-analysis of controlled trials of the response to the traditional antipsychotics (phenothiazines, butyrophenones) in controlling agitation have concluded that the use of neuroleptics results in a response rate of 18%. Clearly neuroleptic therapy for behavior control should be limited with frequent attempts to withdraw the agent given for behavior control.

This medication is considered to be potentially inappropriate in this patient population (Beers Criteria: Quality of evidence - moderate; Strength of recommendation - strong).

Dosage Forms Excipient information presented when available (limited, particularly for generics); consult specific product labeling.
Tablet, oral: 2 mg, 4 mg, 8 mg, 16 mg

- ◆ **Persantine®** see Dipyridamole on page 572
- ◆ **Pethidine Hydrochloride** see Meperidine on page 1208
- ◆ **Pexeva®** see PARoxetine on page 1475
- ◆ **Pfizerpen®** see Penicillin G (Parenteral/Aqueous) on page 1500
- ◆ **PGE₁** see Alprostadil on page 70
- ◆ **Phazyme® Ultra Strength [OTC]** see Simethicone on page 1776
- ◆ **Phenadoz®** see Promethazine on page 1615
- ◆ **Phenazo [OTC]** see Phenazopyridine on page 1516

Phenazopyridine (fen az oh PEER i deen)

Medication Safety Issues
Sound-alike/look-alike issues:
Phenazopyridine may be confused with phenoxybenzamine
Pyridium® may be confused with Dyrenium®, Perdiem®, pyridoxine, pyrithione
Brand Names: U.S. AZO Standard® Maximum Strength [OTC] [DSC]; AZO Standard® [OTC] [DSC]; AZO Urinary Pain Relief™ Maximum Strength [OTC]; AZO Urinary Pain Relief™ [OTC]; Azo-Gesic™ [OTC]; Baridium [OTC]; Phenazo [OTC]; Pyridium®; Urinary Pain Relief [OTC]
Index Terms Phenazopyridine Hydrochloride; Phenylazo Diamino Pyridine Hydrochloride
Generic Availability (U.S.) Yes
Pharmacologic Category Analgesic, Urinary
Use Symptomatic relief of urinary burning, itching, frequency, and urgency in association with urinary tract infection or following urologic procedures
Contraindications Hypersensitivity to phenazopyridine or any component of the formulation; kidney or liver disease; patients with a Cl$_{cr}$ <50 mL/minute
Warnings/Precautions Does not treat urinary infection, acts only as an analgesic; drug should be discontinued if skin or sclera develop a yellow color; use with caution in patients with renal impairment. Use of this agent in the elderly is limited since accumulation of phenazopyridine can occur in patients with renal insufficiency. Use is contraindicated in patients with a Cl$_{cr}$ <50 mL/minute.
Adverse Reactions (Reflective of adult population; not specific for elderly) 1% to 10%:
Central nervous system: Headache, dizziness
Gastrointestinal: Stomach cramps
Drug Interactions
Metabolism/Transport Effects None known.
Avoid Concomitant Use There are no known interactions where it is recommended to avoid concomitant use.
Increased Effect/Toxicity
Phenazopyridine may increase the levels/effects of: Prilocaine
Decreased Effect There are no known significant interactions involving a decrease in effect.
Mechanism of Action An azo dye which exerts local anesthetic or analgesic action on urinary tract mucosa through an unknown mechanism
Pharmacodynamics/Kinetics
Metabolism: Hepatic and via other tissues
Excretion: Urine (65% as unchanged drug)

Dosage
  Geriatric & Adult Urinary analgesic: Oral: 100-200 mg 3 times/day after meals for 2 days when used concomitantly with an antibacterial agent
  Renal Impairment
    Cl_{cr} 50-80 mL/minute: Administer every 8-16 hours.
    Cl_{cr} <50 mL/minute: Avoid use.
Administration Administer after meals.
Monitoring Parameters Relief of urinary discomfort
Test Interactions Phenazopyridine may cause delayed reactions with glucose oxidase reagents (Clinistix®, Tes-Tape®); occasional false-positive tests occur with Tes-Tape®; cupric sulfate tests (Clinitest®) are not affected; interference may also occur with urine ketone tests (Acetest®, Ketostix®) and urinary protein tests; tests for urinary steroids and porphyrins may also occur
Special Geriatric Considerations Use of this agent in older adults is limited since accumulation of phenazopyridine can occur in patients with renal insufficiency.
Dosage Forms Excipient information presented when available (limited, particularly for generics); consult specific product labeling. [DSC] = Discontinued product
  Tablet, oral, as hydrochloride: 100 mg, 200 mg
    AZO Standard®: 95 mg [DSC] [gluten free]
    AZO Standard® Maximum Strength: 97.5 mg [DSC] [gluten free]
    AZO Urinary Pain Relief™: 95 mg [gluten free]
    AZO Urinary Pain Relief™ Maximum Strength: 97.5 mg [gluten free]
    Azo-Gesic™: 95 mg
    Baridium: 97.2 mg [contains sodium 0.184 mg/tablet]
    Phenazo: 95 mg
    Pyridium®: 100 mg, 200 mg
    Urinary Pain Relief: 95 mg

♦ **Phenazopyridine Hydrochloride** see Phenazopyridine on page 1516

Phenelzine (FEN el zeen)

Related Information
  Antidepressant Agents on page 2097
Medication Safety Issues
  Sound-alike/look-alike issues:
    Phenelzine may be confused with phenytoin
    Nardil® may be confused with Norinyl®
Brand Names: U.S. Nardil®
Brand Names: Canada Nardil®
Index Terms Phenelzine Sulfate
Generic Availability (U.S.) Yes
Pharmacologic Category Antidepressant, Monoamine Oxidase Inhibitor
Use Symptomatic treatment of atypical, nonendogenous, or neurotic depression
Medication Guide Available Yes
Contraindications Hypersensitivity to phenelzine or any component of the formulation; congestive heart failure; pheochromocytoma; abnormal liver function tests or history of hepatic disease; renal disease or severe renal disease/impairment
  Concurrent use of sympathomimetics (including amphetamines, cocaine, dopamine, epinephrine, methylphenidate, norepinephrine, or phenylephrine) and related compounds (methyldopa, levodopa, phenylalanine, tryptophan, or tyrosine), ophthalmic alpha$_2$-agonists (apraclonidine, brimonidine), CNS depressants, cyclobenzaprine, dextromethorphan, ethanol, meperidine, bupropion, or buspirone
  At least 2 weeks should elapse between the discontinuation of serotoninergic agents (including SNRIs, SSRIs, and tricyclics) and other MAO inhibitors and the initiation of phenelzine. At least 5 weeks should elapse between the discontinuation of fluoxetine and the initiation of phenelzine. In all cases, a sufficient amount of time must be allowed for the clearance of the serotoninergic agent and any active metabolites prior to the initiation of phenelzine.
  At least 2 weeks should elapse between the discontinuation of phenelzine and the initiation of the following agents: Serotoninergic agents (including SNRIs, SSRIs, fluoxetine, and tricyclics), bupropion, buspirone, and other antidepressants.
  General anesthesia, spinal anesthesia (hypotension may be exaggerated). Use caution with local anesthetics containing sympathomimetic agents. Phenelzine should be discontinued ≥10 days prior to elective surgery.
  Foods high in tyramine or dopamine content; foods and/or supplements containing tyrosine, phenylalanine, tryptophan, or caffeine

Warnings/Precautions [U.S. Boxed Warning]: Antidepressants increase the risk of suicidal thinking and behavior in children, adolescents, and young adults (18-24 years of age) with major depressive disorder (MDD) and other psychiatric disorders; consider risk prior to prescribing. Short-term studies did not show an increased risk in patients >24 years of age and showed a decreased risk in patients ≥65 years. Closely monitor for clinical worsening, suicidality, or unusual changes in behavior; the patient's family or caregiver should be instructed to closely observe the patient and communicate condition with healthcare provider. Such observation would generally include at least weekly face-to-face contact with patients or their family members or caregivers during the first 4 weeks of treatment, then every other week visits for the next 4 weeks, then at 12 weeks, and as clinically indicated beyond 12 weeks. Additional contact by telephone may be appropriate between face-to-face visits. Adults treated with antidepressants should be observed similarly for clinical worsening and suicidality, especially during the initial few months of a course of drug therapy, or at times of dose changes, either increases or decreases. A medication guide should be dispensed with each prescription. Phenelzine is not generally considered a first-line agent for the treatment of depression; phenelzine is typically used in patients who have failed to respond to other treatments.

The possibility of a suicide attempt is inherent in major depression and may persist until remission occurs. Monitor for worsening of depression or suicidality, especially during initiation of therapy (generally first 1-2 months) or with dose increases or decreases. Worsening depression and severe abrupt suicidality that are not part of the presenting symptoms may require discontinuation or modification of drug therapy. Use caution in high-risk patients during initiation of therapy. Prescriptions should be written for the smallest quantity consistent with good patient care. The patient's family or caregiver should be alerted to monitor patients for the emergence of suicidality and associated behaviors such as anxiety, agitation, panic attacks, insomnia, irritability, hostility, impulsivity, akathisia, hypomania, and mania; patients should be instructed to notify their healthcare provider if any of these symptoms or worsening depression occur.

May worsen psychosis in some patients or precipitate a shift to mania or hypomania in patients with bipolar disorder. Monotherapy in patients with bipolar disorder should be avoided. Patients presenting with depressive symptoms should be screened for bipolar disorder. Phenelzine is not FDA approved for the treatment of bipolar depression.

Sensitization to the effects of insulin may occur; monitor blood glucose closely in patients with diabetes. Use with caution in patients who have glaucoma, or hyperthyroidism. Cases of hypertensive crisis (sometimes fatal) have occurred; symptoms include: severe headache, nausea/vomiting, neck stiffness/soreness, photophobia, and sweating. Monitor blood pressure closely in all patients. Hypertensive crisis may occur with tyramine-, tryptophan-, or dopamine-containing foods. Phentolamine is recommended for the treatment of hypertensive crisis. Do not use with other MAO inhibitors or antidepressants. Do not use within 5 weeks of fluoxetine discontinuation or 2 weeks of other antidepressant discontinuation. Avoid products containing sympathomimetic stimulants or dextromethorphan. Concurrent use with antihypertensive agents may lead to exaggeration of hypotensive effects. May cause orthostatic hypotension; use with caution in patients with hypotension or patients who would not tolerate transient hypotensive episodes (cardiovascular or cerebrovascular disease); effects may be additive with other agents which cause orthostasis. Use with caution in patients at risk of seizures, or in patients receiving other drugs which may lower seizure threshold. Discontinue at least 48 hours prior to myelography. May increase the risks associated with electroconvulsive therapy. Consider discontinuing, when possible, prior to elective surgery. Pyridoxine deficiency has occurred; symptoms include numbness and edema of hands; may respond to supplementation.

Adverse Reactions (Reflective of adult population; not specific for elderly) Frequency not defined.

Cardiovascular: Edema, orthostatic hypotension

Central nervous system: Anxiety (acute), ataxia, coma, delirium, dizziness, drowsiness, euphoria, fatigue, fever, headache, hyper-reflexia, hypersomnia, insomnia, mania, schizophrenia, seizure, twitching

Dermatologic: Pruritus, rash

Endocrine & metabolic: Decreased sexual ability (anorgasmia, ejaculatory disturbances, impotence), hypermetabolic syndrome, hypernatremia

Gastrointestinal: Constipation, weight gain, xerostomia

Genitourinary: Urinary retention

Hematologic: Leukopenia

Hepatic: Jaundice, necrotizing hepatocellular necrosis (rare), transaminases increased

Neuromuscular & skeletal: Myoclonia, paresthesia, tremor, weakness

Ocular: Blurred vision, glaucoma, nystagmus

Respiratory: Edema (glottis)

Miscellaneous: Diaphoresis, Lupus-like syndrome, transient cardiac or respiratory depression (following ECT), withdrawal syndrome (nausea, vomiting, malaise)

Drug Interactions

Metabolism/Transport Effects Inhibits Monoamine Oxidase

Avoid Concomitant Use

Avoid concomitant use of Phenelzine with any of the following: Alpha-/Beta-Agonists (Indirect-Acting); Alpha1-Agonists; Alpha2-Agonists (Ophthalmic); Amphetamines; Anilido-piperidine Opioids; Antidepressants (Serotonin Reuptake Inhibitor/Antagonist); AtoMOXetine; Bezafibrate; Buprenorphine; BuPROPion; BusPIRone; CarBAMazepine; Cyclobenzaprine; Dexmethylphenidate; Dextromethorphan; Diethylpropion; HYDROmorphone; Linezolid; Maprotiline; Meperidine; Methyldopa; Methylene Blue; Methylphenidate; Mirtazapine; Oxymorphone; Pizotifen; Selective Serotonin Reuptake Inhibitors; Serotonin 5-HT1D Receptor Agonists; Serotonin/Norepinephrine Reuptake Inhibitors; Tapentadol; Tetrabenazine; Tetrahydrozoline; Tetrahydrozoline (Nasal); Tricyclic Antidepressants; Tryptophan

Increased Effect/Toxicity

Phenelzine may increase the levels/effects of: Alpha-/Beta-Agonists (Direct-Acting); Alpha-/Beta-Agonists (Indirect-Acting); Alpha1-Agonists; Alpha2-Agonists (Ophthalmic); Amphetamines; Anticholinergics; Antidepressants (Serotonin Reuptake Inhibitor/Antagonist); Antihypertensives; AtoMOXetine; Beta2-Agonists; Bezafibrate; BuPROPion; Dexmethylphenidate; Dextromethorphan; Diethylpropion; Doxapram; HYDROmorphone; Hypoglycemic Agents; Linezolid; Lithium; Meperidine; Methadone; Methyldopa; Methylene Blue; Methylphenidate; Metoclopramide; Mirtazapine; Orthostatic Hypotension Producing Agents; Pizotifen; Reserpine; Selective Serotonin Reuptake Inhibitors; Serotonin 5-HT1D Receptor Agonists; Serotonin Modulators; Serotonin/Norepinephrine Reuptake Inhibitors; Succinylcholine; Tetrahydrozoline; Tetrahydrozoline (Nasal); Tricyclic Antidepressants

The levels/effects of Phenelzine may be increased by: Altretamine; Anilidopiperidine Opioids; Antipsychotics; Buprenorphine; BusPIRone; CarBAMazepine; COMT Inhibitors; Cyclobenzaprine; Levodopa; MAO Inhibitors; Maprotiline; Oxymorphone; Pramlintide; Tapentadol; Tetrabenazine; TraMADol; Tryptophan

Decreased Effect

Phenelzine may decrease the levels/effects of: Acetylcholinesterase Inhibitors (Central)

The levels/effects of Phenelzine may be decreased by: Acetylcholinesterase Inhibitors (Central)

Ethanol/Nutrition/Herb Interactions

Ethanol: Ethanol may increase CNS depression. Beverages containing tyramine (eg, hearty red wine and beer) may increase toxic effects. Management: Avoid ethanol and beverages containing tyramine.

Food: Concurrent ingestion of foods rich in tyramine, dopamine, tyrosine, phenylalanine, tryptophan, or caffeine may cause sudden and severe high blood pressure (hypertensive crisis or serotonin syndrome). Management: Avoid tyramine-containing foods (aged or matured cheese, air-dried or cured meats including sausages and salamis; fava or broad bean pods, tap/draft beers, Marmite concentrate, sauerkraut, soy sauce, and other soybean condiments). Food's freshness is also an important concern; improperly stored or spoiled food can create an environment in which tyramine concentrations may increase. Avoid foods containing dopamine, tyrosine, phenylalanine, tryptophan, or caffeine.

Herb/Nutraceutical: Kava kava, valerian, St John's wort, and SAMe may increase risk of serotonin syndrome and/or excessive sedation. Supplements containing caffeine, tyrosine, tryptophan, or phenylalanine may increase the risk of severe side effects like hypertensive reactions or serotonin syndrome. Management: Avoid kava kava, valerian, St John's wort, SAMe, and supplements containing caffeine, tyrosine, tryptophan, or phenylalanine.

Stability Store at 20°C to 25°C (68°F to 77°F). Protect from heat and light.

Mechanism of Action Thought to act by increasing endogenous concentrations of norepinephrine, dopamine, and serotonin through inhibition of the enzyme (monoamine oxidase) responsible for the breakdown of these neurotransmitters

Pharmacodynamics/Kinetics

Onset of action: Therapeutic: 2-4 weeks; geriatric patients receiving an average of 55 mg/day developed a mean platelet MAO activity inhibition of about 85%.

Duration: May continue to have a therapeutic effect and interactions 2 weeks after discontinuing therapy

Absorption: Well absorbed

Metabolism: Oxidized via monoamine oxidase (primary pathway) and acetylation (minor pathway)

Half-life elimination: 12 hours

Excretion: Urine (73% as metabolites)

◄ **Dosage**

Geriatric Depression: Oral: Select dose with caution; generally initiating at the lower end of the dosing range; some clinicians recommend an initial dose of 7.5 mg, with dose increases of 7.5 mg/day every 4-8 days as tolerated to a usual therapeutic dose of 22.5-60 mg/day in older adults (Alexopoulos, 2004).

Adult Depression: Oral: Initial: 15 mg 3 times/day

Early phase: Increase rapidly, based on patient tolerance, to 60-90 mg/day (may take 4 weeks of 60 mg/day therapy before clinical response)

Maintenance: After maximum benefit is obtained, slowly reduce dose over several weeks; dose may be as low as 15 mg/day to 15 mg every other day

Monitoring Parameters Blood pressure, heart rate; diet, weight; mood (if depressive symptoms), suicide ideation (especially during the initial months of therapy or when doses are increased or decreased)

Special Geriatric Considerations The MAO inhibitors are effective and generally well tolerated by elderly patients. It is their potential interactions with tyramine or tryptophan-containing food and other drugs and their effects on blood pressure that have limited their use. Phenelzine is less stimulating than tranylcypromine.

A systematic review and meta-analysis of antidepressant placebo-controlled trials in persons with depression and dementia found evidence "suggestive" of efficacy but not of sufficient strength to "confirm" efficacy. Antidepressant trials in this patient population are small and underpowered. Older patients with depression being treated with an antidepressant should be closely monitored for response and adverse effects. Treatment should be switched or augmented when response is inadequate with a therapeutic dose. Antidepressants that are not tolerated should be discontinued and an alternative agent should be started.

Dosage Forms Excipient information presented when available (limited, particularly for generics); consult specific product labeling.

Tablet, oral: 15 mg

Nardil®: 15 mg

◆ **Phenelzine Sulfate** *see* Phenelzine *on page 1517*

◆ **Phenergan** *see* Promethazine *on page 1615*

◆ **Pheniramine and Naphazoline** *see* Naphazoline and Pheniramine *on page 1338*

PHENobarbital (fee noe BAR bi tal)

Related Information

Beers Criteria – Potentially Inappropriate Medications for Geriatrics *on page 2183*

Medication Safety Issues

Sound-alike/look-alike issues:

PHENobarbital may be confused with PENTobarbital, Phenergan®, phenytoin

BEERS Criteria medication:

This drug may be potentially inappropriate for use in geriatric patients (Quality of evidence - high; Strength of recommendation - strong).

Brand Names: Canada PMS-Phenobarbital

Index Terms Luminal Sodium; Phenobarbital Sodium; Phenobarbitone; Phenylethylmalony-lurea

Generic Availability (U.S.) Yes

Pharmacologic Category Anticonvulsant, Barbiturate; Barbiturate

Use Management of generalized tonic-clonic (grand mal), status epilepticus, and partial seizures; sedative/hypnotic

Note: Use to treat insomnia is not recommended (Schutte-Rodin, 2008)

Unlabeled Use Management of sedative/hypnotic withdrawal

Contraindications Hypersensitivity to barbiturates or any component of the formulation; marked hepatic impairment; dyspnea or airway obstruction; porphyria (manifest and latent); intra-arterial administration, subcutaneous administration (not recommended); use in patients with a history of sedative/hypnotic addiction is not recommended; nephritic patients (large doses)

Warnings/Precautions Potential for drug dependency exists, abrupt cessation may precipitate withdrawal, including status epilepticus in epileptic patients. Do not administer to patients in acute pain. Use caution in debilitated, renal or hepatic dysfunction. May cause paradoxical responses, including agitation and hyperactivity. Avoid use in the eldely due to risk of overdose with low dosages, tolerance to sleep effects, and increased risk of physical dependence (Beers Criteria). Use with caution in patients with depression or suicidal tendencies, or in patients with a history of drug abuse. Tolerance, psychological and physical dependence may occur with prolonged use. May cause CNS depression, which may impair physical or mental abilities. Effects with other sedative drugs or ethanol may be potentiated.

May cause respiratory depression or hypotension, particularly when administered intravenously. Use with caution in hemodynamically unstable patients (hypovolemic shock, CHF) or patients with respiratory disease. Due to its long half-life and risk of dependence, phenobarbital is not recommended as a sedative in the elderly. Use with caution in patients with hypoadrenalism. Intra-arterial administration may cause reactions ranging from transient pain to gangrene and is contraindicated. Subcutaneous administration may cause tissue irritation (eg, redness, tenderness, necrosis) and is not recommended.

Adverse Reactions (Reflective of adult population; not specific for elderly) Frequency not defined.

Cardiovascular: Bradycardia, hypotension, syncope

Central nervous system: Agitation, anxiety, ataxia, CNS excitation or depression, confusion, dizziness drowsiness, hallucinations, "hangover" effect, headache, hyperkinesia, impaired judgment, insomnia, lethargy, nervousness, nightmares, somnolence

Dermatologic: Exfoliative dermatitis, rash, Stevens-Johnson syndrome

Gastrointestinal: Nausea, vomiting, constipation

Hematologic: Agranulocytosis, thrombocytopenia, megaloblastic anemia

Local: Pain at injection site, thrombophlebitis with I.V. use

Renal: Oliguria

Respiratory: Laryngospasm, respiratory depression, apnea (especially with rapid I.V. use), hypoventilation

Miscellaneous: Gangrene with inadvertent intra-arterial injection

Drug Interactions

Metabolism/Transport Effects Substrate of CYP2C19 (major), CYP2C9 (minor), CYP2E1 (minor); **Note:** Assignment of Major/Minor substrate status based on clinically relevant drug interaction potential; **Induces** CYP1A2 (strong), CYP2A6 (strong), CYP2B6 (strong), CYP2C8 (strong), CYP2C9 (strong), CYP3A4 (strong)

Avoid Concomitant Use

Avoid concomitant use of PHENobarbital with any of the following: Axitinib; Azelastine; Azelastine (Nasal); Boceprevir; Bortezomib; Crizotinib; Darunavir; Dronedarone; Etravirine; Everolimus; Itraconazole; Lapatinib; Lurasidone; Methadone; Mifepristone; Mirtazapine; Nilotinib; Paraldehyde; Pazopanib; Praziquantel; Ranolazine; Rilpivirine; Rivaroxaban; Roflumilast; RomiDEPsin; SORAfenib; Telaprevir; Ticagrelor; Tolvaptan; Toremifene; Vandetanib; Voriconazole

Increased Effect/Toxicity

PHENobarbital may increase the levels/effects of: Alcohol (Ethyl); Azelastine; Azelastine (Nasal); Buprenorphine; Clarithromycin; CNS Depressants; Fosphenytoin; Ifosfamide; Meperidine; Methadone; Metyrosine; Mirtazapine; Paraldehyde; Prilocaine; QuiNIDine; Selective Serotonin Reuptake Inhibitors; Thiazide Diuretics; Zolpidem

The levels/effects of PHENobarbital may be increased by: Carbonic Anhydrase Inhibitors; Chloramphenicol; Clarithromycin; CYP2C19 Inhibitors (Moderate); CYP2C19 Inhibitors (Strong); Dexmethylphenidate; Divalproex; Droperidol; Felbamate; Fosphenytoin; HydrOXYzine; Methylphenidate; Phenytoin; Primidone; QuiNINE; Rufinamide; Telaprevir; Valproic Acid

Decreased Effect

PHENobarbital may decrease the levels/effects of: Acetaminophen; Apixaban; ARIPiprazole; Axitinib; Bendamustine; Beta-Blockers; Boceprevir; Bortezomib; Brentuximab Vedotin; Calcium Channel Blockers; Chloramphenicol; Clarithromycin; Contraceptives (Estrogens); Contraceptives (Progestins); Corticosteroids (Systemic); Crizotinib; CycloSPORINE; CycloSPORINE (Systemic); CYP1A2 Substrates; CYP2B6 Substrates; CYP2C8 Substrates; CYP2C9 Substrates; CYP3A4 Substrates; Darunavir; Dasatinib; Deferasirox; Diclofenac; Disopyramide; Divalproex; Doxycycline; Dronedarone; Etoposide; Etoposide Phosphate; Etravirine; Everolimus; Exemestane; Felbamate; Fosphenytoin; Gefitinib; Griseofulvin; GuanFACINE; Imatinib; Irinotecan; Itraconazole; Ixabepilone; Lacosamide; LamoTRIgine; Lapatinib; Linagliptin; Lopinavir; Lurasidone; Maraviroc; MetroNIDAZOLE; MetroNIDAZOLE (Systemic); Mifepristone; Nilotinib; OXcarbazepine; Pazopanib; Phenytoin; Praziquantel; Propafenone; QuiNIDine; QuiNINE; Ranolazine; Rilpivirine; Rivaroxaban; Roflumilast; RomiDEPsin; Rufinamide; Saxagliptin; SORAfenib; SUNItinib; Tadalafil; Telaprevir; Teniposide; Theophylline Derivatives; Ticagrelor; Tipranavir; Tolvaptan; Toremifene; Treprostinil; Tricyclic Antidepressants; Ulipristal; Valproic Acid; Vandetanib; Vemurafenib; Vitamin K Antagonists; Voriconazole; Zonisamide; Zuclopenthixol

The levels/effects of PHENobarbital may be decreased by: Amphetamines; Cholestyramine Resin; CYP2C19 Inducers (Strong); Folic Acid; Ketorolac; Ketorolac (Nasal); Ketorolac (Systemic); Leucovorin Calcium-Levoleucovorin; Levomefolate; Mefloquine; Methylfolate; Pyridoxine; Rifamycin Derivatives; Telaprevir; Tipranavir

Ethanol/Nutrition/Herb Interactions
Ethanol: May increase CNS depression; monitor for increased effects with coadministration. Caution patients about effects.
Food: May cause decrease in vitamin D and calcium.
Herb/Nutraceutical: Avoid evening primrose (seizure threshold decreased). Avoid valerian, St John's wort, kava kava, gotu kola (may increase CNS depression).

Stability Protect elixir from light. Not stable in aqueous solutions; use only clear solutions. Do not add to acidic solutions; precipitation may occur.

Mechanism of Action Long-acting barbiturate with sedative, hypnotic, and anticonvulsant properties. Barbiturates depress the sensory cortex, decrease motor activity, alter cerebellar function, and produce drowsiness, sedation, and hypnosis. In high doses, barbiturates exhibit anticonvulsant activity; barbiturates produce dose-dependent respiratory depression.

Pharmacodynamics/Kinetics
Onset of action: Oral: Hypnosis: 20-60 minutes; I.V.: ~5 minutes
Peak effect: I.V.: ~30 minutes
Duration: Oral: 6-10 hours; I.V.: 4-10 hours
Absorption: Oral: 70% to 90%
Protein binding: 20% to 45%
Metabolism: Hepatic via hydroxylation and glucuronide conjugation
Half-life elimination: Adults: 53-140 hours
Time to peak, serum: Oral: 1-6 hours
Excretion: Urine (20% to 50% as unchanged drug)

Dosage
Geriatric Geriatric patients should be started at the lowest recommended dose. Refer to adult dosing.
Adult
Sedation: Oral, I.M.: 30-120 mg/day in 2-3 divided doses
Preoperative sedation: I.M.: 100-200 mg 1-1.5 hours before procedure
Anticonvulsant/status epilepticus:
Loading dose: I.V.: 10-20 mg/kg (maximum rate ≤60 mg/minute in patients ≥60 kg); may repeat dose in 20-minute intervals as needed (maximum total dose: 30 mg/kg)
Maintenance dose: Oral, I.V.: 1-3 mg/kg/day in divided doses or 50-100 mg 2-3 times/day
Sedative/hypnotic withdrawal (unlabeled use): Initial daily requirement is determined by substituting phenobarbital 30 mg for every 100 mg pentobarbital used during tolerance testing; then daily requirement is decreased by 10% of initial dose.

Renal Impairment
Cl$_{cr}$ <10 mL/minute: Administer every 12-16 hours.
Moderately dialyzable (20% to 50%)
Hepatic Impairment Reduce dose in patients with hepatic impairment.

Administration May be administered I.V., I.M. or orally. Avoid rapid I.V. administration >60 mg/minute in adults; intra-arterial injection is contraindicated; avoid subcutaneous administration; parenteral solutions are highly alkaline; avoid extravasation. For I.M. administration, inject deep into muscle. Do not exceed 5 mL per injection site due to potential for tissue irritation

Monitoring Parameters Phenobarbital serum concentrations, mental status, CBC, LFTs, seizure activity

Reference Range
Therapeutic: Adults: 20-40 mcg/mL (SI: 86-172 micromole/L)
Toxic: >40 mcg/mL (SI: >172 micromole/L)
Toxic concentration: Slowness, ataxia, nystagmus: 35-80 mcg/mL (SI: 150-344 micromole/L)
Coma with reflexes: 65-117 mcg/mL (SI: 279-502 micromole/L)
Coma without reflexes: >100 mcg/mL (SI: >430 micromole/L)

Test Interactions Assay interference of LDH
Pharmacotherapy Pearls Injectable solutions contain propylene glycol.

Phenobarbital tablets are also available from some generic manufacturers in strengths that are exactly equivalent to fractional grain strengths: 16.2 mg (1/4 grain), 32.4 mg (1/2 grain), 64.8 mg (1 grain). To avoid medication errors, do not prescribe phenobarbital in grains.

Special Geriatric Considerations Using barbiturates in elderly may induce paradoxical stimulation, cause or aggravate depression and confusion. Due to its long half-life and risk of dependence, phenobarbital is not recommended as a sedative or hypnotic in the elderly. Interpretive guidelines from the Centers for Medicare and Medicaid Services (CMS) discourage the use of this agent as a sedative/hypnotic in long-term care residents.

This medication is considered to be potentially inappropriate in this patient population (Beers Criteria: Quality of evidence - high; Strength of recommendation - strong).

Controlled Substance C-IV

Dosage Forms Excipient information presented when available (limited, particularly for generics); consult specific product labeling. [DSC] = Discontinued product
Elixir, oral: 20 mg/5 mL (5 mL [DSC], 7.5 mL, 15 mL, 473 mL, 480 mL)
Injection, solution, as sodium: 65 mg/mL (1 mL); 130 mg/mL (1 mL)
Tablet, oral: 15 mg, 16.2 mg, 30 mg, 32.4 mg, 60 mg, 100 mg

Extemporaneously Prepared An alcohol-free phenobarbital 10 mg/mL suspension can be prepared as follows: Levigate ten phenobarbital 60 mg tablets in a glass mortar into a fine powder. Mix 30 mL of Ora-Plus® and 30 mL of either Ora-Sweet® or Ora-Sweet® SF; stir vigorously. Add 15 mL of the Ora-Plus®/Ora-Sweet® (or Ora-Sweet® SF) mixture to the powder; triturate well. Transfer to a 2 ounce amber plastic bottle; qs to a final volume of 60 mL. Stable for up to 115 days at room temperature. Shake well prior to use.

May mix dose with chocolate syrup (1:1 volume) immediately before administration to mask the bitter aftertaste.

Cober M and Johnson CE, "Stability of an Extemporaneously Prepared Alcohol-Free Phenobarbital Suspension," *Am J Health Syst Pharm*, 2007, 64(6):644-6.

◆ **Phenobarbital, Hyoscyamine, Atropine, and Scopolamine** *see* Hyoscyamine, Atropine, Scopolamine, and Phenobarbital *on page 963*
◆ **Phenobarbital Sodium** *see* PHENobarbital *on page 1520*
◆ **Phenobarbitone** *see* PHENobarbital *on page 1520*

Phenoxybenzamine (fen oks ee BEN za meen)

Medication Safety Issues
Sound-alike/look-alike issues:
Phenoxybenzamine may be confused with phenazopyridine
Brand Names: U.S. Dibenzyline®
Index Terms Phenoxybenzamine Hydrochloride
Generic Availability (U.S.) No
Pharmacologic Category Alpha$_1$ Blocker; Antidote
Use Symptomatic management of pheochromocytoma
Unlabeled Use Micturition problems associated with neurogenic bladder, functional outlet obstruction, and partial prostate obstruction; treatment of hypertensive crisis caused by sympathomimetic amines
Dosage
Geriatric & Adult
Pheochromocytoma, hypertension: Oral: Initial: 10 mg twice daily, increase by 10 mg every other day until optimal blood pressure response is achieved; usual range: 20-40 mg 2-3 times/day. Doses up to 240 mg/day have been reported (Kinney, 2000).
Micturition disorders (unlabeled use): Oral: 10-20 mg 1-2 times/day
Special Geriatric Considerations Because of the risk of adverse effects, avoid the use of this medication in the elderly if possible.
Dosage Forms Excipient information presented when available (limited, particularly for generics); consult specific product labeling.
Capsule, oral, as hydrochloride:
Dibenzyline®: 10 mg

◆ **Phenoxybenzamine Hydrochloride** *see* Phenoxybenzamine *on page 1523*
◆ **Phenoxymethyl Penicillin** *see* Penicillin V Potassium *on page 1504*
◆ **Phenylalanine Mustard** *see* Melphalan *on page 1199*
◆ **Phenylazo Diamino Pyridine Hydrochloride** *see* Phenazopyridine *on page 1516*

Phenylephrine (Systemic) (fen il EF rin)

Medication Safety Issues
Sound-alike/look-alike issues:
Sudafed PE® may be confused with Sudafed®
High alert medication:
The Institute for Safe Medication Practices (ISMP) includes this medication among its list of drugs which have a heightened risk of causing significant patient harm when used in error.
Brand Names: U.S. Medi-First® Sinus Decongestant [OTC]; Medi-Phenyl [OTC]; Pedia-Care® Children's Decongestant [OTC]; Sudafed PE® Children's [OTC]; Sudafed PE® Congestion [OTC]; Sudafed PE™ Nasal Decongestant [OTC]; Sudogest™ PE [OTC]; Triaminic Thin Strips® Children's Cold with Stuffy Nose [OTC]
Index Terms Phenylephrine Hydrochloride
Generic Availability (U.S.) Yes: Excludes liquid, strips
Pharmacologic Category Alpha-Adrenergic Agonist

Use Treatment of hypotension, vascular failure in shock; as a vasoconstrictor in regional analgesia; supraventricular tachycardia (**Note:** Not for routine use in treatment of supraventricular tachycardias); as a decongestant [OTC]

Contraindications Hypersensitivity to phenylephrine or any component of the formulation
Injection: Severe hypertension; ventricular tachycardia
Oral: Use with or within 14 days of MAO inhibitor therapy

Warnings/Precautions Some products contain sulfites which may cause allergic reactions in susceptible individuals. Use with extreme caution in patients taking MAO inhibitors.

Intravenous: Use with caution in the elderly, patients with hyperthyroidism, bradycardia, partial heart block, myocardial disease, or severe CAD. Avoid or use with extreme caution in patients with heart failure or cardiogenic shock; increased systemic vascular resistance may significantly reduce cardiac output. Assure adequate circulatory volume to minimize need for vasoconstrictors. Avoid use in patients with hypertension (contraindicated in severe hypertension); monitor blood pressure closely and adjust infusion rate. Avoid extravasation; infuse into a large vein if possible. Avoid infusion into leg veins. Watch I.V. site closely. If extravasation occurs, infiltrate the area subcutaneously with diluted phentolamine (5-10 mg in 10 mL of saline) with a fine hypodermic needle. **Phentolamine should be administered as soon as possible after extravasation is noted. [U.S. Boxed Warning]: Should be administered by adequately trained individuals familiar with its use.**

Oral: When used for self-medication (OTC), use caution with asthma, bowel obstruction/narrowing, hyperthyroidism, diabetes mellitus, cardiovascular disease, ischemic heart disease, hypertension, increased intraocular pressure, prostatic hyperplasia or in the elderly. Notify healthcare provider if symptoms do not improve within 7 days or are accompanied by fever. Discontinue and contact healthcare provider if nervousness, dizziness, or sleeplessness occur.

Adverse Reactions (Reflective of adult population; not specific for elderly) Frequency not defined.
Injection:
Cardiovascular: Arrhythmia (rare), decreased cardiac output, hypertension, pallor, precordial pain or discomfort, reflex bradycardia, severe peripheral and visceral vasoconstriction
Central nervous system: Anxiety, dizziness, excitability, giddiness, headache, insomnia, nervousness, restlessness
Endocrine & metabolic: Metabolic acidosis
Gastrointestinal: Gastric irritation, nausea
Local: I.V.: Extravasation which may lead to necrosis and sloughing of surrounding tissue, blanching of skin
Neuromuscular & skeletal: Paresthesia, pilomotor response, tremor, weakness
Renal: Decreased renal perfusion, reduced urine output
Respiratory: Respiratory distress
Miscellaneous: Hypersensitivity reactions (including rash, urticaria, leukopenia, agranulocytosis, thrombocytopenia)
Oral: Central nervous system: Anxiety, dizziness, excitability, giddiness, headache, insomnia, nervousness, restlessness

Drug Interactions
Metabolism/Transport Effects None known.
Avoid Concomitant Use
Avoid concomitant use of Phenylephrine (Systemic) with any of the following: Ergot Derivatives; Hyaluronidase; Iobenguane I 123; MAO Inhibitors
Increased Effect/Toxicity
Phenylephrine (Systemic) may increase the levels/effects of: Sympathomimetics

The levels/effects of Phenylephrine (Systemic) may be increased by: AtoMOXetine; Cannabinoids; Ergot Derivatives; Hyaluronidase; MAO Inhibitors; Tricyclic Antidepressants
Decreased Effect
Phenylephrine (Systemic) may decrease the levels/effects of: Benzylpenicilloyl Polylysine; FentaNYL; Iobenguane I 123

Ethanol/Nutrition/Herb Interactions Herb/Nutraceutical: Avoid ephedra, yohimbe (may cause CNS stimulation).

Stability
Solution for injection: Store vials at controlled room temperature of 15°C to 30°C (59°F to 86°F). Protect from light. Do not use solution if brown or contains a precipitate.
I.V. infusion: May dilute 10 mg in 500 mL NS or D_5W. May also dilute 50 mg in 500 mL NS or 100 mg in 500 mL NS; both concentrations are stable for at least 14 days at room temperature of 25°C (77°F) (Gupta, 2004). Dilution of 1250 mg in 500 mL NS retained potency for at least 24 hours at 22°C (Weber, 1970).
I.V. injection: May dilute with SWFI to a concentration of 1 mg/mL.

Stability in syringes (Kiser, 2007): Concentration of 0.1 mg/mL in NS (polypropylene syringes) is stable for at least 30 days at -20°C (-4°F), 3°C to 5°C (37°F to 41°F), or 23°C to 25°C (73.4°F to 77°F).

Oral: Store at controlled room temperature of 15°C to 25°C (59°F to 77°F). Protect from light.

Mechanism of Action Potent, direct-acting alpha-adrenergic agonist with virtually no beta-adrenergic activity; produces systemic arterial vasoconstriction. Such increases in systemic vascular resistance result in dose dependent increases in systolic and diastolic blood pressure and reductions in heart rate and cardiac output especially in patients with heart failure.

Pharmacodynamics/Kinetics

Onset of action:

Blood pressure increase/vasoconstriction: I.M., SubQ: 10-15 minutes; I.V.: Immediate

Nasal decongestant: Oral: 15-30 minutes (Kollar, 2007)

Duration:

Blood pressure increase/vasoconstriction: I.M.: 1-2 hours; I.V.: ~15-20 minutes; SubQ: 50 minutes

Nasal decongestant: Oral: ≤4 hours (Kollar, 2007)

Absorption: Oral: Rapid and complete (Kanfer, 1993)

Distribution: V_d: Initial: 26-61 L; V_{dss}: 184-543 L (mean: 340 L) (Hengstmann, 1982)

Metabolism: Hepatic via oxidative deamination (Oral: 24%; I.V.: 50%); Undergoes sulfation (Oral [mostly within gut wall]: 46%; I.V.: 8%) and some glucuronidation; forms inactive metabolites (Kanfer, 1993)

Bioavailability: Oral: ≤38% (Hengstmann, 1982; Kanfer, 1993)

Half-life elimination: Alpha phase: ~5 minutes; Terminal phase: 2-3 hours (Hengstmann, 1982; Kanfer, 1993)

Time to peak: Oral: 0.75-2 hours (Kanfer, 1993)

Excretion: Urine (mostly as inactive metabolites)

Dosage

Geriatric & Adult

Hypotension/shock:

I.V. bolus: 100-500 mcg/dose every 10-15 minutes as needed (initial dose should not exceed 500 mcg)

I.V. infusion: Initial dose: 100-180 mcg/minute, **or alternatively**, 0.5 mcg/kg/minute; titrate to desired response. Dosing ranges between 0.4-9.1 mcg/kg/minute have been reported when treating septic shock (Gregory, 1991).

Nasal congestion: *Oral:* OTC labeling: 10 mg every 4 hours as needed for ≤7 days (maximum: 60 mg/24 hours)

Paroxysmal supraventricular tachycardia (Note: Not recommended for routine use in treatment of supraventricular tachycardias): *I.V.:* 250-500 mcg/dose over 20-30 seconds

Administration I.V.: May cause necrosis or sloughing tissue if extravasation occurs during I.V. administration or SubQ administration.

Extravasation management: Use phentolamine as antidote; mix 5-10 mg with 10 mL of NS. Inject a small amount of this dilution subcutaneously into extravasated area. Blanching should reverse immediately. Monitor site. If blanching should recur, additional injections of phentolamine may be needed.

Monitoring Parameters Blood pressure (or mean arterial pressure), heart rate; cardiac output (as appropriate), intravascular volume status, pulmonary capillary wedge pressure (as appropriate); monitor infusion site closely

Special Geriatric Considerations Elderly are more predisposed to the adverse effects of sympathomimetics since they frequently have cardiovascular disease and diabetes mellitus as well as multiple drug therapies. Elderly patients should be counseled about the proper use of OTC products and in what disease states they should be avoided.

Dosage Forms Excipient information presented when available (limited, particularly for generics); consult specific product labeling.

Injection, solution, as hydrochloride: 1% [10 mg/mL] (1 mL, 5 mL, 10 mL)

Liquid, oral, as hydrochloride:

PediaCare® Children's Decongestant: 2.5 mg/5 mL (118 mL) [contains sodium 14 mg/5 mL, sodium benzoate; raspberry flavor]

Sudafed PE® Children's: 2.5 mg/5 mL (118 mL) [ethanol free, sugar free; contains sodium 14 mg/5 mL, sodium benzoate; raspberry flavor]

Strip, orally disintegrating, oral, as hydrochloride:

Triaminic Thin Strips® Children's Cold with Stuffy Nose: 2.5 mg (14s) [raspberry flavor]

Tablet, oral, as hydrochloride: 10 mg

Medi-First® Sinus Decongestant: 10 mg

Medi-Phenyl: 5 mg

Sudafed PE® Congestion: 10 mg

Sudafed PE™ Nasal Decongestant: 10 mg

Sudogest™ PE: 10 mg

Phenylephrine (Nasal) (fen il EF rin)

Medication Safety Issues
Sound-alike/look-alike issues:
Neo-Synephrine® (phenylephrine, nasal) may be confused with Neo-Synephrine® (oxymetazoline)
Brand Names: U.S. 4 Way® Fast Acting [OTC]; 4 Way® Menthol [OTC]; Little Noses® Decongestant [OTC]; Neo-Synephrine® Extra Strength [OTC]; Neo-Synephrine® Mild Formula [OTC]; Neo-Synephrine® Regular Strength [OTC]; Rhinall® [OTC]
Brand Names: Canada Neo-Synephrine®
Index Terms Phenylephrine Hydrochloride
Pharmacologic Category Alpha-Adrenergic Agonist; Decongestant
Use For OTC use as symptomatic relief of nasal and nasopharyngeal mucosal congestion
Dosage
Geriatric & Adult Nasal congestion: Intranasal: 0.25% to 1% solution: Instill 2-3 sprays or 2-3 drops in each nostril every 4 hours as needed for ≤3 days
Special Geriatric Considerations Evaluate the patient's or caregiver's ability to safely administer the correct dose of nasal medication.
Dosage Forms Excipient information presented when available (limited, particularly for generics); consult specific product labeling.
Solution, intranasal, as hydrochloride [drops]:
Little Noses® Decongestant: 0.125% (15 mL) [ethanol free; contains benzalkonium chloride]
Rhinall®: 0.25% (30 mL) [contains benzalkonium chloride, sodium bisulfite]
Solution, intranasal, as hydrochloride [spray]:
4 Way® Fast Acting: 1% (15 mL, 30 mL, 37 mL) [contains benzalkonium chloride]
4 Way® Menthol: 1% (15 mL, 30 mL) [contains benzalkonium chloride, menthol]
Neo-Synephrine® Extra Strength: 1% (15 mL) [contains benzalkonium chloride]
Neo-Synephrine® Mild Formula: 0.25% (15 mL) [contains benzalkonium chloride]
Neo-Synephrine® Regular Strength: 0.5% (15 mL) [contains benzalkonium chloride]
Rhinall®: 0.25% (40 mL) [contains benzalkonium chloride, sodium bisulfite]

Phenylephrine (Ophthalmic) (fen il EF rin)

Medication Safety Issues
Sound-alike/look-alike issues:
Mydfrin® may be confused with Midrin®
Brand Names: U.S. AK-Dilate™; Altafrin; Mydfrin®; Neofrin
Brand Names: Canada Dionephrine®; Mydfrin®
Index Terms Phenylephrine Hydrochloride
Generic Availability (U.S.) Yes
Pharmacologic Category Alpha-Adrenergic Agonist; Ophthalmic Agent, Antiglaucoma; Ophthalmic Agent, Mydriatic
Use Used as a mydriatic in ophthalmic procedures and treatment of wide-angle glaucoma; OTC use as symptomatic relief of redness of the eye due to irritation
Dosage
Geriatric
Ophthalmic preparations for pupil dilation: Instill 1 drop of 2.5% solution; may repeat in 1 hour if necessary
Other indications: Refer to adult dosing.
Adult
Ocular procedures: Ophthalmic: Instill 1 drop of 2.5% or 10% solution; may repeat in 10-60 minutes as needed
Ophthalmic irritation (OTC formulation): Ophthalmic: Instill 1-2 drops 0.12% solution into affected eye up to 4 times/day; do not use for >72 hours
Special Geriatric Considerations Evaluate the patient's or caregiver's ability to safely administer the correct dose of ophthalmic medication.
Dosage Forms Excipient information presented when available (limited, particularly for generics); consult specific product labeling.
Solution, ophthalmic, as hydrochloride [drops]: 2.5% (2 mL, 3 mL, 5 mL, 15 mL)
AK-Dilate™: 2.5% (2 mL, 15 mL); 10% (5 mL) [contains benzalkonium chloride]
Altafrin: 2.5% (15 mL); 10% (5 mL) [contains benzalkonium chloride]
Mydfrin®: 2.5% (3 mL, 5 mL) [contains benzalkonium chloride, sodium bisulfite]
Neofrin: 2.5% (15 mL); 10% (5 mL)

Phenylephrine (Topical) (fen il EF rin)

Brand Names: U.S. Anu-Med [OTC]; Formulation R™ [OTC]; Medicone® Suppositories [OTC]; Preparation H® [OTC]; Rectacaine [OTC]; Tronolane® Suppository [OTC]
Index Terms Phenylephrine Hydrochloride
Generic Availability (U.S.) Yes
Pharmacologic Category Alpha-Adrenergic Agonist
Use For OTC use as treatment of hemorrhoids
Dosage
  Geriatric & Adult Hemorrhoids: Rectal:
    Ointment: Apply to clean, dry area up to 4 times/day
    Suppository: Insert 1 suppository rectally up to 4 times/day
Special Geriatric Considerations Since topical phenylephrine products can be obtained OTC, elderly patients should be counseled about their proper use and in what disease states they should be avoided.
Dosage Forms Excipient information presented when available (limited, particularly for generics); consult specific product labeling.
  Ointment, rectal, as hydrochloride: 0.25% (60 g)
    Formulation R™: 0.25% (30 g, 60 g) [contains benzoic acid]
    Preparation H®: 0.25% (30 g, 60 g) [contains benzoic acid]
  Suppository, rectal, as hydrochloride: 0.25% (1s); 0.25% (12s)
    Anu-Med: 0.25% (12s)
    Medicone® Suppositories: 0.25% (12s, 24s)
    Preparation H®: 0.25% (12s, 24s, 48s)
    Rectacaine: 0.25% (12s)
    Tronolane® Suppository: 0.25% (12s, 24s)

♦ **Phenylephrine Hydrochloride** *see* Phenylephrine (Nasal) *on page 1526*
♦ **Phenylephrine Hydrochloride** *see* Phenylephrine (Ophthalmic) *on page 1526*
♦ **Phenylephrine Hydrochloride** *see* Phenylephrine (Systemic) *on page 1523*
♦ **Phenylephrine Hydrochloride** *see* Phenylephrine (Topical) *on page 1527*
♦ **Phenylephrine Hydrochloride and Acetaminophen** *see* Acetaminophen and Phenylephrine *on page 37*
♦ **Phenylethylmalonylurea** *see* PHENobarbital *on page 1520*
♦ **Phenytek®** *see* Phenytoin *on page 1527*

Phenytoin (FEN i toyn)

Medication Safety Issues
  Sound-alike/look-alike issues:
    Phenytoin may be confused with phenelzine, phentermine, PHENobarbital
    Dilantin® may be confused with Dilaudid®, diltiazem, Dipentum®
  High alert medication:
    The Institute for Safe Medication Practices (ISMP) includes this medication (I.V. formulation) among its list of drug classes which have a heightened risk of causing significant patient harm when used in error.
  International issues:
    Dilantin [U.S., Canada, and multiple international markets] may be confused with Dolantine brand name for pethidine [Belgium]
Brand Names: U.S. Dilantin-125®; Dilantin®; Phenytek®
Brand Names: Canada Dilantin®; Novo-Phenytoin; Taro-Phenytoin; Tremtoine Inj
Index Terms Diphenylhydantoin; DPH; Phenytoin Sodium; Phenytoin Sodium, Extended; Phenytoin Sodium, Prompt
Generic Availability (U.S.) Yes: Excludes chewable tablet
Pharmacologic Category Anticonvulsant, Hydantoin
Use Management of generalized tonic-clonic (grand mal), complex partial seizures; prevention of seizures following neurosurgery
Unlabeled Use Prevention of early (within 1 week) post-traumatic seizures (PTS) following traumatic brain injury
Medication Guide Available Yes
Contraindications Hypersensitivity to phenytoin, other hydantoins, or any component of the formulation

Warnings/Precautions Antiepileptics are associated with an increased risk of suicidal behavior/thoughts with use (regardless of indication); patients should be monitored for signs/symptoms of depression, suicidal tendencies, and other unusual behavior changes during therapy and instructed to inform their healthcare provider immediately if symptoms occur.

[U.S. Boxed Warning]: Phenytoin must be administered slowly. Intravenous administration should not exceed 50 mg/minute in adult patients. Hypotension may occur with rapid administration. I.V. form may cause skin necrosis at I.V. site; avoid I.V. administration in small veins; may increase frequency of petit mal seizures; use with caution in patients with porphyria; discontinue if rash or lymphadenopathy occurs; a spectrum of hematologic effects have been reported with use (eg, neutropenia, leukopenia, thrombocytopenia, pancytopenia, and anemias); use with caution in patients with hepatic dysfunction, sinus bradycardia, S-A block, or AV block; use with caution in elderly or debilitated patients, or in any condition associated with low serum albumin levels, which will increase the free fraction of phenytoin in the serum and, therefore, the pharmacologic response. Sedation, confusional states, or cerebellar dysfunction (loss of motor coordination) may occur at higher total serum concentrations, or at lower total serum concentrations when the free fraction of phenytoin is increased. Effects with other sedative drugs or ethanol may be potentiated. Abrupt withdrawal may precipitate status epilepticus. Severe reactions, including toxic epidermal necrolysis and Stevens-Johnson syndromes, although rarely reported, have resulted in fatalities; drug should be discontinued if there are any signs of rash. Patients of Asian descent with the variant *HLA-B*1502* may be at an increased risk of developing Stevens-Johnson syndrome and/or toxic epidermal necrolysis.

Adverse Reactions (Reflective of adult population; not specific for elderly) I.V. effects: Hypotension, bradycardia, cardiac arrhythmia, cardiovascular collapse (especially with rapid I.V. use), venous irritation and pain, thrombophlebitis

Effects not related to plasma phenytoin concentrations: Hypertrichosis, gingival hypertrophy, thickening of facial features, carbohydrate intolerance, folic acid deficiency, peripheral neuropathy, vitamin D deficiency, osteomalacia, systemic lupus erythematosus

Concentration-related effects: Nystagmus, blurred vision, diplopia, ataxia, slurred speech, dizziness, drowsiness, lethargy, coma, rash, fever, nausea, vomiting, gum tenderness, confusion, mood changes, folic acid depletion, osteomalacia, hyperglycemia

Related to elevated concentrations:
>20 mcg/mL: Far lateral nystagmus
>30 mcg/mL: 45° lateral gaze nystagmus and ataxia
>40 mcg/mL: Decreased mentation
>100 mcg/mL: Death

Cardiovascular: Bradycardia, cardiac arrhythmia, cardiovascular collapse, hypotension
Central nervous system: Dizziness, drowsiness, headache, insomnia, psychiatric changes, slurred speech
Dermatologic: Rash
Gastrointestinal: Constipation, gingival hyperplasia, enlargement of lips, nausea, taste disturbance, vomiting
Genitourinary: Peyronie's disease
Hematologic: Agranulocytosis, granulocytopenia, leukopenia, pancytopenia, thrombocytopenia
Hepatic: Hepatitis
Local: I.V. administration: Inflammation, irritation, necrosis, sloughing, tenderness, thrombophlebitis
Neuromuscular & skeletal: Paresthesia, peripheral neuropathy, tremor
Ocular: Blurred vision, diplopia, nystagmus
Rarely seen effects: Anaphylaxis, blood dyscrasias, coarsening of facial features, DRESS, dyskinesias, hepatitis, Hodgkin lymphoma, hypertrichosis, immunoglobulin abnormalities, lymphadenopathy, lymphoma, macrocytosis, megaloblastic anemia, periarteritis nodosa, pseudolymphoma, SLE-like syndrome, Stevens-Johnson syndrome, toxic epidermal necrolysis, venous irritation and pain

Drug Interactions
Metabolism/Transport Effects Substrate of CYP2C19 (major), CYP2C9 (major), CYP3A4 (minor); **Note:** Assignment of Major/Minor substrate status based on clinically relevant drug interaction potential; **Induces** CYP2B6 (strong), CYP2C19 (strong), CYP2C8 (strong), CYP2C9 (strong), CYP3A4 (strong)

Avoid Concomitant Use
Avoid concomitant use of Phenytoin with any of the following: Axitinib; Azelastine; Azelastine (Nasal); Boceprevir; Bortezomib; Crizotinib; Darunavir; Delavirdine; Dronedarone; Etravirine; Everolimus; Lapatinib; Lurasidone; Mifepristone; Mirtazapine; Nilotinib; Paraldehyde;

Pazopanib; Praziquantel; Ranolazine; Rilpivirine; Rivaroxaban; Roflumilast; RomiDEPsin; SORAfenib; Telaprevir; Ticagrelor; Tolvaptan; Toremifene; Vandetanib

Increased Effect/Toxicity

Phenytoin may increase the levels/effects of: Azelastine; Azelastine (Nasal); Barbiturates; Buprenorphine; Clarithromycin; CNS Depressants; Fosamprenavir; Ifosfamide; Lithium; Methotrimeprazine; Metyrosine; Mirtazapine; Paraldehyde; Prilocaine; Selective Serotonin Reuptake Inhibitors; Vecuronium; Vitamin K Antagonists; Zolpidem

The levels/effects of Phenytoin may be increased by: Alcohol (Ethyl); Allopurinol; Amiodarone; Antifungal Agents (Azole Derivatives, Systemic); Benzodiazepines; Calcium Channel Blockers; Capecitabine; CarBAMazepine; Carbonic Anhydrase Inhibitors; CeFAZolin; Chloramphenicol; Cimetidine; Clarithromycin; CYP2C19 Inhibitors (Moderate); CYP2C19 Inhibitors (Strong); CYP2C9 Inhibitors (Moderate); CYP2C9 Inhibitors (Strong); Delavirdine; Dexmethylphenidate; Disulfiram; Droperidol; Efavirenz; Ethosuximide; Felbamate; Floxuridine; Fluconazole; Fluorouracil; Fluorouracil (Systemic); Fluorouracil (Topical); FLUoxetine; FluvoxaMINE; Halothane; HydrOXYzine; Isoniazid; Methotrimeprazine; Methylphenidate; MetroNIDAZOLE; MetroNIDAZOLE (Systemic); Mifepristone; OXcarbazepine; Proton Pump Inhibitors; Rufinamide; Sertraline; Sulfonamide Derivatives; Tacrolimus; Tacrolimus (Systemic); Telaprevir; Ticlopidine; Topiramate; TraZODone; Trimethoprim; Vitamin K Antagonists

Decreased Effect

Phenytoin may decrease the levels/effects of: Acetaminophen; Amiodarone; Antifungal Agents (Azole Derivatives, Systemic); Apixaban; ARIPiprazole; Axitinib; Boceprevir; Bortezomib; Brentuximab Vedotin; Busulfan; CarBAMazepine; Caspofungin; Chloramphenicol; Clarithromycin; CloZAPine; Contraceptives (Estrogens); Contraceptives (Progestins); Crizotinib; CycloSPORINE; CycloSPORINE (Systemic); CYP2B6 Substrates; CYP2C19 Substrates; CYP2C8 Substrates; CYP2C9 Substrates; CYP3A4 Substrates; Darunavir; Dasatinib; Deferasirox; Delavirdine; Diclofenac; Disopyramide; Divalproex; Doxycycline; Dronedarone; Efavirenz; Ethosuximide; Etoposide; Etoposide Phosphate; Etravirine; Everolimus; Exemestane; Felbamate; Flunarizine; Gefitinib; GuanFACINE; HMG-CoA Reductase Inhibitors; Imatinib; Irinotecan; Ixabepilone; Lacosamide; LamoTRIgine; Lapatinib; Levodopa; Linagliptin; Loop Diuretics; Lopinavir; Lurasidone; Maraviroc; Mebendazole; Meperidine; Methadone; MethylPREDNISolone; MetroNIDAZOLE; MetroNIDAZOLE (Systemic); Metyrapone; Mexiletine; Mifepristone; Nilotinib; OXcarbazepine; Pazopanib; Praziquantel; PrednisoLONE; PrednisoLONE (Systemic); PredniSONE; Primidone; QUEtiapine; QuiNIDine; QuiNINE; Ranolazine; Rilpivirine; Ritonavir; Rivaroxaban; Roflumilast; RomiDEPsin; Rufinamide; Saxagliptin; Sertraline; Sirolimus; SORAfenib; SUNItinib; Tacrolimus; Tacrolimus (Systemic); Tadalafil; Telaprevir; Temsirolimus; Teniposide; Theophylline Derivatives; Thyroid Products; Ticagrelor; Tipranavir; Tolvaptan; Topiramate; Toremifene; TraZODone; Treprostinil; Ulipristal; Valproic Acid; Vandetanib; Vecuronium; Vemurafenib; Zonisamide; Zuclopenthixol

The levels/effects of Phenytoin may be decreased by: Alcohol (Ethyl); Amphetamines; Antacids; Barbiturates; CarBAMazepine; Ciprofloxacin; Ciprofloxacin (Systemic); CISplatin; Colesevelam; CYP2C19 Inducers (Strong); CYP2C9 Inducers (Strong); Diazoxide; Divalproex; Folic Acid; Fosamprenavir; Ketorolac; Ketorolac (Nasal); Ketorolac (Systemic); Leucovorin Calcium-Levoleucovorin; Levomefolate; Lopinavir; Mefloquine; Methylfolate; Nelfinavir; Peginterferon Alfa-2b; Pyridoxine; Rifamycin Derivatives; Ritonavir; Telaprevir; Theophylline Derivatives; Tipranavir; Tocilizumab; Valproic Acid; Vigabatrin

Ethanol/Nutrition/Herb Interactions

Ethanol:

Acute use: Ethanol inhibits metabolism of phenytoin and may also increase CNS depression. Management: Avoid or limit ethanol. Caution patients about effects.

Chronic use: Ethanol stimulates metabolism of phenytoin. Management: Avoid or limit ethanol.

Food: Phenytoin serum concentrations may be altered if taken with food. If taken with enteral nutrition, phenytoin serum concentrations may be decreased. Tube feedings decrease bioavailability. Phenytoin may decrease calcium, folic acid, and vitamin D levels. Supplementing folic acid may lower the seizure threshold. Management: Hold tube feedings 1-2 hours before and 1-2 hours after phenytoin administration. Do not supplement folic acid. Consider vitamin D supplementation. Take preferably on an empty stomach.

Herb/Nutraceutical: Evening primrose may decrease the seizure threshold; other herbal medications may increase CNS depression. Management: Avoid evening primrose, valerian, St John's wort, kava kava, and gotu kola.

Stability

Capsule, tablet: Store at 20°C to 25°C (68°F to 77°F). Protect capsules from light. Protect capsules and tablets from moisture.

Oral suspension: Store at room temperature of 20°C to 25°C (68°F to 77°F); do not freeze. Protect from light.

Solution for injection: Store at room temperature of 15°C to 30°C (59°F to 86°F). Use only clear solutions free of precipitate and haziness; slightly yellow solutions may be used. Precipitation may occur if solution is refrigerated and may dissolve at room temperature.

Further dilution of the solution for I.V. infusion is controversial and no consensus exists as to the optimal concentration and length of stability. Stability is concentration and pH dependent. Based on limited clinical consensus, NS or LR are recommended diluents (Pfeifle, 1981). Dilutions of 1-10 mg/mL have been used and should be administered as soon as possible after preparation (some recommend to discard if not used within 4 hours). Do not refrigerate.

Mechanism of Action Stabilizes neuronal membranes and decreases seizure activity by increasing efflux or decreasing influx of sodium ions across cell membranes in the motor cortex during generation of nerve impulses; prolongs effective refractory period and suppresses ventricular pacemaker automaticity, shortens action potential in the heart

Pharmacodynamics/Kinetics

Onset of action: I.V.: ~0.5-1 hour

Absorption: Oral: Slow

Distribution: V_d: Adults: 0.6-0.7 L/kg

Protein binding:

Adults: 90% to 95%

Others: Decreased protein binding

Disease states resulting in a decrease in serum albumin concentration: Burns, hepatic cirrhosis, nephrotic syndrome, cystic fibrosis

Disease states resulting in an apparent decrease in affinity of phenytoin for serum albumin: Renal failure, jaundice (severe), other drugs (displacers), hyperbilirubinemia (total bilirubin >15 mg/dL), Cl_{cr} <25 mL/minute (unbound fraction is increased two- to threefold in uremia)

Metabolism: Follows dose-dependent capacity-limited (Michaelis-Menten) pharmacokinetics; major metabolite (via oxidation), HPPA, undergoes enterohepatic recirculation

Bioavailability: Form dependent

Half-life elimination: Oral: 22 hours (range: 7-42 hours)

Time to peak, serum (form dependent): Oral: Extended-release capsule: 4-12 hours; Immediate release preparation: 2-3 hours

Excretion: Urine (<5% as unchanged drug); as glucuronides

Clearance: Highly variable, dependent upon intrinsic hepatic function and dose administered; increased clearance and decreased serum concentrations with febrile illness

Dosage

Geriatric & Adult Note: Phenytoin base (eg, oral suspension, chewable tablets) contains ~8% more drug than phenytoin sodium (~92 mg base is equivalent to 100 mg phenytoin sodium). Dosage adjustments and closer serum monitoring may be necessary when switching dosage forms.

Status epilepticus: I.V.: Loading dose: Manufacturer recommends 10-15 mg/kg, however, 15-20 mg/kg at a maximum rate of 50 mg/minute is generally recommended (Kalvianines, 2007; Lowenstein, 2005); initial maintenance dose: I.V. or Oral: 100 mg every 6-8 hours

Anticonvulsant: Oral: Loading dose: 15-20 mg/kg; consider prior phenytoin serum concentrations and/or recent dosing history if available; administer oral loading dose in 3 divided doses given every 2-4 hours to decrease GI adverse effects and to ensure complete oral absorption; initial maintenance dose: 300 mg/day in 3 divided doses; may also administer in 1-2 divided doses using extended release formulation; adjust dosage based on individual requirements; usual maintenance dose range: 300-600 mg/day

Dosage adjustment in obesity: Loading dose: Use adjusted body weight (ABW) correction based on a pharmacokinetic study of phenytoin loading doses in obese patients (Abernethy, 1985). The larger correction factor (ie, 1.33) is due to a doubling of V_d estimated in these obese patients.

ABW = [(Actual body weight − IBW) x 1.33] + IBW

Maximum loading dose: I.V.: 2000 mg (Erstad, 2004)

Maintenance doses should be based on ideal body weight, conventional daily doses with adjustments based upon therapeutic drug monitoring and clinical effectiveness (Abernethy, 1985; Erstad, 2002; Erstad, 2004).

Renal Impairment Phenytoin level in serum may be difficult to interpret in renal failure. Monitoring of free (unbound) concentrations or adjustment to allow interpretation is recommended.

Hepatic Impairment Safe in usual doses in mild liver disease; clearance may be substantially reduced in cirrhosis and plasma level monitoring with dose adjustment advisable. Free phenytoin levels should be monitored closely.

Administration

Oral: Suspension: Shake well prior to use. Absorption is impaired when phenytoin suspension is given concurrently to patients who are receiving continuous nasogastric feedings. A method to resolve this interaction is to divide the daily dose of phenytoin and withhold the administration of nutritional supplements for 1-2 hours before and after each phenytoin dose.

I.M.: **Avoid** this route (manufacturer recommends I.M. administration) due to severe risk of local tissue destruction and necrosis; use **fos**phenytoin if I.M. administration necessary (Boucher, 1996; Meek, 1999).

I.V.: Vesicant. Fosphenytoin may be considered for loading in patients who are in status epilepticus, hemodynamically unstable, or develop hypotension/bradycardia with I.V. administration of phenytoin. Although, phenytoin may be administered by direct I.V. injection, it is preferable that phenytoin be administered via infusion pump either undiluted or diluted in normal saline as an I.V. piggyback (IVPB) to prevent exceeding the maximum infusion rate (monitor closely for extravasation during infusion). The maximum rate of I.V. administration is 50 mg/minute in adults. Highly sensitive patients (eg, elderly, patients with pre-existing cardiovascular conditions) should receive phenytoin more slowly (eg, 20 mg/minute) (Meek, 1999). An in-line 0.22-5 micron filter is recommended for IVPB solutions due to the high potential for precipitation of the solution. Avoid extravasation. Following I.V. administration, NS should be injected through the same needle or I.V. catheter to prevent irritation. pH: 10.0-12.3

SubQ: SubQ administration is not recommended because of the possibility of local tissue damage (due to high pH).

Monitoring Parameters CBC, liver function; suicidality (eg, suicidal thoughts, depression, behavioral changes); plasma phenytoin concentrations (if available, free phenytoin concentrations should be obtained in patients with renal impairment and/or hypoalbuminemia; if free phenytoin concentrations are unavailable, the adjusted total concentration may be determined based upon equations in adult patients). Trough concentrations are generally recommended for routine monitoring.

Additional monitoring with I.V. use: Continuous cardiac monitoring (rate, rhythm, blood pressure) and observation during administration recommended; blood pressure and pulse should be monitored every 15 minutes for 1 hour after administration (Meek, 1999); infusion site reactions

Reference Range Timing of serum samples: Because it is slowly absorbed, peak blood levels may occur 4-8 hours after ingestion of an oral dose. The serum half-life varies with the dosage and the drug follows Michaelis-Menten kinetics. The average adult half-life is about 24 hours. Steady-state concentrations are reached in 5-10 days.

Adults: Toxicity is measured clinically, and some patients require levels outside the suggested therapeutic range

Therapeutic range:

Total phenytoin: 10-20 mcg/mL

Concentrations of 5-10 mcg/mL may be therapeutic for some patients but concentrations <5 mcg/mL are not likely to be effective

50% of patients show decreased frequency of seizures at concentrations >10 mcg/mL

86% of patients show decreased frequency of seizures at concentrations >15 mcg/mL

Add another anticonvulsant if satisfactory therapeutic response is not achieved with a phenytoin concentration of 20 mcg/mL

Free phenytoin: 1-2.5 mcg/mL

Total phenytoin:

Toxic: >30 mcg/mL (SI: >119 micromole/L)

Lethal: >100 mcg/mL (SI: >400 micromole/L)

When to draw levels: This is dependent on the disease state being treated and the clinical condition of the patient

Key points:

Slow absorption of extended capsules and prolonged half-life minimize fluctuations between peak and trough concentrations, timing of sampling not crucial

Trough concentrations are generally recommended for routine monitoring. Daily levels are not necessary and may result in incorrect dosage adjustments. If it is determined essential to monitor free phenytoin concentrations, concomitant monitoring of total phenytoin concentrations is not necessary and expensive.

After a loading dose: If rapid therapeutic levels are needed, initial levels may be drawn after 1 hour (I.V. loading dose) or within 24 hours (oral loading dose) to aid in determining maintenance dose or need to reload.

Rapid achievement: Draw within 2-3 days of therapy initiation to ensure that the patient's metabolism is not remarkably different from that which would be predicted by average literature-derived pharmacokinetic parameters; early levels should be used cautiously in design of new dosing regimens

Second concentration: Draw within 6-7 days with subsequent doses of phenytoin adjusted accordingly

If plasma concentrations have not changed over a 3- to 5-day period, monitoring interval may be increased to once weekly in the acute clinical setting

In stable patients requiring long-term therapy, generally monitor levels at 3- to 12-month intervals

Adjustment of serum concentration: See tables.

Note: Although it is ideal to obtain free phenytoin concentrations to assess serum concentrations in patients with hypoalbuminemia or renal failure (Cl_{cr} ≤10 mL/minute), it may not always be possible. If free phenytoin concentrations are unavailable, the following equations may be utilized in adult patients.

Adjustment of Serum Concentration in Adults With Low Serum Albumin

Measured Total Phenytoin Concentration (mcg/mL)	Patient's Serum Albumin (g/dL)			
	3.5	3	2.5	2
	Adjusted Total Phenytoin Concentration (mcg/mL)[1]			
5	6	7	8	10
10	13	14	17	20
15	19	21	25	30

[1]Adjusted concentration = measured total concentration divided by [(0.2 x albumin) + 0.1].

Adjustment of Serum Concentration in Adults With Renal Failure (Cl_{cr} ≤10 mL/min)

Measured Total Phenytoin Concentration (mcg/mL)	Patient's Serum Albumin (g/dL)				
	4	3.5	3	2.5	2
	Adjusted Total Phenytoin Concentration (mcg/mL)[1]				
5	10	11	13	14	17
10	20	22	25	29	33
15	30	33	38	43	50

[1]Adjusted concentration = measured total concentration divided by [(0.1 x albumin) + 0.1].

Special Geriatric Considerations Elderly may have reduced hepatic clearance due to age decline in phase I metabolism. Elderly may have low albumin which will increase free fraction and, therefore, pharmacologic response. Monitor closely in those who are hypoalbuminemic. Free fraction measurements advised, also elderly may display a higher incidence of adverse effects (cardiovascular) when using the I.V. loading regimen; therefore, recommended to decrease loading I.V. dose to 25 mg/minute.

Dosage Forms Excipient information presented when available (limited, particularly for generics); consult specific product labeling.

Capsule, extended release, oral, as sodium: 100 mg, 200 mg, 300 mg
  Dilantin®: 30 mg, 100 mg
  Phenytek®: 200 mg, 300 mg
Injection, solution, as sodium: 50 mg/mL (2 mL, 5 mL)
Suspension, oral: 100 mg/4 mL (4 mL); 125 mg/5 mL (237 mL, 240 mL)
  Dilantin-125®: 125 mg/5 mL (240 mL) [contains ethanol ≤0.6%, sodium benzoate; orange-vanilla flavor]
Tablet, chewable, oral:
  Dilantin®: 50 mg [scored]

◆ **Phenytoin Sodium** see Phenytoin on page 1527
◆ **Phenytoin Sodium, Extended** see Phenytoin on page 1527
◆ **Phenytoin Sodium, Prompt** see Phenytoin on page 1527
◆ **Phillips'® M-O [OTC]** see Magnesium Hydroxide and Mineral Oil on page 1179
◆ **Phillips'® Laxative Dietary Supplement Cramp-Free [OTC]** see Magnesium Oxide on page 1181
◆ **Phillips'® Liquid-Gels® [OTC]** see Docusate on page 583
◆ **Phillips'® Milk of Magnesia [OTC]** see Magnesium Hydroxide on page 1177
◆ **Phillips'® Stool Softener Laxative [OTC]** see Docusate on page 583
◆ **Phos-Flur®** see Fluoride on page 806
◆ **Phos-Flur® Rinse [OTC]** see Fluoride on page 806
◆ **PhosLo®** see Calcium Acetate on page 259

Physostigmine (fye zoe STIG meen)

Medication Safety Issues
Sound-alike/look-alike issues:
Physostigmine may be confused with Prostigmin®, pyridostigmine

Index Terms Eserine Salicylate; Physostigmine Salicylate; Physostigmine Sulfate

Generic Availability (U.S.) Yes

Pharmacologic Category Acetylcholinesterase Inhibitor

Use Reverse toxic, life-threatening delirium caused by atropine, diphenhydramine, dimenhydrinate, *Atropa belladonna* (deadly nightshade), or jimson weed (*Datura* spp)

Contraindications Hypersensitivity to physostigmine or any component of the formulation; GI or GU obstruction; asthma; gangrene; diabetes, cardiovascular disease; any vagotonic state; coadministration of choline esters and depolarizing neuromuscular-blocking agents

Warnings/Precautions Hazardous agent - use appropriate precautions for handling and disposal. Patient must have a normal QRS interval, as measured by ECG, in order to receive; use caution in poisoning with agents known to prolong intraventricular conduction. Concomitant administration of choline esters or depolarizing neuromuscular-blocking agents (ie, succinylcholine) are contraindicated. Use with caution in patients with epilepsy, asthma, diabetes, gangrene, cardiovascular disease, bradycardia. Discontinue if excessive salivation or emesis, frequent urination or diarrhea occur. Reduce dosage if excessive sweating or nausea occurs. Administer slowly over 5 minutes to prevent respiratory distress and seizures. Continuous infusions should never be used. Due to the possibility of hypersensitivity or overdose/cholinergic crisis, atropine should be readily available; not intended as a first-line agent for anticholinergic toxicity or Parkinson's disease. Asystole and seizures have been reported when physostigmine was administered to TCA poisoned patients. Physostigmine is not recommended in patients with known or suspected TCA intoxication. Products may contain benzyl alcohol. Products may contain sodium bisulfate.

Adverse Reactions (Reflective of adult population; not specific for elderly) Frequency not defined.
Cardiovascular: Asystole, bradycardia, palpitation
Central nervous system: Hallucinations, nervousness, restlessness, seizure
Gastrointestinal: Diarrhea, nausea, salivation, stomach pain
Genitourinary: Urinary frequency
Neuromuscular & skeletal: Twitching
Ocular: Lacrimation, miosis
Respiratory: Bronchospasm, dyspnea, pulmonary edema, respiratory paralysis
Miscellaneous: Diaphoresis

Drug Interactions
Metabolism/Transport Effects None known.
Avoid Concomitant Use There are no known interactions where it is recommended to avoid concomitant use.
Increased Effect/Toxicity
Physostigmine may increase the levels/effects of: Beta-Blockers; Cholinergic Agonists; Succinylcholine

The levels/effects of Physostigmine may be increased by: Corticosteroids (Systemic)
Decreased Effect
Physostigmine may decrease the levels/effects of: Neuromuscular-Blocking Agents (Nondepolarizing)

The levels/effects of Physostigmine may be decreased by: Dipyridamole
Ethanol/Nutrition/Herb Interactions Herb/Nutraceutical: Ginkgo biloba may enhance the adverse/toxic effect of physostigmine; monitor.
Stability Do not use solution if cloudy or dark brown.

PHYSOSTIGMINE

Mechanism of Action Inhibits destruction of acetylcholine by acetylcholinesterase which facilitates transmission of impulses across myoneural junction and prolongs the central and peripheral effects of acetylcholine

Pharmacodynamics/Kinetics
Onset of action: ~5 minutes
Duration: 1-2 hours
Absorption: I.M.: Readily absorbed
Distribution: Crosses blood-brain barrier readily and reverses both central and peripheral anticholinergic effects
Metabolism: Hepatic and via hydrolysis by cholinesterases
Half-life elimination: 15-40 minutes

Dosage
Geriatric & Adult Reversal of toxic anticholinergic effects: Note: Administer slowly over 5 minutes to prevent respiratory distress and seizures. Continuous infusions of physostigmine should never be used.
I.M., I.V.: 0.5-2 mg to start; repeat every 20 minutes until response occurs or adverse effect occurs; repeat 1-4 mg every 30-60 minutes as life-threatening symptoms recur

Administration Injection: Infuse slowly I.V. over 5 minutes. Too rapid administration can cause bradycardia and hypersalivation leading to respiratory distress and seizures.

Monitoring Parameters ECG, vital signs

Test Interactions Increased aminotransferase [ALT/AST] (S), increased amylase (S)

Special Geriatric Considerations No specific information for use in elderly.

Dosage Forms Excipient information presented when available (limited, particularly for generics); consult specific product labeling.
Injection, solution, as salicylate: 1 mg/mL (2 mL)

◆ **Physostigmine Salicylate** *see* Physostigmine *on page 1533*
◆ **Physostigmine Sulfate** *see* Physostigmine *on page 1533*
◆ **Phytomenadione** *see* Phytonadione *on page 1534*

Phytonadione (fye toe na DYE one)

Medication Safety Issues
Sound-alike/look-alike issues:
Mephyton® may be confused with melphalan, methadone

Brand Names: U.S. Mephyton®
Brand Names: Canada AquaMEPHYTON®; Konakion; Mephyton®
Index Terms Methylphytyl Napthoquinone; Phylloquinone; Phytomenadione; Vitamin K₁
Generic Availability (U.S.) Yes
Pharmacologic Category Vitamin, Fat Soluble
Use Prevention and treatment of hypoprothrombinemia caused by coumarin derivative-induced or other drug-induced vitamin K deficiency, hypoprothrombinemia caused by malabsorption or inability to synthesize vitamin K
Unlabeled Use Treatment of hypoprothrombinemia caused by anticoagulant rodenticides
Contraindications Hypersensitivity to phytonadione or any component of the formulation
Warnings/Precautions [U.S. Boxed Warning]: Severe reactions resembling hypersensitivity (eg, anaphylaxis) reactions have occurred rarely during or immediately after I.V. administration. Allergic reactions have also occurred with I.M. and SubQ injections; oral administration is the safest. In obstructive jaundice or with biliary fistulas concurrent administration of bile salts is necessary. Manufacturers recommend the SubQ route over other parenteral routes. SubQ is less predictable when compared to the oral route. The American College of Chest Physicians recommends the I.V. route in patients with serious or life-threatening bleeding secondary to warfarin. The I.V. route should be restricted to emergency situations where oral phytonadione cannot be used. Efficacy is delayed regardless of route of administration; patient management may require other treatments in the interim. Administer a dose that will quickly lower the INR into a safe range without causing resistance to warfarin. High phytonadione doses may lead to warfarin resistance for at least one week. In liver disease, if initial doses do not reverse coagulopathy then higher doses are unlikely to have any effect. Ineffective in hereditary hypoprothrombinemia. Use caution with renal dysfunction. Injectable products may contain aluminum; may result in toxic levels following prolonged administration. Product may contain polysorbate 80.
Adverse Reactions (Reflective of adult population; not specific for elderly) Parenteral administration: Frequency not defined.
Cardiovascular: Cyanosis, flushing, hypotension
Central nervous system: Dizziness
Dermatologic: Scleroderma-like lesions
Endocrine & metabolic: Hyperbilirubinemia (newborn; greater than recommended doses)

Gastrointestinal: Abnormal taste
Local: Injection site reactions
Respiratory: Dyspnea
Miscellaneous: Anaphylactoid reactions, diaphoresis, hypersensitivity reactions

Drug Interactions

Metabolism/Transport Effects None known.

Avoid Concomitant Use There are no known interactions where it is recommended to avoid concomitant use.

Increased Effect/Toxicity There are no known significant interactions involving an increase in effect.

Decreased Effect

Phytonadione may decrease the levels/effects of: Vitamin K Antagonists

The levels/effects of Phytonadione may be decreased by: Mineral Oil; Orlistat

Stability

Injection: Store at 15°C to 30°C (59°F to 86°F). Dilute in preservative-free NS, D_5W, or D_5NS. To reduce the incidence of anaphylactoid reaction upon I.V. administration, dilute dose in a minimum of 50 mL of compatible solution and administer using an infusion pump over at least 20 minutes (Ageno, 2012).

Note: Store Hospira product at 20°C to 25°C (68°F to 77°F).

Oral: Store tablets at 15°C to 30°C (59°F to 86°F). Protect from light.

Mechanism of Action Promotes liver synthesis of clotting factors (II, VII, IX, X); however, the exact mechanism as to this stimulation is unknown. Menadiol is a water soluble form of vitamin K; phytonadione has a more rapid and prolonged effect than menadione; menadiol sodium diphosphate (K_4) is half as potent as menadione (K_3).

Pharmacodynamics/Kinetics

Onset of action: Increased coagulation factors: Oral: 6-10 hours; I.V.: 1-2 hours

Peak effect: INR values return to normal: Oral: 24-48 hours; I.V.: 12-14 hours

Absorption: Oral: From intestines in presence of bile; SubQ: Variable

Metabolism: Rapidly hepatic

Excretion: Urine and feces

Dosage

Geriatric & Adult Note: According to the manufacturer, SubQ is the preferred parenteral route; I.M. route should be avoided due to the risk of hematoma formation; I.V. route should be restricted for emergency use only. The American College of Chest Physicians (ACCP) recommends the I.V. route in patients with major bleeding secondary to use of vitamin K antagonists.

Adequate intake: Males: 120 mcg/day; Females: 90 mcg/day

Hypoprothrombinemia due to drugs (other than coumarin derivatives) or factors limiting absorption or synthesis: Oral, SubQ, I.M., I.V.: Initial: 2.5-25 mg (rarely up to 50 mg)

Vitamin K deficiency (supratherapeutic INR) secondary to coumarin derivative:

If INR above therapeutic range to <4.5 (no evidence of bleeding): Lower or hold next dose and monitor frequently; when INR approaches desired range, resume dosing with a lower dose (Patriquin, 2011).

If INR 4.5-10 (no evidence of bleeding): The 2012 ACCP guidelines recommend against routine vitamin K administration in this setting (Guyatt, 2012). Previously, the 2008 ACCP guidelines recommended if no risk factors for bleeding exist, to omit next 1 or 2 doses, monitor INR more frequently, and resume with an appropriately adjusted dose when INR in desired range; may consider administering vitamin K orally 1-2.5 mg if other risk factors for bleeding exist (Hirsh, 2008). Others have recommended consideration of vitamin K 1 mg orally or 0.5 mg I.V. (Patriquin, 2011).

If INR >10 (no evidence of bleeding): The 2012 ACCP guidelines recommend administration of oral vitamin K (dose not specified) in this setting (Guyatt, 2012). Previously, the 2008 ACCP guidelines recommended to hold warfarin, administer vitamin K orally 2.5-5 mg, expect INR to be reduced within 24-48 hours, monitor INR more frequently and give additional vitamin K at an appropriate dose if necessary; resume warfarin at an appropriately adjusted dose when INR is in desired range (Hirsh, 2008). Others have recommended consideration of vitamin K 2-2.5 mg orally or 0.5-1 mg I.V. (Patriquin, 2011).

If minor bleeding at any INR elevation: Hold warfarin, may administer vitamin K orally 2.5-5 mg, monitor INR more frequently, may repeat dose after 24 hours if INR correction incomplete; resume warfarin at an appropriately adjusted dose when INR is in desired range (Patriquin, 2011).

If major bleeding at any INR elevation: The 2012 ACCP guidelines recommend administration of four-factor prothrombin complex concentrate (PCC) and I.V. vitamin K 5-10 mg in this setting (Guyatt, 2012); however, in the U.S., the available PCCs (Bebulin®VH and Profilnine® SD) are **three**-factor PCCs and do not contain adequate levels of factor VII. Four-factor PCCs include Beriplex® P/N, Cofact®, Konyne®, or Octaplex® all of which are **not** available in the U.S. Previously, the 2008 ACCP guidelines recommended to hold warfarin, administer vitamin K 10 mg by slow I.V. infusion and supplement with PCC depending on the urgency of the situation; I.V. vitamin K may be repeated every 12 hours (Hirsh, 2008).

Note: Use of high doses of vitamin K (eg, 10-15 mg) may cause warfarin resistance for ≥1 week. During this period of resistance, heparin or low-molecular-weight heparin (LMWH) may be given until INR responds (Ansell, 2008).

Preprocedural/surgical INR normalization in patients receiving warfarin (routine use): Oral: 1-2.5 mg once administered on the day before surgery; recheck INR on day of procedure/surgery (Douketis, 2012). Others have recommended the use of vitamin K 1 mg orally for mild INR elevations (ie, INR 3.0-4.5) (Patriquin, 2011).

Administration

I.V. administration: Infuse slowly; rate of infusion should not exceed 1 mg/minute. Alternatively, dilute dose in a minimum of 50 mL of compatible solution and administer using an infusion pump over at least 20 minutes (Ageno, 2012). The injectable route should be used only if the oral route is not feasible or there is a greater urgency to reverse anticoagulation.

Oral: The parenteral formulation may also be used for small oral doses (eg, 1 mg) or situations in which tablets cannot be swallowed (Crowther, 2000; O'Connor, 1986).

Monitoring Parameters PT, INR

Dosage Forms Excipient information presented when available (limited, particularly for generics); consult specific product labeling.

Injection, aqueous colloidal: 1 mg/0.5 mL (0.5 mL) [contains benzyl alcohol]; 10 mg/mL (1 mL) [contains benzyl alcohol]

Injection, aqueous colloidal [preservative free]: 1 mg/0.5 mL (0.5 mL) [contains polysorbate 80, propylene glycol 10.4 mg/0.5 mL]

Tablet, oral: 100 mcg

Mephyton®: 5 mg [scored]

◆ **Picato®** see Ingenol Mebutate on page 1004

Pilocarpine (Ophthalmic) (pye loe KAR peen)

Related Information

Glaucoma Drug Therapy on page 2115

Medication Safety Issues

Sound-alike/look-alike issues:

Isopto® Carpine may be confused with Isopto® Carbachol

Brand Names: U.S. Isopto® Carpine; Pilopine HS®

Brand Names: Canada Diocarpine; Isopto® Carpine; Pilopine HS®

Index Terms Pilocarpine Hydrochloride

Generic Availability (U.S.) Yes: Excludes gel

Pharmacologic Category Ophthalmic Agent, Antiglaucoma; Ophthalmic Agent, Miotic

Use Management of chronic simple glaucoma, chronic and acute angle-closure glaucoma

Unlabeled Use Counter effects of cycloplegics

Dosage

Geriatric & Adult

Glaucoma: Ophthalmic:

Solution: Instill 1-2 drops up to 6 times/day; adjust the concentration and frequency as required to control elevated intraocular pressure.

Gel: Instill 0.5" ribbon into lower conjunctival sac once daily at bedtime.

To counteract the mydriatic effects of sympathomimetic agents (unlabeled use): Ophthalmic: *Solution:* Instill 1 drop of a 1% solution in the affected eye.

Special Geriatric Considerations Evaluate the patient's or caregiver's ability to safely administer the correct dose of ophthalmic medication.

Dosage Forms Excipient information presented when available (limited, particularly for generics); consult specific product labeling.

Gel, ophthalmic, as hydrochloride:

Pilopine HS®: 4% (4 g) [contains benzalkonium chloride]

Solution, ophthalmic, as hydrochloride [drops]: 1% (15 mL); 2% (15 mL); 4% (15 mL)

Isopto® Carpine: 1% (15 mL); 2% (15 mL); 4% (15 mL) [contains benzalkonium chloride]

◆ **Pilocarpine Hydrochloride** see Pilocarpine (Ophthalmic) on page 1536

◆ **Pilopine HS®** see Pilocarpine (Ophthalmic) on page 1536

◆ **Pimaricin** see Natamycin on page 1345

Pimozide (PI moe zide)

Related Information
Antipsychotic Agents *on page 2103*
Beers Criteria – Potentially Inappropriate Medications for Geriatrics *on page 2183*

Medication Safety Issues
BEERS Criteria medication:
This drug may be potentially inappropriate for use in geriatric patients (Quality of evidence - moderate; Strength of recommendation - strong).

Brand Names: U.S. Orap®
Brand Names: Canada Apo-Pimozide®; Orap®; PMS-Pimozide
Generic Availability (U.S.) No
Pharmacologic Category Antipsychotic Agent, Typical
Use Suppression of severe motor and phonic tics in patients with Tourette's disorder who have failed to respond satisfactorily to standard treatment
Unlabeled Use Psychosis; reported use in individuals with delusions focused on physical symptoms (ie, preoccupation with parasitic infestation); Huntington's chorea
Contraindications Hypersensitivity to pimozide or any component of the formulation; severe toxic CNS depression; coma; history of cardiac arrhythmias; congenital long QT syndrome; concurrent use with QT_c-prolonging agents; hypokalemia or hypomagnesemia; concurrent use of drugs that are inhibitors of CYP3A4, including concurrent use of the azole antifungals itraconazole and ketoconazole, macrolide antibiotics (eg, clarithromycin or erythromycin [Note: The manufacturer lists azithromycin and dirithromycin in its list of contraindicated macrolides; however, azithromycin does not inhibit CYP3A4, but may interact with pimozide on the basis of QT_c prolongation]), protease inhibitors (ie, atazanavir, indinavir, nelfinavir, ritonavir, saquinavir), citalopram, escitalopram, nefazodone, sertraline, and other less potent inhibitors of CYP3A4 (eg, fluvoxamine, zileuton); concurrent use with strong CYP2D6 inhibitors (eg, paroxetine); concurrent use with medications that may cause motor or phonic tics (eg, amphetamines, methylphenidate, pemoline) until it is determined if medications or Tourette's is causing tics; treatment of simple tics or tics other than Tourette's
Warnings/Precautions [U.S. Boxed Warning]: Elderly patients with dementia-related psychosis treated with antipsychotics are at an increased risk of death compared to placebo. Most deaths appeared to be either cardiovascular (eg, heart failure, sudden death) or infectious (eg, pneumonia) in nature. Pimozide is not approved for the treatment of dementia-related psychosis.

May alter cardiac conduction; life-threatening arrhythmias have occurred with therapeutic doses of antipsychotics. Contraindicated in patients with underlying QT prolongation, in those taking medicines that prolong the QT interval, or cause polymorphic ventricular tachycardia; monitor ECG closely for dose-related QT effects. Sudden unexplained deaths have occurred in patients taking high doses (>10 mg).

Leukopenia, neutropenia, and agranulocytosis (sometimes fatal) have been reported in clinical trials and postmarketing reports with antipsychotic use; presence of risk factors (eg, pre-existing low WBC or history of drug-induced leuko-/neutropenia) should prompt periodic blood count assessment. Discontinue therapy at first signs of blood dyscrasias or if absolute neutrophil count <1000/mm^3

Antipsychotic use has been associated with esophageal dysmotility and aspiration; use with caution in patients at risk of pneumonia (ie, Alzheimer's disease). May cause extrapyramidal symptoms (EPS), including pseudoparkinsonism, acute dystonic reactions, akathisia, and tardive dyskinesia. Risk of dystonia (and possibly other EPS) may be greater with increased doses, use of conventional antipsychotics, males, and younger patients. The risk for tardive dyskinesia (may be irreversible) increases with long-term treatment and higher cumulative doses. Use may be associated with NMS; monitor for mental status changes, fever, muscle rigidity, and/or autonomic instability; may also be associated with increased CPK, myoglobinuria, and acute renal failure. Discontinue use; may recur upon rechallenge. May be associated with pigmentary retinopathy. Impaired core body temperature regulation may occur; caution with strenuous exercise, heat exposure, dehydration, and concomitant medication possessing anticholinergic effects.

May be sedating, use with caution in disorders where CNS depression is a feature; patients must be cautioned about performing tasks which require mental alertness (eg, operating machinery or driving). Effects may be potentiated when used with other sedative drugs or ethanol. May cause anticholinergic effects (constipation, xerostomia, blurred vision, urinary retention); use with caution in patients with decreased gastrointestinal motility, paralytic ileus, urinary retention, BPH, xerostomia, or visual problems. Relative to neuroleptics, pimozide has a moderate potency of cholinergic blockade. Antipsychotics are associated with increased prolactin levels; clinical significance of hyperprolactinemia in patients with breast cancer or other prolactin-dependent tumors is unknown.

Use with caution in patients with severe cardiovascular disease, narrow-angle glaucoma, hepatic impairment, myasthenia gravis, Parkinson's disease, renal impairment, or seizure disorder. Use with caution in the elderly and in CYP2D6 poor metabolizers (dose adjustment required).

Use in patients with dementia is associated with an increased risk of mortality and cerebrovascular accidents; avoid antipsychotic use for behavioral problems associated with dementia unless alternative nonpharmacologic therapies have failed and patient may harm self or others. In addition, use may cause or exacerbate syndrome of inappropriate antidiuretic hormone secretion or hyponatremia; monitor sodium closely with initiation or dosage adjustments in older adults. May also be inappropriate in older adults depending on comorbidities (eg, dementia, delirium) due to its potent anticholinergic effects (Beers Criteria). Increased risk for developing tardive dyskinesia, particularly elderly women.

Adverse Reactions (Reflective of adult population; not specific for elderly)

Frequencies as reported in adults (limited data) and/or children with Tourette's disorder:

>10%:

Central nervous system: Sedation (70%), akathisia (40%), akinesia (40%), drowsiness (35%), behavior changes (22% to 25%), somnolence (up to 25% in children)

Gastrointestinal: Xerostomia (25%), constipation (20%)

Genitourinary: Impotence (15%)

Neuromuscular & skeletal: Muscle tightness (15%), weakness (14%)

Ocular: Accommodation decreased (20%), visual disturbance (3% to 20%)

1% to 10%:

Cardiovascular: Abnormal ECG (3%)

Central nervous system: Depression (10%), insomnia (10%), speech disorder (10%), nervousness (5% to 6%), headache (3% to 5%), dreams abnormal (3%), hyperkinesias (3%)

Dermatologic: Rash (3%)

Gastrointestinal: Salivation increased (6%), appetite increased (5%), diarrhea (5%), taste disturbance (5%), thirst (5%), dysphagia (3%)

Neuromuscular & skeletal: Rigidity (10%), stooped posture (10%), handwriting change (5%), myalgia (3%), torticollis (3%), tremor (3%)

Ocular: Photophobia (5%)

Frequency not defined, postmarketing, and/or case reports (some reported for disorders other than Tourette's disorder): Anorexia, blurred vision, cataracts, chest pain, diaphoresis, dizziness, excitement; extrapyramidal symptoms (dystonia, pseudoparkinsonism, tardive dyskinesia); GI distress, gingival hyperplasia (case report), hemolytic anemia, hyper-/hypotension, hyponatremia, libido decreased, nausea, neuroleptic malignant syndrome, nocturia, orthostatic hypotension, palpitation, periorbital edema, polyuria, QT_c prolongation, seizure, skin irritation, syncope, tachycardia, ventricular arrhythmia, vomiting, weight gain/loss

Drug Interactions

Metabolism/Transport Effects Substrate of CYP1A2 (major), CYP3A4 (major); **Note:** Assignment of Major/Minor substrate status based on clinically relevant drug interaction potential; **Inhibits** CYP2C19 (weak), CYP2D6 (weak), CYP2E1 (weak), CYP3A4 (weak)

Avoid Concomitant Use

Avoid concomitant use of Pimozide with any of the following: Antifungal Agents (Azole Derivatives, Systemic); Aprepitant; Azelastine; Azelastine (Nasal); Boceprevir; Crizotinib; CYP2D6 Inhibitors (Strong); CYP3A4 Inhibitors (Moderate); CYP3A4 Inhibitors (Strong); CYP3A4 Inhibitors (Weak); Efavirenz; Fosaprepitant; Grapefruit Juice; Highest Risk QTc-Prolonging Agents; Macrolide Antibiotics; Metoclopramide; Mifepristone; Moderate Risk QTc-Prolonging Agents; Nefazodone; Paraldehyde; Protease Inhibitors; Selective Serotonin Reuptake Inhibitors; Telaprevir; Zileuton

Increased Effect/Toxicity

Pimozide may increase the levels/effects of: Alcohol (Ethyl); Anticholinergics; ARIPiprazole; Azelastine; Azelastine (Nasal); Buprenorphine; CNS Depressants; Highest Risk QTc-Prolonging Agents; Methylphenidate; Paraldehyde; Serotonin Modulators; Zolpidem

The levels/effects of Pimozide may be increased by: Abiraterone Acetate; Acetylcholinesterase Inhibitors (Central); Antifungal Agents (Azole Derivatives, Systemic); Aprepitant; Boceprevir; Crizotinib; CYP1A2 Inhibitors (Moderate); CYP1A2 Inhibitors (Strong); CYP2D6 Inhibitors (Strong); CYP3A4 Inhibitors (Moderate); CYP3A4 Inhibitors (Strong); CYP3A4 Inhibitors (Weak); Deferasirox; Efavirenz; Fosaprepitant; Grapefruit Juice; HydrOXYzine; Ivacaftor; Lithium formulations; Macrolide Antibiotics; Methylphenidate; Metoclopramide; Metyrosine; Mifepristone; Moderate Risk QTc-Prolonging Agents; Nefazodone; Pramlintide;

Protease Inhibitors; QTc-Prolonging Agents (Indeterminate Risk and Risk Modifying); Selective Serotonin Reuptake Inhibitors; Telaprevir; Tetrabenazine; Zileuton

Decreased Effect

Pimozide may decrease the levels/effects of: Amphetamines; Anti-Parkinson's Agents (Dopamine Agonist); Quinagolide

The levels/effects of Pimozide may be decreased by: Anti-Parkinson's Agents (Dopamine Agonist); CYP1A2 Inducers (Strong); CYP3A4 Inducers (Strong); Cyproterone; Deferasirox; Lithium formulations; Tocilizumab

Ethanol/Nutrition/Herb Interactions

Ethanol: Ethanol may increase CNS depression. Management: Monitor for increased effects with coadministration. Caution patients about effects.

Food: Pimozide serum concentration may be increased when taken with grapefruit juice due to CYP3A4 inhibition. Management: Avoid concurrent use with grapefruit juice.

Herb/Nutraceutical: St John's wort may decrease pimozide levels through induction of CYP3A4. Kava kava, gotu kola, and valerian may increase CNS depression. Management: Avoid St John's wort, kava kava, gotu kola, and valerian.

Stability Store at 25°C (77°F); excursion permitted to 15°C to 30°C (59°F to 86°F).

Mechanism of Action Pimozide, a diphenylbutylperidine conventional antipsychotic, is a potent centrally-acting dopamine-receptor antagonist resulting in its characteristic neuroleptic effects

Pharmacodynamics/Kinetics

Absorption: ≥50%

Protein binding: 99%

Metabolism: Hepatic via N-dealkylation primarily by CYP3A4, but with contributions by CYP1A2 and CYP2D6; significant first-pass effect

Half-life elimination: ~55 hours

Time to peak, serum: 6-8 hours (range: 4-12 hours)

Excretion: Urine

Dosage

Geriatric Recommend initial dose of 1 mg/day; periodically attempt gradual reduction of dose to determine if tic persists; follow up for 1-2 weeks before concluding the tic is a persistent disease phenomenon and not a manifestation of drug withdrawal. **Note:** An ECG should be performed baseline and periodically thereafter, especially during dosage adjustment.

Adult

Tourette's disorder: Oral: Initial: 1-2 mg/day in divided doses, then increase dosage as needed every other day; maximum dose: 10 mg/day or 0.2 mg/kg/day (whichever is less); **Note:** If therapy requires exceeding dose of 4 mg/day, CYP2D6 geno-/phenotyping should be performed; CYP2D6 poor metabolizers should be dose titrated in ≥14-day increments and should not receive doses in excess of 4 mg/day.

Note: An ECG should be performed baseline and periodically thereafter, especially during dosage adjustment.

Monitoring Parameters ECG should be performed baseline and periodically thereafter, especially during dosage adjustment; vital signs; electrolytes, lipid profile, fasting blood glucose/Hgb A$_{1c}$; BMI; mental status, abnormal involuntary movement scale (AIMS), extrapyramidal symptoms (EPS); CYP2D6 genotyping or phenotyping

Test Interactions Increased prolactin (S)

Pharmacotherapy Pearls Causes less sedation, but is more likely to cause acute extrapyramidal symptoms than chlorpromazine.

Special Geriatric Considerations No specific clinical studies in the use of this drug in elderly; use with extreme caution in elderly due to cardiovascular effects. Consider cardiovascular effects of drugs an elderly patient may be receiving.

In the treatment of agitated, demented, older adult patients, authors of meta-analysis of controlled trials of the response to the traditional antipsychotics (phenothiazines, butyrophenones) in controlling agitation have concluded that the use of neuroleptics results in a response rate of 18%. Clearly neuroleptic therapy for behavior control should be limited with frequent attempts to withdraw the agent given for behavior control.

This medication is considered to be potentially inappropriate in this patient population (Beers Criteria: Quality of evidence - moderate; Strength of recommendation - strong).

Dosage Forms Excipient information presented when available (limited, particularly for generics); consult specific product labeling.

Tablet, oral:

Orap®: 1 mg, 2 mg [scored]

Pindolol (PIN doe lole)

Related Information
Beta-Blockers *on page* 2108
Medication Safety Issues
Sound-alike/look-alike issues:
Pindolol may be confused with Parlodel®, Plendil®
Visken® may be confused with Visine®, Viskazide®
Brand Names: Canada Apo-Pindol®; Dom-Pindolol; Mylan-Pindolol; Novo-Pindol; Nu-Pindol; PMS-Pindolol; Sandoz-Pindolol; Teva-Pindolol; Visken®
Generic Availability (U.S.) Yes
Pharmacologic Category Beta-Blocker With Intrinsic Sympathomimetic Activity
Use Treatment of hypertension, alone or in combination with other agents
Unlabeled Use Potential augmenting agent for antidepressants; treatment of ventricular arrhythmias/tachycardia, antipsychotic-induced akathisia, situational anxiety, aggressive behavior associated with dementia
Contraindications Bronchial asthma; cardiogenic shock; heart block (2nd or 3rd degree) except in patients with a functioning artificial pacemaker; overt cardiac failure; severe bradycardia
Warnings/Precautions Consider pre-existing conditions such as sick sinus syndrome before initiating. Use with caution in patients with inadequate myocardial function, bronchospastic disease, myasthenia gravis, peripheral vascular disease, renal impairment, psychiatric disease (may cause CNS depression) or impaired hepatic function. Use with caution in patients with diabetes mellitus; may potentiate hypoglycemia and/or mask signs and symptoms. May mask signs of hyperthyroidism (eg, tachycardia); if hyperthyroidism is suspected, carefully manage and monitor; abrupt withdrawal may exacerbate symptoms of hyperthyroidism or precipitate thyroid storm. Bradycardia may be observed more frequently in elderly patients (>65 years of age); dosage reductions may be necessary. Beta-blockers with intrinsic sympathomimetic activity (including pindolol) do not appear to be of benefit in HF. If use is warranted with compensated HF, use with caution and monitor for a worsening of the condition. If condition worsens, consider temporary discontinuation or dosage reduction of pindolol. Beta-blocker therapy should not be withdrawn abruptly (particularly in patients with CAD), but gradually tapered to avoid acute tachycardia, hypertension, and/or ischemia. Chronic beta-blocker therapy should not be routinely withdrawn prior to major surgery. Adequate alpha-blockade is required prior to use of any beta-blocker for patients with untreated pheochromocytoma. Use caution with history of severe anaphylaxis to allergens; patients taking beta-blockers may become more sensitive to repeated challenges. Treatment of anaphylaxis (eg, epinephrine) in patients taking beta-blockers may be ineffective or promote undesirable effects. Use with caution in patients on concurrent digoxin, verapamil, or diltiazem; bradycardia or heart block may occur. Use with caution in patients receiving inhaled anesthetic agents known to depress myocardial contractility.
Adverse Reactions (Reflective of adult population; not specific for elderly)
1% to 10%:
Cardiovascular: Edema (6%), chest pain (3%), bradycardia (≤2%), heart block (≤2%), hypotension (≤2%), syncope (≤2%), tachycardia (≤2%), palpitation (≤1%)
Central nervous system: Insomnia (10%), dizziness (9%), fatigue (8%), nervousness (7%), nightmares/vivid dreams (5%), anxiety (≤2%), lethargy (≤2%)
Dermatologic: Hyperhidrosis (≤2%), pruritus (1%)
Gastrointestinal: Nausea (5%), diarrhea (≤2%), vomiting (≤2%), weight gain (≤2%)
Genitourinary: Impotence (≤2%)
Hematologic: Claudication (≤2%)
Hepatic: ALT increased (7%), AST increased (7%)
Neuromuscular & skeletal: Muscle pain (10%), arthralgia (7%), weakness (4%), paresthesia (3%), muscle cramps (3%)
Ocular: Burning eyes (≤2%), visual disturbances (≤2%), eye discomfort (≤2%)
Renal: Polyuria (≤2%)
Respiratory: Dyspnea (5%), wheezing (≤2%)
Miscellaneous: Cold extremities (≤2%)
Other adverse reactions (noted with other beta-adrenergic-blocking agents that should be considered potential adverse events with pindolol): Agranulocytosis, alopecia, catatonia, clouded sensorium, disorientation, emotional lability, fever, intensification of pre-existing AV block, ischemic colitis, laryngospasm, mental depression, mesenteric artery thrombosis, nonthrombocytopenic purpura, Peyronie's disease, rash (erythematous), respiratory distress, short-term memory loss, thrombocytopenic purpura

Drug Interactions

Metabolism/Transport Effects Substrate of CYP2D6 (minor); **Note:** Assignment of Major/Minor substrate status based on clinically relevant drug interaction potential; **Inhibits** CYP2D6 (weak)

Avoid Concomitant Use

Avoid concomitant use of Pindolol with any of the following: Beta2-Agonists; Floctafenine; Methacholine

Increased Effect/Toxicity

Pindolol may increase the levels/effects of: Alpha-/Beta-Agonists (Direct-Acting); Alpha1-Blockers; Alpha2-Agonists; Amifostine; Antihypertensives; Antipsychotic Agents (Phenothiazines); ARIPiprazole; Bupivacaine; Cardiac Glycosides; Cholinergic Agonists; Fingolimod; Hypotensive Agents; Insulin; Lidocaine; Lidocaine (Systemic); Lidocaine (Topical); Mepivacaine; Methacholine; Midodrine; RiTUXimab; Sulfonylureas

The levels/effects of Pindolol may be increased by: Acetylcholinesterase Inhibitors; Aminoquinolines (Antimalarial); Amiodarone; Anilidopiperidine Opioids; Antipsychotic Agents (Phenothiazines); Calcium Channel Blockers (Dihydropyridine); Calcium Channel Blockers (Nondihydropyridine); Diazoxide; Dipyridamole; Disopyramide; Dronedarone; Floctafenine; Herbs (Hypotensive Properties); MAO Inhibitors; Pentoxifylline; Phosphodiesterase 5 Inhibitors; Propafenone; Prostacyclin Analogues; QuiNIDine; Reserpine; Selective Serotonin Reuptake Inhibitors

Decreased Effect

Pindolol may decrease the levels/effects of: Beta2-Agonists; Theophylline Derivatives

The levels/effects of Pindolol may be decreased by: Barbiturates; Herbs (Hypertensive Properties); Methylphenidate; Nonsteroidal Anti-Inflammatory Agents; Peginterferon Alfa-2b; Rifamycin Derivatives; Yohimbine

Ethanol/Nutrition/Herb Interactions Herb/Nutraceutical: Avoid bayberry, blue cohosh, cayenne, ephedra, ginger, ginseng (American), kola, and licorice (may worsen hypertension). Avoid black cohosh, california poppy, coleus, golden seal, hawthorn, mistletoe, periwinkle, quinine, and shepherd's purse (may increase antihypertensive effect).

Stability Store below 30°C (86°F). Protect from light.

Mechanism of Action Blocks both beta$_1$- and beta$_2$-receptors and has mild intrinsic sympathomimetic activity; pindolol has negative inotropic and chronotropic effects and can significantly slow AV nodal conduction. Augmentive action of antidepressants thought to be mediated via a serotonin 1A autoreceptor antagonism.

Pharmacodynamics/Kinetics

Absorption: Rapid, 50% to 95%

Distribution: V_d: ~2 L/kg

Protein binding: 40%

Metabolism: Hepatic (60% to 65%) to conjugates

Half-life elimination: 3-4 hours; prolonged with advanced age, and cirrhosis (range: 2.5-30 hours)

Time to peak, serum: ~1 hour

Excretion: Urine (35% to 40% as unchanged drug); feces (6% to 9%)

Dosage

Geriatric Oral: Initial: 5 mg once daily; increase as necessary by 5 mg/day every 3-4 weeks.

Adult

Hypertension: Oral: Initial: 5 mg twice daily, increase as necessary by 10 mg/day every 3-4 weeks (maximum daily dose: 60 mg); usual dose range (JNC 7): 10-40 mg twice daily.

Antidepressant augmentation (unlabeled use): Oral: 2.5 mg 3 times/day

Renal Impairment Use with caution. Clearance significantly decreased in uremic patients. Dosage reduction may be necessary.

Hepatic Impairment Use with caution. Elimination half-life in cirrhotic patients may be 10 times as long compared to normal patients. Dosage reduction is necessary in severely impaired.

Administration May be administered without regard to meals.

Monitoring Parameters Blood pressure, heart rate, respiratory function

Special Geriatric Considerations Due to alterations in the beta-adrenergic autonomic nervous system, beta-adrenergic blockade may result in less hemodynamic response than seen in younger adults. Studies indicate that despite decreased sensitivity to the chronotropic effects of beta-blockade with age, there appears to be an increased myocardial sensitivity to the negative inotropic effect during stress (eg, exercise). Controlled trials have shown the overall response rate for propranolol to be only 20% to 50% in elderly populations. Therefore, all beta-adrenergic blocking drugs may result in a decreased response as compared to younger adults.

Dosage Forms Excipient information presented when available (limited, particularly for generics); consult specific product labeling.
Tablet, oral: 5 mg, 10 mg

◆ **Pink Bismuth** *see* Bismuth *on page 216*

Pioglitazone (pye oh GLI ta zone)

Related Information
Diabetes Mellitus Management, Adults *on page 2193*
Medication Safety Issues
 Sound-alike/look-alike issues:
  Actos® may be confused with Actidose®, Actonel®
 High alert medication:
  The Institute for Safe Medication Practices (ISMP) includes this medication among its list of drug classes which have a heightened risk of causing significant patient harm when used in error.
 International issues:
  Tiazac: Brand name for pioglitazone [Chile], but also the brand name for diltiazem [U.S, Canada]
Brand Names: U.S. Actos®
Brand Names: Canada Accel-Pioglitazone; Actos®; Apo-Pioglitazone®; Ava-Pioglitazone; CO Pioglitazone; Dom-Pioglitazone; JAMP-Pioglitazone; Mint-Pioglitazone; Mylan-Pioglitazone; Novo-Pioglitazone; PHL-Pioglitazone; PMS-Pioglitazone; PRO-Pioglitazone; ratio-Pioglitazone; Sandoz-Pioglitazone; Teva-Pioglitazone; ZYM-Pioglitazone
Generic Availability (U.S.) Yes
Pharmacologic Category Antidiabetic Agent, Thiazolidinedione
Use
 Type 2 diabetes mellitus (noninsulin dependent, NIDDM), monotherapy: Adjunct to diet and exercise, to improve glycemic control
 Type 2 diabetes mellitus (noninsulin dependent, NIDDM), combination therapy with sulfonylurea, metformin, or insulin: When diet, exercise, and a single agent alone does not result in adequate glycemic control
Medication Guide Available Yes
Contraindications Hypersensitivity to pioglitazone or any component of the formulation; NYHA Class III/IV heart failure (initiation of therapy)

 Canadian labeling: Additional contraindications (not in U.S. labeling): Any stage of heart failure (eg, NYHA Class I, II, III, IV); serious hepatic impairment
Warnings/Precautions [U.S. Boxed Warning]: Thiazolidinediones, including pioglitazone, may cause or exacerbate heart failure; closely monitor for signs and symptoms of heart failure (eg, rapid weight gain, dyspnea, edema), particularly after initiation or dose increases. Not recommended for use in any patient with symptomatic heart failure. In the U.S., initiation of therapy is contraindicated in patients with NYHA class III or IV heart failure. If used in patients with NYHA class II (systolic heart failure), initiate at lowest dosage and monitor closely. In Canada, use in any stage of heart failure (NYHA I, II, III, IV) is contraindicated. Use with caution in patients with edema; may increase plasma volume and/or cause fluid retention. Dose reduction or discontinuation is recommended if heart failure suspected. Dose-related weight gain observed with use; mechanism unknown but likely associated with fluid retention and fat accumulation.

 Should not be used in diabetic ketoacidosis. Mechanism requires the presence of insulin; therefore use in type 1 diabetes is not recommended. Use with caution in patients with anemia (may reduce hemoglobin and hematocrit). Increased incidence of bone fractures in females treated with pioglitazone; majority of fractures occurred in the lower limb and distal upper limb.

 Use with caution in patients with elevated transaminases (AST or ALT); do not initiate in patients with active liver disease of ALT >2.5 times the upper limit of normal at baseline. During therapy, if ALT >3 times the upper limit of normal, re-evaluate levels promptly and discontinue if elevation persists or if jaundice occurs at any time during use. Idiosyncratic hepatotoxicity has been reported with another thiazolidinedione agent (troglitazone); avoid use in patients who previously experienced jaundice during troglitazone therapy. Monitoring should include periodic determinations of liver function. Use caution with pre-existing macular edema or diabetic retinopathy. Postmarketing reports of new-onset or worsening diabetic macular edema with decreased visual acuity has been reported.

 Canadian labeling (not in U.S. labeling) states use with insulin **or** as part of triple therapy (pioglitazone in combination with a sulfonylurea and metformin) is not indicated.

Adverse Reactions (Reflective of adult population; not specific for elderly)

>10%:

Cardiovascular: Edema (5%; in combination trials with sulfonlyureas or insulin, the incidence of edema was as high as 15%)

Respiratory: Upper respiratory tract infection (13%)

1% to 10%:

Cardiovascular: Heart failure (requiring hospitalization; up to 6% in patients with prior macrovascular disease)

Central nervous system: Headache (9%), fatigue (4%)

Hematologic: Anemia (≤2%)

Neuromuscular & skeletal: Myalgia (5%)

Respiratory: Sinusitis (6%), pharyngitis (5%)

Frequency not defined: HDL-cholesterol increased, hematocrit/hemoglobin decreased, hypoglycemia (in combination trials with sulfonylureas or insulin), serum triglycerides decreased, weight gain/loss

Drug Interactions

Metabolism/Transport Effects Substrate of CYP2C8 (major), CYP3A4 (minor); **Note:** Assignment of Major/Minor substrate status based on clinically relevant drug interaction potential; **Inhibits** CYP2C19 (weak), CYP2C8 (moderate), CYP2C9 (weak); **Induces** CYP3A4 (weak/moderate)

Avoid Concomitant Use

Avoid concomitant use of Pioglitazone with any of the following: Axitinib

Increased Effect/Toxicity

Pioglitazone may increase the levels/effects of: CYP2C8 Substrates; Hypoglycemic Agents

The levels/effects of Pioglitazone may be increased by: CYP2C8 Inhibitors (Moderate); CYP2C8 Inhibitors (Strong); Deferasirox; Gemfibrozil; Herbs (Hypoglycemic Properties); Insulin; MAO Inhibitors; Mifepristone; Pegvisomant; Pregabalin; Salicylates; Selective Serotonin Reuptake Inhibitors; Trimethoprim

Decreased Effect

Pioglitazone may decrease the levels/effects of: ARIPiprazole; Axitinib; Saxagliptin

The levels/effects of Pioglitazone may be decreased by: Bile Acid Sequestrants; Corticosteroids (Orally Inhaled); Corticosteroids (Systemic); CYP2C8 Inducers (Strong); Loop Diuretics; Luteinizing Hormone-Releasing Hormone Analogs; Rifampin; Somatropin; Thiazide Diuretics; Tocilizumab

Ethanol/Nutrition/Herb Interactions

Ethanol: Caution with ethanol (may cause hypoglycemia).

Food: Peak concentrations are delayed when administered with food, but the extent of absorption is not affected. Pioglitazone may be taken without regard to meals.

Herb/Nutraceutical: Caution with alfalfa, aloe, bilberry, bitter melon, burdock, celery, damiana, fenugreek, garcinia, garlic, ginger, ginseng (American), gymnema, marshmallow, and stinging nettle (may cause hypoglycemia).

Mechanism of Action Thiazolidinedione antidiabetic agent that lowers blood glucose by improving target cell response to insulin, without increasing pancreatic insulin secretion. It has a mechanism of action that is dependent on the presence of insulin for activity. Pioglitazone is a potent and selective agonist for peroxisome proliferator-activated receptor-gamma (PPAR-gamma). Activation of nuclear PPARgamma receptors influences the production of a number of gene products involved in glucose and lipid metabolism. PPARgamma is abundant in the cells within the renal collecting tubules; fluid retention results from stimulation by thiazolidinediones which increases sodium reabsorption.

Pharmacodynamics/Kinetics

Onset of action: Delayed

Peak effect: Glucose control: Several weeks

Distribution: V_{ss} (apparent): 0.63 L/kg

Protein binding: Pioglitazone >99% and active metabolites >98%; primarily to albumin

Metabolism: Hepatic (99%) via CYP2C8 and 3A4 to both active and inactive metabolites

Half-life elimination: Parent drug: 3-7 hours; Total: 16-24 hours

Time to peak: ~2 hours; delayed with food

Excretion: Urine (15% to 30%) and feces as metabolites

Dosage

Geriatric & Adult Type 2 diabetes: Oral:

Monotherapy: Initial: 15-30 mg once daily; if response is inadequate, the dosage may be increased in increments up to 45 mg once daily; maximum recommended dose: 45 mg once daily

Combination therapy:

Note: Maximum recommended dose: 45 mg/day

With sulfonylureas: Initial: 15-30 mg once daily; dose of sulfonylurea should be reduced if the patient reports hypoglycemia

With metformin: Initial: 15-30 mg once daily; it is unlikely that the dose of metformin will need to be reduced due to hypoglycemia

With insulin: Initial: 15-30 mg once daily; dose of insulin should be reduced by 10% to 25% if the patient reports hypoglycemia or if the plasma glucose falls to below 100 mg/dL.

Dosage adjustment in patients with CHF (NYHA Class II) in mono- or combination therapy: Oral: Initial: 15 mg once daily; may be increased after several months of treatment, with close attention to heart failure symptoms

Renal Impairment No adjustment is necessary.

Hepatic Impairment Clearance is significantly lower in hepatic impairment (Child-Pugh Grade B/C). Therapy should not be initiated if the patient exhibits active liver disease or increased transaminases (>2.5 times ULN) at baseline. During treatment if ALT levels elevate >3 times ULN, the test should be repeated as soon as possible. If ALT levels remain >3 times ULN or if the patient is jaundiced, therapy should be discontinued.

Administration May be administered without regard to meals

Monitoring Parameters Hemoglobin A$_{1c}$, serum glucose; signs and symptoms of heart failure; liver enzymes prior to initiation and periodically during treatment (per clinician judgment). If the ALT is increased to >2.5 times the upper limit of normal, liver function testing should be performed more frequently until the levels return to normal or pretreatment values. Patients with an elevation in ALT >3 times the upper limit of normal should be rechecked as soon as possible. If the ALT levels remain >3 times the upper limit of normal, therapy with pioglitazone should be discontinued. Routine ophthalmic exams are recommended; patients reporting visual deterioration should have a prompt referral to an ophthalmologist and consideration should be given to discontinuing pioglitazone.

Reference Range Recommendations for glycemic control in adults with diabetes:

Hb A$_{1c}$: <7%

Preprandial capillary plasma glucose: 70-130 mg/dL

Peak postprandial capillary blood glucose: <180 mg/dL

Special Geriatric Considerations Intensive glucose control (Hb A$_{1c}$ <6.5%) has been linked to increased all-cause and cardiovascular mortality, hypoglycemia requiring assistance, and weight gain in adult type 2 diabetes. How "tightly" to control a geriatric patient's blood glucose needs to be individualized. Such a decision should be based on several factors, including the patient's functional and cognitive status, how well he/she recognizes hypoglycemic or hyperglycemic symptoms, and how to respond to them and other disease states. An Hb A$_{1c}$ <7.5% is an acceptable endpoint for a healthy older adult, while <8% is acceptable for frail elderly patients, those with a duration of illness >10 years, or those with comorbid conditions and requiring combination diabetes medications. For elderly patients with diabetes who are relatively healthy, attaining target goals for aspirin use, blood pressure, lipids, smoking cessation, and diet and exercise may be more important than normalized glycemic control. In elderly patients with heart failure, this medication is considered potentially inappropriate (Beers Criteria, 2012).

Dosage Forms Excipient information presented when available (limited, particularly for generics); consult specific product labeling.

Tablet, oral: 15 mg, 30 mg, 45 mg

Actos®: 15 mg, 30 mg, 45 mg

Pioglitazone and Glimepiride (pye oh GLI ta zone & GLYE me pye ride)

Related Information

Glimepiride *on page* 877

Pioglitazone *on page* 1542

Medication Safety Issues

High alert medication:

The Institute for Safe Medication Practices (ISMP) includes this medication among its list of drugs which have a heightened risk of causing significant patient harm when used in error.

Brand Names: U.S. Duetact™

Index Terms Glimepiride and Pioglitazone; Glimepiride and Pioglitazone Hydrochloride

Generic Availability (U.S.) No

Pharmacologic Category Antidiabetic Agent, Sulfonylurea; Antidiabetic Agent, Thiazolidinedione; Hypoglycemic Agent, Oral

Use Management of type 2 diabetes mellitus (noninsulin dependent, NIDDM) as an adjunct to diet and exercise

Medication Guide Available Yes

Dosage
Geriatric Initial: Glimepiride 1 mg/day prior to initiating Duetact™; dose titration and maintenance dosing should be conservative to avoid hypoglycemia. Refer to adult dosing.

Adult Type 2 diabetes mellitus: Oral: Initial dose should be based on current dose of pioglitazone and/or sulfonylurea.

Patients inadequately controlled on **glimepiride** alone: Initial dose: 30 mg/2 mg or 30 mg/4 mg once daily

Patients inadequately controlled on **pioglitazone** alone: Initial dose: 30 mg/2 mg once daily

Patients with systolic dysfunction (eg, NYHA Class I and II): Initiate only after patient has been safely titrated to 30 mg of pioglitazone. Initial dose: 30 mg/2 mg or 30 mg/4 mg once daily.

Note: No exact dosing relationship exists between glimepiride and other sulfonlyureas. Dosing should be limited to less than or equal to the maximum initial dose of glimepiride (2 mg). When converting patients from other sulfonylureas with longer half-lives (eg, chlorpropamide) to glimepiride, observe patient carefully for 1-2 weeks due to overlapping hypoglycemic effects.

Dosing adjustment: Dosage may be increased up to max dose and formulation strengths available; tablet should not be given more than once daily; see individual agents for frequency of adjustments. Dosage adjustments in patients with systolic dysfunction should be done carefully and patient monitored for symptoms of worsening heart failure.

Maximum dose: Pioglitazone 45 mg/glimepiride 8 mg daily

Renal Impairment Cl_{cr} <22 mL/minute: Initial dose should be 1 mg of glimepiride and dosage increments should be based on fasting blood glucose levels.

Hepatic Impairment Do not initiate treatment with active liver disease or ALT >2.5 times ULN. During treatment, if ALT levels elevate >3 times ULN, the test should be repeated as soon as possible. If ALT levels remain >3 times ULN or if the patient is jaundiced, Duetact™ should be discontinued.

Special Geriatric Considerations See individual agents. Combination products are not recommended as first-line treatment. Use only if doses of individual agents correspond to the combination available.

Dosage Forms Excipient information presented when available (limited, particularly for generics); consult specific product labeling.

Tablet:

Duetact™:
30 mg/2 mg: Pioglitazone 30 mg and glimepiride 2 mg
30 mg/4 mg: Pioglitazone 30 mg and glimepiride 4 mg

Pioglitazone and Metformin (pye oh GLI ta zone & met FOR min)

Related Information
MetFORMIN *on page 1222*
Pioglitazone *on page 1542*

Medication Safety Issues
High alert medication:
The Institute for Safe Medication Practices (ISMP) includes this medication among its list of drug classes which have a heightened risk of causing significant patient harm when used in error.

Brand Names: U.S. Actoplus Met®; Actoplus Met® XR
Index Terms Metformin Hydrochloride and Pioglitazone Hydrochloride
Generic Availability (U.S.) Yes: Excludes variable release tablet
Pharmacologic Category Antidiabetic Agent, Biguanide; Antidiabetic Agent, Thiazolidine-dione
Use Management of type 2 diabetes mellitus (noninsulin dependent, NIDDM)
Medication Guide Available Yes
Dosage
Geriatric Refer to adult dosing. The initial and maintenance dosing should be conservative, due to the potential for decreased renal function (monitor). Generally, elderly patients should not be titrated to the maximum; do not use in patients ≥80 years of age unless normal renal function has been established.

Adult Type 2 diabetes mellitus: Oral: Initial dose should be based on current dose of pioglitazone and/or metformin; metformin dose may be titrated every 1-2 weeks and pioglitazone dose may be titrated every 2-3 months as necessary to achieve goals

Immediate release tablet: **Note:** Daily doses higher than pioglitazone 15 mg plus metformin 850 mg should be divided. Initial: Pioglitazone 15 mg plus metformin 500 mg **or** pioglitazone 15 mg plus metformin 850 mg tablets once or twice daily. Maximum daily dose: Pioglitazone 45 mg/metformin 2550 mg

Variable release tablet: Pioglitazone 15 mg plus metformin 1000 mg tablet **or** pioglitazone 30 mg plus metformin 1000 mg tablet once daily with evening meal. Maximum daily dose: Pioglitazone 45 mg/metformin 2000 mg

Renal Impairment Do not use with renal disease or renal dysfunction (serum creatinine ≥1.5 mg/dL in males or ≥1.4 mg/dL in females or abnormal clearance).

Hepatic Impairment Do not initiate treatment with active liver disease or ALT >2.5 times ULN. During treatment, if ALT concentrations increase >3 times ULN, the test should be repeated as soon as possible. If ALT concentrations remain >3 times ULN or if the patient is jaundiced, therapy should be discontinued.

Special Geriatric Considerations See individual agents. Combination products are not recommended as first-line treatment. Use only if doses of individual agents correspond to the combination available.

Dosage Forms Excipient information presented when available (limited, particularly for generics); consult specific product labeling.

Tablet, oral: 15/500: Pioglitazone 15 mg and metformin hydrochloride 500 mg; 15/850: Pioglitazone 15 mg and metformin hydrochloride 850 mg

Actoplus Met®:

15/500: Pioglitazone 15 mg and metformin hydrochloride 500 mg
15/850: Pioglitazone 15 mg and metformin hydrochloride 850 mg

Tablet, variable release, oral:

Actoplus Met® XR:

15/1000: Pioglitazone 15 mg [immediate release] and metformin hydrochloride 1000 mg [extended release]
30/1000: Pioglitazone 30 mg [immediate release] and metformin hydrochloride 1000 mg [extended release]

Piperacillin (pi PER a sil in)

Related Information
Antimicrobial Drugs of Choice *on page 2163*
Brand Names: Canada Piperacillin for Injection, USP
Index Terms Piperacillin Sodium
Pharmacologic Category Antibiotic, Penicillin
Use Treatment of susceptible infections such as septicemia, acute and chronic respiratory tract infections, skin and soft tissue infections, and urinary tract infections due to susceptible strains of *Pseudomonas*, *Proteus*, and *Escherichia coli* and *Enterobacter*; active against some streptococci and some anaerobic bacteria; febrile neutropenia (as part of combination regimen)
Contraindications Hypersensitivity to piperacillin, other beta-lactam antibiotics (penicillins or cephalosporins), or any component of the formulation
Warnings/Precautions Serious and occasionally severe or fatal hypersensitivity (anaphylactoid) reactions have been reported in patients on penicillin therapy, especially with a history of beta-lactam hypersensitivity, history of sensitivity to multiple allergens, or previous IgE-mediated reactions (eg, anaphylaxis, angioedema, urticaria). Use with caution in asthmatic patients. Bleeding disorders have been observed, particularly in patients with renal impairment; discontinue if thrombocytopenia or bleeding occurs. Due to sodium load and adverse effects (anemia, neuropsychological changes), use with caution and modify dosage in patients with renal impairment. Use caution in patients with history of seizure activity. Leukopenia and neutropenia have been reported (during prolonged therapy). An increased frequency of fever and rash has been reported in patients with cystic fibrosis. Prolonged use may result in fungal or bacterial superinfection, including *C. difficile*-associated diarrhea (CDAD) and pseudomembranous colitis; CDAD has been observed >2 months postantibiotic treatment.
Adverse Reactions (Reflective of adult population; not specific for elderly) Frequency not defined.
Central nervous system: Confusion, convulsions, drowsiness, fever, Jarisch-Herxheimer reaction
Dermatologic: Rash, toxic epidermal necrolysis, urticaria
Endocrine & metabolic: Electrolyte imbalance, hypokalemia
Hematologic: Abnormal platelet aggregation and prolonged PT (high doses), agranulocytosis, Coombs' reaction (positive), hemolytic anemia, pancytopenia
Local: Thrombophlebitis
Neuromuscular & skeletal: Myoclonus
Renal: Acute interstitial nephritis, acute renal failure
Miscellaneous: Anaphylaxis, hypersensitivity reactions

Drug Interactions

Metabolism/Transport Effects None known.

Avoid Concomitant Use

Avoid concomitant use of Piperacillin with any of the following: BCG

Increased Effect/Toxicity

Piperacillin may increase the levels/effects of: Methotrexate; Vitamin K Antagonists

The levels/effects of Piperacillin may be increased by: Probenecid

Decreased Effect

Piperacillin may decrease the levels/effects of: Aminoglycosides; BCG; Mycophenolate; Typhoid Vaccine

The levels/effects of Piperacillin may be decreased by: Fusidic Acid; Tetracycline Derivatives

Stability Reconstituted solution is stable (I.V. infusion) in NS or D_5W for 24 hours at room temperature, 7 days when refrigerated, or 4 weeks when frozen. After freezing, thawed solution is stable for 24 hours at room temperature or 48 hours when refrigerated. 40 g bulk vial should **not** be frozen after reconstitution.

Mechanism of Action Inhibits bacterial cell wall synthesis by binding to one or more of the penicillin-binding proteins (PBPs); which in turn inhibits the final transpeptidation step of peptidoglycan synthesis in bacterial cell walls, thus inhibiting cell wall biosynthesis. Bacteria eventually lyse due to ongoing activity of cell wall autolytic enzymes (autolysins and murein hydrolases) while cell wall assembly is arrested.

Pharmacodynamics/Kinetics

Absorption: I.M.: 70% to 80%

Protein binding: ~16%

Bioavailability: Not well absorbed when given orally

Half-life elimination (dose dependent; prolonged with moderately severe renal or hepatic impairment): 36-80 minutes

Time to peak, serum: I.M.: 30-50 minutes

Excretion: Primarily urine; partially feces

Dosage

Geriatric Adjust dose for renal impairment:

I.M.: 1-2 g every 8-12 hours

I.V.: 2-4 g every 6-8 hours

Adult

Usual dosage range:

I.M.: 2-3 g/dose every 6-12 hours; maximum: 24 g/24 hours

I.V.: 3-4 g/dose every 4-6 hours; maximum: 24 g/24 hours

Burn wound sepsis: I.V.: 4 g every 4 hours with vancomycin and amikacin

Cholangitis, acute: I.V.: 4 g every 6 hours

Keratitis *(Pseudomonas):* Ophthalmic: 6-12 mg/mL every 15-60 minutes around the clock for 24-72 hours, then slow reduction

Malignant otitis externa: I.V.: 4-6 g every 4-6 hours with tobramycin

Moderate infections: I.M., I.V.: 2-3 g/dose every 6-12 hours (maximum: 2 g I.M./site)

Prosthetic joint *(Pseudomonas):* I.V.: 3 g every 6 hours with aminoglycoside

Pseudomonas **infections:** I.V.: 4 g every 4 hours

Severe infections: I.M., I.V.: 3-4 g/dose every 4-6 hours (maximum: 24 g/24 hours)

Urinary tract infections: I.V.: 2-3 g/dose every 6-12 hours

Uncomplicated gonorrhea: I.M.: 2 g in a single dose accompanied by 1 g probenecid 30 minutes prior to injection

Renal Impairment

Cl_{cr} 10-50 mL/minute: Administer every 6-8 hours.

Cl_{cr} <10 mL/minute: Administer every 8 hours.

Moderately dialyzable (20% to 50%)

Continuous arteriovenous or venovenous hemofiltration: Dose as for Cl_{cr} 10-50 mL/minute.

Administration Administer around-the-clock to promote less variation in peak and trough serum levels. Give at least 1 hour apart from aminoglycosides. Rapid administration can lead to seizures. Administer direct I.V. over 3-5 minutes. Intermittently infusion over 30 minutes. Do not administer more than 2 g per I.M. injection site.

Some penicillins (eg, carbenicillin, ticarcillin, and piperacillin) have been shown to inactivate aminoglycosides *in vitro*. This has been observed to a greater extent with tobramycin and gentamicin, while amikacin has shown greater stability against inactivation. Concurrent use of these agents may pose a risk of reduced antibacterial efficacy *in vivo*, particularly in the setting of profound renal impairment. However, definitive clinical evidence is lacking. If combination penicillin/aminoglycoside therapy is desired in a patient with renal dysfunction, separation of doses (if feasible), and routine monitoring of aminoglycoside levels, CBC, and clinical response should be considered.

Monitoring Parameters Observe for signs and symptoms of anaphylaxis during first dose

Test Interactions May interfere with urinary glucose tests using cupric sulfate (Benedict's solution, Clinitest®); false-positive urinary and serum proteins, positive Coombs' test [direct]. False-positive Platelia® *Aspergillus* EIA test (Bio-Rad Laboratories) has been reported.
Some penicillin derivatives may accelerate the degradation of aminoglycosides *in vitro*, leading to a potential underestimation of aminoglycoside serum concentration.

Pharmacotherapy Pearls Sodium content of 1 g: 1.85 mEq. Administer 1 hour apart from aminoglycosides.

Special Geriatric Considerations Because of piperacillin's lower sodium content, it is preferred over ticarcillin in patients with a history of heart failure and/or renal or hepatic disease. Adjust dose for renal function.

Piperacillin and Tazobactam (pi PER a sil in & ta zoe BAK tam)

Related Information
Antimicrobial Drugs of Choice *on page 2163*
Community-Acquired Pneumonia in Adults *on page 2171*
Piperacillin *on page 1546*

Medication Safety Issues
Sound-alike/look-alike issues:
Zosyn® may be confused with Zofran®, Zyvox®
International issues:
Tazact [India] may be confused with Tazac brand name for nizatidine [Australia]; Tiazac brand name for diltiazem [U.S., Canada]

Brand Names: U.S. Zosyn®

Brand Names: Canada Piperacillin and Tazobactam for Injection; Tazocin®

Index Terms Piperacillin and Tazobactam Sodium; Piperacillin Sodium and Tazobactam Sodium; Tazobactam and Piperacillin

Generic Availability (U.S.) Yes: Excludes infusion

Pharmacologic Category Antibiotic, Penicillin

Use Treatment of moderate-to-severe infections caused by susceptible organisms, including infections of the lower respiratory tract (community-acquired pneumonia, nosocomial pneumonia); uncomplicated and complicated skin and skin structures (including diabetic foot infections); gynecologic (endometritis, pelvic inflammatory disease); and intra-abdominal infections (appendicitis with rupture/abscess, peritonitis). Tazobactam expands activity of piperacillin to include beta-lactamase producing strains of *S. aureus, H. influenzae, E. coli, Bacteroides* spp and other gram-positive and gram-negative aerobic and anaerobic bacteria.

Unlabeled Use Treatment of moderate-to-severe infections caused by susceptible organisms, including urinary tract infections, bone and joint infections, septicemia, endocarditis, and cystic fibrosis exacerbations

Contraindications Hypersensitivity to penicillins, cephalosporins, beta-lactamase inhibitors, or any component of the formulation

Warnings/Precautions Serious and occasionally severe or fatal hypersensitivity (anaphylactic/anaphylactoid) reactions have been reported in patients on penicillin therapy, especially with a history of beta-lactam hypersensitivity, history of sensitivity to multiple allergens, or previous IgE-mediated reactions (eg, anaphylaxis, angioedema, urticaria). Bleeding disorders have been observed, particularly in patients with renal impairment; discontinue if thrombocytopenia or bleeding occurs. Due to sodium load and to the adverse effects of high serum concentrations of penicillins, dosage modification is required in patients with impaired or underdeveloped renal function; use with caution in patients with seizures or in patients with history of beta-lactam allergy; associated with an increased incidence of rash and fever in cystic fibrosis patients. Use may result in fungal or bacterial superinfection, including *C. difficile*-associated diarrhea (CDAD) and pseudomembranous colitis; CDAD has been observed >2 months postantibiotic treatment.

Adverse Reactions (Reflective of adult population; not specific for elderly)
>10%: Gastrointestinal: Diarrhea (7% to 11%)
1% to 10%:
Cardiovascular: Hypertension (2%), chest pain (1%), edema (1%)
Central nervous system: Insomnia (7%), headache (8%), fever (2% to 5%), agitation (2%), pain (2%), anxiety (1% to 2%), dizziness (1% to 2%)
Dermatologic: Rash (4%), pruritus (3%)
Gastrointestinal: Constipation (1% to 8%), nausea (7%), vomiting (3% to 4%), dyspepsia (3%), stool changes (2%), abdominal pain (1% to 2%)
Hepatic: AST increased (1%)
Local: Local reaction (3%), phlebitis (1%)
Respiratory: Pharyngitis (2%), dyspnea (1%), rhinitis (1%)
Miscellaneous: Moniliasis (2%), sepsis (2%), infection (2%)

Drug Interactions

Metabolism/Transport Effects None known.

Avoid Concomitant Use

Avoid concomitant use of Piperacillin and Tazobactam with any of the following: BCG

Increased Effect/Toxicity

Piperacillin and Tazobactam may increase the levels/effects of: Methotrexate; Vitamin K Antagonists

The levels/effects of Piperacillin and Tazobactam may be increased by: Probenecid

Decreased Effect

Piperacillin and Tazobactam may decrease the levels/effects of: Aminoglycosides; BCG; Mycophenolate; Typhoid Vaccine

The levels/effects of Piperacillin and Tazobactam may be decreased by: Fusidic Acid; Tetracycline Derivatives

Stability

Vials: Store at controlled room temperature of 20°C to 25°C (68°F to 77°F). Use single-dose vials immediately after reconstitution (discard unused portions after 24 hours at room temperature and 48 hours if refrigerated). Reconstitute with 5 mL of diluent per 1 g of piperacillin and then further dilute. After reconstitution, vials or solution are stable in NS or D_5W for 24 hours at room temperature and 48 hours (vials) or 7 days (solution) when refrigerated.

Premixed solution: Store frozen at -20°C (-4°F). Thawed solution is stable for 24 hours at room temperature or 14 days under refrigeration; do not refreeze.

Mechanism of Action Piperacillin inhibits bacterial cell wall synthesis by binding to one or more of the penicillin-binding proteins (PBPs); which in turn inhibits the final transpeptidation step of peptidoglycan synthesis in bacterial cell walls, thus inhibiting cell wall biosynthesis. Bacteria eventually lyse due to ongoing activity of cell wall autolytic enzymes (autolysins and murein hydrolases) while cell wall assembly is arrested. Piperacillin exhibits time-dependent killing. Tazobactam inhibits many beta-lactamases, including staphylococcal penicillinase and Richmond-Sykes types 2, 3, 4, and 5, including extended spectrum enzymes; it has only limited activity against class 1 beta-lactamases other than class 1C types.

Pharmacodynamics/Kinetics Both AUC and peak concentrations are dose proportional; hepatic impairment does not affect kinetics

Distribution: Well into lungs, intestinal mucosa, uterus, ovary, fallopian tube, interstitial fluid, gallbladder, and bile; penetration into CSF is low in subjects with noninflamed meninges

Protein binding: Piperacillin and tazobactam: ~30%

Metabolism:

Piperacillin: 6% to 9% to desethyl metabolite (weak activity)

Tazobactam: ~26% to inactive metabolite

Bioavailability:

Piperacillin: I.M.: 71%

Tazobactam: I.M.: 84%

Half-life elimination: Piperacillin and tazobactam: 0.7-1.2 hours (unaffected by dose or duration of infusion)

Time to peak, plasma: Immediately following completion of 30-minute infusion

Excretion: Clearance of both piperacillin and tazobactam are directly proportional to renal function

Piperacillin: Urine (68% as unchanged drug); feces (10% to 20%)

Tazobactam: Urine (80% as unchanged drug; remainder as inactive metabolite)

Dialysis: Hemodialysis removes 30% to 40% of a piperacillin/tazobactam dose; peritoneal dialysis removes 6% of piperacillin and 21% of tazobactam

Dosage

Geriatric & Adult Note: Dosing presented is based on traditional infusion method (I.V. infusion over 30 minutes) unless otherwise specified as the extended infusion method (I.V. infusion over 4 hours [unlabeled method]).

Usual dosage range: I.V.: 3.375 g every 6 hours **or** 4.5 g every 6-8 hours; maximum: 18 g/day

Extended infusion method (unlabeled dosing): 3.375-4.5 g I.V. over 4 hours every 8 hours (Kim, 2007; Shea, 2009); an alternative regimen of 4.5 g I.V. over 3 hours every 6 hours has also been described (Kim, 2007)

Indication-specific dosing: I.V.: **Note:** Dosing based on piperacillin component:

Diverticulitis, intra-abdominal abscess, peritonitis: I.V.: 3.375 g every 6 hours; **Note:** Some clinicians use 4.5 g every 8 hours for empiric coverage since the %time>MIC is similar between the regimens for most pathogens; however, this regimen is NOT recommended for nosocomial pneumonia or Pseudomonas coverage.

Intra-abdominal infection, complicated: I.V.: 3.375 g every 6 hours for 4-7 days (provided source controlled). **Note:** Increase to 3.375 g every 4 hours or 4.5 g every 6 hours if *P. aeruginosa* is suspected. Not recommended for mild-to-moderate, community-acquired intra-abdominal infections due to risk of toxicity and the development of resistant organisms (Solomkin, 2010).

Pneumonia (nosocomial): I.V.: 4.5 g every 6 hours for 7-14 days (when used empirically, combination with an aminoglycoside or antipseudomonal fluoroquinolone is recommended; consider discontinuation of additional agent if *P. aeruginosa* is not isolated)

Severe infections: I.V.: 3.375 g every 6 hours for 7-10 days; **Note:** Some clinicians use 4.5 g every 8 hours for empiric coverage since the %time>MIC is similar between the regimens for most pathogens; however, this regimen is NOT recommended for nosocomial pneumonia or *Pseudomonas* coverage.

Skin and soft tissue infection: I.V.: 3.375 g every 6-8 hours for 7-14 days. **Notes:** When used for necrotizing infection of skin, fascia, or muscle, combination with clindamycin and ciprofloxacin is recommended (Stevens, 2005); for severe diabetic foot infections, recommended treatment duration is up to 4 weeks depending on severity of infection and response to therapy (Lipsky, 2012).

Renal Impairment

Traditional infusion method (ie, I.V. infusion over 30 minutes): Manufacturer's labeling:

Cl_{cr} >40 mL/minute: No dosage adjustment required.

Cl_{cr} 20-40 mL/minute: Administer 2.25 g every 6 hours (3.375 g every 6 hours for nosocomial pneumonia)

Cl_{cr} <20 mL/minute: Administer 2.25 g every 8 hours (2.25 g every 6 hours for nosocomial pneumonia)

Note: Some clinicians suggest adjusting the dose at Cl_{cr} ≤20 mL/minute (rather than Cl_{cr} <40 mL/minute) in patients receiving either traditional or extended-infusion methods, particularly if treating serious gram-negative infections (empirically or definitively) (Patel, 2010).

Extended infusion method (unlabeled dosing): Cl_{cr} ≤20 mL/minute: 3.375 g I.V. over 4 hours every 12 hours (Patel, 2010)

Intermittent hemodialysis (IHD)/peritoneal dialysis (PD): 2.25 g every 12 hours (2.25 g every 8 hours for nosocomial pneumonia). **Note:** Dosing dependent on the assumption of 3 times/week, complete IHD sessions. Administer scheduled doses after hemodialysis on dialysis days; if next regularly scheduled dose is not due right after dialysis session, administer an additional dose of 0.75 g after the dialysis session.

Continuous renal replacement therapy (CRRT) (Heintz, 2009; Trotman, 2005): Drug clearance is highly dependent on the method of renal replacement, filter type, and flow rate. Appropriate dosing requires close monitoring of pharmacologic response, signs of adverse reactions due to drug accumulation, as well as drug concentrations in relation to target trough (if appropriate). The following are general recommendations only (based on dialysate flow/ultrafiltration rates of 1-2 L/hour and minimal residual renal function) and should not supersede clinical judgment (Trotman, 2005):

CVVH: 2.25-3.375 g every 6-8 hours

CVVHD: 2.25-3.375 g every 6 hours

CVVHDF: 3.375 g every 6 hours

Note: Higher dose of 3.375 g should be considered when treating resistant pathogens (especially *Pseudomonas* spp); alternative recommendations suggest dosing of 4.5 g every 8 hours (Valtonen, 2001); regardless of regimen, there is some concern of tazobactam (TAZ) accumulation, given its lower clearance relative to piperacillin (PIP). Some clinicians advocate dosing with PIP to alternate with PIP/TAZ, particularly in CVVH-dependent patients, to lessen this concern.

Hepatic Impairment No dosage adjustment necessary.

Administration Administer by I.V. infusion over 30 minutes. For extended infusion administration (unlabeled dosing), administer over 3-4 hours (Kim 2007; Shea, 2009).

Some penicillins (eg, carbenicillin, ticarcillin, and piperacillin) have been shown to inactivate aminoglycosides *in vitro*. This has been observed to a greater extent with tobramycin and gentamicin, while amikacin has shown greater stability against inactivation. Concurrent use of these agents may pose a risk of reduced antibacterial efficacy *in vivo*, particularly in the setting of profound renal impairment. However, definitive clinical evidence is lacking. If combination penicillin/aminoglycoside therapy is desired in a patient with renal dysfunction, separation of doses (if feasible), and routine monitoring of aminoglycoside levels, CBC, and clinical response should be considered. **Note:** Reformulated Zosyn® containing EDTA (applies only to specific concentrations and diluents and varies by product; consult manufacturer's labeling) has been shown to be compatible *in vitro* for Y-site infusion with amikacin and gentamicin, but not compatible with tobramycin.

Monitoring Parameters Creatinine, BUN, CBC with differential, PT, PTT, serum electrolytes, LFTs, urinalysis; signs of bleeding; monitor for signs of anaphylaxis during first dose

Test Interactions Positive Coombs' [direct] test; false positive reaction for urine glucose using copper-reduction method (Clinitest®); may result in false positive results with the Platelia® *Aspergillus* enzyme immunoassay (EIA)

Some penicillin derivatives may accelerate the degradation of aminoglycosides *in vitro*, leading to a potential underestimation of aminoglycoside serum concentration. **Note:** Reformulated Zosyn® containing EDTA (applies only to specific concentrations and diluents and varies by product; consult manufacturer's labeling) has been shown to be compatible *in vitro* for Y-site infusion with amikacin and gentamicin, but not compatible with tobramycin.

Special Geriatric Considerations Has not been studied exclusively in the elderly. Adjust dose for renal function.

Dosage Forms Excipient information presented when available (limited, particularly for generics); consult specific product labeling.

Note: 8:1 ratio of piperacillin sodium/tazobactam sodium

Infusion [premixed iso-osmotic solution]:

Zosyn®: 2.25 g: Piperacillin 2 g and tazobactam 0.25 g (50 mL) [contains edetate disodium, sodium 128 mg (5.58 mEq)]

Zosyn®: 3.375 g: Piperacillin 3 g and tazobactam 0.375 g (50 mL) [contains edetate disodium, sodium 192 mg (8.38 mEq)]

Zosyn®: 4.5 g: Piperacillin 4 g and tazobactam 0.5 g (100 mL) [contains edetate disodium, sodium 256 mg (11.17 mEq)]

Injection, powder for reconstitution: 2.25 g: Piperacillin 2 g and tazobactam 0.25 g; 3.375 g: Piperacillin 3 g and tazobactam 0.375 g; 4.5 g: Piperacillin 4 g and tazobactam 0.5 g; 40.5 g: Piperacillin 36 g and tazobactam 4.5 g

Zosyn®: 2.25 g: Piperacillin 2 g and tazobactam 0.25 g [contains edetate disodium, sodium 128 mg (5.58 mEq)]

Zosyn®: 3.375 g: Piperacillin 3 g and tazobactam 0.375 g [contains edetate disodium, sodium 192 mg (8.38 mEq)]

Zosyn®: 4.5 g: Piperacillin 4 g and tazobactam 0.5 g [contains edetate disodium, sodium 256 mg (11.17 mEq)]

Zosyn®: 40.5 g: Piperacillin 36 g and tazobactam 4.5 g [contains edetate disodium, sodium 2304 mg (100.4 mEq); bulk pharmacy vial]

◆ **Piperacillin and Tazobactam Sodium** *see* Piperacillin and Tazobactam *on page 1548*
◆ **Piperacillin Sodium** *see* Piperacillin *on page 1546*
◆ **Piperacillin Sodium and Tazobactam Sodium** *see* Piperacillin and Tazobactam *on page 1548*

Pirbuterol (peer BYOO ter ole)

Related Information

Inhalant Agents *on page 2117*

Brand Names: U.S. Maxair® Autohaler®

Index Terms Pirbuterol Acetate

Generic Availability (U.S.) No

Pharmacologic Category Beta$_2$ Agonist

Use Prevention and treatment of reversible bronchospasm including asthma

Contraindications Hypersensitivity to pirbuterol, albuterol, or any component of the formulation

Warnings/Precautions Optimize anti-inflammatory treatment before initiating maintenance treatment with pirbuterol. Do not use as a component of chronic therapy without an anti-inflammatory agent. Only the mildest form of asthma (Step 1 and/or exercise-induced) would not require concurrent use based upon asthma guidelines. Patient must be instructed to seek medical attention in cases where acute symptoms are not relieved or a previous level of response is diminished. The need to increase frequency of use may indicate deterioration of asthma, and treatment must not be delayed.

Use caution in patients with cardiovascular disease (arrhythmia or hypertension or CHF), convulsive disorders, diabetes, glaucoma, hyperthyroidism, or hypokalemia. Beta-agonists may cause elevation in blood pressure, heart rate, and result in CNS stimulation/excitation. Beta$_2$-agonists may increase risk of arrhythmia, increase serum glucose, or decrease serum potassium.

Do not exceed recommended dose; serious adverse events including fatalities, have been associated with excessive use of inhaled sympathomimetics. Rarely, paradoxical bronchospasm may occur with use of inhaled bronchodilating agents; this should be distinguished from inadequate response. All patients should utilize a spacer device when using a metered-dose inhaler.

Adverse Reactions (Reflective of adult population; not specific for elderly)
>10%:
Central nervous system: Nervousness (7%)
Endocrine & metabolic: Serum glucose increased, serum potassium decreased
Neuromuscular & skeletal: Trembling (6%)
1% to 10%:
Cardiovascular: Palpitation (2%), tachycardia (1%)
Central nervous system: Headache (2%), dizziness (1%)
Gastrointestinal: Nausea (2%)
Respiratory: Cough (1%)

Drug Interactions
Metabolism/Transport Effects None known.
Avoid Concomitant Use
Avoid concomitant use of Pirbuterol with any of the following: Beta-Blockers (Nonselective); Iobenguane I 123
Increased Effect/Toxicity
Pirbuterol may increase the levels/effects of: Loop Diuretics; Sympathomimetics; Thiazide Diuretics

The levels/effects of Pirbuterol may be increased by: AtoMOXetine; Cannabinoids; MAO Inhibitors; Tricyclic Antidepressants
Decreased Effect
Pirbuterol may decrease the levels/effects of: Iobenguane I 123

The levels/effects of Pirbuterol may be decreased by: Alpha-/Beta-Blockers; Beta-Blockers (Beta1 Selective); Beta-Blockers (Nonselective); Betahistine
Stability Store between 15°C and 30°C (59°F and 86°F).
Mechanism of Action Pirbuterol is a beta$_2$-adrenergic agonist with a similar structure to albuterol, specifically a pyridine ring has been substituted for the benzene ring in albuterol. The increased beta$_2$ selectivity of pirbuterol results from the substitution of a tertiary butyl group on the nitrogen of the side chain, which additionally imparts resistance of pirbuterol to degradation by monoamine oxidase and provides a lengthened duration of action in comparison to the less selective previous beta-agonist agents.
Pharmacodynamics/Kinetics
Onset of action: Peak effect: Therapeutic: Oral: 2-3 hours with peak serum concentration of 6.2-9.8 mcg/L; Inhalation: 0.5-1 hour
Half-life elimination: 2-3 hours
Metabolism: Hepatic
Excretion: Urine (10% as unchanged drug)
Dosage
Geriatric & Adult Bronchospasm: Inhalation: 2 inhalations every 4-6 hours for prevention; 2 inhalations at an interval of at least 1-3 minutes, followed by a third inhalation in treatment of bronchospasm, not to exceed 12 inhalations/day
Administration Inhalation: Shake inhaler well before use.
Monitoring Parameters Respiratory rate; FEV$_1$, peak flow, and/or other pulmonary function tests; blood pressure, heart rate; CNS stimulation; serum glucose, serum potassium
Special Geriatric Considerations Elderly patients may find it beneficial to utilize a spacer device when using a metered dose inhaler. Difficulty in using the inhaler often limits its effectiveness. The Maxair™ Autohaler™ may be easier for the elderly to use.
Dosage Forms Excipient information presented when available (limited, particularly for generics); consult specific product labeling.
Aerosol, for oral inhalation, as acetate:
Maxair® Autohaler®: 200 mcg/actuation (14 g) [contains chlorofluorocarbon; 400 actuations]

◆ **Pirbuterol Acetate** *see* Pirbuterol *on page 1551*

Piroxicam (peer OKS i kam)

Related Information
Beers Criteria – Potentially Inappropriate Medications for Geriatrics *on page 2183*
Medication Safety Issues
Sound-alike/look-alike issues:
Feldene® may be confused with FLUoxetine
Piroxicam may be confused with PARoxetine

BEERS Criteria medication:
This drug may be potentially inappropriate for use in geriatric patients (Quality of evidence - moderate; Strength of recommendation - strong).

International issues:
Flogene [Brazil] may be confused with Flogen brand name for naproxen [Mexico]; Florone brand name for diflorasone [Germany, Greece]; Flovent brand name for fluticasone [U.S., Canada]

Brand Names: U.S. Feldene®

Brand Names: Canada Apo-Piroxicam®; Dom-Piroxicam; Novo-Pirocam; Nu-Pirox; PMS-Piroxicam

Generic Availability (U.S.) Yes

Pharmacologic Category Nonsteroidal Anti-inflammatory Drug (NSAID), Oral

Use Symptomatic treatment of acute and chronic rheumatoid arthritis and osteoarthritis

Canadian labeling: Additional use (not in U.S. labeling): Symptomatic treatment of ankylosing spondylitis

Medication Guide Available Yes

Contraindications Hypersensitivity or asthma-type reactions to piroxicam, aspirin, other NSAIDs or any component of the formulation; perioperative pain in the setting of coronary artery bypass graft (CABG) surgery; active peptic ulcer; severe renal and hepatic failure; severe heart failure

Canadian labeling: Additional contraindications (not in U.S. labeling): Recent or recurrent history of GI bleeding; active GI inflammatory disease; inflammatory bowel disease; cerebrovascular bleeding or other bleeding disorders; active liver disease; deteriorating renal disease; known hyperkalemia

Warnings/Precautions [U.S. Boxed Warning]: NSAIDs are associated with an increased risk of adverse cardiovascular thrombotic events, including MI and stroke. Risk may be increased with duration of use or pre-existing cardiovascular risk factors or disease. Carefully evaluate individual cardiovascular risk profiles prior to prescribing. May cause new-onset hypertension or worsening of existing hypertension. Use caution with fluid retention or heart failure. Use is contraindicated in severe heart failure. Concurrent administration of ibuprofen, and potentially other nonselective NSAIDs, may interfere with aspirin's cardioprotective effect. **[U.S. Boxed Warning]: Use is contraindicated for treatment of perioperative pain in the setting of coronary artery bypass graft (CABG) surgery.** Risk of MI and stroke may be increased with use following CABG surgery.

Platelet adhesion and aggregation may be decreased; may prolong bleeding time; patients with coagulation disorders or who are receiving anticoagulants should be monitored closely. Anemia may occur; patients on long-term NSAID therapy should be monitored for anemia. Rarely, NSAID use may cause severe blood dyscrasias (eg, agranulocytosis, aplastic anemia, thrombocytopenia).

NSAID use may compromise existing renal function; dose-dependent decreases in prostaglandin synthesis may result from NSAID use, reducing renal blood flow which may cause renal decompensation. NSAID use may increase the risk for hyperkalemia. Patients with impaired renal function, dehydration, heart failure, liver dysfunction, those taking diuretics, and ACE inhibitors, and the elderly are at greater risk of renal toxicity and hyperkalemia. Rehydrate patient before starting therapy; monitor renal function closely. Use is contraindicated in severe renal failure (Canadian labeling also contraindicates use in patients with deteriorating renal disease or known hyperkalemia). Long-term NSAID use may result in renal papillary necrosis.

[U.S. Boxed Warning]: NSAIDs may increase risk of gastrointestinal irritation, inflammation, ulceration, bleeding, and perforation. These events may occur at any time during therapy and without warning. Use caution with a history of GI disease (bleeding or ulcers), concurrent therapy with aspirin, anticoagulants and/or corticosteroids, smoking, use of alcohol, the elderly or debilitated patients. When used concomitantly with ≤325 mg of aspirin, a substantial increase in the risk of gastrointestinal complications (eg, ulcer) occurs; concomitant gastroprotective therapy (eg, proton pump inhibitors) is recommended (Bhatt, 2008). Use is contraindicated with active peptic ulcers.

Use the lowest effective dose for the shortest duration of time, consistent with individual patient goals, to reduce risk of cardiovascular or GI adverse events. Alternate therapies should be considered for patients at high risk.

NSAIDs may cause serious skin adverse events including exfoliative dermatitis, Stevens-Johnson syndrome (SJS) and toxic epidermal necrolysis (TEN); discontinue use at first sign of skin rash or hypersensitivity. Anaphylactoid reactions may occur, even without prior exposure;

◄ patients with "aspirin triad" (bronchial asthma, aspirin intolerance, rhinitis) may be at increased risk. Do not use in patients who experience bronchospasm, asthma, rhinitis, or urticaria with NSAID or aspirin therapy. Use caution with other forms of asthma. A serum sickness-like reaction can rarely occur; watch for arthralgias, pruritus, fever, fatigue, and rash.

Use with caution in patients with decreased hepatic function (contraindicated in severe hepatic impairment). Closely monitor patients with any abnormal LFT. Severe hepatic reactions (eg, fulminant hepatitis, liver failure) have occurred with NSAID use, rarely; discontinue if signs or symptoms of liver disease develop, or if systemic manifestations occur. Use with caution in poor CYP2C9 metabolizers as hepatic metabolism may be reduced resulting in elevated serum concentrations.

NSAIDS may cause drowsiness, dizziness, blurred vision and other neurologic effects which may impair physical or mental abilities; patients must be cautioned about performing tasks which require mental alertness (eg, operating machinery or driving). Discontinue use with blurred or diminished vision and perform ophthalmologic exam. Monitor vision with long-term therapy.

In the elderly, avoid chronic use (unless alternative agents ineffective and patient can receive concomitant gastroprotective agent); nonselective oral NSAID use is associated with an increased risk of GI bleeding and peptic ulcer disease in older adults in high risk category (eg, >75 years or age or receiving concomitant oral/parenteral corticosteroids, anticoagulants, or antiplatelet agents) (Beers Criteria).

Withhold for at least 4-6 half-lives prior to surgical or dental procedures.

Adverse Reactions (Reflective of adult population; not specific for elderly)
Reported with piroxicam or other NSAIDS:
1% to 10%:
Cardiovascular: Edema
Central nervous system: Dizziness, headache
Dermatologic: Pruritus, rash
Gastrointestinal: Abdominal pain, anorexia, bleeding, constipation, diarrhea, dyspepsia, flatulence, heartburn, nausea, perforation, ulcer, vomiting
Hematologic: Anemia, bleeding time increased
Hepatic: Liver enzymes increased
Otic: Tinnitus
Renal: Renal function abnormal

Drug Interactions
Metabolism/Transport Effects Substrate of CYP2C9 (major); **Note:** Assignment of Major/Minor substrate status based on clinically relevant drug interaction potential; **Inhibits** CYP2C9 (weak)

Avoid Concomitant Use
Avoid concomitant use of Piroxicam with any of the following: Floctafenine; Ketorolac; Ketorolac (Nasal); Ketorolac (Systemic)

Increased Effect/Toxicity
Piroxicam may increase the levels/effects of: Aliskiren; Aminoglycosides; Anticoagulants; Antiplatelet Agents; Bisphosphonate Derivatives; Collagenase (Systemic); CycloSPORINE; CycloSPORINE (Systemic); Dabigatran Etexilate; Deferasirox; Desmopressin; Digoxin; Drotrecogin Alfa (Activated); Eplerenone; Haloperidol; Ibritumomab; Lithium; Methotrexate; Nonsteroidal Anti-Inflammatory Agents; PEMEtrexed; Porfimer; Potassium-Sparing Diuretics; PRALAtrexate; Quinolone Antibiotics; Rivaroxaban; Salicylates; Thrombolytic Agents; Tositumomab and Iodine I 131 Tositumomab; Vancomycin; Vitamin K Antagonists

The levels/effects of Piroxicam may be increased by: ACE Inhibitors; Angiotensin II Receptor Blockers; Antidepressants (Tricyclic, Tertiary Amine); Corticosteroids (Systemic); CycloSPORINE; CycloSPORINE (Systemic); CYP2C9 Inhibitors (Moderate); CYP2C9 Inhibitors (Strong); Dasatinib; Floctafenine; Glucosamine; Herbs (Anticoagulant/Antiplatelet Properties); Ketorolac; Ketorolac (Nasal); Ketorolac (Systemic); Mifepristone; Nonsteroidal Anti-Inflammatory Agents; Omega-3-Acid Ethyl Esters; Pentosan Polysulfate Sodium; Pentoxifylline; Probenecid; Prostacyclin Analogues; Selective Serotonin Reuptake Inhibitors; Serotonin/Norepinephrine Reuptake Inhibitors; Sodium Phosphates; Tipranavir; Treprostinil; Vitamin E

Decreased Effect
Piroxicam may decrease the levels/effects of: ACE Inhibitors; Aliskiren; Angiotensin II Receptor Blockers; Antiplatelet Agents; Beta-Blockers; Eplerenone; HydrALAZINE; Loop Diuretics; Potassium-Sparing Diuretics; Salicylates; Selective Serotonin Reuptake Inhibitors; Thiazide Diuretics

The levels/effects of Piroxicam may be decreased by: Bile Acid Sequestrants; CYP2C9 Inducers (Strong); Nonsteroidal Anti-Inflammatory Agents; Peginterferon Alfa-2b; Salicylates

Ethanol/Nutrition/Herb Interactions

Ethanol: Avoid ethanol (may enhance gastric mucosal irritation).

Food: Onset of effect may be delayed if piroxicam is taken with food.

Herb/Nutraceutical: Avoid alfalfa, anise, bilberry, bladderwrack, bromelain, cat's claw, celery, chamomile, coleus, cordyceps, dong quai, evening primrose, fenugreek, feverfew, garlic, ginger, ginkgo biloba, ginseng (American, Panax, Siberian), grapeseed, green tea, guggul, horse chestnut seed, horseradish, licorice, prickly ash, red clover, reishi, SAMe (S-adenosylmethionine), sweet clover, turmeric, white willow (all have additional antiplatelet activity).

Stability Store at 15°C to 30°C (59°F to 86°F)

Mechanism of Action Reversibly inhibits cyclooxygenase-1 and 2 (COX-1 and 2) enzymes, which results in decreased formation of prostaglandin precursors; has antipyretic, analgesic, and anti-inflammatory properties

Other proposed mechanisms not fully elucidated (and possibly contributing to the anti-inflammatory effect to varying degrees), include inhibiting chemotaxis, altering lymphocyte activity, inhibiting neutrophil aggregation/activation, and decreasing proinflammatory cytokine levels.

Pharmacodynamics/Kinetics

Distribution: V_d: 0.14 L/kg

Protein binding: 99%

Metabolism: Hepatic predominantly via CYP2C9; metabolites are inactive

Half-life elimination: 50 hours

Time to peak: 3-5 hours

Excretion: Primarily urine and feces (small amounts) as unchanged drug (5%) and metabolites

Dosage

Geriatric Refer to adult dosing. Initiate therapy cautiously at low end of dosing range.

Adult Osteoarthritis, rheumatoid arthritis: Oral: 10-20 mg/day in 1-2 divided doses (maximum dose: 20 mg/day)

Ankylosing spondylitis (Canadian labeling; not an approved use in U.S. labeling): Oral: 10-20 mg/day in 1-2 divided doses (maximum dose: 20 mg/day)

Renal Impairment Use is contraindicated in severe renal failure (**Note:** Canadian labeling also contraindicates use in patients with deteriorating renal disease).

Mild-to-moderate impairment: U.S. labeling suggests that dosing adjustments may not be required. Canadian labeling suggests that dose reductions may be necessary although the manufacturer's labeling does not provide specific dose recommendations.

Hepatic Impairment Use is contraindicated in severe hepatic failure. Dose reductions may be necessary with lesser degrees of hepatic impairment although the manufacturer's labeling does not provide specific dose recommendations.

Administration May administer with food or milk to decrease GI upset.

Monitoring Parameters Occult blood loss, hemoglobin, hematocrit, electrolytes, and periodic renal and hepatic function tests; periodic ophthalmologic exams with chronic use

Test Interactions Increased bleeding time

Special Geriatric Considerations Elderly are a high-risk population for adverse effects from NSAIDs. As much as 60% of elderly can develop peptic ulceration and/or hemorrhage asymptomatically. The concomitant use of H_2 blockers and sucralfate is not generally effective as prophylaxis with the exception of NSAID-induced duodenal ulcers which may be prevented by the use of ranitidine. Misoprostol and proton pump inhibitors are the only agents proven to help prevent the development of NSAID-induced ulcers. Also, concomitant disease and drug use contribute to the risk for GI adverse effects. Use lowest effective dose for shortest period possible. Consider renal function decline with age. Use of NSAIDs can compromise existing renal function especially when Cl_{cr} is ≤30 mL/minute. Tinnitus may be a difficult and unreliable indication of toxicity due to age-related hearing loss or eighth cranial nerve damage. CNS adverse effects such as confusion, agitation, and hallucination are generally seen in overdose or high dose situations, but elderly may demonstrate these adverse effects at lower doses than younger adults.

This medication is considered to be potentially inappropriate in this patient population (Beers Criteria: Quality of evidence - moderate; Strength of recommendation - strong).

Dosage Forms Excipient information presented when available (limited, particularly for generics); consult specific product labeling.

Capsule, oral: 10 mg, 20 mg

Feldene®: 10 mg, 20 mg

◆ *p*-Isobutylhydratropic Acid *see* Ibuprofen *on page 966*

Pitavastatin (pi TA va sta tin)

Related Information
Hyperlipidemia Management *on page 2130*

Medication Safety Issues
Sound-alike/look-alike issues:
Pitavastatin may be confused with atorvaSTATin, fluvastatin, lovastatin, nystatin, pravastatin, rosuvastatin, simvastatin

Brand Names: U.S. Livalo®

Index Terms Pitavastatin Calcium

Generic Availability (U.S.) No

Pharmacologic Category Antilipemic Agent, HMG-CoA Reductase Inhibitor

Use Adjunct to dietary therapy to reduce elevations in total cholesterol (TC), LDL-C, apolipoprotein B (Apo B), and triglycerides (TG), and to increase low HDL-C in patients with primary hyperlipidemia and mixed dyslipidemia

Contraindications Hypersensitivity to pitavastatin or any component of the formulation; active liver disease including unexplained persistent elevations of hepatic transaminases; concurrent use with cyclosporine

Warnings/Precautions Secondary causes of hyperlipidemia should be ruled out prior to therapy. Pitavastatin has not been studied when the primary lipid abnormality is chylomicron elevation (Fredrickson types I and V) or in familial dysbetalipoproteinemia (Fredrickson type III). May cause hepatic dysfunction; in all patients, liver function must be monitored prior to initiation of therapy; repeat LFTs if clinically indicated thereafter; routine periodic monitoring of liver enzymes is not necessary. Use with caution in patients who consume large amounts of ethanol or have a history of liver disease; use is contraindicated in patients with active liver disease or unexplained persistent elevations of serum transaminases. If serious hepatotoxicity with clinical symptoms and/or hyperbilirubinemia or jaundice occurs during treatment, interrupt therapy. If an alternate etiology is not identified, do not restart pitavastatin.

Myopathy and rhabdomyolysis with acute renal failure have occurred with use. Risk is dose related and is increased with concurrent use of lipid-lowering agents which may cause rhabdomyolysis (fibric acid derivatives or niacin at doses ≥1 g/day) or during concurrent use with erythromycin or protease inhibitors. Use caution in patients with renal impairment, inadequately treated hypothyroidism, and those taking other drugs associated with myopathy (eg, colchicine); these patients are predisposed to myopathy. Monitor closely if used with other drugs associated with myopathy. Weigh the risk versus benefit when combining any of these drugs with pitavastatin. The manufacturer recommends temporary discontinuation for elective major surgery, acute medical or surgical conditions, or in any patient experiencing an acute or serious condition predisposing to renal failure (eg, sepsis, hypotension, trauma, uncontrolled seizures). However, based upon current evidence, HMG-CoA reductase inhibitor therapy should be continued in the perioperative period unless risk outweighs cardioprotective benefit. Patients should be instructed to report unexplained muscle pain, tenderness, weakness, or brown urine. Concurrent use with cyclosporine is contraindicated. Ensure patient is on the lowest effective pitavastatin dose. Use with caution in elderly patients, as these patients are predisposed to myopathy. Increases in Hb A_{1c} and fasting blood glucose have been reported with HMG-CoA reductase inhibitors; however, the benefits of statin therapy far outweigh the risk of dysglycemia.

Adverse Reactions (Reflective of adult population; not specific for elderly)
2% to 10%:
Gastrointestinal: Constipation (2% to 4%), diarrhea (2% to 3%)
Neuromuscular & skeletal: Back pain (1% to 4%), myalgia (2% to 3%), pain in extremities (1% to 2%)
Additional class-related events or case reports (not necessarily reported with pitavastatin therapy): Cataracts, cirrhosis, dermatomyositis, eosinophilia, extraocular muscle movement impaired, fulminant hepatic necrosis, gynecomastia, hypersensitivity syndrome (symptoms may include anaphylaxis, angioedema, arthralgia, erythema multiforme, eosinophilia, hemolytic anemia, interstitial lung disease, lupus syndrome, photosensitivity, polymyalgia rheumatica, positive ANA, purpura, Stevens-Johnson syndrome, toxic epidermal necrolysis, urticaria, vasculitis), ophthalmoplegia, peripheral nerve palsy, rhabdomyolysis, renal failure (secondary to rhabdomyolysis), thyroid dysfunction, tremor, vertigo

Drug Interactions
Metabolism/Transport Effects Substrate of SLCO1B1, UGT1A3, UGT2B7

Avoid Concomitant Use
Avoid concomitant use of Pitavastatin with any of the following: CycloSPORINE; CycloSPORINE (Systemic); Gemfibrozil; Red Yeast Rice

Increased Effect/Toxicity

Pitavastatin may increase the levels/effects of: DAPTOmycin; Pazopanib; Trabectedin; Vitamin K Antagonists

The levels/effects of Pitavastatin may be increased by: Atazanavir; Colchicine; Cyclo-SPORINE; CycloSPORINE (Systemic); Danazol; Eltrombopag; Fenofibrate; Fenofibric Acid; Gemfibrozil; Macrolide Antibiotics; Niacin; Niacinamide; Red Yeast Rice; Rifamycin Derivatives; Sildenafil

Decreased Effect

Pitavastatin may decrease the levels/effects of: Lanthanum

The levels/effects of Pitavastatin may be decreased by: Antacids; Bosentan; St Johns Wort

Ethanol/Nutrition/Herb Interactions

Ethanol: Avoid excessive ethanol consumption (due to potential hepatic effects).
Food: Red yeast rice contains an estimated 2.4 mg lovastatin per 600 mg rice.

Stability Store at controlled room temperature of 15°C to 30°C (59°F to 86°F). Protect from light.

Mechanism of Action Inhibitor of 3-hydroxy-3-methylglutaryl coenzyme A (HMG-CoA) reductase, the rate-limiting enzyme in cholesterol synthesis (reduces the production of mevalonic acid from HMG-CoA); this then results in a compensatory increase in the expression of LDL receptors on hepatocyte membranes and a stimulation of LDL catabolism

Pharmacodynamics/Kinetics

Distribution: V_d: ~148 L
Protein binding: >99%
Metabolism: Hepatic, via UGT1A3 and UGT 2B7; minimal metabolism via CYP2C9 and CYP2C8
Bioavailability: 51%
Half-life elimination: ~12 hours
Time to peak, plasma: ~1 hour
Excretion: Feces (79%); urine (15%)

Dosage

Geriatric & Adult

Primary hyperlipidemia and mixed dyslipidemia: Oral: Initial: 2 mg once daily; may be increased to maximum 4 mg once daily

Note: Doses should be individualized according to the baseline LDL-cholesterol levels, the recommended goal of therapy, and patient response; adjustments should be made at intervals of 4 weeks.

Dosage adjustment with concomitant medications:

Erythromycin: Pitavastatin dose should not exceed 1 mg once daily
Rifampin: Pitavastatin dose should not exceed 2 mg once daily

Renal Impairment

Cl_{cr} 15-60 mL/minute/1.73 m² (not receiving hemodialysis): Initial: 1 mg once daily; maximum: 2 mg once daily
ESRD: Initial: 1 mg once daily; maximum: 2 mg once daily

Hepatic Impairment Contraindicated in active liver disease or in patients with unexplained persistent elevations of serum transaminases.

Administration May be administered with or without food; may take without regard to time of day.

Monitoring Parameters Baseline CPK (recheck CPK in any patient with symptoms suggestive of myopathy; discontinue therapy if markedly elevated); renal function; baseline liver function tests (LFTs) and repeat when clinically indicated thereafter. Patients with elevated transaminase levels should have a second (confirmatory) test and frequent monitoring until values normalize; discontinue if increase in ALT/AST is persistently >3 times ULN (NCEP, 2002).

Lipid panel (total cholesterol, HDL, LDL, triglycerides):

ATP III recommendations (NCEP, 2002): Baseline; 6-8 weeks after initiation of drug therapy; if dose increased, then at 6-8 weeks until final dose determined. Once treatment goal achieved, follow up intervals may be reduced to every 4-6 months. Lipid panel should be assessed at least annually, and preferably at each clinic visit.

Manufacturer recommendation: Upon initiation or titration, lipid panel should be analyzed after 4 weeks of therapy.

Special Geriatric Considerations The definition of and, therefore, when to treat hyperlipidemia in the elderly is a controversial issue. The National Cholesterol Education Program recommends that all adults maintain a plasma cholesterol <160 mg/dL. For elderly patients with one additional risk factor, goal LDL would be <130 mg/dL. It is the authors' belief that pharmacologic treatment be reserved for those who are unable to obtain a desirable plasma cholesterol concentration by diet alone and for whom the benefits of treatment are believed to outweigh the potential adverse effects, drug interactions, and cost of treatment. Age ≥65 years is a risk factor for myopathy.

Dosage Forms Excipient information presented when available (limited, particularly for generics); consult specific product labeling.

Tablet, oral:

Livalo®: 1 mg, 2 mg, 4 mg

Pneumococcal Polysaccharide Vaccine (Polyvalent)

(noo moe KOK al pol i SAK a ride vak SEEN, pol i VAY lent)

Related Information
Immunization Administration Recommendations *on page 2144*
Immunization Recommendations *on page 2149*

Medication Safety Issues

Sound-alike/look-alike issues:

Pneumococcal 23-Valent Polysaccharide Vaccine (Pneumovax® 23) may be confused with Pneumococcal 7-Valent Conjugate Vaccine (Prevnar®) or with Pneumococcal 13-Valent Conjugate Vaccine (Prevnar 13®)

Brand Names: U.S. Pneumovax® 23

Brand Names: Canada Pneumo 23™; Pneumovax® 23

Index Terms 23-Valent Pneumococcal Polysaccharide Vaccine; 23PS; PPSV; PPSV23; PPV23

Generic Availability (U.S.) No

Pharmacologic Category Vaccine, Inactivated (Bacterial)

Use Immunization against pneumococcal disease caused by serotypes included in the vaccine. Routine vaccination is recommended for persons ≥50 years of age and persons ≥2 years in certain situations.

The Advisory Committee on Immunization Practices (ACIP) recommends routine vaccination for the following (CDC, 59[34], 2010; CDC, 59[11], 2010):

Patients ≥65 years of age without a history of vaccination (CDC, 61[4], 2012)

Patients 2-18 years of age with certain high-risk condition(s):
- Chronic heart disease (particularly cyanotic congenital heart disease and cardiac failure)
- Chronic lung disease (including asthma if treated with high-dose oral corticosteroids)

Patients 2-64 years of age with certain high-risk condition(s):
- Diabetes mellitus
- Cochlear implants
- Cerebrospinal fluid leaks
- Functional or anatomic asplenia (including sickle cell disease and other hemoglobino-pathies, splenic dysfunction, or splenectomy)
- Immunocompromising conditions including congenital immunodeficiency (includes B- or T-lymphocyte deficiency, complement deficiencies, and phagocytic disorders [excluding chronic granulomatous disease]); HIV infection; leukemia, lymphoma, Hodgkin's disease, multiple myeloma, generalized malignancy; chronic renal failure, nephrotic syndrome; patients requiring treatment with immunosuppressive therapy, including chemotherapy, long-term systemic corticosteroids, or radiation therapy; patients who have received a solid organ transplant

Patients 19-64 years of age with certain high-risk condition(s):
- Chronic heart disease (including heart failure and cardiomyopathy, and excluding hypertension)
- Chronic lung disease (including COPD, emphysema, and asthma)
- Persons who smoke cigarettes
- Alcoholism
- Chronic liver disease (including cirrhosis)
- Residents of nursing homes or long term care facilities (CDC, 61[4], 2012)

Routine vaccination is not recommended for Alaska Natives or American Indian persons unless they have underlying conditions which are indications for vaccination; in special situations, vaccination may be recommended when living in an area at increased risk of invasive pneumococcal disease.

Contraindications Hypersensitivity to pneumococcal vaccine or any component of the formulation

Warnings/Precautions Use caution in patients with severely compromised cardiovascular function or pulmonary disease where a systemic reaction may pose a significant risk. May cause relapse in patients with stable idiopathic thrombocytopenia purpura. Epinephrine injection (1:1000) must be immediately available in the case of anaphylaxis. Syncope has been reported with use of injectable vaccines and may be accompanied by transient visual disturbances, weakness, or tonic-clonic movements. Procedures should be in place to avoid injuries from falling and to restore cerebral perfusion if syncope occurs.

Patients who will be receiving immunosuppressive therapy (including Hodgkin's disease, cancer chemotherapy, or transplantation) should be vaccinated at least 2 weeks prior to the initiation of therapy. Immune responses may be impaired for several months following intensive immunosuppressive therapy (up to 2 years in Hodgkin's disease patients). Vaccination may not result in effective immunity in all patients. Response depends upon multiple factors (eg, type of vaccine, age of patient) and may be improved by administering the vaccine at the recommended dose, route, and interval. Vaccines may not be effective if administered during periods of altered immune competence (CDC, 2011). Patients who will undergo splenectomy should also be vaccinated 2 weeks prior to surgery, if possible. In general, household and close contacts of persons with altered immunocompetence may receive all age appropriate vaccines. Patients with HIV should be vaccinated as soon as possible (following confirmation of the diagnosis). The decision to administer or delay vaccination because of current or recent febrile illness depends on the severity of symptoms and the etiology of the disease. Immunization should be delayed during the course of an acute febrile illness or other active infection. In order to maximize vaccination rates, the ACIP recommends simultaneous administration of all age-appropriate vaccines (live or inactivated) for which a person is eligible at a single clinic visit, unless contraindications exist. If a person has not received any pneumococcal vaccine or if pneumococcal vaccination status is unknown, PPSV23 should be administered as indicated. Postmarketing reports of adverse effects in the elderly, especially those with comorbidities, have been significant enough to require hospitalization.

Adverse Reactions (Reflective of adult population; not specific for elderly) All serious adverse reactions must be reported to the U.S. Department of Health and Human Services (DHHS) Vaccine Adverse Event Reporting System (VAERS) 1-800-822-7967 or online at https://vaers.hhs.gov/esub/index.

Frequency not defined.

Central nervous system: Chills, Guillain-Barré syndrome, fever ≤102°F*, fever >102°F, headache, malaise, pain, radiculoneuropathy, seizure (febrile)

Dermatologic: Angioneurotic edema, cellulitis, rash, urticaria

Gastrointestinal: Nausea, vomiting

Hematologic: Hemolytic anemia (in patients with other hematologic disorders), leukocytosis, thrombocytopenia (in patients with stabilized ITP)

Local: Injection site reaction* (erythema, induration, swelling, soreness, warmth); peripheral edema in injected extremity

Neuromuscular & skeletal: Arthralgia, arthritis, limb mobility decreased, myalgia, paresthesia, weakness

Miscellaneous: Anaphylactoid reaction, C-reactive protein increased, lymphadenitis, lymphadenopathy, serum sickness

*Reactions most commonly reported in clinical trials.

Drug Interactions

Metabolism/Transport Effects None known.

Avoid Concomitant Use There are no known interactions where it is recommended to avoid concomitant use.

Increased Effect/Toxicity There are no known significant interactions involving an increase in effect.

Decreased Effect

Pneumococcal Polysaccharide Vaccine (Polyvalent) may decrease the levels/effects of: Zoster Vaccine

The levels/effects of Pneumococcal Polysaccharide Vaccine (Polyvalent) may be decreased by: Belimumab; Fingolimod; Immunosuppressants

Stability Store under refrigeration at 2°C to 8°C (36°F to 46°F).

Mechanism of Action Although there are more than 80 known pneumococcal capsular types, pneumococcal disease is mainly caused by only a few types of pneumococci. Pneumococcal vaccine contains capsular polysaccharides of 23 pneumococcal types of *Streptococcal pneumoniae* which represent at least 85% to 90% of pneumococcal disease isolates in the United States. The 23 capsular pneumococcal vaccine contains purified

PNEUMOCOCCAL POLYSACCHARIDE VACCINE (POLYVALENT)

capsular polysaccharides of pneumococcal types 1, 2, 3, 4, 5, 6B, 7F, 8, 9N, 9V, 10A, 11A, 12F, 14, 15B, 17F, 18C, 19F, 19A, 20, 22F, 23F, and 33F.

Dosage

Geriatric

Primary immunization: I.M., SubQ: Refer to adult dosing.

Revaccination: I.M., SubQ: ≥65 years: One revaccination if ≥5 years after first dose of PPSV23 and if <65 years of age at the time of the initial vaccination (CDC, September 3, 2010).

Adult Immunization: I.M., SubQ: 0.5 mL

Revaccination: I.M., SubQ:

Immunocompetent individuals: Revaccination generally not recommended

Adults at highest risk for pneumococcal disease: One revaccination ≥5 years after first dose of PPSV23. Patients at highest risk for infection include those with asplenia or immunocompromising conditions (eg, sickle cell anemia, HIV infection, leukemia, lymphoma, Hodgkin's disease, multiple myeloma, generalized malignancy, chronic renal failure, nephrotic syndrome, solid organ transplant, and patients on immunosuppressive therapy [including corticosteroids]) (CDC, September 3, 2010; CDC, December 10, 2010).

Administration Do not inject I.V.; avoid intradermal administration (may cause severe local reactions); administer SubQ or I.M. (deltoid muscle or lateral midthigh)

For patients at risk of hemorrhage following intramuscular injection, the ACIP recommends "it should be administered intramuscularly if, in the opinion of the physician familiar with the patient's bleeding risk, the vaccine can be administered by this route with reasonable safety. If the patient receives antihemophilia or other similar therapy, intramuscular vaccination can be scheduled shortly after such therapy is administered. A fine needle (23 gauge or smaller) can be used for the vaccination and firm pressure applied to the site (without rubbing) for at least 2 minutes. The patient should be instructed concerning the risk of hematoma from the injection." Patients on anticoagulant therapy should be considered to have the same bleeding risks and treated as those with clotting factor disorders (CDC, 2011).

Antipyretics have not been shown to prevent febrile seizures. Antipyretics may be used to treat fever or discomfort following vaccination (CDC, 2011). One study reported that routine prophylactic administration of acetaminophen to prevent fever prior to vaccination decreased the immune response of some vaccines; the clinical significance of this reduction in immune response has not been established (Prymula, 2009).

Simultaneous administration of vaccines helps ensure the patients will be fully vaccinated by the appropriate age. Simultaneous administration of vaccines is defined as administering >1 vaccine on the same day at different anatomic sites. Separate vaccines should not be combined in the same syringe unless indicated by product specific labeling. Separate needles and syringes should be used for each injection. The ACIP prefers each dose of a specific vaccine in a series come from the same manufacturer when possible. Adolescents and adults should be vaccinated while seated or lying down. In general, preterm infants should be vaccinated at the same chronological age as full-term infants (CDC, 2011).

Monitoring Parameters Monitor for syncope for 15 minutes following administration. If seizure-like activity associated with syncope occurs, maintain patient in supine or Trendelenburg position to reestablish adequate cerebral perfusion.

Pharmacotherapy Pearls U.S. federal law requires that the name of medication, date of administration, the vaccine manufacturer, lot number of vaccine, and the administering person's name, title, and address be entered into the patient's permanent medical record.

Special Geriatric Considerations Elderly have ~3 times the incidence of pneumococcal pneumonia than younger adults and 30% of all pneumococcal meningitis occurs in persons >50 years of age with a 20% mortality. Limited data on the elderly; however, elderly, compared to young adults, develop slightly lower antibody titers; provides 60% to 70% protection for bacterial pneumonia. 90% protection for pneumococcal pneumonia strains; 20% of the elderly with pneumococcal pneumonia have an associated bacteremia with a 17% to 40% fatality. All persons ≥65 years of age should receive the pneumococcal vaccine including previously unvaccinated persons and persons who have not been vaccinated within 5 years. All persons of unknown vaccination status should receive one dose of vaccine. Postmarketing reports of adverse effects in the elderly, especially those with comorbidities, have been significant enough to require hospitalization.

Dosage Forms Excipient information presented when available (limited, particularly for generics); consult specific product labeling.

Injection, solution:

Pneumovax® 23: 25 mcg each of 23 capsular polysaccharide isolates/0.5 mL (0.5 mL, 2.5 mL)

◆ **Pneumovax® 23** *see* Pneumococcal Polysaccharide Vaccine (Polyvalent) *on page 1558*

- **Podactin Cream [OTC]** *see* Miconazole (Topical) *on page 1276*
- **Podactin Powder [OTC]** *see* Tolnaftate *on page 1930*
- **Polio Vaccine** *see* Poliovirus Vaccine (Inactivated) *on page 1561*
- **Poliovirus, Inactivated (IPV)** *see* Diphtheria and Tetanus Toxoids, Acellular Pertussis, and Poliovirus Vaccine *on page 565*

Poliovirus Vaccine (Inactivated) (POE lee oh VYE rus vak SEEN, in ak ti VAY ted)

Related Information
Immunization Administration Recommendations *on page 2144*
Immunization Recommendations *on page 2149*

Medication Safety Issues
Administration issues:
Poliovirus vaccine (inactivated) may be confused with tuberculin products. Medication errors have occurred when poliovirus vaccine (IPV) has been inadvertently administered instead of ttuberculin skin tests (PPD). These products are refrigerated and often stored in close proximity to each other.

Brand Names: U.S. IPOL®
Brand Names: Canada Imovax® Polio
Index Terms Enhanced-Potency Inactivated Poliovirus Vaccine; IPV; Polio Vaccine; Salk Vaccine
Generic Availability (U.S.) No
Pharmacologic Category Vaccine, Inactivated (Viral)
Use Active immunization against poliomyelitis caused by poliovirus types 1, 2 and 3. **Note:** Combination products containing polio vaccine are also available and may be preferred in certain age groups if recipients are likely to be susceptible to the agents contained within each vaccine.

The Advisory Committee on Immunization Practices (ACIP) recommends routine vaccination for the following:
- All children (first dose given at 2 months of age)

Routine immunization of adults in the United States is generally not recommended. Adults with previous wild poliovirus disease, who have never been immunized, or those who are incompletely immunized may receive inactivated poliovirus vaccine if they fall into one of the following categories:
- Travelers to regions or countries where poliomyelitis is endemic or epidemic
- Healthcare workers in close contact with patients who may be excreting poliovirus
- Laboratory workers handling specimens that may contain poliovirus
- Members of communities or specific population groups with diseases caused by wild poliovirus
- Incompletely vaccinated or unvaccinated adults in a household or with other close contact with children receiving oral poliovirus (may be at increased risk of vaccine associated paralytic poliomyelitis)

Contraindications Hypersensitivity to any component of the vaccine
Warnings/Precautions Patients with prior clinical poliomyelitis, incomplete immunization with oral poliovirus vaccine (OPV), HIV infection, severe combined immunodeficiency, hypogammaglobulinemia, agammaglobulinemia, or altered immunity (due to corticosteroids, alkylating agents, antimetabolites or radiation) may receive inactivated poliovirus vaccine (IPV). In general, household and close contacts of persons with altered immunocompetence may receive all age appropriate vaccines. Immune response may be decreased in patients receiving immune globulin. Vaccination may be deferred with an acute febrile illness; minor illnesses with or without a low-grade fever are not reasons to postpone vaccination. Vaccination may not result in effective immunity in all patients. Response depends upon multiple factors (eg, type of vaccine, age of patient) and may be improved by administering the vaccine at the recommended dose, route, and interval. Vaccines may not be effective if administered during periods of altered immune competence (CDC, 2011). Immediate treatment for anaphylactic/anaphylactoid reaction should be available during vaccine use. In order to maximize vaccination rates, the ACIP recommends simultaneous administration of all age-appropriate vaccines (live or inactivated) for which a person is eligible at a single clinic visit, unless contraindications exist. The use of combination vaccines is generally preferred over separate injections, taking into consideration provider assessment, patient preference, and adverse events. Syncope has been reported with use of injectable vaccines and may be accompanied by transient visual disturbances, weakness, or tonic-clonic movements. Procedures should be in place to avoid injuries from falling and to restore cerebral perfusion if syncope occurs.

The injection contains 2-phenoxyethanol, calf serum protein, formaldehyde, neomycin, streptomycin, and polymyxin B; the packaging contains natural latex rubber. Use of the minimum age and minimum intervals during the first 6 months of life should only be done when the vaccine recipient is at risk for imminent exposure to circulating poliovirus (shorter intervals and earlier start dates may lead to lower seroconversion).

Adverse Reactions (Reflective of adult population; not specific for elderly) All serious adverse reactions must be reported to the U.S. Department of Health and Human Services (DHHS) Vaccine Adverse Event Reporting System (VAERS) 1-800-822-7967 or online at https://vaers.hhs.gov/esub/index. In Canada, adverse reactions may be reported to local provincial/territorial health agencies or to the Vaccine Safety Section at Public Health Agency of Canada (1-866-844-0018).

Percentages noted with concomitant administration of DTP or DTaP vaccine and observed within 48 hours of injection.

>10%:
  Central nervous system: Irritability (7% to 65%), tiredness (4% to 61%), fever ≥39°C (≤38%)
  Gastrointestinal: Anorexia (1% to 17%)
  Local: Injection Site: Tenderness (≤29%), swelling (≤11%)

1% to 10%:
  Central nervous system: Fever >39°C (≤4%)
  Gastrointestinal: Vomiting (1% to 3%)
  Local: Injection site: Erythema (≤3%)
  Miscellaneous: Persistent crying (up to 1% reported within 72 hours)

Drug Interactions

Metabolism/Transport Effects None known.

Avoid Concomitant Use There are no known interactions where it is recommended to avoid concomitant use.

Increased Effect/Toxicity There are no known significant interactions involving an increase in effect.

Decreased Effect
  The levels/effects of Poliovirus Vaccine (Inactivated) may be decreased by: Belimumab; Fingolimod; Immunosuppressants

Stability Store under refrigeration 2°C to 8°C (35°F to 46°F); do not freeze.

Dosage

Geriatric & Adult Immunization: I.M., SubQ:
  Previously unvaccinated: Two 0.5 mL doses administered at 1- to 2-month intervals, followed by a third dose 6-12 months later. If <3 months, but at least 2 months are available before protection is needed, 3 doses may be administered at least 1 month apart. If administration must be completed within 1-2 months, give 2 doses at least 1 month apart. If <1 month is available, give 1 dose.
  Incompletely vaccinated: Adults with at least 1 previous dose of OPV, <3 doses of IPV, or a combination of OPV and IPV equaling <3 doses, administer at least one 0.5 mL dose of IPV. Additional doses to complete the series may be given if time permits.
  Completely vaccinated and at increased risk of exposure: One 0.5 mL dose

Administration Do not administer I.V.; for I.M. or SubQ administration. Administer in the deltoid area to adults.

Simultaneous administration of vaccines helps ensure the patients will be fully vaccinated by the appropriate age. Simultaneous administration of vaccines is defined as administering >1 vaccine on the same day at different anatomic sites. The use of licensed combination vaccines is generally preferred over separate injections of the equivalent components. Separate vaccines should not be combined in the same syringe unless indicated by product specific labeling. Separate needles and syringes should be used for each injection. The ACIP prefers each dose of a specific vaccine in a series come from the same manufacturer when possible. Adolescents and adults should be vaccinated while seated or lying down. In general, preterm infants should be vaccinated at the same chronological age as full-term infants (CDC, 2011).

Antipyretics have not been shown to prevent febrile seizures. Antipyretics may be used to treat fever or discomfort following vaccination (CDC, 2011). One study reported that routine prophylactic administration of acetaminophen to prevent fever prior to vaccination decreased the immune response of some vaccines; the clinical significance of this reduction in immune response has not been established (Prymula, 2009).

Monitoring Parameters Monitor for syncope for 15 minutes following administration. If seizure-like activity associated with syncope occurs, maintain patient in supine or Trendelenburg position to reestablish adequate cerebral perfusion.

Test Interactions May temporarily suppress tuberculin skin test sensitivity (4-6 weeks)

Pharmacotherapy Pearls Federal law requires that the name of medication, date of administration, the vaccine manufacturer, lot number of vaccine, and the administering person's name, title, and address be entered into the patient's permanent medical record.

Currently, the primary risk for paralytic polio in U.S. residents is through travel to countries where polio remains endemic or where polio outbreaks are occurring. Unvaccinated persons traveling to countries that use OPV should be aware of the risk caused by OPV and should consider polio vaccination prior to travel.

Special Geriatric Considerations For the elderly who cannot document a primary immunization series or at risk due to contact or travel, administer the initial series. Boosters may be necessary for travel since antibody titers may diminish with age.

Dosage Forms Excipient information presented when available (limited, particularly for generics); consult specific product labeling.

Injection, suspension:

IPOL®: Type 1 poliovirus 40 D-antigen units, type 2 poliovirus 8 D-antigen units, and type 3 poliovirus 32 D-antigen units per 0.5 mL (0.5 mL, 5 mL) [contains 2-phenoxyethanol, formaldehyde, calf serum protein, neomycin (may have trace amounts), streptomycin (may have trace amounts), and polymyxin B (may have trace amounts)]

Polycarbophil (pol i KAR boe fil)

Brand Names: U.S. Equalactin® [OTC]; Fiber-Lax [OTC]; Fiber-Tabs™ [OTC]; FiberCon® [OTC]; Fibertab [OTC]; Konsyl® Fiber [OTC]

Generic Availability (U.S.) Yes

Pharmacologic Category Antidiarrheal; Fiber Supplement; Laxative, Bulk-Producing

Use Treatment of constipation or diarrhea

Warnings/Precautions Use caution in patients who have difficulty swallowing; taking products without adequate fluid may cause it to swell and block throat or esophagus.

Adverse Reactions (Reflective of adult population; not specific for elderly) Frequency not defined: Gastrointestinal: Abdominal fullness

Drug Interactions

Metabolism/Transport Effects None known.

Avoid Concomitant Use

Avoid concomitant use of Polycarbophil with any of the following: Calcium Acetate

Increased Effect/Toxicity

Polycarbophil may increase the levels/effects of: Calcium Acetate; Vitamin D Analogs

The levels/effects of Polycarbophil may be increased by: Thiazide Diuretics

Decreased Effect

Polycarbophil may decrease the levels/effects of: Bisphosphonate Derivatives; Calcium Channel Blockers; Deferiprone; DOBUTamine; Eltrombopag; Estramustine; Phosphate Supplements; Quinolone Antibiotics; Tetracycline Derivatives; Thyroid Products; Trientine

The levels/effects of Polycarbophil may be decreased by: Trientine

Mechanism of Action Restoring a more normal moisture level and providing bulk in the patient's intestinal tract

Dosage

Geriatric & Adult Constipation or diarrhea: General dosing guidelines (OTC labeling): Oral: 1250 mg calcium polycarbophil 1-4 times/day

Administration Patient should drink adequate fluids (8 oz of water or other fluids) with each dose.

Monitoring Parameters Monitor for diarrhea, abdominal pain, bowel obstruction, or impaction

Pharmacotherapy Pearls Each calcium polycarbophil tablet contains ~100 mg of absorbable elemental calcium; chewable tablets are available

Special Geriatric Considerations Elderly may have insufficient fluid intake which may predispose them to fecal impaction and bowel obstruction. Bloating and flatulence may be a problem when used short-term. Use cautiously in patients with a history of bowel impaction/ obstruction.

Dosage Forms Excipient information presented when available (limited, particularly for generics); consult specific product labeling.

Caplet, oral: Calcium polycarbophil 625 mg [equivalent to polycarbophil 500 mg], Calcium polycarbophil 625 mg

FiberCon®: Calcium polycarbophil 625 mg [scored; contains calcium 140 mg/caplet, magnesium 10 mg/caplet; equivalent to polycarbophil 500 mg]

Konsyl® Fiber: Calcium polycarbophil 625 mg [sugar free; contains calcium 125 mg/caplet; equivalent to polycarbophil 500 mg]

Captab, oral:
Fiber-Lax: Calcium polycarbophil 625 mg [contains calcium 170 mg/caplet; equivalent to polycarbophil 500 mg]
Tablet, oral:
Fiber-Tabs™: Calcium polycarbophil 625 mg [scored; equivalent to polycarbophil 500 mg]
Fibertab: Calcium polycarbophil 625 mg [equivalent to polycarbophil 500 mg]
Tablet, chewable, oral:
Equalactin®: Calcium polycarbophil 625 mg [citrus flavor; equivalent to polycarbophil 500 mg]

◆ Polycitra see Citric Acid, Sodium Citrate, and Potassium Citrate on page 391

Polyethylene Glycol 3350 (pol i ETH i leen GLY kol 3350)

Related Information
Laxatives, Classification and Properties on page 2121
Medication Safety Issues
Sound-alike/look-alike issues:
MiraLax® may be confused with Mirapex®
Polyethylene glycol 3350 may be confused with polyethylene glycol electrolyte solution
International issues:
MiraLax may be confused with Murelax brand name for oxazepam [Australia]
Brand Names: U.S. Dulcolax Balance® [OTC]; MiraLAX® [OTC]
Index Terms PEG
Generic Availability (U.S.) Yes
Pharmacologic Category Laxative, Osmotic
Use Treatment of occasional constipation in adults
Unlabeled Use Bowel preparation before colonoscopy
Contraindications Hypersensitivity to polyethylene glycol or any component of the formulation
Warnings/Precautions Evaluate patients with symptoms of bowel obstruction (nausea, vomiting, abdominal pain, or distension) prior to use; avoid use in patients with known or suspected bowel obstruction. Use with caution in patients with renal impairment. Do not use for longer than 1 week; 2-4 days may be required to produce bowel movement. Prolonged, frequent, or excessive use may lead to electrolyte imbalance. When using for self medication, patients should consult healthcare provider prior to use if they have nausea, vomiting, or abdominal pain, irritable bowel syndrome, kidney disease, or a sudden change in bowel habits for >2 weeks. Patients should be instructed to discontinue use and consult healthcare provider if they have diarrhea, rectal bleeding, if abdominal pain, bloating, cramping, or nausea gets worse, or if need to use for >1 week.
Adverse Reactions (Reflective of adult population; not specific for elderly) Frequency not defined.
Dermatologic: Urticaria
Gastrointestinal: Abdominal bloating, cramping, diarrhea, flatulence, nausea
Drug Interactions
Metabolism/Transport Effects None known.
Avoid Concomitant Use There are no known interactions where it is recommended to avoid concomitant use.
Increased Effect/Toxicity There are no known significant interactions involving an increase in effect.
Decreased Effect There are no known significant interactions involving a decrease in effect.
Stability Store at room temperature before reconstitution. Dissolve powder in 4-8 ounces of water, juice, cola, or tea.
Mechanism of Action An osmotic agent, polyethylene glycol 3350 causes water retention in the stool; increases stool frequency.
Pharmacodynamics/Kinetics
Onset of action: Oral: 24-96 hours
Absorption: Minimal
Bioavailability: 0.2%
Excretion: Feces (93%); urine (0.2%)
Dosage
Geriatric & Adult
Occasional constipation: Oral: 17 g of powder (~1 heaping tablespoon) dissolved in 4-8 ounces of beverage, once daily; do not use for >1 week unless directed by healthcare provider

Bowel preparation before colonoscopy (unlabeled use): Oral: Mix 17 g of powder (~1 heaping tablespoon) in 8 ounces of clear liquid and administer the entire mixture every 10 minutes until 2 L are consumed (start within 6 hours after administering 20 mg bisacodyl delayed-release tablets) (Wexner, 2006).

Administration

Occasional constipation: Stir powder in 4-8 ounces of water, juice, soda, coffee or tea until dissolved and drink.

Bowel preparation for colonoscopy: Stir powder in 8 ounces of clear liquid until dissolved and drink.

Special Geriatric Considerations Elderly are more likely to show CNS signs of dehydration and electrolyte loss than younger adults. Therefore, monitor closely for fluid and electrolyte loss with chronic use.

Dosage Forms Excipient information presented when available (limited, particularly for generics); consult specific product labeling.

Powder for solution, oral: 17 g/dose (119 g, 238 g, 255 g, 510 g, 527 g); 17 g/packet (14s, 30s)

Dulcolax Balance®: 17 g/dose (119 g, 238 g, 510 g)

MiraLAX®: 17 g/dose (119 g, 238 g, 510 g); 17 g/packet (10s)

♦ **Polyethylene Glycol-Conjugated Uricase** see Pegloticase on page 1490

Polyethylene Glycol-Electrolyte Solution and Bisacodyl

(pol i ETH i leen GLY kol ee LEK troe lite soe LOO shun & bis a KOE dil)

Related Information

Bisacodyl on page 214

Brand Names: U.S. HalfLytely® and Bisacodyl

Index Terms Bisacodyl and Polyethylene Glycol-Electrolyte Solution; Electrolyte Lavage Solution

Generic Availability (U.S.) No

Pharmacologic Category Laxative, Bowel Evacuant; Laxative, Stimulant

Use Bowel cleansing prior to colonoscopy

Medication Guide Available Yes

Contraindications Gastrointestinal obstruction; bowel perforation; toxic colitis; toxic mega-colon; gastric retention; ileus

Warnings/Precautions Serious arrhythmias have been reported (rarely) with the use of ionic osmotic laxative products. Use with caution in patients who may be at risk of cardiac arrhythmias (e.g. patients with a history of prolonged QT, uncontrolled arrhythmias, recent MI, unstable angina, CHF, or cardiomyopathy). Consider pre-dose and post-colonoscopy ECGs in these patients. Evaluate patients with symptoms of bowel obstruction or perforation prior to use. Correct electrolyte abnormalities in patients prior to use. Fluid and electrolyte disturbances can lead to arrhythmias, seizures, and renal impairment. Advise patients to maintain adequate hydration before, during, and after treatment. If patient becomes dehydrated or experiences significant vomiting after treatment, consider post-colonoscopy lab tests (electrolytes, creatinine, and BUN).

No additional ingredients or flavors (other than the flavor packs provided) should be added to the polyethylene glycol-electrolyte solution. Use with caution in patients with severe ulcerative colitis, or renal impairment. Observe unconscious or semiconscious patients with impaired gag reflex or those who are prone to regurgitation or aspiration during administration. Closely monitor patients with impaired renal function who develop nausea and vomiting. Generalized tonic-clonic seizures have occurred in patients without a prior history of seizures (4 L solution); use caution in patients taking medications which increase the risk for electrolyte abnormalities (eg, diuretics) and/or patients with pre-existing electrolyte abnormalities. Evaluation of electro-lytes pre- and post-colonoscopy is warranted in this population. Rare cases of ischemic colitis have been reported; development of severe abdominal pain or rectal bleeding should prompt further evaluation.

Adverse Reactions (Reflective of adult population; not specific for elderly)

>10%:

Gastrointestinal: Fullness (40%), cramping (38%), nausea (34%)

Miscellaneous: Overall discomfort (57%)

1% to 10%: Gastrointestinal: Vomiting (10%)

Drug Interactions

Metabolism/Transport Effects None known.

Avoid Concomitant Use There are no known interactions where it is recommended to avoid concomitant use.

Increased Effect/Toxicity There are no known significant interactions involving an increase in effect.

Decreased Effect
The levels/effects of Polyethylene Glycol-Electrolyte Solution and Bisacodyl may be decreased by: Antacids

Ethanol/Nutrition/Herb Interactions Food: Take clear liquid diet the day of and during the bowel preparation; after consuming the solution, avoid drinking large quantities of clear liquids until colonoscopy.

Stability Store at 20°C to 25°C (68°F to 77°F); excursions permitted to 15°C to 30°C (59°F to 86°F). Fill the container with water to the fill mark; may add flavor packet provided in kit to the solution; no other ingredients should be added to the solution. Shake well. When polyethylene glycol-electrolyte solution is reconstituted, may refrigerate. Use within 48 hours.

Mechanism of Action Bisacodyl acts on the colonic mucosa to increase peristalsis throughout the large intestine. Polyethylene glycol-electrolyte solution induces catharsis through strong electrolyte and osmotic effects.

Pharmacodynamics/Kinetics See individual agents.

Dosage
  Geriatric & Adult Bowel cleansing: Oral:
    Bisacodyl: 5 mg as a single dose. After bowel movement or 6 hours (whichever occurs first), initiate polyethylene glycol-electrolyte solution
    Polyethylene glycol-electrolyte solution: 8 ounces every 10 minutes until 2 L are consumed

Administration Administer bisacodyl tablet with water; do not chew or crush tablet. Do not take antacids within 1 hour of taking bisacodyl. Rapidly drinking the polyethylene glycol-electrolyte solution is preferred to drinking small amount continuously. If severe bloating, distention, or abdominal pain occurs, administration should be slowed or temporarily discontinued until symptoms resolve.

Monitoring Parameters Bowel movements; electrolytes, renal function

Special Geriatric Considerations Studies of this combination preparation drug included 28% of patients >65 years of age with 7% being >75 years. Rates of success appear to be lower in patients >65 years. No adjustments in dose are necessary.

Dosage Forms Excipient information presented when available (limited, particularly for generics); consult specific product labeling. [DSC] = Discontinued product
  Kit [each kit contains]:
    HalfLytely® and Bisacodyl [DSC]:
      Powder for solution, oral (HalfLytely®): PEG 3350 210 g, sodium bicarbonate 2.86 g, sodium chloride 5.6 g, potassium chloride 0.74 g (2000 mL) [sulfate-free; cherry, lemon-lime, orange flavor] [DSC]
      Tablet, delayed release (Bisacodyl): 5 mg (2s) [DSC]
    HalfLytely® and Bisacodyl:
      Powder for solution, oral (HalfLytely®): PEG 3350 210 g, sodium bicarbonate 2.86 g, sodium chloride 5.6 g, potassium chloride 0.74 g (2000 mL) [contains 4 flavor packs (each 1 g) cherry, lemon-lime, orange, pineapple flavors]
      Tablet, delayed release (Bisacodyl): 5 mg (1s)

◆ **Polyethylene Glycol Interferon Alfa-2b** *see* Peginterferon Alfa-2b *on page 1485*
◆ **Poly-Iron 150 Forte** *see* Polysaccharide-Iron Complex, Vitamin B12, and Folic Acid *on page 1566*
◆ **Polymyxin B and Neomycin** *see* Neomycin and Polymyxin B *on page 1354*
◆ **Polymyxin B, Neomycin, and Dexamethasone** *see* Neomycin, Polymyxin B, and Dexamethasone *on page 1355*
◆ **Polymyxin B, Neomycin, and Gramicidin** *see* Neomycin, Polymyxin B, and Gramicidin *on page 1357*
◆ **Polysaccharide Iron 150 Forte** *see* Polysaccharide-Iron Complex, Vitamin B12, and Folic Acid *on page 1566*

Polysaccharide-Iron Complex, Vitamin B12, and Folic Acid
(pol i SAK a ride-EYE ern KOM pleks, VYE ta min bee twelve & FOE lik AS id)

Related Information
  Folic Acid *on page 836*
Brand Names: U.S. Ferrex™ 150 Forte; Ferrex™ 150 Forte Plus; Maxaron® Forte; Poly-Iron 150 Forte; Polysaccharide Iron 150 Forte
Index Terms Iron-Polysaccharide Complex, Vitamin B12, and Folic Acid
Generic Availability (U.S.) No
Pharmacologic Category Iron Salt
Use Prevention and treatment of iron-deficiency anemias and/or nutritional megaloblastic anemias

Warnings/Precautions [U.S. Boxed Warning]: Accidental overdose of iron-containing products is a leading cause of fatal poisoning in children under 6 years of age. Keep this product out of the reach of children. In case of accidental overdose call the poison control center immediately. Not appropriate for with pernicious, aplastic, or normocytic anemias when anemia is present with vitamin B_{12} deficiency. Folate doses >0.1 mg/day may obscure pernicious anemia.

Adverse Reactions (Reflective of adult population; not specific for elderly) Frequency not defined.

Gastrointestinal: Abdominal pain, constipation, dark stools, diarrhea, epigastric pain, GI irritation, nausea, stomach cramping, vomiting

Genitourinary: Discolored urine

Miscellaneous: Hypersensitivity reaction

Drug Interactions

Metabolism/Transport Effects None known.

Avoid Concomitant Use

Avoid concomitant use of Polysaccharide-Iron Complex, Vitamin B12, and Folic Acid with any of the following: Dimercaprol; Raltitrexed

Increased Effect/Toxicity

The levels/effects of Polysaccharide-Iron Complex, Vitamin B12, and Folic Acid may be increased by: Dimercaprol

Decreased Effect

Polysaccharide-Iron Complex, Vitamin B12, and Folic Acid may decrease the levels/effects of: Bisphosphonate Derivatives; Cefdinir; Deferiprone; Eltrombopag; Fosphenytoin; Levodopa; Levothyroxine; Methyldopa; PenicillAMINE; PHENobarbital; Phenytoin; Phosphate Supplements; Primidone; Quinolone Antibiotics; Raltitrexed; Tetracycline Derivatives; Trientine

The levels/effects of Polysaccharide-Iron Complex, Vitamin B12, and Folic Acid may be decreased by: Antacids; Green Tea; H2-Antagonists; Pancrelipase; Proton Pump Inhibitors; Trientine

Stability Store at 25°C (77°F); excursions permitted to 15°C to 30°C (59°F to 86°F). Poly-Iron 150 Forte: Store at 15°C to 30°C (59°F to 86°F).

Dosage

Geriatric & Adult Iron deficiency (prevention/treatment): Oral: 1-2 capsules daily

Dosage Forms Excipient information presented when available (limited, particularly for generics); consult specific product labeling.

Capsule, oral:

Ferrex™ 150 Forte: Elemental iron 150 mg, cyanocobalamin 25 mcg, and folic acid 1 mg

Ferrex™ 150 Forte Plus: Elemental iron 150 mg (50 mg as ferrous asparto glycinate), cyanocobalamin 25 mcg, and folic acid 1 mg [contains ascorbic acid 60 mg and succinic acid 50 mg]

Maxaron® Forte: Elemental iron 150 mg (80 mg as ferrous bisglycinate), cyanocobalamin 25 mcg, and folic acid 1 mg [contains ascorbic acid 60 mg]

Poly-Iron 150 Forte: Elemental iron 150 mg, cyanocobalamin 25 mcg, and folic acid 1 mg

Polysaccharide Iron 150 Forte: Elemental iron 150 mg, cyanocobalamin 25 mcg, and folic acid 1 mg

♦ **Polyvinyl Alcohol** *see* Artificial Tears *on page 148*
♦ **P-OM3** *see* Omega-3-Acid Ethyl Esters *on page 1416*
♦ **Ponstel®** *see* Mefenamic Acid *on page 1194*

Posaconazole (poe sa KON a zole)

Medication Safety Issues

Sound-alike/look-alike issues:

Noxafil® may be confused with minoxidil

International issues:

Noxafil [U.S. and multiple international markets] may be confused with Noxidil brand name for minoxidil [Thailand]

Brand Names: U.S. Noxafil®

Brand Names: Canada Posanol™

Index Terms SCH 56592

Generic Availability (U.S.) No

Pharmacologic Category Antifungal Agent, Oral

Use Prophylaxis of invasive *Aspergillus* and *Candida* infections in severely-immunocompromised patients [eg, hematopoietic stem cell transplant (HSCT) recipients with graft-versus-host disease (GVHD) or those with prolonged neutropenia secondary to chemotherapy for

POSACONAZOLE

hematologic malignancies]; treatment of oropharyngeal candidiasis (including patients refractory to itraconazole and/or fluconazole)

Unlabeled Use Salvage therapy of refractory or relapsed invasive fungal infections; mucormycosis; pulmonary infection (nonimmunosuppressed)

Contraindications Hypersensitivity to posaconazole, other azole antifungals, or any component of the formulation; coadministration of cisapride, ergot alkaloids, pimozide, quinidine, simvastatin, or sirolimus

Warnings/Precautions Hepatic dysfunction has occurred, ranging from reversible mild/moderate increases of ALT, AST, alkaline phosphatase, total bilirubin, and/or clinical hepatitis to severe reactions (cholestasis, hepatic failure including death). Consider discontinuation of therapy in patients who develop clinical evidence of liver disease that may be secondary to posaconazole. Use caution in patients with an increased risk of arrhythmia (long QT syndrome, concurrent QT$_c$-prolonging drugs, hypokalemia). Correct electrolyte abnormalities (eg, potassium, magnesium, and calcium) before initiating therapy. Concurrent use with cyclosporine or tacrolimus may significantly increase cyclosporine/tacrolimus concentrations and may result in rare serious adverse events (eg, nephrotoxicity, leukoencephalopathy, and death); dose reduction and close monitoring are recommended with initiation of posaconazole therapy. Concurrent use with midazolam may increase midazolam concentrations and potentiate midazolam-related adverse effects.

Use caution in hypersensitivity with other azole antifungal agents; cross-reaction may occur, but has not been established. Consider alternative therapy or closely monitor for breakthrough fungal infections in patients receiving drugs that decrease absorption or increase the metabolism of posaconazole or in any patient unable to eat or tolerate an oral liquid nutritional supplement. Use caution in severe renal impairment or GI disturbances; monitor for breakthrough fungal infections.

Adverse Reactions (Reflective of adult population; not specific for elderly) Note: Percentages reflect data from use in comparator trials with multiple concomitant conditions and medications; some adverse reactions may be due to underlying condition(s).
>10%:
Cardiovascular: Hypertension (18%), edema (9% to 15%), hypotension (14%), tachycardia (12%)
Central nervous system: Fever (6% to 45%), headache (8% to 28%), fatigue (3% to 17%), insomnia (1% to 17%), dizziness (11%), pain (1% to 11%)
Endocrine & metabolic: Hypokalemia (≤30%), hypomagnesemia (18%), dehydration (1% to 11%), hyperglycemia (11%)
Gastrointestinal: Diarrhea (10% to 42%), nausea (9% to 38%), vomiting (7% to 29%), abdominal pain (5% to 27%), constipation (21%), anorexia (2% to 19%), mucositis (17%), weight loss (1% to 14%), oral candidiasis (1% to 12%)
Hematologic: Thrombocytopenia (29%), anemia (2% to 25%), neutropenia (4% to 23%), neutropenic fever (20%)
Hepatic: ALT increased (6% to 17%)
Neuromuscular & skeletal: Rigors (≤20%), musculoskeletal pain (16%), weakness (2% to 13%), arthralgia (11%)
Respiratory: Cough (3% to 25%), dyspnea (1% to 20%), epistaxis (14%), pharyngitis (12%)
Miscellaneous: Bacteremia (18%), herpes simplex (3% to 15%), CMV infection (14%)
1% to 10%:
Central nervous system: Anxiety (9%)
Endocrine & metabolic: Hypocalcemia (9%)
Gastrointestinal: Dyspepsia (10%)
Genitourinary: Vaginal hemorrhage (10%)
Hepatic: Hyperbilirubinemia (7% to 10%), AST increased (3% to 4%), alkaline phosphatase increased (1% to 3%)
Neuromuscular & skeletal: Back pain (10%)
Respiratory: Pneumonia (3% to 10%), upper respiratory infection (7%)
Miscellaneous: Diaphoresis (2% to 10%)

Drug Interactions
Metabolism/Transport Effects Inhibits CYP3A4 (strong)
Avoid Concomitant Use
Avoid concomitant use of Posaconazole with any of the following: Alfuzosin; Apixaban; Avanafil; Axitinib; Cisapride; Conivaptan; Crizotinib; Dihydroergotamine; Dofetilide; Dronedarone; Efavirenz; Eplerenone; Ergoloid Mesylates; Ergonovine; Ergotamine; Everolimus; Fluticasone (Oral Inhalation); Halofantrine; Lapatinib; Lovastatin; Lurasidone; Methadone; Methylergonovine; Nilotinib; Nisoldipine; Pimozide; Proton Pump Inhibitors; QuiNIDine; Ranolazine; Red Yeast Rice; Rivaroxaban; RomiDEPsin; Salmeterol; Silodosin; Simvastatin; Sirolimus; Tamsulosin; Ticagrelor; Tolvaptan; Toremifene

Increased Effect/Toxicity

Posaconazole may increase the levels/effects of: Alfentanil; Alfuzosin; Almotriptan; Alosetron; Antineoplastic Agents (Vinca Alkaloids); Apixaban; Aprepitant; ARIPiprazole; AtorvaSTATin; Avanafil; Axitinib; Benzodiazepines (metabolized by oxidation); Boceprevir; Bortezomib; Bosentan; Brentuximab Vedotin; Brinzolamide; Budesonide (Nasal); Budesonide (Systemic, Oral Inhalation); BusPIRone; Busulfan; Calcium Channel Blockers; CarBAMazepine; Cardiac Glycosides; Ciclesonide; Cilostazol; Cinacalcet; Cisapride; Colchicine; Conivaptan; Corticosteroids (Orally Inhaled); Corticosteroids (Systemic); Crizotinib; CycloSPORINE; CycloSPORINE (Systemic); CYP3A4 Substrates; Dienogest; Dihydroergotamine; DOCEtaxel; Dofetilide; Dronedarone; Dutasteride; Eletriptan; Eplerenone; Ergoloid Mesylates; Ergonovine; Ergotamine; Erlotinib; Eszopiclone; Etravirine; Everolimus; FentaNYL; Fesoterodine; Fluticasone (Nasal); Fluticasone (Oral Inhalation); Fosamprenavir; Fosaprepitant; Fosphenytoin; Gefitinib; GlipiZIDE; GuanFACINE; Halofantrine; Iloperidone; Imatinib; Irinotecan; Ivacaftor; Ixabepilone; Lapatinib; Losartan; Lovastatin; Lumefantrine; Lurasidone; Macrolide Antibiotics; Maraviroc; Methadone; Methylergonovine; MethylPREDNISolone; Mifepristone; Nilotinib; Nisoldipine; Paricalcitol; Pazopanib; Phenytoin; Pimecrolimus; Pimozide; Propafenone; Protease Inhibitors; QuiNIDine; Ramelteon; Ranolazine; Red Yeast Rice; Repaglinide; Rifamycin Derivatives; Rivaroxaban; RomiDEPsin; Ruxolitinib; Salmeterol; Saxagliptin; Sildenafil; Silodosin; Simvastatin; Sirolimus; Solifenacin; SORAfenib; SUNItinib; Tacrolimus; Tacrolimus (Systemic); Tacrolimus (Topical); Tadalafil; Tamsulosin; Telaprevir; Temsirolimus; Ticagrelor; Tolterodine; Tolvaptan; Toremifene; Vardenafil; Vemurafenib; Vilazodone; Vitamin K Antagonists; Ziprasidone; Zolpidem; Zuclopenthixol

The levels/effects of Posaconazole may be increased by: Boceprevir; Etravirine; Grapefruit Juice; Macrolide Antibiotics; Protease Inhibitors; Tacrolimus; Telaprevir

Decreased Effect

Posaconazole may decrease the levels/effects of: Amphotericin B; Ifosfamide; Prasugrel; Saccharomyces boulardii; Ticagrelor

The levels/effects of Posaconazole may be decreased by: Didanosine; Efavirenz; Etravirine; Fosamprenavir; Fosphenytoin; H2-Antagonists; Metoclopramide; Phenytoin; Proton Pump Inhibitors; Rifamycin Derivatives; Sucralfate

Ethanol/Nutrition/Herb Interactions Food: Bioavailability increased ~3 times when posaconazole is administered with a nonfat meal or an oral liquid nutritional supplement; increased ~4 times when administered with a high-fat meal. Grapefruit juice may decrease the levels/effects of posaconazole. Management: Must be administered with or within 20 minutes of a full meal or an oral liquid nutritional supplement, or may be administered with an acidic carbonated beverage (eg, ginger ale). Consider alternative antifungal therapy in patients with inadequate oral intake or severe diarrhea/vomiting. Avoid concurrent use of grapefruit juice.

Stability Store at 25°C (77°F); excursions permitted to 15°C to 30°C (59°F to 86°F). Do not freeze.

Mechanism of Action Interferes with fungal cytochrome P450 (latosterol-14α-demethylase) activity, decreasing ergosterol synthesis (principal sterol in fungal cell membrane) and inhibiting fungal cell membrane formation.

Pharmacodynamics/Kinetics

Absorption: Coadministration with food, liquid nutritional supplements, and/or acidic carbonated beverages (eg, ginger ale) increases absorption; fasting states do not provide sufficient absorption to ensure adequate plasma concentrations.

Distribution: V_d: 465-1774 L

Protein binding: >98%; predominantly bound to albumin

Metabolism: Not significantly metabolized; ~15% to 17% undergoes non-CYP-mediated metabolism, primarily via hepatic glucuronidation into metabolites

Half-life elimination: 35 hours (range: 20-66 hours)

Time to peak, plasma: ~3-5 hours

Excretion: Feces 71% to 77% (~66% of the total dose as unchanged drug); urine 13% to 14% (<0.2% of the total dose as unchanged drug)

Dosage

Geriatric & Adult

Aspergillosis, invasive: Oral:

Prophylaxis: 200 mg 3 times/day; duration of therapy is based is based on recovery from neutropenia or immunosuppression

Salvage treatment of refractory infection (unlabeled use): 200 mg 4 times/day initially; after disease stabilization may decrease frequency to 400 mg 2 times/day (Walsh, 2007). **Note:** Duration of therapy should be a minimum of 6-12 weeks or throughout period of immunosuppression (Walsh, 2008).

Candidal infections: Oral:

Prophylaxis: 200 mg 3 times/day; duration of therapy is based on recovery from neutropenia or immunosuppression

Treatment of oropharyngeal infection: Initial: 100 mg 2 times/day for 1 day; maintenance: 100 mg once daily for 13 days

Treatment of refractory oropharyngeal infection: 400 mg 2 times/day; duration of therapy is based on underlying disease and clinical response

Mucormycosis (unlabeled use): Oral: 800 mg/day in 2 or 4 divided doses; duration of therapy is based on response and risk of relapse due to immunosuppression (Greenburg, 2006)

Cryptococcal infections: Oral:

Pulmonary, nonimmunosuppressed (unlabeled use): 400 mg 2 times/day. **Note:** Fluconazole is considered first-line treatment (Perfect, 2010).

Salvage treatment of relapsed infection (unlabeled use): 400 mg 2 times/day (or 200 mg 4 times/day) for 10-12 weeks. **Note:** Salvage treatment should only be started after an appropriate course of an induction regimen (Perfect, 2010).

Renal Impairment

Mild-to-moderate renal insufficiency (Cl$_{cr}$ 20-80 mL/minute/1.73 m^2): No adjustment necessary

Severe renal insufficiency (Cl$_{cr}$ <20 mL/minute/1.73 m^2): No adjustment necessary; however, monitor for breakthrough fungal infections due to variability in posaconazole exposure.

Hepatic Impairment

Mild-to-severe hepatic insufficiency (Child-Pugh class A, B, or C): No adjustment necessary. Clinical signs and symptoms of liver disease due to posaconazole: Consider discontinuing therapy.

Administration Oral: Shake well before use. Must be administered during or within 20 minutes following a full meal or an oral liquid nutritional supplement; alternatively, posaconazole may be administered with an acidic carbonated beverage (eg, ginger ale). In patients able to swallow, administer oral suspension using dosing spoon provided by the manufacturer; spoon should be rinsed clean with water after each use and before storage.

Monitoring Parameters Hepatic function (eg, AST/ALT, alkaline phosphatase and bilirubin) prior to initiation and during treatment; renal function; electrolyte disturbances (eg, calcium, magnesium, potassium); CBC

Special Geriatric Considerations Dosage adjustment not necessary.

Dosage Forms Excipient information presented when available (limited, particularly for generics); consult specific product labeling.

Suspension, oral:

Noxafil®: 40 mg/mL (123 mL) [contains sodium benzoate; cherry flavor; delivers 105 mL of suspension]

◆ **Posture® [OTC]** *see* Calcium Phosphate (Tribasic) *on page 274*

Potassium Acid Phosphate (poe TASS ee um AS id FOS fate)

Brand Names: U.S. K-Phos® Original

Generic Availability (U.S.) No

Pharmacologic Category Urinary Acidifying Agent

Use Acidifies urine and lowers urinary calcium concentration; reduces odor and rash caused by ammoniacal urine; increases the antibacterial activity of methenamine

Contraindications Severe renal impairment; hyperkalemia, hyperphosphatemia; infected magnesium ammonium phosphate stones

Warnings/Precautions Use with caution in patients receiving concomitant medications or therapies that increase potassium (eg, ACEI, potassium-sparing diuretics, potassium containing salt substitutes). Use caution in patients with renal insufficiency or severe tissue breakdown (eg, chemotherapy or hemodialysis). May cause GI upset (eg, nausea, vomiting, diarrhea, abdominal pain, discomfort) and lead to GI ulceration, bleeding, perforation and/or obstruction. Close monitoring of serum potassium concentrations is needed to avoid hyperkalemia.

Adverse Reactions (Reflective of adult population; not specific for elderly)

>10%: Gastrointestinal: Diarrhea, nausea, stomach pain, flatulence, vomiting

1% to 10%:

Cardiovascular: Bradycardia

Endocrine & metabolic: Hyperkalemia

Local: Local tissue necrosis with extravasation

Neuromuscular & skeletal: Weakness

Respiratory: Dyspnea

Drug Interactions

Metabolism/Transport Effects None known.

Avoid Concomitant Use There are no known interactions where it is recommended to avoid concomitant use.

Increased Effect/Toxicity

Potassium Acid Phosphate may increase the levels/effects of: ACE Inhibitors; Angiotensin II Receptor Blockers; Potassium-Sparing Diuretics; Salicylates

The levels/effects of Potassium Acid Phosphate may be increased by: Eplerenone

Decreased Effect There are no known significant interactions involving a decrease in effect.

Mechanism of Action The principal intracellular cation; involved in transmission of nerve impulses, muscle contractions, enzyme activity, and glucose utilization

Pharmacodynamics/Kinetics

Absorption: Well absorbed from upper GI tract

Distribution: Enters cells via active transport from extracellular fluid

Excretion: Primarily urine; skin and feces (small amounts); most intestinal potassium reabsorbed

Dosage

Geriatric & Adult Urine acidification: Oral: 1000 mg dissolved in 6-8 oz of water 4 times/day with meals and at bedtime; for best results, soak tablets in water for 2-5 minutes, then stir and swallow

Monitoring Parameters Serum potassium, sodium, phosphate, calcium; serum salicylates (if taking salicylates); signs of muscle weakness, cramps

Reference Range Note: Reference ranges may vary depending on the laboratory

Serum phosphorus: Both low and high ends of the normal range are higher in children than in adults.

Adults: 2.5-4.5 mg/dL (0.81-1.45 mmol/L)

Urinary pH: 4.6-8.0

Test Interactions Decreased ammonia (B)

Special Geriatric Considerations A complete drug history should be taken to rule out potential drug interactions since the elderly frequently may be taking potassium and potassium-sparing diuretics, salicylates, or antacids. Use with caution in renal impairment (low Cl_{cr}).

Dosage Forms Excipient information presented when available (limited, particularly for generics); consult specific product labeling.

Tablet, oral:

K-Phos® Original: 500 mg [scored; phosphorus 114 mg and potassium 144 mg (3.7 mEq) per tablet]

Potassium Chloride (poe TASS ee um KLOR ide)

Related Information

Calculations *on page 2087*

Medication Safety Issues

Sound-alike/look-alike issues:

Kaon-Cl-10® may be confused with kaolin

KCl may be confused with HCl

Klor-Con® may be confused with Klaron®

microK® may be confused with Macrobid®, Micronase

High alert medication:

The Institute for Safe Medication Practices (ISMP) includes this medication (I.V. formulation) among its list of drugs which have a heightened risk of causing significant patient harm when used in error.

Other safety concerns:

Per JCAHO recommendations, concentrated electrolyte solutions should not be available in patient care areas.

Consider special storage requirements for intravenous potassium salts; I.V. potassium salts have been administered IVP in error, leading to fatal outcomes.

Brand Names: U.S. Epiklor™; Epiklor™/25; K-Tab®; Kaon-CL® 10; Klor-Con®; Klor-Con® 10; Klor-Con® 8; Klor-Con® M10; Klor-Con® M15; Klor-Con® M20; Klor-Con®/25; microK®; microK® 10

Brand Names: Canada Apo-K®; K-10®; K-Dur®; Micro-K Extencaps®; Roychlor®; Slo-Pot; Slow-K®

Index Terms KCl; Kdur

Generic Availability (U.S.) Yes: Excludes powder for solution

Pharmacologic Category Electrolyte Supplement, Oral; Electrolyte Supplement, Parenteral ▶

Use Treatment or prevention of hypokalemia

Contraindications Hypersensitivity to any component of the formulation; hyperkalemia. In addition, solid oral dosage forms are contraindicated in patients in whom there is a structural, pathological, and/or pharmacologic cause for delay or arrest in passage through the GI tract.

Warnings/Precautions Close monitoring of serum potassium concentrations is needed to avoid hyperkalemia. Use with caution in patients with renal impairment, cardiac disease, acid/base disorders, or potassium-altering conditions/disorders. Use with caution in digitalized patients or patients receiving concomitant medications or therapies that increase potassium (eg, ACEI, potassium-sparing diuretics, potassium containing salt substitutes). Do **NOT** administer undiluted or I.V. push; inappropriate parenteral administration may be fatal. Always administer potassium further diluted; refer to appropriate dilution and administration rate recommendations. Pain and phlebitis may occur during parenteral infusion requiring a decrease in infusion rate or potassium concentration. Avoid administering potassium diluted in dextrose solutions during initial therapy; potential for transient decreases in serum potassium due to intracellular shift of potassium from dextrose-stimulated insulin release. May cause GI upset (eg, nausea, vomiting, diarrhea, abdominal pain, discomfort) and lead to GI ulceration, bleeding, perforation, and/or obstruction. Oral liquid preparations (not solid) should be used in patients with esophageal compression or delayed gastric emptying.

Adverse Reactions (Reflective of adult population; not specific for elderly) Frequency not defined.

Dermatologic: Rash

Endocrine & metabolic: Hyperkalemia

Gastrointestinal: Abdominal pain/discomfort, diarrhea, flatulence, GI bleeding (oral), GI obstruction (oral), GI perforation (oral), nausea, vomiting

Drug Interactions

Metabolism/Transport Effects None known.

Avoid Concomitant Use

Avoid concomitant use of Potassium Chloride with any of the following: Glycopyrrolate

Increased Effect/Toxicity

Potassium Chloride may increase the levels/effects of: ACE Inhibitors; Angiotensin II Receptor Blockers; Potassium-Sparing Diuretics

The levels/effects of Potassium Chloride may be increased by: Anticholinergic Agents; Eplerenone; Glycopyrrolate

Decreased Effect There are no known significant interactions involving a decrease in effect.

Stability

Capsule: MicroK®: Store between 20°C to 25°C (68°F to 77°F).

Powder for oral solution: Klor-Con®: Store at room temperature of 15°C to 30°C (59°F to 86°F).

Solution for injection: Store at room temperature; do not freeze. Use only clear solutions. Use admixtures within 24 hours.

Tablet: K-Tab®: Store below 30°C (86°F).

Mechanism of Action Potassium is the major cation of intracellular fluid and is essential for the conduction of nerve impulses in heart, brain, and skeletal muscle; contraction of cardiac, skeletal and smooth muscles; maintenance of normal renal function, acid-base balance, carbohydrate metabolism, and gastric secretion

Pharmacodynamics/Kinetics

Absorption: Well absorbed from upper GI tract

Distribution: Enters cells via active transport from extracellular fluid

Excretion: Primarily urine; skin and feces (small amounts); most intestinal potassium reabsorbed

Dosage

Geriatric & Adult I.V. doses should be incorporated into the patient's maintenance I.V. fluids; intermittent I.V. potassium administration should be reserved for severe depletion situations in patients undergoing ECG monitoring. Doses expressed as mEq of potassium.

Normal daily requirements: Oral, I.V.: 40-80 mEq/day

Prevention of hypokalemia: Oral: 20-40 mEq/day in 1-2 divided doses

Treatment of hypokalemia:

Oral:

Asymptomatic, mild hypokalemia: Usual dosage range: 40-100 mEq/day divided in 2-5 doses; generally recommended to limit doses to 20-25 mEq/dose to avoid GI discomfort.

Mild-to-moderate hypokalemia: Some clinicians may administer up to 120-240 mEq/day divided in 3-4 doses; generally recommended to limit doses to 40-60 mEq/dose. If deficits are severe or ongoing losses are great, I.V. route should be considered.

I.V. intermittent infusion: Peripheral or central line: ≤10 mEq/hour; repeat as needed based on frequently obtained lab values; central line infusion and continuous ECG monitoring highly recommended for infusions >10 mEq/hour.

Potassium dosage/rate of infusion general guidelines (per product labeling): **Note:** High variability exists in dosing/infusion rate recommendations; therapy guided by patient condition and specific institutional guidelines.

Serum potassium >2.5 mEq/L: Maximum infusion rate: 10 mEq/hour; maximum concentration: 40 mEq/L; maximum 24-hour dose: 200 mEq

Serum potassium <2 mEq/L and symptomatic (excluding emergency treatment of cardiac arrest): Maximum infusion rate (central line only): 40 mEq/hour in presence of continuous ECG monitoring and frequent lab monitoring; In selected situations, patients may require up to 400 mEq/24 hours.

Administration

Parenteral: Potassium must be diluted prior to parenteral administration. Do not administer I.V. push. In general, the dose, concentration of infusion and rate of administration may be dependent on patient condition and specific institution policy. Some clinicians recommend that the maximum concentration for peripheral infusion is 10 mEq/100 mL and maximum rate of administration for peripheral infusion is 10 mEq/hour. ECG monitoring is recommended for peripheral or central infusions >10 mEq/hour in adults. Concentrations and rates of infusion may be greater with central line administration. Some clinicians recommend that the maximum concentration for central infusion is 20-40 mEq/100 mL and maximum rate of administration for central infusion is 40 mEq/hour.

Oral: Oral dosage forms should be taken with meals and a full glass of water or other liquid to minimize the risk of GI irritation. Prescribing information for the various oral preparations recommend that no more than 20 mEq or 25 mEq should be given as single dose.

Capsule: MicroK®: Swallow whole, do not chew. Capsules may also be opened and contents sprinkled on a spoonful of applesauce or pudding and should be swallowed immediately without chewing.

Powder: Klor-Con®: Dissolve one packet in 4-5 ounces of water or other beverage prior to administration.

Tablet:

K-Tab®, Kaon-Cl®, Klor-Con®: Swallow tablets whole; do not crush, chew, or suck on tablet.

Klor-Con® M: Swallow tablets whole; do not crush, chew, or suck on tablet. Tablet may also be broken in half and each half swallowed separately; the whole tablet may be dissolved in ~4 ounces of water (allow ~2 minutes to dissolve, stir well and drink immediately)

Monitoring Parameters Serum potassium, chloride, magnesium (to facilitate potassium repletion), cardiac monitor (if intermittent infusion or potassium infusion rates >10 mEq/hour in adults); to assess adequate replacement, repeat serum potassium level 2-4 hours after dose

Reference Range Note: Reference ranges may vary depending on the laboratory

Serum potassium: 3.5-5.2 mEq/L

Special Geriatric Considerations Elderly may require less potassium than younger adults due to decreased renal function. For the elderly who do not respond to replacement therapy, check serum magnesium. Long-term use of diuretics may result in hypomagnesemic.

Dosage Forms Excipient information presented when available (limited, particularly for generics); consult specific product labeling. [DSC] = Discontinued product

Capsule, extended release, microencapsulated, oral: 8 mEq, 10 mEq

microK®: 8 mEq [600 mg]

microK® 10: 10 mEq [750 mg]

Infusion, premixed in 1/2 NS: 20 mEq (1000 mL)

Infusion, premixed in D_{10} 1/4 NS: 5 mEq (250 mL [DSC])

Infusion, premixed in D_5 1/2 NS: 10 mEq (500 mL, 1000 mL); 20 mEq (1000 mL); 30 mEq (1000 mL); 40 mEq (1000 mL)

Infusion, premixed in D_5 1/3 NS: 20 mEq (1000 mL)

Infusion, premixed in D_5 1/4 NS: 5 mEq (250 mL); 10 mEq (500 mL, 1000 mL [DSC]); 20 mEq (1000 mL); 30 mEq (1000 mL [DSC]); 40 mEq (1000 mL [DSC])

Infusion, premixed in D_5LR: 20 mEq (1000 mL)

Infusion, premixed in D_5NS: 20 mEq (1000 mL); 40 mEq (1000 mL)

Infusion, premixed in D_5W: 20 mEq (1000 mL); 40 mEq (1000 mL)

Infusion, premixed in NS: 20 mEq (1000 mL); 40 mEq (1000 mL)

Infusion, premixed in water for injection [highly concentrated]: 10 mEq (50 mL, 100 mL); 20 mEq (50 mL, 100 mL); 30 mEq (100 mL); 40 mEq (100 mL)

Injection, solution [concentrate]: 2 mEq/mL (5 mL, 10 mL, 15 mL, 20 mL, 30 mL, 250 mL, 500 mL [DSC])

Injection, solution [concentrate, preservative free]: 2 mEq/mL (5 mL, 10 mL, 15 mL [DSC], 20 mL)

Powder for solution, oral:
  Epiklor™: 20 mEq/packet (30s, 100s) [sugar free; orange flavor]
  Epiklor™/25: 25 mEq/packet (30s, 100s) [sugar free; orange flavor]
  Klor-Con®: 20 mEq/packet (30s, 100s) [sugar free; fruit flavor]
  Klor-Con®/25: 25 mEq/packet (30s, 100s) [sugar free; fruit flavor]
Solution, oral: 20 mEq/15 mL (15 mL, 30 mL, 473 mL, 480 mL); 40 mEq/15 mL (15 mL, 473 mL, 480 mL)
Tablet, extended release, oral: 10 mEq
Tablet, extended release, microencapsulated, oral: 8 mEq, 10 mEq, 20 mEq
  Klor-Con® M10: 10 mEq [750 mg]
  Klor-Con® M15: 15 mEq [scored; 1125 mg]
  Klor-Con® M20: 20 mEq [scored; 1500 mg]
Tablet, extended release, wax matrix, oral: 8 mEq, 10 mEq
  K-Tab®: 10 mEq [750 mg]
  Kaon-CL® 10: 10 mEq [750 mg]
  Klor-Con® 8: 8 mEq [600 mg]
  Klor-Con® 10: 10 mEq [750 mg]

◆ **Potassium Citrate, Citric Acid, and Sodium Citrate** *see* Citric Acid, Sodium Citrate, and Potassium Citrate *on page 391*

Potassium Gluconate (poe TASS ee um GLOO coe nate)

Generic Availability (U.S.) Yes
Pharmacologic Category Electrolyte Supplement, Oral
Use Dietary supplement
Contraindications Hyperkalemia
Warnings/Precautions Use caution in patients with acid/base disorders, cardiovascular disease, potassium-altering conditions/disorders, or renal impairment. Use with caution in patients receiving concomitant medications or therapies that increase potassium (eg, ACEI, potassium-sparing diuretics, potassium containing salt substitutes). Close monitoring of serum potassium concentrations is needed to avoid hyperkalemia. May cause GI upset (eg, nausea, vomiting, diarrhea, abdominal pain, discomfort) and lead to GI ulceration, bleeding, perforation and/or obstruction. Oral liquid preparations (not solid) should be used in patients with esophageal compression or delayed gastric emptying.
Drug Interactions
  Metabolism/Transport Effects None known.
  Avoid Concomitant Use There are no known interactions where it is recommended to avoid concomitant use.
  Increased Effect/Toxicity
    Potassium Gluconate may increase the levels/effects of: ACE Inhibitors; Angiotensin II Receptor Blockers; Potassium-Sparing Diuretics

    The levels/effects of Potassium Gluconate may be increased by: Eplerenone
  Decreased Effect There are no known significant interactions involving a decrease in effect.
Stability Store at room temperature.
Mechanism of Action Potassium is the major cation of intracellular fluid and is essential for the conduction of nerve impulses in heart, brain, and skeletal muscle; contraction of cardiac, skeletal and smooth muscles; maintenance of normal renal function, acid-base balance, carbohydrate metabolism, and gastric secretion
Pharmacodynamics/Kinetics
  Absorption: Well absorbed from upper GI tract
  Distribution: Enters cells via active transport from extracellular fluid
  Excretion: Primarily urine; skin and feces (small amounts); most intestinal potassium reabsorbed
Dosage
  Geriatric & Adult Dietary supplement: Oral: One tablet daily
Monitoring Parameters Serum potassium, blood pressure, pulse, ECG (as needed), signs of muscle weakness, cramps; serum magnesium for failure to respond to replacement
Reference Range Note: Reference ranges may vary depending on the laboratory
  Serum potassium: 3.5-5.2 mEq/L
Test Interactions Decreased ammonia (B)
Pharmacotherapy Pearls 9.4 g potassium gluconate is approximately equal to 40 mEq potassium (4.3 mEq potassium/g salt)

Special Geriatric Considerations Elderly may require less potassium than younger adults due to decreased renal function. For the elderly who do not respond to replacement therapy, check serum magnesium. Long-term use of diuretics may result in hypomagnesemia.

Dosage Forms Excipient information presented when available (limited, particularly for generics); consult specific product labeling.

Caplet, oral: 595 mg [equivalent to potassium 99 mg]

Capsule, oral [strength expressed as base]: 99 mg

Tablet, oral: 550 mg [equivalent to potassium 90 mg], 595 mg [equivalent to potassium 99 mg]

Tablet, oral [strength expressed as base]: 99 mg

Tablet, timed release, oral [strength expressed as base]: 95 mg

---

Potassium Iodide and Iodine (poe TASS ee um EYE oh dide & EYE oh dine)

Medication Safety Issues
Sound-alike/look-alike issues:
Potassium iodide and iodine (Strong Iodide Solution or Lugol's solution) may be confused with potassium iodide products, including saturated solution of potassium iodide (SSKI®)

Index Terms Iodine and Potassium Iodide; Lugol's Solution; Strong Iodine Solution

Generic Availability (U.S.) Yes

Pharmacologic Category Antithyroid Agent

Use Topical antiseptic

Unlabeled Use Reduce thyroid vascularity prior to thyroidectomy and management of thyrotoxic crisis; block thyroidal uptake of radioactive isotopes of iodine in a radiation emergency or after therapeutic/diagnostic use of radioactive iodine

Dosage

Geriatric & Adult RDA: 150 mcg (iodine)

Preparation for thyroidectomy (unlabeled use): Oral: 5-7 drops (0.25-0.35 mL) 3 times/day; administer for 10 days before surgery; if not euthyroid prior to surgery, consider concurrent beta-blockade (eg, propranolol) in the immediate preoperative period to reduce the risk of thyroid storm (Bahn, 2011)

Thyrotoxic crisis (unlabeled use): Oral: 4-8 drops every 6-8 hours; begin administration ≥1 hour following the initial dose of either propylthiouracil or methimazole (Nayak, 2006)

Thyroid gland protection during radiopharmaceutical use (unlabeled use): Oral: 1 drop/kg/day; (maximum: 40 drops/day or 20 drops twice daily) (Giammarile, 2008); alternatively, 20 drops 3 times/day has also been used (Bexxar® prescribing information, 2005)

Note: Initiate 1-48 hours prior to radiopharmaceutical exposure and continue after radiopharmaceutical administration until risk of exposure has diminished (treatment initiation time and duration is dependent on the radiopharmaceutical agent used, consult specific protocol or labeling.

Special Geriatric Considerations Elderly may have reduced renal function and require close monitoring of serum potassium. May be also recommended to check serum magnesium.

Dosage Forms Excipient information presented when available (limited, particularly for generics); consult specific product labeling.

Solution, oral: Potassium iodide 100 mg/mL and iodine 50 mg/mL (473 mL)

Solution, topical: Potassium iodide 100 mg/mL and iodine 50 mg/mL (8 mL)

Potassium Phosphate (poe TASS ee um FOS fate)

Medication Safety Issues
High alert medication:
The Institute for Safe Medication Practices (ISMP) includes this medication (I.V. formulation) among its list of drugs which have a heightened risk of causing significant patient harm when used in error.

Other safety concerns:
Per JCAHO recommendations, concentrated electrolyte solutions should not be available in patient care areas.

Consider special storage requirements for intravenous potassium salts; I.V. potassium salts have been administered IVP in error, leading to fatal outcomes.

Safe Prescribing: Because inorganic phosphate exists as monobasic and dibasic anions, with the mixture of valences dependent on pH, ordering by mEq amounts is unreliable and may lead to large dosing errors. In addition, I.V. phosphate is available in the sodium and potassium salt; therefore, the content of these cations must be considered when ordering phosphate. The most reliable method of ordering I.V. phosphate is by millimoles, then specifying the potassium or sodium salt. For example, an order for 15 mmol of phosphate as potassium phosphate in one liter of normal saline.

Brand Names: U.S. Neutra-Phos®-K [OTC] [DSC]

Index Terms Phosphate, Potassium

Generic Availability (U.S.) Yes: Injection

Pharmacologic Category Electrolyte Supplement, Parenteral

Use Treatment and prevention of hypophosphatemia; **Note:** The concomitant amount of potassium must be calculated into the total electrolyte content. For each 1 mmol of phosphate, ~1.5 mEq of potassium will be administered. Therefore, if ordering 30 mmol of potassium phosphate, the patient will receive ~45 mEq of potassium.

Contraindications Hyperphosphatemia, hyperkalemia, hypocalcemia, hypomagnesemia, renal failure (oral product)

Warnings/Precautions Close monitoring of serum potassium concentrations is needed to avoid hyperkalemia. Use with caution in patients with renal insufficiency, cardiac disease, metabolic alkalosis. Use with caution in digitalized patients and patients receiving concomitant potassium-altering therapies. Parenteral potassium may cause pain and phlebitis, requiring a decrease in infusion rate or potassium concentration. Solutions for injection may contain aluminum; toxic levels may occur following prolonged administration in patients with renal impairment.

Adverse Reactions (Reflective of adult population; not specific for elderly) Frequency not defined.

Cardiovascular: Arrhythmia, bradycardia, chest pain, ECG changes, edema, heart block, hypotension

Central nervous system: Listlessness, mental confusion, tetany (with large doses of phosphate)

Endocrine & metabolic: Hyperkalemia

Gastrointestinal: Diarrhea, nausea, stomach pain, vomiting

Genitourinary: Urine output decreased

Local: Phlebitis

Neuromuscular & skeletal: Paralysis, paresthesia, weakness

Renal: Acute renal failure

Respiratory: Dyspnea

Drug Interactions

Metabolism/Transport Effects None known.

Avoid Concomitant Use There are no known interactions where it is recommended to avoid concomitant use.

Increased Effect/Toxicity

Potassium Phosphate may increase the levels/effects of: ACE Inhibitors; Angiotensin II Receptor Blockers; Potassium-Sparing Diuretics

The levels/effects of Potassium Phosphate may be increased by: Bisphosphonate Derivatives; Eplerenone

Decreased Effect There are no known significant interactions involving a decrease in effect.

Ethanol/Nutrition/Herb Interactions Food: Avoid administering with oxalate (berries, nuts, chocolate, beans, celery, tomato) or phytate-containing foods (bran, whole wheat).

Stability Store at room temperature; do not freeze. Use only clear solutions. Up to 10-15 mEq of calcium may be added per liter before precipitate may occur.

Stability of parenteral admixture at room temperature (25°C) is 24 hours.

Phosphate salts may precipitate when mixed with calcium salts. Solubility is improved in amino acid parenteral nutrition solutions. Check with a pharmacist to determine compatibility.

Dosage

Geriatric & Adult Caution: The concomitant amount of potassium must be calculated into the total electrolyte content. For each 1 mmol of phosphate, ~1.5 mEq of potassium will be administered. Therefore, if ordering 30 mmol of potassium phosphate, the patient will receive ~45 mEq of potassium. With orders for I.V. phosphate, there is considerable confusion associated with the use of millimoles (mmol) versus milliequivalents (mEq) to express the phosphate requirement. The most reliable method of ordering I.V. phosphate is by millimoles, then specifying the potassium or sodium salt. Doses listed as mmol of phosphate.

Acute treatment of hypophosphatemia: Repletion of severe hypophosphatemia should be done I.V. because large doses of oral phosphate may cause diarrhea and intestinal absorption may be unreliable. Reserve intermittent I.V. infusion for severe depletion situations; may require continuous cardiac monitoring depending on potassium administration rate. Guidelines differ based on degree of illness, need/use of parenteral nutrition, and severity of hypophosphatemia. If potassium >4.0 mEq/L consider phosphate replacement strategy without potassium (eg, sodium phosphates). Patients with severe renal impairment were excluded from phosphate supplement trials. **Note:** 1 mmol phosphate = 31 mg phosphorus; 1 mg phosphorus = 0.032 mmol phosphate.

General replacement guidelines (Lentz, 1978):
  Low dose, if serum phosphate losses are recent and uncomplicated: 0.08 mmol/kg over 6 hours
  Intermediate dose, if serum phosphorus level 0.5-1 mg/dL (0.16-0.32 mmol/L): 0.16-0.24 mmol/kg over 4-6 hours
  Note: The initial dose may be increased by 25% to 50% if the patient is symptomatic secondary to hypophosphatemia and lowered by 25% to 50% if the patient is hypercalcemic.

Critically-ill adult patients receiving concurrent enteral/parenteral nutrition (Brown, 2006; Clark, 2006): Note: Round doses to the nearest 7.5 mmol for ease of preparation. If administering with phosphate-containing parenteral nutrition, do not exceed 15 mmol/L within parenteral nutrition. May use adjusted body weight for patients weighing >130% of ideal body weight (and BMI<40 kg/m^2) by using [IBW + 0.25 (ABW-IBW)]:
  Low dose, serum phosphorus level 2.3-3 mg/dL (0.74-0.96 mmol/L): 0.16-0.32 mmol/kg over 4-6 hours
  Intermediate dose, serum phosphorus level 1.6-2.2 mg/dL (0.51-0.71 mmol/L): 0.32-0.64 mmol/kg over 4-6 hours
  High dose, serum phosphorus <1.5 mg/dL (<0.5 mmol/L): 0.64-1 mmol/kg over 8-12 hours

Parenteral nutrition: I.V.: 10-15 mmol/1000 kcal (Hicks, 2001) **or** 20-40 mmol/24 hours (Mirtallo, 2004 [ASPEN guidelines])

Administration Injection must be diluted in appropriate I.V. solution and volume prior to administration. In general, the dose, concentration of infusion, and rate of administration may be dependent on patient condition and specific institution policy. Must consider administration precautions for phosphate and potassium when prescribing.

For adult patients with severe symptomatic hypophosphatemia (ie, <1.5 mg/dL), may admin­ister at rates up to 15 mmol phosphate/hour (this rate will deliver potassium at 22.5 mEq/hour) (Rosen, 1995, Charron, 2003). Potassium infusion rates >10 mEq/hour should be administered via central line (minimizes burning and phlebitis). ECG monitoring is recommended for potassium infusions >10 mEq/hour in adults. In patients with renal dysfunction and/or less severe hypophosphatemia, slower administration rates (eg, over 4-6 hours) or oral repletion is recommended.

Intermittent infusion doses of potassium phosphate are typically prepared in 100-250 mL of NS or D$_5$W (usual phosphate concentration range: 0.15 - 0.6 mmol/mL) (Rosen, 1995, Charron, 2003). Suggested maximum concentrations:
  Peripheral line administration: 6.7 mmoL potassium phosphate/100 mL (10 mEq potassium/100 mL)
  Central line administration: 26.8 mmoL potassium phosphate/100 mL (40 mEq potassium/100 mL)

Monitoring Parameters Serum potassium, calcium, phosphorus, magnesium (to facilitate potassium repletion); cardiac monitor (if intermittent infusion or potassium infusion rates 0.5 mEq/kg/hour in children or >10 mEq/hour in adults); to assess adequate replacement, repeat serum potassium and phosphorus levels 2-4 hours after dose

Reference Range Note: Reference ranges may vary depending on the laboratory
  Serum calcium: 8.4-10.2 mg/dL
  Serum phosphorus: Both low and high ends of the normal range are higher in children than in adults.
  Adults: 2.5-4.5 mg/dL (0.81-1.45 mmol/L)
  Serum potassium: 3.5-5.2 mEq/L

Special Geriatric Considerations Elderly may require less potassium than younger adults due to decreased renal function. Elderly who do not respond to replacement therapy, check serum magnesium. Long-term use of diuretics may result in hypomagnesemia. Monitor closely in elderly with Cl$_{cr}$ <30 mL/minute.

Dosage Forms Excipient information presented when available (limited, particularly for generics); consult specific product labeling.
  Injection, solution: Potassium 4.4 mEq and phosphorus 3 mmol per mL (5 mL, 15 mL, 50 mL) [equivalent to potassium 170 mg and elemental phosphorus 93 mg per mL]

Potassium Phosphate and Sodium Phosphate
(poe TASS ee um FOS fate & SOW dee um FOS fate)

Related Information
Potassium Phosphate *on page 1575*
Sodium Phosphates *on page 1791*

Medication Safety Issues
Sound-alike/look-alike issues:
K-Phos® Neutral may be confused with Neutra-Phos-K®

Brand Names: U.S. K-Phos® MF; K-Phos® Neutral; K-Phos® No. 2; Phos-NaK; Phospha 250™ Neutral

Index Terms Neutra-Phos; Sodium Phosphate and Potassium Phosphate

Generic Availability (U.S.) Yes

Pharmacologic Category Electrolyte Supplement, Oral

Use Treatment of conditions associated with excessive renal phosphate loss or inadequate GI absorption of phosphate; to acidify the urine to lower calcium concentrations; to increase the antibacterial activity of methenamine; reduce odor and rash caused by ammonia in urine

Contraindications Addison's disease, hyperkalemia, hyperphosphatemia, infected urolithiasis or struvite stone formation, patients with severely impaired renal function

Warnings/Precautions Use with caution in patients with renal disease, cardiac disease, metabolic alkalosis, acute dehydration, hepatic impairment, hypernatremia, and hypotension.

Adverse Reactions (Reflective of adult population; not specific for elderly) Frequency not defined.
Cardiovascular: Bradycardia, arrhythmia, chest pain, edema, tachycardia
Central nervous system: Mental confusion, tetany (with large doses of phosphate), headache, dizziness, seizure
Endocrine & metabolic: Hyperkalemia, alkalosis
Gastrointestinal: Diarrhea, nausea, stomach pain, flatulence, vomiting, throat pain, weight gain
Genitourinary: Urine output decreased
Local: Phlebitis
Neuromuscular & skeletal: Weakness, arthralgia, bone pain, paralysis, paresthesia, pain/weakness of extremities, muscle cramps
Renal: Acute renal failure
Respiratory: Dyspnea
Miscellaneous: Thirst

Drug Interactions
Metabolism/Transport Effects None known.
Avoid Concomitant Use There are no known interactions where it is recommended to avoid concomitant use.
Increased Effect/Toxicity
Potassium Phosphate and Sodium Phosphate may increase the levels/effects of: ACE Inhibitors; Angiotensin II Receptor Blockers; Potassium-Sparing Diuretics

The levels/effects of Potassium Phosphate and Sodium Phosphate may be increased by: Bisphosphonate Derivatives; Eplerenone

Decreased Effect There are no known significant interactions involving a decrease in effect.

Pharmacodynamics/Kinetics Excretion: Urine

Dosage
Geriatric & Adult Phosphate supplement: Oral: Elemental phosphorus 250-500 mg 4 times/day after meals and at bedtime

Administration
Powder: Following dilution of powder, solution may be chilled to increase palatability.
Tablet: Should be taken with a full glass of water.

Monitoring Parameters Serum potassium, sodium, magnesium (failure to respond to replacement), calcium, phosphate, ECG; signs of muscle weakness, cramps

Reference Range Note: Reference ranges may vary depending on the laboratory
Serum potassium: 3.5-5.2 mEq/L
Serum phosphorus: Both low and high ends of the normal range are higher in children than in adults.
Adults: 2.5-4.5 mg/dL (0.81-1.45 mmol/L)

Pharmacotherapy Pearls Each mmol of phosphate contains 31 mg elemental phosphorus
Additional terminology for the potassium and sodium salts:
Sodium phosphate monobasic = Sodium acid phosphate
Sodium phosphate dibasic = Disodium phosphate
Potassium phosphate monobasic = Potassium acid phosphate
Potassium phosphate dibasic = Dipotassium phosphate

Special Geriatric Considerations A complete drug history should be taken to rule out potential drug interactions since elderly frequently may be taking potassium and potassium-sparing diuretics or salicylates as antacids. Elderly may require less potassium than younger adults due to decreased renal function. Elderly who do not respond to replacement therapy, check serum magnesium. Long-term use of diuretics may result in hypomagnesemia.

Dosage Forms Excipient information presented when available (limited, particularly for generics); consult specific product labeling.

Powder for solution, oral:

Phos-NaK: Dibasic potassium phosphate, monobasic potassium phosphate, dibasic sodium phosphate, and monobasic sodium phosphate per packet (100s) [sugar free; equivalent to elemental phosphorus 250 mg (8 mmol), sodium 160 mg (6.9 mEq), and potassium 280 mg (7.1 mEq) per packet; fruit flavor]

Tablet, oral:

K-Phos® MF: Potassium acid phosphate 155 mg and sodium acid phosphate 350 mg [equivalent to elemental phosphorus 125.6 mg (4 mmol), sodium 67 mg (2.9 mEq), and potassium 44.5 mg (1.1 mEq)]

K-Phos® Neutral: Monobasic potassium phosphate 155 mg, dibasic sodium phosphate 852 mg, and monobasic sodium phosphate 130 mg [equivalent to elemental phosphorus 250 mg (8 mmol), sodium 298 mg (13 mEq), and potassium 45 mg (1.1 mEq)]

K-Phos® No. 2: Potassium acid phosphate 305 mg and sodium acid phosphate 700 mg [equivalent to elemental phosphorus 250 mg (8 mmol), sodium 134 mg (5.8 mEq), and potassium 88 mg (2.3 mEq)]

Phospha 250™ Neutral: Monobasic potassium phosphate 155 mg, dibasic sodium phosphate 852 mg, and monobasic sodium phosphate 130 mg [equivalent to elemental phosphorus 250 mg (8 mmol), sodium 298 mg (13 mEq), and potassium 45 mg (1.1 mEq)]

◆ **Potiga™** see Ezogabine on page 740
◆ **PPD** see Tuberculin Tests on page 1980
◆ **PPI-0903** see Ceftaroline Fosamil on page 326
◆ **PPI-0903M** see Ceftaroline Fosamil on page 326
◆ **PPSV** see Pneumococcal Polysaccharide Vaccine (Polyvalent) on page 1558
◆ **PPSV23** see Pneumococcal Polysaccharide Vaccine (Polyvalent) on page 1558
◆ **PPV23** see Pneumococcal Polysaccharide Vaccine (Polyvalent) on page 1558
◆ **Pradaxa®** see Dabigatran Etexilate on page 469

Pramipexole (pra mi PEKS ole)

Related Information
Antiparkinsonian Agents on page 2101
Medication Safety Issues
Sound-alike/look-alike issues:
Mirapex® may be confused with Hiprex®, Mifeprex®, MiraLax®
Brand Names: U.S. Mirapex®; Mirapex® ER®
Brand Names: Canada Apo-Pramipexole®; Ava-Pramipexole; CO Pramipexole; Mirapex®; PMS-Pramipexole; Sandoz-Pramipexole; Teva-Pramipexole
Index Terms Pramipexole Dihydrochloride Monohydrate
Generic Availability (U.S.) Yes: Excludes extended release tablet
Pharmacologic Category Anti-Parkinson's Agent, Dopamine Agonist
Use
Immediate release: Treatment of the signs and symptoms of idiopathic Parkinson's disease; treatment of moderate-to-severe primary Restless Legs Syndrome (RLS)
Extended release: Treatment of the signs and symptoms of idiopathic Parkinson's disease
Unlabeled Use Treatment of depression; treatment of fibromyalgia
Contraindications Hypersensitivity to pramipexole or any component of the formulation
Warnings/Precautions Caution should be taken in patients with renal insufficiency; dose adjustment necessary. May cause or exacerbate dyskinesias; use caution in patients with pre-existing dyskinesias. May cause orthostatic hypotension; Parkinson's disease patients appear to have an impaired capacity to respond to a postural challenge. Use with caution in patients at risk of hypotension or where transient hypotensive episodes would be poorly tolerated. Parkinson's patients being treated with dopaminergic agonists ordinarily require careful monitoring for signs and symptoms of postural hypotension, especially during dose escalation. May cause hallucinations.

Dopamine agonists have been associated with compulsive behaviors and/or loss of impulse control, which has manifested as pathological gambling, libido increases (hypersexuality), and/or binge eating. Causality has not been established, and controversy exists as to whether this phenomenon is related to the underlying disease, prior behaviors/addictions and/or drug therapy. Dose reduction or discontinuation of therapy has been reported to reverse these behaviors in some, but not all cases. Risk for melanoma development is increased in Parkinson's disease patients; drug causation or factors contributing to risk have not been established. Patients should be monitored closely and periodic skin examinations should be performed.

Taper gradually over a period of 1 week when discontinuing therapy; dopaminergic agents have been associated with a syndrome resembling neuroleptic malignant syndrome on abrupt withdrawal or significant dosage reduction after long-term use. Ergot-derived dopamine agonists have been associated with fibrotic complications (eg, retroperitoneal fibrosis, pleural thickening, and pulmonary infiltrates). Although pramipexole is not an ergot, there have been postmarketing reports of possible fibrotic complications with pramipexole; monitor closely for signs and symptoms of fibrosis.

Pramipexole has been associated with somnolence, particularly at higher dosages (>1.5 mg/day). In addition, patients have been reported to fall asleep during activities of daily living, including driving, while taking this medication. Whether these patients exhibited somnolence prior to these events is not clear. Patients should be advised of this issue and factors which may increase risk (sleep disorders, other sedating medications, or concomitant medications which increase pramipexole concentrations) and instructed to report daytime somnolence or sleepiness to the prescriber. Patients should use caution in performing activities which require alertness (driving or operating machinery), and to avoid other medications which may cause CNS depression, including ethanol. Use caution in the elderly as they may be more sensitive to these adverse drug reactions.

Pathologic degenerative changes were observed in the retinas of albino rats during studies with this agent, but were not observed in the retinas of albino mice or in other species. The significance of these data for humans remains uncertain. Augmentation (earlier onset of symptoms in the evening/afternoon, increase and/or spread of symptoms to other extremities) or rebound (shifting of symptoms to early morning hours) may occur in some RLS patients.

Adverse Reactions (Reflective of adult population; not specific for elderly)

Parkinson's disease: Actual frequency may be dependent on dose and/or formulation:

>10%:
  Cardiovascular: Orthostatic hypotension (dose related; ≤53%)
  Central nervous system: Somnolence (dose related; 9% to 36%), extrapyramidal syndrome (28%), insomnia (4% to 27%), dizziness (2% to 26%), hallucinations (5% to 17%), abnormal dreams (11%), headache (4% to 7%)
  Gastrointestinal: Nausea (dose related; 11% to 28%), constipation (dose related; 6% to 14%)
  Neuromuscular & skeletal: Dyskinesia (17% to 47%), weakness (1% to 14%)
  Miscellaneous: Accidental injury (17%)

1% to 10%:
  Cardiovascular: Edema (2% to 8%), chest pain (3%)
  Central nervous system: Confusion (4% to 10%), dystonia (2% to 8%), fatigue (6%), amnesia (dose related; 4% to 6%), sudden onset of sleep (3% to 6%), vertigo (2% to 4%), hypesthesia (3%), abnormal thinking (2% to 3%), akathisia (2% to 3%), malaise (2% to 3%), paranoia (2%), sleep disorder (1% to 3%), depression (≤2%), delusions (1%), fever (1%), myoclonus (1%)
  Endocrine & metabolic: Libido decreased (1%)
  Gastrointestinal: Xerostomia (4% to 7%), anorexia (1% to 5%), vomiting (4%), abdominal discomfort/pain (1% to 4%), dyspepsia (3%), appetite increased (2% to 3%), dysphagia (2%), weight loss (2%), salivary hypersecretion (≤2%), diarrhea (1% to 2%)
  Genitourinary: Urinary frequency (6%), urinary tract infection (4%), impotence (2%), urinary incontinence (2%)
  Neuromuscular & skeletal: Gait abnormalities (7%), hypertonia (7%), muscle spasm (3% to 5%), falls (4%), arthritis (3%), tremor (3%), back pain (2% to 3%), bursitis (2%), muscle twitching (2%), balance abnormalities (≤2%), CPK increased (1%), myasthenia (1%)
  Ocular: Accommodation abnormalities (4%), vision abnormalities (3%), diplopia (1%)
  Respiratory: Dyspnea (4%), cough (3%), rhinitis (3%), pneumonia (2%)

Restless legs syndrome: Actual frequency may be dependent on dose:

>10%:
  Central nervous system: Headache (16%), insomnia (9% to 13%)
  Gastrointestinal: Nausea (11% to 27%)

1% to 10%:
  Central nervous system: Fatigue (3% to 9%), abnormal dreams (1% to 8%), somnolence (6%)
  Gastrointestinal: Diarrhea (1% to 7%), constipation (4%), xerostomia (3%)
  Neuromuscular & skeletal: Limb pain (3% to 7%)

Respiratory: Nasal congestion (≤6%)
Miscellaneous: Influenza (1% to 7%)

Drug Interactions

Metabolism/Transport Effects None known.

Avoid Concomitant Use

Avoid concomitant use of Pramipexole with any of the following: Azelastine; Azelastine (Nasal); Methadone; Mirtazapine; Paraldehyde

Increased Effect/Toxicity

Pramipexole may increase the levels/effects of: Alcohol (Ethyl); Azelastine; Azelastine (Nasal); Buprenorphine; CNS Depressants; Methadone; Metyrosine; Mirtazapine; Paraldehyde; Selective Serotonin Reuptake Inhibitors; Zolpidem

The levels/effects of Pramipexole may be increased by: Cimetidine; HydrOXYzine; MAO Inhibitors; Methylphenidate

Decreased Effect

Pramipexole may decrease the levels/effects of: Antipsychotics (Typical)

The levels/effects of Pramipexole may be decreased by: Antipsychotics (Atypical); Antipsychotics (Typical); Metoclopramide

Ethanol/Nutrition/Herb Interactions

Ethanol: May increase CNS depression; monitor for increased effects with coadministration. Caution patients about effects.

Food: Food intake does not affect the extent of drug absorption although the time to maximal plasma concentration is delayed when taken with a meal.

Herb/Nutraceutical: Avoid valerian, St John's wort, SAMe, kava kava (may increase risk of serotonin syndrome and/or excessive sedation).

Stability Store at 25°C (77°F); excursions permitted to 15°C to 30°C (59°F to 86°F). Protect from light and high humidity.

Mechanism of Action Pramipexole is a nonergot dopamine agonist with specificity for the D_2 subfamily dopamine receptor, and has also been shown to bind to D_3 and D_4 receptors. By binding to these receptors, it is thought that pramipexole can stimulate dopamine activity on the nerves of the striatum and substantia nigra.

Pharmacodynamics/Kinetics

Absorption: Rapid

Distribution: V_d: 500 L

Metabolism: Minimal

Bioavailability: >90%

Half-life: Adults: 8 hours; older adults: 12 hours

Elimination: 90% eliminated unchanged in the urine

Clearance is decreased in older adults, likely due to decreased renal function. Clearance in Parkinson's patients was 30% less than healthy older adult volunteers. Clearance is decreased 60% when creatinine clearance is 40 mL/minute; 75% when clearance is 20 mL/minute.

Dosage

Geriatric & Adult

Parkinson's disease: Oral:

Immediate release formulation: Initial: 0.375 mg/day given in 3 divided doses; increase gradually every 5-7 days; range: 1.5-4.5 mg/day.

Extended release formulation (Mirapex® ER™): Initial: 0.375 mg once daily; increase gradually to 0.75 mg once daily. If necessary, may increase by 0.75 mg/dose not more frequently than every 5-7 days; maximum recommended dose 4.5 mg/day.

Note: Converting from immediate release to extended release: May initiate extended release preparation the morning after the last immediate release evening tablet is taken. The total daily dose should remain the same.

Restless legs syndrome: Oral: Initial: 0.125 mg once daily 2-3 hours before bedtime. Dose may be doubled every 4-7 days up to 0.5 mg/day. Maximum dose: 0.5 mg/day (manufacturer's recommendation).

Note: Most patients require <0.5 mg/day, but higher doses have been used (2 mg/day). If augmentation occurs, dose earlier in the day.

Depression (unlabeled use): Initial: 0.25-0.375 mg/day given in 2-3 divided doses with a gradual titration; mean dose: 1.6-1.7 mg/day (Aiken, 2007; Goldberg, 2004)

Fibromyalgia (unlabeled use): Initial: 0.25 mg once daily at bedtime; may be increased weekly by 0.25 mg/day increments up to 4.5 mg/day (Holman, 2005)

Renal Impairment Use caution; renally-eliminated

Parkinson's disease: Immediate release formulation:

Cl_{cr} 35-59 mL/minute: Initial: 0.125 mg twice daily (maximum dose: 1.5 mg twice daily)

Cl_{cr} 15-34 mL/minute: Initial: 0.125 mg once daily (maximum dose: 1.5 mg once daily)

Cl_{cr} <15 mL/minute: Not adequately studied

Hemodialysis: Not adequately studied; a negligible amount of pramipexole is removed by dialysis

Parkinson's disease: Extended release formulation:
Cl_{cr} >50 mL/minute: Dosing adjustment not necessary

Cl_{cr} 30-50 mL/minute: Initial: 0.375 mg every other day; may increase to 0.375 mg once daily no sooner than 1 week after initiation. If necessary, may increase by 0.375 mg/dose not more frequently than every 7 days; maximum recommended dose: 2.25 mg/day

Cl_{cr} <30 mL/minute: Not recommended

Hemodialysis: Not recommended; a negligible amount of pramipexole is removed by dialysis

Restless legs syndrome: Immediate release formulation:
Cl_{cr} 20-60 mL/minute: Duration between titration should be increased to 14 days

Cl_{cr} <20 mL/minute: Not adequately studied

Administration Doses should be titrated gradually in all patients to avoid the onset of intolerable side effects. The dosage should be increased to achieve a maximum therapeutic effect, balanced against the side effects of dyskinesia, hallucinations, somnolence, and dry mouth. May be administered with or without food; may be administered with food to decrease nausea. Extended release tablets should be swallowed whole and not chewed, crushed, or divided.

Monitoring Parameters Blood pressure, heart rate; body weight changes; CNS depression, fall risk

Special Geriatric Considerations Since the dose is titrated to clinical response, no specific dosage adjustment is necessary in the elderly.

Dosage Forms Excipient information presented when available (limited, particularly for generics); consult specific product labeling.

Tablet, oral, as dihydrochloride monohydrate: 0.125 mg, 0.25 mg, 0.5 mg, 0.75 mg, 1 mg, 1.5 mg

Mirapex®: 0.125 mg
Mirapex®: 0.25 mg, 0.5 mg [scored]
Mirapex®: 0.75 mg
Mirapex®: 1 mg, 1.5 mg [scored]

Tablet, extended release, oral, as dihydrochloride monohydrate:
Mirapex® ER®: 0.375 mg, 0.75 mg, 1.5 mg, 2.25 mg, 3 mg, 3.75 mg, 4.5 mg

◆ **Pramipexole Dihydrochloride Monohydrate** *see* Pramipexole *on page 1579*

Pramlintide (PRAM lin tide)

Related Information
Diabetes Mellitus Management, Adults *on page 2193*

Medication Safety Issues
High alert medication:
The Institute for Safe Medication Practices (ISMP) includes this medication among its list of drug classes which have a heightened risk of causing significant patient harm when used in error.

Administration issues:
Use caution when drawing up doses from the vial (concentration 600 micrograms (mcg)/mL). Manufacturer recommended dosing ranges from 15 mcg to 120 mcg, which corresponds to injectable volumes of 0.025 mL to 0.2 mL. Patients and healthcare providers should exercise caution when administering this product to avoid inadvertent calculation of the dose based on "units," which could result in a sixfold overdose.

Brand Names: U.S. SymlinPen®; Symlin® [DSC]

Index Terms Pramlintide Acetate

Generic Availability (U.S.) No

Pharmacologic Category Amylinomimetic; Antidiabetic Agent

Use
Adjunctive treatment with mealtime insulin in type 1 diabetes mellitus (insulin dependent, IDDM) patients who have failed to achieve desired glucose control despite optimal insulin therapy

Adjunctive treatment with mealtime insulin in type 2 diabetes mellitus (noninsulin dependent, NIDDM) patients who have failed to achieve desired glucose control despite optimal insulin therapy, with or without concurrent sulfonylurea and/or metformin

Medication Guide Available Yes

Contraindications Hypersensitivity to pramlintide or any component of the formulation; confirmed diagnosis of gastroparesis; hypoglycemia unawareness

Warnings/Precautions [U.S. Boxed Warning]: Coadministration with insulin may induce severe hypoglycemia (usually within 3 hours following administration); coadministration with insulin therapy is an approved indication but does require an initial dosage reduction of insulin and frequent pre and post blood glucose monitoring to reduce risk of severe hypoglycemia. Concurrent use of other glucose-lowering agents may increase risk of hypoglycemia. Avoid use in patients with poor compliance with their insulin regimen and/or blood glucose monitoring. Do not use in patients with Hb A_{1c} levels >9% or recent, recurrent episodes of hypoglycemia; obtain detailed history of glucose control (eg, Hb A_{1c}, incidence of hypoglycemia, glucose monitoring, and medication compliance) and body weight before initiating therapy. Use caution in patients with visual or dexterity impairment. Use caution when driving or operating heavy machinery until effects on blood sugar are known. Use caution with certain antihypertensive agents (eg, beta-adrenergic blockers) or neuropathic conditions which may mask signs/symptoms of hypoglycemia. Use caution in patients with history of nausea; avoid use in patients with conditions or concurrent medications likely to impair gastric motility (eg, anticholinergics); do not use in patients requiring medication(s) to stimulate gastric emptying.

Adverse Reactions (Reflective of adult population; not specific for elderly)
>10%:
Central nervous system: Headache (5% to 13%)
Gastrointestinal: Nausea (28% to 48%), vomiting (7% to 11%), anorexia (≤17%)
Endocrine & metabolic: Severe hypoglycemia (type 1 diabetes ≤17%)
Miscellaneous: Inflicted injury (8% to 14%)
1% to 10%:
Central nervous system: Fatigue (3% to 7%), dizziness (2% to 6%)
Endocrine & metabolic: Severe hypoglycemia (type 2 diabetes ≤8%)
Gastrointestinal: Abdominal pain (2% to 8%)
Respiratory: Pharyngitis (3% to 5%), cough (2% to 6%)
Neuromuscular & skeletal: Arthralgia (2% to 7%)
Miscellaneous: Allergic reaction (≤6%)

Drug Interactions
Metabolism/Transport Effects None known.
Avoid Concomitant Use There are no known interactions where it is recommended to avoid concomitant use.
Increased Effect/Toxicity
Pramlintide may increase the levels/effects of: Anticholinergics
Decreased Effect There are no known significant interactions involving a decrease in effect.

Ethanol/Nutrition/Herb Interactions
Ethanol: Use caution with ethanol (may increase hypoglycemia).
Herb/Nutraceutical: Use caution with garlic, chromium, gymnema (may increase hypoglycemia).

Stability Store unopened vials at 2°C to 8°C (36°F to 46°F); do not freeze. Opened vials may be kept refrigerated or at room temperature ≤30°C (≤86°F). Discard opened vial after 30 days. Protect from light.

Mechanism of Action Synthetic analog of human amylin cosecreted with insulin by pancreatic beta cells; reduces postprandial glucose increases via the following mechanisms: 1) prolongation of gastric emptying time, 2) reduction of postprandial glucagon secretion, and 3) reduction of caloric intake through centrally-mediated appetite suppression

Pharmacodynamics/Kinetics Note: Pharmacokinetic studies have not been conducted in the elderly.
Protein binding: 60%
Metabolism: Primarily renal to des-lys^1 pramlintide (active metabolite)
Bioavailability: 30% to 40%
Half-life elimination: 48 minutes
Time to peak, plasma: 20 minutes
Excretion: Primarily urine

Dosage
Geriatric & Adult Note: When initiating pramlintide, reduce current insulin dose (including rapidly- and mixed-acting preparations) by 50% to avoid hypoglycemia. If pramlintide is discontinued for any reason, restart therapy with same initial titration protocol.
Type 1 diabetes mellitus (insulin dependent, IDDM): SubQ: Initial: 15 mcg immediately prior to meals; titrate in 15 mcg increments every 3 days (if no significant nausea occurs) to target dose of 30-60 mcg (consider discontinuation if intolerant of 30 mcg dose)
Type 2 diabetes mellitus (noninsulin dependent, NIDDM): SubQ: Initial: 60 mcg immediately prior to meals; after 3-7 days, increase to 120 mcg prior to meals if no significant nausea occurs (if nausea occurs at 120 mcg dose, reduce to 60 mcg)
Renal Impairment No dosage adjustment required; not evaluated in dialysis patients

◄ **Administration** Do not mix with insulins; administer subcutaneously into abdominal or thigh areas at sites distinct from concomitant insulin injections (do not administer into arm due to variable absorption); rotate injection sites frequently. For oral medications in which a rapid onset of action is desired, administer 1 hour before, or 2 hours after pramlintide, if possible.

Monitoring Parameters Prior to initiating therapy: Hb A$_{1c}$, hypoglycemic history, body weight. During therapy: urine sugar and acetone, pre- and postprandial and bedtime serum glucose, electrolytes, Hb A$_{1c}$, lipid profile

Special Geriatric Considerations Patients must be able to adhere to their insulin regimen and self-monitor their blood glucose. In premarketing studies, the change in the Hb A$_{1c}$ values and hypoglycemia frequencies did not differ by age. Monitor regimen closely. Intensive glucose control (Hb A$_{1c}$ <6.5%) has been linked to increased all-cause and cardiovascular mortality, hypoglycemia requiring assistance, and weight gain in adult type 2 diabetes. How "tightly" to control a geriatric patient's blood glucose needs to be individualized. Such a decision should be based on several factors, including the patient's functional and cognitive status, how well he/she recognizes hypoglycemic or hyperglycemic symptoms, and how to respond to them and other disease states. An Hb A$_{1c}$ <7.5% is an acceptable endpoint for a healthy older adult, while <8% is acceptable for frail elderly patients, those with a duration of illness >10 years, or those with comorbid conditions and requiring combination diabetes medications. For elderly patients with diabetes who are relatively healthy, attaining target goals for aspirin use, blood pressure, lipids, smoking cessation, and diet and exercise may be more important than normalized glycemic control.

Dosage Forms Excipient information presented when available (limited, particularly for generics); consult specific product labeling. [DSC] = Discontinued product

Injection, solution, as acetate:
SymlinPen®: 1000 mcg/mL (2.7 mL) [120 pen-injector]
SymlinPen®: 1000 mcg/mL (1.5 mL) [60 pen-injector]
Symlin®: 600 mcg/mL (5 mL [DSC])

◆ **Pramlintide Acetate** see Pramlintide on page 1582
◆ **PrandiMet®** see Repaglinide and Metformin on page 1687
◆ **Prandin®** see Repaglinide on page 1684

Prasugrel (PRA soo grel)

Related Information
Beers Criteria – Potentially Inappropriate Medications for Geriatrics on page 2183
Perioperative/Periprocedural Management of Anticoagulant and Antiplatelet Therapy on page 2209

Medication Safety Issues
Sound-alike/look-alike issues:
Prasugrel may be confused with pravastatin, propranolol
BEERS Criteria medication:
This drug may be potentially inappropriate for use in geriatric patients (Quality of evidence - moderate; Strength of recommendation - weak).

Brand Names: U.S. Effient®
Brand Names: Canada Effient®
Index Terms CS-747; LY-640315; Prasugrel Hydrochloride
Generic Availability (U.S.) No
Pharmacologic Category Antiplatelet Agent; Antiplatelet Agent, Thienopyridine
Use Reduces rate of thrombotic cardiovascular events (eg, stent thrombosis) in patients who are to be managed with percutaneous coronary intervention (PCI) for unstable angina (UA), non-ST-segment elevation MI (NSTEMI), or ST-elevation MI (STEMI)

Unlabeled Use In patients with allergy or major gastrointestinal intolerance to aspirin, initial treatment of UA/NSTEMI; **Note:** Dual antiplatelet therapy with another P2Y$_{12}$ receptor inhibitor is not recommended in this situation (Jneid, 2012).

Medication Guide Available Yes
Contraindications Hypersensitivity (eg, anaphylaxis) to prasugrel or any component of the formulation; active pathological bleeding such as peptic ulcer disease (PUD) or intracranial hemorrhage; history of transient ischemic attack (TIA) or stroke

Warnings/Precautions [U.S. Boxed Warning]: May cause significant or fatal bleeding. Use is contraindicated in patients with active pathological bleeding or history of TIA or stroke. Use with caution in patients who may be at risk of increased bleeding, including patients with active PUD, recent or recurrent GI bleeding, severe hepatic impairment, trauma, or surgery. Additional risk factors include body weight <60 kg, CABG or other surgical procedure, concomitant use of medications that increase risk of bleeding.

[U.S. Boxed Warning]: In patients ≥75 years of age, use is not recommended due to increased risk of fatal and intracranial bleeding and uncertain benefit; use may be considered in high-risk situations (eg, patients with diabetes or history of MI). Risk of bleeding is increased in older adults (Beers Criteria). **[U.S. Boxed Warning]: Do not initiate therapy in patients likely to undergo urgent CABG surgery; when possible, discontinue ≥7 days prior to any surgery; increased risk of bleeding.** The American College of Chest Physicians (ACCP) recommends discontinuing prasugrel 5 days before surgery (Guyatt, 2012). When urgent CABG is necessary, the ACCF/AHA CABG guidelines suggest that it may be reasonable to perform surgery within 7 days of discontinuing prasugrel (Hillis, 2011).

Because of structural similarities, cross-reactivity is possible among the thienopyridines (clopidogrel, prasugrel, and ticlopidine); use with caution or avoid in patients with previous thienopyridine hypersensitivity. Use of prasugrel is contraindicated in patients with hypersensitivity (eg, anaphylaxis) to prasugrel. If necessary, discontinue therapy for active bleeding, elective surgery, stroke, or TIA; reinitiate therapy as soon as possible unless patient suffers stroke or TIA where subsequent use is contraindicated. If possible, manage bleeding without discontinuing prasugrel. Use caution in concurrent treatment with oral anticoagulants (eg, warfarin), NSAIDs, or fibrinolytic agents; bleeding risk is increased. Use with caution in patients with severe liver impairment or end-stage renal disease (experience is limited). Cases of thrombotic thrombocytopenic purpura (TTP) (usually occurring within the first 2 weeks of therapy), resulting in some fatalities, have been reported with prasugrel; urgent plasmapheresis is required. In patients <60 kg, risk of bleeding increased; consider lower maintenance dose.

Adverse Reactions (Reflective of adult population; not specific for elderly) As with all drugs which may affect hemostasis, bleeding is associated with prasugrel. Hemorrhage may occur at virtually any site. Risk is dependent on multiple variables, including patient susceptibility and concurrent use of multiple agents which alter hemostasis.

2% to 10%:

Cardiovascular: Hypertension (8%), hypotension (4%), atrial fibrillation (3%), bradycardia (3%), noncardiac chest pain (3%), peripheral edema (3%)

Central nervous system: Headache (6%), dizziness (4%), fatigue (4%), fever (3%), extremity pain (3%)

Dermatologic: Rash (3%)

Endocrine & metabolic: Hypercholesterolemia/hyperlipidemia (7%)

Gastrointestinal: Nausea (5%), diarrhea (2%), gastrointestinal hemorrhage (2%)

Hematologic: Leukopenia (3%), anemia (2%)

Neuromuscular & skeletal: Back pain (5%)

Respiratory: Epistaxis (6%), dyspnea (5%), cough (4%)

Drug Interactions

Metabolism/Transport Effects Substrate of CYP2B6 (minor), CYP3A4 (minor); **Note:** Assignment of Major/Minor substrate status based on clinically relevant drug interaction potential; **Inhibits** CYP2B6 (weak)

Avoid Concomitant Use There are no known interactions where it is recommended to avoid concomitant use.

Increased Effect/Toxicity

Prasugrel may increase the levels/effects of: Anticoagulants; Antiplatelet Agents; Collagenase (Systemic); Dabigatran Etexilate; Drotrecogin Alfa (Activated); Ibritumomab; Rivaroxaban; Salicylates; Thrombolytic Agents; Tositumomab and Iodine I 131 Tositumomab

The levels/effects of Prasugrel may be increased by: Dasatinib; Glucosamine; Herbs (Anticoagulant/Antiplatelet Properties); Nonsteroidal Anti-Inflammatory Agents; Omega-3-Acid Ethyl Esters; Pentosan Polysulfate Sodium; Pentoxifylline; Prostacyclin Analogues; Tipranavir; Vitamin E

Decreased Effect

The levels/effects of Prasugrel may be decreased by: CYP3A4 Inhibitors (Strong); Nonsteroidal Anti-Inflammatory Agents; Ranitidine; Rifampin; Tocilizumab

Stability Store at 25°C (77°F); excursions permitted to 15°C to 30°C (59°F to 86°F).

Mechanism of Action Prasugrel is a prodrug that is metabolized to both active (R-138727) and inactive metabolites. The active metabolite irreversibly blocks the $P2Y_{12}$ component of ADP receptors on the platelet, which prevents activation of the GPIIb/IIIa receptor complex, thereby reducing platelet activation and aggregation. Platelet aggregation returns to baseline within 5-9 days of discontinuation.

Pharmacodynamics/Kinetics

Onset of action: Inhibition of platelet aggregation (IPA): Dose dependent: 60 mg loading dose: <30 minutes; median time to reach 20% IPA: 30 minutes (Brandt, 2007)

Peak effect: Time to maximal IPA: Dose-dependent: **Note:** Degree of IPA based on adenosine diphosphate (ADP) concentration used during light aggregometry: 60 mg loading dose: Occurs 4 hours post administration; mean IPA (ADP 5 µmol/L): 78.8%: mean IPA (ADP 20 micromole/L): 84.1%

Duration of effect: >3 days; platelet aggregation gradually returns to baseline values over 5-9 days after discontinuation; reflective of new platelet production

Absorption: Rapid; ≥79%

Distribution: V_d: 44-68 L

Protein binding: Active metabolite: ~98%

Metabolism: Rapid intestinal and serum metabolism via esterase-mediated hydrolysis to a thiolactone (inactive), which is then converted, via CYP450-mediated (primarily CYP3A4 and CYP2B6) oxidation, to an active metabolite (R-138727)

Half-life elimination: Active metabolite: ~7 hours (range 2-15 hours)

Time to peak, plasma: Active metabolite: ~30 minutes (peak plasma levels begin to decrease at ~24 hours); with high-fat/high-calorie meal: 1.5 hours

Excretion: Urine (~68% inactive metabolites); feces (27% inactive metabolites)

Dosage

Geriatric Refer to adult dosing. Patients ≥75 years: Use not recommended; may be considered in high-risk situations (eg, patients with diabetes or history of MI).

Adult Acute coronary syndrome managed with PCI: Oral: Loading dose: 60 mg administered promptly (as soon as coronary anatomy is known or before if risk for bleeding is low and need for CABG considered unlikely) and no later than 1 hour after PCI; Maintenance dose: 10 mg once daily (in combination with aspirin 81-325 mg/day; 81 mg/day recommended [Levine, 2011]). **Note:** In patients weighing <60 kg, the manufacturer suggests to consider decreasing maintenance dose to 5 mg once daily; however, prospective clinical trial data does not exist to support this recommendation and may place some patients at risk of thrombotic complications (eg, stent thrombosis); consider use of full dose while monitoring closely for bleeding complications or administration of an alternative agent (eg, clopidogrel).

Duration of prasugrel (in combination with aspirin) after stent placement: **Premature interruption of therapy may result in stent thrombosis with subsequent fatal and nonfatal MI.** Those with ACS receiving either stent type (bare metal [BMS] or drug-eluting stent [DES]) or those receiving a DES for a non-ACS indication, prasugrel for at least 12 months is recommended. Those receiving a BMS for a non-ACS indication should be given at least 1 month and ideally up to 12 months; if patient is at increased risk of bleeding, give for a minimum of 2 weeks. A duration >12 months, regardless of indication, may be considered in patients with DES placement (Jneid, 2012; Levine, 2011).

Renal Impairment No dosage adjustment necessary.

Hepatic Impairment No dosage adjustment necessary for mild-to-moderate hepatic impairment; use in severe hepatic impairment has not been evaluated.

Administration Administer without regard to meals. Tablets may be chewed and swallowed (bitter to taste) or crushed and mixed in food or liquid (eg, applesauce, juice, or water) and immediately administered by mouth or gastric tube. **Note:** Administration via an enteral tube that bypasses the acidic environment of the stomach may result in reduced bioavailability of prasugrel (data on file, Daiichi Sankyo-Lilly, 2012).

Monitoring Parameters Hemoglobin and hematocrit periodically; may consider platelet function testing to determine platelet inhibitory response if results of testing may alter management (Jneid, 2012).

Special Geriatric Considerations See Warnings/Precautions. Not recommended for use in elderly ≥75 years due to risk of fatal intracranial bleeding and lack of certain benefit in this age group. Exceptions may be high-risk patients (eg, diabetics or patients with a history of myocardial infarction). In the TRITON-TIMI 38 study, the AUC of the active metabolite was 19% higher in those ≥75 years of age compared to those participants <75 years.

This medication is considered to be potentially inappropriate in this patient population (Beers Criteria: Quality of evidence - moderate; Strength of recommendation - weak).

Dosage Forms Excipient information presented when available (limited, particularly for generics); consult specific product labeling.

Tablet, oral:

Effient®: 5 mg, 10 mg

◆ **Prasugrel Hydrochloride** *see* Prasugrel *on page 1584*

◆ **Pravachol®** *see* Pravastatin *on page 1587*

Pravastatin (prav a STAT in)

Related Information
Hyperlipidemia Management *on page 2130*

Medication Safety Issues

Sound-alike/look-alike issues:

Pravachol® may be confused with atorvaSTATin, Prevacid®, Prinivil®, propranolol

Pravastatin may be confused with nystatin, pitavastatin, prasugrel

Brand Names: U.S. Pravachol®

Brand Names: Canada Apo-Pravastatin®; CO Pravastatin; Dom-Pravastatin; JAMP-Pravastatin; Mint-Pravastatin; Mylan-Pravastatin; Novo-Pravastatin; Nu-Pravastatin; PHL-Pravastatin; PMS-Pravastatin; Pravachol®; RAN™-Pravastatin; ratio-Pravastatin; Riva-Pravastatin; Sandoz-Pravastatin; Teva-Pravastatin; ZYM-Pravastatin

Index Terms Pravastatin Sodium

Generic Availability (U.S.) Yes

Pharmacologic Category Antilipemic Agent, HMG-CoA Reductase Inhibitor

Use Use with dietary therapy for the following:

Primary prevention of coronary events: In hypercholesterolemic patients without established coronary heart disease to reduce cardiovascular morbidity (myocardial infarction, coronary revascularization procedures) and mortality.

Secondary prevention of cardiovascular events in patients with established coronary heart disease: To slow the progression of coronary atherosclerosis; to reduce cardiovascular morbidity (myocardial infarction, coronary vascular procedures) and to reduce mortality; to reduce the risk of stroke and transient ischemic attacks

Hyperlipidemias: Reduce elevations in total cholesterol, LDL-C, apolipoprotein B, and triglycerides (elevations of 1 or more components are present in Fredrickson type IIa, IIb, III, and IV hyperlipidemias)

Contraindications Hypersensitivity to pravastatin or any component of the formulation; active liver disease; unexplained persistent elevations of serum transaminases

Warnings/Precautions Secondary causes of hyperlipidemia should be ruled out prior to therapy. Liver function must be monitored by periodic laboratory assessment. Rhabdomyolysis with acute renal failure has occurred. Risk may be increased with concurrent use of other drugs which may cause rhabdomyolysis (including colchicine, gemfibrozil, fibric acid derivatives, or niacin at doses ≥1 g/day). Temporarily discontinue in any patient experiencing an acute or serious condition predisposing to renal failure secondary to rhabdomyolysis. Based upon current evidence, HMG-CoA reductase inhibitor therapy should be continued in the perioperative period unless risk outweighs cardioprotective benefit. Use with caution in patients with advanced age, these patients are predisposed to myopathy. Use caution in patients with previous liver disease or heavy ethanol use.

Adverse Reactions (Reflective of adult population; not specific for elderly) As reported in short-term trials; safety and tolerability with long-term use were similar to placebo 1% to 10%:

Cardiovascular: Chest pain (4%)

Central nervous system: Headache (2% to 6%), fatigue (4%), dizziness (1% to 3%)

Dermatologic: Rash (4%)

Gastrointestinal: Nausea/vomiting (7%), diarrhea (6%), heartburn (3%)

Hepatic: Transaminases increased (>3x normal on two occasions: 1%)

Neuromuscular & skeletal: Myalgia (2%)

Respiratory: Cough (3%)

Miscellaneous: Influenza (2%)

Additional class-related events or case reports (not necessarily reported with pravastatin therapy): Angioedema, blood glucose increased, cataracts, depression, diabetes mellitus (new onset), dyspnea, eosinophilia, erectile dysfunction, facial paresis, glycosylated hemoglobin (Hb A_{1c}) increased, hypersensitivity reaction, impaired extraocular muscle movement, impotence, interstitial lung disease, leukopenia, malaise, memory loss, ophthalmoplegia, paresthesia, peripheral neuropathy, photosensitivity, psychic disturbance, skin discoloration, thrombocytopenia, thyroid dysfunction, toxic epidermal necrolysis, transaminases increased, vomiting

Drug Interactions

Metabolism/Transport Effects Substrate of CYP3A4 (minor), P-glycoprotein, SLCO1B1; **Note:** Assignment of Major/Minor substrate status based on clinically relevant drug interaction potential; **Inhibits** CYP2C9 (weak), CYP2D6 (weak), CYP3A4 (weak)

Avoid Concomitant Use

Avoid concomitant use of Pravastatin with any of the following: Gemfibrozil; Pimozide; Red Yeast Rice

Increased Effect/Toxicity

Pravastatin may increase the levels/effects of: ARIPiprazole; CycloSPORINE; CycloSPOR-INE (Systemic); DAPTOmycin; PARoxetine; Pazopanib; Pimozide; Trabectedin; Vitamin K Antagonists

The levels/effects of Pravastatin may be increased by: Boceprevir; Colchicine; Cyclo-SPORINE; CycloSPORINE (Systemic); Darunavir; Eltrombopag; Fenofibrate; Fenofibric Acid; Gemfibrozil; Itraconazole; Niacin; Niacinamide; P-glycoprotein/ABCB1 Inhibitors; Red Yeast Rice

Decreased Effect

Pravastatin may decrease the levels/effects of: Lanthanum

The levels/effects of Pravastatin may be decreased by: Antacids; Bile Acid Sequestrants; Efavirenz; Fosphenytoin; Nelfinavir; P-glycoprotein/ABCB1 Inducers; Phenytoin; Rifamycin Derivatives; Saquinavir; Tocilizumab

Ethanol/Nutrition/Herb Interactions

Ethanol: Consumption of large amounts of ethanol may increase the risk of liver damage with HMG-CoA reductase inhibitors.

Food: Red yeast rice contains an estimated 2.4 mg lovastatin per 600 mg rice.

Herb/Nutraceutical: St John's wort may decrease pravastatin levels.

Stability Store at 25°C (77°F); excursions permitted to 15°C to 30°C (59°F to 86°F). Protect from moisture and light.

Mechanism of Action Pravastatin is a competitive inhibitor of 3-hydroxy-3-methylglutaryl coenzyme A (HMG-CoA) reductase, which is the rate-limiting enzyme involved in *de novo* cholesterol synthesis.

Pharmacodynamics/Kinetics

Onset of action: Several days

Peak effect: 4 weeks

Absorption: Rapidly absorbed; average absorption 34%

Protein binding: 50%

Metabolism: Hepatic multiple metabolites; primary metabolite is 3α-hydroxy-iso-pravastatin (2.5% to 10% activity of parent drug)

Bioavailability: 17%

Half-life elimination: 77 hours (including all metabolites); pravastatin: ~2-3 hours (Pan, 1990); 3α-hydroxy-iso-pravastatin: ~1.5 hours (Gustavson, 2005)

Time to peak, serum: 1-1.5 hours

Excretion: Feces (70%); urine (≤20%, 8% as unchanged drug)

Dosage

Geriatric & Adult

Hyperlipidemias, primary prevention of coronary events, secondary prevention of cardiovascular events: Oral: Initial: 40 mg once daily; titrate dosage to response (usual range: 10-80 mg) (maximum dose: 80 mg once daily)

Dosage adjustment for pravastatin with concomitant medications:

Clarithromycin: Limit daily pravastatin dose to 40 mg/day

Cyclosporine: Initial: 10 mg pravastatin daily, titrate with caution (maximum dose: 20 mg/day)

Note: Doses should be individualized according to the baseline LDL-cholesterol levels, the recommended goal of therapy, and patient response; adjustments should be made at intervals of 4 weeks or more; doses may need adjusted based on concomitant medications

Renal Impairment Significant impairment: Initial dose: 10 mg/day

Hepatic Impairment Contraindicated in active liver disease or in patients with unexplained persistent elevations of serum transaminases.

Administration May be administered without regard to meals.

Monitoring Parameters Baseline CPK (recheck CPK in any patient with symptoms suggestive of myopathy; discontinue therapy if markedly elevated); baseline liver function tests (LFTs) and repeat when clinically indicated thereafter. Patients with elevated transaminase levels should have a second (confirmatory) test and frequent monitoring until values normalize; discontinue if increase in ALT/AST is persistently >3 times ULN (NCEP, 2002).

Lipid panel (total cholesterol, HDL, LDL, triglycerides):

ATP III recommendations (NCEP, 2002): Baseline; 6-8 weeks after initiation of drug therapy; if dose increased, then at 6-8 weeks until final dose determined. Once treatment goal achieved, follow up intervals may be reduced to every 4-6 months. Lipid panel should be assessed at least annually, and preferably at each clinic visit.

Manufacturer recommendation: Upon initiation or titration, lipid panel should be analyzed at intervals of 4 weeks or more.

Special Geriatric Considerations Effective and well tolerated in the elderly. No specific dosage recommendations. Clearance is reduced in the elderly, resulting in an increase in AUC between 25% to 50%; however, substantial accumulation is not expected.

The definition of and, therefore, when to treat hyperlipidemia in elderly is a controversial issue. The National Cholesterol Education Program recommends that all adults maintain a plasma cholesterol <160 mg/dL. For the elderly with one additional risk factor, goal LDL would be <130 mg/dL. It is the authors' belief that pharmacologic treatment be reserved for those who are unable to obtain a desirable plasma cholesterol concentration by diet alone and for whom the benefits of treatment are believed to outweigh the potential adverse effects, drug interactions, and cost of treatment. Age ≥65 years is a risk factor for myopathy.

Dosage Forms Excipient information presented when available (limited, particularly for generics); consult specific product labeling.
Tablet, oral, as sodium: 10 mg, 20 mg, 40 mg, 80 mg
Pravachol®: 10 mg, 20 mg, 40 mg, 80 mg

◆ **Pravastatin Sodium** see Pravastatin on page 1587

Prazosin (PRAZ oh sin)

Related Information
Beers Criteria – Potentially Inappropriate Medications for Geriatrics on page 2183
Medication Safety Issues
Sound-alike/look-alike issues:
Prazosin may be confused with predniSONE
BEERS Criteria medication:
This drug may be potentially inappropriate for use in geriatric patients (Quality of evidence - moderate; Strength of recommendation - strong).
Brand Names: U.S. Minipress®
Brand Names: Canada Apo-Prazo®; Minipress®; Novo-Prazin; Nu-Prazo; Teva-Prazosin
Index Terms Furazosin; Prazosin Hydrochloride
Generic Availability (U.S.) Yes
Pharmacologic Category Alpha₁ Blocker
Use Treatment of hypertension
Unlabeled Use Post-traumatic stress disorder (PTSD) related nightmares and sleep disruption; benign prostatic hyperplasia; Raynaud's syndrome
Contraindications Hypersensitivity to prazosin, quinazolines (eg, doxazosin, terazosin) or any component of the formulation
Warnings/Precautions May cause significant orthostatic hypotension and syncope, especially with first dose; anticipate a similar effect if therapy is interrupted for a few days, if dosage is rapidly increased, or if another antihypertensive drug (particularly vasodilators) or a PDE-5 inhibitor is introduced. Intraoperative floppy iris syndrome (IFIS) has been observed during cataract surgery in some patients treated with alpha₁-blockers. Patients should be cautioned about performing hazardous tasks when starting new therapy or adjusting dosage upward. Discontinue if symptoms of angina occur or worsen. Should rule out prostatic carcinoma before beginning therapy. In the elderly, avoid use as an antihypertensive due to high risk of orthostatic hypotension; alternative agents preferred due to a more favorable risk/benefit profile (Beers Criteria).
Adverse Reactions (Reflective of adult population; not specific for elderly)
>4%:
Cardiovascular: Palpitation (5%)
Central nervous system: Dizziness (10%), headache (8%), drowsiness (8%)
Endocrine & metabolic: Decreased energy (7%)
Gastrointestinal: Nausea (5%)
Neuromuscular & skeletal: Weakness (7%)
1% to 4%:
Cardiovascular: Edema, orthostatic hypotension, syncope
Central nervous system: Depression, nervousness, vertigo
Dermatologic: Rash
Gastrointestinal: Constipation, diarrhea, vomiting, xerostomia
Genitourinary: Urinary frequency
Ocular: Blurred vision, reddened sclera
Respiratory: Dyspnea, epistaxis, nasal congestion

◀ **Drug Interactions**
Metabolism/Transport Effects Induces P-glycoprotein
Avoid Concomitant Use
Avoid concomitant use of Prazosin with any of the following: Alpha1-Blockers; Dabigatran Etexilate
Increased Effect/Toxicity
Prazosin may increase the levels/effects of: Alpha1-Blockers; Amifostine; Antihypertensives; Calcium Channel Blockers; Hypotensive Agents; RiTUXimab

The levels/effects of Prazosin may be increased by: Beta-Blockers; Diazoxide; Herbs (Hypotensive Properties); MAO Inhibitors; Pentoxifylline; Phosphodiesterase 5 Inhibitors; Prostacyclin Analogues
Decreased Effect
Prazosin may decrease the levels/effects of: Dabigatran Etexilate; Linagliptin; P-glycoprotein/ABCB1 Substrates

The levels/effects of Prazosin may be decreased by: Herbs (Hypertensive Properties); Methylphenidate; Yohimbine
Ethanol/Nutrition/Herb Interactions
Ethanol: Avoid ethanol (may increase vasodilation).
Food: Food has variable effects on absorption.
Herb/Nutraceutical: Avoid dong quai if using for hypertension (has estrogenic activity). Avoid ephedra, yohimbe, ginseng (may worsen hypertension). Avoid saw palmetto (due to limited experience with this combination). Avoid garlic (may have increased antihypertensive effect).
Stability Store in airtight container. Protect from light.
Mechanism of Action Competitively inhibits postsynaptic alpha-adrenergic receptors which results in vasodilation of veins and arterioles and a decrease in total peripheral resistance and blood pressure
Pharmacodynamics/Kinetics
Onset of action: Anithypertensive: ~2 hours
 Peak effect: Antihypertensive: 2-4 hours
Duration: 10-24 hours
Distribution: Hypertensive adults: V_d: 0.5 L/kg
Protein binding: 92% to 97%
Metabolism: Extensively hepatic
Bioavailability: 43% to 82%
Time to peak, plasma: ~3 hours
Half-life elimination: 2-3 hours; prolonged with congestive heart failure
Excretion: Feces; urine (6% to 10% as unchanged drug)
Dosage
Geriatric Refer to adult dosing. In the management of hypertension, consider lower initial doses and titrate to response (Aronow, 2011).
Adult
Hypertension: Oral: Initial: 1 mg/dose 2-3 times/day; usual maintenance dose: 2-20 mg/day in divided doses 2-3 times/day (JNC 7); maximum daily dose: 20 mg
PTSD-related nightmares and sleep disruption (unlabeled use): Oral: Initial: 1 mg at bedtime (Raskind, 2002; Raskind, 2007); titrate as tolerated to 2-15 mg at bedtime (Benedek, 2009)
Raynaud's (unlabeled use): Oral: Dosage range: 1-5 mg twice daily (Bakst, 2008)
Benign prostatic hyperplasia (unlabeled use): Oral: Initial: 0.5 mg twice daily; titrate as tolerated to 2 mg twice daily (Moran, 2001)
Monitoring Parameters Blood pressure, standing and sitting/supine
Test Interactions Increased urinary VMA 17%, norepinephrine metabolite 42%; therefore, false positives may occur in screening for pheochromocytoma. If elevated VMA is found, discontinue prazosin and retest after one month.
Special Geriatric Considerations Adverse effects such as orthostatic hypotension, dry mouth, and urinary problems can be particularly bothersome in the elderly.

This medication is considered to be potentially inappropriate in this patient population (Beers Criteria: Quality of evidence - moderate; Strength of recommendation - strong).
Dosage Forms Excipient information presented when available (limited, particularly for generics); consult specific product labeling.
Capsule, oral: 1 mg, 2 mg, 5 mg
Minipress®: 1 mg, 2 mg, 5 mg

◆ **Prazosin Hydrochloride** *see* Prazosin *on page 1589*
◆ **Precose®** *see* Acarbose *on page 26*
◆ **Pred Forte®** *see* PrednisoLONE (Ophthalmic) *on page 1594*

◆ **Pred-G®** *see* Prednisolone and Gentamicin *on page 1594*
◆ **Pred Mild®** *see* PrednisoLONE (Ophthalmic) *on page 1594*

Prednicarbate (pred ni KAR bate)

Related Information
Topical Corticosteroids *on page 2113*
Medication Safety Issues
Sound-alike/look-alike issues:
Dermatop® may be confused with Dimetapp®
Brand Names: U.S. Dermatop®
Brand Names: Canada Dermatop®
Generic Availability (U.S.) Yes
Pharmacologic Category Corticosteroid, Topical
Use Relief of the inflammatory and pruritic manifestations of corticosteroid-responsive dermatoses (medium potency topical corticosteroid)
Dosage
Geriatric & Adult Steroid-responsive dermatoses: Topical: Cream, ointment: Apply a thin film to affected area twice daily. Therapy should be discontinued when control is achieved; if no improvement is seen within 2 weeks, reassessment of diagnosis may be necessary.
Special Geriatric Considerations Due to age-related changes in skin, limit use of topical corticosteroids.
Dosage Forms Excipient information presented when available (limited, particularly for generics); consult specific product labeling.
Cream, topical: 0.1% (15 g, 60 g)
Dermatop®: 0.1% (60 g)
Ointment, topical: 0.1% (15 g, 60 g)
Dermatop®: 0.1% (60 g)

PrednisoLONE (Systemic) (pred NISS oh lone)

Related Information
Corticosteroids Systemic Equivalencies *on page 2112*
Medication Safety Issues
Sound-alike/look-alike issues:
PrednisoLONE may be confused with predniSONE
Pediapred® may be confused with Pediazole®
Prelone® may be confused with PROzac®
Brand Names: U.S. Flo-Pred™; Millipred™; Millipred™ DP; Orapred ODT®; Orapred®; Pediapred®; Veripred™ 20
Brand Names: Canada Hydeltra T.B.A.®; Novo-Prednisolone; Pediapred®
Index Terms Prednisolone Sodium Phosphate
Generic Availability (U.S.) Yes: Excludes orally disintegrating tablet, oral suspension, tablet
Pharmacologic Category Corticosteroid, Systemic
Use Treatment of endocrine disorders, rheumatic disorders, collagen diseases, allergic states, respiratory diseases, hematologic disorders, neoplastic diseases, edematous states, and gastrointestinal diseases; resolution of acute exacerbations of multiple sclerosis; management of fulminating or disseminated tuberculosis and trichinosis; acute or chronic solid organ rejection
Unlabeled Use Severe alcoholic hepatitis
Contraindications Hypersensitivity to prednisolone or any component of the formulation; acute superficial herpes simplex keratitis; live or attenuated virus vaccines (with immunosuppressive doses of corticosteroids); systemic fungal infections; varicella
Warnings/Precautions May cause hypercorticism or suppression of hypothalamic-pituitary-adrenal (HPA) axis, particularly in patients receiving high doses for prolonged periods. HPA axis suppression may lead to adrenal crisis. Withdrawal and discontinuation of a corticosteroid should be done slowly and carefully. Particular care is required when patients are transferred from systemic corticosteroids to inhaled products due to possible adrenal insufficiency or withdrawal from steroids, including an increase in allergic symptoms. Patients receiving >20 mg per day of prednisone (or equivalent) may be most susceptible. Fatalities have occurred due to adrenal insufficiency in asthmatic patients during and after transfer from systemic corticosteroids to aerosol steroids; aerosol steroids do **not** provide the systemic steroid needed to treat patients having trauma, surgery, or infections.

Acute myopathy has been reported with high dose corticosteroids, usually in patients with neuromuscular transmission disorders; may involve ocular and/or respiratory muscles; monitor creatine kinase; recovery may be delayed. Corticosteroid use may cause psychiatric disturbances, including depression, euphoria, insomnia, mood swings, and personality changes. Pre-existing psychiatric conditions may be exacerbated by corticosteroid use. Prolonged use of corticosteroids may also increase the incidence of secondary infection, mask acute infection (including fungal infections), prolong or exacerbate viral infections, or limit response to vaccines. Exposure to chickenpox should be avoided; corticosteroids should not be used to treat ocular herpes simplex. Corticosteroids should not be used for cerebral malaria or viral hepatitis. Close observation is required in patients with latent tuberculosis and/or TB reactivity; restrict use in active TB (only in conjunction with antituberculosis treatment). Prolonged use of corticosteroids may result in glaucoma; cataract formation may occur. Prolonged treatment with corticosteroids has been associated with the development of Kaposi's sarcoma (case reports); if noted, discontinuation of therapy should be considered.

Use with caution in patients with thyroid disease, hepatic impairment, renal impairment, cardiovascular disease, diabetes, glaucoma, cataracts, myasthenia gravis, patients at risk for osteoporosis, patients at risk for seizures, or GI diseases (diverticulitis, peptic ulcer, ulcerative colitis) due to perforation risk. Use caution following acute MI (corticosteroids have been associated with myocardial rupture). Because of the risk of adverse effects, systemic corticosteroids should be used cautiously in the elderly in the smallest possible effective dose for the shortest duration. Withdraw therapy with gradual tapering of dose.

Adverse Reactions (Reflective of adult population; not specific for elderly) Frequency not defined.

Cardiovascular: Cardiomyopathy, CHF, edema, facial edema, hypertension

Central nervous system: Headache, insomnia, malaise, nervousness, pseudotumor cerebri, psychic disorders, seizure, vertigo

Dermatologic: Bruising, facial erythema, hirsutism, petechiae, skin test reaction suppression, thin fragile skin, urticaria

Endocrine & metabolic: Carbohydrate tolerance decreased, Cushing's syndrome, diabetes mellitus, growth suppression, hyperglycemia, hypernatremia, hypokalemia, hypokalemic alkalosis, menstrual irregularities, negative nitrogen balance, pituitary adrenal axis suppression

Gastrointestinal: Abdominal distention, increased appetite, indigestion, nausea, pancreatitis, peptic ulcer, ulcerative esophagitis, weight gain

Hepatic: LFTs increased (usually reversible)

Neuromuscular & skeletal: Arthralgia, aseptic necrosis (humeral/femoral heads), fractures, muscle mass decreased, muscle weakness, osteoporosis, steroid myopathy, tendon rupture, weakness

Ocular: Cataracts, exophthalmus, eyelid edema, glaucoma, intraocular pressure increased, irritation

Respiratory: Epistaxis

Miscellaneous: Diaphoresis increased, impaired wound healing

Drug Interactions

Metabolism/Transport Effects Substrate of CYP3A4 (minor); **Note:** Assignment of Major/Minor substrate status based on clinically relevant drug interaction potential; **Inhibits** CYP3A4 (weak)

Avoid Concomitant Use

Avoid concomitant use of PrednisoLONE (Systemic) with any of the following: Aldesleukin; BCG; Mifepristone; Natalizumab; Pimecrolimus; Pimozide; Tacrolimus (Topical)

Increased Effect/Toxicity

PrednisoLONE (Systemic) may increase the levels/effects of: Acetylcholinesterase Inhibitors; Amphotericin B; ARIPiprazole; CycloSPORINE; CycloSPORINE (Systemic); Deferasirox; Leflunomide; Loop Diuretics; Natalizumab; NSAID (COX-2 Inhibitor); NSAID (Nonselective); Pimozide; Thiazide Diuretics; Vaccines (Live); Warfarin

The levels/effects of PrednisoLONE (Systemic) may be increased by: Antifungal Agents (Azole Derivatives, Systemic); Aprepitant; Calcium Channel Blockers (Nondihydropyridine); CycloSPORINE; CycloSPORINE (Systemic); Denosumab; Estrogen Derivatives; Fluconazole; Fosaprepitant; Indacaterol; Macrolide Antibiotics; Mifepristone; Neuromuscular-Blocking Agents (Nondepolarizing); Pimecrolimus; Quinolone Antibiotics; Roflumilast; Salicylates; Tacrolimus (Topical); Telaprevir; Trastuzumab

Decreased Effect

PrednisoLONE (Systemic) may decrease the levels/effects of: Aldesleukin; Antidiabetic Agents; BCG; Calcitriol; Coccidioidin Skin Test; Corticorelin; CycloSPORINE; CycloSPORINE (Systemic); Hyaluronidase; Isoniazid; Salicylates; Sipuleucel-T; Telaprevir; Vaccines (Inactivated)

The levels/effects of PrednisoLONE (Systemic) may be decreased by: Aminoglutethimide; Antacids; Barbiturates; Bile Acid Sequestrants; Echinacea; Fosphenytoin; Mifepristone; Mitotane; Phenytoin; Primidone; Rifamycin Derivatives; Tocilizumab

Ethanol/Nutrition/Herb Interactions

Ethanol: Avoid ethanol (may increase gastric mucosal irritation).

Food: Prednisolone interferes with calcium absorption. Limit caffeine.

Herb/Nutraceutical: St John's wort may decrease prednisolone levels. Avoid cat's claw, echinacea (have immunostimulant properties).

Stability

Flo-Pred™: Store at 20°C to 25°C (68°F to 77°F). Flo-Pred™ should be dispensed in the original container (to avoid loss of formulation during transfer).

Millipred™: Store at 20°C to 25°C (68°F to 77°F).

Orapred ODT®: Store at 20°C to 25°C (68°F to 77°F) in blister pack. Protect from moisture.

Orapred®, Veripred™ 20: 2°C to 8°C (36°F to 46°F).

Pediapred®: 4°C to 25°C (39°F to 77°F); may be refrigerated.

Mechanism of Action Decreases inflammation by suppression of migration of polymorpho-nuclear leukocytes and reversal of increased capillary permeability; suppresses the immune system by reducing activity and volume of the lymphatic system

Pharmacodynamics/Kinetics

Duration: 18-36 hours

Protein binding (concentration dependent): 65% to 91%; decreased in elderly

Metabolism: Primarily hepatic, but also metabolized in most tissues, to inactive compounds

Half-life elimination: 3.6 hours; End-stage renal disease: 3-5 hours

Excretion: Primarily urine (as glucuronides, sulfates, and unconjugated metabolites)

Dosage

Geriatric Use lowest effective adult dose. Dose depends upon condition being treated and response of patient; alternate day dosing may be attempted in some disease states.

Adult Dose depends upon condition being treated and response of patient. Oral dosage expressed in terms of prednisolone base. Consider alternate day therapy for long-term therapy. Discontinuation of long-term therapy requires gradual withdrawal by tapering the dose. Patients undergoing unusual stress while receiving corticosteroids, should receive increased doses prior to, during, and after the stressful situation.

Usual dose (range): Oral: 5-60 mg/day

Rheumatoid arthritis: Oral: Initial: 5-7.5 mg/day, adjust dose as necessary

Multiple sclerosis: Oral: 200 mg/day for 1 week followed by 80 mg every other day for 1 month

Severe alcoholic hepatitis (Maddrey Discriminant Function [MDF] score ≥32) (unlabeled use): Oral: 40 mg/day for 28 days, followed by a 2-week taper (O'Shea, 2010)

Dosing adjustment in hyperthyroidism: Prednisolone dose may need to be increased to achieve adequate therapeutic effects.

Renal Impairment

Hemodialysis: Slightly dialyzable (5% to 20%); administer dose posthemodialysis

Peritoneal dialysis: Supplemental dose is not necessary

Administration Administer oral formulation with food or milk to decrease GI effects.

Flo-Pred™: Administer using the provided calibrated syringe (supplied by manufacturer) to accurately measure the dose. Syringe should be washed prior to next use.

Orapred ODT®: Do not break or use partial tablet. Remove tablet from blister pack just prior to use. May swallow whole or allow to dissolve on tongue.

Monitoring Parameters Blood pressure; blood glucose, electrolytes; intraocular pressure (use >6 weeks); bone mineral density

Test Interactions Response to skin tests

Special Geriatric Considerations Useful in patients with inability to activate prednisone (liver disease). Because of the risk of adverse effects, systemic corticosteroids should be used cautiously in the elderly, in the smallest possible dose, and for the shortest possible time. For long-term use, monitor bone mineral density and institute fracture prevention strategies.

Dosage Forms Excipient information presented when available (limited, particularly for generics); consult specific product labeling.

Solution, oral, as base: 15 mg/5 mL (240 mL, 480 mL)

Solution, oral, as sodium phosphate [strength expressed as base]: 5 mg/5 mL (120 mL); 15 mg/5 mL (237 mL, 473 mL)

Millipred™: 10 mg/5 mL (237 mL) [dye free, ethanol free; grape flavor]

Orapred®: 15 mg/5 mL (20 mL, 237 mL) [dye free; contains ethanol 2%, sodium benzoate; grape flavor]

Pediapred®: 5 mg/5 mL (120 mL) [dye free; raspberry flavor]
Veripred™ 20: 20 mg/5 mL (237 mL) [dye free, ethanol free; grape flavor]
Suspension, oral, as acetate [strength expressed as base]:
Flo-Pred™: 15 mg/5 mL (52 mL) [contains propylene glycol; cherry flavor]
Tablet, oral, as base:
Millipred™: 5 mg [scored]
Tablet, oral, as base [dose-pack]:
Millipred™ DP: 5 mg [scored; 12-day pack/48s]
Millipred™ DP: 5 mg [scored; 6-day pack/21s]
Tablet, orally disintegrating, oral, as sodium phosphate [strength expressed as base]:
Orapred ODT®: 10 mg, 15 mg, 30 mg [grape flavor]

PrednisoLONE (Ophthalmic) (pred NISS oh lone)

Medication Safety Issues
Sound-alike/look-alike issues:
PrednisoLONE may be confused with predniSONE
Brand Names: U.S. Omnipred™; Pred Forte®; Pred Mild®
Brand Names: Canada Diopred®; Ophtho-Tate®; Pred Forte®; Pred Mild®
Index Terms Econopred; Prednisolone Acetate, Ophthalmic; Prednisolone Sodium Phosphate, Ophthalmic
Generic Availability (U.S.) Yes
Pharmacologic Category Corticosteroid, Ophthalmic
Use Treatment of palpebral and bulbar conjunctivitis; corneal injury from chemical, radiation, thermal burns, or foreign body penetration; steroid-responsive inflammatory ophthalmic diseases
Dosage
Geriatric & Adult Conjunctivitis: Ophthalmic (suspension/solution): Instill 1-2 drops in the eye 2-4 times daily
Special Geriatric Considerations Evaluate the patient's or caregiver's ability to safely administer the correct dose of ophthalmic medication.
Dosage Forms Excipient information presented when available (limited, particularly for generics); consult specific product labeling. [DSC] = Discontinued product
Solution, ophthalmic, as sodium phosphate [drops]: 1% (5 mL [DSC], 10 mL, 15 mL [DSC])
Suspension, ophthalmic, as acetate [drops]: 1% (5 mL, 10 mL, 15 mL)
Omnipred™: 1% (5 mL, 10 mL) [contains benzalkonium chloride]
Pred Forte®: 1% (1 mL, 5 mL, 10 mL, 15 mL) [contains benzalkonium chloride, sodium bisulfite]
Pred Mild®: 0.12% (5 mL, 10 mL) [contains benzalkonium chloride, sodium bisulfite]

◆ **Prednisolone Acetate, Ophthalmic** see PrednisoLONE (Ophthalmic) on page 1594

Prednisolone and Gentamicin (pred NIS oh lone & jen ta MYE sin)

Related Information
Gentamicin (Ophthalmic) on page 876
PrednisoLONE (Ophthalmic) on page 1594
Brand Names: U.S. Pred-G®
Index Terms Gentamicin and Prednisolone
Generic Availability (U.S.) No
Pharmacologic Category Antibiotic/Corticosteroid, Ophthalmic
Use Treatment of steroid responsive inflammatory conditions where either a superficial bacterial ocular infection or the risk of bacterial ocular infection exists
Dosage
Geriatric & Adult Inflammatory conditions and superficial ocular infections: Ophthalmic:
Ointment: Apply 1/2 inch ribbon into the conjunctival sac of the affected eye(s) 1-3 times/day
Suspension: Instill 1 drop into the conjunctival sac of the affected eye(s) 2-4 times/day; during the initial 24-48 hours, the dosing frequency may be increased if necessary up to 1 drop every hour
Note: If signs and symptoms do not improve after 2 days of treatment, the patient should be re-evaluated.
Special Geriatric Considerations Evaluate the patient's or caregiver's ability to safely administer the correct dose of ophthalmic medication.

Dosage Forms Excipient information presented when available (limited, particularly for generics); consult specific product labeling. [DSC] = Discontinued product
Ointment, ophthalmic:
  Pred-G®: Prednisolone acetate 0.6% and gentamicin sulfate 0.3% (3.5 g)
Suspension, ophthalmic:
  Pred-G®: Prednisolone acetate 1% and gentamicin sulfate 0.3% (5 mL, 10 mL [DSC]) [contains benzalkonium chloride]

◆ **Prednisolone and Sulfacetamide** *see* Sulfacetamide and Prednisolone *on page 1812*
◆ **Prednisolone Sodium Phosphate** *see* PrednisoLONE (Systemic) *on page 1591*
◆ **Prednisolone Sodium Phosphate, Ophthalmic** *see* PrednisoLONE (Ophthalmic) *on page 1594*

PredniSONE (PRED ni sone)

Related Information
  Corticosteroids Systemic Equivalencies *on page 2112*
Medication Safety Issues
  Sound-alike/look-alike issues:
    PredniSONE may be confused with methylPREDNISolone, Pramosone®, prazosin, predni-soLONE, PriLOSEC®, primidone, promethazine
Brand Names: U.S. PredniSONE Intensol™
Brand Names: Canada Apo-Prednisone®; Novo-Prednisone; Winpred™
Index Terms Deltacortisone; Deltadehydrocortisone; Rayos®
Generic Availability (U.S.) Yes
Pharmacologic Category Corticosteroid, Systemic
Use Treatment of a variety of diseases, including:
  Allergic states (including adjunctive treatment of anaphylaxis)
  Autoimmune disorders (including systemic lupus erythematosus [SLE])
  Collagen diseases
  Dermatologic conditions/diseases
  Edematous states (including nephrotic syndrome)
  Endocrine disorders
  Gastrointestinal diseases
  Hematologic disorders (including idiopathic thrombocytopenia purpura [ITP])
  Multiple sclerosis exacerbations
  Neoplastic diseases
  Ophthalmic diseases
  Respiratory diseases (including acute asthma exacerbation)
  Rheumatic disorders (including rheumatoid arthritis)
  Trichinosis with neurologic or myocardial involvement
  Tuberculous meningitis
Unlabeled Use Adjunctive therapy for *Pneumocystis jirovecii* (formerly *carinii*) pneumonia (PCP); autoimmune hepatitis; adjunctive therapy for pain management in immunocompetent patients with herpes zoster; tuberculosis (severe, paradoxical reactions); Takayasu arteritis; giant cell arteritis; Grave's ophthalmopathy prophylaxis; subacute thyroiditis; thyrotoxicosis (type II amiodarone-induced)
Contraindications Hypersensitivity to any component of the formulation; systemic fungal infections; administration of live or live attenuated vaccines with immunosuppressive doses of prednisone
Warnings/Precautions May cause hypercorticism or suppression of hypothalamic-pituitary-adrenal (HPA) axis, particularly in patients receiving high doses for prolonged periods. HPA axis suppression may lead to adrenal crisis. Withdrawal and discontinuation of a corticosteroid should be done slowly and carefully. Particular care is required when patients are transferred from systemic corticosteroids to inhaled products due to possible adrenal insufficiency or withdrawal from steroids, including an increase in allergic symptoms. Patients receiving >20 mg per day of prednisone (or equivalent) may be most susceptible. Fatalities have occurred due to adrenal insufficiency in asthmatic patients during and after transfer from systemic corticosteroids to aerosol steroids; aerosol steroids do **not** provide the systemic steroid needed to treat patients having trauma, surgery, or infections.

Acute myopathy has been reported with high dose corticosteroids, usually in patients with neuromuscular transmission disorders; may involve ocular and/or respiratory muscles; monitor creatine kinase; recovery may be delayed. Prolonged use of corticosteroids may increase the incidence of secondary infection, mask acute infection (including fungal infections), prolong or exacerbate viral infections, or limit response to vaccines. Exposure to chickenpox should be avoided. Corticosteroids should not be used to treat ocular herpes

PREDNISONE

simplex or cerebral malaria. Close observation is required in patients with latent tuberculosis and/or TB reactivity; restrict use in active TB (only in conjunction with antituberculosis treatment). Prolonged treatment with corticosteroids has been associated with the development of Kaposi's sarcoma (case reports); if noted, discontinuation of therapy should be considered. Prolonged use may cause posterior subcapsular cataracts, glaucoma (with possible nerve damage) and may increase the risk for ocular infections. Corticosteroid use may cause psychiatric disturbances, including depression, euphoria, insomnia, mood swings, and personality changes. Pre-existing psychiatric conditions may be exacerbated by corticosteroid use.

Use with caution in patients with HF, diabetes, GI diseases (diverticulitis, peptic ulcer, ulcerative colitis; due to risk of perforation); hepatic impairment, myasthenia gravis, MI, patients with or who are at risk for osteoporosis, seizure disorders or thyroid disease.

Prior to use, the dose and duration of treatment should be based on the risk versus benefit for each individual patient. In general, use the smallest effective dose for the shortest duration of time to minimize adverse events. A gradual tapering of dose may be required prior to discontinuing therapy.

Adverse Reactions (Reflective of adult population; not specific for elderly) Frequency not defined.

Cardiovascular: Congestive heart failure (in susceptible patients), hypertension

Central nervous system: Emotional instability, headache, intracranial pressure increased (with papilledema), psychic derangements (including euphoria, insomnia, mood swings, personality changes, severe depression), seizure, vertigo

Dermatologic: Bruising, facial erythema, petechiae, thin fragile skin, urticaria, wound healing impaired

Endocrine & metabolic: Adrenocortical and pituitary unresponsiveness (in times of stress), carbohydrate intolerance, Cushing's syndrome, diabetes mellitus, fluid retention, hypokalemic alkalosis, hypothyroidism enhanced, menstrual irregularities, negative nitrogen balance due to protein catabolism, potassium loss, sodium retention

Gastrointestinal: Abdominal distension, pancreatitis, peptic ulcer (with possible perforation and hemorrhage), ulcerative esophagitis

Hepatic: ALT increased, AST increased, alkaline phosphatase increased

Neuromuscular & skeletal: Aseptic necrosis of femoral and humeral heads, muscle mass loss, muscle weakness, osteoporosis, pathologic fracture of long bones, steroid myopathy, tendon rupture (particularly Achilles tendon), vertebral compression fractures

Ocular: Exophthalmos, glaucoma, intraocular pressure increased, posterior subcapsular cataracts

Miscellaneous: Allergic reactions, anaphylactic reactions, diaphoresis, hypersensitivity reactions, infections, Kaposi's sarcoma

Drug Interactions

Metabolism/Transport Effects Substrate of CYP3A4 (minor); **Note:** Assignment of Major/Minor substrate status based on clinically relevant drug interaction potential; **Induces** CYP2C19 (weak/moderate), CYP3A4 (weak/moderate)

Avoid Concomitant Use

Avoid concomitant use of PredniSONE with any of the following: Aldesleukin; Axitinib; BCG; Mifepristone; Natalizumab; Pimecrolimus; Tacrolimus (Topical)

Increased Effect/Toxicity

PredniSONE may increase the levels/effects of: Acetylcholinesterase Inhibitors; Amphotericin B; CycloSPORINE; CycloSPORINE (Systemic); Deferasirox; Leflunomide; Loop Diuretics; Natalizumab; NSAID (COX-2 Inhibitor); NSAID (Nonselective); Thiazide Diuretics; Vaccines (Live); Warfarin

The levels/effects of PredniSONE may be increased by: Antifungal Agents (Azole Derivatives, Systemic); Aprepitant; Calcium Channel Blockers (Nondihydropyridine); CycloSPORINE; CycloSPORINE (Systemic); Denosumab; Estrogen Derivatives; Fluconazole; Fosaprepitant; Indacaterol; Macrolide Antibiotics; Mifepristone; Neuromuscular-Blocking Agents (Nondepolarizing); Pimecrolimus; Quinolone Antibiotics; Ritonavir; Roflumilast; Salicylates; Tacrolimus (Topical); Telaprevir; Trastuzumab

Decreased Effect

PredniSONE may decrease the levels/effects of: Aldesleukin; Antidiabetic Agents; ARIPiprazole; Axitinib; BCG; Calcitriol; Coccidioidin Skin Test; Corticorelin; CycloSPORINE; CycloSPORINE (Systemic); Hyaluronidase; Isoniazid; Salicylates; Sipuleucel-T; Telaprevir; Vaccines (Inactivated)

The levels/effects of PredniSONE may be decreased by: Aminoglutethimide; Antacids; Barbiturates; Bile Acid Sequestrants; Echinacea; Fosphenytoin; Mifepristone; Mitotane; Phenytoin; Primidone; Rifamycin Derivatives; Somatropin; Tesamorelin; Tocilizumab

Ethanol/Nutrition/Herb Interactions
Ethanol: Avoid ethanol (may increase gastric mucosal irritation)
Food: Prednisone interferes with calcium absorption. Limit caffeine.
Herb/Nutraceutical: St John's wort may decrease prednisone levels. Avoid cat's claw, echinacea (have immunostimulant properties).

Mechanism of Action Decreases inflammation by suppression of migration of polymorpho-nuclear leukocytes and reversal of increased capillary permeability; suppresses the immune system by reducing activity and volume of the lymphatic system; suppresses adrenal function at high doses. Antitumor effects may be related to inhibition of glucose transport, phosphor-ylation, or induction of cell death in immature lymphocytes. Antiemetic effects are thought to occur due to blockade of cerebral innervation of the emetic center via inhibition of prosta-glandin synthesis.

Pharmacodynamics/Kinetics
Absorption: 50% to 90% (may be altered in IBS or hyperthyroidism)
Protein binding (concentration dependent): 65% to 91%
Metabolism: Hepatically converted from prednisone (inactive) to prednisolone (active); may be impaired with hepatic dysfunction
Half-life elimination: Normal renal function: ~3.5 hours
Excretion: Urine (small portion)

Dosage
Geriatric Refer to adult dosing; use the lowest effective dose. Oral dose depends upon condition being treated and response of patient. Alternate day dosing may be attempted.

Adult General dosing range: Oral: Initial: 5-60 mg/day; **Note:** Dose depends upon condition being treated and response of patient. Consider alternate day therapy for long-term therapy. Discontinuation of long-term therapy requires gradual withdrawal by tapering the dose.
Prednisone taper (other regimens also available):
Day 1: 30 mg divided as 10 mg before breakfast, 5 mg at lunch, 5 mg at dinner, 10 mg at bedtime
Day 2: 5 mg at breakfast, 5 mg at lunch, 5 mg at dinner, 10 mg at bedtime
Day 3: 5 mg 4 times/day (with meals and at bedtime)
Day 4: 5 mg 3 times/day (breakfast, lunch, bedtime)
Day 5: 5 mg 2 times/day (breakfast, bedtime)
Day 6: 5 mg before breakfast

Indication-specific dosing:
Acute asthma (NIH guidelines, 2007): Oral: 40-60 mg per day for 3-10 days; administer as single or 2 divided doses
Anaphylaxis, adjunctive treatment (Lieberman, 2005): Oral: 0.5 mg/kg
Antineoplastic: Oral: Usual range: 10 mg/day to 100 mg/m^2/day (depending on indica-tion). **Note:** Details concerning dosing in combination regimens should also be consulted.
Autoimmune hepatitis (unlabeled use; Czaja, 2002): Oral: Initial treatment: 60 mg/day for 1 week, *followed by* 40 mg/day for 1 week, *then* 30 mg/day for 2 weeks, *then* 20 mg/day. Half this dose should be given when used in combination with azathioprine
Dermatomyositis/polymyositis: Oral: 1 mg/kg daily (range: 0.5-1.5 mg/kg/day), often in conjunction with steroid-sparing therapies; depending on response/tolerance, consider slow tapering after 2-8 weeks depending on response; taper regimens vary widely, but often involve 5-10 mg decrements per week and may require 6-12 months to reach a low once-daily or every-other-day dose to prevent disease flare (Briemberg, 2003; Hengst-man, 2009; Iorizzo, 2008; Wiendl, 2008)
Giant cell arteritis (unlabeled use): Oral: Initial: 40-60 mg/day; typically requires 1-2 years of treatment, but may begin to taper after 2-3 months; alternative dosing of 30-40 mg/day has demonstrated similar efficacy (Hiratzka, 2010)
Graves' ophthalmopathy prophylaxis (unlabeled use): Oral: 0.4-0.5 mg/kg/day, starting 1-3 days after radioactive iodine treatment, and continued for 1 month, then gradually taper over 2 months (Bahn, 2011)
Herpes zoster (unlabeled use; Dworkin, 2007): Oral: 60 mg/day for 7 days, *followed by* 30 mg/day for 7 days, *then* 15 mg/day for 7 days
Idiopathic thrombocytopenia purpura (American Society of Hematology, 1997): Oral: 1-2 mg/kg/day
PCP pneumonia (AIDS*info* guidelines, 2008): **Note:** Begin within 72 hours of PCP therapy: 40 mg twice daily for 5 days, *followed by* 40 mg once daily for 5 days, *followed by* 20 mg daily for 11 days or until antimicrobial regimen is completed
Rheumatoid arthritis (American College of Rheumatology, 2002): Oral: ≤10 mg/day
Subacute thyroiditis (unlabeled use): Oral: 40 mg/day for 1-2 weeks; gradually taper over 2-4 weeks or longer depending on clinical response. **Note:** NSAIDs should be considered first-line therapy in such patients (Bahn, 2011).

Systemic lupus erythematosus (American College of Rheumatology, 1999): Oral: Mild SLE: ≤10 mg/day

Refractory or severe organ-threatening disease: 20-60 mg/day

Takayasu arteritis (unlabeled use): Oral: Initial: 40-60 mg/day; taper to lowest effective dose when ESR and CRP levels are normal; usual duration: 1-2 years (Hiratzka, 2010)

Thyrotoxicosis (type II amiodarone-induced; unlabeled use): Oral: 40 mg/day for 14-28 days; gradually taper over 2-3 months depending on clinical response (Bahn, 2011)

Tuberculosis, severe, paradoxical reactions (unlabeled use, AIDS*info* guidelines, 2008): Oral: 1 mg/kg/day, gradually reduce after 1-2 weeks

Renal Impairment Hemodialysis effects: Supplemental dose is not necessary.

Administration Administer with food to decrease gastrointestinal upset

Monitoring Parameters Blood pressure, blood glucose, electrolytes

Following prolonged use: Bone mass density, signs and symptoms of infection, cataract formation, intraocular pressure (use >6 weeks)

Test Interactions Decreased response to skin tests

Pharmacotherapy Pearls Tapering of corticosteroids after a short course of therapy (<7-10 days) is generally not required unless the disease/inflammatory process is slow to respond. Tapering after prolonged exposure is dependent upon the individual patient, duration of corticosteroid treatments, and size of steroid dose. Recovery of the HPA axis may require several months. Subtle but important HPA axis suppression may be present for as long as several months after a course of as few as 10-14 days duration. Testing of HPA axis (cosyntropin) may be required, and signs/symptoms of adrenal insufficiency should be monitored in patients with a history of use.

Special Geriatric Considerations Because of the risk of adverse effects, systemic corticosteroids should be used cautiously in the elderly, in the smallest possible dose, and for the shortest possible time. For long-term use, monitor bone mineral density and institute fracture prevention strategies.

Product Availability Rayos® (prednisone delayed-release tablets): FDA approved July 2012; availability anticipated September 2012. Please consult prescribing information for additional information.

Dosage Forms Excipient information presented when available (limited, particularly for generics); consult specific product labeling.

Solution, oral: 1 mg/mL (5 mL, 120 mL, 500 mL)

Solution, oral [concentrate]:

PredniSONE Intensol™: 5 mg/mL (30 mL) [dye free, sugar free; contains ethanol 30%, propylene glycol]

Tablet, oral: 1 mg, 2.5 mg, 5 mg, 10 mg, 20 mg, 50 mg

◆ **PredniSONE Intensol™** see PredniSONE on page 1595
◆ **Prefest™** see Estradiol and Norgestimate on page 692

Pregabalin (pre GAB a lin)

Medication Safety Issues

Sound-alike/look-alike issues:

Lyrica® may be confused with Lopressor®

Brand Names: U.S. Lyrica®

Brand Names: Canada Lyrica®

Index Terms CI-1008; S-(+)-3-isobutylgaba

Generic Availability (U.S.) No

Pharmacologic Category Analgesic, Miscellaneous; Anticonvulsant, Miscellaneous

Use Management of pain associated with diabetic peripheral neuropathy; management of postherpetic neuralgia; adjunctive therapy for partial-onset seizure disorder in adults; management of fibromyalgia

Medication Guide Available Yes

Contraindications Hypersensitivity to pregabalin or any component of the formulation

Warnings/Precautions Antiepileptics are associated with an increased risk of suicidal behavior/thoughts with use (regardless of indication); patients should be monitored for signs/symptoms of depression, suicidal tendencies, and other unusual behavior changes during therapy and instructed to inform their healthcare provider immediately if symptoms occur.

Angioedema has been reported; may be life threatening; use with caution in patients with a history of angioedema episodes. Concurrent use with other drugs known to cause angioedema (eg, ACE inhibitors) may increase risk. Hypersensitivity reactions, including skin redness, blistering, hives, rash, dyspnea, and wheezing have been reported; discontinue treatment of hypersensitivity occurs. May cause CNS depression and/or dizziness, which may impair physical or mental abilities. Patients must be cautioned about performing tasks which require mental alertness (eg, operating machinery or driving). Effects with other sedative drugs or ethanol may be potentiated. Visual disturbances (blurred vision, decreased acuity and visual field changes) have been associated with pregabalin therapy; patients should be instructed to notify their physician if these effects are noted.

Pregabalin has been associated with increases in CPK and rare cases of rhabdomyolysis. Patients should be instructed to notify their prescriber if unexplained muscle pain, tenderness, or weakness, particularly if fever and/or malaise are associated with these symptoms. Use may be associated with weight gain and peripheral edema; use caution in patients with congestive heart failure, hypertension, or diabetes. Effect on weight gain/edema may be additive to thiazolidinedione antidiabetic agent; particularly in patients with prior cardiovascular disease. May decrease platelet count or prolong PR interval.

Has been noted to be tumorigenic (increased incidence of hemangiosarcoma) in animal studies; significance of these findings in humans is unknown. Pregabalin has been associated with discontinuation symptoms following abrupt cessation, and increases in seizure frequency (when used as an antiepileptic) may occur. Should not be discontinued abruptly; dosage tapering over at least 1 week is recommended. Use caution in renal impairment; dosage adjustment required.

Adverse Reactions (Reflective of adult population; not specific for elderly) Note: Frequency of adverse effects may be influenced by dose or concurrent therapy. In add-on trials in epilepsy, frequency of CNS and visual adverse effects were higher than those reported in pain management trials. Range noted below is inclusive of all trials.

>10%:

Cardiovascular: Peripheral edema (up to 16%)

Central nervous system: Dizziness (8% to 45%), somnolence (4% to 28%), ataxia (up to 20%), headache (up to 14%)

Gastrointestinal: Weight gain (up to 16%), xerostomia (1% to 15%)

Neuromuscular & skeletal: Tremor (up to 11%)

Ocular: Blurred vision (1% to 12%), diplopia (up to 12%)

Miscellaneous: Infection (up to 14%), accidental injury (2% to 11%)

1% to 10%:

Cardiovascular: Chest pain (up to 4%), edema (up to 6%)

Central nervous system: Neuropathy (up to 9%), thinking abnormal (up to 9%), fatigue (up to 8%), confusion (up to 7%), euphoria (up to 7%), speech disorder (up to 7%), attention disturbance (up to 6%), incoordination (up to 6%), amnesia (up to 6%), pain (up to 5%), memory impaired (up to 4%), vertigo (up to 4%), feeling abnormal (up to 3%), hypoesthesia (up to 3%), anxiety (up to 2%), depression (up to 2%), disorientation (up to 2%), lethargy (up to 2%), fever (≥1%), depersonalization (≥1%), hypertonia (≥1%), stupor (≥1%), nervousness (up to 1%)

Dermatologic: Facial edema (up to 3%), bruising (≥1%), pruritus (≥1%)

Endocrine & metabolic: Fluid retention (up to 3%), hypoglycemia (up to 3%), libido decreased (≥1%)

Gastrointestinal: Constipation (up to 10%), appetite increased (up to 7%), flatulence (up to 3%), vomiting (up to 3%), abdominal distension (up to 2%), abdominal pain (≥1%), gastroenteritis (≥1%)

Genitourinary: Incontinence (up to 2%), anorgasmia (≥1%), impotence (≥1%), urinary frequency (≥1%)

Hematologic: Thrombocytopenia (3%)

Neuromuscular & skeletal: Balance disorder (up to 9%), abnormal gait (up to 8%), weakness (up to 7%), arthralgia (up to 6%), twitching (up to 5%), back pain (up to 4%), muscle spasm (up to 4%), myoclonus (up to 4%), paresthesia (>2%), CPK increased (2%), leg cramps (≥1%), myalgia (≥1%), myasthenia (up to 1%)

Ocular: Visual abnormalities (up to 5%), visual field defect (≥2%), eye disorder (up to 2%), nystagmus (>2%), conjunctivitis (≥1%)

Otic: Otitis media (≥1%), tinnitus (≥1%)

Respiratory: Sinusitis (up to 7%), dyspnea (up to 3%), bronchitis (up to 3%), pharyngolaryngeal pain (up to 3%)

Miscellaneous: Flu-like syndrome (up to 2%), allergic reaction (≥1%)

Drug Interactions

Metabolism/Transport Effects None known.

Avoid Concomitant Use

Avoid concomitant use of Pregabalin with any of the following: Azelastine; Azelastine (Nasal); Methadone; Mirtazapine; Paraldehyde

Increased Effect/Toxicity

Pregabalin may increase the levels/effects of: Alcohol (Ethyl); Antidiabetic Agents (Thiazolidinedione); Azelastine; Azelastine (Nasal); Buprenorphine; CNS Depressants; Methadone; Methotrimeprazine; Metyrosine; Mirtazapine; Paraldehyde; Selective Serotonin Reuptake Inhibitors; Zolpidem

The levels/effects of Pregabalin may be increased by: Droperidol; HydrOXYzine; Methotrimeprazine

Decreased Effect

The levels/effects of Pregabalin may be decreased by: Ketorolac; Ketorolac (Nasal); Ketorolac (Systemic); Mefloquine

Ethanol/Nutrition/Herb Interactions

Ethanol: May increase CNS depression; monitor for increased effects with coadministration. Caution patients about effects.

Herb/Nutraceutical: Avoid valerian, St John's wort, kava kava, gotu kola (may increase CNS depression).

Stability Store at 15°C to 30°C (59°F to 86°F).

Mechanism of Action Binds to alpha$_2$-delta subunit of voltage-gated calcium channels within the CNS, inhibiting excitatory neurotransmitter release. Although structurally related to GABA, it does not bind to GABA or benzodiazepine receptors. Exerts antinociceptive and anticonvulsant activity. Decreases symptoms of painful peripheral neuropathies and, as adjunctive therapy in partial seizures, decreases the frequency of seizures.

Pharmacodynamics/Kinetics

Onset of action: Pain management: Effects may be noted as early as the first week of therapy.

Distribution: V_d: 0.5 L/kg

Protein binding: 0%

Metabolism: Negligible

Bioavailability: >90%

Half-life elimination: 6.3 hours

Time to peak, plasma: 1.5 hours (3 hours with food)

Excretion: Urine (90% as unchanged drug; minor metabolites)

Dosage

Geriatric & Adult

Fibromyalgia: Oral: Initial: 150 mg/day in divided doses (75 mg 2 times/day); may be increased to 300 mg/day (150 mg 2 times/day) within 1 week based on tolerability and effect; may be further increased to 450 mg/day (225 mg 2 times/day). Maximum dose: 450 mg/day (dosages up to 600 mg/day were evaluated with no significant additional benefit and an increase in adverse effects)

Neuropathic pain (diabetes-associated): Oral: Initial: 150 mg/day in divided doses (50 mg 3 times/day); may be increased within 1 week based on tolerability and effect; maximum dose: 300 mg/day (dosages up to 600 mg/day were evaluated with no significant additional benefit and an increase in adverse effects)

Postherpetic neuralgia: Oral: Initial: 150 mg/day in divided doses (75 mg 2 times/day or 50 mg 3 times/day); may be increased to 300 mg/day within 1 week based on tolerability and effect; further titration (to 600 mg/day) after 2-4 weeks may be considered in patients who do not experience sufficient relief of pain provided they are able to tolerate pregabalin. Maximum dose: 600 mg/day

Partial onset seizures (adjunctive therapy): Oral: Initial: 150 mg per day in divided doses (75 mg 2 times/day or 50 mg 3 times/day); may be increased based on tolerability and effect (optimal titration schedule has not been defined). Maximum dose: 600 mg/day

Note: Discontinuing therapy: Pregabalin should not be abruptly discontinued; taper dosage over at least 1 week

Renal Impairment Renal function may be estimated using the Cockcroft-Gault formula. Then determine recommended dosage regimen based on the indication-specific total daily dose for normal renal function (Cl$_{cr}$ ≥60 mL/minute). For example, if the indication-specific daily dose is 450 mg/day for normal renal function, the daily dose should be reduced to 225 mg/day (in 2-3 divided doses) for a creatinine clearance of 30-60 mL/minute (see table on next page).

Pregabalin Renal Impairment Dosing

Cl_cr (mL/minute)	Total Pregabalin Daily Dose (mg/day)				Dosing Frequency
≥60 (normal renal function)	150	300	450	600	2-3 divided doses
30-60	75	150	225	300	2-3 divided doses
15-30	25-50	75	100-150	150	1-2 divided doses
<15	25	25-50	50-75	75	Single daily dose

Posthemodialysis supplementary dosage (as a single additional dose):
25 mg/day schedule: Single supplementary dose of 25 mg **or** 50 mg
25-50 mg/day schedule: Single supplementary dose of 50 mg **or** 75 mg
50-75 mg/day schedule: Single supplementary dose of 75 mg **or** 100 mg
75 mg/day schedule: Single supplementary dose of 100 mg **or** 150 mg

Administration May be administered with or without food.

Monitoring Parameters Measures of efficacy (pain intensity/seizure frequency); degree of sedation; symptoms of myopathy or ocular disturbance; weight gain/edema; CPK; skin integrity (in patients with diabetes); suicidality (eg, suicidal thoughts, depression, behavioral changes)

Special Geriatric Considerations In clinical studies, no differences in safety and efficacy were noted between elderly. Since pregabalin is primarily excreted renally, dosage adjustment, based on Cl_cr, is necessary.

Product Availability Lyrica® oral solution: FDA approved December 2009; anticipated availability is currently undetermined

Controlled Substance C-V

Dosage Forms Excipient information presented when available (limited, particularly for generics); consult specific product labeling.
Capsule, oral:
Lyrica®: 25 mg, 50 mg, 75 mg, 100 mg, 150 mg, 200 mg, 225 mg, 300 mg

- ◆ **Pregnenedione** *see* Progesterone *on page 1612*
- ◆ **Premarin®** *see* Estrogens (Conjugated/Equine, Systemic) *on page 703*
- ◆ **Premarin®** *see* Estrogens (Conjugated/Equine, Topical) *on page 707*
- ◆ **Premjact®** *see* Lidocaine (Topical) *on page 1128*
- ◆ **Premphase®** *see* Estrogens (Conjugated/Equine) and Medroxyprogesterone *on page 711*
- ◆ **Prempro®** *see* Estrogens (Conjugated/Equine) and Medroxyprogesterone *on page 711*
- ◆ **Preparation H® [OTC]** *see* Phenylephrine (Topical) *on page 1527*
- ◆ **Preparation H® Hydrocortisone [OTC]** *see* Hydrocortisone (Topical) *on page 943*
- ◆ **Pretz® [OTC]** *see* Sodium Chloride *on page 1787*
- ◆ **Prevacid®** *see* Lansoprazole *on page 1093*
- ◆ **Prevacid® 24 HR [OTC]** *see* Lansoprazole *on page 1093*
- ◆ **Prevacid® SoluTab™** *see* Lansoprazole *on page 1093*
- ◆ **Prevalite®** *see* Cholestyramine Resin *on page 367*
- ◆ **PreviDent®** *see* Fluoride *on page 806*
- ◆ **PreviDent® 5000 Booster** *see* Fluoride *on page 806*
- ◆ **PreviDent® 5000 Dry Mouth** *see* Fluoride *on page 806*
- ◆ **PreviDent® 5000 Plus®** *see* Fluoride *on page 806*
- ◆ **PreviDent® 5000 Sensitive** *see* Fluoride *on page 806*
- ◆ **Prialt®** *see* Ziconotide *on page 2048*
- ◆ **Priftin®** *see* Rifapentine *on page 1700*
- ◆ **PriLOSEC®** *see* Omeprazole *on page 1417*
- ◆ **PriLOSEC OTC® [OTC]** *see* Omeprazole *on page 1417*
- ◆ **Primaclone** *see* Primidone *on page 1601*
- ◆ **Primatene® Mist [OTC] [DSC]** *see* EPINEPHrine (Systemic, Oral Inhalation) *on page 645*
- ◆ **Primaxin® I.M. [DSC]** *see* Imipenem and Cilastatin *on page 975*
- ◆ **Primaxin® I.V.** *see* Imipenem and Cilastatin *on page 975*

Primidone (PRI mi done)

Medication Safety Issues
Sound-alike/look-alike issues:
Primidone may be confused with predniSONE, primaquine, pyridoxine
Brand Names: U.S. Mysoline®
Brand Names: Canada Apo-Primidone®

Index Terms Desoxyphenobarbital; Primaclone
Generic Availability (U.S.) Yes
Pharmacologic Category Anticonvulsant, Miscellaneous; Barbiturate
Use Management of grand mal, psychomotor, and focal seizures
Unlabeled Use Benign familial tremor (essential tremor)
Medication Guide Available Yes
Contraindications Hypersensitivity to phenobarbital; porphyria
Warnings/Precautions Antiepileptics are associated with an increased risk of suicidal behavior/thoughts with use (regardless of indication); patients should be monitored for signs/symptoms of depression, suicidal tendencies, and other unusual behavior changes during therapy and instructed to inform their healthcare provider immediately if symptoms occur.

Use with caution in patients with renal or hepatic impairment, pulmonary insufficiency; abrupt withdrawal may precipitate status epilepticus. Potential for drug dependency exists. Do not administer to patients in acute pain. Use caution in elderly or debilitated patients - may cause paradoxical responses. May cause CNS depression, which may impair physical or mental abilities. Patients must cautioned about performing tasks which require mental alertness (eg, operating machinery or driving). Effects with other sedative drugs or ethanol may be potentiated. Use with caution in patients with depression or suicidal tendencies, or in patients with a history of drug abuse. Tolerance or psychological and physical dependence may occur with prolonged use. Use with caution in patients with hypoadrenalism.

Adverse Reactions (Reflective of adult population; not specific for elderly) Frequency not defined.
Central nervous system: Ataxia, drowsiness, emotional disturbances, fatigue, hyperirritability, suicidal ideation, vertigo
Dermatologic: Morbilliform skin eruptions
Gastrointestinal: Anorexia, nausea, vomiting
Genitourinary: Impotence
Hematologic: Agranulocytosis, granulocytopenia, megaloblastic anemia (idiosyncratic), red cell aplasia/hypoplasia
Ocular: Diplopia, nystagmus

Drug Interactions
Metabolism/Transport Effects Induces CYP1A2 (strong), CYP2B6 (strong), CYP2C8 (strong), CYP2C9 (strong), CYP3A4 (strong)
Avoid Concomitant Use
Avoid concomitant use of Primidone with any of the following: Axitinib; Azelastine; Azelastine (Nasal); Boceprevir; Bortezomib; Crizotinib; Dienogest; Dronedarone; Everolimus; Itraconazole; Lapatinib; Lurasidone; Methadone; Mifepristone; Mirtazapine; Nilotinib; Nisoldipine; Paraldehyde; Pazopanib; Praziquantel; Ranolazine; Rilpivirine; Rivaroxaban; Roflumilast; RomiDEPsin; SORAfenib; Ticagrelor; Tolvaptan; Toremifene; Vandetanib
Increased Effect/Toxicity
Primidone may increase the levels/effects of: Alcohol (Ethyl); Azelastine; Azelastine (Nasal); Barbiturates; Buprenorphine; Clarithromycin; CNS Depressants; Ifosfamide; Methadone; Methotrimeprazine; Metyrosine; Mirtazapine; Paraldehyde; Selective Serotonin Reuptake Inhibitors; Zolpidem

The levels/effects of Primidone may be increased by: Carbonic Anhydrase Inhibitors; Clarithromycin; Dexmethylphenidate; Divalproex; Droperidol; Felbamate; HydrOXYzine; Methotrimeprazine; Methylphenidate; Valproic Acid
Decreased Effect
Primidone may decrease the levels/effects of: Apixaban; ARIPiprazole; Axitinib; Bendamustine; Boceprevir; Bortezomib; Brentuximab Vedotin; Clarithromycin; Corticosteroids (Systemic); Crizotinib; CYP1A2 Substrates; CYP2B6 Substrates; CYP2C8 Substrates; CYP2C9 Substrates; CYP3A4 Substrates; Dasatinib; Diclofenac; Dienogest; Divalproex; Dronedarone; Everolimus; Exemestane; Felbamate; Gefitinib; GuanFACINE; Imatinib; Itraconazole; Ixabepilone; LamoTRIgine; Lapatinib; Linagliptin; Lurasidone; Maraviroc; Mifepristone; NIFEdipine; Nilotinib; Nisoldipine; Pazopanib; Praziquantel; QuiNIDine; Ranolazine; Rilpivirine; Rivaroxaban; Roflumilast; RomiDEPsin; Rufinamide; Saxagliptin; SORAfenib; SUNItinib; Tadalafil; Ticagrelor; Tolvaptan; Toremifene; Treprostinil; Ulipristal; Valproic Acid; Vandetanib; Vemurafenib; Zuclopenthixol

The levels/effects of Primidone may be decreased by: Carbonic Anhydrase Inhibitors; Folic Acid; Fosphenytoin; Ketorolac; Ketorolac (Nasal); Ketorolac (Systemic); Leucovorin Calcium-Levoleucovorin; Levomefolate; Mefloquine; Methylfolate; Phenytoin
Ethanol/Nutrition/Herb Interactions
Ethanol: May increase CNS depression; monitor for increased effects with coadministration. Caution patients about effects.

Food: Protein-deficient diets increase duration of action of primidone.

Herb/Nutraceutical: Avoid valerian, St John's wort, kava kava, gotu kola (may increase CNS depression).

Stability Store at 20°C to 25°C (68°F to 77°F).

Mechanism of Action Decreases neuron excitability, raises seizure threshold similar to phenobarbital; primidone has two active metabolites, phenobarbital and phenylethylmalonamide (PEMA); PEMA may enhance the activity of phenobarbital

Pharmacodynamics/Kinetics

Absorption: 60% to 80%

Distribution: Adults: V_d: 0.6 L/kg

Protein binding: 30%

Metabolism: Hepatic to phenobarbital (active) by oxidation and to phenylethylmalonamide (PEMA; active) by scission of the heterocyclic ring

Half-life elimination (age dependent): Primidone: Mean: 5-15 hours (variable); PEMA: 16 hours (variable)

Time to peak, serum: ~3 hours (variable)

Excretion: Urine (40% as unchanged drug; the remainder is unconjugated PEMA, phenobarbital and its metabolites)

Dosage

Geriatric & Adult

Seizure disorders (grand mal, psychomotor, and focal): Oral: Days 1-3: 100-125 mg/day at bedtime; days 4-6: 100-125 twice daily; days 7-9: 100-125 mg 3 times daily; usual dose: 750-1500 mg/day in divided doses 3-4 times/day with maximum dosage of 2 g/day

Patients already receiving other anticonvulsants: Initial: 100-125 mg at bedtime; gradually increase to maintenance dose as other drug is gradually decreased, continue until desired level obtained or other drug completely withdrawn. If goal is monotherapy, conversion should be completed over ≥2 weeks.

Essential tremor (unlabeled use): Oral: Initial 12.5-25 mg/day at bedtime; titrate up to 250 mg/day in 1-2 divided doses; doses up to 750 mg/day may be beneficial

Renal Impairment

Adults (Aronoff, 2007): **Note:** Avoid in renal failure if possible; due to active metabolites with long half-lives and complex kinetics:

Cl_{cr} ≥50 mL/minute: Administer every 12 hours

Cl_{cr} 10-50 mL/minute: Administer every 12-24 hours

Cl_{cr} <10 mL/minute: Administer every 24 hours

Hemodialysis: Administer dose postdialysis

Hepatic Impairment Increased side effects may occur in severe liver disease. Monitor plasma levels and adjust dose accordingly.

Monitoring Parameters Serum primidone and phenobarbital concentration, neurological status. Due to CNS effects, monitor closely when initiating drug in elderly. Monitor CBC and sequential multiple analysis-12 (SMA-12) at 6-month intervals to compare with baseline obtained at start of therapy. Monitor for suicidality (eg, suicidal thoughts, depression, behavioral changes). Since elderly metabolize phenobarbital at a slower rate than younger adults, it is suggested to measure both primidone and phenobarbital levels together.

Reference Range Therapeutic: Adults: 5-12 mcg/mL (SI: 23-55 μmol/L); toxic effects rarely present with levels <10 mcg/mL (SI: 46 μmol/L) if phenobarbital concentrations are low. Dosage of primidone is adjusted with reference mostly to the phenobarbital level; Toxic: >15 mcg/mL (SI: >69 μmol/L)

Pharmacotherapy Pearls Bioequivalence problems have been noted with primidone from one manufacturer to another, therefore, brand interchange is not recommended

Special Geriatric Considerations Due to CNS effects, monitor closely when initiating drug in elderly. Monitor CBC at 6-month intervals to compare with baseline obtained at start of therapy. Since elderly metabolize phenobarbital at a slower rate than younger adults, it is suggested to measure both primidone and phenobarbital serum concentrations together. Adjust dose for renal function in elderly when initiating or changing dose.

Dosage Forms Excipient information presented when available (limited, particularly for generics); consult specific product labeling.

Tablet, oral: 50 mg, 250 mg

Mysoline®: 50 mg, 250 mg [scored]

Dosage Forms: Canada Excipient information presented when available (limited, particularly for generics); consult specific product labeling.

Tablet, oral:

Apo-Primidone®: 125 mg, 250 mg

◆ **Primlev™** see Oxycodone and Acetaminophen on page 1449
◆ **Primsol®** see Trimethoprim on page 1971
◆ **Prinivil®** see Lisinopril on page 1146
◆ **Prinzide®** see Lisinopril and Hydrochlorothiazide on page 1149

- **Pristiq®** *see* Desvenlafaxine *on page 514*
- **Privigen®** *see* Immune Globulin *on page 982*
- **Privine® [OTC]** *see* Naphazoline (Nasal) *on page 1337*
- **ProAir® HFA** *see* Albuterol *on page 49*
- **ProAmatine** *see* Midodrine *on page 1282*

Probenecid (proe BEN e sid)

Medication Safety Issues
Sound-alike/look-alike issues:
Probenecid may be confused with Procanbid
Brand Names: Canada Benuryl™
Index Terms Benemid [DSC]
Generic Availability (U.S.) Yes
Pharmacologic Category Uricosuric Agent
Use Treatment of hyperuricemia associated with gout or gouty arthritis; prolongation and elevation of beta-lactam plasma levels (eg, uncomplicated gonococcal infection)
Unlabeled Use Prolongation and elevation of beta-lactam plasma levels (eg, neurosyphilis, pelvic inflammatory disease)
Contraindications Hypersensitivity to probenecid or any component of the formulation; small- or large-dose aspirin therapy; blood dyscrasias; uric acid kidney stones; initiation during an acute gout attack
Warnings/Precautions Use with caution in patients with peptic ulcer. Salicylates may diminish the therapeutic effect of probenecid. This effect may be more pronounced with high, chronic doses, however, the manufacturer recommends the use of an alternative analgesic even in place of small doses of aspirin. Use of probenecid with penicillin in patients with renal insufficiency is not recommended. Probenecid monotherapy may not be effective in patients with a creatinine clearance <30 mL/minute. Probenecid may increase the serum concentration of methotrexate. Avoid concomitant use of probenecid and methotrexate if possible. If used together, consider lower methotrexate doses and monitor for methotrexate toxicity. May cause exacerbation of acute gouty attack. If hypersensitivity reaction or anaphylaxis occurs, discontinue medication. Use caution in patients with G6PD deficiency; may increase risk for hemolytic anemia.
Adverse Reactions (Reflective of adult population; not specific for elderly) Frequency not defined.
Cardiovascular: Flushing
Central nervous system: Dizziness, fever, headache
Dermatologic: Alopecia, dermatitis, pruritus, rash
Gastrointestinal: Anorexia, dyspepsia, gastroesophageal reflux, nausea, sore gums, vomiting
Genitourinary: Hematuria, polyuria
Hematologic: Anemia, aplastic anemia, hemolytic anemia (in G6PD deficiency), leukopenia
Hepatic: Hepatic necrosis
Neuromuscular & skeletal: Costovertebral pain, gouty arthritis (acute)
Renal: Nephrotic syndrome, renal colic
Miscellaneous: Anaphylaxis, hypersensitivity
Drug Interactions
Metabolism/Transport Effects Inhibits CYP2C19 (weak), UGT1A6
Avoid Concomitant Use
Avoid concomitant use of Probenecid with any of the following: Doripenem; Ketorolac; Ketorolac (Nasal); Ketorolac (Systemic); Meropenem
Increased Effect/Toxicity
Probenecid may increase the levels/effects of: Acetaminophen; Cefotaxime; Cephalosporins; Dapsone; Dapsone (Systemic); Deferiprone; Doripenem; Ertapenem; Ganciclovir-Valganciclovir; Gemifloxacin; Imipenem; Ketoprofen; Ketorolac; Ketorolac (Nasal); Ketorolac (Systemic); Loop Diuretics; LORazepam; Meropenem; Methotrexate; Mycophenolate; Nitrofurantoin; Nonsteroidal Anti-Inflammatory Agents; Oseltamivir; Penicillins; PRALAtrexate; Quinolone Antibiotics; Sodium Benzoate; Sodium Phenylacetate; Sulfonylureas; Theophylline Derivatives; Zidovudine
Decreased Effect
Probenecid may decrease the levels/effects of: Loop Diuretics

The levels/effects of Probenecid may be decreased by: Salicylates
Stability Store at 20°C to 25°C (68°F to 77°F). Protect from light.
Mechanism of Action Competitively inhibits the reabsorption of uric acid at the proximal convoluted tubule, thereby promoting its excretion and reducing serum uric acid levels; increases plasma levels of weak organic acids (penicillins, cephalosporins, or other beta-lactam antibiotics) by competitively inhibiting their renal tubular secretion

Pharmacodynamics/Kinetics

Onset of action: Effect on penicillin levels: 2 hours

Absorption: Rapid and complete

Metabolism: Hepatic

Half-life elimination (dose dependent): Normal renal function: 6-12 hours

Time to peak, serum: 2-4 hours

Excretion: Urine

Dosage

Geriatric & Adult

Hyperuricemia with gout: Oral: 250 mg twice daily for 1 week; may increase to 500 mg twice daily; if needed, may increase to a maximum of 2 g/day (increase dosage in 500 mg increments every 4 weeks). If serum uric acid levels are within normal limits and gout attacks have been absent for 6 months, daily dosage may be reduced by 500 mg every 6 months.

Prolong penicillin serum levels: Oral: 500 mg 4 times/day. **Note:** Dosing per manufacturer, see indication-specific dosing.

Gonorrhea, uncomplicated infections of cervix, urethra, and rectum: Oral: 1 g once with cefoxitin 2 g I.M. (CDC, 2010)

Pelvic inflammatory disease (unlabeled use): Oral: 1 g once with cefoxitin 2 g I.M. plus doxycycline (CDC, 2010)

Neurosyphilis (unlabeled use): Oral: 500 mg 4 times/day with procaine penicillin 2.4 million units/day I.M for 10-14 days (CDC, 2010). **Note:** Penicillin G aqueous I.V. is the preferred agent.

Renal Impairment Cl_{cr} <30 mL/minute: Avoid use.

Administration Administer with food or antacids to minimize GI effects.

Monitoring Parameters Uric acid, renal function, CBC

Reference Range

Adults:

Males: 3.4-7 mg/dL or slightly more

Females: 2.4-6 mg/dL or slightly more

Target: <6 mg/dL

Values >7 mg/dL are sometimes arbitrarily regarded as hyperuricemia, but there is no sharp line between normals and the serum uric acid of those with clinical gout. Normal ranges cannot be adjusted for purine ingestion, but high-purine diet increases uric acid. Uric acid may be increased with body size, exercise, and stress.

Test Interactions False-positive glucosuria with Clinitest®, a falsely high determination of theophylline has occurred and the renal excretion of phenolsulfonphthalein 17-ketosteroids and bromsulfophthalein (BSP) may be inhibited

Pharmacotherapy Pearls Avoid fluctuation in uric acid (increase or decrease); may precipitate gout attack. The manufacturer recommends the use of sodium bicarbonate (3-7.5 g daily) or potassium citrate (7.5 g daily) is suggested until serum uric acid normalizes and tophaceous deposits disappear.

Special Geriatric Considerations Since probenecid loses its effectiveness when the Cl_{cr} is <30 mL/minute, its usefulness in the elderly is limited.

Dosage Forms Excipient information presented when available (limited, particularly for generics); consult specific product labeling.

Tablet, oral: 500 mg

◆ **Probenecid and Colchicine** see Colchicine and Probenecid on page 440

Procainamide (pro KANE a mide)

Related Information

Beers Criteria – Potentially Inappropriate Medications for Geriatrics on page 2183

Medication Safety Issues

Sound-alike/look-alike issues:

Procanbid may be confused with probenecid, Procan SR®

Pronestyl may be confused with Ponstel®

PROCAINAMIDE

◀

High alert medication:
The Institute for Safe Medication Practices (ISMP) includes this medication among its list of drugs which have a heightened risk of causing significant patient harm when used in error.

BEERS Criteria medication:
This drug may be potentially inappropriate for use in geriatric patients (Quality of evidence - high; Strength of recommendation - strong).

Administration issues:
Procainamide hydrochloride is available in 10 mL vials of 100 mg/mL and in 2 mL vials with 500 mg/mL. Note that **BOTH** vials contain 1 gram of drug; confusing the strengths can lead to massive overdoses or underdoses.

Other safety concerns:
PCA is an error-prone abbreviation (mistaken as patient controlled analgesia)

Brand Names: Canada Apo-Procainamide®; Procainamide Hydrochloride Injection, USP; Procan SR®

Index Terms PCA (error-prone abbreviation); Procainamide Hydrochloride; Procaine Amide Hydrochloride; Procanbid; Pronestyl

Generic Availability (U.S.) Yes

Pharmacologic Category Antiarrhythmic Agent, Class Ia

Use
Intravenous: Treatment of life-threatening ventricular arrhythmias
Oral (Canadian labeling; not available in U.S.): Treatment of supraventricular arrhythmias.
Note: In the treatment of atrial fibrillation, use only when preferred treatment is ineffective or cannot be used. Use in paroxysmal atrial tachycardia when reflex stimulation or other measures are ineffective.

Unlabeled Use
Paroxysmal supraventricular tachycardia (PSVT); prevent recurrence of ventricular tachycardia; symptomatic premature ventricular contractions
ACLS guidelines: I.V.: Treatment of the following arrhythmias in patients with preserved left ventricular function: Stable monomorphic VT; pre-excited atrial fibrillation; stable wide complex regular tachycardia (likely VT)
PALS guidelines: I.V.: Tachycardia with pulses and poor perfusion (probable SVT [unresponsive to vagal maneuvers and adenosine or synchronized cardioversion]; probable VT [unresponsive to synchronized cardioversion or adenosine])

Contraindications Hypersensitivity to procainamide, procaine, other ester-type local anesthetics, or any component of the formulation; complete heart block; second-degree AV block or various types of hemiblock (without a functional artificial pacemaker); SLE; torsade de pointes

Warnings/Precautions Monitor and adjust dose to prevent QT$_c$ prolongation. Watch for proarrhythmic effects. Avoid use in patients with QT prolongation (ACLS, 2010). May precipitate or exacerbate HF due to negative inotropic actions; use with caution or avoid (ACLS, 2010) in patients with HF. Correct electrolyte disturbances, especially hypokalemia or hypomagnesemia, prior to use and throughout therapy. Reduce dosage in renal impairment. May increase ventricular response rate in patients with atrial fibrillation or flutter; control AV conduction before initiating. Correct hypokalemia before initiating therapy; hypokalemia may worsen toxicity. Reduce dose if first-degree heart block occurs. Use caution with concurrent use of other antiarrhythmics; may exacerbate or increase the risk of conduction disturbances. Avoid concurrent use with other drugs known to prolong QT$_c$ interval. Avoid use in myasthenia gravis (may worsen condition).

Use caution and dose cautiously in older adults; renal clearance of procainamide/NAPA declines in patients ≥50 years of age (independent of creatinine clearance reductions) and in the presence of concomitant renal impairment. In the treatment of atrial fibrillation, avoid antiarrhythmics as first-line treatment. In older adults, data suggests rate control may provide more benefits than risks compared to rhythm control for most patients (Beers Criteria).

This product contains sodium metabisulfite which may cause allergic-type reactions, including anaphylactic symptoms and life-threatening asthmatic episodes in susceptible people; this is seen more frequently in asthmatics.

[U.S. Boxed Warning]: Potentially fatal blood dyscrasias (eg, agranulocytosis) have occurred with therapeutic doses; weekly monitoring is recommended during the first 3 months of therapy and periodically thereafter. Discontinue procainamide if this occurs.

[U.S. Boxed Warning]: Long-term administration leads to the development of a positive antinuclear antibody (ANA) test in 50% of patients which may result in a drug-induced lupus erythematosus-like syndrome (in 20% to 30% of patients); discontinue procainamide with rising ANA titers or with SLE symptoms and choose an alternative agent.

[U.S. Boxed Warning] In the Cardiac Arrhythmia Suppression Trial (CAST), recent (>6 days but <2 years ago) myocardial infarction patients with asymptomatic, non-life-threatening ventricular arrhythmias did not benefit and may have been harmed by attempts to suppress the arrhythmia with flecainide or encainide. An increased mortality or nonfatal cardiac arrest rate (7.7%) was seen in the active treatment group compared with patients in the placebo group (3%). The applicability of the CAST results to other populations is unknown. Procainamide should be reserved for patients with life-threatening ventricular arrhythmias.

Adverse Reactions (Reflective of adult population; not specific for elderly) >1%:

Cardiovascular: Hypotension (I.V. up to 5%)

Dermatologic: Rash

Gastrointestinal: Diarrhea (oral: 3% to 4%), nausea (oral: 3% to 4%), taste disorder (oral: 3% to 4%), vomiting (oral: 3% to 4%)

Miscellaneous: Positive ANA (≤50%), SLE-like syndrome (≤30%, increased incidence with long-term therapy or slow acetylators; syndrome may include abdominal pain, arthralgia, arthritis, chills, fever, hepatomegaly, myalgia, pericarditis, pleural effusion, pulmonary infiltrates, rash)

Drug Interactions

Metabolism/Transport Effects Substrate of CYP2D6 (major); **Note:** Assignment of Major/Minor substrate status based on clinically relevant drug interaction potential

Avoid Concomitant Use

Avoid concomitant use of Procainamide with any of the following: Fingolimod; Highest Risk QTc-Prolonging Agents; Mifepristone; Moderate Risk QTc-Prolonging Agents; Propafenone

Increased Effect/Toxicity

Procainamide may increase the levels/effects of: Highest Risk QTc-Prolonging Agents; Neuromuscular-Blocking Agents

The levels/effects of Procainamide may be increased by: Abiraterone Acetate; Amiodarone; Cimetidine; CYP2D6 Inhibitors (Moderate); CYP2D6 Inhibitors (Strong); Darunavir; EriBU-Lin; Fingolimod; LamoTRIgine; Lurasidone; Mifepristone; Moderate Risk QTc-Prolonging Agents; Propafenone; QTc-Prolonging Agents (Indeterminate Risk and Risk Modifying); Ranitidine; Trimethoprim

Decreased Effect

The levels/effects of Procainamide may be decreased by: Peginterferon Alfa-2b

Ethanol/Nutrition/Herb Interactions

Ethanol: Avoid ethanol (acute ethanol administration reduces procainamide serum concentrations).

Herb/Nutraceutical: Avoid ephedra (may worsen arrhythmia).

Stability Store undiluted vials at room temperature of 15°C to 30°C (59°F to 86°F). The solution is initially colorless but may turn slightly yellow on standing. Injection of air into the vial causes solution to darken. Discard solutions darker than light amber. Color formation may occur upon refrigeration.

When admixed in NS or D_5W to a final concentration of 2-4 mg/mL, solution is stable at room temperature for 24 hours and for 7 days under refrigeration.

Mechanism of Action Decreases myocardial excitability and conduction velocity and may depress myocardial contractility, by increasing the electrical stimulation threshold of ventricle, His-Purkinje system and through direct cardiac effects

Pharmacodynamics/Kinetics

Onset of action: I.M. 10-30 minutes

Distribution: V_d: Adults: 2 L/kg; decreased with congestive heart failure or shock

Protein binding: 15% to 20%

Metabolism: Hepatic via acetylation to produce N-acetyl procainamide (NAPA) (active metabolite)

Half-life elimination:

Procainamide (hepatic acetylator, phenotype, cardiac and renal function dependent): Adults: 2.5-4.7 hours; Anephric: 11 hours

NAPA (dependent upon renal function): Adults: 6-8 hours; Anephric: 42 hours

Time to peak, serum: I.M.: 15-60 minutes

Excretion: Urine (30% to 60% unchanged procainamide; 6% to 52% as NAPA); feces (<5% unchanged procainamide. **Note:** >80% of formed NAPA is renally eliminated in contrast to procainamide which is ~50% renally eliminated (Gibson, 1977).

Dosage

Geriatric Refer to adult dosing. Initiate doses at lower end of dosage range.

Adult Dose must be titrated to patient's response.

Antiarrhythmic:

I.M.: 50 mg/kg/day divided every 3-6 hours **or** 0.5-1 g every 4-8 hours (Koch-Weser, 1971)

I.V.:

Loading dose: 15-18 mg/kg administered as slow infusion over 25-30 minutes **or** 100 mg/dose at a rate not to exceed 50 mg/minute repeated every 5 minutes as needed to a total dose of 1 g.

Hemodynamically stable monomorphic VT or pre-excited atrial fibrillation (ACLS, 2010): Loading dose: Infuse 20-50 mg/minute **or** 100 mg every 5 minutes until arrhythmia controlled, hypotension occurs, QRS complex widens by 50% of its original width, or total of 17 mg/kg is given. Follow with a continuous infusion of 1-4 mg/minute. **Note:** Not recommended for use in ongoing ventricular fibrillation (VF) or pulseless ventricular tachycardia (VT) due to prolonged administration time and uncertain efficacy.

Maintenance dose: 1-4 mg/minute by continuous infusion. Maintenance infusions should be reduced by one-third in patients with moderate renal or cardiac impairment and by two-thirds in patients with severe renal or cardiac impairment.

Oral (not available in the U.S.; Canadian labeling): Sustained release formulation (Procan SR®): Maintenance: 50 mg/kg/24 hours given in divided doses every 6 hours

Suggested Procan SR® maintenance dose:

<55 kg: 500 mg every 6 hours

55-91 kg: 750 mg every 6 hours

>91 kg: 1000 mg every 6 hours

Renal Impairment

Oral:

Cl_{cr} 10-50 mL/minute: Administer every 6-12 hours.

Cl_{cr} <10 mL/minute: Administer every 8-24 hours.

I.V.:

Loading dose: Reduce dose to 12 mg/kg in severe renal impairment.

Maintenance infusion: Reduce dose by one-third in patients with mild renal impairment. Reduce dose by two-thirds in patients with severe renal impairment.

Dialysis:

Procainamide: Moderately hemodialyzable (20% to 50%): Monitor procainamide/N-acetyl-procainamide (NAPA) concentrations; supplementation may be necessary.

NAPA: Not dialyzable (0% to 5%)

Procainamide/NAPA: Not peritoneal dialyzable (0% to 5%)

Procainamide/NAPA: Replace according to blood concentration monitoring during continuous arteriovenous or venovenous hemofiltration.

Hepatic Impairment Reduce dose by 50%.

Administration

Oral: Do **not** crush or chew sustained release drug products (not available in the U.S.).

I.V.: Must dilute prior to I.V. administration. Dilute loading dose to a maximum concentration of 20 mg/mL; administer loading dose at a maximum rate of 50 mg/minute

Monitoring Parameters ECG, blood pressure, renal function; with prolonged use monitor CBC with differential, platelet count; procainamide and NAPA blood concentrations in patients with hepatic impairment, renal impairment, or receiving constant infusion >3 mg/minute for longer than 24 hours; ANA titers

Reference Range

Timing of serum samples: Draw 6-12 hours after I.V. infusion has started; half-life is 2.5-5 hours

Therapeutic concentrations: Procainamide: 4-10 mcg/mL; NAPA 15-25 mcg/mL; Combined: 10-30 mcg/mL

Toxic concentration: Procainamide: >10-12 mcg/mL

Test Interactions In the presence of propranolol or suprapharmacologic concentrations of lidocaine or meprobamate, tests which depend on fluorescence to measure procainamide/NAPA concentrations may be affected.

Special Geriatric Considerations Monitor closely since clearance is reduced in those >60 years of age. If clinically possible, start doses at lowest recommended dose. Also, elderly frequently have drug therapy which may interfere with the use of procainamide. Adjust dose for renal function in the elderly.

This medication is considered to be potentially inappropriate in this patient population (Beers Criteria: Quality of evidence - high; Strength of recommendation - strong).

Dosage Forms Excipient information presented when available (limited, particularly for generics); consult specific product labeling.

Injection, solution, as hydrochloride: 100 mg/mL (10 mL); 500 mg/mL (2 mL)

Dosage Forms: Canada Excipient information presented when available (limited, particularly for generics); consult specific product labeling.

Tablet, sustained release, oral, as hydrochloride:

Procan SR®: 250 mg, 500 mg, 750 mg

♦ **Procainamide Hydrochloride** see Procainamide on page 1605
♦ **Procaine Amide Hydrochloride** see Procainamide on page 1605
♦ **Procaine Benzylpenicillin** see Penicillin G Procaine on page 1502
♦ **Procaine Penicillin G** see Penicillin G Procaine on page 1502
♦ **Procanbid** see Procainamide on page 1605
♦ **Procardia®** see NIFEdipine on page 1375
♦ **Procardia XL®** see NIFEdipine on page 1375
♦ **Procetofene** see Fenofibrate on page 752

Prochlorperazine (proe klor PER a zeen)

Related Information

Beers Criteria – Potentially Inappropriate Medications for Geriatrics on page 2183

Medication Safety Issues

Sound-alike/look-alike issues:

Prochlorperazine may be confused with chlorproMAZINE

Compazine may be confused with Copaxone®, Coumadin®

BEERS Criteria medication:

This drug may be potentially inappropriate for use in geriatric patients (Quality of evidence - varies based on comorbidity; Strength of recommendation - varies based on comorbidity)

Other safety concerns:

CPZ (occasional abbreviation for Compazine) is an error-prone abbreviation (mistaken as chlorpromazine)

Brand Names: U.S. Compro®

Brand Names: Canada Apo-Prochlorperazine®; Nu-Prochlor; PMS-Prochlorperazine; Sandoz-Prochlorperazine

Index Terms Chlormeprazine; Compazine; Prochlorperazine Edisylate; Prochlorperazine Maleate; Prochlorperazine Mesylate

Generic Availability (U.S.) Yes

Pharmacologic Category Antiemetic; Antipsychotic Agent, Typical; Phenothiazine

Use Management of nausea and vomiting; psychotic disorders, including schizophrenia and anxiety; nonpsychotic anxiety

Unlabeled Use Behavioral syndromes in dementia; psychosis/agitation related to Alzheimer's dementia

Contraindications Hypersensitivity to prochlorperazine or any component of the formulation (cross-reactivity between phenothiazines may occur); severe CNS depression; coma; Reye's syndrome

Warnings/Precautions [U.S. Boxed Warning]: Elderly patients with dementia-related psychosis treated with antipsychotics are at an increased risk of death compared to placebo. Most deaths appeared to be either cardiovascular (eg, heart failure, sudden death) or infectious (eg, pneumonia) in nature. Prochlorperazine is not approved for the treatment of dementia-related psychosis.

Leukopenia, neutropenia, and agranulocytosis (sometimes fatal) have been reported in clinical trials and postmarketing reports with antipsychotic use; presence of risk factors (eg, pre-existing low WBC or history of drug-induced leuko-/neutropenia) should prompt periodic blood count assessment. Discontinue therapy at first signs of blood dyscrasias or if absolute neutrophil count <1000/mm^3.

May be sedating; use with caution in disorders where CNS depression is a feature. May obscure intestinal obstruction or brain tumor. May impair physical or mental abilities. Effects with other sedative drugs or ethanol may be potentiated. Use with caution in Parkinson's disease; hemodynamic instability; predisposition to seizures; subcortical brain damage; and in severe cardiac, hepatic, or renal disease. May alter temperature regulation or mask toxicity of other drugs. Use caution with exposure to heat. May alter cardiac conduction. May cause orthostatic hypotension. Hypotension may occur following administration, particularly when parenteral form is used or in high dosages. Antipsychotic use has been associated with esophageal dysmotility and aspiration; use with caution in patients at risk of pneumonia (ie, Alzheimer's disease).

PROCHLORPERAZINE

May cause pigmentary retinopathy, and lenticular and corneal deposits, particularly with prolonged therapy. Use associated with increased prolactin levels; clinical significance of hyperprolactinemia in patients with breast cancer or other prolactin-dependent tumors is unknown.

May be inappropriate in older adults depending on comorbidities (eg, dementia, delirium) due to its potent anticholinergic effects (Beers Criteria). Use with caution in the elderly; increased risk for developing tardive dyskinesia, particularly elderly women.

Phenothiazines may cause anticholinergic effects; therefore, they should be used with caution in patients with decreased gastrointestinal motility, urinary retention, BPH, xerostomia, or visual problems. Conditions which also may be exacerbated by cholinergic blockade include narrow-angle glaucoma and worsening of myasthenia gravis. May cause extrapyramidal symptoms (EPS), including pseudoparkinsonism, acute dystonic reactions, akathisia, and tardive dyskinesia. Risk of dystonia (and possibly other EPS) may be greater with increased doses, use of conventional antipsychotics, males, and younger patients. May be associated with neuroleptic malignant syndrome (NMS)

Adverse Reactions (Reflective of adult population; not specific for elderly)

Reported with prochlorperazine or other phenothiazines. Frequency not defined.

Cardiovascular: Cardiac arrest, cerebral edema, hypotension, peripheral edema, Q-wave distortions, sudden death, T-wave distortions

Central nervous system: Agitation, altered cerebrospinal fluid proteins, catatonia, coma, cough reflex suppressed, dizziness, drowsiness, fever (mild [I.M.]), headache, hyperpyrexia, impairment of temperature regulation, insomnia, neuroleptic malignant syndrome (NMS), oculogyric crisis, opisthotonos, restlessness, seizure, somnolence, tremulousness

Dermatologic: Angioedema, contact dermatitis, epithelial keratopathy, erythema, eczema, exfoliative dermatitis, itching, photosensitivity, skin pigmentation, urticaria

Endocrine & metabolic: Amenorrhea, galactorrhea, gynecomastia, glucosuria, hyper-/hypo-glycemia, lactation, libido (changes in), menstrual irregularity

Gastrointestinal: Appetite increased, atonic colon, constipation, ileus, nausea, obstipation, vomiting, weight gain, xerostomia

Genitourinary: Ejaculating dysfunction, ejaculatory disturbances, impotence, priapism, urinary retention

Hematologic: Agranulocytosis, aplastic anemia, eosinophilia, hemolytic anemia, leukopenia, pancytopenia, thrombocytopenic purpura

Hepatic: Biliary stasis, cholestatic jaundice, hepatotoxicity

Neuromuscular & skeletal: Dystonias (torticollis, carpopedal spasm, trismus, protrusion of tongue); extrapyramidal symptoms (pseudoparkinsonism, akathisia, dystonias, tardive dyskinesia, hyperreflexia); SLE-like syndrome, tremor

Ocular: Blurred vision, lenticular/corneal deposits, miosis, mydriasis, pigmentary retinopathy

Respiratory: Asthma, laryngeal edema, nasal congestion

Miscellaneous: Allergic reactions, asphyxia, diaphoresis

Drug Interactions

Metabolism/Transport Effects None known.

Avoid Concomitant Use

Avoid concomitant use of Prochlorperazine with any of the following: Azelastine; Azelastine (Nasal); Dofetilide; Metoclopramide; Paraldehyde

Increased Effect/Toxicity

Prochlorperazine may increase the levels/effects of: Alcohol (Ethyl); Analgesics (Opioid); Anticholinergics; Antidepressants (Serotonin Reuptake Inhibitor/Antagonist); Azelastine; Azelastine (Nasal); Beta-Blockers; CNS Depressants; Dofetilide; Methotrimeprazine; Methylphenidate; Paraldehyde; Porfimer; Serotonin Modulators; Zolpidem

The levels/effects of Prochlorperazine may be increased by: Acetylcholinesterase Inhibitors (Central); Antidepressants (Serotonin Reuptake Inhibitor/Antagonist); Antimalarial Agents; Beta-Blockers; Deferoxamine; Droperidol; HydrOXYzine; Lithium formulations; Methotrimeprazine; Methylphenidate; Metoclopramide; Metyrosine; Pramlintide; Tetrabenazine

Decreased Effect

Prochlorperazine may decrease the levels/effects of: Amphetamines; Anti-Parkinson's Agents (Dopamine Agonist); Quinagolide

The levels/effects of Prochlorperazine may be decreased by: Antacids; Anti-Parkinson's Agents (Dopamine Agonist); Lithium formulations

Ethanol/Nutrition/Herb Interactions

Ethanol: May increase CNS depression; monitor for increased effects with coadministration. Caution patients about effects.

Herb/Nutraceutical: Avoid dong quai, St John's wort (may also cause photosensitization). Avoid kava kava, gotu kola, valerian, St John's wort (may increase CNS depression).

Stability

Injection:

Edisylate: Store at 20°C to 25°C (68°F to 77°F); do not freeze. Protect from light. Clear or slightly yellow solutions may be used.

Mesylate (Canadian availability; not available in U.S.): Store at 15°C to 30°C (59°F to 86°F). Protect from light. Do not use if solution is discolored or hazy.

I.V. infusion: Injection may be diluted in 50-100 mL NS or D_5W.

Suppository: Store at 20°C to 25°C (68°F to 77°F). Protect from light.

Tablet: Store at 20°C to 25°C (68°F to 77°F). Protect from light.

Mechanism of Action Prochlorperazine is a piperazine phenothiazine antipsychotic which blocks postsynaptic mesolimbic dopaminergic D_1 and D_2 receptors in the brain, including the chemoreceptor trigger zone; exhibits a strong alpha-adrenergic and anticholinergic blocking effect and depresses the release of hypothalamic and hypophyseal hormones; believed to depress the reticular activating system, thus affecting basal metabolism, body temperature, wakefulness, vasomotor tone and emesis

Pharmacodynamics/Kinetics

Onset of action: Oral: 30-40 minutes; I.M.: 10-20 minutes; Rectal: ~60 minutes

Peak antiemetic effect: I.V.: 30-60 minutes

Duration: Rectal: 12 hours; Oral: 3-4 hours; I.M., I.V.: Adults: 4-6 hours

Distribution: V_d: 1400-1548 L

Metabolism: Primarily hepatic; N-desmethyl prochlorperazine (major active metabolite)

Bioavailability: Oral: 12.5%

Half-life elimination: Oral: 6-10 hours (single dose), 14-22 hours (repeated dosing); I.V.: 6-10 hours

Dosage

Geriatric Initiate at lower end of dosage range; titrate slowly and cautiously. Refer to adult dosing.

Adult Note: Injection solution mesylate formulation has Canadian availability (not available in U.S.).

Antiemetic:

Oral (tablet): 5-10 mg 3-4 times/day; usual maximum: 40 mg/day; larger doses may rarely be required

I.M. (as edisylate): 5-10 mg every 3-4 hours; usual maximum: 40 mg/day

I.M. (as mesylate): 5-10 mg 2-3 times/day; usual maximum: 40 mg/day

I.V. (as edisylate): 2.5-10 mg; maximum: 10 mg/dose or 40 mg/day; may repeat dose every 3-4 hours as needed

Rectal:

U.S. labeling: 25 mg twice daily

Canadian labeling: 5-10 mg 3-4 times/day

Surgical nausea/vomiting: Note: Should not exceed 40 mg/day

I.M. (as edisylate): 5-10 mg 1-2 hours before anesthesia induction or to control symptoms during or after surgery; may repeat once if necessary

I.M. (as mesylate): 5-10 mg 1-2 hours before anesthesia induction; may repeat once if needed during surgery; postoperatively: 5-10 mg every 3-4 hours as needed up to maximum of 40 mg daily

I.V. (as edisylate): 5-10 mg 15-30 minutes before anesthesia induction or to control symptoms during or after surgery; may repeat once if necessary

I.V. (as mesylate): 20 mg/L of I.V. solution during surgery or postoperatively; usual maximum: 30 mg daily

Rectal (unlabeled use; Golembiewski, 2005): 25 mg

Antipsychotic:

Oral: 5-10 mg 3-4 times/day; titrate dose slowly every 2-3 days; doses up to 150 mg/day may be required in some patients for treatment of severe disturbances

I.M. (as edisylate): Initial: 10-20 mg; if necessary repeat initial dose every 2-4 hours to gain control; more than 3-4 doses are rarely needed. If parenteral administration is still required; give 10-20 mg every 4-6 hours; convert to oral therapy as soon as possible.

I.M. (as mesylate): Initial: 10-20 mg; if necessary repeat initial dose every 2-4 hours to gain control; more than 3-4 doses are rarely needed; convert to oral therapy as soon as possible.

Nonpsychotic anxiety: *Oral (tablet):* Usual dose: 5 mg 3-4 times/day; do not exceed 20 mg/day or administer >12 weeks

Renal Impairment

U.S. labeling: No dosage adjustment provided in manufacturer's labeling.

Canadian labeling: Use is contraindicated.

Hepatic Impairment

U.S. labeling: No dosage adjustment provided in manufacturer's labeling; systemic exposure may be increased as drug undergoes hepatic metabolism.

Canadian labeling: Use is contraindicated.

Administration
I.M.: Inject by deep I.M. into outer quadrant of buttocks.
I.V.: May be administered by slow I.V. push at a rate not exceeding 5 mg/minute or by I.V. infusion. Do not administer as a bolus injection. To reduce the risk of hypotension, patients receiving I.V. prochlorperazine must remain lying down and be observed for at least 30 minutes following administration. Avoid skin contact with injection solution, contact dermatitis has occurred. Do not dilute with any diluent containing parabens as a preservative.
Oral: Administer tablet without regard to meals.

Monitoring Parameters Vital signs; CBC (baseline, frequently during first few months of therapy, periodically thereafter); lipid profile; fasting blood glucose/Hgb A_{1c}; BMI; mental status; abnormal involuntary movement scale (AIMS); periodic ophthalmic exams (if chronically used); extrapyramidal symptoms (EPS)

Test Interactions False-positives for phenylketonuria, urinary amylase, uroporphyrins, urobilinogen

Pharmacotherapy Pearls Not recommended as an antipsychotic due to inferior efficacy compared to other phenothiazines.

Special Geriatric Considerations Due to side effect profile (dystonias, EPS) this is not a preferred drug in the elderly for antiemetic therapy.

Many elderly patients receive antipsychotic medications for inappropriate nonpsychotic behavior. Before initiating antipsychotic medication, the clinician should investigate any possible reversible cause; any stress or stress from any disease can cause acute "confusion" or worsening of baseline nonpsychotic behavior. Most commonly acute changes in behavior are due to increases in drug dose or addition of new drug to regimen, fluid electrolyte loss, infections, and changes in environment.

Any changes in disease status in any organ system can result in behavior changes.

In the treatment of agitated, demented, older adult patients, authors of meta-analysis of controlled trials of the response to the traditional antipsychotics (phenothiazines, butyrophenones) in controlling agitation have concluded that the use of neuroleptics results in a response rate of 18%. Clearly neuroleptic therapy for behavior control should be limited with frequent attempts to withdraw the agent given for behavior control.

This medication is considered to be potentially inappropriate in this patient population (Beers Criteria: Quality of evidence - varies based on comorbidity; Strength of recommendation - varies based on comorbidity).

Dosage Forms Excipient information presented when available (limited, particularly for generics); consult specific product labeling.
Injection, solution, as edisylate [strength expressed as base]: 5 mg/mL (2 mL, 10 mL)
Suppository, rectal: 25 mg (12s)
  Compro®: 25 mg (12s) [contains coconut oil, palm oil]
Tablet, oral, as maleate [strength expressed as base]: 5 mg, 10 mg

Dosage Forms: Canada Excipient information presented when available (limited, particularly for generics); consult specific product labeling.
Injection, solution, as mesylate [strength expressed as base]: 5 mg/mL (2 mL)
Suppository, rectal: 10 mg (10s)

Progesterone (proe JES ter one)

Brand Names: U.S. Crinone®; Endometrin®; First™-Progesterone VGS 100; First™-Progesterone VGS 200; First™-Progesterone VGS 25; First™-Progesterone VGS 400; First™-Progesterone VGS 50; Prometrium®
Brand Names: Canada Crinone®; Prometrium®
Index Terms Pregnenedione; Progestin
Generic Availability (U.S.) Yes: Capsule, injection
Pharmacologic Category Progestin

Use

Oral: Prevention of endometrial hyperplasia in nonhysterectomized, postmenopausal women who are receiving conjugated estrogen tablets

I.M.: Abnormal uterine bleeding due to hormonal imbalance

Contraindications Hypersensitivity to progesterone or any component of the formulation; undiagnosed abnormal vaginal bleeding; history of or current thrombophlebitis or venous thromboembolic disorders (including DVT, PE); history of, active or recent (within 1 year) arterial thromboembolic disease (eg, stroke, MI); history of or known or suspected carcinoma of the breast or genital organs; hepatic dysfunction or disease

Warnings/Precautions [U.S. Boxed Warning]: Estrogens with or without progestin should not be used to prevent cardiovascular disease. Using data from the Women's Health Initiative (WHI) studies, an increased risk of deep vein thrombosis (DVT) and stroke has been reported with CE and an increased risk of DVT, stroke, pulmonary emboli (PE) and myocardial infarction (MI) has been reported with CE with MPA in postmenopausal women. Additional risk factors include diabetes mellitus, hypercholesterolemia, hypertension, SLE, obesity, tobacco use, and/or history of venous thromboembolism (VTE). Risk factors should be managed appropriately; discontinue use if adverse cardiovascular events occur or are suspected.

[U.S. Boxed Warning]: Estrogens with or without progestin should not be used to prevent dementia. In the Women's Health Initiative Memory Study (WHIMS), an increased incidence of dementia was observed in women ≥65 years of age taking CE alone or in combination with MPA.

[U.S. Boxed Warning]: Based on data from the Women's Health Initiative (WHI) studies, an increased risk of invasive breast cancer was observed in postmenopausal women using conjugated estrogens (CE) in combination with medroxyprogesterone acetate (MPA). This risk may be associated with duration of use and declines once combined therapy is discontinued (Chlebowski, 2009). The risk of invasive breast cancer was decreased in postmenopausal women with a hysterectomy using CE only, regardless of weight. However, the risk was not significantly decreased in women at high risk for breast cancer (family history of breast cancer, personal history of benign breast disease) (Anderson, 2012). An increase in abnormal mammogram findings has also been reported with estrogen alone or in combination with progestin therapy. Use is contraindicated in patients with known or suspected breast cancer.

Progesterone is used to reduce the risk of endometrial hyperplasia in nonhysterectomized postmenopausal women receiving conjugated estrogens. The use of unopposed estrogen in women with an intact uterus is associated with an increased risk of endometrial cancer. The addition of a progestin to estrogen therapy may decrease the risk of endometrial hyperplasia, a precursor to endometrial cancer. Adequate diagnostic measures, including endometrial sampling if indicated, should be performed to rule out malignancy in postmenopausal women with undiagnosed abnormal vaginal bleeding.

Estrogens may exacerbate endometriosis. Malignant transformation of residual endometrial implants has been reported posthysterectomy with unopposed estrogen therapy. Consider adding a progestin in women with residual endometriosis posthysterectomy. Postmenopausal estrogen therapy and combined estrogen/progesterone therapy may increase the risk of ovarian cancer; however, the absolute risk to an individual woman is small. Although results from various studies are not consistent, risk does not appear to be significantly associated with the duration, route, or dose of therapy. In one study, the risk decreased after 2 years following discontinuation of therapy (Mørch, 2009). Although the risk of ovarian cancer is rare, women who are at an increased risk (eg, family history) should be counseled about the association (NAMS, 2012).

Discontinue pending examination in cases of sudden partial or complete vision loss, sudden onset of proptosis, diplopia, or migraine; discontinue permanently if papilledema or retinal vascular lesions are observed on examination. Use with caution in patients with diseases that may be exacerbated by fluid retention, including asthma, epilepsy, migraine, diabetes or renal dysfunction. Use caution with history of depression. Patients should be warned that progesterone might cause transient dizziness or drowsiness during initial therapy. Whenever possible, progestins in combination with estrogens should be discontinued at least 4-6 weeks prior to surgeries associated with an increased risk of thromboembolism or during periods of prolonged immobilization.

[U.S. Boxed Warning]: Estrogens with or without progestin should be used for the shortest duration possible at the lowest effective dose consistent with treatment goals. Before prescribing estrogen therapy to postmenopausal women, the risks and benefits must be weighed for each patient. Women should be informed of these risks and benefits, as well as possible effects of progestin when added to estrogen therapy. Patients should be reevaluated as clinically appropriate to determine if treatment is still necessary. Available data related to treatment risks are from Women's Health Initiative (WHI) studies, which evaluated oral CE 0.625 mg with or without MPA 2.5 mg relative to placebo in postmenopausal women. Other combinations and dosage forms of estrogens and progestins were not studied. **Outcomes reported from clinical trials using CE with or without MPA should be assumed to be similar for other doses and other dosage forms of estrogens and progestins until comparable data becomes available.**

Products may contain palm oil, peanut oil, sesame oil, or benzyl alcohol. Not for use prior to menarche.

Adverse Reactions (Reflective of adult population; not specific for elderly)

Injection (I.M.):
Cardiovascular: Cerebral edema, cerebral thrombosis, edema
Central nervous system: Depression, fever, insomnia, somnolence
Dermatologic: Acne, allergic rash (rare), alopecia, hirsutism, pruritus, rash, urticaria
Endocrine & metabolic: Amenorrhea, breakthrough bleeding, breast tenderness, galactorrhea, menstrual flow changes, spotting
Gastrointestinal: Nausea, weight gain/loss
Genitourinary: Cervical erosion changes, cervical secretion changes
Hepatic: Cholestatic jaundice
Local: Injection site: Irritation, pain, redness
Ocular: Optic neuritis, retinal thrombosis
Respiratory: Pulmonary embolism
Miscellaneous: Anaphylactoid reactions

Oral capsule (percentages reported when used in combination with or cycled with conjugated estrogens):
>10%:
Central nervous system: Headache (16% to 31%), dizziness (15% to 24%), depression (19%)
Endocrine & metabolic: Breast tenderness (27%), breast pain (6% to 16%)
Gastrointestinal: Abdominal pain (10% to 20%), abdominal bloating (8% to 12%)
Genitourinary: Urinary problems (11%)
Neuromuscular & skeletal: Joint pain (20%), musculoskeletal pain (12%)
Miscellaneous: Viral infection (12%)
5% to 10%:
Cardiovascular: Chest pain (7%)
Central nervous system: Fatigue (8%), irritability (8%), worry (8%)
Gastrointestinal: Nausea/vomiting (8%), diarrhea (7% to 8%)
Genitourinary: Vaginal discharge (10%)
Respiratory: Cough (8%)
<5%: Breast biopsy, breast cancer, cholecystectomy, constipation

Drug Interactions
Metabolism/Transport Effects Substrate of CYP1A2 (minor), CYP2A6 (minor), CYP2C19 (major), CYP2C9 (minor), CYP2D6 (minor), CYP3A4 (major); **Note:** Assignment of Major/Minor substrate status based on clinically relevant drug interaction potential; **Inhibits** CYP2C19 (weak), CYP2C9 (weak), CYP3A4 (weak), P-glycoprotein

Avoid Concomitant Use
Avoid concomitant use of Progesterone with any of the following: Pimozide; Silodosin; Topotecan

Increased Effect/Toxicity
Progesterone may increase the levels/effects of: ARIPiprazole; Colchicine; Dabigatran Etexilate; Everolimus; P-glycoprotein/ABCB1 Substrates; Pimozide; Prucalopride; Rivaroxaban; Silodosin; Topotecan

The levels/effects of Progesterone may be increased by: Herbs (Progestogenic Properties)

Decreased Effect
The levels/effects of Progesterone may be decreased by: Aminoglutethimide; CYP2C19 Inducers (Strong); CYP3A4 Inducers (Strong); Deferasirox; Herbs (CYP3A4 Inducers); Peginterferon Alfa-2b; Tocilizumab

Ethanol/Nutrition/Herb Interactions
Food: Food increases oral bioavailability.
Herb/Nutraceutical: St John's wort may decrease progesterone levels. Herbs with progestogenic properties may enhance the adverse/toxic effects of progestin; example herbs include bloodroot, chasteberry, damiana, oregano, yucca.

Stability Store at controlled room temperature. Protect capsules from excessive moisture.

Mechanism of Action Natural steroid hormone that induces secretory changes in the endometrium, promotes mammary gland development, relaxes uterine smooth muscle

Pharmacodynamics/Kinetics

Absorption: Vaginal gel: Prolonged

Absorption half-life: 25-50 hours

Protein binding: Albumin (50% to 54%) and cortisol-binding protein (43% to 48%)

Metabolism: Hepatic to metabolites

Half-life elimination: Vaginal gel: 5-20 minutes

Time to peak: Oral: Within 3 hours; I.M.: ~8 hours; Vaginal tablet: ~17-24 hours

Excretion: Urine, bile, feces

Dosage

Geriatric & Adult Females:

Endometrial hyperplasia prevention (in postmenopausal women with a uterus who are receiving daily conjugated estrogen tablets): Oral: 200 mg as a single daily dose every evening for 12 days sequentially per 28-day cycle

Functional uterine bleeding: I.M.: 5-10 mg/day for 6 doses

Administration

I.M.: Administer deep I.M. only

Oral capsule: For patients who experience difficulty swallowing the capsules, taking with a full glass of water in the standing position may be beneficial.

Monitoring Parameters Routine physical examination that includes blood pressure and Papanicolaou smear, breast exam, mammogram. Adequate diagnostic measures, including endometrial sampling, if indicated, should be performed to rule out malignancy in all cases of undiagnosed abnormal vaginal bleeding. Signs and symptoms of thromboembolic disorders, vision changes

Test Interactions Thyroid function, metyrapone, liver function, coagulation tests, endocrine function tests

Special Geriatric Considerations Not a progestin of choice in the elderly for hormonal cycling.

Dosage Forms Excipient information presented when available (limited, particularly for generics); consult specific product labeling.

Capsule:

Prometrium®: 100 mg, 200 mg [contains peanut oil]

Injection, oil: 50 mg/mL (10 mL) [contains benzyl alcohol 10%, sesame oil]

◆ **Progestin** see Progesterone on page 1612
◆ **Prolia™** see Denosumab on page 502

Promethazine (proe METH a zeen)

Related Information

Beers Criteria − Potentially Inappropriate Medications for Geriatrics on page 2183

Medication Safety Issues

Sound-alike/look-alike issues:

Promethazine may be confused with chlorproMAZINE, predniSONE

Phenergan® may be confused with PHENobarbital, Phrenilin®, Theragran

High alert medication:

The Institute for Safe Medication Practices (ISMP) includes this medication (I.V. formulation) among its list of drugs which have a heightened risk of causing significant patient harm when used in error.

BEERS Criteria medication:

This drug may be potentially inappropriate for use in geriatric patients (Quality of evidence - high; Strength of recommendation - strong).

Administration issues:

To prevent or minimize tissue damage during I.V. administration, the Institute for Safe Medication Practices (ISMP) has the following recommendations:

- Limit concentration available to the 25 mg/mL product
- Consider limiting initial doses to 6.25-12.5 mg
- Further dilute the 25 mg/mL strength into 10-20 mL NS
- Administer through a large bore vein (not hand or wrist)
- Administer via running I.V. line at port farthest from patient's vein
- Consider administering over 10-15 minutes
- Instruct patients to report immediately signs of pain or burning

International issues:

Sominex: Brand name for promethazine in Great Britain, but also is a brand name for diphenhydrAMINE in the U.S.

Brand Names: U.S. Phenadoz®; Phenergan; Promethegan™

Brand Names: Canada Bioniche Promethazine; Histantil; Phenergan; PMS-Promethazine

Index Terms Promethazine Hydrochloride

PROMETHAZINE

Generic Availability (U.S.) Yes

Pharmacologic Category Antiemetic; Histamine H$_1$ Antagonist; Histamine H$_1$ Antagonist, First Generation; Phenothiazine Derivative

Use Symptomatic treatment of various allergic conditions; antiemetic; motion sickness; sedative; adjunct to postoperative analgesia and anesthesia

Contraindications Hypersensitivity to promethazine or any component of the formulation (cross-reactivity between phenothiazines may occur); coma; treatment of lower respiratory tract symptoms, including asthma; intra-arterial or subcutaneous administration

Warnings/Precautions [U.S. Boxed Warning]: Promethazine injection can cause severe tissue injury (including gangrene) regardless of the route of administration. Tissue irritation and damage may result from perivascular extravasation, unintentional intra-arterial administration, and intraneuronal or perineuronal infiltration. In addition to gangrene, adverse events reported include tissue necrosis, abscesses, burning, pain, erythema, edema, paralysis, severe spasm of distal vessels, phlebitis, thrombophlebitis, venous thrombosis, sensory loss, paralysis, and palsies. Surgical intervention including fasciotomy, skin graft, and/or amputation have been necessary in some cases. The preferred route of administration is by deep intramuscular (I.M.) injection. Subcutaneous administration is contraindicated. Discontinue intravenous injection immediately with onset of pain and evaluate for arterial injection or perivascular extravasation. Although there is no proven successful management of unintentional intra-arterial injection or perivascular extravasation, sympathetic block and heparinization have been used in the acute management of unintentional intra-arterial injection based on results from animal studies.

May be sedating; use with caution in disorders where CNS depression is a feature. May impair physical or mental abilities; patients must be cautioned about performing tasks which require mental alertness. Use with caution in hemodynamic instability; bone marrow suppression; subcortical brain damage; and in severe cardiac, hepatic or respiratory disease. Avoid use in Reye's syndrome. May lower seizure threshold; use caution in persons with seizure disorders or in persons using narcotics or local anesthetics which may also affect seizure threshold. May alter temperature regulation or mask toxicity of other drugs due to antiemetic effects. May alter cardiac conduction (life-threatening arrhythmias have occurred with therapeutic doses of phenothiazines). May cause orthostatic hypotension; use with caution in patients at risk of hypotension or where transient hypotensive episodes would be poorly tolerated (cardiovascular disease or cerebrovascular disease).

Phenothiazines may cause anticholinergic effects; therefore, they should be used with caution in patients with decreased gastrointestinal motility, GI or GU obstruction, urinary retention, BPH, xerostomia, or visual problems. Conditions which also may be exacerbated by cholinergic blockade include narrow-angle glaucoma (screening is recommended) and worsening of myasthenia gravis. Use with caution in Parkinson's disease. May cause extrapyramidal symptoms, including pseudoparkinsonism, acute dystonic reactions, akathisia, and tardive dyskinesia. May be associated with neuroleptic malignant syndrome (NMS). May cause photosensitivity. In the elderly, avoid use of this potent anticholinergic agent due to increased risk of confusion, dry mouth, constipation, and other anticholinergic effects; clearance decreases in patients of advanced age (Beers Criteria). Injection may contain sodium metabisulfite.

Adverse Reactions (Reflective of adult population; not specific for elderly) Frequency not defined.

Cardiovascular: Bradycardia, hyper-/hypotension, nonspecific QT changes, orthostatic hypotension, tachycardia,

Central nervous system: Agitation akathisia, catatonic states, confusion, delirium, disorientation, dizziness, drowsiness, dystonias, euphoria, excitation, extrapyramidal symptoms, faintness, fatigue, hallucinations, hysteria, insomnia, lassitude, pseudoparkinsonism, tardive dyskinesia, nervousness, neuroleptic malignant syndrome, nightmares, sedation, seizure, somnolence

Dermatologic: Angioneurotic edema, dermatitis, photosensitivity, skin pigmentation (slate gray), urticaria

Endocrine & metabolic: Amenorrhea, breast engorgement, gynecomastia, hyperglycemia, lactation

Gastrointestinal: Constipation, nausea, vomiting, xerostomia

Genitourinary: Ejaculatory disorder, impotence, urinary retention

Hematologic: Agranulocytosis, leukopenia, thrombocytopenia, thrombocytopenic purpura

Hepatic: Jaundice

Local: Abscess, distal vessel spasm, gangrene, injection site reactions (burning, edema, erythema, pain), palsies, paralysis, phlebitis, sensory loss, thrombophlebitis, tissue necrosis, venous thrombosis

Neuromuscular & skeletal: Incoordination, tremor

Ocular: Blurred vision, corneal and lenticular changes, diplopia, epithelial keratopathy, pigmentary retinopathy

Otic: Tinnitus

Respiratory: Apnea, asthma, nasal congestion, respiratory depression

Drug Interactions

Metabolism/Transport Effects Substrate of CYP2B6 (major), CYP2D6 (major); **Note:** Assignment of Major/Minor substrate status based on clinically relevant drug interaction potential; **Inhibits** CYP2D6 (weak)

Avoid Concomitant Use

Avoid concomitant use of Promethazine with any of the following: Azelastine; Azelastine (Nasal); Methadone; Metoclopramide; Paraldehyde

Increased Effect/Toxicity

Promethazine may increase the levels/effects of: Alcohol (Ethyl); Anticholinergics; Azelastine; Azelastine (Nasal); Buprenorphine; CNS Depressants; Methadone; Metoclopramide; Paraldehyde; Serotonin Modulators; Zolpidem

The levels/effects of Promethazine may be increased by: Abiraterone Acetate; Antipsychotics; CYP2B6 Inhibitors (Moderate); CYP2B6 Inhibitors (Strong); CYP2D6 Inhibitors (Moderate); CYP2D6 Inhibitors (Strong); Darunavir; HydrOXYzine; MAO Inhibitors; Metoclopramide; Metyrosine; Pramlintide; Quazepam

Decreased Effect

Promethazine may decrease the levels/effects of: Acetylcholinesterase Inhibitors (Central); EPINEPHrine; EPINEPHrine (Nasal); Epinephrine (Racemic); EPINEPHrine (Systemic, Oral Inhalation)

The levels/effects of Promethazine may be decreased by: Acetylcholinesterase Inhibitors (Central); CYP2B6 Inducers (Strong); Peginterferon Alfa-2b

Ethanol/Nutrition/Herb Interactions

Ethanol: Avoid ethanol (may increase CNS depression).

Herb/Nutraceutical: Avoid valerian, St John's wort, kava kava, gotu kola (may increase CNS depression).

Stability

Injection: Prior to dilution, store at 20°C to 25°C (68°F to 77°F). Protect from light. Solutions in NS or D_5W are stable for 24 hours at room temperature.

Oral solution: Store at 15°C to 25°C (59°F to 77°F). Protect from light.

Suppositories: Store refrigerated at 2°C to 8°C (36°F to 46°F).

Tablets: Store at 20°C to 25°C (68°F to 77°F). Protect from light.

Mechanism of Action Phenothiazine derivative; blocks postsynaptic mesolimbic dopaminergic receptors in the brain; exhibits a strong alpha-adrenergic blocking effect and depresses the release of hypothalamic and hypophyseal hormones; competes with histamine for the H_1-receptor; muscarinic-blocking effect may be responsible for antiemetic activity; reduces stimuli to the brainstem reticular system

Pharmacodynamics/Kinetics

Onset of action: Oral, I.M.: ~20 minutes; I.V.: ~5 minutes

Duration: Usually 4-6 hours (up to 12 hours)

Absorption: Oral: Rapid and complete; large first pass effect limits systemic bioavailability (Sharma, 2003)

Distribution: V_d: Syrup: 98 L/kg (range: 17-277 L/kg) (Strenkoski-Nox, 2000)

Metabolism: Hepatic; hydroxylation via CYP2D6 and N-demethylation via CYP2B6; significant first-pass effect (Sharma, 2003)

Bioavailability: Oral: ~25% (Sharma, 2003)

Half-life elimination: I.M.: ~10 hours; I.V.: 9-16 hours; Suppositories, syrup: 16-19 hours (range: 4-34 hours) (Strenkoski-Nox, 2000)

Time to maximum serum concentration: Suppositories: 6.7-8.6 hours; Syrup: 4.4 hours (Strenkoski-Nox, 2000)

Excretion: Urine

Dosage

Geriatric & Adult

Allergic conditions (including allergic reactions to blood or plasma):

Oral, rectal: 25 mg at bedtime **or** 12.5 mg before meals and at bedtime (range: 6.25-12.5 mg 3 times/day)

I.M., I.V.: 25 mg, may repeat in 2 hours when necessary; switch to oral route as soon as feasible

Antiemetic: Oral, I.M., I.V., rectal: 12.5-25 mg every 4-6 hours as needed

Motion sickness: Oral, rectal: 25 mg 30-60 minutes before departure, then every 12 hours as needed

Obstetrics (labor) analgesia adjunct: I.M., I.V.: Early labor: 50 mg; Established labor: 25-75 mg in combination with analgesic at reduced dosage; may repeat every 4 hours for up to 2 additional doses (maximum: 100 mg/day while in labor)

Pre-/postoperative analgesia/hypnotic adjunct: I.M., I.V.: 25-50 mg in combination with analgesic or hypnotic (at reduced dosage)

Sedation: Oral, I.M., I.V., rectal: 12.5-50 mg/dose

Administration Formulations available for oral, rectal, I.M./I.V.; not for SubQ or intra-arterial administration. Administer I.M. into deep muscle (preferred route of administration). I.V. administration is **not** the preferred route; severe tissue damage may occur. Solution for injection should be administered in a maximum concentration of 25 mg/mL (more dilute solutions are recommended). Administer via running I.V. line at port farthest from patient's vein, or through a large bore vein (not hand or wrist). Consider administering over 10-15 minutes (maximum: 25 mg/minute). Discontinue immediately if burning or pain occurs with administration.

Monitoring Parameters Relief of symptoms, mental status; signs and symptoms of tissue injury (burning or pain at injection site, phlebitis, edema) with I.V. administration

Test Interactions May interfere with urine detection of amphetamine/methamphetamine (false-positive); alters the flare response in intradermal allergen tests

Special Geriatric Considerations Because promethazine is a phenothiazine (and can, therefore, cause side effects such as extrapyramidal symptoms), it is not considered an antihistamine of choice in the elderly.

This medication is considered to be potentially inappropriate in this patient population (Beers Criteria: Quality of evidence - high; Strength of recommendation - strong).

Dosage Forms Excipient information presented when available (limited, particularly for generics); consult specific product labeling.

Injection, solution, as hydrochloride: 25 mg/mL (1 mL); 50 mg/mL (1 mL)

Phenergan: 25 mg/mL (1 mL); 50 mg/mL (1 mL) [contains edetate disodium, sodium metabisulfite]

Suppository, rectal, as hydrochloride: 12.5 mg (12s); 25 mg (12s)

Phenadoz®: 12.5 mg (12s); 25 mg (12s)

Promethegan™: 12.5 mg (12s); 25 mg (12s); 50 mg (12s)

Syrup, oral, as hydrochloride: 6.25 mg/5 mL (118 mL, 473 mL)

Tablet, oral, as hydrochloride: 12.5 mg, 25 mg, 50 mg

◆ **Promethazine Hydrochloride** see Promethazine on page 1615
◆ **Promethegan™** see Promethazine on page 1615
◆ **Prometrium®** see Progesterone on page 1612
◆ **Pronestyl** see Procainamide on page 1605

Propafenone (pro PAF en one)

Related Information

Beers Criteria – Potentially Inappropriate Medications for Geriatrics on page 2183

Medication Safety Issues

BEERS Criteria medication:

This drug may be potentially inappropriate for use in geriatric patients (Quality of evidence - high; Strength of recommendation - strong).

Brand Names: U.S. Rythmol®; Rythmol® SR

Brand Names: Canada Apo-Propafenone®; Mylan-Propafenone; PMS-Propafenone; Rythmol® Gen-Propafenone

Index Terms Propafenone Hydrochloride

Generic Availability (U.S.) Yes

Pharmacologic Category Antiarrhythmic Agent, Class Ic

Use Treatment of life-threatening ventricular arrhythmias; treatment of paroxysmal atrial fibrillation/flutter (PAF) or paroxysmal supraventricular tachycardia (PSVT) in patients with disabling symptoms and without structural heart disease

Extended release capsule: Prolong the time to recurrence of symptomatic atrial fibrillation in patients without structural heart disease

Unlabeled Use Cardioversion of recent-onset atrial fibrillation (single dose); supraventricular tachycardia in patients with Wolff-Parkinson-White syndrome

Contraindications Hypersensitivity to propafenone or any component of the formulation; sinoatrial, AV, and intraventricular disorders of impulse generation and/or conduction (except in patients with a functioning artificial pacemaker); sinus bradycardia; cardiogenic shock; uncompensated cardiac failure; hypotension; bronchospastic disorders or severe obstructive pulmonary disease; uncorrected electrolyte abnormalities; concurrent use of ritonavir

Warnings/Precautions [U.S. Boxed Warning]: In the Cardiac Arrhythmia Suppression Trial (CAST), recent (>6 days but <2 years ago) myocardial infarction patients with asymptomatic, non-life-threatening ventricular arrhythmias did not benefit and may have been harmed by attempts to suppress the arrhythmia with flecainide or encainide. An increased mortality or nonfatal cardiac arrest rate (7.7%) was seen in the active treatment group compared with patients in the placebo group (3%). The applicability of the CAST results to other populations is unknown. Antiarrhythmic agents should be reserved for patients with life-threatening ventricular arrhythmias.

Can cause life-threatening drug-induced arrhythmias, including ventricular fibrillation, ventricular tachycardia, asystole, and torsade de pointes (Hii, 1991). The manufacturer notes that propafenone may increase the QT interval; however, due to QRS prolongation; changes in the QT interval are difficult to interpret. In an evaluation of propafenone (450 mg/day) in healthy individuals compared to other selected antiarrhythmic agents, propafenone did not affect repolarization time (eg, QT, QTc, JT, JTc) only depolarization time (ie, QRS interval) (Sarubbi, 1998). Monitor for proarrhythmic effects, and when necessary, adjust dose to prevent QT_c prolongation.

In the treatment of atrial fibrillation in the elderly, avoid antiarrhythmics as first-line treatment. In older adults, data suggests rate control may provide more benefits than risks compared to rhythm control for most patients (Beers Criteria).

Concurrent use of propafenone with QT-prolonging agents has not been extensively evaluated. The manufacturer recommends withholding Class Ia or Class III antiarrhythmics for at least 5 half-lives prior to starting propafenone. Slows atrioventricular conduction, potentially leading to first degree AV block; degree of PR interval prolongation and increased QRS duration are dose and concentration related. Avoid in patients with conduction disturbances (unless functioning pacemaker present).

May alter pacing and sensing thresholds of artificial pacemakers. The use of propafenone is not recommended in patients with obstructive lung disease (eg, chronic bronchitis, COPD, emphysema) (Fuster, 2006). Use in patients with bronchospastic disease or severe obstructive lung disease is contraindicated.

Avoid use in patients with heart failure; similar agents have been shown to increase mortality in this population; may precipitate or exacerbate condition. Correct electrolyte disturbances, especially hypokalemia or hypomagnesemia, prior to use and throughout therapy. Administer cautiously in significant hepatic or renal dysfunction. Use with caution in patients with myasthenia gravis; may exacerbate condition. Avoid the concurrent use a CYP2D6 inhibitor and CYP3A4 inhibitor; may result in an increased risk of proarrhythmia or exaggerated beta-adrenergic blocking activity Agranulocytosis has been reported; generally occurring within the first 2 months of therapy. Upon therapy discontinuation, WBC usually normalized by 14 days. Positive ANA titers have been reported. Titers have decreased with and without propafenone discontinuation. Positive titers have not usually been associated with clinical symptoms, although at least one case of drug induced lupus erythematosus has been reported. Consider therapy discontinuation in symptomatic patients with positive ANA titers.

Adverse Reactions (Reflective of adult population; not specific for elderly) 1% to 10%:

Cardiovascular: New or worsened arrhythmia (proarrhythmic effect) (2% to 10%), angina (2% to 5%), CHF (1% to 4%), ventricular tachycardia (1% to 3%), palpitation (1% to 3%), AV block (first-degree) (1% to 3%), syncope (1% to 2%), increased QRS interval (1% to 2%), chest pain (1% to 2%), PVCs (1% to 2%), bradycardia (1% to 2%), edema (0% to 1%), bundle branch block (0% to 1%), atrial fibrillation (1%), hypotension (0% to 1%), intraventricular conduction delay (0% to 1%)

Central nervous system: Dizziness (4% to 15%), fatigue (2% to 6%), headache (2% to 5%), ataxia (0% to 2%), insomnia (0% to 2%), anxiety (1% to 2%), drowsiness (1%)

Dermatologic: Rash (1% to 3%)

Gastrointestinal: Nausea/vomiting (2% to 11%), unusual taste (3% to 23%), constipation (2% to 7%), dyspepsia (1% to 3%), diarrhea (1% to 3%), xerostomia (1% to 2%), anorexia (1% to 2%), abdominal pain (1% to 2%), flatulence (0% to 1%)

Neuromuscular & skeletal: Tremor (0% to 1%), arthralgia (0% to 1%), weakness (1% to 2%)

Ocular: Blurred vision (1% to 6%)

Respiratory: Dyspnea (2% to 5%)

Miscellaneous: Diaphoresis (1%)

Drug Interactions

Metabolism/Transport Effects Substrate of CYP1A2 (minor), CYP2D6 (major), CYP3A4 (minor); **Note:** Assignment of Major/Minor substrate status based on clinically relevant drug interaction potential; **Inhibits** CYP1A2 (weak), CYP2D6 (weak)

◀ **Avoid Concomitant Use**

Avoid concomitant use of Propafenone with any of the following: Amiodarone; Antiarrhythmic Agents (Class Ia); Antiarrhythmic Agents (Class III); Fosamprenavir; Highest Risk QTc-Prolonging Agents; Mifepristone; QuiNIDine; Ritonavir; Saquinavir; Tipranavir

Increased Effect/Toxicity

Propafenone may increase the levels/effects of: Antiarrhythmic Agents (Class Ia); Antiarrhythmic Agents (Class III); ARIPiprazole; Beta-Blockers; Cardiac Glycosides; CYP2D6 Inhibitors (Moderate); Highest Risk QTc-Prolonging Agents; Moderate Risk QTc-Prolonging Agents; Propranolol; Theophylline Derivatives; Venlafaxine; Vitamin K Antagonists

The levels/effects of Propafenone may be increased by: Abiraterone Acetate; Amiodarone; Boceprevir; Cimetidine; CYP2D6 Inhibitors (Strong); CYP3A4 Inhibitors (Moderate); CYP3A4 Inhibitors (Strong); FLUoxetine; FluvoxaMINE; Fosamprenavir; Mifepristone; PARoxetine; QTc-Prolonging Agents (Indeterminate Risk and Risk Modifying); QuiNIDine; Ritonavir; Saquinavir; Telaprevir; Tipranavir

Decreased Effect

The levels/effects of Propafenone may be decreased by: Barbiturates; Etravirine; Orlistat; Peginterferon Alfa-2b; Rifamycin Derivatives; Tocilizumab

Ethanol/Nutrition/Herb Interactions

Food: Propafenone serum concentrations may be increased if taken with food.

Herb/Nutraceutical: St John's wort may decrease propafenone levels. Avoid ephedra (may worsen arrhythmia).

Stability Store at 25°C (77°F); excursions permitted to 15°C to 30°C (59°F to 86°F).

Mechanism of Action Propafenone is a class 1c antiarrhythmic agent which possesses local anesthetic properties, blocks the fast inward sodium current, and slows the rate of increase of the action potential. Prolongs conduction and refractoriness in all areas of the myocardium, with a slightly more pronounced effect on intraventricular conduction; it prolongs effective refractory period, reduces spontaneous automaticity and exhibits some beta-blockade activity.

Pharmacodynamics/Kinetics

Absorption: Well absorbed

Distribution: V_d: Adults: 252 L

Protein binding: 95% to alpha$_1$-acid glycoprotein

Metabolism: Hepatic via CYP2D6, CYP3A4 and CYP1A2 to two active metabolites (5-hydroxypropafenone and N-depropylpropafenone) then ultimately to glucuronide or sulfate conjugates. Two genetically determined metabolism groups exist (extensive and poor metabolizers); 10% of Caucasians are poor metabolizers. Exhibits nonlinear pharmacokinetics; when dose is increased from 300-900 mg/day, serum concentrations increase tenfold; this nonlinearity is thought to be due to saturable first-pass effect.

Bioavailability: Immediate release (IR): 150 mg: 3.4%; 300 mg: 10.6%; relative bioavailability of extended release (ER) capsule is less than IR tablet; the bioavailability of an ER capsule regimen of 325 mg twice-daily regimen approximates an IR tablet regimen of 150 mg 3 times/day.

Half-life elimination: Extensive metabolizers: 2-10 hours; Poor metabolizers: 10-32 hours

Time to peak, serum: IR: 3.5 hours; ER: 3-8 hours

Excretion: Urine (<1% unchanged; remainder as glucuronide or sulfate conjugates); feces

Dosage

Geriatric & Adult Note: Patients who exhibit significant widening of QRS complex or second- or third-degree AV block may need dose reduction.

Atrial fibrillation (to prevent recurrence): Oral: *Extended release capsule:* Initial: 225 mg every 12 hours; dosage increase may be made at a minimum of 5-day intervals; may increase to 325 mg every 12 hours; if further increase is necessary, may increase to 425 mg every 12 hours

Paroxysmal atrial fibrillation/flutter, paroxysmal supraventricular tachycardia, ventricular arrhythmias: Oral: *Immediate release tablet:* Initial: 150 mg every 8 hours; dosage increase may be made at minimum of 3- to 4-day intervals, may increase to 225 mg every 8 hours; if further increase is necessary, may increase to 300 mg every 8 hours

Atrial fibrillation, pharmacologic cardioversion (unlabeled use): Oral: **Note:** To prevent rapid AV conduction, start an AV nodal-blocking agent (eg, beta-blocker, nondihydropyridine calcium channel blocker) prior to pharmacologic cardioversion. Effect occurs between 2-6 hours after administration.

Immediate release tablet: 600 mg as single dose (Fuster, 2006)

Renal Impairment No dosage adjustments provided in manufacturer's labeling; however, 50% of propafenone metabolites (active) are excreted in the urine; use with caution in renal impairment.

Hepatic Impairment
Immediate release tablet: Reduce dose by 70% to 80% in patients with hepatic impairment

Extended release capsule: Specific dosage adjustments are not provided in manufacturer's labeling; however, dosage reduction should be considered as drug undergoes hepatic metabolism.

Administration Capsules should be swallowed whole; do not crush or chew; may be taken without regard to meals.

Monitoring Parameters ECG, blood pressure, pulse (particularly at initiation of therapy)

Special Geriatric Considerations Elderly may have age-related decreases in hepatic Phase I metabolism. Propafenone is dependent upon liver metabolism, therefore, monitor closely in the elderly and adjust dose more gradually during initial treatment. No differences in clearance noted with impaired renal function and, therefore, no adjustment for renal function in the elderly is necessary.

This medication is considered to be potentially inappropriate in this patient population (Beers Criteria: Quality of evidence - high; Strength of recommendation - strong).

Dosage Forms Excipient information presented when available (limited, particularly for generics); consult specific product labeling.

Capsule, extended release, oral, as hydrochloride: 225 mg, 325 mg, 425 mg
  Rythmol® SR: 225 mg, 325 mg, 425 mg [contains soy lecithin]
Tablet, oral, as hydrochloride: 150 mg, 225 mg, 300 mg
  Rythmol®: 150 mg, 225 mg [scored]

◆ **Propafenone Hydrochloride** see Propafenone on page 1618

Propantheline (proe PAN the leen)

Related Information
Beers Criteria – Potentially Inappropriate Medications for Geriatrics on page 2183
Pharmacotherapy of Urinary Incontinence on page 2141

Medication Safety Issues
BEERS Criteria medication:
This drug may be potentially inappropriate for use in geriatric patients (Quality of evidence - moderate; Strength of recommendation - strong).

Index Terms Propantheline Bromide

Generic Availability (U.S.) Yes

Pharmacologic Category Anticholinergic Agent

Use Adjunctive treatment of peptic ulcer

Unlabeled Use Decreased salivation and drooling

Contraindications Severe ulcerative colitis, toxic megacolon, obstructive disease of the GI or urinary tract; glaucoma; myasthenia gravis; unstable cardiovascular adjustment in acute hemorrhage; intestinal atony of elderly or debilitated patients

Warnings/Precautions May cause drowsiness and/or blurred vision, which may impair physical or mental abilities; patients must be cautioned about performing tasks which require mental alertness (eg, operating machinery or driving). Use with caution in patients with hyperthyroidism, hiatal hernia with reflux esophagitis, autonomic neuropathy, hepatic, cardiac, or renal disease, hypertension, GI infections, or other endocrine diseases. Avoid use in the elderly due to potent anticholinergic adverse effects and uncertain effectiveness (Beers Criteria). Heat prostration may occur in the presence of increased environmental temperature; use caution in hot weather and/or exercise. Diarrhea may be a sign of incomplete intestinal obstruction, treatment should be discontinued if this occurs.

Adverse Reactions (Reflective of adult population; not specific for elderly) Frequency not defined.

Cardiovascular: Palpitation, tachycardia
Central nervous system: Confusion, dizziness, drowsiness, headache, insomnia, nervousness
Endocrine & metabolic: Suppression of lactation
Gastrointestinal: Bloated feeling, constipation, loss of taste, nausea, vomiting, xerostomia
Genitourinary: Impotence, urinary hesitancy, urinary retention
Neuromuscular & skeletal: Weakness
Ocular: Blurred vision, cycloplegia, mydriasis, ocular tension increased
Miscellaneous: Allergic reactions, anaphylaxis, diaphoresis decreased

Drug Interactions
Metabolism/Transport Effects None known.
Avoid Concomitant Use There are no known interactions where it is recommended to avoid concomitant use.

Increased Effect/Toxicity
Propantheline may increase the levels/effects of: AbobotulinumtoxinA; Anticholinergics; Cannabinoids; OnabotulinumtoxinA; Potassium Chloride; RimabotulinumtoxinB

The levels/effects of Propantheline may be increased by: MAO Inhibitors; Pramlintide

Decreased Effect
Propantheline may decrease the levels/effects of: Acetylcholinesterase Inhibitors (Central); Secretin

The levels/effects of Propantheline may be decreased by: Acetylcholinesterase Inhibitors (Central)

Stability Store at 20°C to 25°C (68°F to 77°F).

Mechanism of Action Competitively blocks the action of acetylcholine at postganglionic parasympathetic receptor sites

Pharmacodynamics/Kinetics
Onset of action: 30-45 minutes
Duration: 4-6 hours
Half-life elimination, serum: Average: 1.6 hours

Dosage
Geriatric Antisecretory (unlabeled use): 7.5 mg 3 times/day before meals and at bedtime; increase as necessary to a maximum of 30 mg 3 times/day
Adult Antisecretory (unlabeled use), antispasmodic: Oral: 15 mg 3 times/day before meals or food and 30 mg at bedtime

Administration Administer 30 minutes before meals and at bedtime.

Special Geriatric Considerations The primary use of propantheline in the geriatric population was for treatment of urinary incontinence due to detrusor instability. It is rarely used presently since newer agents, with fewer side effects, have been introduced. Even though it does not cross the blood-brain barrier, CNS effects have been reported. Orthostatic hypotension may also occur.

This medication is considered to be potentially inappropriate in this patient population (Beers Criteria: Quality of evidence - moderate; Strength of recommendation - strong).

Dosage Forms Excipient information presented when available (limited, particularly for generics); consult specific product labeling.
Tablet, oral, as bromide: 15 mg

◆ **Propantheline Bromide** *see* Propantheline *on page 1621*
◆ **Propecia®** *see* Finasteride *on page 789*

Propranolol (proe PRAN oh lole)

Related Information
Beta-Blockers *on page 2108*

Medication Safety Issues
Sound-alike/look-alike issues:
Propranolol may be confused with prasugrel, Pravachol®, Propulsid®
Inderal® may be confused with Adderall®, Enduron, Imdur®, Imuran®, Inderide, Isordil®, Toradol®

High alert medication:
The Institute for Safe Medication Practices (ISMP) includes this medication among its list of drugs which have a heightened risk of causing significant patient harm when used in error.

Administration issues:
Significant differences exist between oral and I.V. dosing. Use caution when converting from one route of administration to another.

International issues:
Inderal [Canada and multiple international markets] and Inderal LA [U.S.] may be confused with Indiaral brand name for loperamide [France]

Brand Names: U.S. Inderal® LA; InnoPran XL®

Brand Names: Canada Apo-Propranolol®; Dom-Propranolol; Inderal®; Inderal® LA; Novo-Pranol; Nu-Propranolol; PMS-Propranolol; Propranolol Hydrochloride Injection, USP; Teva-Propranolol

Index Terms Propranolol Hydrochloride

Generic Availability (U.S.) Yes

Pharmacologic Category Antianginal Agent; Antiarrhythmic Agent, Class II; Beta-Adrenergic Blocker, Nonselective

Use Management of hypertension; angina pectoris; pheochromocytoma; essential tremor; supraventricular arrhythmias (such as atrial fibrillation and flutter, AV nodal re-entrant tachycardias), ventricular tachycardias (catecholamine-induced arrhythmias, digoxin toxicity);

prevention of myocardial infarction; migraine headache prophylaxis; symptomatic treatment of hypertrophic subaortic stenosis (hypertrophic obstructive cardiomyopathy)

Unlabeled Use Tremor due to Parkinson's disease; aggressive behavior (not recommended for dementia-associated aggression), anxiety, schizophrenia; antipsychotic-induced akathisia; primary and secondary prophylaxis of variceal hemorrhage; acute panic; thyrotoxicosis; tetralogy of Fallot (TOF) hypercyanotic spells

Contraindications Hypersensitivity to propranolol, beta-blockers, or any component of the formulation; uncompensated congestive heart failure (unless the failure is due to tachyarrhythmias being treated with propranolol), cardiogenic shock, severe sinus bradycardia or heart block greater than first-degree (except in patients with a functioning artificial pacemaker), severe hyperactive airway disease (asthma or COPD)

Warnings/Precautions Consider pre-existing conditions such as sick sinus syndrome before initiating. Administer cautiously in compensated heart failure and monitor for a worsening of the condition (efficacy of propranolol in HF has not been demonstrated). **[U.S. Boxed Warning]: Beta-blocker therapy should not be withdrawn abruptly (particularly in patients with CAD), but gradually tapered to avoid acute tachycardia, hypertension, and/or ischemia.** Chronic beta-blocker therapy should not be routinely withdrawn prior to major surgery. May precipitate or aggravate symptoms of arterial insufficiency in patients with PVD and Raynaud's disease; use with caution and monitor for progression of arterial obstruction. Bradycardia may be observed more frequently in elderly patients (>65 years of age); dosage reductions may be necessary. Use caution with concurrent use of digoxin, verapamil, or diltiazem; bradycardia or heart block can occur. Avoid concurrent I.V. use of both agents. Use with caution in patients receiving inhaled anesthetic agents known to depress myocardial contractility.

Use cautiously in patients with diabetes because it can mask prominent hypoglycemic symptoms. May mask signs of hyperthyroidism (eg, tachycardia); if hyperthyroidism is suspected, carefully manage and monitor; abrupt withdrawal may exacerbate symptoms of hyperthyroidism or precipitate thyroid storm. May alter thyroid-function tests. Use with caution in myasthenia gravis or psychiatric disease (may cause CNS depression). Use cautiously in renal and hepatic dysfunction; dosage adjustment required in hepatic impairment. In general, patients with bronchospastic disease should not receive beta-blockers; if used at all, should be used cautiously with close monitoring. Adequate alpha-blockade is required prior to use of any beta-blocker for patients with untreated pheochromocytoma. May induce or exacerbate psoriasis. Use caution with history of severe anaphylaxis to allergens; patients taking beta-blockers may become more sensitive to repeated challenges. Treatment of anaphylaxis (eg, epinephrine) in patients taking beta-blockers may be ineffective or promote undesirable effects.

Adverse Reactions (Reflective of adult population; not specific for elderly) Frequency not defined.

Cardiovascular: Angina, arterial insufficiency, AV conduction disturbance increased, bradycardia, cardiogenic shock, CHF, hypotension, impaired myocardial contractility, mesenteric arterial thrombosis (rare), Raynaud's syndrome, syncope

Central nervous system: Amnesia, catatonia, cognitive dysfunction, confusion, depression, dizziness, emotional lability, fatigue, hallucinations, hypersomnolence, insomnia, lethargy, lightheadedness, psychosis, vertigo, vivid dreams

Dermatologic: Alopecia, contact dermatitis, cutaneous ulcers, eczematous eruptions, erythema multiforme, exfoliative dermatitis, hyperkeratosis, nail changes, oculomucocutaneous reactions, pruritus, psoriasiform eruptions, rash, Stevens-Johnson syndrome, toxic epidermal necrolysis, ulcers, ulcerative lichenoid, urticaria

Endocrine & metabolic: Hyper-/hypoglycemia, hyperkalemia, hyperlipidemia

Gastrointestinal: Anorexia, cramping, constipation, diarrhea, ischemic colitis, nausea, stomach discomfort, vomiting

Genitourinary: Impotence, interstitial nephritis (rare), oliguria (rare), Peyronie's disease, proteinuria (rare)

Hematologic: Agranulocytosis, nonthrombocytopenic purpura, thrombocytopenia, thrombocytopenic purpura

Hepatic: Alkaline phosphatase increased, transaminases increased

Neuromuscular & skeletal: Arthropathy, carpal tunnel syndrome (rare), myotonus, paresthesia, polyarthritis, weakness

Ocular: Hyperemia of the conjunctiva, mydriasis, visual acuity decreased, visual disturbances, xerophthalmia

Renal: BUN increased

Respiratory: Bronchospasm, dyspnea, laryngospasm, pharyngitis, pulmonary edema, respiratory distress, wheezing

Miscellaneous: Anaphylactic/anaphylactoid allergic reaction, cold extremities, lupus-like syndrome (rare)

◀ **Drug Interactions**

Metabolism/Transport Effects Substrate of CYP1A2 (major), CYP2C19 (minor), CYP2D6 (major), CYP3A4 (minor); **Note:** Assignment of Major/Minor substrate status based on clinically relevant drug interaction potential; **Inhibits** CYP1A2 (weak), CYP2D6 (weak), P-glycoprotein

Avoid Concomitant Use

Avoid concomitant use of Propranolol with any of the following: Beta2-Agonists; Floctafenine; Methacholine; Topotecan

Increased Effect/Toxicity

Propranolol may increase the levels/effects of: Alpha-/Beta-Agonists (Direct-Acting); Alpha1-Blockers; Alpha2-Agonists; Amifostine; Antihypertensives; Antipsychotic Agents (Phenothiazines); ARIPiprazole; Bupivacaine; Cardiac Glycosides; Cholinergic Agonists; Colchicine; Dabigatran Etexilate; Everolimus; Fingolimod; Hypotensive Agents; Insulin; Lidocaine; Lidocaine (Systemic); Lidocaine (Topical); Mepivacaine; Methacholine; Midodrine; P-glycoprotein/ABCB1 Substrates; Prucalopride; RiTUXimab; Rivaroxaban; Rizatriptan; Sulfonylureas; Topotecan; ZOLMitriptan

The levels/effects of Propranolol may be increased by: Abiraterone Acetate; Acetylcholinesterase Inhibitors; Alcohol (Ethyl); Aminoquinolines (Antimalarial); Amiodarone; Anilidopiperidine Opioids; Antipsychotic Agents (Phenothiazines); Calcium Channel Blockers (Dihydropyridine); Calcium Channel Blockers (Nondihydropyridine); CYP1A2 Inhibitors (Moderate); CYP1A2 Inhibitors (Strong); CYP2D6 Inhibitors (Moderate); CYP2D6 Inhibitors (Strong); Darunavir; Deferasirox; Diazoxide; Dipyridamole; Disopyramide; Dronedarone; Floctafenine; FluvoxaMINE; Herbs (Hypotensive Properties); Lacidipine; MAO Inhibitors; Pentoxifylline; Phosphodiesterase 5 Inhibitors; Propafenone; Prostacyclin Analogues; QuiNIDine; Reserpine; Selective Serotonin Reuptake Inhibitors; Zileuton

Decreased Effect

Propranolol may decrease the levels/effects of: Beta2-Agonists; Lacidipine; Theophylline Derivatives

The levels/effects of Propranolol may be decreased by: Alcohol (Ethyl); Barbiturates; Bile Acid Sequestrants; CYP1A2 Inducers (Strong); Cyproterone; Herbs (Hypertensive Properties); Methylphenidate; Nonsteroidal Anti-Inflammatory Agents; Peginterferon Alfa-2b; Rifamycin Derivatives; Tocilizumab; Yohimbine

Ethanol/Nutrition/Herb Interactions

Cigarette: Smoking may decrease plasma levels of propranolol by increasing metabolism. Management: Avoid smoking.

Ethanol: Ethanol may increase or decrease plasma levels of propranolol. Reports are variable and have shown both enhanced as well as inhibited hepatic metabolism (of propranolol). Management: Caution advised with consumption of ethanol and monitor for heart rate and/or blood pressure changes.

Food: Propranolol serum levels may be increased if taken with food. Protein-rich foods may increase bioavailability; a change in diet from high carbohydrate/low protein to low carbohydrate/high protein may result in increased oral clearance. Management: Tablets (immediate release) should be taken on an empty stomach. Capsules (extended release) may be taken with or without food, but be consistent with regard to food.

Herb/Nutraceutical: Dong quai has estrogenic activity. Some herbal medications may worsen hypertension (eg, licorice); others may enhance the antihypertensive effect of propranolol (eg, shepherd's purse). Management: Avoid dong quai if using for hypertension. Avoid bayberry, blue cohosh, cayenne, ephedra, ginger, ginseng (American), gotu kola, licorice, and yohimbe. Avoid black cohosh, california poppy, coleus, garlic, golden seal, hawthorn, mistletoe, periwinkle, quinine, and shepherd's purse.

Stability

Injection: Store at 20°C to 25°C (68°F to 77°F); protect from freezing or excessive heat. Once diluted, propranolol is stable for 24 hours at room temperature in D_5W or NS. Protect from light. Solution has a maximum stability at pH of 3 and decomposes rapidly in alkaline pH.

Capsule, tablet: Store at 20°C to 25°C (68°F to 77°F); protect from freezing or excessive heat. Protect from light and moisture.

Mechanism of Action Nonselective beta-adrenergic blocker (class II antiarrhythmic); competitively blocks response to beta$_1$- and beta$_2$-adrenergic stimulation which results in decreases in heart rate, myocardial contractility, blood pressure, and myocardial oxygen demand. Nonselective beta-adrenergic blockers (propranolol, nadolol) reduce portal pressure by producing splanchnic vasoconstriction (beta$_2$ effect) thereby reducing portal blood flow.

Pharmacodynamics/Kinetics

Onset of action: Beta-blockade: Oral: 1-2 hours

Duration: Immediate release: 6-12 hours; Extended-release formulations: ~24-27 hours

Absorption: Oral: Rapid and complete

Distribution: V_d: 4 L/kg in adults

Protein binding: Adults: ~90% (S-isomer primarily to alpha$_1$-acid glycoprotein; R-isomer primarily to albumin)

Metabolism: Hepatic via CYP2D6, and CYP1A2 to 4-hydroxypropranolol (active) and inactive compounds; extensive first-pass effect

Bioavailability: ~25% reaches systemic circulation due to high first-pass metabolism; protein-rich foods increase bioavailability by ~50%

Half-life elimination: Adults: Immediate release formulation: 3-6 hours; Extended-release formulations: 8-10 hours

Time to peak: Immediate release: 1-4 hours; Extended-release formulations: ~6-14 hours

Excretion: Metabolites are excreted primarily in urine (96% to 99%); <1% excreted in urine as unchanged drug

Dosage

Geriatric

I.V.: Use caution; initiate at lower end of the dosing range.

Oral:

Hypertension: Consider lower initial doses and titrate to response (Aronow, 2011)

Tachyarrhythmias: Initial: 10 mg twice daily; increase dosage every 3-7 days; usual dose range: 10-320 mg/day given in 1-2 divided doses.

Refer to adult dosing for additional uses.

Adult

Akathisia (unlabeled use): Oral: 30-120 mg/day in 2-3 divided doses

Essential tremor: Oral: 40 mg twice daily initially; maintenance doses: Usually 120-320 mg/day

Hypertension: Initial: Oral: 40 mg twice daily; increase dosage every 3-7 days; usual dose: 120-240 mg divided in 2-3 doses/day; maximum daily dose: 640 mg; usual dosage range (JNC 7): 40-160 mg/day in 2 divided doses

Extended release formulations:

Inderal® LA: Initial: 80 mg once daily; usual maintenance: 120-160 mg once daily; maximum daily dose: 640 mg; usual dosage range (JNC 7): 60-180 mg/day once daily

InnoPran XL®: Initial: 80 mg once daily at bedtime; if initial response is inadequate, may be increased at 2-3 week intervals to a maximum dose of 120 mg

Hypertrophic subaortic stenosis: Oral: 20-40 mg 3-4 times/day

Inderal® LA: 80-160 mg once daily

Migraine headache prophylaxis: Oral: Initial: 80 mg/day divided every 6-8 hours; increase by 20-40 mg/dose every 3-4 weeks to a maximum of 160-240 mg/day given in divided doses every 6-8 hours; if satisfactory response not achieved within 6 weeks of starting therapy, drug should be withdrawn gradually over several weeks

Inderal® LA: Initial: 80 mg once daily; effective dose range: 160-240 mg once daily

Pheochromocytoma: Oral: 30-60 mg/day in divided doses

Post-MI mortality reduction: Oral: 180-240 mg/day in 3-4 divided doses

Stable angina: Oral: 80-320 mg/day in doses divided 2-4 times/day

Inderal® LA: Initial: 80 mg once daily; maximum dose: 320 mg once daily

Tachyarrhythmias:

Oral: 10-30 mg/dose every 6-8 hours

I.V.: 1-3 mg/dose slow IVP; repeat every 2-5 minutes up to a total of 5 mg; titrate initial dose to desired response

or

0.5-1 mg over 1 minute; may repeat, if necessary, up to a total maximum dose of 0.1 mg/kg (ACLS guidelines, 2010)

Note: Once response achieved or maximum dose administered, additional doses should not be given for at least 4 hours.

Thyroid storm (unlabeled use):

Oral: 60-80 mg every 4 hours; may consider the use of an intravenous shorter-acting beta-blocker (ie, esmolol) (Bahn, 2011)

I.V.: 0.5-1 mg administered over 10 minutes every 3 hours (Gardner, 2011)

Thyrotoxicosis (unlabeled use): Oral: 10-40 mg/dose every 6-8 hours; may also consider administering extended or sustained release formulations (Bahn, 2011)

Variceal hemorrhage prophylaxis (unlabeled use) (Garcia-Tsao, 2007): Oral:

Primary prophylaxis: Initial: 20 mg twice daily; adjust to maximal tolerated dose. **Note:** Risk factors for hemorrhage include Child-Pugh class B/C or variceal red wale markings on endoscopy.

Secondary prophylaxis: Initial: 20 mg twice daily; adjust to maximal tolerated dose

Renal Impairment

Not dialyzable (0% to 5%); supplemental dose is not necessary.

Peritoneal dialysis effects: Supplemental dose is not necessary.

Hepatic Impairment Marked slowing of heart rate may occur in chronic liver disease with conventional doses; low initial dose and regular heart rate monitoring.

◄ **Administration** I.V. dose is much smaller than oral dose. When administered acutely for cardiac treatment, monitor ECG and blood pressure. May administer by rapid infusion (I.V. push) at a rate of 1 mg/minute or by slow infusion over ~30 minutes. Necessary monitoring for surgical patients who are unable to take oral beta-blockers (prolonged ileus) has not been defined. Some institutions require monitoring of baseline and postinfusion heart rate and blood pressure when a patient's response to beta-blockade has not been characterized (ie, the patient's initial dose or following a change in dose). Consult individual institutional policies and procedures. Do not crush long-acting oral forms.

Monitoring Parameters Acute cardiac treatment: Monitor ECG, heart rate, and blood pressure with I.V. administration; heart rate and blood pressure with oral administration

Reference Range Therapeutic: 50-100 ng/mL (SI: 190-390 nmol/L) at end of dose interval

Special Geriatric Considerations Since bioavailability increased in about twofold in elderly patients, geriatrics may require lower maintenance doses. Also, as serum and tissue concentrations increase beta$_1$ selectivity diminishes. Beta-adrenergic blockade may result in less hemodynamic response than seen in younger adults due to alterations in the beta-adrenergic autonomic system. Studies indicate that despite decreased sensitivity to the chronotropic effects of beta-blockade with age, there appears to be an increased myocardial sensitivity to the negative inotropic effect during stress (ie, exercise). Controlled trials have shown the overall response rate for propranolol to be only 20% to 50% in elderly populations. Therefore, all beta-adrenergic blocking drugs may result in a decreased response as compared to younger adults. Due to propranolol's CNS penetration and nonselective action, it may not be the beta-blocker of choice for use in elderly.

Dosage Forms Excipient information presented when available (limited, particularly for generics); consult specific product labeling.
Capsule, extended release, oral, as hydrochloride: 60 mg, 80 mg, 120 mg, 160 mg
InnoPran XL®: 80 mg, 120 mg
Capsule, sustained release, oral, as hydrochloride:
Inderal® LA: 60 mg, 80 mg, 120 mg, 160 mg
Injection, solution, as hydrochloride: 1 mg/mL (1 mL)
Injection, solution, as hydrochloride [preservative free]: 1 mg/mL (1 mL)
Solution, oral, as hydrochloride: 4 mg/mL (500 mL); 8 mg/mL (500 mL)
Tablet, oral, as hydrochloride: 10 mg, 20 mg, 40 mg, 60 mg, 80 mg

Propranolol and Hydrochlorothiazide
(proe PRAN oh lole & hye droe klor oh THYE a zide)

Related Information
Hydrochlorothiazide *on page 933*
Propranolol *on page 1622*

Medication Safety Issues
Sound-alike/look-alike issues:
Inderide may be confused with Inderal®

Index Terms Hydrochlorothiazide and Propranolol; Inderide

Generic Availability (U.S.) Yes

Pharmacologic Category Beta-Blocker, Nonselective; Diuretic, Thiazide

Use Management of hypertension

Dosage
Geriatric & Adult
Hypertension: Oral: Dose is individualized; typical dosages of **hydrochlorothiazide**: 12.5-50 mg/day; initial dose of **propranolol** 80 mg/day
Note: Daily dose of tablet form should be divided into 2 daily doses; may be used to maximum dosage of up to 160 mg of propranolol; higher dosages would result in higher than optimal thiazide dosages.

Special Geriatric Considerations See individual agents. Combination products are not recommended as first-line treatment. Use only if doses of individual agents correspond to the combination available.

Divided doses of diuretics may increase the incidence of nocturia in the elderly.

Dosage Forms Excipient information presented when available (limited, particularly for generics); consult specific product labeling.
Tablet: Propranolol hydrochloride 40 mg and hydrochlorothiazide 25 mg; propranolol hydrochloride 80 mg and hydrochlorothiazide 25 mg

◆ **Propranolol Hydrochloride** *see* Propranolol *on page 1622*
◆ **Proprinal® [OTC]** *see* Ibuprofen *on page 966*
◆ **2-Propylpentanoic Acid** *see* Valproic Acid *on page 1991*

Propylthiouracil (proe pil thye oh YOOR a sil)

Medication Safety Issues
Sound-alike/look-alike issues:
Propylthiouracil may be confused with Purinethol®
PTU is an error-prone abbreviation (mistaken as mercaptopurine [Purinethol®; 6-MP])
Brand Names: Canada Propyl-Thyracil®
Index Terms PTU (error-prone abbreviation)
Generic Availability (U.S.) Yes
Pharmacologic Category Antithyroid Agent; Thioamide
Use Adjunctive therapy in patients intolerant of methimazole to ameliorate hyperthyroidism
symptoms in preparation for surgical treatment or radioactive iodine therapy; treatment of
hyperthyroidism in patients intolerant of methimazole and not candidates for surgical/radio-
therapy
Unlabeled Use Management of Graves' disease, thyrotoxic crisis, or thyroid storm
Medication Guide Available Yes
Contraindications Hypersensitivity to propylthiouracil or any component of the formulation
**Warnings/Precautions [U.S. Boxed Warning]: Severe liver injury (some fatal) and acute
liver failure (some cases requiring transplantation) have been reported.** Patients should
be counseled to recognize and report symptoms suggestive of hepatic dysfunction (especially
in first 6 months of treatment), which should prompt immediate discontinuation. Routine liver
function test monitoring may not reduce risk due to unpredictable and rapid onset.

Has been associated with significant bone marrow depression. The most severe manifestation is agranulocytosis (commonly within first 3 months of therapy). Aplastic anemia,
thrombocytopenia, and leukopenia may also occur. Use with caution in patients receiving
other drugs known to cause myelosuppression particularly agranulocytosis. Discontinue if
significant bone marrow suppression occurs, particularly agranulocytosis or aplastic anemia.

Rare hypersensitivity reactions have been reported, including the development of ANCA-
positive vasculitis, drug fever, interstitial pneumonitis, exfoliative dermatitis, glomerulonephritis, leukocytoclastic vasculitis, and a lupus-like syndrome; prompt discontinuation is warranted in patients who develop symptoms consistent with a form of autoimmunity or other
hypersensitivity during therapy. May cause hypoprothrombinemia and bleeding.
Adverse Reactions (Reflective of adult population; not specific for elderly) Frequency not defined.
Cardiovascular: Periarteritis, vasculitis (ANCA-positive, cutaneous, leukocytoclastic)
Central nervous system: Drowsiness, drug fever, fever, headache, neuritis, vertigo
Dermatologic: Alopecia, erythema nodosum, exfoliative dermatitis, pruritus, skin pigmentation,
skin rash, skin ulcers, urticaria
Endocrine & metabolic: Goiter, weight gain
Gastrointestinal: Constipation, loss of taste, nausea, sialoadenopathy, splenomegaly, stom-
ach pain, taste perversion, vomiting
Hematologic: Agranulocytosis, aplastic anemia, bleeding, granulopenia, hypoprothrombine-
mia, leukopenia, thrombocytopenia
Hepatic: Acute liver failure, cholestatic jaundice, hepatitis
Neuromuscular & skeletal: Arthralgia, myalgia, paresthesia
Renal: Acute renal failure, glomerulonephritis, nephritis
Respiratory: Alveolar hemorrhage, interstitial pneumonitis
Miscellaneous: Lymphadenopathy, SLE-like syndrome
Drug Interactions
Metabolism/Transport Effects None known.
Avoid Concomitant Use
Avoid concomitant use of Propylthiouracil with any of the following: CloZAPine; Sodium
Iodide I131
Increased Effect/Toxicity
Propylthiouracil may increase the levels/effects of: Cardiac Glycosides; CloZAPine; Theo-
phylline Derivatives
Decreased Effect
Propylthiouracil may decrease the levels/effects of: Sodium Iodide I131; Vitamin K Antag-
onists
Ethanol/Nutrition/Herb Interactions Food: Propylthiouracil serum levels may be altered if
taken with food.
Stability Store at 25°C (77°F); excursions permitted to 15°C to 30°C (59°F to 86°F).
Mechanism of Action Inhibits the synthesis of thyroid hormones by blocking the oxidation of
iodine in the thyroid gland; blocks synthesis of thyroxine and triiodothyronine

Pharmacodynamics/Kinetics
Duration: 12-24 hours
Distribution: Concentrated in the thyroid gland
Protein binding: 80% to 85%
Metabolism: Hepatic
Bioavailability: 53% to 88%
Half-life elimination: ~1 hour
Time to peak, serum: 1-2 hours
Excretion: Urine (35%; primarily as metabolites)

Dosage

Adult

Hyperthyroidism: Oral: Initial: 300 mg/day in 3 divided doses; 400 mg/day in patients with severe hyperthyroidism and/or very large goiters; an occasional patient will require 600-900 mg/day; usual maintenance: 100-150 mg/day

Graves' disease (unlabeled use): Oral: Initial: 50-150 mg (depending on severity) 3 times daily to restore euthyroidism; maintenance: 50 mg 2-3 times daily for a total of 12-18 months, then tapered or discontinued if TSH is normal at that time (Bahn, 2011)

Thyrotoxic crisis/thyroid storm (unlabeled use): Oral: **Note:** Recommendations vary widely and have not been evaluated in comparative trials. Typical dosing is 800-1200 mg/day given as 200-300 mg every 4-6 hours; some clinicians advocate an initial loading dose of 600-1000 mg. After initial response, dose may be reduced gradually to a maintenance dosage (100-600 mg/day in divided doses) (Goldberg, 2003; Nayak, 2006). The American Thyroid Association and the American Association of Clinical Endocrinologists recommend 500-1000 mg loading dose followed by 250 mg every 4 hours (Bahn, 2011).

Duration of therapy: Clinical improvement generally occurs in 1-3 months, after which dosage reduction may be employed (to prevent hypothyroidism), with discontinuation considered after 12-18 months of therapy. Thyroid function should be monitored every 2 months thereafter for 6 months until remission is confirmed, followed by annual evaluations (Cooper, 2005).

Renal Impairment Adjustment is not necessary.

Administration Administer at the same time in relation to meals each day, either always with meals or always between meals.

Monitoring Parameters CBC with differential, prothrombin time, liver function tests (bilirubin, alkaline phosphatase, transaminases), and thyroid function tests (TSH, T_3, T_4) every 4-6 weeks until euthyroid; periodic blood counts are recommended for chronic therapy

Reference Range Normal laboratory values:
Total T_4: 5-12 mcg/dL
Serum T_3: 90-185 ng/dL
Free thyroxine index (FT_4 I): 6-10.5
TSH: 0.5-4.0 microunits/mL

Pharmacotherapy Pearls Preferred over methimazole in thyroid storm due to inhibition of peripheral conversion as well as synthesis of thyroid hormone.

Graves' hyperthyroidism: Elevated T_3 may be the sole indicator of inadequate treatment. Elevated TSH indicates excessive antithyroid treatment. Monitoring of TSH is a poor indicator of treatment effectiveness, as levels may remain suppressed for months, despite euthyroid state (Cooper, 2005).

A potency ratio of methimazole to propylthiouracil of at least 20-30:1 is recommended when changing from one drug to another (eg, 300 mg of propylthiouracil would be roughly equivalent to 10-15 mg of methimazole) (Bahn, 2011).

Special Geriatric Considerations The use of antithyroid thioamides is as effective in the elderly as they are in younger adults.

Dosage Forms Excipient information presented when available (limited, particularly for generics); consult specific product labeling.
Tablet, oral: 50 mg

Protriptyline (proe TRIP ti leen)

Related Information
Antidepressant Agents *on page 2097*
Beers Criteria – Potentially Inappropriate Medications for Geriatrics *on page 2183*
Medication Safety Issues
Sound-alike/look-alike issues:
Vivactil® may be confused with Vyvanse®
BEERS Criteria medication:
This drug may be potentially inappropriate for use in geriatric patients (SIADH: Quality of evidence - moderate; Strength of recommendation - strong).
Brand Names: U.S. Vivactil®
Index Terms Protriptyline Hydrochloride
Generic Availability (U.S.) Yes
Pharmacologic Category Antidepressant, Tricyclic (Secondary Amine)
Use Treatment of depression
Medication Guide Available Yes
Contraindications Hypersensitivity to protriptyline (cross-reactivity to other cyclic antidepressants may occur) or any component of the formulation; use of MAO inhibitors within 14 days; use of cisapride; use in a patient during the acute recovery phase of MI
Warnings/Precautions [U.S. Boxed Warning]: Antidepressants increase the risk of suicidal thinking and behavior in children, adolescents, and young adults (18-24 years of age) with major depressive disorder (MDD) and other psychiatric disorders; consider risk prior to prescribing. Short-term studies did not show an increased risk in patients >24 years of age and showed a decreased risk in patients ≥65 years. Closely monitor for clinical worsening, suicidality, or unusual changes in behavior; the patient's family or caregiver should be instructed to closely observe the patient and communicate condition with healthcare provider. A medication guide should be dispensed with each prescription.

The possibility of a suicide attempt is inherent in major depression and may persist until remission occurs. Monitor for worsening of depression or suicidality, especially during initiation of therapy (generally first 1-2 months) or with dose increases or decreases. Use caution in high-risk patients. Worsening depression and severe abrupt suicidality that are not part of the presenting symptoms may require discontinuation or modification of drug therapy. The patient's family or caregiver should be alerted to monitor patients for the emergence of suicidality and associated behaviors (such as agitation, irritability, hostility, impulsivity, and hypomania) and call healthcare provider.

May worsen psychosis in some patients or precipitate a shift to mania or hypomania in patients with bipolar disorder. Patients presenting with depressive symptoms should be screened for bipolar disorder. Monotherapy in patients with bipolar disorder should be avoided. **Protriptyline is not FDA approved for the treatment of bipolar depression.**

TCAs may rarely cause bone marrow suppression; monitor for any signs of infection and obtain CBC if symptoms (eg, fever, sore throat) evident. Although the degree of sedation is low relative to other antidepressant agents, protriptyline may cause sedation, resulting in impaired performance of tasks requiring alertness (eg, operating machinery or driving). Sedative effects may be additive with other CNS depressants and/or ethanol. Protriptyline may aggravate aggressive behavior. Consider discontinuing, when possible, prior to elective surgery. Therapy should not be abruptly discontinued in patients receiving high doses for prolonged periods. May alter glucose regulation - use with caution in patients with diabetes.

May cause orthostatic hypotension or conduction abnormalities (risks are moderate relative to other antidepressants). Use with caution in patients with a history of cardiovascular disease (including previous MI, stroke, tachycardia, or conduction abnormalities). The degree of anticholinergic blockade produced by this agent is moderate relative to other cyclic antidepressants; however, caution should still be used in patients with urinary retention, benign prostatic hyperplasia, narrow-angle glaucoma, xerostomia, visual problems, constipation, or history of bowel obstruction.

Hyperpyrexia has been observed with TCAs in combination with anticholinergics and/or neuroleptics, particularly during hot weather. Use caution in patients with a previous seizure disorder or condition predisposing to seizures such as brain damage, alcoholism, or concurrent therapy with other drugs which lower the seizure threshold. May increase the risks associated with electroconvulsive therapy. Use with caution in hyperthyroid patients or those receiving thyroid supplementation. Use with caution in patients with hepatic or renal dysfunction.

Use caution in elderly patients; may cause or exacerbate syndrome of inappropriate antidiuretic hormone secretion or hyponatremia; monitor sodium closely with initiation or dosage adjustments in older adults. May be inappropriate in older adults depending on comorbidities (eg, dementia, delirium) due to its potent anticholinergic effects (Beers Criteria).

Adverse Reactions (Reflective of adult population; not specific for elderly) Frequency not defined.

Cardiovascular: Arrhythmias, heart block, hyper-/hypotension, MI, palpitation, stroke, tachycardia

Central nervous system: Agitation, anxiety, ataxia, confusion, delirium, delusions, dizziness, drowsiness, EPS, exacerbation of psychosis, fatigue, hallucinations, headache, hypomania, incoordination, insomnia, nightmares, panic, restlessness, seizure

Dermatologic: Alopecia, itching, petechiae, photosensitivity, rash, urticaria

Endocrine & metabolic: Breast enlargement, galactorrhea, gynecomastia, increased or decreased libido, syndrome of inappropriate ADH secretion (SIADH)

Gastrointestinal: Anorexia, constipation, decreased lower esophageal sphincter tone may cause GE reflux, diarrhea, heartburn, increased appetite, nausea, trouble with gums, unpleasant taste, vomiting, weight gain/loss, xerostomia

Genitourinary: Difficult urination, impotence, testicular edema

Hematologic: Agranulocytosis, eosinophilia, leukopenia, purpura, thrombocytopenia

Hepatic: Cholestatic jaundice, increased liver enzymes

Neuromuscular & skeletal: Fine muscle tremor, numbness, tingling, tremor, weakness

Ocular: Blurred vision, eye pain, increased intraocular pressure

Otic: Tinnitus

Miscellaneous: Allergic reactions, excessive diaphoresis

Drug Interactions

Metabolism/Transport Effects Substrate of CYP2D6 (major); **Note:** Assignment of Major/ Minor substrate status based on clinically relevant drug interaction potential

Avoid Concomitant Use

Avoid concomitant use of Protriptyline with any of the following: Cisapride; Iobenguane I 123; MAO Inhibitors; Methylene Blue

Increased Effect/Toxicity

Protriptyline may increase the levels/effects of: Alpha-/Beta-Agonists (Direct-Acting); Alpha1-Agonists; Amphetamines; Anticholinergics; Beta2-Agonists; Cisapride; Desmopressin; Highest Risk QTc-Prolonging Agents; Methylene Blue; Metoclopramide; Moderate Risk QTc-Prolonging Agents; QuiNIDine; Serotonin Modulators; Sodium Phosphates; Sulfonylureas; TraMADol; Vitamin K Antagonists; Yohimbine

The levels/effects of Protriptyline may be increased by: Abiraterone Acetate; Altretamine; Antipsychotics; Cimetidine; Cinacalcet; CYP2D6 Inhibitors (Moderate); CYP2D6 Inhibitors (Strong); Dexmethylphenidate; Divalproex; DULoxetine; Linezolid; Lithium; MAO Inhibitors; Methylphenidate; Metoclopramide; Metyrosine; Mifepristone; Pramlintide; Protease Inhibitors; QuiNIDine; Selective Serotonin Reuptake Inhibitors; Terbinafine; Terbinafine (Systemic); Valproic Acid

Decreased Effect

Protriptyline may decrease the levels/effects of: Acetylcholinesterase Inhibitors (Central); Alpha2-Agonists; Iobenguane I 123

The levels/effects of Protriptyline may be decreased by: Acetylcholinesterase Inhibitors (Central); Barbiturates; CarBAMazepine; Peginterferon Alfa-2b; St Johns Wort

Ethanol/Nutrition/Herb Interactions

Ethanol: May increase CNS depression; monitor for increased effects with coadministration. Caution patients about effects.

Food: Grapefruit juice may inhibit the metabolism of some TCAs and clinical toxicity may result.

Herb/Nutraceutical: Avoid valerian, St John's wort, SAMe, kava kava (may increase risk of serotonin syndrome and/or excessive sedation).

Mechanism of Action Increases the synaptic concentration of serotonin and/or norepinephrine in the central nervous system by inhibition of their reuptake by the presynaptic neuronal membrane

Pharmacodynamics/Kinetics

Protein binding: 92%

Metabolism: Extensively hepatic via N-oxidation, hydroxylation, and glucuronidation; first-pass effect (10% to 25%)

Half-life elimination: 54-92 hours (average: 74 hours)

Time to peak, serum: 24-30 hours

Excretion: Urine

Dosage

Geriatric Oral: Initial: 5-10 mg/day; increase every 3-7 days by 5-10 mg; usual dose: 15-20 mg/day

Adult Depression: Oral: 15-60 mg/day in 3-4 divided doses

Administration Make any dosage increase in the morning dose

Monitoring Parameters Monitor for cardiac abnormalities in elderly patients receiving doses >20 mg; suicide ideation (especially at the beginning of therapy or when doses are increased or decreased)

Reference Range Therapeutic: 70-250 ng/mL (SI: 266-950 nmol/L); Toxic: >500 ng/mL (SI: >1900 nmol/L)

Special Geriatric Considerations Little data on its use in the elderly. Strong anticholinergic properties which may limit its use; more often stimulating rather than sedating.

A systematic review and meta-analysis of antidepressant placebo-controlled trials in persons with depression and dementia found evidence "suggestive" of efficacy but not of sufficient strength to "confirm" efficacy. Antidepressant trials in this patient population are small and underpowered. Older patients with depression being treated with an antidepressant should be closely monitored for response and adverse effects. Treatment should be switched or augmented when response is inadequate with a therapeutic dose. Antidepressants that are not tolerated should be discontinued and an alternative agent should be started.

This medication is considered to be potentially inappropriate in this patient population (Beers Criteria: SIADH: Quality of evidence - moderate; Strength of recommendation - strong).

Dosage Forms Excipient information presented when available (limited, particularly for generics); consult specific product labeling.

Tablet, oral, as hydrochloride: 5 mg, 10 mg
Vivactil®: 5 mg, 10 mg

- ◆ **Protriptyline Hydrochloride** *see* Protriptyline *on page 1629*
- ◆ **Provenge®** *see* Sipuleucel-T *on page 1780*
- ◆ **Proventil® HFA** *see* Albuterol *on page 49*
- ◆ **Provera®** *see* MedroxyPROGESTERone *on page 1190*
- ◆ **Provigil®** *see* Modafinil *on page 1299*
- ◆ **PROzac®** *see* FLUoxetine *on page 808*
- ◆ **PROzac® Weekly™** *see* FLUoxetine *on page 808*

Prucalopride (proo KAL oh pride)

Medication Safety Issues

Sound-alike/look-alike issues:
Resotran™ may be confused with Restoril™

Brand Names: Canada Resotran™

Index Terms Prucalopride Succinate; R093877; R108512

Pharmacologic Category Serotonin 5-HT$_4$ Receptor Agonist

Use Treatment of chronic idiopathic constipation in adult females with inadequate response to laxatives

Unlabeled Use Opioid-induced constipation in chronic pain (noncancer) patients

Contraindications Hypersensitivity to prucalopride or any component of the formulation; renal impairment requiring dialysis; intestinal perforation or obstruction due to structural or functional disorder of the gut wall, obstructive ileus, severe inflammatory conditions of the GI tract (eg, Crohn's disease, ulcerative colitis, toxic megacolon).

Warnings/Precautions Use with caution in patients with a history of arrhythmias, ischemic cardiovascular disease, pre-excitation syndromes (eg, Wolff-Parkinson-White syndrome), or A-V nodal rhythm disorders. Slight increases in heart rate and shortened PR intervals were observed in healthy subjects during clinical trials; treatment-related effects on QRS duration or QTc interval were not observed. Palpitations have also been observed; monitoring of cardiovascular status is recommended. Instruct patients to report severe or persistent palpitations.

Use with caution in renal impairment; manufacturer's labeling recommends a dose reduction in severe impairment; contraindicated in patients requiring dialysis. Use with caution in patients with severe and unstable concomitant disease (eg, cancer, AIDS, psychiatric, hepatic, pulmonary, insulin-dependent diabetes mellitus); has not been studied. Patients with severe or persistent diarrhea should discontinue therapy and consult healthcare provider. Ischemic colitis has not observed during clinical trials but is a potential concern with treatment; instruct patients with onset of severe or worsening GI symptoms, bloody diarrhea or rectal bleeding to discontinue treatment and consult healthcare provider.

Dizziness and fatigue have been observed with initiation of therapy (generally the first day of therapy); caution patients in regards to operating dangerous machinery or driving. May contain lactose; do not use in patients with galactose intolerance, Lapp lactase deficiency, or glucose-galactose malabsorption syndromes. Use with caution in the elderly (limited data); dose reductions may be necessary. Efficacy not established in males.

Adverse Reactions (Reflective of adult population; not specific for elderly)

>10%:
  Central nervous system: Headache (22%)
  Gastrointestinal: Nausea (17%), abdominal pain (12%), diarrhea (12%)

1% to 10%:
  Cardiovascular: Palpitation (1%; similar to placebo)
  Central nervous system: Dizziness (4%), fatigue (3%), fever (1%), malaise (1%)
  Genitourinary: Pollakiuria (1%)
  Gastrointestinal: Upper abdominal pain (5%), flatulence (5%), vomiting (5%), dyspepsia (3%), bowel sounds abnormal (2%), anorexia (1%), gastroenteritis (1%)
  Neuromuscular & skeletal: Muscle spasms (2%)

Drug Interactions

Metabolism/Transport Effects Substrate of P-glycoprotein

Avoid Concomitant Use There are no known interactions where it is recommended to avoid concomitant use.

Increased Effect/Toxicity
  The levels/effects of Prucalopride may be increased by: P-glycoprotein/ABCB1 Inhibitors

Decreased Effect
  Prucalopride may decrease the levels/effects of: Contraceptives (Estrogens); Contraceptives (Progestins)

Stability Store at 15°C to 30°C (59°F to 86°F). Store in original container to protect from moisture.

Mechanism of Action Prucalopride is a selective, high affinity 5-HT$_4$ receptor agonist whose action at the receptor site promotes cholinergic and nonadrenergic, noncholinergic neurotransmission by enteric neurons leading to stimulation of the peristaltic reflex, intestinal secretions, and gastrointestinal motility.

Pharmacodynamics/Kinetics
  Absorption: Rapid
  Distribution: V_d: 567 L
  Protein binding: ~30%
  Metabolism: Minor route of elimination; 8 metabolites produced (*in vitro* data suggest that 4 of 8 metabolites have lower or similar affinity to prucalopride for 5-HT$_4$ receptor)
  Bioavailability: >90%
  Half-life elimination: ~24 hours; terminal half-life increases to 34, 43, and 47 hours in mild, moderate, and severe renal impairment, respectively
  Time to peak: 2-3 hours
  Excretion: Primarily as unchanged drug: Urine (55% to 74%); feces (4% to 8%)

Dosage

Geriatric Chronic idiopathic constipation: Females >65 years: Oral: Initial: 1 mg once daily; may increase to 2 mg once daily if necessary; **Note:** If no bowel movement within 3-4 days, consider adjunctive laxative therapy for acute treatment. Discontinue use if therapy is not effective within 4 weeks of initiation.

Adult Chronic idiopathic constipation: Females (≥18 years): Oral: 2 mg once daily; **Note:** If no bowel movement within 3-4 days, consider adjunctive laxative therapy for acute treatment. Discontinue use if therapy is not effective within 4 weeks of initiation.

Renal Impairment
  Mild-moderate impairment: No dosage adjustment necessary.
  Severe impairment (GFR <30 mL/minute/1.73m^2): 1 mg once daily.
  Dialysis: Use is contraindicated.

Hepatic Impairment No dosage adjustment necessary.

Administration May administer without regard to meals. If a dose is missed, do not double to make up for a missed dose.

Monitoring Parameters Cardiovascular symptoms (eg, palpitations) particularly in patients with cardiovascular disease; frequency of bowel movements

Special Geriatric Considerations
  Limited data suggest there is no difference in prucalopride's safety profile in older patients compared to younger patients. Clinical trials included 564 patients ≥65 years.

Product Availability Not available in U.S.

Dosage Forms: Canada Excipient information presented when available (limited, particularly for generics); consult specific product labeling.
  Tablet, oral:
    Resotran™: 1 mg, 2 mg [contains lactose]

◆ **Prucalopride Succinate** *see* Prucalopride *on page 1631*
◆ **Prudoxin™** *see* Doxepin (Topical) *on page 603*
◆ **P&S® [OTC]** *see* Salicylic Acid *on page 1743*
◆ **23PS** *see* Pneumococcal Polysaccharide Vaccine (Polyvalent) *on page 1558*

Pseudoephedrine (soo doe e FED rin)

Medication Safety Issues
Sound-alike/look-alike issues:
Sudafed® may be confused with sotalol, Sudafed PE®, Sufenta®

Brand Names: U.S. Children's Nasal Decongestant [OTC]; Contac® Cold + Flu Maximum Strength Non-Drowsy [OTC]; Oranyl [OTC]; Silfedrine Children's [OTC]; Sudafed® 12 Hour [OTC]; Sudafed® 24 Hour [OTC]; Sudafed® Children's [OTC]; Sudafed® Maximum Strength Nasal Decongestant [OTC]; Sudo-Tab® [OTC]; SudoGest 12 Hour [OTC]; SudoGest Children's [OTC] [DSC]; SudoGest [OTC]

Brand Names: Canada Balminil Decongestant; Benylin® D for Infants; Contac® Cold 12 Hour Relief Non Drowsy; Drixoral® ND; Eltor®; PMS-Pseudoephedrine; Pseudofrin; Robidrine®; Sudafed® Decongestant

Index Terms d-Isoephedrine Hydrochloride; Pseudoephedrine Hydrochloride; Pseudoephedrine Sulfate; Sudafed

Generic Availability (U.S.) Yes: Excludes extended release products

Pharmacologic Category Alpha/Beta Agonist; Decongestant

Use Temporary symptomatic relief of nasal congestion due to common cold, upper respiratory allergies, and sinusitis; also promotes nasal or sinus drainage

Contraindications Hypersensitivity to pseudoephedrine or any component of the formulation; with or within 14 days of MAO inhibitor therapy

Warnings/Precautions Use with caution in the elderly; may be more sensitive to adverse effects; administer with caution to patients with hypertension, hyperthyroidism, diabetes mellitus, cardiovascular disease, ischemic heart disease, increased intraocular pressure, prostatic hyperplasia, seizure disorders, or renal impairment. When used for self-medication (OTC), notify healthcare provider if symptoms do not improve within 7 days or are accompanied by fever. Discontinue and contact healthcare provider if nervousness, dizziness, or sleeplessness occur. Some products may contain sodium.

Adverse Reactions (Reflective of adult population; not specific for elderly) Frequency not defined.
Cardiovascular: Arrhythmia, cardiovascular collapse with hypotension, hypertension, palpitation, tachycardia
Central nervous system: Chills, confusion, coordination impaired, dizziness, drowsiness, excitability, fatigue, hallucination, headache, insomnia, nervousness, neuritis, restlessness, seizure, transient stimulation, vertigo
Dermatologic: Photosensitivity, rash, urticaria
Gastrointestinal: Anorexia, constipation, diarrhea, dry throat, ischemic colitis, nausea, vomiting, xerostomia
Genitourinary: Difficult urination, dysuria, polyuria, urinary retention
Hematologic: Agranulocytosis, hemolytic anemia, thrombocytopenia
Neuromuscular & skeletal: Tremor, weakness
Ocular: Blurred vision, diplopia
Otic: Tinnitus
Respiratory: Chest/throat tightness, dry nose, dyspnea, nasal congestion, thickening of bronchial secretions, wheezing
Miscellaneous: Anaphylaxis, diaphoresis

Drug Interactions
Metabolism/Transport Effects None known.
Avoid Concomitant Use
Avoid concomitant use of Pseudoephedrine with any of the following: Ergot Derivatives; Iobenguane I 123; MAO Inhibitors
Increased Effect/Toxicity
Pseudoephedrine may increase the levels/effects of: Bromocriptine; Sympathomimetics

The levels/effects of Pseudoephedrine may be increased by: Antacids; AtoMOXetine; Cannabinoids; Carbonic Anhydrase Inhibitors; Ergot Derivatives; MAO Inhibitors; Serotonin/Norepinephrine Reuptake Inhibitors
Decreased Effect
Pseudoephedrine may decrease the levels/effects of: Benzylpenicilloyl Polylysine; FentaNYL; Iobenguane I 123

The levels/effects of Pseudoephedrine may be decreased by: Spironolactone

Ethanol/Nutrition/Herb Interactions
Food: Onset of effect may be delayed if pseudoephedrine is taken with food.
Herb/Nutraceutical: Avoid ephedra, yohimbe (may cause hypertension).

Mechanism of Action Directly stimulates alpha-adrenergic receptors of respiratory mucosa causing vasoconstriction; directly stimulates beta-adrenergic receptors causing bronchial relaxation, increased heart rate and contractility

Pharmacodynamics/Kinetics
Onset of action: Decongestant: Oral: 30 minutes (Chua, 1989)
Peak effect: Decongestant: Oral: ~1-2 hours (Chua, 1989)
Duration: Immediate release tablet: 3-8 hours (Chua, 1989)
Absorption: Rapid (Simons, 1996)
Distribution: Adults: 2.64-3.51 L/kg (Kanfer, 1993)
Metabolism: Undergoes n-demethylation to norpseudoephedrine (active) (Chua, 1989, Kanfer, 1993); Hepatic (<1%) (Kanfer, 1993)
Half-life elimination: Varies by urine pH and flow rate; alkaline urine decreases renal elimination of pseudoephedrine (Kanfer, 1993)
Adults: 9-16 hours (pH 8); 3-6 hours (pH 5) (Chua, 1989)
Time to peak:
Adults (immediate release): 1-3 hours (dose dependent) (Kanfer, 1993)
Excretion: Urine (43% to 96% as unchanged drug, 1% to 6% as active norpseudoephedrine); dependent on urine pH and flow rate; alkaline urine decreases renal elimination of pseudoephedrine (Kanfer, 1993)

Dosage
Geriatric Nasal congestion: Use caution in this population; initiate using immediate release formulation: 30-60 mg every 6 hours as needed
Adult Nasal congestion: General dosing guidelines: Oral: Immediate release: 60 mg every 4-6 hours; Extended release: 120 mg every 12 hours **or** 240 mg every 24 hours; maximum: 240 mg/24 hours
Renal Impairment Consider reducing dose.

Administration Do not crush extended release drug product, swallow whole. May administer with or without food. Sudafed® 24 Hour tablet may not completely dissolve and appear in stool

Test Interactions Interferes with urine detection of amphetamine (false-positive)

Special Geriatric Considerations Elderly patients should be counseled about the proper use of over-the-counter cough and cold preparations. Elderly are more predisposed to adverse effects of sympathomimetics since they frequently have cardiovascular diseases and diabetes mellitus as well as multiple drug therapies. It may be advisable to treat with a short-acting/immediate-release formulation before initiating sustained-release/long-acting formulations.

Dosage Forms Excipient information presented when available (limited, particularly for generics); consult specific product labeling. [DSC] = Discontinued product
Caplet, oral:
Contac® Cold + Flu Maximum Strength Non-Drowsy: Acetaminophen 500 mg and phenylephrine hydrochloride 5 mg
Caplet, extended release, oral, as hydrochloride:
Sudafed® 12 Hour: 120 mg
Liquid, oral, as hydrochloride: 30 mg/5 mL (473 mL)
Children's Nasal Decongestant: 30 mg/5 mL (118 mL) [contains sodium benzoate; raspberry flavor]
Silfedrine Children's: 15 mg/5 mL (118 mL, 237 mL) [ethanol free, sugar free; grape flavor]
Sudafed® Children's: 15 mg/5 mL (118 mL) [ethanol free, sugar free; contains menthol, sodium 5 mg/5 mL, sodium benzoate; grape flavor]
Syrup, oral, as hydrochloride: 30 mg/5 mL (118 mL)
SudoGest Children's: 15 mg/5 mL (118 mL [DSC]) [ethanol free, sugar free; contains sodium 5 mg/5 mL, sodium benzoate; grape flavor]
Tablet, oral, as hydrochloride: 30 mg
Oranyl: 30 mg [sugar free]
Sudafed® Maximum Strength Nasal Decongestant: 30 mg [contains sodium benzoate]
Sudo-Tab®: 30 mg [contains sodium benzoate]
SudoGest: 30 mg
SudoGest: 60 mg [scored]
Tablet, extended release, oral, as hydrochloride:
Sudafed® 24 Hour: 240 mg
SudoGest 12 Hour: 120 mg

◆ **Pseudoephedrine and Triprolidine** see Triprolidine and Pseudoephedrine on page 1975
◆ **Pseudoephedrine Hydrochloride** see Pseudoephedrine on page 1633
◆ **Pseudoephedrine Sulfate** see Pseudoephedrine on page 1633
◆ **Pseudomonic Acid A** see Mupirocin on page 1324

Psyllium (SIL i yum)

Related Information
Laxatives, Classification and Properties *on page 2121*

Medication Safety Issues
Sound-alike/look-alike issues:
Fiberall® may be confused with Feverall®

Brand Names: U.S. Bulk-K [OTC]; Fiberall® [OTC]; Fibro-Lax [OTC]; Fibro-XL [OTC]; Hydrocil® Instant [OTC]; Konsyl-D™ [OTC]; Konsyl® Easy Mix™ [OTC]; Konsyl® Orange [OTC]; Konsyl® Original [OTC]; Konsyl® [OTC]; Metamucil® Plus Calcium [OTC]; Metamucil® Smooth Texture [OTC]; Metamucil® [OTC]; Natural Fiber Therapy Smooth Texture [OTC]; Natural Fiber Therapy [OTC]; Reguloid [OTC]

Brand Names: Canada Metamucil®

Index Terms Plantago Seed; Plantain Seed; Psyllium Husk; Psyllium Hydrophilic Mucilloid

Generic Availability (U.S.) Yes: Excludes wafers

Pharmacologic Category Antidiarrheal; Fiber Supplement; Laxative, Bulk-Producing

Use OTC labeling: Dietary fiber supplement; treatment of occasional constipation; reduce risk of coronary heart disease (CHD)

Unlabeled Use Treatment of diarrhea, chronic constipation, irritable bowel syndrome, inflammatory bowel disease, colon cancer, or diabetes

Contraindications Hypersensitivity to psyllium or any component of the formulation; fecal impaction; GI obstruction

Warnings/Precautions Use with caution in patients with esophageal strictures, ulcers, stenosis, intestinal adhesions, or difficulty swallowing. Use with caution in the elderly; may have insufficient fluid intake which may predispose them to fecal impaction and bowel obstruction. Products must be taken with at least 8 ounces of fluid in order to prevent choking. To reduce the risk of CHD, the soluble fiber from psyllium should be used in conjunction with a diet low in saturated fat and cholesterol. Some products may contain calcium, potassium, sodium, soy lecithin, or phenylalanine.

When used for self-medication (OTC), do not use in the presence of abdominal pain, nausea, or vomiting. Notify healthcare provider in case of sudden changes of bowel habits which last >2 weeks or in case of rectal bleeding. Not for self-treatment of constipation lasting >1 week

Adverse Reactions (Reflective of adult population; not specific for elderly) Frequency not defined.
Gastrointestinal: Abdominal cramps, constipation, diarrhea, esophageal or bowel obstruction
Respiratory: Bronchospasm
Miscellaneous: Anaphylaxis upon inhalation in susceptible individuals, rhinoconjunctivitis

Drug Interactions
Metabolism/Transport Effects None known.
Avoid Concomitant Use There are no known interactions where it is recommended to avoid concomitant use.
Increased Effect/Toxicity There are no known significant interactions involving an increase in effect.
Decreased Effect There are no known significant interactions involving a decrease in effect.

Mechanism of Action Psyllium is a soluble fiber. It absorbs water in the intestine to form a viscous liquid which promotes peristalsis and reduces transit time.

Pharmacodynamics/Kinetics
Onset of action: Relief of constipation: 12-72 hours
Absorption: None; small amounts of grain extracts present in the preparation have been reportedly absorbed following colonic hydrolysis

Dosage
Geriatric & Adult General dosing guidelines; consult specific product labeling.
Adequate intake for total fiber: Oral: **Note:** The definition of "fiber" varies, however, the soluble fiber in psyllium is only one type of fiber which makes up the daily recommended intake of total fiber.
Adults ≥51 years: Male: 30 g/day; Female: 21 g/day
Constipation: Oral: Psyllium: 2.5-30 g per day in divided doses
Reduce risk of CHD: Oral: Soluble fiber ≥7 g (psyllium seed husk ≥10.2 g) per day

Administration Inhalation of psyllium dust may cause sensitivity to psyllium (eg, runny nose, watery eyes, wheezing). Drink at least 8 ounces of liquid with each dose. Powder must be mixed in a glass of water or juice. Capsules should be swallowed one at a time. When more than one dose is required, they should be divided throughout the day. Separate dose by at least 2 hours from other drug therapies.

Monitoring Parameters Monitor for diarrhea, abdominal pain, bowel obstruction, or impaction

◀ **Pharmacotherapy Pearls** 3.4 g psyllium hydrophilic mucilloid per 7 g powder is equivalent to a rounded teaspoonful or one packet; fiber therapy results in increased frequency of defecation. Diabetic patients may need or prefer sugar-free products; psyllium using aspartame is available for diabetic patients. Bloating and flatulence are mostly a problem in first 4 weeks of therapy.

Special Geriatric Considerations Elderly may have insufficient fluid intake which may predispose them to fecal impaction and bowel obstruction. Patients should have a 1 month trial, with at least 14 g/day, before effects in bowel function are determined. Bloating and flatulence are mostly a problem in first 4 weeks of therapy. See Warnings/Precautions.

Dosage Forms Excipient information presented when available (limited, particularly for generics); consult specific product labeling.

Capsule, oral: 500 mg

Fibro-XL: 0.675 g [sugar free; provides dietary fiber 3.8 g and soluble fiber 3 g per 7 capsules]

Konsyl®: 0.52 g [sugar free; contains calcium 8 mg/capsule, potassium <11 mg/capsule, sodium 1 mg/capsule; provides dietary fiber 3 g and soluble fiber 2 g per 5 capsules]

Metamucil®: 0.52 g [contains potassium 5 mg/capsule; provides dietary fiber 3 g and soluble fiber 2.1 g per 6 capsules]

Metamucil® Plus Calcium: 0.52 g [contains calcium 60 mg/capsule, potassium 6 mg/capsule; provides dietary fiber 3 g and soluble fiber 2.1 g per 5 capsules]

Reguloid: 0.52 g [provides dietary fiber 3 g and soluble fiber 2 g per 6 capsules]

Powder, oral: (454 g)

Bulk-K: (392 g)

Fiberall®: (454 g) [sugar free; contains phenylalanine; orange flavor; psyllium is in combination with other fiber sources; also contains vitamins and minerals]

Fibro-Lax: (140 g, 392 g)

Hydrocil® Instant: (300 g) [sugar free]

Hydrocil® Instant: 3.5 g/packet (30s, 500s) [sugar free; provides dietary fiber 3 g and soluble fiber 2.4 g per packet]

Konsyl-D™: (325 g, 397 g, 500 g) [contains calcium, dextrose, potassium, sodium]

Konsyl-D™: 3.4 g/packet (100s, 500s) [contains calcium 6 mg/packet, dextrose 3.1 g/packet, potassium 31 mg/packet, sodium 3 mg/packet; provides dietary fiber 3 g and soluble fiber 2 g per packet]

Konsyl® Easy Mix™: (250 g) [sugar free; contains calcium, potassium, sodium]

Konsyl® Easy Mix™: 6 g/packet (500s) [sugar free; contains calcium 10 mg/packet, potassium 55 mg/packet, sodium 5 mg/packet; provides dietary fiber 5 g and soluble fiber 3 g per packet]

Konsyl® Orange: (538 g) [contains calcium, potassium, sodium, sucrose; orange flavor]

Konsyl® Orange: 3.4 g/packet (30s) [contains calcium 6 mg/packet, potassium 31 mg/packet, sodium 3 mg/packet, sucrose 8 g/packet; orange flavor; provides dietary fiber 3 g and soluble fiber 2 g per packet]

Konsyl® Orange: (425 g) [sugar free; contains calcium, phenylalanine, potassium, sodium; orange flavor]

Konsyl® Original: (300 g, 450 g) [sugar free; contains calcium, potassium, sodium]

Konsyl® Original: 6 g/packet (30s, 100s, 500s) [sugar free; contains calcium 10 mg/packet, potassium 55 mg/packet, sodium 5 mg/packet; provides dietary fiber 5 g and soluble fiber 3 g per packet]

Metamucil®: (390 g, 570 g, 870 g) [contains potassium, sodium; unflavored]

Metamucil®: (570 g, 870 g, 1254 g) [contains potassium, sodium; orange flavor]

Metamucil® Smooth Texture: (609 g, 912 g, 1368 g) [contains potassium, sodium; orange flavor]

Metamucil® Smooth Texture: 3.4 g/packet (30s) [contains potassium 30 mg/packet, sodium 5 mg/packet; orange flavor; provides dietary fiber 3 g and soluble fiber ~2 g per packet]

Metamucil® Smooth Texture: (283 g, 425 g, 660 g) [sugar free; contains phenylalanine, potassium, sodium; berry burst flavor]

Metamucil® Smooth Texture: (173 g, 300 g, 450 g, 660 g, 1020 g) [sugar free; contains phenylalanine, potassium, sodium; orange flavor]

Metamucil® Smooth Texture: (288 g, 432 g, 684 g) [sugar free; contains phenylalanine, potassium, sodium; pink lemonade flavor]

Metamucil® Smooth Texture: (300 g, 450 g, 690 g) [sugar free; contains potassium, sodium; unflavored]

Metamucil® Smooth Texture: 3.4 g/packet (30s) [sugar free; contains phenylalanine 16 mg/packet, potassium 30 mg/packet, sodium 5 mg/packet; berry burst flavor; provides dietary fiber 3 g and soluble fiber ~2 g per packet]

Metamucil® Smooth Texture: 3.4 g/packet (30s) [sugar free; contains phenylalanine 25 mg/packet, potassium 30 mg/packet, sodium 5 mg/packet; orange flavor; provides dietary fiber 3 g and soluble fiber ~2 g per packet]

Natural Fiber Therapy: (390 g, 539 g) [natural flavor]

Natural Fiber Therapy: (390 g, 539 g) [contains sodium; orange flavor]
Natural Fiber Therapy Smooth Texture: (300 g) [sugar free; orange flavor]
Reguloid: (369 g, 540 g) [contains sodium; orange flavor]
Reguloid: (369 g, 540 g) [contains sodium; regular flavor]
Reguloid: (284 g, 426 g) [sugar free; contains phenylalanine, sodium; orange flavor]
Reguloid: (284 g, 426 g) [sugar free; contains phenylalanine, sodium; regular flavor]
Wafer, oral:
  Metamucil®: 3.4 g/2 wafers (24s) [contains potassium 60 mg/2 wafers, sodium 20 mg/2 wafers, soya lecithin; apple flavor; provides dietary fiber 6 g and soluble fiber 3 g per 2 wafers]
  Metamucil®: 3.4 g/2 wafers (24s) [contains potassium 60 mg/2 wafers, sodium 20 mg/2 wafers, soya lecithin; cinnamon-spice flavor; provides dietary fiber 6 g and soluble fiber 3 g per 2 wafers]

- ◆ **Psyllium Husk** *see* Psyllium *on page 1635*
- ◆ **Psyllium Hydrophilic Mucilloid** *see* Psyllium *on page 1635*
- ◆ **Pteroylglutamic Acid** *see* Folic Acid *on page 836*
- ◆ **PTU (error-prone abbreviation)** *see* Propylthiouracil *on page 1627*
- ◆ **Pulmicort Flexhaler®** *see* Budesonide (Systemic, Oral Inhalation) *on page 227*
- ◆ **Pulmicort Respules®** *see* Budesonide (Systemic, Oral Inhalation) *on page 227*
- ◆ **Purified Chick Embryo Cell** *see* Rabies Vaccine *on page 1663*
- ◆ **Purinethol®** *see* Mercaptopurine *on page 1212*

Pyrazinamide (peer a ZIN a mide)

Related Information
  Antimicrobial Drugs of Choice *on page 2163*
Brand Names: Canada Tebrazid™
Index Terms Pyrazinoic Acid Amide
Generic Availability (U.S.) Yes
Pharmacologic Category Antitubercular Agent
Use Adjunctive treatment of tuberculosis in combination with other antituberculosis agents
Contraindications Hypersensitivity to pyrazinamide or any component of the formulation; acute gout; severe hepatic damage
Warnings/Precautions Use with caution in patients with a history of alcoholism, renal failure, chronic gout, diabetes mellitus, or porphyria. Dose-related hepatotoxicity ranging from transient ALT/AST elevations to jaundice, hepatitis and/or liver atrophy (rare) has occurred. Use with caution in patients receiving concurrent medications associated with hepatotoxicity (particularly with rifampin).
Adverse Reactions (Reflective of adult population; not specific for elderly) 1% to 10%:
  Central nervous system: Malaise
  Gastrointestinal: Anorexia, nausea, vomiting
  Neuromuscular & skeletal: Arthralgia, myalgia
Drug Interactions
  Metabolism/Transport Effects None known.
  Avoid Concomitant Use There are no known interactions where it is recommended to avoid concomitant use.
  Increased Effect/Toxicity
    Pyrazinamide may increase the levels/effects of: CycloSPORINE (Systemic); Rifampin
  Decreased Effect
    Pyrazinamide may decrease the levels/effects of: CycloSPORINE
Stability Store at controlled room temperature of 15°C to 30°C (59°F to 86°F).
Mechanism of Action Converted to pyrazinoic acid in susceptible strains of *Mycobacterium* which lowers the pH of the environment; exact mechanism of action has not been elucidated
Pharmacodynamics/Kinetics Bacteriostatic or bactericidal depending on drug's concentration at infection site

Absorption: Well absorbed
Distribution: Widely into body tissues and fluids including liver, lung, and CSF
  Relative diffusion from blood into CSF: Adequate with or without inflammation (exceeds usual MICs)
  CSF:blood level ratio: Inflamed meninges: 100%
Protein binding: 50%
Metabolism: Hepatic
Half-life elimination: 9-10 hours
Time to peak, serum: Within 2 hours
Excretion: Urine (4% as unchanged drug)

Dosage

Adult Tuberculosis treatment: Oral: **Note:** Used as part of a multidrug regimen. Treatment regimens consist of an initial 2-month phase, followed by a continuation phase of 4 or 7 additional months; pyrazinamide is administered in the initial phase of treatment.

Suggested dosing based on lean body weight (Blumberg, 2003; CDC, 2003):

Daily therapy:
40-55 kg: 1000 mg
56-75 kg: 1500 mg
76-90 kg: 2000 mg (maximum dose regardless of weight)

Twice weekly directly observed therapy (DOT):
40-55 kg: 2000 mg
56-75 kg: 3000 mg
76-90 kg: 4000 mg (maximum dose regardless of weight)

Three times/week DOT:
40-55 kg: 1500 mg
56-75 kg: 2500 mg
76-90 kg: 3000 mg (maximum dose regardless of weight)

Renal Impairment Adults: Cl_{cr} <30 mL/minute or receiving hemodialysis: Treatment of TB: 25-35 mg/kg/dose 3 times per week administered after dialysis (Blumberg, 2003; CDC, 2003)

Monitoring Parameters Periodic liver function tests, serum uric acid, sputum culture, chest x-ray 2-3 months into treatment and at completion

Test Interactions Reacts with Acetest® and Ketostix® to produce pinkish-brown color

Special Geriatric Considerations Most elderly acquired their *Mycobacterium tuberculosis* infection before effective chemotherapy was available; however, older persons with new infections (not reactivation), or who are from areas where drug-resistant *M. tuberculosis* is endemic, or who are HIV-infected should receive 3-4 drug therapies including pyrazinamide.

Dosage Forms Excipient information presented when available (limited, particularly for generics); consult specific product labeling.
Tablet, oral: 500 mg

◆ **Pyrazinoic Acid Amide** *see* Pyrazinamide *on page 1637*

◆ **Pyri-500 [OTC]** *see* Pyridoxine *on page 1640*

◆ **Pyridium®** *see* Phenazopyridine *on page 1516*

Pyridostigmine (peer id oh STIG meen)

Medication Safety Issues
Sound-alike/look-alike issues:
Pyridostigmine may be confused with physostigmine
Regonol® may be confused with Reglan®, Renagel®

Brand Names: U.S. Mestinon®; Mestinon® Timespan®; Regonol®

Brand Names: Canada Mestinon®; Mestinon®-SR

Index Terms Pyridostigmine Bromide

Generic Availability (U.S.) Yes: Tablet

Pharmacologic Category Acetylcholinesterase Inhibitor

Use Symptomatic treatment of myasthenia gravis; antagonism of nondepolarizing neuromuscular blockers
Military use: Pretreatment for Soman nerve gas exposure

Contraindications Hypersensitivity to pyridostigmine, bromides, or any component of the formulation; GI or GU obstruction

Warnings/Precautions Use with caution in patients with epilepsy, bradycardia, hyperthyroidism, cardiac arrhythmias, or peptic ulcer; use with extreme caution in patients with asthma or bronchospastic disease; adequate facilities should be available for cardiopulmonary resuscitation when testing and adjusting dose for myasthenia gravis; have atropine and epinephrine ready to treat hypersensitivity reactions; overdosage may result in cholinergic crisis, this must be distinguished from myasthenic crisis; anticholinesterase insensitivity can develop for brief or prolonged periods. Regonol® injection contains 1% benzyl alcohol as the preservative.
[U.S. Boxed Warning]: Regonol® injection must be administered by trained personnel.

Adverse Reactions (Reflective of adult population; not specific for elderly) Frequency not defined.
Cardiovascular: Arrhythmias (especially bradycardia), AV block, cardiac arrest, decreased carbon monoxide, flushing, hypotension, nodal rhythm, nonspecific ECG changes, syncope, tachycardia
Central nervous system: Convulsions, dizziness, drowsiness, dysphonia, headache, loss of consciousness

Dermatologic: Skin rash, thrombophlebitis (I.V.), urticaria

Gastrointestinal: Abdominal pain, diarrhea, dysphagia, flatulence, hyperperistalsis, nausea, salivation, stomach cramps, vomiting

Genitourinary: Urinary urgency

Neuromuscular & skeletal: Arthralgia, dysarthria, fasciculations, muscle cramps, myalgia, spasms, weakness

Ocular: Amblyopia, lacrimation, small pupils

Respiratory: Bronchial secretions increased, bronchiolar constriction, bronchospasm, dyspnea, laryngospasm, respiratory arrest, respiratory depression, respiratory muscle paralysis

Miscellaneous: Allergic reactions, anaphylaxis, diaphoresis increased

Drug Interactions

Metabolism/Transport Effects None known.

Avoid Concomitant Use There are no known interactions where it is recommended to avoid concomitant use.

Increased Effect/Toxicity

Pyridostigmine may increase the levels/effects of: Beta-Blockers; Cholinergic Agonists; Succinylcholine

The levels/effects of Pyridostigmine may be increased by: Corticosteroids (Systemic)

Decreased Effect

Pyridostigmine may decrease the levels/effects of: Neuromuscular-Blocking Agents (Non-depolarizing)

The levels/effects of Pyridostigmine may be decreased by: Dipyridamole; Methocarbamol

Stability

Injection: Protect from light.

Tablet:

30 mg: Store under refrigeration at 2°C to 8°C (36°F to 46°F). Protect from light. Stable at room temperature for up to 3 months.

Mestinon®: Store at 25°C (77°F). Protect from moisture.

Mechanism of Action Inhibits destruction of acetylcholine by acetylcholinesterase which facilitates transmission of impulses across myoneural junction

Pharmacodynamics/Kinetics

Onset of action: Oral, I.M.: 15-30 minutes; I.V. injection: 2-5 minutes

Duration: Oral: Up to 6-8 hours (due to slow absorption); I.V.: 2-3 hours

Absorption: Oral: Very poor

Distribution: 19 ± 12 L

Metabolism: Hepatic

Bioavailability: 10% to 20%

Half-life elimination: 1-2 hours; Renal failure: ≤6 hours

Excretion: Urine (80% to 90% as unchanged drug)

Dosage

Geriatric & Adult

Myasthenia gravis:

Oral: Highly individualized dosing ranges: 60-1500 mg/day, usually 600 mg/day divided into 5-6 doses, spaced to provide maximum relief

Sustained release formulation: Highly individualized dosing ranges: 180-540 mg once or twice daily (doses separated by at least 6 hours); **Note:** Most clinicians reserve sustained release dosage form for bedtime dose only.

I.M. or slow I.V. Push: To supplement oral dosage pre- and postoperatively, during myasthenic crisis, or when oral therapy is impractical): ~1/30th of oral dose; observe patient closely for cholinergic reactions

I.V. infusion: To supplement oral dosage pre- and postoperatively, during myasthenic crisis, or when oral therapy is impractical): Initial: 2 mg/hour with gradual titration in increments of 0.5-1 mg/hour, up to a maximum rate of 4 mg/hour

Pretreatment for Soman nerve gas exposure (military use): Oral: 30 mg every 8 hours beginning several hours prior to exposure; discontinue at first sign of nerve agent exposure, then begin atropine and pralidoxime

Reversal of nondepolarizing muscle relaxants: I.V.: 0.1-0.25 mg/kg/dose; 10-20 mg is usually sufficient (full recovery usually occurs ≤15 minutes, but ≥30 minutes may be required).

Note: Atropine sulfate (0.6-1.2 mg) I.V. immediately prior to pyridostigmine to minimize side effects:

Renal Impairment Lower dosages may be required due to prolonged elimination; no specific recommendations have been published.

Administration When giving for reversal of neuromuscular blockade, keep patient well ventilated until recovered

Monitoring Parameters Observe for cholinergic reactions, particularly when administered I.V.

Test Interactions Increased aminotransferase [ALT/AST] (S), increased amylase (S)

Pharmacotherapy Pearls Myasthenia gravis: Not a cure; patient may develop resistance to the drug; normally, sustained release dosage form is used at bedtime for patients who complain of morning weakness

Special Geriatric Considerations Many elderly may have pulmonary or cardiovascular diseases which will require cautious use of pyridostigmine.

Dosage Forms Excipient information presented when available (limited, particularly for generics); consult specific product labeling.

Injection, solution, as bromide:
Regonol®: 5 mg/mL (2 mL) [contains benzyl alcohol]
Syrup, oral, as bromide:
Mestinon®: 60 mg/5 mL (480 mL) [contains ethanol 5%, sodium benzoate; raspberry flavor]
Tablet, oral, as bromide: 60 mg
Mestinon®: 60 mg [scored]
Tablet, sustained release, oral, as bromide:
Mestinon® Timespan®: 180 mg [scored]

◆ **Pyridostigmine Bromide** see Pyridostigmine on page 1638

Pyridoxine (peer i DOKS een)

Medication Safety Issues
Sound-alike/look-alike issues:
Pyridoxine may be confused with paroxetine, pralidoxime, Pyridium®
International issues:
Doxal [Brazil] may be confused with Doxil brand name for DOXOrubicin [U.S.]
Doxal: Brand name for pyridoxine/thiamine combination [Brazil], but also the brand name for doxepin [Finland]

Brand Names: U.S. Aminoxin® [OTC]; Pyri-500 [OTC]

Index Terms B6; B$_6$; Pyridoxine Hydrochloride; Vitamin B$_6$

Generic Availability (U.S.) Yes

Pharmacologic Category Vitamin, Water Soluble

Use Prevention and treatment of vitamin B$_6$ deficiency

Unlabeled Use Treatment and prophylaxis of neurological toxicities (ie, seizures, coma) associated with isoniazid and Gyromitrin-containing mushroom (false morel) overdose/toxicity

Contraindications Hypersensitivity to pyridoxine or any component of the formulation

Warnings/Precautions Severe, permanent peripheral neuropathies have been reported; neurotoxicity is more common with long-term administration of large doses (>2 g/day). Dependence and withdrawal may occur with doses >200 mg/day. Single vitamin deficiency is rare; evaluate for other deficiencies. Some parenteral products contain aluminum; use caution in patients with impaired renal function.

Pharmacy supply of emergency antidotes: Guidelines suggest that at least 8-24 g be stocked. This is enough to treat 1 patient weighing 100 kg for an initial 8- to 24-hour period. In areas where tuberculosis is common, hospitals should consider stocking 24 g. This is enough to treat 1 patient for 24 hours (Dart, 2009).

Adverse Reactions (Reflective of adult population; not specific for elderly) Frequency not defined.
Central nervous system: Headache, seizure (following very large I.V. doses), somnolence
Endocrine & metabolic: Acidosis, folic acid decreased
Gastrointestinal: Nausea
Hepatic: AST increased
Neuromuscular & skeletal: Neuropathy, paresthesia
Miscellaneous: Allergic reactions

Drug Interactions
Metabolism/Transport Effects None known.
Avoid Concomitant Use There are no known interactions where it is recommended to avoid concomitant use.
Increased Effect/Toxicity There are no known significant interactions involving an increase in effect.
Decreased Effect
Pyridoxine may decrease the levels/effects of: Altretamine; Barbiturates; Fosphenytoin; Levodopa; Phenytoin

Stability Injection: Store at 20°C to 25°C (68°F to 77°F). Protect from light.

Mechanism of Action Precursor to pyridoxal, which functions in the metabolism of proteins, carbohydrates, and fats; pyridoxal also aids in the release of liver and muscle-stored glycogen and in the synthesis of GABA (within the central nervous system) and heme

Pharmacodynamics/Kinetics
Absorption: Enteral, parenteral: Well absorbed
Metabolism: Hepatic to 4-pyridoxic acid (active form) and other metabolites
Half-life elimination: Biologic: 15-20 days
Excretion: Urine

Dosage
Geriatric & Adult
Recommended daily allowance (RDA): Oral (IOM, 1998):
19-50 years: 1.3 mg
≥51 years:
Females: 1.5 mg
Males: 1.7 mg
Dietary deficiency: I.M., I.V.: 10-20 mg/day for 3 weeks, followed by oral therapy. Doses up to 600 mg/day may be needed with pyridoxine dependency syndrome.
Prevention of peripheral neuropathy associated with isoniazid therapy for *Mycobacterium tuberculosis*: Oral: Adults: 25-50 mg/day (CDC, 2009)
Treatment of isoniazid-induced seizures and/or coma (unlabeled use): I.V.:
Acute ingestion of known amount: Initial: A total dose of pyridoxine equal to the amount of isoniazid ingested (maximum dose: 5 g); administer at a rate of 0.5-1 g/minute until seizures stop or the maximum initial dose has been administered; may repeat every 5-10 minutes as needed to control persistent seizure activity and/or CNS toxicity. If seizures stop prior to the administration of the calculated initial dose, infuse the remaining pyridoxine over 4-6 hours (Howland, 2006; Morrow, 2006).
Acute ingestion of unknown amount: Initial: 5 g; administer at a rate of 0.5-1 g/minute; may repeat every 5-10 minutes as needed to control persistent seizure activity and/or CNS toxicity (Howland, 2006; Morrow, 2006)
Prevention of isoniazid-induced seizures and/or coma (unlabeled use): I.V.: Asymptomatic patients who present within 2 hours of ingesting a potentially toxic amount of isoniazid should receive a prophylactic dose of pyridoxine (Boyer, 2006). Dosing recommendations are the same as for the treatment of symptomatic patients.
Treatment of seizures from acute Gyromitrin-containing mushroom toxicity (unlabeled use; Diaz, 2005): I.V.: 25 mg/kg over 15-30 minutes; repeat dose as needed to control seizures

Administration Burning may occur at the injection site after I.M. or SubQ administration; seizures have occurred following I.V. administration of very large doses.

Isoniazid toxicity (unlabeled use): Initial doses should be administered at a rate of 0.5-1 g/minute. If the parenteral formulation is not available, anecdotal reports suggest that pyridoxine tablets may be crushed and made into a slurry and given at the same dose orally or via nasogastric (NG) tube (Boyer, 2006). Oral administration is not recommended for acutely poisoned patients with seizure activity.

Monitoring Parameters For treatment of isoniazid or Gyromitrin-containing mushroom toxicity: Anion gap, arterial blood gases, electrolytes, neurological exam, seizure activity

Reference Range Over 50 ng/mL (SI: 243 nmol/L) (varies considerably with method). A broad range is ~25-80 ng/mL (SI: 122-389 nmol/L). HPLC method for pyridoxal phosphate has normal range of 3.5-18 ng/mL (SI: 17-88 nmol/L).

Test Interactions False positive urobilinogen spot test using Ehrlich's reagent

Special Geriatric Considerations Use with caution in patients with Parkinson's disease treated with levodopa.

Dosage Forms Excipient information presented when available (limited, particularly for generics); consult specific product labeling.
Capsule, oral, as hydrochloride: 50 mg, 250 mg
Aminoxin®: 20 mg
Injection, solution, as hydrochloride: 100 mg/mL (1 mL)
Liquid, oral, as hydrochloride: 200 mg/5 mL (120 mL)
Tablet, oral, as hydrochloride: 25 mg, 50 mg, 100 mg, 250 mg, 500 mg
Tablet, sustained release, oral, as hydrochloride:
Pyri-500: 500 mg

◆ **Pyridoxine Hydrochloride** see Pyridoxine on page 1640
◆ **QAB149** see Indacaterol on page 989
◆ **Q-dryl [OTC]** see DiphenhydrAMINE (Systemic) on page 556
◆ **Qnasl™** see Beclomethasone (Nasal) on page 192
◆ **Q-Pap [OTC]** see Acetaminophen on page 31
◆ **Q-Pap Children's [OTC]** see Acetaminophen on page 31

QUAZEPAM

- ◆ **Q-Pap Extra Strength [OTC]** *see* Acetaminophen *on page* 31
- ◆ **Q-Pap Infant's [OTC]** *see* Acetaminophen *on page* 31
- ◆ **Q-Tussin [OTC]** *see* GuaiFENesin *on page* 904
- ◆ **Q-Tussin DM [OTC]** *see* Guaifenesin and Dextromethorphan *on page* 906
- ◆ **Qualaquin®** *see* QuiNINE *on page* 1655

Quazepam (KWAZ e pam)

Related Information
Anxiolytic, Sedative/Hypnotic, and Miscellaneous Benzodiazepines *on page* 2106
Beers Criteria – Potentially Inappropriate Medications for Geriatrics *on page* 2183

Medication Safety Issues
Sound-alike/look-alike issues:
Quazepam may be confused with oxazepam
BEERS Criteria medication:
This drug may be potentially inappropriate for use in geriatric patients (Quality of evidence - high; Strength of recommendation - strong).

Brand Names: U.S. Doral®
Brand Names: Canada Doral®
Generic Availability (U.S.) No
Pharmacologic Category Benzodiazepine
Use Treatment of insomnia
Medication Guide Available Yes
Contraindications Hypersensitivity to quazepam, other benzodiazepines, or any component of the formulation; sleep apnea

Note: Product labeling does not include narrow-angle glaucoma; however, use in narrow-angle glaucoma is contraindicated with other benzodiazepines.

Warnings/Precautions Should be used only after evaluation of potential causes of sleep disturbance. Failure of sleep disturbance to resolve after 7-10 days may indicate psychiatric or medical illness. A worsening of insomnia or the emergence of new abnormalities of thought or behavior may represent unrecognized psychiatric or medical illness and requires immediate and careful evaluation. Use with caution in elderly or debilitated patients, patients with hepatic disease (including alcoholics), or renal impairment. Use with caution in patients with respiratory disease or impaired gag reflex. Avoid use in patients with sleep apnea.

Causes CNS depression (dose related) resulting in sedation, dizziness, confusion, or ataxia which may impair physical and mental capabilities. Patients must be cautioned about performing tasks which require mental alertness (operating machinery or driving). Use with caution in patients receiving other CNS depressants or psychoactive agents. Postmarketing studies have indicated that the use of hypnotic/sedative agents for sleep has been associated with hypersensitivity reactions including anaphylaxis as well as angioedema. An increased risk for hazardous sleep-related activities such as sleep-driving; cooking and eating food, and making phone calls while asleep have also been noted. Effects with other sedative drugs or ethanol may be potentiated. Benzodiazepines have been associated with falls and traumatic injury and should be used with extreme caution in patients who are at risk of these events. In older adults, benzodiazepines increase the risk of impaired cognition, delirium, falls, fractures, and motor vehicle accidents. Due to increased sensitivity in this age group and slower metabolism of long-acting agents (such as quazepam), avoid use for treatment of insomnia, agitation, or delirium (Beers Criteria).

Use caution in patients with depression, particularly if suicidal risk may be present. Use with caution in patients with a history of drug dependence. Benzodiazepines have been associated with dependence and acute withdrawal symptoms on discontinuation or reduction in dose. Acute withdrawal, including seizures, may be precipitated after administration of flumazenil to patients receiving long-term benzodiazepine therapy.

Benzodiazepines have been associated with anterograde amnesia. Paradoxical reactions, including hyperactive or aggressive behavior have been reported with benzodiazepines, particularly in psychiatric patients. Does not have analgesic, antidepressant, or antipsychotic properties. Use lowest effective dose.

Adverse Reactions (Reflective of adult population; not specific for elderly)
>10%: Central nervous system: Daytime drowsiness (12%)
<10%:
  Central nervous system: Headache (5%), dizziness (2%), fatigue (2%)
  Gastrointestinal: Xerostomia (2%), dyspepsia (1%)

Frequency not defined. **Note:** Asterisked (*) reactions are those reported with benzodiaze-pines.

Cardiovascular: Palpitation

Central nervous system: Abnormal thinking, agitation, amnesia, anxiety, apathy, ataxia, confusion, depression, dystonia*, euphoria, hallucinations*, hyper-/hypokinesia, incoordination, irritability*, malaise, nervousness, nightmare, paranoid reaction, sleep disturbances*, slurred speech*, speech disorder, stimulation*

Dermatologic: Pruritus, rash

Endocrine & metabolic: Libido decreased, menstrual irregularities*

Gastrointestinal: Abdominal pain, abnormal taste perception, anorexia, constipation, diarrhea, nausea

Genitourinary: Impotence, incontinence, urinary retention*

Hepatic: Jaundice*

Neuromuscular & skeletal: Dysarthria*, muscle spasticity*, tremor, weakness

Ocular: Abnormal vision, cataract

Miscellaneous: Drug dependence, withdrawal*

Drug Interactions

Metabolism/Transport Effects Substrate of CYP3A4 (minor); **Note:** Assignment of Major/Minor substrate status based on clinically relevant drug interaction potential; **Inhibits** CYP2B6 (moderate)

Avoid Concomitant Use

Avoid concomitant use of Quazepam with any of the following: Azelastine; Azelastine (Nasal); Methadone; Mirtazapine; OLANZapine; Paraldehyde

Increased Effect/Toxicity

Quazepam may increase the levels/effects of: Alcohol (Ethyl); Azelastine; Azelastine (Nasal); Buprenorphine; CloZAPine; CNS Depressants; CYP2B6 Substrates; Fosphenytoin; Methadone; Methotrimeprazine; Metyrosine; Mirtazapine; Paraldehyde; Phenytoin; Selective Serotonin Reuptake Inhibitors; Zolpidem

The levels/effects of Quazepam may be increased by: Aprepitant; Calcium Channel Blockers (Nondihydropyridine); Cimetidine; Contraceptives (Estrogens); Contraceptives (Progestins); Droperidol; Fosaprepitant; Grapefruit Juice; HydrOXYzine; Isoniazid; Macrolide Antibiotics; Methotrimeprazine; OLANZapine; Proton Pump Inhibitors; Selective Serotonin Reuptake Inhibitors

Decreased Effect

The levels/effects of Quazepam may be decreased by: CarBAMazepine; Rifamycin Derivatives; St Johns Wort; Theophylline Derivatives; Tocilizumab; Yohimbine

Ethanol/Nutrition/Herb Interactions

Ethanol: Ethanol may increase CNS depression. Management: Avoid ethanol.

Food: Grapefruit juice may decrease the metabolism of quazepam. Management: Avoid grapefruit juice.

Herb/Nutraceutical: St John's wort may increase the metabolism of quazepam. Management: Avoid St John's wort.

Stability Store at controlled room temperature of 20°C to 25°C (68°F to 77°F).

Mechanism of Action Binds to stereospecific benzodiazepine receptors on the postsynaptic GABA neuron at several sites within the central nervous system, including the limbic system, reticular formation. Enhancement of the inhibitory effect of GABA on neuronal excitability results by increased neuronal membrane permeability to chloride ions. This shift in chloride ions results in hyperpolarization (a less excitable state) and stabilization.

Pharmacodynamics/Kinetics

Absorption: Rapid

Protein binding: >95%

Metabolism: Hepatic; forms metabolites (active)- 2-oxoquasepam and N-desalkyl-2-oxoquazepam

Half-life elimination, serum: Quazepam, 2-oxoquasepam: 39 hours; N-desalkyl-2-oxoquazepam: 73 hours

Time to peak, plasma: ~2 hours

Excretion: Urine (31%, only trace amounts as unchanged drug); feces (23%)

Dosage

Geriatric Dosing should be cautious; begin at lower end of dosing range (ie, 7.5 mg)

Adult Hypnotic: Oral: Initial: 15 mg at bedtime; in some patients, the dose may be reduced to 7.5 mg after a few nights

Renal Impairment Use caution; monitor for signs of excessive sedation or impaired coordination.

Hepatic Impairment Use caution; monitor for signs of excessive sedation or impaired coordination.

Monitoring Parameters Respiratory status; mental status

Pharmacotherapy Pearls More likely than short-acting benzodiazepine to cause daytime sedation and fatigue. Classified as a long-acting benzodiazepine hypnotic (eg, flurazepam), this long duration of action may prevent withdrawal symptoms when therapy is discontinued. Abrupt discontinuation after sustained use (generally >10 days) may cause withdrawal symptoms.

Special Geriatric Considerations Because of the long half-life of one of its active metabolites, quazepam is not a drug of choice in the elderly. Long-acting benzodiazepines have been associated with falls in the elderly and are not recommended for use in older patients.

This medication is considered to be potentially inappropriate in this patient population (Beers Criteria: Quality of evidence - high; Strength of recommendation - strong).

Controlled Substance C-IV

Dosage Forms Excipient information presented when available (limited, particularly for generics); consult specific product labeling.

Tablet, oral:

Doral®: 15 mg

◆ **Quenalin [OTC]** *see* DiphenhydrAMINE (Systemic) *on page* 556
◆ **Questran®** *see* Cholestyramine Resin *on page* 367
◆ **Questran® Light** *see* Cholestyramine Resin *on page* 367

QUEtiapine (kwe TYE a peen)

Related Information

Antipsychotic Agents *on page* 2103
Atypical Antipsychotics *on page* 2107
Beers Criteria – Potentially Inappropriate Medications for Geriatrics *on page* 2183

Medication Safety Issues

Sound-alike/look-alike issues:

QUEtiapine may be confused with OLANZapine

SEROquel® may be confused with Serzone, SINEquan®

BEERS Criteria medication:

This drug may be potentially inappropriate for use in geriatric patients (Quality of evidence - moderate; Strength of recommendation - strong).

Brand Names: U.S. SEROquel XR®; SEROquel®

Brand Names: Canada Apo-Quetiapine®; CO Quetiapine; Dom-Quetiapine; JAMP-Quetiapine; Mylan-Quetiapine; PHL-Quetiapine; PMS-Quetiapine; PRO-Quetiapine; ratio-Quetiapine; Riva-Quetiapine; Sandoz-Quetiapine; Seroquel XR®; Seroquel®; Teva-Quetiapine

Index Terms Quetiapine Fumarate

Generic Availability (U.S.) Yes: Excludes extended release tablet

Pharmacologic Category Antipsychotic Agent, Atypical

Use Treatment of schizophrenia; treatment of acute manic or mixed episodes associated with bipolar I disorder (as monotherapy or in combination with lithium or divalproex); maintenance treatment of bipolar I disorder (in combination with lithium or divalproex); treatment of acute depressive episodes associated with bipolar disorder; adjunctive treatment of major depressive disorder

Unlabeled Use Autism; delirium in the critically-ill patient; psychosis/agitation related to Alzheimer's dementia

Medication Guide Available Yes

Contraindications There are no contraindications listed in manufacturer's labeling.

Canadian labeling: Hypersensitivity to quetiapine or any component of the formulation

Warnings/Precautions [U.S. Boxed Warning]: Antidepressants increase the risk of suicidal thinking and behavior in children, adolescents, and young adults (18-24 years of age) with major depressive disorder (MDD) and other psychiatric disorders; consider risk prior to prescribing. Short-term studies did not show an increased risk in patients >24 years of age and showed a decreased risk in patients ≥65 years. Closely monitor all patients for clinical worsening, suicidality, or unusual changes in behavior; particularly during the initial 1-2 months of therapy or during periods of dosage adjustments (increased or decreases); the patient's family or caregiver should be instructed to closely observe the patient and communicate condition with healthcare provider. A medication guide concerning the use of antidepressants should be dispensed with each prescription.

[U.S. Boxed Warning]: Elderly patients with dementia-related psychosis treated with antipsychotics are at an increased risk of death compared to placebo. Most deaths appeared to be either cardiovascular (eg, heart failure, sudden death) or infectious (eg, pneumonia) in nature. Quetiapine is not approved for the treatment of dementia-related psychosis.

Leukopenia, neutropenia, and agranulocytosis (sometimes fatal) have been reported in clinical trials and postmarketing reports with antipsychotic use; presence of risk factors (eg, pre-existing low WBC or history of drug-induced leuko-/neutropenia) should prompt periodic blood count assessment. Discontinue therapy at first signs of blood dyscrasias or if absolute neutrophil count <1000/mm^3.

May be sedating, use with caution in disorders where CNS depression is a feature. Use with caution in Parkinson's disease. May induce orthostatic hypotension associated with dizziness, tachycardia, and, in some cases, syncope, especially during the initial dose titration period. Should be used with particular caution in patients with known cardiovascular disease (history of MI or ischemic heart disease, heart failure, or conduction abnormalities), cerebrovascular disease, or conditions that predispose to hypotension. Use has been associated with QT prolongation; postmarketing reports have occurred in patients with concomitant illness, quetiapine overdose, or who were receiving concomitant therapy known to affect QT interval or cause electrolyte imbalance. Esophageal dysmotility and aspiration have been associated with antipsychotic use; use with caution in patients at risk of aspiration pneumonia (eg, Alzheimer's disease). May cause dose-related decreases in thyroid levels, including cases requiring thyroid replacement therapy. Development of cataracts has been observed in animal studies; lens changes have been observed in humans during long-term treatment. Lens examination on initiation of therapy and every 6 months thereafter is recommended.

Due to anticholinergic effects, use with caution in patients with decreased gastrointestinal motility, urinary retention, BPH, xerostomia, visual problems, and narrow-angle glaucoma. Relative to other antipsychotics, quetiapine has a moderate potency of cholinergic blockade. May cause extrapyramidal symptoms (EPS), pseudoparkinsonism, and/or tardive dyskinesia. Risk of dystonia (and probably other EPS) may be greater with increased doses, use of conventional antipsychotics, males, and younger patients. Impaired core body temperature regulation may occur; caution with strenuous exercise, heat exposure, dehydration, and concomitant medication possessing anticholinergic effects. Neuroleptic malignant syndrome (NMS) is a potentially fatal symptom complex that has been reported in association with administration of antipsychotic drugs. Clinical manifestations of NMS are hyperpyrexia, muscle rigidity, altered mental status, and evidence of autonomic instability (irregular pulse or blood pressure, tachycardia, diaphoresis, and cardiac dysrhythmia). Management of NMS should include immediate discontinuation of antipsychotic drugs and other drugs not essential to concurrent therapy, intensive symptomatic treatment and medication monitoring, and treatment of any concomitant medical problems for which specific treatment are available.

Use caution in patients with a history of seizures. May cause decreases in total free thyroxine, elevations of liver enzymes, cholesterol levels, and/or triglyceride increases. Rare cases of priapism have been reported. May increase prolactin levels; clinical significance of hyperprolactinemia in patients with breast cancer or other prolactin-dependent tumors is unknown.

Use in elderly patients with dementia is associated with an increased risk of mortality and cerebrovascular accidents; avoid antipsychotic use for behavioral problems associated with dementia unless alternative nonpharmacologic therapies have failed and patient may harm self or others. In addition, use may cause or exacerbate syndrome of inappropriate antidiuretic hormone secretion or hyponatremia; monitor sodium closely with initiation or dosage adjustments in older adults (Beers Criteria).

May cause hyperglycemia; in some cases may be extreme and associated with ketoacidosis, hyperosmolar coma, or death. Use with caution in patients with diabetes or other disorders of glucose regulation; monitor for worsening of glucose control. Significant weight gain has been observed with antipsychotic therapy; incidence varies with product. Monitor waist circumference and BMI. Patients using immediate release tablets may be switched to extended release tablets at the same total daily dose taken once daily. Dosage adjustments may be necessary based on response and tolerability. May cause withdrawal symptoms (rare) with abrupt cessation; gradually taper dose during discontinuation.

Adverse Reactions (Reflective of adult population; not specific for elderly) Actual frequency may be dependent upon dose and/or indication. Unless otherwise noted, frequency of adverse effects is reported for adult patients; spectrum and incidence of adverse effects similar in children (with significant exceptions noted).

>10%:

Cardiovascular: Diastolic blood pressure increased (children and adolescents, 41%), systolic blood pressure increased (children and adolescents, 15%)

Central nervous system: Somnolence (18% to 57%), headache (7% to 21%), agitation (5% to 20%), dizziness (1% to 18%), fatigue (3% to 14%), extrapyramidal symptoms (1% to 13%)

Endocrine & metabolic: Triglycerides increased (≥200 mg/dL, 8% to 22%), HDL cholesterol decreased (≤40 mg/dL, 6% to 19%), total cholesterol increased (≥240 mg/dL, 7% to 18%), LDL cholesterol increased (≥160 mg/dL, 4% to 17%), hyperglycemia (≥200 mg/dL post glucose challenge or fasting glucose ≥126 mg/dL, 2% to 12%)

Gastrointestinal: Xerostomia (9% to 44%), weight gain (dose related; 3% to 23%), appetite increased (2% to 12%), constipation (6% to 11%)

1% to 10%:

Cardiovascular: Orthostatic hypotension (2% to 7%; children and adolescents <1%), tachycardia (1% to 6%), syncope (<5%), palpitation (4%), peripheral edema (4%), hypotension (3%), hypertension (1% to 2%)

Central nervous system: Insomnia (9%), akathisia (≤8%), pain (1% to 7%), dystonia (≤6%), lethargy (1% to 5%), tardive dyskinesia (<5%), anxiety (2% to 4%), irritability (1% to 4%), parkinsonism (≤4%), abnormal dreams (2% to 3%), depression (1% to 3%), hypersomnia (1% to 3%), abnormal thinking (2%), ataxia (2%), attention disturbance (2%), coordination impaired (2%), disorientation (2%), hypoesthesia (2%), mental impairment (2%), migraine (2%), sluggishness (2%), vertigo (2%), confusion (1% to 2%), restlessness (1% to 2%), fever (1% to 2%), chills (1%)

Dermatologic: Rash (4%), hyperhidrosis (2%)

Endocrine & metabolic: Hyperprolactinemia (4%), libido decreased (≤2%), hypothyroidism (≤2%), female lactation (1%)

Gastrointestinal: Nausea (7% to 8%), abdominal pain (dose related; 4% to 7%), dyspepsia (dose related; 2% to 7%), vomiting (1% to 6%), drooling (<5%), gastroenteritis (2% to 4%), toothache (2% to 3%), appetite decreased (2%), dysphagia (2%), flatulence (2%), GERD (2%), anorexia (≥1%), abnormal taste (1%), abdominal distension (≤1%)

Genitourinary: Pollakiuria (2%), urinary tract infection (2%), impotence (1%)

Hematologic: Neutropenia (≤2%), leukopenia (≥1%), hemorrhage (1%)

Hepatic: Transaminases increased (1% to 6%), GGT increased (1%)

Neuromuscular & skeletal: Weakness (2% to 10%), tremor (2% to 8%), back pain (3% to 5%), dysarthria (1% to 5%), hypertonia (4%), twitching (4%), dyskinesia (≤4%), arthralgia (1% to 4%), paresthesia (3%), muscle spasm (1% to 3%), limb pain (2%), myalgia (2%), neck pain (2%), neck rigidity (1%)

Ocular: Blurred vision (1% to 4%), amblyopia (2% to 3%)

Otic: Ear pain (1% to 2%)

Respiratory: Pharyngitis (4% to 6%), nasal congestion (5%), rhinitis (3% to 4%), upper respiratory tract infection (2% to 3%), sinus congestion (2%), sinus headache (2%), sinusitis (2%), cough (3%), dyspnea (≥1%), dry throat (1%)

Miscellaneous: Diaphoresis (2%), restless legs syndrome (2%), flu-like syndrome (1% to 2%), lymphadenopathy (1%)

Drug Interactions

Metabolism/Transport Effects Substrate of CYP2D6 (minor), CYP3A4 (major); **Note:** Assignment of Major/Minor substrate status based on clinically relevant drug interaction potential

Avoid Concomitant Use

Avoid concomitant use of QUEtiapine with any of the following: Azelastine; Azelastine (Nasal); Conivaptan; Highest Risk QTc-Prolonging Agents; Metoclopramide; Mifepristone; Moderate Risk QTc-Prolonging Agents; Paraldehyde

Increased Effect/Toxicity

QUEtiapine may increase the levels/effects of: Alcohol (Ethyl); Anticholinergics; Azelastine; Azelastine (Nasal); Buprenorphine; CNS Depressants; Highest Risk QTc-Prolonging Agents; Methylphenidate; Paraldehyde; Serotonin Modulators; Zolpidem

The levels/effects of QUEtiapine may be increased by: Acetylcholinesterase Inhibitors (Central); Conivaptan; CYP3A4 Inhibitors (Moderate); CYP3A4 Inhibitors (Strong); HydrOX-Yzine; Ivacaftor; Lithium formulations; Methylphenidate; Metoclopramide; Metyrosine; Mifepristone; Moderate Risk QTc-Prolonging Agents; Pramlintide; QTc-Prolonging Agents (Indeterminate Risk and Risk Modifying); Tetrabenazine

Decreased Effect

QUEtiapine may decrease the levels/effects of: Amphetamines; Anti-Parkinson's Agents (Dopamine Agonist); Quinagolide

The levels/effects of QUEtiapine may be decreased by: CYP3A4 Inducers (Strong); Deferasirox; Fosphenytoin; Lithium formulations; Peginterferon Alfa-2b; Phenytoin; Tocilizumab

Ethanol/Nutrition/Herb Interactions

Ethanol: May increase CNS depression; monitor for increased effects with coadministration. Caution patients about effects.

Food: In healthy volunteers, administration of quetiapine (immediate release) with food resulted in an increase in the peak serum concentration and AUC by 25% and 15%, respectively, compared to the fasting state. Administration of the extended release formulation with a high-fat meal (~800-1000 calories) resulted in an increase in peak serum concentration by 44% to 52% and AUC by 20% to 22% for the 50 mg and 300 mg tablets; administration with a light meal (≤300 calories) had no significant effect on the C_{max} or AUC.

Herb/Nutraceutical: St John's wort may decrease quetiapine levels. Avoid valerian, St John's wort, kava kava, gotu kola (may increase CNS depression).

Stability Store at controlled room temperature of 25°C (77°F); excursions permitted to 15°C to 30°C (59°F to 86°F).

Mechanism of Action Quetiapine is a dibenzothiazepine atypical antipsychotic. It has been proposed that this drug's antipsychotic activity is mediated through a combination of dopamine type 2 (D_2) and serotonin type 2 (5-HT_2) antagonism. It is an antagonist at multiple neurotransmitter receptors in the brain: Serotonin 5-HT_{1A} and 5-HT_2, dopamine D_1 and D_2, histamine H_1, and adrenergic alpha$_1$- and alpha$_2$-receptors; but appears to have no appreciable affinity at cholinergic muscarinic and benzodiazepine receptors. Norquetiapine, an active metabolite, differs from its parent molecule by exhibiting high affinity for muscarinic M1 receptors.

Antagonism at receptors other than dopamine and 5-HT_2 with similar receptor affinities may explain some of the other effects of quetiapine. The drug's antagonism of histamine H_1-receptors may explain the somnolence observed. The drug's antagonism of adrenergic alpha$_1$-receptors may explain the orthostatic hypotension observed.

Pharmacodynamics/Kinetics

Absorption: Rapidly absorbed following oral administration

Distribution: V_d: 6-14 L/kg

Protein binding, plasma: 83%

Metabolism: Primarily hepatic; via CYP3A4; forms the metabolite N-desalkyl quetiapine (active) and two inactive metabolites

Bioavailability: 100% (relative to oral solution)

Half-life elimination:

Mean: Terminal: Quetiapine: ~6 hours; Extended release: ~7 hours

Metabolite: N-desalkyl quetiapine: 9-12 hours

Time to peak, plasma: Immediate release: 1.5 hours; Extended release: 6 hours

Excretion: Urine (73% as metabolites, <1% of total dose as unchanged drug); feces (20%)

Dosage

Geriatric Adults >65 years: 40% lower mean oral clearance of quetiapine in adults >65 years of age; higher plasma levels expected and, therefore, dosage adjustment may be needed; elderly patients usually require 50-200 mg/day of immediate release tablets or 50 mg/day of extended release tablets with a slower titration schedule. Increase immediate release dose by 25-50 mg/day or extended release dose by 50 mg/day to effective dose, based on clinical response and tolerability. If initiated with immediate release tablets, patient may transition to extended release formulation (at equivalent total daily dose) when effective dose has been reached. See "Note" in adult dosing.

Psychosis/agitation related to Alzheimer's dementia (unlabeled use): Initial: 12.5-50 mg/day; if necessary, gradually increase as tolerated not to exceed 200-300 mg/day (Rabins, 2007)

Adult

Bipolar disorder: Oral:

Depression:

Immediate release tablet: Initial: 50 mg once daily the first day; increase to 100 mg once daily on day 2, further increasing by 100 mg/day each day until a target dose of 300 mg once daily is reached by day 4. Further increases up to 600 mg once daily by day 8 have been evaluated in clinical trials, but no additional antidepressant efficacy was noted.

Extended release tablet: Initial: 50 mg/day the first day; increase to 100 mg on day 2, further increasing by 100 mg/day each day until a target dose of 300 mg/day is reached by day 4.

Mania:

Immediate release tablet: Initial: 50 mg twice daily on day 1, increase dose in increments of 100 mg/day to 200 mg twice daily on day 4; may increase to a target dose of 800 mg/day by day 6 at increments ≤200 mg/day. Usual dosage range: 400-800 mg/day.

Extended release tablet: Initial: 300 mg on day 1; increase to 600 mg on day 2 and adjust dose to 400-800 mg once daily on day 3, depending on response and tolerance.

Maintenance therapy: Immediate release tablet: 200-400 mg twice daily with lithium or divalproex; **Note:** Average time of stabilization was 15 weeks in clinical trials.

Major depressive disorder (adjunct to antidepressants): Oral: Extended release tablet: Initial: 50 mg once daily; may be increased to 150 mg on day 3. Usual dosage range: 150-300 mg/day

Schizophrenia/psychoses: Oral:

Immediate release tablet: Initial: 25 mg twice daily; followed by increases in the total daily dose on the second and third day in increments of 25-50 mg divided 2-3 times/day, if tolerated, to a target dose of 300-400 mg/day in 2-3 divided doses by day 4. Make further adjustments as needed at intervals of at least 2 days in adjustments of 25-50 mg divided twice daily. Usual maintenance range: 300-800 mg/day.

Extended-release tablet: Initial: 300 mg once daily; increase in increments of up to 300 mg/day (in intervals of ≥1 day). Usual maintenance range: 400-800 mg/day.

Note: Dose reductions should be attempted periodically to establish lowest effective dose in patients with psychosis. Patients being restarted after 1 week of no drug need to be titrated as above.

ICU delirium: Oral: Initial: 50 mg twice daily; may increase as necessary on a daily basis in increments of 50 mg twice daily to a maximum dose of 400 mg/day (Devlin, 2010)

Renal Impairment No dosage adjustment required: 25% lower mean oral clearance of quetiapine than normal subjects; however, plasma concentrations similar to normal subjects receiving the same dose.

Hepatic Impairment Lower clearance in hepatic impairment (30%), may result in higher concentrations. Dosage adjustment may be required.

Immediate release tablet: Oral: Initial: 25 mg/day, increase dose by 25-50 mg/day to effective dose, based on clinical response and tolerability to patient. If initiated with immediate-release formulation, patient may transition to extended-release formulation (at equivalent total daily dose) when effective dose has been reached.

Extended release tablet Oral: Initial: 50 mg/day; increase dose by 50 mg/day to effective dose, based on clinical response and tolerability to patient.

Administration

Oral:

Immediate release tablet: May be administered with or without food.

Extended release tablet: Administer without food or with a light meal (≤300 calories), preferably in the evening. Swallow tablet whole; do not break, crush, or chew.

Nasogastric/enteral tube (unlabeled route): Hold tube feeds for 30 minutes before administration; flush with 25 mL of sterile water. Crush dose using immediate-release formulation, mix in 10 mL water and administer via NG/enteral tube; follow with a 50 mL flush of sterile water (Devlin, 2010).

Monitoring Parameters Vital signs; fasting lipid profile and fasting blood glucose/Hgb A_{1c} (prior to treatment, at 3 months, then annually); CBC frequently during first few months of therapy in patients with pre-existing low WBC or a history of drug-induced leukopenia/neutropenia; BMI, personal/family history of obesity, waist circumference; mental status, abnormal involuntary movement scale (AIMS). Weight should be assessed prior to treatment, at 4 weeks, 8 weeks, 12 weeks, and then at quarterly intervals. Consider titrating to a different antipsychotic agent for a weight gain ≥5% of the initial weight. Patients should have eyes checked for cataracts every 6 months while on this medication. Observe for new or worsening depression, anxiety, irritability, aggression, or other symptoms of unusual behavior, mood, or suicide ideation (especially at the beginning of therapy or when doses are increased or decreased).

Test Interactions May interfere with urine detection of methadone (false-positives); may cause false-positive serum TCA screen

Special Geriatric Considerations Any changes in disease status in any organ system can result in behavior changes. Evaluation of disease status should be done before initiating psychotropic drug therapy for behavior changes.

Extrapyramidal syndrome symptoms occur less often than with traditional antipsychotics from the phenothiazine and butyrophenone classes. Many elderly patients receive antipsychotic medications for inappropriate nonpsychotic behavior. Before initiating antipsychotic medication, the clinician should investigate any possible reversible cause; any stress or stress from any disease can cause acute "confusion" or worsening of baseline nonpsychotic behavior. Most commonly acute changes in behavior are due to increases in drug dose or addition of new drug to regimen, fluid electrolyte loss, infections, and changes in environment.

In the treatment of agitated, demented elderly patients, authors of meta-analyses of controlled trials of the response to the traditional antipsychotics (eg, phenothiazines, butyrophenones) in controlling agitation, have concluded that the use of neuroleptics results in a response rate of

18%. Clearly neuroleptic therapy for behavior control should be limited with frequent attempts to withdraw the agent given for behavior control. In light of significant risks and adverse effects in the elderly population compared with limited data demonstrating efficacy in the treatment of dementia related psychosis, aggression, and agitation, an extensive risk:benefit analysis should be performed prior to use.

This medication is considered to be potentially inappropriate in this patient population (Beers Criteria: Quality of evidence - moderate; Strength of recommendation - strong).

Dosage Forms Excipient information presented when available (limited, particularly for generics); consult specific product labeling.
Tablet, oral: 25 mg, 50 mg, 100 mg, 150 mg, 200 mg, 300 mg, 400 mg
SEROquel®: 25 mg, 50 mg, 100 mg, 200 mg, 300 mg, 400 mg
Tablet, extended release, oral:
SEROquel XR®: 50 mg, 150 mg, 200 mg, 300 mg, 400 mg
Dosage Forms: Canada Excipient information presented when available (limited, particularly for generics); consult specific product labeling.
Tablet:
Seroquel®: 25 mg, 50 mg, 100 mg, 200 mg, 300 mg, 400 mg
Tablet, extended release:
Seroquel XR®: 50 mg, 150 mg, 200 mg, 300 mg, 400 mg

◆ **Quetiapine Fumarate** see QUEtiapine on page 1644

Quinapril (KWIN a pril)

Related Information
Angiotensin Agents on page 2093
Heart Failure (Systolic) on page 2203
Medication Safety Issues
Sound-alike/look-alike issues:
Accupril® may be confused with Accolate®, Accutane®, AcipHex®, Monopril®
International issues:
Accupril [U.S., Canada] may be confused with Acepril which is a brand name for captopril [Great Britain]; enalapril [Hungary, Switzerland]; lisinopril [Malaysia]
Brand Names: U.S. Accupril®
Brand Names: Canada Accupril®
Index Terms Quinapril Hydrochloride
Generic Availability (U.S.) Yes
Pharmacologic Category Angiotensin-Converting Enzyme (ACE) Inhibitor
Use Treatment of hypertension; treatment of heart failure
Unlabeled Use Treatment of left ventricular dysfunction after myocardial infarction; to delay the progression of nephropathy and reduce risks of cardiovascular events in hypertensive patients with type 1 or 2 diabetes mellitus
Contraindications Hypersensitivity to quinapril or any component of the formulation; angioedema related to previous treatment with an ACE inhibitor
Warnings/Precautions Anaphylactic reactions may occur rarely with ACE inhibitors. At any time during treatment (especially following first dose) angioedema may occur rarely with ACE inhibitors; it may involve the head and neck (potentially compromising airway) or the intestine (presenting with abdominal pain). African-Americans and patients with idiopathic or hereditary angioedema may be at an increased risk. Prolonged frequent monitoring may be required especially if tongue, glottis, or larynx are involved as they are associated with airway obstruction. Patients with a history of airway surgery may have a higher risk of airway obstruction. Aggressive early and appropriate management is critical. Use in patients with previous angioedema associated with ACE inhibitor therapy is contraindicated. Severe anaphylactoid reactions may be seen during hemodialysis (eg, CVVHD) with high-flux dialysis membranes (eg, AN69), and rarely, during low density lipoprotein apheresis with dextran sulfate cellulose. Rare cases of anaphylactoid reactions have been reported in patients undergoing sensitization treatment with hymenoptera (bee, wasp) venom while receiving ACE inhibitors.

Symptomatic hypotension with or without syncope can occur with ACE inhibitors (usually with the first several doses); effects are most often observed in volume-depleted patients; close monitoring of patient is required especially with initial dosing and dosing increases; blood pressure must be lowered at a rate appropriate for the patient's clinical condition. Initiation of therapy in patients with ischemic heart disease or cerebrovascular disease warrants close observation due to the potential consequences posed by falling blood pressure (eg, MI, stroke). Use with caution in hypertrophic cardiomyopathy with outflow tract obstruction, severe aortic stenosis, or before, during, or immediately after major surgery.

QUINAPRIL

Hyperkalemia may occur with ACE inhibitors; risk factors include renal dysfunction, diabetes mellitus, concomitant use of potassium-sparing diuretics, potassium supplements, and/or potassium-containing salts. Use cautiously, if at all, with these agents and monitor potassium closely. Cough may occur with ACE inhibitors. Other causes of cough should be considered (eg, pulmonary congestion in patients with heart failure) and excluded prior to discontinuation.

May be associated with deterioration of renal function and/or increases in serum creatinine, particularly in patients with low renal blood flow (eg, renal artery stenosis, heart failure) whose glomerular filtration rate (GFR) is dependent on efferent arteriolar vasoconstriction by angiotensin II; deterioration may result in oliguria, acute renal failure, and progressive azotemia. Small increases in serum creatinine may occur following initiation; consider discontinuation only in patients with progressive and/or significant deterioration in renal function. Use with caution in patients with unstented unilateral/bilateral renal artery stenosis. When unstented bilateral renal artery stenosis is present, use is generally avoided due to the elevated risk of deterioration in renal function unless possible benefits outweigh risks. Concurrent use of angiotensin receptor blockers may increase the risk of clinically-significant adverse events (eg, renal dysfunction, hyperkalemia).

Rare toxicities associated with ACE inhibitors include cholestatic jaundice (which may progress to fulminant hepatic necrosis), agranulocytosis, neutropenia, or leukopenia with myeloid hypoplasia. Patients with collagen vascular diseases (especially with concomitant renal impairment) or renal impairment alone may be at increased risk for hematologic toxicity; periodically monitor CBC with differential in these patients.

Adverse Reactions (Reflective of adult population; not specific for elderly) Note: Frequency ranges include data from hypertension and heart failure trials. Higher rates of adverse reactions have generally been noted in patients with CHF. However, the frequency of adverse effects associated with placebo is also increased in this population.

1% to 10%:
Cardiovascular: Hypotension (3%), chest pain (2%), first-dose hypotension (up to 3%)
Central nervous system: Dizziness (4% to 8%), headache (2% to 6%), fatigue (3%)
Dermatologic: Rash (1%)
Endocrine & metabolic: Hyperkalemia (2%)
Gastrointestinal: Vomiting/nausea (1% to 2%), diarrhea (2%)
Neuromuscular & skeletal: Myalgias (2% to 5%), back pain (1%)
Renal: BUN/serum creatinine increased (2%, transient elevations may occur with a higher frequency), worsening of renal function (in patients with bilateral renal artery stenosis or hypovolemia)
Respiratory: Upper respiratory symptoms, cough (2% to 4%; up to 13% in some studies), dyspnea (2%)

Drug Interactions

Metabolism/Transport Effects None known.

Avoid Concomitant Use There are no known interactions where it is recommended to avoid concomitant use.

Increased Effect/Toxicity
Quinapril may increase the levels/effects of: Allopurinol; Amifostine; Antihypertensives; AzaTHIOprine; CycloSPORINE; CycloSPORINE (Systemic); Ferric Gluconate; Gold Sodium Thiomalate; Hypotensive Agents; Iron Dextran Complex; Lithium; Nonsteroidal Anti-Inflammatory Agents; RiTUXimab; Sodium Phosphates

The levels/effects of Quinapril may be increased by: Alfuzosin; Aliskiren; Angiotensin II Receptor Blockers; Diazoxide; DPP-IV Inhibitors; Eplerenone; Everolimus; Herbs (Hypotensive Properties); Loop Diuretics; MAO Inhibitors; Pentoxifylline; Phosphodiesterase 5 Inhibitors; Potassium Salts; Potassium-Sparing Diuretics; Prostacyclin Analogues; Sirolimus; Temsirolimus; Thiazide Diuretics; TiZANidine; Tolvaptan; Trimethoprim

Decreased Effect
Quinapril may decrease the levels/effects of: Quinolone Antibiotics; Tetracycline Derivatives

The levels/effects of Quinapril may be decreased by: Antacids; Aprotinin; Herbs (Hypertensive Properties); Icatibant; Lanthanum; Methylphenidate; Nonsteroidal Anti-Inflammatory Agents; Salicylates; Yohimbine

Ethanol/Nutrition/Herb Interactions
Food: Potassium supplements and/or potassium-containing salts may cause or worsen hyperkalemia. Management: Consult prescriber before consuming a potassium-rich diet, potassium supplements, or salt substitutes.

Herb/Nutraceutical: Some herbal medications may worsen hypertension (eg, licorice); others may increase the antihypertensive effects of quinapril (eg, shepherd's purse). Management: Avoid bayberry, blue cohosh, cayenne, ephedra, ginger, ginseng (American), kola, licorice, and yohimbe. Avoid black cohosh, California poppy, coleus, golden seal, hawthorn, mistletoe, periwinkle, quinine, and shepherd's purse.

Stability Store at room temperature. To prepare solution for oral administration, mix prior to administration and use within 10 minutes.

Mechanism of Action Competitive inhibitor of angiotensin-converting enzyme (ACE); prevents conversion of angiotensin I to angiotensin II, a potent vasoconstrictor; results in lower levels of angiotensin II which causes an increase in plasma renin activity and a reduction in aldosterone secretion; a CNS mechanism may also be involved in hypotensive effect as angiotensin II increases adrenergic outflow from CNS; vasoactive kallikreins may be decreased in conversion to active hormones by ACE inhibitors, thus reducing blood pressure

Pharmacodynamics/Kinetics

Onset of action: 1 hour

Duration: 24 hours

Absorption: Quinapril: ≥60%

Protein binding: Quinapril: 97%; Quinaprilat: 97%

Metabolism: Rapidly hydrolyzed to quinaprilat, the active metabolite

Half-life elimination: Quinapril: 0.8 hours; Quinaprilat: 3 hours; increases as Cl_{cr} decreases

Time to peak, serum: Quinapril: 1 hour; Quinaprilat: ~2 hours

Excretion: Urine (50% to 60% primarily as quinaprilat)

Dosage

Geriatric Oral: Initial: 2.5-5 mg/day; increase dosage at increments of 2.5-5 mg at 1- to 2-week intervals; adjust for renal impairment.

Adult

Heart failure: Oral: Initial: 5 mg once or twice daily, titrated at weekly intervals to 20-40 mg daily in 2 divided doses; target dose (heart failure): 20 mg twice daily (ACC/AHA 2009 Heart Failure Guidelines)

Hypertension: Oral: Initial: 10-20 mg once daily, adjust according to blood pressure response at peak and trough blood levels; initial dose may be reduced to 5 mg in patients receiving diuretic therapy if the diuretic is continued.

Usual dose range (JNC 7): 10-40 mg once daily

Renal Impairment Lower initial doses should be used; after initial dose (if tolerated), administer initial dose twice daily; may be increased at weekly intervals to optimal response:

Heart failure: Oral: Initial:

Cl_{cr} >30 mL/minute: Administer 5 mg/day

Cl_{cr} 10-30 mL/minute: Administer 2.5 mg/day

Hypertension: Oral: Initial:

Cl_{cr} >60 mL/minute: Administer 10 mg/day

Cl_{cr} 30-60 mL/minute: Administer 5 mg/day

Cl_{cr} 10-30 mL/minute: Administer 2.5 mg/day

Hepatic Impairment In patients with alcoholic cirrhosis, hydrolysis of quinapril to quinaprilat is impaired; however, the subsequent elimination of quinaprilat is unaltered.

Monitoring Parameters Blood pressure; serum creatinine and potassium; if patient has collagen vascular disease and/or renal impairment, periodically monitor CBC with differential

Pharmacotherapy Pearls Patients taking diuretics are at risk for developing hypotension on initial dosing; to prevent this, discontinue diuretics 2-3 days prior to initiating quinapril; may restart diuretics if blood pressure is not controlled by quinapril alone

Special Geriatric Considerations Due to frequent decreases in glomerular filtration (also creatinine clearance) with aging, elderly patients may have exaggerated responses to ACE inhibitors; differences in clinical response due to hepatic changes are not observed. ACE inhibitors may be preferred agents in elderly patients with CHF and diabetes mellitus. Diabetic proteinuria is reduced and insulin sensitivity is enhanced. In general, the side effect profile is favorable in elderly and causes little or no CNS confusion; use lowest dose recommendations initially. Adjust for renal function. Many elderly may be volume depleted due to diuretic use and/or blunted thirst reflex resulting in inadequate fluid intake.

Dosage Forms Excipient information presented when available (limited, particularly for generics); consult specific product labeling.

Tablet, oral: 5 mg, 10 mg, 20 mg, 40 mg

Accupril®: 5 mg [scored]

Accupril®: 10 mg, 20 mg, 40 mg

Quinapril and Hydrochlorothiazide (KWIN a pril & hye droe klor oh THYE a zide)

Related Information
Hydrochlorothiazide *on page 933*
Quinapril *on page 1649*
Brand Names: U.S. Accuretic®
Brand Names: Canada Accuretic®
Index Terms Hydrochlorothiazide and Quinapril; Quinaretic
Generic Availability (U.S.) Yes
Pharmacologic Category Angiotensin-Converting Enzyme (ACE) Inhibitor; Diuretic, Thiazide
Use Treatment of hypertension (not for initial therapy)
Dosage
Geriatric If previous response to individual components is unknown, initial dose selection should be cautious, at the low end of adult dosage range; titration should occur at 1- to 2-week intervals.
Adult
Hypertension: Oral:
Patients with inadequate response to quinapril monotherapy: Quinapril 10 mg/hydrochlorothiazide 12.5 mg **or** quinapril 20 mg/hydrochlorothiazide 12.5 mg once daily
Patients with adequate blood pressure control on hydrochlorothiazide 25 mg/day, but significant potassium loss: Quinapril 10 mg/hydrochlorothiazide 12.5 mg **or** quinapril 20 mg/hydrochlorothiazide 12.5 mg once daily
Note: Clinical trials of quinapril/hydrochlorothiazide combinations used quinapril doses of 2.5-40 mg/day and hydrochlorothiazide doses of 6.25-25 mg/day.
Renal Impairment Cl_{cr} <30 mL/minute/1.73 m^2 or serum creatinine ≥3 mg/dL: Use is not recommended.
Special Geriatric Considerations See individual agents. Combination products are not recommended as first-line treatment. Use only if doses of individual agents correspond to the combination available.
Dosage Forms Excipient information presented when available (limited, particularly for generics); consult specific product labeling.
Tablet, oral:
10/12.5: Quinapril 10 mg and hydrochlorothiazide 12.5 mg
20/12.5: Quinapril 20 mg and hydrochlorothiazide 12.5 mg
20/25: Quinapril 20 mg and hydrochlorothiazide 25 mg
Accuretic® 10/12.5: Quinapril 10 mg and hydrochlorothiazide 12.5 mg [scored]
Accuretic® 20/12.5: Quinapril 20 mg and hydrochlorothiazide 12.5 mg [scored]
Accuretic® 20/25: Quinapril 20 mg and hydrochlorothiazide 25 mg

◆ **Quinapril Hydrochloride** *see* Quinapril *on page 1649*
◆ **Quinaretic** *see* Quinapril and Hydrochlorothiazide *on page 1652*

QuiNIDine (KWIN i deen)

Related Information
Beers Criteria – Potentially Inappropriate Medications for Geriatrics *on page 2183*
Medication Safety Issues
Sound-alike/look-alike issues:
QuiNIDine may be confused with cloNIDine, quiNINE
High alert medication:
The Institute for Safe Medication Practices (ISMP) includes this medication (I.V. formulation) among its list of drug classes which have a heightened risk of causing significant patient harm when used in error.
BEERS Criteria medication:
This drug may be potentially inappropriate for use in geriatric patients (Quality of evidence - high; Strength of recommendation - strong).
Brand Names: Canada Apo-Quinidine®; BioQuin® Durules™; Novo-Quinidin; Quinate®
Index Terms Quinidine Gluconate; Quinidine Polygalacturonate; Quinidine Sulfate
Generic Availability (U.S.) Yes
Pharmacologic Category Antiarrhythmic Agent, Class Ia; Antimalarial Agent
Use
Quinidine gluconate and sulfate salts: Conversion and prevention of relapse into atrial fibrillation and/or flutter; suppression of ventricular arrhythmias. **Note:** Due to proarrhythmic effects, use should be reserved for life-threatening arrhythmias. Moreover, the use of

quinidine has largely been replaced by more effective/safer antiarrhythmic agents and/or nonpharmacologic therapies (eg, radiofrequency ablation).

Quinidine gluconate (I.V. formulation): Conversion of atrial fibrillation/flutter and ventricular tachycardia. **Note:** The use of I.V. quinidine gluconate for these indications has been replaced by more effective/safer antiarrhythmic agents (eg, amiodarone and procainamide).

Quinidine gluconate (I.V. formulation) and quinidine sulfate: Treatment of malaria (*Plasmodium falciparum*)

Unlabeled Use Paroxysmal supraventricular tachycardia, paroxysmal AV junctional rhythm, and symptomatic atrial or ventricular premature contractions; short QT syndrome; Brugada syndrome

Contraindications Hypersensitivity to quinidine or any component of the formulation; thrombocytopenia; thrombocytopenic purpura; myasthenia gravis; heart block greater than first degree; idioventricular conduction delays (except in patients with a functioning artificial pacemaker); those adversely affected by anticholinergic activity; concurrent use of quinolone antibiotics which prolong QT interval, cisapride, amprenavir, or ritonavir

Warnings/Precautions Watch for proarrhythmic effects; may cause QT prolongation and subsequent torsade de pointes. Monitor and adjust dose to prevent QT_c prolongation. Avoid use in patients with diagnosed or suspected congenital long QT syndrome. Correct hypokalemia before initiating therapy. Hypokalemia may worsen toxicity. **[U.S. Boxed Warning]: Antiarrhythmic drugs have not been shown to enhance survival in non-life-threatening ventricular arrhythmias and may increase mortality; the risk is greatest with structural heart disease. Quinidine may increase mortality in treatment of atrial fibrillation/flutter.** May precipitate or exacerbate HF. Reduce dosage in hepatic impairment. Use may cause digoxin-induced toxicity (adjust digoxin's dose). Use caution with concurrent use of other antiarrhythmics. Hypersensitivity reactions can occur. Can unmask sick sinus syndrome (causes bradycardia); use with caution in patients with heart block. In the treatment of atrial fibrillation in the elderly, avoid antiarrhythmics as first-line treatment. In older adults, data suggests rate control may provide more benefits than risks compared to rhythm control for most patients (Beers Criteria).

Has been associated with severe hepatotoxic reactions, including granulomatous hepatitis. Hemolysis may occur in patients with G6PD (glucose-6-phosphate dehydrogenase) deficiency. Different salt products are not interchangeable.

Adverse Reactions (Reflective of adult population; not specific for elderly)
Frequency not defined: Hypotension, syncope

>10%:

Cardiovascular: QT_c prolongation (modest prolongation is common, however, excessive prolongation is rare and indicates toxicity)

Central nervous system: Lightheadedness (15%)

Gastrointestinal: Diarrhea (35%), upper GI distress, bitter taste, diarrhea, anorexia, nausea, vomiting, stomach cramping (22%)

1% to 10%:

Cardiovascular: Angina (6%), palpitation (7%), new or worsened arrhythmia (proarrhythmic effect)

Central nervous system: Syncope (1% to 8%), headache (7%), fatigue (7%), sleep disturbance (3%), tremor (2%), nervousness (2%), incoordination (1%)

Dermatologic: Rash (5%)

Neuromuscular & skeletal: Weakness (5%)

Ocular: Blurred vision

Otic: Tinnitus

Respiratory: Wheezing

Note: Cinchonism, a syndrome which may include tinnitus, high-frequency hearing loss, deafness, vertigo, blurred vision, diplopia, photophobia, headache, confusion, and delirium has been associated with quinidine use. Usually associated with chronic toxicity, this syndrome has also been described after brief exposure to a moderate dose in sensitive patients. Vomiting and diarrhea may also occur as isolated reactions to therapeutic quinidine levels.

Drug Interactions

Metabolism/Transport Effects Substrate of CYP2C9 (minor), CYP2E1 (minor), CYP3A4 (major), P-glycoprotein; **Note:** Assignment of Major/Minor substrate status based on clinically relevant drug interaction potential; **Inhibits** CYP2C9 (weak), CYP2D6 (strong), CYP3A4 (weak), P-glycoprotein

Avoid Concomitant Use

Avoid concomitant use of QuiNIDine with any of the following: Antifungal Agents (Azole Derivatives, Systemic); Conivaptan; Crizotinib; Fingolimod; Highest Risk QTc-Prolonging Agents; Mefloquine; Mifepristone; Moderate Risk QTc-Prolonging Agents; Propafenone; Protease Inhibitors; Silodosin; Topotecan

Increased Effect/Toxicity
QuiNIDine may increase the levels/effects of: ARIPiprazole; AtoMOXetine; Beta-Blockers; Calcium Channel Blockers (Dihydropyridine); Cardiac Glycosides; Colchicine; CYP2D6 Substrates; Dabigatran Etexilate; Dalfampridine; Dextromethorphan; Everolimus; Fesoterodine; Haloperidol; Highest Risk QTc-Prolonging Agents; Mefloquine; Neuromuscular-Blocking Agents; P-glycoprotein/ABCB1 Substrates; Propafenone; Prucalopride; Rivaroxaban; Silodosin; Topotecan; Tricyclic Antidepressants; Verapamil; Vitamin K Antagonists

The levels/effects of QuiNIDine may be increased by: Amiodarone; Antacids; Antifungal Agents (Azole Derivatives, Systemic); Barbiturates; Boceprevir; Calcium Channel Blockers (Dihydropyridine); Carbonic Anhydrase Inhibitors; Cimetidine; Conivaptan; Crizotinib; CYP3A4 Inhibitors (Moderate); CYP3A4 Inhibitors (Strong); Diltiazem; EriBULin; Fingolimod; Fluconazole; Haloperidol; Ivacaftor; Lurasidone; Macrolide Antibiotics; Mifepristone; Moderate Risk QTc-Prolonging Agents; P-glycoprotein/ABCB1 Inhibitors; Propafenone; Protease Inhibitors; QTc-Prolonging Agents (Indeterminate Risk and Risk Modifying); Reserpine; Selective Serotonin Reuptake Inhibitors; Telaprevir; Tricyclic Antidepressants; Verapamil

Decreased Effect
QuiNIDine may decrease the levels/effects of: Codeine; Dihydrocodeine; Hydrocodone; TraMADol

The levels/effects of QuiNIDine may be decreased by: Barbiturates; Calcium Channel Blockers (Dihydropyridine); CYP3A4 Inducers (Strong); Deferasirox; Etravirine; Fosphenytoin; Herbs (CYP3A4 Inducers); Kaolin; P-glycoprotein/ABCB1 Inducers; Phenytoin; Potassium-Sparing Diuretics; Primidone; Rifamycin Derivatives; Sucralfate; Tocilizumab

Ethanol/Nutrition/Herb Interactions
Food: Changes in dietary salt intake may alter the rate and extent of quinidine absorption. Quinidine serum levels may be increased if taken with food. Food has a variable effect on absorption of sustained release formulation. The rate of absorption of quinidine may be decreased following the ingestion of grapefruit juice. Excessive intake of fruit juice or vitamin C may decrease urine pH and result in increased clearance of quinidine with decreased serum concentration. Alkaline foods may result in increased quinidine serum concentrations. Management: Avoid changes in dietary salt intake. Grapefruit juice should be avoided. Take around-the-clock to avoid variation in serum levels and with food or milk to avoid GI irritation.

Herb/Nutraceutical: St John's wort may decrease quinidine levels. Ephedra may worsen arrhythmia. Management: Avoid St John's wort and ephedra.

Stability
Solution for injection: Store at room temperature of 25°C (77°F).
Tablets: Store at controlled room temperature of 20°C to 25°C (68°F to 77°F). Protect from light.

Mechanism of Action
Class Ia antiarrhythmic agent; depresses phase O of the action potential; decreases myocardial excitability and conduction velocity, and myocardial contractility by decreasing sodium influx during depolarization and potassium efflux in repolarization; also reduces calcium transport across cell membrane

Pharmacodynamics/Kinetics
Distribution: V_d: Adults: 2-3 L/kg, decreased with congestive heart failure (0.5 L/kg), malaria; increased with cirrhosis

Protein binding: Adults: 80% to 88%
Binds mainly to alpha$_1$-acid glycoprotein and to a lesser extent albumin; protein-binding changes may occur in periods of stress due to increased alpha$_1$-acid glycoprotein concentrations (eg, acute myocardial infarction) or in certain disease states due to decreased alpha$_1$-acid glycoprotein concentrations (eg, cirrhosis, hyperthyroidism, malnutrition)

Metabolism: Extensively hepatic (50% to 90%) to inactive compounds
Bioavailability: Sulfate: ~70% with wide variability between patients (45% to 100%); Gluconate: 70% to 80%

Half-life elimination, plasma: Adults: 6-8 hours; prolonged with elderly, cirrhosis, and congestive heart failure

Time to peak, serum: Sulfate: 2 hours; Gluconate: 3-6 hours
Excretion: Urine (15% to 25% as unchanged drug)

Dosage
Geriatric & Adult
Note: Dosage expressed in terms of the salt: 267 mg of quinidine gluconate = 200 mg of quinidine sulfate.

Antiarrhythmic: Oral:
Immediate release formulations: Quinidine sulfate: Initial: 200-400 mg/dose every 6 hours the dose may be increased cautiously to desired effect

Extended release formulations:

Quinidine sulfate: Initial: 300 mg every 8-12 hours; the dose may be increased cautiously to desired effect

Quinidine gluconate: Initial: 324 mg every 8-12 hours; the dose may be increased cautiously to desired effect

Severe malaria, treatment: I.V. (quinidine gluconate): 10 mg/kg infused over 60-120 minutes followed by 0.02 mg/kg/minute continuous infusion for ≥24 hours; alternatively, may administer 24 mg/kg loading dose over 4 hours, followed by 12 mg/kg over 4 hours every 8 hours (beginning 8 hours after initiation of the loading dose); complete treatment with oral quinine once parasite density <1% and patient can receive oral medication; total duration of treatment (quinidine/quinine): 3 days (Africa or South America) or 7 days (Southeast Asia); use in combination with doxycycline, tetracycline or clindamycin (CDC malaria guidelines, 2009). **Note:** Close monitoring, including telemetry, required.

Renal Impairment The FDA-approved labeling recommends that caution should be used in patients with renal impairment; however, no specific dosage adjustment guidelines are available. The following guidelines have been used by some clinicians (Aronoff, 2007): Oral: Cl_{cr} ≥10 mL/minute: No adjustment required.

Cl_{cr} <10 mL/minute: Administer 75% of normal dose.

Hemodialysis: Dose following hemodialysis.

Peritoneal dialysis: Supplemental dose is not necessary.

CRRT: No dosage adjustment required; monitor serum concentrations.

Hepatic Impairment Use caution; hepatic impairment decreases clearance; dosage adjustments are not provided in the manufacturers' labeling although toxicity may occur if the dose is not appropriately adjusted.

Administration Administer around-the-clock to promote less variation in peak and trough serum levels

Oral: Do not crush, chew, or break sustained release dosage forms. Some preparations of quinidine gluconate extended release tablets may be split in half to facilitate dosage titration; tablets are not scored.

Parenteral: Minimize use of PVC tubing to enhance bioavailability; shorter tubing lengths are recommended by the manufacturer

Monitoring Parameters Cardiac monitor required during I.V. administration; CBC, liver and renal function tests, should be routinely performed during long-term administration

Reference Range Therapeutic: 2-5 mcg/mL (SI: 6.2-15.4 micromole/L). Patient-dependent therapeutic response occurs at levels of 3-6 mcg/mL (SI: 9.2-18.5 micromole/L). Optimal therapeutic level is method dependent; >6 mcg/mL (SI: >18 micromole/L).

Special Geriatric Considerations Clearance may be decreased with a resultant increased half-life. Must individualize dose. Bioavailability and half-life are increased in the elderly due to decreases in both renal and hepatic function with age.

This medication is considered to be potentially inappropriate in this patient population (Beers Criteria: Quality of evidence - high; Strength of recommendation - strong).

Dosage Forms Excipient information presented when available (limited, particularly for generics); consult specific product labeling.

Injection, solution, as gluconate: 80 mg/mL (10 mL) [equivalent to quinidine base 50 mg/mL]

Tablet, oral, as sulfate: 200 mg [equivalent to quinidine base 166 mg], 300 mg [equivalent to quinidine base 249 mg]

Tablet, extended release, oral, as gluconate: 324 mg [equivalent to quinidine base 202 mg]

Tablet, extended release, oral, as sulfate: 300 mg [equivalent to quinidine base 249 mg]

◆ **Quinidine Gluconate** *see* QuiNIDine *on page 1652*
◆ **Quinidine Polygalacturonate** *see* QuiNIDine *on page 1652*
◆ **Quinidine Sulfate** *see* QuiNIDine *on page 1652*

QuiNINE (KWYE nine)

Medication Safety Issues
Sound-alike/look-alike issues:
QuiNINE may be confused with quiNIDine

Brand Names: U.S. Qualaquin®

Brand Names: Canada Apo-Quinine®; Novo-Quinine; Quinine-Odan

Index Terms Quinine Sulfate

Generic Availability (U.S.) Yes

Pharmacologic Category Antimalarial Agent

Use In conjunction with other antimalarial agents, treatment of uncomplicated chloroquine-resistant *P. falciparum* malaria

QUININE

Unlabeled Use Treatment of *Babesia microti* infection in conjunction with clindamycin; treatment of uncomplicated chloroquine-resistant *P. vivax* malaria (in conjunction with other antimalarial agents)

Medication Guide Available Yes

Contraindications Hypersensitivity to quinine or any component of the formulation; hypersensitivity to mefloquine or quinidine (cross sensitivity reported); history of potential hypersensitivity reactions (including black water fever, thrombotic thrombocytopenia purpura [TTP], hemolytic uremic syndrome [HUS], or thrombocytopenia) associated with prior quinine use; prolonged QT interval; myasthenia gravis; optic neuritis; G6PD deficiency

Warnings/Precautions [U.S. Boxed Warning]: Quinine is not recommended for the prevention/treatment of nocturnal leg cramps due to the potential for severe and/or life-threatening side effects (eg, cardiac arrhythmias, thrombocytopenia, HUS/TTP, severe hypersensitivity reactions). These risks, as well as the absence of clinical effectiveness, do not justify its use in the unapproved/unlabeled prevention and/or treatment of leg cramps.

Quinine may cause QT interval prolongation, with maximum increase corresponding to maximum plasma concentration. Use caution with medications or clinical conditions which may further prolong the QT interval or cause cardiac arrhythmias. Use caution with atrial fibrillation or flutter, renal or hepatic impairment. Quinine interacts with many medications due to its hepatic metabolism; use caution with other medications metabolized via the CYP3A4 isoenzyme system. Severe hypersensitivity reactions (eg, Stevens-Johnson syndrome, anaphylactic shock) have occurred; discontinue following any signs of sensitivity. Other events (including acute interstitial nephritis, neutropenia, and granulomatous hepatitis) may also be attributed to hypersensitivity reactions. Immune-mediated thrombocytopenia, including life-threatening cases and hemolytic uremic syndrome/thrombotic thrombocytopenic purpura (HUS/TTP), has occurred with use. Chronic renal failure associated with TTP has also been reported. Thrombocytopenia generally resolves within a week upon discontinuation. Re-exposure may result in increased severity of thrombocytopenia and faster onset.

Use may cause significant hypoglycemia due to quinine-induced insulin release. Use with caution in patients with hepatic impairment. Use with caution in patients with renal impairment; dosage adjustment recommended. Quinine should not be used for the prevention of malaria or in the treatment of complicated or severe *P. falciparum* malaria (oral antimalarial agents are not appropriate for initial therapy of severe malaria).

Adverse Reactions (Reflective of adult population; not specific for elderly)
Frequency not defined.

Cardiovascular: Atrial fibrillation, atrioventricular block, bradycardia, cardiac arrest, chest pain, hypotension, irregular rhythm, nodal escape beats, orthostatic hypotension, palpitation, QT prolongation, syncope, tachycardia, torsade de pointes, unifocal premature ventricular contractions, U waves, vasodilation, ventricular fibrillation, ventricular tachycardia

Central nervous system: Aphasia, ataxia, chills, coma, confusion, disorientation, dizziness, dystonic reaction, fever, flushing, headache, mental status altered, restlessness, seizure, suicide, vertigo

Dermatologic: Acral necrosis, allergic contact dermatitis, bullous dermatitis, bruising, cutaneous rash (urticaria, papular, scarlatinal), cutaneous vasculitis, exfoliative dermatitis, erythema multiforme, petechiae, photosensitivity, pruritus, Stevens-Johnson syndrome, toxic epidermal necrolysis

Endocrine & metabolic: Hypoglycemia

Gastrointestinal: Abdominal pain, anorexia, diarrhea, esophagitis, gastric irritation, nausea, vomiting

Hematologic: Agranulocytosis, aplastic anemia, coagulopathy, disseminated intravascular coagulation, hemolytic anemia, hemolytic uremic syndrome, hemorrhage, hypoprothrombinemia, idiopathic thrombocytopenic purpura, leukopenia, neutropenia, pancytopenia, thrombocytopenia, thrombotic thrombocytopenia purpura

Hepatic: Granulomatous hepatitis, hepatitis, jaundice, liver function test abnormalities

Neuromuscular & skeletal: Myalgia, tremor, weakness

Ocular: Blindness, blurred vision (with or without scotomata), color vision disturbance, diminished visual fields, diplopia, night blindness, optic neuritis, photophobia, pupillary dilation, vision loss (sudden)

Otic: Deafness, hearing impaired, tinnitus

Renal: Acute interstitial nephritis, hemoglobinuria, renal failure, renal impairment

Respiratory: Asthma, dyspnea, pulmonary edema

Miscellaneous: Black water fever, diaphoresis, hypersensitivity reaction, lupus anticoagulant, lupus-like syndrome

Drug Interactions

Metabolism/Transport Effects Substrate of CYP1A2 (minor), CYP2C19 (minor), CYP3A4 (major), P-glycoprotein; **Note:** Assignment of Major/Minor substrate status based on clinically relevant drug interaction potential; **Inhibits** CYP2C8 (moderate), CYP2C9 (moderate), CYP2D6 (moderate), CYP3A4 (weak), P-glycoprotein

Avoid Concomitant Use

Avoid concomitant use of QuiNINE with any of the following: Antacids; Artemether; Conivaptan; Halofantrine; Highest Risk QTc-Prolonging Agents; Lopinavir; Lumefantrine; Macrolide Antibiotics; Mefloquine; Mifepristone; Moderate Risk QTc-Prolonging Agents; Neuromuscular-Blocking Agents; Rifampin; Ritonavir; Silodosin; Topotecan

Increased Effect/Toxicity

QuiNINE may increase the levels/effects of: Antihypertensives; Antipsychotic Agents (Phenothiazines); ARIPiprazole; CarBAMazepine; Cardiac Glycosides; Carvedilol; Colchicine; CYP2C8 Substrates; CYP2C9 Substrates; CYP2D6 Substrates; Dabigatran Etexilate; Dapsone; Dapsone (Systemic); Dapsone (Topical); Everolimus; Fesoterodine; Halofantrine; Herbs (Hypotensive Properties); Highest Risk QTc-Prolonging Agents; HMG-CoA Reductase Inhibitors; Lumefantrine; Mefloquine; Nebivolol; Neuromuscular-Blocking Agents; P-glycoprotein/ABCB1 Substrates; PHENobarbital; Prilocaine; Prucalopride; Ritonavir; Rivaroxaban; Silodosin; Theophylline Derivatives; Topotecan; Vitamin K Antagonists

The levels/effects of QuiNINE may be increased by: Alkalinizing Agents; Artemether; Cimetidine; Conivaptan; CYP3A4 Inhibitors (Moderate); CYP3A4 Inhibitors (Strong); Dapsone; Dapsone (Systemic); Ivacaftor; Macrolide Antibiotics; Mefloquine; Mifepristone; Moderate Risk QTc-Prolonging Agents; P-glycoprotein/ABCB1 Inhibitors; QTc-Prolonging Agents (Indeterminate Risk and Risk Modifying); Ritonavir

Decreased Effect

QuiNINE may decrease the levels/effects of: Codeine; TraMADol

The levels/effects of QuiNINE may be decreased by: Antacids; CarBAMazepine; CYP3A4 Inducers (Strong); Deferasirox; Fosphenytoin; Herbs (CYP3A4 Inducers); Lopinavir; P-glycoprotein/ABCB1 Inducers; PHENobarbital; Phenytoin; Rifampin; Ritonavir; Tocilizumab

Ethanol/Nutrition/Herb Interactions Herb/Nutraceutical: St John's wort may decrease quinine levels. Black cohosh, California poppy, coleus, golden seal, hawthorn, mistletoe, periwinkle, and shepherd's purse may cause excessive decreases in blood pressure.

Stability Store at 20°C to 25°C (68°F to 77°F).

Mechanism of Action Depresses oxygen uptake and carbohydrate metabolism; intercalates into DNA, disrupting the parasite's replication and transcription; cardiovascular effects similar to quinidine

Pharmacodynamics/Kinetics

Absorption: Readily, mainly from upper small intestine

Distribution: Adults: 2.5-7.1 L/kg (varies with severity of infection)

Intraerythrocytic levels are ~30% to 50% of the plasma concentration; distributes poorly to the CSF (~2% to 7% of plasma concentration)

Protein binding: 69% to 92% in healthy subjects; 78% to 95% with malaria

Metabolism: Hepatic via CYP450 enzymes, primarily CYP3A4; forms metabolites; major metabolite, 3-hydroxyquinine, is less active than parent

Bioavailability: 76% to 88% in healthy subjects; increased with malaria

Half-life elimination:

Healthy adults: 10-13 hours

Healthy elderly subjects: 18 hours

Time to peak, serum: Adults: 2-4 hours in healthy subjects; 1-11 hours with malaria

Excretion: Urine (<20% as unchanged drug)

Dosage

Geriatric & Adult Note: Actual duration of quinine treatment for malaria may be dependent upon the geographic region or pathogen. Dosage expressed in terms of the salt; 1 capsule Qualaquin® = 324 mg of quinine sulfate = 269 mg of base.

Treatment of uncomplicated chloroquine-resistant *P. falciparum* malaria (CDC guidelines): 648 mg every 8 hours for 3-7 days. Tetracycline, doxycycline, or clindamycin should also be given.

Treatment of uncomplicated chloroquine-resistant *P. vivax* malaria (unlabeled use; CDC guidelines): 648 mg every 8 hours for 3-7 days. Tetracycline or doxycycline plus primaquine should also be given.

Babesiosis (unlabeled use): 650 mg every 8 hours for 7-10 days with clindamycin

Renal Impairment

Cl_{cr} 10-50 mL/minute: Administer every 8-12 hours

Cl_{cr} <10 mL/minute: Administer every 24 hours

Severe chronic renal failure not on dialysis: Initial dose: 648 mg followed by 324 mg every 12 hours

Dialysis: Administer dose after dialysis. **Note:** Clearance of ~6.5% achieved with 1 hour of hemodialysis.

Not removed by hemo- or peritoneal dialysis; dose as for Cl_{cr} <10 mL/minute.

Continuous arteriovenous or hemodialysis: Dose as for Cl_{cr} 10-50 mL/minute.

Hepatic Impairment
Mild-to-moderate impairment: No dosing adjustment required; monitor closely.
Severe impairment (Child-Pugh class C): Data not available.

Administration Avoid use of aluminum- or magnesium-containing antacids because of drug absorption problems. Swallow dose whole to avoid bitter taste. May be administered with food.

Monitoring Parameters Monitor CBC with platelet count, liver function tests, blood glucose, ophthalmologic examination

Test Interactions May interfere with urine detection of opioids (false-positive); positive Coombs' [direct]; false elevation of urinary steroids (when assayed by Zimmerman method) and catecholamines

Special Geriatric Considerations Quinine's efficacy as a treatment for nocturnal leg cramps is not well supported in the medical and pharmacy literature. The FDA's decision to remove all quinine products (except one that is indicated for the treatment of malaria) indicates that quinine's benefits for nocturnal leg cramps do not outweigh its risks.

Dosage Forms Excipient information presented when available (limited, particularly for generics); consult specific product labeling.
Capsule, oral, as sulfate: 324 mg
Qualaquin®: 324 mg

◆ **Quinine Sulfate** see QuiNINE on page 1655

Quinupristin and Dalfopristin (kwi NYOO pris tin & dal FOE pris tin)

Related Information
Antibiotic Treatment of Adults With Infective Endocarditis on page 2157
Antimicrobial Drugs of Choice on page 2163
Brand Names: U.S. Synercid®
Brand Names: Canada Synercid®
Index Terms Dalfopristin and Quinupristin; RP-59500
Generic Availability (U.S.) No
Pharmacologic Category Antibiotic, Streptogramin
Use Treatment of complicated skin and skin structure infections caused by methicillin-susceptible *Staphylococcus aureus* or *Streptococcus pyogenes*
Unlabeled Use Treatment of persistent MRSA bacteremia associated with vancomycin failure
Contraindications Hypersensitivity to quinupristin, dalfopristin, pristinamycin, or virginiamycin, or any component of the formulation
Warnings/Precautions Use with caution in patients with hepatic or renal dysfunction. May cause pain and phlebitis when infused through a peripheral line (not relieved by hydrocortisone or diphenhydramine). Prolonged use may result in fungal or bacterial superinfection, including *C. difficile*-associated diarrhea (CDAD) and pseudomembranous colitis; CDAD has been observed >2 months postantibiotic treatment. May cause arthralgias, myalgias, and hyperbilirubinemia. May inhibit the metabolism of many drugs metabolized by CYP3A4. Concurrent therapy with cisapride (which may prolong QT_c interval and lead to arrhythmias) should be avoided.

Adverse Reactions (Reflective of adult population; not specific for elderly)
>10%:
Hepatic: Hyperbilirubinemia (3% to 35%)
Local: Local pain (40% to 44%), inflammation at infusion site (38% to 42%), local edema (17% to 18%), infusion site reaction (12% to 13%)
Neuromuscular & skeletal: Arthralgia (up to 47%), myalgia (up to 47%)
1% to 10%:
Central nervous system: Pain (2% to 3%), headache (2%)
Dermatologic: Rash (3%), pruritus (2%)
Endocrine & metabolic: Hyperglycemia (1%)
Gastrointestinal: Nausea (3% to 5%), vomiting (3% to 4%), diarrhea (3%)
Hematologic: Anemia (3%)
Hepatic: GGT increased (2%), LDH increased (3%)
Local: Thrombophlebitis (2%)
Neuromuscular & skeletal: CPK increased (2%)

Drug Interactions
Metabolism/Transport Effects Refer to individual components.
Avoid Concomitant Use
Avoid concomitant use of Quinupristin and Dalfopristin with any of the following: Pimozide
Increased Effect/Toxicity
Quinupristin and Dalfopristin may increase the levels/effects of: ARIPiprazole; CycloSPOR-INE; CycloSPORINE (Systemic); Pimozide
Decreased Effect There are no known significant interactions involving a decrease in effect.
Stability Store unopened vials under refrigeration at 2°C to 8°C (36°F to 46°F). The following stability information has also been reported: May be stored at room temperature for up to 7 days (Cohen, 2007).

Reconstitute single dose vial with 5 mL of 5% dextrose in water or sterile water for injection. Swirl gently to dissolve; do not shake (to limit foam formation). The reconstituted solution should be diluted within 30 minutes. Stability of the diluted solution prior to the infusion is established as 5 hours at room temperature or 54 hours if refrigerated at 2°C to 8°C (36°F to 46°F). Reconstituted solution should be added to at least 250 mL of 5% dextrose in water for peripheral administration (increase to 500 mL or 750 mL if necessary to limit venous irritation). An infusion volume of 100 mL may be used for central line infusions. Do not freeze solution.
Mechanism of Action Quinupristin/dalfopristin inhibits bacterial protein synthesis by binding to different sites on the 50S bacterial ribosomal subunit thereby inhibiting protein synthesis
Pharmacodynamics/Kinetics
Distribution: Quinupristin: 0.45 L/kg; Dalfopristin: 0.24 L/kg
Metabolism: To active metabolites via nonenzymatic reactions
Half-life elimination: Quinupristin: 0.85 hour; Dalfopristin: 0.7 hour (mean elimination half-lives, including metabolites: 3 and 1 hours, respectively)
Excretion: Feces (75% to 77% as unchanged drug and metabolites); urine (15% to 19%)
Dosage
Geriatric & Adult
Complicated skin and skin structure infection: I.V.: 7.5 mg/kg every 12 hours for at least 7 days
Bacteremia, MRSA (persistent, vancomycin failure) (unlabeled use): I.V.: 7.5 mg/kg every 8 hours (Liu, 2011)
Renal Impairment No adjustment is necessary in renal failure, hemodialysis, or peritoneal dialysis.
Hepatic Impairment Pharmacokinetic data suggest dosage adjustment may be necessary; however, specific recommendations have not been proposed.
Administration Line should be flushed with 5% dextrose in water prior to and following administration. Infusion should be completed over 60 minutes (toxicity may be increased with shorter infusion). If severe venous irritation occurs following peripheral administration of quinupristin/dalfopristin diluted in 250 mL 5% dextrose in water, consideration should be given to increasing the infusion volume to 500 mL or 750 mL, changing the infusion site, or infusing by a peripherally-inserted central catheter (PICC) or a central venous catheter.
Monitoring Parameters Culture and sensitivity
Special Geriatric Considerations No pharmacokinetic changes in the elderly in one study. No dose adjustment necessary.
Dosage Forms Excipient information presented when available (limited, particularly for generics); consult specific product labeling.
Injection, powder for reconstitution:
Synercid®: 500 mg: Quinupristin 150 mg and dalfopristin 350 mg

RABEprazole (ra BEP ra zole)

Related Information
H. pylori Treatment in Adult Patients *on page 2116*
Medication Safety Issues
Sound-alike/look-alike issues:
AcipHex® may be confused with Acephen™, Accupril®, Aricept®, pHisoHex®

RABEprazole may be confused with ARIPiprazole, donepezil, lansoprazole, omeprazole, raloxifene

Brand Names: U.S. AcipHex®

Brand Names: Canada Apo-Rabeprazole®; Pariet®; Pat-Rabeprazole; PMS-Rabeprazole EC; PRO-Rabeprazole; Rabeprazole EC; RAN™-Rabeprazole; Riva-Rabeprazole EC; Sandoz-Rabeprazole; Teva-Rabeprazole EC

Index Terms Pariprazole

Generic Availability (U.S.) No

Pharmacologic Category Proton Pump Inhibitor; Substituted Benzimidazole

Use Short-term (4-8 weeks) treatment and maintenance of erosive or ulcerative gastroesophageal reflux disease (GERD); symptomatic GERD; short-term (up to 4 weeks) treatment of duodenal ulcers; long-term treatment of pathological hypersecretory conditions, including Zollinger-Ellison syndrome; *H. pylori* eradication (in combination therapy)

Canadian labeling: Additional uses (not in U.S. labeling): Treatment of nonerosive reflux disease (NERD); treatment of gastric ulcers

Unlabeled Use Maintenance of duodenal ulcer

Contraindications Hypersensitivity to rabeprazole, substituted benzimidazoles (ie, esomeprazole, lansoprazole, omeprazole, pantoprazole), or any component of the formulation

Warnings/Precautions Use of proton pump inhibitors (PPIs) may increase the risk of gastrointestinal infections (eg, *Salmonella, Campylobacter*). Use caution in severe hepatic impairment. Relief of symptoms with rabeprazole does not preclude the presence of a gastric malignancy. Decreased *H. pylori* eradication rates have been observed with short-term (≤7 days) combination therapy. The American College of Gastroenterology recommends 10-14 days of therapy (triple or quadruple) for eradication of *H. pylori* (Chey, 2007).

PPIs may diminish the therapeutic effect of clopidogrel, thought to be due to reduced formation of the active metabolite of clopidogrel. The manufacturer of clopidogrel recommends either avoidance of omeprazole or use of a PPI with less potent CYP2C19 inhibition (eg, pantoprazole); given the potency of CYP2C19 inhibitory activity, avoidance of rabeprazole would appear prudent. Others have recommended the continued use of PPIs, regardless of the degree of inhibition, in patients with a history of GI bleeding or multiple risk factors for GI bleeding who are also receiving clopidogrel since no evidence has established clinically meaningful differences in outcome; however, a clinically-significant interaction cannot be excluded in those who are poor metabolizers of clopidogrel (Abraham, 2010; Levine, 2011). Concomitant use of rabeprazole with some drugs may require cautious use, may not be recommended, or may require dosage adjustments.

Increased incidence of osteoporosis-related bone fractures of the hip, spine, or wrist may occur with PPI therapy. Patients on high-dose (multiple daily doses) or long-term therapy (≥1 year) should be monitored. Use the lowest effective dose for the shortest duration of time, use vitamin D and calcium supplementation, and follow appropriate guidelines to reduce risk of fractures in patients at risk.

Hypomagnesemia, reported rarely, usually with prolonged PPI use of >3 months (most cases >1 year of therapy); may be symptomatic or asymptomatic; severe cases may cause tetany, seizures, and cardiac arrhythmias. Consider obtaining serum magnesium concentrations prior to beginning long-term therapy, especially if taking concomitant digoxin, diuretics, or other drugs known to cause hypomagnesemia; and periodically thereafter. Hypomagnesemia may be corrected by magnesium supplementation, although discontinuation of rabeprazole may be necessary; magnesium levels typically return to normal within 1 week of stopping.

Adverse Reactions (Reflective of adult population; not specific for elderly) 1% to 10%:

Central nervous system: Pain (3%), headache (2% to 5%)

Gastrointestinal: Diarrhea (3%), flatulence (3%), constipation (2%), nausea (2%)

Respiratory: Pharyngitis (3%)

Miscellaneous: Infection (2%)

Drug Interactions

Metabolism/Transport Effects Substrate of CYP2C19 (major), CYP3A4 (major); **Note:** Assignment of Major/Minor substrate status based on clinically relevant drug interaction potential; **Inhibits** CYP2C19 (moderate), CYP2C8 (moderate), CYP2D6 (weak), CYP3A4 (weak)

Avoid Concomitant Use

Avoid concomitant use of RABEprazole with any of the following: Delavirdine; Erlotinib; Nelfinavir; Pimozide; Posaconazole; Rilpivirine

Increased Effect/Toxicity

RABEprazole may increase the levels/effects of: Amphetamines; ARIPiprazole; Citalopram; CYP2C19 Substrates; CYP2C8 Substrates; Dexmethylphenidate; Methotrexate; Methylphenidate; Pimozide; Raltegravir; Saquinavir; Tacrolimus; Tacrolimus (Systemic); Voriconazole

The levels/effects of RABEprazole may be increased by: Fluconazole; Ketoconazole; Ketoconazole (Systemic)

Decreased Effect

RABEprazole may decrease the levels/effects of: Atazanavir; Bisphosphonate Derivatives; Cefditoren; Clopidogrel; Dabigatran Etexilate; Dasatinib; Delavirdine; Erlotinib; Gefitinib; Indinavir; Iron Salts; Itraconazole; Ketoconazole; Ketoconazole (Systemic); Mesalamine; Mycophenolate; Nelfinavir; Nilotinib; Posaconazole; Rilpivirine; Vismodegib

The levels/effects of RABEprazole may be decreased by: CYP2C19 Inducers (Strong); CYP3A4 Inducers (Strong); Deferasirox; Herbs (CYP3A4 Inducers); Tipranavir; Tocilizumab

Ethanol/Nutrition/Herb Interactions

Ethanol: Avoid ethanol (may cause gastric mucosal irritation).

Food: High-fat meals may delay absorption, but C_{max} and AUC are not altered.

Herb/Nutraceutical: St John's wort may increase the metabolism and thus decrease the levels/effects of rabeprazole.

Stability Store at 25°C (77°F). Protect from moisture.

Mechanism of Action Potent proton pump inhibitor; suppresses gastric acid secretion by inhibiting the parietal cell H+/K+ ATP pump

Pharmacodynamics/Kinetics

Onset of action: Within 1 hour

Duration: 24 hours

Absorption: Oral: Well absorbed within 1 hour

Protein binding, serum: ~96%

Metabolism: Hepatic via CYP3A and 2C19 to inactive metabolites

Bioavailability: Oral: ~52%

Half-life elimination (dose dependent): 1-2 hours

Time to peak, plasma: 2-5 hours

Excretion: Urine (90% primarily as thioether carboxylic acid metabolites); remainder in feces

Dosage

Geriatric & Adult

GERD, erosive/ulcerative: Oral: Treatment: 20 mg once daily for 4-8 weeks; if inadequate response, may repeat up to an additional 8 weeks; maintenance: 20 mg once daily

Canadian labeling: Oral: 20 mg once daily for 4 weeks; if inadequate response, may repeat for an additional 4 weeks (lack of symptom control after 4 weeks warrants further evaluation); maintenance: 10 mg once daily (maximum: 20 mg once daily)

GERD, symptomatic: Oral: Treatment: 20 mg once daily for 4 weeks; if inadequate response, may repeat for an additional 4 weeks

Canadian labeling: Oral: 10 mg once daily (maximum: 20 mg once daily) for 4 weeks; lack of symptom control after 4 weeks warrants further evaluation

Duodenal ulcer: Oral: 20 mg/day before breakfast for 4 weeks; additional therapy may be required for some patients

Gastric ulcers (*Canadian labeling*): Oral: 20 mg once daily up to 6 weeks; additional therapy may be required for some patients

***Helicobacter pylori* eradication:** Oral:

Manufacturer's labeling: 20 mg twice daily administered with amoxicillin 1000 mg *and* clarithromycin 500 mg twice daily for 7 days

American College of Gastroenterology guidelines (Chey, 2007):

Nonpenicillin allergy: 20 mg twice daily administered with amoxicillin 1000 mg *and* clarithromycin 500 mg twice daily for 10-14 days

Penicillin allergy: 20 mg twice daily administered with clarithromycin 500 mg *and* metronidazole 500 mg twice daily for 10-14 days **or** 20 mg once or twice daily administered with bismuth subsalicylate 525 mg *and* metronidazole 250 mg *plus* tetracycline 500 mg 4 times/day for 10-14 days

Hypersecretory conditions: Oral: 60 mg once daily; dose may need to be adjusted as necessary. Doses as high as 100 mg once daily and 60 mg twice daily have been used, and continued as long as necessary (up to 1 year in some patients).

NERD (*Canadian labeling*): Oral: Treatment: 10 mg (maximum: 20 mg once daily) for 4 weeks; lack of symptom control after 4 weeks warrants further evaluation

Renal Impairment No dosage adjustment required.

Hepatic Impairment

Mild-to-moderate: Elimination decreased; no dosage adjustment required.

Severe: Use caution.

Administration May be administered without regard to meals; best if taken before breakfast. Do not crush, split, or chew tablet. May be administered with an antacid.

Special Geriatric Considerations No difference in efficacy or safety was noted in elderly subjects as compared to younger subjects. No dosage adjustment is necessary in the elderly.

An increased risk of fractures of the hip, spine, or wrist has been observed in epidemiologic studies with proton pump inhibitor (PPI) use, primarily in older adults ≥50 years of age. The greatest risk was seen in patients receiving high doses or on long-term therapy (≥1 year). Calcium and vitamin D supplementation and close monitoring are recommended to reduce the risk of fracture in high-risk patients. Additionally, long-term use of proton pump inhibitors has resulted in reports of hypomagnesemia and *Clostridium difficile* infections.

Dosage Forms Excipient information presented when available (limited, particularly for generics); consult specific product labeling.

Tablet, delayed release, enteric coated, oral, as sodium:

AcipHex®: 20 mg

Dosage Forms: Canada Excipient information presented when available (limited, particularly for generics); consult specific product labeling.

Tablet, delayed release, enteric coated, as sodium:

Pariet®: 10 mg, 20 mg

Rabies Immune Globulin (Human) (RAY beez i MYUN GLOB yoo lin, HYU man)

Related Information

Immunization Administration Recommendations *on page 2144*
Immunization Recommendations *on page 2149*

Brand Names: U.S. HyperRAB® S/D; Imogam® Rabies-HT

Brand Names: Canada HyperRAB® S/D; Imogam® Rabies Pasteurized

Index Terms HRIG; RIG

Generic Availability (U.S.) No

Pharmacologic Category Blood Product Derivative; Immune Globulin

Use Part of postexposure prophylaxis of persons with rabies exposure. Provides passive immunity until active immunity with rabies vaccine is established. Not for use in persons with a history of pre-exposure vaccination, history of postexposure prophylaxis, or previous vaccination with rabies vaccine and documentation of antibody response.

Contraindications There are no contraindications listed within the FDA-approved manufacturer's labeling.

Warnings/Precautions Hypersensitivity and anaphylactic reactions can occur; immediate treatment (including epinephrine 1:1000) should be available. Use with caution in patients with isolated immunoglobulin A deficiency or a history of systemic hypersensitivity to human immunoglobulins. Use with caution in patients with thrombocytopenia or coagulation disorders; I.M. injections may be contraindicated. Product of human plasma; may potentially contain infectious agents which could transmit disease. Screening of donors, as well as testing and/or inactivation or removal of certain viruses, reduces the risk. Infections thought to be transmitted by this product should be reported to the manufacturer. Not for intravenous administration.

Adverse Reactions (Reflective of adult population; not specific for elderly) Frequency not defined.

Central nervous system: Fever (mild), headache, malaise

Dermatologic: Angioneurotic edema, rash

Local: Injection site: Pain, stiffness, soreness, tenderness

Renal: Nephrotic syndrome

Miscellaneous: Anaphylaxis

Drug Interactions

Metabolism/Transport Effects None known.

Avoid Concomitant Use There are no known interactions where it is recommended to avoid concomitant use.

Increased Effect/Toxicity There are no known significant interactions involving an increase in effect.

Decreased Effect

Rabies Immune Globulin (Human) may decrease the levels/effects of: Vaccines (Live)

Stability Store between 2°C to 8°C (36°F to 46°F); do not freeze. Discard product exposed to freezing. The following stability information has also been reported for HyperRAB® S/D: May be exposed to room temperature for a cumulative 7 days (Cohen, 2007).

Mechanism of Action Rabies immune globulin is a solution of globulins dried from the plasma or serum of selected adult human donors who have been immunized with rabies vaccine and have developed high titers of rabies antibody. It generally contains 10% to 18% of protein of which not less than 80% is monomeric immunoglobulin G.

Dosage

Geriatric & Adult Postexposure prophylaxis: Local wound infiltration: 20 units/kg in a single dose, RIG should always be administered as part of rabies vaccine regimen. If anatomically feasible, the full rabies immune globulin dose should be infiltrated around and into the wound(s); remaining volume should be administered I.M. at a site distant from the vaccine administration site. If rabies vaccine was initiated without rabies immune globulin, rabies immune globulin may be administered through the seventh day after the administration of the first dose of the vaccine. Administration of RIG is not recommended after the seventh day post vaccine since an antibody response to the vaccine is expected during this time period.

Note: Not for use in persons with a history of pre-exposure vaccination, history of postexposure prophylaxis, or previous vaccination with rabies vaccine and documentation of antibody response.

Administration Do not administer I.V.

Postexposure wound infiltration: If anatomically feasible, the full rabies immune globulin dose should be infiltrated around and into the wound(s); remaining volume should be administered I.M. in the deltoid muscle of the upper arm or lateral thigh muscle. The gluteal area should be avoided to reduce the risk of sciatic nerve damage. Do not administer rabies vaccine in the same syringe or at the same administration site as RIG.

Monitoring Parameters Monitor for adverse effects

Special Geriatric Considerations No special considerations are needed for initiating therapy. No specific data relevant to the elderly to date.

Dosage Forms Excipient information presented when available (limited, particularly for generics); consult specific product labeling.

Injection, solution [preservative free]:

HyperRAB® S/D: 150 units/mL (2 mL, 10 mL) [solvent/detergent treated]

Imogam® Rabies-HT: 150 units/mL (2 mL, 10 mL) [heat treated]

Rabies Vaccine (RAY beez vak SEEN)

Related Information

Immunization Administration Recommendations *on page 2144*

Immunization Recommendations *on page 2149*

Brand Names: U.S. Imovax® Rabies; RabAvert®

Brand Names: Canada Imovax® Rabies; RabAvert®

Index Terms HDCV; Human Diploid Cell Cultures Rabies Vaccine; PCEC; Purified Chick Embryo Cell

Generic Availability (U.S.) No

Pharmacologic Category Vaccine, Inactivated (Viral)

Use Pre-exposure and postexposure vaccination against rabies

The Advisory Committee on Immunization Practices (ACIP) recommends a primary course of prophylactic immunization (pre-exposure vaccination) for the following:

- Persons with continuous risk of infection, including rabies research laboratory and biologics production workers
- Persons with frequent risk of infection in areas where rabies is enzootic, including rabies diagnostic laboratory workers, cavers, veterinarians and their staff, and animal control and wildlife workers; persons who frequently handle bats
- Persons with infrequent risk of infection, including veterinarians and animal control staff with terrestrial animals in areas where rabies infection is rare, veterinary students, and travelers visiting areas where rabies is enzootic and immediate access to medical care and biologicals is limited

The ACIP recommends the use of postexposure vaccination for a particular person be assessed by the severity and likelihood versus the actual risk of acquiring rabies. Consideration should include the type of exposure, epidemiology of rabies in the area, species of the animal, circumstances of the incident, and the availability of the exposing animal for observation or rabies testing. Postexposure vaccination is used in both previously vaccinated and previously unvaccinated individuals.

Contraindications

Pre-exposure prophylaxis: Hypersensitivity to rabies vaccine or any component of the formulation

Postexposure prophylaxis: There are no contraindications listed within the FDA-approved manufacturer's labeling.

Warnings/Precautions Rabies vaccine should not be used in persons with a confirmed diagnosis of rabies; use after the onset of symptoms may be detrimental. Postexposure vaccination may begin regardless of the length of time from documented or likely exposure, as long as clinical signs of rabies are not present. Immediate treatment (including epinephrine 1:1000) for anaphylactoid and/or hypersensitivity reactions should be available during vaccine use. Once postexposure prophylaxis has begun, administration should generally not be interrupted or discontinued due to local or mild adverse events. Continuation of vaccination following severe systemic reactions should consider the persons risk of developing rabies. Report serious reactions to the State Health Department or the manufacturer/distributor. An immune complex reaction is possible 2-21 days following booster doses of HDCV. Symptoms may include arthralgia, arthritis, angioedema, fever, generalized urticaria, malaise, nausea, and vomiting. Syncope has been reported with use of injectable vaccines and may be accompanied by transient visual disturbances, weakness, or tonic-clonic movements. Procedures should be in place to avoid injuries from falling and to restore cerebral perfusion if syncope occurs. Vaccination may not result in effective immunity in all patients. Response depends upon multiple factors (eg, type of vaccine, age of patient) and may be improved by administering the vaccine at the recommended dose, route, and interval. Vaccines may not be effective if administered during periods of altered immune competence (CDC, 2011). Use with caution in severely immunocompromised patients (eg, patients receiving chemo/radiation therapy or other immunosuppressive therapy [including high-dose corticosteroids]); may have a reduced response to vaccination. Withhold nonessential immunosuppressive agents during postexposure prophylaxis; if possible postpone pre-exposure prophylaxis until the immunocompromising condition is resolved. Persons with altered immunocompetence should receive the five-dose postexposure vaccine regimen. In general, household and close contacts of persons with altered immunocompetence may receive all age appropriate vaccines. Imovax® Rabies contains albumin and neomycin. RabAvert® contains amphotericin B, bovine gelatin, chicken protein, chlortetracycline, and neomycin. For I. M. administration only.

Adverse Reactions (Reflective of adult population; not specific for elderly) All serious adverse reactions must be reported to the U.S. Department of Health and Human Services (DHHS) Vaccine Adverse Event Reporting System (VAERS) 1-800-822-7967 or online at https://vaers.hhs.gov/esub/index. In Canada, adverse reactions may be reported to local provincial/territorial health agencies or to the Vaccine Safety Section at Public Health Agency of Canada (1-866-844-0018).

>10%:
  Central nervous system: Dizziness, headache, malaise
  Gastrointestinal: Abdominal pain, nausea
  Local: Erythema, itching, pain, swelling
  Neuromuscular & skeletal: Myalgia
  Miscellaneous: Lymphadenopathy
Uncommon, frequency not defined, postmarketing, and/or case reports:
  Cardiovascular: Circulatory reactions, edema, palpitation
  Central nervous system: Chills, fatigue, fever >38°C (100°F), Guillain-Barré syndrome, encephalitis, meningitis, multiple sclerosis, myelitis, neuroparalysis, vertigo
  Dermatologic: Pruritus, urticaria, urticaria pigmentosa
  Endocrine & metabolic: Hot flashes
  Local: Limb swelling (extensive)
  Neuromuscular & skeletal: Limb pain, monoarthritis, paralysis (transient), paresthesias (transient)
  Ocular: Retrobulbar neuritis, visual disturbances
  Respiratory: Bronchospasm
  Miscellaneous: Allergic reactions, anaphylaxis, hypersensitivity reactions, swollen lymph nodes

Drug Interactions
  Metabolism/Transport Effects None known.
  Avoid Concomitant Use There are no known interactions where it is recommended to avoid concomitant use.
  Increased Effect/Toxicity There are no known significant interactions involving an increase in effect.
  Decreased Effect
    The levels/effects of Rabies Vaccine may be decreased by: Belimumab; Chloroquine; Fingolimod; Immunosuppressants

Stability Prior to reconstitution, store under refrigeration at 2°C to 8°C (36°F to 46°F); do not freeze. Protect from light. Reconstitute with provided diluent; gently swirl to dissolve. Use immediately after reconstitution.
Imovax®: Suspension will appear pink to red
RabAvert®: Suspension will appear clear to slightly opaque

Mechanism of Action Rabies vaccine is an inactivated virus vaccine which promotes immunity by inducing an active immune response. The production of specific antibodies requires about 7-10 days to develop. Rabies immune globulin or antirabies serum, equine (ARS) is given in conjunction with rabies vaccine to provide immune protection until an antibody response can occur.

Pharmacodynamics/Kinetics
Onset of action: I.M.: Rabies antibody: ~7-10 days
Peak effect: ~30-60 days
Duration: ≥1 year

Dosage

Geriatric & Adult

Pre-exposure vaccination: I.M.: A total of 3 doses, 1 mL each, on days 0, 7, and 21-28.
Note: Prolonging the interval between doses does not interfere with immunity achieved after the concluding dose of the basic series.

Postexposure vaccination: All postexposure treatment should begin with immediate cleansing of the wound with soap and water

Persons not previously immunized as above: I.M.: 5 doses (1 mL each) on days 0, 3, 7, 14, 28. In addition, patients should receive rabies immune globulin with the first dose (day 0).
Note: A regimen of 4 doses (1 mL each) on days 0, 3, 7, 14 may be used in persons who are not immunosuppressed (ACIP recommendations, 2010).

Persons who have previously received postexposure prophylaxis with rabies vaccine, received a recommended I.M. pre-exposure series of rabies vaccine or have a previously documented rabies antibody titer considered adequate: I.M.: Two doses (1 mL each) on days 0 and 3; do not administer rabies immune globulin

Booster (for persons with continuous or frequent risk of infection): I.M.: 1 mL based on antibody titers

Administration For I.M. administration only; this rabies vaccine product must not be administered intradermally; in adults, administer I.M. injections in the deltoid muscle, not the gluteal. Postexposure prophylaxis should begin with immediate cleansing of wounds with soap and water; if available, a virucidal agent (eg povidone-iodine solution) should be used to irrigate the wounds.

For patients at risk of hemorrhage following intramuscular injection, the ACIP recommends "it should be administered intramuscularly if, in the opinion of the physician familiar with the patients bleeding risk, the vaccine can be administered by this route with reasonable safety. If the patient receives antihemophilia or other similar therapy, intramuscular vaccination can be scheduled shortly after such therapy is administered. A fine needle (23 gauge or smaller) can be used for the vaccination and firm pressure applied to the site (without rubbing) for at least 2 minutes. The patient should be instructed concerning the risk of hematoma from the injection." Patients on anticoagulant therapy should be considered to have the same bleeding risks and treated as those with clotting factor disorders (CDC, 2011).

Simultaneous administration of vaccines helps ensure the patients will be fully vaccinated by the appropriate age. Simultaneous administration of vaccines is defined as administering >1 vaccine on the same day at different anatomic sites. The use of licensed combination vaccines is generally preferred over separate injections of the equivalent components. Separate vaccines should not be combined in the same syringe unless indicated by product specific labeling. Separate needles and syringes should be used for each injection. The ACIP prefers each dose of a specific vaccine in a series come from the same manufacturer when possible. Adolescents and adults should be vaccinated while seated or lying down. In general, preterm infants should be vaccinated at the same chronological age as full-term infants (CDC, 2011).

Antipyretics have not been shown to prevent febrile seizures. Antipyretics may be used to treat fever or discomfort following vaccination (CDC, 2011). One study reported that routine prophylactic administration of acetaminophen to prevent fever prior to vaccination decreased the immune response of some vaccines; the clinical significance of this reduction in immune response has not been established (Prymula, 2009).

Monitoring Parameters Monitor for syncope for 15 minutes following administration. If seizure-like activity associated with syncope occurs, maintain patient in supine or Trendelenburg position to reestablish adequate cerebral perfusion.

Antibody response to vaccination is not recommended for otherwise healthy persons who complete the pre-exposure or postexposure regimen. Serologic testing to determine if the antibody titer is at an acceptable level is required for the following persons (booster vaccination recommended if titer is below the acceptable level):

Persons with continuous risk of infection: Serologic testing every 6 months
Persons with frequent risk of infection: Serologic testing every 2 years
Persons who are immunocompromised: Serologic testing after completion of pre-exposure or postexposure prophylaxis series

Monitoring of antibody response to vaccination is not recommended for otherwise healthy persons who complete the pre-exposure or postexposure regimen.

Reference Range Adequate adaptive immune response: antibody titers of 0.5 units/mL [WHO] or complete virus neutralization at a 1:5 serum dilution by the rapid fluorescent focus inhibition test (RFFIT) [ACIP]

Pharmacotherapy Pearls U.S. federal law requires that the name of medication, date of administration, the vaccine manufacturer, lot number of vaccine, and the administering person's name, title, and address be entered into the patient's permanent medical record.

Special Geriatric Considerations No specific data for use in the elderly. Use as recommended in elderly patients for whom this vaccine would be indicated.

Dosage Forms Excipient information presented when available (limited, particularly for generics); consult specific product labeling.

Injection, powder for reconstitution [preservative free]:

Imovax® Rabies: ≥2.5 units [contains albumin (human), neomycin (may have trace amounts); HDCV; grown in human diploid cell culture; supplied with diluent]

RabAvert®: ≥2.5 units [contains albumin (human), amphotericin B (may have trace amounts), bovine gelatin, chicken egg protein, chlortetracycline (may have trace amounts), neomycin (may have trace amounts); PCEC; grown in chicken fibroblast culture; supplied with diluent]

◆ **Racemic Epinephrine** see EPINEPHrine (Systemic, Oral Inhalation) on page 645
◆ **Racepinephrine** see EPINEPHrine (Systemic, Oral Inhalation) on page 645
◆ **R-albuterol** see Levalbuterol on page 1106

Raloxifene (ral OKS i feen)

Related Information
Osteoporosis Management on page 2136

Medication Safety Issues
Sound-alike/look-alike issues:
Evista® may be confused with AVINza®, Eovist®

Brand Names: U.S. Evista®

Brand Names: Canada Apo-Raloxifene®; Evista®; Novo-Raloxifene; Teva-Raloxifene

Index Terms Keoxifene Hydrochloride; Raloxifene Hydrochloride

Generic Availability (U.S.) No

Pharmacologic Category Selective Estrogen Receptor Modulator (SERM)

Use Prevention and treatment of osteoporosis in postmenopausal women; risk reduction for invasive breast cancer in postmenopausal women with osteoporosis and in postmenopausal women with high risk for invasive breast cancer

Medication Guide Available Yes

Contraindications History of or current venous thromboembolic disorders (including DVT, PE, and retinal vein thrombosis)

Warnings/Precautions Hazardous agent - use appropriate precautions for handling and disposal. **[U.S. Boxed Warning]: May increase the risk for DVT or PE; use contraindicated in patients with history of or current venous thromboembolic disorders.** Use with caution in patients at high risk for venous thromboembolism; the risk for DVT and PE are higher in the first 4 months of treatment. Discontinue at least 72 hours prior to and during prolonged immobilization (postoperative recovery or prolonged bedrest). **[U.S. Boxed Warning]: The risk of death due to stroke may be increased in women with coronary heart disease or in women at risk for coronary events;** use with caution in patients with cardiovascular disease. Not be used for the prevention of cardiovascular disease. Use caution with moderate-to-severe renal dysfunction, hepatic impairment, unexplained uterine bleeding, and in women with a history of elevated triglycerides in response to treatment with oral estrogens (or estrogen/progestin). Safety with concomitant estrogen therapy has not been established. Safety and efficacy in premenopausal women or men have not been established. Not indicated for treatment of invasive breast cancer, to reduce the risk of recurrence of invasive breast cancer or to reduce the risk of noninvasive breast cancer. The efficacy (for breast cancer risk reduction) in women with inherited BRCA1 and BRCA1 mutations has not been established.

Adverse Reactions (Reflective of adult population; not specific for elderly) Note: Raloxifene has been associated with increased risk of thromboembolism (DVT, PE) and superficial thrombophlebitis; risk is similar to reported risk of HRT

>10%:
Cardiovascular: Peripheral edema (3% to 14%)
Endocrine & metabolic: Hot flashes (8% to 29%)
Neuromuscular & skeletal: Arthralgia (11% to 16%), leg cramps/muscle spasm (6% to 12%)
Miscellaneous: Flu syndrome (14% to 15%), infection (11%)

1% to 10%:
Cardiovascular: Chest pain (3%), venous thromboembolism (1% to 2%)
Central nervous system: Insomnia (6%)
Dermatologic: Rash (6%)
Endocrine & metabolic: Breast pain (4%)

Gastrointestinal: Weight gain (9%), abdominal pain (7%), vomiting (5%), flatulence (2% to 3%), cholelithiasis (≤3%), gastroenteritis (≤3%)

Genitourinary: Vaginal bleeding (6%), leukorrhea (3%), urinary tract disorder (3%), uterine disorder (3%), vaginal hemorrhage (3%), endometrial disorder (≤3%)

Neuromuscular & skeletal: Myalgia (8%), tendon disorder (4%)

Respiratory: Bronchitis (10%), sinusitis (10%), pharyngitis (8%), pneumonia (3%), laryngitis (≤2%)

Miscellaneous: Diaphoresis (3%)

Drug Interactions

Metabolism/Transport Effects None known.

Avoid Concomitant Use There are no known interactions where it is recommended to avoid concomitant use.

Increased Effect/Toxicity There are no known significant interactions involving an increase in effect.

Decreased Effect

Raloxifene may decrease the levels/effects of: Levothyroxine

The levels/effects of Raloxifene may be decreased by: Bile Acid Sequestrants

Ethanol/Nutrition/Herb Interactions Ethanol: Avoid ethanol (may increase risk of osteoporosis).

Stability Store at controlled room temperature of 20°C to 25°C (68°F to 77°F); excursions permitted to 15°C to 30°C (59°F to 86°F).

Mechanism of Action A selective estrogen receptor modulator (SERM), meaning that it affects some of the same receptors that estrogen does, but not all, and in some instances, it antagonizes or blocks estrogen; it acts like estrogen to prevent bone loss and has the potential to block some estrogen effects in the breast and uterine tissues. Raloxifene decreases bone resorption, increasing bone mineral density and decreasing fracture incidence.

Pharmacodynamics/Kinetics

Onset of action: 8 weeks

Absorption: Rapid; ~60%

Distribution: 2348 L/kg

Protein binding: >95% to albumin and α-glycoprotein; does not bind to sex-hormone-binding globulin

Metabolism: Hepatic, extensive first-pass effect; metabolized to glucuronide conjugates

Bioavailability: ~2%

Half-life elimination: 28-33 hours

Excretion: Primarily feces; urine (<0.2% as unchanged drug; <6% as glucuronide conjugates)

Dosage

Geriatric & Adult

Osteoporosis: Females: Oral: 60 mg once daily

Invasive breast cancer risk reduction: Female: Oral: 60 mg once daily for 5 years per ASCO guidelines (Visvanathan, 2009)

Renal Impairment Moderate-to-severe impairment: Use caution; safety and efficacy have not been established.

Hepatic Impairment Mild impairment (Child-Pugh class A): Plasma concentrations were higher and correlated with total bilirubin. Safety and efficacy in hepatic insufficiency have not been established.

Administration May be administered any time of the day without regard to meals.

Monitoring Parameters Bone mineral density (BMD), lipid profile; adequate diagnostic measures, including endometrial sampling, if indicated, should be performed to rule out malignancy in all cases of undiagnosed abnormal vaginal bleeding

Pharmacotherapy Pearls The decrease in estrogen-related adverse effects with the selective estrogen-receptor modulators in general and raloxifene in particular should improve compliance and decrease the incidence of cardiovascular events and fractures while not increasing breast cancer.

Oncology Comment: The American Society of Clinical Oncology (ASCO) guidelines for breast cancer risk reduction (Visvanathan, 2009) recommend raloxifene (for 5 years) as an option to reduce the risk of ER-positive invasive breast cancer in postmenopausal women with a 5-year projected risk (based on NCI trial model) of ≥1.66%, or with lobular carcinoma *in situ*. Raloxifene should not be used in premenopausal women. Women with osteoporosis may use raloxifene beyond 5 years of treatment. According to the NCCN breast cancer risk reduction guidelines (v.2.2009), raloxifene is only recommended for postmenopausal women (≥35 years of age), and is equivalent to tamoxifen although, raloxifene has a better adverse event profile; however, tamoxifen is superior in reducing the risk on noninvasive breast cancer.

Special Geriatric Considerations Raloxifene has only been shown to lower the risk of vertebral fractures. Women may experience hot flushes, leg cramps, and peripheral edema. Avoid in bedbound patients due to increased risk of thromboembolism. The U.S. Preventive Services Task Force (USPSTF) recommends against routine use of raloxifene (or tamoxifen) for the primary prevention of breast cancer in women at low or average risk.

Dosage Forms Excipient information presented when available (limited, particularly for generics); consult specific product labeling.

Tablet, oral, as hydrochloride:

Evista®: 60 mg

♦ **Raloxifene Hydrochloride** see Raloxifene on page 1666

Ramelteon (ra MEL tee on)

Medication Safety Issues
Sound-alike/look-alike issues:
Ramelteon may be confused with Remeron®
Rozerem® may be confused with Razadyne®, Remeron®

Brand Names: U.S. Rozerem®

Index Terms TAK-375

Generic Availability (U.S.) No

Pharmacologic Category Hypnotic, Miscellaneous

Use Treatment of insomnia characterized by difficulty with sleep onset

Medication Guide Available Yes

Contraindications History of angioedema with previous ramelteon therapy (do not rechallenge); concurrent use with fluvoxamine

Warnings/Precautions Symptomatic treatment of insomnia should be initiated only after careful evaluation of potential causes of sleep disturbance. Failure of sleep disturbance to resolve after a reasonable period of treatment may indicate psychiatric and/or medical illness. Because of the rapid onset of action, administer immediately prior to bedtime or after the patient has gone to bed and is having difficulty falling asleep. Hypnotics/sedatives have been associated with abnormal thinking and behavior changes including decreased inhibition, aggression, bizarre behavior, agitation, hallucinations, and depersonalization. These changes may occur unpredictably and may indicate previously unrecognized psychiatric disorders; evaluate appropriately. Postmarketing studies have indicated that the use of hypnotic/sedative agents (including ramelteon) for sleep has been associated with hypersensitivity reactions including anaphylaxis as well as angioedema. Do not rechallenge patients who have developed angioedema with ramelteon therapy. An increased risk for hazardous sleep-related activities such as sleep-driving; cooking and eating food, and making phone calls while asleep have also been noted. Use caution with pre-existing depression or other psychiatric conditions. Caution when using with other CNS depressants; avoid engaging in hazardous activities or activities requiring mental alertness. Not recommended for use in patients with severe sleep apnea or COPD. Use caution with moderate hepatic impairment; not recommended in patients with severe impairment. May cause disturbances of hormonal regulation. Use caution when administered concomitantly with strong CYP1A2 inhibitors.

Adverse Reactions (Reflective of adult population; not specific for elderly) 1% to 10%:
Central nervous system: Dizziness (4% to 5%), somnolence (3% to 5%), fatigue (3% to 4%), insomnia worsened (3%), depression (2%)
Endocrine & metabolic: Serum cortisol decreased (1%)
Gastrointestinal: Nausea (3%), taste perversion (2%)
Neuromuscular & skeletal: Myalgia (2%), arthralgia (2%)
Respiratory: Upper respiratory infection (3%)
Miscellaneous: Influenza (1%)

Drug Interactions
Metabolism/Transport Effects Substrate of CYP1A2 (major), CYP2C19 (minor), CYP3A4 (minor); **Note:** Assignment of Major/Minor substrate status based on clinically relevant drug interaction potential

Avoid Concomitant Use
Avoid concomitant use of Ramelteon with any of the following: Azelastine; Azelastine (Nasal); FluvoxaMINE; Methadone; Mirtazapine; Paraldehyde

Increased Effect/Toxicity
Ramelteon may increase the levels/effects of: Alcohol (Ethyl); Azelastine; Azelastine (Nasal); Buprenorphine; CNS Depressants; Methadone; Methotrimeprazine; Metyrosine; Mirtazapine; Paraldehyde; Selective Serotonin Reuptake Inhibitors; Zolpidem

The levels/effects of Ramelteon may be increased by: Abiraterone Acetate; Antifungal Agents (Azole Derivatives, Systemic); CYP1A2 Inhibitors (Moderate); CYP1A2 Inhibitors (Strong); Deferasirox; Droperidol; Fluconazole; FluvoxaMINE; HydrOXYzine; Methotrimeprazine

Decreased Effect

The levels/effects of Ramelteon may be decreased by: Rifamycin Derivatives; Tocilizumab

Ethanol/Nutrition/Herb Interactions

Ethanol: May increase CNS depression. Management: Avoid or limit ethanol.

Food: Taking with high-fat meal delays T_{max} and increases AUC (~31%). Management: Do not take with a high-fat meal.

Herb/Nutraceutical: Some herbal medications may increase CNS depression. Management: Avoid valerian, St John's wort, kava kava, and gotu kola.

Stability Store at 25°C (77°F); excursions permitted to 15°C to 30°C (59°F to 86°F). Protect from moisture.

Mechanism of Action Potent, selective agonist of melatonin receptors MT_1 and MT_2 (with little affinity for MT_3) within the suprachiasmic nucleus of the hypothalamus, an area responsible for determination of circadian rhythms and synchronization of the sleep-wake cycle. Agonism of MT_1 is thought to preferentially induce sleepiness, while MT_2 receptor activation preferentially influences regulation of circadian rhythms. Ramelteon is eightfold more selective for MT_1 than MT_2 and exhibits nearly sixfold higher affinity for MT_1 than melatonin, presumably allowing for enhanced effects on sleep induction.

Pharmacodynamics/Kinetics

Onset of action: 30 minutes

Absorption: Rapid; high-fat meal delays T_{max} and increases AUC (~31%)

Distribution: 74 L

Protein binding: ~82%

Metabolism: Extensive first-pass effect; oxidative metabolism primarily through CYP1A2 and to a lesser extent through CYP2C and CYP3A4; forms active metabolite (M-II)

Bioavailability: Absolute: 1.8%

Half-life elimination: Ramelteon: 1-2.6 hours; M-II: 2-5 hours

Time to peak, plasma: Median: 0.5-1.5 hours

Excretion: Primarily as metabolites: Urine (84%); feces (4%)

Dosage

Geriatric & Adult Insomnia: Oral: One 8 mg tablet within 30 minutes of bedtime

Renal Impairment No dosage adjustment required

Hepatic Impairment No adjustment required for mild-to-moderate impairment; use caution. Not recommended with severe impairment.

Administration Do not administer with a high-fat meal. Swallow tablet whole; do not break.

Monitoring Parameters Mental status

Special Geriatric Considerations Although the C_{max} and AUC of ramelteon were increased in elderly patients, in clinical trials there were no significant differences in safety or efficacy between elderly and younger adult subjects.

Dosage Forms Excipient information presented when available (limited, particularly for generics); consult specific product labeling.

Tablet, oral:

Rozerem®: 8 mg

Ramipril (RA mi pril)

Related Information

Angiotensin Agents on page 2093
Heart Failure (Systolic) on page 2203

Medication Safety Issues

Sound-alike/look-alike issues:

Ramipril may be confused with enalapril, Monopril®

Altace® may be confused with Altace® HCT, alteplase, Amaryl®, Amerge®, Artane

Brand Names: U.S. Altace®

Brand Names: Canada Altace®; Apo-Ramipril®; Ava-Ramipril; CO Ramipril; Dom-Ramipril; JAMP-Ramipril; Mylan-Ramipril; PHL-Ramipril; PMS-Ramipril; RAN™-Ramipril; ratio-Ramipril; Sandoz-Ramipril; Teva-Ramipril

Generic Availability (U.S.) Yes

Pharmacologic Category Angiotensin-Converting Enzyme (ACE) Inhibitor

Use Treatment of hypertension, alone or in combination with thiazide diuretics; treatment of left ventricular dysfunction after MI; to reduce risk of MI, stroke, and death in patients at increased risk for these events

Unlabeled Use Treatment of heart failure; to delay the progression of nephropathy and reduce risks of cardiovascular events in hypertensive patients with type 1 or 2 diabetes mellitus

Contraindications Hypersensitivity to ramipril or any component of the formulation; prior hypersensitivity (including angioedema) to ACE inhibitors

Warnings/Precautions Anaphylactic reactions may occur rarely with ACE inhibitors. At any time during treatment (especially following first dose) angioedema may occur rarely with ACE inhibitors; it may involve the head and neck (potentially compromising airway) or the intestine (presenting with abdominal pain). African-Americans and patients with idiopathic or hereditary angioedema may be at an increased risk. Prolonged frequent monitoring may be required especially if tongue, glottis, or larynx are involved as they are associated with airway obstruction. Patients with a history of airway surgery may have a higher risk of airway obstruction. Aggressive early and appropriate management is critical. Use in patients with previous angioedema associated with ACE inhibitor therapy is contraindicated. Severe anaphylactoid reactions may be seen during hemodialysis (eg, CVVHD) with high-flux dialysis membranes (eg, AN69), and rarely, during low density lipoprotein apheresis with dextran sulfate cellulose. Rare cases of anaphylactoid reactions have been reported in patients undergoing sensitization treatment with hymenoptera (bee, wasp) venom while receiving ACE inhibitors.

Symptomatic hypotension with or without syncope can occur with ACE inhibitors (usually with the first several doses); effects are most often observed in volume-depleted patients; close monitoring of patient is required especially with initial dosing and dosing increases; blood pressure must be lowered at a rate appropriate for the patient's clinical condition. Initiation of therapy in patients with ischemic heart disease or cerebrovascular disease warrants close observation due to the potential consequences posed by falling blood pressure (eg, MI, stroke). Use with caution in hypertrophic cardiomyopathy with outflow tract obstruction, severe aortic stenosis, or before, during, or immediately after major surgery.

Hyperkalemia may occur with ACE inhibitors; risk factors include renal dysfunction, diabetes mellitus, concomitant use of potassium-sparing diuretics, potassium supplements, and/or potassium containing salts. Use cautiously, if at all, with these agents and monitor potassium closely. Cough may occur with ACE inhibitors. Other causes of cough should be considered (eg, pulmonary congestion in patients with heart failure) and excluded prior to discontinuation.

May be associated with deterioration of renal function and/or increases in serum creatinine, particularly in patients with low renal blood flow (eg, renal artery stenosis, heart failure) whose glomerular filtration rate (GFR) is dependent on efferent arteriolar vasoconstriction by angiotensin II; deterioration may result in oliguria, acute renal failure, and progressive azotemia. Small increases in serum creatinine may occur following initiation; consider discontinuation only in patients with progressive and/or significant deterioration in renal function. Use with caution in patients with unstented unilateral/bilateral renal artery stenosis. When unstented bilateral renal artery stenosis is present, use is generally avoided due to the elevated risk of deterioration in renal function unless possible benefits outweigh risks. Concurrent use of angiotensin receptor blockers may increase the risk of clinically-significant adverse events (eg, renal dysfunction, hyperkalemia). Concurrent use with telmisartan is not recommended.

Rare toxicities associated with ACE inhibitors include cholestatic jaundice (which may progress to fulminant hepatic necrosis), agranulocytosis, neutropenia, or leukopenia with myeloid hypoplasia. Patients with collagen vascular diseases (especially with concomitant renal impairment) or renal impairment alone may be at increased risk for hematologic toxicity; periodically monitor CBC with differential in these patients.

Adverse Reactions (Reflective of adult population; not specific for elderly) Note: Frequency ranges include data from hypertension and heart failure trials. Higher rates of adverse reactions have generally been noted in patients with CHF. However, the frequency of adverse effects associated with placebo is also increased in this population.

>10%: Respiratory: Cough increased (7% to 12%)
1% to 10%:
  Cardiovascular: Hypotension (11%), angina (up to 3%), orthostatic hypotension (2%), syncope (up to 2%)
  Central nervous system: Headache (1% to 5%), dizziness (2% to 4%), fatigue (2%), vertigo (up to 2%)
  Endocrine & metabolic: Hyperkalemia (1% to 10%)
  Gastrointestinal: Nausea/vomiting (1% to 2%)
  Neuromuscular & skeletal: Chest pain (noncardiac) (1%)
  Renal: Renal dysfunction (1%), serum creatinine increased (1% to 2%), BUN increased (<1% to 3%); transient increases of creatinine and/or BUN may occur more frequently
  Respiratory: Cough (estimated 1% to 10%)

Worsening of renal function may occur in patients with bilateral renal artery stenosis or in hypovolemia. In addition, a syndrome which may include fever, myalgia, arthralgia, interstitial nephritis, vasculitis, rash, eosinophilia and positive ANA, and elevated ESR has been reported with ACE inhibitors. Risk of pancreatitis and agranulocytosis may be increased in patients with collagen vascular disease or renal impairment.

Drug Interactions

Metabolism/Transport Effects None known.

Avoid Concomitant Use There are no known interactions where it is recommended to avoid concomitant use.

Increased Effect/Toxicity

Ramipril may increase the levels/effects of: Allopurinol; Amifostine; Antihypertensives; AzaTHIOprine; CycloSPORINE; CycloSPORINE (Systemic); Ferric Gluconate; Gold Sodium Thiomalate; Hypotensive Agents; Iron Dextran Complex; Lithium; Nonsteroidal Anti-Inflammatory Agents; RiTUXimab; Sodium Phosphates

The levels/effects of Ramipril may be increased by: Alfuzosin; Aliskiren; Angiotensin II Receptor Blockers; Diazoxide; DPP-IV Inhibitors; Eplerenone; Everolimus; Herbs (Hypotensive Properties); Loop Diuretics; MAO Inhibitors; Pentoxifylline; Phosphodiesterase 5 Inhibitors; Potassium Salts; Potassium-Sparing Diuretics; Prostacyclin Analogues; Sirolimus; Telmisartan; Temsirolimus; Thiazide Diuretics; TiZANidine; Tolvaptan; Trimethoprim

Decreased Effect

The levels/effects of Ramipril may be decreased by: Aprotinin; Herbs (Hypertensive Properties); Icatibant; Lanthanum; Methylphenidate; Nonsteroidal Anti-Inflammatory Agents; Salicylates; Yohimbine

Ethanol/Nutrition/Herb Interactions Herb/Nutraceutical: Avoid bayberry, blue cohosh, cayenne, ephedra, ginger, ginseng (American), kola, licorice (may worsen hypertension). Avoid black cohosh, California poppy, coleus, golden seal, hawthorn, mistletoe, periwinkle, quinine, shepherd's purse (may have increased antihypertensive effect).

Stability Store at controlled room temperature.

Mechanism of Action Ramipril is an ACE inhibitor which prevents the formation of angiotensin II from angiotensin I and exhibits pharmacologic effects that are similar to captopril. Ramipril must undergo enzymatic saponification by esterases in the liver to its biologically active metabolite, ramiprilat. The pharmacodynamic effects of ramipril result from the high-affinity, competitive, reversible binding of ramiprilat to angiotensin-converting enzyme, thus preventing the formation of the potent vasoconstrictor angiotensin II. This isomerized enzyme-inhibitor complex has a slow rate of dissociation, which results in high potency and a long duration of action; a CNS mechanism may also be involved in the hypotensive effect as angiotensin II increases adrenergic outflow from CNS; vasoactive kallikreins may be decreased in conversion to active hormones by ACE inhibitors, thus reducing blood pressure

Pharmacodynamics/Kinetics

Onset of action: 1-2 hours

Duration: 24 hours

Absorption: Well absorbed (50% to 60%)

Distribution: Plasma levels decline in a triphasic fashion; rapid decline is a distribution phase to peripheral compartment, plasma protein and tissue ACE (half-life: 2-4 hours); second phase is an apparent elimination phase representing the clearance of free ramiprilat (half-life: 9-18 hours); and final phase is the terminal elimination phase representing the equilibrium phase between tissue binding and dissociation

Protein binding: Ramipril: 73%; Ramiprilat: 56%

Metabolism: Hepatic to the active form, ramiprilat

Bioavailability: Ramipril: 28%; Ramiprilat: 44%

Half-life elimination: Ramiprilat: Effective: 13-17 hours; Terminal: >50 hours

Time to peak, serum: Ramipril: ~1 hour; Ramiprilat: 2-4 hours

Excretion: Urine (60%) and feces (40%) as parent drug and metabolites

Dosage

Geriatric Refer to adult dosing. Adjust for renal function for elderly since glomerular filtration rates are decreased; may see exaggerated hypotensive effects if renal clearance is not considered.

In the management of hypertension, consider lower initial doses and titrate to response (Aronow, 2011).

Adult

Heart failure (unlabeled use): Initial: 1.25-2.5 mg once daily; target dose: 10 mg once daily (ACC/AHA 2009 Heart Failure Guidelines)

Hypertension: Oral: 2.5-5 mg once daily, maximum: 20 mg/day

LV dysfunction postmyocardial infarction: Oral: Initial: 2.5 mg twice daily titrated upward, if possible, to 5 mg twice daily

To reduce the risk of MI, stroke, and death from cardiovascular causes: Oral: Initial: 2.5 mg once daily for 1 week, then 5 mg once daily for the next 3 weeks, then increase as tolerated to 10 mg once daily (may be given as divided dose)

Note: The dose of any concomitant diuretic should be reduced. If the diuretic cannot be discontinued, initiate therapy with 1.25 mg. After the initial dose, the patient should be monitored carefully until blood pressure has stabilized.

Renal Impairment

Cl_{cr} <40 mL/minute: Administer 25% of normal dose.

Renal failure and heart failure: Administer 1.25 mg once daily, increasing to 1.25 mg twice daily up to 2.5 mg twice daily as tolerated.

Renal failure and hypertension: Administer 1.25 mg once daily, titrated upward as possible; maximum daily dose 5 mg.

Administration Capsule is usually swallowed whole, but contents may be mixed in water, apple juice, or applesauce.

Monitoring Parameters Blood pressure; serum creatinine and potassium; if patient has collagen vascular disease and/or renal impairment, periodically monitor CBC with differential

Test Interactions Positive Coombs' [direct]; may cause false-positive results in urine acetone determinations using sodium nitroprusside reagent

Pharmacotherapy Pearls Some patients may have a decreased hypotensive effect between 12 and 16 hours; consider dividing total daily dose into 2 doses 12 hours apart. If patient is receiving a diuretic, a potential for first-dose hypotension is increased. To decrease this potential, stop diuretic for 2-3 days prior to initiating ramipril. If diuretic cannot be stopped temporarily, then initiate therapy with 1.25 mg daily. Continue diuretic if needed to control blood pressure. Capsules should be swallowed whole; if this cannot be done, capsule contents may be mixed with applesauce; also, contents may be mixed with apple juice or water. Mixtures in juice and water are stable for 24 hours at room temperature or 48 hours in refrigeration.

Special Geriatric Considerations Due to frequent decreases in glomerular filtration (also creatinine clearance) with aging, elderly patients may have exaggerated responses to ACE inhibitors; differences in clinical response due to hepatic changes are not observed. ACE inhibitors may be preferred agents in elderly patients with CHF and diabetes mellitus. Diabetic proteinuria is reduced and insulin sensitivity is enhanced. In general, the side effect profile is favorable in the elderly and causes little or no CNS confusion; use lowest dose recommendations initially. Many elderly may be volume depleted due to diuretic use and/or blunted thirst reflex resulting in inadequate fluid intake.

Dosage Forms Excipient information presented when available (limited, particularly for generics); consult specific product labeling.

Capsule, oral: 1.25 mg, 2.5 mg, 5 mg, 10 mg

Altace®: 1.25 mg, 2.5 mg, 5 mg, 10 mg

Ramipril and Hydrochlorothiazide (RA mi pril & hye droe klor oh THYE a zide)

Related Information

Hydrochlorothiazide on page 933
Ramipril on page 1669

Medication Safety Issues

Sound-alike/look-alike issues:

Altace® HCT may be confused with alteplase, Artane, Altace®

Brand Names: Canada Altace® HCT; PMS-Ramipril HCTZ

Index Terms Hydrochlorothiazide and Ramipril

Pharmacologic Category Angiotensin-Converting Enzyme (ACE) Inhibitor; Diuretic, Thiazide

Use Treatment of essential hypertension (not for initial therapy)

Dosage

Geriatric & Adult Note: Not for initial therapy. Dose is individualized; may be substituted for individual components in patients currently maintained on both agents separately or in patients not controlled with monotherapy.

Hypertension: Oral: Usual dosage: Ramipril 2.5 mg/hydrochlorothiazide 12.5 mg once daily; titrate to maximum ramipril 10 mg/hydrochlorothiazide 50 mg once daily

Renal Impairment

Cl_{cr} 30-60 mL/minute/1.73 m²: Maximum dose: Ramipril 5 mg/hydrochlorothiazide 25 mg once daily

Cl_{cr} <30 mL/minute: Hydrochlorothiazide is usually ineffective

Hepatic Impairment There are no dosage adjustments provided in the manufacturer's labeling.

Special Geriatric Considerations See individual agents. Combination products are not recommended as first-line treatment. Use only if doses of individual agents correspond to the combination available.

Product Availability Not available in U.S.

Dosage Forms: Canada Excipient information presented when available (limited, particularly for generics); consult specific product labeling.

Tablet, oral:

Altace® HCT 2.5/12.5: Ramipril 2.5 mg and hydrochlorothiazide 12.5 mg

Altace® HCT 5/12.5: Ramipril 5 mg and hydrochlorothiazide 12.5 mg

Altace® HCT 5/25: Ramipril 5 mg and hydrochlorothiazide 25 mg

Altace® HCT 10/12.5: Ramipril 10 mg and hydrochlorothiazide 12.5 mg

Altace® HCT 10/25: Ramipril 10 mg and hydrochlorothiazide 25 mg

◆ **Ranexa®** see Ranolazine on page 1678

Ranibizumab (ra ni BIZ oo mab)

Brand Names: U.S. Lucentis®

Brand Names: Canada Lucentis®

Index Terms rhuFabV2

Generic Availability (U.S.) No

Pharmacologic Category Angiogenesis Inhibitor; Monoclonal Antibody; Ophthalmic Agent; Vascular Endothelial Growth Factor (VEGF) Inhibitor

Use Treatment of neovascular (wet) age-related macular degeneration (AMD); treatment of macular edema following retinal vein occlusion (RVO)

Canadian labeling: Additional use (not in in U.S. labeling): Treatment of visual impairment associated with diabetic macular edema (DME)

Contraindications Hypersensitivity to ranibizumab or any component of the formulation; ocular or periocular infection

Canadian labeling: Additional contraindications (not in U.S. labeling): Active intraocular inflammation

Warnings/Precautions Intravitreous injections may be associated with endophthalmitis and retinal detachments. Proper aseptic injection techniques should be used and patients should be instructed to report any signs of infection immediately. Intraocular pressure may increase following injection. Intravitreal injections of ranibizumab may induce temporary visual disturbances that impair the ability to drive or operate machinery. Affected patients should be advised to abstain from driving or using machinery until resolution of disturbances. Use for >24 months has not been evaluated.

Risk of thromboembolic events, particularly stroke, may be increased following intravitreal administration of VEGF inhibitors. Use caution in patients with known risk factors (eg, history of stroke, TIA). Rare hypersensitivity reactions (including anaphylaxis) have been associated with another VEGF inhibitor, pegaptanib, occurring within several hours of use; monitor closely. Equipment and appropriate personnel should be available for monitoring and treatment of anaphylaxis.

Adverse Reactions (Reflective of adult population; not specific for elderly) Note: Rates of ocular adverse reactions reported for control group when percentages overlapped with treatment group.

As reported with AMD or RVO:

>10%:

Central nervous system: Headache (3% to 12%)

Neuromuscular & skeletal: Arthralgia (2% to 11%)

Ocular: Conjunctival hemorrhage (48% to 74%; control: 37% to 60%), eye pain (17% to 35%; control 12% to 30%), vitreous floaters (7% to 27%), intraocular pressure increased (7% to 24%), blurred vision/visual disturbance (5% to 18%), intraocular inflammation (1% to 18%; control 3% to 8%), blepharitis (≤12%), maculopathy (6% to 11%; control 6% to 9%), ocular hyperemia (5% to 11%; control 3% to 8%)

Note: Cataract, dry eye, eye irritation, foreign body sensation, lacrimation increased, pruritus, and vitreous detachment occurred in >10% of patients, but also occurred in similar percentages to the control; visual acuity blurred/decreased occurred more often in the control.

Respiratory: Nasopharyngitis (5% to 16%), bronchitis (≤11%)

1% to 10%:
  Cardiovascular: Atrial fibrillation (1% to 5%), arterial thromboembolic events (4%; stroke ≤3%)
  Gastrointestinal: Nausea (1% to 9%), viral gastroenteritis (1% to 4%)
  Hematologic: Anemia (1% to 8%; control up to 7%)
  Ocular: Retinal disorder (2% to 10%), retinal degeneration (1% to 8%), posterior capsule opacification (≤7%), injection site hemorrhage (≤5%)
    Note: Conjunctival hyperemia and ocular discomfort occurred in 1% to 10% of patients, but also occurred in similar percentages to the control; retinal exudates occurred more often in the control.
  Respiratory: Cough (2% to 9%), upper respiratory tract infection (≤9%), sinusitis (3% to 8%), chronic obstructive pulmonary disease (COPD) (≤6%), dyspnea (≤4%)
  Miscellaneous: Ranibizumab antibodies (1% to 8%), influenza (3% to 7%)

As reported with DME:
>10%: Ocular: Intraocular pressure increased (≤28%), conjunctival hemorrhage (7% to 26%), vitreous floaters (2% to 14%)
1% to 10%:
  Cardiovascular: Arrhythmia (2% to 4%), arterial thromboembolic events (≤4%), hypertension exacerbated (≤2%)
  Gastrointestinal: Nausea (≤2%)
  Local: Facial pain (≤2%)
  Ocular: Conjunctival hyperemia (2% to 7%), foreign body sensation (4%), lacrimation increased (2% to 6%), eye irritation (2%to 6%), eye pruritus (4%), endophthalmitis (2% to 4%), vision blurred (2% to 4%), vitreous hemorrhage (2% to 4%), ocular hyperemia (1% to 4%), visual impairment (3%), eye discharge (2%), allergic blepharitis (≤2%), conjunctival edema (≤2%), corneal disorder (≤2%), eyelid edema (≤2%), eyelid erythema (≤2%), hypopyon (≤2%), lenticular opacities (≤2%), retinal artery occlusion (≤2%), retinal disorder (≤2%), retinal exudates (≤2%), ulcerative keratitis (≤2%)

Drug Interactions
Metabolism/Transport Effects None known.
Avoid Concomitant Use There are no known interactions where it is recommended to avoid concomitant use.
Increased Effect/Toxicity There are no known significant interactions involving an increase in effect.
Decreased Effect There are no known significant interactions involving a decrease in effect.
Stability Store in original carton under refrigeration at 2°C to 8°C (36°F to 46°F); protect from light. Do not freeze.
Mechanism of Action Ranibizumab is a recombinant humanized monoclonal antibody fragment which binds to and inhibits human vascular endothelial growth factor A (VEGF-A). Ranibizumab inhibits VEGF from binding to its receptors and thereby suppressing neo-vascularization and slowing vision loss.

Pharmacodynamics/Kinetics
Absorption: Low levels are detected in the serum following intravitreal injection
Half-life elimination: Vitreous: ~9 days

Dosage
Geriatric & Adult
Age-related macular degeneration (AMD): Intravitreal injection:
  U.S. labeling: 0.5 mg (0.05 mL) once a month. **Note:** Frequency may be reduced after the first 4 injections to once every 3 months if monthly injections are not feasible.
  Canadian labeling: 0.5 mg (0.05 mL) once a month. Frequency may be reduced after the first 3 injections to once every 3 months if monthly injections are not feasible.
  Note: Every-3-month dosing regimen has reportedly resulted in a ~5 letter (1 line) loss of visual acuity over 9 months, as compared to monthly dosing.
Macular edema following retinal vein occlusion (RVO): Intravitreal injection: 0.5 mg (0.05 mL) once a month. **Note:** Canadian labeling recommends continuing therapy until achieve-ment of stable visual acuity for 3 consecutive months; upon discontinuation, may resume monthly therapy with loss of visual acuity.
Visual impairment associated with diabetic macular edema (DME): Intravitreal injection: *Canadian labeling (not in U.S. labeling):* 0.5 mg (0.05 mL) once a month until achievement of stable visual acuity for 3 consecutive months. Upon discontinuation, may resume monthly therapy with loss of visual acuity.
Renal Impairment Dose adjustment not expected.
Hepatic Impairment Dose adjustment not expected.
Administration For ophthalmic intravitreal injection only. Remove contents from vial using a 5 micron 19-gauge filter needle attached to a tuberculin syringe. Discard filter needle and replace with a sterile 30 gauge ½ inch needle for injection (do not use filter needle for

intravitreal injection). Adequate anesthesia and a broad-spectrum antimicrobial agent should be administered prior to the procedure. Canadian labeling recommends administering ranibizumab at least 30 minutes after laser photocoagulation therapy when administered on the same day.

Monitoring Parameters Intraocular pressure (within 30 minutes and between 2-7 days following administration); signs of infection/inflammation (for first week following injection); retinal perfusion, endophthalmitis; visual acuity

Special Geriatric Considerations In clinical trials, ~94% of the patients were >65 years and 68% were >75 years of age. No differences were seen in efficacy with increasing age. After correcting for creatinine clearance, age did not affect systemic exposure of ranibizumab.

Dosage Forms Excipient information presented when available (limited, particularly for generics); consult specific product labeling.

Injection, solution [preservative free]:
Lucentis®: 10 mg/mL (0.2 mL)

Dosage Forms: Canada Excipient information presented when available (limited, particularly for generics); consult specific product labeling.

Injection, solution [preservative free]:
Lucentis®: 10 mg/mL (0.3 mL)

Ranitidine (ra NI ti deen)

Medication Safety Issues
Sound-alike/look-alike issues:
Ranitidine may be confused with amantadine, rimantadine
Zantac® may be confused with Xanax®, Zarontin®, Zofran®, ZyrTEC®

Brand Names: U.S. Zantac 150® [OTC]; Zantac 75® [OTC]; Zantac®; Zantac® EFFER-dose®

Brand Names: Canada Acid Reducer; Apo-Ranitidine®; CO Ranitidine; Dom-Ranitidine; Myl-Ranitidine; Mylan-Ranitidine; Nu-Ranit; PHL-Ranitidine; PMS-Ranitidine; Ranitidine Injection, USP; RAN™-Ranitidine; ratio-Ranitidine; Riva-Ranitidine; Sandoz-Ranitidine; Schein-Pharm Ranitidine; Teva-Ranitidine; Zantac 75®; Zantac Maximum Strength Non-Prescription; Zantac®

Index Terms Ranitidine Hydrochloride

Generic Availability (U.S.) Yes: Excludes effervescent tablet, premixed infusion

Pharmacologic Category Histamine H_2 Antagonist

Use
Zantac®: Short-term and maintenance therapy of duodenal ulcer, gastric ulcer, gastroesophageal reflux disease (GERD), active benign ulcer, erosive esophagitis, and pathological hypersecretory conditions; as part of a multidrug regimen for *H. pylori* eradication to reduce the risk of duodenal ulcer recurrence

Zantac 75® [OTC]: Relief of heartburn, acid indigestion, and sour stomach

Unlabeled Use Treatment of recurrent postoperative ulcer, upper GI bleeding; prevention of acid-aspiration pneumonitis during surgery, stress-induced ulcers

Contraindications Hypersensitivity to ranitidine or any component of the formulation

Warnings/Precautions Ranitidine has been associated with confusional states (rare). Use with caution in patients with hepatic impairment; use with caution in renal impairment, dosage modification required. Avoid use in patients with history of acute porphyria (may precipitate attacks); long-term therapy may be associated with vitamin B_{12} deficiency. Symptoms of GI distress may be associated with a variety of conditions; symptomatic response to H_2 antagonists does not rule out the potential for significant pathology (eg, malignancy). EFFERdose® formulation contains phenylalanine.

Adverse Reactions (Reflective of adult population; not specific for elderly) Frequency not defined.
Cardiovascular: Asystole, atrioventricular block, bradycardia (with rapid I.V. administration), premature ventricular beats, tachycardia, vasculitis
Central nervous system: Agitation, dizziness, depression, hallucinations, headache, insomnia, malaise, mental confusion, somnolence, vertigo
Dermatologic: Alopecia, erythema multiforme, rash
Endocrine & metabolic: Prolactin levels increased
Gastrointestinal: Abdominal discomfort/pain, constipation, diarrhea, nausea, necrotizing enterocolitis (VLBW neonates; Guillet, 2006), pancreatitis, vomiting
Hematologic: Acquired immune hemolytic anemia, acute porphyritic attack, agranulocytosis, aplastic anemia, granulocytopenia, leukopenia, pancytopenia, thrombocytopenia
Hepatic: Cholestatic hepatitis, hepatic failure, hepatitis, jaundice
Local: Transient pain, burning or itching at the injection site
Neuromuscular & skeletal: Arthralgia, involuntary motor disturbance, myalgia

Ocular: Blurred vision
Renal: Acute interstitial nephritis, serum creatinine increased
Respiratory: Pneumonia (causal relationship not established)
Miscellaneous: Anaphylaxis, angioneurotic edema, hypersensitivity reactions (eg, broncho-spasm, fever, eosinophilia)

Drug Interactions

Metabolism/Transport Effects Substrate of CYP1A2 (minor), CYP2C19 (minor), CYP2D6 (minor), P-glycoprotein; **Note:** Assignment of Major/Minor substrate status based on clinically relevant drug interaction potential; **Inhibits** CYP1A2 (weak), CYP2D6 (weak)

Avoid Concomitant Use
Avoid concomitant use of Ranitidine with any of the following: Delavirdine

Increased Effect/Toxicity
Ranitidine may increase the levels/effects of: ARIPiprazole; Dexmethylphenidate; Methyl-phenidate; Procainamide; Saquinavir; Sulfonylureas; Varenicline; Warfarin

The levels/effects of Ranitidine may be increased by: P-glycoprotein/ABCB1 Inhibitors

Decreased Effect
Ranitidine may decrease the levels/effects of: Atazanavir; Cefditoren; Cefpodoxime; Cefur-oxime; Dasatinib; Delavirdine; Erlotinib; Fosamprenavir; Gefitinib; Indinavir; Iron Salts; Itraconazole; Ketoconazole; Ketoconazole (Systemic); Mesalamine; Nelfinavir; Nilotinib; Posaconazole; Prasugrel; Rilpivirine; Vismodegib

The levels/effects of Ranitidine may be decreased by: Peginterferon Alfa-2b; P-glycoprotein/ABCB1 Inducers

Ethanol/Nutrition/Herb Interactions

Ethanol: Avoid ethanol (may cause gastric mucosal irritation).
Food: Does not interfere with absorption of ranitidine.

Stability

Injection: Vials: Store between 4°C to 25°C (39°F to 77°F); excursion permitted to 30°C (86°F). Protect from light. Solution is a clear, colorless to yellow solution; slight darkening does not affect potency.
Premixed bag: Store between 2°C to 25°C (36°F to 77°F). Protect from light.
EFFERdose® formulations: Store between 2°C to 30°C (36°F to 86°F).
Syrup: Store between 4°C to 25°C (39°F to 77°F). Protect from light.
Tablet: Store in dry place, between 15°C to 30°C (59°F to 86°F). Protect from light.

Vials can be mixed with NS or D$_5$W; solutions are stable for 48 hours at room temperature.
Intermittent bolus injection, continuous infusion: Dilute to maximum of 2.5 mg/mL.
Intermittent infusion: Dilute to maximum of 0.5 mg/mL.

Mechanism of Action Competitive inhibition of histamine at H$_2$-receptors of the gastric parietal cells, which inhibits gastric acid secretion, gastric volume, and hydrogen ion concentration are reduced. Does not affect pepsin secretion, pentagastrin-stimulated intrinsic factor secretion, or serum gastrin.

Pharmacodynamics/Kinetics

Absorption: Oral: 50%
Distribution: Normal renal function: V$_d$: ~1.4 L/kg; Cl$_{cr}$ 25-35 mL/minute: 1.76 L/kg minimally penetrates the blood-brain barrier
Protein binding: 15%
Metabolism: Hepatic to N-oxide, S-oxide, and N-desmethyl metabolites
Bioavailability: Oral: 48% to 50%; I.M.: 90% to 100%
Half-life elimination:
  Oral: Normal renal function: 2.5-3 hours; Cl$_{cr}$ 25-35 mL/minute: 4.8 hours
  I.V.: Normal renal function: 2-2.5 hours
Time to peak, serum: Oral: 2-3 hours; I.M.: ≤15 minutes
Excretion: Urine: Oral: 30%, I.V.: 70% (as unchanged drug); feces (as metabolites)

Dosage

Geriatric & Adult

Duodenal ulcer: Oral: Treatment: 150 mg twice daily, or 300 mg once daily after the evening meal or at bedtime; maintenance: 150 mg once daily at bedtime

Eradication of *Helicobacter pylori*: Oral: 150 mg twice daily; requires combination therapy

Pathological hypersecretory conditions:
  Oral: 150 mg twice daily; adjust dose or frequency as clinically indicated; doses of up to 6 g/day have been used
  I.V.: Continuous infusion for Zollinger-Ellison: Initial: 1 mg/kg/hour; measure gastric acid output at 4 hours, if >10 mEq or if patient is symptomatic, increase dose in increments of 0.5 mg/kg/hour; doses of up to 2.5 mg/kg/hour (or 220 mg/hour) have been used

Gastric ulcer, benign: *Oral:* 150 mg twice daily; maintenance: 150 mg once daily at bedtime

GERD: *Oral:* 150 mg twice daily

Erosive esophagitis: *Oral:* Treatment: 150 mg 4 times/day; maintenance: 150 mg twice daily

Prevention of heartburn: *Oral:* Zantac 75® [OTC]: 75 mg 30-60 minutes before eating food or drinking beverages which cause heartburn; maximum: 150 mg in 24 hours; do not use for more than 14 days

Patients not able to take oral medication:
I.M.: 50 mg every 6-8 hours
I.V.: Intermittent bolus or infusion: 50 mg every 6-8 hours
Continuous I.V. infusion: 6.25 mg/hour

Renal Impairment Adults: Cl_{cr} <50 mL/minute:
Oral: 150 mg every 24 hours; adjust dose cautiously if needed
I.V.: 50 mg every 18-24 hours; adjust dose cautiously if needed
Hemodialysis: Adjust dosing schedule so that dose coincides with the end of hemodialysis.

Hepatic Impairment Patients with hepatic impairment may have minor changes in ranitidine half-life, distribution, clearance, and bioavailability; dosing adjustments are not necessary; monitor patient.

Administration

Ranitidine injection may be administered I.M. or I.V.:
I.M.: Injection is administered undiluted
I.V.: Must be diluted; may be administered I.V. push, intermittent I.V. infusion, or continuous I.V. infusion
I.V. push: Ranitidine (usually 50 mg) should be diluted to a total of 20 mL (or a concentration not exceeding 2.5 mg/mL) with NS or D_5W and administered over at least 5 minutes or a maximum rate of 10 mg/minute
Intermittent I.V. infusion: Dilute to a maximum concentration of 0.5 mg/mL; administer over 15-20 minutes
Continuous I.V. infusion: Dilute to a maximum concentration of 2.5 mg/mL. Titrate dosage based on gastric pH.
EFFERdose®: Should not be chewed, swallowed whole, or dissolved on tongue: 25 mg tablet: Dissolve in at least 5 mL (1 teaspoonful) of water; wait until completely dissolved before administering

Monitoring Parameters AST, ALT, serum creatinine; when used to prevent stress-related GI bleeding, measure the intragastric pH and try to maintain pH >4; signs and symptoms of peptic ulcer disease, occult blood with GI bleeding, monitor renal function to correct dose

Test Interactions False-positive urine protein using Multistix®; gastric acid secretion test; skin test allergen extracts. May also interfere with urine detection of amphetamine/methamphetamine (false-positive).

Pharmacotherapy Pearls Giving dose at 6 PM may be better than 10 PM bedtime, the highest acid production usually starts at approximately 7 PM, thus giving at 6 PM controls acid secretion better; administer I.V. administration over a 30 minute period to avoid bradycardia; causes fewer adverse reactions and interactions than cimetidine; most patient's ulcers have healed within 4 weeks, however, older adults require 12 weeks of therapy; long-term therapy may cause vitamin B_{12} deficiency

Special Geriatric Considerations Ulcer healing rates and incidence of adverse effects are similar in the elderly, when compared to younger patients; dosing adjustments not necessary based on age alone. Always adjust dose based upon creatinine clearance. Serum half-life is increased to 3-4 hours in elderly patients. H_2 blockers are the preferred drugs for treating PUD in the elderly due to cost and ease of administration. These agents are no less or more effective than any other therapy. The preferred agents, due to side effects and drug interaction profile and pharmacokinetics are ranitidine, famotidine, and nizatidine. Treatment for PUD in the elderly is recommended for 12 weeks since their lesions are larger; therefore, take longer to heal. This drug is substantially cleared renally, and elderly, having decreased renal function in general, should be monitored closely for adverse effects, especially CNS.

Dosage Forms Excipient information presented when available (limited, particularly for generics); consult specific product labeling. [DSC] = Discontinued product
Capsule, oral: 150 mg, 300 mg
Infusion, premixed in 1/2 NS [preservative free]:
  Zantac®: 50 mg (50 mL)
Injection, solution: 25 mg/mL (2 mL, 6 mL, 40 mL)
  Zantac®: 25 mg/mL (2 mL, 6 mL, 40 mL)
Syrup, oral: 15 mg/mL (1 mL, 5 mL, 10 mL, 120 mL, 473 mL, 474 mL, 480 mL)
  Zantac®: 15 mg/mL (480 mL) [contains ethanol 7.5%; peppermint flavor]
Tablet, oral: 75 mg, 150 mg, 300 mg
  Zantac 150®: 150 mg [DSC]
  Zantac 150®: 150 mg [DSC] [cool mint flavor]
  Zantac 150®: 150 mg [sodium free, sugar free]

Zantac 150®: 150 mg [sodium free, sugar free; cool mint flavor]
Zantac 75®: 75 mg [DSC]
Zantac 75®: 75 mg [sodium free, sugar free]
Zantac 75®: 75 mg [DSC] [sugar free]
Zantac®: 150 mg, 300 mg
Tablet for solution, oral [effervescent]:
Zantac® EFFERdose®: 25 mg [contains phenylalanine 2.81 mg/tablet, sodium 30.52 mg (1.33 mEq)/tablet, sodium benzoate]

◆ **Ranitidine Hydrochloride** see Ranitidine on page 1675

Ranolazine (ra NOE la zeen)

Medication Safety Issues
Sound-alike/look-alike issues:
Ranexa® may be confused with CeleXA®
Brand Names: U.S. Ranexa®
Generic Availability (U.S.) No
Pharmacologic Category Antianginal Agent; Cardiovascular Agent, Miscellaneous
Use Treatment of chronic angina
Contraindications Hepatic cirrhosis; concurrent strong CYP3A inhibitors; concurrent CYP3A inducers
Warnings/Precautions Ranolazine does not relieve acute angina attacks. Has been shown to prolong QT interval in a dose/plasma concentration-related manner; assess risk versus benefit of use in patients with potential for prolonged QT including a family history. Hepatically-impaired patients may have a more significant increase in QT interval. Use is contraindicated in patients with cirrhosis (Child-Pugh class ≥A). Use caution in patients ≥75 years of age; they may experience more adverse events. Use caution and monitor blood pressure in patients with renal dysfunction; has not been evaluated in patients requiring dialysis.

Ranolazine is a substrate for and a moderate inhibitor of P-glycoprotein. Inhibitors of P-glycoprotein may increase serum concentrations of ranolazine. Ranolazine may increase serum concentrations of substrates for P-glycoprotein (eg, digoxin). Ranolazine is primarily metabolized by CYP3A; use is contraindicated with inducers and strong inhibitors of CYP3A. Ranolazine has potential to prolong the QT-interval; use caution when administered concomitantly with QT-prolonging drugs. Use caution when administering ranolazine to patients with a history of malignant neoplasms or adenomatous polyps.

Adverse Reactions (Reflective of adult population; not specific for elderly) >0.5% to 10%:
Cardiovascular: Bradycardia (≤4%), hypotension (≤4%), orthostatic hypotension (≤4%), palpitation (≤4%), peripheral edema (≤4%), QT_c prolongation (>500 msec: ≤1%)
Central nervous system: Headache (≤6%), dizziness (1% to 6%), confusion (≤4%), vasovagal attacks (≤4%), vertigo (≤4%)
Dermatologic: Hyperhidrosis (≤4%)
Gastrointestinal: Constipation (≤9%), abdominal pain (≤4%), anorexia (≤4%), dyspepsia (≤4%), nausea (≤4%; dose related), vomiting (≤4%), xerostomia (≤4%)
Neuromuscular: Weakness (≤4%)
Ocular: Blurred vision (≤4%)
Otic: Tinnitus (≤4%)
Renal: Hematuria (≤4%)
Respiratory: Dyspnea (≤4%)

Drug Interactions
Metabolism/Transport Effects Substrate of CYP2D6 (minor), CYP3A4 (major), P-glycoprotein; **Note:** Assignment of Major/Minor substrate status based on clinically relevant drug interaction potential; **Inhibits** CYP2D6 (weak), CYP3A4 (weak), P-glycoprotein

Avoid Concomitant Use
Avoid concomitant use of Ranolazine with any of the following: Antifungal Agents (Azole Derivatives, Systemic); CYP3A4 Inducers (Strong); CYP3A4 Inhibitors (Strong); Highest Risk QTc-Prolonging Agents; Mifepristone; Rifampin; Silodosin; St Johns Wort; Topotecan

Increased Effect/Toxicity
Ranolazine may increase the levels/effects of: ARIPiprazole; Colchicine; Dabigatran Etexilate; Digoxin; Everolimus; Highest Risk QTc-Prolonging Agents; Lovastatin; Moderate Risk QTc-Prolonging Agents; P-glycoprotein/ABCB1 Substrates; Prucalopride; Rivaroxaban; Silodosin; Simvastatin; Tacrolimus; Tacrolimus (Systemic); Topotecan

The levels/effects of Ranolazine may be increased by: Antifungal Agents (Azole Derivatives, Systemic); Calcium Channel Blockers (Nondihydropyridine); CYP3A4 Inhibitors (Moderate);

CYP3A4 Inhibitors (Strong); Ivacaftor; Mifepristone; P-glycoprotein/ABCB1 Inhibitors; QTc-Prolonging Agents (Indeterminate Risk and Risk Modifying)

Decreased Effect

The levels/effects of Ranolazine may be decreased by: CYP3A4 Inducers (Strong); Deferasirox; Peginterferon Alfa-2b; P-glycoprotein/ABCB1 Inducers; Rifampin; St Johns Wort; Tocilizumab

Ethanol/Nutrition/Herb Interactions

Food: Grapefruit, grapefruit juice, or grapefruit-containing products may increase the serum concentration of ranolazine. Management: Avoid grapefruit-containing products or dose adjustment of ranolazine may be required.

Herb/Nutraceutical: St John's wort may decrease the serum concentration of ranolazine. Management: Avoid St John's wort.

Stability Store at 25°C (77°F); excursions permitted to 15°C to 30°C (59°F to 86°F).

Mechanism of Action Ranolazine exerts antianginal and anti-ischemic effects without changing hemodynamic parameters (heart rate or blood pressure). At therapeutic levels, ranolazine inhibits the late phase of the inward sodium channel (late I_{Na}) in ischemic cardiac myocytes during cardiac repolarization reducing intracellular sodium concentrations and thereby reducing calcium influx via Na^+-Ca^{2+} exchange. Decreased intracellular calcium reduces ventricular tension and myocardial oxygen consumption. It is thought that ranolazine produces myocardial relaxation and reduces anginal symptoms through this mechanism although this is uncertain. At higher concentrations, ranolazine inhibits the rapid delayed rectifier potassium current (I_{Kr}) thus prolonging the ventricular action potential duration and subsequent prolongation of the QT interval.

Pharmacodynamics/Kinetics

Absorption: Highly variable; ranolazine is a substrate of P-glycoprotein; concurrent use of P-glycoprotein inhibitors may increase absorption

Protein binding: ~62%

Metabolism: Hepatic via CYP3A (major) and 2D6 (minor); gut

Bioavailability: 35% to 55%

Half-life elimination: Ranolazine: Terminal: 7 hours; Metabolites (activity undefined): 6-22 hours

Time to peak, plasma: 2-5 hours

Excretion: Primarily urine (75% mostly as metabolites); feces (25% mostly as metabolites); in feces and urine, <5% to 7% excreted unchanged

Dosage

Geriatric Refer to adult dosing. Select dose cautiously, starting at the lower end of the dosing range.

Adult

Chronic angina: Oral: Initial: 500 mg twice daily; maximum recommended dose: 1000 mg twice daily

Dosage adjustment for ranolazine with concomitant medications:

Diltiazem, erythromycin, verapamil, and other moderate CYP3A inhibitors: Ranolazine dose should not exceed 500 mg twice daily

P-glycoprotein inhibitors (eg, cyclosporine): Titrate ranolazine based on clinical response

Dosage adjustment for concomitant medications with ranolazine: *Simvastatin:* Simvastatin dose should not exceed 20 mg/day

Renal Impairment There is no dosage adjustments provided in manufacturer's labeling. However, plasma ranolazine levels increased ~50% in patients with varying degrees of renal dysfunction. Patients with severe renal dysfunction had an increase in mean diastolic blood pressure of 10-15 mm Hg. Ranolazine has not been evaluated in patients requiring dialysis.

Hepatic Impairment Use is contraindicated with any degree of hepatic cirrhosis.

Administration May be taken with or without meals. Swallow tablet whole; do not crush, break, or chew.

Monitoring Parameters Baseline and follow up ECG to evaluate QT interval; blood pressure in patients with renal dysfunction; correct and maintain serum potassium in normal limits

Special Geriatric Considerations Elderly comprised 48% of study group participants. For those elderly, no overall difference in efficacy was observed between younger and older adults. There was, however, a higher incidence of adverse effects for those ≥75 years of age, resulting in drug discontinuations. The most common adverse effects were constipation (19%), nausea (6%), and dizziness (6%). Therefore, start dosing at lower end of dosing range recommended.

Dosage Forms Excipient information presented when available (limited, particularly for generics); consult specific product labeling.

Tablet, extended release, oral:

Ranexa®: 500 mg, 1000 mg

◆ **Rapaflo®** *see* Silodosin *on page 1773*

♦ **RapiMed® Children's [OTC]** *see* Acetaminophen *on page* 31
♦ **RapiMed® Junior [OTC]** *see* Acetaminophen *on page* 31

Rasagiline (ra SA ji leen)

Related Information
Antiparkinsonian Agents *on page* 2101
Medication Safety Issues
Sound-alike/look-alike issues:
Azilect® may be confused with Aricept®
Brand Names: U.S. Azilect®
Brand Names: Canada Azilect®
Index Terms AGN 1135; Rasagiline Mesylate; TVP-1012
Generic Availability (U.S.) No
Pharmacologic Category Anti-Parkinson's Agent, MAO Type B Inhibitor
Use Treatment of idiopathic Parkinson's disease (initial monotherapy or as adjunct to levodopa)
Contraindications Concomitant use of cyclobenzaprine, dextromethorphan, methadone, propoxyphene, St John's wort, or tramadol; concomitant use of meperidine or an MAO inhibitor (including selective MAO-B inhibitors) within 14 days of rasagiline
Warnings/Precautions Hazardous agent - use appropriate precautions for handling and disposal.

Cardiovascular system: May cause orthostatic hypotension, particularly in combination with levodopa; use with caution in patients with hypotension or patients who would not tolerate transient hypotensive episodes (cardiovascular or cerebrovascular disease); orthostasis is usually most problematic during first 2 months of therapy and tends to abate thereafter. Due to the potential for hemodynamic instability, patients should not undergo elective surgery requiring general anesthesia and should avoid local anesthesia containing sympathomimetic vasoconstrictors within 14 days of discontinuing rasagiline. If surgery is required, benzodiazepines, mivacurium, fentanyl, morphine or codeine may be used cautiously. In patients taking recommended doses of rasagiline, dietary restriction of most tyramine-containing products is not necessary; however, certain foods (eg, aged cheeses) may contain high amounts (>150 mg) of tyramine and could lead to hypertensive crisis. Avoid concomitant use with foods high in tyramine.

Central nervous system: Serotonin syndrome (SS)/neuroleptic malignant syndrome (NMS)-like reactions may occur rarely, particularly when used at doses exceeding recommendations or when used in combination with an antidepressant (eg, SSRI, SNRI, TCA). May cause hallucinations; signs of severe CNS toxicity (some fatal), including hyperpyrexia, hyperthermia, rigidity, altered mental status, seizure and coma have been reported with selective and nonselective MAO inhibitor use in combination with antidepressants. Do not use within 5 weeks of fluoxetine discontinuation; do not initiate tricyclic, SSRI, or SNRI therapy within 2 weeks of discontinuing rasagiline. Addition to levodopa therapy may result in exacerbation of dyskinesias, requiring a reduction in levodopa dosage.

Dermatologic: Risk of melanoma may be increased with rasagiline, although increased risk has been associated with Parkinson's disease itself; patients should have regular and frequent skin examinations.

Organ dysfunction: Use caution in mild hepatic impairment; dose reduction recommended. Do not use with moderate-to-severe hepatic impairment.
Adverse Reactions (Reflective of adult population; not specific for elderly) Unless otherwise noted, the following adverse reactions are as reported for monotherapy. Spectrum of adverse events was generally similar with adjunctive (levodopa) therapy, though the incidence tended to be higher.
>10%:
Cardiovascular: Orthostatic hypotension (6% to 13% adjunct therapy, dose dependent)
Central nervous system: Dyskinesia (18% adjunct therapy), headache (14%)
Gastrointestinal: Nausea (10% to 12% adjunct therapy)
1% to 10%:
Cardiovascular: Angina, bundle branch block, chest pain, syncope
Central nervous system: Depression (5%), hallucinations (4% to 5% adjunct therapy), fever (3%), malaise (2%), vertigo (2%), anxiety, dizziness
Dermatologic: Bruising (2%), alopecia, skin carcinoma, vesiculobullous rash
Endocrine & metabolic: Impotence, libido decreased

Gastrointestinal: Constipation (4% to 9% adjunct therapy), weight loss (2% to 9% adjunct therapy; dose dependent), dyspepsia (7%), xerostomia (2% to 6% adjunct therapy; dose dependent), gastroenteritis (3%), anorexia, diarrhea, gastrointestinal hemorrhage, vomiting

Genitourinary: Hematuria, urinary incontinence

Hematologic: Leukopenia

Hepatic: Liver function tests increased

Neuromuscular & skeletal: Arthralgia (7%), neck pain (2%), arthritis (2%), paresthesia (2%), abnormal gait, hyperkinesias, hypertonia, neuropathy, tremor, weakness

Ocular: Conjunctivitis (3%)

Renal: Albuminuria

Respiratory: Rhinitis (3%), asthma, cough increased

Miscellaneous: Fall (5%), flu-like syndrome (5%), allergic reaction

Drug Interactions

Metabolism/Transport Effects Substrate of CYP1A2 (major); **Note:** Assignment of Major/Minor substrate status based on clinically relevant drug interaction potential; **Inhibits** Monoamine Oxidase

Avoid Concomitant Use

Avoid concomitant use of Rasagiline with any of the following: Alpha-/Beta-Agonists (Indirect-Acting); Alpha1-Agonists; Alpha2-Agonists (Ophthalmic); Amphetamines; Anilidopiperidine Opioids; Antidepressants (Serotonin Reuptake Inhibitor/Antagonist); AtoMOXetine; Bezafibrate; Buprenorphine; BuPROPion; BusPIRone; CarBAMazepine; Cyclobenzaprine; Dexmethylphenidate; Dextromethorphan; Diethylpropion; HYDROmorphone; Linezolid; Maprotiline; Meperidine; Methyldopa; Methylene Blue; Methylphenidate; Mirtazapine; Oxymorphone; Pizotifen; Selective Serotonin Reuptake Inhibitors; Serotonin 5-HT1D Receptor Agonists; Serotonin/Norepinephrine Reuptake Inhibitors; Tapentadol; Tetrabenazine; Tetrahydrozoline; Tetrahydrozoline (Nasal); Tricyclic Antidepressants; Tryptophan

Increased Effect/Toxicity

Rasagiline may increase the levels/effects of: Alpha-/Beta-Agonists (Direct-Acting); Alpha-/Beta-Agonists (Indirect-Acting); Alpha1-Agonists; Alpha2-Agonists (Ophthalmic); Amphetamines; Antidepressants (Serotonin Reuptake Inhibitor/Antagonist); Antihypertensives; AtoMOXetine; Beta2-Agonists; Bezafibrate; BuPROPion; Dexmethylphenidate; Dextromethorphan; Diethylpropion; Doxapram; HYDROmorphone; Hypoglycemic Agents; Linezolid; Lithium; Meperidine; Methadone; Methyldopa; Methylene Blue; Methylphenidate; Metoclopramide; Mirtazapine; Orthostatic Hypotension Producing Agents; Pizotifen; Reserpine; Selective Serotonin Reuptake Inhibitors; Serotonin 5-HT1D Receptor Agonists; Serotonin Modulators; Serotonin/Norepinephrine Reuptake Inhibitors; Tetrahydrozoline; Tetrahydrozoline (Nasal); Tricyclic Antidepressants

The levels/effects of Rasagiline may be increased by: Abiraterone Acetate; Altretamine; Anilidopiperidine Opioids; Antipsychotics; Buprenorphine; BusPIRone; CarBAMazepine; COMT Inhibitors; Cyclobenzaprine; CYP1A2 Inhibitors (Moderate); CYP1A2 Inhibitors (Strong); Deferasirox; Levodopa; MAO Inhibitors; Maprotiline; Oxymorphone; Tapentadol; Tetrabenazine; TraMADol; Tryptophan

Decreased Effect

The levels/effects of Rasagiline may be decreased by: CYP1A2 Inducers (Strong); Cyproterone

Ethanol/Nutrition/Herb Interactions

Ethanol: Management: Avoid ethanol.

Food: Concurrent ingestion of foods rich in tyramine may cause sudden and severe high blood pressure (hypertensive crisis). Management: Avoid foods containing high amounts (>150 mg) of tyramine (aged or matured cheese, air-dried or cured meats including sausages and salamis; fava or broad bean pods, tap/draft beers, Marmite concentrate, sauerkraut, soy sauce, and other soybean condiments). Food's freshness is also an important concern; improperly stored or spoiled food can create an environment in which tyramine concentrations may increase. Avoid these foods during and for 2 weeks after discontinuation of medication.

Herb/Nutraceutical: Some herbal medications may cause excessive sedation; others may increase the risk of serotonin syndrome or hypertensive reactions. Management: Avoid valerian, St John's wort, SAMe, and kava kava; avoid supplements containing caffeine, tyrosine, tryptophan, or phenylalanine.

Stability Store at 25°C (77°F); excursions permitted to 15°C to 30°C (59°F to 86°F).

Mechanism of Action Potent, irreversible and selective inhibitor of brain monoamine oxidase (MAO) type B, which plays a major role in the catabolism of dopamine. Inhibition of dopamine depletion in the striatal region of the brain reduces the symptomatic motor deficits of Parkinson's disease. There is also experimental evidence of rasagiline conferring neuroprotective effects (antioxidant, antiapoptotic), which may delay onset of symptoms and progression of neuronal deterioration.

◀ **Pharmacodynamics/Kinetics**
Onset of action: Therapeutic: Within 1 hour
Duration: ~1 week (irreversible inhibition); may require ~14-40 days for complete restoration of (brain) MAO-B activity
Absorption: Rapid
Protein binding: 88% to 94%, primarily to albumin
Metabolism: Hepatic N-dealkylation and/or hydroxylation via CYP1A2 to multiple inactive metabolites (nonamphetamine derivatives)
Distribution: V_{dss}: 87 L
Bioavailability: ~36%
Half-life elimination: ~1.3-3 hours (no correlation with biologic effect due to irreversible inhibition)
Time to peak, plasma: ~1 hour
Excretion: Urine (62%, <1% of total dose as unchanged drug); feces (7%)

Dosage
Geriatric & Adult Parkinson's disease: Oral:
Monotherapy: 1 mg once daily
Adjunctive therapy with levodopa: Initial: 0.5 mg once daily; may increase to 1 mg once daily based on response and tolerability
Note: When added to existing levodopa therapy, a dose reduction of levodopa may be required to avoid exacerbation of dyskinesias; typical dose reductions of ~9% to 13% were employed in clinical trials.

Dose reduction with concomitant ciprofloxacin or other CYP1A2 inhibitors: 0.5 mg once daily

Renal Impairment
Mild-to-moderate impairment: No adjustment necessary.
Severe impairment: Not studied.

Hepatic Impairment
Mild impairment (Child-Pugh ≤6): 0.5 mg once daily
Moderate-to-severe impairment: Not recommended.

Administration Administer without regard to meals.

Monitoring Parameters Blood pressure; symptoms of parkinsonism; general mood and behavior (increased anxiety, or presence of mania or agitation); skin examination for presence of melanoma (higher incidence in Parkinson's patients- drug causation not established)

Pharmacotherapy Pearls When adding rasagiline to levodopa/carbidopa, the dose of the latter can usually be decreased. Studies are investigating the use of rasagiline in early Parkinson's disease to slow the progression of the disease.

Special Geriatric Considerations In clinical trials, no significant differences in the safety profile were seen between elderly and younger adults.

Dosage Forms Excipient information presented when available (limited, particularly for generics); consult specific product labeling.
Tablet, oral:
Azilect®: 0.5 mg, 1 mg

Regadenoson (re ga DEN of son)

Brand Names: U.S. Lexiscan®
Index Terms CVT-3146
Generic Availability (U.S.) No
Pharmacologic Category Diagnostic Agent
Use Radionuclide myocardial perfusion imaging (MPI) in patients unable to undergo adequate exercise stress testing
Contraindications Second- or third-degree heart block or sinus node dysfunction in patients without a functioning artificial pacemaker
Warnings/Precautions Equipment for resuscitation and trained personnel experienced in handling cardiac emergencies, bronchoconstriction, and serious hypersensitivity reactions should always be immediately available prior to administration. Pharmacological stress agents may produce myocardial ischemia resulting in life threatening ventricular arrhythmias, MI, and fatal cardiac arrest. Regadenoson decreases conduction through the AV node and may produce first-, second-, or third-degree heart block, or sinus bradycardia. Third-degree heart block and asystole within minutes of administration have been observed. Use caution in patients with first-degree AV block or bundle branch block. Functional pacemaker must be in place to use in patients with second- or third-degree AV block or sinus node dysfunction. May produce profound vasodilation with subsequent hypotension. Syncope and transient ischemic attacks have been reported. Use with caution in patients with autonomic dysfunction, carotid stenosis (with cerebrovascular insufficiency), uncorrected hypovolemia, left main coronary artery stenosis, pericarditis, pericardial effusion and/or stenotic valvular heart disease. Anaphylaxis, angioedema, cardiac and respiratory arrest, and other hypersensitivity reactions have occurred with regadenoson use. May produce hypertension; typically within minutes of administration and usually resolves within 10-15 minutes. Effects may persist; in some patients hypertension continued for 45 minutes after administration. Use with caution in patients with underlying hypertension, especially when low-level exercise is used during MPI. May cause bronchoconstriction in patients with asthma; should be used cautiously in patients with obstructive lung disease not associated with bronchoconstriction (eg, COPD/emphysema, bronchitis). When possible, dipyridamole should be withheld for at least 2 days prior to regadenoson administration. Patients should avoid consumption of any products containing theophylline derivatives (eg, aminophylline, caffeine) for at least 12 hours prior to regadenoson administration.

Adverse Reactions (Reflective of adult population; not specific for elderly)
>10%:
  Cardiovascular: Tachycardia (22%), flushing (16%), premature ventricular contractions (14%), chest discomfort (13%), angina or ST segment depression (12%)
  Central nervous system: Headache (26%)
  Respiratory: Dyspnea (11% to 28%), bronchoconstriction
1% to 10%:
  Cardiovascular: Chest pain (7%), premature atrial contractions (7%), systolic blood pressure decreased >35 mm Hg (7%), systolic blood pressure increased ≥180 mm Hg and ≥20 mm Hg from baseline (5%), ventricular conduction abnormalities (6%), diastolic blood pressure decreased >25 mm Hg (4%), first-degree AV block (PR prolongation >220 msec; 3%), diastolic blood pressure increased ≥30 mm Hg (1%)
  Central nervous system: Dizziness (8%)
  Gastrointestinal: Nausea (6%), abdominal discomfort (5%), abnormal taste (5%)
  Respiratory: Wheezing (<1%; 1% to 3% in patients with asthma or COPD); respiratory adverse reactions overall (includes obstructive airway disorder, exertional dyspnea, tachypnea) (13% to 19% in patients with asthma or COPD)
  Miscellaneous: Feeling hot (5%)
Drug Interactions
  Metabolism/Transport Effects None known.
  Avoid Concomitant Use There are no known interactions where it is recommended to avoid concomitant use.
  Increased Effect/Toxicity
    The levels/effects of Regadenoson may be increased by: Dipyridamole
  Decreased Effect
    The levels/effects of Regadenoson may be decreased by: Aminophylline; Caffeine; Theophylline
Ethanol/Nutrition/Herb Interactions Food: Regadenoson's diagnostic effect may be decreased if used concurrently with caffeine. Management: Avoid food or drugs with caffeine for at least 12 hours prior to pharmacologic stress testing.
Stability Store at controlled room temperature of 25°C (77°F); excursions permitted to 15°C to 30°C (59°F to 86°F).

◀ **Mechanism of Action** Regadenoson, a low affinity agonist of the A_{2A} adenosine receptor, increases coronary blood flow (CBF) and mimics the increase in CBF caused by exercise. Myocardial uptake of the radiopharmaceutical is proportional to CBF creating the contrast required to identify stenotic coronary arteries.

Pharmacodynamics/Kinetics

Distribution: 11.5 L

Metabolism: Unknown

Half-life elimination: Initial phase: 2-4 minutes; Intermediate phase: 30 minutes; Terminal phase: 2 hours

Time to peak, plasma: 1-4 minutes

Excretion: Urine (57% as unchanged drug)

Dosage

Geriatric & Adult Myocardial perfusion imaging: I.V.: 0.4 mg (5 mL) over ~10 seconds, followed immediately by a 5 mL saline flush. Wait 10-20 seconds, then administer the radionuclide myocardial perfusion imaging agent.

Renal Impairment No dosage adjustment necessary.

Hepatic Impairment No dosage adjustment necessary.

Administration Administer over approximately 10 seconds into a peripheral vein using a ≥22-gauge catheter or needle, followed immediately by a 5 mL saline flush. Wait 10-20 seconds, then administer the radionuclide myocardial perfusion imaging agent. The radionuclide may be injected directly into the same catheter as regadenoson.

Monitoring Parameters Heart rate, blood pressure, continuous cardiac monitoring, oxygen saturation

Special Geriatric Considerations In initial studies, elderly had a higher incidence of hypotension (2% vs <1%).

Dosage Forms Excipient information presented when available (limited, particularly for generics); consult specific product labeling.

Injection, solution [preservative free]:

Lexiscan®: 0.08 mg/mL (5 mL) [contains edetate disodium, propylene glycol 150 mg/mL]

◆ **Regenecare®** see Lidocaine (Topical) on page 1128
◆ **Regenecare® HA [OTC]** see Lidocaine (Topical) on page 1128
◆ **Reglan®** see Metoclopramide on page 1258
◆ **Regonol®** see Pyridostigmine on page 1638
◆ **Regranex®** see Becaplermin on page 188
◆ **Regular Insulin** see Insulin Regular on page 1025
◆ **Reguloid [OTC]** see Psyllium on page 1635
◆ **Relafen** see Nabumetone on page 1326
◆ **Relenza®** see Zanamivir on page 2045
◆ **Relistor®** see Methylnaltrexone on page 1246
◆ **Relpax®** see Eletriptan on page 629
◆ **Remeron®** see Mirtazapine on page 1294
◆ **Remeron SolTab®** see Mirtazapine on page 1294
◆ **Renagel®** see Sevelamer on page 1768
◆ **Renvela®** see Sevelamer on page 1768

Repaglinide (re PAG li nide)

Related Information

Diabetes Mellitus Management, Adults on page 2193

Medication Safety Issues

Sound-alike/look-alike issues:

Prandin® may be confused with Avandia®

High alert medication:

The Institute for Safe Medication Practices (ISMP) includes this medication among its list of drug classes which have a heightened risk of causing significant patient harm when used in error.

Brand Names: U.S. Prandin®

Brand Names: Canada CO-Repaglinide; GlucoNorm®; PMS-Repaglinide; Sandoz-Repaglinide

Generic Availability (U.S.) No

Pharmacologic Category Antidiabetic Agent, Meglitinide Derivative

Use Management of type 2 diabetes mellitus (noninsulin dependent, NIDDM) as an adjunct to diet and exercise; may be used in combination with metformin or thiazolidinediones

Contraindications Hypersensitivity to repaglinide or any component of the formulation; diabetic ketoacidosis, with or without coma; type 1 diabetes (insulin dependent, IDDM); concurrent gemfibrozil therapy

Warnings/Precautions Use with caution in patients with hepatic impairment. Use caution in severe renal dysfunction, elderly, malnourished, or patients with adrenal/pituitary dysfunction; may be more susceptible to glucose-lowering effects. May cause hypoglycemia; appropriate patient selection, dosage, and patient education are important to avoid hypoglycemic episodes. It may be necessary to discontinue repaglinide and administer insulin if the patient is exposed to stress (fever, trauma, infection, surgery). Theoretically, repaglinide may increase cardiovascular events as observed in some studies using sulfonylureas, but there are no long-term studies assessing this concern. Not indicated for use in combination with NPH insulin as there have been case reports of myocardial ischemia; further evaluation required to assess the safety of this combination.

Adverse Reactions (Reflective of adult population; not specific for elderly)
>10%:
Central nervous system: Headache (9% to 11%)
Endocrine & metabolic: Hypoglycemia (16% to 31%)
Respiratory: Upper respiratory tract infection (10% to 16%)
1% to 10%:
Cardiovascular: Ischemia (4%), chest pain (2% to 3%)
Gastrointestinal: Diarrhea (4% to 5%), constipation (2% to 3%)
Genitourinary: Urinary tract infection (2% to 3%)
Neuromuscular & skeletal: Back pain (5% to 6%), arthralgia (3% to 6%)
Respiratory: Sinusitis (3% to 6%), bronchitis (2% to 6%)
Miscellaneous: Allergy (1% to 2%)

Drug Interactions

Metabolism/Transport Effects Substrate of CYP2C8 (major), CYP3A4 (major), SLCO1B1; **Note:** Assignment of Major/Minor substrate status based on clinically relevant drug interaction potential

Avoid Concomitant Use

Avoid concomitant use of Repaglinide with any of the following: Conivaptan; Gemfibrozil

Increased Effect/Toxicity

Repaglinide may increase the levels/effects of: Hypoglycemic Agents

The levels/effects of Repaglinide may be increased by: Antifungal Agents (Azole Derivatives, Systemic); Conivaptan; CycloSPORINE; CycloSPORINE (Systemic); CYP2C8 Inhibitors (Moderate); CYP2C8 Inhibitors (Strong); CYP3A4 Inhibitors (Moderate); CYP3A4 Inhibitors (Strong); Dasatinib; Deferasirox; Eltrombopag; Gemfibrozil; Herbs (Hypoglycemic Properties); Ivacaftor; Macrolide Antibiotics; MAO Inhibitors; Mifepristone; Pegvisomant; Salicylates; Selective Serotonin Reuptake Inhibitors; Trimethoprim

Decreased Effect

The levels/effects of Repaglinide may be decreased by: Corticosteroids (Orally Inhaled); Corticosteroids (Systemic); CYP2C8 Inducers (Strong); CYP3A4 Inducers (Strong); Herbs (CYP3A4 Inducers); Loop Diuretics; Luteinizing Hormone-Releasing Hormone Analogs; Rifamycin Derivatives; Somatropin; Thiazide Diuretics; Tocilizumab

Ethanol/Nutrition/Herb Interactions
Ethanol: Ethanol may increase risk of hypoglycemia. Management: Avoid ethanol.
Food: When given with food, the AUC of repaglinide is decreased. Taking medication without eating may cause hypoglycemia. Management: Administer 15-30 minutes prior to a meal. If a meal is skipped, skip dose for that meal.
Herb/Nutraceutical: St John's wort may decrease the levels/effect of repaglinide. Other herbal medications may enhance the hypoglycemic effects of repaglinide. Management: Avoid St John's wort, alfalfa, aloe, bilberry, bitter melon, burdock, celery, damiana, fenugreek, garcinia, garlic, ginger, ginseng (American), gymnema, marshmallow, and stinging nettle.

Stability Do not store above 25°C (77°F). Protect from moisture.

Mechanism of Action Nonsulfonylurea hypoglycemic agent which blocks ATP-dependent potassium channels, depolarizing the membrane and facilitating calcium entry through calcium channels. Increased intracellular calcium stimulates insulin release from the pancreatic beta cells. Repaglinide-induced insulin release is glucose-dependent.

Pharmacodynamics/Kinetics
Onset of action: Single dose: Increased insulin levels: ~15-60 minutes
Duration: 4-6 hours
Absorption: Rapid and complete
Distribution: V_d: 31 L
Protein binding, plasma: >98% to albumin
Metabolism: Hepatic via CYP3A4 and CYP2C8 isoenzymes and glucuronidation to inactive metabolites
Bioavailability: ~56%
Half-life elimination: ~1 hour
Time to peak, plasma: ~1 hour
Excretion: Feces (~90%, <2% as unchanged drug); Urine (~8%, 0.1% as unchanged drug)

◀ **Dosage**

Geriatric & Adult

Type 2 diabetes: Oral:

Patients not previously treated or whose Hb A_{1c} is <8%: Initial: 0.5 mg before each meal

Patients previously treated with blood glucose-lowering agents whose Hb A_{1c} is ≥8%: Initial: 1 or 2 mg before each meal.

Dose adjustment: Determine dosing adjustments by blood glucose response, usually fasting blood glucose. Double the prandial dose up to 4 mg until satisfactory blood glucose response is achieved. At least 1 week should elapse to assess response after each dose adjustment.

Dose range: 0.5-4 mg taken with meals. Repaglinide may be dosed preprandially 2, 3, or 4 times/day in response to changes in the patient's meal pattern. Maximum recommended daily dose: 16 mg.

Patients receiving other oral hypoglycemic agents: When repaglinide is used to replace therapy with other oral hypoglycemic agents, it may be started the day after the final dose is given. Observe patients carefully for hypoglycemia because of potential overlapping of drug effects. When transferred from longer half-life sulfonylureas (eg, chlorpropamide), close monitoring may be indicated for up to ≥1 week.

Note: Combination therapy: If repaglinide monotherapy does not result in adequate glycemic control, metformin or a thiazolidinedione may be added. Or, if metformin or thiazolidinedione therapy does not provide adequate control, repaglinide may be added. The starting dose and dose adjustments for combination therapy are the same as repaglinide monotherapy. Carefully adjust the dose of each drug to determine the minimal dose required to achieve the desired pharmacologic effect. Failure to do so could result in an increase in the incidence of hypoglycemic episodes. Use appropriate monitoring of FPG and Hb A_{1c} measurements to ensure that the patient is not subjected to excessive drug exposure or increased probability of secondary drug failure. If glucose is not achieved after a suitable trial of combination therapy, consider discontinuing these drugs and using insulin.

Renal Impairment

Cl_{cr} 40-80 mL/minute (mild-to-moderate renal dysfunction): Initial dosage adjustment does not appear to be necessary.

Cl_{cr} 20-40 mL/minute (severe renal impairment): Initial: 0.5 mg with meals; titrate carefully.

Cl_{cr} <20 mL/minute: Not studied.

Hemodialysis: Not studied

Hepatic Impairment Use conservative initial and maintenance doses. Use longer intervals between dosage adjustments.

Administration Administer 15 minutes before meals; however, time may vary from immediately preceding a meal to as long as 30 minutes before a meal. If the patient misses a meal or is unable to take anything by mouth, repaglinide should not be administered to avoid hypoglycemia. Patients consuming extra meals should be instructed to add a dose for the extra meal.

Monitoring Parameters Monitor fasting blood glucose (periodically) and glycosylated hemoglobin (Hb A_{1c}) levels (every 3 months) with a goal of decreasing these levels towards the normal range. During dose adjustment, fasting glucose can be used to determine response.

Reference Range

Recommendations for glycemic control in adults with diabetes:

Hb A_{1c}: <7%

Preprandial capillary plasma glucose: 70-130 mg/dL

Peak postprandial capillary blood glucose: <180 mg/dL

Blood pressure: <130/80 mm Hg

Recommendations for glycemic control in older adults with diabetes:

Relatively healthy, cognitively intact, and with a ≥5-year life expectancy: See Adults

Frail, life expectancy <5-years or those for whom the risks of intensive glucose control outweigh the benefits:

Hb A_{1c}: <8% to 9%

Blood pressure: <140/80 mm Hg or <130/80 mm Hg if tolerated

Special Geriatric Considerations Repaglinide has not been studied exclusively in the elderly; information from the manufacturer states that no differences in its effectiveness or adverse effects had been identified between persons younger than and older than 65 years of age. Intensive glucose control (Hb A_{1c} <6.5%) has been linked to increased all-cause and cardiovascular mortality, hypoglycemia requiring assistance, and weight gain in adult type 2 diabetes. How "tightly" to control a geriatric patient's blood glucose needs to be individualized. Such a decision should be based on several factors, including the patient's functional and cognitive status, how well he/she recognizes hypoglycemic or hyperglycemic symptoms, and how to respond to them and other disease states. An Hb A_{1c} <7.5% is an acceptable endpoint for a healthy older adult, while <8% is acceptable for frail elderly patients, those with a duration of illness >10 years, or those with comorbid conditions and requiring combination diabetes medications. For elderly patients with diabetes who are relatively healthy, attaining target goals for aspirin use, blood pressure, lipids, smoking cessation, and diet and exercise may be more important than normalized glycemic control.

Dosage Forms Excipient information presented when available (limited, particularly for generics); consult specific product labeling.

Tablet, oral:

Prandin®: 0.5 mg, 1 mg, 2 mg

Repaglinide and Metformin (re PAG li nide & met FOR min)

Related Information

Diabetes Mellitus Management, Adults *on page 2193*
MetFORMIN *on page 1222*
Repaglinide *on page 1684*

Medication Safety Issues

Sound-alike/look-alike issues:

PrandiMet® may be confused with Avandamet®, Prandin®

High alert medication:

The Institute for Safe Medication Practices (ISMP) includes this medication among its list of drug classes which have a heightened risk of causing significant patient harm when used in error.

Brand Names: U.S. PrandiMet®

Index Terms Metformin and Repaglinide; Repaglinide and Metformin Hydrochloride

Generic Availability (U.S.) No

Pharmacologic Category Antidiabetic Agent, Biguanide; Antidiabetic Agent, Meglitinide Derivative; Hypoglycemic Agent, Oral

Use Management of type 2 diabetes mellitus (noninsulin dependent, NIDDM), as an adjunct to diet and exercise, in patients currently receiving or not adequately controlled on metformin and/or a meglitinide

Dosage

Geriatric & Adult Type 2 diabetes mellitus: Oral: **Note:** Daily doses should be divided and given 2-3 times daily with meals (maximum single dose: 4 mg/dose [repaglinide], 1000 mg/dose [metformin]; maximum daily dose: 10 mg/day [repaglinide], 2500 mg/day [metformin])

Patients currently taking repaglinide and metformin: Initial doses should be based on (but not exceeding) the patient's current doses of repaglinide and metformin; titrate as needed to the maximum daily dose to achieve targeted glycemic control

Patients inadequately controlled on metformin alone: Initial dose: repaglinide 1 mg/ metformin 500 mg twice daily with meals. Titrate slowly to reduce the risk of repaglinide-induced hypoglycemia.

Patients inadequately controlled on a meglitinide alone: Initial dose: metformin 500 mg twice daily plus repaglinide at a dose similar to (but not exceeding) the patient's current dose. Titrate slowly to reduce the risk of metformin-induced gastrointestinal adverse effects.

Renal Impairment Do not use in renal impairment; metformin use is contraindicated in patients with renal impairment (serum creatinine ≥1.5 mg/dL in males or ≥1.4 mg/dL in females).

Hepatic Impairment Avoid use in patients with impaired liver function.

Special Geriatric Considerations See individual agents. Combination products are not recommended as first-line treatment. Use only if doses of individual agents correspond to the combination available.

Dosage Forms Excipient information presented when available (limited, particularly for generics); consult specific product labeling.

Tablet:

PrandiMet®:

1/500: Repaglinide 1 mg and metformin hydrochloride 500 mg

2/500: Repaglinide 2 mg and metformin hydrochloride 500 mg

◆ **Repaglinide and Metformin Hydrochloride** *see* Repaglinide and Metformin *on page 1687*
◆ **Requip®** *see* ROPINIRole *on page 1724*
◆ **Requip® XL™** *see* ROPINIRole *on page 1724*

Reserpine (re SER peen)

Related Information
Beers Criteria – Potentially Inappropriate Medications for Geriatrics *on page 2183*
Medication Safety Issues
Sound-alike/look-alike issues:
Reserpine may be confused with RisperDAL®, risperiDONE
BEERS Criteria medication:
This drug may be potentially inappropriate for use in geriatric patients (Quality of evidence - low; Strength of recommendation - strong).
Generic Availability (U.S.) Yes
Pharmacologic Category Central Monoamine-Depleting Agent; Rauwolfia Alkaloid
Use Management of mild-to-moderate hypertension; treatment of agitated psychotic states (schizophrenia)
Unlabeled Use Management of tardive dyskinesia
Dosage
Geriatric Oral: Initial: 0.05 mg once daily increasing by 0.05 mg every week as necessary; full antihypertensive effects may take as long as 3 weeks (Beers Criteria: Avoid doses >0.25 mg daily)
Adult
Hypertension:
Manufacturer's labeling: Initial: 0.5 mg/day for 1-2 weeks; maintenance: 0.1-0.25 mg/day
Note: Clinically, the need for a "loading" period (as recommended by the manufacturer) is not well supported, and alternative dosing is preferred.
Alternative dosing (unlabeled): Initial: 0.1 mg once daily; adjust as necessary based on response.
Usual dose range (JNC 7): 0.05-0.25 mg once daily; 0.1 mg every other day may be given to achieve 0.05 mg once daily
Schizophrenia (labeled use) or tardive dyskinesia (unlabeled use): Dosing recommendations vary; initial dose recommendations generally range from 0.05-0.25 mg (although manufacturer recommends 0.5 mg once daily initially in schizophrenia). May be increased in increments of 0.1-0.25 mg; maximum dose in tardive dyskinesia: 5 mg/day.
Renal Impairment
Cl_{cr} <10 mL/minute: Avoid use.
Not removed by hemo- or peritoneal dialysis; supplemental dose is not necessary.
Special Geriatric Considerations Some older studies advocated the use of reserpine because of its low cost, long half-life, and efficacy, but it is generally not considered a first-line drug.

This medication is considered to be potentially inappropriate in this patient population (Beers Criteria: Quality of evidence - low; Strength of recommendation - strong).
Dosage Forms Excipient information presented when available (limited, particularly for generics); consult specific product labeling.
Tablet, oral: 0.1 mg, 0.25 mg

◆ **Resistant Dextrin** *see* Wheat Dextrin *on page 2039*
◆ **Resistant Maltodextrin** *see* Wheat Dextrin *on page 2039*
◆ **Restasis®** *see* CycloSPORINE (Ophthalmic) *on page 467*
◆ **Restoril™** *see* Temazepam *on page 1850*

Retapamulin (re te PAM ue lin)

Brand Names: U.S. Altabax™
Generic Availability (U.S.) No
Pharmacologic Category Antibiotic, Pleuromutilin; Antibiotic, Topical
Use Treatment of impetigo caused by susceptible strains of *S. pyogenes* or methicillin-susceptible *S. aureus*
Contraindications Hypersensitivity to retapamulin or any component of the formulation
Warnings/Precautions For treatment of impetigo covering up to 100 cm^2 total area in adults. For external use only; not for intranasal, intravaginal, ophthalmic, oral, or mucosal application. May cause superinfection. Concomitant use with other topical products to the same treatment area has not been evaluated. If skin irritation occurs, discontinue use.

Adverse Reactions (Reflective of adult population; not specific for elderly) 1% to 10%:

Central nervous system: Headache (1% to 2%), pyrexia (1%)

Dermatologic: Pruritus (2%), eczema (1%)

Gastrointestinal: Diarrhea (1% to 2%), nausea (1%)

Local: Application site irritation (2%), application site pruritus (2%)

Respiratory: Nasopharyngitis (1% to 2%)

Drug Interactions

Metabolism/Transport Effects None known.

Avoid Concomitant Use There are no known interactions where it is recommended to avoid concomitant use.

Increased Effect/Toxicity There are no known significant interactions involving an increase in effect.

Decreased Effect There are no known significant interactions involving a decrease in effect.

Stability Store at room temperature of 15°C to 30°C (59°F to 86°F).

Mechanism of Action Primarily bacteriostatic. Inhibits normal bacterial protein biosynthesis by binding at a unique site (protein L3) on the ribosomal 50S subunit; prevents formation of active 50S ribosomal subunits by inhibiting peptidyl transfer and blocking P-site interactions at this site

Pharmacodynamics/Kinetics

Absorption: Topical: Low; increased when applied to abraded skin

Protein binding: 94%

Metabolism: Hepatic via CYP 3A4; extensively metabolized by mono-oxygenation and di-oxygenation to multiple metabolites

Dosage

Adult Impetigo: Topical: Apply to affected area twice daily for 5 days. Total treatment area should not exceed 100 cm² total body surface area.

Administration Topical: May cover treatment area with sterile bandage or gauze dressing if needed. Concomitant use with other topical products to the same treatment area has not been evaluated.

Special Geriatric Considerations Evaluate the patient's or caregiver's ability to safely administer the correct dose of ophthalmic medication.

Dosage Forms Excipient information presented when available (limited, particularly for generics); consult specific product labeling. [DSC] = Discontinued product

Ointment, topical:

Altabax™: 1% (5 g [DSC], 10 g [DSC], 15 g)

♦ **Retavase® Half-Kit** see Reteplase on page 1689
♦ **Retavase® Kit** see Reteplase on page 1689

Reteplase (RE ta plase)

Medication Safety Issues

High alert medication:

The Institute for Safe Medication Practices (ISMP) includes this medication (I.V.) among its list of drugs which have a heightened risk of causing significant patient harm when used in error.

Brand Names: U.S. Retavase® Half-Kit; Retavase® Kit

Brand Names: Canada Retavase®

Index Terms r-PA; Recombinant Plasminogen Activator

Generic Availability (U.S.) No

Pharmacologic Category Thrombolytic Agent

Use Management of ST-elevation myocardial infarction (STEMI); improvement of ventricular function; reduction of the incidence of CHF and the reduction of mortality following AMI

Recommended criteria for treatment (Antman, 2004): STEMI: Chest pain ≥20 minutes duration, onset of chest pain within 12 hours of treatment (or within prior 12-24 hours in patients with continuing ischemic symptoms), and ST-segment elevation >0.1 mV in at least two contiguous precordial leads or two adjacent limb leads on ECG or new or presumably new left bundle branch block (LBBB)

Contraindications Active internal bleeding; history of cerebrovascular accident; recent intracranial or intraspinal surgery or trauma; intracranial neoplasm, arteriovenous malformations, or aneurysm; known bleeding diathesis; severe uncontrolled hypertension

Warnings/Precautions Concurrent heparin anticoagulation can contribute to bleeding; careful attention to all potential bleeding sites. I.M. injections and nonessential handling of the patient should be avoided. Venipunctures should be performed carefully and only when necessary. If arterial puncture is necessary, use an upper extremity vessel that can be manually compressed. If serious bleeding occurs then the infusion of anistreplase and heparin should be stopped.

For the following conditions the risk of bleeding is higher with use of reteplase and should be weighed against the benefits of therapy: recent major surgery (eg, CABG, obstetrical delivery, organ biopsy, previous puncture of noncompressible vessels), cerebrovascular disease, recent gastrointestinal or genitourinary bleeding, recent trauma including CPR, hypertension (systolic BP >180 mm Hg and/or diastolic BP >110 mm Hg), high likelihood of left heart thrombus (eg, mitral stenosis with atrial fibrillation), acute pericarditis, subacute bacterial endocarditis, hemostatic defects including ones caused by severe renal or hepatic dysfunction, significant hepatic dysfunction, diabetic hemorrhagic retinopathy or other hemorrhagic ophthalmic conditions, septic thrombophlebitis or occluded AV cannula at seriously infected site, advanced age (eg, >75 years), patients receiving oral anticoagulants, any other condition in which bleeding constitutes a significant hazard or would be particularly difficult to manage because of location.

Coronary thrombolysis may result in reperfusion arrhythmias. Follow standard MI management. Rare anaphylactic reactions can occur.

Adverse Reactions (Reflective of adult population; not specific for elderly) Bleeding is the most frequent adverse effect associated with reteplase. Heparin and aspirin have been administered concurrently with reteplase in clinical trials. The incidence of adverse events is a reflection of these combined therapies, and is comparable to comparison thrombolytics.

>10%: Local: Injection site bleeding (5% to 49%)
1% to 10%:
  Gastrointestinal: Bleeding (2% to 9%)
  Genitourinary: Bleeding (1% to 10%)
  Hematologic: Anemia (1% to 3%)
Other adverse effects noted are frequently associated with MI (and therefore may or may not be attributable to Retavase®) and include arrhythmia, AV block, cardiac arrest, cardiogenic shock, embolism, heart failure, hypotension, myocardial rupture, mitral regurgitation, pericardial effusion, pericarditis, pulmonary edema, recurrent ischemia, reinfarction, tamponade, thrombosis

Drug Interactions
Metabolism/Transport Effects None known.
Avoid Concomitant Use There are no known interactions where it is recommended to avoid concomitant use.
Increased Effect/Toxicity
Reteplase may increase the levels/effects of: Anticoagulants; Dabigatran Etexilate; Drotrecogin Alfa (Activated)

The levels/effects of Reteplase may be increased by: Antiplatelet Agents; Herbs (Anticoagulant/Antiplatelet Properties); Nonsteroidal Anti-Inflammatory Agents; Salicylates
Decreased Effect
The levels/effects of Reteplase may be decreased by: Aprotinin
Stability Dosage kits should be stored at 2°C to 25°C (36°F to 77°F) and remain sealed until use in order to protect from light. Reteplase should be reconstituted using the diluent, syringe, needle, and dispensing pin provided with each kit. Do not shake while reconstituting; swirl gently. Once reconstituted, use within 4 hours.
Mechanism of Action Reteplase is a nonglycosylated form of tPA produced by recombinant DNA technology using *E. coli*; it initiates local fibrinolysis by binding to fibrin in a thrombus (clot) and converts entrapped plasminogen to plasmin
Pharmacodynamics/Kinetics
Onset of action: Thrombolysis: 30-90 minutes
Half-life elimination: 13-16 minutes
Excretion: Feces and urine
Clearance: Plasma: 250-450 mL/minute
Dosage
Geriatric & Adult
  STEMI: I.V.: 10 units I.V. over 2 minutes, followed by a second dose 30 minutes later of 10 units I.V. over 2 minutes; withhold second dose if serious bleeding or anaphylaxis occurs.
  Note: All patients should receive 162-325 mg of chewable nonenteric coated aspirin as soon as possible and then daily. Administer concurrently with heparin 60 units/kg bolus (maximum: 4000 units) followed by continuous infusion of 12 units/kg/hour (maximum: 1000 units/hour) and adjust to aPTT target of 50-70 seconds (or 1.5-2 times the upper limit of control).
Administration Reteplase should be reconstituted using the diluent, syringe, needle and dispensing pin provided with each kit and the each reconstituted dose should be administered I.V. over 2 minutes; no other medication should be added to the injection solution

RIBAVIRIN

Monitoring Parameters Monitor for signs of bleeding (hematuria, GI bleeding, gingival bleeding); CBC, PTT; ECG monitoring

Test Interactions Altered results of coagulation and fibrinolytic activity tests

Pharmacotherapy Pearls The dosage of reteplase in clinical trials was expressed in terms of million unit (MU); however, reteplase is being marketed in units (U) with 1 unit equivalent to 1 million units, reteplase units are expressed using a reference standard specific for reteplase and are not comparable with units used for other thrombolytic agents, 10 units is equivalent to 17.4 mg

Special Geriatric Considerations No specific changes in use in the elderly are necessary.

Dosage Forms Excipient information presented when available (limited, particularly for generics); consult specific product labeling.

Injection, powder for reconstitution [preservative free]:

Retavase® Half-Kit: 10.4 units [contains polysorbate 80, sucrose 364 mg/vial; equivalent to reteplase 18.1 mg; one Reteplase® vial; supplied with diluent]

Retavase® Kit: 10.4 units [contains polysorbate 80, sucrose 364 mg/vial; equivalent to reteplase 18.1 mg; two Retavase® vials; supplied with diluents]

- ◆ **Retigabine** see Ezogabine on page 740
- ◆ **Retisert®** see Fluocinolone (Ophthalmic) on page 803
- ◆ **Revatio®** see Sildenafil on page 1770
- ◆ **Revonto®** see Dantrolene on page 483
- ◆ **Rexolate®** see Salicylates (Various Salts) on page 1742
- ◆ **Rheumatrex®** see Methotrexate on page 1236
- ◆ **Rhinall® [OTC]** see Phenylephrine (Nasal) on page 1526
- ◆ **Rhinaris® [OTC]** see Sodium Chloride on page 1787
- ◆ **Rhinocort Aqua®:** see Budesonide (Nasal) on page 231
- ◆ **r-Hirudin** see Desirudin on page 508
- ◆ **rhPTH(1-34)** see Teriparatide on page 1859
- ◆ **rHuEPO** see Epoetin Alfa on page 651
- ◆ **rhuFabV2** see Ranibizumab on page 1673
- ◆ **Ribasphere®** see Ribavirin on page 1691
- ◆ **Ribasphere® RibaPak®** see Ribavirin on page 1691

Ribavirin (rye ba VYE rin)

Medication Safety Issues

Sound-alike/look-alike issues:

Ribavirin may be confused with riboflavin, rifampin, Robaxin®

Brand Names: U.S. Copegus®; Rebetol®; Ribasphere®; Ribasphere® RibaPak®; Virazole®

Brand Names: Canada Virazole®

Index Terms RTCA; Tribavirin

Generic Availability (U.S.) Yes: Capsule, tablet

Pharmacologic Category Antiviral Agent

Use

Inhalation: Specially indicated for treatment of severe lower respiratory tract RSV infections in patients with an underlying compromising condition (prematurity, cardiopulmonary disease, or immunosuppression)

Oral capsule:

In combination with interferon alfa-2b (Intron® A) injection for the treatment of chronic hepatitis C in patients with compensated liver disease who have relapsed after alpha interferon therapy or were previously untreated with alpha interferons

In combination with peginterferon alfa-2b (PEG-Intron®) injection for the treatment of chronic hepatitis C in patients with compensated liver disease who were previously untreated with alpha interferons

Oral solution: In combination with interferon alfa-2b (Intron® A) injection for the treatment of chronic hepatitis C in patients with compensated liver disease who were previously untreated with alpha interferons or patients who have relapsed after alpha interferon therapy

Oral tablet: In combination with peginterferon alfa-2a (Pegasys®) injection for the treatment of chronic hepatitis C in patients with compensated liver disease who were previously untreated with alpha interferons (includes patients with histological evidence of cirrhosis [Child-Pugh class A] and patients with clinically-stable HIV disease)

Unlabeled Use

Inhalation: Treatment for RSV in adult hematopoietic stem cell or heart/lung transplant recipients

Used in other viral infections including influenza A and B and adenovirus

Medication Guide Available Yes

Contraindications Hypersensitivity to ribavirin or any component of the formulation

Additional contraindications for oral formulation: Male partners of pregnant women; hemoglobinopathies (eg, thalassemia major, sickle cell anemia); patients with autoimmune hepatitis; ribavirin tablets are contraindicated in patients with hepatic decompensation (Child-Pugh class B and C); concomitant use of didanosine

Warnings/Precautions Oral: Safety and efficacy have not been established in patients who have failed other alfa interferon therapy, received organ transplants, or been coinfected with hepatitis B or HIV (Copegus® may be used in HIV coinfected patients unless CD4+ cell count is <100 cells/microL). Oral products should not be used for HIV infection, adenovirus, RSV, or influenza infections.

[U.S. Boxed Warning]: Monotherapy not effective for chronic hepatitis C infection. Severe psychiatric events have occurred including depression and suicidal behavior during combination therapy. Avoid use in patients with a psychiatric history; discontinue if severe psychiatric symptoms occur. Acute hypersensitivity reactions (eg, anaphylaxis, angioedema, bronchoconstriction, and urticaria) have been observed (rarely) with ribavirin and alfa interferon combination therapy. Severe cutaneous reactions, including Stevens-Johnson syndrome and exfoliative dermatitis have been reported (rarely) with ribavirin and alfa interferon combination therapy; discontinue with signs or symptoms of severe skin reactions. Use with caution in patients with renal impairment; dosage adjustment or discontinuation may be required. Elderly patients are more susceptible to adverse effects; use caution.

[U.S. Boxed Warning]: Hemolytic anemia is the primary toxicity of oral therapy; usually occurring within 1-2 weeks of therapy initiation; observed in ~10% to 13% of patients when alfa interferons were combined with ribavirin. Assess cardiac disease before initiation. Anemia may worsen underlying cardiac disease; avoid use in patients with significant/unstable cardiac disease. If deterioration in cardiovascular status occurs, discontinue therapy. Patients with renal dysfunction and/or those >50 years of age should be carefully assessed for development of anemia. Pancytopenia and bone marrow suppression have been reported with the combination of ribavirin, interferon, and azathioprine. Use caution in pulmonary disease; pulmonary symptoms have been associated with administration. Discontinue therapy if evidence of hepatic decompensation (Child-Pugh score ≥6) is observed. Use caution in patients with sarcoidosis (exacerbation reported). Dental and periodontal disorders have been reported with ribavirin and interferon therapy; patients should be instructed to brush teeth twice daily and have regular dental exams. Serious ophthalmologic disorders have occurred with combination therapy. All patients require an eye exam at baseline; those with pre-existing ophthalmologic disorders (eg, diabetic or hypertensive retinopathy) require periodic follow up.

Inhalation: **[U.S. Boxed Warning]: Use with caution in patients requiring assisted ventilation because precipitation of the drug in the respiratory equipment may interfere with safe and effective patient ventilation; sudden deterioration of respiratory function has been observed;** monitor carefully in patients with COPD and asthma for deterioration of respiratory function. Ribavirin is potentially mutagenic, tumor-promoting, and gonadotoxic. Although anemia has not been reported with inhalation therapy, consider monitoring for anemia 1-2 weeks post-treatment. Pregnant healthcare workers may consider unnecessary occupational exposure; ribavirin has been detected in healthcare workers' urine. Healthcare professionals or family members who are pregnant (or may become pregnant) should be counseled about potential risks of exposure and counseled about risk reduction strategies. Hazardous agent - use appropriate precautions for handling and disposal.

Adverse Reactions (Reflective of adult population; not specific for elderly)
Inhalation:
1% to 10%:
Central nervous system: Fatigue, headache, insomnia
Gastrointestinal: Nausea, anorexia
Hematologic: Anemia
<1%: Hypotension, cardiac arrest, digitalis toxicity, conjunctivitis, mild bronchospasm, worsening of respiratory function, apnea
Note: Incidence of adverse effects (approximate) in healthcare workers: Headache (51%); conjunctivitis (32%); rhinitis, nausea, rash, dizziness, pharyngitis, and lacrimation (10% to 20%); bronchospasm and/or chest pain (case reports in individuals with underlying airway disease)

Oral (all adverse reactions are documented while receiving combination therapy with alfa interferons; percentages as reported in adults); asterisked (*) percentages are those similar to interferon therapy alone:

>10%:

Central nervous system: Fatigue (60% to 70%)*, headache (43% to 66%)*, fever (32% to 55%)*, insomnia (26% to 41%), depression (20% to 36%)*, irritability (23% to 33%), dizziness (14% to 26%), impaired concentration (10% to 21%)*, emotional lability (7% to 12%)*

Dermatologic: Alopecia (27% to 36%), pruritus (13% to 29%), rash (5% to 28%), dry skin (10% to 24%), dermatitis (≤16%)

Endocrine and metabolic: Hyperuricemia (33% to 38%)

Gastrointestinal: Nausea (25% to 47%), anorexia (21% to 32%), weight decrease (10% to 29%), vomiting (9% to 25%)*, diarrhea (10% to 22%), dyspepsia (6% to 16%), abdominal pain (8% to 13%), xerostomia (≤12%), RUQ pain (≤12%)

Hematologic: Leukopenia (6% to 45%), neutropenia (8% to 42%; grade 4: 2% to 11%; 40% with HIV coinfection), hemoglobin decreased (11% to 35%), anemia (11% to 17%), thrombocytopenia (<1% to 15%), lymphopenia (12% to 14%), hemolytic anemia (10% to 13%)

Hepatic: Bilirubin increase (10% to 32%)

Neuromuscular & skeletal: Myalgia (40% to 64%)*, rigors (25% to 48%), arthralgia (22% to 34%)*, musculoskeletal pain (19% to 28%)

Respiratory: Dyspnea (13% to 26%), cough (7% to 23%), pharyngitis (≤13%), sinusitis (≤12%)*

Miscellaneous: Flu-like syndrome (13% to 18%)*, viral infection (≤12%), diaphoresis (≤11%)

1% to 10%:

Cardiovascular: Chest pain (5% to 9%)*, flushing (≤4%)

Central nervous system: Pain (≤10%), mood alteration (≤6%; 9% with HIV coinfection), agitation (5% to 8%), nervousness (6%)*, memory impairment (≤6%), malaise (≤6%), suicidal ideation (adolescents: 2%; adults: 1%)

Dermatologic: Eczema (4% to 5%)

Endocrine & metabolic: Menstrual disorder (≤7%), hypothyroidism (≤5%)

Gastrointestinal: Taste perversion (4% to 9%), constipation (5%)

Hepatic: Hepatomegaly (4%), transaminases increased (1% to 3%), hepatic decompensation (2% with HIV coinfection)

Neuromuscular & skeletal: Weakness (9% to 10%), back pain (5%)

Ocular: Blurred vision (≤6%), conjunctivitis (≤5%)

Respiratory: Rhinitis (≤8%), exertional dyspnea (≤7%)

Miscellaneous: Fungal infection (≤6%), bacterial infection (3% to 5%)

Note: Incidence of anorexia, headache, fever, suicidal ideation, and vomiting are higher in children.

Drug Interactions

Metabolism/Transport Effects None known.

Avoid Concomitant Use

Avoid concomitant use of Ribavirin with any of the following: Didanosine

Increased Effect/Toxicity

Ribavirin may increase the levels/effects of: AzaTHIOprine; Didanosine; Reverse Transcriptase Inhibitors (Nucleoside)

The levels/effects of Ribavirin may be increased by: Interferons (Alfa); Zidovudine

Decreased Effect

Ribavirin may decrease the levels/effects of: Influenza Virus Vaccine (Live/Attenuated)

Ethanol/Nutrition/Herb Interactions Food: Oral: High-fat meal increases the AUC and C$_{max}$. Management: Capsule (in combination with peginterferon alfa-2b) and tablet should be administered with food. Other dosage forms and combinations should be taken consistently in regards to food.

Stability

Inhalation: Store vials in a dry place at 15°C to 30°C (59°F to 86°F). Do not use any water containing an antimicrobial agent to reconstitute drug. Reconstituted solution is stable for 24 hours at room temperature. Should not be mixed with other aerosolized medication.

Oral: Store at controlled room temperature of 25°C (77°F). Solution may also be refrigerated at 2°C to 8°C (36°F to 46°F).

Mechanism of Action Inhibits replication of RNA and DNA viruses; inhibits influenza virus RNA polymerase activity and inhibits the initiation and elongation of RNA fragments resulting in inhibition of viral protein synthesis

Pharmacodynamics/Kinetics

Absorption: Inhalation: Systemic; dependent upon respiratory factors and method of drug delivery; maximal absorption occurs with the use of aerosol generator via endotracheal tube; highest concentrations in respiratory tract and erythrocytes

Distribution: Oral capsule: Single dose: V$_d$: 2825 L; distribution significantly prolonged in the erythrocyte (16-40 days), which can be used as a marker for intracellular metabolism

Protein binding: Oral: None

◄ Metabolism: Hepatically and intracellularly (forms active metabolites); may be necessary for drug action

Bioavailability: Oral: 64%

Half-life elimination, plasma:

Adults: Oral:

Capsule, single dose (Rebetol®, Ribasphere®): 24 hours in healthy adults, 44 hours with chronic hepatitis C infection (increases to ~298 hours at steady state)

Tablet, single dose (Copegus®): ~120-170 hours

Time to peak, serum: Inhalation: At end of inhalation period; Oral capsule: Multiple doses: 3 hours; Tablet: 2 hours

Excretion: Inhalation: Urine (40% as unchanged drug and metabolites); Oral capsule: Urine (61%), feces (12%)

Dosage

Geriatric & Adult

Chronic hepatitis C (in combination with peginterferon alfa-2a): Oral: Tablet (Copegus®):

Monoinfection, genotype 1,4:

<75 kg: 1000 mg/day, in 2 divided doses for 48 weeks

≥75 kg: 1200 mg/day, in 2 divided doses for 48 weeks

Monoinfection, genotype 2,3: 800 mg/day, in 2 divided doses for 24 weeks

Coinfection with HIV: 800 mg/day in 2 divided doses for 48 weeks (regardless of genotype)

Chronic hepatitis C (in combination with interferon alfa-2b): Oral: Capsule (Rebetol®, Ribasphere®):

≤75 kg: 400 mg in the morning, then 600 mg in the evening

>75 kg: 600 mg in the morning, then 600 mg in the evening

Chronic hepatitis C (in combination with peginterferon alfa-2b): Oral: Capsule (Rebetol®, Ribasphere®): 400 mg twice daily

Note: *American Association for the Study of Liver Diseases (AASLD) guidelines recommendation:* Adults with chronic HCV infection (Ghany, 2009): Treatment of choice: Ribavirin plus **peginterferon**; clinical condition and ability of patient to tolerate therapy should be evaluated to determine length and/or likely benefit of therapy. Recommended treatment duration (AASLD guidelines): Genotypes 1,4: 48 weeks; Genotypes 2,3: 24 weeks; Coinfection with HIV: 48 weeks.

RSV Infection in hematopoietic cell or heart/lung transplant recipients (unlabeled use): Aerosol inhalation: 2 g (over 2 hours) every 8 hours

Note: Heart/lung transplant recipients also received IVIG, methylprednisolone and palivizumab. Dosage and protocol may be institution specific. (Boeckh, 2007; Chemaly, 2006; Liu, 2010).

Renal Impairment Oral:

Rebetol® capsules/solution, Ribasphere® capsules:

Cl_{cr} ≥50 mL/minute: No dosage adjustments are recommended.

Cl_{cr} <50 mL/minute: Use is contraindicated.

Ribasphere® tablets:

Cl_{cr} ≥50 mL/minute: No dosage adjustments are recommended.

Cl_{cr} <50 mL/minute: Use is not recommended.

Copegus® tablets:

Cl_{cr} >50 mL/minute: No dosage adjustments are recommended.

Cl_{cr} 30-50 mL/minute: Alternate 200 mg and 400 mg every other day.

Cl_{cr} <30 mL/minute: 200 mg once daily.

ESRD requiring hemodialysis: 200 mg once daily.

Hepatic Impairment Hepatic decompensation (Child-Pugh class B or C): Use of ribavirin tablets is contraindicated.

Administration

Inhalation: Ribavirin should be administered in well-ventilated rooms (at least 6 air changes/hour). In mechanically-ventilated patients, ribavirin can potentially be deposited in the ventilator delivery system depending on temperature, humidity, and electrostatic forces; this deposition can lead to malfunction or obstruction of the expiratory valve, resulting in inadvertently high positive end-expiratory pressures. The use of one-way valves in the inspiratory lines, a breathing circuit filter in the expiratory line, and frequent monitoring and filter replacement have been effective in preventing these problems. Solutions in SPAG-2 unit should be discarded at least every 24 hours and when the liquid level is low before adding newly reconstituted solution. Should not be mixed with other aerosolized medication.

Oral: Administer concurrently with interferon alfa injection. Capsule should not be opened, crushed, chewed, or broken. Use oral solution for those who cannot swallow capsules.

Capsule, in combination with interferon alfa-2b: May be administered with or without food, but always in a consistent manner in regard to food intake.

Capsule, in combination with peginterferon alfa-2b: Administer with food.

Solution, in combination with interferon alfa-2b: May be administered with or without food, but always in a consistent manner in regard to food intake.

Tablet: Should be administered with food.

Monitoring Parameters

Inhalation: Respiratory function, hemoglobin, reticulocyte count, CBC with differential, I & O

Oral: Clinical studies tested as follows: CBC (including hemoglobin, WBC, and platelets) and chemistries (including liver function tests and uric acid) measured at weeks 1, 2, 4, 6, and 8, and then every 4 weeks; TSH measured every 12 weeks

Baseline values used in clinical trials:

Platelet count $\geq$90,000/mm^3 (75,000/mm^3 for cirrhosis or 70,000/mm^3 for coinfection with HIV)

ANC $\geq$1500/mm^3

Hemoglobin $\geq$12 g/dL for women and $\geq$13 g/dL for men (11 g/dL for HIV coinfected women and 12 g/dL for HIV coinfected men)

TSH and T_4 within normal limits or adequately controlled

CD4$^+$ cell count $\geq$200 cells/microL or CD4$^+$ cell count 100-200 cells/microL and HIV-1 RNA <5000 copies/mL for coinfection with HIV

Serum HCV RNA (pretreatment, week 12 and week 24, and 24 weeks after completion of therapy). **Note:** Discontinuation of therapy may be considered after 12 weeks in patients with HCV (genotypes 1,4) who fail to achieve an early virologic response (EVR) (defined as $\geq$2-log decrease in HCV RNA compared to pretreatment) or after 24 weeks with detectable HCV RNA. Treat patients with HCV (genotypes 2,3) for 24 weeks (if tolerated) and then evaluate HCV RNA levels (Ghany, 2009).

Pretreatment ECG in patients with pre-existing cardiac disease; dental exams; ophthalmic exam pretreatment (all patients) and periodically for those with pre-existing ophthalmologic disorders.

Reference Range

Rapid virological response (RVR): Absence of detectable HCV RNA after 4 weeks of treatment

Early viral response (EVR): $\geq$2-log decrease in HCV RNA after 12 weeks of treatment

End of treatment response (ETR): Absence of detectable HCV RNA at end of the recommended treatment period

Sustained treatment response (STR): Absence of HCV RNA in the serum 6 months following completion of full treatment course

Special Geriatric Considerations No specific recommendations are necessary in the elderly; however, in patients with creatinine clearance <50 mL/minute, the oral route not recommended; dosage adjustment or discontinuation may be necessary. Many elderly will fall into this category.

Dosage Forms Excipient information presented when available (limited, particularly for generics); consult specific product labeling.

Capsule, oral: 200 mg

Rebetol®: 200 mg

Ribasphere®: 200 mg

Powder for solution, for nebulization:

Virazole®: 6 g [reconstituted product contains ribavirin 20 mg/mL]

Solution, oral:

Rebetol®: 40 mg/mL (100 mL) [contains propylene glycol, sodium benzoate; bubblegum flavor]

Tablet, oral: 200 mg

Copegus®: 200 mg

Ribasphere®: 200 mg, 400 mg, 600 mg

Tablet, oral:

Ribasphere® RibaPak® 600: 200 mg AM dose (7s) [light blue tablets], 400 mg PM dose (7s) [medium blue tablets] (14s, 56s)

Ribasphere® RibaPak® 1000: 600 mg AM dose (7s) [dark blue], 400 mg PM dose (7s) [medium blue tablets] (14s, 56s)

◆ **Rid® [OTC]** see Permethrin on page 1512

◆ **Ridaura®** see Auranofin on page 170

Rifabutin (rif a BYOO tin)

Related Information
Antimicrobial Drugs of Choice *on page 2163*

Medication Safety Issues
Sound-alike/look-alike issues:
Rifabutin may be confused with rifampin

Brand Names: U.S. Mycobutin®
Brand Names: Canada Mycobutin®
Index Terms Ansamycin
Generic Availability (U.S.) No
Pharmacologic Category Antibiotic, Miscellaneous; Antitubercular Agent

Use Prevention of disseminated *Mycobacterium avium* complex (MAC) in patients with advanced HIV infection

Unlabeled Use Utilized in multidrug regimens for treatment of MAC; alternative to rifampin as prophylaxis for latent tuberculosis infection (LTBI) or part of multidrug regimen for treatment active tuberculosis infection

Contraindications Hypersensitivity to rifabutin, any other rifamycins, or any component of the formulation

Warnings/Precautions Rifabutin must not be administered for MAC prophylaxis to patients with active tuberculosis since its use may lead to the development of tuberculosis that is resistant to both rifabutin and rifampin. May be associated with neutropenia and/or thrombocytopenia (rarely). Dosage reduction recommended in severe impairment (Cl$_{cr}$ <30 mL/minute). Prolonged use may result in fungal or bacterial superinfection, including *C. difficile*-associated diarrhea (CDAD) and pseudomembranous colitis; CDAD has been observed >2 months postantibiotic treatment. May cause brown/orange discoloration of urine, feces, saliva, sweat, tears, and skin. Remove soft contact lenses during therapy since permanent staining may occur.

Adverse Reactions (Reflective of adult population; not specific for elderly)
>10%:
Dermatologic: Rash (11%)
Genitourinary: Discoloration of urine (30%)
Hematologic: Neutropenia (25%), leukopenia (17%)
1% to 10%:
Central nervous system: Headache (3%), fever (2%)
Gastrointestinal: Nausea (3% to 6%), abdominal pain (4%), dyspepsia (3%), eructation (3%), taste perversion (3%), vomiting (3%), flatulence (2%)
Hematologic: Thrombocytopenia (5%)
Hepatic: ALT increased (7% to 9%; incidence less than placebo), AST increased (7% to 9%; incidence less than placebo)
Neuromuscular & skeletal: Myalgia (2%)

Drug Interactions
Metabolism/Transport Effects Substrate of CYP1A2 (minor), CYP3A4 (major); **Note:** Assignment of Major/Minor substrate status based on clinically relevant drug interaction potential; **Induces** CYP3A4 (strong)

Avoid Concomitant Use
Avoid concomitant use of Rifabutin with any of the following: Axitinib; BCG; Boceprevir; Bortezomib; Crizotinib; Dronedarone; Everolimus; Lapatinib; Lurasidone; Mifepristone; Mycophenolate; Nilotinib; Pazopanib; Praziquantel; Ranolazine; Rilpivirine; Rivaroxaban; Roflumilast; RomiDEPsin; SORAfenib; Telaprevir; Ticagrelor; Tolvaptan; Toremifene; Vandetanib; Voriconazole

Increased Effect/Toxicity
Rifabutin may increase the levels/effects of: Clopidogrel; Darunavir; Fosamprenavir; Ifosfamide; Isoniazid; Lopinavir; Pitavastatin

The levels/effects of Rifabutin may be increased by: Antifungal Agents (Azole Derivatives, Systemic); Atazanavir; Boceprevir; Darunavir; Delavirdine; Fluconazole; Fosamprenavir; Indinavir; Lopinavir; Macrolide Antibiotics; Nelfinavir; Nevirapine; Ritonavir; Saquinavir; Telaprevir; Tipranavir; Voriconazole

Decreased Effect
Rifabutin may decrease the levels/effects of: Alfentanil; Amiodarone; Angiotensin II Receptor Blockers; Antiemetics (5HT3 Antagonists); Antifungal Agents (Azole Derivatives, Systemic); Apixaban; Aprepitant; ARIPiprazole; Atovaquone; Axitinib; Barbiturates; BCG; Benzodiazepines (metabolized by oxidation); Boceprevir; Bortezomib; Brentuximab Vedotin; BusPIRone; Calcium Channel Blockers; Contraceptives (Estrogens); Contraceptives (Progestins); Corticosteroids (Systemic); Crizotinib; CycloSPORINE; CycloSPORINE (Systemic);

CYP3A4 Substrates; Dapsone; Dapsone (Systemic); Dasatinib; Delavirdine; Disopyramide; Dronedarone; Efavirenz; Etravirine; Everolimus; Exemestane; FentaNYL; Fluconazole; Fosphenytoin; Gefitinib; GuanFACINE; HMG-CoA Reductase Inhibitors; Imatinib; Indinavir; Ixabepilone; Lapatinib; Linagliptin; Lurasidone; Maraviroc; Mifepristone; Morphine (Systemic); Morphine Sulfate; Mycophenolate; Nelfinavir; Nevirapine; Nilotinib; Pazopanib; Phenytoin; Praziquantel; Propafenone; QuiNIDine; Ramelteon; Ranolazine; Repaglinide; Rilpivirine; Rivaroxaban; Roflumilast; RomiDEPsin; Saxagliptin; SORAfenib; SUNItinib; Tacrolimus; Tacrolimus (Systemic); Tadalafil; Tamoxifen; Telaprevir; Temsirolimus; Terbinafine (Systemic); Ticagrelor; Tolvaptan; Toremifene; Typhoid Vaccine; Ulipristal; Vandetanib; Vemurafenib; Vitamin K Antagonists; Voriconazole; Zaleplon; Zolpidem; Zuclopenthixol

The levels/effects of Rifabutin may be decreased by: CYP3A4 Inducers (Strong); Deferasirox; Efavirenz; Herbs (CYP3A4 Inducers); Nevirapine; Tocilizumab

Ethanol/Nutrition/Herb Interactions Food: High-fat meal may decrease the rate but not the extent of absorption.

Stability Store at 25°C (77°F); excursions permitted to 15°C to 30°C (59°F to 86°F).

Mechanism of Action Inhibits DNA-dependent RNA polymerase at the beta subunit which prevents chain initiation

Pharmacodynamics/Kinetics
Absorption: Readily, 53%
Distribution: V_d: 9.32 L/kg; distributes to body tissues including the lungs, liver, spleen, eyes, and kidneys
Protein binding: 85%
Metabolism: To 5 metabolites; predominantly 25-O-desacetyl-rifabutin (antimicrobial activity equivalent to parent drug; serum AUC 10% of parent drug) and 31-hydroxy-rifabutin (serum AUC 7% of parent drug)
Bioavailability: Absolute: HIV: 20%
Half-life elimination: Terminal: 45 hours (range: 16-69 hours)
Time to peak, serum: 2-4 hours
Excretion: Urine (53% as metabolites); feces (30%)

Dosage
Geriatric & Adult
Disseminated MAC in advanced HIV infection: Oral:
Prophylaxis: 300 mg once daily or 150 mg twice daily to reduce gastrointestinal upset
Treatment (unlabeled use; AIDSinfo guidelines): 300 mg once daily as an optional add-on to primary therapy of clarithromycin and ethambutol
Tuberculosis (unlabeled use as alternative to rifampin; AIDS *info* guidelines): Oral:
Prophylaxis of LTBI: 300 mg once daily for 4 months
Treatment of active TB: 300 mg once daily or intermittently 2-3 times weekly as part of multidrug regimen

Dosage adjustment for concurrent nelfinavir, amprenavir, indinavir: Reduce rifabutin dose to 150 mg/day; no change in dose if administered twice weekly
Dosage adjustment for concurrent efavirenz (no concomitant protease inhibitor): Increase rifabutin dose to 450-600 mg daily, or 600 mg 3 times/week
Renal Impairment Cl_{cr} <30 mL/minute: Reduce dose by 50%
Administration May be mixed with food (ie, applesauce)
Monitoring Parameters Periodic liver function tests, CBC with differential, platelet count
Special Geriatric Considerations No specific recommendations for the elderly.
Dosage Forms Excipient information presented when available (limited, particularly for generics); consult specific product labeling.
Capsule, oral:
Mycobutin®: 150 mg

◆ **Rifadin®** *see* Rifampin *on page 1697*
◆ **Rifampicin** *see* Rifampin *on page 1697*

Rifampin (rif AM pin)

Related Information
Antibiotic Treatment of Adults With Infective Endocarditis *on page 2157*
Antimicrobial Drugs of Choice *on page 2163*
Medication Safety Issues
Sound-alike/look-alike issues:
Rifadin® may be confused with Rifater®, Ritalin®
Rifampin may be confused with ribavirin, rifabutin, Rifamate®, rifapentine, rifaximin
Brand Names: U.S. Rifadin®
Brand Names: Canada Rifadin®; Rofact™

◀ **Index Terms** Rifampicin

Generic Availability (U.S.) Yes

Pharmacologic Category Antibiotic, Miscellaneous; Antitubercular Agent

Use Management of active tuberculosis in combination with other agents; elimination of meningococci from the nasopharynx in asymptomatic carriers

Unlabeled Use Prophylaxis of *Haemophilus influenzae* type b infection; *Legionella* pneumonia; used in combination with other anti-infectives in the treatment of staphylococcal infections; treatment of *M. leprae* infections

Contraindications Hypersensitivity to rifampin, any rifamycins, or any component of the formulation; concurrent use of amprenavir, saquinavir/ritonavir (possibly other protease inhibitors)

Warnings/Precautions Use with caution and modify dosage in patients with liver impairment; observe for hyperbilirubinemia; discontinue therapy if this in conjunction with clinical symptoms or any signs of significant hepatocellular damage develop. Use with caution in patients receiving concurrent medications associated with hepatotoxicity. Use with caution in patients with a history of alcoholism (even if ethanol consumption is discontinued during therapy). Since rifampin since rifampin has enzyme-inducing properties, porphyria exacerbation is possible; use with caution in patients with porphyria; do not use for meningococcal disease, only for short-term treatment of asymptomatic carrier states

Regimens of >600 mg once or twice weekly have been associated with a high incidence of adverse reactions including a flu-like syndrome, hypersensitivity, thrombocytopenia, leukopenia, and anemia. Urine, feces, saliva, sweat, tears, and CSF may be discolored to red/orange; remove soft contact lenses during therapy since permanent staining may occur. Do not administer I.V. form via I.M. or SubQ routes; restart infusion at another site if extravasation occurs. Prolonged use may result in fungal or bacterial superinfection, including *C. difficile*-associated diarrhea (CDAD) and pseudomembranous colitis; CDAD has been observed >2 months postantibiotic treatment. Monitor for compliance in patients on intermittent therapy.

Adverse Reactions (Reflective of adult population; not specific for elderly)

1% to 10%:
  Dermatologic: Rash (1% to 5%)
  Gastrointestinal (1% to 2%): Anorexia, cramps, diarrhea, epigastric distress, flatulence, heartburn, nausea, pseudomembranous colitis, pancreatitis, vomiting
  Hepatic: LFTs increased (up to 14%)
Frequency not defined:
  Cardiovascular: Edema, flushing
  Central nervous system: Ataxia, behavioral changes, concentration impaired, confusion, dizziness, drowsiness, fatigue, fever, headache, numbness, psychosis
  Dermatologic: Pemphigoid reaction, pruritus, urticaria
  Endocrine & metabolic: Adrenal insufficiency, menstrual disorders
  Hematologic: Agranulocytosis (rare), DIC, eosinophilia, hemoglobin decreased, hemolysis, hemolytic anemia, leukopenia, thrombocytopenia (especially with high-dose therapy)
  Hepatic: Hepatitis (rare), jaundice
  Neuromuscular & skeletal: Myalgia, osteomalacia, weakness
  Ocular: Exudative conjunctivitis, visual changes
  Renal: Acute renal failure, BUN increased, hemoglobinuria, hematuria, interstitial nephritis, uric acid increased
  Miscellaneous: Flu-like syndrome

Drug Interactions

Metabolism/Transport Effects Substrate of P-glycoprotein, SLCO1B1; **Induces** CYP1A2 (strong), CYP2A6 (strong), CYP2B6 (strong), CYP2C19 (strong), CYP2C8 (strong), CYP2C9 (strong), CYP3A4 (strong), P-glycoprotein

Avoid Concomitant Use

Avoid concomitant use of Rifampin with any of the following: Atazanavir; Axitinib; BCG; Boceprevir; Bortezomib; Crizotinib; Dabigatran Etexilate; Darunavir; Dronedarone; Esomeprazole; Etravirine; Everolimus; Fosamprenavir; Indinavir; Lapatinib; Lopinavir; Lurasidone; Mifepristone; Mycophenolate; Nelfinavir; Nilotinib; Omeprazole; Pazopanib; Praziquantel; QuiNINE; Ranolazine; Rilpivirine; Ritonavir; Rivaroxaban; Roflumilast; RomiDEPsin; Saquinavir; SORAfenib; Telaprevir; Ticagrelor; Tipranavir; Tolvaptan; Toremifene; Vandetanib; Voriconazole

Increased Effect/Toxicity

Rifampin may increase the levels/effects of: Bosentan; Clopidogrel; Ifosfamide; Isoniazid; Leflunomide; Lopinavir; Pitavastatin; Saquinavir

The levels/effects of Rifampin may be increased by: Antifungal Agents (Azole Derivatives, Systemic); Delavirdine; Eltrombopag; Fluconazole; Macrolide Antibiotics; P-glycoprotein/ABCB1 Inhibitors; Pyrazinamide; Voriconazole

Decreased Effect

Rifampin may decrease the levels/effects of: Alfentanil; Amiodarone; Angiotensin II Receptor Blockers; Antidiabetic Agents (Thiazolidinedione); Antiemetics (5HT3 Antagonists); Antifungal Agents (Azole Derivatives, Systemic); Apixaban; Aprepitant; ARIPiprazole; Atazanavir; Atovaquone; Axitinib; Barbiturates; BCG; Bendamustine; Benzodiazepines (metabolized by oxidation); Beta-Blockers; Boceprevir; Bortezomib; Bosentan; Brentuximab Vedotin; BusPIRone; Calcium Channel Blockers; Caspofungin; Chloramphenicol; Contraceptives (Estrogens); Contraceptives (Progestins); Corticosteroids (Systemic); Crizotinib; Cyclo-SPORINE; CycloSPORINE (Systemic); CYP1A2 Substrates; CYP2B6 Substrates; CYP2C19 Substrates; CYP2C8 Substrates; CYP2C9 Substrates; CYP3A4 Substrates; Dabigatran Etexilate; Dapsone; Dapsone (Systemic); Darunavir; Dasatinib; Deferasirox; Delavirdine; Diclofenac; Disopyramide; Divalproex; Dronedarone; Efavirenz; Erlotinib; Esomeprazole; Etravirine; Everolimus; Exemestane; FentaNYL; Fexofenadine; Fluconazole; Fosamprenavir; Fosaprepitant; Fosphenytoin; Gefitinib; GuanFACINE; HMG-CoA Reductase Inhibitors; Imatinib; Indinavir; Ixabepilone; LamoTRIgine; Lapatinib; Linagliptin; Lopinavir; Lurasidone; Maraviroc; Methadone; Mifepristone; Morphine (Systemic); Morphine Sulfate; Mycophenolate; Nelfinavir; Nevirapine; Nilotinib; Omeprazole; OxyCODONE; Pazopanib; P-glycoprotein/ABCB1 Substrates; Phenytoin; Prasugrel; Praziquantel; Propafenone; QuiNIDine; QuiNINE; Raltegravir; Ramelteon; Ranolazine; Repaglinide; Rilpivirine; Ritonavir; Rivaroxaban; Roflumilast; RomiDEPsin; Saquinavir; Saxagliptin; Sirolimus; SORAfenib; Sulfonylureas; SUNItinib; Tacrolimus; Tacrolimus (Systemic); Tadalafil; Tamoxifen; Telaprevir; Temsirolimus; Terbinafine; Terbinafine (Systemic); Thyroid Products; Ticagrelor; Tipranavir; Tolvaptan; Toremifene; Treprostinil; Typhoid Vaccine; Ulipristal; Valproic Acid; Vandetanib; Vemurafenib; Vitamin K Antagonists; Voriconazole; Zaleplon; Zidovudine; Zolpidem; Zuclopenthixol

The levels/effects of Rifampin may be decreased by: P-glycoprotein/ABCB1 Inducers

Ethanol/Nutrition/Herb Interactions

Ethanol: Avoid ethanol (may increase risk of hepatotoxicity).

Food: Food decreases the extent of absorption; rifampin concentrations may be decreased if taken with food.

Herb/Nutraceutical: St John's wort may decrease rifampin levels.

Stability Rifampin powder is reddish brown. Intact vials should be stored at room temperature and protected from excessive heat and light. Reconstitute powder for injection with SWFI. Prior to injection, dilute in appropriate volume of compatible diluent (eg, 100 mL D_5W). Reconstituted vials are stable for 24 hours at room temperature.

Stability of parenteral admixture at room temperature (25°C) is 4 hours for D_5W and 24 hours for NS.

Mechanism of Action Inhibits bacterial RNA synthesis by binding to the beta subunit of DNA-dependent RNA polymerase, blocking RNA transcription

Pharmacodynamics/Kinetics

Duration: ≤24 hours

Absorption: Oral: Well absorbed; food may delay or slightly reduce peak

Distribution: Highly lipophilic; crosses blood-brain barrier well

Relative diffusion from blood into CSF: Adequate with or without inflammation (exceeds usual MICs)

CSF:blood level ratio: Inflamed meninges: 25%

Protein binding: 80%

Metabolism: Hepatic; undergoes enterohepatic recirculation

Half-life elimination: 3-4 hours; prolonged with hepatic impairment; End-stage renal disease: 1.8-11 hours

Time to peak, serum: Oral: 2-4 hours

Excretion: Feces (60% to 65%) and urine (~30%) as unchanged drug

Dosage

Geriatric & Adult

Tuberculosis, active: Oral, I.V.: **Note:** A four-drug regimen (isoniazid, rifampin, pyrazinamide, and ethambutol) is preferred for the initial, empiric treatment of TB. When the drug susceptibility results are available, the regimen should be altered as appropriate.

Daily therapy: 10 mg/kg/day (maximum: 600 mg/day)

Directly observed therapy (DOT): 10 mg/kg (maximum: 600 mg) administered 2 or 3 times/week (*MMWR*, 2003)

Tuberculosis, latent infection (LTBI): As an alternative to isoniazid: Oral, I.V.: 10 mg/kg/day (maximum: 600 mg/day) for 4 months. **Note:** Combination with pyrazinamide should not generally be offered (*MMWR*, Aug 8, 2003).

Endocarditis, prosthetic valve due to MRSA (unlabeled use): Oral, I.V.: 300 mg every 8 hours for at least 6 weeks (combine with vancomycin for the entire duration of therapy and gentamicin for the first 2 weeks) (Liu, 2011)

◄ *H. influenzae* prophylaxis (unlabeled use): Oral, I.V.: 600 mg every 24 hours for 4 days

Leprosy (unlabeled use): Oral, I.V.:

Multibacillary: 600 mg once monthly for 24 months in combination with ofloxacin and minocycline

Paucibacillary: 600 mg once monthly for 6 months in combination with dapsone

Single lesion: 600 mg as a single dose in combination with ofloxacin 400 mg and minocycline 100 mg

Meningococcal meningitis prophylaxis (unlabeled use): Oral, I.V.: 600 mg every 12 hours for 2 days

Meningitis *(Pneumococcus* or *Staphylococcus)* (unlabeled use): Oral, I.V.: 600 mg once daily

Nasal carriers of *Staphylococcus aureus* (unlabeled use): Oral, I.V.: 600 mg/day for 5-10 days; **Note: Must use in combination with at least one other systemic antistaphylococcal antibiotic.** Not recommended as first-line drug for decolonization; evidence is weak for use in patients with recurrent infections (Liu, 2011).

Nontuberculous mycobacterium *(M. kansasii)* (unlabeled use): Oral, I.V.: 10 mg/kg/day (maximum: 600 mg/day) for duration to include 12 months of culture-negative sputum; typically used in combination with ethambutol and isoniazid

***Staphylococcus aureus* infections, adjunctive therapy (unlabeled use):** Oral, I.V.: 600 mg once daily or 300-450 mg every 12 hours with other antibiotics. **Note:** Must be used in combination with another antistaphylococcal antibiotic to avoid rapid development of resistance (Liu, 2011).

Renal Impairment No dosage adjustment required in renal impairment.

Poorly dialyzed; no supplemental dose or dosage adjustment necessary, including patients on intermittent hemodialysis, peritoneal dialysis, or continuous renal replacement therapy (eg, CVVHD).

Hepatic Impairment Dose reductions are necessary to reduce hepatotoxicity.

Administration

I.V.: Administer I.V. preparation by slow I.V. infusion over 30 minutes to 3 hours at a final concentration not to exceed 6 mg/mL.

Oral: Administer on an empty stomach (ie, 1 hour prior to, or 2 hours after meals or antacids) to increase total absorption. The compounded oral suspension must be shaken well before using. May mix contents of capsule with applesauce or jelly.

Monitoring Parameters Periodic (baseline and every 2-4 weeks during therapy) monitoring of liver function (AST, ALT, bilirubin), CBC, mental status, sputum culture, chest x-ray 2-3 months into treatment

Test Interactions May interfere with urine detection of opiates (false-positive); positive Coombs' reaction [direct], rifampin inhibits standard assay's ability to measure serum folate and B_{12}; transient increase in LFTs and decreased biliary excretion of contrast media

Special Geriatric Considerations Since most older patients acquired their *Mycobacterium tuberculosis* infection before effective chemotherapy was available, either a 9-month regimen of isoniazid and rifampin or a 6-month regimen of isoniazid and rifampin with pyrazinamide (the first 2 months) should be effective.

Dosage Forms Excipient information presented when available (limited, particularly for generics); consult specific product labeling.

Capsule, oral: 150 mg, 300 mg
Rifadin®: 150 mg, 300 mg
Injection, powder for reconstitution: 600 mg
Rifadin®: 600 mg

Rifapentine (rif a PEN teen)

Medication Safety Issues
Sound-alike/look-alike issues:
Rifapentine may be confused with rifampin

Brand Names: U.S. Priftin®

Brand Names: Canada Priftin®

Generic Availability (U.S.) No

Pharmacologic Category Antitubercular Agent

Use Treatment of pulmonary tuberculosis; rifapentine must always be used in conjunction with at least one other antituberculosis drug to which the isolate is susceptible; it may also be necessary to add a third agent (either streptomycin or ethambutol) until susceptibility is known.

Contraindications Hypersensitivity to rifapentine, rifampin, rifabutin, any rifamycin analog, or any component of the formulation

Warnings/Precautions Patients with abnormal liver tests and/or liver disease should only be given rifapentine when absolutely necessary and under strict medical supervision. Monitoring of liver function tests should be carried out prior to therapy and then every 2-4 weeks during therapy if signs of liver disease occur or worsen, rifapentine should be discontinued. All patients treated with rifapentine should have baseline measurements of liver function tests and enzymes, bilirubin, and a complete blood count. Patients should be seen monthly and specifically questioned regarding symptoms associated with adverse reactions. Routine laboratory monitoring in people with normal baseline measurements is generally not necessary. Use with caution in patients with porphyria; exacerbation is possible.

Rifapentine may produce a red-orange discoloration of body tissues/fluids including skin, teeth, tongue, urine, feces, saliva, sputum, tears, sweat, and cerebral spinal fluid. Contact lenses may become permanently stained. Prolonged use may result in fungal or bacterial superinfection, including *C. difficile*-associated diarrhea (CDAD) and pseudomembranous colitis; CDAD has been observed >2 months postantibiotic treatment. Experience in treating TB in HIV-infected patients is limited. Compliance with dosing regimen is absolutely necessary for successful drug therapy.

Adverse Reactions (Reflective of adult population; not specific for elderly)
>10%: Endocrine & metabolic: Hyperuricemia (most likely due to pyrazinamide from initiation phase combination therapy)

1% to 10%:
  Cardiovascular: Hypertension
  Central nervous system: Headache, dizziness
  Dermatologic: Rash, pruritus, acne
  Gastrointestinal: Anorexia, nausea, vomiting, dyspepsia, diarrhea
  Hematologic: Neutropenia, lymphopenia, anemia, leukopenia, thrombocytosis
  Hepatic: ALT increased, AST increased
  Neuromuscular & skeletal: Arthralgia, pain
  Renal: Pyuria, proteinuria, hematuria, urinary casts
  Respiratory: Hemoptysis

Drug Interactions
Metabolism/Transport Effects Induces CYP2C8 (strong), CYP2C9 (strong), CYP3A4 (strong)

Avoid Concomitant Use
Avoid concomitant use of Rifapentine with any of the following: Axitinib; Bortezomib; Crizotinib; Dronedarone; Etravirine; Everolimus; Lapatinib; Lurasidone; Mifepristone; Mycophenolate); Nilotinib; Pazopanib; Praziquantel; Ranolazine; Rilpivirine; Rivaroxaban; Roflumilast; RomiDEPsin; SORAfenib; Ticagrelor; Tolvaptan; Toremifene; Vandetanib; Voriconazole

Increased Effect/Toxicity
Rifapentine may increase the levels/effects of: Clarithromycin; Clopidogrel; Ifosfamide; Isoniazid; Pitavastatin

The levels/effects of Rifapentine may be increased by: Antifungal Agents (Azole Derivatives, Systemic); Clarithromycin; Delavirdine; Fluconazole; Voriconazole

Decreased Effect
Rifapentine may decrease the levels/effects of: Alfentanil; Amiodarone; Angiotensin II Receptor Blockers; Antiemetics (5HT3 Antagonists); Antifungal Agents (Azole Derivatives, Systemic); Apixaban; Aprepitant; ARIPiprazole; Atovaquone; Axitinib; Barbiturates; Benzodiazepines (metabolized by oxidation); Beta-Blockers; Boceprevir; Bortezomib; Brentuximab Vedotin; BusPIRone; Calcium Channel Blockers; Clarithromycin; Contraceptives (Estrogens); Contraceptives (Progestins); Corticosteroids (Systemic); Crizotinib; CycloSPORINE; CycloSPORINE (Systemic); CYP2C8 Substrates; CYP2C9 Substrates; CYP3A4 Substrates; Dapsone; Dapsone (Systemic); Dasatinib; Delavirdine; Diclofenac; Disopyramide; Dronedarone; Etravirine; Everolimus; Exemestane; FentaNYL; Fluconazole; Fosphenytoin; Gefitinib; GuanFACINE; HMG-CoA Reductase Inhibitors; Imatinib; Ixabepilone; Lapatinib; Linagliptin; Lurasidone; Maraviroc; Methadone; Mifepristone; Morphine (Systemic); Morphine Sulfate; Mycophenolate; Nilotinib; Pazopanib; Phenytoin; Praziquantel; Propafenone; QuiNIDine; Ramelteon; Ranolazine; Repaglinide; Rilpivirine; Rivaroxaban; Roflumilast; RomiDEPsin; Saxagliptin; SORAfenib; SUNItinib; Tacrolimus; Tacrolimus (Systemic); Tadalafil; Tamoxifen; Temsirolimus; Terbinafine (Systemic); Ticagrelor; Tolvaptan; Toremifene; Treprostinil; Ulipristal; Vandetanib; Vemurafenib; Vitamin K Antagonists; Voriconazole; Zaleplon; Zidovudine; Zolpidem; Zuclopenthixol

Ethanol/Nutrition/Herb Interactions Food: Food increases AUC and maximum serum concentration by 43% and 44% respectively as compared to fasting conditions.

Stability Store at room temperature (15°C to 30°C; 59°F to 86°F). Protect from excessive heat and humidity.

Mechanism of Action Inhibits DNA-dependent RNA polymerase in susceptible strains of *Mycobacterium tuberculosis* (but not in mammalian cells). Rifapentine is bactericidal against both intracellular and extracellular MTB organisms. MTB resistant to other rifamycins including rifampin are likely to be resistant to rifapentine. Cross-resistance does not appear between rifapentine and other nonrifamycin antimycobacterial agents.

Pharmacodynamics/Kinetics

Absorption: Food increases AUC and C_{max} by 43% and 44% respectively.

Distribution: V_d: ~70.2 L; rifapentine and metabolite accumulate in human monocyte-derived macrophages with intracellular/extracellular ratios of 24:1 and 7:1 respectively

Protein binding: Rifapentine and 25-desacetyl metabolite: 97.7% and 93.2%, primarily to albumin

Metabolism: Hepatic; hydrolyzed by an esterase and esterase enzyme to form the active metabolite 25-desacetyl rifapentine

Bioavailability: ~70%

Half-life elimination: Rifapentine: 14-17 hours; 25-desacetyl rifapentine: 13 hours

Time to peak, serum: 5-6 hours

Excretion: Urine (17% primarily as metabolites)

Dosage

Geriatric & Adult Note: Rifapentine should not be used alone; initial phase should include a 3- to 4-drug regimen.

Tuberculosis, intensive phase (initial 2 months) of short-term therapy: 600 mg (four 150 mg tablets) given twice weekly (with an interval of not less than 72 hours between doses); following the intensive phase, treatment should continue with rifapentine 600 mg once weekly for 4 months in combination with INH or appropriate agent for susceptible organisms.

Monitoring Parameters Patients with pre-existing hepatic problems should have liver function tests monitored every 2-4 weeks during therapy

Test Interactions Rifampin has been shown to inhibit standard microbiological assays for serum folate and vitamin B_{12}; this should be considered for rifapentine; therefore, alternative assay methods should be considered.

Pharmacotherapy Pearls Rifapentine has only been studied in patients with tuberculosis receiving a 6-month short-course intensive regimen approval; outcomes have been based on 6-month follow-up treatment observed in clinical trial 008 as a surrogate for the 2-year follow-up generally accepted as evidence for efficacy in the treatment of pulmonary tuberculosis

Special Geriatric Considerations

A single dose pharmacokinetic comparison study of men ages 65-82 years found a modest decrease in oral clearance and a modest increase maximum concentration; neither which were considered great enough to warrant a dose adjustment (Keung, 1998).

Dosage Forms Excipient information presented when available (limited, particularly for generics); consult specific product labeling.

Tablet, oral:

Priftin® 150 mg

Rifaximin (rif AX i min)

Medication Safety Issues

Sound-alike/look-alike issues:

Rifaximin may be confused with rifampin

Brand Names: U.S. Xifaxan®

Generic Availability (U.S.) No

Pharmacologic Category Antibiotic, Miscellaneous

Use Treatment of travelers' diarrhea caused by noninvasive strains of *E. coli*; reduction in the risk of overt hepatic encephalopathy (HE) recurrence

Unlabeled Use Treatment of hepatic encephalopathy; alternative treatment for *Clostridium difficile*-associated diarrhea (CDAD)

Dosage

Geriatric & Adult

Hepatic encephalopathy: Oral:

Reduction of overt hepatic encephalopathy recurrence: 550 mg 2 times/day. **Note:** Supporting clinical trial evaluated efficacy over 6-month treatment period.

Treatment of hepatic encephalopathy (unlabeled use): 400 mg every 8 hours for 5-10 days (Mas, 2003)

Travelers' diarrhea: Oral: 200 mg 3 times/day for 3 days

***Clostridium difficile*-associated diarrhea (unlabeled use):** Oral: 200-400 mg 2-3 times/day for 14 days (Johnson, 2007)

Renal Impairment Not studied; no dosing recommendation available.

Hepatic Impairment No adjustment necessary, but use with caution in severe impairment (Child-Pugh class C) as systemic absorption does occur and pharmacokinetic parameters are highly variable.

Special Geriatric Considerations In one clinical trial, ~20% of subjects assigned to rifaximin (n=27) or placebo (n=31) were ≥65 years. The risk of a breakthrough episode of hepatic encephalopathy over 6 months was reduced with rifaximin, similar to younger subjects. Adverse drug events were not stratified by age.

Dosage Forms Excipient information presented when available (limited, particularly for generics); consult specific product labeling.

Tablet, oral:

Xifaxan®: 200 mg, 550 mg

♦ **rIFN beta-1b** see Interferon Beta-1b on page 1032
♦ **RIG** see Rabies Immune Globulin (Human) on page 1662
♦ **Rilutek®** see Riluzole on page 1703

Riluzole (RIL yoo zole)

Brand Names: U.S. Rilutek®
Brand Names: Canada Rilutek®
Index Terms 2-Amino-6-Trifluoromethoxy-benzothiazole; RP-54274
Generic Availability (U.S.) No
Pharmacologic Category Glutamate Inhibitor
Use Treatment of amyotrophic lateral sclerosis (ALS); riluzole can extend survival or time to tracheostomy
Contraindications Severe hypersensitivity reactions to riluzole or any component of the formulation
Warnings/Precautions Among 4000 patients given riluzole for ALS, there were 3 cases of marked neutropenia (ANC <500/mm^3), all seen within the first 2 months of treatment. Interstitial lung disease (primarily hypersensitivity pneumonitis) has occurred, requires prompt evaluation and possible discontinuation. Use with caution in patients with concomitant renal insufficiency. Use with caution in patients with current evidence or history of abnormal liver function; do not administer if baseline liver function tests are elevated. May cause elevations in transaminases (usually transient). May cause elevations in transaminases (usually transient) within first 3 months of therapy; discontinue if ALT levels are ≥5 times upper limit of normal or if jaundice develops. The elderly or female patients may have decreased clearance of riluzole; use with caution. May cause dizziness or somnolence; caution should be used performing tasks which require alertness (operating machinery or driving).

Adverse Reactions (Reflective of adult population; not specific for elderly)
>10%:
Gastrointestinal: Nausea (16%)
Neuromuscular & skeletal: Weakness (19%)
1% to 10%:
Cardiovascular: Hypertension (5%), peripheral edema (3%), tachycardia (3%)
Central nervous system: Dizziness (4%), somnolence (2%), vertigo (2%), malaise (1%)
Dermatologic: Pruritus (4%), eczema (2%), exfoliative dermatitis (1%)
Gastrointestinal: Abdominal pain (5%), vomiting (4%), flatulence (3%), oral moniliasis (1%), stomatitis (1%), tooth caries (1%)
Genitourinary: Urinary tract infection (3%), dysuria (1%)
Hepatic: Liver function tests increased (8% >3 x ULN; 2% >5 x ULN)
Neuromuscular & skeletal: Arthralgia (4%), paresthesia (circumoral; 2%), tremor (1%)
Respiratory: Lung function decreased (10%), cough increased (3%)

Drug Interactions
Metabolism/Transport Effects Substrate of CYP1A2 (major); **Note:** Assignment of Major/Minor substrate status based on clinically relevant drug interaction potential
Avoid Concomitant Use There are no known interactions where it is recommended to avoid concomitant use.
Increased Effect/Toxicity There are no known significant interactions involving an increase in effect.
Decreased Effect
The levels/effects of Riluzole may be decreased by: CYP1A2 Inducers (Strong); Cyproterone

Ethanol/Nutrition/Herb Interactions
Ethanol: Avoid ethanol (due to CNS depression and possible risk of liver toxicity).
Food: A high-fat meal decreases absorption of riluzole (decreasing AUC by 20% and peak blood levels by 45%). Charbroiled food may increase riluzole elimination.
Stability Store at 20°C to 25°C (68°F to 77°F). Protect from bright light.

Mechanism of Action Mechanism of action is not known. Pharmacologic properties include inhibitory effect on glutamate release, inactivation of voltage-dependent sodium channels; and ability to interfere with intracellular events that follow transmitter binding at excitatory amino acid receptors

Pharmacodynamics/Kinetics

Absorption: ~90%; high-fat meal decreases AUC by 20% and peak blood levels by 45%

Protein binding, plasma: 96%, primarily to albumin and lipoproteins

Metabolism: Extensively hepatic to six major and a number of minor metabolites via CYP1A2 dependent hydroxylation and glucuronidation

Bioavailability: Oral: Absolute: ~60%

Half-life elimination: 12 hours

Excretion: Urine (90%; 85% as metabolites, 2% as unchanged drug) and feces (5%) within 7 days

Dosage

Geriatric & Adult

ALS treatment: Oral: 50 mg every 12 hours; no increased benefit can be expected from higher daily doses, but adverse events are increased.

Dosage adjustment in smoking: Cigarette smoking is known to induce CYP1A2; patients who smoke cigarettes would be expected to eliminate riluzole faster. There is no information, however, on the effect of, or need for, dosage adjustment in these patients.

Renal Impairment No specific dosage adjustments recommended by manufacturer; use caution.

Hepatic Impairment No specific dosage adjustments recommended by manufacturer; use caution.

Administration Administer at the same time each day, 1 hour before or 2 hours after a meal.

Monitoring Parameters Monitor serum aminotransferases including ALT levels before and during therapy. Evaluate serum ALT levels every month during the first 3 months of therapy, every 3 months during the remainder of the first year and periodically thereafter. Evaluate ALT levels more frequently in patients who develop elevations. Maximum increases in serum ALT usually occurred within 3 months after the start of therapy and were usually transient when <5 times ULN (upper limits of normal). Discontinue therapy if ALT levels are ≥5 times upper limit of normal or if jaundice develops.

In trials, if ALT levels were <5 times ULN, treatment continued and ALT levels usually returned to below 2 times ULN within 2-6 months. There is no experience with continued treatment of ALS patients once ALT values exceed 5 times ULN.

Special Geriatric Considerations In clinical trials, no difference was demonstrated between elderly and younger adults. However, renal and hepatic changes with age can be expected to result in higher serum concentrations of the parent drug and its metabolites.

Dosage Forms Excipient information presented when available (limited, particularly for generics); consult specific product labeling.

Tablet, oral:

Rilutek®: 50 mg

RimabotulinumtoxinB (rime uh BOT yoo lin num TOKS in bee)

Medication Safety Issues

Other safety concerns:

Botulinum products are not interchangeable; potency differences may exist between the products.

Brand Names: U.S. Myobloc®

Index Terms Botulinum Toxin Type B

Generic Availability (U.S.) No

Pharmacologic Category Neuromuscular Blocker Agent, Toxin

Use Treatment of cervical dystonia (spasmodic torticollis)

Unlabeled Use Treatment of cervical dystonia in patients who have developed resistance to botulinum toxin type A

Medication Guide Available Yes

Dosage

Geriatric & Adult Cervical dystonia: I.M.: Initial: 2500-5000 units divided among the affected muscles in patients **previously treated** with botulinum toxin; initial dose in **previously untreated** patients should be lower. Subsequent dosing should be optimized according to patient's response.

Renal Impairment No adjustment is recommended.
Hepatic Impairment No adjustment necessary.
Special Geriatric Considerations No dosage adjustments required, but limited experience in patients ≥75 years of age.
Dosage Forms Excipient information presented when available (limited, particularly for generics); consult specific product labeling.
Injection, solution [preservative free]:
Myobloc®: 5000 units/mL (0.5 mL, 1 mL, 2 mL) [contains albumin (human)]

Rimantadine (ri MAN ta deen)

Medication Safety Issues
Sound-alike/look-alike issues:
Rimantadine may be confused with amantadine, ranitidine, Rimactane
Flumadine® may be confused with fludarabine, flunisolide, flutamide
Brand Names: U.S. Flumadine®
Brand Names: Canada Flumadine®
Index Terms Rimantadine Hydrochloride
Generic Availability (U.S.) Yes
Pharmacologic Category Antiviral Agent; Antiviral Agent, Adamantane
Use Prophylaxis and treatment of influenza A viral infection (per manufacturer's labeling; also refer to current ACIP guidelines for recommendations during current flu season)

Note: In certain circumstances, the ACIP recommends use of rimantadine in combination with oseltamivir for the treatment or prophylaxis of influenza A infection when resistance to oseltamivir is suspected.
Contraindications Hypersensitivity to drugs of the adamantine class, including rimantadine and amantadine, or any component of the formulation
Warnings/Precautions Use with caution in patients with renal and hepatic dysfunction; avoid use, if possible, in patients with uncontrolled psychosis or severe psychoneurosis. An increase in seizure incidence may occur in patients with seizure disorders; discontinue drug if seizures occur; resistance may develop during treatment; viruses exhibit cross-resistance between amantadine and rimantadine. Due to increased resistance, the ACIP has recommended that rimantadine and amantadine no longer be used for the treatment or prophylaxis of influenza A in the United States until susceptibility has been re-established; consult current guidelines. Rimantadine is not effective in the prevention or treatment of influenza B virus infections. The elderly are at higher risk for CNS (eg, dizziness, headache, weakness) and gastrointestinal (eg, nausea/vomiting, abdominal pain) adverse events; dosage adjustment is recommended in elderly patients >65 years of age.
Adverse Reactions (Reflective of adult population; not specific for elderly) 1% to 10%:
Central nervous system: Insomnia (2% to 3%), concentration impaired (≤2%), dizziness (1% to 2%), nervousness (1% to 2%), fatigue (1%), headache (1%)
Gastrointestinal: Nausea (3%), anorexia (2%), vomiting (2%), xerostomia (2%), abdominal pain (1%)
Neuromuscular & skeletal: Weakness (1%)
Drug Interactions
Metabolism/Transport Effects None known.
Avoid Concomitant Use There are no known interactions where it is recommended to avoid concomitant use.
Increased Effect/Toxicity
The levels/effects of Rimantadine may be increased by: MAO Inhibitors
Decreased Effect
Rimantadine may decrease the levels/effects of: Influenza Virus Vaccine (Live/Attenuated)
Ethanol/Nutrition/Herb Interactions Food: Food does not affect rate or extent of absorption
Stability Store at 25°C (77°F); excursions permitted to 15°C to 30°C (59°F to 86°F).
Mechanism of Action Exerts its inhibitory effect on three antigenic subtypes of influenza A virus (H1N1, H2N2, H3N2) early in the viral replicative cycle, possibly inhibiting the uncoating process; it has no activity against influenza B virus and is two- to eightfold more active than amantadine
Pharmacodynamics/Kinetics
Onset of action: Antiviral activity: No data exist establishing a correlation between plasma concentration and antiviral effect
Protein Binding: ~40%, primarily to albumin
Metabolism: Extensively hepatic

Half-life elimination: 25.4 hours; prolonged in elderly, severe liver and severe renal impairment

Time to peak: 6 hours

Excretion: Urine (<25% as unchanged drug)

Clearance: Hemodialysis does not contribute to clearance

Dosage

Geriatric Prophylaxis or treatment of influenza A: Oral: 100 mg daily in the elderly (≥65 years), including elderly nursing home patients.

Adult

Prophylaxis of influenza A: Oral: 100 mg twice daily

Note: Prophylaxis (institutional outbreak): In order to control outbreaks in institutions, if influenza A virus subtyping is unavailable and oseltamivir resistant viruses are circulating, rimantadine may be used in combination with oseltamivir if zanamivir cannot be used. Treatment should continue for ≥2 weeks and until ~10 days after illness onset in the last patient (CDC, 2011; Harper, 2009).

Treatment of influenza A: Oral: 100 mg twice daily

Renal Impairment

Cl$_{cr}$ ≥30 mL/minute: Dose adjustment not required.

Cl$_{cr}$ <30 mL/minute: 100 mg daily

Hepatic Impairment Severe dysfunction: 100 mg daily

Administration Initiation of rimantadine within 48 hours of the onset of influenza A illness halves the duration of illness and significantly reduces the duration of viral shedding and increased peripheral airways resistance; continue therapy for 5-7 days after symptoms begin; discontinue as soon as clinically warranted to reduce the emergence of antiviral drug resistant viruses

Monitoring Parameters Monitor for CNS or GI effects in elderly or patients with renal or hepatic impairment

Special Geriatric Considerations No longer recommended for the treatment or prevention of influenza in the United States because of concerns about resistance and CNS adverse effects. Refer to current CDC guidelines. Monitor GI effects in the elderly or patients with renal or hepatic impairment. Dosing must be individualized (100 mg 1-2 times/day). It is recommended that nursing home patients receive 100 mg/day.

Dosage Forms Excipient information presented when available (limited, particularly for generics); consult specific product labeling.

Tablet, oral, as hydrochloride: 100 mg

Flumadine®: 100 mg

◆ **Rimantadine Hydrochloride** *see* Rimantadine *on page 1705*

Rimexolone (ri MEKS oh lone)

Medication Safety Issues

Sound-alike/look-alike issues:

Vexol® may be confused with VoSoL®

Brand Names: U.S. Vexol®

Brand Names: Canada Vexol®

Generic Availability (U.S.) No

Pharmacologic Category Corticosteroid, Ophthalmic

Use Treatment of inflammation after ocular surgery and the treatment of anterior uveitis

Contraindications Hypersensitivity to rimexolone or any component of the formulation; fungal, mycobacterial, viral (including dendritic keratitis, vaccinia, varicella), or untreated pus-forming bacterial ocular infections

Warnings/Precautions Prolonged use has been associated with the development of corneal or scleral perforation and posterior subcapsular cataracts; may delay healing after cataract surgery; Intraocular pressure should be monitored if this product is used >10 days. Prolonged use of corticosteroids may increase the incidence of secondary infection, mask acute infection (including fungal infections), or prolong or exacerbate viral infections. Corticosteroids should not be used to treat ocular herpes simplex. Fungal infection should be suspected in any patient with persistent corneal ulceration who has received corticosteroids.

Adverse Reactions (Reflective of adult population; not specific for elderly)

1% to 5%: Ocular: Blurred vision, discharge, discomfort, pain, increased intraocular pressure, foreign body sensation, hyperemia, pruritus

<2%:

Cardiovascular: Hypotension

Central nervous system: Headache

Gastrointestinal: Taste perversion

Respiratory: Pharyngitis, rhinitis

Frequency not defined: Cataracts, damage to the optic nerve, defects in visual activity, perforation of globe, secondary ocular infection

Drug Interactions

Metabolism/Transport Effects None known.

Avoid Concomitant Use

Avoid concomitant use of Rimexolone with any of the following: Aldesleukin

Increased Effect/Toxicity

Rimexolone may increase the levels/effects of: Deferasirox

The levels/effects of Rimexolone may be increased by: Telaprevir

Decreased Effect

Rimexolone may decrease the levels/effects of: Aldesleukin; Corticorelin; Hyaluronidase; Telaprevir

Mechanism of Action Decreases inflammation by suppression of migration of polymorphonuclear leukocytes and reversal of increased capillary permeability

Pharmacodynamics/Kinetics

Absorption: Through aqueous humor

Metabolism: Hepatic for any amount of drug absorbed

Excretion: Urine and feces

Dosage

Geriatric & Adult

Anti-inflammatory: Ophthalmic: Instill 1-2 drops in conjunctival sac of affected eye 4 times/day beginning 24 hours after surgery and continuing through the first 2 weeks of the postoperative period

Anterior uveitis: Ophthalmic: Instill 1-2 drops in conjunctival sac of affected eye every hour during waking hours for the first week, then 1 drop every 2 hours during waking hours of the second week, and then taper until uveitis is resolved

Monitoring Parameters Intraocular pressure and periodic examination of lens (with prolonged use)

Special Geriatric Considerations No special considerations; must limit the time steroids are used to prevent adverse effects.

Dosage Forms Excipient information presented when available (limited, particularly for generics); consult specific product labeling.

Suspension, ophthalmic [drops]:

Vexol®: 1% (5 mL, 10 mL) [contains benzalkonium chloride]

◆ **Riomet®** see MetFORMIN on page 1222
◆ **Riopan Plus** see Magaldrate and Simethicone on page 1175
◆ **RisaQuad™ [OTC]** see Lactobacillus on page 1084
◆ **RisaQuad®-2 [OTC]** see Lactobacillus on page 1084

Risedronate (ris ED roe nate)

Related Information

Osteoporosis Management on page 2136

Medication Safety Issues

Sound-alike/look-alike issues:

Actonel® may be confused with Actos®

Risedronate may be confused with alendronate

Brand Names: U.S. Actonel®; Atelvia™

Brand Names: Canada Actonel®; Actonel® DR; Apo-Risedronate®; Dom-Risedronate; Novo-Risedronate; PMS-Risedronate; ratio-Risedronate; Riva-Risedronate; Sandoz-Risedronate; Teva-Risedronate

Index Terms Risedronate Sodium

Generic Availability (U.S.) No

Pharmacologic Category Bisphosphonate Derivative

Use

Actonel®: Treatment of Paget's disease of the bone; treatment and prevention of glucocorticoid-induced osteoporosis; treatment and prevention of osteoporosis in postmenopausal women; treatment of osteoporosis in men

Atelvia™: Treatment of osteoporosis in postmenopausal women

Medication Guide Available Yes

Contraindications Hypersensitivity to risedronate, bisphosphonates, or any component of the formulation; hypocalcemia; inability to stand or sit upright for at least 30 minutes; abnormalities of the esophagus which delay esophageal emptying, such as stricture or achalasia

◀ **Warnings/Precautions** Bisphosphonates may cause upper gastrointestinal disorders such as dysphagia, esophagitis, esophageal ulcer, and gastric ulcer; risk increases in patients unable to comply with dosing instructions. Use with caution in patients with dysphagia, esophageal disease, gastritis, duodenitis, or ulcers (may worsen underlying condition). Discontinue if new or worsening symptoms occur. Use caution in patients with renal impairment (not recommended in patients with a Cl_{cr} <30 mL/minute). Hypocalcemia must be corrected before therapy initiation with risedronate. Ensure adequate calcium and vitamin D intake, especially for patients with Paget's disease in whom the pretreatment rate of bone turnover may be greatly elevated.

Bisphosphonate therapy has been associated with osteonecrosis, primarily of the jaw. Risk factors for osteonecrosis of the jaw (ONJ) include invasive dental procedures (eg, tooth extraction, dental implants, boney surgery); a diagnosis of cancer, with concomitant chemotherapy or corticosteroids; poor oral hygiene, ill-fitting dentures; and comorbid disorders (anemia, coagulopathy, infection, pre-existing dental disease). Most reported cases occurred after I.V. bisphosphonate therapy; however, cases have been reported following oral therapy. A dental exam and preventative dentistry should be performed prior to placing patients with risk factors on chronic bisphosphonate therapy. The manufacturer's labeling states that discontinuing bisphosphonates in patients requiring invasive dental procedures may reduce the risk of ONJ. However, other experts suggest that there is no evidence that discontinuing therapy reduces the risk of developing ONJ (Assael, 2009). The benefit/risk must be assessed by the treating physician and/or dentist/surgeon prior to any invasive dental procedure. Patients developing ONJ while on bisphosphonates should receive care by an oral surgeon.

Atypical femur fractures have been reported in patients receiving bisphosphonates for treatment/prevention of osteoporosis. The fractures include subtrochanteric femur (bone just below the hip joint) and diaphyseal femur (long segment of the thigh bone). Some patients experience prodromal pain weeks or months before the fracture occurs. It is unclear if bisphosphonate therapy is the cause for these fractures, although the majority have been reported in patients taking bisphosphonates. Patients receiving long-term (>3-5 years) therapy may be at an increased risk. Discontinue bisphosphonate therapy in patients who develop femoral shaft fracture.

Infrequently, severe (and occasionally debilitating) bone, joint, and/or muscle pain have been reported during bisphosphonate treatment. The onset of pain ranged from a single day to several months. Consider discontinuing therapy in patients who experience severe symptoms; symptoms usually resolve upon discontinuation. Some patients experienced recurrence when rechallenged with same drug or another bisphosphonate; avoid use in patients with a history of these symptoms in association with bisphosphonate therapy.

When using for glucocorticoid-induced osteoporosis, evaluate sex steroid hormonal status prior to treatment initiation; consider appropriate hormone replacement if necessary.

Adverse Reactions (Reflective of adult population; not specific for elderly) Frequency may vary with product, dose, and indication.

>10%:
  Cardiovascular: Hypertension (11%)
  Central nervous system: Headache (3% to 18%)
  Dermatologic: Rash (8% to 12%)
  Endocrine & metabolic: Serum PTH levels increased (transient; <30%)
  Gastrointestinal: Diarrhea (5% to 20%), nausea (4% to 13%), constipation (3% to 13%), abdominal pain (2% to 12%), dyspepsia (4% to 11%)
  Genitourinary: Urinary tract infection (11%)
  Neuromuscular & skeletal: Arthralgia (7% to 33%), back pain (6% to 28%)
  Miscellaneous: Infection (≤31%)
1% to 10%:
  Cardiovascular: Peripheral edema (8%), chest pain (5% to 7%), arrhythmia (2%)
  Central nervous system: Depression (7%), dizziness (3% to 7%)
  Endocrine & metabolic: Hypocalcemia (≤5%), hypophosphatemia (<3%)
  Gastrointestinal: Vomiting (2% to 5%), gastritis (3%), duodenitis (≤1%), glossitis (≤1%)
  Genitourinary: Prostatic hyperplasia (5%; benign), nephrolithiasis (3%)
  Neuromuscular & skeletal: Joint disorder (7%), myalgia (2% to 7%), neck pain (5%), muscle spasm (1% to 2%)
  Ocular: Cataract (7%)
  Respiratory: Bronchitis (3% to 10%), pharyngitis (6%), rhinitis (6%), dyspnea (4%)
  Miscellaneous: Flu-like syndrome (10%), acute phase reaction (≤8%; includes fever, influenza-like illness)

Drug Interactions
  Metabolism/Transport Effects None known.
  Avoid Concomitant Use There are no known interactions where it is recommended to avoid concomitant use.
  Increased Effect/Toxicity
    Risedronate may increase the levels/effects of: Deferasirox; Phosphate Supplements; SUNItinib

    The levels/effects of Risedronate may be increased by: Aminoglycosides; Nonsteroidal Anti-Inflammatory Agents
  Decreased Effect
    The levels/effects of Risedronate may be decreased by: Antacids; Calcium Salts; Iron Salts; Magnesium Salts; Proton Pump Inhibitors
Ethanol/Nutrition/Herb Interactions
  Ethanol: Avoid ethanol (may increase risk of osteoporosis).
  Food: Food reduces absorption (similar to other bisphosphonates); mean oral bioavailability is decreased when given with food.
Stability Store at room temperature of 20°C to 25°C (68°F to 77°F).
Mechanism of Action A bisphosphonate which inhibits bone resorption via actions on osteoclasts or on osteoclast precursors; decreases the rate of bone resorption, leading to an indirect increase in bone mineral density. In Paget's disease, characterized by disordered resorption and formation of bone, inhibition of resorption leads to an indirect decrease in bone formation; but the newly-formed bone has a more normal architecture.
Pharmacodynamics/Kinetics
  Onset of action: May require weeks
  Absorption: Rapid
  Distribution: V_d: 13.8 L/kg
  Protein binding: ~24%
  Metabolism: None
  Bioavailability: Poor, ~0.54% to 0.75%
  Half-life elimination: Initial: 1.5 hours; Terminal: 480-561 hours
  Time to peak, serum: 1-3 hours
  Excretion: Urine (up to 85%); feces (as unabsorbed drug)
Dosage
  Geriatric & Adult Note: Patients should receive supplemental calcium and vitamin D if dietary intake is inadequate.
    Paget's disease of bone: Oral: *Immediate release tablet:* 30 mg once daily for 2 months
      Note: Retreatment may be considered (following post-treatment observation of at least 2 months) if relapse occurs, or if treatment fails to normalize serum alkaline phosphatase. For retreatment, the dose and duration of therapy are the same as for initial treatment. No data are available on more than one course of retreatment.
    Osteoporosis (postmenopausal): Oral:
      Immediate release tablet: Prevention and treatment: 5 mg once daily **or** 35 mg once weekly **or** 150 mg once a month
      Delayed release tablet: Treatment: 35 mg once weekly
    Osteoporosis (males) treatment: Oral: *Immediate release tablet:* 35 mg once weekly
    Osteoporosis (glucocorticoid-induced) prevention and treatment: Oral: *Immediate release tablet:* 5 mg once daily
  Renal Impairment
    Cl_{cr} ≥30 mL/minute: No adjustment required
    Cl_{cr} <30 mL/minute: Use is not recommended
  Hepatic Impairment No studies performed in hepatic impairment; no dosage adjustment necessary due to lack of hepatic metabolism.
Administration Note: Avoid administration of oral calcium supplements, antacids, magnesium supplements/laxatives, and iron preparations within 30 minutes of risedronate administration.
  Immediate release tablet: Risedronate immediate release tablets must be taken on an empty stomach with a full glass (6-8 oz) of **plain water** (not mineral water) at least 30 minutes before any food, drink, or other medications orally to avoid interference with absorption. Patient must remain sitting upright or standing for at least 30 minutes after taking (to reduce esophageal irritation). Tablet should be swallowed whole; do not crush or chew.
  Delayed release tablet: Risedronate delayed release tablets must be taken with at least 4 oz of **plain water** (not mineral water) immediately after breakfast. Patient must remain sitting upright or standing for at least 30 minutes after taking (to reduce esophageal irritation). Tablet should be swallowed whole; do not cut, split, crush, or chew.

Monitoring Parameters
Osteoporosis: Bone mineral density as measured by central dual-energy x-ray absorptiometry (DXA) of the hip or spine prior to initiation of therapy and at least every 2 years thereafter (6-12 months post-baseline if combined glucocorticoid and risedronate treatment, then every 2 years thereafter); annual measurements of height and weight, assessment of chronic back pain; serum calcium and 25(OH)D; consider measuring biochemical markers of bone turnover
Paget's disease: Alkaline phosphatase; pain; serum calcium and 25(OH)D

Test Interactions Bisphosphonates may interfere with diagnostic imaging agents such as technetium-99m-diphosphonate in bone scans.

Special Geriatric Considerations The elderly are frequently treated long-term for osteoporosis. Elderly patients should be advised to report any lower extremity, jaw (osteonecrosis), or muscle pain that cannot be explained or lasts longer than 2 weeks. Additionally, elderly often receive concomitant diuretic therapy and therefore their electrolyte status (eg, calcium, phosphate) should be periodically evaluated.

Due to the reports of atypical femur fractures and osteonecrosis of the jaw, recommendations for duration of bisphosphonate use in osteoporosis have been modified. Based on available data, consider discontinuing bisphosphonates after 5 years of use in low-risk patients, since the risk of nonvertebral fracture is the same as those patients taking bisphosphonates for 10 years. Those patients with high risk (fracture history) may be continued for a longer period, taking into consideration the risks vs benefits associated with continued therapy.

Dosage Forms Excipient information presented when available (limited, particularly for generics); consult specific product labeling.
Tablet, oral, as sodium:
  Actonel®: 5 mg, 30 mg, 35 mg, 150 mg
Tablet, delayed release, oral, as sodium:
  Atelvia™: 35 mg

♦ **Risedronate Sodium** *see* Risedronate *on page 1707*
♦ **RisperDAL®** *see* RisperiDONE *on page 1710*
♦ **Risperdal M-Tab** *see* RisperiDONE *on page 1710*
♦ **RisperDAL® M-Tab®** *see* RisperiDONE *on page 1710*
♦ **RisperDAL® Consta®** *see* RisperiDONE *on page 1710*

RisperiDONE (ris PER i done)

Related Information
Antipsychotic Agents *on page 2103*
Atypical Antipsychotics *on page 2107*
Beers Criteria – Potentially Inappropriate Medications for Geriatrics *on page 2183*

Medication Safety Issues
Sound-alike/look-alike issues:
RisperiDONE may be confused with reserpine, rOPINIRole
RisperDAL® may be confused with lisinopril, reserpine, Restoril™

BEERS Criteria medication:
This drug may be potentially inappropriate for use in geriatric patients (Quality of evidence - moderate; Strength of recommendation - strong).

Brand Names: U.S. RisperDAL®; RisperDAL® Consta®; RisperDAL® M-Tab®
Brand Names: Canada Apo-Risperidone®; Ava-Risperidone; CO Risperidone; Dom-Risperidone; JAMP-Risperidone; Mint-Risperidon; Mylan-Risperidone; Novo-Risperidone; PHL-Risperidone; PMS-Risperidone; PMS-Risperidone ODT; PRO-Risperidone; RAN™-Risperidone; ratio-Risperidone; Risperdal®; Risperdal® Consta®; Risperdal® M-Tab®; Riva-Risperidone; Sandoz-Risperidone

Index Terms Risperdal M-Tab
Generic Availability (U.S.) Yes: Excludes injection
Pharmacologic Category Antimanic Agent; Antipsychotic Agent, Atypical

Use
Oral: Treatment of schizophrenia; treatment of acute mania or mixed episodes associated with bipolar I disorder (as monotherapy in adults, or in combination with lithium or valproate in adults); treatment of irritability/aggression associated with autistic disorder
Injection: Treatment of schizophrenia; maintenance treatment of bipolar I disorder in adults as monotherapy or in combination with lithium or valproate

Unlabeled Use Treatment of Tourette's syndrome; psychosis/agitation related to Alzheimer's dementia; post-traumatic stress disorder (PTSD)
Contraindications Hypersensitivity to risperidone or any component of the formulation

Warnings/Precautions Hazardous agent - use appropriate precautions for handling and disposal. **[U.S. Boxed Warning]: Elderly patients with dementia-related psychosis treated with antipsychotics are at an increased risk of death compared to placebo.** Most deaths appeared to be either cardiovascular (eg, heart failure, sudden death) or infectious (eg, pneumonia) in nature. In addition, an increased incidence of cerebrovascular effects (eg, transient ischemic attack, cerebrovascular accidents) has been reported in studies of placebo-controlled trials of risperidone in elderly patients with dementia-related psychosis. Risperidone is not approved for the treatment of dementia-related psychosis.

Leukopenia, neutropenia, and agranulocytosis (sometimes fatal) have been reported in clinical trials and postmarketing reports with antipsychotic use; presence of risk factors (eg, pre-existing low WBC or history of drug-induced leuko-/neutropenia) should prompt periodic blood count assessment. Discontinue therapy at first signs of blood dyscrasias or if absolute neutrophil count <1000/mm^3.

Low to moderately sedating, use with caution in disorders where CNS depression is a feature. Use with caution in Parkinson's disease. Caution in patients with predisposition to seizures. Use with caution in renal or hepatic dysfunction; dose reduction recommended. Esophageal dysmotility and aspiration have been associated with antipsychotic use; use with caution in patients at risk of aspiration pneumonia (ie, Alzheimer's disease). Risperidone is associated with greater increases in prolactin levels as compared to other antipsychotic agents; clinical significance of hyperprolactinemia in patients with breast cancer or other prolactin-dependent tumors is unknown. May alter temperature regulation. May mask toxicity of other drugs or conditions (eg intestinal obstruction, Reyes syndrome, brain tumor) due to antiemetic effects. Neutropenia has been reported with antipsychotic use, including fatal cases of agranulocytosis. Pre-existing myelosuppression (disease or drug-induced) increases risk and these patients should have frequent CBC monitoring; decreased blood counts in absence of other causative factors should prompt discontinuation of therapy.

Use with caution in patients with cardiovascular diseases (eg, heart failure, history of myocardial infarction or ischemia, cerebrovascular disease, conduction abnormalities). May cause orthostatic hypotension; use with caution in patients at risk of this effect (eg, concurrent medication use which may predispose to hypotension/bradycardia or presence of hypovolemia) or in those who would not tolerate transient hypotensive episodes. May alter cardiac conduction (low risk relative to other neuroleptics); life-threatening arrhythmias have occurred with therapeutic doses of neuroleptics.

May cause anticholinergic effects (confusion, agitation, constipation, xerostomia, blurred vision, urinary retention); therefore, they should be used with caution in patients with decreased gastrointestinal motility, urinary retention, BPH, xerostomia, or visual problems (including narrow-angle glaucoma). Relative to other neuroleptics, risperidone has a low potency of cholinergic blockade.

May cause extrapyramidal symptoms (EPS), including pseudoparkinsonism, acute dystonic reactions, akathisia, and tardive dyskinesia (risk of these reactions is low relative to other neuroleptics, and is dose dependent). Risk of dystonia (and probably other EPS) may be greater with increased doses, use of conventional antipsychotics, males, and younger patients. Risk of neuroleptic malignant syndrome (NMS) may be increased in patients with Parkinson's disease or Lewy body dementia; monitor for symptoms of confusion, obtundation, postural instability and extrapyramidal symptoms. May cause hyperglycemia; in some cases may be extreme and associated with ketoacidosis, hyperosmolar coma, or death. Use with caution in patients with diabetes or other disorders of glucose regulation; monitor for worsening of glucose control. Dyslipidemia has been reported with atypical antipsychotics; risk profile may differ between agents. Discrepant results have been reported in clinical trials, regarding lipid changes associated with risperidone (American Diabetes Association, 2004). Significant weight gain has been observed with antipsychotic therapy; incidence varies with product. Monitor waist circumference and BMI. Rare cases of priapism have been reported.

Use in elderly patients with dementia is associated with an increased risk of mortality and cerebrovascular accidents; avoid antipsychotic use for behavioral problems associated with dementia unless alternative nonpharmacologic therapies have failed and patient may harm self or others. In addition, use may cause or exacerbate syndrome of inappropriate antidiuretic hormone secretion or hyponatremia; monitor sodium closely with initiation or dosage adjustments in older adults (Beers Criteria).

The possibility of a suicide attempt is inherent in psychotic illness or bipolar disorder; use caution in high-risk patients during initiation of therapy. Prescriptions should be written for the smallest quantity consistent with good patient care. Long-term effects on growth or sexual maturation have not been evaluated. Vehicle used in injectable (polylactide-co-glycolide microspheres) has rarely been associated with retinal artery occlusion in patients with abnormal arteriovenous anastomosis.

◄ Adverse Reactions (Reflective of adult population; not specific for elderly) The frequency of adverse effects is reported as absolute percentages and is not based upon net frequencies as compared to placebo. Actual frequency may be dependent upon dose and/or indication. Events are reported from placebo-controlled studies. Unless otherwise noted, frequency of adverse effects is reported for the oral formulation in adults.

>10%:

Central nervous system: Somnolence (children 12% to 67%; adults 5% to 14%; I.M. injection 5% to 6%), fatigue (children 18% to 42%; adults 1% to 3%), headache (I.M. injection 15% to 21%), fever (children 20%; adults 1% to 2%), dystonia (children 9% to 18%; adults 5% to 11%), anxiety (children ≤16%; adults 2% to 16%), dizziness (children 7% to 16%; adults 4% to 10%), Parkinsonism (children 2% to 16%; adults 12% to 20%)

Dermatologic: Rash (children ≤11%; adults 2% to 4%)

Gastrointestinal: Appetite increased (children 4% to 49%), weight gain (≥7% kg increase from baseline: children 33%; adults 9% to 21%), vomiting (children 10% to 25%), salivation increased (children ≤22%; adults 1% to 3%), constipation (children 21%; adults 8% to 9%), abdominal pain (children 15% to 18%; adults 3% to 4%), nausea (children 8% to 16%; adults 4% to 9%), dyspepsia (children 5% to 16%; adults 4% to 10%), xerostomia (children 13%; adults ≤4%)

Genitourinary: Urinary incontinence (children 5% to 22%; adults <2%)

Neuromuscular & skeletal: Tremor (adults 6%; children 10% to 12%)

Respiratory: Rhinitis (children 13% to 36%; adults 7% to 11%), upper respiratory infection (children 34%; adults 2% to 3%), cough (children 34%; adults 3%)

1% to 10%:

Cardiovascular: Tachycardia (children ≤7%; adults 1% to 5%), hypertension (I.M. injection 3%), chest pain (1% to 3%), creatine phosphokinase increased (≤2%), orthostatic hypotension (≤2%), arrhythmia (≤1%), edema (≤1%), hypotension (≤1%), syncope (≤1%)

Central nervous system: Akathisia (children ≤10%; adults 5% to 9%), automatism (children 7%), confusion (children 5%)

Dermatologic: Seborrhea (up to 2%), acne (1%)

Endocrine & metabolic: Lactation nonpuerperal (children 2% to 5%; adults 1%), ejaculation failure (≤1%)

Gastrointestinal: Diarrhea (children 7% to 8%; adults ≤3%), anorexia (children 8%; adults ≤2%), toothache (I.M. injection 1% to 3%)

Genitourinary: Urinary tract infection (≤3%)

Hematologic: Neutropenia (I.M. injection <2%), anemia (I.M. injection <2%; oral ≤1%)

Hepatic: Transaminases increased (I.M. injection ≥1%; oral 1%)

Neuromuscular & skeletal: Dyskinesia (children 7%; adults 1%), arthralgia (2% to 3%), back pain (2% to 3%), myalgia (≤2%), weakness (1%)

Ocular: Abnormal vision (children 4% to 7%; adults 1% to 3%), blurred vision (I.M. injection 2% to 3%)

Otic: Earache (1%)

Respiratory: Dyspnea (children 2% to 5%; adults 2%), epistaxis (≤2%)

Drug Interactions

Metabolism/Transport Effects Substrate of CYP2D6 (major), CYP3A4 (minor), P-glycoprotein; **Note:** Assignment of Major/Minor substrate status based on clinically relevant drug interaction potential; **Inhibits** CYP2D6 (weak), CYP3A4 (weak)

Avoid Concomitant Use

Avoid concomitant use of RisperiDONE with any of the following: Azelastine; Azelastine (Nasal); Highest Risk QTc-Prolonging Agents; Metoclopramide; Mifepristone; Paraldehyde

Increased Effect/Toxicity

RisperiDONE may increase the levels/effects of: Alcohol (Ethyl); Anticholinergics; ARIPiprazole; Azelastine; Azelastine (Nasal); Buprenorphine; CNS Depressants; Highest Risk QTc-Prolonging Agents; Methylphenidate; Moderate Risk QTc-Prolonging Agents; Paliperidone; Paraldehyde; Serotonin Modulators; Zolpidem

The levels/effects of RisperiDONE may be increased by: Abiraterone Acetate; Acetylcholinesterase Inhibitors (Central); CYP2D6 Inhibitors (Moderate); CYP2D6 Inhibitors (Strong); Darunavir; Divalproex; HydrOXYzine; Lithium formulations; Loop Diuretics; Methylphenidate; Metoclopramide; Metyrosine; Mifepristone; P-glycoprotein/ABCB1 Inhibitors; Pramlintide; QTc-Prolonging Agents (Indeterminate Risk and Risk Modifying); Selective Serotonin Reuptake Inhibitors; Tetrabenazine; Valproic Acid; Verapamil

Decreased Effect

RisperiDONE may decrease the levels/effects of: Amphetamines; Anti-Parkinson's Agents (Dopamine Agonist); Quinagolide

The levels/effects of RisperiDONE may be decreased by: CarBAMazepine; Lithium formulations; Peginterferon Alfa-2b; P-glycoprotein/ABCB1 Inducers; Tocilizumab

Ethanol/Nutrition/Herb Interactions
Ethanol: Ethanol may increase CNS depression. Management: Limit or avoid ethanol.

Food: Oral solution is not compatible with beverages containing tannin or pectinate (cola or tea). Management: Administer oral solution with water, coffee, orange juice, or low-fat milk.

Herb/Nutraceutical: Some herbal medications may increase CNS depression. Management: Avoid kava kava, gotu kola, valerian, and St John's wort.

Stability
Injection: Risperdal® Consta®: Store in refrigerator at 2°C to 8°C (36°F to 46°F) and protect from light. May be stored at room temperature of 25°C (77°F) for up to 7 days prior to administration. Bring to room temperature prior to reconstitution. Reconstitute with provided diluent only. Shake vigorously to mix; will form thick, milky suspension. Following reconstitution, store at room temperature and use within 6 hours. Suspension settles in ~2 minutes; shake vigorously to resuspend prior to administration.

Oral solution, tablet: Store at 15°C to 25°C (59°F to 77°F). Protect from light and moisture. Keep orally-disintegrating tablets sealed in foil pouch until ready to use. Do not freeze solution.

Mechanism of Action
Risperidone is a benzisoxazole atypical antipsychotic with mixed serotonin-dopamine antagonist activity that binds to 5-HT_2-receptors in the CNS and in the periphery with a very high affinity; binds to dopamine-D_2 receptors with less affinity. The binding affinity to the dopamine-D_2 receptor is 20 times lower than the 5-HT_2 affinity. The addition of serotonin antagonism to dopamine antagonism (classic neuroleptic mechanism) is thought to improve negative symptoms of psychoses and reduce the incidence of extrapyramidal side effects. Alpha$_1$, alpha$_2$ adrenergic, and histaminergic receptors are also antagonized with high affinity. Risperidone has low to moderate affinity for 5-HT_{1C}, 5-HT_{1D}, and 5-HT_{1A} receptors, weak affinity for D_1 and no affinity for muscarinics or beta$_1$ and beta$_2$ receptors

Pharmacodynamics/Kinetics
Absorption:

Oral: Rapid and well absorbed; food does not affect rate or extent

Injection: <1% absorbed initially; main release occurs at ~3 weeks and is maintained from 4-6 weeks

Distribution: V_d: 1-2 L/kg

Protein binding, plasma: Risperidone 90%; 9-hydroxyrisperidone: 77%

Metabolism: Extensively hepatic via CYP2D6 to 9-hydroxyrisperidone (similar pharmacological activity as risperidone); N-dealkylation is a second minor pathway

Bioavailability: Oral: 70%; Tablet (relative to solution): 94%; orally-disintegrating tablets and oral solution are bioequivalent to tablets

Half-life elimination: Active moiety (risperidone and its active metabolite 9-hydroxyrisperidone)

Oral: 20 hours (mean)

Extensive metabolizers: Risperidone: 3 hours; 9-hydroxyrisperidone: 21 hours

Poor metabolizers: Risperidone: 20 hours; 9-hydroxyrisperidone: 30 hours

Injection: 3-6 days; related to microsphere erosion and subsequent absorption of risperidone

Time to peak, plasma: Oral: Risperidone: Within 1 hour; 9-hydroxyrisperidone: Extensive metabolizers: 3 hours; Poor metabolizers: 17 hours

Excretion: Urine (70%); feces (14%)

Dosage

Geriatric
Oral: Initial: 0.5 mg twice daily; titration should progress slowly in increments of no more than 0.5 mg twice daily; increases to dosages >1.5 mg twice daily should occur at intervals of ≥1 week.

Note: Additional monitoring of renal function and orthostatic blood pressure may be warranted. If once-a-day dosing in the elderly or debilitated patient is considered, a twice daily regimen should be used to titrate to the target dose, and this dose should be maintained for 2-3 days prior to attempts to switch to a once-daily regimen.

Psychosis/agitation related to Alzheimer's dementia (unlabeled use): Initial: 0.25-1 mg/day; if necessary, gradually increase as tolerated not to exceed 1.5-2 mg/day; doses >1 mg/day are associated with higher rates of extrapyramidal symptoms (Rabins, 2007)

I.M. (Risperdal® Consta®): 25 mg every 2 weeks; a lower initial dose of 12.5 mg may be appropriate in some patients.

Note: Oral risperidone (or other antipsychotic) should be administered with the initial injection of Risperdal® Consta® and continued for 3 weeks (then discontinued) to maintain adequate therapeutic plasma concentrations prior to main release phase of risperidone from injection site. When switching from depot administration to a short-acting formulation, administer short-acting agent in place of the next regularly-scheduled depot injection.

◄ **Adult Note:** When reinitiating treatment after discontinuation, the initial titration schedule should be followed.

Bipolar mania: *Oral:* Recommended starting dose: 2-3 mg once daily; if needed, adjust dose by 1 mg/day in intervals ≥24 hours; dosing range: 1-6 mg/day.

Maintenance: No dosing recommendation available for treatment >3 weeks duration

Bipolar I maintenance: *I.M. (Risperdal® Consta®):* 25 mg every 2 weeks; if unresponsive, some may benefit from larger doses (37.5-50 mg); maximum dose: 50 mg every 2 weeks. Dosage adjustments should not be made more frequently than every 4 weeks. A lower initial dose of 12.5 mg may be appropriate in some patients (eg, demonstrated poor tolerability to other psychotropic medications).

Note: Oral risperidone (or other antipsychotic) should be administered with the initial injection of Risperdal® Consta® and continued for 3 weeks (then discontinued) to maintain adequate therapeutic plasma concentrations prior to main release phase of risperidone from injection site. When switching from depot administration to a short-acting formulation, administer short-acting agent in place of the next regularly-scheduled depot injection.

Schizophrenia:

Oral: Initial: 2 mg/day in 1-2 divided doses; may be increased by 1-2 mg/day at intervals ≥24 hours to a recommended dosage range of 4-8 mg/day; may be given as a single daily dose once maintenance dose is achieved; daily dosages >6 mg do not appear to confer any additional benefit, and the incidence of extrapyramidal symptoms is higher than with lower doses. Further dose adjustments should be made in increments/decrements of 1-2 mg/day on a weekly basis. Dose range studied in clinical trials: 4-16 mg/day. Maintenance: Recommended dosage range: 2-8 mg/day

I.M. (Risperdal® Consta®): Initial: 25 mg every 2 weeks; if unresponsive, some may benefit from larger doses (37.5-50 mg); maximum dose: 50 mg every 2 weeks. Dosage adjustments should not be made more frequently than every 4 weeks. A lower initial dose of 12.5 mg may be appropriate in some patients (eg, demonstrated poor tolerability to other psychotropic medications).

Note: Oral risperidone (or other antipsychotic) should be administered with the initial injection of Risperdal® Consta® and continued for 3 weeks (then discontinued) to maintain adequate therapeutic plasma concentrations prior to main release phase of risperidone from injection site. When switching from depot administration to a short-acting formulation, administer short-acting agent in place of the next regularly-scheduled depot injection.

Post-traumatic stress disorder (PTSD) (unlabeled use): *Oral:* 0.5-8 mg/day (Bandelow, 2008; Benedek, 2009)

Tourette's syndrome (unlabeled use): *Oral:* Initial: 0.25 mg once daily for 2 days, then 0.25 mg twice daily for 3 days, then 0.5 mg twice daily for 2 days; titrate slowly thereafter in increments/decrements ≤0.5 mg twice daily and at intervals ≥3 days; maximum dose: 6 mg/day (Dion, 2002)

Renal Impairment

Oral: Starting dose of 0.5 mg twice daily; titration should progress slowly in increments of no more than 0.5 mg twice daily; increases to dosages >1.5 mg twice daily should occur at intervals of ≥1 week. Clearance of the active moiety is decreased by 60% in patients with moderate-to-severe renal disease compared to healthy subjects.

I.M.: Initiate with **oral** dosing (0.5 mg twice daily for 1 week then 2 mg/day for 1 week); if tolerated, begin 25 mg **I.M.** every 2 weeks; continue oral dosing for 3 weeks after the first I.M. injection. An initial I.M. dose of 12.5 mg may also be considered.

Hepatic Impairment

Oral: Starting dose of 0.5 mg twice daily; titration should progress slowly in increments of no more than 0.5 mg twice daily; increases to dosages >1.5 mg twice daily should occur at intervals of ≥1 week. The mean free fraction of risperidone in plasma was increased by 35% in patients with hepatic impairment compared to healthy subjects.

I.M.: Initiate with **oral** dosing (0.5 mg twice daily for 1 week then 2 mg/day for 1 week); if tolerated, begin 25 mg **I.M.** every 2 weeks; continue oral dosing for 3 weeks after the first I.M. injection. An initial I.M. dose of 12.5 mg may also be considered.

Administration

Oral: May be administered without regard to meals.

Oral solution can be administered directly from the provided pipette or may be mixed with water, coffee, orange juice, or low-fat milk, but is **not compatible** with cola or tea.

Risperdal® M-Tab® should not be removed from blister pack until administered. Using dry hands, place immediately on tongue. Tablet will dissolve within seconds, and may be swallowed with or without liquid. Do not split or chew.

I.M.: Risperdal® Consta® should be administered into either the deltoid muscle or the upper outer quadrant of the gluteal area. Avoid inadvertent injection into vasculature. Injection should alternate between the two arms or buttocks. Do not combine two different dosage strengths into one single administration. Do not substitute any components of the dose-pack; administer with needle provided (1-inch needle for deltoid administration or 2-inch needle for gluteal administration).

Monitoring Parameters Vital signs; fasting lipid profile and fasting blood glucose/Hgb A_{1c} (prior to treatment, at 3 months, then annually); CBC; BMI, personal/family history of obesity, waist circumference; blood pressure; mental status, abnormal involuntary movement scale (AIMS), extrapyramidal symptoms; orthostatic blood pressure changes for 3-5 days after starting or increasing dose. Weight should be assessed prior to treatment, at 4 weeks, 8 weeks, 12 weeks, and then at quarterly intervals. Consider titrating to a different antipsychotic agent for a weight gain ≥5% of the initial weight.

Pharmacotherapy Pearls Risperdal® Consta® is an injectable formulation of risperidone using the extended release Medisorb® drug-delivery system; small polymeric microspheres degrade slowly, releasing the medication at a controlled rate.

Special Geriatric Considerations Acute changes in mental status and/or behavior from baseline are often caused by changes in fluid/electrolytes, infections, addition or increases in CNS active medications, changes in the environment (eg, moving, remodeling, new room-mate, etc.), and changes in disease status of any organ system. These changes in behavior need to be assessed before initiating or increasing antipsychotic therapy.

Extrapyramidal syndrome symptoms occur less with this agent when total daily dose remains <6 mg as compared with phenothiazines and butyrophenone classes of antipsychotics. Many elderly patients receive antipsychotic medications for inappropriate nonpsychotic behavior. Before initiating antipsychotic medication, the clinician should investigate any possible reversible cause; any stress or stress from any disease can cause acute "confusion" or worsening of baseline nonpsychotic behavior. Most commonly acute changes in behavior are due to increases in drug dose or addition of new drug to regimen, fluid electrolyte loss, infections, and changes in environment.

In the treatment of agitated, demented, elderly patients, authors of meta-analysis of controlled trials of the response to the traditional antipsychotics (phenothiazines, butyrophenones) in controlling agitation have concluded that the use of neuroleptics results in a response rate of 18%. Clearly, neuroleptic therapy for behavior control should be limited with frequent attempts to withdraw the agent given for behavior control. In light of significant risks and adverse effects in elderly population compared with limited data demonstrating efficacy in the treatment of dementia-related psychosis, aggression, and agitation, an extensive risk:benefit analysis should be performed prior to use.

This medication is considered to be potentially inappropriate in this patient population (Beers Criteria: Quality of evidence - moderate; Strength of recommendation - strong).

Dosage Forms Excipient information presented when available (limited, particularly for generics); consult specific product labeling.

Injection, microspheres for reconstitution, extended release:
  RisperDAL® Consta®: 12.5 mg, 25 mg, 37.5 mg, 50 mg [contains polylactide-co-glycolide; supplied in a dose-pack containing vial with active ingredient in microsphere formulation, prefilled syringe with diluent, needle-free vial access device, and 2 safety needles (a 21 G UTW 1-inch and a 20 G TW 2-inch)]
Solution, oral: 1 mg/mL (30 mL)
  RisperDAL®: 1 mg/mL (30 mL) [contains benzoic acid]
Tablet, oral: 0.25 mg, 0.5 mg, 1 mg, 2 mg, 3 mg, 4 mg
  RisperDAL®: 0.25 mg, 0.5 mg
  RisperDAL®: 1 mg [scored]
  RisperDAL®: 2 mg, 3 mg, 4 mg
Tablet, orally disintegrating, oral: 0.25 mg, 0.5 mg, 1 mg, 2 mg, 3 mg, 4 mg
  RisperDAL® M-Tab®: 0.5 mg [contains phenylalanine 0.14 mg/tablet]
  RisperDAL® M-Tab®: 1 mg [contains phenylalanine 0.28 mg/tablet]
  RisperDAL® M-Tab®: 2 mg [contains phenylalanine 0.42 mg/tablet]
  RisperDAL® M-Tab®: 3 mg [contains phenylalanine 0.63 mg/tablet]
  RisperDAL® M-Tab®: 4 mg [contains phenylalanine 0.84 mg/tablet]

◆ **Ritalin®** see Methylphenidate on page 1247
◆ **Ritalin LA®** see Methylphenidate on page 1247
◆ **Ritalin-SR®** see Methylphenidate on page 1247

Rivaroxaban (riv a ROX a ban)

Medication Safety Issues
High alert medication:
The Institute for Safe Medication Practices (ISMP) includes this medication among its list of drug classes which have a heightened risk of causing significant patient harm when used in error.

Brand Names: U.S. Xarelto®
Brand Names: Canada Xarelto®
Index Terms BAY 59-7939
Pharmacologic Category Factor Xa Inhibitor
Use Postoperative thromboprophylaxis in patients who have undergone hip or knee replacement surgery; prevention of stroke and systemic embolism in patients with nonvalvular atrial fibrillation

Canadian labeling: Additional use (not in U.S. labeling): Treatment of deep vein thrombosis (DVT) without symptomatic pulmonary embolism
Unlabeled Use Symptomatic pulmonary embolism
Medication Guide Available Yes
Contraindications Hypersensitivity to rivaroxaban or any component of the formulation; active pathological bleeding

Canadian labeling: Additional contraindications (not in U.S. labeling): Hepatic disease (including Child-Pugh classes B and C) associated with coagulopathy and clinically relevant bleeding risk; clinically significant active bleeding, including hemorrhagic manifestations and bleeding diathesis; lesions at increased risk of clinically significant bleeding (eg, hemorrhagic or ischemic cerebral infarction) within previous 6 months; spontaneous hemostasis impairment; concomitant systemic treatment with strong CYP3A4 and P-glycoprotein (P-gp) inhibitors

Warnings/Precautions Most common complication is bleeding; major hemorrhages (eg, intracranial, GI, retinal, epidural hematoma, adrenal bleeding) have been reported. Certain patients are at increased risk of bleeding; risk factors include bacterial endocarditis, congenital or acquired bleeding disorders, thrombocytopenia, recent puncture of large vessels or organ biopsy, stroke, intracerebral surgery, or other neuraxial procedure, severe uncontrolled hypertension, renal impairment, recent major surgery, recent major bleeding (intracranial, GI, intraocular, or pulmonary), concomitant use of drugs that affect hemostasis. Monitor for signs and symptoms of bleeding. Prompt clinical evaluation is warranted with any unexplained decrease in hemoglobin or blood pressure. Avoid use with direct thrombin inhibitors (eg, bivalirudin), unfractionated heparin or heparin derivatives, low molecular weight heparins (eg, enoxaparin), aspirin, coumarin derivatives, and sulfinpyrazone. NSAIDs and other platelet aggregation inhibitors (eg, clopidogrel) should be used cautiously.

[U.S. Boxed Warning]: Spinal or epidural hematomas, including subsequent paralysis, may occur with neuraxial anesthesia (epidural or spinal anesthesia) or spinal puncture in patients who are anticoagulated; the risk is increased with concomitant administration of other drugs that affect hemostasis (eg, NSAIDS, platelet inhibitors, other anticoagulants), in patients with a history of traumatic or repeated epidural or spinal punctures, or a history of spinal deformity or surgery. In patients who receive both rivaroxaban and neuraxial anesthesia, avoid removal of epidural catheter for at least 18 hours following last rivaroxaban dose; avoid rivaroxaban administration for at least 6 hours following epidural catheter removal; if traumatic puncture occurs, avoid rivaroxaban administration for at least 24 hours. Monitor for signs of neurologic impairment (eg, numbness/weakness of legs, bowel/bladder dysfunction); prompt diagnosis and treatment are necessary.

[U.S. Boxed Warning]: An increased risk of stroke was noted upon discontinuation of rivaroxaban in clinical trials of patients with atrial fibrillation; consider the addition of alternative anticoagulant therapy when discontinuing rivaroxaban for reasons other than bleeding.

Avoid use in patients with moderate-to-severe hepatic impairment (Child-Pugh classes B and C) or in patients with any hepatic disease associated with coagulopathy; use in this patient population is contraindicated in the Canadian labeling. Use with caution in patients with moderate renal impairment (Cl_{cr} 30-49 mL/minute) when used for postoperative thromboprophylaxis including patients receiving concomitant drug therapy that may increase rivaroxaban systemic exposure and those with deteriorating renal function. Monitor for any signs or symptoms of blood loss. Avoid use in severe renal impairment (postoperative thromboprophylaxis: Cl_{cr} <30 mL/minute; nonvalvular atrial fibrillation: Cl_{cr} <15 mL/minute); discontinue use in patients who develop acute renal failure.

Concomitant use with combined P-gp and strong CYP3A4 inducers should be avoided. Concomitant use with combined P-gp and strong CYP3A4 inhibitors should be avoided; concurrent use is contraindicated in the Canadian labeling. In patients with renal impairment, concomitant use of rivaroxaban with combined P-gp and weak or moderate CYP3A4 inhibitors should only occur if the potential benefit outweighs the risk of bleeding. Formulation contains lactose; use is not recommended in patients with lactose or galactose intolerance (eg, Lapp lactase deficiency, glucose-galactose malabsorption).

Discontinue rivaroxaban at least 24 hours prior to surgery/invasive procedures; reinitiate when adequate hemostasis has been achieved unless oral therapy cannot be administered then consider administration of a parenteral anticoagulant.

Adverse Reactions (Reflective of adult population; not specific for elderly) 1% to 10%:

Cardiovascular: Peripheral edema (2%)

Central nervous system: Headache (3% to 5%), pyrexia (1% to 3%), dizziness (1% to 2%), fatigue (1%), syncope (1%)

Dermatologic: Bruising (3%), pruritus (≤2%), rash (1% to 2%), blister (1%)

Gastrointestinal: Constipation (1% to 3%), diarrhea (1% to 3%), abdominal pain (≤2%), nausea (1% to 3%), dyspepsia (1%), vomiting (1%)

Genitourinary: Hematuria (2%)

Hematologic: Bleeding (atrial fibrillation: 21% [major: 6%]; DVT prophylaxis: 6% [major: <1%]; DVT treatment: 6% to 8% [major: 1%]), thrombocytopenia (<100,000/mm^3 or <50% baseline: 3%), hematoma (1% to 2%), anemia (≤2%)

Hepatic: GGT increased (>3 times ULN: 7%), ALT increased (>3 times ULN: 3%), AST increased (>3 times ULN: 3%), bilirubin increase (>1.5 times ULN: 3%)

Local: Wound secretion (3%)

Neuromuscular & skeletal: Extremity pain (2% to 5%), muscle spasm (1%)

Respiratory: Epistaxis (4% to 5%), hemoptysis (≤1%)

Drug Interactions

Metabolism/Transport Effects Substrate of CYP3A4 (major), P-glycoprotein; **Note:** Assignment of Major/Minor substrate status based on clinically relevant drug interaction potential

Avoid Concomitant Use

Avoid concomitant use of Rivaroxaban with any of the following: Anticoagulants; CYP3A4 Inducers (Strong); CYP3A4 Inhibitors (Strong); St Johns Wort

Increased Effect/Toxicity

Rivaroxaban may increase the levels/effects of: Collagenase (Systemic); Dabigatran Etexilate; Deferasirox; Ibritumomab; Tositumomab and Iodine I 131 Tositumomab

The levels/effects of Rivaroxaban may be increased by: Anticoagulants; Antiplatelet Agents; Azithromycin; Azithromycin (Systemic); Clarithromycin; CYP3A4 Inhibitors (Strong); Dasatinib; Diltiazem; Erythromycin; Erythromycin (Systemic); Herbs (Anticoagulant/Antiplatelet Properties); Nonsteroidal Anti-Inflammatory Agents; Pentosan Polysulfate Sodium; P-glycoprotein/ABCB1 Inhibitors; Prostacyclin Analogues; Salicylates; Thrombolytic Agents; Tipranavir; Verapamil

Decreased Effect

The levels/effects of Rivaroxaban may be decreased by: CYP3A4 Inducers (Strong); Deferasirox; P-glycoprotein/ABCB1 Inducers; St Johns Wort; Tocilizumab

Ethanol/Nutrition/Herb Interactions

Food: Grapefruit juice may increase levels/effects of rivaroxaban; use caution.

Herb/Nutraceutical: Avoid concomitant use of St John's wort if possible (may decrease levels/effects of rivaroxaban; use with caution and consider dosage adjustment of rivaroxaban if concomitant use cannot be avoided).

Stability Store at 25°C (77°F); excursions permitted to 15°C to 30°C (59°F to 86°F).

Mechanism of Action Inhibits platelet activation and fibrin clot formation via direct, selective and reversible inhibition of factor Xa (FXa) in both the intrinsic and extrinsic coagulation pathways. FXa, as part of the prothrombinase complex consisting also of factor Va, calcium ions, factor II and phospholipid, catalyzes the conversion of prothrombin to thrombin. Thrombin both activates platelets and catalyzes the conversion of fibrinogen to fibrin.

Pharmacodynamics/Kinetics

Absorption: Rapid

Distribution: V_{dss}: ~50 L

Protein binding: ~92% to 95% (primarily to albumin)

Metabolism: Hepatic via CYP3A4/5 and CYP2J2

Bioavailability: Absolute bioavailability: 10 mg dose: ~80% to 100%; 20 mg dose: ~66% (fasting; increased with food)

Half-life elimination: Terminal: 5-9 hours; Elderly: 11-13 hours

Time to peak, plasma: 2-4 hours

Excretion: Urine (66% primarily via active tubular secretion [36% as unchanged drug; 30% as inactive metabolites]); feces (28% [7% as unchanged drug; 21% as inactive metabolites])

Dosage

Geriatric & Adult Note: Extremes of body weight (<50 kg or >120 kg) did not significantly influence rivaroxaban exposure (Kubitza, 2007). Clinical outcomes in postoperative thromboprophylaxis trials were also not affected by weight (range: 37-190 kg) (Turpie, 2011).

DVT (without symptomatic pulmonary embolism) (Canadian labeling; EINSTEIN Investigators, 2010; unlabeled use in U.S.): Oral: Initial: 15 mg twice daily for 3 weeks followed by 20 mg once daily. Continue treatment for at least 3 months if first episode of provoked DVT (ie, secondary to transient risk factors) and for at least 6 months if first episode of unprovoked DVT. **Note:** The American College of Chest Physicians (ACCP) recommends anticoagulant treatment for 3 months in patients with provoked DVT or ≥3 months with unprovoked DVT (duration depends on bleeding risk) (Guyatt, 2012).

Nonvalvular atrial fibrillation (to prevent stroke and systemic embolism): Oral: 20 mg once daily

Conversion from warfarin: Discontinue warfarin and initiate rivaroxaban as soon as INR falls to <3.0 (U.S. labeling) or ≤2.5 (Canadian labeling)

Conversion to warfarin: **Note:** Rivaroxaban affects INR; therefore, initial INR measurements after initiating warfarin may be unreliable.

U.S. labeling: Initiate warfarin and a parenteral anticoagulant 24 hours after discontinuation of rivaroxaban (other approaches to conversion may be acceptable).

Canadian labeling: Continue rivaroxaban concomitantly with warfarin until INR ≥2.0 and then discontinue rivaroxaban. **Note:** Caution must be employed with this strategy given the lack of an antidote for rivaroxaban reversal. During concomitant therapy, measure INR daily at least 24 hours after previous rivaroxaban dose and just prior to the next scheduled rivaroxaban dose.

Conversion from continuous infusion unfractionated heparin: Initiate rivaroxaban at the time of heparin discontinuation

Conversion to continuous infusion unfractionated heparin: Initiate continuous infusion unfractionated heparin 24 hours after discontinuation of rivaroxaban

Conversion from anticoagulants (other than warfarin and continuous infusion unfractionated heparin): Discontinue current anticoagulant and initiate rivaroxaban ≤2 hours prior to the next regularly scheduled evening dose of the discontinued anticoagulant.

Conversion to other anticoagulants (other than warfarin): Initiate the anticoagulant 24 hours after discontinuation of rivaroxaban

Postoperative thromboprophylaxis: Oral: **Note:** Initiate therapy after hemostasis has been established, 6-10 hours postoperatively.

Knee replacement: 10 mg once daily; recommended total duration of therapy: 12-14 days; ACCP recommendation: Minimum of 10-14 days; extended duration of up to 35 days suggested (Guyatt, 2012).

Hip replacement: 10 mg once daily; total duration of therapy: 35 days; ACCP recommendation: Minimum of 10-14 days; extended duration of up to 35 days suggested (Guyatt, 2012).

Pulmonary embolism, symptomatic (unlabeled use): Oral: 15 mg twice daily for 3 weeks, followed by 20 mg once daily (The EINSTEIN-PE Investigators, 2012)

Renal Impairment Note: Clinical trials evaluating safety and efficacy utilized the Cockcroft-Gault formula with the use of actual body weight (data on file; Janssen Pharmaceuticals Inc, 2012).

DVT treatment: Canadian labeling (not in U.S. labeling):

Cl_{cr} ≥50 mL/minute: No dosage adjustment necessary.

Cl_{cr} 30-49 mL/minute: 15 mg twice daily for 3 weeks then 15 mg once daily.

Cl_{cr} <30 mL/minute: Avoid use.

Nonvalvular atrial fibrillation:

U.S. labeling:

Cl_{cr} >50 mL/minute: No dosage adjustment necessary.

Cl_{cr} 15-50 mL/minute: 15 mg once daily

Cl_{cr} <15 mL/minute: Avoid use.

ESRD requiring hemodialysis: Avoid use.

Canadian labeling:

Cl_{cr} ≥50 mL/minute: No dosage adjustment necessary.

Cl_{cr} 30-49 mL/minute: 15 mg once daily

Cl_{cr} <30 mL/minute: Avoid use.

Postoperative thromboprophylaxis:

Cl_{cr} >50 mL/minute: No dosage adjustment necessary.

Cl_{cr} 30-50 mL/minute: No dosage adjustment provided in manufacturer's labeling; use with caution.

Cl_{cr} <30 mL/minute: Avoid use.

ESRD requiring hemodialysis: Avoid use.

Hepatic Impairment

Mild hepatic impairment: No dosage adjustment provided in manufacturer's labeling. Limited data indicates pharmacokinetics and pharmacodynamic response were similar to healthy subjects.

Moderate-to-severe hepatic impairment (Child-Pugh class B or C) and patients with any hepatic disease associated with coagulopathy: Avoid use. **Note:** The Canadian labeling contraindicates use in these patient populations.

Administration Administer doses ≥15 mg/day with food; dose of 10 mg/day may be administered without regard to meals.

A decrease in the AUC and C_{max} (29% and 56%, respectively) was observed when rivaroxaban was delivered to the proximal small intestine; further decreases may be seen with delivery to the distal small intestine or ascending colon. Avoid administering via a feeding tube that delivers the rivaroxaban directly into the small intestine or ascending colon.

Patients receiving once-daily dosing and who miss a dose should take a dose as soon as possible on the same day, and then resume therapy the following day as previously taken. Canadian labeling recommends patients receiving twice-daily dosing (DVT treatment) and who miss a dose, should take a dose as soon as possible or if necessary, take both doses at the same time. Patients should resume twice daily dosing the following day.

Monitoring Parameters Routine monitoring of coagulation tests not required; in major clinical trials, monitoring of aPTT, PT/INR, or antifactor Xa levels did not occur. Measurement of prothrombin time (PT) (not intended to be used for dosage adjustment) may be used to detect presence of rivaroxaban (correlates well with rivaroxaban concentrations) (Kubitza, 2005); therapeutic PT range has not been defined and dosage adjustment based on PT results has not been established; CBC with differential, renal function, hepatic function

Test Interactions Prolongs activated partial thromboplastin time (aPTT), HepTest®, and Russell viper venom time

Special Geriatric Considerations Greater than 50% of patients in the RECORD trials were ≥65 years; 15% were >75 years of age. Efficacy was found to be similar in younger and older patients. Rivaroxaban's mean AUC was found to be 52% greater in older men and 39% greater in older women compared to their younger counterparts. The mean AUC was 41% greater in persons >75 years of age. Rivaroxaban's half-life in older adults was 11-13 hours. These pharmacokinetic differences are thought to be due to decreased renal clearance.

Dosage Forms Excipient information presented when available (limited, particularly for generics); consult specific product labeling.
Tablet, oral:
Xarelto®: 10 mg, 15 mg, 20 mg

Rivastigmine (ri va STIG meen)

Brand Names: U.S. Exelon®
Brand Names: Canada Apo-Rivastigmine®; Exelon®; Mylan-Rivastigmine; Novo-Rivastigmine; PMS-Rivastigmine; ratio-Rivastigmine; Sandoz-Rivastigmine
Index Terms ENA 713; Rivastigmine Tartrate; SDZ ENA 713
Generic Availability (U.S.) Yes: Capsule
Pharmacologic Category Acetylcholinesterase Inhibitor (Central)
Use Treatment of mild-to-moderate dementia associated with Alzheimer's disease or Parkinson's disease
Unlabeled Use Severe dementia associated with Alzheimer's disease; Lewy body dementia
Contraindications Hypersensitivity to rivastigmine, other carbamate derivatives (eg, neostigmine, pyridostigmine, physostigmine), or any component of the formulation

Canadian labeling: Additional contraindications (not in U.S. labeling): Severe hepatic impairment

Warnings/Precautions Significant nausea, vomiting, anorexia, and weight loss are associated with use; occurs more frequently in women and during the titration phase. Nausea and/or vomiting may be severe, particularly at doses higher than recommended. Monitor weight during therapy. Therapy should be initiated at lowest dose and titrated; if treatment is interrupted for more than several days, reinstate at the lowest daily dose. Cholinesterase inhibitors may have vagotonic effects which may cause bradycardia and/or heart block with or without a history of cardiac disease. Alzheimer's treatment guidelines consider bradycardia to be a relative contraindication for use of centrally-active cholinesterase inhibitors. Postmarket cases of overdose (including a few fatalities) have been reported in association with medication errors/improper use of rivastigmine transdermal patches. No more than 1 patch should be applied daily and existing patch must be removed prior to applying new patch.

Use caution in patients with a history of peptic ulcer disease or concurrent NSAID use. Use caution in patients undergoing anesthesia who will receive succinylcholine-type muscle relaxation, patients with sick-sinus syndrome, bradycardia or supraventricular conduction conditions, urinary obstruction, seizure disorders, or pulmonary conditions such as asthma or COPD. May exacerbate or induce extrapyramidal symptoms; worsening of symptoms (eg, tremor) in patients with Parkinson's disease has been observed. May cause dizziness or fatigue; caution patients in regards to driving or operating machinery. Use with caution in patients with low body weight (<50 kg) due to increased risk of adverse reactions.

Adverse Reactions (Reflective of adult population; not specific for elderly) Note: Many concentration-related effects are reported at a lower frequency by transdermal route.

>10%:
  Central nervous system: Dizziness (2% to 21%), headache (3% to 17%)
  Gastrointestinal: Nausea (7% to 47%), vomiting (6% to 31%), diarrhea (5% to 19%), anorexia (3% to 17%), abdominal pain (1% to 13%)

1% to 10%:
  Cardiovascular: Syncope (3%), hypertension (3%)
  Central nervous system: Fatigue (2% to 9%), insomnia (1% to 9%), confusion (8%), depression (4% to 6%), anxiety (2% to 5%), malaise (5%), somnolence (4% to 5%), hallucinations (4%), aggressiveness (3%), parkinsonism symptoms worsening (2% to 3%), vertigo (≤2%), agitation (>1%), paranoia (>1%)
  Gastrointestinal: Dyspepsia (9%), constipation (5%), flatulence (4%), weight loss (3% to 8%), eructation (2%), dehydration (2%)
  Genitourinary: Urinary tract infection (1% to 7%)
  Neuromuscular & skeletal: Weakness (2% to 6%), tremor (1%; up to 10% in Parkinson's patients), back pain (>1%)
  Respiratory: Rhinitis (4%)
  Miscellaneous: Accidental trauma (10%), diaphoresis (4%), flu-like syndrome (3%)

Drug Interactions
  Metabolism/Transport Effects None known.
  Avoid Concomitant Use There are no known interactions where it is recommended to avoid concomitant use.
  Increased Effect/Toxicity
    Rivastigmine may increase the levels/effects of: Antipsychotics; Beta-Blockers; Cholinergic Agonists; Succinylcholine

    The levels/effects of Rivastigmine may be increased by: Corticosteroids (Systemic)
  Decreased Effect
    Rivastigmine may decrease the levels/effects of: Anticholinergics; Neuromuscular-Blocking Agents (Nondepolarizing)

    The levels/effects of Rivastigmine may be decreased by: Anticholinergics; Dipyridamole

Ethanol/Nutrition/Herb Interactions
  Smoking: Nicotine increases the clearance of rivastigmine by 23%.
  Ethanol: Avoid ethanol (due to risk of sedation; may increase GI irritation).
  Food: Food delays absorption by 90 minutes, lowers C_{max} by 30% and increases AUC by 30%.
  Herb/Nutraceutical: Avoid ginkgo biloba (may increase cholinergic effects).

Stability
  Oral: Store at 15°C to 30°C (59°F to 86°F); do not freeze. Store solution in an upright position.
  Transdermal patch: Store at 15°C to 30°C (59°F to 86°F). Patches should be kept in sealed pouch until use.

Mechanism of Action A deficiency of cortical acetylcholine is thought to account for some of the symptoms of Alzheimer's disease and the dementia of Parkinson's disease; rivastigmine increases acetylcholine in the central nervous system through reversible inhibition of its hydrolysis by cholinesterase

Pharmacodynamics/Kinetics
  Duration: Anticholinesterase activity (CSF): ~10 hours (6 mg oral dose)
  Absorption: Oral: Fasting: Rapid and complete within 1 hour
  Distribution: V_d: 1.8-2.7 L/kg; penetrates blood-brain barrier (CSF levels are ~40% of plasma levels following oral administration)
  Protein binding: 40%
  Metabolism: Extensively via cholinesterase-mediated hydrolysis in the brain; metabolite undergoes N-demethylation and/or sulfate conjugation hepatically; CYP minimally involved; linear kinetics at 3 mg twice daily, but nonlinear at higher doses
  Bioavailability: Oral: 36% to 40%
  Half-life elimination: Oral: 1.5 hours; Transdermal patch: 3 hours (after removal)
  Time to peak: Oral: 1 hour; Transdermal patch: 10-16 hours following first dose
  Excretion: Urine (97% as metabolites); feces (0.4%)

Dosage

Geriatric Following oral administration, clearance is significantly lower in patients >60 years of age, but dosage adjustments are not recommended. Age was not associated with exposure in patients treated transdermally. Titrate dose to individual's tolerance. Refer to adult dosing. **Note:** Canadian labeling recommends an initial oral dose of 1.5 mg/day in patients >85 years of age (with low body weight [<50 kg] or serious comorbidities, with a slower titration rate than used for adults.

Adult Note: Exelon® oral solution and capsules are bioequivalent.

Mild-to-moderate Alzheimer's dementia:

Oral: Initial: 1.5 mg twice daily; may increase by 3 mg/day (1.5 mg/dose) every 2 weeks based on tolerability (maximum recommended dose: 6 mg twice daily)

Note: If GI adverse events occur, discontinue treatment for several doses then restart at the same or next lower dosage level; antiemetics have been used to control GI symptoms. If treatment is interrupted for longer than several days, restart the treatment at the lowest dose and titrate as previously described.

Transdermal patch: Initial: 4.6 mg/24 hours; if well tolerated, may be increased (after at least 4 weeks) to 9.5 mg/24 hours (recommended effective dose). Maintenance: 9.5 mg/24 hours (maximum dose: 9.5 mg/24 hours).

Note: If intolerance is noted (nausea, vomiting), patch should be removed and treatment interrupted for several days and restarted at the same or lower dosage. If interrupted for more than 3 days, reinitiate at lowest dosage and increase to maintenance dose after 4 weeks.

Conversion from oral therapy: If oral daily dose <6 mg, switch to 4.6 mg/24 hours patch; if oral daily dose 6-12 mg, switch to 9.5 mg/24 hours patch. Apply patch on the next day following last oral dose.

Mild-to-moderate Parkinson's-related dementia:

Oral: Initial: 1.5 mg twice daily; may increase by 3 mg/day (1.5 mg/dose) every 4 weeks based on tolerability (maximum recommended dose: 6 mg twice daily)

Transdermal patch: See transdermal dosing for Alzheimer's dementia.

Renal Impairment

U.S. labeling: No dosage adjustment provided in manufacturer's labeling; however, the dose should be titrated to the individual's tolerance.

Canadian labeling:

Oral: Initial dose: 1.5 mg once daily; titrate dose at a rate slower than recommended for healthy adults

Transdermal: No dosage adjustment provided in manufacturer's labeling; titrate dose cautiously (has not been studied).

Hepatic Impairment

U.S. labeling: No dosage adjustment provided in manufacturer's labeling; clearance is reduced in mildly- to moderately-impaired patients. Dose should be titrated to the individual's tolerance.

Canadian labeling:

Oral: Initial dose: 1.5 mg once daily; titrate dose at a rate slower than recommended for healthy adults

Transdermal: No dosage adjustment provided in manufacturer's labeling; titrate dose cautiously

Administration

Oral: Should be administered with meals (breakfast or dinner). Capsule should be swallowed whole. Liquid form, which is available for patients who cannot swallow capsules, can be swallowed directly from syringe or mixed with water, soda, or cold fruit juice. Stir well and drink within 4 hours of mixing.

Topical: Apply transdermal patch to upper or lower back (alternatively, may apply to upper arm or chest). Avoid reapplication to same spot of skin for 14 days (may rotate sections of back, for example). Do not apply to red, irritated, or broken skin. Avoid areas of recent application of lotion or powder. After removal, fold patch to press adhesive surfaces together, and discard. Avoid eye contact; wash hands after handling patch. Replace patch every 24 hours. Avoid exposing the patch to external sources of heat (eg, sauna, excessive light) for prolonged periods of time. No more than 1 patch should be applied daily and existing patch must be removed prior to applying new patch.

Monitoring Parameters Cognitive function at periodic intervals, symptoms of GI intolerance, weight

Special Geriatric Considerations Titrate dose to tolerance.

◀ **Dosage Forms** Excipient information presented when available (limited, particularly for generics); consult specific product labeling.
Capsule, oral: 1.5 mg, 3 mg, 4.5 mg, 6 mg
  Exelon®: 1.5 mg, 3 mg, 4.5 mg, 6 mg
Patch, transdermal:
  Exelon®: 4.6 mg/24 hours (30s) [5 cm^2; total rivastigmine 9 mg]
  Exelon®: 9.5 mg/24 hours (30s) [10 cm^2; total rivastigmine 18 mg]
Solution, oral:
  Exelon®: 2 mg/mL (120 mL) [contains sodium benzoate]

♦ **Rivastigmine Tartrate** see Rivastigmine on page 1719

Rizatriptan (rye za TRIP tan)

Brand Names: U.S. Maxalt-MLT®; Maxalt®
Brand Names: Canada CO Rizatriptan ODT; JAMP-Rizatriptan; Maxalt RPD™; Maxalt™; Sandoz-Rizatriptan ODT
Index Terms MK462
Generic Availability (U.S.) No
Pharmacologic Category Antimigraine Agent; Serotonin 5-HT$_{1B, 1D}$ Receptor Agonist
Use Acute treatment of migraine with or without aura
Contraindications Hypersensitivity to rizatriptan or any component of the formulation; documented ischemic heart disease or other significant cardiovascular disease; coronary artery vasospasm (including Prinzmetal's angina); history of stroke or transient ischemic attack; peripheral vascular disease; ischemic bowel disease; uncontrolled hypertension; basilar or hemiplegic migraine; during or within 2 weeks of MAO inhibitors; during or within 24 hours of treatment with another 5-HT$_1$ agonist, or an ergot-containing or ergot-type medication (eg, methysergide, dihydroergotamine)
Warnings/Precautions Only indicated for treatment of acute migraine; not for the prevention of migraines or the treatment of cluster headache. If a patient does not respond to the first dose, the diagnosis of migraine should be reconsidered. Coronary artery vasospasm, transient ischemia, myocardial infarction, ventricular tachycardia/fibrillation, cardiac arrest, and death have been reported with 5-HT$_1$ agonist administration. Patients who experience sensations of chest pain/pressure/tightness or symptoms suggestive of angina following dosing should be evaluated for coronary artery disease or Prinzmetal's angina before receiving additional doses; if dosing is resumed and similar symptoms recur, monitor with ECG. Should not be given to patients who have risk factors for CAD (eg, hypertension, hypercholesterolemia, smoker, obesity, diabetes, strong family history of CAD, menopause, male >40 years of age) without adequate cardiac evaluation. Patients with suspected CAD should have cardiovascular evaluation to rule out CAD before considering use; if cardiovascular evaluation is "satisfactory," first dose should be given in the healthcare provider's office (consider ECG monitoring). Periodic evaluation of cardiovascular status should be done in all patients. Significant elevation in blood pressure, including hypertensive crisis, has also been reported on rare occasions in patients with and without a history of hypertension. Cerebral/subarachnoid hemorrhage, stroke, peripheral vascular ischemia, gastrointestinal ischemia/infarction, splenic infarction and Raynaud's syndrome have been reported with 5-HT$_1$ agonist administration. Use is contraindicated in patients with a history of stroke or transient ischemic attack. Rarely, partial vision loss and blindness (transient and permanent) have been reported with 5-HT$_1$ agonists.

Use with caution in elderly or patients with hepatic or renal impairment (including dialysis patients). Symptoms of agitation, confusion, hallucinations, hyper-reflexia, myoclonus, shivering, and tachycardia may occur with concomitant proserotonergic drugs (eg, SSRIs/SNRIs or triptans) or agents which reduce rizatriptan's metabolism. Concurrent use of serotonin precursors (eg, tryptophan) is not recommended. If concomitant administration with SSRIs is warranted, monitor closely, especially at initiation and with dose increases. Overuse of medications for acute migraine, including 5-HT$_1$ agonists, may lead to headache exacerbation. Maxalt-MLT® tablets contain phenylalanine.
Adverse Reactions (Reflective of adult population; not specific for elderly) 1% to 10%:
Cardiovascular: Chest pain (<2% to 3%), flushing (>1%), palpitation (>1%)
Central nervous system: Dizziness (4% to 9%), somnolence (4% to 8%), fatigue (adults 4% to 7%; children >1%), pain (3%), headache (≤2%), euphoria (>1%), hypoesthesia (>1%)
Dermatologic: Skin flushing
Gastrointestinal: Nausea (4% to 6%), xerostomia (3%), abdominal discomfort (children >1%), diarrhea (>1%), vomiting (>1%)
Neuromuscular & skeletal: Weakness (4% to 7%), paresthesia (3% to 4%); neck, throat, and jaw pain/tightness/pressure (≤2%), tremor (>1%)

Respiratory: Dyspnea (>1%)
Miscellaneous: Feeling of heaviness (<1% to 2%)

Drug Interactions
Metabolism/Transport Effects None known.
Avoid Concomitant Use
Avoid concomitant use of Rizatriptan with any of the following: Ergot Derivatives; MAO Inhibitors
Increased Effect/Toxicity
Rizatriptan may increase the levels/effects of: Ergot Derivatives; Metoclopramide; Serotonin Modulators

The levels/effects of Rizatriptan may be increased by: Antipsychotics; Ergot Derivatives; MAO Inhibitors; Propranolol
Decreased Effect There are no known significant interactions involving a decrease in effect.
Ethanol/Nutrition/Herb Interactions Food: Food delays absorption.
Stability Store at room temperature of 15°C to 30°C (59°F to 86°F); orally disintegrating tablets should be stored in blister pack until administration.
Mechanism of Action Selective agonist for serotonin (5-HT$_{1B}$ and 5-HT$_{1D}$ receptors) in cranial arteries; causes vasoconstriction and reduces sterile inflammation associated with antidromic neuronal transmission correlating with relief of migraine

Pharmacodynamics/Kinetics
Onset of action: Most patients have response to treatment within 2 hours
Distribution: V$_d$: Females: 110 L; Males 140 L
Protein binding: 14%
Metabolism: Via monoamine oxidase-A; forms metabolites; significant first-pass metabolism
Bioavailability: ~45%
Half-life elimination: 2-3 hours
Time to peak: Maxalt®: 1-1.5 hours (delayed up to 0.7 hour with Maxalt-MLT®)
Excretion: Urine (82%, 14% as unchanged drug); feces (12%)

Dosage
Geriatric & Adult Note: In patients with risk factors for coronary artery disease, following adequate evaluation to establish the absence of coronary artery disease, the initial dose should be administered in a setting where response may be evaluated (physician's office or similarly staffed setting). ECG monitoring may be considered.

Migraine: Oral: 5-10 mg, repeat after 2 hours if significant relief is not attained; maximum: 30 mg/24 hours
Dose adjustment with concomitant propranolol therapy: 5 mg/dose (maximum: 15 mg/24 hours)

Renal Impairment No dosage adjustment provided in manufacturer's labeling; however, the AUC was 44% greater in patients on hemodialysis.
Hepatic Impairment No dosage adjustment provided in manufacturer's labeling; however, plasma concentrations are increased by 30% in patients with moderate hepatic dysfunction.
Administration May be administered with or without food. For orally-disintegrating tablets (Maxalt-MLT®), patient should be instructed to place tablet on tongue and allow to dissolve. Dissolved tablet will be swallowed with saliva.
Monitoring Parameters Headache severity, signs/symptoms suggestive of angina; consider monitoring blood pressure, heart rate, and/or ECG with first dose in patients with likelihood of unrecognized coronary disease, such as patients with significant hypertension, hypercholesterolemia, obese patients, patients with diabetes, smokers with other risk factors or strong family history of coronary artery disease
Special Geriatric Considerations Since the elderly often have cardiovascular disease, careful evaluation of the use of 5-HT agonists is needed to avoid complications with the use of these agents. The pharmacokinetic disposition of these agents is similar to that seen in younger adults.
Dosage Forms Excipient information presented when available (limited, particularly for generics); consult specific product labeling.
Tablet, oral:
  Maxalt®: 5 mg, 10 mg
Tablet, orally disintegrating, oral:
  Maxalt-MLT®: 5 mg [contains phenylalanine 1.05 mg/tablet; peppermint flavor]
  Maxalt-MLT®: 10 mg [contains phenylalanine 2.1 mg/tablet; peppermint flavor]

◆ **R-modafinil** *see* Armodafinil *on page 147*
◆ **RoActemra®** *see* Tocilizumab *on page 1918*
◆ **Robafen [OTC]** *see* GuaiFENesin *on page 904*
◆ **Robafen AC** *see* Guaifenesin and Codeine *on page 906*
◆ **Robafen Cough [OTC]** *see* Dextromethorphan *on page 525*

- **Robafen DM [OTC]** *see* Guaifenesin and Dextromethorphan *on page 906*
- **Robafen DM Clear [OTC]** *see* Guaifenesin and Dextromethorphan *on page 906*
- **Robaxin®** *see* Methocarbamol *on page 1234*
- **Robaxin®-750** *see* Methocarbamol *on page 1234*
- **Robinul®** *see* Glycopyrrolate *on page 892*
- **Robinul® Forte** *see* Glycopyrrolate *on page 892*
- **Robitussin AC** *see* Guaifenesin and Codeine *on page 906*
- **Robitussin® Children's Cough Long-Acting [OTC]** *see* Dextromethorphan *on page 525*
- **Robitussin® CoughGels™ Long-Acting [OTC] [DSC]** *see* Dextromethorphan *on page 525*
- **Robitussin® Cough Long Acting [OTC] [DSC]** *see* Dextromethorphan *on page 525*
- **Robitussin® Lingering Cold Long-Acting Cough [OTC]** *see* Dextromethorphan *on page 525*
- **Robitussin® Lingering Cold Long-Acting CoughGels® [OTC]** *see* Dextromethorphan *on page 525*
- **Robitussin® Peak Cold Cough + Chest Congestion DM [OTC]** *see* Guaifenesin and Dextromethorphan *on page 906*
- **Robitussin® Peak Cold Maximum Strength Cough + Chest Congestion DM [OTC]** *see* Guaifenesin and Dextromethorphan *on page 906*
- **Robitussin® Peak Cold Nasal Relief [OTC]** *see* Acetaminophen and Phenylephrine *on page 37*
- **Robitussin® Peak Cold Sugar-Free Cough + Chest Congestion DM [OTC]** *see* Guaifenesin and Dextromethorphan *on page 906*
- **Rocaltrol®** *see* Calcitriol *on page 256*
- **Rocephin®** *see* CefTRIAXone *on page 332*
- **Rolaids® Extra Strength [OTC]** *see* Calcium Carbonate *on page 262*

ROPINIRole (roe PIN i role)

Related Information
Antiparkinsonian Agents *on page 2101*

Medication Safety Issues
Sound-alike/look-alike issues:
Requip® may be confused with Reglan®
ROPINIRole may be confused with RisperDAL®, risperiDONE, ropivacaine

Brand Names: U.S. Requip®; Requip® XL™

Brand Names: Canada CO Ropinirole; JAMP-Ropinirole; PMS-Ropinirole; RAN™-Ropinirole; Requip®

Index Terms Ropinirole Hydrochloride

Generic Availability (U.S.) Yes

Pharmacologic Category Anti-Parkinson's Agent, Dopamine Agonist

Use Treatment of idiopathic Parkinson's disease; in patients with early Parkinson's disease who were not receiving concomitant levodopa therapy as well as in patients with advanced disease on concomitant levodopa; treatment of moderate-to-severe primary Restless Legs Syndrome (RLS)

Contraindications Hypersensitivity to ropinirole or any component of the formulation

Warnings/Precautions Syncope, sometimes associated with bradycardia, was observed in association with ropinirole in both early Parkinson's disease (without levodopa) patients and advanced Parkinson's disease (with levodopa) patients. Dopamine agonists appear to impair the systemic regulation of blood pressure resulting in postural hypotension, especially during dose escalation. Parkinson's disease patients appear to have an impaired capacity to respond to a postural challenge; use with caution in patients at risk of hypotension (ie, those receiving antihypertensive or antiarrhythmic drugs) or where transient hypotensive episodes would be poorly tolerated (cardiovascular disease or cerebrovascular disease). Parkinson's patients being treated with dopaminergic agonists ordinarily require careful monitoring for signs and symptoms of postural hypotension, especially during dose escalation, and should be informed of this risk.

May cause hallucinations (dose dependent); risk may be increased in the elderly. Use with caution in patients with pre-existing dyskinesia, hepatic or severe renal dysfunction (use in patients with severe renal impairment and who are not undergoing regular hemodialysis is not recommended in the Canadian labeling). Avoid use in patients with a major psychotic disorder; may exacerbate psychosis.

Patients treated with ropinirole have reported falling asleep while engaging in activities of daily living; this has been reported to occur without significant warning signs. Monitor for daytime somnolence or pre-existing sleep disorder; caution with concomitant sedating medication;

discontinue if significant daytime sleepiness or episodes of falling asleep occur. Patients must be cautioned about performing tasks which require mental alertness (eg, operating machinery or driving). Use with caution in patients receiving other CNS depressants or psychoactive agents. Effects with other sedative drugs or ethanol may be potentiated.

Dopamine agonists have been associated with compulsive behaviors and/or loss of impulse control, which has manifested as pathological gambling, libido increases (hypersexuality), and/or binge eating. Causality has not been established, and controversy exists as to whether this phenomenon is related to the underlying disease, prior behaviors/addictions and/or drug therapy. Dose reduction or discontinuation of therapy has been reported to reverse these behaviors in some, but not all cases. Risk for melanoma development is increased in Parkinson's disease patients; drug causation or factors contributing to risk have not been established. Patients should be monitored closely and periodic skin examinations should be performed.

Some patients treated for RLS may experience worsening of symptoms in the early morning hours (rebound) or an increase and/or spread of daytime symptoms (augmentation); clinical management of these phenomena has not been evaluated in controlled clinical trials. Pathologic degenerative changes were observed in the retinas of albino rats during studies with this agent, but were not observed in the retinas of albino mice or in other species. The significance of these data for humans remains uncertain.

Other dopaminergic agents have been associated with a syndrome resembling neuroleptic malignant syndrome on withdrawal or significant dosage reduction after long-term use. Risk of fibrotic complications (eg, pleural effusion/fibrosis, interstitial lung disease) and melanoma has been reported in patients receiving ropinirole; drug causation has not been established.

Adverse Reactions (Reflective of adult population; not specific for elderly)
Data inclusive of trials in early Parkinson's disease (without levodopa) and Restless Legs Syndrome:
>10%:
Cardiovascular: Syncope (1% to 12%)
Central nervous system: Somnolence (11% to 40%), dizziness (6% to 40%), fatigue (8% to 11%)
Gastrointestinal: Nausea (immediate release: 40% to 60%; extended release: 19%), vomiting (11% to 12%)
Miscellaneous: Viral infection (11%)
1% to 10%:
Cardiovascular: Dependent/leg edema (2% to 7%), orthostasis (1% to 6%), hypertension (5%), chest pain (4%), flushing (3%), palpitation (3%), peripheral ischemia (2% to 3%), atrial fibrillation (2%), extrasystoles (2%), hypotension (2%), tachycardia (2%)
Central nervous system: Pain (3% to 8%), headache (extended release: 6%), confusion (5%), hallucinations (up to 5%; dose related), hypoesthesia (4%), amnesia (3%), malaise (3%), yawning (3%), concentration impaired (2%), vertigo (2%)
Dermatologic: Hyperhidrosis (3%)
Gastrointestinal: Dyspepsia (4% to 10%), abdominal pain (3% to 7%), constipation (≥5%), xerostomia (3% to 5%), diarrhea (5%), anorexia (4%), flatulence (3%)
Genitourinary: Urinary tract infection (5%), impotence (3%)
Hepatic: Alkaline phosphatase increased (3%)
Neuromuscular & skeletal: Weakness (6%), arthralgia (4%), muscle cramps (3%), paresthesia (3%), hyperkinesia (2%)
Ocular: Abnormal vision (6%), xerophthalmia (2%)
Respiratory: Pharyngitis (6% to 9%), rhinitis (4%), sinusitis (4%), bronchitis (3%), dyspnea (3%), influenza (3%), cough (3%), nasal congestion (2%)
Miscellaneous: Diaphoresis increased (3% to 6%)

Advanced Parkinson's disease (with levodopa):
>10%:
Central nervous system: Dizziness (immediate release: 26%; extended-release: 8%), somnolence (immediate release: 20%, extended release: 17%)
Gastrointestinal: Nausea (immediate release: 30%; extended-release: 11%)
Neuromuscular & skeletal: Dyskinesias (immediate release: 34%; extended-release: 13%; dose related)
1% to 10%:
Cardiovascular: Hypotension (2% to 5%; including orthostatic), peripheral edema (4%), syncope (3%), hypertension (3%; dose related)
Central nervous system: Hallucinations (7% to 10%; dose related), confusion (9%), anxiety (2% to 6%), amnesia (5%), nervousness (5%), pain (5%), vertigo (4%), abnormal dreaming (3%), paresis (3%), aggravated parkinsonism, insomnia

Gastrointestinal: Abdominal pain (6% to 9%), vomiting (7%), constipation (4% to 6%), diarrhea (3% to 5%), xerostomia (2% to 5%), dysphagia (2%), flatulence (2%), salivation increased (2%), weight loss (2%)

Genitourinary: Urinary tract infection (6%), pyuria (2%), urinary incontinence (2%)

Hematologic: Anemia (2%)

Neuromuscular & skeletal: Falls (2% to 10%; dose related), arthralgia (7%), tremor (6%), hypokinesia (5%), paresthesia (5%), arthritis (3%), back pain (3%)

Ocular: Diplopia (2%)

Respiratory: Upper respiratory tract infection (9%), dyspnea (3%)

Miscellaneous: Injury, diaphoresis increased (7%), viral infection, increased drug level (7%)

Other adverse effects (all phase 2/3 trials for Parkinson's disease and Restless Leg Syndrome): ≥1%: Asthma, BUN increased, depression, gastroenteritis, gastrointestinal reflux, irritability, migraine, muscle spasm, myalgia, neck pain, neuralgia, osteoarthritis, pharyngolaryngeal pain, rash, rigors, sleep disorder, tendonitis

Drug Interactions

Metabolism/Transport Effects Substrate of CYP1A2 (major), CYP3A4 (minor); **Note:** Assignment of Major/Minor substrate status based on clinically relevant drug interaction potential; **Inhibits** CYP1A2 (weak), CYP2D6 (weak)

Avoid Concomitant Use There are no known interactions where it is recommended to avoid concomitant use.

Increased Effect/Toxicity

The levels/effects of ROPINIRole may be increased by: Abiraterone Acetate; Ciprofloxacin; Ciprofloxacin (Systemic); CYP1A2 Inhibitors (Moderate); CYP1A2 Inhibitors (Strong); Deferasirox; Estrogen Derivatives; MAO Inhibitors; Methylphenidate

Decreased Effect

ROPINIRole may decrease the levels/effects of: Antipsychotics (Typical)

The levels/effects of ROPINIRole may be decreased by: Antipsychotics (Atypical); Antipsychotics (Typical); CYP1A2 Inducers (Strong); Cyproterone; Metoclopramide; Tocilizumab

Ethanol/Nutrition/Herb Interactions

Ethanol: Avoid ethanol (may increase CNS depression).

Herb/Nutraceutical: Avoid kava kava, gotu kola, valerian, St John's wort (may increase CNS depression).

Stability Store at controlled room temperature of 20°C to 25°C (68°F to 77°F). Protect from light.

Mechanism of Action Ropinirole has a high relative *in vitro* specificity and full intrinsic activity at the D_2 and D_3 dopamine receptor subtypes, binding with higher affinity to D_3 than to D_2 or D_4 receptor subtypes; relevance of D_3 receptor binding in Parkinson's disease is unknown. Ropinirole has moderate *in vitro* affinity for opioid receptors. Ropinirole and its metabolites have negligible *in vitro* affinity for dopamine D_1, $5-HT_1$, $5-HT_2$, benzodiazepine, GABA, muscarinic, alpha$_1$-, alpha$_2$-, and beta-adrenoreceptors. Although precise mechanism of action of ropinirole is unknown, it is believed to be due to stimulation of postsynaptic dopamine D_2-type receptors within the caudate putamen in the brain. Ropinirole caused decreases in systolic and diastolic blood pressure at doses >0.25 mg. The mechanism of ropinirole-induced postural hypotension is believed to be due to D_2-mediated blunting of the noradrenergic response to standing and subsequent decrease in peripheral vascular resistance.

Pharmacodynamics/Kinetics

Absorption: Not affected by food

Distribution: V_d: 525 L

Protein binding: 40%

Metabolism: Extensively hepatic via CYP1A2 to inactive metabolites; first-pass effect

Bioavailability: Absolute: 45% to 55%

Half-life elimination: ~6 hours

Time to peak: Immediate release: ~1-2 hours; Extended release: 6-10 hours; T_{max} increased by 2.5-3 hours when drug taken with food

Excretion: Urine (<10% as unchanged drug, 60% as metabolites)

Clearance: Reduced by 15% to 30% in patients >65 years of age

Dosage

Geriatric Clearance is reduced; however, no dosage adjustment necessary. Titrate dose to clinical response. Refer to adult dosing.

Adult

Parkinson's disease: Oral:

Immediate release tablet: The dosage should be increased to achieve a maximum therapeutic effect, balanced against the principal side effects of nausea, dizziness, somnolence and dyskinesia. Recommended starting dose is 0.25 mg 3 times/day; based on individual patient response, the dosage should be titrated with weekly increments as described below:

- Week 1: 0.25 mg 3 times/day; total daily dose: 0.75 mg
- Week 2: 0.5 mg 3 times/day; total daily dose: 1.5 mg
- Week 3: 0.75 mg 3 times/day; total daily dose: 2.25 mg
- Week 4: 1 mg 3 times/day; total daily dose: 3 mg

   Note: After week 4, if necessary, daily dosage may be increased by 1.5 mg/day on a weekly basis up to a dose of 9 mg/day, and then by up to 3 mg/day weekly to a total of 24 mg/day

Parkinson's disease discontinuation taper: Ropinirole should be gradually tapered over 7 days as follows: reduce frequency of administration from 3 times daily to twice daily for 4 days, then reduce to once daily for remaining 3 days.

Extended release tablet: Initial: 2 mg once daily for 1-2 weeks, followed by increases of 2 mg/day at weekly or longer intervals based on therapeutic response and tolerability (maximum: 24 mg/day); **Note:** When discontinuing gradually taper over 7 days.

Restless legs syndrome: Oral: Immediate release tablets: Initial: 0.25 mg once daily 1-3 hours before bedtime. Dose may be increased after 2 days to 0.5 mg daily, and after 7 days to 1 mg daily. Dose may be further titrated upward in 0.5 mg increments every week until reaching a daily dose of 3 mg during week 6. If symptoms persist or reappear, the daily dose may be increased to a maximum of 4 mg beginning week 7.

   Note: Doses up to 4 mg per day may be discontinued without tapering.

Converting from ropinirole immediate release tablets to ropinirole extended-release tablets: Choose a once daily extended-release dose that most closely matches current immediate-release daily dose.

Renal Impairment

Moderate renal impairment (Cl_{cr} 30-50 mL/minute): No adjustment needed

Severe renal impairment (Cl_{cr} <30 mL/minute): Use with caution; has not been studied in this patient population. **Note:** The Canadian labeling recommends to avoid use in patients with severe renal impairment and who are not undergoing regular hemodialysis.

Hemodialysis: Canadian labeling (not in U.S. labeling): Initial: 0.25 mg 3 times daily; may titrate dose upward based on tolerability and efficacy (maximum dose: 18 mg/day); postdialysis supplemental doses are not required

Hepatic Impairment Titrate with caution; has not been studied.

Administration May be administered with or without food; taking with food may reduce nausea. Swallow extended-release tablet whole; do not crush, split, or chew.

Monitoring Parameters Blood pressure (orthostatic); daytime alertness

Pharmacotherapy Pearls If therapy with a drug known to be a potent inhibitor of CYP1A2 is stopped or started during treatment with ropinirole, adjustment of ropinirole dose may be required. Ropinirole binds to melanin-containing tissues (ie, eyes, skin) in pigmented rats. After a single dose, long-term retention of drug was demonstrated, with a half-life in the eye of 20 days; not known if ropinirole accumulates in these tissues over time.

Special Geriatric Considerations Since the dose is titrated to clinical response, no specific dosage adjustment is necessary in the elderly.

Dosage Forms Excipient information presented when available (limited, particularly for generics); consult specific product labeling.

Tablet, oral: 0.25 mg, 0.5 mg, 1 mg, 2 mg, 3 mg, 4 mg, 5 mg

   Requip®: 0.25 mg, 0.5 mg, 1 mg, 2 mg, 3 mg, 4 mg, 5 mg

Tablet, extended release, oral: 2 mg, 4 mg, 6 mg, 8 mg, 12 mg

   Requip® XL™: 2 mg, 4 mg, 6 mg, 8 mg, 12 mg

◆ **Ropinirole Hydrochloride** *see* ROPINIRole *on page 1724*

◆ **Rosadan™** *see* MetroNIDAZOLE (Topical) *on page 1271*

Rosiglitazone (roh si GLI ta zone)

Related Information
Diabetes Mellitus Management, Adults *on page 2193*

Medication Safety Issues
Sound-alike/look-alike issues:
Avandia® may be confused with Avalide®, Coumadin®, Prandin®
High alert medication:
The Institute for Safe Medication Practices (ISMP) includes this medication among its list of drug classes which have a heightened risk of causing significant patient harm when used in error.
International issues:
Avandia [U.S., Canada, and multiple international markets] may be confused with Avanza brand name for mirtazapine [Australia]

Brand Names: U.S. Avandia®
Brand Names: Canada Avandia®
Generic Availability (U.S.) No
Pharmacologic Category Antidiabetic Agent, Thiazolidinedione
Use Type 2 diabetes mellitus (noninsulin dependent, NIDDM):
Monotherapy: Improve glycemic control as an adjunct to diet and exercise
Note: Canadian labeling approves use as monotherapy only when metformin is contra-indicated or not tolerated.
Combination therapy: **Note:** Use when diet, exercise, and a single agent do not result in adequate glycemic control.
U.S. labeling: In combination with a sulfonylurea, metformin, or sulfonylurea plus metformin
Canadian labeling: In combination with metformin; in combination with a sulfonylurea only when metformin use is contraindicated or not tolerated

Prescribing and Access Restrictions
As a requirement of the REMS program, the prescribing and dispensing of any rosiglitazone-containing medication in the U.S. requires physician and patient enrollment in the Avandia-Rosiglitazone Medicines Access Program™. Complete program details are available at www.avandia.com or by calling the program Coordinating Center at 800-282-6342.

Health Canada requires written informed consent for new and current patients receiving rosiglitazone.

Medication Guide Available Yes
Contraindications
U.S. labeling: NYHA Class III/IV heart failure (initiation of therapy)
Canadian labeling: Hypersensitivity to rosiglitazone or any component of the formulation; any stage of heart failure (eg, NYHA Class I, II, III, IV); serious hepatic impairment

Warnings/Precautions [U.S. Boxed Warning]: Thiazolidinediones, including rosiglitazone, may cause or exacerbate congestive heart failure; closely monitor for signs/symptoms of congestive heart failure (eg, rapid weight gain, dyspnea, edema), particularly after initiation or dose increases. Not recommended for use in any patient with symptomatic heart failure. In the U.S., initiation of therapy is contraindicated in patients with NYHA class III or IV heart failure; in Canada use is contraindicated in patients with any stage of heart failure (NYHA Class I, II, III, IV). Use with caution in patients with edema; may increase plasma volume and/or cause fluid retention, leading to heart failure. Dose-related weight gain observed with use; mechanism unknown but likely associated with fluid retention and fat accumulation. Use may also be associated with an increased risk of angina and MI. Use caution in patients at risk for cardiovascular events and monitor closely. Discontinue if any deterioration in cardiac status occurs.

[U.S. Boxed Warning]: Due to cardiovascular risks, rosiglitazone-containing medications are only available through the Avandia-Rosiglitazone Medicines Access Program™. Patients and prescribers must be registered with and meet conditions of the program. Call 1-800-282-6342 or visit www.avandia.com for more information.

Should not be used in diabetic ketoacidosis. Mechanism requires the presence of insulin; therefore, use in type 1 diabetes (insulin dependent, IDDM) is not recommended. Combination therapy with other hypoglycemic agents may increase risk for hypoglycemic events; dose reduction with the concomitant agent may be warranted. Concomitant use with nitrates is not recommended due to increased risk of myocardial ischemia. Avoid use with insulin due to an increased risk of edema, congestive heart failure, and myocardial ischemic events.

Use with caution in patients with elevated transaminases (AST or ALT); do not initiate in patients with active liver disease or ALT >2.5 times ULN at baseline; evaluate patients with ALT ≤2.5 times ULN at baseline or during therapy for cause of enzyme elevation; during therapy, if ALT >3 times ULN, reevaluate levels promptly and discontinue if elevation persists or if jaundice occurs at any time during use. Idiosyncratic hepatotoxicity has been reported with another thiazolidinedione agent (troglitazone); avoid use in patients who previously experienced jaundice during troglitazone therapy. Monitoring should include periodic determinations of liver function. Increased incidence of bone fractures in females treated with rosiglitazone observed during analysis of long-term trial; majority of fractures occurred in the upper arm, hand, and foot (differing from the hip or spine fractures usually associated with postmenopausal osteoporosis). May decrease hemoglobin/hematocrit and/or WBC count (slight); effects may be related to increased plasma volume and/or dose related; use with caution in patients with anemia.

Rosiglitazone has been associated with new onset and/or worsening of macular edema in patients with diabetes. Rosiglitazone should be used with caution in patients with a pre-existing macular edema or diabetic retinopathy. Discontinuation of rosiglitazone should be considered in any patient who reports visual deterioration. In addition, ophthalmological consultation should be initiated in these patients.

Additional Canadian warnings (not included in U.S. labeling): If glycemic control is inadequate, rosiglitazone may be added to metformin or a sulfonylurea (if metformin use is contraindicated or not tolerated); use of triple therapy (rosiglitazone in combination with both metformin and a sulfonylurea) is not indicated due to increased risks of heart failure and fluid retention.

Adverse Reactions (Reflective of adult population; not specific for elderly) Note: The rate of certain adverse reactions (eg, anemia, edema, hypoglycemia) may be higher with some combination therapies.

>10%: Endocrine & metabolic: HDL-cholesterol increased, LDL-cholesterol increased, total cholesterol increased, weight gain

1% to 10%:
Cardiovascular: Edema (5%), hypertension (4%); heart failure/CHF (up to 2% to 3% in patients receiving insulin; incidence likely higher in patients with pre-existing HF; myocardial ischemia (3%; incidence likely higher in patients with preexisting CAD)

Central nervous system: Headache (6%)

Endocrine & metabolic: Hypoglycemia (1% to 3%; combination therapy with insulin: 12% to 14%)

Gastrointestinal: Diarrhea (3%)

Hematologic: Anemia (2%)

Neuromuscular & skeletal: Fractures (up to 9%; incidence greater in females; usually upper arm, hand, or foot), arthralgia (5%), back pain (4% to 5%)

Respiratory: Upper respiratory tract infection (4% to 10%), nasopharyngitis (6%)

Miscellaneous: Injury (8%)

Drug Interactions

Metabolism/Transport Effects Substrate of CYP2C8 (major), CYP2C9 (minor); **Note:** Assignment of Major/Minor substrate status based on clinically relevant drug interaction potential; **Inhibits** CYP2C19 (weak), CYP2C8 (moderate), CYP2C9 (weak)

Avoid Concomitant Use There are no known interactions where it is recommended to avoid concomitant use.

Increased Effect/Toxicity

Rosiglitazone may increase the levels/effects of: CYP2C8 Substrates; Hypoglycemic Agents

The levels/effects of Rosiglitazone may be increased by: CYP2C8 Inhibitors (Moderate); CYP2C8 Inhibitors (Strong); Deferasirox; Gemfibrozil; Herbs (Hypoglycemic Properties); Insulin; MAO Inhibitors; Mifepristone; Pegvisomant; Pregabalin; Salicylates; Selective Serotonin Reuptake Inhibitors; Trimethoprim; Vasodilators (Organic Nitrates)

Decreased Effect

The levels/effects of Rosiglitazone may be decreased by: Bile Acid Sequestrants; Corticosteroids (Orally Inhaled); Corticosteroids (Systemic); CYP2C8 Inducers (Strong); Loop Diuretics; Luteinizing Hormone-Releasing Hormone Analogs; Rifampin; Somatropin; Thiazide Diuretics

Ethanol/Nutrition/Herb Interactions

Ethanol: Avoid ethanol (may cause hypoglycemia).

Food: Peak concentrations are lower by 28% and delayed when administered with food, but these effects are not believed to be clinically significant.

Herb/Nutraceutical: Avoid alfalfa, aloe, bilberry, bitter melon, burdock, celery, damiana, fenugreek, garcinia, garlic, ginger, ginseng (American), gymnema, marshmallow, stinging nettle (may cause hypoglycemia).

Stability Store at 15°C to 30°C (59°F to 86°F). Protect from light.

ROSIGLITAZONE

Mechanism of Action Thiazolidinedione antidiabetic agent that lowers blood glucose by improving target cell response to insulin, without increasing pancreatic insulin secretion. It has a mechanism of action that is dependent on the presence of insulin for activity. Rosiglitazone is an agonist for peroxisome proliferator-activated receptor-gamma (PPARgamma). Activation of nuclear PPARgamma receptors influences the production of a number of gene products involved in glucose and lipid metabolism. PPARgamma is abundant in the cells within the renal collecting tubules; fluid retention results from stimulation by thiazolidinediones which increases sodium reabsorption.

Pharmacodynamics/Kinetics

Onset of action: Delayed; Maximum effect: Up to 12 weeks

Distribution: V_{dss} (apparent): 17.6 L

Protein binding: 99.8%; primarily albumin

Metabolism: Hepatic (99%) via CYP2C8; minor metabolism via CYP2C9

Bioavailability: 99%

Half-life elimination: 3-4 hours

Time to peak, plasma: 1 hour; delayed with food

Excretion: Urine (~64%) and feces (~23%) as metabolites

Dosage

Geriatric & Adult Type 2 diabetes: Oral: **Note:** All patients should be initiated at the lowest recommended dose.

Monotherapy: Initial: 4 mg daily as a single daily dose or in divided doses twice daily. If response is inadequate after 8-12 weeks of treatment, the dosage may be increased to 8 mg daily as a single daily dose or in divided doses twice daily. In clinical trials, the 4 mg twice-daily regimen resulted in the greatest reduction in fasting plasma glucose and Hb A_{1c}.

Combination therapy: When adding rosiglitazone to existing therapy, continue current dose(s) of previous agents:

U.S. labeling: With sulfonylureas or metformin (or sulfonylurea plus metformin): Initial: 4 mg daily as a single daily dose or in divided doses twice daily. If response is inadequate after 8-12 weeks of treatment, the dosage may be increased to 8 mg daily as a single daily dose or in divided doses twice daily. Reduce dose of sulfonylurea if hypoglycemia occurs. It is unlikely that the dose of metformin will need to be reduced due to hypoglycemia.

Canadian labeling:

With metformin: Initial: 4 mg daily as a single daily dose or in divided doses twice daily. If response is inadequate after 8-12 weeks of treatment, the dosage may be increased to 8 mg daily as a single daily dose or in divided doses twice daily.

With a sulfonylurea: 4 mg daily as a single daily dose or in divided doses twice daily. Dose should not exceed 4 mg daily when using in combination with a sulfonylurea. Reduce dose of sulfonylurea if hypoglycemia occurs.

Renal Impairment No adjustment is necessary.

Hepatic Impairment Clearance is significantly lower in hepatic impairment. Therapy should not be initiated if the patient exhibits active liver disease or increased transaminases (ALT >2.5 times the upper limit of normal) at baseline.

Administration May be administered without regard to meals.

Monitoring Parameters Hemoglobin A_{1c}, fasting serum glucose; signs and symptoms of fluid retention or heart failure; liver enzymes (prior to initiation of therapy, then periodically thereafter); ophthalmic exams. Evaluate patients with ALT ≤2.5 times ULN at baseline or during therapy for cause of enzyme elevation. Patients with an elevation in ALT >3 times ULN should be rechecked as soon as possible. If the ALT levels remain >3 times ULN, therapy with rosiglitazone should be discontinued.

Reference Range Recommendations for glycemic control in adults with diabetes:

Hb A_{1c}: <7%

Preprandial capillary plasma glucose: 70-130 mg/dL

Peak postprandial capillary blood glucose: <180 mg/dL

Special Geriatric Considerations Intensive glucose control (Hb A_{1c} <6.5%) has been linked to increased all-cause mortality and cardiovascular mortality, hypoglycemia requiring assistance, and weight gain in adult type 2 diabetes. How "tightly" to control a geriatric patient's blood glucose needs to be individualized. Such a decision should be based on several factors, including the patient's functional and cognitive status, how well he/she recognizes hypoglycemic or hyperglycemic symptoms, and how to respond to them and other disease states. An Hb A_{1c} <7.5% is an acceptable endpoint for a healthy older adult, while <8% is acceptable for frail elderly patients, those with a duration of illness >10 years, or those with comorbid conditions and requiring combination diabetes medications. For elderly patients with diabetes who are relatively healthy, attaining target goals for aspirin use, blood pressure, lipids, smoking cessation, and diet and exercise may be more important than normalized glycemic control. In elderly patients with heart failure, this medication is considered potentially inappropriate (Beers Criteria, 2012).

Dosage Forms Excipient information presented when available (limited, particularly for generics); consult specific product labeling.

Tablet, oral:

Avandia®: 2 mg, 4 mg, 8 mg

Rosiglitazone and Glimepiride (roh si GLI ta zone & GLYE me pye ride)

Related Information

Glimepiride *on page 877*

Rosiglitazone *on page 1728*

Medication Safety Issues

High alert medication:

The Institute for Safe Medication Practices (ISMP) includes this medication among its list of drugs which have a heightened risk of causing significant patient harm when used in error.

Brand Names: U.S. Avandaryl®

Brand Names: Canada Avandaryl®

Index Terms Glimepiride and Rosiglitazone Maleate

Generic Availability (U.S.) No

Pharmacologic Category Antidiabetic Agent, Sulfonylurea; Antidiabetic Agent, Thiazolidinedione

Use Management of type 2 diabetes mellitus (noninsulin dependent, NIDDM) as an adjunct to diet and exercise

Prescribing and Access Restrictions

As a requirement of the REMS program, the prescribing and dispensing of any rosiglitazone-containing medication in the U.S. requires physician and patient enrollment in the Avandia-Rosiglitazone Medicines Access Program™. Complete program details are available at www.avandia.com or by calling the program Coordinating Center at 800-282-6342.

Health Canada requires written informed consent for new and current patients receiving rosiglitazone.

Medication Guide Available Yes

Dosage

Geriatric Rosiglitazone 4 mg and glimepiride 1 mg once daily. Carefully titrate dose.

Adult Type 2 diabetes mellitus: Oral: Initial: Rosiglitazone 4 mg and glimepiride 1 mg once daily **or** rosiglitazone 4 mg and glimepiride 2 mg once daily (for patients previously treated with sulfonylurea or thiazolidinedione monotherapy)

Patients switching from combination rosiglitazone and glimepiride as separate tablets: Use current dose.

Titration:

Dose adjustment in patients previously on sulfonylurea monotherapy: May take 2 weeks to observe decreased blood glucose and 2-3 months to see full effects of rosiglitazone component. If not adequately controlled after 8-12 weeks, increase daily dose of rosiglitazone component.

Dose adjustment in patients previously on thiazolidinedione monotherapy: If not adequately controlled after 1-2 weeks, increase daily dose of glimepiride component in ≤2 mg increments in 1-2 week intervals.

Maximum dose:

U.S. labeling: Rosiglitazone 8 mg and glimepiride 4 mg once daily

Canadian labeling: Rosiglitazone 4 mg and glimepiride 4 mg once daily

Renal Impairment Rosiglitazone 4 mg and glimepiride 1 mg once daily. Carefully titrate dose.

Hepatic Impairment Rosiglitazone 4 mg and glimepiride 1 mg once daily. Carefully titrate dose.

ALT ≤2.5 times ULN: Use with caution.

ALT >2.5 times ULN: Do not initiate therapy.

ALT >3 times ULN or jaundice: Discontinue.

Special Geriatric Considerations See individual agents. Combination products are not recommended as first-line treatment. Use only if doses of individual agents correspond to the combination available.

Dosage Forms Excipient information presented when available (limited, particularly for generics); consult specific product labeling.
Tablet:
Avandaryl® 4 mg/1 mg: Rosiglitazone maleate 4 mg and glimepiride 1 mg
Avandaryl® 4 mg/2 mg: Rosiglitazone maleate 4 mg and glimepiride 2 mg
Avandaryl® 4 mg/4 mg: Rosiglitazone maleate 4 mg and glimepiride 4 mg
Avandaryl® 8 mg/2 mg: Rosiglitazone maleate 8 mg and glimepiride 2 mg
Avandaryl® 8 mg/4 mg: Rosiglitazone maleate 8 mg and glimepiride 4 mg

Rosiglitazone and Metformin (roh si GLI ta zone & met FOR min)

Related Information
MetFORMIN on page 1222
Rosiglitazone on page 1728

Medication Safety Issues
Sound-alike/look-alike issues:
Avandamet® may be confused with Anzemet®
High alert medication:
The Institute for Safe Medication Practices (ISMP) includes this medication among its list of drug classes which have a heightened risk of causing significant patient harm when used in error.

Brand Names: U.S. Avandamet®
Brand Names: Canada Avandamet®
Index Terms Metformin and Rosiglitazone; Metformin Hydrochloride and Rosiglitazone Maleate; Rosiglitazone Maleate and Metformin Hydrochloride
Generic Availability (U.S.) No
Pharmacologic Category Antidiabetic Agent, Biguanide; Antidiabetic Agent, Thiazolidinedione
Use Management of type 2 diabetes mellitus (noninsulin dependent, NIDDM) as an adjunct to diet and exercise in patients where dual rosiglitazone and metformin therapy is appropriate
Prescribing and Access Restrictions As a requirement of the REMS program, the prescribing and dispensing of any rosiglitazone-containing medication in the U.S. requires physician and patient enrollment in the Avandia-Rosiglitazone Medicines Access Program™. Complete program details are available at www.avandia.com or by calling the program Coordinating Center at 800-282-6342.

Health Canada requires written informed consent for new and current patients receiving rosiglitazone.

Medication Guide Available Yes
Dosage
Geriatric The initial and maintenance dosing should be conservative, due to the potential for decreased renal function (monitor). Generally, elderly patients should not be titrated to the maximum. Do not use in patients ≥80 years unless normal renal function has been established.

Adult Type 2 diabetes mellitus: Oral:
First-line therapy (drug-naive patients): Initial: Rosiglitazone 2 mg and metformin 500 mg once or twice daily; may increase by 2 mg/500 mg per day after 4 weeks to a maximum of 8 mg/2000 mg per day.
Second-line therapy:
Patients inadequately controlled on metformin alone: Initial dose: Rosiglitazone 4 mg/day plus current dose of metformin
Patients inadequately controlled on rosiglitazone alone: Initial dose: Metformin 1000 mg/day plus current dose of rosiglitazone
Note: When switching from combination rosiglitazone and metformin as separate tablets: Use current dose
Dose adjustment: Doses may be increased as increments of rosiglitazone 4 mg and/or metformin 500 mg, up to the maximum dose; doses should be titrated gradually.
After a change in the metformin dosage, titration can be done after 1-2 weeks
After a change in the rosiglitazone dosage, titration can be done after 8-12 weeks
Maximum dose: Rosiglitazone 8 mg/metformin 2000 mg daily
Renal Impairment Do not use with renal disease or renal dysfunction (serum creatinine ≥1.5 mg/dL in males or ≥1.4 mg/dL in females or abnormal clearance).
Hepatic Impairment Do not initiate therapy with active liver disease or ALT >2.5 times the upper limit of normal.
Special Geriatric Considerations See individual agents. Combination products are not recommended as first-line treatment. Use only if doses of individual agents correspond to the combination available.

Dosage Forms Excipient information presented when available (limited, particularly for generics); consult specific product labeling.
Tablet:
Avandamet®: 2/500: Rosiglitazone 2 mg and metformin hydrochloride 500 mg
Avandamet®: 4/500: Rosiglitazone 4 mg and metformin hydrochloride 500 mg
Avandamet®: 2/1000: Rosiglitazone 2 mg and metformin hydrochloride 1000 mg
Avandamet®: 4/1000: Rosiglitazone 4 mg and metformin hydrochloride 1000 mg

◆ **Rosiglitazone Maleate and Metformin Hydrochloride** see Rosiglitazone and Metformin on page 1732

Rosuvastatin (roe soo va STAT in)

Related Information
Hyperlipidemia Management on page 2130
Medication Safety Issues
Sound-alike/look-alike issues:
Rosuvastatin may be confused with atorvaSTATin, nystatin, pitavastatin
Brand Names: U.S. Crestor®
Brand Names: Canada Apo-Rosuvastatin; CO Rosuvastatin; Crestor®; Mylan-Rosuvastatin; PMS-Rosuvastatin; RAN™-Rosuvastatin; Sandoz-Rosuvastatin; Teva-Rosuvastatin
Index Terms Rosuvastatin Calcium
Generic Availability (U.S.) No
Pharmacologic Category Antilipemic Agent, HMG-CoA Reductase Inhibitor
Use
Treatment of dyslipidemias: Used with dietary therapy for hyperlipidemias to reduce elevations in total cholesterol (TC), LDL-C, apolipoprotein B, nonHDL-C, and triglycerides (TG) in patients with primary hypercholesterolemia (elevations of 1 or more components are present in Fredrickson type IIa, IIb, and IV hyperlipidemias); increase HDL-C; treatment of primary dysbetalipoproteinemia (Fredrickson type III hyperlipidemia); treatment of homozygous familial hypercholesterolemia (FH); to slow progression of atherosclerosis as an adjunct to diet to lower TC and LDL-C
Primary prevention of cardiovascular disease: To reduce the risk of stroke, myocardial infarction, or arterial revascularization procedures in patients without clinically evident coronary heart disease or lipid abnormalities but with all of the following: 1) an increased risk of cardiovascular disease based on age ≥50 years old in men and ≥60 years old in women, 2) hsCRP ≥2 mg/L, and 3) the presence of at least one additional cardiovascular disease risk factor such as hypertension, low HDL-C, smoking, or a family history of premature coronary heart disease.
Secondary prevention of cardiovascular disease: To slow progression of atherosclerosis
Contraindications Hypersensitivity to rosuvastatin or any component of the formulation; active liver disease; unexplained persistent elevations of serum transaminases (>3 times ULN)

Canadian labeling: Additional contraindications (not in U.S. labeling): Concomitant administration of cyclosporine; use of 40 mg dose in Asian patients, patients with predisposing risk factors for myopathy/rhabdomyolysis (eg, hereditary muscle disorders, history of myotoxicity with other HMG-CoA reductase inhibitors, concomitant use with fibrates or niacin, severe hepatic impairment, severe renal impairment [Cl_{cr} <30 mL/minute/1.73 m^2], hypothyroidism, alcohol abuse)

Warnings/Precautions Secondary causes of hyperlipidemia should be ruled out prior to therapy. Rosuvastatin has not been studied when the primary lipid abnormality is chylomicron elevation (Fredrickson types I and V). Liver enzyme tests should be obtained at baseline and as clinically indicated; routine periodic monitoring of liver enzymes is not necessary. Use with caution in patients who consume large amounts of ethanol or have a history of liver disease; use is contraindicated with active liver disease or unexplained transaminase elevations. Hematuria (microscopic) and proteinuria have been observed; more commonly reported in patients receiving rosuvastatin 40 mg daily, but typically transient and not associated with a decrease in renal function. Consider dosage reduction if unexplained hematuria and proteinuria persists. HMG-CoA reductase inhibitors may cause rhabdomyolysis with acute renal failure and/or myopathy. Discontinue in any patient in which CPK levels are markedly elevated (>10 times ULN) or if myopathy is suspected/diagnosed. This risk is dose-related and is increased with concurrent use of other lipid-lowering medications (fibric acid derivatives or niacin doses ≥1 g/day), other interacting drugs, drugs associated with myopathy (eg, colchicine), age ≥65 years, female gender, certain subgroups of Asian ancestry, uncontrolled hypothyroidism, and renal dysfunction. Dose reductions may be necessary.

The manufacturer recommends temporary discontinuation for elective major surgery, acute medical or surgical conditions, or in any patient experiencing an acute or serious condition predisposing to renal failure (eg, sepsis, hypotension, trauma, uncontrolled seizures). However, based upon current evidence, HMG-CoA reductase inhibitor therapy should be continued in the perioperative period unless risk outweighs cardioprotective benefit. Patients should be instructed to report unexplained muscle pain, tenderness, weakness, or brown urine; in Canada, concomitant use with cyclosporine or niacin is contraindicated, and rosuvastatin at a dose of 40 mg/day in Asian patients is contraindicated. Small increases in Hb A_{1c} (mean: ~0.1%) and fasting blood glucose have been reported with rosuvastatin; however, the benefits of statin therapy far outweigh the risk of dysglycemia.

Adverse Reactions (Reflective of adult population; not specific for elderly)
>10%: Neuromuscular & skeletal: Myalgia (3% to 13%)

2% to 10%:
Central nervous system: Headache (6%), dizziness (4%)
Gastrointestinal: Nausea (3%), abdominal pain (2%), constipation (2%)
Hepatic: ALT increased (2%; >3 times ULN)
Neuromuscular & skeletal: Arthralgia (4% to 10%), CPK increased (3%; >10 x ULN: Children 3%), weakness (3%)

Adverse reactions reported with other HMG-CoA reductase inhibitors (not necessarily reported with rosuvastatin therapy) include a hypersensitivity syndrome (symptoms may include anaphylaxis, angioedema, arthralgia, erythema multiforme, eosinophilia, hemolytic anemia, interstitial lung disease, lupus syndrome, photosensitivity, polymyalgia rheumatica, positive ANA, purpura, Stevens-Johnson syndrome, toxic epidermal necrolysis, urticaria, vasculitis)

Drug Interactions
Metabolism/Transport Effects Substrate of CYP2C9 (minor), CYP3A4 (minor), SLCO1B1; **Note:** Assignment of Major/Minor substrate status based on clinically relevant drug interaction potential

Avoid Concomitant Use
Avoid concomitant use of Rosuvastatin with any of the following: Gemfibrozil; Red Yeast Rice

Increased Effect/Toxicity
Rosuvastatin may increase the levels/effects of: DAPTOmycin; Pazopanib; Trabectedin; Vitamin K Antagonists

The levels/effects of Rosuvastatin may be increased by: Amiodarone; Colchicine; CycloSPORINE; CycloSPORINE (Systemic); Eltrombopag; Fenofibrate; Fenofibric Acid; Gemfibrozil; Niacin; Niacinamide; Protease Inhibitors; Red Yeast Rice

Decreased Effect
Rosuvastatin may decrease the levels/effects of: Lanthanum

The levels/effects of Rosuvastatin may be decreased by: Antacids; Tocilizumab

Ethanol/Nutrition/Herb Interactions
Ethanol: Avoid excessive ethanol consumption (due to potential hepatic effects).
Food: Red yeast rice contains an estimated 2.4 mg lovastatin per 600 mg rice.

Stability Store between 20°C and 25°C (68°F to 77°F). Protect from moisture.

Mechanism of Action Inhibitor of 3-hydroxy-3-methylglutaryl coenzyme A (HMG-CoA) reductase, the rate-limiting enzyme in cholesterol synthesis (reduces the production of mevalonic acid from HMG-CoA); this then results in a compensatory increase in the expression of LDL receptors on hepatocyte membranes and a stimulation of LDL catabolism

Pharmacodynamics/Kinetics
Onset of action: Within 1 week; maximal at 4 weeks
Distribution: V_d: 134 L
Protein binding: 88%
Metabolism: Hepatic (10%), via CYP2C9 (1 active metabolite identified: N-desmethyl rosuvastatin, one-sixth to one-half the HMG-CoA reductase activity of the parent compound)
Bioavailability: 20% (high first-pass extraction by liver)
Asian patients have been noted to have increased bioavailability.
Half-life elimination: 19 hours
Time to peak, plasma: 3-5 hours
Excretion: Feces (90%), primarily as unchanged drug

Dosage
Geriatric & Adult Note: Doses should be individualized according to the baseline LDL-cholesterol levels, the recommended goal of therapy, and patient response; adjustments should be made at intervals of 4 weeks or more.

Hyperlipidemia, mixed dyslipidemia, hypertriglyceridemia, primary dysbetalipoproteinemia, slowing progression of atherosclerosis: Oral:

Initial dose:

General dosing: 10 mg once daily; 20 mg once daily may be used in patients with severe hyperlipidemia (LDL >190 mg/dL) and aggressive lipid targets

Conservative dosing: Patients requiring less aggressive treatment or predisposed to myopathy (including patients of Asian descent): 5 mg once daily

Titration: After 2 weeks, may be increased by 5-10 mg once daily; dosing range: 5-40 mg/day (maximum dose: 40 mg once daily)

Note: The 40 mg dose should be reserved for patients who have not achieved goal cholesterol levels on a dose of 20 mg/day, including patients switched from another HMG-CoA reductase inhibitor.

Homozygous familial hypercholesterolemia (FH): Oral: Initial: 20 mg once daily (maximum dose: 40 mg/day)

Dosage adjustment with concomitant medications: Oral:

U.S. labeling:

Cyclosporine: Rosuvastatin dose should not exceed 5 mg/day

Gemfibrozil: Avoid concurrent use; if unable to avoid concurrent use, rosuvastatin dose should not exceed 10 mg/day

Atazanavir/ritonavir or lopinavir/ritonavir: Rosuvastatin dose should not exceed 10 mg/day

Canadian labeling:

Cyclosporine: Concomitant use is contraindicated

Gemfibrozil: Rosuvastatin dose should not exceed 20 mg/day

Dosage adjustment for hematuria and/or persistent, unexplained proteinuria while on 40 mg/day: Reduce dose and evaluate causes.

Renal Impairment

Mild-to-moderate impairment: No dosage adjustment required.

Cl_{cr} <30 mL/minute/1.73 m^2: Initial: 5 mg/day; do not exceed 10 mg once daily

Hepatic Impairment

U.S. labeling: Active hepatic disease, including unexplained persistent transaminase elevations: Use is contraindicated.

Canadian labeling:

Active hepatic disease or unexplained persistent transaminase >3 x ULN: Use is contraindicated.

Mild-to-moderate impairment: No dosage adjustment required.

Severe impairment: Initial: 5 mg/day; do not exceed 20 mg once daily.

Administration May be administered with or without food. May be taken at any time of the day.

Monitoring Parameters Baseline CPK (recheck CPK in any patient with symptoms suggestive of myopathy; discontinue therapy if markedly elevated); baseline liver function tests (LFTs) and repeat when clinically indicated thereafter. Patients with elevated transaminase levels should have a second (confirmatory) test and frequent monitoring until values normalize; discontinue if increase in ALT/AST is persistently >3 times ULN (NCEP, 2002).

Lipid panel (total cholesterol, HDL, LDL, triglycerides):

ATP III recommendations (NCEP, 2002): Baseline; 6-8 weeks after initiation of drug therapy; if dose increased, then at 6-8 weeks until final dose determined. Once treatment goal achieved, follow up intervals may be reduced to every 4-6 months. Lipid panel should be assessed at least annually, and preferably at each clinic visit.

Manufacturer recommendation: Upon initiation or titration, lipid panel should be analyzed within 2-4 weeks.

Special Geriatric Considerations Effective and well tolerated in the elderly. The definition of and, therefore, when to treat hyperlipidemia in geriatrics is a controversial issue. The National Cholesterol Education Program recommends that all adults maintain a plasma cholesterol <160 mg/dL. For elderly patients with one additional risk factor, goal LDL would be <130 mg/dL. It is the authors' belief that pharmacologic treatment be reserved for those who are unable to obtain a desirable plasma cholesterol concentration by diet alone and for whom the benefits of treatment are believed to outweigh the potential adverse effects, drug interactions, and cost of treatment. Age ≥65 years is a risk factor for myopathy.

Dosage Forms Excipient information presented when available (limited, particularly for generics); consult specific product labeling.

Tablet, oral:

Crestor®: 5 mg, 10 mg, 20 mg, 40 mg

◆ **Rosuvastatin Calcium** *see* Rosuvastatin *on page 1733*

Rotigotine (roe TIG oh teen)

Medication Safety Issues
Sound-alike/look-alike issues:
Neupro® may be confused with Neupogen®

Transdermal patch contains metal (eg, aluminum); remove patch prior to MRI or cardioversion

Brand Names: U.S. Neupro®

Index Terms N-0923

Generic Availability (U.S.) No

Pharmacologic Category Anti-Parkinson's Agent, Dopamine Agonist

Use Treatment of the signs and symptoms of idiopathic Parkinson's disease (early-stage to advanced-stage disease); treatment of moderate-to-severe primary restless legs syndrome (RLS)

Contraindications Hypersensitivity to rotigotine or any component of the formulation

Warnings/Precautions Use is commonly associated with somnolence. In addition, falling asleep during activities of daily living, including while driving, has also been reported and may occur without significant warning signs. Monitor for daytime somnolence or pre-existing sleep disorder. Patients must be cautioned about performing tasks which require mental alertness (eg, operating machinery or driving). Use with caution in patients receiving other CNS depressants or psychoactive agents; discontinue if significant daytime sleepiness or episodes of falling asleep occur. Effects with other sedative drugs or ethanol may be potentiated.

Dopamine agonists may cause orthostatic hypotension and syncope; Parkinson's disease patients appear to have an impaired capacity to respond to a postural challenge. Use with caution in patients at risk of hypotension (such as those receiving antihypertensive drugs) or where transient hypotensive episodes would be poorly tolerated (cardiovascular disease or cerebrovascular disease). Parkinson's and restless legs syndrome (RLS) patients being treated with dopaminergic agonists ordinarily require careful monitoring for signs and symptoms of postural hypotension, especially during dose escalation, and should be informed of this risk. Weight gain and fluid retention have been reported, primarily associated with development of peripheral edema in Parkinson's disease patients; use caution in patients with heart failure or renal insufficiency. Therapy has also been associated with increases in blood pressure (may be significant), and increased heart rate; use caution in pre-existing cardiovascular disease.

Dopamine agonists have been associated with compulsive behaviors and/or loss of impulse control, which has manifested as pathological gambling, libido increases (hypersexuality), and/or binge eating. Causality has not been established, and controversy exists as to whether this phenomenon is related to the underlying disease, prior behaviors/addictions and/or drug therapy. Dose reduction or discontinuation of therapy has been reported to reverse these behaviors in some, but not all cases.

In RLS patents, augmentation (earlier onset of symptoms each day and/or an overall increase in symptom severity) or rebound (considered to be an end of dose effect) may occur.

Use with caution in patients with pre-existing dyskinesia; therapy may exacerbate. Therapy may also cause hallucinations (dose-related) and other psychotic like behaviors (eg, agitation, delirium, delusions, aggression); in general, avoid use in patients with pre-existing major psychotic disorders. Risk for melanoma development is increased in Parkinson's disease patients; drug causation or factors contributing to risk have not been established. Patients receiving therapy for any indication should be monitored closely and periodic skin examinations should be performed. Other dopaminergic agents have been associated with a syndrome resembling neuroleptic malignant syndrome on withdrawal and/or significant dosage reduction. Taper treatment when discontinuing therapy; do not stop abruptly. Rare cases of pleural effusion, pleural thickening, pulmonary infiltrates, retroperitoneal fibrosis, pericarditis and/or cardiac valvulopathy have been reported in patients treated with ergot-derived dopamine agonists, generally with prolonged use. The potential of rotigotine, a nonergot-derived dopamine agonist, to cause similar fibrotic complications is unknown.

Patch contains aluminum; remove patch prior to magnetic resonance imaging or cardioversion to avoid skin burns. Patch also contains sodium metabisulfite which may cause allergic reaction in susceptible individuals. Dose-dependent application site reactions, potentially severe, have been observed; daily rotation of application sites has been shown to decrease incidence of reactions. If a generalized (nonapplication site) skin reaction occurs; discontinue therapy. Avoid exposure of application site to any direct external heat sources (eg, hair dryers, heating pads, electric blankets, saunas, hot tubs, direct sunlight); heat exposure has not been studied with the rotigotine patch, but an increase in the rate and extent of absorption has been observed with other transdermal products.

Adverse Reactions (Reflective of adult population; not specific for elderly)
>10%:

Cardiovascular: Peripheral edema (dose related; 2% to 14%)

Central nervous system: Somnolence (dose related; 5% to 32%), dizziness (5% to 23%), headache (8% to 18%), fatigue (6% to 18%), orthostatic hypotension (1% to 18%), sleep disorder (disturbance in initiating/maintaining sleep; dose related; 2% to 14%), hallucinations (dose related; 7% to 14%), insomnia (5% to 11%)

Dermatologic: Application site reactions (dose related; 27% to 46%), hyperhidrosis (dose related; 1% to 11%)

Gastrointestinal: Nausea (dose related; 15% to 48%), vomiting (dose related; 2% to 20%)

Neuromuscular & skeletal: Dyskinesia (dose related; 14% to 17%), arthralgia (8% to 11%)

1% to 10%:

Cardiovascular: Hypertension (dose related; 1% to 5%), T-wave abnormalities on ECG (≤3%), syncope

Central nervous system: Abnormal dreams (dose related; 1% to 7%), nightmare (dose related; 3% to 5%), depression (≤5%), vertigo (1% to 4%), early morning awakening (dose related; ≤3%), balance disorder (2% to 3%), lethargy (1% to 2%), postural dizziness (1% to 2%), sleep attacks (dose related; ≤2%)

Dermatologic: Pruritus (3% to 7%), erythema (dose related; ≤6%), pruritic rash (dose related; ≤3%)

Endocrine & metabolic: Hot flash (≤3%), serum ferritin decreased (dose related; 1% to 2%), serum glucose decreased

Gastrointestinal: Constipation (2% to 9%), weight gain (2% to 9%), diarrhea (5% to 7%), anorexia (≤8%), xerostomia (dose related; 3% to 7%), appetite decreased (≤3%), dyspepsia (dose related; ≤3%), weight loss (dose related; ≤3%)

Genitourinary: Erectile dysfunction (dose related; ≤3%), urinary WBC positive (≤3%)

Hematologic: Contusion (dose related; ≤4%), hemoglobin decreased, hematocrit decreased

Neuromuscular & skeletal: Paresthesia (dose related 5% to 6%), tremor (3% to 4%), weakness (3% to 4%), muscle spasms (dose related; 1% to 4%), musculoskeletal pain (2%)

Ocular: Vision changes

Otic: Tinnitus (≤3%)

Renal: BUN increased

Respiratory: Nasopharyngitis (7% to 10%), upper respiratory tract infection (≤5%), cough (3%), nasal congestion (3%), sinus congestion (2% to 3%), sinusitis (dose related; ≤3%), pharyngolaryngeal pain (≤2%)

Miscellaneous: Hiccups (dose related; 2% to 3%)

Drug Interactions

Metabolism/Transport Effects None known.

Avoid Concomitant Use

Avoid concomitant use of Rotigotine with any of the following: Azelastine; Azelastine (Nasal); Methadone; Mirtazapine; Paraldehyde

Increased Effect/Toxicity

Rotigotine may increase the levels/effects of: Alcohol (Ethyl); Azelastine; Azelastine (Nasal); Buprenorphine; CNS Depressants; Methadone; Metyrosine; Mirtazapine; Paraldehyde; Selective Serotonin Reuptake Inhibitors; Zolpidem

The levels/effects of Rotigotine may be increased by: HydrOXYzine; MAO Inhibitors; Methylphenidate

Decreased Effect

Rotigotine may decrease the levels/effects of: Antipsychotics (Typical)

The levels/effects of Rotigotine may be decreased by: Antipsychotics (Atypical); Antipsychotics (Typical); Metoclopramide

Ethanol/Nutrition/Herb Interactions Ethanol: Avoid ethanol (may increase CNS depression).

Stability Store at 20°C to 25°C (68°F to 77°F). Store in original pouch until application.

Mechanism of Action Rotigotine is a nonergot dopamine agonist with specificity for D_3-, D_2-, and D_1-dopamine receptors. Although the precise mechanism of action of rotigotine is unknown, it is believed to be due to stimulation of postsynaptic dopamine D_2-type auto receptors within the substantia nigra in the brain, leading to improved dopaminergic transmission in the motor areas of the basal ganglia, notably the caudate nucleus/putamen regions.

Pharmacodynamics/Kinetics

Distribution: V_d: 84 L/kg

Protein binding: ~90%

Metabolism: Extensive via conjugation and N-dealkylation; multiple CYP isoenzymes, sulfotransferases, and two UDP-glucuronosyltransferases involved in catalyzing the metabolism

Half-life elimination: After removal of patch: ~5-7 hours

Time to peak, plasma: 15-18 hours; can occur 4-27 hours post application

Excretion: Urine (~71% as inactive conjugates and metabolites, <1% as unchanged drug); feces (~23%)

Dosage

Geriatric & Adult

Parkinson's disease: Topical: Transdermal:

Early-stage: Initial: Apply 2 mg/24 hours patch once daily; may increase by 2 mg/24 hours weekly, based on clinical response and tolerability; lowest effective dose: 4 mg/24 hours (maximum dose: 6 mg/24 hours)

Advanced-stage: Initial: Apply 4 mg/24 hours patch once daily; may increase by 2 mg/24 hours weekly, based on clinical response and tolerability (maximum dose: 8 mg/24 hours)

Discontinuation of treatment in Parkinson's disease: Decrease by ≤2 mg/24 hours preferably every other day until withdrawal complete

Restless legs syndrome (RLS): Topical: Transdermal: Initial: Apply 1 mg/24 hours patch once daily; may increase by 1 mg/24 hours weekly, based on clinical response and tolerability; lowest effective dose: 1 mg/24 hours (maximum dose: 3 mg/24 hours)

Discontinuation of treatment for RLS: Decrease by 1 mg/24 hours preferably every other day until withdrawal complete

Renal Impairment Mild-to-severe impairment (Cl_{cr} ≥15 mL/minute): No dosage adjustment necessary.

Hepatic Impairment

Mild-to-moderate hepatic impairment (Child-Pugh class A or B): No dosage adjustment necessary.

Severe hepatic impairment: No dosage adjustment provided in manufacturer's labeling (has not been studied).

Administration Transdermal patch: Apply patch to clean, dry, hairless area of intact healthy skin on the front of the abdomen, thigh, hip, flank, shoulder, or upper arm at approximately the same time daily. Remove from pouch immediately before use and press patch firmly in place on skin for 30 seconds. Application sites should be rotated on a daily basis. Do not apply to same application site more than once every 14 days or apply patch to oily, irritated or damaged skin. Avoid exposing patch to external heat sources (eg, heating pad, electric blanket, heat lamp, hot tub, direct sunlight). If applied to hairy area, shave ≥3 days prior to applying patch. If patch falls off, immediately apply a new one to a new site.

Monitoring Parameters Blood pressure (including orthostatic); daytime alertness; periodic skin evaluations (melanoma development)

Pharmacotherapy Pearls In April 2008, Neupro® was removed from the market following a recall due to the formation of rotigotine crystals (resembling snowflakes) on the patch. The crystallization resulted in decreased drug available for absorption and altered efficacy. Reintroduction of a reformulated Neupro® into the U.S. market was announced in 2012.

Special Geriatric Considerations In clinical trials, no differences in efficacy or safety were seen in younger and older patients. Plasma concentrations of rotigotine in patients 65-80 years of age were similar to younger patients. Plasma concentrations were not measured in patients >80 years of age; however, use caution in this population due to potential for age-related skin changes, which may result in increased exposure.

Dosage Forms Excipient information presented when available (limited, particularly for generics); consult specific product labeling.

Patch, transdermal [once-daily patch]:

Neupro®: 1 mg/24 hours (30s) [contains metal, sodium metabisulfite; 5 cm^2, total rotigotine 2.25 mg]

Neupro®: 2 mg/24 hours (30s) [contains metal, sodium metabisulfite; 10 cm^2, total rotigotine 4.5 mg]

Neupro®: 3 mg/24 hours (30s) [contains metal, sodium metabisulfite; 15 cm^2, total rotigotine 6.75 mg]

Neupro®: 4 mg/24 hours (30s) [contains metal, sodium metabisulfite; 20 cm^2, total rotigotine 9 mg]

Neupro®: 6 mg/24 hours (30s) [contains metal, sodium metabisulfite; 30 cm^2, total rotigotine 13.5 mg]

Neupro®: 8 mg/24 hours (30s) [contains metal, sodium metabisulfite; 40 cm^2, total rotigotine 18 mg]

◆ **Rowasa®** see Mesalamine on page 1217
◆ **Roxanol** see Morphine (Systemic) on page 1312
◆ **Roxicet™** see Oxycodone and Acetaminophen on page 1449
◆ **Roxicet™ 5/500** see Oxycodone and Acetaminophen on page 1449
◆ **Roxicodone®** see OxyCODONE on page 1446
◆ **Rozerem®** see Ramelteon on page 1668
◆ **RP-54274** see Riluzole on page 1703
◆ **RP-59500** see Quinupristin and Dalfopristin on page 1658

- **r-PA** *see* Reteplase *on page* 1689
- **rPDGF-BB** *see* Becaplermin *on page* 188
- **(R,R)-Formoterol L-Tartrate** *see* Arformoterol *on page* 141
- **RTCA** *see* Ribavirin *on page* 1691
- **RTG** *see* Ezogabine *on page* 740
- **RU 0211** *see* Lubiprostone *on page* 1170
- **RU-23908** *see* Nilutamide *on page* 1378
- **Rubella, Measles and Mumps Vaccines** *see* Measles, Mumps, and Rubella Virus Vaccine *on page* 1184
- **RUF 331** *see* Rufinamide *on page* 1739

Rufinamide (roo FIN a mide)

Brand Names: U.S. Banzel®
Brand Names: Canada Banzel™
Index Terms CGP 33101; E 2080; RUF 331; Xilep
Generic Availability (U.S.) No
Pharmacologic Category Anticonvulsant, Triazole Derivative
Use Adjunctive therapy in the treatment of generalized seizures of Lennox-Gastaut syndrome
Medication Guide Available Yes
Contraindications Patients with familial short QT syndrome

Canadian labeling: Additional contraindications (not in U.S. labeling): Family history of short QT syndrome; presence or history of short QT interval; hypersensitivity to rufinamide, triazole derivatives, or any component of the formulation

Warnings/Precautions Has been associated with shortening of the QT interval. Use caution in patients receiving concurrent medications that shorten the QT interval. Contraindicated in patients with familial short-QT syndrome (Canadian labeling also contraindicates use in patients with a family history of short QT syndrome or presence or history of short QT interval). Use has been associated with CNS-related adverse events, most significant of these were cognitive symptoms (including somnolence or fatigue) and coordination abnormalities (including ataxia, dizziness, and gait disturbances). Caution patients about performing tasks which require mental alertness (eg, operating machinery or driving). Effects with other sedative drugs or ethanol may be potentiated. Potentially serious, sometimes fatal, multiorgan hypersensitivity reactions have been reported with some antiepileptic drugs, including rufinamide; monitor for signs and symptoms of possible disparate manifestations associated with lymphatic, hepatic, renal, and/or hematologic organ systems; gradual discontinuation and conversion to alternate therapy may be required. Closely monitor any patient who develops a rash; instruct patients to report any rash associated with fever.

Antiepileptics are associated with an increased risk of suicidal behavior/thoughts with use (regardless of indication); patients should be monitored for signs/symptoms of depression, suicidal tendencies, and other unusual behavior changes during therapy and instructed to inform their healthcare provider immediately if symptoms occur. Use with caution in patients with mild-to-moderate hepatic impairment; use in not recommended in patients with severe hepatic impairment. Concurrent use with hormonal contraceptives may lead to contraceptive failure. Anticonvulsants should not be discontinued abruptly because of the possibility of increasing seizure frequency; therapy should be withdrawn gradually to minimize the potential of increased seizure frequency, unless safety concerns require a more rapid withdrawal. Reducing dose by ~25% every two days was effective in trials.

Adverse Reactions (Reflective of adult population; not specific for elderly)
>10%:
  Cardiovascular: QT shortening (46% to 65%; dose related)
  Central nervous system: Headache (16% to 27%), somnolence (11% to 24%), dizziness (3% to 19%), fatigue (9% to 16%)
  Gastrointestinal: Vomiting (5% to 17%), nausea (7% to 12%)
1% to 10%:
  Central nervous system: Ataxia (4% to 5%), seizure (children 5%), status epilepticus (≤4%), aggression (children 3%), anxiety (adults 3%), attention disturbance (children 3%), hyperactivity (children 3%), vertigo (adults 3%)
  Dermatologic: Rash (children 4%), pruritus (children 3%)
  Gastrointestinal: Appetite decreased (≥1% to 5%), abdominal pain (3%), constipation (adults 3%), dyspepsia (adults 3%), appetite increased (≥1%)
  Hematologic: Leukopenia (≤4%), anemia (≥1%)
  Neuromuscular & skeletal: Tremor (adults 6%), back pain (adults 3%), gait disturbance (1% to 3%)
  Ocular: Diplopia (4% to 9%), blurred vision (adults 6%), nystagmus (adults 6%)

◀ Otic: Otitis media (children 3%)
Renal: Pollakiuria (≥1%)
Respiratory: Nasopharyngitis (children 5%), bronchitis (children 3%), sinusitis (children 3%)
Miscellaneous: Influenza (children 5%)

Drug Interactions

Metabolism/Transport Effects Inhibits CYP2E1 (weak); **Induces** CYP3A4 (weak/moderate)

Avoid Concomitant Use
Avoid concomitant use of Rufinamide with any of the following: Axitinib

Increased Effect/Toxicity
Rufinamide may increase the levels/effects of: Fosphenytoin; PHENobarbital; Phenytoin

The levels/effects of Rufinamide may be increased by: Divalproex; Valproic Acid

Decreased Effect
Rufinamide may decrease the levels/effects of: ARIPiprazole; Axitinib; CarBAMazepine; Ethinyl Estradiol; Norethindrone; Saxagliptin

The levels/effects of Rufinamide may be decreased by: CarBAMazepine; Fosphenytoin; PHENobarbital; Phenytoin; Primidone

Ethanol/Nutrition/Herb Interactions
Ethanol: Ethanol may increase CNS depression. Management: Avoid ethanol.
Food: Food increases the absorption of rufinamide. Management: Take with food.
Herb/Nutraceutical: Evening primrose may decrease seizure threshold. Management: Avoid evening primrose.

Stability Store at 25°C (77°F); excursions permitted to 15°C to 30°C (59°F to 86°F). Protect tablets from moisture. The cap to the oral suspension bottle fits over the adapter.

Mechanism of Action A triazole-derivative antiepileptic whose exact mechanism is unknown. In vitro, it prolongs the inactive state of the sodium channels, thereby limiting repetitive firing of sodium-dependent action potentials mediating anticonvulsant effects.

Pharmacodynamics/Kinetics
Absorption: Slow; extensive ≥85%; increased with food
Distribution: V_d: ~50 L
Protein binding: 34%, primarily to albumin
Metabolism: Extensively via carboxylesterase-mediated hydrolysis of the carboxylamide group to CGP 47292 (inactive metabolite); weak inhibitor of CYP2E1 and weak inducer of CYP3A4
Bioavailability: Extent decreased with increased dose; oral tablets and oral suspension are bioequivalent
Half-life elimination: ~6-10 hours
Time to peak, plasma: 4-6 hours
Excretion: Urine (85%, ~66% as CGP 47292, <2% as unchanged drug)

Dosage

Geriatric & Adult Lennox-Gastaut (adjunctive): Oral:
U.S. labeling: Initial: 400-800 mg/day in 2 equally divided doses; increase dose by 400-800 mg/day every other day to a maximum dose of 3200 mg/day in 2 equally divided doses
Canadian labeling:
<30 kg: Initial: 100 mg twice daily; increase dose by 5 mg/kg/day every 2 weeks until satisfactory control (maximum dose: 1300 mg/day)
≥30 kg: Initial: 200 mg twice daily; increase dose by 5 mg/kg/day every 2 weeks until satisfactory control (maximum dose: 30-50 kg: 1800 mg/day; 50.1-70 kg: 2400 mg/day; ≥70.1 kg: 3200 mg/day). **Note:** Dose was increased as frequently as every other day in clinical trials.

Dosage adjustment for concomitant medications: Valproate:
U.S. labeling: Initial rufinamide dose should be <400 mg/day
Canadian labeling: Initial rufinamide dose should be less than the initial daily recommended dosage; however, a specific dosage recommendation is not included in the manufacturer's labeling.

Renal Impairment
Cl_{cr} <30 mL/minute: No dosage adjustment needed.
Hemodialysis: No specific guidelines available; consider dosage adjustment for loss of drug.

Hepatic Impairment
Mild-to-moderate impairment: Use caution.
Severe impairment: Use in severe impairment has not been studied and is not recommended.

Administration Administer with food. Tablets may be swallowed whole, split in half, or crushed. Oral suspension should be administered using the provided adapter and oral syringe; shake well before every administration.

Monitoring Parameters Seizure (frequency and duration); serum levels of concurrent anticonvulsants; suicidality (eg, suicidal thoughts, depression, behavioral changes)

Special Geriatric Considerations Limited study in the elderly; however, to date, no data to demonstrate differences in pharmacokinetic between elderly and young adults. No dosage adjustment necessary.

Dosage Forms Excipient information presented when available (limited, particularly for generics); consult specific product labeling.

Suspension, oral:

Banzel®: 40 mg/mL (460 mL) [dye free, gluten free; contains propylene glycol; orange flavor]

Tablet, oral:

Banzel®: 200 mg, 400 mg [scored]

Dosage Forms: Canada Excipient information presented when available (limited, particularly for generics); consult specific product labeling.

Tablet, oral:

Banzel™: 100 mg [scored]

- ◆ **Rulox [OTC]** *see* Aluminum Hydroxide, Magnesium Hydroxide, and Simethicone *on page 82*
- ◆ **Rybix™ ODT** *see* TraMADol *on page 1942*
- ◆ **Rythmol®** *see* Propafenone *on page 1618*
- ◆ **Rythmol® SR** *see* Propafenone *on page 1618*
- ◆ **Ryzolt™** *see* TraMADol *on page 1942*
- ◆ **S2® [OTC]** *see* EPINEPHrine (Systemic, Oral Inhalation) *on page 645*
- ◆ **S-(+)-3-isobutylgaba** *see* Pregabalin *on page 1598*
- ◆ **6(S)-5-methyltetrahydrofolate** *see* Methylfolate *on page 1245*
- ◆ **6(S)-5-MTHF** *see* Methylfolate *on page 1245*
- ◆ **S-4661** *see* Doripenem *on page 594*
- ◆ **Sabril®** *see* Vigabatrin *on page 2021*

Saccharomyces boulardii (sak roe MYE sees boo LAR dee)

Medication Safety Issues

International issues:

Codex: Brand name for *saccharomyces boulardii* [Italy], but also the brand name for acetaminophen/codeine [Brazil]

Codex [Italy] may be confused with Cedax brand name for ceftibuten [U.S. and multiple international markets]; Clobex brand name for clobetasol [U.S., Canada, and multiple international markets]

Precosa [Finland, Norway, Sweden] may be confused with Precose brand name for acarbose [U.S.]

Brand Names: U.S. Florastor® Kids [OTC]; Florastor® [OTC]

Index Terms *S. boulardii; Saccharomyces boulardii lyo*

Generic Availability (U.S.) No

Pharmacologic Category Dietary Supplement; Probiotic

Use Promote maintenance of normal microflora in the gastrointestinal tract; used in management of bloating, gas, and diarrhea, particularly to decrease the incidence of diarrhea associated with antibiotic use

Contraindications Hypersensitivity to *Saccharomyces boulardii* or any component of the formulation

Warnings/Precautions *S. boulardii*, a nonpathogenic yeast, has been associated with case reports of invasive fungemias in immunocompromised, debilitated, or critically ill patients; use caution or avoid use in these patients, particularly those with a central venous catheter and/or previous or current antibiotic therapy. Use caution in patients allergic to yeast; *S. boulardii* is a live yeast preparation and a subtype of the species, *S. cervasiae*, which is also referred to as "baker's yeast" or "brewer's yeast." Avoid use in patients on systemic antifungal therapy; *S. boulardii* may be susceptible. Probiotic products are classified as dietary supplements; therefore, there are no safety reviews or approved therapeutic indications by the FDA. There is no conclusive evidence to support widespread use in the treatment of diarrhea. Significant differences may exist from one preparation of *S. boulardii* compared to another with respect to biologic activity and composition. Some products may contain lactose.

Adverse Reactions (Reflective of adult population; not specific for elderly) Frequency not defined.

Gastrointestinal: Constipation, flatulence

Miscellaneous: Thirst

Drug Interactions
  Metabolism/Transport Effects None known.
  Avoid Concomitant Use There are no known interactions where it is recommended to avoid concomitant use.
  Increased Effect/Toxicity There are no known significant interactions involving an increase in effect.
  Decreased Effect
    The levels/effects of Saccharomyces boulardii may be decreased by: Antifungal Agents
Stability Some preparations may need to be refrigerated or stored in freezer; consult individual product labeling.
  Florastor®, Florastor® Kids: Store at ≤25°C (≤77°F); refrigeration not necessary.
Mechanism of Action S. boulardii, a nonpathogenic live yeast probiotic, acts as temporary flora to help re-establish the normal gastrointestinal microflora. May also modulate the immune system by inducing cytokines and suppress pathogenic bacteria growth.
Pharmacodynamics/Kinetics
  Onset of action: Yeast cell release from capsules/powder: 30 minutes
  Duration: Yeast cells cleared in 5-7 days
Dosage
  Geriatric Refer to adult dosing. Use caution in debilitated patients.
  Adult Dietary supplement: Oral: Dosing varies by manufacturer; consult product labeling.
    Florastor®: 250 mg twice daily
Administration
  Florastor®: Swallow capsule whole or capsules may be opened and emptied on tongue (wash down with water or juice) or sprinkled on semi-solid food (eg, applesauce, sour cream, yogurt) or added to a drink (eg, water, apple or orange juice, milk or formula); may be administered with or without food.
  Florastor® Kids: Add powder to a drink or sprinkle on semi-solid food; may be administered with or without food.
Special Geriatric Considerations Use caution in debilitated patients.
Dosage Forms Excipient information presented when available (limited, particularly for generics); consult specific product labeling.
  Capsule, oral:
    Florastor®: S. boulardii lyo 250 mg [contains lactose 32.5 mg/capsule, magnesium 2.85 mg/capsule; provides 5 billion live cells]
  Powder, oral:
    Florastor® Kids: S. boulardii lyo 250 mg/packet (10s) [contains lactose 32.5 mg/packet, magnesium 2.85 mg/packet; tutti frutti flavor; provides 5 billion live cells]

◆ *Saccharomyces boulardii lyo* see Saccharomyces boulardii on page 1741
◆ *Safe Tussin® DM [OTC]* see Guaifenesin and Dextromethorphan on page 906
◆ *Safe Wash™ [OTC]* see Sodium Chloride on page 1787
◆ *Salactic® [OTC]* see Salicylic Acid on page 1743
◆ *Salbutamol* see Albuterol on page 49
◆ *Salbutamol and Ipratropium* see Ipratropium and Albuterol on page 1037
◆ *Salbutamol Sulphate* see Albuterol on page 49
◆ *Salex®* see Salicylic Acid on page 1743

Salicylates (Various Salts) (sa LIS i lates)

Brand Names: U.S. Arthropan®; Asproject®; Extra Strength Doan's® [OTC]; Magan®; Mobidin®; Original Doan's® [OTC]; Rexolate®; Tusal®
Index Terms Choline Salicylate; Magnesium Salicylate; Sodium Salicylate; Sodium Thiosalicylate
Generic Availability (U.S.) Yes
Pharmacologic Category Analgesic, Nonopioid; Anti-inflammatory Agent; Antiplatelet Agent; Antipyretic; Nonsteroidal Anti-inflammatory Drug (NSAID), Oral; Salicylate
Use Treatment of mild to moderate pain, inflammation and fever; may be used as a prophylaxis of myocardial infarction and transient ischemic attacks (TIA)
Contraindications Bleeding disorders, hypersensitivity to salicylates or other nonsteroidal anti-inflammatory drugs (NSAIDs)
Stability Keep suppositories in refrigerator, do not freeze; hydrolysis of aspirin occurs upon exposure to water or moist air, resulting in salicylate and acetate, which possess a vinegar-like odor; do not use if a strong odor is present
Mechanism of Action Inhibits prostaglandin synthesis, acts on the hypothalamus heat-regulating center to reduce fever, blocks prostaglandin synthetase action which prevents formation of the platelet-aggregating substance thromboxane A_2; inhibits both vitamin K-dependent and independent clotting factors

Pharmacodynamics/Kinetics

Absorption: From the stomach and small intestine

Distribution: Readily into most body fluids and tissues

Aspirin is hydrolyzed to salicylate (active) by esterases in the GI mucosa, red blood cells, synovial fluid and blood

Metabolism: Metabolism of salicylate occurs primarily by hepatic microsomal enzymes

Half-life, aspirin: 15-20 minutes; metabolic pathways are saturable such that salicylate half-life is dose-dependent ranging from 3 hours at lower doses (300-600 mg), 5-6 hours (after 1 g) and 15-30 hours with higher doses; in therapeutic anti-inflammatory doses, half-lives generally range from 6-12 hours

Time to peak plasma concentration: ~1-2 hours

Monitoring Parameters Serum concentrations, renal function; hearing changes or tinnitus; monitor for response (ie, pain, inflammation, range of motion, grip strength); observe for abnormal bleeding, bruising, weight gain

Reference Range

Sample size: 1.5-2 mL blood (lavender top (EDTA) tube)

Timing of serum samples: Peak levels usually occur 2 hours after ingestion; half-life increases with dosage (eg, the half-life after 300 mg is 3 hours, and after 1 g is 5-6 hours, and after 8-10 g is 10 hours)

Salicylate serum concentrations correlate with the pharmacological actions and adverse effects observed.

Test Interactions False-negative results for glucose oxidase urinary glucose tests (Clinistix®); false-positives using the cupric sulfate method (Clinitest®); also, interferes with Gerhardt test (urinary ketone analysis), VMA determination; 5-HIAA, xylose tolerance test, and T_3 and T_4; increased PBI; increased uric acid

Pharmacotherapy Pearls Liquid dosage form may be useful for those who have difficulty swallowing tablets or caplets. These agents do not appear to inhibit platelet aggregation. Nonacetylated salicylates have less GI toxicity and renal effects than aspirin and other NSAIDs. They also do not cause reactions in aspirin sensitive patients.

Choline salicylate: Arthropan®

Sodium thiosalicylate: Asproject®; Rexolate®; Tusal®

Magnesium salicylate: Extra Strength Doan's® [OTC]; Magan®; Mobidin®; Original Doan's® [OTC]

Special Geriatric Considerations Elderly are a high-risk population for adverse effects from NSAIDs. As much as 60% of elderly can develop peptic ulceration and/or hemorrhage asymptomatically. The concomitant use of H_2 blockers, omeprazole, and sucralfate is not effective as prophylaxis with the exception of NSAID-induced duodenal ulcers which may be prevented by the use of ranitidine. Misoprostol and proton pump inhibitors are the only agents proven to help prevent the development of NSAID-induced ulcers. Also, concomitant disease and drug use contribute to the risk for GI adverse effects. Use lowest effective dose for shortest period possible. Consider renal function decline with age. Use of NSAIDs can compromise existing renal function especially when Cl_{cr} is ≤30 mL/minute. Tinnitus may be a difficult and unreliable indication of toxicity due to age-related hearing loss or eighth cranial nerve damage. CNS adverse effects such as confusion, agitation, and hallucination are generally seen in overdose or high dose situations, but elderly may demonstrate these adverse effects at lower doses than younger adults.

Dosage Forms

Injection: 50 mg/mL

Liquid: 870 mg/mL (choline salicylate)

Tablet, enteric coated: 325 mg, 545 mg, 600 mg, 650 mg

◆ **Salicylazosulfapyridine** see SulfaSALAzine on page 1817

Salicylic Acid (sal i SIL ik AS id)

Medication Safety Issues

Sound-alike/look-alike issues:

Occlusal™-HP may be confused with Ocuflox®

Other safety concerns:

Transdermal patch may contain conducting metal (eg, aluminum); remove patch prior to MRI.

Brand Names: U.S. Aliclen™; Beta Sal® [OTC]; Clean & Clear® Advantage® Acne Cleanser [OTC]; Clean & Clear® Advantage® Acne Spot Treatment [OTC]; Clean & Clear® Advantage® Invisible Acne Patch [OTC]; Clean & Clear® Advantage® Oil-Free Acne [OTC]; Clean & Clear® Blackhead Clearing Daily Cleansing [OTC]; Clean & Clear® Blackhead Clearing Scrub [OTC]; Clean & Clear® Deep Cleaning [OTC]; Clean & Clear® Dual Action Moisturizer [OTC]; Clean & Clear® Invisible Blemish Treatment [OTC]; Compound W® One Step Invisible

Strip [OTC]; Compound W® One Step Wart Remover for Feet [OTC]; Compound W® One-Step Wart Remover for Kids [OTC]; Compound W® One-Step Wart Remover [OTC]; Compound W® [OTC]; Curad® Mediplast® [OTC]; Denorex® Extra Strength Protection 2-in-1 [OTC]; Denorex® Extra Strength Protection [OTC]; Dermarest® Psoriasis Medicated Moisturizer [OTC]; Dermarest® Psoriasis Medicated Scalp Treatment [OTC]; Dermarest® Psoriasis Medicated Shampoo/Conditioner [OTC]; Dermarest® Psoriasis Medicated Skin Treatment [OTC]; Dermarest® Psoriasis Overnight Treatment [OTC]; DHS™ Sal [OTC]; Dr. Scholl's® Callus Removers [OTC]; Dr. Scholl's® Clear Away® One Step Wart Remover [OTC]; Dr. Scholl's® Clear Away® Plantar Wart Remover For Feet [OTC]; Dr. Scholl's® Clear Away® Wart Remover Fast-Acting [OTC]; Dr. Scholl's® Clear Away® Wart Remover Invisible Strips [OTC]; Dr. Scholl's® Clear Away® Wart Remover [OTC]; Dr. Scholl's® Corn Removers [OTC]; Dr. Scholl's® Corn/Callus Remover [OTC]; Dr. Scholl's® Extra Thick Corn Removers [OTC]; Dr. Scholl's® Extra-Thick Callus Removers [OTC]; Dr. Scholl's® For Her Corn Removers [OTC]; Dr. Scholl's® OneStep Callus Removers [OTC]; Dr. Scholl's® OneStep Corn Removers [OTC]; Dr. Scholl's® Small Corn Removers [OTC]; Dr. Scholl's® Ultra-Thin Corn Removers [OTC]; DuoFilm® [OTC]; Freezone® [OTC]; Fung-O® [OTC]; Gets-It® [OTC]; Gordofilm [OTC]; Hydrisalic® [OTC]; Ionil Plus® [OTC]; Ionil® [OTC]; Keralyt®; Keralyt® [OTC]; LupiCare® Dandruff [OTC]; LupiCare® Psoriasis [OTC]; MG217® Sal-Acid [OTC]; Mosco® Callus & Corn Remover [OTC]; Mosco® One Step Corn Remover [OTC]; Neutrogena® Acne Stress Control [OTC]; Neutrogena® Advanced Solutions™ [OTC]; Neutrogena® Blackhead Eliminating™ 2-in-1 Foaming Pads [OTC]; Neutrogena® Blackhead Eliminating™ Daily Scrub [OTC]; Neutrogena® Blackhead Eliminating™ [OTC]; Neutrogena® Body Clear® [OTC]; Neutrogena® Clear Pore™ Oil-Controlling Astringent [OTC]; Neutrogena® Maximum Strength T/Sal® [OTC]; Neutrogena® Oil-Free Acne Stress Control [OTC]; Neutrogena® Oil-Free Acne Wash 60 Second Mask Scrub [OTC]; Neutrogena® Oil-Free Acne Wash Cream Cleanser [OTC]; Neutrogena® Oil-Free Acne Wash Foam Cleanser [OTC]; Neutrogena® Oil-Free Acne Wash [OTC]; Neutrogena® Oil-Free Acne [OTC]; Neutrogena® Oil-Free Anti-Acne [OTC]; Neutrogena® Rapid Clear® Acne Defense [OTC]; Neutrogena® Rapid Clear® Acne Eliminating [OTC]; Neutrogena® Rapid Clear® [OTC]; OXY® Body Wash [OTC]; OXY® Chill Factor® [OTC]; OXY® Daily Cleansing [OTC]; OXY® Daily [OTC]; OXY® Face Wash [OTC]; OXY® Maximum Daily Cleansing [OTC]; OXY® Maximum [OTC]; OXY® Post-Shave [OTC]; OXY® Spot Treatment [OTC]; OXY® [OTC]; P&S® [OTC]; Palmer's® Skin Success Acne Cleanser [OTC]; Sal-Plant® [OTC]; Salactic® [OTC]; Salex®; Salvax; Scalpicin® Anti-Itch [OTC]; Selsun blue® Deep Cleaning Micro-Bead Scrub [OTC]; Selsun blue® Naturals Island Breeze [OTC]; Selsun blue® Naturals Itchy Dry Scalp [OTC]; Stridex® Essential Care® [OTC]; Stridex® Facewipes To Go® [OTC]; Stridex® Maximum Strength [OTC]; Stridex® Sensitive Skin [OTC]; Thera-Sal [OTC] [DSC]; Tinamed® Corn and Callus Remover [OTC]; Tinamed® Wart Remover [OTC]; Trans-Ver-Sal® [OTC]; Virasal®; Wart-Off® Maximum Strength [OTC]; Zapzyt® Acne Wash [OTC]; Zapzyt® Pore Treatment [OTC]

Brand Names: Canada Duofilm®; Duoforte® 27; Occlusal™-HP; Sebcur®; Soluver®; Soluver® Plus; Trans-Plantar®; Trans-Ver-Sal®

Generic Availability (U.S.) Yes: Foam, Bar, Cream, gel, lotion, shampoo, soap

Pharmacologic Category Acne Products; Keratolytic Agent; Topical Skin Product, Acne

Use Topically for its keratolytic effect in controlling seborrheic dermatitis or psoriasis of body and scalp, dandruff, and other scaling dermatoses; also used to remove warts, corns, and calluses; acne

Contraindications Hypersensitivity to salicylic acid or any component of the formulation

Additional contraindications: Virasal®: Impaired circulation (eg, diabetes, peripheral vascular disease); moles, birthmarks; warts with hair growth or on face

Warnings/Precautions Prior to OTC use, consult with healthcare provider if you have diabetes or poor circulation. Not for application to areas that are irritated, infected, reddened, birthmarks, genital or facial warts, or mucous membranes. Avoid contact with eyes.

Adverse Reactions (Reflective of adult population; not specific for elderly) Frequency not defined.

Central nervous system: Dizziness, headache, mental confusion

Local: Burning and irritation at site of exposure on normal tissue, peeling, scaling

Otic: Tinnitus

Respiratory: Hyperventilation

Drug Interactions

Metabolism/Transport Effects None known.

Avoid Concomitant Use There are no known interactions where it is recommended to avoid concomitant use.

Increased Effect/Toxicity There are no known significant interactions involving an increase in effect.

Decreased Effect There are no known significant interactions involving a decrease in effect.

Mechanism of Action Produces desquamation of hyperkeratotic epithelium via dissolution of the intercellular cement which causes the cornified tissue to swell, soften, macerate, and desquamate. Salicylic acid is keratolytic at concentrations of 3% to 6%; it becomes destructive to tissue at concentrations >6%. Concentrations of 6% to 60% are used to remove corns and warts and in the treatment of psoriasis and other hyperkeratotic disorders.

Pharmacodynamics/Kinetics

Absorption: Percutaneous; systemic toxicity unlikely with normal use

Time to peak, serum: Within 5 hours of application with occlusion

Dosage

Geriatric & Adult

Acne: Topical:

Cream, cloth, foam, or liquid cleansers (2%): Use to cleanse skin once or twice daily. Massage gently into skin, work into lather and rinse thoroughly. Cloths should be wet with water prior to using and disposed of (not flushed) after use.

Gel (0.5% or 2%): Apply small amount to face in the morning or evening; if peeling occurs, may be used every other day. Some products may be labeled for OTC use up to 3 or 4 times per day. Apply to clean, dry skin

Pads (0.5% or 2%): Use pad to cover affected area with thin layer of salicylic acid 1-3 times/day. Apply to clean, dry skin. Do not leave pad on skin.

Patch (2%): At bedtime, after washing face, allow skin to dry at least 5 minutes. Apply patch directly over pimple being treated. Remove in the morning.

Shower/bath gels or soap (2%): Use once daily in shower or bath to massage over skin prone to acne. Rinse well.

Callus, corns, or warts: Topical: Note: For warts: Before applying product, soak area in warm water for 5 minutes; remove loosened wart tissue with a brush, wash cloth, or emery board; dry area thoroughly, then apply medication.

Foam: Apply to affected area twice daily; rub into skin until completely absorbed.

Gel or liquid (17%): Apply to each wart and allow to dry. May repeat once or twice daily, up to 12 weeks. Apply to clean dry area.

Gel (6%): Apply to affected area once daily, generally used at night and rinsed off in the morning.

Liquid (27.5%): Apply to each wart; allow to dry then apply a second application. May repeat two-application process once or twice daily, up to 6 weeks

Transdermal patch (15%): Apply directly over affected area at bedtime, leave in place overnight and remove in the morning. Patch should be trimmed to cover affected area. May repeat daily for up to 12 weeks.

Transdermal patch (40%): Apply directly over affected area, leave in place for 48 hours. Some products may be cut to fit area or secured with adhesive strips. May repeat procedure for up to 12 weeks. Apply to clean, dry skin

Dandruff, psoriasis, or seborrheic dermatitis: Topical:

Cream (2.5%): Apply to affected area 3-4 times daily. Apply to clean, dry skin. Some products may be left in place overnight.

Foam: Apply to affected area twice daily; rub into skin until completely absorbed.

Ointment (3%): Apply to scales or plaques on skin up to 4 times per day (not for scalp or face)

Shampoo (1.8% to 3%): Massage into wet hair or affected area; leave in place for several minutes; rinse thoroughly. Labeled for OTC use 2-3 times a week, or as directed by healthcare provider. Some products may be left in place overnight.

Special Geriatric Considerations No specific considerations are needed if used according to recommended doses and duration of use. Many elderly may have diabetes or impaired circulation and avoidance of topical salicylic acid would be advised.

Dosage Forms Excipient information presented when available (limited, particularly for generics); consult specific product labeling. [DSC] = Discontinued product

Aerosol, foam, topical: 6% (70 g)

Salvax: 6% (70 g, 200 g) [ethanol free]

Bar, topical [soap]: 2% (113 g)

OXY®: 0.5% (119 g)

Cloth, topical:

Neutrogena® Oil-Free Acne Wash: 2% (30s)

Cream, topical: 6% (400 g, 480 g)

Clean & Clear® Advantage® Acne Cleanser: 2% (148 mL)

Clean & Clear® Advantage® Acne Spot Treatment: 2% (22 g) [contains benzalkonium chloride, ethanol 14%]

Clean & Clear® Blackhead Clearing Scrub: 2% (141 g, 226 g) [contains ethanol]

Clean & Clear® Dual Action Moisturizer: 0.5% (120 mL) [contains ethanol]

LupiCare® Psoriasis: 2% (227 g)

Neutrogena® Acne Stress Control: 2% (125 g) [with microbeads]

◄

    Neutrogena® Oil-Free Acne: 2% (125 mL) [contains ethanol, tartrazine; with microbeads]
    Neutrogena® Oil-Free Acne Wash Cream Cleanser: 2% (200 mL) [contains ethanol]
    Neutrogena® Oil-Free Anti-Acne: 0.5% (50 g) [contains aloe]
    Salex®: 6% (454 g)
    Salitop™: 6% (400 g) [contains ethanol]

Cream, topical [wash]:
    Neutrogena® Oil-Free Acne Stress Control: 2% (172 g)

Gel, topical: 6% (40 g)
    Clean & Clear® Advantage® Invisible Acne Patch: 2% (1.9 mL) [contains ethanol]
    Clean & Clear® Invisible Blemish Treatment: 2% (22 mL) [contains ethanol 28%]
    Compound W®: 17.6% (7 g) [contains ethanol 67.5%]
    Dermarest® Psoriasis Medicated Scalp Treatment: 3% (118 mL)
    Dermarest® Psoriasis Medicated Skin Treatment: 3% (118 mL)
    Dermarest® Psoriasis Overnight Treatment: 3% (56.7 g)
    Hydrisalic®: 6% (28 g) [contains ethanol]
    Keralyt®: 3% (30 g); 6% (40 g, 100 g) [contains ethanol 21%]
    Neutrogena® Oil-Free Acne Wash: 2% (177 mL, 296 mL) [contains tartrazine]
    Neutrogena® Rapid Clear® Acne Eliminating: 2% (15 mL) [contains ethanol 38%]
    OXY®: 2% (355 mL) [contains aloe]
    OXY® Body Wash: 2% (355 mL)
    OXY® Body Wash: 2% (355 mL) [contains aloe]
    OXY® Chill Factor®: 2% (142 g)
    OXY® Face Wash: 2% (177 mL) [contains aloe]
    OXY® Maximum: 2% (142 g)
    OXY® Spot Treatment: 1% (14.7 g) [contains aloe]
    Sal-Plant®: 17% (14 g) [contains isopropyl alcohol]
    Zapzyt® Acne Wash: 2% (188.5 g) [ethanol free]
    Zapzyt® Pore Treatment: 2% (22 mL) [ethanol free]

Gel, topical [peel]:
    Neutrogena® Advanced Solutions™: 2% (40 g)

Liquid, topical:
    Clean & Clear® Advantage® Oil-Free Acne: 0.5% (120 mL) [contains benzalkonium chloride]
    Clean & Clear® Deep Cleaning: 2% (240 mL) [contains benzoic acid, ethanol]
    Compound W®: 17.6% (9 mL) [contains ethanol 21.2%]
    Dr. Scholl's® Clear Away® Wart Remover Fast-Acting: 17% (9.8 mL) [contains ethanol 18% w/w; includes 20 cover-up discs]
    Dr. Scholl's® Corn/Callus Remover: 12.6% (9.8 mL)
    Dr. Scholl's® Corn/Callus Remover: 12.6% (9.8 mL) [contains ethanol 18% w/w]
    DuoFilm®: 17% (9.8 mL) [contains ethanol]
    Freezone®: 17.6% (9.3 mL) [contains ethanol]
    Fung-O®: 17% (15 mL) [contains ethanol 2%]
    Gets-It®: 13.9% (15 mL)
    Gordofilm: 16.7% (15 mL)
    Mosco® Callus & Corn Remover: 17.6% (9 mL) [contains ethanol 27%]
    Neutrogena® Blackhead Eliminating™ Daily Scrub: 2% (125 mL)
    Neutrogena® Clear Pore™ Oil-Controlling Astringent: 2% (236 mL) [contains ethanol 45%]
    Neutrogena® Oil-Free Acne Stress Control: 2% (50 mL)
    Palmer's® Skin Success Acne Cleanser: 0.5% (240 mL) [contains aloe, vitamin E]
    Salactic®: 17% (15 mL) [contains isopropyl alcohol]
    Scalpicin® Anti-Itch: 3% (44 mL, 74 mL) [contains aloe]
    Tinamed® Corn and Callus Remover: 17% (15 mL)
    Tinamed® Wart Remover: 17% (15 mL)
    Virasal®: 27.5% (10 mL) [contains isopropyl alcohol]
    Wart-Off® Maximum Strength: 17.5% (14.8 mL) [contains ethanol]

Liquid, topical [body scrub with microbeads]:
    Neutrogena® Body Clear®: 2% (250 mL) [contains tartrazine]

Liquid, topical [body wash]:
    Neutrogena® Body Clear®: 2% (250 mL) [contains tartrazine]

Liquid, topical [foam]:
    Neutrogena® Oil-Free Acne Wash Foam Cleanser: 2% (150 mL)

Liquid, topical [foam/wash]:
    Neutrogena® Oil-Free Acne Stress Control: 0.5% (177 mL)

Liquid, topical [mask/wash]:
    Neutrogena® Oil-Free Acne Wash 60 Second Mask Scrub: 1% (170 g) [ethanol free]

Lotion, topical: 6% (414 mL); 6% (400 g)
    Dermarest® Psoriasis Medicated Moisturizer: 2% (118 mL)
    Neutrogena® Rapid Clear® Acne Defense: 2% (50 mL) [contains ethanol]

OXY® Post-Shave: 0.5% (50 g) [contains aloe]
Salex®: 6% (237 mL)
Salitop™: 6% (414 mL) [contains ethanol]
Ointment, topical:
MG217® Sal-Acid: 3% (57 g) [contains vitamin E]
Pad, topical:
Clean & Clear® Blackhead Clearing Daily Cleansing: 1% (70s) [contains ethanol 39%]
Curad® Mediplast®: 40% (25s)
Neutrogena® Blackhead Eliminating™: 0.5% (28s)
Neutrogena® Blackhead Eliminating™ 2-in-1 Foaming Pads: 0.5% (28s)
Neutrogena® Rapid Clear®: 2% (60s) [contains benzalkonium chloride, ethanol 35%]
OXY® Chill Factor®: 2% (90s) [contains ethanol 46% v/v]
OXY® Daily: 0.2% (90s) [contains ethanol 46% v/v]
OXY® Daily Cleansing: 0.5% (90s) [contains ethanol 34% v/v]
OXY® Maximum Daily Cleansing: 2% (55s, 90s) [contains ethanol 46% v/v]
Stridex® Essential Care®: 1% (55s) [ethanol free; contains vitamin A, vitamin E]
Stridex® Facewipes To Go®: 0.5% (32s) [contains aloe, ethanol 28%]
Stridex® Maximum Strength: 2% (55s, 90s) [ethanol free]
Stridex® Sensitive Skin: 0.5% (55s, 90s) [ethanol free]
Patch, topical:
Compound W® One Step Invisible Strip: 14% (14s)
Compound W® One Step Wart Remover for Feet: 40% (20s)
Compound W® One-Step Wart Remover: 40% (14s)
Compound W® One-Step Wart Remover for Kids: 40% (12s)
Dr. Scholl's® Callus Removers: 40% (4s)
Dr. Scholl's® Callus Removers: 40% (4s) [includes 6 cushions]
Dr. Scholl's® Clear Away® One Step Wart Remover: 40% (14s)
Dr. Scholl's® Clear Away® Plantar Wart Remover For Feet: 40% (24s)
Dr. Scholl's® Clear Away® Wart Remover: 40% (18s)
Dr. Scholl's® Clear Away® Wart Remover Invisible Strips: 40% (18s)
Dr. Scholl's® Corn Removers: 40% (9s)
Dr. Scholl's® Corn Removers: 40% (9s) [includes 9 cushions]
Dr. Scholl's® Extra Thick Corn Removers: 40% (9s)
Dr. Scholl's® Extra-Thick Callus Removers: 40% (4s)
Dr. Scholl's® Extra-Thick Callus Removers: 40% (4s) [includes 4 cushions]
Dr. Scholl's® For Her Corn Removers: 40% (6s) [includes 6 cushions]
Dr. Scholl's® OneStep Callus Removers: 40% (4s)
Dr. Scholl's® OneStep Corn Removers: 40% (6s)
Dr. Scholl's® Small Corn Removers: 40% (9s)
Dr. Scholl's® Ultra-Thin Corn Removers: 40% (9s) [includes 9 covers]
Mosco® One Step Corn Remover: 40% (8s)
Trans-Ver-Sal®: 15% (10s, 25s) [20 mm PlantarPatch]
Trans-Ver-Sal®: 15% (15s, 40s) [contains propylene glycol]
Trans-Ver-Sal®: 15% (12s, 40s) [contains propylene glycol; 12 mm AdultPatch]
Shampoo, topical: 6% (177 mL)
Aliclen™: 6% (177 mL)
Beta Sal®: 3% (480 mL)
Denorex® Extra Strength Protection: 3% (118 mL, 355 mL)
DHS™ Sal: 3% (120 mL)
Ionil Plus®: 2% (240 mL) [conditioning shampoo]
Ionil®: 2% (120 mL)
LupiCare® Dandruff: 2% (237 mL)
LupiCare® Psoriasis: 2% (237 mL)
Neutrogena® Maximum Strength T/Sal®: 3% (135 mL)
P&S®: 2% (118 mL, 236 mL)
Salex®: 6% (177 mL)
Selsun blue® Deep Cleaning Micro-Bead Scrub: 3% (325 mL) [contains aloe, benzyl alcohol, moisturizers]
Selsun blue® Naturals Island Breeze: 3% (325 mL) [contains aloe, benzyl alcohol]
Selsun blue® Naturals Itchy Dry Scalp: 3% (207 mL, 325 mL) [contains aloe, benzyl alcohol, moisturizers]
Thera-Sal: 3% (180 mL [DSC])
Shampoo/Conditioner, topical:
Denorex® Extra Strength Protection 2-in-1: 3% (118 mL, 355 mL)
Dermarest® Psoriasis Medicated Shampoo/Conditioner: 3% (236 mL)

◆ **Salicylsalicylic Acid** see Salsalate on page 1751
◆ **Saline** see Sodium Chloride on page 1787

SALIVA SUBSTITUTE

◆ **Saline Mist [OTC]** *see* Sodium Chloride *on page 1787*

Saliva Substitute (sa LYE va SUB stee tute)

Brand Names: U.S. Aquoral™; Biotene® Moisturizing Mouth Spray [OTC]; Biotene® Oral Balance® [OTC]; Caphosol®; Entertainer's Secret® [OTC]; Moi-Stir® [OTC]; Mouth Kote® [OTC]; NeutraSal®; Numoisyn™; Oasis®; SalivaSure™ [OTC]
Index Terms Artificial Saliva
Generic Availability (U.S.) No
Pharmacologic Category Gastrointestinal Agent, Miscellaneous
Use Relief of dry mouth and throat in xerostomia or hyposalivation; adjunct to standard oral care in relief of symptoms associated with chemotherapy or radiation therapy-induced mucositis
Dosage
Geriatric & Adult
Mucositis (due to high-dose chemotherapy or radiation therapy): Oral:
Caphosol®, NeutraSal®: Swish and spit 4-10 doses daily (use for the duration of chemo- or radiation therapy)
Xerostomia: Oral: Use as needed, or product-specific dosing:
Aquoral™: 2 sprays 3-4 times daily
Biotene® Oral Balance® gel: Apply one-half inch length onto tongue and spread evenly; repeat as often as needed
Caphosol®, NeutraSal®: Swish and spit 2-10 doses daily
Entertainer's Secret®: Spray as often as needed
Mouth Kote® spray: Spray 3-5 times, swish for 8-10 seconds, then spit or swallow; use as often as needed
Numoisyn™ liquid: Use 2 mL as needed
Numoisyn™ lozenges: Dissolve 1 lozenge slowly; maximum 16 lozenges daily
Oasis® mouthwash: Rinse mouth with ~30 mL twice daily or as needed; do not swallow
Oasis® spray: 1-2 sprays as needed; maximum 60 sprays daily
SalivaSure™: Dissolve 1 lozenge slowly as needed; for severe symptoms, 1 lozenge per hour is recommended
Special Geriatric Considerations Saliva production has not been shown to change with aging; however, many drugs used by elderly can cause dry mouth. These patients may benefit from a saliva substitute.
Dosage Forms Excipient information presented when available (limited, particularly for generics); consult specific product labeling.
Liquid, oral:
Biotene® Oral Balance®: Water, starch, sunflower oil, propylene glycol, xylitol, glycerine, purified milk extract (45 mL) [sugar-free]
Numoisyn™: Water, sorbitol, linseed extract, *Chondrus crispus*, methylparaben, sodium benzoate, potassium sorbate, dipotassium phosphate, propylparaben (300 mL)
Lozenge, oral:
Numoisyn™: Sorbitol 0.3 g/lozenge, polyethylene glycol, malic acid, sodium citrate, calcium phosphate dibasic, hydrogenated cottonseed oil, citric acid, magnesium stearate, silicon dioxide (100s)
SalivaSure™: Xylitol, citric acid, apple acid, sodium citrate dihydrate, sodium carboxyme-thylcellulose, dibasic calcium phosphate, silica colloidal, magnesium stearate, stearic acid (90s)
Powder, for reconstitution, oral:
NeutraSal®: Sodium, phosphates, calcium, chloride, bicarbonate, silicon dioxide (30s, 120s)
Solution, oral:
Caphosol®: Dibasic sodium phosphate 0.032%, monobasic sodium phosphate 0.009%, calcium chloride 0.052%, sodium chloride 0.569%, purified water (30 mL) [packaged in two 15 mL ampuls when mixed together provide one 30 mL dose]
Entertainer's Secret®: Sodium carboxymethylcellulose, aloe vera gel, glycerin (60 mL) [ethanol free; honey-apple flavor]
Solution, oral [mouthwash/gargle]:
Oasis®: Water, glycerin, sorbitol, poloxamer 338, PEG-60, hydrogenated castor oil, copo-vidone, sodium benzoate, carboxymethylcellulose (473 mL) [ethanol free, sugar free; mild mint flavor]
Solution, oral [spray]:
Aquoral™: Oxidized glycerol triesters and silicon dioxide (40 mL) [contains aspartame; delivers 400 sprays, citrus flavor]
Biotene® Moisturizing Mouth Spray: Water, polyglycitol, propylene glycol, sunflower oil, xylitol, milk protein extract, potassium sorbate, acesulfame K, potassium thiocyanate, lysozyme, lactoferrin, lactoperoxidase (45 mL)

Moi-Stir®: Water, sorbitol, sodium carboxymethylcellulose, methylparaben, propylparaben, potassium chloride, dibasic sodium phosphate, calcium chloride, magnesium chloride, sodium chloride (120 mL)

Mouth Kote®: Water, xylitol, sorbitol, yerba santa, citric acid, ascorbic acid, sodium saccharin, sodium benzoate (5 mL, 60 mL, 240 mL) [ethanol free, sugar free; lemon-lime flavor]

Oasis®: Glycerin, cetylpyridinium, copovidone (30 mL) [ethanol free, sugar free; contains sodium benzoate; delivers ~150 sprays, mild mint flavor]

♦ **SalivaSure™ [OTC]** *see* Saliva Substitute *on page 1748*
♦ **Saljet® [OTC]** *see* Sodium Chloride *on page 1787*
♦ **Salk Vaccine** *see* Poliovirus Vaccine (Inactivated) *on page 1561*

Salmeterol (sal ME te role)

Related Information
Inhalant Agents *on page 2117*
Medication Safety Issues
Sound-alike/look-alike issues:
Salmeterol may be confused with Salbutamol, Solu-Medrol®
Serevent® may be confused with Atrovent®, Combivent®, sertraline, Sinemet®, Spiriva®, Zoloft®
Brand Names: U.S. Serevent® Diskus®
Brand Names: Canada Serevent® Diskhaler® Disk; Serevent® Diskus®
Index Terms Salmeterol Xinafoate
Generic Availability (U.S.) No
Pharmacologic Category Beta$_2$ Agonist; Beta$_2$-Adrenergic Agonist, Long-Acting
Use Maintenance treatment of asthma and prevention of bronchospasm (as concomitant therapy) in patients with reversible obstructive airway disease, including patients with symptoms of nocturnal asthma; prevention of exercise-induced bronchospasm (monotherapy may be indicated in patients without persistent asthma); maintenance treatment of bronchospasm associated with COPD
Medication Guide Available Yes
Contraindications Hypersensitivity to salmeterol or any component of the formulation (milk proteins); monotherapy in the treatment of asthma (ie, use without a concomitant long-term asthma control medication, such as an inhaled corticosteroid); status asthmaticus or other acute episodes of asthma or COPD
Warnings/Precautions Asthma treatment: **[U.S. Boxed Warning]: Long-acting beta$_2$-agonists (LABAs) increase the risk of asthma-related deaths. Salmeterol should only be used in asthma patients as adjuvant therapy in patients who are currently receiving but are not adequately controlled on a long-term asthma control medication (ie, an inhaled corticosteroid).** Monotherapy with an LABA is contraindicated in the treatment of asthma. In a large, randomized, placebo-controlled U.S. clinical trial (SMART, 2006), salmeterol was associated with an increase in asthma-related deaths (when added to usual asthma therapy); risk is considered a class effect among all LABAs. Data are not available to determine if the addition of an inhaled corticosteroid lessens this increased risk of death associated with LABA use. Assess patients at regular intervals once asthma control is maintained on combination therapy to determine if step-down therapy is appropriate and the LABA can be discontinued (without loss of asthma control), and the patient can be maintained on an inhaled corticosteroid. LABAs are not appropriate in patients whose asthma is adequately controlled on low- or medium-dose inhaled corticosteroids. Do **not** use for acute bronchospasm. Short-acting beta$_2$-agonist (eg, albuterol) should be used for acute symptoms and symptoms occurring between treatments. Do **not** initiate in patients with significantly worsening or acutely deteriorating asthma; reports of severe (sometimes fatal) respiratory events have been reported when salmeterol has been initiated in this situation. Corticosteroids should not be stopped or reduced when salmeterol is initiated. During initiation, watch for signs of worsening asthma. Patients must be instructed to use short-acting beta$_2$-agonists (eg, albuterol) for acute asthmatic or COPD symptoms and to seek medical attention in cases where acute symptoms are not relieved or a previous level of response is diminished. The need to increase frequency of use of short-acting beta$_2$-agonist may indicate deterioration of asthma, and treatment must not be delayed. Because LABAs may disguise poorly controlled persistent asthma, frequent or chronic use of LABAs for exercise-induced bronchospasm is discouraged by the NIH Asthma Guidelines (NIH, 2007). Salmeterol should not be used more than twice daily; do not use with other long-acting beta$_2$-agonists.

COPD treatment: Appropriate use: Do **not** use for acute episodes of COPD. Do **not** initiate in patients with significantly worsening or acutely deteriorating COPD. Data are not available to determine if LABA use increases the risk of death in patients with COPD.

Concurrent diseases: Use caution in patients with cardiovascular disease (eg, arrhythmia, hypertension, or HF), seizure disorders, diabetes, hyperthyroidism, hepatic impairment, or hypokalemia. Beta-agonists may cause elevation in blood pressure, heart rate, CNS stimulation/excitation, increased risk of arrhythmia, increase serum glucose, or decrease serum potassium.

Adverse events: Immediate hypersensitivity reactions (urticaria, angioedema, rash, bronchospasm) have been reported. There have been reports of laryngeal spasm, irritation, swelling (stridor, choking) with use. Salmeterol should not be used more than twice daily; do not exceed recommended dose; do not use with other long-acting beta$_2$-agonists; serious adverse events have been associated with excessive use of inhaled sympathomimetics. Rarely, paradoxical bronchospasm may occur with use of inhaled bronchodilating agents; this should be distinguished from inadequate response. Use with strong CYP3A4 inhibitors (see Drug Interactions) is not recommended due to potential for an increased risk of cardiovascular events. Powder for oral inhalation contains lactose; very rare anaphylactic reactions have been reported in patients with severe milk protein allergy.

Adverse Reactions (Reflective of adult population; not specific for elderly)

>10%:
  Central nervous system: Headache (13% to 17%)
  Neuromuscular & skeletal: Pain (1% to 12%)
1% to 10%:
  Cardiovascular: Hypertension (4%), edema (1% to 3%), pallor
  Central nervous system: Dizziness (4%), sleep disturbance (1% to 3%), fever (1% to 3%), anxiety (1% to 3%), migraine (1% to 3%)
  Dermatologic: Rash (1% to 4%), contact dermatitis (1% to 3%), eczema (1% to 3%), urticaria (3%), photodermatitis (1% to 2%)
  Endocrine & metabolic: Hyperglycemia (1% to 3%)
  Gastrointestinal: Throat irritation (7%), nausea (1% to 3%), dyspepsia (1% to 3%), dental pain (1% to 3%), gastrointestinal infection (1% to 3%), oropharyngeal candidiasis (1% to 3%), xerostomia (1% to 3%)
  Hepatic: Liver enzymes increased
  Neuromuscular & skeletal: Muscular cramps/spasm (3%), articular rheumatism (1% to 3%), arthralgia (1% to 3%), joint pain (1% to 3%), muscular stiffness (1% to 3%), paresthesia (1% to 3%), rigidity (1% to 3%)
  Ocular: Keratitis/conjunctivitis (1% to 3%)
  Respiratory: Nasal congestion (4% to 9%), tracheitis/bronchitis (7%), pharyngitis (≤6%), cough (5%), influenza (5%), viral respiratory tract infection (5%), sinusitis (4% to 5%), rhinitis (4% to 5%), asthma (3% to 4%)

Drug Interactions

Metabolism/Transport Effects Substrate of CYP3A4 (major); **Note:** Assignment of Major/Minor substrate status based on clinically relevant drug interaction potential

Avoid Concomitant Use
Avoid concomitant use of Salmeterol with any of the following: Beta-Blockers (Nonselective); CYP3A4 Inhibitors (Strong); Iobenguane I 123; Telaprevir

Increased Effect/Toxicity
Salmeterol may increase the levels/effects of: Loop Diuretics; Sympathomimetics; Thiazide Diuretics

The levels/effects of Salmeterol may be increased by: AtoMOXetine; Cannabinoids; CYP3A4 Inhibitors (Moderate); CYP3A4 Inhibitors (Strong); Dasatinib; Ivacaftor; MAO Inhibitors; Mifepristone; Telaprevir; Tricyclic Antidepressants

Decreased Effect
Salmeterol may decrease the levels/effects of: Iobenguane I 123

The levels/effects of Salmeterol may be decreased by: Alpha-/Beta-Blockers; Beta-Blockers (Beta1 Selective); Beta-Blockers (Nonselective); Betahistine; Tocilizumab

Stability Inhalation powder: Store at controlled room temperature 20°C to 25°C (68°F to 77°F) in a dry place away from direct heat or sunlight. Stable for 6 weeks after removal from foil pouch.

Mechanism of Action Relaxes bronchial smooth muscle by selective action on beta$_2$-receptors with little effect on heart rate; salmeterol acts locally in the lung.

Pharmacodynamics/Kinetics
  Onset of action: Asthma: 30-48 minutes, COPD: 2 hours
  Peak effect: Asthma: 3 hours, COPD: 2-5 hours
  Duration: 12 hours
  Absorption: Systemic: Inhalation: Undetectable to poor
  Protein binding: 96%
  Metabolism: Hepatic; hydroxylated via CYP3A4

Half-life elimination: 5.5 hours
Time to peak, serum: ~20 minutes
Excretion: Feces (60%); urine (25%)

Dosage

Geriatric & Adult

Asthma, maintenance and prevention: Inhalation, powder (50 mcg/inhalation): One inhalation twice daily (~12 hours apart); maximum: 1 inhalation twice daily. **Note:** For asthma control, long acting beta$_2$-agonists (LABAs) should be used in combination with inhaled corticosteroids and not as monotherapy.

Exercise-induced asthma, prevention: Inhalation, powder (50 mcg/inhalation): One inhalation at least 30 minutes prior to exercise; additional doses should not be used for 12 hours; should not be used in individuals already receiving salmeterol twice daily. **Note:** Because LABAs may disguise poorly controlled persistent asthma, frequent or chronic use of LABAs for exercise-induced bronchospasm is discouraged by the NIH Asthma Guidelines (NIH, 2007).

COPD maintenance: Inhalation, powder (50 mcg/inhalation): One inhalation twice daily (~12 hours apart); maximum: 1 inhalation twice daily

Hepatic Impairment No dosage adjustment required; manufacturer suggests close monitoring of patients with hepatic impairment.

Administration Inhalation: **Not** to be used for the relief of acute attacks. Not for use with a spacer device. Administer with Diskus® in a level, horizontal position. Do not wash mouthpiece; Diskus® should be kept dry. Discard device 6 weeks after removal from foil pouch or when the dose counter reads "0" (whichever comes first).

Monitoring Parameters FEV$_1$, peak flow, and/or other pulmonary function tests; blood pressure, heart rate; CNS stimulation. Monitor for increased use of short-acting beta$_2$-agonist inhalers; may be marker of a deteriorating asthma condition.

Special Geriatric Considerations Geriatric patients were included in four clinical studies of salmeterol; no apparent differences in efficacy and safety were noted in geriatric patients compared to younger adults. Because salmeterol is only to be used for prevention of bronchospasm, patients also need a short-acting beta-agonist to treat acute attacks. Elderly patients should be carefully counseled about which inhaler to use and the proper scheduling of doses.

Dosage Forms Excipient information presented when available (limited, particularly for generics); consult specific product labeling.
Powder, for oral inhalation:
Serevent® Diskus®: 50 mcg (28s, 60s) [contains lactose]

Dosage Forms: Canada Excipient information presented when available (limited, particularly for generics); consult specific product labeling.
Powder for oral inhalation:
Serevent® Diskhaler® Disk: Salmeterol xinafoate 50 mcg (60s) [delivers 50 mcg/inhalation; contains lactose]

♦ **Salmeterol and Fluticasone** see Fluticasone and Salmeterol on page 827
♦ **Salmeterol Xinafoate** see Salmeterol on page 1749
♦ **Salonpas® Gel-Patch Hot [OTC]** see Capsaicin on page 280
♦ **Salonpas® Hot [OTC]** see Capsaicin on page 280
♦ **Sal-Plant® [OTC]** see Salicylic Acid on page 1743

Salsalate (SAL sa late)

Medication Safety Issues
Sound-alike/look-alike issues:
Salsalate may be confused with sucralfate, sulfaSALAzine

Brand Names: Canada Amigesic®; Salflex®

Index Terms Disalicylic Acid; Salicylsalicylic Acid

Generic Availability (U.S.) Yes

Pharmacologic Category Salicylate

Use Treatment of rheumatoid arthritis, osteoarthritis, and related rheumatic disorders

Contraindications Hypersensitivity to salsalate or any component of the formulation; GI ulcer or bleeding

Warnings/Precautions Use with caution in patients with platelet and bleeding disorders, dehydration, renal dysfunction, erosive gastritis, or peptic ulcer disease; patients with sensitivity to tartrazine dyes, nasal polyps, and asthma may have an increased risk of salicylate sensitivity, previous nonreaction does not guarantee future safe taking of medication.

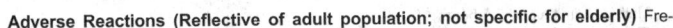

Adverse Reactions (Reflective of adult population; not specific for elderly) Frequency not defined.

Cardiovascular: Hypotension

Central nervous system: Vertigo

Dermatologic: Angioedema, rash, Stevens-Johnson syndrome, toxic epidermal necrolysis, urticaria

Gastrointestinal: Abdominal pain, diarrhea, GI bleeding, GI perforation, GI ulceration, nausea

Hematologic: Anemia

Hepatic: Hepatitis, liver function abnormal

Otic: Hearing impairment, tinnitus

Renal: Creatinine clearance decreased, nephritis

Respiratory: Bronchospasm

Miscellaneous: Anaphylactic shock

Drug Interactions

Metabolism/Transport Effects None known.

Avoid Concomitant Use

Avoid concomitant use of Salsalate with any of the following: Influenza Virus Vaccine (Live/Attenuated)

Increased Effect/Toxicity

Salsalate may increase the levels/effects of: Anticoagulants; Carbonic Anhydrase Inhibitors; Corticosteroids (Systemic); Divalproex; Drotrecogin Alfa (Activated); Hypoglycemic Agents; Methotrexate; PRALAtrexate; Salicylates; Thrombolytic Agents; Valproic Acid; Varicella Virus-Containing Vaccines

The levels/effects of Salsalate may be increased by: Ammonium Chloride; Antiplatelet Agents; Calcium Channel Blockers (Nondihydropyridine); Ginkgo Biloba; Herbs (Anticoagulant/Antiplatelet Properties); Influenza Virus Vaccine (Live/Attenuated); Loop Diuretics; NSAID (Nonselective); Potassium Acid Phosphate; Treprostinil

Decreased Effect

Salsalate may decrease the levels/effects of: ACE Inhibitors; Hyaluronidase; Loop Diuretics; NSAID (Nonselective); Probenecid

The levels/effects of Salsalate may be decreased by: Corticosteroids (Systemic); NSAID (Nonselective)

Ethanol/Nutrition/Herb Interactions

Ethanol: Avoid ethanol (may enhance gastric mucosal irritation).

Food: Salsalate peak serum levels may be delayed if taken with food.

Herb/Nutraceutical: Avoid cat's claw, dong quai, evening primrose, feverfew, garlic, ginger, ginkgo, red clover, horse chestnut, green tea, ginseng (all have additional antiplatelet activity).

Mechanism of Action Weakly inhibits cyclooxygenase enzymes, which results in decreased formation of prostaglandin precursors; has antipyretic, analgesic, and anti-inflammatory properties

Other proposed mechanisms not fully elucidated (and possibly contributing to the anti-inflammatory effect to varying degrees) include inhibiting chemotaxis, altering lymphocyte activity, inhibiting neutrophil aggregation/activation, and decreasing proinflammatory cytokine levels.

Pharmacodynamics/Kinetics

Onset of action: Therapeutic: 3-4 days of continuous dosing

Absorption: Complete from small intestine

Metabolism: Hepatically hydrolyzed to two moles of salicylic acid (active)

Half-life elimination: 7-8 hours

Excretion: Primarily urine

Dosage

Geriatric Refer to adult dosing. May require lower dosage.

Adult Pain, inflammation (arthritis): Oral: 3 g/day in 2-3 divided doses

Administration May be administered with food to decrease GI distress.

Monitoring Parameters Serum concentrations, renal function; hearing changes or tinnitus; monitor for response (ie, pain, inflammation, range of motion, grip strength); observe for abnormal bleeding, bruising, weight gain

Test Interactions False-negative results for glucose oxidase urinary glucose tests (Clinistix®); false-positives using the cupric sulfate method (Clinitest®); also, interferes with Gerhardt test, VMA determination; 5-HIAA, xylose tolerance test and T_3 and T_4

Pharmacotherapy Pearls Does not appear to inhibit platelet aggregation; salsalate causes less GI and renal toxicity than aspirin and other NSAIDs

Special Geriatric Considerations Elderly are a high-risk population for adverse effects from NSAIDs. As much as 60% of the elderly can develop peptic ulceration and/or hemorrhage asymptomatically. The concomitant use of H_2 blockers and sucralfate is not effective as prophylaxis with the exception of NSAID-induced duodenal ulcers which may be prevented by the use of ranitidine. Misoprostol and proton pump inhibitors are the only agents proven to help prevent the development of NSAID-induced ulcers. Also, concomitant disease and drug use contribute to the risk for GI adverse effects. Use lowest effective dose for shortest period possible. Consider renal function decline with age. Use of NSAIDs can compromise existing renal function especially when Cl_{cr} is ≤30 mL/minute. Tinnitus may be a difficult and unreliable indication of toxicity due to age-related hearing loss or eighth cranial nerve damage. CNS adverse effects such as confusion, agitation, and hallucinations are generally seen in overdose or high dose situations, but elderly may demonstrate these adverse effects at lower doses than younger adults.

Dosage Forms Excipient information presented when available (limited, particularly for generics); consult specific product labeling.
Tablet, oral: 500 mg, 750 mg

- **Salt** see Sodium Chloride on page 1787
- **Salvax** see Salicylic Acid on page 1743
- **Samsca™** see Tolvaptan on page 1933
- **Sanctura®** see Trospium on page 1978
- **Sanctura® XR** see Trospium on page 1978
- **Sancuso®** see Granisetron on page 900
- **SandIMMUNE®** see CycloSPORINE (Systemic) on page 460
- **Sani-Supp® [OTC]** see Glycerin on page 891
- **Santyl®** see Collagenase (Topical) on page 443
- **Saphris®** see Asenapine on page 151
- **Sarafem®** see FLUoxetine on page 808
- **Savella®** see Milnacipran on page 1286

Saxagliptin (sax a GLIP tin)

Related Information
Diabetes Mellitus Management, Adults on page 2193

Medication Safety Issues
Sound-alike/look-alike issues:
Saxagliptin may be confused with sitaGLIPtin, SUMAtriptan

High alert medication:
The Institute for Safe Medication Practices (ISMP) includes this medication among its list of drug classes which have a heightened risk of causing significant patient harm when used in error.

Brand Names: U.S. Onglyza™
Brand Names: Canada Onglyza™
Index Terms BMS-477118
Generic Availability (U.S.) No
Pharmacologic Category Antidiabetic Agent, Dipeptidyl Peptidase IV (DPP-IV) Inhibitor
Use Treatment of type 2 diabetes mellitus (noninsulin dependent, NIDDM) as an adjunct to diet and exercise as monotherapy or in combination therapy with other antidiabetic agents to improve glycemic control
Medication Guide Available Yes
Contraindications Hypersensitivity to saxagliptin or any component of the formulation.
Warnings/Precautions Use with caution in patients with moderate-to-severe renal dysfunction, end-stage renal disease (ESRD) requiring hemodialysis, and in patients taking strong CYP3A4/5 inhibitors (eg, atazanavir, clarithromycin, indinavir, itraconazole, nefazodone, nelfinavir, ritonavir, saquinavir, telithromycin [also see Drug Interactions]); dosing adjustment required. Use caution when used in conjunction with insulin or insulin secretagogues (eg, sulfonylureas); risk of hypoglycemia is increased. Monitor blood glucose closely; dosage adjustments of insulin or the insulin secretagogue may be necessary. Rare hypersensitivity reactions, including anaphylaxis, angioedema, and/or exfoliative dermatologic reactions have been reported; discontinue if signs/symptoms of severe hypersensitivity reactions occur. Cases of acute pancreatitis have been reported; discontinue immediately if suspected.
Adverse Reactions (Reflective of adult population; not specific for elderly) Note: Frequencies and adverse reactions reported with monotherapy unless otherwise noted.
1% to 10%:
Cardiovascular: Peripheral edema (≤4%; incidence increased in conjunction with thiazolidinediones: ≤8%)
Central nervous system: Headache (7%)

Endocrine & metabolic: Hypoglycemia (≤6%; incidence increased in conjunction with insulin secretagogues: ≤15%)

Gastrointestinal: Abdominal pain (2%), gastroenteritis (2%), vomiting (2%)

Genitourinary: Urinary tract infection (7%)

Hematologic: Lymphopenia (≤2%; dose related)

Respiratory: Sinusitis (3%)

Miscellaneous: Hypersensitivity reactions (2%; including urticaria and facial edema)

Drug Interactions

Metabolism/Transport Effects Substrate of CYP3A4 (major), P-glycoprotein; **Note:** Assignment of Major/Minor substrate status based on clinically relevant drug interaction potential

Avoid Concomitant Use There are no known interactions where it is recommended to avoid concomitant use.

Increased Effect/Toxicity

Saxagliptin may increase the levels/effects of: ACE Inhibitors; Hypoglycemic Agents

The levels/effects of Saxagliptin may be increased by: CYP3A4 Inhibitors (Moderate); CYP3A4 Inhibitors (Strong); Dasatinib; Herbs (Hypoglycemic Properties); Ivacaftor; MAO Inhibitors; Mifepristone; Pegvisomant; P-glycoprotein/ABCB1 Inhibitors; Salicylates; Selective Serotonin Reuptake Inhibitors

Decreased Effect

The levels/effects of Saxagliptin may be decreased by: Corticosteroids (Orally Inhaled); Corticosteroids (Systemic); CYP3A4 Inducers; Loop Diuretics; Luteinizing Hormone-Releasing Hormone Analogs; P-glycoprotein/ABCB1 Inducers; Somatropin; Thiazide Diuretics; Tocilizumab

Stability Store at 20°C to 25°C (68°F to 77°F); excursions permitted between 15°C to 30°C (59°F to 86°F).

Mechanism of Action Saxagliptin inhibits dipeptidyl peptidase IV (DPP-IV) enzyme resulting in prolonged active incretin levels. Incretin hormones (eg, glucagon-like peptide-1 [GLP-1] and glucose-dependent insulinotropic polypeptide [GIP]) regulate glucose homeostasis by increasing insulin synthesis and release from pancreatic beta cells and decreasing glucagon secretion from pancreatic alpha cells. Decreased glucagon secretion results in decreased hepatic glucose production. Under normal physiologic circumstances, incretin hormones are released by the intestine throughout the day and levels are increased in response to a meal; incretin hormones are rapidly inactivated by the DPP-IV enzyme.

Pharmacodynamics/Kinetics

Duration: 24 hours

Protein binding: Negligible

Metabolism: Hepatic via CYP3A4/5 to 5-hydroxy saxagliptin (active; ~50% potency of the parent compound)

Half-life elimination: Saxagliptin: 2.5 hours; 5-hydroxy saxagliptin: 3.1 hours

Time to peak, plasma: Saxagliptin: 2 hours; 5-hydroxy saxagliptin: 4 hours

Excretion: Urine (75%, 24% of the total dose as saxagliptin, 36% of the total dose as 5-hydroxy saxagliptin); feces (22%)

Dosage

Geriatric & Adult Type 2 diabetes: Oral: 2.5-5 mg once daily

Concomitant use with strong CYP3A4/5 inhibitors: 2.5 mg once daily

Concomitant use with insulin or insulin secretagogues: Reduced dose of insulin or insulin secretagogues (eg, sulfonylureas) may be needed

Renal Impairment Note: Renal function may be estimated using the Cockcroft-Gault formula or the MDRD formula for dosage adjustment purposes.

Cl_{cr} >50 mL/minute: No dosage adjustment necessary.

Cl_{cr} ≤50 mL/minute: 2.5 mg once daily.

ESRD requiring hemodialysis: 2.5 mg once daily; administer postdialysis.

Peritoneal dialysis: Not studied.

Hepatic Impairment No dosage adjustment necessary.

Administration May be administered without regard to meals. Swallow whole; do not split or cut tablets.

Monitoring Parameters Plasma glucose, Hb A_{1c}, renal function

Reference Range

Recommendations for glycemic control in adults with diabetes mellitus (ADA, 2009):

Hb A_{1c}: <7%

Preprandial capillary plasma glucose: 70-130 mg/dL

Peak postprandial capillary blood glucose: <180 mg/dL

Recommendations for glycemic control in older adults with diabetes:

Relatively healthy, cognitively intact, and with a ≥5-year life expectancy: See Adults

Frail, life expectancy <5-years or those for whom the risks of intensive glucose control outweigh the benefits:

Hb A$_{1c}$: <8% to 9%

Blood pressure: <140/80 mm Hg or <130/80 mm Hg if tolerated

Special Geriatric Considerations Persons up to age 77 years were eligible for clinical trials with saxagliptin; ~15% of subjects were 65 years and older. Intensive glucose control (Hb A$_{1c}$ <6.5%) has been linked to increased all-cause and cardiovascular mortality, hypoglycemia requiring assistance, and weight gain in adult type 2 diabetes. How "tightly" to control a geriatric patient's blood glucose needs to be individualized. Such a decision should be based on several factors, including the patient's functional and cognitive status, how well he/she recognizes hypoglycemic or hyperglycemic symptoms, and how to respond to them and other disease states. An Hb A$_{1c}$ <7.5% is an acceptable endpoint for a healthy older adult, while <8% is acceptable for frail elderly patients, those with a duration of illness >10 years, or those with comorbid conditions and requiring combination diabetes medications. For elderly patients with diabetes who are relatively healthy, attaining target goals for aspirin use, blood pressure, lipids, smoking cessation, and diet and exercise may be more important than normalized glycemic control.

Dosage Forms Excipient information presented when available (limited, particularly for generics); consult specific product labeling.

Tablet, oral:

Onglyza™: 2.5 mg, 5 mg

Saxagliptin and Metformin (sax a GLIP tin & met FOR min)

Related Information

Diabetes Mellitus Management, Adults *on page 2193*

MetFORMIN *on page 1222*

Saxagliptin *on page 1753*

Medication Safety Issues

Sound-alike/look-alike issues:

Saxagliptin and Metformin may be confused with sitaGLIPtin and Metformin

High alert medication:

The Institute for Safe Medication Practices (ISMP) includes this medication among its list of drug classes which have a heightened risk of causing significant patient harm when used in error.

Brand Names: U.S. Kombiglyze™ XR

Index Terms Metformin and Saxagliptin; Metformin Hydrochloride and Saxagliptin; Saxagliptin and Metformin Hydrochloride

Pharmacologic Category Antidiabetic Agent, Biguanide; Antidiabetic Agent, Dipeptidyl Peptidase IV (DPP-IV) Inhibitor

Use Management of type 2 diabetes mellitus (noninsulin dependent, NIDDM) as an adjunct to diet and exercise when treatment with both saxagliptin and metformin is appropriate

Medication Guide Available Yes

Dosage

Geriatric Refer to adult dosing. The initial and maintenance dosing should be conservative, due to the potential for decreased renal function (monitor). Do not use in patients ≥80 years of age unless normal renal function has been established.

Adult

Type 2 diabetes mellitus: Oral: Initial doses should be based on current dose of saxagliptin and metformin; daily doses should be given once daily with the evening meal. Maximum: Saxagliptin 5 mg/metformin 2000 mg daily

Patients inadequately controlled on metformin alone: Initial dose: Saxagliptin 2.5-5 mg/day plus current dose of metformin. **Note:** Patients who require saxagliptin 2.5 mg (eg, dose adjusted for concomitant use of strong CYP3A4/5 inhibitors) and metformin >1000 mg should not be switched to the combination product.

Patients inadequately controlled on saxagliptin alone: Initial dose: Metformin 500 mg/day plus saxagliptin 5 mg/day. **Note:** Metformin-naïve patients currently receiving saxagliptin 2.5 mg daily (eg, dose adjusted for concomitant use of strong CYP3A4/5 inhibitors) should not be switched to the combination product.

Concomitant use with strong CYP3A4/5 inhibitors: Maximum: Saxagliptin 2.5 mg/metformin 1000 mg daily

Concomitant use with insulin or insulin secretagogues: Reduced dose of insulin or insulin secretagogues (eg, sulfonylureas) may be needed.

Renal Impairment Do not use in patients with renal disease or renal dysfunction (serum creatinine ≥1.5 mg/dL [≥136 micromole/L] in males or ≥1.4 mg/dL [≥124 micromole/L] in females or abnormal clearance).

Hepatic Impairment Avoid metformin; liver disease is a risk factor for the development of lactic acidosis during metformin therapy.

Special Geriatric Considerations See individual agents. Combination products are not recommended as first-line treatment. Use only if doses of individual agents correspond to the combination available.

Dosage Forms Excipient information presented when available (limited, particularly for generics); consult specific product labeling.

Tablet, variable release, oral:

Kombiglyze™ XR 2.5/1000: Saxagliptin 2.5 mg [immediate release] and metformin hydrochloride 1000 mg [extended release]

Kombiglyze™ XR 5/500: Saxagliptin 5 mg [immediate release] and metformin hydrochloride 500 mg [extended release]

Kombiglyze™ XR 5/1000: Saxagliptin 5 mg [immediate release] and metformin hydrochloride 1000 mg [extended release]

◆ **Saxagliptin and Metformin Hydrochloride** see Saxagliptin and Metformin on page 1755
◆ **SB-265805** see Gemifloxacin on page 871
◆ **SB659746-A** see Vilazodone on page 2024
◆ **S. boulardii** see Saccharomyces boulardii on page 1741
◆ **Scalpana [OTC]** see Hydrocortisone (Topical) on page 943
◆ **Scalpicin® Anti-Itch [OTC]** see Salicylic Acid on page 1743
◆ **SCH 13521** see Flutamide on page 821
◆ **SCH 56592** see Posaconazole on page 1567
◆ **SCIG** see Immune Globulin on page 982
◆ **S-Citalopram** see Escitalopram on page 670

Scopolamine (Systemic) (skoe POL a meen)

Related Information

Beers Criteria – Potentially Inappropriate Medications for Geriatrics on page 2183

Medication Safety Issues

BEERS Criteria medication:

This drug may be potentially inappropriate for use in geriatric patients (Quality of evidence - moderate; Strength of recommendation - strong).

Other safety concerns:

Transdermal patch may contain conducting metal (eg, aluminum); remove patch prior to MRI.

Brand Names: U.S. Transderm Scōp®

Brand Names: Canada Buscopan®; Scopolamine Hydrobromide Injection; Transderm-V®

Index Terms Hyoscine Butylbromide; Scopolamine Base; Scopolamine Butylbromide; Scopolamine Hydrobromide

Generic Availability (U.S.) Yes: Injection

Pharmacologic Category Anticholinergic Agent

Use

Scopolamine base: Transdermal: Prevention of nausea/vomiting associated with motion sickness and recovery from anesthesia and surgery

Scopolamine hydrobromide: Injection: Preoperative medication to produce amnesia, sedation, tranquilization, antiemetic effects, and decrease salivary and respiratory secretions

Scopolamine butylbromide [not available in the U.S.]: Oral/injection: Treatment of smooth muscle spasm of the genitourinary or gastrointestinal tract; injection may also be used prior to radiological/diagnostic procedures to prevent spasm

Unlabeled Use Scopolamine base: Transdermal: Breakthrough treatment of nausea and vomiting associated with chemotherapy

Contraindications

Transdermal, oral: Hypersensitivity to scopolamine, other belladonna alkaloids, or any component of the formulation; narrow-angle glaucoma

Injection: Hypersensitivity to scopolamine, other belladonna alkaloids, or any component of the formulation; narrow-angle glaucoma; chronic lung disease (repeated administration)

Canadian labeling: Additional contraindications (not in U.S. labeling):

Oral: Glaucoma, megacolon, myasthenia gravis, obstructive prostatic hypertrophy

Injection:

Hyoscine butylbromide: Untreated narrow-angle glaucoma; megacolon, prostatic hypertrophy with urinary retention; stenotic lesions of the GI tract; myasthenia gravis;

tachycardia, angina, or heart failure; I.M. administration in patients receiving anticoagulant therapy

Scopolamine hydrobromide: Glaucoma or predisposition to narrow-angle glaucoma; paralytic ileus; prostatic hypertrophy; pyloric obstruction; tachycardia secondary to cardiac insufficiency or thyrotoxicosis

Warnings/Precautions Use with caution in patients with coronary artery disease, tachyarrhythmias, heart failure, hypertension, or hyperthyroidism; evaluate tachycardia prior to administration. Use caution in hepatic or renal impairment; adverse CNS effects occur more often in these patients. Use injectable and transdermal products with caution in patients with prostatic hyperplasia or urinary retention. Discontinue if patient reports unusual visual disturbances or pain within the eye. Use caution in GI obstruction, hiatal hernia, reflux esophagitis, and ulcerative colitis. Use with caution in patients with a history of seizure or psychosis; may exacerbate these conditions.

Anaphylaxis including episodes of shock has been reported following parenteral administration; observe for signs/symptoms of hypersensitivity following parenteral administration. Patients with a history of allergies or asthma may be at increased risk of hypersensitivity reactions. Adverse events (including dizziness, headache, nausea, vomiting) may occur following abrupt discontinuation of large doses or in patients with Parkinson's disease; adverse events may also occur following removal of the transdermal patch although symptoms may not appear until ≥24 hours after removal.

Idiosyncratic reactions may rarely occur; patients may experience acute toxic psychosis, agitation, confusion, delusions, hallucinations, paranoid behavior, and rambling speech. May cause CNS depression, which may impair physical or mental abilities; patients must be cautioned about performing tasks which require mental alertness (eg, operating machinery or driving).

Transdermal patch may contain conducting metal (eg, aluminum); remove patch prior to MRI. Use of the transdermal product in patients with open-angle glaucoma may necessitate adjustments in glaucoma therapy.

Scopolamine (hyoscine) hydrobromide should not be interchanged with scopolamine butylbromide formulations; dosages are not equivalent.

Avoid use in the elderly due to potent anticholinergic adverse effects and uncertain effectiveness (Beers Criteria). Tablets may contain sucrose; avoid use of tablets in patients who are fructose intolerant.

Adverse Reactions (Reflective of adult population; not specific for elderly) Frequency not defined.

Cardiovascular: Bradycardia, flushing, orthostatic hypotension, tachycardia

Central nervous system: Acute toxic psychosis (rare), agitation (rare), ataxia, confusion, delusion (rare), disorientation, dizziness, drowsiness, fatigue, hallucination (rare), headache, irritability, loss of memory, paranoid behavior (rare), restlessness, sedation

Dermatologic: Drug eruptions, dry skin, dyshidrosis, erythema, pruritus, rash, urticaria

Endocrine & metabolic: Thirst

Gastrointestinal: Constipation, diarrhea, dry throat, dysphagia, nausea, vomiting, xerostomia

Genitourinary: Dysuria, urinary retention

Neuromuscular & skeletal: Tremor, weakness

Ocular: Accommodation impaired, blurred vision, conjunctival infection, cycloplegia, dryness, glaucoma (narrow-angle), increased intraocular pain, itching, photophobia, pupil dilation, retinal pigmentation

Respiratory: Dry nose, dyspnea

Miscellaneous: Anaphylaxis (rare), anaphylactic shock (rare), angioedema, diaphoresis decreased, heat intolerance, hypersensitivity reactions

Drug Interactions

Metabolism/Transport Effects None known.

Avoid Concomitant Use

Avoid concomitant use of Scopolamine (Systemic) with any of the following: Azelastine; Azelastine (Nasal); Methadone; Mirtazapine; Paraldehyde

Increased Effect/Toxicity

Scopolamine (Systemic) may increase the levels/effects of: AbobotulinumtoxinA; Alcohol (Ethyl); Anticholinergics; Azelastine; Azelastine (Nasal); Buprenorphine; Cannabinoids; CNS Depressants; Methadone; Methotrimeprazine; Metyrosine; Mirtazapine; OnabotulinumtoxinA; Paraldehyde; Potassium Chloride; RimabotulinumtoxinB; Selective Serotonin Reuptake Inhibitors; Zolpidem

The levels/effects of Scopolamine (Systemic) may be increased by: Droperidol; HydrOXYzine; Methotrimeprazine; Pramlintide

Decreased Effect
Scopolamine (Systemic) may decrease the levels/effects of: Acetylcholinesterase Inhibitors (Central); Secretin

The levels/effects of Scopolamine (Systemic) may be decreased by: Acetylcholinesterase Inhibitors (Central)

Ethanol/Nutrition/Herb Interactions Ethanol: May increase CNS depression; monitor for increased effects with coadministration. Caution patients about effects.

Stability
Injection:
Butylbromide (Canadian availability): Store at room temperature. Do not freeze. Protect from light and heat. Stable in D_5W, $D_{10}W$, NS, Ringer's solution, and LR for up to 8 hours.
Hydrobromide: Store at room temperature of 20°C to 25°C (68°F to 77°F). Protect from light. Avoid acid solutions; hydrolysis occurs at pH <3.
Tablet (Canadian availability): Store at room temperature. Protect from light and heat.
Transdermal system: Store at 20°C to 25°C (68°F to 77°F).

Mechanism of Action Blocks the action of acetylcholine at parasympathetic sites in smooth muscle, secretory glands and the CNS; increases cardiac output, dries secretions, antagonizes histamine and serotonin

Pharmacodynamics/Kinetics
Onset of action: Oral, I.M.: 0.5-1 hour; I.V.: 10 minutes; Transdermal: 6-8 hours
Duration: I.M., I.V., SubQ: 4 hours
Absorption: I.M., SubQ: Rapid; Oral: Quaternary salts (butylbromide) are poorly absorbed (local concentrations in the GI tract following oral dosing may be high)
Distribution: V_d: Butylbromide: 128 L
Protein binding: Butylbromide: ~4% (albumin)
Metabolism: Hepatic
Bioavailability: Oral: 8%
Half-life elimination: Butylbromide: ~5-11 hours; Hydrobromide: ~1-4 hours; Scopolamine base: 9.5 hours
Time to peak: Hydrobromide: I.M.: ~20 minutes, SubQ: ~15 minutes; Butylbromide: Oral: ~2 hours; Scopolamine base: Transdermal: 24 hours
Excretion: Urine (<10%, as parent drug and metabolites); I.V.: Butylbromide: Urine (42% to 61% [half as parent drug]), feces (28% to 37%)

Dosage
Geriatric Lower dosages may be required. Refer to adult dosing.
Adult Note: Scopolamine (hyoscine) hydrobromide should not be interchanged with scopolamine butylbromide formulations. Dosages are not equivalent.
Scopolamine base:
Preoperative: Transdermal patch: Apply 1 patch to hairless area behind ear the night before surgery; remove 24 hours after surgery
Motion sickness: Transdermal patch: Apply 1 patch to hairless area behind the ear at least 4 hours prior to exposure and every 3 days as needed; effective if applied as soon as 2-3 hours before anticipated need, best if 12 hours before
Chemotherapy-induced nausea and vomiting, breakthrough (unlabeled use): Apply 1 patch every 72 hours (NCCN Antiemesis guidelines v.1.2012)
Scopolamine hydrobromide:
Antiemetic: SubQ: 0.6-1 mg
Preoperative: I.M., I.V., SubQ: 0.3-0.65 mg
Sedation, tranquilization: I.M., I.V., SubQ:
U.S. labeling: 0.6 mg 3-4 times/day
Canadian labeling: 0.3-0.6 mg 3-4 times/day
Scopolamine butylbromide: *Gastrointestinal/genitourinary spasm* (Buscopan® [CAN]; not available in the U.S.):
Oral: Acute therapy: 10-20 mg daily (1-2 tablets); prolonged therapy: 10 mg (1 tablet) 3-5 times/day; maximum: 60 mg/day
I.M., I.V., SubQ: 10-20 mg; maximum: 100 mg/day
Renal Impairment There are no dosage adjustments in the manufacturer's labeling; however, caution is recommended due to increased risks of adverse effects.
Hepatic Impairment There are no dosage adjustments in the manufacturer's labeling; however, caution is recommended due to increased risks of adverse effects.
Administration Note: Butylbromide or hydrobromide may be administered by I.M., I.V., or SubQ injection.
I.M.: **Butylbromide:** Intramuscular injections should be administered 10-15 minutes prior to radiological/diagnostic procedures.

I.V.:

Butylbromide: No dilution is necessary prior to injection; inject at a rate of 1 mL/minute

Hydrobromide: Dilute with an equal volume of sterile water and administer by direct I.V.; inject over 2-3 minutes

Oral: Tablet should be swallowed whole and taken with a full glass of water.

Transdermal: Apply to hairless area of skin behind the ear. Wash hands before and after applying the disc to avoid drug contact with eyes. Do not use any patch that has been damaged, cut, or manipulated in any way. Topical patch is programmed to deliver 1 mg over 3 days. Once applied, do not remove the patch for 3 full days (motion sickness). When used postoperatively for nausea/vomiting, the patch should be removed 24 hours after surgery. If patch becomes displaced, discard and apply a new patch.

Monitoring Parameters Body temperature, heart rate, urinary output, intraocular pressure

Test Interactions Interferes with gastric secretion test

Special Geriatric Considerations Anticholinergic agents are not well tolerated in the elderly and their use should be avoided when possible.

This medication is considered to be potentially inappropriate in this patient population (Beers Criteria: Quality of evidence - moderate; Strength of recommendation - strong).

Dosage Forms Excipient information presented when available (limited, particularly for generics); consult specific product labeling.

Injection, solution, as hydrobromide: 0.4 mg/mL (1 mL)

Patch, transdermal:

Transderm Scōp®: 1.5 mg (4s, 10s, 24s) [contains metal; releases ~1 mg over 72 hours]

Dosage Forms: Canada Excipient information presented when available (limited, particularly for generics); consult specific product labeling.

Tablet, oral, as butylbromide:

Buscopan®: 10 mg

Scopolamine (Ophthalmic) (skoe POL a meen)

Brand Names: U.S. Isopto® Hyoscine

Index Terms Hyoscine Hydrobromide; Scopolamine Hydrobromide

Generic Availability (U.S.) No

Pharmacologic Category Anticholinergic Agent; Anticholinergic Agent, Ophthalmic; Ophthalmic Agent, Mydriatic

Use Produce cycloplegia and mydriasis; treatment of iridocyclitis

Dosage

Geriatric & Adult Scopolamine hydrobromide:

Refraction: Ophthalmic: Instill 1-2 drops to eye(s) 1 hour before procedure

Iridocyclitis: Ophthalmic: Instill 1-2 drops to eye(s) up to 4 times/day

Special Geriatric Considerations Evaluate the patient's or caregiver's ability to safely administer the correct dose of ophthalmic medication.

Because of its long duration of action as a mydriatic agent, it should be avoided in elderly patients.

Dosage Forms Excipient information presented when available (limited, particularly for generics); consult specific product labeling.

Solution, ophthalmic, as hydrobromide [drops]:

Isopto® Hyoscine: 0.25% (5 mL) [contains benzalkonium chloride]

◆ **Scopolamine Base** *see* Scopolamine (Systemic) *on page 1756*
◆ **Scopolamine Butylbromide** *see* Scopolamine (Systemic) *on page 1756*
◆ **Scopolamine Hydrobromide** *see* Scopolamine (Ophthalmic) *on page 1759*
◆ **Scopolamine Hydrobromide** *see* Scopolamine (Systemic) *on page 1756*
◆ **Scopolamine, Hyoscyamine, Atropine, and Phenobarbital** *see* Hyoscyamine, Atropine, Scopolamine, and Phenobarbital *on page 963*
◆ **Scot-Tussin® Diabetes [OTC]** *see* Dextromethorphan *on page 525*
◆ **Scot-Tussin® Expectorant [OTC]** *see* GuaiFENesin *on page 904*
◆ **Scot-Tussin® Senior [OTC]** *see* Guaifenesin and Dextromethorphan *on page 906*
◆ **SD/01** *see* Pegfilgrastim *on page 1481*
◆ **SDZ ENA 713** *see* Rivastigmine *on page 1719*
◆ **Sea Soft Nasal Mist [OTC]** *see* Sodium Chloride *on page 1787*
◆ **Seb-Prev™ [DSC]** *see* Sulfacetamide (Topical) *on page 1812*
◆ **Sectral®** *see* Acebutolol *on page 28*
◆ **Secura® Antifungal Extra Thick [OTC]** *see* Miconazole (Topical) *on page 1276*
◆ **Secura® Antifungal Greaseless [OTC]** *see* Miconazole (Topical) *on page 1276*

Selegiline (se LE ji leen)

Related Information

Antidepressant Agents *on page 2097*

Antiparkinsonian Agents *on page 2101*

Parkinson's Disease Management *on page 2140*

Medication Safety Issues

Sound-alike/look-alike issues:

Selegiline may be confused with Salagen®, sertraline, Serzone, Stelazine

Eldepryl® may be confused with Elavil®, enalapril

Zelapar® may be confused with zaleplon, Zemplar®, zolpidem, ZyPREXA® Zydis®

Brand Names: U.S. Eldepryl®; Emsam®; Zelapar®

Brand Names: Canada Apo-Selegiline®; Gen-Selegiline; Mylan-Selegiline; Novo-Selegiline; Nu-Selegiline

Index Terms Deprenyl; L-Deprenyl; Selegiline Hydrochloride

Generic Availability (U.S.) Yes: Capsule, tablet

Pharmacologic Category Anti-Parkinson's Agent, MAO Type B Inhibitor; Antidepressant, Monoamine Oxidase Inhibitor

Use Adjunct in the management of parkinsonian patients in which levodopa/carbidopa therapy is deteriorating (oral products); treatment of major depressive disorder (transdermal product)

Unlabeled Use Early Parkinson's disease; attention-deficit/hyperactivity disorder (ADHD)

Medication Guide Available Yes

Contraindications Hypersensitivity to selegiline or any component of the formulation; concomitant use of meperidine

Orally disintegrating tablet: Additional contraindications: Concomitant use of dextromethorphan, methadone, propoxyphene, tramadol, oral selegiline, other MAO inhibitors

Transdermal: Additional contraindications: Pheochromocytoma; concomitant use of bupropion, selective or dual serotonin reuptake inhibitors (including SSRIs and SNRIs), tricyclic antidepressants, tramadol, propoxyphene, methadone, dextromethorphan, St. John's wort, mirtazapine, cyclobenzaprine, oral selegiline and other MAO inhibitors; carbamazepine, and oxcarbazepine; elective surgery requiring general anesthesia, local anesthesia containing sympathomimetic vasoconstrictors; sympathomimetics (and related compounds); foods high in tyramine content; supplements containing tyrosine, phenylalanine, tryptophan, or caffeine

Warnings/Precautions

Oral: MAO-B selective inhibition should not pose a problem with tyramine-containing products as long as the typical oral doses are employed, however, rare reactions have been reported. Increased risk of nonselective MAO inhibition occurs with oral capsule/tablet doses >10 mg/day or orally disintegrating tablet doses >2.5 mg/day. Use of oral selegiline with tricyclic antidepressants and SSRIs has also been associated with rare reactions and should generally be avoided. Addition to levodopa therapy may result in exacerbation of levodopa adverse effects, requiring a reduction in levodopa dosage. Dopaminergic agents used for Parkinson's disease or restless legs syndrome have been associated with compulsive behaviors and/or loss of impulse control, which has manifested as pathological gambling, libido increases (hypersexuality), and/or binge eating. Causality has not been established, and controversy exists as to whether this phenomenon is related to the underlying disease, prior behaviors/addictions and/or drug therapy. Dose reduction or discontinuation of therapy has been reported to reverse these behaviors in some, but not all cases. Use caution in patients with hepatic or renal impairment. Incidence of orthostatic hypotension may be increased in older adults and when titrating to the 2.5 mg dosage in patients taking the orally disintegrating tablet. Risk for melanoma development is increased in Parkinson's disease patients; drug causation or factors contributing to risk have not been established. Patients should be monitored closely and periodic skin examinations should be performed. Orally disintegrating tablet may cause oral mucosa edema, irritation, pain, ulceration and/or swallowing pain. Do not use orally disintegrating tablet concurrently with other selegiline products; wait at least 14 days from discontinuation before initiating treatment with another selegiline dosage form. Some products may contain phenylalanine.

Transdermal: Nonselective MAO inhibition occurs with transdermal delivery and is necessary for antidepressant efficacy. Hypertensive crisis as a result of ingesting tyramine-rich foods is always a concern with nonselective MAO inhibition. Although transdermal delivery minimizes inhibition of MAO-A in the gut, there is limited data with higher transdermal doses; dietary modifications are recommended with doses >6 mg/24 hours.

Transdermal patch: May cause orthostatic hypotension; use with caution in patients at risk of this effect or in those who would not tolerate transient hypotensive episodes (cerebrovascular disease, cardiovascular disease, hypovolemia, or concurrent medication use which may predispose to hypotension/bradycardia). Discontinue transdermal product at least 10 days prior to elective surgery. May contain conducting metal (eg, aluminum); remove patch prior to MRI. Avoid exposure of application site and surrounding area to direct external heat sources.

Transdermal: **[U.S. Boxed Warning]: Antidepressants increase the risk of suicidal thinking and behavior in children, adolescents, and young adults (18-24 years of age) with major depressive disorder (MDD) and other psychiatric disorders;** consider risk prior to prescribing. Short-term studies did not show an increased risk in patients >24 years of age and showed a decreased risk in patients ≥65 years. Closely monitor patients for worsening of depression, suicidality and/or associated behaviors, particularly during the initial 1-2 months of therapy or during periods of dosage adjustments (increases or decreases); the patient's family or caregiver should be instructed to closely observe the patient and communicate condition with healthcare provider. A medication guide concerning the use of antidepressants should be dispensed with each prescription.

Transdermal: The possibility of a suicide attempt is inherit in major depression and may persist until remission occurs. Patients treated with antidepressants (for any indication) should be observed for clinical worsening and suicidality, especially during the initial few months of a course of drug therapy, or at times of dose changes, either increases or decreases. Use caution in high-risk patients. Worsening depression and severe abrupt suicidality that are not part of the presenting symptoms may require discontinuation or modification of drug therapy. Use caution in high-risk patients during initiation of therapy. The patient's family or caregiver should be alerted to monitor patients for the emergence of suicidality and associated behaviors (such as agitation, irritability, hostility, and hypomania) and call healthcare provider.

Transdermal selegiline may worsen psychosis in some patients or precipitate a shift to mania or hypomania in patients with bipolar disorder. Monotherapy in patients with bipolar disorder should be avoided. Patients presenting with depressive symptoms should be screened for bipolar disorder. **Selegiline is not FDA approved for the treatment of bipolar depression.**

Adverse Reactions (Reflective of adult population; not specific for elderly) Unless otherwise noted, the percentage of adverse events is reported for the transdermal patch (**Note:** ODT = orally disintegrating tablet, Oral = capsule/tablet)

>10%:
  Central nervous system: Headache (18%; ODT 7%; oral 4%), insomnia (12%; ODT 7%), dizziness (oral 14%; ODT 11%)
  Gastrointestinal: Nausea (oral 20%; ODT 11%)
  Local: Application site reaction (24%)
1% to 10%:
  Cardiovascular: Hypotension (including postural 3% to 10%), palpitation (oral 2%), chest pain (≥1%; ODT 2%), hypertension (≥1%; ODT 3%), peripheral edema (≥1%)
  Central nervous system: Pain (ODT 8%; oral 2%), hallucinations (oral 6%; ODT 4%), confusion (oral 6%; ODT 4%), vivid dreams (oral 4%), ataxia (ODT 3%), somnolence (ODT 3%), lethargy (oral 2%), agitation (≥1%), amnesia (≥1%), paresthesia (≥1%), thinking abnormal (≥1%), depression (<1%; ODT 2%)
  Dermatologic: Rash (4%), bruising (≥1%; ODT 2%), pruritus (≥1%), acne (≥1%)
  Endocrine & metabolic: Weight loss (5%; oral 2%), hypokalemia (ODT 2%), sexual side effects (≤1%)
  Gastrointestinal: Diarrhea (9%; ODT 2%; oral 2%), xerostomia (8%; oral 6%; ODT 4%), stomatitis (ODT 5%), abdominal pain (oral 8%), dyspepsia (4%; ODT 5%), dysphagia (ODT 2%), dental caries (ODT 2%), constipation (≥1%; ODT 4%), flatulence (≥1%; ODT 2%), anorexia (≥1%), gastroenteritis (≥1%), taste perversion (≥1%; ODT 2%), vomiting (≥1%; ODT 3%)
  Genitourinary: Urinary retention (oral 2%), dysmenorrhea (≥1%), metrorrhagia (≥1%), UTI (≥1%), urinary frequency (≥1%)
  Neuromuscular & skeletal: Dyskinesia (ODT 6%), back pain (ODT 5%; oral 2%), ataxia (<1%; ODT 3%; oral 2%), leg cramps (ODT 3%; oral 2%), myalgia (≥1%; ODT 3%), neck pain (≥1%), tremor (<1%; ODT 3%)
  Otic: Tinnitus (≥1%)
  Respiratory: Rhinitis (ODT 7%), pharyngitis (3%; ODT 4%), sinusitis (3%), cough (≥1%; bronchitis (≥1%), dyspnea (<1%; ODT 3%)
  Miscellaneous: Diaphoresis (≥1%)

Drug Interactions
  Metabolism/Transport Effects Substrate of CYP1A2 (minor), CYP2A6 (minor), CYP2B6 (major), CYP2C8 (minor), CYP2D6 (minor), CYP3A4 (minor); **Note:** Assignment of Major/Minor substrate status based on clinically relevant drug interaction potential; **Inhibits** CYP1A2 (weak), CYP2A6 (weak), CYP2C19 (weak), CYP2D6 (weak), CYP2E1 (weak), CYP3A4 (weak), Monoamine Oxidase

  Avoid Concomitant Use
  Avoid concomitant use of Selegiline with any of the following: Alpha-/Beta-Agonists (Indirect-Acting); Alpha1-Agonists; Alpha2-Agonists (Ophthalmic); Amphetamines; Anilidopiperidine

Opioids; Antidepressants (Serotonin Reuptake Inhibitor/Antagonist); AtoMOXetine; Bezafibrate; Buprenorphine; BuPROPion; CarBAMazepine; Cyclobenzaprine; Dexmethylphenidate; Dextromethorphan; Diethylpropion; HYDROmorphone; Linezolid; Maprotiline; Meperidine; Methyldopa; Methylene Blue; Methylphenidate; Mirtazapine; OXcarbazepine; Oxymorphone; Pizotifen; Selective Serotonin Reuptake Inhibitors; Serotonin 5-HT1D Receptor Agonists; Serotonin/Norepinephrine Reuptake Inhibitors; Tapentadol; Tetrabenazine; Tetrahydrozoline; Tetrahydrozoline (Nasal); Tricyclic Antidepressants; Tryptophan

Increased Effect/Toxicity

Selegiline may increase the levels/effects of: Alpha-/Beta-Agonists (Direct-Acting); Alpha-/Beta-Agonists (Indirect-Acting); Alpha1-Agonists; Alpha2-Agonists (Ophthalmic); Amphetamines; Antidepressants (Serotonin Reuptake Inhibitor/Antagonist); Antihypertensives; AtoMOXetine; Beta2-Agonists; Bezafibrate; BuPROPion; Dexmethylphenidate; Dextromethorphan; Diethylpropion; Doxapram; HYDROmorphone; Hypoglycemic Agents; Linezolid; Lithium; Meperidine; Methadone; Methyldopa; Methylene Blue; Methylphenidate; Metoclopramide; Mirtazapine; Orthostatic Hypotension Producing Agents; Pizotifen; Reserpine; Selective Serotonin Reuptake Inhibitors; Serotonin 5-HT1D Receptor Agonists; Serotonin Modulators; Serotonin/Norepinephrine Reuptake Inhibitors; Tetrahydrozoline; Tetrahydrozoline (Nasal); Tricyclic Antidepressants

The levels/effects of Selegiline may be increased by: Altretamine; Anilidopiperidine Opioids; Antipsychotics; Buprenorphine; BusPIRone; CarBAMazepine; COMT Inhibitors; Contraceptives (Estrogens); Contraceptives (Progestins); Cyclobenzaprine; CYP2B6 Inhibitors (Moderate); CYP2B6 Inhibitors (Strong); Levodopa; MAO Inhibitors; Maprotiline; OXcarbazepine; Oxymorphone; Quazepam; Tapentadol; Tetrabenazine; TraMADol; Tryptophan

Decreased Effect

Selegiline may decrease the levels/effects of: Ioflupane I 123

The levels/effects of Selegiline may be decreased by: CYP2B6 Inducers (Strong); Peginterferon Alfa-2b; Tocilizumab

Ethanol/Nutrition/Herb Interactions

Ethanol: Ethanol may enhance the adverse/toxic effects of selegiline. Beverages containing tyramine (eg, hearty red wine and beer) may increase toxic effects. Management: Avoid ethanol and beverages containing tyramine.

Food: Concurrent ingestion of foods rich in tyramine, dopamine, tyrosine, phenylalanine, tryptophan, or caffeine may cause sudden and severe high blood pressure (hypertensive crisis or serotonin syndrome). Management: Avoid tyramine-containing foods (aged or matured cheese, air-dried or cured meats including sausages and salamis; fava or broad bean pods, tap/draft beers, Marmite concentrate, sauerkraut, soy sauce, and other soybean condiments). Food's freshness is also an important concern; improperly stored or spoiled food can create an environment in which tyramine concentrations may increase. Avoid foods containing dopamine, tyrosine, phenylalanine, tryptophan, or caffeine.

Herb/Nutraceutical: Kava kava, valerian, St John's wort, and SAMe may increase risk of serotonin syndrome and/or excessive sedation. Supplements containing caffeine, tyrosine, tryptophan, or phenylalanine may increase the risk of severe side effects like hypertensive reactions or serotonin syndrome. Management: Avoid kava kava, valerian, St John's wort, SAMe, and supplements containing caffeine, tyrosine, tryptophan, or phenylalanine.

Stability

Capsule, tablet, transdermal: Store at 20°C to 25°C (68°F to 77°F). Store patch in sealed pouch and apply immediately after removal.

Orally disintegrating tablet: Store at controlled room temperature 25°C (77°F); excursions permitted to 15°C to 30°C (59°F to 86°F). Use within 3 months of opening pouch and immediately after opening individual blister.

Mechanism of Action Potent, irreversible inhibitor of monoamine oxidase (MAO). Plasma concentrations achieved via administration of oral dosage forms in recommended doses confer selective inhibition of MAO type B, which plays a major role in the metabolism of dopamine; selegiline may also increase dopaminergic activity by interfering with dopamine reuptake at the synapse. When administered transdermally in recommended doses, selegiline achieves higher blood levels and effectively inhibits both MAO-A and MAO-B, which blocks catabolism of other centrally-active biogenic amine neurotransmitters.

Pharmacodynamics/Kinetics

Onset of action: Therapeutic: Oral: Within 1 hour

Duration: Oral: 24-72 hours

Absorption:

Orally disintegrating tablet: Rapid; greater bioavailability than capsule/tablet

Transdermal: 25% to 30% (of total selegiline content) over 24 hours

Protein binding: ~90%

Metabolism: Hepatic, primarily via CYP2B6 to active (N-desmethylselegiline, amphetamine, methamphetamine) and inactive metabolites
Half-life elimination: Oral: 10 hours; Transdermal: 18-25 hours
Excretion: Urine (primarily metabolites); feces

Dosage

Geriatric

Parkinson's disease:
Capsule/tablet: ≤5 mg/day (when combined with levodopa) is recommended by some clinicians to decrease the enhanced dopaminergic side effects (Olanow, 2001)
Orally disintegrating tablet (Zelapar®): Refer to adult dosing
Depression: Transdermal (Emsam®): 6 mg/24 hours

Adult

Parkinson's disease:
Capsule/tablet: 5 mg twice daily with breakfast and lunch
Orally disintegrating tablet (Zelapar®): Initial 1.25 mg daily for at least 6 weeks; may increase to 2.5 mg daily based on clinical response (maximum: 2.5 mg daily)
Depression: Transdermal (Emsam®): Initial: 6 mg/24 hours once daily; may titrate based on clinical response in increments of 3 mg/day every 2 weeks up to a maximum of 12 mg/24 hours

Renal Impairment

Oral: Use caution, has not been studied.
Transdermal: No adjustment required in patients with mild-to-moderate impairment.

Hepatic Impairment

Oral: Use caution, has not been studied.
Transdermal: No adjustment required in patients with mild-to-moderate impairment.

Administration

Oral: Orally disintegrating tablet (Zelapar®): Take in morning before breakfast; place on top of tongue and allow to dissolve. Avoid food or liquid 5 minutes before and after administration.
Topical: Transdermal (Emsam®): Apply to clean, dry, intact skin to the upper torso (below the neck and above the waist), upper thigh, or outer surface of the upper arm. Avoid exposure of application site to external heat source, which may increase the amount of drug absorbed. Apply at the same time each day and rotate application sites. Wash hands with soap and water after handling. Avoid touching the sticky side of the patch.

Monitoring Parameters Blood pressure; symptoms of parkinsonism; general mood and behavior (increased anxiety, presence of mania or agitation); suicidal ideation (especially at the beginning of therapy or when doses are increased or decreased)

Test Interactions May interfere with urine detection of amphetamine/methamphetamine (false-positive).

Pharmacotherapy Pearls When adding selegiline to levodopa/carbidopa, the dose of the latter can usually be decreased.

Special Geriatric Considerations Do not use capsule/tablet at doses >10 mg/day or orally disintegrating tablet at doses >2.5 mg/day because of the risks associated with nonselective inhibition of MAO.

Orally-disintegrating tablets: In clinical trials, adverse effects were seen more frequently in the elderly compared to younger adults. This is particularly of concern for hypertension, orthostatic hypotension, dizziness, and somnolence. If using the orally disintegrating tablets, administer at the lowest dose and monitor for side effects.

Dosage Forms Excipient information presented when available (limited, particularly for generics); consult specific product labeling.
Capsule, oral, as hydrochloride: 5 mg
Eldepryl®: 5 mg
Patch, transdermal:
Emsam®: 6 mg/24 hours (30s) [20 cm², total selegiline 20 mg]
Emsam®: 9 mg/24 hours (30s) [30 cm², total selegiline 30 mg]
Emsam®: 12 mg/24 hours (30s) [40 cm², total selegiline 40 mg]
Tablet, oral, as hydrochloride: 5 mg
Tablet, orally disintegrating, oral, as hydrochloride:
Zelapar®: 1.25 mg [contains phenylalanine 1.25 mg/tablet; grapefruit flavor]

◆ **Selegiline Hydrochloride** see Selegiline on page 1760
◆ **Selsun blue® Deep Cleaning Micro-Bead Scrub [OTC]** see Salicylic Acid on page 1743
◆ **Selsun blue® Naturals Island Breeze [OTC]** see Salicylic Acid on page 1743
◆ **Selsun blue® Naturals Itchy Dry Scalp [OTC]** see Salicylic Acid on page 1743
◆ **Senexon [OTC]** see Senna on page 1764
◆ **Senexon-S [OTC]** see Docusate and Senna on page 585

Senna (SEN na)

Related Information
Laxatives, Classification and Properties *on page 2121*
Treatment Options for Constipation *on page 2142*

Medication Safety Issues
Sound-alike/look-alike issues:
Perdiem® may be confused with Pyridium®
Senexon® may be confused with Cenestin®
Senokot® may be confused with Depakote®

Brand Names: U.S. Black Draught® [OTC]; Evac-U-Gen® [OTC]; ex-lax® Maximum Strength [OTC]; ex-lax® [OTC]; Fleet® Pedia-Lax™ Quick Dissolve [OTC]; Fletcher's® [OTC]; Geri-kot [OTC]; Little Tummys® Laxative [OTC]; Perdiem® Overnight Relief [OTC]; Senexon [OTC]; Senna-Lax [OTC]; SennaGen [OTC]; Senokot® [OTC]

Index Terms Sennosides

Generic Availability (U.S.) Yes

Pharmacologic Category Laxative, Stimulant

Use Short-term treatment of constipation; evacuate the colon for bowel or rectal examinations

Contraindications Per Commission E: Intestinal obstruction, acute intestinal inflammation (eg, Crohn's disease), colitis ulcerosa, appendicitis, abdominal pain of unknown origin

Warnings/Precautions Not recommended for over-the-counter (OTC) use in patients experiencing stomach pain, nausea, vomiting, or a sudden change in bowel movements which lasts >2 weeks.

Adverse Reactions (Reflective of adult population; not specific for elderly) Frequency not defined: Gastrointestinal: Abdominal cramps, diarrhea, nausea, vomiting

Drug Interactions
Metabolism/Transport Effects None known.
Avoid Concomitant Use There are no known interactions where it is recommended to avoid concomitant use.
Increased Effect/Toxicity There are no known significant interactions involving an increase in effect.
Decreased Effect There are no known significant interactions involving a decrease in effect.

Pharmacodynamics/Kinetics
Metabolism: In the liver
Elimination: In feces (via bile) and urine

Dosage
Geriatric & Adult
Bowel evacuation: Oral: OTC labeling: Usual dose: Sennosides 130 mg between 2-4 PM the afternoon of the day prior to procedure
Constipation: Oral: OTC ranges: Sennosides 15 mg once daily (maximum: 70-100 mg/day, divided twice daily)

Administration Oral: Once daily doses should be taken at bedtime. Granules may be eaten plain, sprinkled on food, or mixed in liquids

Monitoring Parameters Monitor stools daily for consistency, occult or gross blood; also with chronic use, monitor serum electrolytes; monitor for dehydration and hypotension

Pharmacotherapy Pearls Some products that may have previously been labeled as standardized senna concentrate are now labeled as sennosides. For example, Senokot® tablets, previously labeled as standardized senna concentrate 187 mg, are now labeled as sennosides 8.6 mg. The actual content of senna in this product did not change. Individual product labeling should be consulted prior to dosing.

Special Geriatric Considerations Elderly are often predisposed to constipation due to disease, immobility, drugs, and a decreased "thirst reflex" with age enhancing the possibility of dehydration. Avoid stimulant cathartic use on a chronic basis if possible. Use osmotic, lubricant, stool softeners, and bulk agents as prophylaxis. Patients should be instructed for proper dietary fiber and fluid intake as well as regular exercise. Monitor closely for fluid/electrolyte imbalance, CNS signs of fluid/electrolyte loss, and hypotension.

Dosage Forms Excipient information presented when available (limited, particularly for generics); consult specific product labeling. [DSC] = Discontinued product
Liquid, oral:
Senexon: Sennosides 8.8 mg/5 mL (237 mL) [contains propylene glycol]
Liquid, oral [concentrate]:
Fletcher's®: Senna concentrate 33.3 mg/mL (75 mL) [ethanol free; contains sodium benzoate; rootbeer flavor]

Liquid, oral [concentrate/drops]:
Little Tummys® Laxative: Sennosides 8.8 mg/mL (30 mL) [dye free, ethanol free; contains propylene glycol, soya lecithin; chocolate flavor]
Strip, orally disintegrating, oral:
Fleet® Pedia-Lax™ Quick Dissolve: Sennosides 8.6 mg (12s) [grape flavor]
Syrup, oral: Sennosides 8.8 mg/5 mL (237 mL, 240 mL [DSC])
Tablet, oral: Sennosides 8.6 mg, Sennosides 15 mg, Sennosides 25 mg
ex-lax®: Sennosides USP 15 mg
ex-lax® Maximum Strength: Sennosides USP 25 mg
Geri-kot: Sennosides 8.6 mg
Perdiem® Overnight Relief: Sennosides USP 15 mg
Senexon: Sennosides 8.6 mg
Senna-Lax: Sennosides 8.6 mg [contains calcium 50 mg/tablet]
SennaGen: Sennosides 8.6 mg
Senokot®: Sennosides 8.6 mg
Tablet, chewable, oral:
Black Draught®: Sennosides 10 mg
Evac-U-Gen®: Sennosides 10 mg
ex-lax®: Sennosides USP 15 mg [chocolate flavor]

◆ **Senna and Docusate** see Docusate and Senna on page 585
◆ **SennaGen [OTC]** see Senna on page 1764
◆ **Senna-Lax [OTC]** see Senna on page 1764
◆ **SennaLax-S [OTC]** see Docusate and Senna on page 585
◆ **Senna Plus [OTC]** see Docusate and Senna on page 585
◆ **Senna-S** see Docusate and Senna on page 585
◆ **Sennosides** see Senna on page 1764
◆ **Senokot® [OTC]** see Senna on page 1764
◆ **Senokot-S® [OTC]** see Docusate and Senna on page 585
◆ **SenoSol™-SS [OTC]** see Docusate and Senna on page 585
◆ **Sensipar®** see Cinacalcet on page 379
◆ **Septra** see Sulfamethoxazole and Trimethoprim on page 1813
◆ **Septra® DS** see Sulfamethoxazole and Trimethoprim on page 1813
◆ **Serax** see Oxazepam on page 1438
◆ **Serevent® Diskus®** see Salmeterol on page 1749
◆ **Seromycin®** see CycloSERINE on page 459
◆ **SEROquel®** see QUEtiapine on page 1644
◆ **SEROquel XR®** see QUEtiapine on page 1644

Sertraline (SER tra leen)

Related Information
Antidepressant Agents on page 2097
Medication Safety Issues
Sound-alike/look-alike issues:
Sertraline may be confused with selegiline, Serevent®, Soriatane®
Zoloft® may be confused with Zocor®
BEERS Criteria medication:
This drug may be potentially inappropriate for use in geriatric patients (Quality of evidence - moderate; Strength of recommendation - strong).
Brand Names: U.S. Zoloft®
Brand Names: Canada Apo-Sertraline®; CO Sertraline; Dom-Sertraline; GD-Sertraline; Mylan-Sertraline; Nu-Sertraline; PHL-Sertraline; PMS-Sertraline; ratio-Sertraline; Riva-Sertraline; Sandoz-Sertraline; Teva-Sertraline; Zoloft®
Index Terms Sertraline Hydrochloride
Generic Availability (U.S.) Yes
Pharmacologic Category Antidepressant, Selective Serotonin Reuptake Inhibitor
Use Treatment of major depression; obsessive-compulsive disorder (OCD); panic disorder; post-traumatic stress disorder (PTSD); social anxiety disorder
Unlabeled Use Eating disorders; generalized anxiety disorder (GAD); impulse control disorders; treatment of mild dementia-associated agitation in nonpsychotic patients
Medication Guide Available Yes
Contraindications Hypersensitivity to sertraline or any component of the formulation; use of MAO inhibitors within 14 days; concurrent use of pimozide; concurrent use of sertraline oral concentrate with disulfiram

◀ **Warnings/Precautions** Short-term studies did not show an increased risk in patients >24 years of age and showed a decreased risk in patients ≥65 years. Closely monitor patients for clinical worsening, suicidality, or unusual changes in behavior, particularly during the initial 1-2 months of therapy or during periods of dosage adjustments (increases or decreases); the patient's family or caregiver should be instructed to closely observe the patient and communicate condition with healthcare provider. A medication guide concerning the use of antidepressants should be dispensed with each prescription.

The possibility of a suicide attempt is inherent in major depression and may persist until remission occurs. Use caution in high-risk patients. Worsening depression and severe abrupt suicidality that are not part of the presenting symptoms may require discontinuation or modification of drug therapy. The patient's family or caregiver should be alerted to monitor patients for the emergence of suicidality and associated behaviors (such as agitation, irritability, hostility, impulsivity, and hypomania) and call healthcare provider.

May worsen psychosis in some patients or precipitate a shift to mania or hypomania in patients with bipolar disorder. Patients presenting with depressive symptoms should be screened for bipolar disorder. Monotherapy in patients with bipolar disorder should be avoided. **Sertraline is not FDA approved for the treatment of bipolar depression.**

Serotonin syndrome and neuroleptic malignant syndrome (NMS)-like reactions have occurred with serotonin/norepinephrine reuptake inhibitors (SNRIs) and selective serotonin reuptake inhibitors (SSRIs) when used alone, and particularly when used in combination with serotonergic agents (eg, triptans) or antidopaminergic agents (eg, antipsychotics). Concurrent use with MAO inhibitors is contraindicated. Has a very low potential to impair cognitive or motor performance. However, caution patients regarding activities requiring alertness until response to sertraline is known. Does not appear to potentiate the effects of alcohol, however, ethanol use is not advised.

Use caution in patients with a previous seizure disorder or condition predisposing to seizures such as brain damage, alcoholism, or concurrent therapy with other drugs which lower the seizure threshold. May increase the risks associated with electroconvulsive therapy. Use with caution in patients with hepatic or renal dysfunction and in elderly patients. May cause hyponatremia/SIADH (elderly at increased risk); volume depletion (diuretics may increase risk). Use with caution in patients with renal insufficiency or other concurrent illness (due to limited experience). Use caution in elderly patients; may cause or exacerbate syndrome of inappropriate antidiuretic hormone secretion or hyponatremia; monitor sodium closely with initiation or dosage adjustments in older adults (Beers Criteria). Sertraline acts as a mild uricosuric; use with caution in patients at risk of uric acid nephropathy. Use caution with concomitant use of NSAIDs, ASA, or other drugs that affect coagulation; the risk of bleeding may be potentiated. Use with caution in patients where weight loss is undesirable. May cause or exacerbate sexual dysfunction.

Use oral concentrate formulation with caution in patients with latex sensitivity; dropper dispenser contains dry natural rubber. Discontinuation symptoms (eg, dysphoric mood, irritability, agitation, confusion, anxiety, insomnia, hypomania) may occur upon abrupt discontinuation. Taper dose when discontinuing therapy.

Adverse Reactions (Reflective of adult population; not specific for elderly)
>10%:
  Central nervous system: Dizziness, fatigue, headache, insomnia, somnolence
  Endocrine & metabolic: Libido decreased
  Gastrointestinal: Anorexia, diarrhea, nausea, xerostomia
  Genitourinary: Ejaculatory disturbances
  Neuromuscular & skeletal: Tremors
  Miscellaneous: Diaphoresis
1% to 10%:
  Cardiovascular: Chest pain, palpitation
  Central nervous system: Agitation, anxiety, hypoesthesia, malaise, nervousness, pain
  Dermatologic: Rash
  Endocrine & metabolic: Impotence
  Gastrointestinal: Appetite increased, constipation, dyspepsia, flatulence, vomiting, weight gain
  Neuromuscular & skeletal: Back pain, hypertonia, myalgia, paresthesia, weakness
  Ocular: Visual difficulty, abnormal vision
  Otic: Tinnitus
  Respiratory: Rhinitis
  Miscellaneous: Yawning

  Pediatric patients: Additional adverse reactions reported in pediatric patients (frequency >2%):
  Aggressiveness, epistaxis, hyperkinesia, purpura, sinusitis, urinary incontinence

Drug Interactions

Metabolism/Transport Effects **Substrate** of CYP2B6 (minor), CYP2C19 (minor), CYP2C9 (minor), CYP2D6 (major), CYP3A4 (minor); **Note:** Assignment of Major/Minor substrate status based on clinically relevant drug interaction potential; **Inhibits** CYP1A2 (weak), CYP2B6 (moderate), CYP2C19 (moderate), CYP2C8 (weak), CYP2C9 (weak), CYP2D6 (moderate), CYP3A4 (moderate)

Avoid Concomitant Use

Avoid concomitant use of Sertraline with any of the following: Clopidogrel; Disulfiram; Iobenguane I 123; MAO Inhibitors; Methylene Blue; Pimozide; Tolvaptan; Tryptophan

Increased Effect/Toxicity

Sertraline may increase the levels/effects of: Alpha-/Beta-Blockers; Anticoagulants; Antidepressants (Serotonin Reuptake Inhibitor/Antagonist); Antiplatelet Agents; Aspirin; Avanafil; Beta-Blockers; Budesonide (Systemic, Oral Inhalation); BusPIRone; CarBAMazepine; CloZAPine; Colchicine; Collagenase (Systemic); CYP2B6 Substrates; CYP2C19 Substrates; CYP2D6 Substrates; CYP3A4 Substrates; Dabigatran Etexilate; Desmopressin; Dextromethorphan; Drotrecogin Alfa (Activated); Eplerenone; Everolimus; Fesoterodine; Fosphenytoin; Galantamine; Highest Risk QTc-Prolonging Agents; Hypoglycemic Agents; Ibritumomab; Ivacaftor; Lithium; Methadone; Methylene Blue; Metoclopramide; Moderate Risk QTc-Prolonging Agents; NSAID (COX-2 Inhibitor); NSAID (Nonselective); Phenytoin; Pimecrolimus; Pimozide; RisperiDONE; Rivaroxaban; Salicylates; Salmeterol; Saxagliptin; Serotonin Modulators; Thrombolytic Agents; Tolvaptan; Tositumomab and Iodine I 131 Tositumomab; TraMADol; Tricyclic Antidepressants; Vitamin K Antagonists

The levels/effects of Sertraline may be increased by: Abiraterone Acetate; Alcohol (Ethyl); Analgesics (Opioid); Antipsychotics; BusPIRone; Cimetidine; CNS Depressants; CYP2D6 Inhibitors (Moderate); CYP2D6 Inhibitors (Strong); Disulfiram; Glucosamine; Herbs (Anticoagulant/Antiplatelet Properties); Linezolid; Macrolide Antibiotics; MAO Inhibitors; Metoclopramide; Metyrosine; Mifepristone; Omega-3-Acid Ethyl Esters; Pentosan Polysulfate Sodium; Pentoxifylline; Prostacyclin Analogues; Tipranavir; TraMADol; Tryptophan; Vitamin E

Decreased Effect

Sertraline may decrease the levels/effects of: Clopidogrel; Ifosfamide; Iobenguane I 123; Ioflupane I 123

The levels/effects of Sertraline may be decreased by: CarBAMazepine; Cyproheptadine; Darunavir; Efavirenz; Fosphenytoin; NSAID (COX-2 Inhibitor); NSAID (Nonselective); Peginterferon Alfa-2b; Phenytoin; Tocilizumab

Ethanol/Nutrition/Herb Interactions

Ethanol: May increase CNS depression; monitor for increased effects with coadministration. Caution patients about effects.

Food: Sertraline average peak serum levels may be increased if taken with food.

Herb/Nutraceutical: Avoid valerian, St John's wort, kava kava, gotu kola (may increase CNS depression).

Stability Tablets and oral solution should be stored at controlled room temperature of 15°C to 30°C (59°F to 86°F).

Mechanism of Action Antidepressant with selective inhibitory effects on presynaptic serotonin (5-HT) reuptake and only very weak effects on norepinephrine and dopamine neuronal uptake. In vitro studies demonstrate no significant affinity for adrenergic, cholinergic, GABA, dopaminergic, histaminergic, serotonergic, or benzodiazepine receptors.

Pharmacodynamics/Kinetics

Onset of action: Depression: The onset of action is within a week, however, individual response varies greatly and full response may not be seen until 8-12 weeks after initiation of treatment.

Absorption: Slow

Protein binding: 98%

Metabolism: Hepatic; may involve CYP2C19 and CYP2D6; extensive first pass metabolism; forms metabolite N-desmethylsertraline

Bioavailability: Bioavailability of tablets and solution are equivalent

Half-life elimination: Sertraline: 26 hours; N-desmethylsertraline: 66 hours (range: 62-104 hours)

Time to peak, plasma: Sertraline: 4.5-8.4 hours

Excretion: Urine and feces

Dosage

Geriatric Oral: Initial: 25 mg/day in the morning; increase by 25 mg/day increments every 2-3 days if tolerated to 50-100 mg/day; additional increases may be necessary; maximum: 200 mg/day. **Note:** Patients with Alzheimer's dementia-related depression may require a lower starting dosage of 12.5 mg/day, with titration intervals of 1-2 weeks, up to 150-200 mg/day maximum.

Adult

Depression/obsessive-compulsive disorder: Oral: Initial: 50 mg/day

Note: May increase daily dose, at intervals of not less than 1 week, to a maximum of 200 mg/day. If somnolence is noted, give at bedtime.

Panic disorder, post-traumatic stress disorder, social anxiety disorder: Oral: Initial: 25 mg once daily; increased after 1 week to 50 mg once daily; maximum dose: 200 mg/day

Renal Impairment Multiple-dose pharmacokinetics are unaffected by renal impairment. Hemodialysis effect: Not removed by hemodialysis

Hepatic Impairment Sertraline is extensively metabolized by the liver. Caution should be used in patients with hepatic impairment. A lower dose or less frequent dosing should be used.

Administration Oral concentrate: Must be diluted before use. Immediately before administration, use the dropper provided to measure the required amount of concentrate; mix with 4 ounces (1/2 cup) of water, ginger ale, lemon/lime soda, lemonade, or orange juice only. Do not mix with any other liquids than these. The dose should be taken immediately after mixing; do not mix in advance. A slight haze may appear after mixing; this is normal. Note: Use with caution in patients with latex sensitivity; dropper dispenser contains dry natural rubber.

Monitoring Parameters Monitor nutritional intake and weight; mental status for depression, suicide ideation (especially at the beginning of therapy or when doses are increased or decreased), anxiety, social functioning, mania, panic attacks; akathisia

Test Interactions Increased (minor) serum triglycerides, LFTs; decreased serum uric acid; may interfere with urine detection of benzodiazepines (false-positive)

Pharmacotherapy Pearls Buspirone (15-60 mg/day) may be useful in treatment of sexual dysfunction during treatment with a selective serotonin reuptake inhibitor. May exacerbate tics in Tourette's syndrome.

Special Geriatric Considerations Sertraline's favorable side effect profile makes it a preferred SSRI in older adults. It has the shortest half-life of the currently marketed serotonin-reuptake inhibitors. The elderly are more prone to SSRI/SNRI-induced hyponatremia.

A systematic review and meta-analysis of antidepressant placebo-controlled trials in persons with depression and dementia found evidence "suggestive" of efficacy but not of sufficient strength to "confirm" efficacy. Antidepressant trials in this patient population are small and underpowered. Older patients with depression being treated with an antidepressant should be closely monitored for response and adverse effects. Treatment should be switched or augmented when response is inadequate with a therapeutic dose. Antidepressants that are not tolerated should be discontinued and an alternative agent should be started.

This medication is considered to be potentially inappropriate in this patient population (Beers Criteria: Quality of evidence - moderate; Strength of recommendation - strong).

Dosage Forms Excipient information presented when available (limited, particularly for generics); consult specific product labeling.

Solution, oral [concentrate]: 20 mg/mL (60 mL)

Zoloft®: 20 mg/mL (60 mL) [contains ethanol 12%, menthol, natural rubber/natural latex in packaging]

Tablet, oral: 25 mg, 50 mg, 100 mg

Zoloft®: 25 mg, 50 mg, 100 mg [scored]

◆ **Sertraline Hydrochloride** see Sertraline on page 1765

◆ **Serzone** see Nefazodone on page 1351

Sevelamer (se VEL a mer)

Medication Safety Issues

Sound-alike/look-alike issues:

Renagel® may be confused with Reglan®, Regonol®, Renvela®

Renvela® may be confused with Reglan®, Regonol®, Renagel®

Sevelamer may be confused with Savella®

International issues:

Renagel [U.S., Canada, and multiple international markets] may be confused with Remegel brand name for aluminium hydroxide and magnesium carbonate [Netherlands] and for calcium carbonate [Hungary, Great Britain and Ireland] and with Remegel Wind Relief brand name for calcium carbonate and simethicone [Great Britain]

Brand Names: U.S. Renagel®; Renvela®

Brand Names: Canada Renagel®

Index Terms Sevelamer Carbonate; Sevelamer Hydrochloride

Generic Availability (U.S.) No

Pharmacologic Category Phosphate Binder

Use Reduction or control of serum phosphorous in patients with chronic kidney disease on hemodialysis

Contraindications Bowel obstruction

Warnings/Precautions Use with caution in patients with gastrointestinal disorders including dysphagia, swallowing disorders, severe gastrointestinal motility disorders (including constipation), or major gastrointestinal surgery. May cause reductions in vitamin D, E, K, or folic acid absorption. May bind to some drugs in the gastrointestinal tract and decrease their absorption; when changes in absorption of oral medications may have significant clinical consequences (such as antiarrhythmic and antiseizure medications), these medications should be taken at least 1 hour before or 3 hours after a dose of sevelamer. Tablets should not be taken apart or chewed; broken or crushed tablets will rapidly expand in water/saliva and may be a choking hazard.

Adverse Reactions (Reflective of adult population; not specific for elderly)
>10%: Gastrointestinal: Vomiting (22%), nausea (20%), diarrhea (19%), dyspepsia (16%)
1% to 10%:
    Endocrine & metabolic: Hypercalcemia (5% to 7%)
    Gastrointestinal: Abdominal pain (9%), flatulence (8%), constipation (8%)
    Miscellaneous: Peritonitis (peritoneal dialysis: 8%)

Drug Interactions

  Metabolism/Transport Effects None known.

  Avoid Concomitant Use There are no known interactions where it is recommended to avoid concomitant use.

  Increased Effect/Toxicity There are no known significant interactions involving an increase in effect.

  Decreased Effect
    Sevelamer may decrease the levels/effects of: Calcitriol; Levothyroxine; Mycophenolate; Quinolone Antibiotics

Ethanol/Nutrition/Herb Interactions Food: May cause reductions in vitamin D, E, K, or folic acid absorption. Management: Must be administered with meals. Consider vitamin supplementation.

Stability Store at controlled room temperature of 25°C (77°F); excursions permitted to 15°C to 30°C (59°F to 86°F). Protect from moisture.

Mechanism of Action Sevelamer (a polymeric compound) binds phosphate within the intestinal lumen, limiting absorption and decreasing serum phosphate concentrations without altering calcium, aluminum, or bicarbonate concentrations.

Pharmacodynamics/Kinetics
  Absorption: Not systemically absorbed
  Excretion: Feces

Dosage

  Geriatric & Adult Note: The dosing of sevelamer carbonate and sevelamer hydrochloride are similar; when switching from one product to another, the same dose (on a mg per mg basis) should be utilized.

  Control of serum phosphorous: Oral:
  Patients not taking a phosphate binder: 800-1600 mg 3 times/day with meals; the initial dose may be based on serum phosphorous levels:
    >5.5 mg/dL to <7.5 mg/dL: 800 mg 3 times/day
    ≥7.5 mg/dL to <9.0 mg/dL: 1200-1600 mg 3 times/day
    ≥9.0 mg/dL: 1600 mg 3 times/day
  Maintenance dose adjustment based on serum phosphorous concentration (goal range of 3.5-5.5 mg/dL; maximum dose studied was equivalent to 13 g/day [sevelamer hydrochloride] or 14 g/day [sevelamer carbonate]):
    >5.5 mg/dL: Increase by 400-800 mg per meal at 2-week intervals
    3.5-5.5 mg/dL: Maintain current dose
    <3.5 mg/dL: Decrease by 400-800 mg per meal

  Dosage adjustment when switching between phosphate-binder products: 667 mg of calcium acetate is equivalent to ~800 mg sevelamer (carbonate or hydrochloride)
  Conversion based on dose per meal:
    Calcium acetate 667 mg: Convert to 800 mg Renagel® / Renvela®
    Calcium acetate 1334 mg: Convert to 1600 mg Renagel® 800 mg/ Renvela® **or** 1200 mg Renagel® 400 mg
    Calcium acetate 2001 mg: Convert to 2400 mg Renagel® 800 mg / Renvela® **or** 2000 mg Renagel® 400 mg

◄ **Administration** Must be administered with meals.

Powder for oral suspension: Mix powder with water prior to administration. The 0.8 g packet should be mixed with 30 mL of water and the 2.4 g packet should be mixed with 60 mL of water (multiple packets may be mixed together using the appropriate amount of water). Stir vigorously to suspend mixture just prior to drinking; powder does not dissolve. Drink within 30 minutes of preparing and resuspend just prior to drinking.

Tablets: Swallow whole; do not crush, chew, or break

Monitoring Parameters

Serum chemistries, including bicarbonate and chloride

Serum calcium and phosphorus: Frequency of measurement may be dependent upon the presence and magnitude of abnormalities, the rate of progression of CKD, and the use of treatments for CKD-mineral and bone disorders (KDIGO, 2009):

CKD stage 3: Every 6-12 months

CKD stage 4: Every 3-6 months

CKD stage 5 and 5D: Every 1-3 months

Periodic 24-hour urinary calcium and phosphorus; magnesium; alkaline phosphatase every 12 months or more frequently in the presence of elevated PTH; creatinine, BUN, albumin; intact parathyroid hormone (iPTH) every 3-12 months depending on CKD severity

Reference Range

Corrected total serum calcium (K/DOQI, 2003): CKD stages 3 and 4: 8.4-10.2 mg/dL (2.1-2.6 mmol/L); CKD stage 5: 8.4-9.5 mg/dL (2.1-2.37 mmol/L); KDIGO guidelines recommend maintaining normal ranges for all stages of CKD (3-5D) (KDIGO, 2009)

Phosphorus (K/DOQI, 2003):

CKD stages 3 and 4: 2.7-4.6 mg/dL (0.87-1.48 mmol/L) (adults)

CKD stage 5 (including those treated with dialysis): 3.5-5.5 mg/dL (1.13-1.78 mmol/L) (adults)

KDIGO guidelines recommend maintaining normal ranges for CKD stages 3-5 and lowering elevated phosphorus levels toward the normal range for CKD stage 5D (KDIGO, 2009)

Serum calcium-phosphorus product (K/DOQI, 2003): CKD stage 3-5: <55 mg^2/dL^2 (adults)

PTH: Whole molecule, immunochemiluminometric assay (ICMA): 1.0-5.2 pmol/L; whole molecule, radioimmunoassay (RIA): 10.0-65.0 pg/mL; whole molecule, immunoradiometric, double antibody (IRMA): 1.0-6.0 pmol/L

Target ranges by stage of chronic kidney disease (KDIGO, 2009): CKD stage 3-5: Optimal iPTH is unknown; maintain normal range (assay-dependent); CKD stage 5D: Maintain iPTH within 2-9 times the upper limit of normal for the assay used

Special Geriatric Considerations No specific dose changes needed for the elderly. Since electrolyte changes (ie, phosphorus, calcium) can have dramatic effects in the elderly, monitor closely.

Dosage Forms Excipient information presented when available (limited, particularly for generics); consult specific product labeling.

Powder for suspension, oral, as carbonate:

Renvela®: 0.8 g/packet (90s); 2.4 g/packet (90s) [contains propylene glycol; citrus-cream flavor]

Tablet, oral, as carbonate:

Renvela®: 800 mg

Tablet, oral, as hydrochloride:

Renagel®: 400 mg, 800 mg

◆ **Sevelamer Carbonate** *see* Sevelamer *on page 1768*

◆ **Sevelamer Hydrochloride** *see* Sevelamer *on page 1768*

◆ **sfRowasa™** *see* Mesalamine *on page 1217*

◆ **Shingles Vaccine** *see* Zoster Vaccine *on page 2071*

◆ **Shohl's Solution (Modified)** *see* Sodium Citrate and Citric Acid *on page 1790*

◆ **Silace [OTC]** *see* Docusate *on page 583*

◆ **Siladryl Allergy [OTC]** *see* DiphenhydrAMINE (Systemic) *on page 556*

◆ **Silafed [OTC]** *see* Triprolidine and Pseudoephedrine *on page 1975*

◆ **Silapap Children's [OTC]** *see* Acetaminophen *on page 31*

◆ **Silapap Infant's [OTC]** *see* Acetaminophen *on page 31*

Sildenafil (sil DEN a fil)

Medication Safety Issues

Sound-alike/look-alike issues:

Revatio® may be confused with ReVia®, Revonto®

Sildenafil may be confused with silodosin, tadalafil, vardenafil

Viagra® may be confused with Allegra®, Vaniqa®

Brand Names: U.S. Revatio®; Viagra®

Brand Names: Canada ratio-Sildenafil R; Revatio®; Viagra®
Index Terms Sildenafil Citrate; UK92480
Generic Availability (U.S.) No
Pharmacologic Category Phosphodiesterase-5 Enzyme Inhibitor
Use
  Revatio®: Treatment of pulmonary arterial hypertension (PAH) (WHO Group I) to improve
  exercise ability and delay clinical worsening
  Viagra®: Treatment of erectile dysfunction (ED)
Unlabeled Use No geriatric-specific information.
Contraindications Hypersensitivity to sildenafil or any component of the formulation; con-
current use (regularly/intermittently) of organic nitrates in any form (eg, nitroglycerin, isosorbide dinitrate); concurrent use with a protease inhibitor regimen when sildenafil used for
pulmonary artery hypertension (eg, Revatio®)
Warnings/Precautions Decreases in blood pressure may occur due to vasodilator effects;
use with caution in patients with left ventricular outflow obstruction (aortic stenosis or
hypertrophic obstructive cardiomyopathy); may be more sensitive to hypotensive actions.
Concurrent use with alpha-adrenergic antagonist therapy may cause symptomatic hypotension; patients should be hemodynamically stable prior to initiating therapy at the lowest
possible dose. Avoid or limit concurrent substantial alcohol consumption as this may increase
the risk of symptomatic hypotension. Use with caution in patients with hypotension (<90/50
mm Hg); uncontrolled hypertension (>170/110 mm Hg); life-threatening arrhythmias, stroke or
MI within the last 6 months; cardiac failure or coronary artery disease causing unstable
angina; safety and efficacy have not been studied in these patients. There is a degree of
cardiac risk associated with sexual activity; therefore, physicians should consider the
cardiovascular status of their patients prior to initiating any treatment for erectile dysfunction.
If pulmonary edema occurs when treating pulmonary arterial hypertension (PAH), consider the
possibility of pulmonary veno-occlusive disease (PVOD); continued use is not recommended
in patient with PVOD.

Sildenafil should be used with caution in patients with anatomical deformation of the penis
(angulation, cavernosal fibrosis, or Peyronie's disease) and in patients who have conditions
which may predispose them to priapism (sickle cell anemia, multiple myeloma, leukemia). All
patients should be instructed to seek medical attention if erection persists >4 hours.

Vision loss may occur rarely and be a sign of nonarteritic anterior ischemic optic neuropathy
(NAION). Risk may be increased with history of vision loss. Other risk factors for NAION
include low cup-to-disc ratio ("crowded disc"), coronary artery disease, diabetes, hypertension, hyperlipidemia, smoking, and age >50 years. May cause dose-related impairment
of color discrimination. Use caution in patients with retinitis pigmentosa; a minority have
genetic disorders of retinal phosphodiesterases (no safety information available). Sudden
decrease or loss of hearing has been reported rarely; hearing changes may be accompanied
by tinnitus and dizziness. A direct relationship between therapy and vision or hearing loss has
not been determined.

The potential underlying causes of erectile dysfunction should be evaluated prior to treatment.
The safety and efficacy of sildenafil with other treatments for erectile dysfunction have not
been established; use is not recommended. Efficacy with concurrent bosentan therapy has
not been evaluated; use with caution. Use with caution in patients taking strong CYP3A4
inhibitors or alpha-blockers. Concomitant use with all forms of nitrates is contraindicated. If
nitrate administration is medically necessary, it is not known when nitrates can be safely
administered following the use of sildenafil (per manufacturer); the ACC/AHA 2007 guidelines
supports administration of nitrates only if 24 hours have elapsed.

Avoid abrupt discontinuation, especially if used as monotherapy in PAH as exacerbation may
occur. Use caution in patients with bleeding disorders or with active peptic ulcer disease;
safety and efficacy have not been established. Efficacy has not been established for treatment of
pulmonary hypertension associated with sickle cell disease. Use with caution in the elderly, or
patients with renal or hepatic dysfunction; dose adjustment may be needed.
Adverse Reactions (Reflective of adult population; not specific for elderly) Based
upon normal doses for either indication or route. (Adverse effects such as flushing, diarrhea,
myalgia, and visual disturbances may be increased with adult doses >100 mg/24 hours.)
>10%:
  Central nervous system: Headache (16% to 46%)
  Gastrointestinal: Dyspepsia (7% to 17%; dose related)
2% to 10%:
  Cardiovascular: Flushing (10%)
  Central nervous system: Insomnia (≤7%), pyrexia (6%), dizziness (2%)
  Dermatologic: Erythema (6%), rash (2%)
  Gastrointestinal: Diarrhea (3% to 9%), gastritis (≤3%)

Genitourinary: Urinary tract infection (3%)

Hepatic: LFTs increased

Neuromuscular & skeletal: Myalgia (≤7%), paresthesia (≤3%)

Ocular: Abnormal vision (color changes, blurred vision, or increased sensitivity to light 3% to 11%; dose related)

Respiratory: Epistaxis (9% to 13%), dyspnea exacerbated (≤7%), nasal congestion (4%), rhinitis (4%), sinusitis (3%)

Drug Interactions

Metabolism/Transport Effects Substrate of CYP1A2 (minor), CYP2C19 (minor), CYP2C9 (minor), CYP2D6 (minor), CYP2E1 (minor), CYP3A4 (major); **Note:** Assignment of Major/Minor substrate status based on clinically relevant drug interaction potential; **Inhibits** CYP2C9 (weak), CYP3A4 (weak)

Avoid Concomitant Use

Avoid concomitant use of Sildenafil with any of the following: Alprostadil; Amyl Nitrite; Boceprevir; Phosphodiesterase 5 Inhibitors; Pimozide; Telaprevir; Vasodilators (Organic Nitrates)

Increased Effect/Toxicity

Sildenafil may increase the levels/effects of: Alpha1-Blockers; Alprostadil; Amyl Nitrite; Antihypertensives; ARIPiprazole; Bosentan; HMG-CoA Reductase Inhibitors; Phosphodiesterase 5 Inhibitors; Pimozide; Vasodilators (Organic Nitrates)

The levels/effects of Sildenafil may be increased by: Alcohol (Ethyl); Boceprevir; CYP3A4 Inhibitors (Moderate); CYP3A4 Inhibitors (Strong); Dasatinib; Erythromycin; Fluconazole; Itraconazole; Ivacaftor; Ketoconazole (Systemic); Mifepristone; Posaconazole; Protease Inhibitors; Sapropterin; Telaprevir; Voriconazole

Decreased Effect

The levels/effects of Sildenafil may be decreased by: Bosentan; CYP3A4 Inducers (Strong); Deferasirox; Etravirine; Herbs (CYP3A4 Inducers); Peginterferon Alfa-2b; Tocilizumab

Ethanol/Nutrition/Herb Interactions Ethanol: Substantial consumption of ethanol may increase the risk of hypotension and orthostasis. Lower ethanol consumption has not been associated with significant changes in blood pressure or increase in orthostatic symptoms. Management: Avoid or limit ethanol consumption.

Food: Avoid grapefruit juice.

Herb/Nutraceutical: St John's wort may decrease sildenafil levels. Management: Avoid St John's wort.

Stability Store at controlled room temperature of 25°C (77°F); excursions permitted to 15°C to 30°C (59°F to 86°F).

Mechanism of Action

Erectile dysfunction: Does not directly cause penile erections, but affects the response to sexual stimulation. The physiologic mechanism of erection of the penis involves release of nitric oxide (NO) in the corpus cavernosum during sexual stimulation. NO then activates the enzyme guanylate cyclase, which results in increased levels of cyclic guanosine monophosphate (cGMP), producing smooth muscle relaxation and inflow of blood to the corpus cavernosum. Sildenafil enhances the effect of NO by inhibiting phosphodiesterase type 5 (PDE-5), which is responsible for degradation of cGMP in the corpus cavernosum; when sexual stimulation causes local release of NO, inhibition of PDE-5 by sildenafil causes increased levels of cGMP in the corpus cavernosum, resulting in smooth muscle relaxation and inflow of blood to the corpus cavernosum; at recommended doses, it has no effect in the absence of sexual stimulation.

Pulmonary arterial hypertension (PAH): Inhibits phosphodiesterase type 5 (PDE-5) in smooth muscle of pulmonary vasculature where PDE-5 is responsible for the degradation of cyclic guanosine monophosphate (cGMP). Increased cGMP concentration results in pulmonary vasculature relaxation; vasodilation in the pulmonary bed and the systemic circulation (to a lesser degree) may occur.

Pharmacodynamics/Kinetics

Onset of action: ~60 minutes

Duration: 2-4 hours

Absorption: Rapid; slower with a high-fat meal

Distribution: V_{dss}: 105 L

Protein binding, plasma: ~96%

Metabolism: Hepatic via CYP3A4 (major) and CYP2C9 (minor route); forms N-desmethyl metabolite (active)

Bioavailability: 40% (25% to 63%)

Half-life elimination: ~4 hours; the elderly and those with severe renal impairment have reduced clearance of sildenafil and its active N-desmethyl metabolite

Time to peak: 30-120 minutes; delayed by 60 minutes with a high-fat meal

Excretion: Feces (~80%); urine (~13%)

Dosage

Geriatric Elderly >65 years: Use with caution.
Revatio®: Refer to adult dosing.
Viagra®: Starting dose of 25 mg should be considered.

Adult

Erectile dysfunction (Viagra®): Oral: Usual dose: 50 mg once daily 1 hour (range: 30 minutes to 4 hours) before sexual activity; dosing range: 25-100 mg once daily.

Pulmonary arterial hypertension (PAH) (Revatio®):
I.V.: 10 mg 3 times/day
Oral: 20 mg 3 times/day, taken 4-6 hours apart. **Note:** A delay in clinical worsening was observed in a short-term trial in which most patients achieved a target dose of 80 mg 3 times daily (unlabeled dose). The patients had an incremental dosage escalation while on a stable epoprostenol regimen (Simonneau, 2008).

Dosage considerations for patients stable on alpha-blockers: Viagra®: Initial: 25 mg

Dosage adjustment for concomitant use of potent CYP34A inhibitors:
Revatio®:
Erythromycin: No dosage adjustment
Itraconazole, ketoconazole: Not recommended
Viagra®:
Erythromycin, itraconazole, ketoconazole: Starting dose of 25 mg should be considered
Protease inhibitors: Maximum sildenafil dose: 25 mg every 48 hours

Renal Impairment
Revatio®: Dose adjustment not necessary
Viagra®: Cl_{cr} <30 mL/minute: Starting dose of 25 mg should be considered.

Hepatic Impairment
Revatio®: Child-Pugh class A or B: Dose adjustment not necessary; not studied in severe impairment (Child-Pugh class C).
Viagra®: Child-Pugh class A or B: Starting dose of 25 mg should be considered; not studied in severe impairment (Child-Pugh class C).

Administration

Revatio®: Administer tablets without regard to meals at least 4-6 hours apart. Administer injection as an I.V. bolus.

Viagra®: Administer orally 30 minutes to 4 hours before sexual activity

Pharmacotherapy Pearls Sildenafil is ~10 times more selective for PDE-5 as compared to PDE6. This enzyme is found in the retina and is involved in phototransduction. At higher plasma levels, interference with PDE6 is believed to be the basis for changes in color vision noted in some patients.

Special Geriatric Considerations Since the elderly often have concomitant diseases, many of which may contraindicate the use of sildenafil, a thorough knowledge of diseases and medications used must be assessed. Adjust dose for renal/hepatic function.

Dosage Forms Excipient information presented when available (limited, particularly for generics); consult specific product labeling.

Injection, solution:
Revatio®: 0.8 mg/mL (12.5 mL)
Tablet, oral:
Revatio®: 20 mg
Viagra®: 25 mg, 50 mg, 100 mg

♦ **Sildenafil Citrate** see Sildenafil on page 1770
♦ **Silenor®** see Doxepin (Systemic) on page 601
♦ **Silexin [OTC]** see Guaifenesin and Dextromethorphan on page 906
♦ **Silfedrine Children's [OTC]** see Pseudoephedrine on page 1633

Silodosin (SI lo doe sin)

Related Information
Pharmacotherapy of Urinary Incontinence on page 2141

Medication Safety Issues
Sound-alike/look-alike issues:
Rapaflo® may be confused with Rapamune®
Silodosin may be confused with sildenafil

Brand Names: U.S. Rapaflo®

Brand Names: Canada Rapaflo®

Index Terms KMD 3213

Generic Availability (U.S.) No

Pharmacologic Category Alpha₁ Blocker

SILODOSIN

Use Treatment of signs and symptoms of benign prostatic hyperplasia (BPH)

Contraindications Concurrent use with strong CYP3A4 inhibitors (eg, clarithromycin, itraconazole, ketoconazole, ritonavir); severe renal impairment (Cl_{cr} <30 mL/minute); severe hepatic impairment (Child-Pugh class C)

Warnings/Precautions Not intended for use as an antihypertensive drug. May cause significant orthostatic hypotension and syncope, especially with first dose; anticipate a similar effect if therapy is interrupted for a few days, if dosage is rapidly increased, or if another antihypertensive drug (particularly vasodilators) or a PDE-5 inhibitor (eg, sildenafil, tadalafil, vardenafil) is introduced. "First-dose" orthostatic hypotension may occur 4-8 hours after dosing; may be dose related. Patients should be cautioned about performing hazardous tasks when starting new therapy or adjusting dosage upward. Rule out prostatic carcinoma before beginning therapy with silodosin. Intraoperative floppy iris syndrome has been observed in cataract surgery patients who were on or were previously treated with alpha$_1$-blockers; causality has not been established and there appears to be no benefit in discontinuing alpha-blocker therapy prior to surgery. Use with caution in patients with mild-to-moderate hepatic impairment; contraindicated with severe impairment; not studied. Use with caution in patients with moderate renal impairment; dosage adjustment recommended. Contraindicated in patients with severe impairment (Cl_{cr} <30 mL/minute). Not indicated for use in women.

Adverse Reactions (Reflective of adult population; not specific for elderly)

>10%: Miscellaneous: Retrograde ejaculation (28%)

1% to 10%:
Cardiovascular: Orthostatic hypotension (3%)
Central nervous system: Dizziness (3%), headache (2%), insomnia (1% to 2%)
Gastrointestinal: Diarrhea (3%), abdominal pain (1% to 2%)
Genitourinary: PSA increased (1% to 2%)
Neuromuscular & skeletal: Weakness (1% to 2%)
Respiratory: Nasal congestion (2%), nasopharyngitis (2%), rhinorrhea (1% to 2%), sinusitis (1% to 2%)

Drug Interactions

Metabolism/Transport Effects Substrate of CYP3A4 (major), P-glycoprotein, UGT2B7; **Note:** Assignment of Major/Minor substrate status based on clinically relevant drug interaction potential

Avoid Concomitant Use
Avoid concomitant use of Silodosin with any of the following: Alpha1-Blockers; CYP3A4 Inhibitors (Strong); P-glycoprotein/ABCB1 Inhibitors

Increased Effect/Toxicity
Silodosin may increase the levels/effects of: Alpha1-Blockers; Calcium Channel Blockers

The levels/effects of Silodosin may be increased by: Beta-Blockers; CYP3A4 Inhibitors (Moderate); CYP3A4 Inhibitors (Strong); Dasatinib; Ivacaftor; MAO Inhibitors; Mifepristone; P-glycoprotein/ABCB1 Inhibitors; Phosphodiesterase 5 Inhibitors

Decreased Effect
The levels/effects of Silodosin may be decreased by: CYP3A4 Inducers (Strong); Deferasirox; Herbs (CYP3A4 Inducers); P-glycoprotein/ABCB1 Inducers; Tocilizumab

Ethanol/Nutrition/Herb Interactions
Food: AUC decrease by 4% to 49% and C_{max} decreased by ~18% to 43% with moderate calorie/fat meal. Management: Take once daily with a meal.
Herb/Nutraceutical: St John's wort may decrease the levels/effects of silodosin; other herbal medications may have hypotensive properties. There is limited data regarding use with saw palmetto. Management: Avoid St John's wort, black cohosh, California poppy, coleus, golden seal, hawthorn, mistletoe, periwinkle, quinine, and shepherd's purse. Avoid saw palmetto.

Stability Store at room temperature of 25°C (77°F); excursions permitted to 15°C to 30°C (59°F to 86°F). Protect from light. Protect from moisture.

Mechanism of Action Silodosin is a selective antagonist of alpha$_{1A}$-adrenoreceptors in the prostate and bladder. Smooth muscle tone in the prostate is mediated by alpha$_{1A}$-adrenoreceptors; blocking them leads to relaxation of smooth muscle in the bladder neck and prostate causing an improvement of urine flow and decreased symptoms of BPH. Approximately 75% of the alpha1-receptors in the prostate are of the alpha$_{1A}$ subtype.

Pharmacodynamics/Kinetics
Distribution: V_d: 49.5 L
Protein binding: ~97%
Metabolism: Extensive, via CYP3A4, glucuronidation, and alcohol and aldehyde dehydrogenase pathways; KMD-3213G (active in vitro) and KMD-3293 (not significant) metabolites formed
Bioavailability: ~32%
Half-life elimination: Healthy volunteers: Silodosin: 5-21 hours; KMD-3213G: ~24 hours
Time to peak, plasma: ~3 hours
Excretion: Feces (55%); urine (34%)

Dosage
   Geriatric & Adult BPH: Oral: 8 mg once daily with a meal
   Renal Impairment
      Cl$_{cr}$ >50 mL/minute: No adjustment needed.
      Cl$_{cr}$ 30-50 mL/minute: 4 mg once daily.
      Cl$_{cr}$ <30 mL/minute: Use is contraindicated.
   Hepatic Impairment
      Mild-to-moderate impairment (Child-Pugh class A or B): No adjustment needed.
      Severe impairment (Child-Pugh class C): Use is contraindicated.
   Administration Administer once daily with a meal.
   Monitoring Parameters Blood pressure; urinary symptoms
   Special Geriatric Considerations See Dosage: Renal Impairment. In clinical studies, older men had a higher incidence of orthostatic hypotension when using silodosin.
   Dosage Forms Excipient information presented when available (limited, particularly for generics); consult specific product labeling.
      Capsule, oral:
         Rapaflo®: 4 mg, 8 mg

◆ **Silphen [OTC]** see DiphenhydrAMINE (Systemic) on page 556
◆ **Silphen-DM [OTC]** see Dextromethorphan on page 525
◆ **Siltussin DM [OTC]** see Guaifenesin and Dextromethorphan on page 906
◆ **Siltussin DM DAS [OTC]** see Guaifenesin and Dextromethorphan on page 906
◆ **Siltussin SA [OTC]** see GuaiFENesin on page 904
◆ **Silvadene®** see Silver Sulfadiazine on page 1775

Silver Sulfadiazine (SIL ver sul fa DYE a zeen)

Related Information
   Pressure Ulcer Treatment on page 2246
Brand Names: U.S. Silvadene®; SSD AF™ [DSC]; SSD™; Thermazene®
Brand Names: Canada Flamazine®
Generic Availability (U.S.) Yes
Pharmacologic Category Antibiotic, Topical
Use Prevention and treatment of infection in second and third degree burns
Contraindications Hypersensitivity to silver sulfadiazine or any component of the formulation
Warnings/Precautions Use with caution in patients with G6PD deficiency, renal impairment, or history of allergy to other sulfonamides; sulfadiazine may accumulate in patients with impaired hepatic or renal function. Prolonged use may result in fungal or bacterial super-infection, including C. difficile-associated diarrhea (CDAD) and pseudomembranous colitis; CDAD has been observed >2 months postantibiotic treatment. Use of analgesic might be needed before application; systemic absorption may be significant and adverse reactions may occur
Adverse Reactions (Reflective of adult population; not specific for elderly) Frequency not defined.
   Dermatologic: Discoloration of skin, erythema multiforme, itching, photosensitivity, rash
   Hematologic: Agranulocytosis, aplastic anemia, hemolytic anemia, leukopenia
   Hepatic: Hepatitis
   Renal: Interstitial nephritis
   Miscellaneous: Allergic reactions may be related to sulfa component
Drug Interactions
   Metabolism/Transport Effects None known.
   Avoid Concomitant Use
      Avoid concomitant use of Silver Sulfadiazine with any of the following: BCG
   Increased Effect/Toxicity There are no known significant interactions involving an increase in effect.
   Decreased Effect
      Silver Sulfadiazine may decrease the levels/effects of: BCG
Stability Silvadene® cream will occasionally darken either in the jar or after application to the skin. This color change results from a light catalyzed reaction which is a common characteristic of all silver salts. A similar analogy is the oxidation of silverware. The product of this color change reaction is silver oxide which ranges in color from gray to black. Silver oxide has rarely been associated with permanent skin discoloration. Additionally, the antimicrobial activity of the product is not substantially diminished because the color change reaction involves such a small amount of the active drug and is largely a surface phenomenon.

◀ **Mechanism of Action** Acts upon the bacterial cell wall and cell membrane. Bactericidal for many gram-negative and gram-positive bacteria and is effective against yeast. Active against *Pseudomonas aeruginosa, Pseudomonas maltophilia, Enterobacter* species, *Klebsiella* species, *Serratia* species, *Escherichia coli, Proteus mirabilis, Morganella morganii, Providencia rettgeri, Proteus vulgaris, Providencia* species, *Citrobacter* species, *Acinetobacter calcoaceticus, Staphylococcus aureus, Staphylococcus epidermidis, Enterococcus* species, *Candida albicans, Corynebacterium diphtheriae,* and *Clostridium perfringens*

Pharmacodynamics/Kinetics

Absorption: Significant percutaneous absorption of silver sulfadiazine can occur especially when applied to extensive burns

Half-life elimination: 10 hours; prolonged with renal impairment

Time to peak, serum: 3-11 days of continuous therapy

Excretion: Urine (~50% as unchanged drug)

Dosage

Geriatric & Adult Antiseptic, burns: Topical: Apply once or twice daily

Administration Apply with a sterile-gloved hand. Apply to a thickness ¹/₁₆". Burned area should be covered with cream at all times.

Monitoring Parameters Serum electrolytes, urinalysis, renal function tests, CBC in patients with extensive burns on long-term treatment

Pharmacotherapy Pearls Contains methylparaben and propylene glycol

Special Geriatric Considerations No specific recommendations for use in the elderly.

Dosage Forms Excipient information presented when available (limited, particularly for generics); consult specific product labeling. [DSC] = Discontinued product

Cream, topical: 1% (25 g, 50 g, 85 g, 400 g)

Silvadene®: 1% (20 g, 50 g, 85 g, 400 g, 1000 g)

SSD AF™: 1% (50 g [DSC], 400 g [DSC])

SSD™: 1% (25 g, 50 g, 85 g, 400 g)

Thermazene®: 1% (20 g, 25 g, 50 g, 85 g, 400 g, 1000 g)

◆ **Simcor®** *see* Niacin and Simvastatin *on page 1367*

Simethicone (sye METH i kone)

Medication Safety Issues

Sound-alike/look-alike issues:

Simethicone may be confused with cimetidine

Mylanta® may be confused with Mynatal®

Mylicon® may be confused with Modicon®, Myleran®

Brand Names: U.S. Equalizer Gas Relief [OTC]; Gas Free Extra Strength [OTC]; Gas Relief Ultra Strength [OTC]; Gas-X® Children's Tongue Twisters™ [OTC]; Gas-X® Extra Strength [OTC]; Gas-X® Maximum Strength [OTC]; Gas-X® Thin Strips™ [OTC]; Gas-X® [OTC]; Gas-X® Infant [OTC]; Infantaire Gas [OTC]; Infants Gas Relief Drops [OTC] [DSC]; Little Tummys® Gas Relief [OTC]; Mi-Acid Gas Relief [OTC]; Mylanta® Gas Maximum Strength [OTC]; Mylicon® Infants' [OTC]; Mytab Gas Maximum [OTC]; Mytab Gas [OTC]; Phazyme® Ultra Strength [OTC]

Brand Names: Canada Ovol®; Phazyme™

Index Terms Activated Dimethicone; Activated Methylpolysiloxane

Generic Availability (U.S.) Yes: Excludes orally disintegrating strip

Pharmacologic Category Antiflatulent

Use Postoperative gas pain or for use in endoscopic examination; relief of bloating, pressure, and discomfort of gas

Contraindications Hypersensitivity to simethicone or any component of the formulation

Adverse Reactions (Reflective of adult population; not specific for elderly) No data reported

Drug Interactions

Metabolism/Transport Effects None known.

Avoid Concomitant Use There are no known interactions where it is recommended to avoid concomitant use.

Increased Effect/Toxicity There are no known significant interactions involving an increase in effect.

Decreased Effect There are no known significant interactions involving a decrease in effect.

Ethanol/Nutrition/Herb Interactions Food: Avoid carbonated beverages and gas-forming foods.

Stability Store at room temperature. Avoid high humidity and excessive heat.

Mechanism of Action Decreases the surface tension of gas bubbles thereby disperses and prevents gas pockets in the GI system

Pharmacodynamics/Kinetics Elimination: In feces
Dosage
Geriatric & Adult Flatulence/bloating: Oral: 40-360 mg after meals and at bedtime, as needed
Administration Shake oral suspension (drops) before using; mix with water or other liquids.
Monitoring Parameters Monitor for feelings of relief, decreased pain, bloating
Special Geriatric Considerations Before treating excess gas or pain due to gas accumulation, a thorough evaluation must be made to determine cause since many bowel diseases may present with flatulence and bloating.
Dosage Forms Excipient information presented when available (limited, particularly for generics); consult specific product labeling. [DSC] = Discontinued product
Capsule, softgel, oral: 125 mg, 180 mg
    Gas Free Extra Strength: 125 mg
    Gas Relief Ultra Strength: 180 mg
    Gas-X® Extra Strength: 125 mg
    Gas-X® Maximum Strength: 166 mg
    Mylanta® Gas Maximum Strength: 125 mg
    Phazyme® Ultra Strength: 180 mg
Strip, orally disintegrating, oral:
    Gas-X® Children's Tongue Twisters™: 40 mg (16s) [cinnamon flavor]
    Gas-X® Thin Strips™: 62.5 mg (18s) [cinnamon flavor]
    Gas-X® Thin Strips™: 62.5 mg (18s, 32s) [peppermint flavor]
Suspension, oral [drops]: 40 mg/0.6 mL (30 mL)
    Equalizer Gas Relief: 40 mg/0.6 mL (30 mL) [contains sodium 0.15 mg/0.6 mL]
    Gax-X® Infant: 40 mg/0.6 mL (30 mL) [ethanol free; contains sodium benzoate]
    Infantaire Gas: 40 mg/0.6 mL (30 mL)
    Infants Gas Relief Drops: 40 mg/0.6 mL (30 mL [DSC]) [vanilla flavor]
    Little Tummys® Gas Relief: 40 mg/0.6 mL (30 mL, 45 mL) [dye free, ethanol free; contains sodium benzoate; strawberry flavor]
    Mylicon® Infants': 40 mg/0.6 mL (15 mL, 30 mL) [dye free, ethanol free; contains sodium benzoate; non-staining formula]
    Mylicon® Infants': 40 mg/0.6 mL (15 mL, 30 mL) [ethanol free; contains sodium benzoate]
Tablet, chewable, oral: 80 mg, 125 mg
    Gas-X®: 80 mg [scored; contains calcium 30 mg/tablet; cherry crème flavor]
    Gas-X®: 80 mg [contains calcium 30 mg/tablet; peppermint crème flavor]
    Gas-X® Extra Strength: 125 mg [contains calcium 45 mg/tablet; cherry crème flavor]
    Gas-X® Extra Strength: 125 mg [contains calcium 45 mg/tablet; peppermint crème flavor]
    Mi-Acid Gas Relief: 80 mg
    Mylanta® Gas Maximum Strength: 125 mg [scored; cherry flavor]
    Mylanta® Gas Maximum Strength: 125 mg [mint flavor]
    Mytab Gas: 80 mg [peppermint flavor]
    Mytab Gas Maximum: 125 mg

◆ **Simethicone, Aluminum Hydroxide, and Magnesium Hydroxide** *see* Aluminum Hydroxide, Magnesium Hydroxide, and Simethicone *on page 82*
◆ **Simethicone and Loperamide Hydrochloride** *see* Loperamide and Simethicone *on page 1154*
◆ **Simethicone and Magaldrate** *see* Magaldrate and Simethicone *on page 1175*
◆ **Simply Saline® [OTC]** *see* Sodium Chloride *on page 1787*
◆ **Simply Saline® Baby [OTC]** *see* Sodium Chloride *on page 1787*
◆ **Simply Sleep® [OTC]** *see* DiphenhydrAMINE (Systemic) *on page 556*
◆ **Simponi®** *see* Golimumab *on page 895*

Simvastatin (sim va STAT in)

Related Information
Hyperlipidemia Management *on page 2130*
Medication Safety Issues
Sound-alike/look-alike issues:
    Simvastatin may be confused with atorvasSTATin, nystatin, pitavastatin
    Zocor® may be confused with Cozaar®, Lipitor®, Zoloft®, ZyrTEC®
International issues:
    Cardin [Poland] may be confused with Cardem brand name for celiprolol [Spain]; Cardene brand name for nicardipine [U.S., Great Britain, Netherlands]
Brand Names: U.S. Zocor®

SIMVASTATIN

Brand Names: Canada Apo-Simvastatin®; Ava-Simvastatin; CO Simvastatin; Dom-Simvastatin; JAMP-Simvastatin; Mint-Simvastatin; Mylan-Simvastatin; Nu-Simvastatin; PHL-Simvastatin; PMS-Simvastatin; Q-Simvastatin; RAN™-Simvastatin; ratio-Simvastatin; Riva-Simvastatin; Sandoz-Simvastatin; Simvastatin-Odan; Taro-Simvastatin; Teva-Simvastatin; Zocor®; ZYM-Simvastatin

Generic Availability (U.S.) Yes

Pharmacologic Category Antilipemic Agent, HMG-CoA Reductase Inhibitor

Use Used with dietary therapy for the following:

Secondary prevention of cardiovascular events in hypercholesterolemic patients with established coronary heart disease (CHD) or at high risk for CHD: To reduce cardiovascular morbidity (myocardial infarction, coronary/noncoronary revascularization procedures) and mortality; to reduce the risk of stroke

Hyperlipidemias: To reduce elevations in total cholesterol (total-C), LDL-C, apolipoprotein B, triglycerides, and VLDL-C, and to increase HDL-C in patients with primary hypercholesterolemia (elevations of 1 or more components are present in Fredrickson type IIa, IIb, III, and IV hyperlipidemias); treatment of homozygous familial hypercholesterolemia

Contraindications Hypersensitivity to simvastatin or any component of the formulation; active liver disease; unexplained persistent elevations of serum transaminases; concomitant use of strong CYP3A4 inhibitors (eg, clarithromycin, erythromycin, itraconazole, ketoconazole, nefazodone, posaconazole, protease inhibitors [including boceprevir and telaprevir], telithromycin), cyclosporine, danazol, and gemfibrozil

Warnings/Precautions Secondary causes of hyperlipidemia should be ruled out prior to therapy. Liver enzyme tests should be obtained at baseline and as clinically indicated; routine periodic monitoring of liver enzymes is not necessary. Use with caution in patients who consume large amounts of ethanol or have a history of liver disease; use is contraindicated with active liver disease and with unexplained transaminase elevations. Rhabdomyolysis with acute renal failure has occurred. Risk of rhabdomyolysis is dose-related and increased with high doses (80 mg), concurrent use of lipid-lowering agents which may also cause rhabdomyolysis (other fibrates or niacin doses ≥1 g/day), or moderate-to-strong CYP3A4 inhibitors (eg, amiodarone, grapefruit juice in large quantities, or verapamil), age ≥65 years, female gender, uncontrolled hypothyroidism, and renal dysfunction. In Chinese patients, do not use high-dose simvastatin (80 mg) if concurrently taking niacin ≥1 g/day; may increase risk of myopathy. Concomitant use of simvastatin with some drugs may require cautious use, may not be recommended, may require dosage adjustments, or may be contraindicated. If concurrent use of a contraindicated interacting medication is unavoidable, treatment with simvastatin should be suspended during use or consider the use of an alternative HMG-CoA reductase inhibitor void of CYP3A4 metabolism. Monitor closely if used with other drugs associated with myopathy (eg, colchicine). Increases in Hb A_{1c} and fasting blood glucose have been reported with HMG-CoA reductase inhibitors; however, the benefits of statin therapy far outweigh the risk of dysglycemia. The manufacturer recommends temporary discontinuation for elective major surgery, acute medical or surgical conditions, or in any patient experiencing an acute or serious condition predisposing to renal failure (eg, sepsis, hypotension, trauma, uncontrolled seizures). However, based upon current evidence, HMG-CoA reductase inhibitor therapy should be continued in the perioperative period unless risk outweighs cardioprotective benefit. Use with caution in patients with severe renal impairment; initial dosage adjustment is necessary; monitor closely.

Adverse Reactions (Reflective of adult population; not specific for elderly)

1% to 10%:

Cardiovascular: Atrial fibrillation (6%; placebo 5%), edema (3%; placebo 2%)

Central nervous system: Headache (3% to 7%), vertigo (5%)

Dermatologic: Eczema (5%)

Gastrointestinal: Abdominal pain (7%), constipation (2% to 7%), gastritis (5%), nausea (5%)

Hepatic: Transaminases increased (>3 x ULN; 1%)

Neuromuscular & skeletal: CPK increased (>3 x normal; 5%), myalgia (4%)

Respiratory: Upper respiratory infections (9%), bronchitis (7%)

Additional class-related events or case reports (not necessarily reported with simvastatin therapy): Alteration in taste, anorexia, anxiety, bilirubin increased, cataracts, cholestatic jaundice, cirrhosis, decreased libido, depression, erectile dysfunction/impotence, facial paresis, fatty liver, fulminant hepatic necrosis, gynecomastia, hepatoma, hyperbilirubinemia, impaired extraocular muscle movement, increased CPK (>10 x normal), interstitial lung disease, ophthalmoplegia, peripheral nerve palsy, psychic disturbance, renal failure (secondary to rhabdomyolysis), thyroid dysfunction, tremor, vertigo

Drug Interactions

Metabolism/Transport Effects Substrate of CYP3A4 (major), SLCO1B1; **Note:** Assignment of Major/Minor substrate status based on clinically relevant drug interaction potential; **Inhibits** CYP2C8 (weak), CYP2C9 (weak), CYP2D6 (weak)

Avoid Concomitant Use

Avoid concomitant use of Simvastatin with any of the following: Boceprevir; CycloSPORINE; CycloSPORINE (Systemic); CYP3A4 Inhibitors (Strong); Erythromycin; Gemfibrozil; Mifepristone; Protease Inhibitors; Red Yeast Rice; Telaprevir

Increased Effect/Toxicity

Simvastatin may increase the levels/effects of: ARIPiprazole; DAPTOmycin; Diltiazem; Pazopanib; Trabectedin; Vitamin K Antagonists

The levels/effects of Simvastatin may be increased by: Amiodarone; AmLODIPine; Boceprevir; Colchicine; CycloSPORINE; CycloSPORINE (Systemic); CYP3A4 Inhibitors (Moderate); CYP3A4 Inhibitors (Strong); Cyproterone; Danazol; Dasatinib; Diltiazem; Dronedarone; Eltrombopag; Erythromycin; Fenofibrate; Fenofibric Acid; Fluconazole; Fusidic Acid; Gemfibrozil; Grapefruit Juice; Green Tea; Imatinib; Ivacaftor; Macrolide Antibiotics; Mifepristone; Niacin; Niacinamide; Protease Inhibitors; QuiNINE; Ranolazine; Red Yeast Rice; Sildenafil; Telaprevir; Ticagrelor; Verapamil

Decreased Effect

Simvastatin may decrease the levels/effects of: Lanthanum

The levels/effects of Simvastatin may be decreased by: Antacids; Bosentan; CYP3A4 Inducers (Strong); Deferasirox; Efavirenz; Etravirine; Fosphenytoin; Phenytoin; Rifamycin Derivatives; St Johns Wort; Tocilizumab

Ethanol/Nutrition/Herb Interactions

Ethanol: Excessive ethanol consumption has the potential to cause hepatic effects. Management: Avoid or limit ethanol consumption.

Food: Simvastatin serum concentration may be increased when taken with grapefruit juice. Red yeast rice contains an estimated 2.4 mg lovastatin per 600 mg rice. Management: Avoid concurrent intake of large quantities of grapefruit juice (>1 quart/day).

Herb/Nutraceutical: St John's wort may decrease simvastatin levels. Management: Avoid St John's wort.

Stability Tablets should be stored in tightly-closed containers at temperatures between 5°C to 30°C (41°F to 86°F).

Mechanism of Action Simvastatin is a methylated derivative of lovastatin that acts by competitively inhibiting 3-hydroxy-3-methylglutaryl-coenzyme A (HMG-CoA) reductase, the enzyme that catalyzes the rate-limiting step in cholesterol biosynthesis

Pharmacodynamics/Kinetics

Onset of action: >3 days

Peak effect: 2 weeks

Absorption: 85%

Protein binding: ~95%

Metabolism: Hepatic via CYP3A4; extensive first-pass effect

Bioavailability: <5%

Half-life elimination: Unknown

Time to peak: 1.3-2.4 hours

Excretion: Feces (60%); urine (13%)

Dosage

Geriatric Oral: Initial: Maximum reductions in LDL-cholesterol may be achieved with daily dose ≤20 mg.

Adult Note: Doses should be individualized according to the baseline LDL-cholesterol levels, the recommended goal of therapy, and the patient's response; adjustments should be made at intervals of 4 weeks or more; doses may need adjusted based on concomitant medications

Note: Dosing limitation: Simvastatin 80 mg is limited to patients that have been taking this dose for >12 consecutive months without evidence of myopathy and are not currently taking or beginning to take a simvastatin dose-limiting or contraindicated interacting medication. If patient is unable to achieve low-density lipoprotein-cholesterol (LDL-C) goal using the 40 mg dose of simvastatin, increasing to 80 mg dose is not recommended. Instead, switch patient to an alternative LDL-C-lowering treatment providing greater LDL-C reduction.

Homozygous familial hypercholesterolemia: Oral: 40 mg once daily in the evening

Prevention of cardiovascular events, hyperlipidemias: Oral: 10-20 mg once daily in the evening; range: 5-40 mg/day

Patients requiring only moderate reduction of LDL-C: May be started at 5-10 mg once daily in the evening; adjust to achieve recommended LDL-C goal.

Patients requiring reduction of >40% of LDL-C: May be started at 40 mg once daily in the evening; adjust to achieve recommended LDL-C goal.

Patients with CHD or at high risk for cardiovascular events (patients with diabetes, PVD, history of stroke or other cerebrovascular disease): Dosing should be started at 40 mg once daily in the evening; start simultaneously with diet therapy.

Dosage adjustment for simvastatin with concomitant medications: Note: Patients currently tolerating and requiring a dose of simvastatin 80 mg who require initiation of an interacting drug with a dose cap for simvastatin should be switched to an alternative statin with less potential for drug-drug interaction.

Amiodarone, amlodipine, or ranolazine: Simvastatin dose should **not** exceed 20 mg/day

Diltiazem or verapamil: Simvastatin dose should **not** exceed 10 mg/day

Dosage adjustment in Chinese patients on niacin doses ≥1 g/day: Use caution with simvastatin doses exceeding 20 mg/day; because of an increased risk of myopathy, do not administer simvastatin 80 mg concurrently.

Renal Impairment

Manufacturer's recommendations:

Mild-to-moderate renal impairment: No dosage adjustment necessary; simvastatin does not undergo significant renal excretion.

Severe renal impairment: Cl_{cr} <30 mL/minute: Initial: 5 mg/day with close monitoring

Alternative recommendation: No dosage adjustment necessary for any degree of renal impairment (Aronoff, 2007).

Administration May be administered without regard to meals. Administer in the evening for maximal efficacy.

Monitoring Parameters Baseline CPK (recheck CPK in any patient with symptoms suggestive of myopathy; discontinue therapy if markedly elevated); baseline liver function tests (LFTs) and repeat when clinically indicated thereafter. Patients with elevated transaminase levels should have a second (confirmatory) test and frequent monitoring until values normalize; discontinue if increase in ALT/AST is persistently >3 times ULN (NCEP, 2002).

Lipid panel (total cholesterol, HDL, LDL, triglycerides):

ATP III recommendations (NCEP, 2002): Baseline; 6-8 weeks after initiation of drug therapy; if dose increased, then at 6-8 weeks until final dose determined. Once treatment goal achieved, follow-up intervals may be reduced to every 4-6 months. Lipid panel should be assessed at least annually, and preferably at each clinic visit.

Manufacturer recommendation: Lipid panel should be analyzed after 4 weeks of therapy and periodically thereafter.

Special Geriatric Considerations Effective and well tolerated in the elderly. The definition of and, therefore, when to treat hyperlipidemia in the elderly is a controversial issue. The National Cholesterol Education Program recommends that all adults maintain a plasma cholesterol <160 mg/dL. In elderly patients with one additional risk factor, goal LDL would be <130 mg/dL. It is the authors' belief that pharmacologic treatment be reserved for those who are unable to obtain a desirable plasma cholesterol concentration by diet alone and for whom the benefits of treatment are believed to outweigh the potential adverse effects, drug interactions, and cost of treatment. Age ≥65 years is a risk factor for myopathy.

Dosage Forms Excipient information presented when available (limited, particularly for generics); consult specific product labeling.

Tablet, oral: 5 mg, 10 mg, 20 mg, 40 mg, 80 mg

Zocor®: 5 mg, 10 mg, 20 mg, 40 mg, 80 mg

Sipuleucel-T (si pu LOO sel tee)

Medication Safety Issues

Other safety concerns:

For autologous use only; patient identity must be matched to the patient identifiers on the infusion bag and on the "Cell Product Disposition Form" prior to infusion. Healthcare providers should apply universal precautions when handling both the initial leukapheresis product and the activated product.

Brand Names: U.S. Provenge®

Index Terms APC8015; Prostate Cancer Vaccine, Cell-Based

Generic Availability (U.S.) No

Pharmacologic Category Cellular Immunotherapy, Autologous

Use Treatment of metastatic hormone-refractory prostate cancer in patients who are asymptomatic or minimally symptomatic

Prescribing and Access Restrictions Patients may currently receive Sipuleucel-T at one of the ~50 sites that participated in the clinical trials until the program is expanded to additional sites. Physicians must go through an inservice and register to prescribe the treatment; patients must also complete an enrollment form. Information on registration and enrollment is available at 1-877-336-3736.

Dosage

Geriatric & Adult Note: Premedicate with oral acetaminophen 650 mg and an antihistamine (eg, diphenhydramine 50 mg) ~30 minutes prior to infusion. For autologous use only.

Prostate cancer, metastatic: I.V.: Each dose contains ≥50 million autologous CD54+ cells (obtained through leukapheresis) activated with PAP-GM-CSF; administer doses at ~2 week intervals for a total of 3 doses

Special Geriatric Considerations No specific information for use in elderly.

Dosage Forms Excipient information presented when available (limited, particularly for generics); consult specific product labeling.

Infusion, premixed in LR [preservative free]:

Provenge®: ≥50 million autologous CD54$^+$ cells activated with PAP-GM-CSF (250 mL)

◆ **Sirdalud®** *see* TiZANidine *on page 1910*

SitaGLIPtin (sit a GLIP tin)

Related Information

Diabetes Mellitus Management, Adults *on page 2193*

Medication Safety Issues

Sound-alike/look-alike issues:

Januvia® may be confused with Enjuvia™, Janumet®, Jantoven®

SitaGLIPtin may be confused with saxagliptin, SUMAtriptan

High alert medication:

The Institute for Safe Medication Practices (ISMP) includes this medication among its list of drug classes which have a heightened risk of causing significant patient harm when used in error.

Brand Names: U.S. Januvia®

Brand Names: Canada Januvia®

Index Terms MK-0431; Sitagliptin Phosphate

Generic Availability (U.S.) No

Pharmacologic Category Antidiabetic Agent, Dipeptidyl Peptidase IV (DPP-IV) Inhibitor

Use Management of type 2 diabetes mellitus (noninsulin dependent, NIDDM) as an adjunct to diet and exercise as monotherapy or in combination therapy with other antidiabetic agents

Medication Guide Available Yes

Contraindications Serious hypersensitivity (eg, anaphylaxis, angioedema) to sitagliptan or any component of the formulation

Warnings/Precautions Avoid use in type 1 diabetes mellitus (insulin dependent, IDDM) and diabetic ketoacidosis (DKA) due to lack of efficacy in these populations. Use caution when used in conjunction with insulin or insulin secretagogues; risk of hypoglycemia is increased. Monitor blood glucose closely; dosage adjustments of insulin or insulin secretagogues may be necessary. Use with caution in patients with moderate-to-severe renal dysfunction and end-stage renal disease (ESRD) requiring hemodialysis or peritoneal dialysis; dosing adjustment required. Safety and efficacy have not been established in severe hepatic dysfunction.

Rare hypersensitivity reactions, including anaphylaxis, angioedema, and/or severe dermatologic reactions (such as Stevens-Johnson syndrome), have been reported in postmarketing surveillance; discontinue if signs/symptoms of hypersensitivity reactions occur. Use with caution if patient has experienced angioedema with other DPP-IV inhibitor use. Cases of acute pancreatitis (including hemorrhagic and necrotizing with some fatalities) have been reported with use; monitor for signs/symptoms of pancreatitis. Discontinue use immediately if pancreatitis is suspected and initiate appropriate management. Use with caution in patients with a history of pancreatitis (not known if this population is at greater risk).

Clinical trials included only a limited number of patients with heart failure (HF). No specific recommendations regarding this population are provided in the approved U.S. labeling (Canadian labeling recommends against use in this population). Diabetes self-management education (DSME) is essential to maximize the effectiveness of therapy.

Adverse Reactions (Reflective of adult population; not specific for elderly) As reported with monotherapy: 1% to 10%:

Cardiovascular: Peripheral edema (2%)

Endocrine & metabolic: Hypoglycemia (1%)

Gastrointestinal: Diarrhea (4%), constipation (3%), nausea (2%)

Neuromuscular & skeletal: Osteoarthritis (1%)

Respiratory: Nasopharyngitis (5%), pharyngitis (1%), upper respiratory tract infection (viral; 1%)

Drug Interactions
Metabolism/Transport Effects Substrate of P-glycoprotein

Avoid Concomitant Use There are no known interactions where it is recommended to avoid concomitant use.

Increased Effect/Toxicity
SitaGLIPtin may increase the levels/effects of: ACE Inhibitors; Digoxin; Hypoglycemic Agents

The levels/effects of SitaGLIPtin may be increased by: Herbs (Hypoglycemic Properties); MAO Inhibitors; Pegvisomant; P-glycoprotein/ABCB1 Inhibitors; Salicylates; Selective Serotonin Reuptake Inhibitors

Decreased Effect
The levels/effects of SitaGLIPtin may be decreased by: Corticosteroids (Orally Inhaled); Corticosteroids (Systemic); Loop Diuretics; Luteinizing Hormone-Releasing Hormone Analogs; P-glycoprotein/ABCB1 Inducers; Somatropin; Thiazide Diuretics

Stability Store at 20°C to 25°C (68°F to 77°F); excursions permitted to 15°C to 30°C (59°F to 86°F).

Mechanism of Action Sitagliptin inhibits dipeptidyl peptidase IV (DPP-IV) enzyme resulting in prolonged active incretin levels. Incretin hormones (eg, glucagon-like peptide-1 [GLP-1] and glucose-dependent insulinotropic polypeptide [GIP]) regulate glucose homeostasis by increasing insulin synthesis and release from pancreatic beta cells and decreasing glucagon secretion from pancreatic alpha cells. Decreased glucagon secretion results in decreased hepatic glucose production. Under normal physiologic circumstances, incretin hormones are released by the intestine throughout the day and levels are increased in response to a meal; incretin hormones are rapidly inactivated by the DPP-IV enzyme.

Pharmacodynamics/Kinetics
Absorption: Rapid

Distribution: ~198 L

Protein binding: 38%

Metabolism: Not extensively metabolized; minor metabolism via CYP3A4 and 2C8 to metabolites (inactive) suggested by *in vitro* studies

Bioavailability: ~87%

Half-life elimination: 12 hours

Time to peak, plasma: 1-4 hours

Excretion: Urine 87% (79% as unchanged drug, 16% as metabolites); feces 13%

Dosage
Adult Type 2 diabetes: Oral: 100 mg once daily
Concomitant use with insulin and/or insulin secretagogues (eg, sulfonylureas): Reduced dose of insulin and/or insulin secretagogues may be needed.

Renal Impairment Note: Renal function may be estimated using the Cockcroft-Gault formula for dosage adjustment purposes.

Cl_{cr} ≥50 mL/minute: No dosage adjustment necessary.

Cl_{cr} ≥30 to <50 mL/minute (approximate S_{cr} of >1.7 to ≤3.0 mg/dL [males] or >1.5 to ≤2.5 mg/dL [females]): 50 mg once daily

Cl_{cr} <30 mL/minute (approximate S_{cr} of >3.0 mg/dL [males] or >2.5 mg/dL [females]): 25 mg once daily

ESRD requiring hemodialysis or peritoneal dialysis: 25 mg once daily; administered without regard to timing of hemodialysis

Hepatic Impairment
Mild-to-moderate impairment (Child-Pugh score 7-9): No dosage adjustment required
Severe impairment (Child-Pugh score >9): Not studied

Administration May be administered with or without food. Swallow tablets whole; do not crush, chew, or split.

Monitoring Parameters Hb A$_{1c}$, serum glucose; renal function prior to initiation and periodically during treatment

Reference Range
Recommendations for glycemic control in adults with diabetes:
Hb A$_{1c}$: <7%
Preprandial capillary plasma glucose: 70-130 mg/dL
Peak postprandial capillary blood glucose: <180 mg/dL
Blood pressure: <130/80 mm Hg

Recommendations for glycemic control in older adults with diabetes:
Relatively healthy, cognitively intact, and with a ≥5-year life expectancy: See Adults
Frail, life expectancy <5-years or those for whom the risks of intensive glucose control outweigh the benefits:
Hb A$_{1c}$: <8% to 9%
Blood pressure: <140/80 mm Hg or <130/80 mm Hg if tolerated

Special Geriatric Considerations Sitagliptin has not been studied exclusively in the elderly. The manufacturer reports that 725 out of 3884 patients in clinical trials were >65 years (only 61 were age 75 years and older), with no difference in safety or efficacy compared to younger patients. Intensive glucose control (Hb A_{1c} <6.5%) has been linked to increased all-cause and cardiovascular mortality, hypoglycemia requiring assistance, and weight gain in adult type 2 diabetes. How "tightly" to control a geriatric patient's blood glucose needs to be individualized. Such a decision should be based on several factors, including the patient's functional and cognitive status, how well he/she recognizes hypoglycemic or hyperglycemic symptoms, and how to respond to them and other disease states. An Hb A_{1c} <7.5% is an acceptable endpoint for a healthy older adult, while <8% is acceptable for frail elderly patients, those with a duration of illness >10 years, or those with comorbid conditions and requiring combination diabetes medications. For elderly patients with diabetes who are relatively healthy, attaining target goals for aspirin use, blood pressure, lipids, smoking cessation, and diet and exercise may be more important than normalized glycemic control.

Dosage Forms Excipient information presented when available (limited, particularly for generics); consult specific product labeling.

Tablet, oral:

Januvia®: 25 mg, 50 mg, 100 mg

Sitagliptin and Metformin (sit a GLIP tin & met FOR min)

Related Information

Diabetes Mellitus Management, Adults *on page 2193*
MetFORMIN *on page 1222*
SitaGLIPtin *on page 1781*

Medication Safety Issues

Sound-alike/look-alike issues:

Janumet® may be confused with Jantoven®, Januvia®
Sitagliptin and Metformin may be confused with Linagliptin and Metformin
Sitagliptin and Metformin may be confused with Saxagliptin and Metformin

High alert medication:

The Institute for Safe Medication Practices (ISMP) includes this medication among its list of drug classes which have a heightened risk of causing significant patient harm when used in error.

Brand Names: U.S. Janumet®; Janumet® XR

Brand Names: Canada Janumet®

Index Terms Metformin and Sitagliptin; Sitagliptin Phosphate and Metformin Hydrochloride

Generic Availability (U.S.) No

Pharmacologic Category Antidiabetic Agent, Biguanide; Antidiabetic Agent, Dipeptidyl Peptidase IV (DPP-IV) Inhibitor; Hypoglycemic Agent, Oral

Use Management of type 2 diabetes mellitus (noninsulin dependent, NIDDM) as an adjunct to diet and exercise in patients not adequately controlled on metformin or sitagliptin monotherapy

Medication Guide Available Yes

Dosage

Geriatric Refer to adult dosing. The initial and maintenance dosing should be conservative, due to the potential for decreased renal function (monitor). Do not use in patients ≥80 years of age unless normal renal function has been established.

Adult Note: Patients receiving concomitant insulin and/or insulin secretagogues (eg, sulfonylureas) may require dosage adjustments of these agents.

Type 2 diabetes mellitus: Oral: Initial doses should be based on current dose of sitagliptin and metformin.

Patients inadequately controlled on metformin alone: Initial dose:

Immediate release: Sitagliptin 100 mg/day plus current daily dose of metformin given in 2 equally divided doses; maximum: sitagliptin 100 mg/metformin 2000 mg daily. **Note:** The U.S. labeling recommends patients currently receiving metformin 850 mg twice daily receive an initial dose of sitagliptin 50 mg and metformin 1000 mg twice daily.

Extended release: Sitagliptin 100 mg/day plus current daily dose of metformin given once daily; maximum: sitagliptin 100 mg/metformin 2000 mg daily. **Note:** The U.S. labeling recommends patients currently receiving immediate release metformin 850-1000 mg twice daily receive an initial dose of sitagliptin 100 mg and metformin 2000 mg once daily.

Patients inadequately controlled on sitagliptin alone: Initial dose: **Note:** Patients currently receiving a renally-adjusted dose of sitagliptin should not be switched to a combination product.

Immediate release: Metformin 1000 mg/day plus sitagliptin 100 mg/day given in 2 equally divided doses

Extended release: Metformin 1000 mg and sitagliptin 100 mg once daily

Conversion from immediate release to extended release: Convert using same total daily dose (up to the maximum recommended dose), but adjust frequency as indicated for immediate (twice daily) or extended (once daily) release products.

Dosing adjustment: Metformin component may be gradually increased up to the maximum dose. Maximum dose: Sitagliptin 100 mg/metformin 2000 mg daily

Renal Impairment Do not use with renal disease or renal dysfunction (serum creatinine ≥1.5 mg/dL [≥136 micromole/L] in males or ≥1.4 mg/dL [≥124 micromole/L] in females or abnormal clearance).

Hepatic Impairment Avoid metformin; liver disease is a risk factor for the development of lactic acidosis during metformin therapy.

Special Geriatric Considerations See individual agents. Combination products are not recommended as first-line treatment. Use only if doses of individual agents correspond to the combination available.

Dosage Forms Excipient information presented when available (limited, particularly for generics); consult specific product labeling.

Tablet, oral:

Janumet® 50/500: Sitagliptin 50 mg and metformin hydrochloride 500 mg

Janumet® 50/1000: Sitagliptin 50 mg and metformin hydrochloride 1000 mg

Tablet, extended release, oral:

Janumet® XR: 50/500: Sitagliptin 50 mg and metformin hydrochloride 500 mg

Janumet® XR: 50/1000: Sitagliptin 50 mg and metformin hydrochloride 1000 mg

Janumet® XR: 100/1000: Sitagliptin 100 mg and metformin hydrochloride 1000 mg

Dosage Forms: Canada Excipient information presented when available (limited, particularly for generics); consult specific product labeling.

Tablet, oral:

Janumet® 50/850: Sitagliptin 50 mg and metformin hydrochloride 850 mg

Sitagliptin and Simvastatin (sit a GLIP tin & sim va STAT in)

Medication Safety Issues

High alert medication:

The Institute for Safe Medication Practices (ISMP) includes this medication among its list of drug classes which have a heightened risk of causing significant patient harm when used in error.

Brand Names: U.S. Juvisync™

Index Terms Simvastatin and Sitagliptin; Sitagliptin Phosphate and Simvastatin

Generic Availability (U.S.) No

Pharmacologic Category Antidiabetic Agent, Dipeptidyl Peptidase IV (DPP-IV) Inhibitor; Antilipemic Agent, HMG-CoA Reductase Inhibitor

Use For use when treatment with both sitagliptin and simvastatin is appropriate:

Sitagliptin: Management of type 2 diabetes mellitus (noninsulin dependent, NIDDM) as an adjunct to diet and exercise as monotherapy or in combination therapy with other antidiabetic agents

Simvastatin: Used with dietary therapy for the following:

Secondary prevention of cardiovascular events in hypercholesterolemic patients with established coronary heart disease (CHD) or at high risk for CHD: To reduce cardiovascular morbidity (myocardial infarction, coronary/noncoronary revascularization procedures) and mortality; to reduce the risk of stroke

Hyperlipidemias: To reduce elevations in total cholesterol (total-C), LDL-C, apolipoprotein B, triglycerides, and VLDL-C, and to increase HDL-C in patients with primary hypercholesterolemia (elevations of 1 or more components are present in Fredrickson type IIa, IIb, III, and IV hyperlipidemias); treatment of homozygous familial hypercholesterolemia

Medication Guide Available Yes

Dosage

Adult Hyperlipidemia and type 2 diabetes: Oral: Initial dose: Sitagliptin 100 mg and simvastatin 40 mg once daily. **Note:** Patients already taking simvastatin <40 mg/day (with or without sitagliptin 100 mg daily) can be converted to the comparable equivalent of the combination product. Dose adjustments should be made at intervals of ≥4 weeks.

Concomitant use with insulin and/or insulin secretagogues (eg, sulfonylureas): Reduced dose of insulin and/or insulin secretagogues may be needed.

Dosage adjustment for simvastatin with concomitant medications:
Diltiazem or verapamil: Simvastatin dose should **not** exceed 10 mg/day
Amiodarone, amlodipine, or ranolazine: Simvastatin dose should **not** exceed 20 mg/day
Dosage adjustment for simvastatin in Chinese patients on niacin doses ≥1 g/day: Use caution with simvastatin doses of 40 mg/day because of an increased risk of myopathy
Renal Impairment Renal function may be estimated using Cockcroft-Gault formula for dosage adjustment purposes.
Cl_{cr} ≥50 mL/minute: No dosage adjustment necessary.
Cl_{cr} <50 mL/minute: Use is not recommended.
End-stage renal disease (ESRD): Use is not recommended.
Hepatic Impairment Use is contraindicated.
Special Geriatric Considerations See individual agents. Combination products are not recommended as first-line treatment. Use only if doses of individual agents correspond to the combination available.
Dosage Forms Excipient information presented when available (limited, particularly for generics); consult specific product labeling.
Tablet, oral:
Juvisync™ 100/10: Sitagliptin 100 mg and simvastatin 10 mg
Juvisync™ 100/20: Sitagliptin 100 mg and simvastatin 20 mg
Juvisync™ 100/40: Sitagliptin 100 mg and simvastatin 40 mg

Sodium Bicarbonate (SOW dee um bye KAR bun ate)

Related Information
Calculations *on page 2087*
Brand Names: U.S. Brioschi® [OTC]; Neut®
Index Terms Baking Soda; $NaHCO_3$; Sodium Acid Carbonate; Sodium Hydrogen Carbonate
Generic Availability (U.S.) Yes: Excludes granules
Pharmacologic Category Alkalinizing Agent; Antacid; Electrolyte Supplement, Oral; Electrolyte Supplement, Parenteral
Use Management of metabolic acidosis; gastric hyperacidity; as an alkalinization agent for the urine; treatment of hyperkalemia; management of overdose of certain drugs, including tricyclic antidepressants and aspirin
Unlabeled Use Prevention of contrast-induced nephropathy (CIN)
Contraindications Alkalosis, hypernatremia, severe pulmonary edema, hypocalcemia, unknown abdominal pain
Warnings/Precautions Use of I.V. $NaHCO_3$ should be reserved for documented metabolic acidosis and for hyperkalemia-induced cardiac arrest. Routine use in cardiac arrest is not recommended. Avoid extravasation, tissue necrosis can occur due to the hypertonicity of $NaHCO_3$. May cause sodium retention especially if renal function is impaired; not to be used in treatment of peptic ulcer; use with caution in patients with HF, edema, cirrhosis, or renal failure. Not the antacid of choice for the elderly because of sodium content and potential for systemic alkalosis.

SODIUM BICARBONATE

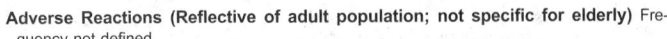

Adverse Reactions (Reflective of adult population; not specific for elderly) Frequency not defined.

Cardiovascular: Cerebral hemorrhage, CHF (aggravated), edema

Central nervous system: Tetany

Gastrointestinal: Belching, flatulence (with oral), gastric distension

Endocrine & metabolic: Hypernatremia, hyperosmolality, hypocalcemia, hypokalemia, increased affinity of hemoglobin for oxygen-reduced pH in myocardial tissue necrosis when extravasated, intracranial acidosis, metabolic alkalosis, milk-alkali syndrome (especially with renal dysfunction)

Respiratory: Pulmonary edema

Drug Interactions

Metabolism/Transport Effects None known.

Avoid Concomitant Use There are no known interactions where it is recommended to avoid concomitant use.

Increased Effect/Toxicity

Sodium Bicarbonate may increase the levels/effects of: Alpha-/Beta-Agonists; Amphetamines; Calcium Polystyrene Sulfonate; Dexmethylphenidate; Flecainide; Memantine; Methylphenidate; QuiNIDine; QuiNINE

The levels/effects of Sodium Bicarbonate may be increased by: AcetaZOLAMIDE

Decreased Effect

Sodium Bicarbonate may decrease the levels/effects of: ACE Inhibitors; Anticonvulsants (Hydantoin); Antipsychotic Agents (Phenothiazines); Atazanavir; Bisacodyl; Cefditoren; Cefpodoxime; Cefuroxime; Chloroquine; Corticosteroids (Oral); Dabigatran Etexilate; Dasatinib; Delavirdine; Erlotinib; Flecainide; Gabapentin; HMG-CoA Reductase Inhibitors; Iron Salts; Isoniazid; Itraconazole; Ketoconazole; Ketoconazole (Systemic); Lithium; Mesalamine; Methenamine; Nilotinib; PenicillAMINE; Phosphate Supplements; Protease Inhibitors; Rilpivirine; Tetracycline Derivatives; Trientine; Vismodegib

Ethanol/Nutrition/Herb Interactions Herb/Nutraceutical: Concurrent doses with iron may decrease iron absorption.

Stability Store injection at room temperature; do not freeze. Protect from heat. Use only clear solutions.

Prevention of contrast-induced nephropathy (unlabeled use): Remove 154 mL from 1000 mL bag of D_5W; replace with 154 mL of 8.4% sodium bicarbonate; resultant concentration is 154 mEq/L (Merten, 2004); more practically, institutions may remove 150 mL from 1000 mL bag of D_5W and replace with 150 mL of 8.4% sodium bicarbonate; resultant concentration is 150 mEq/L

Mechanism of Action Dissociates to provide bicarbonate ion which neutralizes hydrogen ion concentration and raises blood and urinary pH

Pharmacodynamics/Kinetics

Onset of action: Oral: Rapid; I.V.: 15 minutes

Duration: Oral: 8-10 minutes; I.V.: 1-2 hours

Absorption: Oral: Well absorbed

Excretion: Urine (<1%)

Dosage

Geriatric & Adult

Cardiac arrest (ACLS, 2010): I.V.: Initial: 1 mEq/kg/dose; repeat doses should be guided by arterial blood gases

Routine use of $NaHCO_3$ is not recommended. May be considered in the setting of prolonged cardiac arrest only after adequate alveolar ventilation has been established and effective cardiac compressions. **Note:** In some cardiac arrest situations (eg, metabolic acidosis, hyperkalemia, or tricyclic antidepressant overdose), sodium bicarbonate may be beneficial.

Metabolic acidosis: I.V.: Dosage should be based on the following formula if blood gases and pH measurements are available:

HCO_3^-(mEq) = 0.5 x weight (kg) x [24 - serum HCO_3^-(mEq/L)] **or** HCO_3^-(mEq) = 0.5 x weight (kg) x [desired increase in serum HCO_3^-(mEq/L)]

Administer 1/2 dose initially, then remaining 1/2 dose over the next 24 hours; monitor pH, serum HCO_3^-, and clinical status. **Note:** These equations provide an estimated replacement dose. The underlying cause and degree of acidosis may result in the need for larger or smaller replacement doses. In most cases, the initial goal of therapy is to target a pH of ~7.2 and a plasma bicarbonate level of ~10 mEq/L to prevent overalkalinization.

Note: If acid-base status is not available: 2-5 mEq/kg I.V. infusion over 4-8 hours; subsequent doses should be based on patient's acid-base status

Hyperkalemia (ACLS, 2010): I.V.: 50 mEq over 5 minutes (as appropriate, consider methods of enhancing potassium removal/excretion)

Chronic renal failure: Oral: Initiate when plasma HCO_3^- <15 mEq/L Start with 20-36 mEq/day in divided doses, titrate to bicarbonate level of 18-20 mEq/L

Renal tubular acidosis: Oral:

Distal: 0.5-2 mEq/kg/day in 4-5 divided doses

Proximal: Initial: 5-10 mEq/kg/day; maintenance: Increase as required to maintain serum bicarbonate in the normal range

Urine alkalinization: Oral: Initial: 48 mEq (4 g), then 12-24 mEq (1-2 g) every 4 hours; dose should be titrated to desired urinary pH; doses up to 16 g/day (200 mEq) in patients <60 years and 8 g (100 mEq) in patients >60 years

Antacid: Oral: 325 mg to 2 g 1-4 times/day

Prevention of contrast-induced nephropathy (unlabeled use): I.V. infusion: 154 mEq/L sodium bicarbonate in D_5W solution: 3 mL/kg/hour for 1 hour immediately before contrast injection, then 1mL/kg/hour during contrast exposure and for 6 hours after procedure

To prepare solution, remove 154 mL from 1000 mL bag of D_5W; replace with 154 mL of 8.4% sodium bicarbonate; resultant concentration is 154 mEq/L (Merten, 2004); more practically, institutions may remove 150 mL from 1000 mL bag of D_5W and replace with 150 mL of 8.4% sodium bicarbonate; resultant concentration is 150 mEq/L

Administration For infusion, dilute to a maximum concentration of 0.5 mEq/mL in dextrose solution and infuse over 2 hours (maximum rate of administration: 1 mEq/kg/hour)

Oral product should be administered 1-3 hours after meals.

Special Geriatric Considerations Not the antacid of choice for the elderly because of sodium content and potential for systemic alkalosis (see maximum daily dose under Dosage).

Dosage Forms Excipient information presented when available (limited, particularly for generics); consult specific product labeling.

Granules for suspension, oral [effervescent]:

Brioschi®: 2.69 g/capful (120 g, 240 g) [contains sodium 770 mg/capful; lemon flavor]

Brioschi®: 2.69 g/packet (12s) [contains sodium 770 mg/packet; lemon flavor]

Injection, solution: 4.2% [5 mEq/10 mL] (10 mL); 8.4% [10 mEq/10 mL] (50 mL)

Neut®: 4% [2.4 mEq/5 mL] (5 mL) [contains edetate disodium]

Injection, solution [preservative free]: 4.2% [5 mEq/10 mL] (5 mL); 7.5% [8.92 mEq/10 mL] (50 mL); 8.4% [10 mEq/10 mL] (10 mL, 50 mL)

Powder, oral: USP: 100% (120 g, 480 g)

Tablet, oral: 325 mg [3.8 mEq], 650 mg [7.6 mEq]

◆ **Sodium Bicarbonate and Omeprazole** *see* Omeprazole and Sodium Bicarbonate *on page 1420*

Sodium Chloride (SOW dee um KLOR ide)

Related Information

Calculations *on page 2087*

Medication Safety Issues

High alert medication:

The Institute for Safe Medication Practices (ISMP) includes this medication (I.V. formulation >0.9% concentration) among its list of drugs which have a heightened risk of causing significant patient harm when used in error.

Other safety concerns:

Per The Joint Commission (TJC) recommendations, concentrated electrolyte solutions (eg, NaCl >0.9%) should not be available in patient care areas.

Brand Names: U.S. 4-Way® Saline Moisturizing Mist [OTC]; Altachlore [OTC]; Altamist [OTC]; Ayr® Allergy & Sinus [OTC]; Ayr® Baby Saline [OTC]; Ayr® Saline Nasal Gel [OTC]; Ayr® Saline No-Drip [OTC]; Ayr® Saline [OTC]; Deep Sea [OTC]; Entsol® [OTC]; HuMist® [OTC]; HyperSal®; Little Noses® Saline [OTC]; Little Noses® Sterile Saline Nasal Mist [OTC]; Little Noses® Stuffy Nose Kit [OTC]; Muro 128® [OTC]; Na-Zone® [OTC]; NebuSal™; Ocean® for Kids [OTC]; Ocean® [OTC]; Pretz® [OTC]; Rhinaris® [OTC]; Safe Wash™ [OTC]; Saline Mist [OTC]; Saljet® [OTC]; Sea Soft Nasal Mist [OTC]; Simply Saline® Baby [OTC]; Simply Saline® [OTC]; Sochlor™ [OTC]; Syrex; Wound Wash Saline™ [OTC]

Index Terms Hypertonic Saline; NaCl; Normal Saline; Saline; Salt

Generic Availability (U.S.) Yes: Excludes aerosol, gel, powder for solution, swab

Pharmacologic Category Electrolyte Supplement, Parenteral; Genitourinary Irrigant; Irrigant; Lubricant, Ocular; Sodium Salt

◀ **Use**

Parenteral: Restores sodium ion in patients with restricted oral intake (especially hyponatremia states or low salt syndrome).

Concentrated sodium chloride: Additive for parenteral fluid therapy

Hypertonic sodium chloride: For severe hyponatremia and hypochloremia

Hypotonic sodium chloride: Hydrating solution

Normal saline: Restores water/sodium losses

Ophthalmic: Reduces corneal edema

Inhalation: Restores moisture to pulmonary system; loosens and thins congestion caused by colds or allergies; diluent for bronchodilator solutions that require dilution before inhalation

Intranasal: Restores moisture to nasal membranes

Irrigation: Wound cleansing, irrigation, and flushing

Unlabeled Use Traumatic brain injury (hypertonic sodium chloride)

Dosage

Geriatric & Adult

Refractory elevated ICP due to various etiologies (eg, subarachnoid hemorrhage, trauma, neoplasm), transtentorial herniation syndromes (unlabeled use): I.V.: Hypertonic saline: 23.4% (30-60 mL) given over 2-20 minutes administered via central venous access only (Koenig, 2008; Suarez, 1998; Ware, 2005)

Subarachnoid hemorrhage with hyponatremia (ie, ≤135 mEq/L) to enhance cerebral perfusion (unlabeled use): I.V.: Hypertonic saline: 3% sodium chloride/acetate (50:50 mixture) 100-200 mL/hour administered via central venous catheter; titrate to clinical response up to a maximum serum sodium between 150-160 mEq/L (achieved at a rate of 0.5-1 mEq/L/hour) (Suarez, 1999)

Traumatic brain injury with elevated ICP (unlabeled use): I.V.: Hypertonic saline: **Note:** Optimal dose has not been established; due to insufficient evidence, the Brain Trauma Foundation guidelines (Bratton, 2007) do not make specific recommendations on the use of hypertonic saline for the treatment of traumatic intracranial hypertension. Clinical trials are small; few are prospective. **Some concentrations may not be commercially available; administer via central venous catheter;** protocols include:

3%: 300 mL administered over 20 minutes when ICP values exceed 20 mm Hg (Huang, 2006)

7.2%: 1.5 mL/kg administered over 15 minutes when ICP values exceed 15 mm Hg (Munar, 2000)

7.5%: 2 mL/kg administered over 20 minutes when ICP values exceed 25 mm Hg (Vialet, 2003)

23.4%: 30 mL administered over 2 minutes (Ware, 2005) **or** over >30 minutes when ICP values exceed 20 mm Hg (Kerwin, 2009)

GU irrigant: Irrigation: 1-3 L/day by intermittent irrigation

Replacement: I.V.: Determined by laboratory determinations mEq

Hyponatremia: Sodium deficiency (mEq/kg) = [% dehydration (L/kg)/100 x 70 (mEq/L)] + [0.6 (L/kg) x (140 - serum sodium) (mEq/L)]

To correct acute, serious hyponatremia: mEq sodium = [desired sodium (mEq/L) - actual sodium (mEq/L)] x [0.6 x wt (kg)]; for acute correction use 125 mEq/L as the desired serum sodium; acutely correct serum sodium in 5 mEq/L/dose increments; more gradual correction in increments of 10 mEq/L/day is indicated in the asymptomatic patient

Approximate Deficits of Water and Electrolytes in Moderately Severe Dehydration[1]

Condition	Water (mL/kg)	Sodium (mEq/kg)
Fasting and thirsting	100-120	5-7
Diarrhea		
isonatremic	100-120	8-10
hypernatremic	100-120	2-4
hyponatremic	100-120	10-12
Pyloric stenosis	100-120	8-10
Diabetic acidosis	100-120	9-10

[1]A **negative** deficit indicates total body **excess** prior to treatment.

Adapted from Behrman RE, Kleigman RM, Nelson WE, et al, eds, *Nelson Textbook of Pediatrics*, 14th ed, WB Saunders Co, 1992.

Ophthalmic:

Ointment: Apply once daily or more often

Solution: Instill 1-2 drops into affected eye(s) every 3-4 hours

Bronchodilator diluent: Inhalation: 1-3 sprays (1-3 mL) to dilute bronchodilator solution in nebulizer before administration

Nasal congestion: Intranasal: 2-3 sprays in each nostril as needed

Irrigation: Spray affected area

Special Geriatric Considerations No specific information for use in elderly.

Dosage Forms Excipient information presented when available (limited, particularly for generics); consult specific product labeling. [DSC] = Discontinued product

Aerosol, spray, intranasal [preservative free]:
Entsol®: 3% (100 mL) [chlorofluorocarbon free]
Little Noses® Sterile Saline Nasal Mist: 0.9% (50 mL) [ethanol free]

Aerosol, spray, topical [preservative free]:
Safe Wash™: 0.9% (210 mL) [chlorofluorocarbon free]

Gel, intranasal:
Ayr® Saline: <0.5% (14 g) [contains aloe, soybean oil]
Entsol®: 3% (20 g [DSC]) [contains aloe, benzalkonium chloride, vitamin E]
Rhinaris®: 0.2% (28.4 g) [contains benzalkonium chloride]

Gel, intranasal [spray]:
Ayr® Saline No-Drip: <0.5% (22 mL) [contains aloe, benzalkonium chloride, benzyl alcohol, soybean oil]

Injection, solution: 0.45% (50 mL, 100 mL, 250 mL, 500 mL, 1000 mL); 0.9% (25 mL, 50 mL, 100 mL, 150 mL, 250 mL, 500 mL, 1000 mL); 3% (500 mL); 5% (500 mL)

Injection, solution [preservative free]: 0.9% (2 mL, 3 mL, 5 mL, 10 mL, 20 mL, 50 mL, 100 mL)

Injection, solution [I.V. flush, preservative free]: 0.9% (1 mL, 2 mL, 2.5 mL, 3 mL, 5 mL, 10 mL, 50 mL, 125 mL)
Syrex: 0.9% (2.5 mL, 3 mL, 5 mL, 10 mL)

Injection, solution [bacteriostatic]: 0.9% (10 mL, 20 mL, 30 mL)

Injection, solution [concentrate]: 14.6% (20 mL, 40 mL); 23.4% (100 mL, 250 mL)

Injection, solution [concentrate, preservative free]: 14.6% (20 mL, 40 mL); 23.4% (30 mL, 100 mL, 200 mL)

Ointment, ophthalmic: 5% (3.5 g)
Altachlore: 5% (3.5 g)
Sochlor™: 5% (3.5 g)

Ointment, ophthalmic [preservative free]:
Muro 128®: 5% (3.5 g)

Powder for solution, intranasal [concentrate, preservative free]:
Pretz®: 1 teaspoon/dose (360 g) [with yerba santa]

Solution, for blood processing [not for injection]: 0.9% (3000 mL)

Solution, for inhalation [preservative free]: 0.9% (3 mL, 5 mL, 15 mL); 3% (15 mL); 10% (15 mL)

Solution, for irrigation: 0.9% (250 mL, 500 mL, 1000 mL, 1500 mL, 2000 mL, 3000 mL, 4000 mL, 5000 mL)

Solution, for irrigation [preservative free]: 0.9% (250 mL, 500 mL, 1000 mL, 1500 mL, 2000 mL, 3000 mL)

Solution, for irrigation [slush solution]: 0.9% (1000 mL)

Solution, for nebulization [preservative free]: 3% (4 mL); 7% (4 mL)
HyperSal®: 3.5% (4 mL); 7% (4 mL)
NebuSal™: 6% (4 mL)

Solution, intranasal [preservative free]:
Simply Saline®: 3% (44 mL)

Solution, intranasal [buffered/spray, preservative free]:
Pretz®: 0.75% (20 mL) [chlorofluorocarbon free; with yerba santa]

Solution, intranasal [drops]:
Ayr® Saline: 0.65% (50 mL) [ethanol free; contains benzalkonium chloride]

Solution, intranasal [drops/mist/spray]:
HuMist®: 0.65% (45 mL) [ethanol free; contains chlorobutanol]
Ocean®: 0.65% (45 mL, 473 mL) [contains benzalkonium chloride, benzyl alcohol]
Ocean® for Kids: 0.65% (37.5 mL) [ethanol free; contains benzalkonium chloride]

Solution, intranasal [drops/spray]:
Ayr® Baby Saline: 0.65% (30 mL) [ethanol free; contains benzalkonium chloride]
Little Noses® Saline: 0.65% (30 mL) [contains benzalkonium chloride]
Little Noses® Stuffy Nose Kit: 0.65% (15 mL) [contains benzalkonium chloride]

Solution, intranasal [irrigation]:
Pretz®: 0.75% (960 mL) [contains benzalkonium chloride, sodium benzoate; with yerba santa]

Solution, intranasal [isotonic, buffered/spray]:
Pretz®: 0.75% (50 mL) [contains benzalkonium chloride, sodium benzoate; with yerba santa]

Solution, intranasal [mist]:
4-Way® Saline Moisturizing Mist: 0.74% (29.6 mL) [ethanol free; contains benzalkonium chloride, menthol]
Ayr® Allergy & Sinus: 2.65% (50 mL) [ethanol free; contains benzalkonium chloride]
Ayr® Saline: 0.65% (50 mL) [ethanol free; contains benzalkonium chloride]
Entsol®: 3% (30 mL [DSC]) [contains benzalkonium chloride]
Rhinaris®: 0.2% (30 mL) [contains benzalkonium chloride]
Saline Mist: 0.65% (45 mL) [contains benzalkonium chloride]
Sea Soft Nasal Mist: 0.65% (45 mL)
Solution, intranasal [mist, preservative free]:
Simply Saline®: 0.9% (44 mL, 90 mL)
Simply Saline® Baby: 0.9% (45 mL)
Solution, intranasal [nasal wash, preservative free]:
Entsol®: 3% (240 mL [DSC])
Solution, intranasal [spray]: 0.65% (44 mL, 88 mL)
Altamist: 0.65% (60 mL) [contains benzalkonium chloride]
Deep Sea: 0.65% (44 mL) [contains benzalkonium chloride, benzyl alcohol]
Na-Zone®: 0.65% (60 mL) [contains benzalkonium chloride]
Solution, ophthalmic [drops]: 5% (15 mL)
Altachlore: 5% (15 mL, 30 mL [DSC])
Muro 128®: 2% (15 mL); 5% (15 mL, 30 mL)
Sochlor™: 5% (15 mL)
Solution, topical [preservative free]:
Saljet®: 0.9% (30 mL)
Wound Wash Saline™: 0.9% (90 mL, 210 mL)
Swab, intranasal:
Ayr® Saline Nasal Gel: 0.65% (20s) [contains aloe, benzalkonium chloride]
Tablet, oral: 1 g
Tablet for solution, topical: 1000 mg

Sodium Citrate and Citric Acid (SOW dee um SIT rate & SI trik AS id)

Related Information
Calculations on page 2087
Medication Safety Issues
Sound-alike/look-alike issues:
Bicitra may be confused with Polycitra
Brand Names: U.S. Cytra-2; Oracit®; Shohl's Solution (Modified)
Brand Names: Canada PMS-Dicitrate
Index Terms Bicitra; Citric Acid and Sodium Citrate; Modified Shohl's Solution
Generic Availability (U.S.) Yes
Pharmacologic Category Alkalinizing Agent, Oral
Use Treatment of metabolic acidosis; alkalinizing agent in conditions where long-term maintenance of an alkaline urine is desirable
Contraindications Hypersensitivity to sodium citrate, citric acid, or any component of the formulation; severe renal insufficiency; sodium-restricted diet
Warnings/Precautions Conversion to bicarbonate may be impaired in patients with hepatic failure, in shock, or who are severely ill. Use caution with cardiac failure, hypertension, impaired renal function, and peripheral or pulmonary edema; contains sodium.
Adverse Reactions (Reflective of adult population; not specific for elderly) Frequency not defined. Generally well tolerated with normal renal function.
Central nervous system: Tetany
Endocrine & metabolic: Metabolic alkalosis
Gastrointestinal: Diarrhea, nausea, vomiting
Drug Interactions
Metabolism/Transport Effects None known.
Avoid Concomitant Use There are no known interactions where it is recommended to avoid concomitant use.
Increased Effect/Toxicity
Sodium Citrate and Citric Acid may increase the levels/effects of: Aluminum Hydroxide
Decreased Effect There are no known significant interactions involving a decrease in effect.
Stability Store at controlled room temperature of 15°C to 30°C (59°F to 86°F); do not freeze. Protect from excessive heat.
Pharmacodynamics/Kinetics
Metabolism: Oxidized to sodium bicarbonate
Excretion: Urine (<5% as sodium citrate)

Dosage

Geriatric & Adult Systemic alkalization: Oral: 10-30 mL with water after meals and at bedtime

Administration Administer after meals. Dilute with 30-90 mL of water to enhance taste. Chilling solution prior to dosing helps to enhance palatability.

Monitoring Parameters Blood gas for pH and bicarbonate; serum bicarbonate

Reference Range Note: Reference ranges may vary depending on the laboratory
Urinary pH: 4.6-8.0

Pharmacotherapy Pearls 1 mL of solution contains 1 mEq of sodium and is metabolized to form the equivalent of 1 mEq of bicarbonate/mL

Special Geriatric Considerations
No specific information for use in elderly.

Dosage Forms Excipient information presented when available (limited, particularly for generics); consult specific product labeling. **Note:** Contains sodium 1 mEq/mL and is equivalent to bicarbonate 1 mEq/mL

Solution, oral: Sodium citrate 500 mg and citric acid 334 mg per 5 mL (480 mL)

Cytra-2: Sodium citrate 500 mg and citric acid 334 mg per 5 mL (480 mL) [alcohol free, dye free, sugar free; contains propylene glycol and sodium benzoate; grape flavor]

Oracit®: Sodium citrate 490 mg and citric acid 640 mg per 5 mL (15 mL, 30 mL, 500 mL, 3840 mL)

Shohl's Solution (Modified): Sodium citrate 500 mg and citric acid 300 mg per 5 mL (480 mL) [contains alcohol]

◆ **Sodium Citrate, Citric Acid, and Potassium Citrate** see Citric Acid, Sodium Citrate, and Potassium Citrate on page 391

◆ **Sodium Diuril®** see Chlorothiazide on page 356

◆ **Sodium Edecrin®** see Ethacrynic Acid on page 722

◆ **Sodium Etidronate** see Etidronate on page 728

◆ **Sodium Ferric Gluconate** see Ferric Gluconate on page 774

◆ **Sodium Fluoride** see Fluoride on page 806

◆ **Sodium Hydrogen Carbonate** see Sodium Bicarbonate on page 1785

◆ **Sodium Nafcillin** see Nafcillin on page 1330

◆ **Sodium Nitroferricyanide** see Nitroprusside on page 1389

◆ **Sodium Nitroprusside** see Nitroprusside on page 1389

◆ **Sodium PAS** see Aminosalicylic Acid on page 95

◆ **Sodium Phosphate and Potassium Phosphate** see Potassium Phosphate and Sodium Phosphate on page 1578

Sodium Phosphates (SOW dee um FOS fates)

Related Information
Laxatives, Classification and Properties on page 2121
Treatment Options for Constipation on page 2142

Medication Safety Issues
Sound-alike/look-alike issues:
Visicol® may be confused with Asacol®, VESIcare®

Administration issues:
Enemas and oral solution are available in pediatric and adult sizes; prescribe by "volume" not by "bottle."

Because inorganic phosphate exists as monobasic and dibasic anions, with the mixture of valences dependent on pH, ordering by mEq amounts is unreliable and may lead to large dosing errors. In addition, I.V. phosphate is available in the sodium and potassium salt; therefore, the content of these cations must be considered when ordering phosphate. The most reliable method of ordering I.V. phosphate is by millimoles, then specifying the potassium or sodium salt.

Brand Names: U.S. Fleet® Enema Extra® [OTC]; Fleet® Enema [OTC]; Fleet® Pedia-Lax™ Enema [OTC]; LaCrosse Complete [OTC]; OsmoPrep®; Visicol®

Brand Names: Canada Fleet Enema®

Index Terms Phosphates, Sodium

Generic Availability (U.S.) Yes: Enema, injection, oral solution

Pharmacologic Category Cathartic; Electrolyte Supplement, Parenteral; Laxative, Bowel Evacuant

Use
Oral solution, rectal: Short-term treatment of constipation
Oral tablets (OsmoPrep®, Visicol®): Bowel cleansing prior to colonoscopy
I.V.: Source of phosphate in large volume I.V. fluids and parenteral nutrition; treatment and prevention of hypophosphatemia

◄ **Medication Guide Available** Yes

Contraindications Hypersensitivity to sodium phosphate salts or any component of the formulation; additional contraindications vary by product:

Enema: Ascites, clinically significant renal impairment, heart failure, imperforate anus, known or suspected GI obstruction, megacolon (congenital or acquired)

Intravenous preparation: Diseases with hyperphosphatemia, hypocalcemia, or hypernatremia

Oral preparation: Acute phosphate nephropathy (biopsy proven), bowel obstruction, congenital megacolon, toxic megacolon

Warnings/Precautions [U.S. Boxed Warning]: Acute phosphate nephropathy has been reported (rarely) with use of oral products as a colon cleanser prior to colonoscopy. Some cases have resulted in permanent renal impairment (some requiring dialysis). Risk factors for acute phosphate nephropathy may include increased age (>55 years of age), pre-existing renal dysfunction, bowel obstruction, active colitis, or dehydration, and the use of medicines that affect renal perfusion or function (eg, ACE inhibitors, angiotensin receptor blockers, diuretics, and possibly NSAIDs), although some cases have been reported in patients without apparent risk factors. Other preventive measures may include avoid exceeding maximum recommended doses and concurrent use of other laxatives containing sodium phosphate; encourage patients to adequately hydrate before, during, and after use; obtain baseline and postprocedure labs in patients at risk; consider hospitalization and intravenous hydration during bowel cleansing for patients unable to hydrate themselves (eg, frail patients).

Use with caution in patients with impaired renal dysfunction, pre-existing electrolyte imbalances, risk of electrolyte disturbance (hypocalcemia, hyperphosphatemia, hypernatremia), or dehydration. If using as a bowel evacuant, correct electrolyte abnormalities before administration. Use caution in patients with unstable angina, history of myocardial infarction arrhythmia, cardiomyopathy; use caution in patients with or at risk for arrhythmias (eg, cardiomyopathy, prolonged QT interval, history of uncontrolled arrhythmias, recent MI) or with concurrent use of other QT-prolonging medications; pre-/postdose ECGs should be considered in high-risk patients.

Use caution in inflammatory bowel disease; may induce colonic aphthous ulceration. Use caution in patients with any of the following: Bowel obstruction (including pseudo) or perforation, gastric retention or hypomotility, ileus, severe, chronic constipation, colitis, gastric bypass or bariatric surgery.

Use with caution in patients with a history of seizures and those at higher risk of seizures. Inadequate fluid intake may lead to dehydration. Use with caution in debilitated patients; consider each patient's ability to hydrate properly. Use with caution in geriatric patients. Laxatives and purgatives have the potential for abuse by bulimia nervosa patients. Other oral medications may not be well absorbed when given during bowel evacuation because of rapid intestinal peristalsis. Solutions for injection may contain aluminum; toxic levels may occur following prolonged administration in patients with renal impairment. Enemas and oral solution are available in pediatric and adult sizes; prescribe by "volume" not by "bottle."

Visicol®: Use caution with history of swallowing difficulties or esophageal narrowing. Tablet particles may be seen in the stool.

Adverse Reactions (Reflective of adult population; not specific for elderly) Frequency not defined.

Cardiovascular: Edema, hypotension

Central nervous system: Dizziness, headache

Endocrine & metabolic: Hypocalcemia, hypernatremia, hyperphosphatemia, calcium phosphate precipitation

Gastrointestinal: Nausea, vomiting, diarrhea, abdominal bloating, abdominal pain, mucosal bleeding, superficial mucosal ulcerations

Renal: Acute renal failure

Postmarketing and/or case reports: Acute phosphate nephropathy, anaphylaxis, arrhythmia, atrial fibrillation (following severe vomiting [tablet formulation]), BUN increased, creatinine increased, nephrocalcinosis (oral solution), pruritus, rash, renal tubular necrosis, swelling (face, lips, tongue), urticaria, seizure

Drug Interactions

Metabolism/Transport Effects None known.

Avoid Concomitant Use There are no known interactions where it is recommended to avoid concomitant use.

Increased Effect/Toxicity

Sodium Phosphates may increase the levels/effects of: Nonsteroidal Anti-Inflammatory Agents

The levels/effects of Sodium Phosphates may be increased by: ACE Inhibitors; Angiotensin II Receptor Blockers; Bisphosphonate Derivatives; Diuretics; Tricyclic Antidepressants

Decreased Effect

The levels/effects of Sodium Phosphates may be decreased by: Antacids; Calcium Salts; Iron Salts; Magnesium Salts; Sucralfate

Stability Store at 15°C to 30°C (59°F to 86°F).

Mechanism of Action As a laxative, exerts osmotic effect in the small intestine by drawing water into the lumen of the gut, producing distention and promoting peristalsis and evacuation of the bowel; phosphorous participates in bone deposition, calcium metabolism, utilization of B complex vitamins, and as a buffer in acid-base equilibrium

Pharmacodynamics/Kinetics

Onset of action: Cathartic: 3-6 hours; Rectal: 2-5 minutes

Absorption: Oral: ~1% to 20%

Excretion: Urine

Dosage

Geriatric & Adult Caution: With orders for I.V. phosphate, there is considerable confusion associated with the use of millimoles (mmol) versus milliequivalents (mEq) to express the phosphate requirement. The most reliable method of ordering I.V. phosphate is by millimoles, then specifying the potassium or sodium salt. Intravenous doses listed as mmol of phosphate.

Acute treatment of hypophosphatemia: I.V.: It is difficult to provide concrete guidelines for the treatment of severe hypophosphatemia because the extent of total body deficits and response to therapy are difficult to predict. Aggressive doses of phosphate may result in a transient serum elevation followed by redistribution into intracellular compartments or bone tissue. It is recommended that repletion of severe hypophosphatemia be done I.V. because large doses of oral phosphate may cause diarrhea and intestinal absorption may be unreliable. Intermittent I.V. infusion should be reserved for severe depletion situations; requires continuous cardiac monitoring. Guidelines differ based on degree of illness, need/ use of TPN, and severity of hypophosphatemia. If hypokalemia exists (some clinicians recommend threshold of <4 mmol/L), consider phosphate replacement strategy with potassium (eg, potassium phosphates). Obese patients and/or severe renal impairment were excluded from phosphate supplement trials. **Note:** 1 mmol phosphate = 31 mg phosphorus; 1 mg phosphorus = 0.032 mmol phosphate.

General replacement guidelines (Lentz, 1978):

Low dose, serum phosphorus losses are recent and uncomplicated: 0.08 mmol/kg over 6 hours

Intermediate dose, serum phosphorus level 0.5-1 mg/dL (0.16-0.32 mmol/L): 0.16-0.24 mmol/kg over 6 hours

Note: The initial dose may be increased by 25% to 50% if the patient is symptomatic secondary to hypophosphatemia and lowered by 25% to 50% if the patient is hypercalcemic.

Critically-ill adult patients receiving concurrent enteral/parenteral nutrition (Brown, 2006; Clark, 1995): **Note:** Round doses to the nearest 7.5 mmol for ease of preparation. If administering with phosphate-containing parenteral nutrition, do not exceed 15 mmol/L within parenteral nutrition. May use adjusted body weight for patients weighing >130% of ideal body weight (and BMI <40 kg/m^2) by using [IBW + 0.25 (ABW-IBW)]:

Low dose, serum phosphorus level 2.3-3 mg/dL (0.74-0.96 mmol/L): 0.16-0.32 mmol/kg over 4-6 hours

Intermediate dose, serum phosphorus level 1.6-2.2 mg/dL (0.51-0.71 mmol/L): 0.32-0.64 mmol/kg over 4-6 hours

High dose, serum phosphorus <1.5 mg/dL (<0.5 mmol/L): 0.64-1 mmol/kg over 8-12 hours

Parenteral nutrition: I.V.: 10-15 mmol/1000 kcal (Hicks, 2001) **or** 20-40 mmol/24 hours (Mirtallo, 2004 [ASPEN guidelines])

Laxative (Fleet®): Rectal: Contents of one 4.5 oz enema as a single dose

Laxative: Oral solution: 15 mL as a single dose; maximum single daily dose: 45 mL

Bowel cleansing prior to colonoscopy: Oral tablets: **Note:** Do not use additional agents, especially sodium phosphate products.

Visicol®: A total of 40 tablets divided as follows:

Evening before colonoscopy: 3 tablets every 15 minutes for 6 doses, then 2 additional tablets in 15 minutes (total of 20 tablets)

3-5 hours prior to colonoscopy: 3 tablets every 15 minutes for 6 doses, then 2 additional tablets in 15 minutes (total of 20 tablets)

OsmoPrep®: A total of 32 tablets divided as follows:

Evening before colonoscopy: 4 tablets every 15 minutes for 5 doses (total of 20 tablets)

3-5 hours prior to colonoscopy: 4 tablets every 15 minutes for 3 doses (total of 12 tablets)

◄ **Renal Impairment** Use with caution; ionized inorganic phosphate is excreted by the kidneys. Oral solution is contraindicated in patients with kidney disease.

Hepatic Impairment Not expected to be metabolized in the liver.

Administration

Intermittent I.V. infusion; do **not** administer I.V. push. Must be diluted prior to parenteral administration. In general, the dose, concentration of infusion, and rate of administration may be dependent on patient condition and specific institution policy. Intermittent infusion doses are typically prepared in 100-250 mL of NS or D_5W (usual concentration range: 0.15-0.6 mmol/mL). For adult patients with severe symptomatic hypophosphatemia (ie, <1.5 mg/dL), may administer at rates up to 15 mmol/hour (Charron, 2003; Rosen, 1995). In patients with renal dysfunction and/or less severe hypophosphatemia, slower administration rates (eg, over 4-6 hours) or oral repletion is recommended.

Bowel cleansing: Have patient drink ~8 ounces of water with each dose of sodium phosphate (total of 2 quarts/64 ounces); have patient rehydrate before and after colonoscopy

Constipation: Take on an empty stomach; dilute dose with 8 ounces cool water, then follow dose with 8 ounces water; **do not repeat dose within 24 hours**

Monitoring Parameters

I.V.: Serum calcium, sodium and phosphorus levels; renal function; after I.V. phosphate repletion, repeat serum phosphorus level should be checked 2-4 hours later

Oral: Bowel cleansing: Baseline and postprocedure labs (electrolytes, calcium, phosphorus, BUN, creatinine) in patients at risk for acute renal nephropathy, seizure, or who have a history of electrolyte abnormality; ECG in patients with risks for prolonged QT or arrhythmias. Ensure euvolemia before initiating bowel preparation.

Reference Range Note: Reference ranges may vary depending on the laboratory

Serum calcium: 8.4-10.2 mg/dL

Serum phosphorus: Both low and high ends of the normal range are higher in children than in adults.

Adults: 2.5-4.5 mg/dL (0.81-1.45 mmol/L)

Pharmacotherapy Pearls Phosphate salts may precipitate when mixed with calcium salts; solubility is improved in amino acid parenteral nutrition solutions; check with a pharmacist to determine compatibility.

Special Geriatric Considerations The use of laxatives should be limited in the elderly since abuse could lead to fluid/electrolyte deficiencies. Since elderly often have reduced renal function, or disease that could predispose them to adverse effects, caution must be used with parenteral sodium phosphate.

Dosage Forms Excipient information presented when available (limited, particularly for generics); consult specific product labeling.

Injection, solution [concentrate; preservative free]: Phosphorus 3 mmol and sodium 4 mEq per 1 mL (5 mL, 15 mL, 50 mL) [equivalent to phosphorus 93 mg and sodium 92 mg per 1 mL; source of electrolytes: monobasic and dibasic sodium phosphate]

Solution, oral: Monobasic sodium phosphate monohydrate 2.4 g and dibasic sodium phosphate heptahydrate 0.9 g per 5 mL (45 mL) [sugar free; contains sodium 556 mg/5 mL, sodium benzoate; ginger-lemon flavor]

Solution, rectal [enema]: Monobasic sodium phosphate monohydrate 19 g and dibasic sodium phosphate heptahydrate 7 g per 118 mL delivered dose (133 mL)

Fleet® Enema: Monobasic sodium phosphate monohydrate 19 g and dibasic sodium phosphate heptahydrate 7 g per 118 mL delivered dose (133 mL) [contains sodium 4.4 g/118 mL]

Fleet® Enema Extra®: Monobasic sodium phosphate monohydrate 19 g and dibasic sodium phosphate heptahydrate 7 g per 197 mL delivered dose (230 mL) [contains sodium 4.4 g/197 mL]

Fleet® Pedia-Lax™ Enema: Monobasic sodium phosphate monohydrate 9.5 g and dibasic sodium phosphate heptahydrate 3.5 g per 59 mL delivered dose (66 mL) [contains sodium 2.2 g/59 mL]

LaCrosse Complete: Monobasic sodium phosphate monohydrate 19 g and dibasic sodium phosphate heptahydrate 7 g per 118 mL delivered dose (133 mL) [contains sodium 4.4 g/118 mL]

Tablet, oral [scored]:

OsmoPrep®, Visicol®: Monobasic sodium phosphate monohydrate 1.102 g and dibasic sodium phosphate anhydrous 0.398 g [sodium phosphate 1.5 g per tablet; gluten free]

Sodium Polystyrene Sulfonate (SOW dee um pol ee STYE reen SUL fon ate)

Medication Safety Issues

Sound-alike/look-alike issues:

Kayexalate® may be confused with Kaopectate®

Sodium polystyrene sulfonate may be confused with calcium polystyrene sulfonate

Administration issues:
Always prescribe either one-time doses or as a specific number of doses (eg, 15 g q6h x 2 doses). Scheduled doses with no dosage limit could be given for days leading to dangerous hypokalemia.

International issues:
Kionex [U.S.] may be confused with Kinex brand name for biperiden [Mexico]

Brand Names: U.S. Kalexate; Kayexalate®; Kionex®; SPS®

Brand Names: Canada Kayexalate®; PMS-Sodium Polystyrene Sulfonate

Generic Availability (U.S.) Yes: Powder for suspension

Pharmacologic Category Antidote

Use Treatment of hyperkalemia

Contraindications Hypersensitivity to sodium polystyrene sulfonate or any component of the formulation; hypokalemia; obstructive bowel disease

Additional contraindications: Sodium polystyrene sulfonate suspension (**with** sorbitol): Any postoperative patient until normal bowel function resumes

Warnings/Precautions Intestinal necrosis (including fatalities) and other serious gastrointestinal events (eg, bleeding, ischemic colitis, perforation) have been reported, especially when administered with sorbitol. Increased risk may be associated with a history of intestinal disease or surgery, hypovolemia, and renal insufficiency or failure; use with sorbitol is not recommended. Avoid use in any postoperative patient until normal bowel function resumes or in patients at risk for constipation or impaction; discontinue use if constipation occurs. Use with caution in patients with severe HF, hypertension, or edema; sodium load may exacerbate condition. Effective lowering of serum potassium from sodium polystyrene sulfonate may take hours to days after administration; consider alternative measures (eg, dialysis) or concomitant therapy (eg, I.V. sodium bicarbonate) in situations where rapid correction of severe hyperkalemia is required. Severe hypokalemia may occur; frequent monitoring of serum potassium is recommended within each 24-hour period; ECG monitoring may be appropriate in select patients. In addition to serum potassium-lowering effects, cation-exchange resins may also affect other cation concentrations possibly resulting in decreased serum magnesium and calcium. Large oral doses may cause fecal impaction (especially in elderly).

Concomitant administration of oral sodium polystyrene sulfonate with nonabsorbable cation-donating antacids or laxatives (eg, magnesium hydroxide) may result in systemic alkalosis and may diminish ability to reduce serum potassium concentrations; use with such agents is not recommended. In addition, intestinal obstruction has been reported with concomitant administration of aluminum hydroxide due to concretion formation. Enema will reduce the serum potassium faster than oral administration, but the oral route will result in a greater reduction over several hours.

Adverse Reactions (Reflective of adult population; not specific for elderly) Frequency not defined.

Endocrine & metabolic: Hypernatremia, hypocalcemia, hypokalemia, hypomagnesemia, sodium retention

Gastrointestinal: Anorexia, constipation, diarrhea, fecal impaction, intestinal necrosis (rare), intestinal obstruction (due to concretions in association with aluminum hydroxide), nausea, vomiting

Drug Interactions

Metabolism/Transport Effects None known.

Avoid Concomitant Use
Avoid concomitant use of Sodium Polystyrene Sulfonate with any of the following: Laxatives; Meloxicam; Sorbitol

Increased Effect/Toxicity
Sodium Polystyrene Sulfonate may increase the levels/effects of: Aluminum Hydroxide; Digoxin

The levels/effects of Sodium Polystyrene Sulfonate may be increased by: Antacids; Laxatives; Meloxicam; Sorbitol

Decreased Effect
Sodium Polystyrene Sulfonate may decrease the levels/effects of: Lithium; Thyroid Products

Ethanol/Nutrition/Herb Interactions Food: Some liquids may contain potassium: Management: Do not mix in orange juice or in any fruit juice known to contain potassium.

Stability Store at 25°C (77°F); excursions permitted to 15°C to 30°C (59°F to 86°F). Store repackaged product in refrigerator and use within 14 days. Freshly prepared suspensions should be used within 24 hours. Do not heat resin suspension.

SODIUM POLYSTYRENE SULFONATE

Mechanism of Action Removes potassium by exchanging sodium ions for potassium ions in the intestine (especially the large intestine) before the resin is passed from the body; exchange capacity is 1 mEq/g *in vivo*, and *in vitro* capacity is 3.1 mEq/g, therefore, a wide range of exchange capacity exists such that close monitoring of serum electrolytes is necessary

Pharmacodynamics/Kinetics

Onset of action: 2-24 hours

Absorption: None

Excretion: Completely feces (primarily as potassium polystyrene sulfonate)

Dosage

Geriatric & Adult Hyperkalemia:

Oral: 15 g 1-4 times/day

Rectal: 30-50 g every 6 hours

Administration

Oral: Shake suspension well prior to administration. Administer orally (or via NG tube) as a suspension. **Do not mix in orange juice.** Chilling the oral mixture will increase palatability. Powder for suspension: For each 1 g of the powdered resin, add 3-4 mL of water or syrup (amount of fluid usually ranges from 20-100 mL)

Rectal: Enema route is less effective than oral administration. Administer cleansing enema first. Each dose of the powder for suspension should be suspended in 100 mL of aqueous vehicle and administered as a warm emulsion (body temperature). The commercially available suspension should also be warmed to body temperature. During administration, the solution should be agitated gently. Retain enema in colon for at least 30-60 minutes and for several hours, if possible. Once retention time is complete, irrigate colon with a non-sodium-containing solution to remove resin.

Monitoring Parameters Serum electrolytes (potassium, sodium, calcium, magnesium); ECG in select patients

Reference Range Serum potassium: Adults: 3.5-5.2 mEq/L

Pharmacotherapy Pearls 1 g of resin binds approximately 1 mEq of potassium

Historically, sorbitol was often recommended as a cathartic agent to be administered with sodium polystyrene sulfonate (SPS) to prevent SPS-induced fecal impaction. However, SPS, particularly when used with sorbitol, has been associated with cases of intestinal necrosis and other serious GI adverse events. Due to the concern that sorbitol may increase the risk of intestinal necrosis, concomitant use of sorbitol is no longer recommended.

Sodium polystyrene sulfonate is commercially available in a liquid suspension containing 33% sorbitol (~20 g sorbitol per 60 mL suspension).

Special Geriatric Considerations Large doses in the elderly may cause fecal impaction and intestinal obstruction.

Dosage Forms Excipient information presented when available (limited, particularly for generics); consult specific product labeling.

Powder for suspension, oral/rectal: (454 g)

Kalexate: (454 g) [contains sodium 100 mg (4.1 mEq)/g]

Kayexalate®: (454 g) [contains sodium 100 mg (4.1 mEq)/g]

Kionex®: (454 g) [contains sodium 100 mg (4.1 mEq)/g]

Suspension, oral/rectal:

Kionex®: 15 g/60 mL (60 mL, 480 mL) [contains ethanol 0.2%, propylene glycol, sodium 1500 mg (65 mEq)/60 mL, sorbitol; raspberry flavor]

SPS®: 15 g/60 mL (60 mL, 120 mL, 473 mL) [contains ethanol 0.3%, propylene glycol, sodium 1500 mg (65 mEq)/60 mL, sorbitol; cherry flavor]

◆ **Sodium Salicylate** *see* Salicylates (Various Salts) *on page 1742*

◆ **Sodium Sulfacetamide** *see* Sulfacetamide (Ophthalmic) *on page 1811*

◆ **Sodium Sulfacetamide** *see* Sulfacetamide (Topical) *on page 1812*

◆ **Sodium Thiosalicylate** *see* Salicylates (Various Salts) *on page 1742*

◆ **Solaraze®** *see* Diclofenac (Topical) *on page 536*

◆ **Solarcaine® cool aloe Burn Relief [OTC]** *see* Lidocaine (Topical) *on page 1128*

Solifenacin (sol i FEN a sin)

Related Information

Beers Criteria – Potentially Inappropriate Medications for Geriatrics *on page 2183*
Pharmacotherapy of Urinary Incontinence *on page 2141*

Medication Safety Issues

Sound-alike/look-alike issues:
VESIcare® may be confused with Visicol®

BEERS Criteria medication:
This drug may be potentially inappropriate for use in geriatric patients (Quality of evidence - varies based on comorbidity; Strength of recommendation - varies based on comorbidity)

Brand Names: U.S. VESIcare®

Index Terms Solifenacin Succinate; YM905

Generic Availability (U.S.) No

Pharmacologic Category Anticholinergic Agent

Use Treatment of overactive bladder with symptoms of urinary frequency, urgency, or urge incontinence

Contraindications Hypersensitivity to solifenacin or any component of the formulation; urinary retention; gastric retention; uncontrolled narrow-angle glaucoma.

Warnings/Precautions Cases of angioedema involving the face, lips, tongue, and/or larynx have been reported. Immediately discontinue if tongue, hypopharynx, or larynx are involved. May cause drowsiness and/or blurred vision, which may impair physical or mental abilities; patients must be cautioned about performing tasks which require mental alertness (eg, operating machinery or driving). Heat prostration may occur in the presence of increased environmental temperature; use caution in hot weather and/or exercise. Use with caution in patients with bladder outflow obstruction, gastrointestinal obstructive disorders, and decreased gastrointestinal motility. Use with caution in patients with a known history of QT prolongation or other risk factors for QT prolongation (eg, concomitant use of medications known to prolong QT interval and/or electrolyte abnormalities); the risk for QT prolongation is dose-related. Use with caution in patients with controlled (treated) narrow-angle glaucoma; use is contraindicated with uncontrolled narrow-angle glaucoma. Dosage adjustment is required for patients with severe renal impairment (Cl_{cr} <30 mL/minute) or moderate (Child-Pugh class B) hepatic impairment; use is not recommended with severe hepatic impairment (Child-Pugh class C). Patients on potent CYP3A4 inhibitors require the lower dose of solifenacin. This medication is associated with potent anticholinergic properties which may be inappropriate in older adults depending on comorbidities (eg, dementia, delirium) (Beers Criteria).

Adverse Reactions (Reflective of adult population; not specific for elderly)

>10%: Gastrointestinal: Xerostomia (11% to 28%; dose-related), constipation (5% to 13%; dose-related)

1% to 10%:
Cardiovascular: Edema (≤1%), hypertension (≤1%)
Central nervous system: Headache (3% to 6%), fatigue (1% to 2%), depression (≤1%)
Gastrointestinal: Dyspepsia (1% to 4%), nausea (2% to 3%), upper abdominal pain (1% to 2%)
Genitourinary: Urinary tract infection (3% to 5%), urinary retention (≤1%)
Ocular: Blurred vision (4% to 5%), dry eyes (≤2%)
Respiratory: Cough (≤1%)
Miscellaneous: Influenza (≤2%)

Drug Interactions

Metabolism/Transport Effects Substrate of CYP3A4 (major); **Note:** Assignment of Major/Minor substrate status based on clinically relevant drug interaction potential

Avoid Concomitant Use
Avoid concomitant use of Solifenacin with any of the following: Conivaptan

Increased Effect/Toxicity
Solifenacin may increase the levels/effects of: AbobotulinumtoxinA; Anticholinergics; Cannabinoids; Highest Risk QTc-Prolonging Agents; Moderate Risk QTc-Prolonging Agents; OnabotulinumtoxinA; Potassium Chloride; RimabotulinumtoxinB

The levels/effects of Solifenacin may be increased by: Antifungal Agents (Azole Derivatives, Systemic); Conivaptan; CYP3A4 Inhibitors (Moderate); CYP3A4 Inhibitors (Strong); Ivacaftor; Mifepristone; Pramlintide

Decreased Effect

Solifenacin may decrease the levels/effects of: Acetylcholinesterase Inhibitors (Central); Secretin

The levels/effects of Solifenacin may be decreased by: Acetylcholinesterase Inhibitors (Central); CYP3A4 Inducers (Strong); Deferasirox; Herbs (CYP3A4 Inducers); Tocilizumab

Ethanol/Nutrition/Herb Interactions

Food: Grapefruit juice may increase the serum level effects of solifenacin.

Herb/Nutraceutical: St John's wort (*Hypericum*) may decrease the levels/effects of solifenacin.

Stability Store at controlled room temperature of 25°C (77°F); excursions permitted to 15°C to 30°C (59°F to 86°F).

Mechanism of Action Inhibits muscarinic receptors resulting in decreased urinary bladder contraction, increased residual urine volume, and decreased detrusor muscle pressure.

Pharmacodynamics/Kinetics

Distribution: V_d: 600 L

Protein binding: ~98% bound primarily to alpha$_1$-acid glycoprotein

Metabolism: Extensively hepatic; via N-oxidation and 4 R-hydroxylation, forms 1 active and 3 inactive metabolites; primary pathway for elimination is via CYP3A4

Bioavailability: ~90%

Half-life elimination: 45-68 hours following chronic dosing; prolonged in severe renal (Cl_{cr} <30 mL/minute) or moderate hepatic (Child-Pugh class B) impairment

Time to peak, plasma: 3-8 hours

Excretion: Urine 69% (<15% as unchanged drug); feces 23%

Dosage

Geriatric Base dosing on renal/hepatic function.

Adult Overactive bladder: Oral: 5 mg once daily; if tolerated, may increase to 10 mg once daily

Dosage adjustment with concomitant CYP3A4 inhibitors: Maximum solifenacin dose: 5 mg/day

Renal Impairment Use with caution in reduced renal function; Cl_{cr} <30 mL/minute: Maximum dose: 5 mg/day

Hepatic Impairment Use with caution in reduced hepatic function:

Moderate (Child-Pugh class B): Maximum dose: 5 mg/day

Severe (Child-Pugh class C): Use is not recommended

Administration Swallow tablet whole; administer with liquids; may be administered without regard to meals.

Monitoring Parameters Anticholinergic effects (eg, fixed and dilated pupils, blurred vision, tremors, or dry skin); creatinine clearance (prior to treatment for dosing adjustment); liver function

Special Geriatric Considerations In patients with Cl_{cr} <30 mL/minute, doses >5 mg/day are not recommended. Similar safety and effectiveness were observed in elderly and younger patients.

This medication is considered to be potentially inappropriate in this patient population (Beers Criteria: Quality of evidence - varies based on comorbidity; Strength of recommendation - varies based on comorbidity)

Dosage Forms Excipient information presented when available (limited, particularly for generics); consult specific product labeling.

Tablet, oral, as succinate:

VESIcare®: 5 mg, 10 mg

- ◆ **Solifenacin Succinate** *see* Solifenacin *on page 1797*
- ◆ **Solodyn®** *see* Minocycline *on page 1289*
- ◆ **Solu-CORTEF®** *see* Hydrocortisone (Systemic) *on page 940*
- ◆ **Solumedrol** *see* MethylPREDNISolone *on page 1252*
- ◆ **Solu-MEDROL®** *see* MethylPREDNISolone *on page 1252*
- ◆ **Solzira** *see* Gabapentin Enacarbil *on page 861*
- ◆ **Soma®** *see* Carisoprodol *on page 298*
- ◆ **Sominex® [OTC]** *see* DiphenhydrAMINE (Systemic) *on page 556*
- ◆ **Sominex® Maximum Strength [OTC]** *see* DiphenhydrAMINE (Systemic) *on page 556*
- ◆ **Somnote®** *see* Chloral Hydrate *on page 349*
- ◆ **Sonata®** *see* Zaleplon *on page 2043*
- ◆ **Soothe® [OTC]** *see* Artificial Tears *on page 148*
- ◆ **Soothe® Hydration [OTC]** *see* Artificial Tears *on page 148*

Sorbitol (SOR bi tole)

Related Information

Laxatives, Classification and Properties *on page 2121*
Treatment Options for Constipation *on page 2142*

Generic Availability (U.S.) Yes

Pharmacologic Category Genitourinary Irrigant; Laxative, Osmotic

Use Genitourinary irrigant in transurethral prostatic resection or other transurethral resection or other transurethral surgical procedures; diuretic; humectant; sweetening agent; hyperosmotic laxative; facilitate the passage of sodium polystyrene sulfonate through the intestinal tract

Contraindications Anuria

Warnings/Precautions Use with caution in patients with severe cardiopulmonary or renal impairment and in patients unable to metabolize sorbitol; large volumes may result in fluid overload and/or electrolyte changes.

Adverse Reactions (Reflective of adult population; not specific for elderly) Frequency not defined.

Cardiovascular: Edema

Endocrine & metabolic: Fluid and electrolyte losses, hyperglycemia, lactic acidosis

Gastrointestinal: Abdominal discomfort, diarrhea, dry mouth, nausea, vomiting, xerostomia

Drug Interactions

Metabolism/Transport Effects None known.

Avoid Concomitant Use

Avoid concomitant use of Sorbitol with any of the following: Calcium Polystyrene Sulfonate; Sodium Polystyrene Sulfonate

Increased Effect/Toxicity

Sorbitol may increase the levels/effects of: Calcium Polystyrene Sulfonate; Sodium Polystyrene Sulfonate

Decreased Effect There are no known significant interactions involving a decrease in effect.

Stability Avoid storage in temperatures >150°F; do not freeze.

Mechanism of Action A polyalcoholic sugar with osmotic cathartic actions

Pharmacodynamics/Kinetics

Onset of action: 0.25-1 hour

Absorption: Oral, rectal: Poor

Metabolism: Primarily hepatic to fructose

Dosage

Geriatric & Adult

Hyperosmotic laxative (as single dose, at infrequent intervals):

Oral: 30-150 mL (as 70% solution)

Rectal enema: 120 mL as 25% to 30% solution

Adjunct to sodium polystyrene sulfonate: 15 mL as 70% solution orally until diarrhea occurs (10-20 mL/2 hours) or 20-100 mL as an oral vehicle for the sodium polystyrene sulfonate resin

When administered with charcoal:

Oral: 4.3 mL/kg of 70% sorbitol with 1 g/kg of activated charcoal every 4 hours until first stool containing charcoal is passed

Transurethral surgical procedures: Irrigation: Topical: 3% to 3.3% as transurethral surgical procedure irrigation

Monitoring Parameters Monitor for fluid overload and/or electrolyte disturbances following large volumes; changes may be delayed due to slow absorption

Special Geriatric Considerations Causes for constipation must be evaluated prior to initiating treatment. Nonpharmacological dietary treatment should be initiated before laxative use. Sorbitol is as effective as lactulose but is much less expensive.

Dosage Forms Excipient information presented when available (limited, particularly for generics); consult specific product labeling.

Solution, genitourinary irrigation [preservative free]: 3% (3000 mL); 3.3% (2000 mL, 4000 mL)

Solution, oral: 70% (30 mL, 473 mL, 480 mL, 3840 mL)

◆ **Sorilux™** *see* Calcipotriene *on page 253*
◆ **Sorine®** *see* Sotalol *on page 1800*

Sotalol (SOE ta lole)

Related Information
Beers Criteria – Potentially Inappropriate Medications for Geriatrics *on page* 2183
Beta-Blockers *on page* 2108

Medication Safety Issues
Sound-alike/look-alike issues:
Sotalol may be confused with Stadol, Sudafed®
Betapace® may be confused with Betapace AF®

High alert medication:
The Institute for Safe Medication Practices (ISMP) includes this medication (I.V. formulation) among its list of drugs which have a heightened risk of causing significant patient harm when used in error.

BEERS Criteria medication:
This drug may be potentially inappropriate for use in geriatric patients (Quality of evidence - high; Strength of recommendation - strong).

Brand Names: U.S. Betapace AF®; Betapace®; Sorine®

Brand Names: Canada Apo-Sotalol®; CO Sotalol; Dom-Sotalol; Med-Sotalol; Mylan-Sotalol; Novo-Sotalol; Nu-Sotalol; PHL-Sotalol; PMS-Sotalol; PRO-Sotalol; ratio-Sotalol; Rhoxal-sotalol; Riva-Sotalol; Rylosol; Sandoz-Sotalol; ZYM-Sotalol

Index Terms Sotalol Hydrochloride

Generic Availability (U.S.) Yes

Pharmacologic Category Antiarrhythmic Agent, Class II; Antiarrhythmic Agent, Class III; Beta-Adrenergic Blocker, Nonselective

Use Treatment of documented ventricular arrhythmias (ie, sustained ventricular tachycardia), that in the judgment of the physician are life-threatening; maintenance of normal sinus rhythm in patients with symptomatic atrial fibrillation and atrial flutter who are currently in sinus rhythm. Manufacturer states substitutions should not be made for Betapace AF® since Betapace AF® is distributed with a patient package insert specific for atrial fibrillation/flutter.

Injection: Substitution for oral sotalol in those who are unable to take sotalol orally

Unlabeled Use Fetal tachycardia; alternative antiarrhythmic for the treatment of atrial fibrillation in patients with hypertrophic cardiomyopathy (HCM)

Contraindications Hypersensitivity to sotalol or any component of the formulation; bronchial asthma; sinus bradycardia; second- or third-degree AV block (unless a functioning pacemaker is present); congenital or acquired long QT syndromes; cardiogenic shock; uncontrolled heart failure

Additional contraindications: Betapace AF® and the injectable formulation: Baseline QT_c interval >450 msec; bronchospastic conditions; Cl_{cr} <40 mL/minute; serum potassium <4 mEq/L; sick sinus syndrome

Warnings/Precautions [U.S. Boxed Warning] Manufacturer recommends initiation (or reinitiation) and doses increased in a hospital setting with continuous monitoring and staff familiar with the recognition and treatment of life-threatening arrhythmias. Some experts will initiate therapy on an outpatient basis in a patient without heart disease or bradycardia, who has a baseline uncorrected QT interval <450 msec, and normal serum potassium and magnesium levels; close ECG monitoring during this time is necessary. ACC/AHA guidelines for management of atrial fibrillation also recommend that for outpatient initiation the patient not have risk factors predisposing to drug-induced ventricular proarrhythmia (Fuster, 2006). Dosage should be adjusted gradually with 3 days between dosing increments to achieve steady-state concentrations, and to allow time to monitor QT intervals. **[U.S. Boxed Warning]: Adjust dosing interval based on creatinine clearance to decrease risk of proarrhythmia; QT interval prolongation is directly related to sotalol concentration.** Creatinine clearance must be calculated with dose initiation and dose increases. Use cautiously in the renally-impaired (dosage adjustment required). Betapace AF® and the injectable formulation are contraindicated in patients with Cl_{cr} <40 mL/minute.

[U.S. Boxed Warning]: Sotalol injection: Sotalol can cause life-threatening ventricular tachycardia associated with QT-interval prolongation (ie, torsade de pointes). Do not initiate if baseline QTc interval is >450 msec. If QT_c exceeds 500 msec during therapy, reduce the dose, prolong the infusion duration, or discontinue use. If while on oral sotalol therapy baseline QT_c interval is >500 msec, use I.V. sotalol with particular caution; serious consideration should be given to reducing the dose or discontinuing I.V. sotalol when QT_c exceeds 520 msec. QT_c prolongation is directly related to the concentration of sotalol; reduced creatinine clearance, female gender, and large doses increase the risk of QT_c prolongation and subsequent torsade de pointes. Monitor and adjust dose to prevent QT_c prolongation. Concurrent use with other QT_c-prolonging drugs (including Class I and Class III antiarrhythmics) and use within 3 months of discontinuing amiodarone is generally not recommended. To reduce the chance of excessive QT_c-prolongation, withhold QT_c-prolonging drugs for at least 3 half-lives (or 3 months for amiodarone) before initiating sotalol.

Correct electrolyte imbalances before initiating (especially hypokalemia and hypomagnesemia). Consider pre-existing conditions such as sick sinus syndrome before initiating. Conduction abnormalities can occur particularly sinus bradycardia. Use cautiously within the first 2 weeks post-MI especially in patients with markedly impaired ventricular function (experience limited). Administer cautiously in compensated heart failure and monitor for a worsening of the condition. May precipitate or aggravate symptoms of arterial insufficiency in patients with PVD and Raynaud's disease; use with caution and monitor for progression of arterial obstruction. Bradycardia may be observed more frequently in elderly patients (>65 years of age); dosage reductions may be necessary. In the treatment of atrial fibrillation, avoid antiarrhythmics as first-line treatment. In older adults, data suggests rate control may provide more benefits than risks compared to rhythm control for most patients (Beers Criteria). Beta-blocker therapy should not be withdrawn abruptly (particularly in patients with CAD), but gradually tapered to avoid acute tachycardia, hypertension, and/or ischemia. Chronic beta-blocker therapy should not be routinely withdrawn prior to major surgery. Use caution with concurrent use of digoxin, verapamil, or diltiazem; bradycardia or heart block can occur. Use with caution in patients receiving inhaled anesthetic agents known to depress myocardial contractility. Use cautiously in diabetics because it can mask prominent hypoglycemic symptoms. Use with caution in patients with bronchospastic disease, myasthenia gravis or psychiatric disease. Adequate alpha-blockade is required prior to use of any beta-blocker for patients with untreated pheochromocytoma. May mask signs of hyperthyroidism (eg, tachycardia); if hyperthyroidism is suspected, carefully manage and monitor; abrupt withdrawal may exacerbate symptoms of hyperthyroidism or precipitate thyroid storm. Use caution with history of severe anaphylaxis to allergens; patients taking beta-blockers may become more sensitive to repeated challenges. Treatment of anaphylaxis (eg, epinephrine) in patients taking beta-blockers may be ineffective or promote undesirable effects.

[U.S. Boxed Warning]: Betapace® should not be substituted for Betapace® AF; Betapace® AF is distributed with an educational insert specifically for patients with atrial fibrillation/flutter.

Adverse Reactions (Reflective of adult population; not specific for elderly) Note: No clinical experience with I.V. sotalol; however, since exposure is similar between I.V. and oral sotalol, adverse reactions are expected to be similar.
>10%:
Cardiovascular: Bradycardia (13% to 16%), chest pain (3% to 16%), palpitation (14%)
Central nervous system: Fatigue (20%), dizziness (20%), lightheadedness (12%)
Neuromuscular & skeletal: Weakness (13%)
Respiratory: Dyspnea (21%)
1% to 10%:
Cardiovascular: Edema (8%), abnormal ECG (7%), hypotension (6%), proarrhythmia (5%), syncope (5%), CHF (5%), torsade de pointes (dose related; 1% to 4%), peripheral vascular disorders (3%), ventricular tachycardia worsened (1%), QT_c interval prolongation (dose related)
Central nervous system: Headache (8%), sleep problems (8%), mental confusion (6%), anxiety (4%), depression (4%)
Dermatologic: Itching/rash (5%)
Endocrine & metabolic: Sexual ability decreased (3%)
Gastrointestinal: Nausea/vomiting (10%), diarrhea (7%), stomach discomfort (3% to 6%), flatulence (2%)
Genitourinary: Impotence (2%)
Hematologic: Bleeding (2%)
Neuromuscular & skeletal: Extremity pain (7%), paresthesia (4%), back pain (3%)
Ocular: Visual problems (5%)
Respiratory: Upper respiratory problems (5% to 8%), asthma (2%)
Drug Interactions
Metabolism/Transport Effects None known.
Avoid Concomitant Use
Avoid concomitant use of Sotalol with any of the following: Beta2-Agonists; Fingolimod; Floctafenine; Highest Risk QTc-Prolonging Agents; Methacholine; Mifepristone; Moderate Risk QTc-Prolonging Agents; Propafenone
Increased Effect/Toxicity
Sotalol may increase the levels/effects of: Alpha-/Beta-Agonists (Direct-Acting); Alpha1-Blockers; Alpha2-Agonists; Amifostine; Antihypertensives; Antipsychotic Agents (Phenothiazines); Bupivacaine; Cardiac Glycosides; Cholinergic Agonists; Fingolimod; Highest Risk

QTc-Prolonging Agents; Hypotensive Agents; Insulin; Lidocaine; Lidocaine (Systemic); Lidocaine (Topical); Mepivacaine; Methacholine; Midodrine; RiTUXimab; Sulfonylureas

The levels/effects of Sotalol may be increased by: Acetylcholinesterase Inhibitors; Aminoquinolines (Antimalarial); Amiodarone; Anilidopiperidine Opioids; Antipsychotic Agents (Phenothiazines); Calcium Channel Blockers (Dihydropyridine); Calcium Channel Blockers (Nondihydropyridine); Diazoxide; Dipyridamole; Disopyramide; Dronedarone; EriBULin; Fingolimod; Floctafenine; Herbs (Hypotensive Properties); Lidocaine (Topical); MAO Inhibitors; Mifepristone; Moderate Risk QTc-Prolonging Agents; Pentoxifylline; Phosphodiesterase 5 Inhibitors; Propafenone; Prostacyclin Analogues; QTc-Prolonging Agents (Indeterminate Risk and Risk Modifying); QuiNIDine; Reserpine

Decreased Effect

Sotalol may decrease the levels/effects of: Beta2-Agonists; Theophylline Derivatives

The levels/effects of Sotalol may be decreased by: Barbiturates; Herbs (Hypertensive Properties); Methylphenidate; Nonsteroidal Anti-Inflammatory Agents; Rifamycin Derivatives; Yohimbine

Ethanol/Nutrition/Herb Interactions

Food: Sotalol peak serum concentrations may be decreased if taken with food.

Herb/Nutraceutical: Avoid ephedra (may worsen arrhythmia).

Stability Store at 25°C (77°F); excursions permitted to 15°C to 30°C (59°F to 86°F). To prepare sotalol infusion, see manufacturer's prescribing information.

Mechanism of Action

Beta-blocker which contains both beta-adrenoreceptor-blocking (Vaughan Williams Class II) and cardiac action potential duration prolongation (Vaughan Williams Class III) properties

Class II effects: Increased sinus cycle length, slowed heart rate, decreased AV nodal conduction, and increased AV nodal refractoriness Sotalol has both beta$_1$- and beta$_2$-receptor blocking activity. The beta-blocking effect of sotalol is a noncardioselective (half maximal at about 80 mg/day and maximal at doses of 320-640 mg/day). Significant beta-blockade occurs at oral doses as low as 25 mg/day.

Class III effects: Prolongation of the atrial and ventricular monophasic action potentials, and effective refractory prolongation of atrial muscle, ventricular muscle, and atrioventricular accessory pathways in both the antegrade and retrograde directions. Sotalol is a racemic mixture of *d*- and *l*-sotalol; both isomers have similar Class III antiarrhythmic effects while the *l*-isomer is responsible for virtually all of the beta-blocking activity. The Class III effects are seen only at oral doses ≥160 mg/day

Pharmacodynamics/Kinetics

Onset of action: Oral: Rapid, 1-2 hours; when administered I.V. for ongoing VT over 5 minutes, onset of action is ~5-10 minutes (Ho, 1994)

Duration: 8-16 hours

Absorption: Oral: Decreased 20% to 30% by meals compared to fasting

Distribution: V_d: 1.2-2.4 L/kg

Protein binding: None

Metabolism: None

Bioavailability: Oral: 90% to 100%

Half-life elimination: 12 hours; increases with renal dysfunction

Time to peak, serum: Oral: 2.5-4 hours

Excretion: Urine (as unchanged drug)

Dosage

Geriatric & Adult Baseline QT_c interval and creatinine clearance must be determined prior to initiation. Sotalol should be initiated and doses increased in a hospital with facilities for cardiac rhythm monitoring and assessment. Proarrhythmic events can occur after initiation of therapy and with each upward dosage adjustment.

Conversion from oral sotalol to I.V. sotalol:

80 mg oral equivalent to 75 mg I.V.

120 mg oral equivalent to 112.5 mg I.V.

160 mg oral equivalent to 150 mg I.V.

Ventricular arrhythmias:

I.V.: **Note:** The effects of the initial I.V. dose must be monitored and the dose titrated either upward or downward, if needed, based on clinical effect, QT_c interval, or adverse reactions. Substitution for oral sotalol: Initial dose: 75 mg infused over 5 hours twice daily

Dose adjustment: If the frequency of relapse does not reduce and excessive QT_c prolongation does not occur, may increase to 112.5 mg twice daily. For ventricular arrhythmias, may increase dose every 3 days in increments of 75 mg/day.

Dose range: Usual therapeutic dose: 75-150 mg twice daily; maximum dose: 300 mg twice daily.

Hemodynamically stable monomorphic VT, ongoing (unlabeled use): 1.5 mg/kg over 5 minutes (ACLS, 2010); **Note:** Clinical trial employed standard dose of 100 mg (Ho, 1994).

Oral (Betapace®, Sorine®):

Initial: 80 mg twice daily; dose may be increased gradually to 240-320 mg/day; allow 3 days between dosing increments (to attain steady-state plasma concentrations and to allow monitoring of QT_c intervals).

Usual range: Most patients respond to 160-320 mg/day in 2-3 divided doses.

Maximum: Some patients, with life-threatening refractory ventricular arrhythmias, may require doses as high as 480-640 mg/day; prescribed ONLY when the potential benefit outweighs the increased of adverse events.

Atrial fibrillation or atrial flutter:

I.V.: **Note:** The effects of the initial I.V. dose must be monitored and the dose titrated either upward or downward, if needed, based on clinical effect, QT_c interval, or adverse reactions. Substitution for oral sotalol: Initial dose: 75 mg infused over 5 hours twice daily

Dose adjustment: If the frequency of relapse does not reduce and excessive QT_c prolongation does not occur, may increase to 112.5 mg twice daily. For ventricular arrhythmias, may increase dose every 3 days in increments of 75 mg/day.

Dose range: Usual therapeutic dose: 112.5 mg twice daily; maximum dose: 150 mg twice daily

Oral (Betapace AF®): Initial: 80 mg twice daily. If the frequency of relapse does not reduce and excessive QT_c prolongation does not occur after 3 days, the dose may be increased to 120 mg twice daily; may further increase to 160 mg twice daily if response is inadequate and QT_c prolongation is not excessive.

Renal Impairment Adults: Impaired renal function can increase the terminal half-life, resulting in increased drug accumulation. Sotalol (Betapace AF®, injectable formulation) is contraindicated per the manufacturers for treatment of atrial fibrillation/flutter in patients with a Cl_{cr} <40 mL/minute.

Ventricular arrhythmias (Betapace®, Sorine®):

Cl_{cr} >60 mL/minute: Administer every 12 hours.

Cl_{cr} 30-60 mL/minute: Administer every 24 hours.

Cl_{cr} 10-29 mL/minute: Administer every 36-48 hours.

Cl_{cr} <10 mL/minute: Individualize dose.

Atrial fibrillation/flutter (Betapace AF®):

Cl_{cr} >60 mL/minute: Administer every 12 hours.

Cl_{cr} 40-60 mL/minute: Administer every 24 hours.

Cl_{cr} <40 mL/minute: Use is contraindicated.

Note: The manufacturer of the injectable formulation recommends adjustment similar to that used for Betapace AF®. However, the injectable formulation may be used for either indication.

Dialysis: Hemodialysis would be expected to reduce sotalol plasma concentrations because sotalol is not bound to plasma proteins and does not undergo extensive metabolism. Administer dose postdialysis or administer supplemental 80 mg dose. Peritoneal dialysis does not remove sotalol; supplemental dose is not necessary.

Administration

Oral: Administer without regard to meals.

I.V.:

Substitution for oral: Administer over 5 hours.

Hemodynamically stable monomorphic VT: Administer I.V. push over 5 minutes; use with caution due to increased risk of adverse events (eg, bradycardia, hypotension, torsade de pointes) (ACLS, 2010)

Monitoring Parameters Serum creatinine, magnesium, potassium; heart rate, blood pressure; ECG (eg, QT_c interval, PR interval). If baseline QT_c >450 msec (or JT interval >330 msec if QRS over 100 msec), sotalol is contraindicated.

For oral use (Betapace AF®) during initiation period, monitor QT_c interval 2-4 hours after each dose. If QT_c interval ≥500 msec, discontinue use; if QT_c interval <500 msec after 3 days (after fifth or sixth dose if patient receiving once-daily dosing), patient may be discharged on current regimen. Monitor QT_c interval periodically thereafter.

For I.V. use, measure QT_c interval after completion of each infusion.

Test Interactions May falsely increase urinary metanephrine values when fluorimetric or photometric methods are used; does not interact with HPLC assay with solid phase extraction for determination of urinary catecholamines

Special Geriatric Considerations Since elderly frequently have Cl_{cr} <60 mL/minute, attention to dose, creatinine clearance, and monitoring is important. Make dosage adjustments at 3-day intervals or after 5-6 doses at any dosage.

This medication is considered to be potentially inappropriate in this patient population (Beers Criteria: Quality of evidence - high; Strength of recommendation - strong).

◀ **Dosage Forms** Excipient information presented when available (limited, particularly for generics); consult specific product labeling.

Injection, solution, as hydrochloride: 15 mg/mL (10 mL)

Tablet, oral, as hydrochloride: 80 mg [atrial fibrillation], 80 mg, 120 mg [atrial fibrillation], 120 mg, 160 mg [atrial fibrillation], 160 mg, 240 mg

Betapace AF®: 80 mg, 120 mg, 160 mg [scored; atrial fibrillation]

Betapace®: 80 mg, 120 mg, 160 mg [scored]

Sorine®: 80 mg, 120 mg, 160 mg, 240 mg [scored]

Extemporaneously Prepared To make a 5 mg/mL oral solution, using a 6-ounce amber plastic prescription bottle, add five sotalol 120 mg tablets to 120 mL of simple syrup containing 0.1% sodium benzoate (tablets do not need to be crushed). Shake well. Allow tablets to hydrate for ~2 hours; shake intermittently until tablets completely disintegrate. Store at room temperature; shake well before use. Stable for 3 months. (Refer to manufacturer's current labeling.)

◆ **Sotalol Hydrochloride** see Sotalol on page 1800
◆ **SPD417** see CarBAMazepine on page 286
◆ **Spectracef®** see Cefditoren on page 313
◆ **SPI 0211** see Lubiprostone on page 1170

Spinosad (SPIN oh sad)

Brand Names: U.S. Natroba™

Index Terms NatrOVA

Pharmacologic Category Antiparasitic Agent, Topical; Pediculocide

Use Topical treatment of head lice (*Pediculosis capitis*) infestation

Contraindications There are no contraindications listed in the manufacturer's labeling

Warnings/Precautions For topical use on scalp and scalp hair only; avoid contact with eyes. Wash hands after application. The suspension contains benzyl alcohol.

Adverse Reactions (Reflective of adult population; not specific for elderly) 1% to 10%:

Dermatologic: Application site erythema (3%), application site irritation (1%), skin irritation

Ocular: Erythema (2%), hyperemia (2%), irritation

Drug Interactions

Metabolism/Transport Effects None known.

Avoid Concomitant Use There are no known interactions where it is recommended to avoid concomitant use.

Increased Effect/Toxicity There are no known significant interactions involving an increase in effect.

Decreased Effect There are no known significant interactions involving a decrease in effect.

Stability Store at 25°C (77°F); excursions permitted between 15°C to 30°C (59°F to 86°F).

Mechanism of Action Insect paralysis and death is caused by central nervous system excitation and involuntary muscle contractions. Spinosad is thought to be both pediculocidal and ovicidal (Stough, 2009).

Pharmacodynamics/Kinetics Absorption: Not absorbed topically (not detectable in a pediatric patient plasma sampling study); absorption of the benzyl alcohol was not analyzed in this study.

Dosage

Geriatric & Adult Head lice: Topical: Apply sufficient amount to cover dry scalp and completely cover dry hair; 120 mL may be necessary depending on the length of hair. If live lice are seen 7 days after first treatment, repeat with second application.

Administration Topical suspension. For external use only. Shake bottle well. Apply to dry scalp and rub gently until the scalp is thoroughly moistened, then apply to dry hair; completely covering scalp and hair. Leave on for 10 minutes (start timing treatment after the scalp and hair have been completely covered). The hair should then be rinsed thoroughly with warm water. Shampoo may be used immediately after the product is completely rinsed off. If live lice are seen 7 days after the first treatment, repeat with second application. Avoid contact with the eyes. Nit combing is not required, although a fine-tooth comb may be used to remove treated lice and nits.

Spinosad should be a portion of a whole lice removal program, which should include washing or dry cleaning all clothing, hats, bedding and towels recently worn or used by the patient and washing combs, brushes and hair accessories in hot water.

Monitoring Parameters Monitor scalp for lice

Special Geriatric Considerations Specific information on the safety and efficacy of spinosad in persons ≥65 years of age is not available as this age group was not sufficiently represented in clinical trials.

Dosage Forms Excipient information presented when available (limited, particularly for generics); consult specific product labeling.
Suspension, topical:
Natroba™: 0.9% (120 mL) [contains benzyl alcohol, isopropyl alcohol]

♦ **Spiriva® HandiHaler®** see Tiotropium on page 1907

Spironolactone (speer on oh LAK tone)

Related Information
Beers Criteria − Potentially Inappropriate Medications for Geriatrics on page 2183
Medication Safety Issues
Sound-alike/look-alike issues:
Aldactone® may be confused with Aldactazide®
BEERS Criteria medication:
This drug may be potentially inappropriate for use in geriatric patients (Quality of evidence - moderate; Strength of recommendation - strong).
International issues:
Aldactone: Brand name for spironolactone [U.S., Canada, multiple international markets], but also the brand name for potassium canrenoate [Austria, Czech Republic, Germany, Hungary, Poland]
Brand Names: U.S. Aldactone®
Brand Names: Canada Aldactone®; Novo-Spiroton; Teva-Spironolactone
Generic Availability (U.S.) Yes
Pharmacologic Category Diuretic, Potassium-Sparing; Selective Aldosterone Blocker
Use Management of edema associated with excessive aldosterone excretion; hypertension; primary hyperaldosteronism; hypokalemia; cirrhosis of liver accompanied by edema or ascites; nephrotic syndrome; severe heart failure (NYHA class III-IV) to increase survival and reduce hospitalization when added to standard therapy
Unlabeled Use Female acne (adjunctive therapy); hirsutism
Contraindications Anuria; acute renal insufficiency; significant impairment of renal excretory function; hyperkalemia
Warnings/Precautions Monitor serum potassium closely in patients being treated for heart failure. Avoid potassium supplements, potassium-containing salt substitutes, a diet rich in potassium, or other drugs that can cause hyperkalemia. Excess amounts can lead to profound diuresis with fluid and electrolyte loss; close medical supervision and dose evaluation are required. Watch for and correct electrolyte disturbances; adjust dose to avoid dehydration. In cirrhosis, avoid electrolyte and acid/base imbalances that might lead to hepatic encephalopathy. Gynecomastia is related to dose and duration of therapy. Discontinue use prior to adrenal vein catheterization. When evaluating a heart failure patient for spironolactone treatment, creatinine should be ≤2.5 mg/dL in men or ≤2 mg/dL in women and potassium <5 mEq/L. Discontinue or interrupt therapy if serum potassium >5 mEq/L or serum creatinine >4 mg/dL. **[U.S. Boxed Warning]: Shown to be a tumorigen in chronic toxicity animal studies. Avoid unnecessary use.**

In the elderly, avoid use of doses >25 mg/day in patients with heart failure or in patients with reduced renal function (Cl_{cr} <30 mL/minute); risk of hyperkalemia is increased for heart failure patients receiving >25 mg/day, particularly if taking concomitant medications such as NSAIDS, ACE inhibitor, angiotensin receptor blocker, or potassium supplements (Beers Criteria).

Adverse Reactions (Reflective of adult population; not specific for elderly) Frequency not defined.
Cardiovascular: Vasculitis
Central nervous system: Ataxia, confusion, drowsiness, fever, headache, lethargy
Dermatologic: Drug rash with eosinophilia and systemic symptoms (DRESS), maculopapular or erythematous cutaneous eruptions, Stevens-Johnson syndrome, toxic epidermal necrolysis, urticaria
Endocrine & metabolic: Amenorrhea, gynecomastia, hyperkalemia, impotence, irregular menses, postmenopausal bleeding
Gastrointestinal: Cramps, diarrhea, gastritis, gastric bleeding, nausea, ulceration, vomiting
Hematologic: Agranulocytosis
Hepatic: Cholestatic/hepatocellular toxicity
Renal: BUN increased, renal dysfunction, renal failure
Miscellaneous: Anaphylactic reaction, breast cancer

Drug Interactions

Metabolism/Transport Effects None known.

Avoid Concomitant Use

Avoid concomitant use of Spironolactone with any of the following: CycloSPORINE; Cyclo-SPORINE (Systemic); Tacrolimus; Tacrolimus (Systemic)

Increased Effect/Toxicity

Spironolactone may increase the levels/effects of: ACE Inhibitors; Amifostine; Ammonium Chloride; Antihypertensives; Cardiac Glycosides; CycloSPORINE; CycloSPORINE (Systemic); Digoxin; Hypotensive Agents; Neuromuscular-Blocking Agents (Nondepolarizing); RiTUXimab; Sodium Phosphates; Tacrolimus; Tacrolimus (Systemic)

The levels/effects of Spironolactone may be increased by: Alfuzosin; Angiotensin II Receptor Blockers; Diazoxide; Drospirenone; Eplerenone; Herbs (Hypotensive Properties); MAO Inhibitors; Nitrofurantoin; Nonsteroidal Anti-Inflammatory Agents; Pentoxifylline; Phosphodiesterase 5 Inhibitors; Potassium Salts; Prostacyclin Analogues; Tolvaptan; Trimethoprim

Decreased Effect

Spironolactone may decrease the levels/effects of: Alpha-/Beta-Agonists; Cardiac Glycosides; Mitotane; QuiNIDine

The levels/effects of Spironolactone may be decreased by: Herbs (Hypertensive Properties); Methylphenidate; Nonsteroidal Anti-Inflammatory Agents; Yohimbine

Ethanol/Nutrition/Herb Interactions

Ethanol: Increases risk of orthostasis.

Food: Food increases absorption.

Herb/Nutraceutical: Avoid natural licorice (due to mineralocorticoid activity)

Stability Store below 25°C (77°F).

Mechanism of Action Competes with aldosterone for receptor sites in the distal renal tubules, increasing sodium chloride and water excretion while conserving potassium and hydrogen ions; may block the effect of aldosterone on arteriolar smooth muscle as well

Pharmacodynamics/Kinetics

Duration: 2-3 days

Protein binding: 91% to 98%

Metabolism: Hepatic to multiple metabolites, including active metabolites canrenone and 7-alpha-spirolactone

Half-life elimination: Spironolactone: 78-84 minutes; Canrenone: 10-23 hours; 7-alpha-spirolactone: 7-20 hours

Time to peak, serum: 3-4 hours (primarily as the active metabolite)

Excretion: Urine and feces

Dosage

Geriatric Oral: Indication specific: Initial: 25-50 mg/day in 1-2 divided doses; increase by 25-50 mg every 5 days as needed. Adjust for renal impairment.

Adult To reduce delay in onset of effect, a loading dose of 2 or 3 times the daily dose may be administered on the first day of therapy.

Edema: Oral: 25-200 mg/day in 1-2 divided doses

Hypokalemia: Oral: 25-100 mg daily

Hypertension (JNC 7): Oral: 25-50 mg/day in 1-2 divided doses

Diagnosis of primary aldosteronism: Oral: Long test: 400 mg daily for 3-4 weeks; short test: 400 mg daily for 4 days; maintenance until surgical correction: 100-400 mg/day in 1-2 divided doses

Heart failure, severe (NYHA class III-IV; with ACE inhibitor and a loop diuretic ± digoxin): 12.5-25 mg/day; maximum daily dose: 50 mg. If 25 mg once daily not tolerated, reduce to 25 mg every other day was the lowest maintenance dose possible.

Note: If potassium >5 mEq/L or serum creatinine >4 mg/dL, discontinue or interrupt therapy.

Acne in women (unlabeled use): Oral: 25-200 mg once daily

Hirsutism in women (unlabeled use): Oral: 50-200 mg/day in 1-2 divided doses (Koulouri, 2008; Martin, 2008)

Renal Impairment Heart failure:

Cl_{cr} 31-50 mL/minute: Decrease initial dose to 12.5 mg once daily.

Cl_{cr} <30 mL/minute: Not recommended.

Monitoring Parameters Blood pressure, serum electrolytes (potassium, sodium), renal function, I & O ratios and daily weight throughout therapy

HF: Potassium levels and renal function should be checked in 3 days and 1 week after initiation or increase in dose, then every 2-4 weeks for 3 months, then quarterly for a year, then every 6 months thereafter.

Test Interactions May interfere with the radioimmunoassay for digoxin.

Pharmacotherapy Pearls Maximum diuretic effect may be delayed 2-3 days and maximum hypertensive effects may be delayed 2-3 weeks.

Special Geriatric Considerations When used in combination with ACE inhibitors, monitor patient for hyperkalemia.

This medication is considered to be potentially inappropriate in this patient population (Beers Criteria: Quality of evidence - moderate; Strength of recommendation - strong).

Dosage Forms Excipient information presented when available (limited, particularly for generics); consult specific product labeling.
Tablet, oral: 25 mg, 50 mg, 100 mg
Aldactone®: 25 mg
Aldactone®: 50 mg, 100 mg [scored]

Streptomycin (strep toe MYE sin)

Related Information
Antimicrobial Drugs of Choice on page 2163
Medication Safety Issues
Sound-alike/look-alike issues:
Streptomycin may be confused with streptozocin
Brand Names: Canada Streptomycin for Injection
Index Terms Streptomycin Sulfate
Generic Availability (U.S.) Yes
Pharmacologic Category Antibiotic, Aminoglycoside; Antitubercular Agent
Use Part of combination therapy of active tuberculosis; used in combination with other agents for treatment of bacteremia caused by susceptible gram-negative bacilli, brucellosis, chancroid granuloma inguinale, *H. influenzae* (respiratory, endocardial, meningeal infections), *K. pneumoniae*, plague, streptococcal or enterococcal endocarditis, tularemia, urinary tract infections (caused by *A. aerogenes, E. coli, E. faecalis, K. pneumoniae, Proteus* spp)
Unlabeled Use Buruli ulcer (*Mycobacterium ulcerans*), Ménière's disease, *Mycobacterium kansasii* infection
Contraindications Hypersensitivity to streptomycin or any component of the formulation
Warnings/Precautions [U.S. Boxed Warnings]: May cause neurotoxicity, nephrotoxicity, and/or neuromuscular blockade and respiratory paralysis; usual risk factors include pre-existing renal impairment, concomitant neuro-/nephrotoxic medications, advanced age and dehydration. The drug's neurotoxicity can result in respiratory paralysis from neuromuscular blockade, especially when the drug is given soon after anesthesia or muscle relaxants. Use with caution in patients with pre-existing vertigo, tinnitus, hearing loss, neuromuscular disorders, or renal impairment; modify dosage in patients with renal impairment; ototoxicity is directly proportional to the amount of drug given and the duration of treatment; tinnitus or vertigo are indications of vestibular injury and impending bilateral irreversible damage; renal ▶

damage is usually reversible. Monitor renal function closely; peak serum concentrations should not surpass 20-25 mcg/mL in patients with renal impairment. Formulation contains metabisulfite; may cause allergic reactions in patients with sulfite sensitivity. **[U.S. Boxed Warning]: Parenteral form should be used only where appropriate audiometric and laboratory testing facilities are available.** Prolonged use may result in fungal or bacterial superinfection, including *C. difficile*-associated diarrhea (CDAD) or pseudomembranous colitis; CDAD has been observed >2 months postantibiotic treatment. I.M. injections should be administered in a large muscle well within the body to avoid peripheral nerve damage and local skin reactions.

Adverse Reactions (Reflective of adult population; not specific for elderly) Frequency not defined.

Cardiovascular: Hypotension

Central nervous system: Drug fever, headache, neurotoxicity, paresthesia of face

Dermatologic: Angioedema, exfoliative dermatitis, skin rash, urticaria

Gastrointestinal: Nausea, vomiting

Hematologic: Eosinophilia, hemolytic anemia, leukopenia, pancytopenia, thrombocytopenia

Neuromuscular & skeletal: Arthralgia, tremor, weakness

Ocular: Amblyopia

Otic: Ototoxicity (auditory), ototoxicity (vestibular)

Renal: Azotemia, nephrotoxicity

Respiratory: Difficulty in breathing

Miscellaneous: Anaphylaxis

Drug Interactions

Metabolism/Transport Effects None known.

Avoid Concomitant Use

Avoid concomitant use of Streptomycin with any of the following: BCG; Gallium Nitrate

Increased Effect/Toxicity

Streptomycin may increase the levels/effects of: AbobotulinumtoxinA; Bisphosphonate Derivatives; CARBOplatin; Colistimethate; CycloSPORINE; CycloSPORINE (Systemic); Gallium Nitrate; Neuromuscular-Blocking Agents; OnabotulinumtoxinA; RimabotulinumtoxinB

The levels/effects of Streptomycin may be increased by: Amphotericin B; Capreomycin; Cephalosporins (2nd Generation); Cephalosporins (3rd Generation); Cephalosporins (4th Generation); CISplatin; Loop Diuretics; Nonsteroidal Anti-Inflammatory Agents; Vancomycin

Decreased Effect

Streptomycin may decrease the levels/effects of: BCG; Typhoid Vaccine

The levels/effects of Streptomycin may be decreased by: Penicillins

Stability

Lyophilized powder: Store dry powder at controlled room temperature 20°C to 25°C (68°F to 77°F). Protect from light.

Solution: Store in refrigerator at 2°C to 8°C (36°F to 46°F).

Depending upon manufacturer, reconstituted solution remains stable for 24 hours at room temperature. Exposure to light causes darkening of solution without apparent loss of potency.

Mechanism of Action Inhibits bacterial protein synthesis by binding directly to the 30S ribosomal subunits causing faulty peptide sequence to form in the protein chain

Pharmacodynamics/Kinetics

Absorption: Oral: Poorly absorbed; I.M.: Well absorbed

Distribution: To extracellular fluid including serum, abscesses, ascitic, pericardial, pleural, synovial, lymphatic, and peritoneal fluids; poorly distributed into CSF

Half-life elimination: Adults: ~5 hours

Time to peak: I.M.: Within 1 hour

Excretion: Urine (29% to 89% as unchanged drug); feces, saliva, sweat, and tears (minimal)

Dosage

Geriatric I.M.: Manufacturer states dose reductions are necessary in patients >60 years.

Adult Note: For I.M. administration; I.V. use is not recommended.

Usual dosage range: I.M.: 15-30 mg/kg/day or 1-2 g daily

Indication-specific dosing:

Brucellosis: I.M.: 1 g daily in 2-4 divided doses for 14-21 days (with doxycycline) (Skalsky, 2008)

Endocarditis:

Enterococcal: I.M.: 1 g every 12 hours for 2 weeks, 500 mg every 12 hours for 4 weeks in combination with penicillin

Streptococcal: I.M.: 1 g every 12 hours for 1 week, 500 mg every 12 hours for 1 week in combination with penicillin. **Note:** For patients >60 years, 500 mg every 12 hours for 2 weeks is recommended.

***Mycobacterium avium* complex:** I.M.: Adjunct therapy (with macrolide, rifamycin, and ethambutol): 8-25 mg/kg 3 times weekly for first 2-3 months for severe disease (maximum single dose for age ≥50 years: 500 mg) (Griffith, 2007)

***Mycobacterium kansasii* disease (rifampin-resistant):** I.M.: 750 mg to 1 g daily (as part of a three-drug regimen based on susceptibilities) (Campbell, 2000; Griffith, 2007)

***Mycobacterium ulcerans* (Buruli ulcers):** I.M.: 15 mg/kg once daily for 8 weeks (WHO, 2004)

Plague: I.M.: 30 mg/kg/day (or 2 g) divided every 12 hours until the patient is afebrile for at least 3 days. **Note:** Full course is considered 10 days (WHO, 2010).

Tuberculosis: I.M.:

Daily therapy: 15 mg/kg/day (maximum: 1 g)

Directly observed therapy (DOT), twice weekly: 25-30 mg/kg (maximum: 1.5 g)

Directly observed therapy (DOT), 3 times weekly: 25-30 mg/kg (maximum: 1.5 g)

Tularemia: I.M.:

Manufacturer's labeling: 1-2 g daily in divided doses every 12 hours (maximum: 2 g daily) for 7-14 days until the patients is afebrile for 5-7 days

Alternative regimen: 2 g daily in 2 divided doses (maximum: 2 g daily) for 10 days (WHO, 2007)

Renal Impairment The following adjustments have been recommended (Aronoff, 2007):

Cl_{cr} 10-50 mL/minute: Administer every 24-72 hours.

Cl_{cr} <10 mL/minute: Administer every 72-96 hours.

Intermittent hemodialysis (IHD): One-half the dose administered after hemodialysis on dialysis days. **Note:** Dosing dependent on the assumption of 3 times weekly complete IHD sessions.

Peritoneal dialysis (PD): Administration via PD fluid: 20-40 mg/L (20-40 mcg/mL) of PD fluid

Continuous renal replacement therapy (CRRT): Administer every 24-72 hours; monitor levels (Aronoff, 2007). **Note:** Drug clearance is highly dependent on the method of renal replacement, filter type, and flow rate. Appropriate dosing requires close monitoring of pharmacologic response, signs of adverse reactions due to drug accumulation, as well as drug concentrations in relation to target trough (if appropriate).

Administration Inject deep I.M. into large muscle mass; I.V. administration is not recommended

Monitoring Parameters Hearing (audiogram), BUN, creatinine; serum concentration of the drug should be monitored in all patients; eighth cranial nerve damage is usually preceded by high-pitched tinnitus, roaring noises, sense of fullness in ears, or impaired hearing and may persist for weeks after drug is discontinued

Reference Range Therapeutic: Peak: 20-30 mcg/mL; Trough: <5 mcg/mL; Toxic: Peak: >50 mcg/mL; Trough: >10 mcg/mL

Pharmacotherapy Pearls Eighth cranial nerve damage is usually preceded by high-pitched tinnitus, roaring noises, sense of fullness in ears, or impaired hearing and may persist for weeks after drug is discontinued.

Special Geriatric Considerations Streptomycin is indicated for persons from endemic areas of drug-resistant *Mycobacterium tuberculosis* or who are HIV infected. Since most older patients acquired the *M. tuberculosis* infection prior to the availability of effective chemotherapy, isoniazid and rifampin are usually effective unless resistant organisms are suspected or the patient is HIV infected. Adjust dose interval for renal function.

Dosage Forms Excipient information presented when available (limited, particularly for generics); consult specific product labeling.

Injection, powder for reconstitution: 1 g

◆ **Streptomycin Sulfate** *see* Streptomycin *on page 1807*
◆ **Striant®** *see* Testosterone *on page 1861*
◆ **Stridex® Essential Care® [OTC]** *see* Salicylic Acid *on page 1743*
◆ **Stridex® Facewipes To Go® [OTC]** *see* Salicylic Acid *on page 1743*
◆ **Stridex® Maximum Strength [OTC]** *see* Salicylic Acid *on page 1743*
◆ **Stridex® Sensitive Skin [OTC]** *see* Salicylic Acid *on page 1743*
◆ **Strong Iodine Solution** *see* Potassium Iodide and Iodine *on page 1575*
◆ **Subsys®** *see* FentaNYL *on page 761*
◆ **Subutex® [DSC]** *see* Buprenorphine *on page 237*

Sucralfate (soo KRAL fate)

Medication Safety Issues
Sound-alike/look-alike issues:
Sucralfate may be confused with salsalate
Carafate® may be confused with Cafergot®
Brand Names: U.S. Carafate®
Brand Names: Canada Apo-Sucralfate; Dom-Sucralfate; Novo-Sucralate; Nu-Sucralate; PMS-Sucralate; Sucralfate-1; Sulcrate®; Sulcrate® Suspension Plus; Teva-Sucralfate
Index Terms Aluminum Sucrose Sulfate, Basic
Generic Availability (U.S.) Yes
Pharmacologic Category Gastrointestinal Agent, Miscellaneous
Use Short-term (≤8 weeks) management of duodenal ulcers; maintenance therapy for duodenal ulcers
Unlabeled Use Treatment of gastric ulcers, stomatitis due to cancer chemotherapy and other causes of esophageal and gastric erosions (suspension), GERD, esophagitis, NSAID mucosal damage; prevention of stress ulcers; postsclerotherapy for esophageal variceal bleeding
Contraindications Hypersensitivity to sucralfate or any component of the formulation
Warnings/Precautions Because sucralfate acts locally at the ulcer site, successful therapy with sucralfate should not be expected to alter the posthealing frequency of recurrence or the severity of duodenal ulceration. Use with caution in patients with chronic renal failure; sucralfate is an aluminum complex, small amounts of aluminum are absorbed following oral administration. Excretion of aluminum may be decreased in patients with chronic renal failure. Because of the potential for sucralfate to alter the absorption of some drugs, separate administration (take other medication 2 hours before sucralfate) should be considered when alterations in bioavailability are believed to be critical.
Adverse Reactions (Reflective of adult population; not specific for elderly) 1% to 10%: Gastrointestinal: Constipation (2%)
Drug Interactions
Metabolism/Transport Effects None known.
Avoid Concomitant Use
Avoid concomitant use of Sucralfate with any of the following: Vitamin D Analogs
Increased Effect/Toxicity
The levels/effects of Sucralfate may be increased by: Vitamin D Analogs
Decreased Effect
Sucralfate may decrease the levels/effects of: Antifungal Agents (Azole Derivatives, Systemic); Digoxin; Eltrombopag; Furosemide; Levothyroxine; Phosphate Supplements; QuiNIDine; Quinolone Antibiotics; Tetracycline Derivatives; Vitamin K Antagonists
Ethanol/Nutrition/Herb Interactions Food: Sucralfate may interfere with absorption of vitamin A, vitamin D, vitamin E, and vitamin K.
Stability Suspension: Shake well. Store at 20°C to 25°C (68°F to 77°F); do **not** freeze.
Mechanism of Action Forms a complex by binding with positively charged proteins in exudates, forming a viscous paste-like, adhesive substance. This selectively forms a protective coating that acts locally to protect the gastric lining against peptic acid, pepsin, and bile salts.
Pharmacodynamics/Kinetics
Onset of action: Paste formation and ulcer adhesion: 1-2 hours
Duration: Up to 6 hours
Absorption: Oral: <5%
Distribution: Acts locally at ulcer sites; unbound in GI tract to aluminum and sucrose octasulfate
Metabolism: None
Excretion: Urine (small amounts as unchanged compounds)
Dosage
Geriatric & Adult
Stress ulcer prophylaxis (unlabeled use): Oral: 1 g 4 times/day
Stress ulcer treatment (unlabeled use): Oral: 1 g every 4 hours
Treatment of duodenal ulcer: Oral:
Initial treatment: 1 g 4 times/day, 1 hour before meals or food and at bedtime for 4-8 weeks, or alternatively 2 g twice daily; treatment is recommended for 4-8 weeks in adults
Maintenance/prophylaxis of duodenal ulcer: 1 g twice daily
Stomatitis (unlabeled use): Oral: 10 mL (1 g/10 mL suspension); swish and spit or swish and swallow 4 times/day.

Renal Impairment Aluminum salt is minimally absorbed (<5%), however, may accumulate in renal failure.

Administration Tablet may be broken or dissolved in water before ingestion. Administer with water on an empty stomach.

Monitoring Parameters Monitor signs and symptoms of disease process and adverse effects; evaluate by endoscopic examination or x-ray

Pharmacotherapy Pearls May decrease gastric emptying; many trials have demonstrated sucralfate is equivalent in efficacy to antacids and H_2 blockers; equivalence of sucralfate suspension to sucralfate tablets has not been established in studies

Special Geriatric Considerations Caution should be used in the elderly due to reduced renal function. Patients with Cl_{cr} <30 mL/minute may be at risk for aluminum intoxication. Due to low side effect profile, this may be an agent of choice in the elderly with PUD.

Dosage Forms Excipient information presented when available (limited, particularly for generics); consult specific product labeling.

Suspension, oral: 1 g/10 mL (10 mL)
  Carafate®: 1 g/10 mL (420 mL)
Tablet, oral: 1 g
  Carafate®: 1 g [scored]

◆ **Sudafed** see Pseudoephedrine on page 1633
◆ **Sudafed® 12 Hour [OTC]** see Pseudoephedrine on page 1633
◆ **Sudafed® 24 Hour [OTC]** see Pseudoephedrine on page 1633
◆ **Sudafed® Children's [OTC]** see Pseudoephedrine on page 1633
◆ **Sudafed® Maximum Strength Nasal Decongestant [OTC]** see Pseudoephedrine on page 1633
◆ **Sudafed PE® Children's [OTC]** see Phenylephrine (Systemic) on page 1523
◆ **Sudafed PE® Congestion [OTC]** see Phenylephrine (Systemic) on page 1523
◆ **Sudafed PE™ Nasal Decongestant [OTC]** see Phenylephrine (Systemic) on page 1523
◆ **Sudafed PE® Pressure + Pain [OTC]** see Acetaminophen and Phenylephrine on page 37
◆ **SudoGest [OTC]** see Pseudoephedrine on page 1633
◆ **SudoGest 12 Hour [OTC]** see Pseudoephedrine on page 1633
◆ **SudoGest Children's [OTC] [DSC]** see Pseudoephedrine on page 1633
◆ **Sudogest™ PE [OTC]** see Phenylephrine (Systemic) on page 1523
◆ **Sudo-Tab® [OTC]** see Pseudoephedrine on page 1633
◆ **Sulamyd** see Sulfacetamide (Ophthalmic) on page 1811
◆ **Sulamyd** see Sulfacetamide (Topical) on page 1812
◆ **Sular®** see Nisoldipine on page 1381
◆ **Sulbactam and Ampicillin** see Ampicillin and Sulbactam on page 130

Sulfacetamide (Ophthalmic) (sul fa SEE ta mide)

Medication Safety Issues
Sound-alike/look-alike issues:
  Bleph®-10 may be confused with Blephamide®

Brand Names: U.S. Bleph®-10; Sulfamide

Brand Names: Canada AK Sulf Liq; Bleph 10 DPS; Diosulf™; PMS-Sulfacetamide; Sodium Sulamyd

Index Terms Sodium Sulfacetamide; Sulamyd; Sulfacetamide Sodium

Generic Availability (U.S.) Yes

Pharmacologic Category Antibiotic, Ophthalmic

Use Treatment and prophylaxis of conjunctivitis and other superficial ocular infections due to susceptible organisms; adjunctive treatment with systemic sulfonamides for therapy of trachoma

Dosage
Geriatric & Adult
Conjunctivitis: Ophthalmic:
  Ointment: Instill ½" (1.25 cm) ribbon into the conjunctival sac of affected eye(s) every 3-4 hours and at bedtime; increase dosing interval as condition responds. Usual duration of treatment: 7-10 days.
  Solution: Instill 1-2 drops several times daily up to every 2-3 hours in lower conjunctival sac during waking hours and less frequently at night; increase dosing interval as condition responds. Usual duration of treatment: 7-10 days
Trachoma: Ophthalmic: Solution: Instill 2 drops into the conjunctival sac every 2 hours; must be used in conjunction with systemic therapy

Special Geriatric Considerations Evaluate the patient's or caregiver's ability to safely administer the correct dose of ophthalmic medication.

◀ **Dosage Forms** Excipient information presented when available (limited, particularly for generics); consult specific product labeling.
Ointment, ophthalmic, as sodium: 10% (3.5 g)
Solution, ophthalmic, as sodium [drops]: 10% (15 mL)
  Bleph®-10: 10% (5 mL) [contains benzalkonium chloride]
  Sulfamide: 10% (15 mL)

Sulfacetamide (Topical) (sul fa SEE ta mide)

Medication Safety Issues
  Sound-alike/look-alike issues:
    Klaron® may be confused with Klor-Con®
Brand Names: U.S. Klaron®; Ovace®; Ovace® Plus; Seb-Prev™ [DSC]
Brand Names: Canada Sulfacet-R
Index Terms Sodium Sulfacetamide; Sulamyd; Sulfacetamide Sodium
Generic Availability (U.S.) Yes: Lotion, pad, suspension
Pharmacologic Category Acne Products; Antibiotic, Sulfonamide Derivative; Topical Skin Product, Acne
Use
  Cleansing gel, wash: Scaling dermatoses (seborrheic dermatitis and seborrhea sicca [dandruff]); bacterial infections of the skin
  Lotion: Acne vulgaris
  Shampoo: Scaling dermatoses (seborrheic dermatitis and seborrhea sicca [dandruff])
Dosage
  Geriatric & Adult
    Acne: Topical: Lotion: Apply thin film to affected area twice daily
    Seborrheic dermatitis: Topical:
      Cleansing gel, wash: Wash affected areas twice daily; repeat application for 8-10 days. Dosing interval may be increased as eruption subsides. Applications once or twice weekly, or every other week may be used for prevention. If treatment needs to be reinitiated, start therapy as a twice daily regimen.
      Shampoo: Wash hair at least twice weekly
    Secondary cutaneous bacterial infections: Topical: Cleansing gel, wash: Apply to affected areas daily; duration of therapy is usually for 8-10 days
Special Geriatric Considerations Assess whether patient can adequately use topically.
Dosage Forms Excipient information presented when available (limited, particularly for generics); consult specific product labeling. [DSC] = Discontinued product
  Aerosol, foam, topical, as sodium:
    Ovace®: 10% (70 g [DSC])
  Cream, topical, as sodium:
    Seb-Prev™: 10% (30 g [DSC], 60 g [DSC]) [contains benzyl alcohol]
  Gel, topical, as sodium:
    Seb-Prev™: 10% (30 g [DSC], 60 g [DSC])
  Gel, topical, as sodium [emulsion-based/wash]:
    Ovace® Plus: 10% (355 mL)
  Lotion, topical, as sodium: 10% (118 mL)
    Klaron®: 10% (118 mL) [contains sodium metabisulfite]
  Lotion, topical, as sodium [wash]: 10% (177 mL, 354.8 mL)
    Ovace®: 10% (180 mL [DSC], 355 mL, 360 mL [DSC])
  Pad, topical, as sodium: 10% (30s)
  Shampoo, topical, as sodium:
    Ovace® Plus: 10% (237 mL)
  Soap, topical, as sodium [wash]:
    Seb-Prev™: 10% (170 mL [DSC], 340 mL [DSC])
  Suspension, topical, as sodium: 10% (118 mL)

Sulfacetamide and Prednisolone (sul fa SEE ta mide & pred NIS oh lone)

Related Information
  PrednisoLONE (Ophthalmic) *on page 1594*
  Sulfacetamide (Ophthalmic) *on page 1811*
Medication Safety Issues
  Sound-alike/look-alike issues:
    Blephamide® may be confused with Bleph®-10
Brand Names: U.S. Blephamide®
Brand Names: Canada AK Cide Oph; Blephamide®; Dioptimyd®

Index Terms Prednisolone and Sulfacetamide

Generic Availability (U.S.) Yes: Solution

Pharmacologic Category Antibiotic/Corticosteroid, Ophthalmic

Use Steroid-responsive inflammatory ocular conditions in which a corticosteroid is indicated and where infection is present or there is a risk of infection

Dosage

Geriatric & Adult Conjunctivitis: Ophthalmic:

Ointment: Apply ~1/2 inch ribbon to lower conjunctival sac 3-4 times/day and 1-2 times at night

Solution: Instill 2 drops every 4 hours

Suspension: Instill 2 drops every 4 hours during the day and at bedtime

Special Geriatric Considerations Evaluate the patient's or caregiver's ability to safely administer the correct dose of ophthalmic medication.

Dosage Forms Excipient information presented when available (limited, particularly for generics); consult specific product labeling.

Ointment, ophthalmic:

Blephamide®: Sulfacetamide sodium 10% and prednisolone acetate 0.2% (3.5 g)

Solution, ophthalmic [drops]: Sulfacetamide sodium 10% and prednisolone sodium phosphate 0.25% (5 mL, 10 mL)

Suspension, ophthalmic [drops]:

Blephamide®: Sulfacetamide sodium 10% and prednisolone acetate 0.2% (5 mL, 10 mL) [contains benzalkonium chloride]

- ◆ **Sulfacetamide Sodium** *see* Sulfacetamide (Ophthalmic) *on page 1811*
- ◆ **Sulfacetamide Sodium** *see* Sulfacetamide (Topical) *on page 1812*

Sulfamethoxazole and Trimethoprim
(sul fa meth OKS a zole & trye METH oh prim)

Related Information

Antimicrobial Drugs of Choice *on page 2163*
Trimethoprim *on page 1971*

Medication Safety Issues

Sound-alike/look-alike issues:

Bactrim™ may be confused with bacitracin, Bactine®, Bactroban®

Co-trimoxazole may be confused with clotrimazole

Septra® may be confused with Ceptaz, Sectral®

Septra® DS may be confused with Semprex®-D

Brand Names: U.S. Bactrim™; Bactrim™ DS; Septra® DS

Brand Names: Canada Apo-Sulfatrim®; Apo-Sulfatrim® DS; Apo-Sulfatrim® Pediatric; Novo-Trimel; Novo-Trimel D.S.; Nu-Cotrimox; Septra® Injection

Index Terms Co-Trimoxazole; Septra; SMX-TMP; SMZ-TMP; Sulfatrim; TMP-SMX; TMP-SMZ; Trimethoprim and Sulfamethoxazole

Generic Availability (U.S.) Yes

Pharmacologic Category Antibiotic, Miscellaneous; Antibiotic, Sulfonamide Derivative

Use

Oral treatment of urinary tract infections due to *E. coli*, *Klebsiella* and *Enterobacter* sp, *M. morganii*, *P. mirabilis* and *P. vulgaris*; acute exacerbations of chronic bronchitis in adults due to susceptible strains of *H. influenzae* or *S. pneumoniae*; treatment and prophylaxis of *Pneumocystis jirovecii* pneumonia (PCP); traveler's diarrhea due to enterotoxigenic *E. coli*; treatment of enteritis caused by *Shigella flexneri* or *Shigella sonnei*

I.V. treatment of severe or complicated infections when oral therapy is not feasible, for documented PCP, empiric treatment of PCP in immune compromised patients; treatment of documented or suspected shigellosis, typhoid fever, or other infections caused by susceptible bacteria

Unlabeled Use Cholera and *Salmonella*-type infections and nocardiosis; chronic prostatitis; as prophylaxis in neutropenic patients with *P. jirovecii* infections, in leukemia patients, and in patients following renal transplantation, to decrease incidence of PCP; treatment of *Cyclospora* infection, typhoid fever, *Nocardia asteroides* infection; prophylaxis against urinary tract infection; alternative treatment for MRSA infections

Contraindications Hypersensitivity to any sulfa drug, trimethoprim, or any component of the formulation; megaloblastic anemia due to folate deficiency; marked hepatic damage or severe renal disease (if patient not monitored)

Warnings/Precautions Use with caution in patients with G6PD deficiency, impaired renal or hepatic function or potential folate deficiency (malnourished, chronic anticonvulsant therapy, or elderly); maintain adequate hydration to prevent crystalluria; adjust dosage in patients with renal impairment. Injection vehicle contains benzyl alcohol and sodium metabisulfite.

Chemical similarities are present among sulfonamides, sulfonylureas, carbonic anhydrase inhibitors, thiazides, and loop diuretics (except ethacrynic acid). Use in patients with sulfonamide allergy is specifically contraindicated in product labeling, however, a risk of cross-reaction exists in patients with allergy to any of these compounds; avoid use when previous reaction has been severe.

Fatalities associated with severe reactions including Stevens-Johnson syndrome, toxic epidermal necrolysis, hepatic necrosis, agranulocytosis, aplastic anemia, and other blood dyscrasias; discontinue use at first sign of rash or serious adverse reactions. Elderly patients appear at greater risk for more severe adverse reactions. May cause hypoglycemia, particularly in malnourished, or patients with renal or hepatic impairment. Use with caution in patients with porphyria or thyroid dysfunction. Slow acetylators may be more prone to adverse reactions. Caution in patients with allergies or asthma. May cause hyperkalemia (associated with high doses of trimethoprim). Incidence of adverse effects appears to be increased in patients with AIDS. Prolonged use may result in fungal or bacterial super-infection, including *C. difficile*-associated diarrhea (CDAD) and pseudomembranous colitis; CDAD has been observed >2 months postantibiotic treatment.

Adverse Reactions (Reflective of adult population; not specific for elderly) The most common adverse reactions include gastrointestinal upset (nausea, vomiting, anorexia) and dermatologic reactions (rash or urticaria). Rare, life-threatening reactions have been associated with co-trimoxazole, including severe dermatologic reactions, blood dyscrasias, and hepatotoxic reactions. Most other reactions listed are rare, however, frequency cannot be accurately estimated.

Cardiovascular: Allergic myocarditis

Central nervous system: Apathy, aseptic meningitis, ataxia, chills, depression, fatigue, fever, hallucinations, headache, insomnia, kernicterus (in neonates), nervousness, peripheral neuritis, seizure, vertigo

Dermatologic: Photosensitivity, pruritus, rash, skin eruptions, urticaria; rare reactions include erythema multiforme, exfoliative dermatitis, Henoch-Schönlein purpura, Stevens-Johnson syndrome, and toxic epidermal necrolysis

Endocrine & metabolic: Hyperkalemia (generally at high dosages), hypoglycemia (rare), hyponatremia

Gastrointestinal: Abdominal pain, anorexia, diarrhea, glottitis, nausea, pancreatitis, pseudomembranous colitis, stomatitis, vomiting

Hematologic: Agranulocytosis, aplastic anemia, eosinophilia, hemolysis (with G6PD deficiency), hemolytic anemia, hypoprothrombinemia, leukopenia, megaloblastic anemia, methemoglobinemia, neutropenia, thrombocytopenia

Hepatic: Hepatotoxicity (including hepatitis, cholestasis, and hepatic necrosis), hyperbilirubinemia, transaminases increased

Neuromuscular & skeletal: Arthralgia, myalgia, rhabdomyolysis, weakness

Otic: Tinnitus

Renal: BUN increased, crystalluria, diuresis (rare), interstitial nephritis, nephrotoxicity (in association with cyclosporine), renal failure, serum creatinine increased, toxic nephrosis (with anuria and oliguria)

Respiratory: Cough, dyspnea, pulmonary infiltrates

Miscellaneous: Allergic reaction, anaphylaxis, angioedema, periarteritis nodosa (rare), serum sickness, systemic lupus erythematosus (rare)

Drug Interactions

Metabolism/Transport Effects Refer to individual components.

Avoid Concomitant Use

Avoid concomitant use of Sulfamethoxazole and Trimethoprim with any of the following: BCG; Dofetilide; Methenamine; Potassium P-Aminobenzoate; Procaine

Increased Effect/Toxicity

Sulfamethoxazole and Trimethoprim may increase the levels/effects of: ACE Inhibitors; Amantadine; Angiotensin II Receptor Blockers; Antidiabetic Agents (Thiazolidinedione); AzaTHIOprine; Carvedilol; CycloSPORINE; CycloSPORINE (Systemic); CYP2C8 Substrates; CYP2C9 Substrates; Dapsone; Dapsone (Systemic); Dapsone (Topical); Dofetilide; Eplerenone; Fosphenytoin; Highest Risk QTc-Prolonging Agents; LamiVUDine; Memantine; Mercaptopurine; Methotrexate; Moderate Risk QTc-Prolonging Agents; Phenytoin; Porfimer; PRALAtrexate; Prilocaine; Procainamide; Repaglinide; Spironolactone; Sulfonylureas; Varenicline; Vitamin K Antagonists

The levels/effects of Sulfamethoxazole and Trimethoprim may be increased by: Amantadine; CYP2C9 Inhibitors (Moderate); CYP2C9 Inhibitors (Strong); Dapsone; Dapsone (Systemic); Memantine; Methenamine; Mifepristone

Decreased Effect

Sulfamethoxazole and Trimethoprim may decrease the levels/effects of: BCG; CycloSPOR-INE; CycloSPORINE (Systemic); Typhoid Vaccine

The levels/effects of Sulfamethoxazole and Trimethoprim may be decreased by: CYP2C9 Inducers (Strong); CYP3A4 Inducers (Strong); Deferasirox; Herbs (CYP3A4 Inducers); Leucovorin Calcium-Levoleucovorin; Peginterferon Alfa-2b; Potassium P-Aminobenzoate; Procaine; Tocilizumab

Ethanol/Nutrition/Herb Interactions Herb/Nutraceutical: Avoid dong quai; St John's wort (may diminish effects and also cause photosensitization).

Stability

Injection: Store at room temperature; do not refrigerate. Less soluble in more alkaline pH. Protect from light. Solution must be diluted prior to administration. Following dilution, store at room temperature; do not refrigerate. Manufacturer recommended dilutions and stability of parenteral admixture at room temperature (25°C):

5 mL/125 mL D_5W; stable for 6 hours.

5 mL/100 mL D_5W; stable for 4 hours.

5 mL/75 mL D_5W; stable for 2 hours.

Studies have also confirmed limited stability in NS; detailed references should be consulted. Suspension, tablet: Store at controlled room temperature of 15°C to 25°C (59°F to 77°F). Protect from light.

Mechanism of Action Sulfamethoxazole interferes with bacterial folic acid synthesis and growth via inhibition of dihydrofolic acid formation from para-aminobenzoic acid; trimethoprim inhibits dihydrofolic acid reduction to tetrahydrofolate resulting in sequential inhibition of enzymes of the folic acid pathway

Pharmacodynamics/Kinetics

Absorption: Oral: Almost completely, 90% to 100%

Protein binding: SMX: 68%, TMP: 45%

Metabolism: SMX: N-acetylated and glucuronidated; TMP: Metabolized to oxide and hydroxy-lated metabolites

Half-life elimination: SMX: 9 hours, TMP: 6-17 hours; both are prolonged in renal failure

Time to peak, serum: Within 1-4 hours

Excretion: Both are excreted in urine as metabolites and unchanged drug

Effects of aging on the pharmacokinetics of both agents has been variable; increase in half-life and decreases in clearance have been associated with reduced creatinine clearance

Dosage

Geriatric & Adult Dosage recommendations are based on the trimethoprim component. double-strength tablets are equivalent to sulfamethoxazole 800 mg and trimethoprim 160 mg.

General dosing guidelines:

Oral: 1-2 double-strength tablets (sulfamethoxazole 800 mg; trimethoprim 160 mg) every 12-24 hours

I.V.: 8-20 mg TMP/kg/day divided every 6-12 hours

Chronic bronchitis (acute): Oral: One double-strength tablet every 12 hours for 10-14 days

Cyclosporiasis (unlabeled use): Oral, I.V.: 160 mg TMP twice daily for 7-10 days. **Note:** AIDS patients: Oral: One double-strength tablet 2-4 times/day for 10 days, then 1 double-strength tablet 3 times/week for 10 weeks (Pape, 1994; Verdier, 2000).

Granuloma inguinale (donovanosis) (unlabeled use): Oral: One double-strength tablet every 12 hours for at least 3 weeks and until lesions have healed (CDC, 2010)

Isosporiasis (*Isospora belli* infection) in HIV-positive patients (unlabeled use; CDC, 2009):

Treatment: Oral, I.V.: 160 mg TMP 4 times/day for 10 days **or** 160 mg TMP 2 times/day for 7-10 days. May increase dose and/or duration up to 3-4 weeks if symptoms worsen or persist

Secondary prophylaxis (in patients with CD4+ count <200 /microL): Oral: 160 mg TMP 3 times/week (preferred) **or** alternatively, 160 mg TMP daily **or** 320 mg TMP 3 times/week

Meningitis (bacterial): I.V.: 10-20 mg TMP/kg/day in divided doses every 6-12 hours

Nocardia (unlabeled use): Oral, I.V.:

Cutaneous infections: 5-10 mg TMP/kg/day in 2-4 divided doses

Severe infections (pulmonary/cerebral): 15 mg TMP/kg/day in 2-4 divided doses for 3-4 weeks, then 10 mg TMP/kg/day in 2-4 divided doses. Treatment duration is controversial; an average of 7 months has been reported.

Note: Therapy for severe infection may be initiated I.V. and converted to oral therapy (frequently converted to approximate dosages of oral solid dosage forms: 2 DS tablets every 8-12 hours). Although not widely available, sulfonamide levels should be considered in patients with questionable absorption, at risk for dose-related toxicity, or those with poor therapeutic response.

Osteomyelitis due to MRSA (unlabeled use): Oral, I.V.: 3.5-4 mg TMP/kg/dose every 8-12 hours for a minimum of 8 weeks with rifampin 600 mg once daily (Liu, 2011)

***Pneumocystis jirovecii* pneumonia (PCP):** Oral: Manufacturer's labeling:

Prophylaxis: 160 mg TMP daily

Treatment: 15-20 mg TMP/kg/day divided every 6 hours for 14-21 days

***Pneumocystis jirovecii* pneumonia (PCP) prophylaxis and treatment in HIV-positive patients (CDC, 2009): Note:** Sulfamethoxazole and trimethoprim is the preferred regimen for this indication.

Prophylaxis: Oral: 80-160 mg TMP daily **or** alternatively, 160 mg TMP 3 times/week

Treatment:

Mild-to-moderate: Oral: 15-20 mg TMP/kg/day in 3 divided doses for 21 days **or** alternatively, 320 mg TMP 3 times/day for 21 days

Moderate-to-severe: Oral, I.V.: 15-20 mg TMP/kg/day in 3-4 divided doses for 21 days

Sepsis: I.V.: 20 TMP/kg/day divided every 6 hours

Septic arthritis due to MRSA (unlabeled use): Oral, I.V.: 3.5-4 mg TMP/kg/dose every 8-12 hours for 3-4 weeks (some experts combine with rifampin) (Liu, 2011)

Shigellosis:

Oral: One double-strength tablet every 12 hours for 5 days

I.V.: 8-10 mg TMP/kg/day in divided doses every 6, 8, or 12 hours for up to 5 days

Skin/soft tissue infection due to community-acquired MRSA (unlabeled use): Oral: 1-2 double-strength tablets every 12 hours for 5-10 days (Liu, 2011); **Note:** If beta-hemolytic *Streptococcus* spp are also suspected, a beta-lactam antibiotic should be added to the regimen (Liu, 2011)

***Stenotrophomonas maltophilia* (ventilator-associated pneumonia):** I.V.: Most clinicians have utilized 12-15 mg TMP/kg/day for the treatment of VAP caused by *Stenotrophomonas maltophilia*. Higher doses (up to 20 mg TMP/kg/day) have been mentioned for treatment of severe infection in patients with normal renal function (Looney, 2009; Vartivarian, 1989; Wood, 2010)

***Toxoplasma gondii* encephalitis (unlabeled use; CDC, 2009):** Oral:

Primary prophylaxis: Oral: 160 mg TMP daily (preferred) **or** 160 mg TMP 3 times/week **or** 80 mg TMP daily

Treatment (alternative to sulfadiazine, pyrimethamine and leucovorin calcium): Oral, I.V.: 5 mg/kg TMP twice daily

Travelers' diarrhea: Oral: One double-strength tablet every 12 hours for 5 days

Urinary tract infection:

Oral: One double-strength tablet every 12 hours

Duration of therapy: Uncomplicated: 3-5 days; Complicated: 7-10 days

Pyelonephritis: 14 days

Prostatitis: Acute: 2 weeks; Chronic: 2-3 months

I.V.: 8-10 mg TMP/kg/day in divided doses every 6, 8, or 12 hours for up to 14 days with severe infections

Renal Impairment Oral, I.V.:

Manufacturer's recommendation: Adults:

Cl_{cr} >30 mL/minute: No dosage adjustment required

Cl_{cr} 15-30 mL/minute: Administer 50% of recommended dose

Cl_{cr} <15 mL/minute: Use is not recommended

Alternate recommendations:

Cl_{cr} 15-30 mL/minute:

Treatment: Administer full daily dose (divided every 12 hours) for 24-48 hours, then decrease daily dose by 50% and administer every 24 hours (**Note:** For serious infections including *Pneumocystis jirovecii* pneumonia (PCP), full daily dose is given in divided doses every 6-8 hours for 2 days, followed by reduction to 50% daily dose divided every 12 hours) (Nahata, 1995).

PCP prophylaxis: One-half single-strength tablet (40 mg trimethoprim) daily **or** 1 single-strength tablet (80 mg trimethoprim) daily or 3 times weekly (Masur, 2002).

Cl_{cr} <15 mL/minute:

Treatment: Administer full daily dose every 48 hours (Nahata, 1995)

PCP prophylaxis: One-half single-strength tablet (40 mg trimethoprim) daily **or** 1 single-strength tablet (80 mg trimethoprim) 3 times weekly (Masur, 2002). While the guidelines do acknowledge the alternative of giving 1 single-strength tablet daily, this may be inadvisable in the uremic/ESRD patient.

Intermittent Hemodialysis (IHD) (administer after hemodialysis on dialysis days):

Treatment: Full daily dose before dialysis and 50% dose after dialysis (Nahata, 1995)

PCP prophylaxis: One single-strength tablet (80 mg trimethoprim) after each dialysis session (Masur, 2002)

Note: Dosing dependent on the assumption of 3 times/week, complete IHD sessions.

Peritoneal dialysis (PD):
  Use Cl_{cr} <15 mL/minute dosing recommendations. Not significantly removed by PD; supplemental dosing is not required (Aronoff, 2007):
    Exit-site and tunnel infections: Oral: One single-strength tablet daily (Li, 2010)
    Peritonitis: Oral: One double-strength tablet twice daily (Li, 2010)
  Continuous renal replacement therapy (CRRT) (Heintz, 2009; Trotman, 2005): Drug clearance is highly dependent on the method of renal replacement, filter type, and flow rate. Appropriate dosing requires close monitoring of pharmacologic response, signs of adverse reactions due to drug accumulation, as well as drug concentrations in relation to target trough (if appropriate). The following are general recommendations only (based on dialysate flow/ultrafiltration rates of 1-2 L/hour and minimal residual renal function) and should not supersede clinical judgment:
    CVVH/CVVHD/CVVHDF: 2.5-7.5 mg/kg of TMP every 12 hours. **Note:** Dosing regimen dependent on clinical indication. Critically-ill patients with *P. jirovecii* pneumonia receiving CVVHDF may require up to 10 mg/kg every 12 hours (Heintz, 2009).

Administration
  I.V.: Infuse over 60-90 minutes, must dilute well before giving (ie, 1:15 to 1:25, which equates to 5 mL of drug solution diluted in 75-125 mL base solution); not for I.M. injection
  Oral: Administer without regard to meals. Administer with at least 8 ounces of water.

Monitoring Parameters Perform culture and sensitivity testing prior to initiating therapy; CBC, serum potassium, creatinine, BUN

Test Interactions Increased creatinine (Jaffé alkaline picrate reaction); increased serum methotrexate by dihydrofolate reductase method

Special Geriatric Considerations Elderly patients appear at greater risk for more severe adverse reactions.

Dosage Forms Excipient information presented when available (limited, particularly for generics); consult specific product labeling. **Note:** The 5:1 ratio (SMX:TMP) remains constant in all dosage forms.
  Injection, solution: Sulfamethoxazole 80 mg and trimethoprim 16 mg per mL (5 mL, 10 mL, 30 mL) [contains benzyl alcohol, ethanol 12.2%, propylene glycol 400 mg/mL, sodium metabisulfite]
  Suspension, oral: Sulfamethoxazole 200 mg and trimethoprim 40 mg per 5 mL (480 mL)
  Tablet: Sulfamethoxazole 400 mg and trimethoprim 80 mg
    Bactrim™: Sulfamethoxazole 400 mg and trimethoprim 80 mg
  Tablet, double-strength: Sulfamethoxazole 800 mg and trimethoprim 160 mg
    Bactrim™ DS: Sulfamethoxazole 800 mg and trimethoprim 160 mg
    Septra® DS: Sulfamethoxazole 800 mg and trimethoprim 160 mg

◆ **Sulfamide** see Sulfacetamide (Ophthalmic) on page 1811

Sulfanilamide (sul fa NIL a mide)

Brand Names: U.S. AVC™
Index Terms p-amino-benzenesulfonamide
Pharmacologic Category Antifungal Agent, Vaginal
Use Treatment of vulvovaginitis caused by *Candida albicans*
Dosage
  Adult Vulvovaginitis due to *Candida albicans*: Intravaginal: Insert one applicatorful intravaginally once or twice daily; treatment should continue for a period of 30 days
Special Geriatric Considerations Localized fungal infections frequently follow broad-spectrum antimicrobial therapy, specifically, oral and vaginal infections due to *Candida*.
Dosage Forms Excipient information presented when available (limited, particularly for generics); consult specific product labeling.
  Cream, vaginal:
    AVC™: 15% (120 g) [~6 g/applicator]

SulfaSALAzine (sul fa SAL a zeen)

Medication Safety Issues
  Sound-alike/look-alike issues:
    SulfaSALAzine may be confused with salsalate, sulfADIAZINE, sulfiSOXAZOLE
    Azulfidine® may be confused with Augmentin®, azaTHIOprine
Brand Names: U.S. Azulfidine EN-tabs®; Azulfidine®; Sulfazine; Sulfazine EC
Brand Names: Canada Alti-Sulfasalazine; Salazopyrin En-Tabs®; Salazopyrin®
Index Terms Salicylazosulfapyridine
Generic Availability (U.S.) Yes

Pharmacologic Category 5-Aminosalicylic Acid Derivative

Use Treatment of mild-to-moderate ulcerative colitis or as adjunctive therapy in severe ulcerative colitis; enteric coated tablets are also used for rheumatoid arthritis (including juvenile idiopathic arthritis [JIA]) in patients who inadequately respond to analgesics and NSAIDs

Unlabeled Use Ankylosing spondylitis, Crohn's disease, psoriasis, psoriatic arthritis

Contraindications Hypersensitivity to sulfasalazine, sulfa drugs, salicylates, or any component of the formulation; porphyria; GI or GU obstruction

Warnings/Precautions Use with extreme caution in patients with renal impairment, impaired hepatic function or blood dyscrasias. Use caution in patients with severe allergies or asthma, or G6PD deficiency; may cause folate deficiency (consider providing 1 mg/day folate supplement). Deaths from irreversible neuromuscular or central nervous system changes, fibrosing alveolitis, agranulocytosis, aplastic anemia, and other blood dyscrasias have been reported. In males, oligospermia (rare) has been reported. Chemical similarities are present among sulfonamides, sulfonylureas, carbonic anhydrase inhibitors, thiazides, and loop diuretics (except ethacrynic acid). Nausea, vomiting, and abdominal discomfort commonly occur; titration of dose and/or using the enteric coated formulation may decrease GI adverse effects. Use in patients with sulfonamide allergy is specifically contraindicated in product labeling, however, a risk of cross-reaction exists in patients with allergy to any of these compounds; avoid use when previous reaction has been severe. Slow acetylators may be more prone to adverse reactions.

Adverse Reactions (Reflective of adult population; not specific for elderly)

>10%:
  Central nervous system: Headache
  Dermatologic: Rash
  Gastrointestinal: Anorexia, dyspepsia, gastric distress, nausea, vomiting
  Genitourinary: Oligospermia (reversible)

1% to 10%:
  Cardiovascular: Cyanosis
  Central nervous system: Dizziness, fever
  Dermatologic: Pruritus, urticaria
  Gastrointestinal: Abdominal pain, stomatitis
  Hematologic: Heinz body anemia, hemolytic anemia, leukopenia, thrombocytopenia
  Hepatic: Liver function tests abnormal

Drug Interactions

  Metabolism/Transport Effects None known.

  Avoid Concomitant Use There are no known interactions where it is recommended to avoid concomitant use.

  Increased Effect/Toxicity
    SulfaSALAzine may increase the levels/effects of: Heparin; Heparin (Low Molecular Weight); Methotrexate; Prilocaine; Thiopurine Analogs; Varicella Virus-Containing Vaccines

  Decreased Effect
    SulfaSALAzine may decrease the levels/effects of: Cardiac Glycosides; Methylfolate

Ethanol/Nutrition/Herb Interactions
  Food: May impair folate absorption.
  Herb/Nutraceutical: Avoid dong quai, St John's wort (may also cause photosensitization)

Stability Store at 25°C (77°F); excursions permitted to 15°C to 30°C (59°F to 86°F).

Mechanism of Action Acts locally in the colon to decrease the inflammatory response and systemically interferes with secretion by inhibiting prostaglandin synthesis

Pharmacodynamics/Kinetics
  Absorption: ≤15% as unchanged drug from small intestine
  Metabolism: Via colonic intestinal flora to sulfapyridine and 5-aminosalicylic acid (5-ASA). Following absorption, sulfapyridine undergoes acetylation to form AcSP and ring hydroxylation while 5-ASA undergoes N-acetylation (non-acetylation phenotype dependent process); rate of metabolism via acetylation dependent on acetylation phenotype
  Bioavailability: Sulfasalazine: <15%; sulfapyridine: ~60%; 5-aminosalicylic acid: ~10% to 30%
  Half-life elimination: 5.7-10 hours (prolonged in elderly); sulfapyridine half-life prolonged in slow acetylators (14.8 hours)
  Time to peak: Sulfasalazine: 3-12 hours (mean: 6 hours); metabolites: ~10 hours
  Excretion: Primarily urine (as unchanged drug, components, and acetylated metabolites)

Dosage

  Geriatric & Adult

    Ulcerative colitis: Oral:
      Initial: 3-4 g/day in evenly divided doses at ≤8-hour intervals. **Note:** American College of Gastroenterology guideline recommendations: Titrate to 4-6 g/day in 4 divided doses (Kornbluth, 2010).

Maintenance dose: 2 g/day in evenly divided doses at ≤8-hour intervals; may initiate therapy with 1-2 g/day to reduce GI intolerance

Rheumatoid arthritis: Oral (enteric coated tablet): Initial: 0.5-1 g/day; increase weekly to maintenance dose of 2 g/day in 2 divided doses; maximum: 3 g/day (if response to 2 g/day is inadequate after 12 weeks of treatment)

Renal Impairment Use not recommended; weigh risk vs benefit.

Hepatic Impairment Use not recommended; weigh risk vs benefit.

Administration GI intolerance is common during the first few days of therapy (administer with meals). Do not crush enteric coated tablets.

Monitoring Parameters CBC with differential and liver function tests (prior to therapy, then every other week for first 3 months of therapy, followed by every month for the second 3 months, then once every 3 months thereafter); periodic urinalysis and renal function tests; stool frequency; signs of infection

Pharmacotherapy Pearls This drug should be administered after food to reduce GI irritation. Sulfasalazine can be used as a disease-modifying agent (DMARD) in the treatment of progressive rheumatoid arthritis that has not responded adequately to anti-inflammatory agents.

Special Geriatric Considerations Adjust dose for renal function. Elderly with rheumatoid arthritis have demonstrated an increased half-life; however, the clinical significance is not known.

Dosage Forms Excipient information presented when available (limited, particularly for generics); consult specific product labeling.

Tablet, oral: 500 mg
  Azulfidine®: 500 mg [scored]
  Sulfazine: 500 mg [scored]
Tablet, delayed release, enteric coated, oral: 500 mg
  Azulfidine EN-tabs®: 500 mg
  Sulfazine EC: 500 mg

- ◆ **Sulfatrim** see Sulfamethoxazole and Trimethoprim on page 1813
- ◆ **Sulfazine** see SulfaSALAzine on page 1817
- ◆ **Sulfazine EC** see SulfaSALAzine on page 1817
- ◆ **Sulfisoxazole and Erythromycin** see Erythromycin and Sulfisoxazole on page 668

Sulindac (SUL in dak)

Related Information
  Beers Criteria − Potentially Inappropriate Medications for Geriatrics on page 2183

Medication Safety Issues
  Sound-alike/look-alike issues:
    Clinoril® may be confused with Cleocin®, Clozaril®
  BEERS Criteria medication:
    This drug may be potentially inappropriate for use in geriatric patients (Quality of evidence - moderate; Strength of recommendation - strong).

Brand Names: U.S. Clinoril®

Brand Names: Canada Apo-Sulin®; Novo-Sundac; Nu-Sulindac; Nu-Sundac; Teva-Sulindac

Generic Availability (U.S.) Yes

Pharmacologic Category Nonsteroidal Anti-inflammatory Drug (NSAID), Oral

Use Management of inflammatory diseases including osteoarthritis, rheumatoid arthritis, acute gouty arthritis, ankylosing spondylitis, acute painful shoulder (bursitis/tendonitis)

Unlabeled Use Management of preterm labor

Medication Guide Available Yes

Contraindications Hypersensitivity or allergic-type reactions to sulindac, aspirin, other NSAIDs, or any component of the formulation; perioperative pain in the setting of coronary artery bypass graft (CABG) surgery

Warnings/Precautions [U.S. Boxed Warning]: NSAIDs are associated with an increased risk of adverse cardiovascular thrombotic events, including MI and stroke. Use caution with fluid retention. Avoid use in heart failure. Concurrent administration of ibuprofen, and potentially other nonselective NSAIDs, may interfere with aspirin's cardioprotective effect. May cause new-onset hypertension or worsening of existing hypertension. NSAID use may compromise existing renal function; dose-dependent decreases in prostaglandin synthesis may result from NSAID use, reducing renal blood flow which may cause renal decompensation. NSAID use may increase the risk for hyperkalemia. Patients with impaired renal function, dehydration, heart failure, liver dysfunction, those taking diuretics, and ACE inhibitors, and the elderly are at greater risk of renal toxicity and hyperkalemia. Rehydrate patient before starting therapy; monitor renal function closely. Not recommended for use in patients with advanced renal disease. Long-term NSAID use may result in renal papillary necrosis. Use caution in

SULINDAC

patients with renal lithiasis; sulindac metabolites have been reported as components of renal stones. Maintain adequate hydration in patients with a history of renal stones. Use with caution in patients with decreased hepatic function. May require dosage adjustment in hepatic dysfunction; sulfide and sulfone metabolites may accumulate. The elderly are at increased risk for adverse effects. **[U.S. Boxed Warning]: Use is contraindicated for treatment of perioperative pain in the setting of coronary artery bypass graft (CABG) surgery.** Risk of MI and stroke may be increased with use following CABG surgery.

[U.S. Boxed Warning]: NSAIDs may increase risk of gastrointestinal irritation, inflammation, ulceration, bleeding, and perforation. Use the lowest effective dose for the shortest duration of time, consistent with individual patient goals, to reduce risk of cardiovascular or GI adverse events. When used concomitantly with ≤325 mg of aspirin, a substantial increase in the risk of gastrointestinal complications (eg, ulcer) occurs; concomitant gastroprotective therapy (eg, proton pump inhibitors) is recommended (Bhatt, 2008). Pancreatitis has been reported; discontinue with suspected pancreatitis.

Avoid chronic use in the elderly (unless alternative agents ineffective and patient can receive concomitant gastroprotective agent); nonselective oral NSAID use is associated with an increased risk of GI bleeding and peptic ulcer disease in older adults in high risk category (eg, >75 years or age or receiving concomitant oral/parenteral corticosteroids, anticoagulants, or antiplatelet agents) (Beers Criteria).

NSAIDS may cause drowsiness, dizziness, blurred vision and other neurologic effects which may impair physical or mental abilities; patients must be cautioned about performing tasks which require mental alertness (eg, operating machinery or driving). Discontinue use with blurred or diminished vision and perform ophthalmologic exam. Monitor vision with long-term therapy.

Platelet adhesion and aggregation may be decreased, may prolong bleeding time; patients with coagulation disorders or who are receiving anticoagulants should be monitored closely. Anemia may occur; patients on long-term NSAID therapy should be monitored for anemia. Rarely, NSAID use may cause severe blood dyscrasias (eg, agranulocytosis, aplastic anemia, thrombocytopenia). NSAIDs may cause serious skin adverse events including exfoliative dermatitis, Stevens-Johnson syndrome (SJS) and toxic epidermal necrolysis (TEN); discontinue use at first sign of skin rash or hypersensitivity. Anaphylactoid reactions may occur. Do not use in patients who experience bronchospasm, asthma, rhinitis, or urticaria with NSAID or aspirin therapy. Use caution in other forms of asthma. May increase the risk of aseptic meningitis, especially in patients with systemic lupus erythematosus (SLE) and mixed connective tissue disorders.

Withhold for at least 4-6 half-lives prior to surgical or dental procedures.

Adverse Reactions (Reflective of adult population; not specific for elderly) 1% to 10%:

Cardiovascular: Edema (1% to 3%)

Central nervous system: Dizziness (3% to 9%), headache (3% to 9%), nervousness (1% to 3%)

Dermatologic: Rash (3% to 9%), pruritus (1% to 3%)

Gastrointestinal: GI pain (10%), constipation (3% to 9%), diarrhea (3% to 9%), dyspepsia (3% to 9%), nausea (3% to 9%), abdominal cramps (1% to 3%), anorexia (1% to 3%), flatulence (1% to 3%), vomiting (1% to 3%)

Otic: Tinnitus (1% to 3%)

Drug Interactions

Metabolism/Transport Effects None known.

Avoid Concomitant Use

Avoid concomitant use of Sulindac with any of the following: Floctafenine; Ketorolac; Ketorolac (Nasal); Ketorolac (Systemic)

Increased Effect/Toxicity

Sulindac may increase the levels/effects of: Aliskiren; Aminoglycosides; Anticoagulants; Antiplatelet Agents; Bisphosphonate Derivatives; Collagenase (Systemic); CycloSPORINE; CycloSPORINE (Systemic); Dabigatran Etexilate; Deferasirox; Desmopressin; Digoxin; Drotrecogin Alfa (Activated); Eplerenone; Haloperidol; Ibritumomab; Methotrexate; Nonsteroidal Anti-Inflammatory Agents; PEMEtrexed; Porfimer; Potassium-Sparing Diuretics; PRALAtrexate; Quinolone Antibiotics; Rivaroxaban; Salicylates; Thrombolytic Agents; Tositumomab and Iodine I 131 Tositumomab; Vancomycin; Vitamin K Antagonists

The levels/effects of Sulindac may be increased by: ACE Inhibitors; Angiotensin II Receptor Blockers; Antidepressants (Tricyclic, Tertiary Amine); Corticosteroids (Systemic); CycloSPORINE; CycloSPORINE (Systemic); Dasatinib; Dimethyl Sulfoxide; Floctafenine; Glucosamine; Herbs (Anticoagulant/Antiplatelet Properties); Ketorolac; Ketorolac (Nasal); Ketorolac (Systemic); Nonsteroidal Anti-Inflammatory Agents; Omega-3-Acid Ethyl Esters;

Pentosan Polysulfate Sodium; Pentoxifylline; Probenecid; Prostacyclin Analogues; Selective Serotonin Reuptake Inhibitors; Serotonin/Norepinephrine Reuptake Inhibitors; Sodium Phosphates; Tipranavir; Treprostinil; Vitamin E

Decreased Effect

Sulindac may decrease the levels/effects of: ACE Inhibitors; Aliskiren; Angiotensin II Receptor Blockers; Antiplatelet Agents; Beta-Blockers; Eplerenone; HydrALAZINE; Loop Diuretics; Potassium-Sparing Diuretics; Salicylates; Selective Serotonin Reuptake Inhibitors; Thiazide Diuretics

The levels/effects of Sulindac may be decreased by: Bile Acid Sequestrants; Nonsteroidal Anti-Inflammatory Agents; Salicylates

Ethanol/Nutrition/Herb Interactions

Ethanol: Avoid ethanol (may enhance gastric mucosal irritation).

Herb/Nutraceutical: Avoid alfalfa, anise, bilberry, bladderwrack, bromelain, cat's claw, celery, chamomile, coleus, cordyceps, dong quai, evening primrose, fenugreek, feverfew, garlic, ginger, ginkgo biloba, ginseng (American, Panax, Siberian), grapeseed, green tea, guggul, horse chestnut seed, horseradish, licorice, prickly ash, red clover, reishi, SAMe (S-adenosylmethionine), sweet clover, turmeric, white willow (all have additional antiplatelet activity).

Stability Store at room temperature of 15°C to 30°C (59°F to 86°F).

Mechanism of Action Reversibly inhibits cyclooxygenase-1 and 2 (COX-1 and 2) enzymes, which results in decreased formation of prostaglandin precursors; has antipyretic, analgesic, and anti-inflammatory properties

Other proposed mechanisms not fully elucidated (and possibly contributing to the anti-inflammatory effect to varying degrees), include inhibiting chemotaxis, altering lymphocyte activity, inhibiting neutrophil aggregation/activation, and decreasing proinflammatory cytokine levels.

Pharmacodynamics/Kinetics

Absorption: 90%

Distribution: Crosses blood-brain barrier (brain concentrations <4% of plasma concentrations)

Protein binding: Sulindac: 93%, sulfone metabolite: 95%, sulfide metabolite: 98%; primarily to albumin

Metabolism: Hepatic; prodrug metabolized to sulfide metabolite (active) for therapeutic effects and to sulfone metabolites (inactive); parent and inactive sulfone metabolite undergo extensive enterohepatic recirculation

Half-life elimination: Sulindac: ~8 hours; Sulfide metabolite: ~16 hours

Time to peak: Sulindac: 3-4 hours; Sulfide and sulfone metabolites: 5-6 hours

Excretion: Urine (~50%, primarily as inactive metabolites, <1% as active metabolite); feces (~25%, primarily as metabolites)

Dosage

Geriatric & Adult Note: Maximum daily dose: 400 mg

Osteoarthritis, rheumatoid arthritis, ankylosing spondylitis: 150 mg twice daily

Acute painful shoulder (bursitis/tendonitis): 200 mg twice daily; usual treatment: 7-14 days

Acute gouty arthritis: 200 mg twice daily; usual treatment: 7 days

Renal Impairment Not recommended with advanced renal impairment; if required, decrease dose and monitor closely.

Hepatic Impairment Dose reduction is necessary; discontinue if abnormal liver function tests occur.

Administration Should be administered with food or milk.

Monitoring Parameters Liver enzymes, BUN, serum creatinine, CBC, blood pressure; signs and symptoms of GI bleeding; ophthalmic exam (if ocular complaints develop during treatment)

Test Interactions Increased chloride (S), increased sodium (S), increased bleeding time

Special Geriatric Considerations Elderly are a high-risk population for adverse effects from NSAIDs. As much as 60% of the elderly who develop GI complications can develop peptic ulceration and/or hemorrhage asymptomatically. The concomitant use of H_2 blockers and sucralfate is not effective as prophylaxis with the exception of NSAID-induced duodenal ulcers which may be prevented by the use of ranitidine. Misoprostol and proton pump inhibitors are the only agents proven to help prevent the development of NSAID-induced ulcers. Also, concomitant disease and drug use contribute to the risk for GI adverse effects. Use lowest effective dose for shortest period possible. Consider renal function decline with age. Use of NSAIDs can compromise existing renal function especially when Cl_{cr} is ≤30 mL/minute. Tinnitus may be a difficult and unreliable indication of toxicity due to age-related hearing loss or eighth cranial nerve damage. CNS adverse effects such as confusion, agitation, and hallucination are generally seen in overdose or high-dose situations, but the elderly may demonstrate these adverse effects at lower doses than younger adults.

This medication is considered to be potentially inappropriate in this patient population (Beers Criteria: Quality of evidence - moderate; Strength of recommendation - strong).

Dosage Forms Excipient information presented when available (limited, particularly for generics); consult specific product labeling.

Tablet, oral: 150 mg, 200 mg

Clinoril®: 200 mg [scored]

SUMAtriptan (soo ma TRIP tan)

Medication Safety Issues

Sound-alike/look-alike issues:

SUMAtriptan may be confused with saxagliptin, sitaGLIPtin, somatropin, ZOLMitriptan

Brand Names: U.S. Alsuma™; Imitrex®; Sumavel® DosePro®

Brand Names: Canada Apo-Sumatriptan®; Ava-Sumatriptan; CO Sumatriptan; Dom-Sumatriptan; Imitrex®; Imitrex® DF; Imitrex® Injection; Imitrex® Nasal Spray; Mylan-Sumatriptan; PHL-Sumatriptan; PMS-Sumatriptan; Riva-Sumatriptan; Sandoz-Sumatriptan; Sumatriptan Injection; Sumatriptan Sun Injection; Sumatryx; Teva-Sumatriptan; Teva-Sumatriptan DF

Index Terms Sumatriptan Succinate

Generic Availability (U.S.) Yes

Pharmacologic Category Antimigraine Agent; Serotonin 5-HT$_{1B, 1D}$ Receptor Agonist

Use

Intranasal, Oral, SubQ: Acute treatment of migraine with or without aura

SubQ: Acute treatment of cluster headache episodes

Contraindications Hypersensitivity to sumatriptan or any component of the formulation; patients with ischemic heart disease or signs or symptoms of ischemic heart disease (including Prinzmetal's angina, angina pectoris, myocardial infarction, silent myocardial ischemia); cerebrovascular syndromes (including strokes, transient ischemic attacks); peripheral vascular disease (including ischemic bowel disease); uncontrolled hypertension; use within 24 hours of ergotamine derivatives; use within 24 hours of another 5-HT$_1$ agonist; concurrent administration or within 2 weeks of discontinuing an MAO type A inhibitors (oral and nasal sumatriptan only; see Warnings/Precautions); management of hemiplegic or basilar migraine; severe hepatic impairment (oral and nasal sumatriptan, and injectable Imitrex® only); not for I.V. administration

Warnings/Precautions Sumatriptan is only indicated for the acute treatment of migraine or cluster headache (product dependent); not indicated for migraine prophylaxis, or for the treatment of hemiplegic or basilar migraine. If a patient does not respond to the first dose, the diagnosis of migraine or cluster headache should be reconsidered; rule out underlying neurologic disease in patients with atypical headache and in patients with no prior history of migraine or cluster headache. Cardiac events (coronary artery vasospasm, transient ischemia, myocardial infarction, ventricular tachycardia/fibrillation, cardiac arrest and death), cerebral/subarachnoid hemorrhage, and stroke have been reported with 5-HT$_1$ agonist administration. Patients who experience sensations of chest pain/pressure/tightness or symptoms suggestive of angina following dosing should be evaluated for coronary artery disease or Prinzmetal's angina before receiving additional doses; if dosing is resumed and similar symptoms recur, monitor with ECG. Do not give to patients with risk factors for CAD until a cardiovascular evaluation has been performed; if evaluation is satisfactory, the healthcare provider should administer the first dose (consider ECG monitoring) and cardiovascular status should be periodically evaluated.

Significant elevation in blood pressure, including hypertensive crisis, has also been reported on rare occasions in patients with and without a history of hypertension; use is contraindicated in patients with uncontrolled hypertension. Vasospasm-related reactions have been reported other than coronary artery vasospasm. Peripheral vascular ischemia and colonic ischemia with abdominal pain and bloody diarrhea have occurred. Transient and permanent blindness and significant partial vision loss have been very rarely reported. Use with caution in patients with a history of seizure disorder or in patients with a lowered seizure threshold. Use the oral formulation with caution (and with dosage limitations) in patients with hepatic impairment where treatment is necessary and advisable. Presystemic clearance of orally administered sumatriptan is reduced in hepatic impairment, leading to increased plasma concentrations; dosage reduction of the oral product is recommended. Non-oral routes of administration (nasal, subcutaneous formulations) do not undergo similar hepatic first-pass metabolism and are not expected to result in significantly altered pharmacokinetics in patients with hepatic impairment. Use of the oral, nasal, or Imitrex® injectable is contraindicated in severe hepatic impairment.

Symptoms of agitation, confusion, hallucinations, hyper-reflexia, myoclonus, shivering, and tachycardia (serotonin syndrome) may occur with concomitant proserotonergic drugs (ie, SSRIs/SNRIs or triptans) or agents which reduce sumatriptan's metabolism. Concurrent use of serotonin precursors (eg, tryptophan) is not recommended. If concomitant administration with SSRIs is warranted, monitor closely, especially at initiation and with dose increases. Concurrent use with an MAO inhibitor may result in increased sumatriptan concentrations and increased risk for dose-related adverse effects (eg, serotonin syndrome); use with oral or nasal sumatriptan is contraindicated. Although generally not recommended, if concomitant use of MAO inhibitors with injectable sumatriptan is deemed necessary, careful monitoring and appropriate dosage adjustments are required. I.V. administration is contraindicated due to the potential to cause coronary vasospasm. Not recommended for use in elderly patients; older adults are at a higher risk for coronary artery disease and may be more likely to have reduced hepatic function.

Adverse Reactions (Reflective of adult population; not specific for elderly)
Injection:
>10%:
Central nervous system: Dizziness (12%), warm/hot sensation (11%)
Local: Injection site reaction (≤86%; includes bleeding, bruising, edema, and erythema)
Neuromuscular & skeletal: Paresthesia (5% to 14%)
1% to 10%:
Cardiovascular: Chest discomfort/tightness/pressure (2% to 5%)
Central nervous system: Burning sensation (7%), feeling of heaviness (7%), flushing (7%), pressure sensation (7%), feeling of tightness (5%), drowsiness (3%), feeling strange (2%), headache (2%), tight feeling in head (2%), anxiety (1%), cold sensation (1%), malaise/fatigue (1%)
Gastrointestinal: Nausea/vomiting (4%), abdominal discomfort (1%), dysphagia (1%)
Neuromuscular & skeletal: Neck pain/stiffness (5%), numbness (5%), weakness (5%), jaw discomfort (2%), myalgia (2%), muscle cramps (1%)
Ocular: Vision alterations (1%)
Respiratory: Throat discomfort (3%), nasal disorder/discomfort (2%), bronchospasm (1%)
Miscellaneous: Diaphoresis (2%)

Nasal spray:
>10%: Gastrointestinal: Bad taste (13% to 24%), nausea (11% to 13%), vomiting (11% to 13%)
1% to 10%:
Central nervous system: Dizziness (1% to 2%)
Respiratory: Nasal disorder/discomfort (2% to 4%), throat discomfort (1% to 2%)

Tablet:
1% to 10%:
Cardiovascular: Chest pain/tightness/heaviness/pressure (1% to 2%), palpitation (1%), syncope (1%)
Central nervous system: Burning (1%), dizziness (>1%), drowsiness (>1%), malaise/fatigue (2% to 3%), headache (>1%), nonspecified pain (1% to 2%, placebo 1%), vertigo (<1% to 2%), migraine (>1%), sleepiness (>1%)
Gastrointestinal: Diarrhea (1%), nausea (>1%), vomiting (>1%), hyposalivation (>1%)
Hematologic: Hemolytic anemia (1%)
Neuromuscular & skeletal: Neck, throat, and jaw pain/tightness/pressure (2% to 3%), paresthesia (3% to 5%), myalgia (1%), numbness (1%)
Otic: Ear hemorrhage (1%), hearing loss (1%), sensitivity to noise (1%), tinnitus (1%)
Renal: Hematuria (1%)
Respiratory: Allergic rhinitis (1%), dyspnea (1%), nasal inflammation (1%), nose/throat hemorrhage (1%), sinusitis (1%), upper respiratory inflammation (1%)
Miscellaneous: Hypersensitivity reactions (1%), nonspecified pressure/tightness/heaviness (1% to 3%, placebo 2%); warm/cold sensation (2% to 3%, placebo 2%)

Drug Interactions
Metabolism/Transport Effects None known.
Avoid Concomitant Use
Avoid concomitant use of SUMAtriptan with any of the following: Ergot Derivatives; MAO Inhibitors
Increased Effect/Toxicity
SUMAtriptan may increase the levels/effects of: Ergot Derivatives; Metoclopramide; Serotonin Modulators

The levels/effects of SUMAtriptan may be increased by: Antipsychotics; Ergot Derivatives; MAO Inhibitors
Decreased Effect There are no known significant interactions involving a decrease in effect.
Stability
Alsuma™: Store at 25°C (77°F); excursions permitted between 15°C and 30°C (59°F and 86°F); do not refrigerate. Protect from light.

Imitrex® injectable, tablet, nasal spray: Store at 2°C to 30°C (36°F to 86°F). Protect from light.
Sumavel® DosePro®: Store at 20°C to 25°C (68°F to 77°F); excursions permitted between 15°C and 30°C (59°F and 86°F); do not freeze.

Mechanism of Action Selective agonist for serotonin (5-HT$_{1B}$ and 5-HT$_{1D}$ receptors) in cranial arteries; causes vasoconstriction and reduces neurogenic inflammation associated with antidromic neuronal transmission correlating with relief of migraine

Pharmacodynamics/Kinetics

Onset of action: Oral: ~30 minutes; Nasal: ~15-30 minutes; SubQ: ~10 minutes

Distribution: V_d: 2.4 L/kg

Protein binding: 14% to 21%

Metabolism: Hepatic, primarily via MAO-A isoenzyme; extensive first-pass metabolism following oral administration

Bioavailability: Nasal: 17% (compared to SubQ); Oral: 15%; SubQ: 97% ± 16%

Half-life elimination: ~2-2.5 hours

Time to peak, serum: Oral: 2-2.5 hours; SubQ: 12 minutes (range: 4-20 minutes)

Excretion:

Nasal spray: Urine (42% of total dose as indole acetic acid metabolite; 3% of total dose as unchanged drug)

Oral: Urine (~60% of total dose, mostly as indole acetic acid metabolite; 3% of total dose as unchanged drug); feces (~40%)

SubQ: Urine (38% of total dose as indole acetic acid metabolite; 22% of total dose as unchanged drug)

Dosage

Geriatric Use is not recommended (due to increased potential for adverse effects).

Adult

Migraine:

Oral: A single dose of 25 mg, 50 mg, or 100 mg (taken with fluids). If a satisfactory response has not been obtained at 2 hours, a second dose may be administered. Results from clinical trials show that initial doses of 50 mg and 100 mg are more effective than doses of 25 mg, and that 100 mg doses do not provide a greater effect than 50 mg and may have increased incidence of side effects. Although doses of up to 300 mg/day have been studied, the total daily dose should not exceed 200 mg. The safety of treating an average of >4 headaches in a 30-day period have not been established.

Intranasal: A single dose of 5 mg, 10 mg, or 20 mg administered in one nostril. A 10 mg dose may be achieved by administering a single 5 mg dose in each nostril. If headache returns, the dose may be repeated once after 2 hours, not to exceed a total daily dose of 40 mg. In clinical trials, a greater number of patients responded to initial doses of 20 mg versus 5 or 10 mg. The safety of treating an average of >4 headaches in a 30-day period has not been established.

SubQ: Initial: Up to 6 mg; may repeat if needed ≥1 hour after initial dose (maximum: Two 6 mg injections per 24-hour period). However, controlled clinical trials have failed to document a benefit with administration of a second 6 mg dose in nonresponders.

Cluster headache: SubQ: Initial: Up to 6 mg; may repeat if needed ≥1 hour after initial dose (maximum: Two 6 mg injections per 24-hour period)

Renal Impairment No dosage adjustments are recommended.

Hepatic Impairment

Mild-to-moderate hepatic impairment:

Oral: Bioavailability of oral sumatriptan is increased with liver disease. If treatment is needed, do not exceed single doses of 50 mg.

Nasal spray: Has not been studied in patients with hepatic impairment, however, because the spray does not undergo first-pass metabolism, levels would not be expected to be altered.

Subcutaneous: Has been studied and pharmacokinetics were not altered in patients with hepatic impairment compared to healthy patients.

Severe hepatic impairment: Oral, nasal, and subcutaneous (limited to Imitrex® injection, per prescribing information) formulations are contraindicated with severe hepatic impairment.

Administration Should be administered as soon as symptoms appear.

Intranasal: Each nasal spray unit is preloaded with 1 dose; **do not** test the spray unit before use; remove unit from plastic pack when ready to use; while sitting down, gently blow nose to clear nasal passages; keep head upright and close one nostril gently with index finger; hold container with other hand, with thumb supporting bottom and index and middle fingers on either side of nozzle; insert nozzle into nostril about 1/2 inch; close mouth; take a breath through nose while releasing spray into nostril by pressing firmly on blue plunger; remove nozzle from nostril; keep head level for 10-20 seconds and gently breathe in through nose and out through mouth; **do not breathe deeply**

SubQ: Not for I.M. or I.V. use. Needle penetrates $1/4$ inch of skin; use in areas of the body with adequate skin and subcutaneous thickness. Alsuma™ is a prefilled single-use autoinjector device.

Needleless administration (Sumavel® DosePro®): Administer to the abdomen (>2 inches from the navel) or thigh; not for I.M. or I.V. administration. Do not administer to other areas of the body (eg, arm). Device is for single use only, discard after use; do not use if the tip of the device is tilted or broken.

Special Geriatric Considerations Use is not recommended in the elderly, particularly since many elderly have cardiovascular disease which would put them at risk for cardiovascular adverse effects. Safety and efficacy in the elderly (>65 years) have not been established. Pharmacokinetic disposition is, however, similar to that in young adults.

Dosage Forms Excipient information presented when available (limited, particularly for generics); consult specific product labeling.

Injection, solution, as succinate [strength expressed as base]: 4 mg/0.5 mL (0.5 mL); 6 mg/0.5 mL (0.5 mL)

Alsuma™: 6 mg/0.5 mL (0.5 mL) [autoinjector]

Imitrex®: 4 mg/0.5 mL (0.5 mL); 6 mg/0.5 mL (0.5 mL) [cartridge]

Imitrex®: 6 mg/0.5 mL (0.5 mL) [vial]

Sumavel® DosePro®: 6 mg/0.5 mL (0.5 mL) [needleless autoinjector]

Injection, solution, as succinate [strength expressed as base, preservative free]: 6 mg/0.5 mL (0.5 mL)

Solution, intranasal [spray]: 5 mg/0.1 mL (6s); 20 mg/0.1 mL (6s)

Imitrex®: 5 mg/0.1 mL (6s); 20 mg/0.1 mL (6s)

Tablet, oral, as succinate [strength expressed as base]: 25 mg, 50 mg, 100 mg

Imitrex®: 25 mg, 50 mg, 100 mg

Sumatriptan and Naproxen (soo ma TRIP tan & na PROKS en)

Related Information
Naproxen on page 1338
SUMAtriptan on page 1822

Medication Safety Issues
Sound-alike/look-alike issues:
Naproxen may be confused with Natacyn®, Nebcin, neomycin, niacin
SUMAtriptan may be confused with somatropin, ZOLMitriptan
Treximet® may be confused with Trexall™

Brand Names: U.S. Treximet®

Index Terms Naproxen and Sumatriptan; Naproxen Sodium and Sumatriptan; Naproxen Sodium and Sumatriptan Succinate; Sumatriptan Succinate and Naproxen; Sumatriptan Succinate and Naproxen Sodium

Generic Availability (U.S.) No

Pharmacologic Category Antimigraine Agent; Nonsteroidal Anti-inflammatory Drug (NSAID), Oral; Serotonin 5-HT$_{1B, 1D}$ Receptor Agonist

Use Acute treatment of migraine with or without aura

Medication Guide Available Yes

Dosage

Geriatric & Adult Migraine: Oral: 1 tablet (sumatriptan 85 mg and naproxen 500 mg). If a satisfactory response has not been obtained at 2 hours, a second dose may be administered (maximum: 2 tablets/24 hours). **Note:** The safety of treating an average of >5 migraine headaches in a 30-day period has not been established.

Renal Impairment
Cl_{cr} ≥30 mL/minute Dosage adjustment not necessary.
Cl_{cr} <30 mL/minute: Use not recommended.

Hepatic Impairment Mild-to-severe impairment: Use is contraindicated by the manufacturer.

Special Geriatric Considerations See individual agents.

Dosage Forms Excipient information presented when available (limited, particularly for generics); consult specific product labeling.

Tablet, oral:

Treximet® 85/500: Sumatriptan 85 mg and naproxen sodium 500 mg [contains sodium 61.2 mg/tablet (~2.7 mEq/tablet)]

◆ **Sumatriptan Succinate** see SUMAtriptan on page 1822
◆ **Sumatriptan Succinate and Naproxen** see Sumatriptan and Naproxen on page 1825
◆ **Sumatriptan Succinate and Naproxen Sodium** see Sumatriptan and Naproxen on page 1825
◆ **Sumavel® DosePro®** see SUMAtriptan on page 1822

Tadalafil (tah DA la fil)

Medication Safety Issues

Sound-alike/look-alike issues:
Tadalafil may be confused with sildenafil, vardenafil
Adcirca® may be confused with Advair® Diskus®, Advair® HFA, Advicor®

Brand Names: U.S. Adcirca®; Cialis®

Brand Names: Canada Adcirca®; Cialis®

Index Terms GF196960

Generic Availability (U.S.) No

Pharmacologic Category Phosphodiesterase-5 Enzyme Inhibitor

Use
Adcirca®: Treatment of pulmonary arterial hypertension (PAH) (WHO Group I) to improve exercise ability
Cialis®: Treatment of erectile dysfunction (ED); treatment of signs and symptoms of benign prostatic hyperplasia (BPH)

Contraindications Known serious hypersensitivity to tadalafil or any component of the formulation; concurrent use (regularly/intermittently) of organic nitrates in any form (eg, nitroglycerin, isosorbide dinitrate)

Warnings/Precautions There is a degree of cardiac risk associated with sexual activity; therefore, physicians should consider the cardiovascular status of their patients prior to initiation. Use is not recommended in patients with hypotension (<90/50 mm Hg), uncontrolled hypertension (>170/100 mm Hg), NYHA class II-IV heart failure within the last 6 months, uncontrolled arrhythmias, stroke within the last 6 months, MI within the last 3 months, unstable angina or angina during sexual intercourse; safety and efficacy have not been evaluated in these patients. Safety and efficacy in PAH have not been evaluated in patients with clinically significant aortic and/or mitral valve disease, life-threatening arrhythmias, hypotension (<90/50 mm Hg), uncontrolled hypertension, significant left ventricular dysfunction, pericardial constriction, restrictive or congestive cardiomyopathy, symptomatic coronary artery disease. Use caution in patients with left ventricular outflow obstruction (eg, aortic stenosis, hypertrophic obstructive cardiomyopathy); may be more sensitive to vasodilator effects.

Patients experiencing anginal chest pain after tadalafil administration should seek immediate medical attention. Concomitant use (regularly/intermittently) with all forms of nitrates is contraindicated. When used for BPH, erectile dysfunction, or PAH and nitrate administration is medically necessary following use, at least 48 hours should elapse after the tadalafil dose and nitrate administration. When used for PAH, per the manufacturer, nitrate may be administered within 48 hours of tadalafil. For both situations, administration of nitrates should only be done under close medical supervision with hemodynamic monitoring.

Concurrent use with alpha-adrenergic antagonist therapy may cause symptomatic hypotension; patients should be hemodynamically stable prior to initiating tadalafil therapy at the lowest possible dose. Avoid or limit concurrent substantial alcohol consumption as this may increase the risk of symptomatic hypotension. When used for BPH or erectile dysfunction, use caution in patients receiving strong CYP3A4 inhibitors. When used for PAH, avoid use in patients taking strong CYP3A4 inducers/inhibitors. Use in patients receiving or about to receive ritonavir requires dosage adjustment or interruption of therapy, respectively. Canadian labeling does not recommend use of tadalafil in patients with PAH who are also receiving protease inhibitors.

Pulmonary vasodilators may exacerbate the cardiovascular status in patients with pulmonary veno-occlusive disease (PVOD); use is not recommended. In patients with unrecognized PVOD, signs of pulmonary edema should prompt investigation into this diagnosis. Use with caution in patients with mild-to-moderate hepatic impairment; dosage adjustment/limitation is needed. Use is not recommended in patients with severe hepatic impairment or cirrhosis. Use with caution in patients with renal impairment; dosage adjustment/limitation is needed. Safety and efficacy with other tadalafil brands or other PDE-5 inhibitors (ie, sildenafil and vardenafil) have not been established. Patients should be informed not to take with other tadalafil brands or other PDE-5 inhibitors. Use caution in patients with bleeding disorders or peptic ulcer disease due to effect on platelets (bleeding).

When used to treat BPH or erectile dysfunction, potential underlying causes of BPH or erectile dysfunction should be evaluated prior to treatment. Use with caution in patients with anatomical deformation of the penis (angulation, cavernosal fibrosis, or Peyronie's disease), or who have conditions which may predispose them to priapism (sickle cell anemia, multiple myeloma, leukemia). Instruct patients to seek immediate medical attention if erection persists >4 hours. Safety and efficacy with other tadalafil brands or other PDE-5 inhibitors (ie, sildenafil and vardenafil) have not been established. Patients should be informed not to take with other tadalafil brands or other PDE-5 inhibitors. The safety and efficacy of tadalafil with other treatments for erectile dysfunction have not been studied and are, therefore, not recommended as combination therapy.

Rare cases of nonarteritic anterior ischemic optic neuropathy (NAION) have been reported; risk may be increased with history of vision loss or NAION in one eye. Other risk factors for NAION include heart disease, diabetes, hypertension, smoking, age >50 years, or history of certain eye problems. Sudden decrease or loss of hearing has been reported rarely; hearing changes may be accompanied by tinnitus and dizziness. A direct relationship between therapy and vision or hearing loss has not been determined. Instruct patients to seek medical assistance for sudden loss of vision in one or both eyes, sudden decrease in hearing, or sudden loss of hearing.

Patients with genetic retinal disorders (eg, retinitis pigmentosa) were not evaluated in clinical trials; use is not recommended. Use with caution in the elderly.

Adverse Reactions (Reflective of adult population; not specific for elderly) Based upon usual doses for either indication. For erectile dysfunction, similar adverse events are reported with once-daily versus intermittent dosing, but are generally lower than with doses used intermittently.

>10%:
  Cardiovascular: Flushing (1% to 13%; dose related)
  Central nervous system: Headache (3% to 42%; dose related)
  Gastrointestinal: Dyspepsia (1% to 13%), nausea (10% to 11%)
  Neuromuscular & skeletal: Myalgia (1% to 14%; dose related), back pain (2% to 12%), extremity pain (1% to 11%)
  Respiratory: Respiratory tract infection (3% to 13%), nasopharyngitis (2% to 13%)
2% to 10%:
  Cardiovascular: Hypertension (1% to 3%)
  Gastrointestinal: Gastroenteritis (viral; 3% to 5%), GERD (1% to 3%), abdominal pain (1% to 2%), diarrhea (1% to 2%)
  Genitourinary: Urinary tract infection (≤2%)
  Respiratory: Nasal congestion (≤9%), cough (2% to 4%), bronchitis (≤2%)
  Miscellaneous: Flu-like syndrome (2% to 5%)

Drug Interactions

  Metabolism/Transport Effects Substrate of CYP3A4 (major); **Note:** Assignment of Major/Minor substrate status based on clinically relevant drug interaction potential

  Avoid Concomitant Use

  Avoid concomitant use of Tadalafil with any of the following: Alprostadil; Amyl Nitrite; Boceprevir; Phosphodiesterase 5 Inhibitors; Telaprevir; Vasodilators (Organic Nitrates)

  Increased Effect/Toxicity

  Tadalafil may increase the levels/effects of: Alpha1-Blockers; Alprostadil; Amyl Nitrite; Antihypertensives; Bosentan; Phosphodiesterase 5 Inhibitors; Vasodilators (Organic Nitrates)

TADALAFIL

The levels/effects of Tadalafil may be increased by: Alcohol (Ethyl); Boceprevir; CYP3A4 Inhibitors (Moderate); CYP3A4 Inhibitors (Strong); Dasatinib; Fluconazole; Itraconazole; Ivacaftor; Ketoconazole (Systemic); Mifepristone; Posaconazole; Ritonavir; Sapropterin; Telaprevir; Voriconazole

Decreased Effect

The levels/effects of Tadalafil may be decreased by: Bosentan; CYP3A4 Inducers (Strong); Etravirine; Tocilizumab

Ethanol/Nutrition/Herb Interactions Ethanol: Substantial consumption of ethanol may increase the risk of hypotension and orthostasis. Lower ethanol consumption has not been associated with significant changes in blood pressure or increase in orthostatic symptoms. Management: Avoid or limit ethanol consumption.

Food: Rate and extent of absorption are not affected by food. Grapefruit juice may increase serum levels/toxicity of tadalafil. Management: Use of grapefruit juice should be limited or avoided.

Herb/Nutraceutical: St John's wort may decrease the levels/effectiveness of tadalafil. Management: Avoid or use caution with concomitant use.

Stability Store at 25°C (77°F); excursions permitted to 15°C to 30°C (59°F to 86°F).

Mechanism of Action

BPH: Exact mechanism unknown; effects likely due to PDE-5 mediated reduction in smooth muscle and endothelial cell proliferation, decreased nerve activity, and increased smooth muscle relaxation and tissue perfusion of the prostate and bladder

Erectile dysfunction: Does not directly cause penile erections, but affects the response to sexual stimulation. The physiologic mechanism of erection of the penis involves release of nitric oxide (NO) in the corpus cavernosum during sexual stimulation. NO then activates the enzyme guanylate cyclase, which results in increased levels of cyclic guanosine monophosphate (cGMP), producing smooth muscle relaxation and inflow of blood to the corpus cavernosum. Tadalafil enhances the effect of NO by inhibiting phosphodiesterase type 5 (PDE-5), which is responsible for degradation of cGMP in the corpus cavernosum; when sexual stimulation causes local release of NO, inhibition of PDE-5 by tadalafil causes increased levels of cGMP in the corpus cavernosum, resulting in smooth muscle relaxation and inflow of blood to the corpus cavernosum. At recommended doses, it has no effect in the absence of sexual stimulation.

PAH: Inhibits phosphodiesterase type 5 (PDE-5) in smooth muscle of pulmonary vasculature where PDE-5 is responsible for the degradation of cyclic guanosine monophosphate (cGMP). Increased cGMP concentration results in pulmonary vasculature relaxation; vasodilation in the pulmonary bed and the systemic circulation (to a lesser degree) may occur.

Pharmacodynamics/Kinetics

Onset of action: Within 1 hour

Peak effect (pulmonary artery vasodilation): 75-90 minutes (Ghofrani, 2004)

Duration: Erectile dysfunction: Up to 36 hours

Distribution: V_d: 63-77 L

Protein binding: 94%

Metabolism: Hepatic, via CYP3A4 to metabolites (inactive)

Half-life elimination: 15-17.5 hours; Pulmonary hypertension (not receiving bosentan): 35 hours

Time to peak, plasma: ~2-4 hours (range: 30 minutes to 8 hours)

Excretion: Feces (~61%, predominantly as metabolites); urine (~36%, predominantly as metabolites)

Dosage

Geriatric Refer to adult dosing. No dose adjustment for patients >65 years of age in the absence of renal or hepatic impairment.

Adult

Benign prostatic hyperplasia (with or without concomitant erectile dysfunction) (Cialis®): Oral: 5 mg once daily

Dosing adjustment with concomitant medications: CYP3A4 inhibitors (strong): 2.5 mg once daily; maximum: 2.5 mg once daily

Erectile dysfunction (Cialis®): Oral:

As-needed dosing: 10 mg (U.S. labeling) or 20 mg (Canadian labeling) at least 30 minutes prior to anticipated sexual activity (dosing range: 5-20 mg); to be given as one single dose and not given more than once daily. **Note:** Erectile function may be improved for up to 36 hours following a single dose; adjust dose.

Once-daily dosing: 2.5 mg once daily (U.S. labeling) or 5 mg once daily (Canadian labeling) to be given at approximately the same time daily without regard to timing of sexual activity. Dose may be adjusted based on tolerability (dosage range: 2.5-5 mg/day).

Dosing adjustment with concomitant medications:

U.S. labeling: Alpha₁-blockers: If stabilized on either alpha-blockers or tadalafil therapy, initiate new therapy with the other agent at the lowest possible dose.

Canadian labeling: Nonselective alpha-blockers (eg, doxazosin): *As-needed dosing:* 10 mg at least 30 minutes prior to anticipated sexual activity

CYP3A4 inhibitors (strong):

As-needed dosing:

U.S. labeling: Maximum: 10 mg, not to be given more frequently than every 72 hours

Canadian labeling: 10 mg, not to be given more frequently than every 48 hours (maximum 3 doses/week); may increase to 20 mg if lower dose is tolerated but ineffective. Discontinue use if 10 mg dose is not tolerated.

Once-daily dosing:

U.S. labeling: 2.5 mg once daily; maximum: 2.5 mg once daily

Canadian labeling: 2.5-5 mg once daily

Pulmonary arterial hypertension (Adcirca®): Oral: 40 mg once daily

Dosing adjustment with concomitant medications: *Coadministration with protease inhibitor regimen:*

Concurrent use with atazanavir/ritonavir, darunavir/ritonavir, fosamprenavir, ritonavir, saquinavir/ritonavir, tipranavir/ritonavir:

Coadministration of tadalafil in patients currently receiving one of these protease inhibitor regimens for at least 1 week: Initiate tadalafil at 20 mg once daily; increase to 40 mg once daily based on individual tolerability.

Coadministration of one of these protease inhibitor regimens in patients currently receiving tadalafil: Discontinue tadalafil at least 24 hours prior to the initiation of the protease inhibitor regimen. After at least 1 week of the protease inhibitor regimen, resume tadalafil at 20 mg once daily; increase to 40 mg once daily based on individual tolerability.

Concurrent use with indinavir or nelfinavir:

Patient receiving indinavir/nelfinavir when initiating tadalafil: Initiate tadalafil at 20 mg once daily; increase to 40 mg once daily based on individual tolerability

Patient receiving tadalafil when initiating indinavir/nelfinavir: Adjust tadalafil to 20 mg once daily; increase to 40 mg once daily based on individual tolerability

Renal Impairment

Benign prostatic hyperplasia (with or without concomitant erectile dysfunction) (Cialis®):

Cl_{cr} ≥51 mL/minute: No dosage adjustment necessary.

Cl_{cr} 30-50 mL/minute: Initial: 2.5 mg once daily; maximum: 5 mg once daily.

Cl_{cr} <30 mL/minute: Use not recommended.

ESRD requiring hemodialysis: Use not recommended.

Erectile dysfunction (Cialis®):

As-needed use:

U.S. labeling:

Cl_{cr} ≥51 mL/minute: No dosage adjustment necessary.

Cl_{cr} 30-50 mL/minute: Initial: 5 mg once daily; maximum: 10 mg (not to be given more frequently than every 48 hours).

Cl_{cr} <30 mL/minute: Maximum: 5 mg (not to be given more frequently than every 72 hours).

ESRD requiring hemodialysis: Maximum: 5 mg (not to be given more frequently than every 72 hours).

Canadian labeling:

Cl_{cr} >80 mL/minute: No dosage adjustment necessary.

Cl_{cr} ≥31-80 mL/minute: 10 mg, not to be given more frequently than every 48 hours (maximum: 3 doses/week); may increase to 20 mg if lower dose is tolerated but ineffective. Discontinue use if 10 mg dose is not tolerated.

Cl_{cr} <30 mL/minute: Use with extreme caution; has not been adequately studied.

ESRD requiring hemodialysis: Use with extreme caution; has not been adequately studied.

Once-daily use:

Cl_{cr} ≥31 mL/minute: No dosage adjustment necessary.

Cl_{cr} <30 mL/minute: Use not recommended.

ESRD requiring hemodialysis: Use not recommended.

◄ **Pulmonary arterial hypertension (Adcirca®):**
Cl_{cr} >80 mL/minute: No dosage adjustment necessary.
Cl_{cr} 31-80 mL/minute: Initial: 20 mg once daily; increase to 40 mg once daily based on individual tolerability.
Cl_{cr} ≤30 mL/minute: Avoid use due to increased tadalafil exposure, limited clinical experience, and lack of ability to influence clearance by dialysis.

Hepatic Impairment
Benign prostatic hyperplasia (with or without concomitant erectile dysfunction) (Cialis®):
Mild-to-moderate hepatic impairment (Child-Pugh class A or B): Use with caution.
Severe hepatic impairment (Child-Pugh class C): Use is not recommended.

Erectile dysfunction (Cialis®):
As-needed use:
U.S. labeling:
Mild-to-moderate impairment (Child-Pugh class A or B): Use with caution; dose should not exceed 10 mg once daily.
Severe impairment (Child-Pugh class C): Use is not recommended.
Canadian labeling:
Mild-to-moderate impairment (Child-Pugh class A or B): 10 mg, not to be given more frequently than every 48 hours (maximum 3 doses/week); may increase to 20 mg if lower dose is tolerated but ineffective. Discontinue use if 10 mg dose is not tolerated.
Severe impairment (Child-Pugh class C): Use with extreme caution; has not been adequately studied.
Once-daily use:
U.S. labeling:
Mild-to-moderate impairment (Child-Pugh class A or B): Use with caution.
Severe impairment (Child-Pugh class C): Use is not recommended.
Canadian labeling:
Mild-to-moderate impairment (Child-Pugh class A or B): No dosage adjustment necessary.
Severe impairment (Child-Pugh class C): Use with extreme caution; has not been adequately studied.

Pulmonary arterial hypertension (Adcirca®):
Mild-to-moderate hepatic impairment (Child-Pugh class A or B): Use with caution; consider initial dose of 20 mg once daily.
Severe hepatic impairment (Child-Pugh class C): Avoid use; has not been studied in patients with severe hepatic cirrhosis.

Administration May be administered with or without food.
Adcirca®: Administer daily dose all at once; dividing doses throughout the day is not advised.
Cialis®: When used on an as-needed basis, should be taken at least 30 minutes prior to sexual activity. When used on a once-daily basis, should be taken at the same time each day, without regard to timing of sexual activity.

Monitoring Parameters Blood pressure, response and adverse effects; urine flow, PSA

Special Geriatric Considerations No significant differences in pharmacokinetics were seen in elderly men versus younger men. Dosing should be adjusted for renal function. Since older adults often have concomitant diseases, many of which may be contraindicated with the use of tadalafil, prescriber should complete a thorough review of diseases and medications prior to prescribing tadalafil.

Dosage Forms Excipient information presented when available (limited, particularly for generics); consult specific product labeling.
Tablet, oral:
Adcirca®: 20 mg
Cialis®: 2.5 mg, 5 mg, 10 mg, 20 mg

◆ **Tagamet HB 200® [OTC]** *see* Cimetidine *on page* 376
◆ **TAK-375** *see* Ramelteon *on page* 1668
◆ **TAK-390MR** *see* Dexlansoprazole *on page* 523
◆ **TAK-599** *see* Ceftaroline Fosamil *on page* 326
◆ **Talwin®** *see* Pentazocine *on page* 1505
◆ **Tambocor™** *see* Flecainide *on page* 793
◆ **Tamiflu®** *see* Oseltamivir *on page* 1431

Tamoxifen (ta MOKS i fen)

Medication Safety Issues

Sound-alike/look-alike issues:

Tamoxifen may be confused with pentoxifylline, Tambocor™, tamsulosin, temazepam

Brand Names: Canada Apo-Tamox®; Mylan-Tamoxifen; Nolvadex®-D; PMS-Tamoxifen; Teva-Tamoxifen

Index Terms ICI-46474; Nolvadex; Tamoxifen Citras; Tamoxifen Citrate

Generic Availability (U.S.) Yes

Pharmacologic Category Antineoplastic Agent, Estrogen Receptor Antagonist; Selective Estrogen Receptor Modulator (SERM)

Use Treatment of metastatic (female and male) breast cancer; adjuvant treatment of breast cancer after primary treatment with surgery and radiation; reduce risk of invasive breast cancer in women with ductal carcinoma *in situ* (DCIS) after surgery and radiation; reduce the incidence of breast cancer in women at high risk

Unlabeled Use Treatment of mastalgia, gynecomastia, ovarian cancer, endometrial cancer, uterine sarcoma, and desmoid tumors; risk reduction in women with Paget's disease of the breast (with DCIS or without associated cancer)

Medication Guide Available Yes

Contraindications Hypersensitivity to tamoxifen or any component of the formulation; concurrent warfarin therapy or history of deep vein thrombosis or pulmonary embolism (when tamoxifen is used for cancer risk reduction in women at high risk for breast cancer and in women with DCIS)

Warnings/Precautions Hazardous agent - use appropriate precautions for handling and disposal. **[U.S. Boxed Warning]: Serious and life-threatening events (including stroke, pulmonary emboli, and uterine malignancy) have occurred at an incidence greater than placebo during use for breast cancer risk reduction in women at high-risk for breast cancer and in women with DCIS;** these events are rare, but require consideration in risk: benefit evaluation. An increased incidence of thromboembolic events, including DVT and pulmonary embolism, has been associated with use for breast cancer; risk is increased with concomitant chemotherapy; use with caution in individuals with a history of thromboembolic events. Thrombocytopenia and/or leukopenia may occur; neutropenia and pancytopenia have been reported rarely. Although the relationship to tamoxifen therapy is uncertain, rare hemorrhagic episodes have occurred in patients with significant thrombocytopenia. Use with caution in patients with hyperlipidemias; infrequent postmarketing cases of hyperlipidemias have been reported. Decreased visual acuity, retinal vein thrombosis, retinopathy, corneal changes, color perception changes, and increased incidence of cataracts (and the need for cataract surgery), have been reported. Hypercalcemia has occurred in patients with bone metastasis, usually within a few weeks of therapy initiation; institute appropriate hyper-calcemia management; discontinue if severe. Local disease flare and increased bone and tumor pain may occur in patients with metastatic breast cancer; may be associated with (good) tumor response.

Tamoxifen is associated with a high potential for drug interactions, including CYP- and Pgp-mediated interactions. Decreased efficacy and an increased risk of breast cancer recurrence has been reported with concurrent moderate or strong CYP2D6 inhibitors (Aubert, 2009; Dezentje, 2009). Concomitant use with select SSRIs may result in decreased tamoxifen efficacy. Strong CYP2D6 inhibitors (eg, fluoxetine, paroxetine) and moderate CYP2D6 inhibitors (eg, sertraline) are reported to interfere with transformation to the active metabolite endoxifen. Weak CYP2D6 inhibitors (eg, venlafaxine, citalopram) have minimal effect on the conversion to endoxifen (Jin, 2005; NCCN Breast Cancer Risk Reduction Guidelines v.2.2010); escitalopram is also a weak CYP2D6 inhibitor. Lower plasma concentrations of endoxifen (active metabolite) have been observed in patients associated with reduced CYP2D6 activity (Jin, 2005) and may be associated with reduced efficacy. In a retrospective analysis of breast cancer patients taking tamoxifen and SSRIs, concomitant use of paroxetine and tamoxifen was associated with an increased risk of death due to breast cancer (Kelly, 2010).

Tamoxifen use may be associated with changes in bone mineral density (BMD) and the effects may be dependent upon menstrual status. In postmenopausal women, tamoxifen use is associated with a protective effect on bone mineral density (BMD), preventing loss of BMD which lasts over the 5-year treatment period. In premenopausal women, a decline (from baseline) in BMD mineral density has been observed in women who continued to menstruate; may be associated with an increased risk of fractures. Liver abnormalities such as cholestasis, fatty liver, hepatitis, and hepatic necrosis have occurred. Hepatocellular carcinomas have been reported in some studies; relationship to treatment is unclear. Tamoxifen is associated with an increased incidence of uterine or endometrial cancers. Endometrial hyperplasia,

1831

TAMOXIFEN

polyps, endometriosis, uterine fibroids, and ovarian cysts have occurred. Monitor and promptly evaluate any report of abnormal vaginal bleeding. Amenorrhea and menstrual irregularities have been reported with tamoxifen use.

Adverse Reactions (Reflective of adult population; not specific for elderly)

>10%:

Cardiovascular: Vasodilation (41%), flushing (33%), hypertension (11%), peripheral edema (11%)

Central nervous system: Mood changes (12% to 18%), pain (3% to 16%), depression (2% to 12%)

Dermatologic: Skin changes (6% to 19%), rash (13%)

Endocrine & metabolic: Hot flashes (3% to 80%), fluid retention (32%), altered menses (13% to 25%), amenorrhea (16%)

Gastrointestinal: Nausea (5% to 26%), weight loss (23%), vomiting (12%)

Genitourinary: Vaginal discharge (13% to 55%), vaginal bleeding (2% to 23%)

Neuromuscular & skeletal: Weakness (18%), arthritis (14%), arthralgia (11%)

Respiratory: Pharyngitis (14%)

Miscellaneous: Lymphedema (11%)

1% to 10%:

Cardiovascular: Chest pain (5%), venous thrombotic events (5%), edema (4%), cardiovascular ischemia (3%), angina (2%), deep venous thrombus (≤2%), MI (1%)

Central nervous system: Insomnia (9%), dizziness (8%), headache (8%), anxiety (6%), fatigue (4%)

Dermatologic: Alopecia (≤5%)

Endocrine & metabolic: Oligomenorrhea (9%), breast pain (6%), menstrual disorder (6%), breast neoplasm (5%), hypercholesterolemia (4%)

Gastrointestinal: Abdominal pain (9%), weight gain (9%), constipation (4% to 8%), diarrhea (7%), dyspepsia (6%), throat irritation (oral solution 5%), abdominal cramps (1%), anorexia (1%)

Genitourinary: Urinary tract infection (10%), leukorrhea (9%), vaginal hemorrhage (6%), vaginitis (5%), vulvovaginitis (5%), ovarian cyst (3%)

Hematologic: Thrombocytopenia (≤10%), anemia (5%)

Hepatic: AST increased (5%), serum bilirubin increased (2%)

Neuromuscular & skeletal: Back pain (10%), bone pain (6% to 10%), osteoporosis (7%), fracture (7%), arthrosis (5%), joint disorder (5%), myalgia (5%), paresthesia (5%), musculoskeletal pain (3%)

Ocular: Cataract (7%)

Renal: Serum creatinine increased (≤2%)

Respiratory: Cough (4% to 9%), dyspnea (8%), bronchitis (5%), sinusitis (5%)

Miscellaneous: Infection/sepsis (≤9%), diaphoresis (6%), flu-like syndrome (6%), cyst (5%), neoplasm (5%), allergic reaction (3%)

Drug Interactions

Metabolism/Transport Effects Substrate of CYP2A6 (minor), CYP2B6 (minor), CYP2C9 (major), CYP2D6 (major), CYP2E1 (minor), CYP3A4 (major); **Note:** Assignment of Major/Minor substrate status based on clinically relevant drug interaction potential; **Inhibits** CYP2B6 (weak), CYP2C8 (moderate), CYP2C9 (weak), CYP3A4 (weak), P-glycoprotein

Avoid Concomitant Use

Avoid concomitant use of Tamoxifen with any of the following: Conivaptan; CYP2D6 Inhibitors (Strong); Silodosin; Topotecan; Vitamin K Antagonists

Increased Effect/Toxicity

Tamoxifen may increase the levels/effects of: ARIPiprazole; Colchicine; CYP2C8 Substrates; Dabigatran Etexilate; Everolimus; Highest Risk QTc-Prolonging Agents; Moderate Risk QTc-Prolonging Agents; P-glycoprotein/ABCB1 Substrates; Prucalopride; Rivaroxaban; Silodosin; Topotecan; Vitamin K Antagonists

The levels/effects of Tamoxifen may be increased by: Abiraterone Acetate; Conivaptan; CYP2C9 Inhibitors (Moderate); CYP2C9 Inhibitors (Strong); CYP3A4 Inhibitors (Moderate); CYP3A4 Inhibitors (Strong); Darunavir; Ivacaftor; Mifepristone

Decreased Effect

Tamoxifen may decrease the levels/effects of: Anastrozole; Letrozole

The levels/effects of Tamoxifen may be decreased by: Aminoglutethimide; CYP2C9 Inducers (Strong); CYP2D6 Inhibitors (Moderate); CYP2D6 Inhibitors (Strong); CYP3A4 Inducers (Strong); Deferasirox; Herbs (CYP3A4 Inducers); Peginterferon Alfa-2b; Rifamycin Derivatives; Tocilizumab

Ethanol/Nutrition/Herb Interactions

Food: Grapefruit juice may decrease the metabolism of tamoxifen. Management: Avoid grapefruit juice.

Herb/Nutraceutical: Black cohosh and dong quai have estrogenic properties. St John's wort may decrease levels/effects of tamoxifen. Management: Avoid black cohosh and dong quai in estrogen-dependent tumors. Avoid St John's wort.

Stability Store at room temperature of 20°C to 25°C (68°F to 77°F). Protect from light.

Mechanism of Action Competitively binds to estrogen receptors on tumors and other tissue targets, producing a nuclear complex that decreases DNA synthesis and inhibits estrogen effects; nonsteroidal agent with potent antiestrogenic properties which compete with estrogen for binding sites in breast and other tissues; cells accumulate in the G_0 and G_1 phases; therefore, tamoxifen is cytostatic rather than cytocidal.

Pharmacodynamics/Kinetics

Absorption: Well absorbed

Distribution: High concentrations found in uterus, endometrial and breast tissue

Protein binding: 99%

Metabolism: Hepatic; via CYP2D6 to 4-hydroxytamoxifen and via CYP3A4/5 to N-desmethyl-tamoxifen. Each is then further metabolized into endoxifen (4-hydroxy-tamoxifen via CYP3A4/5 and N-desmethyl-tamoxifen via CYP2D6); both 4-hydroxy-tamoxifen and endoxifen are 30- to 100-fold more potent than tamoxifen

Half-life elimination: Tamoxifen: ~5-7 days; N-desmethyl tamoxifen: ~14 days

Time to peak, serum: ~5 hours

Excretion: Feces (26% to 51%); urine (9% to 13%)

Dosage

Geriatric & Adult Note: For the treatment of breast cancer, patients receiving both tamoxifen and chemotherapy, should receive treatment sequentially, with tamoxifen following completion of chemotherapy.

Breast cancer treatment:

Adjuvant therapy (females): 20 mg once daily for 5 years

Metastatic (males and females): 20-40 mg/day (doses >20 mg should be given in 2 divided doses). Note: Although the FDA-approved labeling recommends dosing up to 40 mg/day, clinical benefit has not been demonstrated with doses above 20 mg/day (Bratherton, 1984).

Premenopausal women: Duration of treatment is 5 years (NCCN Breast Cancer guidelines v.1.2011)

Postmenopausal women: Duration of tamoxifen treatment is 2-3 years followed by an aromatase inhibitor (AI) to complete 5 years; if contraindications or intolerant to AI, may take tamoxifen for the full 5 years **or** extended therapy: 4.5-6 years of tamoxifen followed by 5 years of an AI (NCCN Breast Cancer guidelines v.1.2011)

DCIS (females), to reduce the risk for invasive breast cancer: 20 mg once daily for 5 years

Breast cancer risk reduction (pre- and postmenopausal high-risk females): 20 mg once daily for 5 years

Paget's disease of the breast (risk reduction; with DCIS or without associated cancer): 20 mg once daily for 5 years (NCCN Breast Cancer Guidelines, v.1.2011)

Dosage adjustment for DVT, pulmonary embolism, cerebrovascular accident, or prolonged immobilization: Discontinue tamoxifen (NCCN Breast Cancer Risk Reduction Guidelines, v.2.2010)

Administration Administer orally with or without food.

Monitoring Parameters CBC with platelets, serum calcium, LFTs; triglycerides and cholesterol (in patients with pre-existing hyperlipidemias); INR and PT (in patients on vitamin K antagonists); abnormal vaginal bleeding; breast and gynecologic exams (baseline and routine), mammogram (baseline and routine); signs/symptoms of DVT (leg swelling, tenderness) or PE (shortness of breath); ophthalmic exam (if vision problem or cataracts); bone mineral density (premenopausal women)

Test Interactions T_4 elevations (which may be explained by increases in thyroid-binding globulin) have been reported; not accompanied by clinical hyperthyroidism

Pharmacotherapy Pearls Estrogen receptor status may predict if adjuvant treatment with tamoxifen is of benefit. In metastatic breast cancer, patients with estrogen receptor positive tumors are more likely to benefit from tamoxifen treatment. With tamoxifen use to reduce the incidence of breast cancer in high risk-women, high risk is defined as women ≥35 years of age with a 5 year NCI Gail model predicted risk of breast cancer ≥1.67%.

Oncology Comment: The American Society of Clinical Oncology (ASCO) guidelines for adjuvant endocrine therapy in postmenopausal women with HR-positive breast cancer (Burstein, 2010) recommend considering aromatase inhibitor (AI) therapy at some point in the treatment course (primary, sequentially, or extended). Optimal duration at this time is not known; however, treatment with an AI should not exceed 5 years in primary and extended therapies, and 2-3 years if followed by tamoxifen in sequential therapy (total of 5 years). If initial therapy with AI has been discontinued before the 5 years, consideration should be taken to receive tamoxifen for a total of 5 years. The optimal time to switch to an AI is also not known; but data supports switching after 2-3 years of tamoxifen (sequential) or after 5 years of tamoxifen (extended). If patient becomes intolerant or has poor adherence, consideration should be made to switch to another AI or initiate tamoxifen.

The adjuvant endocrine therapy of choice is tamoxifen for men with breast cancer and for pre- or perimenopausal women at diagnosis. CYP2D6 genotyping is not recommended, however, due to the potential for drug-drug interactions use caution and consider avoiding concomitant therapy with tamoxifen and known CYP2D6 inhibitors.

Special Geriatric Considerations Studies have shown tamoxifen to be effective in the treatment of primary breast cancer in elderly women. Comparative studies with other antineoplastic agents in elderly women with breast cancer had more favorable survival rates with tamoxifen. Initiation of hormone therapy rather than chemotherapy is justified for elderly patients with metastatic breast cancer who are responsive.

Dosage Forms Excipient information presented when available (limited, particularly for generics); consult specific product labeling.

Tablet, oral: 10 mg, 20 mg

◆ **Tamoxifen Citras** *see* Tamoxifen *on page 1831*
◆ **Tamoxifen Citrate** *see* Tamoxifen *on page 1831*

Tamsulosin (tam SOO loe sin)

Related Information
Pharmacotherapy of Urinary Incontinence *on page 2141*
Medication Safety Issues
Sound-alike/look-alike issues:
Flomax® may be confused with Flonase®, Flovent®, Foltx®, Fosamax®
Tamsulosin may be confused with tacrolimus, tamoxifen, terazosin
International issues:
Flomax [U.S., Canada, and multiple international markets] may be confused with Flomox brand name for cefcapene [Japan]; Volmax brand name for salbutamol [multiple international markets]
Flomax: Brand name for tamsulosin [U.S., Canada, and multiple international markets], but also the brand name for morniflumate [Italy]
Brand Names: U.S. Flomax®
Brand Names: Canada Ava-Tamsulosin CR; Flomax® CR; JAMP-Tamsulosin; Mylan-Tamsulosin; RAN™-Tamsulosin; ratio-Tamsulosin; Sandoz-Tamsulosin; Sandoz-Tamsulosin CR; Teva-Tamsulosin
Index Terms Tamsulosin Hydrochloride
Generic Availability (U.S.) Yes
Pharmacologic Category Alpha$_1$ Blocker
Use Treatment of signs and symptoms of benign prostatic hyperplasia (BPH)
Unlabeled Use Symptomatic treatment of bladder outlet obstruction or dysfunction; facilitation of expulsion of ureteral stones
Contraindications Hypersensitivity to tamsulosin or any component of the formulation
Warnings/Precautions Not intended for use as an antihypertensive drug. May cause significant orthostatic hypotension and syncope, especially with first dose; anticipate a similar effect if therapy is interrupted for a few days, if dosage is rapidly increased, or if another antihypertensive drug (particularly vasodilators) or a PDE-5 inhibitor (eg, sildenafil, tadalafil, vardenafil) is introduced. "First-dose" orthostatic hypotension may occur 4-8 hours after dosing; may be dose related. Patients should be cautioned about performing hazardous tasks when starting new therapy or adjusting dosage upward. Discontinue if symptoms of angina occur or worsen. Rule out prostatic carcinoma before beginning therapy with tamsulosin. Intraoperative floppy iris syndrome has been observed in cataract surgery patients who were on or were previously treated with alpha$_1$-blockers; causality has not been established and there appears to be no benefit in discontinuing alpha-blocker therapy prior to surgery; instruct patients to inform ophthalmologist of tamsulosin use when considering eye surgery. Priapism has been associated with use (rarely). Rarely, patients with a sulfa allergy have also developed an allergic reaction to tamsulosin; avoid use when previous reaction has been severe.
Adverse Reactions (Reflective of adult population; not specific for elderly)
>10%:
Cardiovascular: Orthostatic hypotension (6% to 19%)
Central nervous system: Headache (19% to 21%), dizziness (15% to 17%)
Genitourinary: Abnormal ejaculation (8% to 18%)
Respiratory: Rhinitis (13% to 18%)
Miscellaneous: Infection (9% to 11%)

1% to 10%:
Cardiovascular: Chest pain (4%)
Central nervous system: Somnolence (3% to 4%), insomnia (1% to 2%), vertigo (≤1%)
Endocrine & metabolic: Libido decreased (1% to 2%)
Gastrointestinal: Diarrhea (4% to 6%), nausea (3% to 4%), gum pain, toothache
Neuromuscular & skeletal: Weakness (8% to 9%), back pain (7% to 8%)
Ocular: Blurred vision (≤2%)
Respiratory: Pharyngitis (5% to 6%), cough (3% to 5%), sinusitis (2% to 4%)

Drug Interactions

Metabolism/Transport Effects Substrate of CYP2D6 (minor), CYP3A4 (major); **Note:** Assignment of Major/Minor substrate status based on clinically relevant drug interaction potential

Avoid Concomitant Use
Avoid concomitant use of Tamsulosin with any of the following: Alpha1-Blockers; CYP3A4 Inhibitors (Strong)

Increased Effect/Toxicity
Tamsulosin may increase the levels/effects of: Alpha1-Blockers; Calcium Channel Blockers

The levels/effects of Tamsulosin may be increased by: Beta-Blockers; CYP3A4 Inhibitors (Moderate); CYP3A4 Inhibitors (Strong); Dasatinib; Ivacaftor; MAO Inhibitors; Mifepristone; Phosphodiesterase 5 Inhibitors

Decreased Effect
The levels/effects of Tamsulosin may be decreased by: CYP3A4 Inducers (Strong); Deferasirox; Herbs (CYP3A4 Inducers); Peginterferon Alfa-2b; Tocilizumab

Ethanol/Nutrition/Herb Interactions

Food: Fasting increases bioavailability by 30% and peak concentration 40% to 70%. Management: Administer 30 minutes after the same meal each day.

Herb/Nutraceutical: St John's wort may decrease the levels/effects of tamsulosin. Some herbal medications have hypotensive properties or may increase the hypotensive effect of tamsulosin. Limited information is available regarding combination with saw palmetto. Management: Avoid St John's wort, black cohosh, California poppy, coleus, golden seal, hawthorn, mistletoe, periwinkle, quinine, and shepherd's purse. Avoid saw palmetto.

Stability Store at room temperature of 25°C (77°F); excursions permitted to 15°C to 30°C (59°F to 86°F).

Mechanism of Action Tamsulosin is an antagonist of alpha$_{1A}$-adrenoreceptors in the prostate. Smooth muscle tone in the prostate is mediated by alpha$_{1A}$-adrenoreceptors; blocking them leads to relaxation of smooth muscle in the bladder neck and prostate causing an improvement of urine flow and decreased symptoms of BPH. Approximately 75% of the alpha$_1$-receptors in the prostate are of the alpha$_{1A}$ subtype.

Pharmacodynamics/Kinetics

Absorption: >90%
Distribution: V_d: 16 L
Protein binding: 94% to 99%, primarily to alpha$_1$ acid glycoprotein (AAG)
Metabolism: Hepatic (extensive) via CYP3A4 and 2D6; metabolites undergo extensive conjugation to glucuronide or sulfate
Bioavailability: Fasting: 30% increase
Steady-state: By the fifth day of once-daily dosing
Half-life elimination: Healthy volunteers: 9-13 hours; Target population: 14-15 hours
Time to peak: Fasting: 4-5 hours; With food: 6-7 hours
Excretion: Urine (76%, <10% as unchanged drug); feces (21%)

Dosage

Geriatric & Adult
Benign prostatic hyperplasia (BPH): Oral: 0.4 mg once daily ~30 minutes after the same meal each day; dose may be increased after 2-4 weeks to 0.8 mg once daily in patients who fail to respond. If therapy is interrupted for several days, restart with 0.4 mg once daily.
Bladder outlet obstruction symptoms (unlabeled use): Oral: 0.4 mg once daily (Rossi, 2001)
Ureteral stones, expulsion (unlabeled use): Oral: 0.4 mg once daily, discontinue after successful expulsion (average time to expulsion was 1-2 weeks) (Agrawal, 2009; Ahmed, 2010). **Note:** Patients with stones >10 mm were excluded from studies.

Renal Impairment
Cl_{cr} ≥10 mL/minute: No adjustment needed.
Cl_{cr} <10 mL/minute: Not studied.

Hepatic Impairment
Mild-to-moderate impairment: No adjustment needed
Severe impairment: Not studied

Administration Administer 30 minutes after the same meal each day. Capsules should be swallowed whole; do not crush, chew, or open.

Special Geriatric Considerations Metabolism of tamsulosin may be slower, and older patients may be more sensitive to the orthostatic hypotension caused by this medication. A 40% higher exposure (AUC) is anticipated in patients between 55 and 75 years of age as compared to younger subjects (20-32 years).

Dosage Forms Excipient information presented when available (limited, particularly for generics); consult specific product labeling.
Capsule, oral, as hydrochloride: 0.4 mg
Flomax®: 0.4 mg

◆ **Tamsulosin and Dutasteride** *see* Dutasteride and Tamsulosin *on page 625*
◆ **Tamsulosin Hydrochloride** *see* Tamsulosin *on page 1834*
◆ **Tamsulosin Hydrochloride and Dutasteride** *see* Dutasteride and Tamsulosin *on page 625*
◆ **TAP-144** *see* Leuprolide *on page 1103*
◆ **Tapazole®** *see* Methimazole *on page 1232*

Tapentadol (ta PEN ta dol)

Medication Safety Issues
Sound-alike/look-alike issues:
Tapentadol may be confused with traMADol
High alert medication:
The Institute for Safe Medication Practices (ISMP) includes this medication among its list of drug classes which have a heightened risk of causing significant patient harm when used in error.
Brand Names: U.S. Nucynta®; Nucynta® ER
Brand Names: Canada Nucynta™ CR
Index Terms CG5503; Tapentadol Hydrochloride
Generic Availability (U.S.) No
Pharmacologic Category Analgesic, Opioid
Use
Immediate release formulation: Relief of moderate-to-severe acute pain
Long acting formulation: Relief of moderate-to-severe chronic pain when continuous, around-the-clock analgesia is necessary for an extended period of time
Medication Guide Available Yes
Contraindications Hypersensitivity to tapentadol or any component of the formulation; impaired pulmonary function (severe respiratory depression, acute or severe asthma or hypercapnia) in unmonitored settings or in absence of resuscitative equipment or ventilatory support; paralytic ileus; use of MAO inhibitors within 14 days

Canadian labeling: Additional contraindications (not in U.S. labeling): Hypersensitivity to opioids; any disease/condition that affects bowel transit (eg, ileus of any type, strictures); severe renal impairment (Cl$_{cr}$ <30 mL/minute); severe hepatic impairment (Child-Pugh class C); mild, intermittent, or short-duration pain that can be managed with alternative pain medication; management of perioperative pain; acute alcoholism, delirium tremens, and seizure disorders; severe CNS depression, increased cerebrospinal or intracranial pressure or head injury

Warnings/Precautions Extended release tablets: **[U.S. Boxed Warning]: Use of alcohol or alcohol-containing medications should be avoided;** concomitant use with alcohol may increase tapentadol systemic exposure which may lead to possible fatal overdose. **[U.S. Boxed warning]: NOT intended for use as an as-needed analgesic; NOT intended for the management of acute or postoperative pain;** approved for the treatment of chronic pain only (not an as-needed basis). **[U.S. Boxed Warning]: Extended-release tablets must be swallowed whole and should NOT be split, crushed, broken, chewed or dissolved. [U.S. Boxed Warning]: Healthcare provider should be alert to problems of abuse, misuse, and diversion.** May cause severe hypotension; use with caution in patients with risk factors (eg, hypovolemia, concomitant use of other hypotensive agents).

Use with caution in patients with respiratory disease or respiratory compromise (eg, asthma, chronic obstructive pulmonary disease [COPD], cor pulmonale, sleep apnea, severe obesity, kyphoscoliosis, hypoxia, hypercapnia); critical respiratory depression may occur, even at therapeutic dosages. May cause CNS depression, which may impair physical or mental abilities; patients must be cautioned about performing tasks which require mental alertness (eg, operating machinery or driving). Use with caution in patients with CNS depression or coma. Effects may be potentiated when used with other sedative drugs or ethanol. Use with caution in patients with adrenal insufficiency, hypothyroidism or prostatic hyperplasia/urinary stricture.

Serotonin syndrome (SS) may occur with serotonin/norepinephrine reuptake inhibitors (SNRIs), including tapentadol. Signs of SS may include agitation, tachycardia, hyperthermia, nausea, and vomiting. Avoid use with serotonergic agents such as TCAs, triptans, venlafaxine, trazodone, lithium, sibutramine, meperidine, dextromethorphan, St John's wort, SNRIs, and SSRIs; concomitant use has been associated with the development of serotonin syndrome. Contraindicated with MAO inhibitor use within 14 days.

Use caution in patients with biliary tract dysfunction or acute pancreatitis; opioids may cause spasm of the sphincter of Oddi. Opioid use may obscure diagnosis or clinical course of patients with acute abdominal conditions. Use with extreme caution in patients with head injury, intracranial lesions, or elevated intracranial pressure (ICP); exaggerated elevation of ICP may occur. Serum concentrations are increased in hepatic impairment; use with caution in patients with moderate hepatic impairment (dosage adjustment required). Not recommended for use in severe hepatic impairment (not studied). Use with caution in patients with mild-to-moderate renal impairment (no dosage adjustment recommended). Not recommended for use in severe renal impairment (not studied). Use caution in patients with a history of seizures or conditions predisposing patients to seizures; patients with a history of seizures were excluded in clinical trials of tapentadol. Tramadol, an analgesic with similar pharmacologic properties to tapentadol, has been associated with seizures, particularly in patients with predisposing factors.

Prolonged use increases risk of abuse, addiction, and withdrawal symptoms. An opioid-containing regimen should be tailored to each patient's needs with respect to degree of tolerance for opioids (naïve versus chronic user), age, weight, and medical condition. Healthcare provider should be alert to problems of abuse, misuse, and diversion. Abrupt discontinuation may lead to withdrawal symptoms. Symptoms may be decreased by tapering prior to discontinuation. Use opioids with caution in elderly; consider decreasing initial dose. Use caution in debilitated patients; there is a greater potential for critical respiratory depression, even at therapeutic dosages.

During dosage adjustments, the Canadian labeling recommends that immediate release tramadol may be used as rescue medication (maximum dose: 400 mg/day) and that fentanyl should not be used as rescue medication.

Adverse Reactions (Reflective of adult population; not specific for elderly)
Immediate release:
>10%:
Central nervous system: Dizziness (24%), somnolence (15%)
Gastrointestinal: Nausea (30%), vomiting (18%), constipation (8%)
≤1% to 10%:
Central nervous system: Fatigue (3%), insomnia (2%), anxiety (1%), confusion (1%), dreams abnormal (1%), lethargy (1%), attention disturbances (<1%), headache (<1%)
Dermatologic: Pruritus (3% to 5%), hyperhidrosis (3%), rash (1%)
Endocrine & metabolic: Hot flushes (1%)
Gastrointestinal: Xerostomia (4%), appetite decreased (2%), dyspepsia (2%)
Genitourinary: Urinary tract infection (1%)
Neuromuscular & skeletal: Arthralgia (1%), tremor (1%)
Respiratory: Nasopharyngitis (1%), upper respiratory tract infection (1%), dyspnea (<1%)

Extended release:
>10%:
Central nervous system: Dizziness (17%), headache (15%), somnolence (12%)
Gastrointestinal: Nausea (21%), constipation (17%), vomiting (8%)
1% to 10%:
Central nervous system: Fatigue (9%), insomnia (4%), anxiety (2%), lethargy (2%), vertigo (2%), attention disturbances (1%), chills (1%), depression/depressed mood (1%)
Dermatologic: Hyperhidrosis (5%), pruritus (5%), rash (1%)
Endocrine & metabolic: Hot flushes (2%)
Gastrointestinal: Xerostomia (7%), dyspepsia (3%), appetite decreased (2%)
Genitourinary: Erectile dysfunction (1%)
Neuromuscular & skeletal: Weakness (2%), tremor (1%)
Ocular: Vision blurred (1%)
Respiratory: Dyspnea (1%)

Drug Interactions
Metabolism/Transport Effects Substrate of CYP2C9 (minor), CYP2D6 (minor); **Note:** Assignment of Major/Minor substrate status based on clinically relevant drug interaction potential
Avoid Concomitant Use
Avoid concomitant use of Tapentadol with any of the following: Alcohol (Ethyl); Azelastine; Azelastine (Nasal); MAO Inhibitors; Methadone; Paraldehyde

TAPENTADOL

Increased Effect/Toxicity
Tapentadol may increase the levels/effects of: Alvimopan; Azelastine; Azelastine (Nasal); CNS Depressants; Desmopressin; MAO Inhibitors; Methadone; Metoclopramide; Metyrosine; Paraldehyde; Selective Serotonin Reuptake Inhibitors; Serotonin Modulators; Thiazide Diuretics; Zolpidem

The levels/effects of Tapentadol may be increased by: Alcohol (Ethyl); Amphetamines; Antipsychotic Agents (Phenothiazines); Antipsychotics; HydrOXYzine; Succinylcholine

Decreased Effect
Tapentadol may decrease the levels/effects of: Pegvisomant

The levels/effects of Tapentadol may be decreased by: Ammonium Chloride; Antiemetics (5HT3 Antagonists); Mixed Agonist / Antagonist Opioids; Peginterferon Alfa-2b

Ethanol/Nutrition/Herb Interactions
Ethanol: May increase CNS depression; monitor for increased effects with coadministration. Caution patients about effects. Bioavailability of extended release tablets may be increased by alcohol; combined use should be avoided.

Food: When administered after a high fat/calorie meal, the AUC and C_{max} increased by 25% and 16%, respectively; may administer without regard to meals.

Herb/Nutraceutical: Avoid St John's wort (may increase CNS depression and risk of serotonin syndrome).

Stability Store at room temperature up to 25°C (77°F); excursions permitted to 15°C to 30°C (59°F to 86°F). Protect from moisture.

Mechanism of Action Binds to μ-opiate receptors in the CNS causing inhibition of ascending pain pathways, altering the perception of and response to pain; also inhibits the reuptake of norepinephrine, which also modifies the ascending pain pathway

Pharmacodynamics/Kinetics
Absorption: Rapid and complete

Distribution: V_d: I.V.: 442-638 L

Protein binding: ~20%

Metabolism: Extensive metabolism, including first pass metabolism; metabolized primarily via phase 2 glucuronidation to glucuronides (major metabolite: tapentadol-O-glucuronide); minimal phase 1 oxidative metabolism; also metabolized to a lesser degree by CYP2C9, CYP2C19, and CYP2D6; all metabolites pharmacologically inactive

Bioavailability: ~32%

Half-life elimination: Immediate release: ~4 hours; Long acting formulations: ~5-6 hours

Time to peak, plasma: Immediate release: 1.25 hours; Long acting formulations: 3-6 hours

Excretion: Urine (99%: 70% conjugated metabolites; 3% unchanged drug)

Dosage
Geriatric Initial: Consider initiating at lower range of dosing. Refer to adult dosing.

Adult Dose and dosage intervals should be individualized according to pain severity with respect to patient's previous experience with similar opioid analgesics. To reduce the risk of withdrawal symptoms, it is recommended to taper the dose when discontinuing therapy.

Acute moderate-severe pain: Oral: *U.S. labeling (immediate release):* Day 1: 50-100 mg every 4-6 hours as needed; may administer a second dose ≥1 hour after the initial dose (maximum dose on first day: 700 mg/day); Day 2 and subsequent dosing: 50-100 mg every 4-6 hours as needed (maximum: 600 mg/day)

Chronic moderate-severe pain: Oral:

U.S. labeling (extended release):
Opioid naive: Initial: 50 mg twice daily (recommended interval: ~12 hours); titrate in increments of 50 mg no more frequently than twice daily every 3 days to effective dose (therapeutic range: 100-250 mg twice daily) (maximum dose: 500 mg/day)

Opioid experienced: Initial: 50 mg titrated to an effective dose; titrate in increments of 50 mg no more frequently than twice daily every 3 days (therapeutic range: 100-250 mg twice daily) (maximum dose: 500 mg/day). **Note:** No adequate data on converting patients from other opioids to tapentadol extended release.

Conversion from Nucynta® immediate release to extended release: Convert using same total daily dose but divide into two equal doses and administer twice daily (recommended interval: ~12 hours) (maximum dose: 500 mg/day).

Canadian labeling (controlled release):
Opioid naive: Initial: 50 mg twice daily (recommended interval: ~12 hours); titrate to effective dose (therapeutic range: 100-250 mg twice daily)

Opioid experienced (**Note:** Decrease initial dose by 50% when switching from other opioid analgesics): Titrate in increments of 50 mg twice daily every 3 days to recommended dosing range of 100-250 mg twice daily (maximum dose should not exceed 500 mg/day)

Renal Impairment
Mild-moderate renal impairment: No adjustment necessary.
Severe renal impairment: Not recommended (not studied); use is contraindicated in the Canadian labeling.

Hepatic Impairment
Mild hepatic impairment: No adjustment necessary.
Moderate hepatic impairment:
   U.S. labeling:
     Immediate release: Initial: 50 mg every 8 hours or longer (maximum: 3 doses/24 hours). Further treatment for maintenance of analgesia may be achieved by either shortening or lengthening the dosing interval.
     Extended release: Initial: 50 mg every 24 hours; maximum: 100 mg once daily
   Canadian labeling (controlled release): Initial: 50 mg every 24 hours; titrate dose cautiously; manufacturer's labeling does not provide specific recommendations.
Severe hepatic impairment: Not recommended (not studied); use is contraindicated in the Canadian labeling.

Administration Administer orally with or without food. Long acting formulations must be swallowed whole and should **not** be split, crushed, broken, chewed, or dissolved.

Special Geriatric Considerations In clinical studies, patients ≥65 years had a higher incidence of constipation as compared to younger patients. See Dosage: Geriatric.

Controlled Substance C-II

Dosage Forms Excipient information presented when available (limited, particularly for generics); consult specific product labeling.
Tablet, oral:
   Nucynta®: 50 mg, 75 mg, 100 mg
Tablet, extended release, oral:
   Nucynta® ER: 50 mg, 100 mg, 150 mg, 200 mg, 250 mg

Dosage Forms: Canada Excipient information presented when available (limited, particularly for generics); consult specific product labeling.
Tablet, controlled release, oral, as hydrochloride:
   Nucynta™ CR: 50 mg, 100 mg, 150 mg, 200 mg, 250 mg

Tegaserod (teg a SER od)

Brand Names: U.S. Zelnorm®
Brand Names: Canada Zelnorm® [DSC]
Index Terms HTF919; Tegaserod Maleate
Generic Availability (U.S.) No
Pharmacologic Category Serotonin 5-HT$_4$ Receptor Agonist
Use Emergency treatment of irritable bowel syndrome with constipation (IBS-C) and chronic idiopathic constipation (CIC) in women (<55 years of age) in which no alternative therapy exists

Prescribing and Access Restrictions Available in U.S. under an emergency investigational new drug (IND) process. Emergency situations are defined as immediately life-threatening or requiring hospitalization. Physicians with patients who may qualify can contact the FDA's Division of Drug Information via email (druginfo@fda.hhs.gov). The FDA may either deny the request or authorize shipment of Zelnorm® by Novartis. Additional information can ▶

◄ be found at http://www.fda.gov/Drugs/DrugSafety/PostmarketDrugSafetyInformationforPatientsandProviders/ucm103223.htm.

Contraindications Per product labeling: Hypersensitivity to tegaserod or any component of the formulation; severe renal impairment; moderate or severe hepatic impairment; history of bowel obstruction, symptomatic gallbladder disease, suspected sphincter of Oddi dysfunction, or abdominal adhesions. Treatment should not be started in patients with diarrhea or in those who experience diarrhea frequently.

Exclusion criteria under the emergency-IND process: Unstable angina, history of MI or stroke, hypertension, hyperlipidemia, diabetes, age ≥55 years, smoking, obesity, depression, anxiety, or suicidal ideation.

Warnings/Precautions Serious cardiovascular events (eg, MI, stroke, unstable angina) may occur; patients should seek emergency care following any sign and symptom suggestive of a serious cardiac event. Use under the emergency IND process will not be permitted in patients with unstable angina, a history of MI or stroke, cigarette smoking, hypertension, hyperlipidemia, obesity, or diabetes. In addition, use will not be permitted in patients with depression, anxiety, or with any signs of suicidal ideation or behavior. Use has been associated with rare intestinal ischemic events. Discontinue immediately with new or sudden worsening abdominal pain or rectal bleeding. Diarrhea may occur after the start of treatment, most cases reported as a single episode within the first week of therapy, and may resolve with continued dosing. However, serious consequences of diarrhea (hypovolemia, syncope) have been reported. Patients should be warned to contact healthcare provider immediately if they develop severe diarrhea, or diarrhea with severe cramping, abdominal pain, or dizziness. Use caution with mild hepatic impairment; not recommended with moderate or severe impairment. Potential benefits should be weighed against potential risks in patients eligible for emergency-IND use. Safety and efficacy have not been established in males with IBS. Use in elderly women (≥55 years of age) is contraindicated.

Adverse Reactions (Reflective of adult population; not specific for elderly)
>10%:
  Central nervous system: Headache (15%)
  Gastrointestinal: Abdominal pain (12%)
1% to 10%:
  Central nervous system: Dizziness (4%), migraine (2%)
  Gastrointestinal: Diarrhea (9%; severe <1%), nausea (8%), flatulence (6%)
  Neuromuscular & skeletal: Back pain (5%), arthropathy (2%), leg pain (1%)

Drug Interactions
  Metabolism/Transport Effects None known.
  Avoid Concomitant Use There are no known interactions where it is recommended to avoid concomitant use.
  Increased Effect/Toxicity There are no known significant interactions involving an increase in effect.
  Decreased Effect There are no known significant interactions involving a decrease in effect.
Ethanol/Nutrition/Herb Interactions Food: Bioavailability is decreased by 40% to 65% and C_{max} is decreased by 20% to 40% when taken with food. T_{max} is prolonged from 1 hour up to 2 hours when taken following a meal, but decreased to 0.7 hours when taken 30 minutes before a meal. Management: Take on an empty stomach 30 minutes before meals.
Stability Store at controlled room temperature of 15°C to 30°C (59°F to 86°F). Protect from moisture.
Mechanism of Action Tegaserod is a partial neuronal 5-HT$_4$ receptor agonist. Its action at the receptor site leads to stimulation of the peristaltic reflex and intestinal secretion, and moderation of visceral sensitivity.
Pharmacodynamics/Kinetics
  Distribution: V_d: 368 ± 223 L
  Protein binding: 98% primarily to α_1-acid glycoprotein
  Metabolism: GI: Hydrolysis in the stomach; Hepatic: Oxidation, conjugation, and glucuronidation; metabolite (negligible activity); significant first-pass effect
  Bioavailability: Fasting: 10%
  Half-life elimination: I.V.: 11 ± 5 hours
  Time to peak: 1 hour
  Excretion: Feces (~66% as unchanged drug); urine (~33% as metabolites)
Dosage
  Geriatric Use in elderly women (≥55 years of age) is contraindicated.
  Adult
    IBS with constipation: Females <55 years of age: Oral: 6 mg twice daily, before meals, for 4-6 weeks; may consider continuing treatment for an additional 4-6 weeks in patients who respond initially

Chronic idiopathic constipation: Females <55 years of age: Oral: 6 mg twice daily, before meals; the need for continued therapy should be reassessed periodically

Renal Impairment C_{max} and AUC of the inactive metabolite are increased with renal impairment.
Mild-to-moderate impairment: No dosage adjustment recommended
Severe impairment: Use is contraindicated

Hepatic Impairment C_{max} and AUC of tegaserod are increased with hepatic impairment.
Mild impairment: No dosage adjustment recommended; however, use caution
Moderate-to-severe impairment: Use is contraindicated

Administration Administer 30 minutes before meals.

Special Geriatric Considerations Use in elderly women (≥55 years of age) is contra-indicated.

Dosage Forms Excipient information presented when available (limited, particularly for generics); consult specific product labeling.
Tablet, oral:
Zelnorm®: 2 mg, 6 mg

◆ **Tegaserod Maleate** *see* Tegaserod *on page 1839*
◆ **TEGretol®** *see* CarBAMazepine *on page 286*
◆ **TEGretol®-XR** *see* CarBAMazepine *on page 286*
◆ **TEI-6720** *see* Febuxostat *on page 747*
◆ **Tekamlo™** *see* Aliskiren and Amlodipine *on page 61*
◆ **Tekturna®** *see* Aliskiren *on page 58*

Telavancin (tel a VAN sin)

Medication Safety Issues
Sound-alike/look-alike issues:
Telavancin may be confused with telithromycin
Vibativ™ may be confused with Viactiv®, Vibramycin®, vigabatrin

Brand Names: U.S. Vibativ™

Index Terms TD-6424; Telavancin Hydrochloride

Generic Availability (U.S.) No

Pharmacologic Category Glycopeptide

Use Treatment of complicated skin and skin structure infections caused by susceptible gram-positive organisms including methicillin-susceptible or -resistant *Staphylococcus aureus*, vancomycin-susceptible *Enterococcus faecalis*, and *Streptococcus pyogenes*, *Streptococcus agalactiae*, or *Streptococcus anginosus* group

Medication Guide Available Yes

Contraindications There are no contraindications listed within the manufacturer's labeling.

Warnings/Precautions May prolong QT_c interval; avoid use in patients with a history of QT_c prolongation, uncompensated heart failure, severe left ventricular hypertrophy, or concurrent administration of other medications known to prolong the QT interval (including Class Ia and Class III antiarrhythmics, cisapride, erythromycin, antipsychotics, and tricyclic antidepressants). Clinical studies indicate mean maximal QT_c prolongation of 12-15 msec at the end of 10 mg/kg infusion. Use with caution in patients with renal impairment or those receiving other nephrotoxic drugs; dosage modification required and efficacy may be reduced in patients with Cl_{cr} ≤50 mL/minute. May cause nephrotoxicity; usual risk factors include pre-existing renal impairment, concomitant nephrotoxic medications, advanced age, and dehydration. Monitor renal function prior to, during, and following therapy. Contains solubilizer cyclodextrin (hydroxypropyl-beta-cyclodextrin) which may accumulate in patients with renal dysfunction. Prolonged use may result in fungal or bacterial superinfection, including *C. difficile*-associated diarrhea (CDAD) and pseudomembranous colitis; CDAD has been observed >2 months postantibiotic treatment.

May interfere with tests used to monitor coagulation (eg, prothrombin time, INR, activated partial thromboplastin time, activated clotting time, coagulation based factor Xa tests) when samples drawn ≤18 hours after drug administration. Blood samples should be collected as close to the next dose of telavancin as possible. Rapid I.V. administration may result in flushing, rash, urticaria, and/or pruritus; slowing or stopping the infusion may alleviate these symptoms. In the elderly, lower doses are often required secondary to age-related decreases in renal function.

Adverse Reactions (Reflective of adult population; not specific for elderly)
>10%:
Central nervous system: Insomnia (13%), psychiatric disorder (12%), headache (11%)
Gastrointestinal: Metallic/soapy taste (33%), nausea (27%), vomiting (14%)
Genitourinary: Foamy urine (13%)

1% to 10%:
Central nervous system: Dizziness (6%)
Dermatologic: Pruritus (3% to 6%), rash (4%)
Endocrine & metabolic: Hypokalemia (7%)
Gastrointestinal: Diarrhea (7%), appetite decreased (3%), abdominal pain (2%)
Hematologic: Thrombocytopenia (7%)
Local: Infusion site pain (4%), infusion site erythema (3%)
Neuromuscular & skeletal: Paresthesia (5%), rigors (4%)
Renal: Serum creatinine increased (8%), microalbuminuria (7%)
Respiratory: Dyspnea (8%)

Drug Interactions

Metabolism/Transport Effects None known.

Avoid Concomitant Use
Avoid concomitant use of Telavancin with any of the following: BCG

Increased Effect/Toxicity
Telavancin may increase the levels/effects of: Highest Risk QTc-Prolonging Agents; Moderate Risk QTc-Prolonging Agents

The levels/effects of Telavancin may be increased by: Mifepristone

Decreased Effect
Telavancin may decrease the levels/effects of: BCG; Typhoid Vaccine

Stability Use appropriate precautions for handling and disposal. Store at 2°C to 8°C (35°F to 46°F); excursions permitted up to 25°C (77°F); avoid excess heat. **Note:** Vials contain no bacteriostatic agent.
Reconstitute 250 mg vial with 15 mL of D_5W, NS, or SWFI to yield 15 mg/mL (total volume of ~17 mL). Reconstitute 750 mg vial with 45 mL of D_5W, NS, or SWFI to yield 15 mg/mL (total volume of ~50 mL). Reconstitution may take 2-20 minutes. Discard vial if vacuum did not pull the diluent into the vial. Prior to administration, dilute dose in 100-250 mL D_5W, LR, or NS to a final concentration of 0.6-8 mg/mL.
Reconstituted solution in the vial or admixed in either D_5W, NS, or SWFI are stable at room temperature for 4 hours or under refrigeration for 72 hours. Total time in vial **plus** time in infusion bag should not exceed 4 hours at room temperature or 72 hours if refrigerated at 2°C to 8°C (35°F to 46°F).

Mechanism of Action Exerts concentration-dependent bactericidal activity; inhibits bacterial cell wall synthesis by blocking polymerization and cross-linking of peptidoglycan by binding to D-Ala-D-Ala portion of cell wall. Unlike vancomycin, additional mechanism involves disruption of membrane potential and changes cell permeability due to presence of lipophilic side chain moiety.

Pharmacodynamics/Kinetics
Distribution: V_{ss}: 0.13 L/kg
Protein binding: ~90%; primarily to albumin
Half-life elimination: 6.6-9.6 hours
Excretion: Urine (~76%); feces (<1%)

Dosage
Geriatric & Adult Complicated skin and skin structure Infection: I.V.: 10 mg/kg every 24 hours for 1-2 weeks
Renal Impairment *Note: Renal function may be estimated using the Cockcroft-Gault formula for dosage adjustment purposes.*
Cl_{cr} 30-50 mL/minute: 7.5 mg/kg every 24 hours.
Cl_{cr} 10 to <30 mL/minute: 10 mg/kg every 48 hours.
Cl_{cr} <10 mL/minute and hemodialysis patients: Dosage adjustment recommendations are not available; use caution or avoid.

Hepatic Impairment
Mild-to-moderate hepatic impairment: no dosage adjustment necessary.
Severe hepatic impairment: Has not been evaluated.

Administration Administer I.V. over 60 minutes. Other medications should not be infused simultaneously through the same I.V. line. When the same intravenous line is used for sequential infusion of other medications, flush line with D_5W, LR, or NS before and after infusing telavancin.
Red-man syndrome may occur if the infusion is too rapid. It is not an allergic reaction, but may be characterized by hypotension and/or a maculopapular rash appearing on the face, neck, trunk, and/or upper extremities. If this should occur, discontinuing or slowing the infusion rate may eliminate these reactions.

Monitoring Parameters Renal function

Test Interactions Interferes with the following coagulation assessments (causes artificially increased clotting times): PT, INR, aPTT, ACT, Xa; interferes with urine protein via qualitative dipstick and quantitative dye methods

Special Geriatric Considerations Of the more than 900 patients treated with telavancin in clinical trials to treat complicated skin and skin-structure infections, 18.7% were ≥65 years of age and 9.4% were ≥75 years of age. The results of subgroup, post-hoc analyses found lower cure rates with telavancin in patients ≥65 years compared to those <65 years of age, 72.1% vs 86.6%, respectively. Lower cure rates were also noted in patients with a Cl_{cr} ≤50 mL/minute. The frequency of adverse events in patients ≥65 years of age was 75% compared to 83% in patients >65 years of age. Renal adverse events were reported in 8.6% of patients ≥65 years and 1.9% of patients <65 years. Common comorbidities in these patients include pre-existing kidney disease, diabetes mellitus, heart failure or hypertension. Concomitant medications that affect kidney function were commonly used, such as NSAIDs, ACE inhibitors, and loop diuretics.

Product Availability Vibativ™: Temporarily not commercially available; anticipated date of availability is unknown.

Dosage Forms Excipient information presented when available (limited, particularly for generics); consult specific product labeling.

Injection, powder for reconstitution:

  Vibativ™: 250 mg, 750 mg [contains cyclodextrin]

♦ **Telavancin Hydrochloride** see Telavancin on page 1841

Telbivudine (tel BI vyoo deen)

Brand Names: U.S. Tyzeka®
Brand Names: Canada Sebivo®
Index Terms L-Deoxythymidine; LdT
Generic Availability (U.S.) No
Pharmacologic Category Antiretroviral Agent, Reverse Transcriptase Inhibitor (Nucleoside)
Use Treatment of chronic hepatitis B with evidence of viral replication and either persistent transaminase elevations or histologically-active disease
Medication Guide Available Yes
Contraindications Concurrent use with peginterferon alfa-2a

Canadian labeling: Additional contraindications (not in U.S. labeling): Hypersensitivity to telbivudine or any component of the formulation

Warnings/Precautions [U.S. Boxed Warnings]: Cases of lactic acidosis and severe hepatomegaly with steatosis, some fatal, have been reported with the use of nucleoside analogues. Severe, acute exacerbation of hepatitis B may occur upon discontinuation. Monitor liver function several months after stopping treatment; reinitiation of antihepatitis B therapy may be required. Myopathy (eg, unexplained muscle aches and/or muscle weakness in conjunction with increases serum creatine kinase) has been reported with telbivudine initiation after several weeks to months; therapy should be interrupted if myopathy suspected and discontinued if diagnosed. Patients taking concomitant medications associated with myopathy should be monitored closely. Peripheral neuropathy may occur alone or in combination with pegylated interferon alfa-2a (concurrent use is contraindicated) or possibly other interferons. Symptoms have been observed within 3 months after initiation of therapy. Interrupt treatment for suspected peripheral neuropathy and discontinue if confirmed; symptoms may be reversible with discontinuation. Use caution in patients with renal impairment or patients receiving concomitant therapy which may reduce renal function; dosage adjustment required (Cl_{cr} <50 mL/minute). Monitor renal function before and during treatment in liver transplant patients receiving concurrent therapy of cyclosporine or tacrolimus; telbivudine may need to be adjusted. Safety and efficacy have not been established in liver transplant patients, Black/African-American patients, or Hispanic patients.

Not recommended as first-line therapy of chronic HBV due to high rate of resistance; use may be appropriate in short-term treatment of acute HBV (Lok, 2009). Cross-resistance among other antivirals for hepatitis B may occur; use caution in patients failing previous therapy with lamivudine. Telbivudine does not exhibit any clinically-relevant activity against human immunodeficiency virus (HIV type 1). Safety and efficacy have not been studied in patients coinfected with HIV, hepatitis C virus (HCV), or hepatitis D virus (HDV).

Adverse Reactions (Reflective of adult population; not specific for elderly)
>10%:
  Central nervous system: Fatigue (13%)
  Neuromuscular & skeletal: CPK increased (79%; grades 3/4: 13%)
1% to 10%:
  Central nervous system: Headache (10%), dizziness (4%), fever (4%), insomnia (3%)
  Dermatologic: Rash (4%), pruritus (2%)
  Endocrine & metabolic: Lipase increased (grades 3/4: 2%)

Gastrointestinal: Abdominal pain (3% to 6%), diarrhea (6%), nausea (5%), abdominal distension (3%), dyspepsia (3%)

Hematologic: Neutropenia (grades 3/4: 2%)

Hepatic: ALT increased (grades 3/4: 5% to 7%), AST increased (grades 3/4: 6%)

Neuromuscular & skeletal: Arthralgia (4%), back pain (4%), myalgia (3%)

Respiratory: Cough (6%), pharyngolaryngeal pain (5%)

Drug Interactions

Metabolism/Transport Effects None known.

Avoid Concomitant Use

Avoid concomitant use of Telbivudine with any of the following: Interferon Alfa-2b; Peginterferon Alfa-2a; Peginterferon Alfa-2b

Increased Effect/Toxicity

The levels/effects of Telbivudine may be increased by: Interferon Alfa-2b; Peginterferon Alfa-2a; Peginterferon Alfa-2b

Decreased Effect There are no known significant interactions involving a decrease in effect.

Ethanol/Nutrition/Herb Interactions

Ethanol: Should be avoided in hepatitis B infection due to potential hepatic toxicity.

Food: Does not have a significant effect on telbivudine absorption.

Stability Store at 25°C (77°F); excursions permitted to 15°C to 30°C (59°F to 86°F).

Mechanism of Action Telbivudine, a synthetic thymidine nucleoside analogue (L-enantiomer of thymidine), is intracellularly phosphorylated to the active triphosphate form, which competes with the natural substrate, thymidine 5'-triphosphate, to inhibit hepatitis B viral DNA polymerase; enzyme inhibition blocks reverse transcriptase activity thereby reducing viral DNA replication.

Pharmacodynamics/Kinetics

Distribution: V_d: >total body water

Protein binding: ~3%

Metabolism: No metabolites detected

Half-life elimination: Terminal: 40-49 hours

Time to peak, plasma: 1-4 hours

Excretion: Urine (~42% as unchanged drug)

Dosage

Adult Chronic hepatitis B: Oral: 600 mg once daily.

Treatment duration (AASLD practice guidelines [Lok, 2009]):

Hepatitis Be antigen (HBeAg) positive chronic hepatitis: Treat ≥1 year until HBeAg seroconversion and undetectable serum HBV DNA; continue therapy for ≥6 months after HBeAg seroconversion.

HBeAg negative chronic hepatitis: Treat >1 year until hepatitis B surface antigen (HBsAg) clearance.

Note: Patients not achieving <2 log decrease in serum HBV DNA after at least 6 months of therapy should either receive additional treatment or be switched to an alternative therapy should either receive additional treatment or be switched to an alternative therapy.

Renal Impairment

Cl_{cr} ≥50 mL/minute: No dosage adjustment is necessary.

Cl_{cr} 30-49 mL/minute: 600 mg every 48 hours

Cl_{cr} <30 mL/minute (not requiring dialysis): 600 mg every 72 hours

End-stage renal disease: 600 mg every 96 hours

Hemodialysis: Administer after dialysis session

Hepatic Impairment No dosage adjustment is necessary.

Administration May be administered without regard to food.

Monitoring Parameters LFTs (eg, AST and ALT) periodically during therapy and for several months following discontinuation of therapy; renal function prior to initiation and periodically during treatment; signs and symptoms of peripheral neuropathy (eg, weakness, paresthesia, leg pain) or myopathy (eg, unexplained muscle pain, tenderness or weakness); serum creatine kinase; HBV DNA (every 3-6 months during therapy); HBeAg and anti-HBe signs/symptoms of HBV relapse/exacerbation after discontinuation of therapy.

Pharmacotherapy Pearls Telbivudine is the L-enantiomer of thymidine

Special Geriatric Considerations Insufficient clinical data in elderly to determine differences between aged patients and younger patients. Since elderly often have Cl_{cr} <50 mL/minute, dosage should be determined accordingly.

Product Availability Tyzeka® oral solution: FDA approved April 2009; anticipated availability is currently undetermined

Dosage Forms Excipient information presented when available (limited, particularly for generics); consult specific product labeling.

Tablet, oral:

Tyzeka®: 600 mg

Telithromycin (tel ith roe MYE sin)

Medication Safety Issues
Sound-alike/look-alike issues:
Telithromycin may be confused with telavancin
Brand Names: U.S. Ketek®
Brand Names: Canada Ketek®
Index Terms HMR 3647
Generic Availability (U.S.) No
Pharmacologic Category Antibiotic, Ketolide
Use Treatment of community-acquired pneumonia (mild-to-moderate) caused by susceptible strains of *Streptococcus pneumoniae* (including multidrug-resistant isolates), *Haemophilus influenzae*, *Chlamydophila pneumoniae*, *Moraxella catarrhalis*, and *Mycoplasma pneumoniae*
Medication Guide Available Yes
Contraindications Hypersensitivity to telithromycin, macrolide antibiotics, or any component of the formulation; myasthenia gravis; history of hepatitis and/or jaundice associated with telithromycin or other macrolide antibiotic use; concurrent use of cisapride or pimozide
Warnings/Precautions Acute hepatic failure and severe liver injury, including hepatitis and hepatic necrosis (leading to some fatalities) have been reported, in some cases after only a few doses; if signs/symptoms of hepatitis or liver damage occur, discontinue therapy and initiate liver function tests. **[U.S. Boxed Warning]: Life-threatening (including fatal) respiratory failure has occurred in patients with myasthenia gravis;** use in these patients is contraindicated. May prolong QT$_c$ interval, leading to a risk of ventricular arrhythmias; closely-related antibiotics have been associated with malignant ventricular arrhythmias and torsade de pointes. Avoid in patients with prolongation of QTc interval due to congenital causes, history of long QT syndrome, uncorrected electrolyte disturbances (hypokalemia or hypomagnesemia), significant bradycardia (<50 bpm), or concurrent therapy with QT$_c$-prolonging drugs (eg, class Ia and class III antiarrhythmics). Avoid use in patients with a prior history of confirmed cardiogenic syncope or ventricular arrhythmias while receiving macrolide antibiotics or other QT$_c$-prolonging drugs. May cause severe visual disturbances (eg, changes in accommodation ability, diplopia, blurred vision). May cause loss of consciousness (possibly vagal-related); caution patients that these events may interfere with ability to operate machinery or drive, and to use caution until effects are known. Use caution in renal impairment; severe impairment (Cl$_{cr}$ <30 mL/minute) requires dosage adjustment. Pseudomembranous colitis has been reported.
Adverse Reactions (Reflective of adult population; not specific for elderly)
>10%: Gastrointestinal: Diarrhea (10% to 11%)
2% to 10%:
Central nervous system: Headache (2% to 6%), dizziness (3% to 4%)
Gastrointestinal: Nausea (7% to 8%), vomiting (2% to 3%), loose stools (2%), dysgeusia (2%)
≥0.2% to <2%:
Central nervous system: Fatigue, insomnia, somnolence, vertigo
Dermatologic: Rash
Gastrointestinal: Abdominal distension, abdominal pain, anorexia, constipation, dyspepsia, flatulence, gastritis, gastroenteritis, GI upset, glossitis, stomatitis, watery stools, xerostomia
Genitourinary: Vaginal candidiasis
Hematologic: Platelets increased
Hepatic: Transaminases increased
Ocular: Blurred vision, accommodation delayed, diplopia
Miscellaneous: Candidiasis, diaphoresis increased
Drug Interactions
Metabolism/Transport Effects Substrate of CYP1A2 (minor), CYP3A4 (major); **Note:** Assignment of Major/Minor substrate status based on clinically relevant drug interaction potential; **Inhibits** CYP2D6 (weak), CYP3A4 (strong)
Avoid Concomitant Use
Avoid concomitant use of Telithromycin with any of the following: Alfuzosin; Avanafil; Axitinib; BCG; Cisapride; Conivaptan; Crizotinib; Disopyramide; Dronedarone; Eplerenone; Everolimus; Fluticasone (Oral Inhalation); Halofantrine; Highest Risk QTc-Prolonging Agents; Lapatinib; Lovastatin; Lurasidone; Mifepristone; Moderate Risk QTc-Prolonging Agents; Nilotinib; Nisoldipine; Pimozide; QuiNINE; Ranolazine; Red Yeast Rice; Rivaroxaban; RomiDEPsin; Salmeterol; Silodosin; Simvastatin; Tamsulosin; Terfenadine; Ticagrelor; Tolvaptan; Toremifene

Increased Effect/Toxicity

Telithromycin may increase the levels/effects of: Alfentanil; Alfuzosin; Almotriptan; Alosetron; Antifungal Agents (Azole Derivatives, Systemic); Antineoplastic Agents (Vinca Alkaloids); ARIPiprazole; Avanafil; Axitinib; Benzodiazepines (metabolized by oxidation); Bortezomib; Brentuximab Vedotin; Brinzolamide; Budesonide (Nasal); Budesonide (Systemic, Oral Inhalation); BusPIRone; Calcium Channel Blockers; CarBAMazepine; Cardiac Glycosides; Ciclesonide; Cilostazol; Cisapride; CloZAPine; Colchicine; Conivaptan; Corticosteroids (Orally Inhaled); Corticosteroids (Systemic); Crizotinib; CycloSPORINE; CycloSPORINE (Systemic); CYP3A4 Substrates; Dienogest; Disopyramide; Dronedarone; Dutasteride; Eletriptan; Eplerenone; Ergot Derivatives; Everolimus; FentaNYL; Fesoterodine; Fluticasone (Nasal); Fluticasone (Oral Inhalation); GuanFACINE; Halofantrine; Highest Risk QTc-Prolonging Agents; HMG-CoA Reductase Inhibitors; Iloperidone; Ivacaftor; Ixabepilone; Lapatinib; Lovastatin; Lumefantrine; Lurasidone; Maraviroc; MethylPREDNISolone; Mifepristone; Nilotinib; Nisoldipine; Paricalcitol; Pazopanib; Pimecrolimus; Pimozide; Propafenone; QuiNIDine; QuiNINE; Ranolazine; Red Yeast Rice; Repaglinide; Rifamycin Derivatives; Rivaroxaban; RomiDEPsin; Ruxolitinib; Salmeterol; Saxagliptin; Selective Serotonin Reuptake Inhibitors; Sildenafil; Silodosin; Simvastatin; Sirolimus; SORAfenib; Tacrolimus; Tacrolimus (Systemic); Tacrolimus (Topical); Tadalafil; Tamsulosin; Telaprevir; Temsirolimus; Terfenadine; Ticagrelor; Tolterodine; Tolvaptan; Toremifene; Vardenafil; Vemurafenib; Verapamil; Vilazodone; Vitamin K Antagonists; Zopiclone; Zuclopenthixol

The levels/effects of Telithromycin may be increased by: Antifungal Agents (Azole Derivatives, Systemic); CYP3A4 Inhibitors (Moderate); CYP3A4 Inhibitors (Strong); Mifepristone; Moderate Risk QTc-Prolonging Agents; QTc-Prolonging Agents (Indeterminate Risk and Risk Modifying); Telaprevir

Decreased Effect

Telithromycin may decrease the levels/effects of: BCG; Clopidogrel; Ifosfamide; Prasugrel; Ticagrelor; Typhoid Vaccine

The levels/effects of Telithromycin may be decreased by: CYP3A4 Inducers (Strong); Deferasirox; Etravirine; Herbs (CYP3A4 Inducers); Tocilizumab

Ethanol/Nutrition/Herb Interactions Herb/Nutraceutical: St John's wort: May decrease the levels/effects of telithromycin.

Stability Store at 15°C to 30°C (59°F to 86°F).

Mechanism of Action Inhibits bacterial protein synthesis by binding to two sites on the 50S ribosomal subunit. Telithromycin has also been demonstrated to alter secretion of IL-1alpha and TNF-alpha; the clinical significance of this immunomodulatory effect has not been evaluated.

Pharmacodynamics/Kinetics

Absorption: Rapid

Distribution: 2.9 L/kg

Protein binding: 60% to 70%; primarily to albumin

Metabolism: Hepatic, via CYP3A4 (50%) and non-CYP-mediated pathways

Bioavailability: 57% (significant first-pass metabolism)

Half-life elimination: 10 hours

Time to peak, plasma: 1 hour

Excretion: Urine (13% unchanged drug, remainder as metabolites); feces (7%)

Dosage

Geriatric & Adult

Community-acquired pneumonia: Oral: 800 mg once daily for 7-10 days

Renal Impairment

Cl_{cr} <30 mL/minute, including dialysis:

U.S. product labeling: 600 mg once daily; when renal impairment is accompanied by hepatic impairment, reduce dosage to 400 mg once daily

Canadian product labeling: Reduce dose to 400 mg once daily

Hemodialysis: Administer following dialysis

Hepatic Impairment No adjustment recommended, unless concurrent severe renal impairment is present.

Administration May be administered with or without food.

Monitoring Parameters Liver function tests; signs/symptoms of liver failure (eg, jaundice, fatigue, malaise, anorexia, nausea, bilirubinemia, acholic stools, liver tenderness, hepatomegaly); visual acuity

Special Geriatric Considerations Bioavailability (57%) equivalent in persons ≥65 years compared to younger adults; although a 1.4- to 2-fold increase in AUC found in older adults. No dosage adjustment required.

Dosage Forms Excipient information presented when available (limited, particularly for generics); consult specific product labeling.
Tablet, oral:
Ketek®: 300 mg, 400 mg

Dosage Forms: Canada Excipient information presented when available (limited, particularly for generics); consult specific product labeling.
Tablet:
Ketek®: 400 mg

Telmisartan (tel mi SAR tan)

Related Information
Angiotensin Agents *on page 2093*
Brand Names: U.S. Micardis®
Brand Names: Canada Micardis®; Mylan-Telmisartan; Teva-Telmisartan
Generic Availability (U.S.) No
Pharmacologic Category Angiotensin II Receptor Blocker
Use Treatment of hypertension (may be used alone or in combination with other antihypertensive agents); cardiovascular risk reduction in patients ≥55 years of age unable to take ACE inhibitors and who are at high risk of major cardiovascular events (eg, MI, stroke, death)
Contraindications Hypersensitivity to telmisartan or any component of the formulation.

Canadian labeling: Additional contraindications: Fructose intolerance
Warnings/Precautions May cause hyperkalemia; avoid potassium supplementation unless specifically required by healthcare provider. Avoid use or use a smaller dose in patients who are volume depleted; correct depletion first. May be associated with deterioration of renal function and/or increases in serum creatinine, particularly in patients with low renal blood flow (eg, renal artery stenosis, heart failure) whose glomerular filtration rate (GFR) is dependent on efferent arteriolar vasoconstriction by angiotensin II. Use with caution in unstented unilateral/bilateral renal artery stenosis. When unstented bilateral renal artery stenosis is present, use is generally avoided due to the elevated risk of deterioration in renal function unless possible benefits outweigh risks. Use with caution with pre-existing renal insufficiency; significant aortic/mitral stenosis. Concurrent use of ACE inhibitors may increase the risk of clinically-significant adverse events (eg, renal dysfunction, hyperkalemia). Concurrent use with ramipril is not recommended. Use with caution in patients who have biliary obstructive disorders or hepatic dysfunction. Product contains sorbitol. The Canadian labeling (not in U.S. labeling) contraindicates use in fructose intolerant patients.
Adverse Reactions (Reflective of adult population; not specific for elderly) May be associated with worsening of renal function in patients dependent on renin-angiotensin-aldosterone system.

1% to 10%:
Cardiovascular: Intermittent claudication (7%; placebo 6%), chest pain (≥1%), hypertension (≥1%), peripheral edema (≥1%)
Central nervous system: Dizziness (≥1%), fatigue (≥1%), headache (≥1%), pain (≥1%)
Dermatologic: Skin ulcer (3%; placebo 2%)
Gastrointestinal: Diarrhea (3%), abdominal pain (≥1%), dyspepsia (≥1%), nausea (≥1%)
Genitourinary: Urinary tract infection (≥1%)
Neuromuscular & skeletal: Back pain (3%), myalgia (≥1%)
Respiratory: Upper respiratory infection (7%), sinusitis (3%), cough (≥1%), pharyngitis (1%)
Drug Interactions
Metabolism/Transport Effects Inhibits CYP2C19 (weak)
Avoid Concomitant Use There are no known interactions where it is recommended to avoid concomitant use.
Increased Effect/Toxicity
Telmisartan may increase the levels/effects of: ACE Inhibitors; Amifostine; Antihypertensives; Cardiac Glycosides; Hypotensive Agents; Lithium; Nonsteroidal Anti-Inflammatory Agents; Potassium-Sparing Diuretics; Ramipril; RiTUXimab; Sodium Phosphates

The levels/effects of Telmisartan may be increased by: Alfuzosin; Aliskiren; Diazoxide; Eplerenone; Herbs (Hypotensive Properties); MAO Inhibitors; Pentoxifylline; Phosphodiesterase 5 Inhibitors; Potassium Salts; Prostacyclin Analogues; Tolvaptan; Trimethoprim
Decreased Effect
The levels/effects of Telmisartan may be decreased by: Herbs (Hypertensive Properties); Methylphenidate; Nonsteroidal Anti-Inflammatory Agents; Yohimbine

Ethanol/Nutrition/Herb Interactions Herb/Nutraceutical: Some herbal medications may have hypertensive or hypotensive properties; others may increase or decrease the anti-hypertensive effect of telmisartan. Management: Avoid bayberry, blue cohosh, cayenne, ephedra, ginger, ginseng (American), kola, licorice, and yohimbe. Avoid black cohosh, California poppy, coleus, golden seal, hawthorn, mistletoe, periwinkle, quinine, and shepherd's purse.

Stability Store at 25°C (77°F); excursions between 15°C to 30°C (59°F to 86°F) permitted. Protect from moisture and do not remove from blister pack until immediately before use.

Mechanism of Action Angiotensin II acts as a vasoconstrictor. In addition to causing direct vasoconstriction, angiotensin II also stimulates the release of aldosterone. Once aldosterone is released, sodium as well as water are reabsorbed. The end result is an elevation in blood pressure. Telmisartan is a nonpeptide AT1 angiotensin II receptor antagonist. This binding prevents angiotensin II from binding to the receptor thereby blocking the vasoconstriction and the aldosterone secreting effects of angiotensin II.

Pharmacodynamics/Kinetics Orally active, not a prodrug
Onset of action: 1-2 hours
Duration: Up to 24 hours
Distribution: V_d: 500 L
Protein binding: >99.5%; primarily to albumin and alpha$_1$-acid glycoprotein
Metabolism: Hepatic via conjugation to inactive metabolites; not metabolized via CYP
Bioavailability (dose dependent): 42% to 58%; Hepatic impairment: Approaches 100%
Half-life elimination: Terminal: 24 hours
Time to peak, plasma: 0.5-1 hours
Excretion: Feces (97%)
Clearance: Total body: 800 mL/minute

Dosage
Geriatric
Hypertension: Oral: Initial: 20 mg/day; usual maintenance dose range: 20-80 mg/day
Cardiovascular risk reduction: Oral: Initial 80 mg once daily

Adult
Hypertension: Oral: Initial: 40 mg once daily; usual maintenance dose range: 20-80 mg/day. Patients with volume depletion should be initiated on the lower dosage with close supervision.
Cardiovascular risk reduction: Oral: Initial: 80 mg once daily. **Note:** It is unknown whether doses <80 mg/day are associated with a reduction in risk of cardiovascular morbidity or mortality.

Renal Impairment No adjustment required; hemodialysis patients are more susceptible to orthostatic hypotension

Hepatic Impairment Initiate therapy with low dose; titrate slowly and monitor closely.
Canadian labeling: Recommended initial dose: 40 mg/day

Administration May be administered without regard to meals.

Monitoring Parameters Blood pressure; electrolytes, serum creatinine, BUN

Special Geriatric Considerations No initial dose adjustment is required. There appear to be no significant differences in response between the elderly and younger adults (limited data available). Monitor closely during initiation phase. Many elderly may be volume depleted due to diuretics and/or blunted thirst reflex resulting in inadequate fluid intake.

Dosage Forms Excipient information presented when available (limited, particularly for generics); consult specific product labeling.
Tablet, oral:
Micardis®: 20 mg
Micardis®: 40 mg, 80 mg [scored]

Telmisartan and Amlodipine (tel mi SAR tan & am LOE di peen)

Related Information
AmLODIPine on page 104
Telmisartan on page 1847
Brand Names: U.S. Twynsta®
Brand Names: Canada Twynsta®
Index Terms Amlodipine and Telmisartan; Amlodipine Besylate and Telmisartan
Generic Availability (U.S.) No
Pharmacologic Category Angiotensin II Receptor Blocker; Antianginal Agent; Calcium Channel Blocker; Calcium Channel Blocker, Dihydropyridine
Use Treatment of hypertension, including initial treatment in patients who will require multiple antihypertensives for adequate control

Dosage

Geriatric Not recommended for initial therapy in patients ≥75 years of age. For add-on/replacement therapy, initiate amlodipine therapy at 2.5 mg once daily and titrate slowly. **Note:** Use of individual agents may be necessary if the appropriate combination dose is not available. **Note:** Use as initial therapy is not an approved indication in the Canadian labeling.

Adult Dose is individualized; combination product may be substituted for individual components in patients currently maintained on both agents separately or in patients not adequately controlled with monotherapy (using one of the agents or an agent within the same antihypertensive class). May also be used as initial therapy in patients who are likely to need >1 antihypertensive to control blood pressure. **Note:** Use as initial therapy is not an approved indication in the Canadian labeling.

Hypertension: Oral:

Initial therapy (antihypertensive naive): Telmisartan 40 mg/amlodipine 5 mg once daily; dose may be increased after 2 weeks of therapy. Patients requiring larger blood pressure reductions may be started on telmisartan 80 mg/amlodipine 5 mg once daily. Maximum recommended dose: Telmisartan 80 mg/day, amlodipine 10 mg/day

Add-on/replacement therapy: Telmisartan 40-80 mg and amlodipine 5-10 mg once daily depending upon previous doses, current control, and goals of therapy; dose may be titrated after 2 weeks of therapy. Maximum recommended dose: Telmisartan 80 mg/day; amlodipine 10 mg/day

Renal Impairment

Mild-to-moderate impairment: No dosage adjustments are recommended.

Severe impairment: No dosage adjustments are recommended; titrate slowly.

Hepatic Impairment Not recommended for initial therapy. For add-on/replacement therapy, initiate amlodipine at 2.5 mg once daily with low-dose telmisartan and titrate slowly; **Note:** Use of individual agents is necessary as the appropriate combination dose is not available. Upon titration to therapeutic dose, may initiate combination dose if available. Canadian labeling contraindicates use in severe hepatic impairment or with biliary obstructive disorders.

Special Geriatric Considerations See individual agents. Combination products are not recommended as first-line treatment. Use only if doses of individual agents correspond to the combination available.

Dosage Forms Excipient information presented when available (limited, particularly for generics); consult specific product labeling.

Tablet, oral:

Twynsta® 40/5: Telmisartan 40 mg and amlodipine 5 mg

Twynsta® 40/10: Telmisartan 40 mg and amlodipine 10 mg

Twynsta® 80/5: Telmisartan 80 mg and amlodipine 5 mg

Twynsta® 80/10: Telmisartan 80 mg and amlodipine 10 mg

Telmisartan and Hydrochlorothiazide
(tel mi SAR tan & hye droe klor oh THYE a zide)

Related Information

Hydrochlorothiazide *on page 933*

Telmisartan *on page 1847*

Brand Names: U.S. Micardis® HCT

Brand Names: Canada Micardis® Plus; Mylan-Telmisartan HCTZ; Teva-Telmisartan HCTZ

Index Terms Hydrochlorothiazide and Telmisartan

Generic Availability (U.S.) No

Pharmacologic Category Angiotensin II Receptor Blocker; Diuretic, Thiazide

Use Treatment of hypertension; combination product should not be used for initial therapy

Dosage

Geriatric Refer to adult dosing. Monitor renal function.

Adult Hypertension: Oral: Replacement therapy: Combination product can be substituted for individual titrated agents. Initiation of combination therapy when monotherapy has failed to achieve desired effects:

Patients currently on telmisartan: Initial dose if blood pressure is not currently controlled on monotherapy of 80 mg telmisartan: Telmisartan 80 mg/hydrochlorothiazide 12.5 mg once daily; may titrate up to telmisartan 160 mg/hydrochlorothiazide 25 mg if needed.

Patients currently on hydrochlorothiazide: Initial dose if blood pressure is not currently controlled on monotherapy of 25 mg once daily: Telmisartan 80 mg/hydrochlorothiazide 12.5 mg once daily or telmisartan 80 mg/hydrochlorothiazide 25 mg once daily; may titrate up to telmisartan 160 mg/hydrochlorothiazide 25 mg if blood pressure remains uncontrolled after 2-4 weeks of therapy. Patients who develop hypokalemia while on hydrochlorothiazide 25 mg may be switched to telmisartan 80 mg/hydrochlorothiazide 12.5 mg.

Renal Impairment

Cl$_{cr}$ >30 mL/minute: No dosage adjustment necessary.

Cl$_{cr}$ ≤30 mL/minute: Not recommended.

Hepatic Impairment

Mild-to-moderate hepatic impairment or biliary obstructive disorders: Initial: Telmisartan 40 mg/hydrochlorothiazide 12.5 mg.

Severe hepatic impairment: Not recommended.

Special Geriatric Considerations See individual agents. Combination products are not recommended as first-line treatment. Use only if doses of individual agents correspond to the combination available.

Dosage Forms Excipient information presented when available (limited, particularly for generics); consult specific product labeling.

Tablet, oral:

Micardis® HCT:

40/12.5: Telmisartan 40 mg and hydrochlorothiazide 12.5 mg

80/12.5: Telmisartan 80 mg and hydrochlorothiazide 12.5 mg

80/25: Telmisartan 80 mg and hydrochlorothiazide 25 mg

Dosage Forms: Canada Excipient information presented when available (limited, particularly for generics); consult specific product labeling.

Tablet, oral:

Micardis® Plus: 80/25: Telmisartan 80 mg and hydrochlorothiazide 25 mg

---

Temazepam (te MAZ e pam)

Related Information

Anxiolytic, Sedative/Hypnotic, and Miscellaneous Benzodiazepines *on page 2106*

Beers Criteria – Potentially Inappropriate Medications for Geriatrics *on page 2183*

Medication Safety Issues

Sound-alike/look-alike issues:

Temazepam may be confused with flurazepam, LORazepam, tamoxifen

Restoril™ may be confused with Resotran™, RisperDAL®, Vistaril®, Zestril®

BEERS Criteria medication:

This drug may be potentially inappropriate for use in geriatric patients (Quality of evidence - high; Strength of recommendation - strong).

Brand Names: U.S. Restoril™

Brand Names: Canada Apo-Temazepam®; CO Temazepam; Dom-Temazepam; Gen-Temazepam; Novo-Temazepam; Nu-Temazepam; PHL-Temazepam; PMS-Temazepam; ratio-Temazepam; Restoril™

Generic Availability (U.S.) Yes

Pharmacologic Category Benzodiazepine

Use Short-term treatment of insomnia

Unlabeled Use Treatment of anxiety

Medication Guide Available Yes

Contraindications Hypersensitivity to temazepam or any component of the formulation (cross-sensitivity with other benzodiazepines may exist); narrow-angle glaucoma (not in product labeling, however, benzodiazepines are contraindicated)

Warnings/Precautions As a hypnotic, should be used only after evaluation of potential causes of sleep disturbance. Failure of sleep disturbance to resolve after 7-10 days may indicate psychiatric or medical illness. A worsening of insomnia or the emergence of new abnormalities of thought or behavior may represent unrecognized psychiatric or medical illness and requires immediate and careful evaluation.

Use with caution in debilitated patients, patients with hepatic disease (including alcoholics), or renal impairment. In older adults, benzodiazepines increase the risk of impaired cognition, delirium, falls, fractures, and motor vehicle accidents. Due to increased sensitivity in this age group, avoid use for treatment of insomnia, agitation, or delirium. (Beers Criteria). Use with caution in patients with respiratory disease, or impaired gag reflex. Avoid use in patients with sleep apnea.

Causes CNS depression (dose-related) resulting in sedation, dizziness, confusion, or ataxia which may impair physical and mental capabilities. Patients must be cautioned about performing tasks which require mental alertness (eg, operating machinery or driving). Use with caution in patients receiving other CNS depressants or psychoactive agents. Postmarketing studies have indicated that the use of hypnotic/sedative agents for sleep has been associated with hypersensitivity reactions including anaphylaxis as well as angioedema. An increased risk for hazardous sleep-related activities such as sleep-driving; cooking and eating food, and making phone calls while asleep have also been noted. Effects with other sedative drugs or ethanol may be potentiated. Benzodiazepines have been associated with falls and traumatic injury and should be used with extreme caution in patients who are at risk of these events.

Use caution in patients with suicidal risk. Use with caution in patients with a history of drug dependence. Benzodiazepines have been associated with dependence and acute withdrawal symptoms on discontinuation or reduction in dose (may occur after as little as 10 days). Acute withdrawal, including seizures, may be precipitated after administration of flumazenil to patients receiving long-term benzodiazepine therapy.

Benzodiazepines have been associated with anterograde amnesia. Paradoxical reactions, including hyperactive or aggressive behavior, have been reported with benzodiazepines, particularly in psychiatric patients. Does not have analgesic, antidepressant, or antipsychotic properties.

Adverse Reactions (Reflective of adult population; not specific for elderly) 1% to 10%:

Central nervous system: Anxiety, confusion, dizziness, drowsiness, euphoria, fatigue, hangover, headache, lethargy, vertigo

Dermatologic: Rash

Endocrine & metabolic: Libido decreased

Gastrointestinal: Diarrhea

Neuromuscular & skeletal: Dysarthria, weakness

Ocular: Blurred vision

Miscellaneous: Diaphoresis

Drug Interactions

Metabolism/Transport Effects Substrate of CYP2B6 (minor), CYP2C19 (minor), CYP2C9 (minor), CYP3A4 (minor); **Note:** Assignment of Major/Minor substrate status based on clinically relevant drug interaction potential

Avoid Concomitant Use

Avoid concomitant use of Temazepam with any of the following: Azelastine; Azelastine (Nasal); Methadone; Mirtazapine; OLANZapine; Paraldehyde

Increased Effect/Toxicity

Temazepam may increase the levels/effects of: Alcohol (Ethyl); Azelastine; Azelastine (Nasal); Buprenorphine; CloZAPine; CNS Depressants; Fosphenytoin; Methadone; Methotrimeprazine; Metyrosine; Mirtazapine; Paraldehyde; Phenytoin; Selective Serotonin Reuptake Inhibitors; Zolpidem

The levels/effects of Temazepam may be increased by: Droperidol; HydrOXYzine; Methotrimeprazine; OLANZapine

Decreased Effect

The levels/effects of Temazepam may be decreased by: Theophylline Derivatives; Tocilizumab; Yohimbine

Ethanol/Nutrition/Herb Interactions

Ethanol: May increase CNS depression; monitor for increased effects with coadministration. Caution patients about effects.

Food: Serum levels may be increased by grapefruit juice.

Herb/Nutraceutical: St John's wort may decrease temazepam levels. Avoid valerian, St John's wort, kava kava, gotu kola (may increase CNS depression).

Mechanism of Action Binds to stereospecific benzodiazepine receptors on the postsynaptic GABA neuron at several sites within the central nervous system, including the limbic system, reticular formation. Enhancement of the inhibitory effect of GABA on neuronal excitability results by increased neuronal membrane permeability to chloride ions. This shift in chloride ions results in hyperpolarization (a less excitable state) and stabilization.

Pharmacodynamics/Kinetics

Distribution: V_d: 1.4 L/kg

Protein binding: 96%

Metabolism: Hepatic

Half-life elimination: 9.5-12.4 hours

Time to peak, serum: 2-3 hours

Excretion: Urine (80% to 90% as inactive metabolites)

Dosage

Geriatric Initial: 7.5 mg in elderly or debilitated patients at bedtime

Adult Insomnia: Oral: Usual dose: 15-30 mg at bedtime; some patients may respond to 7.5 mg in transient insomnia

Monitoring Parameters Respiratory and cardiovascular status

Reference Range Therapeutic: 26 ng/mL after 24 hours

Pharmacotherapy Pearls Abrupt discontinuation after sustained use (generally >10 days) may cause withdrawal symptoms.

Special Geriatric Considerations Hypnotic use should be limited to 10-14 days. If insomnia persists, the patient should be evaluated for etiology.

This medication is considered to be potentially inappropriate in this patient population (Beers Criteria: Quality of evidence - high; Strength of recommendation - strong).

Controlled Substance C-IV

Dosage Forms Excipient information presented when available (limited, particularly for generics); consult specific product labeling.

Capsule, oral: 7.5 mg, 15 mg, 22.5 mg, 30 mg
Restoril™: 7.5 mg, 15 mg, 22.5 mg, 30 mg

- **Temovate®** see Clobetasol on page 406
- **Temovate E®** see Clobetasol on page 406
- **Tenex®** see GuanFACINE on page 908
- **Tenivac™** see Diphtheria and Tetanus Toxoids on page 562
- **Tenormin®** see Atenolol on page 161
- **Terazol® 3** see Terconazole on page 1858
- **Terazol® 7** see Terconazole on page 1858

Terazosin (ter AY zoe sin)

Related Information
Beers Criteria – Potentially Inappropriate Medications for Geriatrics on page 2183
Pharmacotherapy of Urinary Incontinence on page 2141

Medication Safety Issues
BEERS Criteria medication:
This drug may be potentially inappropriate for use in geriatric patients (Quality of evidence - moderate; Strength of recommendation - strong).

Brand Names: Canada Apo-Terazosin®; Dom-Terazosin; Hytrin®; Nu-Terazosin; PHL-Terazosin; PMS-Terazosin; ratio-Terazosin; Teva-Terazosin

Index Terms Hytrin

Generic Availability (U.S.) Yes

Pharmacologic Category Alpha$_1$ Blocker

Use Management of mild-to-moderate hypertension; alone or in combination with other agents such as diuretics or beta-blockers; benign prostate hyperplasia (BPH)

Contraindications Hypersensitivity to terazosin or any component of the formulation

Warnings/Precautions Can cause significant orthostatic hypotension and syncope, especially with first dose; anticipate a similar effect if therapy is interrupted for a few days, if dosage is rapidly increased, or if another antihypertensive drug (particularly vasodilators) or a PDE-5 inhibitor is introduced. Discontinue if symptoms of angina occur or worsen. Patients should be cautioned about performing hazardous tasks when starting new therapy or adjusting dosage upward. Prostate cancer should be ruled out before starting for BPH. Intraoperative floppy iris syndrome has been observed in cataract surgery patients who were on or were previously treated with alpha$_1$-blockers. Causality has not been established and there appears to be no benefit in discontinuing alpha-blocker therapy prior to surgery. Priapism has been associated with use (rarely). In the elderly, avoid use as an antihypertensive due to high risk of orthostatic hypotension; alternative agents preferred due to a more favorable risk/benefit profile (Beers Criteria).

Adverse Reactions (Reflective of adult population; not specific for elderly)
>10%:
Central nervous system: Dizziness (9% to 19%)
Neuromuscular & skeletal: Muscle weakness (7% to 11%)
1% to 10%:
Cardiovascular: Peripheral edema (1% to 6%), orthostatic hypotension (1% to 4%), palpitation (≤4%), tachycardia (≤2%), syncope (≤1%)
Central nervous system: Somnolence (4% to 5%), vertigo (1%)
Gastrointestinal: Nausea (2% to 4%), weight gain (≤1%)
Genitourinary: Impotence (≤2%), libido decreased (≤1%)
Neuromuscular & skeletal: Extremity pain (≤4%), paresthesia (≤3%), back pain (≤2%)
Ocular: Blurred vision (≤2%)
Respiratory: Nasal congestion (2% to 6%), dyspnea (2% to 3%), sinusitis (≤3%)

Drug Interactions
Metabolism/Transport Effects None known.
Avoid Concomitant Use
Avoid concomitant use of Terazosin with any of the following: Alpha1-Blockers

Increased Effect/Toxicity

Terazosin may increase the levels/effects of: Alpha1-Blockers; Amifostine; Antihypertensives; Calcium Channel Blockers; Hypotensive Agents; RiTUXimab

The levels/effects of Terazosin may be increased by: Beta-Blockers; Diazoxide; Herbs (Hypotensive Properties); MAO Inhibitors; Pentoxifylline; Phosphodiesterase 5 Inhibitors; Prostacyclin Analogues

Decreased Effect

The levels/effects of Terazosin may be decreased by: Herbs (Hypertensive Properties); Methylphenidate; Yohimbine

Ethanol/Nutrition/Herb Interactions Herb/Nutraceutical: Avoid dong quai if using for hypertension (has estrogenic activity). Avoid ephedra, yohimbe, ginseng (may worsen hypertension). Avoid saw palmetto. Avoid garlic (may have increased antihypertensive effect).

Stability Store below 30°C (86°F).

Mechanism of Action Alpha$_1$-specific blocking agent with minimal alpha$_2$ effects; this allows peripheral postsynaptic blockade, with the resultant decrease in arterial tone, while preserving the negative feedback loop which is mediated by the peripheral presynaptic alpha$_2$-receptors; terazosin relaxes the smooth muscle of the bladder neck, thus reducing bladder outlet obstruction

Pharmacodynamics/Kinetics

Onset of action: 1-2 hours

Absorption: Rapid and complete

Protein binding: 90% to 95%

Metabolism: Hepatic; minimal first-pass

Half-life elimination: ~12 hours

Time to peak, serum: ~1 hour

Excretion: Feces (~60%, ~20% as unchanged drug); urine (~40%, ~10% as unchanged drug)

Dosage

Geriatric Refer to adult dosing. In the management of hypertension, consider lower initial doses (eg, immediate release: 0.5 mg once daily) and titrate to response (Aronow, 2011).

Adult Note: If drug is discontinued for greater than several days, consider beginning with initial dose and retitrate as needed.

Hypertension: Oral: Initial: 1 mg at bedtime; slowly increase dose to achieve desired blood pressure, up to 20 mg/day; usual dose range (JNC 7): 1-20 mg once daily. **Note:** Dosage may be given on a twice daily regimen if response is diminished at 24 hours and hypotension is observed at 2-4 hours following a dose.

Benign prostatic hyperplasia: Oral: Initial: 1 mg at bedtime; thereafter, titrate upwards, if needed, over several weeks, balancing therapeutic benefit with terazosin-induced postural hypotension; most patients require 10 mg day; if no response after 4-6 weeks of 10 mg/day, may increase to 20 mg/day

Dosage adjustment with concurrent medication:

Concurrent use with a diuretic or other antihypertensive agent (especially verapamil): Dosage reduction may be needed when adding

Concurrent use with PDE-5 inhibitors: Initiate PDE-5 inhibitor therapy at the lowest dose due to additive orthostatic and blood pressure lowering effects

Administration Administer without regard to meals at the same time each day.

Monitoring Parameters Standing and sitting/supine blood pressure, especially following the initial dose at 2-4 hours following the dose and thereafter at the trough point to ensure adequate control throughout the dosing interval; urinary symptoms

Special Geriatric Considerations Adverse reactions such as orthostatic hypotension, dry mouth, and urinary problems can be particularly bothersome in the elderly.

This medication is considered to be potentially inappropriate in this patient population (Beers Criteria: Quality of evidence - moderate; Strength of recommendation - strong).

Dosage Forms Excipient information presented when available (limited, particularly for generics); consult specific product labeling.

Capsule, oral: 1 mg, 2 mg, 5 mg, 10 mg

Terbinafine (Systemic) (TER bin a feen)

Medication Safety Issues

Sound-alike/look-alike issues:

Terbinafine may be confused with terbutaline

LamISIL® may be confused with LaMICtal®, Lomotil®

Brand Names: U.S. LamISIL®; Terbinex™

Brand Names: Canada Apo-Terbinafine®; Auro-Terbinafine; CO Terbinafine; Dom-Terbinafine; GD-Terbinafine; JAMP-Terbinafine; Lamisil®; Mylan-Terbinafine; Nu-Terbinafine; PHL-Terbinafine; PMS-Terbinafine; Q-Terbinafine; Riva-Terbinafine; Sandoz-Terbinafine; Teva-Terbinafine

Index Terms Terbinafine Hydrochloride

Generic Availability (U.S.) Yes: Tablet

Pharmacologic Category Antifungal Agent, Oral

Use Treatment of onychomycosis of the toenail or fingernail due to susceptible dermatophytes; treatment of tinea capitis

Canadian labeling: Additional use (not in U.S. labeling): Severe tineal skin infections unresponsive to topical therapy

Contraindications Hypersensitivity to terbinafine or any component of the formulation

Warnings/Precautions Due to potential toxicity, confirmation of diagnostic testing of nail or skin specimens prior to treatment of onychomycosis or dermatomycosis is recommended. Use caution in patients sensitive to allylamine antifungals (eg, naftifine, butenafine); cross sensitivity to terbinafine may exist. Transient decreases in absolute lymphocyte counts were observed in clinical trials; severe neutropenia (reversible upon discontinuation) has also been reported. Monitor CBC in patients with pre-existing immunosuppression if therapy is to continue >6 weeks and discontinue therapy if ANC ≤1000/mm^3.

While rare, the following complications have been reported and may require discontinuation of therapy; changes in the ocular lens and retina, Stevens-Johnson syndrome, toxic epidermal necrolysis. Precipitation or exacerbation of cutaneous or systemic lupus erythematosus has been observed; discontinue if signs and/or symptoms develop. Rare cases of hepatic failure, including fatal cases, have been reported following treatment of onychomycosis. Not recommended for use in patients with active or chronic liver disease. Discontinue if symptoms or signs of hepatobiliary dysfunction or cholestatic hepatitis develop. Products are not recommended for use with pre-existing renal disease (Cl$_{cr}$ ≤50 mL/minute). Use caution in patients sensitive to allylamine antifungals (eg, naftifine, butenafine); cross-sensitivity to terbinafine may exist. Depression has been reported with use; instruct patients to report depressive symptoms/mood changes.

Disturbances of taste and/or smell may occur; resolution may be delayed (eg, >1 year) following discontinuation of therapy or in some cases, disturbance may be permanent. Discontinue therapy in patients with symptoms of taste or smell disturbance. Some tablet formulations may contain lactose and should be avoided in patients with galactose intolerance, Lapp lactase deficiency, or glucose-galactose malabsorption syndromes.

Adverse Reactions (Reflective of adult population; not specific for elderly) Adverse events listed for tablets unless otherwise specified. Granules were studied in patients 4-12 years of age.

>10%: Central nervous system: Headache (13%; granules 7%)

1% to 10%:

Central nervous system: Fever (granules 7%)

Dermatologic: Rash (6%; granules 2%), pruritus (3%; granules 1%), urticaria (1%)

Gastrointestinal: Diarrhea (6%; granules 3%), vomiting (<1%; granules 5%), dyspepsia (4%), taste disturbance (3%), abdominal pain (2%; granules 2% to 4%), nausea (granules 2%), toothache (granules 1%)

Hepatic: Liver enzyme abnormalities (3%)

Respiratory: Nasopharyngitis (granules 10%), cough (granules 6%), upper respiratory tract infection (granules 5%), nasal congestion (granules 2%), pharyngeal pain (granules 2%), rhinorrhea (granules 2%)

Miscellaneous: Influenza (granules 2%)

Drug Interactions

Metabolism/Transport Effects Substrate of CYP1A2 (minor), CYP2C19 (minor), CYP2C9 (minor), CYP3A4 (minor); **Note:** Assignment of Major/Minor substrate status based on clinically relevant drug interaction potential; **Inhibits** CYP2D6 (strong); **Induces** CYP3A4 (weak/moderate).

Avoid Concomitant Use

Avoid concomitant use of Terbinafine (Systemic) with any of the following: Axitinib; Pimozide; Tamoxifen; Thioridazine

Increased Effect/Toxicity

Terbinafine (Systemic) may increase the levels/effects of: ARIPiprazole; AtoMOXetine; CYP2D6 Substrates; Fesoterodine; Iloperidone; Nebivolol; Pimozide; Propafenone; Tetrabenazine; Thioridazine; Tricyclic Antidepressants

Decreased Effect

Terbinafine (Systemic) may decrease the levels/effects of: ARIPiprazole; Axitinib; Codeine; CycloSPORINE; Iloperidone; Saccharomyces boulardii; Saxagliptin; Tamoxifen; TraMADol

The levels/effects of Terbinafine (Systemic) may be decreased by: Rifamycin Derivatives; Tocilizumab

Stability

Granules: Store at 25°C (77°F).

Tablet: Store below 25°C (77°F). Protect from light.

Mechanism of Action Synthetic allylamine derivative which inhibits squalene epoxidase, a key enzyme in sterol biosynthesis in fungi. This results in a deficiency in ergosterol within the fungal cell wall and results in fungal cell death.

Pharmacodynamics/Kinetics

Absorption: >70%

Distribution: Distributed to sebum and skin predominantly

Protein binding: Plasma: >99%

Metabolism: Hepatic predominantly via CYP1A2, 3A4, 2C8, 2C9, and 2C19 to inactive metabolites

Bioavailability: ~40%

Half-life elimination: Terminal half-life: 200-400 hours; very slow release of drug from skin and adipose tissues occurs; effective half-life: ~36 hours

Time to peak, plasma: Within 2 hours

Excretion: Urine (~70%)

Dosage

Geriatric Use with caution; refer to adult dosing.

Adult

U.S. labeling: **Onychomycosis:** Oral: Tablet: Fingernail: 250 mg once daily for 6 weeks; Toenail: 250 mg once daily for 12 weeks

Canadian labeling: Oral: Tablet: **Note:** Mycologic cure may precede complete resolution of symptoms by several weeks (skin infections) or by several months (onychomycosis).

Onychomycosis (finger or toenail): 250 mg/day in 1-2 divided doses for 6 weeks to 3 months (≥6 months may be necessary in some patients with infections of the big toenail)

Tinea corporis, tinea cruris: 250 mg/day in 1-2 divided doses for 2-4 weeks

Tinea pedis (interdigital and plantar/moccasin type): 250 mg/day in 1-2 divided doses for 2-6 weeks

Sporotrichosis, lymphocutaneous and cutaneous (unlabeled use): Oral: 500 mg twice daily as alternative therapy; treat for 2-4 weeks after resolution of all lesions (usual duration: 3-6 months) (Kauffman, 2007)

Renal Impairment

U.S. labeling: No dosage adjustment provided in manufacturer's U.S. labeling; however, clearance is decreased 50% in patients with Cl_{cr} ≤50 mL/minute.

Canadian labeling: Use is not recommended in patients with Cl_{cr} ≤50 mL/minute.

Hepatic Impairment Hepatic cirrhosis: Use is not recommended in chronic or active hepatic disease.

Administration Tablets may be administered without regard to meals. Granules should be sprinkled on a spoonful of pudding or other soft, nonacidic food (eg, mashed potatoes) and swallowed without chewing; do not mix granules with applesauce or other fruit-based foods.

Monitoring Parameters AST/ALT prior to initiation, repeat if used >6 weeks; CBC

Special Geriatric Considerations No specific information on use in the elderly is available; however, since many elderly will have creatinine clearances <50 mL/minute, this drug is not a drug of choice for elderly with onychomycosis.

Dosage Forms Excipient information presented when available (limited, particularly for generics); consult specific product labeling.

Granules, oral:

LamISIL®: 125 mg/packet (42s); 187.5 mg/packet (14s, 42s)

Tablet, oral: 250 mg

LamISIL®: 250 mg

Terbinex™: 250 mg [kit includes Terbinex™ tablets (30s) and Eco-Formula™ nail enhancer]

Terbinex™: 250 mg [kit includes Terbinex™ tablets (42s) and Eco-Formula™ nail enhancer]

Dosage Forms: Canada Excipient information presented when available (limited, particularly for generics); consult specific product labeling.

Tablet, oral:

LamISIL®: 125 mg [contains lactose]

Terbinafine (Topical) (TER bin a feen)

Medication Safety Issues
Sound-alike/look-alike issues:
Terbinafine may be confused with terbutaline
Brand Names: U.S. LamISIL AT® [OTC]
Brand Names: Canada Lamisil®
Index Terms Terbinafine Hydrochloride
Generic Availability (U.S.) Yes: Cream
Pharmacologic Category Antifungal Agent, Topical
Use Antifungal for the treatment of tinea pedis (athlete's foot), tinea cruris (jock itch), and tinea corporis (ringworm) [OTC/prescription formulations]; tinea versicolor [prescription formulations]
Dosage
Geriatric & Adult
Athlete's foot (tinea pedis): Topical:
Cream: Apply to affected area once daily for at least 1 week, not to exceed 4 weeks [OTC/Canadian/prescription formulations]
Gel: Apply to affected area once daily for at least 1 week, not to exceed 4 weeks [OTC/Canadian/prescription formulations]
Solution: Apply to affected area once daily for at least 1 week, not to exceed 4 weeks [OTC/Canadian/prescription formulations]
Cutaneous candidiasis: Topical:
Cream: Apply to affected area once or twice daily for 7-14 days
Gel: Apply to affected area once or twice daily for 7-14 days
Solution: Apply to affected area once or twice daily for 7-14 days
Ringworm and jock itch (tinea corporis/tinea versicolor, tinea cruris): Topical:
Cream: Apply to affected area once daily for at least 1 week, not to exceed 4 weeks [OTC formulations]; apply to affected area once or twice daily for 2 weeks in tinea versicolor [Canadian/prescription formulation]
Gel: Apply to affected area once daily for 7 days [OTC formulations]
Solution: Apply to affected area once daily for 7 days in tinea corporis and tinea cruris [OTC formulations]; apply to affected area once or twice daily for 2 weeks in tinea versicolor [Canadian/prescription formulation]
Special Geriatric Considerations Instruct patient or caregiver on appropriate use of topical terbinafine products.
Dosage Forms Excipient information presented when available (limited, particularly for generics); consult specific product labeling. [DSC] = Discontinued product
Cream, topical, as hydrochloride: 1% (12 g [DSC], 15 g, 24 g [DSC], 30 g)
LamISIL AT®: 1% (12 g, 15 g, 24 g, 30 g, 36 g) [contains benzyl alcohol]
Gel, topical:
LamISIL AT®: 1% (6 g, 12 g) [contains benzyl alcohol]
Solution, topical, as hydrochloride [spray]:
LamISIL AT®: 1% (30 mL) [contains ethanol]
Dosage Forms: Canada Excipient information presented when available (limited, particularly for generics); consult specific product labeling.
Cream, topical, as hydrochloride: 1% (12 g, 24 g)
Lamisil®: 1% (15 g, 30 g)
Solution, topical, as hydrochloride [spray]:
Lamisil®: 1% (30 mL)

♦ **Terbinafine Hydrochloride** *see* Terbinafine (Systemic) *on page 1853*
♦ **Terbinafine Hydrochloride** *see* Terbinafine (Topical) *on page 1856*
♦ **Terbinex™** *see* Terbinafine (Systemic) *on page 1853*

Terbutaline (ter BYOO ta leen)

Medication Safety Issues
Sound-alike/look-alike issues:
Brethine may be confused with Methergine®
Terbutaline may be confused with terbinafine, TOLBUTamide
Terbutaline and methylergonovine parenteral dosage forms look similar. Due to their contrasting indications, use care when administering these agents.

Brand Names: Canada Bricanyl®
Index Terms Brethaire [DSC]; Brethine; Bricanyl [DSC]
Generic Availability (U.S.) Yes
Pharmacologic Category Beta$_2$ Agonist
Use Bronchodilator in reversible airway obstruction and bronchial asthma
Unlabeled Use Injection: Tocolytic agent (short-term [≤72 hours] prevention or management of preterm labor
Contraindications Hypersensitivity to terbutaline or any component of the formulation; cardiac arrhythmias associated with tachycardia; tachycardia caused by digitalis intoxication

Injection: Additional contraindications: Prolonged (>72 hours) prevention or management of preterm labor

Oral: Additional contraindications: Prevention or treatment of preterm labor
Warnings/Precautions Use caution in patients with cardiovascular disease (arrhythmia or hypertension or HF), convulsive disorders, diabetes, glaucoma, hyperthyroidism, or hypokalemia. Beta-agonists may cause elevation in blood pressure, heart rate, and result in CNS stimulation/excitation. Beta$_2$-agonists may increase risk of arrhythmia, increase serum glucose, or decrease serum potassium.

When used as a bronchodilator, optimize anti-inflammatory treatment before initiating maintenance treatment with terbutaline. Do not use as a component of chronic therapy without an anti-inflammatory agent. Only the mildest form of asthma (Step 1 and/or exercise-induced) would not require concurrent use based upon asthma guidelines. Patient must be instructed to seek medical attention in cases where acute symptoms are not relieved or a previous level of response is diminished. The need to increase frequency of use may indicate deterioration of asthma, and treatment must not be delayed.

Immediate hypersensitivity reactions (urticaria, angioedema, rash, bronchospasm) have been reported. Do not exceed recommended dose; serious adverse events including fatalities, have been associated with excessive use of inhaled sympathomimetics. Rarely, paradoxical bronchospasm may occur with use of inhaled bronchodilating agents; this should be distinguished from inadequate response.
Adverse Reactions (Reflective of adult population; not specific for elderly)
>10%:
  Central nervous system: Nervousness, restlessness
  Endocrine & metabolic: Serum glucose increased, serum potassium decreased
  Neuromuscular & skeletal: Trembling
1% to 10%:
  Cardiovascular: Tachycardia, hypertension
  Central nervous system: Dizziness, drowsiness, headache, insomnia
  Gastrointestinal: Xerostomia, nausea, vomiting, bad taste in mouth
  Neuromuscular & skeletal: Muscle cramps, weakness
  Miscellaneous: Diaphoresis
Drug Interactions
  Metabolism/Transport Effects None known.
  Avoid Concomitant Use
    Avoid concomitant use of Terbutaline with any of the following: Beta-Blockers (Nonselective); Iobenguane I 123
  Increased Effect/Toxicity
    Terbutaline may increase the levels/effects of: Loop Diuretics; Sympathomimetics; Thiazide Diuretics

    The levels/effects of Terbutaline may be increased by: AtoMOXetine; Cannabinoids; MAO Inhibitors; Tricyclic Antidepressants
  Decreased Effect
    Terbutaline may decrease the levels/effects of: Iobenguane I 123

    The levels/effects of Terbutaline may be decreased by: Alpha-/Beta-Blockers; Beta-Blockers (Beta1 Selective); Beta-Blockers (Nonselective); Betahistine
Ethanol/Nutrition/Herb Interactions Herb/Nutraceutical: Avoid ephedra, yohimbe (may cause CNS stimulation).
Stability Store injection at room temperature; do not freeze. Protect from heat and light. Use only clear solutions. Store powder for inhalation (Bricanyl® Turbuhaler [CAN]) at room temperature between 15°C and 30°C (58°F and 86°F).
Mechanism of Action Relaxes bronchial and uterine smooth muscle by action on beta$_2$-receptors with less effect on heart rate

Pharmacodynamics/Kinetics
Onset of action: Oral: 30-45 minutes; SubQ: 6-15 minutes
Protein binding: 25%
Metabolism: Hepatic to inactive sulfate conjugates
Bioavailability: SubQ doses are more bioavailable than oral
Half-life elimination: 11-16 hours
Excretion: Urine

Dosage
Geriatric & Adult
Asthma or bronchoconstriction:
Oral: 5 mg/dose every 6 hours 3 times/day; if side effects occur, reduce dose to 2.5 mg every 6 hours; not to exceed 15 mg in 24 hours.
SubQ:
Manufacturer's labeling: 0.25 mg/dose; may repeat in 15-30 minutes (maximum: 0.5 mg/ 4-hour period)
Unlabeled dose: 0.25 mg/dose; may repeat every 20 minutes for 3 doses (maximum: 0.75 mg/1-hour period) (NIH Guidelines, 2007)
Bronchospasm (acute): *Inhalation* (Bricanyl® [CAN] MDI: 500 mcg/puff, *not labeled for use in the U.S.*): One puff as needed; may repeat with 1 inhalation (after 5 minutes); more than 6 inhalations should not be necessary in any 24 hour period. **Note:** If a previously effective dosage regimen fails to provide the usual relief, or the effects of a dose last for >3 hours, medical advice should be sought immediately; this is a sign of seriously worsening asthma that requires reassessment of therapy.
Premature labor (acute; short-term [≤72 hours] tocolysis; unlabeled use):
I.V.: 2.5-5 mcg/minute; increased gradually every 20-30 minutes by 2.5-5 mcg/minute; effective maximum dosages from 17.5-30 mcg/minute have been used with caution. Duration of infusion is at least 12 hours (Travis, 1993).
SubQ: 0.25 mg every 20 minutes to 3 hours; hold for pulse >120 beats per minute. Terbutaline has not been approved for and should not be used for prolonged tocolysis (beyond 48-72 hours) (ACOG, 2012; Hearne, 2000).

Renal Impairment
Cl_{cr} 10-50 mL/minute: Administer 50% of normal dose.
Cl_{cr} <10 mL/minute: Avoid use.

Administration
I.V.: Use infusion pump.
Oral: Administer around-the-clock to promote less variation in peak and trough serum levels

Monitoring Parameters Serum potassium, glucose; intake/output; heart rate, blood pressure, respiratory rate; chest pain, shortness of breath; monitor for signs and symptoms of pulmonary edema (when used as a tocolytic); monitor FEV_1, peak flow, and/or other pulmonary function tests (when used as bronchodilator)

Special Geriatric Considerations Oral terbutaline should be avoided in the elderly due to the increased incidence of adverse effects as compared to the inhaled form.

Dosage Forms Excipient information presented when available (limited, particularly for generics); consult specific product labeling.
Injection, solution, as sulfate: 1 mg/mL (1 mL)
Tablet, oral, as sulfate: 2.5 mg, 5 mg

Dosage Forms: Canada Excipient information presented when available (limited, particularly for generics); consult specific product labeling.
Powder for oral inhalation:
Bricanyl® Turbuhaler: 500 mcg/actuation [50 or 200 metered actuations]

Terconazole (ter KONE a zole)

Medication Safety Issues
Sound-alike/look-alike issues:
Terconazole may be confused with tioconazole
International issues:
Terazol [U.S., Canada] may be confused with Theradol brand name for tramadol [Netherlands]
Brand Names: U.S. Terazol® 3; Terazol® 7
Brand Names: Canada Terazol®
Index Terms Triaconazole
Generic Availability (U.S.) Yes
Pharmacologic Category Antifungal Agent, Vaginal
Use Local treatment of vulvovaginal candidiasis
Contraindications Hypersensitivity to terconazole or any component of the formulation

Warnings/Precautions Should be discontinued if sensitization or irritation occurs. Microbiological studies (KOH smear and/or cultures) should be repeated in patients not responding to terconazole in order to confirm the diagnosis and rule out other pathogens. Petrolatum-based vaginal products may damage rubber or latex condoms or diaphragms; separate use by 3 days.

Adverse Reactions (Reflective of adult population; not specific for elderly)
>10%: Central nervous system: Headache
1% to 10%:
  Central nervous system: Chills, fever, pain
  Gastrointestinal: Abdominal pain
  Genitourinary: Dysmenorrhea; vulvar/vaginal burning, irritation, or itching

Drug Interactions

Metabolism/Transport Effects None known.

Avoid Concomitant Use There are no known interactions where it is recommended to avoid concomitant use.

Increased Effect/Toxicity There are no known significant interactions involving an increase in effect.

Decreased Effect There are no known significant interactions involving a decrease in effect.

Stability Store at room temperature of 15°C to 30°C (59°F to 86°F).

Mechanism of Action Triazole ketal antifungal agent; involves inhibition of fungal cytochrome P450. Specifically, terconazole inhibits cytochrome P450-dependent 14-alpha-demethylase which results in accumulation of membrane disturbing 14-alpha-demethylsterols and ergosterol depletion.

Pharmacodynamics/Kinetics Absorption: Extent of systemic absorption after vaginal administration may be dependent on presence of a uterus; 5% to 8% in women who had a hysterectomy versus 12% to 16% in nonhysterectomy women

Dosage

Geriatric & Adult Vulvovaginal candidiasis: Intravaginal:
  Terazol® 3 (0.8%) vaginal cream: Insert 1 applicatorful intravaginally at bedtime for 3 consecutive days.
  Terazol® 7 (0.4%) vaginal cream: Insert 1 applicatorful intravaginally at bedtime for 7 consecutive days.
  Terazol® 3 vaginal suppository: Insert 1 suppository intravaginally at bedtime for 3 consecutive days.

Administration

Vaginal cream: Use applicator provided by manufacturer. Insertion should be as far as possible into the vagina without causing discomfort. Wash applicator after each use; allow to dry thoroughly before putting back together.

Vaginal suppository: Remove foil package prior to use. Insertion should be as far as possible into the vagina without causing discomfort. If the provided applicator is used for insertion, wash and dry thoroughly prior to additional use.

Pharmacotherapy Pearls Watch for local irritation; assist patient in administration, if necessary; assess patient's ability to self-administer, may be difficult in patients with arthritis or limited range of motion

Special Geriatric Considerations Assess patient's ability to self-administer; may be difficult in patients with arthritis or limited range of motion.

Dosage Forms Excipient information presented when available (limited, particularly for generics); consult specific product labeling.
  Cream, vaginal: 0.4% (45 g); 0.8% (20 g)
    Terazol® 7: 0.4% (45 g)
    Terazol® 3: 0.8% (20 g)
  Suppository, vaginal: 80 mg (3s)
    Terazol® 3: 80 mg (3s) [contains coconut oil (may have trace amounts), palm kernel oil (may have trace amounts)]

Teriparatide (ter i PAR a tide)

Related Information
  Osteoporosis Management *on page 2136*
Brand Names: U.S. Forteo®
Brand Names: Canada Forteo®
Index Terms Parathyroid Hormone (1-34); Recombinant Human Parathyroid Hormone (1-34); rhPTH(1-34)
Generic Availability (U.S.) No
Pharmacologic Category Parathyroid Hormone Analog

TERIPARATIDE

Use Treatment of osteoporosis in postmenopausal women at high risk of fracture; treatment of primary or hypogonadal osteoporosis in men at high risk of fracture; treatment of glucocorticoid-induced osteoporosis in men and women at high risk for fracture

Medication Guide Available Yes

Contraindications Hypersensitivity to teriparatide or any component of the formulation

Canadian labeling: Additional contraindications (not in U.S. labeling): Pre-existing hypercalcemia; severe renal impairment; metabolic bone diseases other than primary osteoporosis (including hyperparathyroidism and Paget's disease of the bone); unexplained elevations of alkaline phosphatase; prior external beam or implant radiation therapy involving the skeleton; bone metastases or history of skeletal malignancies

Warnings/Precautions [U.S. Boxed Warning]: In animal studies, teriparatide has been associated with an increase in osteosarcoma; risk was dependent on both dose and duration. Avoid use in patients with an increased risk of osteosarcoma (including Paget's disease, prior radiation, unexplained elevation of alkaline phosphatase, or in patients with open epiphyses). Do not use in patients with a history of skeletal metastases, hyperparathyroidism, or pre-existing hypercalcemia. Not for use in patients with metabolic bone disease other than osteoporosis. Use caution in patients with active or recent urolithiasis. Use caution in patients at risk of orthostasis (including concurrent antihypertensive therapy), or in patients who may not tolerate transient hypotension (cardiovascular or cerebrovascular disease). Use caution in patients with cardiac, renal or hepatic impairment (limited data available concerning safety and efficacy). Use of teriparatide for longer than 2 years is not recommended.

Adverse Reactions (Reflective of adult population; not specific for elderly)
>10%: Endocrine & metabolic: Hypercalcemia (transient increases noted 4-6 hours postdose [women 11%; men 6%])

1% to 10%:
Cardiovascular: Orthostatic hypotension (5%; transient), chest pain (3%), syncope (3%)
Central nervous system: Dizziness (8%), insomnia (4% to 5%), anxiety (≤4%), depression (4%), vertigo (4%)
Dermatologic: Rash (5%)
Endocrine & metabolic: Hyperuricemia (3%)
Gastrointestinal: Nausea (9% to 14%), gastritis (≤7%), dyspepsia (5%), vomiting (3%)
Neuromuscular & skeletal: Arthralgia (10%), weakness (9%), leg cramps (3%)
Respiratory: Rhinitis (10%), pharyngitis (6%), dyspnea (4% to 6%), pneumonia (4% to 6%)
Miscellaneous: Antibodies to teriparatide (3% of women in long-term treatment; hypersensitivity reactions or decreased efficacy were not associated in preclinical trials), herpes zoster (≤3%)

Drug Interactions
Metabolism/Transport Effects None known.
Avoid Concomitant Use There are no known interactions where it is recommended to avoid concomitant use.
Increased Effect/Toxicity There are no known significant interactions involving an increase in effect.
Decreased Effect There are no known significant interactions involving a decrease in effect.

Ethanol/Nutrition/Herb Interactions
Ethanol: Excessive intake may increase risk of osteoporosis.
Herb/Nutraceutical: Ensure adequate calcium and vitamin D intake.

Stability Store at 2°C to 8°C (36°F to 46°F); do not freeze. Protect from light. Discard pen 28 days after first injection. Do not use if solution is cloudy, colored or contains solid particles.

Mechanism of Action Teriparatide is a recombinant formulation of endogenous parathyroid hormone (PTH), containing a 34-amino-acid sequence which is identical to the N-terminal portion of this hormone. The pharmacologic activity of teriparatide, which is similar to the physiologic activity of PTH, includes stimulating osteoblast function, increasing gastrointestinal calcium absorption, and increasing renal tubular reabsorption of calcium. Treatment with teriparatide results in increased bone mineral density, bone mass, and strength. In postmenopausal women, teriparatide has been shown to decrease osteoporosis-related fractures.

Pharmacodynamics/Kinetics
Distribution: V_d: ~0.12 L/kg
Metabolism: Hepatic (nonspecific proteolysis)
Bioavailability: 95%
Half-life elimination: I.V.: 5 minutes; SubQ: ~1 hour
Time to peak, serum: ~30 minutes
Excretion: Urine (as metabolites)

Dosage
Geriatric & Adult Osteoporosis: SubQ: 20 mcg once daily; **Note:** Initial administration should occur under circumstances in which the patient may sit or lie down, in the event of orthostasis.

Renal Impairment No dosage adjustment required. Bioavailability and half-life increase with Cl_{cr} <30 mL/minute. Use in severe renal impairment is contraindicated in the Canadian labeling.

Administration Administer by subcutaneous injection into the thigh or abdominal wall. Initial administration should occur under circumstances in which the patient may sit or lie down, in the event of orthostasis. **Note:** The 3 mL prefilled pen (Canadian availability; not available in U.S.) must be primed prior to each dose.

Monitoring Parameters Serum calcium, serum phosphorus, uric acid; blood pressure; bone mineral density

Test Interactions Transiently increases serum calcium; maximal effect 4-6 hours postdose; generally returns to baseline ~16 hours postdose

Pharmacotherapy Pearls Teriparatide was formerly marketed as a diagnostic agent (Perithar™); that agent was withdrawn from the market in 1997. Teriparatide (Forteo®) is manufactured through recombinant DNA technology using a strain of *E. coli*.

Patients are encouraged to enroll in the Forteo® Patient Registry which is designed to monitor the potential risk of osteosarcoma and teriparatide treatment. Enrollment information may be found at www.forteoregistry.rti.org or by calling 1-866-382-6813.

Special Geriatric Considerations No age-related differences in pharmacokinetics have been seen. In studies, no significant difference was seen in either efficacy or adverse effects between older patients and younger patients. Teriparatide should be considered an alternative in patients who cannot tolerate or have not responded to other treatments for osteoporosis.

Dosage Forms Excipient information presented when available (limited, particularly for generics); consult specific product labeling.
Injection, solution:
Forteo®: 250 mcg/mL (2.4 mL) [delivers teriparatide 20 mcg/dose]

Dosage Forms: Canada Excipient information presented when available (limited, particularly for generics); consult specific product labeling.
Injection, solution:
Forteo®: 250 mcg/mL (3 mL) [delivers teriparatide 20 mcg/dose]

◆ **Tessalon®** *see* Benzonatate *on page 200*
◆ **Tessalon Perles** *see* Benzonatate *on page 200*
◆ **Testim®** *see* Testosterone *on page 1861*
◆ **Testopel®** *see* Testosterone *on page 1861*

Testosterone (tes TOS ter one)

Related Information
Beers Criteria – Potentially Inappropriate Medications for Geriatrics *on page 2183*

Medication Safety Issues
Sound-alike/look-alike issues:
Testosterone may be confused with testolactone
Testoderm may be confused with Estraderm®
AndroGel® 1% may be confused with AndroGel® 1.62%
Bio-T-Gel may be confused with T-Gel

BEERS Criteria medication:
This drug may be potentially inappropriate for use in geriatric patients (Quality of evidence - moderate; Strength of recommendation - weak).

Other safety concerns:
Transdermal patch may contain conducting metal (eg, aluminum); remove patch prior to MRI.

Brand Names: U.S. Androderm®; AndroGel®; Axiron®; Delatestryl®; Depo®-Testosterone; First®-Testosterone; First®-Testosterone MC; Fortesta™; Striant®; Testim®; Testopel®

Brand Names: Canada Andriol®; Androderm®; AndroGel®; Andropository®; Delatestryl®; Depotest® 100; Everone® 200; PMS-Testosterone; Testim®

Index Terms Axiron®; Testosterone Cypionate; Testosterone Enanthate

Generic Availability (U.S.) Yes: Injection, powder

Pharmacologic Category Androgen

Use
Injection: Male hypogonadism (primary or hypogonadotropic); inoperable metastatic female breast cancer (enanthate only)
Pellet: Male hypogonadism (primary or hypogonadotropic)
Buccal system, topical gel, topical solution, transdermal system: Male hypogonadism (primary or hypogonadotropic)
Capsule (not available in U.S.): Conditions associated with a deficiency or absence of endogenous testosterone

Unlabeled Use Androgen deficiency in men with AIDS wasting; postmenopausal women (short-term use in select cases)

Medication Guide Available Yes

Contraindications Hypersensitivity to testosterone or any component of the formulation; males with known or suspected carcinoma of the breast or prostate; specific products are contraindicated in women

Depo®-Testosterone: Also contraindicated in serious hepatic, renal, or cardiac disease

Warnings/Precautions May cause hypercalcemia in patients with prolonged immobilization or cancer. May accelerate bone maturation without producing compensating gain in linear growth. Has both androgenic and anabolic activity, the anabolic action may enhance hypoglycemia. May alter serum cholesterol; use caution with history of MI or coronary artery disease. Use caution in elderly patients or patients with other demographic factors which may increase the risk of prostatic carcinoma; careful monitoring is required. Urethral obstruction may develop in patients with BPH; treatment should be discontinued if this should occur (use lower dose if restarted). Withhold treatment pending urological evaluation in patients with palpable prostate nodule or induration, PSA >4 ng/mL, or PSA >3 ng/mL in men at high risk of prostate cancer (Bhasin, 2010). Use with caution in patients with conditions influenced by edema (eg, cardiovascular disease, migraine, seizure disorder, renal or hepatic impairment) or medications that enhance edema formation (eg, corticosteroids); testosterone may cause fluid retention. May cause gynecomastia. Large doses may suppress spermatogenesis. During treatment for metastatic breast cancer, women should be monitored for signs of virilization; discontinue if mild virilization is present to prevent irreversible symptoms.

May be inappropriate in the elderly due to potential risk of cardiac problems and contra-indication for use in men with prostate cancer; in general, avoid use in older adults except in the setting of moderate-to-severe hypogonadism (Beers Criteria). In addition, elderly patients may be at greater risk for prostatic hyperplasia, prostate cancer, fluid retention, and trans-aminase elevations.

Prolonged use of high doses of androgens has been associated with serious hepatic effects (peliosis hepatis, hepatic neoplasms, cholestatic hepatitis, jaundice). May potentiate sleep apnea in some male patients (obesity or chronic lung disease). May increase hematocrit requiring dose adjustment or discontinuation; monitor.

[U.S. Boxed Warning]: Virilization in children has been reported following contact with unwashed or unclothed application sites of men using topical testosterone. Patients should strictly adhere to instructions for use in order to prevent secondary exposure. Virilization of female sexual partners has also been reported with male use of topical testosterone. Symptoms of virilization generally regress following removal of exposure. Signs of inappropriate virilization in women following secondary exposure to topical testosterone should be brought to the attention of a healthcare provider. Axiron® and Fortesta™ are not interchangeable with other topical testosterone products; AndroGel® 1% and AndroGel® 1.62% are not interchangeable. Transdermal patch may contain conducting metal (eg, aluminum); remove patch prior to MRI. Some testosterone products may be chemically synthesized from soy. Some products may contain benzyl alcohol. Use of Axiron® in males with BMI >35 kg/m^2 has not been established.

Adverse Reactions (Reflective of adult population; not specific for elderly) Frequency not always defined.

Cardiovascular: Deep venous thrombosis, edema, hypertension, vasodilation

Central nervous system: Abnormal dreams, aggressive behavior, anger, amnesia, anxiety, blood pressure increased/decreased, chills, depression, dizziness, emotional lability, excitation, fatigue, headache, hostility, insomnia, malaise, memory loss, mood swings, nervousness, seizure, sleep apnea, sleeplessness

Dermatologic: Acne, alopecia, contact dermatitis, dry skin, erythema, folliculitis, hair discoloration, hirsutism (increase in pubic hair growth), pruritus, rash, seborrhea

Endocrine & metabolic: Breast pain/soreness, gonadotropin secretion decreased, growth acceleration, gynecomastia, hot flashes, hypercalcemia, hyperchloremia, hypercholesterolemia, hyper-/hypoglycemia, hyper-/hypokalemia, hyperlipidemia, hypernatremia, inorganic phosphate retention, libido changes, menstrual problems (including amenorrhea), virilism, water retention

Gastrointestinal: Appetite increased, diarrhea, gastroesophageal reflux, GI bleeding, GI irritation, nausea, taste disorder, vomiting, weight gain

Following buccal administration (most common): Bitter taste, gum edema, gum or mouth irritation, gum pain, gum tenderness, taste perversion

Genitourinary: Bladder irritability, impotence, oligospermia, penile erections (spontaneous), priapism, prostatic carcinoma, prostatic hyperplasia, prostatitis, PSA increased, testicular atrophy, urination impaired

Hepatic: Bilirubin increased, cholestatic hepatitis, cholestatic jaundice, hepatic dysfunction, hepatic necrosis, hepatocellular neoplasms, liver function test changes, peliosis hepatis

Hematologic: Anemia, bleeding, hematocrit/hemoglobin increased, leukopenia, polycythemia, suppression of clotting factors

Local: Application site reaction (gel, solution), injection site inflammation/pain

Transdermal system: Pruritus at application site (17% to 37%), burn-like blisters under system (12%), erythema at application site (≤7%), vesicles at application site (6%), allergic contact dermatitis to system (4%), burning at application site (3%), induration at application site (3%), exfoliation at application site (<3%)

Neuromuscular & skeletal: Back pain, hemarthrosis, hyperkinesias, paresthesia, weakness

Ocular: Lacrimation increased

Renal: Creatinine increased, hematuria, polyuria

Respiratory: Dyspnea, nasopharyngitis

Miscellaneous: Anaphylactoid reactions, diaphoresis, hypersensitivity reactions, smell disorder

Drug Interactions

Metabolism/Transport Effects Substrate of CYP2B6 (minor), CYP2C19 (minor), CYP2C9 (minor), CYP3A4 (minor); **Note:** Assignment of Major/Minor substrate status based on clinically relevant drug interaction potential

Avoid Concomitant Use There are no known interactions where it is recommended to avoid concomitant use.

Increased Effect/Toxicity

Testosterone may increase the levels/effects of: CycloSPORINE; CycloSPORINE (Systemic); Vitamin K Antagonists

Decreased Effect

The levels/effects of Testosterone may be decreased by: Tocilizumab

Ethanol/Nutrition/Herb Interactions Herb/Nutraceutical: St John's wort may decrease testosterone levels.

Stability

Androderm®: Store at room temperature. Do not store outside of pouch. Excessive heat may cause system to burst.

AndroGel® 1%, AndroGel® 1.62%, Axiron®, Delatestryl®, Striant®, Testim®: Store at room temperature.

Depo® Testosterone: Store at room temperature. Protect from light.

Fortesta™: Store at room temperature; do not freeze

Testopel®: Store in a cool location.

Mechanism of Action Principal endogenous androgen responsible for promoting the growth and development of the male sex organs and maintaining secondary sex characteristics in androgen-deficient males

Pharmacodynamics/Kinetics

Duration (route and ester dependent): I.M.: Cypionate and enanthate esters have longest duration, ≤2-4 weeks; gel: 24-48 hours

Absorption: Transdermal gel: ~10% of applied dose

Protein binding: 98%; bound to sex hormone-binding globulin (40%) and albumin

Metabolism: Hepatic; forms metabolites, including dihydrotestosterone (DHT) and estradiol (both active)

Half-life elimination: Variable: 10-100 minutes

Excretion: Urine (90%); feces (6%)

Dosage

Geriatric & Adult

Conditions associated with a deficiency or absence of endogenous testosterone: *Oral capsule (Andriol®; not available in U.S.):* Initial: 120-160 mg/day in 2 divided doses for 2-3 weeks; adjust according to individual response; usual maintenance dose: 40-120 mg/day (in divided doses)

Inoperable metastatic breast cancer (females): *I.M. (testosterone enanthate):* 200-400 mg every 2-4 weeks

Hypogonadism or hypogonadotropic hypogonadism (males):

I.M. (testosterone enanthate or testosterone cypionate): 50-400 mg every 2-4 weeks (FDA-approved dosing range); 75-100 mg/week or 150-200 mg every 2 weeks (Bhasin, 2010)

Pellet (for subcutaneous implantation): 150-450 mg every 3-6 months

Topical:

Buccal: 30 mg twice daily (every 12 hours) applied to the gum region above the incisor tooth

Gel: Apply to clean, dry, intact skin. **Do not apply testosterone gel to the genitals.**

AndroGel® 1%, Testim®: 5 g (to deliver 50 mg of testosterone with 5 mg systemically absorbed) applied once daily (preferably in the morning) to the shoulder and upper arms. AndroGel® 1% may also be applied to the abdomen. Dosage may be increased to a maximum of 10 g (100 mg).

Dose adjustment based on testosterone levels:
Less than normal range: Increase dose from 5 g to 7.5 g to 10 g
Greater than normal range: Decrease dose. Discontinue if consistently above normal at 5 g/day

AndroGel® 1.62%: 40.5 mg applied once daily in the morning to the shoulder and upper arms. Dosage may be increased to a maximum of 81 mg.

Dose adjustment based on testosterone levels:
>750 ng/dL: Decrease dose by 20.25 mg/day
≥350 ng/dL to ≤750 ng/dL: Maintain current dose
<350 ng/dL: Increase dose by 20.25 mg/day

Fortesta™: 40 mg once daily in the morning. Apply to the thighs. Dosing range: 10-70 mg/day

Dose adjustment based on serum testosterone levels:
≥2500 ng/dL: Decrease dose by 20 mg/day
≥1250 to <2500 ng/dL: Decrease dose by 10 mg/day
≥500 and <1250 ng/dL: Maintain current dose
<500 ng/dL: Increase dose by 10 mg/day

Solution (Axiron®): 60 mg once daily. (Dosage range 30-120 mg/day). Apply to the axilla at the same time each morning; do not apply to other parts of the body. Apply to clean, dry, intact skin. **Do not apply testosterone solution to the genitals.**

Dose adjustment based on serum testosterone levels:
>1050 ng/dL: Decrease 60 mg/day dose to 30 mg/day; if levels >1050 ng/dL persist after dose reduction discontinue therapy
<300 ng/dL: Increase 60 mg/day dose to 90 mg/day, or increase 90 mg/day dose to 120 mg/day

Transdermal system (Androderm®): **Note:** Patches are available in 2 mg, 2.5 mg, 4 mg, and 5 mg strengths. Initial dose is either 4 mg/day or 5 mg/day and dose adjustment varies as follows:
Initial: 4 mg/day (as one 4 mg/day patch; do **not** use two 2 mg/day patches)

Dose adjustment based on testosterone levels:
>930 ng/dL: Decrease dose to 2 mg/day
400-930 ng/dL: Continue 4 mg/day
<400 ng/dL: Increase dose to 6 mg/day (as one 4 mg/day and one 2 mg/day patch)

Initial: 5 mg/day (as one 5 mg/day or two 2.5 mg/day patches)

Dose adjustment based on testosterone levels:
>1030 ng/dL: Decrease dose to 2.5 mg/day
300-1030 ng/dL: Continue 5 mg/day
<300 ng/dL: Increase dose to 7.5 mg/day (as one 5 mg/day and one 2.5 mg/day patch)

Dosing conversion: If needed, patients may be switched from the 2.5 mg/day, 5 mg/day, and 7.5 mg/day patches as follows. Patch change should occur at their next scheduled dosing. Measure early morning testosterone concentrations ~2 weeks after switching therapy:
From 2.5 mg/day patch to 2 mg/day patch
From 5 mg/day patch to 4 mg/day patch
From 7.5 mg/day patch to 6 mg/day patch (one 2 mg/day and one 4 mg/day patch)

Renal Impairment No dosage adjustment provided in manufacturer's labeling (has not been studied). Use with caution; may enhance edema formation.

Hepatic Impairment No dosage adjustment provided in manufacturer's labeling (has not been studied). Use with caution; may enhance edema formation.

Administration

I.M.: Warm to room temperature; shaking vial will help redissolve crystals that have formed after storage. Administer by deep I.M. injection into the upper outer quadrant of the gluteus maximus.

Oral, buccal application (Striant®): One mucoadhesive for buccal application (buccal system) should be applied to a comfortable area above the incisor tooth. Apply flat side of system to gum. Rotate to alternate sides of mouth with each application. Hold buccal system firmly in place for 30 seconds to ensure adhesion. The buccal system should adhere to gum for 12 hours. If the buccal system falls out, replace with a new system. If the system falls out within 4 hours of next dose, the new buccal system should remain in place until the time of the following scheduled dose. System will soften and mold to shape of gum as it absorbs moisture from mouth. Do not chew or swallow the buccal system. The buccal system will not dissolve; gently remove by sliding downwards from gum; avoid scratching gum.

Oral, capsule (Andriol®; not available in the U.S.): Should be administered with meals. Should be swallowed whole; do not crush or chew.

Transdermal patch (Androderm®): Apply patch to clean, dry area of skin on the back, abdomen, upper arms, or thigh. Do not apply to bony areas or parts of the body that are subject to prolonged pressure while sleeping or sitting. **Do not apply to the scrotum.** Avoid showering, washing the site, or swimming for 3 hours after application. Following patch removal, mild skin irritation may be treated with OTC hydrocortisone cream. A small amount of triamcinolone acetonide 0.1% cream may be applied under the system to decrease irritation; do not use ointment. Patch should be applied nightly. Rotate administration sites, allowing 7 days between applying to the same site.

Topical gel and solution: Apply to clean, dry, intact skin. Application sites should be allowed to dry for a few minutes prior to dressing. Hands should be washed with soap and water after application. **Do not apply testosterone gel or solution to the genitals.** Alcohol-based gels and solutions are flammable; avoid fire or smoking until dry. Testosterone may be transferred to another person following skin-to-skin contact with the application site. Strict adherence to application instructions is needed in order to decrease secondary exposure. Thoroughly wash hands after application and cover application site with clothing (ie, shirt) once gel or solution has dried, or clean application site thoroughly with soap and water prior to contact in order to minimize transfer. In addition to skin-to-skin contact, secondary exposure has also been reported following exposure to secondary items (eg, towel, shirt, sheets). If secondary exposure occurs, the other person should thoroughly wash the skin with soap and water as soon as possible.

AndroGel® 1%, AndroGel® 1.62%, Testim®: Apply (preferably in the morning) to clean, dry, intact skin of the shoulder and upper arms. AndroGel® 1% may also be applied to the abdomen; do not apply AndroGel® 1.62% or Testim® to the abdomen. Area of application should be limited to what will be covered by a short sleeve t-shirt. Apply at the same time each day. Upon opening the packet(s), the entire contents should be squeezed into the palm of the hand and immediately applied to the application site(s). Alternatively, a portion may be squeezed onto palm of hand and applied, repeating the process until entire packet has been applied. Application site should not be washed for ≥2 hours following application of AndroGel® 1.62% or Testim®, or >5 hours for AndroGel® 1%.

AndroGel® 1% multidose pump: Prime pump 3 times (and discard this portion of product) prior to initial use. Each actuation delivers 1.25 g of gel (4 actuations = 5 g; 6 actuations = 7.5 g; 8 actuations = 10 g); each actuation may be applied individually or all at the same time.

AndroGel® 1.62% multidose pump: Prime pump 3 times (and discard this portion of product) prior to initial use. Each actuation delivers 20.25 mg of gel (2 actuations = 40.5 mg; 3 actuations = 60.75 mg; 4 actuations = 81 mg); each actuation may be applied individually or all at the same time.

Axiron®: Apply using the applicator to the axilla at the same time each morning. Do not apply to other parts of the body (eg, abdomen, genitals, shoulders, upper arms). Avoid washing the site or swimming for 2 hours after application. Prior to first use, prime the applicator pump by depressing it 3 times (discard this portion of the product). After priming, position the nozzle over the applicator cup and depress pump fully one time; ensure liquid enters cup. Each pump actuation delivers testosterone 30 mg. No more than 30 mg (one pump) should be added to the cup at one time. The total dose should be divided between axilla (example, 30 mg/day: apply to one axilla only; 60 mg/day: apply 30 mg to each axilla; 90 mg/day: apply 30 mg to each axilla, allow to dry, then apply an additional 30 mg to one axilla; etc). To apply dose, keep applicator upright and wipe into the axilla; if solution runs or drips, use cup to wipe. Do not rub into skin with fingers or hand. If more than one 30 mg dose is needed, repeat process. Apply roll-on or stick antiperspirants or deodorants prior to testosterone. Once application site is dry, cover with clothing. After use, rinse applicator under running water and pat dry with a tissue. The application site and dose of this product are not interchangeable with other topical testosterone products.

Fortesta™: Apply to skin of front and inner thighs. Do not apply to other parts of the body. Use one finger to rub gel evenly onto skin of each thigh. Avoid showering, washing the site, or swimming for 2 hours after application. Prior to first dose, prime the pump by holding canister upright and fully depressing the pump 8 times (discard this portion of the product). Each pump actuation delivers testosterone 10 mg. The total dose should be divided between thighs (example, 10 mg/day: apply 10 mg to one thigh only; 20 mg/day: apply 10 mg to each thigh; 30 mg/day: apply 20 mg to one thigh and 10 mg to the other thigh; etc). Once application site is dry, cover with clothing. The application site and dose of this product are not interchangeable with other topical testosterone products.

Monitoring Parameters Periodic liver function tests, cholesterol, hemoglobin and hematocrit (prior to therapy, at 3-6 months, then annually). Withhold initial treatment with hematocrit >50%, hyperviscosity, untreated obstructive sleep apnea, or uncontrolled severe heart failure. Monitor urine and serum calcium and signs of virilization in women treated for breast cancer. Serum glucose (may be decreased by testosterone, monitor patients with diabetes). Evaluate males for response to treatment and adverse events 3-6 months after initiation and then annually.

◄ Bone mineral density: Monitor after 1-2 years of therapy in hypogonadal men with osteoporosis or low trauma fracture (Bhasin, 2010)

PSA: In men >40 years of age with baseline PSA >0.6 ng/mL, PSA and prostate exam (prior to therapy, at 3-6 months, then as based on current guidelines). Withhold treatment pending urological evaluation in patients with palpable prostate nodule or induration or PSA >4 ng/mL or if PSA >3 ng/mL in men at high risk of prostate cancer (Bhasin, 2010).

Do not treat with severe untreated BPH with IPSS symptom score >19.

Serum testosterone: After initial dose titration (if applicable), monitor 3-6 months after initiating treatment, then annually.

Injection: Measure midway between injections. Adjust dose or frequency if testosterone concentration is <400 ng/dL or >700 ng/dL (Bhasin, 2010).

AndroGel® 1%, Testim®: Morning serum testosterone levels ~14 days after start of therapy or dose adjustments

AndroGel® 1.62%: Morning serum testosterone levels after 14 and 28 days of starting therapy or dose adjustments and periodically thereafter

Androderm®: Morning serum testosterone levels (following application the previous evening) ~14 days after start of therapy or dose adjustments

Axiron®: Serum testosterone levels can be measured 2-8 hours after application and after 14 days of starting therapy or dose adjustments

Fortesta™: Serum testosterone levels can be measured 2 hours after application and after 14 and 35 days of starting therapy or dose adjustments

Striant®: Application area of gums; total serum testosterone 4-12 weeks after initiating treatment, prior to morning dose

Testopel®: Measure at the end of the dosing interval (Bhasin, 2010)

Reference Range
Total testosterone, males:
- 12-13 years: <800 ng/dL
- 14 years: <1200 ng/dL
- 15-16 years: 100-1200ng/dL
- 17-18 years: 300-1200 ng/dL
- 19-40 years: 300-950 ng/dL
- >40 years: 240-950 ng/dL

Free testosterone, males: 9-30 ng/dL

Test Interactions Testosterone may decrease thyroxine-binding globulin, resulting in decreased total T_4; free thyroid hormone levels are not changed.

Special Geriatric Considerations Elderly males treated with androgens may be at increased risk of developing prostatic hyperplasia and prostatic carcinoma. Increase in libido may occur.

This medication is considered to be potentially inappropriate in this patient population (Beers Criteria: Quality of evidence - moderate; Strength of recommendation - weak).

Controlled Substance C-III

Dosage Forms Excipient information presented when available (limited, particularly for generics); consult specific product labeling. [DSC] = Discontinued product

Cream, topical [compounding kit]:
First®-Testosterone MC: 2% (60 g) [contains benzyl alcohol, sesame oil]

Gel, topical:
AndroGel®: 1% [5 g gel/packet] (30s); 1% [2.5 g gel/packet] (30s); 1% [1.25 g gel/actuation] (75 g) [contains ethanol 67%; may be chemically synthesized from soy]
AndroGel®: 1.62% [1.25 g gel/actuation] (75 g) [contains ethanol]
Fortesta™: 10 mg/actuation (60 g) [contains ethanol; 0.5 g gel/actuation; 120 metered actuations]
Testim®: 1% [5 g gel/tube] (30s) [contains ethanol 74%; may be chemically synthesized from soy]

Implant, subcutaneous:
Testopel®: 75 mg (10s, 24s, 100s)

Injection, oil, as cypionate: 100 mg/mL (10 mL [DSC]); 200 mg/mL (1 mL, 10 mL)
Depo®-Testosterone: 100 mg/mL (10 mL); 200 mg/mL (1 mL, 10 mL) [contains benzyl alcohol, benzyl benzoate, cottonseed oil]

Injection, oil, as enanthate: 200 mg/mL (5 mL)
Delatestryl®: 200 mg/mL (5 mL) [contains chlorobutanol, sesame oil]

Mucoadhesive, for buccal application [buccal system]:
Striant®: 30 mg (60s) [may be chemically synthesized from soy]

Ointment, topical [compounding kit]:
First®-Testosterone: 2% (60 g) [contains benzyl alcohol, sesame oil]

Patch, transdermal:
Androderm®: 2 mg/24 hours (60s); 2.5 mg/24 hours (60s [DSC]); 4 mg/24 hours (30s); 5 mg/24 hours (30s [DSC]) [contains ethanol, metal]

Powder, for prescription compounding [micronized]: USP: 100% (5 g, 25 g)
Powder, for prescription compounding, as propionate: USP: 100% (5 g, 25 g)
Solution, topical:
  Axiron®: 30 mg/actuation (110 mL) [contains ethanol, isopropyl alcohol; 60 metered actuations]
Dosage Forms: Canada Excipient information presented when available (limited, particularly for generics); consult specific product labeling.
  Capsule, gelatin, as undecanoate:
    Andriol™: 40 mg (10s)

♦ **Testosterone Cypionate** see Testosterone on page 1861
♦ **Testosterone Enanthate** see Testosterone on page 1861
♦ **Testred®** see MethylTESTOSTERone on page 1256
♦ **Tetanus and Diphtheria Toxoid** see Diphtheria and Tetanus Toxoids on page 562

Tetanus Immune Globulin (Human) (TET a nus i MYUN GLOB yoo lin HYU man)

Related Information
  Immunization Administration Recommendations on page 2144
  Immunization Recommendations on page 2149
Brand Names: U.S. HyperTET™ S/D
Brand Names: Canada HyperTET™ S/D
Index Terms TIG
Generic Availability (U.S.) No
Pharmacologic Category Immune Globulin
Use Prophylaxis against tetanus following injury in patients where immunization status is not known or uncertain
  The Advisory Committee on Immunization Practices (ACIP) recommends passive immunization with TIG for the following:
  • Persons with a wound that is not clean or minor and in whom contraindications to a tetanus-toxoid containing vaccine exist and they have not completed a primary series of tetanus toxoid immunization.
  • Persons who are wounded in bombings or similar mass casualty events who have penetrating injuries or nonintact skin exposure and who cannot confirm receipt of a tetanus booster within the previous 5 years. In case of shortage, use should be reserved for persons ≥60 years of age.
Warnings/Precautions Hypersensitivity and anaphylactic reactions can occur; immediate treatment (including epinephrine 1:1000) should be available. Use caution in patients with isolated immunoglobulin A deficiency or a history of systemic hypersensitivity to human immunoglobulins. Use with caution in patients with thrombocytopenia or coagulation disorders; I.M. injections may be contraindicated. Product of human plasma; may potentially contain infectious agents which could transmit disease. Screening of donors, as well as testing and/or inactivation or removal of certain viruses, reduces the risk. Infections thought to be transmitted by this product should be reported to the manufacturer. Skin testing should not be performed as local irritation can occur and be misinterpreted as a positive reaction. Not for intravenous administration.
Adverse Reactions (Reflective of adult population; not specific for elderly) Frequency not defined.
  Central nervous system: Temperature increased
  Dermatologic: Angioneurotic edema (rare)
  Local: Injection site: Pain, soreness, tenderness
  Renal: Nephritic syndrome (rare)
  Miscellaneous: Anaphylactic shock (rare)
Drug Interactions
  Metabolism/Transport Effects None known.
  Avoid Concomitant Use There are no known interactions where it is recommended to avoid concomitant use.
  Increased Effect/Toxicity There are no known significant interactions involving an increase in effect.
  Decreased Effect
  Tetanus Immune Globulin (Human) may decrease the levels/effects of: Vaccines (Live)
Stability Store at 2°C to 8°C (26°F to 46°F). Do not use if frozen. The following stability information has also been reported for HyperTET™ S/D: May be exposed to room temperature for a cumulative 7 days (Cohen, 2007).
Mechanism of Action Passive immunity toward tetanus
Pharmacodynamics/Kinetics Absorption: Well absorbed

◄ **Dosage**
  Geriatric & Adult
   Prophylaxis of tetanus: I.M.: 250 units
   Tetanus prophylaxis in wound management: I.M.: Tetanus prophylaxis in patients with wounds should consider if the wound is clean or contaminated, the immunization status of the patient, proper use of tetanus toxoid and/or tetanus immune globulin (TIG), wound cleaning, and (if required) surgical debridement and the proper use of antibiotics. Patients with an uncertain or incomplete tetanus immunization status should have additional follow up to ensure a series is completed. Patients with a history of Arthus reaction following a previous dose of a tetanus toxoid-containing vaccine should not receive a tetanus toxoid-containing vaccine until >10 years after the most recent dose even if they have a wound that is neither clean nor minor. See table.

Tetanus Prophylaxis in Wound Management

History of Tetanus Immunization Doses	Clean, Minor Wounds		All Other Wounds[1]	
	Tetanus Toxoid[2]	TIG	Tetanus Toxoid[2]	TIG
Uncertain or <3 doses	Yes	No	Yes	Yes
3 or more doses	No[3]	No	No[4]	No

[1]Such as, but not limited to, wounds contaminated with dirt, feces, soil, and saliva; puncture wounds; wounds from crushing, tears, burns, and frostbite.

[2]Tetanus toxoid in this chart refers to a tetanus toxoid-containing vaccine. For children <7 years of age, DTaP (DT, if pertussis vaccine contraindicated) is preferred to tetanus toxoid alone. For children ≥7 years and Adults, Td preferred to tetanus toxoid alone; Tdap may be preferred if the patient has not previously been vaccinated with Tdap.

[3]Yes, if ≥10 years since last dose.

[4]Yes, if ≥5 years since last dose.

Adapted from CDC "Yellow Book" (*Health Information for International Travel 2010*), "Routine Vaccine-Preventable Diseases, Tetanus" (available at http://www.cdc.gov/yellowbook) and *MMWR* 2006, 55(RR-17).

Abbreviations: **DT** = Diphtheria and Tetanus Toxoids (formulation for age ≤6 years); **DTaP** = Diphtheria and Tetanus Toxoids, and Acellular Pertussis (formulation for age ≤6 years; Daptacel®, Infanrix®); **Td** = Diphtheria and Tetanus Toxoids (formulation for age ≥7 years; Decavac®,Tenivac™); **TT**= Tetanus toxoid (adsorbed [formulation for age ≥7 years]); **Tdap** = Diphtheria and Tetanus Toxoids, and Acellular Pertussis (Adacel® or Boostrix® [formulations for age ≥7 years]); **TIG** = Tetanus Immune Globulin

   Treatment of tetanus: I.M.: 500-6000 units. Infiltration of part of the dose around the wound is recommended.
  Administration Do not administer I.V.; I.M. use only
  Monitoring Parameters Monitor for hypersensitivity reactions
  Pharmacotherapy Pearls Tetanus immune globulin (TIG) must not contain <50 units/mL. Protein makes up 10% to 18% of TIG preparations. The great majority of this (≥90%) is IgG. TIG has almost no color or odor and it is a sterile, nonpyrogenic, concentrated preparation of immunoglobulins that has been derived from the plasma of adults hyperimmunized with tetanus toxoid. The pooled material from which the immunoglobulin is derived may be from fewer than 1000 donors. This plasma has been shown to be free of hepatitis B surface antigen.
  Special Geriatric Considerations Tetanus is a rare disease in the U.S. with <50 cases annually; 40% of cases occurred in persons ≥60 years of age; protective tetanus and diphtheria antibodies decline with age; it is estimated that <50% of the elderly are protected.

   Elderly are at risk because:
     Many lack proper immunization maintenance
     Higher case fatality ratio
     Immunizations are not available from childhood
   Indications for vaccination:
     Primary series with combined tetanus-diphtheria (Td) should be given to all elderly lacking a clear history of vaccination
     Boosters with Td (may substitute a single dose of Tdap for a single dose of Td as a one-time replacement) should be given at 10-year intervals (earlier for wounds)
     Elderly are more likely to require tetanus immune globulin with infection of tetanus due to lower antibody titer.
  Dosage Forms Excipient information presented when available (limited, particularly for generics); consult specific product labeling.
   Injection, solution [preservative free]:
     HyperTET™ S/D: 250 units/mL (~1 mL)

Tetanus Toxoid (Adsorbed) (TET a nus TOKS oyd, ad SORBED)

Related Information

Immunization Administration Recommendations *on page 2144*
Immunization Recommendations *on page 2149*

Medication Safety Issues

Sound-alike/look-alike issues:

Tetanus toxoid products may be confused with influenza virus vaccine and tuberculin products. Medication errors have occurred when tetanus toxoid products have been inadvertently administered instead of tuberculin skin tests (PPD) and influenza virus vaccine. These products are refrigerated and often stored in close proximity to each other.

Index Terms TT

Generic Availability (U.S.) No

Pharmacologic Category Vaccine, Inactivated (Bacterial)

Use Active immunization against tetanus when combination antigen preparations are not indicated; tetanus prophylaxis in wound management. **Note:** Tetanus and diphtheria toxoids for adult use (Td) is the preferred immunizing agent for most adults and for children after their seventh birthday. Young children should receive trivalent DTaP (diphtheria/tetanus/acellular pertussis) as part of their childhood immunization program, unless pertussis is contra-indicated, then DT is warranted.

Contraindications Hypersensitivity to tetanus toxoid or any component of the formulation

Warnings/Precautions Avoid injection into a blood vessel; allergic reactions may occur; epinephrine 1:1000 must be available. Patients who are immunocompromised may have reduced response; may be used in patients with HIV infection. In general, household and close contacts of persons with altered immunocompetence may receive all age appropriate vaccines. May defer elective immunization during febrile illness or acute infection. In patients with a history of severe local reaction (Arthus-type) following previous dose, do not give further routine or emergency doses of tetanus and diphtheria toxoids for 10 years. Use caution in patients on anticoagulants, with thrombocytopenia, or bleeding disorders (bleeding may occur following intramuscular injection). Use with caution if Guillain-Barré syndrome occurred within 6 weeks of prior tetanus toxoid. Syncope has been reported with use of injectable vaccines and may be accompanied by transient visual disturbances, weakness, or tonic-clonic move-ments. Procedures should be in place to avoid injuries from falling and to restore cerebral perfusion if syncope occurs. Contains thimerosal. In order to maximize vaccination rates, the ACIP recommends simultaneous administration of all age-appropriate vaccines (live or inactivated) for which a person is eligible at a single clinic visit, unless contraindications exist. The use of combination vaccines is generally preferred over separate injections, taking into consideration provider assessment, patient preference, and adverse events. When using combination vaccines, the minimum age for administration is the oldest minimum age for any individual component; the minimum interval between dosing is the greatest minimum interval between any individual component.

Adverse Reactions (Reflective of adult population; not specific for elderly) All serious adverse reactions must be reported to the U.S. Department of Health and Human Services (DHHS) Vaccine Adverse Event Reporting System (VAERS) 1-800-822-7967 or online at https://vaers.hhs.gov/esub/index.

Frequency not defined.

Cardiovascular: Hypotension

Central nervous system: Brachial neuritis, fever, malaise, pain

Gastrointestinal: Nausea

Local: Edema, induration (with or without tenderness), rash, redness, urticaria, warmth

Neuromuscular: Arthralgia, Guillain-Barré syndrome

Miscellaneous: Anaphylactic reaction, Arthus-type hypersensitivity reaction

Drug Interactions

Metabolism/Transport Effects None known.

Avoid Concomitant Use There are no known interactions where it is recommended to avoid concomitant use.

Increased Effect/Toxicity There are no known significant interactions involving an increase in effect.

Decreased Effect

The levels/effects of Tetanus Toxoid (Adsorbed) may be decreased by: Belimumab; Fingolimod; Immunosuppressants

Stability Store at 2°C to 8°C (26°F to 46°F); do not freeze.

TETANUS TOXOID (ADSORBED)

Mechanism of Action Tetanus toxoid preparations contain the toxin produced by virulent tetanus bacilli (detoxified growth products of *Clostridium tetani*). The toxin has been modified by treatment with formaldehyde so that it has lost toxicity but still retains ability to act as antigen and produce active immunity; the aluminum salt, a mineral adjuvant, delays the rate of absorption and prolongs and enhances its properties; duration ~10 years.

Pharmacodynamics/Kinetics Duration: Primary immunization: ~10 years

Dosage

Geriatric & Adult Note: In most patients, Td is the recommended product for primary immunization, booster doses, and tetanus immunization in wound management (refer to Diphtheria and Tetanus Toxoids monograph).

Primary immunization: I.M.: 0.5 mL; repeat 0.5 mL at 4-8 weeks after first dose and at 6-12 months after second dose

Routine booster dose: Recommended every 10 years

Tetanus prophylaxis in wound management: Tetanus prophylaxis in patients with wounds should consider if the wound is clean or contaminated, the immunization status of the patient, proper use of tetanus toxoid and/or tetanus immune globulin (TIG), wound cleaning, and (if required) surgical debridement and the proper use of antibiotics. Patients with an uncertain or incomplete tetanus immunization status should have additional follow up to ensure a series is completed. Patients with a history of Arthus reaction following a previous dose of a tetanus toxoid-containing vaccine should not receive a tetanus toxoid-containing vaccine until >10 years after the most recent dose even if they have a wound that is neither clean nor minor. See table.

Tetanus Prophylaxis in Wound Management

History of Tetanus Immunization Doses	Clean, Minor Wounds		All Other Wounds[1]	
	Tetanus Toxoid[2]	TIG	Tetanus Toxoid[2]	TIG
Uncertain or <3 doses	Yes	No	Yes	Yes
3 or more doses	No[3]	No	No[4]	No

[1]Such as, but not limited to, wounds contaminated with dirt, feces, soil, and saliva; puncture wounds; wounds from crushing, tears, burns, and frostbite.

[2]Tetanus toxoid in this chart refers to a tetanus toxoid-containing vaccine. For children <7 years of age, DTaP (DT, if pertussis vaccine contraindicated) is preferred to tetanus toxoid alone. For children ≥7 years and Adults, Td preferred to tetanus toxoid alone; Tdap may be preferred if the patient has not previously been vaccinated with Tdap.

[3]Yes, if ≥10 years since last dose.

[4]Yes, if ≥5 years since last dose.

Adapted from CDC "Yellow Book" (*Health Information for International Travel 2010*), "Routine Vaccine-Preventable Diseases, Tetanus" (available at http://www.cdc.gov/yellowbook) and *MMWR* 2006, 55(RR-17).

Abbreviations: **DT** = Diphtheria and Tetanus Toxoids (formulation for age ≤6 years); **DTaP** = Diphtheria and Tetanus Toxoids, and Acellular Pertussis (formulation for age ≤6 years; Daptacel®, Infanrix®); **Td** = Diphtheria and Tetanus Toxoids (formulation for age ≥7 years; Decavac®,Tenivac™); **TT** = Tetanus toxoid (adsorbed [formulation for age ≥7 years]); **Tdap** = Diphtheria and Tetanus Toxoids, and Acellular Pertussis (Adacel® or Boostrix® [formulations for age ≥7 years]); **TIG** = Tetanus Immune Globulin

Administration Inject intramuscularly in the area of the vastus lateralis (midthigh laterally) or deltoid. Do not inject into gluteal area. Shake well prior to withdrawing dose; do not use if product does not form a suspension.

For patients at risk of hemorrhage following intramuscular injection, the ACIP recommends "it should be administered intramuscularly if, in the opinion of the physician familiar with the patient's bleeding risk, the vaccine can be administered by this route with reasonable safety. If the patient receives antihemophilia or other similar therapy, intramuscular vaccination can be scheduled shortly after such therapy is administered. A fine needle (23 gauge or smaller) can be used for the vaccination and firm pressure applied to the site (without rubbing) for at least 2 minutes. The patient should be instructed concerning the risk of hematoma from the injection." Patients on anticoagulant therapy should be considered to have the same bleeding risks and treated as those with clotting factor disorders (CDC, 2011).

Simultaneous administration of vaccines helps ensure the patients will be fully vaccinated by the appropriate age. Simultaneous administration of vaccines is defined as administering >1 vaccine on the same day at different anatomic sites. The use of licensed combination vaccines is generally preferred over separate injections of the equivalent components. Separate vaccines should not be combined in the same syringe unless indicated by product specific labeling. Separate needles and syringes should be used for each injection. The ACIP prefers each dose of a specific vaccine in a series come from the same manufacturer when possible. Adolescents and adults should be vaccinated while seated or lying down. In general, preterm infants should be vaccinated at the same chronological age as full-term infants (CDC, 2011).

Antipyretics have not been shown to prevent febrile seizures. Antipyretics may be used to treat fever or discomfort following vaccination (CDC, 2011). One study reported that routine prophylactic administration of acetaminophen to prevent fever prior to vaccination decreased the immune response of some vaccines; the clinical significance of this reduction in immune response has not been established (Prymula, 2009).

Monitoring Parameters Monitor for syncope for 15 minutes following administration. If seizure-like activity associated with syncope occurs, maintain patient in supine or Trendelen-burg position to reestablish adequate cerebral perfusion.

Pharmacotherapy Pearls U.S. federal law requires that the name of medication, date of administration, the vaccine manufacturer, lot number of vaccine, and the administering person's name, title and address be entered into the patient's permanent medical record.

Special Geriatric Considerations Tetanus is a rare disease in the U.S. with <50 cases annually; 40% of cases occurred in persons ≥60 years of age; protective tetanus and diphtheria antibodies decline with age; it is estimated that <50% of the elderly are protected.

Elderly are at risk because:
  Many lack proper immunization maintenance
  Higher case fatality ratio
  Immunizations are not available from childhood
Indications for vaccination:
  Primary series with combined tetanus-diphtheria (Td) should be given to all elderly lacking a clean history of vaccination
  Boosters with Td (may substitute a single dose of Tdap for a single dose of Td as a one-time replacement) should be given at 10-year intervals (earlier for wounds)
  Elderly are more likely to require tetanus immune globulin with infection of tetanus due to lower antibody titer.

Dosage Forms Excipient information presented when available (limited, particularly for generics); consult specific product labeling.
Injection, suspension: 5 Lf units/0.5 mL (0.5 mL) [contains aluminum and thimerosal (may have trace amounts)]

◆ **Tetanus Toxoid, Reduced Diphtheria Toxoid, and Acellular Pertussis, Adsorbed** *see* Diphtheria and Tetanus Toxoids, and Acellular Pertussis Vaccine *on page* 567

Tetrabenazine (tet ra BEN a zeen)

Brand Names: U.S. Xenazine®
Brand Names: Canada Nitoman™
Pharmacologic Category Central Monoamine-Depleting Agent
Use Treatment of chorea associated with Huntington's disease

Canadian labeling: Treatment of hyperkinetic movement disorders, including Huntington's chorea, hemiballismus, senile chorea, Tourette syndrome, and tardive dyskinesia

Prescribing and Access Restrictions Xenazine® is available only through specialty pharmacies. For more information regarding the procurement of Xenazine®, healthcare providers, patients, and caregivers may contact the Xenazine® Information Center (XIC) at 1-888-882-6013 or at:
  Healthcare providers: http://www.xenazineusa.com/HCP/PrescribingXenazine/Default.aspx
  Patients and caregivers: http://www.xenazineusa.com/AboutXenazine/Getting-Your-Prescription.aspx
Medication Guide Available Yes
Dosage
  Geriatric Canadian labeling: Elderly and/or debilitated patients: Consider initiation at lower doses; must be titrated slowly to individualize dosage.
  Adult Dose should be individualized; titrate slowly
    Chorea associated with Huntington's disease: Oral:
      Initial: 12.5 mg once daily, may increase to 12.5 mg twice daily after 1 week
      Maintenance: May be increased by 12.5 mg/day at weekly intervals; doses >37.5 mg/day should be divided into 3 doses (maximum single dose: 25 mg)
      Patients requiring doses >50 mg/day: Genotype for CYP2D6:
        Extensive/intermediate metabolizers: Maximum: 100 mg/day; 37.5 mg/dose
        Poor metabolizers: Maximum: 50 mg/day; 25 mg/dose
      Concomitant use with strong CYP2D6 inhibitors (eg, fluoxetine, paroxetine, quinidine): Dose of tetrabenazine should be reduced by 50% in patients receiving strong CYP2D6

inhibitors, follow dosing for poor CYP2D6 metabolizers. Use caution when adding a CYP2D6 inhibitor to patients already taking tetrabenazine.

Note: If treatment is interrupted for >5 days, retitration is recommended. If treatment is interrupted for <5 days resume at previous maintenance dose.

Canadian labeling: Hyperkinetic movement disorders: Initial: 12.5 mg twice daily (may be given 3 times/day); may be increased by 12.5 mg/day every 3-5 days; should be titrated slowly to maximal tolerated and effective dose (dose is individualized)

Usual maximum tolerated dosage: 25 mg 3 times/day; maximum recommended dose: 200 mg/day

Note: If there is no improvement at the maximum tolerated dose after 7 days, improvement is unlikely; discontinuation should be considered.

Hepatic Impairment Use is contraindicated.

Special Geriatric Considerations No specific geriatric information is available.

Dosage Forms Excipient information presented when available (limited, particularly for generics); consult specific product labeling.

Tablet, oral:

Xenazine®: 12.5 mg

Xenazine®: 25 mg [scored]

Dosage Forms: Canada Excipient information presented when available (limited, particularly for generics); consult specific product labeling.

Tablet:

Nitoman™: 25 mg

◆ **Tetracaine and Lidocaine** *see* Lidocaine and Tetracaine *on page* 1130

Tetracycline (tet ra SYE kleen)

Related Information

Antimicrobial Drugs of Choice *on page* 2163

H. pylori Treatment in Adult Patients *on page* 2116

Medication Safety Issues

Sound-alike/look-alike issues:

Tetracycline may be confused with tetradecyl sulfate

Achromycin may be confused with actinomycin, Adriamycin®

Brand Names: Canada Apo-Tetra®; Nu-Tetra

Index Terms Achromycin; TCN; Tetracycline Hydrochloride

Generic Availability (U.S.) Yes: Capsule

Pharmacologic Category Antibiotic, Tetracycline Derivative

Use Treatment of susceptible bacterial infections of both gram-positive and gram-negative organisms; also infections due to *Mycoplasma*, *Chlamydia*, and *Rickettsia*; indicated for acne, exacerbations of chronic bronchitis, and treatment of gonorrhea and syphilis in patients who are allergic to penicillin; as part of a multidrug regimen for *H. pylori* eradication to reduce the risk of duodenal ulcer recurrence

Unlabeled Use Treatment of periodontitis associated with presence of *Actinobacillus actinomycetemcomitans* (AA)

Contraindications Hypersensitivity to tetracycline or any component of the formulation

Warnings/Precautions Hazardous agent - use appropriate precautions for handling and disposal. Use with caution in patients with renal or hepatic impairment (eg, elderly); dosage modification required in patients with renal impairment since it may increase BUN as an antianabolic agent. Hepatotoxicity has been reported rarely; risk may be increased in patients with pre-existing hepatic or renal impairment. Pseudotumor cerebri has been reported with tetracycline use (usually resolves with discontinuation); outdated drug can cause nephropathy; use protective measure to avoid photosensitivity. Prolonged use may result in fungal or bacterial superinfection, including *C. difficile*-associated diarrhea (CDAD) and pseudomembranous colitis; CDAD has been observed >2 months postantibiotic treatment. May cause tissue hyperpigmentation, enamel hypoplasia, or permanent tooth discoloration. In addition to affecting tooth development, tetracycline use has been associated with retardation of skeletal development and reduced bone growth.

Adverse Reactions (Reflective of adult population; not specific for elderly) Frequency not defined.

Cardiovascular: Pericarditis

Central nervous system: Bulging fontanels in infants, increased intracranial pressure, paresthesia, pseudotumor cerebri

Dermatologic: Exfoliative dermatitis, photosensitivity, pigmentation of nails, pruritus

Gastrointestinal: Abdominal cramps, anorexia, antibiotic-associated pseudomembranous colitis, diarrhea, discoloration of teeth and enamel hypoplasia (young children), esophagitis, nausea, pancreatitis, staphylococcal enterocolitis, vomiting

Hematologic: Thrombophlebitis

Hepatic: Hepatotoxicity

Renal: Acute renal failure, azotemia, renal damage

Miscellaneous: Anaphylaxis, candidal superinfection, hypersensitivity reactions, superinfection

Drug Interactions

Metabolism/Transport Effects Substrate of CYP3A4 (major); **Note:** Assignment of Major/Minor substrate status based on clinically relevant drug interaction potential; **Inhibits** CYP3A4 (moderate)

Avoid Concomitant Use

Avoid concomitant use of Tetracycline with any of the following: BCG; Pimozide; Retinoic Acid Derivatives; Tolvaptan

Increased Effect/Toxicity

Tetracycline may increase the levels/effects of: ARIPiprazole; Avanafil; Budesonide (Systemic, Oral Inhalation); Colchicine; CYP3A4 Substrates; Eplerenone; Everolimus; FentaNYL; Halofantrine; Ivacaftor; Lurasidone; Neuromuscular-Blocking Agents; Pimecrolimus; Pimozide; Porfimer; Propafenone; Ranolazine; Retinoic Acid Derivatives; Salmeterol; Saxagliptin; Tolvaptan; Vilazodone; Vitamin K Antagonists; Zuclopenthixol

Decreased Effect

Tetracycline may decrease the levels/effects of: Atovaquone; BCG; Ifosfamide; Penicillins; Typhoid Vaccine

The levels/effects of Tetracycline may be decreased by: Antacids; Bile Acid Sequestrants; Bismuth; Bismuth Subsalicylate; Calcium Salts; CYP3A4 Inducers (Strong); Deferasirox; Herbs (CYP3A4 Inducers); Iron Salts; Lanthanum; Magnesium Salts; Quinapril; Sucralfate; Tocilizumab; Zinc Salts

Ethanol/Nutrition/Herb Interactions

Food: Serum concentrations may be decreased if taken with dairy products. Take on an empty stomach 1 hour before or 2 hours after meals to increase total absorption. Administer around-the-clock to promote less variation in peak and trough serum levels.

Herb/Nutraceutical: Dong quai and St John's wort may also cause photosensitization. Management: Avoid dong quai and St John's wort.

Stability Outdated tetracyclines have caused a Fanconi-like syndrome. Protect oral dosage forms from light.

Mechanism of Action Inhibits bacterial protein synthesis by binding with the 30S and possibly the 50S ribosomal subunit(s) of susceptible bacteria; may also cause alterations in the cytoplasmic membrane

Pharmacodynamics/Kinetics

Absorption: Oral: 75%

Distribution: Small amount appears in bile

Relative diffusion from blood into CSF: Good only with inflammation (exceeds usual MICs)

CSF:blood level ratio: Inflamed meninges: 25%

Protein binding: ~65%

Half-life elimination: Normal renal function: 8-11 hours; End-stage renal disease: 57-108 hours

Time to peak, serum: Oral: 2-4 hours

Excretion: Urine (60% as unchanged drug); feces (as active form)

Dosage

Geriatric & Adult

Usual dosage range: Oral: 250-500 mg every 6 hours

Acne: Oral: 250-500 twice daily

Chronic bronchitis, acute exacerbation: Oral: 500 mg 4 times/day

Erlichiosis: Oral: 500 mg 4 times/day for 7-14 days

Malaria, severe, treatment (unlabeled use): Oral: 250 mg 4 times/day for 7 days with quinidine gluconate. **Note:** Quinidine gluconate duration is region specific; consult CDC for current recommendations (CDC, 2009).

Malaria, uncomplicated, treatment (unlabeled use): Oral: 250 mg 4 times/day for 7 days with quinine sulfate. **Note:** Quinine sulfate duration is region specific; consult CDC for current recommendations (CDC, 2009).

Peptic ulcer disease: Eradication of *Helicobacter pylori*: Oral: 500 mg 2-4 times/day depending on regimen; requires combination therapy with at least one other antibiotic and an acid-suppressing agent (proton pump inhibitor or H$_2$ blocker)

Periodontitis (unlabeled use): Oral: 250 mg every 6 hours until improvement (usually 10 days)

Vibrio cholerae: Oral: 500 mg 4 times/day for 3 days

Renal Impairment

Cl$_{cr}$ 50-80 mL/minute: Administer every 8-12 hours.

Cl$_{cr}$ 10-50 mL/minute: Administer every 12-24 hours.

Cl$_{cr}$ <10 mL/minute: Administer every 24 hours.

Slightly dialyzable (5% to 20%) via hemo- and peritoneal dialysis or via continuous arteriovenous or venovenous hemofiltration; supplemental dose is not necessary.

Hepatic Impairment Use caution; no dosing adjustment required

Administration Should be administered on an empty stomach (ie, 1 hour prior to, or 2 hours after meals) to increase total absorption. Administer at least 1-2 hours prior to, or 4 hours after antacid because aluminum and magnesium cations may chelate with tetracycline and reduce its total absorption.

Monitoring Parameters Renal, hepatic, and hematologic function test, temperature, WBC, cultures and sensitivity, appetite, mental status

Special Geriatric Considerations The role of tetracycline has decreased because of the emergence of resistant organisms. Doxycycline is the tetracycline of choice when one is indicated because of its better GI absorption, less interactions with divalent cations, longer half-life, and the fact that the majority is cleared by nonrenal mechanisms.

Dosage Forms Excipient information presented when available (limited, particularly for generics); consult specific product labeling.

Capsule, oral, as hydrochloride: 250 mg, 500 mg

◆ **Tetracycline Hydrochloride** see Tetracycline on page 1872
◆ **Tetrahydrocannabinol** see Dronabinol on page 610

Tetrahydrozoline (Nasal) (tet ra hye DROZ a leen)

Brand Names: U.S. Tyzine®; Tyzine® Pediatric

Index Terms Tetrahydrozoline Hydrochloride; Tetryzoline

Generic Availability (U.S.) No

Pharmacologic Category Adrenergic Agonist Agent; Decongestant; Imidazoline Derivative

Use Symptomatic relief of nasal congestion

Dosage

Geriatric & Adult Nasal congestion: Intranasal: Instill 2-4 drops or 3-4 sprays of 0.1% solution into each nostril every 3-4 hours as needed, no more frequently than every 3 hours

Special Geriatric Considerations Evaluate the patient's or caregiver's ability to safely administer the correct dose of nasal medication. Use with caution in patients with cardiovascular disease.

Dosage Forms Excipient information presented when available (limited, particularly for generics); consult specific product labeling.

Solution, intranasal, as hydrochloride [drops]:

Tyzine®: 0.1% (30 mL) [contains benzalkonium chloride]

Tyzine® Pediatric: 0.05% (15 mL) [contains benzalkonium chloride]

Solution, intranasal, as hydrochloride [spray]:

Tyzine®: 0.1% (15 mL) [contains benzalkonium chloride]

Tetrahydrozoline (Ophthalmic) (tet ra hye DROZ a leen)

Medication Safety Issues

Sound-alike/look-alike issues:

Visine® may be confused with Visken®

Brand Names: U.S. Murine® Tears Plus [OTC]; Opti-Clear [OTC]; Visine® Advanced Relief [OTC]; Visine® Original [OTC]

Index Terms Tetrahydrozoline Hydrochloride; Tetryzoline

Pharmacologic Category Adrenergic Agonist Agent; Imidazoline Derivative; Ophthalmic Agent, Vasoconstrictor

Use Symptomatic relief of conjunctival congestion

Contraindications Hypersensitivity to tetrahydrozoline or any component of the formulation.

Warnings/Precautions For ophthalmic use only. Stop use if vision changes, condition worsens, or symptoms persist >72 hours. Use with caution in patients with cardiovascular disease, including hypertension and coronary artery disease. Use with caution in patients with endocrine disorders, including diabetes and hyperthyroidism.

Adverse Reactions (Reflective of adult population; not specific for elderly) Frequency not established

Cardiovascular: Hypertension, palpitation, tachycardia

Central nervous system: Headache

Local: Transient stinging

Neuromuscular & skeletal: Tremor

Ocular: Blurred vision

Drug Interactions

Metabolism/Transport Effects None known.

Avoid Concomitant Use There are no known interactions where it is recommended to avoid concomitant use.

Increased Effect/Toxicity There are no known significant interactions involving an increase in effect.

Decreased Effect There are no known significant interactions involving a decrease in effect.

Stability Do not use if solution changes color or becomes cloudy.

Mechanism of Action Stimulates alpha-adrenergic receptors in the arterioles of the conjunctiva to produce vasoconstriction

Pharmacodynamics/Kinetics Duration: Vasoconstriction: 2-3 hours

Dosage

Geriatric & Adult Conjunctival congestion: Ophthalmic: Instill 1-2 drops in each eye 2-4 times/day

Monitoring Parameters Blood pressure, heart rate

Special Geriatric Considerations Use with caution in patients with cardiovascular disease. Evaluate the patient's or caregiver's ability to safely administer the correct dose of ophthalmic medication.

Dosage Forms Excipient information presented when available (limited, particularly for generics); consult specific product labeling.

Solution, ophthalmic, as hydrochloride [drops]: 0.05% (15 mL); 0.5% (15 mL)

Murine® Tears Plus: 0.05% (15 mL) [contains benzalkonium chloride]

Opti-Clear: 0.05% (15 mL)

Visine® Advanced Relief: 0.05% (15 mL, 30 mL) [contains benzalkonium chloride; contains polyethylene glycol]

Visine® Original: 0.05% (15 mL, 30 mL) [contains benzalkonium chloride]

◆ **Tetrahydrozoline Hydrochloride** *see* Tetrahydrozoline (Nasal) *on page 1874*

◆ **Tetrahydrozoline Hydrochloride** *see* Tetrahydrozoline (Ophthalmic) *on page 1874*

◆ **Tetraiodothyronine and Triiodothyronine** *see* Thyroid, Desiccated *on page 1885*

◆ **Tetryzoline** *see* Tetrahydrozoline (Nasal) *on page 1874*

◆ **Tetryzoline** *see* Tetrahydrozoline (Ophthalmic) *on page 1874*

◆ **Teveten®** *see* Eprosartan *on page 655*

◆ **Teveten® HCT** *see* Eprosartan and Hydrochlorothiazide *on page 657*

◆ **Texacort™** *see* Hydrocortisone (Topical) *on page 943*

◆ **Thalitone®** *see* Chlorthalidone *on page 364*

◆ **THC** *see* Dronabinol *on page 610*

◆ **Theo-24®** *see* Theophylline *on page 1875*

Theophylline (thee OFF i lin)

Brand Names: U.S. Elixophyllin® Elixir; Theo-24®

Brand Names: Canada Apo-Theo LA®; Novo-Theophyl SR; PMS-Theophylline; Pulmophylline; ratio-Theo-Bronc; Teva-Theophylline SR; Theo ER; Theolair; Uniphyl

Index Terms Theophylline Anhydrous

Generic Availability (U.S.) Yes: Extended release tablet, infusion, solution

Pharmacologic Category Phosphodiesterase Enzyme Inhibitor, Nonselective

Use Treatment of symptoms and reversible airway obstruction due to chronic asthma, or other chronic lung diseases

Note: The Global Initiative for Asthma Guidelines (2009) and the National Heart, Lung and Blood Institute Guidelines (2007) do not recommend theophylline for the treatment of exacerbations of asthma.

The Global Initiative for Chronic Obstructive Lung Disease Guidelines (2009) suggest that while higher doses of slow release formulations of theophylline have been proven to be effective for use in COPD, it is not a preferred agent due to its potential for toxicity.

Contraindications Hypersensitivity to theophylline or any component of the formulation; premixed injection may contain corn-derived dextrose and its use is contraindicated in patients with allergy to corn-related products

Warnings/Precautions If a patient develops signs and symptoms of theophylline toxicity (eg, persistent, repetitive vomiting), a serum theophylline level should be measured and subsequent doses held. Serum theophylline monitoring may be lessened as lower therapeutic ranges are established. More intense monitoring may be required during acute illness or when interacting drugs are introduced into the regimen. Use with caution in patients with peptic ▶

ulcer, hyperthyroidism, seizure disorders, and patients with tachyarrhythmias (eg, sinus tachycardia, atrial fibrillation); use may exacerbate these conditions. Theophylline-induced nonconvulsive status epilepticus has been reported (rarely) and should be considered in patients who develop CNS abnormalities. Theophylline clearance may be decreased in patients with acute pulmonary edema, congestive heart failure, cor-pulmonale, fever, hepatic disease, acute hepatitis, cirrhosis, hypothyroidism, sepsis with multiorgan failure, and shock; clearance may also be decreased in the elderly >60 years, and patients following cessation of smoking.

Adverse Reactions (Reflective of adult population; not specific for elderly) Frequency not defined. Adverse events observed at therapeutic serum levels:

Cardiovascular: Flutter, tachycardia

Central nervous system: Headache, hyperactivity (children), insomnia, restlessness, seizures, status epilepticus (nonconvulsive)

Endocrine & metabolic: Hypercalcemia (with concomitant hyperthyroid disease)

Gastrointestinal: Nausea, reflux or ulcer aggravation, vomiting

Genitourinary: Difficulty urinating (elderly males with prostatism)

Neuromuscular & skeletal: Tremor

Renal: Diuresis (transient)

Drug Interactions

Metabolism/Transport Effects Substrate of CYP1A2 (major), CYP2C9 (minor), CYP2D6 (minor), CYP2E1 (major), CYP3A4 (major); **Note:** Assignment of Major/Minor substrate status based on clinically relevant drug interaction potential; **Inhibits** CYP1A2 (weak)

Avoid Concomitant Use

Avoid concomitant use of Theophylline with any of the following: Conivaptan; Deferasirox; Iobenguane I 123

Increased Effect/Toxicity

Theophylline may increase the levels/effects of: Formoterol; Indacaterol; Pancuronium; Sympathomimetics

The levels/effects of Theophylline may be increased by: Abiraterone Acetate; Allopurinol; Antithyroid Agents; AtoMOXetine; Cannabinoids; Cimetidine; Conivaptan; Contraceptives (Estrogens); CYP1A2 Inhibitors (Moderate); CYP1A2 Inhibitors (Strong); CYP3A4 Inhibitors (Moderate); CYP3A4 Inhibitors (Strong); Dasatinib; Deferasirox; Disulfiram; Febuxostat; FluvoxaMINE; Interferons; Isoniazid; Ivacaftor; Linezolid; Macrolide Antibiotics; Methotrexate; Mexiletine; Mifepristone; Pentoxifylline; Propafenone; QuiNINE; Quinolone Antibiotics; Thiabendazole; Ticlopidine; Zafirlukast; Zileuton

Decreased Effect

Theophylline may decrease the levels/effects of: Adenosine; Benzodiazepines; CarBAMazepine; Fosphenytoin; Iobenguane I 123; Lithium; Pancuronium; Phenytoin; Regadenoson; Zafirlukast

The levels/effects of Theophylline may be decreased by: Aminoglutethimide; Barbiturates; Beta-Blockers (Beta1 Selective); Beta-Blockers (Nonselective); CarBAMazepine; CYP1A2 Inducers (Strong); CYP3A4 Inducers (Strong); Cyproterone; Fosphenytoin; Herbs (CYP3A4 Inducers); Isoproterenol; Phenytoin; Protease Inhibitors; Thyroid Products; Tocilizumab

Ethanol/Nutrition/Herb Interactions Food: Food does not appreciably affect the absorption of liquid, fast-release products, and most sustained release products; however, food may induce a sudden release (dose-dumping) of once-daily sustained release products resulting in an increase in serum drug levels and potential toxicity. Changes in diet may affect the elimination of theophylline; charbroiled foods may increase elimination, reducing half-life by 50%. Management: Should be taken with water 1 hour before or 2 hours after meals. Avoid excessive amounts of caffeine. Avoid extremes of dietary protein and carbohydrate intake.

Stability Tablet, premixed infusion, solution: Store at controlled room temperature of 25°C (77°F).

Mechanism of Action Causes bronchodilatation, diuresis, CNS and cardiac stimulation, and gastric acid secretion by blocking phosphodiesterase which increases tissue concentrations of cyclic adenine monophosphate (cAMP) which in turn promotes catecholamine stimulation of lipolysis, glycogenolysis, and gluconeogenesis and induces release of epinephrine from adrenal medulla cells

Pharmacodynamics/Kinetics

Absorption: Oral: Dosage form dependent

Distribution: 0.45 L/kg (range: 0.3-0.7 L/kg) based on ideal body weight; distributes poorly into body fat; V_d may increase in patients with hepatic cirrhosis, acidemia (uncorrected), the elderly

Metabolism: Adults: Hepatic; involves CYP1A2, 2E1 and 3A4; forms active metabolites (caffeine and 3-methylxanthine)

Protein binding: 40%, primarily to albumin

Half-life elimination: Highly variable and dependent upon age, liver function, cardiac function, lung disease, and smoking history

Adults 16-60 years with asthma, nonsmoking, otherwise healthy: 8.7 hours (range: 6.1-12.8 hours)

Time to peak, serum:
Oral: Liquid: 1 hour
I.V.: Within 30 minutes

Excretion: Urine: Adults: ~10% as unchanged theophylline

Dosage

Geriatric

Acute symptoms: Adults >60 years:

Loading dose: Oral, I.V.: Refer to adult dosing.

Maintenance dose: I.V.: 0.3 mg/kg/hour; maximum 400 mg/day unless serum levels indicate need for larger dose

Chronic conditions: Oral: Adults >60 years: Do not exceed a dose of 400 mg/day

Cardiac decompensation, cor pulmonale, hepatic dysfunction, sepsis with multiorgan failure, shock: Refer to adult dosing.

Adult Doses should be individualized based on steady-state serum concentrations and ideal body weight.

Acute symptoms: Loading dose: Oral, I.V.:

Asthma exacerbations: While theophylline may be considered for relief of asthma symptoms, the role of treating exacerbations is not supported by current practice.

COPD treatment: Theophylline is currently considered second-line intravenous therapy in the emergency department or hospital setting when there is inadequate or insufficient response to short acting bronchodilators (Global Initiative for COPD Guidelines, 2009).

If no theophylline received within the previous 24 hours: 4.6 mg/kg loading dose (~5.8 mg/kg hydrous aminophylline) I.V. or 5 mg/kg orally. Loading dose intended to achieve a serum level of approximately 10 mcg/mL; loading doses should be given intravenously (preferred) or with a rapidly absorbed oral product (not an extended-release product). **Note:** On the average, for every 1 mg/kg theophylline given, blood levels will rise 2 mcg/mL.

If theophylline has been administered in the previous 24 hours: A loading dose is not recommended without obtaining a serum theophylline concentration. The loading dose should be calculated as follows:

Dose = (desired serum theophylline concentration - measured serum theophylline concentration) (V_d)

Acute symptoms: Maintenance dose: I.V.: **Note:** To achieve a target concentration of 10 mcg/mL unless otherwise noted. Lower initial doses may be required in patients with reduced theophylline clearance. Dosage should be adjusted according to serum level measurements during the first 12- to 24-hour period.

Adults 16-60 years (otherwise healthy, nonsmokers): 0.4 mg/kg/hour; maximum 900 mg/day unless serum levels indicate need for larger dose

Adults >60 years: 0.3 mg/kg/hour; maximum 400 mg/day unless serum levels indicate need for larger dose

Treatment of chronic conditions:

Oral solution: Initial dose: 300 mg/day administered in divided doses every 6-8 hours; Maintenance: 400-600 mg/day (maximum: 600 mg/day)

Oral extended release formulations: Initial dose: 300-400 mg once daily; Maintenance: 400-600 mg once daily (maximum: 600 mg/day)

Dosage adjustment after serum theophylline measurement: Asthma: Within normal limits: Adults: 5-15 mcg/mL: Maintain dosage if tolerated. Recheck serum theophylline concentration at 24-hour intervals (for acute I.V. dosing) or at 6- to 12-month intervals (for oral dosing). Finer adjustments in dosage may be needed for some patients. If levels ≥15 mcg/mL, consider 10% dose reduction to improve safety margin.

Note: Recheck serum theophylline levels after 3 days when using oral dosing, or after 24 hours (adults) when dosing intravenously. Patients maintained with oral therapy may be reassessed at 6- to 12-month intervals.

Administration

I.V.: Administer loading dose over 30 minutes; follow with a continuous infusion as appropriate

Oral: Long-acting preparations should be taken with a full glass of water, swallowed whole, or cut in half if scored. Do **not** crush. Extended release capsule forms may be opened and the contents sprinkled on soft foods; do **not** chew beads.

◀ **Monitoring Parameters** Monitor heart rate, CNS effects (insomnia, irritability); respiratory rate (COPD patients often have resting controlled respiratory rates in low 20s); arterial or capillary blood gases (if applicable)

Theophylline levels: Serum theophylline levels should be monitored prior to making dose increases; in the presence of signs or symptoms of toxicity; or when a new illness, worsening of a present illness, or medication changes occur that may change theophylline clearance

I.V. loading dose: Measure serum concentrations 30 minutes after the end of an I.V. loading dose

I.V. infusion: Measure serum concentrations one half-life after starting a continuous infusion, then every 12-24 hours

Reference Range Therapeutic levels: Asthma: Adults: 5-15 mcg/mL

Test Interactions Plasma glucose, uric acid, free fatty acids, total cholesterol, HDL, HDL/LDL ratio, and urinary free cortisol excretion may be increased by theophylline. Theophylline may decrease triiodothyronine.

Special Geriatric Considerations Although there is a great intersubject variability for half-lives of methylxanthines (2-10 hours), elderly as a group have slower hepatic clearance. Therefore, use lower initial doses and monitor closely for response and adverse reactions. Additionally, elderly are at greater risk for toxicity due to concomitant disease (eg, CHF, arrhythmias), and drug use (eg, cimetidine, ciprofloxacin).

Dosage Forms Excipient information presented when available (limited, particularly for generics); consult specific product labeling.

Capsule, extended release, oral:

Theo-24®: 100 mg, 200 mg, 300 mg, 400 mg [24 hours]

Infusion, premixed in D_5W: 400 mg (500 mL); 800 mg (500 mL)

Solution, oral: 80 mg/15 mL (15 mL, 473 mL)

Elixophyllin® Elixir: 80 mg/15 mL (473 mL) [contains ethanol 20%; mixed fruit flavor]

Tablet, extended release, oral: 100 mg, 200 mg, 300 mg, 400 mg, 450 mg, 600 mg

- ◆ **Theophylline Anhydrous** see Theophylline on page 1875
- ◆ **Theophylline Ethylenediamine** see Aminophylline on page 92
- ◆ **Theraflu® Thin Strips® Multi Symptom [OTC]** see DiphenhydrAMINE (Systemic) on page 556
- ◆ **Thera-Sal [OTC] [DSC]** see Salicylic Acid on page 1743
- ◆ **Thermazene®** see Silver Sulfadiazine on page 1775
- ◆ **Thiamazole** see Methimazole on page 1232
- ◆ **Thiamin** see Thiamine on page 1878

Thiamine (THYE a min)

Medication Safety Issues

Sound-alike/look-alike issues:

Thiamine may be confused with Tenormin®, Thalomid®, Thorazine

International issues:

Doxal [Brazil] may be confused with Doxil brand name for doxorubicin [U.S.]

Doxal: Brand name for pyridoxine/thiamine [Brazil], but also the brand name for doxepin [Finland]

Brand Names: Canada Betaxin®

Index Terms Aneurine Hydrochloride; Thiamin; Thiamine Hydrochloride; Thiaminium Chloride Hydrochloride; Vitamin B_1

Generic Availability (U.S.) Yes

Pharmacologic Category Vitamin, Water Soluble

Use Treatment of thiamine deficiency including beriberi, Wernicke's encephalopathy, Korsakoff's syndrome, or in alcoholic patients; dietary supplement

Contraindications Hypersensitivity to thiamine or any component of the formulation

Warnings/Precautions Use with caution with parenteral route (especially I.V.) of administration. Hypersensitivity reactions have been reported following repeated parenteral doses; consider skin test in individuals with history of allergic reactions. Single vitamin deficiency is rare; evaluate for other deficiencies. Dextrose administration may precipitate acute symptoms of thiamine deficiency; use caution when thiamine status is marginal or suspect. Some parenteral products contain aluminum; use caution in patients with impaired renal function.

Adverse Reactions (Reflective of adult population; not specific for elderly) Adverse reactions reported with injection. Frequency not defined.

Cardiovascular: Cyanosis

Central nervous system: Restlessness

Dermatologic: Angioneurotic edema, pruritus, urticaria

Gastrointestinal: Hemorrhage into GI tract, nausea, tightness of the throat

Local: Induration and/or tenderness at the injection site (following I.M. administration)

Neuromuscular & skeletal: Weakness

Respiratory: Pulmonary edema

Miscellaneous: Anaphylactic/hypersensitivity reactions (following I.V. administration), diaphoresis, warmth

Drug Interactions

Metabolism/Transport Effects None known.

Avoid Concomitant Use There are no known interactions where it is recommended to avoid concomitant use.

Increased Effect/Toxicity There are no known significant interactions involving an increase in effect.

Decreased Effect There are no known significant interactions involving a decrease in effect.

Ethanol/Nutrition/Herb Interactions

Ethanol: May decrease thiamine absorption.

Food: High carbohydrate diets may increase thiamine requirement.

Stability Injection: Store at 15°C to 30°C (59°F to 86°F). Protect from light

Mechanism of Action An essential coenzyme in carbohydrate metabolism by combining with adenosine triphosphate to form thiamine pyrophosphate

Pharmacodynamics/Kinetics

Absorption: Oral: Adequate; I.M.: Rapid and complete

Distribution: Highest concentrations found in brain, heart, kidney, liver

Excretion: Urine (as unchanged drug and as pyrimidine after body storage sites become saturated)

Dosage

Geriatric & Adult

Recommended daily intake: Female: 1.1 mg; Male: 1.2 mg

Parenteral nutrition supplementation: 6 mg/day; may be increased to 25-50 mg/day with history of alcohol abuse

Thiamine deficiency (beriberi): 5-30 mg/dose I.M. or I.V. 3 times/day (if critically ill); then orally 5-30 mg/day in single or divided doses 3 times/day for 1 month

Alcohol withdrawal syndrome: 100 mg/day I.M. or I.V. for several days, followed by 50-100 mg/day orally

Wernicke's encephalopathy: Treatment (manufacturer's labeling): Initial: 100 mg I.V., then 50-100 mg/day I.M. or I.V. until consuming a regular, balanced diet. However, larger doses may be required based on failure of lower doses to produce clinical improvement in some patients.

Alternate dosage: The Royal College of Physicians (U.K.) has recommended the use of higher doses of thiamine (in combination with other B vitamins, ascorbic acid, potassium, phosphate, and magnesium) for the management of Wernicke's encephalopathy (Thomson, 2002):

Prophylaxis: 250 mg I.V. once daily for 3-5 days

Treatment: Initial: 500 mg I.V. 3 times/day for 3 days. If response to thiamine after 3 days, continue with 250 mg I.M. or I.V. once daily for an additional 5 days or until clinical improvement.

Administration Parenteral form may be administered by I.M. or I.V. injection. Various rates of administration have been reported. Local injection reactions may be minimized by slow administration (~30 minutes) into larger, more proximal veins. Thiamine should be administered prior to parenteral glucose solutions to prevent precipitation of acute symptoms of thiamine deficiency in the poorly nourished.

Reference Range Normal, serum: 1.1-1.6 mg/dL

Test Interactions False-positive for uric acid using the phosphotungstate method and for urobilinogen using the Ehrlich's reagent; large doses may interfere with the spectrophotometric determination of serum theophylline concentration

Pharmacotherapy Pearls Thiamine (vitamin B_1) is unstable in alkaline or neutral solutions, therefore, do not mix with carbonates, citrates, barbiturates. Also, any solution containing sulfites is incompatible with thiamine. Recommended thiamine intake is 0.5 mg/1000 Kcal.

Special Geriatric Considerations No special recommendations are necessary. Elderly are treated the same as younger adults.

Dosage Forms Excipient information presented when available (limited, particularly for generics); consult specific product labeling.

Injection, solution, as hydrochloride: 100 mg/mL (2 mL)

Tablet, oral, as hydrochloride: 50 mg, 100 mg, 250 mg, 500 mg

◆ **Thiamine Hydrochloride** see Thiamine on page 1878
◆ **Thiaminium Chloride Hydrochloride** see Thiamine on page 1878

Thioridazine (thye oh RID a zeen)

Related Information

Antipsychotic Agents *on page 2103*

Beers Criteria – Potentially Inappropriate Medications for Geriatrics *on page 2183*

Medication Safety Issues

Sound-alike/look-alike issues:

Thioridazine may be confused with thiothixene, Thorazine

Mellaril may be confused with Elavil, Mebaral®

BEERS Criteria medication:

This drug may be potentially inappropriate for use in geriatric patients (Quality of evidence - moderate; Strength of recommendation - strong).

Index Terms Mellaril; Thioridazine Hydrochloride

Generic Availability (U.S.) Yes

Pharmacologic Category Antipsychotic Agent, Typical, Phenothiazine

Use Management of schizophrenic patients who fail to respond adequately to treatment with other antipsychotic drugs, either because of insufficient effectiveness or the inability to achieve an effective dose due to intolerable adverse effects from those medications

Unlabeled Use Depressive disorders/dementia (adults); behavioral symptoms associated with dementia (elderly); psychosis/agitation related to Alzheimer's dementia

Contraindications Severe CNS depression; severe hyper-/hypotensive heart disease; coma; in combination with other drugs that are known to prolong the QT_c interval and/or CYP2D6 inhibitors; in patients with congenital long QT syndrome or a history of cardiac arrhythmias; concurrent use with medications that inhibit the metabolism of thioridazine (fluoxetine, paroxetine, fluvoxamine, propranolol, pindolol); patients known to have genetic defect leading to reduced levels of activity of CYP2D6

Warnings/Precautions [U.S. Boxed Warning]: Thioridazine has dose-related effects on ventricular repolarization leading to QT_c prolongation, a potentially life-threatening effect. Therefore, it should be reserved for patients with schizophrenia who have failed to respond to adequate levels of other antipsychotic drugs. Due to potential for QT_c prolongation; use contraindicated with concomitant CYP2D6 inhibitors and/or concomitant use with other agents that prolong the QT_c interval. May cause orthostatic hypotension; use with caution in patients at risk of this effect or those who would tolerate transient hypotensive episodes (cerebrovascular disease, cardiovascular disease, or other medications which may predispose). **[U.S. Boxed Warning]: Elderly patients with dementia-related psychosis treated with antipsychotics are at an increased risk of death compared to placebo.** Most deaths appeared to be either cardiovascular (eg, heart failure, sudden death) or infectious (eg, pneumonia) in nature. Thioridazine is not approved for the treatment of dementia-related psychosis.

Leukopenia, neutropenia, and agranulocytosis (sometimes fatal) have been reported in clinical trials and postmarketing reports with antipsychotic use; presence of risk factors (eg, pre-existing low WBC or history of drug-induced leuko-/neutropenia) should prompt periodic blood count assessment. Discontinue therapy at first signs of blood dyscrasias or if absolute neutrophil count <1000/mm^3.

Highly sedating, use with caution in disorders where CNS depression is a feature. Use with caution in Parkinson's disease. Use caution in patients with hemodynamic instability; predisposition to seizures; subcortical brain damage; severe cardiac, hepatic, or renal disease. Esophageal dysmotility and aspiration have been associated with antipsychotic use; use with caution in patients at risk of pneumonia (ie, Alzheimer's disease). Use associated with increased prolactin levels; clinical significance of hyperprolactinemia in patients with breast cancer or other prolactin-dependent tumors is unknown. May alter temperature regulation or mask toxicity of other drugs due to antiemetic effects.

Phenothiazines may cause anticholinergic effects (confusion, agitation, constipation, xerostomia, blurred vision, urinary retention); therefore, they should be used with caution in patients with decreased gastrointestinal motility, urinary retention, BPH, xerostomia, or visual problems. Conditions which also may be exacerbated by cholinergic blockade include narrowangle glaucoma and worsening of myasthenia gravis. Relative to other neuroleptics, thioridazine has a high potency of cholinergic blockade.

May cause extrapyramidal symptoms (EPS), including pseudoparkinsonism, acute dystonic reactions, akathisia, and tardive dyskinesia. Risk of dystonia (and possibly other EPS) may be greater with increased doses, use of conventional antipsychotics, males, and younger patients. In the elderly, avoid use; potent anticholinergic agent with potential to cause QT-interval prolongation. Use in elderly patients with dementia is associated with an increased risk of mortality and cerebrovascular accidents; avoid antipsychotic use for behavioral problems associated with dementia unless alternative nonpharmacologic therapies have failed and patient may harm self or others. In addition, use may cause or exacerbate syndrome of inappropriate antidiuretic hormone secretion or hyponatremia; monitor sodium closely with initiation or dosage adjustments in older adults (Beers Criteria). May be associated with neuroleptic malignant syndrome (NMS). May cause pigmentary retinopathy, and lenticular and corneal deposits, particularly with prolonged therapy.

Adverse Reactions (Reflective of adult population; not specific for elderly) Frequency not defined.

Cardiovascular: Hypotension, orthostatic hypotension, peripheral edema, ECG changes

Central nervous system: EPS (pseudoparkinsonism, akathisia, dystonias, tardive dyskinesia), dizziness, drowsiness, neuroleptic malignant syndrome (NMS), impairment of temperature regulation, lowering of seizure threshold, seizure

Dermatologic: Increased sensitivity to sun, rash, discoloration of skin (blue-gray)

Endocrine & metabolic: Changes in menstrual cycle, libido (changes in), breast pain, galactorrhea, amenorrhea

Gastrointestinal: Constipation, weight gain, nausea, vomiting, stomach pain, xerostomia, nausea, vomiting, diarrhea

Genitourinary: Difficulty in urination, ejaculatory disturbances, urinary retention, priapism

Hematologic: Agranulocytosis, leukopenia

Hepatic: Cholestatic jaundice, hepatotoxicity

Neuromuscular & skeletal: Tremor

Ocular: Pigmentary retinopathy, blurred vision, cornea and lens changes

Respiratory: Nasal congestion

Drug Interactions

Metabolism/Transport Effects Substrate of CYP2C19 (minor), CYP2D6 (major); **Note:** Assignment of Major/Minor substrate status based on clinically relevant drug interaction potential; **Inhibits** CYP1A2 (weak), CYP2C9 (weak), CYP2D6 (strong), CYP2E1 (weak)

Avoid Concomitant Use

Avoid concomitant use of Thioridazine with any of the following: Azelastine; Azelastine (Nasal); CYP2D6 Inhibitors; FluvoxaMINE; Highest Risk QTc-Prolonging Agents; Metoclopramide; Mifepristone; Moclobemide; Moderate Risk QTc-Prolonging Agents; Paraldehyde

Increased Effect/Toxicity

Thioridazine may increase the levels/effects of: Alcohol (Ethyl); Analgesics (Opioid); Anticholinergics; Antidepressants (Serotonin Reuptake Inhibitor/Antagonist); ARIPiprazole; AtoMOXetine; Azelastine; Azelastine (Nasal); Beta-Blockers; CNS Depressants; CYP2D6 Substrates; Fesoterodine; Highest Risk QTc-Prolonging Agents; Methylphenidate; Paraldehyde; Porfimer; Serotonin Modulators; Zolpidem

The levels/effects of Thioridazine may be increased by: Abiraterone Acetate; Acetylcholinesterase Inhibitors (Central); Antidepressants (Serotonin Reuptake Inhibitor/Antagonist); Antimalarial Agents; Beta-Blockers; CYP2D6 Inhibitors; Darunavir; FluvoxaMINE; HydrOXYzine; Lithium formulations; Methylphenidate; Metoclopramide; Metyrosine; Mifepristone; Moclobemide; Moderate Risk QTc-Prolonging Agents; Pramlintide; QTc-Prolonging Agents (Indeterminate Risk and Risk Modifying); Tetrabenazine

Decreased Effect

Thioridazine may decrease the levels/effects of: Amphetamines; Anti-Parkinson's Agents (Dopamine Agonist); Quinagolide

The levels/effects of Thioridazine may be decreased by: Antacids; Anti-Parkinson's Agents (Dopamine Agonist); Lithium formulations; Peginterferon Alfa-2b

Ethanol/Nutrition/Herb Interactions

Ethanol: May increase CNS depression; monitor for increased effects with coadministration. Caution patients about effects.

Herb/Nutraceutical: Avoid kava kava, valerian, St John's wort, gotu kola (may increase CNS depression). Avoid dong quai, St John's wort (may also cause photosensitization).

Stability Protect from light.

Mechanism of Action Thioridazine is a piperidine phenothiazine which blocks postsynaptic mesolimbic dopaminergic receptors in the brain; exhibits a strong alpha-adrenergic blocking effect and depresses the release of hypothalamic and hypophyseal hormones

Pharmacodynamics/Kinetics

Duration: 4-5 days

Half-life elimination: 21-25 hours

Time to peak, serum: ~1 hour

Dosage

Geriatric Behavioral symptoms associated with dementia (unlabeled use): Oral: Initial: 10-25 mg 1-2 times/day; increase at 4- to 7-day intervals by 10-25 mg/day; increase dose intervals (once daily, twice daily, etc) as necessary to control response or side effects.

◄ Maximum daily dose: 400 mg; gradual increases (titration) may prevent some side effects or decrease their severity.

Adult

Schizophrenia/psychosis: Oral: Initial: 50-100 mg 3 times/day with gradual increments as needed and tolerated; maximum: 800 mg/day in 2-4 divided doses

Depressive disorders, dementia (unlabeled use): Oral: Initial: 25 mg 3 times/day; maintenance dose: 20-200 mg/day

Renal Impairment Not dialyzable (0% to 5%)

Administration Do not take antacid within 2 hours of taking drug.

Monitoring Parameters Baseline and periodic ECG; vital signs; serum potassium, lipid profile, fasting blood glucose and Hgb A_{1c}; BMI; mental status, abnormal involuntary movement scale (AIMS); periodic eye exam; do not initiate if QT_c >450 msec

Reference Range Toxic: >1 mg/mL; lethal: 2-8 mg/dL

Test Interactions False-positives for phenylketonuria, urinary amylase, uroporphyrins, urobilinogen; may interfere with urine detection of methadone and PCP (false-positives)

Special Geriatric Considerations Any changes in disease status in any organ system can result in behavior changes.

Many elderly patients receive antipsychotic medications for inappropriate nonpsychotic behavior. Before initiating antipsychotic medication, the clinician should investigate any possible reversible cause; any stress or stress from any disease can cause acute "confusion" or worsening of baseline nonpsychotic behavior. Most commonly acute changes in behavior are due to increases in drug dose or addition of new drug to regimen; fluid electrolyte loss; infections; and changes in environment.

In the treatment of agitated, demented, older adult patients, authors of meta-analysis of controlled trials of the response to the traditional antipsychotics (phenothiazines, butyrophenones) in controlling agitation have concluded that the use of neuroleptics results in a response rate of 18%. Clearly neuroleptic therapy for behavior control should be limited with frequent attempts to withdraw the agent given for behavior control.

This medication is considered to be potentially inappropriate in this patient population (Beers Criteria: Quality of evidence - moderate; Strength of recommendation - strong).

Dosage Forms Excipient information presented when available (limited, particularly for generics); consult specific product labeling.

Tablet, oral, as hydrochloride: 10 mg, 25 mg, 50 mg, 100 mg

◆ **Thioridazine Hydrochloride** see Thioridazine on page 1880

Thiothixene (thye oh THIKS een)

Related Information

Antipsychotic Agents on page 2103

Beers Criteria – Potentially Inappropriate Medications for Geriatrics on page 2183

Medication Safety Issues

Sound-alike/look-alike issues:

Thiothixene may be confused with FLUoxetine, thioridazine

Navane® may be confused with Norvasc®, Nubain

BEERS Criteria medication:

This drug may be potentially inappropriate for use in geriatric patients (Quality of evidence - moderate; Strength of recommendation - strong).

Brand Names: U.S. Navane® [DSC]

Brand Names: Canada Navane®

Index Terms Tiotixene

Generic Availability (U.S.) Yes

Pharmacologic Category Antipsychotic Agent, Typical

Use Management of schizophrenia

Unlabeled Use Nonpsychotic patient, dementia behavior (elderly); psychosis/agitation related to Alzheimer's dementia

Contraindications Hypersensitivity to thiothixene or any component of the formulation; severe CNS depression; circulatory collapse; blood dyscrasias; coma

Warnings/Precautions [U.S. Boxed Warning]: Elderly patients with dementia-related psychosis treated with antipsychotics are at an increased risk of death compared to placebo. Most deaths appeared to be either cardiovascular (eg, heart failure, sudden death) or infectious (eg, pneumonia) in nature. Thiothixene is not approved for the treatment of dementia-related psychosis.

May alter cardiac conduction; life-threatening arrhythmias have occurred with therapeutic doses of antipsychotics. Avoid use in patients with underlying QT prolongation, in those taking medicines that prolong the QT interval, or cause polymorphic ventricular tachycardia; monitor ECG closely for dose-related QT effects.

Leukopenia, neutropenia, and agranulocytosis (sometimes fatal) have been reported in clinical trials and postmarketing reports with antipsychotic use; presence of risk factors (eg, pre-existing low WBC or history of drug-induced leuko-/neutropenia) should prompt periodic blood count assessment. Discontinue therapy at first signs of blood dyscrasias or if absolute neutrophil count <1000/mm^3.

Antipsychotic use has been associated with esophageal dysmotility and aspiration; use with caution in patients at risk of pneumonia (ie, Alzheimer's disease). May cause extrapyramidal symptoms (EPS), including pseudoparkinsonism, acute dystonic reactions, akathisia, and tardive dyskinesia. Risk of dystonia (and possibly other EPS) may be greater with increased doses, use of conventional antipsychotics, males, and younger patients. Use may be associated with NMS; monitor for mental status changes, fever, muscle rigidity, and/or autonomic instability. May cause orthostatic hypotension; use with caution in patients at risk of this effect or in those who would not tolerate transient hypotensive episodes (cerebrovascular disease, cardiovascular disease, hypovolemia, or concurrent medication use which may predispose to hypotension/bradycardia). May rarely cause pigmentary retinopathy and lenticular pigmentation. Impaired core body temperature regulation may occur; caution with strenuous exercise, heat exposure, dehydration, and concomitant medication possessing anticholinergic effects.

May be sedating, use with caution in disorders where CNS depression is a feature; patients must be cautioned about performing tasks which require mental alertness (eg, operating machinery or driving). Effects may be potentiated when used with other sedative drugs or ethanol. May cause anticholinergic effects (constipation, xerostomia, blurred vision, urinary retention); use with caution in patients with decreased gastrointestinal motility, paralytic ileus, urinary retention, BPH, xerostomia, or visual problems. Relative to other neuroleptics, thiothixene has a low potency of cholinergic blockade. May mask toxicity of other drugs or conditions (eg, intestinal obstruction, Reye's syndrome, brain tumor) due to antiemetic effects. Use is associated with increased prolactin levels; clinical significance of hyperprolactinemia in patients with breast cancer or other prolactin-dependent tumors is unknown.

Use with caution in patients with severe cardiovascular disease, narrow-angle glaucoma, hepatic impairment, myasthenia gravis, Parkinson's disease, renal impairment, or seizure disorder.

Use in elderly patients with dementia is associated with an increased risk of mortality and cerebrovascular accidents; avoid antipsychotic use for behavioral problems associated with dementia unless alternative nonpharmacologic therapies have failed and patient may harm self or others. In addition, use may cause or exacerbate syndrome of inappropriate antidiuretic hormone secretion or hyponatremia; monitor sodium closely with initiation or dosage adjustments in older adults May also be inappropriate in older adults depending on comorbidities (eg, dementia, delirium) due to its potent anticholinergic effects (Beers Criteria). Increased risk for developing tardive dyskinesia, particularly elderly women.

Adverse Reactions (Reflective of adult population; not specific for elderly) Frequency not defined.

Cardiovascular: Hypotension, nonspecific ECG changes, syncope, tachycardia

Central nervous system: Agitation, dizziness, drowsiness, extrapyramidal symptoms (akathisia, dystonias, lightheadedness, pseudoparkinsonism, tardive dyskinesia), insomnia restlessness

Dermatologic: Discoloration of skin (blue-gray), photosensitivity, pruritus, rash, urticaria

Endocrine & metabolic: Amenorrhea, breast pain, libido (changes in), changes in menstrual cycle, galactorrhea, gynecomastia, hyper-/hypoglycemia, hyperprolactinemia, lactation

Gastrointestinal: Constipation, nausea, salivation increased, stomach pain, vomiting, weight gain, xerostomia

Genitourinary: Difficulty in urination, ejaculatory disturbances, impotence

Hematologic: Leukocytes, leukopenia

Neuromuscular & skeletal: Tremors

Ocular: Blurred vision, pigmentary retinopathy

Respiratory: Nasal congestion

Miscellaneous: Diaphoresis

Drug Interactions

Metabolism/Transport Effects Substrate of CYP1A2 (major); **Note:** Assignment of Major/Minor substrate status based on clinically relevant drug interaction potential; **Inhibits** CYP2D6 (weak)

Avoid Concomitant Use
Avoid concomitant use of Thiothixene with any of the following: Azelastine; Azelastine (Nasal); Metoclopramide; Paraldehyde

Increased Effect/Toxicity
Thiothixene may increase the levels/effects of: Alcohol (Ethyl); Anticholinergics; ARIPiprazole; Azelastine; Azelastine (Nasal); Buprenorphine; CNS Depressants; Highest Risk QTc-Prolonging Agents; Methylphenidate; Moderate Risk QTc-Prolonging Agents; Paraldehyde; Serotonin Modulators; Zolpidem

The levels/effects of Thiothixene may be increased by: Abiraterone Acetate; Acetylcholinesterase Inhibitors (Central); CYP1A2 Inhibitors (Moderate); CYP1A2 Inhibitors (Strong); Deferasirox; HydrOXYzine; Lithium formulations; Methylphenidate; Metoclopramide; Metyrosine; Mifepristone; Pramlintide; Tetrabenazine

Decreased Effect
Thiothixene may decrease the levels/effects of: Amphetamines; Anti-Parkinson's Agents (Dopamine Agonist); Quinagolide

The levels/effects of Thiothixene may be decreased by: Anti-Parkinson's Agents (Dopamine Agonist); CYP1A2 Inducers (Strong); Cyproterone; Lithium formulations

Ethanol/Nutrition/Herb Interactions
Ethanol: May increase CNS depression; monitor for increased effects with coadministration. Caution patients about effects.
Herb/Nutraceutical: Avoid kava kava, valerian, St John's wort, gotu kola (may increase CNS depression).

Mechanism of Action
Thiothixene is a thioxanthene antipsychotic which elicits antipsychotic activity by postsynaptic blockade of CNS dopamine receptors resulting in inhibition of dopamine-mediated effects; also has alpha-adrenergic blocking activity

Pharmacodynamics/Kinetics
Metabolism: Extensively hepatic
Half-life elimination: >24 hours with chronic use

Dosage
Geriatric Nonpsychotic patient, dementia behavior (unlabeled use): Initial: 1-2 mg 1-2 times/day; increase dose at 4- to 7-day intervals by 1-2 mg/day. Increase dosing intervals (bid, tid, etc) as necessary to control response or side effects; maximum daily dose: 30 mg. Gradual increases in dose may prevent some side effects or decrease their severity.

Adult
Mild-to-moderate psychosis: Oral: 2 mg 3 times/day, up to 20-30 mg/day; more severe psychosis: Initial: 5 mg 2 times/day, may increase gradually, if necessary; maximum: 60 mg/day
Rapid tranquilization of the agitated patient (administered every 30-60 minutes): Oral: 5-10 mg; average total dose for tranquilization: 15-30 mg
Renal Impairment Not dialyzable (0% to 5%)

Monitoring Parameters
Vital signs; lipid profile, fasting blood glucose/Hgb A_{1c}; BMI; mental status, abnormal involuntary movement scale (AIMS), extrapyramidal symptoms (EPS)

Special Geriatric Considerations
Any changes in disease status in any organ system can result in behavior changes.

Many elderly patients receive antipsychotic medications for inappropriate nonpsychotic behavior. Before initiating antipsychotic medication, the clinician should investigate any possible reversible cause; any stress or stress from any disease can cause acute "confusion" or worsening of baseline nonpsychotic behavior. Most commonly acute changes in behavior are due to increases in drug dose or addition of new drug to regimen; fluid electrolyte loss; infections; and changes in environment.

In the treatment of agitated, demented, elderly patients, authors of meta-analysis of controlled trials of the response to the traditional antipsychotics (phenothiazines, butyrophenones) in controlling agitation have concluded that the use of neuroleptics results in a response rate of 18%. Clearly neuroleptic therapy for behavior control should be limited with frequent attempts to withdraw the agent given for behavior control.

This medication is considered to be potentially inappropriate in this patient population (Beers Criteria: Quality of evidence - moderate; Strength of recommendation - strong).

Dosage Forms
Excipient information presented when available (limited, particularly for generics); consult specific product labeling. [DSC] = Discontinued product
Capsule, oral: 1 mg, 2 mg, 5 mg, 10 mg
Navane®: 2 mg [DSC], 10 mg [DSC], 20 mg [DSC]

◆ **Thonzonium, Neomycin, Colistin, and Hydrocortisone** *see* Neomycin, Colistin, Hydrocortisone, and Thonzonium *on page 1355*
◆ **Thorazine** *see* ChlorproMAZINE *on page 359*

◆ Thrive™ [OTC] *see* Nicotine *on page 1372*

Thyroid, Desiccated (THYE roid DES i kay tid)

Related Information

Beers Criteria – Potentially Inappropriate Medications for Geriatrics *on page 2183*

Medication Safety Issues

BEERS Criteria medication:

This drug may be potentially inappropriate for use in geriatric patients (Quality of evidence - low; Strength of recommendation - strong).

Brand Names: U.S. Armour® Thyroid; Nature-Throid™; Westhroid™

Index Terms Desiccated Thyroid; Levothyroxine and Liothyronine; Tetraiodothyronine and Triiodothyronine; Thyroid Extract; Thyroid USP

Generic Availability (U.S.) Yes

Pharmacologic Category Thyroid Product

Use Replacement or supplemental therapy in hypothyroidism; pituitary TSH suppressants (thyroid nodules, thyroiditis, multinodular goiter, thyroid cancer)

Contraindications Hypersensitivity to beef or pork or any component of the formulation; untreated thyrotoxicosis; uncorrected adrenal insufficiency

Warnings/Precautions [U.S. Boxed Warning]: In euthyroid patients, thyroid supplements are ineffective and potentially toxic for weight reduction. High doses may produce serious or even life-threatening toxic effects particularly when used with some anorectic drugs. Thyroid supplements are not recommended for the treatment of female or male infertility, unless associated with hypothyroidism. Use with caution and reduce dosage in patients with angina pectoris or other cardiovascular disease and elderly since they may be more likely to have compromised cardiovascular function (Beers Criteria); chronic hypothyroidism predisposes patients to coronary artery disease. Use with caution in patients with adrenal insufficiency (contraindicated with uncorrected adrenal insufficiency), diabetes mellitus or insipidus, and myxedema; symptoms may be exaggerated or aggravated; initial dosage reduction is recommended in patients with long-standing myxedema. Desiccated thyroid contains variable amounts of T_3, T_4, and other triiodothyronine compounds which are more likely to cause cardiac signs or symptoms due to fluctuating levels. Avoid use in the elderly due to risk of cardiac effects and the availability of safer alternatives (Beers Criteria). Many clinicians consider levothyroxine to be the drug of choice for thyroid replacement.

Drug Interactions

Metabolism/Transport Effects None known.

Avoid Concomitant Use

Avoid concomitant use of Thyroid, Desiccated with any of the following: Sodium Iodide I131

Increased Effect/Toxicity

Thyroid, Desiccated may increase the levels/effects of: Vitamin K Antagonists

Decreased Effect

Thyroid, Desiccated may decrease the levels/effects of: Sodium Iodide I131; Theophylline Derivatives

The levels/effects of Thyroid, Desiccated may be decreased by: Bile Acid Sequestrants; Calcium Polystyrene Sulfonate; Calcium Salts; CarBAMazepine; Estrogen Derivatives; Fosphenytoin; Lanthanum; Phenytoin; Rifampin; Sodium Polystyrene Sulfonate

Ethanol/Nutrition/Herb Interactions Food: Management: Take in the morning before breakfast on an empty stomach.

Mechanism of Action The primary active compound is T_3 (triiodothyronine), which may be converted from T_4 (thyroxine) and then circulates throughout the body to influence growth and maturation of various tissues; exact mechanism of action is unknown; however, it is believed the thyroid hormone exerts its many metabolic effects through control of DNA transcription and protein synthesis; involved in normal metabolism, growth, and development; promotes gluconeogenesis, increases utilization and mobilization of glycogen stores and stimulates protein synthesis, increases basal metabolic rate

Pharmacodynamics/Kinetics

Onset of action: Liothyronine (T_3): ~3 hours

Absorption: Thyroxine (T_4): 40% to 80%; T_3: 95%; desiccated thyroid contains T_4, T_3, and iodine (primarily bound)

Protein binding: T_4: >99% bound to plasma proteins including thyroxine-binding globulin, thyroxine-binding prealbumin, and albumin

Metabolism: Hepatic to triiodothyronine (active); ~80% T_4 deiodinated in kidney and periphery; glucuronidation/conjugation also occurs; undergoes enterohepatic recirculation

Half-life elimination, serum:

T_4: Euthyroid: 6-7 days; Hyperthyroid: 3-4 days; Hypothyroid: 9-10 days

T_3: 2.5 days

Time to peak: Serum: T_4: 2-4 hours; T_3: 2-3 days
Excretion: Urine (major route of elimination); partially feces

Dosage
Geriatric Not recommended for use in the elderly.
Adult Note: The American Association of Clinical Endocrinologists does not recommend the use of desiccated thyroid for thyroid replacement therapy for hypothyroidism (Baskin, 2002).
Hypothyroidism: Oral: Initial: 15-30 mg; increase with 15 mg increments every 2-3 weeks; use 15 mg in patients with cardiovascular disease or long-standing myxedema. Maintenance dose: Usually 60-120 mg/day; monitor TSH and clinical symptoms.

Administration Administer on an empty stomach. Take in the morning before breakfast.

Monitoring Parameters T_4, TSH; heart rate, blood pressure; clinical signs of hypo- and hyperthyroidism; TSH is the most reliable guide for evaluating adequacy of thyroid replacement dosage. TSH may be elevated during the first few months of thyroid replacement despite patients being clinically euthyroid. In cases where T_4 remains low and TSH is within normal limits, an evaluation of "free" (unbound) T_4 is needed to evaluate further increase in dosage.

Pharmacotherapy Pearls Equivalent doses: The following statement on relative potency of thyroid products is included in a joint statement by American Thyroid Association (ATA), American Association of Clinical Endocrinologists (AACE) and The Endocrine Society (TES): For purposes of conversion, levothyroxine sodium (T_4) 100 mcg is usually considered equivalent to desiccated thyroid 60 mg, thyroglobulin 60 mg, or liothyronine sodium (T_3) 25 mcg. However, these are rough guidelines only and do not obviate the careful re-evaluation of a patient when switching thyroid hormone preparations, including a change from one brand of levothyroxine to another. Joint position statement is available at http://www.thyroid.org/professionals/advocacy/04_12_08_thyroxine.html.

Special Geriatric Considerations Desiccated thyroid contains variable amounts of T_3, T_4, and other triiodothyronine compounds which are more likely to cause cardiac signs or symptoms due to fluctuating levels. Should avoid use in the elderly for this reason. Many clinicians consider levothyroxine to be the drug of choice.

This medication is considered to be potentially inappropriate in this patient population (Beers Criteria: Quality of evidence - low; Strength of recommendation - strong).

Dosage Forms Excipient information presented when available (limited, particularly for generics); consult specific product labeling. [DSC] = Discontinued product
Tablet, oral: 30 mg [DSC], 60 mg [DSC], 120 mg [DSC]
  Armour® Thyroid: 15 mg, 30 mg, 60 mg, 90 mg, 120 mg
  Armour® Thyroid: 180 mg [scored]
  Armour® Thyroid: 240 mg
  Armour® Thyroid: 300 mg [scored]
  Nature-Throid™: 16.25 mg, 32.5 mg, 65 mg, 130 mg, 195 mg
  Westhroid™: 32.5 mg, 65 mg, 130 mg

◆ **Thyroid Extract** see Thyroid, Desiccated on page 1885
◆ **Thyroid USP** see Thyroid, Desiccated on page 1885
◆ **Thyrolar®** see Liotrix on page 1142
◆ **Tiacumicin B** see Fidaxomicin on page 786

TiaGABine (tye AG a been)

Medication Safety Issues
  Sound-alike/look-alike issues:
    TiaGABine may be confused with tiZANidine
Brand Names: U.S. Gabitril®
Index Terms Tiagabine Hydrochloride
Generic Availability (U.S.) No
Pharmacologic Category Anticonvulsant, Miscellaneous
Use Adjunctive therapy in the treatment of partial seizures
Medication Guide Available Yes
Contraindications Hypersensitivity to tiagabine or any component of the formulation
Warnings/Precautions Antiepileptics are associated with an increased risk of suicidal behavior/thoughts with use (regardless of indication); patients should be monitored for signs/symptoms of depression, suicidal tendencies, and other unusual behavior changes during therapy and instructed to inform their healthcare provider immediately if symptoms occur. New-onset seizures and status epilepticus have been associated with tiagabine use when taken for unlabeled indications. Often these seizures have occurred shortly after the initiation of treatment or shortly after a dosage increase. Seizures have also occurred with very low doses or after several months of therapy. In most cases, patients were using concomitant medications (eg, antidepressants, antipsychotics, stimulants, narcotics). In these

instances, the discontinuation of tiagabine, followed by an evaluation for an underlying seizure disorder, is suggested. Use for unapproved indications, however, has not been proven to be safe or effective and is not recommended. When tiagabine is used as an adjunct in partial seizures (an FDA-approved indication), it should not be abruptly discontinued because of the possibility of increasing seizure frequency, unless safety concerns require a more rapid withdrawal. Rarely, nonconvulsive status epilepticus has been reported following abrupt discontinuation or dosage reduction.

Use with caution in patients with hepatic impairment. Experience in patients not receiving enzyme-inducing drugs has been limited; caution should be used in treating any patient who is not receiving one of these medications (decreased dose and slower titration may be required). Weakness, sedation, and confusion may occur with tiagabine use. Patients must be cautioned about performing tasks which require mental alertness (eg, operating machinery or driving). Effects with other sedative drugs or ethanol may be potentiated. May cause serious rash, including Stevens-Johnson syndrome.

Adverse Reactions (Reflective of adult population; not specific for elderly)
>10%:
Central nervous system: Concentration decreased, dizziness, nervousness, somnolence
Gastrointestinal: Nausea
Neuromuscular & skeletal: Weakness, tremor
1% to 10%:
Cardiovascular: Chest pain, edema, hypertension, palpitation, peripheral edema, syncope, tachycardia, vasodilation
Central nervous system: Agitation, ataxia, chills, confusion, difficulty with memory, confusion, depersonalization, depression, euphoria, hallucination, hostility, insomnia, malaise, migraine, paranoid reaction, personality disorder, speech disorder
Dermatologic: Alopecia, bruising, dry skin, pruritus, rash
Gastrointestinal: Abdominal pain, diarrhea, gingivitis, increased appetite, mouth ulceration, stomatitis, vomiting, weight gain/loss
Neuromuscular & skeletal: Abnormal gait, arthralgia, dysarthria, hyper-/hypokinesia, hyper-/hypotonia, myasthenia, myalgia, myoclonus, neck pain, paresthesia, reflexes decreased, stupor, twitching, vertigo
Ocular: Abnormal vision, amblyopia, nystagmus
Otic: Ear pain, hearing impairment, otitis media, tinnitus
Respiratory: Bronchitis, cough, dyspnea, epistaxis, pneumonia
Miscellaneous: Allergic reaction, cyst, diaphoresis, flu-like syndrome, lymphadenopathy

Drug Interactions
Metabolism/Transport Effects Substrate of CYP3A4 (major); **Note:** Assignment of Major/Minor substrate status based on clinically relevant drug interaction potential
Avoid Concomitant Use
Avoid concomitant use of TiaGABine with any of the following: Azelastine; Azelastine (Nasal); Conivaptan; Methadone; Mirtazapine; Paraldehyde
Increased Effect/Toxicity
TiaGABine may increase the levels/effects of: Alcohol (Ethyl); Azelastine; Azelastine (Nasal); Buprenorphine; CNS Depressants; Methadone; Methotrimeprazine; Metyrosine; Mirtazapine; Paraldehyde; Selective Serotonin Reuptake Inhibitors; Zolpidem

The levels/effects of TiaGABine may be increased by: Conivaptan; CYP3A4 Inhibitors (Moderate); CYP3A4 Inhibitors (Strong); Dasatinib; Droperidol; HydrOXYzine; Ivacaftor; Methotrimeprazine; Mifepristone
Decreased Effect
The levels/effects of TiaGABine may be decreased by: CYP3A4 Inducers (Strong); Deferasirox; Herbs (CYP3A4 Inducers); Ketorolac; Ketorolac (Nasal); Ketorolac (Systemic); Mefloquine; Tocilizumab

Ethanol/Nutrition/Herb Interactions
Ethanol: May increase CNS depression; monitor for increased effects with coadministration. Caution patients about effects.
Food: Food reduces the rate but not the extent of absorption.
Herb/Nutraceutical: St John's wort may decrease tiagabine levels. Avoid valerian, St John's wort, kava kava, gotu kola (may increase CNS depression).

Mechanism of Action
The exact mechanism by which tiagabine exerts antiseizure activity is not definitively known; however, *in vitro* experiments demonstrate that it enhances the activity of gamma aminobutyric acid (GABA), the major neuroinhibitory transmitter in the nervous system; it is thought that binding to the GABA uptake carrier inhibits the uptake of GABA into presynaptic neurons, allowing an increased amount of GABA to be available to postsynaptic neurons; based on *in vitro* studies, tiagabine does not inhibit the uptake of dopamine, norepinephrine, serotonin, glutamate, or choline

Pharmacodynamics/Kinetics

Absorption: Rapid (45 minutes); prolonged with food

Protein binding: 96%, primarily to albumin and α_1-acid glycoprotein

Metabolism: Hepatic via CYP (primarily 3A4)

Bioavailability: Oral: Absolute: 90%

Half-life elimination: 2-5 hours when administered with enzyme inducers; 7-9 hours when administered without enzyme inducers

Time to peak, plasma: 45 minutes

Excretion: Feces (63%); urine (25%); 2% as unchanged drug; primarily as metabolites

Dosage

Geriatric & Adult Partial seizures (adjunct): Oral:

Patients receiving enzyme-inducing AED regimens: 4 mg once daily for 1 week; may increase by 4-8 mg weekly to response or up to 56 mg daily in 2-4 divided doses; usual maintenance: 32-56 mg/day

Patients **not** receiving enzyme-inducing AED regimens: The estimated plasma concentrations of tiagabine in patients not taking enzyme-inducing medications is twice that of patients receiving enzyme-inducing AEDs. Lower doses are required; slower titration may be necessary.

Monitoring Parameters A reduction in seizure frequency is indicative of therapeutic response to tiagabine in patients with partial seizures; complete blood counts, renal function tests, liver function tests, and routine blood chemistry should be monitored periodically during therapy; suicidality (eg, suicidal thoughts, depression, behavioral changes)

Reference Range Maximal plasma level after a 24 mg/dose: 552 ng/mL

Pharmacotherapy Pearls Animal studies suggest that tiagabine may bind to retina and uvea; however, no treatment-related ophthalmoscopic changes were seen long-term; periodic monitoring may be considered.

Special Geriatric Considerations No special recommendations are made for the elderly; dose according to response.

Dosage Forms Excipient information presented when available (limited, particularly for generics); consult specific product labeling.

Tablet, oral, as hydrochloride:

Gabitril®: 2 mg, 4 mg, 12 mg, 16 mg

♦ **Tiagabine Hydrochloride** *see* TiaGABine *on page 1886*

♦ **Tiazac®** *see* Diltiazem *on page 550*

Ticagrelor (tye KA grel or)

Related Information

Perioperative/Periprocedural Management of Anticoagulant and Antiplatelet Therapy *on page 2209*

Brand Names: U.S. Brilinta™

Brand Names: Canada Brilinta™

Index Terms AZD6140

Pharmacologic Category Antiplatelet Agent; Antiplatelet Agent, Cyclopentyltriazolopyrimidine

Use Used in conjunction with aspirin for secondary prevention of thrombotic events in patients with unstable angina (UA), non-ST-elevation myocardial infarction (NSTEMI), or ST-elevation myocardial infarction (STEMI) managed medically or with percutaneous coronary intervention (PCI) and/or coronary artery bypass graft (CABG)

Unlabeled Use In patients with allergy or major gastrointestinal intolerance to aspirin, initial treatment of UA/NSTEMI; **Note:** Dual antiplatelet therapy with another $P2Y_{12}$ receptor inhibitor is not recommended in this situation (Jneid, 2012).

Medication Guide Available Yes

Contraindications Active pathological bleeding (eg, peptic ulcer or intracranial hemorrhage); history of intracranial hemorrhage; hepatic impairment

Canadian labeling: Additional contraindications (not in U.S. labeling): Hypersensitivity to ticagrelor or any component of the formulation; moderate hepatic impairment; concomitant use of strong CYP3A4 inhibitors (eg, ketoconazole, clarithromycin, ritonavir, atazanavir, nefazodone)

Warnings/Precautions [U.S. Boxed Warning]: Ticagrelor increases the risk of bleeding including significant and sometimes fatal bleeding. Use is contraindicated in patients with active pathological bleeding and presence or history of intracranial hemorrhage. Additional risk factors for bleeding include propensity to bleed (eg, recent trauma or surgery, recent or recurrent GI bleeding, active PUD, moderate-to-severe hepatic impairment), CABG or other surgical procedure, concomitant use of medications that increase risk of bleeding (eg, warfarin, NSAIDs), and advanced age. Bleeding should be suspected if patient becomes hypotensive after undergoing recent coronary angiography, PCI, CABG, or other surgical procedure even if overt signs of bleeding do not exist. **Where possible, manage bleeding without discontinuing ticagrelor as the risk of cardiovascular events is increased upon discontinuation.** If discontinuation of ticagrelor is necessary, resume as soon as possible after the bleeding source is identified and controlled. Hemostatic benefits of platelet transfusions are not known; may inhibit transfused platelets. Premature discontinuation of therapy may increase the risk of cardiac events (eg, stent thrombosis with subsequent fatal or nonfatal MI). Duration of therapy, in general, is determined by the type of stent placed (bare metal or drug eluting) and whether an ACS event was ongoing at the time of placement. Use with caution in patients who are at an increased risk of bradycardia (eg, second- or third-degree AV block, sick sinus syndrome) or taking other bradycardic-inducing agents (eg, beta blockers, nondihydropyridine calcium channel blockers). Ventricular pauses ≥3 seconds were noted more frequently with ticagrelor than with clopidogrel in a substudy of the Platelet Inhibition and Patient Outcomes (PLATO) trial. Dyspnea (often mild-to-moderate and transient) was observed more frequently in patients receiving ticagrelor than clopidogrel during clinical trials. Ticagrelor-related dyspnea does not require specific treatment nor does it warrant therapy interruption (Canadian labeling recommends discontinuing therapy in patients unable to tolerate ticagrelor-related dyspnea).

[U.S. Boxed Warning]: Maintenance doses of aspirin greater than 100 mg/day reduce the efficacy of ticagrelor and should be avoided. Use of higher maintenance doses of aspirin (ie, >100 mg/day) was associated with relatively unfavorable outcomes for ticagrelor versus clopidogrel in the PLATO trial (Gaglia, 2011; Wallentin, 2009). Canadian labeling recommends a maximum maintenance aspirin dose of 150 mg/day.

[U.S. Boxed Warning]: Avoid initiation of ticagrelor when urgent CABG surgery is planned; when possible discontinue use at least 5 days before any surgery. Discontinue 5 days before elective surgery (except in patients with cardiac stents that have not completed their full course of dual antiplatelet therapy; patient-specific situations need to be discussed with cardiologist). When urgent CABG is necessary, the ACCF/AHA CABG guidelines recommend discontinuation for at least 24 hours prior to surgery (Hillis, 2011).

Use is contraindicated in patients with severe hepatic impairment (Canadian labeling also contraindicates use in moderate-to-severe hepatic impairment). Use with caution in patients with renal impairment, a history of hyperuricemia or gouty arthritis. Canadian labeling does not recommend use in patients with uric acid nephropathy. Avoid concomitant use with strong CYP3A4 inhibitors (eg, ketoconazole, ritonavir, nefazodone) or strong CYP3A4 inducers (eg, rifampin, carbamazepine, dexamethasone, phenobarbital, phenytoin). Canadian labeling contraindicates use with strong CYP3A4 inhibitors.

Adverse Reactions (Reflective of adult population; not specific for elderly) Note: As with all drugs which may affect hemostasis, bleeding is associated with ticagrelor. Hemorrhage may occur at virtually any site. Risk is dependent on multiple variables, including the concurrent use of multiple agents which alter hemostasis and patient susceptibility. Frequencies as reported in PLATO trial versus clopidogrel:

>10%: Respiratory: Dyspnea (≤14%)

1% to 10%:

Cardiovascular: Ventricular pauses (6%; 2% after 1 month of therapy), atrial fibrillation (4%), hypertension (4%), angina (3%), hypotension (3%), bradycardia (1% to 3%), cardiac failure (2%), peripheral edema (2%), ventricular tachycardia (2%), palpitation (1%), syncope (1%), ventricular extrasystoles (1%), ventricular fibrillation (1%)

Central nervous system: Headache (7%), dizziness (5%), fatigue (3%), fever (3%), anxiety (2%), insomnia (2%), vertigo (2%), depression (1%)

Dermatologic: Bruising (2% to 4%), rash (2%), pruritus (1%), subcutaneous or dermal bleeding

Endocrine & metabolic: Hypokalemia (2%), diabetes mellitus (1%), dyslipidemia (1%), hypercholesterolemia (1%)

Gastrointestinal: Diarrhea (4%), nausea (4%), vomiting (3%), abdominal pain (2%), constipation (2%), dyspepsia (2%), GI hemorrhage

Genitourinary: Urinary tract infection (2%), urinary tract bleeding

Hematologic: Major bleeding (12%; composite of major fatal/life threatening and other major bleeding events), minor bleeding (~5%), anemia (2%), hematoma (2%), postprocedural hemorrhage (2%)

Local: Puncture site hematoma (2%)

Neuromuscular & skeletal: Back pain (4%), noncardiac chest pain (4%), extremity pain (2%), arthralgia (2%), musculoskeletal pain (2%), weakness (2%), myalgia (1%)

Renal: Creatinine increased (7%; mechanism undetermined), hematuria (2%), renal failure (1%)

Respiratory: Epistaxis (6%), cough (5%), nasopharyngitis (2%), bronchitis (1%), pneumonia (1%)

Drug Interactions

Metabolism/Transport Effects Substrate of CYP3A4 (major); **Note:** Assignment of Major/Minor substrate status based on clinically relevant drug interaction potential; **Inhibits** CYP2B6 (weak), CYP2C9 (moderate), CYP2D6 (weak)

Avoid Concomitant Use

Avoid concomitant use of Ticagrelor with any of the following: CYP3A4 Inducers (Strong); CYP3A4 Inhibitors (Strong)

Increased Effect/Toxicity

Ticagrelor may increase the levels/effects of: Anticoagulants; Antiplatelet Agents; ARIPiprazole; Carvedilol; Collagenase (Systemic); CYP2C9 Substrates; Dabigatran Etexilate; Digoxin; Drotrecogin Alfa (Activated); Ibritumomab; Lovastatin; Rivaroxaban; Salicylates; Simvastatin; Thrombolytic Agents; Tositumomab and Iodine I 131 Tositumomab

The levels/effects of Ticagrelor may be increased by: Aspirin; CYP3A4 Inhibitors (Strong); Dasatinib; Glucosamine; Herbs (Anticoagulant/Antiplatelet Properties); Nonsteroidal Anti-Inflammatory Agents; Omega-3-Acid Ethyl Esters; Pentosan Polysulfate Sodium; Pentoxifylline; Prostacyclin Analogues; Tipranavir; Vitamin E

Decreased Effect

The levels/effects of Ticagrelor may be decreased by: Aspirin; CYP3A4 Inducers (Strong); CYP3A4 Inhibitors (Strong); Deferasirox; Herbs (CYP3A4 Inducers); Nonsteroidal Anti-Inflammatory Agents; Tocilizumab

Stability Store in the original container at 25°C (77°F); excursions permitted to 15°C to 30°C (59°F to 86°F).

Mechanism of Action Reversibly and noncompetitively binds the adenosine diphosphate (ADP) $P2Y_{12}$ receptor on the platelet surface which prevents ADP-mediated activation of the GPIIb/IIIa receptor complex thereby reducing platelet aggregation. Due to the reversible antagonism of the $P2Y_{12}$ receptor, recovery of platelet function is likely to depend on serum concentrations of ticagrelor and its active metabolite.

Pharmacodynamics/Kinetics

Onset of inhibition of platelet aggregation (IPA): 180 mg loading dose: ~41% within 30 minutes (similar to clopidogrel 600 mg at 8 hours)

Peak effect: Time to maximal IPA: 180 mg loading dose: IPA ~88% at 2 hours post administration

Duration of IPA: 180 mg loading dose: 87% to 89% maintained from 2-8 hours; 24 hours after the last maintenance dose, IPA is 58% (similar to maintenance clopidogrel)

Time after discontinuation when IPA is 30%: ~56 hours; IPA 10%: ~110 hours (Gurbel, 2009). Mean IPA observed with ticagrelor at 3 days post-discontinuation was comparable to that observed with clopidogrel at 5 days post discontinuation.

Absorption: Rapid

Distribution: 88 L

Protein binding: >99% (parent drug and active metabolite)

Metabolism: Hepatic via CYP3A4/5 to active metabolite (AR-C124910XX)

Bioavailability: ~36% (range: 30% to 42%)

Half-life elimination: Parent drug: ~7 hours; active metabolite: ~9 hours

Time to peak: Parent drug: ~1.5 hours; active metabolite (AR-C124910XX): ~2.5 hours

Excretion: Feces (58%); urine (26%); actual amount of parent drug and active metabolite excreted in urine was <1% of total dose administered

Dosage

Geriatric & Adult

Acute coronary syndrome: Unstable angina, non-ST-segment elevation myocardial infarction (NSTEMI), ST-segment elevation myocardial infarction (STEMI): Initial: 180 mg loading dose (with a loading dose of aspirin [eg, 325 mg] if not already receiving); Maintenance: 90 mg twice daily; initiated 12 hours after initial loading dose (with low-dose aspirin 75-100 mg/day or 81 mg/day in patients with UA/NSTEMI as recommended by the ACC/AHA [Jneid, 2012]). For UA/NSTEMI patients managed medically, continue ticagrelor for up to 12 months (Jneid, 2012). **Note:** Canadian labeling recommends a maintenance aspirin dose of 75-150 mg/day. Safety and efficacy of therapy beyond 12 months has not been established.

Duration of ticagrelor (in combination with aspirin) after stent placement: **Premature interruption of therapy may result in stent thrombosis with subsequent fatal and nonfatal MI.** Those with ACS receiving either stent type (bare metal [BMS] or drug-eluting stent [DES]) or those receiving a DES for a non-ACS indication, ticagrelor for at least 12 months is recommended. A duration >12 months may be considered in patients with DES placement. Those receiving a BMS for a non-ACS indication should be given at least 1 month and ideally up to 12 months; if patient is at increased risk of bleeding, give for a minimum of 2 weeks (Levine, 2011). A duration >12 months, regardless of indication, may be considered in patients with DES placement (Jneid, 2012; Levine, 2011).

Conversion from clopidogrel to ticagrelor: May initiate ticagrelor 90 mg twice daily beginning 24 hours after last clopidogrel dose (loading or maintenance); patients who are in the acute phase of an acute coronary syndrome, especially if determined to be clopidogrel non-responsive, may be considered for administration of ticagrelor 180 mg loading dose followed by 90 mg twice daily regardless of previous clopidogrel exposure, taking into consideration the administration of other antiplatelet agents (eg, GP IIb/IIIa inhibitors) (Gurbel, 2010; Wallentin, 2009). **Note:** In general, conversion to ticagrelor results in an absolute inhibition of platelet aggregation (IPA) increase of 26.4%.

Renal Impairment No dosage adjustments are recommended.

Hemodialysis: Use caution; drug is thought to be nondialyzable.

Hepatic Impairment

Mild hepatic impairment: No dosage adjustments are recommended.

Moderate hepatic impairment: Use has not been studied; however, undergoes hepatic metabolism; use caution. The manufacturer's labeling does not provide specific dosing recommendations. Use is contraindicated in the Canadian labeling.

Severe hepatic impairment: Use is contraindicated.

Administration May be administered without regard to meals. Missed doses should be taken at their next regularly scheduled time.

Monitoring Parameters Signs of bleeding; hemoglobin and hematocrit periodically; renal function; uric acid levels (patients with gout or at risk of hyperuricemia); signs/symptoms of dyspnea; may consider platelet function testing to determine platelet inhibitory response if results of testing may alter management (Jneid, 2012).

Pharmacotherapy Pearls Unlike thienopyridines (eg, clopidogrel, prasugrel) which are prodrugs and require metabolic transformation to their active metabolites for their activity, ticagrelor and its active metabolite both exhibit antiplatelet activity by reversibly and non-competitively binding to the adenosine diphosphate (ADP) $P2Y_{12}$ receptor on the platelet surface. Due to the reversible antagonism of the $P2Y_{12}$ receptor, recovery of platelet function is faster than with use of irreversible $P2Y_{12}$ receptor antagonists such as clopidogrel or prasugrel.

Special Geriatric Considerations In the PLATO study, 43% of the participants were ≥65 years and 15% were ≥75 years of age. The relative risk of bleeding was similar in both elderly groups. Additionally, there was no overall difference observed in safety and efficacy in the elderly compared to younger adults in the PLATO study, although insufficient data exists to exclude potential for clinical differences in response or safety between elderly and younger adults. Use with caution in the elderly and monitor closely while initiating this agent.

Dosage Forms Excipient information presented when available (limited, particularly for generics); consult specific product labeling.

Tablet, oral:

Brilinta™: 90 mg

Dosage Forms: Canada Excipient information presented when available (limited, particularly for generics); consult specific product labeling.

Tablet, oral:

Brilinta®: 90 mg

Ticarcillin and Clavulanate Potassium

(tye kar SIL in & klav yoo LAN ate poe TASS ee um)

Related Information

Antimicrobial Drugs of Choice *on page 2163*

Brand Names: U.S. Timentin®

Brand Names: Canada Timentin®

Index Terms Ticarcillin and Clavulanic Acid

Generic Availability (U.S.) No

Pharmacologic Category Antibiotic, Penicillin

Use Treatment of lower respiratory tract, urinary tract, skin and skin structures, bone and joint, gynecologic (endometritis) and intra-abdominal (peritonitis) infections, and septicemia caused by susceptible organisms. Clavulanate expands activity of ticarcillin to include beta-lactamase producing strains of *S. aureus, H. influenzae, Bacteroides* species, and some other gram-negative bacilli

Contraindications Hypersensitivity to ticarcillin, clavulanate, any penicillin, or any component of the formulation

Warnings/Precautions Use with caution and modify dosage in patients with renal impairment; serious and occasionally severe or fatal hypersensitivity (anaphylactoid) reactions have been reported in patients on penicillin therapy (especially with a history of beta-lactam hypersensitivity and/or a history of sensitivity to multiple allergens); use with caution in patients with seizures and in patients with HF due to high sodium load. Particularly in patients with renal impairment, bleeding disorders have been observed; discontinue if thrombocytopenia or bleeding occurs. Prolonged use may result in fungal or bacterial superinfection, including *C. difficile*-associated diarrhea (CDAD) and pseudomembranous colitis; CDAD has been observed >2 months postantibiotic treatment.

Adverse Reactions (Reflective of adult population; not specific for elderly) Frequency not defined.

Central nervous system: Confusion, drowsiness, fever, headache, Jarisch-Herxheimer reaction, seizure

Dermatologic: Erythema multiforme, pruritus, rash, Stevens-Johnson syndrome, toxic epidermal necrolysis, urticaria

Endocrine & metabolic: Electrolyte imbalance

Gastrointestinal: *Clostridium difficile* colitis, diarrhea, nausea, vomiting

Hematologic: Bleeding, eosinophilia, hemolytic anemia, leukopenia, neutropenia, positive Coombs' reaction, prothrombin time prolonged, thrombocytopenia

Hepatic: Hepatotoxicity, jaundice

Local: Injection site reaction (pain, burning, induration); thrombophlebitis

Neuromuscular & skeletal: Myoclonus

Renal: BUN increased, interstitial nephritis (acute), serum creatinine increased

Miscellaneous: Anaphylaxis, hypersensitivity reactions

Drug Interactions

Metabolism/Transport Effects None known.

Avoid Concomitant Use

Avoid concomitant use of Ticarcillin and Clavulanate Potassium with any of the following: BCG

Increased Effect/Toxicity

Ticarcillin and Clavulanate Potassium may increase the levels/effects of: Methotrexate; Vitamin K Antagonists

The levels/effects of Ticarcillin and Clavulanate Potassium may be increased by: Probenecid

Decreased Effect

Ticarcillin and Clavulanate Potassium may decrease the levels/effects of: Aminoglycosides; BCG; Mycophenolate; Typhoid Vaccine

The levels/effects of Ticarcillin and Clavulanate Potassium may be decreased by: Fusidic Acid; Tetracycline Derivatives

Stability

Vials: Store intact vials at <24°C (<75°F). Reconstituted solution is stable for 6 hours at room temperature and 72 hours when refrigerated. I.V. infusion in NS or LR is stable for 24 hours at room temperature, 7 days when refrigerated, or 30 days when frozen. I.V. infusion in D_5W solution is stable for 24 hours at room temperature, 3 days when refrigerated, or 7 days when frozen. After freezing, thawed solution is stable for 8 hours at room temperature. Darkening of drug indicates loss of potency of clavulanate potassium.

Premixed solution: Store frozen at ≤-20°C (-4°F). Thawed solution is stable for 24 hours at room temperature or 7 days under refrigeration; do not refreeze.

Mechanism of Action Inhibits bacterial cell wall synthesis by binding to one or more of the penicillin-binding proteins (PBPs); which in turn inhibits the final transpeptidation step of peptidoglycan synthesis in bacterial cell walls, thus inhibiting cell wall biosynthesis. Bacteria eventually lyse due to ongoing activity of cell wall autolytic enzymes (autolysins and murein hydrolases) while cell wall assembly is arrested.

Pharmacodynamics/Kinetics

Absorption: Ticarcillin: Not absorbed orally

Protein binding: Ticarcillin: ~45%; Clavulanic acid: ~25%

Metabolism: Clavulanic acid: Hepatic

Half-life elimination: Ticarcillin: 1.1 hours; Clavulanic acid: 1.1 hours

Excretion: Ticarcillin: Urine (60% to 70%); Clavulanic acid: Urine (35% to 45% as unchanged drug)

Clearance: Clavulanic acid does not affect clearance of ticarcillin

Dosage

Geriatric I.V.: 3.1 g every 4-6 hours; adjust for renal function.

Adult Note: Timentin® (ticarcillin/clavulanate) is a combination product; each 3.1 g dosage form contains 3 g ticarcillin disodium and 0.1 g clavulanic acid.

Systemic infections: I.V.: 3.1 g (ticarcillin 3 g plus clavulanic acid 0.1 g) every 4-6 hours (maximum: 24 g of ticarcillin component/day)

Amnionitis, cholangitis, diverticulitis, endometritis, epididymo-orchitis, mastoiditis, orbital cellulitis, peritonitis, pneumonia (aspiration): I.V.: 3.1 g every 6 hours

Intra-abdominal infection, complicated, community-acquired, mild-to-moderate: I.V.: 3.1 g every 6 hours for 4-7 days (provided source controlled)

Liver abscess, parafascial space infections, septic thrombophlebitis: I.V.: 3.1 g every 4 hours

***Pseudomonas* infections:** I.V.: 3.1 g every 4 hours

Urinary tract infections: I.V.: 3.1 g every 6-8 hours

Renal Impairment

Loading dose: I.V.: 3.1 g one dose, followed by maintenance dose based on creatinine clearance:

Cl_{cr} 30-60 mL/minute: Administer 2 g of ticarcillin component every 4 hours or 3.1 g every 8 hours

Cl_{cr} 10-30 mL/minute: Administer 2 g of ticarcillin component every 8 hours or 3.1 g every 12 hours

Cl_{cr} <10 mL/minute: Administer 2 g of ticarcillin component every 12 hours

Cl_{cr} <10 mL/minute with concomitant hepatic dysfunction: 2 g of ticarcillin component every 24 hours

Intermittent hemodialysis (IHD) (administer after hemodialysis on dialysis days): Dialyzable (20% to 50%): 2 g of ticarcillin component every 12 hours; supplemented with 3.1 g (ticarcillin/clavulanate) after each dialysis session. Alternatively, administer 2 g every 8 hours without a supplemental dose for deep-seated infections (Heintz, 2009). **Note:** Dosing dependent on the assumption of 3 times/week, complete IHD sessions.

Peritoneal dialysis (PD): 3.1 g every 12 hours

Continuous renal replacement therapy (CRRT) (Heintz, 2009; Trotman, 2005): Drug clearance is highly dependent on the method of renal replacement, filter type, and flow rate. Appropriate dosing requires close monitoring of pharmacologic response, signs of adverse reactions due to drug accumulation, as well as drug concentrations in relation to target trough (if appropriate). The following are general recommendations only (based on dialysate flow/ultrafiltration rates of 1-2 L/hour and minimal residual renal function) and should not supersede clinical judgment:

CVVH: Loading dose of 3.1g followed by 2 g every 6-8 hours

CVVHD: Loading dose of 3.1 g followed by 3.1 g every 6-8 hours

CVVHDF: Loading dose of 3.1 g followed by 3.1 g every 6 hours

Note: Do not administer in intervals exceeding every 8 hours. Clavulanate component is hepatically eliminated; extending the dosing interval beyond 8 hours may result in loss of beta-lactamase inhibition.

Hepatic Impairment With concomitant renal dysfunction (Cl_{cr} <10 mL/minute): 2 g of ticarcillin component every 24 hours.

Administration Infuse over 30 minutes. Administer 1 hour apart from aminoglycosides. Give around-the-clock. Rapid administration may lead to seizures.

Monitoring Parameters Observe for signs and symptoms of anaphylaxis during first dose; serum electrolytes, bleeding time, and periodic tests of renal, hepatic, and hematologic function

Test Interactions Positive Coombs' test, false-positive urinary proteins

Some penicillin derivatives may accelerate the degradation of aminoglycosides *in vitro*, leading to a potential underestimation of aminoglycoside serum concentration.

Special Geriatric Considerations When used as empiric therapy or for a documented pseudomonal pneumonia, it is best to combine with an aminoglycoside such as gentamicin or tobramycin. High sodium content may limit use in patients with congestive heart failure. Adjust dose for renal function.

Dosage Forms Excipient information presented when available (limited, particularly for generics); consult specific product labeling.

Infusion [premixed, frozen]: Ticarcillin 3 g and clavulanic acid 0.1 g (100 mL) [contains sodium 4.51 mEq and potassium 0.15 mEq per g]

Injection, powder for reconstitution: Ticarcillin 3 g and clavulanic acid 0.1 g (3.1 g, 31 g) [contains sodium 4.51 mEq and potassium 0.15 mEq per g]

♦ **Ticarcillin and Clavulanic Acid** *see* Ticarcillin and Clavulanate Potassium *on page 1891*

Ticlopidine (tye KLOE pi deen)

Related Information
Beers Criteria − Potentially Inappropriate Medications for Geriatrics *on page 2183*

Medication Safety Issues
BEERS Criteria medication:
This drug may be potentially inappropriate for use in geriatric patients (Quality of evidence - moderate; Strength of recommendation - strong).

Brand Names: Canada Apo-Ticlopidine®; Dom-Ticlopidine; Gen-Ticlopidine; Mylan-Ticlopidine; Novo-Ticlopidine; Nu-Ticlopidine; PMS-Ticlopidine; Sandoz-Ticlopidine; Teva-Ticlopidine

Index Terms Ticlopidine Hydrochloride

Generic Availability (U.S.) Yes

Pharmacologic Category Antiplatelet Agent; Antiplatelet Agent, Thienopyridine

Use Platelet aggregation inhibitor that reduces the risk of thrombotic stroke in patients who have had a stroke or stroke precursors. **Note:** Due to its association with life-threatening hematologic disorders, ticlopidine should be reserved for patients who are intolerant to aspirin, or who have failed aspirin therapy. Adjunctive therapy (with aspirin) following successful coronary stent implantation to reduce the incidence of subacute stent thrombosis.

Unlabeled Use Protection of aortocoronary bypass grafts, diabetic microangiopathy, ischemic heart disease, prevention of postoperative DVT, reduction of graft loss following renal transplant

Contraindications Hypersensitivity to ticlopidine or any component of the formulation; active pathological bleeding such as peptic ulcer disease (PUD) or intracranial hemorrhage; severe liver dysfunction; hematopoietic disorders (neutropenia, thrombocytopenia, a past history of TTP or aplastic anemia)

Warnings/Precautions Use with caution in patients who may be at risk of increased bleeding (eg, PUD, trauma, or surgery). Consider discontinuing 10-14 days before elective surgery (except in patients with cardiac stents that have not completed their full course of dual antiplatelet therapy; patient-specific situations need to be discussed with cardiologist; AHA/ACC/SCAI/ACS/ADA Science Advisory provides recommendations). Use caution in concurrent treatment with anticoagulants (eg, heparin, warfarin) or other antiplatelet drugs; bleeding risk is increased.

Because of structural similarities, cross-reactivity is possible among the thienopyridines (clopidogrel, prasugrel, and ticlopidine); use with caution or avoid in patients with previous thienopyridine hypersensitivity. Use of ticlopidine is contraindicated in patients with hypersensitivity to ticlopidine.

Use with caution in patients with mild-to-moderate hepatic impairment; use is contraindicated with severe hepatic impairment. Use with caution in patients with moderate-to-severe renal impairment (experience is limited); bleeding times may be significantly prolonged and the risk of hematologic adverse effects (eg, neutropenia) may be increased. **[U.S. Boxed Warning]: May cause life-threatening hematologic reactions, including neutropenia, agranulocytosis, thrombotic thrombocytopenia purpura (TTP), and aplastic anemia.** Routine monitoring is required (see Monitoring Parameters). Monitor for signs and symptoms of neutropenia including WBC count. Discontinue if the absolute neutrophil count falls to <1200/mm^3 or if the platelet count falls to <80,000/mm^3. Avoid use in the elderly due to availability of safer alternative agents (Beers Criteria).

Adverse Reactions (Reflective of adult population; not specific for elderly) As with all drugs which may affect hemostasis, bleeding is associated with ticlopidine. Hemorrhage may occur at virtually any site. Risk is dependent on multiple variables, including the use of multiple agents which alter hemostasis and patient susceptibility.

>10%:
Endocrine & metabolic: Total cholesterol increased (increases of ~8% to 10% within 1 month of therapy), triglycerides increased
Gastrointestinal: Diarrhea (13%)

1% to 10%:
Central nervous system: Dizziness (1%)
Dermatologic: Rash (5%), purpura (2%), pruritus (1%)
Gastrointestinal: Nausea (7%), dyspepsia (7%), gastrointestinal pain (4%), vomiting (2%), flatulence (2%), anorexia (1%)
Hematologic: Neutropenia (2%)
Hepatic: Alkaline phosphatase increased (>2 x upper limit of normal; 8%), abnormal liver function test (1%)

Drug Interactions

Metabolism/Transport Effects Substrate of CYP3A4 (major); **Note:** Assignment of Major/ Minor substrate status based on clinically relevant drug interaction potential; **Inhibits** CYP1A2 (weak), CYP2B6 (moderate), CYP2C19 (strong), CYP2C9 (weak), CYP2D6 (moderate), CYP2E1 (weak), CYP3A4 (weak)

Avoid Concomitant Use

Avoid concomitant use of Ticlopidine with any of the following: Clopidogrel; Pimozide; Thioridazine

Increased Effect/Toxicity

Ticlopidine may increase the levels/effects of: Anticoagulants; Antiplatelet Agents; ARIPiprazole; Citalopram; Collagenase (Systemic); CYP2B6 Substrates; CYP2C19 Substrates; CYP2D6 Substrates; Dabigatran Etexilate; Drotrecogin Alfa (Activated); Fesoterodine; Fosphenytoin; Ibritumomab; Nebivolol; Phenytoin; Pimozide; Rivaroxaban; Salicylates; Theophylline Derivatives; Thioridazine; Thrombolytic Agents; Tositumomab and Iodine I 131 Tositumomab

The levels/effects of Ticlopidine may be increased by: Dasatinib; Glucosamine; Herbs (Anticoagulant/Antiplatelet Properties); Nonsteroidal Anti-Inflammatory Agents; Omega-3-Acid Ethyl Esters; Pentosan Polysulfate Sodium; Pentoxifylline; Propafenone; Prostacyclin Analogues; Tipranavir; Vitamin E

Decreased Effect

Ticlopidine may decrease the levels/effects of: Clopidogrel; Codeine; Tamoxifen; TraMADol

The levels/effects of Ticlopidine may be decreased by: CYP3A4 Inducers (Strong); Deferasirox; Herbs (CYP3A4 Inducers); Nonsteroidal Anti-Inflammatory Agents; Tocilizumab

Ethanol/Nutrition/Herb Interactions

Food: Ticlopidine bioavailability may be increased (20%) if taken with food. High-fat meals increase absorption, antacids decrease absorption. May cause upset stomach. Management: Take with food to reduce stomach upset.

Herb/Nutraceutical: Some herbal medications have additional antiplatelet activity. Management: Avoid alfalfa, anise, bilberry, bladderwrack, bromelain, cat's claw, chamomile, coleus, cordyceps, dong quai, evening primrose oil, fenugreek, feverfew, garlic, ginger, ginkgo biloba, ginseng (American), ginseng (Panax), ginseng (Siberian), grapeseed, green tea, guggul, horse chestnut seed, horseradish, licorice, prickly ash, red clover, reishi, SAMe (S-adenosylmethionine), sweet clover, turmeric, and white willow.

Mechanism of Action Ticlopidine requires *in vivo* biotransformation to an unidentified active metabolite. This active metabolite irreversibly blocks the P2Y12 component of ADP receptors, which prevents activation of the GPIIb/IIIa receptor complex, thereby reducing platelet aggregation. Platelets blocked by ticlopidine are affected for the remainder of their lifespan.

Pharmacodynamics/Kinetics

Onset of action: ~6 hours

Peak effect: 3-5 days; serum levels do not correlate with clinical antiplatelet activity

Absorption: Well absorbed

Protein binding: Parent drug: 98%; <15% bound to alpha$_1$-acid glycoprotein

Metabolism: Extensively hepatic; has at least 1 active metabolite

Half-life elimination: 13 hours

Time to peak, serum: ~2 hours

Excretion: Urine (60%); feces (23%)

Dosage

Geriatric 250 mg twice daily with food; dosage in older patients has not been determined; however, in two large clinical trials, the average age of subjects was 63 and 66 years. A dosage decrease may be necessary if bleeding develops.

Adult

Stroke prevention: Oral: 250 mg twice daily

Coronary artery stenting (initiate after successful implantation): Oral: 250 mg twice daily (in combination with antiplatelet doses of aspirin) for up to 30 days

Unstable angina, non-ST-segment elevation myocardial infarction (UA/NSTEMI) undergoing percutaneous coronary intervention (PCI) in patients unable to receive clopidogrel (unlabeled dosing): Initial: 500 mg loading dose given at least 6 hours prior to PCI, followed by 250 mg twice daily (in combination with aspirin 75-325 mg once daily). Duration of therapy dependent upon type of stent implanted during PCI and whether an ACS event was ongoing at the time of placement (Anderson, 2011; Levine, 2011).

Renal Impairment No adjustment is necessary.

Hepatic Impairment No specific guidelines for patients with hepatic impairment; use with caution. Use is contraindicated with severe hepatic impairment.

Administration Administer with food.

Monitoring Parameters Signs of bleeding; CBC with differential every 2 weeks starting the second week through the third month of treatment; more frequent monitoring is recommended for patients whose absolute neutrophil counts have been consistently declining or are 30% less than baseline values. The peak incidence of TTP occurs between 3-4 weeks, the peak incidence of neutropenia occurs at approximately 4-6 weeks, and the incidence of aplastic anemia peaks after 4-8 weeks of therapy. Few cases have been reported after 3 months of treatment. Liver function tests (alkaline phosphatase and transaminases) should be performed in the first 4 months of therapy if liver dysfunction is suspected.

Special Geriatric Considerations Because of the risk of neutropenia and its relative expense as compared with aspirin, ticlopidine should only be used in patients with a documented intolerance to aspirin.

This medication is considered to be potentially inappropriate in this patient population (Beers Criteria: Quality of evidence - moderate; Strength of recommendation - strong).

Dosage Forms Excipient information presented when available (limited, particularly for generics); consult specific product labeling.

Tablet, oral, as hydrochloride: 250 mg

◆ **Ticlopidine Hydrochloride** see Ticlopidine on page 1894
◆ **TIG** see Tetanus Immune Globulin (Human) on page 1867
◆ **Tigan®** see Trimethobenzamide on page 1970

Tigecycline (tye ge SYE kleen)

Related Information
Antimicrobial Drugs of Choice on page 2163
Brand Names: U.S. Tygacil®
Brand Names: Canada Tygacil®
Index Terms GAR-936
Generic Availability (U.S.) No
Pharmacologic Category Antibiotic, Glycylcycline
Use Treatment of complicated skin and skin structure infections caused by susceptible organisms, including methicillin-resistant *Staphylococcus aureus* and vancomycin-sensitive *Enterococcus faecalis*; complicated intra-abdominal infections (cIAI); community-acquired pneumonia

Contraindications Hypersensitivity to tigecycline or any component of the formulation

Canadian labeling: Additional contraindications (not in U.S. labeling): Hypersensitivity to tetracycline class of antibiotics

Warnings/Precautions In Phase 3 and 4 clinical trials, an increase in all-cause mortality was observed in patients treated with tigecycline compared to those treated with comparator antibiotics; cause has not been established. In general, deaths were the result of worsening infection, complications of infection, or underlying comorbidity. May cause life-threatening anaphylaxis/anaphylactoid reactions. Due to structural similarity with tetracyclines, use caution in patients with prior hypersensitivity and/or severe adverse reactions associated with tetracycline use. Due to structural similarities with tetracyclines, may be associated with photosensitivity, pseudotumor cerebri, pancreatitis, and antianabolic effects (including increased BUN, azotemia, acidosis, and hyperphosphatemia) observed with this class. Acute pancreatitis (including fatalities) has been reported, including patients without known risk factors; discontinue use when suspected.

Use caution in hepatic impairment; dosage adjustment recommended in severe hepatic impairment. Abnormal liver function tests (increased total bilirubin, prothrombin time, transaminases) have been reported. Isolated cases of significant hepatic dysfunction and hepatic failure have occurred. Closely monitor for worsening hepatic function in patients that develop abnormal liver function tests during therapy. Adverse hepatic effects may occur after drug discontinuation.

Prolonged use may result in fungal or bacterial superinfection, including *C. difficile*-associated diarrhea (CDAD) and pseudomembranous colitis; CDAD has been observed >2 months postantibiotic treatment. Use with caution if using as monotherapy for patients with intestinal perforation (in the small sample of available cases, septic shock occurred more frequently than patients treated with imipenem/cilastatin comparator). Demonstrated inferior efficacy (versus comparator antibiotic), including lower cure rates and increased mortality in the subgroup of patients with VAP (particularly those with VAP and concurrent bacteremia at baseline).

Adverse Reactions (Reflective of adult population; not specific for elderly) Note: Frequencies relative to placebo are not available; some frequencies are lower than those experienced with comparator drugs.

>10%: Gastrointestinal: Nausea (26%; severe: 1%), vomiting (18%; severe: 1%), diarrhea (12%)

2% to 10%:

Central nervous system: Headache (6%), dizziness (3%)

Dermatologic: Rash (3%)

Endocrine & metabolic: Hypoproteinemia (5%)

Gastrointestinal: Abdominal pain (6%), dyspepsia (2%)

Hematologic: Anemia (4%)

Hepatic: ALT increased (5%), AST increased (4%), alkaline phosphatase increased (4%), amylase increased (3%), bilirubin increased (2%)

Local: Phlebitis (3%)

Neuromuscular & skeletal: Weakness (3%)

Renal: BUN increased (3%)

Miscellaneous: Infection (8%), abnormal healing (4%), abscess (3%)

Drug Interactions

Metabolism/Transport Effects None known.

Avoid Concomitant Use There are no known interactions where it is recommended to avoid concomitant use.

Increased Effect/Toxicity

Tigecycline may increase the levels/effects of: Warfarin

Decreased Effect There are no known significant interactions involving a decrease in effect.

Stability Prior to reconstitution, store at 20°C to 25°C (68°F to 77°F); excursions permitted to 15°C to 30°C (59°F to 86°F). Add 5.3 mL NS, D_5W, or LR to each 50 mg vial. Swirl gently to dissolve. Resulting solution is 10 mg/mL. Reconstituted solution must be further diluted to allow I.V. administration. Transfer to 100 mL I.V. bag for infusion (final concentration should not exceed 1 mg/mL). Reconstituted solution may be stored at room temperature for up to 6 hours or up to 24 hours if further diluted in a compatible I.V. solution. Alternatively, may be stored refrigerated at 2°C to 8°C (36°F to 46°F) for up to 48 hours following immediate transfer of the reconstituted solution into NS or D_5W. Reconstituted solution should be yellow-orange; discard if not this color.

Mechanism of Action A glycylcycline antibiotic that binds to the 30S ribosomal subunit of susceptible bacteria, thereby, inhibiting protein synthesis. Generally considered bacteriostatic; however, bactericidal activity has been demonstrated against isolates of *S. pneumoniae* and *L. pneumophila*. Tigecycline is a derivative of minocycline (9-t-butylglycylamido minocycline), and while not classified as a tetracycline, it may share some class-associated adverse effects. Tigecycline has demonstrated activity against a variety of gram-positive and -negative bacterial pathogens including methicillin-resistant staphylococci.

Pharmacodynamics/Kinetics Note: Systemic clearance is reduced by 55% and half-life increased by 43% in severe hepatic impairment.

Distribution: V_d: 7-9 L/kg; extensive tissue distribution

Protein binding: 71% to 89%

Metabolism: Hepatic, via glucuronidation, N-acetylation, and epimerization to several metabolites, each <10% of the dose

Half-life elimination: Single dose: 27 hours; following multiple doses: 42 hours

Excretion: Feces (59%, primarily as unchanged drug); urine (33%, with 22% of the total dose as unchanged drug)

Dosage

Geriatric & Adult Note: Duration of therapy dependent on severity/site of infection and clinical status and response to therapy.

Pneumonia, community-acquired: I.V.: Initial: 100 mg as a single dose; Maintenance dose: 50 mg every 12 hours for 7-14 days

Intra-abdominal infections, complicated (cIAI): I.V.: Initial: 100 mg as a single dose; Maintenance dose: 50 mg every 12 hours for 5-14 days; **Note:** 2010 IDSA guidelines recommend a treatment duration of 4-7 days (provided source controlled) for community-acquired, mild-to-moderate IAI

Skin/skin structure infections, complicated: I.V.: Initial: 100 mg as a single dose; Maintenance dose: 50 mg every 12 hours for 5-14 days

Renal Impairment No dosage adjustment required in renal impairment.

Poorly dialyzed; no supplemental dose or dosage adjustment necessary, including patients on intermittent hemodialysis, peritoneal dialysis, or continuous renal replacement therapy (eg, CVVHD).

Hepatic Impairment
Mild-to-moderate hepatic impairment (Child-Pugh class A or B): No dosage adjustment required.
Severe hepatic impairment (Child-Pugh class C): Initial: 100 mg single dose; Maintenance: 25 mg every 12 hours.

Administration Infuse over 30-60 minutes through dedicated line or via Y-site

Special Geriatric Considerations The manufacturer reports no significant differences in tigecycline's pharmacokinetics in small numbers of healthy older adults 65-75 years of age and >75 years compared to younger adults following a single 100 mg dose. No dosage adjustment is recommended.

Dosage Forms Excipient information presented when available (limited, particularly for generics); consult specific product labeling.
Injection, powder for reconstitution:
Tygacil®: 50 mg [contains lactose 100 mg]

◆ **Tikosyn®** see Dofetilide on page 586

Tiludronate (tye LOO droe nate)

Brand Names: U.S. Skelid®
Index Terms Tiludronate Disodium
Generic Availability (U.S.) No
Pharmacologic Category Bisphosphonate Derivative
Use Treatment of Paget's disease of the bone (osteitis deformans) in patients who have a level of serum alkaline phosphatase (SAP) at least twice the upper limit of normal, or who are symptomatic, or who are at risk for future complications of their disease
Contraindications Hypersensitivity to tiludronate, bisphosphonates, or any component of the formulation; inability to stand or sit upright for at least 30 minutes
Warnings/Precautions Not recommended in patients with severe renal impairment (Cl_{cr} <30 mL/minute). Use with caution in patients with active upper GI problems (eg, dysphagia, symptomatic esophageal diseases, gastritis, duodenitis, ulcers); discontinue use if new or worsening symptoms develop.

Osteonecrosis of the jaw (ONJ) has been reported in patients receiving bisphosphonates. Risk factors include invasive dental procedures (eg, tooth extraction, dental implants, boney surgery); a diagnosis of cancer, with concomitant chemotherapy or corticosteroids; poor oral hygiene, ill-fitting dentures; and comorbid disorders (anemia, coagulopathy, infection, pre-existing dental disease). Most reported cases occurred after I.V. bisphosphonate therapy; however, cases have been reported following oral therapy. A dental exam and preventative dentistry should be performed prior to placing patients with risk factors on chronic bisphosphonate therapy. The manufacturer's labeling states that discontinuing bisphosphonates in patients requiring invasive dental procedures may reduce the risk of ONJ. However, other experts suggest that there is no evidence that discontinuing therapy reduces the risk of developing ONJ (Assael, 2009). The benefit/risk must be assessed by the treating physician and/or dentist/surgeon prior to any invasive dental procedure. Patients developing ONJ while on bisphosphonates should receive care by an oral surgeon.

Infrequently, severe (and occasionally debilitating) bone, joint, and/or muscle pain have been reported during bisphosphonate treatment. The onset of pain ranged from a single day to several months. Consider discontinuing therapy in patients who experience severe symptoms; symptoms usually resolve upon discontinuation. Some patients experienced recurrence when rechallenged with same drug or another bisphosphonate; avoid use in patients with a history of these symptoms in association with bisphosphonate therapy.

Adverse Reactions (Reflective of adult population; not specific for elderly) 1% to 10%:
Cardiovascular: Chest pain (3%), edema (3%), peripheral edema (3%), flushing, hypertension, syncope
Central nervous system: Anxiety, fatigue, insomnia, nervousness, somnolence, vertigo
Dermatologic: Rash (3%), skin disorder (3%), pruritus
Endocrine & metabolic: Hyperparathyroidism (3%)
Gastrointestinal: Nausea (9%), diarrhea (9%), dyspepsia (5%), vomiting (4%), flatulence (3%), abdominal pain, anorexia, constipation, gastritis, xerostomia
Genitourinary: Urinary tract infection
Neuromuscular & skeletal: Paresthesia (4%), arthrosis (3%), fractures, muscle spasm, weakness
Ocular: Cataract (3%), conjunctivitis (3%), glaucoma (3%)
Respiratory: Rhinitis (5%), sinusitis (5%), pharyngitis (3%), bronchitis
Miscellaneous: Accidental injury (4%), infection (3%), diaphoresis

Drug Interactions

Metabolism/Transport Effects None known.

Avoid Concomitant Use There are no known interactions where it is recommended to avoid concomitant use.

Increased Effect/Toxicity

Tiludronate may increase the levels/effects of: Deferasirox; Phosphate Supplements; SUNItinib

The levels/effects of Tiludronate may be increased by: Aminoglycosides; Indomethacin; Nonsteroidal Anti-Inflammatory Agents

Decreased Effect

The levels/effects of Tiludronate may be decreased by: Antacids; Aspirin; Calcium Salts; Iron Salts; Magnesium Salts; Proton Pump Inhibitors

Ethanol/Nutrition/Herb Interactions Food: In single-dose studies, the bioavailability of tiludronate was reduced by 90% when an oral dose was administered with, or 2 hours after, a standard breakfast compared to the same dose administered after an overnight fast and 4 hours before a standard breakfast. Management: Administer as a single oral dose with 6-8 oz of plain water. Should not be taken with beverages containing minerals (eg, mineral water), food, or with other medications. Do not take within 2 hours of food. Take calcium or mineral supplements at least 2 hours before or after tiludronate.

Stability Store at 25°C (77°F); excursions permitted to 15°C to 30°C (59°F to 86°F). Do not remove tablets from foil strips until they are to be used.

Mechanism of Action Inhibition of normal and abnormal bone resorption. Inhibits osteoclasts through at least two mechanisms: disruption of the cytoskeletal ring structure, possibly by inhibition of protein-tyrosine-phosphatase, thus leading to the detachment of osteoclasts from the bone surface area and the inhibition of the osteoclast proton pump.

Pharmacodynamics/Kinetics

Onset of action: Delayed, may require several weeks

Absorption: Rapid

Distribution: Widely to bone and soft tissue

Protein binding: ~90%, primarily to albumin

Metabolism: Little, if any

Bioavailability: ~6% (range: 2% to 11%); reduced by 90% when given with food

Half-life elimination: Healthy volunteers: Single dose: 50 hours; Cl_{cr} 11-18 mL/minute: 205 hours; Pagetic patients: Repeated dosing: 150 hours

Time to peak, plasma: Within 2 hours

Excretion: Urine (~60%, as tiludronic acid within 13 days)

Dosage

Geriatric & Adult Paget's disease: Oral: 400 mg (2 tablets of tiludronic acid) daily for a period of 3 months

Renal Impairment Tiludronate is excreted renally. It is not recommended for use in patients with severe renal impairment (Cl_{cr} <30 mL/minute) and is not removed by dialysis.

Administration Administer as a single oral dose, take with 6-8 oz of plain water. Should not be taken with beverages containing minerals (eg, mineral water), food, or with other medications (may reduce absorption). Do not take within 2 hours of food. Take calcium or mineral supplements at least 2 hours before or after tiludronate. Take aluminum- or magnesium-containing antacids at least 2 hours after taking tiludronate. Patients should be instructed to stay upright (not to lie down) for at least 30 minutes and until after first food of the day (to reduce esophageal irritation).

Monitoring Parameters Alkaline phosphatase; pain; serum calcium and 25(OH)D

Test Interactions Bisphosphonates may interfere with diagnostic imaging agents such as technetium-99m-diphosphonate in bone scans.

Special Geriatric Considerations Elderly patients should be advised to report any lower extremity, jaw (osteonecrosis), or muscle pain that cannot be explained or lasts longer than 2 weeks. Additionally, elderly often receive concomitant diuretic therapy and therefore their electrolyte status (eg, calcium, phosphate) should be periodically evaluated.

Dosage Forms Excipient information presented when available (limited, particularly for generics); consult specific product labeling.

Tablet, oral, as tiludronic acid:

Skelid®: 200 mg [equivalent tiludronate disodium 240 mg]

◆ **Tiludronate Disodium** *see* Tiludronate *on page 1898*

◆ **Time-C® [OTC]** *see* Ascorbic Acid *on page 149*

◆ **Timentin®** *see* Ticarcillin and Clavulanate Potassium *on page 1891*

Timolol (Systemic) (TIM oh lol)

Related Information
Beta-Blockers *on page 2108*
Medication Safety Issues
  Sound-alike/look-alike issues:
    Timolol may be confused with atenolol, Tylenol®
Brand Names: Canada Apo-Timol®; Nu-Timolol; Teva-Timolol
Index Terms Timolol Maleate
Generic Availability (U.S.) Yes
Pharmacologic Category Beta-Blocker, Nonselective
Use Treatment of hypertension and angina; to reduce mortality following myocardial infarction; prophylaxis of migraine
Contraindications Hypersensitivity to timolol or any component of the formulation; sinus bradycardia; sinus node dysfunction; heart block greater than first degree (except in patients with a functioning artificial pacemaker); cardiogenic shock; uncompensated cardiac failure; bronchospastic disease
Warnings/Precautions Consider pre-existing conditions, such as sick sinus syndrome before initiating. Administer cautiously in compensated heart failure and monitor for a worsening of the condition. **[U.S. Boxed Warning]: Beta-blocker therapy should not be withdrawn abruptly (particularly in patients with CAD), but gradually tapered to avoid acute tachycardia, hypertension, and/or ischemia.** Chronic beta-blocker therapy should not be routinely withdrawn prior to major surgery. Use caution with concurrent use of digoxin, verapamil or diltiazem; bradycardia or heart block can occur. Use with caution in patients receiving inhaled anesthetic agents known to depress myocardial contractility. May precipitate or aggravate symptoms of arterial insufficiency in patients with PVD and Raynaud's disease; use with caution and monitor for progression of arterial obstruction. Patients with bronchospastic disease should generally not receive beta-blockers - monitor closely if used in patients with potential risk of bronchospasm. Use cautiously in patients with diabetes because it can mask prominent hypoglycemic symptoms.

May mask signs of hyperthyroidism (eg, tachycardia); if hyperthyroidism is suspected, carefully manage and monitor; abrupt withdrawal may exacerbate symptoms of hyperthyroidism or precipitate thyroid storm. Bradycardia may be observed more frequently in elderly patients (>65 years of age); dosage reductions may be necessary. Use cautiously in severe renal impairment: marked hypotension can occur in patients maintained on hemodialysis. Can worsen myasthenia gravis. Use with caution in patients with a history of psychiatric illness; may cause or exacerbate CNS depression. Adequate alpha-blockade is required prior to use of any beta-blocker for patients with untreated pheochromocytoma. May induce or exacerbate psoriasis. Use caution with history of severe anaphylaxis to allergens; patients taking beta-blockers may become more sensitive to repeated challenges. Treatment of anaphylaxis (eg, epinephrine) in patients taking beta-blockers may be ineffective or promote undesirable effects.

Adverse Reactions (Reflective of adult population; not specific for elderly) 1% to 10%:
Cardiovascular: Bradycardia
Central nervous system: Fatigue, dizziness
Respiratory: Dyspnea

Frequency not defined:
  Cardiovascular: Angina pectoris, arrhythmia, cardiac failure, cardiac arrest, cerebral vascular accident, cerebral ischemia, edema, hypotension, heart block, palpitation, Raynaud's phenomenon
  Central nervous system: Anxiety, confusion, depression, disorientation, hallucinations, insomnia, memory loss, nervousness, nightmares, somnolence
  Dermatologic: Alopecia, angioedema, pseudopemphigoid, psoriasiform rash, psoriasis exacerbation, rash, urticaria
  Endocrine & metabolic: Hypoglycemia masked, libido decreased
  Gastrointestinal: Anorexia, diarrhea, dyspepsia, nausea, xerostomia
  Genitourinary: Impotence, retoperitoneal fibrosis
  Hematologic: Claudication
  Neuromuscular & skeletal: Myasthenia gravis exacerbation, paresthesia
  Ocular: Blepharitis, conjunctivitis, corneal sensitivity decreased, cystoid macular edema, diplopia, dry eyes, foreign body sensation, keratitis, ocular discharge, ocular pain, ptosis, refractive changes, tearing, visual disturbances
  Otic: Tinnitus
  Respiratory: Bronchospasm, cough, nasal congestion, pulmonary edema, respiratory failure

Miscellaneous: Allergic reactions, cold hands/feet, Peyronie's disease, systemic lupus erythematosus

Drug Interactions

Metabolism/Transport Effects Substrate of CYP2D6 (major); **Note:** Assignment of Major/Minor substrate status based on clinically relevant drug interaction potential; **Inhibits** CYP2D6 (weak)

Avoid Concomitant Use

Avoid concomitant use of Timolol (Systemic) with any of the following: Beta2-Agonists; Floctafenine; Methacholine

Increased Effect/Toxicity

Timolol (Systemic) may increase the levels/effects of: Alpha-/Beta-Agonists (Direct-Acting); Alpha1-Blockers; Alpha2-Agonists; Amifostine; Antihypertensives; Antipsychotic Agents (Phenothiazines); ARIPiprazole; Bupivacaine; Cardiac Glycosides; Cholinergic Agonists; Fingolimod; Hypotensive Agents; Insulin; Lidocaine; Lidocaine (Systemic); Lidocaine (Topical); Mepivacaine; Methacholine; Midodrine; RiTUXimab; Sulfonylureas

The levels/effects of Timolol (Systemic) may be increased by: Abiraterone Acetate; Acetylcholinesterase Inhibitors; Aminoquinolines (Antimalarial); Amiodarone; Anilidopiperidine Opioids; Antipsychotic Agents (Phenothiazines); Calcium Channel Blockers (Dihydropyridine); Calcium Channel Blockers (Nondihydropyridine); CYP2D6 Inhibitors (Moderate); CYP2D6 Inhibitors (Strong); Darunavir; Diazoxide; Dipyridamole; Disopyramide; Dronedarone; Floctafenine; Herbs (Hypotensive Properties); MAO Inhibitors; Pentoxifylline; Phosphodiesterase 5 Inhibitors; Propafenone; Prostacyclin Analogues; QuiNIDine; Reserpine; Selective Serotonin Reuptake Inhibitors

Decreased Effect

Timolol (Systemic) may decrease the levels/effects of: Beta2-Agonists; Theophylline Derivatives

The levels/effects of Timolol (Systemic) may be decreased by: Barbiturates; Herbs (Hypertensive Properties); Methylphenidate; Nonsteroidal Anti-Inflammatory Agents; Peginterferon Alfa-2b; Rifamycin Derivatives; Yohimbine

Mechanism of Action Blocks both beta$_1$- and beta$_2$-adrenergic receptors; reduces blood pressure by blocking adrenergic receptors and decreasing sympathetic outflow, produces a negative chronotropic and inotropic activity through an unknown mechanism

Pharmacodynamics/Kinetics

Onset of action: Hypotensive: 15-45 minutes
  Peak effect: 0.5-2.5 hours
Duration: ~4 hours
Absorption: Rapid and complete (~90%)
Distribution: V_d: 1.7 L/kg
Protein binding: 60%
Metabolism: Extensively hepatic via CYP2D6; extensive first-pass effect
Bioavailability: 50%
Half-life elimination: 2-2.7 hours; prolonged with renal impairment
Time to peak, plasma: 1-2 hours
Excretion: Urine (15% to 20% as unchanged drug)

Dosage

Geriatric & Adult

Hypertension: Oral: Initial: 10 mg twice daily, increase gradually every 7 days, usual dosage: 20-40 mg/day in 2 divided doses; maximum: 60 mg/day.

Prevention of myocardial infarction: Oral: 10 mg twice daily initiated within 1-4 weeks after infarction.

Migraine prophylaxis: Oral: Initial: 10 mg twice daily, increase to maximum of 30 mg/day.

Monitoring Parameters Blood pressure, apical and radial pulses, fluid I & O, daily weight, respirations, mental status, and circulation in extremities before and during therapy; monitor for systemic effect of beta-blockade

Special Geriatric Considerations Since bioavailability increased in about twofold in elderly patients, geriatrics may require lower maintenance doses. Also, as serum and tissue concentrations increase beta$_1$ selectivity diminishes. Beta-adrenergic blockade may result in less hemodynamic response than seen in younger adults due to alterations in the beta-adrenergic autonomic system. Studies indicate that despite decreased sensitivity to the chronotropic effects of beta-blockade with age, there appears to be an increased myocardial sensitivity to the negative inotropic effect during stress (ie, exercise). Controlled trials have shown the overall response rate for propranolol to be only 20% to 50% in elderly populations. Therefore, all beta-adrenergic blocking drugs may result in a decreased response as compared to younger adults.

Dosage Forms Excipient information presented when available (limited, particularly for generics); consult specific product labeling.

Tablet, oral, as maleate: 5 mg, 10 mg, 20 mg

Timolol (Ophthalmic) (TIM oh lol)

Related Information
Glaucoma Drug Therapy *on page 2115*
Medication Safety Issues
Sound-alike/look-alike issues:
Timolol may be confused with atenolol, Tylenol®
Timoptic® may be confused with Betoptic S®, Talacen, Viroptic®
Other safety concerns:
Bottle cap color change: Timoptic®: Both the 0.25% and 0.5% strengths are now packaged in bottles with yellow caps; previously, the color of the cap on the product corresponded to different strengths.
International issues:
Betimol [U.S.] may be confused with Betanol brand name for metipranolol [Monaco]
Brand Names: U.S. Betimol®; Istalol®; Timolol GFS; Timoptic-XE®; Timoptic®; Timoptic® in OcuDose®
Brand Names: Canada Apo-Timop®; Dom-Timolol; Mylan-Timolol; Novo-Timol; PMS-Timolol; Sandoz-Timolol; Tim-AK; Timolol Maleate-EX; Timoptic-XE®; Timoptic®
Index Terms Timolol Hemihydrate; Timolol Maleate
Generic Availability (U.S.) Yes: Excludes solution as maleate (preservative free), solution as hemihydrate
Pharmacologic Category Beta-Blocker, Nonselective; Ophthalmic Agent, Antiglaucoma
Use Treatment of elevated intraocular pressure such as glaucoma or ocular hypertension
Dosage
Geriatric & Adult Glaucoma: Ophthalmic:
Solution: Initial: 0.25% solution, instill 1 drop twice daily into affected eye(s); increase to 0.5% solution if response not adequate; decrease to 1 drop/day if controlled; do not exceed 1 drop twice daily of 0.5% solution.
Istalol®: Instill 1 drop (0.5% solution) once daily in the morning.
Gel-forming solution (Timolol GFS, Timoptic-XE®): Instill 1 drop (either 0.25% or 0.5%) once daily
Special Geriatric Considerations Evaluate the patient's or caregiver's ability to safely administer the correct dose of ophthalmic medication.
Dosage Forms Excipient information presented when available (limited, particularly for generics); consult specific product labeling.
Gel forming solution, ophthalmic, as maleate [strength expressed as base, drops]: 0.25% (5 mL); 0.5% (5 mL)
Timolol GFS: 0.25% (5 mL); 0.5% (5 mL)
Timoptic-XE®: 0.25% (5 mL); 0.5% (5 mL)
Solution, ophthalmic, as hemihydrate [strength expressed as base, drops]:
Betimol®: 0.25% (5 mL); 0.5% (5 mL, 10 mL, 15 mL) [contains benzalkonium chloride]
Solution, ophthalmic, as maleate [strength expressed as base, drops]: 0.25% (5 mL, 10 mL, 15 mL); 0.5% (5 mL, 10 mL, 15 mL)
Istalol®: 0.5% (2.5 mL, 5 mL) [contains benzalkonium chloride]
Timoptic®: 0.25% (5 mL); 0.5% (5 mL, 10 mL) [contains benzalkonium chloride]
Solution, ophthalmic, as maleate [strength expressed as base, drops, preservative free]:
Timoptic® in OcuDose®: 0.25% (0.2 mL); 0.5% (0.2 mL)

Tinzaparin (tin ZA pa rin)

Related Information
Injectable Heparins/Heparinoids Comparison Table *on page 2119*

Medication Safety Issues
High alert medication:
The Institute for Safe Medication Practices (ISMP) includes this medication among its list of drug classes which have a heightened risk of causing significant patient harm when used in error.

Brand Names: Canada Innohep®

Index Terms Tinzaparin Sodium

Pharmacologic Category Low Molecular Weight Heparin

Use Treatment of deep vein thrombosis (DVT) and/or pulmonary embolism (PE) (except in patients with severe hemodynamic instability); prevention of venous thromboembolism (VTE) following orthopedic surgery or following general surgery in patients at high risk of VTE; prevention of clotting in indwelling intravenous lines and extracorporeal circuit during hemodialysis (in patients without high bleeding risk)

Contraindications Hypersensitivity to tinzaparin sodium, heparin or other low molecular weight heparins (LMWH), or any component of the formulation; active bleeding; heparin-induced thrombocytopenia (current or history of) or positive *in vitro* platelet-aggregation test in the presence of tinzaparin; acute or subacute endocarditis; generalized hemorrhage tendency and other conditions involving increased risks of hemorrhage (eg, severe hepatic insufficiency, imminent abortion); hemophilia or major blood clotting disorders; acute cerebral insult or hemorrhagic cerebrovascular accidents without systemic emboli; uncontrolled severe hypertension; diabetic or hemorrhagic retinopathy; injury or surgery involving the brain, spinal cord, eyes or ears; spinal/epidural anesthesia in patients requiring treatment dosages of tinzaparin

Warnings/Precautions Spinal or epidural hematomas, including subsequent paralysis, may occur with recent or anticipated neuraxial anesthesia (epidural or spinal) or spinal puncture in patients anticoagulated with low molecular weight heparin (LMWH) or heparinoids. Consider risk versus benefit prior to spinal procedures; risk is increased by the use of concomitant agents which may alter hemostasis, the use of indwelling epidural catheters for analgesia, a history of spinal deformity or spinal surgery, as well as traumatic or repeated epidural or spinal punctures. Avoid invasive spinal procedures for 12 hours following tinzaparin administration and withhold the next tinzaparin dose for at least 2 hours after the spinal procedure. Patient should be observed closely for signs and symptoms of neurological impairment. Not to be used interchangeably (unit for unit) with heparin or any other LMWHs.

Monitor patient closely for signs or symptoms of bleeding. Certain patients are at increased risk of bleeding. Risk factors include bacterial endocarditis; congenital or acquired bleeding disorders; active ulcerative or angiodysplastic GI diseases; severe uncontrolled hypertension; history of hemorrhagic stroke; use shortly after brain, spinal, or ophthalmologic surgery; those concomitantly treated with drugs that increase bleeding risk (eg, antiplatelet agents, anticoagulants); recent GI bleeding; thrombocytopenia or platelet defects; severe liver disease; hypertensive or diabetic retinopathy; or in patients undergoing invasive procedures. Monitor platelet count closely. Withhold or discontinue for minor bleeding. Protamine infusion may be necessary for serious bleeding. Rare cases of thrombocytopenia have occurred. Rare cases of thrombocytopenia with thrombosis have occurred. Asymptomatic thrombocytosis has been observed with use, particularly in patients undergoing orthopedic surgery or with concurrent inflammatory process; discontinue use with increased platelet counts and evaluate the risks/necessity of further therapy. Prosthetic valve thrombosis has been reported in patients receiving thromboprophylaxis therapy with LMWHs.

Use with caution in hepatic impairment; associated with transient, dose-dependent increases in AST/ALT which typically resolve within 2-4 weeks of therapy discontinuation. Use with caution in patients with renal insufficiency. Reduced tinzaparin clearance has been observed in patients with moderate-to-severe renal impairment; Consider dosage reduction in patients with Cl_{cr} <30 mL/minute. Use with caution in the elderly (delayed elimination may occur). Use is not recommended in patients >70 years of age with renal impairment. An increase in all-cause mortality has been observed in patients ≥70 years (mean age: >82 years) with Cl_{cr} ≤60 mL/minute treated with tinzaparin compared to unfractionated heparin for acute DVT (Leizorovicz, 2011).

Heparin can cause hyperkalemia by suppressing aldosterone production; similar reactions could occur with LMWHs. Monitor for hyperkalemia which most commonly occurs in patients with risk factors for the development of hyperkalemia (eg, renal dysfunction, concomitant use of potassium-sparing diuretics or potassium supplements, hematoma in body tissues). For subcutaneous use only; do not administer intramuscularly or intravenously. Use with caution in patients <45 kg or >120 kg; limited experience in these patients. Individualized clinical and laboratory monitoring are recommended. Derived from porcine intestinal mucosa. Some dosage forms may contain benzyl alcohol or sodium metabisulfite.

Adverse Reactions (Reflective of adult population; not specific for elderly) As with all anticoagulants, bleeding is the major adverse effect of tinzaparin. Hemorrhage may occur at virtually any site. Risk is dependent on multiple variables. **Note:** Incidence not always reported.

>10%:
Hepatic: ALT increased (≤13%)
Local: Injection site hematoma

1% to 10%:
Cardiovascular: Chest pain (2%), angina pectoris (≥1%), arrhythmia (≥1%), coronary thrombosis/MI (≥1%), dependent edema (≥1%), thromboembolism (≥1%)
Central nervous system: Fever (2%), headache (2%), pain (2%)
Dermatologic: Bullous eruption (≥1%), erythematous rash (≥1%), maculopapular rash (≥1%), skin necrosis (≥1%)
Gastrointestinal: Nausea (2%), abdominal pain (1%), constipation (1%), diarrhea (1%), vomiting (1%)
Genitourinary: Urinary tract infection (4%)
Hematologic: Bleeding events (major events including intracranial, retroperitoneal, or bleeding into a major prosthetic joint: ≤3%; hemorrhage site not specified (2%); other bleeding events reported at an incidence of ≥1% include anorectal bleeding, GI hemorrhage, hemarthrosis, hematemesis, hematuria, hemopericardium, injection site bleeding, melena, purpura, intra-abdominal bleeding, vaginal bleeding, wound hemorrhage), granulocytopenia (≥1%), thrombocytopenia (≥1%)
Hepatic: AST increased (9%)
Local: Injection site cellulitis (≥1%)
Neuromuscular & skeletal: Back pain (2%)
Respiratory: Epistaxis (2%), dyspnea (1%)
Miscellaneous: Allergic reaction (≥1%), neoplasm (≥1%)

Drug Interactions
Metabolism/Transport Effects None known.
Avoid Concomitant Use
Avoid concomitant use of Tinzaparin with any of the following: Rivaroxaban
Increased Effect/Toxicity
Tinzaparin may increase the levels/effects of: Anticoagulants; Collagenase (Systemic); Dabigatran Etexilate; Deferasirox; Drotrecogin Alfa (Activated); Ibritumomab; Palifermin; Rivaroxaban; Tositumomab and Iodine I 131 Tositumomab

The levels/effects of Tinzaparin may be increased by: 5-ASA Derivatives; Antiplatelet Agents; Dasatinib; Herbs (Anticoagulant/Antiplatelet Properties); Nonsteroidal Anti-Inflammatory Agents; Pentosan Polysulfate Sodium; Pentoxifylline; Prostacyclin Analogues; Salicylates; Thrombolytic Agents; Tipranavir
Decreased Effect There are no known significant interactions involving a decrease in effect.
Stability Store at 15°C to 25°C (59°F to 77°F).
Mechanism of Action Tinzaparin is a low molecular weight heparin (average molecular weight ranges between 5500 and 7500 daltons, distributed as <2000 daltons [<10%], 2000-8000 daltons [60% to 72%], and >8000 daltons [22% to 36%]) that binds antithrombin III, enhancing the inhibition of several clotting factors, particularly factor Xa. Tinzaparin anti-Xa activity (70-120 units/mg) is greater than anti-IIa activity (~55 units/mg) and it has a higher ratio of antifactor Xa to antifactor IIa activity compared to unfractionated heparin. Low molecular weight heparins have a small effect on the activated partial thromboplastin time.
Pharmacodynamics/Kinetics Note: Values reflective of anti-Xa activity.
Onset of action: 2-3 hours
Duration: Detectable anti-Xa activity persists for 24 hours
Absorption: Slow; absorption half-life ~3 hours after subcutaneous administration
Distribution: 4 L
Metabolism: Does not undergo hepatic metabolism
Bioavailability: SubQ: ~90%
Half-life elimination: 82 minutes; prolonged in renal impairment
Time to peak: 4-6 hours
Excretion: Urine

Dosage
Geriatric Refer to adult dosing. Increased sensitivity to tinzaparin in elderly patients may be possible due to a decline in renal function. Use is not recommended in patients >70 years of age with renal impairment.
Adult Note: 1 mg of tinzaparin equals 70-120 units of anti-Xa activity

Note: A pharmacokinetic study confirmed that weight-based dosing (single doses of 75 or 175 units/kg) using actual body weight in heavy/obese patients between 100 and 165 kg led to achievement of similar anti-Xa activity levels compared to normal-weight patients (Hainer, 2002). However, there is limited clinical experience in patients with a BMI >40 kg/m^2.

DVT and/or PE treatment: SubQ: 175 anti-Xa units/kg once daily (maximum: 18,000 anti-Xa units/day). The 2012 *Chest* guidelines recommend starting warfarin on the first or second treatment day and continuing tinzaparin until INR is ≥2 for at least 24 hours (usually 5-7 days) (Guyatt, 2012). Body weight dosing using prefilled syringes may also be considered. Refer to manufacturer's labeling for detailed dosing recommendations.

DVT prophylaxis: SubQ:

Hip replacement surgery: **Note:** The American College of Chest Physicians recommends initiation of LMWH ≥12 hours preoperatively **or** ≥12 hours postoperatively; extended duration up to 35 days suggested (Guyatt, 2012).

Preoperative regimen: 50 anti-Xa units/kg given 2 hours preoperatively followed by 50 anti-Xa units/kg once daily for 7-10 days

Postoperative regimen: 75 anti-Xa units/kg once daily, with initial dose given postoperatively and continued for 7-10 days

Knee replacement surgery: 75 anti-Xa units/kg once daily, with initial dose given postoperatively and continued for 7-10 days. **Note:** The American College of Chest Physicians recommends initiation of LMWH ≥12 hours preoperatively **or** ≥12 hours postoperatively; extended duration of up to 35 days suggested (Guyatt, 2012). Body weight dosing using prefilled syringes may also be considered. Refer to manufacturer's labeling for detailed dosing recommendations.

General surgery: 3500 anti-Xa units once daily, with initial dose given 2 hours prior to surgery and then continued postoperatively for 7-10 days

Anticoagulant in extracorporeal circuit during hemodialysis (recommendations apply to stable patients with chronic renal failure): I.V.:

Dialysis session ≤4 hours (no hemorrhage risk): Initial bolus (via arterial side of circuit or I.V.): 4500 anti-Xa units at beginning of dialysis; typically achieves plasma concentrations of 0.5-1 anti-Xa units/mL; may give larger bolus for dialysis sessions >4 hours. For subsequent dialysis sessions, may adjust dose as necessary in increments of 500 anti-Xa units based on previous outcome.

Dialysis session ≤4 hours (hemorrhage risk): Initial bolus (I.V. only): 2250 anti-Xa units at beginning of dialysis (do not add to dialysis circuit). A smaller second I.V. dose may be administered during dialysis sessions >4 hours. For subsequent dialysis sessions, adjust dose as necessary to achieve plasma concentrations of 0.2-0.4 anti-Xa units/mL.

Renal Impairment

Cl_{cr} ≥30 mL/minute: No dosage adjustment provided in manufacturer's labeling; however, primarily undergoes renal elimination. Clearance is decreased in renal impairment; use with caution.

Cl_{cr} <30 mL/minute: Manufacturer's labeling suggests that a reduction in dose be considered but does not provide specific dose recommendations. Use with caution.

Hepatic Impairment No dosage adjustment provided in manufacturer's labeling. Does not undergo hepatic metabolism; however, has been associated with transient increases in transaminase levels; use with caution.

Administration Patient should be lying down or sitting. Administer by deep SubQ injection into the lower abdomen, outer thigh, lower back, or upper arm. Injection site should be varied daily. To minimize bruising, do not rub the injection site. In hemodialysis patients, may be administered I.V. (patients with high or low hemorrhage risk) or added to the dialyzer circuit (patients with low hemorrhage risk).

Monitoring Parameters CBC (at baseline then twice weekly throughout therapy); renal function (use Cockcroft-Gault formula); hepatic function; potassium (baseline in patients at risk for hyperkalemia, monitor regularly if duration >7 days); stool for occult blood. Routine monitoring of anti-Xa levels is generally not recommended; however, anti-Xa levels may be beneficial in certain patients (eg, children, obese patients, patients with severe renal insufficiency receiving therapeutic doses, and possibly pregnant women receiving therapeutic doses) (Guyatt, 2012). Peak anti-Xa levels are measured 4-6 hours after administration. Monitoring of PT and/or aPTT is not of clinical benefit.

Reference Range Anti-Xa level (measured 4 hours after administration): Fixed-dose (3500 units): 0.15 anti-Xa units/mL; weight-based (75-175 units/kg): 0.34-0.70 anti-Xa units/mL; in treatment of venous thromboembolism, a target of 0.85 anti-Xa units/mL has been recommended (Garcia, 2012)

Special Geriatric Considerations No significant differences in safety or response were seen when used in patients ≥65 years of age. However, increased sensitivity to tinzaparin in elderly patients may be possible due to a decline in renal function. Results from the Innohep in Renal Insufficiency Study (IRIS) study showed an increase in all-cause mortality in elderly patients receiving tinzaparin compared to unfractionated heparin for treatment of DVT and/or PE. The at-risk population has defined as patients ≥70 years of age with Cl_{cr} ≤30 mL/minute or ≥75 years of age and Cl_{cr} ≤60 mL/minute.

Dosage Forms: Canada Excipient information presented when available (limited, particularly for generics); consult specific product labeling. [DSC] = Discontinued product

Injection, solution, as sodium:
Innohep®: 10,000 anti-Xa units/mL (2 mL) [contains benzyl alcohol, sodium metabisulfite]
Innohep®: 20,000 anti-Xa units/mL (0.5 mL, 0.7 mL, 0.9 mL) [contains sodium metabisulfite]
Innohep®: 20,000 anti-Xa units/mL (2 mL) [contains benzyl alcohol, sodium metabisulfite]
Injection, solution, as sodium [preservative free]:
Innohep®: 10,000 anti-Xa units/mL (0.25 mL, 0.35 mL, 0.45 mL)

◆ **Tinzaparin Sodium** see Tinzaparin on page 1903

Tioconazole (tye oh KONE a zole)

Medication Safety Issues
Sound-alike/look-alike issues:
Tioconazole may be confused with terconazole
Brand Names: U.S. 1-Day™ [OTC]; Vagistat®-1 [OTC]
Generic Availability (U.S.) No
Pharmacologic Category Antifungal Agent, Vaginal
Use Local treatment of vulvovaginal candidiasis
Contraindications Hypersensitivity to tioconazole or any component of the formulation
Warnings/Precautions If irritation or sensitization occurs, discontinue use. Petrolatum-based vaginal products may damage rubber or latex condoms or diaphragms. Separate use by 3 days.
Adverse Reactions (Reflective of adult population; not specific for elderly) Frequency not defined.
Central nervous system: Headache
Gastrointestinal: Abdominal pain
Dermatologic: Burning, desquamation
Genitourinary: Discharge, dyspareunia, dysuria, irritation, itching, nocturia, vaginal pain, vaginitis, vulvar swelling
Drug Interactions
Metabolism/Transport Effects Inhibits CYP1A2 (weak), CYP2A6 (weak), CYP2C19 (weak), CYP2C9 (weak), CYP2D6 (weak), CYP2E1 (weak)
Avoid Concomitant Use There are no known interactions where it is recommended to avoid concomitant use.
Increased Effect/Toxicity
Tioconazole may increase the levels/effects of: ARIPiprazole
Decreased Effect There are no known significant interactions involving a decrease in effect.
Stability Store at room temperature.
Mechanism of Action A 1-substituted imidazole derivative with a broad antifungal spectrum against a wide variety of dermatophytes and yeasts, including *Trichophyton mentagrophytes*, *T. rubrum*, *T. erinacei*, *T. tonsurans*, *Microsporum canis*, *Microsporum gypseum*, and *Candida albicans*. Both agents appear to be similarly effective against *Epidermophyton floccosum*.
Pharmacodynamics/Kinetics
Onset of action: Some improvement: Within 24 hours; Complete relief: Within 7 days
Absorption: Intravaginal: Systemic (small amounts)
Distribution: Vaginal fluid: 24-72 hours
Excretion: Urine and feces
Dosage
Geriatric & Adult Vulvovaginal candidiasis: Vaginal: Insert 1 applicatorful in vagina, just prior to bedtime, as a single dose
Administration Insert high into vagina
Special Geriatric Considerations Assess patient's ability to self-administer; may be difficult in patients with arthritis or limited range of motion.
Dosage Forms Excipient information presented when available (limited, particularly for generics); consult specific product labeling.
Ointment, vaginal:
1-Day™: 6.5% (4.6 g)
Vagistat®-1: 6.5% (4.6 g) [applicator delivers approximately 300 mg of tioconazole]

◆ **Tiotixene** see Thiothixene on page 1882

Tiotropium (ty oh TRO pee um)

Related Information
Inhalant Agents *on page 2117*

Medication Safety Issues
Sound-alike/look-alike issues:
Spiriva® may be confused with Inspra™, Serevent®
Tiotropium may be confused with ipratropium
Administration issues:
Spiriva® capsules for inhalation are for administration via HandiHaler® device and are **not** for oral use

Brand Names: U.S. Spiriva® HandiHaler®
Brand Names: Canada Spiriva®
Index Terms Tiotropium Bromide Monohydrate
Generic Availability (U.S.) No
Pharmacologic Category Anticholinergic Agent
Use Maintenance treatment of bronchospasm associated with COPD (including bronchitis and emphysema); reduction of COPD exacerbations
Contraindications Hypersensitivity to tiotropium or ipratropium, or any component of the formulation (contains lactose)
Warnings/Precautions Rarely, paradoxical bronchospasm may occur with use of inhaled bronchodilating agents; discontinue use and consider other therapy if bronchospasm occurs.

Not indicated for the initial (rescue) treatment of acute episodes of bronchospasm. Use with caution in patients with myasthenia gravis, narrow-angle glaucoma, prostatic hyperplasia, moderate-severe renal impairment (Cl_{cr} ≤50 mL/minute), or bladder neck obstruction; avoid inadvertent instillation of powder into the eyes. Immediate hypersensitivity reactions may occur; discontinue immediately if signs/symptoms occur. Use with caution in patients with a history of hypersensitivity to atropine.

The contents of Spiriva® capsules are for inhalation only via the HandiHaler® device. There have been reports of incorrect administration (swallowing of the capsules). Capsule for oral inhalation contains lactose; use with caution in patients with severe milk protein allergy.

Adverse Reactions (Reflective of adult population; not specific for elderly)
>10%:
Gastrointestinal: Xerostomia (5% to 16%)
Respiratory: Upper respiratory tract infection (41%), pharyngitis (9% to 13%), sinusitis (7% to 11%)
1% to 10%:
Cardiovascular: Chest pain (1% to 7%), edema (dependent, 5%)
Central nervous system: Headache (6%), insomnia (4%), depression (1% to 4%), dysphonia (1% to 3%)
Dermatologic: Rash (4%)
Endocrine & metabolic: Hypercholesterolemia (1% to 3%), hyperglycemia (1% to 3%)
Gastrointestinal: Dyspepsia (6%), abdominal pain (5%), constipation (4% to 5%), vomiting (4%), gastroesophageal reflux (1% to 3%), stomatitis (including ulcerative; 1% to 3%)
Genitourinary: Urinary tract infection (7%)
Neuromuscular & skeletal: Arthralgia (4%), myalgia (4%), arthritis (≥3%), leg pain (1% to 3%), paresthesia (1% to 3%), skeletal pain (1% to 3%)
Ocular: Cataract (1% to 3%)
Respiratory: Rhinitis (6%), epistaxis (4%), cough (≥3%), laryngitis (1% to 3%)
Miscellaneous: Infection (4%), moniliasis (4%), flu-like syndrome (≥3%), allergic reaction (1% to 3%), herpes zoster (1% to 3%)

Drug Interactions
Metabolism/Transport Effects Substrate of CYP2D6 (minor), CYP3A4 (minor); **Note:** Assignment of Major/Minor substrate status based on clinically relevant drug interaction potential
Avoid Concomitant Use There are no known interactions where it is recommended to avoid concomitant use.
Increased Effect/Toxicity
Tiotropium may increase the levels/effects of: AbobotulinumtoxinA; Anticholinergics; Cannabinoids; OnabotulinumtoxinA; Potassium Chloride; RimabotulinumtoxinB

The levels/effects of Tiotropium may be increased by: Pramlintide

Decreased Effect

Tiotropium may decrease the levels/effects of: Acetylcholinesterase Inhibitors (Central); Secretin

The levels/effects of Tiotropium may be decreased by: Acetylcholinesterase Inhibitors (Central); Peginterferon Alfa-2b; Tocilizumab

Stability Store at 25°C (77°F); excursions permitted to 15°C to 30°C (59°F to 86°F). Avoid excessive temperatures and moisture. Do not store capsules in HandiHaler® device. Capsules should be stored in the blister pack and only removed immediately before use. Once protective foil is peeled back and/or removed the capsule should be used immediately; if capsule is not used immediately it should be discarded.

Mechanism of Action Competitively and reversibly inhibits the action of acetylcholine at type 3 muscarinic (M$_3$) receptors in bronchial smooth muscle causing bronchodilation

Pharmacodynamics/Kinetics

Absorption: Poorly absorbed from GI tract, systemic absorption may occur from lung

Distribution: V$_d$: 32 L/kg

Protein binding: 72%

Metabolism: Hepatic (minimal), via CYP2D6 and CYP3A4

Bioavailability: Following inhalation, 19.5%; oral solution: 2% to 3%

Half-life elimination: 5-6 days

Time to peak, plasma: 5 minutes (following inhalation)

Excretion: Urine (14% of an inhaled dose); feces (primarily nonabsorbed drug)

Dosage

Geriatric & Adult COPD: Oral inhalation: Contents of 1 capsule (18 mcg) inhaled once daily using HandiHaler® device. **Note:** To ensure drug delivery the contents of each capsule should be inhaled twice.

Renal Impairment Plasma concentrations may increase in renal impairment. Use caution in moderate-to-severe impairment (Cl$_{cr}$ ≤50 mL/minute); although no dosage adjustment is required, monitor closely.

Administration Administer once daily at the same time each day. Remove capsule from foil blister immediately before use. Place capsule in the capsule-chamber in the base of the HandiHaler® Inhaler. Must only use the HandiHaler® Inhaler. Close mouthpiece until a click is heard, leaving dustcap open. Exhale fully. Do not exhale into inhaler. Tilt head slightly back and inhale (rapidly, steadily and deeply); the capsule vibration may be heard within the device. Hold breath as long as possible. If any powder remains in capsule, exhale and inhale again. Repeat until capsule is empty. Throw away empty capsule; do not leave in inhaler. Do not use a spacer with the HandiHaler® Inhaler. Always keep capsules and inhaler dry.

Delivery of dose: Instruct patient to place mouthpiece gently between teeth, closing lips around inhaler. Instruct patient to inhale deeply and hold breath held for 5-10 seconds. The amount of drug delivered is small, and the individual will not sense the medication as it is inhaled. Remove mouthpiece prior to exhalation. Patient should not breathe out through the mouthpiece.

Monitoring Parameters FEV$_1$, peak flow (or other pulmonary function studies)

Special Geriatric Considerations Assess patient's ability to use the HandiHaler®. In elderly patients, renal clearance of tiotropium was decreased and plasma concentrations were increased, due to decreased renal function. In clinical trials, the incidence of constipation, UTIs and xerostomia increased with age. No dosage adjustments are recommended due to age or renal function. However, the manufacturer recommends monitoring patients with moderate-to-severe renal impairment. Monitor urinary function in men with benign prostatic hyperplasia while on this medication.

Dosage Forms Excipient information presented when available (limited, particularly for generics); consult specific product labeling.

Powder, for oral inhalation:

Spiriva® HandiHaler®: 18 mcg/capsule (5s, 30s, 90s) [contains lactose]

Dosage Forms: Canada Excipient information presented when available (limited, particularly for generics); consult specific product labeling.

Powder, for oral inhalation:

Spiriva®: 18 mcg/capsule (10s) [contains lactose]

◆ **Tiotropium Bromide Monohydrate** *see* Tiotropium *on page 1907*

Tirofiban (tye roe FYE ban)

Medication Safety Issues

Sound-alike/look-alike issues:

Aggrastat® may be confused with Aggrenox®, argatroban

High alert medication:

The Institute for Safe Medication Practices (ISMP) includes this medication among its list of drugs which have a heightened risk of causing significant patient harm when used in error.

Brand Names: U.S. Aggrastat®

Brand Names: Canada Aggrastat®

Index Terms MK383; Tirofiban Hydrochloride

Generic Availability (U.S.) No

Pharmacologic Category Antiplatelet Agent, Glycoprotein IIb/IIIa Inhibitor

Use Treatment of acute coronary syndrome (ie, unstable angina/non-ST-elevation myocardial infarction [UA/NSTEMI]) in combination with heparin

Unlabeled Use To support PCI (administered at the time of PCI) for ST-elevation myocardial infarction (STEMI), UA/NSTEMI, and stable ischemic heart disease (ie, elective PCI)

Contraindications Hypersensitivity to tirofiban or any component of the formulation; active internal bleeding or a history of bleeding diathesis within the previous 30 days; history of intracranial hemorrhage, intracranial neoplasm, arteriovenous malformation, or aneurysm; history of thrombocytopenia following prior exposure; history of CVA within 30 days or any history of hemorrhagic stroke; major surgical procedure or severe physical trauma within the previous month; history, symptoms, or findings suggestive of aortic dissection; severe hypertension (systolic BP >180 mm Hg and/or diastolic BP >110 mm Hg); concomitant use of another parenteral GP IIb/IIIa inhibitor; acute pericarditis

Warnings/Precautions Bleeding is the most common complication encountered during this therapy; most major bleeding occurs at the arterial access site for cardiac catheterization. Caution in patients with platelets <150,000/mm³; patients with hemorrhagic retinopathy; chronic dialysis patients; when used in combination with other drugs impacting on coagulation. Prior to pulling the sheath, heparin should be discontinued for 3-4 hours and ACT <180 seconds or aPTT <45 seconds. Use standard compression techniques after sheath removal. Watch the site closely afterwards for further bleeding. Sheath hemostasis should be achieved at least 4 hours before hospital discharge. Other trauma and vascular punctures should be minimized. Avoid obtaining vascular access through a noncompressible site (eg, subclavian or jugular vein). Discontinue at least 2-4 hours prior to coronary artery bypass graft surgery (Hillis, 2011). Patients with severe renal insufficiency require dosage reduction.

Adverse Reactions (Reflective of adult population; not specific for elderly) Bleeding is the major drug-related adverse effect. Patients received background treatment with aspirin and heparin. Major bleeding was reported in 1.4% to 2.2%; minor bleeding in 10.5% to 12%; transfusion was required in 4% to 4.3%.

>1% (nonbleeding adverse events):

Cardiovascular: Coronary artery dissection (5%), bradycardia (4%), edema (2%)

Central nervous system: Dizziness (3%), vasovagal reaction (2%), fever (>1%), headache (>1%)

Gastrointestinal: Nausea (>1%)

Genitourinary: Pelvic pain (6%)

Hematologic: Thrombocytopenia: <90,000/mm³ (1.5%), <50,000/mm³ (0.3%)

Neuromuscular & skeletal: Leg pain (3%)

Miscellaneous: Diaphoresis (2%)

Drug Interactions

Metabolism/Transport Effects None known.

Avoid Concomitant Use There are no known interactions where it is recommended to avoid concomitant use.

Increased Effect/Toxicity

Tirofiban may increase the levels/effects of: Anticoagulants; Antiplatelet Agents; Collagenase (Systemic); Dabigatran Etexilate; Drotrecogin Alfa (Activated); Ibritumomab; Rivaroxaban; Salicylates; Thrombolytic Agents; Tositumomab and Iodine I 131 Tositumomab

The levels/effects of Tirofiban may be increased by: Dasatinib; Glucosamine; Herbs (Anticoagulant/Antiplatelet Properties); Nonsteroidal Anti-Inflammatory Agents; Omega-3-Acid Ethyl Esters; Pentosan Polysulfate Sodium; Pentoxifylline; Prostacyclin Analogues; Tipranavir; Vitamin E

Decreased Effect

The levels/effects of Tirofiban may be decreased by: Nonsteroidal Anti-Inflammatory Agents

Stability Store at 25°C (77°F); do not freeze. Protect from light during storage.

Mechanism of Action A reversible antagonist of fibrinogen binding to the GP IIb/IIIa receptor, the major platelet surface receptor involved in platelet aggregation. When administered intravenously, it inhibits *ex vivo* platelet aggregation in a dose- and concentration-dependent manner. When given according to the recommended regimen, >90% inhibition is attained by the end of the 30-minute infusion. Platelet aggregation inhibition is reversible following cessation of the infusion.

Pharmacodynamics/Kinetics

Distribution: 35% unbound

Metabolism: Minimally hepatic

Half-life elimination: 2 hours

Excretion: Urine (65%) and feces (25%) primarily as unchanged drug

   Clearance: Elderly: Reduced by 19% to 26%

Dosage

Geriatric & Adult

   Unstable angina/non-ST-elevation myocardial infarction (UA/NSTEMI): I.V.: Initial rate of 0.4 mcg/kg/minute for 30 minutes and then continued at 0.1 mcg/kg/minute. Dosing should be continued through angiography and for 12-24 hours after angioplasty or atherectomy.

   Percutaneous coronary intervention (PCI) (unlabeled use): I.V.: Loading dose: 25 mcg/kg over 3 minutes at the time of PCI; Maintenance infusion: 0.15 mcg/kg/minute continued for up to 18-24 hours (Levine, 2011; Valgimigli, 2008; Van't Hof, 2008)

Renal Impairment Cl_{cr} <30 mL/minute: Reduce dose to 50% of normal rate.

Administration Intended for intravenous delivery using sterile equipment and technique. Do not add other drugs or remove solution directly from the bag with a syringe. Do not use plastic containers in series connections; such use can result in air embolism by drawing air from the first container if it is empty of solution. Discard unused solution 24 hours following the start of infusion. May be administered through the same catheter as heparin. Tirofiban injection must be diluted to a concentration of 50 mcg/mL (premixed solution does not require dilution). For unstable angina/non-ST-elevation MI (UA/NSTEMI), infuse loading dose over 30 minutes, followed by continuous infusion. When used during percutaneous coronary intervention (PCI), may administer loading dose over 3 minutes, followed by continuous infusion.

Monitoring Parameters Platelet count. Hemoglobin and hematocrit should be monitored prior to treatment, within 6 hours following loading infusion, and at least daily thereafter during therapy. Platelet count may need to be monitored earlier in patients who received prior glycoprotein IIb/IIIa antagonists. Persistent reductions of platelet counts <90,000/mm^3 may require interruption or discontinuation of infusion. Because tirofiban requires concurrent heparin therapy, aPTT levels should also be followed. Monitor vital signs and laboratory results prior to, during, and after therapy. Assess infusion insertion site during and after therapy (every 15 minutes or as institutional policy). Observe and teach patient bleeding precautions (avoid invasive procedures and activities that could result in injury). Monitor closely for signs of unusual or excessive bleeding (eg, CNS changes, blood in urine, stool, or vomitus, unusual bruising or bleeding).

Special Geriatric Considerations Elderly patients receiving tirofiban with heparin or heparin alone had a higher incidence of bleeding in clinical trials. Caution must be used when using other drugs affecting hemostasis, which are commonly used in elderly.

Dosage Forms Excipient information presented when available (limited, particularly for generics); consult specific product labeling. [DSC] = Discontinued product

Infusion, premixed in NS [preservative free]:

   Aggrastat®: 50 mcg/mL (100 mL [DSC], 250 mL)

◆ **Tirofiban Hydrochloride** *see* Tirofiban *on page 1909*

◆ **Tirosint®** *see* Levothyroxine *on page 1122*

◆ **Titralac™ [OTC]** *see* Calcium Carbonate *on page 262*

◆ **TIV** *see* Influenza Virus Vaccine (Inactivated) *on page 997*

TiZANidine (tye ZAN i deen)

Related Information

Beers Criteria – Potentially Inappropriate Medications for Geriatrics *on page 2183*

Medication Safety Issues

   Sound-alike/look-alike issues:

      TiZANidine may be confused with tiaGABine

      Zanaflex® may be confused with Xiaflex®

BEERS Criteria medication:
This drug may be potentially inappropriate for use in geriatric patients (Quality of evidence - varies based on comorbidity; Strength of recommendation - varies based on comorbidity)
Other safety concerns:
Zanaflex® capsules and Zanaflex® tablets (or generic tizanidine tablets) are not interchangeable in the fed state

Brand Names: U.S. Zanaflex Capsules®; Zanaflex®

Brand Names: Canada Apo-Tizanidine®; Gen-Tizanidine; Mylan-Tizanidine; Zanaflex®

Index Terms Sirdalud®

Generic Availability (U.S.) Yes

Pharmacologic Category Alpha$_2$-Adrenergic Agonist

Use Skeletal muscle relaxant used for treatment of muscle spasticity

Unlabeled Use Tension headaches, acute low back pain

Contraindications Hypersensitivity to tizanidine or any component of the formulation; concomitant therapy with ciprofloxacin or fluvoxamine (potent CYP1A2 inhibitors)

Warnings/Precautions Significant hypotension (possibly with bradycardia or orthostatic hypotension) and sedation may occur; use caution in patients with cardiac disease or those at risk for severe hypotensive (eg, patients taking concurrent medications which may predispose to hypotension/bradycardia) or sedative effects (patients must be cautioned about performing tasks which require mental alertness [eg, operating machinery or driving]). Should not be used with other alpha$_2$-adrenergic agonists. Avoid concomitant administration with CYP1A2 inhibitors; increased tizanidine levels/effects (severe hypotension and sedation) may occur. Concomitant use of ciprofloxacin or fluvoxamine is contraindicated. These effects may also be increased with concomitant administration with other CNS depressants and/or antihypertensives; use caution. In general, avoid concomitant use of oral contraceptives with tizanidine; clearance of tizanidine may be decreased by 50%; if taken concomitantly, decrease initial tizanidine dose and titration rate. Elderly patients are at risk due to decreased clearance, particulary in elderly patients with renal insufficiency (Cl$_{cr}$ <25 mL/minute) compared to healthy elderly subjects; this may lead to an increased risk of adverse effects and/or a longer duration of effects. Use caution in any patient with renal impairment. Clearance decreased significantly in patients with severe impairment (Cl$_{cr}$<25 mL/minute); dose reductions recommended. Use with extreme caution or avoid in hepatic impairment due to extensive hepatic metabolism and potential hepatotoxicity; AST/ALT elevations (>3 times ULN) and rarely hepatic failure have occurred; monitoring recommended.

May be inappropriate in older adults depending on comorbidities (eg, dementia, delirium) due to its potent anticholinergic effects (Beers Criteria).

Use has been associated with visual hallucinations or delusions, generally in first 6 weeks of therapy; use caution in patients with psychiatric disorders. Withdrawal resulting in rebound hypertension, tachycardia, and hypertonia may occur upon discontinuation; doses should be decreased slowly, particularly in patients receiving high doses for prolonged periods. Pharmacokinetics and bioequivalence between capsules and tablets altered by nonfasting vs fasting conditions (capsules and tablets are bioequivalent under fasting conditions, but not under nonfasting conditions). Limited data exist for chronic use of single doses >8 mg and multiple doses >24 mg/day.

Adverse Reactions (Reflective of adult population; not specific for elderly) Frequency percentages below reported during multiple-dose studies, unless specified otherwise.
>10%:
Cardiovascular: Hypotension (16% to 33%)
Central nervous system: Somnolence (48%), dizziness (16%)
Gastrointestinal: Xerostomia (49%)
Neuromuscular & skeletal: Weakness (41%)
1% to 10%:
Cardiovascular: Bradycardia (2% to 10%)
Central nervous system: Nervousness (3%), speech disorder (3%), visual hallucinations/delusions (3%), anxiety (1%), depression (1%), fever (1%)
Dermatologic: Rash (1%), skin ulcer (1%)
Gastrointestinal: Constipation (4%), vomiting (3%), abdominal pain (1%), diarrhea (1%), dyspepsia (1%)
Genitourinary: UTI (10%), urinary frequency (3%)
Hepatic: Liver enzymes increased (3% to 5%)
Neuromuscular & skeletal: Dyskinesia (3%), back pain (1%), myasthenia (1%), paresthesia (1%)
Ocular: Blurred vision (3%)
Respiratory: Pharyngitis (3%), rhinitis (3%)
Miscellaneous: Infection (6%), flu-like syndrome (3%), diaphoresis (1%)

Drug Interactions

Metabolism/Transport Effects Substrate of CYP1A2 (major); **Note:** Assignment of Major/Minor substrate status based on clinically relevant drug interaction potential

Avoid Concomitant Use

Avoid concomitant use of TiZANidine with any of the following: Azelastine; Azelastine (Nasal); Ciprofloxacin; Ciprofloxacin (Systemic); FluvoxaMINE; Iobenguane I 123; Paraldehyde

Increased Effect/Toxicity

TiZANidine may increase the levels/effects of: ACE Inhibitors; Alcohol (Ethyl); Azelastine; Azelastine (Nasal); Buprenorphine; CNS Depressants; Highest Risk QTc-Prolonging Agents; Hypotensive Agents; Lisinopril; Metyrosine; Moderate Risk QTc-Prolonging Agents; Paraldehyde; Selective Serotonin Reuptake Inhibitors; Zolpidem

The levels/effects of TiZANidine may be increased by: Abiraterone Acetate; Beta-Blockers; Ciprofloxacin; Ciprofloxacin (Systemic); Contraceptives (Estrogens); CYP1A2 Inhibitors (Moderate); CYP1A2 Inhibitors (Strong); Deferasirox; FluvoxaMINE; HydrOXYzine; MAO Inhibitors; Mifepristone

Decreased Effect

TiZANidine may decrease the levels/effects of: Iobenguane I 123

The levels/effects of TiZANidine may be decreased by: Antidepressants (Alpha2-Antagonist); Serotonin/Norepinephrine Reuptake Inhibitors; Tricyclic Antidepressants

Ethanol/Nutrition/Herb Interactions

Ethanol: May increase CNS depression; monitor for increased effects with coadministration. Caution patients about effects.

Food: The tablet and capsule dosage forms are not bioequivalent when administered with food. Food increases both the time to peak concentration and the extent of absorption for both the tablet and capsule. However, maximal concentrations of tizanidine achieved when administered with food were increased by 30% for the tablet, but decreased by 20% for the capsule. Under fed conditions, the capsule is approximately 80% bioavailable relative to the tablet.

Herb/Nutraceutical: Avoid valerian, St John's wort, kava kava, gotu kola (may increase CNS depression). Avoid black cohosh, California poppy, coleus, golden seal, hawthorn, mistletoe, periwinkle, quinine, shepherd's purse (may increase hypotensive effects).

Stability Store at 25°C (77°F); excursions permitted to 15°C to 30°C (59°F to 86°F).

Mechanism of Action An alpha$_2$-adrenergic agonist agent which decreases excitatory input to alpha motor neurons; an imidazole derivative chemically-related to clonidine, is a centrally acting muscle relaxant with alpha$_2$-adrenergic agonist properties; acts on the level of the spinal cord

Pharmacodynamics/Kinetics

Onset: Single dose (8 mg): Peak effect: 1-2 hours

Duration: Single dose (8 mg): 3-6 hours

Absorption: Tablets and capsules are bioequivalent under fasting conditions, but not under nonfasting conditions.

Tablets administered with food: Peak plasma concentration is increased by ~30%; time to peak increased by 25 minutes; extent of absorption increased by ~30%.

Capsules administered with food: Peak plasma concentration decreased by 20%; time to peak increased by 2 hours; extent of absorption increased by ~10%.

Capsules opened and sprinkled on applesauce are not bioequivalent to administration of intact capsules under fasting conditions. Peak plasma concentration and AUC are increased by 15% to 20%.

Distribution: 2.4 L/kg

Protein binding: ~30%

Metabolism: Extensively hepatic via CYP1A2 to inactive metabolites

Bioavailability: ~40% (extensive first-pass metabolism)

Half-life elimination: 2.5 hours

Time to peak, serum:

Fasting state: Capsule, tablet: 1 hour

Fed state: Capsule: 3-4 hours, Tablet: 1.5 hours

Excretion: Urine (60%); feces (20%)

Dosage

Geriatric Use with caution; clearance is decreased. Refer to adult dosing.

Adult Spasticity: Oral: Initial: 4 mg up to 3 times daily (at 6- to 8-hour intervals); may titrate to optimal effect in 2-4 mg increments as needed to a maximum of 3 doses in 24 hours (at 6- to 8-hour intervals); maximum: 36 mg daily. **Note:** Limited experience with single doses >8 mg and daily doses >24 mg.

Renal Impairment

Cl$_{cr}$ ≥25 mL/minute: No dosage adjustment provided in manufacturer's labeling; however, caution may be needed as creatinine clearance decreases.

Cl$_{cr}$ <25 mL/minute: Use with caution; clearance reduced >50%. During initial dose titration, use reduced doses. If higher doses are necessary, increase dose instead of increasing dosing frequency.

Hepatic Impairment Avoid use in hepatic impairment; if used, lowest possible dose should be used initially with close monitoring for adverse effects (eg, hypotension).

Administration Capsules may be opened and contents sprinkled on food; however, extent of absorption is increased up to 20% relative to administration of the capsule under fasted conditions.

Monitoring Parameters Monitor liver function (aminotransferases) at baseline, 1, 3, 6 months and periodically thereafter; blood pressure; renal function

Special Geriatric Considerations Since elderly commonly have renal function of Cl$_{cr}$ <30 mL/minute, creatinine clearance should be estimated before dosing this medication. Low doses should be started initially because of the possibility of CNS effects.

This medication is considered to be potentially inappropriate in this patient population (Beers Criteria: Quality of evidence - varies based on comorbidity; Strength of recommendation - varies based on comorbidity)

Dosage Forms Excipient information presented when available (limited, particularly for generics); consult specific product labeling.

Capsule, oral: 2 mg, 4 mg, 6 mg

Zanaflex Capsules®: 2 mg, 4 mg, 6 mg

Tablet, oral: 2 mg, 4 mg

Zanaflex®: 4 mg [scored]

◆ **TMP** see Trimethoprim on page 1971
◆ **TMP-SMX** see Sulfamethoxazole and Trimethoprim on page 1813
◆ **TMP-SMZ** see Sulfamethoxazole and Trimethoprim on page 1813
◆ **TMX-67** see Febuxostat on page 747
◆ **TOBI®** see Tobramycin (Systemic, Oral Inhalation) on page 1913
◆ **TobraDex®** see Tobramycin and Dexamethasone on page 1918
◆ **TobraDex® ST** see Tobramycin and Dexamethasone on page 1918

Tobramycin (Systemic, Oral Inhalation) (toe bra MYE sin)

Related Information

Antimicrobial Drugs of Choice on page 2163

Medication Safety Issues

Sound-alike/look-alike issues:

Tobramycin may be confused with Trobicin®, vancomycin

International issues:

Nebcin [Multiple international markets] may be confused with Naprosyn brand name for naproxen [U.S., Canada, and multiple international markets]; Nubain brand name for nalbuphine [Multiple international markets]

High alert medication:

The Institute for Safe Medication Practices (ISMP) includes this medication (intrathecal administration) among its list of drug classes which have a heightened risk of causing significant patient harm when used in error.

Brand Names: U.S. TOBI®

Brand Names: Canada TOBI®; TOBI® Podhaler®; Tobramycin Injection, USP

Index Terms Tobramycin Sulfate

Generic Availability (U.S.) Yes: Excludes solution for nebulization

Pharmacologic Category Antibiotic, Aminoglycoside

Use Treatment of documented or suspected infections caused by susceptible gram-negative bacilli, including Pseudomonas aeruginosa.

Contraindications Hypersensitivity to tobramycin, other aminoglycosides, or any component of the formulation

Warnings/Precautions [U.S. Boxed Warning]: Aminoglycosides may cause neurotoxicity and/or nephrotoxicity; usual risk factors include pre-existing renal impairment, concomitant neuro-/nephrotoxic medications, advanced age, and dehydration. Ototoxicity may be directly proportional to the amount of drug given and the duration of treatment; tinnitus or vertigo are indications of vestibular injury and impending hearing loss; renal damage is usually reversible. May cause neuromuscular blockade and respiratory paralysis, especially when given soon after anesthesia or muscle relaxants.

TOBRAMYCIN (SYSTEMIC, ORAL INHALATION)

Not intended for long-term therapy due to toxic hazards associated with extended administration; use caution in pre-existing renal insufficiency, vestibular or cochlear impairment, myasthenia gravis, hypocalcemia, and conditions which depress neuromuscular transmission. Dosage modification required in patients with impaired renal function. Prolonged use may result in fungal or bacterial superinfection, including *C. difficile*-associated diarrhea (CDAD) and pseudomembranous colitis; CDAD has been observed >2 months postantibiotic treatment. Solution may contain sodium metabisulfate; use caution in patients with sulfite allergy.

Adverse Reactions (Reflective of adult population; not specific for elderly)

Injection: Frequency not defined:

Central nervous system: Confusion, disorientation, dizziness, fever, headache, lethargy, vertigo

Dermatologic: Exfoliative dermatitis, itching, rash, urticaria

Endocrine & metabolic: Serum calcium, magnesium, potassium, and/or sodium decreased

Gastrointestinal: Diarrhea, nausea, vomiting

Hematologic: Anemia, eosinophilia, granulocytopenia, leukocytosis, leukopenia, thrombocytopenia

Hepatic: ALT increased, AST increased, bilirubin increased, LDH increased

Local: Pain at the injection site

Otic: Hearing loss, tinnitus, ototoxicity (auditory), ototoxicity (vestibular), roaring in the ears

Renal: BUN increased, cylindruria, serum creatinine increased, oliguria, proteinuria

Inhalation (as reported for solution for inhalation unless otherwise noted):

>10%:

Gastrointestinal: Sputum discoloration (21%)

Respiratory: Cough (22% [powder for inhalation]), voice alteration (13%)

1% to 10%:

Cardiovascular: Chest discomfort (3% [powder for inhalation])

Central nervous system: Malaise (6%), pyrexia (1% [powder for inhalation])

Gastrointestinal: Abnormal taste (5% [powder for inhalation]), xerostomia (2% [powder for inhalation])

Otic: Tinnitus (3%)

Respiratory: Dyspnea (4% [powder for inhalation]), oropharyngeal pain (4% [powder for inhalation]), throat irritation (3% [powder for inhalation]), FEV decreased (2% [powder for inhalation]), pulmonary function decreased (2% [powder for inhalation]), bronchospasm (1% [powder for inhalation]), upper respiratory tract infection (1% [powder for inhalation])

Drug Interactions

Metabolism/Transport Effects None known.

Avoid Concomitant Use

Avoid concomitant use of Tobramycin (Systemic, Oral Inhalation) with any of the following: BCG; Gallium Nitrate

Increased Effect/Toxicity

Tobramycin (Systemic, Oral Inhalation) may increase the levels/effects of: AbobotulinumtoxinA; Bisphosphonate Derivatives; CARBOplatin; Colistimethate; CycloSPORINE; CycloSPORINE (Systemic); Gallium Nitrate; Neuromuscular-Blocking Agents; OnabotulinumtoxinA; RimabotulinumtoxinB

The levels/effects of Tobramycin (Systemic, Oral Inhalation) may be increased by: Amphotericin B; Capreomycin; Cephalosporins (2nd Generation); Cephalosporins (3rd Generation); Cephalosporins (4th Generation); CISplatin; Loop Diuretics; Nonsteroidal Anti-Inflammatory Agents; Vancomycin

Decreased Effect

Tobramycin (Systemic, Oral Inhalation) may decrease the levels/effects of: BCG; Typhoid Vaccine

The levels/effects of Tobramycin (Systemic, Oral Inhalation) may be decreased by: Penicillins

Stability

Injection: Stable at room temperature both as the clear, colorless solution and as the dry powder. Reconstituted solutions remain stable for 24 hours at room temperature and 96 hours when refrigerated. Dilute in 50-100 mL NS, D_5W for I.V. infusion.

Powder, for inhalation (TOBI® Podhaler®) [Canadian availability; not available in the U.S.]): Store in original package at 15°C to 30°C (59°F to 86°F). Protect from moisture.

Solution, for inhalation (TOBI®): Store under refrigeration at 2°C to 8°C (36°F to 46°F). May be stored in foil pouch at room temperature of 25°C (77°F) for up to 28 days. Avoid intense light. Solution may darken over time; however, do not use if cloudy or contains particles.

Mechanism of Action Interferes with bacterial protein synthesis by binding to 30S and 50S ribosomal subunits, resulting in a defective bacterial cell membrane

Pharmacodynamics/Kinetics

Absorption:

Oral: Poorly absorbed

I.M.: Rapid and complete

Inhalation: Peak serum concentrations are ~1 mcg/mL following a 300 mg dose

Distribution: V_d: 0.2-0.3 L/kg; to extracellular fluid, including serum, abscesses, ascitic, pericardial, pleural, synovial, lymphatic, and peritoneal fluids; poor penetration into CSF, eye, bone, prostate

Inhalation: Tobramycin remains concentrated primarily in the airways

Protein binding: <30%

Half-life elimination:

Adults: 2-3 hours; directly dependent upon glomerular filtration rate

Adults with impaired renal function: 5-70 hours

Time to peak, serum: I.M.: 30-60 minutes; I.V.: ~30 minutes

Excretion: Normal renal function: Urine (~90% to 95%) within 24 hours

Dosage

Geriatric Dosage should be based on an estimate of ideal body weight.

I.M., I.V.: 1.5-5 mg/kg/day in 1-2 divided doses

I.V.: Once daily or extended interval: 5-7 mg/kg/dose given every 24, 36, or 48 hours based on creatinine clearance

Adult Note: Individualization is **critical** because of the low therapeutic index.

Use of ideal body weight (IBW) for determining the mg/kg/dose appears to be more accurate than dosing on the basis of total body weight (TBW). In morbid obesity, dosage requirement may best be estimated using a dosing weight of IBW + 0.4 (TBW - IBW).

Initial and periodic plasma drug levels (eg, peak and trough with conventional dosing) should be determined, particularly in critically-ill patients with serious infections or in disease states known to significantly alter aminoglycoside pharmacokinetics (eg, cystic fibrosis, burns, or major surgery).

Severe life-threatening infections: I.M., I.V.:

Conventional: 1-2.5 mg/kg/dose every 8-12 hours; to ensure adequate peak concentrations early in therapy, higher initial dosage may be considered in selected patients when extracellular water is increased (edema, septic shock, postsurgical, and/or trauma)

Once-daily: 4-7 mg/kg/dose once daily; some clinicians recommend this approach for all patients with normal renal function; this dose is at least as efficacious with similar, if not less, toxicity than conventional dosing.

Brucellosis: I.M., I.V.: 240 mg (I.M.) daily or 5 mg/kg (I.V.) daily for 7 days; either regimen recommended in combination with doxycycline

Cholangitis: I.M., I.V.: 4-6 mg/kg once daily with ampicillin

CNS shunt infection: Intrathecal (unlabeled route): 5-20 mg/day (Tunkel, 2004)

Diverticulitis, complicated: I.M., I.V.: 1.5-2 mg/kg every 8 hours (with ampicillin and metronidazole)

Infective endocarditis or synergy (for gram-positive infections): I.M., I.V.: 1 mg/kg every 8 hours (with ampicillin)

Meningitis *(Enterococcus or Pseudomonas aeruginosa)*: I.V.: 5 mg/kg/day in divided doses every 8 hours (administered with another bacteriocidal drug)

Pelvic inflammatory disease: I.M., I.V.: Loading dose: 2 mg/kg, then 1.5 mg/kg every 8 hours **or** 4.5 mg/kg once daily

Plague *(Yersinia pestis):* I.M., I.V.: Treatment: 5 mg/kg/day, followed by postexposure prophylaxis with doxycycline

Pneumonia, hospital- or ventilator-associated: I.M., I.V.: 7 mg/kg/day (with antipseudomonal beta-lactam or carbapenem)

Prophylaxis against endocarditis (dental, oral, upper respiratory procedures, GI/GU procedures): I.M., I.V.: 1.5 mg/kg with ampicillin (50 mg/kg) 30 minutes prior to procedure. **Note:** AHA guidelines now recommend prophylaxis only in patients undergoing invasive procedures and in whom underlying cardiac conditions may predispose to a higher risk of adverse outcomes should infection occur. As of April 2007, routine prophylaxis no longer recommended by the AHA.

Tularemia: I.M., I.V.: 5 mg/kg/day divided every 8 hours for 1-2 weeks

Urinary tract infection: I.M., I.V.: 1.5 mg/kg/dose every 8 hours

Renal Impairment I.M., I.V.:

Conventional dosing:

Cl_{cr} ≥60 mL/minute: Administer every 8 hours.

Cl_{cr} 40-60 mL/minute: Administer every 12 hours.

Cl_{cr} 20-40 mL/minute: Administer every 24 hours.

Cl_{cr} 10-20 mL/minute: Administer every 48 hours.

Cl_{cr} <10 mL/minute: Administer every 72 hours.

High-dose therapy: Interval may be extended (eg, every 48 hours) in patients with moderate renal impairment (Cl$_{cr}$ 30-59 mL/minute) and/or adjusted based on serum level determinations.

Intermittent hemodialysis (IHD) (administer after hemodialysis on dialysis days) (Heintz, 2009): Dialyzable (25% to 70%; variable; dependent on filter, duration, and type of HD): I.V.:

Loading dose of 2-3 mg/kg, followed by:

Mild UTI or synergy: I.V.: 1 mg/kg every 48-72 hours; consider redosing for pre-HD or post-HD concentrations <1 mg/L

Moderate-to-severe UTI: I.V. 1-1.5 mg/kg every 48-72 hours; consider redosing for pre-HD concentrations <1.5-2 mg/L or post-HD concentrations <1 mg/L

Systemic gram-negative infection: I.V.: 1.5-2 mg/kg every 48-72 hours; consider redosing for pre-HD concentrations <3-5 mg/L or post-HD concentrations <2 mg/L

Note: Dosing dependent on the assumption of 3 times/week, complete IHD sessions.

Peritoneal dialysis (PD):

Administration via peritoneal dialysis (PD) fluid:

Gram-negative infection: 4-8 mg/L (4-8 mcg/mL) of PD fluid

Gram-positive infection (ie, synergy): 3-4 mg/L (3-4 mcg/mL) of PD fluid

Administration IVPB/I.M.: Dose as for Cl$_{cr}$ <10 mL/minute and follow levels

Continuous renal replacement therapy (CRRT) (Heintz, 2009; Trotman, 2005): Drug clearance is highly dependent on the method of renal replacement, filter type, and flow rate. Appropriate dosing requires close monitoring of pharmacologic response, signs of adverse reactions due to drug accumulation, as well as drug concentrations in relation to target trough (if appropriate). The following are general recommendations only (based on dialysate flow/ultrafiltration rates of 1-2 L/hour and minimal residual renal function) and should not supersede clinical judgment:

CVVH/CVVHD/CVVHDF: I.V.: Loading dose of 2-3 mg/kg, followed by:

Mild UTI or synergy: I.V. 1 mg/kg every 24-36 hours (redose when concentration <1 mg/L)

Moderate-severe UTI: I.V.: 1-1.5 mg/kg every 24-36 hours (redose when concentration <1.5-2 mg/L)

Systemic gram-negative infection: I.V.: 1.5-2.5 mg/kg every 24-48 hours (redose when concentration <3-5 mg/L)

Hepatic Impairment No dosage adjustment necessary in hepatic impairment; monitor plasma concentrations as appropriate.

Administration

I.V.: Infuse over 30-60 minutes. Flush with saline before and after administration.

Inhalation:

TOBI®: To be inhaled over ~15 minutes using a handheld nebulizer (PARI-LC PLUS™). If multiple different nebulizer treatments are required, administer bronchodilator first, followed by chest physiotherapy, any other nebulized medications, and then TOBI® last. Do not mix with other nebulizer medications.

TOBI® Podhaler® (Canadian availability; not available in the U.S.): Capsules should be administered by oral inhalation via Podhaler® device following manufacturer recommendations for use and handling. Capsules should not be swallowed. Patients requiring bronchodilator therapy should administer the bronchodilator 15-90 minutes prior to TOBI® Podhaler®. The sequence of chest physiotherapy and additional inhaled therapies is at the discretion of the healthcare provider however TOBI® Podhaler® should always be administered last.

Some penicillins (eg, carbenicillin, ticarcillin, and piperacillin) have been shown to inactivate aminoglycosides in vitro. This has been observed to a greater extent with tobramycin and gentamicin, while amikacin has shown greater stability against inactivation. Concurrent use of these agents may pose a risk of reduced antibacterial efficacy in vivo, particularly in the setting of profound renal impairment. However, definitive clinical evidence is lacking. If combination penicillin/aminoglycoside therapy is desired in a patient with renal dysfunction, separation of doses (if feasible), and routine monitoring of aminoglycoside levels, CBC, and clinical response should be considered.

Monitoring Parameters Urinalysis, urine output, BUN, serum creatinine, peak and trough plasma tobramycin levels; be alert to ototoxicity; hearing should be tested before and during treatment

Some penicillin derivatives may accelerate the degradation of aminoglycosides in vitro. This may be clinically-significant for certain penicillin (ticarcillin, piperacillin, carbenicillin) and aminoglycoside (gentamicin, tobramycin) combination therapy in patients with significant renal impairment. Close monitoring of aminoglycoside levels is warranted.

Reference Range

Timing of serum samples: Draw peak 30 minutes after 30-minute infusion has been completed or 1 hour following I.M. injection or beginning of infusion; draw trough immediately before next dose

Therapeutic levels:

Peak:

Serious infections: 6-8 mcg/mL (SI: 12-17 micromole/L)

Life-threatening infections: 8-10 mcg/mL (SI: 17-21 micromole/L)

Urinary tract infections: 4-6 mcg/mL (SI: 7-12 micromole/L)

Synergy against gram-positive organisms: 3-5 mcg/mL

Trough:

Serious infections: 0.5-1 mcg/mL

Life-threatening infections: 1-2 mcg/mL

The American Thoracic Society (ATS) recommends trough levels of <1 mcg/mL for patients with hospital-acquired pneumonia.

Monitor serum creatinine and urine output; obtain drug levels after the third dose unless otherwise directed

Inhalation: Serum levels are ~1 mcg/mL one hour following a 300 mg dose in patients with normal renal function.

Test Interactions Some penicillin derivatives may accelerate the degradation of aminoglycosides *in vitro*, leading to a potential underestimation of aminoglycoside serum concentration.

Pharmacotherapy Pearls Once-daily dosing: Higher peak serum drug concentration to MIC ratios, demonstrated aminoglycoside postantibiotic effect, decreased renal cortex drug uptake, and improved cost-time efficiency are supportive reasons for the use of once daily dosing regimens for aminoglycosides. Current research indicates these regimens to be as effective for nonlife-threatening infections, with no higher incidence of nephrotoxicity, than those requiring multiple daily doses. Doses are determined by calculating the entire day's dose via usual multiple dose calculation techniques and administering this quantity as a single dose. Doses are then adjusted to maintain mean serum concentrations above the MIC(s) of the causative organism(s). (Example: 2.5-5 mg/kg as a single dose; expected Cp_{max}: 10-20 mcg/mL and Cp_{min}: <1 mcg/mL). Further research is needed for universal recommendation in all patient populations and gram-negative disease; exceptions may include those with known high clearance (eg, patients with burns who may require shorter dosage intervals) and patients with renal function impairment for whom longer than conventional dosage intervals are usually required.

Special Geriatric Considerations The aminoglycosides are an important therapeutic intervention for susceptible organisms and as empiric therapy in seriously ill patients. Their use is not without risks; these risks can be minimized if initial dosing is adjusted for estimated renal function and appropriate monitoring is performed. High dose, once daily aminoglycosides have been advocated as an alternative to traditional dosing regimens. Once daily or extended interval dosing is as effective and may be safer than traditional dosing. Interval must be adjusted for renal function.

Dosage Forms Excipient information presented when available (limited, particularly for generics); consult specific product labeling.

Infusion, premixed in NS: 80 mg (100 mL)

Injection, powder for reconstitution: 1.2 g

Injection, solution: 10 mg/mL (2 mL); 40 mg/mL (2 mL, 30 mL, 50 mL)

Solution, for nebulization [preservative free]:

TOBI®: 300 mg/5 mL (56s)

Dosage Forms: Canada Excipient information presented when available (limited, particularly for generics); consult specific product labeling.

Powder, for oral inhalation [capsule]:

TOBI® Podhaler®: 28 mg/capsule (224s)

Tobramycin (Ophthalmic) (toe bra MYE sin)

Medication Safety Issues

Sound-alike/look-alike issues:

Tobramycin may be confused with Trobicin®, vancomycin

Tobrex® may be confused with TobraDex®

Brand Names: U.S. AK-Tob™; Tobrex®

Brand Names: Canada PMS-Tobramycin; Sandoz-Tobramycin; Tobrex®

Index Terms Tobramycin Sulfate

Generic Availability (U.S.) Yes: Solution

Pharmacologic Category Antibiotic, Aminoglycoside; Antibiotic, Ophthalmic

Use Treatment of superficial ophthalmic infections caused by susceptible bacteria

Dosage
Adult Ocular infections: Ophthalmic:
Ointment: Instill ½" (1.25 cm) 2-3 times/day; for severe infections, apply every 3-4 hours
Solution: Instill 1-2 drops every 2-4 hours; for severe infections, instill up to 2 drops every hour until improved, then reduce to less frequent intervals
Special Geriatric Considerations Evaluate the patient's or caregiver's ability to safely administer the correct dose of ophthalmic medication.
Dosage Forms Excipient information presented when available (limited, particularly for generics); consult specific product labeling.
Ointment, ophthalmic:
Tobrex®: 0.3% (3.5 g) [contains chlorobutanol]
Solution, ophthalmic [drops]: 0.3% (5 mL)
AK-Tob™: 0.3% (5 mL) [contains benzalkonium chloride]
Tobrex®: 0.3% (5 mL) [contains benzalkonium chloride]

Tobramycin and Dexamethasone (toe bra MYE sin & deks a METH a sone)

Related Information
Dexamethasone (Ophthalmic) *on page 521*
Tobramycin (Ophthalmic) *on page 1917*
Medication Safety Issues
Sound-alike/look-alike issues:
TobraDex® may be confused with Tobrex®
Brand Names: U.S. TobraDex®; TobraDex® ST
Brand Names: Canada Tobradex®
Index Terms Dexamethasone and Tobramycin
Generic Availability (U.S.) Yes: Suspension (0.3%/0.1%)
Pharmacologic Category Antibiotic/Corticosteroid, Ophthalmic
Use Treatment of external ocular infection caused by susceptible gram-negative bacteria and steroid responsive inflammatory conditions of the palpebral and bulbar conjunctiva, cornea, and anterior segment of the globe
Dosage
Geriatric & Adult Ocular infection/inflammation: Ophthalmic:
Ointment: Apply a small amount (~½-inch ribbon of ointment) up to 3-4 times/day
Suspension: Instill 1-2 drops every 4-6 hours; may be increased to 1-2 drops every 2 hours for the first 24-48 hours, then reduce to less frequent intervals
Special Geriatric Considerations Evaluate the patient's or caregiver's ability to safely administer the correct dose of ophthalmic medication.
Dosage Forms Excipient information presented when available (limited, particularly for generics); consult specific product labeling.
Ointment, ophthalmic:
TobraDex®: Tobramycin 0.3% and dexamethasone 0.1% (3.5 g) [contains chlorobutanol]
Suspension, ophthalmic: Tobramycin 0.3% and dexamethasone 0.1% (2.5 mL, 5 mL, 10 mL)
TobraDex®: Tobramycin 0.3% and dexamethasone 0.1% (2.5 mL, 5 mL, 10 mL) [contains benzalkonium chloride]
TobraDex® ST: Tobramycin 0.3% and dexamethasone 0.05% (5 mL) [contains benzalkonium chloride]

◆ **Tobramycin and Loteprednol Etabonate** *see* Loteprednol and Tobramycin *on page 1164*
◆ **Tobramycin Sulfate** *see* Tobramycin (Ophthalmic) *on page 1917*
◆ **Tobramycin Sulfate** *see* Tobramycin (Systemic, Oral Inhalation) *on page 1913*
◆ **Tobrex®** *see* Tobramycin (Ophthalmic) *on page 1917*

Tocilizumab (toe si LIZ oo mab)

Brand Names: U.S. Actemra®
Brand Names: Canada Actemra®
Index Terms Atlizumab; MRA; R-1569; RoActemra®
Generic Availability (U.S.) No
Pharmacologic Category Antirheumatic, Disease Modifying; Interleukin-6 Receptor Antagonist
Use Treatment of moderately- to severely-active rheumatoid arthritis in adult patients who have had an inadequate response to one or more TNF antagonists (as monotherapy or in combination with nonbiological disease-modifying antirheumatic drugs [DMARDs]); treatment of active systemic juvenile idiopathic arthritis (SJIA) (as monotherapy or in combination with methotrexate)

Medication Guide Available Yes

Contraindications Hypersensitivity to tocilizumab or any component of the formulation

Warnings/Precautions [U.S. Boxed Warning]: Serious and potentially fatal infections (including tuberculosis, invasive fungal, bacterial, viral, protozoal, and other opportunistic infections) have been reported in patients receiving tocilizumab. Most of the serious infections have occurred in patients on concomitant immunosuppressive therapy. Do not administer tocilizumab to a patient with an active infection, including localized infection. Caution should be exercised when considering use in patients with chronic or recurrent infections, previous exposure to tuberculosis, previous residence or travel in an area of endemic tuberculosis or mycoses, or predisposition to infection. Patients should be closely monitored for signs and symptoms of infection during and after treatment. If a patient develops a serious infection, therapy should be discontinued. **[U.S. Boxed Warning]: Tuberculosis (disseminated or extrapulmonary) has been reported in patients receiving tocilizumab; both reactivation of latent infection and new infections have been reported.** Patients should be evaluated for latent tuberculosis infection with a tuberculin skin test prior to starting therapy. Treatment of latent tuberculosis should be initiated before therapy is used. Some patients who test negative prior to therapy may develop active infection; monitor for signs and symptoms of tuberculosis in all patients. Rare reactivation of herpes zoster has been reported. Patients should be brought up to date with all immunizations before initiating therapy. Live vaccines should not be given concurrently; there is no data available concerning secondary transmission of infection from live vaccines in patients receiving therapy.

Impact on the development and course of malignancies is not fully defined, however, malignancies were observed in clinical trials. Use with caution in patients with pre-existing or recent onset CNS demyelinating disorders; rare cases of CNS demyelinating disorders (eg, multiple sclerosis) have occurred. All patients should be monitored for signs and symptoms of demyelinating disorders. May cause hypersensitivity, anaphylaxis, or anaphylactoid reactions; permanently discontinue treatment in patients who develop a hypersensitivity reaction to tocilizumab. Medications for the treatment of hypersensitivity reactions should be available for immediate use. Use is not recommended in patients with active hepatic disease or hepatic impairment; use with caution in patients at increased risk for gastrointestinal perforation.

Use may cause increases in total cholesterol, triglycerides, LDL and HDL cholesterol; hyperlipidemia should be managed according to current guidelines. Therapy should not be initiated in patients with an ANC <2000/mm^3, platelet count <100,000/mm^3, or ALT/AST >1.5 times the upper limit of normal (ULN); discontinue treatment in patients who develop an ANC <500/mm^3, platelet count <50,000/mm^3, or ALT/AST >5 x ULN.

Due to higher incidence of serious infections, concomitant use with other biological DMARDs (eg, TNF blockers, IL-1 receptor blockers, anti-CD20 monoclonal antibodies, selective costimulation modulators) should be avoided. Cautious use is recommended in elderly patients due to an increased incidence of serious infections.

Adverse Reactions (Reflective of adult population; not specific for elderly) Incidence as reported for monotherapy, except where noted. Combination therapy refers to use in rheumatoid arthritis with nonbiological DMARDs or use in SJIA in trials where most patients (~70%) were taking methotrexate at baseline.

>10%: Hepatic: ALT increased (≤36%; grades 3/4: <1%), AST increased (≤22%; grades 3/4: <1%)

1% to 10%:

Cardiovascular: Hypertension (1% to 6%), peripheral edema (<2%)

Central nervous system: Headache (1% to 7%), dizziness (3%)

Dermatologic: Rash (2%), skin reaction (combination therapy; 1% [includes pruritus, urticaria])

Endocrine & metabolic: LDL cholesterol increased (>1.5-2 x ULN; combination therapy; children 2%), total cholesterol increased (>1.5-2 x ULN; combination therapy; children 2%), hypothyroidism (<2%)

Gastrointestinal: Diarrhea (children ≤5%), abdominal pain (2%), mouth ulceration (2%), gastric ulcer (<2%), stomatitis (<2%), weight gain (<2%), gastritis (1%)

Hematologic: Neutropenia (combination therapy; grade 3: 2% to 7%; grade 4: <1%), thrombocytopenia (combination therapy; 1% to 2%), leukopenia (<2%)

Hepatic: Bilirubin increased (<2%)

Local: Infusion-related reactions (combination therapy; 4% to 16%)

Ocular: Conjunctivitis (<2%)

Renal: Nephrolithiasis (<2%)

Respiratory: Upper respiratory tract infection (7%), nasopharyngitis (7%), bronchitis (3%), cough (<2%), dyspnea (<2%)

Miscellaneous: Anti-tocilizumab antibody formation (2%), herpes simplex (<2%)

TOCILIZUMAB

Drug Interactions
Metabolism/Transport Effects None known.
Avoid Concomitant Use
Avoid concomitant use of Tocilizumab with any of the following: BCG; Belimumab; Natalizumab; Pimecrolimus; Tacrolimus (Topical); Vaccines (Live)
Increased Effect/Toxicity
Tocilizumab may increase the levels/effects of: Belimumab; Leflunomide; Natalizumab; Vaccines (Live)

The levels/effects of Tocilizumab may be increased by: Abciximab; Denosumab; Pimecrolimus; Roflumilast; Tacrolimus (Topical); Trastuzumab
Decreased Effect
Tocilizumab may decrease the levels/effects of: BCG; Coccidioidin Skin Test; CYP3A4 Substrates; Sipuleucel-T; Vaccines (Inactivated); Vaccines (Live)

The levels/effects of Tocilizumab may be decreased by: Echinacea
Stability Store unopened vials at 2°C to 8°C (36°F to 46°F); do not freeze. Protect from light. Prior to administration, dilute to 50 mL (children <30 kg) or 100 mL (children ≥30 kg and adults) using 0.9% sodium chloride. Diluted solutions may be stored under refrigeration or at room temperature for up to 24 hours and are compatible with polypropylene, polyethylene (PE), polyvinyl chloride (PVC), and glass infusion containers.
Mechanism of Action Antagonist of the interleukin-6 (IL-6) receptor. Endogenous IL-6 is induced by inflammatory stimuli and mediates a variety of immunological responses. Inhibition of IL-6 receptors by tocilizumab leads to a reduction in cytokine and acute phase reactant production.
Pharmacodynamics/Kinetics
Distribution: V_{dss}: Adults: 6.4 L
Half life elimination: Terminal, single dose: 6.3 days (concentration-dependent; may be increased up to 13 days [adults] at steady state)
Dosage
Adult Rheumatoid arthritis: I.V.: Initial: 4 mg/kg every 4 weeks; may be increased to 8 mg/kg based on clinical response (maximum: 800 mg per infusion).
Renal Impairment
Mild renal impairment: No dosage adjustment required.
Moderate-to-severe renal impairment: Limited experience; no specific dosage adjustment recommended by the manufacturer.
Hepatic Impairment Not recommended for use in patients with active hepatic disease or hepatic impairment.
Administration I.V.: Allow diluted solution to reach room temperature prior to administration; infuse over 60 minutes using a dedicated I.V. line. Do not infuse other agents through same I.V. line. Do not administer I.V. push or I.V. bolus. Do not use if opaque particles or discoloration is visible.
Monitoring Parameters Signs and symptoms of infection (prior to and during therapy); latent TB screening prior to therapy initiation; CBC with differential (prior to and every 2-4 weeks [SJIA] or 4-8 weeks [RA] during therapy); ALT/AST (prior to and every 2-4 weeks [SJIA] or 4-8 weeks [RA] during therapy); additional liver function tests (eg, bilirubin) as clinically indicated; lipid panel (prior to, at 4-8 weeks following initiation, and every ~6 months during therapy); signs and symptoms of CNS demyelinating disorders
Special Geriatric Considerations Due to higher infection rate in elderly, this medication should be used cautiously and patients should be monitored closely for infection. In clinical studies, patients over the age of 65 had a higher infection rate than those younger than 65 years of age.
Dosage Forms Excipient information presented when available (limited, particularly for generics); consult specific product labeling.
Injection, solution [preservative free]:
Actemra®: 20 mg/mL (4 mL, 10 mL, 20 mL) [contains polysorbate 80, sucrose 50 mg/mL]

♦ **Tofranil®** *see* Imipramine *on page 979*
♦ **Tofranil-PM®** *see* Imipramine *on page 979*

TOLAZamide (tole AZ a mide)

Related Information
Diabetes Mellitus Management, Adults *on page 2193*
Medication Safety Issues
Sound-alike/look-alike issues:
TOLAZamide may be confused with TOLBUTamide
Tolinase® may be confused with Orinase

High alert medication:
The Institute for Safe Medication Practices (ISMP) includes this medication among its list of drugs which have a heightened risk of causing significant patient harm when used in error.

Generic Availability (U.S.) Yes

Pharmacologic Category Antidiabetic Agent, Sulfonylurea

Use Adjunct to diet for the management of mild-to-moderately severe, stable, type 2 diabetes mellitus (noninsulin dependent, NIDDM)

Contraindications Hypersensitivity to tolazamide, sulfonylureas, or any component of the formulation; type 1 diabetes mellitus (insulin dependent, IDDM) therapy; diabetic ketoacidosis

Warnings/Precautions All sulfonylurea drugs are capable of producing severe hypoglycemia. Hypoglycemia is more likely to occur when caloric intake is deficient, after severe or prolonged exercise, when ethanol is ingested, or when more than one glucose-lowering drug is used. It is also more likely in elderly patients, malnourished patients and in patients with impaired renal or hepatic function; use with caution.

Loss of efficacy may be observed following prolonged use as a result of the progression of type 2 diabetes mellitus which results in continued beta cell destruction. In patients who were previously responding to sulfonylurea therapy, consider additional factors which may be contributing to decreased efficacy (eg, inappropriate dose, nonadherence to diet and exercise regimen). If no contributing factors can be identified, consider discontinuing use of the sulfonylurea due to secondary failure of treatment. Additional antidiabetic therapy (eg, insulin) will be required. It may be necessary to discontinue therapy and administer insulin if the patient is exposed to stress (fever, trauma, infection, surgery).

Chemical similarities are present among sulfonamides, sulfonylureas, carbonic anhydrase inhibitors, thiazides, and loop diuretics (except ethacrynic acid). Use in patients with sulfonylurea allergy is specifically contraindicated in product labeling, however, a risk of cross-reaction exists in patients with allergy to any of these compounds; avoid use when previous reaction has been severe. Patients with G6PD deficiency may be at an increased risk of sulfonylurea-induced hemolytic anemia; however, cases have also been described in patients without G6PD deficiency during postmarketing surveillance. Use with caution and consider a nonsulfonylurea alternative in patients with G6PD deficiency.

Product labeling states oral hypoglycemic drugs may be associated with an increased cardiovascular mortality as compared to treatment with diet alone or diet plus insulin. Data to support this association are limited, and several studies, including a large prospective trial (UKPDS) have not supported an association.

Adverse Reactions (Reflective of adult population; not specific for elderly) Frequency not defined.

Central nervous system: Dizziness, fatigue, headache, malaise, vertigo

Dermatologic: Maculopapular eruptions, morbilliform eruptions, photosensitivity, pruritus, rash, urticaria

Endocrine & metabolic: Disulfiram-like reaction, hypoglycemia, hyponatremia, SIADH

Gastrointestinal: Anorexia, constipation, diarrhea, epigastric fullness, heartburn, nausea, vomiting

Hematologic: Agranulocytosis, aplastic anemia, hemolytic anemia, leukopenia, pancytopenia, porphyria cutanea tarda, thrombocytopenia

Hepatic: Cholestatic jaundice, hepatic porphyria

Neuromuscular & skeletal: Weakness

Renal: Diuretic effect

Drug Interactions

Metabolism/Transport Effects None known.

Avoid Concomitant Use There are no known interactions where it is recommended to avoid concomitant use.

Increased Effect/Toxicity

TOLAZamide may increase the levels/effects of: Alcohol (Ethyl); Hypoglycemic Agents; Porfimer; Vitamin K Antagonists

The levels/effects of TOLAZamide may be increased by: Beta-Blockers; Chloramphenicol; Cimetidine; Cyclic Antidepressants; Fibric Acid Derivatives; Fluconazole; GLP-1 Agonists; Herbs (Hypoglycemic Properties); MAO Inhibitors; Pegvisomant; Probenecid; Quinolone Antibiotics; Ranitidine; Salicylates; Selective Serotonin Reuptake Inhibitors; Sulfonamide Derivatives; Vitamin K Antagonists; Voriconazole

Decreased Effect

The levels/effects of TOLAZamide may be decreased by: Corticosteroids (Orally Inhaled); Corticosteroids (Systemic); Loop Diuretics; Luteinizing Hormone-Releasing Hormone Analogs; Quinolone Antibiotics; Rifampin; Somatropin; Thiazide Diuretics

Ethanol/Nutrition/Herb Interactions

Ethanol: Avoid ethanol (possible disulfiram-like reaction).

Herb/Nutraceutical: Herbs with hypoglycemic properties may enhance the hypoglycemic effect of tolazamide. This includes alfalfa, aloe, bilberry, bitter melon, burdock, celery, damiana, fenugreek, garcinia, garlic, ginger, ginseng (American), gymnema, marshmallow, stinging nettle.

Mechanism of Action Stimulates insulin release from the pancreatic beta cells; reduces glucose output from the liver; insulin sensitivity is increased at peripheral target sites

Pharmacodynamics/Kinetics

Onset of hypoglycemic effect: 20 minutes

Peak hypoglycemic effect: 4-6 hours

Duration: 10-24 hours

Absorption: Rapid

Protein binding: 94%

Metabolism: Extensively hepatic to 5 metabolites (activity 0% to 70%)

Half-life elimination: 7 hours

Time to peak, serum: 3-4 hours

Excretion: Urine (85%); feces (7%)

Dosage

Geriatric & Adult

Type 2 diabetes: Oral (doses >500 mg/day should be given in 2 divided doses):

Initial: 100-250 mg/day with breakfast or the first main meal of the day

Fasting blood sugar <200 mg/dL: 100 mg/day

Fasting blood sugar >200 mg/dL: 250 mg/day

Patient is malnourished, underweight, elderly, or not eating properly: 100 mg/day

Adjustment/titration: Increase in increments of 100-250 mg/day at weekly intervals to response; maximum daily dose: 1 g (doses >1 g/day are not likely to improve control)

Conversion from insulin to tolazamide:

<20 units day = 100 mg/day

21-<40 units/day = 250 mg/day

≥40 units/day = 250 mg/day and 50% of insulin dose

Renal Impairment Conservative initial and maintenance doses are recommended because tolazamide is metabolized to active metabolites, which are eliminated in the urine.

Hepatic Impairment Conservative initial and maintenance doses and careful monitoring of blood glucose are recommended.

Monitoring Parameters Signs and symptoms of hypoglycemia (fatigue, sweating, numbness of extremities); blood glucose; hemoglobin A_{1c}

Reference Range

Recommendations for glycemic control in adults with diabetes:

Hb A_{1c}: <7%

Preprandial capillary plasma glucose: 70-130 mg/dL

Peak postprandial capillary blood glucose: <180 mg/dL

Blood pressure: <130/80 mm Hg

Recommendations for glycemic control in older adults with diabetes:

Relatively healthy, cognitively intact, and with a ≥5-year life expectancy: See Adults

Frail, life expectancy <5-years or those for whom the risks of intensive glucose control outweigh the benefits:

Hb A_{1c}: <8% to 9%

Blood pressure: <140/80 mm Hg or <130/80 mm Hg if tolerated

Pharmacotherapy Pearls Transferring a patient from one sulfonylurea to another does not require a priming dose; doses >1000 mg/day normally do not improve diabetic control.

Special Geriatric Considerations Has not been studied in elderly patients; however, except for drug interactions, it appears to have a safe profile and decline in renal function does not affect its pharmacokinetics. Intensive glucose control (Hb A_{1c} <6.5%) has been linked to increased all-cause and cardiovascular mortality, hypoglycemia requiring assistance, and weight gain in adult type 2 diabetes. How "tightly" to control a geriatric patient's blood glucose needs to be individualized. Such a decision should be based on several factors, including the patient's functional and cognitive status, how well he/she recognizes hypoglycemic or hyperglycemic symptoms, and how to respond to them and other disease states. An Hb A_{1c} <7.5% is an acceptable endpoint for a healthy older adult, while <8% is acceptable for frail elderly patients, those with a duration of illness >10 years, or those with comorbid conditions and requiring combination diabetes medications. For elderly patients with diabetes who are relatively healthy, attaining target goals for aspirin use, blood pressure, lipids, smoking cessation, and diet and exercise may be more important than normalized glycemic control.

Dosage Forms Excipient information presented when available (limited, particularly for generics); consult specific product labeling.

Tablet, oral: 250 mg, 500 mg

TOLBUTamide (tole BYOO ta mide)

Related Information
Diabetes Mellitus Management, Adults on page 2193
Medication Safety Issues
.**Sound-alike/look-alike issues:**
TOLBUTamide may be confused with terbutaline, TOLAZamide
Orinase may be confused with Orabase®, Ornex®, Tolinase®
High alert medication:
The Institute for Safe Medication Practices (ISMP) includes this medication among its list of drugs which have a heightened risk of causing significant patient harm when used in error.
Brand Names: Canada Apo-Tolbutamide®
Index Terms Orinase; Tolbutamide Sodium
Generic Availability (U.S.) Yes
Pharmacologic Category Antidiabetic Agent, Sulfonylurea
Use Adjunct to diet for the management of type 2 diabetes mellitus (noninsulin dependent, NIDDM)
Contraindications Hypersensitivity to tolbutamide, sulfonylureas, or any component of the formulation; treatment of type 1 diabetes; diabetic ketoacidosis
Warnings/Precautions All sulfonylurea drugs are capable of producing severe hypoglycemia. Hypoglycemia is more likely to occur when caloric intake is deficient, after severe or prolonged exercise, when ethanol is ingested, or when more than one glucose-lowering drug is used. It is also more likely in elderly patients, malnourished patients and in patients with impaired renal or hepatic function; use with caution.

Loss of efficacy may be observed following prolonged use as a result of the progression of type 2 diabetes mellitus which results in continued beta cell destruction. In patients who were previously responding to sulfonylurea therapy, consider additional factors which may be contributing to decreased efficacy (eg, inappropriate dose, nonadherence to diet and exercise regimen). If no contributing factors can be identified, consider discontinuing use of the sulfonylurea due to secondary failure of treatment. Additional antidiabetic therapy (eg, insulin) will be required. It may be necessary to discontinue therapy and administer insulin if the patient is exposed to stress (fever, trauma, infection, surgery).

Chemical similarities are present among sulfonamides, sulfonylureas, carbonic anhydrase inhibitors, thiazides, and loop diuretics (except ethacrynic acid). Use in patients with sulfonylurea allergy is specifically contraindicated in product labeling, however, a risk of cross-reaction exists in patients with allergy to any of these compounds; avoid use when previous reaction has been severe. Patients with G6PD deficiency may be at an increased risk of sulfonylurea-induced hemolytic anemia; however, cases have also been described in patients without G6PD deficiency during postmarketing surveillance. Use with caution and consider a nonsulfonylurea alternative in patients with G6PD deficiency.

Product labeling states oral hypoglycemic drugs may be associated with an increased cardiovascular mortality as compared to treatment with diet alone or diet plus insulin. Data to support this association are limited, and several studies, including a large prospective trial (UKPDS) have not supported an association.
Adverse Reactions (Reflective of adult population; not specific for elderly) Frequency not defined.
Central nervous system: Headache
Dermatologic: Erythema, maculopapular rash, morbilliform rash, pruritus, urticaria, photosensitivity
Endocrine & metabolic: Disulfiram-like reactions, hypoglycemia, hyponatremia, SIADH
Gastrointestinal: Epigastric fullness, heartburn, nausea, taste alteration
Hematologic: Agranulocytosis, aplastic anemia, hemolytic anemia, leukopenia, pancytopenia, thrombocytopenia
Hepatic: Cholestatic jaundice, hepatic porphyria, porphyria cutanea tarda
Miscellaneous: Hypersensitivity reaction
Drug Interactions
Metabolism/Transport Effects Substrate of CYP2C19 (minor), CYP2C9 (major); **Note:** Assignment of Major/Minor substrate status based on clinically relevant drug interaction potential; **Inhibits** CYP2C8 (weak), CYP2C9 (strong)
Avoid Concomitant Use There are no known interactions where it is recommended to avoid concomitant use.
Increased Effect/Toxicity
TOLBUTamide may increase the levels/effects of: Alcohol (Ethyl); CYP2C9 Substrates; Diclofenac; Hypoglycemic Agents; Leflunomide; Porfimer; Vitamin K Antagonists

TOLBUTAMIDE

The levels/effects of TOLBUTamide may be increased by: Beta-Blockers; Chloramphenicol; Cimetidine; Cyclic Antidepressants; CYP2C9 Inhibitors (Moderate); CYP2C9 Inhibitors (Strong); Fibric Acid Derivatives; Fluconazole; GLP-1 Agonists; Herbs (Hypoglycemic Properties); Leflunomide; MAO Inhibitors; Mifepristone; Pegvisomant; Probenecid; Quinolone Antibiotics; Ranitidine; Salicylates; Selective Serotonin Reuptake Inhibitors; Sulfonamide Derivatives; Vitamin K Antagonists; Voriconazole

Decreased Effect

The levels/effects of TOLBUTamide may be decreased by: Aprepitant; Corticosteroids (Orally Inhaled); Corticosteroids (Systemic); CYP2C9 Inducers (Strong); Fosaprepitant; Loop Diuretics; Luteinizing Hormone-Releasing Hormone Analogs; Peginterferon Alfa-2b; Quinolone Antibiotics; Rifampin; Somatropin; Thiazide Diuretics

Ethanol/Nutrition/Herb Interactions

Ethanol: Avoid ethanol (possible disulfiram-like reaction).

Herb/Nutraceutical: Herbs with hypoglycemic properties may enhance the hypoglycemic effect of tolbutamide. This includes alfalfa, aloe, bilberry, bitter melon, burdock, celery, damiana, fenugreek, garcinia, garlic, ginger, ginseng (American), gymnema, marshmallow, stinging nettle.

Mechanism of Action Stimulates insulin release from the pancreatic beta cells; reduces glucose output from the liver; insulin sensitivity is increased at peripheral target sites, suppression of glucagon may also contribute

Pharmacodynamics/Kinetics

Onset of action: 1 hour

Duration: Oral: 6-24 hours

Absorption: Oral: Rapid

Distribution: V_d: 0.15 L/kg

Protein binding: ~95% (concentration dependent)

Metabolism: Hepatic via CYP2C9 to hydroxymethyltolbutamide (mildly active) and carboxytolbutamide (inactive); metabolism does not appear to be affected by age

Half-life elimination: 4.5-6.5 hours (range: 4-25 hours)

Time to peak, serum: 3-4 hours

Excretion: Urine (75% to 85% primarily as metabolites); feces

Dosage

Geriatric Initial: 250 mg 1-3 times/day; usual: 500-2000 mg; maximum: 3 g/day

Adult Type 2 diabetes: Oral: Initial: 1-2 g/day as a single dose in the morning or in divided doses throughout the day. Maintenance dose: 0.25-3 g/day; however, a maintenance dose >2 g/day is seldom required. **Note:** Divided doses may improve gastrointestinal tolerance

Renal Impairment Adjustment is not necessary.

Hemodialysis: Not dialyzable (0% to 5%)

Hepatic Impairment Reduced dose may be necessary.

Administration Oral: Entire dose can be administered in AM, divided doses may improve GI tolerance

Monitoring Parameters Blood glucose, hemoglobin A_{1c}; signs and symptoms of hypoglycemia

Reference Range

Recommendations for glycemic control in adults with diabetes:

Hb A_{1c}: <7%

Preprandial capillary plasma glucose: 70-130 mg/dL

Peak postprandial capillary blood glucose: <180 mg/dL

Blood pressure: <130/80 mm Hg

Recommendations for glycemic control in older adults with diabetes:

Relatively healthy, cognitively intact, and with a ≥5-year life expectancy: See Adults

Frail, life expectancy <5-years or those for whom the risks of intensive glucose control outweigh the benefits:

Hb A_{1c}: <8% to 9%

Blood pressure: <140/80 mm Hg or <130/80 mm Hg if tolerated

Special Geriatric Considerations Because of its low potency and short duration, it is a useful agent in the elderly if drug interactions can be avoided. Intensive glucose control (Hb A_{1c} <6.5%) has been linked to increased all-cause and cardiovascular mortality, hypoglycemia requiring assistance, and weight gain in adult type 2 diabetes. How "tightly" to control a geriatric patient's blood glucose needs to be individualized. Such a decision should be based on several factors, including the patient's functional and cognitive status, how well he/she recognizes hypoglycemic or hyperglycemic symptoms, and how to respond to them and other disease states. An Hb A_{1c} <7.5% is an acceptable endpoint for a healthy older adult, while <8% is acceptable for frail elderly patients, those with a duration of illness >10 years, or those with comorbid conditions and requiring combination diabetes medications. For elderly patients with diabetes who are relatively healthy, attaining target goals for aspirin use, blood pressure, lipids, smoking cessation, and diet and exercise may be more important than normalized glycemic control.

Dosage Forms Excipient information presented when available (limited, particularly for generics); consult specific product labeling.

Tablet, oral: 500 mg

◆ **Tolbutamide Sodium** see TOLBUTamide on page 1923

Tolcapone (TOLE ka pone)

Related Information

Antiparkinsonian Agents on page 2101

Brand Names: U.S. Tasmar®

Generic Availability (U.S.) No

Pharmacologic Category Anti-Parkinson's Agent, COMT Inhibitor

Use Adjunct to levodopa and carbidopa for the treatment of signs and symptoms of idiopathic Parkinson's disease in patients with motor fluctuations not responsive to other therapies

Prescribing and Access Restrictions A patient signed consent form acknowledging the risks of hepatic injury should be obtained by the treating physician.

Contraindications Hypersensitivity to tolcapone or any component of the formulation; history of liver disease or tolcapone-induced hepatocellular injury; nontraumatic rhabdomyolysis or hyperpyrexia and confusion

Warnings/Precautions [U.S. Boxed Warning]: Due to reports of fatal liver injury associated with use of this drug, the manufacturer is advising that tolcapone be reserved for patients who are experiencing inadequate symptom control or who are not appropriate candidates for other available treatments. Patients must provide written consent acknowledging the risks of hepatic injury. Liver disease should be excluded prior to initiation; laboratory monitoring is recommended. Discontinue if signs and/or symptoms of hepatic injury are noted (eg, transaminases >2 times upper limit of normal) or if clinical improvement is not evident after 3 weeks of therapy. Use with caution in patients with pre-existing dyskinesias; exacerbation of pre-existing dyskinesia and severe rhabdomyolysis has been reported. Levodopa dosage reduction may be required, particularly in patients with levodopa dosages >600 mg daily or with moderate-to-severe dyskinesia prior to initiation.

May cause orthostatic hypotension and syncope; Parkinson's disease patients appear to have an impaired capacity to respond to a postural challenge; use with caution in patients at risk of hypotension (such as those receiving antihypertensive drugs) or where transient hypotensive episodes would be poorly tolerated (cardiovascular disease or cerebrovascular disease). Parkinson's patients being treated with dopaminergic agonists ordinarily require careful monitoring for signs and symptoms of postural hypotension, especially during dose escalation, and should be informed of this risk. May cause hallucinations, which may improve with reduction in levodopa therapy. Use with caution in patients with lower gastrointestinal disease or an increased risk of dehydration; tolcapone has been associated with delayed development of diarrhea (onset after 2-12 weeks).

Tolcapone, in conjunction with other drug therapy that alters brain biogenic amine concentrations (eg, MAO inhibitors, SSRIs), has been associated with a syndrome resembling neuroleptic malignant syndrome (hyperpyrexia and confusion - some fatal) on abrupt withdrawal or dosage reduction. Concomitant use of tolcapone and nonselective MAO inhibitors should be avoided. Selegiline is a selective MAO type B inhibitor (when given orally at ≤10 mg/day) and can be taken with tolcapone. Dopaminergic agents have been associated with compulsive behaviors and/or loss of impulse control, which has manifested as pathological gambling, libido increases (hypersexuality), and/or binge eating. Causality has not been established, and controversy exists as to whether this phenomenon is related to the underlying disease, prior behaviors/addictions and/or drug therapy. Dose reduction or discontinuation of therapy has been reported to reverse these behaviors in some, but not all cases. Risk for melanoma development is increased in Parkinson's disease patients; drug causation or factors contributing to risk have not been established. Patients should be monitored closely and periodic skin examinations should be performed. Dopaminergic agents from the ergot class have also been associated with fibrotic complications, such as retroperitoneal fibrosis, pulmonary infiltrates or effusion and pleural thickening. It is unknown whether non-ergot, pro-dopaminergic agents like tolcapone confer this risk. Use caution in patients with hepatic impairment or severe renal impairment.

Adverse Reactions (Reflective of adult population; not specific for elderly)

>10%:

Cardiovascular: Orthostatic hypotension (17%)

Central nervous system: Somnolence (14% to 32%), sleep disorder (24% to 25%), hallucinations (8% to 24%), excessive dreaming (16% to 21%), dizziness (6% to 13%), headache (10% to 11%), confusion (10% to 11%)

Gastrointestinal: Nausea (28% to 50%), diarrhea (16% to 34%; approximately 3% to 4% severe), anorexia (19% to 23%)

Neuromuscular & skeletal: Dyskinesia (42% to 51%), dystonia (19% to 22%), muscle cramps (17% to 18%)

1% to 10%:

Cardiovascular: Syncope (4% to 5%), chest pain (1% to 3%), hypotension (2%), palpitation

Central nervous system: Fatigue (3% to 7%), loss of balance (2% to 3%), agitation (1%), euphoria (1%), hyperactivity (1%), malaise (1%), panic reaction (1%), irritability (1%), mental deficiency (1%), fever (1%), depression, hypoesthesia, tremor, speech disorder, vertigo, emotional lability, hyperkinesia

Dermatologic: Alopecia (1%), bleeding (1%), tumor (1%), rash

Gastrointestinal: Vomiting (8% to 10%), constipation (6% to 8%), xerostomia (5% to 6%), abdominal pain (5% to 6%), dyspepsia (3% to 4%), flatulence (2% to 4%)

Genitourinary: UTI (5%), hematuria (4% to 5%), urine discoloration (2% to 3%), urination disorder (1% to 2%), uterine tumor (1%), incontinence, impotence

Hepatic: Transaminases increased (1% to 3%; 3 times ULN, usually with first 6 months of therapy)

Neuromuscular & skeletal: Paresthesia (1% to 3%), hyper-/hypokinesia (1% to 3%), arthritis (1% to 2%), neck pain (2%), stiffness (2%), myalgia, rhabdomyolysis

Ocular: Cataract (1%), eye inflammation (1%)

Otic: Tinnitus

Respiratory: Upper respiratory infection (5% to 7%), dyspnea (3%), sinus congestion (1% to 2%), bronchitis, pharyngitis

Miscellaneous: Diaphoresis (4% to 7%), influenza (3% to 4%), burning (1% to 2%), flank pain, injury, infection

Drug Interactions

Metabolism/Transport Effects Inhibits COMT, CYP2C9 (weak)

Avoid Concomitant Use

Avoid concomitant use of Tolcapone with any of the following: Azelastine; Azelastine (Nasal); Methadone; Mirtazapine; Paraldehyde

Increased Effect/Toxicity

Tolcapone may increase the levels/effects of: Alcohol (Ethyl); Azelastine; Azelastine (Nasal); Buprenorphine; CNS Depressants; COMT Substrates; MAO Inhibitors; Methadone; Methotrimeprazine; Metyrosine; Mirtazapine; Paraldehyde; Selective Serotonin Reuptake Inhibitors; Zolpidem

The levels/effects of Tolcapone may be increased by: Droperidol; HydrOXYzine; MAO Inhibitors; Methotrimeprazine

Decreased Effect There are no known significant interactions involving a decrease in effect.

Ethanol/Nutrition/Herb Interactions

Ethanol: May increase CNS depression; monitor for increased effects with coadministration. Caution patients about effects.

Food: Tolcapone, taken with food within 1 hour before or 2 hours after the dose, decreases bioavailability by 10% to 20%.

Avoid valerian, St John's wort, kava kava, gotu kola (may increase CNS depression).

Stability Store at 20°C to 25°C (68°F to 77°F).

Mechanism of Action Tolcapone is a selective and reversible inhibitor of catechol-o-methyltransferase (COMT). In the presence of a decarboxylase inhibitor (eg, carbidopa), COMT is the major degradation pathway for levodopa. Inhibition of COMT leads to more sustained plasma levels of levodopa and enhanced central dopaminergic activity.

Pharmacodynamics/Kinetics

Absorption: Rapid

Distribution: 9 L

Protein binding: >99.0%

Metabolism: Hepatic, via glucuronidation, to inactive metabolite (>99%)

Bioavailability: 65%

Half-life elimination: 2-3 hours

Time to peak: ~2 hours

Excretion: Urine (60% as metabolites, 0.5% as unchanged drug); feces (40%)

Dosage

Geriatric & Adult Note: If clinical improvement is not observed after 3 weeks of therapy (regardless of dose), tolcapone treatment should be discontinued.

Parkinson's Disease: Oral: Initial: 100 mg 3 times/day; may increase as tolerated to 200 mg 3 times/day. **Note:** Levodopa dose may need to be decreased upon initiation of tolcapone (average reduction in clinical trials was 30%). As many as 70% of patients receiving levodopa doses >600 mg daily required levodopa dosage reduction in clinical trials. Patients with moderate-to-severe dyskinesia prior to initiation are also more likely to require dosage reduction.

Renal Impairment No adjustment necessary for mild-moderate impairment. Use caution with severe impairment; no safety information available in patients with Cl_{cr} <25 mL/minute.

Hepatic Impairment Do not use. Discontinue immediately if signs/symptoms of hepatic impairment develop.

Administration May be administered with or without food. In clinical studies, the first dose of the day was given with levodopa/carbidopa and the subsequent doses were given 6 hours and 12 hours later.

Monitoring Parameters Blood pressure, symptoms of Parkinson's disease, liver enzymes at baseline and then every 2-4 weeks for the first 6 months of therapy; thereafter, periodic monitoring should be conducted as deemed clinically relevant. If the dose is increased to 200 mg 3 times/day, reinitiate LFT monitoring every 2-4 weeks for 6 months, and then resume periodic monitoring. Discontinue therapy if the ALT or AST exceeds 2 times ULN or if the clinical signs and symptoms suggest the onset of liver failure.

Pharmacotherapy Pearls If no significant response in 3 weeks, discontinue tolcapone. Patient informed consent forms can be obtained from the manufacturer.

Special Geriatric Considerations No specific data in elderly patients, but based on the pharmacokinetic profile, no dosage adjustment appears necessary.

Dosage Forms Excipient information presented when available (limited, particularly for generics); consult specific product labeling. [DSC] = Discontinued product
Tablet, oral:
Tasmar®: 100 mg, 200 mg [DSC]

◆ **Tolectin** see Tolmetin on page 1927

Tolmetin (TOLE met in)

Related Information

Beers Criteria – Potentially Inappropriate Medications for Geriatrics on page 2183

Medication Safety Issues

BEERS Criteria medication:
This drug may be potentially inappropriate for use in geriatric patients (Quality of evidence - moderate; Strength of recommendation - strong).

Index Terms Tolectin; Tolmetin Sodium

Generic Availability (U.S.) Yes

Pharmacologic Category Nonsteroidal Anti-inflammatory Drug (NSAID), Oral

Use Treatment of rheumatoid arthritis and osteoarthritis, juvenile idiopathic arthritis (JIA)

Medication Guide Available Yes

Contraindications Hypersensitivity to tolmetin, aspirin, other NSAIDs, or any component of the formulation; perioperative pain in the setting of coronary artery bypass graft (CABG) surgery

Warnings/Precautions [U.S. Boxed Warning]: NSAIDs are associated with an increased risk of adverse cardiovascular thrombotic events, including MI and stroke. Risk may be increased with duration of use or pre-existing cardiovascular risk factors or disease. Carefully evaluate individual cardiovascular risk profiles prior to prescribing. May cause new-onset hypertension or worsening of existing hypertension. Use caution with fluid retention. Avoid use in heart failure. Concurrent administration of ibuprofen, and potentially other nonselective NSAIDs, may interfere with aspirin's cardioprotective effect. **[U.S. Boxed Warning]: Use is contraindicated for treatment of perioperative pain in the setting of coronary artery bypass graft (CABG) surgery.** Risk of MI and stroke may be increased with use following CABG surgery.

Platelet adhesion and aggregation may be decreased; may prolong bleeding time; patients with coagulation disorders or who are receiving anticoagulants should be monitored closely. Anemia may occur; patients on long-term NSAID therapy should be monitored for anemia. Rarely, NSAID use may cause severe blood dyscrasias (eg, agranulocytosis, aplastic anemia, thrombocytopenia).

NSAID use may compromise existing renal function; dose-dependent decreases in prostaglandin synthesis may result from NSAID use, reducing renal blood flow which may cause renal decompensation. NSAID use may increase the risk for hyperkalemia. Patients with impaired renal function, dehydration, heart failure, liver dysfunction, those taking diuretics, and ACE inhibitors, and the elderly are at greater risk of renal toxicity and hyperkalemia. Rehydrate patient before starting therapy; monitor renal function closely. Not recommended for use in patients with advanced renal disease. Long-term NSAID use may result in renal papillary necrosis. Acute interstitial nephritis and nephritic syndrome have been reported with tolmetin.

In the elderly, avoid chronic use (unless alternative agents ineffective and patient can receive concomitant gastroprotective agent); nonselective oral NSAID use is associated with an increased risk of GI bleeding and peptic ulcer disease in older adults in high risk category (eg, >75 years or age or receiving concomitant oral/parenteral corticosteroids, anticoagulants, or antiplatelet agents) (Beers Criteria).

[U.S. Boxed Warning]: NSAIDs may increase risk of gastrointestinal irritation, inflammation, ulceration, bleeding, and perforation. These events may occur at any time during therapy and without warning. Use caution with a history of GI disease (bleeding or ulcers), concurrent therapy with aspirin, anticoagulants and/or corticosteroids, smoking, use of alcohol, the elderly or debilitated patients. When used concomitantly with ≤325 mg of aspirin, a substantial increase in the risk of gastrointestinal complications (eg, ulcer) occurs; concomitant gastroprotective therapy (eg, proton pump inhibitors) is recommended (Bhatt, 2008).

Use the lowest effective dose for the shortest duration of time, consistent with individual patient goals, to reduce risk of cardiovascular or GI adverse events. Alternate therapies should be considered for patients at high risk.

NSAIDs may cause serious skin adverse events including exfoliative dermatitis, Stevens-Johnson syndrome (SJS) and toxic epidermal necrolysis (TEN); discontinue use at first sign of skin rash or hypersensitivity. Anaphylactoid reactions may occur, even without prior exposure; patients with "aspirin triad" (bronchial asthma, aspirin intolerance, rhinitis) may be at increased risk. Do not use in patients who experience bronchospasm, asthma, rhinitis, or urticaria with NSAID or aspirin therapy.

Use with caution in patients with decreased hepatic function. Closely monitor patients with any abnormal LFT. Severe hepatic reactions (eg, fulminant hepatitis, liver failure) have occurred with NSAID use, rarely; discontinue if signs or symptoms of liver disease develop, or if systemic manifestations occur.

NSAIDS may cause drowsiness, dizziness, blurred vision, and other neurologic effects which may impair physical or mental abilities; patients must be cautioned about performing tasks which require mental alertness (eg, operating machinery or driving). Discontinue use with blurred or diminished vision and perform ophthalmologic exam. Monitor vision with long-term therapy.

The elderly are at increased risk for adverse effects (especially peptic ulceration, CNS effects, renal toxicity) from NSAIDs even at low doses.

Withhold for at least 4-6 half-lives prior to surgical or dental procedures.

Adverse Reactions (Reflective of adult population; not specific for elderly)
>10%: Gastrointestinal: Nausea (11%)
1% to 10%:
 Cardiovascular: Edema (3% to 9%), hypertension (3% to 9%), chest pain (1% to 3%)
 Central nervous system: Dizziness (3% to 9%), headache (3% to 9%), depression (1% to 3%), drowsiness (1% to 3%)
 Dermatologic: Skin irritation (1% to 3%)
 Endocrine & metabolic: Weight gain/loss (3% to 9%)
 Gastrointestinal: Abdominal pain (3% to 9%), diarrhea (3% to 9%), dyspepsia (3% to 9%), flatulence (3% to 9%), gastrointestinal distress (3% to 9%), vomiting (3% to 9%), constipation (1% to 3%), gastritis (1% to 3%), peptic ulcer (1% to 3%)
 Genitourinary: Urinary tract infection (1% to 3%)
 Hematologic: Hemoglobin/hematocrit decreased (transient; 1% to 3%)
 Neuromuscular & skeletal: Weakness (3% to 9%)
 Ocular: Visual disturbances (1% to 3%)
 Otic: Tinnitus (1% to 3%)
 Renal: BUN increased (1% to 3%)
Drug Interactions
 Metabolism/Transport Effects None known.

Avoid Concomitant Use

Avoid concomitant use of Tolmetin with any of the following: Floctafenine; Ketorolac; Ketorolac (Nasal); Ketorolac (Systemic)

Increased Effect/Toxicity

Tolmetin may increase the levels/effects of: Aliskiren; Aminoglycosides; Anticoagulants; Antiplatelet Agents; Bisphosphonate Derivatives; Collagenase (Systemic); CycloSPORINE; CycloSPORINE (Systemic); Dabigatran Etexilate; Deferasirox; Desmopressin; Digoxin; Drotrecogin Alfa (Activated); Eplerenone; Haloperidol; Ibritumomab; Lithium; Methotrexate; Nonsteroidal Anti-Inflammatory Agents; PEMEtrexed; Porfimer; Potassium-Sparing Diuretics; PRALAtrexate; Quinolone Antibiotics; Rivaroxaban; Salicylates; Thrombolytic Agents; Tositumomab and Iodine I 131 Tositumomab; Vancomycin; Vitamin K Antagonists

The levels/effects of Tolmetin may be increased by: ACE Inhibitors; Angiotensin II Receptor Blockers; Antidepressants (Tricyclic, Tertiary Amine); Corticosteroids (Systemic); CycloSPORINE; CycloSPORINE (Systemic); Dasatinib; Floctafenine; Glucosamine; Herbs (Anticoagulant/Antiplatelet Properties); Ketorolac; Ketorolac (Nasal); Ketorolac (Systemic); Nonsteroidal Anti-Inflammatory Agents; Omega-3-Acid Ethyl Esters; Pentosan Polysulfate Sodium; Pentoxifylline; Probenecid; Prostacyclin Analogues; Selective Serotonin Reuptake Inhibitors; Serotonin/Norepinephrine Reuptake Inhibitors; Sodium Phosphates; Tipranavir; Treprostinil; Vitamin E

Decreased Effect

Tolmetin may decrease the levels/effects of: ACE Inhibitors; Aliskiren; Angiotensin II Receptor Blockers; Antiplatelet Agents; Beta-Blockers; Eplerenone; HydrALAZINE; Loop Diuretics; Potassium-Sparing Diuretics; Salicylates; Selective Serotonin Reuptake Inhibitors; Thiazide Diuretics

The levels/effects of Tolmetin may be decreased by: Bile Acid Sequestrants; Nonsteroidal Anti-Inflammatory Agents; Salicylates

Ethanol/Nutrition/Herb Interactions

Ethanol: Avoid ethanol (may enhance gastric mucosal irritation).

Food: Tolmetin peak serum concentrations may be decreased if taken with food or milk.

Herb/Nutraceutical: Avoid alfalfa, anise, bilberry, bladderwrack, bromelain, cat's claw, celery, chamomile, coleus, cordyceps, dong quai, evening primrose, fenugreek, feverfew, fenugreek, garlic, ginger, ginkgo biloba, ginseng (American, Panax, Siberian), grapeseed, green tea, guggul, horse chestnut seed, horseradish, licorice, prickly ash, red clover, reishi, SAMe (S-adenosylmethionine), sweet clover, turmeric, white willow (all have additional antiplatelet activity).

Stability Store at 15°C to 30°C (59°F to 86°F). Protect from light.

Mechanism of Action Reversibly inhibits cyclooxygenase-1 and 2 (COX-1 and 2) enzymes, which results in decreased formation of prostaglandin precursors; has antipyretic, analgesic, and anti-inflammatory properties.

Other proposed mechanisms not fully elucidated (and possibly contributing to the anti-inflammatory effect to varying degrees) include inhibiting chemotaxis, altering lymphocyte activity, inhibiting neutrophil aggregation/activation, and decreasing proinflammatory cytokine levels.

Pharmacodynamics/Kinetics

Onset of action: Analgesic: 1-2 hours; Anti-inflammatory: Days to weeks

Absorption: Well absorbed, rapid

Bioavailability: Reduced 16% with food or milk

Half-life elimination: Biphasic: Rapid: 1-2 hours; Slow: 5 hours

Time to peak, serum: 30-60 minutes

Excretion: Urine (as inactive metabolites or conjugates) within 24 hours

Dosage

Geriatric & Adult Inflammation, arthritis: Oral: 400 mg 3 times/day; usual dose: 600 mg to 1.8 g/day; maximum: 1.8 g/day

Monitoring Parameters Monitor CBC, liver enzymes, occult blood loss; monitor urine output and BUN/ serum creatinine in patients receiving diuretics and ACE inhibitors, monitor blood pressure in patients receiving antihypertensives

Test Interactions Increased protein, bleeding time; may interfere with urine detection of cannabinoids (false-positive)

Special Geriatric Considerations Elderly are a high-risk population for adverse effects from NSAIDs. As much as 60% of the elderly can develop peptic ulceration and/or hemorrhage asymptomatically. The concomitant use of H_2 blockers and sucralfate is not effective as prophylaxis with the exception of NSAID-induced duodenal ulcers which may be prevented by the use of ranitidine. Misoprostol and proton pump inhibitors are the only agents proven to help prevent the development of NSAID-induced ulcers. Also, concomitant disease and drug use contribute to the risk for GI adverse effects. Use lowest effective dose for shortest period possible. Consider renal function decline with age. Use of NSAIDs can compromise existing renal function especially when Cl_{cr} is ≤30 mL/minute. Tinnitus may be a difficult and unreliable indication of toxicity due to age-related hearing loss or eighth cranial nerve damage. CNS adverse effects such as confusion, agitation, and hallucination are generally seen in overdose or high dose situations, but elderly may demonstrate these adverse effects at lower doses than younger adults.

This medication is considered to be potentially inappropriate in this patient population (Beers Criteria: Quality of evidence - moderate; Strength of recommendation - strong).

Dosage Forms Excipient information presented when available (limited, particularly for generics); consult specific product labeling.

Capsule, oral: 400 mg

Tablet, oral: 200 mg, 600 mg

◆ **Tolmetin Sodium** *see* Tolmetin *on page* 1927

Tolnaftate (tole NAF tate)

Medication Safety Issues

Sound-alike/look-alike issues:

Tinactin® may be confused with Talacen

Brand Names: U.S. Blis-To-Sol® [OTC]; Mycocide® NS [OTC]; Podactin Powder [OTC]; Tinactin® Antifungal Deodorant [OTC]; Tinactin® Antifungal Jock Itch [OTC]; Tinactin® Antifungal [OTC]; Tinaderm [OTC]; Ting® Cream [OTC]; Ting® Spray Liquid [OTC]

Brand Names: Canada Pitrex

Generic Availability (U.S.) Yes: Cream, powder, solution

Pharmacologic Category Antifungal Agent, Topical

Use Treatment of tinea pedis, tinea cruris, tinea corporis

Contraindications Hypersensitivity to tolnaftate or any component of the formulation; nail and scalp infections

Warnings/Precautions For topical use only; avoid contact with eyes. Apply to clean, dry skin. When used for self-medication (OTC use), contact healthcare provider if condition does not improve within 4 weeks. Discontinue if sensitivity or irritation occurs.

Adverse Reactions (Reflective of adult population; not specific for elderly) Frequency not defined.

Dermatologic: Contact dermatitis, pruritus

Local: Irritation, stinging

Drug Interactions

Metabolism/Transport Effects None known.

Avoid Concomitant Use There are no known interactions where it is recommended to avoid concomitant use.

Increased Effect/Toxicity There are no known significant interactions involving an increase in effect.

Decreased Effect There are no known significant interactions involving a decrease in effect.

Mechanism of Action Distorts the hyphae and stunts mycelial growth in susceptible fungi

Pharmacodynamics/Kinetics Onset of action: 24-72 hours

Dosage

Geriatric & Adult Tinea infection: Topical: Wash and dry affected area; spray aerosol or apply 1-3 drops of solution or a small amount of cream, or powder and rub into the affected areas 2 times/day

Note: May use for up to 4 weeks for tinea pedis or tinea corporis, and up to 2 weeks for tinea cruris.

Monitoring Parameters Resolution of skin infection

Pharmacotherapy Pearls Usually not effective alone for the treatment of infections involving hair follicles or nails

Special Geriatric Considerations No specific recommendations for use in the elderly.

Dosage Forms Excipient information presented when available (limited, particularly for generics); consult specific product labeling.

Aerosol, powder, topical:

Tinactin® Antifungal: 1% (133 g) [contains ethanol 11% v/v, talc]

Tinactin® Antifungal Deodorant: 1% (133 g) [contains ethanol 11% v/v, talc]

Tinactin® Antifungal Jock Itch: 1% (133 g) [contains ethanol 11% v/v, talc]

Aerosol, spray, topical:

Tinactin® Antifungal: 1% (150 g) [contains ethanol 29% v/v]

Ting® Spray Liquid: 1% (128 g) [contains ethanol 41% w/w]

Cream, topical: 1% (15 g, 30 g, 114 g)
  Tinactin® Antifungal: 1% (15 g, 30 g)
  Tinactin® Antifungal Jock Itch: 1% (15 g)
  Ting® Cream: 1% (15 g)
Liquid, topical:
  Blis-To-Sol®: 1% (30 mL, 55 mL)
Liquid, topical [spray]:
  Tinactin® Antifungal: 1% (59 mL) [contains ethanol 70% v/v]
Powder, topical: 1% (45 g)
  Podactin Powder: 1% (60 g)
  Tinactin® Antifungal: 1% (108 g)
Solution, topical:
  Mycocide® NS: 1% (30 mL)
  Tinaderm: 1% (10 mL)

Tolterodine (tole TER oh deen)

Related Information
Beers Criteria – Potentially Inappropriate Medications for Geriatrics *on page 2183*
Pharmacotherapy of Urinary Incontinence *on page 2141*

Medication Safety Issues
Sound-alike/look-alike issues:
Tolterodine may be confused with fesoterodine
Detrol® may be confused with Ditropan

BEERS Criteria medication:
This drug may be potentially inappropriate for use in geriatric patients (Quality of evidence - varies based on comorbidity; Strength of recommendation - varies based on comorbidity)

Brand Names: U.S. Detrol®; Detrol® LA
Brand Names: Canada Detrol®; Detrol® LA; Unidet®
Index Terms Tolterodine Tartrate
Generic Availability (U.S.) Yes: Tablet
Pharmacologic Category Anticholinergic Agent
Use Treatment of patients with an overactive bladder with symptoms of urinary frequency, urgency, or urge incontinence
Contraindications Hypersensitivity to tolterodine or fesoterodine (both are metabolized to 5-hydroxymethyl tolterodine) or any component of the formulation; urinary retention; gastric retention; uncontrolled narrow-angle glaucoma
Warnings/Precautions Cases of angioedema have been reported with oral tolterodine; some cases have occurred after a single dose. Discontinue immediately if develops. May cause drowsiness and/or blurred vision, which may impair physical or mental abilities; patients must be cautioned about performing tasks which require mental alertness (eg, operating machinery or driving). Use with caution in patients with bladder flow obstruction, may increase the risk of urinary retention. Use with caution in patients with gastrointestinal obstructive disorders (ie, pyloric stenosis), may increase the risk of gastric retention. Use with caution in patients with myasthenia gravis and controlled (treated) narrow-angle glaucoma; metabolized in the liver and excreted in the urine and feces, dosage adjustment is required for patients with renal or hepatic impairment. Tolterodine has been associated with QT$_c$ prolongation at high (supratherapeutic) doses. The manufacturer recommends caution in patients with congenital prolonged QT or in patients receiving concurrent therapy with QT$_c$-prolonging drugs (class Ia or III antiarrhythmics). However, the mean change in QT$_c$ even at supratherapeutic dosages was less than 15 msec. Individuals who are CYP2D6 poor metabolizers or in the presence of inhibitors of CYP2D6 and CYP3A4 may be more likely to exhibit prolongation. Dosage adjustment is recommended in patients receiving CYP3A4 inhibitors (a lower dose of tolterodine is recommended). This medication is associated with potent anticholinergic properties which may be inappropriate in older adults depending on comorbidities (eg, dementia, delirium) (Beers Criteria).
Adverse Reactions (Reflective of adult population; not specific for elderly) As reported with immediate release tablet, unless otherwise specified
>10%: Gastrointestinal: Dry mouth (35%; extended release capsules 23%)
1% to 10%:
  Cardiovascular: Chest pain (2%)
  Central nervous system: Headache (7%; extended release capsules 6%), somnolence (3%; extended release capsules 3%), fatigue (4%; extended release capsules 2%), dizziness (5%; extended release capsules 2%), anxiety (extended release capsules 1%)
  Dermatologic: Dry skin (1%)

Gastrointestinal: Abdominal pain (5%; extended release capsules 4%), constipation (7%; extended release capsules 6%), dyspepsia (4%; extended release capsules 3%), diarrhea (4%), weight gain (1%)

Genitourinary: Dysuria (2%; extended release capsules 1%)

Neuromuscular & skeletal: Arthralgia (2%)

Ocular: Abnormal vision (2%; extended release capsules 1%), dry eyes (3%; extended release capsules 3%)

Respiratory: Bronchitis (2%), sinusitis (extended release capsules 2%)

Miscellaneous: Flu-like syndrome (3%), infection (1%)

Drug Interactions

Metabolism/Transport Effects Substrate of CYP2C19 (minor), CYP2C9 (minor), CYP2D6 (major), CYP3A4 (major); **Note:** Assignment of Major/Minor substrate status based on clinically relevant drug interaction potential

Avoid Concomitant Use There are no known interactions where it is recommended to avoid concomitant use.

Increased Effect/Toxicity

Tolterodine may increase the levels/effects of: AbobotulinumtoxinA; Anticholinergics; Cannabinoids; OnabotulinumtoxinA; Potassium Chloride; RimabotulinumtoxinB; Warfarin

The levels/effects of Tolterodine may be increased by: Abiraterone Acetate; Antifungal Agents (Azole Derivatives, Systemic); CYP2D6 Inhibitors (Moderate); CYP2D6 Inhibitors (Strong); CYP3A4 Inhibitors (Moderate); CYP3A4 Inhibitors (Strong); Dasatinib; Fluconazole; Ivacaftor; Mifepristone; Pramlintide; VinBLAStine

Decreased Effect

Tolterodine may decrease the levels/effects of: Acetylcholinesterase Inhibitors (Central); Secretin

The levels/effects of Tolterodine may be decreased by: Acetylcholinesterase Inhibitors (Central); CYP3A4 Inducers (Strong); Deferasirox; Herbs (CYP3A4 Inducers); Peginterferon Alfa-2b; Tocilizumab

Ethanol/Nutrition/Herb Interactions

Food: Increases bioavailability (~53% increase) of tolterodine tablets (dose adjustment not necessary); does not affect the pharmacokinetics of tolterodine extended release capsules. As a CYP3A4 inhibitor, grapefruit juice may increase the serum level and/or toxicity of tolterodine, but unlikely secondary to high oral bioavailability.

Herb/Nutraceutical: St John's wort (*Hypericum*) appears to induce CYP3A enzymes.

Stability Store at 25°C (77°F); excursions permitted to 15°C to 30°C (59°F to 86°F). Protect from light.

Mechanism of Action Tolterodine is a competitive antagonist of muscarinic receptors. In animal models, tolterodine demonstrates selectivity for urinary bladder receptors over salivary receptors. Urinary bladder contraction is mediated by muscarinic receptors. Tolterodine increases residual urine volume and decreases detrusor muscle pressure.

Pharmacodynamics/Kinetics

Absorption: Immediate release tablet: Rapid; ≥77%

Distribution: I.V.: V_d: 113 ± 27 L

Protein binding: >96% (primarily to alpha$_1$-acid glycoprotein)

Metabolism: Extensively hepatic, primarily via CYP2D6 to 5-hydroxymethyltolterodine (active) and 3A4 usually (minor pathway). In patients with a genetic deficiency of CYP2D6, metabolism via 3A4 predominates.

Bioavailability: Immediate release tablet: Increased 53% with food

Half-life elimination:

Immediate release tablet: Extensive metabolizers: ~2 hours; Poor metabolizers: ~10 hours

Extended release capsule: Extensive metabolizers: ~7 hours; Poor metabolizers: ~18 hours

Time to peak: Immediate release tablet: 1-2 hours; Extended release tablet: 2-6 hours

Excretion: Urine (77%); feces (17%); primarily as metabolites (<1% unchanged drug) of which the active 5-hydroxymethyl metabolite accounts for 5% to 14% (<1% in poor metabolizers); as unchanged drug (<1%; <2.5% in poor metabolizers)

Dosage

Geriatric & Adult Treatment of overactive bladder: Oral:

Immediate release tablet: 2 mg twice daily; the dose may be lowered to 1 mg twice daily based on individual response and tolerability

Dosing adjustment in patients concurrently taking CYP3A4 inhibitors: 1 mg twice daily

Extended release capsule: 4 mg once a day; dose may be lowered to 2 mg daily based on individual response and tolerability

Dosing adjustment in patients concurrently taking CYP3A4 inhibitors: 2 mg daily

Renal Impairment Use with caution (studies conducted in patients with Cl_{cr} 10-30 mL/minute):

Immediate release tablet: 1 mg twice daily
Extended release capsule: 2 mg daily

Hepatic Impairment

Immediate release tablet: 1 mg twice daily
Extended release capsule: 2 mg daily

Administration Extended release capsule: Swallow whole; do not crush, chew, or open

Monitoring Parameters Renal function (BUN, creatinine); hepatic function

Special Geriatric Considerations No difference in safety has been noted between elderly and younger patients, therefore, no dosage adjustment is recommended.

This medication is considered to be potentially inappropriate in this patient population (Beers Criteria: Quality of evidence - varies based on comorbidity; Strength of recommendation - varies based on comorbidity)

Dosage Forms Excipient information presented when available (limited, particularly for generics); consult specific product labeling.

Capsule, extended release, oral, as tartrate:
Detrol® LA: 2 mg, 4 mg
Tablet, oral, as tartrate: 1 mg, 2 mg
Detrol®: 1 mg, 2 mg

◆ **Tolterodine Tartrate** *see* Tolterodine *on page 1931*

Tolvaptan (tol VAP tan)

Brand Names: U.S. Samsca™
Brand Names: Canada Samsca™
Index Terms OPC-41061
Generic Availability (U.S.) No
Pharmacologic Category Vasopressin Antagonist

Use Treatment of clinically significant hypervolemic or euvolemic hyponatremia (associated with heart failure, cirrhosis, or SIADH) with either a serum sodium <125 mEq/L or less marked hyponatremia that is symptomatic and resistant to fluid restriction

Medication Guide Available Yes

Contraindications Hypovolemic hyponatremia; urgent need to raise serum sodium acutely; use in patients unable to sense or appropriately respond to thirst; anuria; concurrent use with strong CYP3A inhibitors (eg, ketoconazole, itraconazole, ritonavir, indinavir, nelfinavir, saquinavir, nefazodone, telithromycin, clarithromycin)

Canadian labeling: Additional contraindications (not in U.S. labeling): Hypersensitivity to tolvaptan or any component of the formulation

Warnings/Precautions [U.S. Boxed Warning]: Tolvaptan should be initiated and reinitiated in patients only in a hospital where serum sodium can be closely monitored. Too rapid correction of hyponatremia (ie, >12 mEq/L/24 hours) can cause osmotic demyelination resulting in dysarthria, mutism, dysphagia, lethargy, affective changes, spastic quadriparesis, seizures, coma, and death. In susceptible patients (including those with severe malnutrition, alcoholism, or advanced liver disease), slower rates of correction may be advisable. Patients with SIADH or very low baseline serum sodium concentrations may be at greater risk for overly-rapid correction.

Interrupt or discontinue therapy in patients who develop medically significant signs or symptoms of hypovolemia. Patients should ingest fluids in response to thirst. Gastrointestinal bleeding can occur in patients with cirrhosis; use only if the need to treat outweighs the risk. Reductions in extracellular fluid volumes may cause hyperkalemia. Patients with a pretreatment serum potassium >5 mEq/L should be monitored after initiation of therapy.

Use in patients with creatinine clearance <10 mL/minute has not been studied. Do not use in anuric patients. Use with hypertonic saline is not recommended. Use contraindicated in patients taking strong CYP3A inhibitors; avoid use in patients taking moderate CYP3A4 inhibitors. If possible, avoid use with CYP3A4 inducers; if administered with CYP3A4 inducers, dose increases may be necessary. Dose reductions may be necessary if administered with P-gp inhibitors. Consider alternative agents that avoid or lessen the potential for CYP- or P-gp mediated interactions. Patients receiving medications known to increase potassium should be monitored for hyperkalemia.

Monitor closely for rate of serum sodium increase and neurological status; rapid serum sodium correction (>12 mEq/L/24 hours) can lead to permanent neurological damage. Discontinue use if rate of serum sodium increase is undesirable; fluid restriction during the first 24 hours of sodium correction can increase the risk of overly-rapid correction and should generally be avoided; not intended for urgent correction of serum sodium to prevent or treat serious neurologic symptoms; it has not been demonstrated that raising serum sodium with tolvaptan provides a symptomatic benefit.

Adverse Reactions (Reflective of adult population; not specific for elderly)

>10%:
  Gastrointestinal: Nausea (21%), xerostomia (7% to 13%)
  Renal: Pollakiuria (4% to 11%), polyuria (4% to 11%)
  Miscellaneous: Thirst (12% to 16%)
2% to 10%:
  Central nervous system: Pyrexia (4%)
  Endocrine & metabolic: Hyperglycemia (6%)
  Gastrointestinal: Constipation (7%), anorexia (4%)
  Neuromuscular & skeletal: Weakness (9%)

Drug Interactions

Metabolism/Transport Effects Substrate of CYP3A4 (major), P-glycoprotein; **Note:** Assignment of Major/Minor substrate status based on clinically relevant drug interaction potential; **Inhibits** CYP3A4 (weak)

Avoid Concomitant Use
  Avoid concomitant use of Tolvaptan with any of the following: CYP3A4 Inducers (Strong); CYP3A4 Inhibitors (Moderate); CYP3A4 Inhibitors (Strong); Pimozide; Sodium Chloride

Increased Effect/Toxicity
  Tolvaptan may increase the levels/effects of: ACE Inhibitors; Angiotensin II Receptor Blockers; ARIPiprazole; Digoxin; Pimozide; Potassium-Sparing Diuretics

  The levels/effects of Tolvaptan may be increased by: CYP3A4 Inhibitors (Moderate); CYP3A4 Inhibitors (Strong); Dasatinib; Ivacaftor; Mifepristone; P-glycoprotein/ABCB1 Inhibitors; Sodium Chloride

Decreased Effect
  The levels/effects of Tolvaptan may be decreased by: CYP3A4 Inducers (Strong); Deferasirox; Herbs (CYP3A4 Inducers); P-glycoprotein/ABCB1 Inducers; Tocilizumab

Ethanol/Nutrition/Herb Interactions

Food: Tolvaptan exposure may be doubled when taken with grapefruit juice. Management: Avoid grapefruit juice.
Herb/Nutraceutical: St John's wort may decrease tolvaptan serum concentrations. Management: Avoid St John's wort.

Stability Store at 25°C (77°F); excursions permitted between 15°C and 30°C (59°F and 86°F).

Mechanism of Action An arginine vasopressin (AVP) receptor antagonist with affinity for AVP receptor subtypes V_2 and V_{1a} in a ratio of 29:1. Antagonism of the V_2 receptor by tolvaptan promotes the excretion of free water (without loss of serum electrolytes) resulting in net fluid loss, increased urine output, decreased urine osmolality, and subsequent restoration of normal serum sodium levels.

Pharmacodynamics/Kinetics

Onset of action: 2-4 hours
  Peak effect: 4-8 hours
Duration: 60% peak serum sodium elevation is retained at 24 hours; urinary excretion of free water is no longer elevated
Distribution: V_d: 3 L/kg
Protein binding: 99%
Metabolism: Hepatic via CYP3A4
Bioavailability: ~40%
Half-life elimination: 5-12 hours; dominant half-life <12 hours
Time to peak, plasma: 2-4 hours
Excretion: Feces

Dosage

Geriatric & Adult Hyponatremia: Oral: Initial: 15 mg once daily; after at least 24 hours, may increase to 30 mg once daily to a maximum of 60 mg once daily titrating at 24-hour intervals to desired serum sodium concentration.

Renal Impairment
  Cl_{cr} ≥10 mL/minute: No dosage adjustment necessary.
  Cl_{cr} <10 mL/minute: Use not recommended (not studied); contraindicated in anuria (no benefit expected).

Hepatic Impairment No dosage adjustment necessary.

Administration Treatment should be initiated or reinitiated in a hospital. May be administered without regards to meals.

Nasogastric (NG) tube: Administration via NG tube resulted in an ~25% reduction in AUC and a modest reduction in C_{max} in one study; 24-hour urine output was reduced by only 2.8%. Therefore, until further studies are done to determine a bioequivalent dose when administering via NG tube, NG tube administration of a crushed 15 mg tablet appears to be a viable alternative method of administration (McNeely, 2012).

Monitoring Parameters Serum sodium concentration, rate of serum sodium increase, serum potassium concentration (if >5 mEq/L prior to administration or receiving medications known to elevate serum potassium); volume status

Special Geriatric Considerations Age had no effect on plasma concentrations. In clinical trials, there was no significant difference in safety or efficacy in elderly versus younger patients.

Dosage Forms Excipient information presented when available (limited, particularly for generics); consult specific product labeling.

Tablet, oral:
Samsca™: 15 mg, 30 mg

Dosage Forms: Canada Excipient information presented when available (limited, particularly for generics); consult specific product labeling.

Tablet, oral:
Samsca™: 15 mg, 30 mg, 60 mg

◆ **Topamax®** see Topiramate on page 1935
◆ **TopCare® Junior Strength [OTC]** see Ibuprofen on page 966
◆ **Topicaine® [OTC]** see Lidocaine (Topical) on page 1128

Topiramate (toe PYRE a mate)

Medication Safety Issues
Sound-alike/look-alike issues:
Topamax® may be confused with Sporanox®, TEGretol®, TEGretol®-XR, Toprol-XL®

Brand Names: U.S. Topamax®

Brand Names: Canada Apo-Topiramate®; CO Topiramate; Dom-Topiramate; Mint-Topiramate; Mylan-Topiramate; Novo-Topiramate; PHL-Topiramate; PMS-Topiramate; PRO-Topiramate; ratio-Topiramate; Sandoz-Topiramate; Topamax®; ZYM-Topiramate

Generic Availability (U.S.) Yes

Pharmacologic Category Anticonvulsant, Miscellaneous

Use Monotherapy or adjunctive therapy for partial onset seizures and primary generalized tonic-clonic seizures; adjunctive treatment of seizures associated with Lennox-Gastaut syndrome; prophylaxis of migraine headache

Unlabeled Use Diabetic neuropathy, neuropathic pain; prophylaxis of cluster headache

Medication Guide Available Yes

Contraindications There are no contraindications listed in the manufacturers' labeling.

Canadian labeling (not in U.S. labeling): Hypersensitivity to topiramate or any component of the formulation or container

Warnings/Precautions Antiepileptics are associated with an increased risk of suicidal behavior/thoughts with use (regardless of indication); patients should be monitored for signs/symptoms of depression, suicidal tendencies, and other unusual behavior changes during therapy and instructed to inform their healthcare provider immediately if symptoms occur. Use with caution in patients with hepatic, respiratory, or renal impairment. Topiramate may decrease serum bicarbonate concentrations (up to 67% of patients); treatment-emergent metabolic acidosis is less common. Risk may be increased in patients with a predisposing condition (organ dysfunction, ketogenic diet, or concurrent treatment with other drugs which may cause acidosis). Metabolic acidosis may occur at dosages as low as 50 mg/day. Monitor serum bicarbonate as well as potential complications of chronic acidosis (nephrolithiasis and osteomalacia). Kidney stones have been reported; the risk of kidney stones is about 2-4 times that of the untreated population; the risk of this event may be reduced by increasing fluid intake.

Cognitive dysfunction, psychiatric disturbances (mood disorders), and sedation (somnolence or fatigue) may occur with topiramate use; incidence may be related to rapid titration and higher doses. Patients must be cautioned about performing tasks which require mental alertness (eg, operating machinery or driving). Topiramate may also cause paresthesia, dizziness, and ataxia. Topiramate has been associated with acute myopia and secondary angle-closure glaucoma in adults and children, typically within 1 month of initiation; discontinue in patients with acute onset of decreased visual acuity or ocular pain. Hyperammonemia with or without encephalopathy may occur with or without concomitant valproate adminis-tration; valproic acid dose-dependency was observed in limited pediatric studies; use with caution in patients with inborn errors of metabolism or decreased hepatic mitochondrial activity. Hypothermia (core body temperature <35°C [95°F]) has been reported with concom-itant use of topiramate and valproic acid; may occur with or without associated hyper-ammonemia and may develop after topiramate initiation or dosage increase; discontinuation of topiramate or valproic acid may be necessary. Topiramate may be associated (rarely) with severe oligohydrosis and hyperthermia, most frequently in children; use caution and monitor closely during strenuous exercise, during exposure to high environ-mental temperature, or in patients receiving receiving other carbonic anhydrase inhibitors and drugs with anticholinergic activity. Concurrent use of topiramate and hydrochlorothiazide may increase the risk for hypokalemia; monitor potassium closely.

Avoid abrupt withdrawal of topiramate therapy, it should be withdrawn/tapered slowly to minimize the potential of increased seizure frequency. Doses were also gradually withdrawn in migraine prophylaxis studies. Effects with other sedative drugs or ethanol may be potentiated.

Adverse Reactions (Reflective of adult population; not specific for elderly) Adverse events are reported for placebo-controlled trials of adjunctive therapy in adult and pediatric patients. Unless otherwise noted, the percentages refer to incidence in epilepsy trials. **Note:** A wide range of dosages were studied; incidence of adverse events was frequently lower in the pediatric population studied.

>10%:
  Central nervous system: Somnolence (15% to 29%), dizziness (4% to 25%; dose depend-ent), fatigue (9% to 16%; dose-dependent), nervousness (9% to 18%), ataxia (6% to 16%), psychomotor slowing (3% to 13%; dose dependent), speech problems (2% to 13%), memory difficulties (2% to 12%), behavior problems (children 11%), confusion (4% to 11%)
  Endocrine & metabolic: Serum bicarbonate decreased (dose related: 7% to 67%; marked reductions [to <17 mEq/L] 1% to 11%)
  Gastrointestinal: Anorexia (4% to 24%; dose dependent), nausea (6% to 10%; migraine trial: 9% to 14%)
  Neuromuscular & skeletal: Paresthesia (1% to 11%; migraine trial: 35% to 51%)
  Ocular: Abnormal vision (2% to 13%)
  Respiratory: Upper respiratory infection (migraine trial: 12% to 14%)
  Miscellaneous: Injury (14%)
1% to 10%:
  Cardiovascular: Chest pain (2% to 4%), edema (2%), hypertension (1% to 2%), bradycardia (1%), pallor (1%), syncope (1%)
  Central nervous system: Difficulty concentrating (5% to 10%), aggressive reactions (2% to 9%), depression (5% to 9%; dose dependent), insomnia (4% to 8%), mood problems (≤6%), abnormal coordination (4%), agitation (3%), cognitive problems (3%), emotional lability (3%), anxiety (2% to 3%; dose dependent), hypoesthesia (2%; migraine trial: 6% to 8%), stupor (2%), vertigo (2%), fever (migraine trial: 1% to 2%), apathy (1%), hallucination (1%), neurosis (1%), psychosis (1%), seizure (1%), suicide attempt (1%)
  Dermatologic: Pruritus (migraine trial: 2% to 4%), skin disorder (2% to 3%), alopecia (2%), dermatitis (2%), hypertrichosis (2%), rash erythematous (1% to 2%), eczema (1%), seborrhea (1%), skin discoloration (1%)
  Endocrine & metabolic: Breast pain (4%), hot flashes (1% to 2%), libido decreased (<1% to 2%), menstrual irregularities (1% to 2%), hypoglycemia (1%), metabolic acidosis (hyper-chloremia, nonanion gap)
  Gastrointestinal: Weight loss (4% to 9%), dyspepsia (2% to 7%), abdominal pain (5% to 6%), salivation increased (6%), constipation (4% to 5%), gastroenteritis (2% to 3%), vomiting (migraine trial: 1% to 3%), diarrhea (2%; migraine trial: 9% to 11%), dysgeusia (2%; migraine trial: 8% to 15%), xerostomia (2%), loss of taste (migraine trial: ≤2%), appetite increased (1%), dysphagia (1%), fecal incontinence (1%), flatulence (1%), GERD (1%), gingivitis (1%), glossitis (1%), gum hyperplasia (1%), weight gain (1%)
  Genitourinary: Incontinence (2% to 4%), UTI (2%), premature ejaculation (migraine trial: ≤3%), cystitis (2%), leukorrhea (2%), impotence (1%), nocturia (1%)
  Hematologic: Purpura (8%), leukopenia (2%), anemia (1%), hematoma (1%), prothrombin time increased (1%), thrombocytopenia (1%)
  Neuromuscular & skeletal: Tremor (3% to 9%), gait abnormal (3% to 8%), arthralgia (migraine trial: 1% to 7%), weakness (6%), hyperkinesia (5%), back pain (1% to 5%), involuntary muscle contractions (2%; migraine trial: 2% to 4%), leg cramps (2%), leg pain (2%), myalgia (2%), hyporeflexia (2%), rigors (1%), skeletal pain (1%)
  Ocular: Diplopia (1% to 10%), nystagmus (10%), conjunctivitis (1%), lacrimation abnormal (1%), myopia (1%)
  Otic: Hearing decreased (2%), tinnitus (2%), otitis media (migraine trial: 1% to 2%)

Renal: Hematuria (2%), renal calculus (migraine trial ≤2%)

Respiratory: Rhinitis (4% to 7%), pharyngitis (6%), sinusitis (5%; migraine trial: 6% to 10%), pneumonia (5%), epistaxis (2% to 4%), cough (migraine trial: 2% to 4%), bronchitis (migraine trial: 3%), dyspnea (migraine trial: 1% to 3%)

Miscellaneous: Viral infection (2% to 7%: migraine trial: 3% to 4%), flu-like syndrome (3%), allergy (2%), infection (2%), thirst (2%), body odor (1%), diaphoresis (1%), moniliasis (1%)

Drug Interactions

Metabolism/Transport Effects Inhibits CYP2C19 (weak); **Induces** CYP3A4 (weak/moderate)

Avoid Concomitant Use

Avoid concomitant use of Topiramate with any of the following: Axitinib; Azelastine; Azelastine (Nasal); Carbonic Anhydrase Inhibitors; Methadone; Mirtazapine; Paraldehyde

Increased Effect/Toxicity

Topiramate may increase the levels/effects of: Alcohol (Ethyl); Alpha-/Beta-Agonists; Amphetamines; Anticonvulsants (Barbiturate); Anticonvulsants (Hydantoin); Azelastine; Azelastine (Nasal); Buprenorphine; CarBAMazepine; Carbonic Anhydrase Inhibitors; CNS Depressants; Flecainide; Fosphenytoin; Lithium; Memantine; MetFORMIN; Methadone; Methotrimeprazine; Metyrosine; Mirtazapine; Paraldehyde; Phenytoin; Primidone; QuiNIDine; Selective Serotonin Reuptake Inhibitors; Valproic Acid; Zolpidem

The levels/effects of Topiramate may be increased by: Divalproex; Droperidol; HydrOXYzine; Methotrimeprazine; Salicylates; Thiazide Diuretics

Decreased Effect

Topiramate may decrease the levels/effects of: ARIPiprazole; Axitinib; Contraceptives (Estrogens); Contraceptives (Progestins); Lithium; Methenamine; Primidone; Saxagliptin

The levels/effects of Topiramate may be decreased by: CarBAMazepine; Fosphenytoin; Ketorolac; Ketorolac (Nasal); Ketorolac (Systemic); Mefloquine; Phenytoin

Ethanol/Nutrition/Herb Interactions

Ethanol: May increase CNS depression; monitor for increased effects with coadministration. Caution patients about effects.

Food: Ketogenic diet may increase the possibility of acidosis and/or kidney stones.

Herb/Nutraceutical: Avoid evening primrose (seizure threshold decreased).

Stability Store at room temperature of 15°C to 30°C (59°F to 86°F). Protect from moisture.

Mechanism of Action Anticonvulsant activity may be due to a combination of potential mechanisms: Blocks neuronal voltage-dependent sodium channels, enhances GABA(A) activity, antagonizes AMPA/kainate glutamate receptors, and weakly inhibits carbonic anhydrase.

Pharmacodynamics/Kinetics

Absorption: Good, rapid; unaffected by food

Protein binding: 15% to 41% (inversely related to plasma concentrations)

Metabolism: Minor amounts metabolized in liver via hydroxylation, hydrolysis, and glucuronidation; percentage of dose metabolized in liver and clearance are increased in patients receiving enzyme inducers (eg, carbamazepine, phenytoin)

Bioavailability: ~80%

Half-life elimination: Mean: Adults: Normal renal function: 21 hours; Elderly: ~24 hours

Time to peak, serum: ~1-4 hours

Excretion: Urine (~70% to 80% as unchanged drug)

Dialyzable: Significantly hemodialyzed; dialysis clearance: 120 mL/minute (4-6 times higher than in adults with normal renal function); supplemental doses may be required

Dosage

Geriatric Most older adults have creatinine clearances <70 mL/minute/1.73 m^2; obtain a serum creatinine and calculate creatinine clearance prior to initiation of therapy. An initial dose of 25 mg/day may be recommended, followed by incremental increases of 25 mg at weekly intervals until an effective dose is reached; refer to adult dosing for titration schedule.

Adult Note: Do not abruptly discontinue therapy; taper dosage gradually to prevent rebound effects. (In clinical trials, adult doses were withdrawn by decreasing in weekly intervals of 50-100 mg/day gradually over 2-8 weeks for seizure treatment, and by decreasing in weekly intervals by 25-50 mg/day for migraine prophylaxis.)

Epilepsy, monotherapy:

Partial onset seizure and primary generalized tonic-clonic seizure: Oral: Initial: 25 mg twice daily; may increase weekly by 50 mg/day up to 100 mg twice daily (week 4 dose); thereafter, may further increase weekly by 100 mg/day up to the recommended maximum of 200 mg twice daily

Canadian labeling: Oral: Initial: 25 mg once daily (in evening); may increase to 25 mg twice daily in weeks 2 or 3 and up to 50 mg twice daily by weeks 3 or 4; may further increase weekly in increments of 50 mg/day up to recommended maximum of 200 mg twice daily

TOPIRAMATE

Epilepsy, adjunctive therapy:
Partial onset seizure: Oral: Initial: 25 mg once or twice daily for 1 week; may increase weekly by 25-50 mg/day until response; usual maintenance dose: 100-200 mg twice daily. Doses >1600 mg/day have not been studied

Primary generalized tonic-clonic seizure: Oral: Use initial dose as listed above for partial onset seizures, but use slower initial titration rate; titrate upwards to recommended dose by the end of 8 weeks; usual maintenance dose: 200 mg twice daily. Doses >1600 mg/day have not been studied.

Canadian labeling: Oral: Initial: 25 mg once or twice daily; may increase weekly by 50 mg/day up to the recommended dose of 100-200 mg twice daily (maximum recommended dose: 800 mg/day; doses >400 mg/day have shown no additional benefit)

Migraine prophylaxis: Oral: Initial: 25 mg once daily (in evening); may increase weekly by 25 mg/day up to the recommended dose of 100 mg/day given in 2 divided doses. Doses >100 mg/day have shown no additional benefit.

Cluster headache prophylaxis (unlabeled use): Oral: Initial: 25 mg/day, titrated at weekly intervals in 25 mg increments, up to 200 mg/day (Pascual, 2007)

Diabetic neuropathy (unlabeled use): Oral: Initial: 25 mg/day, titrated at weekly intervals in 25-50 mg increments to target dose of 400 mg daily in 2 divided doses (Raskin, 2004; Thienel, 2004)

Renal Impairment Cl_{cr} <70 mL/minute/1.73 m²: Administer 50% dose and titrate more slowly.
Hemodialysis: Supplemental dose may be needed during hemodialysis

Hepatic Impairment Clearance may be reduced; however the manufacturer's labeling provides no specific dosing recommendations.

Administration Oral: May be administered without regard to meals
Capsule sprinkles: May be swallowed whole or opened to sprinkle the contents on a small amount (~1 teaspoon) of soft food (drug/food mixture should not be chewed; swallow immediately).
Tablet: Because of bitter taste, tablets should not be broken or chewed.

Monitoring Parameters Seizure frequency, hydration status; electrolytes (recommended monitoring includes serum bicarbonate at baseline and periodically during treatment), serum creatinine; monitor for symptoms of acute acidosis and complications of long-term acidosis (nephrolithiasis, osteomalacia); ammonia level in patients with unexplained lethargy, vomiting, or mental status changes; intraocular pressure, symptoms of secondary angle closure glaucoma; suicidality (eg, suicidal thoughts, depression, behavioral changes)

Pharmacotherapy Pearls May be associated with weight loss in some patients

Special Geriatric Considerations This drug may not be a drug of choice in the elderly until all other therapies for seizures have been exhausted. Follow the recommended titration schedule and adjust time intervals to meet patient's needs. Since most elderly will have a Cl_{cr} <70 mL/minute, it is important to either measure or estimate by calculation the Cl_{cr} prior to initiating therapy.

Dosage Forms Excipient information presented when available (limited, particularly for generics); consult specific product labeling.
Capsule, sprinkle, oral: 15 mg, 25 mg
  Topamax®: 15 mg, 25 mg
Tablet, oral: 25 mg, 50 mg, 100 mg, 200 mg
  Topamax®: 25 mg, 50 mg, 100 mg, 200 mg

◆ **Toprol-XL®** *see* Metoprolol *on page 1263*
◆ **Toradol** *see* Ketorolac (Systemic) *on page 1069*

Toremifene (tore EM i feen)

Brand Names: U.S. Fareston®
Brand Names: Canada Fareston®
Index Terms FC1157a; Toremifene Citrate
Generic Availability (U.S.) No
Pharmacologic Category Antineoplastic Agent, Estrogen Receptor Antagonist; Selective Estrogen Receptor Modulator (SERM)
Use Treatment of metastatic breast cancer in postmenopausal women with estrogen receptor positive or estrogen receptor status unknown
Unlabeled Use Treatment of soft tissue sarcoma (desmoid tumors)
Contraindications Hypersensitivity to toremifene or any component of the formulation; long QT syndrome (congenital or acquired QT prolongation), uncorrected hypokalemia, uncorrected hypomagnesemia
Warnings/Precautions Hazardous agent - use appropriate precautions for handling and disposal.

[U.S. Boxed Warning]: May prolong the QT interval; QT$_c$ prolongation is dose-dependent and concentration dependent. Torsade de pointes, syncope, seizure and/or sudden death may occur. Use is contraindicated in patients with congenital or acquired long QT syndrome, uncorrected hypokalemia, or uncorrected hypomagnesemia. Avoid use with other medications known to prolong the QT interval and with strong CYP3A4 inhibitors. Use with caution in patients with heart failure, hepatic impairment, or electrolyte abnormalities. Monitor electrolytes; correct hypokalemia and hypomagnesemia prior to treatment. Obtain ECG at baseline and as clinically indicated in patients at risk for QT prolongation

Hypercalcemia and tumor flare have been reported during the first weeks of treatment in some breast cancer patients with bone metastases; monitor closely for hypocalcemia. Institute appropriate measures if hypercalcemia occurs, and if severe, discontinue treatment. Tumor flare consists of diffuse musculoskeletal pain and erythema with initial increased size of tumor lesions that later regress; is often accompanied by hypercalcemia. Tumor flare does not imply treatment failure or represent tumor progression. Drugs that decrease renal calcium excretion (eg, thiazide diuretics) may increase the risk of hypercalcemia in patients receiving toremifene. Leukopenia and thrombocytopenia have been reported rarely; monitor leukocyte and platelet counts. Endometrial hyperplasia has been reported; some patients have developed endometrial cancer, although a role of toremifene in endometrial cancer development has not been established. Avoid long-term use in patients with pre-existing endometrial hyperplasia. Use with caution in patients with hepatic failure. Avoid use in patients with a history of thromboembolic disease.

Adverse Reactions (Reflective of adult population; not specific for elderly)
>10%:
  Endocrine & metabolic: Hot flashes (35%)
  Gastrointestinal: Nausea (14%)
  Genitourinary: Vaginal discharge (13%)
  Hepatic: Alkaline phosphatase increased (8% to 19%), AST increased (5% to 19%)
  Miscellaneous: Diaphoresis (20%)
1% to 10%:
  Cardiovascular: Edema (5%), arrhythmia (≤2%), CVA/TIA (≤2%), thrombosis (≤2%), cardiac failure (≤1%), MI (≤1%)
  Central nervous system: Dizziness (9%)
  Endocrine & metabolic: Hypercalcemia (≤3%)
  Gastrointestinal: Vomiting (4%)
  Genitourinary: Vaginal bleeding (2%)
  Hepatic: Bilirubin increased (1% to 2%)
  Local: Thrombophlebitis (≤2%)
  Ocular: Cataracts (≤10%), xerophthalmia (≤9%), visual field abnormal (≤4%), corneal keratopathy (≤2%), glaucoma (≤2%), vision abnormal/diplopia (≤2%)
  Respiratory: Pulmonary embolism (≤2%)

Drug Interactions
Metabolism/Transport Effects Substrate of CYP1A2 (minor), CYP3A4 (major); **Note:** Assignment of Major/Minor substrate status based on clinically relevant drug interaction potential

Avoid Concomitant Use
Avoid concomitant use of Toremifene with any of the following: CYP3A4 Inducers (Strong); CYP3A4 Inhibitors (Strong); Highest Risk QTc-Prolonging Agents; Mifepristone; Moderate Risk QTc-Prolonging Agents

Increased Effect/Toxicity
Toremifene may increase the levels/effects of: Highest Risk QTc-Prolonging Agents; Vitamin K Antagonists

The levels/effects of Toremifene may be increased by: CYP3A4 Inhibitors (Strong); Mifepristone; Moderate Risk QTc-Prolonging Agents; QTc-Prolonging Agents (Indeterminate Risk and Risk Modifying); Thiazide Diuretics

Decreased Effect
The levels/effects of Toremifene may be decreased by: CYP3A4 Inducers (Strong); Deferasirox; Herbs (CYP3A4 Inducers); Tocilizumab

Ethanol/Nutrition/Herb Interactions
Food: Grapefruit juice may increase toremifene levels. Management: Avoid grapefruit juice. Herb/Nutraceutical: St John's wort may decrease toremifene levels. Management: Avoid St John's wort.

Stability Store at 25°C (77°F); excursions permitted to 15°C to 30°C (59°F to 86°F); protect from heat. Protect from light.

Mechanism of Action Nonsteroidal, triphenylethylene derivative with potent antiestrogenic properties (also has estrogenic effects). Competitively binds to estrogen receptors on tumors and other tissue targets, producing a nuclear complex that decreases DNA synthesis and inhibits estrogen effects. Competes with estrogen for binding sites in breast and other tissues; cells accumulate in the G_0 and G_1 phases; therefore, toremifene is cytostatic rather than cytocidal.

Pharmacodynamics/Kinetics

Absorption: Well absorbed

Distribution: V_d: 580 L (range: 457-958 L)

Protein binding, plasma: >99.5%, primarily to albumin

Metabolism: Extensively hepatic, principally by CYP3A4 to N-demethyltoremifene (a weak antiestrogen)

Bioavailability: Not affected by food

Half-life elimination: Toremifene: ~5 days; N-demethyltoremifene: 6 days

Time to peak, serum: ≤3 hours

Excretion: Primarily feces; urine (10%) during a 1-week period

Dosage

Geriatric & Adult Metastatic breast cancer (postmenopausal): Oral: 60 mg once daily, continue until disease progression

Administration Administer orally, as a single daily dose, with or without food.

Monitoring Parameters CBC with differential, electrolytes (calcium, magnesium, and potassium), hepatic function. Obtain ECG in patients at risk for QT prolongation. In patients with bone metastases, monitor closely for hypercalcemia during the first few weeks of treatment.

Special Geriatric Considerations No specific information concerning elderly patients.

Dosage Forms Excipient information presented when available (limited, particularly for generics); consult specific product labeling.

Tablet, oral:
  Fareston®: 60 mg

◆ **Toremifene Citrate** see Toremifene on page 1938

Torsemide (TORE se mide)

Medication Safety Issues

Sound-alike/look-alike issues:
  Torsemide may be confused with furosemide
  Demadex® may be confused with Denorex®

Brand Names: U.S. Demadex®

Generic Availability (U.S.) Yes

Pharmacologic Category Diuretic, Loop

Use Management of edema associated with heart failure and hepatic or renal disease (including chronic renal failure); treatment of hypertension

Contraindications Hypersensitivity to torsemide, any component of the formulation, or any sulfonylurea; anuria

Warnings/Precautions Loop diuretics are potent diuretics; excess amounts can lead to profound diuresis with fluid and electrolyte loss; close medical supervision and dose evaluation are required. Potassium supplementation and/or use of potassium-sparing diuretics may be necessary to prevent hypokalemia. Use with caution in patients with cirrhosis; avoid sudden changes in fluid and electrolyte balance and acid/base status which may lead to hepatic encephalopathy. Administration with an aldosterone antagonist or potassium-sparing diuretic may provide additional diuretic efficacy and maintain normokalemia. Coadministration of antihypertensives may increase the risk of hypotension.

Monitor fluid status and renal function in an attempt to prevent oliguria, azotemia, and reversible increases in BUN and creatinine; close medical supervision of aggressive diuresis required. Ototoxicity has been demonstrated following oral administration of torsemide and following rapid I.V. administration of other loop diuretics. Other possible risk factors may include use in renal impairment, excessive doses, and concurrent use of other ototoxins (eg, aminoglycosides).

Chemical similarities are present among sulfonamides, sulfonylureas, carbonic anhydrase inhibitors, thiazides, and loop diuretics (except ethacrynic acid). Use in patients with sulfonylurea allergy is specifically contraindicated in product labeling; a risk of cross-reaction exists in patients with allergy to any of these compounds; avoid use when previous reaction has been severe. Discontinue if signs of hypersensitivity are noted.

Adverse Reactions (Reflective of adult population; not specific for elderly) 1% to 10%:

Cardiovascular: ECG abnormality (2%), chest pain (1%)

Central nervous system: Nervousness (1%)

Gastrointestinal: Constipation (2%), diarrhea (2%), dyspepsia (2%), nausea (2%), sore throat (2%)

Genitourinary: Excessive urination (7%)

Neuromuscular & skeletal: Arthralgia (2%), myalgia (2%), weakness (2%)

Respiratory: Rhinitis (3%), cough (2%)

Drug Interactions

Metabolism/Transport Effects Substrate of CYP2C8 (minor), CYP2C9 (major), SLCO1B1; **Note:** Assignment of Major/Minor substrate status based on clinically relevant drug interaction potential; **Inhibits** CYP2C19 (weak)

Avoid Concomitant Use There are no known interactions where it is recommended to avoid concomitant use.

Increased Effect/Toxicity

Torsemide may increase the levels/effects of: ACE Inhibitors; Allopurinol; Amifostine; Aminoglycosides; Antihypertensives; Cardiac Glycosides; CISplatin; Dofetilide; Hypotensive Agents; Lithium; Methotrexate; Neuromuscular-Blocking Agents; RisperiDONE; RiTUXimab; Salicylates; Sodium Phosphates; Warfarin

The levels/effects of Torsemide may be increased by: Alfuzosin; Beta2-Agonists; Corticosteroids (Orally Inhaled); Corticosteroids (Systemic); CycloSPORINE (Systemic); CYP2C9 Inhibitors (Moderate); CYP2C9 Inhibitors (Strong); Diazoxide; Eltrombopag; Herbs (Hypotensive Properties); Licorice; MAO Inhibitors; Methotrexate; Mifepristone; Pentoxifylline; Phosphodiesterase 5 Inhibitors; Probenecid; Prostacyclin Analogues

Decreased Effect

Torsemide may decrease the levels/effects of: Hypoglycemic Agents; Lithium; Neuromuscular-Blocking Agents

The levels/effects of Torsemide may be decreased by: Bile Acid Sequestrants; CYP2C9 Inducers (Strong); Fosphenytoin; Herbs (Hypertensive Properties); Methotrexate; Methylphenidate; Nonsteroidal Anti-Inflammatory Agents; Peginterferon Alfa-2b; Phenytoin; Probenecid; Salicylates; Yohimbine

Ethanol/Nutrition/Herb Interactions Herb/Nutraceutical: Avoid herbs with *hypertensive* properties (bayberry, blue cohosh, cayenne, ephedra, ginger, ginseng [American], kola, licorice); may diminish the antihypertensive effect of torsemide. Avoid herbs with *hypotensive* properties (black cohosh, California poppy, coleus, golden seal, hawthorn, mistletoe, periwinkle, quinine, shepherd's purse); may enhance the hypotensive effect of torsemide.

Stability

I.V.: Store at 15°C to 30°C (59°F to 86°F). If torsemide is to be administered via continuous infusion, stability has been demonstrated through 24 hours at room temperature in plastic containers for the following fluids and concentrations:

200 mg torsemide (10 mg/mL) added to 250 mL D_5W, 250 mL NS or 500 mL 0.45% sodium chloride

50 mg torsemide (10 mg/mL) added to 500 mL D_5W, 500 mL NS, or 500 mL 0.45% sodium chloride

Tablets: Store at 15°C to 30°C (59°F to 86°F).

Mechanism of Action Inhibits reabsorption of sodium and chloride in the ascending loop of Henle and distal renal tubule, interfering with the chloride-binding cotransport system, thus causing increased excretion of water, sodium, chloride, magnesium, and calcium; does not alter GFR, renal plasma flow, or acid-base balance

Pharmacodynamics/Kinetics

Onset of action: Diuresis: Oral: Within 1hour

Peak effect: Diuresis: Oral: 1-2 hours; Antihypertensive: Oral: 4-6 weeks (up to 12 weeks)

Duration: Diuresis: Oral: ~6-8 hours

Absorption: Oral: Rapid

Distribution: V_d: 12-15 L; Cirrhosis: Approximately doubled

Protein binding: >99%

Metabolism: Hepatic (~80%) via CYP

Bioavailability: ~80%

Half-life elimination: ~3.5 hours; Cirrhosis: 7-8 hours

Time to peak, plasma: Oral: 1 hour; delayed ~30 minutes when administered with food

Excretion: Urine (~20% as unchanged drug)

Dosage

Geriatric & Adult Note: I.V. and oral dosing are equivalent.

Edema:

Chronic renal failure: Oral, I.V.: Initial: 20 mg once daily; may increase gradually by doubling dose until the desired diuretic response is obtained (maximum recommended daily dose: 200 mg)

Heart failure:
Oral: Initial: 10-20 mg once daily; may increase gradually by doubling dose until the desired diuretic response is obtained. **Note:** ACC/AHA 2009 guidelines for heart failure maximum daily dose: 200 mg (Hunt, 2009)

I.V.: Initial: 10-20 mg; may repeat every 2 hours with double the dose as needed. **Note:** ACC/AHA 2009 guidelines for heart failure recommend maximum single dose: 100-200 mg (Hunt, 2009)

Continuous I.V. infusion (unlabeled dose): Initial: 20 mg I.V. load, then 5-20 mg/hour (Hunt, 2009)

Hepatic cirrhosis: Oral: Initial: 5-10 mg once daily; may increase gradually by doubling dose until the desired diuretic response is obtained (maximum recommended single dose: 40 mg). **Note:** Administer with an aldosterone antagonist or a potassium-sparing diuretic.

Hypertension: Oral: Initial: 5 mg once daily; may increase to 10 mg once daily after 4-6 weeks if adequate antihypertensive response is not apparent; if still not effective, an additional antihypertensive agent may be added. Usual dosage range (JNC 7): 2.5-10 mg once daily. **Note:** Thiazide-type diuretics are preferred in the treatment of hypertension (Chobanian, 2003)

Administration Administer the I.V. dose slowly over 2 minutes

Monitoring Parameters Renal function, electrolytes, and fluid status (weight and I & O), blood pressure

Pharmacotherapy Pearls 10-20 mg torsemide is approximately equivalent to:
Furosemide 40 mg
Bumetanide 1 mg

Special Geriatric Considerations Loop diuretics are potent diuretics; excess amounts can lead to profound diuresis with fluid and electrolyte loss. Close medical supervision and dose evaluation is required, particularly in the elderly. Severe loss of sodium and/or increase in BUN can cause confusion; for any change in mental status, monitor electrolytes and renal function.

Dosage Forms Excipient information presented when available (limited, particularly for generics); consult specific product labeling.
Injection, solution: 10 mg/mL (2 mL, 5 mL)
Tablet, oral: 5 mg, 10 mg, 20 mg, 100 mg
Demadex®: 5 mg, 10 mg, 20 mg, 100 mg [scored]

◆ **Toviaz™** *see* Fesoterodine *on page* 782
◆ **tPA** *see* Alteplase *on page* 73
◆ **Tradjenta™** *see* Linagliptin *on page* 1130
◆ **Trajenta** *see* Linagliptin *on page* 1130

TraMADol (TRA ma dole)

Medication Safety Issues
Sound-alike/look-alike issues:
TraMADol may be confused with tapentadol, Toradol®, Trandate®, traZODone, Voltaren® Ultram® may be confused with Ultane®, Ultracet®, Voltaren®

International issues:
Theradol [Netherlands] may be confused with Foradil brand name for formoterol [U.S., Canada, and multiple international markets], Terazol brand name for terconazole [U.S. and Canada], and Toradol brand name for ketorolac [Canada and multiple international markets]

Trexol [Mexico] may be confused with Trexall brand name for methotrexate [U.S.]; Truxal brand name for chlorprothixene [multiple international markets]

Brand Names: U.S. ConZip™; Rybix™ ODT; Ryzolt™; Ultram®; Ultram® ER
Brand Names: Canada Durela™; Ralivia™; Tridural™; Ultram®; Zytram® XL
Index Terms Tramadol Hydrochloride
Generic Availability (U.S.) Yes: Excludes tablet (orally disintegrating)
Pharmacologic Category Analgesic, Opioid
Use Relief of moderate to moderately-severe pain
Extended release formulations are indicated for patients requiring around-the-clock management of moderate to moderately-severe pain for an extended period of time

Contraindications Hypersensitivity to tramadol, opioids, or any component of the formulation
Additional contraindications for Ultram®, Rybix™ ODT, and Ultram® ER: Any situation where opioids are contraindicated, including acute intoxication with alcohol, hypnotics, centrally-acting analgesics, opioids, or psychotropic drugs

Additional contraindications for ConZip™, Ryzolt™: Severe/acute bronchial asthma, hypercapnia, or significant respiratory depression in the absence of appropriately monitored setting and/or resuscitative equipment

Canadian product labeling:

Tramadol is contraindicated during or within 14 days following MAO inhibitor therapy

Extended release formulations (Ralivia™ ER [CAN], Tridural™[CAN], and Zytram® XL [CAN]): Additional contraindications: Severe (Cl$_{cr}$ <30 mL/minute) renal dysfunction, severe (Child-Pugh class C) hepatic dysfunction

Warnings/Precautions Rare but serious anaphylactoid reactions (including fatalities) often following initial dosing have been reported. Pruritus, hives, bronchospasm, angioedema, toxic epidermal necrolysis (TEN) and Stevens-Johnson syndrome also have been reported with use. Previous anaphylactoid reactions to opioids may increase risks for similar reactions to tramadol. Caution patients to swallow extended release tablets whole. Rapid release and absorption of tramadol from extended release tablets that are broken, crushed, or chewed may lead to a potentially lethal overdose. May cause CNS depression, which may impair physical or mental abilities; patients must be cautioned about performing tasks which require mental alertness (eg, operating machinery or driving). May cause CNS depression and/or respiratory depression, particularly when combined with other CNS depressants. Use with caution and reduce dosage when administered to patients receiving other CNS depressants. An increased risk of seizures may occur in patients receiving serotonin reuptake inhibitors (SSRIs or anorectics), tricyclic antidepressants or other cyclic compounds (including cyclo-benzaprine, promethazine), neuroleptics, drugs which may lower seizure threshold, or drugs which impair metabolism of tramadol (ie, CYP2D6 and 3A4 inhibitors). Patients with a history of seizures, or with a risk of seizures (head trauma, metabolic disorders, CNS infection, or malignancy, or during ethanol/drug withdrawal) are also at increased risk. Avoid use, if possible, with serotonergic agents such as TCAs, MAO inhibitors (use with extreme caution; contraindicated in Canadian product labeling), triptans, venlafaxine, trazodone, lithium, sibutramine, meperidine, dextromethorphan, St John's wort, SNRIs, and SSRIs; use caution with drugs which impair metabolism of tramadol (ie, CYP2D6 and 3A4 inhibitors); concomitant may increase the risk of serotonin syndrome.

Elderly (particularly >75 years of age), debilitated patients and patients with chronic respiratory disorders may be at greater risk of adverse events. Use with caution in patients with increased intracranial pressure or head injury. Avoid use in patients who are suicidal or addiction prone; use with caution in patients taking tranquilizers and/or antidepressants, or those with an emotional disturbance including depression. Healthcare provider should be alert to problems of abuse, misuse, and diversion. Use caution in heavy alcohol users. Use caution in treatment of acute abdominal conditions; may mask pain. Use tramadol with caution and reduce dosage in patients with liver disease or renal dysfunction. Avoid using extended release tablets in severe hepatic impairment. Do not use Ryzolt™ in any degree of hepatic impairment. Tolerance or drug dependence may result from extended use (withdrawal symptoms have been reported); abrupt discontinuation should be avoided. Tapering of dose at the time of discontinuation limits the risk of withdrawal symptoms. Some products may contain phenylalanine.

Adverse Reactions (Reflective of adult population; not specific for elderly)

>10%:

Cardiovascular: Flushing (8% to 16%)

Central nervous system: Dizziness (10% to 33%), headache (4% to 32%), somnolence (7% to 25%), insomnia (2% to 11%)

Dermatologic: Pruritus (3% to 12%)

Gastrointestinal: Constipation (9% to 46%), nausea (15% to 40%), vomiting (5% to 17%), dyspepsia (1% to 13%)

Neuromuscular & skeletal: Weakness (4% to 12%)

1% to 10%:

Cardiovascular: Orthostatic hypotension (2% to 5%), chest pain (1% to <5%), hypertension (1% to <5%), peripheral edema (1% to <5%), vasodilation (1% to <5%)

Central nervous system: Agitation (1% to <5%), anxiety (1% to <5%), apathy (1% to <5%), chills (1% to <5%), confusion (1% to <5%), coordination impaired (1% to <5%), depersonalization (1% to <5%), depression (1% to <5%), euphoria (1% to <5%), fever (1% to <5%), hypoesthesia (1% to <5%), lethargy (1% to <5%), nervousness (1% to <5%), pain (1% to <5%), pyrexia (1% to <5%), restlessness (1% to <5%), malaise (<1% to <5%), fatigue (2%), vertigo (2%)

Dermatologic: Dermatitis (1% to <5%), rash (1% to <5%)

Endocrine & metabolic: Hot flashes (2% to 9%), hyperglycemia (1% to <5%), menopausal symptoms (1% to <5%)

Gastrointestinal: Diarrhea (5% to 10%), xerostomia (3% to 13%), anorexia (1% to 6%), abdominal pain (1% to <5%), appetite decreased (1% to <5%), weight loss (1% to <5%), flatulence (<1% to <5%)

Genitourinary: Pelvic pain (1% to <5%), prostatic disorder (1% to <5%), urine abnormalities (1% to <5%), urinary tract infection (1% to <5%), urinary frequency (<1% to <5%), urinary retention (<1% to <5%)

Neuromuscular & skeletal: Arthralgia (1% to 5%), back pain (1% to <5%), creatine phosphokinase increased (1% to <5%), myalgia (1% to <5%), hypertonia (1% to <5%), neck pain (1% to <5%), rigors (1% to <5%), paresthesia (1% to <5%), tremor (1% to <5%)

Ocular: Blurred vision (1% to <5%), miosis (1% to <5%)

Respiratory: Bronchitis (1% to <5%), congestion (nasal/sinus) (1% to <5%), cough (1% to <5%), dyspnea (1% to <5%), nasopharyngitis (1% to <5%), pharyngitis (1% to <5%), rhinitis (1% to <5%), rhinorrhea (1% to <5%), sinusitis (1% to <5%), sneezing (1% to <5%), sore throat (1% to <5%), upper respiratory infection (1% to <5%)

Miscellaneous: Diaphoresis (2% to 9%), flu-like syndrome (1% to <5%), withdrawal syndrome (1% to <5%), shivering (<1% to <5%)

A withdrawal syndrome may include anxiety, diarrhea, hallucinations (rare), nausea, pain, piloerection, rigors, sweating, and tremor. Uncommon discontinuation symptoms may include severe anxiety, panic attacks, or paresthesia.

Drug Interactions

Metabolism/Transport Effects Substrate of CYP2B6 (minor), CYP2D6 (major), CYP3A4 (major); **Note:** Assignment of Major/Minor substrate status based on clinically relevant drug interaction potential

Avoid Concomitant Use

Avoid concomitant use of TraMADol with any of the following: Azelastine; Azelastine (Nasal); CarBAMazepine; Conivaptan; Methadone; Paraldehyde

Increased Effect/Toxicity

TraMADol may increase the levels/effects of: Alcohol (Ethyl); Alvimopan; Azelastine; Azelastine (Nasal); CarBAMazepine; CNS Depressants; Desmopressin; MAO Inhibitors; Methadone; Metoclopramide; Metyrosine; Paraldehyde; Selective Serotonin Reuptake Inhibitors; Serotonin Modulators; Thiazide Diuretics; Vitamin K Antagonists; Zolpidem

The levels/effects of TraMADol may be increased by: Amphetamines; Antipsychotic Agents (Phenothiazines); Antipsychotics; Conivaptan; CYP2D6 Inhibitors (Moderate); CYP3A4 Inhibitors (Strong); Dasatinib; HydrOXYzine; Ivacaftor; Mifepristone; Selective Serotonin Reuptake Inhibitors; Succinylcholine; Tricyclic Antidepressants

Decreased Effect

TraMADol may decrease the levels/effects of: CarBAMazepine; Pegvisomant

The levels/effects of TraMADol may be decreased by: Ammonium Chloride; Antiemetics (5HT3 Antagonists); CarBAMazepine; CYP2D6 Inhibitors (Moderate); CYP2D6 Inhibitors (Strong); CYP3A4 Inducers (Strong); Deferasirox; Mixed Agonist / Antagonist Opioids; Tocilizumab

Ethanol/Nutrition/Herb Interactions

Ethanol: May increase CNS depression; monitor for increased effects with coadministration. Caution patients about effects.

Food:

Immediate release tablet: Rate and extent of absorption were not significantly affected.

Extended release:

ConZip™: Rate and extent of absorption were unaffected.

Ryzolt™: Increased C_{max}; no effect on AUC.

Ultram® ER: High-fat meal reduced C_{max} and AUC, and increased T_{max} by 3 hours.

Orally disintegrating tablet: Food delays the time to peak serum concentration by 30 minutes; extent of absorption was not significantly affected.

Herb/Nutraceutical: Avoid valerian, St John's wort, kava kava, gotu kola (may increase CNS depression).

Stability Store at 25°C (77°F); excursions permitted to 15°C to 30°C (59°F to 86°F).

Mechanism of Action Tramadol and its active metabolite (M1) binds to μ-opiate receptors in the CNS causing inhibition of ascending pain pathways, altering the perception of and response to pain; also inhibits the reuptake of norepinephrine and serotonin, which also modifies the ascending pain pathway

Pharmacodynamics/Kinetics

Onset of action: Immediate release: ~1 hour

Duration: 9 hours

Absorption: Immediate release formulation: Rapid and complete; Extended release formulation: Delayed

Distribution: V_d: 2.5-3 L/kg

Protein binding, plasma: ~20%

Metabolism: Extensively hepatic via demethylation (mediated by CYP3A4 and CYP2B6), glucuronidation, and sulfation; has pharmacologically active metabolite formed by CYP2D6 (M1; O-desmethyl tramadol)

Bioavailability: Immediate release: 75%; Extended release: Ultram® ER: 85% to 90% (as compared to immediate release), Zytram® XL, Tridural™: 70%, Ryzolt™: ~95% (as compared to immediate release)

Half-life elimination: Tramadol: ~6-8 hours; Active metabolite: 7-9 hours; prolonged in elderly, hepatic or renal impairment; Zytram® XL: ~16 hours; Ralivia™ ER, Ryzolt™, Tridural™: ~5-9 hours

Time to peak: Immediate release: ~2 hours; Extended release: ConZip™: ~10-12 hours, Ryzolt™: ~4 hours, Tridural™: ~4 hours, Ultram® ER: ~12 hours

Excretion: Urine (30% as unchanged drug; 60% as metabolites)

Dosage

Geriatric Elderly >65 years: Oral: Use caution and initiate at the lower end of the dosing range. Refer to adult dosing.

Elderly >75 years:

Immediate release: Do not exceed 300 mg/day; see Dosage: Renal Impairment and Dosage: Hepatic Impairment.

Extended release: Use with great caution; see Dosage: Adult, Dosage: Renal Impairment, and Dosage: Hepatic Impairment.

Adult Moderate-to-severe pain: Oral:

Immediate release: 50-100 mg every 4-6 hours (not to exceed 400 mg/day). For patients not requiring rapid onset of effect, tolerability may be improved by starting dose at 25 mg/day and titrating dose by 25 mg every 3 days, until reaching 25 mg 4 times/day. The total daily dose may then be increased by 50 mg every 3 days as tolerated, to reach dose of 50 mg 4 times/day. After titration, 50-100 mg may be given every 4-6 hours as needed up to a maximum 400 mg/day.

Orally-disintegrating tablet (Rybix™ ODT): 50-100 mg every 4-6 hours (not to exceed 400 mg/day); for patients not requiring rapid onset of effect, tolerability may be improved by starting dose at 50 mg/day and titrating dose by 50 mg every 3 days, until reaching 50 mg 4 times/day. After titration, 50-100 mg may be given every 4-6 hours as needed up to a maximum 400 mg/day.

Extended release:

ConZip™, Ultram® ER:

Patients not currently on immediate-release: 100 mg once daily; titrate every 5 days (maximum: 300 mg/day)

Patients currently on immediate-release: Calculate 24-hour immediate release total dose and initiate total extended release daily dose (round dose to the next lowest 100 mg increment); titrate as tolerated to desired effect (maximum: 300 mg/day)

Ryzolt™:

Patients not currently on immediate-release: 100 mg once daily; titrate every 2-3 days by 100 mg/day increments; usual daily dose: 200-300 mg/day (maximum: 300 mg/day)

Patients currently on immediate-release: Calculate 24 hour immediate release total dose and initiate total extended release daily dose (round dose to the next lowest 100 mg increment); titrate as tolerated to desired effect (maximum: 300 mg/day)

Ralivia™ ER (Canadian labeling, not available in U.S.): 100 mg once daily; titrate every 5 days as needed based on clinical response and severity of pain (maximum: 300 mg/day)

Tridural™ (Canadian labeling, not available in U.S.): 100 mg once daily; titrate by 100 mg/day every 2 days as needed based on clinical response and severity of pain (maximum: 300 mg/day)

Zytram® XL (Canadian labeling, not available in U.S.): 150 mg once daily; if pain relief is not achieved may titrate by increasing dosage incrementally, with sufficient time to evaluate effect of increased dosage; generally not more often than every 7 days (maximum: 400 mg/day)

Renal Impairment

Immediate release: Cl$_{cr}$ <30 mL/minute: Administer 50-100 mg dose every 12 hours (maximum: 200 mg/day).

Extended release: Should not be used in patients with Cl$_{cr}$ <30 mL/minute.

Hepatic Impairment

Immediate release: Cirrhosis: Recommended dose: 50 mg every 12 hours.

Extended release: Should not be used in patients with severe (Child-Pugh class C) hepatic dysfunction; Ryzolt™ should not be used in any degree of hepatic impairment

Administration

Immediate release: Administer without regard to meals.

Extended release: Swallow whole; do not crush, chew, or split.

ConZip™, Zytram® XL (Canadian labeling, not available in U.S.): May administer without regard to meals.

Ultram® ER, Ralivia™ ER (Canadian labeling, not available in U.S.), Tridural™ (Canadian labeling, not available in U.S.): May administer without regard to meals, but administer in a consistent manner of either with or without meals.

Orally-disintegrating tablet: Remove from foil blister by peeling back (do not push tablet through the foil). Place tablet on tongue and allow to dissolve (may take ~1 minute); water is not needed, but may be administered with water. Do not chew, break, or split tablet.

◀ **Monitoring Parameters** Pain relief, respiratory rate, blood pressure, and pulse; signs of tolerance, abuse, or suicidal ideation

Reference Range 100-300 ng/mL; however, serum level monitoring is not required

Test Interactions May interfere with urine detection of PCP (false-positive).

Special Geriatric Considerations One study in the elderly found that tramadol 50 mg was similar in efficacy as acetaminophen 300 mg with codeine 30 mg. In Ultram® ER trials, elderly patients experienced more adverse effects than younger adults, particularly constipation, fatigue, weakness, postural hypotension, and dyspepsia. In Conzip™ trials, elderly patients also experienced more side effects than younger adults. For this reason, the extended release formulations should probably be avoided in the elderly, or only used with great caution.

Dosage Forms Excipient information presented when available (limited, particularly for generics); consult specific product labeling.

Capsule, variable release, oral, as hydrochloride: 150 mg [37.5 mg (immediate release) and 112.5 mg (extended release)]

ConZip™: 100 mg [25 mg (immediate release) and 75 mg (extended release)]
ConZip™: 200 mg [50 mg (immediate release) and 150 mg (extended release)]
ConZip™: 300 mg [50 mg (immediate release) and 250 mg (extended release)]

Tablet, oral, as hydrochloride: 50 mg
Ultram®: 50 mg [scored]

Tablet, extended release, oral, as hydrochloride: 100 mg, 200 mg, 300 mg
Ryzolt™: 100 mg, 200 mg, 300 mg
Ultram® ER: 100 mg, 200 mg, 300 mg

Tablet, orally disintegrating, oral, as hydrochloride:
Rybix™ ODT: 50 mg [contains aspartame; mint flavor]

Dosage Forms: Canada Excipient information presented when available (limited, particularly for generics); consult specific product labeling.

Tablet, extended release, as hydrochloride
Ralivia™ ER: 100 mg, 200 mg, 300 mg
Tridural™: 100 mg, 200 mg, 300 mg
Zytram® XL: 75 mg, 150 mg, 200 mg, 300 mg, 400 mg

◆ **Tramadol Hydrochloride** *see* TraMADol *on page 1942*
◆ **Trandate®** *see* Labetalol *on page 1078*

Trandolapril (tran DOE la pril)

Related Information
Angiotensin Agents *on page 2093*
Heart Failure (Systolic) *on page 2203*

Brand Names: U.S. Mavik®

Brand Names: Canada Mavik®

Generic Availability (U.S.) Yes

Pharmacologic Category Angiotensin-Converting Enzyme (ACE) Inhibitor

Use Treatment of hypertension alone or in combination with other antihypertensive agents; treatment of heart failure (HF) or left ventricular (LV) dysfunction after myocardial infarction (MI)

Unlabeled Use To delay the progression of nephropathy and reduce risks of cardiovascular events in hypertensive patients with type 1 or 2 diabetes mellitus

Contraindications Hypersensitivity to trandolapril or any component of the formulation; history of angioedema related to previous treatment with an ACE inhibitor; patients with idiopathic or hereditary angioedema

Warnings/Precautions Anaphylactic reactions may occur rarely with ACE inhibitors. At any time during treatment (especially following first dose) angioedema may occur rarely with ACE inhibitors; it may involve the head and neck (potentially compromising the airway) or the intestine (presenting with abdominal pain). African-Americans and patients with idiopathic or hereditary angioedema may be at an increased risk. Prolonged frequent monitoring may be required especially if tongue, glottis, or larynx are involved as they are associated with airway obstruction. Patients with a history of airway surgery may have a higher risk of airway obstruction. Aggressive early and appropriate management is critical. Use in patients with previous angioedema associated with ACE inhibitor therapy is contraindicated. Severe anaphylactoid reactions may be seen during hemodialysis (eg, CVVHD) with high-flux dialysis membranes (eg, AN69). Rare cases of anaphylactoid reactions have been reported in patients undergoing sensitization treatment with hymenoptera (bee, wasp) venom while receiving ACE inhibitors.

Symptomatic hypotension with or without syncope can occur with ACE inhibitors (usually with the first several doses); effects are most often observed in volume-depleted patients; correct volume depletion prior to initiation; close monitoring of patient is required especially with initial dosing and dosing increases; blood pressure must be lowered at a rate appropriate for the patient's clinical condition. Initiation of therapy in patients with ischemic heart disease or cerebrovascular disease warrants close observation due to the potential consequences posed by falling blood pressure (eg, MI, stroke). Use with caution in hypertrophic cardiomyopathy with outflow tract obstruction, severe aortic stenosis, or before, during, or immediately after major surgery.

Hyperkalemia may occur with ACE inhibitors; risk factors include renal dysfunction, diabetes mellitus, concomitant use of potassium-sparing diuretics, potassium supplements, and/or potassium-containing salts. Use cautiously, if at all, with these agents and monitor potassium closely. Cough may occur with ACE inhibitors. Other causes of cough should be considered (eg, pulmonary congestion in patients with heart failure) and excluded prior to discontinuation.

Dosage adjustment needed in severe renal dysfunction (Cl_{cr} <30 mL/minute) or hepatic cirrhosis. May be associated with deterioration of renal function and/or increases in serum creatinine, particularly in patients with low renal blood flow (eg, renal artery stenosis, heart failure) whose glomerular filtration rate (GFR) is dependent on efferent arteriolar vaso-constriction by angiotensin II; deterioration may result in oliguria, acute renal failure, and progressive azotemia. Small increases in serum creatinine may occur following initiation; consider discontinuation only in patients with progressive and/or significant deterioration in renal function. Use with caution in patients with unstented unilateral/bilateral renal artery stenosis. When unstented bilateral renal artery stenosis is present, use is generally avoided due to the elevated risk of deterioration in renal function unless possible benefits outweigh risks. Concurrent use of angiotensin receptor blockers may increase the risk of clinically-significant adverse events (eg, renal dysfunction, hyperkalemia).

Rare toxicities associated with ACE inhibitors include cholestatic jaundice (which may progress to fulminant hepatic necrosis), agranulocytosis, neutropenia, or leukopenia with myeloid hypoplasia. Patients with collagen vascular diseases (especially with concomitant renal impairment) or renal impairment alone may be at increased risk for hematologic toxicity; periodically monitor CBC with differential in these patients.

Adverse Reactions (Reflective of adult population; not specific for elderly) Note: Frequency ranges include data from hypertension and heart failure trials. Higher rates of adverse reactions have generally been noted in patients with CHF. However, the frequency of adverse effects associated with placebo is also increased in this population.

>1%:
  Cardiovascular: Hypotension (<1% to 11%), syncope (6%), bradycardia (<1% to 5%), cardiogenic shock (4%), intermittent claudication (4%)
  Central nervous system: Dizziness (1% to 23%), stroke (3%)
  Endocrine & metabolic: Uric acid increased (15%), hyperkalemia (5%), hypocalcemia (5%)
  Gastrointestinal: Gastritis (4%), diarrhea (1%)
  Neuromuscular & skeletal: Myalgia (5%), weakness (3%)
  Renal: BUN increased (9%), serum creatinine increased (1% to 5%)
  Respiratory: Cough (2% to 35%)

Worsening of renal function may occur in patients with bilateral renal artery stenosis or hypovolemia. In addition, a syndrome which may include fever, myalgia, arthralgia, interstitial nephritis, vasculitis, rash, eosinophilia and positive ANA, and elevated ESR has been reported with ACE inhibitors. Eosinophilic pneumonitis has also been reported with other ACE inhibitors.

Drug Interactions

Metabolism/Transport Effects None known.

Avoid Concomitant Use There are no known interactions where it is recommended to avoid concomitant use.

Increased Effect/Toxicity

Trandolapril may increase the levels/effects of: Allopurinol; Amifostine; Antihypertensives; AzaTHIOprine; CycloSPORINE; CycloSPORINE (Systemic); Ferric Gluconate; Gold Sodium Thiomalate; Hypotensive Agents; Iron Dextran Complex; Lithium; Nonsteroidal Anti-Inflammatory Agents; RiTUXimab; Sodium Phosphates

The levels/effects of Trandolapril may be increased by: Alfuzosin; Aliskiren; Angiotensin II Receptor Blockers; Diazoxide; DPP-IV Inhibitors; Eplerenone; Everolimus; Herbs (Hypotensive Properties); Loop Diuretics; MAO Inhibitors; Pentoxifylline; Phosphodiesterase 5 Inhibitors; Potassium Salts; Potassium-Sparing Diuretics; Prostacyclin Analogues; Sirolimus; Temsirolimus; Thiazide Diuretics; TiZANidine; Tolvaptan; Trimethoprim

◄ **Decreased Effect**
The levels/effects of Trandolapril may be decreased by: Antacids; Aprotinin; Herbs (Hypertensive Properties); Icatibant; Lanthanum; Methylphenidate; Nonsteroidal Anti-Inflammatory Agents; Salicylates; Yohimbine

Ethanol/Nutrition/Herb Interactions Herb/Nutraceutical: Some herbal medications may worsen hypertension (eg, licorice); others may increase the antihypertensive effects of trandolapril (eg, shepherd's purse). Management: Avoid bayberry, blue cohosh, cayenne, ephedra, ginger, ginseng (American), kola, licorice, and yohimbe. Avoid black cohosh, California poppy, coleus, golden seal, hawthorn, mistletoe, periwinkle, quinine, and shepherd's purse.

Stability Store at controlled room temperature of 20°C to 25°C (68°F to 77°F).

Mechanism of Action Trandolapril is an ACE inhibitor which prevents the formation of angiotensin II from angiotensin I. Trandolapril must undergo enzymatic hydrolysis, mainly in liver, to its biologically active metabolite, trandolaprilat. A CNS mechanism may also be involved in the hypotensive effect as angiotensin II increases adrenergic outflow from the CNS. Vasoactive kallikrein's may be decreased in conversion to active hormones by ACE inhibitors, thus reducing blood pressure.

Pharmacodynamics/Kinetics
Onset of action: 1-2 hours
  Peak effect: Reduction in blood pressure: 6 hours
Duration: Prolonged; 72 hours after single dose
Absorption: Rapid
Distribution:
  Trandolapril: ~18L
  Trandolaprilat (active metabolite) is very lipophilic in comparison to other ACE inhibitors
Protein binding:
  Trandolapril: ~80%
  Trandolaprilat: 65% to 94% (concentration dependent)
Metabolism: Hepatically hydrolyzed to active metabolite, trandolaprilat
Bioavailability:
  Trandolapril: 10%
  Trandolaprilat: 70%
Half-life elimination:
  Trandolapril: 6 hours; Trandolaprilat: Effective: 22.5 hours
Time to peak: Parent: 1 hour; Active metabolite trandolaprilat: 4-10 hours
Excretion: Urine (33%); feces (66%)
  Clearance: Reduce dose in renal failure; creatinine clearances ≤30 mL/minute result in accumulation of active metabolite

Dosage
Geriatric & Adult
  Hypertension: Initial dose in patients not receiving a diuretic: Oral: 1 mg once daily (2 mg/day in black patients). Adjust dosage at intervals of ≥1 week according to blood pressure response; most patients require 2-4 mg/day. There is little experience with doses >8 mg/day. Patients inadequately treated with once daily dosing at 4 mg may be treated with twice daily dosing. If blood pressure is not adequately controlled with trandolapril monotherapy, a diuretic may be added.
    Usual dose range (JNC 7): 1-4 mg once daily
  Post-MI heart failure or LV dysfunction: Oral: Initial: 1 mg once daily; titrate (as tolerated) towards target dose of 4 mg/day. If 4 mg dose is not tolerated, patients may continue therapy with the greatest tolerated dose.

Renal Impairment Cl$_{cr}$ <30 mL/minute: Recommended starting dose: 0.5 mg once daily.
Hepatic Impairment Cirrhosis: Recommended starting dose: 0.5 mg once daily.
Monitoring Parameters Blood pressure; serum creatinine and potassium; if patient has collagen vascular disease and/or renal impairment, periodically monitor CBC with differential
Special Geriatric Considerations Due to frequent decreases in glomerular filtration (also creatinine clearance) with aging, elderly patients may have exaggerated responses to ACE inhibitors; differences in clinical response due to hepatic changes are not observed. ACE inhibitors may be preferred agents in elderly patients with CHF and diabetes mellitus. Diabetic proteinuria is reduced and insulin sensitivity is enhanced. In general, the side effect profile is favorable in the elderly and causes little or no CNS confusion; use lowest dose recommendations initially. Adjust for renal function. Many elderly may be volume depleted due to diuretic use and/or blunted thirst reflex resulting in inadequate fluid intake.
Dosage Forms Excipient information presented when available (limited, particularly for generics); consult specific product labeling.
  Tablet, oral: 1 mg, 2 mg, 4 mg
    Mavik®: 1 mg [scored]
    Mavik®: 2 mg, 4 mg

Trandolapril and Verapamil (tran DOE la pril & ver AP a mil)

Related Information
Trandolapril *on page 1946*
Verapamil *on page 2014*
Brand Names: U.S. Tarka®
Brand Names: Canada Tarka®
Index Terms Verapamil and Trandolapril
Generic Availability (U.S.) Yes
Pharmacologic Category Angiotensin-Converting Enzyme (ACE) Inhibitor; Calcium Channel Blocker
Use Treatment of hypertension; however, not indicated for initial treatment of hypertension
Dosage
Geriatric Refer to dosing in individual monographs.
Adult Hypertension: Oral: Individualize dose. Patients receiving trandolapril (up to 8 mg) and verapamil (up to 240 mg) in separate tablets may wish to receive Tarka® at equivalent dosages once daily.
Renal Impairment Usual regimen need not be adjusted unless patient's creatinine clearance is <30 mL/minute. Titration of individual components must be done prior to switching to combination product
Hepatic Impairment Has not been evaluated in hepatic impairment. Verapamil is hepatically metabolized, adjustment of dosage in hepatic impairment is recommended.
Special Geriatric Considerations See individual agents. Combination products are not recommended as first-line treatment. Use only if doses of individual agents correspond to the combination available.
Dosage Forms Excipient information presented when available (limited, particularly for generics); consult specific product labeling.
Tablet, variable release: Trandolapril 2 mg [immediate release] and verapamil hydrochloride 180 mg [sustained release]; Trandolapril 2 mg [immediate release] and verapamil hydrochloride 240 mg [sustained release]; Trandolapril 4 mg [immediate release] and verapamil hydrochloride 240 mg [sustained release]
Tarka®:
1/240: Trandolapril 1 mg [immediate release] and verapamil hydrochloride 240 mg [sustained release]
2/180: Trandolapril 2 mg [immediate release] and verapamil hydrochloride 180 mg [sustained release]
2/240: Trandolapril 2 mg [immediate release] and verapamil hydrochloride 240 mg [sustained release]
4/240: Trandolapril 4 mg [immediate release] and verapamil hydrochloride 240 mg [sustained release]

◆ **Transamine Sulphate** *see* Tranylcypromine *on page 1949*
◆ **Transderm Scōp®** *see* Scopolamine (Systemic) *on page 1756*
◆ **Trans-Ver-Sal® [OTC]** *see* Salicylic Acid *on page 1743*
◆ **Tranxene T-Tab** *see* Clorazepate *on page 423*
◆ **Tranxene® T-Tab®** *see* Clorazepate *on page 423*

Tranylcypromine (tran il SIP roe meen)

Related Information
Antidepressant Agents *on page 2097*
Brand Names: U.S. Parnate®
Brand Names: Canada Parnate®
Index Terms Transamine Sulphate; Tranylcypromine Sulfate
Generic Availability (U.S.) No
Pharmacologic Category Antidepressant, Monoamine Oxidase Inhibitor
Use Treatment of major depressive episode without melancholia
Unlabeled Use Treatment of post-traumatic stress disorder
Medication Guide Available Yes
Contraindications
Cardiovascular disease (including hypertension); cerebrovascular defect; history of headache; history of hepatic disease or abnormal liver function tests; pheochromocytoma
Concurrent use of antihistamines, antihypertensives, antiparkinson drugs, bupropion, buspirone, caffeine (excessive use), CNS depressants (including ethanol and narcotics), dextromethorphan, diuretics, elective surgery requiring general anesthesia (discontinue

tranylcypromine ≥10 days prior to elective surgery), local vasoconstrictors, meperidine, MAO inhibitors or dibenzazepine derivatives (eg, amitriptyline, clomipramine, desipramine, imipramine, nortriptyline, protriptyline, doxepin, carbamazepine, cyclobenzaprine, amoxapine, maprotiline, trimipramine), SSRIs or SNRIs, spinal anesthesia (hypotension may be exaggerated), sympathomimetics (including amphetamines, cocaine, phenylephrine, pseudoephedrine) or related compounds (methyldopa, reserpine, levodopa, tryptophan), or foods high in tyramine content

Bupropion: At least 14 days should elapse between MAO inhibitor discontinuation and bupropion initiation.

Buspirone: At least 10 days should elapse between tranylcypromine discontinuation and buspirone initiation.

MAO inhibitors or dibenzazepine derivatives: At least 1-2 weeks should elapse between the use of another MAO inhibitor or dibenzazepine derivative and tranylcypromine use.

Meperidine: At least 2-3 weeks should elapse between MAO inhibitor discontinuation and meperidine use.

SSRIs or SNRIs: At least 2 weeks should elapse between the discontinuation of sertraline or paroxetine and the initiation of tranylcypromine. At least 5 weeks should elapse between the discontinuation of fluoxetine and the initiation of tranylcypromine. At least 1 week should elapse between discontinuation of a SNRI and the initiation of tranylcypromine. At least 2 weeks should elapse between the discontinuation of tranylcypromine and the initiation of SNRIs and SSRIs.

Warnings/Precautions Risk of suicide: [U.S. Boxed Warning]: Antidepressants increase the risk of suicidal thinking and behavior in children, adolescents, and young adults (18-24 years of age) with major depressive disorder (MDD) and other psychiatric disorders; consider risk prior to prescribing. Short-term studies did not show an increased risk in patients >24 years of age and showed a decreased risk inpatients >65 years. Closely monitor for clinical worsening, suicidality, or unusual changes in behavior such as anxiety, agitation, panic attacks, insomnia, irritability, hostility, impulsivity, akathisia, hypomania, and mania. The patient's family or caregiver should be instructed to closely observe the patient and communicate condition with healthcare provider. Such observation would generally include at least weekly face-to-face contact with patients or their family members or caregivers during the first 4 weeks of treatment, then every other week visits for the next 4 weeks, then at 12 weeks, and as clinically indicated beyond 12 weeks. Additional contact by telephone may be appropriate between face-to-face visits. A medication guide should be dispensed with each prescription.

All patients treated with antidepressants should be observed similarly for clinical worsening and suicidality, especially during the initial few months of a course of drug therapy, or at times of dose changes, either increases or decreases. The possibility of a suicide attempt is inherent in major depression and may persist until remission occurs. Worsening depression and severe abrupt suicidality that are not part of the presenting symptoms may require discontinuation or modification of drug therapy. Use caution in high-risk patients during initiation of therapy. Prescriptions should be written for the smallest quantity consistent with good patient care.

Hypertensive crisis may occur with foods/supplements high in tyramine, tryptophan, phenylalanine, or tyrosine content; treatment with phentolamine is recommended for hypertensive crisis. Use with caution in patients who have glaucoma, hyperthyroidism, diabetes or hypotension. May cause orthostatic hypotension (especially at dosages >30 mg/day). Use with caution in patients at risk of seizures, or in patients receiving other drugs which may lower seizure threshold. Use with caution in patients with a history of drug abuse or acute alcoholism; potential for drug dependency exists especially in patients using excessive doses. Discontinue at least 48 hours prior to myelography. May increase the risks associated with electroconvulsive therapy. Consider discontinuing, when possible, prior to elective surgery. Use with caution in patients with renal impairment. Do not use with other MAO inhibitors or antidepressants. Avoid products containing sympathomimetic stimulants or dextromethorphan. Concurrent use with antihypertensive agents may lead to exaggeration of hypotensive effects. Tranylcypromine is not generally considered a first-line agent for the treatment of depression; tranylcypromine is typically used in patients who have failed to respond to other treatments. May worsen psychosis in some patients or precipitate a shift to mania or hypomania in patients with bipolar disorder. **Tranylcypromine is not FDA approved for the treatment of bipolar depression.**

Adverse Reactions (Reflective of adult population; not specific for elderly) Frequency not defined.

Cardiovascular: Edema, orthostatic hypotension, palpitation, tachycardia

Central nervous system: Agitation, anxiety, chills, dizziness, drowsiness, headache, insomnia, mania, restlessness

Dermatologic: Alopecia (rare), rash (rare), urticaria

Endocrine & metabolic: Sexual dysfunction (anorgasmia, ejaculatory disturbances, impotence); SIADH

Gastrointestinal: Abdominal pain, anorexia, constipation, diarrhea, nausea, xerostomia

Genitourinary: Urinary retention

Hematologic: Agranulocytosis, anemia, leukopenia, thrombocytopenia

Hepatic: Hepatitis (rare)

Neuromuscular & skeletal: Muscle spasm, myoclonus, numbness, paresthesia, tremor, weakness

Ocular: Blurred vision

Otic: Tinnitus

Miscellaneous: Diaphoresis

Drug Interactions

Metabolism/Transport Effects Inhibits CYP1A2 (moderate), CYP2A6 (strong), CYP2C19 (moderate), CYP2C8 (weak), CYP2C9 (weak), CYP2D6 (moderate), CYP2E1 (weak), CYP3A4 (weak), Monoamine Oxidase

Avoid Concomitant Use

Avoid concomitant use of Tranylcypromine with any of the following: Alpha-/Beta-Agonists (Indirect-Acting); Alpha1-Agonists; Alpha2-Agonists (Ophthalmic); Amphetamines; Anilidopiperidine Opioids; Antidepressants (Serotonin Reuptake Inhibitor/Antagonist); AtoMOXetine; Bezafibrate; Buprenorphine; BuPROPion; BusPIRone; CarBAMazepine; Clopidogrel; Cyclobenzaprine; Dexmethylphenidate; Dextromethorphan; Diethylpropion; HYDROmorphone; Linezolid; Maprotiline; Meperidine; Methyldopa; Methylene Blue; Methylphenidate; Mirtazapine; Oxymorphone; Pizotifen; Selective Serotonin Reuptake Inhibitors; Serotonin 5-HT1D Receptor Agonists; Serotonin/Norepinephrine Reuptake Inhibitors; Tapentadol; Tetrabenazine; Tetrahydrozoline; Tetrahydrozoline (Nasal); Tricyclic Antidepressants; Tryptophan

Increased Effect/Toxicity

Tranylcypromine may increase the levels/effects of: Alpha-/Beta-Agonists (Direct-Acting); Alpha-/Beta-Agonists (Indirect-Acting); Alpha1-Agonists; Alpha2-Agonists (Ophthalmic); Amphetamines; Anticholinergics; Antidepressants (Serotonin Reuptake Inhibitor/Antagonist); Antihypertensives; AtoMOXetine; Beta2-Agonists; Bezafibrate; BuPROPion; CYP1A2 Substrates; CYP2A6 Substrates; CYP2C19 Substrates; CYP2D6 Substrates; Dexmethylphenidate; Dextromethorphan; Diethylpropion; Doxapram; Fesoterodine; HYDROmorphone; Hypoglycemic Agents; Linezolid; Lithium; Meperidine; Methadone; Methyldopa; Methylene Blue; Methylphenidate; Metoclopramide; Mirtazapine; Orthostatic Hypotension Producing Agents; Pizotifen; Reserpine; Selective Serotonin Reuptake Inhibitors; Serotonin 5-HT1D Receptor Agonists; Serotonin Modulators; Serotonin/Norepinephrine Reuptake Inhibitors; Tetrahydrozoline; Tetrahydrozoline (Nasal); Tricyclic Antidepressants

The levels/effects of Tranylcypromine may be increased by: Altretamine; Anilidopiperidine Opioids; Antipsychotics; Buprenorphine; BusPIRone; CarBAMazepine; COMT Inhibitors; Cyclobenzaprine; Levodopa; MAO Inhibitors; Maprotiline; Oxymorphone; Pramlintide; Propafenone; Tapentadol; Tetrabenazine; TraMADol; Tryptophan

Decreased Effect

Tranylcypromine may decrease the levels/effects of: Acetylcholinesterase Inhibitors (Central); Clopidogrel; Codeine; Tamoxifen

The levels/effects of Tranylcypromine may be decreased by: Acetylcholinesterase Inhibitors (Central)

Ethanol/Nutrition/Herb Interactions

Ethanol: Ethanol may increase CNS depression. Beverages containing tyramine (eg, hearty red wine and beer) may increase toxic effects. Management: Avoid ethanol and beverages containing tyramine.

Food: Concurrent ingestion of foods rich in tyramine, dopamine, tyrosine, phenylalanine, tryptophan, or caffeine may cause sudden and severe high blood pressure (hypertensive crisis or serotonin syndrome). Management: Avoid tyramine-containing foods (aged or matured cheese, air-dried or cured meats including sausages and salamis; fava or broad bean pods, tap/draft beers, Marmite concentrate, sauerkraut, soy sauce, and other soybean condiments). Food's freshness is also an important concern; improperly stored or spoiled food can create an environment in which tyramine concentrations may increase. Avoid foods containing dopamine, tyrosine, phenylalanine, tryptophan, or caffeine.

Herb/Nutraceutical: Kava kava, valerian, St John's wort, and SAMe may increase risk of serotonin syndrome and/or excessive sedation. Supplements containing caffeine, tyrosine, tryptophan, or phenylalanine may increase the risk of severe side effects like hypertensive reactions or serotonin syndrome. Management: Avoid kava kava, valerian, St John's wort, SAMe, and supplements containing caffeine, tyrosine, tryptophan, or phenylalanine.

Stability Store at room temperature of 15°C to 30°C (59°F to 86°F).

◄ **Mechanism of Action** Tranylcypromine is a nonhydrazine monoamine oxidase inhibitor. It increases endogenous concentrations of epinephrine, norepinephrine, dopamine, and serotonin through inhibition of the enzyme (monoamine oxidase) responsible for the breakdown of these neurotransmitters.

Pharmacodynamics/Kinetics
Onset of action: Therapeutic: 2 days to 3 weeks continued dosing
Duration: MAO inhibition may persist for up to 10 days following discontinuation
Half-life elimination: 90-190 minutes
Time to peak, serum: ~2 hours
Excretion: Urine

Dosage
Geriatric & Adult Depression: Oral: Usual effective dose: 30 mg/day in divided doses; if symptoms don't improve after 2 weeks, increase by 10 mg increments at 1- to 3-week intervals; maximum: 60 mg/day

Transitioning from another MAO inhibitor or dibenzazepine derivative (eg, TCAs, carbamazepine, cyclobenzaprine) to tranylcypromine therapy: Allow at least 1 medication-free week, then initiate tranylcypromine at 50% of usual starting dose for at least 1 week.

Administration Administer second dose before 4 PM to avoid insomnia

Monitoring Parameters Blood glucose; blood pressure, mental status, suicide ideation (especially at the beginning of therapy or when doses are increased or decreased)

Pharmacotherapy Pearls Has a more rapid onset of therapeutic effect than other MAO inhibitors, but causes more severe hypertensive reactions

Special Geriatric Considerations MAO inhibitors are effective and generally well tolerated by older patients. Potential interactions with tyramine- or tryptophan-containing foods, other drugs, and adverse effects on blood pressure have limited use of MAO inhibitors. They are usually reserved for patients who do not tolerate or respond to traditional "cyclic" or "second generation" antidepressants. Tranylcypromine is the preferred MAO inhibitor because its enzymatic-blocking effects are more rapidly reversed.

Dosage Forms Excipient information presented when available (limited, particularly for generics); consult specific product labeling.
Tablet, oral: 10 mg
Parnate®: 10 mg

◆ **Tranylcypromine Sulfate** *see* Tranylcypromine *on page 1949*
◆ **Trav-L-Tabs® [OTC]** *see* Meclizine *on page 1186*
◆ **Travatan Z®** *see* Travoprost *on page 1952*

Travoprost (TRA voe prost)

Related Information
Glaucoma Drug Therapy *on page 2115*
Medication Safety Issues
Sound-alike/look-alike issues:
Travatan® may be confused with Xalatan®
Brand Names: U.S. Travatan Z®
Brand Names: Canada Travatan Z®
Generic Availability (U.S.) No
Pharmacologic Category Ophthalmic Agent, Antiglaucoma; Prostaglandin, Ophthalmic
Use Reduction of elevated intraocular pressure in patients with open-angle glaucoma or ocular hypertension who are intolerant of the other IOP-lowering medications or insufficiently responsive (failed to achieve target IOP determined after multiple measurements over time) to another IOP-lowering medication
Contraindications Hypersensitivity to travoprost or any component of the formulation
Warnings/Precautions May permanently change/increase brown pigmentation of the iris, the eyelid skin, and eyelashes. In addition, may increase the length and/or number of eyelashes (may vary between eyes); changes occur slowly and may not be noticeable for months or years. Bacterial keratitis, caused by inadvertent contamination of multiple-dose ophthalmic solutions, has been reported. Use caution in patients with intraocular inflammation, aphakic patients, pseudophakic patients with a torn posterior lens capsule, or patients with risk factors for macular edema. Contact with contents of vial should be avoided in women who are pregnant or attempting to become pregnant; in case of accidental exposure to the skin, wash the exposed area with soap and water immediately. Safety and efficacy have not been determined for use in patients with renal or hepatic impairment, angle-closure-, inflammatory-, or neovascular glaucoma.

Adverse Reactions (Reflective of adult population; not specific for elderly)
>10%: Ocular: Hyperemia (30% to 50%)
1% to 10%:
  Cardiovascular: Angina pectoris (1% to 5%), bradycardia (1% to 5%), hyper-/hypotension (1% to 5%)
  Central nervous system: Anxiety (1% to 5%), depression (1% to 5%), headache (1% to 5%), pain (1% to 5%)
  Endocrine & metabolic: Hypercholesterolemia (1% to 5%)
  Gastrointestinal: Dyspepsia (1% to 5%), gastrointestinal symptoms (1% to 5%)
  Genitourinary: Prostate disorder (1% to 5%), urinary incontinence (1% to 5%), urinary tract infection (1% to 5%)
  Miscellaneous: Allergic reaction (1% to 5%), flu-like syndrome (1% to 5%), infection (1% to 5%)
  Neuromuscular & skeletal: Arthritis (1% to 5%), back pain (1% to 5%), chest pain (1% to 5%)
  Ocular: Decreased visual acuity (5% to 10%), eye discomfort (5% to 10%), foreign body sensation (5% to 10%), pain (5% to 10%), pruritus (5% to 10%), abnormal vision (1% to 4%), blepharitis (1% to 4%), blurred vision (1% to 4%), cataract (1% to 4%), conjunctivitis (1% to 4%), corneal staining (1% to 4%), dry eye (1% to 4%), eyelash darkening (1% to 4%), eyelash growth increased (1% to 4%), inflammation (1% to 4%), iris discoloration (1% to 4%), keratitis (1% to 4%), lid margin crusting (1% to 4%), periorbital skin discoloration (darkening) (1% to 4%), photophobia (1% to 4%), subconjunctival hemorrhage (1% to 4%), tearing (1% to 4%)
  Respiratory: Bronchitis (1% to 5%), sinusitis (1% to 5%)
Drug Interactions
  Metabolism/Transport Effects None known.
  Avoid Concomitant Use There are no known interactions where it is recommended to avoid concomitant use.
  Increased Effect/Toxicity There are no known significant interactions involving an increase in effect.
  Decreased Effect There are no known significant interactions involving a decrease in effect.
Stability Store between 2°C to 25°C (36°F to 77°F).
Mechanism of Action A selective FP prostanoid receptor agonist which lowers intraocular pressure by increasing trabecular meshwork and outflow
Pharmacodynamics/Kinetics
  Onset of action: ~2 hours
    Peak effect: 12 hours
  Duration: Plasma levels decrease to <10 pg/mL within 1 hour
  Absorption: Absorbed via cornea
  Metabolism: Hydrolyzed by esterases in the cornea to active free acid; systemically; the free acid is metabolized to inactive metabolites
Dosage
  Geriatric & Adult Glaucoma (open angle) or ocular hypertension: Ophthalmic: Instill 1 drop into affected eye(s) once daily in the evening; do not exceed once-daily dosing (may decrease IOP-lowering effect). If used with other topical ophthalmic agents, separate administration by at least 5 minutes.
Administration May be used with other eye drops to lower intraocular pressure. If using more than one ophthalmic product, wait at least 5 minutes in between application of each medication.
Pharmacotherapy Pearls The IOP-lowering effect was shown to be 7-8 mm Hg in clinical studies. The mean IOP reduction in African-American patients was up to 1.8 mm Hg greater than in non-African-American patients. The reason for this effect is unknown.
Special Geriatric Considerations Evaluate the patient's or caregiver's ability to safely administer the correct dose of ophthalmic medication.
Dosage Forms Excipient information presented when available (limited, particularly for generics); consult specific product labeling.
  Solution, ophthalmic [drops]:
    Travatan Z®: 0.004% (2.5 mL, 5 mL)

TraZODone (TRAZ oh done)

Related Information
  Antidepressant Agents *on page 2097*
Medication Safety Issues
  Sound-alike/look-alike issues:
    Desyrel may be confused with deferoxamine, Demerol®, Delsym®, Zestril®
    TraZODone may be confused with traMADol, ziprasidone

International issues:
Desyrel [Canada, Turkey] may be confused with Deseril brand name for methysergide [Australia, Belgium, Great Britain, Netherlands]

Brand Names: U.S. Oleptro™

Brand Names: Canada Apo-Trazodone D®; Apo-Trazodone®; Dom-Trazodone; Mylan-Trazodone; Novo-Trazodone; Nu-Trazodone; Nu-Trazodone D; Oleptro™; PHL-Trazodone; PMS-Trazodone; ratio-Trazodone; Teva-Trazodone; Trazorel®; ZYM-Trazodone

Index Terms Desyrel; Trazodone Hydrochloride

Generic Availability (U.S.) Yes: Excludes extended release tablet

Pharmacologic Category Antidepressant, Serotonin Reuptake Inhibitor/Antagonist

Use Treatment of major depressive disorder

Unlabeled Use Potential augmenting agent for antidepressants, hypnotic

Medication Guide Available Yes

Contraindications Hypersensitivity to trazodone or any component of the formulation

Warnings/Precautions [U.S. Boxed Warning]: Antidepressants increase the risk of suicidal thinking and behavior in children, adolescents, and young adults (18-24 years of age) with major depressive disorder (MDD) and other psychiatric disorders; consider risk prior to prescribing. Short-term studies did not show an increased risk in patients >24 years of age and showed a decreased risk in patients ≥65 years of age. Closely monitor for clinical worsening, suicidality, or unusual changes in behavior; the patient's family or caregiver should be instructed to closely observe the patient and communicate condition with healthcare provider. A medication guide should be dispensed with each prescription.

The possibility of a suicide attempt is inherent in major depression and may persist until remission occurs. Monitor for worsening of depression or suicidality, especially during initiation of therapy (generally first 1-2 months) or with dose increases or decreases. Use caution in high-risk patients. Worsening depression and severe abrupt suicidality that are not part of the presenting symptoms may require discontinuation or modification of drug therapy. The patient's family or caregiver should be alerted to monitor patients for the emergence of suicidality and associated behaviors (such as agitation, irritability, hostility, impulsivity, and hypomania) and call healthcare provider.

May worsen psychosis in some patients or precipitate a shift to mania or hypomania in patients with bipolar disorder. Patients presenting with depressive symptoms should be screened for bipolar disorder. Monotherapy in patients with bipolar disorder should be avoided. **Trazodone is not FDA approved for the treatment of bipolar depression.**

Priapism, including cases resulting in permanent dysfunction, has occurred with the use of trazodone. Instruct patient to seek medical assistance for erection lasting >4 hours; use with caution in patients who have conditions which may predispose them to priapism (eg, sickle cell anemia, multiple myeloma, leukemia). Not recommended for use in a patient during the acute recovery phase of MI. The risks of sedation, postural hypotension, and/or syncope are high relative to other antidepressants. Trazodone frequently causes sedation, which may result in impaired performance of tasks requiring alertness (eg, operating machinery or driving). Sedative effects may be additive with other CNS depressants and ethanol.

Use with caution in patients with a history of cardiovascular disease (including previous MI, stroke, tachycardia, or conduction abnormalities). Although the risk of conduction abnormalities with this agent is low relative to other antidepressants, QT prolongation (with or without torsade de pointes), ventricular tachycardia, and other arrhythmias have been observed with the use of trazodone (reports limited to immediate-release formulation); use with caution in patients with pre-existing cardiac disease. Concurrent use of CYP3A4 inhibitors may increase the risk of QT prolongation and/or proarrhythmia. Concurrent use with other drugs known to prolong QT_c interval is not recommended. May impair platelet aggregation resulting in increased risk of bleeding events (eg, epistaxis, life threatening bleeding), particularly if used concomitantly with aspirin, NSAIDs, warfarin or other anticoagulants. Trazodone should be initiated with caution in patients who are receiving concurrent or recent therapy with a MAO inhibitor. Oleptro™: Avoid use in combination with or within 14 days of an MAO inhibitor.

Serotonin syndrome (SS)/neuroleptic malignant syndrome (NMS)-like reactions may occur with trazodone when used alone, particularly if used with other serotonergic agents (eg, serotonin/norepinephrine reuptake inhibitors [SNRIs], selective serotonin reuptake inhibitors [SSRIs], or triptans), drugs that impair serotonin metabolism (eg, MAO inhibitors), or antidopaminergic agents (eg, antipsychotics). If concurrent use is clinically warranted, carefully observe patient during treatment initiation and dose increases. Do not use concurrently with serotonin precursors (eg, tryptophan).

May cause SIADH and hyponatremia, predominantly in the elderly; volume depletion and/or concurrent use of diuretics likely increases risk. Use with caution in patients taking antihypertensives; may increase the risk of hypotension or syncope. Use with caution in patients taking strong CYP3A4 inhibitors and moderate or strong CYP3A4 inducers; monitor or consider alternative agents that avoid or lessen the potential for CYP-mediated interactions.

Therapy should not be abruptly discontinued in patients receiving high doses for prolonged periods; gradually reduce dosage prior to complete discontinuation to avoid withdrawal symptoms (eg, anxiety, agitation, sleep disturbance). Use caution in patients with a previous seizure disorder or condition predisposing to seizures such as brain damage, alcoholism, or concurrent therapy with other drugs which lower the seizure threshold. Use with caution in patients with hepatic or renal dysfunction and in elderly patients.

Adverse Reactions (Reflective of adult population; not specific for elderly)
>10%:
Central nervous system: Sedation (≤46%), headache (10% to 33%), dizziness (20% to 28%), fatigue (6% to 15%)
Gastrointestinal: Xerostomia (15% to 34%), nausea (10% to 21%)
Ocular: Blurred vision (5% to 15%)
1% to 10%:
Cardiovascular: Edema (3% to 7%), hypotension (≤7%), syncope (≤5%), hypertension (1% to 2%)
Central nervous system: Confusion (5% to 6%), incoordination (2% to 5%), concentration decreased (1% to 3%), disorientation (≤2%), memory impairment (≤1%), agitation, migraine
Endocrine & metabolic: Libido decreased (1% to 2%)
Gastrointestinal: Diarrhea (5% to 9%), constipation (7% to 8%), abdominal pain, abnormal taste, flatulence, vomiting, weight gain/loss
Genitourinary: Ejaculation disorder (2%), urinary urgency
Neuromuscular & skeletal: Back pain (≤5%), tremor (1% to 5%), paresthesia (≤1%), myalgia
Ocular: Visual disturbance
Respiratory: Nasal congestion (3% to 6%), dyspnea
Miscellaneous: Night sweats

Drug Interactions
Metabolism/Transport Effects Substrate of CYP2D6 (minor), CYP3A4 (major); **Note:** Assignment of Major/Minor substrate status based on clinically relevant drug interaction potential; **Inhibits** CYP3A4 (weak); **Induces** P-glycoprotein

Avoid Concomitant Use
Avoid concomitant use of TraZODone with any of the following: Conivaptan; Dabigatran Etexilate; Highest Risk QTc-Prolonging Agents; MAO Inhibitors; Methylene Blue; Mifepristone; Saquinavir

Increased Effect/Toxicity
TraZODone may increase the levels/effects of: Antipsychotic Agents (Phenothiazines); Fosphenytoin; Highest Risk QTc-Prolonging Agents; Methylene Blue; Metoclopramide; Moderate Risk QTc-Prolonging Agents; Phenytoin; Serotonin Modulators

The levels/effects of TraZODone may be increased by: Antipsychotic Agents (Phenothiazines); Antipsychotics; Boceprevir; BusPIRone; Conivaptan; CYP3A4 Inhibitors (Moderate); CYP3A4 Inhibitors (Strong); Ivacaftor; Linezolid; MAO Inhibitors; Mifepristone; Protease Inhibitors; QTc-Prolonging Agents (Indeterminate Risk and Risk Modifying); Saquinavir; Selective Serotonin Reuptake Inhibitors; Telaprevir; Venlafaxine

Decreased Effect
TraZODone may decrease the levels/effects of: Dabigatran Etexilate; Linagliptin; P-glycoprotein/ABCB1 Substrates; Warfarin

The levels/effects of TraZODone may be decreased by: CYP3A4 Inducers (Strong); Deferasirox; Fosphenytoin; Peginterferon Alfa-2b; Phenytoin; Tocilizumab

Ethanol/Nutrition/Herb Interactions
Ethanol: May increase CNS depression; monitor for increased effects with coadministration. Caution patients about effects.
Food: Time to peak serum levels may be increased if immediate release trazodone is taken with food.
Herb/Nutraceutical: Avoid valerian, St John's wort, SAMe, kava kava (may increase risk of serotonin syndrome and/or excessive sedation).

Stability
Immediate release tablet: Store at room temperature; avoid temperatures >40°C (>104°F). Protect from light.
Extended release tablet: Store at room temperature of 15°C to 30°C (59°F to 86°F). Protect from light.

TRAZODONE

Mechanism of Action Inhibits reuptake of serotonin, causes adrenoreceptor subsensitivity, and induces significant changes in 5-HT presynaptic receptor adrenoreceptors. Trazodone also significantly blocks histamine (H_1) and alpha$_1$-adrenergic receptors.

Pharmacodynamics/Kinetics

Onset of action: Therapeutic (antidepressant): Up to 6 weeks; sleep aid: 1-3 hours

Absorption: Well absorbed; Extended release: C_{max} increases ~86% when taken shortly after ingestion of a high-fat meal compared to fasting conditions

Protein binding: 85% to 95%

Metabolism: Hepatic via CYP3A4 (extensive) to an active metabolite (mCPP)

Half-life elimination: 7-10 hours

Time to peak, serum:

Immediate release: 30-100 minutes; delayed with food (up to 2.5 hours)

Extended release: 9 hours; not significantly affected by food

Excretion: Primarily urine (<1% excreted unchanged); secondarily feces

Dosage

Geriatric

Immediate release: Oral: 25-50 mg at bedtime with 25-50 mg/day dose increase every 3 days for inpatients and weekly for outpatients, if tolerated; usual dose: 75-150 mg/day

Extended release: Refer to adult dosing. Use with caution in the elderly; clinical experience is limited.

Adult

Depression: Oral: Initial: 150 mg/day in 3 divided doses (may increase by 50 mg/day every 3-7 days); maximum dose: 600 mg/day

Extended release formulation: Initial: 150 mg once daily at bedtime (may increase by 75 mg/day every 3 days); maximum dose: 375 mg/day; once adequate response obtained, gradually reduce with adjustment based on therapeutic response

Note: Therapeutic effects may take up to 6 weeks. Therapy is normally maintained for 6-12 months after optimum response is reached to prevent recurrence of depression.

Sedation/hypnotic (unlabeled use): Oral: 25-50 mg at bedtime (often in combination with daytime SSRIs). May increase up to 200 mg at bedtime.

Administration

Immediate release tablet: Dosing after meals may decrease lightheadedness and postural hypotension

Extended release tablet: Take on an empty stomach; swallow whole or as a half tablet without food. Tablet may be broken along the score line, but do not crush or chew.

Monitoring Parameters Baseline liver function prior to and periodically during therapy; suicide ideation (especially at the beginning of therapy or when doses are increased or decreased)

Reference Range

Plasma levels do not always correlate with clinical effectiveness

Therapeutic: 0.5-2.5 mcg/mL

Potentially toxic: >2.5 mcg/mL

Toxic: >4 mcg/mL

Test Interactions May interfere with urine detection of amphetamine/methamphetamine (false-positive).

Special Geriatric Considerations Very sedating, but little anticholinergic effects.

Dosage Forms Excipient information presented when available (limited, particularly for generics); consult specific product labeling.

Tablet, oral: 50 mg, 100 mg

Tablet, oral, as hydrochloride: 50 mg, 100 mg, 150 mg, 300 mg

Tablet, extended release, oral, as hydrochloride:

Oleptro™: 150 mg, 300 mg [scored]

Triamcinolone (Systemic) (trye am SIN oh lone)

Related Information
Corticosteroids Systemic Equivalencies *on page 2112*

Medication Safety Issues
Sound-alike/look-alike issues:
Kenalog® may be confused with Ketalar®
Other safety concerns:
TAC (occasional abbreviation for triamcinolone) is an error-prone abbreviation (mistaken as tetracaine-adrenaline-cocaine)

Brand Names: U.S. Aristospan®; Kenalog®-10; Kenalog®-40

Brand Names: Canada Aristospan®

Index Terms Triamcinolone Acetonide, Parenteral; Triamcinolone Hexacetonide

Generic Availability (U.S.) No

Pharmacologic Category Corticosteroid, Systemic

Use
Intra-articular (soft tissue): Acute gouty arthritis, acute/subacute bursitis, acute tenosynovitis, epicondylitis, rheumatoid arthritis, synovitis of osteoarthritis

Intralesional: Alopecia areata, discoid lupus erythematosus, keloids, granuloma annulare lesions (localized hypertrophic, infiltrated, or inflammatory), lichen planus plaques, lichen simplex chronicus plaques, psoriatic plaques, necrobiosis lipoidica diabeticorum, cystic tumors of aponeurosis or tendon (ganglia)

Systemic: Adrenocortical insufficiency, dermatologic diseases, endocrine disorders, gastrointestinal diseases, hematologic and neoplastic disorders, nervous system disorders, nephrotic syndrome, rheumatic disorders, allergic states, respiratory diseases, systemic lupus erythematosus (SLE), and other diseases requiring anti-inflammatory or immunosuppressive effects

Contraindications Hypersensitivity to triamcinolone or any component of the formulation; systemic fungal infections; cerebral malaria; idiopathic thrombocytopenic purpura (I.M. injection)

Warnings/Precautions May cause hypercorticism or suppression of hypothalamic-pituitary-adrenal (HPA) axis, particularly in patients receiving high doses for prolonged periods. HPA axis suppression may lead to adrenal crisis. Withdrawal and discontinuation of a corticosteroid should be done slowly and carefully.

Acute myopathy has been reported with high-dose corticosteroids, usually in patients with neuromuscular transmission disorders; may involve ocular and/or respiratory muscles; monitor creatine kinase; recovery may be delayed. Corticosteroid use may cause psychiatric disturbances, including depression, euphoria, insomnia, mood swings, and personality changes. Pre-existing psychiatric conditions may be exacerbated by corticosteroid use. Prolonged use of corticosteroids may also increase the incidence of secondary infection, mask acute infection (including fungal infections), prolong or exacerbate viral infections, or limit response to vaccines. Exposure to chickenpox should be avoided; corticosteroids should not be used to treat ocular herpes simplex. Corticosteroids should not be used for cerebral malaria or viral hepatitis. Close observation is required in patients with latent tuberculosis and/or TB reactivity; restrict use in active TB (only in conjunction with antituberculosis treatment). Use with caution in patients with threadworm infection; may cause serious hyperinfection. Prolonged treatment with corticosteroids has been associated with the development of Kaposi's sarcoma (case reports); if noted, discontinuation of therapy should be considered. Avoid use in head injury patients.

Use with caution in patients with thyroid disease, hepatic impairment, renal impairment, cardiovascular disease, diabetes, myasthenia gravis, patients at risk for osteoporosis, patients at risk for seizures, or GI diseases (diverticulitis, peptic ulcer, ulcerative colitis) due to perforation risk. Avoid use in head injury patients. Use caution following acute MI (corticosteroids have been associated with myocardial rupture). Because of the risk of adverse effects, systemic corticosteroids should be used cautiously in the elderly in the smallest possible effective dose for the shortest duration. Patients should not be immunized with live, viral vaccines while receiving immunosuppressive doses of corticosteroids. The ability to respond to dead viral vaccines is unknown.

Withdraw therapy with gradual tapering of dose. There have been reports of systemic corticosteroid withdrawal symptoms (eg, joint/muscle pain, lassitude, depression) when withdrawing oral inhalation therapy. Injection suspension contains benzyl alcohol. Administer products only via recommended route (depending on product used). Do **not** administer any triamcinolone product via the epidural or intrathecal route; serious adverse events, including fatalities, have been reported.

Adverse Reactions (Reflective of adult population; not specific for elderly) Frequency not defined; reactions reported with corticosteroid therapy in general:

Cardiovascular: Arrhythmia, bradycardia, cardiac arrest, cardiac enlargement, CHF, circulatory collapse, edema, hypertension, hypertrophic cardiomyopathy (premature infants), myocardial rupture (following recent MI), syncope, tachycardia, thromboembolism, vasculitis

Central nervous system: Arachnoiditis (I.T.), depression, emotional instability, euphoria, headache, insomnia, intracranial pressure increased, malaise, meningitis (I.T.), mood changes, neuritis, neuropathy, personality change, pseudotumor cerebri (with discontinuation), seizure, spinal cord infarction, stroke, vertigo

Dermatologic: Abscess (sterile), acne, allergic dermatitis, angioedema, atrophy (cutaneous/subcutaneous), bruising, dry skin, erythema, hair thinning, hirsutism, hyper-/hypopigmentation, hypertrichosis, impaired wound healing, lupus erythematosus-like lesions, petechiae, purpura, rash, skin test suppression, striae, thin skin

Endocrine & metabolic: Carbohydrate intolerance, Cushingoid state, diabetes mellitus, fluid retention, glucose intolerance, growth suppression (children), hypokalemia, hypokalemic alkalosis, menstrual irregularities, negative nitrogen balance, sodium retention, sperm motility altered

Gastrointestinal: Abdominal distention, appetite increased, GI hemorrhage, GI perforation, nausea, pancreatitis, peptic ulcer, ulcerative esophagitis, weight gain

Hepatic: Hepatomegaly, liver function tests increased

Local: Thrombophlebitis

Neuromuscular & skeletal: Aseptic necrosis of femoral and humeral heads, calcinosis, Charcot-like arthropathy, fractures, joint tissue damage, muscle mass loss, myopathy, osteoporosis, parasthesia, paraplegia, quadriplegia, tendon rupture, vertebral compression fractures, weakness

Ocular: Cataracts, cortical blindness, exophthalmos, glaucoma, ocular pressure increased, papilledema

Renal: Glycosuria

Respiratory: Pulmonary edema

Miscellaneous: Abnormal fat deposits, anaphylactoid reaction, anaphylaxis, diaphoresis, hiccups, infection, moon face

Drug Interactions

Metabolism/Transport Effects None known.

Avoid Concomitant Use

Avoid concomitant use of Triamcinolone (Systemic) with any of the following: Aldesleukin; BCG; Mifepristone; Natalizumab; Pimecrolimus; Tacrolimus (Topical)

Increased Effect/Toxicity

Triamcinolone (Systemic) may increase the levels/effects of: Acetylcholinesterase Inhibitors; Amphotericin B; Deferasirox; Leflunomide; Loop Diuretics; Natalizumab; NSAID (COX-2 Inhibitor); NSAID (Nonselective); Thiazide Diuretics; Vaccines (Live); Warfarin

The levels/effects of Triamcinolone (Systemic) may be increased by: Antifungal Agents (Azole Derivatives, Systemic); Aprepitant; Calcium Channel Blockers (Nondihydropyridine); Denosumab; Estrogen Derivatives; Fluconazole; Fosaprepitant; Indacaterol; Macrolide Antibiotics; Mifepristone; Neuromuscular-Blocking Agents (Nondepolarizing); Pimecrolimus; Quinolone Antibiotics; Roflumilast; Salicylates; Tacrolimus (Topical); Telaprevir; Trastuzumab

Decreased Effect

Triamcinolone (Systemic) may decrease the levels/effects of: Aldesleukin; Antidiabetic Agents; BCG; Calcitriol; Coccidioidin Skin Test; Corticorelin; Hyaluronidase; Isoniazid; Salicylates; Sipuleucel-T; Telaprevir; Vaccines (Inactivated)

The levels/effects of Triamcinolone (Systemic) may be decreased by: Aminoglutethimide; Barbiturates; Echinacea; Mifepristone; Mitotane; Primidone; Rifamycin Derivatives

Stability Injection, suspension:

Acetonide injectable suspension: Kenalog®: Store at 20°C to 25°C (68°F to 77°F); avoid freezing. Protect from light.

Hexacetonide injectable suspension: Store at 20°C to 25°C (68°F to 77°F); avoid freezing. Protect from light. Avoid diluents containing parabens, phenol, or other preservatives (may cause flocculation). Diluted suspension stable up to 1 week. Suspension for intralesional use may be diluted with D$_5$NS, D$_{10}$NS, NS, or SWFI to a 1:1, 1:2, or 1:4 concentration. Solutions for intra-articular use, may be diluted with lidocaine 1% or 2%.

Mechanism of Action Decreases inflammation by suppression of migration of polymorphonuclear leukocytes and reversal of increased capillary permeability; suppresses the immune system by reducing activity and volume of the lymphatic system; suppresses adrenal function at high doses

Pharmacodynamics/Kinetics
Distribution: V_d: 99.5 L
Protein binding: ~68%
Half-life elimination: Biologic: 18-36 hours
Time to peak: I.M.: 8-10 hours
Excretion: Urine (~40%); feces (~60%)

Dosage
Geriatric & Adult The lowest possible dose should be used to control the condition; when dose reduction is possible, the dose should be reduced gradually.

Dermatoses (steroid-responsive, including contact/atopic dermatitis): Injection:
Acetonide: Intradermal: Initial: 1 mg
Hexacetonide: Intralesional, sublesional: Up to 0.5 mg/square inch of affected skin; range: 2-48 mg/day

Hay fever/pollen asthma: I.M.: 40-100 mg as a single injection/season

Multiple sclerosis (acute exacerbation): I.M.: 160 mg daily for 1 week, followed by 64 mg every other day for 1 month

Rheumatic or arthritic disorders:
Intra-articular (or similar injection as designated):
Acetonide: Intra-articular, intrabursal, tendon sheaths: Initial: Smaller joints: 2.5-5 mg, larger joints: 5-15 mg; may require up to 10 mg for small joints and up to 40 mg for large joints; maximum dose/treatment (several joints at one time): 20-80 mg
Hexacetonide: Intra-articular: Average dose: 2-20 mg; smaller joints: 2-6 mg; larger joints: 10-20 mg. Frequency of injection into a single joint is every 3-4 weeks as necessary; to avoid possible joint destruction use as infrequently as possible.
I.M.: Acetonide: Range: 2.5-100 mg/day; Initial: 60 mg
See table.

Triamcinolone Dosing

	Acetonide	Hexacetonide
Intrasynovial	5-40 mg	
Intralesional	1-30 mg (usually 1 mg per injection site); 10 mg/mL suspension usually used	Up to 0.5 mg/sq inch affected area
Sublesional	1-30 mg	
Systemic I.M.	2.5-60 mg/dose (usual adult dose: 60 mg; may repeat with 20-100 mg dose when symptoms recur)	
Intra-articular	2.5-40 mg	2-20 mg average
large joints	5-15 mg	10-20 mg
small joints	2.5-5 mg	2-6 mg
Tendon sheaths	2.5-10 mg	
Intradermal	1 mg/site	

Administration Shake well before use to ensure suspension is uniform. Inspect visually to ensure no clumping; administer immediately after withdrawal so settling does not occur in the syringe. Do **not** administer any product I.V. or via the epidural or intrathecal route.
Aristospan® (20 mg/mL concentration): For intra-articular and soft tissue administration only; a ≥23-gauge needle is preferred.
Aristospan® (5 mg/mL concentration): For intralesional or sublesional administration only; a ≥23-gauge needle is preferred.
Kenalog®-10 injection: For intra-articular or intralesional administration only. When administered intralesionally, inject directly into the lesion (ie, intradermally or subcutaneously). Tuberculin syringes with a 23- to 25-gauge needle are preferable for intralesional injections.
Kenalog®-40 injection: For intra-articular, soft tissue or I.M. administration. When administered I.M., inject deep into the gluteal muscle using a minimum needle length of 1½ inches for adults. Obese patients may require a longer needle. Alternate sites for subsequent injections.

Special Geriatric Considerations Because of the risk of adverse effects, corticosteroids should be used cautiously in the elderly, in the smallest possible dose, and for the shortest possible time.

◀ **Dosage Forms** Excipient information presented when available (limited, particularly for generics); consult specific product labeling.

Injection, suspension, as acetonide:

Kenalog®-10: 10 mg/mL (5 mL) [contains benzyl alcohol, polysorbate 80; **not** for I.V., I.M., intraocular, epidural, or intrathecal use]

Kenalog®-40: 40 mg/mL (1 mL, 5 mL, 10 mL) [contains benzyl alcohol, polysorbate 80; **not** for I.V., intradermal, intraocular, intraocular, epidural, or intrathecal use]

Injection, suspension, as hexacetonide:

Aristospan®: 5 mg/mL (5 mL); 20 mg/mL (1 mL, 5 mL) [contains benzyl alcohol, polysorbate 80; **not** for I.V. use]

Triamcinolone (Nasal) (trye am SIN oh lone)

Medication Safety Issues
Sound-alike/look-alike issues:
Nasacort® may be confused with NasalCrom®
Other safety concerns:
TAC (occasional abbreviation for triamcinolone) is an error-prone abbreviation (mistaken as tetracaine-adrenaline-cocaine)

Brand Names: U.S. Nasacort® AQ

Brand Names: Canada Nasacort® AQ; Trinasal®

Index Terms Triamcinolone Acetonide

Generic Availability (U.S.) Yes

Pharmacologic Category Corticosteroid, Nasal

Use Management of seasonal and perennial allergic rhinitis

Unlabeled Use Adjunct to antibiotics in empiric treatment of acute bacterial rhinosinusitis (ABRS) (Chow, 2012)

Dosage

Geriatric & Adult Allergic rhinitis (perennial or seasonal):

Nasal spray: 220 mcg/day as 2 sprays in each nostril once daily; once symptoms controlled reduce to 110 mcg/day

Nasal inhaler: Initial: 220 mcg/day as 2 sprays in each nostril once daily; may increase dose to 440 mcg/day (given once daily or divided and given 2 or 4 times/day)

Special Geriatric Considerations Evaluate the patient's or caregiver's ability to safely administer the correct dose of nasal medication.

Dosage Forms Excipient information presented when available (limited, particularly for generics); consult specific product labeling.

Suspension, intranasal, as acetonide [spray]: 55 mcg/inhalation (16.5 g)

Nasacort® AQ: 55 mcg/inhalation (16.5 g) [chlorofluorocarbon free; contains benzalkonium chloride; 120 actuations]

Triamcinolone (Ophthalmic) (trye am SIN oh lone)

Medication Safety Issues
Other safety concerns:
TAC (occasional abbreviation for triamcinolone) is an error-prone abbreviation (mistaken as tetracaine-adrenaline-cocaine)

Brand Names: U.S. Triesence™

Index Terms Triamcinolone acetonide

Generic Availability (U.S.) No

Pharmacologic Category Corticosteroid, Ophthalmic

Use

Intavitreal: Treatment of sympathetic ophthalmia, temporal arteritis, uveitis, ocular inflammatory conditions unresponsive to topical corticosteroids

Triesence™: Visualization during vitrectomy

Dosage

Geriatric & Adult

Ocular disease: Intravitreal: Initial: 4 mg as a single dose; additional doses may be given as needed

Visualization during vitrectomy: Intravitreal (Triesence™): 1-4 mg

Special Geriatric Considerations Evaluate the patient's or caregiver's ability to safely administer the correct dose of ophthalmic medication.

Dosage Forms Excipient information presented when available (limited, particularly for generics); consult specific product labeling.
Injection, suspension, ophthalmic, as acetonide:
Triesence™: 40 mg/mL (1 mL) [contains polysorbate 80; not for I.V. use]

Triamcinolone (Topical) (trye am SIN oh lone)

Related Information
Topical Corticosteroids *on page 2113*
Medication Safety Issues
Sound-alike/look-alike issues:
Kenalog® may be confused with Ketalar®
Other safety concerns:
TAC (occasional abbreviation for triamcinolone) is an error-prone abbreviation (mistaken as tetracaine-adrenaline-cocaine)
Brand Names: U.S. Kenalog®; Oralone®; Pediaderm™ TA; Trianex™; Triderm®; Zytopic™
Brand Names: Canada Kenalog®; Oracort; Triaderm
Generic Availability (U.S.) Yes: Excludes spray
Pharmacologic Category Corticosteroid, Topical
Use
Oral topical: Adjunctive treatment and temporary relief of symptoms associated with oral inflammatory lesions and ulcerative lesions resulting from trauma
Topical: Inflammatory dermatoses responsive to steroids
Dosage
Geriatric & Adult
Dermatoses (steroid-responsive, including contact/atopic dermatitis): Topical:
Cream, Ointment:
0.025% or 0.05%: Apply thin film to affected areas 2-4 times/day
0.1% or 0.5%: Apply thin film to affected areas 2-3 times/day
Spray: Apply to affected area 3-4 times/day
Oral inflammatory lesions/ulcers: Oral topical: Press a small dab (about ¼ inch) to the lesion until a thin film develops; a larger quantity may be required for coverage of some lesions. For optimal results, use only enough to coat the lesion with a thin film; do not rub in.
Special Geriatric Considerations Instruct patient or caregiver on appropriate use of topical triamcinolone products.
Dosage Forms Excipient information presented when available (limited, particularly for generics); consult specific product labeling.
Aerosol, spray, topical, as acetonide:
Kenalog®: 0.2 mg/2-second spray (63 g, 100 g) [contains dehydrated ethanol 10.3%]
Cream, topical, as acetonide: 0.025% (15 g, 80 g, 454 g); 0.1% (15 g, 30 g, 80 g, 454 g); 0.5% (15 g)
Triderm®: 0.1% (30 g, 85 g)
Cream, topical, as acetonide [kit]:
Pediaderm™ TA: 0.1% (30 g) [packaged with protective emollient]
Zytopic™: 0.1% (85 g) [packaged with cleanser and moisturizer]
Lotion, topical, as acetonide: 0.025% (60 mL); 0.1% (60 mL); 0.1%
Ointment, topical, as acetonide: 0.025% (15 g, 80 g, 454 g); 0.05% (430 g); 0.1% (15 g, 80 g, 454 g); 0.5% (15 g)
Trianex™: 0.05% (17 g, 85 g)
Paste, oral topical, as acetonide: 0.1% (5 g)
Oralone®: 0.1% (5 g)

◆ **Triamcinolone Acetonide** *see* Triamcinolone (Nasal) *on page 1960*
◆ **Triamcinolone acetonide** *see* Triamcinolone (Ophthalmic) *on page 1960*
◆ **Triamcinolone Acetonide, Parenteral** *see* Triamcinolone (Systemic) *on page 1957*
◆ **Triamcinolone and Nystatin** *see* Nystatin and Triamcinolone *on page 1400*
◆ **Triamcinolone Hexacetonide** *see* Triamcinolone (Systemic) *on page 1957*
◆ **Triaminic® Children's Cough Long Acting [OTC]** *see* Dextromethorphan *on page 525*
◆ **Triaminic™ Children's Fever Reducer Pain Reliever [OTC]** *see* Acetaminophen *on page 31*
◆ **Triaminic Thin Strips® Children's Cold with Stuffy Nose [OTC]** *see* Phenylephrine (Systemic) *on page 1523*
◆ **Triaminic Thin Strips® Children's Cough & Runny Nose [OTC]** *see* DiphenhydrAMINE (Systemic) *on page 556*
◆ **Triaminic Thin Strips® Children's Long Acting Cough [OTC]** *see* Dextromethorphan *on page 525*

Triamterene (trye AM ter een)

Medication Safety Issues
Sound-alike/look-alike issues:
Triamterene may be confused with trimipramine

Dyrenium® may be confused with Pyridium®

Brand Names: U.S. Dyrenium®

Generic Availability (U.S.) No

Pharmacologic Category Diuretic, Potassium-Sparing

Use Alone or in combination with other diuretics in treatment of edema and hypertension; decreases potassium excretion caused by kaliuretic diuretics

Contraindications Hypersensitivity to triamterene or any component of the formulation; patients receiving other potassium-sparing diuretics; anuria; severe hepatic disease; hyperkalemia or history of hyperkalemia; severe or progressive renal disease

Warnings/Precautions [U.S. Boxed Warning]: Hyperkalemia can occur; patients at risk include those with renal impairment, diabetes, the elderly, and the severely ill. Serum potassium levels must be monitored at frequent intervals especially when dosages are changed or with any illness that may cause renal dysfunction. Avoid potassium supplements, potassium-containing salt substitutes, a diet rich in potassium, or other drugs that can cause hyperkalemia. Monitor for fluid and electrolyte imbalances. Diuretic therapy should be carefully used in severe hepatic dysfunction; electrolyte and fluid shifts can cause or exacerbate encephalopathy. Use cautiously in patients with history of kidney stones and diabetes. Can cause photosensitivity.

Adverse Reactions (Reflective of adult population; not specific for elderly) 1% to 10%:

Cardiovascular: Hypotension, edema, CHF, bradycardia

Central nervous system: Dizziness, headache, fatigue

Gastrointestinal: Constipation, nausea

Respiratory: Dyspnea

Drug Interactions
Metabolism/Transport Effects None known.

Avoid Concomitant Use

Avoid concomitant use of Triamterene with any of the following: CycloSPORINE; CycloSPORINE (Systemic); Tacrolimus; Tacrolimus (Systemic)

Increased Effect/Toxicity

Triamterene may increase the levels/effects of: ACE Inhibitors; Amifostine; Ammonium Chloride; Antihypertensives; Cardiac Glycosides; CycloSPORINE; CycloSPORINE (Systemic); Dofetilide; Hypotensive Agents; RiTUXimab; Sodium Phosphates; Tacrolimus; Tacrolimus (Systemic)

The levels/effects of Triamterene may be increased by: Alfuzosin; Angiotensin II Receptor Blockers; Diazoxide; Drospirenone; Eplerenone; Herbs (Hypotensive Properties); Indomethacin; MAO Inhibitors; Nonsteroidal Anti-Inflammatory Agents; Pentoxifylline; Phosphodiesterase 5 Inhibitors; Potassium Salts; Prostacyclin Analogues; Tolvaptan

Decreased Effect

Triamterene may decrease the levels/effects of: Cardiac Glycosides; QuiNIDine

The levels/effects of Triamterene may be decreased by: Herbs (Hypertensive Properties); Methylphenidate; Nonsteroidal Anti-Inflammatory Agents; Yohimbine

Mechanism of Action Blocks epithelial sodium channels in the late distal convoluted tubule (DCT) and collecting duct which inhibits sodium reabsorption from the lumen. This effectively reduces intracellular sodium, decreasing the function of Na+/K+ ATPase, leading to potassium retention and decreased calcium, magnesium, and hydrogen excretion. As sodium uptake capacity in the DCT/collecting duct is limited, the natriuretic, diuretic, and antihypertensive effects are generally considered weak.

Pharmacodynamics/Kinetics
Onset of action: Diuresis: 2-4 hours

Duration: 7-9 hours

Absorption: Unreliable

Dosage
Geriatric Refer to adult dosing. In the management of hypertension, consider lower initial doses and titrate to response (Aronow, 2011).

Adult Edema, hypertension: Oral: 100-300 mg/day in 1-2 divided doses; maximum dose: 300 mg/day; usual dosage range (JNC 7): 50-100 mg/day

Renal Impairment Cl_{cr} <10 mL/minute: Avoid use.

Hepatic Impairment Dose reduction is recommended in patients with cirrhosis.

Administration May be administered with food.

Monitoring Parameters Blood pressure; serum electrolytes (especially potassium), renal function; weight, I & O

Test Interactions Interferes with fluorometric assay of quinidine

Special Geriatric Considerations Monitor serum potassium.

Dosage Forms Excipient information presented when available (limited, particularly for generics); consult specific product labeling.

Capsule, oral:

Dyrenium®: 50 mg, 100 mg

♦ **Triamterene and Hydrochlorothiazide** *see* Hydrochlorothiazide and Triamterene *on page 936*

♦ **Trianex™** *see* Triamcinolone (Topical) *on page 1961*

Triazolam (trye AY zoe lam)

Related Information

Anxiolytic, Sedative/Hypnotic, and Miscellaneous Benzodiazepines *on page 2106*

Beers Criteria − Potentially Inappropriate Medications for Geriatrics *on page 2183*

Medication Safety Issues

Sound-alike/look-alike issues:

Triazolam may be confused with alPRAZolam

Halcion® may be confused with halcinonide, Haldol®

BEERS Criteria medication:

This drug may be potentially inappropriate for use in geriatric patients (Quality of evidence - high; Strength of recommendation - strong).

Brand Names: U.S. Halcion®

Brand Names: Canada Apo-Triazo®; Gen-Triazolam; Halcion®; Mylan-Triazolam

Generic Availability (U.S.) Yes

Pharmacologic Category Benzodiazepine

Use Short-term treatment of insomnia

Unlabeled Use Treatment of anxiety before dental procedures

Medication Guide Available Yes

Contraindications Hypersensitivity to triazolam or any component of the formulation (cross-sensitivity with other benzodiazepines may exist); concurrent therapy with itraconazole, ketoconazole, nefazodone, and other moderate/strong CYP3A4 inhibitors

Warnings/Precautions As a hypnotic, should be used only after evaluation of potential causes of sleep disturbance. Failure of sleep disturbance to resolve after 7-10 days may indicate psychiatric or medical illness. A worsening of insomnia or the emergence of new abnormalities of thought or behavior may represent unrecognized psychiatric or medical illness and requires immediate and careful evaluation. Prescription should be written for a maximum of 7-10 days and should not be prescribed in quantities exceeding a 1-month supply. Abrupt discontinuation after sustained use (generally >10 days) may cause withdrawal symptoms.

An increase in daytime anxiety may occur after as few as 10 days of continuous use, which may be related to withdrawal reaction in some patients. Anterograde amnesia may occur at a higher rate with triazolam than with other benzodiazepines. Use with caution in elderly or debilitated patients, patients with hepatic disease (including alcoholics), or renal impairment. Use with caution in patients with respiratory disease or impaired gag reflex. Avoid use in patients with sleep apnea.

In older adults, benzodiazepines increase the risk of impaired cognition, delirium, falls, fractures, and motor vehicle accidents. Due to increased sensitivity in this age group, avoid use for treatment of insomnia, agitation, or delirium. (Beers Criteria).

Causes CNS depression (dose-related) resulting in sedation, dizziness, confusion, or ataxia which may impair physical and mental capabilities. Patients must be cautioned about performing tasks which require mental alertness (eg, operating machinery or driving). Use with caution in patients receiving other CNS depressants or psychoactive agents. Postmarketing studies have indicated that the use of hypnotic/sedative agents for sleep has been associated with hypersensitivity reactions including anaphylaxis as well as angioedema. An increased risk for hazardous sleep-related activities such as sleep-driving; cooking and eating food, and making phone calls while asleep have also been noted. Effects with other sedative drugs or ethanol may be potentiated. Benzodiazepines have been associated with falls and traumatic injury and should be used with extreme caution in patients who are at risk of these events (especially the elderly).

Use caution with potent CYP3A4 inhibitors, as they may significantly decreased the clearance of triazolam. Use caution in patients with suicidal risk. Use with caution in patients with a history of drug dependence. Benzodiazepines have been associated with dependence and acute withdrawal symptoms on discontinuation or reduction in dose. Acute withdrawal, including seizures, may be precipitated after administration of flumazenil to patients receiving long-term benzodiazepine therapy.

Paradoxical reactions, including hyperactive or aggressive behavior have been reported with benzodiazepines, particularly in psychiatric patients. Does not have analgesic, antidepressant, or antipsychotic properties.

Adverse Reactions (Reflective of adult population; not specific for elderly)
>10%: Central nervous system: Drowsiness (14%)
1% to 10%:
  Central nervous system: Headache (10%), dizziness (8%), nervousness (5%), lightheadedness (5%), ataxia (5%)
  Gastrointestinal: Nausea (5%), vomiting (5%)

Drug Interactions
  Metabolism/Transport Effects Substrate of CYP3A4 (major); **Note:** Assignment of Major/Minor substrate status based on clinically relevant drug interaction potential; **Inhibits** CYP2C8 (weak), CYP2C9 (weak)
  Avoid Concomitant Use
    Avoid concomitant use of Triazolam with any of the following: Azelastine; Azelastine (Nasal); Boceprevir; Conivaptan; Efavirenz; Methadone; Mirtazapine; OLANZapine; Paraldehyde; Protease Inhibitors; Telaprevir
  Increased Effect/Toxicity
    Triazolam may increase the levels/effects of: Alcohol (Ethyl); Azelastine; Azelastine (Nasal); Buprenorphine; CloZAPine; CNS Depressants; Fosphenytoin; Methadone; Methotrimeprazine; Metyrosine; Mirtazapine; Paraldehyde; Phenytoin; Selective Serotonin Reuptake Inhibitors; Zolpidem

    The levels/effects of Triazolam may be increased by: Antifungal Agents (Azole Derivatives, Systemic); Aprepitant; Boceprevir; Calcium Channel Blockers (Nondihydropyridine); Cimetidine; Conivaptan; Contraceptives (Estrogens); Contraceptives (Progestins); CYP3A4 Inhibitors (Moderate); CYP3A4 Inhibitors (Strong); Dasatinib; Droperidol; Efavirenz; Fosaprepitant; Grapefruit Juice; HydrOXYzine; Isoniazid; Ivacaftor; Macrolide Antibiotics; Methotrimeprazine; Mifepristone; OLANZapine; Protease Inhibitors; Proton Pump Inhibitors; Selective Serotonin Reuptake Inhibitors; Telaprevir
  Decreased Effect
    The levels/effects of Triazolam may be decreased by: CarBAMazepine; CYP3A4 Inducers (Strong); Deferasirox; Rifamycin Derivatives; St Johns Wort; Theophylline Derivatives; Tocilizumab; Yohimbine

Ethanol/Nutrition/Herb Interactions
  Ethanol: Ethanol may increase CNS depression. Management: Limit or avoid ethanol consumption.
  Food: Food may decrease the rate of absorption. Benzodiazepine serum concentrations may be increased by grapefruit juice. Management: Limit or avoid grapefruit juice.
  Herb/Nutraceutical: St John's wort may decrease levels/effects of benzodiazepines. Other herbal medications may increase CNS depression. Management: Avoid St John's wort, valerian, kava kava, and gotu kola.

Stability Store at controlled room temperature of 20°C to 25°C (68°F to 77°F).

Mechanism of Action Binds to stereospecific benzodiazepine receptors on the postsynaptic GABA neuron at several sites within the central nervous system, including the limbic system, reticular formation. Enhancement of the inhibitory effect of GABA on neuronal excitability results by increased neuronal membrane permeability to chloride ions. This shift in chloride ions results in hyperpolarization (a less excitable state) and stabilization.

Pharmacodynamics/Kinetics
  Onset of action: Hypnotic: 15-30 minutes
  Duration: 6-7 hours
  Distribution: V_d: 0.8-1.8 L/kg
  Protein binding: 89%
  Metabolism: Extensively hepatic
  Half-life elimination: 1.5-5.5 hours
  Excretion: Urine as unchanged drug and metabolites

Dosage
  Geriatric Oral: Insomnia (short-term use): Initial: 0.125 mg at bedtime; maximum dose: 0.25 mg/day
  Adult Note: Onset of action is rapid, patient should be in bed when taking medication.
    Insomnia (short-term): Oral: 0.125-0.25 mg at bedtime (maximum dose: 0.5 mg/day)

Dental (preprocedure) (unlabeled use): Oral: 0.25 mg taken the evening before oral surgery; or 0.25 mg 1 hour before procedure

Hepatic Impairment Reduce dose or avoid use in cirrhosis.

Administration May take with food. Tablet may be crushed or swallowed whole. Onset of action is rapid, patient should be in bed when taking medication.

Monitoring Parameters Respiratory and cardiovascular status

Special Geriatric Considerations Due to the higher incidence of CNS adverse reactions and its short half-life, this benzodiazepine is not a drug of first choice. For short-term only.

This medication is considered to be potentially inappropriate in this patient population (Beers Criteria: Quality of evidence - high; Strength of recommendation - strong).

Controlled Substance C-IV

Dosage Forms Excipient information presented when available (limited, particularly for generics); consult specific product labeling.

Tablet, oral: 0.125 mg, 0.25 mg

Halcion®: 0.25 mg [scored]

Trifluoperazine (trye floo oh PER a zeen)

Related Information

Antipsychotic Agents on page 2103

Beers Criteria – Potentially Inappropriate Medications for Geriatrics on page 2183

Medication Safety Issues

Sound-alike/look-alike issues:

Trifluoperazine may be confused with trihexyphenidyl

Stelazine may be confused with selegiline

BEERS Criteria medication:

This drug may be potentially inappropriate for use in geriatric patients (Quality of evidence - moderate; Strength of recommendation - strong).

Brand Names: Canada Apo-Trifluoperazine®; Novo-Trifluzine; PMS-Trifluoperazine; Terfluzine

Index Terms Stelazine; Trifluoperazine Hydrochloride

Generic Availability (U.S.) Yes

Pharmacologic Category Antipsychotic Agent, Typical, Phenothiazine

Use Treatment of schizophrenia; short-term treatment of generalized nonpsychotic anxiety

Unlabeled Use Management of psychotic disorders; behavioral symptoms associated with dementia behavior (elderly); psychosis/agitation related to Alzheimer's dementia

Contraindications Hypersensitivity to trifluoperazine or any component of the formulation (cross-reactivity between phenothiazines may occur); severe CNS depression; bone marrow suppression; blood dyscrasias; severe hepatic disease; coma

Warnings/Precautions [U.S. Boxed Warning]: Elderly patients with dementia-related psychosis treated with antipsychotics are at an increased risk of death compared to placebo. Most deaths appeared to be either cardiovascular (eg, heart failure, sudden death) or infectious (eg, pneumonia) in nature. Trifluoperazine is not approved for the treatment of dementia-related psychosis.

Leukopenia, neutropenia, and agranulocytosis (sometimes fatal) have been reported in clinical trials and postmarketing reports with antipsychotic use; presence of risk factors (eg, pre-existing low WBC or history of drug-induced leuko-/neutropenia) should prompt periodic blood count assessment. Discontinue therapy at first signs of blood dyscrasias or if absolute neutrophil count <1000/mm^3.

May be sedating, use with caution in disorders where CNS depression is a feature. Use with caution in Parkinson's disease. Caution in patients with hemodynamic instability; predisposition to seizures; subcortical brain damage; severe cardiac or renal disease. Liver damage and jaundice of the cholestatic type of hepatitis have been reported with use; use is contraindicated in patients with pre-existing hepatic disease. Esophageal dysmotility and aspiration have been associated with antipsychotic use - use with caution in patients at risk of pneumonia (ie, Alzheimer's disease). Use associated with increased prolactin levels; clinical significance of hyperprolactinemia in patients with breast cancer or other prolactin-dependent tumors is unknown. May alter temperature regulation or mask toxicity of other drugs due to antiemetic effects. May alter cardiac conduction - life-threatening arrhythmias have occurred with therapeutic doses of phenothiazines. May cause orthostatic hypotension - use with caution in patients at risk of this effect or those who would tolerate transient hypotensive episodes (cerebrovascular disease, cardiovascular disease or other medications which may predispose).

Due to anticholinergic effects, should be used with caution in patients with decreased gastrointestinal motility, urinary retention, BPH, xerostomia, visual problems, narrow-angle glaucoma, and myasthenia gravis. Relative to other antipsychotics, trifluoperazine has a low potency of cholinergic blockade.

Use in elderly patients with dementia is associated with an increased risk of mortality and cerebrovascular accidents; avoid antipsychotic use for behavioral problems associated with dementia unless alternative nonpharmacologic therapies have failed and patient may harm self or others. In addition, use may cause or exacerbate syndrome of inappropriate antidiuretic hormone secretion or hyponatremia; monitor sodium closely with initiation or dosage adjustments in older adults. May also be inappropriate in older adults depending on comorbidities (eg, dementia, delirium) due to its potent anticholinergic effects (Beers Criteria). Increased risk for developing tardive dyskinesia, particularly elderly women.

May cause extrapyramidal symptoms (EPS), including pseudoparkinsonism, acute dystonic reactions, akathisia, and tardive dyskinesia. Risk of dystonia (and possibly other EPS) may be greater with increased doses, use of conventional antipsychotics, males, and younger patients. Use caution in the elderly. May be associated with neuroleptic malignant syndrome (NMS) or pigmentary retinopathy.

Adverse Reactions (Reflective of adult population; not specific for elderly) Frequency not defined.

Cardiovascular: Cardiac arrest, hypotension, orthostatic hypotension

Central nervous system: Dizziness; extrapyramidal symptoms (akathisia, dystonias, pseudoparkinsonism, tardive dyskinesia); headache, impairment of temperature regulation, lowering of seizure threshold, neuroleptic malignant syndrome (NMS)

Dermatologic: Discoloration of skin (blue-gray), increased sensitivity to sun, photosensitivity, rash

Endocrine & metabolic: Breast pain, galactorrhea, gynecomastia, hyperglycemia, hypoglycemia, lactation, libido (changes in), menstrual cycle (changes in)

Gastrointestinal: Constipation, nausea, stomach pain, vomiting, weight gain, xerostomia

Genitourinary: Difficulty in urination, ejaculatory disturbances, priapism, urinary retention

Hematologic: Agranulocytosis, aplastic anemia, eosinophilia, hemolytic anemia, leukopenia, pancytopenia, thrombocytopenic purpura

Hepatic: Cholestatic jaundice, hepatotoxicity

Neuromuscular & skeletal: Tremor

Ocular: Cornea and lens changes, pigmentary retinopathy

Respiratory: Nasal congestion

Drug Interactions

Metabolism/Transport Effects Substrate of CYP1A2 (major); **Note:** Assignment of Major/Minor substrate status based on clinically relevant drug interaction potential

Avoid Concomitant Use

Avoid concomitant use of Trifluoperazine with any of the following: Azelastine; Azelastine (Nasal); Metoclopramide; Paraldehyde

Increased Effect/Toxicity

Trifluoperazine may increase the levels/effects of: Alcohol (Ethyl); Analgesics (Opioid); Anticholinergics; Antidepressants (Serotonin Reuptake Inhibitor/Antagonist); Azelastine; Azelastine (Nasal); Beta-Blockers; CNS Depressants; Methotrimeprazine; Methylphenidate; Paraldehyde; Porfimer; Serotonin Modulators; Zolpidem

The levels/effects of Trifluoperazine may be increased by: Abiraterone Acetate; Acetylcholinesterase Inhibitors (Central); Antidepressants (Serotonin Reuptake Inhibitor/Antagonist); Antimalarial Agents; Beta-Blockers; CYP1A2 Inhibitors (Moderate); CYP1A2 Inhibitors (Strong); Deferasirox; Droperidol; HydrOXYzine; Lithium formulations; Methotrimeprazine; Methylphenidate; Metoclopramide; Metyrosine; Pramlintide; Tetrabenazine

Decreased Effect

Trifluoperazine may decrease the levels/effects of: Amphetamines; Anti-Parkinson's Agents (Dopamine Agonist); Quinagolide

The levels/effects of Trifluoperazine may be decreased by: Antacids; Anti-Parkinson's Agents (Dopamine Agonist); CYP1A2 Inducers (Strong); Cyproterone; Lithium formulations

Ethanol/Nutrition/Herb Interactions

Ethanol: May increase CNS depression; monitor for increased effects with coadministration. Caution patients about effects.

Herb/Nutraceutical: Avoid kava kava, gotu kola, valerian, St John's wort (may increase CNS depression). Avoid dong quai, St John's wort (may also cause photosensitization).

Mechanism of Action Trifluoperazine is a piperazine phenothiazine antipsychotic which blocks postsynaptic mesolimbic dopaminergic receptors in the brain; exhibits alpha-adrenergic blocking effect and depresses the release of hypothalamic and hypophyseal hormones

Pharmacodynamics/Kinetics

Metabolism: Extensively hepatic

Half-life elimination: >24 hours with chronic use

Dosage

Geriatric

Schizophrenia/psychoses: Oral: Refer to adult dosing. Dose selection should start at the low end of the dosage range and titration must be gradual.

Behavioral symptoms associated with dementia behavior (unlabeled use): Oral: Initial: 0.5-1 mg 1-2 times/day; increase dose at 4- to 7-day intervals by 0.5-1 mg/day; increase dosing intervals (bid, tid, etc) as necessary to control response or side effects. Maximum daily dose: 40 mg. Gradual increases (titration) may prevent some side effects or decrease their severity.

Adult

Schizophrenia/psychoses: Oral:

Outpatients: 1-2 mg twice daily

Hospitalized or well supervised patient: Initial: 2-5 mg twice daily with optimum response in the 15-20 mg/day range; do not exceed 40 mg/day.

Nonpsychotic anxiety: Oral: 1-2 mg twice daily; maximum: 6 mg/day; therapy for anxiety should not exceed 12 weeks; do not exceed 6 mg/day for longer than 12 weeks when treating anxiety; agitation, jitteriness, or insomnia may be confused with original neurotic or psychotic symptoms.

Renal Impairment Not dialyzable (0% to 5%)

Monitoring Parameters Vital signs; lipid profile, fasting blood glucose/Hgb A_{1c}; BMI; mental status, abnormal involuntary movement scale (AIMS)

Reference Range Therapeutic response and blood levels have not been established

Test Interactions False-positive for phenylketonuria

Pharmacotherapy Pearls Do not exceed 6 mg/day for longer than 12 weeks when treating anxiety. Agitation, jitteriness, or insomnia may be confused with original neurotic or psychotic symptoms.

Special Geriatric Considerations Elderly are more susceptible to hypotension and neuromuscular reactions.

Many elderly patients receive antipsychotic medications for inappropriate nonpsychotic behavior. Before initiating antipsychotic medication, the clinician should investigate any possible reversible cause; any stress or stress from any disease can cause acute "confusion" or worsening of baseline nonpsychotic behavior. Most commonly acute changes in behavior are due to increases in drug dose or addition of new drug to regimen; fluid electrolyte loss; infections; and changes in environment.

Any changes in disease status in any organ system can result in behavior changes.

In the treatment of agitated, demented, elderly patients, authors of meta-analysis of controlled trials of the response to the traditional antipsychotics (phenothiazines, butyrophenones) in controlling agitation have concluded that the use of neuroleptics results in a response rate of 18%. Clearly neuroleptic therapy for behavior control should be limited with frequent attempts to withdraw the agent given for behavior control.

This medication is considered to be potentially inappropriate in this patient population (Beers Criteria: Quality of evidence - moderate; Strength of recommendation - strong).

Dosage Forms Excipient information presented when available (limited, particularly for generics); consult specific product labeling.

Tablet, oral: 1 mg, 2 mg, 5 mg, 10 mg

♦ **Trifluoperazine Hydrochloride** *see* Trifluoperazine *on page 1965*

♦ **Trifluorothymidine** *see* Trifluridine *on page 1968*

Trifluridine (trye FLURE i deen)

Medication Safety Issues
Sound-alike/look-alike issues:
Viroptic® may be confused with Timoptic®
Brand Names: U.S. Viroptic®
Brand Names: Canada Sandoz-Trifluridine; Viroptic®
Index Terms F_3T; Trifluorothymidine
Generic Availability (U.S.) Yes
Pharmacologic Category Antiviral Agent, Ophthalmic
Use Treatment of primary keratoconjunctivitis and recurrent epithelial keratitis caused by herpes simplex virus types I and II
Dosage
Geriatric & Adult Herpes keratoconjunctivitis, keratitis: Ophthalmic: Instill 1 drop into affected eye every 2 hours while awake, to a maximum of 9 drops/day, until re-epithelialization of corneal ulcer occurs. Then use 1 drop every 4 hours for another 7 days. Do **not** exceed 21 days of treatment. If improvement has not taken place in 7-14 days, consider another form of therapy.
Special Geriatric Considerations Evaluate the patient's or caregiver's ability to safely administer the correct dose of ophthalmic medication.
Dosage Forms Excipient information presented when available (limited, particularly for generics); consult specific product labeling.
Solution, ophthalmic [drops]: 1% (7.5 mL)
Viroptic®: 1% (7.5 mL)

◆ **Triglide®** see Fenofibrate on page 752

Trihexyphenidyl (trye heks ee FEN i dil)

Related Information
Antiparkinsonian Agents on page 2101
Beers Criteria – Potentially Inappropriate Medications for Geriatrics on page 2183
Medication Safety Issues
Sound-alike/look-alike issues:
Trihexyphenidyl may be confused with trifluoperazine
BEERS Criteria medication:
This drug may be potentially inappropriate for use in geriatric patients (Quality of evidence - moderate; Strength of recommendation - strong).
Brand Names: Canada PMS-Trihexyphenidyl; Trihexyphen; Trihexyphenidyl
Index Terms Artane; Benzhexol Hydrochloride; Trihexyphenidyl Hydrochloride
Generic Availability (U.S.) Yes
Pharmacologic Category Anti-Parkinson's Agent, Anticholinergic; Anticholinergic Agent
Use Adjunctive treatment of Parkinson's disease; treatment of drug-induced extrapyramidal symptoms
Contraindications There are no contraindications listed within the manufacturer's labeling.
Warnings/Precautions Use with caution in hot weather or during exercise, especially when administered concomitantly with other atropine-like drugs to chronically-ill patients, alcoholics, patients with CNS disease, or persons doing manual labor in a hot environment. Use with caution in patients with cardiovascular disease (including hypertension), glaucoma, prostatic hyperplasia or any tendency toward urinary retention, liver or kidney disorders, and obstructive disease of the GI tract. May exacerbate mental symptoms when used to treat extrapyramidal symptoms. When given in large doses or to susceptible patients, may cause weakness. May impair physical or mental abilities; patients must be cautioned about performing tasks which require mental alertness (eg, operating machinery or driving). Does not improve symptoms of tardive dyskinesias. Avoid use in older adults; not recommended for prevention of extrapyramidal symptoms with antipsychotics; alternative agents preferred in the treatment of Parkinson disease. May be inappropriate in older adults depending on comorbidities(eg, dementia, delirium) due to its potent anticholinergic effects (Beers Criteria).
Adverse Reactions (Reflective of adult population; not specific for elderly) Frequency not defined.
Cardiovascular: Tachycardia
Central nervous system: Agitation, confusion, delusions, dizziness, drowsiness, euphoria, hallucinations, headache, nervousness, paranoia, psychiatric disturbances
Dermatologic: Rash
Gastrointestinal: Constipation, dilatation of colon, ileus, nausea, parotitis, vomiting, xerostomia

Genitourinary: Urinary retention

Neuromuscular & skeletal: Weakness

Ocular: Blurred vision, glaucoma, intraocular pressure increased, mydriasis

Drug Interactions

Metabolism/Transport Effects None known.

Avoid Concomitant Use There are no known interactions where it is recommended to avoid concomitant use.

Increased Effect/Toxicity

Trihexyphenidyl may increase the levels/effects of: AbobotulinumtoxinA; Anticholinergics; Cannabinoids; OnabotulinumtoxinA; Potassium Chloride; RimabotulinumtoxinB

The levels/effects of Trihexyphenidyl may be increased by: Pramlintide

Decreased Effect

Trihexyphenidyl may decrease the levels/effects of: Acetylcholinesterase Inhibitors (Central); Secretin

The levels/effects of Trihexyphenidyl may be decreased by: Acetylcholinesterase Inhibitors (Central)

Ethanol/Nutrition/Herb Interactions Ethanol: Avoid ethanol (may increase CNS depression).

Stability Store at 20°C to 25°C (68°F to 77°F).

Mechanism of Action Exerts a direct inhibitory effect on the parasympathetic nervous system. It also has a relaxing effect on smooth musculature; exerted both directly on the muscle itself and indirectly through parasympathetic nervous system (inhibitory effect)

Pharmacodynamics/Kinetics

Metabolism: Hydroxylation of the alicyclic groups

Half-life elimination: 33 hours

Time to peak, serum: 1.3 hours

Excretion: Urine and bile

Dosage

Geriatric Parkinson's disease: Refer to adult dosing. **Note:** Conservative initial doses and gradual titration is especially important in patients >60 years of age.

Adult

Parkinson's disease: Oral: Initial: 1 mg/day, increase by 2 mg increments at intervals of 3-5 days; usual dose: 6-10 mg/day in 3-4 divided doses; doses of 12-15 mg/day may be required

Drug-induced EPS: Oral: Initial: 1 mg/day; increase as necessary to usual range: 5-15 mg/day in 3-4 divided doses

Use in combination with levodopa: Usual range: 3-6 mg/day in divided doses

Administration May be administered before or after meals; tolerated best if given in 3 daily doses and with food. High doses (>10 mg/day) may be divided into 4 doses, at meal times and at bedtime.

Monitoring Parameters IOP monitoring and gonioscopic evaluations should be performed periodically

Pharmacotherapy Pearls Incidence and severity of side effects are dose related. Patients may be switched to sustained-action capsules when stabilized on conventional dosage forms.

Special Geriatric Considerations Anticholinergic agents are generally not well tolerated in the elderly (eg, confusion, constipation, urinary retention) and their use should be avoided when possible. In elderly, anticholinergic agents should not be used as prophylaxis against extrapyramidal symptoms.

This medication is considered to be potentially inappropriate in this patient population (Beers Criteria: Quality of evidence - moderate; Strength of recommendation - strong).

Dosage Forms Excipient information presented when available (limited, particularly for generics); consult specific product labeling.

Elixir, oral, as hydrochloride: 2 mg/5 mL (473 mL)

Tablet, oral, as hydrochloride: 2 mg, 5 mg

◆ **Trihexyphenidyl Hydrochloride** see Trihexyphenidyl on page 1968
◆ **Trilafon** see Perphenazine on page 1513
◆ **Trileptal®** see OXcarbazepine on page 1440
◆ **TriLipix®** see Fenofibric Acid on page 755
◆ **Trilisate** see Choline Magnesium Trisalicylate on page 369

Trimethobenzamide (trye meth oh BEN za mide)

Related Information
Beers Criteria – Potentially Inappropriate Medications for Geriatrics *on page 2183*
Medication Safety Issues
Sound-alike/look-alike issues:
Tigan® may be confused with Tiazac®, Ticlid
Trimethobenzamide may be confused with metoclopramide, trimethoprim
BEERS Criteria medication:
This drug may be potentially inappropriate for use in geriatric patients (Quality of evidence - moderate; Strength of recommendation - strong).
Brand Names: U.S. Tigan®
Brand Names: Canada Tigan®
Index Terms Trimethobenzamide Hydrochloride
Generic Availability (U.S.) Yes
Pharmacologic Category Antiemetic
Use Treatment of postoperative nausea and vomiting; treatment of nausea associated with gastroenteritis
Contraindications Hypersensitivity to trimethobenzamide or any component of the formulation
Warnings/Precautions May mask emesis due to Reye's syndrome or mimic CNS effects of Reye's syndrome in patients with emesis of other etiologies. Antiemetic effects may mask toxicity of other drugs or conditions (eg, intestinal obstruction). May cause drowsiness; patient should avoid tasks requiring alertness (eg, driving, operating machinery). May cause extrapyramidal symptoms (EPS) which may be confused with CNS symptoms of primary disease responsible for emesis. Avoid use in the elderly due to the risk of EPS adverse effects combined with lower efficacy, as compared to other antiemetics (Beers Criteria). Risk of CNS adverse effects (eg, coma, EPS, seizure) may be increased in patients with acute febrile illness, dehydration, electrolyte imbalance, encephalitis, or gastroenteritis; use caution. Allergic-type skin reactions have been reported with use; discontinue with signs of sensitization. Trimethobenzamide clearance is predominantly renal; dosage reductions may be recommended in patient with renal impairment. Limit antiemetic use to prolonged vomiting of known etiology.
Adverse Reactions (Reflective of adult population; not specific for elderly) Frequency not defined.
Cardiovascular: Hypotension (I.V. administration)
Central nervous system: Coma, depression, disorientation, dizziness, drowsiness, EPS, headache, Parkinson-like symptoms, seizure
Dermatologic: Allergic-type skin reactions
Gastrointestinal: Diarrhea
Hematologic: Blood dyscrasias
Hepatic: Jaundice
Local: Injection site burning, pain, redness, stinging, or swelling
Neuromuscular & skeletal: Muscle cramps, opisthotonos
Ocular: Blurred vision
Miscellaneous: Hypersensitivity reactions
Drug Interactions
Metabolism/Transport Effects None known.
Avoid Concomitant Use There are no known interactions where it is recommended to avoid concomitant use.
Increased Effect/Toxicity
Trimethobenzamide may increase the levels/effects of: AbobotulinumtoxinA; Anticholinergics; Cannabinoids; OnabotulinumtoxinA; Potassium Chloride; RimabotulinumtoxinB

The levels/effects of Trimethobenzamide may be increased by: Pramlintide
Decreased Effect
Trimethobenzamide may decrease the levels/effects of: Acetylcholinesterase Inhibitors (Central); Secretin

The levels/effects of Trimethobenzamide may be decreased by: Acetylcholinesterase Inhibitors (Central)
Ethanol/Nutrition/Herb Interactions Ethanol: Concomitant use should be avoided (sedative effects may be additive).
Stability Store capsules and injection solution at room temperature of 25°C (77°F); excursions permitted to 15°C to 30°C (59°F to 86°F).
Mechanism of Action Acts centrally to inhibit the medullary chemoreceptor trigger zone by blocking emetic impulses to the vomiting center

Pharmacodynamics/Kinetics

Onset of action: Antiemetic: Oral: 10-40 minutes; I.M.: 15-35 minutes

Duration: 3-4 hours

Metabolism: Via oxidation, forms metabolite trimethobenzamide N-oxide

Bioavailability: Oral: 60% to 100%

Half-life elimination: 7-9 hours

Time to peak: Oral: ~45 minutes; I.M.: ~30 minutes

Excretion: Urine (30% to 50%, as unchanged drug)

Dosage

Geriatric Refer to adult dosing. Consider dosage reduction or increasing dosing interval in elderly patients with renal impairment (specific adjustment guidelines are not provided in the manufacturer's labeling).

Adult

Nausea, vomiting:

Oral: 300 mg 3-4 times/day

I.M.: 200 mg 3-4 times/day

Postoperative nausea and vomiting (PONV): I.M.: 200 mg, followed 1 hour later by a second 200 mg dose

Renal Impairment Cl_{cr} ≤70 mL/minute: Consider dosage reduction or increasing dosing interval (specific adjustment guidelines are not provided in the manufacturer's labeling)

Administration

Injection: Administer I.M. only; not for I.V. administration. Inject deep into upper outer quadrant of gluteal muscle.

Capsule: Administer capsule orally without regard to meals.

Monitoring Parameters Renal function (at baseline)

Special Geriatric Considerations No specific data for use in the elderly have been established; as with any drug which has EPS adverse effects and possibility of confusion, caution should be used when administering to elderly.

This medication is considered to be potentially inappropriate in this patient population (Beers Criteria: Quality of evidence - moderate; Strength of recommendation - strong).

Dosage Forms Excipient information presented when available (limited, particularly for generics); consult specific product labeling.

Capsule, oral, as hydrochloride: 300 mg

Tigan®: 300 mg

Injection, solution, as hydrochloride: 100 mg/mL (20 mL)

Tigan®: 100 mg/mL (20 mL)

Injection, solution, as hydrochloride [preservative free]: 100 mg/mL (2 mL)

Tigan®: 100 mg/mL (2 mL)

◆ **Trimethobenzamide Hydrochloride** see Trimethobenzamide on page 1970

Trimethoprim (trye METH oh prim)

Brand Names: U.S. Primsol®

Brand Names: Canada Apo-Trimethoprim®

Index Terms TMP

Generic Availability (U.S.) Yes: Tablet

Pharmacologic Category Antibiotic, Miscellaneous

Use Treatment of urinary tract infections due to susceptible strains of *E. coli, P. mirabilis, K. pneumoniae, Enterobacter* spp and coagulase-negative *Staphylococcus* including *S. saprophyticus*

Unlabeled Use Alternative agent for *Pneumocystis jirovecii* pneumonia (in combination with dapsone)

Contraindications Hypersensitivity to trimethoprim or any component of the formulation; megaloblastic anemia due to folate deficiency

Warnings/Precautions Use with caution in patients with impaired renal or hepatic function or with possible folate deficiency. Prolonged use may result in fungal or bacterial superinfection, including *C. difficile*-associated diarrhea (CDAD) and pseudomembranous colitis; CDAD has been observed >2 months postantibiotic treatment.

Adverse Reactions (Reflective of adult population; not specific for elderly) Frequency not defined.

Central nervous system: Aseptic meningitis (rare), fever

Dermatologic: Maculopapular rash (3% to 7% at 200 mg/day; incidence higher with larger daily doses), erythema multiforme (rare), exfoliative dermatitis (rare), pruritus (common), phototoxic skin eruptions, Stevens-Johnson syndrome (rare), toxic epidermal necrolysis (rare)

Endocrine & metabolic: Hyperkalemia, hyponatremia

Gastrointestinal: Epigastric distress, glossitis, nausea, vomiting

Hematologic: Leukopenia, megaloblastic anemia, methemoglobinemia, neutropenia, thrombocytopenia

Hepatic: Cholestatic jaundice (rare), liver enzymes increased

Renal: BUN and creatinine increased

Miscellaneous: Anaphylaxis, hypersensitivity reactions

Drug Interactions

Metabolism/Transport Effects Substrate of CYP2C9 (major), CYP3A4 (major); **Note:** Assignment of Major/Minor substrate status based on clinically relevant drug interaction potential; **Inhibits** CYP2C8 (moderate), CYP2C9 (moderate)

Avoid Concomitant Use

Avoid concomitant use of Trimethoprim with any of the following: BCG; Dofetilide

Increased Effect/Toxicity

Trimethoprim may increase the levels/effects of: ACE Inhibitors; Amantadine; Angiotensin II Receptor Blockers; Antidiabetic Agents (Thiazolidinedione); AzaTHIOprine; Carvedilol; CYP2C8 Substrates; CYP2C9 Substrates; Dapsone; Dapsone (Systemic); Dapsone (Topical); Dofetilide; Eplerenone; Fosphenytoin; Highest Risk QTc-Prolonging Agents; LamiVUDine; Memantine; Mercaptopurine; Methotrexate; Moderate Risk QTc-Prolonging Agents; Phenytoin; PRALAtrexate; Procainamide; Repaglinide; Spironolactone; Varenicline

The levels/effects of Trimethoprim may be increased by: Amantadine; CYP2C9 Inhibitors (Moderate); CYP2C9 Inhibitors (Strong); Dapsone; Dapsone (Systemic); Memantine; Mifepristone

Decreased Effect

Trimethoprim may decrease the levels/effects of: BCG; Typhoid Vaccine

The levels/effects of Trimethoprim may be decreased by: CYP2C9 Inducers (Strong); CYP3A4 Inducers (Strong); Deferasirox; Herbs (CYP3A4 Inducers); Leucovorin Calcium-Levoleucovorin; Peginterferon Alfa-2b; Tocilizumab

Stability

Solution: Store between 15°C to 25°C (59°F to 77°F). Protect from light.

Tablets: Store at 20°C to 25°C (68°F to 77°F). Protect from light.

Mechanism of Action Inhibits folic acid reduction to tetrahydrofolate, and thereby inhibits microbial growth

Pharmacodynamics/Kinetics

Absorption: Oral: Readily and extensively

Protein binding: 42% to 46%

Metabolism: Partially in the liver

Half-life: 8-14 hours, prolonged with renal impairment

Time to peak serum concentration: Within 1-4 hours

Elimination: Significantly in urine (60% to 80% as unchanged drug); in older adults, the area under the curve and peak concentration have been reported to be greater compared to younger subjects

Dosage

Geriatric & Adult

Pneumocystis jirovecii pneumonia, mild-to-moderate (unlabeled use) (CDC, 2009): Oral: 15 mg/kg/day in 3 divided doses in combination with dapsone

Susceptible infections: Oral: 100 mg every 12 hours or 200 mg every 24 hours for 10 days

Urinary tract infection, uncomplicated (unlabeled duration): Oral:

Treatment: 100 mg every 12 hours for 3 days (Gupta, 2011)

Prophylaxis: 100 mg once daily (Kodner, 2010)

Renal Impairment

Cl$_{cr}$ 15-30 mL/minute: Administer 50 mg every 12 hours.

Cl$_{cr}$ <15 mL/minute: Not recommended.

Moderately dialyzable (20% to 50%)

Administration Administer with milk or food.

Monitoring Parameters Periodic CBC and serum potassium during long-term therapy

Reference Range Therapeutic: Peak: 5-15 mg/L; Trough: 2-8 mg/L

Test Interactions May falsely increase creatinine determination measured by the Jaffé alkaline picrate assay; may interfere with determination of serum methotrexate when measured by methods that use a bacterial dihydrofolate reductase as the binding protein (eg, the competitive binding protein technique); does **not** interfere with RIA for methotrexate

Special Geriatric Considerations Trimethoprim is often used in combination with sulfamethoxazole; it can be used alone in patients who are allergic to sulfonamides; adjust dose for renal function (see Pharmacodynamics/Kinetics and Dosage).

Dosage Forms Excipient information presented when available (limited, particularly for generics); consult specific product labeling.
Solution, oral:
   Primsol®: 50 mg (base)/5 mL (473 mL) [dye free, ethanol free; contains propylene glycol, sodium benzoate; bubblegum flavor]
Tablet, oral: 100 mg

◆ **Trimethoprim and Sulfamethoxazole** *see* Sulfamethoxazole and Trimethoprim *on page 1813*

Trimipramine (trye MI pra meen)

Related Information
Antidepressant Agents *on page 2097*
Beers Criteria – Potentially Inappropriate Medications for Geriatrics *on page 2183*

Medication Safety Issues
Sound-alike/look-alike issues:
Trimipramine may be confused with triamterene
BEERS Criteria medication:
This drug may be potentially inappropriate for use in geriatric patients (Quality of evidence - high [moderate for SIADH]; Strength of recommendation - strong).

Brand Names: U.S. Surmontil®
Brand Names: Canada Apo-Trimip®; Nu-Trimipramine; Rhotrimine®; Surmontil®
Index Terms Trimipramine Maleate
Generic Availability (U.S.) Yes
Pharmacologic Category Antidepressant, Tricyclic (Tertiary Amine)
Use Treatment of depression
Medication Guide Available Yes
Contraindications Hypersensitivity to trimipramine, any component of the formulation, or other dibenzodiazepines; use of MAO inhibitors within 14 days; use in a patient during the acute recovery phase of MI

Warnings/Precautions [U.S. Boxed Warning]: Antidepressants increase the risk of suicidal thinking and behavior in children, adolescents, and young adults (18-24 years of age) with major depressive disorder (MDD) and other psychiatric disorders; consider risk prior to prescribing. Short-term studies did not show an increased risk in patients >24 years of age and showed a decreased risk in patients ≥65 years. Closely monitor for clinical worsening, suicidality, or unusual changes in behavior; the patient's family or caregiver should be instructed to closely observe the patient and communicate condition with healthcare provider. A medication guide should be dispensed with each prescription.

The possibility of a suicide attempt is inherent in major depression and may persist until remission occurs. Monitor for worsening of depression or suicidality, especially during initiation of therapy (generally first 1-2 months) or with dose increases or decreases. Use caution in high-risk patients. Worsening depression and severe abrupt suicidality that are not part of the presenting symptoms may require discontinuation or modification of drug therapy. The patient's family or caregiver should be alerted to monitor patients for the emergence of suicidality and associated behaviors (such as agitation, irritability, hostility, impulsivity, and hypomania) and call healthcare provider.

May worsen psychosis in some patients or precipitate a shift to mania or hypomania in patients with bipolar disorder. Patients presenting with depressive symptoms should be screened for bipolar disorder. Monotherapy in patients with bipolar disorder should be avoided. **Trimipramine is not FDA approved for the treatment of bipolar depression.**

The degree of sedation, anticholinergic effects, orthostasis, and conduction abnormalities are high relative to other antidepressants. Trimipramine often causes drowsiness/sedation, resulting in impaired performance of tasks requiring alertness (eg, operating machinery or driving). Sedative effects may be additive with other CNS depressants and/or ethanol. Use with caution in patients with a history of cardiovascular disease (including previous MI, stroke, tachycardia, or conduction abnormalities). Use with caution in patients with urinary retention, benign prostatic hyperplasia, narrow-angle glaucoma, xerostomia, visual problems, constipation, or a history of bowel obstruction.

May alter glucose control - use with caution in patients with diabetes. Consider discontinuing, when possible, prior to elective surgery. Therapy should not be abruptly discontinued in patients receiving high doses for prolonged periods. May lower seizure threshold - use caution in patients with a previous seizure disorder or condition predisposing to seizures such as brain damage, alcoholism, or concurrent therapy with other drugs which lower the seizure threshold. May increase the risks associated with electroconvulsive therapy. Use with caution in hyperthyroid patients or those receiving thyroid supplementation. Use with caution in patients with hepatic or renal dysfunction. Avoid use in the elderly due to its potent anticholinergic and sedative properties, and potential to cause orthostatic hypotension. May also cause or exacerbate syndrome of inappropriate antidiuretic hormone secretion or hyponatremia; monitor sodium closely with initiation or dosage adjustments in older adults (Beers Criteria).

Adverse Reactions (Reflective of adult population; not specific for elderly) Frequency not defined.

Cardiovascular: Arrhythmias, facial edema, flushing, heart block, hyper-/hypotension, MI, palpitation, stroke, tachycardia

Central nervous system: Agitation, anxiety, confusion, delusions, disorientation, dizziness, drowsiness, EEG abnormalities, exacerbation of psychosis, fatigue, hallucinations, headache, hypomania, insomnia, nightmares, restlessness, seizure

Dermatologic: Alopecia, itching, petechiae, photosensitivity, rash, urticaria

Endocrine & metabolic: Breast enlargement, galactorrhea, gynecomastia, hyper-/hypoglycemia, libido (changes in), parotid swelling, syndrome of inappropriate ADH secretion (SIADH)

Gastrointestinal: Abdominal cramps, anorexia, black tongue, constipation, diarrhea, epigastric distress, nausea, paralytic ileus, stomatitis, tongue edema, unpleasant taste, tongue edema, vomiting, weight gain/loss, xerostomia

Genitourinary: Delayed/difficult urination, impotence, polyuria, testicular edema, urinary retention

Hematologic: Agranulocytosis, eosinophilia, purpura, thrombocytopenia

Hepatic: Cholestatic jaundice, liver enzymes increased

Neuromuscular & skeletal: Ataxia, extrapyramidal symptoms, incoordination, numbness, paresthesia, peripheral neuropathy, tingling, tremor, weakness

Ocular: Blurred vision, disturbances in accommodation, mydriasis

Otic: Tinnitus

Miscellaneous: Diaphoresis, withdrawal syndrome

Drug Interactions

Metabolism/Transport Effects Substrate of CYP2C19 (major), CYP2D6 (major), CYP3A4 (major); **Note:** Assignment of Major/Minor substrate status based on clinically relevant drug interaction potential

Avoid Concomitant Use

Avoid concomitant use of Trimipramine with any of the following: Conivaptan; Iobenguane I 123; MAO Inhibitors; Methylene Blue

Increased Effect/Toxicity

Trimipramine may increase the levels/effects of: Alpha-/Beta-Agonists (Direct-Acting); Alpha1-Agonists; Amphetamines; Anticholinergics; Aspirin; Beta2-Agonists; Desmopressin; Highest Risk QTc-Prolonging Agents; Methylene Blue; Metoclopramide; Moderate Risk QTc-Prolonging Agents; NSAID (COX-2 Inhibitor); NSAID (Nonselective); QuiNIDine; Serotonin Modulators; Sodium Phosphates; Sulfonylureas; TraMADol; Vitamin K Antagonists; Yohimbine

The levels/effects of Trimipramine may be increased by: Abiraterone Acetate; Altretamine; Antipsychotics; BuPROPion; Cimetidine; Cinacalcet; Conivaptan; CYP2C19 Inhibitors (Moderate); CYP2C19 Inhibitors (Strong); CYP2D6 Inhibitors (Moderate); CYP2D6 Inhibitors (Strong); CYP3A4 Inhibitors (Moderate); CYP3A4 Inhibitors (Strong); Dexmethylphenidate; Divalproex; DULoxetine; Ivacaftor; Linezolid; Lithium; MAO Inhibitors; Methylphenidate; Metoclopramide; Metyrosine; Mifepristone; Pramlintide; Protease Inhibitors; QuiNIDine; Selective Serotonin Reuptake Inhibitors; Terbinafine; Terbinafine (Systemic); Valproic Acid

Decreased Effect

Trimipramine may decrease the levels/effects of: Acetylcholinesterase Inhibitors (Central); Alpha2-Agonists; Iobenguane I 123

The levels/effects of Trimipramine may be decreased by: Acetylcholinesterase Inhibitors (Central); Barbiturates; CarBAMazepine; CYP2C19 Inducers (Strong); CYP3A4 Inducers (Strong); Deferasirox; Peginterferon Alfa-2b; St Johns Wort; Tocilizumab

Ethanol/Nutrition/Herb Interactions

Ethanol: May increase CNS depression; monitor for increased effects with coadministration. Caution patients about effects.

Food: Grapefruit juice may inhibit the metabolism of some TCAs and clinical toxicity may result.

Herb/Nutraceutical: Avoid valerian, St John's wort, SAMe, kava kava (may increase risk of serotonin syndrome and/or excessive sedation).

Stability Solutions stable at a pH of 4-5. Turns yellowish or reddish on exposure to light. Slight discoloration does not affect potency; marked discoloration is associated with loss of potency. Capsules stable for 3 years following date of manufacture.

Mechanism of Action Increases the synaptic concentration of serotonin and/or norepinephrine in the central nervous system by inhibition of their reuptake by the presynaptic neuronal membrane

Pharmacodynamics/Kinetics

Distribution: V_d: 17-48 L/kg

Protein binding: 95%; free drug: 3% to 7%

Metabolism: Hepatic; significant first-pass effect

Bioavailability: 18% to 63%

Half-life elimination: 16-40 hours

Excretion: Urine

Dosage

Geriatric Oral: 50 mg/day; gradually increase dose to 100 mg/day

Adult Depression: Oral:

Outpatients: Initial: 75 mg/day in divided doses; may increase to 150 mg/day; Maintenance: 50-150 mg/day as a single bedtime dose; maximum: 200 mg/day

Inpatients: Initial: 100 mg/day in divided doses; may increase to 200 mg/day; if no improvement after 2-3 weeks, dose may be increased to 250-300 mg/day

Monitoring Parameters Blood pressure and pulse rate prior to and during initial therapy; evaluate mental status, suicide ideation (especially at the beginning of therapy or when doses are increased or decreased); monitor weight; ECG in older adults

Pharmacotherapy Pearls May cause alterations in bleeding time.

Special Geriatric Considerations Similar to doxepin in its side effect profile; has not been well studied in the elderly; strong anticholinergic properties and, therefore, not considered a drug of first choice in the elderly when selecting an antidepressant.

A systematic review and meta-analysis of antidepressant placebo-controlled trials in persons with depression and dementia found evidence "suggestive" of efficacy but not of sufficient strength to "confirm" efficacy. Antidepressant trials in this patient population are small and underpowered. Older patients with depression being treated with an antidepressant should be closely monitored for response and adverse effects. Treatment should be switched or augmented when response is inadequate with a therapeutic dose. Antidepressants that are not tolerated should be discontinued and an alternative agent should be started.

This medication is considered to be potentially inappropriate in this patient population (Beers Criteria: Quality of evidence - high [moderate for SIADH]; Strength of recommendation - strong).

Dosage Forms Excipient information presented when available (limited, particularly for generics); consult specific product labeling.

Capsule, oral: 25 mg, 50 mg

Surmontil®: 25 mg, 50 mg, 100 mg

◆ **Trimipramine Maleate** see Trimipramine on page 1973

◆ **Triostat®** see Liothyronine on page 1139

◆ **Tripedia** see Diphtheria and Tetanus Toxoids, and Acellular Pertussis Vaccine on page 567

Triprolidine and Pseudoephedrine (trye PROE li deen & soo doe e FED rin)

Related Information

Pseudoephedrine on page 1633

Medication Safety Issues

BEERS Criteria medication:

This drug may be potentially inappropriate for use in geriatric patients (Quality of evidence - moderate; Strength of recommendation - strong).

Brand Names: U.S. Aprodine [OTC]; Pediatex® TD; Silafed [OTC]

Brand Names: Canada Actifed®

Index Terms Pseudoephedrine and Triprolidine

Generic Availability (U.S.) Yes

Pharmacologic Category Alkylamine Derivative; Alpha/Beta Agonist; Decongestant; Histamine H_1 Antagonist; Histamine H_1 Antagonist, First Generation

Use Temporary relief of nasal congestion, decongest sinus openings, running nose, sneezing, itching of nose or throat and itchy, watery eyes due to common cold, hay fever, or other upper respiratory allergies

Dosage

Geriatric & Adult Cold, allergy symptoms: Oral:

Liquid (Pediatex® TD): 2.67 mL every 6 hours (maximum: 4 doses/24 hours)

Syrup (Aprodine®): 10 mL every 4-6 hours; do not exceed 4 doses in 24 hours

Tablet (Aprodine®): One tablet every 4-6 hours; do not exceed 4 doses in 24 hours

Special Geriatric Considerations Use with caution in patients with cardiovascular disease; the anticholinergic action of triprolidine may cause confusion, constipation, or urinary retention in the elderly. Also refer to Pseudoephedrine on page 1633.

This medication is considered to be potentially inappropriate in this patient population (Beers Criteria: Quality of evidence - moderate; Strength of recommendation - strong).

Dosage Forms Excipient information presented when available (limited, particularly for generics); consult specific product labeling. [DSC] = Discontinued product

Liquid, oral:
Pediatex® TD: Triprolidine hydrochloride 0.938 mg and pseudoephedrine hydrochloride 10 mg per 1 mL (30 mL) [cotton candy flavor]

Syrup, oral: Triprolidine hydrochloride 1.25 mg and pseudoephedrine hydrochloride 30 mg per 5 mL (120 mL) [DSC]
Aprodine: Triprolidine hydrochloride 1.25 mg and pseudoephedrine hydrochloride 30 mg per 5 mL (120 mL)
Silafed: Triprolidine hydrochloride 1.25 mg and pseudoephedrine hydrochloride 30 mg per 5 mL (120 mL, 240 mL)

Tablet, oral:
Aprodine: Triprolidine hydrochloride 2.5 mg and pseudoephedrine hydrochloride 60 mg

◆ **TripTone® [OTC]** see DimenhyDRINATE on page 554

Triptorelin (trip toe REL in)

Brand Names: U.S. Trelstar®
Brand Names: Canada Trelstar®
Index Terms AY-25650; CL-118,532; D-Trp(6)-LHRH; Detryptoreline; Triptorelin Pamoate; Tryptoreline
Generic Availability (U.S.) No
Pharmacologic Category Gonadotropin Releasing Hormone Agonist
Use Palliative treatment of advanced prostate cancer
Unlabeled Use Uterine sarcoma
Contraindications Hypersensitivity to triptorelin or any component of the formulation, other GnRH agonists or GnRH
Warnings/Precautions Hazardous agent - use appropriate precautions for handling and disposal. Transient increases in testosterone can lead to worsening symptoms (bone pain, hematuria, bladder outlet obstruction, neuropathy, spinal cord compression) of prostate cancer during the first few weeks of therapy. Androgen-deprivation therapy may increase the risk for cardiovascular disease (Levine, 2010). Hyperglycemia has been reported with androgen deprivation therapy (in prostate cancer) and may manifest as diabetes or worsening of pre-existing diabetes; monitor blood glucose and/or Hb A$_{1c}$. Cases of spinal cord compression have been reported with GnRH agonists. Closely observe (during the first 2 weeks of treatment) patients with metastatic vertebral lesions or urinary tract obstruction. Hypersensitivity reactions including angioedema, anaphylaxis and anaphylactic shock have rarely occurred; discontinue if severe reaction occurs. Rare cases of pituitary apoplexy (frequently secondary to pituitary adenoma) have been observed with GnRH agonist administration (onset from 1 hour to usually <2 weeks); may present as sudden headache, vomiting, visual or mental status changes, and infrequently cardiovascular collapse; immediate medical attention required.
Adverse Reactions (Reflective of adult population; not specific for elderly) As reported with all strengths; frequency of effect may vary by strength:
>10%:
Endocrine & metabolic: Hot flashes (59% to 73%), glucose increased, testosterone levels increased (peak: days 2-4; decline to low levels by weeks 3-4)
Hematologic: Hemoglobin decreased, RBC count decreased
Hepatic: Alkaline phosphatase increased (2% to >10%), ALT increased, AST increased
Neuromuscular & skeletal: Skeletal pain (12% to 13%)
Renal: BUN increased
1% to 10%:
Cardiovascular: Leg edema (6%), hypertension (1% to 4%), chest pain (2%), edema (2%), peripheral edema (≤1%)
Central nervous system: Headache (2% to 7%), pain (2% to 3%), dizziness (1% to 3%), fatigue (2%), insomnia (1% to 2%), emotional lability (1%)
Dermatologic: Rash (2%), pruritus (1%)
Endocrine & metabolic: Breast pain (2%), gynecomastia (2%), libido decreased (2%)
Gastrointestinal: Nausea (3%), anorexia (2%), constipation (2%), dyspepsia (2%), vomiting (2%), abdominal pain (1%), diarrhea (1%)

Genitourinary: Erectile dysfunction (10%), testicular atrophy (8%), impotence (2% to 7%), dysuria (5%), urinary retention (≤1%), urinary tract infection (≤1%)

Hematologic: Anemia (1%)

Local: Injection site pain (4%)

Neuromuscular & skeletal: Leg pain (2% to 5%), back pain (1% to 3%), leg cramps (2%), arthralgia (1% to 2%), extremity pain (1%), myalgia (1%), weakness (1%)

Ocular: Conjunctivitis (1%), eye pain (1%)

Respiratory: Cough (2%), dyspnea (1%), pharyngitis (1%)

Drug Interactions

Metabolism/Transport Effects None known.

Avoid Concomitant Use There are no known interactions where it is recommended to avoid concomitant use.

Increased Effect/Toxicity There are no known significant interactions involving an increase in effect.

Decreased Effect

Triptorelin may decrease the levels/effects of: Antidiabetic Agents

Stability Store at 20°C to 25°C (68°F to 77°F). Do not freeze MIXJECT® system. Reconstitute with 2 mL sterile water for injection. Shake well to obtain a uniform suspension. Solution will appear milky. Administer immediately after reconstitution.

MIXJECT® System: Follow manufacturer's instructions for mixing prior to use.

Mechanism of Action Causes suppression of ovarian and testicular steroidogenesis due to decreased levels of LH and FSH with subsequent decrease in testosterone (male) and estrogen (female) levels. After chronic and continuous administration, usually 2-4 weeks after initiation, a sustained decrease in LH and FSH secretion occurs.

Pharmacodynamics/Kinetics

Distribution: V_d: 30-33 L

Protein binding: None

Metabolism: Unknown; unlikely to involve CYP; no known metabolites

Half-life elimination: 2.8 ± 1.2 hours

Moderate-to-severe renal impairment: 6.5-7.7 hours

Hepatic impairment: 7.6 hours

Time to peak: 1-3 hours

Excretion: Urine (42% as intact peptide); hepatic

Dosage

Geriatric & Adult Advanced prostate carcinoma: I.M.:

3.75 mg once every 4 weeks **or**

11.25 mg once every 12 weeks **or**

22.5 mg once every 24 weeks

Administration Administer by I.M. injection into the buttock; alternate injection sites. Administer immediately after reconstitution.

Monitoring Parameters Serum testosterone levels, prostate-specific antigen

Test Interactions Pituitary-gonadal function may be suppressed with chronic administration and for up to 8 weeks after triptorelin therapy has been discontinued.

Special Geriatric Considerations No dosage adjustments are needed in the elderly. Monitoring for bone density changes, serum lipid, hemoglobin A_{1c}, blood pressure, and serum calcium changes is recommended.

Dosage Forms Excipient information presented when available (limited, particularly for generics); consult specific product labeling.

Injection, powder for reconstitution:

Trelstar®: 3.75 mg, 11.25 mg, 22.5 mg [contains polylactide-co-glycolide, polysorbate 80]

◆ **Triptorelin Pamoate** *see* Triptorelin *on page 1976*

◆ **Trivalent Inactivated Influenza Vaccine** *see* Influenza Virus Vaccine (Inactivated) *on page 997*

◆ **Trixaicin [OTC]** *see* Capsaicin *on page 280*

◆ **Trixaicin HP [OTC]** *see* Capsaicin *on page 280*

◆ **Trocal® [OTC] [DSC]** *see* Dextromethorphan *on page 525*

◆ **Tronolane® Suppository [OTC]** *see* Phenylephrine (Topical) *on page 1527*

Trospium (TROSE pee um)

Related Information
Beers Criteria – Potentially Inappropriate Medications for Geriatrics *on page 2183*
Pharmacotherapy of Urinary Incontinence *on page 2141*

Medication Safety Issues
BEERS Criteria medication:
This drug may be potentially inappropriate for use in geriatric patients (Quality of evidence - varies based on comorbidity; Strength of recommendation - varies based on comorbidity)

Brand Names: U.S. Sanctura®; Sanctura® XR
Brand Names: Canada Sanctura® XR; Trosec
Index Terms Trospium Chloride
Generic Availability (U.S.) Yes: Tablet
Pharmacologic Category Anticholinergic Agent
Use Treatment of overactive bladder with symptoms of urgency, incontinence, and urinary frequency
Contraindications Hypersensitivity to trospium or any component of the formulation; urinary retention; gastric retention; uncontrolled narrow-angle glaucoma
Warnings/Precautions Cases of angioedema involving the face, lips, tongue, and/or larynx have been reported. Immediately discontinue if tongue, hypopharynx, or larynx are involved. May cause drowsiness and/or blurred vision, which may impair physical or mental abilities; patients must be cautioned about performing tasks which require mental alertness (eg, operating machinery or driving). May occur in the presence of increased environmental temperature; use caution in hot weather and/or exercise. Use with caution in patients with bladder flow obstruction, may increase the risk of urinary retention. Use with caution in patients with gastrointestinal obstructive disorders (eg, pyloric stenosis); may increase the risk of gastric retention. Use caution in patients with decreased GI motility (eg, myasthenia gravis, ulcerative colitis). Avoid use of extended release formulation in severe renal impairment (Cl_{cr} <30 mL/minute). Use immediate release formulation with caution in renal dysfunction; dosage adjustment is required. Ethanol should not be ingested within 2 hours of the administration of the extended release formulation. Concurrent ethanol use may increase the incidence of drowsiness. Active tubular secretion (ATS) is a route of elimination; use caution with other medications that are eliminated by ATS (eg, procainamide, pancuronium, vancomycin, morphine, metformin, and tenofovir). Use with extreme caution in patients with controlled (treated) narrow-angle glaucoma. Use caution in patients with moderate or severe hepatic dysfunction. Use caution in Alzheimer's patients. Use caution in the elderly (≥65 years of age); increased anticholinergic side effects are seen. This medication is associated with potent anticholinergic properties which may be inappropriate in older adults depending on comorbidities (eg, dementia, delirium) (Beers Criteria).

Adverse Reactions (Reflective of adult population; not specific for elderly)
>10%: Gastrointestinal: Xerostomia (9% to 22%)
1% to 10%:
Cardiovascular: Tachycardia
Central nervous system: Headache (4% to 7%), fatigue (2%)
Dermatologic: Dry skin
Gastrointestinal: Constipation (9% to 10%), abdominal pain (1% to 3%), dyspepsia (1% to 2%), flatulence (1% to 2%), nausea (1%), abdominal distention (<2%), taste abnormal, vomiting
Genitourinary: Urinary tract infection (1% to 7%), urinary retention (≤1%)
Ocular: Dry eyes (1% to 2%), blurred vision (1%)
Respiratory: Nasopharyngitis (3%), nasal dryness (1%)
Miscellaneous: Influenza (2%)

Drug Interactions
Metabolism/Transport Effects None known.
Avoid Concomitant Use There are no known interactions where it is recommended to avoid concomitant use.
Increased Effect/Toxicity
Trospium may increase the levels/effects of: AbobotulinumtoxinA; Anticholinergics; Cannabinoids; OnabotulinumtoxinA; Potassium Chloride; RimabotulinumtoxinB

The levels/effects of Trospium may be increased by: Alcohol (Ethyl); Pramlintide
Decreased Effect
Trospium may decrease the levels/effects of: Acetylcholinesterase Inhibitors (Central); Secretin

The levels/effects of Trospium may be decreased by: Acetylcholinesterase Inhibitors (Central); MetFORMIN

Ethanol/Nutrition/Herb Interactions

Ethanol: Ethanol may enhance the sedative effects of trospium. Ethanol may increase the peak (maximum) serum concentration of trospium when consumed within 2 hours of taking extended release trospium. Management: Avoid use of ethanol. Avoid consuming any alcohol within 2 hours of taking a dose of extended release trospium.

Food: Administration with a fatty meal reduces the absorption and bioavailability of trospium. Management: Administer 1 hour prior to meals or an empty stomach. Administer extended release capsules in the morning with a full glass of water.

Stability Store at 20°C to 25°C (68°F to 77°F).

Mechanism of Action Trospium antagonizes the effects of acetylcholine on muscarinic receptors in cholinergically innervated organs. It reduces the smooth muscle tone of the bladder.

Pharmacodynamics/Kinetics

Absorption: <10%; decreased with food

Distribution: V_d: 395 - >600 L, primarily in plasma

Protein binding: 48% to 85% *in vitro*

Metabolism: Hypothesized to be via esterase hydrolysis and conjugation; forms metabolites

Bioavailability: Immediate release formulation: ~10% (range: 4% to 16%)

Half-life elimination: Immediate release formulation: 20 hours
  Severe renal insufficiency (Cl_{cr} <30 mL/minute): ~33 hours; extended release formulation: ~35 hours

Time to peak, plasma: 5-6 hours

Excretion: Feces (85%); urine (~6%; mostly as unchanged drug) primarily via active tubular secretion

Dosage

Geriatric ≥75 years: Immediate release formulation: Consider initial dose of 20 mg once daily (based on tolerability) at bedtime

Adult Overactive bladder: Oral: Immediate release formulation: 20 mg twice daily; extended release formulation: 60 mg once daily

Renal Impairment Cl_{cr} ≤30 mL/minute: Immediate release formulation: 20 mg once daily at bedtime; Extended release formulation: Use not recommended

Administration Administer 1 hour prior to meals or an empty stomach. Administer extended release capsules in the morning with a full glass of water.

Special Geriatric Considerations In studies, the incidence of anticholinergic side effects was higher in patients ≥65 years of age as compared to younger adults. The extended release formulation should be avoided in patients with Cl_{cr} <30 mL/minute.

This medication is considered to be potentially inappropriate in this patient population (Beers Criteria: Quality of evidence - varies based on comorbidity; Strength of recommendation - varies based on comorbidity)

Dosage Forms Excipient information presented when available (limited, particularly for generics); consult specific product labeling.

Capsule, extended release, oral, as chloride:
  Sanctura® XR: 60 mg
Tablet, oral, as chloride: 20 mg
  Sanctura®: 20 mg

◆ **Trospium Chloride** see Trospium on page 1978
◆ **Trusopt®** see Dorzolamide on page 596

Trypsin, Balsam Peru, and Castor Oil

(TRIP sin, BAL sam pe RUE, & KAS tor oyl)

Related Information

Castor Oil on page 305

Medication Safety Issues

Sound-alike/look-alike issues:
  Granulex® may be confused with Regranex®

Brand Names: U.S. Granulex®; Optase™; TBC; Vasolex™; Xenaderm®

Index Terms Balsam Peru, Castor Oil, and Trypsin; Castor Oil, Trypsin, and Balsam Peru

Generic Availability (U.S.) No

Pharmacologic Category Protectant, Topical

Use Treatment of decubitus ulcers, varicose ulcers, debridement of eschar, dehiscent wounds and sunburn; promote wound healing; reduce odor from necrotic wounds

Contraindications There are no contraindications listed in the manufacturer's labeling.

Warnings/Precautions For external use only; avoid contact with eyes. Do not apply to fresh arterial clots. Wound healing may be retarded in the presence of hemoglobin or zinc deficiency. Aerosol product is flammable; do not expose to high temperatures or flame.

Adverse Reactions (Reflective of adult population; not specific for elderly) Frequency not defined: Local: Temporary stinging at application site

Drug Interactions

Metabolism/Transport Effects None known.

Avoid Concomitant Use There are no known interactions where it is recommended to avoid concomitant use.

Increased Effect/Toxicity There are no known significant interactions involving an increase in effect.

Decreased Effect There are no known significant interactions involving a decrease in effect.

Stability

Aerosol spray: Store at room temperature; do not expose to fire, open flame, or temperatures >120°F.

Gel, ointment: Store at 25°C (77°F): excursions permitted to 15°C to 30°C (59°F to 86°F). Do not freeze.

Mechanism of Action Trypsin is used to debride necrotic tissue; balsam peru stimulates circulation at the wound site and may be mildly bactericidal; castor oil improves epithelialization, acts as a protectant covering and helps reduce pain

Dosage

Geriatric & Adult Dermatologic conditions: Topical: Apply a minimum of twice daily or as often as necessary

Administration Clean wound prior to application and at each redressing; shake well before spraying; hold can upright ~12" from area to be treated.

Monitoring Parameters Size of the ulcer, skin integrity

Special Geriatric Considerations Preventive skin care should be instituted in all elderly patients at high risk for decubitus ulcers. Practical experience with Granulex® has found that it is not as effective in debriding wounds as compared to other enzymatic products. Therefore, Granulex® may be more appropriately used on stage 1 and 2 decubiti.

Dosage Forms Excipient information presented when available (limited, particularly for generics); consult specific product labeling.

Aerosol, spray, topical:

Granulex®: Trypsin 0.12 mg, balsam Peru 87 mg, and castor oil 788 mg per gram (60 g, 120 g)

TBC: Trypsin 0.1 mg, balsam Peru 72.5 mg, and castor oil 650 mg per 0.82 mL (60 g, 120 g)

Gel, topical:

Optase™: Trypsin 0.12 mg, balsam Peru 87 mg, and castor oil 788 mg per gram (95 g)

Ointment, topical:

Vasolex™: Trypsin 90 USP units, balsam Peru 87 mg, and castor oil 788 mg per gram (5 g, 30 g, 60 g)

Xenaderm®: Trypsin 90 USP units, balsam Peru 87 mg, and castor oil 788 mg per gram (30 g, 60 g)

◆ **Tryptoreline** see Triptorelin on page 1976
◆ **TST** see Tuberculin Tests on page 1980
◆ **TT** see Tetanus Toxoid (Adsorbed) on page 1869
◆ **Tuberculin Purified Protein Derivative** see Tuberculin Tests on page 1980
◆ **Tuberculin Skin Test** see Tuberculin Tests on page 1980

Tuberculin Tests (too BER kyoo lin tests)

Medication Safety Issues

Sound-alike/look-alike issues:

Aplisol® may be confused with Anusol®

Administration issues:

Tuberculin products may be confused with tetanus toxoid products, poliovirus vaccine (inactivated), and influenza virus vaccine. Medication errors have occurred when tuberculin skin tests (PPD) have been inadvertently administered instead of tetanus toxoid products and influenza virus vaccine. These products are refrigerated and often stored in close proximity to each other.

Brand Names: U.S. Aplisol®; Tubersol®

Index Terms Mantoux; PPD; TB Skin Test; TST; Tuberculin Purified Protein Derivative; Tuberculin Skin Test

Generic Availability (U.S.) No

Pharmacologic Category Diagnostic Agent

Use Skin test in diagnosis of tuberculosis

Contraindications Hypersensitivity to tuberculin purified protein derivative (PPD) or any component of the formulation; previous severe reaction to tuberculin PPD skin test (TST)

Warnings/Precautions Patients with a previous severe reaction to TST (vesiculation, ulceration, necrosis) at the injection site should not receive tuberculin PPD again. Do not administer to persons with documented tuberculosis or a clear history of treatment for tuberculosis; persons with extensive burns or eczema. Skin testing may be deferred with major viral infections or live-virus vaccination within 1 month. Tuberculous or other bacterial infections, viral infection, live virus vaccination, malignancy, immunosuppressive agents, and conditions which impair immune response may cause a decreased response to test. For intradermal administration only; do not administer I.V., I.M., or SubQ. Epinephrine (1:1000) should be available to treat possible allergic reactions.

Adverse Reactions (Reflective of adult population; not specific for elderly) Suspected adverse reactions should be reported to the Food and Drug Administration (FDA) MedWatch Program at 1-800-332-1088

Frequency not defined:

Dermatologic: Rash

Local: Injection site reactions: Bleeding, bruising, discomfort, erythematous reaction, hematoma, necrosis, pain, pruritus, redness, scarring, ulceration, vesiculation

Miscellaneous: Anaphylaxis

Drug Interactions

Metabolism/Transport Effects None known.

Avoid Concomitant Use There are no known interactions where it is recommended to avoid concomitant use.

Increased Effect/Toxicity There are no known significant interactions involving an increase in effect.

Decreased Effect

The levels/effects of Tuberculin Tests may be decreased by: Vaccines (Live)

Stability Aplisol®, Tubersol®: Store under refrigeration at 2°C to 8°C (36°F to 46°F); do not freeze. Protect from light. Opened vials should be discarded after 30 days.

Mechanism of Action Tuberculosis results in individuals becoming sensitized to certain antigenic components of the *M. tuberculosis* organism. Culture extracts called tuberculins are contained in tuberculin skin test preparations. Upon intracutaneous injection of these culture extracts, a classic delayed (cellular) hypersensitivity reaction occurs. This reaction is characteristic of a delayed course (peak occurs >24 hours after injection, induration of the skin secondary to cell infiltration, and occasional vesiculation and necrosis). Delayed hypersensitivity reactions to tuberculin may indicate infection with a variety of nontuberculosis mycobacteria, or vaccination with the live attenuated mycobacterial strain of *M. bovis* vaccine, BCG, in addition to previous natural infection with *M. tuberculosis*.

Pharmacodynamics/Kinetics

Onset of action: Delayed hypersensitivity reactions: 5-6 hours

Peak effect: 48-72 hours

Duration: Reactions subside over a few days

Dosage

Geriatric & Adult

Diagnosis of tuberculosis, cell-mediated immunodeficiencies: Intradermal: 0.1 mL

TST interpretation: Criteria for positive TST read at 48-72 hours (see Note for healthcare workers):

Induration ≥5 mm: Persons with HIV infection (or risk factors for HIV infection, but unknown status), recent close contact to person with known active TB, persons with chest x-ray consistent with healed TB, persons who are immunosuppressed

Induration ≥10 mm: Persons with clinical conditions which increase risk of TB infection, recent immigrants, I.V. drug users, residents and employees of high-risk settings

Induration ≥15 mm: Persons who do not meet any of the above criteria (no risk factors for TB)

Note: A two-step test is recommended when testing will be performed at regular intervals (eg, for healthcare workers). If the first test is negative, a second TST should be administered 1-3 weeks after the first test was read.

TST interpretation (CDC guidelines) in a healthcare setting:

Baseline test: ≥10 mm is positive (either first or second step)

Serial testing without known exposure: Increase of ≥10 mm is positive

Known exposure:

≥5 mm is positive in patients with baseline of 0 mm

≥10 mm is positive in patients with negative baseline or previous screening result of ≥0mm

Read test at 48-72 hours following placement. Test results with 0 mm induration or measured induration less than the defined cutoff point are considered to signify absence of infection with *M. tuberculosis*. Test results should be documented in millimeters even if classified as negative. Erythema and redness of skin are not indicative of a positive test result.

Administration For intradermal administration only. Administer to upper third of forearm (palm up) ≥2 inches from elbow, wrist, or other injection site. If neither arm can be used, may administer to back of shoulder. Administer using inch ¼ to ½ inch 27-gauge needle or finer tuberculin syringe. Should form wheal (6-10 mm in diameter) as liquid is injected which will remain ~10 minutes. Avoid pressure or bandage at injection site. Document date and time of injection, person placing TST, location of injection site and lot number of solution.

Monitoring Parameters Monitor for immediate hypersensitivity reactions for ~15 minutes following injection.

Test Interactions False-positive reactions may occur with BCG vaccination or previous mycobacteria (nonTB) infection (previous BCG vaccination is not a contraindication to testing). False-negative reactions may occur with impaired cell mediated immunity.

Pharmacotherapy Pearls Situations where risk of tuberculosis infection may be increased are with contacts of recently-diagnosed persons with active disease, contact with immigrants from countries where tuberculosis is still common, or reactivation with impaired immunity (HIV infection, diabetes, renal failure, immunosuppressant use, pulmonary silicosis). Healthcare workers, staff of correctional facilities, and travelers at high risk of exposure should have routine testing. Patients with HIV infection should be tested as soon as possible following diagnosis.

The date of administration, the product manufacturer, and lot number of product must be entered into the patient's permanent medical record. Results should be recorded in millimeters (even if 0), not "negative" or "positive".

Special Geriatric Considerations Due to changes in the immune system with age, skin test response may be delayed or reduced in magnitude; therefore when testing, use a two-step test procedure; repeat test 2-4 weeks after reading first test dose; this elicits a "booster effect".

Dosage Forms Excipient information presented when available (limited, particularly for generics); consult specific product labeling.

Injection, solution:

Aplisol®: 5 TU/0.1 mL (1 mL, 5 mL) [contains polysorbate 80]

Tubersol®: 5 TU/0.1 mL (1 mL, 5 mL) [contains polysorbate 80]

Typhoid and Hepatitis A Vaccine (TYE foid & hep a TYE tis aye vak SEEN)

Related Information
Immunization Administration Recommendations *on page 2144*
Medication Safety Issues
  Sound-alike/look-alike issues:
    ViVAXIM® may be confused with Vyvanse™
Brand Names: Canada ViVAXIM®
Index Terms HA; Hepatitis A and Typhoid Vaccine; Typh-1
Pharmacologic Category Vaccine, Inactivated (Bacterial); Vaccine, Inactivated (Viral)
Use Active immunization against typhoid fever caused by *Salmonella typhi* and against disease caused by hepatitis A virus (HAV)

National Advisory Committee on Immunizations (NACI) does not recommend use for routine vaccination but does recommend that immunization be considered in the following groups:
- Travelers to areas with a prolonged risk (>4 weeks) of exposure to *S. typhi* or travelers to areas with endemic hepatitis A
- Persons with intimate exposure to a *S. typhi* carrier or who are residing in communities with high endemic rates of hepatitis A virus or at risk of outbreaks
- Laboratory technicians with frequent exposure to *S. typhi* or individuals involved in hepatitis A research or production of hepatitis A vaccine
- Travelers with achlorhydria or hypochlorhydria
- Military personnel, relief workers, or others relocated to areas with high rates of hepatitis A infection
- Persons with lifestyle risks for hepatitis A infection (eg, drug abusers, homosexual men), chronic liver disease, receiving hepatotoxic medication or with disease(s) which may necessitate use of hepatotoxic medications
- Persons with hemophilia A or B treated with plasma-derived clotting factors
- Zookeepers, veterinarians, and researchers who handle nonhuman primates

Contraindications Hypersensitivity to typhoid vaccine, hepatitis A vaccine or any component of the formulation

Warnings/Precautions Immediate treatment (including epinephrine 1:1000) for anaphylactoid and/or hypersensitivity reactions should be available during vaccine use. Defer administration in patients with acute or febrile illness; may administer to patients with mild acute illness with low-grade fever. Use with caution in patients with a history of bleeding disorders (including thrombocytopenia) and/or patients on anticoagulant therapy; bleeding/hematoma may occur from I.M. administration. Syncope has been reported with use of injectable vaccines and may be accompanied by transient visual disturbances, weakness, or tonic-clonic movements. Procedures should be in place to avoid injuries from falling and to restore cerebral perfusion if syncope occurs.

Vaccination may not result in effective immunity in all patients. Response depends upon multiple factors (eg, type of vaccine, age of patient) and is improved by administering the vaccine at the recommended dose, route, and interval. Vaccines may not be effective if administered during periods of altered immune competence (CDC, 2011). Due to the long incubation period for hepatitis, unrecognized hepatitis A infection may be present at time of vaccination; immunization may not prevent infection in these patients. Patients with chronic liver disease may have decreased antibody response. Should not be used to treat typhoid fever. Not all recipients of typhoid vaccine will be fully protected against typhoid fever. Travelers should take all necessary precautions to avoid contact or ingestion of potentially contaminated food or water sources.

Simultaneous administration of other vaccines at different injection sites is not likely to affect immune response. Hepatitis A seroconversion rates are not lower when simultaneous administration of immune globulins (at separate sites) however hepatitis A antibody titers may be lower. The NACI recommends simultaneous administration of all age-appropriate vaccines for which a person is eligible at a single clinic visit, unless contraindications exist.

◄ Use with caution in severely immunocompromised patients (eg, patients receiving chemo/ radiation therapy or other immunosuppressive therapy (including high dose corticosteroids); may have a reduced response to vaccination. If appropriate, consider delaying administration until after completion of immunosuppressive therapy. In general, household and close contacts of persons with altered immunocompetence may receive all age appropriate vaccines. Formulation may contain polysorbate 80 or neomycin.

Adverse Reactions (Reflective of adult population; not specific for elderly) In Canada, adverse reactions may be reported to local provincial/territorial health agencies or to the Vaccine Safety Section at Public Health Agency of Canada (1-866-844-0018).

>10%:
Central nervous system: Headache (15%)
Local: Injection site: Pain (90%), induration/edema (28%), erythema (10%)
Neuromuscular & skeletal: Weakness (17%), myalgia (16%)

1% to 10%:
Central nervous system: Fever (5%), malaise (3%), dizziness (1%)
Gastrointestinal: Diarrhea (3%), nausea (3%)

Drug Interactions

Metabolism/Transport Effects None known.

Avoid Concomitant Use There are no known interactions where it is recommended to avoid concomitant use.

Increased Effect/Toxicity There are no known significant interactions involving an increase in effect.

Decreased Effect
The levels/effects of Typhoid and Hepatitis A Vaccine may be decreased by: Belimumab; Fingolimod; Immunosuppressants

Stability Store between 2°C to 8°C (35°F to 46°F); do not freeze. Discard if frozen. Administer vaccine immediately after mixing.

Mechanism of Action Provides active immunization against typhoid fever through production of antibodies (predominantly IgG) and against hepatitis A infection through production of antihepatitis A virus antibodies.

Pharmacodynamics/Kinetics
Onset: Seroprotection rate at 14 days: Hepatitis A: ~96%, typhoid: ~89%; Seroprotection at 28 days: Hepatitis A: ~100%, typhoid: ~90%
Duration: Kinetic models suggest antihepatitis A antibodies may persist ≥20 years (NACI, 2006); Typhoid: 3 years

Dosage

Geriatric & Adult
Immunization: I.M.: 1 mL single dose at least 2 weeks prior to expected exposure
Booster: May administer 1 mL booster dose 3 years after previous dose in individuals requiring a booster dose

Administration Mix vaccine components immediately before administration according to manufacturer's labeling instructions. Shake well until white, cloudy suspension is achieved. **Do not administer intravascularly or intradermally.** Intramuscular administration into deltoid muscle is preferred. Do not administer to gluteal region. May consider subcutaneous administration in individuals at risk of hemorrhage (eg, thrombocytopenia, hemophilia). Subcutaneous administration may be associated with greater risk of injection site reactions. **Note:** For patients at risk of hemorrhage following intramuscular injection, the NACI recommends weighing the benefits and risks of intramuscular vaccination. If the patient receives antihemophilia or other similar therapy, intramuscular vaccination can be scheduled shortly after such therapy is administered. A fine needle can be used for the vaccination and firm pressure applied to the site (without rubbing) for at least 5 minutes. Patients on low-dose aspirin or long-term anticoagulant therapy (warfarin, heparin) are not considered to be at greater risk of complications and should receive scheduled vaccinations (NACI, 2006).

Simultaneous administration of vaccines helps ensure patients will be fully vaccinated by the appropriate age. Simultaneous administration of vaccines is defined as administering >1 vaccine on the same day at different anatomic sites. Antipyretics have not been shown to prevent febrile seizures. Antipyretics may be used to treat fever or discomfort following vaccination (CDC, 2011). One study reported that routine prophylactic administration of acetaminophen to prevent fever prior to vaccination decreased the immune response of some vaccines; the clinical significance of this reduction in immune response has not been established (Prymula, 2009).

Monitoring Parameters Monitor for syncope for 15 minutes following administration. If seizure-like activity associated with syncope occurs, maintain patient in supine or Trendelenburg position to reestablish adequate cerebral perfusion.

Pharmacotherapy Pearls Name of medication, date of administration, the vaccine manufacturer, lot number of vaccine, should be entered into the patient's permanent medical record.

Product Availability Not available in the U.S.

Dosage Forms: Canada Excipient information presented when available (limited, particularly for generics); consult specific product labeling.

Injection, solution:

ViVAXIM®: Purified Vi capsular polysaccharide 25 mcg and hepatitis A virus 160 antigen units per 1 mL [contains polysorbate 80 and neomycin]

Typhoid Vaccine (TYE foid vak SEEN)

Related Information
Immunization Administration Recommendations *on page 2144*
Immunization Recommendations *on page 2149*

Brand Names: U.S. Typhim Vi®; Vivotif®
Brand Names: Canada Typherix®; Typhim Vi®; Vivotif®
Index Terms Ty21a Vaccine; Typhoid Vaccine Live Oral Ty21a; Vi Vaccine
Generic Availability (U.S.) No
Pharmacologic Category Vaccine, Inactivated (Bacterial); Vaccine, Live (Bacterial)
Use Active immunization against typhoid fever caused by *Salmonella typhi*
Not for routine vaccination. In the United States and Canada, use should be limited to:
– Travelers to areas with a prolonged risk of exposure to *S. typhi*
– Persons with intimate exposure to a *S. typhi* carrier
– Laboratory technicians with exposure to *S. typhi*
– Travelers with achlorhydria or hypochlorhydria (Canadian recommendation)

Dosage
Geriatric & Adult Immunization:
Oral:

Primary immunization: One capsule on alternate days (day 1, 3, 5, and 7) for a total of 4 doses; all doses should be complete at least 1 week prior to potential exposure
Booster immunization (with repeated or continued exposure to typhoid fever):
U.S. labeling: Repeat full course of primary immunization every 5 years
Canadian labeling: Repeat full course of primary immunization every 7 years

I.M.:
Initial: 0.5 mL given at least 2 weeks prior to expected exposure
Reimmunization:
Typhim Vi®: 0.5 mL; optimal schedule has not been established; a single dose every 2 years is currently recommended for repeated or continued exposure
Typherix® (Canadian labeling; not available in U.S.): 0.5 mL every 3 years

Special Geriatric Considerations Vaccinating elderly is often overlooked; if no record of immunization can be recalled, repeat primary series.

Dosage Forms Excipient information presented when available (limited, particularly for generics); consult specific product labeling.

Capsule, enteric coated [live]:

Vivotif®: Viable *S. typhi* Ty21a 2-6.8 x 10^9 colony-forming units and nonviable *S. typhi* Ty21a 5-50 x 10^9 bacterial cells [contains lactose 100-180 mg/capsule and sucrose 26-130 mg/capsule]

Injection, solution [inactivated]:

Typhim Vi®: Purified Vi capsular polysaccharide 25 mcg/0.5 mL (0.5 mL, 10 mL) [derived from *S. typhi* Ty2 strain]

Dosage Forms: Canada Excipient information presented when available (limited, particularly for generics); consult specific product labeling.

Injection, solution:

Typherix®: Vi capsular polysaccharide 25 mcg/0.5 mL (0.5 mL) [derived from *S. typhi* Ty2 strain]

- ◆ **Ultravate®** *see* Halobetasol *on page 910*
- ◆ **Ultresa™** *see* Pancrelipase *on page 1466*
- ◆ **Unasyn®** *see* Ampicillin and Sulbactam *on page 130*
- ◆ **Unburn® [OTC]** *see* Lidocaine (Topical) *on page 1128*
- ◆ **Unisom® SleepGels® Maximum Strength [OTC]** *see* DiphenhydrAMINE (Systemic) *on page 556*
- ◆ **Unisom® SleepMelts™ [OTC]** *see* DiphenhydrAMINE (Systemic) *on page 556*
- ◆ **Unithroid®** *see* Levothyroxine *on page 1122*
- ◆ **Univasc®** *see* Moexipril *on page 1301*
- ◆ **Urate Oxidase, Pegylated** *see* Pegloticase *on page 1490*
- ◆ **Urea Peroxide** *see* Carbamide Peroxide *on page 291*
- ◆ **Urecholine®** *see* Bethanechol *on page 209*
- ◆ **Urex** *see* Methenamine *on page 1231*
- ◆ **Urinary Pain Relief [OTC]** *see* Phenazopyridine *on page 1516*
- ◆ **Urispas** *see* FlavoxATE *on page 792*
- ◆ **Uro-Mag® [OTC]** *see* Magnesium Oxide *on page 1181*
- ◆ **Uroxatral®** *see* Alfuzosin *on page 56*
- ◆ **Urso 250®** *see* Ursodiol *on page 1986*
- ◆ **Ursodeoxycholic Acid** *see* Ursodiol *on page 1986*

Ursodiol (ur soe DYE ol)

Medication Safety Issues
Sound-alike/look-alike issues:
Ursodiol may be confused with ulipristal
Brand Names: U.S. Actigall®; Urso 250®; Urso Forte®
Brand Names: Canada Dom-Ursodiol C; PHL-Ursodiol C; PMS-Ursodiol C; Urso®; Urso® DS
Index Terms Ursodeoxycholic Acid
Generic Availability (U.S.) Yes
Pharmacologic Category Gallstone Dissolution Agent
Use
Actigall®: Gallbladder stone dissolution; prevention of gallstones in obese patients experiencing rapid weight loss
Urso®, Urso Forte®: Primary biliary cirrhosis
Unlabeled Use Liver transplantation
Contraindications Hypersensitivity to ursodiol or any component of the formulation; not to be used with cholesterol, radiopaque, bile pigment stones; patients with unremitting acute cholecystitis, cholangitis, biliary obstruction, gallstone pancreatitis, or biliary-gastrointestinal fistula; allergy to bile acids
Warnings/Precautions Gallbladder stone dissolution may take several months of therapy. Complete dissolution may not occur and recurrence of stones within 5 years has been observed in 50% of patients. Use with caution in patients with a nonvisualizing gallbladder and those with chronic liver disease.
Adverse Reactions (Reflective of adult population; not specific for elderly)
>10%:
Central nervous system: Headache (up to 25%), dizziness (17%)
Gastrointestinal: Diarrhea (up to 27%), constipation (up to 26%), dyspepsia (17%), nausea (up to 17%), vomiting (up to 14%)
Neuromuscular & skeletal: Back pain (up to 12%)
Respiratory: Upper respiratory tract infection (up to 16%)
1% to 10%:
Dermatologic: Alopecia (5%), rash (3%)
Endocrine & metabolic: Hyperglycemia (1%)
Gastrointestinal: Flatulence (up to 8%), peptic ulcer (1%)
Genitourinary: Urinary tract infection (7%)
Hematologic: Leukopenia (3%), thrombocytopenia (1%)
Hepatic: Cholecystitis (5%)
Neuromuscular & skeletal: Arthritis (6%), myalgia (6%)
Renal: Serum creatinine increased (1%)
Respiratory: Pharyngitis (up to 8%), bronchitis (7%), cough (7%)
Miscellaneous: Viral infection (9%), flu-like syndrome (7%), allergy (5%)
Drug Interactions
Metabolism/Transport Effects None known.
Avoid Concomitant Use There are no known interactions where it is recommended to avoid concomitant use.

Increased Effect/Toxicity There are no known significant interactions involving an increase in effect.

Decreased Effect

Ursodiol may decrease the levels/effects of: Nitrendipine

The levels/effects of Ursodiol may be decreased by: Aluminum Hydroxide; Bile Acid Sequestrants; Estrogen Derivatives; Fibric Acid Derivatives

Stability

Actigall®: Store at 25°C (77°F); excursions permitted to 15°C to 30°C (59°F to 86°F).

Urso®: Store at 20°C to 25°C (68°F to 77°F).

Urso Forte®: Store at 20°C to 25°C (68°F to 77°F). When broken in half, scored Urso Forte® 500 mg tablets maintain quality for up to 28 days when kept in current packaging and stored at 20°C to 25°C (68°F to 77°F). Split tablets should be stored separately from whole tablets due to bitter taste.

Mechanism of Action Decreases the cholesterol content of bile and bile stones by reducing the secretion of cholesterol from the liver and the fractional reabsorption of cholesterol by the intestines. Mechanism of action in primary biliary cirrhosis is not clearly defined.

Pharmacodynamics/Kinetics

Protein binding: ~70%

Metabolism: Undergoes extensive enterohepatic recycling; following hepatic conjugation and biliary secretion, the drug is hydrolyzed to active ursodiol, where it is recycled or transformed to lithocholic acid by colonic microbial flora

Excretion: Feces; urine (<1%)

Dosage

Geriatric & Adult

Gallstone dissolution (Actigall®): Oral: 8-10 mg/kg/day in 2-3 divided doses; use beyond 24 months is not established

Gallstone prevention (Actigall®): Oral: 300 mg twice daily

Primary biliary cirrhosis (Urso®, Urso Forte®): Oral: 13-15 mg/kg/day in 2-4 divided doses (with food)

Administration Oral: Do not administer with aluminum-based antacids. If aluminum-based antacids are needed, administer 2 hours after ursodiol.

Monitoring Parameters

Gallstone disease: ALT, ALP, AST at initiation, 1 and 3 months and every 6 months thereafter, sonogram

Hepatic disease: Monitor hepatic function tests frequently

Special Geriatric Considerations No specific clinical studies in the elderly. Would recommend starting at lowest recommended dose with scheduled monitoring.

Dosage Forms Excipient information presented when available (limited, particularly for generics); consult specific product labeling.

Capsule, oral: 300 mg

Actigall®: 300 mg

Tablet, oral: 250 mg, 500 mg

Urso 250®: 250 mg

Urso Forte®: 500 mg [scored]

♦ **Urso Forte®** *see* Ursodiol *on page 1986*

Ustekinumab (yoo stek in YOO mab)

Medication Safety Issues

Sound-alike/look-alike issues:

Stelara™ may be confused with Aldara®

Ustekinumab may be confused with infliximab, rituximab

Brand Names: U.S. Stelara™

Brand Names: Canada Stelara™

Index Terms CNTO 1275

Generic Availability (U.S.) No

Pharmacologic Category Antipsoriatic Agent; Interleukin-12 Inhibitor; Interleukin-23 Inhibitor; Monoclonal Antibody

Use Treatment of moderate-to-severe plaque psoriasis

Medication Guide Available Yes

Contraindications Hypersensitivity to ustekinumab or any component of the formulation

Canadian labeling: Additional contraindications (not in U.S. labeling): Severe infections such as sepsis, tuberculosis, and opportunistic infections

Warnings/Precautions May increase the risk for malignancy although the impact on the development and course of malignancies is not fully defined. In clinical trials, the incidence of malignancy associated with therapy was comparable to that of the general population. Use with caution in patients with prior malignancy (use not studied in this population).

Infrequent, but serious bacterial, fungal, and viral infections have been observed with use. Avoid use in patients with clinically important active infection. Caution should be exercised when considering use in patients with a history of new/recurrent infections, with conditions that predispose them to infections (eg, diabetes or residence/travel from areas of endemic mycoses), or with chronic, latent, or localized infections. Patients who develop a new infection while undergoing treatment should be monitored closely. If a patient develops a serious infection, therapy should be discontinued or withheld until successful resolution of infection.

Avoid use in patients with active tuberculosis (TB). Patients should be evaluated for latent tuberculosis infection with a tuberculin skin test prior to starting therapy. Treatment of latent TB should be initiated before ustekinumab therapy is used.

Antibody formation to ustekinumab has been observed with therapy and has been associated with decreased serum levels and therapeutic response in some patients. Discontinue immediately with signs/symptoms of hypersensitivity reaction and treat appropriately as indicated. Use in combination with other immunosuppressive drugs or phototherapy has not been studied. Patients should be brought up to date with all immunizations before initiating therapy. **Live vaccines should not be given concurrently;** inactivated or nonlive vaccines may be given concurrently. BCG vaccines should not be given 1 year prior to, during, or 1 year following treatment. Patients >100 kg may require higher dose to achieve adequate serum levels. Use in hepatic or renal impairment has not been studied.

The packaging may contain latex. Product may contain polysorbate 80.

Adverse Reactions (Reflective of adult population; not specific for elderly)
>10%: Miscellaneous: Infection (27% to 61%)
1% to 10%:
Central nervous system: Headache (5%), fatigue (3%), dizziness (1% to 2%), depression (1%)
Dermatologic: Pruritus (1% to 2%)
Local: Injection site erythema (1% to 2%)
Neuromuscular & skeletal: Back pain (1% to 2%)
Respiratory: Pharyngolaryngeal pain (1% to 2%)
Miscellaneous: Antibody formation (3% to 5%)

Drug Interactions
Metabolism/Transport Effects None known.
Avoid Concomitant Use
Avoid concomitant use of Ustekinumab with any of the following: BCG; Belimumab; Natalizumab; Pimecrolimus; Tacrolimus (Topical); Vaccines (Live)
Increased Effect/Toxicity
Ustekinumab may increase the levels/effects of: Belimumab; Leflunomide; Natalizumab; Vaccines (Live)

The levels/effects of Ustekinumab may be increased by: Abciximab; Denosumab; Pimecrolimus; Roflumilast; Tacrolimus (Topical); Trastuzumab
Decreased Effect
Ustekinumab may decrease the levels/effects of: BCG; Coccidioidin Skin Test; Sipuleucel-T; Vaccines (Inactivated); Vaccines (Live)

The levels/effects of Ustekinumab may be decreased by: Echinacea

Stability Store vials refrigerated at 2°C to 8°C (36°F to 46°F); do not freeze. Do not shake. Protect from light; store in original container. Discard any unused portion.

Mechanism of Action Ustekinumab is a human monoclonal antibody that binds to and interferes with the proinflammatory cytokines, interleukin (IL)-12 and IL-23. Biological effects of IL-12 and IL-23 include natural killer (NK) cell activation, CD4+ T-cell differentiation and activation. Ustekinumab also interferes with the expression of monocyte chemotactic protein-1 (MCP-1), tumor necrosis factor-alpha (TNF-α), interferon-inducible protein-10 (IP-10), and interleukin-8 (IL-8). Significant clinical improvement in psoriasis patients is seen in association with reduction of these proinflammatory signalers.

Pharmacodynamics/Kinetics
Distribution: V_d (terminal elimination phase): 0.096-0.264 L/kg
Bioavailability: Absolute bioavailability: SubQ: ~57%
Half-life elimination: 10-126 days
Time to peak, plasma: 7-13.5 days

Dosage

Geriatric & Adult Plaque psoriasis: SubQ:

Initial and maintenance: **Note:** Following an interruption in therapy, retreatment may be initiated at the initial dosing interval. Consider therapy discontinuation in any patient failing to demonstrate a response after 12 weeks of therapy.

≤100 kg: 45 mg at 0- and 4 weeks, and then every 12 weeks thereafter

>100 kg: 45 mg or 90 mg at 0- and 4 weeks, and then every 12 weeks thereafter

Per Canadian labeling, if response inadequate on every 12 week therapy, may increase to every 8 weeks.

Renal Impairment Use has not been studied in renal dysfunction.

Hepatic Impairment Use has not been studied in hepatic dysfunction.

Administration Do not use if cloudy or discolored. Administer by subcutaneous injection into the top of the thigh, abdomen, upper arms, or buttocks. Rotate sites. Avoid areas of skin where psoriasis is present.

Monitoring Parameters Place and read PPD prior to initiating therapy; monitor for signs/symptoms of infection; CBC; Ustekinumab-antibody formation

Special Geriatric Considerations Studies to date have not had sufficient numbers of elderly to demonstrate differences in safety and efficacy between elderly and younger adults.

Dosage Forms Excipient information presented when available (limited, particularly for generics); consult specific product labeling.

Injection, solution [preservative free]:

Stelara™: 45 mg/0.5 mL (0.5 mL) [contains natural rubber/natural latex in packaging, polysorbate 80, sucrose 38 mg/syringe]

Stelara™: 90 mg/mL (1 mL) [contains natural rubber/natural latex in packaging, polysorbate 80, sucrose 76 mg/syringe]

Dosage Forms: Canada Excipient information presented when available (limited, particularly for generics); consult specific product labeling.

Injection, solution [preservative free]:

Stelara™: 45 mg/0.5 mL (0.5 mL)

◆ **Vagifem®** *see* Estradiol (Topical) *on page* 689

◆ **Vagistat®-1 [OTC]** *see* Tioconazole *on page* 1906

ValACYclovir (val ay SYE kloe veer)

Medication Safety Issues

Sound-alike/look-alike issues:

Valtrex® may be confused with Keflex®, Valcyte®, Zovirax®

ValACYclovir may be confused with acyclovir, valGANciclovir, vancomycin

Brand Names: U.S. Valtrex®

Brand Names: Canada Apo-Valacyclovir®; CO Valacyclovir; DOM-Valacyclovir; Mylan-Valacyclovir; PHL-Valacyclovir; PMS-Valacyclovir; PRO-Valacyclovir; Riva-Valacyclovir; Valtrex®

Index Terms Valacyclovir Hydrochloride

Generic Availability (U.S.) Yes

Pharmacologic Category Antiviral Agent; Antiviral Agent, Oral

Use Treatment of herpes zoster (shingles) in immunocompetent patients; treatment of first-episode and recurrent genital herpes; suppression of recurrent genital herpes and reduction of heterosexual transmission of genital herpes in immunocompetent patients; suppression of genital herpes in HIV-infected individuals; treatment of herpes labialis (cold sores)

Unlabeled Use Prophylaxis of cancer-related HSV, VZV, and CMV infections; treatment of cancer-related HSV, VZV infection

Contraindications Hypersensitivity to valacyclovir, acyclovir, or any component of the formulation

Warnings/Precautions Thrombotic thrombocytopenic purpura/hemolytic uremic syndrome has occurred in immunocompromised patients (at doses of 8 g/day). Safety and efficacy have not been established for treatment/suppression of recurrent genital herpes or disseminated herpes in patients with profound immunosuppression (eg, advanced HIV with CD4 <100 cells/mm^3). CNS adverse effects (including agitation, hallucinations, confusion, delirium, seizures, and encephalopathy) have been reported. Use caution in patients with renal impairment, the elderly, and/or those receiving nephrotoxic agents. Acute renal failure has been observed in patients with renal dysfunction; dose adjustment may be required. Decreased precipitation in renal tubules may occur leading to urinary precipitation; adequately hydrate patient. For cold sores, treatment should begin at with earliest symptom (tingling, itching, burning). For genital herpes, treatment should begin as soon as possible after the first signs and symptoms (within 72 hours of onset of first diagnosis or within 24 hours of onset of recurrent episodes). For herpes zoster, treatment should begin within 72 hours of onset of rash. For chickenpox,

VALACYCLOVIR

treatment should begin with earliest sign or symptom. Use with caution in the elderly; CNS effects have been reported. Safety and efficacy have not been established in patients <2 years of age.

Adverse Reactions (Reflective of adult population; not specific for elderly)

>10%:
Central nervous system: Headache (13% to 38%)
Gastrointestinal: Nausea (5% to 15%), abdominal pain (1% to 11%)
Hematologic: Neutropenia (≤18%)
Hepatic: ALT increased (≤14%), AST increased (2% to 16%)
Respiratory: Nasopharyngitis (≤16%)

1% to 10%:
Central nervous system: Fatigue (≤8%), depression (≤7%), fever (children 4%), dizziness (2% to 4%)
Dermatologic: Rash (≤8%)
Endocrine: Dysmenorrhea (≤1% to 8%), dehydration (children 2%)
Gastrointestinal: Vomiting (<1% to 6%), diarrhea (children 5%; adults <1%)
Hematologic: Thrombocytopenia (≤3%)
Hepatic: Alkaline phosphatase increased (≤4%)
Neuromuscular & skeletal: Arthralgia (<1 to 6%)
Respiratory: Rhinorrhea (children 2%)
Miscellaneous: Herpes simplex (children 2%)

Drug Interactions

Metabolism/Transport Effects None known.

Avoid Concomitant Use
Avoid concomitant use of ValACYclovir with any of the following: Zoster Vaccine

Increased Effect/Toxicity
ValACYclovir may increase the levels/effects of: Mycophenolate; Tenofovir; Zidovudine

The levels/effects of ValACYclovir may be increased by: Mycophenolate

Decreased Effect
ValACYclovir may decrease the levels/effects of: Zoster Vaccine

Stability Store at 15°C to 25°C (59°F to 77°F).

Mechanism of Action Valacyclovir is rapidly and nearly completely converted to acyclovir by intestinal and hepatic metabolism. Acyclovir is converted to acyclovir monophosphate by virus-specific thymidine kinase then further converted to acyclovir triphosphate by other cellular enzymes. Acyclovir triphosphate inhibits DNA synthesis and viral replication by competing with deoxyguanosine triphosphate for viral DNA polymerase and being incorporated into viral DNA.

Pharmacodynamics/Kinetics
Absorption: Rapid
Distribution: Acyclovir is widely distributed throughout the body including brain, kidney, lungs, liver, spleen, muscle, uterus, vagina, and CSF
Protein binding: ~14% to 18%
Metabolism: Hepatic; valacyclovir is rapidly and nearly completely converted to acyclovir and L-valine by first-pass effect; acyclovir is hepatically metabolized to a very small extent by aldehyde oxidase and by alcohol and aldehyde dehydrogenase (inactive metabolites)
Bioavailability: ~55% once converted to acyclovir
Half-life elimination: Normal renal function: Adults: Acyclovir: 2.5-3.3 hours, Valacyclovir: ~30 minutes; End-stage renal disease: Acyclovir: 14-20 hours; During hemodialysis: 4 hours
Excretion: Urine, primarily as acyclovir (89%); **Note:** Following oral administration of radiolabeled valacyclovir, 46% of the label is eliminated in the feces (corresponding to non-absorbed drug), while 47% of the radiolabel is eliminated in the urine.

Dosage
Geriatric & Adult
CMV prophylaxis in allogeneic HSCT recipients (unlabeled use): 2 g 4 times daily
Herpes labialis (cold sores): Oral: 2 g twice daily for 1 day (separate doses by ~12 hours)
Herpes zoster (shingles): Oral: 1 g 3 times daily for 7 days
HSV, VZV in cancer patients (unlabeled use):
Prophylaxis: 500 mg 2-3 times daily
Treatment: 1 g 3 times daily
Genital herpes: Oral:
Initial episode: 1 g twice daily for 10 days
Recurrent episode: 500 mg twice daily for 3 days
Reduction of transmission: 500 mg once daily (source partner)

Suppressive therapy:
Immunocompetent patients: 1 g once daily (500 mg once daily in patients with <9 recurrences per year)
HIV-infected patients (CD4 ≥100 cells/mm^3): 500 mg twice daily

Renal Impairment
Herpes zoster: Adults:
Cl_{cr} 30-49 mL/minute: 1 g every 12 hours
Cl_{cr} 10-29 mL/minute: 1 g every 24 hours
Cl_{cr} <10 mL/minute: 500 mg every 24 hours
Genital herpes: Adults:
Initial episode:
Cl_{cr} 10-29 mL/minute: 1 g every 24 hours
Cl_{cr} <10 mL/minute: 500 mg every 24 hours
Recurrent episode: Cl_{cr} <29 mL/minute: 500 mg every 24 hours
Suppressive therapy: Cl_{cr} <29 mL/minute:
For usual dose of 1 g every 24 hours, decrease dose to 500 mg every 24 hours
For usual dose of 500 mg every 24 hours, decrease dose to 500 mg every 48 hours
HIV-infected patients: 500 mg every 24 hours
Herpes labialis:
Cl_{cr} 30-49 mL/minute: 1 g every 12 hours for 2 doses
Cl_{cr} 10-29 mL/minute: 500 mg every 12 hours for 2 doses
Cl_{cr} <10 mL/minute: 500 mg as a single dose
Hemodialysis: Dialyzable (~33% removed during 4-hour session); administer dose post-dialysis
Chronic ambulatory peritoneal dialysis/continuous arteriovenous hemofiltration dialysis: Pharmacokinetic parameters are similar to those in patients with ESRD; supplemental dose not needed following dialysis

Hepatic Impairment No adjustment required.

Administration If GI upset occurs, administer with meals.

Monitoring Parameters Urinalysis, BUN, serum creatinine, liver enzymes, and CBC

Special Geriatric Considerations More convenient dosing and increased bioavailability, without increasing side effects, make valacyclovir a favorable choice compared to acyclovir. Has been shown to accelerate resolution of postherpetic pain. Adjust dose for renal impairment.

Dosage Forms Excipient information presented when available (limited, particularly for generics); consult specific product labeling.
Caplet, oral: 500 mg, 1 g
Valtrex®: 500 mg
Valtrex®: 1 g [scored]
Tablet, oral: 500 mg, 1 g

Extemporaneously Prepared
To prepare a valacyclovir 25 mg/mL oral suspension, crush five valacyclovir 500 mg caplets (10 caplets for 50 mg/mL suspension) into a fine powder in a mortar. Gradually add 5 mL aliquots of Suspension Structured Vehicle USP-NF (SSV) to powder and triturate until a paste is formed. Continue adding 5 mL aliquots of SSV to the mortar until a suspension is formed (minimum 20 mL SSV and maximum 40 mL SSV). Transfer to 100 mL bottle. Add the cherry flavor (amount recommended on package) to the mortar and dissolve in ~5 mL of SSV. Add to bottle once dissolved. Rinse the mortar at least 3 times with ~5 mL of SSV, transferring contents between additions of SSV. Continue to add the SSV to bring final volume to 100 mL. The preparation is stable for 28 days under refrigeration; shake well before using. (Refer to manufacturer's current labeling.)

♦ **Valacyclovir Hydrochloride** *see* ValACYclovir *on page 1989*
♦ **23-Valent Pneumococcal Polysaccharide Vaccine** *see* Pneumococcal Polysaccharide Vaccine (Polyvalent) *on page 1558*
♦ **Valium®** *see* Diazepam *on page 527*
♦ **Valorin [OTC]** *see* Acetaminophen *on page 31*
♦ **Valorin Extra [OTC]** *see* Acetaminophen *on page 31*
♦ **Valproate Semisodium** *see* Divalproex *on page 577*
♦ **Valproate Semisodium** *see* Valproic Acid *on page 1991*
♦ **Valproate Sodium** *see* Valproic Acid *on page 1991*

Valproic Acid (val PROE ik AS id)

Medication Safety Issues
Sound-alike/look-alike issues:
Depakene® may be confused with Depakote®
Valproate sodium may be confused with vecuronium

VALPROIC ACID

Brand Names: U.S. Depacon®; Depakene®; Stavzor™

Brand Names: Canada Apo-Valproic®; Depakene®; Epival® I.V.; Mylan-Valproic; PHL-Valproic Acid; PHL-Valproic Acid E.C.; PMS-Valproic Acid; PMS-Valproic Acid E.C.; ratio-Valproic; ratio-Valproic ECC; Rhoxal-valproic; Sandoz-Valproic

Index Terms 2-Propylpentanoic Acid; 2-Propylvaleric Acid; Dipropylacetic Acid; DPA; Valproate Semisodium; Valproate Sodium

Generic Availability (U.S.) Yes: Excludes delayed release capsule

Pharmacologic Category Anticonvulsant, Miscellaneous; Antimanic Agent; Histone Deacetylase Inhibitor

Use Monotherapy and adjunctive therapy in the treatment of patients with complex partial seizures; monotherapy and adjunctive therapy of simple and complex absence seizures; adjunctive therapy in patients with multiple seizure types that include absence seizures Stavzor™: Mania associated with bipolar disorder; migraine prophylaxis

Unlabeled Use Status epilepticus, diabetic neuropathy

Contraindications Hypersensitivity to valproic acid, derivatives, or any component of the formulation; hepatic disease or significant impairment; urea cycle disorders

Warnings/Precautions [U.S. Boxed Warning]: Hepatic failure resulting in fatalities has occurred in patients. Other risk factors include organic brain disease, mental retardation with severe seizure disorders, congenital metabolic disorders, and patients on multiple anticonvulsants. Hepatotoxicity has usually been reported within 6 months of therapy initiation. Monitor patients closely for appearance of malaise, weakness, facial edema, anorexia, jaundice, and vomiting; discontinue immediately with signs/symptom of significant or suspected impairment. Liver function tests should be performed at baseline and at regular intervals after initiation of therapy, especially within the first 6 months. Hepatic dysfunction may progress despite discontinuing treatment. Should only be used as monotherapy in patients at high risk for hepatotoxicity. Contraindicated with severe impairment.

[U.S. Boxed Warning]: Cases of life-threatening pancreatitis, occurring at the start of therapy or following years of use, have been reported in adults and children. Some cases have been hemorrhagic with rapid progression of initial symptoms to death. Promptly evaluate symptoms of abdominal pain, nausea, vomiting, and/or anorexia; should generally be discontinued if pancreatitis is diagnosed.

May cause severe thrombocytopenia, inhibition of platelet aggregation, and bleeding. Tremors may indicate overdosage; use with caution in patients receiving other anticonvulsants. Hypersensitivity reactions affecting multiple organs have been reported in association with valproic acid use; may include dermatologic and/or hematologic changes (eosinophilia, neutropenia, thrombocytopenia) or symptoms of organ dysfunction.

Hyperammonemia and/or encephalopathy, sometimes fatal, have been reported following the initiation of valproic acid therapy and may be present with normal transaminase levels. Ammonia levels should be measured in patients who develop unexplained lethargy and vomiting, changes in mental status, or in patients who present with hypothermia (unintentional drop in core body temperature to <35°C/95°F). Discontinue therapy if ammonia levels are increased and evaluate for possible urea cycle disorder (UCD); contraindicated in patients with UCD. Evaluation of UCD should be considered for the following patients prior to the start of therapy: History of unexplained encephalopathy or coma; encephalopathy associated with protein load; unexplained mental retardation; history of elevated plasma ammonia or glutamine; history of cyclical vomiting and lethargy; episodic extreme irritability, ataxia; low BUN or protein avoidance; family history of UCD or unexplained infant deaths (particularly male); or signs or symptoms of UCD (hyperammonemia, encephalopathy, respiratory alkalosis). Hypothermia has been reported with valproic acid therapy; may or may not be associated with hyperammonemia; may also occur with concomitant topiramate therapy.

In vitro studies have suggested valproic acid stimulates the replication of HIV and CMV viruses under experimental conditions. The clinical consequence of this is unknown, but should be considered when monitoring affected patients.

Antiepileptics are associated with an increased risk of suicidal behavior/thoughts with use (regardless of indication); patients should be monitored for signs/symptoms of depression, suicidal tendencies, and other unusual behavior changes during therapy and instructed to inform their healthcare provider immediately if symptoms occur.

Use of Depacon® injection is not recommended for post-traumatic seizure prophylaxis following acute head trauma. Anticonvulsants should not be discontinued abruptly because of the possibility of increasing seizure frequency; valproic acid should be withdrawn gradually to minimize the potential of increased seizure frequency, unless safety concerns require a more rapid withdrawal. Concomitant use with carbapenem antibiotics may reduce valproic acid levels to subtherapeutic levels; monitor levels frequently and consider alternate therapy if levels drop significantly or lack of seizure control occurs. Concomitant use with clonazepam may induce absence status. Patients treated for bipolar disorder should be monitored closely for clinical worsening or suicidality; prescriptions should be written for the smallest quantity consistent with good patient care.

CNS depression may occur with valproic acid use. Patients must be cautioned about performing tasks which require mental alertness (operating machinery or driving). Effects with other sedative drugs or ethanol may be potentiated. Use with caution in the elderly.

Adverse Reactions (Reflective of adult population; not specific for elderly)

>10%:

Central nervous system: Headache (≤31%), somnolence (≤30%), dizziness (12% to 25%), insomnia (>1% to 15%), nervousness (>1% to 11%), pain (1% to 11%)

Dermatologic: Alopecia (>1% to 24%)

Gastrointestinal: Nausea (15% to 48%), vomiting (7% to 27%), diarrhea (7% to 23%), abdominal pain (7% to 23%), dyspepsia (7% to 23%), anorexia (>1% to 12%)

Hematologic: Thrombocytopenia (1% to 24%; dose related)

Neuromuscular & skeletal: Tremor (≤57%), weakness (6% to 27%)

Ocular: Diplopia (>1% to 16%), amblyopia/blurred vision (≤12%)

Miscellaneous: Infection (≤20%), flu-like syndrome (12%)

1% to 10%:

Cardiovascular: Peripheral edema (>1% to 8%), chest pain (>1% to <5%), edema (>1% to <5%), facial edema (>1% to <5%), hypertension (>1% to <5%), hypotension (>1% to <5%), orthostatic hypotension (>1% to <5%), palpitation (>1% to <5%), tachycardia (>1% to <5%), vasodilation (>1% to <5%), arrhythmia

Central nervous system: Ataxia (>1% to 8%), amnesia (>1% to 7%), emotional lability (>1% to 6%), fever (>1% to 6%), abnormal thinking (≤6%), depression (>1% to 5%), abnormal dreams (>1% to <5%), agitation (>1% to <5%), anxiety (>1% to <5%), catatonia (>1% to <5%), chills (>1% to <5%), confusion (>1% to <5%), coordination abnormal (>1% to <5%), hallucination (>1% to <5%), malaise (>1% to <5%), personality disorder (>1% to <5%), speech disorder (>1% to <5%), tardive dyskinesia (>1% to <5%), vertigo (>1% to <5%), euphoria (1%), hypoesthesia (1%)

Dermatologic: Rash (>1% to 6%), bruising (>1% to 5%), discoid lupus erythematosus (>1% to <5%), dry skin (>1% to <5%), furunculosis (>1% to <5%), petechia (>1% to <5%), pruritus (>1% to <5), seborrhea (>1% to <5%)

Endocrine & metabolic: Amenorrhea (>1% to <5%), dysmenorrhea (>1% to <5%), metrorrhagia (>1% to <5%), hypoproteinemia

Gastrointestinal: Weight gain (4% to 9%), weight loss (6%), appetite increased (≤6%), constipation (>1% to 5%), xerostomia (>1% to 5%), eructation (>1% to <5%), fecal incontinence (>1% to <5%), flatulence (>1% to <5%), gastroenteritis (>1% to <5%), glossitis (>1% to <5%), hematemesis (>1% to <5%), pancreatitis (>1% to <5%), periodontal abscess (>1% to <5%), stomatitis (>1% to <5%), taste perversion (>1% to <5%), dysphagia, gum hemorrhage, mouth ulceration

Genitourinary: Cystitis (>1% to 5%), dysuria (>1% to 5%), urinary frequency (>1% to <5%), urinary incontinence (>1% to <5%), vaginal hemorrhage (>1% to 5%), vaginitis (>1% to <5%)

Hepatic: ALT increased (>1% to <5%), AST increased (>1% to <5%)

Local: Injection site pain (3%), injection site reaction (2%), injection site inflammation (1%)

Neuromuscular & skeletal: Back pain (≤8%), abnormal gait (>1% to <5%), arthralgia (>1% to <5%), arthrosis (>1% to <5%), dysarthria (>1% to <5%), hypertonia (>1% to <5%), hypokinesia (>1% to <5%), leg cramps (>1% to <5%), myalgia (>1% to <5%), myasthenia (>1% to <5%), neck pain (>1% to <5%), neck rigidity (>1% to <5%), paresthesia (>1% to <5%), reflex increased (>1% to <5%), twitching (>1% to <5%)

Ocular: Nystagmus (1% to 8%), dry eyes (>1% to 5%), eye pain (>1% to 5%), abnormal vision (>1% to <5%), conjunctivitis (>1% to <5%)

Otic: Tinnitus (1% to 7%), ear pain (>1% to 5%), deafness (>1% to <5%), otitis media (>1% to <5%)

Respiratory: Pharyngitis (2% to 8%), bronchitis (5%), rhinitis (>1% to 5%), dyspnea (1% to 5%), cough (>1% to <5%), epistaxis (>1% to <5%), pneumonia (>1% to <5%), sinusitis (>1% to <5%)

Miscellaneous: Diaphoresis (1%), hiccups

Drug Interactions

Metabolism/Transport Effects Substrate of CYP2A6 (minor), CYP2B6 (minor), CYP2C19 (minor), CYP2C9 (minor), CYP2E1 (minor); **Note:** Assignment of Major/Minor substrate status based on clinically relevant drug interaction potential; **Inhibits** CYP2C9 (weak); **Induces** CYP2A6 (weak/moderate)

Avoid Concomitant Use There are no known interactions where it is recommended to avoid concomitant use.

◄ **Increased Effect/Toxicity**

Valproic Acid may increase the levels/effects of: Barbiturates; Ethosuximide; LamoTRIgine; LORazepam; Paliperidone; Primidone; RisperiDONE; Rufinamide; Temozolomide; Tricyclic Antidepressants; Vorinostat; Zidovudine

The levels/effects of Valproic Acid may be increased by: ChlorproMAZINE; Felbamate; GuanFACINE; Salicylates; Topiramate

Decreased Effect

Valproic Acid may decrease the levels/effects of: CarBAMazepine; Fosphenytoin; OXcarbazepine; Phenytoin

The levels/effects of Valproic Acid may be decreased by: Barbiturates; CarBAMazepine; Carbapenems; Ethosuximide; Fosphenytoin; Methylfolate; Phenytoin; Primidone; Protease Inhibitors; Rifampin

Ethanol/Nutrition/Herb Interactions

Ethanol: Avoid ethanol (may increase CNS depression).

Food: Food may delay but does not affect the extent of absorption. Valproic acid serum concentrations may be decreased if taken with food. Milk has no effect on absorption.

Herb/Nutraceutical: Avoid evening primrose (seizure threshold decreased).

Stability Use appropriate precautions for handling and disposal (hazardous agent).

Depakene® solution: Store below 30°C (86°F).

Stavzor™: Store at controlled room temperature of 25°C (77°F).

Depakene® capsule: Store at controlled room temperature of 15°C to 25°C (59°F to 77°F).

Depacon®: Store vial at room temperature of 15°C to 30°C (59°F to 86°F). Injection should be diluted in 50 mL of a compatible diluent. Stable in D_5W, NS, and LR for at least 24 hours when stored in glass or PVC.

Mechanism of Action Causes increased availability of gamma-aminobutyric acid (GABA), an inhibitory neurotransmitter, to brain neurons or may enhance the action of GABA or mimic its action at postsynaptic receptor sites

Pharmacodynamics/Kinetics

Distribution: Total valproate: 11 L/1.73 m²; free valproate 92 L/1.73 m²

Protein binding (dose dependent): 80% to 90%; decreased in the elderly and with hepatic or renal dysfunction

Metabolism: Extensively hepatic via glucuronide conjugation and mitochondrial beta-oxidation. The relationship between dose and total valproate concentration is nonlinear; concentration does not increase proportionally with the dose, but increases to a lesser extent due to saturable plasma protein binding. The kinetics of unbound drug are linear.

Half-life elimination (increased with liver disease): Adults: 9-16 hours

Time to peak, serum: Stavzor™: 2 hours

Excretion: Urine (30% to 50% as glucuronide conjugate, 3% as unchanged drug)

Dosage

Geriatric Initiate at lower doses; dose escalation should be managed more slowly (in persons of advanced age). Refer to adult dosing.

Adult

Seizures: Administer doses >250 mg/day in divided doses.

Oral:

Simple and complex absence seizure: Initial: 15 mg/kg/day; increase by 5-10 mg/kg/day at weekly intervals until therapeutic levels are achieved; maximum: 60 mg/kg/day.

Complex partial seizure: Initial: 10-15 mg/kg/day; increase by 5-10 mg/kg/day at weekly intervals until therapeutic levels are achieved; maximum: 60 mg/kg/day.

Note: Regular release and delayed release formulations are usually given in 2-4 divided doses/day

I.V.: Administer as a 60-minute infusion (≤20 mg/minute) with the same frequency as oral products; switch patient to oral products as soon as possible. Rapid infusions ≤45 mg/kg over 5-10 minutes (1.5-6 mg/kg/minute) were generally well tolerated in clinical trials.

Rectal (unlabeled): Dilute syrup 1:1 with water for use as a retention enema; loading dose: 17-20 mg/kg one time; maintenance: 10-15 mg/kg/dose every 8 hours

Status epilepticus (unlabeled use):

Loading dose: I.V.: 15-45 mg/kg administered at ≤6 mg/kg/minute

Maintenance dose: I.V. infusion: 1-4 mg/kg/hour; titrate dose as needed based upon patient response and evaluation of drug-drug interactions

Mania (Stavzor™): Oral: Initial: 750 mg/day in divided doses; dose should be adjusted as rapidly as possible to desired clinical effect; maximum recommended dosage: 60 mg/kg/day

Migraine prophylaxis (Stavzor™): *Oral:* 250 mg twice daily; adjust dose based on patient response, up to 1000 mg/day

Diabetic neuropathy (unlabeled use): *Oral:* 500-1200 mg/day (Bril, 2011)

Renal Impairment A 27% reduction in clearance of unbound valproate is seen in patients with Cl$_{cr}$ <10 mL/minute. Hemodialysis reduces valproate concentrations by 20%, therefore, no dose adjustment is needed in patients with renal failure. Protein binding is reduced, monitoring only total valproate concentrations may be misleading.

Hepatic Impairment Dosage reduction is required. Clearance is decreased with liver impairment. Hepatic disease is also associated with decreased albumin concentrations and 2- to 2.6-fold increase in the unbound fraction. Free concentrations of valproate may be elevated while total concentrations appear normal. Use is contraindicated in severe impairment.

Administration

Depacon®: Following dilution to final concentration, administer over 60 minutes at a rate ≤20 mg/minute. Alternatively, single doses up to 45 mg/kg have been administered as a rapid infusion over 5-10 minutes (1.5-6 mg/kg/minute).

Depakene® capsule, Stavzor™: Swallow whole; do not chew.

Monitoring Parameters Liver enzymes (at baseline and during therapy), CBC with platelets (baseline and periodic intervals), PT/PTT (especially prior to surgery), serum ammonia (with symptoms of lethargy, mental status change), serum valproate levels (trough for therapeutic levels); suicidality (eg, suicidal thoughts, depression, behavioral changes)

Reference Range Note: In general, trough concentrations should be used to assess adequacy of therapy; peak concentrations may also be drawn if clinically necessary (eg, concentration-related toxicity). Within 2-4 days of initiation or dose adjustment, trough concentrations should be drawn just before the next dose (extended-release preparations) or before the morning dose (for immediate-release preparations). Patients with epilepsy should **not** delay taking their dose for >2-3 hours. Additional patient-specific factors must be taken into consideration when interpreting drug levels, including indication, age, clinical response, adherence, comorbidities, adverse effects, and concomitant medications (Patsalos, 2008; Reed, 2006).

Therapeutic:

Epilepsy: 50-100 mcg/mL (SI: 350-700 micromole/L); although seizure control may improve at levels >100 mcg/mL (SI: 700 micromole/L), toxicity may occur at levels of 100-150 mcg/mL (SI: 700-1040 micromole/L)

Mania: 50-125 mcg/mL (SI: 350-875 micromole/L)

Toxic: Some laboratories may report >200 mcg/mL (SI: >1390 micromole/L) as a toxic threshold, although clinical toxicity can occur at lower concentrations. Probability of thrombocytopenia increases with total valproate levels ≥110 mcg/mL in females or ≥135 mcg/mL in males.

Epilepsy: Although seizure control may improve at levels >100 mcg/mL (SI: 700 micromole/L), toxicity may occur at levels of 100-150 mcg/mL (SI: 700-1050 micromole/L)

Mania: Clinical response seen with trough levels between 50-125 mcg/mL (SI: 350-875 micromole/L); risk of toxicity increases at levels >125 mcg/mL (SI: 875 micromole/L)

Test Interactions False-positive result for urine ketones; altered thyroid function tests

Special Geriatric Considerations Although there is little data in elderly for the use of valproic acid in the treatment of seizures, there are a number of studies which demonstrate its benefit in the treatment of agitation and dementia and other psychiatric disorders. It is important that the clinician understand that serum concentrations do not correlate with behavior response; likewise, it is imperative to monitor LFTs and CBC during the first 6 months of therapy. See Warnings/Precautions and Monitoring Parameters.

Elimination is decreased in elderly. Studies of older adults with dementia show a high incidence of somnolence (which is usually transient); cognitive side effects generally minimal. In some patients, this was associated with weight loss. Starting doses should be lower and increased slowly, with careful monitoring of nutritional intake and dehydration. Safety and efficacy for use in patients >65 years of age have not been studied for migraine prophylaxis.

Dosage Forms Excipient information presented when available (limited, particularly for generics); consult specific product labeling.

Capsule, softgel, oral: 250 mg [strength expressed as valproic acid]

Depakene®: 250 mg [strength expressed as valproic acid]

Capsule, softgel, delayed release, oral:

Stavzor™: 125 mg, 250 mg, 500 mg [strength expressed as valproic acid]

Injection, solution, as valproate sodium: 100 mg/mL (5 mL) [strength expressed as valproic acid]

Injection, solution, as valproate sodium [preservative free]: 100 mg/mL (5 mL) [strength expressed as valproic acid]

Depacon®: 100 mg/mL (5 mL) [contains edetate disodium; strength expressed as valproic acid]

Solution, oral, as valproate sodium: 250 mg/5 mL (5 mL, 473 mL, 480 mL) [strength expressed as valproic acid]; 250 mg/5 mL (5 mL, 473 mL, 480 mL)

Syrup, oral, as valproate sodium: 250 mg/5 mL (5 mL, 10 mL, 473 mL, 480 mL) [strength expressed as valproic acid]

Depakene®: 250 mg/5 mL (473 mL) [strength expressed as valproic acid]

♦ **Valproic Acid Derivative** see Divalproex on page 577

Valsartan (val SAR tan)

Related Information
Angiotensin Agents on page 2093
Heart Failure (Systolic) on page 2203
Medication Safety Issues
Sound-alike/look-alike issues:
Valsartan may be confused with losartan, Valstar®, Valturna®
Diovan® may be confused with Zyban®
International issues:
Diovan [U.S., Canada, and multiple international markets] may be confused with Dianben, a brand name for metformin [Spain]
Brand Names: U.S. Diovan®
Brand Names: Canada CO Valsartan; Diovan®; Ran-Valsartan; Sandoz-Valsartan; Teva-Valsartan
Generic Availability (U.S.) No
Pharmacologic Category Angiotensin II Receptor Blocker
Use Alone or in combination with other antihypertensive agents in the treatment of essential hypertension; reduction of cardiovascular mortality in patients with left ventricular dysfunction postmyocardial infarction; treatment of heart failure (NYHA Class II-IV)
Contraindications There are no contraindications listed in manufacturer's labeling.

Canadian labeling: Hypersensitivity to valsartan or any component of the formulation

Warnings/Precautions May cause hyperkalemia; avoid potassium supplementation unless specifically required by healthcare provider. During the initiation of therapy, hypotension may occur, particularly in patients with heart failure or post-MI patients. Use extreme caution with concurrent administration of potassium-sparing diuretics or potassium supplements, in patients with mild-to-moderate hepatic dysfunction (adjust dose), in those who may be sodium/water depleted (eg, on high-dose diuretics), and in the elderly; correct depletion first.

Use caution with unstented unilateral/bilateral renal artery stenosis. When unstented bilateral renal artery stenosis is present, use is generally avoided due to the elevated risk of deterioration in renal function unless possible benefits outweigh risks. Use with caution with preexisting renal insufficiency; significant aortic/mitral stenosis. May be associated with deterioration of renal function and/or increases in serum creatinine, particularly in patients with low renal blood flow (eg, renal artery stenosis, heart failure) whose glomerular filtration rate (GFR) is dependent on efferent arteriolar vasoconstriction by angiotensin II. Use caution in patients with severe renal impairment or significant hepatic dysfunction. Monitor renal function closely in patients with severe heart failure; changes in renal function should be anticipated and dosage adjustments of valsartan or concomitant medications may be needed. Concurrent use of ACE inhibitors may increase the risk of clinically-significant adverse events (eg, renal dysfunction, hyperkalemia).

Adverse Reactions (Reflective of adult population; not specific for elderly)
>10%:
Central nervous system: Dizziness (heart failure trials 17%)
Renal: BUN increased >50% (heart failure trials 17%)
1% to 10%:
Cardiovascular: Hypotension (heart failure trials 7%; MI trial 1%), orthostatic hypotension (heart failure trials 2%), syncope (up to >1%)
Central nervous system: Dizziness (hypertension trial 2% to 8%), fatigue (heart failure trials 3%; hypertension trial 2%), postural dizziness (heart failure trials 2%), headache (heart failure trials >1%), vertigo (up to >1%)
Endocrine & metabolic: Serum potassium increased by >20% (4% to 10%), hyperkalemia (heart failure trials 2%)
Gastrointestinal: Diarrhea (heart failure trials 5%), abdominal pain (2%), nausea (heart failure trials >1%), upper abdominal pain (heart failure trials >1%)
Hematologic: Neutropenia (2%)
Neuromuscular & skeletal: Arthralgia (heart failure trials 3%), back pain (up to >3%)

Ocular: Blurred vision (heart failure trials >1%)

Renal: Creatinine doubled (MI trial 4%), creatinine increased >50% (heart failure trials 4%), renal dysfunction (up to >1%)

Respiratory: Cough (1% to 3%)

Miscellaneous: Viral infection (3%)

Drug Interactions

Metabolism/Transport Effects Substrate of SLCO1B1; **Inhibits** CYP2C9 (weak)

Avoid Concomitant Use There are no known interactions where it is recommended to avoid concomitant use.

Increased Effect/Toxicity

Valsartan may increase the levels/effects of: ACE Inhibitors; Amifostine; Antihypertensives; Hydrochlorothiazide; Hypotensive Agents; Lithium; Nonsteroidal Anti-Inflammatory Agents; Potassium-Sparing Diuretics; RiTUXimab; Sodium Phosphates

The levels/effects of Valsartan may be increased by: Alfuzosin; Aliskiren; Diazoxide; Eltrombopag; Eplerenone; Herbs (Hypotensive Properties); Hydrochlorothiazide; MAO Inhibitors; Pentoxifylline; Phosphodiesterase 5 Inhibitors; Potassium Salts; Prostacyclin Analogues; Tolvaptan; Trimethoprim

Decreased Effect

The levels/effects of Valsartan may be decreased by: Herbs (Hypertensive Properties); Methylphenidate; Nonsteroidal Anti-Inflammatory Agents; Yohimbine

Ethanol/Nutrition/Herb Interactions

Food: Decreases the peak plasma concentration and extent of absorption by 50% and 40%, respectively. Potassium supplements and/or potassium-containing salts may cause or worsen hyperkalemia. Management: Take consistently with regard to food. Consult prescriber before consuming a potassium-rich diet, potassium supplements, or salt substitutes.

Herb/Nutraceutical: Some herbal medications may worsen hypertension (eg, licorice); others may increase the antihypertensive effect of valsartan (eg, shepherd's purse). Management: Avoid bayberry, blue cohosh, cayenne, ephedra, ginger, ginseng (American), kola, licorice, and yohimbe. Avoid black cohosh, California poppy, coleus, golden seal, hawthorn, mistletoe, periwinkle, quinine, and shepherd's purse.

Stability Store at 25°C (77°F); excursions permitted to 15°C to 30°C (59°F to 86°F). Protect from moisture.

Mechanism of Action Valsartan produces direct antagonism of the angiotensin II (AT2) receptors, unlike the ACE inhibitors. It displaces angiotensin II from the AT1 receptor and produces its blood pressure-lowering effects by antagonizing AT1-induced vasoconstriction, aldosterone release, catecholamine release, arginine vasopressin release, water intake, and hypertrophic responses. This action results in more efficient blockade of the cardiovascular effects of angiotensin II and fewer side effects than the ACE inhibitors.

Pharmacodynamics/Kinetics

Onset of action: ~2 hours

Duration: 24 hours

Distribution: V_d: 17 L (adults)

Protein binding: 95%, primarily albumin

Metabolism: To inactive metabolite

Bioavailability: Tablet: 25% (range: 10% to 35%); suspension: ~40% (~1.6 times more than tablet)

Half-life elimination: ~6 hours

Time to peak, serum: 2-4 hours

Excretion: Feces (83%) and urine (13%) as unchanged drug

Dosage

Geriatric & Adult

Hypertension: Initial: 80 mg or 160 mg once daily (in patients who are not volume depleted); dose may be increased to achieve desired effect; maximum recommended dose: 320 mg/day

Heart failure: Initial: 40 mg twice daily; titrate dose to 80-160 mg twice daily, as tolerated; maximum daily dose: 320 mg

Left ventricular dysfunction after MI: Initial: 20 mg twice daily; titrate dose to target of 160 mg twice daily as tolerated; may initiate ≥12 hours following MI

Renal Impairment

No dosage adjustment necessary if Cl_{cr} >10 mL/minute.

Dialysis: Not significantly removed.

Hepatic Impairment In mild-to-moderate liver disease no adjustment is needed. Use caution in patients with liver disease. Patients with mild-to-moderate chronic disease have twice the exposure as healthy volunteers.

Administration Administer with or without food.

Monitoring Parameters Baseline and periodic electrolyte panels, renal function, BP; in CHF, serum potassium during dose escalation and periodically thereafter

Pharmacotherapy Pearls Valsartan may have an advantage over losartan due to minimal metabolism requirements and consequent use in mild-to-moderate hepatic impairment.

Special Geriatric Considerations No dosage adjustment is necessary when initiating angiotensin II receptor antagonists in the elderly. In clinical studies, no differences between younger adults and elderly were demonstrated. Many elderly may be volume depleted due to diuretic use and/or blunted thirst reflex resulting in inadequate fluid intake.

Dosage Forms Excipient information presented when available (limited, particularly for generics); consult specific product labeling.

Tablet, oral:
  Diovan®: 40 mg [scored]
  Diovan®: 80 mg, 160 mg, 320 mg

Extemporaneously Prepared To prepare valsartan suspension, add 80 mL of Ora-Plus® to an 8-ounce amber glass bottle containing eight (8) valsartan 80 mg tablets. Shake well ≥2 minutes. Allow the suspension to stand for a minimum of 1 hour then shake for 1 minute. Then add 80 mL of Ora-Sweet SF® to the bottle and shake for at least 10 seconds. Resulting 160 mL suspension will contain valsartan 4 mg/mL. Store for either up to 30 days at room temperature (below 30°C/86°F) or up to 75 days under refrigeration (2°C to 8°C/35°F to 46°F) in the glass bottle. Shake well before use.

Product information, December, 2007; Novartis Pharmaceuticals Corp.

◆ **Valsartan and Aliskiren** *see* Aliskiren and Valsartan *on page 62*
◆ **Valsartan and Amlodipine** *see* Amlodipine and Valsartan *on page 107*

Valsartan and Hydrochlorothiazide (val SAR tan & hye droe klor oh THYE a zide)

Related Information
  Hydrochlorothiazide *on page 933*
  Valsartan *on page 1996*

Medication Safety Issues
  Sound-alike/look-alike issues:
    Diovan® may be confused with Zyban®

Brand Names: U.S. Diovan HCT®

Brand Names: Canada Diovan HCT®; Sandoz Valsartan HCT; Teva-Valsartan HCTZ; Valsartan-HCTZ

Index Terms Hydrochlorothiazide and Valsartan

Generic Availability (U.S.) No

Pharmacologic Category Angiotensin II Receptor Blocker; Diuretic, Thiazide

Use Treatment of hypertension

Dosage
  Geriatric & Adult Note: Dose is individualized; combination product may be used as initial therapy or substituted for individual components in patients currently maintained on both agents separately or in patients not adequately controlled with monotherapy (using one of the agents or an agent within same antihypertensive class).

  Hypertension: Oral:
    Initial therapy: Valsartan 160 mg and hydrochlorothiazide 12.5 mg once daily; dose may be titrated after 1-2 weeks of therapy. Maximum recommended daily doses: Valsartan 320 mg; hydrochlorothiazide 25 mg.
    Add-on/replacement therapy: Valsartan 80-160 mg and hydrochlorothiazide 12.5-25 mg once daily; dose may be titrated after 3-4 weeks of therapy. Maximum recommended daily dose: Valsartan 320 mg; hydrochlorothiazide 25 mg.

  Renal Impairment
    Cl_{cr} >30 mL/minute: No adjustment needed
    Cl_{cr} ≤30 mL/minute: Use of combination not recommended. Contraindicated in patients with anuria.

  Hepatic Impairment Use with caution; initiate at lower dose and titrate slowly.

  Special Geriatric Considerations See individual agents. Combination products are not recommended as first-line treatment. Use only if doses of individual agents correspond to the combination available.

  Dosage Forms Excipient information presented when available (limited, particularly for generics); consult specific product labeling.
    Tablet:
      Diovan HCT® 80 mg/12.5 mg: Valsartan 80 mg and hydrochlorothiazide 12.5 mg
      Diovan HCT® 160 mg/12.5 mg: Valsartan 160 mg and hydrochlorothiazide 12.5 mg
      Diovan HCT® 160 mg/25 mg: Valsartan 160 mg and hydrochlorothiazide 25 mg
      Diovan HCT® 320 mg/12.5 mg: Valsartan 320 mg and hydrochlorothiazide 12.5 mg
      Diovan HCT® 320 mg/25 mg: Valsartan 320 mg and hydrochlorothiazide 25 mg

♦ **Valsartan, Hydrochlorothiazide, and Amlodipine** *see* Amlodipine, Valsartan, and Hydro-chlorothiazide *on page 108*

♦ **Valtrex®** *see* ValACYclovir *on page 1989*

♦ **Valturna® [DSC]** *see* Aliskiren and Valsartan *on page 62*

♦ **Vanceril** *see* Beclomethasone (Oral Inhalation) *on page 189*

♦ **Vancocin®** *see* Vancomycin *on page 1999*

Vancomycin (van koe MYE sin)

Related Information
Antibiotic Treatment of Adults With Infective Endocarditis *on page 2157*
Antimicrobial Drugs of Choice *on page 2163*
Community-Acquired Pneumonia in Adults *on page 2171*

Medication Safety Issues
Sound-alike/look-alike issues:
I.V. vancomycin may be confused with INVanz®
Vancomycin may be confused with clindamycin, gentamicin, tobramycin, valACYclovir, vecuronium, Vibramycin®

High alert medication:
The Institute for Safe Medication Practices (ISMP) includes this medication (intrathecal administration) among its list of drug classes which have a heightened risk of causing significant patient harm when used in error.

Brand Names: U.S. Vancocin®

Brand Names: Canada PMS-Vancomycin; Sterile Vancomycin Hydrochloride, USP; Val-Vancomycin; Vancocin®; Vancomycin Hydrochloride for Injection, USP

Index Terms Vancomycin Hydrochloride

Generic Availability (U.S.) Yes

Pharmacologic Category Glycopeptide

Use
I.V.: Treatment of patients with infections caused by staphylococcal species and streptococcal species

Oral: Treatment of *C. difficile*-associated diarrhea and treatment of enterocolitis caused by *Staphylococcus aureus* (including methicillin-resistant strains)

Unlabeled Use Bacterial endophthalmitis; treatment of infections caused by gram-positive organisms in patients who have serious allergies to beta-lactam agents; treatment of beta-lactam resistant gram-positive infections; surgical prophylaxis

Contraindications Hypersensitivity to vancomycin or any component of the formulation

Warnings/Precautions May cause nephrotoxicity although limited data suggest direct causal relationship; usual risk factors include pre-existing renal impairment, concomitant nephrotoxic medications, advanced age, and dehydration (nephrotoxicity has also been reported following treatment with oral vancomycin, typically in patients >65 years of age). If multiple sequential (≥2) serum creatinine concentrations demonstrate an increase of 0.5 mg/dL or ≥50% increase from baseline (whichever is greater) in the absence of an alternative explanation, the patient should be identified as having vancomycin-induced nephrotoxicity (Rybak, 2009). Discontinue treatment if signs of nephrotoxicity occur; renal damage is usually reversible.

May cause neurotoxicity; usual risk factors include pre-existing renal impairment, concomitant neuro-/nephrotoxic medications, advanced age, and dehydration. Ototoxicity, although rarely associated with monotherapy, is proportional to the amount of drug given and the duration of treatment. Tinnitus or vertigo may be indications of vestibular injury and impending bilateral irreversible damage. Discontinue treatment if signs of ototoxicity occur. Prolonged therapy (>1 week) or total doses exceeding 25 g may increase the risk of neutropenia; prompt reversal of neutropenia is expected after discontinuation of therapy. Prolonged use may result in fungal or bacterial superinfection, including *C. difficile*-associated diarrhea (CDAD) and pseudomem-branous colitis; CDAD has been observed >2 months postantibiotic treatment. Use with caution in patients with renal impairment or those receiving other nephrotoxic or ototoxic drugs; dosage modification required in patients with impaired renal function (especially elderly). Accumulation may occur after multiple oral doses of vancomycin in patients with renal impairment; consider monitoring trough concentrations in this circumstance.

Rapid I.V. administration may result in hypotension, flushing, erythema, urticaria, and/or pruritus. Oral vancomycin is only indicated for the treatment of pseudomembranous colitis due to *C. difficile* and enterocolitis due to *S. aureus* and is not effective for systemic infections; parenteral vancomycin is not effective for the treatment of colitis due to *C. difficile* and enterocolitis due to *S. aureus*. Clinically significant serum concentrations have been reported in patients with inflammatory disorders of the intestinal mucosa who have taken oral vancomycin (multiple doses) for the treatment of *C. difficile*-associated diarrhea. Although use may be warranted, the risk for adverse reactions may be higher in this situation; consider monitoring serum trough concentrations, especially with renal insufficiency, severe colitis, concurrent rectal vancomycin administration, and/or concomitant I.V. aminoglycosides. The IDSA suggests that it is appropriate to obtain trough concentrations when a patient is receiving long courses of ≥2 g/day (Cohen, 2010). **Note:** The Infectious Disease Society of America (IDSA) recommends the use of oral metronidazole for initial treatment of mild-to-moderate *C. difficile* infection and the use of oral vancomycin for initial treatment of severe *C. difficile* infection (Cohen, 2010).

Adverse Reactions (Reflective of adult population; not specific for elderly)

Injection:
>10%:
Cardiovascular: Hypotension accompanied by flushing
Dermatologic: Erythematous rash on face and upper body (red neck or red man syndrome - infusion rate related)
1% to 10%:
Central nervous system: Chills, drug fever
Dermatologic: Rash
Hematologic: Eosinophilia, reversible neutropenia
Local: Phlebitis

Oral:
>10%: Gastrointestinal: Abdominal pain, bad taste (with oral solution), nausea
1% to 10%:
Cardiovascular: Peripheral edema
Central nervous system: Fatigue, fever, headache
Gastrointestinal: Diarrhea, flatulence, vomiting
Genitourinary: Urinary tract infection
Neuromuscular & skeletal: Back pain

Drug Interactions

Metabolism/Transport Effects None known.

Avoid Concomitant Use
Avoid concomitant use of Vancomycin with any of the following: BCG; Gallium Nitrate

Increased Effect/Toxicity
Vancomycin may increase the levels/effects of: Aminoglycosides; Colistimethate; Gallium Nitrate; Neuromuscular-Blocking Agents

The levels/effects of Vancomycin may be increased by: Nonsteroidal Anti-Inflammatory Agents

Decreased Effect
Vancomycin may decrease the levels/effects of: BCG; Typhoid Vaccine

The levels/effects of Vancomycin may be decreased by: Bile Acid Sequestrants

Stability
Capsules: Store at controlled room temperature of 15°C to 30°C (59°F to 86°F).
Injection: Reconstituted 500 mg and 1 g vials are stable at either room temperature or under refrigeration for 14 days. **Note:** Vials contain no bacteriostatic agent. Solutions diluted for administration in either D_5W or NS are stable under refrigeration for 14 days or at room temperature for 7 days. Reconstitute vials with 20 mL of SWFI for each 1 g of vancomycin (10 mL/500 mg vial; 20 mL/1 g vial; 100 mL/5 g vial; 200 mL/10 g vial). The reconstituted solution must be further diluted with at least 100 mL of a compatible diluent per 500 mg of vancomycin prior to parenteral administration.
Intrathecal (unlabeled route): Vancomycin is available as a powder for injection and may be diluted to 1-5 mg/mL concentration in preservative free 0.9% sodium chloride for administration into the CSF.

Mechanism of Action Inhibits bacterial cell wall synthesis by blocking glycopeptide polymerization through binding tightly to D-alanyl-D-alanine portion of cell wall precursor

Pharmacodynamics/Kinetics
Absorption: Oral: Poor; may be enhanced with bowel inflammation; I.M.: Erratic; Intraperitoneal: ~38%
Distribution: V_d: 0.4-1 L/kg; Distributes widely in body tissue and fluids, except for CSF
Relative diffusion from blood into CSF: Good only with inflammation (exceeds usual MICs)
Uninflamed meninges: 0-4 mcg/mL; serum concentration dependent
Inflamed meninges: 6-11 mcg/mL; serum concentration dependent
CSF:blood level ratio: Normal meninges: Nil; Inflamed meninges: 20% to 30%
Protein binding: ~50%

Half-life elimination: Biphasic: Terminal:
  Adults: 5-11 hours; significantly prolonged with renal impairment
  End-stage renal disease: 200-250 hours
Time to peak, serum: I.V.: Immediately after completion of infusion
Excretion: I.V.: Urine (80% to 90% as unchanged drug); Oral: Primarily feces

Dosage

Geriatric & Adult

Usual dosage range: Initial intravenous dosing should be based on actual body weight; subsequent dosing adjusted based on serum trough vancomycin concentrations.
  I.V.: 2000-3000 mg/day (or 30-60 mg/kg/day) in divided doses every 8-12 hours (Rybak, 2009); **Note:** Dose requires adjustment in renal impairment
  Oral: 500-2000 mg/day in divided doses every 6 hours

Indication-specific dosing:

Catheter-related infections: Antibiotic lock technique (Mermel, 2009): 2 mg/mL ± 10 units heparin/mL **or** 2.5 mg/mL ± 2500 **or** 5000 units heparin/mL **or** 5 mg/mL ± 5000 units heparin/mL (preferred regimen); instill into catheter port with a volume sufficient to fill the catheter (2-5 mL). **Note:** May use SWFI/NS or D_5W as diluents. Do not mix with any other solutions. Dwell times generally should not exceed 48 hours before renewal of lock solution. Remove lock solution prior to catheter use, then replace.

C. difficile -associated diarrhea (CDAD):
  Oral:
    Manufacturer recommendations: 125 mg 4 times/day for 10 days
    IDSA guideline recommendations: Severe infection: 125 mg every 6 hours for 10-14 days; Severe, complicated infection: 500 mg every 6 hours with or without concurrent I.V. metronidazole. May consider vancomycin retention enema (in patients with complete ileus) (Cohen, 2010).
  Rectal (unlabeled route): Retention enema (in patients with complete ileus): SHEA/IDSA guideline recommendations: Severe, complicated infection in patients with ileus: 500 mg every 6 hours (in 100 mL 0.9% sodium chloride) with oral vancomycin with or without concurrent I.V. metronidazole (Cohen, 2010)

Complicated infections in seriously-ill patients: I.V.: Loading dose: 25-30 mg/kg (based on actual body weight) may be used to rapidly achieve target concentration; then 15-20 mg/kg/dose every 8-12 hours (Rybak, 2009)

Enterocolitis *(S. aureus):* Oral: 500-2000 mg/day in 3-4 divided doses for 7-10 days (usual dose: 125-500 mg every 6 hours)

Meningitis:
  I.V.: 30-60 mg/kg/day in divided doses every 8-12 hours (Rybak, 2009) **or** 500-750 mg every 6 hours (with third-generation cephalosporin for PCN-resistant *Streptococcus pneumoniae*)
  Alternate regimen: *S. aureus* (methicillin-resistant) (unlabeled use; Liu, 2011): 15-20 mg/kg/dose every 8-12 hours for 2 weeks (some experts combine with rifampin
  Intrathecal, intraventricular (unlabeled route): 5-20 mg/day

Pneumonia: I.V.:
  Community-acquired pneumonia (CAP): S. aureus (methicillin-resistant): 45-60 mg/kg/day divided every 8-12 hours (maximum: 2000 mg/dose) for 7-21 days depending on severity (Liu, 2011)
  Healthcare-associated pneumonia (HAP): S. aureus (methicillin-resistant): 45-60 mg/kg/day divided every 8-12 hours (maximum: 2000 mg/dose) for 7-21 days depending on severity (American Thoracic Society [ATS], 2005; Liu, 2011; Rybak 2009)

Prophylaxis against infective endocarditis: I.V.:
  Dental, oral, or upper respiratory tract surgery: 1000 mg 1 hour before surgery. **Note:** AHA guidelines now recommend prophylaxis only in patients undergoing invasive procedures and in whom underlying cardiac conditions may predispose to a higher risk of adverse outcomes should infection occur
  GI/GU procedure: 1000 mg plus 1.5 mg/kg gentamicin 1 hour prior to surgery. **Note:** As of April 2007, routine prophylaxis no longer recommended by the AHA.

Susceptible (MIC ≤1 mcg/mL) gram-positive infections: I.V.: 15-20 mg/kg/dose (usual: 750-1500 mg) every 8-12 hours (Rybak, 2009). **Note:** If MIC ≥2 mcg/mL, alternative therapies are recommended.

Bacteremia (*S. aureus* [methicillin-resistant]) (unlabeled use; Liu, 2011): I.V.: 15-20 mg/kg/dose every 8-12 hours for 2-6 weeks depending on severity

Brain abscess, subdural empyema, spinal epidural abscess (*S. aureus* [methicillin-resistant]) (unlabeled use; Liu, 2011): I.V.: 15-20 mg/kg/dose every 8-12 hours for 4-6 weeks (some experts combine with rifampin)

Endocarditis:
  Native valve (*Enterococcus*, vancomycin MIC ≤4 mg/L) (unlabeled use; Gould, 2012): I.V.: 1000 mg every 12 hours for 4-6 weeks (combine with gentamicin for 4-6 weeks)

Native valve (*S. aureus* [methicillin-resistant]) (unlabeled use; Liu, 2011): I.V.: 15-20 mg/kg/dose every 8-12 hours for 6 weeks (European guidelines support the entire duration of therapy to be 4 weeks and in combination with rifampin [Gould, 2012])

Native or prosthetic valve (streptococcal [penicillin MIC >0.5 mg/L or patient intolerant to penicillin]) (unlabeled use; Gould, 2012): I.V.: 1000 mg every 12 hours for 4-6 weeks (combine with gentamicin for at least the first 2 weeks); **Note:** The longer duration of treatment (ie, 6 weeks) should be used for patients with prosthetic valve endocarditis.

Prosthetic valve (*Enterococcus*, vancomycin MIC ≤4 mg/L) (unlabeled use; Gould, 2012): I.V.: 1000 mg every 12 hours for 6 weeks (combine with gentamicin for 4-6 weeks)

Prosthetic valve (*S. aureus* [methicillin-resistant]) (unlabeled use; Liu, 2011): I.V.: 15-20 mg/kg/dose every 8-12 hours for at least 6 weeks (combine with rifampin for the entire duration of therapy and gentamicin for the first 2 weeks)

Endophthalmitis (unlabeled use): Intravitreal: Usual dose: 1 mg/0.1 mL NS instilled into vitreum; may repeat administration if necessary in 3-4 days, usually in combination with ceftazidime or an aminoglycoside. **Note:** Some clinicians have recommended using a lower dose of 0.2 mg/0.1 mL, based on concerns for retinotoxicity.

Osteomyelitis (*S. aureus* [methicillin-resistant]) (unlabeled use; Liu, 2011): I.V.: 15-20 mg/kg/dose every 8-12 hours for a minimum of 8 weeks (some experts combine with rifampin)

Septic arthritis (*S. aureus* [methicillin-resistant]) (unlabeled use; Liu, 2011): I.V.: 15-20 mg/kg/dose every 8-12 hours for 3-4 weeks

Septic thrombosis of cavernous or dural venous sinus (*S. aureus* [methicillin-resistant]) (unlabeled use; Liu, 2011): I.V.: 15-20 mg/kg/dose every 8-12 hours for 4-6 weeks (some experts combine with rifampin)

Skin and skin structure infections, complicated (*S. aureus* [methicillin-resistant]) (unlabeled use; Liu, 2011): I.V.: 15-20 mg/kg/dose every 8-12 hours for 7-14 days

Surgical prophylaxis (unlabeled use): I.V.: 1000 mg or 10-15 mg/kg over 60 minutes (longer infusion time if dose >1000 mg) (Bratzler, 2004)

The Society of Thoracic Surgeons recommends 1000-1500 mg or 15 mg/kg over 60 minutes with completion within 1 hour of skin incision. Although not well established, a second dose of 7.5 mg/kg may be considered during cardiopulmonary bypass (Engelman, 2007).

Renal Impairment Vancomycin levels should be monitored in patients with any renal impairment: I.V.:

Cl_{cr} >50 mL/minute: Start with 15-20 mg/kg/dose (usual: 750-1500 mg) every 8-12 hours

Cl_{cr} 20-49 mL/minute: Start with 15-20 mg/kg/dose (usual: 750-1500 mg) every 24 hours

Cl_{cr} <20 mL/minute: Will need longer intervals; determine by serum concentration monitoring

Note: In the critically-ill patient with renal insufficiency, the initial loading dose (25-30 mg/kg) should not be reduced. However, subsequent dosage adjustments should be made based on renal function and trough serum concentrations.

Poorly dialyzable by intermittent hemodialysis (0% to 5%); however, use of high-flux membranes and continuous renal replacement therapy (CRRT) increases vancomycin clearance, and generally requires replacement dosing.

Intermittent hemodialysis (IHD) (administer after hemodialysis on dialysis days): Following loading dose of 15-25 mg/kg, give either 500-1000 mg **or** 5-10 mg/kg after each dialysis session. (Heintz, 2009). **Note:** Dosing dependent on the assumption of 3 times/week, complete IHD sessions.

Redosing based on pre-HD concentrations:

<10 mg/L: Administer 1000 mg after HD

10-25 mg/L: Administer 500-750 mg after HD

>25 mg/L: Hold vancomycin

Redosing based on post-HD concentrations: <10-15 mg/L: Administer 500-1000 mg

Peritoneal dialysis (PD):

Administration via PD fluid: 15-30 mg/L (15-30 mcg/mL) of PD fluid

Systemic: Loading dose of 1000 mg, followed by 500-1000 mg every 48-72 hours with close monitoring of levels

Continuous renal replacement therapy (CRRT) (Heintz, 2009; Trotman, 2005): Drug clearance is highly dependent on the method of renal replacement, filter type, and flow rate. Appropriate dosing requires close monitoring of pharmacologic response, signs of adverse reactions due to drug accumulation, as well as drug concentrations in relation to target trough (if appropriate). The following are general recommendations only (based on dialysate flow/ultrafiltration rates of 1-2 L/hour and minimal residual renal function) and should not supersede clinical judgment:

CVVH: Loading dose of 15-25 mg/kg, followed by either 1000 mg every 48 hours **or** 10-15 mg/kg every 24-48 hours

CVVHD: Loading dose of 15-25 mg/kg, followed by either 1000 mg every 24 hours **or** 10-15 mg/kg every 24 hours

CVVHDF: Loading dose of 15-25 mg/kg, followed by either 1000 mg every 24 hours **or** 7.5-10 mg/kg every 12 hours

Note: Consider redosing patients receiving CRRT for vancomycin concentrations <10-15 mg/L.

Hepatic Impairment Degrees of hepatic dysfunction do not affect the pharmacokinetics of vancomycin (Marti, 1996).

Oral: No adjustment provided in the manufacturer's labeling.

Administration

Intravenous: Administer vancomycin with a final concentration not to exceed 5 mg/mL by I.V. intermittent infusion over at least 60 minutes (recommended infusion period of ≥30 minutes for every 500 mg administered).

If a maculopapular rash appears on the face, neck, trunk, and/or upper extremities (red man syndrome), slow the infusion rate to over 1½ to 2 hours and increase the dilution volume. Hypotension, shock, and cardiac arrest (rare) have also been reported with too rapid of infusion. Reactions are often treated with antihistamines and steroids.

Intrathecal (unlabeled route): Vancomycin is available as a powder for injection and may be diluted to 1-5 mg/mL concentration in preservative free 0.9% sodium chloride for intrathecal administration.

Intravitreal: May be administered by intravitreal injection (unlabeled use).

Oral: Vancomycin powder for injection may be reconstituted and used for oral administration (Cohen, 2010). Reconstituted powder for injection (not premixed solution) may be administered orally by diluting the reconstituted solution in 30 mL of water; common flavoring syrups may be added to improve taste. The unflavored, diluted solution may also be administered via nasogastric tube.

Rectal (unlabeled route): May be administered as a retention enema per rectum (Cohen, 2010)

Not for I.M. administration.

Extravasation treatment: Monitor I.V. site closely; extravasation will cause serious injury with possible necrosis and tissue sloughing. Rotate infusion site frequently.

Monitoring Parameters Periodic renal function tests, urinalysis, WBC; serum trough vancomycin concentrations in select patients (eg, aggressive dosing, unstable renal function, concurrent nephrotoxins, prolonged courses)

Suggested frequency of trough vancomycin concentration monitoring (Rybak, 2009):

Hemodynamically stable patients: Draw trough concentrations at least once-weekly.

Hemodynamically unstable patients: Draw trough concentrations more frequently or in some instances daily.

Prolonged courses (>3-5 days): Draw at least one steady-state trough concentration; repeat as clinically appropriate.

Note: Drawing >1 trough concentration prior to the fourth dose for short course (<3 days) or lower intensity dosing (target trough concentrations <15 mcg/mL) is not recommended.

Reference Range

Timing of serum samples: Draw trough just before next dose at steady-state conditions (approximately after the fourth dose). Drawing peak concentrations is no longer recommended.

Therapeutic levels: Trough: ≥10 mcg/mL. For pathogens with an MIC ≤1 mcg/mL, the minimum trough concentration should be 15 mcg/mL to meet target AUC/MIC of ≥400 (see "Note"). For complicated infections (eg, bacteremia, endocarditis, osteomyelitis, meningitis, and hospital-acquired pneumonia caused by *S. aureus*), trough concentrations of 15-20 mcg/mL are recommended to improve penetration and improve clinical outcomes (Liu, 2011; Rybak, 2009). The American Thoracic Society (ATS) guidelines for hospital-acquired pneumonia and the Infectious Disease Society of America (IDSA) meningitis guidelines also recommend trough concentrations of 15-20 mcg/mL.

Note: Although AUC/MIC is the preferred pharmacokinetic-pharmacodynamic parameter used to determine clinical effectiveness, trough serum concentrations may be used as a surrogate marker for AUC and are recommended as the most accurate and practical method of vancomycin monitoring (Liu, 2011; Rybak, 2009).

Toxic: >80 mcg/mL (SI: >54 micromole/L)

Pharmacotherapy Pearls Because of its long half-life, vancomycin should be dosed on an every 8- to 12-hour basis. Monitoring of trough serum concentrations is advisable in certain situations. "Red man syndrome", characterized by skin rash and hypotension, is not an allergic reaction but rather is associated with too rapid infusion of the drug. To alleviate or prevent the reaction, infuse vancomycin at a rate of ≥30 minutes for each 500 mg of drug being administered (eg, 1 g over ≥60 minutes; 1.5 g over ≥90 minutes.

Special Geriatric Considerations As a result of age-related changes in renal function and volume of distribution, accumulation and toxicity are a risk in the elderly with I.V. administration. Careful monitoring and dosing adjustment is necessary.

VANCOMYCIN

◀ **Dosage Forms** Excipient information presented when available (limited, particularly for generics); consult specific product labeling.
Capsule, oral: 125 mg, 250 mg
Vancocin®: 125 mg, 250 mg
Infusion, premixed iso-osmotic dextrose solution: 500 mg (100 mL); 750 mg (150 mL); 1 g (200 mL)
Injection, powder for reconstitution: 500 mg, 750 mg, 1 g, 5 g, 10 g

- ◆ **Vancomycin Hydrochloride** *see* Vancomycin *on page 1999*
- ◆ **Vandazole®** *see* MetroNIDAZOLE (Topical) *on page 1271*
- ◆ **Vanos®** *see* Fluocinonide *on page 804*
- ◆ **Vantin** *see* Cefpodoxime *on page 323*
- ◆ **Vaprisol®** *see* Conivaptan *on page 444*
- ◆ **VAQTA®** *see* Hepatitis A Vaccine *on page 921*

Vardenafil (var DEN a fil)

Medication Safety Issues
Sound-alike/look-alike issues:
Vardenafil may be confused with sildenafil, tadalafil
Levitra® may be confused with Kaletra®, Lexiva®
Brand Names: U.S. Levitra®; Staxyn™
Brand Names: Canada Levitra®; Staxyn™
Index Terms Vardenafil Hydrochloride
Generic Availability (U.S.) No
Pharmacologic Category Phosphodiesterase-5 Enzyme Inhibitor
Use Treatment of erectile dysfunction (ED)
Contraindications Hypersensitivity to vardenafil or any component of the formulation; concurrent (regular or intermittent) use of organic nitrates in any form (eg, nitroglycerin, isosorbide dinitrate)
Warnings/Precautions There is a degree of cardiac risk associated with sexual activity; therefore, physicians may wish to consider the patient's cardiovascular status prior to initiating any treatment for erectile dysfunction. Use caution in patients with anatomical deformation of the penis (angulation, cavernosal fibrosis, or Peyronie's disease) and in patients who have conditions which may predispose them to priapism (sickle cell anemia, multiple myeloma, leukemia). Instruct patients to seek immediate medical attention if erection persists >4 hours.

Use is not recommended in patients with hypotension (<90/50 mm Hg); uncontrolled hypertension (>170/100 mm Hg); unstable angina or angina during intercourse; life-threatening arrhythmias, stroke, or MI within the last 6 months; cardiac failure or coronary artery disease causing unstable angina. Safety and efficacy have not been studied in these patients. Use caution in patients with left ventricular outflow obstruction (eg, aortic stenosis). Use caution with alpha-blockers, effective CYP3A4 inhibitors, the elderly, or those with hepatic impairment (Child-Pugh class B); dosage adjustment is needed. Concurrent use with alpha-adrenergic antagonist therapy may cause symptomatic hypotension; patients should be hemodynamically stable prior to initiating tadalafil therapy at the lowest possible dose. Avoid or limit concurrent substantial alcohol consumption as this may increase the risk of symptomatic hypotension.

Rare cases of nonarteritic ischemic optic neuropathy (NAION) have been reported; risk may be increased with history of vision loss. Other risk factors for NAION include heart disease, diabetes, hypertension, smoking, age >50 years, or history of certain eye problems. Sudden decrease or loss of hearing has been reported rarely; hearing changes may be accompanied by tinnitus and dizziness.

Safety and efficacy have not been studied in patients with the following conditions, therefore, use in these patients is not recommended at this time: Congenital QT prolongation, patients taking medications known to prolong the QT interval (avoid use in patients taking Class Ia or III antiarrhythmics); severe hepatic impairment (Child-Pugh class C); end-stage renal disease requiring dialysis; retinitis pigmentosa or other degenerative retinal disorders. The safety and efficacy of vardenafil with other treatments for erectile dysfunction have not been studied and are not recommended as combination therapy. Concomitant use with all forms of nitrates is contraindicated. If nitrate administration is medically necessary, it is not known when nitrates can be safely administered following the use of vardenafil; the ACC/AHA 2007 guidelines support administration of nitrates only if 24 hours have elapsed. Potential underlying causes of erectile dysfunction should be evaluated prior to treatment. Some products may contain phylalanine. Some products may contain sorbitol; do not use in patients with fructose intolerance.

Adverse Reactions (Reflective of adult population; not specific for elderly)

>10%:

Cardiovascular: Flushing (8% to 11%)

Central nervous system: Headache (14% to 15%)

2% to 10%:

Central nervous system: Dizziness (2%)

Gastrointestinal: Dyspepsia (3% to 4%), nausea (2%)

Neuromuscular & skeletal: Back pain (2%), CPK increased (2%)

Respiratory: Rhinitis (9%), nasal congestion (3%), sinusitis (3%)

Miscellaneous: Flu-like syndrome (3%)

Drug Interactions

Metabolism/Transport Effects Substrate of CYP3A4 (major); **Note:** Assignment of Major/ Minor substrate status based on clinically relevant drug interaction potential

Avoid Concomitant Use

Avoid concomitant use of Vardenafil with any of the following: Alprostadil; Amyl Nitrite; Phosphodiesterase 5 Inhibitors; Vasodilators (Organic Nitrates)

Increased Effect/Toxicity

Vardenafil may increase the levels/effects of: Alpha1-Blockers; Alprostadil; Amyl Nitrite; Antihypertensives; Bosentan; Highest Risk QTc-Prolonging Agents; Moderate Risk QTc-Prolonging Agents; Phosphodiesterase 5 Inhibitors; Vasodilators (Organic Nitrates)

The levels/effects of Vardenafil may be increased by: Alcohol (Ethyl); Boceprevir; Clari-thromycin; CYP3A4 Inhibitors (Moderate); CYP3A4 Inhibitors (Strong); Erythromycin; Flu-conazole; Itraconazole; Ivacaftor; Ketoconazole (Systemic); Mifepristone; Posaconazole; Protease Inhibitors; Sapropterin; Telaprevir; Voriconazole

Decreased Effect

The levels/effects of Vardenafil may be decreased by: Bosentan; Etravirine; Tocilizumab

Ethanol/Nutrition/Herb Interactions Ethanol: Substantial consumption of ethanol may increase the risk of hypotension and orthostasis. Lower ethanol consumption has not been associated with significant changes in blood pressure or increase in orthostatic symptoms. Management: Avoid or limit ethanol consumption.

Food: High-fat meals decrease maximum serum concentration 18% to 50%. Serum concentrations/toxicity may be increased with grapefruit juice. Management: Do not take with a high-fat meal. Avoid grapefruit juice.

Stability Store at controlled room temperature of 25°C (77°F); excursions permitted to 15°C to 25°C (59°F to 86°F). Keep oral disintegrating tablets sealed in blisterpack until ready to use.

Mechanism of Action Does not directly cause penile erections, but affects the response to sexual stimulation. The physiologic mechanism of erection of the penis involves release of nitric oxide (NO) in the corpus cavernosum during sexual stimulation. NO then activates the enzyme guanylate cyclase, which results in increased levels of cyclic guanosine mono-phosphate (cGMP), producing smooth muscle relaxation and inflow of blood to the corpus cavernosum. Vardenafil enhances the effect of NO by inhibiting phosphodiesterase type 5 (PDE-5), which is responsible for degradation of cGMP in the corpus cavernosum; when sexual stimulation causes local release of NO, inhibition of PDE-5 by vardenafil causes increased levels of cGMP in the corpus cavernosum, resulting in smooth muscle relaxation and inflow of blood to the corpus cavernosum; at recommended doses, it has no effect in the absence of sexual stimulation.

Pharmacodynamics/Kinetics

Onset of action: ~60 minutes

Absorption: Rapid

Distribution: V_d: 208 L

Protein binding: ~95% (parent drug and metabolite)

Metabolism: Hepatic via CYP3A4 (major), CYP2C and 3A5 (minor); forms metabolite (active)

Bioavailability: ~15%

Film-coated tablet: Elderly (≥65 years): AUC increased by 52%; Hepatic impairment (moderate, Child-Pugh class B): AUC increased by 160%

Oral disintegrating tablet: Elderly (≥65 years): AUC increased by 21% more compared to film-coated tablet. When administered with water, AUC decreases by 29%.

Half-life elimination: Terminal: Vardenafil and metabolite: 3-6 hours

Time to peak, plasma: 0.5-2 hours

Excretion: Feces (~91% to 95% as metabolites); urine (~2% to 6%)

Dosage

Geriatric Erectile dysfunction: Elderly ≥65 years: Oral: Initial: 5 mg 60 minutes prior to sexual activity; to be given as one single dose and not given more than once daily.

Adult Note: Oral disintegrating tablets should not be used interchangeably with film-coated tablets; patients requiring a dose other than 10 mg should use the film-coated tablets.

Erectile dysfunction: Oral:
Film-coated tablet (Levitra®): 10 mg 60 minutes prior to sexual activity; dosing range: 5-20 mg; to be given as one single dose and not given more than once daily
Oral disintegrating tablet (Staxyn™): 10 mg 60 minutes prior to sexual activity; maximum: 10 mg/day

Dosing adjustment with concomitant medications:
Alpha-blocker (dose should be stable at time of vardenafil initiation):
Film-coated tablet (Levitra®): Initial vardenafil dose: 5 mg/24 hours; if an alpha-blocker is added to vardenafil therapy, it should be initiated at the smallest possible dose and titrated carefully.
Oral disintegrating tablet (Staxyn™): Do not use to initiate therapy. Initial therapy should be with film-coated tablets at lower doses. Patients who have previously used film-coated tablets may be switched to oral disintegrating tablets as recommended by healthcare provider.
Film-coated tablet (Levitra®):
Atazanavir: Maximum vardenafil dose: 2.5 mg/24 hours
Clarithromycin: Maximum vardenafil dose: 2.5 mg/24 hours
Darunavir: Maximum vardenafil dose: 2.5 mg/72 hours
Erythromycin: Maximum vardenafil dose: 5 mg/24 hours
Fosamprenavir: Maximum vardenafil dose: 2.5 mg/24 hours
Fosamprenavir/ritonavir: Maximum vardenafil dose: 2.5 mg/72 hours
Indinavir: Maximum vardenafil dose: 2.5 mg/24 hours
Itraconazole:
  200 mg/day: Maximum vardenafil dose: 5 mg/24 hours
  400 mg/day: Maximum vardenafil dose: 2.5 mg/24 hours
Ketoconazole:
  200 mg/day: Maximum vardenafil dose: 5 mg/24 hours
  400 mg/day: Maximum vardenafil dose: 2.5 mg/24 hours
Lopinavir/ritonavir: Maximum vardenafil dose: 2.5 mg/72 hours
Nelfinavir: Maximum vardenafil dose: 2.5 mg/24 hours
Ritonavir: Maximum vardenafil dose: 2.5 mg/72 hours
Saquinavir: Maximum vardenafil dose: 2.5 mg/24 hours
Tipranavir: Maximum vardenafil dose: 2.5 mg/72 hours
Oral disintegrating tablet (Staxyn™): Concurrent use not recommended with potent or moderate CYP3A4 inhibitors (atazanavir, clarithromycin, erythromycin, indinavir, itraconazole, ketoconazole, ritonavir, saquinavir)
Renal Impairment Dose adjustment not needed for mild, moderate, or severe impairment; use not recommended in patients on hemodialysis.
Hepatic Impairment
Child-Pugh class A: No adjustment required
Child-Pugh class B:
Film-coated tablet (Levitra®): Initial: 5 mg 60 minutes prior to sexual activity (maximum dose: 10 mg); to be given as one single dose and not given more than once daily
Oral disintegrating tablet (Staxyn™): Use not recommended
Child-Pugh class C: Has not been studied; use is not recommended by the manufacturer
Administration Administer 60 minutes prior to sexual activity.
Monitoring Parameters Monitor for response, adverse reactions, blood pressure, and heart rate.
Special Geriatric Considerations In adults ≥65 years of age, vardenafil plasma concentrations were higher than younger males (mean C_{max} was 34% higher), therefore, initial dose should be lower than the usual adult dose. Since the elderly often have concomitant diseases, many of which may be contraindicated with the use of vardenafil, a thorough knowledge of disease and medications must be accessed.
Dosage Forms Excipient information presented when available (limited, particularly for generics); consult specific product labeling.
Tablet, oral:
Levitra®: 2.5 mg, 5 mg, 10 mg, 20 mg
Tablet, orally disintegrating, oral:
Staxyn™: 10 mg [contains phenylalanine 1.01 mg/tablet; peppermint flavor]

◆ **Vardenafil Hydrochloride** *see* Vardenafil *on page 2004*

Varenicline (var e NI kleen)

Brand Names: U.S. Chantix®
Brand Names: Canada Champix®
Index Terms Varenicline Tartrate

Generic Availability (U.S.) No

Pharmacologic Category Partial Nicotine Agonist; Smoking Cessation Aid

Use Treatment to aid in smoking cessation

Medication Guide Available Yes

Contraindications Known history of serious hypersensitivity or skin reactions to varenicline

Warnings/Precautions [U.S. Boxed Warning]: Serious neuropsychiatric events (including depression, suicidal thoughts, and suicide) have been reported with use; some cases may have been complicated by symptoms of nicotine withdrawal following smoking cessation. Smoking cessation (with or without treatment) is associated with nicotine withdrawal symptoms and the exacerbation of underlying psychiatric illness; however, some of the behavioral disturbances were reported in treated patients who continued to smoke. Neuropsychiatric symptoms (eg, mood disturbances, psychosis, hostility) have occurred in patients with and without pre-existing psychiatric disease; many cases resolved following therapy discontinuation although in some cases, symptoms persisted. Ethanol consumption may increase the risk of psychiatric adverse events. Monitor all patients for behavioral changes and psychiatric symptoms (eg, agitation, depression, suicidal behavior, suicidal ideation); inform patients to discontinue treatment and contact their healthcare provider immediately if they experience any behavioral and/or mood changes. **[U.S. Boxed Warning]: Before prescribing, the risks of serious neuropsychiatric events must be weighed against the immediate and long term benefits of smoking abstinence for each patient.**

Hypersensitivity reactions (including angioedema) and rare cases of serious skin reactions (including Stevens-Johnson syndrome and erythema multiforme) have been reported. Patients should be instructed to discontinue use and contact healthcare provider if signs/symptoms occur. Treatment may increase risk of cardiovascular events (eg, angina pectoris, nonfatal MI, nonfatal stroke, need for coronary revascularization, new diagnosis of or treatment for PVD). Varenicline was not studied in patients with unstable cardiovascular disease or in patients experiencing recent events (<2 months) prior to treatment. Dose-dependent nausea may occur; both transient and persistent nausea has been reported. Dosage reduction may be considered for intolerable nausea. May cause sedation, which may impair physical or mental abilities; patients must be cautioned about performing tasks which require mental alertness (eg, operating machinery or driving).

Use caution in renal dysfunction; dosage adjustment required. Safety and efficacy of varenicline with other smoking cessation therapies have not been established; increased adverse events when used concurrently with nicotine replacement therapy.

Adverse Reactions (Reflective of adult population; not specific for elderly)

>10%:

  Central nervous system: Insomnia (18% to 19%), headache (15% to 19%), abnormal dreams (9% to 13%)

  Gastrointestinal: Nausea (16% to 40%; dose related)

1% to 10%:

  Central nervous system: Malaise (≤7%), sleep disorder (≤5%), somnolence (3%), nightmares (1% to 2%), lethargy (1% to 2%)

  Dermatologic: Rash (≤3%)

  Gastrointestinal: Flatulence (6% to 9%), constipation (5% to 8%), abnormal taste (5% to 8%), abdominal pain (≤7%), xerostomia (≤6%), dyspepsia (5%), vomiting (≤5%), appetite increased (3% to 4%), anorexia (≤2%), gastroesophageal reflux (1%)

  Respiratory: Upper respiratory tract disorder (5% to 7%), dyspnea (≤2%), rhinorrhea (≤1%)

Drug Interactions

Metabolism/Transport Effects None known.

Avoid Concomitant Use There are no known interactions where it is recommended to avoid concomitant use.

Increased Effect/Toxicity

  The levels/effects of Varenicline may be increased by: Alcohol (Ethyl); H2-Antagonists; Quinolone Antibiotics; Trimethoprim

Decreased Effect There are no known significant interactions involving a decrease in effect.

Ethanol/Nutrition/Herb Interactions Ethanol: May increase the risk of psychiatric adverse events. Caution patients about the potential effects of ethanol consumption during therapy.

Stability Store at 25°C (77°F); excursions permitted to 15°C to 30°C (59°F to 86°F).

Mechanism of Action Partial neuronal α_4 β_2 nicotinic receptor agonist; prevents nicotine stimulation of mesolimbic dopamine system associated with nicotine addiction. Also binds to $5HT_3$ receptor (significance not determined) with moderate affinity. Varenicline stimulates dopamine activity but to a much smaller degree than nicotine does, resulting in decreased craving and withdrawal symptoms.

Pharmacodynamics/Kinetics

Absorption: Well absorbed; unaffected by food

Protein binding: ≤20%

Metabolism: Minimal (<10% of clearance is through metabolism)

Half-life elimination: ~24 hours

Time to peak, plasma: ~3-4 hours

Excretion: Urine (92% as unchanged drug)

Dosage

Geriatric & Adult Smoking cessation: Oral:

Initial:

Days 1-3: 0.5 mg once daily

Days 4-7: 0.5 mg twice daily

Maintenance (≥Day 8):

U.S. labeling: 1 mg twice daily for 11 weeks

Canadian labeling: 0.5-1 mg twice daily for 11 weeks

Note: Start 1 week before target quit date. Alternatively, patients may consider setting a quit date up to 35 days after initiation of varenicline (some data suggest that an extended pretreatment regimen may result in higher abstinence rates [Hajek, 2011]). If patient successfully quits smoking at the end of the 12 weeks, may continue for another 12 weeks to help maintain success. If not successful in first 12 weeks, then stop medication and reassess factors contributing to failure.

Renal Impairment

Cl_{cr} ≥30 mL/minute: No adjustment required

Cl_{cr} <30 mL/minute: Initiate: 0.5 mg once daily; maximum dose: 0.5 mg twice daily

Hemodialysis: Maximum dose: 0.5 mg once daily

Hepatic Impairment Dosage adjustment not required

Administration Administer with food and a full glass of water.

Monitoring Parameters Monitor for behavioral changes and psychiatric symptoms (eg, agitation, depression, suicidal behavior, suicidal ideation)

Pharmacotherapy Pearls In all studies, patients received an educational booklet on smoking cessation and received up to 10 minutes of counseling at each weekly visit. Dosing started 1 week before target quit date. Successful cessation of smoking may alter pharmacokinetic properties of other medications (eg, theophylline, warfarin, insulin).

Special Geriatric Considerations Dosage adjustment for renal function may be necessary. Although studies to date do not demonstrate any significant pharmacokinetic differences between elderly (65-75 years of age) and younger adults.

Dosage Forms Excipient information presented when available (limited, particularly for generics); consult specific product labeling.

Combination package, oral [dose-pack]:

Chantix®: Tablet: 0.5 mg (11s) [white tablets] and Tablet: 1 mg (42s) [light blue tablets]

Tablet, oral:

Chantix®: 0.5 mg, 1 mg

◆ **Varenicline Tartrate** see Varenicline on page 2006

◆ **Varicella-Zoster (VZV) Vaccine (Zoster)** see Zoster Vaccine on page 2071

◆ **Vaseretic®** see Enalapril and Hydrochlorothiazide on page 634

◆ **Vasodilan** see Isoxsuprine on page 1054

◆ **Vasolex™** see Trypsin, Balsam Peru, and Castor Oil on page 1979

Vasopressin (vay soe PRES in)

Medication Safety Issues

High alert medication:

The Institute for Safe Medication Practices (ISMP) includes this medication (I.V. or intraosseous administration) among its list of drugs which have a heightened risk of causing significant patient harm when used in error.

Administration issues:

Use care when prescribing and/or administering vasopressin solutions. Close attention should be given to concentration of solution, route of administration, dose, and rate of administration (units/minute, units/kg/minute, units/kg/hour).

Brand Names: U.S. Pitressin®

Brand Names: Canada Pressyn®; Pressyn® AR

Index Terms 8-Arginine Vasopressin; ADH; Antidiuretic Hormone; AVP

Generic Availability (U.S.) Yes

Pharmacologic Category Antidiuretic Hormone Analog; Hormone, Posterior Pituitary

Use Treatment of central diabetes insipidus; differential diagnosis of diabetes insipidus

Unlabeled Use ACLS guidelines: Pulseless arrest (ventricular tachycardia [VT]/ventricular fibrillation [VF], asystole/pulseless electrical activity [PEA]); cardiac arrest secondary to anaphylaxis (unresponsive to epinephrine)

Adjunct in the treatment of GI hemorrhage and esophageal varices; adjunct in the treatment of vasodilatory shock (septic shock); donor management in brain-dead patients (hormone replacement therapy)

Contraindications Hypersensitivity to vasopressin or any component of the formulation

Warnings/Precautions Use with caution in patients with seizure disorders, migraine, asthma, vascular disease, renal disease, cardiac disease; chronic nephritis with nitrogen retention, goiter with cardiac complications, or arteriosclerosis. I.V. infiltration may lead to severe vasoconstriction and localized tissue necrosis, gangrene of extremities, tongue, and ischemic colitis. May cause water intoxication; early signs include drowsiness, listlessness, and headache, these should be recognized to prevent coma and seizures. Elderly patients should be cautioned not to increase their fluid intake beyond that sufficient to satisfy their thirst in order to avoid water intoxication and hyponatremia; under experimental conditions, the elderly have shown to have a decreased responsiveness to vasopressin with respect to its effects on water homeostasis.

Adverse Reactions (Reflective of adult population; not specific for elderly) Frequency not defined.

Cardiovascular: Arrhythmia, asystole (>0.04 units/minute), blood pressure increased, cardiac output decreased (>0.04 units/minute), chest pain, MI, vasoconstriction (with higher doses), venous thrombosis

Central nervous system: Pounding in the head, fever, vertigo

Dermatologic: Ischemic skin lesions, circumoral pallor, urticaria

Gastrointestinal: Abdominal cramps, flatulence, mesenteric ischemia, nausea, vomiting

Genitourinary: Uterine contraction

Neuromuscular & skeletal: Tremor

Respiratory: Bronchial constriction

Miscellaneous: Diaphoresis

Drug Interactions

Metabolism/Transport Effects None known.

Avoid Concomitant Use There are no known interactions where it is recommended to avoid concomitant use.

Increased Effect/Toxicity There are no known significant interactions involving an increase in effect.

Decreased Effect There are no known significant interactions involving a decrease in effect.

Ethanol/Nutrition/Herb Interactions Ethanol: Avoid ethanol (due to effects on ADH).

Stability Store injection at room temperature; do not freeze. Protect from heat. Use only clear solutions.

Mechanism of Action Increases cyclic adenosine monophosphate (cAMP) which increases water permeability at the renal tubule resulting in decreased urine volume and increased osmolality; causes peristalsis by directly stimulating the smooth muscle in the GI tract; direct vasoconstrictor without inotropic or chronotropic effects

Pharmacodynamics/Kinetics

Onset of action: Nasal: 1 hour

Duration: Nasal: 3-8 hours; I.M., SubQ: 2-8 hours

Metabolism: Nasal/Parenteral: Hepatic, renal

Half-life elimination: Nasal: 15 minutes; Parenteral: 10-20 minutes

Excretion: Nasal: Urine; SubQ: Urine (5% as unchanged drug) after 4 hours

Dosage

Geriatric & Adult

Central diabetes insipidus: Note: Dosage is highly variable; titrated based on serum and urine sodium and osmolality in addition to fluid balance and urine output. Use of vasopressin is impractical for chronic therapy.

I.M., SubQ: 5-10 units 2-4 times/day as needed

Continuous I.V. infusion (unlabeled route): Continuous infusion has not been formally evaluated in the post-neurosurgical adult. However, some convert I.M./SubQ requirement to an hourly continuous I.V. infusion rate.

Central diabetes insipidus, post-traumatic (unlabeled use): *I.V.:* Initial: 2.5 units/hour; titrate to adequately reduce urine output (Levitt, 1984)

Donor management in brain-dead patients (hormone replacement therapy) (unlabeled use): *I.V.:* Initial: 1 unit bolus followed by 0.5-4 units/hour (Rosendale, 2003; UNOS Critical Pathway, 2002)

Variceal hemorrhage (unlabeled use): *Continuous I.V. infusion:* Dilute in NS or D$_5$W to 0.1-1 unit/mL. **Note:** Other therapies may be preferred.

◀ [AASLD guidelines, 2007]: *Continuous I.V. infusion:* Initial: 0.2-0.4 units/minute, may titrate dose as needed to a maximum dose of 0.8 units/minute; maximum duration: 24 hours at highest effective dose continuously (to reduce incidence of adverse effects). Patient should also receive I.V. nitroglycerin concurrently to prevent myocardial ischemic complications. Monitor closely for signs/symptoms of ischemia (myocardial, peripheral, bowel).

Pulseless arrest (unlabeled use) [ACLS, 2010]: I.V., I.O.: 40 units; may give 1 dose to replace first or second dose of epinephrine. I.V./I.O. drug administration is preferred, but if no access, may give endotracheally. ACLS guidelines do not recommend a specific endotracheal dose; however, may be given endotracheally using the same I.V. dose (ACLS, 2010; Wenzel, 1997).

Vasodilatory shock/septic shock (unlabeled use): *I.V.:* 0.01-0.03 units/minute for the treatment of septic shock (Russell, 2008). **Note:** Recommended as a second-line vasopressor in addition to norepinephrine (Dellinger, 2008). Doses >0.04 units/minute may have more cardiovascular side effects. Most case reports have used 0.04 units/minute continuous infusion as a fixed dose. To prevent subsequent hypotension after withdrawal of vasopressors, vasopressin should be slowly tapered (eg, titrated down by 0.01 units/minute every 30 minutes) **after** the catecholamine(s) are discontinued until no longer required (Bauer, 2010).

Hepatic Impairment Some patients respond to much lower doses with cirrhosis.

Administration

I.V.: May administer as I.V. push over seconds (ACLS) or as a continuous I.V. infusion; when administered as a continuous I.V. infusion for vasodilatory shock, the use of a central venous catheter is recommended. Use extreme caution to avoid extravasation because of risk of necrosis and gangrene. In treatment of varices, infusions are often supplemented with nitroglycerin infusions to minimize cardiac effects.

Intranasal (topical administration on nasal mucosa): Administer injectable vasopressin on cotton plugs, as nasal spray, or by dropper. Should not be inhaled.

Endotracheal: If no I.V./I.O. access may give endotracheally. ACLS guidelines do not recommend a specific endotracheal dose; however, may be given endotracheally using the same I.V. dose (ACLS, 2010; Wenzel, 1997). Mix with 5-10 mL of water or normal saline, and administer down the endotracheal tube.

Monitoring Parameters Serum and urine sodium, urine specific gravity, urine and serum osmolality; urine output, fluid input and output, blood pressure, heart rate

Pharmacotherapy Pearls Vasopressin increases factor VIII levels and may be useful in hemophiliacs.

Special Geriatric Considerations Elderly patients should be cautioned not to increase their fluid intake beyond that sufficient to satisfy their thirst in order to avoid water intoxication and hyponatremia. Under experimental conditions, the elderly have shown to have a decreased responsiveness to vasopressin with respect to its effects on water homeostasis.

Dosage Forms Excipient information presented when available (limited, particularly for generics); consult specific product labeling.

Injection, solution: 20 units/mL (0.5 mL, 1 mL, 10 mL)

Pitressin®: 20 units/mL (1 mL)

◆ **Vasotec®** *see* Enalapril *on page 631*
◆ **Vectical®** *see* Calcitriol *on page 256*
◆ **VEGF Trap** *see* Aflibercept (Ophthalmic) *on page 48*
◆ **VEGF Trap-Eye** *see* Aflibercept (Ophthalmic) *on page 48*
◆ **Veltin™** *see* Clindamycin and Tretinoin *on page 403*

Venlafaxine (ven la FAX een)

Related Information

Antidepressant Agents *on page 2097*

Medication Safety Issues

Sound-alike/look-alike issues:

Effexor® may be confused with Effexor XR®

BEERS Criteria medication:

This drug may be potentially inappropriate for use in geriatric patients (Quality of evidence - moderate; Strength of recommendation - strong).

Brand Names: U.S. Effexor XR®; Effexor®

Brand Names: Canada CO Venlafaxine XR; Effexor XR®; GD-Venlafaxine XR; Mylan-Venlafaxine XR; PMS-Venlafaxine XR; Ran-Venlafaxine XR; ratio-Venlafaxine XR; Riva-Venlafaxine XR; Sandoz-Venlafaxine XR; Teva-Venlafaxine XR; Venlafaxine XR

Generic Availability (U.S.) Yes

Pharmacologic Category Antidepressant, Serotonin/Norepinephrine Reuptake Inhibitor

Use Treatment of major depressive disorder, generalized anxiety disorder (GAD), social anxiety disorder (social phobia), panic disorder

Unlabeled Use Obsessive-compulsive disorder (OCD); hot flashes; neuropathic pain (including diabetic neuropathy); attention-deficit/hyperactivity disorder (ADHD); post-traumatic stress disorder (PTSD); migraine prophylaxis

Medication Guide Available Yes

Contraindications Hypersensitivity to venlafaxine or any component of the formulation; use of MAO inhibitors within 14 days; should not initiate MAO inhibitor within 7 days of discontinuing venlafaxine

Warnings/Precautions [U.S. Boxed Warning]: Antidepressants increase the risk of suicidal thinking and behavior in children, adolescents, and young adults (18-24 years of age) with major depressive disorder (MDD) and other psychiatric disorders; consider risk prior to prescribing. Short-term studies did not show an increased risk in patients >24 years of age and showed a decreased risk in patients ≥65 years. Closely monitor for clinical worsening, suicidality, or unusual changes in behavior; the patient's family or caregiver should be instructed to closely observe the patient and communicate condition with healthcare provider. Reduced growth rate has been observed with venlafaxine therapy in children. A medication guide should be dispensed with each prescription.

The possibility of a suicide attempt is inherent in major depression and may persist until remission occurs. Monitor for worsening of depression or suicidality, especially during initiation of therapy (generally first 1-2 months) or with dose increases or decreases. Use caution in high-risk patients. Worsening depression and severe abrupt suicidality that are not part of the presenting symptoms may require discontinuation or modification of drug therapy. The patient's family or caregiver should be alerted to monitor patients for the emergence of suicidality and associated behaviors (such as agitation, irritability, hostility, impulsivity, and hypomania) and call healthcare provider.

May worsen psychosis in some patients or precipitate a shift to mania or hypomania in patients with bipolar disorder. Patients presenting with depressive symptoms should be screened for bipolar disorder. Monotherapy in patients with bipolar disorder should be avoided. **Venlafaxine is not FDA approved for the treatment of bipolar depression.**

Serotonin syndrome and neuroleptic malignant syndrome (NMS)-like reactions have occurred with serotonin/norepinephrine reuptake inhibitors (SNRIs) and selective serotonin reuptake inhibitors (SSRIs) when used alone, and particularly when used in combination with serotonergic agents (eg, triptans) or antidopaminergic agents (eg, antipsychotics). Concurrent use with MAO inhibitors is contraindicated. May cause sustained increase in blood pressure or tachycardia; dose related and increases are generally modest (12-15 mm Hg diastolic). Control pre-existing hypertension prior to initiation of venlafaxine. Use caution in patients with recent history of MI, unstable heart disease, or hyperthyroidism; may cause increase in anxiety, nervousness, insomnia; may cause weight loss (use with caution in patients where weight loss is undesirable); may cause increases in serum cholesterol. Use caution with hepatic or renal impairment; dosage adjustments recommended. May cause hyponatremia/SIADH (elderly at increased risk); volume depletion (diuretics may increase risk).

May impair platelet aggregation resulting in increased risk of bleeding events, particularly if used concomitantly with aspirin or NSAIDs. Bleeding related to SSRI or SNRI use has been reported to range from relatively minor bruising and epistaxis to life-threatening hemorrhage. Interstitial lung disease and eosinophilic pneumonia have been rarely reported; may present as progressive dyspnea, cough, and/or chest pain. Prompt evaluation and possible discontinuation of therapy may be necessary. Venlafaxine may increase the risks associated with electroconvulsive therapy. Use cautiously in patients with a history of seizures. The risks of cognitive or motor impairment, as well as the potential for anticholinergic effects are very low. May cause or exacerbate sexual dysfunction.

Use caution in elderly patients; may cause or exacerbate syndrome of inappropriate antidiuretic hormone secretion or hyponatremia; monitor sodium closely with initiation or dosage adjustments in older adults (Beers Criteria).

Abrupt discontinuation or dosage reduction after extended (≥6 weeks) therapy may lead to agitation, dysphoria, nervousness, anxiety, and other symptoms. When discontinuing therapy, dosage should be tapered gradually over at least a 2-week period. If intolerable symptoms occur following a decrease in dosage or upon discontinuation of therapy, then resuming the previous dose with a more gradual taper should be considered. Use caution in patients with increased intraocular pressure or at risk of acute narrow-angle glaucoma.

◀ **Adverse Reactions (Reflective of adult population; not specific for elderly) Note:**
Actual frequency may be dependent upon formulation and/or indication

>10%:

Central nervous system: Headache (25% to 38%), somnolence (12% to 26%), dizziness (11% to 24%), insomnia (15% to 24%), nervousness (6% to 21%), anxiety (2% to 11%),

Gastrointestinal: Nausea (21% to 58%), xerostomia (12% to 22%), anorexia (8% to 17%), constipation (8% to 15%)

Genitourinary: Abnormal ejaculation/orgasm (2% to 19%)

Neuromuscular & skeletal: Weakness (8% to 19%)

Miscellaneous: Diaphoresis (7% to 19%)

1% to 10%:

Cardiovascular: Vasodilation (2% to 6%), hypertension (dose related; 3% in patients receiving <100 mg/day, up to 13% in patients receiving >300 mg/day), palpitation (3%), tachycardia (2%), chest pain (2%), orthostatic hypotension (1%), edema

Central nervous system: Yawning (3% to 8%), abnormal dreams (3% to 7%), chills (2% to 7%), agitation (2% to 5%), confusion (2%), abnormal thinking (2%), depersonalization (1%), depression (1% to 3%), fever, migraine, amnesia, hypoesthesia, vertigo

Dermatologic: Rash (3%), pruritus (1%), bruising

Endocrine & metabolic: Libido decreased (2% to 8%), hypercholesterolemia (5%), triglycerides increased

Gastrointestinal: Abdominal pain (8%), diarrhea (8%), vomiting (3% to 8%), dyspepsia (5% to 7%), weight loss (1% to 6%), flatulence (3% to 4%), taste perversion (2%), appetite increased, belching, weight gain

Genitourinary: Impotence (4% to 6%), urinary frequency (3%), urination impaired (2%), urinary retention (1%), metrorrhagia, prostatic disorder, vaginitis

Neuromuscular & skeletal: Tremor (1% to 10%), hypertonia (3%), paresthesia (2% to 3%), twitching (1% to 3%), arthralgia, neck pain, trismus

Ocular: Accommodation abnormal (6% to 9%), abnormal or blurred vision (4% to 6%), mydriasis (2%)

Otic: Tinnitus (2%)

Renal: Albuminuria

Respiratory: Pharyngitis (7%), sinusitis (2%), bronchitis, cough increased, dyspnea

Miscellaneous: Infection (6%), flu-like syndrome (2%), trauma (2%)

Drug Interactions

Metabolism/Transport Effects Substrate of CYP2C19 (minor), CYP2C9 (minor), CYP2D6 (major), CYP3A4 (major); **Note:** Assignment of Major/Minor substrate status based on clinically relevant drug interaction potential; **Inhibits** CYP2B6 (weak), CYP2D6 (weak), CYP3A4 (weak)

Avoid Concomitant Use

Avoid concomitant use of Venlafaxine with any of the following: Conivaptan; Iobenguane I 123; MAO Inhibitors; Methylene Blue

Increased Effect/Toxicity

Venlafaxine may increase the levels/effects of: Alpha-/Beta-Agonists; Aspirin; Highest Risk QTc-Prolonging Agents; Methylene Blue; Metoclopramide; Moderate Risk QTc-Prolonging Agents; NSAID (Nonselective); Serotonin Modulators; TraZODone; Vitamin K Antagonists

The levels/effects of Venlafaxine may be increased by: Abiraterone Acetate; Alcohol (Ethyl); Antipsychotics; Conivaptan; CYP2D6 Inhibitors (Moderate); CYP2D6 Inhibitors (Strong); CYP3A4 Inhibitors (Moderate); CYP3A4 Inhibitors (Strong); Darunavir; Ivacaftor; Linezolid; MAO Inhibitors; Metoclopramide; Mifepristone; Propafenone; Voriconazole

Decreased Effect

Venlafaxine may decrease the levels/effects of: Alpha2-Agonists; Indinavir; Iobenguane I 123; Ioflupane I 123

The levels/effects of Venlafaxine may be decreased by: CYP3A4 Inducers (Strong); Deferasirox; Peginterferon Alfa-2b; Tocilizumab

Ethanol/Nutrition/Herb Interactions

Ethanol: May increase CNS depression; monitor for increased effects with coadministration. Caution patients about effects.

Herb/Nutraceutical: Avoid valerian, St John's wort, SAMe, kava kava, tryptophan (may increase risk of serotonin syndrome and/or excessive sedation).

Stability Store at controlled room temperature of 20°C to 25°C (68°F to 77°F).

Mechanism of Action Venlafaxine and its active metabolite, O-desmethylvenlafaxine (ODV), are potent inhibitors of neuronal serotonin and norepinephrine reuptake and weak inhibitors of dopamine reuptake. Venlafaxine and ODV have no significant activity for muscarinic cholinergic, H_1-histaminergic, or alpha$_2$-adrenergic receptors. Venlafaxine and ODV do not possess MAO-inhibitory activity.

Pharmacodynamics/Kinetics

Absorption: Oral: ≥92%; food has no significant effect on absorption or formation of active metabolite

Distribution: V_{dss}: Venlafaxine 7.5 ± 3.7 L/kg, ODV 5.7 ± 1.8 L/Kg

Protein binding: Venlafaxine 27% ± 2%, ODV 30% ± 12%

Metabolism: Hepatic via CYP2D6 to active metabolite, O-desmethylvenlafaxine (ODV); other metabolites include N-desmethylvenlafaxine and N,O-didesmethylvenlafaxine

Bioavailability: Oral: ~45%

Half-life elimination: Venlafaxine: 5 ± 2 hours; ODV: 11 ± 2 hours; prolonged with cirrhosis (venlafaxine: ~30%, ODV: ~60%), renal impairment (venlafaxine: ~50%, ODV: ~40%), and during dialysis (venlafaxine: ~180%, ODV: ~142%)

Time to peak:
  Immediate release: Venlafaxine: 2 hours, ODV: 3 hours
  Extended release: Venlafaxine: 5.5 hours, ODV: 9 hours

Excretion: Urine (~87%; 5% of total dose as unchanged drug; 29% of total dose as unconjugated ODV; 26% of total dose as conjugated ODV; 27% of total dose as minor inactive metabolites)

Dosage

Geriatric Refer to adult dosing. No specific recommendations for elderly, but may be best to start lower at 25-50 mg twice daily and increase as tolerated by 25 mg/dose. Extended-release formulation: 37.5 mg once daily, increase by 37.5 mg every 4-7 days as tolerated

Adult

Depression: Oral:

Immediate-release tablets: Initial: 75 mg/day, administered in 2 or 3 divided doses; may increase in ≤75 mg/day increments at intervals of ≥4 days as tolerated (maximum daily dose: 225-375 mg)

Extended-release capsules or tablets: Initial: 37.5-75 mg once daily; in patients who are initiated at 37.5 mg once daily, may increase to 75 mg once daily after 4-7 days; dose may then be increased by ≤75 mg/day increments at intervals of ≥4 days as tolerated (maximum daily dose: 225 mg)

Generalized anxiety disorder: Oral: *Extended-release capsules:* Initial: 37.5-75 mg once daily; in patients who are initiated at 37.5 mg once daily, may increase to 75 mg once daily after 4-7 days; may then be increased by ≤75 mg/day increments at intervals of ≥4 days as tolerated (maximum daily dose: 225 mg)

Panic disorder: Oral: *Extended-release capsules:* Initial: 37.5 mg once daily for 1 week; may increase to 75 mg once daily after 7 days, may then be increased by ≤75 mg/day increments at intervals of ≥7 days (maximum daily dose: 225 mg)

Social anxiety disorder: Oral: *Extended-release capsules or tablets:* 75 mg once daily (maximum daily dose: 75 mg); no evidence that doses >75 mg/day offer any additional benefit

Obsessive-compulsive disorder (unlabeled use): Oral: Titrate to usual dosage range of 150-300 mg/day; however, doses up to 375 mg/day have been used; response may be seen in 4 weeks (Phelps, 2005)

Neuropathic pain (unlabeled use): Oral: Dosages evaluated varied considerably based on etiology of chronic pain, but efficacy has been shown for many conditions in the range of 75-225 mg/day; onset of relief may occur in 1-2 weeks, or take up to 6 weeks for full benefit (Grothe, 2004).

Diabetic neuropathy (unlabeled use): Oral: 75-225 mg/day (Bril, 2011)

Hot flashes (unlabeled use): Oral: Doses of 37.5-75 mg/day have demonstrated significant improvement of vasomotor symptoms after 4-8 weeks of treatment; in one study, doses >75 mg/day offered no additional benefit (Evans, 2005; Loprinzi, 2000); however, higher doses (225 mg/day) may be beneficial in patients with perimenopausal depression.

Attention-deficit disorder (unlabeled use): Oral: Initial: Doses vary between 18.75 to 75 mg/day; may increase after 4 weeks to 150 mg/day; if tolerated, doses up to 225 mg/day have been used (Maidment, 2003)

Post-traumatic stress disorder (PTSD) (unlabeled use): Oral: *Extended release formulation:* 37.5-300 mg/day (Bandelow, 2008; Benedek, 2009)

Note: When discontinuing this medication after more than 1 week of treatment, it is generally recommended that the dose be tapered. If venlafaxine is used for 6 weeks or longer, the dose should be tapered over 2 weeks when discontinuing its use.

Renal Impairment

GFR: 10-70 mL/minute: Reduce total daily dose by 25% to 50%

Hemodialysis: Reduce total daily dose by 50%

Hepatic Impairment Mild-to-moderate hepatic impairment: Reduce total daily dose by 50%; further reductions may be necessary in some patients

Administration Administer with food.

Extended-release formulations: Swallow capsule or tablet whole; do not crush or chew. Contents of capsule may be sprinkled on a spoonful of applesauce and swallowed immediately without chewing; followed with a glass of water to ensure complete swallowing of the pellets.

Monitoring Parameters Blood pressure should be regularly monitored, especially in patients with a high baseline blood pressure; may cause mean increase in heart rate of 4-9 beats/minute; cholesterol; mental status for depression, suicide ideation (especially at the beginning of therapy or when doses are increased or decreased), anxiety, social functioning, mania, panic attacks

Test Interactions May interfere with urine detection of PCP and amphetamine (false-positives).

Special Geriatric Considerations Venlafaxine's low anticholinergic activity, minimal sedation, and hypotension properties makes this a valuable antidepressant in treating elderly with depression or anxiety disorders. No dose adjustment is necessary for age alone; adjust dose for renal function in the elderly. The elderly are more prone to SSRI/SNRI-induced hyponatremia.

A systematic review and meta-analysis of antidepressant placebo-controlled trials in persons with depression and dementia found evidence "suggestive" of efficacy but not of sufficient strength to "confirm" efficacy. Antidepressant trials in this patient population are small and underpowered. Older patients with depression being treated with an antidepressant should be closely monitored for response and adverse effects. Treatment should be switched or augmented when response is inadequate with a therapeutic dose. Antidepressants that are not tolerated should be discontinued and an alternative agent should be started.

This medication is considered to be potentially inappropriate in this patient population (Beers Criteria: Quality of evidence - moderate; Strength of recommendation - strong).

Dosage Forms Excipient information presented when available (limited, particularly for generics); consult specific product labeling.

Capsule, extended release, oral: 37.5 mg, 75 mg, 150 mg
Effexor XR®: 37.5 mg, 75 mg, 150 mg
Tablet, oral: 25 mg, 37.5 mg, 50 mg, 75 mg, 100 mg
Effexor®: 50 mg [scored]
Tablet, extended release, oral: 37.5 mg, 75 mg, 150 mg, 225 mg

◆ **Venofer®** see Iron Sucrose on page 1042
◆ **Ventolin® HFA** see Albuterol on page 49
◆ **Veracolate® [OTC]** see Bisacodyl on page 214
◆ **Veramyst®** see Fluticasone (Nasal) on page 826

Verapamil (ver AP a mil)

Related Information
Calcium Channel Blockers – Comparative Pharmacokinetics on page 2111
Medication Safety Issues
Sound-alike/look-alike issues:
Calan® may be confused with Colace®, diltiazem
Covera-HS® may be confused with Provera®
Isoptin® may be confused with Isopto® Tears
Verelan® may be confused with Voltaren®
High alert medication:
The Institute for Safe Medication Practices (ISMP) includes this medication (I.V. formulation) among its list of drug classes which have a heightened risk of causing significant patient harm when used in error.
Administration issues:
Significant differences exist between oral and I.V. dosing. Use caution when converting from one route of administration to another.
International issues:
Dilacor [Brazil] may be confused with Dilacor XR brand name for diltiazem [U.S.]
Brand Names: U.S. Calan®; Calan® SR; Covera-HS® [DSC]; Isoptin® SR; Verelan®; Verelan® PM
Brand Names: Canada Apo-Verap®; Apo-Verap® SR; Covera-HS®; Covera®; Dom-Verapamil SR; Isoptin® SR; Mylan-Verapamil; Mylan-Verapamil SR; Novo-Veramil; Novo-Veramil SR; Nu-Verap; Nu-Verap SR; PHL-Verapamil SR; PMS-Verapamil SR; PRO-Verapamil SR; Riva-Verapamil SR; Verapamil Hydrochloride Injection, USP; Verapamil SR; Verelan®
Index Terms Iproveratril Hydrochloride; Verapamil Hydrochloride
Generic Availability (U.S.) Yes: Excludes caplet (sustained release) and tablet (extended release, controlled onset)

Pharmacologic Category Antianginal Agent; Antiarrhythmic Agent, Class IV; Calcium Channel Blocker; Calcium Channel Blocker, Nondihydropyridine

Use

Oral: Treatment of hypertension; angina pectoris (vasospastic, chronic stable, unstable) (Calan®, Covera-HS®); supraventricular tachyarrhythmia (PSVT, atrial fibrillation/flutter [rate control])

I.V.: Supraventricular tachyarrhythmia (PSVT, atrial fibrillation/flutter [rate control])

Unlabeled Use Hypertrophic cardiomyopathy; bipolar disorder (manic manifestations)

Contraindications Hypersensitivity to verapamil or any component of the formulation; severe left ventricular dysfunction; hypotension (systolic pressure <90 mm Hg) or cardiogenic shock; sick sinus syndrome (except in patients with a functioning artificial ventricular pacemaker); second- or third-degree AV block (except in patients with a functioning artificial ventricular pacemaker); atrial flutter or fibrillation and an accessory bypass tract (Wolff-Parkinson-White [WPW] syndrome, Lown-Ganong-Levine syndrome)

I.V.: Additional contraindications include concurrent use of I.V. beta-blocking agents; ventricular tachycardia

Warnings/Precautions Avoid use in heart failure; can exacerbate condition; use is contraindicated in severe left ventricular dysfunction. Symptomatic hypotension with or without syncope can rarely occur; blood pressure must be lowered at a rate appropriate for the patient's clinical condition. Rare increases in hepatic enzymes can be observed. Can cause first-degree AV block or sinus bradycardia; use is contraindicated in patients with sick sinus syndrome, second- or third-degree AV block (except in patients with a functioning artificial pacemaker), or an accessory bypass tract (eg, WPW syndrome). Other conduction abnormalities are rare. Use caution when using verapamil together with a beta-blocker. Administration of I.V. verapamil and an I.V. beta-blocker within a few hours of each other may result in asystole and should be avoided; simultaneous administration is contraindicated. Use with caution in patients with hypertrophic cardiomyopathy with outflow tract obstruction (especially those with resting outflow obstruction and severe limiting symptoms); may be used in patients who cannot tolerate beta-blockade.

Decreased neuromuscular transmission has been reported with verapamil; use with caution in patients with attenuated neuromuscular transmission (Duchenne's muscular dystrophy, myasthenia gravis); dosage reduction may be required. Use with caution in renal impairment; monitor hemodynamics and possibly ECG if severe impairment, particularly if concomitant hepatic impairment. Use with caution in patients with hepatic impairment; dosage reduction may be required; monitor hemodynamics and possibly ECG if severe impairment. May prolong recovery from nondepolarizing neuromuscular-blocking agents. Use Covera-HS® (extended-release delivery system) with caution in patients with severe GI narrowing. In patients with extremely short GI transit times (eg, <7 hours), dosage adjustment may be required.

Adverse Reactions (Reflective of adult population; not specific for elderly)

>10%:

Central nervous system: Headache (1% to 12%)

Gastrointestinal: Gingival hyperplasia (≤19%), constipation (7% to 12%)

1% to 10%:

Cardiovascular: Peripheral edema (1% to 4%), hypotension (3%), CHF/pulmonary edema (2%), AV block (1% to 2%), bradycardia (HR <50 bpm: 1%), flushing (1%)

Central nervous system: Fatigue (2% to 5%), dizziness (1% to 5%), lethargy (3%), pain (2%), sleep disturbance (1%)

Dermatologic: Rash (1% to 2%)

Gastrointestinal: Dyspepsia (3%), nausea (1% to 3%), diarrhea (2%)

Hepatic: Liver enzymes increased (1%)

Neuromuscular & skeletal: Myalgia (1%), paresthesia (1%)

Respiratory: Dyspnea (1%)

Miscellaneous: Flu-like syndrome (4%)

Drug Interactions

Metabolism/Transport Effects Substrate of CYP1A2 (minor), CYP2B6 (minor), CYP2C9 (minor), CYP2E1 (minor), CYP3A4 (major), P-glycoprotein; **Note:** Assignment of Major/Minor substrate status based on clinically relevant drug interaction potential; **Inhibits** CYP1A2 (weak), CYP2C9 (weak), CYP2D6 (weak), CYP3A4 (moderate), P-glycoprotein

Avoid Concomitant Use

Avoid concomitant use of Verapamil with any of the following: Conivaptan; Dantrolene; Disopyramide; Dofetilide; Pimozide; Tolvaptan; Topotecan

Increased Effect/Toxicity

Verapamil may increase the levels/effects of: Alcohol (Ethyl); Aliskiren; Amifostine; Amiodarone; Antihypertensives; ARIPiprazole; AtorvaSTATin; Avanafil; Benzodiazepines (metabolized by oxidation); Beta-Blockers; Budesonide (Systemic, Oral Inhalation); BusPIRone;

Calcium Channel Blockers (Dihydropyridine); CarBAMazepine; Cardiac Glycosides; Colchicine; Corticosteroids (Systemic); CycloSPORINE; CycloSPORINE (Systemic); CYP3A4 Substrates; Dabigatran Etexilate; Disopyramide; Dofetilide; Dronedarone; Eletriptan; Eplerenone; Everolimus; Fexofenadine; Fingolimod; Flecainide; Fosphenytoin; Halofantrine; Hypotensive Agents; Ivacaftor; Lithium; Lovastatin; Lurasidone; Magnesium Salts; Midodrine; Neuromuscular-Blocking Agents (Nondepolarizing); Nitroprusside; P-glycoprotein/ABCB1 Substrates; Phenytoin; Pimecrolimus; Pimozide; Propafenone; Prucalopride; QuiNIDine; Ranolazine; Red Yeast Rice; RisperiDONE; RiTUXimab; Rivaroxaban; Salicylates; Salmeterol; Saxagliptin; Simvastatin; Tacrolimus; Tacrolimus (Systemic); Tacrolimus (Topical); Tolvaptan; Topotecan; Vilazodone; Zuclopenthixol

The levels/effects of Verapamil may be increased by: Alpha1-Blockers; Anilidopiperidine Opioids; Antifungal Agents (Azole Derivatives, Systemic); AtorvaSTATin; Calcium Channel Blockers (Dihydropyridine); Cimetidine; Conivaptan; CycloSPORINE; CycloSPORINE (Systemic); CYP3A4 Inhibitors (Moderate); CYP3A4 Inhibitors (Strong); Dantrolene; Dasatinib; Diazoxide; Dronedarone; Fluconazole; Grapefruit Juice; Herbs (Hypotensive Properties); Ivacaftor; Macrolide Antibiotics; Magnesium Salts; MAO Inhibitors; Mifepristone; Pentoxifylline; P-glycoprotein/ABCB1 Inhibitors; Phosphodiesterase 5 Inhibitors; Prostacyclin Analogues; Protease Inhibitors; QuiNIDine; Telithromycin

Decreased Effect

Verapamil may decrease the levels/effects of: Clopidogrel; Ifosfamide

The levels/effects of Verapamil may be decreased by: Barbiturates; Calcium Salts; CarBAMazepine; CYP3A4 Inducers (Strong); Deferasirox; Herbs (CYP3A4 Inducers); Herbs (Hypertensive Properties); Methylphenidate; Nafcillin; P-glycoprotein/ABCB1 Inducers; Rifamycin Derivatives; Tocilizumab; Yohimbine

Ethanol/Nutrition/Herb Interactions

Ethanol: Ethanol may increase ethanol levels. Management: Avoid or limit ethanol.

Food: Grapefruit juice may increase the serum concentration of verapamil. Management: Avoid grapefruit juice or use with caution and monitor for effects. Calan® SR and Isoptin® SR products should be taken with food or milk; other formulations may be administered without regard to meals.

Herb/Nutraceutical: St John's wort may decrease levels of verapamil. Some herbal medications have hypertensive properties (eg, licorice); others may increase or decrease the antihypertensive effect of verapamil. Management: Avoid St John's wort, bayberry, blue cohosh, cayenne, ephedra, ginger, ginseng (American), kola, licorice, and yohimbe. Avoid black cohosh, California poppy, coleus, golden seal, hawthorn, mistletoe, periwinkle, quinine, and shepherd's purse.

Stability Store at controlled room temperature of 15°C to 30°C (59°F to 86°F). Protect from light.

Mechanism of Action Inhibits calcium ion from entering the "slow channels" or select voltage-sensitive areas of vascular smooth muscle and myocardium during depolarization; produces relaxation of coronary vascular smooth muscle and coronary vasodilation; increases myocardial oxygen delivery in patients with vasospastic angina; slows automaticity and conduction of AV node.

Pharmacodynamics/Kinetics

Onset of action: Peak effect: Oral: Immediate release: 1-2 hours; I.V.: 1-5 minutes

Duration: Oral: Immediate release tablets: 6-8 hours; I.V.: 10-20 minutes

Absorption: Well absorbed

Distribution: V_d: 3.89 L/kg (Storstein, 1984)

Protein binding: ~90%

Metabolism: Hepatic (extensive first-pass effect) via multiple CYP isoenzymes; primary metabolite is norverapamil (20% pharmacologic activity of verapamil)

Bioavailability: Oral: 20% to 35%

Half-life elimination: Adults: Single dose: 3-7 hours, Multiple doses: 4.5-12 hours; severe hepatic impairment: 14-16 hours

Time to peak, serum: Oral:

Immediate release: 1-2 hours

Extended release (Covera-HS®, Verelan PM®): ~11 hours, drug release delayed ~4-5 hours

Sustained release: 5.21 hours (Calan® SR, Isoptin® SR); 7-9 hours (Verelan®)

Excretion: Urine (70% as metabolites, 3% to 4% as unchanged drug); feces (16%)

Dosage

Geriatric

Refer to adult dosing.

Hypertension: Oral: **Note:** When switching from immediate release to extended or sustained release formulations, the total daily dose remains the same unless formulation strength does not allow for equal conversion.

Manufacturer's recommendations:

Immediate release: Initial: 40 mg 3 times daily

Sustained release: Calan® SR, Isoptin® SR, Verelan®: Initial: 120 mg once daily in the morning

Extended release:

Covera-HS®: Initial: 180 mg once daily at bedtime

Verelan® PM: Initial: 100 mg once daily at bedtime

ACCF/AHA Expert Consensus recommendations: Consider lower initial doses and titrating to response (Aronow, 2011)

Adult

Angina: Oral: **Note:** When switching from immediate-release to extended/sustained release formulations, the total daily dose remains the same unless formulation strength does not allow for equal conversion.

Immediate release: Initial: 80-120 mg 3 times/day (elderly or small stature: 40 mg 3 times/day); Usual dose range (Gibbons, 2002): 80-160 mg 3 times/day

Extended release (Covera-HS®): Initial: 180 mg once daily at bedtime; if inadequate response, may increase dose at weekly intervals to 240 mg once daily, then 360 mg once daily, then 480 mg once daily; maximum dose: 480 mg/day

Chronic atrial fibrillation (rate-control), PSVT prophylaxis: Oral: Immediate release: 240-480 mg/day in 3-4 divided doses; Usual dose range (Fuster, 2006): 120-360 mg/day in divided doses

Hypertension: Oral: **Note:** When switching from immediate-release to extended/sustained release formulations, the total daily dose remains the same unless formulation strength does not allow for equal conversion.

Immediate release: 80 mg 3 times/day; usual dose range (JNC 7): 80-320 mg/day in 2 divided doses

Sustained release: Usual dose range (JNC 7): 120-480 mg/day in 1-2 divided doses; **Note:** There is no evidence of additional benefit with doses >360 mg/day.

Calan® SR, Isoptin® SR: Initial: 180 mg once daily in the morning (elderly or small stature: 120 mg/day); if inadequate response, may increase dose at weekly intervals to 240 mg once daily, then 180 mg twice daily (or 240 mg in the morning followed by 120 mg in the evening); maximum dose: 240 mg twice daily.

Verelan®: Initial: 180 mg once daily in the morning (elderly or small stature: 120 mg/day); if inadequate response, may increase dose at weekly intervals to 240 mg once daily, then 360 mg once daily, then 480 mg once daily; maximum dose: 480 mg/day

Extended release: Usual dose range (JNC 7): 120-360 mg once daily (once-daily dosing is recommended at bedtime)

Covera-HS®: Initial: 180 mg once daily at bedtime; if inadequate response, may increase dose at weekly intervals to 240 mg once daily, then 360 mg once daily, then 480 mg once daily; maximum dose: 480 mg/day

Verelan® PM: Initial: 200 mg once daily at bedtime (elderly or small stature: 100 mg/day); if inadequate response, may increase dose at weekly intervals to 300 mg once daily, then 400 mg once daily; maximum dose: 400 mg/day

SVT (ACLS, 2010): I.V.: 2.5-5 mg over 2 minutes; second dose of 5-10 mg (~0.15 mg/kg) may be given 15-30 minutes after the initial dose if patient tolerates, but does not respond to initial dose; maximum total dose: 20-30 mg

Renal Impairment Manufacturer recommends caution and additional ECG monitoring in patients with renal insufficiency. The manufacturer of Verelan PM® recommends an initial dose of 100 mg/day at bedtime. **Note:** A multiple dose study in adults suggests reduced renal clearance of verapamil and its metabolite (norverapamil) with advanced renal failure (Storstein, 1984). Additionally, several clinical papers report adverse effects of verapamil in patients with chronic renal failure receiving recommended doses of verapamil (Pritza, 1991; Váquez, 1996). In contrast, a number of single dose studies show no difference in verapamil (or norverapamil metabolite) disposition between chronic renal failure and control patients (Beyerlein, 1990; Hanyok, 1988; Mooy, 1985; Zachariah, 1991).

Dialysis: Not removed by hemodialysis (Mooy, 1985); supplemental dose is not necessary.

Hepatic Impairment In cirrhosis, reduce dose to 20% and 50% of normal for oral and intravenous administration, respectively, and monitor ECG (Somogyi, 1981). The manufacturer of Verelan PM® recommends an initial adult dose of 100 mg/day at bedtime. The manufacturers of Calan®, Calan® SR, Covera-HS®, Isoptin® SR, and Verelan® recommend giving 30% of the normal dose to patients with severe hepatic impairment.

Administration
Oral: Do not crush or chew sustained or extended release products.
  Calan® SR, Isoptin® SR: Administer with food.
  Verelan®, Verelan® PM: Capsules may be opened and the contents sprinkled on 1 tablespoonful of applesauce, then swallowed immediately without chewing. Do not subdivide contents of capsules.
  I.V.: Rate of infusion: Over 2 minutes; over 3 minutes in older patients (ACLS, 2010)

Monitoring Parameters Monitor blood pressure and heart rate; periodic liver function tests; ECG, especially with renal and/or hepatic impairment

Test Interactions May interfere with urine detection of methadone (false-positive).

Pharmacotherapy Pearls Incidence of adverse reactions is most common with I.V. administration; discontinue disopyramide 48 hours before starting therapy, do not restart therapy until 24 hours after verapamil has been discontinued

Special Geriatric Considerations Elderly may experience a greater hypotensive response. Constipation may be more of a problem in the elderly. Calcium channel blockers are no more effective in the elderly than other therapies; however, they do not cause significant CNS effects which is an advantage over some antihypertensive agents. Generic verapamil products which are bioequivalent in young adults may not be bioequivalent in the elderly; use generics cautiously.

Dosage Forms Excipient information presented when available (limited, particularly for generics); consult specific product labeling. [DSC] = Discontinued product
Caplet, sustained release, oral, as hydrochloride:
  Calan® SR: 120 mg
  Calan® SR: 180 mg, 240 mg [scored]
Capsule, extended release, oral, as hydrochloride: 120 mg, 180 mg, 240 mg
Capsule, extended release, controlled onset, oral, as hydrochloride: 100 mg, 200 mg, 300 mg
  Verelan® PM: 100 mg, 200 mg, 300 mg
Capsule, sustained release, oral, as hydrochloride: 120 mg, 180 mg, 240 mg, 360 mg
  Verelan®: 120 mg, 180 mg, 240 mg, 360 mg
Injection, solution, as hydrochloride: 2.5 mg/mL (2 mL, 4 mL)
Tablet, oral, as hydrochloride: 40 mg, 80 mg, 120 mg
  Calan®: 80 mg, 120 mg [scored]
Tablet, extended release, oral, as hydrochloride: 120 mg, 180 mg, 240 mg
Tablet, extended release, controlled onset, oral, as hydrochloride:
  Covera-HS®: 180 mg [DSC], 240 mg [DSC]
Tablet, sustained release, oral, as hydrochloride: 120 mg, 180 mg, 240 mg
  Isoptin® SR: 120 mg
  Isoptin® SR: 180 mg, 240 mg [DSC] [scored]

Extemporaneously Prepared To prepare a verapamil 50 mg/mL liquid, crush 75 verapamil hydrochloride 80 mg tablets into a fine powder. Add ~40 mL of either Ora-Sweet® and Ora-Plus® (1:1 preparation), or Ora-Sweet® SF and Ora-Plus® (1:1 preparation), or cherry syrup. Mix to a uniform paste. Continue to add the vehicle to bring the final volume to 120 mL. The preparation is stable for 60 days; shake well before using and protect from light.
Allen LV and Erickson III MA, "Stability of Labetalol Hydrochloride, Metoprolol Tartrate, Verapamil Hydrochloride, and Spironolactone With Hydrochlorothiazide in Extemporaneously Compounded Oral Liquids," *Am J Health Syst Pharm*, 1996, 53:304-9.

◆ **Verapamil and Trandolapril** see Trandolapril and Verapamil *on page 1949*
◆ **Verapamil Hydrochloride** see Verapamil *on page 2014*
◆ **Verelan®** see Verapamil *on page 2014*
◆ **Verelan® PM** see Verapamil *on page 2014*
◆ **Veripred™ 20** see PrednisoLONE (Systemic) *on page 1591*
◆ **Versed** see Midazolam *on page 1278*

Verteporfin (ver te POR fin)

Brand Names: U.S. Visudyne®
Brand Names: Canada Visudyne®
Index Terms Photodynamic Therapy
Generic Availability (U.S.) No
Pharmacologic Category Ophthalmic Agent
Use Treatment of predominantly classic subfoveal choroidal neovascularization due to age-related macular degeneration, presumed ocular histoplasmosis, or pathologic myopia
Unlabeled Use Predominantly **occult** subfoveal choroidal neovascularization
Contraindications Hypersensitivity to verteporfin or any component of the formulation; porphyria

Warnings/Precautions Avoid exposing skin or eyes to direct sunlight or bright indoor light for 5 days following treatment. In case of emergency surgery within 48 hours of treatment, protect as much of the internal tissue as possible from intense light. Do not retreat patients who experience a decrease of vision ≥4 lines within 1 week of treatment unless vision recovers and the potential benefits and risks are carefully considered. Use of incompatible lasers (which do not provide the required light for photoactivation) can result in incomplete treatment, over-treatment, or damage to normal tissue.

Use in more than one eye has not been studied; however, it is recommended that if required, initial treatment should be applied to the more aggressive lesion first, followed by the second eye a week later (subsequent treatment may be concurrent). Standard precautions should be taken to avoid extravasation (eg free-flowing I.V. line, use of largest arm vein). If extravasation occurs, stop the infusion immediately and protect from direct light until swelling and discoloration have faded; use cold compresses and oral pain medications, if necessary. Chest pain, vasovagal and hypersensitivity reactions have occurred rarely; observation of patient during infusion is suggested.

Use in patients with moderate-to-severe hepatic impairment, biliary obstruction, or under anesthesia has not been studied. Patients with dark irides, occult lesions, <50% classic choroidal neovascularization, or patients ≥75 years of age are less likely to benefit from therapy. Safety and efficacy of use for longer than 2 years have not been established.

Adverse Reactions (Reflective of adult population; not specific for elderly)
>10%:
  Local: Injection site reactions (including injection site discoloration, edema, extravasation, hemorrhage, inflammation, pain, and rash)
  Ocular: Blurred vision, flashes of light, visual acuity decreased, visual field defects (including scotoma)
1% to 10%:
  Cardiovascular: Atrial fibrillation, hypertension, peripheral vascular disorder, varicose veins
  Central nervous system: Fever, hypoesthesia, sleep disturbance, vertigo
  Dermatologic: Eczema, photosensitivity
  Gastrointestinal: Constipation, gastrointestinal cancers, nausea
  Genitourinary: Prostatic disorder
  Hematologic: Anemia, leukocytosis, leukopenia
  Hepatic: Liver function tests increased
  Neuromuscular & skeletal: Arthralgia, arthrosis, back pain (primarily during infusion), myasthenia, weakness
  Ocular: Diplopia, lacrimation disorder
    Treatment site: Blepharitis, cataracts, conjunctivitis/conjunctival injection, dry eyes, ocular itching, severe vision loss with or without subretinal/retinal or vitreous hemorrhage (decrease in 4 lines or more within 7 days of treatment [1% to 5%])
  Otic: Hearing loss
  Renal: Albuminuria, creatinine increased
  Respiratory: Cough, pharyngitis, pneumonia
  Miscellaneous: Flu-like syndrome

Drug Interactions
  Metabolism/Transport Effects None known.
  Avoid Concomitant Use There are no known interactions where it is recommended to avoid concomitant use.
  Increased Effect/Toxicity There are no known significant interactions involving an increase in effect.
  Decreased Effect There are no known significant interactions involving a decrease in effect.

Ethanol/Nutrition/Herb Interactions Ethanol: Ethanol may decrease efficacy of verteporfin.

Stability Store vial at 20°C to 25°C (68°F to 77°F). Each vial should be reconstituted with 7 mL of sterile water for injection, providing a total volume of 7.5 mL. Resulting solution will be 2 mg/mL. Solution should be protected from light and used within 4 hours. Once reconstituted, verteporfin will be an opaque dark green solution. The total volume of solution needed to administer the dose should be withdrawn from the vial and further diluted in D_5W to a total volume of 30 mL (precipitation may occur in saline solutions; only use D_5W for dilution). Infuse at 3 mL/minute over 10 minutes, using syringe pump and in-line filter.

Mechanism of Action Following intravenous administration, verteporfin is transported by lipoproteins to the neovascular endothelium in the affected eye(s), including choroidal neo-vasculature and the retina. Verteporfin then needs to be activated by nonthermal red light, which results in local damage to the endothelium, leading to temporary choroidal vessel occlusion.

Pharmacodynamics/Kinetics
Metabolism: Hepatic and by plasma esterases to diacid metabolite
Half-life elimination: Terminal: 5-6 hours, biexponential
Excretion: Feces

Dosage
Geriatric Refer to adult dosing. Patients ≥75 years were less likely to benefit from therapy in clinical trials.

Adult Therapy is a two-step process; first the infusion of verteporfin, then the activation of verteporfin with a nonthermal diode laser (for light administration details, see Administration).

Subfoveal choroidal neovascularization: I.V.: 6 mg/m^2 body surface area

Note: Treatment in more than one eye: Patients who have lesions in both eyes should be evaluated and treatment should first be done to the more aggressive lesion. Following safe and acceptable treatment, the second eye can be treated one week later. Patients who have had previous verteporfin therapy, with an acceptable safety profile, may then have both eyes treated concurrently. Treat the more aggressive lesion followed immediately with the second eye. The light treatment to the second eye should begin no later than 20 minutes from the start of the infusion.

Renal Impairment No dosage adjustment necessary.

Hepatic Impairment
Mild impairment: No dosage adjustment provided in manufacturer's labeling; however, half-life is increased by 20% with mild hepatic impairment.
Moderate-to-severe impairment: Use caution; no dosage adjustment provided in manufacturer's labeling (has not been studied).

Administration A free-flowing I.V. line should be established prior to starting infusion. Use of the largest arm vein, especially in the elderly, is suggested; avoid small veins in the back of the hand. Reconstituted solution should be given at 3 mL/minute over 10 minutes using a syringe pump and an in-line filter. If extravasation occurs, protect the site from light. Use of rubber gloves and eye protection is recommended. Skin and eye contact should be avoided and all materials should be disposed of properly.

Light administration: Following intravenous infusion, verteporfin must be light activated using a nonthermal diode laser. The system must provide a stable power output at a wavelength of 689 ± 3 nm. Approved laser systems are listed in manufacturer's package insert. Light delivery should begin 15 minutes following the start of the 10-minute infusion. The light dose is J/cm^2 of neovascular lesion administered over 83 seconds at an intensity of 600 mW/cm^2. Instructions for determining lesion size and treatment spot size can also be found in the package insert.

Monitoring Parameters Intravenous site during infusion, to avoid extravasation; fluorescein angiography every 3 months to monitor choroidal neovascular leakage (if detected, repeat therapy)

Special Geriatric Considerations Clinical efficacy trials involved ~90% of patients >65 years of age and showed a decrease in efficacy with increasing age.

Dosage Forms Excipient information presented when available (limited, particularly for generics); consult specific product labeling.
Injection, powder for reconstitution:
Visudyne®: 15 mg [contains egg phosphatidylglycerol]

- ◆ **VertiCalm™ [OTC]** *see* Meclizine *on page 1186*
- ◆ **VESIcare®** *see* Solifenacin *on page 1797*
- ◆ **Vexol®** *see* Rimexolone *on page 1706*
- ◆ **VFEND®** *see* Voriconazole *on page 2029*
- ◆ **Viagra®** *see* Sildenafil *on page 1770*
- ◆ **Vibativ™** *see* Telavancin *on page 1841*
- ◆ **Vibramycin®** *see* Doxycycline *on page 606*
- ◆ **Vicks® 44® Cough Relief [OTC]** *see* Dextromethorphan *on page 525*
- ◆ **Vicks® 44E [OTC]** *see* Guaifenesin and Dextromethorphan *on page 906*
- ◆ **Vicks® Casero™ Chest Congestion Relief [OTC]** *see* GuaiFENesin *on page 904*
- ◆ **Vicks® DayQuil® Cough [OTC]** *see* Dextromethorphan *on page 525*
- ◆ **Vicks® DayQuil® Mucus Control [OTC]** *see* GuaiFENesin *on page 904*
- ◆ **Vicks® DayQuil® Mucus Control DM [OTC]** *see* Guaifenesin and Dextromethorphan *on page 906*
- ◆ **Vicks® DayQuil® Sinex® Daytime Sinus [OTC]** *see* Acetaminophen and Phenylephrine *on page 37*
- ◆ **Vicks® Nature Fusion™ Cough [OTC]** *see* Dextromethorphan *on page 525*
- ◆ **Vicks® Nature Fusion™ Cough & Chest Congestion [OTC]** *see* Guaifenesin and Dextromethorphan *on page 906*
- ◆ **Vicks® Pediatric Formula 44E [OTC]** *see* Guaifenesin and Dextromethorphan *on page 906*

- **Vicks® Sinex® VapoSpray 12-Hour** *see* Oxymetazoline (Nasal) *on page 1452*
- **Vicks® Sinex® VapoSpray 12-Hour UltraFine Mist [OTC]** *see* Oxymetazoline (Nasal) *on page 1452*
- **Vicks® Sinex® VapoSpray Moisturizing 12-Hour UltraFine Mist [OTC]** *see* Oxymetazoline (Nasal) *on page 1452*
- **Vicks® Vitamin C [OTC]** *see* Ascorbic Acid *on page 149*
- **Vicks® ZzzQuil™ [OTC]** *see* DiphenhydrAMINE (Systemic) *on page 556*
- **Vicodin®** *see* Hydrocodone and Acetaminophen *on page 937*
- **Vicodin® ES** *see* Hydrocodone and Acetaminophen *on page 937*
- **Vicodin® HP** *see* Hydrocodone and Acetaminophen *on page 937*
- **Victoza®** *see* Liraglutide *on page 1144*

Vigabatrin (vye GA ba trin)

Medication Safety Issues
Sound-alike/look-alike issues:
Vigabatrin may be confused with Vibativ™
Brand Names: U.S. Sabril®
Brand Names: Canada Sabril®
Generic Availability (U.S.) No
Pharmacologic Category Anticonvulsant, Miscellaneous
Use Treatment of refractory complex partial seizures not controlled by usual treatments

Additional uses in Canadian labeling (not in U.S. labeling): Active management of partial or secondary generalized seizures not controlled by usual treatments
Unlabeled Use Spasticity, tardive dyskinesias
Prescribing and Access Restrictions As a requirement of the REMS program, access to this medication is restricted. Vigabatrin is only available in the U.S. under a special restricted distribution program (SHARE). Under the SHARE program, only prescribers and pharmacies registered with the program are able to prescribe and distribute vigabatrin. Vigabatrin may only be dispensed to patients who are enrolled in and meet all conditions of SHARE. Contact the SHARE program at 1-888-45-SHARE.
Medication Guide Available Yes
Contraindications There are no contraindications listed within the FDA-approved manufacturer's labeling.

Canadian labeling (not in U.S. labeling): Hypersensitivity to vigabatrin or any component of the formulation
Warnings/Precautions Use has been associated with decreased hemoglobin and hematocrit; cases of significantly reduced hemoglobin (<8 g/dL) and/or hematocrit (<24%) have been reported. Somnolence and fatigue can occur with use; patients must be cautioned about performing tasks which require mental alertness (eg, operating machinery or driving). Peripheral edema independent of hypertension, heart failure, weight gain, renal or hepatic dysfunction has been reported. Neurotoxicity: Patients must be closely monitored for potential neurotoxicity (observed in animal models but not established in humans). Peripheral neuropathy and manifesting as numbness or tingling in the toes or feet, reduced distal lower limb vibration or position sensation, or progressive loss of reflexes, starting at the ankles has been reported in adult patients. Pooled analysis of trials involving various antiepileptics (regardless of indication) showed an increased risk of suicidal thoughts/behavior (incidence rate: 0.43% treated patients compared to 0.24% of patients receiving placebo); risk observed as early as 1 week after initiation and continued through duration of trials (most trials ≤24 weeks). Monitor all patients for notable changes in behavior that might indicate suicidal thoughts or depression; notify healthcare provider immediately if symptoms occur. Use has been associated with an average weight gain of 3.5 kg in adults.

[U.S. Boxed Warning]: Vigabatrin causes permanent vision loss in infants, children and adults. Due to the risk of vision loss and because vigabatrin, provides an observable symptomatic benefit when it is effective, the patient who fails to show substantial clinical benefit within a short period of time after initiation of treatment -4 weeks for infantile spasms; <3 months in adults), should be withdrawn from therapy. If in the clinical judgment of the prescriber evidence of treatment failure becomes obvious earlier in treatment, vigabatrin should be discontinued at that time. Patient response to and continued need for treatment should be periodically assessed. The onset of vision loss is unpredictable, and can occur within weeks of starting treatment or sooner, or at any time during treatment, even after months or years. The risk of vision loss increases with increasing dose and cumulative exposure, but there is no dose or exposure known to be free of risk of vision loss. It is possible that vision loss can worsen despite discontinuation. Most data are available in adult patients. Vigabatrin causes permanent bilateral concentric visual field constriction in >30% of patients ranging in severity from mild to severe, including tunnel vision to within 10 degrees of visual fixation, and can result in disability. In some cases, vigabatrin can damage the central retina and may decrease visual acuity. Patient response to and continued need for vigabatrin should be periodically reassessed. Vision loss of milder severity, although potentially unrecognized by the parent or caregiver, may still adversely affect function. Vision should be assessed to the extent possible at baseline (no later than 4 weeks after initiation), at least every 3 months during therapy and at 3-6 months after discontinuation. Once detected, vision loss is not reversible. Vigabatrin should not be used in patients with, or at high risk of, other types of irreversible vision loss unless the benefits of treatment clearly outweigh the risks. The interaction of other types of irreversible vision damage with vision damage from vigabatrin has not been well-characterized, but is likely adverse. Vigabatrin should not be used with other drugs associated with serious adverse ophthalmic effects such as retinopathy or glaucoma unless the benefits clearly outweigh the risks. The lowest dose and shortest exposure should be used that is consistent with clinical objectives.

Use with caution in patients with a history of psychosis (psychotic/agitated reactions may occur more frequently), depression, or behavioral problems. Use with caution in patients with renal impairment; modify dose in renal impairment (Cl_{cr} <80 mL/minute). May cause an increase in seizure frequency in some patients; use with particular caution in patients with myoclonic seizures, which may be more prone to this effect. Effects with other sedative drugs or ethanol may be potentiated. Use with caution in the elderly as severe sedation and confusion have been reported; consider dose and/or frequency adjustments as renal clearance may be decreased.

Abnormal MRI changes have been reported in some infants. Resolution of MRI changes usually occurs with discontinuation of therapy. MRI changes were not seen in older children and adult patients. In the U.S., vigabatrin is only available under a special restricted distribution program (SHARE). Under the SHARE program, only prescribers and pharmacies registered with the program are able to prescribe and distribute vigabatrin. Vigabatrin may only be dispensed to patients who are enrolled in and meet all conditions of SHARE. Anticonvulsants should not be discontinued abruptly because of the possibility of increasing seizure frequency; therapy should be withdrawn gradually to minimize the potential of increased seizure frequency, unless safety concerns require a more rapid withdrawal.

Adverse Reactions (Reflective of adult population; not specific for elderly) Note: Adult and pediatric information presented combined unless significantly different.

>10%:

Central nervous system: Somnolence (adults 17% to 24%; infants 17% to 45%), headache (18% to 33%), fatigue (16% to 28%), fever (adults 4% to 6%; infants 19% to 29%), dizziness (15% to 24%), irritability (adults 7%; infants 16% to 23%), sedation (adults 4%; infants 17% to 19%), nystagmus (7% to 15%), tremor (7% to 15%), insomnia (10% to 12%), seizure (4% to 11%)

Dermatologic: Rash (4% to 11%)

Gastrointestinal: Vomiting (adults 6% to 7%; infants 14% to 20%), weight gain (6% to 17%), constipation (6% to 14%), diarrhea (7% to 13%)

Neuromuscular & skeletal: Tremor (7% to 15%)

Ocular: Blurred vision (6% to 13%)

Otic: Otitis media (infants 7% to 44%)

Respiratory: Upper respiratory tract infection (adults 7% to 10%; infants 46% to 51%), bronchitis (infants 30%), pharyngitis (10% to 14%), pneumonia (infants 11% to 13%), nasal congestion (infants 4% to 13%)

Miscellaneous: Viral infection (infants 19% to 20%)

1% to 10%:

Cardiovascular: Peripheral edema (2% to 5%), chest pain (1%)

Central nervous system: Irritability (adults 7% to 10%; infants 16% to 23%), memory impairment (7% to 10%), coordination impaired (7% to 9%), disturbance in attention (5% to 9%), depression (4% to 8%), lethargy (4% to 7%), confusional state (4% to 6%), hypotonia (4% to 6%), status epilepticus (2% to 6%), weakness (5%), hyporeflexia (4% to 5%), sensory disturbance (4% to 5%), anxiety (4%), hypoesthesia (3% to 4%), abnormal behavior (3%), abnormal thinking (3%), aggression (2%), nervousness (2%), postictal state (2%), vertigo (2%), abnormal dreams (1%), dystonia (1%), expressive language disorder (1%), hypertonia (1%)

Dermatologic: Contusion (3% to 4%)

Endocrine & metabolic: Dysmenorrhea (7% to 9%), fluid retention (2%)

Gastrointestinal: Nausea (7% to 10%), decreased appetite (7% to 9%), viral gastroenteritis (infants 5% to 6%), abdominal pain (3% to 5%), dyspepsia (4%), abdominal distention (2%), hemorrhoidal symptoms (2%), toothache (2%), increased appetite (1% to 2%)

Genitourinary: Urinary tract infection (4% to 6%)

Neuromuscular & skeletal: Arthralgia (8% to 10%), gait disturbance (6%), paresthesia (5% to 7%), pain in extremity (5% to 6%), back pain (4% to 6%), hyper-reflexia (4%), myalgia (3%), muscle spasms (2% to 3%), dysarthria (2%), joint swelling (2%), shoulder pain (2%), joint sprain (1%), muscle strain (1%), muscle twitching (1%)

Ocular: Visual field defect (9%), diplopia (3% to 7%), strabismus (5%), conjunctivitis (2% to 5%), eye strain (2%)

Otic: Tinnitus (2%)

Respiratory: Pharyngolaryngeal pain (7% to 9%), sinusitis (5% to 9%), cough (2% to 8%), sinus headache (4% to 6%), dyspnea (2%)

Miscellaneous: Candidiasis (3% to 8%), influenza (3% to 6%), croup (1% to 5%), thirst (2%)

Drug Interactions

Metabolism/Transport Effects Induces CYP2C9 (weak/moderate)

Avoid Concomitant Use

Avoid concomitant use of Vigabatrin with any of the following: Azelastine; Azelastine (Nasal); Methadone; Mirtazapine; Paraldehyde

Increased Effect/Toxicity

Vigabatrin may increase the levels/effects of: Alcohol (Ethyl); Azelastine; Azelastine (Nasal); Buprenorphine; CNS Depressants; Methadone; Methotrimeprazine; Metyrosine; Mirtazapine; Paraldehyde; Selective Serotonin Reuptake Inhibitors; Zolpidem

The levels/effects of Vigabatrin may be increased by: Droperidol; HydrOXYzine; Methotrimeprazine

Decreased Effect

Vigabatrin may decrease the levels/effects of: Fosphenytoin; Phenytoin

The levels/effects of Vigabatrin may be decreased by: Ketorolac; Ketorolac (Nasal); Ketorolac (Systemic); Mefloquine

Ethanol/Nutrition/Herb Interactions

Ethanol: May increase CNS depression; monitor for increased effects with coadministration. Caution about effects.

Herb/Nutraceutical: Avoid evening primrose (seizure threshold decreased). Avoid valerian, St John's wort, kava kava, gotu kola (may increase CNS depression).

Stability Store tablet and powder for oral solution at 20°C to 25°C (68°F to 77°F).

Mechanism of Action Irreversibly inhibits gamma-aminobutyric acid transaminase (GABA-T), increasing the levels of the inhibitory compound gamma amino butyric acid (GABA) within the brain. Duration of effect is dependent upon rate of GABA-T resynthesis.

Pharmacodynamics/Kinetics

Duration (rate of GABA-T resynthesis dependent): Variable (not strictly correlated to serum concentrations)

Absorption: Rapid

Distribution: V_d: 1.1 L/kg

Metabolism: Insignificant

Half-life elimination: Adults: 7.5 hours; Elderly: 12-13 hours

Time to peak: Adults: 1 hour

Excretion: Urine (80%, as unchanged drug)

Dosage

Geriatric Refractory complex partial seizures: Refer to adult dosing. Initiate at low end of dosage range; monitor closely for sedation and confusion.

Adult Refractory complex partial seizures: Oral: Initial: 500 mg twice daily; increase daily dose by 500 mg at weekly intervals based on response and tolerability. Recommended dose: 3 g/day. (**Note:** Canadian labeling suggests that initial doses up to 2 g/day may be considered in patients with severe seizures.)

Note: To taper, decrease dose by 1 g/day on a weekly basis

Renal Impairment

Cl_{cr} >50-80 mL/minute: Decrease dose by 25%

Cl_{cr} >30-50 mL/minute: Decrease dose by 50%

Cl_{cr} >10-30 mL/minute: Decrease dose by 75%

Hepatic Impairment No dosage adjustment provided in manufacturer's labeling; has not been studied. However, does not undergo appreciable hepatic metabolism.

Administration May be administered without regard to meals.

Packet: Dissolve each 500 mg powder packet in 10 mL of cold or room temperature water to make a 50 mg/mL solution. Use immediately. The appropriate aliquot may be administered using an oral syringe.

Monitoring Parameters Ophthalmologic examination by an ophthalmic professional with expertise in visual field interpretation and the ability to perform dilated indirect ophthalmoscopy of the retina at baseline (no later than 4 weeks after therapy initiation), periodically during therapy (every 3 months), and 3-6 months after discontinuation of therapy; assessment should include visual acuity and visual field whenever possible including mydriatic peripheral

fundus examination and visual field perimetry. Observe patient for excessive sedation, especially when instituting or increasing therapy; hemoglobin and hematocrit

Test Interactions Vigabatrin has been reported to decrease AST and ALT activity in the plasma in up to 90% of patients, causing the enzymes to become undetectable in some patients; this may preclude use of AST and ALT as markers for hepatic injury. Vigabatrin may increase amino acids in the urine leading to false-positive tests for rare genetic metabolic disorders

Special Geriatric Considerations Vigabatrin has not been studied exclusively in the elderly. Clinical trials included an insufficient number of elderly to determine if their response differed from younger adults. Moderate-to-severe sedation and confusion, lasting up to 5 days, was seen in elderly patients with Cl_{cr} <50 mL/minute after a single 1.5 g dose.

Dosage Forms Excipient information presented when available (limited, particularly for generics); consult specific product labeling.
Powder for solution, oral:
  Sabril®: 500 mg/packet (50s)
Tablet, oral:
  Sabril®: 500 mg [scored]

Dosage Forms: Canada Excipient information presented when available (limited, particularly for generics); consult specific product labeling.
Powder for suspension, oral [sachets]:
  Sabril®: 0.5 g

◆ **Vigamox®** see Moxifloxacin (Ophthalmic) *on page 1323*
◆ **Viibryd™** see Vilazodone *on page 2024*

Vilazodone (vil AZ oh done)

Related Information
  Antidepressant Agents *on page 2097*
Brand Names: U.S. Viibryd™
Index Terms EMD 68843; SB659746-A; Vilazodone Hydrochloride
Generic Availability (U.S.) No
Pharmacologic Category Antidepressant, Selective Serotonin Reuptake Inhibitor/5-HT$_{1A}$ Receptor Partial Agonist
Use Treatment of major depressive disorder
Medication Guide Available Yes
Contraindications Concomitant use with MAO inhibitors or within 2 weeks of discontinuing MAO inhibitors
Warnings/Precautions [U.S. Boxed Warning]: Antidepressants increase the risk of suicidal thinking and behavior in children, adolescents, and young adults (18-24 years of age) with major depressive disorder (MDD) and other psychiatric disorders; consider risk prior to prescribing. Short-term studies did not show an increased risk in patients >24 years of age and showed a decreased risk in patients ≥65 years. Closely monitor patients for clinical worsening, suicidality, or unusual changes in behavior, particularly during the initial 1-2 months of therapy or during periods of dosage adjustments (increases or decreases); the patient's family or caregiver should be instructed to closely observe the patient and communicate condition with healthcare provider. A medication guide concerning the use of antidepressants should be dispensed with each prescription.

The possibility of a suicide attempt is inherent in major depression and may persist until remission occurs. Use caution in high-risk patients. Worsening depression and severe abrupt suicidality that are not part of the presenting symptoms may require discontinuation or modification of drug therapy. The patient's family or caregiver should be alerted to monitor patients for the emergence of suicidality and associated behaviors (such as agitation, irritability, hostility, impulsivity, and hypomania) and call healthcare provider.

May worsen psychosis in some patients or precipitate a shift to mania or hypomania in patients with bipolar disorder. Patients presenting with depressive symptoms should be screened for bipolar disorder. Monotherapy in patients with bipolar disorder should be avoided. **Vilazodone is not FDA approved for the treatment of bipolar depression.**

Serotonin syndrome and neuroleptic malignant syndrome (NMS)-like reactions have occurred with serotonin/norepinephrine reuptake inhibitors (SNRIs) and selective serotonin reuptake inhibitors (SSRIs) when used alone, and particularly when used in combination with serotonergic agents (eg, triptans) or antidopaminergic agents (eg, antipsychotics). Concurrent use or use within 2 weeks of discontinuing MAO inhibitors is contraindicated. In addition, allow at least 14 days after stopping vilazodone before starting an MAO inhibitor. High potential for interaction with concomitant medications (see Drug Interactions); monitor closely for toxicity or adverse effects. Dose reductions are recommended with concomitant use of strong or moderate CYP3A4 inhibitors. May increase the risks associated with electroconvulsive therapy. Has a low potential to impair cognitive or motor performance; caution operating hazardous machinery or driving.

Use with caution in patients with hepatic impairment, seizure disorder, in elderly patients, or on concomitant CNS depressants. Use caution with concomitant use of aspirin, NSAIDs, warfarin, or other drugs that affect coagulation; the risk of bleeding may be potentiated. May cause hyponatremia/SIADH (elderly at increased risk); volume depletion and diuretics may increase risk. May cause or exacerbate sexual dysfunction. Upon discontinuation of vilazodone therapy, gradually taper dose. If intolerable symptoms occur following a decrease in dosage or upon discontinuation of therapy, consider resuming the previous dose with a more gradual taper.

Adverse Reactions (Reflective of adult population; not specific for elderly)

>10%:

Gastrointestinal: Diarrhea (28%), nausea (23%)

1% to 10%:

Cardiovascular: Palpitation (2%)

Central nervous system: Dizziness (9%), insomnia (6%), dreams abnormal (4%), fatigue (4%), restlessness (3%), somnolence (3%), migraine (≥1%), sedation (≥1%)

Dermatologic: Hyperhidrosis (≥1%)

Endocrine & metabolic: Libido decreased (3% to 5%), orgasm abnormal (2% to 4%), sexual dysfunction (≤2%)

Gastrointestinal: Xerostomia (8%), vomiting (5%), dyspepsia (3%), flatulence (3%), gastroenteritis (3%), appetite increased (2%), appetite decreased (≥1%)

Genitourinary: Ejaculation delayed (2%), erectile dysfunction (2%)

Neuromuscular & skeletal: Arthralgia (3%), paresthesia (3%), jittery (2%), tremor (2%)

Ocular: Blurred vision (≥1%), dry eyes (≥1%)

Miscellaneous: Night sweats (≥1%)

Drug Interactions

Metabolism/Transport Effects Substrate of CYP2C19 (minor), CYP2D6 (minor), CYP3A4 (major); **Note:** Assignment of Major/Minor substrate status based on clinically relevant drug interaction potential; **Inhibits** CYP2C8 (weak), CYP2D6 (weak); **Induces** CYP2C19 (weak/moderate)

Avoid Concomitant Use

Avoid concomitant use of Vilazodone with any of the following: Iobenguane I 123; MAO Inhibitors; Methylene Blue; Pimozide; Tryptophan

Increased Effect/Toxicity

Vilazodone may increase the levels/effects of: Alpha-/Beta-Blockers; Anticoagulants; Antidepressants (Serotonin Reuptake Inhibitor/Antagonist); Antiplatelet Agents; Aspirin; Benzodiazepines (metabolized by oxidation); Beta-Blockers; BusPIRone; CarBAMazepine; CloZAPine; Collagenase (Systemic); Dabigatran Etexilate; Desmopressin; Dextromethorphan; Drotrecogin Alfa (Activated); Galantamine; Hypoglycemic Agents; Ibritumomab; Lithium; Methadone; Methylene Blue; Metoclopramide; Mexiletine; NSAID (COX-2 Inhibitor); NSAID (Nonselective); Pimozide; RisperiDONE; Rivaroxaban; Salicylates; Serotonin Modulators; Thrombolytic Agents; Tositumomab and Iodine I 131 Tositumomab; TraMADol; Tricyclic Antidepressants; Vitamin K Antagonists

The levels/effects of Vilazodone may be increased by: Alcohol (Ethyl); Analgesics (Opioid); Antipsychotics; BusPIRone; Cimetidine; CNS Depressants; CYP3A4 Inhibitors (Moderate); CYP3A4 Inhibitors (Strong); Dasatinib; Glucosamine; Herbs (Anticoagulant/Antiplatelet Properties); Linezolid; Macrolide Antibiotics; MAO Inhibitors; Metoclopramide; Metyrosine; Omega-3-Acid Ethyl Esters; Pentosan Polysulfate Sodium; Pentoxifylline; Prostacyclin Analogues; Tipranavir; TraMADol; Tryptophan; Vitamin E

Decreased Effect

Vilazodone may decrease the levels/effects of: Iobenguane I 123; Ioflupane I 123

The levels/effects of Vilazodone may be decreased by: CarBAMazepine; CYP3A4 Inducers (Strong); Cyproheptadine; Deferasirox; NSAID (COX-2 Inhibitor); NSAID (Nonselective); Peginterferon Alfa-2b; Tocilizumab

Ethanol/Nutrition/Herb Interactions

Ethanol: Ethanol may increase CNS depression. Management: Avoid or limit use and monitor for increased effects.

Food: Management: Take with food.

Stability Store at 25°C (77°F); excursions permitted to 15°C to 30°C (50°F to 86°F).

Mechanism of Action Vilazodone inhibits CNS neuron serotonin uptake; minimal or no effect on reuptake of norepinephrine or dopamine. It also binds selectively with high affinity to 5-HT$_{1A}$ receptors and is a 5-HT$_{1A}$ receptor partial agonist. 5-HT$_{1A}$ receptor activity may be altered in depression and anxiety.

Pharmacodynamics/Kinetics

Protein binding: ~96% to 99%

Metabolism: Extensively hepatic, via CYP3A4 (major pathway) and 2C19 and 2D6 (minor pathways)

Bioavailability: 72% (with food); blood concentrations (AUC) may be decreased ~50% in the fasted state

Half-life elimination: Terminal: ~25 hours

Time to peak, serum: 4-5 hours

Excretion: Urine (1% as unchanged drug); feces (2% as unchanged drug)

Dosage

Geriatric & Adult Depression: Oral: Initial: 10 mg once daily for 7 days, then increase to 20 mg once daily for 7 days, then to recommended dose of 40 mg once daily

Dosing adjustment for concomitant medications:

Strong CYP3A4 inhibitors: Reduce vilazodone dose to 20 mg once daily

Moderate CYP3A4 inhibitors (eg, erythromycin): Reduce vilazodone dose to 20 mg once daily in patients with intolerable side effects

Hepatic Impairment

Mild-to-moderate impairment (Child-Pugh class A or B): No adjustment needed

Severe impairment (Child-Pugh class C): Not studied

Administration Administer with food.

Monitoring Parameters Monitor patient periodically for symptom resolution, mental status for depression, suicidal ideation (especially at the beginning of therapy or when doses are increased or decreased), anxiety, social functioning, mania, panic attacks, akathisia

Special Geriatric Considerations Results of a single dose pharmacokinetic study suggest that a dose adjustment is not necessary for persons ≥65 years of age; however, there is limited experience with vilazodone in this age group as <2% of subjects in the clinical trials were ≥65 years. The elderly are more prone to SSRI/SNRI-induced hyponatremia.

A systematic review and meta-analysis of antidepressant placebo-controlled trials in persons with depression and dementia found evidence "suggestive" of efficacy but not of sufficient strength to "confirm" efficacy. Antidepressant trials in this patient population are small and underpowered. Older patients with depression being treated with an antidepressant should be closely monitored for response and adverse effects. Treatment should be switched or augmented when response is inadequate with a therapeutic dose. Antidepressants that are not tolerated should be discontinued and an alternative agent should be started.

Dosage Forms Excipient information presented when available (limited, particularly for generics); consult specific product labeling.

Tablet, oral, as hydrochloride:

Viibryd™: 10 mg, 20 mg, 40 mg

◆ **Vitamin D and Calcium Carbonate** *see* Calcium and Vitamin D *on page* 261
◆ **Vitamin D₃ and Alendronate** *see* Alendronate and Cholecalciferol *on page* 55
◆ **Vitamin D2** *see* Ergocalciferol *on page* 657
◆ **Vitamin D3 [OTC]** *see* Cholecalciferol *on page* 365

Vitamin E (VYE ta min ee)

Medication Safety Issues
Sound-alike/look-alike issues:
Aquasol E® may be confused with Anusol®
Brand Names: U.S. Alph-E [OTC]; Alph-E-Mixed [OTC]; Aqua Gem-E™ [OTC]; Aquasol E® [OTC]; d-Alpha Gems™ [OTC]; E-Gems® Elite [OTC]; E-Gems® Plus [OTC]; E-Gems® [OTC]; E-Gem® Lip Care [OTC]; E-Gem® [OTC]; Ester-E™ [OTC]; Gamma E-Gems® [OTC]; Gamma-E PLUS [OTC]; High Gamma Vitamin E Complete™ [OTC]; Key-E® Kaps [OTC]; Key-E® Powder [OTC]; Key-E® [OTC]
Index Terms *d*-Alpha Tocopherol; *dl*-Alpha Tocopherol
Generic Availability (U.S.) Yes
Pharmacologic Category Vitamin, Fat Soluble
Use Dietary supplement
Contraindications Hypersensitivity to vitamin E or any component of the formulation
Warnings/Precautions May induce vitamin K deficiency. Necrotizing enterocolitis has been associated with oral administration of large dosages (eg, >200 units/day) of a hyperosmolar vitamin E preparation in low birth weight infants.
Adverse Reactions (Reflective of adult population; not specific for elderly) Frequency not defined.
Central nervous system: Fatigue, headache
Dermatologic: Contact dermatitis with topical preparation, rash
Endocrine & metabolic: Creatinuria, gonadal dysfunction, hypercholesterolemia, hypertriglyceridemia, serum thyroxine decreased, serum triiodothyronine decreased
Gastrointestinal: Diarrhea, intestinal cramps, nausea, necrotizing enterocolitis (infants)
Neuromuscular & skeletal: CPK increased, weakness
Ocular: Blurred vision
Renal: Serum creatinine increased
Drug Interactions
Metabolism/Transport Effects None known.
Avoid Concomitant Use There are no known interactions where it is recommended to avoid concomitant use.
Increased Effect/Toxicity
Vitamin E may increase the levels/effects of: Antiplatelet Agents; Vitamin K Antagonists

The levels/effects of Vitamin E may be increased by: Tipranavir
Decreased Effect
Vitamin E may decrease the levels/effects of: CycloSPORINE; CycloSPORINE (Systemic)

The levels/effects of Vitamin E may be decreased by: Orlistat
Stability Protect from light.
Mechanism of Action Prevents oxidation of vitamin A and C; protects polyunsaturated fatty acids in membranes from attack by free radicals and protects red blood cells against hemolysis
Pharmacodynamics/Kinetics
Absorption: Oral: Depends on presence of bile; reduced in conditions of malabsorption and as dosage increases; water miscible preparations are better absorbed than oil preparations
Distribution: To all body tissues, especially adipose tissue, where it is stored
Metabolism: Hepatic to glucuronides
Excretion: Feces
Dosage
Geriatric & Adult Vitamin E may be expressed as alpha-tocopherol equivalents (ATE), which refer to the biologically-active (R) stereoisomer content.
Recommended daily allowance (RDA) (IOM, 2000): Oral: 15 mg; upper limit of intake should not exceed 1000 mg/day
Vitamin E deficiency: Oral: 60-75 units/day
Superficial dermatologic irritation: Topical: Apply a thin layer over affected area.
Administration Swallow capsules whole; do not crush or chew.
Monitoring Parameters Plasma tocopherol concentrations (normal range: 6-14 mcg/mL)
Reference Range Therapeutic: 0.8-1.5 mg/dL (SI: 19-35 micromole/L), some method variation

◀ **Pharmacotherapy Pearls** The 2R-stereoisomeric forms of α-tocopherol are used to define vitamin E intake and RDA. While international units are no longer recognized, many fortified foods and supplements continue to use this term although USP units are now used by the pharmaceutical industry when labeling vitamin E supplements. Both IUs and USP units are based on the same equivalency. The following can be used to convert international units (IU) of vitamin E (and esters) to milligrams α-tocopherol in order to meet recommended daily intake:

Synthetic (eg, all-racemic α-tocopherol):
dl-α-tocopherol:
  USP: 1.10 IU / mg; 0.91 mg / IU
  Molar: 2.12 µmol / IU
  α-tocopherol: 0.45 mg / IU
dl-α-tocopherol acetate:
  USP: 1 IU / mg; 1 mg / IU
  Molar: 2.12 µmol / IU
  α-tocopherol: 0.45 mg / IU
dl-α-tocopherol succinate:
  USP: 0.89 IU / mg; 1.12 mg / IU
  Molar: 2.12 µmol / IU
  α-tocopherol: 0.45 mg / IU

Natural (eg, RRR-α-tocopherol):
d-α-tocopherol:
  USP: 1.49 IU / mg; 0.67 mg / IU
  Molar: 1.56 µmol / IU
  α-tocopherol: 0.67 mg / IU
d-α-tocopherol acetate:
  USP: 1.36 IU / mg; 0.74mg / IU
  Molar: 1.56 µmol / IU
  α-tocopherol: 0.67 mg / IU
d-α-tocopherol succinate:
  USP: 1.21 IU / mg; 0.83 mg / IU
  Molar: 1.56 µmol / IU
  α-tocopherol: 0.67 mg / IU

Historically, vitamin E supplements have been labeled (incorrectly) as *d*- or *dl*-tocopherol. Synthetic vitamin E compounds are racemic mixtures, and may be designated as all-racemic (all rac-α-tocopherol). The natural form contains the only RRR-α-tocopherol. All of these compounds may be present in fortified foods and multivitamins. Not all stereoisomers are capable of performing physiological functions in humans; therefore, cannot be considered to meet vitamin E requirements.

Special Geriatric Considerations Elderly may have vitamin E prescribed for those with cardiovascular disease. Elderly should be advised not to take more than prescribed.

Dosage Forms Excipient information presented when available (limited, particularly for generics); consult specific product labeling.
Capsule, oral: 1000 units
  Key-E® Kaps: 200 units, 400 units [derived from or manufactured using soybean oil]
Capsule, liquid, oral: 400 units
Capsule, softgel, oral: 100 units, 200 units, 400 units, 600 units, 1000 units
  Alph-E: 200 units, 400 units
  Alph-E: 400 units [contains soybean oil]
  Alph-E: 1000 units
  Alph-E-Mixed: 200 units, 400 units
  Alph-E-Mixed: 1000 units [sugar free]
  Aqua Gem-E™: 200 units, 400 units
  d-Alpha Gems™: 400 units [derived from or manufactured using soybean oil]
  E-Gems®: 30 units, 100 units, 200 units, 400 units, 600 units, 800 units, 1000 units, 1200 units [derived from or manufactured using soybean oil]
  E-Gems® Elite: 400 units
  E-Gems® Plus: 200 units, 400 units, 800 units [derived from or manufactured using soybean oil]
  Ester-E™: 400 units
  Gamma E-Gems®: 90 units
  Gamma-E PLUS: 200 units [contains soybean oil]
  High Gamma Vitamin E Complete™: 200 units [contains soybean oil]
Cream, topical: 1000 units/120 g (120 g); 100 units/g (57 g, 60 g); 30,000 units/57 g (57 g)
  Key-E®: 30 units/g (57 g, 120 g, 600 g)

Lip balm, topical:
  E-Gem® Lip Care: 1000 units/tube [contains aloe, vitamin A]
Liquid, oral/topical: 1150 units/1.25 mL (30 mL, 60 mL, 120 mL)
Oil, oral/topical: 100 units/0.25 mL (74 mL)
Oil, oral/topical [drops]:
  E-Gem®: 10 units/drop (15 mL, 60 mL)
Oil, topical:
  Alph-E: 28,000 units/30 mL (30 mL)
Ointment, topical:
  Key-E®: 30 units/g (57 g, 113 g, 500 g)
Powder, oral:
  Key-E® Powder: (15 g, 75 g, 1000 g) [derived from or manufactured using soybean oil]
Solution, oral [drops]: 15 units/0.3 mL (30 mL)
  Aquasol E®: 15 units/0.3 mL (12 mL, 30 mL)
Suppository, rectal/vaginal:
  Key-E®: 30 units (12s, 24s) [contains coconut oil]
Tablet, oral: 100 units, 200 units, 400 units, 500 units
  Key-E®: 200 units, 400 units [derived from or manufactured using soybean oil]

- **Vitamin K₁** *see* Phytonadione *on page 1534*
- **Vitrase®** *see* Hyaluronidase *on page 931*
- **Vitrasert®** *see* Ganciclovir (Ophthalmic) *on page 867*
- **Vi Vaccine** *see* Typhoid Vaccine *on page 1985*
- **Vivactil®** *see* Protriptyline *on page 1629*
- **Viva-Drops® [OTC]** *see* Artificial Tears *on page 148*
- **Vivaglobin® [DSC]** *see* Immune Globulin *on page 982*
- **Vivelle-Dot®** *see* Estradiol (Systemic) *on page 681*
- **Vivotif®** *see* Typhoid Vaccine *on page 1985*
- **Voltaren** *see* Diclofenac (Systemic) *on page 531*
- **Voltaren® Gel** *see* Diclofenac (Topical) *on page 536*
- **Voltaren Ophthalmic®** *see* Diclofenac (Ophthalmic) *on page 535*
- **Voltaren®-XR** *see* Diclofenac (Systemic) *on page 531*
- **Voraxaze** *see* Glucarpidase *on page 885*
- **Voraxaze®** *see* Glucarpidase *on page 885*

Voriconazole (vor i KOE na zole)

Medication Safety Issues
Sound-alike/look-alike issues:
Voriconazole may be confused with fluconazole

Brand Names: U.S. VFEND®

Brand Names: Canada VFEND®

Index Terms UK109496

Generic Availability (U.S.) Yes: Excludes powder for suspension

Pharmacologic Category Antifungal Agent, Oral; Antifungal Agent, Parenteral

Use Treatment of invasive aspergillosis; treatment of esophageal candidiasis; treatment of candidemia (in non-neutropenic patients); treatment of disseminated *Candida* infections of the skin and viscera; treatment of serious fungal infections caused by *Scedosporium apiospermum* and *Fusarium* spp (including *Fusarium solani*) in patients intolerant of, or refractory to, other therapy

Unlabeled Use Fungal infection prophylaxis in intermediate or high risk neutropenic cancer patients with myelodysplastic syndrome (MDS) or acute myelogenous leukemia (AML), neutropenic allogeneic hematopoietic stem cell recipients, and patients with significant graft-versus-host disease; empiric antifungal therapy (second-line) for persistent neutropenic fever

Contraindications Hypersensitivity to voriconazole or any component of the formulation (cross-reaction with other azole antifungal agents may occur but has not been established, use caution); coadministration of CYP3A4 substrates which may lead to QT$_c$ prolongation (cisapride, pimozide, or quinidine); coadministration with barbiturates (long acting), carbamazepine, efavirenz (with standard [eg, not adjusted] voriconazole and efavirenz doses), ergot derivatives, rifampin, rifabutin, ritonavir (≥800 mg/day), sirolimus, St John's wort

Warnings/Precautions Visual changes, including blurred vision, changes in visual acuity, color perception, and photophobia, are commonly associated with treatment; postmarketing cases of optic neuritis and papilledema (lasting >1 month) have also been reported. Patients should be warned to avoid tasks which depend on vision, including operating machinery or driving. Changes are reversible on discontinuation following brief exposure/treatment regimens (≤28 days).

Serious hepatic reactions (including hepatitis, cholestasis, and fulminant hepatic failure) have occurred during treatment, primarily in patients with serious concomitant medical conditions. However, hepatotoxicity has occurred in patients with no identifiable risk factors. Use caution in patients with pre-existing hepatic impairment (dose adjustment or discontinuation may be required).

Voriconazole tablets contain lactose; avoid administration in hereditary galactose intolerance, Lapp lactase deficiency, or glucose-galactose malabsorption. Suspension contains sucrose; use caution with fructose intolerance, sucrase-isomaltase deficiency, or glucose-galactose malabsorption. Avoid/limit use of intravenous formulation in patients with renal impairment; intravenous formulation contains excipient cyclodextrin (sulfobutyl ether beta-cyclodextrin), which may accumulate in renal insufficiency. Acute renal failure has been observed in severely ill patients; use with caution in patients receiving concomitant nephrotoxic medications. Anaphylactoid-type infusion-related reactions may occur with intravenous dosing. Consider discontinuation of infusion if reaction is severe.

Use caution in patients taking strong cytochrome P450 inducers, CYP2C9 inhibitors, and major 3A4 substrates (see Drug Interactions); consider alternative agents that avoid or lessen the potential for CYP-mediated interactions. QT interval prolongation has been associated with voriconazole use; rare cases of arrhythmia (including torsade de pointes), cardiac arrest, and sudden death have been reported, usually in seriously ill patients with comorbidities and/or risk factors (eg, prior cardiotoxic chemotherapy, cardiomyopathy, electrolyte imbalance, or concomitant QT_c-prolonging drugs). Use with caution in these patient populations; correct electrolyte abnormalities (eg, hypokalemia, hypomagnesemia, hypocalcemia) prior to initiating therapy. Do not infuse concomitantly with blood products or short-term concentrated electrolyte solutions, even if the two infusions are running in separate intravenous lines (or cannulas).

Rare cases of malignancy (melanoma, squamous cell carcinoma) have been reported in patients (mostly immunocompromised) with prior onset of severe photosensitivity reactions and exposure to long-term voriconazole therapy. Other serious exfoliative cutaneous reactions, including Stevens-Johnson syndrome, have also been reported. Patient should avoid strong, direct exposure to sunlight; may cause photosensitivity, especially with long-term use. Discontinue use in patients who develop an exfoliative cutaneous reaction or a skin lesion consistent with squamous cell carcinoma or melanoma. Periodic total body skin examinations should be performed, particularly with prolonged use.

Monitor pancreatic function in patients at risk for acute pancreatitis (eg, recent chemotherapy or hematopoietic stem cell transplantation); there have been postmarketing reports of pancreatitis in children.

Adverse Reactions (Reflective of adult population; not specific for elderly)

>10%:

Central nervous system: Hallucinations (4% to 12%; auditory and/or visual and likely serum concentration-dependent)

Ocular: Visual changes (dose related; photophobia, color changes, increased or decreased visual acuity, or blurred vision occur in ~21%)

Renal: Creatinine increased (1% to 21%)

2% to 10%:

Cardiovascular: Tachycardia (≤2%)

Central nervous system: Fever (≤6%), chills (≤4%), headache (≤3%)

Dermatologic: Rash (≤7%)

Endocrine & metabolic: Hypokalemia (≤2%)

Gastrointestinal: Nausea (1% to 5%), vomiting (1% to 4%)

Hepatic: Alkaline phosphatase increased (4% to 5%), AST increased (2% to 4%), ALT increased (2% to 3%), cholestatic jaundice (1% to 2%)

Ocular: Photophobia (2% to 3%)

Drug Interactions

Metabolism/Transport Effects Substrate of CYP2C19 (major), CYP2C9 (major), CYP3A4 (minor); **Note:** Assignment of Major/Minor substrate status based on clinically relevant drug interaction potential; **Inhibits** CYP2C19 (moderate), CYP2C9 (moderate), CYP3A4 (strong)

Avoid Concomitant Use

Avoid concomitant use of Voriconazole with any of the following: Alfuzosin; Apixaban; Avanafil; Axitinib; Barbiturates; CarBAMazepine; Cisapride; Clopidogrel; Conivaptan; Crizotinib; Darunavir; Dihydroergotamine; Dofetilide; Dronedarone; Eplerenone; Ergoloid Mesylates; Ergonovine; Ergotamine; Everolimus; Fluconazole; Fluticasone (Oral Inhalation); Halofantrine; Highest Risk QTc-Prolonging Agents; Lapatinib; Lopinavir; Lovastatin; Lurasidone; Methylergonovine; Mifepristone; Nilotinib; Nisoldipine; Pimozide; QuiNIDine; Ranolazine; Red Yeast Rice; Rifamycin Derivatives; Ritonavir; Rivaroxaban; RomiDEPsin;

Salmeterol; Silodosin; Simvastatin; Sirolimus; St Johns Wort; Tamsulosin; Ticagrelor; Tolvaptan; Toremifene

Increased Effect/Toxicity

Voriconazole may increase the levels/effects of: Alfentanil; Alfuzosin; Almotriptan; Alosetron; Antineoplastic Agents (Vinca Alkaloids); Apixaban; Aprepitant; ARIPiprazole; AtorvaSTATin; Avanafil; Axitinib; Benzodiazepines (metabolized by oxidation); Boceprevir; Bortezomib; Bosentan; Brentuximab Vedotin; Brinzolamide; Budesonide (Nasal); Budesonide (Systemic, Oral Inhalation); BusPIRone; Busulfan; Calcium Channel Blockers; CarBAMazepine; Carvedilol; Ciclesonide; Cilostazol; Cinacalcet; Cisapride; Colchicine; Conivaptan; Contraceptives (Estrogens); Contraceptives (Progestins); Corticosteroids (Orally Inhaled); Corticosteroids (Systemic); Crizotinib; CycloSPORINE; CycloSPORINE (Systemic); CYP2C19 Substrates; CYP2C9 Substrates; CYP3A4 Substrates; Diclofenac; Diclofenac (Systemic); Diclofenac (Topical); Dienogest; Dihydroergotamine; DOCEtaxel; Dofetilide; Dronedarone; Dutasteride; Eletriptan; Eplerenone; Ergoloid Mesylates; Ergonovine; Ergotamine; Erlotinib; Eszopiclone; Etravirine; Everolimus; FentaNYL; Fesoterodine; Fluticasone (Nasal); Fluticasone (Oral Inhalation); Fosaprepitant; Fosphenytoin; Gefitinib; GuanFACINE; Halofantrine; Highest Risk QTc-Prolonging Agents; Ibuprofen; Iloperidone; Imatinib; Irinotecan; Ivacaftor; Ixabepilone; Lapatinib; Losartan; Lovastatin; Lumefantrine; Lurasidone; Macrolide Antibiotics; Maraviroc; Meloxicam; Methadone; Methylergonovine; MethylPREDNISolone; Mifepristone; Moderate Risk QTc-Prolonging Agents; Nilotinib; Nisoldipine; OxyCODONE; Paricalcitol; Pazopanib; Phenytoin; Pimecrolimus; Pimozide; Propafenone; Protease Inhibitors; QuiNIDine; Ramelteon; Ranolazine; Red Yeast Rice; Repaglinide; Reverse Transcriptase Inhibitors (Non-Nucleoside); Rifamycin Derivatives; Rivaroxaban; RomiDEPsin; Ruxolitinib; Salmeterol; Saxagliptin; Sildenafil; Silodosin; Simvastatin; Sirolimus; Solifenacin; SORAfenib; Sulfonylureas; SUNItinib; Tacrolimus; Tacrolimus (Systemic); Tacrolimus (Topical); Tadalafil; Tamsulosin; Telaprevir; Ticagrelor; Tolterodine; Tolvaptan; Toremifene; Vardenafil; Vemurafenib; Venlafaxine; Vilazodone; Vitamin K Antagonists; Ziprasidone; Zolpidem; Zuclopenthixol

The levels/effects of Voriconazole may be increased by: Boceprevir; Chloramphenicol; Contraceptives (Estrogens); Contraceptives (Progestins); CYP2C19 Inhibitors (Moderate); CYP2C19 Inhibitors (Strong); CYP2C9 Inhibitors (Moderate); CYP2C9 Inhibitors (Strong); Etravirine; Fluconazole; Grapefruit Juice; Macrolide Antibiotics; Mifepristone; Protease Inhibitors; Proton Pump Inhibitors; QTc-Prolonging Agents (Indeterminate Risk and Risk Modifying); Telaprevir

Decreased Effect

Voriconazole may decrease the levels/effects of: Amphotericin B; Clopidogrel; Ifosfamide; Prasugrel; Saccharomyces boulardii; Ticagrelor

The levels/effects of Voriconazole may be decreased by: Barbiturates; CarBAMazepine; CYP2C19 Inducers (Strong); CYP2C9 Inducers (Strong); Darunavir; Didanosine; Etravirine; Fosphenytoin; Lopinavir; Peginterferon Alfa-2b; Phenytoin; Reverse Transcriptase Inhibitors (Non-Nucleoside); Rifamycin Derivatives; Ritonavir; St Johns Wort; Sucralfate; Telaprevir; Tocilizumab

Ethanol/Nutrition/Herb Interactions

Food: Food may decrease voriconazole absorption. Grapefruit juice may decrease voriconazole levels. Management: Oral voriconazole should be taken 1 hour before or 1 hour after a meal. Avoid grapefruit juice. Maintain adequate hydration unless instructed to restrict fluid intake.

Herb/Nutraceutical: St John's wort may decrease voriconazole levels. Management: Concurrent use of St John's wort with voriconazole is contraindicated.

Stability

Powder for injection: Store at 15°C to 30°C (59°F to 86°F). Reconstitute 200 mg vial with 19 mL of sterile water for injection (use of automated syringe is not recommended). Resultant solution (20 mL) has a concentration of 10 mg/mL. Prior to infusion, must dilute to 0.5-5 mg/mL with NS, LR, D$_5$WLR, D$_5$W^1/$_2$NS, D$_5$W, D$_5$W with KCl 20 mEq, ^{1}/$_2$NS, or D$_5$WNS. Do not dilute with 4.2% sodium bicarbonate infusion. Reconstituted solutions are stable for up to 24 hours under refrigeration at 2°C to 8°C (36°F to 46°F).

Powder for oral suspension: Store at 2°C to 8°C (36°F to 46°F). Add 46 mL of water to the bottle to make 40 mg/mL suspension. Reconstituted oral suspension may be stored at 15°C to 30°C (59°F to 86°F). Discard after 14 days.

Tablets: Store at 15°C to 30°C (59°F to 86°F).

Mechanism of Action Interferes with fungal cytochrome P450 activity (selectively inhibits 14-alpha-lanosterol demethylation), decreasing ergosterol synthesis (principal sterol in fungal cell membrane) and inhibiting fungal cell membrane formation.

VORICONAZOLE

Pharmacodynamics/Kinetics
Absorption: Well absorbed after oral administration; administration of crushed tablets is considered bioequivalent to whole tablets
Distribution: V_d: 4.6 L/kg
Protein binding: 58%
Metabolism: Hepatic, via CYP2C19 (major pathway) and CYP2C9 and CYP3A4 (less significant); saturable (may demonstrate nonlinearity)
Bioavailability: 96%
Half-life elimination: Variable, dose-dependent
Time to peak: Oral: 1-2 hours; 0.5 hours (crushed tablet)
Excretion: Urine (as inactive metabolites; <2% as unchanged drug)

Dosage
Geriatric & Adult
Aspergillosis, invasive, including disseminated and extrapulmonary infection: Duration of therapy should be a minimum of 6-12 weeks or throughout period of immunosuppression (Walsh, 2008):
I.V.: Initial: Loading dose: 6 mg/kg every 12 hours for 2 doses; followed by maintenance dose of 4 mg/kg every 12 hours
Oral: Maintenance dose:
Manufacturer's recommendations:
Patients <40 kg: 100 mg every 12 hours; maximum: 300 mg/day
Patients ≥40 kg: 200 mg every 12 hours; maximum: 600 mg/day
IDSA recommendations (Walsh, 2008): May consider oral therapy in place of I.V. with dosing of 4 mg/kg (rounded up to convenient tablet dosage form) every 12 hours; however, I.V. administration is preferred in serious infections since comparative efficacy with the oral formulation has not been established.

Scedosporiosis, fusariosis:
I.V.: Initial: Loading dose: 6 mg/kg every 12 hours for 2 doses; followed by maintenance dose of 4 mg/kg every 12 hours
Oral: Maintenance dose:
Patients <40 kg: 100 mg every 12 hours; maximum 300 mg/day
Patients ≥40 kg: 200 mg every 12 hours; maximum: 600 mg/day

Candidemia and other deep tissue *Candida* infections: Treatment should continue for a minimum of 14 days following resolution of symptoms or following last positive culture, whichever is longer.
I.V.: Initial: Loading dose 6 mg/kg every 12 hours for 2 doses; followed by maintenance dose of 3-4 mg/kg every 12 hours
Oral:
Manufacturer's recommendations: Maintenance dose:
Patients <40 kg: 100 mg every 12 hours; maximum: 300 mg/day
Patients ≥40 kg: 200 mg every 12 hours; maximum: 600 mg/day
IDSA recommendations (Pappas, 2009): Initial: Loading dose: 400 mg every 12 hours for 2 doses; followed by 200 mg every 12 hours

Endophthalmitis, fungal (unlabeled use; Pappas, 2009): I.V.: 6 mg/kg every 12 hours for 2 doses, then 3-4 mg/kg every 12 hours

Esophageal candidiasis: Oral: Treatment should continue for a minimum of 14 days, and for at least 7 days following resolution of symptoms:
Patients <40 kg: 100 mg every 12 hours; maximum: 300 mg/day
Patients ≥40 kg: 200 mg every 12 hours; maximum: 600 mg/day

Dosage adjustment in patients unable to tolerate treatment:
I.V.: Dose may be reduced to 3 mg/kg every 12 hours
Oral: Dose may be reduced in 50 mg decrements to a minimum dosage of 200 mg every 12 hours in patients weighing ≥40 kg (100 mg every 12 hours in patients <40 kg)

Dosage adjustment in patients receiving concomitant CYP450 enzyme inducers or substrates:
Efavirenz: Oral: Increase maintenance dose of voriconazole to 400 mg every 12 hours and reduce efavirenz dose to 300 mg once daily; upon discontinuation of voriconazole, return to the initial dose of efavirenz
Phenytoin:
I.V.: Increase voriconazole maintenance dosage to 5 mg/kg every 12 hours
Oral: Increase voriconazole dose to 400 mg every 12 hours in patients ≥40 kg (200 mg every 12 hours in patients <40 kg)

Renal Impairment In patients with Cl_{cr} <50 mL/minute, accumulation of the intravenous vehicle (cyclodextrin) occurs. After initial I.V. loading dose, oral voriconazole should be administered to these patients, unless an assessment of the benefit:risk to the patient justifies the use of I.V. voriconazole. Monitor serum creatinine and change to oral voriconazole therapy when possible.

Oral: Poorly dialyzed; no supplemental dose or dosage adjustment necessary, including patients on intermittent hemodialysis, peritoneal dialysis, or continuous renal replacement therapy (eg, CVVHD).

Note: I.V. dosing **NOT** recommended since cyclodextrin vehicle is cleared at half the rate of voriconazole and may accumulate.

Hepatic Impairment

Mild-to-moderate hepatic dysfunction (Child-Pugh class A or B): Following standard loading dose, reduce maintenance dosage by 50%

Severe hepatic impairment: Should only be used if benefit outweighs risk; monitor closely for toxicity

Administration

Oral: Administer 1 hour before or 1 hour after a meal.

I.V.: Infuse over 1-2 hours (rate not to exceed 3 mg/kg/hour). Do not infuse concomitantly into same line or cannula with other drug infusions, including TPN.

Monitoring Parameters Hepatic function at initiation and during course of treatment; renal function; serum electrolytes (particularly calcium, magnesium and potassium) prior to therapy initiation; visual function (visual acuity, visual field and color perception) if treatment course continues >28 days; may consider obtaining voriconazole trough level in patients failing therapy or exhibiting signs of toxicity; pancreatic function (in patients at risk for acute pancreatitis); total body skin examination yearly (more frequently if lesions noted)

Special Geriatric Considerations The manufacturer reports that median voriconazole plasma concentrations were increased in patients 65 years and older compared to those 65 years and younger. The recommendation that a dose adjustment is not needed for the elderly was based on a similar safety profile between young and older patients.

Dosage Forms Excipient information presented when available (limited, particularly for generics); consult specific product labeling.

Injection, powder for reconstitution: 200 mg

VFEND®: 200 mg [contains cyclodextrin]

Powder for suspension, oral:

VFEND®: 40 mg/mL (70 mL) [contains sodium benzoate, sucrose; orange flavor]

Tablet, oral: 50 mg, 200 mg

VFEND®: 50 mg, 200 mg [contains lactose]

◆ **VoSpire ER®** see Albuterol on page 49
◆ **VSL #3® [OTC]** see Lactobacillus on page 1084
◆ **VSL #3®-DS** see Lactobacillus on page 1084
◆ **Vytorin®** see Ezetimibe and Simvastatin on page 739
◆ **VZV Vaccine (Zoster)** see Zoster Vaccine on page 2071

Warfarin (WAR far in)

Related Information

Antithrombotic Therapy in Adult Patients With Prosthetic Heart Valves on page 2182

Injectable Heparins/Heparinoids Comparison Table on page 2119

Perioperative/Periprocedural Management of Anticoagulant and Antiplatelet Therapy on page 2209

Treatment of Elevated INR Due to Warfarin on page 2216

Medication Safety Issues

Sound-alike/look-alike issues:

Coumadin® may be confused with Avandia®, Cardura®, Compazine®, Kemadrin

Jantoven® may be confused with Janumet®, Januvia®

High alert medication:

The Institute for Safe Medication Practices (ISMP) includes this medication among its list of drugs which have a heightened risk of causing significant patient harm when used in error.

National Patient Safety Goals:

The Joint Commission on Accreditation of Healthcare Organizations requires healthcare organizations that provide anticoagulant therapy to have a process in place to reduce the risk of anticoagulant-associated patient harm. Patients receiving anticoagulants should receive individualized care through a defined process that includes standardized ordering, dispensing, administration, monitoring and education. This does not apply to routine short-term use of anticoagulants for prevention of venous thromboembolism when the expectation is that the patient's laboratory values will remain within or close to normal values (NPSG.03.05.01).

Brand Names: U.S. Coumadin®; Jantoven®

Brand Names: Canada Apo-Warfarin®; Coumadin®; Mylan-Warfarin; Novo-Warfarin; Taro-Warfarin

Index Terms Warfarin Sodium

Generic Availability (U.S.) Yes: Tablet

Pharmacologic Category Anticoagulant, Coumarin Derivative; Vitamin K Antagonist

Use Prophylaxis and treatment of thromboembolic disorders (eg, venous, pulmonary) and embolic complications arising from atrial fibrillation or cardiac valve replacement; adjunct to reduce risk of systemic embolism (eg, recurrent MI, stroke) after myocardial infarction

Unlabeled Use Prevention of recurrent transient ischemic attacks

Medication Guide Available Yes

Contraindications Hypersensitivity to warfarin or any component of the formulation; hemorrhagic tendencies; patients bleeding from the GI, respiratory, or GU tract; cerebral aneurysm; cerebrovascular hemorrhage; dissecting aortic aneurysm; spinal puncture and other diagnostic or therapeutic procedures with potential for significant bleeding; history of bleeding diathesis); recent or potential surgery of the eye or CNS; major regional lumbar block anesthesia or traumatic surgery resulting in large, open surfaces; blood dyscrasias; severe uncontrolled or malignant hypertension; pericarditis or pericardial effusion; bacterial endocarditis; unsupervised patients with conditions associated with a high potential for non-compliance

Warnings/Precautions Hazardous agent - use appropriate precautions for handling and disposal. Use care in the selection of patients appropriate for this treatment. Ensure patient cooperation especially from the alcoholic, illicit drug user, demented, or psychotic patient; ability to comply with routine laboratory monitoring is essential. Use with caution in trauma, acute infection, moderate-severe renal insufficiency, prolonged dietary insufficiencies, moderate-severe hypertension, polycythemia vera, vasculitis, open wound, active TB, any disruption in normal GI flora, history of PUD, anaphylactic disorders, indwelling catheters, and severe diabetes. Use with caution in patients with thyroid disease; warfarin responsiveness may increase (Ageno, 2012). Use with caution in protein C deficiency. Use with caution in patients with heparin-induced thrombocytopenia and DVT. Warfarin monotherapy is contraindicated in the initial treatment of active HIT. Reduced liver function, regardless of etiology, may impair synthesis of coagulation factors leading to increased warfarin sensitivity.

[U.S. Boxed Warning]: May cause major or fatal bleeding. Risk factors for bleeding include high intensity anticoagulation (INR >4), age (>65 years), variable INRs, history of GI bleeding, hypertension, cerebrovascular disease, serious heart disease, anemia, malignancy, trauma, renal insufficiency, drug-drug interactions, long duration of therapy, or known genetic deficiency in CYP2C9 activity. Patient must be instructed to report bleeding, accidents, or falls. Unrecognized bleeding sites (eg, colon cancer) may be uncovered by anticoagulation. Patient must also report any new or discontinued medications, herbal or alternative products used, or significant changes in smoking or dietary habits. Necrosis or gangrene of the skin and other tissue can occur, usually in conjunction with protein C or S deficiency. Consider alternative therapies if anticoagulation is necessary. Warfarin therapy may release atheromatous plaque emboli; symptoms depend on site of embolization, most commonly kidneys, pancreas, liver, and spleen. In some cases may lead to necrosis or death. "Purple toes syndrome," due to cholesterol microembolization, may rarely occur. The elderly may be more sensitive to anticoagulant therapy.

Presence of the CYP2C9*2 or *3 allele and/or polymorphism of the vitamin K oxidoreductase (VKORC1) gene may increase the risk of bleeding. Lower doses may be required in these patients; genetic testing may help determine appropriate dosing.

When temporary interruption is necessary before surgery, discontinue for approximately 5 days before surgery; when there is adequate hemostasis, may reinstitute warfarin therapy ~12-24 hours after surgery (evening of or next morning). Decision to safely continue warfarin therapy through the procedure and whether or not bridging of anticoagulation is necessary is dependent upon risk of perioperative bleeding and risk of thromboembolism, respectively. If risk of thromboembolism is elevated, consider bridging warfarin therapy with an alternative anticoagulant (eg, unfractionated heparin, LMWH) (Guyatt, 2012).

Adverse Reactions (Reflective of adult population; not specific for elderly) Bleeding is the major adverse effect of warfarin. Hemorrhage may occur at virtually any site. Risk is dependent on multiple variables, including the intensity of anticoagulation and patient susceptibility.

Cardiovascular: Vasculitis

Central nervous system: Signs/symptoms of bleeding (eg, dizziness, fatigue, fever, headache, lethargy, malaise, pain)

Dermatologic: Alopecia, bullous eruptions, dermatitis, rash, pruritus, urticaria

Gastrointestinal: Abdominal pain, diarrhea, flatulence, gastrointestinal bleeding, nausea, taste disturbance, vomiting

Genitourinary: Hematuria

Hematologic: Anemia, retroperitoneal hematoma, unrecognized bleeding sites (eg, colon cancer) may be uncovered by anticoagulation

Hepatic: Hepatitis (including cholestatic hepatitis), transaminases increased

Neuromuscular & skeletal: Osteoporosis (potential association with long-term use), paralysis, paresthesia, weakness

Respiratory: Respiratory tract bleeding, tracheobronchial calcification

Miscellaneous: Anaphylactic reaction, hypersensitivity/allergic reactions, skin necrosis, gangrene, "purple toes" syndrome

Drug Interactions

Metabolism/Transport Effects Substrate of CYP1A2 (minor), CYP2C19 (minor), CYP2C9 (major), CYP3A4 (minor); **Note:** Assignment of Major/Minor substrate status based on clinically relevant drug interaction potential; **Inhibits** CYP2C19 (weak), CYP2C9 (weak)

Avoid Concomitant Use

Avoid concomitant use of Warfarin with any of the following: Rivaroxaban; Tamoxifen

Increased Effect/Toxicity

Warfarin may increase the levels/effects of: Anticoagulants; Collagenase (Systemic); Dabigatran Etexilate; Deferasirox; Drotrecogin Alfa (Activated); Ethotoin; Fosphenytoin; Phenytoin; Rivaroxaban; Sulfonylureas

The levels/effects of Warfarin may be increased by: Acetaminophen; Allopurinol; Amiodarone; Androgens; Antineoplastic Agents; Antiplatelet Agents; Atazanavir; Bicalutamide; Boceprevir; Capecitabine; Cephalosporins; Chloral Hydrate; Chloramphenicol; Cimetidine; Clopidogrel; Corticosteroids (Systemic); Cranberry; CYP2C9 Inhibitors (Moderate); CYP2C9 Inhibitors (Strong); Desvenlafaxine; Dexmethylphenidate; Disulfiram; Dronedarone; Efavirenz; Erythromycin (Ophthalmic); Esomeprazole; Ethacrynic Acid; Ethotoin; Etoposide; Exenatide; Fenofibrate; Fenofibric Acid; Fenugreek; Fibric Acid Derivatives; Fluconazole; Fluorouracil; Fluorouracil (Systemic); Fluorouracil (Topical); Fosamprenavir; Fosphenytoin; Gefitinib; Ginkgo Biloba; Glucagon; Green Tea; Herbs (Anticoagulant/Antiplatelet Properties); HMG-CoA Reductase Inhibitors; Ifosfamide; Imatinib; Itraconazole; Ivermectin; Ivermectin (Systemic); Ketoconazole; Ketoconazole (Systemic); Lansoprazole; Leflunomide; Macrolide Antibiotics; Methylphenidate; MetroNIDAZOLE; MetroNIDAZOLE (Systemic); Miconazole (Oral); Miconazole (Topical); Mifepristone; Milnacipran; Mirtazapine; Nelfinavir; Neomycin; NSAID (COX-2 Inhibitor); NSAID (Nonselective); Omega-3-Acid Ethyl Esters; Omeprazole; Orlistat; Penicillins; Pentosan Polysulfate Sodium; Pentoxifylline; Phenytoin; Posaconazole; Propafenone; Prostacyclin Analogues; QuiNIDine; QuiNINE; Quinolone Antibiotics; Ranitidine; RomiDEPsin; Salicylates; Saquinavir; Selective Serotonin Reuptake Inhibitors; Sitaxentan; SORAfenib; Sulfinpyrazone [Off Market]; Sulfonamide Derivatives; Sulfonylureas; Tamoxifen; Telaprevir; Tetracycline Derivatives; Thrombolytic Agents; Thyroid Products; Tigecycline; Tipranavir; Tolterodine; Toremifene; Torsemide; TraMADol; Tricyclic Antidepressants; Venlafaxine; Vitamin E; Voriconazole; Vorinostat; Zafirlukast; Zileuton

Decreased Effect

The levels/effects of Warfarin may be decreased by: Aminoglutethimide; Antineoplastic Agents; Antithyroid Agents; Aprepitant; AzaTHIOprine; Barbiturates; Bile Acid Sequestrants; Boceprevir; Bosentan; CarBAMazepine; Coenzyme Q-10; Contraceptives (Estrogens); Contraceptives (Progestins); CYP2C9 Inducers (Strong); Darunavir; Dicloxacillin; Efavirenz; Fosaprepitant; Ginseng (American); Glutethimide; Green Tea; Griseofulvin; Lopinavir; Mercaptopurine; Nafcillin; Nelfinavir; Peginterferon Alfa-2b; Phytonadione; Rifamycin Derivatives; Ritonavir; St Johns Wort; Sucralfate; Telaprevir; Tocilizumab; TraZODone

Ethanol/Nutrition/Herb Interactions

Ethanol: Acute ethanol ingestion (binge drinking) decreases the metabolism of warfarin and increases PT/INR. Chronic daily ethanol use increases the metabolism of warfarin and decreases PT/INR. Management: Avoid ethanol.

Food: The anticoagulant effects of warfarin may be decreased if taken with foods rich in vitamin K. Vitamin E may increase warfarin effect. Cranberry juice may increase warfarin effect. Management: Maintain a consistent diet; consult prescriber before making changes in diet. Take warfarin at the same time each day.

Herb/Nutraceutical: Some herbal medications (eg, St John's wort) may decrease warfarin levels and effects; many others can add additional antiplatelet activity to warfarin therapy. Management: Avoid ginseng (American), coenzyme Q_{10}, and St John's wort. Avoid cranberry, fenugreek, ginkgo biloba, glucosamine, alfalfa, anise, bilberry, bladderwrack, bromelain, cat's claw, celery, chamomile, coleus, cordyceps, dong quai, evening primrose oil, fenugreek, feverfew, garlic, ginger, ginkgo biloba, ginseng (Panax), ginseng (Siberian), grapeseed, green tea, guggul, horse chestnut seed, horseradish, licorice, omega-3-acids, prickly ash, red clover, reishi, SAMe (s-adenosylmethionine), sweet clover, turmeric, and white willow.

Stability

Injection: Prior to reconstitution, store at 15°C to 30°C (59°F to 86°F). Following reconstitution with 2.7 mL of sterile water (yields 2 mg/mL solution), stable for 4 hours at 15°C to 30°C (59°F to 86°F). Protect from light.

Tablet: Store at 15°C to 30°C (59°F to 86°F). Protect from light.

Mechanism of Action
Hepatic synthesis of coagulation factors II, VII, IX, and X, as well as proteins C and S, requires the presence of vitamin K. These clotting factors are biologically activated by the addition of carboxyl groups to key glutamic acid residues within the proteins' structure. In the process, "active" vitamin K is oxidatively converted to an "inactive" form, which is then subsequently reactivated by vitamin K epoxide reductase complex 1 (VKORC1). Warfarin competitively inhibits the subunit 1 of the multi-unit VKOR complex, thus depleting functional vitamin K reserves and hence reduces synthesis of active clotting factors.

Pharmacodynamics/Kinetics

Onset of action: Anticoagulation: Oral: 24-72 hours

Peak effect: Full therapeutic effect: 5-7 days; INR may increase in 36-72 hours

Duration: 2-5 days

Absorption: Oral: Rapid, complete

Distribution: 0.14 L/kg

Protein binding: 99%

Metabolism: Hepatic, primarily via CYP2C9; minor pathways include CYP2C8, 2C18, 2C19, 1A2, and 3A4

Genomic variants: Approximately 37% reduced clearance of S-warfarin in patients heterozygous for 2C9 (*1/*2 or *1/*3), and ~70% reduced in patients homozygous for reduced function alleles (*2/*2, *2/*3, or *3/*3)

Half-life elimination: 20-60 hours; Mean: 40 hours; highly variable among individuals

Time to peak, plasma: Oral: ~4 hours

Excretion: Urine (92%, primarily as metabolites)

Dosage

Geriatric Oral: Initial dose ≤5 mg. Usual maintenance dose: 2-5 mg/day. The elderly tend to require lower dosages to produce a therapeutic level of anticoagulation (due to changes in the pattern of warfarin metabolism).

Adult Note: Labeling identifies genetic factors which may increase patient sensitivity to warfarin. Specifically, genetic variations in the proteins CYP2C9 and VKORC1, responsible for warfarin's primary metabolism and pharmacodynamic activity, respectively, have been identified as predisposing factors associated with decreased dose requirement and increased bleeding risk. Genotyping tests are available, and may provide guidance on initiation of anticoagulant therapy. The American College of Chest Physicians recommends against the use of routine pharmacogenomic testing to guide dosing (Guyatt, 2012). For management of elevated INRs as a result of warfarin therapy, see Pharmacotherapy Pearls for guidance.

Prevention/treatment of thrombosis/embolism:

I.V. (administer as a slow bolus injection): 2-5 mg/day

Oral: Initial dosing must be individualized. Consider the patient (hepatic function, cardiac function, age, nutritional status, concurrent therapy, risk of bleeding) in addition to prior dose response (if available) and the clinical situation. Start 2-5 mg once daily for 2 days **or** for healthy individuals, 10 mg once daily for 2 days; lower doses (eg, 5 mg once daily) recommended for patients with confirmed HIT once platelet recovery has occurred (Guyatt, 2012). In patients with acute venous thromboembolism, initiation may begin on the first or second day of low molecular weight heparin or unfractionated heparin therapy (Guyatt, 2012). Adjust dose according to INR results; usual maintenance dose ranges from 2-10 mg daily (individual patients may require loading and maintenance doses outside these general guidelines).

Note: Lower starting doses may be required for patients with hepatic impairment, poor nutrition, CHF, elderly, high risk of bleeding, or patients who are debilitated, or those with reduced function genomic variants of the catabolic enzymes CYP2C9 (*2 or *3 alleles) or VKORC1 (-1639 polymorphism); see table on next page. Higher initial doses may be reasonable in selected patients (ie, receiving enzyme-inducing agents and with low risk of bleeding).

Range[1] of Expected Therapeutic Maintenance Dose Based on CYP2C9[2] and VKORC1[3] Genotypes

VKORC1	CYP2C9					
	*1/*1	*1/*2	*1/*3	*2/*2	*2/*3	*3/*3
GG	5-7 mg	5-7 mg	3-4 mg	3-4 mg	3-4 mg	0.5-2 mg
AG	5-7 mg	3-4 mg	3-4 mg	3-4 mg	0.5-2 mg	0.5-2 mg
AA	3-4 mg	3-4 mg	0.5-2 mg	0.5-2 mg	0.5-2 mg	0.5-2 mg

Note: Must also take into account other patient related factors when determining initial dose (eg, age, body weight, concomitant medications, comorbidities). The American College of Chest Physicians recommends against the use of routine pharmacogenomic testing to guide dosing (Guyatt, 2012).

[1]Ranges derived from multiple published clinical studies.

[2]Patients with CYP2C9 *1/*3, *2/*2, *2/*3, and *3/*3 alleles may take up to 4 weeks to achieve maximum INR with a given dose regimen.

[3]VKORC1 -1639G>A (rs 9923231) variant is used in this table; other VKORC1 variants may also be important determinants of dose.

Renal Impairment No adjustment required, however, patients with renal failure have an increased risk of bleeding complications. Monitor closely.

Hepatic Impairment Monitor effect at usual doses. The response to oral anticoagulants may be markedly enhanced in obstructive jaundice, hepatitis, and cirrhosis. INR should be closely monitored.

Administration
Oral: Administer with or without food. Take at the same time each day.
I.V.: Administer as a slow bolus injection over 1-2 minutes; avoid all I.M. injections

Monitoring Parameters Prothrombin time, hematocrit; INR (frequency varies depending on INR stability); may consider genotyping of CYP2C9 and VKORC1 prior to initiation of therapy, if available

Reference Range
INR = patient prothrombin time/mean normal prothrombin time
ISI = international sensitivity index
INR should be increased by 2-3.5 times depending upon indication. An INR >4 does not generally add additional therapeutic benefit and is associated with increased risk of bleeding. **Note:** To prevent gastrointestinal bleeding events in patients receiving the combination of warfarin, aspirin, and clopidogrel, an INR of 2-2.5 is recommended unless condition requires a higher INR target (eg, certain mechanical heart valves) (Bhatt, 2008).

Adult Target INR Ranges Based Upon Indication

Indication	Targeted INR	Targeted INR Range
Cardiac		
Anterior myocardial infarction with LV thrombus or high risk for LV thrombus (EF<40%, anteroapical wall motion abnormality)[1,2]	2.5	2-3
Atrial fibrillation or atrial flutter	2.5	2-3
LV systolic dysfunction (without established CAD) with an LV thrombus (eg, Takotsubo cardiomyopathy)	2.5	2-3
Valvular		
Carbomedics or St. Jude Medical bileaflet or Medtronic Hall tilting disk mechanical aortic valve in normal sinus rhythm and normal LA size[3]	2.5	2-3
Bileaflet or tilting disk mechanical mitral valve[3]	3	2.5-3.5
Caged ball or caged disk mechanical valve[3]	3	2.5-3.5
Mechanical aortic valve[4]	2.5	2-3
Mechanical mitral valve **or** mechanical valves in both the aortic and mitral positions[4]	3	2.5-3.5
Bioprosthetic mitral valve[5]	2.5	2-3
Rheumatic mitral valve disease (particularly mitral stenosis) and normal sinus rhythm (LA diameter >5.5 cm), AF, previous systemic embolism, or LA thrombus	2.5	2-3
Thromboembolism Treatment		
Venous thromboembolism[6]	2.5	2-3

(continued)

WARFARIN

Adult Target INR Ranges Based Upon Indication *(continued)*

Indication	Targeted INR	Targeted INR Range
Thromboprophylaxis		
Idiopathic pulmonary artery hypertension (IPAH)[7]	2	1.5-2.5
Antiphospholipid syndrome (no other risk factors)	2.5	2-3
Antiphospholipid syndrome and recurrent thromboembolism	2.5	2-3
Total hip or knee replacement or hip fracture surgery[8]	2.5	2-3
Other Indications		
Ischemic stroke due to AF[9]	2.5	2-3
Cryptogenic stroke (recurrent) and either patent foramen ovale (PFO) or atrial septal aneurysm	2.5	2-3

Note: Unless otherwise noted, all recommendations derived from "Antithrombotic Therapy and Prevention of Thrombosis, 9th ed: American College of Chest Physicians Evidence-Based Clinical Practice Guidelines."

[1]If coronary stent placed, triple therapy (warfarin, low-dose aspirin, and clopidogrel) is recommended for 1 month (bare-metal stent) or 3-6 months (drug-eluting stent) followed by discontinuation of warfarin and use of dual antiplatelet therapy (eg, aspirin and clopidogrel) for up to 12 months.

[2]If coronary stent **not** placed, maintain anticoagulation (in combination with low-dose aspirin) for 3 months followed by discontinuation of warfarin and use of dual antiplatelet therapy (eg, aspirin and clopidogrel) for up to 12 months.

[3]Recommendation from Stein, 2001.

[4]If at low risk of bleeding, combine with aspirin 81 mg/day.

[5]Maintain anticoagulation for 3 months after valve insertion then switch to aspirin 81 mg/day if no other indications for warfarin exist or clinically reassess need for warfarin in patients with prior history of systemic embolism.

[6]Treat for 3 months in patients with provoked VTE due to transient reversible risk factor. Treat for a minimum of 3 months in patients with unprovoked VTE and evaluate for extended anticoagulant therapy (ie, >3 months of therapy without a scheduled stop date). Other risk groups (eg, cancer) may require extended anticoagulant therapy.

[7]Recommendation from the ACCF/AHA 2009 Expert Consensus Document on Pulmonary Hypertension (McLaughlin, 2009)

[8]Continue for at least 10-14 days; up to 35 days after surgery is suggested.

[9]Instead of adjusted dose warfarin, the use of dabigatran has been suggested. In either case, oral anticoagulation should be initiated within 1-2 weeks after stroke onset or earlier in patients at low bleeding risk; bridging with aspirin may be required.

Warfarin levels are not used for monitoring degree of anticoagulation. They may be useful if a patient with unexplained coagulopathy is using the drug surreptitiously or if it is unclear whether clinical resistance is due to true drug resistance or lack of drug intake.

Normal prothrombin time (PT): 10.9-12.9 seconds. Healthy premature newborns have prolonged coagulation test screening results (eg, PT, aPTT, TT) which return to normal adult values at approximately 6 months of age. Healthy prematures, however, do not develop spontaneous hemorrhage or thrombotic complications because of a balance between procoagulants and inhibitors.

Pharmacotherapy Pearls

Pharmacogenomic Testing: The American College of Chest Physicians recommends against the use of routine pharmacogenomic testing to guide dosing (Guyatt, 2012). However, prospective genotyping is available, and may provide guidance on initiation of anticoagulant therapy. Commercial testing with PGxPredict™: WARFARIN is available from PGxHealth™ (Division of Clinical Data, Inc, New Haven, CT). The test genotypes patients for presence of the CYP2C9*2 or *3 alleles and the VKORC1 -1639G>A polymorphism. The results of the test allow patients to be phenotyped as extensive, intermediate, or poor metabolizers (CYP2C9) and as low, intermediate, or high warfarin sensitivity (VKORC1). Ordering information is available at 888-592-7327 or warfarininfo@pgxhealth.com.

Management of Elevated INR:

If INR above therapeutic range to <4.5 (no evidence of bleeding): Lower or hold next dose and monitor frequently; when INR approaches desired range, resume dosing with a lower dose (Patriquin, 2011).

If INR 4.5-10 (no evidence of bleeding): The 2012 ACCP guidelines recommend against routine vitamin K administration in this setting (Guyatt, 2012). Previously, the 2008 ACCP guidelines recommended if no risk factors for bleeding exist, to omit next 1 or 2 doses, monitor INR more frequently, and resume with an appropriately adjusted dose when INR in desired range; may consider administering vitamin K orally 1-2.5 mg if other risk factors for bleeding exist (Hirsh, 2008). Others have recommended consideration of vitamin K 1 mg orally or 0.5 mg I.V. (Patriquin, 2011).

If INR >10 (no evidence of bleeding): The 2012 ACCP guidelines recommend administration of oral vitamin K (dose not specified) in this setting (Guyatt, 2012). Previously, the 2008 ACCP guidelines recommended to hold warfarin, administer vitamin K orally 2.5-5 mg, expect INR to be reduced within 24-48 hours, monitor INR more frequently and give additional vitamin K at an appropriate dose if necessary; resume warfarin at an appropriately adjusted dose when INR is in desired range (Hirsh, 2008). Others have recommended consideration of vitamin K 2-2.5 mg orally or 0.5-1 mg I.V. (Patriquin, 2011).

If minor bleeding at any INR elevation: Hold warfarin, may administer vitamin K orally 2.5-5 mg, monitor INR more frequently, may repeat dose after 24 hours if INR correction incomplete; resume warfarin at an appropriately adjusted dose when INR is in desired range (Patriquin, 2011).

If major bleeding at any INR elevation: The 2012 ACCP guidelines recommend administration of four-factor prothrombin complex concentrate (PCC) and I.V. vitamin K 5-10 mg in this setting (Guyatt, 2012); however, in the U.S., the available PCCs (Bebulin®VH and Profilnine® SD) are three-factor PCCs and do not contain adequate levels of factor VII. Four-factor PCCs include Beriplex® P/N, Cofact®, Konyne®, or Octaplex® all of which are not available in the U.S. Previously, the 2008 ACCP guidelines recommended to hold warfarin, administer vitamin K 10 mg by slow I.V. infusion and supplement with PCC depending on the urgency of the situation; I.V. vitamin K may be repeated every 12 hours (Hirsh, 2008).

Note: Use of high doses of vitamin K (eg, 10-15 mg) may cause warfarin resistance for ≥1 week. During this period of resistance, heparin or low-molecular-weight heparin (LMWH) may be given until INR responds.

Special Geriatric Considerations Before committing an elderly patient to long-term anticoagulation therapy, the risk for bleeding complications secondary to falls, drug interactions, living situation, and cognitive status should be considered. A risk of bleeding complications has been associated with increased age.

Dosage Forms Excipient information presented when available (limited, particularly for generics); consult specific product labeling.

Injection, powder for reconstitution, as sodium:
 Coumadin®: 5 mg
Tablet, oral, as sodium: 1 mg, 2 mg, 2.5 mg, 3 mg, 4 mg, 5 mg, 6 mg, 7.5 mg, 10 mg
 Coumadin®: 1 mg, 2 mg, 2.5 mg, 3 mg, 4 mg, 5 mg, 6 mg, 7.5 mg [scored]
 Coumadin®: 10 mg [scored; dye free]
 Jantoven®: 1 mg, 2 mg, 2.5 mg, 3 mg, 4 mg, 5 mg, 6 mg, 7.5 mg [scored]
 Jantoven®: 10 mg [scored; dye free]

◆ **Warfarin Sodium** *see* Warfarin *on page 2033*
◆ **Wart-Off® Maximum Strength [OTC]** *see* Salicylic Acid *on page 1743*
◆ **Wax Away [OTC]** *see* Carbamide Peroxide *on page 291*
◆ **4-Way® 12 Hour [OTC]** *see* Oxymetazoline (Nasal) *on page 1452*
◆ **4 Way® Fast Acting [OTC]** *see* Phenylephrine (Nasal) *on page 1526*
◆ **4 Way® Menthol [OTC]** *see* Phenylephrine (Nasal) *on page 1526*
◆ **4-Way® Saline Moisturizing Mist [OTC]** *see* Sodium Chloride *on page 1787*
◆ **Welchol®** *see* Colesevelam *on page 440*
◆ **Wellbutrin®** *see* BuPROPion *on page 241*
◆ **Wellbutrin XL®** *see* BuPROPion *on page 241*
◆ **Wellbutrin SR®** *see* BuPROPion *on page 241*
◆ **Westcort®** *see* Hydrocortisone (Topical) *on page 943*
◆ **Westhroid™** *see* Thyroid, Desiccated *on page 1885*

Wheat Dextrin (weet DEKS trin)

Related Information
Laxatives, Classification and Properties *on page 2121*
Brand Names: U.S. Benefiber® Plus Calcium [OTC]; Benefiber® [OTC]
Index Terms Dextrin; Resistant Dextrin; Resistant Maltodextrin
Generic Availability (U.S.) No
Pharmacologic Category Fiber Supplement; Laxative, Bulk-Producing
Use OTC labeling: Dietary fiber supplement
Unlabeled Use Treatment of constipation; aid to enhance LDL lowering to reduce the risk of coronary heart disease
Warnings/Precautions Use with caution in patients with esophageal strictures, ulcers, stenosis, intestinal adhesions, GI obstruction, fecal impaction, or difficulty swallowing. Use with caution in the elderly; may have insufficient fluid intake which may predispose them to fecal impaction and bowel obstruction. To aid in reducing the risk of CHD, the soluble fiber from wheat dextrin should be used in conjunction with a diet low in saturated fat and cholesterol. Some products may contain calcium, potassium, sodium, aspartame, or phenylalanine.
Adverse Reactions (Reflective of adult population; not specific for elderly) Frequency not defined: Gastrointestinal: Bloating, flatulence, GI discomfort

Drug Interactions
Metabolism/Transport Effects None known.
Avoid Concomitant Use There are no known interactions where it is recommended to avoid concomitant use.
Increased Effect/Toxicity There are no known significant interactions involving an increase in effect.
Decreased Effect There are no known significant interactions involving a decrease in effect.
Stability Store at 20°C to 25°C (68°F to 77°F). Protect from moisture.
Mechanism of Action Wheat dextrin is a soluble fiber. It absorbs water in the intestine to form a viscous liquid which promotes peristalsis and reduces transit time.
Dosage
Geriatric & Adult General dosing guidelines; consult specific product labeling.
Adequate intake for total fiber: Oral: **Note:** The definition of "fiber" varies; however, the soluble fiber in wheat dextrin is only one type of fiber which makes up the daily recommended intake of total fiber.
Adults 19-50 years: Male: 38 g/day; Female: 25 g/day
Adults ≥51 years: Male: 30 g/day; Female: 21 g/day
Administration Powder can be mixed into hot or cold beverages (eg, water, coffee, juice), soft foods (eg, applesauce, pudding, yogurt), or cooked into recipes for foods; not recommended for use in carbonated beverages. Caplets should be swallowed with liquid.
Special Geriatric Considerations Elderly may have insufficient fluid intake which may predispose them to fecal impaction and bowel obstruction. Patients should have a 1-month trial, with at least 14 g/day, before effects in bowel function are determined. Bloating and flatulence are mostly a problem in first 4 weeks of therapy.
Dosage Forms Excipient information presented when available (limited, particularly for generics); consult specific product labeling.
Caplet, oral:
Benefiber®: 1.3 g [gluten free, sugar free; provides dietary fiber 3 g and soluble fiber 3 g per 3 caplets]
Powder, oral:
Benefiber®: (80 g, 155 g, 245 g, 350 g, 477 g) [gluten free, sugar free; original flavor]
Benefiber®: (161 g, 267 g, 529 g) [gluten free, sugar free; contains aspartame; orange flavor]
Benefiber®: 3.5 g/packet (28s) [gluten free, sugar free; original flavor; provides dietary fiber 3 g and soluble fiber 3 g per packet]
Benefiber®: 3.5 g/packet (16s) [sugar free; contains phenylalanine; kiwi-strawberry flavor; provides dietary fiber 3 g and soluble fiber 3 g per packet]
Benefiber®: 3.5 g/packet (8s) [sugar free; contains phenylalanine; raspberry tea flavor; provides dietary fiber 3 g and soluble fiber 3 g per packet]
Benefiber®: 3.5 g/packet (8s) [sugar free; contains phenylalanine, sodium 20 mg/packet; cherry-pomegranate flavor; provides dietary fiber 3 g and soluble fiber 3 g per packet]
Benefiber®: 3.5 g/packet (16s) [sugar free; contains phenylalanine, soy; citrus punch flavor; provides dietary fiber 3 g and soluble fiber 3 g per packet]
Benefiber® Plus Calcium: (424 g) [gluten free, sugar free]
Tablet, chewable, oral:
Benefiber®: 2.7 g [gluten free, sugar free; contains phenylalanine, soy; assorted fruit flavor; provides dietary fiber 3 g and soluble fiber 3 g per 3 tablets]
Benefiber®: 2.7 g [gluten free, sugar free; contains phenylalanine, soy; orange créme flavor; provides dietary fiber 3 g and soluble fiber 3 g per 3 tablets]
Benefiber® Plus Calcium: 2.7 g [gluten free, sugar free; contains calcium 100 mg/tablet, phenylalanine, soy; wildberry flavor; provides dietary fiber 3 g and soluble fiber 3 g per 3 tablets]

- ◆ **Xodol® 5/300** *see* Hydrocodone and Acetaminophen *on page 937*
- ◆ **Xodol® 7.5/300** *see* Hydrocodone and Acetaminophen *on page 937*
- ◆ **Xodol® 10/300** *see* Hydrocodone and Acetaminophen *on page 937*
- ◆ **Xolegel®** *see* Ketoconazole (Topical) *on page 1065*
- ◆ **Xopenex®** *see* Levalbuterol *on page 1106*
- ◆ **Xopenex HFA™** *see* Levalbuterol *on page 1106*
- ◆ **XP13512** *see* Gabapentin Enacarbil *on page 861*
- ◆ **Xpect™ [OTC]** *see* GuaiFENesin *on page 904*
- ◆ **Xylocaine®** *see* Lidocaine (Systemic) *on page 1126*
- ◆ **Xylocaine®** *see* Lidocaine (Topical) *on page 1128*
- ◆ **Xylocaine® Dental** *see* Lidocaine (Systemic) *on page 1126*
- ◆ **Xylocaine® MPF** *see* Lidocaine (Systemic) *on page 1126*
- ◆ **Xylocaine Viscous** *see* Lidocaine (Topical) *on page 1128*
- ◆ **Xyzal®** *see* Levocetirizine *on page 1114*

Yellow Fever Vaccine (YEL oh FEE ver vak SEEN)

Related Information
Immunization Administration Recommendations *on page 2144*
Immunization Recommendations *on page 2149*
Brand Names: U.S. YF-VAX®
Brand Names: Canada YF-VAX®
Generic Availability (U.S.) No
Pharmacologic Category Vaccine, Live (Viral)
Use Induction of active immunity against yellow fever virus, primarily among persons traveling or living in areas where yellow fever infection exists and laboratory workers who may be exposed to the virus; vaccination may also be required for some international travelers

The Advisory Committee on Immunization Practices (ACIP) recommends vaccination for:
- Persons traveling to or living in areas at risk for yellow fever transmission
- Persons traveling to countries which require vaccination for international travel
- Laboratory personnel who may be exposed to the yellow fever virus or concentrated preparations of the vaccine

Dosage
Geriatric Refer to adult dosing. Monitor closely due to an increased incidence of serious adverse events in patients ≥60 years of age, particularly in patients receiving their first dose. The ACIP guidelines note that if travel is unavoidable, the decision to vaccinate travelers ≥60 years should be made after weighing the risks vs benefits.
Adult Immunization: SubQ: One dose (0.5 mL) ≥10 days before travel; Booster: Every 10 years for those at continued risk of exposure
Special Geriatric Considerations The rate of serious adverse events is greater in persons aged ≥60 years than in persons aged 19-29 years. The risk for YEL-AND and YEL-AVD also are increased. Use with caution in older travelers who might be receiving vaccine for the first time.

Dosage Forms Excipient information presented when available (limited, particularly for generics); consult specific product labeling.
Injection, powder for reconstitution [17D-204 strain]:
YF-VAX®: ≥4.74 Log_{10} plaque-forming units (PFU) per 0.5 mL dose [single-dose or 5-dose vial; produced in chicken embryos; contains gelatin; packaged with diluent; vial stopper contains latex]

- ◆ **YF-VAX®** *see* Yellow Fever Vaccine *on page 2041*
- ◆ **YM087** *see* Conivaptan *on page 444*
- ◆ **YM905** *see* Solifenacin *on page 1797*
- ◆ **Yodoxin®** *see* Iodoquinol *on page 1034*
- ◆ **Zaditor® [OTC]** *see* Ketotifen (Ophthalmic) *on page 1076*

Zafirlukast (za FIR loo kast)

Medication Safety Issues
Sound-alike/look-alike issues:
Accolate® may be confused with Accupril®, Accutane®, Aclovate®
Brand Names: U.S. Accolate®
Brand Names: Canada Accolate®
Index Terms ICI-204,219
Generic Availability (U.S.) Yes
Pharmacologic Category Leukotriene-Receptor Antagonist

◀ **Use** Prophylaxis and chronic treatment of asthma

Contraindications Hypersensitivity to zafirlukast or any component of the formulation; hepatic impairment (including hepatic cirrhosis)

Canadian labeling: Additional contraindications (not in U.S. labeling): Patients in whom zafirlukast was discontinued due to treatment related hepatotoxicity

Warnings/Precautions Zafirlukast is not approved for use in the reversal of bronchospasm in acute asthma attacks, including status asthmaticus. Therapy with zafirlukast can be continued during acute exacerbations of asthma.

Hepatic adverse events (including hepatitis, hyperbilirubinemia, and hepatic failure) have been reported; female patients may be at greater risk. Periodic testing of liver function may be considered (early detection coupled with therapy discontinuation is generally believed to improve the likelihood of recovery). Advise patients to be alert for and to immediately report symptoms (eg, anorexia, right upper quadrant abdominal pain, nausea). If hepatic dysfunction is suspected (due to clinical signs/symptoms), discontinue use immediately and measure liver function tests (particularly ALT); resolution observed in most but not all cases upon discontinuation of therapy. Do not resume or restart if hepatic function studies indicate dysfunction. Use in patients with hepatic impairment (including hepatic cirrhosis) is contraindicated. Postmarketing reports of behavioral changes (ie, depression, insomnia) have been noted. Instruct patients to report neuropsychiatric symptoms/events during therapy.

Monitor INR closely with concomitant warfarin use. Rare cases of eosinophilic vasculitis (Churg-Strauss) have been reported in patients receiving zafirlukast (usually, but not always, associated with reduction in concurrent steroid dosage). No causal relationship established. Monitor for eosinophilic vasculitis, rash, pulmonary symptoms, cardiac symptoms, or neuropathy.

Clearance is decreased in elderly patients; C_{max} and AUC are increased approximately two- to threefold in adults ≥65 years compared to younger adults; however, no dosage adjustments are recommended in this age group. An increased proportion of zafirlukast patients >55 years of age reported infections as compared to placebo-treated patients. These infections are mostly mild or moderate in intensity and predominantly affected the respiratory tract. Infections occurred equally in both sexes, were dose-proportional to total milligrams of zafirlukast exposure, and were associated with coadministration of inhaled corticosteroids.

Adverse Reactions (Reflective of adult population; not specific for elderly) Incidence reported in children ≥12 years and adults unless otherwise specified.

>10%: Central nervous system: Headache (13%; children 5-11 years: 5%)

1% to 10%:
Central nervous system: Dizziness (2%), pain (2%), fever (2%)
Gastrointestinal: Nausea (3%), diarrhea (3%), abdominal pain (2%; children 5-11 years: 3%), vomiting (2%), dyspepsia (1%)
Hepatic: ALT increased (2%)
Neuromuscular & skeletal: Back pain (2%), myalgia (2%), weakness (2%)
Miscellaneous: Infection (4%)

Drug Interactions

Metabolism/Transport Effects Substrate of CYP2C9 (major); **Note:** Assignment of Major/Minor substrate status based on clinically relevant drug interaction potential; **Inhibits** CYP1A2 (weak), CYP2C19 (weak), CYP2C8 (weak), CYP2C9 (moderate), CYP2D6 (weak), CYP3A4 (weak)

Avoid Concomitant Use
Avoid concomitant use of Zafirlukast with any of the following: Pimozide

Increased Effect/Toxicity
Zafirlukast may increase the levels/effects of: ARIPiprazole; Carvedilol; CYP2C9 Substrates; Pimozide; Theophylline Derivatives; Vitamin K Antagonists

The levels/effects of Zafirlukast may be increased by: CYP2C9 Inhibitors (Moderate); CYP2C9 Inhibitors (Strong); Mifepristone

Decreased Effect
The levels/effects of Zafirlukast may be decreased by: CYP2C9 Inducers (Strong); Erythromycin; Erythromycin (Systemic); Peginterferon Alfa-2b; Theophylline Derivatives

Ethanol/Nutrition/Herb Interactions Food: Food decreases bioavailability of zafirlukast by 40%. Management: Take on an empty stomach 1 hour before or 2 hours after meals.

Stability Store tablets at controlled room temperature of 20°C to 25°C (68°F to 77°F). Protect from light and moisture; dispense in original airtight container.

Mechanism of Action Zafirlukast is a selectively and competitive leukotriene-receptor antagonist (LTRA) of leukotriene D4 and E4 (LTD4 and LTE4), components of slow-reacting substance of anaphylaxis (SRSA). Cysteinyl leukotriene production and receptor occupation have been correlated with the pathophysiology of asthma, including airway edema, smooth muscle constriction, and altered cellular activity associated with the inflammatory process, which contribute to the signs and symptoms of asthma.

Pharmacodynamics/Kinetics
Distribution: V_{dss}: ~70 L
Protein binding: >99%, primarily to albumin
Metabolism: Extensively hepatic via CYP2C9
Bioavailability: Reduced 40% with food
Half-life elimination: ~10 hours
Time to peak, serum: 3 hours
Excretion: Feces (~90%); Urine (~10%)

Dosage
Geriatric & Adult Asthma: Oral: 20 mg twice daily
Renal Impairment No dosage adjustment necessary.
Hepatic Impairment Use is contraindicated.

Administration Administer at least 1 hour before or 2 hours after a meal.

Monitoring Parameters Monitor for improvements in air flow; monitor closely for sign/ symptoms of hepatic injury; periodic monitoring of LFTs may be considered (not proved to prevent serious injury, but early detection may enhance recovery)

Special Geriatric Considerations Clearance is decreased in elderly patients; compared to younger adults, an approximately two- to threefold increase in C_{max} and AUC has been observed in patients ≥65 years of age. In placebo-controlled short-term trials, an overall increase in infection frequency was seen in elderly patients exposed to zafirlukast compared to elderly patients receiving placebo; infections primarily involved the lower respiratory tract and did not require therapy discontinuation. Some studies have demonstrated a higher percentage of elderly reporting adverse effects compared to adolescents and adults (eg, headache [5%], nausea/vomiting [2%], and pharyngitis [1%]). No dosage adjustments are recommended in the elderly.

Dosage Forms Excipient information presented when available (limited, particularly for generics); consult specific product labeling.
Tablet, oral: 10 mg, 20 mg
Accolate®: 10 mg, 20 mg

Zaleplon (ZAL e plon)

Related information
Beers Criteria − Potentially Inappropriate Medications for Geriatrics on page 2183
Medication Safety Issues
Sound-alike/look-alike issues:
Zaleplon may be confused with Soriatane®
Zaleplon may be confused with Zelapar®, Zemplar®, zolpidem, ZyPREXA® Zydis®
BEERS Criteria medication:
This drug may be potentially inappropriate for use in geriatric patients (Quality of evidence - moderate; Strength of recommendation - strong).

Brand Names: U.S. Sonata®
Generic Availability (U.S.) Yes
Pharmacologic Category Hypnotic, Miscellaneous
Use Short-term (7-10 days) treatment of insomnia (has been demonstrated to be effective for up to 5 weeks in controlled trial)
Medication Guide Available Yes
Contraindications Hypersensitivity to zaleplon or any component of the formulation
Warnings/Precautions Symptomatic treatment of insomnia should be initiated only after careful evaluation of potential causes of sleep disturbance. Failure of sleep disturbance to resolve after 7-10 days may indicate psychiatric and/or medical illness.

Use with caution in patients with depression, particularly if suicidal risk may be present. Use with caution in patients with a history of drug dependence. Abrupt discontinuance may lead to withdrawal symptoms. Hypnotics/sedatives have been associated with abnormal thinking and behavior changes including decreased inhibition, aggression, bizarre behavior, agitation, hallucinations, and depersonalization. These changes may occur unpredictably and may indicate previously unrecognized psychiatric disorders; evaluate appropriately. May impair physical and mental capabilities. Patients must be cautioned about performing tasks which require mental alertness (operating machinery or driving). Use with caution in patients receiving other CNS depressants or psychoactive medications. Effects with other sedative drugs or ethanol may be potentiated. Postmarketing studies have indicated that the use of hypnotic/sedative agents for sleep has been associated with hypersensitivity reactions including anaphylaxis as well as angioedema. An increased risk for hazardous sleep-related activities such as sleep-driving, cooking and eating food, and making phone calls while asleep have been noted; amnesia may also occur. Evaluation is recommended in patients who report any sleep-related episodes.

Avoid chronic use (>90 days) in older adults; adverse events, including delirium, falls, fractures, has been observed with nonbenzodiazepine hypnotic use in the elderly similar to events observed with benzodiazepines. Data suggests improvements in sleep duration and latency are minimal (Beers Criteria).

Use with caution in the elderly, those with compromised respiratory function, or hepatic impairment (dosage adjustment recommended in mild-to-moderate hepatic impairment; use is not recommended in patients with severe impairment). Because of the rapid onset of action, zaleplon should be administered immediately prior to bedtime or after the patient has gone to bed and is having difficulty falling asleep. Capsules contain tartrazine (FDC yellow #5); avoid in patients with sensitivity (caution in patients with asthma).

Adverse Reactions (Reflective of adult population; not specific for elderly)
>10%: Central nervous system: Headache (30% to 42%)

1% to 10%:
Cardiovascular: Chest pain (≥1%), peripheral edema (≤1%)
Central nervous system: Dizziness (7% to 9%), somnolence (5% to 6%), amnesia (2% to 4%), depersonalization (<1% to 2%), hypoesthesia (<1% to 2%), malaise (<1% to 2%), abnormal thinking (≥1%), anxiety (≥1%), depression (≥1%), fever (≥1%), migraine (≥1%), nervousness (≥1%), confusion (≤1%), hallucination (≤1%), vertigo (≤1%)
Dermatologic: Pruritus (≥1%), rash (≥1%), photosensitivity reaction (≤1%)
Endocrine & metabolic: Dysmenorrhea (3% to 4%)
Gastrointestinal: Nausea (6% to 8%), abdominal pain (6%), anorexia (<1% to 2%), constipation (≥1%), dyspepsia (≥1%), taste perversion (≥1%), xerostomia (≥1%), colitis (up to 1%)
Neuromuscular & skeletal: Weakness (5% to 7%), paresthesia (3%), tremor (2%), arthralgia (≥1%), arthritis (≥1%), back pain (≥1%), myalgia (≥1%), hypertonia (1%)
Ocular: Eye pain (3% to 4%), abnormal vision (<1% to 2%), conjunctivitis (≥1%)
Otic: Hyperacusis (1% to 2%), ear pain (≤1%)
Respiratory: Bronchitis (≥1%), epistaxis (≤1%)
Miscellaneous: Parosmia (<1% to 2%)

Drug Interactions
Metabolism/Transport Effects Substrate of CYP3A4 (minor); **Note:** Assignment of Major/Minor substrate status based on clinically relevant drug interaction potential

Avoid Concomitant Use
Avoid concomitant use of Zaleplon with any of the following: Azelastine; Azelastine (Nasal); Methadone; Mirtazapine; Paraldehyde

Increased Effect/Toxicity
Zaleplon may increase the levels/effects of: Alcohol (Ethyl); Azelastine; Azelastine (Nasal); Buprenorphine; CNS Depressants; Methadone; Methotrimeprazine; Metyrosine; Mirtazapine; Paraldehyde; Selective Serotonin Reuptake Inhibitors; Zolpidem

The levels/effects of Zaleplon may be increased by: Cimetidine; Droperidol; HydrOXYzine; Methotrimeprazine

Decreased Effect
The levels/effects of Zaleplon may be decreased by: Flumazenil; Rifamycin Derivatives; Tocilizumab

Ethanol/Nutrition/Herb Interactions
Ethanol: Ethanol may increase CNS depression. Management: Avoid or limit use of ethanol and monitor for increased effects.
Food: High-fat meals prolong absorption; delay T_{max} by 2 hours, and reduce C_{max} by 35%. Management: Avoid taking after a high-fat meal.
Herb/Nutraceutical: St John's wort may decrease zaleplon levels. Some herbal medications may increase CNS depression. Management: Avoid St John's wort, valerian, kava kava, and gotu kola.

Stability Store at controlled room temperature of 20°C to 25°C (68°F to 77°F). Protect from light.

Mechanism of Action Zaleplon is unrelated to benzodiazepines, barbiturates, or other hypnotics. However, it interacts with the benzodiazepine GABA receptor complex. Nonclinical studies have shown that it binds selectively to the brain omega-1 receptor situated on the alpha subunit of the GABA-A receptor complex.

Pharmacodynamics/Kinetics
Onset of action: Rapid
Absorption: Rapid and almost complete; high-fat meal delays absorption
Distribution: V_d: ~1.4 L/kg

Protein binding: ~45% to 75%

Metabolism: Extensive, primarily via aldehyde oxidase to form 5-oxo-zaleplon and, to a lesser extent, by CYP3A4 to desethylzaleplon; all metabolites are pharmacologically inactive

Bioavailability: ~30%

Half-life elimination: 1 hour

Time to peak, serum: 1 hour

Excretion: Urine (~70% primarily metabolites, <1% as unchanged drug); feces (~17%)

Clearance: Plasma: Oral: 3 L/hour/kg

Dosage

Geriatric Reduce dose to 5 mg at bedtime; maximum: 10 mg/day

Adult Insomnia (short-term use): Oral: 10 mg at bedtime (range: 5-20 mg)

Renal Impairment No adjustment for mild-to-moderate renal impairment; use in severe renal impairment has not been adequately studied.

Hepatic Impairment Mild-to-moderate impairment: 5 mg; not recommended for use in patients with severe hepatic impairment.

Administration Immediately before bedtime or when the patient is in bed and cannot fall asleep

Pharmacotherapy Pearls Prescription quantities should not exceed a 1-month supply.

Special Geriatric Considerations In clinical trials, elderly responded to the 5 mg dose with decreased sleep latency. As with all hypnotics, assess underlying cause of insomnia.

This medication is considered to be potentially inappropriate in this patient population (Beers Criteria: Quality of evidence - moderate; Strength of recommendation - strong).

Controlled Substance C-IV

Dosage Forms Excipient information presented when available (limited, particularly for generics); consult specific product labeling.

Capsule, oral: 5 mg, 10 mg

Sonata®: 5 mg

Sonata®: 10 mg [contains tartrazine]

◆ **Zamicet™** see Hydrocodone and Acetaminophen on page 937
◆ **Zanaflex®** see TiZANidine on page 1910
◆ **Zanaflex Capsules®** see TiZANidine on page 1910

Zanamivir (za NA mi veer)

Related Information

Community-Acquired Pneumonia in Adults on page 2171

Medication Safety Issues

Sound-alike/look-alike issues:

Relenza® may be confused with Albenza®, Aplenzin™

Brand Names: U.S. Relenza®

Brand Names: Canada Relenza®

Generic Availability (U.S.) No

Pharmacologic Category Antiviral Agent; Neuraminidase Inhibitor

Use Treatment of uncomplicated acute illness due to influenza virus A and B in patients who have been symptomatic for no more than 2 days; prophylaxis against influenza virus A and B

The Advisory Committee on Immunization Practices (ACIP) recommends that **treatment** be considered for the following:

• Persons with severe, complicated or progressive illness

• Hospitalized persons

• Persons at higher risk for influenza complications:

- Adults ≥65 years of age
- Persons with chronic disorders of the pulmonary (including asthma) or cardiovascular systems (except hypertension)
- Persons with chronic metabolic diseases (including diabetes mellitus), hepatic disease, renal dysfunction, hematologic disorders (including sickle cell disease), or immunosuppression (including immunosuppression caused by medications or HIV)
- Persons with neurologic/neuromuscular conditions (including conditions such as spinal cord injuries, seizure disorders, cerebral palsy, stroke, mental retardation, moderate to severe developmental delay, or muscular dystrophy) which may compromise respiratory function, the handling of respiratory secretions, or that can increase the risk of aspiration
- American Indians and Alaskan Natives
- Persons who are morbidly obese (BMI ≥40)
- Residents of nursing homes or other chronic care facilities

- Use may also be considered for previously healthy, nonhigh-risk outpatients with confirmed or suspected influenza based on clinical judgment when treatment can be started within 48 hours of illness onset.

The ACIP recommends that **prophylaxis** be considered for the following:
- Postexposure prophylaxis may be considered for family or close contacts of suspected or confirmed cases, who are at higher risk of influenza complications, and who have not been vaccinated against the circulating strain at the time of the exposure.
- Postexposure prophylaxis may be considered for unvaccinated healthcare workers who had occupational exposure without protective equipment.
- Pre-exposure prophylaxis should only be used for persons at very high risk of influenza complications who cannot be otherwise protected at times of high risk for exposure.
- Prophylaxis should also be administered to all eligible residents of institutions that house patients at high risk when needed to control outbreaks.

Prescribing and Access Restrictions Zanamivir *aqueous solution* intended for nebulization or intravenous (I.V.) administration is **not** currently approved for use. Data on safety and efficacy via these routes of administration are limited. However, limited supplies of zanamivir aqueous solution may be made available through the Zanamivir Compassionate Use Program for qualifying patients for the treatment of serious influenza illness. For information, contact the GlaxoSmithKline Clinical Support Help Desk at 1-866-341-9160 or gskclinicalsupportHD@gsk.com.

Contraindications Hypersensitivity to zanamivir or any component of the formulation (contains milk proteins)

Warnings/Precautions Allergic-like reactions, including anaphylaxis, oropharyngeal edema, and serious skin rashes have been reported. Rare occurrences of neuropsychiatric events (including confusion, delirium, hallucinations, and/or self-injury) have been reported from postmarketing surveillance; direct causation is difficult to establish (influenza infection may also be associated with behavioral and neurologic changes). Patients must be instructed in the use of the delivery system. Antiviral treatment should begin within 48 hours of symptom onset. However, the CDC recommends that treatment may still be beneficial and should be started in hospitalized patients with severe, complicated or progressive illness if >48 hours. Nonhospitalized persons who are not at high risk for developing severe or complicated illness and who have a mild disease are not likely to benefit if treatment is started >48 hours after symptom onset. Nonhospitalized persons who are already beginning to recover do not need treatment. Effectiveness has not been established in patients with significant underlying medical conditions or for prophylaxis of influenza in nursing home patients (per manufacturer). The CDC recommends zanamivir to be used to control institutional outbreaks of influenza when circulating strains are suspected of being resistant to oseltamivir (refer to current guidelines). Not recommended for use in patients with underlying respiratory disease, such as asthma or COPD, due to lack of efficacy and risk of serious adverse effects. Bronchospasm, decreased lung function, and other serious adverse reactions, including those with fatal outcomes, have been reported in patients with and without airway disease; discontinue with bronchospasm or signs of decreased lung function. For a patient with an underlying airway disease where a medical decision has been made to use zanamivir, a fast-acting bronchodilator should be made available, and used prior to each dose. Not a substitute for annual flu vaccination; has not been shown to reduce risk of transmission of influenza to others. Consider primary or concomitant bacterial infections. Powder for oral inhalation contains lactose; use contraindicated in patients allergic to milk proteins. The inhalation powder should only be administered via inhalation using the provided Diskhaler® delivery device. The commercially available formulation is **not** intended to be solubilized or administered via any nebulizer/mechanical ventilator; inappropriate administration has resulted in death. Safety and efficacy of repeated courses or use with hepatic impairment or severe renal impairment have not been established.

Adverse Reactions (Reflective of adult population; not specific for elderly) Most adverse reactions occurred at a frequency which was less than or equal to the control (lactose vehicle).

>10%:
  Central nervous system: Headache (prophylaxis 13% to 24%; treatment 2%)
  Gastrointestinal: Throat/tonsil discomfort/pain (prophylaxis 8% to 19%)
  Respiratory: Nasal signs and symptoms (prophylaxis 12% to 20%; treatment 2%), cough (prophylaxis 7% to 17%; treatment ≤2%)
  Miscellaneous: Viral infection (prophylaxis 3% to 13%)
1% to 10%:
  Central nervous system: Fever/chills (prophylaxis 5% to 9%; treatment <1.5%), fatigue (prophylaxis 5% to 8%; treatment <1.5%), malaise (prophylaxis 5% to 8%; treatment <1.5%), dizziness (treatment 1% to 2%)
  Dermatologic: Urticaria (treatment <1.5%)

Gastrointestinal: Anorexia/appetite decreased (prophylaxis 2% to 4%), appetite increased (prophylaxis 2% to 4%), nausea (prophylaxis 1% to 2%; treatment ≤3%), diarrhea (prophylaxis 2%; treatment 2% to 3%), vomiting (prophylaxis 1% to 2%; treatment 1% to 2%), abdominal pain (treatment <1.5%)

Neuromuscular & skeletal: Muscle pain (prophylaxis 3% to 8%), musculoskeletal pain (prophylaxis 6%), arthralgia/articular rheumatism (prophylaxis 2%), arthralgia (treatment <1.5%), myalgia (treatment <1.5%)

Respiratory: Infection (ear/nose/throat; prophylaxis 2%; treatment 1% to 5%), sinusitis (treatment 3%), bronchitis (treatment 2%), nasal inflammation (prophylaxis 1%)

Drug Interactions

Metabolism/Transport Effects None known.

Avoid Concomitant Use There are no known interactions where it is recommended to avoid concomitant use.

Increased Effect/Toxicity There are no known significant interactions involving an increase in effect.

Decreased Effect

Zanamivir may decrease the levels/effects of: Influenza Virus Vaccine (Live/Attenuated)

Stability Store at 25°C (77°F); excursions permitted to 15°C to 30°C (59°F to 86°F). Do not puncture blister until taking a dose using the Diskhaler®.

Mechanism of Action Zanamivir inhibits influenza virus neuraminidase enzymes, potentially altering virus particle aggregation and release.

Pharmacodynamics/Kinetics

Absorption: Inhalation: Systemic: ~4% to 17%

Protein binding, plasma: <10%

Metabolism: None

Half-life elimination, serum: 2.5-5.1 hours; Mild-to-moderate renal impairment: 4.7 hours; Severe renal impairment: 18.5 hours

Time to peak, plasma: 1-2 hours

Excretion: Urine (as unchanged drug); feces (unabsorbed drug)

Dosage

Geriatric & Adult Influenza virus A and B:

Manufacturer's recommendations: Oral inhalation:

Prophylaxis, household setting: Two inhalations (10 mg) once daily for 10 days. Begin within 36 hours following onset of signs or symptoms of index case.

Prophylaxis, community outbreak: Two inhalations (10 mg) once daily for 28 days. Begin within 5 days of outbreak.

Treatment: Two inhalations (10 mg total) twice daily for 5 days. Doses on first day should be separated by at least 2 hours; on subsequent days, doses should be spaced by ~12 hours. Begin within 2 days of signs or symptoms. Longer treatment may be considered for patients who remain severely ill after 5 days.

Alternate recommendations: Oral inhalation:

Prophylaxis (institutional outbreak, CDC 2011 recommendations): Two inhalations (10 mg) once daily; continue for ≥2 weeks and until ~10 days after identification of illness onset in the last patient. Zanamivir is to be used to control institutional outbreaks of influenza when circulating strains are suspected of being resistant to oseltamivir.

Prophylaxis (community outbreak, IDSA/PIDS, 2011): Two inhalations (10 mg) once daily; continue until influenza activity in community subsides or immunity obtained from immunization

Renal Impairment Adjustment not necessary following a 5-day course of treatment due to low systemic absorption; however the potential for drug accumulation should be considered.

Administration Inhalation: Must be used with Diskhaler® delivery device. The foil blister disk containing zanamivir inhalation powder should not be manipulated, solubilized, or administered via a nebulizer. Patients who are scheduled to use an inhaled bronchodilator should use their bronchodilator prior to zanamivir. With the exception of the initial dose when used for treatment, administer at the same time each day.

Pharmacotherapy Pearls Majority of patients included in clinical trials were infected with influenza A, however, a number of patients with influenza B infections were also enrolled. Patients with lower temperature or less severe symptoms appeared to derive less benefit from therapy. No consistent treatment benefit was demonstrated in patients with chronic underlying medical conditions.

The absence of symptoms does not rule out viral influenza infection and clinical judgment should guide the decision for therapy. Treatment should not be delayed while waiting for the results of diagnostic tests. Treatment should be considered for high-risk patients with symptoms despite a negative rapid influenza test when the illness cannot be contributed to another cause. Use of zanamivir is not a substitute for vaccination (when available); susceptibility to influenza infection returns once therapy is discontinued.

Special Geriatric Considerations A study demonstrated that most elderly were unable to use an inhaler device effectively. Evaluate the patient's or caregiver's ability to safely administer the correct dose of medication.

Dosage Forms Excipient information presented when available (limited, particularly for generics); consult specific product labeling.

Powder, for oral inhalation:

Relenza®: 5 mg/blister (20s) [contains lactose 20 mg/blister; 4 blisters per Rotadisk® foil pack, 5 Rotadisk® per package; packaged with Diskhaler® inhalation device]

Ziconotide (zi KOE no tide)

Medication Safety Issues

High alert medication:

The Institute for Safe Medication Practices (ISMP) includes this medication among its list of drugs which have a heightened risk of causing significant patient harm when used in error.

Brand Names: U.S. Prialt®

Generic Availability (U.S.) No

Pharmacologic Category Analgesic, Nonopioid; Calcium Channel Blocker, N-Type

Use Management of severe chronic pain in patients requiring intrathecal (I.T.) therapy and who are intolerant or refractory to other therapies

Contraindications Hypersensitivity to ziconotide or any component of the formulation; history of psychosis; I.V. administration

I.T. administration is contraindicated in patients with infection at the injection site, uncontrolled bleeding, or spinal canal obstruction that impairs CSF circulation

Warnings/Precautions [U.S Boxed Warning]: Severe psychiatric symptoms and neurological impairment have been reported; interrupt or discontinue therapy if cognitive impairment, hallucinations, mood changes, or changes in consciousness occur. May cause or worsen depression and/or risk of suicide. Cognitive impairment may appear gradually during treatment and is generally reversible after discontinuation (may take up to 2 weeks for cognitive effects to reverse). Use caution in the elderly; may experience a higher incidence of confusion. Patients should be instructed to use caution in performing tasks which require alertness (eg, operating machinery or driving). May have additive effects with opiates or other CNS-depressant medications; may potentiate opioid-induced decreased GI motility; does not interact with opioid receptors or potentiate opiate-induced respiratory depression. Will not prevent or relieve symptoms associated with opiate withdrawal and opiates should not be abruptly discontinued. Unlike opioids, ziconotide therapy can be interrupted abruptly or discontinued without evidence of withdrawal.

Meningitis may occur with use of I.T. pumps; monitor for signs and symptoms of meningitis; treatment of meningitis may require removal of system and discontinuation of intrathecal therapy. Elevated serum creatine kinase can occur, particularly during the first 2 months of therapy; consider dose reduction or discontinuing if combined with new neuromuscular symptoms (myalgias, myasthenia, muscle cramps, weakness) or reduction in physical activity. Safety and efficacy have not been established with renal or hepatic dysfunction. Should not be used in combination with intrathecal opiates.

Adverse Reactions (Reflective of adult population; not specific for elderly)

>10%:

Central nervous system: Dizziness (46%), confusion (15% to 33%), memory impairment (7% to 22%), somnolence (17%), ataxia (14%), speech disorder (14%), headache (13%), aphasia (12%), hallucination (12%; including auditory and visual)

Gastrointestinal: Nausea (40%), diarrhea (18%), vomiting (16%)

Neuromuscular & skeletal: Creatine kinase increased (40%; ≥3 times ULN: 11%), weakness (18%), gait disturbances (14%)

Ocular: Blurred vision (12%)

2% to 10%:

Cardiovascular: Hypotension, orthostatic hypotension, peripheral edema

Central nervous system: Abnormal thinking (8%), amnesia (8%), anxiety (8%), vertigo (7%), insomnia (6%), fever (5%), paranoid reaction (3%), delirium (2%), hostility (2%), stupor (2%), agitation, attention disturbance, balance impaired, burning sensation, coordination abnormal, depression, disorientation, fatigue, fever, hypoesthesia, irritability, lethargy, mental impairment, mood disorder, nervousness, pain, sedation

Dermatologic: Pruritus (7%)

Gastrointestinal: Anorexia (6%), taste perversion (5%), abdominal pain, appetite decreased, constipation, xerostomia

Genitourinary: Urinary retention (9%), dysuria, urinary hesitance

Neuromuscular & skeletal: Dysarthria (7%), paresthesia (7%), rigors (7%), tremor (7%), muscle spasm (6%), limb pain (5%), areflexia, muscle cramp, muscle weakness, myalgia

Ocular: Nystagmus (8%), diplopia, visual disturbance

Respiratory: Sinusitis (5%)

Miscellaneous: Diaphoresis (5%)

Drug Interactions

Metabolism/Transport Effects None known.

Avoid Concomitant Use

Avoid concomitant use of Ziconotide with any of the following: Azelastine; Azelastine (Nasal); Methadone; Mirtazapine; Paraldehyde

Increased Effect/Toxicity

Ziconotide may increase the levels/effects of: Alcohol (Ethyl); Azelastine; Azelastine (Nasal); Buprenorphine; CNS Depressants; Methadone; Methotrimeprazine; Metyrosine; Mirtazapine; Paraldehyde; Selective Serotonin Reuptake Inhibitors; Zolpidem

The levels/effects of Ziconotide may be increased by: Droperidol; HydrOXYzine; Methotrimeprazine

Decreased Effect There are no known significant interactions involving a decrease in effect.

Ethanol/Nutrition/Herb Interactions Ethanol: May increase CNS depression; monitor for increased effects with coadministration. Caution patients about effects.

Stability Prior to use, store vials at 2°C to 8°C (36°F to 46°F). Once diluted, may be stored at 2°C to 8°C (36°F to 46°F) for 24 hours; refrigerate during transit. Do not freeze. Protect from light.

Preservative free NS should be used when dilution is needed.

CADD-Micro® ambulatory infusion pump: Initial fill: Dilute to final concentration of 5 mcg/mL.

Medtronic SynchroMed® EL or SynchroMed® II infusion system: Prior to initial fill, rinse internal pump surfaces with 2 mL ziconotide (25 mcg/mL), repeat twice. Only the 25 mcg/mL concentration (undiluted) should be used for initial pump fill. When using the Medtronic SynchroMed® EL or SynchroMed® II Infusion System, solutions expire as follows:

25 mcg/mL: Undiluted:

Initial fill: Use within 14 days.

Refill: Use within 84 days.

100 mcg/mL:

Undiluted: Refill: Use within 84 days.

Diluted: Refill: Use within 40 days.

Mechanism of Action Ziconotide selectively binds to N-type voltage-sensitive calcium channels located on the nociceptive afferent nerves of the dorsal horn in the spinal cord. This binding is thought to block N-type calcium channels, leading to a blockade of excitatory neurotransmitter release and reducing sensitivity to painful stimuli.

Pharmacodynamics/Kinetics

Distribution: I.T.: V_d: ~140 mL

Protein binding: ~50%

Metabolism: Metabolized via endopeptidases and exopeptidases present on multiple organs including kidney, liver, lung; degraded to peptide fragments and free amino acids

Half-life elimination: I.V.: 1-1.6 hours (plasma); I.T.: 2.9-6.5 hours (CSF)
Excretion: I.V.: Urine (<1%)

Dosage

Geriatric Refer to adult dosing. Use with caution.

Adult Chronic pain: I.T.: Initial dose: ≤2.4 mcg/day (0.1 mcg/hour)

Dose may be titrated by ≤2.4 mcg/day (0.1 mcg/hour) at intervals ≤2-3 times/week to a maximum dose of 19.2 mcg/day (0.8 mcg/hour) by day 21; average dose at day 21: 6.9 mcg/day (0.29 mcg/hour). A faster titration should be used only if the urgent need for analgesia outweighs the possible risk to patient safety.

Administration Not for I.V. administration. For I.T. administration only using Medtronic SynchroMed® EL, SynchroMed® II Infusion System, or CADD-Micro® ambulatory infusion pump.

Medtronic SynchroMed® EL or SynchroMed® II Infusion Systems:

Naive pump priming (first time use with ziconotide): Use 2 mL of undiluted ziconotide 25 mcg/mL solution to rinse the internal surfaces of the pump; repeat twice for a total of 3 rinses

Initial pump fill: Use only undiluted 25 mcg/mL solution and fill pump after priming. Following the initial fill only, adsorption on internal device surfaces will occur, requiring the use of the undiluted solution and refill within 14 days.

Pump refills: Contents should be emptied prior to refill. Subsequent pump refills should occur at least every 40 days if using diluted solution or at least every 84 days if using undiluted solution.

CADD-Micro® ambulatory infusion pump: Refer to manufacturers' manual for initial fill and refill instructions

Monitoring Parameters Monitor for psychiatric or neurological impairment; signs and symptoms of meningitis or other infection; serum CPK (every other week for first month then monthly); pain relief

Special Geriatric Considerations Manufacturer reports that in all trials there was a higher incidence of confusion in the elderly compared to younger adults.

Dosage Forms Excipient information presented when available (limited, particularly for generics); consult specific product labeling.

Infusion, intrathecal, as acetate [preservative free]:

Prialt®: 25 mcg/mL (20 mL); 100 mcg/mL (1 mL, 5 mL)

Zileuton (zye LOO ton)

Brand Names: U.S. Zyflo CR®; Zyflo®

Generic Availability (U.S.) No

Pharmacologic Category 5-Lipoxygenase Inhibitor

Use Prophylaxis and chronic treatment of asthma

Contraindications Hypersensitivity to zileuton or any component of the formulation; active liver disease or transaminase elevations ≥3 times ULN

Warnings/Precautions Not appropriate or indicated for the reversal of bronchospasm in acute asthma attacks, including status asthmaticus; therapy may be continued during acute asthma exacerbations. Hepatic adverse effects have been reported (elevated transaminase levels); females >65 years and patients with pre-existing elevated transaminases may be at greater risk. Serum ALT should be monitored. Discontinue zileuton and follow transaminases until normal if patients develop clinical signs/symptoms of liver dysfunction or with transaminase levels >5 times ULN (use caution with history of liver disease and/or in those patients who consume substantial quantities of ethanol). Postmarketing reports of behavioral changes and sleep disorders have been noted.

Adverse Reactions (Reflective of adult population; not specific for elderly)

>10%: Central nervous system: Headache (23% to 25%)

1% to 10%:

Cardiovascular: Chest pain

Central nervous system: Pain (8%), dizziness, fever, insomnia, malaise, nervousness, somnolence

Dermatologic: Pruritus, rash

Gastrointestinal: Dyspepsia (8%), diarrhea (5%), nausea (5% to 6%), abdominal pain (5%), constipation, flatulence, vomiting

Genitourinary: Urinary tract infection, vaginitis

Hematologic: Leukopenia (1% to 3%)

Hepatic: ALT increased (≥3 x ULN: 2% to 5%), hepatotoxicity

Neuromuscular & skeletal: Myalgia (7%), weakness (4%), arthralgia, hypertonia, neck pain/rigidity

Ocular: Conjunctivitis

Respiratory: Upper respiratory tract infection (9%), sinusitis (7%), pharyngolaryngeal pain (5%)

Miscellaneous: Hypersensitivity reactions, lymphadenopathy

Drug Interactions

Metabolism/Transport Effects Substrate of CYP1A2 (minor), CYP2C9 (minor), CYP3A4 (minor); **Note:** Assignment of Major/Minor substrate status based on clinically relevant drug interaction potential; **Inhibits** CYP1A2 (weak)

Avoid Concomitant Use

Avoid concomitant use of Zileuton with any of the following: Pimozide

Increased Effect/Toxicity

Zileuton may increase the levels/effects of: Pimozide; Propranolol; Theophylline; Warfarin

Decreased Effect

The levels/effects of Zileuton may be decreased by: Tocilizumab

Ethanol/Nutrition/Herb Interactions

Ethanol: Avoid ethanol (may increase CNS depression; may increase risk of hepatic toxicity).

Food: Zyflo CR®: Improved absorption when administered with food.

Herb/Nutraceutical: St John's wort may decrease zileuton levels.

Stability Store tablets at 20°C to 25°C (68°F to 77°F). Protect from light.

Mechanism of Action Specific 5-lipoxygenase inhibitor which inhibits leukotriene formation. Leukotrienes augment neutrophil and eosinophil migration, neutrophil and monocyte aggregation, leukocyte adhesion, increased capillary permeability, and smooth muscle contraction (which contribute to inflammation, edema, mucous secretion, and bronchoconstriction in the airway of the asthmatic.)

Pharmacodynamics/Kinetics

Distribution: 1.2 L/kg

Protein binding: 93%, primarily albumin

Metabolism: Hepatic and gastrointestinal; zileuton and N-dehydroxylated metabolite can be metabolized by CYP1A2, 2C9, and 3A4

Half-life elimination: ~3 hours

Time to peak: Immediate release: 1.7 hours

Excretion: Urine (~95% primarily as metabolites); feces (~2%)

Dosage

Geriatric & Adult Asthma: Oral:

Immediate release: 600 mg 4 times/day

Extended release: 1200 mg twice daily

Renal Impairment Adjustment not necessary in renal dysfunction or with hemodialysis.

Hepatic Impairment Contraindicated with hepatic dysfunction.

Administration

Immediate release: Administer without regard to meals.

Extended release: Do not crush, cut, or chew tablet; administer within 1 hour after morning and evening meals.

Monitoring Parameters Hepatic transaminases (prior to initiation and during therapy), specifically monitor serum ALT (prior to initiation, once-a-month for the first 3 months, every 2-3 months for the remainder of the first year, and periodically thereafter for patients receiving long-term therapy)

Special Geriatric Considerations No differences in the pharmacokinetics found between younger adults and elderly; no dosage adjustments necessary. However, monitor liver effects closely as with any patient regardless of age.

Dosage Forms Excipient information presented when available (limited, particularly for generics); consult specific product labeling.

Tablet, oral:

Zyflo®: 600 mg [scored]

Tablet, extended release, oral:

Zyflo CR®: 600 mg

- ◆ **Zinacef®** *see* Cefuroxime *on page 336*
- ◆ **Zinc 15 [OTC]** *see* Zinc Sulfate *on page 2051*
- ◆ **Zincate® [DSC]** *see* Zinc Sulfate *on page 2051*

Zinc Sulfate (zink SUL fate)

Related Information

Calculations *on page 2087*

Medication Safety Issues

Sound-alike/look-alike issues:

$ZnSO_4$ is an error-prone abbreviation (mistaken as morphine sulfate)

ZINC SULFATE

Brand Names: U.S. Orazinc® 110 [OTC]; Orazinc® 220 [OTC]; Zinc 15 [OTC]; Zincate® [DSC]

Brand Names: Canada Anuzinc; Rivasol

Index Terms $ZnSO_4$ (error-prone abbreviation)

Generic Availability (U.S.) Yes

Pharmacologic Category Trace Element

Use Zinc supplement (oral and parenteral); may improve wound healing in those who are deficient

Contraindications

Injection: Do not administer undiluted into peripheral vein

Warnings/Precautions Use with caution in patients with renal impairment. I.V. administration of zinc without copper may cause a decrease in copper serum concentrations. Solutions may contain aluminum; toxic concentrations may occur following prolonged administration in patients with renal impairment.

Adverse Reactions (Reflective of adult population; not specific for elderly) Frequency not defined.

Central nervous system: Dizziness, headache

Gastrointestinal: Abdominal cramps, diarrhea, nausea, vomiting

Drug Interactions

Metabolism/Transport Effects None known.

Avoid Concomitant Use There are no known interactions where it is recommended to avoid concomitant use.

Increased Effect/Toxicity There are no known significant interactions involving an increase in effect.

Decreased Effect

Zinc Sulfate may decrease the levels/effects of: Cephalexin; Deferiprone; Eltrombopag; Quinolone Antibiotics; Tetracycline Derivatives; Trientine

The levels/effects of Zinc Sulfate may be decreased by: Trientine

Ethanol/Nutrition/Herb Interactions Food: Avoid foods high in calcium or phosphorus.

Stability

Capsule, tablet: Store at room temperature.

Injection: Prior to use, store at room temperature of 20°C to 25°C (68°F to 77°F); excursions permitted to 15°C to 30°C (59°F to 86°F).

Pharmacodynamics/Kinetics

Absorption: Zinc and its salts are poorly absorbed from the gastrointestinal tract (20% to 30%)

Elimination: In feces with only traces appearing in urine

Dosage

Geriatric & Adult

Recommended daily allowance (RDA): Oral (dose expressed as elemental zinc): Adults ≥19 years:

Males: 11 mg/day

Females: 8 mg/day

Parenteral TPN: I.V.:

Acute metabolic states: 4.5-6 mg/day

Metabolically stable: 2.5-4 mg/day

Replacement for small bowel fluid loss (metabolically stable): An additional 12.2 mg zinc/L of fluid lost, or an additional 17.1 mg zinc per kg of stool or ileostomy output

Monitoring Parameters Skin integrity

Pharmacotherapy Pearls Zinc acetate can be used as an alternative to zinc sulfate in patients who cannot tolerate the gastrointestinal irritant effects of the sulfate salt

Special Geriatric Considerations May be useful to promote wound healing in patients with pressure sores.

Dosage Forms Excipient information presented when available (limited, particularly for generics); consult specific product labeling. [DSC] = Discontinued product

Capsule, oral: 220 mg [elemental zinc 50 mg]

Orazinc® 220: 220 mg [elemental zinc 50 mg]

Zincate®: 220 mg [DSC] [elemental zinc 50 mg]

Injection, solution [preservative free]: Elemental zinc 1 mg/mL (10 mL)

Injection, solution [concentrate, preservative free]: Elemental zinc 5 mg/mL (5 mL)

Tablet, oral: 220 mg [elemental zinc 50 mg]

Orazinc® 110: 110 mg [elemental zinc 25 mg]

Zinc 15: 66 mg [elemental zinc 15 mg]

Ziprasidone (zi PRAS i done)

Related Information
Antipsychotic Agents *on page 2103*
Atypical Antipsychotics *on page 2107*
Beers Criteria – Potentially Inappropriate Medications for Geriatrics *on page 2183*

Medication Safety Issues
Sound-alike/look-alike issues:
Ziprasidone may be confused with TraZODone

BEERS Criteria medication:
This drug may be potentially inappropriate for use in geriatric patients (Quality of evidence - moderate; Strength of recommendation - strong).

Brand Names: U.S. Geodon®
Brand Names: Canada Zeldox®
Index Terms Zeldox; Ziprasidone Hydrochloride; Ziprasidone Mesylate
Generic Availability (U.S.) Yes: Capsule
Pharmacologic Category Antipsychotic Agent, Atypical
Use Treatment of schizophrenia; treatment of acute manic or mixed episodes associated with bipolar disorder with or without psychosis; maintenance treatment of bipolar disorder as an adjunct to lithium or valproate; acute agitation in patients with schizophrenia
Unlabeled Use Tourette's syndrome; psychosis/agitation related to Alzheimer's dementia
Contraindications Hypersensitivity to ziprasidone or any component of the formulation; history of (or current) prolonged QT; congenital long QT syndrome; recent myocardial infarction; uncompensated heart failure; concurrent use of other QT$_c$-prolonging agents including arsenic trioxide, chlorpromazine, class Ia antiarrhythmics (eg, disopyramide, quinidine, procainamide), class III antiarrhythmics (eg, amiodarone, dofetilide, ibutilide, sotalol), dolasetron, droperidol, gatifloxacin, levomethadyl, mefloquine, mesoridazine, moxifloxacin, pentamidine, pimozide, probucol, tacrolimus, and thioridazine
Warnings/Precautions Hazardous agent - use appropriate precautions for handling and disposal. **[U.S. Boxed Warning]: Elderly patients with dementia-related behavioral disorders treated with antipsychotics are at an increased risk of death compared to placebo.** Most deaths appeared to be either cardiovascular (eg, heart failure, sudden death) or infectious (eg, pneumonia) in nature. Ziprasidone is not approved for the treatment of dementia-related psychosis.

May result in QT$_c$ prolongation (dose related), which has been associated with the development of malignant ventricular arrhythmias (torsade de pointes) and sudden death. Note contraindications related to this effect. Observed prolongation was greater than with other atypical antipsychotic agents (risperidone, olanzapine, quetiapine), but less than with thioridazine. Correct electrolyte disturbances, especially hypokalemia or hypomagnesemia, prior to use and throughout therapy. Use caution in patients with bradycardia. Discontinue in patients found to have persistent QT$_c$ intervals >500 msec. Patients with symptoms of dizziness, palpitations, or syncope should receive further cardiac evaluation. May cause orthostatic hypotension. Use is contraindicated in patients with recent acute myocardial infarction (MI), QT prolongation, or uncompensated heart failure. Avoid use in patients with a history of cardiac arrhythmias; use with caution in patients with history of MI or unstable heart disease.

Leukopenia, neutropenia, and agranulocytosis (sometimes fatal) have been reported in clinical trials and postmarketing reports with antipsychotic use; presence of risk factors (eg, pre-existing low WBC or history of drug-induced leuko-/neutropenia) should prompt periodic blood count assessment. Discontinue therapy at first signs of blood dyscrasias or if absolute neutrophil count <1000/mm^3.

May cause extrapyramidal symptoms (EPS). Risk of dystonia (and probably other EPS) may be greater with increased doses, use of conventional antipsychotics, males, and younger patients. Impaired core body temperature regulation may occur; caution with strenuous exercise, heat exposure, dehydration, and concomitant medication possessing anticholinergic effects; not reported in premarketing trials of ziprasidone. Antipsychotic use may also be associated with neuroleptic malignant syndrome (NMS). Use with caution in patients at risk of seizures.

Atypical antipsychotics have been associated with development of hyperglycemia. There is limited documentation with ziprasidone and specific risk associated with this agent is not known. Use caution in patients with diabetes or other disorders of glucose regulation; monitor for worsening of glucose control. May increase prolactin levels; clinical significance of hyperprolactinemia in patients with breast cancer or other prolactin-dependent tumors is unknown.

Use in elderly patients with dementia is associated with an increased risk of mortality and cerebrovascular accidents; avoid antipsychotic use for behavioral problems associated with dementia unless alternative nonpharmacologic therapies have failed and patient may harm self or others. In addition, use may cause or exacerbate syndrome of inappropriate antidiuretic hormone secretion or hyponatremia; monitor sodium closely with initiation or dosage adjustments in older adults (Beers Criteria).

Cognitive and/or motor impairment (sedation) is common with ziprasidone. Use with caution in disorders where CNS depression is a feature. Use with caution in Parkinson's disease. Antipsychotic use has been associated with esophageal dysmotility and aspiration; use with caution in patients at risk of pneumonia (ie, Alzheimer's disease). Use caution in hepatic impairment. Ziprasidone has been associated with a fairly high incidence of rash (5%). Significant weight gain has been observed with antipsychotic therapy; incidence varies with product. Monitor waist circumference and BMI. Rare cases of priapism have been reported. Use the intramuscular formulation with caution in patients with renal impairment; formulation contains cyclodextrin, an excipient which may accumulate in renal insufficiency.

The possibility of a suicide attempt is inherent in psychotic illness or bipolar disorder; use caution in high-risk patients during initiation of therapy. Prescriptions should be written for the smallest quantity consistent with good patient care.

Adverse Reactions (Reflective of adult population; not specific for elderly) Note: Although minor QT$_c$ prolongation (mean: 10 msec at 160 mg/day) may occur more frequently (incidence not specified), clinically-relevant prolongation (>500 msec) was rare (0.06%) and less than placebo (0.23%).

>10%:
 Central nervous system: Extrapyramidal symptoms (2% to 31%), somnolence (8% to 31%), headache (3% to 18%), dizziness (3% to 16%)
 Gastrointestinal: Nausea (4% to 12%)

1% to 10%:
 Cardiovascular: Orthostatic hypotension (5%), chest pain (3%), hypertension (2% to 3%), tachycardia (2%), bradycardia (≤2%), facial edema (1%), vasodilation (≤1%)
 Central nervous system: Akathisia (2% to 10%), anxiety (2% to 5%), insomnia (3%), agitation (2%), speech disorder (2%), personality disorder (≥1%), akinesia (≥1%), amnesia (≥1%), ataxia (≥1%), confusion (≥1%), coordination abnormal (≥1%), delirium (≥1%), dystonia (≥1%), hostility (≥1%), oculogyric crisis (≥1%), vertigo (≥1%), chills (1%), fever (1%), hypothermia (1%), psychosis (1%)
 Dermatologic: Rash (4% to 5%), fungal dermatitis (2%), photosensitivity reaction (1%)
 Endocrine & metabolic: Dysmenorrhea (2%)
 Gastrointestinal: Weight gain (6% to 10%), constipation (2% to 9%), dyspepsia (1% to 8%), diarrhea (3% to 5%), vomiting (3% to 5%), xerostomia (1% to 5%), salivation increased (4%), tongue edema (≤3%), anorexia (2%), abdominal pain (≤2%), dysphagia (≤2%), rectal hemorrhage (≤2%), buccoglossal syndrome (≥1%)
 Genitourinary: Priapism (1%)
 Local: Injection site pain (7% to 9%)
 Neuromuscular & skeletal: Weakness (2% to 6%), hypoesthesia (2%), myalgia (2%), paresthesia (2%), abnormal gait (≥1%), choreoathetosis (≥1%), dysarthria (≥1%), dyskinesia (≥1%), hyper-/hypokinesia (≥1%), hypotonia (≥1%), neuropathy (≥1%), tremor (≥1%), twitching (≥1%), back pain (1%), cogwheel rigidity (1%), hypertonia (1%)
 Ocular: Vision abnormal (3% to 6%), diplopia (≥1%)
 Respiratory: Infection (8%), rhinitis (1% to 4%), cough (3%), pharyngitis (3%), dyspnea (2%)
 Miscellaneous: Diaphoresis (2%), furunculosis (2%), withdrawal syndrome (≥1%), flank pain (1%), flu-like syndrome (1%)

Drug Interactions
 Metabolism/Transport Effects Substrate of CYP1A2 (minor), CYP3A4 (minor); **Note:** Assignment of Major/Minor substrate status based on clinically relevant drug interaction potential; **Inhibits** CYP2D6 (weak), CYP3A4 (weak)
 Avoid Concomitant Use
 Avoid concomitant use of Ziprasidone with any of the following: Azelastine; Azelastine (Nasal); Highest Risk QTc-Prolonging Agents; Metoclopramide; Mifepristone; Moderate Risk QTc-Prolonging Agents; Paraldehyde
 Increased Effect/Toxicity
 Ziprasidone may increase the levels/effects of: Alcohol (Ethyl); ARIPiprazole; Azelastine; Azelastine (Nasal); Buprenorphine; CNS Depressants; Highest Risk QTc-Prolonging Agents; Methylphenidate; Paraldehyde; Serotonin Modulators; Zolpidem

The levels/effects of Ziprasidone may be increased by: Acetylcholinesterase Inhibitors (Central); Antifungal Agents (Azole Derivatives, Systemic); HydrOXYzine; Lithium formulations; Methylphenidate; Metoclopramide; Metyrosine; Mifepristone; Moderate Risk QTc-Prolonging Agents; QTc-Prolonging Agents (Indeterminate Risk and Risk Modifying); Tetrabenazine

Decreased Effect

Ziprasidone may decrease the levels/effects of: Amphetamines; Anti-Parkinson's Agents (Dopamine Agonist); Quinagolide

The levels/effects of Ziprasidone may be decreased by: CarBAMazepine; Lithium formulations; Tocilizumab

Ethanol/Nutrition/Herb Interactions

Ethanol: May increase CNS depression; monitor for increased effects with coadministration. Caution patients about effects.

Food: Administration with food increases serum levels twofold. Grapefruit juice may increase serum concentration of ziprasidone.

Herb/Nutraceutical: St John's wort may decrease serum levels of ziprasidone, due to a potential effect on CYP3A4. This has not been specifically studied. Avoid kava kava, chamomile (may increase CNS depression).

Stability Use appropriate precautions for handling and disposal.

Capsule: Store at 25°C (77°F); excursion permitted to 15°C to 30°C (59°F to 86°F).

Vials for injection: Store at 25°C (77°F); excursion permitted to 15°C to 30°C (59°F to 86°F). Protect from light. Each vial should be reconstituted with 1.2 mL SWFI. Shake vigorously; will form a pale, pink solution containing 20 mg/mL ziprasidone. Following reconstitution, injection may be stored at room temperature up to 24 hours or under refrigeration for up to 7 days. Protect from light.

Mechanism of Action Ziprasidone is a benzylisothiazolylpiperazine antipsychotic. The exact mechanism of action is unknown. However, *in vitro* radioligand studies show that ziprasidone has high affinity for D_2, D_3, $5-HT_{2A}$, $5-HT_{1A}$, $5-HT_{2C}$, $5-HT_{1D}$, and alpha$_1$-adrenergic; moderate affinity for histamine H_1 receptors, and no appreciable affinity for alpha$_2$-adrenergic receptors, beta-adrenergic, $5-HT_3$, $5-HT_4$, cholinergic, mu, sigma, or benzodiazepine receptors. Ziprasidone functions as an antagonist at the D_2, $5-HT_{2A}$, and $5-HT_{1D}$ receptors and as an agonist at the $5-HT_{1A}$ receptor. Ziprasidone moderately inhibits the reuptake of serotonin and norepinephrine.

Pharmacodynamics/Kinetics

Absorption: Well absorbed

Distribution: V_d: 1.5 L/kg

Protein binding: >99%, primarily to albumin and alpha$_1$-acid glycoprotein

Metabolism: Extensively hepatic, primarily via aldehyde oxidase; less than $1/3$ of total metabolism via CYP3A4 and CYP1A2 (minor)

Bioavailability: Oral (with food): 60% (up to twofold increase with food); I.M.: 100%

Half-life elimination: 2-7 hours

Time to peak: Oral: 6-8 hours; I.M.: ≤60 minutes

Excretion: Feces (~66%; <4% of total dose as unchanged drug); urine (~20%; <1% of total dose as unchanged drug)

Dosage

Geriatric No dosage adjustment is recommended; consider initiating at a low end of the dosage range, with slower titration.

Adult

Bipolar mania (acute): Oral: Initial: 40 mg twice daily

Adjustment: May increase to 60 mg or 80 mg twice daily on second day of treatment; average dose 40-80 mg twice daily.

Bipolar disorder (maintenance; as adjunct to lithium or valproate): Oral: Continue ziprasidone dose at which the patient was initially stabilized; usual dosage range: 40-80 mg twice daily

Schizophrenia: Oral: Initial: 20 mg twice daily (U.S. labeling) or 20-40 mg twice daily (Canadian labeling)

Adjustment: Increases (if indicated) should be made no more frequently than every 2 days; ordinarily patients should be observed for improvement over several weeks before adjusting the dose.

Maintenance: Range: 20-100 mg twice daily; however, dosages >80 mg twice daily are generally not recommended.

Acute agitation (schizophrenia): I.M.: 10 mg every 2 hours **or** 20 mg every 4 hours (maximum: 40 mg/day). Oral therapy should replace I.M. administration as soon as possible.

Renal Impairment
Oral: No dosage adjustment is recommended

I.M.: Cyclodextrin, an excipient in the I.M. formulation, is cleared by renal filtration; use with caution.

Ziprasidone is not removed by hemodialysis.

Hepatic Impairment
U.S. labeling: No dosage adjustment is recommended; however, drug undergoes extensive hepatic metabolism and systemic exposure may be increased. Use with caution.

Canadian labeling: Manufacturer's labeling suggests that dose reductions should be considered but does not provide specific dosing recommendations.

Administration
Oral: Administer with food.

Injection: For I.M. administration only.

Monitoring Parameters Blood pressure, heart rate; temperature; serum potassium and magnesium; fasting lipid profile and fasting blood glucose/Hgb A_{1c} (prior to treatment, at 3 months, then annually); BMI; waist circumference; mental status, abnormal involuntary movement scale (AIMS), extrapyramidal symptoms. Weight should be assessed prior to treatment, at 4 weeks, 8 weeks, 12 weeks, and then at quarterly intervals. Consider titrating to a different antipsychotic agent for a weight gain ≥5% of the initial weight. The value of routine ECG screening or monitoring has not been established.

Test Interactions Increased cholesterol, triglycerides, eosinophils

Pharmacotherapy Pearls The increased potential to prolong QT_c, as compared to other available antipsychotic agents, should be considered in the evaluation of available alternatives.

Special Geriatric Considerations Extrapyramidal syndrome symptoms occur less with this agent than phenothiazine and butyrophenone classes of antipsychotics.

Many elderly patients receive antipsychotic medications for inappropriate nonpsychotic behavior. Before initiating antipsychotic medication, the clinician should investigate any possible reversible cause; any stress or stress from any disease can cause acute "confusion" or worsening of baseline nonpsychotic behavior. Most commonly, acute changes in behavior are due to increases in drug dose or addition of a new drug to regimen, fluid electrolyte loss, infection, and changes in environment. Any changes in disease status and any organ system can result in behavior changes.

In the treatment of agitated, demented, elderly patients, authors of meta-analysis of controlled trials of the response to the traditional antipsychotics (phenothiazines, butyrophenones) in controlling agitation have concluded that the use of neuroleptics results in a response rate of 18%. Clearly, neuroleptic therapy for behavior control should be limited with frequent attempts to withdraw the agent given for behavior control. In light of significant risks and adverse effects in elderly population compared with limited data demonstrating efficacy in the treatment of dementia related psychosis, aggression, and agitation, an extensive risk:benefit analysis should be performed prior to use.

Since diabetes is prevalent in elderly, monitor closely when using this agent in this population.

This medication is considered to be potentially inappropriate in this patient population (Beers Criteria: Quality of evidence - moderate; Strength of recommendation - strong).

Dosage Forms Excipient information presented when available (limited, particularly for generics); consult specific product labeling.

Capsule, oral, as hydrochloride: 20 mg, 40 mg, 60 mg, 80 mg
   Geodon®: 20 mg, 40 mg, 60 mg, 80 mg

Injection, powder for reconstitution, as mesylate [strength expressed as base]:
   Geodon®: 20 mg [contains cyclodextrin]

- ◆ **Zol 446** *see* Zoledronic Acid *on page 2057*
- ◆ **Zoladex®** *see* Goserelin *on page 898*
- ◆ **Zoledronate** *see* Zoledronic Acid *on page 2057*

Zoledronic Acid (zoe le DRON ik AS id)

Related Information
Osteoporosis Management *on page 2136*

Medication Safety Issues

Sound-alike/look-alike issues:
Zometa® may be confused with Zofran®, Zoladex®

Other safety concerns:
Duplicate therapy issues: Reclast® and Aclasta® contain zoledronic acid, which is the same ingredient contained in Zometa®; patients receiving Zometa® should not be treated with Reclast® or Aclasta®

Brand Names: U.S. Reclast®; Zometa®

Brand Names: Canada Aclasta®; Zometa®

Index Terms CGP-42446; Zol 446; Zoledronate

Generic Availability (U.S.) No

Pharmacologic Category Antidote; Bisphosphonate Derivative

Use

Oncology-related uses: Treatment of hypercalcemia of malignancy (albumin-corrected serum calcium >12 mg/dL); treatment of multiple myeloma; treatment of bone metastases of solid tumors

Nononcology uses: Treatment of Paget's disease of bone; treatment of osteoporosis in postmenopausal women (to reduce the incidence of fractures or to reduce the incidence of new clinical fractures in patients with low-trauma hip fracture); prevention of osteoporosis in postmenopausal women, treatment of osteoporosis in men (to increase bone mass); treatment and prevention of glucocorticoid-induced osteoporosis (in patients initiating or continuing prednisone ≥7.5 mg/day [or equivalent] and expected to remain on glucocorticoids for at least 12 months)

Unlabeled Use Prevention of bone loss associated with aromatase inhibitor therapy in postmenopausal women with breast cancer; prevention of bone loss associated with androgen deprivation therapy in prostate cancer

Medication Guide Available Yes

Contraindications Hypersensitivity to zoledronic acid or any component of the formulation; hypocalcemia (Reclast®); in patients with a creatinine clearance (Cl$_{cr}$) <35 mL/minute and in patients with evidence of acute renal impairment due to an increased risk of renal failure (Reclast®)

Canadian labeling: Hypersensitivity to other bisphosphonates. Aclasta® is also contraindicated with uncorrected hypocalcemia at the time of infusion.

Warnings/Precautions Hazardous agent - use appropriate precautions for handling and disposal. Osteonecrosis of the jaw (ONJ) has been reported in patients receiving bisphosphonates. Risk factors include invasive dental procedures (eg, tooth extraction, dental implants, boney surgery); a diagnosis of cancer, with concomitant chemotherapy, radiotherapy, or corticosteroids; poor oral hygiene, ill-fitting dentures; and comorbid disorders (anemia, coagulopathy, infection, pre-existing dental disease). Most reported cases occurred after I.V. bisphosphonate therapy; however, cases have been reported following oral therapy. A dental exam and preventative dentistry should be performed prior to placing patients with risk factors on chronic bisphosphonate therapy. The manufacturer's labeling states that there are no data to suggest whether discontinuing bisphosphonates in patients requiring invasive dental procedures reduces the risk of ONJ. However, other experts suggest that there is no evidence that discontinuing therapy reduces the risk of developing ONJ (Assael, 2009). The benefit/risk must be assessed by the treating physician and/or dentist/surgeon prior to any invasive dental procedure. Patients developing ONJ while on bisphosphonates should receive care by an oral surgeon.

Atypical, low energy, or low trauma femur fractures have been reported in patients receiving bisphosphonates for treatment/prevention of osteoporosis. The fractures include subtrochanteric femur (bone just below the hip joint) and diaphyseal femur (long segment of the thigh bone). Some patients experience prodromal pain weeks or months before the fracture occurs. It is unclear if bisphosphonate therapy is the cause for these fractures; atypical femur fractures have also been reported in patients not taking bisphosphonates, and in patients receiving glucocorticoids. Patients receiving long-term (>3-5 years) bisphosphonate therapy may be at an increased risk. Patients presenting with thigh or groin pain with a history of receiving bisphosphonates should be evaluated for femur fracture. Consider interrupting ▶

bisphosphonate therapy in patients who develop a femoral shaft fracture; assess for fracture in the contralateral limb.

Infrequently, severe (and occasionally debilitating) musculoskeletal (bone, joint, and/or muscle) pain have been reported during bisphosphonate treatment. The onset of pain ranged from a single day to several months. Consider discontinuing therapy in patients who experience severe symptoms; symptoms usually resolve upon discontinuation. Some patients experienced recurrence when rechallenged with same drug or another bisphosphonate; avoid use in patients with a history of these symptoms in association with bisphosphonate therapy.

May cause a significant risk of hypocalcemia in patients with Paget's disease, in whom the pretreatment rate of bone turnover may be greatly elevated. Hypocalcemia must be corrected before initiation of therapy in patients with Paget's disease and osteoporosis. Ensure adequate calcium and vitamin D intake during therapy. Use caution in patients with disturbances of calcium and mineral metabolism (eg, hypoparathyroidism, thyroid/parathyroid, surgery, malabsorption syndromes, excision of small intestine).

Reclast®: Use is contraindicated in patients with Cl_{cr} <35 mL/minute and in patients with evidence of acute renal impairment due to an increased risk of renal failure. Re-evaluate the need for continued therapy for the treatment of osteoporosis periodically; the optimal duration of treatment has not yet been determined.

Zometa®: Use caution in mild-to-moderate renal dysfunction; dosage adjustment required. In cancer patients, renal toxicity has been reported with doses >4 mg or infusions administered over 15 minutes. Risk factors for renal deterioration include pre-existing renal insufficiency and repeated doses of zoledronic acid and other bisphosphonates. Dehydration and the use of other nephrotoxic drugs which may contribute to renal deterioration should be identified and managed. Use is not recommended in patients with severe renal impairment (serum creatinine >3 mg/dL or Cl_{cr} <30 mL/minute) and bone metastases (limited data); use in patients with hypercalcemia of malignancy and severe renal impairment (serum creatinine >4.5 mg/dL for hypercalcemia of malignancy) should only be done if the benefits outweigh the risks. Renal function should be assessed prior to treatment; if decreased after treatment, additional treatments should be withheld until renal function returns to within 10% of baseline. Diuretics should not be used before correcting hypovolemia. Renal deterioration, resulting in renal failure and dialysis has occurred in patients treated with zoledronic acid after single and multiple infusions at recommended doses of 4 mg over 15 minutes.

Aclasta® [CAN; not available in U.S.]: Use is not recommended in patients with Cl_{cr} <30 mL/minute.

According to the American Society of Clinical Oncology (ASCO) guidelines for bisphosphonates in multiple myeloma, treatment with zoledronic acid is not recommended for asymptomatic (smoldering) or indolent myeloma or with solitary plasmacytoma (Kyle, 2007). The National Comprehensive Cancer Network® (NCCN) multiple myeloma guidelines (v.1.2011) also do not recommend the use of bisphosphonates in stage 1 or smoldering disease, unless part of a clinical trial.

Adequate hydration is required during treatment (urine output ~2 L/day); avoid overhydration, especially in patients with heart failure. Pre-existing renal compromise, severe dehydration, and concurrent use with diuretics or other nephrotoxic drugs may increase the risk for renal impairment. Single and multiple infusions in patients with both normal and impaired renal function have been associated with renal deterioration, resulting in renal failure and dialysis or death (rare). Patients with underlying moderate-to-severe renal impairment, increased age, concurrent use of nephrotoxic or diuretic medications, or severe dehydration prior to or after zoledronic acid administration may have an increased risk of acute renal impairment or renal failure. Others with increased risk include patients with renal impairment or dehydration secondary to fever, sepsis, gastrointestinal losses, or diuretic use. If history or physical exam suggests dehydration, treatment should not be given until the patient is normovolemic. Creatinine clearance (using actual body weight) should be calculated with the Cockcroft-Gault formula prior to each administration. Transient increases in serum creatinine may be more pronounced in patients with impaired renal function; consider monitoring creatinine clearance in at-risk patients taking other renally-eliminated drugs.

Use caution in patients with aspirin-sensitive asthma (may cause bronchoconstriction) and the elderly. Rare cases of urticaria and angioedema and very rare cases of anaphylactic reactions/shock have been reported. Do not administer Zometa® and Reclast® to the same patient for different indications.

Adverse Reactions (Reflective of adult population; not specific for elderly) Note: An acute reaction (eg, arthralgia, fever, flu-like symptoms, myalgia) may occur within the first 3 days following infusion in up to 44% of patients; usually resolves within 3-4 days of onset, although may take up to 14 days to resolve. The incidence may be decreased with acetaminophen (prior to infusion and for 72 hours postinfusion).

Zometa®:
>10%:
Cardiovascular: Leg edema (5% to 21%), hypotension (11%)
Central nervous system: Fatigue (39%), fever (32% to 44%), headache (5% to 19%), dizziness (18%), insomnia (15% to 16%), anxiety (11% to 14%), depression (14%), agitation (13%), confusion (7% to 13%), hypoesthesia (12%)
Dermatologic: Alopecia (12%), dermatitis (11%)
Endocrine & metabolic: Dehydration (5% to 14%), hypophosphatemia (13%), hypokalemia (12%), hypomagnesemia (11%)
Gastrointestinal: Nausea (29% to 46%), vomiting (14% to 32%), constipation (27% to 31%), diarrhea (17% to 24%), anorexia (9% to 22%), abdominal pain (14% to 16%), weight loss (16%), appetite decreased (13%)
Genitourinary: Urinary tract infection (12% to 14%)
Hematologic: Anemia (22% to 33%), neutropenia (12%)
Neuromuscular & skeletal: Bone pain (55%), weakness (5% to 24%), myalgia (23%), arthralgia (5% to 21%), back pain (15%), paresthesia (15%), limb pain (14%), skeletal pain (12%), rigors (11%)
Renal: Renal deterioration (8% to 17%; up to 40% in patients with abnormal baseline creatinine)
Respiratory: Dyspnea (22% to 27%), cough (12% to 22%)
Miscellaneous: Cancer progression (16% to 20%), moniliasis (12%)
1% to 10%:
Cardiovascular: Chest pain (5% to 10%)
Central nervous system: Somnolence (5% to 10%)
Endocrine & metabolic: Hypocalcemia (5% to 10%; grades 3/4: ≤1%), hypermagnesemia (grade 3: 2%)
Gastrointestinal: Dyspepsia (10%), dysphagia (5% to 10%), mucositis (5% to 10%), stomatitis (8%), sore throat (8%)
Hematologic: Granulocytopenia (5% to 10%), pancytopenia (5% to 10%), thrombocytopenia (5% to 10%)
Renal: Serum creatinine increased (grades 3/4: ≤2%)
Respiratory: Upper respiratory tract infection (10%)
Miscellaneous: Infection (nonspecific; 5% to 10%)

Reclast®:
>10%:
Cardiovascular: Hypertension (5% to 13%)
Central nervous system: Pain (2% to 24%), fever (9% to 22%), headache (4% to 20%), chills (2% to 18%), fatigue (2% to 18%)
Endocrine & metabolic: Hypocalcemia (≤3%; Paget's disease 21%)
Gastrointestinal: Nausea (5% to 18%)
Neuromuscular & skeletal: Arthralgia (9% to 27%), myalgia (5% to 23%), back pain (4% to 18%), limb pain (3% to 16%), musculoskeletal pain (≤12%)
Miscellaneous: Acute phase reaction (4% to 25%), flu-like syndrome (1% to 11%)
1% to 10%:
Cardiovascular: Chest pain (1% to 8%), peripheral edema (3% to 6%), atrial fibrillation (1% to 3%), palpitation (≤3%)
Central nervous system: Dizziness (2% to 9%), malaise (1% to 7%), hypoesthesia (≤6%), lethargy (3% to 5%), vertigo (1% to 4%), hyperthermia (≤2%)
Dermatologic: Rash (2% to 3%), hyperhidrosis (≤3%)
Gastrointestinal: Abdominal pain (1% to 9%), diarrhea (5% to 8%), vomiting (2% to 8%), constipation (6% to 7%), dyspepsia (2% to 7%), abdominal discomfort/distension (1% to 2%), anorexia (1% to 2%)
Neuromuscular & skeletal: Bone pain (3% to 9%), arthritis (2% to 9%), rigors (8%), shoulder pain (≤7%), neck pain (1% to 7%), weakness (2% to 6%), muscle spasm (2% to 6%), stiffness (1% to 5%), jaw pain (2% to 4%), joint swelling (≤3%), paresthesia (2%)
Ocular: Eye pain (≤2%)
Renal: Serum creatinine increased (2%)
Respiratory: Dyspnea (5% to 7%)
Miscellaneous: C-reactive protein increased (≤5%)

Drug Interactions
Metabolism/Transport Effects None known.
Avoid Concomitant Use There are no known interactions where it is recommended to avoid concomitant use.

Increased Effect/Toxicity
Zoledronic Acid may increase the levels/effects of: Deferasirox; Phosphate Supplements; SUNItinib

The levels/effects of Zoledronic Acid may be increased by: Aminoglycosides; Nonsteroidal Anti-Inflammatory Agents; Thalidomide

Decreased Effect
The levels/effects of Zoledronic Acid may be decreased by: Proton Pump Inhibitors

Stability Use appropriate precautions for handling and disposal.

Aclasta® [CAN]: Store at room temperature of 15°C to 30°C (59°F to 86°F).

Reclast®: Store at room temperature of 25°C (77°F); excursions permitted to 15°C to 30°C (59°F to 86°F). After opening, stable for 24 hours at 2°C to 8°C (36°F to 46°F).

Zometa®: Store concentrate vials and ready-to-use bottles at 25°C (77°F); excursions permitted to 15°C to 30°C (59°F to 86°F).

Concentrate vials: Further dilute in 100 mL NS or D_5W prior to administration. Solutions for infusion which are not used immediately after preparation should be refrigerated at 2°C to 8°C (36°F to 46°F). Infusion of solution must be completed within 24 hours of preparation.

Ready-to-use bottles: No further preparation necessary; bottles intended for single use only. If reduced doses are necessary for patients with renal impairment, withdraw the appropriate volume of solution and replace with an equal amount of NS or D_5W. The prepared, diluted solution may be refrigerated at 2°C to 8°C (36°F to 46°F) if not used immediately. Infusion of solution must be completed within 24 hours of preparation. The previously withdrawn volume from the ready-to-use solution should be discarded; do not store or reuse.

Mechanism of Action A bisphosphonate which inhibits bone resorption via actions on osteoclasts or on osteoclast precursors; inhibits osteoclastic activity and skeletal calcium release induced by tumors. Decreases serum calcium and phosphorus, and increases their elimination. In osteoporosis, zoledronic acid inhibits osteoclast-mediated resorption, therefore reducing bone turnover.

Pharmacodynamics/Kinetics
Distribution: Binds to bone
Protein binding: 28% to 53%
Half-life elimination: Triphasic; Terminal: 146 hours
Excretion: Urine (39% ± 16% as unchanged drug) within 24 hours; feces (<3%)

Dosage
Geriatric Refer to adult dosing. **Note:** Acetaminophen administration after infusion may reduce symptoms of acute-phase reactions. Patients treated for multiple myeloma, osteoporosis, and Paget's disease should receive a daily calcium supplement with vitamin D.

Adult Note: Acetaminophen administration after the infusion may reduce symptoms of acute-phase reactions. Patients treated for multiple myeloma, osteoporosis, and Paget's disease should receive a daily calcium supplement and multivitamin containing vitamin D (if dietary intake is inadequate).

Hypercalcemia of malignancy (albumin-corrected serum calcium ≥12 mg/dL) (Zometa®): I.V.: 4 mg (maximum) given as a single dose. Wait at least 7 days before considering retreatment. Dosage adjustment may be needed in patients with decreased renal function following treatment.

Multiple myeloma or metastatic bone lesions from solid tumors (Zometa®): I.V.: 4 mg every 3-4 weeks

Osteoporosis, glucocorticoid-induced, treatment and prevention (Reclast®, Aclasta® [CAN]): 5 mg infused over at least 15 minutes once a year

Osteoporosis, prevention (Reclast®): 5 mg infused over at least 15 minutes every 2 years

Osteoporosis, treatment (Reclast®, Aclasta® [CAN]): 5 mg infused over at least 15 minutes once a year

Paget's disease: I.V.: 5 mg infused over at least 15 minutes. **Note:** Data concerning retreatment is not available; retreatment may be considered for relapse (increase in alkaline phosphatase) if appropriate, for inadequate response, or in patients who are symptomatic.

Prevention of aromatase inhibitor-induced bone loss in breast cancer (unlabeled use): 4 mg every 6 months (Brufsky, 2007)

Prevention of androgen deprivation-induced bone loss in nonmetastatic prostate cancer (unlabeled use): 4 mg every 3 months for 1 year (Smith, 2003) or 4 mg every 12 months (Michaelson, 2007)

Renal Impairment
Reclast®:
Cl_{cr} ≥35 mL/minute: No adjustment required.
Cl_{cr} <35 mL/minute: Use is contraindicated.

Zometa®: Multiple myeloma and bone metastases (at treatment initiation):
Cl$_{cr}$ >60 mL/minute: 4 mg
Cl$_{cr}$ 50-60 mL/minute: 3.5 mg
Cl$_{cr}$ 40-49 mL/minute: 3.3 mg
Cl$_{cr}$ 30-39 mL/minute: 3 mg
Cl$_{cr}$ <30 mL/minute: Use is not recommended.
Zometa®: Hypercalcemia of malignancy (at treatment initiation):
Mild-to-moderate impairment: No adjustment necessary.
Severe impairment (serum creatinine >4.5 mg/dL): Evaluate risk versus benefit.
Aclasta® [CAN]:
Cl$_{cr}$ ≥30 mL/minute: No adjustment required.
Cl$_{cr}$ <30 mL/minute: Use is not recommended.

Renal toxicity (during treatment):
Hypercalcemia of malignancy: Evidence of renal deterioration: Evaluate risk versus benefit.
Multiple myeloma and bone metastases: Evidence of renal deterioration: Withhold dose until renal function returns to within 10% of baseline: renal deterioration defined as follows:
Normal baseline creatinine: Increase of 0.5 mg/dL
Abnormal baseline creatinine: Increase of 1 mg/dL
Reinitiate dose at the same dose administered prior to treatment interruption.
Multiple myeloma: Albuminuria >500 mg/24 hours (unexplained): Withhold dose until return to baseline, then re-evaluate every 3-4 weeks; consider reinitiating with a longer infusion time of at least 30 minutes (Kyle, 2007).

Hepatic Impairment Specific guidelines are not available.

Administration Infuse over at least 15 minutes. Flush I.V. line with 10 mL NS flush following infusion. Infuse in a line separate from other medications. Patients should be appropriately hydrated prior to treatment.
Reclast®, Zometa®: If refrigerated, allow to reach room temperature prior to administration. Acetaminophen after administration may reduce the incidence of acute reaction (eg, arthralgia, fever, flu-like symptoms, myalgia).

Monitoring Parameters Prior to initiation of therapy, dental exam and preventative dentistry for patients at risk for osteonecrosis, including all cancer patients
Aclasta® [CAN], Reclast®: Serum creatinine prior to each dose, especially in patients with risk factors, calculate creatinine clearance before each treatment (consider interim monitoring in patients at risk for acute renal failure), evaluate fluid status and adequately hydrate patients prior to and following administration.
Osteoporosis: Bone mineral density as measured by central dual-energy x-ray absorptiometry (DXA) of the hip or spine (prior to initiation of therapy and at least every 2 years; after 6-12 months of combined glucocorticoid and zoledronic acid treatment); annual measurements of height and weight, assessment of chronic back pain; serum calcium and 25(OH)D; phosphorus and magnesium; may consider monitoring biochemical markers of bone turnover
Paget's disease: Alkaline phosphatase; pain; serum calcium and 25(OH)D; phosphorus and magnesium
Zometa®: Serum creatinine prior to each dose; serum electrolytes, phosphate, magnesium, and hemoglobin/hematocrit should be evaluated regularly. Monitor serum calcium to assess response and avoid overtreatment. In patients with multiple myeloma, monitor urine every 3-6 months for albuminuria.

Test Interactions Bisphosphonates may interfere with diagnostic imaging agents such as technetium-99m-diphosphonate in bone scans.

Pharmacotherapy Pearls Oncology Comment:
Metastatic breast cancer: The American Society of Clinical Oncology (ASCO) guidelines on the role of bone-modifying agents (BMAs) in the prevention and treatment of skeletal-related events for metastatic breast cancer patients were updated (Van Poznak, 2011). The guidelines recommend initiating a BMA (denosumab, pamidronate, zoledronic acid) in patients with a diagnosis of metastatic breast cancer to the bone. There is currently no literature indicating the superiority of one particular BMA over another. The optimal duration has yet to be defined; however, the guidelines recommend continuing therapy until substantial decline in patient's performance status. In patients with normal creatinine clearance (>60 mL/minute), no dosage/interval/infusion rate changes for pamidronate or zoledronic acid are necessary. For patients with Cl$_{cr}$ <30 mL/minute, pamidronate and zoledronic acid are not recommended. While no renal dose adjustments are recommended for denosumab, close monitoring is advised for risk of hypocalcemia in patients with Cl$_{cr}$ <30 mL/minute or on dialysis. The ASCO guidelines are in alignment with package insert guidelines for dosing, renal dose adjustments, infusion times, prevention and management of osteonecrosis of the jaw, and monitoring of laboratory parameter recommendations. BMAs are not the first-line therapy for pain. BMAs are to be

used as adjunctive therapy for cancer-related bone pain associated with bone metastasis, demonstrating a modest pain control benefit. BMAs should be used in conjunction with agents such as NSAIDS, opioid and nonopioid analgesics, corticosteroids, radiation/surgery, interventional procedures.

Multiple myeloma: The American Society of Clinical Oncology (ASCO) also has guidelines published on the use of bisphosphonates for prevention and treatment of bone disease in multiple myeloma (Kyle, 2007). Pamidronate or zoledronic acid use is recommended in multiple myeloma patients with lytic bone destruction or compression spine fracture from osteopenia. Clodronate (not available in the U.S.; available in Canada), administered orally or I.V., is an alternative treatment. The use of the bisphosphonates pamidronate and zoledronic acid may be considered in patients with pain secondary to osteolytic disease, adjunct therapy to stabilize fractures or impending fractures, and I.V. bisphosphonates for multiple myeloma patients with osteopenia but no radiographic evidence of lytic bone disease. Bisphosphonates are not recommended in patients with solitary plasmacytoma, smoldering (asymptomatic) or indolent myeloma, or monoclonal gammopathy of undetermined significance. The guidelines recommend monthly treatment for a period of 2 years. At that time, physicians need to consider discontinuing in responsive and stable patients, and reinitiate if new-onset skeletal-related event occurs. The ASCO guidelines are in alignment with package insert guidelines for dosing, renal dose adjustments, infusion times, prevention and management of osteonecrosis of the jaw, and monitoring of laboratory parameter recommendations. The guidelines also state in patients with a serum creatinine >3 mg/dL or Cl_{cr} <30 mL/minute or extensive bone disease, pamidronate at a dose of 90 mg over 4-6 hours is recommended (unless pre-existing renal disease at which a reduced dose should be considered). The ASCO committee also recommends monitoring for the presence of albuminuria every 3-6 months. In patients with albuminuria >500 mg/24 hours, withhold the dose until level returns to baseline, then recheck every 3-4 weeks. Pamidronate may be reinitiated at a dose not to exceed 90 mg every 4 weeks with a longer infusion time of at least 4 hours. The committee also recommends considering increasing the infusion time of zoledronic acid to at least 30 minutes. However, one study has demonstrated that extending the infusion to 30 minutes did not change the safety profile (Berenson, 2011).

Special Geriatric Considerations The elderly are frequently treated long-term for osteoporosis. Elderly patients should be advised to report any lower extremity, jaw (osteonecrosis), or muscle pain that cannot be explained or lasts longer than 2 weeks. Additionally, elderly often receive concomitant diuretic therapy and therefore their electrolyte status (eg, calcium, phosphate) should be periodically evaluated.

Due to the reports of atypical femur fractures and osteonecrosis of the jaw, recommendations for duration of bisphosphonate use in osteoporosis have been modified. Based on available data, consider discontinuing bisphosphonates after 5 years of use in low-risk patients, since the risk of nonvertebral fracture is the same as those patients taking bisphosphonates for 10 years. Those patients with high risk (fracture history) may be continued for a longer period, taking into consideration the risks vs benefits associated with continued therapy.

Dosage Forms Excipient information presented when available (limited, particularly for generics); consult specific product labeling.
Infusion, premixed:
  Reclast®: 5 mg (100 mL)
  Zometa®: 4 mg (100 mL)
Injection, solution [concentrate]:
  Zometa®: 4 mg/5 mL (5 mL)
Dosage Forms: Canada Excipient information presented when available (limited, particularly for generics); consult specific product labeling.
Infusion, solution [premixed]:
  Aclasta®: 5 mg (100 mL)

ZOLMitriptan (zohl mi TRIP tan)

Medication Safety Issues
  Sound-alike/look-alike issues:
    ZOLMitriptan may be confused with SUMAtriptan
Brand Names: U.S. Zomig-ZMT®; Zomig®
Brand Names: Canada Mylan-Zolmitriptan; PMS-Zolmitriptan; PMS-Zolmitriptan ODT; Sandoz-Zolmitriptan; Sandoz-Zolmitriptan ODT; Teva-Zolmitriptan; Teva-Zolmitriptan OD; Zolmitriptan ODT; Zomig®; Zomig® Nasal Spray; Zomig® Rapimelt
Index Terms 311C90
Generic Availability (U.S.) No
Pharmacologic Category Antimigraine Agent; Serotonin 5-HT$_{1B, 1D}$ Receptor Agonist
Use Acute treatment of migraine with or without aura

Unlabeled Use Short-term prevention of menstrually-associated migraines (MAMs)

Contraindications Hypersensitivity to zolmitriptan or any component of the formulation; ischemic heart disease or vasospastic coronary artery disease, including Prinzmetal's angina; signs or symptoms of ischemic heart disease; uncontrolled hypertension; symptomatic Wolff-Parkinson-White syndrome or arrhythmias associated with other cardiac accessory conduction pathway disorders; use with ergotamine derivatives (within 24 hours of); use within 24 hours of another 5-HT$_1$ agonist; concurrent administration or within 2 weeks of discontinuing an MAO inhibitor; management of hemiplegic or basilar migraine

Nasal spray: Additional contraindications with nasal spray: Cerebrovascular syndromes (eg, stroke, TIA); peripheral vascular disease (including ischemic bowel disease)

Warnings/Precautions Zolmitriptan is indicated only in patient populations with a clear diagnosis of migraine. Not for prophylactic treatment of migraine headaches. Cardiac events (coronary artery vasospasm, transient ischemia, myocardial infarction, ventricular tachycardia/fibrillation, cardiac arrest, and death) have been reported with 5-HT$_1$ agonist administration. Patients who experience sensations of chest pain/pressure/tightness or symptoms suggestive of angina following dosing should be evaluated for coronary artery disease or Prinzmetal's angina before receiving additional doses; if dosing is resumed and similar symptoms recur, monitor with ECG. Should not be given to patients who have risk factors for CAD (eg, hypertension, hypercholesterolemia, smoker, obesity, diabetes, strong family history of CAD, menopause, male >40 years of age) without adequate cardiac evaluation. Patients with suspected CAD should have cardiovascular evaluation to rule out CAD before considering zolmitriptan's use; if cardiovascular evaluation negative, first dose would be safest if given in the healthcare provider's office (consider ECG monitoring). Periodic evaluation of those without cardiovascular disease, but with continued risk factors, should be done. Significant elevation in blood pressure, including hypertensive crisis, has also been reported on rare occasions in patients with and without a history of hypertension. Vasospasm-related reactions have been reported other than coronary artery vasospasm. Peripheral vascular ischemia and colonic ischemia with abdominal pain and bloody diarrhea have occurred. Cerebral/subarachnoid hemorrhage and stroke have been reported with 5-HT$_1$ agonist administration; nasal spray contraindicated in patients with cerebrovascular syndromes. Rarely, partial vision loss and blindness (transient and permanent) have been reported with 5-HT$_1$ agonists. Use with caution in patients with hepatic impairment. Zomig-ZMT™ tablets contain phenylalanine. Symptoms of agitation, confusion, hallucinations, hyper-reflexia, myoclonus, shivering, and tachycardia (serotonin syndrome) may occur with concomitant proserotonergic drugs (eg, SSRIs/SNRIs or triptans) or agents which reduce zolmitriptan's metabolism. Concurrent use of serotonin precursors (eg, tryptophan) is not recommended.

Adverse Reactions (Reflective of adult population; not specific for elderly) Percentages noted from oral preparations.

1% to 10%:

  Cardiovascular: Chest pain (2% to 4%), palpitation (up to 2%)

  Central nervous system: Dizziness (6% to 10%), somnolence (5% to 8%), pain (2% to 3%), vertigo (≤2%)

  Gastrointestinal: Nausea (4% to 9%), xerostomia (3% to 5%), dyspepsia (1% to 3%), dysphagia (≤2%)

  Neuromuscular & skeletal: Paresthesia (5% to 9%), weakness (3% to 9%), warm/cold sensation (5% to 7%), hypoesthesia (1% to 2%), myalgia (1% to 2%), myasthenia (up to 2%)

  Miscellaneous: Neck/throat/jaw pain (4% to 10%), diaphoresis (up to 3%), allergic reaction (up to 1%)

Drug Interactions

  Metabolism/Transport Effects Substrate of CYP1A2 (minor); **Note:** Assignment of Major/Minor substrate status based on clinically relevant drug interaction potential

  Avoid Concomitant Use

  Avoid concomitant use of ZOLMitriptan with any of the following: Ergot Derivatives; MAO Inhibitors

  Increased Effect/Toxicity

  ZOLMitriptan may increase the levels/effects of: Ergot Derivatives; Metoclopramide; Serotonin Modulators

  The levels/effects of ZOLMitriptan may be increased by: Antipsychotics; Cimetidine; Ergot Derivatives; MAO Inhibitors; Propranolol

  Decreased Effect There are no known significant interactions involving a decrease in effect.

Ethanol/Nutrition/Herb Interactions Ethanol: Limit use (may have additive CNS toxicity).

Stability Store at 20°C to 25°C (68°F to 77°F). Protect from light and moisture.

Mechanism of Action Selective agonist for serotonin (5-HT$_{1B}$ and 5-HT$_{1D}$ receptors) in cranial arteries; causes vasoconstriction and reduces sterile inflammation associated with antidromic neuronal transmission correlating with relief of migraine

Pharmacodynamics/Kinetics

Onset of action: 0.5-1 hour

Absorption: Well absorbed

Distribution: V_d: 7 L/kg

Protein binding: 25%

Metabolism: Converted to an active N-desmethyl metabolite (2-6 times more potent than zolmitriptan)

Bioavailability: 40%

Half-life elimination: 2.8-3.7 hours

Time to peak, serum: Tablet: 1.5 hours; Orally-disintegrating tablet and nasal spray: 3 hours

Excretion: Urine (~60% to 65% total dose); feces (30% to 40%)

Dosage

Geriatric Refer to adult dosing. No dosage adjustment needed, but elderly patients are more likely to have underlying cardiovascular disease and should have careful evaluation of cardiovascular system before prescribing.

Adult

Migraine headache:

Oral:

Tablet: Initial: ≤2.5 mg at the onset of migraine headache; may break 2.5 mg tablet in half

Orally-disintegrating tablet: Initial: 2.5 mg at the onset of migraine headache

Nasal spray: Initial: 1 spray (5 mg) at the onset of migraine headache

Note: Use the lowest possible dose to minimize adverse events. If the headache returns, the dose may be repeated after 2 hours; do not exceed 10 mg within a 24-hour period. Controlled trials have not established the effectiveness of a second dose if the initial one was ineffective.

Renal Impairment No dosage adjustment recommended. There is a 25% reduction in zolmitriptan's clearance in patients with severe renal impairment (Cl_{cr} 5-25 mL/minute).

Hepatic Impairment Administer with caution in patients with liver disease, generally using doses <2.5 mg (doses <5 mg can only be achieved using oral tablets). Patients with moderate-to-severe hepatic impairment may have decreased clearance of zolmitriptan, and significant elevation in blood pressure was observed in some patients.

Administration Administer as soon as migraine headache starts.

Tablets: May be broken

Orally-disintegrating tablets: Must be taken whole; do not break, crush, or chew; place on tongue and allow to dissolve; administration with liquid is not required

Nasal spray: Blow nose gently prior to use. After removing protective cap, instill device into nostril. Block opposite nostril; breathe in gently through nose while pressing plunger of spray device. One dose (5 mg) is equal to 1 spray in 1 nostril.

Pharmacotherapy Pearls Not recommended if the patient has risk factors for heart disease (high blood pressure, high cholesterol, obesity, diabetes, smoking, strong family history of heart disease, postmenopausal woman, or a male >40 years of age).

This agent is intended to relieve migraine, but not to prevent or reduce the number of attacks. Use only to treat an actual migraine attack.

Special Geriatric Considerations No dosage adjustment needed, but elderly patients are more likely to have underlying cardiovascular disease and should have careful evaluation of the cardiovascular system before prescribing.

Dosage Forms Excipient information presented when available (limited, particularly for generics); consult specific product labeling.

Solution, intranasal [spray]:

Zomig®: 5 mg/0.1 mL (0.1 mL)

Tablet, oral:

Zomig®: 2.5 mg [scored]

Zomig®: 5 mg

Tablet, orally disintegrating, oral:

Zomig-ZMT®: 2.5 mg [contains phenylalanine 2.81 mg/tablet; orange flavor]

Zomig-ZMT®: 5 mg [contains phenylalanine 5.62 mg/tablet; orange flavor]

◆ **Zoloft®** see Sertraline on page 1765

Zolpidem (zole PI dem)

Related Information

Beers Criteria – Potentially Inappropriate Medications for Geriatrics on page 2183

Medication Safety Issues

Sound-alike/look-alike issues:

Ambien® may be confused with Abilify®, Ativan®, Ambi 10®

Sublinox™ may be confused with Suboxone®

Zolpidem may be confused with lorazepam, zaleplon

BEERS Criteria medication:

This drug may be potentially inappropriate for use in geriatric patients (Quality of evidence - moderate; Strength of recommendation - strong).

International issues:

Ambien [U.S., Argentina, Israel] may be confused with Amyben brand name for amiodarone [Great Britain]

Brand Names: U.S. Ambien CR®; Ambien®; Edluar™; Intermezzo®; Zolpimist®

Brand Names: Canada Sublinox™

Index Terms Zolpidem Tartrate

Generic Availability (U.S.) Yes: Excludes oral spray, sublingual tablet

Pharmacologic Category Hypnotic, Miscellaneous

Use

Ambien®, Edluar™, Zolpimist®: Short-term treatment of insomnia (with difficulty of sleep onset)

Ambien CR®: Treatment of insomnia (with difficulty of sleep onset and/or sleep maintenance)

Intermezzo®: "As needed" treatment of middle-of-the-night insomnia with ≥4 hours of sleep time remaining.

Sublinox™ (Canadian availability; not available in U.S.): Short-term treatment of insomnia (with difficulty of sleep onset, frequent awakenings, and/or early awakenings)

Medication Guide Available Yes

Contraindications Hypersensitivity to zolpidem or any component of the formulation

Canadian labeling: Additional contraindications (not in U.S. labeling): Significant obstructive sleep apnea syndrome and acute and/or severe impairment of respiratory function; myasthenia gravis; severe hepatic impairment; personal or family history of sleepwalking

Warnings/Precautions Should be used only after evaluation of potential causes of sleep disturbance. Failure of sleep disturbance to resolve after 7-10 days may indicate psychiatric or medical illness. Hypnotics/sedatives have been associated with abnormal thinking and behavior changes including decreased inhibition, aggression, bizarre behavior, agitation, hallucinations, and depersonalization. These changes may occur unpredictably and may indicate previously unrecognized psychiatric disorders; evaluate appropriately. Sedative/hypnotics may produce withdrawal symptoms following abrupt discontinuation. Use with caution in patients with depression; worsening of depression, including suicide or suicidal ideation has been reported with the use of hypnotics. Intentional overdose may be an issue in this population. The minimum dose that will effectively treat the individual patient should be used. Prescriptions should be written for the smallest quantity consistent with good patient care. Causes CNS depression, which may impair physical and mental capabilities. Zolpidem should only be administered when the patient is able to stay in bed a full night (7-8 hours) before being active again. Effects with other sedative drugs or ethanol may be potentiated. Canadian labeling does not recommend concomitant use with alcohol.

Use caution in patients with myasthenia gravis (contraindicated in the Canadian labeling). Avoid use in patients with sleep apnea or a history of sedative-hypnotic abuse. Postmarketing studies have indicated that the use of hypnotic/sedative agents for sleep has been associated with hypersensitivity reactions including anaphylaxis as well as angioedema. An increased risk for hazardous sleep-related activities such as sleep-driving; cooking and eating food, and making phone calls while asleep have also been noted; amnesia may also occur. Discontinue treatment in patients who report any sleep-related episodes. Canadian labeling recommends avoiding use in patients with disorders (eg, restless legs syndrome, periodic limb movement disorder, sleep apnea) that may disrupt sleep and cause frequent awakenings, potentially increasing the risk of complex sleep-related behaviors.

Use caution with respiratory disease (Canadian labeling contraindicates use with acute and/or severe impairment of respiratory function). Use caution with hepatic impairment (Canadian labeling contraindicates use in severe impairment); dose adjustment required. Because of the rapid onset of action, administer immediately prior to bedtime or after the patient has gone to bed and is having difficulty falling asleep.

Use caution in the elderly; dose adjustment recommended. Closely monitor elderly or debilitated patients for impaired cognitive and/or motor performance, confusion, and potential for falling. Avoid chronic use (>90 days) in older adults; adverse events, including delirium, falls, fractures, have been observed with nonbenzodiazepine hypnotic use in the elderly similar to events observed with benzodiazepines. Data suggests improvements in sleep duration and latency are minimal (Beers Criteria).

◄ Dosage adjustment is recommended for females receiving Intermezzo®; pharmacokinetic studies involving sublingual zolpidem (Intermezzo®) showed a significant increase in maximum concentration and exposure in females compared to males at the same dose.

Adverse Reactions (Reflective of adult population; not specific for elderly) Actual frequency may be dosage form, dose, and/or age dependent

>10%: Central nervous system: Headache (3% to 19%), somnolence (6% to 15%), dizziness (1% to 12%)

1% to 10%:

Cardiovascular: Blood pressure increased, chest discomfort/pain, palpitation

Central nervous system: Abnormal dreams, anxiety, apathy, amnesia, ataxia, attention disturbance, body temperature increased, burning sensation, confusion, depersonalization, depression, disinhibition, disorientation, drowsiness, drugged feeling, euphoria, fatigue, fever, hallucinations, hypoesthesia, insomnia, lethargy, lightheadedness, memory disorder, mood swings, sleep disorder, stress

Dermatologic: Rash, urticaria, wrinkling

Endocrine & metabolic: Menorrhagia

Gastrointestinal: Abdominal discomfort, abdominal pain, abdominal tenderness, appetite disorder, constipation, diarrhea, dyspepsia, flatulence, gastroenteritis, gastroesophageal reflux, hiccup, nausea, vomiting, xerostomia

Genitourinary: Urinary tract infection, vulvovaginal dryness

Neuromuscular & skeletal: Arthralgia, back pain, balance disorder, involuntary muscle contractions, myalgia, neck pain, paresthesia, psychomotor retardation, tremor, weakness

Ocular: Asthenopia, blurred vision, depth perception altered, diplopia, red eye, visual disturbance

Otic: Labyrinthitis, tinnitus, vertigo

Renal: Dysuria

Respiratory: Pharyngitis, sinusitis, throat irritation, upper respiratory tract infection

Miscellaneous: Allergy, binge eating, flu-like syndrome

Drug Interactions

Metabolism/Transport Effects Substrate of CYP1A2 (minor), CYP2C19 (minor), CYP2C9 (minor), CYP2D6 (minor), CYP3A4 (major); **Note:** Assignment of Major/Minor substrate status based on clinically relevant drug interaction potential

Avoid Concomitant Use

Avoid concomitant use of Zolpidem with any of the following: Azelastine; Azelastine (Nasal); Conivaptan; Methadone; Mirtazapine; Paraldehyde

Increased Effect/Toxicity

Zolpidem may increase the levels/effects of: Alcohol (Ethyl); Azelastine; Azelastine (Nasal); Buprenorphine; CarBAMazepine; Methadone; Methotrimeprazine; Metyrosine; Mirtazapine; Paraldehyde; Selective Serotonin Reuptake Inhibitors

The levels/effects of Zolpidem may be increased by: Antifungal Agents (Azole Derivatives, Systemic); CNS Depressants; Conivaptan; CYP3A4 Inhibitors (Moderate); CYP3A4 Inhibitors (Strong); Dasatinib; Droperidol; FluvoxaMINE; HydrOXYzine; Ivacaftor; Methotrimeprazine; Mifepristone

Decreased Effect

The levels/effects of Zolpidem may be decreased by: CarBAMazepine; CYP3A4 Inducers (Strong); Deferasirox; Flumazenil; Herbs (CYP3A4 Inducers); Peginterferon Alfa-2b; Rifamycin Derivatives; Telaprevir; Tocilizumab

Ethanol/Nutrition/Herb Interactions

Ethanol: May enhance the adverse/toxic effects of zolpidem. Management: Avoid use of ethanol.

Food: Maximum plasma concentration and bioavailability are decreased with food; time to peak plasma concentration is increased; half-life remains unchanged. Grapefruit juice may decrease the metabolism of zolpidem. Management: Avoid grapefruit juice.

Herb/Nutraceutical: St John's wort may decrease the levels/effects of zolpidem. Some herbal medications should be avoided due to the risk of increased CNS depression. Management: Avoid concomitant use of St John's wort. Avoid valerian, kava kava, and gotu kola.

Stability

Ambien®, Edluar™, Intermezzo®: Store at 20°C to 25°C (68°F to 77°F). Protect sublingual tablets from light and moisture.

Ambien CR®: Store at 15°C to 25°C (59°F to 77°F); limited excursions permitted up to 30°C (86°F).

Zolpimist®: Store at 25°C (77°F); do not freeze. Avoid prolonged exposure to temperatures >30°C (86°F).

Sublinox™ (Canadian availability; not available in U.S.): Store at 15°C to 30°C (59°F to 86°F); protect from light and moisture.

Mechanism of Action Zolpidem, an imidazopyridine hypnotic that is structurally dissimilar to benzodiazepines, enhances the activity of the inhibitory neurotransmitter, γ-aminobutyric acid (GABA), via selective agonism at the benzodiazepine-1 (BZ_1) receptor; the result is increased chloride conductance, neuronal hyperpolarization, inhibition of the action potential, and a decrease in neuronal excitability leading to sedative and hypnotic effects. Because of its selectivity for the BZ_1 receptor site over the BZ_2 receptor site, zolpidem exhibits minimal anxiolytic, myorelaxant, and anticonvulsant properties (effects largely attributed to agonism at the BZ_2 receptor site).

Pharmacodynamics/Kinetics

Onset of action: Immediate release: 30 minutes

Duration: Immediate release: 6-8 hours

Absorption: Rapid

Sublingual tablet: Intermezzo®: C_{max} and AUC is increased by ~45% in females compared to male subjects

Distribution: V_d: 0.54 L/kg

Protein binding: ~93%

Metabolism: Hepatic methylation and hydroxylation via CYP3A4 (~60%), CYP2C9 (~22%), CYP1A2 (~14%), CYP2D6 (~3%), and CYP2C19 (~3%) to three inactive metabolites

Bioavailability: 70%

Half-life elimination:

Immediate release, Extended release: ~2.5 hours (range 1.4-4.5 hours); Cirrhosis: Up to 9.9 hours; Elderly: Prolonged up to 32%

Spray: ~3 hours (range: 1.7-8.4)

Sublingual tablet (Edluar™, Intermezzo®): ~3 hours (range: 1.4-6.7 hours)

Time to peak, plasma:

Immediate release: 1.6 hours; 2.2 hours with food

Extended release: 1.5 hours; 4 hours with food

Spray: ~0.9 hours

Sublingual tablet: Edluar™: ~1.4 hours, ~1.8 hours with food; Intermezzo®: 0.6-1.3 hours, ~3 hours with food

Excretion: Urine (48% to 67%, primarily as metabolites); feces (29% to 42%, primarily as metabolites)

Dosage

Geriatric Oral:

Immediate release tablet, spray: 5 mg immediately before bedtime

Sublingual tablet:

U.S. labeling:

Edluar™: 5 mg immediately before bedtime

Intermezzo®: Females and males: 1.75 mg once per night as needed (maximum: 1.75 mg/night). **Note:** Take only if ≥4 hours left before waking.

Canadian labeling (Sublinox™): Not recommended; tablet cannot not be split for a reduced dose.

Extended release tablet: 6.25 mg immediately before bedtime

Adult Insomnia: Oral:

Immediate release tablet, spray: 10 mg immediately before bedtime; maximum dose: 10 mg/day

Extended release tablet: 12.5 mg immediately before bedtime

Sublingual tablet:

Edluar™, Sublinox™ (Canadian availability; not available in U.S.): 10 mg immediately before bedtime; maximum dose: 10 mg/day

Intermezzo®: **Note:** Take only if ≥4 hours left before waking

Females: 1.75 mg once per night as needed (maximum: 1.75 mg/night)

Males: 3.5 mg once per night as needed (maximum: 3.5 mg/night)

Dosage adjustment with concomitant CNS depressants: Females and males: 1.75 mg once per night as needed; dose adjustment of concomitant CNS depressant(s) may be necessary.

Renal Impairment No dosage adjustment provided in manufacturer's labeling; however, some zolpidem labeling recommends monitoring patients with renal impairment closely. Not dialyzable

Hepatic Impairment

U.S. labeling:

Immediate release tablet, spray: 5 mg immediately before bedtime

Extended release tablet: 6.25 mg immediately before bedtime

Sublingual tablet:

Edluar™: 5 mg immediately before bedtime

Intermezzo®: Females and males: 1.75 mg once per night as needed. **Note:** Take only if ≥4 hours left before waking.

Canadian labeling: Sublingual tablet: Sublinox®:
Mild-to-moderate impairment: Use is not recommended; tablet cannot be split for reduced dose.
Severe impairment: Use is contraindicated.

Administration Ingest immediately before bedtime due to rapid onset of action. Regardless of dosage form, do not administer with or immediately after a meal.

Ambien CR® tablets should be swallowed whole; do not divide, crush, or chew.

Edluar™, Intermezzo®, or Sublinox™ (Canadian availability; not available in U.S.) sublingual tablets should be placed under the tongue and allowed to disintegrate; do not swallow or administer with water.

Zolpimist® oral spray should be sprayed directly into the mouth over the tongue. Prior to initial use, pump should be primed by spraying 5 times. If pump is not used for at least 14 days, re-prime pump with 1 spray.

Monitoring Parameters Daytime alertness; respiratory rate; behavior profile

Test Interactions Increased aminotransferase [ALT/AST], bilirubin (S); decreased RAI uptake

Pharmacotherapy Pearls Causes fewer disturbances in sleep stages as compared to benzodiazepines. Time spent in sleep stages 3 and 4 are maintained; zolpidem decreases sleep latency; should not be prescribed in quantities exceeding a 1-month supply.

Special Geriatric Considerations In doses >5 mg, there was subjective evidence of impaired sleep on the first post-treatment night. There have been reports of increased hypotension and/or falls in the elderly with this drug. With Ambien CR®, the adverse event profile of 6.25 mg in elderly patients was similar to the 12.5 mg dose in younger adults. Until there is more experience with this dosage form, use with caution in the elderly. For Intermezzo®, it may be advisable to avoid this formulation since elderly patients may not realize if they have >4 more hours to sleep.

This medication is considered to be potentially inappropriate in this patient population (Beers Criteria: Quality of evidence - moderate; Strength of recommendation - strong).

Controlled Substance C-IV

Dosage Forms Excipient information presented when available (limited, particularly for generics); consult specific product labeling.

Solution, oral, as tartrate [spray]:
Zolpimist®: 5 mg/actuation (8.2 g) [contains benzoic acid, propylene glycol; cherry flavor; 60 metered actuations]
Tablet, oral, as tartrate: 5 mg, 10 mg
Ambien®: 5 mg, 10 mg
Tablet, sublingual, as tartrate:
Edluar™: 5 mg, 10 mg
Intermezzo®: 1.75 mg, 3.5 mg [spearmint flavor]
Tablet, extended release, oral, as tartrate: 6.25 mg, 12.5 mg
Ambien CR®: 6.25 mg, 12.5 mg

Dosage Forms: Canada Excipient information presented when available (limited, particularly for generics); consult specific product labeling.

Tablet, sublingual, as tartrate:
Sublinox™: 10 mg

Zonisamide (zoe NIS a mide)

Medication Safety Issues
Sound-alike/look-alike issues:
Zonegran® may be confused with SINEquan®
Zonisamide may be confused with lacosamide

Brand Names: U.S. Zonegran®

Generic Availability (U.S.) Yes

Pharmacologic Category Anticonvulsant, Miscellaneous

Use Adjunct treatment of partial seizures in adults with epilepsy

Unlabeled Use Bipolar disorder

Medication Guide Available Yes

Contraindications Hypersensitivity to zonisamide, sulfonamides, or any component of the formulation

Warnings/Precautions Hazardous agent - use appropriate precautions for handling and disposal. Rare, but potentially fatal sulfonamide reactions have occurred following the use of zonisamide. These reactions include Stevens-Johnson syndrome, fulminant hepatic necrosis, agranulocytosis, aplastic anemia, and toxic epidermal necrolysis, usually appearing within 2-16 weeks of drug initiation. Discontinue zonisamide if rash develops. Chemical similarities are present among sulfonamides, sulfonylureas, carbonic anhydrase inhibitors, thiazides, and loop diuretics (except ethacrynic acid). Use in patients with sulfonamide allergy is specifically contraindicated in product labeling, however, a risk of cross-reaction exists in patients with allergy to any of these compounds; avoid use when previous reaction has been severe. Use may be associated with the development of metabolic acidosis (generally dose-dependent) in certain patients; predisposing conditions/therapies include renal disease, severe respiratory disease, diarrhea, surgery, ketogenic diet, and other medications. Serum bicarbonate should be monitored in all patients prior to and during use; if metabolic acidosis occurs, consider decreasing the dose or tapering the dose to discontinue. If use continued despite acidosis, alkali treatment should be considered. Untreated metabolic acidosis may increase the risk of developing nephrolithiasis, nephrocalcinosis, osteomalacia, or osteoporosis.

Pooled analysis of trials involving various antiepileptics (regardless of indication) showed an increased risk of suicidal thoughts/behavior (incidence rate: 0.43% treated patients compared to 0.24% of patients receiving placebo); risk observed as early as 1 week after initiation and continued through duration of trials (most trials ≤24 weeks). Monitor all patients for notable changes in behavior that might indicate suicidal thoughts or depression; notify healthcare provider immediately if symptoms occur.

Discontinue zonisamide in patients who develop acute renal failure or a significant sustained increase in creatinine/BUN concentration. Kidney stones have been reported. Do not use in patients with renal impairment (GFR <50 mL/minute); use with caution in patients with hepatic impairment.

Significant CNS effects include psychiatric symptoms, psychomotor slowing, and fatigue or somnolence. Fatigue and somnolence occur within the first month of treatment, most commonly at doses of 300-500 mg/day. Effects with other sedative drugs or ethanol may be potentiated. May cause sedation, which may impair physical or mental abilities; patients must be cautioned about performing tasks which require mental alertness (eg, operating machinery or driving). Abrupt withdrawal may precipitate seizures; discontinue or reduce doses gradually.

Adverse Reactions (Reflective of adult population; not specific for elderly) Frequencies noted in patients receiving other anticonvulsants:
>10%:
 Central nervous system: Somnolence (17%), dizziness (13%)
 Gastrointestinal: Anorexia (13%)
1% to 10%:
 Central nervous system: Headache (10%), agitation/irritability (9%), fatigue (8%), tiredness (7%), ataxia (6%), confusion (6%), concentration decreased (6%), memory impairment (6%), depression (6%), insomnia (6%), speech disorders (5%), mental slowing (4%), anxiety (3%), nervousness (2%), schizophrenic/schizophreniform behavior (2%), difficulty in verbal expression (2%), status epilepticus (1%), seizure (1%), hyperesthesia (1%), incoordination (1%)
 Dermatologic: Rash (3%), bruising (2%), pruritus (1%)
 Gastrointestinal: Nausea (9%), abdominal pain (6%), diarrhea (5%), dyspepsia (3%), weight loss (3%), constipation (2%), taste perversion (2%), xerostomia (2%), vomiting (1%)
 Neuromuscular & skeletal: Paresthesia (4%), abnormal gait (1%), tremor (1%), weakness (1%)
 Ocular: Diplopia (6%), nystagmus (4%), amblyopia (1%)
 Otic: Tinnitus (1%)
 Renal: Kidney stones (4%, children 3% to 8%)
 Respiratory: Rhinitis (2%), pharyngitis (1%), increased cough (1%)
 Miscellaneous: Flu-like syndrome (4%) accidental injury (1%)
Drug Interactions
 Metabolism/Transport Effects Substrate of CYP2C19 (minor), CYP3A4 (major); **Note:** Assignment of Major/Minor substrate status based on clinically relevant drug interaction potential
 Avoid Concomitant Use
  Avoid concomitant use of Zonisamide with any of the following: Azelastine; Azelastine (Nasal); Carbonic Anhydrase Inhibitors; Conivaptan; Methadone; Mirtazapine; Paraldehyde ▶

Increased Effect/Toxicity

Zonisamide may increase the levels/effects of: Alcohol (Ethyl); Alpha-/Beta-Agonists; Amphetamines; Anticonvulsants (Barbiturate); Anticonvulsants (Hydantoin); Azelastine; Azelastine (Nasal); Buprenorphine; CarBAMazepine; Carbonic Anhydrase Inhibitors; CNS Depressants; Flecainide; Memantine; MetFORMIN; Methadone; Methotrimeprazine; Metyrosine; Mirtazapine; Paraldehyde; Primidone; QuiNIDine; Selective Serotonin Reuptake Inhibitors; Zolpidem

The levels/effects of Zonisamide may be increased by: Conivaptan; CYP3A4 Inhibitors (Moderate); CYP3A4 Inhibitors (Strong); Dasatinib; Droperidol; HydrOXYzine; Ivacaftor; Methotrimeprazine; Mifepristone; Salicylates

Decreased Effect

Zonisamide may decrease the levels/effects of: Lithium; Methenamine; Primidone

The levels/effects of Zonisamide may be decreased by: CYP3A4 Inducers (Strong); Deferasirox; Fosphenytoin; Herbs (CYP3A4 Inducers); Ketorolac; Ketorolac (Nasal); Ketorolac (Systemic); Mefloquine; PHENobarbital; Phenytoin; Tocilizumab

Ethanol/Nutrition/Herb Interactions

Ethanol: May increase CNS depression; monitor for increased effects with coadministration. Caution patients about effects.

Food: Food delays time to maximum concentration, but does not affect bioavailability.

Stability Store at controlled room temperature 25°C (77°F). Protect from moisture and light.

Mechanism of Action The exact mechanism of action is not known. May stabilize neuronal membranes and suppress neuronal hypersynchronization through action at sodium and calcium channels. Does not affect GABA activity.

Pharmacodynamics/Kinetics

Distribution: V_d: 1.45 L/kg

Protein binding: 40%

Metabolism: Hepatic via CYP3A4; forms N-acetyl zonisamide and 2-sulfamoylacetyl phenol (SMAP)

Half-life elimination: Plasma: ~63 hours

Time to peak: 2-6 hours

Excretion: Urine (62%, 35% as unchanged drug, 65% as metabolites); feces (3%)

Dosage

Geriatric Data from clinical trials is insufficient for patients older than 65. Begin dosing at the low end of the dosing range.

Adult

Adjunctive treatment of partial seizures: Oral: Initial: 100 mg/day. Dose may be increased to 200 mg/day after 2 weeks. Further dosage increases to 300 mg and 400 mg/day can then be made with a minimum of 2 weeks between adjustments, in order to reach steady state at each dosage level. Doses of up to 600 mg/day have been studied, however, there is no evidence of increased response with doses >400 mg/day.

Mania (unlabeled use): Oral: Initial: 100-200 mg/day; maximum: 600 mg/day (Kanba, 1994)

Renal Impairment Slower titration and frequent monitoring are indicated in patients with renal disease. Use is not recommended in patients with GFR <50 mL/minute. Marked renal impairment (Cl_{cr} <20 mL/minute) was associated with a 35% increase in AUC.

Hepatic Impairment Slower titration and frequent monitoring are indicated.

Administration Capsules should be swallowed whole. Dose may be administered once or twice daily. Doses of 300 mg/day and higher are associated with increased side effects. Steady-state levels are reached in 14 days.

Monitoring Parameters Metabolic profile, specifically BUN, serum creatinine; serum bicarbonate (prior to initiation and periodically during therapy); suicidality (eg, suicidal thoughts, depression, behavioral changes)

Special Geriatric Considerations Studies and clinical experience have not demonstrated any clinical differences in response when elderly are compared to younger adults. Since elderly potentially have reduced hepatic and renal function, dosing should be stated at the lowest recommended dose and titrated to response and tolerability. Monitor for the CNS effects commonly encountered (sedation, dizziness, and confusion) initially.

Dosage Forms Excipient information presented when available (limited, particularly for generics); consult specific product labeling.

Capsule, oral: 25 mg, 50 mg, 100 mg

Zonegran®: 25 mg, 100 mg

◆ **ZOS** see Zoster Vaccine on page 2071

◆ **Zostavax®** see Zoster Vaccine on page 2071

Zoster Vaccine (ZOS ter vak SEEN)

Related Information
Immunization Administration Recommendations *on page 2144*
Immunization Recommendations *on page 2149*

Medication Safety Issues
Administration issues:
Both varicella vaccine and zoster vaccine are live, attenuated strains of varicella-zoster virus. Their indications, dosing, and composition are distinct. Varicella vaccine is indicated for the prevention of chickenpox, while zoster vaccine is indicated in older individuals to prevent reactivation of the virus which causes shingles. Zoster vaccine is **not** a substitute for varicella vaccine and should not be used in children.

Brand Names: U.S. Zostavax®

Brand Names: Canada Zostavax®

Index Terms Shingles Vaccine; Varicella-Zoster (VZV) Vaccine (Zoster); VZV Vaccine (Zoster); ZOS

Generic Availability (U.S.) No

Pharmacologic Category Vaccine, Live (Viral)

Use Prevention of herpes zoster (shingles) in patients ≥50 years of age

The Advisory Committee on Immunization Practices (ACIP) recommends routine vaccination of all patients ≥60 years of age, including:
- Patients who report a previous episode of zoster.
- Patients with chronic medical conditions (eg, chronic renal failure, diabetes mellitus, rheumatoid arthritis, chronic pulmonary disease) unless those conditions are contraindications.
- Residents of nursing homes and other long-term care facilities ≥60 years of age, without contraindications.

Although not specifically recommended for their profession, healthcare providers within the recommended age group should also receive the zoster vaccine (CDC, 61[4], 2012)

Contraindications Hypersensitivity to any component of the vaccine; individuals with leukemia, lymphomas, or other malignant neoplasms affecting the bone marrow or lymphatic systems; primary and acquired immunodeficiency states including AIDS or clinical manifestations of HIV; those receiving immunosuppressive therapy (including high-dose corticosteroids)

In addition, ACIP recommends that the following immunocompromised patients should not receive zoster vaccine:

Patients undergoing hematopoietic stem cell transplant (limited data; assess risk:benefit, if needed, administer ≥24 months after transplantation);

Patients receiving recombinant human immune modulators, particularly antitumor necrosis factor agents (eg, adalimumab, infliximab, etanercept). Safety and efficacy of concurrent administration is unknown and not recommended. Defer vaccination for ≥1 month after discontinuation.

Patients with unspecified cellular immunodeficiency (exception, patients with impaired humoral immunity may receive vaccine).

Warnings/Precautions Zoster vaccine is not a substitute for varicella vaccine and should not be used in children. Not for use in the treatment of active zoster outbreak, the treatment of postherpetic neuropathy (PHN), or prevention of primary varicella infection (chickenpox). Vaccination may not result in effective immunity in all patients. Response depends upon multiple factors (eg, type of vaccine, age of patient) and may be improved by administering the vaccine at the recommended dose, route, and interval. Vaccines may not be effective if administered during periods of altered immune competence (CDC, 2011). Avoid administration in patients with acute febrile illness; consider deferral of vaccination; may administer to patients with mild acute illness (with or without fever). Defer treatment in patients with active untreated tuberculosis. May be used in patients with a history of zoster infection.

Medications active against the herpesvirus family (eg, acyclovir, famciclovir, valacyclovir) may interfere with the zoster vaccine. In patients where immunosuppressant therapy is anticipated, zoster vaccine should be given at least 14 days to 1 month prior to beginning therapy when possible Use is contraindicated in severely immunocompromised patients (eg, patients receiving chemo-/radiation therapy or other immunosuppressive therapy [including high-dose corticosteroids]); may have a reduced response to vaccination. Patients receiving corticosteroids in low-to-moderate doses, topical (inhaled, nasal, skin), local injection (intra-articular, bursal, tendon) may receive vaccine. Vaccinated individuals do not need to take precautions against spreading varicella following vaccination; transmission of virus is rare unless rash develops. In case of rash, standard contact precautions should be followed. In general, household and close contacts of persons with altered immunocompetence may receive all age-appropriate vaccines.

Immediate treatment for anaphylactoid reaction should be available during vaccine use. Syncope has been reported with use of injectable vaccines and may be accompanied by transient visual disturbances, weakness, or tonic-clonic movements. Procedures should be in place to avoid injuries from falling and to restore cerebral perfusion if syncope occurs. Contains gelatin and neomycin; do not use in patients with a history of anaphylactic/anaphylactoid reaction. Contact dermatitis to neomycin is not a contraindication to the vaccine. Not for use in patients <50 years of age. The ACIP does not recommend zoster vaccination in patients of any age who have received the varicella vaccine.

Adverse Reactions (Reflective of adult population; not specific for elderly) All serious adverse reactions must be reported to the U.S. Department of Health and Human Services (DHHS) Vaccine Adverse Event Reporting System (VAERS) 1-800-822-7967 or online at https://vaers.hhs.gov/esub/index.

>10%: Local: Injection site reaction (48% to 64%; includes erythema, tenderness, pain, swelling, hematoma, pruritus, and/or warmth)

1% to 10% (**Note:** Rates similar to placebo):

Central nervous system: Fever (2%), headache (1% to 9%)

Dermatologic: Skin disorder (1%)

Gastrointestinal: Diarrhea (2%)

Neuromuscular & skeletal: Weakness (1%)

Respiratory: Respiratory tract infection (2%), rhinitis (1%)

Miscellaneous: Flu-like syndrome (2%)

Drug Interactions

Metabolism/Transport Effects None known.

Avoid Concomitant Use

Avoid concomitant use of Zoster Vaccine with any of the following: Acyclovir-Valacyclovir; Belimumab; Famciclovir; Fingolimod; Immunosuppressants

Increased Effect/Toxicity

The levels/effects of Zoster Vaccine may be increased by: AzaTHIOprine; Belimumab; Corticosteroids (Systemic); Fingolimod; Hydroxychloroquine; Immunosuppressants; Leflunomide; Mercaptopurine; Methotrexate

Decreased Effect

Zoster Vaccine may decrease the levels/effects of: Tuberculin Tests

The levels/effects of Zoster Vaccine may be decreased by: Acyclovir-Valacyclovir; Famciclovir; Fingolimod; Immune Globulins; Immunosuppressants; Pneumococcal Polysaccharide Vaccine (Polyvalent)

Stability To maintain potency, the lypholyzed vaccine must be stored frozen between -50°C to -15°C (-58°F to 5°F). Temperatures below -50°C (-58°F) may occur if stored in dry ice. During shipment, should be maintained at -15°C (5°F) or colder. Store powder in freezer at -15°C (5°F). Protect from light. Store diluent separately at room temperature of 20°C to 25°C (68°F to 77°F) or in refrigerator at 2°C to 8°C (36°F to 46°F). Products with 15-month expiry dating may also be transported/stored under refrigeration at 2°C to 8°C (36°F to 46°F) for up to 72 hours prior to reconstitution; discard if stored under refrigeration and not used within 72 hours.

Withdraw entire contents of the vial containing the provided diluent to reconstitute vaccine. Gently agitate to mix thoroughly. Withdraw entire contents of reconstituted vaccine vial for administration. Discard if reconstituted vaccine is not used within 30 minutes. Do not freeze reconstituted vaccine.

Mechanism of Action As a live, attenuated vaccine (Oka/Merck strain of varicella-zoster virus), zoster virus vaccine stimulates active immunity to disease caused by the varicella-zoster virus. Administration has been demonstrated to protect against the development of herpes zoster, with the highest efficacy in patients 60-69 years of age. It may also reduce the severity of complications, including postherpetic neuralgia, in patients who develop zoster following vaccination.

Pharmacodynamics/Kinetics

Onset of action: Seroconversion: ~6 weeks

Duration: Not established; protection has been demonstrated for at least 4 years

Dosage

Geriatric & Adult Shingles: Adults ≥50 years: SubQ: 0.65 mL administered as a single dose; there are no data to support readministration of the vaccine

Renal Impairment No adjustment required.

Administration Do not administer I.V. or I.M.; inject immediately after reconstitution. Inject SubQ into the deltoid region of the upper arm, if possible. In persons anticipating immuno-suppression, give at least 14 days to 1 month prior to starting immunosuppressant.

Administration with chronic use of acyclovir, famciclovir, or valacyclovir: Discontinue ≥24 hours before administration of zoster vaccine. Do not use for ≥14 days after vaccination.

Simultaneous administration of vaccines helps ensure the patients will be fully vaccinated by the appropriate age. Simultaneous administration of vaccines is defined as administering >1 vaccine on the same day at different anatomic sites. Separate vaccines should not be combined in the same syringe unless indicated by product specific labeling. Separate needles and syringes should be used for each injection. The ACIP prefers each dose of a specific vaccine in a series come from the same manufacturer when possible. Adolescents and adults should be vaccinated while seated or lying down (CDC, 2011).

Antipyretics have not been shown to prevent febrile seizures. Antipyretics may be used to treat fever or discomfort following vaccination (CDC, 2011). One study reported that routine prophylactic administration of acetaminophen to prevent fever prior to vaccination decreased the immune response of some vaccines; the clinical significance of this reduction in immune response has not been established (Prymula, 2009).

Monitoring Parameters Fever, rash; monitor for syncope for 15 minutes following administration. If seizure-like activity associated with syncope occurs, maintain patient in supine or Trendelenburg position to reestablish adequate cerebral perfusion.

Pharmacotherapy Pearls U.S. federal law requires that the name of medication, date of administration, the vaccine manufacturer, lot number of vaccine, and the administering person's name, title, and address be entered into the patient's permanent medical record.

The varicella-zoster virus (VZV) is capable of causing two distinct manifestations of infection. Primary infection results in chickenpox (varicella). These infections tend to occur in young children or younger adults. Reactivation of latent infection (painful vesicular cutaneous eruption usually in a dermatomal pattern) occurs in older patients or in immunosuppressed populations. This is commonly referred to as shingles (herpes zoster). Although the vaccines are directed against the same causative organism, healthcare workers should be aware of differences in indications, dosing, populations, and composition of the vaccine. Neither vaccine is intended for administration during active outbreaks.

Special Geriatric Considerations This vaccine is intended for those ≥50 years of age. This live attenuated vaccine should be used with caution in patients with neoplastic disease or those who are immunosuppressed.

Dosage Forms Excipient information presented when available (limited, particularly for generics); consult specific product labeling.

Injection, powder for reconstitution [preservative free]:

Zostavax®: 19,400 PFU [contains bovine serum, gelatin, neomycin (may have trace amounts), sucrose (31.16 mg/vial); supplied with diluent]

- ◆ **Zostrix® [OTC]** see Capsaicin on page 280
- ◆ **Zostrix® Diabetic Foot Pain [OTC]** see Capsaicin on page 280
- ◆ **Zostrix®-HP [OTC]** see Capsaicin on page 280
- ◆ **Zosyn®** see Piperacillin and Tazobactam on page 1548
- ◆ **Zovirax®** see Acyclovir (Systemic) on page 41
- ◆ **Zovirax®** see Acyclovir (Topical) on page 44
- ◆ **Z-Pak** see Azithromycin (Systemic) on page 180
- ◆ **Zuplenz®** see Ondansetron on page 1425
- ◆ **Zuplenz®** see Ondansetron on page 1425
- ◆ **Zyban®** see BuPROPion on page 241
- ◆ **Zydone®** see Hydrocodone and Acetaminophen on page 937
- ◆ **Zyflo®** see Zileuton on page 2050
- ◆ **Zyflo CR®** see Zileuton on page 2050
- ◆ **Zylet®** see Loteprednol and Tobramycin on page 1164
- ◆ **Zyloprim®** see Allopurinol on page 63
- ◆ **Zymaxid™** see Gatifloxacin on page 868
- ◆ **ZyPREXA®** see OLANZapine on page 1403
- ◆ **ZyPREXA® IntraMuscular** see OLANZapine on page 1403
- ◆ **ZyPREXA® Relprevv™** see OLANZapine on page 1403
- ◆ **Zyprexa Zydis** see OLANZapine on page 1403
- ◆ **ZyPREXA® Zydis®** see OLANZapine on page 1403
- ◆ **ZyrTEC® Allergy [OTC]** see Cetirizine on page 346
- ◆ **ZyrTEC® Children's Allergy [OTC]** see Cetirizine on page 346
- ◆ **ZyrTEC® Children's Hives Relief [OTC]** see Cetirizine on page 346
- ◆ **ZyrTEC® Itchy Eye [OTC]** see Ketotifen (Ophthalmic) on page 1076
- ◆ **Zytiga™** see Abiraterone Acetate on page 22
- ◆ **Zytopic™** see Triamcinolone (Topical) on page 1961
- ◆ **Zyvox®** see Linezolid on page 1136

APPENDIX TABLE OF CONTENTS

ABBREVIATIONS, ACRONYMS, AND SYMBOLS

Abbreviations Which May Be Used in This Reference

Abbreviation	Meaning
½NS	0.45% sodium chloride
5-HT	5-hydroxytryptamine
AAP	American Academy of Pediatrics
AAPC	antibiotic-associated pseudomembranous colitis
ABG	arterial blood gases
ABMT	autologous bone marrow transplant
ABW	adjusted body weight
AACT	American Academy of Clinical Toxicology
ACC	American College of Cardiology
ACE	angiotensin-converting enzyme
ACLS	advanced cardiac life support
ACOG	American College of Obstetricians and Gynecologists
ACTH	adrenocorticotrophic hormone
ADH	antidiuretic hormone
ADHD	attention-deficit/hyperactivity disorder
ADI	adequate daily intake
ADLs	activities of daily living
AED	antiepileptic drug
AHA	American Heart Association
AHCPR	Agency for Health Care Policy and Research
AIDS	acquired immunodeficiency syndrome
AIMS	Abnormal Involuntary Movement Scale
ALL	acute lymphoblastic leukemia
ALS	amyotrophic lateral sclerosis
ALT	alanine aminotransferase (formerly called SGPT)
AMA	American Medical Association
AML	acute myeloblastic leukemia
ANA	antinuclear antibodies
ANC	absolute neutrophil count
ANLL	acute nonlymphoblastic leukemia
aPTT	activated partial thromboplastin time
ARB	angiotensin receptor blocker
ARDS	acute respiratory distress syndrome
ASA-PS	American Society of Anesthesiologists – Physical Status P1: Normal, healthy patient P2: Patient having mild systemic disease P3: Patient having severe systemic disease P4: Patient having severe systemic disease which is a constant threat to life P5: Moribund patient; not expected to survive without the procedure P6: Patient declared brain-dead; organs being removed for donor purposes
AST	aspartate aminotransferase (formerly called SGOT)
ATP	adenosine triphosphate
AUC	area under the curve (area under the serum concentration-time curve)
A-V	atrial-ventricular
BDI	Beck Depression Inventory

Abbreviations Which May Be Used in This Reference *(continued)*

Abbreviation	Meaning
BEC	blood ethanol concentration
BLS	basic life support
BMI	body mass index
BMT	bone marrow transplant
BP	blood pressure
BPD	bronchopulmonary disease or dysplasia
BPH	benign prostatic hyperplasia
BPRS	Brief Psychiatric Rating Scale
BSA	body surface area
BUN	blood urea nitrogen
CABG	coronary artery bypass graft
CAD	coronary artery disease
CADD	computer ambulatory drug delivery
cAMP	cyclic adenosine monophosphate
CAN	Canadian
CAPD	continuous ambulatory peritoneal dialysis
CAS	chemical abstract service
CBC	complete blood count
CBT	cognitive behavioral therapy
Cl_{cr}	creatinine clearance
CDC	Centers for Disease Control and Prevention
CF	cystic fibrosis
CFC	chlorofluorocarbons
CGI	Clinical Global Impression
CHD	coronary heart disease
CHF	congestive heart failure; chronic heart failure
CI	cardiac index
CIE	chemotherapy-induced emesis
C-II	schedule two controlled substance
C-III	schedule three controlled substance
C-IV	schedule four controlled substance
C-V	schedule five controlled substance
CIV	continuous I.V. infusion
Cl_{cr}	creatinine clearance
CLL	chronic lymphocytic leukemia
C_{max}	maximum plasma concentration
C_{min}	minimum plasma concentration
CML	chronic myelogenous leukemia
CMV	cytomegalovirus
CNS	central nervous system or coagulase negative staphylococcus
COLD	chronic obstructive lung disease
COPD	chronic obstructive pulmonary disease
COX	cyclooxygenase
CPK	creatine phosphokinase
CPR	cardiopulmonary resuscitation
CRF	chronic renal failure
CRP	C-reactive protein
CRRT	continuous renal replacement therapy
CSF	cerebrospinal fluid
CSII	continuous subcutaneous insulin infusion

Abbreviations Which May Be Used in This Reference *(continued)*

Abbreviation	Meaning
CT	computed tomography
CVA	cerebrovascular accident
CVP	central venous pressure
CVVH	continuous venovenous hemofiltration
CVVHD	continuous venovenous hemodialysis
CVVHDF	continuous venovenous hemodiafiltration
CYP	cytochrome
$D_5/^1/_4NS$	dextrose 5% in sodium chloride 0.2%
$D_5/^1/_2NS$	dextrose 5% in sodium chloride 0.45%
D_5/LR	dextrose 5% in lactated Ringer's
D_5/NS	dextrose 5% in sodium chloride 0.9%
D_5W	dextrose 5% in water
$D_{10}W$	dextrose 10% in water
DBP	diastolic blood pressure
DEHP	di(3-ethylhexyl)phthalate
DIC	disseminated intravascular coagulation
DL_{co}	pulmonary diffusion capacity for carbon monoxide
DM	diabetes mellitus
DMARD	disease modifying antirheumatic drug
DNA	deoxyribonucleic acid
DSC	discontinued
DSM-IV	Diagnostic and Statistical Manual
DVT	deep vein thrombosis
EBV	Epstein-Barr virus
ECG	electrocardiogram
ECHO	echocardiogram
ECMO	extracorporeal membrane oxygenation
ECT	electroconvulsive therapy
ED	emergency department
EEG	electroencephalogram
EF	ejection fraction
EG	ethylene glycol
EGA	estimated gestational age
EIA	enzyme immunoassay
ELBW	extremely low birth weight
ELISA	enzyme-linked immunosorbent assay
EPS	extrapyramidal side effects
ESR	erythrocyte sedimentation rate
ESRD	end stage renal disease
E.T.	endotracheal
EtOH	alcohol
FDA	Food and Drug Administration (United States)
FEV_1	forced expiratory volume exhaled after 1 second
FSH	follicle-stimulating hormone
FTT	failure to thrive
FVC	forced vital capacity
G-6-PD	glucose-6-phosphate dehydrogenase
GA	gestational age
GABA	gamma-aminobutyric acid
GAD	generalized anxiety disorder

Abbreviations Which May Be Used in This Reference (continued)

Abbreviation	Meaning
GE	gastroesophageal
GERD	gastroesophageal reflux disease
GFR	glomerular filtration rate
GGT	gamma-glutamyltransferase
GI	gastrointestinal
GU	genitourinary
GVHD	graft versus host disease
HAM-A	Hamilton Anxiety Scale
HAM-D	Hamilton Depression Scale
HARS	HIV-associated adipose redistribution syndrome
Hct	hematocrit
HDL-C	high density lipoprotein cholesterol
HF	heart failure
HFA	hydrofluoroalkane
HFSA	Heart Failure Society of America
Hgb	hemoglobin
HIV	human immunodeficiency virus
HMG-CoA	3-hydroxy-3-methylglutaryl-coenzyme A
HOCM	hypertrophic obstructive cardiomyopathy
HPA	hypothalamic-pituitary-adrenal
HPLC	high performance liquid chromatography
HSV	herpes simplex virus
HTN	hypertension
HUS	hemolytic uremic syndrome
IBD	inflammatory bowel disease
IBS	irritable bowel syndrome
IBW	ideal body weight
ICD	implantable cardioverter defibrillator
ICH	intracranial hemorrhage
ICP	intracranial pressure
IDDM	insulin-dependent diabetes mellitus
IDSA	Infectious Diseases Society of America
IgG	immune globulin G
IHSS	idiopathic hypertrophic subaortic stenosis
I.M.	intramuscular
ILCOR	International Liaison Committee on Resuscitation
INR	international normalized ration
Int. unit	international unit
I.O.	intraosseous
I & O	input and output
IOP	intraocular pressure
IQ	intelligence quotient
I.T.	intrathecal
ITP	idiopathic thrombocytopenic purpura
IUGR	intrauterine growth retardation
I.V.	intravenous
IVH	intraventricular hemorrhage
IVP	intravenous push
IVPB	intravenous piggyback
JIA	juvenile idiopathic arthritis

Abbreviation	Meaning
JNC	Joint National Committee
JRA	juvenile rheumatoid arthritis
kg	kilogram
KIU	kallikrein inhibitor unit
KOH	potassium hydroxide
LAMM	L-α-acetyl methadol
LDH	lactate dehydrogenase
LDL-C	low density lipoprotein cholesterol
LE	lupus erythematosus
LFT	liver function test
LGA	large for gestational age
LH	luteinizing hormone
LP	lumbar posture
LR	lactated Ringer's
LV	left ventricular
LVEF	left ventricular ejection fraction
LVH	left ventricular hypertrophy
MAC	*Mycobacterium avium* complex
MADRS	Montgomery Asbery Depression Rating Scale
MAO	monoamine oxidase
MAOIs	monamine oxidase inhibitors
MAP	mean arterial pressure
MDD	major depressive disorder
MDRD	modification of diet in renal disease
MDRSP	multidrug resistant *streptococcus pneumoniae*
MI	myocardial infarction
MMSE	mini mental status examination
MOPP	mustargen (mechlorethamine), Oncovin® (vincristine), procarbazine, and prednisone
M/P	milk to plasma ratio
MPS I	mucopolysaccharidosis I
MRHD	maximum recommended human dose
MRI	magnetic resonance imaging
MRSA	methicillin-resistant *Staphylococcus aureus*
MUGA	multiple gated acquisition scan
NAEPP	National Asthma Education and Prevention Program
NAS	neonatal abstinence syndrome
NCI	National Cancer Institute
ND	nasoduodenal
NF	National Formulary
NFD	Nephrogenic fibrosing dermopathy
NG	nasogastric
NIDDM	noninsulin-dependent diabetes mellitus
NIH	National Institute of Health
NKA	no known allergies
NKDA	No known drug allergies
NMDA	n-methyl-d-aspartate
NMS	neuroleptic malignant syndrome
NNRTI	non-nucleoside reverse transcriptase inhibitor
NRTI	nucleoside reverse transcriptase inhibitor

Abbreviations Which May Be Used in This Reference (continued)

Abbreviation	Meaning
NS	normal saline (0.9% sodium chloride)
NSAID	nonsteroidal anti-inflammatory drug
NSF	nephrogenic systemic fibrosis
NSTEMI	Non-ST-elevation myocardial infarction
NYHA	New York Heart Association
OA	osteoarthritis
OCD	obsessive-compulsive disorder
OHSS	ovarian hyperstimulation syndrome
O.R.	operating room
OTC	over-the-counter (nonprescription)
PABA	para-aminobenzoic acid
PACTG	Pediatric AIDS Clinical Trials Group
PALS	pediatric advanced life support
PAT	paroxysmal atrial tachycardia
PCA	patient-controlled analgesia
PCP	*Pneumocystis jiroveci* pneumonia (also called *Pneumocystis carinii* pneumonia)
PCWP	pulmonary capillary wedge pressure
PD	Parkinson's disease; peritoneal dialysis
PDA	patent ductus arteriosus
PDE-5	phosphodiesterase-5
PE	pulmonary embolism
PEG tube	percutaneous endoscopic gastrostomy tube
P-gp	P-glycoprotein
PHN	post-herpetic neuralgia
PICU	Pediatric Intensive Care Unit
PID	pelvic inflammatory disease
PIP	peak inspiratory pressure
PMA	postmenstrual age
PMDD	premenstrual dysphoric disorder
PNA	postnatal age
PONV	postoperative nausea and vomiting
PPHN	persistent pulmonary hypertension of the neonate
PPN	peripheral parenteral nutrition
PROM	premature rupture of membranes
PSVT	paroxysmal supraventricular tachycardia
PT	prothrombin time
PTH	parathyroid hormone
PTSD	post-traumatic stress disorder
PTT	partial thromboplastin time
PUD	peptic ulcer disease
PVC	premature ventricular contraction
PVD	peripheral vascular disease
PVR	peripheral vascular resistance
QT_c	corrected QT interval
QT_cF	corrected QT interval by Fredricia's formula
RA	rheumatoid arthritis
RAP	right arterial pressure
RDA	recommended daily allowance
REM	rapid eye movement

Abbreviations Which May Be Used in This Reference (continued)

Abbreviation	Meaning
REMS	risk evaluation and mitigation strategies
RIA	radioimmunoassay
RNA	ribonucleic acid
RPLS	reversible posterior leukoencephalopathy syndrome
RSV	respiratory syncytial virus
SA	sinoatrial
SAD	seasonal affective disorder
SAH	subarachnoid hemorrhage
SBE	subacute bacterial endocarditis
SBP	systolic blood pressure
S_{cr}	serum creatinine
SERM	selective estrogen receptor modulator
SGA	small for gestational age
SGOT	serum glutamic oxaloacetic aminotransferase
SGPT	serum glutamic pyruvate transaminase
SI	International System of Units or Systeme international d'Unites
SIADH	syndrome of inappropriate antidiuretic hormone secretion
SLE	systemic lupus erythematosus
SLEDD	sustained low-efficiency daily diafiltration
SNRI	serotonin norepinephrine reuptake inhibitor
SSKI	saturated solution of potassium iodide
SSRIs	selective serotonin reuptake inhibitors
STD	sexually transmitted disease
STEM I	ST-elevation myocardial infarction
SVR	systemic vascular resistance
SVT	supraventricular tachycardia
SWFI	sterile water for injection
SWI	sterile water for injection
$T_{1/2}$	half-life
T_3	triiodothyronine
T_4	thyroxine
TB	tuberculosis
TC	total cholesterol
TCA	tricyclic antidepressant
TD	tardive dyskinesia
TG	triglyceride
TIA	transient ischemic attack
TIBC	total iron binding capacity
TMA	thrombotic microangiopathy
T_{max}	time to maximum observed concentration, plasma
TNF	tumor necrosis factor
TPN	total parenteral nutrition
TSH	thyroid stimulating hormone
TT	thrombin time
TTP	thrombotic thrombocytopenic purpura
UA	urine analysis
UC	ulcerative colitis
ULN	upper limits of normal
URI	upper respiratory infection
USAN	United States Adopted Names

Abbreviations Which May Be Used in This Reference (continued)

Abbreviation	Meaning
USP	United States Pharmacopeia
UTI	urinary tract infection
UV	ultraviolet
V_d	volume of distribution
V_{dss}	volume of distribution at steady-state
VEGF	vascular endothelial growth factor
VF	ventricular fibrillation
VLBW	very low birth weight
VMA	vanillylmandelic acid
VT	ventricular tachycardia
VTE	venous thromboembolism
vWD	von Willebrand disease
VZV	varicella zoster virus
WHO	World Health Organization
w/v	weight for volume
w/w	weight for weight
YBOC	Yale Brown Obsessive-Compulsive Scale
YMRS	Young Mania Rating Scale

Common Weights, Measures, or Apothecary Abbreviations

Abbreviation	Meaning
<[1]	less than
>[1]	greater than
≤	less than or equal to
≥	greater than or equal to
ac	before meals or food
ad	to, up to
ad lib	at pleasure
AM	morning
AMA	against medical advice
amp	ampul
amt	amount
aq	water
aq. dest.	distilled water
ASAP	as soon as possible
a.u.[1]	each ear
bid	twice daily
bm	bowel movement
C	Celsius, centigrade
cal	calorie
cap	capsule
cc[1]	cubic centimeter
cm	centimeter
comp	compound
cont	continue
d	day
d/c[1]	discharge
dil	dilute

Common Weights, Measures, or Apothecary Abbreviations *(continued)*

Abbreviation	Meaning
disp	dispense
div	divide
dtd	give of such a dose
Dx	diagnosis
elix, el	elixir
emp	as directed
et	and
ex aq	in water
F	Fahrenheit
f, ft	make, let be made
g	gram
gr	grain
gtt	a drop
h	hour
hs[1]	at bedtime
kcal	kilocalorie
kg	kilogram
L	liter
liq	a liquor, solution
M	molar
mcg	microgram
m. dict	as directed
mEq	milliequivalent
mg	milligram
microL	microliter
min	minute
mL	milliliter
mm	millimeter
mM	millimole
mm Hg	millimeters of mercury
mo	month
mOsm	milliosmoles
ng	nanogram
nmol	nanomole
no.	number
noc	in the night
non rep	do not repeat, no refills
NPO	nothing by mouth
NV	nausea and vomiting
O, Oct	a pint
o.d.[1]	right eye
o.l.	left eye
o.s.[1]	left eye
o.u.[1]	each eye
pc, post cib	after meals
PM	afternoon or evening
P.O.	by mouth
P.R.	rectally
prn	as needed
pulv	a powder

Common Weights, Measures, or Apothecary Abbreviations *(continued)*

Abbreviation	Meaning
q	every
qad	every other day
qd[1,2]	every day, daily
qh	every hour
qid	four times a day
qod[1,2]	every other day
qs	a sufficient quantity
qs ad	a sufficient quantity to make
Rx	take, a recipe
S.L.	sublingual
stat	at once, immediately
SubQ	subcutaneous
supp	suppository
syr	syrup
tab	tablet
tal	such
tid	three times a day
tr, tinct	tincture
trit	triturate
tsp	teaspoon
u.d.	as directed
ung	ointment
v.o.	verbal order
w.a.	while awake
x3	3 times
x4	4 times
y	year

[1]ISMP error-prone abbreviation

[2]JCAHO Do Not Use list

Additional abbreviations used and defined within a specific monograph or text piece may only apply to that text.

REFERENCES

The Institute for Safe Medication Practices (ISMP) list of Error-Prone Abbreviations, Symbols, and Dose Designations. Available at http://www.ismp.org/Tools/errorproneabbreviations.pdf

The Joint Commission Official "Do Not Use" list. Available at http://www.jointcommission.org/assets/1/18/Official_Do_-Not_Use_List_6_111.PDF

BODY SURFACE AREA (BSA)

$$\text{BSA (m}^2\text{)} = (\text{kg}^{0.425} \times \text{cm}^{0.725} \times 71.84) / 10{,}000$$

or

$$\log \text{BSA (m}^2\text{)} = [(\log \text{kg} \times 0.425) + (\log \text{cm} \times 0.725) + 1.8564] / 10{,}000$$

DuBois D and DuBois EF, "A Formula to Estimate the Approximate Surface Area if Height and Weight Be Known," *Arch Intern Med*, 1916, 17:863-71.

$$\text{BSA (m}^2\text{)} = \sqrt{\frac{\text{ht (in) x wt (lb)}}{3131}} \quad \textbf{\textit{or}} \quad \text{BSA (m}^2\text{)} = \sqrt{\frac{\text{ht (cm) x wt (kg)}}{3600}}$$

Lam TK and Leung DT, "More on Simplified Calculation of Body-Surface Area," *N Engl J Med*, 1988, 318(17):1130.
Mosteller RD, "Simplified Calculation of Body Surface Area," *N Engl J Med*, 1987, 317(17):1098.

BODY MASS INDEX (BMI)

$$\text{BMI} = \frac{\text{weight (kg)}}{[\text{height (m)}]^2}$$

CALCULATIONS

Ideal Body Weight

Adults (18 years and older) (IBW is in kg)
IBW (male) = 50 + (2.3 x height in inches over 5 feet)
IBW (female) = 45.5 + (2.3 x height in inches over 5 feet)

Lean Body Weight

Adults: Determination of lean body weight (LBW) in kg.
LBW = IBW + 0.4(actual body weight - IBW)

Millimoles and Milliequivalent

Definitions

mole	=	gram molecular weight of a substance (aka molar weight)
millimole (mM)	=	milligram molecular weight of a substance (a millimole is 1/1000 of a mole)
equivalent weight	=	gram weight of a substance which will combine with or replace 1 gram (1 mole) of hydrogen; an equivalent weight can be determined by dividing the molar weight of a substance by its ionic valence
milliequivalent (mEq)	=	milligram weight of a substance which will combine with or replace 1 milligram (1 millimole) of hydrogen (a milliequivalent is 1/1000 of an equivalent)

Calculations

moles	=	$\dfrac{\text{weight of a substance (grams)}}{\text{molecular weight of that substance (grams)}}$
millimoles	=	$\dfrac{\text{weight of a substance (milligrams)}}{\text{molecular weight of that substance (milligrams)}}$
equivalents	=	moles x valence of ion
milliequivalents	=	millimoles x valence of ion
moles	=	$\dfrac{\text{equivalents}}{\text{valence of ion}}$
millimoles	=	$\dfrac{\text{milliequivalents}}{\text{valence of ion}}$
millimoles	=	moles x 1000
milliequivalents	=	equivalents x 1000

Note: Use of equivalents and milliequivalents is valid only for those substances which have fixed ionic valences (eg, sodium, potassium, calcium, chlorine, magnesium bromine, etc). For substances with variable ionic valences (eg, phosphorous), a reliable equivalent value cannot be determined. In these instances, one should calculate millimoles (which are fixed and reliable) rather than milliequivalents.

CALCULATIONS

Approximate Milliequivalents — Weights of Selected Ions

Salt	mEq/g Salt	mg Salt/mEq
Calcium carbonate [CaCO$_3$]	20	50
Calcium chloride [CaCl$_2$ • 2H$_2$O]	14	74
Calcium gluceptate [Ca(C$_7$H$_{13}$O$_8$)$_2$]	4	245
Calcium gluconate [Ca(C$_6$H$_{11}$O$_7$)$_2$ • H$_2$O]	5	224
Calcium lactate [Ca(C$_3$H$_5$O$_3$)$_2$ • 5H$_2$O]	7	154
Magnesium gluconate [Mg(C$_6$H$_{11}$O$_7$)$_2$ • H$_2$O]	5	216
Magnesium oxide [MgO]	50	20
Magnesium sulfate [MgSO$_4$]	17	60
Magnesium sulfate [MgSO$_4$ • 7H$_2$O]	8	123
Potassium acetate [K(C$_2$H$_3$O$_2$)]	10	98
Potassium chloride [KCl]	13	75
Potassium citrate [K$_3$(C$_6$H$_5$O$_7$) • H$_2$O]	9	108
Potassium iodide [KI]	6	166
Sodium acetate [Na(C$_2$H$_3$O$_2$)]	12	82
Sodium acetate [Na(C$_2$H$_3$O$_2$) • 3H$_2$O]	7	136
Sodium bicarbonate [NaHCO$_3$]	12	84
Sodium chloride [NaCl]	17	58
Sodium citrate [Na$_3$(C$_6$H$_5$O$_7$) • 2H$_2$O]	10	98
Sodium iodine [NaI]	7	150
Sodium lactate [Na(C$_3$H$_5$O$_3$)]	9	112
Zinc sulfate [ZnSO$_4$ • 7H$_2$O]	7	144

Valences and Atomic Weights of Selected Ions

Substance	Electrolyte	Valence	Molecular Wt
Calcium	Ca^{++}	2	40
Chloride	Cl$^-$	1	35.5
Magnesium	Mg^{++}	2	24
Phosphate	HPO$_4^{--}$ (80%)	1.8	96[1]
pH = 7.4	H$_2$PO$_4^-$ (20%)	1.8	96[1]
Potassium	K$^+$	1	39
Sodium	Na$^+$	1	23
Sulfate	SO$_4^{--}$	2	96[1]

[1]The molecular weight of phosphorus only is 31, and sulfur only is 32.

CONVERSIONS

Apothecary-Metric Exact Equivalents

1 gram (g)	=	15.43 grains		0.1 mg	=	1/600 gr
1 milliliter (mL)	=	16.23 minims		0.12 mg	=	1/500 gr
1 grain (gr)	=	64.8 milligrams		0.15 mg	=	1/400 gr
1 fluid ounce (fl. oz)	=	29.57 mL		0.2 mg	=	1/300 gr
1 pint (pt)	=	473.2 mL		0.3 mg	=	1/200 gr
1 ounce (oz)	=	28.35 grams		0.4 mg	=	1/150 gr
1 pound (lb)	=	453.6 grams		0.5 mg	=	1/120 gr
1 kilogram (kg)	=	2.2 pounds		0.6 mg	=	1/100 gr
1 quart (qt)	=	946.4 mL		0.8 mg	=	1/80 gr
				1 mg	=	1/65 gr

Apothecary-Metric Approximate Equivalents[1]

Liquids			Solids		
1 teaspoonful	=	5 mL	¼ grain	=	15 mg
1 tablespoonful	=	15 mL	½ grain	=	30 mg
			1 grain	=	60 mg
			1½ grain	=	100 mg
			5 grains	=	300 mg
			10 grains	=	600 mg

[1]Use exact equivalents for compounding and calculations requiring a high degree of accuracy.

Pounds-Kilograms

1 pound = 0.45359 kilograms
1 kilogram = 2.2 pounds

Temperature

Celsius to Fahrenheit = (°C x 9/5) + 32 = °F
Fahrenheit to Celsius = (°F - 32) x 5/9 = °C

RENAL FUNCTION ESTIMATION IN ADULT PATIENTS

Evaluation of a patient's renal function often includes the use of equations to estimate glomerular filtration rate (GFR) (eg, estimated GFR [eGFR] creatinine clearance [Cl_{Cr}]) using an endogenous filtration marker (eg, serum creatinine) and other patient variables. For example, the Cockcroft-Gault equation estimates renal function by calculating Cl_{Cr} and is typically used to steer medication dosing. Equations which calculate eGFR are primarily used to categorize chronic kidney disease (CKD) staging. The rate of creatinine clearance does not always accurately represent GFR; creatinine may be cleared by other renal mechanisms in addition to glomerular filtration and serum creatinine concentrations may be affected by non-renal factors (eg, age, gender, race, body habitus, illness, diet). In addition, these equations were developed based on studies in limited populations and may either over- or underestimate the renal function of a specific patient.

Nevertheless, most clinicians estimate renal function using Cl_{Cr} as an indicator of actual renal function for the purpose of adjusting medication doses. For medications that require dose adjustment for renal impairment, utilization of eGFR (ie, Modification of Diet in Renal Disease [MDRD]) may overestimate renal function by up to 40% which may result in supratherapeutic medication doses (Hermsen, 2009). These equations should only be used in the clinical context of patient-specific factors noted during the physical exam/work-up. Decisions regarding drug therapy and doses must be based on clinical judgment.

RENAL FUNCTION ESTIMATION EQUATIONS

Commonly used equations include the Cockcroft-Gault, Jelliffe, four-variable Modification of Diet in Renal Disease (MDRD), and six-variable MDRD (aka, MDRD extended). All of these equations were originally developed using a serum creatinine assay measured by the alkaline picrate-based (Jaffe) method. Many substances, including proteins, can interfere with the accuracy of this assay and overestimate serum creatinine concentration. The National Kidney Foundation and The National Kidney Disease Education Program (NDKEP) advocate for a universal creatinine assay, in order to ensure an accurate estimate of renal function in patients. As a result, a more specific enzymatic assay with an isotope dilution mass spectrometry (IDMS)-traceable international standard has been developed. Compared to the older methods, IDMS-traceable assays may report lower serum creatinine values and may, therefore, overestimate renal function when used in the original equations (eg, Cockcroft-Gault, Jelliffe, original MDRD). Updated four-variable MDRD and six-variable MDRD equations based on serum creatinine measured by the IDMS-traceable method has been proposed for adults (Levey, 2006); the Cockcroft-Gault and Jelliffe equations have not been re-expressed and may overestimate renal function when used with a serum creatinine measured by the IDMS-traceable method. Clinicians should be aware of the serum creatinine assay used by their institution and the ramifications the assay may have on the equations used for renal function estimation.

Regardless of the serum creatinine assay used, the following factors may contribute to an inaccurate estimation of renal function (Stevens, 2006):

- Increased creatinine generation (may underestimate renal function):
    - Black or African American patients
    - Muscular body habitus
    - Ingestion of cooked meats
- Decreased creatinine generation (may overestimate renal function):
    - Increased age
    - Female patients
    - Hispanic patients
    - Asian patients
    - Amputees
    - Malnutrition, inflammation, or deconditioning (eg, cancer, severe cardiovascular disease, hospitalized patients)
    - Neuromuscular disease
    - Vegetarian diet

- Rapidly changing serum creatinine (either up or down): In patients with rapidly rising serum creatinines (ie, increasing by >0.5-0.7 mg/dL/day), it is best to assume that the patient's renal function is severely impaired

Use extreme caution when estimating renal function in the following patient populations:

- Low body weight (actual body weight < ideal body weight)

- Liver transplant

- Elderly (>90 years of age)

- Dehydration

- Recent kidney transplantation (serum creatinine values may decrease rapidly and can lead to renal function underestimation; conversely, delayed graft function may be present)

Note: In most situations, the use of the patient's ideal body weight (IBW) is recommended for estimating renal function, except when the patient's actual body weight (ABW) is less than ideal. Use of actual body weight (ABW) in obese patients (and possibly patients with ascites) may significantly overestimate renal function. Some clinicians prefer to use an adjusted body weight in such cases [eg, IBW + 0.4 (ABW - IBW)]; the adjustment factor may vary based on practitioner and/or institutional preference.

Alkaline picrate-based (Jaffe) methods

Note: These equations have not been updated for use with serum creatinine methods traceable to IDMS. Use with IDMS-traceable serum creatinine methods may overestimate renal function; use with caution.

Method 1: MDRD equation:

$$eGFR = 186 \times (Creatinine)^{-1.154} \times (Age)^{-0.203} \times (Gender) \times (Race)$$
where:
eGFR = estimated GFR; calculated in mL/minute/1.73 m^2
Creatinine is input in mg/dL
Age is input in years
Gender: Females: Gender = 0.742; Males: Gender = 1
Race: Black: Race = 1.212; White or other: Race = 1

Method 2: MDRD Extended equation:

$$eGFR = 170 \times (Creatinine)^{-0.999} \times (Age)^{-0.176} \times (SUN)^{-0.170} \times (Albumin)^{0.318} \times (Gender) \times (Race)$$
where:
eGFR = estimated GFR; calculated in mL/minute/1.73 m^2
Creatinine is input in mg/dL
Age is input in years
SUN = Serum Urea Nitrogen; input in mg/dL
Albumin = Serum Albumin; input in g/dL
Gender: Females: Gender = 0.762; Males: Gender = 1
Race: Black: Race = 1.18; White or other: Race = 1

Method 3: Cockroft-Gault equation[1]

Males: Cl_{Cr} = [(140 - Age) X Weight] / (72 X Creatinine)
Females: Cl_{Cr} = {[(140 - Age) X Weight] / (72 X Creatinine)} X 0.85
where:
Cl_{Cr} = creatinine clearance; calculated in mL/minute
Age is input in years
Weight is input in kg
Creatinine is input in mg/dL

Method 4: Jelliffe equation

Males: Cl_{Cr} = {98 - [0.8 X (Age - 20)]} / (Creatinine)
Females: Cl_{Cr} = Use above equation, then multiply result by 0.9
where:
Cl_{Cr} = creatinine clearance; calculated in mL/minute/1.73m^2
Age is input in years
Creatinine is input in mg/dL

IDMS-traceable methods

Method 1: MDRD equation[2]:

eGFR = 175 X (Creatinine)$^{-1.154}$ X (Age)$^{-0.203}$ X (Gender) X (Race)
where:
eGFR = estimated GFR; calculated in mL/minute/1.73 m^2
Creatinine is input in mg/dL
Age is input in years
Gender: Females: Gender = 0.742; Males: Gender = 1
Race: Black: Race = 1.212; White or other: Race = 1

Method 2: MDRD Extended equation:

eGFR = 161.5 X (Creatinine)$^{-0.999}$ X (Age)$^{-0.176}$ X (SUN)$^{-0.170}$ X (Albumin)$^{0.318}$ X (Gender) X (Race)
where:
eGFR = estimated GFR; calculated in mL/minute/1.73 m^2
Creatinine is input in mg/dL
Age is input in years
SUN = Serum Urea Nitrogen; input in mg/dL
Albumin = Serum Albumin; input in g/dL
Gender: Females: Gender = 0.762; Males: Gender = 1
Race: Black: Race = 1.18; White or other: Race = 1

FOOTNOTES

[1]Equation typically used for adjusting medication doses
[2]Preferred equation for CKD staging National Kidney Disease Education Program

REFERENCES

Cockcroft DW and Gault MH, "Prediction of Creatinine Clearance From Serum Creatinine," *Nephron*, 1976, 16 (1):31-41.

Dowling TC, Matzke GR, Murphy JE, et al, "Evaluation of Renal Drug Dosing: Prescribing Information and Clinical Pharmacist Approaches," *Pharmacotherapy*, 2010, 30(8):776-86.

Hermsen ED, Maiefski M, Florescu MC, et al, "Comparison of the Modification of Diet in Renal Disease and Cockcroft-Gault Equations for Dosing Antimicrobials," *Pharmacotherapy*, 2009, 29(6):649-55.

Jelliffe RW, "Letter: Creatinine Clearance: Bedside Estimate," *Ann Intern Med*, 1973, 79(4):604-5.

Levey AS, Bosch JP, Lewis JB, et al, "A More Accurate Method to Estimate Glomerular Filtration Rate From Serum Creatinine: A New Prediction Equation. Modification of Diet in Renal Disease Study Group," *Ann Intern Med*, 1999, 16;130(6):461–70.

Levey AS, Coresh J, Greene T, et al, "Using Standardized Serum Creatinine Values in the Modification of Diet in Renal Disease Study Equation for Estimating Glomerular Filtration Rate," *Ann Intern Med*, 2006, 145(4):247-54.

National Kidney Disease Education Program, "GFR Calculators." Available at http://www.nkdep.nih.gov/professionals/gfr_calculators. Last accessed January 20, 2011.

Stevens LA, Coresh J, Greene T, et al, "Assessing Kidney Function - Measured and Estimated Glomerular Filtration Rate," *N Engl J Med*, 2006, 354(23):2473-83.

ANGIOTENSIN AGENTS

Comparison of Indications and Adult Dosages

Drug	Hypertension	HF	Renal Dysfunction	Dialyzable	Strengths (mg)
ACE Inhibitors					
Benazepril (Lotensin®)	10-40 mg/day	Not FDA-approved	Cl_{cr} <30 mL/min: 5 mg/day initially Maximum: 40 mg/day	Yes	Tablets 5, 10, 20, 40
Captopril (Capoten®)	25-100 mg/day bid-tid	6.25-100 mg tid Maximum: 450 mg/day	Cl_{cr} 10-50 mL/min: 75% of usual dose Cl_{cr} <10 mL/min: 50% of usual dose	Yes	Tablets 12.5, 25, 50, 100
Cilazapril (Inhibace®) Note: Not available in U.S.	2.5-10 mg/day	0.5-2.5 mg/day	Cl_{cr} 10-40 mL/min: Initial: 0.5 mg/day (0.25-0.5 mg/day for HF) (maximum: 2.5 mg/day) Cl_{cr} <10 mL/minute: 0.25-0.5 mg once or twice weekly	Yes	Tablets 1, 2.5, 5
Enalapril (Vasotec®)	2.5-40 mg/day qd-bid	2.5-20 mg bid Maximum: 20 mg bid	Cl_{cr} 30-80 mL/min: 5 mg/day initially Cl_{cr} <30 mL/min: 2.5 mg/day initially	Yes	Tablets 2.5, 5, 10, 20
Enalaprilat[1]	0.625 mg, 1.25 mg, 2.5 mg q6h Maximum: 5 mg q6h	Not FDA-approved	Cl_{cr} <30 mL/min: 0.625 mg q6h	Yes	1.25 mg/mL (1 mL, 2 mL vials)
Fosinopril (Monopril®)	10-40 mg/day	10-40 mg/day	No dosage reduction necessary	Not well dialyzed	Tablets 10, 20, 40
Lisinopril (Prinivil®, Zestril®)	10-40 mg/day Maximum: 40 mg/day	5-40 mg/day	Cl_{cr} 10-30 mL/min: 5 mg/day initially Cl_{cr} <10 mL/min: 2.5 mg/day initially	Yes	Tablets 2.5, 5, 10, 20, 30, 40
Moexipril (Univasc®)	7.5-30 mg/day qd-bid Maximum: 30 mg/day	LV dysfunction (post-MI): 7.5-30 mg/day	Cl_{cr} <40 mL/min: 3.75 mg/day initially Maximum: 15 mg/day	Unknown	Tablets 7.5, 15
Perindopril (Aceon®)	4-8 mg/day	4-8 mg/day Maximum: 16 mg/day	Cl_{cr} 30-60 mL/min: 2 mg/day Cl_{cr} 15-29 mL/min: 2 mg qod Cl_{cr} <15 mL/min: 2 mg on dialysis days	Yes	Tablets 2, 4, 8
Quinapril (Accupril®)	10-40 mg/day qd-bid	5-20 mg bid	Cl_{cr} 30-60 mL/min: 5 mg/day initially Cl_{cr} <10-30 mL/min: 2.5 mg/day initially	Not well dialyzed	Tablets 5, 10, 20, 40
Ramipril (Altace®)	2.5-20 mg/day qd-bid	2.5-10 mg/day	Cl_{cr} <40 mL/min: 25% of normal dose	Unknown	Capsules 1.25, 2.5, 5, 10

Comparison of Indications and Adult Dosages *continued*

Drug	Hypertension	HF	Renal Dysfunction	Dialyzable	Strengths (mg)
Trandolapril (Mavik®)	1-4 mg/day Maximum: 8 mg/day qd-bid	LV dysfunction (post-MI): 1-4 mg/day	Cl_{cr} <30 mL/min: 0.5 mg/day initially	No	Tablets 1, 2, 4
Angiotensin II Receptor Blockers					
Azilsartan (Edarbi™)	40-80 mg/day	Not FDA-approved	No dosage adjustment necessary	Unknown	Tablets 40, 80
Candesartan (Atacand®)	8-32 mg/day	Target: 32 mg once daily	No dosage adjustment necessary	No	Tablets 4, 8, 16, 32
Eprosartan (Teveten®)	400-800 mg/day qd-bid	Not FDA-approved	No dosage adjustment necessary	Unknown	Tablets 400, 600
Irbesartan (Avapro®)	150-300 mg/day	Not FDA-approved	No dosage reduction necessary	No	Tablets 75, 150, 300
Losartan (Cozaar®)	25-100 mg qd or bid	Not FDA-approved	No dosage adjustment necessary	No	Tablets 25, 50, 100
Olmesartan (Benicar®)	20-40 mg/day	Not FDA-approved	No dosage adjustment necessary	Unknown	Tablets 5, 20, 40
Telmisartan (Micardis®)	20-80 mg/day	Not FDA-approved	No dosage reduction necessary	No	Tablets 20, 40, 80
Valsartan (Diovan®)	80-320 mg/day	Target: 160 mg bid	Decrease dose only if Cl_{cr} <10 mL/minute	No	Tablets 40, 80, 160, 320
Renin Inhibitors					
Aliskiren (Tekturna®)	150-300 mg once daily	Not FDA-approved	No dosage adjustment necessary in mild-to-moderate impairment; not adequately studied in severe impairment	Unknown	Tablets 150, 300

Dosage is based on 70 kg adult with normal hepatic and renal function.

[1]Enalaprilat is the only available ACE inhibitor in a parenteral formulation.

ACE Inhibitors: Comparative Pharmacokinetics

Drug	Prodrug	Absorption (%)	Serum $t_{1/2}$ (h) Normal Renal Function	Serum Protein Binding (%)	Elimination	Onset of BP Lowering Action (h)	Peak BP Lowering Effects (h)	Duration of BP Lowering Effects (h)
Benazepril	Yes	37	10-11 (effective)	~97	Renal (32%), biliary (~12%)	1	2-4	24
Benazeprilat				~95				
Captopril	No	60-75 (fasting)	1.9 (elimination)	25-30	Renal	0.25-0.5	1-1.5	~6
Enalapril	Yes	55-75	2	50-60	Renal (60%-80%), fecal	1	4-6	12-24
Enalaprilat			11 (effective)			0.25	1-4	~6
Fosinopril		36	12 (effective)		Renal (~50%), biliary (~50%)	1		24
Fosinoprilat				>99				
Lisinopril	No	25	11-12	25	Renal	1	6	24
Moexipril	Yes		1	90	Fecal (53%), renal (8%)			>24
Moexiprilat			2-10	50			1-2	
Perindopril	Yes		1.5-3	60	Renal			
Perindoprilat			3-10 (effective)	10-20			3-7	
Quinapril	Yes	>60	0.8	97	Renal (~60%) as metabolite, fecal	1	2-4	24
Quinaprilat			3					
Ramipril	Yes	50-60	1-2	73	Renal (60%), fecal (40%)	1-2	3-6	24
Ramiprilat			13-17 (effective)	56				
Trandolapril	Yes		6	80	Renal (33%), fecal (66%)	1-2		≥24
Trandolaprilat			10	65-94			6	

Angiotensin II Receptor Blockers and Renin Inhibitors: Comparative Pharmacokinetics

Drug	Prodrug	Time to Peak	Bioavailability	Food "Area-Under-the-Curve"	Elimination Half-Life	Elimination Altered in Renal Dysfunction	Precautions in Severe Renal Dysfunction	Elimination Altered in Hepatic Dysfunction	Precautions in Hepatic Dysfunction	Protein Binding (%)
Angiotensin II Receptor Blockers										
Azilsartan (Edarbi™)	Yes	1.5-3 h	60%	No effect	11 h	No	Yes	No	No	>99
Candesartan (Atacand®)	Yes[1]	3-4 h	15%	No effect	9 h	Yes[2]	Yes	No	Yes	>99
Eprosartan (Teveten®)	No	1-2 h	13%	No effect	5-9 h	No	Yes	No	Yes	98
Irbesartan (Avapro®)	No	1.5-2 h	60% to 80%	No effect	11-15 h	No	Yes	No	No	90
Losartan (Cozaar®)	Yes[3]	1 h/3-4 h[3]	33%	9% to 10%	1.5-2 h/6-9 h[3]	No	Yes	Yes	Yes	~99
Olmesartan (Benicar®)	Yes	1-2 h	26%	No effect	13 h	Yes	Yes	Yes	No	99
Telmisartan (Micardis®)	No	0.5-1 h	42% to 58%	9.6% to 20%	24 h	No	Yes	Yes	Yes	>99.5
Valsartan (Diovan®)	No	2-4 h	25%	9% to 40%	6 h	No	Yes	Yes	Yes	95
Renin Inhibitors										
Aliskiren (Tekturna®)	No	1-3 h	~3%	85% (high-fat meal)	16-32 h	Yes[4]	Yes	No	No	?

[1] Candesartan cilexetil: Active metabolite candesartan

[2] Dosage adjustments are not necessary.

[3] Losartan: Active metabolite E-3174

[4] No initial dosage adjustment in mild-to-moderate impairment

ANTIDEPRESSANT AGENTS

Comparison of Usual Adult Dosage, Mechanism of Action, and Adverse Effects

Drug	Initial Adult Dose	Usual Adult Dosage (mg/d)	Dosage Forms	ACH	Drowsiness	Orthostatic Hypotension	Conduction Abnormalities[1]	GI Distress	Weight Gain	Comments
Tricyclic Antidepressants and Related Compounds[1]										
Amitriptyline	25-75 mg qhs	100-300	T	4+	4+	3+	3+	1+	4+	Also used in chronic pain, migraine, and as a hypnotic; contraindicated with cisapride
Amoxapine	50 mg bid	100-400	T	2+	2+	2+	2+	0	2+	May cause extrapyramidal symptom (EPS)
ClomiPRAMINE[2] (Anafranil®)	25-75 mg qhs	100-250	C	4+	4+	2+	3+	1+	4+	Only approved for OCD
Desipramine (Norpramin®)	25-75 mg qhs	100-300	T	1+	2+	2+	2+	0	1+	Blood levels useful for therapeutic monitoring
Doxepin	25-75 mg qhs	100-300	C, L	3+	4+	2+	2+	0	4+	
Imipramine (Tofranil®, Tofranil-PM®)	25-75 mg qhs	100-300	T, C	3+	3+	4+	3+	1+	4+	Blood levels useful for therapeutic monitoring
Maprotiline	25-75 mg qhs	100-225	T	2+	3+	2+	2+	0	2+	
Nortriptyline (Pamelor®)	25-50 mg qhs	50-150	C, L	2+	2+	1+	2+	0	1+	Blood levels useful for therapeutic monitoring
Protriptyline (Vivactil®)	15 mg qAM	15-60	T	2+	1+	2+	3+	1+	1+	
Trimipramine (Surmontil®)	25-75 mg qhs	100-300	C	4+	4+	3+	3+	0	4+	
Selective Serotonin Reuptake Inhibitors[3]										
Citalopram (Celexa®)	20 mg qAM	20-60	T, L	0	0	0	0	3+[4]	1+	
Escitalopram (Lexapro®)	10 mg qAM	10-20	T, L	0	0	0	0	3+	1+	S-enantiomer of citalopram

Comparison of Usual Adult Dosage, Mechanism of Action, and Adverse Effects *continued*

Drug	Initial Adult Dose	Usual Adult Dosage (mg/d)	Dosage Forms	ACH	Drowsiness	Orthostatic Hypotension	Conduction Abnormalities	GI Distress	Weight Gain	Comments
						Adverse Effects				
FLUoxetine (PROzac®, PROzac® Weekly™, Sarafem®, Selfemra®)	10-20 mg qAM	20-80	C, CDR, L, T	0	0	0	0	3+⁴	1+	CYP2B6 and 2D6 inhibitor
FluvoxaMINE[2] (Luvox® CR)	50 mg qhs	100-300	T, CXR	0	0	0	0	3+⁴	1+	Contraindicated with pimozide, thioridazine, mesoridazine, CYP1A2, 2B6, 2C19, and 3A4 inhibitors
PARoxetine (Paxil®, Paxil CR®, Pexeva®)	10-20 mg qAM	20-50	T, CXR, L	1+	1+	0	0	3+⁴	2+	CYP2B6 and 2D6 inhibitor
Sertraline (Zoloft®)	25-50 mg qAM	50-200	T, L	0	0	0	0	3+⁴	1+	CYP2B6 and 2C19 inhibitor
Vilazodone (Viibryd™)	10 mg qAM	10-40	T	0	0	0	0	3+	0	CYP2C8, 2C19, and 2D6 inhibitor; also is a 5-HT₁A partial agonist
Dopamine-Reuptake Blocking Compounds										
BuPROPion (Aplenzin™, Buproban®, Budeprion SR®, Budeprion XL®, Wellbutrin®, Wellbutrin SR®, Wellbutrin XL®, Zyban®)	100 mg bid-tid IR⁵ 150 mg qAM-bid SR⁶	300-450	T, TSR, TXR	0	0	0	1+/0	1+	0	Contraindicated with seizures, bulimia, and anorexia; low incidence of sexual dysfunction IR: A 6-h interval between doses preferred SR: An 8-h interval between doses preferred XL: Administer once daily

Comparison of Usual Adult Dosage, Mechanism of Action, and Adverse Effects *continued*

Drug	Initial Adult Dose	Usual Adult Dosage (mg/d)	Dosage Forms	Adverse Effects						Comments
				ACH	Drowsiness	Orthostatic Hypotension	Conduction Abnormalities[7]	GI Distress	Weight Gain	
Serotonin/Norepinephrine Reuptake Inhibitors[7]										
Desvenlafaxine (Pristiq®)	50 mg/d	50–100	TXR	0	1+	1+	0	3+[4]	0	Active metabolite of venlafaxine
DULoxetine (Cymbalta®)	40–60 mg/d	40–60	CDR	1+	1+	0	1+	3+	0	Also indicated for GAD, management of pain associated with diabetic neuropathy, and management of fibromyalgia
Milnacipran[8] (Savella™)	12.5 mg/d	100–200	T	2+	1+	0	1+	3+	0	Only indicated for fibromyalgia
Venlafaxine (Effexor®, Effexor XR®)	25 mg bid-tid IR 37.5 mg qd XR	75–375 IR 75–225 XR	T, TXR, CXR	1+	1+	0	1+	3+[4]	0	High-dose may be useful to treat refractory depression; frequency of hypertension increases with dosage >225 mg/d
5-HT$_2$ Receptor Antagonist Properties										
Nefazodone	100 mg bid	300–600	T	1+	1+	2+	1+	1+	0	Contraindicated with carbamazepine, pimozide, astemizole, cisapride, and terfenadine; caution with triazolam and alprazolam; low incidence of sexual dysfunction
TraZODone	50 mg tid	150–600	T	0	4+	3+	1+	1+	2+	
Noradrenergic Antagonist										
Mirtazapine (Remeron®, Remeron SolTab®)	15 mg qhs	15–45	T, TOD	1+	3+	1+	1+	0	3+	Dose >15 mg/d less sedating, low incidence of sexual dysfunction

Comparison of Usual Adult Dosage, Mechanism of Action, and Adverse Effects *continued*

Drug	Initial Adult Dose	Usual Adult Dosage (mg/d)	Dosage Forms	Adverse Effects						Comments
				ACH	Drowsiness	Orthostatic Hypotension	Conduction Abnormalities	GI Distress	Weight Gain	
Monoamine Oxidase Inhibitors										
Isocarboxazid (Marplan®)	10 mg tid	10-30	T	2+	2+	2+	1+	1+	2+	Diet must be low in tyramine; contraindicated with sympathomimetics and other antidepressants
Phenelzine (Nardil®)	15 mg tid	15-90	T	2+	2+	2+	0	1+	3+	
Tranylcypromine (Parnate®)	10 mg bid	10-60	T	2+	1+	2+	1+	1+	2+	
Selegiline (EmSam®)	6 mg/d	6-12	Transdermal	2+	1+	2+	0	1+	0	Low tyramine diet not required for 6 mg/d dosage

ACH = anticholinergic effects (dry mouth, blurred vision, urinary retention, constipation); 0 - 4+ = absent or rare - relatively common; T = tablet; TSR = tablet, sustained release; TXR = tablet, extended release; TOD = tablet, orally disintegrating; L = liquid; C = capsule; CDR = capsule, delayed release; CXR = capsule, extended release; IR = immediate release; SR = sustained release; XR = extended release

[1]**Important note:** A 1-week supply taken all at once in a patient receiving the maximum dose can be fatal.

[2]Not approved by FDA for depression; approved for OCD

[3]Flat dose response curve, headache, nausea, and sexual dysfunction are common side effects for SSRIs.

[4]Nausea is usually mild and transient.

[5]IR: 100 mg bid; may be increased to 100 mg bid no sooner than 3 days after beginning therapy

[6]SR: 150 mg qAM; may be increased to 150 mg bid as early as day 4 of dosing. To minimize seizure risk, do not exceed SR 200 mg/dose.

[7]Do not use with sibutramine; relatively safe in overdose

[8]Milnacipran is only approved for fibromyalgia.

ANTIPARKINSONIAN AGENTS

Drugs Used for the Treatment of Parkinsonian Symptoms[1]

Drug	Mechanism	Initial Dose	Titration Schedule	Usual Daily Dosage	Recommended Dosing Schedule
Dopaminergic Agents					
Amantadine (Symmetrel®)	NMDA receptor antagonist and inhibits neuronal reuptake of dopamine	100 mg every other day	100 mg/dose every week, up to 300 mg 3 times/d	100-200 mg	Twice daily
Apomorphine (Apokyn®)	D_2 receptors (caudate-putamen)	1-2 mg	Complex; based on tolerance and response to test dose(s)	Variable; <20 mg	Individualized; 3-5 times/d prn
Bromocriptine (Parlodel®)	Moderate affinity for D_2 and D_3 dopamine receptors	1.25 mg twice daily	2.5 mg/d every 2-4 wk	2.5-100 mg	3 times/d
Carbidopa/levodopa (Sinemet®)	Converts to dopamine; binds to all CNS dopamine receptors	10-25/100 mg 2-4 times/d CR: 50/200 mg 2 times/d	0.5-1 tablet (10 or 25/100 mg) every 1-2 d	50/200 to 200/2000 mg (3-8 tablets)	3 times/d or twice daily (for controlled release)
Entacapone (Comtan®)	COMT enzyme inhibitor	200 mg 3 times/d	Titrate down the doses of carbidopa/levodopa as required	600-1600 mg	3 times/d; up to 8 times/d
Levodopa/carbidopa/ entacapone (Stalevo®)	Converts to dopamine; binds to all CNS dopamine receptors; COMT enzyme inhibitor	1 tablet 3-4 times/d (to replace previous dosing with individual agents)	As tolerated based on response and presence of dyskinesias	3-8 tablets per day	3-4 times/d
Pramipexole (Mirapex®)	High affinity for D_2 and D_3 dopamine receptors	0.125 mg 3 times/d	0.125 mg/dose every 5-7 d	1.5-4.5 mg	3 times/d
Rasagiline (Azilect®)	Inhibits MAO-B	0.5-1 mg once daily	≤1 mg daily	0.5-1 mg	Once daily
Ropinirole (Requip®)	High affinity for D_2 and D_3 dopamine receptors	0.25 mg 3 times/d	0.25 mg/dose weekly for 4 wk, then 1.5 mg/d every week up to 9 mg/d; 3 mg/d up to a max of 24 mg/d	0.75-24 mg	3 times/d
Selegiline (Eldepryl®)	Inhibits MAO-B	5-10 mg twice daily	5-10 mg daily	5-10 mg	Twice daily
Tolcapone (Tasmar®)	COMT enzyme inhibitor	100 mg 3 times/d	Titrate down the doses of carbidopa/levodopa as required	300-600 mg	3 times/d

Drugs Used for the Treatment of Parkinsonian Symptoms[1] *continued*

Drug	Mechanism	Initial Dose	Titration Schedule	Usual Daily Dosage	Recommended Dosing Schedule
Anticholinergic Agents					
Benztropine (Cogentin®)	Blocks cholinergic receptors, also has antihistamine effects	0.5-2 mg/d in 1-4 divided doses	0.5 mg/dose every 5-6 d	2-6 mg	1-2 times/d
Procyclidine (Kemadrin®)	Blocks cholinergic receptors	2.5 mg 3 times/d	Gradually as tolerated	7.5-20 mg	3 times/d
Trihexyphenidyl (Artane)	Blocks cholinergic receptors; also some direct effects	1-2 mg/d	2 mg/d at intervals of 3-5 d	5-15 mg	3-4 times/d

[1]The medications listed in the table represent treatment options for both idiopathic Parkinson's disease, as well as Parkinsonian symptoms resulting from other drug therapy.

[2]Cabergoline is not FDA approved for the treatment of Parkinson's disease.

ANTIPSYCHOTIC AGENTS

Antipsychotic Agent	Dosage Forms	I.M./P.O. Potency	Equiv. Dosages (approx) (mg/d)	Usual Adult Daily Maintenance Dose (mg)	Sedation (Incidence)	Extrapyramidal Side Effects	Anticholinergic Side Effects	Orthostatic Hypotension	Comments
ARIPiprazole (Abilify®)	Solution; tablet; tablet, orally disintegrating; injection		7.5	10-30	Low	Low	Very low	Very low	Low weight gain; activating
Asenapine (Saphris®)	Tablet, sublingual			10-20	Moderate	Low	Very low	Low/moderate	Low weight gain; activating
ChlorproMAZINE	Injection; tablet	4:1	100	200-1000	High	Moderate	Moderate	Moderate/high	
CloZAPine (Clozaril®, FazaClo®)	Tablet, tablet, orally disintegrating		100	75-900	High	Very low	High	High	~1% incidence of agranulocytosis; weekly-biweekly CBC required; potential for weight gain, lipid abnormalities, and diabetes
FluPHENAZine	Solution, concentrate; injection; tablet	2:1	2	0.5-20	Low	High	Low	Low	
	Injection, long-acting			12.5-25*					
Haloperidol (Haldol®)	Solution, concentrate; injection; tablet	2:1	2	0.5-20	Low	High	Low	Low	
(Haldol® Decanoate)	Injection, long-acting			50-200*					
Iloperidone (Fanapt™)	Tablet			12-24	Low	Low	Very low	Low/moderate	
Loxapine (Loxitane®)	Capsule		10	25-250	Moderate	Moderate	Low	Low	

Antipsychotic Agent	Dosage Forms	I.M./P.O. Potency	Equiv. Dosages (approx) (mg/d)	Usual Adult Daily Maintenance Dose (mg)	Sedation (Incidence)	Extrapyramidal Side Effects	Anticholinergic Side Effects	Orthostatic Hypotension	Comments
Lurasidone (Latuda®)	Tablet			40-80	Moderate	Low/moderate	Low	Low	Contraindicated with strong CYP3A4 inducers and inhibitors. Take with food.
OLANZapine (ZyPREXA®)	Injection; tablet; tablet, orally disintegrating		5	5-20	Moderate/ high	Low	Moderate	Moderate	Potential for weight gain, lipid abnormalities, diabetes
(ZyPREXA® Relprew™)	Injection, long-acting			210-405*					
Paliperidone (Invega®)	Tablet, extended release			3-12	Low/ moderate	Low	Very low	Moderate	Active metabolite of risperidone
(Invega® Sustenna®)	Injection, long-acting			39-234*		Moderate			
Perphenazine	Tablet		10	16-64	Low	High	Low	Low	
Pimozide (Orap®)	Tablet		2	1-10	Moderate	Very low	Moderate	Low	Contraindicated with CYP3A inhibitors
QUEtiapine (SEROquel®, SEROquel XR®)	Tablet; tablet, extended release		75	50-800	Moderate/ high	Very low	Moderate	Moderate	Moderate weight gain; potential for lipid abnormalities; diabetes
RisperiDONE (RisperDAL®)	Solution; tablet; tablet, orally disintegrating		2	0.5-6	Low/ moderate	Low	Very low	Moderate	Low to moderate weight gain; potential for diabetes
(RisperDAL® Consta®)	Injection, long-acting			25-50*					

Antipsychotic Agent	Dosage Forms	I.M./P.O. Potency	Equiv. Dosages (approx) (mg/d)	Usual Adult Daily Maintenance Dose (mg)	Sedation (Incidence)	Extrapyramidal Side Effects	Anticholinergic Side Effects	Orthostatic Hypotension	Comments
Thioridazine	Tablet		100	200-800	High	Low	High	Moderate/high	May cause irreversible retinitis pigmentosa at doses >800 mg/d; prolongs QTc; use only in treatment of refractory illness
Thiothixene (Navane®)	Capsule	4:1	4	5-40	Low	High	Low	Low/moderate	
Trifluoperazine	Tablet		5	2-40	Low	High	Low	Low	
Ziprasidone (Geodon®)	Capsule; injection; powder	2:1	60	40-160	Low/ moderate	Low	Very low	Low/moderate	Low weight gain; contraindicated with QTc-prolonging agents. Take with food.

*Administered every 2 or 4 weeks; consult drug monograph for specific dosage details

Woods SW. "Chlorpromazine Equivalent Doses for the Newer Atypical Antipsychotics," *J Clin Psychiatry*, 2003, 64(6):663-7.

ANXIOLYTIC, SEDATIVE/HYPNOTIC, AND MISCELLANEOUS BENZODIAZEPINES

	Peak Blood Concentration (oral) (h)	Protein Binding %	Major Active Metabolite	Half-Life (parent) Adults (h)	Half-Life[1] (metabolite) Adults (h)	Adult Oral Dosage Range	Geriatric Oral Dosage Range
Anxiolytic							
ALPRAZolam (Alprazolam Intensol®, Xanax®)	1-2	80	No	12-15	—	0.75-4 mg/d	0.25-0.75 mg/d
ChlordiazePOXIDE (Librium®)	2-4	90-98	Yes	5-30	24-96	15-100 mg/d	10-20 mg/d[2]
Diazepam (Diastat® Rectal Delivery System, Diazepam Intensol®, Valium®)	0.5-2	98	Yes	20-80	50-100	4-40 mg/d	1-20 mg/d[2]
LORazepam (Ativan®)[3]	1-6	88-92	No	10-20	—	2-4 mg/d	0.5-4 mg/d
Oxazepam (Serax®)	2-4	86-99	No	5-20	—	30-120 mg/d	20-45 mg/d
Sedative/Hypnotic							
Estazolam (ProSom®)	2	93	No	10-24	—	1-2 mg	0.5-1 mg
Flurazepam (Dalmane®)	0.5-2	97	Yes	Not significant	40-114	15-60 mg	15 mg[2]
Quazepam (Doral®)	2	95	Yes	25-41	28-114	7.5-15 mg	7.5 mg[2]
Temazepam (Restoril®)	2-3	96	No	10-40	—	15-30 mg; Transient insomnia: 7.5 mg	7.5-15 mg
Triazolam (Halcion®)	1	89-94	No	2.3	—	0.125-0.5 mg	0.0625-0.25 mg
Miscellaneous							
ClonazePAM (Klonopin®)	1-2	86	No	18-50	—	1.5-20 mg/d	0.5-20 mg/d
Clorazepate (Tranxene®)	1-2	80-95	Yes	Not significant	50-100	15-60 mg/d	7.5-15 mg/d[2]
Midazolam	0.4-0.7[4]	95	No	2-5	—	NA	NA

[1] Significant metabolite

[2] Not recommended for use in geriatric patients

[3] Reliable bioavailability when given I.M.

[4] I.V. only

NA = not available

ATYPICAL ANTIPSYCHOTICS

Drug[1]	DR EPS	PROL	TD[2]	ACH	SZ	OH	LFTs	SED	WT GAIN	NMS	AGRAN	TX REFR	Lipid	DM	QTc
ARIPiprazole (Abilify®)	No	No	Uncommon	Very low	Low	Low	Low	Low	Very low	Yes	?	Maybe	Very low	Very low	Low
Asenapine (Saphris®)	Yes	No	Uncommon	Very low	Low	Low / moderate	Low	Moderate	Low	Yes	?	No	Very low	Very low	Low
CloZAPine (Clozaril®)	No	No	Uncommon	High	DD	High	Low	High	High	Yes	Yes	Yes	High	High	Low
Iloperidone (Fanapt™)	No	No	Uncommon	Very low	Low	Low / moderate	Low	Low	Low / moderate	Yes	?	No	Very low	Very low	Moderate
Lurasidone (Latuda®)	Yes	Yes	Uncommon	Very low	Low	Low	Low	Moderate	Very low	Yes	?	No	Very low	Very low	Low
OLANZapine ZyPREXA®, ZyPREXA®, Zydis®	Yes	Yes	Uncommon	Moderate	Low	Low / moderate	Low / moderate	Moderate	High	Yes	Yes[3]	Maybe	High	High	Low
Paliperidone (Invega™)	Yes	Yes	Uncommon	Very low	Low	Moderate	Low	Low	Low	Yes	?	Maybe	Low	Low	Low
QUEtiapine (SEROquel®)	No	No	Uncommon	Moderate	Low	Moderate	Low / moderate	Moderate	Moderate	Yes	Yes[3]	Maybe	Moderate	Low / moderate	Moderate
RisperiDONE (RisperDAL®)	Yes	Yes	Uncommon	Very low	Low	Moderate	Low	Low	Low / moderate	Yes	Yes[3]	Maybe	Low	Low / moderate	Low
Ziprasidone (Geodon®)	Yes	Yes	Uncommon	Very low	Low	Low	Low	Low	Very low	Yes	Yes[3]	Maybe	Very low	Very low	Moderate[4]

DR EPS = dose related extrapyramidal symptoms; **PROL** = prolactin elevation (may cause amenorrhea, galactorrhea, gynecomastia, impotence); **TD** = tardive dyskinesia; **ACH** = anticholinergic side effects (dry mouth, blurred vision, constipation, urinary hesitancy); **SZ** = seizures; **OH** = orthostatic hypotension (blood pressure drops upon standing); **LFTs** = increased liver function test results; **SED** = sedation; **WT GAIN** = weight gain; **NMS** = neuroleptic malignant syndrome; **AGRAN** = agranulocytosis (without white blood cells to fight infection); **TX REFR** = efficacy in treatment refractory schizophrenia; **Lipid** = lipid abnormalities; cholesterol and/or triglyceride elevations; **DM** = diabetes (based on case reports); **QTc** = QTc prolongation; **DD** = dose dependent

[1] Defined as 1) decrease or no EPS at doses producing antipsychotic effect; 2) minimum or no increase in prolactin; 3) decrease in both positive and negative symptoms of schizophrenia.

[2] Rate of TD ~⅓ that seen with conventional antipsychotics.

[3] Case reports.

[4] Dose related within 40-160 mg dosage range.

BETA-BLOCKERS

Agent	Adrenergic Receptor Blocking Activity	Intrinsic Sympathomimetic Activity (ISA)	Lipid Solubility	Protein Bound (%)	Half-Life (h)	Bioavailability (%)	Primary Site of Metabolism	Primary (Secondary) Route of Elimination	Indications	Usual Dosage
Acebutolol (Sectra®)	beta[1]	Yes	Low	15-25	3-4	40 7-fold[1]	Hepatic	Feces (renal)	Hypertension, arrhythmias	P.O.: 400-1200 mg/d
Atenolol (Tenormin®)	beta[1]	No	Low	<5-10	6-9	50-60 4-fold[1]	Hepatic (limited)	Feces (renal)	Hypertension, angina pectoris, acute MI	P.O.: 50-200 mg/d I.V.: Acute MI: 5 mg x 2 doses
Betaxolol (Kerlone®)	beta[1]	No	Low	50-55	14-22	84-94	Hepatic	Renal	Hypertension	P.O.: 5-20 mg/d
Bisoprolol (Zebeta®)	beta[1]	No	Low	26-33	9-12	80	Hepatic	Renal	Hypertension, heart failure	P.O.: HF: 2.5-10 mg/d HTN: 2.5-20 mg/d
Carvedilol (Coreg®, Coreg CR®)	alpha[1] beta[1] beta[2]	No	ND	98	7-10	25-35	Hepatic	Feces	Hypertension, heart failure (mild to severe)	P.O.: 3.125-25 mg twice daily
Esmolol (Brevibloc)	beta[1]	No	Low	55	0.15	NA 5-fold[1]	Red blood cell esterase	Renal	Supraventricular tachycardia, sinus tachycardia, atrial fibrillation/ flutter, hypertension	I.V. infusion: 25-300 mcg/kg/min
Labetalol (Trandate®)	alpha[1] beta[1] beta[2]	No	Moderate	50	5.5-8	18-30 10-fold[1]	Hepatic	Renal	Hypertension	P.O.: 200-2400 mg/d I.V.: 20-80 mg at 10-min intervals up to a maximum of 300 mg or continuous infusion of 2-6 mg/min

Agent	Adrenergic Receptor Blocking Activity	Intrinsic Sympathomimetic Activity (ISA)	Lipid Solubility	Protein Bound (%)	Half-Life (h)	Bioavailability (%)	Primary Site of Metabolism	Primary (Secondary) Route of Elimination	Indications	Usual Dosage
Metoprolol (Lopressor®, Toprol-XL®)	beta₁	No	Moderate	10-12	3-7	50 7- to 10-fold[1] (Toprol XL®: 77)	Hepatic	Renal	Hypertension, angina pectoris, acute MI, heart failure (mild to moderate; XL formulation only), atrial tachyarrhythmias (rate control)	P.O.: 100-450 mg/d HF: (Toprol-XL®): 12.5-200 mg/d I.V.: Acute MI: 5 mg q2 min x 3 doses AF (rate control): 2.5-5 mg q2-5 min (max total dose: 15 mg over 0-15 min)
Nadolol (Corgard®)	beta₁ beta₂	No	Low	25-30	20-24	30 5- to 8-fold[1]	None	Renal	Hypertension, angina pectoris	P.O.: 40-320 mg/d
Nebivolol (Bystolic®)	beta₁	No	High	98	10-32	12-96	Hepatic	Renal (feces)	Hypertension	P.O.: 5-40 mg/d
Penbutolol (Levatol®)	beta₁ beta₂	Yes	High	80-98	5	~100	Hepatic	Renal	Hypertension	P.O.: 20-80 mg/d
Pindolol	beta₁ beta₂	Yes	Moderate	57	3-4	90 2- to 2.5-fold[1]	Hepatic	Renal (feces)	Hypertension	P.O.: 20-60 mg/d
Propranolol (Inderal®, various)	beta₁ beta₂	No	High	90	3-5	25 2- to 3-fold[1]	Hepatic	Renal	Hypertension, angina pectoris, arrhythmias, prophylaxis (post-MI)	P.O.: 40-480 mg/d I.V.: Tachyarrhythmias: 1-3 mg q2-5 min (max: 5 mg)
Propranolol long-acting (Inderal-LA®, InnoPran XL™)	beta₁ beta₂	No	High	90	9-18	25 2- to 3-fold[1]	Hepatic	Renal	Hypertrophic cardiomyopathy with outflow tract obstruction, prophylaxis (post-MI)	P.O.: 180-240 mg/d

Agent	Adrenergic Receptor Blocking Activity	Intrinsic Sympathomimetic Activity (ISA)	Lipid Solubility	Protein Bound (%)	Half-Life (h)	Bioavailability (%)	Primary Site of Metabolism	Primary (Secondary) Route of Elimination	Indications	Usual Dosage
Sotalol (Betapace®, Betapace AF®, Sorine®)	$beta_1$ $beta_2$	No	Low	0	12	90-100	None	Renal	Atrial and ventricular tachyarrhythmias	P.O. 160-320 mg/d
Timolol (Blocadren®)	$beta_1$ $beta_2$	No	Low to moderate	<10	4	75 7-fold[1]	Hepatic	Renal	Hypertension, prophylaxis (post-MI)	P.O.: 20-60 mg/d

Dosage is based on 70 kg adult with normal hepatic and renal function.

Note: All beta$_1$-selective agents will inhibit beta$_2$ receptors at higher doses.

[1]Interpatient variations in plasma levels

CALCIUM CHANNEL BLOCKERS – COMPARATIVE PHARMACOKINETICS

Comparative Pharmacokinetics

Agent	Bioavailability (%)	Protein Binding (%)	Onset of BP Effect (min)	Duration of BP Effect (h)	Half-Life (h)	Volume of Distribution	Route of Metabolism	Route of Excretion
Dihydropyridines								
AmLODIPine (Norvasc®)	64-90	93-98	30-50	24	30-50	21 L/kg	Hepatic; inactive metabolites	Urine; 10% as parent
Clevidipine (Cleviprex™)		>99.5	2-4	5-15 min	1-15 min	0.17 L/kg	Blood and extravascular tissue esterases	Urine (63% to 74%; as metabolites); feces (7% to 22%)
Felodipine (Plendil)	20	>99	2-5 h	24	11-16	10 L/kg	Hepatic; CYP3A4 substrate (major); inactive metabolites; extensive first pass	Urine (70%; as metabolites); feces 10%
Isradipine (DynaCirc CR®)	15-24	95	20	>12	8	3 L/kg	Hepatic; CYP3A4 substrate (major); inactive metabolites; extensive first pass	Urine as metabolites
NICARdipine (Cardene®)	35	>95	30	≤8	2-4		Hepatic; CYP3A4 substrate (major); saturable first pass	Urine (60%; as metabolites); feces 35%
NIFEdipine (Procardia®)	40-77	92-98	Within 20		2-5		Hepatic; CYP3A4 substrate (major); inactive metabolites	Urine as metabolites
NiMODipine (Nimotop®)	13	>95	ND	4-6	1-2		Hepatic; CYP3A4 substrate (major); metabolites inactive or less active than parent; extensive first pass	Urine (50%; as metabolites); feces 32%
Nisoldipine (Sular®)	5	>99	ND	6-12	7-12		Hepatic; CYP3A4 substrate (major); 1 active metabolite (10% of parent); extensive first pass	Urine as metabolites
Phenylalkylamines								
Verapamil (Calan®, Verelan®)	20-35	90	30	6-8	4.5-12		Hepatic; CYP3A4 substrate (major); 1 active metabolite (20% of parent); extensive first pass	Urine (70%; 3% to 4% as unchanged drug); feces 16%
Benzothiazepines								
Diltiazem (Cardizem®)	~40	70-80	30-60	6-8	3-4.5	3-13 L/kg	Hepatic; CYP3A4 substrate (major); 1 major metabolite (20%-50% of parent); extensive first pass	Urine as metabolites

CORTICOSTEROIDS SYSTEMIC EQUIVALENCIES

Glucocorticoid	Approximate Equivalent Dose (mg)	Routes of Administration	Relative Anti-inflammatory Potency	Relative Mineralocorticoid Potency	Protein Binding (%)	Half-life Plasma (min)
		Short-Acting				
Cortisone	25	P.O., I.M.	0.8	0.8	90	30
Hydrocortisone	20	I.M., I.V.	1	1	90	90
		Intermediate-Acting				
MethylPREDNISolone[1]	4	P.O., I.M., I.V.	5	0	—	180
PrednisoLONE	5	P.O., I.M., I.V., intra-articular, intradermal, soft tissue injection	4	0.8	90-95	200
PredniSONE	5	P.O.	4	0.8	70	60
Triamcinolone[1]	4	I.M. intra-articular, intradermal, intrasynovial, soft tissue injection	5	0	—	300
		Long-Acting				
Betamethasone	0.75	P.O., I.M., intra-articular, intradermal, intrasynovial, soft tissue injection	25	0	64	100-300
Dexamethasone	0.75	P.O., I.M., I.V., intra-articular, intradermal, soft tissue injection	25-30	0	—	100-300
		Mineralocorticoids				
Fludrocortisone	—	P.O.	10	125	42	200

[1]May contain propylene glycol as an excipient in injectable forms

Asare K, "Diagnosis and Treatment of Adrenal Insufficiency in the Critically Ill Patient," *Pharmacotherapy*, 2007, 27(11):1512-28.

TOPICAL CORTICOSTEROIDS

GUIDELINES FOR SELECTION AND USE OF TOPICAL CORTICOSTEROIDS

The quantity prescribed and the frequency of refills should be monitored to reduce the risk of adrenal suppression. In general, short courses of high-potency agents are preferable to prolonged use of low potency. After control is achieved, control should be maintained with a low potency preparation.

1. Low-to-medium potency agents are usually effective for treating thin, acute, inflammatory skin lesions; whereas, high or super-potent agents are often required for treating chronic, hyperkeratotic, or lichenified lesions.

2. Since the stratum corneum is thin on the face and intertriginous areas, low-potency agents are preferred but a higher potency agent may be used for 2 weeks.

3. Because the palms and soles have a thick stratum corneum, high or super-potent agents are frequently required.

4. Low potency agents are preferred for infants and the elderly. Infants have a high body surface area to weight ratio; elderly patients have thin, fragile skin.

5. The vehicle in which the topical corticosteroid is formulated influences the absorption and potency of the drug. Ointment bases are preferred for thick, lichenified lesions; they enhance penetration of the drug. Creams are preferred for acute and subacute dermatoses; they may be used on moist skin areas or intertriginous areas. Solutions, gels, and sprays are preferred for the scalp or for areas where a nonoil-based vehicle is needed.

6. In general, super-potent agents should not be used for longer than 2-3 weeks unless the lesion is limited to a small body area. Medium-to-high potency agents usually cause only rare adverse effects when treatment is limited to 3 months or less, and use on the face and intertriginous areas are avoided. If long-term treatment is needed, intermittent vs continued treatment is recommended.

7. Most preparations are applied once or twice daily. More frequent application may be necessary for the palms or soles because the preparation is easily removed by normal activity and penetration is poor due to a thick stratum corneum. Every-other-day or weekend-only application may be effective for treating some chronic conditions.

Relative Potency of Selected Topical Corticosteroids

	Steroid	Dosage Form
	Very High Potency	
0.05%	Betamethasone dipropionate, augmented	Cream, gel, lotion, ointment
0.05%	Clobetasol propionate	Cream, foam, gel, lotion, ointment, shampoo, spray
0.05%	Diflorasone diacetate	Ointment
0.05%	Halobetasol propionate	Cream, ointment
	High Potency	
0.1%	Amcinonide	Cream, ointment, lotion
0.05%	Betamethasone dipropionate, augmented	Cream
0.05%	Betamethasone dipropionate	Cream, ointment
0.1%	Betamethasone valerate	Ointment
0.05%	Desoximetasone	Gel
0.25%	Desoximetasone	Cream, ointment
0.05%	Diflorasone diacetate	Cream, ointment
0.05%	Fluocinonide	Cream, ointment, gel
0.1%	Halcinonide	Cream, ointment
0.5%	Triamcinolone acetonide	Cream, spray

TOPICAL CORTICOSTEROIDS

Relative Potency of Selected Topical Corticosteroids *(continued)*

	Steroid	Dosage Form
	Intermediate Potency	
0.05%	Betamethasone dipropionate	Lotion
0.1%	Betamethasone valerate	Cream
0.1%	Clocortolone pivalate	Cream
0.05%	Desoximetasone	Cream
0.025%	Fluocinolone acetonide	Cream, ointment
0.05%	Flurandrenolide	Cream, ointment, lotion, tape
0.005%	Fluticasone propionate	Ointment
0.05%	Fluticasone propionate	Cream, lotion
0.1%	Hydrocortisone butyrate[1]	Ointment, solution
0.2%	Hydrocortisone valerate[1]	Cream, ointment
0.1%	Mometasone furoate[1]	Cream, ointment, lotion
0.1%	Prednicarbate	Cream, ointment
0.025%	Triamcinolone acetonide	Cream, ointment, lotion
0.1%	Triamcinolone acetonide	Cream, ointment, lotion
	Low Potency	
0.05%	Alclometasone dipropionate[1]	Cream, ointment
0.05%	Desonide	Cream, ointment
0.01%	Fluocinolone acetonide	Cream, solution
0.5%	Hydrocortisone[1]	Cream, ointment, lotion
0.5%	Hydrocortisone acetate[1]	Cream, ointment
1%	Hydrocortisone acetate[1]	Cream, ointment
1%	Hydrocortisone[1]	Cream, ointment, lotion, solution
2.5%	Hydrocortisone[1]	Cream, ointment, lotion

[1] Not fluorinated

GLAUCOMA DRUG THERAPY

Ophthalmic Agent (Brand)	Reduces Aqueous Humor Production	Increases Aqueous Humor Outflow [1]	Average Duration of Action	Strengths Available
Cholinesterase Inhibitors [1]				
Echothiophate iodide (Phospholine Iodide®)	No data	Significant	2 wk	0.125%
Direct-Acting Cholinergic Miotics				
Carbachol (Isopto® Carbachol)	Some activity	Significant	8 h	1.5%, 3%
Pilocarpine (Isopto® Carpine, Pilopine HS®)	Some activity	Significant	5 h	0.5%, 1%, 2%, 3%, 4%, 6%
Sympathomimetics				
Apraclonidine (Iopidine®)	Moderate	Moderate	4 h	0.5%, 1%
Brimonidine (Alphagan® P)	Moderate	Moderate	8 h	0.1%, 0.15%
Dipivefrin (Propine®)	Some activity	Moderate	12 h	0.1%
Beta-Blockers				
Betaxolol (Betoptic® S, Kerlone®)	Significant	Some activity	≥12 h	0.25%, 0.5%
Carteolol	Yes	No	12 h	1%
Levobunolol (Betagan®)	Significant	Some activity	24 h	0.25%, 0.5%
Metipranolol (OptiPranolol®)	Significant	Some activity	18 h	0.3%
Timolol (Betimol®, Timoptic®)	Significant	Some activity	24 h	0.25%, 0.5%
Carbonic Anhydrase Inhibitors				
Acetazolamide (Diamox® Sequels®)	Significant	No data	10 h	125 mg tab, 250 mg tab; 500 mg cap
Brinzolamide (Azopt®)	Yes	No data	8 h	1%
Dorzolamide (Trusopt®)	Yes	No	8 h	2%
Methazolamide	Significant	No data	14 h	25 mg, 50 mg
Prostaglandin Agonists				
Bimatoprost (Lumigan®)		Yes	≥24 h	0.03%
Latanoprost (Xalatan®)		Yes	≥24 h	0.005%
Tafluprost (Zioptan™)		Yes	≥24 h	0.0015%
Travoprost (Travatan®)		Yes	24 h	0.004%

[1] All miotic drugs significantly affect accommodation.

H. PYLORI TREATMENT IN ADULT PATIENTS

Medication Regimen	Dosages	Duration of Therapy
First-Line Therapy (Option 1)		
H$_2$-Receptor antagonist (H$_2$RA) **or** proton pump inhibitor (PPI)	Standard dose of H$_2$RA or PPI[1]	10-14 days
plus		
Bismuth subsalicylate	525 mg 4 times/day	10-14 days
plus		
MetroNIDAZOLE	250 mg 4 times/day	10-14 days
plus		
Tetracycline	500 mg 4 times/day	10-14 days
First-Line Therapy (Option 2)		
PPI	Standard dose[1]	10-14 days
plus		
Clarithromycin	500 mg 2 times/day	10-14 days
plus		
Amoxicillin	1000 mg 2 times/day	10-14 days
First-Line Therapy (Option 3)		
PPI	Standard dose[1]	10-14 days
plus		
Clarithromycin	500 mg 2 times/day	10-14 days
plus		
MetroNIDAZOLE	500 mg 2 times/day	10-14 days
Salvage Therapy for Persistent Infection (Option 1)		
PPI (once daily), bismuth, metroNIDAZOLE, and tetracycline (4 times/day) for 7-14 days		
Salvage Therapy for Persistent Infection (Option 2)		
PPI (standard dose[1]), levofloxacin 500 mg (once daily), and amoxicillin 1000 mg (2 times/day) for 10 days		

[1]Standard proton pump inhibitor dose: Esomeprazole = 40 mg once daily, lansoprazole = 30 mg 2 times/day, omeprazole = 20 mg 2 times/day, RABEprazole = 20 mg 2 times/day

REFERENCES

Chey WD, Wong BC, and Practice Parameters Committee of the American College of Gastroenterology, "American College of Gastroenterology Guideline on the Management of *Helicobacter pylori* Infection," *Am J Gastroenterol*, 2007, 102(8):1808-25.

Saad RJ, Schoenfeld P, Kim HM, et al, "Levofloxacin-Based Triple Therapy Versus Bismuth-Based Quadruple Therapy for Persistent *Helicobacter pylori* Infection: A Meta-Analysis," *Am J Gastroenterol*, 2006, 101(3):488-96.

INHALANT AGENTS

Medications Commonly Used for Asthma, Bronchospasm, and COPD

Agent	Indications	Onset	Duration	Frequency	Comments
Anticholinergics					
Ipratropium bromide (Atrovent®)	Bronchospasm associated with COPD; severe asthma exacerbation (Asthma Guidelines, 2007)	1-3 min	≤4 h	4 times/day	Asthma: Should be used as adjunct therapy to SABA in severe exacerbations. May not provide further benefit if patient hospitalized.
Tiotropium (Spiriva®)	Bronchospasm associated with COPD			Daily	For COPD only
Short-Acting Beta₂-Agonists (SABA)[1]					
Albuterol (Proventil®, Proventil® HFA, Ventolin® HFA)	Prevention of EIB; relief and prevention of bronchospasm	5 min	6-8 h	q4-6h	
Levalbuterol (Xopenex®)	Relief and prevention of bronchospasm	6-17 min	3-6 h	6-8 h intervals (nebulization); 4-6 h (inhaler)	May be used as SABA in asthma exacerbations
Pirbuterol acetate (Maxair™ Autohaler™)	Treatment and prevention of bronchospasm	Within 5 min	4-6 h	q4-6h	Not studied in severe exacerbations
Long-Acting Beta₂-Agonists (LABA)[2]					
Arformoterol (Brovana™)	Long-term maintenance treatment in COPD	7-20 min	12 h	q12h	Not to be used for treatment of episodes of acute bronchospasm as rescue therapy
Formoterol (Foradil® Aerolizer™)	Long-term maintenance treatment of asthma; prevention of EIB; maintenance treatment of COPD	Within 3 min	12 h	q12h	Not meant to relieve acute asthmatic symptoms
Salmeterol (Serevent® Diskus®)	Long-term maintenance treatment of asthma; prevention of EIB; maintenance treatment of COPD	20 min	12 h	q12h	Not meant to relieve acute asthmatic symptoms

Medications Commonly Used for Asthma, Bronchospasm, and COPD *continued*

Agent	Indications	Onset	Duration	Frequency	Comments
Inhalation Corticosteroids[3]					
Beclomethasone dipropionate (various)	Maintenance and prevention of asthma		6–8 h	Twice daily	Adjustable dose approach may enable reduction in cumulative dose over time without decreasing asthma control
Budesonide (Pulmicort®)	Maintenance and prevention of asthma		12 h	Twice daily	
Flunisolide (various)	Maintenance and prevention of asthma		12 h	Twice daily	
Fluticasone (Flovent®)	Maintenance and prevention of asthma		—	Twice daily	
Mometasone	Maintenance and prevention of asthma		—	Once or twice daily	
Mast Cell Stabilizers[3]					
Nedocromil sodium (Alocril®)	Maintenance treatment of mild-to-moderate asthma		2 h	4 times/day	

EIB = exercise-induced bronchospasm

[1]Asthma: Only selective beta$_2$-agonists are recommended

[2]Asthma: Should not be used for symptom relief or exacerbations; use only with ICS

[3]Asthma: Should not be used for symptom relief or exacerbations
Expert Panel Report 3, "Guidelines for the Diagnosis and Management of Asthma." *Clinical Practice Guidelines*, National Institutes of Health, National Heart, Lung, and Blood Institute. NIH Publication No. 08-4051, prepublication 2007. Available at http://www.nhlbi.nih.gov/guidelines/asthma/asthgdln.htm

INJECTABLE HEPARINS/HEPARINOIDS COMPARISON TABLE

Name	Use	Limitation	Dose (SubQ unless otherwise noted)	Average MW Range (in Daltons)
Low Molecular Weight Heparins				
Dalteparin (Fragmin®) Note: Dose may require adjustment according to renal function	Prophylaxis	Abdominal surgery[1]	2500 int. units/day	2000-9000
	Prophylaxis	Abdominal surgery[2]	5000 int. units/day	
	Prophylaxis	Hip surgery[1]	5000 int. units/day postoperatively	
	Treatment	DVT or PE (in patients with cancer)	Month 1: 200 int. units/kg once daily (max: 18,000 units); Months 2-6: 150 int. units/kg once daily (max: 18,000 units)	
	Treatment	Unstable angina NSTEMI	120 int. units/kg (max: 10,000 int units) q12h	
Enoxaparin (Lovenox®) Note: Dose may require adjustment according to renal function	Prophylaxis	Hip replacement	30 mg q12h or 40 mg once daily	2000-8000
	Prophylaxis	Knee replacement	30 mg q12h	
	Prophylaxis	Abdominal surgery	40 mg once daily	
	Treatment	DVT or PE	1 mg/kg q12h or 1.5 mg/kg once daily	
	Treatment	Unstable angina/NSTEMI	1 mg/kg q12h	
	Treatment	STEMI	<75 years: 1 mg/kg q12h; ≥75 years: 0.75 mg/kg q12h	
Tinzaparin (Innohep®) Note: Dose may require adjustment according to renal function	Treatment	DVT or PE	175 anti-Xa int. units/kg/day	5500-7500
Heparin				
Heparin	Prophylaxis	Risk of thromboembolic disease	5000 units q8-12h	3000-30,000
	Treatment	DVT or PE[3]	80 units/kg (or 5000 units) IVP then 18 units/kg/hour (or 1300 units/hour)	
	Treatment	STEMI/Unstable angina/NSTEMI[4,5]	60 units/kg IVP (max: 4000 units), then 12 units/kg/hour (max: 1000 units/hour)	

Name	Use	Limitation	Dose (SubQ unless otherwise noted)	Average MW Range (in Daltons)
Selective Anti-Xa Inhibitor				
Fondaparinux[6] (Arixtra®) **Note**: Dose may require adjustment according to renal function	Prophylaxis	Abdominal surgery Hip fracture Hip or knee replacement	≥50 kg: 2.5 mg once daily	1728
	Treatment	DVT or PE	<50 kg: 5 mg once daily 50-100 kg: 7.5 mg once daily >100 kg: 10 mg once daily	
Coumarin Derivatives				
Warfarin (Coumadin®)	Prophylaxis	NS	Variable	NS
	Treatment		2-5 mg/day	

NS = not stated in labeling, DVT = Deep venous thrombosis, NSTEMI = Non-ST-elevation MI, STEMI = ST-elevation MI, PE = Pulmonary embolism

[1]Patients with low risk of DVT

[2]Patients with high risk of DVT

[3]Dosing according to current clinical practice guidelines (Kearon, 2008)

[4]Not an FDA-approved indication; dosing according to current clinical practice guidelines (Anderson, 2007; Antman, 2004)

[5]Elderly patients may require a lower bolus dose of heparin.

[6]Synthetic pentasaccharide

Anderson JL, Adams CD, Antman EM, et al, "ACC/AHA 2007 Guidelines for the Management of Patients With Unstable Angina/Non-ST-Elevation Myocardial Infarction: A Report of the American College of Cardiology/American Heart Association Task Force on Practice Guidelines (Writing Committee to Revise the 2002 Guidelines for the Management of Patients With Unstable Angina/Non-ST-Elevation Myocardial Infarction) Developed in Collaboration With the American College of Emergency Physicians, the Society for Cardiovascular Angiography and Interventions, and the Society of Thoracic Surgeons Endorsed by the American Association of Cardiovascular and Pulmonary Rehabilitation and the Society for Academic Emergency Medicine," *J Am Coll Cardiol*, 2007, 50(7):e1-e157.

Antman EM, Anbe DT, Armstrong PW, et al, "ACC/AHA Guidelines for the Management of Patients With ST-Elevation Myocardial Infarction: A Report of the American College of Cardiology/American Heart Association Task Force on Practice Guidelines (Committee to Revise the 1999 Guidelines for the Management of Patients With Acute Myocardial Infarction)," *Circulation*, 2004, 110(9):e82-292.

Kearon C, Kahn SR, Agnelli G, et al, "Antithrombotic Therapy for Venous Thromboembolic Disease: American College of Chest Physicians Evidence-Based Clinical Practice Guidelines (8th Edition)," *Chest*, 2008, 133(6 Suppl):454S-545S.

LAXATIVES, CLASSIFICATION AND PROPERTIES

Laxative	Onset of Action	Site of Action	Mechanism of Action
Saline			
Magnesium citrate Magnesium hydroxide (Phillips'® Milk of Magnesia)	30 min to 3 h	Small and large intestine	Attract/retain water in intestinal lumen increasing intraluminal pressure; cholecystokinin release
Sodium phosphates (Fleet® Enema)	2-15 min	Colon	
Irritant/Stimulant			
Senna (Senokot®)	6-10 h	Colon	Direct action on intestinal mucosa; stimulate myenteric plexus; alter water and electrolyte secretion
Bisacodyl (Dulcolax®) tablets, suppositories	15 min to 1 h	Colon	
Castor oil	2-6 h	Small intestine	
Bulk-Producing			
Methylcellulose (Citrucel®) Psyllium (Metamucil®) Wheat dextrin (Benefiber®)	12-24 h (up to 72 h) 24-48 h	Small and large intestine	Holds water in stool; mechanical distention
Lubricant			
Mineral oil	6-8 h	Colon	Lubricates intestine; retards colonic absorption of fecal water; softens stool
Surfactants/Stool Softener			
Docusate/senna (Peri-Colace®)	8-12 h	Small and large intestine	Senna – mild irritant; docusate – stool softener
Docusate sodium (Colace®) Docusate calcium (Surfak®)	24-72 h	Small and large intestine	Detergent activity; facilitates admixture of fat and water to soften stool
Osmotic Laxatives			
Glycerin suppository	15-30 min	Colon	Local irritation; hyperosmotic action
Lactulose	24-48 h	Colon	Delivers osmotically active molecules to colon
Polyethylene glycol 3350 (GlycoLax™, MiraLax™)	48 h	Small and large intestine	Nonabsorbable solution which acts as an osmotic agent
Sodium sulfate, potassium sulfate, and magnesium sulfate (Suprep®)	24 h	Small and large intestine	Hyperosmotic action
Sorbitol 70%	24-48 h	Colon	Delivers osmotically active molecules to colon
Miscellaneous Laxatives			
Lubiprostone (Amitiza®)	24-48 h	Apical membrane of the GI epithelium	Activates intestinal chloride channels increasing intestinal fluid

OPIOID ANALGESICS

This table serves as a general guide to opioid conversion. Utilization of a direct conversion without a detailed patients and medication assessment is not recommended and may result in over- or underdosing. Chronic administration may alter pharmacokinetics and change parenteral: oral ratio.

Opioid Analgesics – Initial Oral Dosing Commonly Used for Severe Pain

Drug	Equianalgesic Dose (mg)		Initial Oral Dose	
	Oral[1]	Parenteral[2]	Children[3] (mg/kg)	Adults (mg)
Buprenorphine	—	0.4	—	—
Butorphanol	—	2	—	—
FentaNYL	—	0.1	—	—
HYDROmorphone	7.5	1.5	0.06	4-8
Levorphanol	Acute: 4 Chronic: 1	Acute: 2 Chronic: 1	0.04	2-4
Meperidine[4]	300	75	Not recommended	
Methadone[5]	See Guidelines for Conversion to Oral Methadone in Adults	Variable	0.2	5-10
Morphine	30	10	0.3	15-30
Nalbuphine	—	10	—	—
OxyCODONE	20	—	0.2	10-20
Oxymorphone	10	1	—	5-10
Pentazocine	50	30	—	—

Guidelines for Conversion to Oral Methadone in Adults[5]

Oral Morphine Dose or Equivalent (mg/day)	Oral Morphine:Oral Methadone (Conversion Ratio)
<90	4:1
90-300	8:1
>300	12:1

[1]Elderly: Starting dose should be lower for this population group.

[2]Standard parenteral doses (I.M.) for acute pain in adults; can be used to convert doses for I.V. infusions and repeated small I.V. boluses. For single I.V. boluses, use half the I.M. dose.

[3]The pharmacokinetics of opioids in children and infants >6 months old are similar to adults, but infants <6 months old, especially premature or physically compromised ones, are at risk of apnea.

[4]Not recommended for routine use

[5]Conversion of higher doses may be guided by the following (consult a pain or palliative care specialist if unfamiliar with methadone prescribing): As the total daily chronic dose of morphine increases, the equianalgesic dose ratio (morphine:methadone) changes (American Pain Society, 2008). Total daily dose should be divided by 3; delivered every 8 hours. Methadone is significantly more potent with repetitive dosing (due to its active metabolite). Begin methadone at lower doses and gradually titrate. Applicability to pediatric patients is unknown.

REFERENCES

National Cancer Institute, "Pain (PDQ®)," Last Modified 5/7/09. Available at http://www.cancer.gov/cancertopics/pdq/supportivecare/pain/HealthProfessional/page1

National Comprehensive Cancer Network® (NCCN), "Clinical Practice Guidelines in Oncology™: Adult Cancer Pain," Version 1, 2009. Available at http://www.nccn.org/professionals/physician_gls/PDF/pain.pdf

Patanwala AE, Duby J, Waters D, et al, "Opioid Conversions in Acute Care," *Ann Pharmacother*, 2007, 41(2):255-66.

Principles of Analgesic Use in the Treatment of Acute Pain and Cancer Pain, 6th ed, Glenview, IL: American Pain Society, 2008.

SOME POTENTIAL PHOTOSENSITIZING AGENTS

Analgesics
Almotriptan
Nonsteroidal anti-inflammatory drugs[1]
  Celecoxib
  Diclofenac
  Flurbiprofen
  Ibuprofen
  Ketoprofen
  Meloxicam
  Nabumetone
  Naproxen
  Oxaprozin
  Piroxicam
  Tiaprofenic acid
Pentosan polysulfate sodium
SulfaSALAzine
SUMAtriptan
ZOLMitriptan

Antineoplastics
Capecitabine
Dacarbazine
Dasatinib
Epirubicin
Floxuridine
Flucytosine
Fluorouracil
Flutamide
Imatinib
Leuprolide
Methotrexate
Porfimer
Thioguanine
UFT
VinBLAStine

Antimicrobials
Amantadine
Atazanavir
Atovaquone and proguanil
Chloroquine
Dapsone
Demeclocycline[1]
Doxycycline[1]
Gentamicin
Griseofulvin
Interferon alpha-n3
Interferon beta-1b
Itraconazole
Kanamycin
Minocycline
Oxytetracycline
Pyrazinamide
Quinolones[1]
  Ciprofloxacin
  Gemifloxacin
  Levofloxacin
  Lomefloxacin
  Nalidixic acid
  Norfloxacin
  Ofloxacin
  Sparfloxacin
SulfADIAZINE

Sulfadoxine and pyrimethamine
Sulfamethoxazole and trimethoprim
Sulfisoxazole
Tetracycline
Valacyclovir
Voriconazole

Cardiovascular Agents
Antilipemic agents
  Atorvastatin
  Fenofibrate
  Fluvastatin
  Gemfibrozil
  Lovastatin
  Pravastatin
  Simvastatin
ACE inhibitors
  Benazepril
  Enalapril
  Fosinopril
  Lisinopril
  Quinapril
  Ramipril
Beta-Blockers
  Carvedilol
  Metoprolol
  Sotalol
Calcium channel blockers
  Diltiazem
  NIFEdipine
Diuretics
  AcetaZOLAMIDE
  Furosemide
  Methazolamide
  Metolazone
  Thiazides[1]
    Chlorothiazide
    Chlorthalidone
    Hydrochlorothiazide
    Methyclothiazide
    Polythiazide
Miscellaneous cardiovascular agents
  Amiodarone[1]
  Losartan
  QuiNIDine[1]

CNS Agents
Antidepressants, tricyclic[1]
  Amitriptyline
  Amoxapine
  ClomiPRAMINE
  Desipramine
  Doxepin
  Imipramine
  Loxapine
  Maprotiline
  Nortriptyline
  Protriptyline
  Trimipramine
Antidepressants, SSRI
  FLUoxetine
  Sertraline

SOME POTENTIAL PHOTOSENSITIZING AGENTS

◄ Antidepressants, miscellaneous
  BuPROPion
  DULoxetine
  Mirtazapine
  Nefazodone
Antihistamines
  Cetirizine
  Clemastine
  Cyproheptadine
  DiphenhydrAMINE
  Loratadine
  Meclizine
Antipsychotic, miscellaneous
  Flupentixol
  Haloperidol
  Molindone
  QUEtiapine
  RisperiDONE
  Thiothixene
  Ziprasidone
  Zuclopenthixol
Antipsychotic, phenothiazine
  ChlorproMAZINE
  FluPHENAZine
  Methotrimeprazine
  Perphenazine
  Pipotiazine
  Prochlorperazine
  Promethazine
  Trifluoperazine
Antiseizure agents
  CarBAMazepine
  Felbamate
  LamoTRIgine
  OXcarbazepine
  Topiramate
  Valproic acid

Miscellaneous CNS agents
  ChlordiazePOXIDE
  Ropinirole
  Zaleplon

Hypoglycemic Agents
ChlorproPAMIDE
Gliclazide
Glimepiride
GlipiZIDE
GlyBURIDE
TOLAZamide
TOLBUTamide

Skin Agents
Acitretin
Coal tar
Hexachlorophene
Silver sulfADIAZINE
Tretinoin
Triamcinolone

Miscellaneous Agents
Acamprosate
Alendronate
Anagrelide
Cevimeline
Cromolyn
Danazol
Droperidol
Glatiramer
Pilocarpine
Rabeprazole
Sildenafil
Tacrolimus
Thalidomide
Vardenafil
Verteporfin

[1]A 2004 NEJM paper identifies the marked drugs as being established as photosensitizing (Morison WL, "Clinical Practice. Photosensitivity," *N Engl J Med*, 2004, 350[11]:1111-7). In light of sporadic and limited case reports, most other drugs labeled as photosensitizing are apparently only weakly and rarely so.

ASTHMA

MANAGEMENT OF ASTHMA IN ADULTS

Goals of Asthma Treatment

- Prevent chronic and troublesome symptoms: Minimal or no chronic symptoms day or night
- No limitations on activities; no school/work missed
- Minimal use of inhaled short-acting beta$_2$-agonist ($\leq$2 days/week, <1 canister/month) (not including prevention of exercise induced asthma)
- Minimal or no adverse effects from medications
- Maintain (near) normal pulmonary function
- Prevent recurrent exacerbations (ie, trips to emergency department or hospitalizations)

All Patients

- Short-acting bronchodilator: **Inhaled beta$_2$-agonists** as needed for symptoms.
- Intensity of treatment will depend on severity of exacerbation; see "Management of Asthma Exacerbations".
- Use of short-acting inhaled beta$_2$-agonists on a daily basis, or increasing use, indicates the need to initiate or titrate long-term control therapy.

Education

- Teach self-management.
- Teach about controlling environmental factors (avoidance of allergens or other factors that contribute to asthma severity).
- Review administration technique and compliance with patient.
- Use a written action plan to help educate.

Stepwise Approach for Managing Asthma in Adults

Symptoms	Lung Function	Daily Medications
STEP 6: Severe Asthma		
Day: Throughout the day Night: Often 7 times/week SABA use: Several times/ day	FEV$_1$ <60% predicted FEV$_1$/FVC reduced 5%	**Preferred:** High dose ICS plus LABA plus oral corticosteroid AND Consider: Omalizumab (in those with allergies)[1]
STEP 5: Severe Asthma		
Day: Throughout the day Night: Often 7 times/week SABA use: Several times/ day	FEV$_1$ <60% predicted FEV$_1$/FVC reduced 5%	**Preferred:** High dose ICS plus LABA AND Consider: Omalizumab (in those with allergies)[1]
STEP 4: Severe Asthma		
Day: Throughout the day Night: Often 7 times/week SABA use: Several times/ day	FEV$_1$ <60% predicted FEV$_1$/FVC reduced 5%	**Preferred:** Medium dose ICS plus LABA **Alternatives[2]:** Medium dose ICS plus either LTRA, theophylline, or zileuton[3]
STEP 3: Moderate Asthma		
Day: Daily Night: >1 night/week (not nightly) SABA use: Daily	FEV$_1$ >60%, <80% predicted FEV$_1$/FVC reduced 5%	**Preferred:** Low dose ICS plus LABA OR Medium dose ICS **Alternatives[2]:** Low dose ICS plus either LTRA, theophylline, or zileuton[3]

Stepwise Approach for Managing Asthma in Adults *(continued)*

Symptoms	Lung Function	Daily Medications
STEP 2: Mild Asthma		
Day: >2 days/week (not daily) Night: 3-4 times/month SABA use: >2 days/week, no more than once per day (not daily)	FEV_1 <80% FEV_1/FVC normal	**Preferred:** Low dose ICS **Alternatives[2]:** LTRA, nedocromil, or theophylline
STEP 1: Intermittent Asthma		
Day: ≤2 days/week Night: ≤2 nights/month SABA use: ≤2 days/week	FEV_1 normal between exacerbations FEV_1 >80% predicted FEV_1/FVC normal	**Preferred:** SABA as needed

Note: Treatment options within each step are listed in alphabetical order.

Steps 2-4: Consider subcutaneous allergen immunotherapy for patients with allergic asthma.[1]

Consult with asthma specialist if Step 4 or higher care is needed.

FEV_1 = forced expiratory volume in 1 second, FVC = forced vital capacity, ICS = inhaled corticosteroid, LABA = long-acting inhaled beta$_2$-agonist, SABA = short-acting inhaled beta$_2$-agonist, LTRA = leukotriene receptor antagonist

[1]When using immunotherapy or omalizumab, clinicians should be prepared to identify and treat anaphylaxis in the event it occurs.

[2]If alternative treatment is used and response is inadequate, discontinue it and use preferred treatment before stepping up.

[3]Zileuton is less desirable alternative due to limited studies and need to monitor liver function.

Notes:

- **The stepwise approach presents general guidelines to assist clinical decision making; it is not intended to be a specific prescription. Asthma is highly variable; clinicians should tailor specific medication plans to the needs and circumstances of individual patients.**

- Gain control as quickly as possible; then decrease treatment to the least medication necessary to maintain control.

- A rescue course of systemic corticosteroids may be needed at any time and at any step.

- Some patients with intermittent asthma experience severe and life-threatening exacerbations separated by long periods of normal lung function and no symptoms. This may be especially common with exacerbations provoked by respiratory infections.

- At each step, patient education, environmental control, management of comorbidities emphasized.

- Antibiotics are not recommended for treatment of acute asthma exacerbations except where there is evidence or suspicion of bacterial infection.

- Consultation with an asthma specialist is recommended for moderate or severe persistent asthma.

- Peak flow monitoring for patients with moderate-severe persistent asthma and patients who have a history of severe exacerbations should be considered.

Management of Asthma Exacerbations: Home Treatment

Assess Severity

- **Patients at high risk for a fatal attack require immediate medical attention after initial treatment.**

- Symptoms and signs suggestive of a more serious exacerbation such as marked breathlessness, inability to speak more than short phrases, use of accessory muscles, or drowsiness should result in initial treatment while immediately consulting with a clinician.

- If available, measure PEF—values of 50% to 79% predicted or personal best indicate the need for quick-relief mediation. Depending on the response to treatment, contact with a clinician may also be indicated. Values below 50% indicate the need for immediate medical care.

Initial Treatment

- Inhaled SABA: Up to two treatments 20 minutes apart of 2–6 puffs by metered-dose inhaler (MDI) or nebulizer treatments.

- Note: Medication delivery is highly variable. Children and individuals who have exacerbations of lesser severity may need fewer puffs than suggested above.

Good Response

No wheezing or dyspnea (assess tachypnea in young children).

PEF ≥80% predicted or personal best.

- Contact clinician for followup instructions and further management.

- May continue inhaled SABA every 3–4 hours for 24–48 hours.

- Consider short course of oral systemic corticosteroids.

Incomplete Response

Persistent wheezing and dyspnea (tachypnea).

PEF 50% to 79% predicted or personal best.

- Add oral systemic corticosteroid.

- Continue inhaled SABA.

- Contact clinician urgently (this day) for further instruction.

Poor Response

Marked wheezing and dyspñea.

PEF <50% predicted or personal best.

- Add oral systemic corticosteroid

- Repeat inhaled SABA immediately.

- If distress is severe and nonresponsive to initial treatment:

  - Call your doctor AND

  - **PROCEED TO EMERGENCY DEPARTMENT**;

  - Consider calling 911 (ambulance transport).

- To emergency department.

MDI: Metered-dose inhaler; PEF: Peak expiratory flow; SABA: Short-acting beta₂-agonist (quick relief inhaler)

Management of Asthma Exacerbations: Emergency Department and Hospital-Based Care

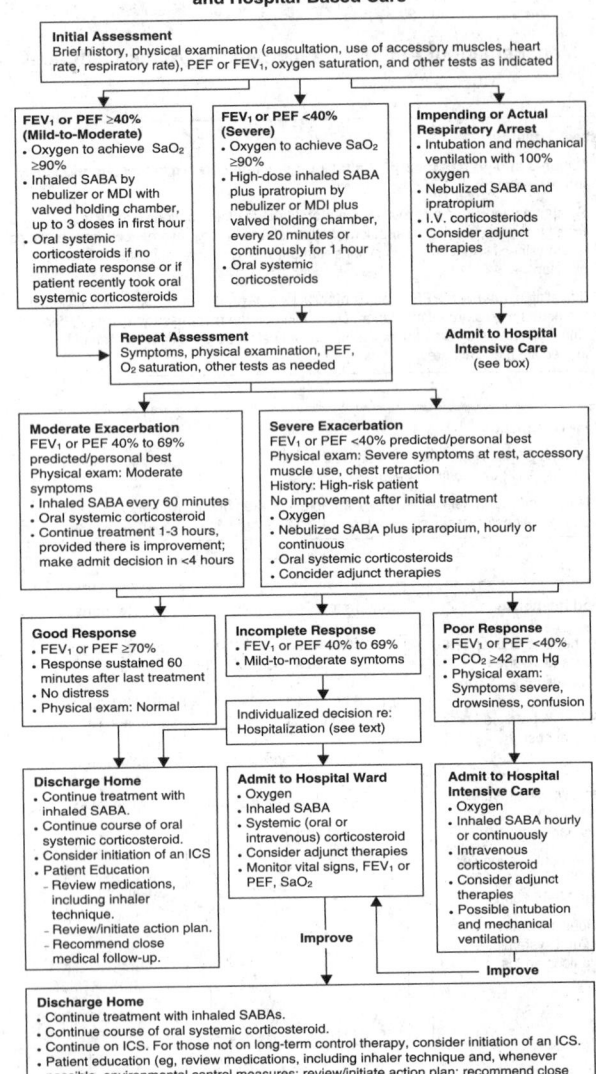

Initial Assessment
Brief history, physical examination (auscultation, use of accessory muscles, heart rate, respiratory rate), PEF or FEV$_1$, oxygen saturation, and other tests as indicated

FEV$_1$ or PEF ≥40% (Mild-to-Moderate)
- Oxygen to achieve SaO$_2$ ≥90%
- Inhaled SABA by nebulizer or MDI with valved holding chamber, up to 3 doses in first hour
- Oral systemic corticosteroids if no immediate response or if patient recently took oral systemic corticosteroids

FEV$_1$ or PEF <40% (Severe)
- Oxygen to achieve SaO$_2$ ≥90%
- High-dose inhaled SABA plus ipratropium by nebulizer or MDI plus valved holding chamber, every 20 minutes or continuously for 1 hour
- Oral systemic corticosteroids

Impending or Actual Respiratory Arrest
- Intubation and mechanical ventilation with 100% oxygen
- Nebulized SABA and ipratropium
- I.V. corticosteroids
- Consider adjunct therapies

Repeat Assessment
Symptoms, physical examination, PEF, O$_2$ saturation, other tests as needed

Admit to Hospital Intensive Care
(see box)

Moderate Exacerbation
FEV$_1$ or PEF 40% to 69% predicted/personal best
Physical exam: Moderate symptoms
- Inhaled SABA every 60 minutes
- Oral systemic corticosteroid
- Continue treatment 1-3 hours, provided there is improvement; make admit decision in <4 hours

Severe Exacerbation
FEV$_1$ or PEF <40% predicted/personal best
Physical exam: Severe symptoms at rest, accessory muscle use, chest retraction
History: High-risk patient
No improvement after initial treatment
- Oxygen
- Nebulized SABA plus ipraropium, hourly or continuous
- Oral systemic corticosteroids
- Concider adjunct therapies

Good Response
- FEV$_1$ or PEF ≥70%
- Response sustained 60 minutes after last treatment
- No distress
- Physical exam: Normal

Incomplete Response
- FEV$_1$ or PEF 40% to 69%
- Mild-to-moderate symtoms

Individualized decision re: Hospitalization (see text)

Poor Response
- FEV$_1$ or PEF <40%
- PCO$_2$ ≥42 mm Hg
- Physical exam: Symptoms severe, drowsiness, confusion

Discharge Home
- Continue treatment with inhaled SABA.
- Continue course of oral systemic corticosteroid.
- Consider initiation of an ICS.
- Patient Education
  - Review medications, including inhaler technique.
  - Review/initiate action plan.
  - Recommend close medical follow-up.

Admit to Hospital Ward
- Oxygen
- Inhaled SABA
- Systemic (oral or intravenous) corticosteroid
- Consider adjunct therapies
- Monitor vital signs, FEV$_1$ or PEF, SaO$_2$

Improve

Admit to Hospital Intensive Care
- Oxygen
- Inhaled SABA hourly or continuously
- Intravenous corticosteroid
- Consider adjunct therapies
- Possible intubation and mechanical ventilation

Improve

Discharge Home
- Continue treatment with inhaled SABAs.
- Continue course of oral systemic corticosteroid.
- Continue on ICS. For those not on long-term control therapy, consider initiation of an ICS.
- Patient education (eg, review medications, including inhaler technique and, whenever possible, environmental control measures; review/initiate action plan; recommend close medical follow-up).
- Before discharge, schedule follow-up appointment with primary care provider and/or asthma specialist in 1-4 weeks.

FEV$_1$ = forced expiratory volume in 1 second; ICS = inhaled corticosteroid; MDI = metered dose inhaler; PCO$_2$ = partial pressure carbon dioxide; PEF = peak expiratory flow; SABA = short-acting beta$_2$-agonist; SaO$_2$ = oxygen saturation

ESTIMATED COMPARATIVE DAILY DOSAGES FOR INHALED CORTICOSTEROIDS

Adults

Drug	Low Daily Dose	Medium Daily Dose	High Daily Dose
Beclomethasone HFA 40 mcg/puff 80 mcg/puff	80-240 mcg	>240-480 mcg	>480 mcg
Budesonide DPI 90 mcg/puff 180 mcg/puff 200 mcg/puff	180-600 mcg	>600-1200 mcg	>1200 mcg
Flunisolide 250 mcg/puff	500-1000 mcg	>1000-2000 mcg	>2000 mcg
Flunisolide HFA 80 mcg/puff	320 mcg	>320-640 mcg	>640 mcg
Fluticasone HFA 44 mcg/puff 110 mcg/puff 220 mcg/puff	88-264 mcg	>264-440 mcg	>440 mcg
Mometasone DPI 220 mcg/puff	220 mcg	440 mcg	>440 mcg

DPI = dry powder inhaler, HFA = hydrofluoroalkane

REFERENCE

Expert Panel Report 3, "Guidelines for the Diagnosis and Management of Asthma," *Clinical Practice Guidelines*, National Institutes of Health, National Heart, Lung, and Blood Institute, NIH Publication No. 08-4051. Available at http://www.nhlbi.nih.gov/guidelines/asthma/asthgdln.htm

HYPERLIPIDEMIA MANAGEMENT

MORTALITY

There is a strong link between serum cholesterol and cardiovascular mortality. This association becomes stronger in patients with established coronary artery disease. Lipid-lowering trials show that reductions in LDL cholesterol are followed by reductions in mortality. In general, each 1% fall in LDL cholesterol confers a 2% reduction in cardiovascular events. The aim of therapy for hyperlipidemia is to decrease cardiovascular morbidity and mortality by lowering cholesterol to a target level using safe and cost-effective treatment modalities. The target LDL cholesterol is determined by the number of patient risk factors (see the following Risk Factors and Goal LDL Cholesterol tables). The goal is achieved through diet, lifestyle modification, and drug therapy. The basis for these recommendations is provided by longitudinal interventional studies, demonstrating that lipid-lowering in patients with prior cardiovascular events (secondary prevention) and in patients with hyperlipidemia but no prior cardiac event (primary prevention) lowers the occurrence of future cardiovascular events, including stroke.

Major Risk Factors That Modify LDL Goals

Positive risk factors	Male ≥45 years
	Female ≥55 years
	Family history of premature coronary heart disease, defined as CHD in male first-degree relative <55 years; CHD in female first-degree relative <65 years
	Cigarette smoking
	Hypertension (blood pressure ≥140/90 mm Hg) or taking antihypertensive medication
	Low HDL (<40 mg/dL [1.03 mmol/L])
Negative risk factors	High HDL (≥60 mg/dL [1.6 mmol/L])[1]

[1]If HDL is ≥60 mg/dL, may subtract one positive risk factor

Adult Treatment Panel (ATP) III LDL-C Goals and Cutpoints for Therapeutic Lifestyle Changes (TLC) and Drug Therapy in Different Risk Categories

Risk Category	LDL-C Goal	Initiate TLC	Consider Drug Therapy[1]
High risk: CHD[2] or CHD risk equivalents[3] (10-year risk >20%)	<100 mg/dL (optional goal: <70 mg/dL)[4]	≥100 mg/dL[5]	≥100 mg/dL[6] (<100 mg/dL: Consider drug options)[1]
Moderately high risk: ≥2 risk factors[7] (10-year risk 10% to 20%)[8]	<130 mg/dL[9]	≥130 mg/dL[5]	≥130 mg/dL (100-120 mg/dL: Consider drug options)[10]
Moderate risk: ≥2 risk factors[7] (10-year risk <10%)[8]	<130 mg/dL	≥130 mg/dL	≥160 mg/dL
Lower risk: 0-1 risk factor[11]	<160 mg/dL	≥160 mg/dL	≥190 mg/dL (160-189 mg/dL: LDL-lowering drug optional)

[1]When LDL-lowering drug therapy is employed, it is advised that intensity of therapy be sufficient to achieve at least a 30% to 40% reduction in LDL-C levels.

[2]CHD includes history of myocardial infarction, unstable angina, stable angina, coronary artery procedures (angioplasty or bypass surgery), or evidence of clinically significant myocardial ischemia.

[3]CHD risk equivalents include clinical manifestations of noncoronary forms of atherosclerotic disease (peripheral arterial disease, abdominal aortic aneurysm, and carotid artery disease [transient ischemic attacks or stroke of carotid origin or >50% obstruction of a carotid artery]), diabetes, and 2+ risk factors with 10-year risk for hard CHD >20%.

[4]Very high risk favors the optional LDL-C goal of <70 mg/dL, and in patients with high triglycerides, non-HDL-C <100 mg/dL

[5]Any person at high risk or moderately high risk who has lifestyle-related risk factors (eg, obesity, physical inactivity, elevated triglyceride, low HDL-C, or metabolic syndrome) is a candidate for therapeutic lifestyle changes to modify these risk factors regardless of LDL-C level.

[6]If baseline LDL-C is <100 mg/dL, institution of an LDL-lowering drug is a therapeutic option on the basis of available clinical trial results. If a high-risk person has high triglycerides or low HDL-C, combining a fibrate or nicotinic acid with an LDL-lowering drug can be considered.

(See additional footnotes on next page.)

(Footnotes continued from previous page.)

[7]Risk factors include cigarette smoking, hypertension (BP ≥140/90 mm Hg or on antihypertensive medication), low HDL cholesterol (<40 mg/dL), family history of premature CHD (CHD in male first-degree relative <55 years of age; CHD in female first-degree relative <65 years of age), and age (men ≥45 years; women ≥55 years).

[8]Electronic 10-year risk calculators are available at www.nhlbi.nih.gov/guidelines/cholesterol.

[9]Optional LDL-C goal <100 mg/dL

[10]For moderately high-risk persons, when LDL-C level is 100-129 mg/dL, at baseline or on lifestyle therapy, initiation of an LDL-lowering drug to achieve an LDL-C level <100 mg/dL is a therapeutic option on the basis of available clinical trial results.

[11]Almost all people with zero or 1 risk factor have a 10-year risk <10%, and 10-year risk assessment in people with zero or 1 risk factor thus not necessary

Any person with elevated LDL cholesterol or other form of hyperlipidemia should undergo evaluation to rule out secondary dyslipidemia. Causes of secondary dyslipidemia include diabetes, hypothyroidism, obstructive liver disease, chronic renal failure, and drugs that increase LDL and decrease HDL (progestins, anabolic steroids, corticosteroids).

Elevated Serum Triglyceride Levels

Elevated serum triglyceride levels may be an independent risk factor for coronary heart disease. Factors that contribute to hypertriglyceridemia include obesity, inactivity, cigarette smoking, excess alcohol intake, high carbohydrate diets (>60% of energy intake), type 2 diabetes, chronic renal failure, nephrotic syndrome, certain medications (corticosteroids, estrogens, retinoids, higher doses of beta-blockers), and genetic disorders. Non-HDL cholesterol (total cholesterol minus HDL cholesterol) is a secondary focus for clinicians treating patients with high serum triglyceride levels (≥200 mg/dL). The goal for non-HDL cholesterol in patients with high serum triglyceride levels can be set 30 mg/dL higher than usual LDL cholesterol goals. Patients with serum triglyceride levels <200 mg/dL should aim for the target LDL cholesterol goal.

ATP classification of serum triglyceride levels:

–   Normal triglycerides: <150 mg/dL

–   Borderline-high: 150-199 mg/dL

–   High: 200-499 mg/dL

–   Very high: ≥500 mg/dL

NONDRUG THERAPY

Dietary therapy and lifestyle modifications should be individualized for each patient. A total lifestyle change is recommended for all patients. Dietary and lifestyle modifications should be tried for 3 months, if deemed appropriate. Nondrug and drug therapy should be initiated simultaneously in patients with highly elevated cholesterol (see LDL Cholesterol Goals and Cutpoints for Therapeutic Lifestyle Changes and Drug Therapy in Different Risk Categories table on previous page). Increasing physical activity and smoking cessation will aid in the treatment of hyperlipidemia and improve cardiovascular health.

Note: Refer to the National Cholesterol Education Program reference for details concerning the calculation of 10-year risk of CHD using Framingham risk scoring. Risk assessment tool is available on-line at http://hin.nhlbi.nih.gov/atpiii/calculator.asp?usertype=prof, last accessed March 14, 2002.

Total Lifestyle Change (TLC) Diet

	Recommended Intake
Total fat	25%-35% of total calories
Saturated fat[1]	<7% of total calories
Polyunsaturated fat	≤10% of total calories
Monounsaturated fat	≤20% of total calories
Carbohydrates[2]	50%-60% of total calories
Fiber	20-30 g/day
Protein	~15% of total calories
Cholesterol	<200 mg/day
Total calories[3]	Balance energy intake and expenditure to maintain desirable body weight/prevent weight gain

[1]*Trans* fatty acids (partially hydrogenated oils) intake should be kept low. These are found in potato chips, other snack foods, margarines and shortenings, and fast-foods.

[2]Complex carbohydrates, including grains (especially whole grains, fruits, and vegetables)

[3]Daily energy expenditure should include at least moderate physical activity.

DRUG THERAPY

Drug therapy should be selected based on the patient's lipid profile, concomitant disease states, and the cost of therapy. The following table lists specific advantages and disadvantages for various classes of lipid-lowering medications. The expected reduction in lipids with therapy is listed in the Lipid-Lowering Agents table. Refer to individual drug monographs for detailed information.

Advantages and Disadvantages of Specific Lipid-Lowering Therapies

	Advantages	Disadvantages
Bile acid sequestrants	Good choice for ↑ LDL, especially when combined with a statin (↓ LDL ≤50%); low potential for systemic side effects; good choice for younger patients	May increase triglycerides; higher incidence of adverse effects; moderately expensive; drug interactions; inconvenient dosing
Niacin	Good choice for almost any lipid abnormality; inexpensive; greatest increase in HDL	High incidence of adverse effects; may adversely affect type 2 DM (with high dose >1.5 g/day) and gout; sustained release niacin may decrease the incidence of flushing and circumvent the need for multiple daily dosing; sustained release niacin may not increase HDL cholesterol or decrease triglycerides as well as immediate release niacin
HMG-CoA reductase inhibitors	Produces greatest ↓ in LDL; generally well-tolerated; convenient once-daily dosing; proven decrease in mortality	Expensive
Fibric acid derivatives	Good choice in patients with ↑ triglycerides where niacin is contraindicated or not well-tolerated	Variable effects on LDL
Ezetimibe	Additional cholesterol-lowering effects when combined with HMG-CoA reductase inhibitors	Effects similar to bile acid sequestrants

Lipid-Lowering Agents

Drug	Dose/Day	Effect on LDL (%)	Effect on HDL (%)	Effect on TG (%)
HMG-CoA Reductase Inhibitors ("Statins")				
Atorvastatin	10 mg 20 mg 40 mg 80 mg	-39 -43 -50 -60	+6 +9 +6 +5	-19 -26 -29 -37
Fluvastatin	20 mg 40 mg 80 mg	-22 -25 -36	+3 +4 +6	-12 -14 -18
Lovastatin	10 mg 20 mg 40 mg 80 mg	-21 -24 -30 -40	+5 +7 +7 +9.5	-10 -10 -14 -19
Pitavastatin	1 mg 2 mg 4 mg	-32 -36 -43	+8 +7 +5	-15 -19 -18
Pravastatin	10 mg 20 mg 40 mg 80 mg	-22 -32 -34 -37	+7 +2 +12 +3	-15 -11 -24 -19
Rosuvastatin	5 mg 10 mg 20 mg 40 mg	-45 -52 -55 -63	+13 +14 +8 +10	-35 -10 -23 -28
Simvastatin	5 mg 10 mg 20 mg 40 mg 80 mg	-26 -30 -38 -41 -47	+10 +12 +8 +13 +16	-12 -15 -19 -28 -33
Bile Acid Sequestrants				
Cholestyramine	4-24 g	-15 to -30	+3 to +5	+0 to +20
Colesevelam	6 tablets 7 tablets	-15 -18	+3 +3	+10 +9
Colestipol	7-30 g	-15 to -30	+3 to +5	+0 to +20
Fibric Acid Derivatives				
Fenofibrate	67-200 mg	-20 to -31	+9 to +14	-30 to -50
Gemfibrozil	600 mg twice daily	-5 to -10[1]	+10 to +20	-40 to -60
Niacin	1.5-6 g	-5 to -25	+15 to +35	-20 to -50
2-Azetidinone				
Ezetimibe	10 mg	-15 to -20	+1 to +4	-5 to -8
Omega-3-Acid Ethyl Esters	4 g	+44.5	+9.1	-44.9
Combination Products				
Ezetimibe and simvastatin	10/10 mg 10/20 mg 10/40 mg 10/80 mg	-45 -52 -55 -60	+8 +10 +6 +6	-23 -24 -23 -31
Niacin and lovastatin	1000/20 mg 1000/40 mg 1500/40 mg 2000/40 mg	-30 -36 -37 -42	+20 +20 +27 +30	-32 -39 -44 -44
Niacin and simvastatin	1000/20 mg 1000/40 mg 2000/20 mg 2000/40 mg	-12 -7 -14 -5	+21 +15 +29 +24	-27 -23 -38 -32

[1] May increase LDL in some patients

Progression of Drug Therapy in Primary Prevention

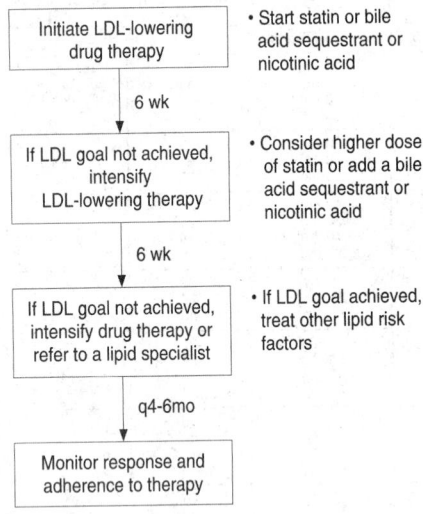

Initiate LDL-lowering drug therapy	• Start statin or bile acid sequestrant or nicotinic acid
↓ 6 wk	
If LDL goal not achieved, intensify LDL-lowering therapy	• Consider higher dose of statin or add a bile acid sequestrant or nicotinic acid
↓ 6 wk	
If LDL goal not achieved, intensify drug therapy or refer to a lipid specialist	• If LDL goal achieved, treat other lipid risk factors
↓ q4-6mo	
Monitor response and adherence to therapy	

DRUG SELECTION

Lipid Profile	Monotherapy	Combination Therapies
Increased LDL with normal HDL and triglycerides (TG)	Resin Niacin[1] Statin	Resin plus niacin[1] or statin Statin plus niacin[1,2]
Increased LDL and increased TG (200-499 mg/dL)[2]	Intensify LDL-lowering therapy	Statin plus niacin[1,3] Statin plus fibrate[3]
Increased LDL and increased TG (≥500 mg/dL)[2]	Consider combination therapy (niacin,[1] fibrates, statin)	
Increased TG	Niacin[1] Fibrates	Niacin[1] plus fibrates
Increased LDL and low HDL	Niacin[1] Statin	Statin plus niacin[1,2]

[1]Avoid in diabetics.

[2]Emphasize weight reduction and increased physical activity.

[3]Risk of myopathy with combination

Resins = bile acid sequestrants, statins = HMG-CoA reductase inhibitors, fibrates = fibric acid derivatives (eg, gemfibrozil, fenofibrate)

COMBINATION DRUG THERAPY

If after at least 6 weeks of therapy at the maximum recommended or tolerated dose, the patient's LDL cholesterol is not at target, consider optimizing nondrug measures, prescribing a higher dose of current lipid-lowering drug, or adding another lipid-lowering medication to the current therapy. Successful drug combinations include statin and niacin, statin and bile acid sequestrant, or niacin and bile acid sequestrant. At maximum recommended doses, LDL cholesterol may be decreased by 50% to 60% with combination therapy. This is the same reduction achieved by atorvastatin 40 mg twice daily. If a bile acid sequestrant is used with other lipid-lowering agents, space doses 1 hour before or 4 hours after the bile acid sequestrant administration. Statins combined with either fenofibrate, gemfibrozil, or niacin increase the risk of rhabdomyolysis. In this situation, patient education (muscle pain/weakness) and careful follow-up are warranted.

REFERENCES

Guidelines

American Diabetes Association, "Standards of Medical Care in Diabetes – 2010," *Diabetes Care*, 2010, 33(Suppl 1): S11-61.

Brunzell JD, Davidson M, Furberg CD, et al, "Lipoprotein Management in Patients With Cardiometabolic Risk: Consensus Statement From the American Diabetes Association and the American College of Cardiology Foundation," *Diabetes Care*, 2008, 31(4):811-22.

Grundy SM, Cleeman JI, Merz CN, et al, "Implications of Recent Clinical Trials for the National Cholesterol Education Program Adult Treatment Panel III Guidelines," *J Am Coll Cardiol*, 2004, 44(3):720-32.

National Cholesterol Education Program, "Third Report of the Expert Panel on Detection, Evaluation, and Treatment of High Blood Cholesterol in Adults (Adult Treatment Panel III)," *JAMA*, 2001, 285(19):2486-97.

Others

Berthold HK, Sudhop T, and von Bergmann K, "Effect of a Garlic Oil Preparation on Serum Lipoproteins and Cholesterol Metabolism: A Randomized Controlled Trial," *JAMA*, 1998, 279(23):1900-2.

Bertolini S, Bon GB, Campbell LM, et al, "Efficacy and Safety of Atorvastatin Compared to Pravastatin in Patients With Hypercholesterolemia," *Atherosclerosis*, 1997, 130(1-2):191-7.

Blankenhorn DH, Nessim SA, Johnson RL, et al, "Beneficial Effects of Combined Colestipol-Niacin Therapy on Coronary Atherosclerosis and Venous Bypass Grafts," *JAMA*, 1987, 257(23):3233-40.

Bradford RH, Shear CL, Chremos AN, et al, "Expanded Clinical Evaluation of Lovastatin (EXCEL) Study Results. I. Efficacy in Modifying Plasma Lipoproteins and Adverse Event Profile in 8245 Patients With Moderate Hypercholesterolemia," *Arch Intern Med*, 1991, 151(1):43-9.

Brown G, Albers JJ, Fisher LD, et al, "Regression of Coronary Artery Disease as a Result of Intensive Lipid-Lowering Therapy in Men With High Levels of Apolipoprotein B," *N Engl J Med*, 1990, 323(19):1289-98.

Capuzzi DM, Guyton JR, Morgan JM, et al, "Efficacy and Safety of an Extended-Release Niacin (Niaspan®): A Long-Term Study," *Am J Cardiol*, 1998, 82(12A):74U-81U.

Coronary Drug Project Research Program, "Clofibrate and Niacin in Coronary Heart Disease," *JAMA*, 1975, 231 (4):360-81.

Dart A, Jerums G, Nicholson G, et al, "A Multicenter, Double-Blind, One-Year Study Comparing Safety and Efficacy of Atorvastatin Versus Simvastatin in Patients With Hypercholesterolemia," *Am J Cardiol*, 1997, 80(1):39-44.

Davidson MH, Dillon MA, Gordon B, et al, "Colesevelam Hydrochloride (Cholestagel): A New Potent Bile Acid Sequestrant Associated With a Low Incidence of Gastrointestinal Side Effects," *Arch Intern Med*, 1999, 159 (16):1893-900.

Davidson M, McKenney J, Stein E, et al, "Comparison of One-Year Efficacy and Safety of Atorvastatin Versus Lovastatin in Primary Hypercholesterolemia," *Am J Cardiol*, 1997, 79(11):1475-81.

Frick MH, Heinonen OP, Huttunen JK, et al, "Helsinki Heart Study: Primary-Prevention Trial With Gemfibrozil in Middle-Aged Men With Dyslipidemia," *N Engl J Med*, 1987, 317(20):1237-45.

Garber AM, Browner WS, and Hulley SB, "Clinical Guideline, Part 2: Cholesterol Screening in Asymptomatic Adults, Revisited," *Ann Intern Med*, 1995, 124(5):518-31.

Johannesson M, Jonsson B, Kjekshus J, et al, "Cost-Effectiveness of Simvastatin Treatment to Lower Cholesterol Levels in Patients With Coronary Heart Disease. Scandinavian Simvastatin Survival Study Group," *N Engl N Med*, 1997, 336(5):332-6.

Jones P, Kafonek S, Laurora I, et al, "Comparative Dose Efficacy Study of Atorvastatin Versus Simvastatin, Pravastatin, Lovastatin, and Fluvastatin in Patients With Hypercholesterolemia," *Am J Cardiol*, 1998, 81(5):582-7.

Kasiske BL, Ma JZ, Kalil RS, et al, "Effects of Antihypertensive Therapy on Serum Lipids," *Ann Intern Med*, 1995, 122 (2):133-41.

Lipid Research Clinics Program, "The Lipid Research Clinics Coronary Primary Prevention Trial Results: I. Reduction in Incidence of Coronary Heart Disease," *JAMA*, 1984, 251(3):351-64.

Mauro VF and Tuckerman CE, "Ezetimibe for Management of Hypercholesterolemia," *Ann Pharmacother*, 2003, 37 (6):839-48.

Multiple Risk Factor Intervention Trial Research Group, "Multiple Risk Factor Intervention Trial: Risk Factor Changes and Mortality Results," *JAMA*, 1982, 248(12):1465-77.

Pitt B, Waters D, Brown WV, et al, "Aggressive Lipid-Lowering Therapy Compared With Angioplasty in Stable Coronary Artery Disease. Atorvastatin Versus Revascularization Treatment Investigators," *N Engl J Med*, 1999, 341(2):70-6.

Ross SD, Allen IE, Connelly JE, et al, "Clinical Outcomes in Statin Treatment Trials: A Meta-Analysis," *Arch Intern Med*, 1999, 159(15):1793-802.

Sacks FM, Pfeffer MA, Moye LA, et al, "The Effect of Pravastatin on Coronary Events After Myocardial Infarction in Patients With Average Cholesterol Levels," *N Engl J Med*, 1996, 335(14):1001-9.

Scandinavian Simvastatin Survival Study, "Randomized Trial of Cholesterol Lowering in 4444 Patients With Coronary Heart Disease: The Scandinavian Simvastatin Survival Study (4S)," *Lancet*, 1994, 344(8934):1383-9.

Schrott HG, Bittner V, Vittinghoff E, et al, "Adherence to National Cholesterol Education Program Treatment Goals in Postmenopausal Women With Heart Disease. The Heart and Estrogen/Progestin Replacement Study (HERS)," *JAMA*, 1997, 277(16):1281-6.

Shepherd J, Cobbe SM, Ford I, et al, "Prevention of Coronary Heart Disease With Pravastatin in Men With Hypercholesterolemia. The West of Scotland Coronary Prevention Study Group," *N Engl J Med*, 1995, 333 (20):1301-7.

Stein EA, Davidson MH, Dobs AS, et al, "Efficacy and Safety of Simvastatin 80 mg/day in Hypercholesterolemic Patients. The Expanded Dose Simvastatin U.S. Study Group," *Am J Cardiol*, 1998, 82(3):311-6.

OSTEOPOROSIS MANAGEMENT

PREVALENCE

Osteoporosis affects more than 10 million Americans. An additional 34 million Americans have low bone density of the hip. An osteoporosis-related fracture will occur in approximately one out of every two Caucasian females at some point in her lifetime, and will occur in approximately one in five men.

CONSEQUENCES

Fractures and the complications resulting from fractures are the clinically significant sequelae of osteoporosis. Fractures may result in pain, physical limitations, lifestyle changes, and decreased quality of life. In particular, hip fractures result in a 10% to 20% excess mortality in one year. In the U.S., osteoporosis-related fractures result in heavy economic burden caused by the >432,000 hospitalizations, almost 2.5 million medical office visits, and ~180,000 nursing home admissions that occur annually as a result.

RISK FACTORS

Conditions, Diseases, and Medications

- Postmenopausal women and men ≥50 years of age
- Endocrine disorders, such as adrenal insufficiency, Cushing's disease, diabetes mellitus, hyperparathyroidism, thyrotoxicosis
- Excessive alcohol intake (≥3 drinks/day)
- Excessive vitamin A intake
- Falls
- Parental history of hip fracture
- Genetic factors, due to conditions such as cystic fibrosis, Ehlers-Danlos, Gaucher's disease, glycogen storage diseases, hemochromatosis, homocystinuria, hypophosphatasia, idiopathic hypercalciuria, Marfan syndrome, Menkes steely hair syndrome, osteogenesis imperfecta, porphyria, Riley-Day syndrome
- Gastrointestinal disorders, such as celiac disease, gastric bypass, GI surgery, inflammatory bowel disease, malabsorption, pancreatic disease, primary biliary cirrhosis
- Hematologic disorders, such as hemophilia, leukemia/lymphoma, multiple myeloma, sickle cell disease, systemic mastocytosis, thalassemia
- High caffeine and/or sodium intake
- Hypogonadal states, due to conditions such as androgen insensitivity, anorexia, athletic amenorrhea, hyperprolactinemia, panhypopituitarism, premature ovarian failure, Turner's and Klinefelter's syndrome
- Low calcium and/or vitamin D intake
- Medications: Aluminum-containing antacids (excessive use), anticoagulants (heparin), anticonvulsants, aromatase inhibitors, barbiturates, chemotherapy, cyclosporine A, depomedroxyprogesterone, glucocorticoids (≥5 mg/day of prednisone or equivalent for ≥3 months), gonadotropin-releasing hormone agonists, heparin, lithium, parenteral nutrition, tacrolimus
- Miscellaneous conditions/diseases, including amyloidosis, chronic metabolic acidosis, depression, emphysema, end-stage renal disease, epilepsy, heart failure, idiopathic scoliosis, multiple sclerosis, muscular dystrophy, post-transplant bone disease, sarcoidosis
- Previous fracture as an adult
- Rheumatic/autoimmune diseases, such as ankylosing spondylitis, lupus, rheumatoid arthritis
- Sedentary lifestyle or immobilization
- Smoking (active or passive)
- Thinness (low body mass index)

DIAGNOSIS/MONITORING

- Bone mineral density (BMD) measurement using Dual-energy x-ray absorptiometry (DXA) bone density scan[1]

- U.S.-adapted WHO Fracture Risk Algorithm (FRAX®; www.nof.org and www.shef.ac.uk/FRAX)[2]

[1]BMD measurement by DXA at the hip or spine is used to establish or confirm an osteoporosis diagnosis.

[2]US-FRAX® is designed to calculate the 10 year probability of a hip fracture and the 10 year probability of a major osteoporotic fracture (vertebral, hip, forearm, or humerus fracture). Application of Frax™ is intended for postmenopausal women and men ≥50 years of age (not for younger adults or pediatrics) and results apply only to previously untreated patients.

Definition of Osteoporosis[1]

Normal: T score at -1.0 and above
Low bone mass or "osteopenia": T score between -1.0 and -2.5
Osteoporosis: T score at -2.5 or below

[1]Based on World Health Organization (WHO) established definition of osteoporosis using BMD measurements by DXA devices at the spine, hip or forearm. T-score values are based on standard deviations (SD) below that of a "young normal" adult. The WHO diagnostic classification only applies to postmenopausal women and men ≥50 years of age; not applicable for premenopausal women, men <50 years of age or pediatrics.

Bone Mineral Density (BMD) Testing

Recommend for the following patients:

- All women ≥65 years and men ≥70 years

- High risk postmenopausal women and men aged 50-69 years

- Women in menopausal transition if increased fracture risk present (eg, low body weight, prior low-trauma fracture, receiving high risk medication)

- Patients with a history of a fracture (occurring after age 50)

- Adults with a predisposing condition associated with low bone mass or loss (see Risk Factors)

- Any patient being considered for pharmacologic therapy for osteoporosis or receiving treatment for osteoporosis (monitoring typically performed every 2 years unless more frequent testing warranted)

- Any patient not receiving therapy but evidence of bone loss would lead to treatment

Consider for the following patients:

- Postmenopausal women discontinuing estrogen

PREVENTION/TREATMENT

- Fall prevention (eg, visual/hearing checks, minimizing pharmacologic agents that contribute to fall risk, checking environment for safety hazards)

- Weight-bearing exercise (eg, walking) and muscle strengthening, as tolerated

- Avoidance of tobacco use and excessive alcohol intake

- Adequate intake of at least 1200 mg **elemental** calcium daily in the form of dietary calcium or calcium supplementation, particularly women ≥50 years of age. Intakes exceeding 1200-1500 mg offer limited additional benefit and may increase the risk for cardiovascular disease or kidney stones. Also refer to table located at the end of appendix piece for selected calcium supplement information.

- Adequate intake of at least 800-1000 int. units of vitamin D for adults ≥50 years of age. Measuring serum vitamin D concentrations may be warranted, particularly in those at greatest risk for deficiency, to allow for the administration of vitamin D replacement. **Note:** Certain patients at risk for vitamin D deficiency (eg, elderly, diseases associated with malabsorption, chronic renal insufficiency) may require higher intakes.

◀ **Pharmacologic Therapy**

- Consider using FDA approved pharmacologic therapy in postmenopausal women and men ≥50 years with a hip or vertebral fracture **or** those with a T score ≤ -2.5 at the femoral neck or spine (after excluding secondary causes) **or** those with low bone mass (T score between -1.0 and -2.5 at the femoral neck or spine) in combination with a 10-year hip fracture probability of ≥3% or a 10-year osteoporosis-related major fracture probability of ≥20% (based on the U.S.-adapted WHO algorithm)

1. Bisphosphonates: Oral bisphosphonates should be administered ≥30 minutes before first food or drink (except water) with 6-8 ounces tap water (**not** mineral water) and patients should remain upright (or raise head of bed to at least a 30° angle) to avoid ulcerative esophagitis. Consult individual monographs for details regarding use, precautions, and dosing and administration of any of the specific drugs mentioned below.

    Osteoporosis prevention: Postmenopausal females:

    - Alendronate: Oral: 5 mg once daily or 35 mg once weekly

    - Ibandronate: Oral: 2.5 mg once daily or 150 mg once per month

    - Risedronate: Oral: 5 mg once daily or 35 mg once weekly or one 75 mg tablet once daily on two consecutive days per month (total of 2 tablets/month) or 150 mg once per month

    - Zoledronic acid (Reclast®): I.V.: 5 mg infused over at least 15 minutes every 2 years

    Osteoporosis treatment:

    - Alendronate: Males and Postmenopausal females: Oral: 10 mg once daily or 70 mg once weekly

    - Ibandronate: Postmenopausal females:

        - Oral: 2.5 mg once daily or 150 mg once per month

        - I.V.: 3 mg every 3 months

    - Risedronate:

        - Postmenopausal females: Oral: 5 mg once daily or 35 mg once weekly or one 75 mg tablet once daily on two consecutive days per month (total of 2 tablets/month) or 150 mg once monthly

        - Males: Oral: 35 mg once weekly

    - Zoledronic acid (Reclast®): Males and Postmenopausal females: I.V.: 5 mg infused over at least 15 minutes every 12 months

    Glucocorticoid-induced osteoporosis prevention:

    - Risedronate: Oral: 5 mg once daily

    - Zoledronic acid (Reclast®): I.V.: 5 mg infused over at least 15 minutes every 12 months (in patients initiating or continuing prednisone ≥7.5 mg/day [or equivalent] and expected to remain on glucocorticoids for at least 12 months)

    Glucocorticoid-induced osteoporosis treatment:

    - Alendronate: Oral: 5 mg once daily; Postmenopausal women not receiving estrogen: 10 mg once daily

    - Risedronate: Oral: 5 mg once daily

    - Zoledronic acid (Reclast®): I.V.: 5 mg infused over at least 15 minutes every 12 months (in patients initiating or continuing prednisone ≥7.5 mg/day [or equivalent] and expected to remain on glucocorticoids for at least 12 months)

2. Estrogen agonist/antagonist (previously known as selective estrogen receptor modulators)

    Osteoporosis prevention and treatment: Postmenopausal females:

    - Raloxifene: Oral: 60 mg once daily; may be taken any time of the day without regard to meals but should be stopped 72 hours prior to or during immobilization due to risk of thromboembolic events.

3. Estrogens/hormone therapy: Should not be considered first agents for preventing osteoporosis due to increased risk of breast cancer, heart disease, stroke, and deep-vein thrombosis (DVT) found in the Women's Health Initiative study. Estrogens, as well as various combination therapies, including ethinyl estradiol and norethindrone (femhrt®) and estradiol and norgestimate (Prefest™), have been approved for the prevention of osteoporosis. The FDA recommends that approved nonestrogen treatments should be considered before the use of estrogen/hormone therapy for the sole purpose of prevention of osteoporosis.

    Note: In women with an intact uterus, administer estrogen with oral progesterone; unopposed estrogen can cause endometrial cancer.

4. Calcitonin: Adequate dietary or supplemental calcium and vitamin D are essential.

    Osteoporosis treatment: Postmenopausal females (>5 years postmenopause):

    *   Calcitonin (Miacalcin®): I.M., SubQ: 100 units every other day (I.M. route is preferred if volume exceeds 2 mL)

    *   Calcitonin (Fortical®, Miacalcin®): Intranasal: 200 units (1 spray) in one nostril daily, alternate right and left nostril daily

5. Parathyroid hormone: Initial administration of teriparatide should occur under circumstances in which the patient may sit or lie down, in the event of orthostasis

    Osteoporosis treatment: Postmenopausal women at high risk of fracture or treatment of primary or hypogonadal osteoporosis in men at high risk of fracture:

    *   Teriparatide: SubQ: 20 mcg once daily

    Glucocorticoid induced osteoporosis treatment: Men and women:

    *   Teriparatide: SubQ: 20 mcg once daily

Calcium Type	Elemental Calcium	Equivalent Elemental Calcium	Example Brands
Acetate	25%	667 mg = 169 mg	Phos-Lo®
Carbonate	40%	364 mg = 145.6 mg	Florical®
		500 mg = 200 mg	Tums® chewable tablets
		1000 mg = 400 mg	Tums® Ultra chewable tablets
		1500 mg = 600 mg	Calcarb 600, Caltrate® 600, Nephro-Calci®
Citrate	21%	950 mg = 200 mg	Citracal®
Glubionate	6.5%	1.8 g/5 mL = 115 mg/5 mL	Various OTC and generic brands available
Gluconate	9%	500 mg = 45 mg	
Lactate	13%	650 mg = 84.5 mg	
Phosphate (tribasic)	39%	1565.2 mg = 600 mg	Posture®

REFERENCES

Ashworth L, "Focus on Alendronate. A Nonhormonal Option for the Treatment of Osteoporosis in Postmenopausal Women," *Formulary*, 1996, 31:23-30.

Barrett-Connor E, Grady D, Sashegyi A, et al, "Raloxifene and Cardiovascular Events in Osteoporotic Postmenopausal Women: Four-Year Results From the MORE (Multiple Outcomes of Raloxifene Evaluation) Randomized Trial," *JAMA*, 2002, 287(7):847-57.

Hully S, Grady D, Bush T, et al, "Randomized Trial of Estrogen Plus Progestin for Secondary Prevention of Coronary Heart Disease in Postmenopausal Women. Heart and Estrogen/Progestin Replacement Study (HERS) Research Group," *JAMA*, 1998, 280(7):605-13.

Johnson SR, "Should Older Women Use Estrogen Replacement," *J Am Geriatr Soc*, 1996, 44(1):89-90.

NIH Consensus Development Panel on Optimal Calcium Intake, *JAMA*, 1994, 272(24):1942-8.

National Osteoporosis Foundation, "Clinician's Guide to Prevention and Treatment of Osteoporosis," Washington, DC: National Osteoporosis Foundation, 2010, 1-44. Available at http://www.nof.org/sites/default/files/pdfs/NOF_ClinicianGuide2009_v7.pdf

Rossouw JE, Anderson GL, Prentice RL, et al, "Risks and Benefits of Estrogen Plus Progestin in Healthy Postmenopausal Women: Principle Results From the Women's Health Initiative Randomized Controlled Trial," *JAMA*, 2002, 288(3):321-33.

PARKINSON'S DISEASE MANAGEMENT

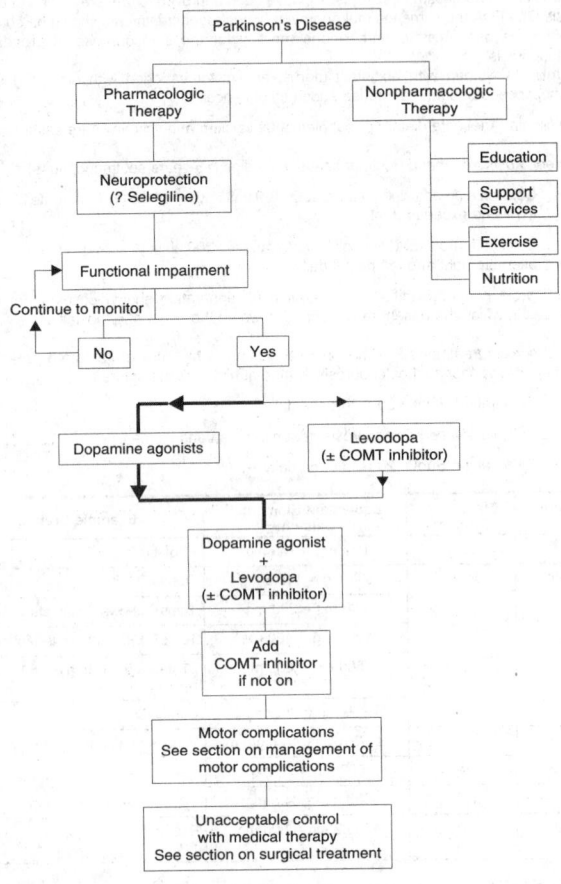

Recommendations for PD management are as follows:
- Ensure that correct diagnosis is made.
- Consider neuroprotective therapy as soon as diagnosis is made.
- Initiate symptomatic therapy with a dopamine agonist as appropriate.
- Supplement with levodopa when dopamine agonist monotherapy no longer provides satisfactory clinical control.
- Consider introducing supplemental levodopa therapy in combination with a COMT inhibitor to extend its elimination half-life.
- Consider surgical intervention when parkonsonism cannot be satisfactorily controlled with medical therapies.

Adapted from Olanow CW, Watts RL, and Koller WC, "An Algorithm (Decision Tree) for the Management of Parkinson's Disease (2001): Treatment Guidelines," *Neurology*, 2001, 56(11; Suppl 5):54.

PHARMACOTHERAPY OF URINARY INCONTINENCE

Incontinence Type	Drug Class	Drug Therapy	Adverse Effects and Precautions	Comments
Urge incontinence	Anticholinergic agents (antimuscarinic effects)	**Oxybutynin** (2.5 mg 2-3 times/day, extended release 5-30 mg once daily, or transdermal 1 patch twice weekly delivering 3.9 mg/day, or topical gel 1 g daily), **propantheline** (15-30 mg 3-5 times/day), **dicyclomine** (10-20 mg 3 times/day), **tolterodine** (1-2 mg twice daily; extended release capsule: 2-4 mg once daily), **trospium** (20 mg twice daily, extended release 60 mg daily), **solifenacin** (5-10 mg once daily), **darifenacin** (7.5-15 mg once daily), **fesoterodine** (4-8 mg once daily)	Dry mouth, blurred vision, constipation, dry skin, decreased cognitive function	Anticholinergics are the first-line drug therapy. Propantheline and dicyclomine are not considered drugs of choice in older adults. Darifenacin and solifenacin may cause less anticholinergic side effects. Trospium may cause less CNS effects.
	Tricyclic antidepressants (TCAs)	Imipramine (10-25 mg 1-4 times/day)	Not recommended for older patients because of anticholinergic and orthostatic effects.	May be used in women with mixed incontinence.
Stress or combined urge/stress incontinence	Estrogen	Topical, intravaginal, dissolving tablets in postmenopausal women; administered with varying dosing intervals (twice weekly to once daily)	Should not be used if suspected or confirmed breast or endometrial cancer, active or past thromboembolism with past oral contraceptive, estrogen, or pregnancy	Medications may not play a strong role in treatment of stress incontinence. Oral estrogen should not be prescribed for this indication; may worsen incontinence.
	Tricyclic antidepressants (TCAs)	Imipramine (10-25 mg 1-4 times/day)	May worsen cardiac conduction abnormalities, postural hypotension, anticholinergic effects	TCAs are generally reserved for patients with an additional indication (eg, depression, neuralgia) at an initial dose of 10-25 mg 1-4 times/day.
Overflow	Alpha-adrenergic antagonists	**Terazosin** (1 mg at bedtime with first dose in supine position and increase by 1 mg every 4 days to maximum 10 mg/day), **doxazosin** (1 mg at bedtime with first dose in supine position and increase by 1 mg every 7-14 days to maximum 8 mg/day), **tamsulosin** (0.4 mg-0.8 mg daily), **alfuzosin** (10 mg daily), **silodosin** (8 mg daily)	Postural hypotension, headache, dizziness	Effective in men with overactive bladder symptoms associated with benign prostatic hypertrophy.

Chapple C, Khullar V, Gabriel Z, et al, "The Effects of Antimuscarinic Treatments in Overactive Bladder: A Systematic Review and Meta-Analysis," *Eur Urol,* 2005, 48(1):5-26.

Herbison P, Hay-Smith J, Ellis G, et al, "Effectiveness of Anticholinergic Drugs Compared With Placebo in the Treatment of Overactive Bladder: Systematic Review," *BMJ,* 2003, 326(7394):841-4.

Resnick NM, "Urinary Incontinence," *Lancet,* 1995, 346(8967):94-9.

Rossouw JE, Anderson GL, Prentice RL, et al, "Risks and Benefits of Estrogen Plus Progestin in Healthy Postmenopausal Women: Principal Results From the Women's Health Initiative Randomized Controlled Trial," *JAMA,* 2002, 288(3):321-33.

TREATMENT OPTIONS FOR CONSTIPATION

- Define constipation as no more than two bowel movements per week, or straining upon defecation 25% of the time or more. If possible, educate resident about this definition to develop cooperation.
- Verify constipation with digital exam and/or x-ray (radiography) if impaction is suspected. Establish baseline and toilet daily 30 minutes after breakfast.

Adequate fluids? — No → Adjust fluid intake to 2-8 (8 oz) glasses per day if no fluid restrictions.

Adequate fiber? — No → Review for decrease in fiber intake. Normally recommended 2-10 g fiber per day (**Note:** 10 g raw bran contains 4 g fiber by weight) if not contraindicated.

↓ Yes

Recent medication changes? — Yes → Review new medications for those which may cause constipation and/or discontinue dose if possible or use alternative. If medication was discontinued, was it a promotility agent or laxative? Consider restarting.

↓ No

Aggravating diseases? — Yes → Rule out disorders of GI tract (tumors, diverticuli, etc), metabolic (diabetes), endocrine (hypothyroid), and neurologic disorders (Parkinson's MS), immobilizing diseases (arthritis), diseases which interfere with breathing (COPD), and those which interfere with use of voluntary muscles (post-stroke). Assure optimum treatment.

↓ No

Recent changes in exercise/activity level? — Yes → Evaluate for possibility of increase in exercise. Also evaluate whether any recent changes in personal schedule has occurred which may be interfering with usual BM habits.

↓

Once constipation is identified and contributing factors are ruled out, determine if any signs or symptoms of fecal impaction are exhibited (distended abdomen, fever, vomiting, confusion).

Not impacted ↓ | Impacted

Manifest by straining > 25% of the time?

No ↓ | Yes →

No — Ambulatory? — Yes

No — Hydrated? — Yes

Bulk-forming laxative +/- increase dietary fiber (if no intestinal stenosis)

↓ Ineffective

Consider hyperosmotic (lactulose or sorbitol 70%)

↓ Ineffective

Senna P.O. or suppositories 3 times/week. Note that suppositories alone are often effective in residents who have difficulty evacuating stool from the rectum, but do not retain stool in the colon.

Stool softeners may be used to help **prevent** straining after recent MI, with crescendo angina, after recent rectal surgery, with painful or bleeding hemorrhoids, or other high-risk conditions. See Stool Softeners on next page.

Otherwise, use glycerin suppository after breakfast. Note that suppositories alone are often effective in residents who have difficulty evacuating stool from the rectum, but do not retain stool in colon.

↓ Ineffective

Stool consistency is hard/dry | Stool consistency is putty-like

Use tap water enema up to 3 times/week. May use saline/phosphate enema if used infrequently and no Na^+ restriction is in place. Alternatively, may use bisacodyl suppositories or oral senna up to 3 times/week.

Consider osmotic laxative (lactulose, sorbitol 70%, polyethylene glycol 3350)

↓ Ineffective → ↓ Ineffective ←

Try sequentialy every 2-3 days PRN:
1. MOM, 2. Senna (P.O.), 3. Bisacodyl (P.O.) and discontinue concurrent stool softener or bulk laxative while using. Also, try to limit continuous therapy to 1 week.

↓ Ineffective

Assess for impaction. If it is high impaction, use oil retention enema followed by tap water enema. Manual disimpaction may precede or follow enemas, but the softening effect of the oil helps with this step. May also use sorbitol 30 mL and senna 30 mg up to 3 times/day until obstruction is cleared (per x-ray). Firm rectal impaction can often simply be resolved with manual disimpaction facilitated by the use of a local anesthetic gel.

One should expect gradual rather than immediate results from a newly instituted laxative regimen. Additionally, nondrug interventions should be maintained during pharmacologic treatment of constipation as this is one of the cornerstones of long-term management.

Constipating Drugs
Aluminum (antacids, sucralfate)
Anticholinergics (antiparkinsons)
Antihistamines
CCBs
Levodopa
Opiates
MAOIs
Tricyclic antidepressants
Aluminum
Calcium (supplements & antacids)
Iron
Phenothiazines
Diuretics
Clonidine
Guanabenz
Guanfacine
Disopyramide
Irritant laxatives (with cathartic colon)
Vinca alkaloids
5-HT$_3$ antagonists
Anticonvulsants

Stool Softeners

Stool softeners have no laxative action and are not helpful in alleviating chronic constipation and may cause fecal incontinence. Short-term use is appropriate to minimize straining caused by hard stools following rectal surgery or recent MI or when defecation causes hemorrhoidal pain, rectal bleeding, crescendo angina, or other high risk condition.

Saline Laxatives

Regular use of saline laxatives is not recommended because their risks outweigh the benefits of the laxative. Saline laxatives are only indicated for acute bowel evacuation for diagnostic procedures. Also, note that use of Milk of Magnesia in renally impaired residents can result in Mg^{++} toxicity (hypotension, muscle weakness, EKG changes, CNS changes).

Combination Laxatives

Use of products containing two or more laxatives is not advised because of a lack of documented therapeutic benefit over use of a single ingredient. Additionally, risks may outweigh benefits.

References

Bosshard W, Dreher R, Schnegg JF, et al, "The Treatment of Chronic Constipation in Elderly People: An Update," *Drugs Aging*, 2004, 21(14):911-30.

Floch MH and Wald A, "Clinical Evaluation and Treatment of Constipation," *Gastrolenterologist*, 1994, 2(1):50-60.

Harari D, Gurwitz JH, and Minaker KL, "Constipation in the Elderly," *JAGS*, 1993; 41:1130-40.

Hsieh C, "Treatment of Constipation in Older Adults," *Am Fam Physician*, 2005, 72(11):2277-84.

Izard MW and Ellison FS, "Treatment of Drug Induced Constipation with a Purified Senna Derivative," *Conn Med*, 1962; 26:589.

Lange RL and DiPiro JT, *Pharmacotherapy*, 2nd ed, Norwalk, CT: Appleton & Lange, 1993.

Maguire LC, Yon JL, and Miller E, "Prevention of Narcotic-Induced Constipation," *N Eng J Med*, 1981; 305:1651.

Ramkumar D and Rao SS, "Efficacy and Safety of Traditional Medical Therapies for Chronic Constipation: Systematic Review," *Am J Gastroenterol*, 2005, 100(4):936-71.

Spinzi G, Amat A, Imperiali G, et al, "Constipation in the Elderly," *Drugs Aging*, 2009, 26(6):469-74.

Tariq SH, "Constipation in Long-Term Care," *J Am Med Dir Assoc*, 2007, 8(4):209-18.

Wald A, "Is Chronic Use of Stimulant Laxatives Harmful to the Colon?" *J Clin Gastroenterol*, 2003, 36(5):386-9.

Wrenn K, "Fecal Impaction," *N Engl J Med*, 1989; 321:658-61.

IMMUNIZATION ADMINISTRATION RECOMMENDATIONS

The following tables are taken from the General Recommendations on Immunization, 2011:

- Guidelines for Spacing of Live and Inactivated Antigens
- Guidelines for Administering Antibody-Containing Products and Vaccines
- Recommended Intervals Between Administration of Antibody-Containing Products and Measles- or Varicella-Containing Vaccine, by Product and Indication for Vaccination
- Vaccination of persons with Primary and Secondary Immunodeficiencies
- Needle length and Injection Site of I.M. injections

Guidelines for Spacing of Live and Inactivated Antigens

Antigen Combination	Recommended Minimum Interval Between Doses
Two or more inactivated[1]	May be administered simultaneously or at any interval between doses
Inactivated and live	May be administered simultaneously or at any interval between doses
Two or more live injectable[2]	28 days minimum interval, if not administered simultaneously

[1]Certain experts suggest a 28-day interval between tetanus toxoid, reduced diphtheria toxoid, and reduced acellular pertussis (Tdap) vaccine and tetravalent meningococcal conjugate vaccine if they are not administered simultaneously.

[2]Live oral vaccines (eg, Ty21a typhoid vaccine and rotavirus vaccine) may be administered simultaneously or at any interval before or after inactivated or live injectable vaccines.

Adapted from American Academy of Pediatrics, "Pertussis," In: Pickering LK, Baker CJ, Kimberlin DW, et al, eds, *Red Book*: 2009 Report of the Committee on Infectious Diseases, 28th ed, Elk Grove Village, IL: American Academy of Pediatrics, 2009, 22.

Guidelines for Administering Antibody-Containing Products[1] and Vaccines

Simultaneous Administration (during the same office visit)

Products Administered	Recommended Minimum Interval Between Doses
Antibody-containing products and inactivated antigen	Can be administered simultaneously at different anatomic sites or at any time interval between doses.
Antibody-containing products and live antigen	Should **not** be administered simultaneously.[2] If simultaneous administration of measles-containing vaccine or varicella vaccine is unavoidable, administer at different sites and revaccinate or test for seroconversion after the recommended interval.

Nonsimultaneous Administration

Products Administered		Recommended Minimum Interval Between Doses
Administered first	Administered second	
Antibody-containing products	Inactivated antigen	No interval necessary
Inactivated antigen	Antibody-containing products	No interval necessary
Antibody-containing products	Live antigen	Dose-related[2,3]
Live antigen	Antibody-containing products	2 weeks[2]

[1]Blood products containing substantial amounts of immune globulin include intramuscular and intravenous immune globulin, specific hyperimmune globulin (eg, hepatitis B immune globulin, tetanus immune globulin, varicella zoster immune globulin, and rabies immune globulin), whole blood, packed red blood cells, plasma, and platelet products.

[2]Yellow fever vaccine, rotavirus vaccine, oral Ty21a typhoid vaccine, live-attenuated influenza vaccine, and zoster vaccine are exceptions to these recommendations. These live-attenuated vaccines can be administered at any time before, after, or simultaneously with an antibody-containing product.

[3]The duration of interference of antibody-containing products with the immune response to the measles component of measles-containing vaccine, and possibly varicella vaccine, is dose-related.

Recommended Intervals Between Administration of Antibody-Containing Products and Measles- or Varicella-Containing Vaccine, by Product and Indication for Vaccination

Product/Indication	Dose (mg IgG/kg) and Route[1]	Recommended Interval Before Measles- or Varicella-Containing Vaccine[2] Administration (mo)
Tetanus IG	I.M.: 250 units (10 mg IgG/kg)	3
Hepatitis A IG		
Contact prophylaxis	I.M.: 0.02 mL/kg (3.3 mg IgG/kg)	3
International travel	I.M.: 0.06 mL/kg (10 mg IgG/kg)	3
Hepatitis B IG	I.M.: 0.06 mL/kg (10 mg IgG/kg)	3
Rabies IG	I.M.: 20 int. units/kg (22 mg IgG/kg)	4
Varicella IG	I.M.: 125 units/10 kg (60-200 mg IgG/kg) (maximum: 625 units)	5
Measles prophylaxis IG		
Standard (ie, nonimmunocompromised) contact	I.M.: 0.25 mL/kg (40 mg IgG/kg)	5
Immunocompromised contact	I.M.: 0.50 mL/kg (80 mg IgG/kg)	6
Blood transfusion		
Red blood cells (RBCs), washed	I.V.: 10 mL/kg (negligible IgG/kg)	None
RBCs, adenine-saline added	I.V.: 10 mL/kg (10 mg IgG/kg)	3
Packed RBCs (hematocrit 65%)[3]	I.V.: 10 mL/kg (60 mg IgG/kg)	6
Whole blood cells (hematocrit 35% to 50%)[3]	I.V.: 10 mL/kg (80-100 mg IgG/kg)	6
Plasma/platelet products	I.V.: 10 mL/kg (160 mg IgG/kg)	7
Cytomegalovirus intravenous immune globulin (IGIV)	150 mg/kg maximum	6
IGIV		
Replacement therapy for immune deficiencies[4]	I.V.: 300-400 mg/kg[4]	8
Immune thrombocytopenic purpura treatment	I.V.: 400 mg/kg	8
Postexposure varicella prophylaxis[5]	I.V.: 400 mg/kg	8
Immune thrombocytopenic purpura treatment	I.V.: 1000 mg/kg	10
Kawasaki disease	I.V.: 2 g/kg	11
Monoclonal antibody to respiratory syncytial virus F protein (Synagis® [Medimmune])[6]	I.M.: 15 mg/kg	None

HIV = human immunodeficiency virus, IG = immune globulin, IgG = immune globulin G, IGIV = intravenous immune globulin, mg IgG/kg = milligrams of immune globulin G per kilogram of body weight, I.M. = intramuscular, I.V. = intravenous, RBCs = red blood cells

[1]This table is not intended for determining the correct indications and dosages for using antibody-containing products. Unvaccinated persons might not be fully protected against measles during the entire recommended interval, and additional doses of IG or measles vaccine might be indicated after measles exposure. Concentrations of measles antibody in an IG preparation can vary by manufacturer's lot. Rates of antibody clearance after receipt of an IG preparation also might vary. Recommended intervals are extrapolated from an estimated half-life of 30 days for passively acquired antibody and an observed interference with the immune response to measles vaccine for 5 months after a dose of 80 mg IgG/kg.

[2]Does not include zoster vaccine. Zoster vaccine may be given with antibody-containing blood products.

[3]Assumes a serum IgG concentration of 16 mg/mL

[4]Measles and varicella vaccinations are recommended for children with asymptomatic or mildly symptomatic HIV infection but are contraindicated for persons with severe immunosuppression from HIV or any other immunosuppressive disorder.

[5]The investigational product VariZIG™, similar to licensed varicella-zoster IG (VZIG), is a purified human IG preparation made from plasma containing high levels of anti-varicella antibodies (IgG). The interval between VariZIG™ and varicella vaccine (Var or MMRV) is 5 months.

[6]Contains antibody only to respiratory syncytial virus

Vaccination of Persons With Primary and Secondary Immunodeficiencies

Category	Specific Immunodeficiency	Contraindicated Vaccines[1]	Risk-Specific Recommended Vaccines[1]	Effectiveness and Comments
		Primary		
B-lymphocyte (humoral)	Severe antibody deficiencies (eg, X-linked agammaglobulinemia and common variable immunodeficiency)	Oral poliovirus (OPV)[2] Smallpox Live-attenuated influenza vaccine (LAIV) BCG Ty21a (live oral typhoid) Yellow fever	Pneumococcal Consider measles and varicella vaccination	The effectiveness of any vaccine is uncertain if it depends only on the humoral response (eg, PPSV or MPSV4) IGIV interferes with the immune response to measles vaccine and possibly varicella vaccine
	Less severe antibody deficiencies (eg, selective IgA deficiency and IgG subclass deficiency)	OPV[2] BCG Yellow Fever Other live-vaccines appear to be safe	Pneumococcal	All vaccines likely effective; immune response may be attenuated
T-lymphocyte (cell-mediated and humoral)	Complete defects (eg, severe combined immunodeficiency [SCID] disease, complete DiGeorge syndrome)	All live vaccines[3,4,5]	Pneumococcal	Vaccines might be ineffective
	Partial defects (eg, most patients with DiGeorge syndrome, Wiskott-Aldrich syndrome, ataxia-telangiectasia)	All live vaccines[3,4,5]	Pneumococcal Meningococcal Hib (if not administered in infancy)	Effectiveness of any vaccine depends on degree of immune suppression
Complement	Persistent complement, properdin, or factor B deficiency	None	Pneumococcal Meningococcal	All routine vaccines likely effective
Phagocytic function	Chronic granulomatous disease, leukocyte adhesion defect, and myeloperoxidase deficiency	Live bacterial vaccines[3]	Pneumococcal[6]	All inactivated vaccines safe and likely effective; live viral vaccines likely safe and effective

Vaccination of Persons With Primary and Secondary Immunodeficiencies *continued*

Category	Specific Immunodeficiency	Contraindicated Vaccines[1]	Risk-Specific Recommended Vaccines[1]	Effectiveness and Comments
		Secondary		
	HIV/AIDS	OPV[2] Smallpox BCG LAIV Withhold MMR and varicella in severely immunocompromised persons Yellow fever vaccine might have a contraindication or a precaution depending on clinical parameters of immune function[9]	Pneumococcal Consider Hib (if not administered in infancy) and meningococcal vaccination.	MMR, varicella, rotavirus, and all inactivated vaccines, including inactivated influenza, might be effective.[7]
	Malignant neoplasm, transplantation, immunosuppressive or radiation therapy	Live viral and bacterial, depending on immune status[3,4]	Pneumococcal	Effectiveness of any vaccine depends on degree of immune suppression
	Asplenia	None	Pneumococcal Meningococcal Hib (if not administered in infancy)	All routine vaccines likely effective
	Chronic renal disease	LAIV	Pneumococcal Hepatitis B[8]	All routine vaccines likely effective

AIDS = acquired immunodeficiency syndrome; BCG = bacille Calmette-Guerin; Hib = *Haemophilus influenzae* type b; HIV = human immunodeficiency virus; IG = immunoglobulin; IGIV = immune globulin intravenous; LAIV = live, attenuated influenza vaccine; MMR = measles, mumps, and rubella; MPSV4 = quadrivalent meningococcal polysaccharide vaccine; OPV = oral poliovirus vaccine (live); PPSV = pneumococcal polysaccharide vaccine; TIV = trivalent inactivated influenza vaccine

[1] Other vaccines that are universally or routinely recommended should be administered if not contraindicated.

[2] OPV is no longer available in the United States.

[3] Live bacterial vaccines: BCG and oral Ty21a *Salmonella typhi* vaccine

[4] Live viral vaccines: MMR, MMRV, OPV, LAIV, yellow fever, zoster, rotavirus, varicella, and vaccinia (smallpox). Smallpox vaccine is not recommended for children or the general public.

[5] Regarding T-lymphocyte immunodeficiency as a contraindication for rotavirus vaccine, data exist only for severe combined immunodeficiency.

[6] Pneumococcal vaccine is not indicated for children with chronic granulomatous disease beyond age-based universal recommendations for PCV. Children with chronic granulomatous disease are not at increased risk for pneumococcal disease.

[7] HIV-infected children should receive IG after exposure to measles and may receive varicella and measles vaccine if CD4[+] lymphocyte count is ≥15%.

[8] Indicated based on the risk from dialysis-based bloodborne transmission

[9] Symptomatic HIV infection or CD4[+] T-lymphocyte count of <200/mm[3] or <15% of total lymphocytes for children aged <6 years is a contraindication to yellow fever vaccine administration. Asymptomatic HIV infection with CD4[+] T-lymphocyte count of 200-499/mm[3] for persons aged 26 years or 15% to 24% of total lymphocytes for children aged <6 years is a precaution for yellow fever vaccine administration. Details of yellow fever vaccine recommendations are available from the CDC. (CDC. "Yellow Fever Vaccine: Recommendations of the Advisory Committee on Immunization Practices [ACIP]." *MMWR Recomm Rep*, 2010, 59[No. RR-7].)

Adapted from American Academy of Pediatrics, "Passive Immunization." In: Pickering LK, Baker CJ, Kimberline DW, et al, eds, *Red Book: 2009 Report of the Committee on Infectious Diseases*, 28th ed, Elk Grove Village, IL: American Academy of Pediatrics, 2009, 74-5.

Needle Length and Injection Site of I.M. for Adults Aged ≥19 years
(by sex and weight)

Age Group	Needle Length	Injection Site
Adults ≥19 y		
Men and women <60 kg (130 lb)	1" (25 mm)[1]	Deltoid muscle of the arm
Men and women 60-70 kg (130-152 lb)	1" (25 mm)	
Men 70-118 kg (152-260 lb)	1-1½" (25-38 mm)	
Women 70-90 kg (152-200 lb)		
Men >118 kg (260 lb)	1½" (38 mm)	
Women >90 kg (200 lb)		

I.M. = intramuscular

[1]Some experts recommend a ⅝" needle for men and women who weigh <60 kg.

Adapted from Poland GA, Borrud A, Jacobsen RM, et al, "Determination of Deltoid Fat Pad Thickness: Implications for Needle Length in Adult Immunization," *JAMA*, 1997, 277:1709-11.

RECOMMENDATIONS FOR TRAVELERS

The Centers for Disease Control and Prevention (CDC) also provides guidance to assist travelers and their healthcare providers in deciding the vaccines, medications, and other measures necessary to prevent illness and injury during international travel. Available at http://wwwnc.-cdc.gov/travel

REFERENCE

Centers for Disease Control, "Recommendations of the Advisory Committee on Immunization Practices (ACIP): General Recommendations on Immunization," *MMWR Recomm Rep*, 2011, 60(2):1-61.

IMMUNIZATION RECOMMENDATIONS

Recommended adult immunization schedule, by vaccine and age group[1] — United States, 2012

VACCINE ▼ AGE GROUP▶	19–21 years	22–26 years	27–49 years	50–59 years	60–64 years	≥65 years
Influenza[2,*]	1 dose annually					
Tetanus, diphtheria, pertussis (Td/Tdap)[3,*]	Substitute 1-time dose of Tdap for Td booster; then boost with Td every 10 years					Td/Tdap
Varicella[4,*]	2 doses					
Human papillomavirus (HPV)[5,*] Female	3 doses					
Human papillomavirus (HPV)[5,*] Male	3 doses					
Zoster[6]					1 dose	
Measles, mumps, rubella (MMR)[7,*]	1 or 2 doses				1 dose	
Pneumococcal (polysaccharide)[8,9]		1 or 2 doses				1 dose
Meningococcal[10,*]	1 or more doses					
Hepatitis A[11,*]	2 doses					
Hepatitis B[12,*]	3 doses					

*Covered by the Vaccine Injury Compensation Program

For all persons in this category who meet the age requirements and who lack documentation of vaccination or have no evidence of previous infection	Recommended if some other risk factor is present (e.g., on the basis of medical, occupational, lifestyle, or other indications)	Tdap recommended for ≥65 if contact with <12 month old child. Either Td or Tdap can be used if no infant contact	No recommendation

Vaccines that might be indicated for adults, based on medical and other indications[1] — United States, 2012

INDICATION▶ VACCINE ▼	Pregnancy	Immunocompromising conditions (excluding human immunodeficiency virus [HIV])[4,6,7,14]	HIV infection[4,7,13,14] CD4+ T lymphocyte count <200 cells/μL	HIV infection[4,7,13,14] CD4+ T lymphocyte count ≥200 cells/μL	Men who have sex with men (MSM)	Heart disease, chronic lung disease, chronic alcoholism	Asplenia[18] (including elective splenectomy and persistent complement component deficiencies)	Chronic liver disease	Diabetes, kidney failure, end-stage renal disease, receipt of hemodialysis	Health-care personnel
Influenza[2,*]	1 dose TIV annually		1 dose TIV or LAIV annually	1 dose TIV annually						1 dose TIV or LAIV annually
Tetanus, diphtheria, pertussis (Td/Tdap)[3,*]	Substitute 1-time dose of Tdap for Td booster; then boost with Td every 10 years									
Varicella[4,*]	Contraindicated			2 doses						
Human papillomavirus (HPV)[5,*] Female	3 doses through age 26 years					3 doses through age 26 years				
Human papillomavirus (HPV)[5,*] Male	3 doses through age 26 years					3 doses through age 21 years				
Zoster[6]	Contraindicated			1 dose						
Measles, mumps, rubella[7,*]	Contraindicated			1 or 2 doses						
Pneumococcal (polysaccharide)[8,9]	1 or 2 doses									
Meningococcal[10,*]	1 or more doses									
Hepatitis A[11,*]	2 doses									
Hepatitis B[12,*]	3 doses									

*Covered by the Vaccine Injury Compensation Program

For all persons in this category who meet the age requirements and who lack documentation of vaccination or have no evidence of previous infection	Recommended if some other risk factor is present (e.g., on the basis of medical, occupational, lifestyle, or other indications)	Contraindicated	No recommendation

◀ Footnotes to Recommended Adult Immunization Schedule

[1]Additional information

- Advisory Committee on Immunization Practices (ACIP) vaccine recommendations and additional information are available at http://www.cdc.gov/vaccines/pubs/acip-list.htm.

- Information on travel vaccine requirements and recommendations (eg, for hepatitis A and B, meningococcal, and other vaccines) are available at http://wwwnc.cdc.gov/travel/page/vaccinations.htm.

[2]Influenza vaccine

- Annual vaccination against influenza is recommended for all persons ≥6 months of age.

- Persons ≥6 months of age, including pregnant women, can receive the trivalent inactivated vaccine (TIV).

- Healthy, nonpregnant adults <50 years of age without high-risk medical conditions can receive either intranasally administered live, attenuated influenza vaccine (LAIV) (Flu-Mist®) or TIV. Healthcare personnel who care for severely immunocompromised persons (ie, those who require care in a protected environment) should receive TIV, rather than LAIV. Other persons should receive TIV.

- The intramuscularly or intradermally administered TIV are options for adults 18-64 years of age.

- Adults ≥65 years of age can receive the standard-dose TIV or the high-dose TIV (Fluzone® High Dose).

[3]Tetanus, diphtheria, and acellular pertussis vaccine (Td/Tdap)

- Administer a one-time dose of Tdap to adults <65 years of age who have not received Tdap previously or for whom vaccine status is unknown to replace one of the 10-year Td boosters.

- Tdap is specifically recommended for the following persons:

  - Pregnant women >20 weeks gestation

  - Adults, regardless of age, who are close contacts of infants <12 months of age (eg, parents, grandparents, or child-care providers), and

  - Healthcare personnel

- Tdap can be administered regardless of interval since the most recent tetanus or diphtheria-containing vaccine.

- Pregnant women not vaccinated during pregnancy should receive Tdap immediately postpartum.

- Adults ≥65 years of age may receive Tdap.

- Adults with unknown or incomplete history of completing a 3-dose primary vaccination series with Td-containing vaccines should begin or complete a primary vaccination series. Tdap should be substituted for a single dose of Td in the vaccination series, with Tdap preferred as the first dose.

- For unvaccinated adults, administer the first 2 doses ≥4 weeks apart and the third dose 6–12 months after the second.

- If incompletely vaccinated (ie, less than 3 doses), administer remaining doses. Refer to the ACIP statement for recommendations for administering Td/Tdap as prophylaxis in wound management (see footnote 1).

[4]Varicella vaccine

- All adults without evidence of immunity to varicella should receive 2 doses of single-antigen varicella vaccine or a second dose if they have received only 1 dose.

- Special consideration should be given to those who:

  - Have close contact with persons at high risk for severe disease (eg, healthcare personnel and family contacts of persons with immunocompromising conditions), or

  - Are at high risk for exposure or transmission (eg, teachers; child-care employees; residents and staff members of institutional settings, including correctional institutions; college students; military personnel; adolescents and adults living in households with children; nonpregnant women of childbearing age; international travelers)

- Pregnant women should be assessed for evidence of varicella immunity. Women who do not have evidence of immunity should receive the first dose of varicella vaccine upon completion or termination of pregnancy and before discharge from the healthcare facility. The second dose should be administered 4–8 weeks after the first dose.

- Evidence of immunity to varicella in adults includes any of the following:

    - Documentation of 2 doses of varicella vaccine ≥4 weeks apart

    - U.S.-born before 1980 (although for healthcare personnel and pregnant women, birth before 1980 should not be considered evidence of immunity)

    - History of varicella based on diagnosis or verification of varicella by a healthcare provider (for a patient reporting a history of or having an atypical case, a mild case, or both, healthcare providers should seek either an epidemiologic link with a typical varicella case or to a laboratory-confirmed case or evidence of laboratory confirmation if it was performed at the time of acute disease)

    - History of herpes zoster based on diagnosis or verification of herpes zoster by a healthcare provider, or

    - Laboratory evidence of immunity or laboratory confirmation of disease

[5]Human papillomavirus vaccine (HPV)

- Two vaccines are licensed for use in females, bivalent HPV vaccine (HPV2) and quadrivalent HPV vaccine (HPV4), and one HPV vaccine for use in males (HPV4).

- For females, either HPV4 or HPV2 is recommended in a 3-dose series for routine vaccination at 11 or 12 years of age, and for those 13-26 years of age, if not previously vaccinated.

- For males, HPV4 is recommended in a 3-dose series for routine vaccination at 11 or 12 years of age, and for those 13-21 years of age, if not previously vaccinated. Males 22-26 years of age may be vaccinated.

- HPV vaccines are not live vaccines and can be administered to persons who are immunocompromised as a result of infection (including HIV infection), disease, or medications. Vaccine is recommended for immunocompromised persons through 26 years of age who did not get any or all doses when they were younger. The immune response and vaccine efficacy might be less than that in immunocompetent persons.

- Men who have sex with men (MSM) might especially benefit from vaccination to prevent condyloma and anal cancer. HPV4 is recommended for MSM through 26 years of age who did not get any or all doses when they were younger.

- Ideally, vaccine should be administered before potential exposure to HPV through sexual activity; however, persons who are sexually active should still be vaccinated consistent with age-based recommendations. HPV vaccine can be administered to persons with a history of genital warts, abnormal Papanicolaou test, or positive HPV DNA test.

- A complete series for either HPV4 or HPV2 consists of 3 doses. The second dose should be administered 1–2 months after the first dose; the third dose should be administered 6 months after the first dose (≥24 weeks after the first dose).

- Although HPV vaccination is not specifically recommended for healthcare personnel (HCP) based on their occupation, HCP should receive the HPV vaccine if they are in the recommended age group.

[6]Zoster vaccine

- A single dose of zoster vaccine is recommended for adults ≥60 years of age, regardless of whether they report a prior episode of herpes zoster. Although the vaccine is licensed by the Food and Drug Administration (FDA) for use among and can be administered to persons ≥50 years of age, ACIP recommendes that vaccination begin at 60 years of age.

- Persons with chronic medical conditions may be vaccinated, unless their condition constitutes a contraindication, such as pregnancy or severe immunodeficiency.

- Although zoster vaccination is not specifically recommended for healthcare personnel (HCP), HCP should receive the vaccine if they are in the recommended age group.

[7]Measles, mumps, rubella vaccine (MMR)

- Adults born before 1957 generally are considered immune to measles and mumps. All adults born in 1957 or later should have documentation of ≥1 dose of MMR vaccine, unless they have a medical contraindication to the vaccine, laboratory evidence of immunity to each of the three diseases, or documentation of provider-diagnosed measles or mumps disease. For rubella, documentation of provider-diagnosed disease is not considered acceptable evidence of immunity.

- *Measles component:*
  - A routine second dose of MMR vaccine, administered a minimum of 28 days after the first dose, is recommended for adults who:
    - Are students in postsecondary educational institutions
    - Work in a healthcare facility, or
    - Plan to travel internationally
  - Persons who received inactivated (killed) measles vaccine or measles vaccine of unknown type during 1963–1967 should be revaccinated with 2 doses of MMR vaccine.

- *Mumps component:*
  - A routine second dose of MMR vaccine, administered a minimum of 28 days after the first dose, is recommended for adults who:
    - Are students in postsecondary educational institutions
    - Work in a healthcare facility, or
    - Plan to travel internationally
  - Persons vaccinated before 1979 with either killed mumps vaccine or mumps vaccine of unknown type who are at high risk for mumps infection (eg, persons who are working in a healthcare facility) should be considered for revaccination with 2 doses of MMR vaccine.

- *Rubella component:* For women of childbearing age, regardless of birth year, rubella immunity should be determined. If there is no evidence of immunity, women who are not pregnant should be vaccinated. Pregnant women who do not have evidence of immunity should receive MMR vaccine upon completion or termination of pregnancy and before discharge from the healthcare facility.

- *Healthcare personnel born before 1957:* For unvaccinated healthcare personnel born before 1957 who lack laboratory evidence of measles, mumps, and/or rubella immunity or laboratory confirmation of disease, healthcare facilities should consider routinely vaccinating personnel with 2 doses of MMR vaccine at the appropriate interval for measles and mumps or 1 dose of MMR vaccine for rubella.

[8]Pneumococcal polysaccharide vaccine (PPSV)

- Vaccinate all persons with the following indications:
  - ≥65 years of age without a history of PPSV vaccination
  - Adults <65 years of age with chronic lung disease (including chronic obstructive pulmonary disease, emphysema, and asthma), chronic cardiovascular diseases, diabetes mellitus, chronic liver diseases (including cirrhosis), alcoholism, cochlear implants, cerebrospinal fluid leaks, immunocompromising conditions, and functional or anatomic asplenia (eg, sickle cell disease and other hemoglobinophathies, congenital or acquired asplenia, splenic dysfunction, or splenectomy [if elective splenectomy is planned, vaccinate ≥2 weeks before surgery])
  - Residents of nursing homes or long-term care facilities, and
  - Adults who smoke cigarettes

- Persons with asymptomatic or symptomatic HIV infection should be vaccinated as soon as possible after their diagonosis.

- When cancer chemotherapy or other immunosuppressive therapy is being considered, the interval between vaccination and initiation of immunosuppresive therapy should be ≥2 weeks. Vaccination during chemotherapy or radiation therapy should be avoided.

- Routine use of PPSV is not recommended for American Indians/Alaska Natives or other persons <65 years of age, unless they have underlying medical conditions that are PPSV indications. However, public health authorities may consider recommending PPSV for American Indians/Alaska Natives who are living in areas where the risk for invasive pneumococcal disease is increased.

[9]Revaccination with PPSV

- One-time revaccination 5 years after the first dose is recommended for persons 19-64 years of age with chronic renal failure or nephrotic syndrome, functional or anatomic asplenia (eg, sickle cell disease or splenectomy), and for persons with immunocompromising conditions.

- Persons who received PPSV before 65 years of age for any indication should receive another dose of the vaccine at ≥65 years of age if ≥5 years have passed since their previous dose.

- No further doses are needed for persons vaccinated with PPSV ≥65 years of age.

[10]Meningococcal vaccine

- Administer 2 doses of meningococcal conjugate vaccine quadrivalent (MCV4) ≥2 months apart to adults with functional asplenia or persistent complement component deficiencies.

- HIV-infected persons who are vaccinated should also receive 2 doses.

- Administer a single dose of meningococcal vaccine to microbiologists routinely exposed to isolates of *Neisseria meningitidis*, military recruits, and persons who travel to or live in countries in which meningococcal disease is hyperendemic or epidemic.

- First-year college students ≤21 years of age who are living in residence halls should be vaccinated if they have not received a dose on or after their 16th birthday.

- MCV4 is preferred for adults with any of the preceding indications who are ≤55 years of age; meningococcal polysaccharide vaccine (MPSV4) is preferred for adults ≥56 years of age.

- Revaccination with MCV4 every 5 years is recommended for adults previously vaccinated with MCV4 or MPSV4 who remain at increased risk for infection (eg, adults with anatomic or functional asplenia or persistent complement component deficiencies).

[11]Hepatitis A vaccine

- Vaccinate any person seeking protection from hepatitis A virus (HAV) infection and persons with any of the following indications:

  - Men who have sex with men and persons who use injection drugs

  - Persons working with HAV-infected primates or with HAV in a research laboratory setting

  - Persons with chronic liver disease and persons who receive clotting factor concentrates

  - Persons traveling to or working in countries that have high or intermediate endemicity of hepatitis A, and

  - Unvaccinated persons who anticipate close personal contatct (eg, household or regular babysitting) with an international adoptee during the first 60 days after arrival in the United States from a country with high or intermediate endemicity (see footnote 1 for more information on travel recommendations). The first dose of the 2-dose hepatitis A vaccine series should be administered as soon as adoption is planned, ideally 2 or more weeks before the arrival of the adoptee.

- Single-antigen vaccine formulations should be administered in a 2-dose schedule at either 0 and 6–12 months (Havrix®), or 0 and 6–18 months (VAQTA®). If the combined hepatitis A and hepatitis B vaccine (Twinrix®) is used, administer 3 doses at 0, 1, and 6 months; alternatively, a 4-dose schedule may be used, administered on days 0, 7, and 21–30, followed by a booster dose at month 12.

[12]Hepatitis B vaccine

- Vaccinate persons with any of the following indications and any person seeking protection from hepatitis B virus (HBV) infection:

  - Sexually active persons who are not in a long-term, mutually monogamous relationship (eg, persons with more than one sex partner during the previous 6 months); persons seeking evaluation or treatment for a sexually transmitted disease (STD); current or recent injection-drug users; and men who have sex with men.

  - Healthcare personnel and public-safety workers who are exposed to blood or other potentially infectious body fluids.

- Persons with diabetes <60 years of age as soon as feasible after diagnosis; persons with diabetes who are ≥60 years of age at the discretion of the treating clinician, based on increased need for assisted blood glucose monitoring in long-term care facilities, likelihood of acquiring hepatitis B infection, its complications, or chronic sequelae, and likelihood of immune response to vaccination

- Persons with end-stage renal disease, including patients receiving hemodialysis; persons with HIV infection; and persons with chronic liver disease

- Household contacts and sex partners of persons with chronic HBV infection; clients and staff members of institutions for persons with developmental disabilities; and international travelers to countries with high or intermediate prevalence of chronic HBV infection; and

- All adults in the following settings: STD treatment facilities, HIV testing and treatment facilities, facilities providing drug-abuse treatment and prevention services, healthcare settings targeting services to injection-drug users or men who have sex with men, correctional facilities, end-stage renal disease programs and facilities for chronic hemodialysis patients, and institutions and nonresidential daycare facilities for persons with developmental disabilities

• Administer missing doses to complete a 3-dose series of hepatitis B vaccine to those persons not vaccinated or not completely vaccinated. The second dose should be administered 1 month after the first dose; the third dose should be given ≥2 months after the second dose (and ≥4 months after the first dose). If the combined hepatitis A and hepatitis B vaccine (Twinrix®) is used, give 3 doses at 0, 1, and 6 months; alternatively, a 4-dose Twinrix® schedule, administered on days 0, 7, and 21-30, followed by a booster dose at month 12, may be used.

• Adult patients receiving hemodialysis or with other immunocompromising conditions should receive 1 dose of 40 µg/mL (Recombivax HB®), administered on a 3-dose schedule, or 2 doses of 20 µg/mL (Engerix-B®), administered simultaneously on a 4-dose schedule at 0, 1, 2, and 6 months.

[13]Selected conditions for which *Haemophilus influenzae* type b (Hib) vaccine may be used

• One dose of Hib vaccine should be considered for persons who have sickle cell disease, leukemia, or HIV infection, or who have anatomic or functional asplenia if they have not previously received Hib vaccine.

[14]Immunocompromising conditions

• Inactivated vaccines generally are acceptable (eg, pneumococcal, meningococcal, influenza [inactivated influenza vaccine]) and live vaccines generally are avoided in persons with immune deficiencies or immunocompromising conditions. Information on specific conditions is available at http://www.cdc.gov/vaccines/pubs/acip-list.htm.

REFERENCE

"Recommended Adult Immunization Schedule – United States, 2012," *MMWR Recomm Rep*, 2012, 61(4):Q1-5. Available at http://www.cdc.gov/mmwr/pdf/rr/rr6002.pdf

These schedules indicate the recommended age groups and medical indications for which administration of currently licensed vaccines is commonly indicated for adults ≥19 years of age, as of January 1, 2011. For all vaccines being recommended on the adult immunization schedule, a vaccine series does not need to be restarted, regardless of the time that has elapsed between doses. Licensed combination vaccines may be used whenever any components of the combination are indicated and when the vaccine's other components are not contraindicated. For detailed recommendations on all vaccines, including those used primarily for travelers or that are issued during the year, consult the manufacturers' package inserts and the complete statements from the Advisory Committee on Immunization Practices (http://www.cdc.gov/vaccines/pubs/acip-list.htm).

Report all clinically significant postvaccination reactions to the Vaccine Adverse Event Reporting System (VAERS). Reporting forms and instructions on filing a VAERS report are available at http://www.vaers.hhs.gov or by telephone, (800) 822-7967.

Information on how to file a Vaccine Injury Compensation Program claim is available at http://www.hrsa.gov/vaccinecompensation or by telephone, (800) 338-2382. Information about filing a claim for vaccine injury is available through the U.S. Court of Federal Claims, 717 Madison Place, N.W., Washington, D.C. 20005; telephone, (202) 357-6400.

Additional information about the vaccines in this schedule, extent of available data, and contraindications for vaccination also is available at http://www.cdc.gov/vaccines or from the CDC-INFO Contact Center at (800) CDC-INFO (800-232-4636) in English and Spanish, 8 a.m. to 8 p.m., Monday through Friday, excluding holidays.

Use of trade names and commercial sources is for identification only and does not imply endorsement by the U.S. Department of Health and Human Services.

U.S. Department of Health and Human Services • Centers for Disease Control and Prevention

VACCINE INJURY TABLE

The Vaccine Injury Table makes it easier for some people to get compensation. The table lists and explains injuries/conditions that are presumed to be caused by vaccines. It also lists time periods in which the first symptom of these injuries/conditions must occur after receiving the vaccine. If the first symptom of these injuries/conditions occurs within the listed time periods, it is presumed that the vaccine was the cause of the injury or condition unless another cause is found. For example, if the patient received the tetanus vaccines and had a severe allergic reaction (anaphylaxis) within 4 hours after receiving the vaccine, then it is presumed that the tetanus vaccine caused the injury if no other cause is found.

If the injury/condition is not on the table or if the injury/condition did not occur within the time period on the table, it must be proven that the vaccine caused the injury/condition. Such proof must be based on medical records or opinion, which may include expert witness testimony.

Vaccine Injury Table[1]

Vaccine	Illness, Disability, Injury, or Condition Covered		Time Period for First Symptom or Manifestation of Onset or of Significant Aggravation After Vaccine Administration
Vaccines containing tetanus toxoid (eg, DTaP, DTP, DT, Td, TT)	A.	Anaphylaxis or anaphylactic shock	4 hours
	B.	Brachial neuritis	2-28 days
	C.	Any acute complication or sequela (including death) of above events	Not applicable
Vaccines containing whole cell pertussis bacteria, extracted or partial cell pertussis bacteria, or specific pertussis antigen(s) (eg, DTP, DTaP, P, DTP-Hib)	A.	Anaphylaxis or anaphylactic shock	4 hours
	B.	Encephalopathy (or encephalitis)	72 hours
	C.	Any acute complication or sequela (including death) of above events	Not applicable
Measles, mumps, and rubella vaccine or any of its components (eg, MMR, MR, M, R)	A.	Anaphylaxis or anaphylactic shock	4 hours
	B.	Encephalopathy (or encephalitis)	5-15 days
	C.	Any acute complication or sequela (including death) of above events	Not applicable
Vaccines containing rubella virus (eg, MMR, MR, R)	A.	Chronic arthritis	7-42 days
	B.	Any acute complication or sequela (including death) of above events	Not applicable
Vaccines containing measles virus (eg, MMR, MR, M)	A.	Thrombocytopenic purpura	7-30 days
	B.	Vaccine-strain measles viral infection in an immunodeficient recipient	6 months
	C.	Any acute complication or sequela (including death) of above events	Not applicable
Vaccines containing polio live virus (OPV)	A.	Paralytic polio	
		• In a nonimmunodeficient recipient	30 days
		• In an immunodeficient recipient	6 months
		• In a vaccine-associated community case	Not applicable
	B.	Vaccine-strain polio viral infection	
		• In a nonimmunodeficient recipient	30 days
		• In an immunodeficient recipient	6 months
		• In a vaccine-associated community case	Not applicable
	C.	Any acute complication or sequela (including death) of above events	Not applicable
Vaccines containing polio inactivated (eg, IPV)	A.	Anaphylaxis or anaphylactic shock	4 hours
	B.	Any acute complication or sequela (including death) of above events	Not applicable

Vaccine Injury Table[1] *(continued)*

Vaccine	Illness, Disability, Injury, or Condition Covered	Time Period for First Symptom or Manifestation of Onset or of Significant Aggravation After Vaccine Administration
Hepatitis B vaccines	A. Anaphylaxis or anaphylactic shock	4 hours
	B. Any acute complication or sequela (including death) of above events	Not applicable
Hemophilus influenzae type b polysaccharide conjugate vaccines	A. No condition specified	Not applicable
Varicella vaccine	A. No condition specified	Not applicable
Rotavirus vaccine	A. No condition specified	Not applicable
Pneumococcal conjugate vaccines	A. No condition specified	Not applicable
Hepatitis A vaccines	A. No condition specified	Not applicable
Trivalent influenza vaccines	A. No condition specified	Not applicable
Meningococcal vaccines	A. No condition specified	Not applicable
Human papillomavirus (HPV) vaccines	A. No condition specified	Not applicable
Any new vaccine recommended by the Centers for Disease Control and Prevention for routine administration to children, after publication by Secretary, HHS of a notice of coverage	A. No condition specified	Not applicable

[1]Effective date: July 22, 2011

ANTIBIOTIC TREATMENT OF ADULTS WITH INFECTIVE ENDOCARDITIS

Table 1. Suggested Regimens for Therapy of Native Valve Endocarditis Due to Penicillin-Susceptible Viridans Streptococci and *Streptococcus bovis*

(Minimum Inhibitory Concentration ≤0.12 mcg/mL)[1]

Antibiotic	Dosage and Route	Duration (wk)	Comments
Aqueous crystalline penicillin G sodium **or**	12-18 million units/24 h I.V. either continuously or in 4-6 equally divided doses	4	Preferred in most patients older than 65 y and in those with impairment of the 8th cranial nerve or renal function
CefTRIAXone sodium	2 g once daily I.V. or I.M.[2]	4	
Either penicillin or cefTRIAXone regimen above with gentamicin sulfate[3]	3 mg/kg/24 h I.M./I.V. as single daily dose	2	When using combination therapy, both β-lactam and aminoglycoside regimen duration is 2 weeks; 2-week regimen not intended if known cardiac or extracardiac abscess, Cl_{cr} <20 mL/min, 8th cranial nerve impairment or *Abiotrophia*, *Granulicatella*, or *Gemella* spp
Vancomycin hydrochloride[4]	30 mg/kg/24 h I.V. in 2 equally divided doses, not to exceed 2 g/24 h unless serum levels are monitored	4	Vancomycin therapy is recommended for patients allergic to β-lactams; peak serum concentrations of vancomycin should be obtained 1 h after completion of the infusion and should be in the range of 30-45 mcg/mL and trough of 10-15 mcg/mL for twice-daily dosing

[1] Dosages recommended are for patients with normal renal function. For nutritionally variant streptococci, see Table 3. I.V. indicates intravenous; I.M., intramuscular.

[2] Patients should be informed that I.M. injection of cefTRIAXone is painful.

[3] Dosing of gentamicin on a mg/kg basis will produce higher serum concentrations in obese patients than in lean patients. Therefore, in obese patients, dosing should be based on ideal body weight. (Ideal body weight for men is 50 kg + 2.3 kg per inch over 5 feet, and ideal body weight for women is 45.5 kg + 2.3 kg per inch over 5 feet.) Relative contraindications to the use of gentamicin are age >65 years, renal impairment, or impairment of the eighth nerve. Other potentially nephrotoxic agents (eg, nonsteroidal anti-inflammatory drugs) should be used cautiously in patients receiving gentamicin.

[4] Vancomycin dosage should be reduced in patients with impaired renal function. Vancomycin given on a mg/kg basis will produce higher serum concentrations in obese patients than in lean patients. Therefore, in obese patients, dosing should be based on ideal body weight. Each dose of vancomycin should be infused over at least 1 hour to reduce the risk of the histamine-release "red man" syndrome.

Table 2. Therapy for Native Valve Endocarditis Due to Strains of Viridans Streptococci and *Streptococcus bovis* Relatively Resistant to Penicillin G (Minimum Inhibitory Concentration >0.12 mcg/mL and ≤0.5 mcg/mL)[1]

Antibiotic	Dosage and Route	Duration (wk)	Comments
Aqueous crystalline penicillin G sodium	24 million units/24 h I.V. either continuously or in 4-6 equally divided doses	4	CeFAZolin or other first-generation cephalosporins may be substituted for penicillin in patients whose penicillin hypersensitivity is not of the immediate type.
With gentamicin sulfate[2]	3 mg/kg/24 h I.M./I.V. as single daily dose	2	
CefTRIAXone sodium	2 g once daily I.V. or I.M.[2]	4	
With gentamicin sulfate[2]	3 mg/kg/24 h I.M./I.V. as single daily dose	2	
Vancomycin hydrochloride[3]	30 mg/kg/24 h I.V. in 2 equally divided doses, not to exceed 2 g/24 h unless serum levels are monitored	4	Vancomycin therapy is recommended for patients allergic to β-lactams

[1]Dosages recommended are for patients with normal renal function. I.V. = intravenous, I.M. = intramuscular

[2]For specific dosing adjustment and issues concerning gentamicin (obese patients, relative contraindications), see Table 1 footnotes.

[3]For specific dosing adjustment and issues concerning vancomycin (obese patients, length of infusion), see Table 1 footnotes.

Table 3. Standard Therapy for Endocarditis Due to Enterococci[1]

Antibiotic	Dosage and Route	Duration (wk)	Comments
Aqueous crystalline penicillin G sodium	18-30 million units/24 h I.V. either continuously or in 6 equally divided doses	4-6	Native valve: 4-week therapy recommended for patients with symptoms ≤3 months in duration; 6-week therapy recommended for patients with symptoms >3 months in duration
With gentamicin sulfate[2]	1 mg/kg I.M. or I.V. every 8 h	4-6	
Ampicillin sodium	12 g/24 h I.V. in 6 equally divided doses	4-6	Prosthetic valve or other prosthetic material: 6-week minimum therapy recommended
With gentamicin sulfate[2]	1 mg/kg I.M. or I.V. every 8 hours	4-6	
			Target gentamicin peak concentration of 3-4 mcg/mL and trough of <1 mcg/mL
Vancomycin hydrochloride[2,3]	30 mg/kg/24 h I.V. in 2 equally divided doses, not to exceed 2 g/24 h unless serum levels are monitored	6	Vancomycin therapy is recommended for patients allergic to β-lactams; cephalosporins are not acceptable alternatives for patients allergic to penicillin
With gentamicin sulfate[2]	1 mg/kg I.M. or I.V. every 8 h	6	

[1]All enterococci causing endocarditis must be tested for antimicrobial susceptibility in order to select optimal therapy. This table is for endocarditis due to penicillin-, gentamicin-, and vancomycin-susceptible enterococci, viridans streptococci with a minimum inhibitory concentration of >0.5 mcg/mL, nutritionally variant viridans streptococci, or prosthetic valve endocarditis caused by viridans streptococci or *Streptococcus bovis*. If penicillin-resistant organisms, use vancomycin/gentamicin regimen above, or may use ampicillin/sulbactam (12 g/24 h in 4 divided doses) with gentamicin for 6 weeks. Antibiotic dosages are for patients with normal renal function. I.V. indicates intravenous; I.M., intramuscular.

[2]For specific dosing adjustment and issues concerning gentamicin (obese patients, relative contraindications), see Table 1 footnotes.

[3]For specific dosing adjustment and issues concerning vancomycin (obese patients, length of infusion), see Table 1 footnotes.

Table 4. Therapy for Native or Prosthetic Valve Endocarditis Due to Enterococci[1] Resistant to Vancomycin, Aminoglycosides, and Penicillin[2]

Antibiotic	Dosage and Route	Duration (wk)	Comments
E. faecium			
Linezolid	1200 mg/24 h P.O./I.V. in 2 divided doses	≥8	May cause severe, but reversible thrombocytopenia, particularly with extended therapy >2 weeks.
Quinupristin-dalfopristin	22.5 mg/kg/24 h I.V. in 3 divided doses	≥8	May cause severe myalgia; not effective against *E. faecalis*.
E. faecalis			
Imipenem/cilastatin	2 g/24 h I.V. in 4 divided doses	≥8	Limited patient experience with these regimens.
With ampicillin sodium	12 g/24 h in 6 divided doses	≥8	
or			
CefTRIAXone sodium	2 g/24 h I.V./I.M.[3] once daily	≥8	Limited patient experience with these regimens.
With ampicillin sodium	12 g/24 h in 6 divided doses	≥8	

[1]Endocarditis caused by the organisms should be treated in consultation with an infectious disease specialist; bacteriologic cure with antimicrobial therapy alone may be <50% and valve replacement may be required.

[2]Dosages recommended are for patients with normal renal function. I.V. = intravenous, I.M. = intramuscular

[3]Patients should be informed that I.M. injection of cefTRIAXone is painful.

Table 5. Therapy for Endocarditis Due to *Staphylococcus* in the Absence of Prosthetic Material[1]

Antibiotic	Dosage and Route	Duration	Comments
Methicillin-Susceptible Staphylococci			
Regimens for non-β-lactam-allergic patients			
Nafcillin sodium or oxacillin sodium	12 g/24 h I.V. in 4-6 divided doses	6 wk	Uncomplicated right side endocarditis may be treated for 2 weeks.
With optional addition of gentamicin sulfate[2]	3 mg/kg/24 h I.M./I.V. in 2-3 divided doses	3-5 d	Benefit of additional aminoglycosides has not been established.
Regimens for β-lactam-allergic patients (nonanaphylactic)			
CeFAZolin (or other first-generation cephalosporins in equivalent dosages)	2 g I.V. every 8 h	6 wk	Cephalosporins should be avoided in patients with immediate-type hypersensitivity to penicillin; if penicillin-sensitive, vancomycin should be used.
With optional addition of gentamicin[2]	3 mg/kg/24 h I.M./I.V. in 2-3 divided doses	3-5 d	Benefit of additional aminoglycosides has not been established.
Methicillin-Resistant Staphylococci			
Vancomycin hydrochloride[3]	30 mg/kg/24 h I.V. in 2 equally divided doses; not to exceed 2 g/24 h unless serum levels are monitored	4-6 wk	Vancomycin therapy is recommended for patients allergic to β-lactams; peak serum concentrations of vancomycin should be obtained 1 h after completion of the infusion and should be in the range of 30-45 mcg/mL and trough of 10-15 mcg/mL for twice-daily dosing.

[1]For treatment of endocarditis due to penicillin-susceptible staphylococci (minimum inhibitory concentration ≤0.1 mcg/mL and non-beta-lactamase producing), aqueous crystalline penicillin G sodium 24 million units/24 h can be used instead of nafcillin or oxacillin. Shorter antibiotic courses have been effective in some drug addicts with right-sided endocarditis due to Staphylococcus aureus. I.V. = intravenous, I.M. = intramuscular

[2]For specific dosing adjustment and issues concerning gentamicin (obese patients, relative contraindications), see Table 1 footnotes.

[3]For specific dosing adjustment and issues concerning vancomycin (obese patients, length of infusion), see Table 1 footnotes.

Table 6. Treatment of Staphylococcal Endocarditis in the Presence of a Prosthetic Valve or Other Prosthetic Material[1]

Antibiotic	Dosage and Route	Duration (wk)	Comments
Methicillin-Susceptible Staphylococci			
Nafcillin sodium or oxacillin sodium[2]	12 g/24 h I.V. in 6 divided doses	≥6	First-generation cephalosporins or vancomycin should be used in patients allergic to β-lactam. Cephalosporins should be avoided in patients with immediate-type hypersensitivity to penicillin or with methicillin-resistant staphylococci.
With rifampin[3]	300 mg P.O./I.V. every 8 h	≥6	–
And with gentamicin sulfate[4,5]	3 mg/kg I.M./I.V. in 2-3 divided doses	2	Aminoglycoside should be administered in close proximity to vancomycin, nafcillin, or oxacillin.
Methicillin-Resistant Staphylococci			
Vancomycin hydrochloride[6]	30 mg/kg/24 h I.V. in 2 equally divided doses, not to exceed 2 g/24 h unless serum levels are monitored	≥6	–
With rifampin[3]	300 mg P.O./I.V. every 8 h	≥6	Rifampin increases the amount of warfarin sodium required for antithrombotic therapy.
And with gentamicin sulfate[4,5]	3 mg/kg I.M./I.V. in 2-3 divided doses	2	Aminoglycoside should be administered in close proximity to vancomycin, nafcillin, or oxacillin.

[1]Dosages recommended are for patients with normal renal function. I.V. = intravenous, I.M. = intramuscular

[2]May use aqueous penicillin G 24 million units/24 h in 4-6 divided doses if strain is penicillin susceptible (MIC ≤0.1 mcg/mL and non-beta-lactamase producing).

[3]Rifampin plays a unique role in the eradication of staphylococcal infection involving prosthetic material; combination therapy is essential to prevent emergence of rifampin resistance.

[4]For a specific dosing adjustment and issues concerning gentamicin (obese patients, relative contraindications), see Table 1 footnotes.

[5]Use during initial 2 weeks.

[6]For specific dosing adjustment and issues concerning vancomycin (obese patients, relative contraindications), see Table 1 footnotes.

Table 7. Therapy for Native or Prosthetic Valve Endocarditis Due to HACEK Microorganisms (*Haemophilus parainfluenzae, Haemophilus aphrophilus, Actinobacillus actinomycetemcomitans, Cardiobacterium hominus, Eikenella corrodens,* and *Kingella kingae*)[1]

Antibiotic	Dosage and Route	Duration (wk)	Comments
CefTRIAXone sodium[2]	2 g once daily I.V. or I.M.[2]	4	Cefotaxime sodium or other third- or fourth-generation cephalosporins may be substituted.
Ampicillin/ sulbactam[3]	12 g/24 h I.V. in 6 equally divided doses	4	
Ciprofloxacin	1000 mg/24 h orally or 800 mg/24 h I.V. in 2 divided doses	4	Use of fluoroquinolone recommended only if patient intolerant to ampicillin or cephalosporins; may substitute fluoroquinolone with equivalent coverage (eg, levofloxacin, moxifloxacin); if prosthetic material involved, treatment duration should be 6 weeks.

[1]Antibiotic dosages are for patients with normal renal function. I.V. = intravenous, I.M. = intramuscular

[2]Patients should be informed that I.M. injection of cefTRIAXone is painful.

[3]Ampicillin should not be used if laboratory tests show β-lactamase production.

REFERENCE

Baddour LM, Wilson WR, Bayer AS, et al, "Infective Endocarditis. Diagnosis, Antimicrobial Therapy, and Management of Complications. A Statement for Healthcare Professionals from the Committee on Rheumatic Fever, Endocarditis, and Kawasaki Disease, Council on Cardiovascular Disease in the Young, and the Councils on Clinical Cardiology, Stroke, and Cardiovascular Surgery and Anesthesia, American Heart Association," *Circulation*, 2005, 111(23): e394-434.

ANTIMICROBIAL DRUGS OF CHOICE

Empirical treatment of some common infecting organisms is listed below. These recommendations are based on results of susceptibility studies, clinical trials, and the opinions of *Medical Letter* consultants. The site and severity of the infection, pharmacokinetic characteristics of antibiotics, local resistance patterns, potential drug interactions, and specific patient factors should be taken into account in choosing an appropriate regimen.

Infecting Organism	Drug of First Choice	Alternative Drugs
GRAM-POSITIVE COCCI		
Enterococcus spp.[1]		
endocarditis or other severe infection	Penicillin G or ampicillin + gentamicin or streptomycin[2]	Vancomycin + gentamicin or streptomycin[2]; linezolid[3]; DAPTOmycin[4]; quinupristin/dalfopristin[5]
uncomplicated urinary tract infection	Ampicillin or amoxicillin	Nitrofurantoin; a fluoroquinolone[6]; fosfomycin
Staphylococcus aureus or *epidermidis*		
methicillin-susceptible	A penicillinase-resistant penicillin[7]	A cephalosporin[8,9]; vancomycin; imipenem or meropenem; clindamycin; linezolid[3]; DAPTOmycin[4]; a fluoroquinolone[6]
methicillin-resistant[10]	Vancomycin ± gentamicin ± rifampin	Linezolid[3]; DAPTOmycin[4]; tigecycline[11]; a fluoroquinolone[6]; trimethoprim/sulfamethoxazole; quinupristin/dalfopristin; a doxycycline[11]
Streptococcus pyogenes (group A[12]) and groups C and G	Penicillin G or V[13]	Clindamycin; erythromycin; a cephalosporin[8,9]; vancomycin; clarithromycin[14]; azithromycin; linezolid[3]; DAPTOmycin[4]
Streptococcus, group B	Penicillin G or ampicillin	A cephalosporin[8,9]; vancomycin; DAPTOmycin[4]; erythromycin
Streptococcus, viridans group[1]	Penicillin G ± gentamicin	A cephalosporin[8,9]; vancomycin
Streptococcus bovis	Penicillin G	A cephalosporin[8,9]; vancomycin
Streptococcus, anaerobic or *Peptostreptococcus*	Penicillin G	Clindamycin; a cephalosporin[8,9]; vancomycin
Streptococcus pneumoniae[15] (pneumococcus)		
penicillin-susceptible (MIC <0.1 mcg/mL)	Penicillin G or V[13]; amoxicillin	A cephalosporin[8,9]; erythromycin; azithromycin; clarithromycin[14]; levofloxacin, gemifloxacin, or moxifloxacin[6]; meropenem, imipenem, or ertapenem; trimethoprim/sulfamethoxazole; clindamycin; a tetracycline[11]; vancomycin
penicillin-intermediate resistance (MIC 0.1-1 mcg/mL)	Penicillin G I.V. (12 million units/day for adults); cefTRIAXone or cefotaxime	Levofloxacin, gemifloxacin, or moxifloxacin[6]; vancomycin; clindamycin

Infecting Organism	Drug of First Choice	Alternative Drugs
penicillin-high level resistance (MIC ≥2 mcg/mL)	**Meningitis:** Vancomycin + cefTRIAXone or cefotaxime, ± rifampin	
	Other Infections: Vancomycin + cefTRIAXone or cefotaxime; levofloxacin, gemifloxacin, or moxifloxacin[6]	Linezolid[3]; quinupristin/dalfopristin
GRAM-NEGATIVE COCCI		
Moraxella (Branhamella) catarrhalis	Cefuroxime[8]; a fluoroquinolone[6]	Trimethoprim/sulfamethoxazole; amoxicillin/clavulanate; erythromycin; clarithromycin[14]; azithromycin; doxycycline[11]; cefotaxime[8]; ceftizoxime[8]; cefTRIAXone[8]; cefpodoxime[8]
*Neisseria gonorrhoeae (gonococcus)[16]	CefTRIAXone[8]	Cefixime[8]; cefotaxime[8]; penicillin G
Neisseria meningitidis[17] (meningococcus)	Penicillin G	Cefotaxime[8]; ceftizoxime[8]; cefTRIAXone[8]; chloramphenicol[18]; a sulfonamide[19]; a fluoroquinolone[6]
GRAM-POSITIVE BACILLI		
*Bacillus anthracis[20] (anthrax)	Ciprofloxacin[6]; a tetracycline[11]	Penicillin G; amoxicillin; erythromycin; imipenem; clindamycin; levofloxacin[6]
Bacillus cereus, subtilis	Vancomycin	Imipenem or meropenem; clindamycin
Clostridium perfringens[21]	Penicillin G; clindamycin	MetroNIDAZOLE; imipenem, meropenem, or ertapenem; chloramphenicol[18]
Clostridium tetani[22]	MetroNIDAZOLE	Penicillin G; a doxycycline[11]
Clostridium difficile[23]	MetroNIDAZOLE (oral)	Vancomycin (oral)
Corynebacterium diphtheriae[24]	Erythromycin	Penicillin G
Corynebacterium, jeikeium	Vancomycin	Penicillin G + gentamicin; erythromycin
*Erysipelothrix rhusiopathiae	Penicillin G	Erythromycin; a cephalosporin[8,9]; a fluoroquinolone[6]
Listeria monocytogenes	Ampicillin ± gentamicin	Trimethoprim/sulfamethoxazole
ENTERIC GRAM-NEGATIVE BACILLI		
*Campylobacter fetus	A third-generation cephalosporin[9]; gentamicin	Ampicillin; imipenem or meropenem
*Campylobacter jejuni	Erythromycin or azithromycin	A fluoroquinolone[6]; a tetracycline[11]; gentamicin
*Citrobacter freundi	Imipenem or meropenem[25]	A fluoroquinolone[6]; ertapenem; amikacin; doxycycline[11]; trimethoprim/sulfamethoxazole; cefotaxime[8,25], ceftizoxime[8,25], cefTRIAXone[8,25], cefepime[8,25] or cefTAZidime[8,25]
*Enterobacter spp.	Imipenem or meropenem[25]; cefepime[8,25]	Gentamicin, tobramycin or amikacin; trimethoprim/sulfamethoxazole; ciprofloxacin[6]; ticarcillin/clavulanate[26] or piperacillin/tazobactam[26]; aztreonam[25]; cefotaxime, ceftizoxime, cefTRIAXone, or cefTAZidime[8,25]; tigecycline[11]

Infecting Organism	Drug of First Choice	Alternative Drugs
*Escherichia coli[27]	Cefotaxime, cefTRIAXone, cefepime, or cefTAZidime[8,25]	Ampicillin ± gentamicin, tobramycin, or amikacin; gentamicin, tobramycin, or amikacin; amoxicillin/clavulanate; ticarcillin/clavulanate[26]; piperacillin/ tazobactam[26]; ampicillin/sulbactam[25]; trimethoprim/sulfamethoxazole; imipenem, meropenem, or ertapenem[25]; aztreonam[25]; a fluoroquinolone[6]; another cephalosporin[8,9]; tigecycline[11]
*Klebsiella pneumoniae[27]	Cefotaxime, cefTRIAXone, cefepime, or cefTAZidime[8,25]	Imipenem, meropenem, or ertapenem[25]; gentamicin, tobramycin, or amikacin; amoxicillin/clavulanate; ticarcillin/clavulanate[26]; piperacillin/ tazobactam[26]; ampicillin/sulbactam[25]; trimethoprim/sulfamethoxazole; aztreonam[25]; a fluoroquinolone[6]; another cephalosporin[8,9]; tigecycline[11]
*Proteus mirabilis[27]	Ampicillin[28]	A cephalosporin[8,9,25]; ticarcillin/ clavulanate or piperacillin/ tazobactam[26]; gentamicin, tobramycin, or amikacin; trimethoprim/sulfamethoxazole; imipenem, meropenem, or ertapenem[25]; aztreonam[25]; a fluoroquinolone[6]; chloramphenicol[18]
*Proteus, indole-positive (includingProvidencia rettgeri, Morganella morganii, and Proteus vulgaris)	Cefotaxime, cefTRIAXone, cefepime, or cefTAZidime[8,25]	Imipenem, meropenem, or ertapenem[25]; gentamicin, tobramycin, or amikacin; amoxicillin/clavulanate; ticarcillin/clavulanate[26]; piperacillin/ tazobactam[26]; ampicillin/sulbactam[25]; aztreonam[25]; trimethoprim/ sulfamethoxazole; a fluoroquinolone[6]
*Providencia stuartii	Cefotaxime, cefTRIAXone, cefepime, or cefTAZidime[8,25]	Imipenem, meropenem, or ertapenem[25]; ticarcillin/clavulanate[26]; piperacillin/tazobactam[26]; gentamicin, tobramycin, or amikacin; aztreonam[25]; trimethoprim/ sulfamethoxazole; a fluoroquinolone[6]
*Salmonella typhi (typhoid fever)[29]	A fluoroquinolone[6] or cefTRIAXone[8]	Chloramphenicol[18]; trimethoprim/ sulfamethoxazole; ampicillin; amoxicillin; azithromycin[30]
*Other Salmonella spp.[31]	Cefotaxime[8] or cefTRIAXone[8] or a fluoroquinolone[6]	Ampicillin or amoxicillin; trimethoprim/ sulfamethoxazole; chloramphenicol[18]
*Serratia spp.	Imipenem or meropenem[25]	Gentamicin or amikacin; cefotaxime, ceftizoxime, cefTRIAXone, cefepime, or cefTAZidime[8,25]; aztreonam[25]; trimethoprim/sulfamethoxazole; a fluoroquinolone[6]
*Shigella spp.	A fluoroquinolone[6]	Azithromycin; trimethoprim/ sulfamethoxazole; ampicillin; cefTRIAXone[8]
*Yersinia enterocolitica	Trimethoprim/ sulfamethoxazole	A fluoroquinolone[6]; gentamicin, tobramycin, or amikacin; cefotaxime[8]
OTHER GRAM-NEGATIVE BACILLI		
*Acinetobacter	Imipenem or meropenem[25]	An aminoglycoside; ciprofloxacin[6]; trimethoprim/sulfamethoxazole; ticarcillin/clavulanate[26] or piperacillin/ tazobactam[26]; cefTAZidime[25]; doxycycline[11]; sulbactam[32]; colistin[18]
*Aeromonas	Trimethoprim/ sulfamethoxazole	Gentamicin or tobramycin; imipenem; a fluoroquinolone[6]

Infecting Organism	Drug of First Choice	Alternative Drugs
*Bacteroides	MetroNIDAZOLE	Imipenem, meropenem, or ertapenem; amoxicillin/clavulanate; ticarcillin/clavulanate; piperacillin/ tazobactam or ampicillin/sulbactam; chloramphenicol[18]
Bartonella henselae or quintana (bacillary angiomatosis, trench fever)	Erythromycin	Azithromycin; doxycycline[11]
Bartonella henselae[33] (cat scratch bacillus)	Azithromycin	Erythromycin; ciprofloxacin[6]; trimethoprim/sulfamethoxazole; gentamicin; rifampin
Bordetella pertussis (whooping cough)	Azithromycin; erythromycin; clarithromycin[14]	Trimethoprim/sulfamethoxazole
*Brucella spp.	A tetracycline[11] + rifampin	A tetracycline[11] + streptomycin or gentamicin; chloramphenicol[18] ± streptomycin; trimethoprim/ sulfamethoxazole ± gentamicin; ciprofloxacin[6] + rifampin
*Burkholderia cepacia	Trimethoprim/ sulfamethoxazole	CefTAZidime[8]; chloramphenicol[18]; imipenem
Burkholderia (Pseudomonas) mallei (glanders)	Streptomycin + a tetracycline[11]	Streptomycin + chloramphenicol[18]; imipenem
*Burkholderia (Pseudomonas) pseudomallei (melioidosis)	Imipenem; ceftazidime[8]	Meropenem; chloramphenicol[18] + doxycycline[11] + trimethoprim/ sulfamethoxazole; amoxicillin/ clavulanate
Calymmatobacterium granulomatis (granuloma inguinale)	Trimethoprim/ sulfamethoxazole	Doxycycline[11] or ciprofloxacin[6] ± gentamicin
Capnocytophaga canimorsus[34]	Penicillin G	Cefotaxime, ceftizoxime, or cefTRIAXone[8]; imipenem or meropenem; vancomycin; a fluoroquinolone[6]; clindamycin
*Eikenella corrodens	Ampicillin	Erythromycin; azithromycin; clarithromycin[14]; doxycycline[11]; amoxicillin/clavulanate; ampicillin/ sulbactam; cefTRIAXone[8]
*Francisella tularensis (tularemia)[35]	Gentamicin (or streptomycin) + a tetracycline[11]	Chloramphenicol[18]; ciprofloxacin[6]
*Fusobacterium	Penicillin G; metroNIDAZOLE	Clindamycin; cefOXitin[8]; chloramphenicol[18]
Gardnerella vaginalis (bacterial vaginosis)	Oral metroNIDAZOLE[36]	Topical clindamycin or metroNIDAZOLE; oral clindamycin
*Haemophilus ducreyi (chancroid)	Azithromycin or cefTRIAXone	Ciprofloxacin[6] or erythromycin
*Haemophilus influenzae		
meningitis, epiglottitis, arthritis, and other serious infections	Cefotaxime or cefTRIAXone[8]	Cefuroxime[8] (not for meningitis); chloramphenicol[18]; meropenem
upper respiratory infections and bronchitis	Trimethoprim/ sulfamethoxazole	Cefuroxime[8]; amoxicillin/clavulanate; cefuroxime axetil[8]; cefpodoxime[8]; cefaclor[8]; cefotaxime[8]; ceftizoxime[8]; cefTRIAXone[8]; cefixime[8]; doxycycline[11]; clarithromycin[14]; azithromycin; a fluoroquinolone[6]; ampicillin or amoxicillin
*Helicobacter pylori[37]	Proton pump inhibitor[38] + clarithromycin[14] + either amoxicillin or metroNIDAZOLE	Bismuth subsalicylate + metroNIDAZOLE + tetracycline HCl[11] + either a proton pump inhibitor[38] or H2-blocker[38]

Infecting Organism	Drug of First Choice	Alternative Drugs
Legionella species	Azithromycin or a fluoroquinolone[6] ± rifampin	Doxycycline[11] ± rifampin; trimethoprim/sulfamethoxazole; erythromycin
Leptotrichia buccalis	Penicillin G	Doxycycline[11]; clindamycin; erythromycin
Pasteurella multocida	Penicillin G	Doxycycline[11]; a second- or third-generation cephalosporin[8,9]; amoxicillin/clavulanate; ampicillin/sulbactam
*Pseudomonas aeruginosa		
urinary tract infection	Ciprofloxacin[6]	Levofloxacin[6]; piperacillin/tazobactam; cefTAZidime[8]; cefepime[8]; imipenem or meropenem; aztreonam; tobramycin; gentamicin or amikacin
other infections	Piperacillin/tazobactam or ticarcillin/clavulanate, **plus/minus** tobramycin, gentamicin, or amikacin[39]	CefTAZidime[8]; ciprofloxacin[6]; imipenem or meropenem; aztreonam; cefepime[8] **plus/minus** tobramycin, gentamicin, or amikacin
Spirillum minus (rat bite fever)	Penicillin G	Doxycycline[11]; streptomycin[18]
*Stenotrophomonas maltophilia	Trimethoprim/sulfamethoxazole	Ticarcillin/clavulanate[26]; minocycline[11]; a fluoroquinolone[6]; tigecycline[11]
Streptobacillus moniliformis (rat bite fever, Haverhill fever)	Penicillin G	Doxycycline[11]; streptomycin[18]
Vibrio cholerae (cholera)[40]	A tetracycline[11]	A fluoroquinolone[6]; trimethoprim/sulfamethoxazole
Vibrio vulnificus	A tetracycline[11]	Cefotaxime[8]; ciprofloxacin[14]
Yersinia pestis (plague)	Streptomycin ± a tetracycline[11]	Chloramphenicol[18]; gentamicin; trimethoprim/sulfamethoxazole; ciprofloxacin[14]
MYCOBACTERIA		
*Mycobacterium tuberculosis[41]	Isoniazid + rifampin + pyrazinamide ± ethambutol or streptomycin[18]	A fluoroquinolone[6]; cycloserine[18]; capreomycin[18] or kanamycin[18] or amikacin[18]; ethionamide[18]; para-aminosalicylic acid[18]
*Mycobacterium kansasii[41]	Isoniazid + rifampin ± ethambutol or streptomycin[18]	Clarithromycin[14] or azithromycin; ethionamide[18]; cycloserine[18]
*Mycobacterium avium complex		
treatment	Clarithromycin[14] or azithromycin + ethambutol ± rifabutin	Ciprofloxacin[6]; amikacin[18]
prophylaxis	Clarithromycin[14] or azithromycin ± rifabutin	
*Mycobacterium fortuitum/chelonae[41] complex	Amikacin + clarithromycin[14]	CefOXitin[8]; rifampin; a sulfonamide; doxycycline[11]; ethambutol; linezolid[3]
Mycobacterium marinum (balnei)[42]	Minocycline[11]	Trimethoprim/sulfamethoxazole; rifampin; clarithromycin[14]; doxycycline[11]
Mycobacterium leprae (leprosy)	Dapsone + rifampin ± clofazimine	Minocycline[11]; ofloxacin[6]; clarithromycin[14]

Infecting Organism	Drug of First Choice	Alternative Drugs
ACTINOMYCETES		
Actinomyces israelii (actinomycosis)	Penicillin G	Doxycycline[11]; erythromycin; clindamycin
Nocardia	Trimethoprim/ sulfamethoxazole	Sulfisoxazole; amikacin[18]; a tetracycline[11]; cefTRIAXone; imipenem or meropenem; cycloserine[18]; linezolid[3]
*Rhodococcus equi	Vancomycin ± a fluoroquinolone,[6] rifampin, imipenem, or meropenem; amikacin	Erythromycin
Tropheryma whippelii[43] (Whipple's disease)	Trimethoprim/ sulfamethoxazole	Penicillin G; a tetracycline[11]; cefTRIAXone
CHLAMYDIAE		
Chlamydia trachomatis		
trachoma	Azithromycin	Doxycycline[11]; a sulfonamide (topical plus oral)
inclusion conjunctivitis	Erythromycin (oral or I.V.)	A sulfonamide
pneumonia	Erythromycin	A sulfonamide
urethritis, cervicitis	Azithromycin or doxycycline[11]	Erythromycin; ofloxacin[6]; amoxicillin
lymphogranuloma venereum	A tetracycline[11]	Erythromycin
Chlamydophilia (formerly *Chlamydia*) *pneumoniae*	Erythromycin; a tetracycline[11]; clarithromycin[14] or azithromycin	A fluoroquinolone[6]
Chlamydophilia (formerly *Chlamydia*) *psittaci* (psittacosis, ornithosis)	A tetracycline[11]	Chloramphenicol[18]
EHRLICHIA		
Anaplasma phagocytophilum (formerly *Ehrlichia phagocytophila*)	Doxycycline[11]	Rifampin
Ehrlichia chaffeensis	Doxycycline[11]	Chloramphenicol[18]
Ehrlichia ewingii	Doxycycline[11]	
MYCOPLASMA		
Mycoplasma pneumoniae	Erythromycin; a tetracycline[11]; clarithromycin[14] or azithromycin	A fluoroquinolone[6]
Ureaplasma urealyticum	Azithromycin	Erythromycin; a tetracycline[11]; clarithromycin[14]; ofloxacin[6]
RICKETTSIOSES		
Rickettsia rickettsii (Rocky Mountain spotted fever)	Doxycycline[11]	A fluoroquinolone[6]; chloramphenicol[18]
Rickettsia typhi (endemic typhus – murine)	Doxycycline[11]	A fluoroquinolone[6]; chloramphenicol[18]
Rickettsia prowazekii (epidemic typhus – louse-borne)	Doxycycline[11]	A fluoroquinolone[6]; chloramphenicol[18]
Orientia tsutsugamushi (scrub typhus)	Doxycycline[11]	A fluoroquinolone[6]; chloramphenicol[18]
Coxiella burnetii (Q fever)	Doxycycline[11]	A fluoroquinolone[6]; chloramphenicol[18]

Infecting Organism	Drug of First Choice	Alternative Drugs
SPIROCHETES		
Borrelia burgdorferi (Lyme disease)[44]	Doxycycline[11]; amoxicillin; cefuroxime axetil[8]	CefTRIAXone[8]; cefotaxime[8]; penicillin G; azithromycin; clarithromycin[14]
Borrelia recurrentis (relapsing fever)	A tetracycline[11]	Penicillin G; erythromycin
Leptospira	Penicillin G	Doxycycline[11]; cefTRIAXone[8,45]
Treponema pallidum (syphilis)	Penicillin G[13]	Doxycycline[11]; cefTRIAXone[8]
Treponema pertenue (yaws)	Penicillin G	Doxycycline[11]

*Resistance may be a problem; susceptibility tests should be used to guide therapy.

[1] Disk sensitivity testing may not provide adequate information; beta-lactamase assays, "E" tests, and dilution tests for susceptibility should be used in serious infections.

[2] Aminoglycoside resistance is increasingly common among enterococci; treatment options include ampicillin 2 g I.V. every 4 hours, continuous infusion of ampicillin, a combination of ampicillin plus a fluoroquinolone, or a combination of ampicillin, imipenem, and vancomycin.

[3] Reversible bone marrow suppression has occurred, especially with therapy for more than 2 weeks. Linezolid is an MAO inhibitor and can interact with serotonergic and adrenergic drugs and with tyramine-containing foods (Taylor JJ, Wilson JW, and Estes LL, "Linezolid and Serotonergic Drug Interactions: A Retrospective Survey," *Clin Infect Dis*, 2006, 43(2):180-7).

[4] Not recommended for use in children or pregnant women.

[5] Quinupristin/dalfopristin is not active against *Enterococcus faecalis*.

[6] Among the fluoroquinolones, levofloxacin, gemifloxacin, and moxifloxacin have excellent *in vitro* activity against *S. pneumoniae*, including penicillin- and cephalosporin-resistant strains. Levofloxacin, gemifloxacin, and moxifloxacin also have good activity against many strains of *S. aureus*, but resistance has become frequent among methicillin-resistant strains. Gemifloxacin is associated with a high rate of rash; other fluoroquinolones are preferred. Ciprofloxacin has the greatest activity against *Pseudomonas aeruginosa*. For urinary tract infections, norfloxacin can be used. For tuberculosis, levofloxacin, ofloxacin, ciprofloxacin, or moxifloxacin could be used ("Drugs for Tuberculosis," *Treat Guidel Med Lett*, 2007, 5(55):15-22). Ciprofloxacin, ofloxacin, levofloxacin, and moxifloxacin are available for I.V. use. None of these agents is recommended for use in children or pregnant women.

[7] For oral use against staphylococci, cloxacillin or dicloxacillin is preferred; for severe infections, a parenteral formulation (nafcillin or oxacillin) should be used. Ampicillin, amoxicillin, carbenicillin, ticarcillin, and piperacillin are not effective against penicillinase-producing staphylococci. The combinations of clavulanate with amoxicillin or ticarcillin, sulbactam with ampicillin, and tazobactam with piperacillin may be active against these organisms.

[8] Cephalosporins have been used as alternatives to penicillins in patients allergic to penicillins, but such patients may also have allergic reactions to cephalosporins.

[9] For parenteral treatment of staphylococcal or nonenterococcal streptococcal infections, a first-generation cephalosporin such as ceFAZolin can be used. For oral therapy, cephalexin or cephradine can be used. The second-generation cephalosporins cefamandole, cefprozil, cefuroxime, cefoTEtan, cefOXitin, and loracarbef are more active than the first-generation drugs against gram-negative bacteria. CefoTEtan and cefamandole are no longer available. Cefuroxime is active against ampicillin-resistant strains of *H. influenzae*. CefOXitin is the most active of the cephalosporins against *B. fragilis*. The third-generation cephalosporins cefotaxime, cefoperazone, ceftizoxime, cefTRIAXone, and cefTAZidime, and the fourth-generation cefepime have greater activity than the second-generation drugs against enteric gram-negative bacilli. CefTAZidime has poor activity against many gram-positive cocci and anaerobes, and ceftizoxime has poor activity against penicillin-resistant *S. pneumoniae*. Cefepime has *in vitro* activity against gram-positive cocci similar to cefotaxime and cefTRIAXone and somewhat greater activity against enteric gram-negative bacilli. The activity of cefepime against *P. aeruginosa* is similar to that of cefTAZidime. Cefixime, cefpodoxime, cefdinir, ceftibuten, and cefditoren are oral cephalosporins with more activity than second-generation cephalosporins against facultative gram-negative bacilli; they have no useful activity against anaerobes or *P. aeruginosa*, and cefixime and ceftibuten have no useful activity against staphylococci. With the exception of cefoperazone (which can cause bleeding), cefTAZidime, and cefepime, the activity of all currently available cephalosporins against *P. aeruginosa* is poor or inconsistent.

[10] Many strains of coagulase-positive and coagulase-negative staphylococci are resistant to penicillinase-resistant penicillins; these strains are also resistant to cephalosporins and carbapenems and are often resistant to fluoroquinolones, trimethoprim/sulfamethoxazole, and clindamycin. Community-acquired MRSA often is susceptible to clindamycin and trimethoprim/sulfamethoxazole.

[11] Tetracyclines and tigecycline, a derivative of minocycline, are generally not recommended for pregnant women or children <8 years of age.

[12] For serious soft-tissue infection due to group A streptococci, clindamycin may be more effective than penicillin. Group A streptococci may, however, be resistant to clindamycin; therefore, some *Medical Letter* consultants suggest using both clindamycin and penicillin, with or without I.V. immune globulin, to treat serious soft-tissue infections. Surgical debridement is usually needed for necrotizing soft tissue infections due to group A streptococci. Group A streptococci may also be resistant to erythromycin, azithromycin, and clarithromycin.

[13] Penicillin V (or amoxicillin) is preferred for oral treatment of infections caused by nonpenicillinase-producing streptococci. For initial therapy of severe infections, penicillin G, administered parenterally, is the first choice. For somewhat longer action in less severe infections due to group A streptococci, pneumococci, or *Treponema pallidum*, procaine penicillin G, an I.M. formulation, can be given once or twice daily, but is seldom used now. Benzathine penicillin G, a slowly absorbed preparation, is usually given in a single monthly injection for prophylaxis of rheumatic fever, once for treatment of group A streptococcal pharyngitis and once or more for treatment of syphilis.

[14] Not recommended for use in pregnancy.

[15] Some strains of *S. pneumoniae* are resistant to erythromycin, clindamycin, trimethoprim/sulfamethoxazole, clarithromycin, azithromycin, and chloramphenicol, and resistance to the newer fluoroquinolones is rare but increasing. Nearly all strains tested so far are susceptible to linezolid and quinupristin/dalfopristin *in vitro*.

[16]Patients with gonorrhea should be treated presumptively for coinfection with *C. trachomatis* with azithromycin or doxycycline. Fluoroquinolones are no longer recommended for treatment (Centers for Disease Control and Prevention [CDC], "Update to CDC's Sexually Transmitted Diseases Treatment Guidelines, 2006: Fluoroquinolones No Longer Recommended for Treatment of Gonococcal Infections," *MMWR Morb Mortal Wkly Rep*, 2007, 56 (14):332-6).

[17]Rare strains of *N. meningitidis* are resistant or relatively resistant to penicillin. A fluoroquinolone or rifampin is recommended for prophylaxis after close contact with infected patients.

[18]Because of the possibility of serious adverse effects, this drug should be used only for severe infections when less hazardous drugs are ineffective.

[19]Sulfonamide-resistant strains are frequent in the U.S; sulfonamides should be used only when susceptibility is established by susceptibility tests.

[20]For postexposure prophylaxis, ciprofloxacin for 4 weeks if given with vaccination, and 60 days if not given with vaccination, might prevent disease; if the strain is susceptible, doxycycline is an alternative (Bartlett JG, Inglesby TV Jr, and Borio L, "Management of Anthrax," *Clin Infect Dis*, 2002, 35(7):851-8).

[21]Debridement is primary. Large doses of penicillin G are required. Hyperbaric oxygen therapy may be a useful adjunct to surgical debridement in management of the spreading, necrotizing type of infection.

[22]For prophylaxis, a tetanus toxoid booster and, for some patients, tetanus immune globulin (human) are required.

[23]In order to decrease the emergence of vancomycin-resistant enterococci in hospitals and to reduce costs, most clinicians now recommend use of metronidazole first in treatment of patients with *C. difficile* associated diarrhea, with oral vancomycin used only for seriously ill patients, or those who do not respond to metronidazole. Patients who are unable to take oral medications can be treated with I.V. metronidazole.

[24]Antitoxin is primary; antimicrobials are used only to halt further toxin production and to prevent the carrier state.

[25]In severely ill patients, most *Medical Letter* consultants would add gentamicin, tobramycin, or amikacin.

[26]In severely ill patients, most *Medical Letter* consultants would add gentamicin, tobramycin, or amikacin (but see footnote 39).

[27]For an acute, uncomplicated urinary tract infection, before the infecting organism is known, the drug of first choice is trimethoprim/sulfamethoxazole. Antibacterial treatment of gastroenteritis due to *E. coli* O157:H7 may increase toxin release and risk of hemolytic uremic syndrome and is not recommended (Centers for Disease Control and Prevention [CDC], "Ongoing Multistate Outbreak of Escherichia coli Serotype O157:H7 Infections Associated With Consumption of Fresh Spinach–United States, September 2006," *MMWR Morb Mortal Wkly Rep*, 2006, 55 (38):1045-6).

[28]Large doses (≥6 g/day) are usually necessary for systemic infections. In severely ill patients, some *Medical Letter* consultants would add gentamicin, tobramycin, or amikacin.

[29]A fluoroquinolone or amoxicillin is the drug of choice for *S. typhi* carriers (Parry CM, Hien TT, Dougan G, "Typhoid Fever," *N Engl J Med*, 2002, 347(22):1770-82).

[30]Frenck RW Jr, Nakhla I, Sultan Y, et al, "Azithromycin Versus Ceftriaxone for the Treatment of Uncomplicated Typhoid Fever in Children," *Clin Infect Dis*, 2000, 31(5):1134-8.

[31]Most cases of *Salmonella* gastroenteritis subside spontaneously without antimicrobial therapy. Immunosuppressed patients, young children, and the elderly may benefit the most from antibacterials.

[32]Sulbactam may be useful to treat multidrug resistant *Acinetobacter*. It is only available in combination with ampicillin as Unasyn®. *Medical Letter* consultants recommend 3 g I.V. every 4 hours.

[33]Role of antibiotics is not clear (Conrad DA, "Treatment of Cat-Scratch Disease," *Curr Opin Pediatr*, 2001, 13(1):56-9).

[34]Pers C, Gahrn-Hansen B, Frederiksen W, et al, "*Capnocytophaga canimorsus* Septicemia in Denmark, 1982-1995: Review of 39 Cases," *Clin Infect Dis*, 1996, 23(1):71-5.

[35]For postexposure prophylaxis, doxycycline or ciprofloxacin begun during the incubation period and continued for 14 days might prevent disease ("Drugs and Vaccines for Biological Weapons," *Med Lett Drugs Ther*, 2001, 43 (1115):87-9).

[36]MetroNIDAZOLE is effective for bacterial vaginosis even though it is not usually active *in vitro* against *Gardnerella*.

[37]Eradication of *H. pylori* with various antibacterial combinations, given concurrently with a proton pump inhibitor or H_2-blocker, has led to rapid healing of active peptic ulcers and low recurrence rates.

[38]Proton pump inhibitors available in the U.S. are omeprazole (PriLOSEC® and others), lansoprazole (Prevacid®), pantoprazole (Protonix®), esomeprazole (Nexium®), and rabeprazole (Aciphex®). Available H_2-blockers include cimetidine (Tagamet® and others), famotidine (Pepcid® and others), nizatidine (Axid® and others), and ranitidine (Zantac® and others).

[39]Neither gentamicin, tobramycin, netilmicin, or amikacin should be mixed in the same bottle with carbenicillin, ticarcillin, mezlocillin, or piperacillin for I.V. administration. When used in high doses or in patients with renal impairment, these penicillins may inactivate the aminoglycosides.

[40]Antibiotic therapy is an adjunct to and not a substitute for prompt fluid and electrolyte replacement.

[41]Multidrug regimens are necessary for successful treatment. Drugs listed as alternatives are substitutions for primary regimens and are meant to be used in combination. For additional treatment recommendations for tuberculosis, see "Drugs for Tuberculosis," *Treat Guidel Med Lett*, 2007, 5(55):15-22.

[42]Most infections are self-limited without drug treatment.

[43]Fenollar F, Puéchal X, and Raoult D, "Whipple's Disease," *N Engl J Med*, 2007, 356(1):55-66.

[44]For treatment of erythema migrans, uncomplicated facial nerve palsy, mild cardiac disease, and arthritis, oral therapy is satisfactory; for other neurologic or more serious cardiac disease, parenteral therapy with cefTRIAXone, cefotaxime, or penicillin G is recommended. For recurrent arthritis after an oral regimen, another course of oral therapy or a parenteral drug may be given ("Treatment of Lyme Disease," *Med Lett Drugs Ther*, 2005, 47 (1209):41-3).

[45]Vinetz JM, "A Mountain Out of a Molehill: Do We Treat Acute Leptospirosis, and If So, With What?" *Clin Infect Dis*, 2003, 36(12):1514-5; Panaphut T, Domrongkitchaiporn S, Vibhagool A, et al, "CefTRIAXone Compared With Sodium Penicillin G for Treatment of Severe Leptospirosis," *Clin Infect Dis*, 2003, 36(12):1507-13.

Reprinted with permission from "Choice of Antibacterial Drugs," *Treat Guidel Med Lett*, 2007, 5(57):33-50.

COMMUNITY-ACQUIRED PNEUMONIA IN ADULTS

Alternative methods exist to facilitate the objective rating of disease severity in community-acquired pneumonia patients in order to guide appropriate site of care and aggressiveness of treatment. The first option, the Pneumonia Severity Index (PSI) was derived from the Pneumonia Patient Outcomes Research Team (PORT). This is a well-validated instrument which stratifies patients based on risk of mortality; however, calculation of the patient's score requires assessment of 19 variables. The second method is referred to as the "Confusion, Uremia, Respiratory rate, Blood pressure, and age >65 years (CURB-65)" score. This system has fewer variables to evaluate and focuses more on assessment of disease severity, but is less well validated. In either case, these measures should not be used in exclusion to appropriate clinical judgement.

PNEUMONIA SEVERITY INDEX (PSI)

The initial site of treatment should be based on a 3-step process:

1. Assessment of pre-existing conditions that compromise safety of home care

2. Calculation of the Pneumonia Severity Index with recommendation for home care for risk classes I, II, and III, and

3. Clinical judgment

Algorithm

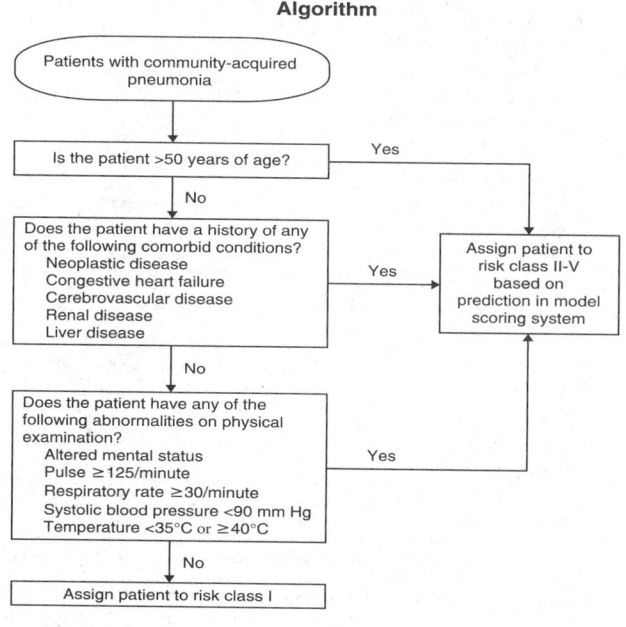

Stratification of Risk Score

Risk	Risk Class	Based on
	I	Algorithm
Low	II	≤70 total points
	III	71-90 total points
Moderate	IV	91-130 total points
High	V	>130 total points

Risk-Class Mortality Rates for Patients With Pneumonia

Risk Class	No. of Points	Validation Cohort		Recommended Site of Care
		No. of Patients	Mortality (%)	
I	No predictors	3034	0.1	Outpatient
II	≤70	5778	0.6	Outpatient
III	71-90	6790	2.8	Outpatient or brief inpatient
IV	91-130	13,104	8.2	Inpatient
V	>130	9333	29.2	Inpatient

Scoring System: Assignment to Risk Classes II-V

Patient Characteristic	Points Assigned[1]
Demographic factors	
Age	
Male	No. of years
Female	No. of years -10
Nursing home resident	+10
Comorbid illnesses	
Neoplastic disease[2]	+30
Liver disease[3]	+20
Congestive heart failure[4]	+10
Cerebrovascular disease[5]	+10
Renal disease[6]	+10
Physical examination findings	
Altered mental status[7]	+20
Respiratory rate >30 breaths/minute	+20
Systolic blood pressure <90 mm Hg	+20
Temperature <35°C or >40°C	+15
Pulse >125 beats/minute	+10
Laboratory or radiographic findings	
Arterial pH <7.35	+30
BUN >30 mg/dL	+20
Sodium <130 mEq/L	+20
Glucose >250 mg/dL	+10
Hematocrit <30%	+10
pO$_2$ <60 mm Hg[8]	+10
Pleural effusion	+10

[1]A total point score for a given patient is obtained by adding the patient's age in years (age -10, for females) and the points for each applicable patient characteristic.

[2]Any cancer, except basal or squamous cell cancer of the skin, that was active at the time of presentation or diagnosed within 1 year of presentation

[3]A clinical or histologic diagnosis of cirrhosis or other form of chronic liver disease, such as chronic active hepatitis

[4]Systolic or diastolic ventricular dysfunction documented by history and physical examination, as well as chest radiography, echocardiography, Muga scanning, or left ventriculography

[5]A clinical diagnosis of stroke, transient ischemic attack, or stroke documented by MRI or computed axial tomography

[6]A history of chronic renal disease or abnormal blood urea nitrogen (BUN) and creatinine values documented in the medical record

[7]Disorientation (to person, place, or time; not known to be chronic), stupor, or coma

[8]In the Pneumonia Patient Outcome Research Team cohort study, an oxygen saturation value <90% on pulse oximetry or intubation before admission was also considered abnormal.

CONFUSION, UREMIA, RESPIRATORY RATE, BLOOD PRESSURE, AND AGE >65 YEARS (CURB-65)

Risk factors:

1. Presence of confusion (based on specific tests or noted disorientation to people, place, or time)

2. Blood urea nitrogen (BUN) of >7mmol/L (20 mg/dL)

3. Respiratory rate >30 breaths/minute

4. Systolic blood pressure <90 mmHg or diastolic <60 mmHg

5. Age >65 years

Number of Risk Factors	30-Day Mortality Risk (%)
0	0.7
1	2.1
2	9.2
3	14.5
4	40
5	57

Scoring:

0-1 risk factors: Treat as outpatient.

2 risk factors: Treat as inpatient.

3-5 risk factors: Treat as inpatient; likely requires more aggressive management, possibly ICU.

Epidemiological Conditions Related to Specific Pathogens in Patients With Selected Community-Acquired Pneumonia

Condition	Commonly Encountered Pathogens
Alcoholism	*Streptococcus pneumoniae*, anaerobes
COPD and/or smoker	*S. pneumoniae, Haemophilus influenzae, Moraxella catarrhalis, Legionella* species
Nursing home residency	*S. pneumoniae*, gram-negative bacilli, *H. influenzae, Staphylococcus aureus*, anaerobes, *Chlamydia pneumoniae*
Poor dental hygiene	Anaerobes
Epidemic Legionnaires' disease	*Legionella* species
Exposure to bats or soil enriched with bird droppings	*Histoplasma capsulatum*
Exposure to birds	*Chlamydia psittaci*
Exposure to rabbits	*Francisella tularensis*
HIV infection (early stage)	*S. pneumoniae, H. influenzae, Mycobacterium tuberculosis*
HIV infection (late stage)	Above plus *P. carinii, Cryptococcus, Histoplasma* species
Travel to southwestern United States	*Coccidioides* species
Exposure to farm animals or parturient cats	*Coxiella burnetii* (Q fever)
Influenza active in community	Influenza, *S. pneumoniae, S. aureus, Streptococcus pyogenes, H. influenzae*
Suspected large-volume aspiration	Anaerobes (chemical pneumonitis, obstruction)
Structural disease of the lung (bronchiectasis, cystic fibrosis, etc)	*Pseudomonas aeruginosa, Burkholderia (Pseudomonas) cepacia, S. aureus*
Injection drug use	*S. aureus*, anaerobes, *M. tuberculosis, S. pneumoniae*
Airway obstruction	Anaerobes, *S. pneumoniae, H. influenzae, S. aureus*

COPD = chronic obstructive pulmonary disease

Initial Empiric Therapy for Suspected Bacterial Community-Acquired Pneumonia (CAP) in Immunocompetent Adults

Patient Variable	Preferred Treatment Options
Outpatient	
Previously healthy	
No recent antibiotic therapy or risk for DRSP	A macrolide[1] or doxycycline
Comorbidities[2]; recent antibiotic therapy[3]; risk factors for DRSP[4]	A respiratory fluoroquinolone[5] alone, or an advanced macrolide[6] plus high-dose amoxicillin,[7] high-dose amoxicillin-clavulanate,[8] cefpodoxime, cefTRIAXone, or cefuroxime
Suspected aspiration with infection	Amoxicillin-clavulanate or clindamycin
Influenza with bacterial superinfection	Antiviral agent oseltamivir or zanamivir, plus a cefotaxime or cefTRIAXone or a respiratory fluoroquinolone[5]
Inpatient	
Non-ICU	A respiratory fluoroquinolone alone or macrolide plus a β-lactam[9]
ICU	
Pseudomonas infection is not an issue	Cefotaxime, cefTRIAXone, or ampicillin-sulbactam plus either azithromycin or a respiratory fluoroquinolone[5]
Pseudomonas infection is not an issue but patient has a β-lactam allergy	A respiratory fluoroquinolone,[5] with aztreonam
Pseudomonas infection is an issue[10]	Either (1) an antipseudomonal agent[11] plus ciprofloxacin or levofloxacin, or (2) an antipseudomonal agent plus an aminoglycoside[12] plus a respiratory fluoroquinolone[5] or azithromycin
Pseudomonas infection is an issue but the patient has a β-lactam allergy	Substitute aztreonam for any β-lactam antipseudomonal agent[11]
Nursing home	
Receiving treatment in nursing home	A respiratory fluoroquinolone[5] alone or amoxicillin-clavulanate plus an advanced macrolide
Suspicion or MRSA	Add vancomycin or linezolid to any suggested regimens

DRSP = drug-resistant *Streptococcus pneumoniae*, ICU = intensive care unit

[1]Erythromycin, azithromycin, or clarithromycin

[2]Chronic heart, lung, liver, and/or renal disease; diabetes; malignancy; or immunosuppressive medication and/or conditions

[3]That is, the patient was given a course of antibiotic(s) for treatment of any infection within the past 3 months, excluding the current episode of infection. Such treatment is a risk factor for drug-resistant *Streptococcus pneumoniae* and possibly for infection with gram-negative bacilli. Depending on the class of antibiotics recently given, one or other of the suggested options may be selected. Recent use of a fluoroquinolone should dictate selection of a nonfluoroquinolone regimen, and vice versa.

[4]Risk factors for β-lactam-resistant *S. pneumoniae* include age <2 or >65 years, recent antimicrobial therapy (within previous 3 months, and especially to repeated courses of same antibiotic class), alcoholism, comorbidities, immunosuppressive illness or therapy, and exposure to child care centers.

[5]Moxifloxacin, levofloxacin, or gemifloxacin

[6]Azithromycin or clarithromycin

[7]Dosage: 1 g P.O. 3 times/day

[8]Dosage: 2 g P.O. twice daily

[9]Cefotaxime, cefTRIAXone, ampicillin (or ampicillin-sulbactam), or ertapenem; ertapenem was recently approved for such use (in once-daily parenteral treatment), but there is still limited experience thus far. **Note:** The 2007 CAP guidelines excluded ampicillin-sulbactam in favor of the single agent without the lactamase inhibitor. While this may be useful in specific situations, the prevalence of beta-lactamase-producing *H. influenzae* should be a concern, and thus the use of ampicillin-sulbactam may be more appropriate for empiric use.

[10]The antipseudomonal agents chosen reflect this concern. Risk factors for *Pseudomonas* infection include severe structural lung disease (eg, bronchiectasis), and recent antibiotic therapy or stay in hospital (especially in the ICU). For patients with CAP in the ICU, coverage for *S. pneumoniae* and *Legionella* species must always be assured. Piperacillin-tazobactam, imipenem, meropenem, and cefepime are excellent β-lactams and are adequate for most *S. pneumoniae* and *Haemophilus influenzae* infections. They may be preferred when there is concern for relatively unusual CAP pathogens, such as *Pseudomonas aeruginosa*, *Klebsiella* species, and other gram-negative bacteria.

[11]Piperacillin-tazobactam, imipenem, meropenem, or cefepime

[12]Data suggest that elderly patients receiving aminoglycosides have worse outcomes.

REFERENCES

Bartlett JG, Breiman RF, Mandell LA, et al, "Community-Acquired Pneumonia in Adults: Guidelines for Management. The Infectious Diseases Society of America," *Clin Infect Dis*, 1998, 26(4):811-38.

Mandell LA, Bartlett JG, Dowell SF, et al, "Update of Practice Guidelines for the Management of Community-Acquired Pneumonia in Immunocompetent Adults," *Clin Infect Dis*, 2003, 37(11):1405-33.

Mandell LA, Wunderink RG, Anzueto A, et al, "Infectious Diseases Society of America/American Thoracic Society Consensus Guidelines on the Management of Community-Acquired Pneumonia in Adults," *Clin Infect Dis*, 2007, 44 (Suppl 2):S27-72.

PREVENTION OF INFECTIVE ENDOCARDITIS

Recommendations by the American Heart Association
(*Circulation*, 2007, 116(15):1736-54.)

Consensus Process – The recommendations were formulated by a writing group under the auspices of the American Heart Association (AHA), and included representation from the Infectious Diseases Society of America (IDSA), the American Academy of Pediatrics (AAP), and the American Dental Association (ADA). Additionally, input was received from both national and international experts on infective endocarditis (IE). These guidelines are based on expert interpretation and review of scientific literature from 1950 through 2006. The consensus statement was subsequently reviewed by outside experts not affiliated with the writing group and by the Science Advisory and Coordinating Committee of the American Heart Association. These guidelines are meant to aid practitioners but are not intended as the standard of care or as a substitute for clinical judgment.

Significant change from the previous 1997 guidelines – The previously published guidelines identified a broad range of cardiac conditions thought to predispose patients to a higher risk of IE. The document stratified these conditions into high-, moderate-, and low-risk categories, based on the likelihood of developing IE. The subsequent recommendations for prophylaxis were based on this classification, in conjunction with specification of numerous invasive procedures which were assumed to confer a higher risk of bacteremia, and therefore a higher risk of endocarditis. However, it is the consensus of the current writing group that existing data fail to show a clear link between many of these procedures, preexisting cardiovascular condition and IE. In the case of dental procedures, it was determined that the cumulative lifetime risk of developing bacteremia as a result of normal hygiene measures (eg, teeth brushing, flossing) vastly exceeded the risk associated with many of the procedures for which prophylaxis was previously recommended. Similarly, the writing group estimated that the absolute risk of developing IE as a result of dental procedures in patients with preexisting cardiac conditions was quite low, and there was little evidence to support the value of prophylactic antimicrobial efficacy in these cases.

In a major departure from the former recommendations, the current guidelines have been greatly simplified to place a much greater emphasis on a very limited number of underlying cardiac conditions (see below). These specific conditions have been associated with the highest risk of adverse outcomes due to IE. Patients should receive IE prophylaxis only if they are undergoing certain invasive procedures (see Table 1 on next page) and have one of the underlying cardiovascular conditions specified below.

Common situations for which routine prophylaxis was previously, but no longer recommended, include mitral valve prolapse, general dental cleanings and local anesthetic administration (noninfected tissue), and bronchoscopy (see Table 1 on next page).

Specific cardiac conditions for which IE antibiotic prophylaxis is recommended:

- Previous infective endocarditis

- Prosthetic cardiac valve or prosthetic material used for cardiac valve repair

- Cardiac transplantation patients who develop valvulopathy

- Congenital heart disease (CHD), only under the following conditions:

    - Unrepaired cyanotic CHD, including palliative shunts and conduits

    - Completely repaired defects (with prosthetic materials/devices), regardless of method of repair, within the first 6 months after the procedure

    - Repaired CHD with residual defects at or adjacent to the site of repair

PREVENTION OF INFECTIVE ENDOCARDITIS

Table 1. Guidance for Use of Prophylactic Antibiotic Therapy Based on Procedure or Condition[1]

Location of Procedure	Prophylaxis Recommended	Prophylaxis NOT Recommended
Dental	All invasive manipulations of the gingival or periapical region or perforation of oral mucosa	Anesthetic injections (through noninfected tissue), radiographs, placement/adjustment/removal prosthodontic/orthodontic appliances or brackets, shedding of deciduous teeth, trauma-induced bleeding from lips, gums, or oral mucosa
Respiratory tract	Biopsy/incision of respiratory mucosa (eg, tonsillectomy/adenoidectomy); drainage of abscess or empyema[2]	Bronchoscopy (unless incision of mucosa required)
Gastrointestinal (GI) or genitourinary (GU) tract	Established GI/GU infection or prevention of infectious sequelae[3]; elective cystoscopy or other urinary tract procedure with established enterococci infection/colonization[3,4]	Routine diagnostic procedures, including esophagogastroduodenoscopy or colonoscopy in the absence of active infection; vaginal delivery and hysterectomy
Skin, skin structure, or musculoskeletal	Any surgical procedure involving infected tissue	Procedures conducted in noninfected tissue; tattoos and ear/body piercing

[1]Patients should receive prophylactic antibiotic therapy if they meet the criteria for a specified procedure/condition in this table and they have a high-risk cardiovascular condition listed in the preceding text.

[2]If treating an infection of known staphylococcal origin, consider antistaphylococcal penicillin or cephalosporin, or vancomycin in beta-lactam-sensitive patients.

[3]Alternative agents with activity against enterococci to consider: Vancomycin (for beta-lactam-sensitive patients) or piperacillin

[4]Eradication of enterococci from the urinary tract should be considered.

Table 2. Prophylactic Regimens for Oral/Dental, Respiratory Tract, Genitoruinary Tract, or Esophageal Procedures

Situation	Agent	Regimen to Be Given 30-60 Minutes Before Procedure	
		Adults	Children[1]
Standard general prophylaxis	Amoxicillin	2 g P.O.	50 mg/kg P.O.
Unable to take oral medications	Ampicillin or	2 g I.M./I.V.	50 mg/kg I.M./I.V.
	CeFAZolin or cefTRIAXone	1 g I.M./I.V.	50 mg/kg I.M./I.V.
Allergic to penicillin	Clindamycin or	600 mg P.O.	20 mg/kg P.O.
	Cephalexin[2] or other dose-equivalent first/second generation cephalosporin or	2 g P.O	50 mg/kg P.O.
	Azithromycin or clarithromycin	500 mg P.O.	15 mg/kg P.O.
Allergic to penicillin and unable to take oral medications	Clindamycin or	600 mg I.V.	20 mg/kg I.V.
	CeFAZolin or cefTRIAXone[2]	1 g I.M./I.V.	50 mg/kg I.M./I.V.

[1]Total children's dose should not exceed adult dose.

[2]Cephalosporins should not be used in individuals with immediate-type hypersensitivity reaction (urticaria, angioedema, or anaphylaxis) to penicillins.

REFERENCE

Wilson W, Taubert KA, Gewitz M, et al, "Prevention of Infective Endocarditis. Guidelines From the American Heart Association. A Guideline From the American Heart Association Rheumatic Fever, Endocarditis, and Kawasaki Disease Committee, Council on Cardiovascular Disease in the Young, and the Council on Clinical Cardiology, Council on Cardiovascular Surgery and Anesthesia, and the Quality of Care and Outcomes Research Interdisciplinary Working Group," *Circulation*, 2007, 116(15):1736-54.

REFERENCE VALUES FOR ADULTS

CHEMISTRY

Test	Values	Remarks
Serum/Plasma		
Acetone	Negative	
Albumin	3.2-5 g/dL	
Alcohol, ethyl	Negative	
Aldolase	1.2-7.6 IU/L	
Ammonia	20-70 mcg/dL	Specimen to be placed on ice as soon as collected.
Amylase	30-110 units/L	
Bilirubin, direct	0-0.3 mg/dL	
Bilirubin, total	0.1-1.2 mg/dL	
Calcium	8.6-10.3 mg/dL	
Calcium, ionized	2.24-2.46 mEq/L	
Chloride	95-108 mEq/L	
Cholesterol, total	≤200 mg/dL	Fasted blood required – normal value affected by dietary habits. This reference range is for a general adult population.
HDL cholesterol	40-60 mg/dL	Fasted blood required – normal value affected by dietary habits.
LDL cholesterol	<160 mg/dL	If triglyceride is >400 mg/dL, LDL cannot be calculated accurately (Friedewald equation). Target LDL-C depends on patient's risk factors.
CO_2	23-30 mEq/L	
Creatine kinase (CK) isoenzymes		
CK-BB	0%	
CK-MB (cardiac)	0% to 3.9%	
CK-MM (muscle)	96% to 100%	
CK-MB levels must be both ≥4% and 10 IU/L to meet diagnostic criteria for CK-MB positive result consistent with myocardial injury.		
Creatine phosphokinase (CPK)	8-150 IU/L	
Creatinine	0.5-1.4 mg/dL	
Ferritin	13-300 ng/mL	
Folate	3.6-20 ng/dL	
GGT (gamma-glutamyltranspeptidase)		
male	11-63 IU/L	
female	8-35 IU/L	
GLDH	To be determined	
Glucose (preprandial)	<115 mg/dL	Goals different for diabetics.
Glucose, fasting	60-110 mg/dL	Goals different for diabetics.
Glucose, nonfasting (2-h postprandial)	<120 mg/dL	Goals different for diabetics.
Hemoglobin A_{1c}	<8	

CHEMISTRY *(continued)*

Test	Values	Remarks
Hemoglobin, plasma free	<2.5 mg/100 mL	
Hemoglobin, total glycosolated (Hb A$_1$)	4% to 8%	
Iron	65-150 mcg/dL	
Iron binding capacity, total (TIBC)	250-420 mcg/dL	
Lactic acid	0.7-2.1 mEq/L	Specimen to be kept on ice and sent to lab as soon as possible.
Lactate dehydrogenase (LDH)	56-194 IU/L	
Lactate dehydrogenase (LDH) isoenzymes		
LD$_1$	20% to 34%	
LD$_2$	29% to 41%	
LD$_3$	15% to 25%	
LD$_4$	1% to 12%	
LD$_5$	1% to 15%	

Flipped LD$_1$/LD$_2$ ratios (>1 may be consistent with myocardial injury) particularly when considered in combination with a recent CK-MB positive result.

Test	Values	Remarks
Lipase	23-208 units/L	
Magnesium	1.6-2.5 mg/dL	Increased by slight hemolysis.
Osmolality	289-308 mOsm/kg	
Phosphatase, alkaline		
adults 25-60 y	33-131 IU/L	
adults ≥61 y	51-153 IU/L	
infancy-adolescence	Values range up to 3-5 times higher than adults	
Phosphate, inorganic	2.8-4.2 mg/dL	
Potassium	3.5-5.2 mEq/L	Increased by slight hemolysis.
Prealbumin	>15 mg/dL	
Protein, total	6.5-7.9 g/dL	
AST	<35 IU/L (20-48)	
ALT (10-35)	<35 IU/L	
Sodium	134-149 mEq/L	
Thyroid stimulating hormone (TSH)		
adults ≤20 y	0.7-6.4 mIU/L	
21-54 y	0.4-4.2 mIU/L	
55-87 y	0.5-8.9 mIU/L	
Transferrin	>200 mg/dL	
Triglycerides	45-155 mg/dL	Fasted blood required.
Troponin I	<1.5 ng/mL	
Urea nitrogen (BUN)	7-20 mg/dL	
Uric acid		
male	2-8 mg/dL	
female	2-7.5 mg/dL	

CHEMISTRY *(continued)*

Test	Values	Remarks
Cerebrospinal Fluid		
Glucose	50-70 mg/dL	
Protein	15-45 mg/dL	CSF obtained by lumbar puncture.

Note: Bloody specimen gives erroneously high value due to contamination with blood proteins

Urine
(24-hour specimen is required for all these tests unless specified)

Test	Values	Remarks
Amylase	32-641 units/L	The value is in units/L and **not** calculated for total volume.
Amylase, fluid (random samples)		Interpretation of value left for physician, depends on the nature of fluid.
Calcium	Depends upon dietary intake	
Creatine		
male	150 mg/24 h	Higher value on children and during pregnancy.
female	250 mg/24 h	
Creatinine	1000-2000 mg/24 h	
Creatinine clearance (endogenous)		
male	85-125 mL/min	A blood sample must accompany urine specimen.
female	75-115 mL/min	
Glucose	1 g/24 h	
5-hydroxyindoleacetic acid	2-8 mg/24 h	
Iron	0.15 mg/24 h	Acid washed container required.
Magnesium	146-209 mg/24 h	
Osmolality	500-800 mOsm/kg	With normal fluid intake.
Oxalate	10-40 mg/24 h	
Phosphate	400-1300 mg/24 h	
Potassium	25-120 mEq/24 h	Varies with diet; the interpretation of urine electrolytes and osmolality should be left for the physician.
Sodium	40-220 mEq/24 h	
Porphobilinogen, qualitative	Negative	
Porphyrins, qualitative	Negative	
Proteins	0.05-0.1 g/24 h	
Salicylate	Negative	
Urea clearance	60-95 mL/min	A blood sample must accompany specimen.
Urea N	10-40 g/24 h	Dependent on protein intake.
Uric acid	250-750 mg/24 h	Dependent on diet and therapy.
Urobilinogen	0.5-3.5 mg/24 h	For qualitative determination on random urine, send sample to urinalysis section in Hematology Lab.
Xylose absorption test		
children	16% to 33% of ingested xylose	

CHEMISTRY (continued)

Test	Values	Remarks
Feces		
Fat, 3-day collection	<5 g/d	Value depends on fat intake of 100 g/d for 3 days preceding and during collection.
Gastric Acidity		
Acidity, total, 12 h	10-60 mEq/L	Titrated at pH 7.

Blood Gases

	Arterial	Capillary	Venous
pH	7.35-7.45	7.35-7.45	7.32-7.42
pCO_2 (mm Hg)	35-45	35-45	38-52
pO_2 (mm Hg)	70-100	60-80	24-48
HCO_3 (mEq/L)	19-25	19-25	19-25
TCO_2 (mEq/L)	19-29	19-29	23-33
O_2 saturation (%)	90-95	90-95	40-70
Base excess (mEq/L)	-5 to +5	-5 to +5	-5 to +5

HEMATOLOGY

Complete Blood Count

Age	Hgb (g/dL)	Hct (%)	RBC (mill/mm³)	RDW
0-3 d	15.0-20.0	45-61	4.0-5.9	<18
1-2 wk	12.5-18.5	39-57	3.6-5.5	<17
1-6 mo	10.0-13.0	29-42	3.1-4.3	<16.5
7 mo to 2 y	10.5-13.0	33-38	3.7-4.9	<16
2-5 y	11.5-13.0	34-39	3.9-5.0	<15
5-8 y	11.5-14.5	35-42	4.0-4.9	<15
13-18 y	12.0-15.2	36-47	4.5-5.1	<14.5
Adult male	13.5-16.5	41-50	4.5-5.5	<14.5
Adult female	12.0-15.0	36-44	4.0-4.9	<14.5

Age	MCV (fL)	MCH (pg)	MCHC (%)	Plts (x 10³/mm³)
0-3 d	95-115	31-37	29-37	250-450
1-2 wk	86-110	28-36	28-38	250-450
1-6 mo	74-96	25-35	30-36	300-700
7 mo to 2 y	70-84	23-30	31-37	250-600
2-5 y	75-87	24-30	31-37	250-550
5-8 y	77-95	25-33	31-37	250-550
13-18 y	78-96	25-35	31-37	150-450
Adult male	80-100	26-34	31-37	150-450
Adult female	80-100	26-34	31-37	150-450

WBC and Differential

Age	WBC (x 10^3/mm³)	Segs	Bands	Lymphs	Monos
0-3 d	9.0-35.0	32-62	<18	19-29	5-7
1-2 wk	5.0-20.0	14-34	<14	36-45	6-10
1-6 mo	6.0-17.5	13-33	<12	41-71	4-7
7 mo to 2 y	6.0-17.0	15-35	<11	45-76	3-6
2-5 y	5.5-15.5	23-45	<11	35-65	3-6
5-8 y	5.0-14.5	32-54	<11	28-48	3-6
13-18 y	4.5-13.0	34-64	<11	25-45	3-6
Adults	4.5-11.0	35-66	<11	24-44	3-6

Age	Eosinophils	Basophils	Atypical Lymphs	No. of NRBCs
0-3 d	0-2	0-1	0-8	0-2
1-2 wk	0-2	0-1	0-8	0
1-6 mo	0-3	0-1	0-8	0
7 mo to 2 y	0-3	0-1	0-8	0
2-5 y	0-3	0-1	0-8	0
5-8 y	0-3	0-1	0-8	0
13-18 y	0-3	0-1	0-8	0
Adults	0-3	0-1	0-8	0

Segs = segmented neutrophils.
Bands = band neutrophils.
Lymphs = lymphocytes.
Monos = monocytes.

Erythrocyte Sedimentation Rates and Reticulocyte Counts

Sedimentation rate, Westergren

Children   0-20 mm/h
Adult male   0-15 mm/h
Adult female   0-20 mm/h

Sedimentation rate, Wintrobe

Children   0-13 mm/h
Adult male   0-10 mm/h
Adult female   0-15 mm/h

Reticulocyte count

Newborns   2% to 6%
1-6 mo   0% to 2.8%
Adults   0.5% to 1.5%

ANTITHROMBOTIC THERAPY IN ADULT PATIENTS WITH PROSTHETIC HEART VALVES

PROSTHETIC HEART VALVES

Patients with mechanical prosthetic valves require life-long anticoagulation therapy with a vitamin K antagonist (eg, warfarin). The optimal intensity of anticoagulation is not established. The risk of thromboembolism is greater in valve patients who have atrial fibrillation (AF); have an enlarged left atrium (>5.5 cm); have a history of systemic embolism, left ventricular systolic dysfunction, coronary artery disease, left atrial thrombus; have ball valve; or have more than one mechanical valve. The risk for thromboembolism is also higher for mechanical valves in the mitral position compared to aortic. These factors should be weighed in each patient before deciding the desired level of anticoagulation to prevent thromboembolism and to avoid bleeding complications. Ranges for anticoagulation intensity in patients with prosthetic valves are described in the following table.

Antithrombotic Management of Mechanical and Bioprosthetic Valves

Valve Type	Location and Specific Valve Type/Clinical Situation	Recommended INR Range/Therapy
Mechanical	Aortic, including bileaflet or tilting disk in normal sinus rhythm and normal LA size[1]	2-3
	Mitral, including bileaflet or tilting disk[1]	2.5-3.5
	Both aortic and mitral[1]	2.5-3.5
	Mitral or aortic – caged ball or disk	2.5-3.5
Bioprosthetic	Mitral valve	2-3; Maintain for 3 months after valve insertion then aspirin 81 mg/day if no other indications for warfarin
	Aortic valve in normal sinus rhythm without other indications for warfarin	Aspirin 81 mg/day
	Transcatheter aortic valve	Aspirin 81 mg/day **plus** clopidogrel 75 mg/day; maintain for 3 months after valve insertion, then aspirin 81 mg/day if no other indications for clopidogrel

AF = atrial fibrillation, EF = ejection fraction, LA = left atrial, MI = myocardial infarction

[1]For patients at low risk of bleeding, combine with aspirin 81 mg/day, if not previously receiving.

As a general rule, concomitant warfarin and aspirin therapy should be avoided, except in special situations. The combination of warfarin and low-dose aspirin in all mechanical valve patients is uncertain; patients at the highest risk (eg, AF, hypercoagulable state, or low EF) for thromboembolism should be considered. In general, patients with mechanical prosthetic valves should be prescribed aspirin in addition to warfarin given a suggestion of reduced mortality and reduced risk of thromboembolism, unless the patient is at a higher risk of bleeding.

In some situations aspirin alone with or without initial treatment with warfarin is appropriate. Patients with bioprosthetic mitral valves should be initially treated with warfarin for 3 months after insertion due to the higher rate of thromboembolism during this time and then switched to low-dose aspirin. For patients with bioprosthetic aortic valves, treatment with warfarin is not recommended at any time since treatment with warfarin in the postoperative period has not shown a reduction in thromboembolism compared to aspirin alone and may increase the risk of bleeding. Therefore, patients with a bioprosthetic aortic valve should be treated with low dose aspirin only unless other indications for warfarin exist.

REFERENCES

Stein PD, Alpert JS, Bussey HI, et al, "Antithrombotic Therapy in Patients With Mechanical and Biological Prosthetic Heart Valves," *Chest*, 2001, 119(1 Suppl):220S-227S.

Whitlock RP, Sun JC, Fremes SE, et al, "Antithrombotic and Thrombolytic Therapy for Valvular Disease: Antithrombotic Therapy and Prevention of Thrombosis, 9th ed: American College of Chest Physicians Evidence-Based Clinical Practice Guidelines," *Chest*, 2012, 141(2 Suppl):e576S-600S.

BEERS CRITERIA – POTENTIALLY INAPPROPRIATE MEDICATIONS FOR GERIATRICS

Criteria for Medications That Should Be Avoided or Used With Caution in Older Adults (Independent of Diagnoses or Conditions)

Applicable Medications	Summary of Prescribing Concerns	Recommendation	Quality of Evidence	Strength of Recommendation
Alpha₁-blockers: Doxazosin, prazosin, terazosin	High risk of orthostatic hypotension; alternative agents preferred due to a more favorable risk:benefit profile	Avoid use as an antihypertensive	Moderate	Strong
Alpha₂-agonists: CloNIDine, guanabenz, guanFACINE, methyldopa Central monoamine-depleting agent: Reserpine (>0.1 mg/day)	High risk of CNS adverse effects; may also cause orthostatic hypotension and bradycardia; not recommended for routine use as an antihypertensive	Avoid clonidine as a first-line antihypertensive. Avoid others as listed.	Low	Strong
Antiarrhythmic drugs (Class Ia, Ic, III): Amiodarone, dofetilide, dronedarone, flecainide, ibutilide, procainamide, propafenone, quinidine, sotalol	In older adults, data suggest rate control may provide more benefits than risks compared to rhythm control for most patients. Amiodarone is associated with numerous toxicities (eg, thyroid disease, QT prolongation, pulmonary disorders).	Avoid antiarrhythmic drugs as first-line treatment of atrial fibrillation	High	Strong
Antihistamines, first generation (alone or in combination products): Brompheniramine, carbinoxamine, chlorpheniramine, clemastine, cyproheptadine, dexchlorpheniramine, diphenhydrAMINE (oral), doxylamine, hydrOXYzine, promethazine, triprolidine	First generation antihistamines have potent anticholinergic properties; older adults are at increased risk for anticholinergic effects and toxicity. Diphenhydramine use may be appropriate in certain situations such as the acute treatment of severe allergic reactions.	Avoid	High (hydroxyzine, promethazine) Moderate (all others)	Strong
Antiparkinson agents: Benztropine (oral), trihexyphenidyl	Alternative, more-efficacious agents preferred for treatment of Parkinson's disease. Not recommended for prevention of extrapyramidal symptoms associated with antipsychotics.	Avoid	Moderate	Strong
Antipsychotics, first generation **and** second generation: ARIPiprazole, asenapine, chlorproMAZINE, cloZAPine, fluPHENAZine, haloperidol, iloperidone, loxapine, lurasidone, olanzapine, paliperidone, perphenazine, pimozide, QUEtiapine, risperiDONE, thioridazine, thiothixene, trifluoperazine, ziprasidone	Increased risk of stroke and mortality in patients with dementia. In addition, use may cause or exacerbate syndrome of inappropriate antidiuretic hormone secretion or hyponatremia; monitor sodium closely with initiation or dosage adjustments in older adults.	Avoid use for behavioral problems of dementia unless nonpharmacological options have failed and patient is threat to self or others; SIADH risk: Use with caution	Moderate	Strong

BEERS CRITERIA – POTENTIALLY INAPPROPRIATE MEDICATIONS FOR GERIATRICS

Criteria for Medications That Should Be Avoided or Used With Caution in Older Adults (Independent of Diagnoses or Conditions) *continued*

Applicable Medications	Summary of Prescribing Concerns	Recommendation	Quality of Evidence	Strength of Recommendation
Antispasmodic drugs: Belladonna alkaloids, clidinium and chlordiazepoxide, dicyclomine, hyoscyamine, propantheline, scopolamine	Potent anticholinergic properties and uncertain efficacy	Avoid except in short-term palliative care to decrease oral secretions	Moderate	Strong
Barbiturates: Amobarbital, butabarbital, butalbital, mephobarbital, PENTobarbital, PHENobarbital, secobarbital	Risk of overdose with low dosages, tolerance to sleep effects, and increased risk of physical dependence	Avoid	High	Strong
Benzodiazepines, long-acting: Amitriptyline and chlordiazepoxide, chlorazepate, chlordiazePOXIDE, clidinium and chlordiazepoxide, clonazePAM, diazepam, flurazepam, quazepam	In older adults, benzodiazepines increase the risk of impaired cognition, delirium, falls, fractures, and motor vehicle accidents. Increased sensitivity to benzodiazepines in this age group and slower metabolism of long-acting agents.	Avoid benzodiazepines (any type) for treatment of insomnia, agitation, or delirium	High	Strong
Benzodiazepines, short-acting: ALPRAZolam, estazolam, LORazepam, oxazepam, temazepam, triazolam	In older adults, benzodiazepines increase the risk of impaired cognition, delirium, falls, fractures, and motor vehicle accidents. Increased sensitivity in this age group to benzodiazepines.	Avoid benzodiazepines (any type) for treatment of insomnia, agitation, or delirium	High	Strong
CarBAMazepine	Use may cause or exacerbate syndrome of inappropriate antidiuretic hormone secretion or hyponatremia; monitor sodium closely with initiation or dosage adjustments in older adults.	Use with caution	Moderate	Strong
CARBOplatin	Use may cause or exacerbate syndrome of inappropriate antidiuretic hormone secretion or hyponatremia; monitor sodium closely with initiation or dosage adjustments in older adults.	Use with caution	Moderate	Strong
Chloral hydrate	Potential risks exceed benefits; doses only 3 times the recommended dose are associated with overdosage potential; in addition, tolerance develops within 10 days of use.	Avoid	Low	Strong
ChlorproPAMIDE	Prolonged half-life in elderly patients which could cause prolonged hypoglycemia. Additionally, causes SIADH.	Avoid	High	Strong
CISplatin	Use may cause or exacerbate syndrome of inappropriate antidiuretic hormone secretion or hyponatremia; monitor sodium closely with initiation or dosage adjustments in older adults.	Use with caution	Moderate	Strong

Criteria for Medications That Should Be Avoided or Used With Caution in Older Adults (Independent of Diagnoses or Conditions) *continued*

Applicable Medications	Summary of Prescribing Concerns	Recommendation	Quality of Evidence	Strength of Recommendation
Dabigatran	Greater risk of bleeding in older adults aged ≥75 years (exceeds warfarin bleeding risk); lack of safety and efficacy in patients with Cl_{cr} <30 mL/minute	Use with caution in adults aged ≥75 years of if Cl_{cr} <30mL/minute	Moderate	Weak
Desiccated thyroid	Concerns about cardiac effects; safer alternatives available	Avoid	Low	Strong
Digoxin >0.125 mg/day	Decreased renal clearance may lead to increased risk of toxic effects. Higher doses are associated with no additional benefit in heart failure patients, and may increase the risk of toxicity.	Avoid	Moderate	Strong
Dipyridamole, oral (short-acting)	May cause orthostatic hypotension; more-efficacious alternative agents available	Avoid	Moderate	Strong
Disopyramide	Potent negative inotrope and therefore may induce heart failure in elderly patients. It is also strongly anticholinergic. Other antiarrhythmic drugs should be used.	Avoid	Low	Strong
Dronedarone	In patient with permanent atrial fibrillation or heart failure, worse outcomes have been reported with use. In general, rate control is preferred over rhythm control for atrial fibrillation.	Avoid in patients with permanent atrial fibrillation or heart failure	Moderate	Strong
Ergot mesylates	Have not been shown to be effective	Avoid	High	Strong
Estrogens (with or without progestins)	Evidence of the carcinogenic (breast and endometrial cancer) potential of these agents and lack of cardioprotective effect in older women Evidence for vaginal estrogens for treatment of vaginal dryness to be safe and effective in women with breast cancer, particularly at estradiol doses <25 mcg twice weekly	Avoid oral and topical patch. Topical vaginal cream: Acceptable to use low-dose intravaginal estrogen for the management of dyspareunia, lower urinary tract infections, and other vaginal symptoms	High (oral and patch formulations) Moderate (topical formulations)	Strong (oral and patch formulations) Weak (topical formulations)
Glyburide	Increased risk of severe, prolonged hypoglycemia in older adults	Avoid	High	Strong

Criteria for Medications That Should Be Avoided or Used With Caution in Older Adults (Independent of Diagnoses or Conditions) *continued*

Applicable Medications	Summary of Prescribing Concerns	Recommendation	Quality of Evidence	Strength of Recommendation
Indomethacin	Of all available NSAIDs, this drug produces the most adverse effects. Non-COX-selective oral NSAID use associated with an increased risk of GI bleeding and peptic ulcer disease in older adults in high-risk category (eg, >75 years or age or receiving concomitant oral/parenteral corticosteroids, anticoagulants, or antiplatelet agents). Proton pump inhibitors or misoprostol use reduces risk, but does not eliminate it. Longer duration of NSAID use correlates with a trend towards increasing incidence GI ulcers, bleeding, or perforation.	Avoid	Moderate	Strong
Insulin, sliding scale	Regardless of care setting, an increased risk of hypoglycemia without improvement in management of hyperglycemia	Avoid	Moderate	Strong
Isoxsuprine	Lack of efficacy	Avoid	High	Strong
Ketorolac (includes parenteral)	Associated with an increased risk of GI bleeding and peptic ulcer disease in older adults in high-risk category (eg, >75 years or age or receiving concomitant oral/parenteral corticosteroids, anticoagulants, or antiplatelet agents). Proton pump inhibitors or misoprostol use reduces risk, but does not eliminate it. Longer duration of NSAID use correlates with a trend towards increasing incidence GI ulcers, bleeding, or perforation.	Avoid	High	Strong
Megestrol	Increased risk of thrombotic events and possibly death; effect on weight is minimal	Avoid	Moderate	Strong
Meperidine	Not an effective oral analgesic in doses commonly used. Safer alternative agents preferred due to potential for neurotoxicity.	Avoid	High	Strong
Meprobamate	Highly sedating anxiolytic with a high rate of physical dependence	Avoid	Moderate	Strong
MethylTESTOSTERone	Potential for cardiac problems; contraindicated in men with prostate cancer	Avoid unless indicated for moderate-to-severe hypogonadism	Moderate	Weak

Criteria for Medications That Should Be Avoided or Used With Caution in Older Adults (Independent of Diagnoses or Conditions) *continued*

Applicable Medications	Summary of Prescribing Concerns	Recommendation	Quality of Evidence	Strength of Recommendation
Metoclopramide	May cause extrapyramidal effects (including tardive dyskinesia), particularly in frail older adults	Avoid, unless for gastroparesis	Moderate	Strong
Mineral oil	Potential for aspiration and adverse effects; safer alternatives available	Avoid	Moderate	Strong
Mirtazapine	Use may cause or exacerbate syndrome of inappropriate antidiuretic hormone secretion or hyponatremia; monitor sodium closely with initiation or dosage adjustments in older adults.	Use with caution	Moderate	Strong
NIFEdipine, short-acting	Potential for hypotension; risk of precipitating myocardial ischemia	Avoid	High	Strong
Nitrofurantoin	Potential for pulmonary toxicity; safer alternatives available; renal impairment (Cl_{cr} <60 mL/minute) results in inadequate drug concentration in urine and lack of efficacy	Avoid for long-term suppression; avoid in patients with Cl_{cr} <60 mL/minute	Moderate	Strong
Nonbenzodiazepine hypnotics: Eszopiclone, zolpidem, zaleplon	Similar adverse events (eg, delirium, falls, fractures) in older adults to events seen with benzodiazepine use; minimal improvement seen with sleep latency and duration	Avoid chronic use (>90 days)	Moderate	Strong
Non-COX-selective NSAIDS (oral): Aspirin (>325 mg/day), diclofenac, diflunisal, etodolac, fenoprofen, ibuprofen, ketoprofen, meclofenamate, mefenamic acid, meloxicam, nabumetone, naproxen, oxaprozin, piroxicam, sulindac, tolmetin	Use associated with an increased risk of GI bleeding and peptic ulcer disease in older adults in high risk category (eg, >75 years or age or receiving concomitant oral/parenteral corticosteroids, anticoagulants, or antiplatelet agents). Proton pump inhibitors or misoprostol use reduce risk, but do not eliminate it. Longer duration of NSAID use correlates with a trend towards increasing incidence GI ulcers, bleeding, or perforation.	Avoid chronic use unless other alternatives are not effective and patient can take gastroprotective agent (proton pump inhibitor or misoprostol)	Moderate	Strong
Pentazocine	Opioid analgesic that causes more CNS adverse effects, including confusion and hallucinations, more commonly than other narcotic drugs. Additionally, it is a mixed agonist and antagonist; safer alternative agents are available.	Avoid	Low	Strong
Prasugrel	Risk of bleeding is increased in older adults; risk may be offset by benefit in older adults at highest risk (eg, prior MI or diabetes)	Use with caution in adults aged ≥75 years	Moderate	Weak

Criteria for Medications That Should Be Avoided or Used With Caution in Older Adults (Independent of Diagnoses or Conditions) *continued*

Applicable Medications	Summary of Prescribing Concerns	Recommendation	Quality of Evidence	Strength of Recommendation
Serotonin-norepinephrine reuptake inhibitors and selective serotonin reuptake inhibitors	Use may cause or exacerbate syndrome of inappropriate antidiuretic hormone secretion or hyponatremia; monitor sodium closely with initiation or dosage adjustments in older adults.	Use with caution	Moderate	Strong
Skeletal muscle relaxants: Carisoprodol, chlorzoxazone, cyclobenzaprine, metaxalone, methocarbamol, orphenadrine	Most muscle relaxants are poorly tolerated by elderly patients, since these cause anticholinergic adverse effects, sedation, and risk of fracture. Additionally, efficacy is questionable at dosages tolerated by elderly patients.	Avoid	Moderate	Strong
Somatropin (growth hormone)	Body composition effects are minimal and use associated with edema, arthralgia, carpal tunnel syndrome, gynecomastia, and impaired fasting glucose.	Avoid, except as hormone replacement after pituitary gland removal	High	Strong
Spironolactone (>25 mg/day)	Risk of hyperkalemia is increased for heart failure patients receiving >25 mg/day, particularly if taking concomitant medications such as NSAIDS, ACE inhibitors, angiotensin receptor blockers, or potassium supplements.	Avoid in patients with heart failure or with a Cl_{cr} <30 mL/minute	Moderate	Strong
Testosterone	Potential for cardiac problems; contraindicated in men with prostate cancer	Avoid unless indicated for moderate-to-severe hypogonadism	Moderate	Weak
Thioridazine	Potent anticholinergic properties; risk of QT-interval prolongation	Avoid	Moderate	Strong

Criteria for Medications That Should Be Avoided or Used With Caution in Older Adults (Independent of Diagnoses or Conditions) *continued*

Applicable Medications	Summary of Prescribing Concerns	Recommendation	Quality of Evidence	Strength of Recommendation
Ticlopidine	Safer, more effective alternatives exist.	Avoid	Moderate	Strong
Tricyclic antidepressants	Use may cause or exacerbate syndrome of inappropriate antidiuretic hormone secretion or hyponatremia; monitor sodium closely with initiation or dosage adjustments in older adults.	Use with caution	High	Strong
Tricyclic antidepressants, tertiary (alone or in combination): Amitriptyline, amitriptyline and chlordiazepoxide, clomiPRAMINE, doxepin >6 mg/day, imipramine, perphenazine and amitriptyline, trimipramine	Potent anticholinergic properties, sedating, and potential for orthostatic hypotension; doxepin at doses ≤6 mg/day has safety profile comparable to placebo	Avoid	High	Strong
Trimethobenzamide	One of the least effective antiemetic drugs and may cause extrapyramidal adverse effects	Avoid	Moderate	Strong
VinCRIStine	Use may cause or exacerbate syndrome of inappropriate antidiuretic hormone secretion or hyponatremia; monitor sodium closely with initiation or dosage adjustments in older adults.	Use with caution	Moderate	Strong

Drugs with Potent Anticholinergic Properties

Class of Drug	Individual Agents
Antihistamines	Brompheniramine, carbinoxamine, chlorpheniramine, clemastine, cyproheptadine, dimenhydrinate, diphenhydrAMINE, hydrOXYzine, loratadine, meclizine
Antidepressants	Amitriptyline, amoxapine, clomiPRAMINE, desipramine, doxepin, imipramine, nortriptyline, PARoxetine, protriptyline, trimipramine
Antimuscarinics (urinary incontinence)	Darifenacin, fesoterodine, flavoxATE, oxybutynin, solifenacin, tolterodine, trospium
Antiparkinson agents	Benztropine, trihexyphenidyl
Antipsychotics	ChlorproMAZINE, cloZAPine, fluPHENAZine, loxapine, OLANZapine, perphenazine, pimozide, prochlorperazine, promethazine, thioridazine, thiothixene, trifluoperazine
Antispasmodics	Atropine products, belladonna alkaloids, dicyclomine, homatropine, hyoscyamine products, propantheline, scopolamine
Skeletal muscle relaxants	Carisoprodol, cyclobenzaprine, orphenadrine, tiZANidine

REFERENCE

American Geriatrics Society 2012 Beers Criteria Update Expert Panel, "American Geriatrics Society Updated Beers Criteria for Potentially Inappropriate Medication Use in Older Adults," *J Am Geriatr Soc*, 2012, 60(4):616-31.

CMS GUIDELINES FOR GRADUAL DOSE REDUCTION OF PSYCHOPHARMACOLOGICAL AGENTS IN NURSING FACILITY RESIDENTS

http://www.cms.hhs.gov/transmittals/downloads/R22SOMA.pdf
Section 483.25(l)

The following is an excerpt from Appendix PP of the Centers for Medicare and Medicaid Services (CMS) State Operations Manual concerning gradual dose reduction in relation to specific classes of psychopharmacologic agents. The reader is referred to Table 1 (Medication Issues of Particular Relevance) in the above document, for further information regarding the use of psychopharmacological agents in nursing facilities.

CONSIDERATIONS SPECIFIC TO ANTIPSYCHOTICS

The regulation addressing the use of antipsychotic medications identifies the process of tapering as a "gradual dose reduction (GDR)" and requires a GDR, unless clinically contraindicated.

Within the first year in which a resident is admitted on an antipsychotic medication or after the facility has initiated an antipsychotic medication, the facility must attempt a GDR in two separate quarters (with at least one month between the attempts), unless clinically contraindicated. After the first year, a GDR must be attempted annually, unless clinically contraindicated.

For any individual who is receiving an antipsychotic medication to treat behavioral symptoms related to dementia, the GDR may be considered clinically contraindicated if:

- The resident's target symptoms returned or worsened after the most recent attempt at a GDR within the facility; and

- The physician has documented the clinical rationale for why any additional attempted dose reduction at that time would be likely to impair the resident's function or increase distressed behavior.

For any individual who is receiving an antipsychotic medication to treat a psychiatric disorder other than behavioral symptoms related to dementia (for example, schizophrenia, bipolar mania, or depression with psychotic features), the GDR may be considered contraindicated, if:

- The continued use is in accordance with relevant current standards of practice and the physician has documented the clinical rationale for why any attempted dose reduction would be likely to impair the resident's function or cause psychiatric instability by exacerbating an underlying psychiatric disorder; or

- The resident's target symptoms returned or worsened after the most recent attempt at a GDR within the facility and the physician has documented the clinical rationale for why any additional attempted dose reduction at that time would be likely to impair the resident's function or cause psychiatric instability by exacerbating an underlying medical or psychiatric disorder.

ATTEMPTED TAPERING RELATIVE TO CONTINUED INDICATION OR OPTIMAL DOSE

As noted, attempted tapering is one way to determine whether a specific medication is still indicated, and whether target symptoms and risks can be managed with a lesser dose of a medication. As noted, many medications in various categories can be tapered safely. The following examples of tapering relate to two common categories of concern: Sedatives/hypnotics and psychopharmacologic medications (other than antipsychotic and sedatives/hypnotics medications).

◀ TAPERING CONSIDERATIONS SPECIFIC TO SEDATIVES/HYPNOTICS

For as long as a resident remains on a sedative/hypnotic that is used routinely and beyond the manufacturer's recommendations for duration of use, the facility should attempt to taper the medication quarterly unless clinically contraindicated. Clinically contraindicated means:

- The continued use is in accordance with relevant current standards of practice and the physician has documented the clinical rationale for why any attempted dose reduction would be likely to impair the resident's function or cause psychiatric instability by exacerbating an underlying medical or psychiatric disorder; or

- The resident's target symptoms returned or worsened after the most recent attempt at tapering the dose within the facility and the physician has documented the clinical rationale for why any additional attempted dose reduction at that time would be likely to impair the resident's function or cause psychiatric instability by exacerbating an underlying medical or psychiatric disorder.

CONSIDERATIONS SPECIFIC TO PSYCHOPHARMACOLOGICAL MEDICATIONS (OTHER THAN ANTIPSYCHOTICS AND SEDATIVES/HYPNOTICS)

During the first year in which a resident is admitted on a psychopharmacological medication (other than an antipsychotic or a sedative/hypnotic), or after the facility has initiated such medication, the facility should attempt to taper the medication during at least two separate quarters (with at least one month between the attempts), unless clinically contraindicated. After the first year, a tapering should be attempted annually, unless clinically contraindicated. The tapering may be considered clinically contraindicated, if:

- The continued use is in accordance with relevant current standards of practice and the physician has documented the clinical rationale for why any attempted dose reduction would be likely to impair the resident's function or cause psychiatric instability by exacerbating an underlying medical or psychiatric disorder; or

- The resident's target symptoms returned or worsened after the most recent attempt at tapering the dose within the facility and the physician has documented the clinical rationale for why any additional attempted dose reduction at that time would be likely to impair the resident's function or cause psychiatric instability by exacerbating an underlying medical or psychiatric disorder.

DIABETES MELLITUS MANAGEMENT, ADULTS

OVERVIEW

Diabetes represents a significant health care problem in the United States and worldwide. Of the nearly 23.6 million Americans (7.8% of the population) with diabetes, the majority (90% to 95%) have type 2 diabetes. Of this number, nearly one-quarter are undiagnosed. The incidence of type 2 diabetes is increasing around the world. There is strong evidence to support an interaction between a genetic predisposition and behavioral or environmental factors, such as obesity and physical inactivity, in the development of this disease. In individuals at high risk of developing type 2 diabetes, it has been shown that the development of diabetes may be prevented or delayed by changes in lifestyle or pharmacologic intervention.

Within the United States, type 1 diabetes is estimated to comprise 5% to 10% of those with diabetes, and therefore represents the minority of individuals with diabetes. In addition to type 1 and type 2 diabetes, approximately 7% of pregnancies are complicated by the development of gestational diabetes. Gestational diabetes mellitus is defined as the first onset or recognition of glucose intolerance during pregnancy. Women who have had gestational diabetes are at an increased risk for later development of type 2 diabetes. In addition to the causes noted above, diabetes may result from genetic syndromes, surgery (pancreatectomy), chemicals and/or drugs, recurrent pancreatitis, malnutrition, and viral infections.

Additional information available at: http://care.diabetesjournals.org/content/34/Supplement_1

COMPLICATIONS OF DIABETES

Diabetes was listed as the seventh leading cause of death in the United States in 2007. Complications of diabetes are often contributing factors in the death of these patients; the most frequently reported diabetes complications on the death certificates of patients with diabetes in 2004 were heart disease and stroke, which were listed as contributing factors in 68% and 16% of diabetes-related deaths, respectively.

In addition to cardiovascular effects, diabetes is the leading cause of new blindness in people 20-74 years of age, and diabetic nephropathy is the most common cause of end-stage renal disease. Mild to severe forms of diabetic neuropathy are common. Neuropathy and circulatory insufficiency combine to make diabetes the most frequent cause of nontraumatic lower-limb amputations (60% of cases). The rate of impotence in diabetic males over 50 years of age has been estimated to be as high as 35% to 50%. Control of hyperglycemia may significantly decrease the rate at which diabetic complications develop; this provides compelling justification for early diagnosis and management of this disorder.

DIAGNOSIS

Diabetes

Diagnosis of diabetes in nonpregnant adults is made by any of the four criteria described below. In the absence of unequivocal hyperglycemia with acute metabolic decompensation, these criteria should be confirmed by repeat testing on a different day. New in the 2010 American Diabetes Association (ADA) Standards of Medical Care is the recommendation for the use of Hb A_{1c} for the diagnosis of diabetes; the method used should be certified by the National Glycohemoglobin Standardization Program (NGSP) and standardized to the Diabetes Control and Complications Trial (DCCT) assay. Screening should be considered in overweight adult patients (BMI ≥25 kg/m^2) who have at least one risk factor for diabetes (eg, physical inactivity, first-degree relative with diabetes, history of cardiovascular disease, etc). In patients without risk factors, testing should begin at age 45. Repeat testing should occur at least every 3 years in patients with normal test results.

Criteria for Diagnosis

1. Hb A$_{1c}$ ≥6.5%

   OR

2. Fasting plasma glucose (no caloric intake for at least 8 hours) ≥126 mg/dL (7 mmol/L)
   OR

3. Casual plasma glucose concentration≥200 mg/dL (11.1 mmol/L) in patients with symptoms of hyperglycemia (polydipsia, polyuria, unexplained weight loss) or hyperglycemic crisis. **Note:** Casual plasma glucose is defined as any time of day without regard to time of last meal.
   OR

4. A 2-hour plasma glucose ≥200 mg/dL (11.1 mmol/L) during an oral glucose tolerance test (OGTT) in accordance with the standards set forth by the World Health Organization (WHO) using a 75 g anhydrous glucose load (or equivalent) dissolved in water. **Note:** OGTT is not recommended for routine clinical use.

Note: In the absence of unequivocal hyperglycemia, criteria 1, 2, and 4 should be confirmed by repeat testing.

Categories of Increased Risk for Diabetes

Patients with impaired fasting glucose (IFG), impaired glucose tolerance (IGT), or an intermediately high Hb A$_{1c}$ are considered to be in a group whose glucose levels do not meet the criteria for diabetes, yet are higher than normal. Patients who meet any of the following criteria are considered to be at high risk for developing diabetes and cardiovascular disease, and are referred to as having "prediabetes":

1. IFG: Fasting plasma glucose (no caloric intake for at least 8 hours) 100-125 mg/dL (5.6-6.9 mmol/L)

   OR

2. IGT: A 2-hour plasma glucose 140-199 mg/dL (7.8-11 mmol/L) during an oral glucose tolerance test (OGTT) in accordance with the standards set forth by the World Health Organization (WHO) using a 75 g anhydrous glucose load (or equivalent) dissolved in water.
   OR

3. Hb A$_{1c}$: 5.7% to 6.4%; **Note:** Patients with an Hb A$_{1c}$ >6% should be considered at very high risk for diabetes and receive intensive interventions and monitoring.

The International Expert Committee consisting of members of the ADA, the European Association for the Study of Diabetes (EASD), and the International Diabetes Federation (IDF) recently recommended that the clinical states "prediabetes," IFG, and IGT be phased out as the Hb A$_{1c}$ becomes the preferred diagnostic test (International Expert Committee, 2009).

GOALS

The goals of diabetes treatment include normalization of hyperglycemia, avoidance of hypoglycemia, and slowing the development of diabetic complications. The following is a summary of recommendations for nonpregnant adults with diabetes.

2011 ADA Summary of Recommendations for Adults With Diabetes

Glycemic control	
Hb A_{1c}	<7%[1]
Preprandial capillary plasma glucose	70-130 mg/dL
Peak postprandial capillary plasma glucose[2]	<180 mg/dL
Blood pressure[7]	<130/80 mm Hg
Lipids[3]	
LDL[4]	<100 mg/dL
Triglycerides	<150 mg/dL
HDL	Male: >40 mg/dL Female: >50 mg/dL
Non-HDL choesterol[5]	<130 mg/dL
Apolipoprotein B[6]	<90 mg/dL

[1]Referenced to a nondiabetic range of 4% to 6% using a DCCT-based assay. **Note:** The Hb A_{1c} goal for patients in general is <7%; an even lower goal may be appropriate for selected individuals (eg, short duration of diabetes, long life expectancy, and no significant cardiovascular disease) so long as a lower goal can be achieved without significant hypoglycemia or other adverse effects. Conversely, a less stringent goal may be appropriate in certain patients (eg, history of severe hypoglycemia, limited life expectancy, advanced micro- or macrovascular complications, extensive comorbid conditions, longstanding diabetes in whom the general goal is difficult to attain despite appropriate diabetes management).

[2]Postprandial glucose measurements should be made 1-2 hours after the beginning of the meal, generally peak levels in patients with diabetes.

[3]Current NCEP/ATP III guidelines suggest that in patients with triglycerides ≥200 mg/dL, the non-HDL cholesterol (total cholesterol minus HDL) be used. The goal is <130 mg/dL.

[4]In patients with overt CVD or cardiometabolic risk factors (eg, central obesity, insulin resistance, hypertension), a lower LDL goal of <70 mg/dL is an option.

[5]In patients with overt CVD or cardiometabolic risk factors (eg, central obesity, insulin resistance, hypertension) with an LDL goal of <70 mg/dL, the non-HDL cholesterol goal is <100 mg/dL

[6]In patients on a statin with an LDL goal of <70 mg/dL or patients with cardiometabolic risk factors (eg, central obesity, insulin resistance, hypertension), the apolipoprotein B goal is <80 mg/dL

[7]Higher or lower systolic blood pressure targets may be appropriate based on individual patient characteristics and response to therapy.

Key concepts in setting glycemic goals:

- Hb A_{1c} is the primary target for glycemic control.

- Goals should be individualized.

- Certain populations (children, pregnant women, and elderly) require special considerations.

- Less intensive glycemic goals may be indicated in patients with severe or frequent hypoglycemia.

- A lower glycemic goal (eg, Hb A_{1c} <6%) may further reduce the risk of microvascular complications at the cost of an increased risk of hypoglycemia (particularly in those with type 1 diabetes). However, recent studies (eg, ACCORD and VADT) have highlighted certain patient populations in which the risks of intensive glycemic control may outweigh the benefits, including patients with a very long duration of diabetes, history of severe hypoglycemia, advanced atherosclerosis, and advanced age or frailty.

- Postprandial glucose may be targeted if Hb A_{1c} goals are not met despite reaching preprandial glucose goals.

MANAGEMENT

Multidisciplinary approach necessary. Patient education:

- Wearing appropriate identification of disease

- Foot care

- Eye care

- Acute illness management

- Hypoglycemia recognition and management

- Weight monitoring and management, including diet and exercise and bariatric surgery options (BMI >35 kg/m^2)

TYPE 1 DIABETES DRUG TREATMENT

Intensive insulin therapy: ≥3 injections/day of basal and prandial insulin or continuous subcutaneous infusion. If hypoglycemia is problematic, the use of insulin analogs may be helpful.

Monitoring

Self-monitoring of blood glucose (SMBG) should be carried out three or more times daily for patients using multiple insulin injections or insulin pump therapy. For patients using less frequent insulin injections, noninsulin therapies, or medical nutrition therapy (MNT) alone, SMBG may be useful as a guide to the success of therapy. To achieve postprandial glucose targets, postprandial SMBG may be appropriate.

Continuous glucose monitoring (CGM) in conjunction with intensive insulin regimens can be a useful tool to lower A_{1C} in selected adults (age ≥25 years) with type 1 diabetes. CGM may be a supplemental tool in those with hypoglycemia episodes.

Insulin

Insulin therapy is required in type 1 diabetes, and may be necessary in some individuals with type 2 diabetes. The general objective of insulin replacement therapy is to approximate the physiologic pattern of insulin secretion which is characterized by two distinct phases. Phase 1 insulin secretion suppresses hepatic glucose production and phase 2 insulin secretion occurs in response to carbohydrate ingestion. This requires a basal level of insulin throughout the day (such as intermediate- or long-acting insulin or continuous insulin infusion administered via an external SubQ insulin infusion pump), supplemented by additional insulin at mealtimes (eg, short- or rapid-acting insulin).

Multiple daily doses guided by blood glucose monitoring are the standard of diabetes care. Combinations of insulin are commonly used. The number and size of daily doses, time of administration, and diet and exercise require continuous medical supervision. In addition, specific formulations may require distinct administration procedures/timing (refer to individual monographs).

There is solid scientific documentation of the benefit of tight glucose control, either by insulin pump or multiple daily injections (4-6 times daily). However, the benefits must be balanced against the risk of hypoglycemia, the patient's ability to adhere to the regimen, and other issues regarding the complexity of management. Diabetes self-management education (DSME) and medical nutrition therapy (MNT) are essential to maximize the effectiveness of therapy. In addition to the educational issues outlined above, patients should be instructed in insulin administration techniques, timing of administration, and sick-day management.

The initial dose of insulin in type 1 diabetes is typically 0.5-1 units/kg/day in divided doses. Conservative initial doses of 0.2-0.4 units/kg/day are often recommended to avoid the potential for hypoglycemia. Generally, one-half to three-fourths of the daily insulin dose is given as an intermediate- or long-acting form of insulin (in 1-2 daily injections). The remaining portion of the 24-hour insulin requirement is divided and administered as a rapid-acting or short-acting form of insulin. These may be given with meals (before or at the time of meals depending on the form of insulin) or at the same time as injections of intermediate forms (some premixed combinations are intended for this purpose). Some patients may benefit from the use of continuous subcutaneous insulin infusion (CSII) which delivers rapid-acting insulin as a continuous infusion throughout the day and as boluses at mealtimes via an external pump device.

Since combinations of agents are frequently used, dosage adjustment must address the individual component of the insulin regimen which most directly influences the blood glucose value in question, based on the known onset and duration of the insulin component (see table). The frequency of doses and monitoring must also be individualized in consideration of the patient's ability to manage therapy.

Types of Insulin	Onset (h)	Peak Glycemic Effect (h)	Duration (h)
Rapid-Acting			
Insulin lispro (HumaLOG®)	0.25-0.5	0.5-2.5	≤5
Insulin aspart (NovoLOG®)	0.2-0.3	1-3	3-5
Insulin glulisine (Apidra®)	0.2-0.5	1.6-2.8	3-4
Short-Acting			
Insulin regular (HumuLIN® R, NovoLIN® R)	0.5	2.5-5	4-12 – U-100 Up to 24 – U-500
Intermediate-Acting			
Insulin NPH (isophane suspension) (HumuLIN® N, NovoLIN® N)	1-2	4-12	14-24
Intermediate- to Long-Acting			
Insulin detemir (Levemir®)	3-4	3-9	6-23 (duration is dose-dependent)
Long-Acting			
Insulin glargine (Lantus®)	3-4	*	10.8-≥24
Combinations			
Insulin aspart protamine suspension and insulin aspart (NovoLOG® Mix 70/30)	0.17-0.33	1-4	18-24
Insulin lispro protamine suspension and insulin lispro (HumaLOG® Mix 75/25™)	0.25-0.5	1-6.5	14-24
Insulin NPH suspension and insulin regular solution (NovoLIN® 70/30)	0.5	2-12	18-24

*Insulin glargine has no pronounced peak.

Maintenance Dosing

Typical maintenance insulin doses are between 0.5 and 1.2 units/kg/day in divided doses. Adolescents may require as much as 1.5 units/kg/day during puberty; whereas prepubescent individuals may only require 0.7-1 unit/kg/day.

As stated above, the general objective of insulin replacement therapy is to approximate the physiologic pattern of insulin secretion. This requires a basal level of insulin throughout the day, supplemented by additional insulin at mealtimes. Combination regimens which exploit differences in the onset and duration of different insulin products are commonly used to approximate physiologic secretion. Frequently, split-mixed or basal-bolus regimens are used to approximate physiologic secretion.

Split-mixed regimens: In split-mixed regimens, an intermediate-acting insulin (eg, NPH insulin) is administered once or twice daily and supplemented by short-acting (regular) or rapid-acting (lispro, aspart, or glulisine) insulin. Blood glucose measurements are completed several times daily. Dosages are adjusted emphasizing the individual component of the regimen which most directly influences the blood sugar in question (either the intermediate-acting component or the shorter-acting component). Fixed-ratio formulations (eg, 70/30 mix) may be used as twice daily injections in this scenario; however, the ability to titrate the dosage of an individual component is limited. An example of a "split-mixed" regimen would be 21 units of NPH plus 9 units of regular in the morning and an evening meal dose consisting of 14 units of NPH plus 6 units of regular insulin.

Basal-bolus regimens: Basal-bolus regimens are designed to more closely mimic physiologic secretion. These regimens employ intermediate- to long-acting insulins (eg, glargine, detemir) or a continuous insulin infusion administered via an external SubQ insulin infusion pump to simulate basal insulin secretion. The basal component is frequently administered at bedtime or in the early morning or as a continuous insulin infusion and then supplemented by multiple daily injections of rapid-acting products (lispro, glulisine, or aspart) immediately prior to a meal; thereby, providing insulin at the time when nutrients are absorbed. An example of a basal-bolus regimen would be 30 units of glargine at bedtime and 12 units of lispro insulin prior to each meal.

◄ ## Adjustment of Insulin Dose

Dosage must be titrated to achieve glucose control and avoid hypoglycemia. In general, dosage is adjusted to maintain recommendations for glycemic control. Since treatment regimens often consist of multiple formulations, dosage adjustments must address the specific phase of insulin release that is primarily contributing to the patient's impaired glycemic control. Treatment and monitoring regimens must be individualized.

Estimation of the effect per unit: A "Rule of 1500" has been frequently used as a means to estimate the change in blood sugar relative to each unit of insulin administered. In fact, the recommended values used in these calculations may vary from 1500-2200 (a value of at least 1800 is recommended for lispro). The higher values lead to more conservative estimates of the effect per unit of insulin, and therefore lead to more cautious adjustments. The effect per unit of insulin (aka, correction factor) is approximated by dividing the selected numerical value (eg, 1500-2200) by the number of units/day received by the patient. The correction factor may be used as a crude approximation of the patient's insulin sensitivity to determine the correction doses of insulin or adjust the current insulin regimen. Each additional unit of insulin added to the corresponding insulin dose may be expected to lower the blood glucose by the value of the correction factor.

To illustrate, in the "basal-bolus" regimen which includes 30 units of glargine at bedtime and 12 units of lispro insulin prior to each meal, the rule of 1800 would indicate an expected change of 27 mg/dL per unit of insulin (the total daily insulin dose is 66 units; using the formula: correction factor = 1800/66 = 27). A patient may be instructed to add additional insulin if the preprandial glucose is >125 mg/dL. For a prelunch glucose of 195 mg/dL (70 mg/dL higher than goal), this would mean the patient would administer the scheduled 12 units of lispro along with an additional "correction dose" of 3 units (70 divided by the correction factor of 27 derived from the formula) for a total of 15 units prior to the meal. If correction doses are required on a consistent basis, an adjustment of the patient's diet and/or scheduled insulin dose may be necessary.

Hypoglycemia

Hypoglycemia is the leading limiting factor in the treatment of diabetes. A patient experiencing an episode of acutely low blood sugar can perceive the event as an inconvenience in milder cases to a real threat of falls, motor vehicle accidents, etc. in severe cases.

Management of hypoglycemia:

- Conscious individual: Oral glucose: 15-20 g (any form of carbohydrate that contains glucose may be used). If a self-measurement of blood glucose (SMBG) 15 minutes after treatment shows continued hypoglycemia, the treatment should be repeated. Once SMBG glucose returns to normal, the individual should consume a meal or snack to prevent recurrence of hypoglycemia.

- Glucagon should be prescribed for all individuals at significant risk of severe hypoglycemia, and caregivers or family members should be instructed in administration.

- Patients with hypoglycemia unawareness or one or more episodes of severe hypoglycemia should be advised to raise their glycemic targets to avoid further hypoglycemia at least for a short period of time.

- Re-enforce education about prevention of hypoglycemia.

TYPE 2 DIABETES DRUG TREATMENT

Insulin Therapy

Several suggested algorithms for management of adult nonpregnant patients may be found (Nathan, 2009; Rodbard, 2009). Insulin may be used in type 2 diabetes as a means to augment response to oral antidiabetic agents or as monotherapy in selected patients. According to a consensus statement developed by the ADA and the European Association for the Study of Diabetes, basal insulin (eg, glargine, detemir) should be considered in patients who have failed to achieve their glycemic goals following lifestyle interventions and the administration of the maximal tolerated dose of metformin (ADA, 2009; Rodbard, 2009). Furthermore, intensive insulin therapy (eg, basal-bolus regimens) should be considered in patients who have failed to achieve their glycemic goals with an optimized two- or three-drug regimen (ADA, 2009; Rodbard, 2009). Augmentation to control postprandial glucose may be accomplished with regular, glulisine, aspart, or lispro insulin. Dosage must be carefully adjusted.

When used as monotherapy, the requirements for insulin are highly variable. An empirically defined scheme for dosage estimation based on fasting plasma glucose and degree of obesity has been published with recommended doses ranging from 6-77 units/day (Holman, 1995). In the setting of glucose toxicity (loss of beta-cell sensitivity to glucose concentrations), insulin therapy may be used for short-term management to restore sensitivity of beta-cells; in these cases, the dose may need to be rapidly reduced/withdrawn when sensitivity is re-established.

Oral Agents

A large number of drugs for oral administration have become available for the management of type 2 diabetes. Oral antidiabetic agents include sulfonylureas, meglitinides, alpha-glucosidase inhibitors, biguanides, thiazolidinediones (TZDs), and dipeptidyl peptidase IV (DPP-IV) inhibitors. The drug classes vary in terms of their magnitude of effect on glycemic control, mechanism of action, and adverse effect profiles. In many cases, the adverse effect profile may influence the selection of a particular drug. The risk of hypoglycemia is higher for drugs which promote insulin secretion (particularly sulfonylureas or insulin secretagogues). Drug selection is based on patient-specific factors and anticipated tolerance of adverse effects.

Metformin is currently the drug of choice if the patient has no contraindications. If lifestyle intervention and the maximal tolerated dose of metformin fail to achieve or sustain the glycemic goals, another medication should be added in several months. Another medication may also be necessary if metformin is contraindicated or not tolerated. Insulin or a sulfonylurea may be considered the next step if metformin and lifestyle changes are not adequate.

Combination therapy may be necessary to achieve glycemic goals. The risk of additive or additional adverse effects must be balanced with the desire to achieve goals of glycemic control as well as normalization of other metabolic parameters. In particular, weight gain and lipid disturbances may complicate drug treatment.

Oral Antidiabetic Agents for Type 2 Diabetes

Generic Name (Brand Name)	Expected Decrease (%) in Hb A$_{1c}$ With Monotherapy	Key Adverse Effects
Alpha-Glucosidase Inhibitors		
Acarbose (Precose®)	0.5-0.8	GI distress, bloating, flatulence
Miglitol (Glyset®)		
Antilipemic Agent (Adjunct Therapy)		
Colesevelam (WelChol®)	0.5-1 (not for use as monotherapy)	Constipation, dyspepsia
Biguanide		
Metformin (Fortamet™; Glucophage® XR; Glucophage®; Glumetza®; Riomet®)	1-2	**Lactic acidosis [BOXED WARNING]**, GI distress, weakness
Dipeptidyl Peptidase IV (DPP-IV) Inhibitors		
Linagliptin (Tradjenta™)	0.4	Headache, nasopharyngitis, arthralgia, back pain
Saxagliptin (Onglyza™)	0.4-0.5	Headache, UTI, sinusitis
Sitagliptin (Januvia™)	0.5-0.8	Nasopharyngitis, GI distress, nausea, peripheral edema, hypoglycemia
Dopamine agonists		
Bromocriptine (Cycloset®)	0.1	Nausea, dizziness, somnolence, postural hypotension, headache
Meglitinide Derivatives		
Nateglinide (Starlix®)	0.5-1.5 (repaglinide may be more effective)	Upper respiratory infection, flu-like syndrome, headache, hypoglycemia
Repaglinide (Prandin®)		
Sulfonylurea, 1st Generation		
ChlorproPAMIDE (Diabinese®)	1-2	Hypoglycemia, dizziness, headache, GI distress, SIADH
Tolazamide		
TOLBUTamide		
Sulfonylurea, 2nd Generation		
Glimepiride (Amaryl®)	1-2	Hypoglycemia, dizziness, headache, GI distress, SIADH
GlipiZIDE (Glucotrol® XL; Glucotrol®)		
GlyBURIDE (DiaBeta®; Glynase® PresTab®; Micronase®)		
Thiazolidinediones		
Pioglitazone (Actos®)	0.5-1.4	**May cause or exacerbate heart failure [BOXED WARNING]**, hepatic dysfunction, weight gain, edema, lipid changes
Rosiglitazone (Avandia®)		

Injectable Agents (Noninsulin)

In addition to insulin and oral agents, three injectable products are available for the management of diabetes. Exenatide (Byetta®) and liraglutide (Victoza®) are GLP-1 receptor agonists FDA-approved for the treatment of type 2 diabetes. Exenatide is used as an adjunct to diet and exercise to improve glycemic control in patients with type 2 diabetes mellitus. The manufacturer of liraglutide states that it is an injectable prescription medicine that may improve blood sugar in adults with type 2 diabetes when used along with diet and exercise. GLP-1 agonists increase insulin secretion, increase B-cell growth/replication, slow gastric emptying, and may decrease food intake.

Pramlintide (Symlin®) is FDA approved for the treatment of type 1 and type 2 diabetes. In type 1 diabetes, it is approved for use in patients who have failed to achieve glucose control despite optimal insulin therapy. When used for type 2 diabetes, pramlintide is approved for use in patients who have failed to achieve desired glucose control despite optimal insulin therapy, with or without concurrent sulfonylurea and/or metformin. Pramlintide is a synthetic analog of human amylin cosecreted with insulin by pancreatic beta cells. It reduces postprandial glucose increases by prolonging gastric emptying time, reducing postprandial glucagon secretion, and reducing caloric intake through centrally-mediated appetite suppression. It should be noted that the concentration of this product is in mcg/mL; patients and healthcare providers should exercise caution when administering this product to avoid inadvertent calculation of the dose based on "units," which could result in a sixfold overdose.

Injectable Agents (Non-Insulin) for Type 2 Diabetes

Generic Name (Brand Name)	Expected Decrease (%) in Hb A_{1c} With Monotherapy	Key Adverse Effects
Glucagon-Like Peptide 1 (GLP-1) Agonist		
Exenatide (Byetta®)	0.5-1	Hypoglycemia, nausea, vomiting, pancreatitis, headache, jittery feeling
Liraglutide (Victoza®)	1	**Thyroid C-cell Tumors [BOXED WARNING]**, nausea, vomiting, diarrhea, constipation, headache, pancreatitis
Amylin Agonists		
Pramlintide (Symlin®)	0.4-0.6	**Coadministration with insulin may induce severe hypoglycemia [BOXED WARNING]**, nausea, vomiting, hypoglycemia, headache, anorexia

Additional Management Issues

Recommendation by the ADA include glycemic control, as well as the following:

- Monitoring: In all patients with diabetes, cardiovascular risk factors should be assessed at least annually.

- Cardiovascular risk management

  - Use an ACEI or ARB in patients with diabetes who have hypertension and micro- or macroalbuminuria to slow the progression of nephropathy, unless contraindicated (eg, pregnancy); additional agents (eg, thiazide or loop diuretics) may be added as needed to achieve blood pressure goals.

  - Consider statin use in all patients with diabetes and cardiovascular disease or in patients with diabetes >40 years of age without cardiovascular disease but have at least one other cardiovascular disease risk factor, irrespective of lipoprotein levels (exception: Statin use is contraindicated in pregnancy). For patients without overt CVD and <40 years of age, statin therapy may be considered if LDL remains >100 mg/dL with lifestyles changes or in those with multiple cardiovascular risk factors. In individuals with overt CVD, lower LDL goals (<70 mg/dL) are suggested.

  - Use of low-dose aspirin (75-162 mg daily) is reasonable for primary prevention in all patients with diabetes at increased cardiovascular disease (CVD) risk (10-year risk >10%), including most men >50 years of age and most women >60 years of age who have at least one additional risk factor (eg, hypertension, smoking, family history of CVD, dyslipidemia, albuminuria), unless contraindicated. Low-dose aspirin may be considered for those at intermediate CVD risk (younger patients with ≥1 risk factor, older patients without risk factors, or patients with 10-year CVD risk of 5% to 10%). Aspirin is not recommended for primary prevention in patients with lower risk for CVD (eg, men <50 years of age and women <60 years of age without additional risk factor; 10-year CVD risk <5%). In secondary prevention, all patients with a history of CVD should receive aspirin (75-162 mg daily). Given the risk of Reye syndrome with the use of aspirin in patients <21 years of age, aspirin is not recommended in this population for primary or secondary prevention. In patients unable to take aspirin (eg, documented allergy), the use of clopidogrel is considered a reasonable alternative.

– Coronary heart disease (CHD): In patients with known cardiovascular disease (CVD), ACE inhibitor therapy and aspirin and statin therapy (if not contraindicated) should be used to reduce the risk of cardiovascular events. In patients with a prior myocardial infarction, beta-blockers should be continued for at least 2 years after the event. Avoid thiazolidinedione (TZD) treatment in patients with symptomatic heart failure. Metformin may be used in patients with stable congestive heart failure (CHF) if renal function is normal; however, it should be avoided in unstable or hospitalized patients with CHF.

- Other preventative actions

  – Immunize against pneumococcal disease in patients ≥2 years of age. One-time revaccination is recommended for individuals >64 years of age if they were <65 years of age when previously immunized >5 years ago.

  – Influenza immunization annually for all diabetic patients ≥6 months old

  – Patients should be advised not to smoke.

  – Patients should be advised to perform at least 150 minutes/week of moderate-intensity aerobic physical activity (50% to 70% of maximal heart rate). In the absence of contradictions, patients with type 2 diabetes should be encouraged to perform resistance training 3 times/week.

  – Eye care: To reduce the risk or slow the progression of retinopathy, optimize glycemic and blood pressure control. Adults and children ≥10 years of age with type 1 diabetes should have an initial dilated and comprehensive eye examination within 5 years after the onset of diabetes (if type 2, exam should occur shortly after the diagnosis of diabetes). Subsequent examinations should be repeated annually. Promptly refer patients with any level of macular edema, severe nonproliferative diabetic retinopathy (NPDR), or any proliferative diabetic retinopathy (PDR) to an ophthalmologist who is knowledgeable and experienced in the management and treatment of diabetic retinopathy.

  – Nephropathy: To reduce the risk or slow the progression of nephropathy, optimize glucose and blood pressure control. In the treatment of the nonpregnant patient with micro- or macroalbuminuria, either ACE inhibitors or ARBs should be used (if one class is not tolerated, the other should be substituted). When estimated GFR (eGFR) is <60 mL/minute/1.73 m^2, evaluate and manage potential complications of CKD. Consider referral to a physician experienced in the care of kidney disease when there is uncertainty about the etiology of the disease (heavy proteinuria, active urine sediment, absence of retinopathy, rapid decline in GFR), difficult management issues, or advanced kidney disease.

  – Neuropathy: All patients should be screened for distal symmetric polyneuropathy (DPN) at diagnosis and at least annually thereafter, using simple clinical tests. Screening for signs and symptoms of cardiovascular autonomic neuropathy should be instituted at diagnosis of type 2 and 5 years after the diagnosis of type 1 diabetes.

  – Foot care: Perform general foot self-care education to all patients with diabetes. For all patients with diabetes, perform an annual comprehensive foot examination. The foot examination should include inspection, assessment of foot pulses, and testing for loss of protective sensation (10 g monofilament, plus testing any one of: Vibration using a 128-Hz tuning fork, pinprick sensation, ankle reflexes, or vibration perception threshold).

  – Thyroid: TSH concentrations should be measured after metabolic control has been established. If normal, they should be rechecked every 1-2 years or if the patient develops symptoms of thyroid dysfunction, thyromegaly, or an abnormal growth rate.

REFERENCES

Action to Control Cardiovascular Risk in Diabetes Study Group, "Effects of Intensive Glucose Lowering in Type 2 Diabetes," *N Engl J Med*, 2008, 358(24):2545-59.

ADVANCE Collaborative Group, "Intensive Blood Glucose Control and Vascular Outcomes in Patients With Type 2 Diabetes," *N Engl J Med*, 2008, 358(24):2560-72.

American Diabetes Association, "Diagnosis and Classification of Diabetes Mellitus," *Diabetes Care*, 2011, 34(Suppl 1): S62-9.

American Diabetes Association, "Standards of Medical Care in Diabetes - 2011," *Diabetes Care*, 2011, 34(Suppl 1): S11-61.

Brunzell JD, Davidson M, Furberg CD, et al, "Lipoprotein Management in Patients With Cardiometabolic Risk: Consensus Statement From the American Diabetes Association and the American College of Cardiology Foundation," *Diabetes Care*, 2008, 31(4):811-22.

Centers for Disease Control (CDC), "National Diabetes Fact Sheet: 2007 General Information," Available at: http://www.cdc.gov/diabetes/pubs/pdf/ndfs_2007.pdf. Accessed January 9, 2009.

Colhoun HM, Betteridge DJ, Durrington PN, et al, "Primary Prevention of Cardiovascular Disease With Atorvastatin in Type 2 Diabetes in the Collaborative Atorvastatin Diabetes Study (CARDS): Multicentre Randomised Placebo-Controlled Trial," *Lancet*, 2004, 364(9435):685-96.

Dailey G, "New Strategies for Basal Insulin Treatment in Type 2 Diabetes Mellitus," *Clin Ther*, 2004, 26(6):889-901.

DeFronzo RA, "Pharmacologic Therapy for Type 2 Diabetes Mellitus," *Ann Intern Med*, 1999, 131(4):281-303.

DeFronzo RA, "Pharmacologic Therapy for Type 2 Diabetes Mellitus," *Ann Intern Med*, 2000, 133(1):73-4.

Duckworth W, Abraira C, Moritz T, et al, "Glucose Control and Vascular Complications in Veterans With Type 2 Diabetes," *N Engl J Med*, 2009, 360(2):129-39.

Holman RR and Turner RC, "Insulin Therapy in Type II Diabetes," *Diabetes Res Clin Pract*, 1995, (28 Suppl):S179-84.

International Expert Committee, "International Expert Committee Report on the Role of the A_{1C} Assay in the Diagnosis of Diabetes," *Diabetes Care*, 2009, 32(7):1327-34.

Kitabchi AE, Umpierrez GE, Murphy MB, et al, "Hyperglycemic Crises in Diabetes," *Diabetes Care*, 2004, 27(Suppl 1): S94-102.

Nathan DM, Buse JB, Davidson MB, et al, "Medical Management of Hyperglycemia in Type 2 Diabetes: A Consensus Algorithm for the Initiation and Adjustment of Therapy: A Consensus Statement of the American Diabetes Association and the European Association for the Study of Diabetes," *Diabetes Care*, 2009, 32(1):193-203.

National Institute of Diabetes and Kigestive and Kidney Diseases, "Erectile Dysfunction," available at http://kidney.niddk.nih.gov/kudiseases/pubs/pdf/ErectileDysfunction.pdf. Accessed January 9, 2009.

Oiknine R, Bernbaum M, and Mooradian AD, "A Critical Appraisal of the Role of Insulin Analogues in the Management of Diabetes Mellitus," *Drugs*, 2005, 65(3):325-40.

Pignone M, Alberts MJ, Colwell JA, et al, "Aspirin for Primary Prevention of Cardiovascular Events in People With Diabetes: A Position Statement of the American Diabetes Association, a Scientific Statement of the American Heart Association, and an Expert Consensus Document of the American College of Cardiology Foundation," *Circulation*, 2010, 121(24):2694-701.

Rodbard HW, Jellinger PS, Davidson JA, et al, "Statement by an American Association of Clinical Endocrinologists/American College of Endocrinology Consensus Panel on Type 2 Diabetes Mellitus: An Algorithm for Glycemic Control," *Endocr Pract*, 2009, 15(6):540-59.

Scheife RT (editor), "Liraglutide: A New Option for the Treatment of Type 2 Diabetes Mellitus," *Pharmacotherapy*, 2009, 29(12 part 2): 23s-67s.

Sherifali D, Nerenberg K, Pullenayegum E, et al, "The Effect of Oral Antidiabetic Agents on A_{1C} Levels: A Systematic Review and Meta-Analysis," *Diabetes Care*, 2010, 33(8):1859-64.

Silverstein J, Klingensmith G, Copeland K, et al, "Care of Children and Adolescents With Type 1 Diabetes: A Statement of the American Diabetes Association," *Diabetes Care*, 2005, 28(1):186-212.

The Diabetes Control and Complications Trial Research Group, "The Effect of Intensive Treatment of Diabetes on the Development and Progression of Long-Term Complications in Insulin-dependent Diabetes Mellitus," *N Engl J Med*, 1993, 329(14):977-86.

Tuomilehto J, Lindstrom J, Eriksson JG, et al, "Prevention of Type 2 Diabetes Mellitus by Changes in Lifestyle Among Subjects With Impaired Glucose Tolerance," *N Engl J Med*, 2001, 344(18):1343-50.

UK Prospective Diabetes Study Group, "Intensive Blood Glucose Control With Sulphonylureas or Insulin Compared With Conventional Treatment and Risk of Complications in Patients With Type 2 Diabetes (UKPDS 33)," *Lancet*, 1998, 352(9131):837-53.

HEART FAILURE (SYSTOLIC)

INTRODUCTORY COMMENTS

This summarizes the pharmacotherapy of patients with systolic heart failure with respect to treating mild-to-moderate exacerbations and chronic therapy. A more detailed discussion is available at http://content.onlinejacc.org/cgi/content/full/j.jacc.2008.11.013.

It should be recognized that the most common cause for exacerbations of patients' heart failure is poor adherence to therapy (medications and diet restriction). Healthcare providers need to educate patients about the importance of adherence to medical regimens.

For many years, therapy of heart failure focused on correcting the hemodynamic imbalances that occurred in heart failure. It is now recognized that heart failure triggers the release of several neurohormones that, in the short-run, help the patient; but, in the long-run, are detrimental. Newer pharmacotherapeutic approaches address countering the actions of these harmful neuro-hormones as well as address hemodynamic issues.

DIURETICS

Although data have yet to demonstrate that diuretics reduce the mortality associated with heart failure, they relieve symptoms seen in heart failure. Diuretics should only be used in patients experiencing congestion with their heart failure. Although not usually the case, some patients do have heart failure without congestion. In such rare instances, diuretic therapy is not indicated since they further stimulate the deleterious neurohormonal responses seen.

Although some heart failure patients with congestion can be controlled with thiazide diuretics, most will require the more potent loop diuretics, either because a strong diuretic effect is needed or renal function is compromised (thus limiting the effectiveness of the thiazide diuretic). When patients with heart failure are discovered to have mild-to-moderate worsening congestion, they often can be controlled by adjusting their oral loop diuretic dose or, if applicable, initiating a loop diuretic regimen. If a more aggressive diuresis is indicated, especially if the patient is suffering from pulmonary congestion, intravenous loop diuretics would be indicated. When loop diuretics are given intravenously, before any diuretic effect occurs, they benefit the patient by dilating veins and reducing preload, thus relieving pulmonary congestion. Intravenous loop diuretics may also be considered in a patient where concerns exist about the ability to absorb orally administered medication.

If already on an oral loop diuretic, the dosage should be increased (generally, 1.5-2 times their current regimen) in an effort for the patient to lose about 1-1.5 liters of fluid per day (about equivalent to 1-1.5 kg of weight per day). If the patient had yet to be started on a diuretic or was previously receiving a thiazide diuretic, initiating furosemide at 20-40 mg once or twice daily is a reasonable consideration. If the initial increase (or initiation) in dosage fails to induce a diuretic response, the dosage may be increased. If the initial increase (or initiation) does induce a diuretic response but the patient fails to lose weight or is not losing more fluids than taking in, the frequency of giving the loop diuretic may be increased. When an effective regimen is achieved, this regimen should be continued until the patient achieves a goal "dry" weight. Once this weight is attained, a decision needs to be made on how to continue the patient on diuretic therapy. If the patient had not been on a diuretic at home, continuation of the loop diuretic at a reduced dose is a worthy consideration. If the exacerbation was related to nonadherence with the diuretic or diet, the previous home dose might be continued with education on adherence to the prescribed diet and medication use. If the exacerbation was caused by an inadequate pharmacotherapeutic regimen (such as vasodilator was not being used), the previous home dose might be continued in conjunction with a more complete pharmacotherapeutic regimen. If the patient was compliant and on an acceptable pharmacotherapeutic regimen, the patient's original diuretic dose would be increased to some dosage greater than their home regimen, yet generally less than what was just used to achieve their dry weight.

The use of loop diuretics can lead to hypokalemia and/or hypomagnesemia. Electrolyte disturbances can predispose a patient to serious cardiac arrhythmias particularly if the patient is concurrently receiving digoxin. Fluid depletion, hypotension, and azotemia can also result from excessive use of diuretics. In contrast to thiazide diuretics, a loop diuretic can also lower serum calcium concentrations. For some patients, despite higher doses of loop diuretic treatment, an adequate diuretic response cannot be attained. Diuretic resistance can usually be overcome by intravenous administration (including continuous infusion), the use of 2 diuretics together (eg, furosemide and metolazone), or the use of a diuretic with a positive inotropic agent. When such combinations are used, serum electrolytes need to be monitored even more closely.

When loop diuretics are used in patients with renal dysfunction, to achieve the desired diuretic response, dosages typically will need to be greater than what is used in patients with normal renal function.

Due to its long existence and inexpensive price, furosemide tends to be the loop diuretic most commonly used. Bumetanide and torsemide are now available as generics and their use, especially bumetanide, has increased. The oral bioavailability of bumetanide and torsemide are nearly 100%; whereas, furosemide's oral bioavailability averages about 50%. A useful rule of thumb for conversion of intravenous loop diuretics is 40 mg of furosemide is equal to 1 mg bumetanide is equal to 20 mg torsemide. A few patients have allergies to diuretics because many contain a sulfur element. The only loop diuretic that lacks a sulfur element is ethacrynic acid.

VASODILATORS

Combination Hydralazine and Isosorbide Dinitrate

Vasodilator therapy, specifically the combination of hydralazine and isosorbide dinitrate, was the first pharmacotherapeutic treatment demonstrated to enhance survival of heart failure patients. The use of hydralazine 75 mg (which reduces afterload) and isosorbide dinitrate 40 mg 4 times a day (which reduces preload) demonstrated enhanced survival compared to placebo and prazosin. Unfortunately, many patients were unable to tolerate this regimen (primarily due to headaches and gastrointestinal disturbances) and the magnitude of benefit in survival dissipated with time.

The African-American Heart Failure Trial (A-HeFT) demonstrated mortality benefit with the use of a fixed combination of hydralazine and isosorbide dinitrate in combination with standard heart failure therapies, including ACE inhibitors, in self-identified African-American heart failure patients. The use of the commercially available combination of hydralazine and isosorbide dinitrate may be cost prohibitive in some patients; therefore, the use of the individually separate products is justifiable.

ACE Inhibitors

A series of investigations demonstrated that enalapril (which reduces both afterload and preload) enhances the survival of heart failure patients. Dosages used in these trials averaged about 10 mg twice daily. Since these trials, other ACE inhibitors were proven to benefit heart failure patients.

This led to the question – which is superior, ACE inhibitor or the combination of hydralazine and isosorbide dinitrate? In a comparative trial, using doses described above, enalapril was superior to the combination of hydralazine and isosorbide dinitrate, making an ACE inhibitor the vasodilator of choice in heart failure patients. An ACE inhibitor can alleviate symptoms, improve clinical status, and enhance a patient's quality of life. In addition an ACE inhibitor can reduce the risk of death and the combined risk of death or hospitalization.

Adverse effects associated with ACE inhibitors include hyperkalemia, rash, dysgeusia, dry cough, and (rarely) angioedema. Patients sometime develop renal dysfunction with the initiation of ACE inhibitors. This is not due to direct nephrotoxicity but is related to the ACE inhibitor dilating the efferent renal artery of the kidney, thus shunting blood away from being filtered in the glomerulus. The risk for renal dysfunction is increased when the ACE inhibitor is introduced to a patient who is hypovolemic, is being aggressively diuresed, is on an NSAID (which should be avoided in heart failure patients), or has bilateral renal artery stenosis (unilateral if only one kidney is present). ACE inhibitors should be avoided in patients with known renal artery stenosis. Monitor renal function and serum potassium within 1-2 weeks of initiation of therapy and routinely thereafter especially in patients with pre-existing hypotension, hyponatremia, diabetes, azotemia, or those taking potassium supplements. Some patients will have an exaggerated hypotensive response following the initial doses (especially the first dose) of an ACE inhibitor.

Angiotensin Receptor Blockers

A major limitation to using ACE inhibitors treatment in heart failure can be the dry cough that some patients develop. Lowering the ACE inhibitor dose sometimes can control it, but this may limit the effectiveness of the ACE inhibitor treatment. The development of angiotensin receptor blockers (ARBs) has helped address this issue. ARBs were demonstrated to enhance survival of heart failure patients. Although they are not the vasodilator of first choice in heart failure, they are a reasonable alternative in patients who cannot tolerate an ACE inhibitor due to the cough or some other adverse effect (with the exception of hyperkalemia and renal dysfunction; ARBs can induce as well). ARBs do not cause an accumulation of kinins as ACE inhibitors do.

Can ARBs be used in patients who suffer angioedema with ACE inhibitors? Reports are available in the literature describing patients who experienced angioedema with both ACE inhibitors and ARBs. These cases do not indicate the safety of an ARB when used in a patient who has experienced ACE inhibitor-induced angioedema. The CHARM-Alternative trial confirmed that only one of 39 patients (~2.6%) who experienced angioedema with an ACE inhibitors also experienced it with an ARB.

Concurrent Use of an ACE Inhibitor and an ARB

In Val-HeFT, valsartan added to conventional treatment (included ACE inhibitor treatment) did not impact survival but did reduce morbidity. Of note, a subgroup analysis of this trial suggested the combination of valsartan and an ACE inhibitor may be detrimental to patients also receiving a beta-blocker. In CHARM-Added, candesartan added to ACE inhibitor therapy was of benefit to heart failure patients (modest reduction in hospitalization; increased risk of hyperkalemia and renal dysfunction), even for those receiving a beta-blocker. As a result, the ACCF/AHA Practice Guidelines do not speak against using the combination of ACE inhibitors and ARBs. However, few patients in these trials were receiving an aldosterone blocker (such as spironolactone), which is now known to be of benefit to heart failure patients. Since there is enhanced risk for hyperkalemia and outcome data are currently unknown, the ACCF/AHA Practice Guidelines for heart failure do not advocate the combined use of ACE inhibitors, ARBs, and an aldosterone inhibitor.

In summary, vasodilator therapy should initially consist of an ACE inhibitor. If such therapy cannot be tolerated due to renal failure or hyperkalemia, the combination of hydralazine and isosorbide dinitrate may be considered as ARBs can also cause renal failure and hyperkalemia. If the ACE inhibitor cannot be tolerated due to adverse effects such as dry cough, an ARB may be considered. If an ACE inhibitor and beta-blocker have been maximized yet heart failure symptoms persist, consider adding hydralazine and isosorbide dinitrate. This approach, in fact, has been demonstrated to enhance the survival of African-American patients with heart failure. Another approach may be to add an ARB to the ACE inhibitor; but caution should occur, due to the risk of hyperkalemia.

BETA-BLOCKERS

Despite being negative inotropes, beta-blockers have been demonstrated to enhance the survival of systolic heart failure patients. Their benefit is attributed to their ability to protect the myocardium from the "bombardment" of catecholamines present in heart failure that can lead to ventricular remodeling. Bisoprolol, metoprolol succinate (extended release), and carvedilol have been demonstrated in trials to improve survival. Carvedilol is also available as a once-a-day extended-release preparation; but, its daily cost is considerably greater than generically-available immediate-release carvedilol that is given twice a day. At present, superiority of a particular beta-blocker over another has not been definitively demonstrated. For patients to be able to tolerate this therapy, beta-blocker treatment needs to be initiated at low doses and titrated slowly (generally, the dose is double every two weeks). Following the initiation of treatment and increase in dosage, patients may feel that their disease is worsening but this should dissipate after a few days. If this ill feeling continues beyond a few days, consideration should be given to regimen adjustments. If the patient is congested, increase the diuretic dosage. If the patient's discomfort is related to hypotension, staggering the beta-blocker dose with the vasodilator dose and/or lowering the vasodilator dosage may be helpful. If these approaches are ineffective or cannot explain the patient's ill feeling, consideration should be given to lowering the beta-blocker dosage and attempt a dose titration increase later on. Sometimes, a patient may not be able to tolerate "goal" doses of both beta-blockers and concurrent vasodilator treatment due to hypotension. It is the consensus opinion that a reduced dose of each agent is better than a goal dose of just one agent. Beta-blockers are not necessarily contraindicated but need to be used cautiously in patients with bronchospastic disease, peripheral arterial disease, or diabetes mellitus.

ALDOSTERONE BLOCKERS

It has been demonstrated, especially in the more severe forms of heart failure, that spirono-lactone, at an average dose of 25 mg daily, enhances the survival of heart failure patients. In patients who suffer hyperkalemia at this relatively low dosage, lowering the dose to 25 mg every other day may be attempted. In patients who remain symptomatic with their heart failure and have maximized the other proven treatments of heart failure and whose potassium concentrations can tolerate increases, the spironolactone dose may be increased to 50 mg daily.

Obviously, hyperkalemia is a concern with this treatment, especially since patients generally will also be receiving an ACE inhibitor or ARB. It has been demonstrated that the number of emergency visits related to hyperkalemia in heart failure has increased with the introduction of aldosterone blocking therapy in treating heart failure. About 10% of patients will experience endocrinological effects with spironolactone. In men, breast tenderness and gynecomastia may occur. In women, menstrual irregularities may be seen. In such instances, the use of eplerenone may be considered. Eplerenone is less apt to induce endocrinological effects but it is more expensive. A typical dose is 25-50 mg daily. Eplerenone has been demonstrated to enhance survival of post-MI patients with reduced ejection fractions. Spironolactone has not been studied in this patient group.

These medications should not be started in patients with renal insufficiency. These medications should be avoided if the serum creatinine exceeds 2.5 mg/dL in men (2 mg/dL in women) or if baseline potassium ≥5 mEq/L.

DIGOXIN

The value of digoxin in heart failure has crossed the spectrum. In the late 1980s, further investigation with digoxin suggested that indeed it may have a role in heart failure treatment, but the methods of these trials were not ideal (digoxin was taken away from stabilized patients to see if the condition of patients worsened – it did). Finally, digoxin was studied in a prospective manner where patients were on known optimal heart failure treatment at the time and randomized to placebo or digoxin. The digoxin dosage used resulted in digoxin steady-state concentrations of 1 mcg/L. This trial revealed that digoxin did not impact survival but reduced the number of patient hospitalizations, suggesting digoxin has a morbidity benefit. Many are of the opinion that digoxin's benefit is unrelated to its positive inotropic activity but related to inhibiting neuro-hormonal activity. Healthcare providers may consider adding digoxin in patients with persistent heart failure symptoms as a fourth line agent.

Digoxin is primarily renally eliminated; therefore, renal function of patients should be closely monitored and the dose adjusted. Digoxin does become difficult to use in patients whose renal function is unstable. In the DIG trial, effective digoxin steady-state concentrations ranged between 0.7-1 mcg/L. Concentrations much beyond 1 mcg/L were associated with worsened outcomes, especially in women. Since digoxin's benefit is long-term, a loading dose is not necessary. When checking a digoxin serum concentration, the sample should not be obtained until 12 hours after a dose, especially if it was oral, since digoxin has a relatively long distribution phase. It should also be assured that the patient is at steady-state (recall that the half-life of digoxin in a patient with normal renal function is approximately 36 hours and that patients with heart failure generally have worsened renal function).

Hypokalemia, hypomagnesia, hypercalcemia, and hypothyroidism can precipitate digoxin toxicity in the presence of a therapeutic digoxin concentration. This toxicity can be alleviated by correcting the electrolyte abnormality. In acute digoxin overdoses, hyperkalemia can occur since digoxin inhibits the sodium-potassium ATPase pump. For this reason, one should not assume potassium is given to just **any** patient with digoxin toxicity. Digoxin toxicity can present as bradyarrhythmias, heart blocks, ventricular tachyarrhythmias, and atrial tachyarrhythmias (PAT with block is pathognomonic). Other toxic manifestations include visual disturbances (including greenish-yellowish vision and halos around lights), gastrointestinal disturbances, anorexia, and altered mental status. Many medications elevate digoxin concentrations and a patient's regimen should be assessed for potential interactions.

OTHER HEART FAILURE THERAPEUTIC CONSIDERATIONS

- If a calcium channel blocker is desired, amlodipine or felodipine are preferred choices.

- To treat arrhythmias, amiodarone and dofetilide are best documented to lack significant proarrhythmic propensity in heart failure patients. Dronedarone, a newer antiarrhythmic agent structurally similar to amiodarone, is contraindicated in patients with NYHA Class IV heart failure or Class II-III heart failure with recent decompensation requiring hospitalization or referral to a specialized heart failure clinic.

- In heart failure patients with diabetes mellitus, metformin should not be used and "glitazones" should not be used in severe heart failure (NYHA III and IV) and used cautiously, if at all, in mild-to-moderate heart failure.

- The use of cilostazol, because it has type III phosphodiesterase-inhibiting properties, is contraindicated in heart failure. This is because the chronic use of oral milrinone and inamrinone, also type III phosphodiesterase inhibitors, resulted in enhanced mortality in heart failure patients (and therefore, these two agents were never FDA-approved for oral use).

- NSAID use should be avoided or used minimally as these agents antagonize the effects of diuretics and ACE inhibitors.

- Retrospective data suggests that daily aspirin may also negate the effects of ACE inhibitors but this has yet to be definitively proven in prospective trials. Using the lowest possible aspirin dose with the highest possible ACE inhibitor dose has been suggested as a way to best circumvent this issue.

- Routine intermittent intravenous infusions of positive inotropes are not recommended; but their use may be considered as palliative therapy in end-stage disease when ordinary therapy is insufficient.

CLASS I RECOMMENDATIONS FOR THE HOSPITALIZED PATIENT WITH ACUTE DECOMPENSATED HEART FAILURE

- Patients presenting to the hospital with fluid overload should be treated immediately with intravenous loop diuretics (eg, furosemide) since earlier treatment may be associated with better outcomes. If chronically receiving oral loop diuretic therapy, the initial intravenous dose should equal or exceed their chronic oral daily dose and titrated to relieve symptoms and reduce fluid excess. If this is inadequate, use of higher doses of loop diuretics, adding a second diuretic (eg, intravenous chlorothiazide), or a continuous infusion of the loop diuretic may improve diuresis.

- If evidence of hypotension with associated hypoperfusion and elevated cardiac filling pressures (eg, increase JVP) exists, intravenous inotropic support (eg, dobutamine) or vasopressor drugs (eg, dopamine) should be administered. Use of intravenous inotropes in patients without evidence of hypoperfusion is not recommended.

- In the absence of hemodynamic instability or contraindications, the use of therapies known to improve outcomes (eg, ACE inhibitors or ARBs, and beta-blockers) should be continued during the hospital stay. When appropriate, these agents should be initiated or reinitiated to stabilized patients prior to hospital discharge. Beta-blockers should only be initiated upon successful discontinuation of intravenous diuretics, vasodilators, and inotropic agents in the stabilized patient; initiate at a low dose and use caution in those patients who required inotropic support during their hospital course.

Dosing of ACE Inhibitors in Heart Failure[1]

ACEI	Initial Dose	Maximum Dose[2]
Captopril	6.25 mg tid	50 mg tid
Enalapril	2.5 mg bid	10-20 mg bid
Fosinopril	5-10 mg daily	40 mg daily
Lisinopril	2.5-5 mg daily	20-40 mg daily
Perindopril	2 mg daily	8-16 mg daily
Quinapril	5 mg bid	20 mg bid
Ramipril	1.25-2.5 mg daily	10 mg daily
Trandolapril	1 mg daily	4 mg daily

[1]From ACCF/AHA Guidelines

[2]Maximum/target dose recommendation may vary between guidelines (also see Heart Failure Society of America, 2010)

Dosing of ARBs in Heart Failure[1]

ARB	Initial Dose	Maximum Dose[2]
Candesartan	4-8 mg daily	32 mg daily
Losartan	25-50 mg daily	50-100 mg daily
Valsartan	20-40 mg bid	160 mg bid

[1]From ACCF/AHA Guidelines

[2]Maximum/target dose recommendation may vary between guidelines (also see Heart Failure Society of America, 2010)

Initial and Target Doses for Beta-Blocker Therapy in Heart Failure[1]

Beta-Blocker	Starting Dose	Target Dose	Comment
Bisoprolol	1.25 mg daily	10 mg daily	β₁-Selective blocker Inconvenient dosage forms for initial dose titration
Carvedilol	3.125 mg bid	25 mg bid (≤85 kg) 50 mg bid (>85 kg)	β-Nonselective blocker α₁-Blocking properties
Carvedilol phosphate, extended release	10 mg daily	80 mg daily[2]	
Metoprolol succinate, extended release	12.5-25 mg daily	200 mg daily	β₁-Selective blocker

[1]From ACCF/AHA Guidelines

[2]Equivalent to carvedilol immediate release 25 mg twice daily

Conversion From Immediate Release to Extended Release Carvedilol (Coreg CR®)

Carvedilol Immediate Release Dose	Carvedilol Phosphate Extended Release Dose
3.125 mg twice daily	10 mg once daily
6.25 mg twice daily	20 mg once daily
12.5 mg twice daily	40 mg once daily
25 mg twice daily	80 mg once daily

REFERENCES

Brater DC, "Diuretic Therapy," N Engl J Med, 1998, 339(6):387-95.

Granger CB, McMurray JJ, Yusuf S, et al, "Effects of Candesartan in Patients With Chronic Heart Failure and Reduced Left-Ventricular Systolic Function Intolerant to Angiotensin-Converting-Enzyme Inhibitors: The CHARM-Alternative Trial," Lancet, 2003, 362(9386):772-6.

Heart Failure Society of America, Lindenfeld J, Albert NM, et al, "HFSA 2010 Comprehensive Heart Failure Practice Guideline," J Card Fail, 2010, 16(6):e1-194.

Hunt SA, Abraham WT, Chin MH, et al, "2009 Focused Update Incorporated Into the ACC/AHA 2005 Guidelines for the Diagnosis and Management of Heart Failure in Adults A Report of the American College of Cardiology Foundation/ American Heart Association Task Force on Practice Guidelines Developed in Collaboration With the International Society for Heart and Lung Transplantation," J Am Coll Cardiol, 2009, 53(15):e1-e90.

McMurray JJ, Ostergren J, Swedberg K, et al, "Effects of Candesartan in Patients With Chronic Heart Failure and Reduced Left-Ventricular Systolic Function Taking Angiotensin-Converting-Enzyme Inhibitors: The CHARM-Added Trial," Lancet, 2003, 362(9386):767-71.

Taylor AL, Ziesche S, Yancy C, et al, "Combination of Isosorbide Dinitrate and Hydralazine in Blacks With Heart Failure," N Engl J Med, 2004, 351(20):2049-57.

PERIOPERATIVE/PERIPROCEDURAL MANAGEMENT OF ANTICOAGULANT AND ANTIPLATELET THERAPY

RISK OF PERIOPERATIVE ARTERIAL OR VENOUS THROMBOEMBOLISM

Perioperative management of patients who may require temporary interruption of antithrombotic therapy is a common challenge in patient care. Interruption of antithrombotic therapy in some patients may cause devastating consequences (eg, MI, stroke, valve thrombosis). It is important to address two questions prior to interrupting antithrombotic therapy. First, is interruption in the perioperative period necessary? Secondly, if interruption is necessary, is bridging anticoagulation necessary? The answers to these questions are determined by the type of surgery or procedure and the risk of thrombosis if antithrombotic therapy is interrupted, respectively. Although a validated risk stratification tool does not exist, the following guidelines (see Table 1 below) may be helpful in identifying those patients who are at risk of arterial or venous thromboembolism. In patients with atrial fibrillation, the CHADS$_2$ (Cardiac failure-Hypertension-Age-Diabetes-Stroke [doubled]) score, which identifies those patients at higher risk of stroke, must be calculated (see Table 2 on next page) to determine level of risk for perioperative arterial or venous thromboembolism.

Table 1. Suggested Risk Stratification for Perioperative Arterial or Venous Thromboembolism (Douketis, 2012)

Indication for Warfarin	High Risk	Moderate Risk	Low Risk
Mechanical Heart Valve	Any mitral valve prosthesis; Older (caged-ball or tilting disc) aortic valve prosthesis Recent (within 6 months) stroke or TIA	Bileaflet aortic valve prosthesis and at least one of the following: • AF • Prior stroke or TIA • Hypertension • Diabetes • Heart failure • Age >75 years	Bileaflet aortic valve prosthesis without AF or other risk factors for stroke
Atrial Fibrillation[1]	CHADS$_2$ score of 5 or 6 Recent (within 3 months) stroke or TIA Rheumatic valvular heart disease	CHADS$_2$ score of 3 or 4	CHADS$_2$ score of 0-2 (no prior stroke or TIA)
Venous Thromboembolism (VTE)	Recent (within 3 months) VTE Protein C or S deficiency, antithrombin or antiphospholipid antibodies, or multiple thrombophilic abnormalities	VTE within in the past 3-12 months Heterozygous factor V Leiden or prothrombin gene mutation Recurrent VTE Cancer (active)	Single VTE occurring >12 months ago (no additional risk factors)

CHADS$_2$ = Cardiac failure-Hypertension-Age-Diabetes-Stroke (doubled), TIA = transient ischemic attack

[1]Calculate CHADS$_2$ score (see Table 2 on next page) to determine level of risk for perioperative thrombosis

Table 2. CHADS$_2$ Index: Stroke Risk in Patients with Nonvalvular AF Not Treated With Antithrombotic Therapy

CHADS$_2$ Risk Criteria	Point(s)
Cardiac failure	1
Hypertension	1
>75 years of age	1
Diabetes mellitus	1
Prior stroke or TIA	2

AF = atrial fibrillation, CHADS$_2$ = Cardiac failure-Hypertension-Age-Diabetes-Stroke (doubled), TIA = transient ischemic attack

The CHADS$_2$ Risk Score is calculated by adding up the points assigned for each individual risk criteria. For example, if a patient has heart failure, is >75 years of age, and has diabetes mellitus, then the patient's CHADS$_2$ risk score is 3. This patient would be considered high-risk with an adjusted stroke rate of 5.9% per year, which assumes no antithrombotic usage (Gage, 2001).

Table 3. Surgeries and Procedures Considered High Risk of Bleeding in the Setting of Perioperative Antithrombotic Use

Surgery or Procedure
Urologic surgery (eg, TURP, bladder resection, tumor ablation, nephrectomy, kidney biopsy)
Pacemaker or ICD implantation
Colonic polyp resection (especially if >1-2 cm long)
Surgery/procedures in high vascular organs (eg, kidney, liver, spleen)
Bowel resection
Major surgery with extensive tissue injury (eg, cancer surgery, joint arthroplasty, reconstructive plastic surgery)
Cardiac, intracranial, or spinal surgery

ICD = implantable cardioverter defibrillator, TURP = transurethral prostate resection

Table 4. Perioperative/Periprocedural Management of Warfarin

Type of Surgery / Procedure / Patient Population	Action	Reinstitution	Comments
Urgent surgery/procedures	Administer I.V. or oral vitamin K low-dose (2.5-5 mg)		Consider FFP or recombinant factor VIIa in addition to vitamin K; however, these effects are temporary and may not last as long as the vitamin K inhibition
Surgery/procedure requiring normalization of INR	Stop ~5 days before surgery	12-24 hours **AFTER** surgery/procedure when adequate hemostasis achieved	Administer low-dose oral vitamin K (1-2 mg); if INR is still elevated (≥1.5) 1-2 days before surgery
HIGH risk of thromboembolism in patients with either a mechanical heart valve, AF, or VTE	Bridge with therapeutic SubQ LMWH or I.V. UFH	*Low to moderate bleeding risk surgery:* Therapeutic SubQ LMWH - 24 hours **AFTER** surgery/procedure when adequate hemostasis achieved *High bleeding risk surgery:* Delay initiation of therapeutic LMWH/UFH for 48-72 hours **AFTER** surgery when adequate hemostasis achieved	Last dose of therapeutic SubQ LMWH should be given 24 hours PRIOR to surgery/procedure (may give half the dose with once daily regimen); for therapeutic I.V. UFH, stop 4-6 hours **BEFORE** surgery/procedure Always consider the anticipated bleeding risk prior to reinstitution of LMWH/UFH instead of resuming at a fixed time.
MODERATE risk of thromboembolism in patients with a mechanical heart valve, AF, or VTE	Depending on patient or surgery-related factors, may choose not to bridge **or** may bridge with therapeutic SubQ LMWH or I.V. UFH or low-dose SubQ LMWH	*Low to moderate bleeding risk surgery:* Therapeutic SubQ LMWH, 24 hours **AFTER** surgery when adequate hemostasis achieved *High bleeding risk surgery:* Delay initiation of therapeutic LMWH/UFH for 48-72 hours **AFTER** surgery when adequate hemostasis achieved; may administer low-dose heparin bridge or warfarin resumption without postoperative bridging	Therapeutic SubQ LMHW preferred over other options; last dose of therapeutic SubQ LMWH should be given 24 hours **PRIOR** to surgery/procedure (may give half the dose); for therapeutic I.V. UFH, stop 4-6 hours **BEFORE** surgery/procedure Always consider the anticipated bleeding risk prior to reinstitution of LMWH/UFH instead of resuming at a fixed time.

Table 4. Perioperative/Periprocedural Management of Warfarin *continued*

Type of Surgery / Procedure / Patient Population	Action	Reinstitution	Comments
LOW risk of thromboembolism in patients with a mechanical heart valve, AF, or VTE	No bridge necessary		
Cataract surgery	Continue through procedure		
Minor dental procedures	Continue and administer oral prohemostatic agent (eg, aminocaproic acid) or stop 2-3 days prior to procedure		
Minor dermatologic procedures	Continue through procedure; optimize local hemostasis		

AF = atrial fibrillation, FFP = fresh frozen plasma, INR = international normalized ratio, LMWH = low molecular weight heparin, SubQ = subcutaneous, UFH = unfractionated heparin, VTE = venous thromboembolism

Table 5. Perioperative/Periprocedural Management of Antiplatelet Therapy[1]

Type of Surgery / Procedure / Patient Population	Action	Reinstitution	Comments
Urgent surgery/procedures	Transfuse with platelets or administer other prohemostatic agents		
Surgery/procedure requiring temporary interruption of aspirin or clopidogrel	Stop 7-10 days PRIOR to surgery/procedure	24 hours AFTER surgery/procedure when adequate hemostasis achieved	
Noncardiac surgery: LOW risk of cardiac events (exclusive of coronary stents)	Aspirin: Stop 7-10 days before surgery Clopidogrel: Stop at least 5 days, preferably 10 days, before surgery		
Noncardiac surgery: MODERATE to HIGH risk of cardiac events (exclusive of coronary stents)	Aspirin: Continue through surgery Clopidogrel: Stop at least 5 days, preferably 10 days, before surgery		
CABG (elective)[2]	Aspirin: Continue through surgery Clopidogrel: Stop at least 5 days before surgery Prasugrel: Stop at least 5 days before surgery; Note: The manufacturer recommends discontinuing at least 7 days before surgery Ticagrelor: Stop at least 5 days before surgery	Aspirin: If stopped, restart 6-48 hours AFTER CABG when adequate hemostasis achieved	Patients referred for urgent CABG (Hillis, 2012): Clopidogrel/ticagrelor: Stop at least 24 hours prior to surgery Prasugrel: Reasonable to perform surgery within 7 days of discontinuation
PCI[3]	Aspirin: Continue through procedure Clopidogrel, prasugrel, ticagrelor: Continue through procedure		It is uncertain whether or not reloading is necessary in patients on a chronic clopidogrel regimen prior to PCI (Di Sciascio, 2010; Mahmoudi, 2011)
Bare metal coronary stent: Surgery required within 6 weeks of stent placement	Continue aspirin and clopidogrel (if currently taking) in the preoperative period		If antiplatelet agent is stopped, do not bridge with UFH, LMWH, direct thrombin inhibitor, or glycoprotein IIb/IIIa inhibitor; no efficacy or safety data to support If increased bleeding is anticipated or procedure is elective with a significant risk of bleeding, then antiplatelet regimen should be completed first (Grines, 2007).

Table 5. Perioperative/Periprocedural Management of Antiplatelet Therapy[1] continued

Type of Surgery / Procedure / Patient Population	Action	Reinstitution	Comments
Drug-eluting coronary stent: Surgery required within 6 months of stent placement	Continue aspirin and clopidogrel in the preoperative period		If antiplatelet agent is stopped, do not bridge with UFH, LMWH, direct thrombin inhibitor, or glycoprotein IIb/IIIa inhibitor; no efficacy or safety data to support If increased bleeding is anticipated or procedure is elective with a significant risk of bleeding, then antiplatelet regimen should be completed first (Grines, 2007).
Minor dental or dermatologic procedures or cataract surgery	Aspirin: Continue through procedure Clopidogrel: See above indications for stent		In patients receiving dual antiplatelet therapy for prevention of stent thrombosis, the American Heart Association and other organizations recommend that aspirin and clopidogrel be continued throughout the procedure. If increased bleeding is anticipated or procedure is elective with a significant risk of bleeding, then antiplatelet regimen should be completed first (Grines, 2007).
Regional/neuraxial anesthesia	Refer to Regional Anesthesia in Patients Receiving Anticoagulant and Antiplatelet Therapy.[4]	**AFTER** catheter removal	NSAIDs (including aspirin) do not appear to increase the risk of spinal hematoma. The actual risk of spinal hematoma with clopidogrel or ticlopidine is unknown.

ACS = acute coronary syndrome, CABG = coronary artery bypass graft, LMWH = subcutaneous low molecular weight heparin, NSAIDs = nonsteroidal anti-inflammatory drugs, PCI = percutaneous coronary intervention, UFH = unfractionated heparin

[1] Recommendations from the American College of Chest Physicians Evidence-Based Clinical Practice Guidelines (Douketis, 2012), unless otherwise noted.

[2] 2011 ACCF/AHA Guideline for Coronary Artery Bypass Graft Surgery (Hillis, 2012)

[3] 2011 ACCF/AHA/SCAI Guideline for Percutaneous Coronary Intervention (Levine, 2011)

[4] Horlocker TT, Wedel DJ, Benzon H, et al, "Regional Anesthesia in the Anticoagulated Patient: Defining the Risks (The Second ASRA Consensus Conference on Neuraxial Anesthesia and Anticoagulation)," *Reg Anesth Pain Med*, 2003, 28(3):172-97.

If patient receiving antiplatelet regimen for prevention of stent thrombosis, contact patient's cardiologist prior to discontinuation (Grines, 2007). Premature interruption of therapy may result in stent thrombosis with subsequent fatal and nonfatal MI. See Table 6 for duration of antiplatelet therapy according to current practice guidelines.

Table 6. Duration of Antiplatelet Therapy According to Current Practice Guidelines

Indication for Antiplatelet Therapy	Recommended Duration of Aspirin	Recommended Duration of P2Y$_{12}$ Inhibition[1]
Acute Coronary Syndrome (ACS)		
NSTEMI	Indefinite	12 months
NSTEMI with subsequent CABG	Indefinite	9-12 months
STEMI with or without fibrinolysis	Indefinite	2-4 weeks
Percutaneous Coronary Intervention (PCI)		
BMS implantation following ACS	Indefinite	At least 12 months
BMS implantation without ongoing ACS	Indefinite	At least 1 month (ideally up to 12 months)[2]
DES implantation with or without ongoing ACS	Indefinite	At least 12 months[3]

BMS = bare metal stent, CABG = coronary artery bypass graft, DES = drug eluting stent, NSTEMI = non-ST-elevation myocardial infarction, STEMI = ST-elevation myocardial infarction

[1] Clopidogrel (and other P2Y$_{12}$ inhibitors) is preferred over ticlopidine due to its lower incidence of serious side effects (eg, neutropenia). **Note:** Prasugrel and ticagrelor, newer P2Y$_{12}$ inhibitors indicated for patients with ACS managed with PCI, may also be used with the same durations.

[2] If patient is at increased risk of bleeding, P2Y$_{12}$ inhibition should be given for at least 2 weeks.

[3] The optimal duration of therapy >1 year has not been established; however, >1 year may be considered in patients with a DES. Clinical predictors of late stent thrombosis during this time period include stenting ostial or bifurcation lesions, prior brachytherapy, advanced age, diabetes mellitus, renal failure, and others.

REFERENCES

Di Sciascio G, Patti G, Pasceri V, et al, "Clopidogrel Reloading in Patients Undergoing Percutaneous Coronary Intervention on Chronic Clopidogrel Therapy: Results of the ARMYDA-4 RELOAD (Antiplatelet Therapy for Reduction of Myocardial Damage During Angioplasty) Randomized Trial," Eur Heart J, 2010, 31(11):1337-43.

Douketis JD, Spyropoulos AC, Spencer FA, et al, "Perioperative Management of Antithrombotic Therapy: Antithrombotic Therapy and Prevention of Thrombosis, 9th ed: American College of Chest Physicians Evidence-Based Clinical Practice Guidelines," Chest, 2012, 141(2 Suppl):326S-50S.

Gage BF, Waterman AD, Shannon W, et al, "Validation of Clinical Classification Schemes for Predicting Stroke: Results From the National Registry of Atrial Fibrillation," JAMA, 2001, 285(22):2864-70.

Grines CL, Bonow RO, Casey DE Jr, et al, "Prevention of Premature Discontinuation of Dual Antiplatelet Therapy in Patients With Coronary Artery Stents: A Science Advisory From the American Heart Association, American College of Cardiology, Society for Cardiovascular Angiography and Interventions, American College of Surgeons, and American Dental Association, With Representation From the American College of Physicians," Circulation, 2007, 115(6):813-8. Available at http://www.acc.org/qualityandscience/clinical/pdfs/Final_Dual_Antiplatelet_Statement_010507.pdf

Hillis LD, Smith PK, Anderson JL, et al, "Special Articles: 2011 ACCF/AHA Guideline for Coronary Artery Bypass Graft Surgery: Executive Summary: A Report of the American College of Cardiology Foundation/American Heart Association Task Force on Practice Guidelines," Anesth Analg, 2012, 114(1):11-45.

Levine GN, Bates ER, Blankenship JC, et al, "2011 ACCF/AHA/SCAI Guideline for Percutaneous Coronary Intervention: A Report of the American College of Cardiology Foundation/American Heart Association Task Force on Practice Guidelines and the Society for Cardiovascular Angiography and Interventions," Circulation, 2011, 124 (23):e574-651.

Mahmoudi M, Syed AI, Ben-Dor I, et al, "Safety and Efficacy of Clopidogrel Reloading in Patients on Chronic Clopidogrel Therapy Who Present With an Acute Coronary Syndrome and Undergo Percutaneous Coronary Intervention," Am J Cardiol, 2011, 107(12):1779-82.

van Walraven C, Hart RG, Wells GA, et al, "A Clinical Prediction Rule to Identify Patients With Atrial Fibrillation and a Low Risk for Stroke While Taking Aspirin," Arch Intern Med, 2003, 163(8):936-43.

Wann LS, Curtis AB, January CT, et al, "2011 ACCF/AHA/HRS Focused Update on the Management of Patients With Atrial Fibrillation (Updating the 2006 Guideline): A Report of the American College of Cardiology Foundation/ American Heart Association Task Force on Practice Guidelines," Circulation, 2011, 123(1):104-23.

TREATMENT OF ELEVATED INR DUE TO WARFARIN

Management of Elevated INR in Patients Taking Warfarin

INR above therapeutic range to <4.5 No evidence of bleeding and rapid reversal unnecessary	INR 4.5 to 10 No evidence of bleeding	INR >10 No evidence of bleeding	Minor bleeding at any INR elevation	Major bleeding at any INR elevation
Lower or hold next dose and monitor frequently; when INR approaches desired range, resume dosing with a lower dose.	The 2012 ACCP guidelines recommend against routine vitamin K administration in this setting. Previously, the 2008 ACCP guidelines recommended if no risk factors for bleeding exist, to omit next 1 or 2 doses, monitor INR more frequently, and resume with an appropriately adjusted dose when INR in desired range; may consider administering vitamin K orally 1-2.5 mg if other risk factors for bleeding exist. Others have recommended consideration of vitamin K 1 mg orally or 0.5 mg I.V.	The 2012 ACCP guidelines recommend administration of oral vitamin K (dose not specified) in this setting. Previously, the 2008 ACCP guidelines recommended to hold warfarin, administer vitamin K orally 2.5-5 mg, expect INR to be reduced within 24-48 hours, monitor INR more frequently, and give additional vitamin K at an appropriate dose if necessary; resume warfarin at an appropriately adjusted dose when INR is in desired range. Others have recommended consideration of vitamin K 2-2.5 mg orally or 0.5-1 mg I.V.	Hold warfarin, may administer vitamin K orally 2.5-5 mg, monitor INR more frequently, may repeat dose after 24 hours if INR correction incomplete; resume warfarin at an appropriately adjusted dose when INR is in desired range.	The 2012 ACCP guidelines recommend administration of vitamin K 5-10 mg by slow I.V. infusion (may repeat in 12 hours if necessary) and four-factor prothrombin complex concentrate (PCC); however, in the U.S., the available PCCs (Bebulin®VH and Profilnine® SD) are three-factor PCCs and do not contain adequate levels of factor VII. Four-factor PCCs include Beriplex® P/N, Cofact®, Konyne®, or Octaplex®, all of which are **not** available in the U.S.

INR = international normalized ratio

Note: Use of high doses of vitamin K (eg, 10-15 mg) may cause warfarin resistance for ≥1 week. During this period of resistance, heparin or low molecular weight heparin may be given until INR responds.

WARFARIN THERAPY

Patients should **not** receive loading doses of warfarin >10 mg as the steady-state INR is not achieved more quickly. In general, most patients should receive doses between 5-10 mg for the first 1-2 days with the addition of heparin or low molecular weight heparin when a more rapid anticoagulant effect is required. Initial warfarin doses of 5 mg usually results in an INR>2 in 4-5 days. Initial doses of 10 mg usually results in a therapeutic INR in 3-4 days; however, 10 mg doses may be associated with more excessive anticoagulation. Patients who are debilitated, malnourished, have heart failure, have had recent surgery, or are taking medications known to increase the effects of warfarin should begin treatment with a dose ≤5 mg. The intensity of anticoagulation therapy should be monitored closely until the patient has reached a stable PT/INR. Once the patient is stabilized on a fixed dose of warfarin, the PT/INR can be monitored on a monthly basis if the patient demonstrates a stable PT/INR on chronic therapy. If dosage adjustments are made, PT/INR should be evaluated in approximately 2 weeks.

Supratherapeutic INR values are managed based on the presence and severity of bleeding (see chart). Determinants of bleeding due to warfarin therapy include intensity of treatment, patient characteristics, concomitant use of drugs that interfere with hemostasis, and the length therapy. The target INR should be established with consideration of these factors. Patients on warfarin should be warned to seek medical evaluation if they develop a very severe headache, abdominal pain, unusual bleeding, backache, or if they experience significant trauma, particularly head injuries. Please refer to the Warfarin monograph on page 2033 for complete drug information.

REFERENCES

Ansell J, Hirsh J, Hylek E, et al, "Pharmacology and Management of the Vitamin K Antagonists: American College of Chest Physicians Evidence-Based Clinical Practice Guidelines (8th Edition)," Chest, 2008, 133(6 Suppl):160S-98S.

Holbrook A, Schulman S, Witt DM, et al, "Evidence-Based Management of Anticoagulant Therapy: Antithrombotic Therapy and Prevention of Thrombosis, 9th ed: American College of Chest Physicians Evidence-Based Clinical Practice Guidelines," Chest, 2012, 141(2 Suppl):e152-84.

Patriquin C and Crowther M, "Treatment of Warfarin-Associated Coagulopathy With Vitamin K," Expert Rev Hematol, 2011, 4(6):657-65.

CYTOCHROME P450 ENZYMES: SUBSTRATES, INHIBITORS, AND INDUCERS

INTRODUCTION

Most drugs are eliminated from the body, at least in part, by being chemically altered to less lipid-soluble products (ie, metabolized), and thus are more likely to be excreted via the kidneys or the bile. Phase I metabolism includes drug hydrolysis, oxidation, and reduction, and results in drugs that are more polar in their chemical structure, while Phase II metabolism involves the attachment of an additional molecule onto the drug (or partially metabolized drug) in order to create an inactive and/or more water soluble compound. Phase II processes include (primarily) glucuronidation, sulfation, glutathione conjugation, acetylation, and methylation.

Virtually any of the Phase I and II enzymes can be inhibited by some xenobiotic or drug. Some of the Phase I and II enzymes can be induced. Inhibition of the activity of metabolic enzymes will result in increased concentrations of the substrate (drug), whereas induction of the activity of metabolic enzymes will result in decreased concentrations of the substrate. For example, the well-documented enzyme-inducing effects of phenobarbital may include a combination of Phase I and II enzymes. Phase II glucuronidation may be increased via induced UDP-glucuronosyl-transferase (UGT) activity, whereas Phase I oxidation may be increased via induced cytochrome P450 (CYP) activity. However, for most drugs, the primary route of metabolism (and the primary focus of drug-drug interaction) is Phase I oxidation.

CYP enzymes may be responsible for the metabolism (at least partial metabolism) of approximately 75% of all drugs, with the CYP3A subfamily responsible for nearly half of this activity. Found throughout plant, animal, and bacterial species, CYP enzymes represent a superfamily of xenobiotic metabolizing proteins. There have been several hundred CYP enzymes identified in nature, each of which has been assigned to a family (1, 2, 3, etc), subfamily (A, B, C, etc), and given a specific enzyme number (1, 2, 3, etc) according to the similarity in amino acid sequence that it shares with other enzymes. Of these many enzymes, only a few are found in humans, and even fewer appear to be involved in the metabolism of xenobiotics (eg, drugs). The key human enzyme subfamilies include CYP1A, CYP2A, CYP2B, CYP2C, CYP2D, CYP2E, and CYP3A. However, the number of distinct isozymes (eg, CYP2C9) found to be functionally active in humans, as well as, the number of genetically variant forms of these isozymes (eg, CYP2C9*2) in individuals continues to expand.

CYP enzymes are found in the endoplasmic reticulum of cells in a variety of human tissues (eg, skin, kidneys, brain, lungs), but their predominant sites of concentration and activity are the liver and intestine. Though the abundance of CYP enzymes throughout the body is relatively equally distributed among the various subfamilies, the relative contribution to drug metabolism is (in decreasing order of magnitude) CYP3A4 (nearly 50%), CYP2D6 (nearly 25%), CYP2C8/9 (nearly 15%), then CYP1A2, CYP2C19, CYP2A6, and CYP2E1. Owing to their potential for numerous drug-drug interactions, those drugs that are identified in preclinical studies as substrates of CYP3A enzymes are often given a lower priority for continued research and development in favor of drugs that appear to be less affected by (or less likely to affect) this enzyme subfamily.

Each enzyme subfamily possesses unique selectivity toward potential substrates. For example, CYP1A2 preferentially binds medium-sized, planar, lipophilic molecules, while CYP2D6 preferentially binds molecules that possess a basic nitrogen atom. Some CYP subfamilies exhibit polymorphism (ie, genetic variation that results in a modified enzyme with small changes in amino acid sequences that may manifest differing catalytic properties). The best described polymorphisms involve CYP2C9, CYP2C19, and CYP2D6. Individuals possessing "wild type" genes exhibit normal functioning CYP capacity. Others, however, possess genetic variants that leave the person with a subnormal level of catalytic potential (so called "poor metabolizers"). Poor metabolizers would be more likely to experience toxicity from drugs metabolized by the affected enzymes (or less effects if the enzyme is responsible for converting a prodrug to it's active form as in the case of codeine). The percentage of people classified as poor metabolizers varies by enzyme and population group. As an example, approximately 7% of Caucasians and only about 1% of Asians appear to be CYP2D6 poor metabolizers.

CYP enzymes can be both inhibited and induced by other drugs, leading to increased or decreased serum concentrations (along with the associated effects), respectively. Induction occurs when a drug causes an increase in the amount of smooth endoplasmic reticulum, secondary to increasing the amount of the affected CYP enzymes in the tissues. This "revving up" of the CYP enzyme system may take several days to reach peak activity, and likewise, may take several days, even months, to return to normal following discontinuation of the inducing agent.

CYP inhibition occurs via several potential mechanisms. Most commonly, a CYP inhibitor competitively (and reversibly) binds to the active site on the enzyme, thus preventing the substrate from binding to the same site, and preventing the substrate from being metabolized. The affinity of an inhibitor for an enzyme may be expressed by an inhibition constant (Ki) or IC50 (defined as the concentration of the inhibitor required to cause 50% inhibition under a given set of conditions). In addition to reversible competition for an enzyme site, drugs may inhibit enzyme activity by binding to sites on the enzyme other than that to which the substrate would bind, and thereby cause a change in the functionality or physical structure of the enzyme. A drug may also bind to the enzyme in an irreversible (ie, "suicide") fashion. In such a case, it is not the concentration of drug at the enzyme site that is important (constantly binding and releasing), but the number of molecules available for binding (once bound, always bound).

Although an inhibitor or inducer may be known to affect a variety of CYP subfamilies, it may only inhibit one or two in a clinically important fashion. Likewise, although a substrate is known to be at least partially metabolized by a variety of CYP enzymes, only one or two enzymes may contribute significantly enough to its overall metabolism to warrant concern when used with potential inducers or inhibitors. Therefore, when attempting to predict the level of risk of using two drugs that may affect each other via altered CYP function, it is important to identify the relative effectiveness of the inhibiting/inducing drug on the CYP subfamilies that significantly contribute to the metabolism of the substrate. The contribution of a specific CYP pathway to substrate metabolism should be considered not only in light of other known CYP pathways, but also other nonoxidative pathways for substrate metabolism (eg, glucuronidation) and transporter proteins (eg, P-glycoprotein) that may affect the presentation of a substrate to a metabolic pathway.

HOW TO USE THIS TABLE

The following table provides a clinically relevant perspective on drugs that are affected by, or affect, cytochrome P450 (CYP) enzymes. Not all human, drug-metabolizing CYP enzymes are specifically (or separately) included in the table. Some enzymes have been excluded because they do not appear to significantly contribute to the metabolism of marketed drugs (eg, CYP2C18). In the case of CYP3A4, the industry routinely uses this single enzyme designation to represent all enzymes in the CYP3A subfamily. CYP3A7 is present in fetal livers. It is effectively absent from adult livers. CYP3A4 (adult) and CYP3A7 (fetal) appear to share similar properties in their respective hosts. The impact of CYP3A7 in fetal and neonatal drug interactions has not been investigated.

An enzyme that appears to play a clinically significant (major) role in a drug's metabolism is indicated by "S". A clinically significant designation is the result of a two-phase review. The first phase considered the contribution of each CYP enzyme to the overall metabolism of the drug. The enzyme pathway was considered potentially clinically relevant if it was responsible for at least 30% of the metabolism of the drug. If so, the drug was subjected to a second phase. The second phase considered the clinical relevance of a substrate's concentration being increased twofold, or decreased by one-half (such as might be observed if combined with an effective CYP inhibitor or inducer, respectively). If either of these changes was considered to present a clinically significant concern, the CYP pathway for the drug was designated "major." If neither change would appear to present a clinically significant concern, or if the CYP enzyme was responsible for a smaller portion of the overall metabolism (ie, <30%), then no association between the enzyme and the drug will appear in the table.

Enzymes that are strongly or moderately inhibited by a drug are indicated by "↓". Enzymes that are weakly inhibited are not identified in the table. The designations are the result of a review of published clinical reports, available Ki data, and assessments published by other experts in the field. As it pertains to Ki values set in a ratio with achievable serum drug concentrations ([I]) under normal dosing conditions, the following parameters were employed: [I]/Ki ≥1 = strong; [I]/Ki 0.1-1 = moderate; [I]/Ki <0.1 = weak.

Enzymes that appear to be effectively induced by a drug are indicated by "↑". This designation is the result of a review of published clinical reports and assessments published by experts in the field.

In general, clinically significant interactions are more likely to occur between substrates ("S") and either inhibitors or inducers of the same enzyme(s), which have been indicated by "↓" and "↑", respectively. However, these assessments possess a degree of subjectivity, at times based on limited indications regarding the significance of CYP effects of particular agents. An attempt has been made to balance a conservative, clinically-sensitive presentation of the data with a desire to avoid the numbing effect of a "beware of everything" approach. It is important to note that information related to CYP metabolism of drugs is expanding at a rapid pace, and thus, the contents of this table should only be considered to represent a "snapshot" of the information available at the time of publication.

SELECTED READINGS

Bjornsson TD, Callaghan JT, Einolf HJ, et al, "The Conduct of *in vitro* and *in vivo* Drug-Drug Interaction Studies: A PhRMA Perspective," *J Clin Pharmacol*, 2003, 43(5):443-69.

Drug-Drug Interactions, Rodrigues AD, ed, New York, NY: Marcel Dekker, Inc, 2002.

Levy RH, Thummel KE, Trager WF, et al, eds, *Metabolic Drug Interactions*, Philadelphia, PA: Lippincott Williams & Wilkins, 2000.

Michalets EL, "Update: Clinically Significant Cytochrome P-450 Drug Interactions," *Pharmacotherapy*, 1998, 18 (1):84-112.

Thummel KE and Wilkinson GR, "*In vitro* and *in vivo* Drug Interactions Involving Human CYP3A," *Annu Rev Pharmacol Toxicol*, 1998, 38:389-430.

Zhang Y and Benet LZ, "The Gut as a Barrier to Drug Absorption: Combined Role of Cytochrome P450 3A and P-Glycoprotein," *Clin Pharmacokinet*, 2001, 40(3):159-68.

SELECTED WEBSITES

http://www.imm.ki.se/CYPalleles
http://medicine.iupui.edu/flockhart
http://www.fda.gov/Drugs/DevelopmentApprovalProcess/DevelopmentResources/DrugInteractionsLabeling/ucm080499.htm

CYP: Substrates, Inhibitors, Inducers

S = substrate; ↓ = inhibitor; ↑ = inducer

Drug	1A2	2A6	2B6	2C8	2C9	2C19	2D6	2E1	3A4
Acenocoumarol	S				S				
Alfentanil									S
Alfuzosin									S
Alosetron	S								
ALPRAZolam									S
Ambrisentan						S			S
Aminophylline	S								
Amiodarone		↓		S	↓		↓		S, ↓
Amitriptyline							S		
AmLODIPine	↓								S
Amobarbital		↑							
Amoxapine							S		
Aprepitant									S, ↓
ARIPiprazole							S		S
Armodafinil						↓			S, ↑
Atazanavir									S, ↓
Atomoxetine							S		
Atorvastatin									S
Benzphetamine									S
Betaxolol	S						S		
Bisoprolol									S
Bortezomib						S, ↓			S
Bosentan					S, ↑				S, ↑
Bromazepam					S				S
Bromocriptine									S
Budesonide									S
Buprenorphine									S
BuPROPion			S						

CYP: Substrates, Inhibitors, Inducers *(continued)*

Drug	1A2	2A6	2B6	2C8	2C9	2C19	2D6	2E1	3A4
BusPIRone									S
Busulfan									S
Caffeine	S								↓
Captopril							S		
CarBAMazepine	↑		↑	↑	↑	↑			S, ↑
Carisoprodol						S			
Carvedilol					S		S		
Celecoxib				↓	S				
ChlordiazePOXIDE									S
Chloroquine							S, ↓		S
Chlorpheniramine									S
ChlorproMAZINE							S, ↓		
Chlorzoxazone								S	
Ciclesonide									S
Cilostazol									S
Cimetidine	↓					↓	↓		↓
Cinacalcet							↓		
Ciprofloxacin	↓								
Cisapride									S
Citalopram						S			S
Clarithromycin									S, ↓
Clobazam						S			S
ClomiPRAMINE	S					S	S, ↓		
ClonazePAM									S
Clorazepate									S
Clotrimazole									↓
CloZAPine	S						↓		
Cocaine							↓		S
Codeine[1]							S		
Colchicine									S
Conivaptan									S, ↓
Cyclobenzaprine	S								
Cyclophosphamide[2]			S						S
CycloSPORINE									S, ↓
Dacarbazine	S							S	
Dantrolene									S
Dapsone					S				S
Darifenacin							↓		S
Darunavir									S
Dasatinib									S
Delavirdine					↓	↓	↓		S, ↓
Desipramine		↓	↓				S, ↓		↓
Desogestrel						S			
Dexamethasone									S, ↑
Dexlansoprazole						S, ↓			S

CYP: Substrates, Inhibitors, Inducers *(continued)*

Drug	1A2	2A6	2B6	2C8	2C9	2C19	2D6	2E1	3A4
Dexmedetomidine		S					↓		
Dextromethorphan							S		
Diazepam						S			S
Diclofenac	↓								
Dihydroergotamine									S
Diltiazem									S, ↓
DiphenhydrAMINE							↓		
Disopyramide									S
Disulfiram								↓	
DOCEtaxel									S
Doxepin							S		
DOXOrubicin			↓				S		S
Doxycycline									↓
DULoxetine	S						S, ↓		
Efavirenz[3]			S		↓	↓			S, ↓, ↑
Eletriptan									S
Enflurane								S	
Eplerenone									S
Ergoloid mesylates									S
Ergonovine									S
Ergotamine									S
Erlotinib									S
Erythromycin									S, ↓
Escitalopram						S			S
Esomeprazole						S, ↓			S
Estradiol	S								S
Estrogens, conjugated A/synthetic	S								S
Estrogens, conjugated equine	S								S
Estrogens, esterified	S								S
Estropipate	S								S
Eszopiclone									S
Ethinyl estradiol									S
Ethosuximide									S
Etoposide									S
Exemestane									S
Felbamate									S
Felodipine					↓				S
FentaNYL									S
Flecainide							S		
Fluconazole					↓	↓			↓
Flunisolide									S
FLUoxetine	↓				S	↓	S, ↓		
FluPHENAZine							S		
Flurazepam									S
Flurbiprofen					↓				

CYP: Substrates, Inhibitors, Inducers *(continued)*

Drug	1A2	2A6	2B6	2C8	2C9	2C19	2D6	2E1	3A4
Flutamide	S								S
Fluticasone									S
Fluvastatin					S, ↓				
FluvoxaMINE	S, ↓					↓	S		
Fosamprenavir (as amprenavir)									S, ↓
Fosaprepitant									S, ↓
Fosphenytoin (as phenytoin)			↑	↑	S, ↑	S, ↑			↑
Fospropofol	↓		S		S	↓			↓
Gefitinib									S
Gemfibrozil	↓			↓	↓	↓			
Glimepiride					S				
GlipiZIDE					S				
Guanabenz	S								
Haloperidol							S, ↓		S, ↓
Halothane								S	
Ibuprofen					↓				
Ifosfamide[4]		S				S			S
Imatinib							↓		S, ↓
Imipramine						S	S, ↓		
Indinavir									S, ↓
Indomethacin					↓				
Irbesartan				↓	↓				
Irinotecan			S						S
Isoflurane								S	
Isoniazid		↓				↓	↓	S, ↓	
Isosorbide dinitrate									S
Isosorbide mononitrate									S
Isradipine									S
Itraconazole									S, ↓
Ixabepilone									S
Ketamine			S		S				S
Ketoconazole	↓	↓			↓	↓	↓		S, ↓
Lansoprazole						S, ↓			S
Lapatinib									S
Letrozole		↓							
Levonorgestrel									S
Lidocaine							S, ↓		S, ↓
Lomustine							S		
Lopinavir									S
Loratadine						↓			
Losartan				↓	S, ↓				S
Lovastatin									S
Maprotiline							S		
Maraviroc									S
MedroxyPROGESTERone									S

CYP: Substrates, Inhibitors, Inducers (continued)

Drug	1A2	2A6	2B6	2C8	2C9	2C19	2D6	2E1	3A4
Mefenamic acid					↓				
Mefloquine									S
Mephobarbital						S			
Mestranol[5]					S				S
Methadone							↓		S
Methamphetamine							S		
Methoxsalen	↓	↓							
Methsuximide						S			
Methylergonovine									S
MethylPREDNISolone									S
Metoprolol							S		
MetroNIDAZOLE									↓
Mexiletine	S, ↓						S		
Miconazole	↓	↓			↓	↓	↓	↓	S, ↓
Midazolam									S
Mirtazapine	S						S		S
Moclobemide						S	S		
Modafinil						↓			S
Montelukast					S				S
Nafcillin									↑
Nateglinide					S				S
Nebivolol							S		
Nefazodone							S		S, ↓
Nelfinavir						S			S, ↓
Nevirapine			↑						S, ↑
NiCARdipine					↓	↓	↓		S, ↓
NIFEdipine	↓								S
Nilotinib									S
Nilutamide					S				
NiMODipine									S
Nisoldipine									S
Norethindrone									S
Norfloxacin	↓								↓
Norgestrel									S
Nortriptyline							S		
Ofloxacin	↓								
OLANZapine	S								
Omeprazole					↓	S, ↓			S
Ondansetron									S
OXcarbazepine									↑
PACLitaxel				S	S				3A4
Pantoprazole						S			
Paricalcitol									S
PARoxetine			↓				S, ↓		
Pazopanib									S

CYP: Substrates, Inhibitors, Inducers *(continued)*

Drug	1A2	2A6	2B6	2C8	2C9	2C19	2D6	2E1	3A4
Pentamidine						S			
PENTobarbital		↑							↑
Perphenazine							S		
PHENobarbital	↑	↑	↑	↑	↑	S			↑
Phenytoin			↑	↑	S, ↑	S, ↑			↑
Pimozide	S								S
Pindolol							S		
Pioglitazone				S, ↓					
Piroxicam					↓				
Posaconazole									↓
Primaquine	↓								S
Primidone	↑		↑	↑	↑				↑
Procainamide							S		
Progesterone						S			S
Promethazine			S				S		
Propafenone							S		
Propofol	↓		S		S	↓			↓
Propranolol	S						S		
Protriptyline							S		
Pyrimethamine					↓				
Quazepam						S			S
QUEtiapine									S
QuiNIDine							↓		S, ↓
QuiNINE				↓	↓		↓		S
RABEprazole				↓		S, ↓			S
Ramelteon	S								
Ranolazine							↓		S
Rasagiline	S								
Repaglinide				S					S
Rifabutin									S, ↑
Rifampin	↑	↑	↑	↑	↑	↑			↑
Rifapentine				↑	↑				↑
Riluzole	S								
RisperiDONE							S		
Ritonavir				↓			S, ↓		S, ↓
ROPINIRole	S								
Ropivacaine	S								
Rosiglitazone				S, ↓					
Salmeterol									S
Saquinavir									S, ↓
Secobarbital		↑			↑	↑			
Selegiline			S						
Sertraline			↓			S, ↓	S, ↓		↓
Sevoflurane								S	
Sibutramine									S

CYP: Substrates, Inhibitors, Inducers *(continued)*

Drug	1A2	2A6	2B6	2C8	2C9	2C19	2D6	2E1	3A4
Sildenafil									S
Simvastatin									S
Sirolimus									S
Sitaxsentan					↓	↓			↓
Solifenacin									S
SORAfenib			↓	↓	↓				
Spiramycin									S
SUFentanil									S
SulfADIAZINE					S, ↓				
Sulfamethoxazole					S, ↓				
SUNItinib									S
Tacrine	S								
Tacrolimus									S
Tadalafil									S
Tamoxifen					↓	S		S	S
Tamsulosin							S		S
Telithromycin									S, ↓
Temsirolimus									S
Teniposide									S
Terbinafine							↓		
Tetracycline									S, ↓
Theophylline	S							S	S
Thiabendazole	↓								
Thioridazine							S, ↓		
Thiotepa			↓						
Thiothixene	S								
TiaGABine									S
Ticlopidine						↓	↓		S
Timolol							S		
Tinidazole									S
Tipranavir									S
TiZANidine	S								
TOLBUTamide					S, ↓				
Tolterodine							S		S
Toremifene									S
Torsemide					S				
TraMADol[1]							S		S
Tranylcypromine	↓	↓					↓	↓	
TraZODone									S
Tretinoin				S					
Triazolam									S
Trifluoperazine	S								
Trimethoprim					↓	S, ↓			S
Trimipramine							S	S	S
Vardenafil									S

CYP: Substrates, Inhibitors, Inducers *(continued)*

Drug	1A2	2A6	2B6	2C8	2C9	2C19	2D6	2E1	3A4
Venlafaxine							S		S
Verapamil									S, ↓
VinBLAStine									S
VinCRIStine									S
Vinorelbine									S
Voriconazole					S	S			↓
Warfarin					S, ↓				
Zafirlukast					S, ↓				
Zileuton	↓								
Zolpidem									S
Zonisamide									S
Zopiclone					S				S
Zuclopenthixol							S		

[1]This opioid analgesic is bioactivated *in vivo* via CYP2D6. Inhibiting this enzyme would decrease the effects of the analgesic. The active metabolite might also affect, or be affected by, CYP enzymes.

[2]Cyclophosphamide is bioactivated *in vivo* to acrolein via CYP2B6 and 3A4. Inhibiting these enzymes would decrease the effects of cyclophosphamide.

[3]Data have shown both induction (*in vivo*) and inhibition (*in vitro*) of CYP3A4.

[4]Ifosfamide is bioactivated *in vivo* to acrolein via CYP3A4. Inhibiting this enzyme would decrease the effects of ifosfamide.

[5]Mestranol is bioactivated *in vivo* to ethinyl estradiol via CYP2C8/9.

DEPRESSION SCALES

Short Form Geriatric Depression Scale*

NAME _____ AGE _____ SEX _____ DATE _____

WING _____ ROOM _____ PHYSICIAN _____

SCORING SYSTEM

Answers indicating depression are highlighted. Each BOLD-FACED answer counts one (1) point. Score greater than 5 indicates probable depression

1.	Are you basically satisfied with your life?	YES / **NO**
2.	Have you dropped any of your activities and interests?	**YES** / NO
3.	Do you feel that your life is empty?	**YES** / NO
4.	Do you often get bored?	**YES** / NO
5.	Are you in good spirits most of the time?	YES / **NO**
6.	Are you afraid that something bad is going to happen to you?	**YES** / NO
7.	Do you feel happy most of the time?	YES / **NO**
8.	Do you often feel helpless?	**YES** / NO
9.	Do you prefer to stay in your room/facility, rather than going out and doing new things?	**YES** / NO
10.	Do you feel you have more problems with memory than most?	**YES** / NO
11.	Do you think it is wonderful to be alive?	YES / **NO**
12.	Do you feel worthless the way you are now?	**YES** / NO
13.	Do you feel full of energy?	YES / **NO**
14.	Do you feel that your situation is hopeless?	**YES** / NO
15.	Do you think that most people are better off than you?	**YES** / NO

SCORE

NOTES / CURRENT MEDICATIONS:

ASSESSOR:

*This scale may be used when evaluating residents who do not have limited cognition.

The following Patient Health Questionnaire - 9 (PHQ-9) is intended to assist clinicians with diagnosing depressive behavior, as well as determining depressive symptom severity for monitoring treatment. The nine items are based directly on the nine signs and symptoms of major depression. Patients should not be diagnosed solely on the basis of a PHQ-9 score. The clinician should corroborate the score with clinical determination that a significant depressive syndrome is present. Scores of 5, 10, 15, and 20 represent cutpoints for mild, moderate, moderately severe, and severe depression, respectively. Table 2 directs the clinician in determining the patient's depression severity and a treatment plan, if necessary, based on the total score of the PHQ-9.

Table 1: Patient Health Questionnaire - 9 (PHQ-9)

Over the last 2 weeks, how often have you been bothered by any of the following problems? (Check to indicate your answer.)	Not at all	Several days	More than half the days	Nearly every day
	(0)	(1)	(2)	(3)
1. Little interest or pleasure in doing things	O	O	O	O
2. Feeling down, depressed, or hopeless	O	O	O	O
3. Trouble falling or staying asleep, or sleeping too much	O	O	O	O
4. Feeling tired or having little energy	O	O	O	O
5. Poor appetite or overeating	O	O	O	O
6. Feeling bad about yourself – or that you are a failure or have let yourself or your family down	O	O	O	O
7. Trouble concentrating on things, such as reading the newspaper or watching television	O	O	O	O
8. Moving or speaking so slowly that other people could have noticed, or the opposite – being so fidgety or restless that you have been moving around a lot more than usual	O	O	O	O
9. Thoughts that you would be better off dead or of hurting yourself in some way	O	O	O	O
For office coding:	O	+ ____	+ ____	+ ____
			= Total score: ____	

If you checked off **any** problems, how **difficult** have these problems made it for you to do your work, take care of things at home, or get along with other people?			
O Not difficult at all	O Somewhat difficult	O Very difficult	O Extremely difficult

Developed by Spitzer RL, Williams JBW, Kroenke K, et al, with an educational grant from Pfizer, Inc. Available at http://www.phqscreeners.com/pdfs/02_PHQ-9/English.pdf

Table 2: PHQ-9 Scores and Proposed Treatment Actions

PHQ-9 Score	Depression Severity	Proposed Treatment Actions
0 - 4	None - minimal	None
5 - 9	Mild	Watchful waiting; repeat PHQ-9 at follow-up
10 - 14	Moderate	Treatment plan; considering counseling, follow-up, and/or pharmacotherapy
15 - 19	Moderately Severe	Active treatment with pharmacotherapy and/or psychotherapy
20 - 27	Severe	Immediate initiation of pharmacotherapy and, if severe impairment or poor response to therapy, expedited referral to a mental health specialist for psychotherapy and/or collaborative management

Developed by Spitzer RL, Williams JBW, Kroenke K, et al, with an educational grant from Pfizer, Inc. Available at http://www.phqscreeners.com/instructions/instructions.pdf

ORAL MEDICATIONS THAT SHOULD NOT BE CRUSHED OR ALTERED

There are a variety of reasons for crushing tablets or capsule contents prior to administering to the patient. Patients may have nasogastric tubes which do not permit the administration of tablets or capsules, an oral solution for a particular medication may not be available from the manufacturer or readily prepared by pharmacy, patients may have difficulty swallowing capsules or tablets, or mixing of powdered medication with food or drink may make the drug more palatable.

Generally, medications which should not be crushed fall into one of the following categories:

- **Extended Release Products:** The formulation of some tablets is specialized as to allow the medication within it to be slowly released into the body. This may be accomplished by centering the drug within the core of the tablet, with a subsequent shedding of multiple layers around the core. Wax melts in the GI tract, releasing drug contained within the wax matrix (eg, OxyCONTIN®). Capsules may contain beads which have multiple layers which are slowly dissolved with time.

  Common Abbreviations for Extended Release Products

CD	Controlled dose
CR	Controlled release
CRT	Controlled release tablet
LA	Long-acting
SR	Sustained release
TR	Timed release
TD	Time delay
SA	Sustained action
XL	Extended release
XR	Extended release

- **Medications Which Are Irritating to the Stomach:** Tablets which are irritating to the stomach may be enteric-coated which delays release of the drug until the time when it reaches the small intestine. Enteric-coated aspirin is an example of this.

- **Foul-Tasting Medication:** Some drugs are quite unpleasant to taste so the manufacturer coats the tablet in a sugar coating to increase its palatability. By crushing the tablet, this sugar coating is lost and the patient tastes the unpleasant tasting medication.

- **Sublingual Medication:** Medication intended for use under the tongue should not be crushed. While it appears to be obvious, it is not always easy to determine if a medication is to be used sublingually. Sublingual medications should indicate on the package that they are intended for sublingual use.

- **Effervescent Tablets:** These are tablets which, when dropped into a liquid, quickly dissolve to yield a solution. Many effervescent tablets, when crushed, lose their ability to quickly dissolve.

- **Potentially Hazardous Substances:** Certain drugs, including antineoplastic agents, hormonal agents, some antivirals, some bioengineered agents, and other miscellaneous drugs, are considered potentially hazardous when used in humans based on their characteristics. Examples of these characteristics include carcinogenicity, teratogenicity, reproductive toxicity, organ toxicity at low doses, genotoxicity, or new drugs with structural and toxicity profiles similar to existing hazardous drugs. Exposure to these substances can result in adverse effects and should be avoided. Crushing or breaking a tablet or opening a capsule of a potentially hazardous substance may increase the risk of exposure to the substance through skin contact, inhalation, or accidental ingestion. The extent of exposure, potency, and toxicity of the hazardous substance determines the health risk. Institutions have policies and procedures to follow when handling any potentially hazardous substance. **Note:** All potentially hazardous substances may not be represented in this table. Refer to institution-specific guidelines for precautions to observe when handling hazardous substances.

RECOMMENDATIONS

1. It is not advisable to crush certain medications.

2. Consult individual monographs prior to crushing capsule or tablet.

3. If crushing a tablet or capsule is contraindicated, consult with your pharmacist to determine whether an oral solution exists or can be compounded.

Drug Product	Dosage Form	Dosage Reasons/Comments
Accutane®	Capsule	Mucous membrane irritant; teratogenic potential
Aciphex®	Tablet	Slow release
Actiq®	Lozenge	Slow release. This lollipop delivery system requires the patient to dissolve it slowly.
Actoplus Met® XR	Tablet	Slow release
Actonel®	Tablet	Irritant. Chewed, crushed, or sucked tablets may cause oropharyngeal irritation.
Adalat® CC	Tablet	Slow release
Adderall XR®	Capsule	Slow release[1]
Adenovirus (Types 4, 7) Vaccine	Tablet	Teratogenic potential; enteric-coated; do not disrupt tablet to avoid releasing live adenovirus in upper respiratory tract
Advicor®	Tablet	Slow release
AeroHist Plus™	Tablet	Slow release[8]
Afeditab® CR	Tablet	Slow release
Afinitor®	Tablet	Mucous membrane irritant; teratogenic potential; hazardous substance[10]
Aggrenox®	Capsule	Slow release. Capsule may be opened; contents include an aspirin tablet that may be chewed and dipyridamole pellets that may be sprinkled on applesauce.
Alavert™ Allergy Sinus 12 Hour	Tablet	Slow release
Allegra-D®	Tablet	Slow release
Alophen®	Tablet	Enteric-coated
ALPRAZolam ER	Tablet	Slow release
Altoprev®	Tablet	Slow release
Ambien CR®	Tablet	Slow release
Amitiza®	Capsule	Slow release
Amnesteem®	Capsule	Mucous membrane irritant; teratogenic potential
Ampyra™	Tablet	Slow release
Amrix®	Capsule	Slow release
Aplenzin™	Tablet	Slow release
Apriso™	Capsule	Slow release[1]
Aptivus®	Capsule	Taste. Oil emulsion within spheres

Drug Product	Dosage Form	Dosage Reasons/Comments
Aricept® 23 mg	Tablet	Film-coated; chewing or crushing may increase rate of absorption
Arava®	Tablet	Teratogenic potential; hazardous substance[10]
Arthrotec®	Tablet	Enteric-coated
Asacol®	Tablet	Slow release
Ascriptin® A/D	Tablet	Enteric-coated
Atelvia™	Tablet	Slow release; tablet coating is an important part of the delayed release
Augmentin XR®	Tablet	Slow release[2, 8]
AVINza™	Capsule	Slow release[1] (applesauce)
Avodart®	Capsule	Capsule should not be handled by pregnant women due to teratogenic potential[9]; hazardous substance[10]
Azulfidine® EN-tabs®	Tablet	Enteric-coated
Bayer® Aspirin EC	Caplet	Enteric-coated
Bayer® Aspirin, Low Adult 81 mg	Tablet	Enteric-coated
Bayer® Aspirin, Regular Strength 325 mg	Caplet	Enteric-coated
Biaxin® XL	Tablet	Slow release
Biltricide®	Tablet	Taste[8]
Biohist LA	Tablet	Slow release[8]
Bisa-Lax	Tablet	Enteric-coacted[3]
Bisac-Evac™	Tablet	Enteric-coated[3]
Bisacodyl	Tablet	Enteric-coated[3]
Boniva®	Tablet	Irritant. Chewed, crushed, or sucked tablets may cause oropharyngeal irritation.
Bontril® Slow-Release	Capsule	Slow release
Bromfed®	Capsule	Slow release
Bromfed®-PD	Capsule	Slow release
Budeprion SR®, Budeprion XL®	Tablet	Slow release
Buproban®	Tablet	Slow release
BuPROPion SR	Tablet	Slow release
Campral®	Tablet	Enteric-coated; slow release
Calan® SR	Tablet	Slow release[8]
Caprelsa®	Tablet	Teratogenic potential; hazardous substance[10]
Carbatrol®	Capsule	Slow release[1]
Cardene® SR	Capsule	Slow release
Cardizem®	Tablet	Not described as slow release but releases drug over 3 hours.
Cardizem® CD	Capsule	Slow release
Cardizem® LA	Tablet	Slow release
Cardura® XL	Tablet	Slow release
Cartia® XT	Capsule	Slow release
Casodex®	Tablet	Teratogenic potential; hazardous substance[10]

ORAL MEDICATIONS THAT SHOULD NOT BE CRUSHED OR ALTERED

Drug Product	Dosage Form	Dosage Reasons/Comments
CeeNU®	Capsule	Teratogenic potential; hazardous substance[10]
Cefaclor extended release	Tablet	Slow release
Ceftin®	Tablet	Taste[2]. Use suspension for children.
Cefuroxime	Tablet	Taste[2]. Use suspension for children.
CellCept®	Capsule, tablet	Teratogenic potential; hazardous substance[10]
Charcoal Plus®	Tablet	Enteric-coated
Chlor-Trimeton® 12-Hour	Tablet	Slow release[2]
Cipro® XR	Tablet	Slow release
Claravis™	Capsule	Mucous membrane irritant; teratogenic potential
Claritin-D® 12-Hour	Tablet	Slow release
Claritin-D® 24-Hour	Tablet	Slow release
Colace®	Capsule	Taste[5]
Colestid®	Tablet	Slow release
Commit®	Lozenge	Integrity compromised by chewing or crushing.
Concerta®	Tablet	Slow release
ConZip™	Capsule	Extended release; tablet disruption may cause overdose
Coreg CR®	Capsule	Slow release[1]
Cotazym-S®	Capsule	Enteric-coated[1]
Covera-HS®	Tablet	Slow release
Creon®	Capsule	Slow release[1]
Crixivan®	Capsule	Taste. Capsule may be opened and mixed with fruit puree (eg, banana).
Cymbalta®	Capsule	Enteric-coated
Cytoxan®	Tablet	Drug may be crushed, but manufacturer recommends using injection; hazardous substance[10]
Depakene®	Capsule	Slow release; mucous membrane irritant[2]; hazardous substance[10]
Depakote®	Tablet	Slow release; hazardous substance[10]
Depakote® ER	Tablet	Slow release; hazardous substance[10]
Detrol® LA	Capsule	Slow release
Dexedrine® Spansule®	Capsule	Slow release
Dexilant™	Capsule	Slow release[1]
Diamox® Sequels®	Capsule	Slow release
Dibenzyline®	Capsule	Hazardous substance[10]
Dilacor® XR	Capsule	Slow release
Dilatrate-SR®	Capsule	Slow release
Dilt-CD	Capsule	Slow release
Dilt-XR	Capsule	Slow release
Diltia XT®	Capsule	Slow release
Ditropan® XL	Tablet	Slow release

Drug Product	Dosage Form	Dosage Reasons/Comments
Divalproex ER	Tablet	Slow release
Donnatal® Extentab®	Tablet	Slow release[2]
Doxidan®	Tablet	Enteric-coated[3]
Drisdol®	Capsule	Liquid filled[4]
Drixoral®	Tablet	Slow release
Droxia®	Capsule	May be opened; wear gloves to handle; hazardous substance[10]
Drysec	Tablet	Slow release[8]
Dulcolax®	Capsule	Liquid-filled
Dulcolax®	Tablet	Enteric-coated[3]
DynaCirc® CR	Tablet	Slow release
Easprin®	Tablet	Enteric-coated
EC-Naprosyn®	Tablet	Enteric-coated
Ecotrin® Adult Low Strength	Tablet	Enteric-coated
Ecotrin® Maximum Strength	Tablet	Enteric-coated
Ecotrin® Regular Strength	Tablet	Enteric-coated
Ed A-Hist™	Tablet	Slow release[2]
E.E.S.® 400	Tablet	Enteric-coated[2]
Effer-K™	Tablet	Effervescent tablet[6]
Effervescent Potassium	Tablet	Effervescent tablet[6]
Effexor® XR	Capsule	Slow release
Embeda™	Capsule	Slow release; can open capsule and sprinkle on applesauce; do not give via NG tube
E-Mycin®	Tablet	Enteric-coated
Enablex®	Tablet	Slow release
Entocort® EC	Capsule	Enteric-coated[1]
Equetro®	Capsule	Slow release[1]
Ergomar®	Tablet	Sublingual form[7]
Ery-Tab®	Tablet	Enteric-coated
Erythromycin Stearate	Tablet	Enteric-coated
Erythromycin Base	Tablet	Enteric-coated
Erythromycin Delayed-Release	Capsule	Enteric-coated pellets[1]
Etoposide	Capsule	Hazardous substance[10]
Evista®	Tablet	Taste; teratogenic potential; hazardous substance[10]
Eviredge™	Capsule	Teratogenic potential[10]
Exalgo™	Tablet	Slow release; breaking, chewing, crushing, or dissolving before ingestion increases the risk of overdose
ExeFen-PD	Tablet	Slow release[8]
Fareston®	Tablet	Teratogenic potential; hazardous substance[10]
Feen-A-Mint®	Tablet	Enteric-coated[3]
Feldene®	Capsule	Mucous membrane irritant
Fentora®	Tablet	Buccal tablet

ORAL MEDICATIONS THAT SHOULD NOT BE CRUSHED OR ALTERED

Drug Product	Dosage Form	Dosage Reasons/Comments
Feosol®	Tablet	Enteric-coated[2]
Feratab®	Tablet	Enteric-coated[2]
Fergon®	Tablet	Enteric-coated
Fero-Grad 500®	Tablet	Slow release
Ferro-Sequels®	Tablet	Slow release
Flagyl ER®	Tablet	Slow release
Flomax®	Capsule	Slow release
Focalin® XR	Capsule	Slow release[1]
Fosamax®	Tablet	Mucous membrane irritant
Fosamax Plus D™	Tablet	Mucous membrane irritant
Gengraf®	Capsule	Teratogenic potential; hazardous substance[10]
Geodon®	Capsule	Hazardous substance[10]
Gleevec®	Tablet	Taste[8]. May be dissolved in water or apple juice; hazardous substance[10]
GlipiZIDE ER	Tablet	Slow release
Glucophage® XR	Tablet	Slow release
Glucotrol® XL	Tablet	Slow release
Glumetza™	Tablet	Slow release
Gralise™	Tablet	Slow release
Guaifenex® GP	Tablet	Slow release[8]
Guaifenex® PSE	Tablet	Slow release[8]
Guaimax-D®	Tablet	Slow release[8]
Halfprin®	Tablet	Enteric coated
Hexalen®	Capsule	Teratogenic potential; hazardous substance[10]
Horizant™	Tablet	Slow release
Hycamtin®	Capsule	Teratogenic potential; hazardous substance[10]
Hydrea®	Capsule	Can be opened and mixed with water; wear gloves to handle; hazardous substance[10]
Imdur®	Tablet	Slow release[8]
Inderal® LA	Capsule	Slow release
Indocin® SR	Capsule	Slow release[1,2]
Inlyta®	Tablet	Teratogenic potential; hazardous substance[10]
InnoPran XL®	Capsule	Slow release
Intelence™	Tablet	Tablet should be swallowed whole and not crushed; tablet may be dispersed in water
Intuniv™	Tablet	Slow release
Invega®	Tablet	Slow release
Ionamin®	Capsule	Slow release
Isochron™	Tablet	Slow release
Isoptin® SR	Tablet	Slow release[8]
Isordil® Sublingual	Tablet	Sublingual form[7]

Drug Product	Dosage Form	Dosage Reasons/Comments
Isosorbide Dinitrate Sublingual	Tablet	Sublingual form[7]
Isosorbide SR	Tablet	Slow release
Jalyn®	Capsule	Capsule should not be handled by pregnant women due to teratogenic potential[9]; hazardous substance[10]
Janumet®	Tablet	Slow release
Januvia®	Tablet	Film coated
Kadian®	Capsule	Slow release[1]. Do not give via NG tubes.
Kaletra®	Tablet	Film coated
Kaon-Cl®	Tablet	Slow release[2]
Kapidex™	Capsule	Slow release[1]
Kapvay™	Tablet	Slow release
K-Dur®	Tablet	Slow release
Keppra®	Tablet	Taste[2]
Keppra® XR	Tablet	Slow release
Ketek®	Tablet	Slow release
Klor-Con®	Tablet	Slow release[2]
Klor-Con® M	Tablet	Slow release[2]; some strengths are scored
Klotrix®	Tablet	Slow release[2]
K-Lyte®	Tablet	Effervescent tablet[6]
K-Lyte/Cl®	Tablet	Effervescent tablet[6]
K-Lyte DS®	Tablet	Effervescent tablet[6]
Kombiglyze™ XR	Tablet	Slow release; tablet matrix may remain in stool
K-Tab®	Tablet	Slow release[2]
LaMICtal® XR™	Tablet	Slow release
Lescol® XL	Tablet	Slow release
Letairis®	Tablet	Film coated; hazardous substance[10]
Leukeran®	Tablet	Teratogenic potential; hazardous substance[10]
Levbid®	Tablet	Slow release[8]
Levsinex® Timecaps®	Capsule	Slow release
Lexxel®	Tablet	Slow release
Lialda™	Tablet	Delayed release, enteric coated
Lipram 4500	Capsule	Enteric-coated[1]
Lipram-PN	Capsule	Slow release[1]
Lipram-UL	Capsule	Slow release[1]
Liquibid-D®	Tablet	Slow release
Lithobid®	Tablet	Slow release
Lodrane® 24	Capsule	Slow release
Lodrane® 24D	Capsule	Slow release
LoHist 12D	Tablet	Slow release

ORAL MEDICATIONS THAT SHOULD NOT BE CRUSHED OR ALTERED

Drug Product	Dosage Form	Dosage Reasons/Comments
Lovaza®	Capsule	Contents of capsule may erode walls of styrofoam or plastic materials
Luvox® CR	Capsule	Slow release
Lysodren®	Tablet	Hazardous substance[10]
Mag-Tab® SR	Tablet	Slow release
Matulane®	Capsule	Teratogenic potential; hazardous substance[10]
Maxifed DMX ER	Tablet	Slow release[8]
Maxifed-G®	Tablet	Slow release
Maxiphen DM	Tablet	Slow release[8]
Medent-DM	Tablet	Slow release
Mestinon® Timespan®	Tablet	Slow release[2]
Metadate® CD	Capsule	Slow release[1]
Metadate® ER	Tablet	Slow release
Methylin® ER	Tablet	Slow release
Metoprolol ER	Tablet	Slow release
MicroK® Extencaps	Capsule	Slow release[1,2]
Minocin	Capsule	Slow release
Morphine sulfate extended-release	Tablet	Slow release
Motrin®	Tablet	Taste[5]
Moxatag™	Tablet	Slow release
MS Contin®	Tablet	Slow release[2]
Mucinex®	Tablet	Slow release
Mucinex® DM	Tablet	Slow release[2]
Multaq®	Tablet	Hazardous substance[10]
Myfortic®	Tablet	Slow release; teratogenic potential; hazardous substance[10]
Naprelan®	Tablet	Slow release
Neoral®	Capsule	Teratogenic potential; hazardous substance[10]
NexIUM®	Capsule	Slow release[1]
Niaspan®	Tablet	Slow release
Nicotinic Acid	Capsule, Tablet	Slow release[8]
Nifediac® CC	Tablet	Slow release
Nifedical® XL	Tablet	Slow release
NIFEdipine ER	Tablet	Slow release
Nitrostat®	Tablet	Sublingual route[7]
Norflex™	Tablet	Slow release
Norpace® CR	Capsule	Slow release
Norvir®	Tablet	Crushing tablets has resulted in decreased bioavailability of drug[2]
Nucynta® ER	Tablet	Slow release; tablet disruption may cause a potentially fatal overdose
Oforta™	Tablet	Teratogenic potential; hazardous substance[10]
Oleptro™	Tablet	Slow release[8]

Drug Product	Dosage Form	Dosage Reasons/Comments
Onglyza®	Tablet	Film coated
Opana® ER	Tablet	Slow release; tablet disruption may cause a potentially fatal overdose
Oracea™	Capsule	Slow release
Oramorph SR®	Tablet	Slow release[2]
Orphenadrine citrate ER	Tablet	Slow release
OxyCONTIN®	Tablet	Slow release; surrounded by wax matrix; tablet disruption may cause a potentially fatal overdose
Pancrease MT®	Capsule	Enteric-coated[1]
Pancreaze™	Capsule	Enteric-coated[1]
Pancrelipase™	Capsule	Enteric-coated[1]
Paxil CR®	Tablet	Slow release
Pentasa®	Capsule	Slow release
Plendil®	Tablet	Slow release
Pradaxa®	Capsule	Bioavailability increases by 75% when the pellets are taken without the capsule shell
Prevacid®	Capsule	Slow release[1]
Prevacid®	Suspension	Slow release. Contains enteric-coated granules. Not for use in NG tubes.
Prevacid® SoluTab™	Tablet	Orally disintegrating. Do not swallow; dissolve in water only and dispense via dosing syringe or NG tube.
PriLOSEC®	Capsule	Slow release
PriLOSEC OTC™	Tablet	Slow release
Pristiq®	Tablet	Slow release
Procardia XL®	Tablet	Slow release
Propecia®	Tablet	Women who are, or may become, pregnant should not handle crushed or broken tablets due to teratogenic potential[9]; hazardous substance[10]
Proquin® XR	Tablet	Slow release
Proscar®	Tablet	Women who are, or may become, pregnant should not handle crushed or broken tablets due to teratogenic potential[9]; hazardous substance[10]
Protonix®	Tablet	Slow release
PROzac® Weekly™	Capsule	Enteric coated
Purinethol®	Tablet	Teratogenic potential[9]; hazardous substance[10]
QuiNIDine ER	Tablet	Slow release[8]; enteric-coated
Ralix	Tablet	Slow release
Ranexa®	Tablet	Slow release
Rapamune®	Tablet	Taste; hazardous substance[10]
Razadyne™ ER	Capsule	Slow release
Renagel®	Tablet	Expands in liquid if broken/crushed.
Renvela	Tablet	Enteric-coated
Requip® XL™	Tablet	Slow release

Drug Product	Dosage Form	Dosage Reasons/Comments
Rescon®	Tablet	Slow release
Rescon-Jr	Tablet	Slow release
Rescriptor®	Tablet	If unable to swallow, may dissolve 100 mg tablets in water and drink; 200 mg tablets must be swallowed whole
Revlimid®	Capsule	Teratogenic potential; hazardous substance[10]; healthcare workers should avoid contact with capsule contents/body fluids
RisperDAL® M-Tab	Tablet	Orally disintegrating. Do not chew or break tablet; after dissolving under tongue, tablet may be swallowed
Ritalin® LA	Capsule	Slow release[1]
Ritalin-SR®	Tablet	Slow release
R-Tanna	Tablet	Slow release[2]
Rybix™ ODT	Tablet	Orally disintegrating. Do not chew, break, or split tablet; after dissolving on the tongue, may swallow.
Rythmol® SR	Capsule	Slow release
Ryzolt™	Tablet	Slow release; tablet disruption may cause overdose
SandIMMUNE®	Capsule	Teratogenic potential; hazardous substance[10]
Saphris®	Tablet	Sublingual form[7]
Sensipar®	Tablet	Tablets are not scored and cutting may cause inaccurate dosage
SEROquel® XR	Tablet	Slow release
Sinemet® CR	Tablet	Slow release
SINUvent® PE	Tablet	Slow release[8]
Slo-Niacin®	Tablet	Slow release[8]
Slow-Mag®	Tablet	Slow release
Solodyn®	Tablet	Slow release
Somnote®	Capsule	Liquid filled
Soriatane®	Capsule	Teratogenic potential; hazardous substance[10]
Sotret®	Capsule	Mucous membrane irritant; teratogenic potential
Sprycel®	Tablet	Film coated. Active ingredients are surrounded by a wax matrix to prevent healthcare exposure. Women who are, or may become pregnant, should not handle crushed or broken tablets; teratogenic potential; hazardous substance[10]
Stavzor™	Capsule	Slow release; hazardous substance[10]
Strattera®	Capsule	Capsule contents can cause ocular irritation.
Sudafed® 12-Hour	Capsule	Slow release[2]
Sudafed® 24-Hour	Capsule	Slow release[2]
Sulfazine EC	Tablet	Delayed release, enteric coated
Sular®	Tablet	Slow release

Drug Product	Dosage Form	Dosage Reasons/Comments
Sustiva®	Tablet	Tablets should not be broken (capsules should be used if dosage adjustment needed)
Symax® Duotab	Tablet	Slow release
Symax® SR	Tablet	Slow release
Syprine®	Capsule	Potential risk of contact dermatitis
Tabloid®	Tablet	Teratogenic potential; hazardous substance[10]
Tamoxifen®	Tablet	Teratogenic potential; hazardous substance[10]
Tasigna®	Capsule	Hazardous substance[10]; altering capsule may lead to high blood levels, increasing the risk of toxicity
Taztia XT®	Capsule	Slow release[1]
TEGretol®-XR	Tablet	Slow release
Temodar®	Capsule	Teratogenic potential; hazardous substance[10]. **Note:** If capsules are accidentally opened or damaged, rigorous precautions should be taken to avoid inhalation or contact of contents with the skin or mucous membranes.
Tessalon®	Capsule	Swallow whole; pharmacologic action may cause choking if chewed or opened and swallowed.
Tetracycline	Capsule	Hazardous substance[10]
Thalomid®	Capsule	Teratogenic potential; hazardous substance[10]
Theo-24®	Tablet	Slow release[2]
Theochron™	Tablet	Slow release[2]
Tiazac®	Capsule	Slow release[1]
Topamax®	Capsule	Taste[1]
Topamax®	Tablet	Taste
Toprol XL®	Tablet	Slow release[8]
Touro® CC/CC-LD	Caplet	Slow release[2,8]
Touro® DM®	Tablet	Slow release[2]
Touro LA®	Caplet	Slow release
Toviaz™	Tablet	Slow release
Tracleer®	Tablet	Teratogenic potential; hazardous substance[9,10]
TRENtal®	Tablet	Slow release
Treximet™	Tablet	Unique formulation enhances rapid drug absorption
Tylenol® Arthritis Pain	Caplet	Slow release
Tylenol® 8 Hour	Caplet	Slow release
Ultram® ER	Tablet	Slow release. Tablet disruption my cause a potentially fatal overdose.
Ultrase®	Capsule	Enteric-coated[1]
Ultrase® MT	Capsule	Enteric-coated[1]
Uniphyl®	Tablet	Slow release
Urocit®-K	Tablet	Wax-coated

Drug Product	Dosage Form	Dosage Reasons/Comments
Uroxatral®	Tablet	Slow release
Valcyte®	Tablet	Irritant potential; teratogenic potential; hazardous substance[10]
Verapamil SR	Tablet	Slow release[8]
Verelan®	Capsule	Slow release[1]
Verelan® PM	Capsule	Slow release[1]
Vesanoid®	Capsule	Teratogenic potential; hazardous substance[10]
VESIcare®	Tablet	Enteric-coated
Videx® EC	Capsule	Slow release
Vimovo™	Tablet	Slow release
Viramune® XR™	Tablet	Slow release[2]
Voltaren®-XR	Tablet	Slow release
VoSpire ER®	Tablet	Slow release
Votrient™	Tablet	Crushing significantly increases AUC and T_{max}; hazardous substance[10]
Wellbutrin SR®	Tablet	Slow release
Wellbutrin XL™	Tablet	Slow release
Xalkori®	Capsule	Teratogenic potential; hazardous substance[10]
Xanax XR®	Tablet	Slow release
Xeloda®	Tablet	Teratogenic potential; hazardous substance[10].
Zegerid OTC™	Capsule	Slow release
Zelboraf™	Tablet	Teratogenic potential; hazardous substance[10]
ZENPEP®	Capsule	Slow release[1]
Zolinza®	Capsule	Irritant; avoid contact with skin or mucous membranes; use gloves to handle; teratogenic potential; hazardous substance[10]
Zomig-ZMT®	Tablet	Sublingual form[7]
ZORprin®	Tablet	Slow release
Zortress®	Tablet	Mucous membrane irritant; teratogenic potential; hazardous substance[10]
Zyban®	Tablet	Slow release
Zyflo CR®	Tablet	Slow release
ZyrTEC-D® Allergy & Congestion	Tablet	Slow release
Zytiga™	Tablet	Teratogenic potential; hazardous substance[10]

[1]Capsule may be opened and the contents taken without crushing or chewing; soft food, such as applesauce or pudding, may facilitate administration; contents may generally be administered via nasogastric tube using an appropriate fluid, provided entire contents are washed down the tube.

[2]Liquid dosage forms of the product are available; however, dose, frequency of administration, and manufacturers may differ from that of the solid dosage form.

[3]Antacids and/or milk may prematurely dissolve the coating of the tablet.

[4]Capsule may be opened and the liquid contents removed for administration.

[5]The taste of this product in a liquid form would likely be unacceptable to the patient; administration via nasogastric tube should be acceptable.

[6]Effervescent tablets must be dissolved in the amount of diluent recommended by the manufacturer.

[7]Tablets are made to disintegrate under (or on) the tongue.

[8]Tablet is scored and may be broken in half without affecting release characteristics.

[9]Prescribing information recommends that women who are, or may become, pregnant should not handle medication, especially if crushed or broken; avoid direct contact.

[10]Potentially hazardous or hazardous substance; refer to institution-specific guidelines for precautions to observe when handling this substance.

REFERENCES

Mitchell JF, "Oral Dosage Forms That Should Not Be Crushed." Available at http://www.ismp.org/tools/DoNotCrush.-pdf. Accessed November 11, 2011.

National Institute for Occupational Safety and Health (NIOSH), "NIOSH List of Antineoplastic and Other Hazardous Drugs in Healthcare Settings 2012," Available at http://www.cdc.gov/niosh/docs/2012-150/pdfs/2012-150.pdf. Accessed July 11, 2012.

PATIENT INFORMATION FOR DISPOSAL OF UNUSED MEDICATIONS

Federal guidelines and the Food and Drug Administration (FDA) recommend that disposal of most unused medications should NOT be accomplished by flushing them down the toilet or drain unless specifically stated in the drug label prescribing information. (See "Disposal of Unused Medications Not Specified to be Flushed".)

However, certain drugs can potentially harm an individual for whom it is not intended, even in a single dose, depending on the size of the individual and strength of the medication. Accidental (or intentional) ingestion of one of these drugs by an unintended individual (eg, child or pet) can cause hypotension, somnolence, respiratory depression, or other severe adverse events that could lead to coma or death. For this reason, certain unused medications **should** be disposed of by flushing them down a toilet or sink.

Disposal by flushing of these medications is not believed to pose a risk to human health or the environment. Trace amounts of medicine in the water system have been noted, mainly from the body's normal elimination through urine or feces, but there has been no evidence of these small amounts being harmful. Disposal by flushing of these select, few medications contributes a small fraction to the amount of medicine in the water system. The FDA believes that the benefit of avoiding a potentially life-threatening overdose by accidental ingestion outweighs the potential risk to the environment by flushing these medications.

Medications Recommended for Disposal by Flushing

Medication	Active Ingredient
Actiq®, oral transmucosal lozenge	FentaNYL citrate
AVINza®, capsule (extended release)	Morphine sulfate
Daytrana™, transdermal patch	Methylphenidate
Demerol®, tablet[1]	Meperidine hydrochloride
Demerol®, oral solution[1]	Meperidine hydrochloride
Diastat® / Diastat® AcuDial™, rectal gel	Diazepam
Dilaudid®, tablet[1]	HYDROmorphone hydrochloride
Dilaudid®, oral liquid[1]	HYDROmorphone hydrochloride
Dolophine®, tablet (as hydrochloride)[1]	Methadone hydrochloride
Duragesic®, patch (extended release)[1]	FentaNYL
Embeda™, capsule (extended release)	Morphine sulfate and naltrexone hydrochloride
Fentora®, tablet (buccal)	FentaNYL citrate
Kadian®, capsule (extended release)	Morphine sulfate
Methadone hydrochloride (oral solution)[1]	Methadone hydrochloride
Methadose®, tablet[1]	Methadone hydrochloride
Morphine sulfate, tablet (immediate release)[1]	Morphine sulfate
Morphine sulfate, oral solution[1]	Morphine sulfate
MS Contin®, tablet (extended release)[1]	Morphine sulfate
Onsolis™, soluble film (buccal)	FentaNYL citrate
Opana®, tablet (immediate release)	Oxymorphone hydrochloride
Opana® ER, tablet (extended release)	Oxymorphone hydrochloride
Oramorph® SR, tablet (sustained release)	Morphine sulfate
OxyCONTIN®, tablet (extended release)[1]	OxyCODONE hydrochloride
Percocet®, tablet[1]	Oxycodone hydrochloride and acetaminophen
Percodan®, tablet[1]	Oxycodone hydrochloride and aspirin
Xyrem®, oral solution	Sodium oxybate

[1]Medications available in generic formulations

DISPOSAL OF UNUSED MEDICATIONS NOT SPECIFIED TO BE FLUSHED

The majority of medications should be disposed of without flushing them down a toilet or drain. These medications should be removed from the original container, mixed with an unappealing substance (eg, coffee grounds, cat litter), sealed in a plastic bag or other closable container, and disposed of in the household trash.

Another option for disposal of unused medications is through drug take-back programs. For information on availability of drug take-back programs in your area, contact city or county trash and recycling service.

For more information on unused medication disposal, see specific drug product labeling information or call the FDA at (888) INFO-FDA (1-888-463-6332).

REFERENCE

U.S. Food and Drug Administration (FDA), "Disposal by Flushing of Certain Unused Medicines: What You Should Know." Available at: http://www.fda.gov/Drugs/ResourcesForYou/Consumers/BuyingUsingMedicineSafely/Ensuring-SafeUseofMedicine/SafeDisposalofMedicines/ucm186187.htm Accessed October 20, 2009.

PRESSURE ULCER TREATMENT

Specific Treatment Options by Category	Description by Category	Advantages by Category	Disadvantages by Category
Surgical/Sharp Debridement Indicated when there is evidence of cellulitis or sepsis	Surgical excision of eschar by physician; may require concomitant treatment with systemic antimicrobials	Rapid removal of necrotic tissue; large wounds may be partially debrided, reducing risk to resident	May require hospitalization for procedure; caution must be used with those who are immunosuppressed, debilitated, or have bleeding disorders; may leave some necrotic debris in place
Autolytic Debriders Uses topical hydrocolloid, hydrogel, and transparent film dressings; indicated in wounds with minimal exudate; do not use in presence of infection	Use of occlusive dressings or dressings which impart moisture to soften and liquefy necrotic tissue	Selective form of debridement (does not harm healing tissue); effective alternative for debridement of small wounds; readily available	May lead to infection in large necrotic wounds; not indicated for clinically infected wounds due to increased bacterial growth beneath dressing
Enzymatic Debriders Uses topical agents, such as collagenase, fibrinolysin, and deoxyribonuclease; **Note:** Papain has been used in the past but is not available in the U.S. due to reports of serious hypersensitivity reactions; enzymatic debriders promote growth of granulation tissue; indicated in patients in long-term care or who cannot tolerate surgery *Examples:* Granulex® Santyl® Xenaderm™	Enzyme topically applied to necrotic surface; usually covered with wet gauze and/or transparent dressing; applying a protectant (ie, moisture barrier cream) to surrounding tissue may be indicated; often require concomitant treatment with topical or systemic antimicrobials; discontinue when wound is red and granulating or if it bleeds easily when cleansed	Less traumatic than surgical debriding; ease of application; cost-effective debridement therapy	Cross-hatching recommended if thick eschar is present; some detergents and antiseptics may inactivate certain products; effect on viable tissue varies by product; take longer than surgical debridement; may need barrier cream around wound to protect healthy skin; require secondary dressing
Mechanical Debriders Wet-to-dry gauze dressings, hydrotherapy, wound irrigation, and scrubbing the wound with gauze; best for wounds with thick exudate, slough on loose necrotic tissue	Removal of eschar using mechanical forces that pull off necrotic tissue; discontinue when wound is red and granulating or if it bleeds easily when cleansed	Promote softening and loosening of eschar; potentially less traumatic than surgical debridement; economical; readily available	Generally not as effective in severely necrotic wounds; must monitor for signs of injury to healthy tissue
Maggot Debridement Therapy Has been used as a method of debridement when other methods have failed to slow the progression of tissue destruction	Maggots excrete collagenases that primarily feed on necrotic or partially decomposed material in the ulcer	Maggot debridement is useful in separating the necrotic tissue from the living tissue (which allows for easier surgical debridement)	Psychological/esthetic concerns by the patient; may cause tickling/itching; may cause increased pain during treatment (can be treated with analgesics); may cause erythema or cellulitis due to digestive enzymes of maggots (wound periphery should be protected to keep maggots localized to wound)
Cleansing Solutions *Examples:* Acetic acid Hydrogen peroxide Lactated Ringer's Normal saline Povidone-iodine (Betadine)®	Cleansing solutions that also hydrate; some products are bactericidal	Cleanse wound; maintain moist environment	Can disturb granulation tissue; can be cytotoxic if not diluted (especially those with antiseptic properties) or used too vigorously

Specific Treatment Options by Category	Description by Category	Advantages by Category	Disadvantages by Category
Topical Antibiotics Indicated for prophylaxis or for treatment of an infected wound *Examples:* Gentamicin MetroNIDAZOLE (Topical) Mupirocin Neosporin® Silvadene®	Antimicrobial solutions, ointments, and creams	Easy to apply; water miscible creams easy to remove; help control bacterial growth until necrotic tissue can be debrided	May have cytotoxic effects, which may delay wound healing; ointments are difficult to remove; allergic reactions may occur; bacteria may become resistant with prolonged use
Calcium Alginate Dressings Used for wounds with significant exudate and infected or noninfected wounds *Examples:* Algicell Carraginate Kaltostat® Sorbsan®	Derived from brown seaweed; form a gel on contact; maintain a moist environment	Conform to wound shape; easy to apply and remove; facilitate autolytic debridement	Require secondary dressing; may dehydrate the wound bed; not recommended for light exudate
Foam Dressings *Examples:* Biatain® Dermalevin® Optifoam®	Provide moist environment, thermal insulation, and high absorbancy	Absorb light-to-heavy exudate; repel contaminants, water, and bacteria; reduce odor; may be used on fragile skin	Maceration may occur in surrounding skin; may require secondary dressing
Gauze Dressings	Fine mesh gauze dressings used as vehicles for soaks, lubricants, or antimicrobials	Economical; readily available; effective delivery of solution if kept moist; cost-effective filler for large wounds	May cause bleeding and pain and may remove healthy granulation tissue if allowed to dry; require increased nursing time to keep dressing moist
Hydrocolloid Dressings *Examples:* Comfeel® Plus DuoDERM® Tegaderm™ Hydrocolloid Dressing Ultec™	Dressings that react with exudate to form a gel; create a physical barrier and maintain a moist/acidic environment	Totally occlusive; protect wound from physical injury and contamination; maintain moist environment; easy removal without adhesion to wound surface; may remain on wound for up to 5 days; waterproof dressings allow resident to shower	Difficult to observe wound (unless transparent); may promote development of infection in deep wounds; may accumulate excess fluid and macerate tissue; dressings may soften and wrinkles may increase pressure on wound base
Nonadherent Dressings *Examples:* ABD Pads Telfa®	Nonocclusive, absorbent dressings; may be used with topical medications	Easy to use; inexpensive; nontraumatic	Nonocclusive; do not physically protect wound site from injury; less absorptive than plain gauze; need secondary dressing
Transparent Film Dressings *Examples:* Bioclusive® Op-Site® Tegaderm® Uniflex®	Adhesive, transparent, thin, film-type semipermeable dressings; semipermeable membranes allow moisture and oxygen exchange	Barriers to contamination that also keep wound moist; allow for easy visual inspection; good adhesive properties; waterproof dressings allow resident to shower; reduce pain; time-saving	May lead to tissue maceration in extremely moist wounds; some products are difficult to apply and wrinkling may occur; may promote infection if necrotic tissue is present; potential for adhesive injury; expensive
Hydrogels Used for ulcers with little or no exudate *Examples:* Aquaflo™ Carrasyn Dermasyn® Tegagel™ Transigel™	Topicals with absorptive and moisturizing properties	Nonadherent; may cool and/or soothe wound; easy to apply; conform to wound bed; facilitate autolytic debridement	Usually require protective outer dressing; may require multiple daily dressing changes; may macerate surrounding tissue; not recommended for wounds with heavy exudate or infection

PRESSURE ULCER TREATMENT

Specific Treatment Options by Category	Description by Category	Advantages by Category	Disadvantages by Category
Pain Control Options:			
Pain Control Pain may be present in pressure ulcers and should be assessed/monitored regularly during treatment	• Topical local anesthetics (eg, lidocaine; lidocaine and prilocaine [EMLA®]) • Topical opioid preparations: Benefit has been seen in small trials using an extemporaneous preparrtion of 1 mL of injectable morphine sulfate 10 mg/1 mL in 8 g of Intrasite® gel applied topically once daily; cover with Tegaderm® dressing • Oral nonopioids: May be necessary for mild pain • Oral opioids: May be necessary for moderate-to-severe pain		

REFERENCES

Bluestein D and Javaheri A, "Pressure Ulcers: Prevention, Evaluation, and Management," *Am Fam Physician*, 2008, 78(10):1186-94.

Cannon BC and Cannon JP, "Management of Pressure Ulcers," *Am J Health Syst Pharm*, 2004, 61(18):1895-905.

Flock P, "Pilot Study to Determine the Effectiveness of Diamorphine Gel to Control Pressure Ulcer Pain," *J Pain Symptom Manage*, 2003, 25(6):547-54.

Lyder CH, "Pressure Ulcer Prevention and Management," *JAMA*, 2003, 289(2):223-6.

Mumcuoglu KY, "Clinical Applications for Maggots in Wound Care," *Am J Clin Dermatol*, 2001, 2(4):219-27.

Pullen R, Popp R, Volkers P, et al, "Prospective Randomized Double-Blind Study of the Wound-Debriding Effects of Collagenase and Fibrinolysin/Deoxyribonuclease in Pressure Ulcers," *Age Ageing*, 2002, 31(2):126-30.

Zeppetella G and Ribeiro MD, "Morphine in Intrasite Gel Applied Topically to Painful Ulcers," *J Pain Symptom Manage*, 2005, 29(2):118-9.

Zeppetella G, Paul J, and Ribeiro MD, "Analgesic Efficacy of Morphine Applied Topically to Painful Ulcers," *J Pain Symptom Manage*, 2003, 25(6):555-8.

PHARMACOLOGIC CATEGORY
INDEX

DECONGESTANT

Other Products Offered by Lexicomp

Anesthesiology & Critical Care Drug Handbook

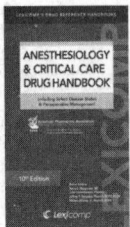

Designed for anesthesiologists, critical care practitioners, and all healthcare professionals involved in the treatment of surgical or ICU patients.

Includes: Comprehensive drug information to ensure appropriate clinical management of patients; Intensivist and Anesthesiologist perspective; Over 2000 medications most commonly used in the preoperative and critical care setting; Special Topics/Issues addressing frequently encountered patient conditions.

Drug Information Handbook

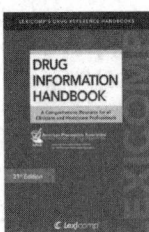

An easy-to-use reference for pharmacists, physicians and other healthcare professionals requiring fast access to comprehensive drug information. This handbook presents over 1400 drug monographs, each with up to 37 fields of information. A valuable appendix includes hundreds of charts and reviews of special topics such as guidelines for treatment and therapy recommendations. A pharmacologic category index is also provided.

Drug Information Handbook with International Trade Names Index

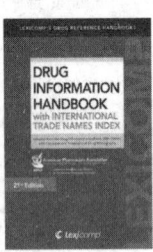

The *Drug Information Handbook with International Trade Names Index* includes the content of our *Drug Information Handbook*, plus international drug monographs for use worldwide! This easy-to-use reference is complied especially for the pharmacist, physician or other healthcare professional seeking quick access to comprehensive drug information.

Drug Information Handbook for Advanced Practice Nursing

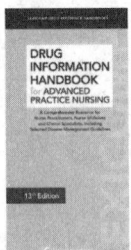

Designed to assist the advanced practice nurse with prescribing for, monitoring and educating patients.

Includes: Over 4800 generic and brand names cross-referenced by page number; generic drug names and cross-references highlighted in RED; Labeled and Investigational indications; Adult, Geriatric and Pediatric dosing; up to 60 fields of information per monograph, including Patient Education and Physical Assessment.

To order, call Customer Service at 1-866-397-3433 or visit www.lexi.com.
Outside of the U.S., call 330-650-6506 or visit www.lexi.com.

Other Products Offered by Lexicomp

Drug Information Handbook for Nursing

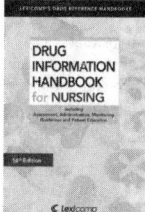

Designed for registered professional nurses and upper-division nursing students requiring dosing, administration, monitoring and patient education information.

Includes: Over 4800 generic and brand name drugs, cross-referenced by page number; drug names and specific nursing fields highlighted in RED for easy reference; Nursing Actions field includes Physical Assessment and Patient Education guidelines.

Drug Information Handbook for Oncology

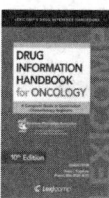

Designed for oncology professionals requiring information on combination chemotherapy regimens and dosing protocols.

Includes: Monographs containing warnings, adverse reaction profiles, drug interactions, dosing for specific indications, vesicant, emetic potential, combination regimens and more; where applicable, a special Combination Chemotherapy field links to specific oncology monographs; Special Topics such as Cancer Treatment Related Complications, Bone Marrow Transplantation and Drug Development.

Pediatric Dosage Handbook

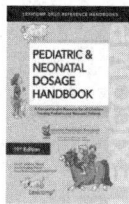

This book is designed for healthcare professionals requiring quick access to comprehensive pediatric drug information. Each monograph contains multiple fields of content, including usual dosage by age group, indication and route of administration. Drug interactions, adverse reactions, extemporaneous preparations, pharmacodynamics/pharmacokinetics data and medication safety issues are covered.

Also available:
Manual de Prescripción Pediátrica (Spanish version)

Pediatric Dosage Handbook with International Trade Names Index

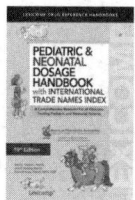

The *Pediatric Dosage Handbook with International Trade Names Index* is the trusted pediatric drug resource of medical professionals worldwide. The International Edition contains all the content of Lexicomp's *Pediatric Dosage Handbook*, plus an International Trade Names Index including trade names from over 100 countries.

Other Products Offered by Lexicomp

Pharmacogenomics Handbook

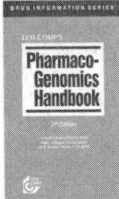

Ideal for any healthcare professional or student wishing to gain insight into the emerging field of pharmacogenomics.

Includes: Information concerning key genetic variations that may influence drug disposition and/or sensitivity; brief introduction to fundamental concepts in genetics and genomics. A foundation for all clinicians who will be called on to integrate rapidly-expanding genomics knowledge into the management of drug therapy.

Rating Scales in Mental Health

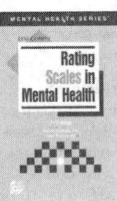

Ideal for clinicians as well as administrators, this book provides an overview of over 100 recommended rating scales for mental assessment.

Includes: Rating scales for conditions such as General Anxiety, Social/Family Functioning, Eating Disorders and Sleep Disorders; Monograph format covering such topics as Overview of Scale, General Applications, Psychometric Properties and References.

Other Products Offered by Lexicomp

Lexicomp® Online™

Fourteen of the top 17 hospitals in *U.S. News & World Report's* 2012-13 Honor Roll ranking rely on Lexicomp products and services. These include Johns Hopkins, Massachusetts General, Cleveland Clinic and others.

Lexicomp Online integrates industry-leading databases and enhanced searching technology, delivering time-sensitive clinical information at the point-of-care. Our easy-to-use interface and concise information eliminate the need to navigate through multiple pages or make unnecessary mouse clicks.

Lexicomp Online includes multiple databases and modules covering the following topic areas:

- Core drug information with specialty fields
- Pediatrics and Geriatrics
- Interaction Analysis
- Pharmacogenomics
- Infectious Diseases
- Laboratory Tests and Diagnostic Procedures
- Natural Products
- Patient Education
- Drug Identification
- Calculations
- I.V. Compatibility: *King® Guide to Parenteral Admixtures®*
- Toxicology

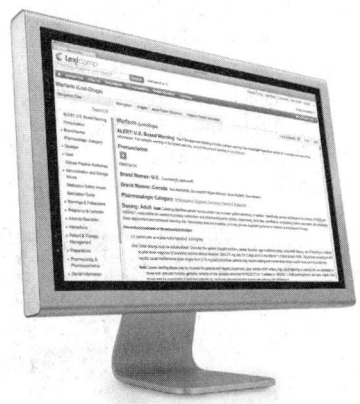

Register for a FREE 45-day trial
Visit www.lexi.com/institutions

Academic and Institutional licenses available.

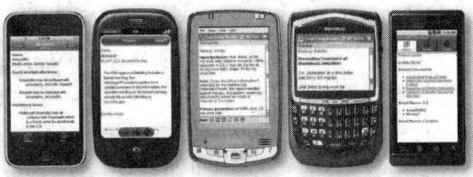